CECIL
TEXTBOOK
of
MEDICINE

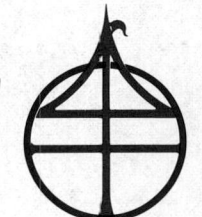

Editor for Neurologic and Behavioral Diseases

FRED PLUM, M.D.

Anne Parrish Titzell Professor and Chairman,
Department of Neurology, Cornell University Medical College;
Neurologist-in-Chief, The New York Hospital–Cornell Medical Center,
New York, New York

The Consulting Editors:

Renal Diseases

THOMAS E. ANDREOLI, M.D.

Professor and Chairman,
Department of Internal Medicine,
University of Arkansas College of Medicine;
Chief of Medicine, University of Arkansas Hospital,
Little Rock, Arkansas

Infectious Diseases

GERALD L. MANDELL, M.D.

Head, Division of Infectious Diseases, and
Professor of Medicine, University of Virginia,
Owen R. Cheatham Professor of the Sciences,
Charlottesville, Virginia

Respiratory Diseases

JOHN F. MURRAY, M.D.

Professor of Medicine,
University of California, San Francisco,
School of Medicine

Hematologic and Hematopoietic Diseases

DAVID G. NATHAN, M.D.

Robert G. Stranahan Professor of Pediatrics,
Harvard Medical School;
Physician-in-Chief, Children's Hospital,
Boston, Massachusetts

Diseases of the Digestive System

ROBERT K. OCKNER, M.D.

Professor of Medicine and Director, Liver Center,
University of California, San Francisco,
School of Medicine,
San Francisco, California

Cardiovascular Diseases

THOMAS W. SMITH, M.D.

Professor of Medicine, Harvard Medical School;
Chief, Cardiovascular Division,
Brigham and Women's Hospital,
Boston, Massachusetts

VOLUME 1

CECIL

TEXTBOOK of MEDICINE

19th edition

Edited by

JAMES B. WYNGAARDEN, M.D.

Professor of Medicine and
Associate Vice-Chancellor for Health Affairs,
Duke University School of Medicine,
Durham, North Carolina

LLOYD H. SMITH, Jr., M.D.

Professor of Medicine and
Associate Dean,
University of California, San Francisco,
School of Medicine,
San Francisco, California

J. CLAUDE BENNETT, M.D.

Professor and Chairman,
Department of Medicine,
University of Alabama at Birmingham,
School of Medicine,
Birmingham, Alabama

W. B. SAUNDERS COMPANY

HARCOURT BRACE JOVANOVICH, INC.

Philadelphia London Toronto Montreal Sydney Tokyo

W. B. SAUNDERS COMPANY
Harcourt Brace Jovanovich, Inc.

The Curtis Center
Independence Square West
Philadelphia, PA 19106

Library of Congress Cataloging-in-Publication Data

Cecil textbook of medicine / edited by James B. Wyngaarden,
Lloyd H. Smith, Jr., J. Claude Bennett.—19th ed.

p. cm

Rev. ed. of: Textbook of medicine / [edited by] Cecil. 18th ed.
1988.

Includes bibliographical references and index.

ISBN 0–7216–2928–8 (single v.).—ISBN 0–7216–2929-6 (v. 1).—
ISBN 0–7216–2930–X (v. 2).—ISBN 0–7216–2931–8 (set)

1. Internal medicine   I. Cecil, Russell L. (Russell La Fayette),
1881–1965.   II. Wyngaarden, James B.   III. Smith,
Lloyd H.   IV. Bennett, J. Claude.   V. Title: Textbook
of Medicine.

[DNLM: 1. Medicine. WB 100 C3888]

RC46.C423 1992

616—dc20

DNLM/DLC   91–31268

Editor: John Dyson
Designer: Lorraine B. Kilmer
Production Manager: Frank Polizzano
Manuscript Editors: Donna Walker and Bonnie Boehme
Illustration Coordinator: Matt Andrews
Indexer: Donna Walker

ISBN 0–7216–2928–8   Single Volume
ISBN 0–7216–2929–6   Volume 1
ISBN 0–7216–2930–X   Volume 2
ISBN 0–7216–2931–8   Set

CECIL TEXTBOOK OF MEDICINE

DOSAGE NOTICE

Every effort has been made by the authors, the editors, and the publisher of this book to ensure that dosage recommendations are precise and in agreement with the standards of practice accepted at the time of publication.

However, dosage schedules are changed from time to time in the light of accumulating clinical experience and continuing laboratory studies. This is most likely to occur in the case of recently introduced products.

We urge, therefore, that you check the package information data for the manufacturer's recommended dosage to be certain that changes have not been made in the recommended dose or in the contraindications for administration. In addition, there are some quite serious situations in which drug therapy must be individualized and expert judgment advises the use of a higher dosage or administration by a different route than is included in the manufacturer's recommendations. Throughout the text examples of such instances are indicated by a footnote.

THE EDITORS

ALSO ASSOCIATED WITH THE *CECIL TEXTBOOK OF MEDICINE*

Review of General Internal Medicine: A Self-Assessment Manual, 5th Edition, 1992

Editors: J. Allen D. Cooper, Jr., M.D.; Peter G. Pappas, M.D.

The fifth edition of this self-assessment book contains approximately 1200 questions covering all the specialty areas of internal medicine. The answers are linked to this edition of the *Cecil Textbook of Medicine*, to the *Cecil Essentials of Medicine,* and to other readily available sources.

Available from W. B. Saunders Company
The Curtis Center
Independence Square West
Philadelphia, PA 19106

Material in the chapters listed below is in the public domain:

PREFACE

The 19th edition of the *Cecil Textbook of Medicine* appears on the one-hundredth anniversary of the publication of William Osler's influential *The Principles and Practice of Medicine*, a monumental single-authored volume notable for its comprehensive clinical coverage, authoritative pathologic descriptions, and literary qualities. Microbiology was then the newest medical science. A tone of therapeutic nihilism was the book's most salutary contribution. At least two generations of physicians would fall under its influence. The textbook ushered in a period of increasingly exact diagnosis, especially in infectious diseases, and an ever more critical evaluation of drugs, remedies, and nostrums in the practice of medicine. It also led to the establishment of the Rockefeller Institute, founded to address the pervasive ignorance of the pathophysiology of disease so abundantly displayed in Osler's textbook, avant garde though it was for its day.

Thirty-five years later, in 1927, Russell Cecil introduced "*A Text-book of Medicine* by American authors." Single-authored textbooks had largely given way to books jointly authored by a small number of writers, but the idea of an edited textbook compiled by multiple authors, each writing on topics of personal interest and experience, was new. Basic biologic sciences were making increasingly important contributions to clinical medicine, and these were to be accorded substantial attention. The maturing sciences were physiology, pharmacology, and biochemistry. With succeeding editions, Cecil's philosophy became more explicit. Cecil believed that ". . . in terms of biological processes, fragmentation of the discussion of disease is artificial" (Preface, 10th edition, 1959). Each chapter was a treatise in which clinical description, pathologic information, pathophysiologic knowledge, diagnostic criteria, and therapeutic measures were well integrated, so that students and physicians consulting the text could secure the most authoritative information available and find it in one place (Beeson and McDermott, Preface, 11th edition, 1963).

Cecil's inaugural philosophy continues into the 19th edition of the *Cecil Textbook*, 65 years later, appropriately adapted to ever-changing circumstances. By 1992, several generations of physicians have learned medicine with the help of *Cecil*. The series spans a period of remarkable progress in biomedical and behavioral sciences, and each new edition has incorporated new insights on disease causation, prevention, and treatment. The pace has quickened as we approach the twenty-first century. New technologies have revolutionized molecular genetics, neurobiology, immunology, cell biology, and structural biology; the application of these disciplines to all branches of the traditional biomedical sciences proceeds apace. The structure of DNA was elucidated less than 40 years ago, and recombinant DNA technology was discovered less than 20 years ago. Today, the leitmotif of biologic science, regardless of its disciplinary name, is increasingly cell and molecular biology. This theme is now permeating medicine and prefiguring the developments of the next few decades. Beyond these contributions from the biologic sciences, applications of the physical and mathematical sciences, especially in diagnostic imaging (CT, MRI, PET, and sonography) and in the information sciences, continue to alter medical practice. In such a climate of change, medical competence itself is fragile. It must be constantly renewed or else it will erode.

To reflect the best in medical practice, a major textbook of medicine must also be constantly renewed. In that spirit, this edition of the *Cecil Textbook of Medicine* has been thoroughly revised. As before, approximately one third of the book is "new" in that different authors have been selected, in this way assuring that their chapters have been completely recast. All other chapters have been revised and updated by their current authors, carefully chosen authorities in their respective subjects. The editors are deeply grateful to all retiring authors for the high standards of their contributions. We have retained the two-color presentation of figures and charts, so well received in the 18th edition, and have expanded the color plates from 8 to 16 pages.

The most extensive change in the 19th edition is the further expansion of space devoted to the acquired immunodeficiency syndrome (AIDS), a still unfolding epidemic. This condition now commands a part of its own (Part XXI, HIV and Associated Disorders), comprising 13 newly written chapters: "Immunology Related to AIDS" (B. D. Walker); "Biology of Human Immunodeficiency Viruses" (G. M. Shaw); "Epidemiology of HIV Infection and AIDS" (J. W. Curran); "Prevention of HIV Infection" (M. S. Saag); "Neurologic Complications of HIV-1 Infection" (R. W. Price); "Pulmonary Manifestations of AIDS: Special Emphasis on Pneumocystosis" (F. R. Sattler); "Gastrointestinal Manifestations of AIDS" (J. G. Bartlett); "Cutaneous Signs of AIDS" (N. S. Penneys); "Ophthalmologic Manifestations of AIDS" (M. A. Jacobson); "Hematology/Oncology in AIDS" (J. E. Groopman and D. T. Scadden); "Renal, Cardiac, Endocrine, and Rheumatologic Manifestations of HIV Infection" (M. S. Saag); "Treatment of AIDS and Related Disorders" (R. Yarchoan and S. Broder); and "Chronic Management and Counseling for Persons with HIV Infection" (J. A. Bartlett). In addition, related chapters on AIDS dementia and on opportunistic infections associated with AIDS, found elsewhere in the book, have been thoroughly updated.

A new chapter, "Human T Cell Lymphotropic Virus Type I–Associated Myelopathy and Tropical Spastic Paraparesis" (R. W. Price), reflects the growing appreciation of other retroviruses as causes of human disease. Oncology (Part XIII) has been strengthened by the addition of two new chapters: "Oncologic Emergencies" (S. M. Hahn and A. Russo) and "Metastatic Cancer, Source Unknown" (D. C. Ihde). In addition, a new chapter, "Ovarian Carcinoma" (H. W. Jones), is included in Part XVI, Endocine and Reproductive Diseases. Part XXIII, Neurology, has been reorganized to increase the depth of focus on problems of the elderly. New chapters include "Neurologic Problems Associated with Aging" (F. Plum) and "Disturbances of Memory and Language" and "Alzheimer's Disease and Related Dementias" (both by A. R. Damasio). Also, "Brief Loss of Consciousness," "Sustained Impairments of Consciousness," and "Brain Death" (all by F. Plum) are now full chapters.

New chapters have also been added elsewhere, including "Zoonoses" (B. McLain), "Liver Transplantation" (J. P. Roberts), and "Erythromelalgia" (E. V. Ball). Part IV, Principles of Diagnosis and Management, is now expanded by a new chapter, "NSAID's: Aspirin and Aspirin-like Drugs" (G. Weissmann), in response to the need for an authoritative discussion of the nature, use, and side effects of these widely employed agents. Also, in this edition "Antimicrobial Therapy" (L. S. Young) and "Antiviral Therapy" (a new chapter by M. Middlebrooks) have been transferred from Part IV to be associated more closely with chapters on specific bacterial and viral diseases in Part XX, Infectious Diseases. As in recent editions of *Cecil*, each chapter lists a limited number of carefully selected, recent references to research or review articles in accessible journals, or to books, that may be consulted for additional information. The particular value of each entry is briefly described in an annotation. Finally, a new chapter entitled "Internal Medicine and Today's Internist" has been contributed by our co-editor, J. Claude Bennett, whom the continuing editors warmly welcome to the task of shepherding the 19th edition of *Cecil*, with its attendant high honor and immense responsibility.

Cecil not only stands alone; it is also the senior member of a trilogy. *Cecil Essentials of Medicine* (edited by T. E. Andreoli, C. C. J. Carpenter, F. Plum, and L. H. Smith, Jr.), now in its 2nd edition, offers a more concentrated guide to what every doctor should know about internal medicine. It is designed primarily for the medical student, for whom the authoritative compendium of *Cecil* may sometimes seem formidable. Nevertheless, it serves in general as a useful point of entry guide. *Cecil Review of General Internal Medicine* (edited by J. A. D. Cooper, Jr., and P. G. Pappas) appears in a 5th edition in parallel with this 19th edition of *Cecil*. As before, its 1200 questions and answers are designed to be of general educational benefit as well as to reinforce the value of *Cecil* as a reference text.

Editing a major textbook is a complex task, as one attempts to balance content, format, style, integration, and innovation. The editors have been privileged to work with an admirable group of colleagues in this shared responsibility. Fred Plum has continued in his role as Editor for Neurology. We welcome two new Consulting Editors: Gerald L. Mandell for Infectious Diseases and Robert K. Ockner for Digestive Diseases. They join a seasoned team of fellow Consulting Editors: Thomas E. Andreoli (Renal Diseases), John F. Murray (Respiratory Diseases), David G. Nathan (Hematologic and Hematopoietic Diseases), and Thomas W. Smith (Cardiovascular Diseases). We thank our retiring Consulting Editors, Robert Lefkowitz, William Paul, and Marvin Sleisenger, for extraordinary contributions to *Cecil*, in one case (M. Sleisenger) extending over eight editions. The Consulting Editors continually review their respective sections of this complex book and bring us their ideas and expertise concerning modifications. Our special gratitude is extended to the 360 contributors who have written the 534 chapters that collectively constitute this 19th edition. The ultimate value and authenticity of *Cecil* lie not with the editors but with the scholarship and experience that these individual physicians and scientists have brought to this joint enterprise.

"Language is the armoury of the human mind; and at once contains the trophies of its past, and the weapons of its future conquests." The weaponry of language, in Coleridge's image above, does not always come fully burnished in submitted manuscripts. As in the 18th edition, we have been most fortunate to work with seasoned editorial assistants in Washington (Margaret Quinlan), San Francisco (Judith Serrell), and Birmingham (Carolyn Thomley), without whose dedication and skill this large project could not have been completed. At W. B. Saunders Company, Lorraine Kilmer, Donna Walker, Frank Polizzano, and Faith Voit carried out with experienced professionalism the intricate task of formatting, editing, and assembling the book. The overall editor at the W. B. Saunders Company for this 19th edition of *Cecil* was again John Dyson, who has been an invaluable guide, colleague, and good friend. We are deeply indebted to him for his extensive contributions in bringing to completion this 19th edition of a venerable book.

JAMES B. WYNGAARDEN, M.D.
LLOYD H. SMITH, JR., M.D.
J. CLAUDE BENNETT, M.D.

CONTRIBUTORS

ROBERT H. ALLEN, M.D.

Professor of Medicine and of Biochemistry and Director, Division of Hematology, University of Colorado Health Sciences Center School of Medicine. Staff Physician, University Hospital, Denver, Colorado.

Megaloblastic Anemia

DAVID H. ALPERS

Professor of Medicine and Chief, Division of Gastroenterology, Washington University School of Medicine. Physician, Barnes Hospital, and Consultant, Jewish Hospital of St. Louis and St. Louis Children's Hospital, St. Louis, Missouri.

Principles of Nutritional Support: Enteral Nutritional Therapy

DAVID F. ALTMAN, M.D.

Professor of Clinical Medicine and Associate Dean, University of California, San Francisco, School of Medicine, San Francisco, California.

Food Poisoning

KARL E. ANDERSON, M.D.

Professor, University of Texas Medical School at Galveston. Full-time Active Member of the Medical Staff, The University of Texas Medical Branch Hospitals, Galveston, Texas.

The Porphyrias

W. FRENCH ANDERSON, M.D.

Adjunct Professor, Graduate Genetics Program, George Washington University School of Medicine and Health, Washington, D.C.; Faculty, Department of Medicine and Physiology, National Institutes of Health Graduate Program. Chief, Molecular Hematology Branch, National Heart, Lung, and Blood Institute, National Institutes of Health, Bethesda, Maryland.

Expectations from Recombinant DNA Research

THOMAS E. ANDREOLI, M.D.

Professor and Chairman, Department of Internal Medicine, University of Arkansas College of Medicine. Chief of Medicine, University Hospital of Arkansas, Little Rock, Arkansas.

Approach to the Patient with Renal Disease; Disorders of Fluid Volume, Electrolyte, and Acid-Base Balance; The Posterior Pituitary

VINCENT T. ANDRIOLE, M.D.

Professor of Medicine, Yale University School of Medicine. Attending Physician, Yale–New Haven Hospital, New Haven, Connecticut.

Urinary Tract Infections and Pyelonephritis

FREDERICK R. APPELBAUM, M.D.

Professor of Medicine, University of Washington School of Medicine. Member, Fred Hutchinson Cancer Research Center, Seattle, Washington.

The Acute Leukemias

FRANK C. ARNETT, M.D.

Professor of Internal Medicine. University of Texas Medical School at Houston. Chief, Division of Rheumatology, Hermann Hospital and Lyndon B. Johnson General Hospital, Houston, Texas.

Rheumatoid Arthritis

WILLIAM J. ARNOLD, M.D.

Clinical Professor of Medicine, University of Chicago Pritzker School of Medicine, Chicago. Chairman, Department of Internal Medicine, Lutheran General Hospital, Park Ridge, Illinois.

Specialized Procedures in the Management of Patients with Rheumatic Diseases

DENNIS A. AUSIELLO, M.D.

Associate Professor of Medicine, Harvard Medical School. Chief, Renal Unit, Massachusetts General Hospital, Boston, Massachusetts.

Natriuretic Hormones

BERNARD M. BABIOR, M.D., Ph.D.

Adjunct Professor of Medicine, University of California, San Diego, School of Medicine. Member and Head, Division of Biochemistry, Department of Molecular and Experimental Medicine, Research Institute of Scripps Clinic. Staff Physician, Division of Hematology/Oncology, Scripps Clinic and Research Foundation, La Jolla, California.

Function of Neutrophils and Mononuclear Phagocytes; Disorders of Neutrophil Function

GROVER C. BAGBY, Jr., M.D.

Professor of Medicine and Medical Genetics, Oregon Health Sciences University School of Medicine. Section Head, Hematology and Medical Oncology, Veterans Affairs Medical Center, Portland, Oregon.

Leukopenia; Leukocytosis and Leukemoid Reactions

EUGENE V. BALL, M.D.

Professor of Medicine, University of Alabama School of Medicine. Staff Physician, University of Alabama Hospital, Birmingham, Alabama.

Behçet's Disease; Systemic Diseases in Which Arthritis Is a Feature; Miscellaneous Forms of Arthritis; Nonarticular Rheumatism; Articular Tumors; Erythromelalgia

ROBERT W. BALOH, M.D.

Professor of Neurology and Surgery (Head and Neck), University of California, Los Angeles, UCLA School of Medicine. Director, Neurotology Laboratories, University of California at Los Angeles Medical Center, Los Angeles, California.

The Special Senses

MURRAY G. BARON, M.D.

Professor and Associate Chairman, Department of Radiology, Emory University School of Medicine. Associate Chairman, Radiology Department, Emory University Hospital; Attending Neurologist, Grady Memorial Hospital and Henrietta Egleston Hospital for Children, Atlanta, Georgia.

Radiology of the Heart

ROBERT B. BARON, M.D., M.S.

Associate Professor of Clinical Medicine, University of California, San Francisco, School of Medicine. Director, Primary Care Internal Medicine Residency Program, and Continuing Medical Education, Department of Medicine, University of California San Francisco Medical Center, San Francisco, California.

Protein-Energy Malnutrition

WILLIAM H. BARRY, M.D.

Nora Eccles Harrison Professor of Cardiology, University of Utah School of Medicine. Attending Cardiologist, University of Utah Hospital and Clinics, Salt Lake City, Utah.

Cardiac Catheterization and Angiography

JOHN A. BARTLETT, M.D.

Assistant Professor of Medicine, Duke University Medical Center, Durham, North Carolina.

Chronic Management and Counseling for Persons with HIV Infection

JOHN G. BARTLETT, M.D.

Professor of Medicine, Johns Hopkins University School of Medicine. Chief, Division of Infectious Diseases, Johns Hopkins Hospital, Baltimore, Maryland.

Lung Abscess; Clostridial Diseases; Gastrointestinal Manifestations of AIDS

NATHAN M. BASS, M.D., Ph.D.

Associate Professor of Medicine, University of California, San Francisco, School of Medicine. Attending Physician, University of California San Francisco Medical Center, San Francisco, California.

Toxic and Drug-Induced Liver Disease

STEPHEN G. BAUM, M.D.

Professor of Medicine, Mount Sinai School of Medicine of the City University of New York. Director, Department of Medicine, Beth Israel Medical Center, New York, New York.

Mycoplasmal Infections; Adenovirus Diseases

JOHN D. BAXTER, M.D.

Professor of Medicine and Director, Metabolic Research Unit, University of California, San Francisco, School of Medicine. Chief, Division of Endocrinology, Moffitt Hospital, San Francisco, California.

Disorders of the Adrenal Cortex

STEPHEN B. BAYLIN, M.D.

Professor of Oncology and Medicine, Johns Hopkins University School of Medicine. Active Staff Member, Johns Hopkins Hospital, Baltimore, Maryland.

Endocrine Manifestations of Tumors: "Ectopic" Hormone Production

CHARLES E. BECKER, M.D.

Professor of Medicine, University of California, San Francisco, School of Medicine. Director, Center for Occupational and Environmental Health, University of California, San Francisco. Chief, Occupational Medicine and Toxicology, San Francisco General Hospital Medical Center, San Francisco, California.

Principles of Occupational Medicine

MICHAEL D. BENDER, M.D.

Associate Clinical Professor of Medicine, University of California, San Francisco, School of Medicine. Director of Medical Education and Attending Physician, Mills-Peninsula Hospitals, Burlingame, and Seton Medical Center, Daly City, California.

Diseases of the Peritoneum, Mesentery, and Omentum

PAUL E. BENDHEIM, M.D.

Associate Professor of Neurology, State University of New York Health Science Center at Brooklyn College of Medicine. Head, Laboratory of Neurodegenerative Diseases, Institute for Basic Research, Staten Island, New York.

Creutzfeldt-Jakob Disease

J. CLAUDE BENNETT, M.D.

Professor and Chairman, University of Alabama School of Medicine. Physician-in-Chief, University of Alabama Hospital, Birmingham, Alabama.

Internal Medicine and Today's Internist; The Immune System: Introduction

EDWARD J. BENZ, Jr., M.D.

Professor of Internal Medicine and Genetics; Chief, Section of Hematology; and Vice Chairman, Department of Internal Medicine, Yale University School of Medicine. Attending Physician and Chief of Hematology, Yale–New Haven Hospital, New Haven, Connecticut.

Structure, Function, and Synthesis of the Human Hemoglobins; Classification and Basic Pathophysiology of the Hemoglobinopathies; Hemoglobinopathies with Altered Solubility or Oxygen Affinity

PAUL D. BERK, M.D.

Lillian and Henry M. Stratton Professor of Molecular Medicine; Professor of Medicine and Biochemistry; and Chief, Division of Liver Diseases (Department of Medicine), Mount Sinai School of Medicine of the City University of New York. Attending Physician, Mount Sinai Medical Center, New York, New York.

Erythrocytosis and Polycythemia; Myeloproliferative Disorders

BRUCE BEUTLER, M.D.

Associate Professor of Internal Medicine, University of Texas Health Science Center at Dallas Southwestern Medical School. Attending Physician, Parkland Memorial Hospital, Dallas, Texas.

The Pathogenesis of Fever

STEVEN M. BEUTLER, M.D.

Clinical Assistant Professor of Medicine, University of California, Irvine, California College of Medicine, Irvine. Director, Division of Infectious Diseases, San Bernadino County Medical Center, and Assistant Chairman, Department of Medicine, St. Bernadine Medical Center, San Bernadino, California.

The Pathogenesis of Fever

J. THOMAS BIGGER, Jr., M.D.

Professor of Medicine and of Pharmacology, Columbia University College of Physicians and Surgeons. Attending Physician and Director, Arrhythmia Control Unit, Presbyterian Hospital in the City of New York, New York.

Cardiac Arrhythmias

DANIEL D. BIKLE, M.D., Ph.D.

Associate Professor, University of California, San Francisco, School of Medicine. Attending Physician, University of California San Francisco Medical Center; Co-Director, Special Diagnostic and Treatment Unit, Department of Veterans Affairs Medical Center, San Francisco, California.

Vitamin D; Osteomalacia and Rickets

J. MICHAEL BISHOP, M.D.

Professor, Microbiology and Immunology, Biochemistry and Biophysics; and Director, The G. W. Hooper Research Foundation, University of California, San Francisco, School of Medicine, San Francisco, California.

Oncogenes

ALAN L. BISNO, M.D.

Professor of Medicine, University of Miami School of Medicine. Chief, Medical Service, Veterans Administration Medical Center, and Attending Physician, Jackson Memorial Hospital, Miami, Florida.

Rheumatic Fever

WILLIAM A. BLATTNER, M.D.

Chief, Viral Epidemiology Section, Environmental Epidemiology Branch, Epidemiology and Biostatistics Program, Division of Cancer Etiology, National Cancer Institute, National Institutes of Health, Rockville, Maryland.

Retroviruses That Cause Human Disease

WILLIAM J. BLOT, Ph.D.

Chief, Biostatistics Branch, National Cancer Institute, National Institutes of Health, Bethesda, Maryland.

The Epidemiology of Cancer

ROGER BONE, M.D.

The Ralph Crissman Brown Professor and Chairman, Department of Internal Medicine, Rush Medical College of Rush University. Chief, Section of Pulmonary and Critical Care Medicine, Rush-Presbyterian-St. Luke's Medical Center, Chicago, Illinois.

Bronchiectasis; Cystic Fibrosis

THOMAS D. BOYER, M.D.

Professor of Medicine and Director, Division of Digestive Diseases, Emory University School of Medicine, Atlanta, Georgia.

Cirrhosis of the Liver and Its Major Sequelae

CHARLES B. BRENDLER, M.D.

Associate Professor of Urology, Johns Hopkins University School of Medicine. Active Full-time Staff Member, Department of Urology, Johns Hopkins Hospital, Baltimore, Maryland.

Diseases of the Prostate

SAMUEL BRODER, M.D.

Director, National Cancer Institute; Attending Physician, Clinical Center, National Institutes of Health, Bethesda, Maryland.

Treatment of AIDS and Related Disorders

PHILIP A. BRUNELL, M.D.

Professor of Pediatrics in Residence, University of California, Los Angeles, UCLA School of Medicine. Director, Pediatric Infectious Diseases, Cedars-Sinai Medical Center, Los Angeles, California.

Measles; Rubella; Varicella

JOHN D. BRUNZELL, M.D.

Professor of Medicine, Division of Metabolism, University of Washington School of Medicine, Seattle, Washington.

The Hyperlipoproteinemias

REBECCA H. BUCKLEY, M.D.

J. Buren Sidbury Professor of Pediatrics and Professor of Immunology, Duke University School of Medicine. Chief, Division of Pediatric Allergy and Immunology, Duke University Hospital, Durham, North Carolina.

Primary Immunodeficiency Diseases

WARD E. BULLOCK, M.D.

Arthur Russell Morgan Professor of Medicine and Director, Division of Infectious Diseases, University of Cincinnati College of Medicine. Attending Physician, University Hospital; Consulting Physician in Infectious Diseases, Department of Veterans Affairs Medical Center and Children's Hospital Medical Center, Cincinnati, Ohio.

Actinomycosis; Nocardiosis

PAUL A. BUNN, Jr., M.D.

Professor of Medicine; Director, University of Colorado Cancer Center; and Head, Division of Medical Oncology, University of Colorado Health Sciences Center School of Medicine. Staff Physician, University Hospital, Denver, Colorado.

Paraneoplastic Syndromes; Tumor Markers

DAVID M. BURNS, M.D.

Associate Professor of Medicine, Department of Medicine, Pulmonary and Critical Care Division, University of California, San Diego, School of Medicine, La Jolla. Medical Director, Department of Respiratory Therapy, University of California San Diego Medical Center, San Diego, California.

Tobacco and Health

THOMAS BUTLER, M.D.

Professor, Texas Tech University Health Sciences Center School of Medicine. Attending Physician, University Medical Center, Lubbock, Texas.

Typhoid Fever; Shigellosis; Yersinia Infections; Nonsyphilitic Treponematoses; Relapsing Fever

JOEL N. BUXBAUM, M.D.

Professor of Medicine, New York University School of Medicine. Chief, Rheumatology Section, Veterans Administration Medical Center; Attending Physician, Bellevue Hospital Center, New York, New York.

The Amyloid Diseases

PETER H. BYERS, M.D.

Professor, Departments of Pathology and Medicine, University of Washington School of Medicine, Seattle, Washington.

The Marfan Syndrome; Ehlers-Danlos Syndrome

ANDREI CALIN, M.D., F.R.C.P.

Consultant Rheumatologist, Royal National Hospital for Rheumatic Diseases, Bath, Ireland.

The Spondylarthropathies

BARTOLOME R. CELLI, M.D.

Associate Professor, Boston University School of Medicine. Chief, Pulmonary Section, Veterans Administration Medical Center; Director, Respiratory Care Center, University Hospital, Boston, Massachusetts.

Diseases of the Diaphragm, Chest Wall, Pleura, and Mediastinum

JOHN P. CELLO, M.D.

Professor of Medicine, University of California, San Francisco, School of Medicine. Attending Physician, Moffitt-Long Hospitals; Chief of Gastroenterology, San Francisco General Hospital Medical Center, San Francisco, California.

Gastrointestinal Hemorrhage

BRUCE A. CHABNER, M.D.

Director, Division of Cancer Treatment, National Cancer Institute, National Institutes of Health, Bethesda, Maryland.

Oncology: Introduction

ROBERT M. CHANOCK, M.D.

Laboratory of Infectious Diseases, National Institute of Allergy and Infectious Diseases, National Institutes of Health, Bethesda, Maryland.

Respiratory Syncytial Virus; Parainfluenza Viral Diseases

SANDY F. S. CHUN, M.D.

Staff Physician, Kaiser Foundation Hospital, Santa Clara, California.

Zygomycosis

LINDA HAWES CLEVER, M.D., F.A.C.P.

Clinical Professor of Medicine, University of California, San Francisco, School of Medicine. Chairman, Department of Occupational Health, and Active Staff Member, California Pacific Medical Center, San Francisco, California.

The Health of the Physician

RAY E. CLOUSE, M.D.

Associate Professor of Medicine, Washington University School of Medicine. Associate Physician, Barnes Hospital; Consulting Physician, The Jewish Hospital of St. Louis and The John Cochran Veterans Administration Medical Center, St. Louis, Missouri.

Parenteral Nutrition

C. GLENN COBBS, M.D.

Professor of Medicine and Vice Chairman for Veterans Affairs, University of Alabama School of Medicine. Chief, Medical Service, Veterans Administration Medical Center, Birmingham, Alabama.

Bartonellosis

MARTIN G. COGAN, M.D.

Professor of Medicine, University of California, San Francisco, School of Medicine. Chief, Nephrology Section, Department of Veterans Affairs Medical Center, San Francisco, California.

Specific Renal Tubular Disorders

JORDAN J. COHEN, M.D.

Dean and Professor of Medicine, State University of New York at Stony Brook Health Sciences Center School of Medicine. President, Medical Staff, and Attending Physician, Department of Medicine, University Hospital, Stony Brook, New York.

Vascular Disorders of the Kidney

LAWRENCE S. COHEN, M.D.

The Ebenezer K. Hunt Professor of Medicine, Yale University School of Medicine. Attending Physician, Yale–New Haven Hospital, New Haven, Connecticut.

Surgical Treatment of Coronary Artery Disease; Diseases of the Aorta

SIDNEY COHEN, M.D.

Chairman, Department of Medicine, and Richard Laylord Evans Professor of Medicine, Temple University School of Medicine, Philadelphia, Pennsylvania.

Diseases of the Esophagus

ZANVIL A. COHN, M.D.

Professor, Laboratory of Cellular Physiology and Immunology, Rockefeller University. Senior Physician, Rockefeller University Hospital, New York, New York.

Leprosy—Hansen's Disease

WILLIAM G. COUSER, M.D.

Professor of Medicine, University of Washington School of Medicine. Head, Division of Nephrology, University of Washington Medical Center, Seattle, Washington.

Glomerular Disorders

PHILIP E. CRYER, M.D.

Professor of Medicine and Director, Division of Endocrinology, Diabetes and Metabolism, Washington University School of Medicine. Physician, Barnes Hospital, St. Louis, Missouri.

The Adrenal Medullae; The Carcinoid Syndrome

RONALD G. CRYSTAL, M.D.

Chief, Pulmonary Branch, National Heart, Lung and Blood Institute, National Institutes of Health, Bethesda, Maryland.

Interstitial Lung Disease

JAMES W. CURRAN, M.D., M.P.H.

Director, Division of HIV/AIDS, Center for Infectious Diseases, Centers for Disease Control, Atlanta, Georgia.

Epidemiology of HIV Infection and AIDS

JOHN J. CURTIS, M.D.

Professor of Medicine, University of Alabama School of Medicine. Staff Physician, University of Alabama Hospital, Birmingham, Alabama.

Treatment of Irreversible Renal Failure: Renal Transplantation

DAVID C. DALE, M.D.

Professor of Medicine, University of Washington School of Medicine. Attending Physician, University of Washington Medical Center, Seattle, Washington.

The Febrile Patient

ANTONIO R. DAMASIO, M.D., Ph.D.

Professor, University of Iowa College of Medicine. Head, Department of Neurology, University of Iowa Hospitals and Clinics, Iowa City, Iowa.

Diagnosis of Regional Cerebral Dysfunction; Disturbances of Memory and Language; Alzheimer's Disease and Related Dementias

TROY E. DANIELS, D.D.S., M.S.

Professor and Chair, Division of Oral Pathology, School of Dentistry, University of California, San Francisco. Attending Dentist, Moffitt-Long Hospitals and University of California San Francisco Medical Center, San Francisco, California.

Diseases of the Mouth and Salivary Glands

MICHAEL DECK, M.B., B.S., F.R.A.C.R., F.R.C.R.

Professor of Radiology, Cornell University Medical College. Attending Radiologist, New York Hospital, New York, New York.

Radiologic Imaging Techniques

LEONARD J. DEFTOS, M.D.

Professor of Medicine, University of California, San Diego, School of Medicine, La Jolla. Staff, Laboratory of Bone and Mineral Research, Department of Veterans Affairs Medical Center, San Diego, California.

Calcitonin and Medullary Thyroid Carcinoma

ANDREW DEISS, M.D.

Associate Professor of Medicine, University of Utah School of Medicine. Associate Chief of Staff for Research and Development, Veterans Affairs Medical Center, Salt Lake City, Utah.

Wilson's Disease

VINCENT W. DENNIS, M.D.

Professor of Medicine and Chief, Division of Nephrology, Duke University School of Medicine, Durham, North Carolina.

Investigations of Renal Function

ROBERT J. DESNICK, Ph.D., M.D.

Arthur J. and Nellie Z. Cohen Professor of Pediatrics and Genetics and Chief, Division of Medical and Molecular Genetics, Mount Sinai School of Medicine of the City University of New York. Attending Physician, Mount Sinai Medical Center, New York, New York.

Fabry's Disease

IVAN DIAMOND, M.D., Ph.D.

Professor and Vice Chairman, Department of Neurology, and Professor of Pediatrics and Pharmacology, University of California, San Francisco, School of Medicine. Director, Ernest Gallo Clinic and Research Center. Attending Neurologist, University of California San Francisco Medical Center, San Francisco General Hospital, and Department of Veterans Affairs Medical Center, San Francisco, California.

Alcoholism and Alcohol Abuse; Nutritional Disorders of the Nervous System

EUGENE P. DIMAGNO, M.D.

Professor of Medicine, Mayo Medical School. Consultant in Internal Medicine and Gastroenterology, Mayo Clinic; Director of GI Diagnostic Unit, Saint Mary's Hospital, Rochester, Minnesota.

Carcinoma of the Pancreas

CHARLES A. DINARELLO, M.D.

Professor of Medicine, Tufts University School of Medicine. Staff Physician, New England Medical Center, Boston, Massachusetts.

The Acute Phase Response

WILLIAM E. DISMUKES, M.D.

Director, Division of Infectious Diseases, and Professor and Vice-Chairman for Educational Programs, Department of Medicine, University of Alabama School of Medicine. Attending Physician, University of Alabama Hospital, Birmingham, Alabama.

The Mycoses: Introduction; Histoplasmosis; Blastomycosis; Paracoccidioidomycosis; Cryptococcosis; Sporotrichosis; Candidiasis

R. GORDON DOUGLAS, Jr., M.D.

Clinical Professor of Medicine, Cornell University Medical College. Attending Physician, New York Hospital, New York, New York.

Introduction to Viral Diseases; Influenza; Arthropod-Borne Viral Encephalitides

JEFFREY M. DRAZEN, M.D.

Parker B. Francis Professor of Medicine, Harvard Medical School. Chief, Combined Pulmonary and Critical Care Divisions, Beth Israel and Brigham and Women's Hospitals, Boston, Massachusetts.

Asthma

DOUGLAS A. DROSSMAN, M.D.

Professor of Medicine and Psychiatry, Division of Digestive Diseases, University of North Carolina at Chapel Hill School of Medicine. Attending Physician, University of North Carolina Hospitals, Chapel Hill, North Carolina.

The Eating Disorders

RICHARD J. DUMA, M.D., Ph.D.

Professor of Medicine, Microbiology, and Pathology, Virginia Commonwealth University Medical College of Virginia School of Medicine. Chairman, Division of Infectious Diseases, Department of Internal Medicine, Medical College of Virginia Hospitals, Richmond, Virginia.

Pneumococcal Pneumonia

DAVID T. DURACK, M.B., D.Phil.

Professor of Medicine and of Microbiology and Immunology, Duke University School of Medicine. Chief, Division of Infectious Diseases, Duke University Hospital, Durham, North Carolina.

Infective Endocarditis

PAUL H. EDELSTEIN, M.D.

Associate Professor of Pathology and Laboratory Medicine and of Medicine, University of Pennsylvania School of Medicine. Director of Clinical Microbiology and Attending Physician in Infectious Diseases, Hospital of the University of Pennsylvania, Philadelphia, Pennsylvania.

Legionellosis

THEODORE C. EICKHOFF, M.D.

Professor of Medicine, University of Colorado Health Sciences Center School of Medicine. Director of Internal Medicine, Presbyterian–Saint Luke's Medical Center, Denver, Colorado.

Colorado Tick Fever

RONALD J. ELIN, M.D., Ph.D.

Clinical Professor of Pathology, Uniformed Services University of the Health Sciences F. Edward Hebert School of Medicine. Pathologist, Clinical Center, National Institutes of Health, Bethesda, Maryland.

Laboratory Reference Interval Values of Clinical Importance

EDWARD A. EMMETT, M.B., S.

Worksafe Australia, National Occupational and Health Safety Commission, Sydney, Australia.

Occupational Diseases of the Skin

ANDREW G. ENGEL, M.D.

William L. McKnight 3M Professor of Neuroscience, Mayo Medical School. Attending Physician, Saint Mary's and Rochester Methodist Hospitals, Rochester, Minnesota.

Diseases of Muscles (Myopathies) and Neuromuscular Junction

JEROME ENGEL, Jr., M.D., Ph.D.

Professor of Neurology and Anatomy and Cell Biology, University of California, Los Angeles, UCLA School of Medicine. Attending Neurologist and Chief of Epilepsy and Clinical Neurophysiology, University of California at Los Angeles Medical Center, Los Angeles, California.

The Epilepsies

DOUGLAS V. FALLER, Ph.D., M.D.

Associate Professor, Harvard Medical School. Staff Physician, Dana Farber Cancer Institute and Children's Hospital, Boston, Massachusetts.

Diseases of the Lymph Nodes and Spleen

BARRY L. FANBURG, M.D.

Professor of Medicine, Tufts University School of Medicine. Chief, Pulmonary Division, New England Medical Center, Boston, Massachusetts.

Sarcoidosis

W. EDMUND FARRAR, M.D.

Professor of Medicine and Microbiology, Infectious Diseases Division, Medical University of South Carolina College of Medicine. Staff Physician, Medical University of South Carolina Hospital, Charleston Memorial Hospital, and Veterans Administration Medical Center, Charleston, South Carolina.

Erysipeloid

MARK FELDMAN, M.D.

Professor and Vice Chairman, Department of Internal Medicine, University of Texas Health Science Center at Dallas Southwestern Medical School. Chief, Medical Service, Department of Veterans Affairs Medical Center, Dallas, Texas.

Peptic Ulcer: Complications

DAVID W. FERGUSON, M.D.

Associate Professor of Medicine, Cardiovascular Division, Department of Internal Medicine, University of Iowa College of Medicine. Director, Cardiovascular Intensive Care Unit, Clinical Cardiovascular Physiology Laboratory, and Heart Failure Clinic, University of Iowa Hospitals and Clinics, Iowa City, Iowa.

Shock

ALFRED P. FISHMAN, M.D.

William Maul Measey Professor of Medicine, University of Pennsylvania School of Medicine. Attending Physician, Hospital of the University of Pennsylvania, Philadelphia, Pennsylvania.

Pulmonary Hypertension

GARRET A. FITZGERALD, M.D.

Professor of Medicine and of Pharmacology; The William Stokes Professor of Experimental Therapeutics; Chief, Division of Clinical Pharmacology, Vanderbilt University School of Medicine. Attending Physician, Hypertension and Clinical Pharmacology, Vanderbilt University Medical Center, Nashville, Tennessee.

Prostaglandins and Related Compounds

SUZANNE W. FLETCHER, M.D.

Adjunct Professor, University of Pennsylvania School of Medicine, Philadelphia, Pennsylvania.

Clinical Approach to the Patient

KATHLEEN M. FOLEY, M.D.

Professor of Neurology and Pharmacology, Cornell University Medical College. Chief, Pain Service, Department of Neurology, Memorial Hospital, New York, New York.

Pain and Its Management

BERNARD G. FORGET, M.D.

Professor of Medicine and Human Genetics, Yale University School of Medicine. Attending Physician, Yale–New Haven Hospital, New Haven, Connecticut.

Sickle Cell Anemia and Associated Hemoglobinopathies

MICHAEL M. FRANK, M.D.

Professor and Chairman, Department of Pediatrics, and Professor, Department of Medicine, Duke University School of Medicine. Staff Physician, Duke University Hospital, Durham, North Carolina.

Urticaria and Angioedema

WILLIAM T. FRIEDEWALD, M.D.

Vice-President and Chief Medical Director, Metropolitan Life Insurance Company, New York, New York.

Epidemiology of Cardiovascular Disease

GARY D. FRIEDMAN, M.D., M.S.

Assistant Director for Epidemiology and Biostatistics, Division of Research, Kaiser Permanente Medical Care Program, Oakland. Associate Clinical Professor of Medicine and of Family and Community Medicine, University of California, San Francisco, School of Medicine, San Francisco; Lecturer in Epidemiology, School of Public Health, University of California, Berkeley, California.

The Preventive Health Examination

JAMES F. FRIES, M.D.

Associate Professor of Medicine, Stanford University School of Medicine. Staff Physician, Stanford University Hospital, Stanford, and Veterans Administration Medical Center, Palo Alto, California.

Approach to the Patient with Musculoskeletal Disease

LAWRENCE A. FROHMAN, M.D.

Professor of Medicine and Director, Division of Endocrinology and Metabolism, University of Cincinnati College of Medicine. Director of Endocrinology, University of Cincinnati Hospital, Cincinnati, Ohio.

Neuroendocrine Regulation and Its Disorders; The Anterior Pituitary

PATRICIA A. GABOW, M.D.

Professor, University of Colorado Health Sciences Center School of Medicine. Director of Medical Services, Denver General Hospital, Denver, Colorado.

Cystic Disease of the Kidney

JOHN N. GALGIANI, M.D.

Professor of Medicine, University of Arizona College of Medicine. Chief, Section of Infectious Diseases, Department of Veterans Affairs Medical Center, Tucson, Arizona.

Coccidioidomycosis

RENATE E. GAY, M.D.

Research Associate Professor of Medicine, University of Alabama School of Medicine, Birmingham, Alabama.

Connective Tissue Structure and Function

STEFFEN GAY, M.D.

Professor of Medicine, University of Alabama School of Medicine, Birmingham, Alabama. Director, WHO Collaborating Centre for the Biochemical Classification and Diagnostic Criteria of Rheumatoid Arthritis and Allied Diseases.

Connective Tissue Structure and Function

GORDON N. GILL, M.D.

Professor of Medicine and Co-Director, Division of Endocrinology and Metabolism, University of California, San Diego, School of Medicine, La Jolla. Attending Physician, University of California San Diego Medical Center, San Diego, California.

Principles of Endocrinology

JOHN W. GITTINGER, Jr., M.D.

Professor of Surgery and Neurology and Chairman, Division of Ophthalmology, University of Massachusetts Medical School. Chief of Ophthalmology, University of Massachusetts Medical Center, Worcester, Massachusetts.

Eye Diseases

JOHN H. GLICK, M.D.

Professor of Medicine and Madlyn and Leonard Abramson Professor of Clinical Oncology, University of Pennsylvania School of Medicine. Director, University of Pennsylvania Cancer Center; Attending Physician, Hospital of the University of Pennsylvania, Philadelphia, Pennsylvania.

Hodgkin's Disease

JOHN W. GNANN, Jr., M.D.

Assistant Professor of Medicine and Microbiology, University of Alabama School of Medicine. Attending Physician, Division of Infectious Diseases, University of Alabama Hospital, Birmingham, Alabama.

Foot-and-Mouth Disease; Mumps

CLEON W. GOODWIN, M.D.

Associate Professor, Department of Surgery, Cornell University Medical College. Associate Attending Surgeon and Director, Burn Center, New York Hospital; Associate Attending Surgeon, Jamaica Hospital, New York, New York.

Electrical Injury

SHERWOOD L. GORBACH, M.D.

Professor of Community Health, Medicine, and Microbiology and Immunology, Tufts University School of Medicine. Attending Physician, New England Medical Center and St. Elizabeth's Hospital, Boston, Massachusetts.

Diseases Caused by Non–Spore-Forming Anaerobic Bacteria

JARED J. GRANTHAM, M.D.

Professor of Medicine, University of Kansas Medical Center School of Medicine. Director of Nephrology, University of Kansas Medical Center, Kansas City, Kansas.

Acute Renal Failure

BRUCE M. GREENE, M.D.

Professor of Medicine and Director, Division of Geographic Medicine, Department of Medicine, University of Alabama College of Medicine. Staff Physician, University of Alabama Hospital and Veterans Administration Medical Center, Birmingham, Alabama.

Advice to Travelers; Enteric Infections: Introduction; Onchocerciasis

HARRY L. GREENE, M.D.

Professor of Pediatrics and Associate Professor of Biochemistry, Vanderbilt University School of Medicine. Director, Clinical Nutrition Center, and Associate Director, Vanderbilt Hospital, Nashville, Tennessee.

The Glycogen Storage Diseases; Fructose Intolerance

JOSEPH C. GREENFIELD, Jr., M.D.

James B. Duke Distinguished Professor, Duke University School of Medicine. Chairman, Department of Medicine, Duke University Hospital, Durham, North Carolina.

Electrocardiography

WILLIAM B. GREENOUGH, III, M.D.

Professor of Medicine and of International Health, Johns Hopkins University School of Medicine. Attending Physician, Francis Scott Key Medical Center and Johns Hopkins Hospital, Baltimore, Maryland.

Cholera

JAMES H. GRENDELL, M.D.

Associate Professor of Medicine and Physiology, University of California, San Francisco, School of Medicine. Chief, Gastroenterology Section, Department of Veterans Affairs Medical Center, San Francisco, California.

Vascular Diseases of the Intestine

JEROME E. GROOPMAN, M.D.

Associate Professor of Medicine, Harvard Medical School. Chief of Hematology/Oncology, New England Deaconess Hospital, Boston, Massachusetts.

Langerhans Cell (Eosinophilic) Granulomatosis; Hematology/Oncology in AIDS

CARL GRUNFELD, M.D., Ph.D.

Associate Professor of Medicine, University of California, San Francisco, School of Medicine. Co-Director, Special Diagnostic and Treatment Unit, Department of Veterans Affairs Medical Center, San Francisco, California.

Pancreatic Islet Cell Tumors

RICHARD L. GUERRANT, M.D.

Thomas H. Hunter Professor of International Medicine and Head, Division of Geographic Medicine, University of Virginia School of Medicine. Attending Physician, University of Virginia Hospital, Charlottesville, Virginia.

Campylobacter *Enteritis; Enteric* Escherichia coli *Infections*

STEPHEN M. HAHN, M.D.

Junior Attending Physician, Medicine/Radiation Oncology Branches, National Cancer Institute, National Institutes of Health, Bethesda, Maryland.

Oncologic Emergencies

JOHN L. HAMERTON, D.Sc.

Professor, Department of Human Genetics, University of Manitoba Faculty of Medicine, Winnipeg, Manitoba, Canada.

Chromosomes and Their Disorders

STEPHEN B. HANAUER, M.D.

Associate Professor of Medicine, University of Chicago Pritzker School of Medicine. Co-Director, Outpatient Gastroenterology Clinic, University of Chicago Hospitals, Chicago, Illinois.

Inflammatory Bowel Disease

WILLIAM L. HASKELL, Ph.D.

Professor of Medicine, Stanford University School of Medicine, Stanford, California.

Exercise and Health

BARTON F. HAYNES, M.D.

Chief, Division of Rheumatology and Immunology and Frederic M. Hanes Professor of Medicine, Duke University School of Medicine. Chief, Division of Rheumatology and Immunology, Duke University Hospital, Durham, North Carolina.

Glucocorticosteroid Therapy; Wegener's Granulomatosis and Midline Granuloma

JOHN P. HAYSLETT, M.D.

Professor of Medicine, Yale University School of Medicine. Attending Physician, Yale–New Haven Hospital, New Haven, Connecticut.

Renal Disease in Pregnancy

BERNADINE P. HEALY, M.D.

Director, National Institutes of Health, Bethesda, Maryland.

Miscellaneous Conditions of the Heart: Tumor, Trauma, and Systemic Disease

DONALD A. HENDERSON, M.D., M.P.H.

Edgar Berman Professor, Johns Hopkins School of Hygiene and Public Health, Baltimore, Maryland.

Variola and Vaccinia

ERIK L. HEWLETT, M.D.

Professor of Medicine and of Pharmacology, University of Virginia School of Medicine. Staff Physician, University of Virginia Hospital, Charlottesville, Virginia.

Diphtheria

EDWARD W. HOLMES, M.D.

Chairman, Department of Medicine, Hospital of the University of Pennsylvania, Philadelphia, Pennsylvania.

Other Disorders of Purine Metabolism

LEWIS B. HOLMES, M.D.

Professor of Pediatrics, Harvard Medical School. Pediatrician and Chief, Embryology-Teratology Unit, Children's Service, Massachusetts General Hospital; Director of Genetic and Birth Defects Evaluation and Counseling, Antenatal Diagnostic Test Center, Brigham and Women's Hospital, Boston, Massachusetts.

Congenital Malformations

PHILIP C. HOPEWELL, M.D.

Professor of Medicine, University of California, San Francisco, School of Medicine. Chief of Chest Service, San Francisco General Hospital Medical Center, San Francisco, California.

Critical Care Medicine

DONALD R. HOPKINS, M.D., M.P.H.

Senior Consultant, Global 2000/Carter Center, Chicago, Illinois.

Dracunculiasis

RICHARD B. HORNICK, M.D.

Clinical Professor of Medicine, University of Florida College of Medicine, Gainesville. Vice President of Medical Education, Orlando Regional Medical Center, Orlando, Florida.

Tularemia; Rickettsial Diseases

DAVID S. HOWELL, M.D.

Professor of Medicine and Director, Arthritis Division, University of Miami School of Medicine. Staff Physician, Jackson Memorial Hospital, Miami, Florida.

Osteoarthritis; The Painful Shoulder; The Painful Back

STEPHEN B. HULLEY, M.D., M.P.H.

Professor and Chief, Division of Clinical Epidemiology, Department of Epidemiology and Biostatistics, University of California, San Francisco, School of Medicine, San Francisco, California.

Principles of Preventive Medicine; Control of Unintended Injuries and Those Due to Violence

GENE HUNDER, M.D.

Professor of Medicine, Mayo Medical School. Chairman, Division of Rheumatology, and Consultant in Internal Medicine and Rheumatology, Mayo Clinic, Rochester, Minnesota.

Polymyalgia Rheumatica and Giant Cell Arteritis

DANIEL C. IHDE, M.D.

Professor of Medicine, Uniformed Services University of the Health Sciences F. Edward Hebert School of Medicine. Deputy Chief, Navy Medical Oncology Branch, National Cancer Institute, National Institutes of Health, Bethesda, Maryland.

Approach to the Patient with Metastatic Cancer, Primary Site Unknown

ROBERT W. IKE, M.D.

Instructor of Internal Medicine, University of Michigan Medical School. Attending Physician, University of Michigan Hospital, and Consultant, Department of Veterans Affairs, Veterans Administration Medical Center, Ann Arbor, Michigan.

Specialized Management Procedures for Rheumatic Diseases

JULIANNE IMPERATO-McGINLEY, M.D.

Associate Professor of Medicine, Cornell University Medical College. Associate Attending Physician in Medicine, New York Hospital–Cornell University Medical Center, New York, New York.

Disorders of Sexual Differentiation

MARK A. JACOBSON, M.D.

Assistant Professor of Medicine in Residence, University of California, San Francisco, School of Medicine. Director, Clinical Research Section, AIDS Program, San Francisco General Hospital Medical Center, San Francisco, California.

Ophthalmologic Manifestations of AIDS

JOSEPH JANKOVIC, M.D.

Professor of Neurology and Director of Parkinson's Disease Center and Movement Disorders Clinic, Baylor College of Medicine. Senior Attending Physician, Methodist Hospital and Texas Medical Center, Houston, Texas.

The Extrapyramidal Disorders

WALDEMAR G. JOHANSON, Jr., M.D.

Professor, Department of Internal Medicine, University of Texas Medical School at Galveston, Galveston, Texas.

Introduction to Pneumonia; Pneumonia Caused by Aerobic Gram-Negative Bacilli; Recurrent Aspiration Pneumonia

RICHARD B. JOHNSTON, Jr., M.D.

William H. Bennett Professor of Pediatrics, University of Pennsylvania School of Medicine. Senior Physician, Children's Hospital of Philadelphia, Philadelphia, Pennsylvania.

Whooping Cough

HOWARD W. JONES, III, M.D.

Professor, Obstetrics and Gynecology, and Director of Gynecologic Oncology, Vanderbilt University School of Medicine. Staff Physician, Vanderbilt University Hospital and Metropolitan Nashville General Hospital, Nashville, Tennessee.

Ovarian Carcinoma

ANTHONY KALES, M.D.

Professor and Chairman, Department of Psychiatry, Pennsylvania State University College of Medicine. Director, Sleep Research and Treatment Center, Milton S. Hershey Medical Center, Hershey, Pennsylvania.

Sleep and Its Disorders

JOHN P. KANE, M.D., Ph.D.

Professor of Medicine and of Biochemistry and Biophysics, University of California, San Francisco, School of Medicine. Attending Physician, Moffitt-Long Hospitals, San Francisco, California.

The Judicious Diet

ALBERT Z. KAPIKIAN, M.D.

Head, Epidemiology Section, Laboratory of Infectious Diseases, National Institute of Allergy and Infectious Diseases, National Institutes of Health, Bethesda, Maryland.

The Common Cold; Viral Gastroenteritis

ALLEN P. KAPLAN, M.D.

Chairman, Department of Medicine, State University of New York at Stony Brook Health Sciences Center School of Medicine. Staff Physician, University Hospital, Stony Brook, and Veterans Administration Medical Center, Northport, New York.

Anaphylaxis

GILLA KAPLAN, Ph.D.

Associate Professor, Laboratory of Cellular Physiology and Immunology, Rockefeller University, New York, New York.

Leprosy—Hansen's Disease

MANUEL E. KAPLAN, M.D.

Professor of Medicine, University of Minnesota Medical School. Chief of Hematology/Oncology, Department of Veterans Affairs Medical Center, Minneapolis, Minnesota.

Hemolytic Disorders: Introduction; Acquired Hemolytic Disorders

SAMUEL KAPLAN, M.D.

Professor of Pediatrics (Cardiology), University of California, Los Angeles, UCLA School of Medicine. Attending Physician, University of Califonia at Los Angeles Medical Center, Los Angeles, California.

Congenital Heart Disease

DONALD KAYE, M.D.

Professor and Chairman, Department of Medicine, Medical College of Pennsylvania. Chief of Medicine, Hospital of the Medical College of Pennsylvania; Consultant, Veterans Affairs Medical Center, Philadelphia, Pennsylvania.

Salmonella Infections Other Than Typhoid Fever

JAMES W. KAZURA, M.D.

Professor of Medicine and International Health, Case Western Reserve University School of Medicine. Physician, University Hospitals of Cleveland, Cleveland, Ohio.

Nematode Infections

MICHAEL J. KEATING, M.B., B.S., F.R.A.C.P.

Professor of Medicine, University of Texas Medical School at Houston. Associate Vice President for Clinical Investigation, University of Texas M. D. Anderson Cancer Center, Houston, Texas.

The Chronic Leukemias

ELLIOT D. KIEFF, M.D., Ph.D.

Albee Professor of Medicine and of Microbiology and Molecular Genetics, Harvard Medical School. Director, Infectious Disease Division, Brigham and Women's Hospital, Boston, Massachusetts.

Infectious Mononucleosis

CHARLES H. KING, M.D.

Associate Professor of Medicine, Case Western Reserve University School of Medicine. Assistant Physician, University Hospitals of Cleveland, Cleveland, Ohio.

Cestode Infections

SAULO KLAHR, M.D.

Joseph Friedman Professor of Renal Disease and Director, Renal Division, Washington University School of Medicine. Physician, Barnes Hospital; Staff Physician and Consultant in Nephrology, Jewish Hospital of St. Louis, St. Louis, Missouri.

Structure and Function of the Kidneys; Obstructive Uropathy

JAMES P. KNOCHEL, M.D.

Professor of Internal Medicine, University of Texas Health Science Center at Dallas Southwestern Medical School. Chairman, Department of Internal Medicine, Presbyterian Hospital; Senior Attending Physician, Parkland Memorial Hospital, Dallas, Texas.

Disorders Due to Heat and Cold

EDWIN H. KOLODNY, M.D.

Professor of Neurology, Harvard Medical School. Associate Neurologist, Massachusetts General Hospital, Boston, Massachusetts.

Gaucher Disease; Niemann-Pick Disease

HERMES A. KONTOS, M.D., Ph.D.

Professor of Medicine; Chairman, Division of Cardiology; and Vice-Chairman, Department of Internal Medicine, Virginia Commonwealth University Medical College of Virginia School of Medicine, Richmond, Virginia.

Vascular Diseases of the Limbs

RICHARD M. KRAUSE, M.D.

Senior Scientific Advisor, Fogarty International Center, National Institutes of Health, Bethesda, Maryland.

Streptococcal Diseases

GUENTER J. KREJS, M.D.

Professor and Chairman, Department of Medicine, Karl-Franzens-Universitat, Graz, Austria.

Diarrhea

WILLIAM L. KRINSKY, M.D., Ph.D.

Associate Clinical Professor of Epidemiology, Section of Medical Entomology, Yale University School of Medicine, New Haven, Connecticut.

Arthropods and Leeches

DONALD J. KROGSTAD, M.D.

Associate Professor of Pathology and Medicine, Washington University School of Medicine. Staff Physician, Barnes Hospital and Jewish Hospital of St. Louis, St. Louis, Missouri.

Malaria

JAMES P. KUSHNER, M.D.

Maxwell M. Wintrobe Professor of Medicine and Chief, Division of Hematology-Oncology, University of Utah School of Medicine. Attending Physician, University of Utah Hospital and Veterans Affairs Medical Center, Salt Lake City, Utah.

Normochromic, Normocytic Anemias; Hypochromic Anemias

ROBERT A. KYLE, M.D.

Professor of Medicine and of Laboratory Medicine, Mayo Medical School. Chair, Division of Hematology and Internal Medicine, Mayo Clinic and Mayo Foundation, Rochester, Minnesota.

Plasma Cell Disorders

DAVID J. LANG, M.D.

Vice-Chair, Department of Pediatrics, University of California, Irvine, California College of Medicine, Irvine. Pediatrician-in-Chief and Director of Medical Education, Research, and Infectious Disease, Children's Hospital of Orange County, Orange, California.

Cytomegalovirus Infection

P. REED LARSEN, M.D.

Professor of Medicine, Harvard Medical School. Chief, Thyroid Division, and Senior Physician, Brigham and Women's Hospital, Boston, Massachusetts.

The Thyroid

ROBERT B. LAYZER, M.D.

Professor of Neurology, University of California, San Francisco, School of Medicine, San Francisco, California.

Degenerative Diseases of the Nervous System

GERALD S. LAZARUS, M.D.

Hartzell Professor and Chairman, Department of Dermatology, University of Pennsylvania School of Medicine. Chief, Department of Dermatology, Hospital of the University of Pennsylvania, Philadelphia, Pennsylvania.

Panniculitis and Disorders of the Subcutaneous Fat

E. CARWILE LeROY, M.D.

Professor of Medicine, Medical University of South Carolina College of Medicine. Attending Physician, Medical University Hospital, Charleston, South Carolina.

Systemic Sclerosis

BERNARD LEVIN, M.D.

Professor of Medicine, University of Texas Medical School at Houston, and Clinical Professor, Baylor College of Medicine. Chief, Section of Gastrointestinal Oncology and Digestive Diseases, University of Texas M. D. Anderson Cancer Center, Houston, Texas.

Neoplasms of the Large and Small Intestine

DAVID E. LEVY, M.D.

Clinical Associate Professor of Neurology, Cornell University Medical College. Associate Attending Neurologist, New York Hospital, New York, New York.

Cerebrovascular Diseases

BRIAN J. LEWIS, M.D.

Clinical Professor of Medicine, University of California, San Francisco, School of Medicine. Staff Physician, The Permanente Medical Group, San Francisco, California.

Breast Cancer

ALFRED J. LEWY, M.D., Ph.D.

Professor of Psychiatry, Ophthalmology, and Pharmacology, Oregon Health Sciences University School of Medicine. Director, Sleep and Mood Disorders Laboratory and Mass Spectrometry Laboratory, Oregon Health Sciences University, Portland, Oregon.

The Pineal Gland

LAWRENCE M. LICHTENSTEIN, M.D.

Professor of Medicine, Johns Hopkins University School of Medicine, Baltimore, Maryland.

Insect Sting Allergy

JOHN LINDENBAUM, M.D.

Professor of Medicine and Acting Chairman, Department of Medicine, Columbia University College of Physicians and Surgeons. Attending Physician and Acting Director, Medical Service, Presbyterian Hospital in the City of New York, New York.

An Approach to the Anemias

IRIS F. LITT, M.D.

Professor of Pediatrics, Stanford University School of Medicine. Director, Division of Adolescent Medicine, Stanford University Hospital and Children's Hospital at Stanford, California.

Adolescent Medicine

JOHN N. LOEB, M.D.

Professor of Medicine, Columbia University College of Physicians and Surgeons. Attending Physician, Presbyterian Hospital in the City of New York, New York.

Polyglandular Disorders

DONALD B. LOURIA, M.D.

Professor and Chairman, Department of Preventive Medicine and Community Health, University of Medicine and Dentistry of New Jersey–New Jersey Medical School, Newark, New Jersey.

Trace Metal Poisoning

JOHN M. LUCE, M.D.

Associate Professor of Medicine and Anesthesia, University of California, San Francisco, School of Medicine. Associate Director, Medical-Surgical Intensive Care Unit, San Francisco General Hospital Medical Center, San Francisco, California.

Critical Care Medicine

ROBERT G. LUKE, M.D.

Chairman, Department of Internal Medicine, University of Cincinnati College of Medicine. Physician-in-Chief, University of Cincinnati Hospital, Cincinnati, Ohio.

Treatment of Irreversible Renal Failure: Dialysis

SAMUEL E. LUX, M.D.

Professor of Pediatrics, Harvard Medical School. Chief, Division of Hematology/Oncology, Children's Hospital, Boston, Massachusetts.

Hereditary Defects in the Membrane or Metabolism of the Red Cell

ADEL A. F. MAHMOUD, M.D., Ph.D.

Chairman, Department of Medicine, Case Western Reserve University School of Medicine. Physician-in-Chief, University Hospitals of Cleveland, Cleveland, Ohio.

Introduction to Protozoan and Helminthic Diseases; Schistosomiasis

STEPHEN E. MALAWISTA, M.D.

Professor of Medicine, Department of Internal Medicine, Yale University School of Medicine. Attending Physician, Yale–New Haven Hospital, New Haven, and Veterans Affairs Medical Center, West Haven, Connecticut.

Infectious Arthritis; Lyme Disease

PETER F. MALET, M.D.

Associate Professor of Medicine, University of Pennsylvania School of Medicine. Director, Gallstone Evaluation and Treatment Center, Hospital of the University of Pennsylvania, Philadelphia, Pennsylvania.

Diseases of the Gallbladder and Bile Ducts

GERALD L. MANDELL, M.D.

Professor of Internal Medicine; Owen R. Cheatham Professor of the Sciences; Head, Division of Infectious Diseases, University of Virginia School of Medicine, Charlottesville, Virginia.

Introduction to Microbial Disease; Introduction to Bacterial Disease

HENRY J. MANKIN, M.D.

Edith M. Ashley Professor of Orthopaedic Surgery, Harvard Medical School. Chief of the Orthopaedic Service, Massachusetts General Hospital, Boston, Massachusetts.

Bone Tumors

DOUGLAS J. MARCHANT, M.D.

Professor of Surgery and of Obstetrics and Gynecology, Tufts University School of Medicine. Senior Gynecologist, New England Medical Center, Boston, Massachusetts.

Nonmalignant Diseases of the Breast

ANDREW M. MARGILETH, M.D.

Professor of Pediatrics, University of Virginia School of Medicine. Attending Associate Consultant in Pediatric Dermatology and Infectious Diseases, University of Virginia Hospital, Charlottesville, and Mary Washington Hospital, Fredericksburg, Virginia.

Cat Scratch Disease

ALEXANDER R. MARGULIS, M.D.

Professor of Radiology, University of California, San Francisco, School of Medicine. Staff Radiologist, Moffitt-Long Hospitals; Consultant, San Francisco General Hospital Medical Center, Mt. Zion Hospital, Department of Veterans Affairs Medical Center, and Letterman Army Medical Center, San Francisco, California.

Overview of Imaging Techniques and Projection for the Future

LAWRENCE F. MARSHALL, M.D.

Professor of Surgery, University of California, San Diego, School of Medicine, La Jolla. Chief, Neurosurgical Services, University of California San Diego Medical Center, San Diego, California.

Injury to the Head and Spinal Cord

STEPHEN J. MARX, M.D.

Chief, Mineral Metabolism Section, National Institute of Diabetes and Digestive and Kidney Diseases, National Institutes of Health, Bethesda, Maryland.

Mineral and Bone Homeostasis

HENRY MASUR, M.D.

Clinical Professor of Medicine, George Washington University School of Medicine and Health Sciences, Washington, D.C. Chief, Critical Care Medicine Department, Clinical Center, National Institutes of Health, Bethesda, Maryland.

Toxoplasmosis

ALVIN M. MATSUMOTO, M.D.

Associate Professor of Medicine, University of Washington School of Medicine. Attending Physician, Geriatric Research, Education and Clinical Center, Veterans Administration Medical Center, Seattle, Washington.

The Testis and Male Sexual Function

RICHARD A. MATTHAY, M.D.

Professor and Associate Chairman, Department of Medicine, Yale University School of Medicine. Associate Director, Winchester Chest Clinic, Yale–New Haven Hospital, New Haven, Connecticut.

Chronic Airways Diseases; Abnormalities of Lung Aeration

JAMES R. McARTHUR, M.D.

Professor of Medicine and Hematology, University of Washington School of Medicine. Director, American Society of Hematology Slide Bank. Attending and Consulting Physician, University of Washington Medical Center, Seattle, Washington.

Selection and Preparation of Slides for Hematology Color Plates

J. BRUCE McCLAIN, M.D.

Associate Professor of Medicine, Uniformed Services University of the Health Sciences F. Edward Hebert School of Medicine, Bethesda, Maryland. Staff Physician, Department of Bacterial Diseases, Walter Reed Army Institute of Research, Washington, D.C.

Leptospirosis; Zoonoses

T. DWIGHT McKINNEY, M.D.

Professor of Medicine and Director, Nephrology Section, Indiana University School of Medicine. Staff Physician, Indiana University Medical Center, Richard L. Roudebush Veterans Administration Medical Center, and Wishard Memorial Hospital, Indianapolis, Indiana.

Tubulointerstitial Diseases and Toxic Nephropathies

JAY E. MENITOVE, M.D.

Clinical Associate Professor of Medicine, Medical College of Wisconsin and University of Wisconsin Medical School. Medical Director, Blood Center of Southeastern Wisconsin, Milwaukee, Wisconsin.

Blood Transfusion

DEAN D. METCALFE, M.D.

Head, Mast Cell Physiology Section, Laboratory of Clinical Investigation, National Institute of Allergy and Infectious Diseases, National Institutes of Health. Staff Physician, Clinical Center, National Institutes of Health, Bethesda, Maryland.

Mastocytosis

MARK MIDDLEBROOKS, M.D.

Associate/Fellow, Department of Medicine, Division of Infectious Diseases, University of Alabama School of Medicine. Staff Physician, University of Alabama Hospital, Birmingham, Alabama.

Antiviral Therapy; Herpes Simplex Virus Infections

DEANE F. MOSHER, M.D.

Professor of Medicine and Physiological Chemistry and Head, Section of Hematology, University of Wisconsin Medical School. Consultant, University of Wisconsin Hospital and Clinics, Madison, Wisconsin.

Disorders of Blood Coagulation

ARNO G. MOTULSKY, M.D., D.Sc.

Professor of Medicine and Genetics, University of Washington School of Medicine. Attending Physician, University of Washington Medical Center, Seattle, Washington.

Hemochromatosis; Hereditary Syndromes Involving Multiple Organ Systems

BALFOUR M. MOUNT, C.M., M.D., F.R.C.S.C.

Professor of Surgery and Director, Division of Palliative Care, McGill University Faculty of Medicine. Attending Physician, Royal Victoria Hospital, Montreal, Quebec, Canada.

Care of Dying Patients and Their Families

S. HARVEY MUDD, M.D.

Guest Worker, Laboratory of General and Comparative Biochemistry, National Institute of Mental Health, National Institutes of Health, Bethesda, Maryland.

Homocystinuria

MAURICE A. MUFSON, M.D.

Professor of Microbiology and Professor and Chairman, Department of Medicine, Marshall University School of Medicine. Associate Chief of Staff for Research, Veterans Administration Medical Center; Staff Physician, Cabell Huntington Hospital and St. Mary's Hospital, Huntington, West Virginia.

Viral Pharyngitis, Laryngitis, Croup, and Bronchitis

JOHN F. MURRAY, M.D.

Professor of Medicine, University of California, San Francisco, School of Medicine. Former Chief of the Chest Service, San Francisco General Hospital Medical Center, San Francisco, California.

Respiratory Diseases: Introduction; Respiratory Structure and Function; Respiratory Failure

BRYAN D. MYERS, M.B., Ch.B., M.R.C.P.(UK)

Professor of Medicine and Chief, Division of Nephrology, Stanford University School of Medicine. Chief of Nephrology, Stanford University Medical Center, Stanford, California.

Diabetes and the Kidney

DAVID G. NATHAN, M.D.

Robert G. Stranahan Professor of Pediatrics, Harvard Medical School. Physician-in-Chief, Children's Hospital, Boston, Massachusetts.

Introduction to Hematologic Diseases

FRANKLIN A. NEVA, M.D.

Chief, Laboratory of Parasitic Diseases, National Institute of Allergy and Infectious Diseases, National Institutes of Health. Attending Physician, Clinical Center, National Institutes of Health, Bethesda, Maryland.

American Trypanosomiasis; Leishmaniasis

ARTHUR W. NIENHUIS, M.D.

Chief, Clinical Hematology Branch, National Heart, Lung and Blood Institute, National Institutes of Health, Bethesda, Maryland.

The Thalassemias

ALAN S. NIES, M.D.

Professor of Medicine and Pharmacology and Head, Division of Clinical Pharmacology, University of Colorado Health Sciences Center School of Medicine. Attending Physician, University Hospital, Denver, Colorado.

Principles of Drug Therapy; Interactions Between Drugs; Adverse Reactions to Drugs

CHARLES P. O'BRIEN, M.D., Ph.D.

Professor and Vice-Chairman of Psychiatry, University of Pennsylvania School of Medicine. Chief of Psychiatry, Veterans Affairs Medical Center, Philadelphia, Pennsylvania.

Drug Abuse and Dependence

ROBERT K. OCKNER, M.D.

Professor of Medicine and Director, Liver Center, University of California, San Francisco, School of Medicine. Attending Physician, Moffitt-Long Hospitals, San Francisco, California.

Introduction to Gastrointestinal Diseases; Clinical Approach to Liver Disease; Acute Viral Hepatitis; Chronic Hepatitis

JERROLD M. OLEFSKY, M.D.

Professor of Medicine, University of California, San Diego, School of Medicine, La Jolla. Staff Member, Medical Research Service, Department of Veterans Affairs Medical Center, San Diego, California.

Diabetes Mellitus

SUZANNE OPARIL, M.D.

Professor of Medicine and Associate Professor of Physiology and Biophysics, University of Alabama School of Medicine. Director, Hypertension Program, Division of Cardiovascular Diseases, and Attending Cardiologist, University Hospital, Birmingham, Alabama.

Arterial Hypertension

WALTER A. ORENSTEIN, M.D.

Director, Division of Immunization, Centers for Disease Control, Atlanta, Georgia.

Immunization

ERIC A. OTTESEN, M.D.

Attending Physician, Clinical Center, National Institutes of Health, Bethesda, Maryland, and Children's Hospital National Medical Center, Washington, D.C.

Filariasis: Introduction; Lymphatic Filariasis; Tropical Eosinophilia; Loiasis; Other Filarial Infections

MICHAEL N. OXMAN, M.D.

Professor of Medicine and Pathology, University of California, San Diego, School of Medicine, La Jolla. Staff Physician, Infectious Diseases Section, Department of Veterans Affairs Medical Center, San Diego, California.

Enteroviral Diseases; Epidemic Pleurodynia; Myocarditis and Pericarditis Caused by Enteroviruses; Mucocutaneous Syndrome Caused by Enteroviruses; Acute Hemorrhagic Conjunctivitis

CHARLES Y. C. PAK, M.D.

University Distinguished Chair in Mineral Metabolism, University of Texas Health Science Center at Dallas Southwestern Medical School, Dallas, Texas.

Renal Calculi

FRANK PARKER, M.D.

Professor and Chairman, Department of Dermatology, Oregon Health Sciences University School of Medicine. Staff Physician, Oregon Health Sciences University Hospital, Portland, Oregon.

Cutaneous Manifestations of Internal Malignancy; Skin Diseases

STEPHEN G. PAUKER, M.D.

Professor of Medicine, Tufts University School of Medicine. Chief, Division of Clinical Decision Making, Department of Medicine, New England Medical Center, Boston, Massachusetts.

Clinical Decision Making

NEAL S. PENNEYS, M.D., Ph.D.

Professor of Dermatology, University of Miami School of Medicine. Attending Physician, Jackson Memorial Hospital, Miami, Florida.

Cutaneous Signs of AIDS

JOSEPH K. PERLOFF, M.D.

Streisand/American Heart Association Professor of Medicine and Pediatrics, University of California, Los Angeles, UCLA School of Medicine, Los Angeles, California.

Diseases of the Myocardium

WALTER L. PETERSON, M.D.

Professor of Medicine, University of Texas Health Science Center at Dallas Southwestern Medical School. Chief of Digestive Diseases, Department of Veterans Affairs Medical Center, Dallas, Texas.

Peptic Ulcer: Medical Therapy

THEODORE L. PHILLIPS, M.D.

Professor and Chairman, Department of Radiation Oncology, University of California, San Francisco, School of Medicine. Attending Physician, Long-Moffitt Hospitals, San Francisco; Chief, Section of Radiation Oncology, University of California Davis Hospital, Davis, California.

Radiation Injury

CLAUDE A. PIANTADOSI, M.D.

Associate Professor of Medicine, Duke University School of Medicine. Attending Physician, Duke University Hospital, Durham, North Carolina.

Physical, Chemical, and Aspiration Injuries of the Lung

F. XAVIER PI-SUNYER, M.D.

Professor of Clinical Medicine, Columbia University College of Physicians and Surgeons. Chief, Division of Endocrinology, Diabetes, and Nutrition; Director, Obesity Research Center, St. Luke's–Roosevelt Hospital Center, New York, New York.

Obesity

PHILIP A. PIZZO, M.D.

Professor of Pediatrics, Uniformed Services University of the Health Sciences F. Edward Hebert School of Medicine. Chief of Pediatrics and Head, Infectious Disease Section, National Cancer Institute, National Institutes of Health, Bethesda, Maryland.

The Compromised Host

FRED PLUM, M.D.

Anne Parrish Titzell Professor and Chairman of Neurology and Neuroscience, Cornell University Medical College. Neurologist-in-Chief, Department of Neurology, New York Hospital–Cornell Medical Center, New York, New York.

Clinical Neurologic Diagnosis; Neurologic Problems Associated with Aging; Disturbances of Consciousness and Arousal; Sustained Impairments of Consciousness; Brain Death; Brief Loss of Consciousness; Disorders of Motor Function

RICHARD L. POPP, M.D.

Professor of Medicine, Stanford University School of Medicine. Associate Chairman, Department of Medicine, Stanford University Hospital, Stanford, California.

Echocardiography

CAROL S. PORTLOCK, M.D.

Associate Professor of Clinical Medicine, Cornell University Medical College. Acting Chief, Lymphoma Service, Memorial Sloan-Kettering Cancer Center, New York, New York.

Introduction to Neoplasms of the Immune System; The Non-Hodgkin's Lymphomas

JEROME B. POSNER, M.D.

Professor of Neurology and Neuroscience, Cornell University Medical College. Attending Neurologist, Memorial Sloan-Kettering Cancer Center, New York, New York.

Nonmetastatic Effects of Cancer on the Nervous System; Clinical Neurologic Diagnosis; Episodic Loss of Motor Function; Disorders of Sensation; Mechanical Lesions of the Spine and Related Structures

RICHARD W. PRICE, M.D.

Professor and Head, Department of Neurology, University of Minnesota Medical School. Chief of Neurology Service, University of Minnesota Hospital, Minneapolis, Minnesota.

Neurologic Complications of HIV-1 Infection; Viral Infections of the Nervous System

WILLIAM A. PULSINELLI, M.D., Ph.D.

Professor of Neurology and Neuroscience, Cornell University Medical College. Attending Neurologist, New York Hospital, New York, New York.

Cerebrovascular Diseases

THOMAS C. QUINN, M.D.

Senior Investigator, National Institute of Allergy and Infectious Diseases, National Institutes of Health; Associate Professor of Medicine and International Health, Johns Hopkins Medical Institutions. Staff Physician, Johns Hopkins Hospital, Baltimore, and Clinical Center, National Institutes of Health, Bethesda, Maryland.

African Trypanosomiasis

CHARLES E. RACKLEY, M.D.

Anton and Margaret Fuisz Professor of Medicine and Director, Lipid Disorder Center, Georgetown University School of Medicine. Attending Physician, Department of Medicine, Georgetown University Medical Center, Washington, D.C.

Valvular Heart Disease

JONATHAN I. RAVDIN, M.D.

Professor and Vice Chairman, Department of Medicine, Case Western Reserve University School of Medicine. Chief, Medical Service, Department of Veterans Affairs Medical Center, Cleveland, Ohio.

Amebiasis

ROBERT W. REBAR, M.D.

George B. Riley Professor and Chairman, Department of Obstetrics and Gynecology, University of Cincinnati College of Medicine. Clinical Director, Department of Obstetrics and Gynecology, University of Cincinnati Hospital, Cincinnati, Ohio.

The Ovaries

CHARLES E. REED, M.D.

Professor of Internal Medicine, Mayo Medical School. Staff Physician, Saint Mary's and Methodist Hospitals, Rochester, Minnesota.

Drug Allergy

ROBERT R. RICH, M.D.

Professor of Microbiology and of Immunology and Medicine and Vice President and Dean of Research, Baylor College of Medicine. Attending Physician, Veterans Affairs Medical Center; Medical Staff Member, Methodist Hospital, Houston, Texas.

Immune Complex Diseases

CHARLES T. RICHARDSON, M.D.

Clinical Professor of Internal Medicine, University of Texas Health Science Center at Dallas Southwestern Medical School. Attending Physician, Baylor University Medical Center, Dallas, Texas.

Peptic Ulcer: Pathogenesis; Zollinger-Ellison Syndrome

B. LAWRENCE RIGGS, M.D.

Purvis and Roberta Tabor Professor of Medical Research, Mayo Medical School, Rochester, Minnesota.

Osteoporosis

ROGER S. RITTMASTER, M.D.

Associate Professor, Dalhousie University Faculty of Medicine. Active Staff Member, Camp Hill Medical Center, Halifax, Nova Scotia, Canada.

Hirsutism

RICHARD S. RIVLIN, M.D.

Professor of Medicine, Cornell University Medical College. Head, Nutrition Research Program, Memorial Sloan-Kettering Cancer Center; Chief, Nutrition Division, New York Hospital–Cornell Medical Center; Visiting Physician, Rockefeller University Hospital, New York, New York.

Disorders of Vitamin Metabolism: Deficiencies, Metabolic Abnormalities, and Excesses

JOHN PAUL ROBERTS, M.D.

Assistant Professor of Surgery, University of California, San Francisco, School of Medicine, San Francisco, California.

Liver Transplantation

WILLIAM O. ROBERTSON, M.D.

Professor of Pediatrics, University of Washington School of Medicine. Medical Director, Washington Poison Network, Children's Hospital and Medical Center, Seattle, Washington.

Common Poisonings

WILLIAM J. ROGERS, M.D.

Professor of Medicine, University of Alabama School of Medicine. Director of Coronary Care Unit, University of Alabama Hospital, Birmingham, Alabama.

Angina Pectoris

JOHN ROSS, Jr., M.D.

Professor of Medicine, University of California, San Diego, School of Medicine, La Jolla. Head, Division of Cardiology, University of California San Diego Medical Center, San Diego, California.

Cardiac Function and Circulatory Control

RUSSELL ROSS, Ph.D.

Professor and Chairman of Pathology, University of Washington School of Medicine, Seattle, Washington.

Atherosclerosis

DAVID A. ROTTENBERG, M.D.

Director, PET Imaging Service, and Chief, Neurology Service, Veterans Administration Medical Center, Minneapolis, Minnesota.

Disorders of Intracranial Pressure

DAVID W. ROWE, M.D.

Professor of Pediatrics, University of Connecticut School of Medicine. Attending Physician, John Dempsey Hospital and University of Connecticut Health Center, Farmington, Connecticut.

Osteogenesis Imperfecta

JOHN W. ROWE, M.D.

President and Professor of Medicine and Geriatrics, Mount Sinai School of Medicine of the City University of New York. President, Mount Sinai Medical Center, New York, New York.

Aging and Geriatric Medicine

ROBERT M. RUSSELL, M.D.

Professor of Medicine and Nutrition, Tufts University Schools of Medicine and Nutrition. Staff Physician, New England Medical Center, Boston, Massachusetts.

Nutrient Requirements; Nutritional Assessment

ANGELO RUSSO, M.D., Ph.D.

Senior Investigator, National Cancer Institute, National Institutes of Health. Staff Physician, Clinical Center, National Institutes of Health, Bethesda, Maryland.

Oncologic Emergencies

MICHAEL S. SAAG, M.D.

Assistant Professor of Medicine, Division of Infectious Diseases, University of Alabama School of Medicine, and Director, University of Alabama AIDS Outpatient Clinic. Associate Director, General Clinical Research Center, and Assistant Chief, Medical Service, Veterans Administration Medical Center, Birmingham, Alabama.

Mycetoma; Dematiaceous Fungal Infections; HIV and Associated Disorders: Introduction; Prevention of HIV Infection; Renal, Cardiac, Endocrine, and Rheumatologic Manifestations of HIV Infection

R. BRADLEY SACK, M.D., Sc.D.

Professor, Department of International Health, Johns Hopkins University School of Hygiene and Public Health. Staff Physician, Department of Medicine, Johns Hopkins Hospital, Baltimore, Maryland.

The Diarrhea of Travelers

ROBERT A. SALATA, M.D.

Assistant Professor of Medicine and International Health, Case Western Reserve University School of Medicine. Attending Physician and Consultant, University Hospitals of Cleveland, Cleveland, Ohio.

Brucellosis

SYDNEY E. SALMON, M.D.

Regents Professor of Medicine, University of Arizona College of Medicine. Director, Arizona Cancer Center; Attending Physician, University Medical Center, Tucson, Arizona.

Principles of Cancer Therapy

JOHN E. SALVAGGIO, M.D.

Henderson Professor of Medicine and Vice Chancellor, Tulane University School of Medicine. Active Staff Member, Tulane University Hospital; Visiting Physician, Charity Hospital and Department of Veterans Affairs Medical Center, New Orleans, Louisiana.

Allergic Rhinitis

JAY P. SANFORD, M.D.

Professor of Medicine Emeritus and Dean Emeritus, Uniformed Services University of the Health Sciences F. Edward Hebert School of Medicine, Bethesda. Attending Physician (Infectious Diseases), Walter Reed Army Medical Center, Washington, D.C., and National Naval Medical Center, Bethesda, Maryland.

Dengue; West Nile Fever; Phlebotomus Fever; Rift Valley Fever; Alphaviruses Associated with Polyarthritis; Snake Bites

CLIFFORD B. SAPER, M.D.

William D. Mabie Professor of Neuroscience and Neurology, University of Chicago Pritzker School of Medicine. Staff Physician, University of Chicago Hospitals, Chicago, Illinois.

Autonomic Disorders and Their Management

FRED R. SATTLER, M.D.

Associate Professor of Medicine, University of Southern California School of Medicine. Coordinator, Interdisciplinary AIDS Service, Los Angeles County–University of Southern California Medical Center, Los Angeles, California. Chairman, Opportunistic Infections Committee, AIDS Clinical Trials Group, Division of AIDS, National Institutes of Allergy and Infectious Disease, National Institutes of Health.

Pulmonary Manifestations of AIDS: Special Emphasis on Pneumocystosis

DAVID T. SCADDEN, M.D.

Instructor in Medicine, Harvard Medical School. Active Staff, New England Deaconess Hospital, Boston, Massachusetts.

Hematology/Oncology in AIDS

WILLIAM SCHAFFNER, M.D.

Professor and Chairman, Department of Preventive Medicine, and Professor of Medicine (Infectious Diseases), Vanderbilt University School of Medicine. Hospital Epidemiologist, Vanderbilt University Hospital, Nashville, Tennessee.

Prevention and Control of Hospital-Acquired Infections

BRUCE F. SCHARSCHMIDT, M.D.

Professor of Medicine and Director, Division of Gastroenterology, University of California, San Francisco, School of Medicine. Attending Hematologist, Liver Transplant Service, and Attending Physician, University of California San Francisco Medical Center, San Francisco, California.

Bilirubin Metabolism and Hyperbilirubinemia; Inherited, Infiltrative, and Metabolic Disorders Involving the Liver; Acute and Chronic Hepatic Failure; Hepatic Tumors

HERBERT H. SCHAUMBURG, M.D.

Professor and Chairman, Department of Neurology, Albert Einstein College of Medicine of Yeshiva University. Director of Neurology, Montefiore Medical Center, Bronx, New York.

Diseases of the Peripheral Nervous System

LAWRENCE R. SCHILLER, M.D.

Clinical Assistant Professor of Internal Medicine, University of Texas Health Science Center at Dallas Southwestern Medical School. Director of Gastrointestinal Physiology Laboratory and Attending Physician, Baylor University Medical Center, Dallas, Texas.

Peptic Ulcer: Epidemiology, Clinical Manifestations, and Diagnosis

STEPHEN C. SCHIMPFF, M.D.

Professor of Medicine, Pharmacology, and Oncology, University of Maryland School of Medicine. Executive Vice President, University of Maryland Medical System, Baltimore, Maryland.

Diseases Caused by Pseudomonads

THEODORE R. SCHROCK, M.D.

Professor of Surgery, University of California, San Francisco, School of Medicine, San Francisco, California.

Diseases of the Rectum and Anus

H. RALPH SCHUMACHER, Jr., M.D.

Professor of Medicine and Acting Chief, Rheumatology Section, University of Pennsylvania School of Medicine. Director, Arthritis-Immunology Center, Veterans Affairs Medical Center, Philadelphia, Pennsylvania.

Crystal Deposition Arthropathies; Relapsing Polychondritis; Multifocal Fibrosclerosis

BENJAMIN D. SCHWARTZ, M.D., Ph.D.

Professor of Medicine (Rheumatology), Washington University School of Medicine. Chief, Division of Rheumatology, Jewish Hospital of St. Louis; Associate Attending Physician, Barnes Hospital, St. Louis, Missouri.

The Major Histocompatibility Complex and Disease Susceptibility

CHARLES H. SCOGGIN, M.D.

President, Somatogen, Broomfield, Colorado.

Pulmonary Neoplasms

CHARLES R. SCRIVER, M.D.C.M., F.R.S.C.

Professor of Biology, Human Genetics, and Pediatrics, McGill University Faculty of Medicine. Physician and Director, DeBelle Laboratory for Biomedical Genetics, Montreal Children's Hospital, Montreal, Quebec, Canada.

Hyperaminoaciduria; The Hyperphenylalaninemias

S. K. K. SEAH, M.D., Ph.D.

Associate Professor of Medicine, McGill University Faculty of Medicine. Attending Physician, Montreal General Hospital, Montreal, Quebec, Canada.

Hermaphroditic Flukes

MARGRETTA R. SEASHORE, M.D.

Professor of Human Genetics and Pediatrics, Yale University School of Medicine. Attending Physician, Yale–New Haven Hospital, New Haven, Connecticut.

Genetic Counseling

STANTON SEGAL, M.D.

Professor of Pediatrics and Medicine, University of Pennsylvania School of Medicine. Director, Division of Biochemical Development and Molecular Diseases, Children's Hospital of Philadelphia, Philadelphia, Pennsylvania.

Galactosemia

ROBERT M. SENIOR, M.D.

Dorothy R. and Hubert C. Moog Professor of Pulmonary Diseases in Medicine, Department of Medicine, Washington University School of Medicine. Director, Respiratory and Critical Care Division, Department of Medicine, Jewish Hospital of St. Louis, St. Louis, Missouri.

Pulmonary Embolism; Fat Embolism Syndrome

F. JOHN SERVICE, M.D., Ph.D.

Professor of Medicine, Mayo Medical School. Consultant, Division of Endocrinology and Metabolism, Department of Internal Medicine, Mayo Clinic, Rochester, Minnesota.

Hypoglycemic Disorders

RALPH SHABETAI, M.D., F.R.C.P.(Edin)

Professor of Medicine, University of California, San Diego, School of Medicine, La Jolla. Chief of Cardiology, Department of Veterans Affairs Medical Center, San Diego, California.

Diseases of the Pericardium

GEORGE M. SHAW, M.D., Ph.D.

Associate Professor of Medicine, Division of Hematology and Oncology, University of Alabama School of Medicine, Birmingham, Alabama.

Biology of Human Immunodeficiency Viruses

JOHN N. SHEAGREN, M.D.

Professor of Medicine, University of Illinois College of Medicine at Chicago. Chairman, Department of Internal Medicine, Illinois Masonic Medical Center, Chicago, Illinois.

Shock Syndromes Related to Sepsis; Staphylococcal Infections

DEAN SHEPPARD, M.D.

Associate Professor of Medicine, University of California, San Francisco, School of Medicine. Attending Physician, Chest Service, San Francisco General Hospital Medical Center, San Francisco, California.

Occupational Pulmonary Disorders

ROBERT E. SHOPE, M.D.

Professor of Epidemiology, Yale University School of Medicine, New Haven, Connecticut.

Arthropod-Borne Viral Diseases: Introduction; Viral Hemorrhagic Fevers

JONAS A. SHULMAN, M.D.

Professor of Medicine (Infectious Diseases), Emory University School of Medicine. Chief of Medicine, Crawford Long Hospital of Emory University, Atlanta, Georgia.

Anthrax

MARC SHUMAN, M.D.

Professor of Medicine and Associate Director, Cancer Research Institute, University of California, San Francisco, School of Medicine. Attending Physician, Moffitt-Long Hospitals, San Francisco, California.

Hemorrhagic Disorders: Abnormalities of Platelet and Vascular Function

MARK SIEGLER, M.D.

Professor of Medicine, University of Chicago Pritzker School of Medicine; Director, Center for Clinical Medical Ethics, University of Chicago. Attending and Consulting Physician, University of Chicago Hospitals, Chicago, Illinois.

Clinical Ethics in the Practice of Medicine

DONALD H. SILBERBERG, M.D.

Professor and Chairman, Department of Neurology, University of Pennsylvania School of Medicine. Chief of Service, Department of Neurology, Hospital of the University of Pennsylvania, Philadelphia, Pennsylvania.

The Demyelinating Diseases

ROGER P. SIMON, M.D.

Professor, Department of Neurology, University of California, San Francisco, School of Medicine. Chief, Neurology Service, San Francisco General Hospital Medical Center, San Francisco, California.

Parameningeal Infections; Neurosyphilis

FREDERICK R. SINGER, M.D.

Professor of Medicine in Residence, University of California, Los Angeles, UCLA School of Medicine. Director, Bone Center, Cedars-Sinai Medical Center, Los Angeles, California.

Paget's Disease of Bone

PETER A. SINGER, M.D., F.R.C.P.C.

Assistant Professor of Medicine and Associate Director, Centre for Bioethics, University of Toronto Faculty of Medicine. Attending Physician, Toronto Hospital (Toronto Western Division), Toronto, Ontario, Canada

Clinical Ethics in the Practice of Medicine

EDUARDO SLATOPOLSKY, M.D.

Professor of Medicine, Washington University School of Medicine. Director, Chromalloy American Kidney Center; Attending Physician, Barnes Hospital; Consultant in Nephrology, Jewish Hospital of St. Louis, St. Louis, Missouri.

Renal Osteodystrophy

MARVIN H. SLEISENGER, M.D.

Professor of Medicine and Director, Cancer Research Institute, University of California, San Francisco, School of Medicine. Attending Physician, Moffitt-Long Hospitals; Consulting Physician, Department of Veterans Affairs Medical Center, San Francisco, California.

Miscellaneous Inflammatory Diseases of the Intestine

WILLIAM S. SLY, M.D.

Professor and Chairman, Edward A. Doisy Department of Biochemistry and Molecular Biology, St. Louis University School of Medicine. Active Staff Member, Cardinal Glennon Children's Hospital, St. Louis, Missouri.

The Mucopolysaccharidoses

LLOYD H. SMITH, Jr., M.D.

Professor of Medicine and Associate Dean, University of California, San Francisco, School of Medicine, San Francisco, California.

Medicine as an Art; Primary Hyperoxaluria; The Hyperprolinemias and Hydroxyprolinemia; Diseases of the Urea Cycle; Branched-Chain Aminoaciduria; Disorders of Pyrimidine Metabolism; Phosphorus Deficiency and Hypophosphatemia; Disorders of Magnesium Metabolism

THOMAS W. SMITH, M.D.

Professor of Medicine, Harvard Medical School. Chief, Cardiovascular Division, Brigham and Women's Hospital, Boston, Massachusetts.

Approach to the Patient with Cardiovascular Disease; Heart Failure

WILLIAM J. SNAPE, Jr., M.D.

Professor of Medicine, University of California, Los Angeles, UCLA School of Medicine. Chief of Gastroenterology, Harbor-UCLA Medical Center, Los Angeles, California.

Disorders of Gastrointestinal Motility

ROSEMARY SOAVE, M.D.

Assistant Professor of Medicine and Public Health, Cornell University Medical College. Associate Attending Physician, New York Hospital–Cornell Medical Center, New York, New York.

Cryptosporidiosis

BURTON E. SOBEL, M.D.

Tobias and Hortense Lewin Distinguished Professor in Cardiovascular Disease, Washington University School of Medicine. Director, Cardiovascular Division, Washington University School of Medicine and Barnes and Wohl Hospitals, St. Louis, Missouri.

Acute Myocardial Infarction

ANDREW H. SOLL, M.D.

Professor of Medicine, University of California, Los Angeles, UCLA School of Medicine. Chief of Gastroenterology, Wadsworth Veterans Administration Medical Center, Los Angeles, California.

Gastritis

ROGER D. SOLOWAY, M.D.

Marie B. Gale Professor of Medicine and Acting Chairman, Department of Internal Medicine, University of Texas Medical School at Galveston, Galveston, Texas.

Diseases of the Gallbladder and Bile Ducts

P. FREDERICK SPARLING, M.D.

Professor and Chairman, Department of Medicine, University of North Carolina at Chapel Hill School of Medicine. Chair, Department of Medicine, University of North Carolina Hospitals, Chapel Hill, North Carolina.

Sexually Transmitted Diseases

ALLEN M. SPIEGEL, M.D.

Chief, Molecular Pathophysiology Branch, National Institute of Diabetes and Digestive and Kidney Diseases, National Institutes of Health, Bethesda, Maryland.

The Parathyroid Glands, Hypercalcemia, and Hypocalcemia

ALAN M. STAMM, M.D.

Associate Professor of Medicine, University of Alabama School of Medicine. Attending Physician, University of Alabama Hospital, Birmingham, Alabama.

Listeriosis

WALTER E. STAMM, M.D.

Professor of Medicine, University of Washington School of Medicine. Head, Infectious Disease Division, Harborview Medical Center, Seattle, Washington.

Diseases Caused by Chlamydiae

ALFRED D. STEINBERG, M.D.

Chief, Cellular Immunology, Arthritis and Rheumatism Branch, National Institute of Arthritis and Musculoskeletal and Skin Diseases, National Institutes of Health. Attending Physician, Clinical Center, National Institutes of Health, Bethesda, Maryland.

Systemic Lupus Erythematosus

WILLIAM M. STEINBERG, M.D.

Professor of Medicine, George Washington University School of Medicine and Health Sciences. Staff Physician, Division of Gastroenterology, George Washington University Hospital, Washington, D.C.

Pancreatitis

DAVID A. STEVENS, M.D.

Professor of Medicine, Stanford University School of Medicine, Stanford. Chief, Division of Infectious Diseases, Department of Medicine, Santa Clara Valley Medical Center, San Jose. Principal Investigator, Infectious Disease Research Laboratory, California Institute for Medical Research, San Jose, California.

Aspergillosis; Zygomycosis

DAVID P. STEVENS, M.D.

Scott R. Inkley Professor of General Internal Medicine and Vice Chairman, Department of Medicine, Case Western Reserve University School of Medicine. Chief, Division of General Internal Medicine, University Hospitals of Cleveland, Cleveland, Ohio.

Giardiasis; Other Protozoan Diseases

DANIEL P. STITES, M.D.

Professor and Vice Chairman, Department of Laboratory Medicine, University of California, San Francisco, School of Medicine. Staff Physician, University of California San Francisco Medical Center, San Francisco, California.

Diseases of the Thymus

RAINER STORB, M.D.

Professor of Medicine, University of Washington School of Medicine. Head, Program in Transplantation Biology, and Member, Fred Hutchinson Cancer Research Center, Seattle, Washington.

Bone Marrow Transplantation

GORDON J. STREWLER, M.D.

Associate Professor of Medicine, University of California, San Francisco, School of Medicine. Chief, Endocrine Unit, Department of Veterans Affairs Medical Center, San Francisco, California.

Osteonecrosis, Osteosclerosis, and Other Disorders of Bone

WADI N. SUKI, M.D.

Professor of Medicine and of Molecular Physiology and Biophysics, and Chief, Renal Section, Department of Medicine, Baylor College of Medicine. Senior Attending Physician and Chief, Renal Service, Methodist Hospital, Houston, Texas.

Hereditary Chronic Nephropathies

MORTON N. SWARTZ, M.D.

Professor of Medicine, Harvard Medical School. Chief, James Jackson Firm Medical Services; Member, Infectious Disease Unit, Massachusetts General Hospital, Boston, Massachusetts.

Bacterial Meningitis; Meningococcal Disease; Infections Caused by Haemophilus *Species*

NORMAN TALAL, M.D.

Professor of Medicine and Microbiology and Head, Division of Clinical Immunology, University of Texas Medical School at San Antonio. Head, Division of Clinical Immunology, Medical Center Hospital; Chief, Division of Clinical Immunology, Audie L. Murphy Veterans Hospital, San Antonio, Texas.

Sjögren's Syndrome

CLIFFORD TASMAN-JONES, M.B., Ch.B., F.R.C.P., F.R.A.C.P.

Head, Section of Gastroenterology and Human Nutrition, University of Auckland Medical School. Senior Physician and Gastroenterologist, Auckland Hospital, Auckland, New Zealand.

Disturbances of Trace Mineral Metabolism

RICHARD C. THIRLBY, M.D.

Clinical Assistant Professor of Surgery, University of Washington School of Medicine. Attending Surgeon, Virginia Mason Medical Center, Seattle, Washington.

Peptic Ulcer: Surgical Therapy

PHILLIP P. TOSKES, M.D.

Professor of Medicine, University of Florida College of Medicine. Director, Division of Gastroenterology, Hepatology and Nutrition, Shands Hospital of the University of Florida College of Medicine; Chief, Gastroenterology Section, Veterans Administration Medical Center, Gainesville, Florida.

Malabsorption

GARY J. TUCKER, M.D.

Professor and Chairman, Department of Psychiatry and Behavioral Sciences, University of Washington School of Medicine. Staff Physician, University of Washington Medical Center, Seattle, Washington.

Psychiatric Disorders in Medical Practice

J. BLAKE TYRRELL, M.D.

Clinical Professor of Medicine and Associate Director, Metabolic Research Unit, University of California, San Francisco, School of Medicine. Director, Endocrine Clinic, Moffitt-Long Hospitals, San Francisco, California.

Disorders of the Adrenal Cortex

JOUNI UITTO, M.D., Ph.D.

Professor and Chairman, Department of Dermatology, Jefferson Medical College of Thomas Jefferson University. Staff Physician, Thomas Jefferson University Hospital, Philadelphia, Pennsylvania.

Pseudoxanthoma Elasticum

JACK A. VENNES, M.D.

Professor of Medicine, University of Minnesota Medical School. Staff Physician, University of Minnesota Hospitals and Clinics, Minneapolis, Minnesota.

Gastrointestinal Endoscopy

NICHOLAS A. VICK, M.D.

Professor of Neurology, Northwestern University Medical School, Chicago. Head, Division of Neurology, Evanston Hospital, Evanston, Illinois.

Intracranial Tumors and States of Altered Intracranial Pressure

JONATHAN D. VICTOR, M.D., Ph.D.

Professor of Neurology and Neuroscience, Cornell University Medical College. Attending Neurologist, New York Hospital, and Associate Attending Physician, Hospital for Special Surgery, New York, New York.

Neurologic Diagnostic Procedures

JOHN E. VOLANAKIS, M.D.

Anna Lois Wares Chair of Medicine in Rheumatology and Professor of Medicine, Microbiology, and Pathology, University of Alabama School of Medicine, Birmingham, Alabama.

Complement

FRANCIS A. WALDVOGEL, M.D.

Professor of Medicine, University of Geneva. Chairman, Department of Medicine, and Physician-in-Chief, Clinique Medical Therapeutique, University Hospital, Geneva, Switzerland.

Osteomyelitis

BRUCE D. WALKER, M.D.

Assistant Professor of Medicine, Harvard Medical School. Attending Physician, Infectious Disease Unit, Massachusetts General Hospital, Boston, Massachusetts.

Immunology Related to AIDS

SUSAN D. WALL, M.D.

Associate Professor of Radiology, University of California, San Francisco, School of Medicine. Assistant Chief of Radiology, Department of Veterans Affairs Medical Center, San Francisco, California.

Diagnostic Imaging Procedures in Gastroenterology

DAVID C. WARNOCK, M.D.

Professor of Medicine and Physiology, University of Alabama School of Medicine, Birmingham, Alabama.

Chronic Renal Failure

STANLEY J. WATSON, Ph.D., M.D.

Professor of Psychiatry, Mental Health Research Institute, University of Michigan, Ann Arbor, Michigan.

The Endorphin Family of Opioid Peptides: Biochemistry, Anatomy, and Physiology

RICHARD A. WEISIGER, M.D., Ph.D.

Associate Professor, Department of Medicine and Liver Center, University of California, San Francisco, School of Medicine. Staff Physician, University of California San Francisco Medical Center and Moffitt Hospital, San Francisco, California.

Hepatic Metabolism in Liver Disease; Laboratory Tests in Liver Disease

GERALD WEISSMANN, M.D.

Professor of Medicine and Director, Division of Rheumatology, New York University School of Medicine. Attending Physician in Medicine, Tisch and Bellevue Hospitals, and Consulting Physician, Veterans Administration Medical Center, New York, New York.

NSAID's: Aspirin and Aspirin-like Drugs; Tissue Injury in Rheumatic Diseases

PETER F. WELLER, M.D.

Associate Professor of Medicine, Harvard Medical School. Associate Physician, Beth Israel and Brigham and Women's Hospitals, Boston, Massachusetts.

Eosinophilic Syndromes

RICHARD J. WHITLEY, M.D.

Professor of Pediatrics, Microbiology, and Medicine, University of Alabama School of Medicine. Staff, Children's Hospital, Birmingham, Alabama.

Antiviral Therapy; Herpes Simplex Virus Infections

RICHARD D. WILLIAMS, M.D.

Professor and Chairman, Department of Urology, University of Iowa College of Medicine. Chairman, Department of Urology, University of Iowa Hospitals and Clinics, Iowa City, Iowa.

Anomalies of the Urinary Tract; Tumors of the Kidney, Ureter, and Bladder

T. FRANKLIN WILLIAMS, M.D.

Director, National Institute on Aging, National Institutes of Health, Bethesda, Maryland.

Management of Common Problems in the Elderly

JOHN WILLIAMSON, B.Sc., M.B., B.S., D.A.(Melb)

Senior Lecturer, Department of Anaesthesia and Intensive Care, and Hyperbaric Medicine, Adelaide University Medical School. Director of Hyperbaric Medicine, Royal Adelaide Hospital, Adelaide, South Australia.

Venomous and Poisonous Marine Animals

SIDNEY J. WINAWER, M.D.

Professor of Clinical Medicine, Cornell University Medical College. Chief, Gastroenterology Service; Head, Laboratory for Gastrointestinal Cancer Research and World Health Organization Collaborating Center for the Prevention of Colorectal Cancer, Memorial Sloan-Kettering Cancer Center, New York, New York.

Neoplasms of the Stomach

SHELDON M. WOLFF, M.D.

Endicott Professor and Chairman, Department of Medicine, Tufts University School of Medicine. Physician-in-Chief, New England Medical Center, Boston, Massachusetts.

The Vasculitic Syndromes; Polyarteritis Nodosa Group

EMANUEL WOLINSKY, M.D.

Professor Emeritus, Medicine and Pathology, Case Western Reserve University School of Medicine. Head, Division of Microbiology, and Physician, Infectious Disease Division, Department of Medicine, Metropolitan Medical Center, Cleveland, Ohio.

Tuberculosis; Other Mycobacterioses

JERRY S. WOLINSKY, M.D.

Professor of Neurology, University of Texas Medical School at Houston. Attending Neurologist, Hermann Hospital, Houston, Texas.

Neurologic Disorders Associated with Altered Immunity or Unexplained Host-Parasitic Alterations

ROBERT L. WORTMANN, M.D.

Professor and Vice Chairman, Department of Medicine, Medical College of Wisconsin. Chief of Medical Service, Clement J. Zablocki Veterans Administration Medical Center, Milwaukee, Wisconsin.

Polymyositis

DANIEL G. WRIGHT, M.D.

Professor of Medicine, Uniformed Services University of the Health Sciences F. Edward Hebert School of Medicine, Bethesda, Maryland. Chief, Department of Hematology, Walter Reed Army Institute of Research, Washington, D.C.

Familial Mediterranean Fever

TERESA L. WRIGHT, B.M., B.S.

Assistant Professor of Medicine, University of California, San Francisco, School of Medicine. Staff Physician, Department of Veterans Affairs Medical Center; Attending Physician, University of California San Francisco Medical Center, San Francisco, California.

Parasitic, Bacterial, Fungal, and Granulomatous Liver Disease

JAMES B. WYNGAARDEN, M.D.

Professor of Medicine and Associate Vice-Chancellor for Health Affairs, Duke University School of Medicine. Physician, Duke University Hospital, Durham, North Carolina.

Medicine as a Science; The Use and Interpretation of Laboratory-Derived Data; Human Heredity; Inborn Errors of Metabolism; Metabolic Diseases: Introduction; Alcaptonuria; Gout

ROBERT YARCHOAN, M.D.

Senior Investigator, Medicine Branch, National Cancer Institute, National Institutes of Health. Attending Physician, Clinical Center, National Institutes of Health, Bethesda, Maryland.

Treatment of AIDS and Related Disorders

LOWELL S. YOUNG, M.D.

Clinical Professor of Medicine, University of California, San Francisco, School of Medicine. Chief, Division of Infectious Diseases, Pacific Presbyterian Medical Center, San Francisco, California.

Antimicrobial Therapy

NEAL S. YOUNG, M.D.

Chief, Clinical Services, and Head, Cell Biology Section, Clinical Hematology Branch, National Heart, Lung, and Blood Institute, National Institutes of Health, Bethesda, Maryland.

Aplastic Anemia and Related Bone Marrow Failure Syndromes

BARRY L. ZARET, M.D.

Robert W. Berliner Professor of Medicine, Professor of Diagnostic Radiology, and Chief of Cardiovascular Medicine, Yale University School of Medicine. Chief of Cardiology, Yale–New Haven Hospital, New Haven, Connecticut.

Nuclear Cardiology

ELIZABETH J. ZIEGLER, M.D.

Professor of Medicine, University of California, San Diego, School of Medicine, La Jolla. Attending Physician, University of California San Diego Medical Center, San Diego, California.

Extraintestinal Infections Caused by Enteric Bacteria

DOUGLAS P. ZIPES, M.D.

Professor of Medicine, Indiana University School of Medicine. Attending Physician, Indiana University Medical Center, Wishard Memorial Hospital, and Richard L. Roudebush Veterans Administration Medical Center, Indianapolis, Indiana.

Sudden Cardiac Death

CONTENTS

(Detailed table of contents begins on page xxxi.)

PART XX INFECTIOUS DISEASES

Section One Introduction

Section Two Bacterial Diseases

Streptococcal Diseases

Endocarditis

Staphylococcal Infections

Bacterial Meningitis, Morton N. Swartz

Osteomyelitis

Whooping Cough

Diphtheria

Clostridial Diseases, John G. Bartlett

Anaerobic Bacteria

Enteric Infections

Other Bacterial Infections

Diseases Due to Mycobacteria

Sexually Transmitted Diseases, P. Frederick Sparling

Spirochetal Diseases Other Than Syphilis

Diseases Caused by Chlamydiae, Walter E. Stamm

Rickettsial Diseases, Richard B. Hornick

Zoonoses

Section Three Viral Diseases

Viral Infections of the Respiratory Tract

COLOR PLATES

The hematology color photomicrographs (which are used with permission) are from the American Society of Hematology Slide Bank, third edition. This edition is supported in part by an educational grant from Ortho Biotech. Specific contributors to these four plates are:

James R. McArthur, *Director*   Marion Dugdale   Mudite Petersons
John R. Bolles, *Assistant Director*   Eugene P. Ewing   Jean Shafer
Marguerite Candler Ballard   Joseph Fanning   Claud Sultan
Ann Bell   N. Frickhofen   Marilyn Winkler
Yvonne Betson   Elaine Jaffe   M. M. Wintrobe
Richard Brunning   Charles L. Johnston   Rose Yoda
L. W. Diggs   Pamela Kidd   Neal S. Young
   Dorothea Zucker-Franklin

Information about slide orders can be obtained from Dr. James R. McArthur.

The following code refers to the approximate magnification of the hematology color photomicrographs.

(L.P.) = Low-power magnification (dry)

(H.P.) = High-power magnification (dry)

(L.O.) = Low oil immersion magnification ($\sim$800–1000$\times$)

(H.O.) = High oil immersion magnification ($\sim$1500$\times$)

(V.H.O.) = Very high oil magnification (significantly in excess of 1500$\times$)

CECIL
TEXTBOOK
of
MEDICINE

PART I

MEDICINE AS A LEARNED AND HUMANE PROFESSION

As originally conceived by Russell Cecil in the 1920's, this textbook aims to provide both an overview of internal medicine and an encyclopedic and up-to-date reference that incorporates recent research. Its audience has grown over the years, ranging from medical students to seasoned practitioners. Although the essays that follow are addressed primarily to the former group, the editors hope that all our readers may find them worthy of at least passing attention. All readers of this book deserve a broader perspective of medicine than is offered by its subject matter alone.

1 Internal Medicine and Today's Internist

J. Claude Bennett

QUESTIONS/PLEAS OF THE PATIENT

"How can I find a good doctor?"

"How can I find a good doctor whom I can afford?"

"How can I find a good doctor who cares about me as a person?"

"How can I find a good doctor who will take the time to listen and understand?"

People who need medical care ask these questions throughout the world every day. They ask them because they face a health care system that is scientifically complex, organizationally overloaded, and generally not oriented to the patient as a *person*. When an individual first becomes ill, regardless of the symptoms, he or she needs most someone who seems to say, "I am a good doctor; I charge a reasonable amount for my services; I care about you, the patient; and I will take the time to listen and understand."

A prominent teacher/physician in a major medical center taught his students to "listen to the patient and he will tell you what is wrong, and he will tell you what he needs." Having found a physician who answers so profoundly to their needs, some patients are extremely grateful—but most are utterly overwhelmed. With the discovery of that relationship, the difference between a superb technician and a true physician really becomes evident to the patient. That physician/teacher was a scholarly gentleman with deep scientific insight and an active and stimulating clinical and research practice. Unfortunately, he developed crippling rheumatoid arthritis in the midst of his career. Beyond question, his own disease sensitized him to the complex mix of expectations, needs, fears, and appreciation that patients feel when facing a physical-mental trial while at the same time looking for that perfect physician to help them. Patients flocked to this doctor—not just for his accurate diagnoses, his correct therapies, or even his warmth, but for the intellect he expressed and the sheer joy of living that he extended in every encounter with another human being. He had a Shakespearean grasp of the qualities of being human and an uncommon ability to transmit love and respect for his fellow human beings. He exhibited the ideal all physicians should emulate. Many readers know a phy-

sician with these characteristics; all should seek to know one and to develop their own professional persona so that human qualities are not lost to technical acumen.

THE SCIENTIFIC AND TECHNOLOGIC BACKGROUND OF A "GOOD DOCTOR"

Since Flexner issued his famous report in 1910, American medical education has striven toward the development of a strong scientific base. This intellectual prerequisite, therefore, has become an integral part of premedical, undergraduate, graduate, and, indeed, continuing medical education. Biomedical science is fundamental to understanding disease, making diagnoses, developing new therapies, and appreciating the complexities and contributions of new technologies. Physicians cannot be satisfied with simply knowing that a certain form of therapy works 80 to 90 per cent of the time. They must understand the basic physiology and pharmacology of any approach they use. They must possess the intellectual tools to follow reports of current research in medical journals so that they can continue to grasp the newest and latest approaches, no matter how complicated the field may become. That is why, in a textbook of medicine like this, strong emphasis is given to how things work, what goes amiss when pathologic processes ensue, and what effect a given therapy has in correcting that defect. We seek to create within the minds of our readers a yearning for a greater depth of understanding and a continuing commitment to stay at the frontier of scientific knowledge. These are, in fact, among the hallmarks of a professional in any scientific field.

We are moving into an era when pharmacotherapeutic agents are no longer merely wonders of organic chemistry, but increasingly often are biologic products. Some of these are isolated from nature; others are developed by recombinant DNA technology. On the horizon is the availability of a true replacement or supplement for defective or deficient biochemical constituents of the body. No physician can with intellectual honesty use these new classes of agents without fully understanding their action, their meaning, and their potential side effects. The diagnostic and therapeutic contributions and potential, in clinical situations, of biocompatible prosthetic devices, nuclear magnetic resonance spectroscopy, high-frequency laser beams, and so on through developments not yet conceived, can be appreciated only by the mind that is disciplined in fundamental science.

THE ORGANIZATION AND FINANCING OF TODAY'S MEDICINE

Patients, as well as their representatives in government, industry, and managed-care organizations, are concerned about the rising cost of medical care. The total bill for health care in America now rises at a rate of about 10 per cent per year, an increase that seems to continue unabated. Federal legislation instituting diagnosis-related groups (DRG's) has clearly moderated the rise of hospital costs, but physician costs continue to rise at an ever-increasing rate. Every student of medicine should ask if this is realistic. Is it sustainable? Is it defensible? What will be the limits? Patients already ask, "Can I really afford the best doctors in the most prestigious practices, in the most famous medical centers?" "Can I afford to be referred to a subspecialist?" "Can I afford to be out of work and in the hospital?" "Can I afford to pay my rising insurance premiums?" "How much deductible on my insurance can I afford?" Worse yet, an increasing number of patients have to make choices between seeking medical and dental care and getting food, clothing, shelter, and other essentials of daily living. These issues have become major concerns in American households and clearly represent one of the most disturbing weaknesses in our economy, of which now nearly 12 per cent (by annual gross national product) is devoted to health care, up from 8 per cent in 1975.

Over the last two to three decades it has been a goal of our nation to promote ever-increasing quality and cost-effectiveness of health care for all. Unfortunately, we have failed miserably. The United States spends more per capita on health care than any other nation in the world. Yet in the major indices of health our population ranks nineteenth! At the same time we continue to see a wasteful maldistribution of physicians both by specialty and geographically and a growing number of medically indigent and medically uninsured people in our nation. Somehow, the costs of what we are trying to achieve—even though the goal is commendable—are not being placed in proper perspective by the medical profession, health-care managers, and representatives of the people in order to provide suitable care for all. Unfortunately, in the present system the real needs of the populace are not always met by affordable services. At the same time, over-utilization of medical services may be the very engine that drives up the total cost of health care delivery. With the passage of the Medicare program for the elderly and the Medicaid plan for the poor by Congress in 1965, we had hoped as a nation that we were moving toward a more just and efficient system. In fact, the opposite has been the trend. This societal goal must now be readdressed, reformulated, and restructured in terms of modern needs, reflecting fairly and fully measured cost/benefit ratios for every form of medical service.

Medical professionals often attribute overutilization to patient behavior. In fact, however, physicians control 70 per cent of health expenditures. A few patients with hypochondriasis, for example, may visit physicians too often, and many older patients may seek medical help at times when a friendly, reassuring chat is their real desire, but in the final analysis utilization of the health care system is in the hands of physicians. Ironically, although physician competence is often equated to mastery of expensive techniques and technologies, physicians are actually at their professional best when listening to the patient and responding to what they hear and see with medicine's most comprehensive armamentarium. Overutilization, when it occurs, is thus most likely to be our fault as physicians. Our responsibility as professionals is to be absolutely certain that our errors in this direction are driven by well-founded concern for the health of our patients, not by the financial interests of our practices or the hospitals where we work.

Individual physicians, then, must take a personal and professional interest in the control of health care costs—not only because it is right for the nation, but because it is right for the patient. In our litigious society, a legalistically defensive approach to medical practice has become too prevalent. The conditions that engender this tendency must be altered. Physicians must use all of their diagnostic skills to focus on the very best approach to medical diagnosis and therapy and to steer away from unnecessary use or repetition of expensive procedures such as computed tomography, magnetic resonance imaging, and cardiac catheterization. The physician must use intellect—scientific knowledge and analytical skills—to best serve the patient without inundating the system with unnecessary costs and the patient with a financial burden he simply cannot continue to bear.

Costs can be controlled only if physicians are convinced of the need and are willing to participate in providing this vital service. One aspect of this control is attention to various possible means of health care finance, including prepaid plans, preferred provider organizations, health maintenance organizations, and other managed care systems. All of these must be carefully explored with a view to making health care accessible where it is most needed. Clearly, multiple tools and programs may be necessary, but they should not be thrust upon the patient simply to satisfy doctrines of free enterprise. To provide the best health care in a finite economy we need systems that provide such care in the most efficient way, regardless of the payment scheme.

Another aspect of our cost-control job is to support and participate in research on outcomes, aiming toward systematic evaluation of cost-effectiveness of the medical procedures we

choose in the light of *all* the interests of our patient. For example, we do not know why treatment of prostatic hypertrophy is more commonly medical in some parts of the nation, surgical in others. Why does the incidence of caesarean sections vary so widely? The costs and benefits of coronary angioplasty versus bypass surgery remain obscure. Every year *billions* of dollars are spent as a result of clinical decisions that may hinge on these or similar issues. Physicians must involve themselves in the processes of change with an eye first to the individual patient and then to society.

THOSE WHO CARE

"How can I find a good doctor who cares about me as a person?"

When speaking of caring, one has to define specifically what is meant. A physician can diagnose and prescribe in a technically correct and scientific but insensitive way, and the patient may be made better—even cured. On the other hand, when the patient asks the question, "Does my physician really care?" the patient means, "Does it matter to the physician what happens to me? Does my doctor show sensitivity and compassion beyond the mere technical qualities of medicine?" It is in this sense that we address ourselves to the nature of those who care.

It may seem odd to talk about caring as a skill, but in a real sense it is just that. Those involved in the education of students realize that at least some forms of compassion have to be learned. The developing physician must see such traits in action in order to acquire and apply them in interaction with patients and their families. Sometimes this involves *learning how* to demonstrate compassion. Kahlil Gibran has taught us, "You give but little when you give of your possessions—it is when you give of yourself that you truly give." Giving of ourselves—with ease, with grace, and with meaning—is for most of us an acquired skill. Sometimes it involves a deep sense of reawakening within, to bring out an innate sensitivity and compassion that perhaps has not expressed itself since childhood. At other times, learning to care may involve a complete transformation of behavior and attitudes toward people, particularly those who are not from our own cultural background. Many believe that the greatest responsibility in medical education today is to foster compassion within the student of medicine.

To receive medical care, patients must trust their bodies and their very lives to physicians, and so to be in an honest position to give medical care, physicians must earn such radical trust. Mere technical treatment of disease does not suffice. Patients must be able reasonably to believe that their physicians care about them in an extraordinarily personal way. This exchange of care for trust, while not identical to friendship or love, is equally binding. From it develops an interdependence that is far from unwholesome; rather, it potentiates care and promotes healing. Our late twentieth century sophistication and technologic orientation have too often cost us warmth, humor, and humanity, leaving us in social isolation. We do far better as professionals to err on the side of being human with our patients than to try to play *deus ex machina*, the god from the machine.

THE SOCIAL RESPONSIBILITIES AND HUMANISTIC QUALITIES OF "THE GOOD DOCTOR"

The patient says, "Take charge, make me well, help me feel comfortable, show me compassion, listen to my problems and I will give you trust." Dag Hammarskjöld reminds us of "the humility which comes from others having faith in you" (*Markings*, 1965). The natural outcome of this giving and receiving of trust is that the physician must accept some degree of obligation to the patient. Of course, the patient, if able, keeps some responsibility for the healing process, but the physician must be willing to answer the patient's needs, however demanding, however changing, however at times unreasonable or falsely perceived. Generalists in internal medicine undertake a long-term commitment to a patient's care. They are reminded daily that this commitment continues beyond a particularly insightful diagnosis or the completion of an endoscopic procedure: that the patient still needs care when the numbers are back from the most recent cardiac catheterization or when the final stitch is completed in a complex procedure and the patient is rolled from the operating suite. The internist continues to care for and nurture the patient through the whole process of healing in a way that requires enormous skill in close personal interaction.

Help with Family Interactions

The woman who comes into her physician's office with a history of fatigue, listlessness, inability to sleep, and irritability may be describing the early symptoms of a morbid disease. She may, however, be showing signs of depression secondary to her inability to cope any longer with an alcoholic husband, with a teenage son addicted to cocaine, or with an elderly mother for whom she must care. The wise physician considers organic pathology but also realizes that presenting symptoms may be only part of what is really troubling the patient. This requires an unusual sensitivity and an ability to pursue in a cautious, understanding, and careful way and to listen to the concerns and needs the patient describes—traits, again, that can and must be developed and practiced. The physician's role is to help the patient understand the connections between unpleasant situations, emotional disturbances, and organic symptoms. Sometimes patients are helped simply by understanding those relationships and being aware that the doctor appreciates them and reassures, listens with a sympathetic ear, and seldom advises in a direct way, but does express concern. In earlier days, when most medical care was delivered at home, the physician was quickly made aware of living situations and family interactions—if he or she did not already know the entire family and their circumstances. Today when the patient comes to the office, generally alone and certainly out of socioeconomic context, it is much more difficult to perceive what is going on. The physician must exercise a much greater degree of skill and understanding in exploring family interrelationships during a history and physical examination or in an even shorter visit.

Help with Obtaining Necessary Additional Professional Services

The warm and intimate relationship that any patient seeks is not one that a typical patient can have with many physicians at the same time. The internist must demonstrate a variety of skills, attitudes, and abilities and a store of diverse information that allows him or her to be the patient's health care *manager* as well as his confidant, keeping in mind that the average patient does not understand the system of medical referrals for subspecialty consultation.

An oncologist/internist recently described for me how she weaves the fabric of health care management for a patient who has been referred with a positive biopsy for a malignant disease. In this situation the oncologist has to view herself as the captain of a rather complicated ship. She has to talk with the referring physician, obtain the biopsy slides, have them re-read by her own consulting pathologist, and review them herself. She then has to review the chart and the radiographs with a consulting radiologist and decide, given all the data, how best to institute therapy. This may require interaction with the surgeon, with the radiation oncologist, and with additional specialists with the skills for exploration, including various techniques for interventional radiology or endoscopy. Having decided on the course to take, she then has to become the patient's advocate and interact with the surgeon, the radiation oncologist, or other consultants on the patient's behalf and with the patient's best interests in mind. It is then necessary to spend time with the patient to explain the disease and what is to be expected and with the family to answer their questions and as much as possible to enlist them as allies for the hard times to come. Further, she has to commit herself to the long-term counseling, reassurance, and constant caring needed by a patient with a chronic and possibly fatal disease. This physician's role is much different from that of a physician-technician who performs a procedure and then sends the patient back to the doctor who will care for the long-term needs. While technicians' roles in this process are often crucial, their interactions with the patient are brief. The health care manager, in this case the oncologist, knits the technical information together and confers with her patient about the best way to proceed.

The physician who takes responsibility for the total oversight of the patient's needs as related to the disease is the one who really must captain the ship and with whom the patient needs a very special, trusting relationship. Too often in modern medicine, with its exquisitely developed technologies, a degree of impersonal behavior creeps in. The skilled cardiac surgeon, the superb master of angioplasty, the excellent endoscopist, the impressive neurosurgeon all touch "our" patients from time to time, exercise their skills in their one intervention, and then go on to the next patient. The general internist must define the need for the procedural intervention, give support during its execution, and most importantly continue to care following the procedure. When the consulting surgeon or specialist is no longer available, the one-on-one interaction between the patient and the internist, *"his or her* doctor," must remain inviolate.

Help with Suffering

Most chronic diseases involve physical, mental, and emotional suffering to some degree during their courses. Some patients do beautifully because of their own intrinsic personalities, strong wills, or deep convictions. Others have great difficulty and sometimes even the toughest break under the severe suffering of a chronic illness. Physicians must develop skills of interpersonal relationship based on familiarity with all sides of life and especially with suffering. They need to *participate* in suffering. They need to be able to relate it to a broad range of experience so that they can deal with an enormous variety of patients at many different stages of coping with their suffering. Students sometimes get a glimpse of this in dealing with patients on inpatient services, but most often in outpatient clinics where they treat chronic diseases that continue unabated for many years. Often the physician has little specific therapy to offer except a kind touch, a gentle presence, and a knowing acknowledgment. Students of medicine learn through experience with patients as their own involvement in the practice of medicine grows through the years. The best physicians are always learning, because each patient teaches something new about the way in which a particular kind of suffering must be considered and ameliorated.

In the last two decades, patient support groups have become more numerous and more widely sought by patients. Many are now associated with major medical centers. These groups play a vitally important role in allowing patients to express their concerns and fears and to hear other patients in similar situations share their concerns and frustrations. As important as these are, as constructive as they are, and as meaningful as they have become in the overall care of patients, physicians still must understand the circumstances and the degree of suffering of each patient. Each one's needs are unique. Merely sharing them does not make them go away, and merely knowing that someone else also carries burdens does not solve the problem. The physician must be both interactive and supportive—even when the ways to change the physical situation may be sadly limited.

Help with Aging

The past several decades have seen a remarkable increase in the proportion of the population over 65, over 75, and even over 85 years of age—the last being the fastest-growing of all age groups. These proportions will continue to increase significantly (Fig. 1–1). Already the average age of the practice population in the offices of many general internists exceeds 70 years. This demographic shift has been accompanied by increasing awareness of the general field of geriatric medicine and expanding knowledge of the biologic processes involved in aging. Projected population trends indicate that every general internist must become experienced in the needs of the geriatric population, as the aging process involves essentially every organ system. However, there are at least two—the nervous system and the musculoskeletal system—with which essentially every person reaching the seventh, eighth, and ninth decades of life will experience trouble to an increasing degree. Much of this is discussed in Ch. 442 and in the chapters involving rheumatologic diseases, especially osteoarthritis.

Memory loss of some degree is essentially universal in the elderly, although it clearly is more pronounced in some than others and may or may not be associated with the true clinical syndrome of Alzheimer's disease. Memory loss affects the individual's self-perception, ability to interact with friends and family,

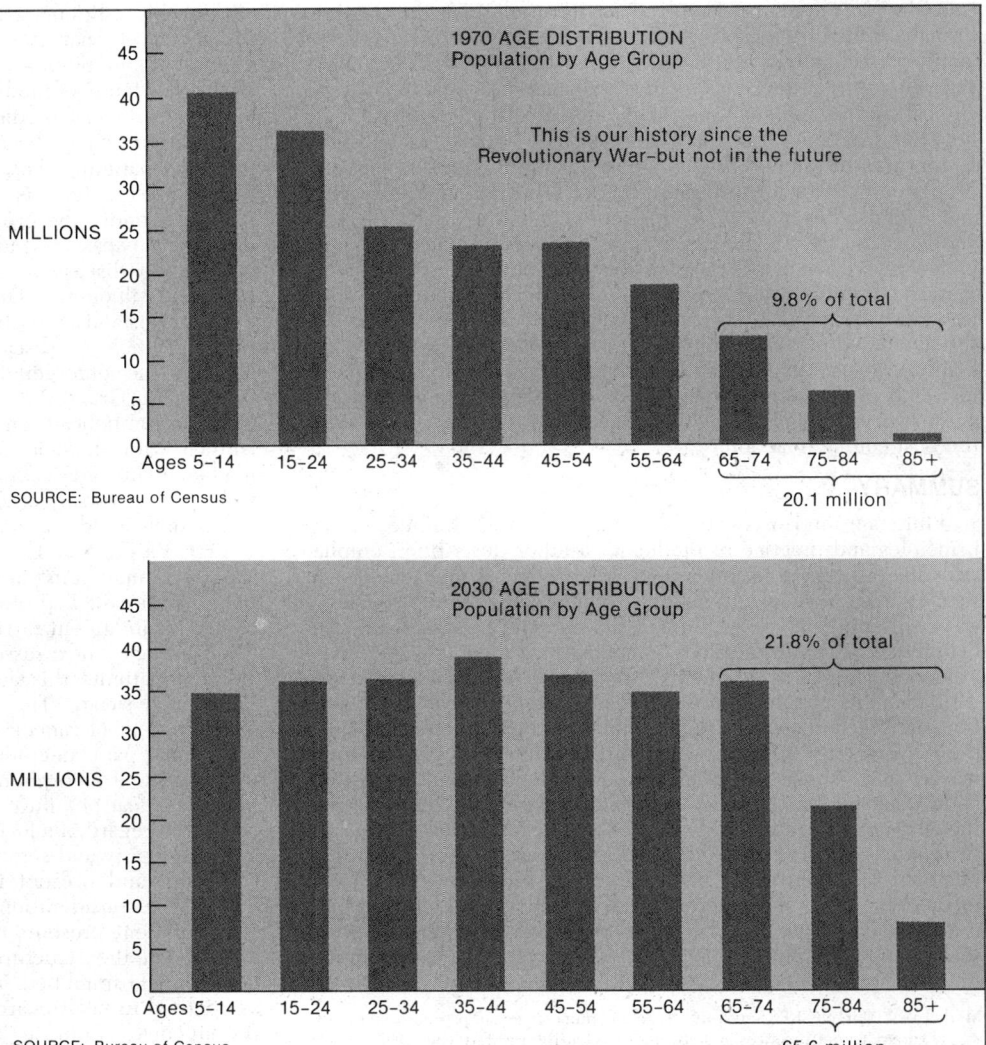

FIGURE 1–1. The Aging of the American population. (From Numbers that make you think. Retirement Systems of Alabama Advisor XV (9):3, 1990; with permission.)

and ability to accommodate to the pressures of our changing world. It can put barriers between the individual and those he or she most needs. This is true even for the very lucky individual who is able to maintain work activities, friends, and family as he or she did in his prime. The same situation develops with osteoarthritis, as gait problems, muscle fatigue, and weakness become more prevalent with advancing age. These effectively limit the individual's ability to get away from home and sustain a normally active lifestyle. Physical difficulties simply prohibit him or her from doing the things he or she likes to do. Much of the focus of the general internist, therefore, is to keep the elderly individual as physically and mentally active and as personally and emotionally interactive with others as possible.

Loneliness, despair, chronic illness, and depression are all prevalent in the geriatric population. Our effort must be to treat individual symptoms and organ system failure as they appear—but, most important, to help aging individuals develop an overall lifestyle that gives them a sense of well-being—of being useful, of being appreciated, and of having meaning in their lives. The internist must devote increasing time and effort to aging patients and must be particularly sensitive to subtle changes in their environments, including the loss of a loved one, shrinking income relative to cost of living, dislocation from their homes, and the despair that comes from being unable to adjust to new surroundings such as a retirement center or nursing home. Each of these profoundly affects the way a patient reacts to physical diseases. The responsibility of the internist extends beyond the usual in this situation and requires a very special integration of medical knowledge and knowledge of how people adjust to their changing needs.

Help with Dying

Rarely does an individual really wish to die, but when the time does come patients want to die with dignity. What most of us desire above all is not just life, but a satisfactory quality of life, and we may sometimes quite rationally risk death to escape an unacceptable life. Issues surrounding dying patients and even the realistic definition of death are topics frequently encountered by today's internist.

It is an often if sometimes faintly praised triumph for modern medicine that we now have the technologic skills and instrumentation to keep essential body functions such as circulation and respiration operating almost indefinitely. The ability to continue these functions regardless of the expected outcome for the patient has produced considerable ethical conflict for many who deal with patients in critical life support areas and intensive care units.

Young people in medical training must make an effort to become "comfortable" with the process and the event of dying. The problems of when to withdraw life support mechanisms or to withhold resuscitation may present deep emotional conflicts for medical students—as well as for many very experienced physicians. Although medical ethics touches almost every aspect of health and the practice of medicine (see Ch. 4), the particular problems related to dying patients, stemming in part from legal considerations and from highly publicized special cases, put the physician in an especially difficult position. Only recently have objective conclusions begun to emerge from clinical investigation of outcomes from intensive care units. Although striking successes do occur, the survival rate with a high quality of life upon discharge from intensive care units is less than one would hope (see Ch. 71). Therefore, the physician frequently may be required to make difficult decisions for or with the patient and his or her family. Ultimately, society at large will have to make policy regarding those decisions, using information based on careful clinical studies and analyses of the costs of sustaining life in truly hopeless situations. But that policy has not yet been established. In this area the skilled internist plays a uniquely personal role in preparing patients for terminal situations, becoming their teacher and confidant as they come to understand the disease process and what to expect. The physician is also called upon to help the patient's loved ones prepare for the outcome.

Each patient must be considered individually, keeping in mind previously expressed wishes, the nature of the terminal illness, the likelihood of recovery with an acceptable quality of life, and family wishes and interactions. Although these factors are difficult to weigh in the care of dying patients, objective evaluation and an unswerving concern for the patient will lead the physician to the best course of action.

SUMMARY

While an internist may be defined as one trained in the principles and practice of medicine, a fuller description emphasizes his possession of uncommon knowledge of biologic science ranging from molecular events to whole organ system physiology, a special appreciation for human life and the needs of suffering people, and a comprehensive perspective on modern society—its influence on our lives and its stresses on our social structure. Although this chapter has emphasized patient/physician interaction, we must recognize that basic biomedical science provides the infrastructure for our profession. We must first and foremost master our science if we are to be good physicians. We must know what is best to offer to correct the disease; then we weave the fabric of the physician's social and ethical responsibilities into the context of current medical care organization. Few physicians function well merely as knowledgeable scientists or talented technicians, but none functions well simply as a crutch on which the patient can lean. The good physician—the one patients seek—must combine working scientific techniques with compassion and social responsibility.

Merkel WT, Margolis RB, Smith RC: Teaching humanistic and psychosocial aspects of care: Current practices and attitudes. J Gen Intern Med 5:34, 1990.
Scherr L, Farber SJ, Hildreth EA, et al.: American College of Physicians Ethics Manual. Part 1: History; the patient; other physicians. Ann Intern Med 111:145, 1989.
Smedira NG, Evans BH, Grais LS: Withholding and withdrawal of life support from the critically ill. N Engl J Med 322:309, 1990.

2 Medicine as an Art

Lloyd H. Smith, Jr.

What is medicine? "Medicine is not a science but a learned profession, deeply rooted in a number of sciences and charged with the obligation to apply them for man's benefit." In this eloquent statement from an earlier edition of this book, Walsh McDermott defined medicine as a human activity undertaken for the benefit of others whether in the area of public health, "statistical compassion," or in the care of the individual patient.

Medicine can also be defined in other terms. It is a mutable body of knowledge, skills, and traditions applicable to the preservation of health, the cure of disease, and the amelioration of suffering. The boundaries of medicine blend into psychology, sociology, economics, and even cultural heritage. Disease may be encoded in the genome; disease may also be encoded by the deprivations of poverty and ignorance. Medicine must therefore be concerned not only with an abnormal molecule but also with an abnormal childhood. As such it is open ended in a way that is both humbling and exhilarating to those who pursue it as a career.

Medicine is continually changing. The honored verities of one generation become the shopworn shibboleths of the next. Much of what we now so confidently espouse, including that compressed within this edition, will amuse our successors as remarkably bizarre in its naiveté. Medical competence is based on the continuing pursuit of ever-changing concepts. It must be renewed as the substance of medicine itself is transformed.

The practice of medicine is far more than the application of scientific principles to a particular biologic aberration. Its focus is on the patient, whose welfare is its continuing purpose. That purpose of medicine is self evident in theory, but more difficult to sustain under the pressures of medical practice. For example, it is tragically easy for the patient to become merely the repository in which a disease or a syndrome has chosen to manifest its particular silhouette. During the training years every physician has subconsciously participated in what might be termed the personification of disease. A case of meningitis is admitted through the emergency room; a pheochromocytoma will be discussed at Grand Rounds. It is perhaps inevitable that a disease becomes symbolically an entity to the physician who must become familiar with all of its manifestations and guises. In the art of medicine the physician must be the advocate of the patient as well as the adversary of disease. It is the patient who is personified rather than the disease.

THE PATIENT. The description of a patient is simply that of a fellow human being in need of help. The patient comes seeking help because of a problem relating to his or her health. This subjective judgment carries with it disquieting concerns, although these may be unexpressed. Anxiety is present even in the most stoical of patients; this fact must never be forgotten or disregarded by the physician. The patient's anxiety may be specific—for example, fear of cancer with all that implies in the public mind concerning pain, degradation, and inexorable death. More often the anxiety is amorphous: fear of loss of independence or employment; fear of failure to meet obligations to one's family or to retain the regard of a loved one; or fear of an inability to maintain a life of dignity and significance. In the rush to crystallize a chief complaint and present illness the physician too often brushes aside these considerations.

The patient presents to the physician on alien and unfamiliar ground—in the structured and artificial setting of an office, a clinic, or a hospital bed. This form of health care of the individual, as opposed to health care in the aggregate, is often described by the unfelicitous phrase "the personal encounter system." Unfortunately it often seems distressingly like confrontation to the patient, who comes after all for comfort, not for encounter. Each human being is unique within a life that is enormously complex—in heredity, early experiences, cultural and psychological environment, education, opportunities, successes, failures, fantasies, emotional commitments, motivations, and in the adjustments and compromises that serve to cripple or to mature. Living, therefore, is the ultimate personal encounter system. With an extensive and diverse experience the patient comes to the physician with "a problem." A chief complaint is requested. Defenses must be lowered and the emotions that spill out may be distressing. The patient's response must be selective and brief; as a result it is not infrequently distorted, perhaps even misleading.

What does the patient want when coming to see a physician? There are certain common hopes and expectations. Patients want to be listened to, so that their fears and concerns can be fully expressed and the burden shared. They want physicians to be interested in them as fellow human beings in a compassionate but nonjudgmental fashion. They expect professional competence incorporating the best in medical science and technology. They want to be reasonably informed as to the probable cause of their concerns and what the future is likely to hold. They want not to be abandoned. To each patient these desires and expectations vary in relative importance. It is notable that not all patients expect to be cured. These expectations are further discussed in the light of how the physician should endeavor to meet them.

TRADITIONAL EXPECTATIONS OF PATIENTS. *Patients want to be listened to and understood.* This has been well expressed by Wilfred Trotter, a great English neurosurgeon:

". . . As long as medicine is an art, its chief and characteristic instrument must be human faculty. We come therefore to the very practical question of what aspects of human faculty it is necessary for the good doctor to cultivate. . . . The first to be named must always be the power of attention, of giving one's whole mind to the patient without the interposition of oneself. It sounds simple but only the very greatest doctors ever fully attain it. It is an active process and not either mere resigned listening or even politely waiting until you can interrupt. Disease often tells its secrets in a casual parenthesis. . . ."

Eventually the medical record must be organized in a logical and consistent fashion. But a history rarely unfolds that way. Patients do not divulge their fears in neat paragraphs or in direct responses to a cascade of queries. It is important to let patients tell their own stories. The manner of formulation and expression of symptoms and anxieties may be as informative as the medical data transmitted. The good physician is an attentive listener, with an ear for Trotter's "casual parenthesis."

Patients want physicians to be interested in them as fellow human beings. This interest cannot be that of the unusual "case" of the carcinoid syndrome or of hairy cell leukemia; the center of interest must be the patient as a person. It is difficult for the physician to feign such an interest, for patients are very perceptive, especially during the vulnerability that illness induces. In the practice of medicine the physician encounters all of the virtues and vices to which mankind is heir. The physician need not be morally neutral in personal judgments, but these must be stringently excluded from professional activities. The response of the physician to human frailty and fallibility should be that of compassion rather than cynicism, of interest in the infinite variety of human experience rather than of repulsion from its aberrations.

Patients expect professional competence in medical science and technology. The physician must be a scholar both to attain professional competence and to sustain it during times of revolutionary changes in science and technology. All of the other attributes of the good physician are of little avail in the absence of sound scholarship. Compassion is no substitute for knowing what should be done. The education of the physician and the role of the physician as a scientist will be discussed more fully below.

Patients want to be kept informed. The physician must listen to and communicate with the patient. Time must be set aside for this. Failure to do so is a serious error, for silence is a form of communication that is usually adverse. The physician should voluntarily answer questions of concern to the patient. The physician must also inform the patient concerning the illness and what it implies. A number of books have been developed to assist in patient education and are often quite effective in translating medical terminology into lay terms. Furthermore, clubs for mutual support and education have been formed by patients who share their common experiences with such chronic disabilities as ileostomies or amputations. Admirable and important as these are, they do not obviate the need for patients to learn from their own physicians about their particular illnesses and what they may mean in and for their future lives. This need extends beyond the legal confines of informed consent, which is now an important issue in medical practice.

Patients want not to be abandoned. Death comes to everyone. There are finite limits to what can be accomplished by medical science and technology in the alleviation of suffering and the prolongation of life. This fact is well known to both patients and physicians. When that limit is reached, the physician often feels powerless and even guilty that no more can be done. As a consequence there is a tendency to withdraw attention and direct it elsewhere. Nothing could be a greater mistake. It is at the margins of medical science that the role of the physician is enhanced. It is here that the art of medicine comes to the forefront in the care of the patient, whether it be by emotional support, relief of pain, small adjustments in medicines or diet, daily conversation and examination, or other methods to show that the patient is still someone of dignity and worth in whom interest has not been lost and for whom hope has not been abandoned. And when no more can be done for the patient, it is time to care for the family. At this stage, as Walsh McDermott has written, "it is up to each of us to follow to the fullest measure the charge laid down long ago for the physician to become himself the treatment."

THE PHYSICIAN. The physician has both chosen and been chosen to enter an arduous and demanding profession, the origins of which stretch back to antiquity. Part priest, part shaman, part mystic, part alchemist, the physician of the past reflected the beliefs and expectations of the time and met a perceived need of

fellow men. The history of medicine is part of the heritage of every physician and reflects the cultural history of each society.

The physician enters a profession with established values and traditions of ethical conduct and responsibilities. But each physician, like each patient, is unique. The physician is not a disembodied instrument that can be passively shaped by the profession, but rather a human being with innate strengths and weaknesses that must be recognized in order to meet the expectations of patients and of the profession, not least of which are those standards established for oneself. The qualities of the ideal physician are easy to state but difficult to attain: compassion, sincere interest in one's fellow man, knowledge of human nature, tact, equanimity, sustained scholarship, curiosity, and high ethical standards. Physical and mental vigor might be added to those traits, for the life of the physician is not for the languid or the disengaged. No one has been endowed with or ever fully achieves excellence in all of these qualities. One must first know oneself and judge how one can most closely approach those ideals in one's professional life.

THE EDUCATION OF THE PHYSICIAN. Barriers are encountered at the very beginning in the initial selection for medical school as many seek entry for few positions. Undergraduate education is sometimes distorted and breadth of personal experience curtailed in a grim and often distasteful race for competitive acceptance. This inadvertent feedback inhibition not infrequently results from erroneous conceptions of what may or may not impress admission committees of medical schools. Nevertheless, the phenomenon remains a concern to all who are interested in the future of our profession. Admission committees of medical schools too often exercise allosteric control over the higher education of those destined to enter our profession.

The Basic Science Years. In the standard curriculum of medical school in the United States two years are largely devoted to the sciences basic to medicine and two years to clinical training. Fortunately there are a number of interesting variations on this thematic progression which diminish its rigidity and permit the student to re-explore basic science after an introductory clinical experience.

In the United States students usually arrive at medical school after an intensive four-year experience at a college or a university. They anticipate a scholarly atmosphere of a graduate school which will prepare them to enter the practice of a profession for which they hold idealistic expectations. Instead they are immediately assailed with a formidable array of "basic sciences" linked to the structure and function of the human organ systems. New facts constitute not so much an intellectual feast as an engorgement. Each discipline is attended by devotees who are passionately persuaded of the seminal role of their segment of science in the future of the profession. This commitment is translated into the basic academic commodity, curricular time, in which these cluttered wares are exhibited. Awed by the dimensionless task, students struggle with uneven success to assimilate and survive, conscious always that their receptor mechanisms are overloaded and of a continuing sense of high output failure. They look forward in hope that subsequent years will reward their endurance in the more congenial atmosphere of the clinic.

This is patently a caricature, as all will recognize. It can be said, as Mark Twain said of Wagner's music, "it is not as bad as it sounds." The quality of basic science in medical schools is often superb; the substance of modern science has a certain grandeur; many faculty members are gifted in imparting a sense of intellectual adventure to their students; finally, many students now arrive at medical school with a mature understanding of one or more of the fundamental disciplines of biology. Nevertheless this caricature contains elements of truth as seen from the perspective of medical students. The central question is not whether basic science is necessary for medical research, since few would deny its importance there, but whether it is relevant in the education of every physician to the degree to which it is currently emphasized. In the real world of patient care, public health, and medical economics, should the student have to struggle with the intricacies of post-transcriptional modifications of messenger RNA, or is this merely a rite of passage prescribed by a science-obsessed faculty? This is a reasonable question and calls for a response other than a simple reference to flexnerian orthodoxy.

A knowledge of the scientific underpinnings of medicine is clearly necessary in order to marshal the basic information required to understand a patient's illness and to be able to reason logically about the problems of diagnosis and therapy. If there were any doubt on that point, it would be quickly dispelled by random perusal of this book. Much of the basic science which seems abstruse and irrelevant today will find its way into clinical practice in the not too distant future. Medical research is only one step removed from patient care.

Beyond the assimilation of scientific information, there is an even more important consideration. Many of you will have most of your professional experience in the twenty-first century. The changes in medical science and technology will be enormous and largely unpredictable. Only the scientific method will remain unaltered as an invaluable instrument with which fallible man can acquire new knowledge and, equally important, discard that which proves fallacious. It is imperative that students learn the scientific method as part of their education if they are to participate critically and effectively in a changing profession. How can this be done? Perhaps the best method is to participate personally, even for a relatively brief period of time, in a research project so that learning comes from first-hand experience. If that does not prove practical, one can pursue some scientific topic in depth and write a critical analysis of it. It is important to learn one area of inquiry in great detail, even though it may have to be a limited area, in order to penetrate to its frontier. It is only there that science can be understood as a process rather than as a repository.

The Clinical Years. Most students enter the clinical years with a sense of relief, but it is relief lined with anxieties. Some of these anxieties cluster around the following questions:

How can I cope with the uncertainties of clinical medicine?

What are the boundaries of clinical medicine? How much and what am I supposed to learn?

How will I function in my interactions with patients?

How will I measure up to the expectations of my colleagues?

How will I be able to maintain my own identity as an individual in a profession that so obsessively dominates my time and energy?

Other questions could be formulated. Each student possesses a unique idiotype of anxieties that cannot be purged by platitudes. Each will arrive at personal answers, or more likely at personal accommodations, through experience.

The Uncertainty Principle of Clinical Medicine. There is an "uncertainty principle" in medicine as there is in physics. The practice of medicine is inexact and will remain so. If it were not, it would be a science or a technology rather than an art. The measuring instrument is personal and unique. Subjective mensuration defies precision. Who can quantify nausea or the severity of pain? Symptoms may be forgotten, suppressed, or amplified when filtered through the grid of personality. Available data are often indirect, incomplete, or even contradictory. Patients respond in varying fashions to treatment across the range from simple reassurance (which is rarely simple) to surgical or pharmaceutical interventions. Clinical medicine is often based on experience and judgment—which are largely euphemisms for a knowledge of probabilities.

The process of formulating a diagnosis or selecting a therapy is not as arbitrary as it first seems. There are rational means for narrowing the range of diagnostic possibilities: a precise description of symptoms; an accurate and thorough characterization of physical findings; selective laboratory studies to evaluate the functions of organ systems; a synthesis of information to define syndromic patterns; a marshaling of information on etiology and pathogenesis. All of this requires attention to detail, consistency of work habits, and good intellect.

Hypotheses are formed and algorithms branch away from various entry points as new data are obtained which support or fail to support a working diagnosis. This process of clinical reasoning is often best displayed in the clinicopathologic conference (CPC). In the absence of certainty, best guesses must be utilized and in making informed guesses, generally dignified as judgments, the clinician actually relies upon subliminal statistics.

Medical decisions based on probabilities are necessary but also perilous. Even the most astute physician is occasionally wrong. The wise physician often recognizes that a decision is erroneous and discards or modifies the hypothesis on which it is based. The best decision may be approached only by successive approximations. Action may have to be taken despite lack of confirmation of a hypothesis (working diagnosis). Chester M. Jones, a noted clinical teacher, used to say: "If you cannot make a diagnosis, make a decision." Despite the remarkable contributions of science and technology, clinical medicine is frequently inexactitude in action. The student entering the clinical years quickly realizes the dangers to the welfare of the patient of dogmatism in clinical practice. The ambiguities and errors that you encounter in your own experience and observe in the work of others should be an antidote to arrogance. Some errors are inevitable and should not humiliate you, but they should teach humility.

What is the role of the *Cecil Textbook of Medicine* in the learning process? This book attempts to provide the student or the physician with succinct but authoritative summaries about diseases or groups of diseases. Essays written by more than 250 acknowledged experts in their respective fields represent collectively a systematic approach to internal medicine. The chapters are designed to give a basic, lucid, and up-to-date consensus concerning the state of the art in our understanding of specific diseases, but they cannot be all inclusive. Many of the topics discussed within a few pages have received more extended treatment elsewhere as separate monographs. Each of the subspecialty areas (cardiology, gastroenterology, endocrinology, etc.) is the subject of textbooks similar in size to this one. The student should therefore cultivate the habit of consulting at least some of the carefully selected references that extend the information supplied in this basic text.

In general it is also wise for students to begin reading medical journals early in their study of clinical medicine. In this way a start can be made toward the regular study of current medical literature and also the foundations of one's own medical library can be laid. Each student may have a personal preference. The most frequently read medical journal by students and practitioners is the *New England Journal of Medicine*. It is particularly useful for the student with its CPC, surveys of medical progress, editorial comments on current topics, original articles, and lively correspondence. In this manner the student establishes an early acquaintance with the frontiers of medicine and with its issues, uncertainties, and controversies.

The Student and the Patient. One of the student's earliest concerns on entering clinical medicine is how to interact with patients and how to assume the traditional role of a physician. The student is concerned that personal insecurities will impair effective communication with patients in whose care he or she is now called upon to participate. Rarely does this turn out in practice to be a serious problem. The expectations of most patients in the physician-patient interaction, discussed above, are realistic ones. Patients are usually aware of the progression of assigned responsibilities in the student-house staff-faculty team and do not expect omniscience or authoritarianism from the student. Not infrequently the patient forms a special attachment to the student, especially if the student has been perceptive enough to listen in the sense described above by Wilfred Trotter. If the student respects the personal dignity of the patient as a fellow human being, and listens in a sensitive manner, the patient responds with gratitude and returns that respect. Even when patients are initially perceived as hostile or belligerent, the student must maintain equanimity and try to understand the sources of these reactions. Do not allow yourself to be drawn into the flippant cynicism that sometimes passes for sophistication in the subculture of student and house staff training. Francis Peabody's sentient summary is still most apt, "for the secret of the care of the patient is in caring for the patient."

Students and Their Colleagues. Beginning in the clinical years the relationships of students with their colleagues in medicine undergo a subtle change. No longer are they merely the passive recipients of data and concepts supplied by the faculty through lectures, conferences, syllabi, or laboratories. They are participating with graduated responsibilities in the practice of medicine. A point in the medical history or a question asked by the student may prove decisive in arriving at the solution of a clinical problem. Frequently the most effective teachers of students are the house staff or more advanced students. Students will find many residents to be splendid teachers who not only make them feel at home in the service but also take the extra time to include them in all of the discussions. On most teaching services there is a certain amount of badinage or gamesmanship which enlivens interactions. If this is recognized as such, and not taken too seriously, it can serve to enhance rather than demean the learning experience. As a student you must not hesitate to ask questions or bring up new points of view and must not be intimidated by your current position in this shifting hierarchy. Even the chief medical resident faced similar qualms only a few years ago. But above all, remember that it is the patient's welfare, and not your own ego, that is paramount.

The Physician as a Nonphysician. Beginning in the basic science years but exacerbated in the clinical years, students often become concerned about the level of commitment demanded of them. How much of a life that is finite in time and energy must be devoted to medicine? What is the boundary between dedication and obsession? After all, one does not really become a physician; one remains a human being who has acquired certain knowledge and skills that allow one to function as a physician during specific periods of time. What should those times be? How and when does one shift roles from being a physician to being a "nonphysician"? This is, of course, a generic question that is as applicable to science, art, business, or any other human activity as it is to medicine.

The student will not readily find an all-embracing answer to this question. Each student will most likely evolve a personal answer and it will be an operational one representing the integral of microcompromises and adjustments made throughout one's subsequent career. The "complete physician," narrowly construed, would be a very poor physician if he were merely an observer rather than a participant in the pageantry of his time. Physicians owe it to themselves, to their families, to society, and to their patients not to become simply skilled but detached automatons. On the other hand, the practice of medicine is not a job but a profession that cannot be sealed off into convenient hours for earning one's living. To attempt to do so smacks of dilettantism. Between these extremes one must decide for oneself where the compromises will be made along the varying border between personal and professional life. Tensions will remain, but properly channeled they can be creative and rewarding.

3 Medicine as a Science

James B. Wyngaarden

It is not my purpose in this chapter to contend that medicine is itself a science, much less merely the application of scientific knowledge to the diagnosis and treatment of human diseases. Rather it is to accord the scientific base of the profession of medicine its proper recognition as the foundation of the intellectual and professional competence that enables a skillful physician to serve other human beings in the preservation of health and the prevention, diagnosis, and amelioration or cure of disease.

In the interactions of physicians with people of extraordinary diversity, whether throughout the full life cycle or in a single encounter, it is difficult to imagine any form of knowledge that does not prove useful at one time or another in the practice of medicine. Yet it is knowledge of humans, in all their biologic, behavioral, and social complexity, and the ability to base one's decisions and actions on that knowledge that distinguish physicians from other professionals. The particular training of the individual physician and extent of his or her knowledge, judgment, wisdom, compassion, and humanity distinguish the truly great physician from others. But the effectiveness of a physician begins with professional competence, without which compassion and humanity are ineffectual. And a major portion of professional competence depends on understanding the scientific principles of the branch or segment of medicine practiced.

I say "branch or segment of medicine practiced" to acknowledge that medicine is far too vast and complex a field to be mastered in all its specialties and techniques by any one physician. Nevertheless, all physicians need a considerable breadth of scientific knowledge of the type acquired during a lengthy

primary and secondary education, a liberal arts college experience, and a medical school curriculum. In addition, each physician needs to acquire a profound understanding of the particular science base of his or her specialty and a comfortable familiarity with it. The neurologist and ophthalmologist must delve deeply into the neurosciences, the rheumatologist into immunology and connective tissue biology, and the psychiatrist into behavioral and social sciences.

The *Cecil Textbook of Medicine* is a comprehensive general textbook of medicine, principally of diseases of young, mature, or aging adults, which stresses medical as contrasted with surgical approaches. It addresses the full expanse of what is usually termed general internal medicine, but with sufficient detail that each part also defines the scope of a major medical subspecialty, albeit in considerably less detail than corresponding subspecialty texts provide. It is intended to speak to the needs of advanced medical students and graduate physicians in training as well as practicing physicians. Accordingly, the *Textbook* extends its taproots into a remarkably large and rich garden of biologic and behavioral science. The practitioners of medicine of the scope addressed in this book thus have need for a broader grasp of scientific principles and specific information than almost any other subgroup of physician. And given the pace of scientific advances and the extraordinary potential of the new biology to explicate life processes and their aberrations, and of the biotechnology industry to develop new agents of remarkable specificity and complexity, the need for continuing scientific currency becomes a daunting challenge to maintaining and extending one's professional competence. Only through continuing attention to one's scientific education can the physician be a critical and independent participant in medical progress and avoid the pitfall of becoming a passive purveyor of medical fashion.

Advances in biologic science and accompanying technologic developments underlie most of the medical progress of the past half century, which has so remarkably advanced the ability of the physician to intervene in illness. Much of this progress has been in fundamental or "basic" science, conducted in the pursuit of understanding for its own sake. Significant progress has also resulted from research conducted by physician-scientists with a specified clinical goal in mind—for example, the elucidation of a disease mechanism or the critical evaluation of a therapeutic practice. Advances in medicine also continue to occur through serendipity or by astute clinical observations concerning patients or groups of patients and their illnesses. Nevertheless, the only rational approach to finding new methods for prevention or treatment is based on scientific explanations of the causes and mechanisms of disease. As Sir William Osler has said of the ambitions of medicine, "To wrest from nature the secrets which have perplexed philosophers in all ages, to track to their sources the causes of disease."[*]

Some years ago, Comroe and Dripps[†] traced the origins of ten major clinical innovations in cardiovascular and pulmonary medicine in an effort to identify the antecedents of these advances. Over 60 per cent of the enabling discoveries were in the category of basic science; over 40 per cent were the result of research carried out without any particular clinical application in mind. These observations are probably representative of medical progress in general.

The ability to control infections with antibiotics, hypertension with antihypertensive agents, and inflammatory reactions with glucocorticoids represents remarkable advances that have contributed to a lengthening of life expectancy. But the agenda is far from being fulfilled. The major health care problems of our time lie in the continued existence of diseases for which we can as yet do little. We have no definitive answers for cancer,

*Bean WB: Sir William Osler Aphorisms. Springfield, Ill., Charles C Thomas, pp 61–62. Quoted by Jackson CE, Norum RA: N Engl J Med 321:1040, 1989.

†Comroe JH, Dripps RD: The top ten clinical advances in cardiovascular-pulmonary medicine and surgery between 1945 and 1975: How they came about. Bethesda, Md., Public Inquiries and Reports Branch, National Heart, Lung, and Blood Institute, National Institutes of Health, 1977.

rheumatoid arthritis, schizophremia, and many other diseases, the descriptions of which constitute the substance of this book —or else we have what Lewis Thomas has called a "halfway technology," measures capable of modifying and ameliorating illness but not of preventing or curing it. Medicine as a science is incomplete and will remain so, for science itself is by its nature incomplete.

The present bioscientific character of medical practice is a relatively recent development. Throughout most of recorded history, medicine was anything but scientific. Diagnoses were inexact, causes of diseases poorly understood, and therapies frivolous and haphazard. Interventions by physicians consisted of myriads of procedures with no scientific foundation. Nor could there be such a foundation, for the scientific base did not yet exist.

Harbingers of change emerged slowly in the early nineteenth century, as new principles of physics and chemistry were applied to medicine. Physiologists stressed functions of organs and tissues. Its exemplars, especially Claude Bernard (1813–1878), emphasized the experimental method in establishing biologic knowledge and the necessity of basing medical practice in such knowledge. Pathologists, led by Virchow (1821–1902), stressed the critical study of normal and abnormal tissues and the correlation of features of disease with precise anatomic observations. Bacteriologists, with Pasteur (1822–1895) and Koch (1843–1910) in the vanguard, began to identify the microorganisms and to implicate specific organisms in specific diseases—the anthrax bacillus in anthrax, the tubercle bacillus in consumption, the pneumococcus in lobar pneumonia, the streptococcus in puerperal fever. The groundwork for future therapies was being laid by these great Western European scientists, but physicians could do relatively little about most illnesses at the time. Their major contributions were diagnostic, prognostic, and supportive. By correct diagnosis they could advise concerning outcome. By common-sense supportive measures they could provide comfort and maximize opportunities for recovery. But interventions were as likely as not to make things worse. The first edition of Osler's *Textbook of Medicine* in 1892 was revolutionary for its skepticism and its therapeutic nihilism, as this outstanding physician and teacher condemned the majority of nostrums and remedies as useless, even harmful.

Slowly, specific therapies—insulin for diabetes, liver extract for pernicious anemia—or specific immunizations—diphtheria antitoxin, pneumococcic antisera—appeared. But it was not until the decade of 1935 to 1945 that the entry of sulfonamides and penicillin into clinical medicine made curable a large number of previously lethal and untreatable diseases. It is customary to date the beginnings of modern medicine from these relatively recent events.

The language of contemporary biologic science has become increasingly biochemical. The compositions of organs, tissues, cells, organelles, and membranes have been defined. The biosynthesis and catabolism of hundreds of compounds have been elucidated. The regulation of body processes has been described at progressively finer levels and in chemical language. Many pharmacologic agents are now understood in terms of specific loci and mechanisms of action. The expansion of new knowledge continues at a pace that is bewildering to all but experts in a given field. Current advances are particularly rapid in immunology, virology, molecular and cellular biology, peptide research, and structural biology. A beginning has been made in explaining human behavior in mechanistic terms, as more and more chemical mediators and pharmacologic modifiers are discovered.

We are in a molecular age of basic biologic science. The molecular influence pervades all the traditional disciplines underlying clinical medicine. Approximately 375 inborn errors are now understood in terms of specific missing or abnormal enzymes or other proteins. There are more than 575 known abnormal human hemoglobins, and for each of these the precise structural defect in the DNA of the mutant gene can be defined. Membrane, cytoplasmic, and nuclear receptors for hormones and drugs are exploding upon us, and old as well as new diseases are being defined in terms of receptor abnormalities—for example, type II hypercholesterolemia and nephrogenic diabetes insipidus. Recognition of opiate receptors has led to the discovery of endogenous

peptides (endorphins) with analgesic activity. Their localization gives promise of further understanding of the limbic system, affective states, and addictions. The number and function of neurotransmitters have greatly increased, and these and other advances in neuroscience portend exciting developments in understanding how the brain works. DNA sequencing techniques and restriction endonucleases now permit precise identification of the exact structural alteration of the gene in an increasing number of hereditary diseases. The complete sequencing of the human genome is now technically possible and is being undertaken. A coordinated international program is being organized in the hope of accomplishing this goal in about 15 years. About 0.5 per cent of it has already been done. Gene therapy—both pharmacologic modification of specific gene action and physical replacement of damaged genetic segments—is now possible in experimental systems (see Ch. 32).

Much of the recent fundamental information in science has been obtained by the process of reductionism—the belief that all living processes can ultimately be explained in biochemical terms. The scientists responsible for our evolving understanding of biologic systems know that the reductionist approach must often precede reconstitutive endeavors. Scientific progress rests on myriads of small observations, tedious measurements, and the findings of investigators asking humble, answerable questions. Instead of reaching for the whole truth, the scientist examines small, defined, and clearly separable phenomena. The pattern of science is a stepwise extension of what came before, with an occasional giant leap forward through great discovery.

The examples of advances in medical science mentioned above have been largely drawn from the areas of ultrastructure, biochemistry, and molecular biology. In biology these disciplines have arbitrary and porous boundaries: physiology, pharmacology, neurosciences, cell biology, molecular biology, biochemistry, immunology, biophysics—all are in a phase of confluence, and the common language is chemistry. Medicine is not only a branch of applied biology, however. It also subsumes many aspects of psychology, sociology, anthropology, and economics. These disciplines, too long neglected or denigrated as "soft science," are now increasingly recognized as germane to medicine as a discipline and the practice of medicine as a profession.

However, not all observers of the evolution of modern medicine are in agreement with the current emphasis on scientific discovery as the motive force of medical advance. Critics of the bioscientific strategy of medicine, especially Ivan Illich, have claimed that the great advances that have dramatically reduced mortality rates consist in the improvement of the environment, the correction of malnutrition, and the control of infectious diseases through immunizations and antimicrobial agents, and that the relevant medical breakthroughs largely occurred before the prodigious expansion of federal support of biomedical science begun in the early 1950's. They contend that the enormous expenditures that have made the United States pre-eminent in biomedical research have produced too little in the way of medical advance to justify their continuation and have instead fostered the development of an extremely costly technology that has had only a minimal effect upon mortality statistics. They propose that the bioscientific strategy of medicine be replaced by an ecologic strategy for health.

No doubt safe water supplies, better sewage disposal, improved nutrition, immunizations, and improved standards of living deserve considerable credit for health improvements. In addition, the current public concern with the environment—with air, water, and food safety—will probably result in further health improvements. These are part of a new ecologic strategy for health. But one does not need to denigrate science in order to support a concomitant environmental concern. A scientific strategy for medicine and an ecologic strategy for health are not mutually exclusive. Furthermore, the medical advances of the past few decades—for example, in the treatment of Hodgkin's disease, childhood leukemias, Parkinson's disease, Wilson's disease, and AIDS, and, more recently, relief of an impending worldwide insulin shortage with rDNA-derived insulin, replacement of potentially virus-contaminated growth hormone with rDNA-derived growth hormone, and production of erythropoietin for treatment of anemia of end-stage renal disease—have all depended on a deeper and clearer understanding of biologic mechanisms and application of basic scientific knowledge to clinical problems.

The list of human diseases for which there are as yet no definitive measures for prevention or cure is still formidable. Fresh insights into the nature of these diseases are needed, insights that can come only from continued basic research. But the expansion of the knowledge bank of the past quarter century justifies great optimism for the eventual control and cure of major diseases and the possible elimination of premature death from illness. The science and the art of medicine must remain intimately linked if physicians are to be maximally effective.

THE PHYSICIAN AS A SCIENTIST. Since medicine is derived from a number of sciences relevant to the health of individuals or of groups, physicians must be trained as scientists to utilize these complex disciplines effectively.

To be a scientist, the physician must be conversant with the processes of scientific inquiry—how data are obtained and evaluated; how hypotheses are framed, modified, or discarded; the uses and limitations of inductive reasoning. In short, they must understand science as an intellectual instrument that has been slowly improved over centuries. Only in this way can they remain attentive to medical progress. Both the spirit and rigor of science are necessary for the physician to become and remain a scholar in medicine. Medical practice itself contains many of the elements of scientific inquiry in the pursuit and evaluation of data (history, physical examination, laboratory studies) and in framing a hypothesis (tentative clinical diagnosis).

As a scientist the physician is the beneficiary of both the fruits of scientific research and the mental discipline of the scientific method. To a greater or lesser degree the physician also has the opportunity to contribute personally to medical progress. Most medical research is now carried out by teams of participating investigators in elaborately equipped laboratories that utilize the advanced instrumentation and technology of modern science. There is still room, however, for scientific contributions made by inquiring physicians based on their own experiences in patient care. Much of medical progress has derived from this kind of curiosity in the past. In addition, this form of clinical research, on whatever modest scale it may be engaged in, adds excitement and zest to professional life. As Thomas Hobbes has written: "Desire to know why, and how, curiosity, which is a lust of the mind, that by a perseverance of delight in the continued and indefatigable generation of knowledge, exceedeth the short vehemence of any carnal pleasure."

4 Clinical Ethics in the Practice of Medicine

Mark Siegler and Peter A. Singer

Clinical medical ethics (CME) is a practical discipline that aims to improve patient care and patient outcomes. It focuses on the doctor-patient relationship and takes explicit account of the ethical and legal issues that patients, physicians, and health care institutions must address in reaching the best decisions for individual patients. CME emphasizes that in practicing good clinical medicine physicians must combine scientific and technical abilities with ethical concerns for the personal preferences and values of the patient who seeks their help. CME also provides a structured approach to decision making that can assist physicians to identify, analyze, and resolve clinical ethical dilemmas.

CME begins with the encounter between patient and physician, an encounter that both establishes the doctor-patient relationship and imposes stringent moral requirements on the physician, including the need for honesty, competence, compassion, and respect for the patient. Beyond these fundamental moral requirements, CME assists physicians to address a wide range of specifically ethical problems—for example, informed consent, end-of-life decisions, allocation of scarce resources, confidentiality, and third party interference with the autonomy of both patients and physicians—problems that arise with increasing frequency in the practice of modern high technology medicine.

For the foreseeable future, the critical problem facing concerned patients and conscientious physicians will be to balance the rights and responsibilities of patients and physicians at a time when societal values and expectations are changing rapidly and relations between patients and physicians are increasingly regulated and legislated. In the light of such changes, CME may assist patients, physicians, and society to achieve an ethically acceptable new arrangement because CME emphasizes the moral dimensions of the encounter between patient and physician, an encounter that remains the central and unchanging event in medicine.

This chapter aims to introduce students and practicing physicians to the field of clinical ethics by describing a framework for approaching ethical problems in clinical practice. The framework proposes that three sets of considerations be taken into account in analyzing ethical problems in clinical medicine: (1) clinical circumstances, (2) patient preferences, and (3) socioeconomic constraints.

DECISION MAKING STRATEGY FOR CLINICAL ETHICAL PROBLEMS

Every aspect of medical practice involves ethical considerations, but during the past 20 years certain issues have become recognized as specifically ethical "issues" or "problems." In recent years, investigators have begun to describe the epidemiology of these ethical problems in clinical practice. A 1981 study found that the incidence of ethical dilemmas recognized in a medical inpatient service was 17 per cent when an internist-ethicist participated on ward rounds. The ethical problems, in order of decreasing frequency, included withholding tests or treatment, informed consent, truth telling, and allocation of limited resources. A 1988 study found that important ethical problems were noted in 30 per cent of patients in an internal medicine office practice. The most common ethical problems in this outpatient study were costs of care, psychological factors that influence patient preferences, competence and capacity to choose, and informed consent.

Experienced clinicians who have faced each of these problems many times before often can respond to them appropriately without analyzing and dissecting each case. Students of medicine, however, may find it useful to consider explicitly three sets of issues when confronted with an ethical problem. These three levels of consideration are (1) the clinical circumstances presented by the patient's case, (2) the patient's wishes regarding treatment, and (3) the socioeconomic factors that tend to constrain individual patient-doctor decision making at levels 1 and 2.

CLINICAL CIRCUMSTANCES

Both the ethical and medical evaluations of a patient's case begin from precisely the same point: an accurate assessment of the patient's clinical circumstances. Data concerning the patient's clinical situation are collected through the traditional methods of history taking, physical examination, and laboratory investigations. From these data, the physician reaches a diagnosis and prognosis and develops options for therapy. Finally, the physician makes a specific recommendation to the patient after taking account of the nature of the medical problem, the values and goals of the patient, and the risks and benefits of various alternative treatment approaches for the particular patient. The physician informs and educates the patient about the anticipated benefits from the clinical recommendation and encourages the patient to accept the proposed treatment or a reasonable alternative. This is usually the critical step in the doctor-patient encounter. In general, patients accept the physician's recommendation because the physician and patient share the same goal—improvement of the patient's health status—and because patients usually trust and have confidence in both the physician's technical abilities and his or her concern for the patient as an individual.

Prior to making recommendations to a patient, the physician is obligated to consider two clinical issues that may influence the process of clinical-ethical decision making: (1) Is the patient competent? (2) Is the treatment proposal "futile"? If the patient is incompetent, the focus of decision making broadens to incorporate the patient's family or other surrogate decision maker (see below, "Incompetent Patients"). If the proposed treatment is futile, the focus of decision making may be narrowed to clinical circumstances alone.

Competency Assessment

The assessment of competency plays a pivotal role in patient care. Whether a doctor finds a patient competent or incompetent often determines whether or not the doctor accepts the patient's stated wishes about treatment or takes steps to review or override the patient's decision. Respect for the ethical and legal rights of patients means that competent patients may accept or reject treatment even if it may result in their death. On the other hand, doctors are obligated to question or even overrule requests to forego treatment made by incompetent patients because they are expected to protect patients from serious harm that the patient would not intend if he or she were competent. With so much at stake, it would be desirable to have well-developed clinical standards for the determination of competency. Unfortunately, at present, there are no clearly stipulated criteria for the determination of competency at the bedside.

The President's Commission for the Study of Ethical Problems in Medicine and Biomedical and Behavioral Research identified three elements of competency: possession of a set of values and goals, the ability to communicate and understand information, and the ability to reason and deliberate about one's choices. The Commission also noted that competency was specific to "the person's actual functioning in situations in which a decision about health care was to be made." More recently, Appelbaum and Grisso have suggested that the competent patient should be able to communicate choices, understand relevant information, appreciate the situation and its consequences, and manipulate information rationally. An effective clinical index of patient competency, however, would require a list of specific questions for the physician to ask the patient, clearly stipulated criteria for the appraisal of patient responses, and a mechanism for combining the responses on individual questions into an overall assessment. Until such an index has been developed and evaluated, physicians and consultants must continue to rely on ad hoc assessments of competency.

At the extremes, doctors can usually establish whether a patient is competent or incompetent. Moreover, the clinician can sometimes restore patients to a state of competency by treating reversible causes of cognitive dysfunction, correcting a wide range of metabolic encephalopathies, or discontinuing psychoactive drugs. If uncertainty remains about the patient's competency, the physician should consult with colleagues, such as psychiatrists, neurologists, institutional ethics committees, ethics consultation services, and hospital attorneys.

Futility

The claim that a treatment is futile is often used to justify a shift in the physician's ethical obligations to patients. In clinical situations in which nonfutile treatments are available, the physician has an obligation to discuss therapeutic alternatives with the patient and to encourage patient choice. By contrast, a physician is under no obligation to offer, or even to discuss, futile therapies. This shift in obligation is supported by moral reasoning in ancient and modern medical ethics, by public policy, and by case law.

Given this shift in ethical obligations, one might expect that physicians would have unambiguous criteria for determining when a therapy is futile. Unfortunately, this is not the case. Ambiguity in determining futility arises from disagreements about the goals of therapy and uncertainty about the probability of attaining those goals. Given the importance of futility claims in clinical practice, physicians must try to separate these two components of futility determinations: the goals of therapy and the chances of attaining them.

In some situations, physicians may acknowledge that therapy is effective but believe that the goals that can be achieved with therapy are not desirable or not compatible with adequate quality of life. Examples are prolonged nutritional support for patients in a persistent vegetative state and the treatment of pneumonia in a patient dying of untreatable pancreatic cancer. In such

situations, physicians should acknowledge that potentially achievable goals exist. Since quality-of-life judgments are best made by the patient, these treatment decisions should be discussed with the patient or the patient's surrogate or be based on the patient's previously expressed goals.

In other situations, physicians may regard the likelihood of therapeutic success as quite remote, for example, cardiopulmonary resuscitation for elderly patients with cancer or sepsis and further chemotherapy for a patient with advanced metastatic cancer. It is not clear exactly how such probability considerations should be factored into clinical decision making, how low a probability (? 10%, 5%, 0.5%) constitutes "futility," or whether determination of probable futility should be made by the patient, the physician, or society (e.g., third-party payers).

"Futility" is an important clinical concept, but physicians should use it with precision. Physicians should stipulate whether they consider the goals of treatment undesirable or the chance of success too low. Unless the specific circumstances are explicitly recognized as "futile" by professional consensus or by legal-administrative guidelines, the physician should review his conclusions with the competent patient or the incompetent patient's surrogate decision maker.

PATIENT PREFERENCES

How patient preferences are incorporated into clinical decision making depends on whether the patient is competent or incompetent; decision making for competent and incompetent patients is the focus of the first two parts of this section. The third part examines the situation that arises when the patient's and physician's preferences conflict.

Competent Patients

Given the medical facts (as organized and presented by the physician), what course of action does the competent patient wish to pursue? This is the pivotal question in the therapeutic alliance between doctor and patient. The doctor should educate the patient regarding clinical condition, prognosis, and therapeutic options. The patient may then choose a course of management based on his preferences, values, and goals.

In the doctor-patient relationship, the doctor has both objective and subjective roles. In conveying the clinical circumstances to the patient, the doctor must be reasonably objective so as not to bias the patient's choice. After this objective information has been presented, however, physicians are entitled to offer their subjective opinion to the patient about which treatment choice the physician would prefer. Such personal opinions should be clearly identified as such, and, whenever possible, the physician should also explain why a particular choice of treatment seems preferable.

The patient's right to participate in treatment decisions is well recognized in law, philosophy, public policy, and clinical practice. Perhaps the clearest *legal* statement of this right was enunciated in 1914 by Justice Cardozo: "Every human being of adult years and sound mind has the right to determine what shall be done with his own body." The *philosophical* right of patients to control their own medical care is based on the principle of individual autonomy. In the 1980's, a Presidential Commission clearly stated that respect for patient preferences should be the basis of *public policy* in medical ethics. Moreover, there is evidence from *clinical* research that empowering patients to participate in their own health care may actually lead to improved functional outcomes in chronic diseases.

Incompetent Patients

As a practical matter, competent adult patients can discuss their treatment preferences directly with their physician; incompetent patients cannot. Since the 1976 Quinlan case, judges and legislators have increasingly permitted others to make decisions on behalf of incompetent patients. Forty states have enacted laws recognizing the authority of "living wills," and 17 states have laws about durable powers of attorney for health care. Since only 15 per cent of Americans have executed a formal advance directive, court opinions in many states also permit a process called surrogate decision making, in which another person known as a surrogate decision maker can make decisions on behalf of an incompetent patient.

Surrogate decision making is a method that physicians can use to care for incompetent patients who lack advance directives. Such decision making relies on two standards: substituted judgment and best interests. The goal of substituted judgment, the preferred standard, is "to reach the decision that the incapacitated person would make if he or she were able to choose." Substituted judgment relies upon a knowledge of the patient's attitudes, values, and aspirations; such information must be supplied by the family or friends of the patient. Recent empiric data that show low rates of agreement between patients and their surrogates in resuscitation and end-of-life decisions raise troubling questions about the adequacy of the substituted judgment approach and argue for broader use of advance directives. In the *Cruzan* decision, the United States Supreme Court ruled that in applying the substituted judgment approach, states may establish standards of evidence for determining a patient's prior wishes.

The best interests test is applied in situations in which the patient's attitudes and values are not known to the physician and cannot be learned in the future because of the patient's irreversible cognitive impairment. The best interests approach encourages a surrogate to balance the benefits and burdens of treatment for a particular patient by applying "objective, societally shared criteria." Since such criteria are difficult to agree upon in a pluralistic society, the best interests standard should be used only as a last resort in reaching decisions for incompetent patients who lack advance directives and whose prior attitudes and preferences are not known.

Conscientious Objection

Sometimes the patient or surrogate chooses a treatment option to which the physician is morally opposed. Examples of such treatment plans might include elective abortion, discontinuation of tube feeding, or the request for physician-assisted euthanasia. The right of individual health care providers to refuse to participate in treatment plans that they find morally objectionable has been well established. The President's Commission noted that a health care professional is not "obligated to accede to the patient in a way that violates . . . the provider's own deeply held moral beliefs." (The health care professional may not refuse to provide emergency care.) If the provider refuses, on grounds of personal conscience, to participate in a patient's legal treatment (or nontreatment) request, he should usually arrange for an alternative source of care for the patient. The prerogative of health care facilities or of the entire medical profession to refuse to participate in a morally objectionable treatment plan is more complex and has been discussed elsewhere (see Miles et al., 1989).

SOCIOECONOMIC CONSIDERATIONS

Many factors influence and constrain the individual decisions made by doctors and patients. These factors include family wishes, institutional policies, laws, scarce resources, and economic costs. Because in the 1990's economic considerations are likely to become increasingly important in individual decisions, we focus here on potential conflicts between medical ethics and medical economics.

The cost of health care raises challenging ethical issues at several levels. At the national and state level, the 12 per cent of gross national product ($661 billion in 1990) spent on health care must be balanced against other priorities such as defense, education, and housing. Moreover, priorities must be set between different health programs, as exemplified by the 1988 decision in Oregon to cut funding for organ transplantation in favor of prenatal care. At the institutional level, health care facilities must choose to emphasize some services, such as burn care or cardiac surgery, at the expense of others. It is, however, at the level of the individual patient-physician relationship that economic-ethical conflicts are of greatest concern to the practicing physician.

From the perspective of individual physicians, the essential ethical dilemma is how to incorporate considerations of costs into the traditional decision making framework that places priority on clinical circumstances and patient preferences. Specifically, is it ethically acceptable for physicians to recommend a "less than optimal" management strategy to a patient because of the cost concerns of third parties such as insurance companies, federal or state payers, or HMO's?

Conflict arises between the physician's obligation to serve the patient's "good" and his obligation to serve the public "good" by controlling health care costs. This conflict admits no easy resolution. Some argue that the physician's obligation to control cost may, at times, outweigh his obligation to the patient. We agree that the physician is not obliged to provide inappropriate or ineffective health services (even at the patient's request). We believe, however, that physicians should not withhold medically indicated and desired services on grounds of cost control.

The physician should serve as the patient's advocate (and not as the payer's gatekeeper) for health services that are likely to benefit the patient. Conversely, in a world of limited resources, the physician has the duty to not expend resources that are medically inappropriate or that the patient does not want. For example, researchers at RAND have found that 14 per cent of coronary artery bypass procedures and 32 per cent of carotid endarterectomies are performed for inappropriate reasons, and the National Leadership Commission on Health Care has estimated that the United States could save as much as $22 billion per year by eliminating inappropriate care. There are, of course, many areas of uncertainty in which solid outcome data do not exist or in which marginal benefits and marginal costs must be given serious consideration. The principles of clinical ethics suggest that such decisions be based primarily on clinical circumstances and patient preferences.

The limitation of health services for reasons of cost is a political decision that a society may choose to make. The principle of justice requires, however, that such decisions not be made capriciously in the context of individual patient-physician relationships, but rather as the openly debated public policy of a democratic society.

CONCLUSIONS

In the last decade, clinical medical ethics has emerged as a new and useful component of medical practice. CME emphasizes that technical and ethical concerns are inseparable in the practice of medicine. CME focuses on the continuing centrality of the doctor-patient relationship and on how patients and physicians work within existing administrative structures to reach mutual agreement on clinical decisions that affect the patient. In addition, CME offers a language of discourse that attempts to broaden the medical model from one that is narrowly technical to one that takes serious account of the needs and wants of individual patients. The language and content of clinical ethics have been adopted not only by patients, physicians, and medical educators, but also by health economists, hospital administrators, legislators, and judges. In this regard, ethical considerations in medicine are likely to remain an important component of medical education, clinical practice, and the political evolution of our health system.

After a century of extraordinary scientific achievements, unparalleled in the history of medicine, medical educators and political leaders have come to acknowledge the importance of combining technical excellence with ethical sensitivity to the individual patient's goals. Plato recognized the importance of this 2500 years ago when, in Book IV of *The Laws*, he described the excellent physician as one who ". . . treats disease by going into things thoroughly from the beginning in a scientific way and takes the patient and family into confidence. Thus he learns something from the sufferer . . . He does not give prescriptions until he has won the patient's support, and when he has done so, he steadfastly aims at providing complete restoration to health by persuading the sufferer into compliance. . . ." The best clinical medicine, Plato tells us, is achieved when patient and physician have established a relationship in which technical and personal aspects of care are integrated. The practice of ethical medicine in the twenty-first century will require nothing more but demand nothing less.

Appelbaum PS, Grisso T: Assessing patients' capacities to consent to treatment. N Engl J Med 319:1635–1638, 1988. *A review of the four factors to consider in assessing patients' decision-making capacity.*

Connelly JE, DalleMura S: Ethical problems in the medical office. JAMA 260:812–815, 1988. *An empirical study of the epidemiology of outpatient clinical-ethical problems.*

Emanuel LL, Emanuel EJ: The medical directive. A new comprehensive advance care document. JAMA 261:3288–3293, 1989. *An expanded version of the "living will" which may prove more useful clinically.*

Ethics Committee, American College of Physicians: American College of Physicians Ethics Manual, 2nd edition. Ann Intern Med 111:245–252, 327–335, 1989. *An official consensus statement by the American College of Physicians on a wide range of ethical issues that relate to internal medicine practice, including decisions to forego life-sustaining treatments and economic-ethical conflicts.*

Jonsen AR, Siegler M, Winslade WJ: Clinical Ethics: A Practical Approach to Ethical Decisions in Clinical Medicine. 3rd ed. New York, Pergamon Press, 1990. *A practical guide to help clinicians deal with ethical problems that occur frequently in medical practice.*

Lantos JD, Singer PA, Walker RM, et al.: The illusion of futility in clinical practice. Am J Med 87:81–84, 1989. *An analysis of how the powerful concept of "futility" is used and misused in clinical medicine.*

Lo B, Schroeder SA: Frequency of ethical dilemmas in a medical inpatient service. Arch Intern Med 141:1062–1064, 1981. *An empirical study of the epidemiology of inpatient clinical-ethical problems.*

Miles SH, Singer PA, Siegler M: Conflicts between patients' requests to forego treatment and the policies of health care facilities. N Engl J Med 321:48–50, 1989. *An approach for resolving conflicts that arise when patient preferences conflict with institutional policy.*

President's Commission for the Study of Ethical Problems in Medicine and Biomedical and Behavioral Research: Making Health Care Decisions: The Ethical and Legal Implications of Informed Consent in the Patient-Practitioner Relationship, Vol. 1. Washington, D.C., U.S. Government Printing Office, 1982. *This important report concluded that ethically valid consent is a process of shared decision making between physicians and patients.*

Siegler M, Singer PA, Schiedermayer DL: Medical Ethics: An Annotated Bibliography. Philadelphia, American College of Physicians, 1988. *A clinically oriented annotated bibliography of the medical ethics literature through July 1988; designed to accompany the second edition of the American College of Physicians Ethics Manual.*

Singer PA, Siegler M: Elective use of life-sustaining treatments. *In* Stollerman GH (ed.): Advances in Internal Medicine, Vol. 36. New York, Year Book, 1991. *Reviews empirical data and provides a clinical approach to the elective use of life-sustaining treatments in internal medicine.*

PART II

HUMAN GROWTH, DEVELOPMENT, AND AGING

5 Adolescent Medicine

Iris F. Litt

The teenager is a psychosocially and physically unique individual, and this uniqueness has important implications for health and health care. In addition to the age-specific features of this period of life, there are significant differences among adolescents, based upon their rates of pubertal development as well as their psychosocial development. The view of the adolescent from the physical standpoint reveals the importance of stage of pubertal development, rather than chronologic age, as an organizing principle, owing to the wide variability in timing of pubertal events. From a psychosocial perspective, early adolescents, middle adolescents, and late adolescents have many psychosocial and cognitive characteristics shared with others in their own age groups. There is a growing tendency to combine these vantage points and recognize the areas of interaction between pubertal and psychosocial development.

PSYCHOSOCIAL DEVELOPMENT

During adolescence, certain tasks must be mastered if the child is going to evolve into a successful adult in our society. These include the "tasks of adolescence": the process of separation from the protective milieu of the family and, with it, development of independence; incorporation of the physical and emotional effects of pubertal hormonal changes into one's self-concept; development of a clear sexual identity and a sense of sexual adequacy; educational and vocational decision making; and achievement of the capacity for intimacy. Accomplishing these goals may, in actuality, take a lifetime, but the physician caring for adolescents may encounter opportunities to assist in the psychosocial development of the adolescent.

The physician may foster development of independence by encouraging the adolescent to make his or her own appointments, by promising confidentiality when appropriate, by handing the prescription directly to the adolescent patient rather than to the parent, and so on. Encouraging the parent of a chronically ill adolescent to assign household chores, to provide an allowance, and to allow going to friends' houses for "overnights" may prevent infantilization at the time when adolescents must be allowed to experience their emerging maturity. Failure to do so often results in "acting-out" behavior. One consequence of the stereotype of adolescents as rebellious patients is that physicians may expect them to be noncompliant with prescribed medication. When this stereotype is examined, however, it is found that the incidence of noncompliance is no different among adolescents than among adult patients, in the range of 40 to 50 per cent. The factors associated with noncompliance among adolescents are, however, different. Self-concept is the single most important predictor of compliance: The teenager who has a positive self-image is likely to follow the physician's advice. Moreover, the risk of noncompliance is great with any medication that affects appearance adversely, such as a systemic corticosteroid. The patient's satisfaction, a valid predictor of compliance for adult patients, is also important for the adolescent patient, but here again its determinants are different. The satisfied adolescent patient is the one whose privacy is respected, who is afforded the courtesy of confidentiality, and who is informed about the reasons for laboratory testing. Self-concept is also related to the risk of pregnancy during adolescence. Poor self-concept may place the young adolescent girl at increased risk of an exploitative relationship or cause her to lack the confidence to set limits within a sexual relationship. Low self-concept is also associated with poor compliance with oral contraceptives, further contributing to pregnancy risk.

Among the many causes of poor self-concept is the timing of pubertal maturation. For males, maturing earlier than the peer group appears to be an advantage, associated with popularity and athletic prowess, whereas a late-maturing male is predisposed to poorer educational performance and lower self-image. For females, the effects vary with the environmental context; for example, early maturers who remain in a kindergarten–through–eighth grade school exhibit no apparent ill effect from being out of synchrony with their peer group, whereas those early maturers who move to a junior high school have a higher incidence of poor self-image, have a lower grade-point average, and date more. Timing of pubertal development may also influence selection of sports involvement. Early-maturing females tend to have more adipose tissue, are more buoyant, and therefore may be channeled into swimming. The late-maturing girl, on the other hand, with her shorter upper to lower body ratio and leaner body may be more likely to become a ballet dancer or runner. An increase in body fat accompanies normal pubertal development in females, who often have difficulty reconciling it with our society's idealized female form of a skinny fashion model. Their dissatisfaction may result in dieting and the risk of nutritional deficiencies. This puberty-associated dieting may be the forerunner of anorexia nervosa in the predisposed individual (see Ch. 12).

The physician may assist the adolescent's development of a healthy sense of sexual identity and adequacy by offering reassurance about the normality of secondary sex characteristics and genitalia during the course of a routine physical examination. This is particularly important when gynecomastia is observed, as this common phenomenon often causes concern to the adolescent male, who is unlikely to have the courage to inquire about it. The female adolescent with asymmetry of her breasts or one who has not gotten pregnant despite having had unprotected intercourse, or the male teenager who has never impregnated his sexual partner, all may be questioning their sexual adequacy and normality. Even more problematic is the male adolescent who has a renal or urologic condition. The separation of reproductive from excretory function and structure may not be known or apparent to the apprehensive patient, although this is often assumed by his physician. A useful method for allaying such fear may be concrete explanations about anatomy and pathogenesis of the condition, prefaced by a comment like the following: "Some other boys who have had this operation have been worried that it may interfere with their ability to have sex. I don't know if you have had this worry, but I want to reassure you that it will not."

COGNITIVE DEVELOPMENT

The issues of counseling and confidentiality in the context of health care delivery to adolescents are complicated by the developmental differences in cognition among them. Piaget classified children and adolescents on the basis of discrete stages of cognitive development (Table 5–1). According to this schema, most early adolescents are at the stage of concrete operational thinking, whereas middle and late adolescents are more likely to have progressed to the highest stage of development, that of formal operations. This stage is distinguished by the ability to generate hypotheses that may be tested without their actual enactment. Moreover, the person in the stage of formal operations can think abstractly, entertain multiple contingencies simultaneously, generalize from one situation to another, and consider potential behavioral consequences logically without actually having to experience them. Piaget's static, categoric approach to cognitive development has been challenged. Newer research in the field stresses "trends" in domain-specific development. For example, the thinking of the younger individual is now regarded as more "empirico-deductive" than that of the older adolescent, who is viewed as more "hypothetico-deductive." Whatever the system used to evaluate cognition, it is important for the physician working with the adolescent patient to be able to assess his or her capacity for understanding the information conveyed and using it in a manner conducive to improving health status. For example, the adolescent female who is not able to think abstractly may have difficulty adhering to a regimen of oral contraceptives designed to prevent pregnancy. Similarly, truly informed consent to participate in a research project may not be obtainable from an adolescent subject unable to consider hypothetic consequences of his or her decision to participate or not.

PUBERTAL DEVELOPMENT

The Endocrinology of Puberty

The signal that initiates puberty remains elusive but it is known that just prior to puberty there is decreasing sensitivity of the hypothalamus and pituitary to circulating estrogen and testosterone and to the restraining influence of the hypothalamic arcuate neuron gonadotropin-releasing hormone. The latter is a pulsatile secretion augmented by sleep. The onset of puberty is marked by increased secretion of luteinizing hormone (LH) by the pituitary during sleep in a pulsatile fashion. The amplitude and frequency of LH pulses increase as puberty progresses. In late puberty, the adult pattern of approximately 12 pulses, evenly distributed over the course of a 24-hour period, is reached. There is a sex difference in gonadotropin secretion during puberty: A dramatic increase in LH levels occurs during early puberty in boys and later in girls. Follicle-stimulating hormone (FSH), on the other hand, rises gradually throughout puberty in boys and manifests an early rise in girls. The effect of the gonadotropin rise in males is to stimulate testicular production of testosterone. In females, the gonadotropin rise (predominantly involving FSH) stimulates the ovary to produce estradiol, with serum levels rising incrementally as puberty progresses. This is manifested by the development of secondary sex characteristics (see p. 17). Cyclic fluctuations in estradiol levels are noted around the time of menarche. Estrone, derived from conversion of estradiol and adrenal androstenedione, reaches its peak at sex maturity rating (SMR) 2 in girls. In boys, both estrone and estradiol (derived from conversion of adrenal and testicular testosterone and androstenedione) contribute to the frequent occurrence (in 30 to 50 per cent) of gynecomastia during SMR 2 and 3. Circulating sex hormones exert a constant or tonic negative feedback effect upon the hypothalamus in both sexes. The female also experiences a cyclic positive feedback loop by which increasing levels of circulating estrogens in the follicular phase cause a surge in LH. Sex hormone binding globulin levels fall in males during puberty. As only unbound sex hormones are physiologically active, this results in levels of free testosterone that are more than twice the female levels. Prolactin secretion by the pituitary is augmented by estrogen, resulting in higher levels in females than males, peaking between SMR 2 and 3. Prolactin response to thyrotropin-releasing hormone (TRH) stimulation, however, peaks at SMR 4 to 5.

Growth Hormone and Somatomedin-C

Growth hormone is also produced in a pulsatile fashion, during sleep stages 3 and 4 in early puberty. Somatomedins are responsible for the anabolic activity of growth hormone. Somatomedin-C (IGF-1) levels are age dependent and rise in conjunction with advancing development of secondary sex characteristics during puberty. Accordingly, their levels correlate better with stage of sexual maturation than chronologic age.

Physical Growth During Puberty

During puberty, a growth spurt is experienced by every organ system in the body, with the exception of the central nervous system, which remains stable in size, and the lymphoid system, which undergoes involution. The most noticeable changes produced by the pubertal growth spurt are in height, weight, and the secondary sex characteristics.

The pubertal height spurt occurs during midpuberty (SMR 3 to 4) in most individuals, with its peak occurring at an average age of 12 years in girls and 14 years in boys. During this height spurt, males gain 10.3 ± 1.54 cm per year and females gain 9.0 ± 1.03 cm per year. The growth velocity is greater the earlier it occurs. There is an orderly pattern of linear growth, beginning with the foot, followed within 6 months by the lower leg and then the thigh. Growth of the upper extremity and of the trunk occurs after that of the lower extremity. The later onset of the growth spurt in males than in females results in a longer period of prepubertal growth and hence longer legs in males. Assessment of height during puberty should be undertaken using a height velocity curve, which records increments in height per year (Fig. 5–1).

Approximately 4 months after the peak of leg-length acceleration, there is an increase in the biacromial and biiliac diameters, the former of greater magnitude in males and the latter in females, resulting in characteristic sex differences in adult physiques. At about the same time, the cranial bones undergo a growth spurt, particularly the jaw, which becomes more prominent, especially in boys. Elongation of the pharynx causes lowering of the hyoid bone. Dentition is another reflection of pubertal development. The cuspids (canines) and first molars of the primary dentition are shed by early adolescence, at which time the permanent cuspids and the first and second premolars erupt in their place. The timing of appearance of the second permanent molar correlates well with that of menarche. The third molars, "wisdom teeth," erupt during late adolescence.

Bone age can be determined from a roentgenogram of the hand, which is compared with standards in an atlas. During puberty, there is close correlation between bone age and stage of sexual maturation (SMR—see below).

Although both sexes experience a weight spurt during puberty, its origin is different in males and females. In males, it is due to increase in muscle mass, and in females, to fat tissue. Eight per cent of body composition is about average fat content in both sexes throughout childhood. At puberty, males experience a loss in fat tissue, whereas it begins to increase in females and reaches approximately 22 per cent when pubertal growth is complete (SMR 5).

Secondary Sex Characteristics

Estrogen and testosterone have a profound effect on a variety of tissues and organs during puberty. These effects are collectively referred to as secondary sex characteristics and include voice change, body and facial hair in males, breast development in females, and axillary and pubic hair in both sexes. Of these changes, those most consistent in pattern and timing are pubic hair in both sexes and breast development in females. Accordingly, these traits have formed the basis for categorization of the

TABLE 5–1. PIAGET'S ERAS AND STAGES OF LOGICAL AND COGNITIVE DEVELOPMENT

Era I	(ages 0–2): The era of sensorimotor intelligence
Era II	(ages 2–5): Symbolic, intuitive, or prelogical thought
Era III	(ages 6–10): Concrete operational thought
Era IV	(ages 11–adulthood): Formal operational thought

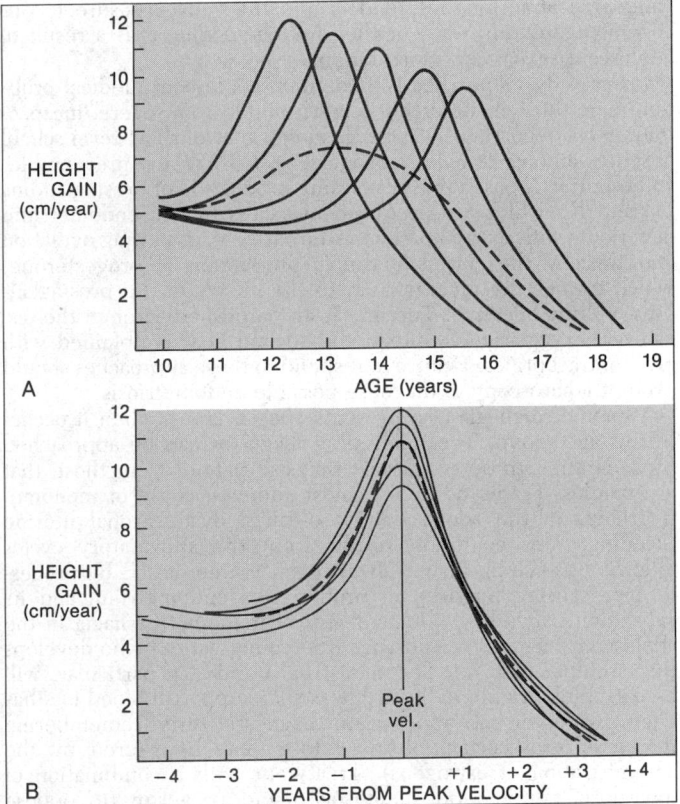

FIGURE 5–1. The relation between individual and mean velocities during the adolescent spurt. *A,* The individual height velocity curves of five boys of the Harpenden Growth Study (solid lines) with the mean curve (dashed) constructed by averaging their values at each age. *B,* The same curves all plotted according to their peak height velocity. (Adapted by permission of the publishers from *Fetus into Man* by J. M. Tanner, Cambridge, Mass.: Harvard University Press, copyright © 1978 by J. M. Tanner.)

stages of pubertal development, generally referred to as sex maturity ratings (SMR's).

STAGES OF PUBERTAL DEVELOPMENT (SMR's): BREAST

SMR 1: Childlike. No breast development.
SMR 2: Appearance of a breast bud.
Increase in diameter of the areola. Average age is 11.2 ± 1.6 years.
SMR 3: Enlargement of the breast. Average age is 12.15 ± 1.09 years.
SMR 4: The areola and papilla enlarge to form a mound above the underlying breast tissue. Average age is 13.11 ± 1.15 years.
SMR 5: Adult configuration with areola and underlying breast tissue in same plane. Average age is 14.5 ± 1.6 years.

STAGES OF PUBERTAL DEVELOPMENT (SMR's): PUBIC HAIR

SMR 1: Childlike. No pubic hair.
SMR 2: Hair is fine, long, silky, and lightly pigmented. Distributed in the midline, along the separation of the labia majora in females and the base of the phallus in males. Average age is 11.9 ± 1.5 years in females and 12.3 ± 0.8 years in males.
SMR 3: Hair is darker and coarser and begins to curl. It extends upward and laterally. Average age is 12.7 ± 0.5 years in females and 13.9 ± 1.04 years in males.
SMR 4: Adult texture and distributed to cover the mons pubis. Average age is 13.4 ± 1.2 in females and 14.36 ± 1.08 years in males.
SMR 5: Adult texture. Distributed beyond the mons to the medial aspect of the thighs. Average age is 14.6 ± 1.1 years in females and 15.3 ± 0.8 years in males.

STAGES OF PUBERTAL DEVELOPMENT (SMR's): MALE GENITALIA

SMR 1: Childlike. Testes average 2 ml in volume.
SMR 2: Scrotal skin begins to redden and thin. Scrotum narrows proximally, testes enlarge, and left testis lowers. Penis begins to lengthen. Mean age is 11.64 ± 1.07 years.
SMR 3: Testes continue to enlarge. Growth of corpora cavernosa penis contributes to widening, as well as lengthening, of penis. Mean age is 12.85 ± 1.04 years.
SMR 4: Further enlargement of testes and penis. Scrotum darkens. The glans becomes prominent. Average age is 13.7 ± 1.02 years.
SMR 5: Testes have reached adult size of approximately 25 ml and weight of 20 gm. Full reproductive capability by this stage. Average age is 15.1 ± 1.1 years.

"Primary" Sex Characteristics

The sine qua non of puberty is attainment of reproductive function. To this end, there is considerable growth of the reproductive organs. As indicated above, this process in the male commences with enlargement of the testes as a result of the growth in size of their seminiferous tubules and the number of Leydig and Sertoli cells. The epididymis, seminal vesicles, and prostate enlarge as well. The capacity for ejaculation is achieved approximately 1 year after testicular growth begins, coincident with appearance of pubic hair (SMR 2). For most, the first ejaculatory episode occurs in the context of masturbation, followed about 1 year later by nocturnal emissions. The median age for appearance of sperm in the first morning urine sample is 13.5 to 14.5 years. The timing of spermarche is asynchronous with other manifestations of puberty, occurring at any SMR from 1 to 5 and antedating the peak height velocity. Although complete reproductive capability is not reached until SMR 5, it is possible for impregnation to occur earlier. Accordingly, anticipatory guidance about pregnancy prevention should commence during early to middle adolescence for males.

Increasing levels of estrogen during pubertal development lead to endometrial thickening, enlargement of the corpus, and increase in cellular content of actomyosin, creatine phosphokinase (CPK), and adenosine triphosphate (ATP). Menarche occurs at a mean age of 13.3 ± 1.3 years, although its timing corresponds better with developmental than chronologic age. Ten per cent of girls have menarche at SMR 2, 20 per cent at SMR 3, 60 per cent at SMR 4, and the remaining 10 per cent at SMR 5. In addition, there is close concordance between menarche and the peak of the weight velocity curve, which follows by approximately 6 months the peak of the height velocity curve. The interrelationships of timing of pubertal events are shown in Figures 5–2

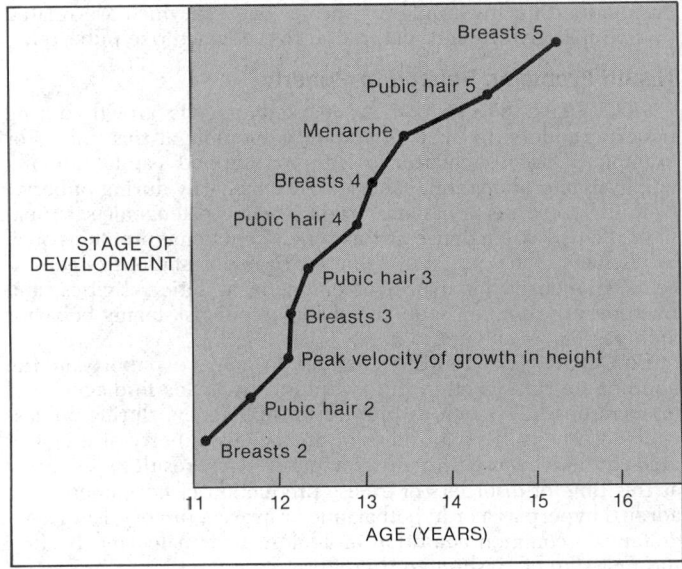

FIGURE 5–2. Sequence of breast and pubic hair development in adolescent girls.

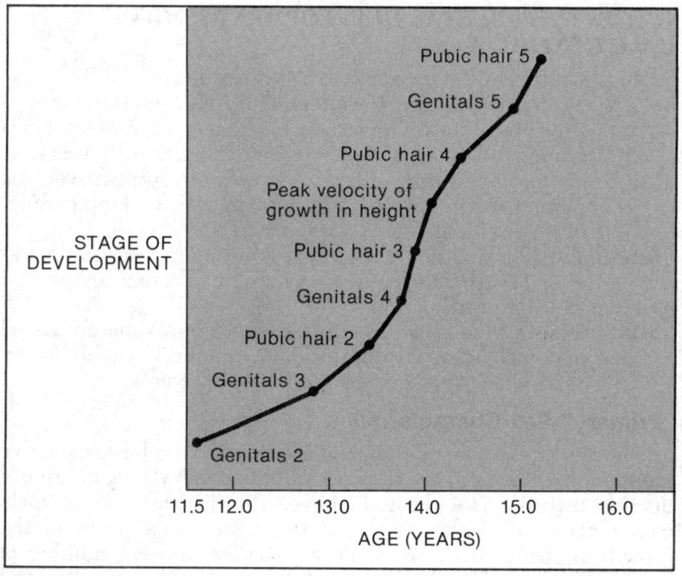

FIGURE 5–3. Sequence of genital and pubic hair development in adolescent boys.

and 5–3. These interrelationships are useful in the clinical assessment of the young adolescent who is concerned about her failure to begin to menstruate. Regardless of her chronologic age, she should be further evaluated if she is more than 1 year older than her mother or siblings at the time they experienced menarche, if she is at SMR 5, or if her bone age is 14.5 years or greater. In addition, failure to begin pubertal development by the age of 11 years should be cause for concern. Menarche occurs earlier in the obese than the lean adolescent female. Moreover, weight loss of as little as 10 per cent of body weight may result in cessation of menstruation, as can vigorous athletic training with or without weight loss. Full reproductive capability is typically reached within a year following menarche, but some adolescents ovulate regularly from the time of menarche, underscoring the need for timely education about pregnancy risk.

HEALTH PROBLEMS OF ADOLESCENTS

The image of adolescents as healthy and therefore not in need of health care has been fostered by a number of factors. Among them is the fact that this age group contributes only 11 per cent of office visits to physicians, the majority for gynecologic or obstetric care or acute injuries. However, data from the National Health Examination Survey of 1966 to 1970 reveal that 20 per cent of presumably healthy 12- to 17-year-olds have previously undiagnosed health problems, the majority of which are related to the rapid growth and maturation that characterize puberty.

Health Problems Related to Puberty

SKELETAL SYSTEM. The marked osseous growth during puberty renders the skeletal system vulnerable at this time. For example, Osgood-Schlatter disease or slipped capital femoral epiphysis and idiopathic scoliosis occur primarily during puberty. Certain neoplasms of osseous origin, such as osteogenic sarcoma, have their peak incidence at this time. Functional problems such as pitcher's elbow or "shin splints" are manifestations of adolescents' propensity for overinvolvement in athletic activities, and fractures are common sequelae of adolescent risk-taking behavior and resultant accidents.

ENDOCRINE SYSTEM. Failure to achieve puberty at the appropriate time is often the symptom that leads to diagnosis of endocrinopathies, such as pituitary insufficiency, during adolescence. Conversely, syndromes of precocious puberty or exaggerated adrenarche (e.g., hirsutism and acne) may result in discovery at this time of disorders of excess production of hormones (e.g., adrenal hyperplasia or hypothalamic or ovarian tumor). Euthyroid goiter is a common condition of adolescent females and is often the first sign of Hashimoto thyroiditis.

GYNECOLOGIC. Gynecologic problems are common during this age period. They may be the result of previously undiagnosed

congenital abnormalities, endocrinopathies, or exposure to oncogenic agents in utero, or they may be acquired as a result of adolescent sexual experimentation.

Primary dysmenorrhea is a common adolescent medical problem. One third of adolescent females suffer from severe, incapacitating dysmenorrhea. It is the leading cause of short-term school absence among female teenagers, yet is easily preventable. Intervention is based on suppressing production of prostaglandins $F_{2\alpha}$ and E_2, which are produced in excess by the endometrium of patients with dysmenorrhea. Alternatively, inhibiting ovulation and thereby the corpus luteum's production of progesterone, which primes the myometrium to the effects of the prostaglandins, will be effective. The first is accomplished through the use of cyclo-oxygenase inhibitors; the second goal is obtained with oral contraceptives. Failure to respond to these approaches should prompt laparoscopy to diagnose possible endometriosis.

Menometrorrhagia also presents special issues when it occurs in this age group. The differential diagnosis can be approached by separating those conditions that are painful from those that are painless (Table 5–2). The most common cause of menometrorrhagia in the adolescent is so-called dysfunctional uterine bleeding. This condition results from the anovulatory cycles following menarche in which estrogen is unopposed by progesterone, causing build-up of proliferative endometrium and its subsequent shedding. Management of menometrorrhagia in the adolescent includes reassurance (the young patient who develops this problem with her first menstrual period, in particular, will be extremely frightened), cardiovascular support if blood loss has been excessive, and appropriate diagnostic tests (remembering that results of certain of these tests may be altered by the administration of estrogens). Treatment with a combination of high-dose estrogen (for hemostasis) and progestin (to oppose endogenous estrogen effect), as may be found in Enovid (mestranol and norethynodrel), is effective except in cases of pregnancy, trauma, or infection.

Another menstrually associated condition of particular importance in adolescents is toxic shock syndrome (see Ch. 300). Forty-two per cent of cases reported during its peak years of 1980 to 1982 were in this age group.

A number of other gynecologic conditions of adolescents result from sexual experimentation. The reported prevalence of sexual intercourse among American girls between 13 and 19 years of age increases from 10 to 50 per cent and sexually transmitted diseases and pregnancy increase correspondingly.

Pregnancy during adolescence continues to be a major problem in the United States, which has the highest rate of any of the developed countries. Close to one-half million 15- to 19-year-olds become pregnant yearly. In addition, over the past two decades, there has been nearly a 200 per cent rise in the rate of out-of-wedlock births in this age group, as well as an increase in the number of unmarried adolescents who elect to keep their babies rather than place them for adoption. Among those under the age

TABLE 5–2. DIFFERENTIAL DIAGNOSIS OF MENOMETRORRHAGIA

Painless	Painful
Systematic	Trauma
Coagulopathy	Threatened abortion
Congenital	Salpingitis
von Willebrand disease	Intrauterine device
Acquired	
Aspirin sensitivity	
Aplastic anemia	
Anticoagulant treatment	
Neoplasm–bone marrow infiltration	
Idiopathic thrombocytopenia	
Endocrine	
Hypothyroidism	
Oral contraceptives–used improperly	
Local	
Gynecologic	
Dysfunctional uterine bleeding	
Neoplasm	

From Litt IF: Menstrual problems during adolescence. Reproduced by permission of Pediatrics in Review, Vol. 4, page 203, copyright 1983.

of 15 years, the pregnancy rate continues to rise, with 31,000 births last year. In addition to the psychosocial sequelae of adolescent births (such as adverse educational, vocational, economic, and marital outcomes), those who become pregnant under the age of 15 years are generally at increased risk for obstetric and perinatal complications such as toxemia, postpartum hemorrhage, postpartum infection, and small-for-gestational age and stillborn infants.

SEXUALLY TRANSMITTED DISEASE (STD). Adolescents have the highest rate of sexually transmitted disease of any age group. The most common of the STD's are gonorrhea, chlamydial and human papilloma virus (HPV) infections. Physicians should routinely test for the presence of other STD's when one is discovered, treat with the shortest effective methods, including parenteral antibiotics when feasible, and extend confidentiality to contacts.

Violence

Accidents, homicides, and suicides together are responsible for 70 per cent of adolescent deaths. Anticipatory guidance, prevention, and identification and referral of the youngster at risk are therefore important interventions by the physician.

ACCIDENTS. Although athletic injuries and accidental drowning contribute significantly to morbidity and mortality, the greatest toll among adolescents is taken by accidents involving motor vehicles. Sixteen- to 19-year-olds constitute 8 per cent of the United States population yet account for 17 per cent of vehicular fatalities. Passengers in cars driven by adolescents account for 63 per cent of automotive deaths. More male than female adolescents are involved as drivers in fatal accidents, and most of these occur between the hours of 8 P.M. and 4 A.M. Aside from failure to use seatbelts in cars and to wear helmets on motorcycles, alcohol abuse is the leading cause of most motor vehicular fatalities. Lowering the drinking age to 18 years has been associated with a 5 per cent increase in fatal automotive accidents. Talking with adolescent patients about their use of automotive safety devices and alcohol use prior to driving should be a routine part of health care. Moreover, physicians may act to improve the well-being of their teenaged patients by influencing legislative efforts such as those directed at requiring seatbelts in school buses and use of motorcycle helmets, raising the drinking age, and imposing late-night curfews for adolescent drivers.

SUICIDE. Suicide currently ranks as the third leading cause of death among the 15- to 19-year-old cohort in the United States. Completed suicides are more likely to occur in males, whereas female adolescents are more likely to make uncompleted attempts. Sex differences also exist regarding the method used in the attempt; males are more likely to use violent methods, such as shooting, hanging, or wrist slashing, whereas females are more prone to ingestion of drugs. Chronically ill adolescents are at high risk for suicide, and their own medication may be ingested in the suicide attempt. Alternatively, the medication is often that of the parent with whom the teenager is in conflict. Assessment of the seriousness of the adolescent's suicide attempt becomes crucial to planning following such an act. The physician may be surprised to learn that the youngster who ingested a bottle of antibiotics was actually expecting to die as a result or, conversely, that the one who took a bottle of acetaminophen resulting in admission to the intensive care unit had erroneously thought the substance harmless and was only trying to get some attention from his or her parents. The adolescent who fails in an initial suicide attempt is at increased risk for a subsequent serious one, if the crisis has not been adequately addressed in the interim. Simply attending to the pharmacologic or surgical sequelae of the attempt does little to resolve the underlying conflict. Short-term hospitalization is often effective in providing a secure setting for the teenager and impressing parents with the need to seek help for the contributing problems.

Identification of the adolescent at risk for suicide prior to an attempt presents an even greater challenge to the physician. Mood swings from deep despair to the heights of elation are not uncommon during adolescence, but persistence of the depressed mood should be regarded as a sign of potential trouble. According to Puig-Antich, depression should be considered persistent if it lasts for at least 3 consecutive hours for three or more periods

TABLE 5–3. THE WELL-ADOLESCENT VISIT: EARLY ADOLESCENCE (TANNER 2)

	Females	Males
Screening		
Physical	Hematocrit	—
	Urine culture screen	—
	Tuberculin test	Tuberculin test
Psychosocial	Self-image	Self-image
	Depression	Depression
	Peer interaction (including sexuality)	Peer interaction (including sexuality)
	School performance	School performance
	Substance abuse	Substance abuse
Health promotion	Self-examination of breasts	Self-examination of scrotum
	Nutrition counseling	Nutrition counseling
Prevention	Smoking	Smoking
	Cycle safety	Cycle safety
	Automotive passenger safety	Automotive passenger safety
	Immunization update	Immunization update
Anticipatory guidance	Developing independence	Developing independence
	Dealing with peer pressure	Dealing with peer pressure
	Confidentiality	Confidentiality
	Variations in growth and development	Variations in growth and development
	Dating	Dating
	Preparation for menarche	
Physical examination with special attention to:	Blood pressure	Blood pressure
	Height, weight	Height, weight
	Skinfold thickness	Skinfold thickness
	—	Grip strength
	Stage of sexual development	Stage of sexual development
	Scoliosis	—
	Goiter	—
	Acne	Acne
	—	Gynecomastia
	Tibial tubercle	Tibial tubercle
	Gait	
Symptomatic treatment (anything revealed by the above +)	Acne	Acne
	Dysmenorrhea	—

From Litt IF: Adolescent health care. *In* Green M, Haggarty RJ (eds.): Ambulatory Pediatrics IV. Philadelphia, W. B. Saunders Company, 1989.

TABLE 5–4. THE WELL-ADOLESCENT VISIT: MID-ADOLESCENCE (TANNER 3–4)

	Females	Males
Screening		
Physical	Vision testing	Vision testing
	Hearing testing	Hearing testing
If sexually active	Pap smear	—
	VDRL	VDRL
	Gonorrhea culture	Gonorrhea culture
Prevention	Automotive safety	Automotive safety
	STD prevention	STD prevention
	Pregnancy prevention	Pregnancy prevention
	Vocational/educational planning	Vocational/educational planning
	Obesity/inactivity	Obesity/inactivity
Physical examination	Breast masses	Gynecomastia
	—	Testicular tumor
	Vaginal discharge	Urethral discharge
	Pregnancy	—

From Litt IF: Adolescent health care. *In* Green M, Haggarty RJ (eds.): Ambulatory Pediatrics IV. Philadelphia, W. B. Saunders Company, 1989.

each week. Expressions of hopelessness and helplessness are also serious signs of depression. Disturbance of eating or sleeping may or may not be found in the depressed adolescent. A family history of depression is a useful predictor of seriousness. Some depressed adolescents may, alternatively, appear perpetually euphoric and may engage in socially self-destructive behavior such as drug use or sexual promiscuity. In evaluating the adolescent suspected of depression, it may be useful to inquire about plans for the future. When none are expressed or when the response is "what does it matter, I won't be here much longer," serious depression is obvious. When there is a suggestion of depression, the physician should not hesitate to inquire if the teenager has ever felt so sad that death was viewed as preferable. If the answer is affirmative, the existence of a suicide plan should be sought and such a patient should be immediately evaluated by a psychiatrist. Such questioning will not prompt suicidal thoughts in a youngster who has not already had them and will be greeted with relief by the one who has.

Substance Abuse

Experimentation with drugs serves a variety of purposes for adolescents in our society. It may symbolize attainment of adult maturity or rejection of parental values, facilitate peer acceptance, reduce stress, and, for some, provide an opportunity to explore the limits of new cognitive abilities through hallucinogenic effects. Intervention strategies for preventing or stopping drug use by adolescents must consider these various developmentally adaptive implications. Since more than 90 per cent of adolescents have experimented with either alcohol or marijuana by the time of high school graduation, the focus of the physician's involvement should be on the functional and physical implications of use rather than on the simple ascertainment of use or non-use.

Overall use of illicit drugs by high school seniors has decreased from a peak of 54 per cent in 1978 to 42 per cent in 1987 (Johnston et al.). Decline of daily marijuana use to 3.0 per cent is largely responsible for this finding. Declines have also been recorded for use of amphetamine, methaqualone, LSD (lysergic acid diethylamide), barbiturates, tranquilizers, heroin, inhalants, and phencyclidine. By contrast, however, cocaine use has doubled and smokeless tobacco is now used by approximately 20 per cent of male adolescents. Other sex differences include the increase in smoking by adolescent females and their 45 per cent lifetime incidence of use of diet pills. Alcohol is the most widely abused substance by this age group, with 93 per cent reporting use at some time and 5.5 per cent citing daily use. The time of greatest risk for initiation of cigarette smoking and alcohol and marijuana use is prior to the age of 20 years. Follow-up studies of adolescent "problem" drinkers demonstrated that one half of the males and one quarter of the females continued to have drinking problems as young adults.

Pubertal growth and development may be adversely affected by the use of drugs during this period of life. That the incidence of menstrual dysfunction resulting from drugs is higher in adolescent than adult women suggests greater vulnerability of the hypothalamic-pituitary-ovarian axis in the young. Heroin appears to block gonadotropin-releasing hormone. Amphetamines interfere with stage 4 sleep and may thus impair secretion of gonadotropins in early puberty. Induction of smooth endoplasmic reticulum of the liver by a variety of abused substances, such as opiates, barbiturates, and tobacco smoke, has the potential for accelerating metabolism of hormones important for pubertal development, such as estrogens.

Regular use of any drug will eventually diminish the youngster's ability to function appropriately in school, to hold a job, or to operate a motor vehicle. An "amotivational" syndrome has been described in chronic marijuana users who lose interest in age-appropriate behavior.

The "infectious disease" model of prevention has little relevance to the problem of adolescent drug or alcohol abuse, nor are "scare" techniques effective. A more realistic approach is one that anticipates that most adolescents will experiment with some drug at some point and is designed to delay that event as long as possible, to limit the extent of use, and to prevent its use in conjunction with operating a motor vehicle. Presentation of

TABLE 5–5. THE WELL-ADOLESCENT VISIT: LATE ADOLESCENCE (TANNER 5)

	Females	Males
Screening		
Physical	Genetically transmitted diseases	Genetically transmitted diseases
If sexually active	Pap smear	—
	VDRL	VDRL
If homosexual or bisexual	Gonorrhea culture	Gonorrhea culture, HIV
	—	
Prevention	Automotive safety	Automotive safety
	STD prevention	STD prevention
	Pregnancy prevention	Pregnancy prevention
	Obesity/inactivity	Obesity/inactivity
Anticipatory guidance	Planning for marriage	Planning for marriage
	Vocational/educational planning	Vocational/educational planning
	Cults	Cults
	Becoming a health care consumer	Becoming a health care consumer
	Leaving home	Leaving home
	Moving into work force/college	Moving into work force/college
	Entering military	Entering military
	Health insurance	Health insurance
Physical examination	Breast masses	Testicular tumor
	Vaginal discharge	Urethral discharge
	Pregnancy	—
Treatment	Corrective surgery (after growth complete)	Corrective surgery (after growth complete)

From Litt IF: Adolescent health care. *In* Green M, Haggarty RJ (eds.): Ambulatory Pediatrics IV. Philadelphia, W. B. Saunders Company, 1989.

factual information about medical complications of drug use by health professionals appears to have some positive impact. Strategies that enable young adolescents to resist peer pressure to smoke, by the use of trained peer counselors using role-playing techniques, have significantly reduced the onset of smoking in a number of studies.

The content of the medical evaluation of the adolescent is outlined in Tables 5–3 to 5–5.

General

Litt IF: Evaluation of the Adolescent Patient. Philadelphia, Hanley and Belfus, 1990. *A symptom-focused guide to assessment of the adolescent patient.*

Growth and Development

Grumbach MM: The neuroendocrinology of puberty. *In* Krieger DT, Hughes JC (eds.): Neuroendocrinology. Sunderland, Mass., Sinauer Associates, 1980. *The intricacies of neuroendocrine pathways and developmental interrelationship are presented in an easily understood manner.*

Kagan J, Coles R (eds.): Twelve to Sixteen: Early Adolescence. New York, W. W. Norton and Company, 1972. *A series of papers on various psychosocial aspects of adolescent development.*

Litt IF: Adolescent health care. *In* Green M, Haggerty RJ (eds.): Ambulatory Pediatrics. IV. Philadelphia, W. B. Saunders Company, 1989. *Useful information and suggestions for approaching and screening adolescents in an ambulatory setting.*

Litt IF: Menstrual problems during adolescence. Pediatr Rev 4:203, 1983. *A review of special issues in care of adolescents with menstrual disorders.*

Litt IF, Martin JA: Development of sexuality and its problems. *In* Levine MD, Carey WB, Crocker AC, et al. (eds.): Developmental-Behavioral Pediatrics. Philadelphia, W. B. Saunders Company, 1983. *Development of sexuality begins at birth and is influenced by a variety of social, psychological, and physical factors thereafter. This article reviews the process.*

Marshall WA, Tanner JM: Puberty. *In* Davis JA, Dobbing J (eds.): Scientific Foundations of Pediatrics. 2nd ed. Baltimore, University Park Press, 1974. *A concise review of the physiology and endocrinology of puberty with excellent charts and tables.*

Vaughan VC III, Litt IF: Child and Adolescent Development: Clinical Implications. Philadelphia, W. B. Saunders Company, 1990. *A comprehensive review and synthesis of biologic, psychosocial, and cognitive development.*

Zacharias L, Wurtman RJ: Age at menarche. N Engl J Med 280:868, 1969. *The multifactorial influences on menarcheal timing are chronicled.*

Depression (Suicide)

Beck AT, Beck R, Kovacs M: Classification of suicidal behaviors: Quantifying intent and medical lethality. Am J Psychiatry 132:285, 1975. *Useful in the assessment of seriousness of a suicidal attempt in patients of any age.*

Mattsson A: Adolescent depression and suicide. *In* Friedman SB, Hoekelman RA (eds.): Behavioral Pediatrics. New York, McGraw-Hill Book Company, 1980. *Useful categorization of manifestations of depression in the adolescent.*

Pugh-Antich J, Rabinovich H: Major child and adolescent psychiatric disorders. *In* Levine MD, Carey WB, Crocker AC, et al. (eds.): Developmental-Behavioral Pediatrics. Philadelphia, W. B. Saunders Company, 1983. *A summary of the psychobiology of adolescent behavioral disorders and their management.*

Adolescent Pregnancy

Alan Guttmacher Institute: Teenage Pregnancy: The Problem That Hasn't Gone Away. New York, Alan Guttmacher Institute, 1981. *Summary of statistics relating to adolescent sexual activity, pregnancy, abortion, and contraceptive use.*

Substance Abuse

Jessor R, Jessor SL: Adolescence to young adulthood: A twelve-year prospective study of problem behavior and psychosocial development. *In* Mednick S, Hornway M (eds.): Longitudinal Research in the United States. New York, Praeger, 1984. *A comprehensive prospective assessment of early psychosocial predictors of drug use during adolescence as well as its implications for adult behavior.*

Johnston LD, O'Malley PM, Bachman JG: Illicit Drug Use, Smoking and Drinking by America's High School Students, College Students and Young Adults, 1975–1987. U. S. Dept. of Health and Human Services, Public Health Service, Alcohol, Drug Abuse and Mental Health Administration, 1988. *A longitudinal study of trends in adolescent drug use.*

Kandel DB, Logan JA: Patterns of drug use from adolescence to young adulthood: 1) Periods of risk for initiation, continued use, and discontinuation. Am J Public Health 74:660, 1984.

6 Aging and Geriatric Medicine

John W. Rowe

THE DEMOGRAPHIC IMPERATIVE

The Longevity Revolution

Over the next several decades, the practice of medicine in North America will be increasingly influenced by the health care needs of our rapidly enlarging elderly population. The portion of our population over age 65 years has grown from 4 per cent in 1900 to its current level of approximately 12.7 per cent. As members of the post–World War II "baby boom" age, projections call for a steady rise in the number of elderly in the United States from 25.5 million in 1980 to 64 million in 2030, when one of every five Americans will be 65 years or older. These changes reflect decreased death rates not only in youth and middle age but also in old age: Life expectancy at age 65 has risen from 11.9 years in 1900 to 16.9 years in 1987.

A second demographic shift of major importance is hidden within the general increase in the number of older persons. The elderly population itself is aging rapidly (Fig. 6–1). The longevity revolution has even affected the very old, as the past three decades have brought a 26 per cent reduction in mortality rates in individuals over age 80 in the United States. This trend will continue and, in fact, accelerate, as the number of persons over age 85 is projected to triple by the year 2020.

Coupling Longevity with Health

These remarkable improvements in life expectancy have focused attention on improving health span and maintaining functional ability in old age. The general health status of older persons is substantially better than is often assumed. Objective health data show a pattern in which vigorous old age predominates. Dependency and institutionalization are the exception rather than the rule, since only 5 per cent of America's elderly reside in nursing homes at any one time. Most community-dwelling older Americans are cognitively intact and fully independent in their activities of daily living.

However, as individuals age they accumulate disabilities and

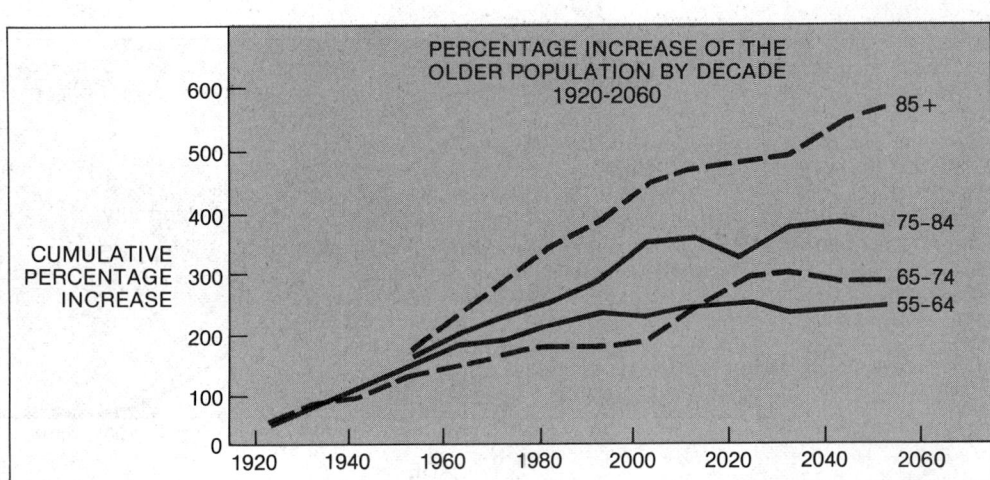

FIGURE 6–1. Past and projected increases in the elderly by decade. (Source: Bureau of the Census, Current Population Reports, Series P-25, No. 952, 1984.)

PERCENTAGE INCREASE OF THE OLDER POPULATION BY DECADE 1920-2060

CUMULATIVE PERCENTAGE INCREASE

85+
75-84
65-74
55-64

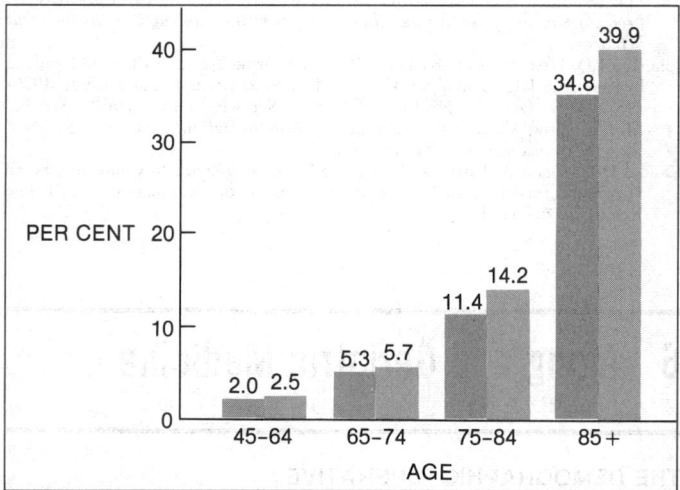

FIGURE 6–2. Percentages of community-dwelling adults, by age group, requiring assistance in basic activities (walking, bathing, dressing, using the toilet, transferring from bed to chair, eating, going outside) and in home-management activities (shopping, chores, meals, handling money) because of chronic disease. Colored bars denote basic activities and gray bars home-management activities.

diseases, and doctor visits increase. A substantial portion of community-dwelling elderly report major activity limitations due to chronic conditions. These functional impairments are clearly age related. The proportion of community-dwelling elderly that requires assistance with basic activities increases from approximately 5 per cent at ages 65 to 74 to nearly 12 per cent at ages 75 to 84 to approximately 35 per cent above the age of 85 (Fig. 6–2). Even if one maintains functional independence into old age, the risk of prolonged frailty is still high. For independent persons between the ages of 65 and 70 years, about 60 per cent of the remaining years will be characterized by independence; this proportion falls to 40 per cent at age 85.

Prolongation of Morbidity

The now familiar mortality curve for a modern aging population (Fig. 6–3C) has beneath it two additional clinically relevant curves, one describing the effect of age on the portion of the population in good health (i.e., morbidity curve, Fig. 6–3A) and another describing the transition of diseased aging individuals from the asymptomatic to the symptomatic or functionally impaired state (disability curve, Fig. 6–3B).

A major health policy issue relates to the relationship between future changes in morbidity and disability in an aging population. The question is whether we will see a prolongation of dependency (i.e., widening of gap between curves of Fig. 6–3B and C) or whether active life expectancy will increase (i.e., compression of morbidity), as health promotion and disease prevention strategies

become increasingly effective and curve 6–3B shifts rightward toward the mortality curve. The initial hope that as mortality declined, morbidity would also decline, has recently been challenged by studies suggesting that the increased lifespan of the oldest old is not accompanied by decreased morbidity and may actually result in more dramatic increases in the need for health care services, unless our understanding of disease in old age, and our capacity to treat it, improve substantially.

BIOLOGIC THEORIES OF AGING
Theories Relating to Alterations in Proteins
ERROR IN PROTEIN SYNTHESIS

This theory holds that age-associated impairments in cellular function result from an accumulation of errors in protein synthesis. It is reasoned that random errors in DNA, transcription, or translation accumulate with aging to a level that markedly impairs cell function. Substantial basic research in aging over the past two decades has shown that both transcription and translation maintain their fidelity with advancing age and that aging is characterized by a remarkable constancy of the composition of a variety of physiologically important proteins. Specific findings inconsistent with the error catastrophe theory include the facts that aged fibroblast cultures infected with viruses do not have a decreased virus yield, that newly synthesized enzymes from tissues in the aged are found to contain no synthetic errors, that experimentally induced errors fail to produce an error catastrophe, and that there is no increase in the infidelity of tRNA's with age and no age-related differences in the accuracy of poly(U)-directed protein synthesis. Thus, the error theory is considered by many to be disproven.

POST-TRANSLATIONAL MODIFICATIONS (CROSS-LINKAGE THEORY)

This theory is based on findings that although transcription and translation are intact with age, *altered* proteins accumulate with advancing age. Thus, post-translational modifications may be important in mediating age-related losses in cell and organ function. A number of physiologically critical enzymes have been shown to undergo post-translational modifications with age, although these changes are by no means universal. One important post-translational modification—glycosylation—appears to be important in age-related development of increasing opacification in crystalline lens protein and eventual development of cataracts. Another modification, increased cross-linking, is central to the major aging modifications in collagen and might have direct clinical consequences for arteriosclerosis and other diseases. Cross-links should not be considered important only in extracellular tissues, since an age-related increase in cross-links has also been shown to occur in DNA. There are a number of criticisms of this theory, including the lack of evidence for varied rates of post-translational change in the same class of molecules in different species despite the remarkable diversity in species specificity of lifespan. Although it is unlikely that post-translational modifications are central to all aging-related biologic decrements, there is general agreement that they may play an important role in the emergence of some clinical consequences of aging.

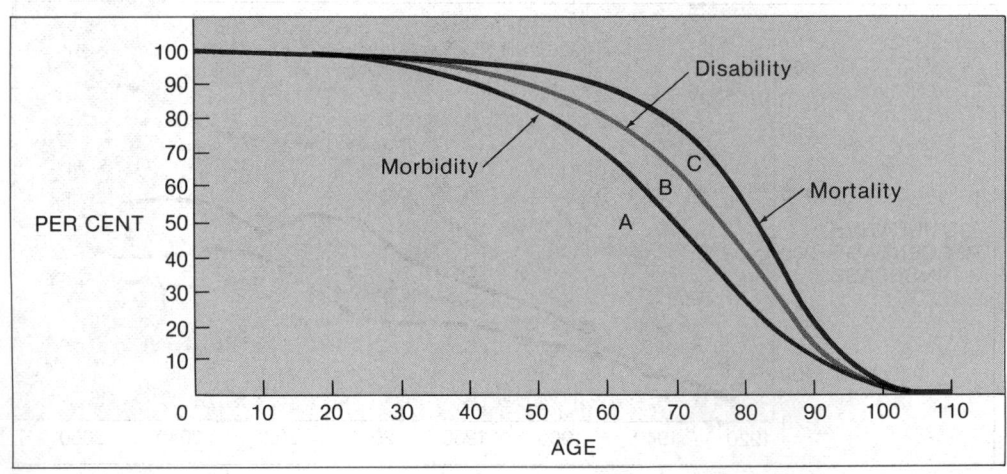

FIGURE 6–3. Mortality (observed), morbidity (hypothetical), and disability (hypothetical) survival curves for females in the United States in 1980.

ALTERED PROTEIN TURNOVER

Another aspect of protein chemistry that has attracted substantial gerontologic attention is alteration with age in the *rate* of protein biosynthesis. Although there appears to be no missynthesis of proteins with age, many proteins are *produced more slowly* in aged cells than in their younger counterparts. Delays have been identified in all of the four major stages of protein synthesis, including amino acylation of tRNA, initiation, elongation, and termination.

In addition, lysosomal pathways for *elimination* of proteins are substantially altered with age, with some proteins being degraded more quickly than in younger cells and others more slowly. Future experiments involving recombinant DNA techniques to correct modifications in these lysosomal pathways may permit evaluation of the impact of these changes on cell aging.

DNA DAMAGE AND REPAIR THEORY

The intact fidelity of protein synthesis with age does not exclude major age-related alterations in DNA, since a substantial portion of DNA is responsible for regulatory rather than synthetic activities. The DNA damage and repair theory focuses on the facts that, throughout life, DNA is constantly damaged and that age-related impairments in the repair mechanisms might be expected to be associated with progressive declines in cellular function. Although modifications in DNA repair capacity with age have been identified, these have generally not been well correlated with lifespan, suggesting either that DNA repair defects are not important in aging or that, to date, investigations have not focused on the critical repair mechanisms.

Free Radical Theory

Free radicals are highly reactive atoms or molecules bearing an unpaired electron, which can cause random damage to structural proteins, enzymes, informational macromolecules, and DNA. In mammals the most important source of free radicals is the reduction of oxygen, with subsequent development of hydrogen peroxide. The free radical theory holds that advancing age is associated with an accumulation of low-level free radical damage, which leads to the physiologic and clinical consequences associated with aging. Normal defense mechanisms against free radical damage include a number of endogenous antioxidants, including selenium-containing glutathione peroxidase, superoxide dismutase, DNA repair mechanisms, and alpha-tocopherol. Preliminary support for this theory rests in studies which indicate that animals whose oxygen consumption is high in proportion to their size have shorter lifespans and that administration of antioxidants results in modest increases in life expectancy. Within primates, the levels of the cellular antioxidant superoxide dismutase correlate well with lifespan. In addition, in lower forms of life, mutations leading to defects in production of free radical quenching enzymes are associated with shorter lifespan.

Organ System Theory (Pacemaker Theory)

This theory holds that certain organs or organ systems decline with advancing age and their loss of function drives the systemic aging process. The organs that have attracted the most attention as the "pacemakers" of aging are the immune system and the neuroendocrine system, particularly the hypothalamus.

With regard to immunosenescence, aging is associated with declines of over 75 per cent in T lymphocyte function as well as a progressive development of autoantibodies, with obvious potential clinical ramifications, such as increased morbidity from infections, increased risk of cancer, and perhaps autoimmune damage as well. Support for the importance of these changes in the aging process is found in studies of mice identical except for the major histocompatibility complex (MHC), which show a close relation between MHC and lifespan.

The neuroendocrine system is another central control complex in which marked age-related changes have been identified and which has been targeted as a possible aging pacemaker. Sympathetic nervous system responsiveness is increased with age, and it has been postulated that this increase might be responsible for a number of age-related changes, such as hypertension, impaired carbohydrate tolerance, and altered sleep architecture. Investigators have also sought to identify the presence of a "death hormone," a substance that is produced in increasing amounts with advancing age and that might regulate the aging process, or perhaps a "Methuselah hormone," which is present in decreasing amounts with advanced age. To date, no firm data are available to support the presence of such substances.

These theories focusing on individual organ systems as major regulators of systemic aging suffer from the weaknesses that not all organisms known to age have well-developed immune or neuroendocrine systems and that such theories would fail to explain the origin of the changes in the pacemaker system itself.

GENETIC ASPECTS OF AGING

Despite the apparent lack of evolutionary value to increases in lifespan beyond the reproductive years, gerontologists have long been attracted to the notion that just as growth and development are clearly regulated by a systematic turning on and off of various genes, so aging might represent a process in which systematic modifications in gene expression result in age-related physiologic and pathologic changes. Several of the theories of aging discussed above are linked by the likelihood that the basic mechanisms of aging—whether they be decreases in the production of antioxidants, impairments in DNA structure or repair, or age-related modifications of protein disposal systems or T lymphocyte function—may all have a genetic basis.

Substantial information exists to support the view that genetic factors are important to the aging process. There is a remarkable species specificity to lifespan. Within an individual species, the life expectancy of identical twins is more similar than that of nonidentical twins, which in turn is more similar than that of siblings. On a more basic level, recent studies in *Caenorhabditis elegans*, a nematode, have identified mutant varieties with lifespans that exceed normal lifespans by 50 per cent. In some of these strains, the lifespan extension appears to be due to a single gene change. These findings suggest that more intensive genetic approaches are promising avenues for future research in aging.

CLINICAL IMPACT OF THE AGING PROCESS

Distinction Between Successful and Usual Aging

A thorough understanding of age-related physiologic changes that occur in humans, in the absence of disease, is critical to diagnosis and management of disease in old age. These physiologic changes influence the presentation of disease, its response to treatment, and the complications that ensue. Cross-sectional and longitudinal studies in carefully screened, community-dwelling groups across the adult age range indicate that increasing age is accompanied by inevitable physiologic changes that are separate from the effects of disease. Growth and development, characterized by rapid increases in many physiologic functions, generally continue into early adulthood, peaking in the late twenties or early thirties. In those variables that change with age after adulthood, and not all do, a linear decline begins at the end of the growth and development phase and continues into old age. There is generally no pleasant plateau during the middle years, during which physiologic function is stable, but rather a progressive age-related reduction in the function of many organs.

The elderly population is characterized by substantial variability in the severity of age-related physiologic changes, as rates of organ aging vary substantially among healthy elderly individuals. Physiologically, it seems that as individuals become older, they become less like each other. For many organs the physiologic losses that accompany "normal" aging now appear to be significantly less than was previously assumed. Thus, the differences between older persons may be due, in part, to lifestyle differences that confound the effects of aging. For instance, although maximal oxygen consumption has repeatedly been shown to decline with age, studies also indicate that oxygen consumption increases in response to exercise training in older persons, with older master athletes achieving levels higher than those seen in normal young adults. As greater attention is paid to the potential beneficial effects of exercise, diet, smoking cessation, moderation in alcohol intake, and so forth, we may encounter increasing numbers of robust elders who demonstrate *successful aging*, i.e., not only lack of disease, but also physiologic performance only moderately below that of healthy young adults. However, the fact remains that most older adults exhibit another syndrome, that of usual aging, in which the effects of aging per se are mixed with adverse effects of confounding environmental, dietary, or lifestyle factors.

Distinction Between Aging and Disease

Since age has an important influence on numerous physiologic variables, and since detection of disease depends upon the determination that an individual is different from what would be expected by virtue of his age, it is important to establish age-adjusted criteria for clinically relevant variables to facilitate differentiation of the physiologic consequences of usual aging from those of concomitant diseases. Such criteria have been in wide clinical use for many years for several clinically important functions. For example, spirometric measures of pulmonary function are commonly expressed as "per cent of expected" for age and body size. Similarly, the validity of an exercise tolerance test as a suitable stress for detection of ischemic heart disease is judged on the basis of age-adjusted achievements of maximum heart rates. Standardized criteria are also available for age-related changes in glomerular filtration rate (GFR) and oral glucose tolerance, although variability of these functions is great among the elderly and individual determinations are required to guide diagnosis or therapy. If measurement of GFR is not available, application of age-related standards of renal function is facilitated by the fact that the age-related decline in creatinine clearance (approximately 10 ml per minute per decade) is balanced by a similar reduction in endogenous creatinine production. Thus, serum creatinine levels remain unchanged in spite of substantially lower GFR's in older patients. Familiarity with age changes in renal function and the hepatic oxidizing system is of particular importance in guiding drug therapy in the elderly (see below).

Interaction of Aging and Disease

There is a wide spectrum of interaction between aging processes and diseases, ranging from a lack of interaction at one extreme to age changes that have direct adverse clinical sequelae. Several specific clinically relevant points along this continuum can be identified.

PHYSIOLOGIC VARIABLES THAT DO NOT CHANGE WITH AGE

Perhaps the most important phenomenon seen in the aged, from a clinical standpoint, is no age-related change at all. Too frequently, clinicians attribute a disability or abnormal physical or laboratory finding to "old age," when the actual cause may be a specific disease process. Often there is no influence of age on the specific variable being evaluated. For example, old patients with low hematocrit values may be incorrectly characterized as having "anemia of old age" and be assured that no diagnostic evaluation or treatment is warranted. Data from several sources clearly indicate that in healthy, community-dwelling elders, there is no age-related change in hematocrit. Thus, a low hematocrit level in an elderly individual cannot be ascribed to normal aging and requires prompt investigation and treatment. Other common clinical measures not strongly influenced by age include fasting blood glucose level, serum electrolyte concentrations, blood pH and carbon dioxide content, and numerous hormone levels, including those of insulin, cortisol, thyroxine, and parathyroid hormone.

IMPAIRED HOMEOSTASIS IN THE ELDERLY

This category encompasses age-related reductions in the function of numerous organs that place the elderly person at special risk of increased morbidity from coincident pathologic changes in those organs. Although usual age-related declines in physiologic function are not so severe as to result in impairments in function under basal circumstances, these declines are of sufficient magnitude to reduce physiologic reserve and thus to move old individuals closer to the clinical threshold for the emergence of symptoms. Declines in basal immune, renal, and pulmonary function and the declines in glucose tolerance and cardiac function during physiologic stress all place the elderly at risk for earlier emergence or greater severity of clinical disease. This fact can be illustrated with several clinically relevant examples:

1. Aging is associated with significant progressive reductions in the dopamine content of the substantia nigra. These decreases may interact with pathophysiologic changes to account for the increasing prevalence of Parkinson's disease in late life and are also consistent with the well-recognized enhanced susceptibility of older individuals to extrapyramidal side effects of neuroleptic agents.

2. Age-related reductions in pulmonary function are so substantial that healthy individuals in the ninth decade of life frequently have only one half of the pulmonary function of their 30-year-old counterparts. Thus, acute bacterial pneumonias of equal initial severity are much more likely to induce a serious clinical manifestation in the elderly. In addition, the marked decline in immune function with age will also be expressed as an impaired capacity to respond to the infecting agent and a subsequent worsening of the clinical picture.

3. Since usual renal function in older persons may be as much as 40 per cent less than in healthy younger adults, the loss of one kidney due to ureteral obstruction, vascular occlusion, or trauma is more likely to result in a clinically significant reduction in overall renal function in an old patient than in a healthy younger individual.

4. The mortality associated with severe burns increases dra-

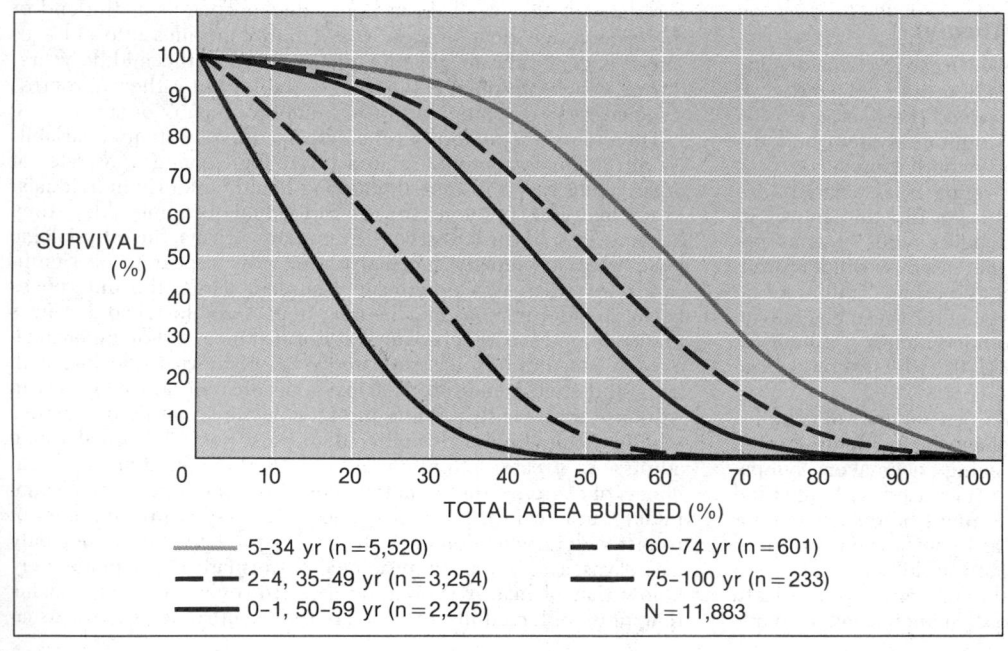

FIGURE 6–4. Survival of patients as a function of the total percentage of body surface burned and age.

matically with advancing age throughout adulthood (Fig. 6–4). This effect, which reflects the multiple parallel reductions in physiologic function during middle age and early senescence, is apparent well before diseases become highly prevalent and exemplifies the impaired homeostasis associated with the physiologic changes with age.

ALTERED PRESENTATION OF DISEASE IN THE ELDERLY

Age-related alterations in disease presentation have long been recognized as being of major importance to the practice of geriatric medicine. Many diseases occurring in both young and old adults have manifestly different clinical presentations and natural histories, depending upon the age of the individual. These disorders should not be regarded as being either more or less severe in the elderly, but just different. One example is hyperthyroidism. Young individuals often present with agitation, anxiety, an elevated heart rate and blood pressure, hyperactive deep tendon reflexes, complaints of weight loss and irritability, hyperkinesis, and a palpable goiter. In the older person with thyroid hormone levels equally elevated, irritability and hyperkinesis are infrequent and goiter is rare. In addition, deep tendon reflexes may be normal or even hypoactive, and the older patient may present a deactivated clinical picture ("apathetic thyrotoxicosis"). Physicians not familiar with presentation of thyroid hormone excess in the elderly may miss the diagnosis early on, thus permitting the adverse sequelae to persist.

Another disorder that is revealed differently in different age groups is uncontrolled diabetes mellitus. In children and young adults, uncontrolled diabetes is generally manifested as diabetic ketoacidosis. By contrast, the elderly with uncontrolled diabetes frequently present with hyperosmolar nonketotic coma, with blood glucose levels markedly higher than in ketoacidosis and a relative or absolute lack of circulating ketones. Thus, the elderly may present with obtundation or in coma secondary to markedly high blood osmolality, whereas younger individuals are more likely to present with severe metabolic acidosis, polyuria, or volume depletion or any combination. The physiologic mechanisms underlying these major effects of age on presentation of common diseases remain unexplained.

HEALTH PROMOTION AND DISEASE PREVENTION IN THE ELDERLY

Not many years ago, it would have seemed paradoxical to discuss health promotion and disease prevention for the elderly. Recently, however, this has become an important theme in geriatrics in view of both the remarkable increases in longevity and the awareness that the physiologic and pathophysiologic changes associated with advancing age may be much more reversible than was previously appreciated. This *plasticity* of the aging process is reflected in findings that moderate exercise (30 minutes three times weekly) retards age-related loss of bone mineral content in elderly women, including individuals in their ninth decade of life living in long-term care facilities. Similarly, even though elderly smokers have a much higher risk of cardiac mortality than nonsmokers, quitting smoking late in life is associated with a rapid and sustained reduction in mortality from coronary disease. Clearly, one should not assume that risk factors are necessarily cumulative in their impact or that little is to be gained by altering long-term habits or treating longstanding disorders in the elderly. This perspective not only is relevant for healthy older persons but can help limit disability and dependence in those suffering from one or more chronic conditions.

A note of caution is required concerning health promotion and disease prevention strategies in the elderly population. Attempts to improve the quality of old age require an understanding of the risk factors for common diseases in the elderly and the efficacy of strategies to decrease the risk of morbidity. Simplistic generalizations of findings in young and middle-aged groups to the elderly are fraught with difficulty. The elderly clearly represent a select group of survivors with physiologic alterations that may influence pathophysiologic processes.

Another aspect of prevention in the care of the elderly is recognition that physiologic or pathologic changes so common in advancing age as to be considered "normal aging" should not be considered to be without risk. Thus, although systolic blood pressure increases with advancing age, it is also clear that rises in systolic pressure are associated with marked increase in the risk of stroke and coronary heart disease. Elevations in blood sugar represent another potentially harmful aging change that is usually considered harmless.

Finally, it should be noted that remarkable beneficial effects can be gained by modest delays in the onset of age-related disorders. For instance, the increase with age in the incidence of hip fracture among the very old is so steep that if preventive strategies, such as calcium supplementation or exercise, delayed clinical expression of osteoporosis for 5 years, without increasing lifespan, the result would be a 50 per cent reduction in the number of hip fractures.

MEDICATION USE IN OLDER PERSONS

Numerous studies have documented that old people have more trouble with medications than do the adult population in general. The aged use an excessive proportion of the prescription and over-the-counter drugs consumed in the United States. Although the elderly represent less than 12 per cent of our population, they purchase 25 per cent of the drugs sold in America. This excess consumption of medications is accompanied, not surprisingly, by higher rates of side effects. Of equal importance is that when older people consume the same drugs with the same frequency as the young, toxicity is still more frequent and severe in the elderly. Often, standards for the use of current therapeutic agents were developed in young adults, and simplistic application of these guidelines to the elderly is often hazardous. Rates of adverse drug reaction rise steadily after age 50, and patients over 60 years old are twice as likely to suffer an adverse drug reaction as younger patients. Those over 80 years have a one in four risk of drug intoxication, twice the rate seen in patients under 50 years. Hospital stays are prolonged for all patients with adverse reactions, but older patients remain hospitalized the longest.

This increased toxicity of medication use in the elderly has three components: special vulnerability due to the physiologic effects of aging (drug-age interaction); modification of drug effects by multiple diseases often present in frail elders (drug-disease interaction); and the interactions of a given pharmacologic agent with the other medications, over the counter or prescribed, that the individual is taking (drug-drug interaction).

With regard to drug-age interactions, the changes with aging that occur in hepatic drug oxidation systems and in renal function have their major clinical impact on alterations in the pharmacokinetics of many medications. Several very commonly used medications such as digitalis and aminoglycoside antibiotics are excreted primarily via renal mechanisms and thus have prolonged half-lives in many elderly compared with younger adults, necessitating an adjustment in treatment schedules. These pharmacokinetic considerations are frequently compounded by parallel changes in pharmacodynamics, inasmuch as the tissues of elderly individuals, especially the central nervous system, become more sensitive to some agents with advancing age. Older persons are more sensitive than younger adults to the sedative effects of benzodiazepines and to the analgesic effects of narcotics. The combination of alterations in pharmacokinetics and pharmacodynamics is often further influenced by changes in body composition in the elderly. The average old individual has more fat and less lean body mass per kilogram of body weight than the younger adult. Thus, the volumes of distributions of many agents, such as diazepam, are altered in the elderly. Similarly, circulating levels of serum albumin fall moderately with age and influence free circulating levels of medications that are highly protein bound, such as phenytoin.

Drug-disease interactions are particularly common in the elderly. It is not uncommon to have five or six major diagnoses exist in as many organ systems of a frail elderly patient. The resulting frequent worsening of one illness by treatment of another leads to disproportionately longer hospital stays and increased frequency of complications. Drug-drug interactions are clearly more common in the elderly in view of the polypharmacy noted above.

Andres R, Bierman EL, Hazzard WR: Principles of Geriatric Medicine. New York, McGraw-Hill Book Company, 1985. *A detailed comprehensive textbook of geriatrics.*

Schneider EL, Rowe JW: Handbook of the Biology of Aging. 3rd ed. San Diego, Academic Press, 1990. *An encyclopedic reference text, very detailed and well referenced, covering all aspects of aging from plants and nematodes through detailed system-by-system discussions of human aging.*

Greenblatt DJ, Seller EM, Shader RI: Drug therapy: Drug disposition in old age. N Engl J Med 306:1081, 1982. *A useful review of the principles of geriatric pharmacology.*

Hayflick L: Theories of biological aging. *In* Andres R, Bierman EL, Hazzard WR (eds.): Principles of Geriatric Medicine. New York, McGraw-Hill Book Company, 1985, pp 9–22. *This chapter provides a detailed review of the major current biologic theories of aging, with a good historical review and balanced perspectives of the evidence for and against each theory.*

Katz S, Branch LG, Branson MH, et al.: Active life expectancy. N Engl J Med 309:1218, 1983. *This important paper coined the phrase "active life expectancy" and provides information on the functional capacity of the elderly.*

Rowe JW: Health care of the elderly. N Engl J Med 312:827, 1985. *A detailed, heavily referenced review of the physiologic changes with age and their clinical influence, with additional updates on several geriatric diseases, including dementia, incontinence, and osteoporosis.*

Rowe JW, Besdine RW: Geriatric Medicine. Boston, Little, Brown and Company, 1988. *A concise, practical textbook of geriatric medicine for students and practitioners. Emphasis on both normal aging and age-related diseases.*

Rowe JW, Kahn RL: Human aging: Usual versus successful. Science 237:143, 1987. *A review of the importance of distinguishing between the effects of intrinsic aging processes and extrinsic, often preventable factors that complicate "normal" aging.*

Salzman C: Clinical Geriatric Psychopharmacology. New York, McGraw-Hill, 1984. *A very concise, practical clinical guide to use of psychotropic medications in the elderly with numerous references and instructive clinical vignettes.*

Schneider EL, Brody JA: Aging, natural death, and the compression of morbidity—another view. N Engl J Med 309:854, 1983. *A detailed update of evidence for and against the compression of morbidity hypothesis.*

7 Management of Common Problems in the Elderly

T. Franklin Williams

A physician must approach the care of elderly persons with an informed, comprehensive, balanced perspective about aging itself and about the diseases and disabilities that commonly occur in older people. The previous chapter has described the physiologic changes that normally occur with aging. From the clinical perspective it is important to keep in mind that most older people are in reasonably good health and, despite some decline in maximum functional ability, can still function well at all ordinary activities. There are many persons in their eighties and nineties who can and do carry on all usual living activities, take long walks, are intellectually sharp with good memories, continue to be sexually active, and most of the time are symptom free. Thus when someone, no matter how old, comes to a physician with a complaint of discomfort or dysfunction, the complaint should not be dismissed as being simply "old age," but should be investigated and treated appropriately.

At the same time, a physician must understand that with increasing age people do accumulate chronic diseases and disabilities. Over the age of 65, 80 per cent have one or more chronic conditions; among the most common are some form of arthritis (present in 40 per cent in national surveys), hearing impairment (30 per cent), and chronic cardiac conditions (20 per cent). One in five persons over the age of 75 may be expected to have diabetes. In those 75 or older, four or more identifiable chronic problems are commonly present.

In addition to recognizing and treating the acute and chronic *diseases* that occur, the physician must give attention to the functional losses, the *disabilities* that are present, and attempt to reverse or minimize them no matter what can or cannot be done about underlying chronic diseases. The ultimate goal of care for elderly persons should be to restore or maintain as much function as possible—to help the patient to maintain as much independence of living, as much of a preferred lifestyle, as possible. Such a rehabilitative approach is an essential part of the therapy.

In those elderly patients who have some irreversible functional losses and thus need regular assistance, an additional part of the plan for care must be identification of who will provide the needed help and where. The extent and quality of family support and the potentials for community or institutional support services must be determined and worked into the overall, ongoing therapeutic program.

SPECIAL FEATURES OF THE WORKUP OF ELDERLY PATIENTS

HISTORY TAKING. Special attention should be given to the history of other (chronic) conditions in addition to the immediate chief complaint and to obtaining additional historical information from close relatives and previous records. An older person, like any patient consulting a physician, is most interested in having the immediate problem addressed and may tend to downplay past history and other chronic but less troubling conditions. It is the interaction of multiple diseases, the necessity to deal simultaneously with these multiple problems, that is one of the distinguishing characteristics of geriatric medicine. A closely related necessity is to obtain complete information on all drugs the patient is taking, both prescribed and over-the-counter medications. The number and variety are often astounding, and unfavorable drug interactions commonly contribute to the patient's discomfort and dysfunctions. A good technique is to have the patient (or responsible family member) bring in all the medications the patient is taking, for review, on each office visit.

Certain common functional problems should be explicitly inquired about: any history of falling; any episodes of urinary incontinence; any disturbances in sleep; and any difficulties with vision, hearing, or sexual function.

One must keep in mind the atypical presentations of common acute problems: pneumonia presenting as confusion, acute myocardial infarction as sudden weakness, or an acute abdomen as refusal to eat.

It is a good practice whenever possible to talk with one or more close family members to obtain their observations on the patient's functional status, mood, and daily routines, including intake of food and medicines. Such additional information is absolutely essential if there is evidence of dementia or depression in the patient—in such circumstances the patient may give quite a misleading story. If the patient is living alone (as a third or more of older women are), then it may be desirable or even necessary to have the benefit of observations from a home visit by the physician or by a visiting nurse or social worker.

The physician should obtain summaries or copies of all previous records, including results of all diagnostic tests. Such information should help both in managing current problems and in reducing the extent of further diagnostic tests that are needed. In particularly complex or unclear situations, there should be direct discussion with physicians who have previously seen the patient.

PHYSICAL EXAMINATION. As part of a regular complete physical examination of an older patient, certain features should receive special attention, depending in part on clues from the history. These include evaluation of mobility, mental status, mood, vision, hearing, and performance of usual activities of daily living. In recent years considerable attention has been given to developing simple, reliable, objective procedures and instruments for assessing these characteristics which may be used practically in physicians' practices. Applegate et al. (1990) provide a summary of such instruments; Lachs et al. (1990) describe a simple sequence for detecting potential problems which should then lead to more thorough investigations.

In light of the frequency of poor eating practices by older persons, particularly those living alone, special attention should be given to any indications of poor nutrition—weight loss, anemia, vitamin deficiency. A careful oral examination is important.

ADDITIONAL DIAGNOSTIC TESTS. The same general principles for choosing diagnostic tests for younger patients should apply in the workup of older patients. The aim is to obtain any information that will help in clarifying the cause of disease or the functional loss, *if* this information will likely lead to effective therapy. Decisions should be weighed in consultation with the patient and close family before diagnostic procedures are embarked on. If the treatment plans will not be changed by the outcome of the procedure, then it should not be done. However, because of the tendency, referred to earlier, to dismiss treatable problems of elderly patients as simply the concomitants of old age, it is important to identify any potentially reversible condition and to use relevant diagnostic aids.

ASSESSMENT OF FAMILY AND COMMUNITY SUPPORTS. A final essential element in the workup of a frail, elderly person, i.e., a patient who may face the necessity of ongoing help with daily activities, is the collection of information about the home environment, the family relationships, the degree of supporting services potentially available, the degree of "burn-out" or exhaustion that may have already occurred, and the availability of home care services and institutional services in the community. A visiting nurse or social worker can be very helpful in obtaining some of these services and in helping to integrate them into an overall plan.

DIAGNOSIS AND MANAGEMENT OF MAJOR COMMON PROBLEMS OF ELDERLY PATIENTS

EPISODES OF ACUTE ILLNESS. Older people with diminished reserves and chronic diseases are more prone to injuries, acute infections (especially respiratory), and other acute illnesses than are younger people, and are also more likely to decompensate at such times. It is a common observation that an old person, previously mentally competent at home, may become quite confused on admission to the strange environment of a hospital under the stresses of an acute illness. Careful attention must be given to every aspect of the patient's status, looking for the appearance of heart failure, overt diabetes, delirium, or increased risk of falling. Drug regimens should be kept simple and the possibility of deleterious effects of overdosage or drug interactions should be continuously reviewed.

Recovery from an acute illness will also take longer than in a younger person, and there is real risk that the previous functional level may not be regained. As early as possible in an episode of acute illness the older patient should be helped to be up and about, to keep joints supple and muscular strength as intact as possible, to retain or regain urinary continence through use of regular toilet facilities, to dress and feed oneself, and to engage in social exchanges in usual ways, i.e., out of bed and dressed, and to return home as quickly as possible. Convalescent and rehabilitative efforts should be continued as long as any progress is being made.

DEMENTIA. The loss of mental competence is one of the most common and most distressing of functional disabilities in older persons, affecting up to 40 to 45 per cent of those over age 80. We now know that dementia is *not* a feature of normal aging but instead is due to one or another of several disease processes. The most common form of dementia in old people is that of the Alzheimer's type, accounting for 50 per cent or more of cases. This is a (usually) progressive dementia associated with considerable cerebral atrophy and characteristic pathologic changes in selected regions of the brain, with neurofibrillary tangles within the neurons and amyloid plaques at end-plates. These damaged neurons are producing far less of the neurotransmitter acetylcholine (and possibly other neurotransmitters also) than normal. Research at an accelerating pace is providing promising clues to causes (both genetic and environmental) and to potentially effective interventions including nerve growth factors and drugs aimed at increasing the supply or persistence of acetylcholine. Thus far, results are inconclusive.

Other causes of dementia in older people include damage from multiple small infarcts or one or more larger infarcts secondary to cerebrovascular disease, metabolic or endocrine disorders such as hypothyroidism and vitamin B_{12} deficiency, brain tumors, brain injury (such as late dementia in professional boxers, which has the same pathologic changes as Alzheimer's disease), Korsakoff's dementia of chronic alcoholism, and the condition known as normal-pressure hydrocephalus. Most importantly, severe depression can present as dementia, reversible with successful treatment of the depression. Indeed, a number of the possible causes are potentially reversible or treatable. Thus it is essential, when confronted by an older person with any signs of dementia, to conduct a thorough differential diagnostic evaluation. This should include comprehensive mental testing to define the extent of the dementia, specific tests for all of the treatable causes, and in most instances, a scan—computed tomographic (CT) or magnetic resonance imaging (MRI)—which can usually identify or exclude infarcts and tumors and can help diagnose normal-

pressure hydrocephalus. Evidence of cerebral atrophy alone would be consistent with, but not diagnostic of, dementia of Alzheimer's type, inasmuch as a significant degree of atrophy occurs in the normal aging process without loss of mental function. However, unequivocal progression in such atrophy, as seen in a repeated scan within 6 to 24 months, does not occur in normal older persons and is strong diagnostic confirmation of Alzheimer's disease.

The physician should be sensitive to the alarm older patients and family members may have at the least sign of any aberration in mentation and should be able to reassure them that "benign forgetfulness" is a common trait at all ages. Benign forgetfulness characteristically is the inability to recall a name or some specific element of a prior experience, when one thinks one should be able to do so. The person can recall many related features of the person or episode and knows precisely what element or name is not being recalled. Usually recall of that element will occur later, unexpectedly. In contrast, a person with progressive dementia will have no recollection of the entire episode, as if it never happened, or can make only feeble, ineffective efforts to reconstruct the identity of the forgotten subject.

If the final diagnosis is dementia of the Alzheimer's type or one of the other irreversible dementias, the physician, nurses, and social workers must treat the family as well as the patient and help them to make the best of a distressing situation. The long-established daily activities of the patient in familiar surroundings should be maintained as much as possible, with avoidance of surprises or new and different decisions to be made. Family members should be helped to accept the services of home support personnel to assist in the care of the patient—housekeeper, personal care aide, home health aide, or nurse—as needed to help prevent "burn-out" on their part; to accept respite care for the patient (day programs or temporary full-time care given in the home or a temporary nursing home admission) so that the family members may get away for a vacation or a special occasion; and to accept permanent nursing home care for the patient if this becomes best for everyone. They should be informed of support groups like the Alzheimer's Association, chapters of which now exist in most larger communities, and should be put in touch with social agencies and legal resources if necessary to help in making various legal and financial arrangements. The physician's involvement in all of these aspects may seem to some to be peripheral to the practice of medicine but in fact is central to the physician's primary goals of maintaining the health and functioning of the patient and the patient's family to the maximum extent possible. In working with problems like these the physician needs the close participation of well-informed nurses and social workers who can take the lead in management of many aspects.

The physician should keep in mind (and the family should be reminded) that any sudden worsening of dementia is not consistent with Alzheimer's disease and is likely a sign of some complicating acute illness.

DEPRESSION. Depressive reactions of varying degrees of severity are more common in elderly persons than has been recognized and warrant more attention in diagnosis and treatment. As a person lives into later years, losses are inevitable—death of family members and friends, usually "loss" of job through retirement, usually less income, often loss of some degree of health, less vigor, possibly loss of familiar home environment through moving. Some degree of grief and reactive depression is to be expected in response to such losses, but emotionally healthy older persons work through such grief and return to their usual level of mood, outlook, and activity. Persistence of depressive symptoms may represent activation of a longer-standing depressed state or appearance of a new disorder.

If depression is suspected, it should be thoroughly evaluated with psychiatric consultation and perhaps treated by therapeutic trials of antidepressant drugs. In severe instances not responsive to drugs, electroshock therapy has been found to be successful in many elderly patients.

FALLS. Falling is common as people become older, occurring as often as once a year or more in half of those over age 75. In addition to the accompanying risk of injury—with up to 5 per cent of falls there may be fracture of the hip or arm—one or more falls may lead to such a fear of further falling that an older person severely limits mobility and activities. Falls are often also a harbinger of other diseases or disabilities.

A number of risk factors contribute to the likelihood of falling, and it is typically the multiplicity of such risk factors in the same person that makes falling highly likely, rather than any one of them. These include diminished distant vision, deafness, disturbances in balance, abnormal gait, weakness in the lower extremities, decreased mental status, orthostatic hypotension, depression, and effects of drugs on alertness. All such factors should be searched for and as many as possible corrected as a part of regular preventive care and especially at the time of any fall.

Environmental hazards also contribute to the risk. A home visit by at least one of the professionals should include observation and recommendations for correcting such environmental hazards as poor lighting, rugs that can slide, objects blocking usual walkways, lack of nonslipping strips and handgrips in bath tubs, and lack of handrails on stairs.

A person who has fallen should be thoroughly examined for subtle signs of injury or fracture and for any underlying or associated disease condition, including a new febrile illness, painless myocardial infarction, and stroke.

URINARY INCONTINENCE. Lack of control of urination is far more common than generally recognized; some studies suggest that up to 30 per cent of older women have this problem. It has been referred to as the "closet disease" of old age because of the high frequency of denial of its presence—out of embarrassment or the mistaken view that nothing can be done about it. Older persons living alone may become oblivious to its presence, unaware of the odors that are obvious to visitors. Frequent urinary incontinence, particularly night-time incontinence, by a person living with family is a major cause of caregiver exhaustion and the precipitating reason for their seeking institutional care.

For all of these reasons it is important for the physician, in evaluating any older patient, to determine (from patient, family, or visiting nurse) whether the patient has any problem with urinary incontinence and, if so, to conduct a thorough diagnostic workup and, based on the findings, to undertake appropriate treatment. In most instances the problem can be eliminated or controlled.

A good first step in evaluating reported or suspected urinary incontinence is to arrange to have an "incontinence diary" kept by the patient or caregiver—a daily record for several days of just when episodes of incontinence occur, roughly how much urine is spilled, the circumstances—while up and about or in bed or while on the way to the bathroom but "didn't quite make it"—and whether the patient is aware of the episode. In some instances simply keeping such a diary leads a previously careless person to achieve satisfactory control. The diary provides information on the magnitude of the problem and clues to possible causes.

Further workup of the incontinence should proceed from simple to more complex tests, as needed. Urinalysis and culture may indicate a urinary tract infection that, if eliminated, will result in restoration of continence. Observing whether there is any urinary spillage with coughing or straining in the upright position (after adequate hydration) may point to stress incontinence. Catheterization after the patient has attempted to void completely can provide evidence for an obstructed or atonic bladder and overflow incontinence.

The most common cause of urinary incontinence in older people is instability of the detrusor system of the bladder—the loss of normal neurologic inhibiting influences as the bladder fills. The detrusor muscle, if uninhibited, will begin to contract spontaneously when filling has reached relatively small volumes, 150 ml or less, and the patient will find it difficult or impossible to suppress the tendency to void. Unequivocal diagnosis of this condition requires cystometric studies and such should be done when needed; some physicians who are thoroughly familiar with the differential diagnosis of incontinence may choose to use first a trial of therapy for the presumptive diagnosis of instability, once other causes such as those referred to above have been eliminated.

In persons with stress incontinence or detrusor instability, the use of biofeedback and other training exercises has been found to help a number of patients to control this problem. Assuring quick access to a toilet, such as use of a bedside toilet at night, can help a person with detrusor instability reach the toilet in time. If stress incontinence in women is associated with major anatomic changes, e.g., severe uterine prolapse, or when prostatic obstruction in men is the apparent cause, surgical intervention may be indicated.

Drugs with anticholinergic effects are successful in decreasing detrusor instability in some patients; their use is often limited by undesirable anticholinergic effects in other organ systems, such as dry mouth and disturbances in gastrointestinal function. At least theoretically, anticholinergic drugs could worsen dementia of the Alzheimer's type (see above). Efforts have been made to identify drugs of this type whose effects are mainly on the bladder. Oxybutynin has smooth muscle-relaxing as well as anticholinergic effects, and imipramine has at least theoretically useful sympathomimetic and anticholinergic actions.

When overflow incontinence is secondary to a distended, atonic bladder (as with diabetic neuropathy), cholinergic drugs may be helpful.

Even if none of the above approaches is effective, acceptable management of the incontinence may be achieved through use of special waterproof pants with absorbent liners, the use of special absorbent pads on the bed, specially fitted collecting devices in women, and in selected patients the use of intermittent straight catheterization. The use of chronic indwelling catheters is rarely indicated.

PRESSURE ULCERS AND CONTRACTURES. These are unfortunate and for the most part preventable common complications of chronic illness in frail older people. Even a few hours of total immobility, as after a stroke or in the recovery period following surgery, will likely result in pressure damage to the skin and subcutaneous tissues; as little as a day or two of immobility in a joint may lead to contracture formation. Once these problems develop, correcting them is a long, tedious, and expensive process.

Preventive measures for any patient at risk of developing pressure (decubitus) ulcers or contractures should include regular, frequent passive or active movement of joints and turning, assiduous skin care, careful attention to avoiding potential damage from wrinkled bed clothes, and care in lifting, not pulling, a patient while changing his or her position.

Ulcers should be kept clean, with scrubbing and soaking three to four times a day; mild antiseptic cleansing solutions such as half-strength providone are better than stronger agents, which may cause further tissue damage. A good practice is to leave wet-to-dry gauze dressings on the wound. Surgical debridement of any necrotic tissue should be done.

As important as local care of the wound is attention to adequate general nutrition and to the treatment of any systemic disease that may cause a general catabolic response. With good wound care in a patient who is adequately nourished and otherwise well or recovering, ulcers will heal rapidly; the presence of chronic infection elsewhere, or poor nutrition, can thwart the effectiveness of even the best wound care. With large ulcers, once the wound surface is thoroughly healthy, skin grafting may be indicated.

Minor degrees of contractures can often be corrected with regular, frequent, careful stretching exercises, following a regimen established for the patient by a physical therapist. More severe and unresponsive contractures may require surgical correction. Such a step can be valuable and justified if it helps to restore mobility and independence or significantly eases nursing care burdens.

DECISIONS ABOUT LONG-TERM CARE. Elderly persons who acquire chronic, irreversible functional losses must have appropriate ongoing supportive services. The goal should be to substitute help only to the extent necessary, thus preserving the maximum possible degree of independence for the patient.

Often the need for decisions arises at a time of crisis. Already borderline functional capabilities of the older person may have further deteriorated owing to a new condition, e.g., injury, stroke, and so on, or the caregiving spouse or child may become ill or unable to continue the previous extent of care. The physician, in collaboration with other professionals (e.g., visiting nurse, social worker) and the patient and family, must weigh the relative merits and feasibility of maintaining the patient at home with support services or arranging care in a nursing home or intermediate care facility. Most older people strongly prefer to continue living in their familiar home settings, and most families desire to help the patient to stay there. Through thoughtful use of various supportive services—Meals on Wheels, housekeeper, personal care or home health aides, day programs—it is possible to maintain many such patients at home whose care needs would have equally well justified nursing home admission.

These features are discussed here because with the continually growing numbers of very elderly persons in our society there will be major increases in the pressures on our long-term care systems, and physicians will continue to be involved at the critical points of decision making where careful efforts to help stabilize and maintain many patients at home will be most important. Comprehensive geriatric evaluation services are becoming available, as ambulatory or inpatient units, in many settings. They have been shown to be valuable for consultative help at these critical points in the lives of many older people and their families.

CARE OF TERMINALLY ILL ELDERLY PERSONS. "Aging" and "dying" are so often thought of as almost synonymous that the problems of how to approach terminal care and how far to go in heroic or extraordinarily expensive diagnosis and treatment are considered by many to be issues that primarily appear in the care of the aged. The actual picture is somewhat different. Almost all of the circumstances in which inevitable death can be predicted in a fairly short time occur in patients with advanced cancer, at any age. For elderly patients with terminal cancer the same principles of care apply as for younger patients: When patient, family, and the responsible physician have agreed that no further efforts at curative therapy are warranted, the primary goal should be comfort care, avoiding heroics.

Similar decisions can be made in instances in which an older person has had such irreversible loss of mental function that he or she has little, if any, remaining apparent contact with surroundings and communication with others, especially family or nursing personnel. If those who are closest to the patient agree on the hopelessness of further curative or extraordinary treatment, including their view that this is also what the patient would say for himself or herself (or perhaps did say earlier, verbally or in writing, such as in a "living will"), then comfort care should be the practice.

The precise details of comfort care will vary with the condition of each individual patient. Overall, the physician should be concerned to see that pain is relieved, that the patient's own preferences for daily routines and activities are respected, including preferred foods, cleanliness, comfortable positioning, visits by family or friends, and outings, and that no diagnostic or treatment efforts are undertaken that may be unpleasant or painful or that will not contribute to comfort. These guidelines do not eliminate all ambiguity. For example, what should the physician decide when confronted with a new infection such as pneumonia in a patient in whom comfort care is the primary goal? If no treatment is given, the patient will likely have several days of very uncomfortable respiratory distress and may or may not survive. Comfort care in this instance would probably include respiratory therapy to help clear the airway and use of an oral antibiotic, avoiding painful injections or intravenous therapy.

Applegate WB, Blass JP, Williams TF: Instruments for the functional assessment of older patients. N Engl J Med 322:1207, 1990. *A good summary of clinically useful instruments for assessing physical, cognitive, and emotional functions.*

Blazer DG: Depression in Late Life. St. Louis, C. V. Mosby, 1982. *A thorough and practically useful presentation of this topic, including information on incidence and prevalence, diagnosis and differential diagnosis, and effective modes of therapy.*

Katzman R: Alzheimer's disease (medical progress). N Engl J Med 314:964, 1986. *An excellent summary of current knowledge of pathophysiology, possible causes, diagnosis, and management of this condition, including references to useful screening tests for dementia.*

Lachs MS, Feinstein AR, Cooney LM Jr, et al.: A simple procedure for general screening for functional disability in elderly patients. Ann Intern Med 112:699, 1990. *A useful guide to detecting evidence for such disabilities as a routine part of the workup.*

NIH Consensus Conference: Urinary incontinence in adults. JAMA 261:2685, 1989. *A careful summary of evidence and recommendations on recognition, evaluation, and treatment of this condition. The background papers (and summary) are published in J Am Geriatr Soc 38:263–386, 1989.*

Radebaugh TS, Hadley E, Suzman R (eds.): Symposium on falls in the elderly: Biological and behavioral aspects. Clin Geriatr Med 1 (3), August, 1985. *This NIH symposium covers the many interrelated risk factors contributing to this major cause of disability among older people.*

Rubenstein LZ, Campbell LJ, Kane RL (eds.): Geriatric assessment. Clin Geriatr Med 3 (1), February, 1987. *With increasing recognition of the value of comprehensive geriatric assessment, this volume provides information on when, where, how, and by whom such assessment may best be done.*

8   Care of Dying Patients and Their Families

Balfour M. Mount

Death calls into question our competence, our unconscious premises regarding the omniscience of modern medical science, and the nature of our role as caregivers. It raises questions concerning meaning, life, death, and immortality. It may undermine communication with our patients and their family members, resulting in increased isolation and despair. It presents us with a therapeutic paradox, since it is both the time when it is said that "nothing more can be done" and a time to relieve suffering and promote reconciliation and growth. The physician has an unparalleled opportunity to act as a catalyst to enable comfort, communication, integration, and healing.

DEFINITION AND GOALS OF PALLIATIVE CARE

Palliative care aims at improving the quality of life when treatment aimed at cure and prolongation of life is no longer appropriate. It offers services designed to address the physical, psychological, social, and spiritual needs of dying patients and their families. Its goals are to relieve suffering, to attain patient comfort without iatrogenic somnolence or change in affect, to assist patient and family in making the most of decreasing resources, and to support those involved in a search for meaning.

SYMPTOM CONTROL

Elimination of pain and the control of other symptoms are the foundation on which competent care of the dying rests. Chapter 26 provides a detailed review of pain and its management.

Table 8–1 offers guidelines for symptom control. Because symptoms may change rapidly, frequent re-evaluation is an essential component of effective care of the dying. Norms of care are redefined in this setting. Only investigations which may lead to a treatment that will improve quality of life are considered. Blood pressure, pulse, and temperature are not routinely monitored, whereas the frequency of bowel movements is!

Skill must be developed in the management of symptoms commonly encountered in terminal care, including insomnia, confusion, anorexia, dry or sore mouth, altered taste, nausea and vomiting, constipation, diarrhea, bowel obstruction, dyspnea, cough, pruritus, decubitus ulcers, and urinary frequency and incontinence.

Attention to detail is required for both assessment and care planning. For one very weak patient, use of a bedside commode or a bedpan and simple acceptance of occasional incontinence of urine and stool enabled conservation of scant energy reserves for eagerly anticipated daily visits with his family. Bowel care for the equally weak, fiercely independent man in the next bed involved planned nonintervention while he laboriously struggled unaided to the toilet some 15 feet from his bed. A gentle offer of assistance was given ("When you wish, just let us know"), and a discussion of his need for autonomy was held with family members. Thus, radically different approaches to the details of bowel care were used for two dying men with divergent needs.

Competent care of the dying involves compulsive care of skin, mouth, and eyes; adaptation of activities of daily living, furniture, and utensils to accommodate progressive weakness (a favorite chair raised on blocks, a padded and raised toilet seat, a spoon with a padded handle to accommodate a weak grip); clean smooth sheets; quiet music, flowers, and a few cherished belongings; the reassuring glow of soft lighting at night; and the reliable availability of both skilled nursing and an interested physician.

TABLE 8–1. GUIDELINES FOR SYMPTOM CONTROL

1. "Nothing matters more than the bowels" (Saunders). Daily assessment needed.
2. Control of one symptom improves control of all symptoms.
3. Most symptoms are caused by multiple factors. Psychological distress may augment all symptoms.
4. "Assessment must precede treatment" (Twycross).
5. Rule out correctable factors underlying each symptom.
6. Clarify who is bothered by symptom: patient, family, or staff.
7. Give simple explanation for each symptom to patient and family. Diagrams helpful.
8. Consider anticipated prognosis, functional status, and the patient's goals in determining appropriate treatment.
9. Discuss treatment options with patient and family and involve them in treatment planning where practical.
10. Determine what was helpful in the past.
11. Use a total-care approach employing nondrug, environmental, and other supportive measures.
12. If needed, utilize combinations of pharmacologic agents when differing mechanisms of action and toxicity permit.
13. Prescribe drugs prophylactically in individually optimized, regular doses for persistent symptoms.
14. Never say "Nothing more can be done." Consult or refer if comfort is not achieved.

Fears and misunderstandings about existing or anticipated symptoms and the effects of medication are common. They are minimized if patient and family are involved in both planning and providing care. Clear explanations of symptoms and treatment options give reassurance that "the doctor understands what's going on" and "there is a plan."

COMMUNICATION ISSUES

Giving bad news is always difficult. The physician should bring to discussions of prognosis not a set of fixed rules concerning whether "to tell" or "not to tell," but an openness to examining with the patient the reality at hand. Communication that is insensitive in the interest of "telling all" or evasive, falsely optimistic, or otherwise misleading in the interest of "protecting" the patient generally risks seriously undermining long-range physician credibility. Studies suggest that the majority of patients with a serious illness sense the possibility of death, whether or not they have been told. Fears are usually diminished if they can be named.

For the patient, integration of "bad news" is usually a process, not an event. Grave tidings are often repressed and simply "not heard" at the first airing. The physician should follow the pace of disclosure set by the patient, being sensitive to all forms of communication: plain language ("I fear I may be dying"), symbolic language ("I keep dreaming of a long tunnel with a candle at the end and I am afraid someone is going to blow the candle out"), and nonverbal communication (depressed facial expression, excessive muscle tension). It has been estimated that 80 per cent of communication is nonverbal. The absence of questions does not mean that questions do not exist for the patient. The physician who says "I never tell patients they have cancer unless they ask me" risks leaving the responsibility of broaching the most sensitive and awesome questions to the one who is most vulnerable, the patient.

Discussions should be positive yet reality oriented. "Am I dying? How long do I have?" may be responded to by "I don't know how long any of us have to live. If you are asking if it is serious enough to warrant getting your affairs in order, I would say yes, get your house in order. While you're doing that, you and I will deal with the medical problems you're experiencing."

Discussions focused on the goals of treatment minimize uncertainty and foster confidence. Involving the family in these discussions facilitates their subsequent mutual support. Sitting together, patient, family, and doctor examine what is still possible rather than what has been lost.

"There are only three aims we can have in treating any illness, Bill. We are not going to be able to cure your tumor, in the sense of making it go away permanently. But, you know, there are many medical problems we can't cure—including diabetes, arthritis, and most types of heart disease—yet many people with these conditions live meaningful lives, sometimes for longer periods than we expect.

"So 'cure' isn't an option. What about the next goal, 'to prolong life'? You could undergo surgery, but there is no sense putting you through something that wouldn't be helpful." (Surgery is often used as the first example, since it presents a concrete, easily grasped image of futility.) "With treatments as they now stand, the same would be said for chemotherapy, radiotherapy, and immunotherapy." (The phrasing focuses on the limitations of current therapy, not the hopelessness of the illness.)

"Does this mean nothing more can be done?" (thus naming the worst fear). "Not at all! It simply means we are at the third goal—that of focusing on the quality of life. How can we make the best of this? Let's examine that. If I understand you, the three complaints you have right now are your backache, that cough, and your loss of appetite. Let's see what we can do about each of these. . . ."

The patient and family are left with a clear understanding that the issue is not "to treat or not to treat," but an appropriate shifting in therapeutic goals by a physician who is interested, involved, and undaunted by the specter of this illness. Hope is contagious. Hope is a way through, not a way out.

Specific estimates of survival should never be given, since they are based on data relevant to populations of patients with the same illness, not to the patient in question. No matter how carefully phrased, such pronouncements always unsheathe a sword of Damocles that heightens anxiety and drains ability to live fully in the moment. "I have only 2 more months."

Acceptance of the present reality, including the increasing weakness, dependence, uncertain future, and impending loss, frees the patient to choose from available options. Acceptance of that kind is not born out of despair and resignation. It is the transcendant alternative to denial. It is a path to meaning which is possible even in the face of physical deterioration and advancing disease.

FAMILY AS THE UNIT OF CARE

Terminal illness is a pressure cooker of family stress. Grief, fear, anger, and guilt abound. Longstanding interpersonal tensions tend to be accentuated. Brief family meetings to discuss treatment plans and identify problems and fears are a time-efficient tool highly effective in preventing impending crises, clarifying misunderstandings, and building bridges of mutual support.

Table 8–2 presents a checklist of areas of inquiry useful in family assessment. Ensure that children and the elderly are informed and involved. Their exclusion often leaves them ill-prepared for loss.

The bereaved are a high-risk population with an increased incidence of impaired function, medical illness, psychological distress, and even death. Some who have been found to have an increased risk of bereavement morbidity are listed in Table 8–3. Referral to programs offering bereavement support may be beneficial.

DYING AT HOME

Death has been moved from the home to the institution in industrial nations, and family members often feel ill-prepared to care for dying loved ones. With careful planning, family education, mobilization of community resources, and continuing support, however, both family and patient may benefit from experiencing this last time together in the home.

TABLE 8–2. FAMILY ASSESSMENT ISSUES

1. Identity of nuclear family, extended family, and social network.
2. Characteristics of family system: roles, relationships, communication patterns.
3. Presence of concurrent life crises.
4. History of coping with past crises.
5. Values and beliefs about death.
6. Response to current illness: changes in roles and relationships.
7. Family resources: physical, emotional, financial, social, spiritual.
8. Immediate family needs.
9. Long-range family needs.

TABLE 8–3. SELECTED BEREAVEMENT RISK INDICATORS

1. Parental grief.
2. Social isolation.
3. Timid, dependent personality; poorly developed coping skills.
4. Short preparation time (duration of illness).
5. Ambivalent or charged relationship with deceased.
6. Concurrent life crisis.
7. Pining and clinging in final illness.
8. Grief expression repressed by cultural or family norms.
9. Disenfranchised grief: mistress, lover, divorcée, loss of a secret relationship.

Home care of the dying begins with careful home assessment performed by an experienced home care team able to direct the family to needed community resources and to recommend modifications in living arrangements and furnishings to simplify care. "You will find it much easier if you rent a hospital bed. They are inexpensive. Try placing it in the living room where she can be quiet, close to the family, and able to see the children passing in the street.

"She is weaker now. You will need a handrail and small bench for the bath tub and a walker. I think you would find a commode for the bedside helpful as well."

An effective palliative home care program implies the involvement of a team. Regularly scheduled nursing visits are supplemented by emergency visits as required. A trusted physician is available to consult in the home when the need arises. A social worker, occupational therapist, chaplain, and volunteers may all play a role. Simple, clear routines for medications and treatments are established. A sense of order and safety is fostered by round-the-clock availability of telephone consultation with experienced staff who are aware of recent changes in the patient's condition and medications. Brief respite admissions before family exhaustion sets in may serve to prolong capability of home care.

A sensitive discussion with the family about what to do when their loved one dies may promote a sense of confidence and preparedness. Acknowledgment of a job well done ("You certainly have done well to keep her at home this long") helps to allay feelings of inadequacy and guilt should admission to hospital become necessary.

AS DEATH APPROACHES

During the final days or weeks of a terminal illness, frequent changes in clinical status may occur. Eventualities such as the need for parenteral or rectal medications should be foreseen and planned for. Common crises include progressive weakness, inability to swallow and aspiration of oral intake, inability or refusal to take medications, changing levels of consciousness and orientation, restlessness, and urinary or fecal incontinence. Careful planning and prompt response to the request for emergency assistance can avoid unnecessary admission to hospital.

Decreasing requirements for most medications are encountered as death approaches. Individualized reductions in dose can prolong an alert, interactive, comfortable state, often to the moment of death.

Noisy upper airway secretions ("death rattle") are troubling to the family, who will need reassurance, but they are generally not troubling to the patient. They may be reduced by early intervention with hyoscine 0.4 mg given subcutaneously at intervals of 2 to 4 hours as needed.

Questions and fears the patient and family have about death should be gently explored. The will, funeral arrangements, and a "life review" may be discussed as a means of completing unfinished business and facilitating closure.

Encourage family members, including the young, the elderly, and those from out of town, to visit earlier rather than later. Assess bereavement risks and arrange follow-up support if indicated.

Decathexis, a protective "separating off" or "turning in" by the patient, is sometimes seen as death approaches. A simple explanation may reassure the concerned family that this is not depression or rejection but a normal protective mechanism. "He doesn't need you to say much now, but your presence will help."

Take premonitions of death seriously, and watch for the need for family members to give their lingering loved one permission to die. "It's all right, John. You can let go. You've taken care of everything. We'll miss you, but thanks to you we'll be O.K."

AT THE TIME OF DEATH

The hours that surround the death of a family member are charged with meaning for the bereaved and are usually remembered for years to come. Caregivers may use this to therapeutic advantage by establishing guidelines for patient and family care that facilitate subsequent grief work.

Endeavor to have someone sitting at the bedside of the imminently dying person. If the bedside companion is a family member, be sensitive to his or her need either for support or for time to be alone with the loved one. Encourage available family members to view the body before it has been moved to the funeral home. Seeing the body facilitates acceptance of the fact of death.

When family members arrive, offer support and quiet hospitality, including a handkerchief, a cup of tea, a listening ear. Acknowledge the support given by the bereaved to the deceased during the illness.

Allow sufficient time with the body for active grieving. It is a helpful role model for a caregiver to unobtrusively touch the body, indicating that there is nothing frightening about physical contact with the body—an experience that may be highly effective in promoting closure.

Discuss whether the family wishes to have an autopsy. Many find the documentation of reality that it provides helpful in the months and years to come.

When death occurs in a hospital, ask the family if they would prefer to collect and pack their loved one's personal effects, particularly if a child has died. A memento of the event such as a lock of hair or a picture may be an aid to bereavement, especially in parental grief.

Respect cultural differences in the expression of acute grief. Mediterranean peoples, some Asian nationalities, and others may be extremely vocal and demonstrative in their grieving. Wails, screams, fainting attacks, and highly dramatic gestures such as throwing themselves across the body of the deceased have therapeutic value for many and may be followed in a remarkably short period of time by a sense of composure and evident relief.

Acknowledge the mystery of death without offering "answers" concerning the unknowable. Honor religious rites and prayers meaningful to the bereaved.

The presence at the death or funeral service of the physician who was involved during the illness assists review of the illness, emphasizes the value of the deceased, underscores respect for the family, and assists the physician's own grief work.

THE PHYSICIAN AND DEATH

In caring for the dying, physicians are challenged in each dimension of their personhood. William James termed death "the worm at the core of man's pretensions to happiness," while La Rochefouchauld observed: "Death and the sun are not to be looked at steadily." What do we do with our accumulated losses as caregivers? How do we establish a new balance in our emotional economy when an important investment has been lost? At what cost? To whom? Do our professional encounters with death leave a need for thicker defensive shells, emotional distancing, intellectualization, and acting out? The risk is minimized if we accept relief of suffering as our mandate rather than the narrower goal of fighting disease and if we attend to our own physical, psychosocial, and spiritual needs. Indeed, confrontation with death may foster insight and enrich life. It has been said that to live is to suffer and to survive is to find meaning in the suffering; that having a "why" to live can enable living with any "how"; that our last freedom, when all others have been stripped away, is the ability to choose our response in a given set of circumstances. It is a privilege to be able to assist our patients in their growing toward an understanding of the truth of these observations. It is a source of personal growth when we recognize their truth ourselves.

Cassel E: The nature of suffering and the goals of medicine. N Engl J Med 306:639, 1982. *A classic examination of the components of personhood and their impact on the experience of illness.*

Doyle D: Palliative Care: The Management of Far Advanced Illness. Philadelphia, The Charles Press, 1984. *Comprehensive review of management strategies in both nonmalignant and malignant advanced disease.*

Frankl V: Man's Search for Meaning. New York, Simon and Schuster, 1963. *A psychiatrist and Auschwitz survivor reflects on motivation, meaning, and quality of life. Moving. Insightful. A classic.*

Saunders C: The Management of Terminal Malignant Disease. 2nd ed. Baltimore, Edward Arnold, 1984. *The principles and practice of palliative medicine by the pioneering founder of the modern hospice movement.*

Twycross RG, Lack SA: Therapeutics in Terminal Cancer. 2nd ed. New York, Churchill Livingstone, 1990. *A useful and authoritative guide to the care of patients with advanced cancer. Pragmatic. Organized for easy reference at the bedside.*

Walsh TD: Symptom Control. Cambridge, Mass., Blackwell Scientific Publications, 1989. *Detailed consideration of symptom control from angina to xerostomia! Additional chapters on ten specific areas of clinical concern including the elderly, stoma care, menopause, multiple sclerosis, pregnancy, and speech disorders.*

Worden JW: Grief Counselling and Grief Therapy. A Handbook for the Mental Health Practitioner. New York, Springer Publishing, 1982. *Mechanisms of grief and approaches to helping the bereaved accomplish the "tasks of mourning." Lucid and informative. An excellent resource for the general physician.*

PART III
PERSONAL HEALTH CARE AND PREVENTIVE MEDICINE

9 PRINCIPLES OF PREVENTIVE MEDICINE

Stephen B. Hulley

In the early part of this century the efforts of preventive medicine were focused on the predominant cause of illness and death at the time, infectious disease. In western countries, governmental provisions to control the spread of disease with modern water and sewage systems complemented the success of the medical profession in the developing science of immunization. These programs combined with improved nutrition, better medical care, and other factors to make death from infectious disease an uncommon event by 1980. Despite a small reversal of this trend in the next decade caused by the AIDS epidemic, life expectancy has risen to unprecedented levels and the noninfectious and chronic diseases have become the major cause of death and disability (Table 9–1). A new set of strategies has evolved to prevent the chief causes of mortality today: coronary heart disease, cancer, stroke, and injury.

Preventive medicine is based on epidemiologic studies that have identified risk factors for these conditions. Many of these risk factors are aspects of individually chosen lifestyles: cigarette smoking (the most important single cause of preventable death), substance abuse, and unhealthy eating and exercising habits. This has changed the nature of the therapeutic relationship. The patient must take on the larger responsibility of making the necessary lifestyle changes, and the physician must now add the role of health counselor to his clinical duties.

RISK MODIFICATION

The process of guiding lifestyle change *begins* with serving as a model. A physician who has healthy habits and provides an appropriate environment (prohibiting smoking in the waiting room, for example) has set the stage for successful intervention. The *second step* is to identify the individual characteristics of the patient, testing for the presence of risk factors and exploring motivations for changing, and for not changing, unhealthy habits. The *third step* is to provide a clear message about the scientific facts on the relationship between risk factors and disease, specifying, for example, the nature and extent of the adverse health consequences of cigarettes.

The *fourth step* is to formulate and apply recommendations that will lead to behavior change. These include (1) involving the patient as a partner in choosing attainable objectives and in making a firm commitment (a written contract may be helpful); (2) adjusting the environment to promote the desired behavior (by discarding ashtrays and not keeping unhealthy food in the home, for example); (3) establishing and rehearsing new behaviors step by step (first eating a healthier breakfast, then incorporating a 10-minute walk in commute, etc.); (4) positively reinforcing desired behavior (through praise, rewards, and risk factor feedback); and (5) involving the family and other social supports. Many clinics include staff with special skills in behavioral medicine, but even in the absence of formal training, physicians can accomplish a great deal just by addressing and lending importance to these activities. In addition to serving as health counselors themselves, physicians can guide the patient's access to other resources for lifestyle changes by providing pamphlets (obtained free from organizations like the American Heart Association) and by referral to appropriate books, support groups, and health professionals.

Whatever the intervention approach, the *fifth step* is a sustained effort to follow up on the risk factor levels. Habits are difficult to change, and health counselors need the tenacity and imagination to try a variety of approaches over the years. This does not mean harassing an unwilling or unsuccessful patient. The best health counselors are sensitive to the preferences of their patients and make wise decisions about when to promote recommendations for change and when to leave the patient alone.

IMPLICATIONS OF CHRONIC DISEASE PREVENTION

If the entire population were fully successful in the lifestyle changes proposed in this second wave of twentieth century preventive medicine efforts, the chief causes of premature death in western countries might become far less common. In addition to further extending life expectancy, the potential reward of fully effective lifestyle intervention is the possibility that most people could live their full lifespan without major illness or disability.

Speculation of this sort is based, in part, on the remarkable decline in mortality observed in the United States over the past

TABLE 9–1. ANNUAL MORTALITY RATES AND YEARS OF LIFE LOST PREMATURELY IN THE UNITED STATES IN 1900 AND IN 1986

Causes of Death*	1900 Annual Mortality (rate/100,000)	1986 Annual Mortality (rate/100,000)	Years of Potential Life Lost Before Age 65 by Persons Dying in 1986
Diseases of the heart	137	319	1,600,000
Malignant neoplasms	64	196	1,800,000
Cerebrovascular disease	107	62	200,000
Injuries	83	61	3,700,000
All others	1330	237	4,700,000
Total	1721	873	12,000,000

*The causes of death are the four most common in 1986. The statistics, which are not age adjusted, are subject to the usual inaccuracies of death certificate attribution. The top three causes of death in 1900 were pneumonia and influenza (202/100,000), tuberculosis (194/100,000), and diarrhea and enteritis (143/100,000).

TABLE 9–2. FIFTEEN AREAS OF ENDEAVOR FOR PREVENTIVE MEDICINE ESTABLISHED BY THE U.S. DEPARTMENT OF HEALTH AND HUMAN SERVICES

Topics that Are Covered in Chapters of this Section
- Smoking and health
- Injury prevention
- Control of stress and violent behavior
- Nutrition
- Physical fitness and exercise
- Misuse of alcohol and drugs
- Immunization

Topics that Are Addressed Elsewhere in this Book
- High blood pressure
- Sexually transmitted diseases
- Toxic agents
- Occupational safety and health
- Infectious diseases

Topics that Are the Concern of Other Specialties
- Family planning
- Pregnancy and infant health
- Fluoridation and dental health

20 years. The chief component of the decline is coronary heart disease, which has decreased more rapidly in the United States (2 per cent per year) than in any other nation. It seems reasonable to attribute this, at least in part, to the changes in lifestyle that are occurring in this country: the substantial decline in the national prevalence of smoking and of inadequately treated hypertension, the decrease in the mean serum cholesterol level, and the movement to become more physically fit.

The extent and thrust of preventive medicine today have been established by formal health goals in 15 areas of endeavor, created by the U.S. Department of Health and Human Services (Table 9–2). For each of these topics, there are specific objectives for the nation to achieve by the year 2000 that address health status, risk factor levels, public and professional awareness, provision of health services, and mechanisms for evaluation. This section of *Cecil Textbook of Medicine* addresses 7 of these 15 topics that are part of personal health care.

SUMMARY

The emergence of chronic and noninfectious disease as the predominant cause of death and disability in western nations has been accompanied by a growing importance of lifestyle factors as causal agents in health and disease. Among these, cigarette smoking is the single most important modifiable health hazard; abuse of alcohol and other substances, sedentary lifestyle, and improper diet are also important. The clinician's role in preventive medicine still begins with immunization and treatment of such medical conditions as hypertension, but it now extends to health counseling: examining a patient's risk factors, educating the patient, listening to preferences for changing (or not changing) lifestyle, implementing the appropriate behavioral interventions, and following up on these personal health care strategies over the years.

Higgins M, Thom T: Trends in coronary heart disease in the U.S. Int J Epidemiol 18(Suppl 1):S58, 1990. *Recent update on the remarkable 20-year decline in CHD mortality.*

Martin AR, Coates TJ: A clinician's guide to helping patients change. West J Med 146:751, 1987. *Practical guidelines in helping patients modify their risks.*

McGinnis JM, Hamburg MA: Opportunities for health promotion and disease prevention in the clinical setting. West J Med 149:468, 1988. *Practical and concise summary of prevention approaches for clinicians.*

Public Health Service, U.S. Dept of Health and Human Services: The 1990 Objectives for the Nation: A mid course review. 1986. *Update on progress in achieving the 1990 objectives for 15 areas of preventive medicine.*

U.S. Dept. of Health, Education and Welfare: Healthy People: The Surgeon General's Report on Health Promotion and Disease Prevention. DHEW Publication No. 79–55071, 1979. *Summary of trends in illness and death rates from 1900 to the 1970's.*

U.S. Preventive Services Task Force: Guide to clinical preventive services. Baltimore, Williams and Wilkins, 1989. *Most comprehensive set of prevention guidelines.*

10 Tobacco and Health

David M. Burns

Cigarette smoking is the largest preventable public health problem in the United States. An estimated 390,000 deaths per year, one sixth of the total mortality in the United States, occur prematurely secondary to the smoking habits of the American population.

Tobacco use, both oral and smoking, was introduced to European settlers by the American Indian, and tobacco was one of the main cash crops in revolutionary America. The invention of a cigarette-making machine in the 1880's and, around the turn of the century, of matches that could be carried safely resulted in a marked shift in tobacco consumption from predominantly pipes, cigars, and chewing tobacco to predominantly cigarettes. Per capita cigarette consumption in the United States increased from 54 in 1900 to a peak of 4336 in 1963. This dramatic switch to cigarette use was followed some 20 to 25 years later by an equally dramatic rise in deaths from lung cancer. The risks associated with tobacco smoking appear to be closely related to the amount of smoke inhaled. Smokers who have used only pipes or cigars tend not to inhale, and therefore the majority of the health risks are correlated with cigarette consumption (Table 10–1).

In the early part of the century, cigarette smoking was largely a male habit, but in the late 1930's and early 1940's women began to smoke in large numbers. Currently, smoking habits in young adults are similar for the two sexes. The prevalence of cigarette smoking is declining in both men and women in the United States population. In contrast, a new marketing effort for smokeless tobacco has led to a major resurgence of snuff use, particularly among adolescent males.

CIGARETTE SMOKE

Tobacco smoke is a complex mixture of some 4000 individual constituents. The smoke is a combination of pyrolysis and distillation products distributed between a particulate phase and a gas phase. Tar, the total particulate matter of the smoke once the water vapor and nicotine have been removed, is the major carcinogen of whole smoke. The gas phase of the smoke has a number of irritating and ciliotoxic agents, as well as high levels of carbon monoxide.

FACTORS DETERMINING RISK

The risks due to cigarette smoking vary with differences in individual smoking habits and with the presence of other risk factors. The risk increases with increasing number of cigarettes

TABLE 10–1. INCREASED RISKS FOR CIGARETTE SMOKERS

Cardiovascular Disease
- Coronary artery disease
- Peripheral vascular disease
- Aortic aneurysm
- Stroke

Cancer
- Lung
- Larynx, oral cavity, esophagus
- Bladder, kidney
- Pancreas

Lung Disorders
- Cancer (as noted above)
- Chronic bronchitis with airflow obstruction
- Emphysema

Complications of Pregnancy
- Infants—small for gestational age, higher perinatal mortality
- Maternal complications—placenta previa, abruptio placentae

Gastrointestinal Complications
- Peptic ulcer
- Esophageal reflux

Other
- Altered drug metabolism

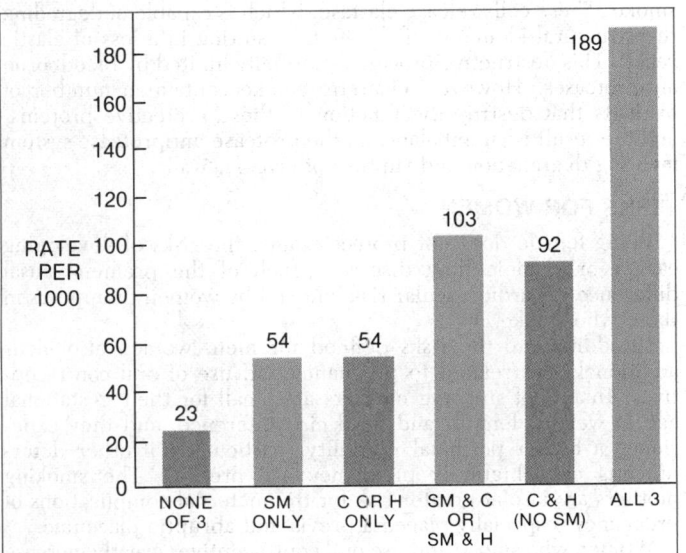

FIGURE 10–1. Major risk factor combinations, 10-year incidence of first major coronary events, men age 30 to 59 at entry, Pooling Project. Risk factor status at entry: Definitions of the three major risk factors and their symbols are hypercholesterolemia (C) = ≥ 250 mg/dl; elevated blood pressure (H) = diastolic pressure ≥ 90 mm Hg; cigarette smoking (SM) = any current use of cigarettes at entry.

smoked per day, depth of inhalation, and duration of the smoking habit. The risk also increases with the younger age at which regular smoking is begun.

A given dose of smoke exposure may interact with other personal characteristics or environmental exposures to magnify the risk of disease greatly. Thus, the risks incurred by cigarette smoking in someone with elevated blood pressure or high levels of asbestos exposure are much larger than the risks for smokers without those characteristics. In addition, the presence of smoking-induced disease in one organ system (e.g., chronic obstructive lung disease) may alter the ability to treat or survive a second disease process (e.g., lung cancer).

CARDIOVASCULAR DISEASE

Cigarette smokers have almost twice the risk of nonsmokers of developing a myocardial infarction or dying of coronary heart disease. This relative risk of heart disease is even greater at younger ages, when the incidence of disease would otherwise be very low. The relative risks for sudden death from coronary disease, peripheral vascular disease, and aneurysm of the aorta are even higher. In contrast, cigarette smokers have only a slightly greater risk of developing angina pectoris.

The magnitude of the risk of coronary heart disease associated with cigarette smoking is equivalent to the risks associated with elevated blood pressure or elevated serum cholesterol. The per cent of the population with smoking as a risk factor is substantially larger than the percentage with either elevated blood pressure or elevated serum cholesterol. As a result, *smoking ranks as the largest avoidable cause of coronary heart disease in the American population.*

Cigarette smoking acts as an independent risk factor for coronary heart disease; that is, its effect is not explained by levels of other risk factors. When more than one risk factor is present, however, smoking interacts with the other major risk factors to increase the risk synergistically (Fig. 10–1). The presence of smoking, or of either of the other risk factors, increases the risk by 31 per 1000, compared with the risk of someone with none of the risk factors. The presence of a second risk factor in someone who smokes results in an increase in risk of 49 per 1000 over the risk when only one risk factor is present, and the addition of a third risk factor increases the risk by 86 per 1000. The actual risk is always greater than the sum of the risks measured independently, suggesting that when multiple risk factors are present, they interact to create more disease. This interaction may occur by accelerating the development of atherosclerosis or by increasing the likelihood or severity of a myocardial infarction for any given level of atherosclerosis.

Smokers have more atherosclerosis than nonsmokers, particularly in the aorta. Smoking a cigarette raises heart rate and blood pressure, necessitating a greater myocardial oxygen delivery, while the carbon monoxide in the smoke increases the blood's carboxyhemoglobin level, thus decreasing its oxygen-carrying capacity. Cigarette smoking also increases platelet adhesiveness and lowers the threshold for ventricular fibrillation and may thereby play a role in the acute events surrounding some thrombotic myocardial infarctions.

Cigarette smoking has a more profound effect on the peripheral vascular bed than on the coronary or cerebral vessels. Over 90 per cent of patients with atherosclerotic peripheral vascular disease are cigarette smokers. Cessation of cigarette smoking is critical to treatment of these patients. In those who fail to quit, there is a higher incidence of amputation, and surgical therapy is dramatically less successful.

The risk of coronary heart disease due to smoking is present at all ages beyond 30, but smoking is responsible for a greater proportion of coronary deaths in younger age groups than in older age groups. This risk declines dramatically with the cessation of cigarette smoking. By 5 years after the last cigarette, the risk in those who had smoked less than one pack per day approximates the risk in lifelong nonsmokers. For those who had smoked more than one pack per day, a small residual risk of coronary heart disease may persist.

CANCER

Lung cancer is the largest cause of death from cancer in men and women (Ch. 68). *Approximately 85 per cent of mortality due to lung cancer is causally attributed to cigarette smoking and is therefore potentially preventable.*

Cigarette smokers are ten times more likely to develop lung cancer than nonsmokers. This risk is proportional to the number of cigarettes smoked per day, increasing to 20 to 25 times the risk of the nonsmoker in those who smoke two or more packs of cigarettes per day. The risk is also increased in those who inhale more deeply or began smoking at a younger age. Lung cancer death rates begin to increase rapidly after age 35 (Fig. 10–2). Cigarette smoking causes all of the major types of lung cancer, including squamous cell, adenocarcinoma, oat cell, and large cell

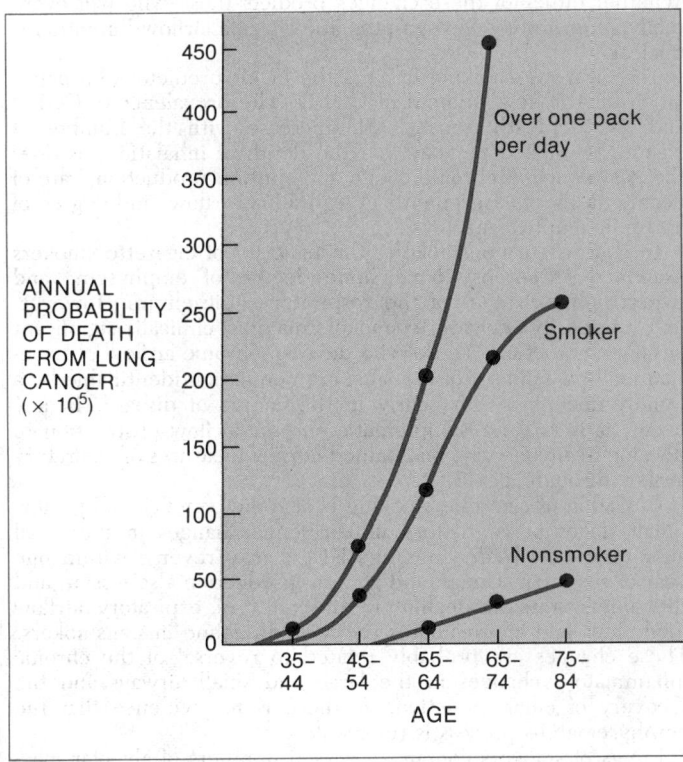

FIGURE 10–2. Annual death rate from lung cancer in nonsmokers, smokers in general, and those who smoke more than one pack per day.

carcinoma. Asbestos exposure and uranium mining interact with cigarette smoking to increase the risk of lung cancer dramatically.

The relative risks of developing *laryngeal cancer* for the cigarette smoker closely track those of lung cancer, but the total number of cases is smaller and the survival better. Cigarette smokers are five times more likely to develop *cancer of the oral cavity and esophagus*, and there appears to be a synergistic interaction between cigarette smoking and alcohol consumption for cancer of the larynx, oral cavity, and esophagus. Cigarette smoking is also a major contributing factor in *cancers of the bladder, kidney, and pancreas*, and an association between cigarette smoking and *gastric and cervical cancers* has been noted. The use of chewing tobacco or snuff can cause cancers of the cheek or gum. Overall, tobacco consumption is responsible for approximately 30 per cent of the total United States cancer mortality.

Cigarette smoking induces changes in the respiratory epithelium that progress from hyperplasia to dysplasia and even to carcinoma in situ. Tobacco smoke contains a variety of tumorigenic agents, including several that can act as complete carcinogens. The impact of these tumorigenic agents may be magnified by the ciliotoxic agents in the smoke that interfere with the normal clearance mechanisms of the lung and result in a prolonged retention of the carcinogenic agents in the lung.

Cessation of cigarette smoking results in a lessening of the risk of cancer in comparison with the risk to the continuing smoker. The risk for light smokers approximates the risk of the nonsmoker by 10 to 15 years after cessation. Heavy smokers have a residual two- to threefold increased risk that is proportional to their lifetime exposure to smoke.

CHRONIC OBSTRUCTIVE PULMONARY DISEASE (COPD)

Cigarette-induced lung injury is characterized by three overlapping syndromes: cough and mucus hypersecretion, bronchitis with airflow obstruction, and emphysema (see Ch. 58). By age 60 most cigarette smokers have changes in the airways and some degree of pathologic emphysema, but only the minority have symptomatic ventilatory limitation. The prevalence of cough increases in cigarette smokers by the early teens, and the small airways are abnormal in many smokers by early adulthood. Whether either of these changes predicts those who will eventually go on to develop symptomatic chronic airflow limitation is unclear.

The cigarette smoking habit is the major predictor in a population for the development of COPD. The prevalence of COPD and risk of death from COPD increase with the number of cigarettes smoked per day and the depth of inhalation, as does the prevalence of chronic cough and sputum production, rate of decline in the measurements of expiratory airflow, and degree of anatomic emphysema.

In contrast to nonsmokers, the majority of cigarette smokers examined at autopsy have some degree of emphysema and hypertrophic changes of the respiratory epithelium. However, only a minority of cigarette smokers manifest clinically significant airflow obstruction. Those who develop chronic airflow obstruction may be a subset of the smoking population identifiable by a rapidly declining FEV_1 early in the course of disease. In any event, it is rare for symptomatic chronic airflow obstruction to develop in anyone who maintained normal measures of expiratory airflow through age 45.

Cessation of cigarette smoking is of some benefit at all preterminal stages of ventilatory impairment. Changes in the small airways and early declines of FEF_{25-75} may reverse within one year of cessation. Cough and sputum production also lessen, and the annual rate of decline in measures of expiratory airflow moderates and approximates the rate of decline in nonsmokers. These changes are probably related to reversal of the chronic inflammatory changes in the large and small airways and the recovery of ciliary function, as there is no evidence that the emphysematous process is reversible.

Lungs of smokers contain increased numbers of alveolar macrophages and polymorphonuclear leukocytes, probably drawn there as part of the inflammatory response to the irritants in the smoke. These cells release elastase, which is capable of degrading the structural elements of the lung, resulting in a loss of elastic recoil. This destructive process is normally limited by bloodborne antiproteases. However, cigarette smoke contains a number of oxidants that destroy the function of these protective proteins, and the result is an imbalance in the protease-antiprotease system favoring degradation and rupture of alveolar walls.

RISKS FOR WOMEN

Being female does not protect against the risks of developing cancer or chronic lung disease. Much of the premenopausal difference in cardiovascular risk enjoyed by women disappears in those who smoke.

In addition to the risks defined for men, women also incur additional risks related to pregnancy and use of oral contraceptives. Infants of smoking mothers are small for their gestational age in weight, length, and head circumference, and they experience a higher perinatal mortality, particularly if other determinants of a high-risk pregnancy are present. The smoking mothers are also at greater risk for the maternal complications of pregnancy, especially placenta previa and abruptio placentae.

Women who smoke and use oral contraceptives greatly increase their risk of cardiovascular disease. They are over 30 times more likely to develop a myocardial infarction, and about 20 times more likely to have a subarachnoid hemorrhage, than their nonsmoking peers who do not use oral contraceptives.

INVOLUNTARY SMOKING

Environmental tobacco smoke contains most of the toxic and carcinogenic compounds identified in mainstream smoke; and therefore the question is not whether these agents can cause disease, but rather whether the dose and mode of exposure experienced in involuntary smoking carry a measurable risk. Absorption of smoke constituents from the environment has been documented in both infants and adults, and a number of epidemiologic studies have demonstrated health effects in humans.

Involuntary smoking can cause lung cancer in nonsmokers. The risk is small in comparison to active smoking but is large in comparison to other carcinogenic exposures experienced by the general population. From 500 to 5000 lung cancers per year have been estimated to result from involuntary smoking.

The majority of nonsmokers express annoyance and experience eye and respiratory tract irritation on exposure to smoke. Individuals with pre-existing disease may become more symptomatic on exposure to smoke, particularly those with allergies, and possibly those with chronic heart and lung disease. Nonsmokers with long-term exposure to environmental tobacco smoke may develop changes in the small airways of the lung.

Infants of smoking parents have a higher incidence of bronchitis and pneumonia in the first year of life, and the children of smoking mothers experience a developmental lag in lung growth.

CIGARETTES WITH LOW TAR AND NICOTINE

The machine-measured yield of tar and nicotine for the average cigarette smoked by the American population has been steadily declining. Smokers of lower yield cigarettes have a slightly lower risk of lung cancer than smokers of the high-yield cigarette, but this benefit disappears if they increase the number of cigarettes they smoke per day. There is also a lower prevalence of cough and phlegm, but probably no major impact on the risk of developing cardiovascular disease or chronic airflow obstruction. There are two major reasons why the decline in machine-measured tar and nicotine yield has not been accompanied by a concomitant reduction in biologic effect: (1) Many smokers may compensate for the decline in yield by increasing the number of cigarettes smoked per day, or by inhaling more deeply, thereby negating any possible reduction in smoke exposure "dose." (2) The machine-measured yield may not correspond to the yield when the cigarette is actually smoked. This is particularly true for the very low-yield cigarettes that have vents or channels designed into the filter so that the machine draws very little smoke through the filter. These vents can be occluded by the smoker, or the volume of the puff increased, with a resultant dramatic rise in the yield. For these cigarettes, the measured tar and nicotine yields have almost no relation to either actual yield or biologic potency.

An additional concern is the wide variety of flavoring and other additives that have been used to compensate for the decline in tobacco content. These additives are considered trade secrets and may be added to the cigarette without informing the public of their presence and without any review for toxic effects. These additives represent a major gap in the understanding of the disease risks associated with smoking the modern cigarette.

OTHER EFFECTS

Cigarette smokers have a greater incidence of gastric and duodenal ulcers and delayed healing of these ulcers. Smoking also relaxes the esophageal sphincter and may contribute to esophageal reflux.

Several of the constituents of tobacco smoke are capable of inducing hepatic microsomal systems, which then alter the metabolism of other drugs. Theophylline, phenacetin, antipyrine, caffeine, and imipramine are metabolized more rapidly by smokers, and adjustment in the dosage may be required with cessation. Smokers have lower blood levels of vitamins C and B_{12} Hematocrit and hemoglobin levels, as well as carboxyhemoglobin levels, are elevated in smokers; and smoking is one cause of an elevated red cell volume. Smokers also have small alterations in the other diagnostic tests, including a higher leukocyte count, but these differences are not usually clinically significant for an individual patient.

Pipe and cigar smokers who have never smoked cigarettes have a lower risk of cardiovascular disease, lung cancer, and chronic airflow obstruction than do cigarette smokers. They have similar risks of cancer of the upper respiratory tract. These differences are due to the tendency of pipe and cigar smokers not to inhale the more irritating smoke of these forms of tobacco. Cigarette smokers who switch to pipes and cigars do tend to inhale, however, and so it is not clear that switching to a pipe or cigars results in a lowering of the risks for the cigarette smoker.

The re-emergence of oral snuff use among male adolescents in the last several years has generated substantial public health concern. Smokeless tobacco use can cause cancer of the cheek and gum and gingival recession. It may also increase the risk of other oral cancers, and regular use of snuff can lead to nicotine addiction.

SMOKING BEHAVIOR AND CESSATION

Regular cigarette smoking begins almost exclusively during adolescence; 90 per cent of smokers begin before age 20. The availability and relatively low cost of cigarettes coupled with peer pressure and the desire to model adult behavior are determinants of adolescent smoking. Tobacco advertising may also influence the initiation of regular smoking by creating an image of the smoker as a secure, confident, successful, in control, and attractive individual. By smoking, adolescents are able to superimpose this positive image created by advertising on their own inadequate self-image and thereby feel better. Those adolescents with the least external validation of their self worth (through academic, athletic, or social achievements) are the ones most in need of manipulation of their internal self-image and, correspondingly, most susceptible to the images presented by advertising.

Addiction to cigarettes depends on nicotine. Beyond the pharmacologic stimulus of nicotine, however, the smoker usually creates a series of learned responses that reduce stress and alter mood. The pattern of tobacco use therefore merges into the way that the smoker learns to deal with the world. Cessation of smoking requires that the smoker give up a major coping mechanism.

Smoking cessation clinics have long-term success in 30 to 40 per cent of the smokers who persevere in their programs, but comparatively few smokers are willing to participate in these clinics. Current tobacco control strategies emphasize altering the environment in which the smoker lives by making smoking socially unacceptable, by increasing the cost of cigarettes, and by limiting the locations in which it is permissible to smoke.

Physicians can effect sustained cessation of smoking in a substantial number of patients if they are willing to treat smoking as a potentially serious medical problem. This requires obtaining information, defining a therapeutic plan, and following the results of that therapy. The information to be obtained includes the smoking status, a history of past cessation attempts and the methods used, as well as the current interest in quitting. In addition, the time from awakening to first cigarette is a measure of the strength of the addiction and may be useful in deciding whether to prescribe pharmacologic aids to the cessation attempt. In their offices physicians can ask the patient to quit, can motivate the attempt, and can negotiate a date for quitting. No smoking patient should leave the office without understanding that his or her smoking is a major health problem. The responsibility of the physician is not to get all patients to quit on a single visit, but to move each smoking patient closer to cessation on each visit. Those who have not thought about quitting should think about it; those who are thinking about it should try; and those who have tried and failed should be motivated to try again. Smokers should be encouraged to quit "cold turkey" rather than tapering down. The follow-up of cessation advice is also critical, not only because it reinforces the importance of cessation for the patient, but also because it improves the likelihood of successful cessation. A simple letter of encouragement from the physician 2 weeks following the quit date may substantially improve patient motivation and success.

The use of nicotine gum increases the chance of successful short-term cessation when utilized with an appropriate behavioral intervention program. Clonidine, particularly when used as a patch, has shown promise as a means of reducing the withdrawal symptoms but remains an investigational drug for this purpose.

Effective smoking intervention by the physician can be delivered in 3 to 5 minutes using the above approach. Physicians should refer patients who need more extensive assistance to programs designed to provide this assistance. A variety of community organizations provide cessation assistance, both in groups and as self-help materials, and these organizations can be located in the telephone directory or by contacting the local heart, lung, or cancer societies.

Fielding JE: Smoking: Health effects and control. N Engl J Med 313:491, 555, 1985. *An overall review of smoking issues.*

Glynn TJ, Manley MW, Pechacek TF: Physician-initiated smoking cessation program: The National Cancer Institute Trials. *In* Engstrom P (ed.): Advances in Cancer Control. New York, Alan R. Liss, in press. *A review of the current state of our knowledge on effective office-based smoking interventions.*

Health and Public Policy Committee, American College of Physicians: Methods for stopping cigarette smoking. Ann Intern Med 105:281, 1986. *A review of smoking cessation methods.*

Janerick DT, Thompson D, Varela LR, et al.: Lung cancer and exposure to tobacco smoke in the household. N Engl J Med 323:632, 1990. *These studies suggest that 17 per cent of lung cancer among nonsmokers may be secondary to exposure to cigarette smoke during childhood and adolescence.*

U.S. Dept. of Health and Human Services: The Health Consequences of Smoking Cessation: A Report of the Surgeon General. Sept., 1990, in press. *A complete review of the benefits of cessation.*

U.S. Dept. of Health and Human Services: The Health Consequences of Smoking: Cardiovascular Disease. DHHS Publication No. (PHS) 84–50204, 1983. *A review of the evidence on smoking and cardiovascular disease.*

U.S. Dept. of Health and Human Services: The Health Consequences of Smoking: Chronic Obstructive Lung Disease. DHHS Publication No. (PHS) 84–50205, 1984. *A review of the evidence on smoking and lung disease.*

U.S. Dept. of Health and Human Services: The Health Consequences of Smoking: Involuntary Smoking. DHHS Publication (CDC) 87–8398, 1986. *A review of the evidence on involuntary smoking.*

U.S. Dept. of Health and Human Services: The Health Consequences of Using Smokeless Tobacco. DHHS Publication No. (PHS) 86–2874, 1986. *A review of the health effects of using snuff.*

11 Control of Unintended Injuries and Those Due to Violence

Stephen B. Hulley

Deaths from injury are the fourth most common cause of death in the United States; they number more than 150,000 each year and are the leading cause of death for young and middle-aged people in the age range 1 to 45. The problem is even larger if *nonfatal* injuries, some of which cause permanent disability, are considered: There are several hundred injury-related emergency room visits for every death from injury. One third of all injury deaths are due to motor vehicles, one third result from other forms of unintended injury (falls are the most common, followed by drowning, fires, and poisoning), and the remaining third are due to violence (homicide and suicide).

Each of these causes of death and disability has risk factors that identify high-risk groups and that are susceptible to physician-mediated efforts to prevent occurrence or recurrence. Yet until recently, injury control has been largely ignored by the medical and public health establishment; it is the sleeping giant of preventive medicine.

THE EPIDEMIOLOGY OF UNINTENDED INJURIES

Motor vehicle fatality rates decreased by one third in the 1970's after automobile safety regulations and the 55 mile per hour national speed limit were instituted, but most of the benefit has since been lost as average speeds have returned to higher levels and smaller cars (which have a twofold higher crash fatality rate) have become more prevalent. Deaths due to motor vehicles rise to alarmingly high levels among young adults, particularly males (Fig. 11–1). The impact of this is brought home by the current projection that 1.4 per cent of all 15-year-old boys in the United States will die of an injury before age 25. The most important modifiable risk factors are excessive alcohol intake, which plays a role in half of all fatal crashes, and the failure to observe speed limits and to use seatbelts.

Half of all deaths from unintended injury are unrelated to traffic. Falls are the most common cause (27 per cent), followed by drowning (15 per cent), fire (12 per cent), poisoning (6 per cent), adverse effects of medical care (5 per cent), unintended firearm use (4 per cent), aspiration of food (4 per cent), airplane crashes (3 per cent), machinery accidents (3 per cent), aspiration other than food (3 per cent), electric current (2 per cent), and other less common causes. These deaths tend to have a common pattern of risk factors, including male sex, old age, low income, and alcohol intake.

Implications for Medical Practice

Injury prevention has assumed an important role in the practice of medicine only in the field of pediatrics. Perhaps it has not received more attention in internal medicine because the term "accident" connotes an event that has occurred by chance and is therefore unavoidable. This is far from the case; there are many lifestyle risk factors for injuries that are suitable for intervention with various behavioral techniques. (For this reason, the term "unintended injury" is now preferred over "accident," and the term "motor vehicle crash" over "motor vehicle accident.") The potential for preventing premature death and disability is substantial, and injury prevention advice should become as important in the general practice of medicine as the more familiar interventions on risk factors for cardiovascular disease and cancer.

Advice on preventing *motor vehicle injuries* begins with widely known precepts such as observing the speed limit and using a diagonal-lap or other well-designed seatbelt. From the medical viewpoint, patients should be warned when drugs that impair performance are prescribed, especially those like diazepam that may interact with alcohol. But the most important concern is alcohol itself. The knowledge that a particular patient drinks heavily should prompt a clinician to point out the danger to that individual and to others. Intervention can include counseling on ways to alter alcohol habits and on the use of other drivers, alternative forms of transportation, or different locations for drinking. The alarming motor vehicle crash rate among teenagers can be approached by counseling parents on the rules that they can establish for when and how their teenage children may drive (e.g., curfews for use of the family car). Society plays an important role in these areas—for example, in setting the penalties for drunken driving and for the minimum age for licensing—and physicians can be an important force behind social legislation of this sort.

Injuries due to *falls* in the elderly can be prevented by designing an environment that makes falls less likely (e.g., by providing handrails and night lights and by removing loose rugs) and that reduces the extent of injury should a fall occur (e.g., through avoiding sharp corners and selecting a home without stairs). The clinician should undertake regular tests and appropriate correction of problems with vision and should identify and treat diseases that impair mobility and balance, advising against heavy alcohol use and not prescribing drugs that contribute to these problems. Hip fracture has received less attention than it deserves (there are more than 200,000 each year, involving one of every three women who reach extreme old age, and half of these die or are permanently disabled). White women are at the greatest risk and should receive treatment to retard osteoporosis (Ch. 238). This may include postmenopausal estrogens for some and should always include advice about calcium intake (1000 to 1500 mg per day in the diet or as calcium carbonate supplements), about not smoking (cigarettes are a risk factor for hip fracture), and about being physically active.

Many of the other causes of unintentional injury can be controlled by discussing the role of excess alcohol and other specific risk factors with patients. *Drowning*, for example, can be made less likely by fencing in swimming pools where there are small children and by instruction in water safety rules. Injury due to *fires* can be reduced by counseling on the dangers of smoking (cigarettes are the most common cause of fire-related deaths) and on the value of smoke detectors and fire extinguishers.

THE EPIDEMIOLOGY OF INJURY DUE TO VIOLENCE

The homicide rate in the United States has doubled in recent years and now exceeds 20,000 per year. One third of all homicides are between family members, and another third involve people

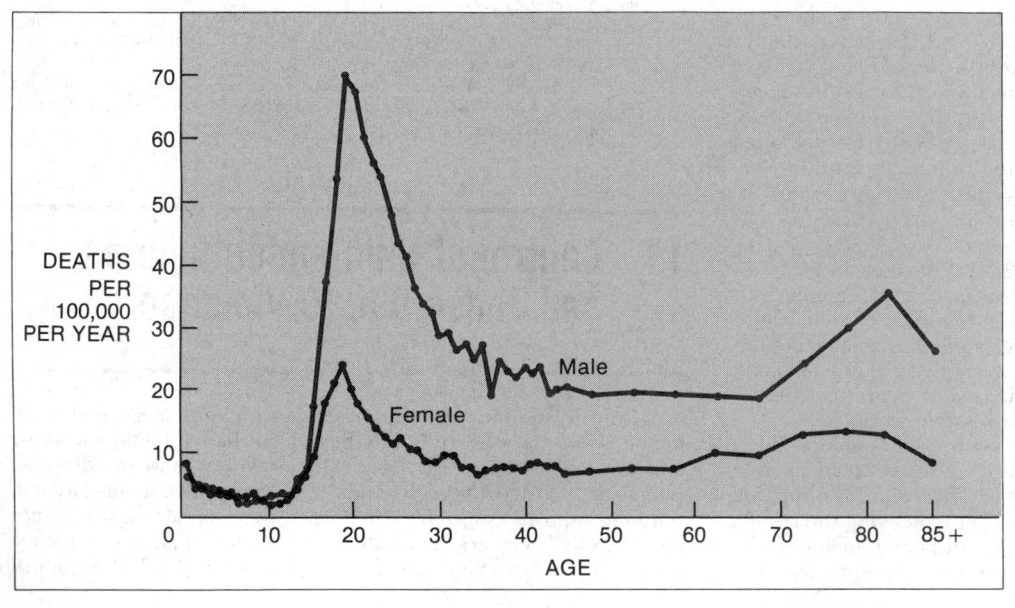

FIGURE 11–1. Age-specific death rates of motor vehicle occupants in the United States in 1976. The very high rates in 16- to 30-year-old males are a major component of the premature loss of life in this country. (From Haddon W, Baker SP: Injury control. *In* Clark D, MacMahon B [eds.]: Preventive and Community Medicine. Boston, Little, Brown & Co, 1981, pp 109–140.)

who know each other. In the United States, more than half of all homicides are carried out with handguns. Countries like England, Sweden, and Japan that have strict handgun ownership laws have handgun homicide rates that are 100-fold lower; these countries also have much lower overall rates of homicide. It is difficult to estimate the rates of nonfatal injury due to violence (assault, wife beating, rape, and child abuse), but each is undoubtedly far more common than homicide. Suicide rates have increased slightly in recent years, particularly in young men. Almost all forms of violent injury are more common in the male sex and in the socioeconomically disadvantaged, and all are commonly associated with excessive alcohol intake.

Implications for Medical Practice

The medical profession's role in dealing with the death and disability that result from violent behavior begins at an individual level. One focus is on preventing the occurrence (primary prevention) or recurrence (secondary prevention) of violent episodes, and the other is on providing medical, psychiatric, and social service care for the victims. Victims of assault and rape may present themselves for treatment of the injury, but those involved in violence within the family, such as wife beating, child abuse, or self-destructive behavior, often do not volunteer the information. The existence of a problem can sometimes be discovered by gentle probing about clues such as unexplained bruises or depressed affect. Interventions to prevent future episodes include psychiatric and social service referral, notification of police and public health authorities (when appropriate), and counseling by the clinician. The management of such problems is a major challenge to a physician's wisdom, courage, and skill.

The medical profession's most effective avenue for preventing violence may be in guiding the evolution of society and its rules. Doctors are important opinion leaders, and their comments on the medical and epidemiologic facts can help mold public opinion and legislation directed at such things as handgun control and violence in the media.

Approaches of this sort are probably the only way that the medical profession can have an effect on the most serious injury control issue of our age: the prevention of nuclear war. In addition to their general civic responsibility to express their views on this problem, some physicians regard it as a professional responsibility to educate community leaders and acquaintances on medical realities such as the false security of civil defense plans that would be inoperable in the event of a nuclear attack.

SUMMARY

Injuries are the most important cause of premature death and disability in western countries. One third of all deaths from injury are due to motor vehicle crashes, one third to other unintended causes (especially falls), and one third to intentional violence. Interventions designed to prevent each of these sources of injury are a useful and neglected focus for preventive medicine.

Physicians can play a major role in counseling individual patients about lifestyle factors that prevent motor vehicle crash injuries (e.g., avoiding alcohol in excess, using seatbelts, and setting curfews for teenage drivers) and about those that prevent other forms of unintended injuries (e.g., avoiding alcohol in excess and various medical and environmental strategies to prevent osteoporosis, falls, drowning, and fire in the home). Physicians need to take a greater role in the primary and secondary prevention of injury due to violence. In addition, medical professionals can contribute to the emergence of societal measures dealing with hazards to health that range from drunken driving to nuclear war.

Baker SP, O'Neill B, Karpf RS: The Injury Fact Book. Lexington, Mass., D. C. Heath & Company, 1984. *A fascinating and readable book that comprehensively describes the epidemiology of injury: who is especially at risk and what are the potentially modifiable risk factors.*

Cassel C, McCally M, Abraham H: Nuclear Weapons and Nuclear War: A Source Book for Health Professionals. New York, Praeger Publishers, 1984. *Reports on the medical, biologic, psychologic, and ethical implications by many of the major medical writers on this topic.*

Lowenstein SR, Hunt D: Injury prevention in primary care. Ann Intern Med 113:261, 1990. *Recent review of the issues and literature.*

National Committee for Injury Prevention and Control: Injury prevention: Meeting the challenges. Am J Preventive Med 5 (Suppl 3), 1989. *Recent and well-balanced review of this developing field.*

Riggs BL, Melton LJ: Involutional osteoporosis. N Engl J Med 314:1676, 1986. *Good review of strategies for preventing osteoporosis.*

Tinetti ME, Speechley M: Prevention of falls among the elderly. N Engl J Med 320:1055, 1989. *Review of causes of falls and practical approaches to prevention.*

12 The Judicious Diet
John P. Kane

The composition of an individual's diet and its relationship to his or her energy needs and to special requirements for growth, repair, or response to stress are among the important variables in the maintenance of health or the advent of disease. In Part XV of this book, there is an extensive discussion of nutritional requirements for calories, amino acids, essential fatty acids, minerals, and vitamins. Obviously, a judicious diet is one that meets these requirements for the individual. An excess of calories leads to obesity, one of the most prevalent nutritional disorders found in the developed countries of the world. This is discussed in detail in Ch. 203. Undernutrition can also produce serious impairment of health (Ch. 201). Deficits or excesses of other nutrients lead to a wide variety of specific disorders. In this chapter, however, we shall be concerned with variables within what would ordinarily be considered an adequate diet but that may influence the susceptibility of the individual to four major classes of disease: atherosclerosis, hypertension, cancer, and urolithiasis.

In few areas relevant to health is there so much misinformation and faddism as surrounds the subject of diet. Billions of dollars are spent in this major national industry to promote an astonishing variety of nostrums and dietary aberrations alleged to promote holistic health, vitality, and attractiveness or to reverse the process of disease. By and large, these programs are ingenious but harmless instruments to defraud the credulous. In some cases, however, they either produce harmful dietary imbalances or delay the patient's seeking effective medical care. Physicians need to be informed about the dimensions of this cultism in order to be able to advise their patients and to participate effectively in the development of controlling public policy.

DIET AND ARTERIOSCLEROSIS

In current models of atherogenesis, cholesterol and its esters enter the artery wall via plasma lipoproteins. These lipoproteins include low density lipoproteins (LDL), intermediate density lipoproteins (IDL), and, perhaps to a lesser extent, very low density lipoproteins (VLDL). More extensive descriptions of these lipoproteins and of their metabolism are given in Ch. 172. Elevated levels of LDL and IDL are strongly associated epidemiologically with accelerated atherogenesis. For instance, the risk of coronary heart disease in the United States, where the average level of serum cholesterol in an adult male is approximately 215 mg per deciliter, is several-fold higher than that in rural Japan, where the average is about 160 mg per deciliter. An inverse relationship between plasma levels of high density lipoprotein (HDL) cholesterol and risk of coronary heart disease has been noted in a number of epidemiologic surveys. This may reflect the efficiency of mechanisms involved in the centripetal (retrieval) pathways of cholesterol transport.

The risk of coronary heart disease correlates with levels of cholesterol as low as 180 mg per deciliter in plasma. The majority of individuals in industrialized Western nations would therefore be expected to benefit from reduction of levels of serum cholesterol, primarily reflecting changes in the content of LDL in plasma. The results of several intervention studies lend support to this contention. Increasing the levels of HDL in plasma in order to increase the mobilization and retrieval of cholesterol might be equally attractive, but no studies have been reported of the effect of such an intervention on heart disease independent of changes in other lipoproteins. The rationale for prevention of atherosclerosis and guidelines for management of hyperlipidemia with diet and drugs have been set forth by a panel of experts in the National Cholesterol Education Program. This program recommends that all patients with LDL cholesterol levels over 159 mg per deciliter be treated and that those with levels between 130 and 159 mg per deciliter be treated if coronary disease or at least two of a group of defined risk factors are present.

A single pattern of dietary modification is appropriate for individuals with nearly all types of primary hyperlipidemia (excepting only primary chylomicronemia), as well as for those individuals in the population at large who have less striking elevations of levels of atherogenic lipoproteins. The elements of this "universal" diet are considered individually.

1. *Reduce body weight to the ideal.* This primarily induces a marked reduction in elevated VLDL levels. It also effects a modest reduction in LDL cholesterol levels and may increase HDL cholesterol levels slightly. Maintenance of ideal body weight is the most effective means of forestalling the appearance of type II diabetes, itself a risk factor for atherosclerosis.

2. *Decrease the intake of saturated fat.* This change effects a potent and uniform lowering of LDL cholesterol. The typical American diet contains approximately 40 per cent or more of calories as fat (15 per cent saturated fat). Levels of 30 per cent of calories as fat (less than 10 per cent saturated fat) can be achieved easily, and an intake of less than 7 per cent saturated fat is attainable with major changes in food selection. To achieve the 30 per cent level of dietary fat, fat-rich meats, dairy products, and items such as certain baked goods must be restricted. To achieve the 20 per cent level, major substitution of vegetable protein sources for meats must be made.

When the intake of saturated fats is decreased, there are several possible sources of replacement calories: polyunsaturated fats, monounsaturated fats, and carbohydrates. Major substitution with polyunsaturated fat may result in lower levels of HDL cholesterol and of the principal HDL protein, apolipoprotein A-I. Furthermore, polyunsaturated fatty acids are susceptible to hydroperoxidation, which could lead to generation of free radical chains and perhaps to carcinogenesis. Monounsaturated fats, abundant in certain vegetable oils such as olive oil, do not increase LDL levels and do not hydroperoxidize readily. HDL cholesterol levels are somewhat higher with use of monounsaturates than with diets that are low in total fat. Trans fatty acids formed during catalytic hydrogenation or prolonged heating exert effects similar to those of saturated fats. Major substitution of carbohydrate for fat is associated with modest elevations of plasma triglyceride levels in the short term, but these levels return to normal after a period of several months. Strict vegetarians tend to have lower levels of both LDL and HDL than individuals on a typical American diet, but the changes in LDL levels are of much greater magnitude. Furthermore, potentially important differences in composition of HDL are seen, with an increased ratio of phospholipid to cholesterol. Vegetarian diets appear to be compatible with good health, provided that the foods selected supply all essential amino acids and adequate amounts of vitamin B_{12}.

Omega-3 fatty acids contained in marine fish oils, appear to have a unique ability to reduce elevated levels of VLDL and chylomicrons in plasma at doses of 15 to 20 grams per day. Plasma levels of LDL may be decreased modestly in some individuals with normal or moderately elevated levels of plasma cholesterol and even increased in some, accompanied by some decrease in HDL cholesterol levels. The marked decreases in plasma triglycerides that occur are due at least in part to inhibition of VLDL secretion. Omega-3 fatty acids moderately reduce formation of thromboxane B_2 in platelets, inhibiting aggregation and adhesion, an effect that may account in part for the low incidence of arteriosclerotic heart disease in populations for whom cold-water marine fish are a major food source.

Overall, a major reduction of saturated fat should be made from levels found in Western diets, and complex carbohydrate should be used to provide the requisite caloric replacement. Small amounts of polyunsaturated fats from plant sources should be used to provide essential fatty acids. The use of fish oils might be considered if hypertriglyceridemia is present.

3. *Decrease the intake of cholesterol.* Reduction of dietary saturated fats automatically eliminates much cholesterol; however, rich sources such as organ meats and egg yolks should be restricted specifically. The effect of restriction of cholesterol on LDL levels varies widely among individuals. This variation appears to reflect two factors: (a) There is an approximately fourfold difference among individuals in the fraction of dietary cholesterol that is absorbed. (b) There are differences in the degree to which dietary cholesterol is capable of suppressing endogenous cholesterogenesis. It is reasonable to presume, however, that reduction of dietary cholesterol is likely to be of benefit. The typical American diet provides 400 mg or more of cholesterol per day, but an intake of 250 to 300 mg per day is relatively easily achieved, and intakes of 100 mg per day can be achieved with more rigorous mixed diets. Strict vegetarian diets contain no cholesterol.

4. *Restrict alcohol.* Alcohol should be limited in all cases to maintain ideal body weight. VLDL secretion is increased dramatically by even limited use of alcohol. Therefore, alcohol should always be restricted in the diet of individuals with elevated serum triglycerides. Increased alcohol intake may be associated with elevated levels of HDL cholesterol, but it is not yet clear whether this change represents subspecies of HDL that participate in centripetal cholesterol transport. No categorical presumption of beneficial effects of alcohol on HDL can yet be made.

5. *Other factors.* Increased dietary fiber appears to have a marginal effect on serum lipoprotein levels, although certain sources of fiber, such as oat or wheat bran, appear to reduce LDL levels slightly. In addition, saponins in foodstuffs such as oats may decrease absorption of cholesterol. The ingestion of lecithin, which is widely suggested by health food advocates, lacks significant effect, as do a number of vitamins and minerals that have been similarly recommended.

Individuals adhering to this regimen may show reductions of plasma cholesterol levels of 10 or even 15 per cent on the basis of reduction of saturated fats. An additional reduction of 1 to 10 per cent may be achieved by restriction of cholesterol. At least a twofold reduction in risk of coronary disease would be expected in the American population if such modifications of lipid levels were uniformly achieved.

DIET AND HYPERTENSION

Essential hypertension has been assumed to result from a constitutional inability to excrete sodium chloride efficiently, because of which calcium ions accumulate in arteriolar smooth muscle cells, increasing tonicity. Indeed, evidence from cross-transplantation studies in animals and from human renal transplants lends credence to the existence of such a mechanism. Cross-cultural studies also have shown, in the aggregate, convincing positive correlation between blood pressure and intake of salt. Patient populations with essential hypertension are heterogeneous with respect to renin levels, plasma calcium concentrations, response to individual antihypertensive drugs, and sensitivity to dietary salt. Normotensive individuals and perhaps half of American patients with hypertension do not show a pressor response to increased dietary salt. Thus, justification for the prescription of reduced salt intake appears to be limited to individuals with salt-sensitive hypertension and members of their kindreds. Most Americans consume 10 to 20 grams of salt per day; an intake of 4 grams is a more reasonable goal for individuals in such kindreds. Increasing calcium intake has been reported to reduce blood pressure. If true, this effect will probably be restricted to a subset of patients. Furthermore, indiscriminate increase in calcium intake could increase urinary calcium excretion in individuals with absorptive hypercalciuria (Ch. 88). Thus, increasing calcium intake to prevent or treat hypertension cannot be recommended as a general measure at this time.

DIET AND CANCER

The consumption of certain major food components is epidemiologically correlated with an increased incidence of some types of cancer. Although the mechanisms of these associations are still largely unknown, a judicious diet at this time involves changes that would be expected to minimize these risks. A number of components that occur in foods naturally or are formed or added during processing are mutagens in bacterial test systems (Ames test) or carcinogens or promoters of carcinogenesis in whole animals. Prudence would dictate elimination of these from human consumption to whatever extent is practicable, because definitive studies demonstrating specific risks of these agents in humans may emerge only slowly.

DIETARY FAT. In multinational studies, the prevalence of cancer of the breast, colon, and prostate correlates with dietary fat intake. Within cultures, however, breast cancer correlates poorly, whereas colon cancer continues to show a positive correlation with fat intake in many, but not all, studies. Also, the incidence of breast cancer changes slowly when women immigrate to countries with a high incidence and high-fat diets, whereas that of colon cancer accommodates within a few years. Enhancement of chemical carcinogenesis by dietary fat occurs in several animal models. Total fat intake correlates best with carcinogenesis at high levels, but polyunsaturated fats appear to be most important at lower levels of intake. Polyunsaturated fats are substrates for hydroperoxidative reactions initiating free radical chains, and therefore they probably should not constitute a major component of the diet. Reduction of total fat intake, with an increased content of complex carbohydrates, is completely compatible with the "prudent" diet for prevention of arteriosclerotic heart disease.

FIBER. Carcinogens formed in the bowel may play a role in the development of carcinoma of the colon. Increased fiber in the diet would decrease the duration of contact of carcinogens with the mucosa and therefore might reduce the risk of cancer. Only minimal epidemiologic support for this view exists. With the possible exception of pentosans from wheat, fiber has not been proven effective in animal models. In many studies, a reduced risk of cancer is more closely correlated with the intake of fruits and vegetables than with fiber per se.

ALCOHOL. Alcohol consumption has long been known to correlate with risk of carcinoma of the mouth, pharynx, and esophagus. Several studies have also shown a strong correlation with risk of breast cancer. Alcohol also appears to be teratogenic in humans and causes congenital malformations, mental dysfunction, and growth retardation in infants born to alcohol-abusing mothers. Alcohol metabolism produces acetaldehyde, which is both mutagenic and carcinogenic, in addition to other mutagenic and carcinogenic compounds.

POSSIBLE RISKS ASSOCIATED WITH LOW LEVELS OF CHOLESTEROL IN PLASMA. An increased risk of cancer has been associated epidemiologically with very low levels of serum cholesterol. When present such an association is always weak and tends to occur only in the lowest range of cholesterol levels. Further, in nearly 20 prospective population studies, half have shown no such correlation, especially in those in which sufficient time elapsed between measurement of serum lipids and detection of cancer to minimize the number of pre-existing cancer cases. Because many cancers reduce levels of LDL, the association may be completely an epiphenomenon. Furthermore, the risk of colon and rectal cancer is positively correlated with serum cholesterol levels. In view of the strong correlation of higher levels of cholesterol in plasma with risk of coronary disease, dietary modifications directed at lowering the risk of coronary disease should not be abandoned on the premise that a significant increase in the risk of cancer would ensue. Two studies have yielded a weak association between extremely low levels of serum cholesterol (less than 130 mg per deciliter) and cerebral hemorrhage, especially when hypertension is present. This suggests that reduction of total cholesterol levels below 150 to 160 mg per deciliter may be contraindicated.

FOOD PREPARATION AND PRESERVATION. Exposure of meats to high temperatures, as in charcoal broiling, may be important in oncogenesis because compounds with very high carcinogenic potential are formed. In addition to benzo(a)pyrene, several mutagenic pyrolysates are formed from amino acids. Components of wood smoke in smoked foods have been linked epidemiologically and from animal studies to carcinoma of the gastrointestinal tract. Nitrites, used as preservatives in meats, react with a number of natural amines and even certain medications to form nitrosamines, which are mutagenic. This reaction is favored by low pH; hence it proceeds readily in the stomach. Clinical observations tend to link nitrites with carcinogenesis of the stomach and esophagus. Vitamin C inhibits the formation of nitrosamines in vitro. Increased intake of this vitamin by the public may account in part for decreases in the incidence of gastric carcinoma observed in recent years. At this time, restriction of nitrites and nitrosamines in the diet would appear reasonable. This is complicated by the presence of large amounts of nitrates, which can be reduced to nitrites, in certain vegetables that have been overfertilized by growers. The average American ingests about 75 mg of nitrate, 0.8 mg of nitrite, and 1 µg of preformed nitrosamines daily.

NATURALLY OCCURRING CARCINOGENS AND MUTAGENS. Several species of *Aspergillus* molds produce aflatoxins, which are among the most potent natural carcinogens. These agents are carcinogenic in a number of animals, chiefly causing carcinoma of the liver. Induction of tumors of colon, lung, and kidney has also been observed. Aflatoxins have been linked strongly to human hepatocellular carcinoma in Africa and Asia, acting in concert with the hepatitis B virus. Aflatoxins have been found chiefly in peanuts, apple products, and grains stored under moist conditions. Efforts to reduce the intake of these agents center on proper storage of foods. Emerging awareness of other naturally occurring mutagens and carcinogens may be expected to lead to an evaluation of their importance in human carcinogenesis. Among these agents are allyl isothiocyanate found in many plant sources; hydrazine derivatives found in many mushrooms; safrol of sassafras; the methyl xanthines of coffee, tea, and cocoa; and phorbol esters and pyrrolizidine alkaloids found in herbal teas.

NATURAL INHIBITORS OF CARCINOGENESIS. Some naturally occurring compounds appear to inhibit carcinogenesis by certain agents. Tocopherols, which interrupt free radical chains, are capable of reducing the carcinogenicity of doxorubicin (Adriamycin) and daunomycin and are protective against oxygen radical damage to tissues. Certain indoles found in cruciferous vegetables (broccoli, cabbage, cauliflower, and the like) inhibit the carcinogenicity of benzo(a)pyrene, and substituted isothiocyanates found in these plants inhibit the carcinogenesis induced by polycyclic aromatic hydrocarbons. Higher intakes of beta-carotene and perhaps other carotenoids have been correlated with reduced risk of cancer of the lung in several studies. Weaker correlations with other tumor types have also been observed. Selenium, a cofactor in the reduction of hydroperoxides, also may confer resistance to free radical-mediated carcinogenesis.

DIET AND UROLITHIASIS

Certain measures that should reduce the risk of urolithiasis are applicable to the general population (also see Ch. 88). Sufficient intake of water to ensure a daily urine volume of 2 to 3 liters is a most important preventive measure and is useful in all forms of urolithiasis. Restriction of dietary purine intake is also desirable because uricosuria can enhance the crystallization of calcium oxalate as well as uric acid. Restriction of the intake of animal proteins reduces the "acid ash" residue of urine, diminishing the urinary excretion of calcium, a stratagem that may also be of value in prevention of osteoporosis.

Moderate restriction of oxalate intake is reasonable in view of the prevalence of oxalate stones. More stringently reduced intake should be advised for individuals who have had one or more oxalate stones, if urinary oxalate is elevated. The oxalate content is particularly high in rhubarb, spinach, chard, beets, citrus pulp, pecans, peanuts, sweet potatoes, and a number of berries and fruits. Citrate appears to inhibit the crystallization of calcium with oxalate. Some patients with calcium oxalate urolithiasis have low levels of citrate in urine. Regular intake of citrate-rich, pulp-free fruit juices appears to be a reasonable intervention. In general, restriction of dietary calcium should be limited to patients with hypercalciuria.

SUMMARY

The following recommendations for dietary modifications can be made for the general population. Caloric intake should be adjusted to achieve and maintain ideal body weight. Fat intake should be reduced to 30 per cent of total calories (7 to 10 per cent as saturated fat) or less, and cholesterol intake to 150 mg, or less, per day. Even moderate use of alcohol should be avoided in individuals with hypertriglyceridemia. Complex carbohydrates should be used to make up the caloric deficits resulting from these changes. Individuals with a predisposition to hypertension should limit salt intake to 4 grams per day. Prudence also suggests reasonable limitation of charcoal-broiled and smoked foods and foods rich in nitrites or nitrates.

Ames BN: Dietary carcinogens and anticarcinogens: Oxygen radicals and degenerative diseases. Science 221:1256, 1983. *A comprehensive review of mutagens and carcinogens in the diet.*

Ames BN: Food constituents as a source of mutagens, carcinogens, and anticarcinogens. *In* Knudsen I (ed.): Genetic Toxicology of the Diet. New York, Alan R. Liss, Inc, 1986, pp 3–32. *A discussion of mechanisms by which food constituents can promote or retard the formation of tumors.*

Committee on Diet, Nutrition, and Cancer. Assembly of Life Sciences, National Research Council: Diet, Nutrition and Cancer. National Academic Press, 1982. *A comprehensive evaluation of the roles of dietary components and additives in carcinogenesis.*

The Expert Panel: Report of the National Cholesterol Education Program Expert Panel on detection, evaluation, and treatment of high blood cholesterol in adults. Arch Intern Med 148:36, 1988. *Guidelines for the detection of hyperlipidemia and its treatment with diet and drugs, proposed by a consensus panel appointed by the National Heart, Lung, and Blood Institute.*

Menkes MS, Comstock GW, Vuilleumier JP, et al.: Serum beta-carotene, vitamins A and E, selenium, and the risk of lung cancer. N Engl J Med 315:1250, 1986. *Epidemiologic evidence relating beta-carotene and vitamin E to a reduced risk of lung cancer.*

Mensink RP, Katan MB: Effect of dietary trans fatty acids on high-density and low-density lipoprotein cholesterol levels in healthy subjects. N Engl J Med 323:439, 1990. *New evidence on the impact of trans fatty acids on plasma lipoproteins.*

Nordy A, Goodnight SH: Dietary lipids and thrombosis. Relationships to atherosclerosis. Arteriosclerosis 10:149, 1990. *A review of the role of diet and thrombogenesis.*

Trock B, Lanza E, Greenwald P: Dietary fiber, vegetables and colon cancer: Critical review and meta analysis of the epidemiologic evidence. J Natl Cancer Inst 82:650, 1990. *A review of dietary factors related to colon cancer.*

Willett WC, Stampfer MJ, Colditz GA, et al.: Moderate alcohol consumption and the risk of breast cancer. N Engl J Med 316:1174, 1987. *Observations on the association of alcohol with breast cancer.*

Willett W: The search for the causes of breast and colon cancer. Nature 338:389, 1989. *A comprehensive review of the relationships of a number of dietary factors to the risk of developing breast or colon cancer.*

13 Exercise and Health

William L. Haskell

The biologic and psychologic benefits ascribed to exercise are extremely diverse and vary substantially with regard to scientific documentation. Some of these benefits have been definitively established and are achievable by anyone who exercises appropriately. Other benefits, frequently promoted by exercise advocates, usually do not occur, and at times inappropriate advice has been given that has placed patients at undue risk for exercise-caused morbidity or mortality. As with many other areas of health promotion, enthusiasm to help others by encouraging them to exercise can easily outstrip the scientific basis for such actions. While the idea that exercise promotes health is not new, many of the details regarding specific health benefits and exercise requirements are still much debated and under investigation.

EXERCISE AND PHYSICAL WORKING CAPACITY

The most effective method of achieving an increase in physical working capacity or "physical fitness" is through a systematic increase in habitual exercise (exercise training). This increase in capacity is an adaptative response by the body to the stress placed on various tissues and biologic functions by the increased metabolic or physical demands of the exercise. If the appropriate type of exercise is performed at the proper intensity, duration, and frequency, sedentary individuals of all ages will achieve significant improvements in physical working capacity. After training, they will be able to exercise at a greater intensity and for a longer duration than before. Also, at the same submaximal exercise intensity they will experience less fatigue. This increase in functional capacity is due to enhanced metabolic capacity and efficiency of skeletal muscle, increased capacity for substrate and oxygen delivery to the muscle, and changes in autonomic nervous system regulation during exercise.

Increases in physical working capacity often are equated inappropriately with improvements in health status or disease prevention. This is an important and often difficult distinction to make: that while a very high level of physical fitness usually requires good health, an improvement in fitness does not ensure an increase in resistance to disease or a reduction in clinical manifestations. For example, patients with disorders such as emphysema, diabetes, or hypertension can significantly increase their working capacity through exercise without necessarily changing the severity of their disease or their medical prognosis. Becoming more physically fit and improving health status are interrelated but not synonymous.

HEALTH BENEFITS OF EXERCISE

Most of the health-related benefits of exercise appear to result from the increase in metabolism required to provide the energy needed for skeletal muscle contraction. This increase in demand for energy triggers a number of adaptations designed to enhance the efficiency and capacity of the skeletal muscle to perform work and minimize fatigue. Adaptations also occur in those systems that support the increased energy requirements of skeletal muscle, including the nervous, endocrine, cardiovascular, respiratory, and skeletal systems.

CORONARY HEART DISEASE. The area of greatest scientific inquiry regarding the health benefits of exercise has been its potential role in the prevention of coronary heart disease (CHD). In classic studies of a generation ago the conductors on double-decker buses in London were shown to develop fewer manifestations of CHD than did the less active bus drivers. Most subsequent studies have confirmed that men and women who select more active jobs or leisure-time pursuits tend to experience fewer fatal and nonfatal CHD events. These studies do not rigorously demonstrate a cause and effect relationship, but the direction of the association is positive and quite consistent, the magnitude of the differences in CHD events is clinically meaningful, and the amount of exercise performed during leisure time associated with lower CHD risk is well within the capacity of most healthy adults. As of yet no randomized trial of adequate design has been performed to determine if an increase in exercise by sedentary adults free of clinically evident CHD on entry into the study would significantly reduce future CHD events.

Patients with ischemic heart disease enrolled in exercise-based cardiac rehabilitation programs experience a significantly lower cardiovascular and all-cause mortality rate than do nonparticipants one to three years following hospitalization. Although other risk factors were also altered in some studies, exercise training appears to have been the essential ingredient. Exercise training also improves clinical status (less angina, shortness of breath, fatigue) and functional capacity. In general, appropriate exercise enhances both the clinical and psychological status of these patients and should be included in a comprehensive treatment program.

There are several mechanisms by which exercise can reduce CHD risk. Exercise may maintain or increase oxygen supply to the myocardium by decreasing the progression of atherosclerosis, increasing coronary collateralization, or enlarging the diameter of proximal coronary arteries, but these changes have not been clearly documented to occur in humans. Potentially beneficial changes in blood clotting–fibrinolysis activity and in plasma lipoprotein profiles often follow training and may improve the coronary blood flow in some individuals.

Endurance exercise training decreases myocardial oxygen demand, primarily by a decrease in heart rate at rest, and decreases in heart rate and systolic blood pressure during submaximal exercise. These changes are most likely produced by a modification in central nervous system regulation of cardiovascular function (decreased sympathetic and increased parasympathetic drive) and an increase in blood volume, with little, if any, change occurring in intrinsic myocardial function.

CARBOHYDRATE METABOLISM. A frequently unrecognized health benefit of exercise is its effect on carbohydrate metabolism. During large-muscle, dynamic exercise of moderate intensity, the glycogen stored in skeletal muscle is used for the production of energy and becomes partially depleted. For the next 24 to 72 hours this glycogen is replaced by the uptake of glucose from the blood. In addition to this acute effect of increased glucose removal, the insulin receptors in skeletal muscle and adipose tissue increase in sensitivity and thus remove glucose more effectively at any given concentration of plasma insulin. This "insulin-sparing" effect of endurance exercise training decreases insulin production and may reduce the risk of insulin deficiency developing with increasing age.

OSTEOPOROSIS. The bone mineral loss that occurs with aging is accelerated by inactivity, especially bed rest (Ch. 238). Exercise will blunt but not prevent all of this loss. For example, in a survey of postmenopausal women, level of habitual activity was one of the major determinants of bone mass as measured by computed tomography. In the more active women, arm and leg bone mass was greater after accounting for the effects of age, body weight, and calcium intake. Also, when a cohort of elderly women exercised three times per week for 30 minutes each session, an increase in bone mineral content was observed (2.3 per cent), while 12 women who remained sedentary during this time showed a decrease of 3.3 per cent ($p < 0.005$). These experiences support the use of moderate intensity exercise requiring the movement of body weight against gravity as part of a comprehensive program of osteoporosis prevention. One note of caution is that young women who become amenorrheic in conjunction with vigorous exercise training experience loss of bone mass that may last for several years after return of normal menstrual function.

WEIGHT CONTROL. More physically active individuals tend to weigh less than their sedentary counterparts and at any given body weight have a greater muscle mass. Even though calorie consumption frequently goes up when sedentary people exercise substantially more, they usually lose adipose tissue. Not only are more calories expended during exercise, but the *resting metabolic rate* may be increased for an extended period after exercise. *Basal metabolic rate* at any given body weight may also increase. People who include exercise as part of their weight loss program are more successful in maintaining optimal weight. For these reasons, exercise, along with proper nutrition, can improve health status by contributing to the maintenance of optimal body composition.

PSYCHOLOGICAL STATUS. Many physically active people state that the major health benefit that keeps them exercising is their improved psychological status. They report less anxiety and depression, more self-confidence, and an increased ability to cope with at-home and job-related stress. How frequently such benefits occur when sedentary people take up exercise is not known, nor is there any understanding of how to design an exercise program to maximize the positive psychological effects. Whether or not this perceived improvement in psychological status has a biologic basis has not been established. Proposed explanations for a biologic basis are the decrease in circulating catecholamines produced by exercise training and the acute increase in beta-endorphins that occurs during and following vigorous exercise. Regardless of the mechanism, consideration should be given to getting sedentary people up and away from chronic stress-producing environments and having them participate in an exercise of their choice.

OTHER DISORDERS. There are a number of other situations in which selected patients with an established disease tend to show some clinical improvement if they exercise properly, but there is no good evidence that exercise prevents these disorders. Diseases included in this category are chronic obstructive lung disease (emphysema and bronchitis), mild or labile hypertension, osteoarthritis, and intermittent claudication. Exercise has not been shown to prevent any infectious disease.

A Comment on Safety

When recommending exercise for health promotion, one does battle with the proverbial two-edged sword. Inappropriate exercise literally can pose dangers to life and limb. Most commonly musculoskeletal discomfort or injury is caused by trauma or overuse. Much less frequently, a major cardiac event is precipitated, usually ventricular fibrillation, but the likelihood that exercise will cause a cardiac arrest in individuals without underlying cardiac disease is remote.

Other health risks of exercise are usually limited to individuals with established disease (e.g., diabetes, asthma, or renal failure) or occur with very extended or competitive exercise. The most important of these risks is the development of severe heat injury (Ch. 532). These injuries cannot be totally prevented if adults increase their exercise, but the risks can be reduced by proper medical evaluation, individualized exercise recommendations, and improved public education.

MEDICAL EVALUATION

Guidelines vary regarding the type of medical evaluation recommended prior to initiating a health-oriented exercise program. Advice depends on the specific exercise to be undertaken, as well as on the person's age and clinical status. For sedentary people who plan to undertake a low-level program such as brisk walking, no special medical examination is recommended unless they currently are under treatment for cardiopulmonary, metabolic, or musculoskeletal disorders. Such patients should be evaluated by a physician prior to an increase in exercise. For persons under age 40 who are free of clinically evident cardiopulmonary, metabolic, or musculoskeletal disorders, no special medical evaluation is considered necessary if they also are free of major cardiopulmonary disease risk factors (hypertension, hypercholesterolemia, or cigarette smoking). All persons under age 40 with disease or increased cardiopulmonary risk or over age 40 should have a medical examination prior to beginning vigorous exercise. An electrocardiographic and blood pressure–monitored exercise tolerance test should be included in the medical evaluation of all patients with cardiopulmonary disorders. Such tests should be symptom limited and monitored by a physician. Similar tests are recommended but not required for clinically healthy persons.

IMPLICATIONS FOR MEDICAL PRACTICE

The *type* of exercise that provides the greatest health benefits and permits the greatest increase in energy expenditure with the least fatigue consists of performing rhythmic contractions of large muscles to move the body over a distance or against gravity. Such exercise frequently is referred to as being endurance or "aerobic," since, if it is performed at an intensity that is moderate relative to the person's capacity, most of the resynthesis of high-

TABLE 13–1. THE EXERCISE PRESCRIPTION

Type of Exercise
  Primarily aerobic
  Stretching for flexibility
  Resistance exercise for muscle tone

Intensity
  Moderate relative to capacity (50%–75%)
  Target heart rate = 60%–85% MHR
  Maximum heart rate (MHR) = 220 − age

Duration
  25–45 minutes per session
  Target of 300 kilocalories per session

Frequency
  Daily if intensity <65% MHR and duration <30 minutes
  Every other day if intensity >65% and duration >30 minutes

Session
  Warm-up, 3 to 5 minutes
  Conditioning, 15 to 40 minutes
  Cool-down, 2 to 5 minutes

Progression
  Use exercise log
  Keep pulse in target range
  Evaluate every 2–4 weeks or each visit

Warning Signs
  Severe musculoskeletal pain
  Claudication
  Chest pressure/pain, discomfort
  Unusual shortness of breath
  Dizziness, nausea, vomiting

energy compounds in the muscle is performed in the presence of oxygen. Examples of this type of exercise are walking, hiking, jogging or running, cycling, cross-country skiing, swimming, active games and sports, selected calisthenics, and vigorous at-home or on-the-job chores. While very specific activities may be required when training for athletic competition, for health purposes any exercise of this type seems to be of benefit if performed frequently enough at the proper intensity (Table 13–1).

The exercise-induced changes that contribute to health are achieved when the exercise *intensity* is somewhat greater than that usually performed by the individual. This increased intensity or overload causes adaptations that allow the metabolic needs of the muscles during exercise to be more readily met. While exercise intensities even slightly greater than usual will produce changes, the usual recommendation is that exercise for optimizing health should be performed at 50 to 75 per cent of the individual's oxygen transport (aerobic) capacity or at 60 to 85 per cent of maximal achievable heart rate during exercise. Using these guidelines, exercise training heart rates for individuals 30 years of age would range from 114 to 162 beats per minute, whereas at age 60 the range would be from 86 to 137 beats per minute. For most people this recommendation produces a substantial intensity overload, since they usually do not exercise at more than about 40 per cent of their aerobic capacity during everyday activities.

The exercise *duration* to be recommended depends on the person's health or fitness goals and exercise capacity as well as on the type of exercise being performed. People who do even a little bit of exercise on a regular basis are better off than those who do almost nothing. A reasonable goal for a sedentary person is an energy expenditure over usual activities of approximately 300 kilocalories per session with a *frequency* of at least every other day. Most clinically healthy adults have the capacity to expend from 400 to 700 kilocalories per hour while performing activity of moderate intensity; thus they can expend 300 kilocalories in 25 to 45 minutes. Activities meeting this goal include walking or jogging 4 kilometers, cycling or swimming for 30 minutes, or playing several sets of singles tennis lasting for 45 minutes. Lower intensity exercise such as walking or gardening will not produce a large increase in exercise capacity, but if performed for longer periods or more frequently, it seems to provide many of the health benefits derived from more vigorous exercise.

SUMMARY

Inactivity does not appear to be the sole cause of any major disease, but a physically active lifestyle improves general health status and retards many of the functional impairments that frequently occur with aging. Success in initiating and maintaining an exercise program is most likely to occur when it is individually designed and takes into account the person's goals, interests, skills, and exercise opportunities, as well as exercise capacity. Patients should be advised to set aside a time for exercise and to fill it with a variety of activities, rather than selecting a single activity as the sole basis for increasing exercise for health purposes. The exercise plan should be convenient to perform, fit within the general lifestyle of the individual, and be considered fun or at least enjoyable. Success at exercise is increased when the individual has acquired the *knowledge* of what is to be done and why, the *confidence* that success can be achieved, and the *patience* to wait for the benefits to accrue.

American College of Sports Medicine: Guidelines for Graded Exercise Testing and Exercise Prescription. 4th ed. Philadelphia, Lea & Febiger, 1990. *Comprehensive guidelines for the exercise testing and training of healthy persons and patients.*
Horton ES: Role and management of exercise in diabetes mellitus. Diabetes Care 11:201, 1988. *A comprehensive review of the biochemical effects of exercise on carbohydrate metabolism and the implication of these data for the use of exercise in the prevention and treatment of diabetes mellitus.*
Oldridge NB, Guyatt GH, Fischer ME, et al.: Cardiac rehabilitation after myocardial infarction: Combined experience of randomized clinical trials. JAMA 260:945, 1988. *Review of major studies of exercise rehabilitation following myocardial infarction demonstrating an overall reduction in cardiovascular and all-cause mortality in program participants.*
Powell KE, Thompson PD, Caspersen CJ, et al.: Physical activity and the incidence of coronary heart disease. Ann Rev Public Health 8:253, 1987. *A critical review of the relationship of habitual physical activity and ischemic heart disease mortality as established by epidemiologic observations.*

14 Alcoholism and Alcohol Abuse
Ivan Diamond

EPIDEMIOLOGY

Nearly two thirds of Americans over age 14 drink alcoholic beverages. Their per capita consumption is the equivalent of 9.7 gallons of whiskey, 89 gallons of beer, or 31 gallons of wine per year. Heavy drinkers, who constitute 10 per cent of the drinking population in the United States (7 per cent of the total adult population), account for half of the alcohol consumed and nearly all of the socioeconomic and medical complications of alcoholism and alcohol abuse. In 1990 the estimated annual cost of these problems to American society was $136 billion. Alcoholism and alcohol abuse are encountered in all socioeconomic classes and cultural groups; it is estimated that the prevalence of alcohol-related problems among hospitalized patients is 25 per cent.

DEFINITIONS

Alcoholism is characterized by addiction to ethanol. Although there are behavioral and socioeconomic definitions of alcoholism, in a medical setting alcoholism refers to a chronic disease in which the alcoholic craves and consumes ethanol without satiation, becomes increasingly *tolerant* to the intoxicating effects of the drug, and, when drinking is discontinued, exhibits the symptoms and signs of withdrawal as evidence of *physical dependence* on ethanol. Alcoholism with ethanol dependence can also develop as a secondary complication of depression, bipolar affective disorder, or schizophrenia, but 80 per cent of alcoholics have alcoholism without prior evidence of major psychiatric problems (*primary alcoholism*). Individuals who drink prodigiously without evidence of physical dependence are considered to have *alcohol abuse*. They often continue excessive drinking, sometimes episodically *(binge drinking)*, despite significant personal socioeconomic hardship and medical complications.

GENETIC FACTORS

While environmental conditions influence drinking habits and the prevalence of alcoholism and alcohol abuse, there is also persuasive evidence that many individuals are at risk to develop alcoholism because of genetic factors. Alcoholism tends to run in families, and studies of alcoholism in identical twins, alcoholic parents and children, and offspring from alcoholic parents adopted into nondrinking families consistently suggest a genetically transmitted susceptibility for alcoholism. This is particularly evident for "male-limited" alcoholism in fathers and sons with antisocial, impulsive, novelty-seeking behavior, who become alcoholics in teenage years; they usually cannot abstain from drinking throughout life. Adoption studies indicate that this type of alcoholism in the biologic father is a much greater predictor for alcoholism in the son than is the environment in which the boy is raised. This is in contrast to other types of familial and nonfamilial alcoholism in which individuals may begin drinking as teenagers but become alcoholic later in life without an apparent genetic predisposition.

Such patients appear to have less difficulty in abstaining from alcohol once they develop motivation to stop drinking.

PHARMACOLOGY OF ETHANOL

ETHANOL ABSORPTION, DISTRIBUTION, AND ELIMINATION. Ethanol is absorbed rapidly and completely from the gastrointestinal tract and is detected in the blood within minutes of ingestion. Clinically significant amounts of vaporized alcohol can also be absorbed directly through the lungs. About 25 per cent of ethanol enters the bloodstream from the stomach and 75 per cent from the intestine, but many factors modify gastrointestinal absorption. These include food, the rate of drinking, the concentration, amount, and type of alcoholic beverage, and variations in gastrointestinal motility. For example, most foods in the stomach delay gastric absorption of ethanol, and pylorospasm due to high concentrations of alcohol in the stomach can slow gastric emptying and retard intestinal absorption. By contrast, rapid gastric emptying or gastrectomy causes increased rates of alcohol absorption from the small intestine.

Because of its solubility properties, ethanol readily crosses biologic membranes and equilibrates rapidly into total body water. Ninety to 98 per cent is removed by metabolism in the liver, and the remainder is excreted by the kidneys, lungs, and skin. Elimination follows zero-order kinetics and is independent of concentration; a 70-kg man can metabolize 5 to 10 grams of ethanol per hour. Since the average drink contains 12 to 15 grams of ethanol, blood alcohol levels continue to rise when an individual drinks at a rate greater than metabolism, but when drinking is discontinued, blood levels fall about 10 to 25 mg per deciliter per hour.

ETHANOL METABOLISM. Ethanol oxidation to acetaldehyde by alcohol dehydrogenase in the liver is the most clinically significant rate-limiting step, accounting for more than 90 per cent of ethanol metabolism in vivo. When blood alcohol concentrations are high, a microsomal ethanol oxidizing system can also generate acetaldehyde. Moreover, this second enzyme system mediates ethanol effects on drug metabolism in the liver (Ch. 118). Acetaldehyde is converted to acetate by aldehyde dehydrogenase, a metabolic step with important clinical ramifications. For example, 50 per cent of Japanese and other Asian people have a mutation in an aldehyde dehydrogenase isoenzyme which results in reduced enzyme activity in vivo. Shortly after drinking alcohol, affected individuals develop increased blood acetaldehyde levels and experience an *alcohol-flush* reaction, characterized by vasodilatation with facial flushing, hot sensations, tachycardia, and hypotension. These unpleasant experiences can act as a deterrent to drinking, and in Japan people with this mutation have a lower rate of alcoholism. Pharmacologic inhibition of aldehyde dehydrogenase causes even more severe aversive symptoms after drinking alcohol and is the reason why disulfiram (Antabuse) has been used to help discourage drinking. Disulfiram inhibits aldehyde dehydrogenase (and other sulfhydryl-containing enzymes), but it is not ordinarily toxic when taken therapeutically without ethanol. After drinking alcohol, however, patients on prophylactic disulfiram therapy have large increases in blood acetaldehyde levels and develop a more severe *acetaldehyde syndrome.* They can experience dysphoria, intense palpitations, sweating, thirst, throbbing headache, dyspnea, nausea and vomiting, weakness, vertigo, and syncope. Disulfiram does not cure alcoholism and is not widely used.

In peripheral tissues, acetate derived from acetaldehyde is converted to acetyl coenzyme A and subsequently to CO_2 and water. Complete oxidation of ethanol yields 7.1 kcal per gram, and some estimate that ethanol accounts for 10 per cent of the total caloric intake in the United States. Alcoholics often obtain 50 per cent of their calories from ethanol, and some develop serious nutritional deficiencies, particularly for protein, thiamine, folate, and pyridoxine (Table 14–1) (Ch. 204). Moreover, as a consequence of ethanol metabolism, alcoholics can develop hypoglycemia (Ch. 219), lactic acidosis (Ch. 75), hyperuricemia (Ch. 183), hypertriglyceridemia (Ch. 172), and ketoacidosis (Ch. 75) (Table 14–1).

ACUTE AND CHRONIC TOLERANCE TO ETHANOL. Tolerance develops after prolonged exposure to ethanol and is characterized by a reduced response to ethanol. When blood

TABLE 14–1. ALCOHOL-RELATED MEDICAL DISORDERS

Affected Organ or System	Disorder
Nutrition	Deficiencies of:
	Folate, thiamine, pyridoxine, niacin, and riboflavin
	Magnesium, zinc, calcium
	Protein
Brain	Hepatic encephalopathy
	Wernicke-Korsakoff syndrome
	Cerebral atrophy
	Amblyopia
	Central pontine myelinolysis
	Marchiafava-Bignami disease
Nerve	Neuropathy
Muscle	Myopathy
Liver	Fatty liver
	Hepatitis
	Cirrhosis
	Hepatoma
Heart	Hypertension
	Cardiomyopathy
	Arrhythmia
Blood	Anemia
	Leukopenia
	Thrombocytopenia
	Macrocytosis
Gut	Esophagitis and gastritis
	Pancreatitis
Metabolite and electrolytes	Hypoglycemia
	Hyperlipidemia
	Hyperuricemia
	Ketoacidosis
	Hypomagnesemia
	Hypophosphatemia
Endocrine	Pseudo-Cushing's syndrome
	Testicular atrophy
	Amenorrhea
Bone	Osteopenia

alcohol levels are no longer rising several hours after a drinking episode, normal subjects can appear to be sober at even higher alcohol concentrations that caused intoxication hours earlier. This phenomenon is known as *acute tolerance.* Similarly, chronic alcoholics have increased resistance to the intoxicating effects of ethanol and can even appear to be sober at blood alcohol levels of 400 to 500 mg per deciliter, concentrations known to produce stupor, coma, or death in naive individuals. This is known as *chronic tolerance.* Indeed, some chronic alcoholics can be so tolerant to ethanol as to survive blood alcohol concentrations as high as 1500 mg per deciliter. Thus, despite legal definitions of intoxication at blood alcohol levels above 100 mg per deciliter, a single blood ethanol determination may not accurately measure the extent of drunkenness.

ACUTE ETHANOL INTOXICATION

There is virtually no blood-brain barrier to ethanol; uptake into the brain is limited primarily by cerebral blood flow and capillary perfusion. Therefore, within a short period of time after drinking, the concentration of ethanol in the brain is nearly the same as the level of alcohol in the blood. In nonalcoholics, rising blood alcohol levels to 50 to 150 mg per deciliter are associated with increasing symptoms of intoxication (Table 14–2). Symptoms vary directly with the rate of drinking and are more severe when the blood alcohol concentration is rising than when it is falling. Most individuals feel euphoric, lose social inhibitions, and manifest expansive, sometimes garrulous behavior, whereas others may become gloomy, belligerent, or even explosively combative. Some people do not experience euphoria but instead become sleepy after moderate drinking; they rarely abuse alcohol. Neurologic signs of intoxication include impaired cognition, slurred

TABLE 14–2. BLOOD ETHANOL LEVELS AND SYMPTOMS

Blood Ethanol Levels (mg/dl)	Symptoms	
	Sporadic Drinkers	*Chronic Drinkers*
50–100	Euphoria Gregariousness Incoordination	Minimal or no effect
100–200	Slurred speech Ataxia Labile mood Drowsiness Nausea	Sobriety or incoordination Euphoria
200–300	Lethargic Combative Stuporous Incoherent speech Vomiting	Mild emotional and motor changes
300–400	Coma	Drowsiness
>500	Respiratory depression Death	Lethargy Stupor Coma

speech, incoordination, mild truncal ataxia, and slow or irregular eye movements. Signs of increased sympathetic activity include mydriasis, tachycardia, and skin flushing. The findings of central nervous system (CNS) depression predominate at higher blood alcohol concentrations. Cerebellar and vestibular function deteriorates, and drunkenness is characterized by dysarthria, more severe ataxia, nystagmus, and diplopia. Patients may become lethargic with bradycardia, reduced blood pressure, and diminished respirations, sometimes complicated by vomiting and pulmonary aspiration. In nonalcoholics, stupor and coma may develop at 400 mg per deciliter, and fatalities ensue at 500 mg per deciliter usually because of respiratory depression with ventilatory acidosis and hypotension. The LD_{30} for ethanol is approximately 450 mg per deciliter.

Alcoholic blackouts sometimes complicate acute alcohol intoxication during consumption of large amounts of ethanol. These episodes, which can occur in alcoholics or sporadic drinkers, are characterized by several hours of amnesia without impaired consciousness during the event. The patient reports an inability to remember new events but has no difficulty with long-term memory or immediate recall. These symptoms resemble the syndrome of transient global amnesia (Ch. 469).

EVALUATION AND MANAGEMENT. Severe acute alcohol intoxication can be fatal and is a medical emergency. The immediate history should include information about the quantity of alcohol consumed, the rate of drinking, use of other drugs including methanol, complicating medical and psychiatric disorders, and prior alcohol abuse or alcoholism. If the patient is stuporous and unable to walk, the airway must be evaluated immediately. Indications for endotracheal intubation and assisted ventilation include marked hypoventilation, accumulating secretions, and coma. In such patients, complications such as hypoglycemia, meningitis, and subdural hematoma must be considered. Evidence of head trauma or focal or lateralizing neurologic signs suggests urgent intracranial pathology, and a computed tomography (CT) scan should be performed immediately. Otherwise, routine CT scans for alcohol intoxication are not indicated. Gastric lavage may be performed if obtundation is due to recent and massive alcohol consumption, but only after endotracheal intubation. Hemodialysis should be considered if the blood ethanol level exceeds 600 mg per deciliter.

After a history and physical examination, patients with adequate vital signs, acceptable mental status, and no evidence of other disorders can be kept under observation until sobriety returns. However, medical information is usually incomplete, and it is often necessary to anticipate complications commonly associated with severe alcohol intoxication or alcoholism (see Table 14–1). Routine blood counts and chemistries will uncover anemia (Ch. 122), hypokalemia, hypophosphatemia, and hypomagnesemia (Ch. 75, 194, and 195). Alcoholic hypoglycemia (Ch. 219) can be evaluated rapidly by a bedside blood glucose determination. If

laboratory results are delayed, 12.5 to 25 grams of glucose should be given intravenously. Alcoholic ketoacidosis (Ch. 75) will be improved by infusion of 5 per cent dextrose in 0.5N saline. Elevated serum ammonia levels support the diagnosis of hepatic encephalopathy (Ch. 123). If the blood alcohol level is too low to account for the patient's obtundation or if improvement does not occur as expected, it is necessary to search for other causes of stupor and coma (Ch. 443).

ETHANOL WITHDRAWAL SYNDROME

Ethanol is a CNS depressant. In alcoholics, the nervous system appears to adapt to chronic ethanol exposure by increasing the activity of neural mechanisms that counteract alcohol's depressant effects. When drinking is abruptly reduced or discontinued, these stimulatory neural mechanisms are left unrestrained by ethanol, and a hyperexcitable *ethanol withdrawal syndrome* develops. This is evidence of *physical dependence* on ethanol. The ethanol withdrawal syndrome consists of several characteristic abnormalities that vary in severity. These include tremulousness, disordered perceptions, seizures, and delirium tremens (Table 14–3).

The general medical evaluation and management are as described for acute ethanol intoxication. One hundred milligrams of thiamine should be given parenterally to all patients undergoing ethanol withdrawal to prevent or treat Wernicke's encephalopathy (Ch. 456), followed by daily multivitamins. It is important to search for evidence of alcohol-related medical disorders (see Table 14–1) and the associated complications of alcohol abuse, as described earlier. The alarming symptoms of ethanol withdrawal are best managed by substituting another CNS depressant. However, alcoholics undergoing withdrawal are very resistant to sedatives (*cross-tolerance*), and large doses are often required to calm their agitation. The more specific forms of treatment are listed under the individual manifestations below.

TREMULOUSNESS. Tremor, the earliest, most common, and most apparent symptom, begins about 6 to 8 hours after the last drink, usually the morning after an overnight abstinence ("morning shakes"). Tremor is generalized, coarse, and rapid and is often accompanied by irritability, nausea, and vomiting. The patient usually senses an inner tremulousness even when tremor is not severe. Self-treatment commonly consists of a morning drink to "quiet the nerves," after which drinking is continued for the rest of the day. If the alcoholic does not resume drinking, tremor becomes much more intense by 24 to 36 hours and is exacerbated by motor activity or stress. It can be so severe as to interfere with walking, eating, or speech. Accompanying symptoms and signs of sympathetic hyperactivity are also apparent. The patient is increasingly anxious and easily startled by minor stimuli and complains of insomnia and anorexia. Increased sweating, facial flushing, mydriasis, tachycardia, and mild hypertension occur. Although most abnormalities subside in a few days, increased arousal and anxiety may persist for 2 weeks.

DISORDERED PERCEPTIONS. Disordered perceptions also accompany the development of tremor and sympathetic hyperactivity in approximately 25 per cent of tremulous patients. These symptoms similarly become most pronounced at 24 to 36 hours, before clearing in a few days. The patient frequently experiences vivid nightmares that interfere with sleep; ordinary visual, auditory, and tactile experiences may become distorted and misinterpreted during waking hours.

Sometimes alcoholics undergoing withdrawal develop isolated and more prolonged auditory hallucinations (*alcoholic hallucinosis*), despite being alert, oriented, and without memory loss. Hallucinations may continue for weeks even though other signs of ethanol withdrawal have improved and the patient is less agitated and tremulous. In the absence of sympathetic hyperactivity, persistent auditory hallucinations may be confused with acute schizophrenia (Ch. 456). However, alcoholic hallucinosis is

TABLE 14–3. ETHANOL WITHDRAWAL SYNDROME

8 hours	Tremulousness, anxiety, irritability, nausea, and vomiting
24 hours	Hyperexcitability, insomnia, disordered perceptions, convulsions
2–5 days	Delirium tremens

closely associated with ethanol withdrawal and usually subsides in weeks to months.

Benzodiazepines are widely used to manage tremulousness and disordered perceptions during ethanol withdrawal. The goal is to suppress symptoms and produce mild sedation, and drug dosage is adjusted to the severity of the withdrawal reaction. Patients with mild tremulousness and few associated symptoms usually respond to oral diazepam, 5 to 10 mg every 4 to 6 hours. Dosage is then reduced by 20 to 25 per cent on successive days, or increased if symptoms of ethanol withdrawal return. Diazepam is used intravenously if symptoms are severe, and some patients may require extraordinarily high doses to achieve mild sedation. Once the symptoms of ethanol withdrawal are suppressed, it is necessary to avoid oversedation and the danger of respiratory depression by carefully titrating the dose of diazepam to just keep the patient calm.

ETHANOL WITHDRAWAL SEIZURES. Five to 33 per cent of alcoholics develop generalized tonic-clonic convulsions, most often within 12 to 24 hours after reducing or discontinuing alcohol consumption. Ethanol withdrawal seizures characterize ethanol dependence in experimental animals, and mice have been bred to be genetically prone to develop convulsions during withdrawal, suggesting that genetic factors could be important in humans. An alternate view is that the first seizure in alcoholics may be a consequence of ethanol toxicity. Ethanol withdrawal seizures are usually associated with a history of chronic daily drinking, but 5- to 7-day episodes of binge drinking can also be followed by convulsions. Seizures may be one to six in number and usually occur within a 6-hour period. Alcoholics who have seizures during one episode of ethanol withdrawal are likely to have convulsions again when alcohol withdrawal is repeated. Focal seizures are less common and should always suggest a focal lesion and an additional diagnosis. Status epilepticus occurs in about 3 per cent of cases, and ethanol withdrawal accounts for about 15 per cent of all patients who present with status epilepticus (Ch. 483).

Most ethanol withdrawal convulsions are brief and self-limited. However, a complete evaluation for a convulsive disorder is indicated (Ch. 483) if there is a clinical suspicion of other CNS disorders, if the patient has focal seizures, if there are more than six seizures, if the convulsions persist beyond 6 hours, or if the postictal state is prolonged. Typical ethanol withdrawal seizures do not require specific anticonvulsant therapy; phenytoin does not prevent recurrent seizures in these patients. However, status epilepticus from any cause is a medical emergency and requires immediate treatment with anticonvulsants as described in Ch. 483.

DELIRIUM TREMENS. Delirium tremens, the most alarming manifestation of the ethanol withdrawal syndrome, occurs in about 5 per cent of such patients. It is characterized by agitated arousal, global confusion and disorientation, insomnia, and vivid, often threatening hallucinations and delusions. Signs of sympathetic hyperactivity include tremor, mydriasis, tachycardia, fever, and intense diaphoresis. In contrast to tremulousness, disordered perceptions, and seizures, which appear earlier after withdrawal, delirium tremens begins abruptly within 2 to 4 days of abstinence, often as a surprising development in unrecognized alcoholics who have been admitted to the hospital for other reasons. These patients are terrified by their hallucinations and can be combative, destructive, and very dangerous. Episodes of delirium tremens last from one to three days and end as abruptly as they begin. However, relapses can occur and the disorder may continue for days to weeks with intervening periods of lucidity.

Delirium tremens requires hospitalization and vigorous emergency treatment. When there are no signs of sympathetic hyperactivity, it may be difficult to distinguish delirium tremens from an acute psychosis. However, the diagnosis is usually suggested by the evolution of symptoms in a chronic alcoholic undergoing withdrawal. The differential diagnosis includes alcoholic hypoglycemia, overdose with anticholinergic agents, intoxication with amphetamines, cocaine, and phencyclidine (PCP), encephalitis, meningitis, thyrotoxicosis, and withdrawal from other sedating drugs. Seizures are unusual in delirium tremens and should be evaluated promptly because of the possibility of meningitis or other diagnoses. Mortality can reach 15 per cent, primarily because of injuries or associated medical disorders complicated by hyperthermia and dehydration. Volume depletion accompanying delirium tremens may cause circulatory collapse, and fluid losses can require replacement of 4 to 10 liters in the first day. The goal of treatment is to control behavior and suppress symptoms without danger to the patient. Five to 10 mg or more of diazepam is given intravenously every 5 to 15 minutes until the patient is calm, and maintenance therapy is continued every 1 to 4 hours, as needed. Initially, as much as 200 mg of diazepam may be required before agitation subsides, and some patients may need up to 1200 mg in the first 3 to 4 days of treatment to keep calm.

RECOGNITION AND REHABILITATION OF ALCOHOLICS

Most alcoholics rarely admit to problem drinking and are often not recognized by their primary care physicians. Instead, alcoholics are usually identified because of the adverse socioeconomic consequences of heavy drinking or the development of medical complications and the alcohol-related disorders (see Table 14–1) which bring them to medical attention. After several days of detoxification under medical supervision, the patient should be referred to a rehabilitation program because alcoholism and alcohol abuse can rarely be treated by the physician alone. The patient needs encouragement to develop a high level of motivation to stop drinking and to adjust to a life without alcohol. The most successful treatment usually requires active participation of family members, friends, and peers, and the prognosis is best for alcoholics who enter treatment programs before the onset of associated medical disorders. Many patients and families find local support groups such as Alcoholics Anonymous and Al-Anon to be very helpful, and about 50 to 70 per cent of socially stable, middle-class alcoholics can achieve abstinence. However, this success rate is not attributable to a specific kind of rehabilitation scheme.

Adinoff B, Bone GHA, Linnoila M: Acute ethanol poisoning and the ethanol withdrawal syndrome. Med Toxicol 3:172, 1988. *An extensive discussion of the presentation and management of ethanol intoxication and withdrawal.*

Goldstein DB: Pharmacology of Alcohol. New York, Oxford University Press, 1983. *An excellent introduction to the principles of ethanol pharmacology.*

Kiianmaa K, Tabakoff B, Saito T (eds.): Genetic Aspects of Alcoholism. Helsinki, The Finnish Foundation for Alcohol Studies, 1989. *This book includes a series of brief presentations about the major issues concerning the genetics of alcoholism and the characteristics of low-risk and high-risk individuals.*

Porter R, Mattson R, Kramer J, et al. (eds.): Alcohol and Seizures: Basic Mechanisms and Clinical Concepts. Philadelphia, F.A. Davis, 1990. *This book focuses on the pathogenesis and management of ethanol withdrawal seizures.*

Seventh Special Report to the U.S. Congress on Alcohol and Health. U.S. Dept. of Health and Human Services. Rockville, Md., National Institute on Alcohol Abuse and Alcoholism, 1990. *An excellent comprehensive discussion of the major socioeconomic and biomedical problems of alcoholism and alcohol abuse.*

15 Drug Abuse and Dependence

Charles P. O'Brien

In the 1990's substance abuse is found in all strata of American society. The average physician is likely to encounter many patients exhibiting behavioral or medical complications of licit or illicit drug use, but the relationship of the symptoms to drugs often goes unrecognized. Early diagnosis, which is critical for effective treatment, is difficult because at an early stage patients rarely fit the addict stereotype.

Clinicians have been mainly concerned with tolerance and physical dependence. *Tolerance* is the result of a homeostatic process in which the body adapts to the repeated effects of a drug. This adaptation tends to compensate for the pharmacologic effects of the drug with the result that higher doses are required to achieve a drug effect. With daily dosing, tolerance increases and a state of physical dependence can occur. *Physical dependence* is diagnosed by the presence of a rebound known as a *withdrawal syndrome* that follows interruption of dosing. Withdrawal phenomena tend to be opposite to the effects of the drugs themselves. Thus a drug that produces sedation is marked by hyperreflexia and irritability during withdrawal, and a stimulant drug is followed by weakness and depression during withdrawal.

Changes in *behavior* are the pivotal diagnostic criteria for drug dependence. While tolerance and physical dependence have been emphasized in the past, *intermittent* use that does not cause tolerance or a withdrawal syndrome may produce behavioral or social consequences urgently requiring treatment. *Drug abuse* is therefore defined as a maladaptive pattern in the use of any substance which persists despite adverse social, psychological, or medical consequences. The pattern of abuse may be intermittent and the condition does not meet the criteria for dependence. *Drug dependence* is a behavioral syndrome that involves compulsive drug-taking, neglect of constructive activities, and adverse social effects and *may* include pharmacologic tolerance and physical dependence.

RECOGNITION. Since early diagnosis is so important, the physician should have a low threshold for including drug abuse in the differential diagnosis of any patient. The abuse pattern that presents the most difficulty is that of a successful middle-class adult whose substance abuse is detected incidental to a routine physical examination or during treatment of an unrelated disorder. Invariably the patient denies that drug or alcohol abuse is a problem. Physicians must be aware that denial of problems and minimizing of the drug or alcohol use are fundamental aspects of the syndrome. These patients usually do not admit to a problem until it becomes so severe that there is no alternative, by which time treatment is much more difficult.

The diagnosis of drug abuse or dependence is basically a clinical diagnosis. The physician should use all available information, including the patient's history, information from relatives or employer, physical examination, and laboratory tests. Blood or urine tests showing the presence of drugs or their metabolites can be useful but also misleading. The toxicologic tests, when properly done and confirmed, indicate use within a varying period of time depending on the drug and its dose. Such tests do not disclose pattern of use or the presence of dependence. Metabolites of some drugs, such as marijuana or cocaine, remain in the urine for at least several days following a single dose. Thus the tests require interpretation and integration with other clinical information.

Clues discovered on the physical examination include the presence of scars from numerous intravenous injections ("tracks") or edema of the arms and veins that are difficult to find. Chronic sinusitis or a scarred and perhaps perforated nasal septum suggests "snorting" of cocaine, a powerful vasoconstrictor. Frequent injuries due to falls or auto accidents are seen in sedative abusers as well as alcoholics. Infections such as abscesses, hepatitis, respiratory infections, and endocarditis are well-known risks of drug abuse. The most devastating disease associated with drug abuse is acquired immunodeficiency syndrome (AIDS), and intravenous drug users now represent more than 25 per cent of cases of HIV infection.

Physicians must also be alert to the signs of drug abuse in order to avoid unwittingly prescribing medication that will perpetuate the dependence. Patients taking sleeping medications, pain medications, or antianxiety agents on a chronic basis may visit several physicians in order to obtain a larger drug supply. Others deliberately feign illness, particularly pain syndromes. Some will have read textbooks and recite classic descriptions of acute renal calculus, migraine headache, or pancreatitis. Physicians should be particularly wary of patients who ask for a specific medication or who claim to have an "allergy" to non-narcotic pain medication.

American Psychiatric Association: Diagnostic and Statistical Manual of Mental Disorders, 3rd ed. rev. Washington, D.C., American Psychiatric Association, 1987, pp 165–186. *Clear summary of the new diagnostic criteria for dependence on alcohol and other drugs.*

Jaffe J: Drug addiction and drug abuse. *In* Gilman AG, Goodman LS, Rall TR, et al. (eds.): The Pharmacological Basis of Therapeutics. 8th ed. New York, Pergamon Press, 1990. *Thorough discussion of pharmacologic and clinical aspects of drug abuse.*

Smith DE (ed.): Addiction medicine. West J Med 152:499, 1990. *A special issue that contains 21 articles covering many general topics relating to drug abuse and dependence.*

SEDATIVES

Examples of sedatives include the following:
Ethanol
Barbiturates
Diazepam (Valium)
Alprazolam (Xanax)
Flurazepam (Dalmane)
Lorazepam (Ativan)
Meprobamate (Miltown)
Glutethimide (Doriden)

These drugs are central nervous system depressants and all are capable of producing abuse, tolerance, and physical dependence. Their withdrawal syndromes are generally similar, although the sedatives come from different chemical categories (e.g., alcohol, barbiturate, benzodiazepine). Their effects are additive, and they are often used in combination. This aspect is particularly important in considering interactions with alcohol (Ch. 14) and in treating patients who are dependent on multiple sedatives with different durations of action.

Patterns of Abuse

There are two basic patterns of sedative drug abuse other than that with alcohol: One is produced inadvertently by taking prescription sedatives without proper concern for their potential to produce dependence, and the second involves deliberate use of sedatives to obtain a "high."

PRESCRIPTION SEDATIVES. The problem of improper use of prescription sedatives is a concern to all physicians because they are among the most widely prescribed of all drugs throughout the world. They have legitimate medical uses in the short-term treatment of insomnia or anxiety and in the long-term treatment of seizure disorders. The chronic use of medication for insomnia, however, often leads to problems because insomnia is merely a symptom. It may signal the presence of an underlying illness, or it may simply require a change in activity patterns, but the chronic use of sedatives simply adds a new problem. After daily use for several weeks, tolerance develops and sleep difficulties may return, often in a modified form. The patient may have become dependent, however, on the daily ingestion of the sedative. If the drug is stopped, a rebound occurs, with the appearance of symptoms worse than those experienced prior to treatment. Sedatives are not equal in their tendency to produce this iatrogenic insomnia. Long-acting benzodiazepines, for example, are unlikely to produce rebound effects at usual doses. Other liabilities are associated with their use, however, such as "hangover" effects, which produce subtle neuropsychological deficits and may mimic dementia in older persons. On balance, insomnia should not be treated with drugs except for brief periods of time.

Another pattern associated with the prescription of sedatives is that found in the treatment of anxiety. Benzodiazepines (e.g., diazepam, alprazolam) are the most effective medications available for the treatment of anxiety, and they produce relatively less sedation than older medications used for this purpose, such as meprobamate or phenobarbital. Symptoms of anxiety are widespread; one survey found that about 15 per cent of all Americans received a prescription for one of these drugs in a single year. While some argue that this suggests overprescribing, it is not out of line with experiences in other western countries.

Approximately 6 per cent of the population take benzodiazepines chronically, and this leads to *tolerance* and *physical dependence*. This does not imply a similar prevalence of *abuse* because the patient may be taking the benzodiazepine for a legitimate anxiety disorder. It does mean, however, that since the patient perceives less sedation, there may be a tendency to increase the dose. It also implies that the patient should be warned about withdrawal symptoms if the drug is terminated abruptly. Occasionally, a patient who allows a prescription for a short-acting benzodiazepine to run out is brought to an emergency room because of benzodiazepine withdrawal seizures. Some of these patients are mislabeled "addicts," even though the patient has never used more of the antianxiety medication than was prescribed. Others, however, become deliberate abusers of sedatives after beginning treatment for anxiety under a doctor's care and may purposely increase their dose while obtaining medication from several different physicians. Benzodiazepines in general have a relatively low abuse potential, but their use should be avoided or severely limited in patients with a history of alcoholism or other forms of drug abuse.

DELIBERATE SEDATIVE ABUSE. Sedatives are used at parties by groups of abusers, usually adolescents and young adults, to obtain a "high." The "high" appears to be a form of disinhibition or release and depends partially on the setting in which the drug is taken. As with alcohol, increasing the dose produces depression and eventual loss of consciousness. A dangerous aspect of sedative abuse is that tolerance to the sought-after subjective effects rapidly develops, but tolerance to the depressant effects on the brain stem remains low. As the experienced user increases the dose to obtain a "high," he or she may unexpectedly reach the dose that depresses vital functions and threatens survival.

Abstinence Syndrome

The withdrawal syndrome following sedative dependence is similar to alcohol withdrawal (described in Ch. 14). Among the sedatives, the syndrome varies in onset, duration, and severity with the dose and duration of action of the drug used and the duration of daily use. The long-acting benzodiazepines, such as diazepam, may have a withdrawal syndrome whose onset is delayed for several days following the termination of the drug. At doses within the therapeutic range, withdrawal symptoms may consist of only mild irritability, complaints of peculiar sensations, diaphoresis, and sleep disturbance accompanied by rebound increases in rapid eye movement (REM) sleep. The symptoms may be similar to the anxiety symptoms for which the drug was initially prescribed. At higher doses, the sedative withdrawal syndrome is more severe and can be life-threatening. Major abnormalities include paroxysmal electroencephalographic (EEG) abnormalities, generalized seizures, and a toxic psychosis similar to delirium tremens. Restlessness, anxiety, tremulousness, and weakness occur, often accompanied by orthostatic hypotension, nausea, cramps, and vomiting. Irritability, anxiety, photophobia, depressive symptoms, and neuropsychological deficits may persist for weeks or months.

Treatment

The acute withdrawal syndrome should be considered a serious medical illness usually requiring inpatient treatment. Close monitoring for cardiac arrhythmias or seizures is necessary. Several detoxification techniques are available, each requiring the substitution of a prescribed sedative with cross-tolerance for the drug on which the patient is dependent. The physician should not simply accept the history but rather determine the level of dependence by giving a test dose of a known sedative, such as diazepam or pentobarbital. If the patient shows no evidence of slurred speech or sedation after a test dose of 20 to 40 mg of diazepam, a higher level of dependence is indicated, and the daily sedative dose should be adjusted accordingly. Gradual detoxification using diazepam can be accomplished over 1 to 3 weeks, although in some treatment centers where diazepam is the object of much drug-seeking behavior and manipulation by patients, phenobarbital is preferred. Patients dependent on both a short-acting sedative, such as alcohol, and a long-acting drug, such as diazepam, should be watched for a biphasic withdrawal. The alcohol withdrawal peaks and subsides during the first week, but the diazepam withdrawal may not be evident until early in the second week. Patients dependent on both an opioid, such as heroin, and a sedative should be maintained on a low dose of methadone until the sedative withdrawal is completed. After detoxification, the patient must be put in a treatment program to prevent recurrence, as described at the end of this chapter.

American Psychiatric Association: Benzodiazepine Dependence, Toxicity and Abuse, APA Task Force Report. Washington, D.C., American Psychiatric Association, 1990. *Excellent review of the data concerning the use and risks of benzodiazepines with practical prescribing guidelines.*

O'Brien CP, Woody GE: Sedative hypnotic and anti-anxiety agents. In Frances AJ, Hales R (eds.): American Psychiatric Association Annual Review, Vol 5, Washington, D.C., APA Press, 1986, pp 186–199. *Review of diagnosis, treatment, and prevention of sedative abuse.*

STIMULANTS

Examples of stimulants include the following:
Cocaine
Dextroamphetamine
Methamphetamine
Methylphenidate (Ritalin)
Phenmetrazine (Preludin)
Diethylpropion (Tepanil)

Patterns of Abuse

Cocaine became the major drug of abuse in the United States, excluding alcohol, during the 1980's. At present, attitudes toward the use of cocaine have become more negative among high school seniors, but overall use has not yet significantly declined. Despite increased efforts at federal interdiction, cocaine supplies in the United States have increased so rapidly that the price has become low. Not only is cocaine available to a wider market, especially children, but its sellers have developed clever new and efficient ways to administer cocaine, increasing its potency and danger.

Until recently, cocaine hydrochloride was available as a white powder through illicit channels in an adulterated form and at a cost so high that only the affluent could afford to use it regularly. The typical mode of administration was "snorting," which consists of application of the powder to the nasal mucous membranes. Intravenous injection of an aqueous solution was also used, resulting in a more rapid onset and greater likelihood of seizures. Inhalation of the "free base" alkaloid form of cocaine has more recently been found to be the most convenient and efficient system for delivering the drug to the brain. During the mid-1980's, dealers began supplying a mass-produced solid form of "free base" called "crack." "Crack" is produced by sodium bicarbonate extraction of cocaine hydrochloride; the agent can be sold in small yellow-white lumps for as little as $5 to $10 per dose. When heated in a small pipe, the resulting cocaine vapor can be inhaled, producing a brief and very intense "high." This drug is clearly the *most addicting substance* yet encountered by clinicians. Dependence in the behavioral sense can be produced very rapidly, perhaps in days and certainly in weeks. Users may administer the drug continuously for several days without eating or sleeping. The widespread availability of "crack," its cheap price, and its tendency to produce dependence have led to problems in all strata of society.

The sought-after effect of cocaine is an intense "high" or euphoria, which is often described in sexual terms but is claimed to be "better than sex." The euphoria may last only a few minutes, depending on the dose and mode of administration. The aftereffect is one of depression and craving for more cocaine. During a period of regular cocaine use, the person becomes irritable and suspicious. High doses may result in persecutory delusions or hallucinations, but these are more common with longer-acting stimulants such as amphetamines. Families and friends of chronic cocaine users often note personality changes not observed by the users themselves. Alcohol, sedatives, opioids, and marijuana are often taken concurrently to combat the anxiety and irritability experienced by those using cocaine regularly. Users deprived of cocaine experience intense craving, depression, apathy, fatigue, and sleepiness.

Amphetamines and related drugs have a longer duration of action than cocaine, but many of the effects are similar. Dextroamphetamine has been used by physicians for a variety of conditions, including weight reduction, narcolepsy, and attention deficit disorder. Amphetamines have not been shown to be of value in weight reduction programs, and their use for all purposes has been curtailed by legal restrictions. In the early 1990's, a new street drug consisting of crystalline methamphetamine ("ice") has been reported. Like "crack," this drug can be heated and inhaled, thus producing a longer-lasting and potentially more dangerous state of intoxication. Because stimulants produce effects that are mostly pleasant, patients have a tendency to increase the dose and to take them longer than the prescribing physician intended. Tolerance develops rapidly to the stimulant effects of amphetamines, but with higher doses, toxic effects are common. These effects can resemble acute paranoid schizophrenia with delusions and hallucinations. Cessation of use of amphetamines produces a withdrawal syndrome similar to that after cocaine use and depressive symptoms that may continue for several months.

The milder stimulants, such as methylphenidate and phenmetrazine, rarely are associated with abuse problems, but they should be prescribed only when specifically indicated and with awareness of their abuse potential.

Lange RA, Cigarroa RG, Yancy CW Jr, et al.: Cocaine-induced coronary-artery vasoconstriction. N Engl J Med 321:1557, 1989. *Excellent study of the effects of cocaine on cardiac function.*

Pharmacology

Cocaine has several effects, but the critical action for abuse potential appears to be the blocking of reuptake of dopamine at central synapses, thus increasing the effects of synaptic dopamine. Systemic effects of cocaine and amphetamine include increased cardiac contraction, increased blood pressure and heart rate, dilated pupils, constriction of peripheral blood vessels, rise in body temperature, relaxation of the bronchial musculature, and increases in central venous pressure, pulmonary arterial pressure, and renal blood flow. Cocaine is an effective topical local anesthetic and vasoconstrictor of mucous membranes. Low doses of stimulants increase alertness and physical and cognitive ability. Stimulants do reduce appetite, but significant tolerance develops to this effect. When stimulants are discontinued, a rebound increase in weight often leaves the person heavier than before the drug was taken.

Heavy users report acute tolerance to the euphorigenic effects of cocaine when the drug is used repeatedly at a single occasion. However, a day or two later, a "high" can again be obtained at approximately the same dose as previously. Tolerance to the respiratory and cardiac stimulatory effects of cocaine does occur. Although abrupt cessation of stimulant use produces a distinct withdrawal syndrome as described above, it is generally limited to *behavioral* evidence of brain dysfunction rather than reflected in the presence of physical signs. During the excessive periods of sleep seen during withdrawal, the EEG shows a significant increase in the proportion of REM sleep and nightmares may occur. Rarely, withdrawal has been marked by headaches, profuse sweating, muscle cramps, disorientation, and confusion.

Adverse Effects

The most common adverse effect of cocaine use is loss of control, so that a severe dependence syndrome occurs with neglect of all constructive activities. *Acute cocaine toxicity* is dose related and is characterized by sympathomimetic effects, including tachycardia, hypertension, hyperthermia, and arrhythmias, and is followed by seizures, brain stem depression, and cardiorespiratory collapse. Stroke, coma, intracranial vasculitis, myocardial infarction, and sudden death have each occasionally occurred as complications of cocaine binges. At lower doses the acute toxic effects may be marked by a brief period of paranoid behavior with hallucinations. *Acute amphetamine toxicity* is also characterized by excessive sympathomimetic stimulation. There may be stereotyped compulsive behavior, tactile hallucinations consisting of "bugs" crawling under the skin, and visual or auditory hallucinations.

Chronic use of intranasal cocaine commonly causes ulceration or perforation of the nasal septum. Chronic users are typically debilitated and subject to infections as a result of neglect of hygiene, lack of sleep, and poor nutrition. There is evidence of neuronal degeneration in dopamine-rich areas of the brains of animals treated chronically with amphetamine. This raises the possibility of an increased risk for later development of Parkinson's disease. Schizophrenic disorders have been reported to be increased in chronic stimulant users. Chronic cocaine use among pregnant women results in a high incidence of premature, low birth weight, and neurologically abnormal infants.

Treatment

Treatment of the anxiety reactions and irritability produced by cocaine or amphetamines can be accomplished with benzodiazepines. Acute psychotic reactions may require haloperidol if amphetamines are involved, but reactions produced by cocaine are usually self-limiting. Withdrawal from stimulant dependence requires a supportive environment and protection from the supply of cocaine. Intense craving for cocaine is the most prominent of the withdrawal symptoms, although severe fatigue and depression may occur. The most difficult aspect of treatment is to prevent relapse when the patient returns to his or her normal environment and is confronted with opportunities to re-establish the habit. This aspect of treatment is discussed at the end of this chapter.

Gawin FH, Ellinwood EH: Cocaine and other stimulants. N Engl J Med 318:1173, 1988. *Review of clinical and pharmacologic aspects of stimulant abuse.*

OPIOIDS

Examples of opioids include the following:

Agonists

Morphine
Methadone
Meperidine (Demerol)
Oxycodone (Percodan)
Propoxyphene (Darvon)
Heroin
Hydromorphone (Dilaudid)
Fentanyl (Sublimaze)
Codeine

Mixed agonist-antagonists

Pentazocine (Talwin)
Nalbuphine (Nubain)
Buprenorphine (Buprenex)
Butorphanol (Stadol)

Antagonists

Naloxone (Narcan)
Naltrexone (Trexan)

Opiates are derivatives of the opium poppy plant, which contains more than 20 alkaloids. Heroin, morphine, and codeine are examples of commonly used *opiates*. Synthetic drugs that act via opiate receptors in the body are called *opioids*. The body also produces peptides that act at these receptors as neurohormones or neurotransmitters and are called *endogenous opioids* (Ch. 209).

Patterns of Abuse

Opioid abuse has been a problem in the United States for well over 100 years. The patterns have changed considerably since the turn of the century, when most opium-dependent persons were either Civil War veterans or users of patent medicines. Currently two abuse patterns exist in this country. The smaller group by far involves those patients initially treated by a physician for a legitimate pain problem with opioid drugs. The pain may become chronic and the dose is increased, usually at the patient's demand. The treatment may have begun with a relatively weak medication, such as propoxyphene or pentazocine, but it tends to progress through to the more potent opioids, such as oxycodone or hydromorphone. Prescriptions may be refilled excessively, and patients may visit more than one physician for medication or frequent emergency rooms. Such individuals vehemently deny being addicts; they are just seeking relief of pain. On closer examination, however, they are usually found to have symptoms of anxiety or depression that are temporarily relieved by opioids.

The second pattern is that of intentional misuse of opioids for their euphoria-producing ability. Intermittent heroin use, primarily among males in the inner city, typically begins during adolescence, and dependence ensues within a year or two of first use. Development in all areas—educational, social, occupational, and even psychosexual—is curtailed by use of heroin. It is not known how many people begin experimenting with heroin and stop using it. Those who continue to use heroin develop tolerance to its euphorigenic effects, continue to increase the dose, and soon find that they must use the drug daily to avoid withdrawal symptoms even while chasing that elusive first "high."

Older users tend to introduce younger ones to heroin and to techniques of crime required to support the "habit." Street heroin available in the United States tends to be diluted many times so that there may be an average of only 4 to 10 mg of heroin in a typical 100-mg bag. Furthermore, the heroin on the street at any given time may be more or less potent, depending on the supply and the pressure from law enforcement agencies. Most street heroin users have relatively mild degrees of physical dependence in terms of number of milligrams of heroin or its equivalent in morphine or methadone per day. Heroin-dependent persons, although they insist that they are seeking a "high," actually fear withdrawal and go to great lengths to obtain sufficient drug to inject themselves one to three times per day.

Some heroin users discover that prescription medications are more reliable than street drugs because the latter have no quality control. Hydromorphone, a very potent opioid, cannot be distinguished from heroin even by experienced users under double-blind conditions. Addicts may visit physicians or emergency rooms and feign pain syndromes to obtain opioids. Occasionally, unscrupulous physicians may simply sell prescriptions for whatever the addict requests. A few addicts have had prescription pads printed with their own name and a false Drug Enforcement Agency (DEA) number in an effort to trick pharmacists. Some of the prescription drugs prized on the street are not even the more potent ones.

In recent years heroin dependence has spread from inner-city to middle-class populations. The same supply system that distributes cocaine and marijuana also makes heroin available. Some educated and employed persons seeking a "thrill" prefer the effects of heroin. Others learn to use heroin to combat some of the unpleasant anxiety and irritability produced by chronic cocaine use.

Pharmacology

Opioids act at specific receptors that are widely distributed throughout the body in virtually all major organ systems. Since these receptors are heavily represented in the endocrine, cardiovascular, gastrointestinal, and nervous systems (Ch. 209), the effects of opioids are many and varied. The potency of individual drugs appears to depend on receptor affinity as well as metabolism. Heroin, for example, is diacetylmorphine, which has high lipid solubility and enters the brain rapidly. It is hydrolyzed to morphine, which is the form active at opiate receptors. Other opioids have similar systemic effects but reach brain receptors less rapidly. The mixed agonist-antagonist drugs, such as pentazocine, butorphanol, and nalbuphine, appear to act as agonists at kappa opiate receptors, but they also act as antagonists at mu (morphine) receptors. Thus, pentazocine can relieve pain on its own but, if given to someone already receiving morphine, displaces the morphine and precipitates withdrawal symptoms. Pure antagonists, such as naloxone and naltrexone, have no opiate-like effects, but they can reverse overdose and precipitate withdrawal if given *after* an opioid and prevent opiate effects if given *before* the opioid.

After heroin injection, traces of morphine can be found in the urine for about 12 to 48 hours, depending on the dose and the laboratory detection technique. Quinine, a common adulterant of street heroin, persists longer, but it is also found in legal substances such as tonic water. Parenteral injections of morphine or methadone have equal analgesic effects and persist for 4 to 6 hours, whereas heroin is three times as potent, and meperidine and codeine are one tenth as potent as morphine. Codeine, meperidine, and methadone remain active when taken orally, and the duration of action of methadone is extended considerably when taken orally. For prevention of withdrawal in dependent persons, methadone remains active for 24 to 30 hours, far longer than its analgesic effect.

Opioids appear to produce a state in which the patient can still feel pain but is less bothered by it. This state is produced, at least in part, by activation of an endogenous pain control system mediated via opiate receptors. Inhibition of pain sensation occurs at the spinal level as well as within the brain. Opioids are much more effective for clinical pain with anxiety than for experimental pain in research subjects. Opioids produce a reduction in anxiety, some sedation, and a feeling of well-being or euphoria. This effect seems important to both their clinical usefulness and their abuse potential. It is this euphoria that is sought by street addicts and that probably leads some medical patients to abuse prescribed opioids.

Tolerance to the euphoric effects of opioids develops rapidly, resulting in a tendency for users to increase their dose if possible. Only partial tolerance develops to other effects, such as pupillary constriction, inhibition of gastrointestinal contractions, and suppression of anterior pituitary function.

Adverse Effects

Acute opioid overdose occurs when a user inadvertently injects a much higher dose than expected. This also can be seen when a previously tolerant person returns to opioid use after a long interval, so that most of his tolerance has been lost. Many of the "overdoses" found with street heroin are now thought to have been due to a reaction to some of the adulterants rather than to the opiate. Acute reactions to adulterants including quinine, allergic reactions, and synergistic interactions among several drugs used simultaneously may produce the *acute heroin reaction*. The syndrome is marked clinically by the rapid development of cyanosis, pulmonary edema, respiratory distress, and altered levels of consciousness progressing to coma. Increased intracranial pressure and occasionally seizures are seen. Fever to 40°C may occur initially and persist for 48 hours in association with leukocytosis. The pupils are usually pinpoint, although dilated, nonreactive pupils may occur with hypoxia or use of multiple drugs. The pathologic picture includes pulmonary congestion and edema and frequently cerebral edema.

Opioids themselves are surprisingly nontoxic even when used in substantial daily doses for many years. Partial tolerance develops to their pharmacologic effects on the endocrine system. Thus females on methadone initially are amenorrheic, but the cycle usually returns in 6 to 12 months. Cortisol, luteinizing hormone, and testosterone are depressed while the patient is on methadone. Sexual response may be delayed; sperm count and ejaculate volume are reduced. Since street heroin users tend to have frequent periods of partial withdrawal, their endocrine systems are in turmoil. In contrast, a level dose of methadone induces some order, and the effects are reversible when the opioid is terminated. Chronic constipation may persist throughout opioid use.

The major adverse effects of opioid use come from the adulterants found in street drugs and the nonsterile practices typically followed by users. Skin abscesses, cellulitis, and thrombophlebitis are the most frequent complications. Pentazocine injection causes chronic ulcers and sclerosis of muscle in the area of injection. Septicemia and bacterial endocarditis with involvement of either or both sides of the heart are seen. *Staphylococcus aureus* is frequently the causative agent in right-sided endocarditis. Peripheral and pulmonary embolic phenomena occur.

Viral hepatitis has long been common among intravenous drug abusers owing to the practice of sharing needles during an injection session. More recently this illness has been overshadowed by the appearance of AIDS. In 1990, up to 60 per cent of patients in methadone programs in some large cities tested positive for HIV antibodies, and it has been suggested that this group is particularly susceptible to the infection because the drugs may suppress host resistance. Intravenous drug abusers tend to persist in high-risk practices such as needle-sharing and unprotected sex despite knowledge of the danger.

Among applicants for drug abuse treatment, 75 to 80 per cent of heroin users have significantly abnormal liver function tests. These findings may be related to persistent chronic hepatitis, but alcohol, malnutrition, allergic phenomena, and the toxic effects of adulterants may contribute. Pulmonary complications include pneumonia, abscess, infarct, and tuberculosis. Disseminated extrapulmonary tuberculosis has been reported. Angiothrombotic pulmonary hypertension and granulomatosis result from the intravenous injection of foreign bodies, including talc or cotton. Other complications include nephropathy, local arterial occlusion, phlebitis, mycotic aneurysms, and necrotizing angiitis.

Neurologic complications of street heroin use include transverse myelitis, acute inflammatory polyneuropathy, peripheral nerve lesions, toxic amblyopia secondary to quinine, and muscle disorders, including acute rhabdomyolysis with myoglobinuria and a fibrosing chronic myopathy. Septic states may lead to bacterial meningitis and brain, subdural, and epidural abscesses. Tetanus may result from dirty needles.

Pregnant addicts have a high incidence of toxemia and premature deliveries. About 50 per cent of their newborns require treatment of withdrawal symptoms.

Treatment

More distinctly different kinds of treatment are available for dependence on opioid drugs than for any other type of drug dependence. As with other drugs, the prevention of relapse to drug-seeking behavior is the most difficult aspect, as described later. The treatment of *acute overdose* is effective and straightforward. In any emergency situation in which opioid overdose is suspected, naloxone should be administered, preferably intravenously. The patient will have constricted pupils, and a dose of 0.4 mg naloxone should cause an increase in pupil size, respiratory rate, and alertness within several minutes. Repeated doses may be necessary if the patient does not respond within several minutes to the first dose. Absence of a response to naloxone excludes the diagnosis of opioid overdose.

There is virtually no risk in giving naloxone, but the potential benefits mean that it should be tried even in doubtful cases. Two pitfalls should be mentioned, however. One is that naloxone not only reverses the overdose but also goes beyond mere reversal and actually precipitates *withdrawal* symptoms in opioid-dependent persons. To avoid this, the dose of naloxone should be titrated according to the level of consciousness and respiratory rate. The second risk is that the more rapid metabolism of naloxone than that of a long-acting drug, such as methadone, may result in a later recurrence of the overdose symptoms. Naloxone should be titrated via an intravenous drip or repeated every 2 to 3 hours with careful monitoring of vital signs for at least 24 hours.

The opioid withdrawal syndrome varies in severity and duration, depending on the specific drug, dose, and duration of use. The typical heroin-dependent person notes the onset of withdrawal 6 to 10 hours after the last injection. Feelings of drug craving, anxiety, restlessness, irritability, sweating, rhinorrhea, and yawning develop early. These are followed by dilated pupils, sneezing, piloerection, anorexia, nausea, vomiting, diarrhea, abdominal cramps, bone pain, myalgias, tremors, sleep disturbance, and, very rarely, convulsions or cardiovascular collapse. Untreated, these symptoms peak at 36 to 48 hours and gradually subside over 5 to 10 days. Withdrawal is generally not life-threatening, and it has been compared with a severe case of the "flu." There is also a protracted abstinence syndrome consisting of mild symptoms of anxiety, sleep disturbance, and autonomic nervous system instability, which may persist for 6 months after acute withdrawal. Longer-acting opioids, such as methadone, produce an abstinence syndrome that develops more slowly and with less intensity but persists much longer.

Medically assisted withdrawal is usually accomplished using methadone, beginning with a test dose of 20 mg. If 20 mg has no appreciable effect on the signs and symptoms within 1 hour, an additional 20 mg can be given. The methadone can be gradually reduced over 7 to 10 days. An alternative is clonidine, an alpha$_2$-adrenergic agonist/partial agonist, which produces complex central effects that result in reduced central adrenergic outflow. Developed for the treatment of hypertension, clonidine has also been found to reduce many of the signs of autonomic hyperactivity during opioid withdrawal. Thus clonidine can be useful in situations in which methadone is not available. Beginning with low doses of 0.1 to 0.2 mg to minimize the possibility of postural hypotension, clonidine can be increased to 1 to 1.5 mg daily in divided doses over 4 to 10 days and then tapered over the next 5 days.

CANNABIS (Marijuana and Hashish)

Cannabis is not a single drug, but a complex preparation containing many biologically active chemicals. Δ-9-Tetrahydrocannabinol (Δ-9-THC) accounts for most of the pharmacologic effects of the complex.

Patterns of Abuse

Cannabis has long been used in many societies as a form of folk medicine and for relaxation. Throughout the 1970's, its use increased explosively in the United States. Surveys indicate that use peaked in 1979 when more than 50 million Americans reported using the drug at least once, and 9 per cent of high school seniors reported daily use. In the 1980's, the popularity of this drug declined, partially due to decreased availability and increased price. Domestic sources of marijuana have recently increased and use is still common, but significantly less than in the past. The vast majority of users smoke marijuana cigarettes or hashish pipes in groups in which the ritual of preparation and sharing is part of the social interaction. Others demonstrate a compulsive pattern of daily use, with lives dominated by the acquisition and use of cannabis.

Pharmacology

Cannabis preparations are three to four times more potent when smoked than when taken orally. After inhalation, effects begin within 3 minutes and peak within 1 hour, and the subject reports feeling "normal" within 3 hours. Psychomotor effects, however, such as impairment on eye-tracking and vigilance tasks, may be evident for up to 11 hours after a single dose.

The acute physiologic effects of cannabis are dose related and include an increase in heart rate, conjunctival vascular congestion, decreased intraocular pressure, bronchodilation, increased airway conductance, and peripheral vasodilation. Dryness of mouth, fine tremors, ataxia, nystagmus, nausea, and vomiting have been noted. Sleep patterns are altered, and orthostatic hypotension occurs infrequently.

Delta-9-tetrahydrocannabinol is the main psychoactive factor in marijuana. A cannabinoid receptor has been located and characterized in rat brain, but no endogenous cannabinoid-like factor has yet been identified. Psychoactive effects depend on the dose, route of administration, personality and experience of the user, and environment in which the drug is used. Enhanced perceptions of colors, sounds, and tastes have been reported. Time seems to pass slowly, and the ability to learn new facts is impaired. There is often some drowsiness and inattentiveness, which may account for some of the poor performance on driving simulators. *Motor vehicular driving performance is definitely impaired by cannabis*, and this impairment may persist for several hours after the period of obvious intoxication. Tolerance and physical dependence have been experimentally demonstrated with regular cannabis use. This is not relevant to the occasional user, but daily heavy users show clinical evidence of withdrawal when deprived of access to cannabis.

Cannabis contains chemicals with unusually high lipid solubility and thus a high affinity for brain tissue. Metabolites may persist for several weeks, although their biologic significance is unknown. Urine tests for marijuana can remain positive for more than a week after a dose and even longer in chronic users. Positive urine tests have also been experimentally demonstrated in subjects who simply sat for several hours in a room where marijuana was being smoked.

Cannabis derivatives have been investigated for their therapeutic potential in several illnesses. The antiemetic effect is useful for some patients in reducing the nausea produced by cancer chemotherapy. The accompanying psychological effects have so far limited its usefulness. Glaucoma, convulsive seizures, asthma, and muscle spasticity are other conditions in which cannabis or a synthetic analogue may eventually prove useful.

Adverse Effects

Most clinicians believe that regular cannabis use by adolescents impairs maturation and often results in poor social and scholastic adjustment. Although there is no way to experimentally demonstrate causality, cannabis use is associated with poor academic performance. Occasional users have fewer problems, but acute panic, paranoid reactions, and frightening distortions of body image are sometimes experienced. Rarely, these reactions are severe enough to require emergency room treatment. Such reactions seem to be more common with higher doses and with oral administration rather than with smoking, which is easier to titrate. Patients with a history of schizophrenia may be particularly sensitive to adverse consequences of cannabis and should be warned to avoid it.

The cardiac stimulatory effects of cannabis may pose a threat to patients with cardiovascular disease. Chronic smoking of cannabis produces inflammatory changes in the bronchi and sinusitis. Experimentally cannabis is carcinogenic, but clinical studies are confounded by the concurrent use of tobacco by virtually all regular cannabis smokers.

Treatment

The acute anxiety reactions produced by cannabis are seldom severe enough to warrant medical attention. Treatment should be supportive and reassuring with frequent reminders of the drug-induced nature of the symptoms. Benzodiazepines may be indicated in more severely agitated states. For the chronic heavy user, treatment is much more difficult. Such patients typically insist that treatment is not necessary, and they feel no need to stop using cannabis on a daily basis. Meanwhile, they are failing in school or employment. Psychotherapy is unlikely to be of value unless the cannabis consumption can be interrupted. Hospitalization or entrance into a therapeutic community may be indicated, if the patient can be so persuaded. Medication is usually not required to treat withdrawal, and the drug-free patient clears mentally over several weeks. Psychotherapy is often necessary in addition to removing the cannabis.

Marijuana and Health. Report of a study by a Committee of the Institute of Medicine: Division of Health Sciences Policy. Washington, D.C., National Academy Press, 1982. *Critical review of the published reports of marijuana's effects on organ systems and behavior.*

PSYCHEDELICS

Psychedelic drugs include the following:
Lysergic acid diethylamide (LSD)
Mescaline
Phencyclidine (PCP)
5-Methoxy-3,4-methylene dioxyamphetamine (MDMA; "ecstasy")
Dimethyltryptamine (DMT)
Psilocybin

Many drugs at some dose produce hallucinations, but the drugs classified here reliably produce distortions in perception or thinking as a primary effect, even at low dose. This category represents several chemical classes and different mechanisms of action. Phencyclidine in particular is quite different from the others in that it produces, in addition to hallucinations, analgesia and amphetamine-like stimulation.

Patterns of Abuse

Hallucinogenic drugs are among the oldest known psychoactive drugs, having long been used as adjuncts to religious practices in some societies. During the 1960's they became well known on college campuses, where they were used in an effort to "gain insight" or to experiment in expanding the potential of the mind. Physicians in emergency rooms were frequently called upon to treat young people suffering from "bad trips" or adverse reactions to these substances. One of the problems with the use of illicit supplies of these drugs is their gross mislabeling. Chemical analyses of samples obtained from street purchases show that phencyclidine ("angel dust," PCP) and by-products of phencyclidine are often the active ingredient in LSD or psilocybin purchases. Thus users often get unexpected and severe effects. Use of phencyclidine as a veterinary anesthetic has been discontinued, and it is now available only from clandestine laboratories where purity is quite variable. The toxic by-products produced during phencyclidine synthesis may cause severe toxic symptoms.

The use of psychedelics declined in the late 1970's and early 1980's, but the use of PCP continues to be a significant problem in some areas. The typical pattern of psychedelic drug use involves intermittent rather than daily use. Recently there has been great interest in MDMA, known as "ecstasy." This drug has been reported to facilitate insight and maturation and thus enhance the effects of psychotherapy. The drug has never been studied rigorously for this use, however, and thus there is no evidence to support these claims. Similar claims were made for LSD in the past and all attempts to demonstrate a beneficial effect failed. Both MDMA and the closely related MDA are toxic to serotonergic nerve cells.

Pharmacology

LSD is the most potent psychedelic drug known. It has marked effects on serotonergic systems in the CNS, but it affects other systems as well; the mechanism for its psychoactive effects is unknown. The usual street dose of LSD is around 200 μg, but doses as low as 20 μg produce psychological effects in susceptible individuals. Central sympathomimetic stimulation occurs within 20 minutes of oral ingestion and is characterized by mydriasis, hyperthermia, tachycardia, elevated blood pressure, piloerection, increased alertness, and facilitation of monosynaptic reflexes. Nausea and vomiting occasionally occur.

Psychoactive effects of LSD, developing within 1 to 2 hours, vary with the subject, dose, setting, expectation, and mood of the subject. Perceptions are heightened and may become overwhelming. Afterimages are prolonged and may overlap with ongoing perceptions. There may be a sense of unusual clarity, and one's thoughts may assume extraordinary importance. Time seems to pass slowly, and body distortions are commonly perceived. True hallucinations, usually visual, may occur in susceptible individuals. Mood is highly variable and labile and may range from expansive reactions characterized by euphoria and self-confidence to a constricted reaction marked by depression and panic.

The syndrome begins to clear after 10 to 12 hours, but fatigue and tension may persist for an additional 24 hours. The duration of action of mescaline is about 12 hours and that of psilocybin 4 to 6 hours. Tolerance develops to repeated daily doses of LSD within 3 to 4 days, but recovery is rapid and weekly use of the same dose is possible.

Phencyclidine comes in various forms (powder, liquid, capsule, tablet) and often is taken inadvertently when the user is expecting something else. It produces a prompt stimulant effect similar to that of amphetamine and usually a feeling of euphoria. Ataxia, slurred speech, nystagmus, and feelings of numbness are commonly observed. At higher doses, frightening and bizarre visual hallucinations can arise. There may be hostile or aggressive behavior and amnesia for the episode. With still higher doses, catatonia and coma occur, with the patient's eyes open and the pupils partially dilated. Heart rate and blood pressure are elevated. Tolerance to the stimulant effects occurs, and some mild withdrawal symptoms have been observed in daily users.

Adverse Effects

The acute reactions such as panic or psychosis ("bad trip") most commonly complicate psychedelic use. With LSD, these reactions vary in intensity and occasionally have led to self-injury or suicide. Phencyclidine is more likely to produce a severe reaction that results in suicide, often by drowning. Assaults and murders have been attributed to the effects of phencyclidine, and aggressive behavior can occur during the psychotic episode.

Prolonged psychotic episodes sometimes occur after psychedelic use. It is not known whether these can occur only in individuals who have pre-existing tendencies toward psychosis. Many clinicians believe that chronic or high-dose use of psychedelics, especially phencyclidine, can produce prolonged psychosis even in healthy individuals. Overdose resulting in death can occur with phencyclidine. The syndrome can progress rapidly from aggressive psychotic behavior to coma with elevated blood pressure, dilated pupils, muscular rigidity, arrhythmias, and seizures.

Another adverse effect of psychedelic use is known as "flashbacks." These are brief reappearances of the hallucinations or distortions experienced during the acute ingestion occurring days or weeks after the last psychedelic dose. "Flashbacks" appear to be more common with heavy use, and they eventually disappear without treatment.

Treatment

The use of medication in an emergency situation with a patient suffering from an unknown drug reaction can be dangerous owing to progression of the street drug effect with further absorption from the gut and to possible drug interactions with any prescribed medications. Thus treatment of acute panic reactions is best accomplished, when possible, by a supportive environment, observation, and reassurance. In severely agitated patients, intramuscular lorazepam or haloperidol can be used. Prolonged psychosis requires hospitalization and treatment with neuroleptics.

Treatment of phencyclidine overdose may require support of vital signs. Gastric lavage with activated charcoal may prevent further absorption of the drug. To enhance the excretion of phencyclidine, acidification of the urine may be accomplished acutely by intravenous ammonium chloride, 75 mg per kilogram per day in four divided doses, or ascorbic acid, 500 mg every 4 hours, with repeated monitoring of blood pH, blood gases, blood urea nitrogen (BUN), blood ammonia, and electrolytes. If symptoms are mild, cranberry juice and 1 or 2 grams of ascorbic acid given orally four times per day may be sufficient.

ANTICHOLINERGIC COMPOUNDS

Effects in some ways similar to those of psychedelic drugs may be produced by ingestion of the alkaloids *atropine, hyoscyamine,* and *scopolamine* in their natural plant forms. These are found in "herbal teas" and a variety of proprietary medications, and several deaths have occurred. Excessive use of *antihistaminic* compounds with anticholinergic effects also occurs. Psychoactive effects are those of an acute toxic delirium with confusion, visual or tactile hallucinations, and amnesia for the episode. Symptoms of the potent peripheral effects of the intoxication include dilated pupils, tachycardia, dry mouth, flushing, and hyperthermia. Treatment is symptomatic and consists of protecting the patient from self-injury, providing fluids, and reducing the fever. Administration of cholinesterase inhibitors and lorazepam intramuscularly may be indicated in severe cases. Phenothiazines are contraindicated because of their anticholinergic effects. Anticholinergic drugs are sometimes sold as hallucinogenics, thus creating a potentially dangerous additive interaction if a phenothiazine is administered in the emergency room to treat a "bad trip."

INHALANTS

Examples of inhalants include the following:

Toluene (airplane glue)
Kerosene
Gasoline
Carbon tetrachloride
Amyl nitrite
Nitrous oxide

Chemicals that are volatile at room temperatures and that produce perceptible changes in brain function when inhaled have been popular among certain groups as a means of producing altered states of consciousness. There are characteristic patterns for each chemical.

Organic solvents, such as toluene, are typically used by children beginning at about age 12. The material is usually placed in a plastic bag, and the vapors are inhaled. Dizziness and intoxication are described after several minutes of inhalation. Inhalant abuse also involves the use of aerosol sprays containing fluorocarbon propellants. Prolonged exposure or daily use may result in toxic effects on several organ systems, including cardiac arrhythmias, bone marrow depression, cerebral degeneration, and damage to liver, kidney, and peripheral nerves. Death has occasionally been attributed to inhalant abuse, probably via the mechanism of cardiac arrhythmias, especially accompanying exercise or associated with upper airway obstruction.

Amyl nitrite is a yellowish, volatile, inflammable liquid with a fruity odor. It produces dilation of smooth muscle and has been used in the past for treatment of angina. In recent years, amyl nitrite has been used to enhance orgasm, particularly by male homosexuals. It is sold in the form of room deodorizers and can produce a feeling of "rush," flushing, and dizziness. Adverse effects include palpitations, postural hypotension, and headache progressing to loss of consciousness.

Nitrous oxide, alone or in combination with oxygen, and *halothane* are sometimes used as intoxicants by medical personnel. Compulsive use and chronic toxicity have not been reported, but there are obvious acute dangers in the unauthorized use of such potent agents.

Treatment

Since the effects of solvents are brief, specific acute treatments are generally not indicated. When inhalant use is chronic or associated with other psychiatric diagnoses, specific psychiatric treatment and measures to prevent relapse are indicated.

Sharp CW, Brehem ML: Review of Inhalants: From Euphoria to Dysfunction. NIDA Research Monograph Series No. 15, National Institute on Drug Abuse, Rockville, MD 20857. *Good review of clinical and toxicologic aspects of the spectrum of inhalant problems.*

NICOTINE

The medical consequences of smoking tobacco products are covered in many chapters of this book because the effects are so widespread. As the dangers of smoking have become so well known, it has become more apparent that smoking cigarettes can produce a very powerful dependence on nicotine, which is clearly an addicting drug. Cessation of smoking may be very difficult even in patients who strongly desire to remain abstinent (see Ch. 10).

ILLICIT SYNTHETIC DRUGS (Designer Drugs)

The so-called designer drugs are produced in clandestine laboratories, and they vary in their composition and purity. Fentanyl analogues have been produced that have extremely potent opioid actions and have resulted in overdose deaths. Other attempts at synthesis of opioids have resulted in toxic compounds. An example is MPTP, a toxic by-product of botched attempts to synthesize a meperidine (Demerol) analogue, which produces an irreversible Parkinson's syndrome in those who have taken it intravenously. Other chemicals found in street samples are phenethylamines, which are analogues of amphetamine, and various analogues of phencyclidine. In evaluating the drug history of any patient, the physician must remember that those who purchase drugs on the street have no way of knowing what they actually take.

TREATMENT OF DRUG DEPENDENCE

The treatment of drug dependence involves four stages (Table 15–1): acknowledgment, detoxification, pharmacotherapy, and psychotherapy.

ACKNOWLEDGMENT OF THE PROBLEM. Rarely does a patient in the early and most treatable phase of drug dependence spontaneously volunteer for treatment. Friends or relatives who observe the signs of a drug problem must confront the patient. Often the family physician is in a good position to notice the problem early and to convince the patient to enter treatment. Confrontation is best accomplished when several concerned people approach the patient together in a firm but supportive way. Even when confronted with evidence of a substance abuse problem, the patient usually continues to deny its existence, making persistence necessary.

DETOXIFICATION. The pharmacologic aspects of detoxification were described in the discussions of specific drug categories. In some cases, hospitalization is mandatory, particularly when there is a large degree of physical dependence. If, however, the drug taking can be interrupted while the individual remains an outpatient, this can be far less expensive and just as effective. "Treatment programs" that advertise a 28-day inpatient treatment of drug dependence are misleading, because the heart of effective treatment is continued therapy, usually lasting months or years, designed to prevent relapse after the patient returns to work or school. Frequently, the patient has so much cognitive impairment during the detoxification period that he or she retains little of therapy or education provided during this first phase.

PHARMACOTHERAPY. This mode of therapy has been dis-

TABLE 15–1. TREATMENT OF DRUG DEPENDENCE

	Confrontation	Detoxification	Pharmacotherapy	Psychotherapy
Sedatives	S	Diazepam or phenobarbital	Antidepressants as needed	S
Stimulants	I	Not usually needed	Antidepressants or neuroleptics	I
Opioids	M	Methadone or clonidine	Methadone, naltrexone, or antidepressants	M
Cannabis	I	None	Antidepressants, as needed	I
Psychedelics	L	None	Neuroleptics as needed	L
Inhalants	A	None	None	A
Nicotine	R	Nicotine gum	None	R

cussed under specific drug categories. For the most part, pharmacotherapy involves treatment of specific psychiatric disorders, such as affective disorders or psychosis commonly associated with a particular form of drug dependence. It must be remembered that patients who have abused one drug have a strong likelihood of abusing a prescribed psychoactive drug. For this reason, antianxiety agents or sedatives should rarely if ever be prescribed in the rehabilitation of drug-dependent persons.

Certain pharmacotherapies are directed at the drug-seeking behavior rather than an associated psychiatric disorder. The use of disulfiram (Antabuse) in the treatment of alcoholics is discussed in Ch. 14. Opioid-dependent patients who have repeatedly relapsed after detoxification can be transferred from the use of illicit drugs to methadone maintenance. The patient can then be maintained on a steady dose of methadone as a substitute for his opioid drug of choice. The advantage is that the patient is stabilized owing to the long duration of action of methadone and, if properly managed, experiences no "highs" or "lows." Patients are able to function well on methadone and perform complex tasks competently. Methadone may enable the patient to participate effectively in a rehabilitation program, including psychotherapy. Methadone may involve several years of maintenance and must be used only in authorized programs in which staff have received specialized training.

Naltrexone (Trexan) is a relatively long-acting opioid antagonist. Before receiving this medication, the patient must be thoroughly detoxified or the naltrexone will precipitate withdrawal. Since naltrexone blocks opiate receptors, the effects of impulsive opioid use are prevented while naltrexone is in the body. This treatment has been successful in conjunction with a comprehensive rehabilitation program, including a wide range of psychotherapies. Naltrexone must be taken at least two or three times per week to protect against relapse, so it requires strong motivation on the part of the patient to remain opioid free.

PSYCHOTHERAPY. Psychotherapy is generally similar across all classes of drugs. It should be started as early as possible in the treatment program, but it is of little value when the patient is still intoxicated or confused. This treatment is, however, completely compatible with pharmacotherapy such as psychoactive medication, methadone, naltrexone, disulfiram, or nicotine chewing gum. Such psychotherapy is broadly defined and involves counseling regarding job-finding or legal problems, family therapy, group therapy, individual therapy, all types of behavioral treatments, and self-help programs such as Narcotics Anonymous. The purpose of these treatments is to teach the patient alternate behaviors to drug ingestion and to enable him or her to deal more effectively with problems of living. The general physician often can convince patients to join a specialized treatment program and can collaborate in the medical aspects of the treatment. Severe forms of drug dependence, however, are best managed by a treatment team specially trained in this area of medicine.

Hayashida M, Alterman A, McLellan AT, et al.: Comparative effectiveness of inpatient and outpatient detoxification of patients with mild to moderate alcohol withdrawal syndrome. N Engl J Med 320:358, 1989. *Controlled study demonstrating that outpatient detoxification is approximately as effective as inpatient detoxification for the majority of alcoholics.*

Woody GE, McLellan AT, Luborsky L, et al.: Psychotherapy for opiate dependence: A twelve-month follow-up. Am J Psychiatry 144:590, 1987. *This study of 112 opiate addicts demonstrated that psychotherapy is effective when combined with methadone treatment.*

16 Immunization

Walter A. Orenstein

Immunization is one of the most cost-effective means of preventing morbidity and mortality from infectious diseases. Routine immunization, particularly of children, has resulted in decreases of 90 per cent or more in reported cases of measles, mumps, rubella, congenital rubella syndrome, polio, tetanus, diphtheria, and pertussis.

General Characteristics of Immunizations

Immunization protects against disease or the sequelae of disease through administration of an immunobiologic: vaccines, toxoids, immune globulin preparations, and antitoxins. Protection induced by immunization can be active or passive.

ACTIVE IMMUNIZATION. Administering a vaccine or toxoid causes the body to produce an immune response against the infectious agent or its toxins. Vaccines consist of suspensions of live (usually attenuated) or inactivated microorganisms or fractions thereof. Toxoids are modified bacterial toxins that retain immunogenic properties but lack toxicity. Active immunization generally results in long-term immunity, although onset of protection may be delayed because it takes time for the body to respond. With live attenuated vaccines small quantities of living organisms multiply within the recipient until an immune response cuts off replication. In contrast, inactivated vaccines and toxoids contain large quantities of antigen. Live vaccines generally induce immune responses more closely paralleling natural infection and are more likely to induce long-term immunity. Most induce active immunity in the majority of recipients after a single dose; killed vaccines, in contrast, often require multiple doses.

PASSIVE IMMUNIZATION. Temporary immunity is provided through administration of preformed antibodies as immune globulins or antitoxins. Immune globulins (IG), obtained from human blood, may contain antibodies to a variety of agents depending on the pool of human plasma used in preparation. Specific immune globulins are made from plasma from donors with high levels of antibodies to specific antigens, such as tetanus immune globulin (TIG). Most immune globulins must be injected intramuscularly. A special preparation for intravenous use is also available. Antitoxins are solutions of antibodies derived from animals immunized with specific antigens (e.g., diphtheria antitoxin). Table 16–1 gives the major indications for currently available immune globulins and antitoxins. Passive immunization is usually used to protect individuals immediately prior to an anticipated exposure or shortly after a known or suspected exposure to an infectious agent.

ROUTE AND TIMING OF VACCINATION. Each immunobiologic has a preferred site and route of administration. Vaccines containing adjuvants should be injected intramuscularly (IM). For adults, most IM injections should be given in the deltoid. Use of the buttocks is discouraged except when large volumes are required both because of the potential for damage to the sciatic nerve and because of diminished immune response to some vaccines such as hepatitis B. Subcutaneous vaccines are also usually administered in the deltoid area, and intradermal vaccines are usually given on the volar surface of the forearm. Many immunobiologics can be given simultaneously to reduce the number of health care visits required for full immunization. In general, inactivated vaccines and toxoids can be given simultaneously at different sites. With vaccines that frequently cause side effects, such as cholera and parenterally administered typhoid vaccines, it may be best to separate administration by at least a week. With the exception of cholera and yellow fever vaccines, which should ideally be administered at least 3 weeks apart, live and inactivated vaccines can be administered at the same time. Measles, mumps, and rubella (MMR) vaccine can be administered with oral polio vaccine (OPV); OPV can be administered with yellow fever vaccine. For theoretical reasons, live vaccines not delivered on the same day should be separated by at least 1 month. Immune globulin may interfere with the take of live vaccines such as measles. Ideally, such vaccines should be administered at least 2 weeks prior to IG or 3 months after IG. IG does not appear to interfere with the response to OPV.

ADVERSE REACTIONS. Hypersensitivity to vaccine components can lead to local and systemic reactions ranging from mild to severe. Responsible components may include animal proteins, antibiotics, preservatives, and stabilizers. Egg proteins, contained in vaccines grown in chicken eggs or chick embryo tissue culture, are common allergens in measles, mumps, influenza, and yellow fever vaccines. In general, persons without anaphylactic type allergies to eggs can be given these vaccines safely. Persons with anaphylactic reactions to eggs, however, should receive these vaccines only with extreme caution under established protocols (see Greenberg and Birx, 1988).

TABLE 16–1. PASSIVE IMMUNIZATIONS FOR ADULTS

Disease	Name of Material	Comments and Use
Tetanus	Tetanus immune globulin human (TIG)	Management of tetanus-prone wounds and treatment of tetanus
Diphtheria	Diphtheria antitoxin equine	Treatment of established disease, high frequency of reactions to serum of nonhuman origin
Rabies	Rabies immune globulin human (RIG) Antirabies, serum equine (ARS)	Postexposure prophylaxis of animal bites
Measles	Immune globulin, human (IG)	Prevention or modification of disease in contacts of cases; not for control of epidemics
Hepatitis A	Immune globulin, human (IG)	Protection of household contacts; control of epidemics; pre-exposure prophylaxis for travelers
Hepatitis B	Hepatitis B immune globulin, human	For needle stick or mucous membrane contact with HBsAG-positive persons; for sexual partners with acute hepatitis B or hepatitis B carriers; for infants born to mothers who are HBsAg-positive; for infants whose mother or primary caregiver has acute hepatitis B
Varicella zoster	Varicella zoster immune globulin (VZIG)	Persons under 15 years of age with underlying disease who have not had varicella and who are exposed to varicella; may be given to known susceptible adults, particularly if antibody-negative
Erythroblastosis fetalis	Rh immune globulin (RIG)	Rh-negative women who give birth to Rh-positive infants or who abort
Hypogammaglobulinemia	Immune globulin, intravenous	Maintenance therapy
Idiopathic thrombocytopenic purpura	Immune globulin, intravenous	Therapy of acute episodes
Botulism	Trivalent A, B, and E antitoxin, equine	Treatment of botulism
Snakebite	Antivenin, equine (North American coral snake antivenin)	Specific for North American coral snake, *Micrurus fulvius*
	Antivenin, equine Crotalidae, polyvalent	Effective for viper and pit viper, including rattlesnakes, copperheads, moccasins
Spider bite	Antivenin, equine	Specific for black widow spider, *Latrodectus mactans*, and other members of the genus

No vaccine is completely safe or completely effective. Recommendations for use are based on an evaluation of the risks and benefits. Two major bodies make recommendations regarding immunization of adults: (1) the Task Force on Adult Immunization of the American College of Physicians, which publishes the *Guide for Adult Immunization*, and (2) the Immunization Practices Advisory Committee (ACIP) of the U.S. Public Health Service. The latter group publishes its information in the *Morbidity and Mortality Weekly Report*. The reader is referred to these sources for comprehensive information on vaccines, including indications, contraindications, precautions, and side effects.

ADVERSE EVENTS. Prior to licensure, vaccines are evaluated in prospective, randomized double-blind, placebo-controlled trials that are capable of detecting common adverse reactions attributable to vaccine. Uncommon and rare adverse events must usually be evaluated in postmarketing studies. Physician reporting of serious events temporally related to vaccination forms the basis for assessing whether such events are actually caused by the vaccine. Such events are usually called "adverse events" as opposed to "adverse reactions," which imply in advance whether the vaccine produced the illness. It must be determined whether the clinical syndrome is distinctive from events not caused by vaccine and, if not, whether the frequency of the illness following vaccination is significantly greater than that expected from chance alone.

GENERAL CONSIDERATIONS. Immunizations for adults depend on age, lifestyle, occupation, and medical conditions. All adults should have a primary series of tetanus and diphtheria toxoids with boosters of combined toxoids (Td) every 10 years. Persons born in or after 1957 should have evidence of immunity to measles and mumps. Rubella vaccine is especially indicated for susceptible females of childbearing age. Pneumococcal vaccine and annual vaccination against influenza are indicated for all adults 65 years of age and older. Health care workers exposed to blood or blood products should receive hepatitis B vaccine. Those caring for patients at high risk of complications from influenza should receive annual vaccination. Health care workers likely to come in contact with persons transmitting measles, mumps, or rubella should be immune to those diseases.

IMMUNOCOMPROMISE. Patients with conditions that compromise their immune systems should not receive live attenuated vaccines. Such patients include those with immunodeficiency diseases, leukemia, lymphoma, and generalized malignancy and those who are immunosuppressed from therapy with corticosteroids, alkylating agents, antimetabolites, and radiation. An exception is infection with human immunodeficiency virus (HIV). Asymptomatic patients should receive MMR vaccine. MMR should be considered for symptomatic patients with HIV. Because of the availability of enhanced potency inactivated polio vaccine (eIPV), all patients known to be infected with HIV should receive eIPV instead of OPV. Patients with leukemia in remission who are off all chemotherapy for at least 3 months may receive live-virus vaccines. Short-course therapy (< 2 weeks) with corticosteroids, alternate-day regimens with low to moderate doses of short-acting corticosteroids, and topical applications or tendon injections do not ordinarily contraindicate live vaccines.

Immunocompromised patients can receive inactivated vaccines and toxoids, although the efficacy of such preparations may be diminished. Patients with known HIV infection should receive pneumococcal vaccine. Those with symptomatic infection should receive annual vaccination against influenza.

PREGNANCY. In general, live vaccines should not be given to pregnant women because of the theoretical concern that such vaccines could adversely affect the fetus. No significant adverse events attributable to vaccination with MMR of pregnant women have been documented, but pregnant women should not receive MMR, and women who do receive MMR should wait 3 months before becoming pregnant. Polio and yellow fever vaccines should not usually be given to pregnant women unless there is substantial risk of disease. Td is especially indicated for pregnant females who are not appropriately vaccinated to prevent neonatal tetanus in their infants. Vaccination is best performed after the first trimester. All pregnant women should be screened for hepatitis B surface antigen (HBsAg). Offspring of carrier mothers should receive HBV and hepatitis B immune globulin (HBIG).

INDIVIDUAL IMMUNOBIOLOGIES (Table 16–2)
Tetanus and Diphtheria (Ch. 310 and 306)

Tetanus toxoid is one of the most effective immunizations, with over 95 per cent protection following a primary series. The adsorbed is preferred over the fluid preparation because it induces protective levels of antitoxin that persist longer after fewer doses. In persons 7 years of age or older, it should always be used in combination with Td, which is more than 85 per cent effective in preventing disease. A primary series consists of three doses (Table 16–2). There is no need to repeat doses if the schedule is interrupted. Boosters are recommended every 10 years. An easy way to remember is to schedule immunization at the middle of each decade (e.g., 25 years, 35 years, etc.).

Following a wound, persons of unknown immunization status or those who have received fewer than three doses of tetanus toxoid should receive a dose of Td regardless of the severity of the wound. Td is also indicated for those who previously received three or more doses if more than 10 years have elapsed, in the case of clean, minor wounds, and if more than 5 years have elapsed for all other wounds. TIG should be administered simultaneously at a separate site to persons who have not received at least three doses of toxoid and who have wounds that are not clean and minor.

Measles (Ch. 367)

Measles immunization is recommended for all persons born in or after 1957 who lack evidence of immunity to measles: prior physician-diagnosed measles, laboratory evidence of immunity, or appropriate vaccination. Prior to 1989, appropriate vaccination consisted of a single dose of live vaccine administered on or after the first birthday. Now, a routine two-dose schedule is recommended: the first dose, which is 95 to 98 per cent effective, at 15 months of age and the second dose either at entry to primary school or at entry to middle or junior high school, depending upon local policy. Most adults are considered to have been appropriately vaccinated if they received one dose of vaccine administered on or after their first birthday. Some adults, however, who are at increased risk of measles (health care workers with direct patient contact, students in colleges, international travelers, etc.) should ideally receive a second dose of vaccine unless they have documentation of prior physician-diagnosed measles or serologic evidence of immunity. Persons embarking on foreign travel should ideally have received two doses or have other evidence of measles immunity. Persons born before 1957 are usually immune as a result of natural infection and do not require vaccination, although there is no contraindication if they are believed to be susceptible.

During outbreaks of measles in institutions, all persons at risk who have not received two doses or who lack other evidence of measles immunity should be vaccinated. Measles vaccine is usually administered as combined measles, mumps, and rubella vaccine (MMR) to ensure immunity against all three diseases. There is no harm if individuals are already immune to one or more of the components.

Measles vaccine is contraindicated for pregnant women on theoretical grounds, for persons with moderate to severe acute febrile illnesses, and for persons with altered immunocompetence except those with HIV infection (Table 16–2). Patients with anaphylactic reactions to eggs should be vaccinated only with caution under established protocols.

Approximately 5 to 15 per cent of susceptible recipients of measles vaccine develop fever of 39.4°C or higher with onset between 5 and 12 days after vaccination and lasting 1 to 2 days. About 5 per cent develop transient rashes. The overall rate of reactions following the second dose of a measles-containing vaccine is substantially lower than after the first dose. Encephalopathy or encephalitis following measles vaccines has been reported at a rate lower than the background or expected rate.

Rubella (Ch. 368)

Rubella vaccine is indicated for adults, particularly women of childbearing age, without a prior history of rubella, vaccination on or after the first birthday, or laboratory evidence of immunity. A single dose of vaccine is 95 per cent or more effective. Many persons receive two doses of rubella vaccine via the two-dose schedule of MMR.

Follow-up of 305 susceptible women who received rubella vaccines within 3 months of the estimated date of conception has failed to reveal any evidence of defects compatible with congenital rubella syndrome in their offspring. Nevertheless, vaccine is contraindicated in pregnant women on theoretical grounds.

Reactions occur only in susceptible persons. Up to 40 per cent of susceptible adults develop arthralgia, usually of the small peripheral joints, and 10 to 20 per cent develop frank arthritis. Joint symptoms usually begin 1 to 3 weeks following vaccination and persist for 1 day to 3 weeks. Very rarely patients have developed chronic recurrent or persistent joint symptoms following vaccination. In fact, such symptoms are considerably more common after the disease than after the vaccine. Other rare adverse events include transient peripheral neuritis and pain in the arms and legs. Rubella vaccine is contraindicated for persons with moderate to severe acute febrile illnesses and for persons with reduced immunocompetence. When given with measles vaccine, it may be administered to those with asymptomatic HIV infection and considered for those with symptomatic infection. Rubella vaccine is grown in human diploid cells and can be administered without problems to persons with allergy to eggs.

Mumps (Ch. 370)

Mumps vaccine is indicated for all persons, especially susceptible males, without a prior history of vaccination on or after the first birthday, physician-diagnosed mumps, or laboratory evidence of immunity. Most persons born prior to 1957 can be considered immune as a result of natural infection, although there is no contraindication if such persons are thought to be susceptible. In clinical trials, a single dose of vaccine has induced seroconversion in more than 90 per cent of recipients.

Adverse events following mumps vaccine are uncommon—fever, parotitis, and allergic manifestations. Mumps vaccine is contraindicated for pregnant women on theoretical grounds, for persons with moderate to severe acute febrile illnesses, and for persons with altered immunocompetence. Combined with measles vaccine, it may be given to those with asymptomatic HIV infection and considered for those with symptomatic infection. Patients with anaphylactic reactions to eggs should be vaccinated only with caution under established protocols.

Hepatitis B

Hepatitis B vaccine is the first vaccine that can prevent cancer (an estimated 800 persons die annually in the United States from hepatitis B–related liver cancer; many times more die in the Third World). It can also prevent acute and chronic complications of hepatitis B, including an estimated 4000 deaths annually from cirrhosis and 250 deaths annually from fulminant hepatic disease in the United States. The original hepatitis vaccine in the United States consisted of purified, inactivated, alum-adsorbed, 22-nm hepatitis B surface antigen (HBsAg) particles obtained from human plasma. Currently produced vaccines are derived from insertion of the gene for HBsAg into *Saccharomyces cerevisiae*. Hepatitis B vaccine, the first licensed vaccine made using recombinant techniques, produces adequate antibody responses in more than 90 per cent of normal adults and more than 95 per cent of normal infants, children, and adolescents when administered in a three-dose series. Dosage depends on the product, the age group, and the underlying clinical condition and can be determined by consulting the package insert. The duration of vaccine-conferred immunity is not known, although follow-up of vaccinees within 7 years indicates persistence of protection against clinically significant infections (i.e., detectable viremia and clinical disease). Booster doses are not currently recommended. Vaccine must be injected intramuscularly, preferably in the deltoid.

Current strategy targets vaccine use to high-risk populations (Table 16–2). Such targeted vaccination has not had a significant impact on hepatitis B incidence, and strategies of universal vaccination are now being considered. Universal infant vaccination is now recommended for populations with highly endemic hepatitis B, including Alaskan natives, Pacific islanders, and infants of mothers born in countries with high endemicity of hepatitis B (e.g., eastern Asia). Universal screening for HBsAg is recommended for all pregnant women, with administration of three doses of vaccine and one dose of HBIG recommended for infants of carrier mothers. Universal vaccination of all infants and/

TABLE 16–2. SELECTED IMMUNIZING AGENTS INDICATED FOR ADULTS*

Disease	Immunizing Agent	Indications	Schedule	Major Contraindications	Comments
Immunizations Indicated for All Adults					
Diphtheria	Tetanus and diphtheria toxoids combined (Td)	All adults	2 doses 4 wk apart; 3rd dose 6–12 mo after 2nd dose; booster every 10 yr; no need to repeat if schedule is interrupted	History of neurologic or severe hypersensitivity reaction following a previous dose	—
Tetanus	Tetanus and diphtheria toxoids combined (TD)	All adults	3 doses needed for primary series; 2 doses 4 wk apart; 3rd dose 6–12 mo after the 2nd dose; booster every 10 yr; no need to repeat if schedule is interrupted.	History of neurologic or severe hypersensitivity reaction following a previous dose	Special recommendations for wound treatment (see text)
Immunizations Recommended for Many Adults					
Influenza	Inactivated influenza virus vaccine	All adults ≥65 yr; other adults with high-risk conditions; adults caring for persons with high-risk conditions, including medical personnel (see text)	Annual vaccination; see annual ACIP recommendation	Anaphylactic hypersensitivity to eggs	—
Pneumococcal disease	23-valent polysaccharide vaccine	Adults with cardiovascular disease, pulmonary disease, diabetes mellitus, alcoholism, cirrhosis, cerebrospinal fluid leaks, splenic dysfunction or anatomic asplenia, Hodgkin's disease, lymphoma, multiple myeloma, chronic renal failure, nephrotic syndrome, immunosuppression, HIV infection; high-risk populations, such as certain native Americans and *all* adults ≥65 yr	1 dose; a second dose should be considered 6 or more years later for adults at high risk of disease (e.g., asplenic patients) as well as those who lose antibody rapidly (e.g., nephrotic syndrome, renal failure, transplant recipients)		—
Measles	Live-virus vaccine	All adults born after 1956 without history of live vaccine on or after 1st birthday, physician-diagnosed measles, or detectable measles antibody; persons born before 1957 can generally be considered immune	1 dose sufficient for most adults; 2 doses at least 1 month apart indicated for persons entering college, medical facility employment, traveling abroad, or at risk of measles during outbreaks	Altered immunity (e.g., leukemia, lymphoma, generalized malignancy, congenital immunodeficiency, immunosuppressive therapy); immune globulin within prior 3 mo; untreated tuberculosis; anaphylactic hypersensitivity to neomycin; pregnancy	May be administered combined with mumps and rubella vaccines for persons who might be susceptible to these other diseases. Persons with anaphylactic allergies to eggs may be vaccinated with extreme caution using established protocols (see text). Vaccine should be administered to persons with asymptomatic HIV infection and should be considered for symptomatic HIV patients.
Rubella	Live-virus vaccine	Adult women of childbearing age who lack history of rubella vaccine and detectable rubella-specific antibodies in serum; both males and females in institutions where rubella outbreaks may occur, such as hospitals, the military, and colleges	1 dose	Pregnancy, altered immunity (e.g., leukemia, lymphoma, generalized malignancy, congenital immunodeficiency, immunosuppressive therapy), immune globulin within the 3 mo prior to vaccination, anaphylactic hypersensitivity to neomycin; administration of blood products should not contraindicate postpartum vaccination; however, in this instance, serologic testing 6–8 wk after vaccination should be performed	Women should be counseled to avoid pregnancy for 3 mo following vaccination; available data on previous and current rubella vaccines indicate that the risk, if any, of causing defects compatible with congenital rubella syndrome is small. The ACIP believes that, although a final decision rests with the patient and her physician, vaccination of a pregnant woman should not ordinarily indicate that an abortion is necessary.
Mumps	Live-virus vaccine	All adults born after 1956 without history of live vaccine on or after 1st birthday, physician-diagnosed mumps, or detectable mumps antibody; persons born before 1957 can generally be considered immune	1 dose	Altered immunity (e.g., leukemia, lymphoma, generalized malignancy, congenital immunodeficiency, immunosuppressive therapy); immune globulin within prior 3 mo; anaphylactic hypersensitivity to neomycin; pregnancy	Although persons born before 1957 are generally immune, vaccine can be given to adults of all ages and may be particularly indicated for postpubertal males, who are thought to be susceptible. Persons with anaphylactic allergies to eggs may be vaccinated with extreme caution using established protocols (see text).

TABLE 16–2. SELECTED IMMUNIZING AGENTS INDICATED FOR ADULTS* Continued

Disease	Immunizing Agent	Indications	Schedule	Major Contraindications	Comments
Hepatitis B	Inactivated virus vaccine	Health care and public safety workers potentially exposed to blood; clients and staff of institutions for the developmentally disabled; hemodialysis patients; sexually active homosexual men; users of illicit injectable drugs; recipients of clotting factors; household and sexual contacts of HBV carriers; inmates of long-term correctional facilities; heterosexuals treated for sexually transmitted diseases or with multiple sexual partners; and travelers with close contact for ≥6 mo with populations with high prevalence of hepatitis B carriage	IM; 3 doses at 0, 1, and 6 mo	—	Pregnancy should not be considered a contraindication if the woman is otherwise eligible. All pregnant women should be screened for hepatitis B surface antigen (HB$_s$Ag), and infants of carrier mothers should be vaccinated at time of delivery with hepatitis B immune globulin and vaccine. Do not administer vaccine subcutaneously.
Immunizations Recommended for Special Situations					
Poliomyelitis	e-IPV (inactivated), OPV (live attenuated)	Certain adults who are at greater risk of exposure to wild poliovirus than the general population, including travelers to countries where polio is epidemic or endemic; members of community or specific population groups with disease caused by wild polioviruses; laboratory workers handling specimens that may contain polioviruses; health care workers in close contact with patients who may be excreting wild polioviruses	For unvaccinated adults, e-IPV is preferred: 2 doses, 4 wk apart; a 3rd dose 6–12 mo after the 2nd; if less than 4 wk available before protection is needed, a single dose of OPV or e-IPV. For incompletely immunized adults, a complete primary series with either vaccine is used; primary series consists of three doses of e-IPV or OPV; no need to restart interrupted series. A single dose of OPV or e-IPV can be given to adults who previously completed a primary series.	For OPV, immunodeficiency diseases; patients with altered immune status (e.g., leukemia); household contacts of immunodeficient patients; household contacts in whom there is a family history of immunodeficiency until the immune status of individuals is established. On theoretical grounds, pregnant women should not receive e-IPV or OPV. However, if immediate protection is needed, OPV can be used.	Adults who have not been adequately immunized against polio are at a very small risk of polio when their children are vaccinated with OPV. The child can be vaccinated with OPV regardless of the immune status of the parents. An acceptable alternative, provided the full immunization of the child is not compromised, is to vaccinate the parents first with e-IPV.
Rabies	Inactivated vaccine; human diploid cell rabies vaccine (HDCV); or rabies vaccine adsorbed (RVA)	High-risk persons, including animal handlers, selected laboratory and field workers, and persons traveling for ≥1 mo to areas at high risk of rabies	Pre-exposure *prophylaxis:* 3 doses of 1.0 ml IM for HDCV or RVA on days 0, 7, and 28; for HDCV only, 3 doses of 0.1 ml ID on days 0, 7, and 21 or 28	History of severe hypersensitivity reaction	Further doses needed after exposure. If to be given concurrently with chloroquine, only the IM route should be used.
Meningococcal disease	Polysaccharide vaccine containing tetravalent A, C, W135 and Y	Terminal complement component deficiencies; anatomic or functional asplenia; and travelers who will live in areas with hyperendemic or epidemic disease; may be useful during localized outbreaks	1 dose	—	—
Typhoid fever	Heat-phenol inactivated vaccine; live attenuated Ty2IA oral vaccine	Travelers to areas where the risk of prolonged exposure to contaminated food and water is high; may be considered for family and intimate contacts of carriers and laboratory workers who work with *Salmonella typhi*	*Inactivated vaccine:* two 0.5-ml doses SC 4 or more wk apart; boosters of 0.5 ml SC or 0.1 ml ID every 3 yr *Oral vaccine:* 4 doses on alternate days; boosters every 4 yr	Severe local or systemic reaction to a prior dose	Efficacy only 50–77%; food and water precautions essential
Yellow fever	Live attenuated virus (17 D strain)	Persons living or traveling in areas where yellow fever exists	1 dose; boosters every 10 yr	Immunocompromised persons; history of anaphylactic allergies to eggs; pregnancy on theoretical grounds, although may be given if risk is high	—
Cholera	Inactivated vaccine	Meeting international travel requirements	Two 0.5-ml doses SC or IM or two 0.2-ml doses ID 1 wk to 1 mo apart; booster doses every 6 mo		

*See text and package inserts for further details, particularly regarding indications, dosage, mode of administration, side effects, and adverse reactions and contraindications. ACIP = Immunization Practices Advisory Committee; e-IPV = enhanced potency inactivated polio vaccine; OPV = live-virus trivalent oral polio vaccine. Adapted with permission from JAMA 248:1607, 1982. Copyright 1982, American Medical Association.

or all adolescents is now being discussed as a means of substantially reducing and even eliminating the considerable health burden of hepatitis B in the United States.

The major side effect is soreness at the injection site. Guillain-Barré syndrome (GBS) among adults following receipt of the plasma-derived vaccine shows borderline statistically significant increased risk after the first dose; however, the overall risk, if real, is very small and is outweighed by the substantial benefits of vaccination. Information about GBS and recombinant vaccines is not available. There is no risk of acquiring HIV infection from either vaccine.

Influenza (Ch. 364)

Annual influenza vaccination is indicated for adults at high risk of complications from the disease: (1) persons with chronic cardiopulmonary disorders, (2) residents of nursing homes or other chronic care facilities, (3) persons 65 years of age or older, (4) patients with other chronic diseases such as metabolic disorders (e.g., diabetes mellitus), kidney dysfunction, hemoglobinopathies, and immunosuppression, and (5) children on long-term aspirin therapy. In addition, transmission of influenza to high-risk patients can be reduced by annual vaccination of health care workers in institutions, offices, and homes who have contact with high-risk patients and immunization of household contacts of such patients.

The efficacy of influenza vaccine varies with host condition and the degree to which antigens in the vaccine match viruses in circulation the following season. Current vaccines contain whole or split inactivated viruses of three major antigenic types—A (H3N2), A (H1N1), and B. Provided that there is a good match, vaccine efficacy is usually 70 to 90 per cent among normal healthy young adults. Efficacy is substantially lower, however, among the institutionalized elderly, often between 20 and 40 per cent. Nevertheless, despite low efficacy at preventing illness, the vaccine appears to protect against pneumonia and death on the order of 60 to 90 per cent. Ideally, vaccines should be administered during November of each year, although earlier in the fall suffices if circumstances require.

Persons with anaphylactic allergies to eggs should not be vaccinated. The most common side effect is soreness at the injection site. Fever, malaise, and myalgia may begin 6 to 12 hours after vaccination and persist for 1 to 2 days, although such reactions are most common in children exposed to vaccine for the first time. Severe allergic reactions are rare. GBS has not been associated with any vaccines used since A/New Jersey (swine flu) in 1976.

Pneumococcal Vaccine (Ch. 292)

Pneumococcal vaccine consists of the purified polysaccharide capsular antigens from the 23 types of *Streptococcus pneumoniae* that are responsible for 88 per cent of the bacteremic disease in the United States. Most healthy adults, including the elderly and patients with alcoholic cirrhosis and diabetes mellitus, develop a twofold or greater rise in type-specific antibodies within 2 to 3 weeks of vaccination. Although serologic response is generally acceptable, estimates of vaccine efficacy in preventing disease vary widely. Efficacy may be lower in some patients, such as those with alcoholic cirrhosis or Hodgkin's disease. Evidence regarding efficacy against pneumonia among high-risk populations is not clear. Regardless, the preponderance of information supports use of pneumococcal vaccine in high-risk populations. Indications for vaccine are shown in Table 16–2.

Immunity may decrease 6 or more years following initial vaccination; boosters should therefore be considered at that time for adults at highest risk of fatal infection (e.g., asplenic patients) as well as for those who lose antibody rapidly such as patients with nephrotic syndrome or renal failure.

Local reactions are frequent. Fewer than 1 per cent of vaccinees experience severe local reactions or systemic illness such as fever and malaise. Severe events such as anaphylaxis are rare.

Special efforts should target hospitalized patients. Approximately two thirds of patients later admitted with pneumococcal disease had been hospitalized for other reasons within the preceding 5 years.

Poliomyelitis (Ch. 475)

The last documented cases of indigenously acquired poliomyelitis caused by wild polio viruses in the United States were reported in 1979. All indigenous cases since 1981, approximately eight per year, have been linked epidemiologically and/or via laboratory tests to OPV exposure. Between 1973 and 1984, the overall risk of vaccine-associated polio was one case for every 2.6 million doses distributed. The risk is higher for immunodeficient persons; an estimated 0.5 per cent of these recipients develop polio. Vaccine polioviruses may spread from recipients to contacts, and cases among the latter account for over half of the total vaccine-associated cases.

Adults are at increased risk of paralytic disease from receipt of OPV; their routine vaccination is not warranted, therefore, given the small risk of exposure to wild virus in the United States. The major indication for adult vaccination is travel to areas where wild polio viruses are endemic or epidemic. For children, OPV is the vaccine of choice; for previously unvaccinated adults, however, eIPV is indicated. Travelers who have histories of partial vaccination should complete a primary series (three doses) of either eIPV or OPV. Persons who formerly completed a primary series should receive a booster of OPV or eIPV. Health care personnel who come in contact with wild viruses should be immune to polio. EIPV is the vaccine of choice in such persons to protect both the recipient and any immunocompromised persons with whom the health care worker has contact from exposure to OPV. Parents of children to be vaccinated with OPV may elect to receive eIPV prior to vaccination of their child. Most providers administer OPV to the child regardless of the parent's immune status.

A primary series of both OPV and eIPV consists of three doses (Table 16–2). There are no known serious side effects of eIPV. OPV should never be given to immunocompromised individuals or to a child living in a household with immunocompromised persons.

Meningococcal Polysaccharide Vaccine (Ch. 302)

A quadrivalent meningococcal polysaccharide vaccine containing serogroups A, C, Y, and W135 is now available. These groups account for approximately 40 to 50 per cent of meningococcal disease in the United States. Serogroups A and C vaccines have had 85 to 95 per cent efficacy in epidemic settings, whereas vaccines for the other groups have documented good immunogenicity in adults. The duration of immunity is unknown, although protection in older children and adults probably persists at least 3 years. Protection in preschool children may be shorter. Routine vaccination is not recommended in the United States because of the low risk of infection. A single dose is indicated for high-risk persons (Table 16–2). Vaccination may also be useful during localized epidemics of serogroups in the vaccine. Meningococcal vaccine may be offered to travelers and persons who will live in areas with hyperendemic or epidemic disease, e.g., the "meningitis belt" of sub-Saharan Africa stretching from Mauritania to Ethiopia.

Booster doses are not currently recommended for adults. The major side effects are local reactions lasting 1 to 2 days.

Rabies (Ch. 477)

Rabies vaccine is indicated for pre-exposure prophylaxis of high-risk persons, including animal handlers, selected laboratory and field workers, and persons traveling for more than 1 month to areas where rabies is a constant threat. The pre-exposure regimen consists of either three 1.0-ml intramuscular injections on days 0, 7, and 28 for all rabies vaccines or, for the human diploid cell vaccine (HDCV) only, three 0.1-ml intradermal injections on days 0, 7, and 21 or 28. Testing for serum antibody or a booster every 2 years is indicated for persons with continuing risk. Postexposure treatment depends on prior exposure to vaccine and is discussed in detail in Ch. 477.

Vaccines Intended Primarily for International Travelers (Ch. 290)

YELLOW FEVER (Ch. 391). Yellow fever now occurs only in areas of South America and Africa. Vaccination with a single dose of the live attenuated 17D strain of virus confers protection to almost all recipients for at least 10 years. Boosters are recommended every 10 years for those at risk. Side effects are uncommon. Yellow fever vaccine should not be given to immunocompromised persons or those with anaphylactic allergies to eggs. The vaccine is contraindicated in pregnant women on theoretical grounds, although if such women must travel to a high-risk area, they may be vaccinated.

TYPHOID VACCINE (Ch. 313). Two types of vaccines, a live attenuated Ty21a oral vaccine and a parenteral heat-phenol–inactivated vaccine, appear to be of comparable efficacy (50 to 77 per cent). Typhoid vaccine is indicated primarily for travelers to areas where the risk of prolonged exposure to contaminated food and water is high. The vaccine is not optimally effective; food and water precautions are still essential. The vaccine may also be considered for family or other intimate contacts of typhoid carriers and for laboratory workers who work with *Salmonella typhi*. For adults and children 6 years of age and older, either vaccine may be used. For Ty21a, one enteric-coated capsule is taken every other day for four doses. Alternatively, two doses of inactivated vaccine separated by 4 or more weeks may be given. The duration of protection with Ty21a is not known; the manufacturer recommends a repeat primary series every 4 to 5 years for persons at risk. Boosters every 3 years are recommended for recipients of the inactivated vaccine if they continue to be at risk.

The parenteral vaccine is often associated with local reactions and fever. Reactions to the oral vaccine appear to be rare.

CHOLERA (Ch. 317). Cholera vaccines offer only about 50 per cent protection after completion of a primary series of two doses 1 week to 1 month apart. Peak protection appears about 2 months after the last dose, and protection wanes by 3 to 6 months. Vaccination often results in significant local reactions accompanied by fever. Neurologic reactions are rare. The major indication is to meet requirements imposed by some countries for entry.

Other Vaccines

A number of other vaccines, used in selected circumstances, include (1) smallpox vaccine, which is used by the military and laboratory workers who handle orthopox viruses; (2) BCG vaccine, a vaccine used to prevent tuberculosis, which has very limited use in the United States; (3) oral adenovirus vaccines types 4 and 7 for use in the military; (4) anthrax vaccine, which is indicated in selected high-risk worker populations; and (5) plague vaccine, which may be considered for workers at risk and for some travelers. In addition, trivalent botulism antitoxin (ABE) is available from the CDC for treatment of suspected cases of botulism. Japanese encephalitis vaccine (with a protective efficacy of greater than 95 per cent) is available in Canada, Australia, and various European and Asian countries. Although not currently licensed in the United States, the vaccine is indicated for persons who live in endemic areas or will travel to rural endemic areas during transmission season.

Although not available today, a number of vaccines are under development and may be licensed in the future. Extensive field trials have occurred with varicella vaccine, which is probably the closest to completing development. Because of the biotechnology revolution, it is likely that many more vaccines will become available in the future.

ACP Task Force on Adult Immunization, Infectious Diseases Society of America. Guide for Adult Immunization, 2nd ed. Philadelphia, American College of Physicians, 1990, pp 1–188. *An excellent comprehensive guide covering all aspects of adult immunization. A must for the physician who cares for adults, whether in primary, secondary, or tertiary care.*

Centers for Disease Control: Adult Immunization. Recommendations of the Immunization Practices Advisory Committee (ACIP). MMWR 33:1S, 1984. *A compendium of ACIP statements on immunizations for adults as well as valuable information on other aspects of immunization. This version is currently being revised. ACIP statements on individual vaccines are published as available in the* Morbidity and Mortality Weekly Report.

Committee on Infectious Diseases, American Academy of Pediatrics: Report of the Committee on Infectious Diseases. 21st ed. Elk Grove Village, Ill., American Academy of Pediatrics, 1988, pp 1–566. *The "Red Book" is published every 2 to 3 years and addresses in a comprehensive manner vaccination of children and adolescents as well as other issues relating to prevention, control, and treatment of infectious diseases.*

Centers for Disease Control: Health Information for International Travel. Washington, D.C., U.S. Government Printing Office, 1989. *A complete guide for the international traveler, including required and recommended vaccinations. Revised annually.*

Centers for Disease Control: Measles prevention: Recommendations of the Immu-

nization Practices Advisory Committee (ACIP) MMWR 38 (S-9):1, 1989. *A thorough review of the current measles situation and the new recommendations for a routine two-dose schedule.*

Centers for Disease Control: Protection against viral hepatitis: Recommendations of the Immunization Practices Advisory Committee (ACIP). MMWR 39 (RR-2):1, 1990. *An extensive document covering all aspects of hepatitis B prevention and control.*

Greenberg MA, Birx DL: Safe administration of mumps-measles-rubella vaccine in egg-allergic children. J Pediatr 113:504, 1988. *A protocol for vaccinating persons with anaphylactic allergies to eggs. Also reviews other protocols.*

17 The Preventive Health Examination

Gary D. Friedman

The primary purpose of preventive health examinations is to maintain or improve health. The rationale is that early detection of disease or of high risk of subsequent disease can lead to treatment or remedial measures that will prevent or postpone morbidity, disability, or mortality.

An "annual physical" for asymptomatic adults was once accepted as good medical practice. In recent years periodic health examinations have become controversial: (1) The costs of a thorough medical history, physical examination, and standard laboratory tests would be enormous if these procedures were annually and universally applied. (2) Many elements of traditional check-ups have not been shown to benefit asymptomatic persons. On the other hand, certain simple procedures and screening tests have the potential of prolonging life and preventing disability.

ROUTINE TESTS AND PROCEDURES OF PROVEN OR PROBABLE VALUE IN PREVENTIVE CARE FOR ADULTS. A test is suitable for routine use if it can detect a serious and relatively common disease at an early stage, or at a predisease high-risk stage, when treatment or intervention would be more effective. Furthermore, the test should be relatively economical in terms of both money and professional time. A few tests or procedures meet these criteria; a few others are of probable value but less universally accepted (Table 17–1). Doubts about tests of probable value revolve primarily around the benefits of treatment compared with the harm of labeling (e.g., mild asymptomatic diabetes mellitus), the high relative frequency and high cost of evaluating false-positive results (e.g., occult blood in the stool), and the low yield of significant disease in the asymptomatic patient (e.g., palpating the abdomen).

Some previously accepted tests are no longer advised. A good example is the routine chest radiograph, which has not proved effective in reducing mortality from lung cancer. Additional tests currently recommended for pregnant women, such as screening for bacteriuria or hepatitis B surface antigen, are discussed in the *Guide to Clinical Preventive Services* (see references). Evidence concerning the efficacy in preserving health and the cost-effectiveness of screening tests is slow to accumulate. As it does, current recommendations may be expected to change.

ADDITIONAL BENEFITS OF PREVENTIVE HEALTH APPRAISALS. Detecting disease or abnormalities is not the only benefit of the preventive health examination. Negative findings are also of value because of the reassurance they provide to the patient, especially if the patient has received what he or she perceives to be a thorough examination. In contemplating cuts in the content of routine checkups, physicians and health care planners must weigh the immediate economic gains against the possible decrease in this reassurance if patients perceive the examinations to be abbreviated or cursory.

A lengthy and thorough examination when a patient is first seen permits collection of baseline data that may be useful when symptoms or findings develop later. Also, the additional time spent in obtaining a medical and social history, examining the patient, and discussing the patient's concerns helps to establish a good doctor-patient relationship. Further, certain valuable information can be obtained during a thorough first examination

TABLE 17-1. STANDARD CONTENT OF THE PREVENTIVE HEALTH EXAMINATION FOR ASYMPTOMATIC, NONPREGNANT ADULTS

Of Accepted Value	Of Probable Value, Especially in High-Risk Individuals
Medical History	
1. Smoking, particularly cigarettes	1. Postmenopausal bleeding
2. Drinking alcohol to excess	2. Immunization status
3. Failure to wear seat belts in cars and safety helmets on motorcycles or bicycles	3. Use of nonmedical drugs other than alcohol, tobacco, and caffeine
4. Unsafe sexual practices	4. Lack of regular physical activity
5. Excessive sun exposure	5. Excessive saturated fat consumption
Physical Examination	
1. Assessment of obesity	1. Search for cancers or precancerous lesions of the skin, mouth, pharynx, thyroid, testes, uterus, prostate, and rectum
2. Measurement of blood pressure	
3. Detection of suspicious breast lumps	2. Palpation of the abdomen for aortic aneurysms in men at least 60 years of age
Laboratory or Diagnostic Studies	
1. Mammography in women at least 50 years of age	1. Mammography in women age 35 or 40 to 49 years
2. Papanicolaou test for cervical cancer	2. Test of stool for occult blood
3. Serum cholesterol concentration	3. Fasting blood glucose (in persons at high risk for diabetes mellitus)
4. Serologic test for latent syphilis, cervical culture for gonorrhea, and serologic test (with counseling) for HIV infection (for persons at high risk)	4. Tuberculin skin test (in high-risk individuals)
	5. Sigmoidoscopy in persons at least 50 years of age
	6. Testing for *Chlamydia* infection (in high-risk individuals)

and need not be sought routinely again. A good example is rheumatic heart disease detected by history and cardiac auscultation.

MULTIPHASIC AND SELECTIVE SCREENING. Screening tests aimed at early disease detection are sometimes offered singly, as in special programs to detect tuberculosis, diabetes mellitus, or breast cancer. Clearly, it is more economical and efficient to test for several diseases at a single visit than for single diseases at several visits. Multiphasic screening provides several tests comparatively economically at one patient visit and can be used as part of a periodic health examination. Components of health screening or health examinations may be used for some patients and not others, depending on previous findings, risk characteristics, medical history, or current symptoms of the patient. This use of screening tests is known as selective or discriminate screening.

FREQUENCY OF EXAMINATIONS. It is not clear how frequently preventive health examinations, either basic or thorough, should be performed. The physician must strike a balance between excessive costs and low yield of too frequent examinations, and the chance that an important and controllable condition will develop and become irreversible if examinations are not provided often enough. Several sets of recommendations have been made recently based on available evidence and "prudent" judgment (see references). A common theme is that the incidence of most disabling and fatal diseases increases with age. Thus, basic examinations containing essential tests such as blood pressure measurement and breast palpation should increase in frequency from once in several years in the patient's twenties to annually in the fifties or sixties and older. As age advances it is advisable to observe the patient for losses in hearing, vision, and mental functioning as well. Even if losses are irreversible, knowledge of these limitations aids in advising the patient and his or her family. Clearly, in our present state of knowledge, clinical

judgment must play an important role both in deciding on the frequency of examinations and in selecting examination components for individual patients based on their age, sex, medical history, and current risk status. Many of the preventive maneuvers can, of course, be incorporated into visits for care of illness.

NEED FOR APPROPRIATE FOLLOW-UP. A *health examination is of little value without appropriate follow-up,* including treatment of early disease if indicated and counseling to encourage favorable changes in risk factors and a healthier lifestyle. For many physicians the latter may require a change in orientation. The training of the physician, particularly the internist, tends to emphasize disease and treatment rather than health and prevention, diseases with complex pathogenesis rather than simple injuries, and technical procedures rather than simple observation and conversation. Time spent detecting and correcting unhealthy habits, such as failure to use seat belts in cars, may in the long run do more for the health of the patient than routinely performing panels of biochemical tests. Complementary changes are required, not only in the system of providing and paying for care, but also in the orientation of many patients. They must be made aware that much of the responsibility for staying healthy is theirs.

American Cancer Society: Report on the cancer-related health checkup. CA 30:194, 1980. *A critical evaluation of methods of early detection of cancer.*

Breslow L, Somers AR: The lifetime health-monitoring program: A practical approach to preventive medicine. N Engl J Med 296:601, 1977. *This review of health examinations contains recommendations that emphasize a changing approach for different age groups and the need for cost-effective preventive measures.*

Canadian Task Force on the Periodic Health Examination (Spitzer W, chairman): The periodic health examination. Can Med Assoc J 121:1193, 1979; 130:1276, 1984; 134:721, 1986; 138:617, 1988. *A summary of various components of preventive health examinations and preventive care. The need for a selective rather than a routine approach is emphasized.*

Council on Scientific Affairs, Division of Scientific Activities, American Medical Association: Medical evaluation of healthy persons. JAMA 249:1626, 1983. *A brief compilation of recommendations concerning health examinations at all ages, reviewed in the context of current and previous positions of the American Medical Association.*

Frame PS: A critical review of adult health maintenance. J Fam Pract 22:341, 417, 511; 23:29, 1986. *An updated and very readable review of major elements of the adult health examination with specific recommendations.*

Guide to clinical preventive services: An assessment of the effectiveness of 169 interventions. Report of the U.S. Preventive Services Task Force, Baltimore, Williams and Wilkins, 1989. *A thorough, well-organized review of a large number of preventive maneuvers in the context of the doctor's office or clinic.*

Medical Practice Committee, American College of Physicians: Periodic health examination: A guide for designing individualized preventive health care in the asymptomatic patient. Ann Intern Med 95:729, 1981. *A diagrammatic summary of recommendations that are considered minimal preventive measures for apparently well asymptomatic individuals at low medical risk.*

Oboler SK, LaForce FM: The periodic physical examination in asymptomatic adults. Ann Intern Med 110:214, 1989. *An up-to-date evaluation of the usefulness in periodic health appraisals of components of the physical examination.*

18 The Health of the Physician

Linda Hawes Clever

Physicians are a singular lot. In some areas, their health habits and health are exemplary, yet in others they are dangerous to themselves and patients. The purpose of this chapter is to review available data about the lives, deaths, and personal health practices of physicians and to make recommendations about health maintenance activities for them.

PHYSICIANS' WORK

Physicians work harder than most people. They work 15 hours per week longer than other professionals; take less vacation time (4 weeks per year versus 8 weeks per year for most other professionals); and work more years than the general population and therefore have a shorter retirement (3.1 years versus 7.8 years). They also have unique responsibilities and duties.

Demands of Training and Practice

Tensions develop early in medicine. Students and house officers may have to contend with information overload, sleep deprivation, sexual harassment and other abuse, time limitations, health risks, lack of faculty support, and chemical dependency. They, and physicians in practice, also cite special pressures generated by patients and patients' families. These include unwarranted but firmly held expectations of cure, relief, or certainty. Physicians are disturbed by inflicting pain during diagnostic tests, coping with their own minor or grievous errors, and dealing with dying patients. Physicians feel angry or guilty about working with "difficult" patients or being unable to answer questions. They dislike medical politics, paperwork, and committee work. Public policy changes spawn concerns about preserving the quality of patient care, competition from other physicians and health practitioners, independence, the funding of both research and graduate medical education, and income maintenance. Professional liability casts a long shadow, with a 10 per cent increase per year in medical malpractice suits. The world changes rapidly; morale wavers.

Family and Lifestyle Tensions and Pleasures

It has been said that physicians have one of the few socially acceptable reasons for abandoning a family. The rigors of being "on call" can interfere with family plans. Intensive focus on professional responsibilities leads to muddled values, constricted relationships, and stunted personal growth. Taxing schedules can clash with parenting and constrict creativity. Even reading for pleasure, attending church, and exercise may be squeezed out by professional pressures. Women face particular demands as they juggle family and work exigencies.

Fairness requires comments on the "other" side. There are numerous intrinsic pleasures in the medical profession. Making precision diagnoses, teaching, counseling, providing support and motivation, ameliorating suffering, treating disease, and saving lives are particularly satisfying. Developing personal relationships with patients and their families and earning a reasonable living have appeal. Working with people during crises and dealing with the most private aspects of their lives and bodies provide staggering yet exhilarating experiences.

PHYSICIANS' HEALTH
Overall Mortality

Unfortunately, data about the health status of physicians are scattered and rarely provide comparisons with other professionals. Despite the complexities and challenges of physicians' work and lives, *they are at least as healthy as the general population in most respects.*

For both male and female physicians in the United States, age-adjusted mortality is less than for their counterparts in almost every 5-year grouping from age 20 to over 85. Life expectancy for male and female physicians is greater by over 3 years and over 1 year respectively, than for the general American population from ages 25 to 80. Firm conclusions about the relative longevity of specialists and nonspecialists await further studies.

Disease-Specific Mortality

TOBACCO-RELATED ILLNESS. About one third of Americans smoke; fewer than 10 per cent of physicians smoke; and fewer than 5 per cent of physicians under 30 years of age smoke. It is not surprising that *smoking-related mortality among physicians is plummeting.* Deaths from lung cancer in male physicians in California halved between 1950 to 1959 and 1970 to 1979; other smoking-related diseases had striking declines (bronchitis, chronic obstructive pulmonary disease, and cancers of the esophagus and mouth). Although the incidence of fatal arteriosclerotic cardiovascular disease among physicians *was* higher than in the general population, it is now lower.

SUICIDES. On the darker side, *early death from suicide* appears to be excessive among physicians. Male physicians probably commit suicide twice as often as the United States white male population. Female physicians take their own lives at a rate slightly more than triple that of white American women. Differences in suicide rates by specialty have not been verified. Professionals in other health sciences such as dentistry and pharmacy have strikingly higher suicide rates than physicians. Overall, however, data are marred by incorrect reporting or underreporting, small numbers, and inadequate comparison groups by age, sex, and profession. It is not surprising that

physicians may have the same sorts of characteristics that drive others to suicide. These include a variety of family-related markers such as (1) death of a close relative during childhood or thereafter, (2) being single, and (3) excessive or incomplete integration into a family unit. Depression is an important element (Ch. 451). Other psychiatric diagnoses such as severe personality disorder or psychosis may also lead to suicide. A history of a prior suicide attempt is a warning of high suicide risk. Financial problems, poor health, and substance abuse often contribute as well. Special problems that may incline physicians toward suicide include professional isolation, the tensions of training or practice, unrealistic expectations, rifts in relationships, and the exhaustion and emotional burdens of patient care.

Morbidity

The age-adjusted death rate of physicians is lower than that of other Americans, but it might be even lower except for several factors. For example, most physicians *do not have their own doctor* who can provide health promotion and surveillance. Fortunately, two thirds of physicians over 50 have routine health examinations. Self-treatment, curbstone consultations, and delays because of embarrassment about professional courtesy can impede diagnosis and treatment. Fear and denial may slow care. A pathologic extension of denial is the "physician invulnerability syndrome," which is characterized by the conviction that the personal and family problems, the aggravations, and the diseases that affect others cannot or will not affect the physician.

Substance Abuse

There is reason for concern about alcohol and drug abuse among physicians. Reliable, recent statistics are scarce, however. Current literature suggests parity between physicians and the general public in the prevalence of alcoholism. Drug abuse may be somewhat more common among physicians than other Americans. Regardless of population comparisons, of course, *substance abuse is a deadly problem for physicians, their families, and their patients.* Damage to patients resulting from confusion, inattention, poor judgment, unavailability, or psychomotor deficits often occurs before the physician seeks, or is forced, into care. Automobile and private plane accidents are associated with intoxication, as are family dissolution and substance abuse in children of abusers (see Ch. 15). Although denial plays a major role at the inception of addiction and denial makes therapy more challenging, physicians seem to have a better prognosis, with treatment, than other middle-class substance abusers.

PERSONAL HEALTH PRACTICES OF PHYSICIANS

Many health promotion efforts for adults target smoking cessation, good nutrition, exercise, moderation of alcohol intake, immunization, and seatbelt use. The regular use of low-dose aspirin to counter cardiovascular disease may become indicated. As with other health care workers, universal precautions for infectious diseases and hazardous chemicals are being emphasized. The exceptional record of physicians in smoking avoidance has already been described, but other health habits seem to be less exemplary. For example, although most physicians report that they are careful about dietary fat, calories, and/or salt, 29 to 58 per cent acknowledge that they are overweight. Thirty-seven to 73 per cent of physicians do not engage in weekly vigorous exercise. Although most are moderate in the frequency and volume of alcohol consumption, 13 to 24 per cent of physicians drink daily, and 20 per cent have at least two drinks when they do drink. Up to 10 per cent of physicians are problem drinkers.

Immunization

By and large, physicians have an abysmal record of immunization for diseases that can affect them or that they can transmit. For example, only 10 to 31 per cent of rubella antibody–negative physicians who work with children, pregnant women, and other patients receive rubella vaccine. At least 84 per cent of physicians are susceptible to hepatitis B (and, therefore, delta hepatitis), but very few house officers or attending physicians receive hepatitis B vaccine. The prevalence of immunization of physicians for tetanus/diphtheria, polio, and influenza is unknown. Since health risks and costs are low, results are favorable, and the professional liability of not being vaccinated is high, wise physicians get vaccinated.

AIDS and Hepatitis B

AIDS is causing widespread tragedy. Among physicians, it can engender fear, dislike, exhaustion, avoidance, a sense of helplessness, and skewed experience (in medical training and practice). It can also bring the distinct satisfactions of making difficult diagnoses, providing treatment and comfort, solving research challenges, and working with respected colleagues. The causative agent, human immunodeficiency virus (HIV), can be transmitted during medical procedures, especially by punctures with hollow needles when visible blood is injected into the health care worker. The risk of transmitting HIV during a needle stick has been estimated at 0.4 per cent. This is small compared to the risk of transmitting hepatitis B virus (HBV) during a similar accident: 25 per cent. To avoid disease and death, it is imperative for physicians and other health care workers to use universal precautions. That is, assume that all patients are infected with all agents. Whenever a procedure may be damp or wet or fluids may fly, gloves, goggles, and masks, as indicated, must be worn. Hepatitis B vaccine and AIDS vaccine (if and when available) must be taken.

Other important measures during the AIDS catastrophe include continuing education, examination of prejudices, and provision of support groups and grief counseling for caregivers.

TABLE 18–1. SUGGESTIONS TO PHYSICIANS ABOUT GOOD HEALTH

Do:
1. Get help when you need it. Don't deny; don't delay.
2. Fasten your seatbelt—always.
3. Get antibody screening and appropriate vaccination for hepatitis B, tetanus/diphtheria, influenza, rubella, pneumonia, polio, and measles.
4. Practice moderation in diet and alcohol intake.
5. Exercise regularly and sensibly.
6. Engage fully in the pageantry of living in activities with your family, friends, and community.
7. Cultivate your creativity; be interested, not just interesting, and use your sense of humor.
8. Start planning for your retirement 25 to 30 years before your goal.
    a. Feel free to relish your profession, and if you don't, consider important changes.
    b. Get reputable, professional help with financial planning.

Do not:
1. Smoke.
2. Use nonprescribed drugs.
3. Ignore your family and friends while serving others or meeting their demands.
4. Ignore your own needs for personal and intellectual growth.

Seatbelt Use

Seatbelt use by physicians is the least well-documented good health habit. One might extrapolate from other factors that correlate with seatbelt use (such as educational level, regular visits to a dentist, and nonsmoking) that physicians buckle up more often than others. Such a practice would be felicitous, since (1) many physicians drive hundreds of miles per week; (2) each American has a one in three chance of being disabled by an automobile injury during his or her lifetime; (3) always using a seatbelt can reduce the risk of serious injury or death by greater than one half.

Effects on Others of Good Health Habits by the Physician

Good health practices not only improve the health and lives of physicians themselves but also can affect others as well. As implied above, moderation of alcohol use and eschewing of drug use by physicians can prevent direct harm to patients. Vaccination of physicians can prevent transmission of infectious diseases. Of great importance is the observation that *physicians' personal health habits help determine the advice that they give to patients.* Physicians with good health habits (regarding smoking, weight, exercise, and alcohol) are far more likely to counsel primary prevention than are others.

RECOMMENDATIONS

Physicians, in concert with their own physicians and families, need to analyze their own health and health behavior (Table 18–1). They need to assess pain and pleasure, risks and benefits. If change is necessary or desirable, a plan needs to be developed. Barriers need to be removed, incentives and rewards incorporated, and progress documented and celebrated.

Hayward RA, Shapiro MF: A national study of AIDS and residency training: Experiences, concerns, and consequences. Ann Intern Med 114:23, 1991. *A cross-sectional, self-administered questionnaire sent to senior internal medicine and family medicine residents revealed their experiences with AIDS patients, plans for providing primary care to them, and impressions about the adequacy of training as well as their concerns about contracting human immunodeficiency virus infection.*

Koran LM, Litt IF: House staff well-being. West J Med 148:97, 1988. *A large number of house officers at a university medical center were surveyed. Results include the incidence of anxiety or depression, drug and alcohol use, and comparisons of men and women as well as married and unmarried house officers by departments.*

Lewis CE, et al.: The counseling practices of internists. Ann Intern Med 114:54, 1991. *This paper combines an analysis of physicians' health education advice to their patients with their own health promotion activities. Areas covered include smoking, seat belt use, alcohol use, and exercise.*

McAuliffe WE, Rohman M, Santangelo S, et al.: Psychoactive drug use among practicing physicians and medical students. N Engl J Med 315:805, 1986. *This well-referenced research paper shows that physicians' use of psychoactive drugs is not very different from that of other professionals. High drug use by younger physicians and poor education of most physicians about drugs and alcohol are danger signals, however.*

Roy A: Suicide in doctors. Psychiatry Clin North Am 8:377, 1985. *Its important topic, incisive commentary, and 44 references make this short paper especially useful.*

PART IV
PRINCIPLES OF DIAGNOSIS AND MANAGEMENT

19 Clinical Approach to the Patient

Suzanne W. Fletcher

When a patient sees a doctor, whether in the office, the hospital ward, the emergency room, or the nursing home, almost always the patient is seeking help—to regain or retain physical, emotional, and/or mental health. The physician's task is to work for the health of the patient. The doctor does so by trying to prevent, cure or ameliorate disease; relieve discomforts such as pain or nausea; help the patient to be as functional as possible; prevent untimely death; and maximize contentment and satisfaction. (Some have summarized these activities as tackling "the five D's" of health— disease, discomfort, disability, death, and dissatisfaction.) Sometimes there is success in all these areas; in the best of circumstances, the doctor is able to prevent disease and help the patient remain healthy. In other cases, disease and death will triumph, and it is possible only to make the patient more comfortable. In some cases, none of the goals is achieved. Regardless of success, it is important that the physician work on the five D's in every encounter with a patient. By doing so, the doctor learns to focus on health outcomes of the patient and to test the myriad activities of clinical medicine against these outcomes.

In most clinical encounters the patient presents one or more basic questions to the doctor: Am I sick? If so, what is causing my sickness? Will it go away? Will it kill me? Can you make me well, or at least better? If I am not sick, can you help me stay well?

The patient's questions set the stage for the clinical activities of making a diagnosis, determining prognosis, carrying out treatment, promoting health, and preventing disease. These activities make up the bulk of daily clinical work. Although young physicians learn them one at a time, the master clinician blends them so skillfully that often it is difficult to discern which is occurring at a given moment. For instance, when obtaining a history or performing a physical examination to determine a diagnosis, the master clinician all the while is considering prognosis and is treating the patient with appropriate attention, words, empathy, and therapeutic and preventive information, thus ensuring that the patient feels and is better just for having been with the doctor.

DIAGNOSIS

Diagnosis is accomplished with history, physical examination, and laboratory tests. Modern medicine has shifted attention toward the laboratory, but even today most of the diagnosis is accomplished by the history and physical examination, which narrow the diagnostic possibilities before laboratory tests are used. Also, through taking the medical history and conducting the physical examination, the doctor humanizes the medical encounter for the patient and sets the stage for successful treatment.

Medical History

There are standard sections to a complete medical history (Table 19–1). It is usually appropriate to obtain the complete history when a physician and patient meet for the first time.

During follow-up visits active medical problems are the focus. If the patient's presenting complaint is urgent, it may not be feasible to obtain a complete medical history—for example, when a patient is admitted to the intensive care unit or is seen in the emergency room or walk-in clinic. In all cases, the doctor should start with what is most important in the history (the present illness), and according to circumstances, adjust the rest of the history taking. The patient's medical history can and should be augmented at each subsequent doctor-patient encounter.

HISTORY OF THE PRESENT ILLNESS. The present illness is like a newspaper story. For each major symptom, the doctor must determine *what* (pain, nausea, weakness, etc.), *where* (part of body), *when* (continuous, intermittent, time of day, etc.), *how much* (severity), *chronologic course* (beginning of symptom, end, improvement, worsening), and what makes the symptom *better or worse*. It is important to determine what medical care the patient has already received for the problem, including laboratory tests previously done, their results, the diagnosis reached, the treatment given, whether the patient adhered to the treatment, and results of the treatment. Finally, the physician must seek answers to questions that narrow the diagnostic possibilities. This step, the most difficult part of obtaining an understanding of the present illness, requires a great deal of diagnostic skill and knowledge. Skilled clinicians form diagnostic hypotheses early in the patient's story and are able to ask specific questions, the answers to which confirm or exclude a given diagnostic possibility. Parts of the history of the present illness (description of symptoms and treatment compliance) are best obtained from the patient, whereas others (details about previously performed laboratory tests and treatment) are best acquired from medical sources.

TABLE 19–1. THE PATIENT'S MEDICAL HISTORY

Description of patient
  Age, gender, race, occupation, and, for women, parity
Chief Complaint
  Four or five words, preferably quoting the patient, stating the
    purpose of the visit and the duration of the complaint. Occasionally
    the patient states a request (e.g., "I need a flu shot") instead of a
    complaint.
Other physicians involved in the patient's care
  Name, address, telephone number, and relationship to the patient
History of the present illness
  For each major symptom, what, where, when, how much,
    chronologic course, what makes the symptom better or worse, past
    medical care, questions to narrow diagnostic possibilities
Past medical history
  Previous illnesses and hospitalizations, immunizations, medications
    the patient takes, allergies, and alcohol, tobacco, and drug habits
Social and occupational history
  Description of a typical day in the patient's life and how the present
    illness affects it, social supports (family, friends, and colleagues)
    available to the patient, and occupational history
Family history
  History of genetically related diseases in the patient's family and
    longevity and cause of death of family members
Review of systems
  Systematic review of major organ systems: skin, hematopoietic system
    (including lymph nodes), head, eyes, ears, nose, mouth, throat,
    neck, breasts, and respiratory, cardiovascular, gastrointestinal,
    genitourinary, musculoskeletal, nervous, endocrine and psychiatric
    systems

THE CLINICAL INTERVIEW TECHNIQUE. The interaction of a doctor and patient during the medical interview is, at its best, a marvelous mixture of art and science. The art is the interaction of two unique human beings; the science is from both the biologic and behavioral sciences.

Each physician must develop an interviewing technique that is comfortable and true to his or her own personality. The interview style must also vary according to the particular patient. Some patients are incredibly long-winded; others, right to the point; and still others, mute. Some patients want to control the encounter, some are passive, some are downright hostile. The doctor should adjust the interview accordingly. At all times, however, the patient must be treated with courtesy and dignity.

Certain principles are emerging from scientific study of the doctor-patient interview. It is the physician's job to manage the pace and direction of the interview. At the beginning, the doctor should introduce himself or herself and address the patient by name. It is reasonable to indicate how long the encounter is likely to last, thereby setting the stage for subsequent activities. The physician should communicate total attention toward the patient. Usually, this is best done by sitting down and looking the patient in the eye. Even a few minutes of full attention are worth 30 minutes of distracted interaction.

Most patients do not follow the order the physician wants in the medical history. A patient may include bits and pieces of social and family history while describing the current complaint. It is the physician's job to fashion order out of the story, while still allowing the patient a chance to tell the story in his or her own way. Giving the patient this chance increases the likelihood of patient satisfaction with the clinical encounter as well as the patient's willingness to follow the doctor's advice about treatment. In addition, many doctors enjoy listening to their patients. Over a lifetime, a physician will meet patients from almost every class, race, educational level, profession, moral persuasion, and personality type. The rich variety of humanity can be gleaned by listening to patients' stories told in their own ways.

After introductions, the physician asks why the patient has come. Then the doctor should listen. If questions are needed to help the patient along, they should be open-ended and nonspecific. After a few minutes, the doctor should begin to direct the interview more actively, by facilitating the patient's story with more directed questions. Often, it helps to summarize the history during the interview. Finally, the doctor must narrow the diagnostic possibilities with appropriate questions.

If time is short, the doctor must take charge of the interview more quickly, but in almost all circumstances, the patient should be given a chance to tell his or her story. If the physician takes charge too quickly, not only does patient satisfaction and cooperation decrease, but the chances for a missed diagnosis increase. This is especially true when the patient is afraid or uncomfortable to speak openly, as with teenage pregnancies or cases of sexual abuse.

PAST MEDICAL HISTORY, SOCIAL HISTORY, FAMILY HISTORY, AND REVIEW OF SYSTEMS. These sections (Table 19–1) are far more rote than the history of the present illness, and the questions in each section are best memorized. The doctor should explain briefly each new section so that the patient understands the shift in topic ("Now I would like to ask you about other illnesses you may have had in the past") and start with general questions ("Have you ever been sick before?").

Usually, the social history is least relevant for diagnosis and therefore is most frequently shortened or omitted by physicians. However, learning about a patient's daily life, how the current illness is affecting it, and what social supports the patient can call on for assistance are particularly important when trying to fashion an effective treatment for the patient.

Because most questions in the latter sections of the medical history are standard, in some cases answers can be obtained by giving the patient a printed questionnaire or by using a computerized questionnaire. Both can be set up in a branching manner, so that affirmative answers can be explored further.

Physical Examination

The physical examination is accomplished with the eyes, ears, hands, and sometimes the nose. Physicians in training should practice the complete physical examination on as many patients as possible to master all parts thoroughly. A complete examination, with a thorough neurologic and pelvic examination, takes even skillful examiners a good deal of time. Sometimes, because of time and setting restraints, or because the visit is a follow-up, the doctor conducts only a partial examination.

Several principles are important every time a physician performs a physical examination. The physician must demonstrate respect for the patient and the patient's modesty, making sure to expose private parts of the body only for as long as necessary for a careful examination. The physical examination should follow a standard order and be carried out in a systematic manner. It should be as comfortable as possible for the patient and require a minimum amount of shifting and changing of position. The more uncomfortable parts of the examination, such as the rectal and pelvic examinations, generally should be performed last.

The physical examination starts with inspection, begun during the interview, and obtaining the vital signs. The physician always should examine carefully those parts of the body that are related or potentially related to the reason for the patient's visit. Whenever possible, objective measurements, such as number and size of nodes, breadth of the liver, or the circumference of the calf, should be taken and recorded, not only for accurate assessment of the clinical course of a medical condition but also for more precise communication with other clinicians who may see the patient. In most cases there is time to perform at least a cursory complete examination as well. The less time spent on the examination, the more intently the physician should use his or her eyes to pick up every possible cue.

Physicians should strive to improve their physical examination skills throughout their careers. One way to do this is to pick out different parts of the examination and practice it on every patient seen during a given period. For example, a few weeks of extra attention to the thyroid will solidify and improve that examination, even if none of the patients so examined has thyroid disease.

Questioning and examining the patient are types of diagnostic tests, subject to scientific investigation just as laboratory tests are. Some questions and examination techniques are more valid than others in making diagnoses. For example, the many different ways of examining the breast are not equally good at detecting lumps. As research develops improved examination techniques, clinicians should master them.

Laboratory Tests

Although laboratory tests have become a standard part of the doctor-patient encounter, their correct use is complex and subject to a number of scientific principles (see Ch. 21). One of the modern physician's most important tasks is to learn these principles and use laboratory tests appropriately. The physician must also explain clearly to the patient the purpose and use of tests, as described below. Although generally used for diagnosis or screening, occasionally a laboratory test is ordered as a therapeutic maneuver. For example, a patient with chest pain may be reassured by a normal chest radiograph.

PROGNOSIS

It is important to tell the patient the diagnosis (writing it down often helps) and discuss what to expect from the clinical course of the condition. For many patients, the prognosis of the illness is their greatest concern. If it is likely that the illness will resolve without sequelae, reassurance is often all that is needed.

The most difficult prognoses to discuss are those for lethal illnesses, especially for most cancers. Most patients want to know even bad prognoses, but how much a physician tells a given patient should be determined primarily by the patient, not the physician. The physician has the duty to make the patient aware of his or her willingness to discuss prognosis. Often detailed discussions are best conducted at follow-up visits, after the two have had a chance to get to know each other. The best physicians blend honest fact and hope together, helping the patient through the complicated steps of shock, denial, depression, and acceptance of a fatal illness. Most importantly, they make it clear that they will not abandon the patient.

Doctors should educate themselves about the clinical course of the medical illnesses they encounter. No matter the import of the disease, they should learn how long, on average, the pain of herpes zoster continues, the headache of sinusitis persists, and the patient with class IV congestive heart failure lives.

TREATMENT AND PREVENTION

Increasingly, patients visit doctors not for diagnosis but for treatment of ongoing medical problems. Even when a doctor must make the diagnosis, it is important to remember that making a diagnosis alone cannot improve the health of the patient. Only treatment and prevention can.

Two general principles should be kept in mind about treatment. First, the physician should treat the patient as well as the disease. With every clinical encounter, the physician should strive to ensure that the patient feels better just for having been with the doctor. When prescribing specific treatment, alleviation of symptoms, especially pain and nausea, is often as important to the patient as, say, antibiotics for an infection. Second, successful treatment for an illness, especially outside the hospital, usually requires the active participation of the patient.

Therapeutic Procedures

Therapeutic procedures like surgery, radiation, angioplasty, and chemotherapy (as well as invasive diagnostic tests) must be explained thoroughly to the patient; in most cases, signed consent must be obtained. The physician must help the patient understand what will happen during the procedure, the hoped-for outcome and its probability, and adverse effects of the procedure and their probabilities. Informed consent is a medical-legal requirement, but just as important, it is a requirement of excellent clinical care. Technologic advances in medicine are complicated, rarely without the potential for adverse complications, and often costly. True informed consent requires a great deal of clinical skill on the doctor's part. The physician should act as the patient's advocate. The patient should be given the necessary facts, but not overwhelmed with incomprehensible technical details or a long list of terrifying yet improbable adverse effects of a procedure. The physician should freely give professional advice but clearly communicate that the final decision is the patient's. If the patient remains undecided about a procedure after a thorough discussion, in most cases it is best to delay the decision. A patient who feels pressured by the doctor to undergo a risky procedure may be particularly upset if complications arise.

Medications

The physician's medication order will usually be carried out in the hospital regardless of the patient's understanding or cooperation, but this is certainly not true outside the hospital. With ambulatory patients it is especially important to explain the medication to the patient, its purpose in simple terms, its dosage schedule, and how long the patient should continue the medicine.

It is useful to ask the patient to bring all medicines to each follow-up visit. Many patients do not know the names of their medicines; discussing pills in bottles is easier than abstract medication names. Often the doctor can make a rough estimate of medication compliance by the level of pills in the bottle (although for ongoing prescriptions patients may combine bottles or refill prescriptions before beginning to take the medication in a particular bottle, thus making accurate compliance measurement impossible). Sometimes the physician discovers that the patient does not have one of the prescribed medicines. The doctor may discover that the patient is taking medication prescribed by another physician. For each medicine discussed, the doctor should ask how often the patient is taking it and if there are any problems. If the patient is taking the medicine incorrectly, the physician can determine whether the problem is misunderstanding of the dosage schedule, forgetfulness, an adverse side effect, the cost of the drug, or some other reason.

To help the patient take prescribed medication, the physician should follow a few common sense rules. The most important determinant of medication compliance is the number of medicines prescribed, so parsimony is key. In general, and especially for a patient on multiple medications, the doctor should strive for simple (once or twice daily) dosage schedules of the least expensive effective medication. At follow-up visits, the fewer the medication changes the better. For patients who have trouble remembering to take their medicines, written instructions or pill containers with alarms can help. Sometimes the physician can

refer the patient to special pharmacy or nursing programs for help with medication compliance.

Prevention

Preventive activities (performing a breast examination and ordering a mammogram on an asymptomatic 55-year-old nurse, administering influenza vaccine to an 80-year-old retired janitor with congestive heart failure, or counseling a 45-year-old truck driver to stop smoking) are periodically performed according to an algorithm based on the patient's age, gender, and clinical status. Prompting systems, such as a prevention checklist, help incorporate appropriate preventive activities into the doctor-patient encounter. If there is no checklist or other system in place, the doctor should briefly consider what preventive activities are indicated in a patient of the given age and sex (see Ch. 17) and perform them.

Doctors perform three types of preventive activities: screening examinations to identify asymptomatic disease or risk factors, immunizations to prevent subsequent disease, and lifestyle counseling to stop harmful habits and promote healthful ones. Physician counseling, especially for smoking cessation and dietary changes, is beginning to receive serious scientific study.

It is much more difficult to get a patient to change daily habits than to agree to screening tests. Physicians who counsel patients to make lifestyle changes should expect many failures. Before beginning counseling, the patient's motivation for change should be determined. If the patient is motivated, and most are, counseling should concentrate on the actual steps the patient should take. Follow-up is key. Most patients fail the first few times they attempt to make a lifestyle change. If that happens, the doctor should encourage the patient to keep trying and avoid being judgmental. Success with even a small percentage of patients can lead to substantial health benefits. If doctors succeed in helping only 10 per cent of their patients who smoke to break the habit, it has been estimated that over 1 million American lives would be saved.

WRAP-UP

After taking the medical history, performing the physical examination, reviewing what laboratory tests are being ordered and why, and discussing recommended treatment and preventive activities, the doctor and patient should discuss follow-up plans and what to do if a problem occurs before the scheduled follow-up visit. The patient should be given the physician's name, *in writing*, and should know how to contact the doctor if the need arises. These steps are particularly important in the practice of internal medicine, in which most patient care involves chronic medical problems rather than episodic illness. The patient should be given a chance to ask any questions he or she may have. At the end of the visit, the doctor should indicate that it was good to see the patient.

CONCLUSION

A successful doctor-patient encounter requires a great deal of work on the doctor's part. The physician must be thinking of many different things at once, not only the diagnostic possibilities, but also the prognostic implications, how and what to communicate to the patient, how to help the patient feel as comfortable as possible, what laboratory tests and therapy to choose, and how to explain them clearly to the patient. These questions must be addressed and updated constantly throughout the interview, often simultaneously. The doctor must translate all the above thought processes into effective interactions with the patient and must work to develop a partnership with the patient so that medically indicated diagnostic tests and treatments that are acceptable to the patient are identified and used. Overriding all of these activities, the doctor must keep asking how to improve and enhance the health of the patient, how to change the five D's.

Paradoxically, modern medicine, with its powerful technologies for diagnosis and treatment, requires more than ever that the physician emphasize one of medicine's most ancient activities, that of being a teacher. Fittingly, society requires that the doctor work with, not on, the patient. Although physicians may come to have a good deal of influence with some of their patients, the best carefully avoid trying to have power over their patients. Like great physicians of old, they know the truth of the classic maxim that the secret of the care of the patient is caring for the patient. By doing so skillfully, the modern physician can help each patient maximize the chances for better health.

Fletcher RH, Fletcher SW, Wagner EH: Clinical Epidemiology—The Essentials. Baltimore, Williams and Wilkins, 1988. *This text outlines the clinical-epidemiologic principles that underlie all doctor-patient encounters.*

Haynes RB, Taylor DW, Sackett DL (eds.): Compliance in Health Care. Baltimore, Johns Hopkins University Press, 1979. *A text with many useful chapters, this book summarizes much of the theory, research findings, and clinical applications of the compliance literature.*

Kottke TE, Battista RN, DeFriese GH, Brekke ML: Attributes of successful smoking cessation interventions in medical practice: A meta-analysis of 39 controlled trials. JAMA. 259:2883–2889, 1988. *The article reviews the techniques found to be effective in physician counseling for smoking cessation.*

Lipkin M, Quill TE, Napadano RJ: The medical interview: A core curriculum for residencies in internal medicine. Ann Intern Med 100:277–284, 1984. *The result of the Working Group on the Model Curriculum of the Task Force on the Medical Interview and Related Skills of the Society for Research and Education in Primary Care Internal Medicine, the curriculum outlines objectives, knowledge, and skills clinicians should master in four areas of the medical interview: (1) patient-centered interviewing and treatment, (2) biopsychosocial approach to clinical reasoning and patient care, (3) personal development of humanistic values, and (4) psychosocial and psychiatric medicine.*

Morgan WL, Engel GL: The Clinical Approach to the Patient. Philadelphia, W. B. Saunders Company, 1969. *This classic text and guide to the medical interview and physical examination is especially good for medical students but has useful insights for physicians at all stages.*

Schneiderman H: Bedside Diagnosis: An Annotated Bibliography of Recent Literature on Interviewing and Physical Examination. Philadelphia, American College of Physicians, 1988. *This annotated bibliography lists references on the medical history and physical diagnosis, collected from a computerized search of the medical literature from 1974 through 1987 and other materials collected by the author.*

20 Clinical Decision Making

Stephen G. Pauker

The primary role of the physician is to make decisions—about what tests to order, what test results mean, what drugs to administer, whether or not to perform surgery. Virtually all medical decisions are made beneath a cloak of uncertainty—about diagnosis, the effectiveness of therapeutic alternatives, prognosis. Classic medical education has rarely included a formal approach to decision making in an uncertain world, despite its central position in medical practice. Over the past two decades, normative prescriptive techniques, borrowed from the military and business worlds, have been applied increasingly to medicine.

The benefits of these approaches rest on their explicit nature, on their unyielding requirements for information, and on the ability to ask "What if?" What if this disease were more likely? What if surgery were more effective but also engendered a higher risk? What if the patient is an octogenarian? What if the optimal time for diagnostic testing has passed and the test's sensitivity has therefore diminished? Of course, these approaches also carry significant cost: They are unfamiliar to most physicians, sometimes require extra effort, and always require the decision maker to confront uncertainty and to be explicit about his or her assumptions and data base.

Clinical decision analyses are often confused with clinical algorithms or flow charts, which have gained increasing popularity as media for representing and communicating management strategies. The latter are compact schemata for summarizing a set of rules of "if-then" statements that can lead the clinician down an established management pathway. It would be possible, for example, to translate many of the management strategies in this book into flow charts. Unfortunately, algorithms do not provide a process for creating such rules; they are most often the implicit product of singular or communal experience, although algorithms are sometimes annotated to describe the rationale that underlies them. Indeed, some investigators have used the decision analytic techniques described in this chapter to help formulate algorithms.

THE INTERPRETATION OF DATA

In making a diagnosis, the physician moves continually between two tasks: data gathering and data interpretation. The former task involves identifying potential data elements and deciding which elements to select. The latter task involves modifying a set of hypotheses based on new data elements; those new elements might be drawn from the patient's history, from the physical examination, from laboratory tests, or from the patient's response to diagnostic or therapeutic maneuvers. In each case, however, the new data may suggest new diagnostic hypotheses and almost always will modify the clinician's strength of belief in existing hypotheses. Those beliefs can be most conveniently represented as *probabilities*, the likelihood of each diagnosis on a scale from 0 to 1, which can be manipulated by several basic rules:

1. The probability of a diagnosis being false ($P_{no\ dis}$) equals $(1 - P_{dis})$ where P_{dis} is the probability of the diagnosis.
2. The list of alternative diagnoses must be exhaustive, and the probabilities must sum to 1.0 (thus, one often includes a category "other" in the list of diagnoses).
3. The various hypotheses must be mutually exclusive (thus, if one hypothesis is that diseases a and b coexist, then the explicit hypothesis "diseases a and b" must be included).
4. Among these mutually exclusive diagnoses, the probability that the patient has at least one of several diagnoses equals the sum of their probabilities [thus, $P_{a\ or\ b}$ equals $(P_a + P_b)$].
5. If events are independent, then their joint probability equals the product of the probabilities (thus, $P_{a\ and\ b}$ equals $P_a \times P_b$).
6. If events are dependent, then their joint probability equals the product of the probability of the first (P_a) and the conditional probability of the second, given the first ($P_{b/a}$).

Bayes' Rule

In this context, data are interpreted using Bayes' rule, a relation among probabilities that allows the clinician to modify his or her level of belief in each hypothesis based on incremental data. The technique begins with the probability of each disease before knowledge of the incremental finding. These probabilities are called the *prior probabilities* and are often estimated by the prevalence of each disease. Next, for each disease the *conditional probability* of the incremental finding ($P_{finding/dis_i}$) is specified. Although these probabilities can be combined using the equation for Bayes' rule

$$P_{dis/finding} = \frac{P_{dis_i} \times P_{finding/dis_i}}{\sum_{i=1}^{n} P_{dis_i} \times P_{finding/dis_i}}$$

it is almost always easier to use the tabular form of the technique (Table 20–1) or the cohort flow form (Fig. 20–1).

In the simplest case, the physician considers a single disease and interprets a diagnostic test result, which is either positive or negative. In that situation, the probability of a positive test result

TABLE 20–1. USING BAYES' RULE TO INTERPRET A SPUTUM CYTOLOGIC STUDY DEMONSTRATING ATYPICAL CELLS IN A NONSMOKER WITH A PULMONARY NODULE

A Diagnosis	B Prior Probability	C Conditional Probability of Observed Test Result	D Product (Col B times Col C)	E Revised or Posterior Probability (Col E/Sum)
Cancer	0.01	0.40	0.004	0.04
No Cancer	0.99	0.10	0.099	0.96
			Sum = 0.103	

Step 1: List diagnoses in Column A.
Step 2: List prior probabilities in Column B.
Step 3: List conditional probabilities of finding in Column C.
Step 4: Multiply Columns B and C and place products in Column D.
Step 5: Divide each entry in Column D by sum of Column D and place quotients in Column E.

in a patient who has the disease, $P_{positive\ test/dis}$, is called the *sensitivity* of the test, and the probability of a negative test result in a patient who does not have the disease, $P_{negative\ test/no\ dis}$, is called *specificity* of the test. The examples in Table 20–1 and Figure 20–1 demonstrate common settings in which implicit test interpretation is fraught with error: (1) In the setting of a low prior probability of disease, a positive finding often does not suggest a very high probability of disease unless the test is extremely specific; and (2) in the setting of a high prior probability of disease, a negative finding often does not suggest a very low probability of disease unless the test is extremely sensitive. Especially in these situations, it would be important to interpret the finding in an explicit and formal manner, using probabilities as described here.

When interpreting several findings, the calculated posterior or revised probabilities based on the first finding become the prior probabilities for interpreting the next finding in a sequential application of Bayes' rule. In such circumstances, the several findings may not be conditionally independent of one another. For example, in the diagnostic evaluation of a patient suspected of having a pulmonary embolism, the chest radiograph and the lung scan are not conditionally independent: In the setting of a normal chest film, a perfusion scan with a segmental defect is far more suggestive of pulmonary embolism than the same scan result in a patient with the radiologic findings of chronic pulmonary disease. In such situations, the probability of the finding must be conditioned on both disease and on the other dependent findings ($P_{finding/dis\ and\ other\ findings}$).

Many findings are innately continuous in nature, e.g., a serum creatine kinase level, the size of the liver, and the size of the left atrium. For a given finding to be positive or negative, one must first establish a *criterion* for defining a positive result. Furthermore, to determine the conditional probabilities of a given finding, one needs a separate *gold standard* to define the presence or absence of each disease. Changing either the gold standard or the test criterion changes the conditional probabilities of the findings. For example, if a positive exercise tolerance test is defined as one with ≥ 1 mm ST depression, then the sensitivity for the diagnosis of coronary disease would be 81 per cent and the specificity would be 85 per cent (see data in Fig. 20–1). On the other hand, if a positive result were defined as > 2 mm ST depression, then the sensitivity would be only 23 per cent but the specificity would be 99 per cent. In general, a more strict criterion (e.g., > 2 mm compared with ≥ 1 mm of ST depression) increases specificity and decreases sensitivity; a more lax criterion increases sensitivity and decreases specificity. The relations among sensitivity, specificity, and the definition of a positive finding are summarized by a *receiver operator characteristic (ROC) curve*, which plots the sensitivity, $P_{positive\ result/dis}$, on the vertical axis against (1 − specificity), $P_{positive\ result/no\ dis}$, on the horizontal axis for a variety of criteria for a positive result.

DECIDING WHICH STRATEGY IS BEST

Whenever the physician manages a patient, he or she must choose among alternative plans. Such decisions often involve balancing risks and benefits. These choices often can be made more explicit and consistent by employing formal *decision analysis*. The technique involves seven basic steps: (1) frame the question; (2) structure the problem; (3) determine the probability of the possible outcomes; (4) assign a value or utility to each possible outcome; (5) calculate the best strategy; (6) vary the assumptions and data over reasonable ranges to see whether the apparently optimal strategy changes; and (7) interpret the analysis.

As an example, consider a 54-year-old man with acute myelogenous leukemia complicating longstanding lymphoma. The patient is immunosuppressed by chemotherapy and develops a persistent fever, pulmonary infiltrates, and respiratory distress

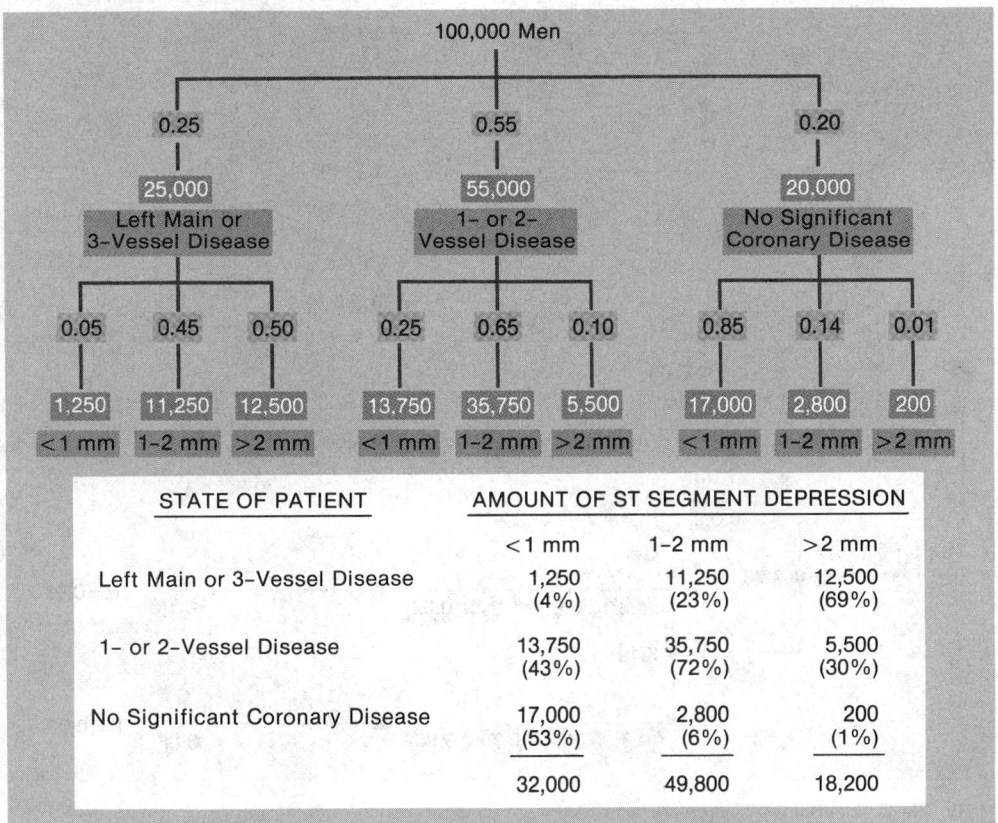

STATE OF PATIENT	AMOUNT OF ST SEGMENT DEPRESSION		
	<1 mm	1–2 mm	>2 mm
Left Main or 3–Vessel Disease	1,250 (4%)	11,250 (23%)	12,500 (69%)
1– or 2–Vessel Disease	13,750 (43%)	35,750 (72%)	5,500 (30%)
No Significant Coronary Disease	17,000 (53%)	2,800 (6%)	200 (1%)
	32,000	49,800	18,200

FIGURE 20–1. Cohort flow model of Bayes' rule used to interpret an exercise tolerance test in a 50-year-old man with typical angina. Consider a cohort of 100,000 such men: 25 per cent have left main or 3-vessel disease, 55 per cent have 1- or 2-vessel disease, and 20 per cent are free of significant coronary disease. If the conditional probabilities of <1 mm, 1–2 mm, and >2 mm of ST depression are as shown and determine how many men from each diagnostic subgroup will have each finding, then of the 1,250 + 13,750 + 17,000 (or 32,000) men with <1 mm of ST depression, 17,000, or 53 per cent, will have no significant coronary disease, 43 per cent will have 1- or 2-vessel disease, and 4 per cent will have left main or 3-vessel disease.

without clear etiology and despite empiric treatment with antibiotics and antituberculosis drugs. The possibilities of empiric therapy with amphotericin and open lung biopsy are raised.

Framing the Question

Formal decision analysis is designed to answer specific questions by evaluating well-specified alternatives and choosing the best. Rather than asking "How should this patient be managed," we shall ask which of three alternatives is best: (1) empiric therapy with amphotericin, (2) conservative therapy, or (3) open lung biopsy with the amphotericin decision being based on the biopsy results.

Structuring the Problem

The typical decision tree contains three basic elements: (1) decision nodes depicting choices, (2) chance nodes depicting events or diagnostic alternatives not under the control of the decision maker, and (3) outcome or terminal nodes summarizing events not explicitly occurring within the time horizon of the decision tree. This problem can be represented by the decision tree shown in Figure 20–2. The three choices are depicted by the decision node at the left. In both the "No Amphotericin" and "Amphotericin" strategies, prognosis is determined by whether or not a fungal infection is present and by the probability of short-term survival, conditioned on the presence or absence of fungal infection and on whether or not specific antifungal therapy is given. In the "Lung Biopsy" strategy, initially there is a chance of dying during the procedure. The biopsy may be either positive or negative, with the likelihood being determined by the prior probability of fungal infection and the sensitivity and specificity of the biopsy. If the biopsy result is positive, then the probability

of fungal infection will increase (the revised probability being calculated by Bayes' rule) and amphotericin will be administered. If the biopsy is negative, then the probability of fungal infection will decrease and amphotericin will be withheld.

Determining the Probabilities

In a decision tree, probabilities describe the present state of the patient (e.g., whether or not fungal disease is present) and the patient's prognosis. In both cases, these estimates can be based on the literature or on expert opinion. In either case, the physician uses descriptions of the past experience of other similar patients to predict the current and future state of the patient at hand.

In this case, we estimated the probability of fungal infection to be 30 per cent; we estimated the chance of dying from untreated fungal infection to be 95 per cent and the chance of dying from treated fungal infection to be 45 per cent. If fungal disease is not present, we estimated that the probability of death during this hospitalization to be 20 per cent. We estimated that, in this setting, lung biopsy would be associated with a 5 per cent mortality, a sensitivity of 80 per cent in diagnosing fungal infection, and a specificity of 98 per cent.

Assigning Utilities

The relative value of each possible outcome is summarized on a single consistent scale by a utility. Such scales can be arbitrary (e.g., 0 being the worst outcome and 100 being the best) or can describe the outcomes in identifiable units (e.g., 5-year survival, years of life, years of disease-free survival, or even dollars spent). One useful metric can be *quality-adjusted life expectancy*, in which average survival is depreciated by long- and short-term morbidities. If such a metric is used, it is sometimes possible for

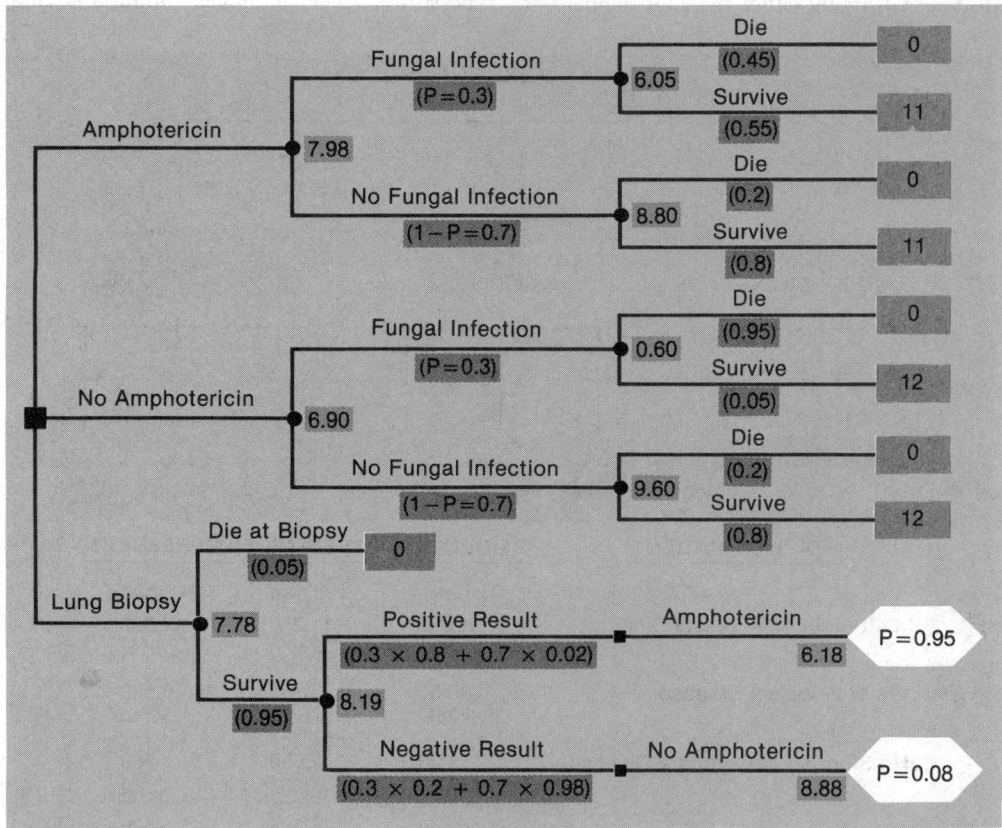

FIGURE 20–2. Decision tree depicting management choices in an immunosuppressed man with fever and pulmonary infiltrates. Decision nodes appear as squares. Chance nodes appear as circles. Outcome or terminal nodes appear as rectangles that contain the assigned utilities (in this case as quality-adjusted months of survival). Probabilities are shown (shaded red) within parentheses on each branch of each chance node. The hexagons at the end of the "Lung Biopsy" strategy represent the use of the "No Amphotericin" and "Amphotericin" subtrees (which are used in the first two branches of the main decision node) with the probability of fungal infection being modified to 0.95 and 0.08 after a positive and negative biopsy, respectively, by the application of Bayes' rule. Calculated expected utilities are shown solid red to the right of each chance node. The sensitivity of the biopsy is taken as 0.8; the specificity is taken as 0.98. P = Probability of fungal infection.

the patient or the patient's family to contribute to the decision by expressing their attitudes about quality of life.

In this case, we shall use average survival modified by the short-term morbidity of amphotericin therapy. We estimated that survival would be 18 months if the patient achieves a remission of his leukemia but only 3 months if he does not. Because we assumed the chance of remission to be 60 per cent, the average survival for this man, if he survived the acute event, would be 60 per cent × 18 plus 40 per cent × 3, or 12 months. Although many physicians are very conservative in using amphotericin, the literature suggests that death and permanent renal failure are extremely rare complications of that drug; most side effects involve short-term toxicity. We assumed that the average duration of amphotericin therapy would be 2 months and that short-term morbidity would, on average, diminish quality of life during that period to half of what it otherwise would have been. Thus, we subtracted 1 month from the life expectancy to account for this morbidity, yielding a quality-adjusted survival of 11 months if amphotericin is administered. We assigned a utility of 0 to death during this acute illness.

Calculating the Expected Utility

In evaluating a tree, the decision maker follows two basic rules: (1) When facing a choice, select the option with the highest utility or expected utility; (2) when evaluating a chance event, the expected utility is the weighted average of the utilities of its outcomes, with the weights being the respective probability of each outcome. In applying these rules, the decision maker begins at the distal outcome nodes of the tree and sequentially calculates the average or expected utility of each node, moving toward the proximal decision node.

In this case, consider first the top branch of the decision node, the "Amphotericin" strategy. The highest distal chance node describes the short-term consequences of a fungal infection treated with specific antifungal therapy. There is a 0.45 probability of dying (utility 0) and 0.55 probability of surviving (utility 11 quality-adjusted months). Thus, the average or expected utility of this chance node is 0.45 × 0 plus 0.55 × 11, or 6.05 quality-adjusted months. Similarly, the expected utility of amphotericin in the absence of a fungal infection (the second distal chance node) is 0.2 × 0 plus 0.8 × 11, or 8.8 quality-adjusted months. The expected utility of the "Amphotericin" strategy is the weighted average of these two expected utilities: 0.3 × 6.05 plus 0.7 × 8.8, or 7.98 quality-adjusted months. In a similar fashion, we calculated the expected utility of "No Amphotericin" to be 6.9 quality-adjusted months.

Next we consider the lowest branch of the main decision node: the "Lung Biopsy" strategy. As depicted at the end of the "Positive" result branch, the expected utility is calculated using the "Amphotericin" subtree, with the probability of fungal infection being increased to 0.95. In that case, the expected utility is 0.95 × 6.05 plus 0.05 × 8.8, or 6.18 quality-adjusted months. Similarly, the expected utility of the "Negative" result branch is calculated with the "No Amphotericin" subtree, with the probability of fungal infection being decreased to 0.08, yielding 0.08 × 0.6 plus 0.92 × 9.6, or 8.88 quality-adjusted months. The weighted average of these expected utilities depends on the probability of a positive result (0.3 × 0.8 plus 0.7 × 0.02, or 0.25). The expected utility of the entire strategy is a weighted average of this result (8.19 quality-adjusted months) and the 5 per cent chance of a procedure-related death (utility 0), providing an expected utility of 7.78 quality-adjusted months.

Performing Sensitivity Analyses

Having calculated the expected utility in the baseline case, we next examine various central assumptions to determine whether reasonable variations in those assumed values will change the conclusions. Such sensitivity analyses initially examine variables one at a time, usually beginning with the "softest" data. Such analyses are often called *one-way sensitivity analyses* (see Fig. 20–3).

Typically, one strategy will be best for all values of the variable below a certain cutoff, and another strategy will be best for all values above that cutoff. The value at which the strategies have equal expected utility is called the *threshold* value for that variable. In addition to finding relevant threshold values, it is

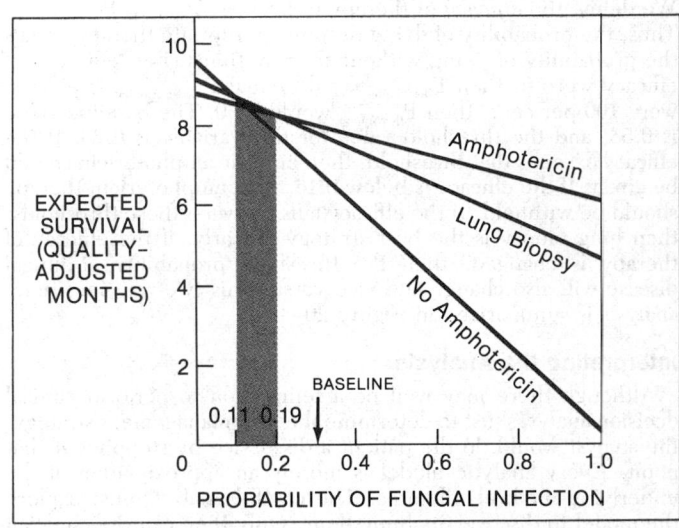

FIGURE 20–3. One-way sensitivity analysis of the effect of changing the probability of fungal infection in the decision tree shown in Figure 20–2. If the probability of fungal infection is zero, then the "No Amphotericin" strategy is best. If the probability of fungal infection is 100 per cent, then empiric amphotericin therapy is best. Lung biopsy is the optimal strategy in the narrow region between the two thresholds (vertical color bar) at 0.11 and 0.19. The baseline value of 0.3 is shown by the arrow.

often important to examine the magnitude of the differences in expected values of the various strategies. If those differences are very small and potentially clinically insignificant, then the decision may well be a *close call*, and there may be relatively little to gain or lose in selecting one management plan over another. With sufficient time and energy or with adequate computational support, the clinician also can examine the effect of simultaneous changes in two or more variables. Such multiway sensitivity analyses are often summarized by decision diagrams that specify the best strategy for each combination of values (see Fig. 20–4).

In this case, the softest piece of data is the likelihood that this patient has a fungal infection. The one-way sensitivity analysis of this variable is summarized in Figure 20–3. Another central variable is the effectiveness of amphotericin in enhancing survival in an immunosuppressed patient known to have fungal disease.

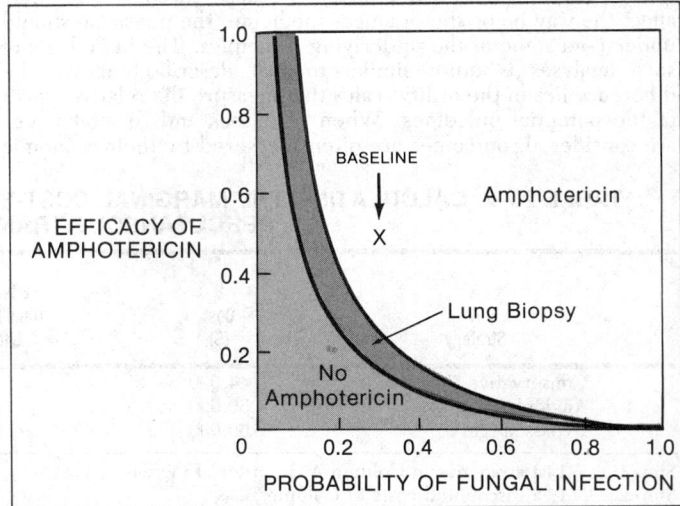

FIGURE 20–4. Two-way sensitivity analysis of the relation between the probability of fungal infection (horizontal axis) and the efficacy of amphotericin (vertical axis). Each combination of values corresponds to a unique point on the graph. All combinations falling in the lighter shaded area correspond to settings in which "no amphotericin" is the best strategy. All combinations falling in the darker shaded area correspond to settings in which "lung biopsy" is best. The baseline values correspond to the bold X, which lies within the settings in which amphotericin is best.

We define the *efficacy* of therapy to be $1 - (P_{die/Ampho}/P_{die/No\ Ampho})$. Thus, the probability of dying despite appropriate therapy equals the probability of dying without therapy times $(1 - \text{efficacy})$. If efficacy were 0, then $P_{die/Ampho}$ would equal $P_{die/No\ Ampho}$; if efficacy were 100 per cent, then $P_{die/Ampho}$ would be 0. The baseline value is 0.53, and the threshold value for this variable is 0.28. If the efficacy exceeds that threshold, then empiric amphotericin should be given. If the efficacy is below 0.15, then amphotericin therapy should be withheld. If the efficacy falls between these thresholds, then lung biopsy is the best strategy. Clearly, if the efficacy of therapy is changed, then the threshold probability of fungal disease will also change and vice versa. This two-way sensitivity analysis is summarized in Figure 20–4.

Interpreting the Analysis

Although there may well be a temptation to perform clinical decision analyses just to determine the best management strategy, the analyst would do the patient a disservice by stopping at that point. Every analytic model is merely an approximation of the underlying medical dilemma. The careful analyst must explore the model to discover its limitations. Only then can the clinician have reasonable confidence in its conclusions. One of the central benefits of a clinical decision analysis should be a better understanding of the clinical problem and a delineation of the settings in which the planned strategy is proper.

In this analysis, we see that empiric therapy with amphotericin is appropriate for any patient who has at least a moderate likelihood (over 20 per cent) of fungal infection. Therapy based on the results of lung biopsy is best only for the narrow wedge of patients falling in the darker shaded region of Figure 20–4. This region would be broadened if lung biopsy had a lower complication rate but would still be limited by the imperfect sensitivity of the test: Some patients with potentially treatable fungal infections would be denied therapy if their biopsy yielded falsely negative results. The major driving force is the surprisingly benign characteristics of amphotericin. Although patients receiving the drug have significant short-term morbidity, very few develop permanent renal insufficiency and even fewer die.

COST-BENEFIT AND COST-EFFECTIVENESS ANALYSES

The practice of medicine in a world of limited resources sometimes leads physicians to consider not only what is "best" for the patient but also the resources that such medical care will use. In such contexts, cost-benefit and cost-effectiveness analyses can be used to establish policies. Because those policies may affect the way he or she practices medicine, the physician should understand some of the underlying principles. The basic logic of such analyses is quite similar to that described above; the difference lies in the utility scales that measure the relative worth of the potential outcomes. When resources and societal issues are considered, outcomes are often measured by their economic impact. Economists argue that the magnitude of a cost depends on, among other things, *when* that cost is incurred. Money saved or spent immediately is worth more than money saved or spent in the future. This principle is called the *discounting* of future benefits and costs: Future costs and benefits are diminished by a fixed proportion for each year into the future when such cost and benefits occur. When several different utilities are considered (e.g., survival and economic costs), some analysts argue that all utility scales should be discounted at the same rate; other analysts argue that discounting should be restricted to monetary factors. When considering the economics of medical care, we should be careful to distinguish actual *costs* from *charges*, which may be quite distorted by particular billing practices or insurance plans. We also should consider *indirect costs* (e.g., heating and cleaning in the hospital and even malpractice insurance) and *induced costs* (e.g., the diagnostic evaluation of patients with falsely positive screening test results and even the medical care for treating cancer that develops years later in a patient who is "saved" from tuberculous pneumonia). Even among true direct costs, we must distinguish between *average* costs and *variable* costs (e.g., if a new policy eliminates the need for 30 creatine phosphokinase tests each day, the hospital may not be able to decrease its laboratory personnel and thus may save only part of the cost of the tests).

In a *cost-benefit analysis*, economic impact is the only utility scale used: All benefits are measured in those terms. Thus, if a strategy increases survival, that benefit is translated into its monetary equivalent: Each year of life saved would be associated with a societal worth, perhaps based on economic productivity. If the benefits minus the costs of a given strategy are positive, the program contributes in the net to society. Presumably, the bigger the difference, the larger the contribution. If the costs of a strategy exceed its benefits, the program should not necessarily be rejected. Society might well wish to underwrite such a program. For example, extending the life of a disabled, elderly nursing home resident might not provide net economic benefit to society, but our ethical values argue strongly against withdrawing care from such individuals.

Because the economic value of life and improved quality of life are difficult to quantify, we often turn to *cost-effectiveness analyses*, in which two separate utility measures are analyzed simultaneously, e.g., monetary costs and years of life saved. The results are expressed as the *ratio* of cost to benefits. That ratio does not measure the overall worth of a single strategy; rather, it is used to compare strategies. Often the strategy that engenders greater resource costs is also the strategy that provides the greater effectiveness. Thus, one usually examines the ratio of the difference in costs to the difference in effectiveness (the *marginal cost-effectiveness ratio*), which might be expressed as additional dollars spent per additional year of life saved or even as additional dollars spent per additional cancer detected (Table 20–2). Such analyses rarely tell the decision maker in an absolute sense which strategy is best: They provide only a measure of cost per unit of gain. Some external standard, perhaps established by society, must be applied to decide how much money is too much to spend to gain

TABLE 20–2. CALCULATING THE MARGINAL COST-EFFECTIVENESS OF CORONARY BYPASS SURGERY AND PERCUTANEOUS TRANSLUMINAL ANGIOPLASTY*

A Strategy	B Cost ($)	C Effectiveness (Quality-Adjusted Life Years)	D Marginal Cost ($)	E Marginal Effectiveness (QALY)	F Marginal C/E Ratio ($/QALY)
Conservative therapy	44,000	5.8			
Angioplasty	50,000	6.7	6,000	0.9	6,667
Bypass surgery	60,000	7.2	10,000	0.5	20,000

Step 1: List strategies in Column A, in order of increasing cost.
Step 2: List discounted costs in Column B.
Step 3: List discounted effectivenesses in Column C.
Step 4: Calculate marginal (additional) cost of each strategy compared to next least expensive alternative (a strategy pair) and record in Colmun D.
Step 5: For each strategy pair, calculate marginal (additional) effectiveness achieved for that marginal cost and record in column E.
Step 6: If entry in Column E is negative, then that next least expensive strategy has higher effectiveness and this strategy is dominated and eliminated from consideration.
Step 7: Divide each value in Column D by corresponding value in Column E and record marginal cost-effectiveness ratio in column F.

*For a 55-year-old man with chronic stable angina in terms of additional cost per quality-adjusted life year gained (three-vessel disease and depressed ejection fraction)

a year of life. Such analyses can also help when we must choose among alternate uses for a fixed amount of resource, i.e., a budget. When we have only another $100,000 to spend, should we "buy" one heart transplant, five coronary bypass operations, or a year of therapy for 1000 hypertensive men? These are difficult decisions, but physicians must now contribute to the discussion, hopefully in a logical, explicit, and useful way.

Diamond GA, Forrester JS: Analysis of probability as an aid in the clinical diagnosis of coronary-artery disease. N Engl J Med 300:1350, 1979. *Provides data and techniques for the interpretation of exercise testing in the context of various clinical presentations of coronary disease.*

Gottlieb JE, Pauker SG: Whether or not to administer amphotericin B to an immunosuppressed patient with hematologic malignancy and undiagnosed fever. Med Decision Making 1:75, 1981. *The detailed clinical decision analysis that forms the basis for the amphotericin decision model.*

Griner PF, Mayessski RJ, Mushlin AI, et al.: Selection and interpretation of diagnostic tests and procedures. Ann Intern Med 94:553, 1981. *Primer on Bayes' rule with many examples.*

Kassirer JP: The principles of clinical decision making: An introduction to decision analysis. Yale J Biol 49:149, 1976. *Conversational introduction to building decision trees for professional football and medicine.*

Kassirer JP, Moskowitz AJ, Lau J, et al.: Decision analysis: A progress report. Ann Intern Med 106:275, 1987. *Review of the literature and classification of techniques and clinical questions.*

Lusted LB: Introduction To Medical Decision Making. Springfield, Ill., Charles C Thomas, 1968. *One of the first monographs suggesting how probability theory could be applied to medicine.*

McNeil BJ, Keeler E, Adelstein SJ: Primer on certain elements of medical decision making. N Engl J Med 293:211, 1975. *General introduction to Bayes' rule, ROC analysis, and information theory.*

Pauker SG, Kassirer JP: Medical progress: Decision analysis. N Engl J Med 316:250, 1987. *A tutorial about new techniques.*

Plante DA, Kassirer JP, Zarin DA, et al.: A clinical decision consultation service. Am J Med 80:1169, 1986. *Description of experience using clinical decision analysis in the care of individual patients.*

Raiffa H: Decision Analysis: Introductory Lectures on Choices Under Uncertainty. Reading, Mass., Addison-Wesley, 1968. *The classic introduction to decision theory for business students.*

Sox HC, Blatt MA, Higgins MC, et al.: Medical Decision Making. Boston, Butterworths, 1988. *Very readable compact introduction for students and practitioners.*

Wong JB, Sonnenberg FA, Salem DN, et al.: Myocardial revascularization for chronic stable angina: An analysis of the role of percutaneous transluminal coronary angioplasty based on data available in 1989. Ann Intern Med (in press). *A detailed cost-effectiveness analysis of revascularization for chronic stable angina.*

Weinstein MC, Fineberg HV, Elstein AS, et al.: Clinical Decision Analysis. Philadelphia, W.B. Saunders Company, 1980. *Overall introduction replete with examples.*

21 The Use and Interpretation of Laboratory-Derived Data

James B. Wyngaarden

The basic workup of a patient begins with the acquisition of information. The experienced clinician will acquire a discerning and sensitive history and perform a thorough physical examination and such laboratory tests as may be necessary to evaluate the general health of the patient, to arrive at a specific diagnosis, to assess the functional status of involved organs, or to provide a basis for monitoring effectiveness of therapy.

Until two decades ago only a few laboratory tests were performed routinely in the workup of a patient. When screening was practiced, the panel of tests was usually limited to hemoglobin (or hematocrit) determination, blood cell counts, urinalysis, stool examination for occult blood, and perhaps a chest radiograph and an electrocardiogram, particularly in adults. Additional tests were ordered only when suggested by the clinical assessment. In this setting an attending physician could evaluate the reasoning process that led a physician in training to order a serum calcium determination or a serum alkaline phosphatase assay. The ordering of laboratory procedures is a consequence of the intellectual discipline of constructing a logical differential diagnosis or of the need to monitor the progress of a patient, e.g., one in diabetic ketoacidosis. Thus it was a vital component of the educational process itself.

In 1966 Thiers published a provocative study comparing the results of a screening battery of 11 tests run by an automated multichannel analyzer with those of tests specifically ordered on the same patients by physicians as part of the admission workup. The screening battery detected twice as many abnormal test results as were uncovered by selective ordering. The most common findings were elevated glucose and uric acid concentrations. Ensuing developments were rapid. Ingenious automated analyzers brought an increasing number and variety of tests within the reach of all practitioners. The cost of such a screening battery fell rapidly until soon one could obtain 12 to 18 test results for no more than the cost of 3 or 4 selected tests run manually a decade earlier.

The inclusion of a panel of chemical tests or enzyme assays of blood (or urine) became a routine component of a basic medical workup. For more than a decade, medical students and resident physicians have been brought up with a dependency upon such screening batteries of chemical measurements. Only a few hospitals resisted the temptation to institute such screening procedures and continued the traditional practice of letting the intellectual evaluation of the patient determine the indications for further laboratory procedures. The pendulum has now begun to swing back, as the limited utility of large panel testing has become more generally recognized. Only a small number of "screening tests" (history, physical examination, stool guaiac test, and blood pressure measurement) have actually been shown to improve the health outcome of asymptomatic outpatients. Admission screening tests, such as a "Chem 12," complete blood count, and sedimentation rate, have a relatively low yield: Fewer than 1 per cent lead to a "new" diagnosis. In fact, fewer than 10 per cent of Chem 12 data are ever used clinically, and as few as 40 per cent of "abnormal" results initiate a follow-up. Furthermore, unnecessary hospitalization has occurred when one laboratory test result of a screening panel was "abnormal" by chance on a statistical basis alone. Whenever 20 procedures are done, whose "normal" range is defined as the central 95 per cent segment, one test result will, on the average, fall outside this range on the basis of chance alone, in 64 per cent of instances $[1 - (0.95^{20} = 0.36) \times 100]$. Statistically, 46 per cent of all Chem 12 panels performed on healthy individuals will result in one "abnormal" result. Repetition of tests showing such aberrant results contributes to the high cost of medical care, but only rarely to the detection of significant dysfunction or disease. As a consequence of this additional experience, some large teaching hospitals have discontinued screening panels. This movement has been accelerated by the exclusion of routine screening procedures from the list of reimbursable expenditures by some third-party payers of medical services.

In order to utilize the results of laboratory tests intelligently (and economically), the physician must be able to evaluate the validity of the test result, understand principles of variation and distribution of values, and integrate the data received from the laboratory with the information acquired from the patient. If the test result deviates from values found in a healthy control population, is the difference trivial, or is it indicative of important dysfunction? Should the test be repeated? How often need a particular measurement be followed up? What additional tests or studies are indicated on the basis of these leads?

The more information the physician has, the more effective the physician should be in caring for the patient. To ensure that this is the result requires knowledge of science and medicine, clinical judgment, and a profound respect for the limitations of the laboratory. One of the best ways of acquiring the constructively critical attitude so essential to the proper evaluation of laboratory data is to work in a laboratory for a while. There is a paradox in the present pattern of medical education: At a time of increasing reliance upon an expanding array of laboratory tests in the practice of medicine, learning experiences in the laboratory have largely been eliminated from the medical curriculum!

SOME LIMITATIONS OF THE LABORATORY

CRITERIA FOR EVALUATION OF LABORATORY METHODS. A trustworthy laboratory test must pass critical evaluations of analytic specificity, sensitivity, accuracy, and precision.

Specificity refers to the detection of the substance in question and no other. It is doubtful that any test is absolutely specific for the substance being measured. There is always some other substance around that is capable of reacting. In biochemical analyses this limitation is most serious in tests dependent upon color development, less in the case of assays dependent upon degradation of the analyte by purified enzymes, and perhaps least in such procedures as atomic absorption spectroscopy.

Sensitivity refers to the ability of the test to detect the substance in question at the required concentrations, namely, those at which the compound exists in body fluids.

Accuracy refers to the quantitative detection of the correct amount of the substance being measured. This property rests upon both specificity and sensitivity. A test may be accurate in the absence of certain interfering drugs, and only in a certain range of values. It may fail this criterion under other conditions.

Precision embodies *repeatability*, the obtaining of the same result on samples analyzed in replicated fashion, and *reproducibility*, representing quality control over time.

THE "LAW OF ERRORS." Early in the nineteenth century, the German mathematician and physicist Johann C. F. Gauss introduced the "law of errors." This law states that in repeated measurements of the *same* object or substance, the random component on the errors will be distributed about the mean as a frequency function. This distribution, which is bell shaped, is often called "normal" or "gaussian." Note that the law applies to repeated measurements of the same item. Its extension to a population of those items is justifiable only under certain circumstances, for not all distributions are bell shaped, and not all bell-shaped distributions are gaussian. The matter of distributions will be discussed further below, when we consider the topic of "normal range" of a biologic variable.

SOURCES OF VARIANCE

These include some factors under the control of the clinician, such as the dietary preparation of the patient and the techniques of collection and handling of samples. Reduction of variance to an acceptable minimum requires compulsive attention to every detail of the process.

LABORATORY ERRORS. There is imprecision in every measurement. In tests run by hand, pipetting, timing, reading, and recording errors occur. They are more frequent when technicians are overworked or fatigued. It is common to find greater scatter of results of replicate tests at the end of the day than at the beginning. Technician fatigue can be largely eliminated by automation, but there will always remain the technical limitations of machines and the human error in the preparation of reagents, in the standardization of instruments, and in the copying of test results. Quality control varies widely from laboratory to laboratory. Split samples submitted to different laboratories may show surprising disparities in results.

DRUG INTERFERENCE. According to Osler, humans are distinguished from all other members of the animal kingdom by their desire to take drugs. Since many patients do not regard proprietary pain remedies or vitamins as drugs, the physician may obtain a negative drug history unless questions are appropriately phrased. Drugs have great potential for interference with laboratory tests. High-resolution chromatography of urine yields about 300 peaks of ultraviolet-absorbing materials. Two hundred and fifty of these disappear when the "normal subject" abstains from salicylates and vitamins for a few days. Salicylates, vitamins, and many other drugs or their metabolites also produce chromogens that interfere with certain analytic methods employed in automated tests, particularly of the urine.

DISTRIBUTIONS OF VALUES

There is widespread belief among medical students and physicians that when the sample of test results from a healthy population is large enough, the distribution will be "normal" (gaussian); that on this assumption one may justifiably determine a mean value ($\bar{x}$) and its standard deviation (s); that the value, $\bar{x} \pm 2s$, will include the central 95 per cent of all measurements; that this segment of the distribution is the "normal range"; and that values that fall outside this range are by definition "abnor-

mal." These assumptions are erroneous in many instances, particularly in the case of organic analytes. The experimental fact is that for about one half of the methods of clinical chemistry, the distribution is smooth, unimodal, and skewed and that $\bar{x} \pm 2s$ does not cut off the desired central 95 per cent. For example, among the distributions of serum calcium, inorganic phosphorus, magnesium, alkaline phosphatase, total proteins, albumin, uric acid, and blood urea, only that of albumin is gaussian. All others are skewed, leptokurtic, or both. In such situations, the value $\pm$ 2s will cut off many more measurements in one tail of the distribution than the other. The uncritical application of principles of normal distributions in situations in which variables are not normally distributed sometimes leads to values of $\bar{x} - 2s$ that are negative, surely a biologic absurdity (see Fig. 21–1).

One can avoid the question of gaussian distribution by use of *nonparametric* methods for estimating the reference range, that is, methods that do not involve any a priori assumption regarding the parental distribution shape except that it is continuous. Two nonparametric methods of normal range estimation are the method of *percentile estimates* with associated nonparametric confidence intervals and the method of nonparametric *tolerance intervals*, which include a specified proportion of the population with a specified probability.

Physicians are familiar with the percentile method of expressing interindividual variation through the use of pediatric growth charts of height and weight. The method avoids the arbitrary distinction of normal and abnormal. It also removes the aura of precision of the standard deviation.

From every laboratory test for which a good normal-value study has been done, the laboratory can report not only the result but also the percentile corresponding to that result and appropriate to the age and sex of the patient under study. With this information the clinician can appreciate just how common or how unusual the test result is. The percentile method is superior to an arbitrary definition of a normal range, such as $\bar{x} \pm 2s$, even in those few cases in which a distribution is gaussian because it indicates for each test result the relationship of that result to the healthy population. The percentile method is also superior to the definition of the normal range as the range of all observed values in a healthy sample population because the latter method seriously underestimates any selected segment, e.g., the central 95 per cent, in small samples.

With the percentile method, if one wishes to cut off the lowest and highest 2.5 per cent, or 5 per cent, one simply orders all values and finds the value that cuts off the desired percentage of observations at either tail of the distribution. Obvious outlier values are discarded. The complete percentile range is readily defined. No assumptions are required about distribution shape except that it is continuous. From the size of the healthy population represented in the distribution, the confidence limits of a given percentile may be ascertained, with known probability, by reference to standard tables.

REFERENCE INTERVALS. From this discussion, it is clear

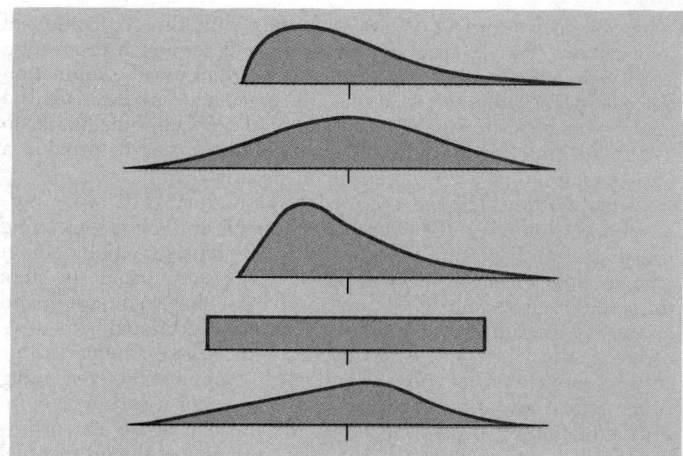

FIGURE 21–1. Five distributions with the same mean and standard deviation ($\bar{x} = 4$, $s = 2.83$). From top to bottom: χ_4^2, normal, lognormal, rectangular, and mixture of two normals. (From Elveback LR: Mayo Clinic Proc 47:93, 1972; with permission.)

that "normal range" is an arbitrary and potentially misleading term. By whatever method it is defined, the normal range excludes observations of the parental distribution of healthy subjects and very likely includes some values of other distributions. What the clinician desires is cut-off points at either end of a distribution that includes nearly all values of healthy individuals in the central segment, and very few values of other distributions, i.e., that the numbers of false-positive and false-negative values are both minimized. Ingrained habits will probably lead us to select the central 95 per cent of the parental distribution as "clinical limits," even though there is no magic in this number. Some clinical investigators advocate use of the central 90 per cent.

The term "normal range" has come in for substantial criticism. The connotation of a sharp demarcation between normal and abnormal values is unfortunate and usually erroneous. A value may fall outside the range, $\bar{x} \pm 2s$, or the central 95 per cent segment, on the basis of chance alone one time in 20 for each test! The present consensus is that laboratory results should be interpreted in relationship to "reference intervals" rather than normal ranges. In the case of inorganic analytes (sodium, potassium, etc.), the quoted reference intervals for a given laboratory test result are about the same as the previously published normal ranges. In the case of organic analytes (glucose, cholesterol, uric acid, bilirubin, etc.), the reference intervals differ considerably from $\bar{x} \pm 2s$ values. The term "reference intervals" emphasizes the manner in which such intervals are determined and avoids an assumption of normality or abnormality of the test result. The newer terminology requires the laboratory to describe what it is using as a reference population to generate the interval values.

Influence of Age. The distributions of values of many plasma constituents vary with age in the apparently healthy population. For example, plasma cholesterol concentrations in men, 90 per cent limits, are 216 mg per deciliter in the 20- to 29-year age group and 258 mg per deciliter in the over 50-year age group.

Influence of Sex. Distributions in men may differ from those in women. For example, in women, cholesterol values analogous to those cited above for men are 208 and 281 mg per deciliter, respectively. Plasma urate concentration values, mean and 90 per cent limits, are 4.9 (2.7 to 7.2) mg per deciliter in men and 4.0 (2.5 to 6.3) mg per deciliter in premenopausal women. Mean serum calcium values in normal men decline 0.0068 mg per deciliter per year from age 20 to age 80. Those of women show no regression against age. This is an important point in the diagnosis of hyperparathyroidism, which is chiefly a disease of the older age group.

Other Influences. These include weight (creatinine values), diet (triglycerides), drugs (diuretics), environment (altitude—hemoglobin), lifestyle (vegetarian diet), habits (alcohol), and the analytic methods themselves.

BIOLOGIC REFERENCE INTERVALS. In a few instances, sufficient data are available to set reference intervals on the basis of risk assessments. For example, Table 21–1 shows reference intervals for total and LDL cholesterol in plasma selected on the basis of low, moderate, and high risk for coronary heart disease, as determined by epidemiologic studies.

Another example concerns urate concentration values. An electrolyte solution with the sodium concentration of plasma is saturated with urate at 6.4 to 6.8 mg per deciliter. In addition, proteins of plasma bind urate equivalent to about 4 per cent of the amount in solution. Values above 7.0 (perhaps 7.2) mg per deciliter represent supersaturation and are associated with increased risk of renal stone and clinical gout. The magnitude of the risk factor increases as urate concentration values rise above

7.0 mg per deciliter. The 95 per cent limits of serum urate values in "healthy" male New Zealand Maoris are 4 to 10 mg per deciliter, and 10 per cent of adult males develop gout. Surely values of serum urate above 7.0 mg per deciliter in this male population cannot be considered "normal," even though they fall within the reference interval as selected by the usual criteria.

DISCONTINUOUS DISTRIBUTIONS. Some traits may be distributed bimodally or trimodally. Such relationships are most likely in families in which there is a monogenetic disease characterized by a chemical abnormality. For example, measurements of galactose-1-phosphate uridyltransferase activity in the families of patients with transferase deficiency galactosemia are distributed trimodally. The effects of two and of one mutant allele are clearly distinguishable from the normal and from each other. Assay values in the three modes are zero, 7.5 to 13.5 units, and 19.5 to 32 units. The intermediate enzyme assay values are found in subjects who are presumed heterozygotes by pedigree analysis. It is common to hear the term "heterozygote value" applied to an enzyme activity value approximately one half of normal. This practice is justifiable only when assay data are combined with pedigree data, for there may be other reasons for a reduced enzyme assay value that have nothing to do with genetics.

An apparently continuous distribution with marked skewing may at times be dissected into two or even three distribution modes by appropriate clinical and pedigree studies. For example, the distribution of plasma cholesterol concentrations in familial hypercholesterolemia displays marked overlap between subjects who are clinically normal and those who are heterozygotes by pedigree analysis. Similarly, there is considerable overlap between heterozygotes and abnormal homozygotes. Only a complete family pedigree permits adequate definition of the range of values in each distribution mode.

THE PHYSICIAN AND THE LABORATORY TEST RESULT

The tables at the end (Part XXVI) of this book contain values that define the reference intervals for a large number of substances commonly measured in clinical medicine. They represent the best data currently available but are subject to all the uncertainties discussed above. In some instances more selective data of an age- and sex-matched control population will need to be consulted by the physician.

Clinical judgment will always be required in the interpretation of laboratory data. For example, a blood urea nitrogen (BUN) concentration of 22 mg per deciliter is not a normal value for a patient on a very low protein diet. Also, electrolyte values of sodium at 145 mEq per liter, potassium at 3.5 mEq per liter, chloride at 98 mEq per liter, and CO_2 at 30 mEq per liter may indicate metabolic alkalosis even though all individual values fall within published reference intervals.

Laboratory tests are critical to the diagnosis of disease and management of patients. The physician must know the limits of reliability and usefulness of each test result in the clinical setting of the individual patient. This is particularly true when all deviant test results have returned to normal but the patient is not improving. It is especially when laboratory data provide little or no help that the patient needs a doctor.

Dales LG, Friedman GD, Collen MF: Evaluating periodic multiphasic health checkups: A controlled trial. J Chronic Dis 32:385, 1979. *Only a limited number of screening tests (history or physical examination, stool test for occult blood, and blood pressure) actually improve health outcome of asymptomatic outpatients.*

TABLE 21–1. CLASSIFICATION OF TOTAL AND LDL-CHOLESTEROL LEVELS AMONG AMERICAN ADULTS ACCORDING TO RISK FOR CORONARY HEART DISEASE

Classification Based on Total Cholesterol	Classification Based on LDL-Cholesterol
<200 mg/dl (<5.17 mmol/L) Desirable blood cholesterol	<130 mg/dl (<3.36 mmol/L) Desirable LDL-cholesterol
200–239 mg/dl (5.17–6.18 mmol/L) Borderline high blood cholesterol	130–159 mg/dl (3.36–4.11 mmol/L) Borderline high-risk LDL-cholesterol
≥240 mg/dl (≥6.21 mmol/L) High blood cholesterol	≥160 mg/dl (≥4.14 mmol/L) High-risk LDL-cholesterol

Source: National Institutes of Health Publication No. 90–2964, 1990.

Dixon RH, Laszlo J: Utilization of clinical chemistry services by medical house staff. Arch Intern Med 134:1064, 1974. *Less than 10 per cent of data obtained from a panel of 12 tests were used clinically.*

Elveback LR, Guillier CL, Keating FR: Health, normality, and the ghost of Gauss. JAMA 211:69, 1970. *Of eight distributions evaluated, only that of serum albumin was "normal" or gaussian.*

Korvin CC, Pearce RH, Stanley J: Admissions screening: Clinical benefits. Ann Intern Med 83:197, 1975. *Admission screening tests have a relatively low benefit. Fewer than 1 per cent lead to new diagnoses of significance to the patient.*

Mainland D: Remarks on clinical "norms." Clin Chem 17:267, 1971. *An excellent article explaining the use of nonparametric methods for establishing reference intervals.*

Parkerson GR, Eisenson HJ: Association of patient and physician characteristics with follow-up of abnormal laboratory results. J Fam Pract 11:943, 1980. *As few as 40 per cent of abnormal results initiate clinical follow-up.*

Recommendations for Improving Cholesterol Measurement. U.S. Department of Health and Human Services, Public Health Service, National Institutes of Health Publication No 90–2964, February, 1990. *This publication presents new reference intervals for serum cholesterol values in adults (total and LDL-cholesterol) based on risk for coronary heart disease.*

Valenstein PN: Evaluating diagnostic tests with imperfect standards. Am J Clin Pathol 93:252, 1990.

Young DS, Pestaner LC, Gibberman V: Effects of drugs on clinical laboratory tests. Clin Chem 21:1D–432D, 1975.

22 Overview of Imaging Techniques and Projection for the Future

Alexander R. Margulis

HISTORICAL PERSPECTIVE

Radiology has undergone tremendous changes in the post–World War II decades. Progress in technologic developments related to medical imaging has been continuously accelerating, making diagnostic radiology one of the most exciting areas of diagnostic medicine during the last few years. Diagnostic imaging has been and continues to be the direct beneficiary of some of the areas of technology that are most heavily subsidized by governments and industry. Space exploration provided miniaturization of imaging equipment components. Extremely high-resolution television techniques used for space exploration and photographing of the earth's surface and advances in computers and techniques of storage of information have contributed to the development of digital radiography, highly advanced x-ray computed tomography (CT) machines, positron emission tomography, and magnetic resonance imaging (MRI). These modalities, although expensive, are eventually cost effective because they significantly reduce invasiveness and permit the performance of many procedures on an outpatient basis. Because of this they have found ready acceptance and have rapidly proliferated, not only in the United States, but throughout the Western world and Japan.

PRESENT STATUS OF RADIOLOGIC IMAGING

Conventional Radiography

The term "conventional radiography" is a misnomer today. Equipment that was considered advanced in the early 1970's is today hopelessly obsolete. Although there have been no breakthroughs in x-ray tube design, the generators and controls have been computerized; the television cameras are smaller and more reliable; and the equipment as a whole has grown more functional and often multipurpose. The highly specialized, extremely expensive rooms used in the past for angiography only are changing, particularly in small hospitals, into rooms that can be used for many different procedures, including digital subtraction fluoroscopy (Fig. 22–1). Even conventional darkrooms are being replaced by daylight developing facilities, which save space, time, and personnel. These trends of saving space, time, and personnel will become even more evident in the future as departments of radiology will have to become smaller and more intensively active

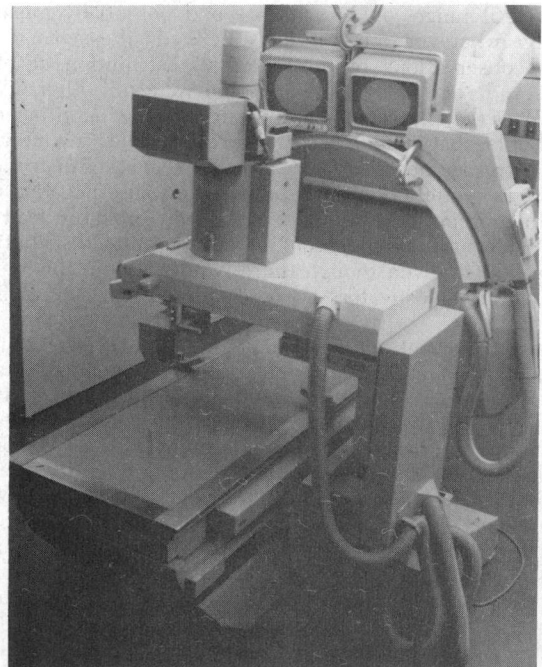

FIGURE 22–1. Photograph of a bi-plane fluoroscopic and radiographic multipurpose room with digital fluoroscopy. Multiple types of procedures are performed in this room: interventional, angiography, biliary procedures (including gallstone removal), gastrointestinal examinations, myelography, etc. Machines of this type, although expensive, are cost efficient because they are in constant use.

and will have to serve inpatients and outpatients with the same equipment over longer hours each day.

As computers improve and the capacity to store data increases, the present halide film will be replaced by laser discs or other similar devices that will significantly reduce the size of filing areas and permit rapid and reliable access to images projected on television monitors. Hard copies from laser cameras will be instantly available in multiple formats similar to CT and MRI.

As videotaping improves and better resolution is obtained, fluoroscopic information will be recorded on tape and diagnostic frames will be recorded on multiformatted hard copy as the only record. This will result in reduced radiation exposure and eventually in cost saving.

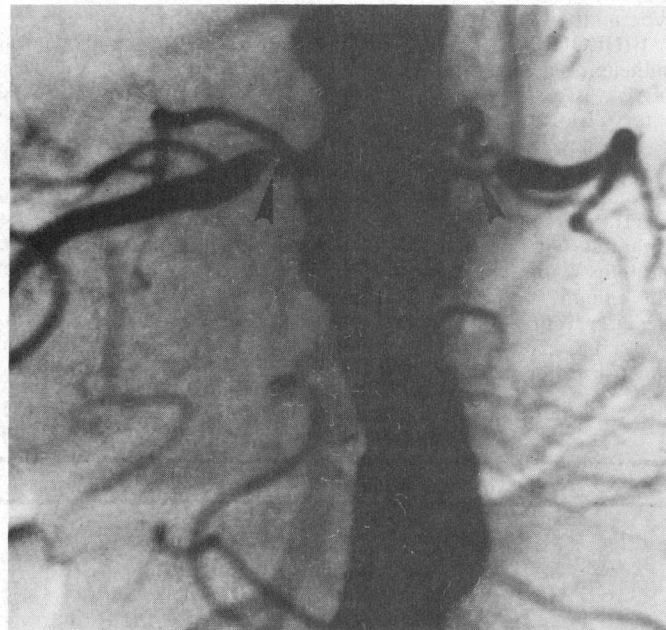

FIGURE 22–2. Intra-arterial digital subtraction aortogram showing bilateral renal artery stenoses (*arrowheads*).

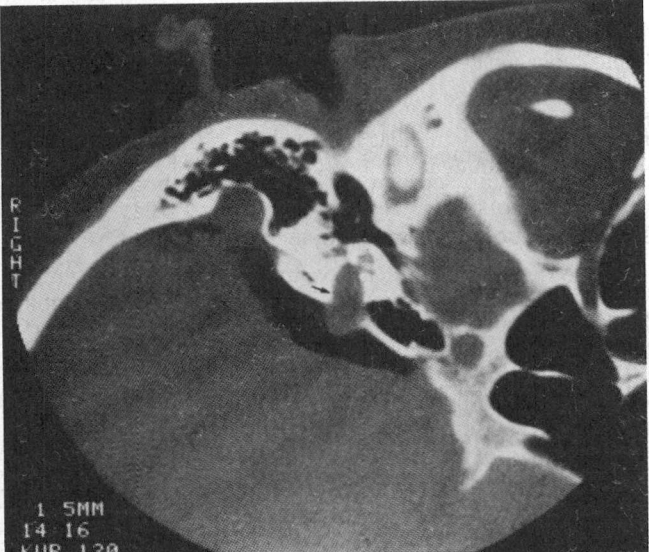

FIGURE 22–3. High-resolution axial view computed tomogram showing an acoustic neuroma widening the internal acoustic meatus. The lesion itself (*arrow*) is seen with outstanding detail.

Digital Radiography and Fluoroscopy

Digital subtraction fluoroscopy did not fulfill all the expectations that greeted its introduction at the end of the 1970's. It was expected then that all arteriography would be performed intravenously, noninvasively, with images showing excellent detail. This has not occurred, and angiography still requires that large amounts of iodine-containing contrast media be injected intravenously through catheters advanced into large veins. Even then, owing to breathing or involuntary motion, blurring detracts from the quality of the images. At this time intra-arterial injections of small amounts of contrast medium appear to be the best method for performing digital subtraction angiography (Fig. 22–2). Further improvements in digital subtraction fluoroscopy will probably occur, but as even digital subtraction angiography is invasive, it is probable that duplex ultrasonography and/or magnetic resonance angiography (MRA) will be the accepted mode of diagnostic angiography as their spatial resolution improves. Digital subtrac-

tion angiography, however, will continue to be indispensable for the performance of vascular interventional radiologic procedures.

Computed Tomography

CT has become an indispensable diagnostic tool in a modern hospital as well as in sophisticated outpatient centers throughout the United States, Canada, most of Western Europe, and particularly Japan. For the last 10 years there has been a steady improvement in the quality of images. The speed of scanning, which indirectly also results in better spatial resolution, has come down to 1 second for conventional CT scanners and is in the 20 msec range for the ultrafast CT scanner, an advanced scanner with no moving parts. CT is still considered an acceptable method for the examination of the brain (Fig. 22–3) and spine. CT is still the modality of choice for the examination of the mediastinum and chest, as well as the upper abdomen and peritoneal cavity. It is a tomographic examination in the axial plane, but it also allows redisplay of images in any plane (Fig. 22–4), and with newer napiol scanners, scans without gaps can be obtained, providing three-dimensional data that can then create images in any plane, including curved oblique planes of the spine. CT numbers accurately reflect the average density of small tissue volume elements and can be used to identify various tissues, fluids, and lesions. CT is of great advantage in showing tumors, abscesses, ruptures of organs, and accumulation of fluid, with high accuracy. Since the introduction of MRI, CT has remained the examination of choice for organs in the peritoneal cavity and the alimentary tube, with MRI rapidly replacing it in most other areas. CT is also the preferred procedure for the guidance of needle biopsies and introduction of tubes for drainage of abcesses. Ultrasound guidance is an alternate approach. A recent application of ultrafast CT has been examination for the detection of coronary arterial calcifications. This test is significantly more sensitive than image-intensified fluoroscopy and appears to be valuable in predicting obstructive coronary disease in the third, fourth, and fifth decades of life.

Ultrasonography

Diagnostic ultrasonography uses a pulse echo device to record reflected waves of a sound beam in two dimensions. The resolution of sonographic images is inferior to the image obtained from CT or MRI, predominantly because of noise in the images. The great advantages of this modality, however, are (1) it is relatively

FIGURE 22–4. Coronal sections through spine showing nerve bundles in the canal. These are computer-generated images obtained with a modern, ultrafast CT scanner generating thin slices without gap. The three-dimensional information can yield direct images in any plane.

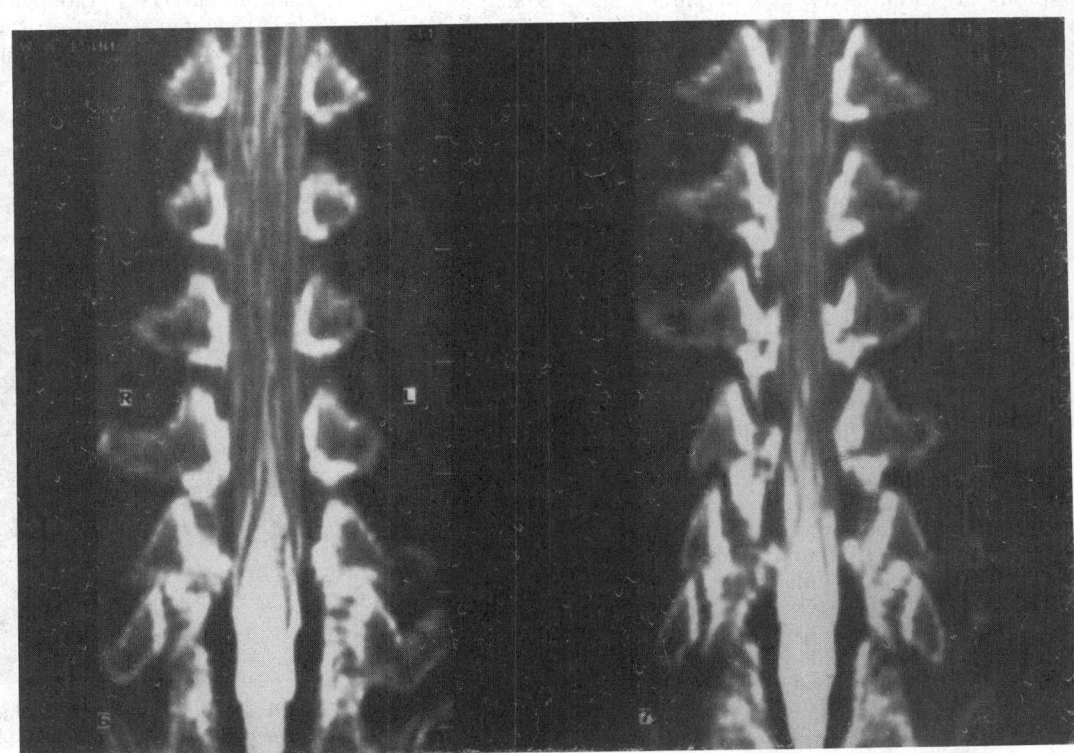

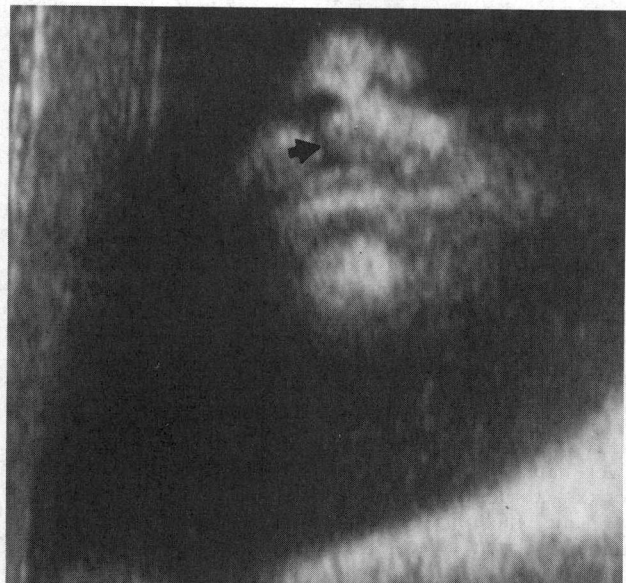

FIGURE 22–5. Ultrasonogram of fetus in uterus showing a cleft palate (*arrow*). Such detail is obtainable only with highly sophisticated equipment.

inexpensive, (2) it is rapid, (3) it can produce images in real time, (4) it can obtain images in any plane without revision of format, (5) because of its speed it is ideal for directing certain interventional procedures, and (6) no biologic hazards have been demonstrated within the diagnostic range. It does not depend on ionizing radiation. The disadvantages of the method are that (1) it is highly dependent on operator skill, (2) its spatial resolution and resolving power lag behind those of CT and MRI, and (3) no good contrast media are available at present. In the diagnostic range, ultrasonography is of no use in examining the lungs, the brain through the intact skull of an adult, the spine, or areas where there is a great deal of gas. Ultrasound images, however, exceed the quality of CT in asthenic or cachectic individuals. It is currently the method of choice in examining the female pelvis, particularly in obstetrics. An entire field of intrauterine diagnosis of fetal abnormalities by ultrasonography has developed, leading also to surgical intrauterine interventions, again guided by ultrasonography (Fig. 22–5). Ultrasonography is also of great use in diagnosis of abnormalities of the neonatal brain through the intact skull and in the intraoperative diagnosis of brain abnormalities through open skull flaps.

Within the last 5 years, intracavitary ultrasonographic procedures have become among the most commonly used examinations, particularly transrectal ultrasonography for the staging and needle biopsy guidance of carcinoma of the prostate. The transrectal approach is also useful in the staging of carcinoma of the rectum. Endovaginal ultrasonography is an excellent procedure for the staging of pelvic malignancies in the female. Transesophageally introduced ultrasound transducers have been used for the study and staging of neoplasms of the esophagus and stomach and are also of value in echocardiography. A more detailed discussion of echocardiography is found in Ch. 39. Ultrasound guidance of needle biopsies and introduction of drainage catheters is in common use and is competing there with CT. Ultrasonography is also used in guiding the introduction of nephrostomy tubes for the direct drainage of the renal pelves or ureters in obstruction.

Duplex ultrasonography, a combination of Doppler and imaging ultrasonography, is becoming a common method for the screening of major vessels for patency and evaluation of flow. It is particularly valuable in the neck and extremities, but it is increasingly applied for the determination of patency of the vessels of transplanted organs and in the follow-up of repair of aneurysms of the aorta and its major branches. Color Doppler ultrasonography, assigning different colors to the vessels according to the direction of flow, is rapidly receiving acceptance.

The many uses of ultrasonography are responsible for the presence of a vast array of equipment varying from relatively simple, inexpensive hand-held units that permit only gross screening and serve as an adjunct to the physical examination, to highly sophisticated, very precise, versatile duplex units capable of rendering excellent images with high spatial resolution. The cost of such equipment can be 10 to 20 times higher than that of the simplest clinical ultrasound apparatus.

Magnetic Resonance Imaging

MRI is an imaging modality that has been derived from chemical magnetic resonance. For imaging, hydrogen protons give the best images. The strength of the signal will indicate the amount of hydrogen modified by tissue relaxation parameters, T1 and T2. T1, also known as the spin lattice parameter, is dependent on the interaction of other nuclei with hydrogen. T2 depends on the influence of protons on each other. It is also referred to as the spin-spin parameter. Other parameters such as diffusion, magnetic susceptibility, and chemical shift also affect the image characteristics and sequences can be devised to enhance, for each, the differences between normal and abnormal tissues. The techniques of MRI are so numerous that it is possible to individualize them according to the problem investigated. By applying the right sequence, a great deal of information about the nature of normal and abnormal tissues can be obtained. MRI has several advantages over other imaging modalities. MRI offers superb resolving power. This is due to contrast resolution that is considerably better than that of CT, with spatial resolution often comparable to that of CT.

MRI is already superior to any other imaging modality in the examination of the brain (Fig. 22–7), spinal cord (Fig. 22–9), cancellous bone, the male and female pelvic organs (Figs. 22–6 and 22–8), and the urinary bladder. With the use of surface or specially designed coils, it is the best method for the examination of large joints (Fig. 22–10). It has in general replaced arthrography of the knee, hip, shoulder, and temporomandibular joint. MRI has been very successful in the examination of the spine. With respiratory suppression techniques, electrocardiographic (ECG) gating, and fast cines sequences, it is providing outstanding images of the heart (Fig. 22–11). Studies of the mediastinum of quality unsurpassed by other modalities are also being obtained. MRI is valuable in the examination of the liver, particularly in the search for metastases, hepatocellular carcinomas, and hemangiomas. With the intravenous injection of gadolinium DTPA (0.5 μmol per kilogram) it has advantages over other techniques in the examination of the kidneys.

Gadolinium-DTPA (gadopentetate dimeglumine, Gd-DTPA) with T_1 weighted sequences is also very useful in improving the sensitivity of MRI in the examination of the brain, particularly

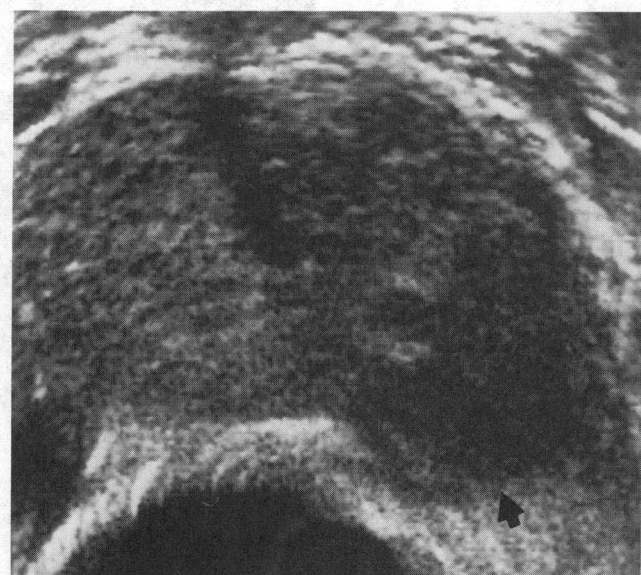

FIGURE 22–6. Transrectal ultrasonogram of prostate showing a carcinoma (*arrow*) that has penetrated through the capsule.

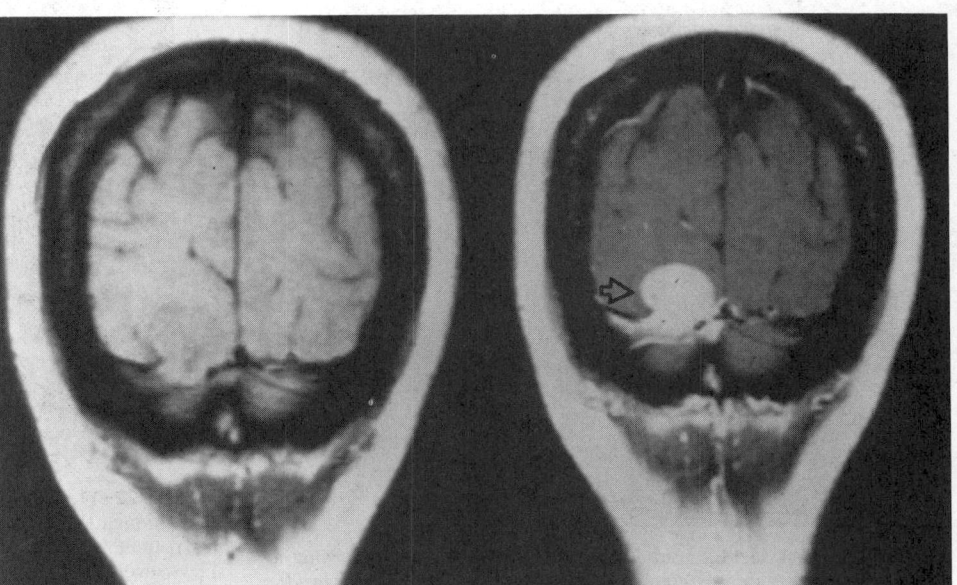

FIGURE 22–7. Coronal MR images of head showing a meningioma before and after gadolinium-DTPA (gadopentetate dimeglumine) injection (*arrow*).

for meningiomas and acoustic neurinomas and for lesions of the spinal cord. Gd-DTPA is also valuable in improving the staging of pelvic tumors. Other contrast media, generally employing firmly chelated paramagnetic metals, are being developed to improve the diagnostic capabilities of MRI in focal diseases of the liver, spleen, and pancreas. Contrast media that would permit MR lymphangiography are also being developed and tested. The drawbacks of paramagnetic contrast media are their cost and the occasional necessity to use sequences before and after contrast media enhancement.

MR angiography, a method of studying vessels and flow through magnetization of the moving column of blood in one direction while the signal of the blood moving in the opposite direction is suppressed by a saturation radiofrequency pulse above the field of view, is evolving very rapidly. It is already a noninvasive screening procedure for vessel patency, and it possesses better spatial resolution than Doppler ultrasonography. It cannot, however, compete with Doppler in price and will need further improvements in spatial resolution before it replaces contrast x-ray digital subtraction selective arteriography. MRI does not show calcifications. It is currently of no value in the examination of the small bowel and its mesentery and has only limited applications in the examination of the pancreas. In the staging of tumors of the rectum and esophagus it is not superior to CT. Further drawbacks are relatively slow scanning (in minutes at present), the expense of the equipment and siting, the large

amounts of space necessary for the facility, and the danger of loose metallic objects flying into the machine. Other disadvantages are the inability to examine patients with cardiac pacemakers, metallic particles in the eyes, or vascular metallic clips in brain vessels. The drawback of slow scanning by MRI is being eliminated by the development of rapid scanning sequences (in seconds), which use different pulses, resulting in reduced flip angles of protons, and imaginative handling of data by the computer. It appears, however, that echoplanar techniques permitting real time imaging by rapid acquisition of data are rapidly improving the quality of images and may become the most useful technique of the future. The use of MRI in the United States has increased by 41 per cent between 1989 and 1990. It is estimated that there are 1500 MR imagers operating clinically in the United States at the start of 1990.

Although MRI has greatly improved the sensitivity of cross-sectional imaging in many areas of the body and the rapid scanning techniques that are being developed promise to make MRI the universal tomographic imaging modality, it has not fulfilled the expectations of significantly improving diagnostic specificity. These expectations may still be met with improvements in localized magnetic resonance spectroscopy (LMRS) and spectroscopic imaging (MRSI). LMRS of ^{31}P has the disadvantages that ^{31}P is not very sensitive for MR and is present in only small quantities in the body. As ^{31}P is very important in energy transfer, it is particularly useful in the study of diseases of muscle and

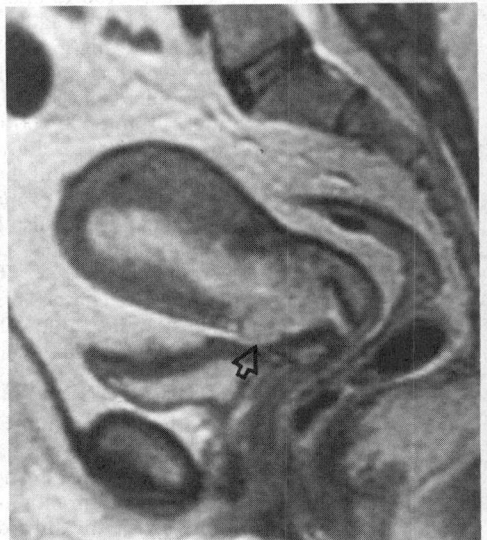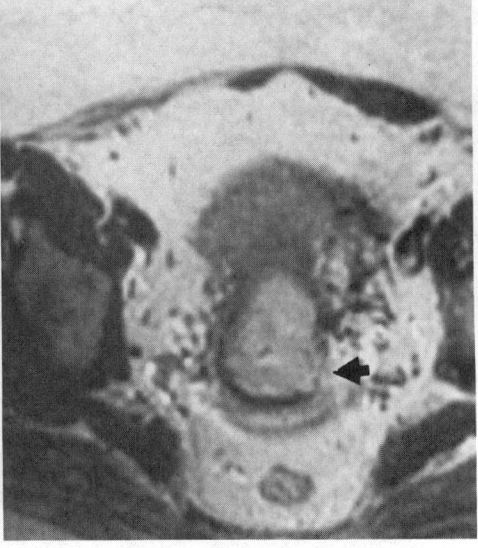

FIGURE 22–8. Sagittal and transverse MR images of the pelvis showing an endometrial carcinoma that has broken through the myometrium anteriorly and laterally (*arrows*) and invaded the left parametrium.

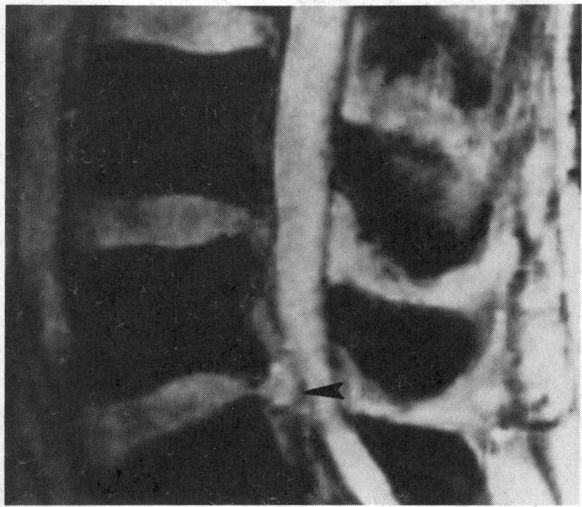

FIGURE 22–9. A sagittal gradient-echo image of the spine showing a ruptured nucleus pulposus compressing the cauda equina (*arrowhead*). With this technique, the vertebral bone marrow is dark (signal void).

brain, but the voxels (volume elements from which signal emanates) are relatively large (2 to 3 cu cm). ^{1}H (protons) LMRS is more promising. The voxels can be 10 times smaller than for ^{31}P, it is most MR-sensitive and is present in all tissues, and it is involved in all physiologic processes. ^{13}C is natively present in only small quantities but can be introduced into the body as a tracer.

The greatest promise for spectroscopy, however, lies in spectroscopic imaging. Data from multiple voxels in one area of the body are acquired simultaneously. Certain peaks are isolated and can either form separate images or can be superimposed in color over a proton image of the same area. An example for the future would be superimposing an image of lactate in red over the grayscale proton image, showing the ischemic area localized in the myocardium. Spectroscopic MR imaging has the highest potential of combining images of abnormal physiology with abnormal morphology.

The Algorithmic Approach

With many different radiologic modalities, the physician is often in a dilemma as to which examination is indicated and, if several are to be requested, in what order they should be performed. The algorithmic approach offers a logical sequence in which one examination follows the previous one, depending on

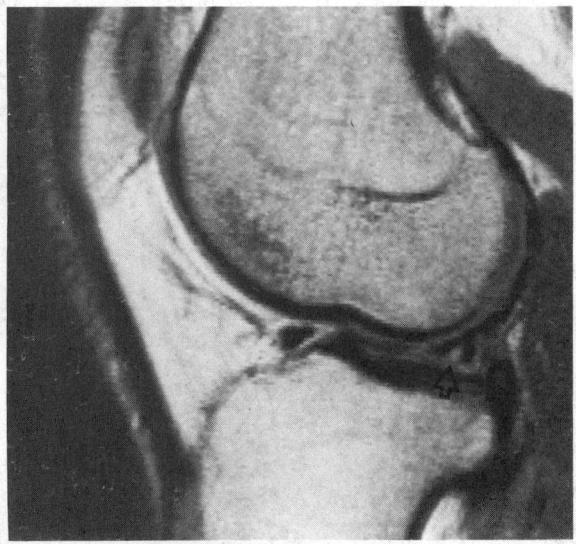

FIGURE 22–10. Sagittal MR image of knee showing a torn posterior meniscus (*arrow*).

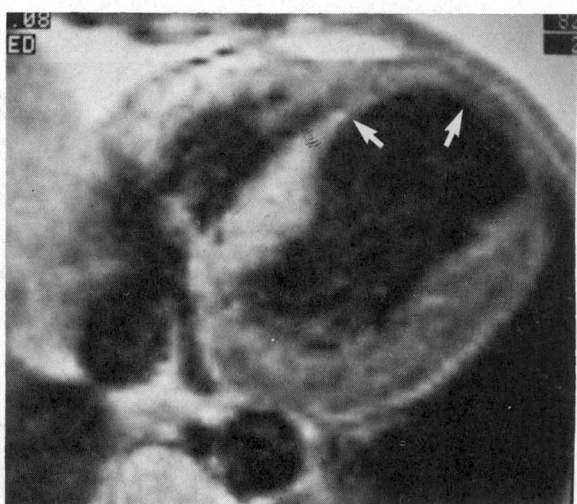

FIGURE 22–11. Gated (ECG) magnetic resonance image at a transverse level through the left ventricle sharply displays the myocardial walls. In this patient with a prior anteroseptal myocardial infarction, the image shows severe thinning of the anterior septum and anterior wall of the left ventricle (*arrows*).

its results, in order to provide a definitive diagnosis. This approach relies very much on the equipment available as well as on the skills of the operators. It is often linked with local experience and sometimes is tinged with prejudice. The best approach for selecting the proper procedures results from a continuing dialogue between the clinician and radiologist in which the two familiarize each other with the newest developments and experiences.

Financial Considerations

The cost of radiologic equipment has soared; in most hospitals modern imaging equipment has overwhelmed equipment budgets. The sophistication and expense of the equipment necessitate an organized referral system to prevent duplication of equipment and to allow utilization of imaging systems to their best advantage. Noninvasive imaging procedures can result in shorter hospital stays, in avoidance of hospitalization altogether, and in almost complete elimination of exploratory surgery. When surgery is necessary, precise preoperative diagnosis shortens the procedure and reduces the number of complications. Properly utilized and properly distributed imaging systems can enhance outpatient diagnostic capabilities, thus shortening hospital stays and greatly reducing the number of acute care hospitals needed. Interventional radiologic procedures are relatively less invasive than surgical procedures. Their advances have already served to avoid or shorten hospitalizations and to reduce significantly the number of complications and expense of open surgery. The elimination of hospital beds resulting from all these procedures should eventually lead to enormous cost savings.

The cost of imaging equipment is still very high and, unit for unit, is the highest in all of the health industry. The price of a fluoroscopic radiography room without siting but with installation varies between $300,000 and $400,000. The cost of a CT scanner ranges from $600,000 to $1.5 million, and MR scanners can cost from $850,000 for a low field permanent magnet to $2.25 million for a 1.5-tesla unit with spectroscopic and advanced imaging options. The cost of magnetic shielding and siting of a 1.5- or 2-tesla magnet may also be a million dollars or more. The cost of a sophisticated biplane computerized angiographic unit with high-resolution (1024 × 1024) TV screens can exceed 1.5 million dollars. The charges of some often-ordered radiologic procedures are listed in Table 22–1. Although costs vary somewhat from hospital to hospital, they are fairly typical.

FUTURE DEVELOPMENTS IN IMAGING

With the continuous advances in the development of computers and television systems, combining increased versatility and decreased cost, diagnostic imaging can expect to make progress in several new directions. It is certain that the departments of radiology of the future in the industrialized world will become

TABLE 22–1. TYPICAL CHARGES OF SOME COMMONLY ORDERED RADIOLOGIC PROCEDURES

Procedure	Technical and Professional
Chest, posteroanterior and lateral	$135.00
Barium enema	$319.00
Upper GI	$314.00
Small bowel	$439.00
Head CT	
without contrast	$756.00
with contrast	$841.00
Abdominal CT	
without contrast	$1004.00
with contrast	$1087.00
MRI: head, abdomen, pelvis	
1 sequence	$907.00
2 sequences	$1054.00
3 sequences	$1202.00
3+ sequences	$1347.00
MRI: lower extremity or upper extremity	
1 sequence	$840.00
2 sequences	$976.00
3 sequences	$1112.00
3+ sequences	$1248.00
Ultrasonography	
Pelvic	$285.00
Abdominal	$314.00
Transrectal	$220.00

totally computerized, integrating into the hospital's general computer system. This means that images themselves as well as reports will be instantly available on television monitors on wards along with laboratory information and information from medical records and pathologic studies. These systems will be expensive but at the same time will be cost effective, saving on personnel, communication, and duration of hospital stay of the patient. Computers will also help to store data correlating clinical information and allowing the most efficient and most rational algorithmic approaches for reaching the correct diagnosis. Computers will therefore help physicians, surgeons, and radiologists to reach the correct, least invasive, and most time-saving sequence of diagnostic studies. Similarly, artificial intelligence based on clinical experience and previous imaging results will also help in selection of the proper techniques for rapid diagnoses. This again will not only improve clinical results but will also make the use of equipment more cost effective and less traumatic for patients.

These remarkable advances in imaging will increasingly attract the interest and collaboration of other physicians (such as internists, neurologists, ophthalmologists, obstetricians, neurosurgeons, and surgeons) with the radiologist in the field of diagnostic imaging in order to optimize progress through the exchange of experience and ideas.

Historical and General References

Grigg ERN: The Train of the Invisible Light. Springfield, Ill., Charles C Thomas, 1965. *An extensive, well-illustrated review of the development of roentgenology from its earliest days.*

Digital Radiography and Fluoroscopy

Carmody RF, Yang PJ, Seeger JF, Capp MP: Digital subtraction angiography: Update 1986. Invest Radiol 21:899–905, 1986. *Good review.*
Enzmann DR, Djang WT, Riederer SJ, et al.: Digital subtraction angiography: Current status and use of intra-arterial injection. Radiology 146:669, 1983. *A clever technical review of two approaches to digital angiography.*
Foley WD, Milde MW: Intra-arterial digital subtraction angiography. Radiol Clin North Am 23:293, 1985. *A clear, objective view of the subject.*
Riederer SJ, Kruger RA: Basic Concepts of Digital Subtraction Angiography. Boston, G. K. Hall Medical Publisher, 1984. *More extensive and more basic discussion of the subject.*
Riederer SJ, Kruger RA: Intravenous digital subtraction: A summary of recent developments. Radiology 147:633, 1983. *An extensive summary of multiple approaches with the advantages and disadvantages of each.*

Computed Tomography

Agatston AS, Janowitz WR, Hildner F, et al.: Quantification of coronary artery calcium using ultrafast CT. J Am Coll Cardiol 15:827–832, 1990. *An excellent article on the importance of coronary artery calcification as shown by ultrafast CT.*

Lee JKT, Sagel SS, Stanley RJ (eds.): Computed Body Tomography with MRI Correlations. 2nd ed. New York, Raven Press, 1989. *A well-illustrated, modern, complete textbook on computed tomography of the body. Particularly good sections on kidney and liver.*
Moss AA, Gamsu G, Genant HK (eds.): Computed Tomography of the Body. Philadelphia, W.B. Saunders Company, 1983. *Still the best.*

Ultrasonography

Callen PW (ed.): Ultrasonography in Obstetrics and Gynecology. 2nd ed. Philadelphia, W. B. Saunders Company, 1988. *Even better than the first edition; a well-illustrated and organized textbook on modern ultrasound applications in the field of obstetrics and gynecology.*
Sarti DA, Sample WF (eds.): Diagnostic Ultrasound. Text and Cases. 2nd ed. Chicago, Year Book Medical Publishers, Inc., 1987. *Still one of the best-illustrated books on ultrasonography, with exquisite illustrations.*

Magnetic Resonance

Higgins CB, Hricak H: Magnetic Resonance Imaging of the Body. New York, Raven Press, 1987. *Superb treatise of MR body imaging. Easily understandable.*
James TL, Margulis AR (eds.): Biomedical Magnetic Resonance. San Francisco, Radiology Research and Education Foundation, 1984. *Multiauthored, still valid.*
Margulis AR, Crooks LE: Present and future status of MR imaging. AJR 150:487–492, 1988. *A good review of the state of MR imaging.*
Pykett IL: NMR imaging in medicine. Sci Am 246:78, 1982. *An imaginative, clear, and well-illustrated explanation of the physics and techniques of NMR.*
Rothschild P, Crooks LE, Margulis AR: Direction of MR imaging. Invest Radiol 25(1):275–281, 1990. *An up-to-date discussion of MRI.*
Stark DD, Bradley WG Jr.: Magnetic Resonance Imaging. St. Louis, The C. V. Mosby Company, 1988. *The most complete update on MR imaging. The physics is simply worded for physicians.*

Economic Data and Benefits

Margulis AR, Shea WJ Jr: Advances in Imaging Technology and Their Impact on Medicine. Mackenzie Davidson Memorial Lecture, April 1986. Br J Radiol 59:309–315, 1986. *A review of the status of imaging.*
Newton DR, Witz S, Norman D, et al.: Economic impact of CT scanning on the evaluation of pituitary adenomas. Am J Neurol Radiol 4:57, 1983. *A carefully designed study showing the economic benefits of computed tomography in one selected condition where controls were available.*
Norman D, Ulloa N, Brant-Zawadzki M, et al.: Intraarterial digital subtraction imaging cost considerations. Radiology 156:33, 1985. *Irrational handling of new technology.*
Sox H, Stern S, Owens D, Abrams HL: Assessment of Diagnostic Technology in Health Care: Rationale, Methods, Problems, and Directions. Washington, D.C., National Academy Press, 1989. *A complete multiauthored review of approaches to diagnostic technology assessment.*

Interventional Radiology

Kadir S: Diagnostic Angiography. Philadelphia, W.B. Saunders, 1986. *Detailed textbook on angiography.*
Castaneda-Zuniga W, Tadavarthy SF: Interventional Radiology. Baltimore, Williams and Wilkins, 1988. *A complete, innovative treatment of the subject.*
Johnsrude IS, Jackson DC, Dunnick NR: A Practical Approach to Angiography. Boston, Little, Brown and Company 1987. *A pratical book.*

23 Principles of Drug Therapy

Alan S. Nies

Because all patients respond differently to drugs, individualization of drug dosages is required so that therapy will be effective and nontoxic. A basic tenet of clinical pharmacology is that a closer relationship exists between the concentration of drug in the blood and the drug's effect than between drug dose and effect. The relationship between drug concentration and effect has fostered the study of the factors influencing drug movement in the body, a science called pharmacokinetics (Fig. 23–1). Rational drug therapy requires a basic understanding of pharmacokinetic principles that can be applied to patient care. In this way the amount of drug delivered to the target tissue can be controlled within a definable and safe range.

ABSORPTION. When a drug is administered, it must first be absorbed into the systemic circulation to produce its effects. In the simplest case, the drug is given intravenously, and absorption is obviously complete and immediate. For all other routes of administration, there is a delay before the drug reaches the circulation, and the absorption may be incomplete. Most drugs

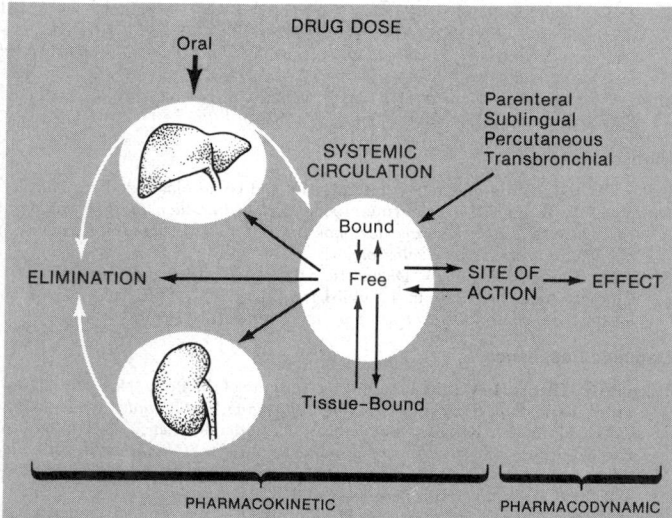

FIGURE 23–1. Drug movement in the body. The variation in effects following a given dose is related to pharmacokinetic and pharmacodynamic factors. The systemic circulation can be sampled to determine the pharmacokinetics.

are absorbed by passive diffusion into the circulation from their site of administration. Since the process of diffusion is dependent upon the concentration of drug contacting the absorbing surface, the rate of absorption can be influenced by affecting the rate of dissolution of the dosage form. Depot intramuscular preparations of some drugs (e.g., penicillin, progesterone) slowly release the active drug into tissue fluids, from which it can be absorbed into the circulation. In this way, drug levels in the blood can be maintained by a continuous absorption process for many hours or days even though the drug may be rapidly eliminated from the body. A similar technique can be used for oral drug administration by producing a dosage form that slowly releases active drug. The duration of sustained absorption from an oral preparation, however, is limited by the gastrointestinal transit time. Drugs that are slowly absorbed from the intestine may be affected by alterations in gut transit time more than drugs that are rapidly absorbed. An increase in gut motility leads to a decrease in the extent of absorption of slowly absorbed drugs (such as digoxin or sustained release preparations of several drugs), whereas a decrease in motility may increase the extent of absorption.

Depending on the drug, absorption can occur from the skin or through the nasal, oral, or bronchial mucous membranes. Nitro-

glycerin can be absorbed percutaneously, buccally, and sublingually. When given as a sublingual tablet or sprayed into the mouth, nitroglycerin is rapidly absorbed into the systemic circulation and produces a transient effect. When applied to the skin, nitroglycerin has a slow but sustained absorption lasting up to 24 hours with a sustained release patch. The transdermal route also can be used for scopolamine, estradiol, and clonidine. However, most drugs are not absorbed well from the skin or oral mucous membrane because of the limited surface utilized for absorption and the solubility characteristics of the drug. Occasionally, unwanted systemic effects follow the absorption of topically applied drugs from the skin (e.g., corticosteroids) or eye (e.g., timolol).

Parenteral, sublingual, transbronchial, and percutaneous routes of absorption have the advantage of delivering the drug directly into the systemic circulation. By contrast, when absorbed by the intestine, the drug enters the portal circulation and is presented to the liver, where a portion of the drug can be eliminated before reaching the systemic circulation (Fig. 23–1). Thus, nitroglycerin can be absorbed readily from the intestine but is rapidly destroyed by the liver so that only a fraction of the orally administered dose reaches the circulation. A similar situation exists for propranolol, in which over half of an orally administered dose is removed by the liver. Hepatic removal during absorption of drug from the gut is called "first-pass" or "presystemic" elimination and, along with poor absorption from the intestine, accounts for the need to give larger oral than parenteral doses of some drugs to achieve equivalent pharmacologic effects. "Bioavailability" is the fraction of the dose that reaches the systemic circulation. Bioavailability ranges from 0 (no drug reaches the systemic circulation) to 1 (all of the ingested dose reaches the systemic circulation). For some drugs, such as lidocaine and morphine, the oral bioavailability is sufficiently low to preclude oral administration. Formulation of oral preparations can affect bioavailability. There are well-documented examples of differences in bioavailability for different brands of the same drug. In addition, sustained-release preparations often show greater interpatient variation in bioavailability than do standard formulations of the same drug. For all pharmacokinetic calculations utilizing the oral dosage, the dosage must be corrected for less than complete bioavailability.

DISTRIBUTION. Once absorbed into the systemic circulation, the drug distributes throughout the body. If the drug is injected intravenously, it is first delivered to the well-perfused tissues and only more slowly distributed to less well-perfused tissues. By measuring drug concentrations in plasma at various times after a drug is administered, a curve can be described from which distribution and elimination can be quantified. For example, if 100 mg of lidocaine is given as an intravenous bolus to an adult, the curve in Figure 23–2 results. This curve of lidocaine concentration versus time can be separated into an early distribution

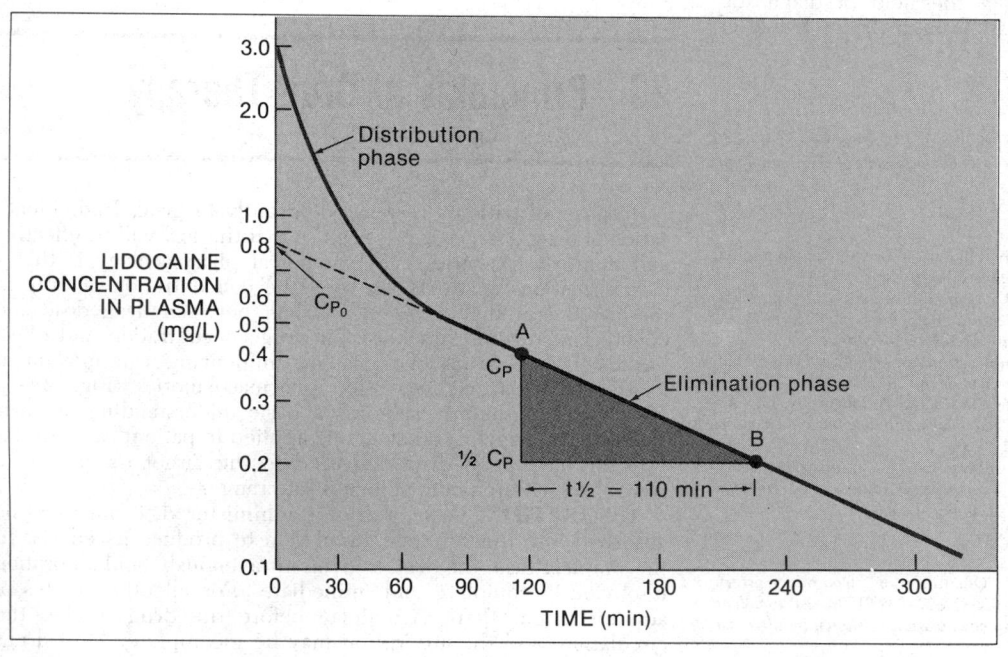

FIGURE 23–2. Lidocaine concentrations on a log scale plotted against time in minutes following a 100-mg bolus given intravenously to a 70-kg person. The C_{P_0} is the concentration of lidocaine in plasma that would be achieved if the dose were distributed instantaneously to the tissues. C_P at point A is twice the concentration of lidocaine at point B. The time between point A and point B is the half-life ($t\frac{1}{2}$).

TABLE 23–1. PHARMACOKINETIC PARAMETERS FOR SOME COMMONLY USED DRUGS

	Cl_r* (ml/min)	Cl_{nr}† (ml/min)	Per Cent‡ Nonrenal	V_D (liter/kg)	$t\frac{1}{2}$ (hours)	Per Cent** Bound
Aminoglycosides	70	3	5	0.3	2–3	<10
Carbamazepine	0	70	100	1.3	15	75
Digitoxin	0	3	100	0.6	165	97
Digoxin§	110	40	30	7	36	25
Disopyramide	60	40	40	0.8	6	20–70
Flecainide	100	400	80	9	15	50
Lidocaine	60	800	95	1.7	1.7	70
Lithium	30	0	0	0.6	15	0
Mexiletine	50	400	90	6	11	65
Penicillin G	350	35	10	0.2	0.5	65
Phenobarbital	1.5	4	70	0.6	86	50
Procainamide	330	120	30	1.6	3	65
Quinidine	100	200	65	2.5	7	75
Theophylline¶	0	55	100	0.5	7	55
Tocainide	70	110	60	3.1	14	10
Valproic Acid	0	8.5	100	0.15	14	93

*Cl_r = renal clearance for an adult with a creatinine clearance of 100 ml per minute.
†Cl_{nr} = nonrenal clearance for an adult.
‡Per cent nonrenal is the nonrenal clearance as a percentage of the total clearance.
§The oral bioavailability of digoxin is 0.7 from the tablet and 0.95 from the capsule.
¶Aminophylline is 85 per cent theophylline.
**Per cent bound to plasma proteins.

phase, during which the drug rapidly disappears from the circulation, and a later elimination phase, during which drug in the blood is in equilibrium with drug in the tissues (Fig. 23–2). The effects of most drugs are related to the plasma concentration during the elimination phase. However, whether the plasma concentration of the drug during the distribution phase is predictive of drug effects depends on the particular drug. For a drug such as lidocaine that quickly reaches its sites of action, the initial concentrations shortly after a bolus of drug can produce therapeutic antiarrhythmic effects and toxic effects on the heart or brain. On the other hand, digoxin requires time to equilibrate with its cardiac receptors. When given intravenously, digoxin does not produce maximal cardiac effects for 4 to 8 hours, during which time the blood levels are falling as the drug equilibrates with tissues. After the equilibration period of 8 hours, digoxin concentrations fall more slowly, and only then does the digoxin concentration correlate with the drug's effects.

Apparent Volume of Distribution. The relationship between the amount of drug in the body and the concentration of drug in the plasma is defined as the "apparent volume of distribution" (V_D) of the drug:

$$V_D = \frac{\text{amount of drug in the body}}{\text{concentration of drug in plasma}}$$

The V_D is the "apparent" volume needed to contain the entire amount of drug if the drug were everywhere at the same concentration as in the plasma. The apparent volume of distribution of a drug during the elimination phase can be determined from a semi-log plot of the plasma drug concentration versus time by extrapolating the elimination phase back to zero time, giving the C_{P_0} (plasma concentration at time 0), an estimate of the concentration of drug in the plasma that would have been achieved by the intravenous dose of drug if the drug had been distributed throughout the tissues instantaneously. Thus:

$$V_D = \frac{\text{IV dose}}{C_{P_0}}$$

In Figure 23–2, the C_{P_0} for lidocaine is 0.84 mg per liter following a 100-mg dose. The V_D for lidocaine, therefore, is 100 mg ÷ 0.84 mg per liter = 119 liters. The V_D for several drugs are shown in Tables 23–1 and 23–2.

The V_D is an empirically determined constant that allows one to relate the plasma concentration to the amount of drug in the body and should not be given a physiologic interpretation relating to real body volumes. For many drugs the V_D is larger than the

entire body. For example, digoxin has a V_D of 7 liters per kilogram or about 500 liters in a 70-kg person. Such a large apparent volume of distribution indicates that most of the drug in the body is not in the plasma but is bound to the tissues at a greater concentration than in the plasma.

LOADING DOSES. A major use of the apparent volume of distribution is to calculate the loading dose required to achieve a desired plasma drug concentration (Table 23–3). From Figure 23–2 the V_D of lidocaine is 119 liters in a 70-kg person. In order to establish rapidly a therapeutic plasma lidocaine concentration of 2 mg per liter, a loading dose of 238 mg (desired concentration × V_D) must be given. After the distribution phase, the loading dose (238 mg) will be contained in an apparent volume of 119 liters, resulting in a plasma concentration of 2 mg per liter. However, because lidocaine and many other drugs can produce toxic effects during the distribution phase, the entire loading dose should not be given in a single bolus; to do so would produce lidocaine concentrations during the distribution phase that would be potentially toxic. The initial high concentrations can be avoided by giving the desired amount of drug in divided doses or as an infusion rather than a bolus. This also allows the loading process to be aborted if early signs of drug toxicity occur. If the drug can be given orally, high initial concentrations are less of a problem after a loading dose because gradual absorption from the intestine allows time for the drug to distribute to the tissues during the absorption process. As an example, the V_D of phenytoin is 0.6 liter per kilogram or 40 liters in a 70-kg adult. To achieve a low therapeutic plasma concentration of 10 mg per liter requires a loading dose of 400 mg. Since phenytoin has an oral bioavailability of 0.8, an oral loading dose of 500 mg (400 ÷ 0.8) will deliver 400 mg to the systemic circulation. Because of its slow absorption the 500 mg of phenytoin can be given safely as a single oral dose even though the 400-mg loading dose given as a bolus intravenously could cause a cardiac arrest. A loading dose also can be used to boost an inadequate drug concentration into the therapeutic range. A patient with a phenytoin level of 5 mg per liter

TABLE 23–2. DRUGS SHOWING DOSE-DEPENDENT KINETICS

	Maximal Metabolic Rate	Volume of Distribution
Salicylate	4000 mg/day	0.2–0.6 liter/kg*
Ethanol	8000 mg/hour	0.6 liter/kg
Phenytoin†	700 mg/day‡	0.6 liter/kg

*The volume of distribution of salicylate increases with increasing dose.
†The oral bioavailability of phenytoin is 0.8.
‡Some individuals have a lower maximal metabolic rate.

TABLE 23–3. CLINICALLY USEFUL EQUATIONS

Loading

$$\text{Dose} = \frac{\text{Desired Concentration} \times V_D}{\text{Bioavailability}}$$

Maintenance

$$\text{I or Dose/t} = \frac{\text{Steady-state Concentration} \times \text{Clearance}}{\text{Bioavailability}}$$

Half-life

$$t_{1/2} = \frac{0.693 \times V_D}{\text{Clearance}} = \frac{0.693 \times V_D \times \text{Steady-state Concentration}}{\text{I or Dose/t}}$$

Renal Function
Creatinine Clearance
(ml/min in males)
$$= \frac{(140 - \text{Age}) \times \text{Weight (kg)}}{72 \times \text{Serum Creatinine (mg/dl)}}$$

or

$$0.81 \times \text{Serum Creatinine (}\mu\text{mol/liter)}$$

(For females multiply calculated value by 0.85)

V_D = Apparent volume of distribution.
t = Dosing interval.
I = Infusion rate.

can be given a 400-mg phenytoin load (or 500 mg orally) to increase his level to 15 mg per liter.

ELIMINATION. *Drug Clearance.* Once in the circulation, drugs are eliminated from the body by two major processes: hepatic metabolism-biliary excretion and renal filtration-secretion into the urine. With a few important exceptions, the rates of hepatic and renal elimination are directly proportional to the concentration of the drug in the plasma, a process mathematically described as "first order." The pharmacokinetic parameter best describing the efficiency of the elimination processes is drug clearance. Drug clearance is defined as the volume of a fluid (usually plasma or blood) from which all drug is removed per unit of time. Clearance is familiar to clinicians defining renal function. Creatinine clearance is the volume of plasma that is completely cleared of creatinine per minute and can be directly determined by relating the rate of creatinine excretion into the urine to the plasma creatinine concentration. *Renal drug clearances* can be determined in the same way by dividing renal excretory rate of the drug by the plasma drug concentration. *Hepatic drug clearance* is, by analogy to renal clearance, the volume of blood or plasma entirely cleared of drug by the liver and is therefore the rate of drug removal by the liver divided by the drug concentration in blood or plasma. *Total drug clearance* (Cl) is the sum of all the individual organ clearances, which consists of renal (Cl$_r$) and nonrenal (Cl$_{nr}$) clearances. Total drug clearance is the rate of drug elimination by all processes (R) divided by the plasma concentration (C$_p$):

$$\text{Cl} = \frac{\dot{R}}{C_p}$$

Drug clearance can be influenced by the blood flow to the clearing organ, the binding of drug to plasma proteins, and the activity of the processes responsible for drug removal, such as hepatic enzyme activity, glomerular filtration rate, and renal secretory processes. In physiologic terms, drug clearance by an organ is the product of organ blood flow (Q) and the fraction of the drug in the blood extracted on a single passage through the organ (E): Cl = QE. The extraction ratio, E, is calculated by dividing the arteriovenous difference in drug concentration (C$_a$ − C$_v$) by the arterial drug concentration (C$_a$):

$$E = \frac{C_a - C_v}{C_a}$$

Clearance is *independent* of the distribution of drugs in the body (i.e., the V$_D$), since the eliminating organs "see" and can remove only the drug present in the blood.

Drug Half-Life. Both the clearance and the distribution of drug in the body influence the amount of time necessary to eliminate drug from the body. The proportion of the apparent volume of distribution cleared of drug per unit of time is a constant called the "first-order elimination rate constant," or k$_e$:

$$k_e = \frac{\text{Cl}}{V_D}$$

This constant describes the exponential disappearance of drug from the plasma with time during the elimination phase. When plotted on semi-log graph paper, as in Figure 23–2, the exponential elimination phase is a straight line with a slope of K$_e$. A conceptually more useful term describing the time required to eliminate drug is the drug's elimination half-life (t½), which is the time required to reduce the plasma concentration of drug (and hence the body load of drug) to half the initial concentration. For drugs with first-order elimination, the t½ is independent of drug concentration. The t½ is frequently determined graphically as in Figure 23–2, and mathematically the half-life is the natural logarithm of 2 (indicating a reduction of drug concentration by half) divided by the elimination rate constant: t½ = ln 2/K$_e$ = 0.693/K$_e$. Since the elimination rate constant is related to both clearance and volume of distribution as independent variables, it can be appreciated that half-life must also be related to these two variables:

$$t\frac{1}{2} = \frac{0.693\,V_D}{\text{Cl}}$$

As the apparent volume of distribution increases, the half-life is prolonged for any given drug clearance, since a greater "volume" must be cleared of drug; as clearance increases, half-life shortens for any given V$_D$. A change in half-life frequently is used as an index of a change in efficiency of drug elimination, but this is true only when the apparent volume of distribution is unchanged. Disease can alter the apparent volume of distribution as well as drug clearance. Half-life, being affected by both V$_D$ and Cl, may be affected to a greater or lesser extent than drug clearance, and therefore t½ may not indicate the degree of abnormality in drug elimination. For example, patients with congestive heart failure have a 50 per cent reduction in the clearance of lidocaine and may, in addition, have a similarly contracted volume of distribution of the drug. Since both Cl and V$_D$ can be reduced by a similar magnitude, the half-life may be unchanged and may not give any clue to the abnormal lidocaine clearance and the need for reduced infusion rates to avoid toxicity. (See "Maintenance Doses" below for discussion of the relationship of clearance to steady-state blood concentration.)

With first-order drug elimination, half the drug is eliminated in the first half-life, half the remaining drug eliminated in the second half-life, and so forth. Thus, by starting with an effective blood level, which we shall call 100 per cent, 50 per cent will be present after one half-life, 25 per cent after two half-lives, 12.5 per cent after three half-lives, 6.25 per cent after four half-lives, and 3.125 per cent after five half-lives, as shown in Figure 23–3 for lidocaine. For practical purposes, most drugs can be considered to have been eliminated completely when less than 10 per cent of the effective concentration remains in the body, requiring three to four half-lives. For lidocaine (Fig. 23–3) this time is about 6 hours.

DRUG ACCUMULATION. When drug is given as a sustained infusion or in repeated doses, drug accumulates in the body until a steady state is achieved, at which time the amount of drug being administered is equal to the amount of drug eliminated so that body stores and plasma levels remain constant. The time course of drug accumulation, like the time course of elimination, is determined by the drug's elimination half-life, these processes being mirror images of each other (Fig. 23–3). Thus, accumulation to half the ultimate steady state occurs in one half-life, 75 per cent in two half-lives, 87.5 per cent in three half-lives, and 93.75 per cent in four half-lives. For practical purposes, the steady state is considered to have been achieved when 90 per cent of the ultimate accumulation occurs, requiring three to four half-lives. For drugs with short half-lives, accumulation occurs rapidly. However, for drugs with long half-lives, accumulation occurs slowly, and loading doses are frequently required to achieve a prompt therapeutic effect. Regardless of whether a loading dose

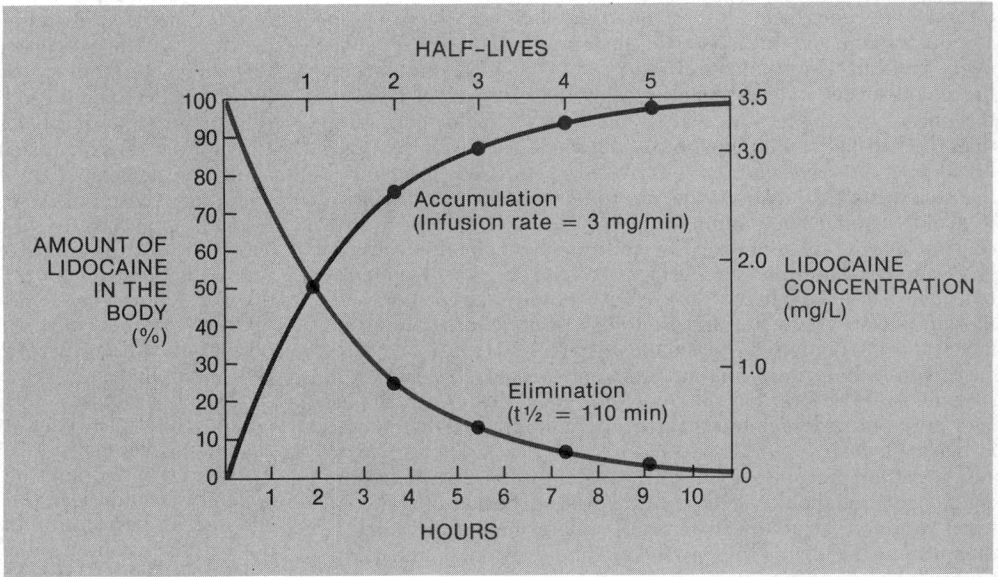

FIGURE 23–3. The accumulation of lidocaine during an infusion of 3 mg per minute and the elimination of lidocaine after the drug is discontinued. Time is indicated in hours and in half-lives and concentration in milligrams per liter. The amount of lidocaine in the body is the percentage remaining after discontinuation of the drug (elimination curve—red) or the percentage of the ultimate steady-state value achieved by the chronic infusion (accumulation curve). The two curves are mirror images of each other.

is given, the ultimate steady-state concentration achieved depends only on the maintenance dose and drug clearance. Figure 23–3 shows the accumulation of lidocaine to a steady state during a constant intravenous infusion of 3 mg per minute. The ultimate steady-state plasma level is approached with a half-life of 110 minutes. A loading dose would be required to achieve therapeutic concentrations more quickly.

When a drug is given intermittently, such as procainamide, illustrated in Figure 23–4, the average concentration approaches steady state with the same time course as during a constant infusion. The more frequently doses are given, the smaller the differences between peak and trough plasma concentrations, and the closer the intermittent dosing approximates an intravenous infusion.

Whenever the drug doses or infusion rates are changed, a new steady state will be achieved. The approach to the new steady state also is dependent on the half-life so that three to four half-lives are required before the plasma concentrations and body stores of drug are at 90 per cent of the new steady state. Therefore, the effects of a dosage adjustment are not immediate and are not fully expressed for a time that is dependent on the drug's half-life.

MAINTENANCE DOSES. Steady state is achieved when the rate of drug administration equals the rate of drug elimination. The rate of drug administration is either the infusion rate (I) or the dose per unit time (D/t), and the rate of drug elimination is the product of drug clearance (Cl) and the drug concentration (C_p). Therefore, during a steady-state infusion, $I = ClC_p$, and during intermittent dosing, $D/t = ClC_p$. Note that there is a direct, linear relationship between the dose and the resulting steady-state plasma concentration, which is independent of the distribution of the drug (Fig. 23–5). The equations for steady state can be used to calculate the infusion rate or the intermittent dose required to achieve a desired plasma concentration, and, conversely, the plasma concentration at steady state produced by a known infusion rate can be used to calculate drug clearance (Table 23–3). With the value for V_D (see Table 23–1), half-life can also be calculated from the steady-state data as $0.693 V_D/Cl$ (Table 23–3). For procainamide with a clearance of 450 ml per minute, an infusion rate of 2 mg per minute will achieve and maintain a steady-state concentration of 4.4 μg per milliliter: $I = 450$ ml per minute × 4.4 μg per milliliter = 2 mg per minute. The half-life of procainamide in this patient is 0.693 (1.6 liters per kilogram × 70 kg)/0.45 liters per minute = 172 minutes, or about 3 hours. If procainamide is given intermittently, the same average concentration will be achieved if 360 mg is infused over 3 hours, is given as a single dose every 3 hours, or is given as 180 mg every 90 minutes (see Fig. 23–4). Obviously, drug concentrations fluctuate when a drug is given intermittently, and the degree of fluctuation depends on the

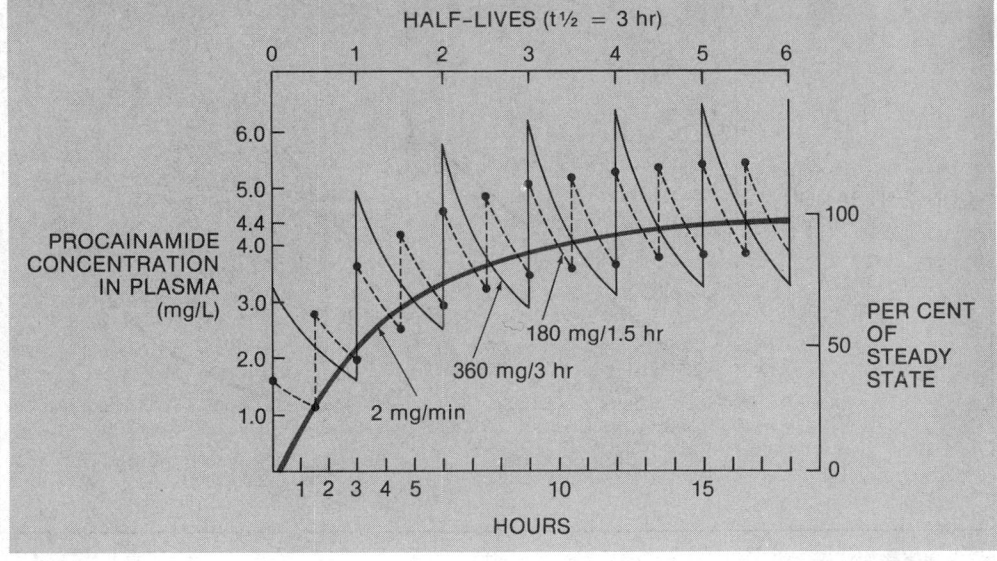

FIGURE 23–4. The accumulation to steady state of procainamide given as an infusion of 2 mg per minute (smooth red curve) or intermittent doses of 180 mg per 1.5 hours (dashed line) or 360 mg per 3 hours (solid line). Regardless of the method of administration, the accumulation follows the same time course and requires three to four half-lives to reach 90 per cent of steady state.

interval between drug doses, the drug half-life, the route of administration, and the speed of absorption. If a dose is given every half-life, the fluctuation is at most 100 per cent; that is, the blood levels and body stores fall to half the initial level by the end of the dosage interval. If the drug is given more often than the half-life, the fluctuations are less. In each case, the drug lost during a dosage interval is replaced by the dose to maintain the steady state. Usually drugs are given at least every half-life to avoid extreme fluctuations of blood levels. Only if very high concentrations are nontoxic or continuously effective plasma levels are not required can a drug be given much less frequently than one half-life. When a dose is given orally, absorption from the gut occurs gradually, and therefore peak concentrations are lower and fluctuations in plasma levels are less than if the same dose were administered as an intravenous bolus. In fact, with sustained-release oral formulations, absorption can be sustained over most of the dosage interval, resulting in minimal fluctuations in plasma levels.

If a patient becomes toxic during an infusion of a necessary drug, the drug should be discontinued for a period of time and then resumed at a lower dose. To determine how long to discontinue the drug, the physician should estimate the $t\frac{1}{2}$ in the individual patient rather than assume an average value. For instance, suppose a patient becomes toxic during an infusion of aminophylline at 0.8 mg per kilogram per hour and is found to have a plasma theophylline concentration of 36 mg per liter. If this is a steady-state concentration, the drug should be discontinued for one half-life and then resumed at an infusion rate of 0.4 mg per kilogram per hour, which should achieve a steady-state plasma theophylline concentration of 18 mg per liter. Since $t\frac{1}{2} = 0.693 \, V_D/Cl$ and $Cl = I/Cp_{ss}$ (Table 23-3) and aminophylline is 85 per cent theophylline, the $t\frac{1}{2}$ in this patient is 15.6 hours, assuming a normal V_D. This relatively long half-life is due to the low clearance in this patient. It would be inappropriate to discontinue the drug for only 7 hours (the average half-life) because this would prolong the toxicity.

DRUG REMOVAL FOLLOWING OVERDOSE. The principles described above can be used to predict the efficacy of hemodialysis or hemoperfusion in removing drug following an overdose. To be a valuable addition to the therapy of overdose, the drug removal process must make a substantial contribution to overall clearance of the drug and the amount of drug removed must be a significant portion of the body load. Consider the case of a digoxin overdose in an adult producing a plasma digoxin level of 8 ng per milliliter. The body load of digoxin is $V_D \times C_p$ or 500 liters $\times$ 8 µg per liter = 4 mg. At a clearance of 100 ml per minute with the hemoperfusion apparatus, the rate of drug removal with a C_p of 8 ng per milliliter is $Cl \times C_p$ = 100 ml per

minute $\times$ 8 ng per milliliter = 800 ng per minute = 48 µg per hour, or only 1 per cent of the body load. Therefore, hemoperfusion cannot be of significant value in reducing the body stores of digoxin. The reason so little drug is removed is related to digoxin's very large V_D, so that very little drug is present in the plasma from which it can be cleared. Recently, digoxin antibodies (Fab fragment) have become available for the treatment of life-threatening digoxin toxicity. These antibodies have such a high affinity for digoxin that the drug is removed from tissue sites, including those areas responsible for toxicity, and becomes trapped as an inactive digoxin-antibody complex in the plasma. This shift of drug from tissue to plasma results in a reduction of the V_D for digoxin by a factor of 10 or more. Thus not only is digoxin reduced by binding to the antibody, but much more digoxin is present in the plasma, from which it can be cleared by normal renal excretory processes. In theory this technique could also be applied to other drugs with a large V_D.

The other circumstance that limits the benefit to be gained by hemoperfusion is when the drug normally has a very large clearance. The clearance of the tricyclic antidepressants, for instance, is in the range of 1000 ml per minute. If a hemoperfusion apparatus could clear the drug at 100 ml per minute, it would add only 10 per cent to the normal clearance and would therefore not be of substantial value.

DOSE-DEPENDENT PHARMACOKINETICS. For a few drugs, the pharmacokinetics do not follow the rules outlined above, and such drugs are said to have dose-dependent, nonlinear, or saturation kinetics (see Table 23-2). For those drugs the amount of drug eliminated is not directly related to the drug concentration (first order), but as the concentration of drug is increased, the relative amount of drug eliminated decreases (i.e., clearance decreases) until a maximal rate of drug metabolism is achieved that is independent of drug concentration, at which point drug elimination is termed zero order. With such drugs, the relationship of maintenance dose to the steady-state plasma concentration is not linear, and a small increment in dose can result in a very large increase in plasma concentration (Fig. 23-5).

Phenytoin is the most important example of a therapeutic agent with dose-dependent kinetics. A dose of 300 mg of phenytoin daily may give a plasma level of 8 mg per liter, and a dose of 400 mg per day, a plasma level of 25 mg per liter. Since patients differ in their ability to eliminate phenytoin, proper dosage adjustments are difficult to predict for an individual patient, and plasma concentration measurements (see below) must be used to establish a proper maintenance dose. High-dose salicylate therapy also behaves in a dose-dependent manner, as does ethanol. However, ethanol is eliminated by zero-order kinetics at all doses, and therefore its elimination is much more predictable than that of phenytoin and salicylate, for which the elimination changes from first order to zero over the therapeutic range.

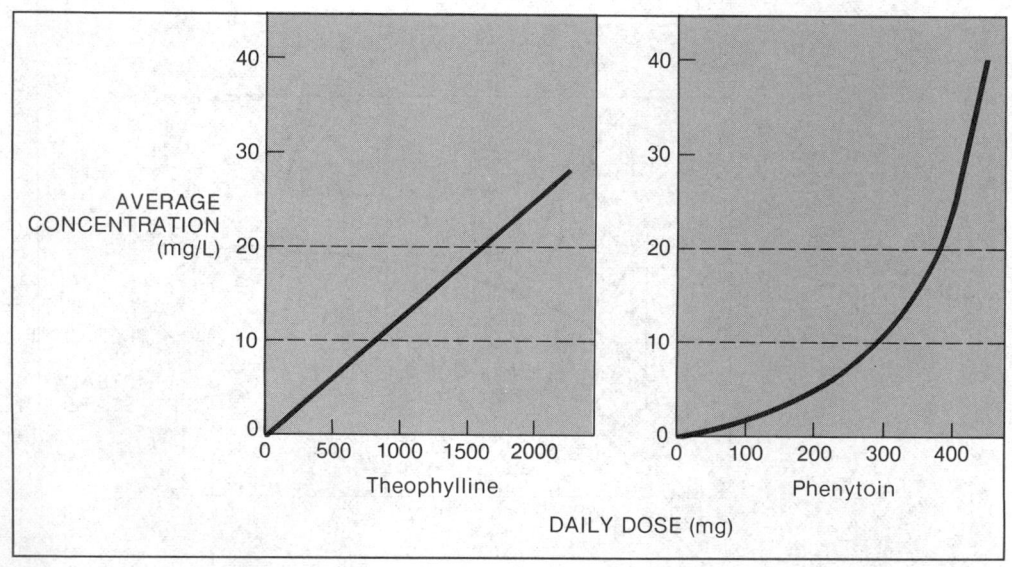

FIGURE 23-5. Average steady-state concentration of theophylline and phenytoin as a function of daily dose. The data for theophylline are from a patient with a metabolic clearance of 55 ml per minute. The data for phenytoin are from a patient with a maximum metabolic rate of 550 mg per day and a half-maximum rate of metabolism occurring at a plasma concentration of 9 mg per liter. The therapeutic ranges are 10 to 20 mg per liter for both drugs as shown. Note that the increase of theophylline concentration is linear with dose, indicating first-order pharmacokinetics. However, the increase of phenytoin dose is not linear except at very low doses. As the plasma concentration of phenytoin approaches the therapeutic range, small increments in dose result in large increases in plasma concentration characteristic of substances that have dose-dependent pharmacokinetics.

AVERAGE CONCENTRATION (mg/L)

DAILY DOSE (mg)

Theophylline

Phenytoin

USE OF PLASMA DRUG CONCENTRATION TO GUIDE THERAPY. The principles outlined above allow the clinician to choose a loading and maintenance dose based on the desired plasma concentration to achieve therapeutic effects and minimize the risk of toxicity. The underlying premise is that following distribution of a dose, the concentration of drug in plasma is in equilibrium with drug at the site of action and therefore is a direct reflection of the drug at the target site (see Fig. 23–1).

However, the published pharmacokinetic data on which initial dosage recommendations are based are averages for a population and usually need modification for the individual patient. Dosage adjustment is best accomplished when the therapeutic effects of the drug are readily quantifiable, such as with antihypertensive drugs and oral anticoagulants. For many drugs, however, the desired endpoint is difficult to assess clinically, either because there is no readily quantifiable measurement to assess drug effect or because the disease being treated has an intermittent expression so that the clinician cannot be certain that a therapeutic effect has been achieved. Two good examples are epilepsy and sporadic cardiac arrhythmias, in which drug dosage adjustments are difficult to make from clinical observation. Frequently, therefore, patients with sporadic arrhythmias or epilepsy receive doses of drugs based on the average patient, and if these doses are ineffective or toxic, the drug is deemed a failure and the patient is "resistant" or "intolerant" to the therapy, in which case other drugs are tried.

Dosage adjustment can be aided by using the plasma concentration when there are no other easily quantifiable endpoints by which the drug's therapeutic effects can be gauged. In order for the plasma concentration to have therapeutic meaning, the drug in plasma must be in equilibrium with the drug at the site of action and the effects must be reversible. If a drug has irreversible effects, such as the effect of aspirin to inhibit platelet aggregation, the plasma level will not correlate with effect. Fortunately, such situations are uncommon.

The sources of variation in drug effects can be divided into pharmacokinetic and pharmacodynamic factors. Those factors that alter the plasma drug concentration resulting from a given dose are the pharmacokinetic variables—absorption, distribution, and clearance. Those factors that alter the response to a given plasma level are the pharmacodynamic variables. If the pharmacodynamic variation among patients is very large, then plasma drug concentrations will not be a helpful guide for therapy. Fortunately, pharmacokinetic factors account for the major variation in response among patients for many drugs, and this variability can be managed with the use of plasma drug level monitoring.

Therapeutic Window. For plasma levels to be a useful guide to therapy, the range of drug concentrations required for optimal therapeutic effects with minimal toxicity must be established. This range is called the "therapeutic window" and is determined experimentally for each drug in a group of patients who are carefully observed for desired and toxic drug effects (Fig. 23–6). The width of the therapeutic window relates to the steepness of the concentration-effect curve and is an index of the pharmacodynamic variability in the population being treated. For procainamide, illustrated in Figure 23–6, the therapeutic window is 4 to 8 mg per liter. The separation between the therapeutic and toxic concentration-effect curves is an index of the toxicity of the drug frequently referred to as the "therapeutic index," which is the toxic dose divided by therapeutic dose. For procainamide the therapeutic index is ~3. With all drugs there is overlap between the therapeutic and toxic ranges. In addition, since the therapeutic window is based on a population of patients, one cannot be certain of the optimal drug concentration for a given patient. Although most patients achieve a therapeutic effect within the therapeutic range, a few patients require concentrations below or above the range. Similarly, toxicity begins to occur in some patients within the therapeutic window, but the incidence of side effects increases sharply as the therapeutic range is exceeded. Therefore, the plasma concentration cannot be an infallible guide to safe and effective therapy, since it controls only the pharmacokinetic variability and not the pharmacodynamic variability. It is undoubtedly better, however, than the use of a standard dose that allows for no variability.

Table 23–4 lists some drugs for which therapeutic windows have been established. These drugs have several common characteristics: First, their pharmacologic effects are not readily quantifiable; second, they are used for therapy of serious or life-threatening illness so that therapeutic inefficacy cannot be tolerated; and third, their toxicity is serious, and the therapeutic index is small. Therapeutic windows are not required for drugs that have a very large therapeutic index and are used for therapy of diseases that do not have serious consequences if undertreated.

Interpretation of Plasma Drug Concentration. **Timing.** Several problems exist in interpretation of plasma drug concentrations. If the blood sample is drawn during the distribution phase shortly after drug administration, the plasma drug concentration is high, may not reflect drug at the site of action, and certainly does not indicate the steady-state drug concentration. The data on which the therapeutic windows are based are concentrations obtained after the distribution phase and frequently are minimal or trough concentrations. Therefore, the best time to draw blood for drug assay is just prior to a dose, during a steady-state infusion, or, for drugs given once or twice daily, at least 8 hours after a dose.

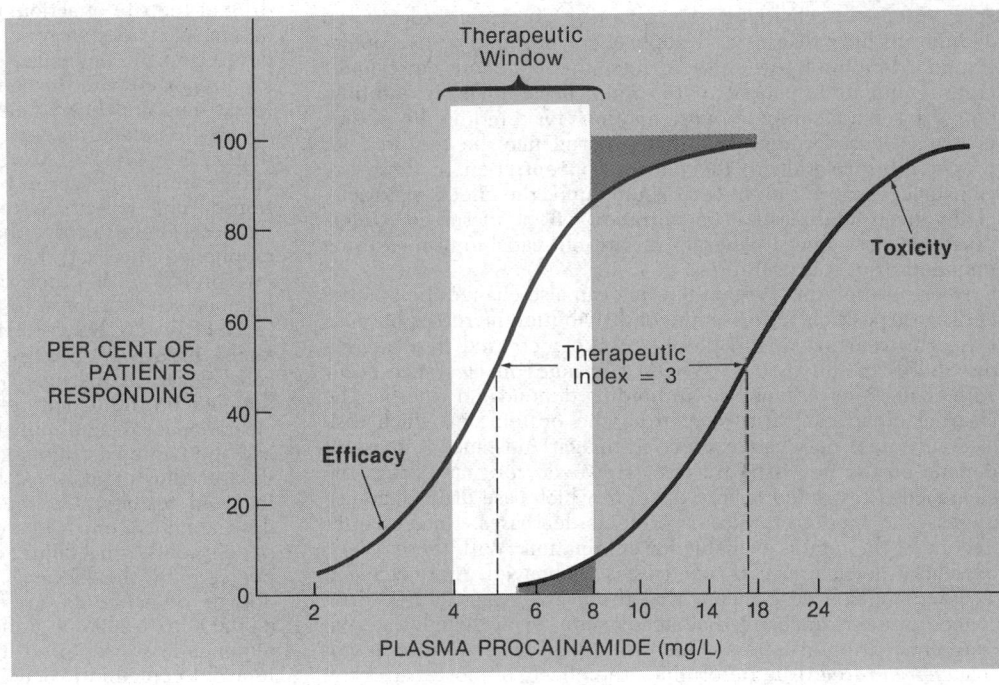

FIGURE 23–6. Population dose-response curves for the antiarrhythmic and acute toxic effects of procainamide. The therapeutic window is the range encompassing most of the therapeutic dose-effect curve and includes less than 10 per cent of the toxic dose-effect curve. The toxic dose divided by the therapeutic dose is the therapeutic index, here shown for 50 per cent of the population. Individual patients may lie anywhere on these curves.

TABLE 23–4. THERAPEUTIC WINDOWS

Drug	Therapeutic Range
Cardiovascular Drugs:	
Digitoxin	10–25 μg/liter
Digoxin	0.8–2 μg/liter
Disopyramide	2–6 mg/liter
Flecainide	0.2–1 mg/liter
Lidocaine	1.5–5 mg/liter
Mexiletine	0.5–2 mg/liter
Procainamide	4–8 mg/liter
Quinidine	2–6 mg/liter
Theophylline	8–20 mg/liter
Tocainide	4–12 mg/liter
Antiseizure Drugs:	
Carbamazepine	6–12 mg/liter
Ethosuximide	40–80 mg/liter
Phenobarbital	15–30 mg/liter
Phenytoin	10–20 mg/liter
Valproic acid	50–100 mg/liter
Antibiotics:*	
Amikacin‡	20–40 mg/liter
Carbenicillin	100–300 mg/liter
Gentamicin‡	5–10 mg/liter
Penicillin G†	1–25 mg/liter
Tobramycin‡	5–10 mg/liter
Others:	
Lithium	0.5–1.5 mEq/liter
Nortriptyline	50–150 μg/liter
Salicylate	<300 mg/liter

*Actual concentration required related to minimal inhibitory concentration for infecting bacterium.
†1 mg of penicillin = 1.6×10^6 units.
‡Peak levels.

Protein Binding. A second potential problem in interpretation of plasma drug concentration is abnormal binding of drugs to plasma proteins. Many drugs are highly bound (> 80 per cent) to plasma protein, and routine assays of plasma for drug concentrations include total (bound plus free) drug. However, only the free drug is in equilibrium with the tissues and the site of action. If the fraction bound is constant, then total drug concentration is an accurate index of the free drug concentration. If binding is altered by other drugs or by disease, then the meaning of a given total concentration of drug is changed, since a greater proportion of the drug is unbound. Both liver and kidney disease can alter the protein binding of some drugs (phenytoin, digitoxin, clofibrate, diazoxide, some sulfonamides, valproic acid, and salicylic acid) either by changing the quantity of protein (decreased albumin in liver disease and nephrotic syndrome) or by competition for binding between the drug and endogenous compounds that accumulate in patients with uremia or jaundice. In addition, one drug may compete with another for binding to plasma proteins. Measurement of unbound drug may be required for proper interpretation of the plasma concentration in these circumstances, since if more drug is unbound, the effects or toxicity of any given total plasma concentration will be increased. Unfortunately, most clinical laboratories are not capable of measuring unbound drug concentrations.

Decreased plasma protein binding can also change the kinetics of drug disposition. The volume of distribution increases because less drug remains in the plasma as the increased free fraction distributes to the tissues. Whether changes in clearance occur with changes in plasma protein binding depends on whether the clearing organ can strip drug from the protein, in which case clearance does not change, since in this circumstance it does not depend on the free drug fraction. However, for many drugs the clearance is restricted to free drug, in which case drug clearance increases as binding to plasma proteins decreases, since a larger fraction of the total is available for elimination. With these drugs, however, the clearance of *free* drug is unchanged. An unchanged clearance of free drug means that the average plasma free drug concentration is unchanged at steady state, even though the total drug concentration is less. Since free drug concentration is not changed and free drug determines the effects of most drugs, the daily dose of drug need not be changed. The best-studied example is that of phenytoin, which is normally >90 per cent bound to plasma albumin. In patients with uremia, phenytoin binding can decrease to 70 per cent so that the unbound fraction increases from 10 to 30 per cent. As a consequence of the increase in free fraction, both the apparent volume of distribution and the clearance increase. The plasma concentration of total phenytoin falls as a result of the increased clearance, but the average free concentration at steady state is unchanged. A therapeutic phenytoin level with 90 per cent protein binding is 10 to 20 mg per liter, corresponding to an unbound drug concentration of 1 to 2 mg per liter. With 30 per cent unbound, the corresponding therapeutic level of total phenytoin would be 3.3 to 6.7 mg per liter to achieve the same free drug concentration. Obviously, if the goal were to attain a total concentration of 10 to 20 mg per liter with 30 per cent unbound phenytoin, toxicity would result, since the free drug concentration would be threefold higher than therapeutic.

Active Metabolites. A third pitfall in interpretation of the plasma concentration of some drugs is the presence of unmeasured but active or toxic drug metabolites. Procainamide is metabolized to acecainide (formerly called N-acetylprocainamide), which has antiarrhythmic activity. The importance of active metabolites depends on their intrinsic activity and toxicity and the extent to which they accumulate relative to the parent compound. In situations in which a metabolite accounts for a significant portion of the drug's activity or toxicity, the metabolite must be measured along with the parent drug for proper interpretation.

Optical Isomers. The majority of drug molecules have an asymmetric center and can exist as two isomers called enantiomers, which are mirror images of each other. Most of these drugs are administered as racemic (equimolar) mixtures of the isomers. Although the enantiomers frequently have different pharmacologic effects, pharmacokinetics, and/or toxicity, clinically available drug assays do not distinguish between them. This leads to a number of potential problems that are only beginning to be appreciated but will be of increasing relevance to the design and testing of new drugs and the interpretation of plasma concentration data.

Pharmacodynamic Changes. A final factor altering the interpretation of plasma levels is a physiologic change that alters the response to a given plasma concentration. For instance, a change in serum potassium, magnesium, or calcium concentration alters the toxic concentration-effect relationship for digoxin such that concentrations not usually associated with adverse effects may now be toxic. The development of tolerance to a drug also distorts the relationship of plasma concentration to effect. Tolerance can be defined as a reduction in response to a given concentration of drug at the site of action and was originally recognized for drugs of abuse, particularly opiates. However, tolerance may also develop to the beneficial effects of therapeutic drugs. The tolerance reported with the continuous use of beta-adrenergic agonists for asthma and heart disease may be due to a reduction in the density of beta-adrenergic receptors during chronic agonist stimulation (see Ch. 25). More recently, tolerance to the therapeutic effects of nitroglycerin has been described with the 24-hour transdermal delivery systems.

These alterations in pharmacodynamics of the drug response emphasize the fact that plasma drug concentrations must be interpreted with other clinical and laboratory data that may influence the response to the drug.

ALTERATIONS OF DRUG DOSES IN DISEASE STATES.
Renal Disease. A decrease in renal function results in a decreased renal clearance of drugs. Whether a dosage adjustment is required depends on the toxicity of the drug and the importance of renal clearance for drug elimination. If the drug has significant toxicity and the kidney accounts for most of the drug's elimination, then dosage adjustments must be made in patients with renal disease to avoid toxicity. On the other hand, if the drug is nontoxic, dosage adjustment is less critical even if the drug accumulates in patients with renal failure. For instance, penicillin is cleared >90 per cent by the kidneys, but because it is relatively nontoxic, dosage adjustments are not required for low-dose therapy (600,000 to 1,200,000 units per day). However, if massive doses of penicillin are required, then dosage adjustments must be made to avoid penicillin toxicity.

TABLE 23–5. THE RENAL ELIMINATION RATE CONSTANTS (k_r), NONRENAL ELIMINATION RATE CONSTANTS (k_{nr}), AND PER CENT NONRENAL ELIMINATION IN A NORMAL INDIVIDUAL FOR SELECTED DRUGS

	k_r (per hour)	k_{nr} (per hour)	Per Cent Non-renal
Group A (>80% renal)			
Acyclovir	0.2	0.02	10
Amantadine	0.05	0.005	10
Amikacin	0.3	0.01	5
Amoxicillin	0.6	0.1	10
Ampicillin	0.5	0.06	10
Atenolol	0.10	0.005	5
Bretylium	0.07	0.01	15
Carbenicillin	0.5	0.05	10
Cefamandole	0.84	0.04	5
Cefazolin	0.3	0.02	5
Cefoxitin	1.0	0.05	5
Cephalexin	0.7	0.03	5
Cephalothin	1.4	0.03	5
Cephradine	0.5	0.05	10
Colistin	0.3	0.02	10
Flucytosine	0.24	0.01	5
Gentamicin	0.3	0.02	5
Kanamycin	0.3	0.01	5
Methicillin	1.2	0.15	10
Methotrexate	0.07	0.007	10
Moxalactam	0.3	0.02	5
Oxypurinol*	0.03	0.003	10
Penicillin G	1.3	0.1	10
Polymyxin B	0.13	0.02	10
Streptomycin	0.24	0.01	5
Tetracycline	0.07	0.01	10
Ticarcillin	0.6	0.06	10
Tobramycin	0.3	0.01	5
Vancomycin	0.12	0.003	5
Group B (50–80% renal)			
Cefotaxime	0.6	0.28	30
Cephapirin	0.9	0.3	25
Cimetidine	0.27	0.09	25
Dicloxacillin	0.6	0.6	50
Erythromycin	0.30	0.15	35
Ethambutol	0.09	0.09	50
Isoniazid (slow acetylators)	0.12	0.12	50
Lincomycin	0.1	0.06	40
Nadolol	0.03	0.01	25
Nafcillin	0.7	0.5	40
Oxacillin	1.1	0.35	25
Oxytetracycline	0.065	0.015	20
Ranitidine	0.25	0.08	25
Trimethoprim	0.03	0.03	50
Group C (<50% renal)			
Amphotericin B	0.01	0.02	70
Chloramphenicol	0.02	0.3	80
Clindamycin	0	0.25	100
Doxycycline	0.005	0.03	80
Flecainide	0.013	0.03	80
Isoniazid (fast acetylators)	0.1	0.4	80
Mexiletine	0.006	0.06	90
Minocycline	0	0.06	100
Rifampin	0	0.25	100
Sulfamethoxazole	0.01	0.06	85
Tocainide	0.02	0.03	60

*Oxypurinol is the major active metabolite of allopurinol.

Fortunately, renal drug clearance is closely correlated with the clearance of creatinine even for those drugs that are eliminated by tubular secretion. For this reason, an adjustment of the average drug dose can be calculated from the creatinine clearance. The process is simple: The calculated renal drug clearance is reduced by the same proportion as the reduction from 100 ml per minute in the creatinine clearance (see Table 23–3). If the drug is cleared by nonrenal (usually hepatic) mechanisms as well

as by renal mechanisms, only the renal clearance (Cl_r) is adjusted; the nonrenal clearance (Cl_{nr}) is assumed to remain normal. The dose is then adjusted in direct proportion to the change in total clearance, since $Cl \times C_p$ = dose/time. Renal and nonrenal clearances for some drugs are listed in Table 23–1. Consider as an example the alteration of digoxin dosage in renal failure. The average renal clearance of digoxin is 110 ml per minute at a creatinine clearance of 100 ml per minute; the nonrenal clearance is 40 ml per minute. If the measured creatinine clearance is 50 ml per minute, or half normal, then the renal clearance of digoxin is reduced by a similar fraction; thus, Cl_r(digoxin) = 55 ml per minute in this patient. If the nonrenal clearance is assumed to be unchanged, the total digoxin clearance is $Cl_{nr} + Cl_r$ = 40 + 55 = 95 ml per minute in the patient with a creatinine clearance of 50 ml per minute, versus a total digoxin clearance of 150 ml per minute in a patient with normal renal function. The total digoxin clearance is therefore reduced by the fraction $^{95}/_{150}$ and the dose should be adjusted using the same fraction. If the average dose is 0.25 mg per day, this would be decreased to $^{95}/_{150}$ × 0.25 mg = 0.16 mg per day. These calculations can give only a first approximation of the appropriate dose for an individual patient, since they are based on the average dose for the average patient. In practice, a dose conveniently close to the calculated dose is administered to the patient, and the patient's response and/or plasma drug concentrations are monitored. With the information provided by either the plasma drug concentrations or clinical observations, the dosage can be adjusted.

If the desired plasma concentration is known, one can calculate the dosage directly from the drug clearance (see Table 23–3). For example, an average procainamide concentration of 5 μg per milliliter is desired in a patient with a creatinine clearance of 50 ml per minute. The total procainamide clearance is $^{50}/_{100}$ × 330 (Cl_r) + 120 (Cl_{nr}) = 285 ml per minute. An infusion of 1.4 mg per minute ($Cl \times C_p$) or a dose of 250 mg every 3 hours will achieve and maintain the desired plasma concentration.

Although drug clearance is the best way to calculate doses for drugs, clearance data are not available for many drugs. For a few drugs, published nomograms are available to guide dosage. It would be preferable, both from a practical and from an intellectual standpoint, to be able to use a more generally applicable method to calculate proper dosage. Two such methods are outlined in the next two paragraphs.

For many drugs, the elimination rate constant (k_e) is known. If the apparent volume of distribution is unchanged in renal disease, then the k_e and Cl are proportional ($k_e = Cl/V_D$) and the change in k_e can be used to adjust the dose in a manner entirely analogous to the use of changes in clearance to adjust dose. Like clearance values, the elimination rate constant can be expressed as the sum of the rate constants for the separate eliminating organs; thus $k_e = k_{renal} + k_{nonrenal}$. Values for k_r and k_{nr} are listed in Table 23–5. To use these values to adjust dosage in renal insufficiency, the procedure is exactly the same as with the clearance calculations used above. Thus, k_e for amikacin in a patient with normal renal function is 0.31, which is made up of k_r = 0.3 and k_{nr} = 0.01. The dose alteration in a patient with a creatinine clearance of 25 ml per minute is calculated as follows: The k_r for the patient is 25/100 × 0.3 = 0.08. The k_e therefore is $k_r + k_{nr}$ = 0.08 + 0.01 = 0.09 versus the normal k_e of 0.31. The dose of amikacin must therefore be reduced to 0.09/0.31 or 30 per cent of the usual dose per unit time. As can be readily appreciated, the dose of amikacin is reduced almost in proportion to the reduction in creatinine clearance, since the nonrenal elimination is negligible until creatinine clearance is reduced to very low values (i.e., <15 ml per minute). Several other drugs that are like amikacin in this regard are in Group A in Table 23–5. For all these drugs, dosage adjustment can be made by multiplying the usual dose by the fraction of the creatinine clearance remaining in the patient. When the patient has essentially no renal function, then the small k_{nr} may be used to calculate doses as illustrated above. For drugs that have nonrenal elimination that is a substantial fraction (e.g., 20 to 50 per cent) of the total elimination, the dosage reduction in renal insufficiency is less than the reduction in creatinine clearance and can be calculated as illustrated above. These drugs are in Group B in Table 23–5. If the nonrenal elimination is greater than 50 per cent of the k_e, then the dosage usually does not need to be adjusted for changes in renal function. In all cases, the calculations adjust only the average dose, and blood level determinations are required to make final dosage adjustments. This is particularly true if nonrenal elimination may also be reduced, as in liver or cardiac disease.

A final method for estimating the average dose in patients with renal failure is to use the per cent nonrenal elimination determined in normal individuals. These values are listed in Tables 23–1 and 23–5 and are frequently available for drugs even if clearances or elimination rate constants are not. This method uses the nomogram in Figure 23–7, in which creatinine clearance is plotted against the drug clearance as a per cent of normal. The black lines intersecting the black ordinate are for drugs that have a nonrenal elimination of 0 to 50 per cent in a normal individual. The nomogram is used by drawing a perpendicular line to the creatinine clearance until it intersects the black line corresponding to the drug of interest. The per cent drug clearance can then be read directly from the red ordinate and the dosage adjusted accordingly. For instance, consider the amikacin example calculated above. Since the per cent nonrenal elimination in a normal individual is ~5 per cent, the clearance values for amikacin fall on the line intersecting the ordinate at 5 per cent in Figure 23–7. The drug clearance as a percentage of normal for a creatinine clearance of 25 ml per minute is ~30 per cent (as indicated by the dotted line), and the dose of this drug in the patient with a creatinine clearance of 25 ml therefore must be 30 per cent normal.

The reduction in dose per unit time can be applied to patient care by giving either the reduced dose at the usual interval or the same dose at a longer interval. The average plasma level is the same by both methods, but the fluctuations in plasma concentration are less when the reduced dose is given at the usual intervals.

Loading doses for most drugs used in patients with renal failure need not be adjusted for creatinine clearance because V_D is usually close to normal. However, since the $t\frac{1}{2}$ of renally cleared drugs is prolonged in these patients, drug accumulation during initiation of therapy with maintenance doses is slower. Because of the slower accumulation, a loading dose may be required in patients with renal failure in order to achieve a therapeutic blood concentration rapidly, whereas patients with normal renal function may not need a loading dose for the same drug. Digoxin, for example, with a half-life of 1.5 days in a patient with normal renal function accumulates to 90 per cent of steady-state levels in 5 days (three to four half-lives), and many patients need not be loaded, since this accumulation is sufficiently rapid to produce the desired therapeutic effects. On the other hand, in a patient without renal function, digoxin half-life increases to 5 days. If the anephric patient is begun on the appropriately reduced maintenance dose of digoxin, accumulation to the same steady-state level takes more than 15 days to occur. In this case, a loading dose may be desired to achieve a more rapid effect without waiting for drug accumulation. However, whether or not a loading dose is given, the ultimate steady-state drug concentration is the same and, as always, depends only on drug dose and drug clearance.

Patients with end-stage renal disease are usually supported with hemodialysis. Dialysis can remove some therapeutic drugs from the circulation and necessitate supplemental dosing to maintain a therapeutic effect. The most important characteristics of the drug that determine the ability of dialysis to remove a significant amount of drug from the body are the V_D, drug binding to plasma proteins, and the nonrenal clearance of the drug. Of these, V_D is the most important parameter, and only if it is less than 1 liter per kilogram can significant amounts of drug be removed by dialysis. Dialysis is also more effective in drug removal if the drug is not highly bound to plasma proteins. Since clearance of drugs by hemodialysis is limited to a maximum of ~ 100 ml per minute, drugs that have a relatively small extrarenal clearance (< 400 ml per minute) may have a significant increment in their removal rate during hemodialysis even if they are not normally cleared by the kidney. For instance, aminoglycosides have a small V_D, low binding to plasma protein, and mostly renal clearance and are therefore removed to a significant extent by hemodialysis. Theophylline, although not normally cleared by the kidneys, has a relatively small V_D, a nonrenal clearance of 55 ml per minute, and moderate protein binding and therefore may be sufficiently removed during a 3- to 6-hour hemodialysis session to require a modest supplemental dosage. For most drugs that require supplemental therapy after hemodialysis to maintain a therapeutic effect, blood level determinations are available as a guide.

Some drugs form metabolites that are active or toxic and are eliminated by the kidneys. In patients with renal insufficiency, these metabolites may accumulate and produce effects. As an example, procainamide is in part excreted unchanged and in part metabolized to acecainide, which has antiarrhythmic effects and can produce toxicity. The metabolite may achieve concentrations in renal failure that are many-fold higher than the parent drug and can contribute to the antiarrhythmic effects and toxicity of procainamide. Drugs with renally excreted active or toxic metabolites include (in addition to procainamide) meperidine, propoxyphene, allopurinol, acetohexamide, clofibrate, nitrofurantoin, and nitroprusside. If alternative drugs are available for the

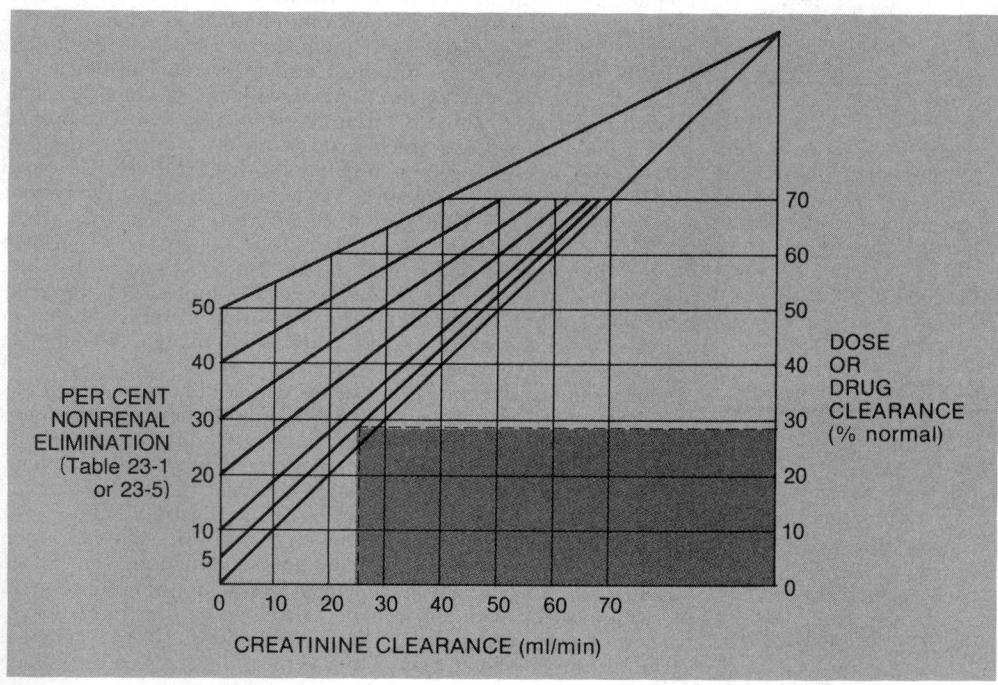

FIGURE 23–7. Nomogram for calculation of drug doses in patients with renal disease. The dose of any drug in a patient with renal disease (as a per cent of normal) is determined by connecting a line from the measured or calculated creatinine clearance to the black line that corresponds to the per cent nonrenal elimination for the drug of interest (from Table 23–1 or 23–5). The point of intersection is then extended to the red axis, where the dose per unit time as a per cent of normal is read directly. The dotted line indicates that in a patient with a creatinine clearance of 25 ml per minute the dose of amikacin, which normally has 5 per cent nonrenal elimination, must be reduced to approximately 30 per cent of normal.

treatment of patients with renal insufficiency, it is probably best to avoid the former drugs when active or toxic metabolites may accumulate.

Hepatic Disease. Although many drugs are biotransformed by the liver, no quantitive predictor of the degree of abnormality in drug metabolism is available for patients with liver disease. If the indices of the liver's capacity to form proteins (serum albumin level and prothrombin time) are abnormal, then it is probable that the clearance of drugs metabolized by the mixed function oxidase (P450) system will be reduced. However, the elimination of drugs metabolized by hepatic conjugation mechanisms is much less affected by chronic liver disease. Acute liver disease has an inconstant and unpredictable effect on drug metabolism, but, in general, drug metabolism is not so abnormal as with chronic liver disease.

With chronic liver disease, portacaval anastomoses may develop. Not only does this decrease the blood flow to the liver with consequent reduction in clearance of some drugs, but the portacaval shunting can allow drug absorbed by the gut to pass directly into the systemic circulation and bypass the liver, thereby avoiding the "first-pass" or "presystemic" elimination. For those drugs that are largely extracted from the blood by the liver (e.g., propranolol, metoprolol, lidocaine), portacaval shunting allows a much greater fraction of an orally administered dose to reach the systemic circulation.

Hemodynamic Disorders. Pharmacokinetics can be affected in several ways by disorders of the circulation. Hypotension and poor cardiac output reduce renal blood flow, glomerular filtration rate, and hepatic blood flow. As with primary renal disease, the impairment in renal drug excretion may be estimated by the change in creatinine clearance and dosage adjustments made accordingly. The effects of reduced hepatic blood flow on drug metabolism are highly dependent on the drug. For drugs that are essentially completely cleared from the blood on a single passage through the liver, i.e., when the extraction from the blood is close to 100 per cent, a reduction in liver blood flow reduces hepatic drug clearance proportionately. On the other hand, many drugs that are metabolized are extracted poorly by the liver, and for these drugs a reduction in liver blood flow has relatively little influence on their hepatic clearance. A complicating factor is that circulatory abnormalities also can result in hepatic congestion or tissue hypoxia that can impair hepatocellular function, so that drug metabolism may be reduced during hypotensive states independent of the effects of blood flow on drug delivery to the liver. Therefore, it is difficult to predict the proper dosage of hepatic metabolized drugs in individual patients with circulatory abnormalities. Certainly a drug such as lidocaine that has a very high hepatic clearance is cleared less well in congestive heart failure or shock, and the maintenance infusion rates must be reduced by about half in these situations to avoid toxicity.

The distribution of some drugs is also affected by hemodynamic changes. For several drugs with large distribution volumes (lidocaine, quinidine, and procainamide), the apparent volume of distribution is decreased in heart failure and shock, and loading doses should also be reduced to avoid toxic plasma concentrations. However, for theophylline, a drug with a relatively small volume of distribution, the apparent volume of distribution is not changed by heart failure. Since data are not available for most drugs, we advise a conservative approach to loading and maintenance doses of toxic drugs in the setting of congestive heart failure or shock, with careful monitoring of the clinical status and plasma levels to guide further dosage adjustments.

USE OF DRUGS IN THE ELDERLY. Elderly persons (over 65 years) comprise 11 to 12 per cent of the United States population, but over 30 per cent of all prescriptions are written for this group of patients, and the trend is for an increased prescribing rate in the elderly in contrast to a decreased rate in younger patients. As an individual ages, changes occur that may affect drug kinetics and drug action. These age-related changes accentuate the normal interindividual variation in drug effects, thus making the elderly the most diverse segment of the adult population in terms of their drug responses. Because of the changes that occur with aging, the number of illnesses present, and the large numbers of drugs used in this population, the elderly are also highly susceptible to serious adverse drug effects and drug interactions.

The pharmacokinetic changes that occur in the elderly are related to changes in body composition as well as to changes in function of pharmacokinetically important organs. In spite of a decrease in gastric acid secretion, a decrease in mucosal absorptive surface of the small bowel by about 30 per cent, and a decrease in splanchnic blood flow by about 40 per cent, very few studies have shown an effect of aging on drug absorption.

The distribution of drugs may change markedly with aging, probably because lean body mass and total body water decrease as the percentage of total body fat increases. In addition, the plasma concentration of albumin decreases, probably as a result of decreased albumin production by the liver, and this may affect those drugs that are bound to plasma albumin. Alpha$_1$-acid glycoprotein, the major plasma protein that binds basic drugs, is not diminished with aging. Because of the changes in body composition, water-soluble drugs that are not bound to plasma proteins may have a reduced apparent volume of distribution. However, for lipid-soluble drugs, such as many psychotropic agents, the volume of distribution relative to body weight may be increased, probably because of the increased percentage of body weight as fat. For water-soluble, albumin-bound drugs, the changes in distribution with aging are not predictable.

The clearance of many drugs is diminished in the elderly. Cardiac output and blood flow to the kidneys and liver may decrease by 30 to 40 per cent with aging, and glomerular filtration rate may be reduced by as much as 50 per cent. However, since older persons have a decreased muscle mass, they have a decreased rate of creatinine production so that a reduced creatinine clearance can coexist with an apparently normal serum creatinine concentration. As a general rule, one should consider that renal elimination of drugs is reduced by 50 per cent in elderly patients without evidence of renal disease and make dosage adjustments accordingly.

Both hepatic blood flow and the intrinsic ability of the liver to metabolize some drugs may be reduced in the elderly, but the interindividual variability in the metabolism of drugs is so large as to preclude any useful predictions. The reduction in hepatic blood flow influences the hepatic elimination of drugs with high extraction ratios, such as lidocaine. The reduction in mixed function oxidase activity in some elderly patients may reduce the clearance of drugs with a low hepatic extraction ratio as well as reduce the presystemic (first-pass) elimination of those drugs with a high hepatic extraction ratio. However, conjugation reactions usually are unaffected by aging.

Elimination half-life of many drugs is increased with aging as a consequence of a larger apparent volume of distribution and/or a smaller metabolic or renal clearance. Frequently, elimination half-life can be prolonged even without changes in drug clearance. This is true with diazepam, which has an increased apparent volume of distribution with no change in metabolic clearance, and this combination of changes produces a prolonged elimination half-life.

Age-related changes in target-organ responsiveness are also important. The antianxiety agents and sedative hypnotic agents produce greater degrees of depression of central nervous system function in the elderly than in the young even at the same plasma levels. The hypotensive side effects of many psychotropic drugs are greater in the elderly because of reduced functioning of baroreceptor reflexes. Hemorrhage with anticoagulants is more common in the elderly even with good control of the clotting parameters. These changes in pharmacodynamics require the use of smaller doses of drugs in the elderly, even if the kinetics of the drug are not altered.

The following general principles derive from studies of drugs in the elderly: (1) Drugs that are eliminated by the kidneys very likely have a reduced clearance, and the doses required to achieve a therapeutic blood concentration may be 50 per cent of those required in a young population. (2) Drugs that are eliminated by the liver may be less affected, but for parenterally given drugs such as lidocaine that have high hepatic clearances, the reduction in liver blood flow would be expected to decrease the clearance of the drug. In addition, some individuals have a reduction in hepatic drug metabolism, and enzyme induction may not occur as readily in the elderly. (3) The sensitivity of target organs to drugs is increased for central nervous system depressants and probably for other drugs as well. Thus, the elderly constitute a population in whom drug use is likely to be marred by enhanced toxicity, and physician awareness of the possibility of altered drug disposition or effects is mandatory. It is a population in which drugs should be used in the lowest effective doses and only in individuals in whom they are absolutely necessary. That this is not commonly done is indicated by the increasing numbers of prescriptions written for elderly patients, frequently without well-defined endpoints or even well-defined therapeutic indications. Frequent reviews of the patient's drug history, including over-the-counter medications, and discontinuation of those drugs that are not necessary would greatly improve medical care for the elderly population.

Benet LZ, Williams RL: Design and optimization of dosage regimens: Pharmacokinetic data. *In* Gilman AG, Rall TW, Nies AS, Taylor P (eds.): Goodman and Gilman's Pharmacological Basis of Therapeutics. 8th ed. New York, Pergamon Press, 1990, pp 1650–1735. *This series of tables lists the pharmacokinetic parameters of over 150 drugs with references to the literature. This represents the most concise and complete listing currently available and is the source for some of the data in Table 23–5.*

Bennett WM, Aronoff GR, Golper TA, et al.: Drug Prescribing in Renal Failure. Dosing Guidelines for Adults. Philadelphia, American College of Physicians, 1987. *A useful paperback manual that recommends dosage adjustments for many drugs in patients with varying degrees of renal dysfunction and those on dialysis.*

Bjornsson TD: Nomogram for drug dosage adjustment in patients with renal failure. Clin Pharmacokin 11:164, 1986. *This review of drug elimination in renal disease uses an approach to dosage adjustment similar to the nomogram in this chapter. There is an extensive compilation of over 130 drugs that can be used as a reference for those drugs not in Table 23–1 or Table 23–5.*

Cartwright A, Smith C: Elderly People, Their Medicines and Their Doctors. London, Routledge, 1988. *A landmark community-based study of medication use by the elderly in the United Kingdom. The findings indicate that although many elderly would rather not take drugs, patient compliance and knowledge of the purpose of their medications are quite good. However, there is a need for additional physician effort to avoid contraindicated and duplicated drugs, to improve the labeling and written instructions for patients, and to review the medications at each visit and discontinue those that are no longer needed.*

Montamat SC, Cusack BJ, Vestal RE: Management of drug therapy in the elderly. N Engl J Med 321:310, 1989. *A review of the use of drugs in the elderly that summarizes the relevant literature.*

Wilkinson GR, Shand DG: A physiological approach to hepatic drug clearance. Clin Pharmacol Ther 18:377, 1975. *This article discusses hepatic drug clearance in relation to blood flow, enzyme activity, and plasma protein binding. The concepts are valuable for physiologically oriented individuals.*

24 Interactions Between Drugs

Alan S. Nies

Good medical practice frequently demands treatment with multiple drugs for a single disease in an attempt to maximize therapeutic effects and minimize side effects. When one is treating multiple diseases, the number of co-administered drugs increases, as does the possibility of undesirable interactions occurring between the drugs. Entire textbooks have been written in an attempt to list all possible drug interactions. It is obviously impossible for a clinician to remember such lists, and frequently the *clinically important* drug interactions are lost in the midst of large listings of interactions that are based on undocumented case reports, animal experimentation, or theory.

Not all drug interactions that occur are clinically important because (1) many drugs have such large therapeutic indices that toxicity does not result when there are moderate increases in drug concentration; (2) the disease being treated may not be serious so that a change of drug concentration to less than therapeutic levels may not be easily recognized; (3) many drugs are given without well-defined therapeutic endpoints, making the drug effect difficult to assess, and therefore changes in drug effect are not recognized; (4) there is a large intersubject variability due to genetic, environmental, and disease factors that may obscure many drug interactions. These comments are not to imply that drug interactions are not important. Drug interactions are important if the drug has easily recognizable toxicity and a low therapeutic index such that small increases in amount of drug

in the body produce significant toxicity. Second, drug interactions are recognized and important if the diseases that are being controlled with the drug are serious or potentially fatal when undertreated. Third, drug interactions are recognized if the therapeutic endpoints for the drug are clearly defined or if drug levels are used to maximize therapy for a given drug. Thus major interactions have been reported with anticoagulants and oral hypoglycemics, both of which have easily recognizable toxicity with low therapeutic indices. Drug interactions are reported with antiseizure medication and antiarrhythmic drugs; not only do these drugs have recognized toxicity, but also the diseases being treated become clinically manifest if the amount of drug is inadequate. Drug interactions have been recognized with cardiac glycosides when blood levels are used to maximize efficacy in some patients.

Clinically important drug interactions are related to (1) changes in the amount of drug or active metabolite available at the site of action, the so-called pharmacokinetic drug interactions, or (2) changes in drug effect without a change in pharmacokinetics, the pharmacodynamic drug interactions. These latter interactions may result from interactions at a receptor site, from independent actions of two drugs either adding to or counteracting the effects of each other, or from one drug altering the cellular milieu, thus changing the effects of another drug.

PHARMACOKINETIC DRUG INTERACTIONS

These interactions involve the processes of absorption, distribution, and elimination such that there is a change in the amount of a drug (or an active metabolite) at the site of action and a corresponding change in drug effect.

Interactions Resulting in Less Drug Available at the Site of Action

DECREASED ABSORPTION. Since drug absorption generally occurs across the gastrointestinal mucosa by passive diffusion, one drug would not be expected to compete with another for absorption. However, drugs may physically interact in the lumen of the gastrointestinal tract so as to cause decreased absorption. Cholestyramine and colestipol, resins used to bind bile acids and to lower serum cholesterol, can also bind a number of drugs if they are simultaneously present in the gastrointestinal lumen. Thus cholestyramine can diminish the absorption of thyroid hormones, cardiac glycosides, warfarin, and corticosteroids. It is likely that other drugs also bind to the steroid-binding resins, so one is advised to separate the administration of the resin from that of other drug doses by at least 2 hours.

Tetracyclines are potent chelating agents that form insoluble complexes with metal ions such as magnesium, calcium, and aluminum, commonly found in antacids, as well as with iron, with the result that the absorption of tetracycline is reduced. Sucralfate used for peptic ulcer disease has been reported to reduce the absorption of warfarin and phenytoin. Kaolin used to halt diarrhea effectively inhibits the absorption of some drugs such as lincomycin and digoxin. In addition, drug products may contain "inert" substances that can interact with other drugs. For instance, para-aminosalicylic acid (PAS) contains bentonite (a kaolin-like substance), which can hamper the absorption of co-administered rifampin.

If a drug is susceptible to degradation at acid pH, anything that delays emptying of the stomach, such as a drug with anticholinergic properties, can result in more degradation of the co-administered acid-sensitive drug, e.g., penicillin G or L-dopa, and thus a decrease in the amount of drug absorbed. Conversely, a drug that speeds gastric emptying, such as metoclopramide, can increase the absorption of acid-unstable drugs. With most other drugs only the time course of absorption is changed so that drug absorption is faster if gastric emptying is enhanced or slower if gastric emptying is delayed, but the total amount of drug absorbed is unchanged. Whether a change in rate of absorption results in any important clinical effects depends on whether rapid absorption is necessary for drug effect, in which case drug effect is diminished. Usually, if total absorption is unchanged, there is no important interaction, particularly during chronic administration of drugs.

The pH of the gastrointestinal fluid can affect the dissolution of drug from the dosage form. Ketoconazole, a weak base, is most soluble in acidic gastric fluid. If gastric pH is increased by antacids or H_2-antihistamines, the dissolution and hence the absorption of ketoconazole are reduced.

ALTERED DISTRIBUTION. A few drugs reach their site of action via active transport. In this case, drugs can compete with each other for the transport mechanism. In order to produce blockade of adrenergic activity, the antihypertensive drugs guanethidine, guanadrel, and bethanidine must be actively transported by an amine transport system into adrenergic neurons. This transport system can be interfered with by tricyclic antidepressants, high doses of phenothiazines, and some sympathomimetic amines. Thus co-administration of guanethidine with one of these other compounds effectively blocks the antihypertensive effects of guanethidine. This is an undesirable interaction with guanethidine; however, with the antiarrhythmic drug bretylium, sympathetic blockade produces orthostatic hypotension as an unwanted side effect. Bretylium also gains access to adrenergic neurons via the same amine transport system used by guanethidine. Therapeutic advantage can be taken of a drug interaction that blocks access of bretylium to its antiadrenergic site of action. Thus tricyclic antidepressants or ephedrine reverses bretylium's sympathetic blocking effects but does not affect the direct antiarrhythmic effects of bretylium.

ENHANCED METABOLISM. Several drugs can increase the ability of the liver to metabolize other drugs by the mixed function oxidase (P450) system. Phenobarbital, other barbiturates, phenytoin, rifampin, glutethimide, griseofulvin, ethanol, phenylbutazone, chronic smoking, certain chlorinated hydrocarbons such as lindane and DDT, carbamazepine, and primidone have all been associated with induction of hepatic microsomal, drug-metabolizing enzymes. The amount of enzyme induction that occurs appears to be under genetic control, and not all individuals experience quantitatively similar effects when taking an inducing agent.

Induction of hepatic metabolizing enzymes can affect many drugs. The effects are greatest when the drugs are given orally, because all of the drug must pass through the liver prior to reaching the systemic circulation. Therefore, even for drugs that have a systemic clearance largely dependent upon hepatic blood flow, the amount of drug that escapes metabolism on the first pass is influenced by enzyme-inducing drugs. Some examples of drugs that can have their metabolism induced are oral anticoagulants, quinidine, digitoxin, corticosteroids, low-dose oral contraceptives, cyclosporine, some beta-adrenergic blockers, mexiletine, and theophylline. The induction of corticosteroid metabolism has produced some interesting effects, including (1) inappropriate interpretation of low-dose dexamethasone suppression tests in which the enhanced metabolism of dexamethasone produced by enzyme induction resulted in too low a dexamethasone concentration to inhibit normal steroidogenesis; (2) exacerbation of steroid-dependent asthma; (3) rejection of a renal transplant by individuals who required steroids and received an enzyme-inducing agent; (4) nonresponsiveness of the nephrotic syndrome to steroid therapy; and (5) increased adrenal corticosteroid replacement dosage in patients with Addison's disease.

Frequently the most critical time occurs when the inducing agent is discontinued. At this time the drug-metabolizing activity gradually decreases, and drug toxicity can occur if dosage adjustments of other co-administered drugs are not made. This phenomenon has been described most frequently with induction of warfarin metabolism and resultant warfarin toxicity when the inducing agent is discontinued.

Interactions Resulting in More Drug Available at the Site of Action

ENHANCED ABSORPTION. In general, absorption is not a common process in which drugs can interact to enhance efficacy. One exception is with acid-unstable drugs and enhanced gastric emptying mentioned above. Another potential interaction is with relatively poorly absorbed drugs, such as tablet formulations of digoxin, with which absorption occurs throughout the gastrointestinal tract. With such a drug a decrease in intestinal motility could enhance the degree of absorption by prolonging contact with the absorbing mucosa.

ALTERED DISTRIBUTION. Many drugs are bound to plasma proteins, and drug so bound is not available for action at

receptors or for distribution throughout the body. In addition, for many compounds only the free drug is available for metabolism or excretion. The drug bound to plasma protein, therefore, acts as an inactive reservoir of drug in the blood. Since drugs can compete with each other for binding to plasma proteins, a potential for interactions exists. Pure plasma protein–binding interactions, however, rarely are clinically significant. The one probable exception to this is the displacement of albumin-bound bilirubin by sulfonamides or salicylates, thus allowing the bilirubin to distribute into the tissues and cause kernicterus in jaundiced infants. However, when a drug is displaced from plasma protein binding, it very rapidly distributes into the apparent volume of distribution so that the increase in free drug concentration in the plasma is always considerably less than suggested by experiments in vitro. The larger the apparent volume of distribution, the less of an impact a displacement from protein binding has. Following the immediate displacement and redistribution of the drug, the free fraction generally is readily available for metabolism or excretion, and the clearance processes in the body reduce the free drug concentration to that which existed prior to the protein-binding interaction (Fig. 24–1). Therefore the effect of such an interaction is small and transient. The relationship of free drug to total drug, however, is changed by such drug interactions, and therefore the interpretation of plasma drug assays that measure total drug in blood may have to be altered (see Ch. 23).

DECREASED METABOLISM. Inhibition of drug metabolism can have a profound effect on drug disposition, resulting in drug toxicity. Inhibition of the metabolism of one drug by another occurs rapidly, and the enhanced effect or toxicity therefore often occurs shortly after the interaction takes place. Some drugs seem to be rather specific for inhibiting the metabolism of other individual drugs. However, there are a few drugs that can inhibit the metabolism of many drugs. The most commonly used such drug is cimetidine, which can inhibit the metabolism of theophylline, warfarin, diazepam, phenytoin, lidocaine, chlordiazepoxide, propranolol, carbamazepine, digitoxin, imipramine, quin-

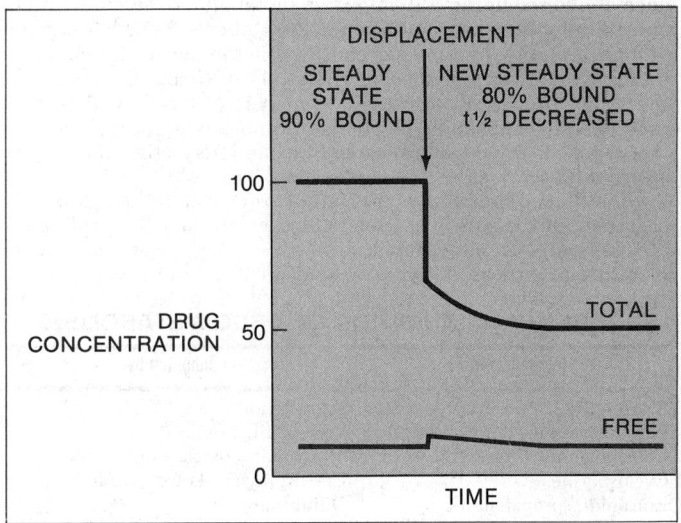

FIGURE 24–1. The effects of altered plasma drug binding on total and free plasma concentrations of the drug. The drug is assumed to be bound 90 per cent to albumin, not bound to tissues, and to have a V_D of 8.5 liters. At the arrow an agent is given that displaces the drug from albumin such that binding is reduced to 80 per cent. The expected changes are an immediate increase in free drug concentration by only 40 per cent, with a fall of total concentration to 70 per cent of the initial value. Since the free drug clearance is not altered by this interaction, a new steady state is achieved with the same free drug concentration and a reduction of total concentration to 50 per cent. For drugs with larger volumes of distribution, i.e., more tissue binding, the immediate increase of free concentration is even less than in this example, but the ultimate steady-state condition of unchanged free drug concentration and a halving of the concentration of total drug is the same. (Adapted from Shand et al.: *In* Handbook of Experimental Pharmacology. Vol 28, No 3, pp 272–314, 1975.)

idine, flecainide, calcium channel blockers, and probably others. The antiarrhythmic drug amiodarone also appears to be a potent inhibitor of the metabolism of many other drugs, including warfarin, phenytoin, flecainide, calcium channel blockers, and quinidine. Since amiodarone has a half-life of 1 to 2 months, inhibition of enzyme activity produced by amiodarone may persist for several months after the drug is discontinued. Other important interactions resulting from decreased metabolism are listed in Table 24–1. As with other interactions resulting in an increased amount of drug at the sites of action, the most important examples are drugs that have a low therapeutic index and easily recognized, serious toxicity.

In addition to inhibition of hepatic drug metabolism via mixed function oxidase, inhibition of metabolism at other enzyme sites can be important. Thus nonselective monoamine oxidase inhibitors can inhibit the metabolism of catecholamines and tyramine at multiple sites, allowing for build-up of these substances and the so-called cheese reaction due to enhanced catecholamine release with the ingestion of tyramine-containing foods. The new MAO inhibitor selegiline (deprenyl), which is selective for the B isozyme of MAO, does not produce this type of interaction at low doses (< 20 mg per day). Allopurinol inhibits xanthine oxidase, which can be important for the metabolism of azathioprine and 6-mercaptopurine. If allopurinol is given, much less azathioprine or 6-mercaptopurine is needed for equivalent effects. As discussed above, ethanol can induce hepatic microsomal drug-metabolizing enzymes. However, if ethanol is present, it can also act as an inhibitor of drug metabolism. Thus drugs given to an individual who is intoxicated may have an enhanced effect, whereas drugs given to an individual who has been drinking chronically but is no longer intoxicated may have diminished effect.

DIMINISHED RENAL EXCRETION. Some important drug interactions occur when active transport of one drug across the renal tubule is inhibited by another drug. Most of the reported interactions occur at the acid transport site. Thus probenecid is given to decrease penicillin clearance and thereby increase penicillin blood levels. Phenylbutazone can inhibit the renal clearance of hydroxyhexamide, an active metabolite of acetohexamide, and thereby increase its hypoglycemic effect. Salicylates, phenylbutazone, and probenecid can inhibit the renal elimination of methotrexate and enhance its effect. Drugs can also interact at the renal tubular site for active transport of bases, which is the probable mechanism by which cimetidine and amiodarone reduce the renal clearance of procainamide and its active metabolite, acecainide.

Quinidine, verapamil, and amiodarone can reduce the renal clearance of digoxin. The exact tubular site at which this interaction occurs is not known, but it is a significant interaction resulting in increased digoxin blood levels and effects.

TABLE 24–1. INHIBITION OF DRUG METABOLISM

Metabolism of	Inhibited by
Azathioprine, 6-mercaptopurine	Allopurinol
Carbamazepine	Verapamil, isoniazid
Catecholamines, tyramine	Monoamine oxidase inhibitors
Cyclosporine	Erythromycin, ketoconazole
Encainide, propafenone, propranolol	Quinidine
Phenobarbital	Valproic acid
Phenytoin	Isoniazid (in slow acetylators), chloramphenicol, cimetidine, clofibrate, phenylbutazone, disulfiram, dicumarol, amiodarone, valproic acid
Theophylline	Cimetidine, erythromycin, troleandomycin
Tolbutamide	Chloramphenicol, phenylbutazone, clofibrate, sulfaphenazole, dicumarol
Warfarin	Phenylbutazone, alcohol, disulfiram, allopurinol, cimetidine, disopyramide, sulfinpyrazone, trimethoprim-sulfamethoxazole, metronidazole, amiodarone

Decreased renal excretion of lithium occurs when proximal tubular reabsorption is enhanced. Since lithium and sodium are handled similarly in the proximal tubule, anything that results in more proximal tubular sodium reabsorption also affects lithium in the same way. Thus dietary salt restriction, salt depletion due to diarrhea, and diuretics acting at more distal segments of the nephron can reduce renal lithium excretion, requiring a reduction in lithium dose. Indomethacin and other nonsteroidal anti-inflammatory drugs also reduce lithium clearance, probably by enhancing proximal tubular reabsorption of the ion.

PHARMACODYNAMIC DRUG INTERACTIONS

Numerous drugs interact with each other at receptor sites or have additive effects by acting at separate sites on cells. Thus vitamin K can inhibit the effects of warfarin. Propranolol can interact with epinephrine by blocking the beta-adrenergic receptors and thus allowing the alpha-adrenergic effects of epinephrine to be unopposed, which can result in severe hypertension. Clonidine has been shown to have its antihypertensive effects in humans inhibited by tricyclic antidepressants. The mechanism for this is not entirely worked out but might be an interaction at an alpha-adrenergic receptor in the brain.

Additive effects of drugs are common. Additive negative cardiac inotropic effects of disopyramide, beta-adrenergic blockers, and calcium channel blocking drugs can produce heart failure. Similarly, the additive negative chronotropic and dromotropic effects of amiodarone, digoxin, beta-adrenergic blockers, and calcium channel blocking drugs can produce bradycardia, sinus arrest, or atrioventricular block. Two drugs that may affect the eighth cranial nerve, such as ethacrynic acid and aminoglycosides, may produce additional ototoxicity if given together. Drugs such as curare have an enhanced effect if given with aminoglycosides, lincomycin, clindamycin, quinidine, or quinine, which also affect neuromuscular function.

One drug may alter the normal homeostatic mechanisms, resulting in a change in the internal milieu and thereby enhancing or diminishing the effect of another drug. The best-studied example of this type of interaction is the effect of diuretics to produce hypokalemia, which enhances the toxicity of cardiac glycosides.

Some drug interactions have not been well characterized, although the interaction is clearly significant. This is true for the interaction of warfarin with clofibrate. Clofibrate has a marked effect to increase the efficacy of warfarin, but sufficient pharmacokinetic changes to account for this effect do not occur even though clofibrate may displace warfarin from plasma protein.

When viewed in perspective, drug interactions are only one of many factors that can alter the response of patients to drugs. Clinicians must be aware of the serious interactions and have well-defined therapeutic goals so that altered amounts or effects of drugs become evident. The only way to accomplish this is to individualize therapy using effects or plasma drug levels when appropriate, particularly for drugs with low therapeutic indices or during treatment of serious illnesses. Care must be used when a drug regimen is changed in any major way. If an interaction is appreciated, dosage adjustments can be made, and the two drugs often can be used together effectively. Drug interactions are an accepted fact of modern medical practice and should not be ignored, nor should they be overly feared.

Hansten PD, Horn JR: Drug Interactions. 6th ed. Philadelphia, Lea and Febiger, 1989. *This frequently revised text is a useful compilation of known drug interactions. The interactions listed are referenced, and an estimate of probable clinical significance of the interaction is given. The 6th edition is available in a loose-leaf format that can be updated periodically with inserts sent by the publisher.*

McInnes GT, Brodie MT: Drug interactions that matter. A critical reappraisal. Drugs 36:83, 1988. *There is no dearth of reviews on this topic trying to sort the clinically important from the unimportant drug interactions. This review is recent and well referenced.*

Shand DG, Mitchell JR, Oates JA: Pharmacokinetic drug interactions. In Gillette JR, Mitchell JR (eds.): Handbook of Experimental Pharmacology. Vol 28, No 3. Concepts in Biochemical Pharmacology. New York, Springer-Verlag, 1975, pp 272–314. *This is a thorough review of pharmacokinetic mechanisms whereby drugs can interact. It is not a complete listing of potential drug interactions, although many illustrative examples for the various mechanisms are given.*

25 Adverse Reactions to Drugs

Alan S. Nies

Although difficult to quantify, adverse reactions to drugs constitute an inevitable consequence of modern therapeutics. No drug is devoid of the potential to do harm, and benefit-versus-risk decisions are made with every decision to start drug therapy. Frequently it is difficult to be certain that an adverse effect is due to an individual drug because of the confounding effects of the underlying disease and the use of multiple drugs.

The overall incidence of significant adverse drug reactions is probably quite low, in the range of 1 to 5 per cent. Nevertheless, adverse drug reactions account for 2 to 10 per cent of admissions to hospital medical departments. An inpatient has a 10 to 20 per cent chance of experiencing a major adverse drug reaction, which is the most common iatrogenic illness in the hospital. Patients at highest risk are those who are receiving the most drugs and who have the most complicated illnesses. Drugs most commonly associated with serious adverse reactions include cardiovascular drugs (especially digitalis), steroidal and nonsteroidal anti-inflammatory drugs, diuretics, theophylline, anticoagulants, CNS active drugs, and antimicrobials.

Recent studies do not indicate that the incidence of adverse drug reactions is decreasing. On the contrary, the risk may be increasing as the number of potent drugs available increases. It is impossible to make a quantitative statement of risk versus benefit of medical therapy. Adverse reactions cannot be completely prevented even under the best of circumstances. Nonetheless, it is important to continue investigation into ways to assess the risk and to reduce both the incidence and severity of these adverse reactions.

MECHANISMS OF ADVERSE DRUG REACTIONS

Unwanted effects of drugs are due to (1) exaggerated responses to the known desired or unwanted pharmacologic effects of the drug; (2) immunologic reactions to the drug or its metabolites; and (3) toxic effects of a drug or its metabolites. "Idiosyncratic" effects may be due to any of these mechanisms. The extension of the normal pharmacology accounts for most adverse drug effects. However, since these effects are predictable, they often may be avoided or treated by careful dosage adjustment without necessarily discontinuing drug treatment. The immunologically mediated and toxic adverse effects of drugs are less predictable and may be so severe as to require discontinuation of the offending drug. These latter effects are the least well understood, but mechanisms of some of the toxic drug effects have been discovered. Any organ system can be affected by drugs, and drug-induced disease should be a consideration in the differential diagnosis of most syndromes that present to an internist.

EXAGGERATED RESPONSES TO DRUGS

Excessive drug effects result from altered pharmacokinetics or altered target-organ response, as discussed in the previous chapters. Thus adverse drug effects are more common in the elderly, in patients with abnormal renal or hepatic function, and in patients receiving other drugs that may result in pharmacokinetic or pharmacodynamic interactions.

An example of a disease exaggerating the unwanted effects of a normally innocuous drug is the reduction in glomerular filtration rate produced by nonsteroidal anti-inflammatory drugs in patients who have activation of their sympathetic nervous system and/or increased plasma renin activity as a result of hepatic, renal, or cardiovascular disease. This adverse effect is a consequence of the same pharmacologic action responsible for the salutary effects of the drug, namely, inhibition of cyclo-oxygenase activity with a reduction in prostaglandin synthesis.

In addition, patients may have genetic abnormalities that make them susceptible to one or another effect of a drug. These genetic differences may be quantitative deviations from the norm or qualitative abnormalities. An example of such quantitative differences is the variability in hepatic drug oxidation that is described by a unimodal frequency distribution. Twin studies have indicated that genetic differences account for much of the variation between individuals in the metabolism of phenytoin, phenylbutazone, warfarin, ethanol, nortriptyline, and salicylate. In addition, an increasing number of drug metabolic processes are now recognized to be controlled by genes at a single locus, such as slow acetylation of isoniazid, some sulfonamides, and procainamide; deficient parahydroxylation of phenytoin; deficient hydroxylation of debrisoquin, or mephenytoin; deficient N-glucosidation of amobarbital; and deficient hydrolysis of succinylcholine. The excessive drug effects resulting from the genetically determined slow metabolic processes reflect an increased concentration of unmetabolized drug available at the site of action.

In addition to these quantitative differences in drug metabolism, genetic abnormalities may result in qualitatively different responses to drugs. These reactions are due to known properties of the drug that are usually not important but become markedly exaggerated owing to the genetic defect. Thus individuals with a deficiency of the enzyme activity of glucose-6-phosphate dehydrogenase (G6PD) are unable to cope with the oxidative stress produced by some drugs, and hemolysis results. Drugs having this effect include primaquine, aspirin, sulfonamides, nitrofurantoin, sulfones, vitamin K, probenecid, quinidine, and quinine. In a similar manner, genetic deficiency of methemoglobin reductase results in inability to maintain hemoglobin in the ferrous form, resulting in methemoglobinemia upon exposure to some oxidizing drugs such as sulfones, sulfonamides, and nitrites. Likewise certain genetically abnormal hemoglobins may be unstable and result in drug-induced hemolysis or methemoglobinemia. Frequently patients with these "pharmacogenetic" syndromes are unaware of any abnormality until they are challenged with a drug that produces the adverse effect.

TOXIC AND IMMUNOLOGIC REACTIONS

Adverse drug reactions in these categories are often lumped together because it is frequently difficult to be certain of the etiology of an individual reaction (Table 25–1). Toxic reactions include direct effects of a drug on a target organ, such as the nephrotoxicity and ototoxicity produced by aminoglycosides. In other cases drugs are metabolized to reactive intermediates that can covalently bind to cellular components, often near the site of metabolism, and produce toxicity. This mechanism is well established for the hepatotoxicity produced by overdoses of acetaminophen. During therapeutic use of acetaminophen the small amount of reactive metabolite formed by oxidative metabolism is rapidly detoxified by interacting with reduced glutathione. With overdose, however, glutathione is depleted, and the reactive metabolite attacks hepatic macromolecules, resulting in liver damage. Sulfhydryl-containing compounds such as N-acetylcysteine or cysteamine can protect the liver by reducing the amount of toxic metabolite that remains unreacted with a sulfhydryl-containing compound. Other drugs may produce liver disease by somewhat similar mechanisms. Isoniazid-induced hepatitis may result from acetylation to acetylisoniazid that can be hydrolyzed to acetylhydrazine, which can be oxidized by the hepatic mixed function oxidase system to a reactive metabolite. One might expect from this theory that individuals who rapidly acetylate isoniazid would be more susceptible to the hepatotoxicity. However, the opposite may be true. This apparent discrepancy may be related to observations that rapid acetylators not only form acetylisoniazid rapidly but also quickly convert this metabolite to diacetylisoniazid, which is nontoxic. Slow acetylators, on the other hand, form acetylisoniazid gradually but are much less able to convert it to diacetylisoniazid. Consequently, more of the acetylisoniazid is available for hydrolysis to acetylhydrazine and subsequent oxidation to the reactive metabolite. However, considerable controversy remains regarding the relevance of this theory to the clinical hepatitis that results from isoniazid, and other factors, such as the patient's age, are also important.

Hepatocellular damage, such as that produced by methyldopa or halothane, is frequently considered to be immunologically produced. However, reactive metabolites could be important for these as well as a variety of other drugs that produce hepatotoxicity on occasion.

Immunologic reactions to drugs account for only 5 to 10 per cent of all adverse drug reactions and probably result from the

TABLE 25–1. "ALLERGIC" DRUG REACTIONS

Type of Reaction	Example (not inclusive)
Definite Immunologically Mediated Syndromes	
1. Immediate hypersensitivity (IgE-mediated) reactions	Penicillin-induced anaphylaxis Insulin-induced wheal and flare
2. Cytotoxic reactions	Drug-induced destruction of formed elements in the blood: Penicillin-induced hemolytic anemia Quinidine- or quinine-induced thrombocytopenia Phenylbutazone-induced granulocytopenia
3. Immune complex–induced vasculitis	Serum sickness–like reactions to penicillin, sulfonamides, and other drugs presenting as fever, rash, palpable purpura, arthralgia, and/or lymphadenopathy
4. Delayed hypersensitivity reactions	Contact dermatitis from topically applied drugs
Possible Immunologically Mediated Syndromes but with Unknown Mechanism	
1. Skin rashes of various types	Many drugs and a variety of skin eruptions
2. Stevens-Johnson syndrome	Sulfonamides, penicillins, phenytoin, phenylbutazone
3. Fever	Antibiotics, quinidine, methyldopa, procainamide, phenytoin, antineoplastic drugs
4. Pneumonitis	Löffler's syndrome
5. Lupus erythematosus–like condition	Procainamide, hydralazine, isoniazid
6. Hepatic dysfunction	Chlorpromazine-induced cholestasis ? Methyldopa-induced hepatitis ? Halothane-induced hepatitis
7. Renal dysfunction	Interstitial nephritis from methicillin, furosemide, allopurinol
8. Lymphadenopathy	Phenytoin, sulfonamides

drug or a reactive metabolite combining with a protein to form an antigenic drug-protein complex that stimulates the immune response. Without such a reaction, most drugs, which have a molecular weight less than 1000, would not be able to elicit an immunologic response. The typical immunologic reaction requires a latent period of 10 to 20 days for stimulation of the production of antibodies and activated immune effector cells that cause the allergic reaction. After the initial exposure, however, the allergic reaction occurs with a much shorter or no latent period after re-exposure to the drug. Drug hypersensitivity can produce mediator release, initiate cell lysis, activate the complement system, or activate cellular hypersensitivity reactions.

The most dramatic allergic reaction is anaphylaxis, or IgE-mediated hypersensitivity. Penicillin is the most common drug to produce anaphylaxis, but many other drugs or diagnostic agents (such as Bromsulphalein) can produce this life-threatening reaction. Although oral therapy is least sensitizing, once sensitization has occurred, anaphylaxis may occur with any route of administration. A history of penicillin allergy increases the risk of this reaction occurring, but most (75 per cent) of the 100 to 300 patients dying of penicillin-induced anaphylaxis each year have no history of penicillin allergy. Skin testing with penicilloyl-polylysine, penicillin G, and penicilloic acid is the best method to identify patients at risk for anaphylaxis and should be used if penicillin therapy is considered mandatory in a patient with a history of penicillin allergy. Patients with a negative skin test can be given penicillin therapy cautiously. Patients with a positive skin test should be desensitized prior to receiving penicillin

therapy. Unfortunately, a negative assay in vitro to detect penicilloyl-specific IgE is less specific than skin testing to rule out the possibility of penicillin anaphylaxis, but a positive test in vitro has the same implications as a positive skin test.

Cytotoxic allergic reactions occur when a drug binds to the surface of a cell and is then attacked by antibody. Penicillin-induced hemolytic anemia is of this type. Immune complexes of drug and antibody may become adsorbed to the cell membrane, resulting in complement-mediated cytotoxicity. Thrombocytopenia and hemolytic anemia due to quinine or quinidine are examples of immune complex–mediated cytotoxicity. Methyldopa-induced Coombs' positivity occurs in up to 20 per cent of patients on therapy for over 6 months and results in antibodies directed at the Rh loci of the red cell. However, the continued presence of methyldopa is not necessary for the immune reaction to continue, and the Coombs' positivity only gradually resolves upon discontinuation of the drug.

Circulating immune complexes of drug and antibody can produce serum sickness (see Ch. 245 and 256), a vasculitic syndrome produced by deposition of immune complexes. Penicillin, sulfonamides, thiouracil, cholecystographic dyes, phenytoin, and other drugs can cause serum sickness.

Drug-induced lupus syndromes as caused by procainamide, hydralazine, and isoniazid may be associated with circulating immune complexes. In this case the drug or a reactive metabolite may interact with nuclear material to allow formation of antinuclear antibodies. The drug-induced systemic lupus erythematosus (SLE) (see Ch. 261) differs from spontaneous lupus by being uncommon in blacks and by only rarely causing nephritis. The acetylator phenotype also is important in drug-induced lupus. Hydralazine-induced lupus is very uncommon in fast acetylators. Procainamide-induced lupus occurs with smaller cumulative doses of drug in slow acetylators, although fast acetylators are also at risk.

In addition to the immune phenomena outlined above, many other syndromes are attributed to drug allergy (Table 25–1). These include a variety of skin rashes, drug fever, pulmonary reactions, hepatocellular or cholestatic reactions, interstitial nephritis, and lymphadenopathy. For most of these reactions, the exact immune mechanism is unknown. One interesting syndrome that is sometimes classified as immune but may involve other mechanisms as well is that of aspirin sensitivity. In some patients this syndrome resembles IgE-mediated allergy with rhinitis, sinusitis, nasal polyps, and asthma. However, other cyclo-oxygenase inhibitors, such as indomethacin and meclofenamate, also produce asthma in many of these patients, suggesting a possible etiologic role for an arachidonic acid metabolite, such as a leukotriene, rather than an immunologic mechanism. It seems likely that several syndromes of aspirin sensitivity exist.

Some adverse drug reactions mimic anaphylactic reactions but are not immune mediated. Such reactions are due to direct release of mediators by drugs and are called anaphylactoid reactions. Reactions to radiocontrast dyes are of this type. The risk of re-exposure to the dye is unpredictable and skin testing is of no value. If re-exposure is absolutely necessary, pretreatment with steroids and H_1-antihistamines is the current practice. Since the newer, low-osmolality radiocontrast media appear to produce fewer anaphylactoid reactions, their use is preferable in patients who give a history of reaction to the older agents.

RECOGNITION AND IDENTIFICATION

Adverse drug effects must first be suspected to be recognized. In some situations, the adverse effect mimics the illness being treated (for instance, arrhythmias caused by antiarrhythmic drugs or antibiotic-induced fever). In other instances, the reaction is more obviously drug induced, as is the case with characteristic skin rashes or anticoagulant-induced bleeding. The first confirmation of an adverse reaction is its disappearance with drug withdrawal. In some cases cautious readministration of the putative offending drug may be warranted if the drug is likely to be required again for therapy. In the case of serious allergic or toxic reactions, however, this may be too dangerous. Tests in vitro are occasionally helpful for drug-induced thrombocytopenia or hemolytic anemia but are not useful for most drug reactions. Skin testing is of value with penicillin, insulin, and horse serum.

Adverse reactions will continue to occur as long as potent drugs are available. Most of the reactions are predictable. The unexpected toxic and immunologic reactions remain a problem that continues to stimulate discussions as to how to detect rare adverse effects. During the process of drug development, reactions occurring less often than 1 per 1000 patients are not detected. In addition, drugs are developed by testing in patients who have well-defined diseases, are not on many other drugs, are not pregnant, and are usually neither in the pediatric nor the geriatric population. After approval, however, all patient populations may be exposed to the drug. Therefore, the adverse effects of a new drug frequently are not discovered until after marketing. Different systems exist for early detection of drug reactions after marketing. A major mechanism is an early warning that results from anecdotal reports by practicing physicians to pharmaceutical companies or drug regulatory agencies or letters published in general medical journals. Following the first alerts, a verification mechanism is required. It is in this area that much remains to be learned. Postmarketing surveillance of patients taking drugs will not be effective for uncommon drug reactions unless sample sizes of more than 100,000 patients are followed. Surveys of patients with certain diseases to determine the incidence of use of the drug suspected to have caused the illness (case-control study) may be a more efficient way to detect drug-induced illness for rare adverse effects. A controversial but promising and potentially powerful new method for detecting or verifying adverse events after drug marketing is the technique of automated record linkage, whereby computerized data bases are used to link prescription records with the medical records of individual patients. However, the alert practitioner has been and will continue to be the primary individual who makes the initial important observation that often provides the first clue to an unsuspected adverse drug reaction.

Anderson J, Adkinson NF Jr: Allergic reactions to drugs and biologic agents. JAMA 258:2891, 1987. *Part of the "primer on allergic and immunologic diseases," this short review outlines the mechanisms of immunologic reactions to drugs. The authors provide relevant references and distinguish between allergic reactions for which the immune mechanisms are established and those that are only conjectured to be immunologically mediated.*

Davies DM (ed.): Textbook of Adverse Drug Reactions. 3rd ed. Oxford, Oxford University Press, 1985. *This well-referenced book is organized by specific syndromes, with a discussion of the drugs that may cause the syndrome. General problems of detecting and verifying adverse reactions are also discussed.*

Edlavitch SA: Adverse drug event reporting. Improving the low US reporting rates. Arch Intern Med 148:1499, 1988. *This editorial discusses the importance of spontaneous reports of drug reactions by physicians in providing an early warning of previously unsuspected drug risks. It accompanies a study indicating that nearly half of the physicians in the United States are unaware of the existence of the FDA reporting system for adverse drug events, and those that are aware report only a low percentage of such events. Suggestions for improving the system are discussed.*

Lewis JH, Zimmerman HJ: Drug-induced liver disease. Med Clin North Am 73:775, 1989. *This is an update discussing the spectrum, pathology, and possible mechanisms of drug-induced liver disease and serves as an entry to the extensive literature on this important adverse drug effect.*

Steel K, Gertman PM, Crescenzi C, et al.: Iatrogenic illness on a general medical service at a university hospital. N Engl J Med 304:638, 1981. *This study of a medical service indicates a 36 per cent incidence of iatrogenic illness, of which 42 per cent were drug related.*

26 Pain and Its Management

Kathleen M. Foley

INTRODUCTION

Pain is the most common symptom for which patients seek medical assistance. To manage pain, the physician must understand its nature—the relationship between its medical, psychologic, and social aspects—and must establish a relationship of mutual trust with the patient. The physician's therapeutic task is twofold: to discover and treat the cause of the pain and to treat the pain itself, whether or not the underlying cause is treatable. Advances in knowledge of the physiology, pharmacology, and psychology of pain perception have led to improved care of patients with both acute and chronic pain (see also Ch. 455), but a lack of generally agreed-upon definitions and classification of pain has hampered communication among physicians. To provide a more common ground for the evaluation and treatment of patients with pain, the International Association for the Study of Pain (IASP) has proposed a working definition: Pain is "an unpleasant sensory and emotional experience associated with either actual or potential tissue damage, or described in terms of such damage." The IASP has also developed a taxonomy of pain syndromes that serves as a universal classification of pain syndromes (see references).

TYPES OF PAIN

Clinically, pain can be classified *temporally* as acute or chronic, *physiologically* as somatic, visceral, or neuropathic, and *etiologically* as medical or psychogenic.

TEMPORAL CHARACTERISTICS. Patients with severe *acute pain* can usually give a clear description of its location, character, and timing. Furthermore, objective signs, particularly of autonomic nervous system hyperactivity, with tachycardia, hypertension, diaphoresis, mydriasis, and pallor are present. The pain is usually self-limited (e.g., postoperative pain, acute traumatic pain). The patient's ability to tolerate acute pain is influenced by the setting of the pain, its duration, and its psychologic significance. Treatment of both the cause of acute pain and the pain itself is usually possible. Pain lasting longer than 3 months is usually considered *chronic*. In patients with chronic pain, the localization, character, and timing of the pain are often more vague, and because the autonomic nervous system adapts, signs of autonomic hyperactivity disappear. Significant changes occur in the psychologic, social, and functional status of patients with chronic pain, often requiring a multidisciplinary approach to treatment, including pharmacologic, behavioral, and rehabilitative therapeutic approaches.

PHYSIOLOGIC CHARACTERISTICS. *Somatic pain* results from activation of peripheral receptors and somatic efferent nerves, without injury to the peripheral nerves or central nervous system. The pain can be either sharp or dull but is typically well localized and intermittent. *Visceral pain* results from activation of visceral nociceptive receptors and visceral efferent nerves and is characterized as a deep aching, cramping sensation, often referred to cutaneous sites. *Neuropathic pain* results from direct injury to peripheral receptors, nerves, or central nervous system. It is typically burning and dysesthetic and often occurs in an area of sensory loss (e.g., postherpetic neuralgia). The autonomic nervous system plays a significant modulatory role in all three types of pain but is most prominent in visceral and neuropathic pain. The somatic and visceral types of pain are readily managed with a wide variety of nonopioid or opioid analgesics, anesthetic blocks, and neurosurgical approaches. In contrast, neuropathic pain has a variable response to nonopioid and opioid analgesics and to anesthetic and neurosurgical procedures.

ETIOLOGIC CHARACTERISTICS. Patients with chronic pain can generally be classified into one of three major etiologic groups, allowing for some overlap. The first group includes patients with chronic pain associated with *structural disease*. Such pain occurs, for example, with rheumatoid arthritis, metastatic cancer, and sickle cell anemia and is usually characterized by prolonged episodes of pain alternating with pain-free intervals or by unremitting pain waxing and waning in severity. Successful treatment of the pain is closely allied with treatment of the disease, but in certain instances treatment of the pain is the only therapeutic goal, e.g., the dying cancer patient with pain. Psychological factors may play an important role in exacerbating or relieving pain, but analgesic drug therapy is the mainstay of therapy while attempting to treat the underlying disease.

The second group comprises patients who suffer from *psychophysiologic disorders* causing pain. In these patients, structural disease such as a herniated disc or torn ligaments may once have been present but psychological factors have caused chronic physiologic alterations, such as muscle spasm, which produce pain long after the underlying defect has healed. Typically, such patients are physically inactive and spend much of their time thinking and talking about their pain, often leading to social and emotional isolation. Patients are more impaired by their "chronic illness behavior" than by a defined pathologic condition. They usually respond poorly to analgesic drugs and often suffer from iatrogenic complications, such as adverse drug reactions and ineffective surgical procedures. They use health care resources excessively. Successful treatment can be expected only through a structured rehabilitation program designed to modify pain behaviors and not through medical intervention designed to correct pathologic conditions. Multidisciplinary pain clinics that diagnose and treat intractable pain exist in many centers and should be utilized to evaluate and treat such patients.

Patients of the third group complain of pain that appears to have neither a structural nor a physiologic basis. These patients probably suffer from *somatic delusions*. Such patients usually have serious psychiatric disorders, and the history of the pain is so vague and bizarre and its distribution so unanatomic as to suggest the diagnosis. These patients respond only to psychiatric therapy.

ASSESSMENT OF PAIN

No objective tests (except observing patient behavior) assess the severity of pain or even its presence. Therefore, the physician must accept the patient's report, taking into consideration his or her age, cultural background, environment, and psychological circumstances known to alter reaction to pain.

A thorough history, general physical examination, and careful neurologic examination are imperative in any patient complaining of pain. The description of the nature and distribution of the pain may be so characteristic (e.g., trigeminal neuralgia or tabetic lightning pains) that it allows no other diagnosis. Inquiry should be made concerning (1) the temporal pattern of pain, (2) its distribution, (3) exacerbating factors, (4) relieving factors, and (5) its meaning to the patient. For example, headache beginning early in the morning before arising suggests increased intracranial pressure, whereas headache occurring late in the day is more suggestive of tension. Back pain and sciatica made worse by sitting or walking suggest disc disease, whereas back pain and sciatica that are worse while the person is in bed indicate intraspinal tumor. All pain is relieved to some extent by distraction and a pleasurable environment and is exacerbated by anxiety or psychological stress. Postoperative pain has positive meaning for the patient undergoing hip replacement but negative meaning for the patient who has been diagnosed with metastatic bone disease to the hip. Clarifying the patient's concept of what the pain implies can improve the physician's understanding of the psychological factors associated with the pain.

A careful psychiatric history, looking particularly for signs and symptoms of depression, should be elicited from all patients. The distinction between pain and suffering should be made by both the physician and the patient. Specifically, physicians should inquire about the degree to which pain has interfered with the patient's activities, whether he or she is having difficulty sleeping, and whether there is a change in appetite or bowel habits. Early morning awakening, anorexia, and constipation are somatic manifestations of depression and may either be caused by chronic pain or exacerbate the effects of the pain. Patients should be questioned about suicidal thoughts associated with the severity and chronicity of the pain.

A general physical examination must be performed. Both the physical and the laboratory examination should begin with the assumption that the site of pathologic change is at the site of pain. The painful areas should be examined for swelling and redness as well as for any obvious deformity. (The pain of herpes zoster usually precedes the rash, and occasionally on examination one may note the faintest reddening of the skin in a dermatomal distribution.) The areas reported as painful should be palpated, the temperature estimated, and points of tenderness sought. (If the site of pain is in a soft tissue, bone, or joint, it should be tender to palpation as well as spontaneously painful.) Joints should be taken through a full range of motion, and the effect of movement on the pain assessed. Nerve trunks going to the extremities should be palpated and stretched by movement of that member (e.g., straight-leg raising, abduction and extension of the arm). Inflamed and compressed nerve roots and nerve plexuses are more painful when stretched. A careful neurologic examination must also be performed. If there are neurologic abnormalities (e.g., weakness, sensory loss, and reflex changes) in the painful part, one can infer that nervous system disease is responsible for the pain. However, the absence of neurologic abnormalities on first examination does not guarantee that the nervous system is free of disease, because the process may simply not have advanced beyond the stage of selectively involving pain pathways. For example, a Pancoast's tumor may cause shoulder and arm pain before other signs of neural involvement, such as Horner's syndrome or motor or sensory loss, appear.

Finally, laboratory examinations are performed. If the site of disease appears to be in bones or joints, radiographs, computed tomography (CT) scans, magnetic resonance imaging (MRI), or radioisotope scans may localize it. First attention should be paid to the local site of pain, but the physician should be familiar with the common referred patterns of pain (e.g., hip disease commonly causes knee pain, cardiac pain is frequently referred to the ulnar aspect of the arm and forearm, the pain of renal colic may be felt primarily in the groin and testicle, and pain resulting from disease of the throat may be referred to the ear).

Referred pain is pain perceived at a site remote from the source of the disturbance. Usually, referred pain is perceived as cutaneous and is evoked by disease of deep structures innervated by the same dermatome. Referred pain may be associated with cutaneous hyperalgesia and even relieved by procaine injection into the area of referral. When pain is referred to the same dermatome or myotome that innervates the diseased structure (e.g., pain down the medial aspect of the arm [T1-T2] produced by myocardial infarction or angina pectoris), it is often helpful in diagnosis. However, pain is sometimes referred a great distance from the primary site to segments not similarly innervated, and in such cases the mechanism is perplexing (e.g., anginal pain referred to the jaw). Various theories, such as division of the same nerve into deep and superficial branches, release of chemical mediators into the nervous system, and convergence of cutaneous and visceral nerves into a common synaptic pool at the spinal cord, all explain the dermatomal referral of pain but fail to explain pain at remote sites.

MANAGEMENT OF PAIN

Recent advances in pain research provide a scientific rationale that has improved treatment. These include better and more effective use of standard drug therapy (non-narcotic, narcotic, and adjuvant analgesic drugs), the development of new drugs and the use of novel routes of drug administration, more selective anesthetic and neurosurgical approaches, and the integration of behavioral approaches to pain control.

General Principles (Table 26–1)

1. Pain is best managed by treating the underlying disorder (e.g., steroids for giant cell arteritis relieve headache; radiation therapy for bone pain caused by cancer is often helpful), but in many patients the pain is chronic and the physician is able neither to treat the underlying disturbances nor to offer specific therapy for that type of pain.

2. Pain should be treated early and promptly. The persistence of untreated pain results in significant psychological morbidity, most commonly anxiety and depression with a sense of loss of control and hopelessness. Early treatment that provides prompt and continuous pain relief is crucial to prevent further compromise of the patient's emotional resources.

3. Multiple therapeutic approaches, often delivered simultaneously, should be utilized because different treatment modalities may be additive or synergistic when used together rather than separately. For example, combinations of narcotic and non-narcotic analgesics provide greater analgesia than either alone. Nonpharmacologic methods, such as relaxation techniques and cognitive coping skills, coupled with physical therapy and vocational rehabilitation, can often help in selected patients with chronic pain, especially when added to judicious drug therapy.

4. Narcotic drugs should be used with discrimination, but they should not be withheld if alternative therapy is ineffective. Long-term use of narcotics produces tolerance and physical dependence. Tolerance is the term used to describe increasing dose requirements to maintain analgesia. *Physical dependence* means

TABLE 26–1. GUIDELINES FOR THE USE OF ANALGESICS IN PAIN MANAGEMENT

1. Tailor drugs to nature and severity of pain
2. Know the pharmacology of the drug prescribed
   a. Know the duration of the analgesic effect
   b. Know the pharmacokinetic properties of the drug (duration of action and half-life)
   c. Know the equianalgesic doses for the drug and its route of administration (Table 26–2)
3. Adjust the route of administration to the patient's needs using oral, rectal, subcutaneous, intramuscular, intravenous, epidural, and intrathecal routes
4. Administer the analgesic on a regular basis after initial titration of the dose
5. Use drug combinations to provide additive analgesia and reduce side effects, e.g., nonsteroidal anti-inflammatory drugs, antihistamine (hydroxyzine), amphetamine (dextroamphetamine)
6. Avoid drug combinations that increase sedation without enhancing analgesia, e.g., benzodiazepine (diazepam) and phenothiazine
7. For narcotics, anticipate and treat side effects
   a. Sedation
   b. Respiratory depression
   c. Nausea and vomiting
   d. Constipation
   e. Multifocal myoclonus and seizures
8. When using narcotics, watch for the development of tolerance
   a. Switch to an alternate narcotic analgesic
   b. Start with one half of the equianalgesic dose and titrate to pain relief
   c. Use adjuvant analgesics and anesthetic and neurosurgical approaches
9. Prevent acute withdrawal
   a. Taper drugs slowly
   b. Use diluted doses of naloxone (0.4 mg in 10 ml of saline) to reverse narcotic-induced respiratory depression in the physically dependent patient and administer cautiously
10. Do not use placebos to assess pain

that the signs and symptoms of withdrawal appear if the narcotic drug is abruptly discontinued. These effects should not be confused with psychological dependence or *"addiction,"* which implies both a craving for the drug for effects other than analgesia and drug abuse behavior. The percentage of patients who actually become psychologically dependent on narcotics when they are given to treat medical illness is unknown, but recent data suggest that psychological dependence is unusual in patients treated for pain when the pain is later relieved by other means.

5. Psychological factors play a major role in chronic pain and must be carefully assessed. However, no patient should be diagnosed as having "psychogenic" pain until an exhaustive examination has ruled out structural disease. Depression should be identified and treated, and since the tricyclic antidepressants have analgesic properties as well, they are useful adjuvant analgesic drugs, particularly in patients with neuropathic pain.

6. Placebo effects are important. A positive analgesic response from intramuscular saline indicates only that the patient is a placebo responder. It does not suggest that the pain is unreal or less severe than reported by the patient. Misuse of placebo creates distrust between the patient and the physician and interferes with adequate pain assessment and management. In most clinical studies, up to one third of patients report relief of pain when given a placebo.

Drug Therapy

Analgesic drugs can be divided into three groups: Group I—the non-narcotic analgesics, such as aspirin and acetaminophen and the nonsteroidal anti-inflammatory drugs (NSAID's), act peripherally, probably on pain receptors; Group II—the narcotic agonist and antagonist drugs activate opiate receptors in the central and peripheral nervous systems; and Group III—the adjuvant analgesic drugs are designed for management of symptoms other than pain but produce relief in certain pain states (carbamazepine for trigeminal neuralgia) or potentiate narcotic analgesics. These three groups represent the mainstay of therapy for patients with acute and chronic pain. Effective use of these drugs requires an understanding of their pharmacologic characteristics and selection of a particular drug and dose geared to the needs of the individual patient.

NON-NARCOTIC ANALGESICS (Table 26–2). Aspirin, acetaminophen, and the NSAID's are the first-line agents for the management of mild to moderate pain, and in patients with severe pain these drugs potentiate the effects of narcotic analgesics. Non-narcotic analgesics have a ceiling effect, and their long-term use is limited by gastrointestinal and hematologic side effects. The choice and use of these drugs must be individualized, with the patient receiving maximal levels of one drug before another is tried. If pain control is ineffective or the non-narcotic agents are poorly tolerated, the use of narcotic analgesics is indicated. In general, the use of narcotics is limited to acute structural or chronic, irreversible structural pain, as in cancer.

NARCOTIC ANALGESICS (Table 26–3). The narcotic analgesics vary in potency, efficacy, and adverse effects. They are classified as agonist or antagonist drugs, depending on their ability to bind to the opiate receptors and produce analgesia. The narcotic *agonist* drugs, such as morphine, bind to specific opiate receptors, resulting in analgesia. These agents are commonly used in the management of chronic pain of structural cause, such as cancer pain. The narcotic *antagonist* drugs block the effect of morphine at its receptor. Included in this category is a group of drugs with analgesic properties referred to as the mixed agonist-antagonist drugs. These drugs are often used in acute postoperative pain management but are of limited use in chronic pain management for several reasons: They produce psychotomimetic effects with increasing doses; only pentazocine is available in oral form and only in combinations with naloxone, aspirin, or acetaminophen; they precipitate withdrawal in narcotic-dependent patients. Effective use of narcotic analgesics requires balancing of the desirable effect of pain relief with the undesirable side effects of nausea, vomiting, mental clouding, sedation, tolerance, and physical dependence. These undesirable effects impose a practical limit on the dose one can give a particular patient.

Much of the difficulty encountered with the clinical use of narcotics arises from individual variation, consisting of differences in response of specific patients to the same drug dose. Thus, although Tables 26–2 to 26–4 can serve as reference points, individualization of drug treatment is the cardinal rule of management. Drugs should be given in sufficient amounts and at close enough intervals to achieve adequate pain relief. "Weak"

TABLE 26–2. ORAL NON-NARCOTIC ANALGESIC DRUGS

Drug	Indications	Equianalgesic Dose	Starting Dose (mg), Range/24 hr	Comments
Aspirin	Often used in combination with narcotics	650	650	Contraindicated in hepatic and renal dysfunction; avoid during pregnancy, in hemolytic disorders, and in combination with steroids
Acetaminophen	Like aspirin	650	650	
Ibuprofen	Higher analgesic potential than aspirin	ND	200–400	Like aspirin
Fenoprofen	Like ibuprofen	ND	200–400	Like aspirin
Diflunisal	Longer duration of action than ibuprofen; higher analgesic potential than aspirin	ND	500–1000	Like aspirin
Naproxen	Like diflunisal	ND	250–500	Like aspirin

ND = not documented.

narcotics, such as codeine, propoxyphene, and oxycodone, are selected to treat moderate pain. If the pain remains unrelieved, the "strong" narcotic analgesics, such as morphine, hydromorphone, levorphanol, and methadone, should be employed. To ensure adequate dosing schedules, one must know the clinical pharmacology of the narcotic analgesics, including their duration of analgesic effect, their half-lives, and the equianalgesic doses for both oral and parenteral routes of administration. For example, the plasma half-lives of the narcotics vary widely and do not correlate with their analgesic time courses. Both methadone, with a half-life of 15 to 30 hours, and levorphanol, with a half-life of 12 to 16 hours, produce analgesia for only 4 to 6 hours. With repeated doses, these drugs accumulate in plasma and can result in excessive sedation and respiratory depression. It is necessary to adjust the dose and schedule, considering both the patient's degree of pain relief and the plasma half-life of the drug when it is introduced.

Knowledge of the equianalgesic doses when a switch is made from one medication to another or from one route of administration to another prevents undermedication. However, cross-tolerance is not complete, and patients tolerant to the analgesic effects of one narcotic can often be given another to provide better analgesia. The usual rule is to begin with one half of the calculated equianalgesic dose of the new drug and increase as required.

Medication should be administered on a regular basis, with the interval between doses based on the duration of the analgesic effect. The pharmacologic objective is to maintain the plasma level of the drug above the "minimal effective concentration for pain relief." The time required to reach steady state after repeated administration depends on the half-life of the drug; full assessment of the analgesic efficacy of a drug regimen may take 24 hours for a drug such as morphine or up to 5 to 7 days for methadone.

Combinations of drugs enable the physician to improve pain relief without escalation of the narcotic dose. Several combinations have been proven effective, including a narcotic plus a non-narcotic (aspirin, acetaminophen, or ibuprofen), a narcotic plus an amphetamine (dextroamphetamine, 10 mg), and a narcotic plus an antihistamine (100 mg of hydroxyzine given intramuscularly). Other drugs such as diazepam and chlorpromazine do not provide additive analgesia and may produce additive sedative effects.

Oral administration of drugs is the most practical route, but the choice must be made according to the needs of the patient. Several alternate methods of drug administration have been developed to maximize pharmacologic effects and minimize the undesirable effects associated with standard methods. The approaches that are most useful in the management of acute or chronic pain with chronic medical illness include slow-release morphine preparations effective for 8 to 12 hours, enabling a full night's rest; continuous subcutaneous and intravenous infusions for patients who are unable to tolerate oral analgesics because of gastrointestinal obstruction or malabsorption and in whom repeated parenteral dosing is difficult because of limited muscle mass or a bleeding diathesis; and epidural and intrathecal narcotic administration via temporary catheters or implanted pumps. This last approach minimizes the distribution of drugs to receptors in the brain stem and cerebral hemispheres, avoids the side effects of systemic administration, and is effective in selected patients with cancer pain who are unable to tolerate the excessive sedation or mental clouding associated with an oral or parenteral route.

Patient-controlled analgesia (PCA) has developed as a useful approach to treat both acute postoperative and chronic cancer-related pain. Parenteral infusion (intravenous or subcutaneous) of opioids can be self-administered by the patient using specially designed computerized pumps that can be set to deliver specific amounts of drugs on demand or by continuous infusions. These devices allow patients control in their own pain management. Studies demonstrate that patients using PCA use less medication than patients who must relay on standard postoperative or chronic pain management approaches.

Side Effects of Narcotics. Side effects of the narcotic analgesics should be anticipated and treated. *Sedation and drowsiness* vary with the drug dose and may occur after either single or repeated

TABLE 26–3. NARCOTIC ANALGESIC DRUGS

Class	Drug	Indications	IM/PO Equianalgesic Dose (mg)*	Starting Dose (mg) Range/24 hr	Comments
Morphine-like agonist, mild to moderate pain	Codeine	Often used in combination with non-narcotic analgesics	32/65	32–65	Commonly used as first drug
	Oxycodone	Shorter acting; combination with non-narcotic analgesics limits dose escalation	5/30	5–10	Fewer side effects than codeine, available alone
	Meperidine	Shorter acting; biotransformed to normeperidine, a toxic metabolite	75/300	50–100	Normeperidine accumulates with repetitive dosing, causing CNS excitation; not for use in patients with renal dysfunction or receiving monoamine oxidase inhibitors
	Proproxyphene hydrochloride (Darvon)	Used in combination with non-narcotic analgesics; long half-life; biotransformed to potentially toxic metabolite (norproproxyphene)	65 PO	65–130	Proproxyphene and metabolite accumulate with repetitive dosing; overdose complicated by convulsions
Mixed-agonist antagonist	Pentazocine	In combination with non-narcotics, in combination with naloxone to discourage parenteral abuse	50 IM	50–100	May cause psychotomimetic effects; may precipitate withdrawal in narcotic-dependent patients
Morphine-like agonists, moderate to severe pain	Morphine	Used for chronic cancer pain, available in oral liquid and tablets and slow-release preparations	10/60	30–60	Standard of comparison for narcotic-type analgesics; morphine-6-glucuronide, active metabolite, accumulates in renal failure
	Hydromorphone (Dilaudid)	Like morphine	1.5/8.0	4–8	Slightly shorter acting, high-potency IM dosage form available for tolerant patients
	Methadone (Dolphine)	Like morphine; may accumulate with repetitive dosing, causing excessive sedation	10/20	10–20	Good oral potency; long plasma half-life
	Levorphanol (Levo-Dromoran)	Like methadone	2/4	2–4	Like methadone

*Dose given intramuscularly or by mouth.
IM = intramuscular; CNS = central nervous system.
Equianalgesic doses are based on single-dose controlled analgesic studies.

administration. Reducing the individual dose and prescribing it more frequently, switching to a drug with a short plasma half-life (hydromorphone), using an amphetamine (dextroamphetamine, 2 to 5 mg) in combination with the narcotic twice daily, and discontinuing all other sedative drugs are useful approaches to counteract the sedative effects.

Respiratory depression is the most serious adverse effect, but tolerance develops rapidly, allowing prolonged use of narcotics for chronic pain. If respiratory depression occurs, it can be reversed by administering the specific narcotic antagonist naloxone in a dose of 0.4 mg per milliliter. In patients who receive narcotics for prolonged periods and develop respiratory depression, diluted doses of naloxone (0.4 mg in 10 ml of saline) should be infused slowly to reverse the respiratory depression but prevent precipitation of severe withdrawal symptoms. The occurrence of *nausea and vomiting* with one drug does not mean that all narcotics will produce similar symptoms. Changing to an alternate narcotic or using an antiemetic in combination commonly obviates this effect. Tolerance rapidly develops to the emetic effect of narcotics so that after a few days antiemetics often are unnecessary. *Constipation* should be prevented by the provision of a regular bowel regimen, including cathartics, stool softeners, and careful attention to diet. *Multifocal myoclonus* may occur with toxic doses of any narcotic. The most common offender is meperidine because of the accumulation of the active metabolite normeperidine, which can cause seizures. Since the half-life of normeperidine is 16 hours, it may take several days for toxic side effects to clear. Patients should be switched to morphine to control their pain and managed symptomatically for seizures.

Tolerance is common when patients receive narcotic analgesics chronically for pain. The earliest sign is a decrease in the duration of effective analgesia. Increasing the frequency of drug administration of the dose provides improved pain relief. There is no limit to tolerance, and the dose of drug should not be the major concern of the prescribing physician. Adjuvant drugs and anesthetic and neurosurgical methods sometimes help to manage pain in the tolerant patient. These guidelines notwithstanding, the management of pain with narcotic analgesics is difficult and requires meticulous attention by the physician.

ADJUVANT ANALGESICS (Table 26–4). The adjuvant analgesics include several different categories of drugs, including anticonvulsants, phenothiazines, tricyclic antidepressants, antihistamines, amphetamines, and steroids (see Table 26–4). Carbamazepine and phenytoin are useful in the management of patients with some neuropathic pain syndromes, e.g., trigeminal neuralgia. The mechanism of action is suppression of the spontaneous neuronal firing that commonly occurs with nerve injury. For both drugs, the minimal effective concentration for analgesia is unknown.

Certain phenothiazines have potent analgesic effects. Methotrimeprazine (Levoprome) has an analgesic potential close to that of morphine (15 mg given intramuscularly is equivalent to 10 mg of morphine given intramuscularly). This drug helps manage severe pain in patients tolerant to narcotic analgesics. The tricyclic antidepressants both enhance the analgesic effects of morphine and have independent analgesic properties. Doses of 10 to 75 mg administered orally are used to treat postherpetic neuralgia. The analgesic effects of these drugs occur independently of their antidepressant properties. The antihistamine hydroxyzine and the amphetamine dextroamphetamine are also sometimes helpful adjuvants. Steroids produce analgesia in patients with acute inflammatory diseases and in patients with tumor infiltration of bone or nerve or both. A series of drugs from other drug classes has been reported to be useful in specific pain states. Baclofen and pimozide in patients with trigeminal neuralgia have demonstrated efficacy in patients refractory to tegretol. Mexiletine, an antiarrhythmic cardiac drug, has analgesic effects in managing patients with painful diabetic neuropathy.

Alternate Methods of Pain Control

A variety of nonpharmacologic therapeutic approaches can be used alone or in combination with the analgesic drugs. These include physical therapy, trigger point injections, transcutaneous nerve stimulation, and certain behavioral approaches, all of which should be familiar to general physicians. Technically demanding anesthetic and neurosurgical approaches require consultation with pain experts. Certain guidelines apply to these procedures:

1. Evaluate thoroughly the nature of the pain and the prognosis of the patient's primary disease. Neurolytic nerve blocks and neuroablative and neurostimulatory surgical procedures often yield only temporary relief in patients with chronic pain and are not useful for neuropathic pain. In contrast, patients with cancer pain of somatic origin who are not expected to live for more than several months are excellent candidates for such procedures.

2. Nondestructive procedures, such as transcutaneous electrical stimulation or temporary blocks with local anesthetics, should be tried first.

3. Start with the least destructive procedure. For example, try

TABLE 26–4. ADJUVANT ANALGESIC DRUGS

Class	Drug	Indications	Starting Dose (mg) Range/24 hr	Comments
Anticonvulsants	Phenytoin (Dilantin)	Neuropathic pain, acute lancinating type (tic)	100, 100–300	Start with low doses; titrate slowly
	Carbamazepine (Tegretol)	Acute lancinating type (tic)	100, 200–800	Useful in paroxysmal nerve pain
Antidepressants	Amitriptyline, imipramine	Neuropathic pain, e.g., postherpetic neuralgia	10, 10–150	Start at low dose and titrate slowly; have analgesic properties
Stimulants	Dextroamphetamine	Somatic and visceral pain, e.g., postoperative	2.5, 10	Additive analgesia in combination with narcotics; reduces sedative effects
Antihistamine	Hydroxyzine	Somatic and visceral pain	25, 100	Additive analgesia in combination with narcotics; antiemetic, antianxiety properties
Phenothiazine	Methotrimeprazine (Levoprome)	Somatic and visceral pain; useful in narcotic-tolerant patients with GI obstruction and pain	10 (IM), 10–40 (IM)	Has antianxiety and antiemetic effects; available only in IM preparation
Steroids	Prednisone	Somatic and neuropathic pain, e.g., inflammatory pain, reflex sympathetic dystrophy	5, 5–60	Anti-inflammatory, antiemetic, analgesic effects
	Dexamethasone		0.5, 0.5–16	Same as prednisone
Miscellaneous	Baclofen	Paroxysmal pain of trigeminal neuralgia and central pain states	10, 10–80	May be used with tegretol
	Pimozide	Refractory trigeminal neuralgia	2, 4–12	Adverse effects include acute dystonia and akathisias
	Mexiletine	Neuropathic pain; useful in diabetic neuropathy	150, 150–600	Dose-response studies have not been done

continuous epidural local anesthetics to manage perineal pain before initiating an intrathecal neurolytic block.

4. Evaluate patients psychologically. If psychological factors play a major role in the pain, such procedures will not help and will often exacerbate the condition.

5. Inform the patient fully of the potential risks and benefits of the planned procedure.

PHYSICAL THERAPY. Chronic pain is commonly associated with reduced physical activity and splinting or immobilization of the injured body part. A graded exercise program with appropriate use of splints and braces and reactivation of the injured part plays a pivotal role in re-establishing the functional status of the patient. Local rubbing and transcutaneous electrical stimulation for "counterirritation" may help to mobilize the patient with a localized pain. Trigger point injections with either saline or a local anesthetic provide dramatic relief of painful muscle spasm.

BEHAVIORAL THERAPY. Behavioral approaches that often improve the patient's coping mechanism include breathing exercises to increase relaxation, coping strategies to integrate pain symptoms into a functioning lifestyle, and improving control over psychological factors of anxiety, fear, and demoralization associated with chronic pain.

ANESTHETIC PROCEDURES (Table 26–5). Local anesthetics and injectable neurolytic agents are sometimes useful in managing both acute and chronic pain that occupies a well-defined anatomic site. Sympathetic blocks, for example, often predict the relief that can be expected from sympathectomy in treating causalgia due to peripheral sensory nerve damage. Blocking nerves with short- or long-acting anesthetics determines in a reversible manner whether semipermanent nerve blocks will be effective and what side effects they might have. In some patients, particularly when muscle spasm plays a major role in pain production, repeated temporary blocks produce long-lasting relief of pain. If an anesthetic nerve block has been effective temporarily and then begins to lose its efficacy, neurolytic agents, such as phenol, alcohol, and freezing (cryoanesthesia), can be used to destroy nerve structures. The principal pathologic effect produced by these neurolytic agents is demyelination with secondary nerve degeneration. Because peripheral nerves and roots have overlapping sensory functions, multiple nerves and roots must be blocked to yield adequate pain control. Since such blocks may paralyze as well as anesthetize, they have a limited role in extremity pain and are most useful to treat thoracic and abdominal pain or perineal and sacral pain in patients with cancer.

Neurolytic agents can be injected into the epidural or intrathecal space as well as into peripheral nerves or roots. However, the limitations of motor weakness and autonomic dysfunction make this technique suitable for only a limited number of

TABLE 26–5. TYPES OF ANESTHETIC PROCEDURES COMMONLY USED IN CHRONIC PAIN

I. Nerve Blocks	
Peripheral	Pain in discrete dermatomes in chest and abdomen
Epidural	Unilateral lumbar or sacral pain
	Midline perineal pain
	Bilateral lumbosacral pain
Intrathecal	Midline perineal pain
	Bilateral lumbosacral pain
Autonomic	Reflex sympathetic dystrophy, e.g.,
Stellate ganglion	frozen shoulder
	Arm pain
Lumbar sympathetic	Reflex sympathetic dystrophy
	Lumbosacral plexopathy
	Vascular insufficiency of the lower extremity
Celiac plexus	Midabdominal pain
II. Continuous Epidural	Unilateral and bilateral lumbosacral
Infusion with Local	pain
Anesthetic	Midline perineal pain
III. Inhalation Therapy	Generalized pain
	Incident pain
IV. Trigger Point Injection	Focal muscle pain

TABLE 26–6. NEUROABLATIVE, NEUROSTIMULATORY, AND NEUROPHARMACOLOGIC PROCEDURES

Site	Neurostimulatory	Neuroablative	Neuropharmacologic
Peripheral nerve	Transcutaneous and percutaneous electrical nerve stimulation	Neurectomy	Local anesthetics
Nerve root		Rhizotomy	Local anesthetics Neurolytic agents*
Spinal cord	Dorsal column stimulation	Dorsal root entry zone lesions Cordotomy Myelotomy	Epidural and intrathecal opiates*
Brain stem	Periaqueductal stimulation	Mesencephalic tractotomy	Intraventricular opiates*
Thalamus	Thalamic stimulation	Thalamotomy	
Cortex		Cingulumotomy Frontal lobotomy	
Pituitary		Trans-sphenoidal hypophysectomy*	Chemical hypophysectomy*

*Procedures restricted for the treatment of chronic cancer-related pain.

patients. Neurolytic blocks find their best use in the management of well-defined localized pain caused by cancer. Their role in managing pain of nonmalignant origin is controversial because they work for only a limited period of time. There is a real risk of adding morbidity without providing pain relief, and they are not effective in managing neuropathic pain.

Blocks of the cervical (stellate ganglion) and lumbar sympathetic chains are most useful in managing limb pain and swelling associated with vascular or peripheral nerve injury, as occurs in diabetic peripheral vascular disease and reflex sympathetic dystrophy. Celiac plexus block is the procedure of choice to manage visceral pain from pancreatic carcinoma.

Intermittent or continuous epidural infusions of local anesthetics are useful for temporary relief of chronic pain involving the lumbosacral plexus and sacrum. This approach is most useful to treat an acute exacerbation of chronic cancer pain. The technique does not result in cross-tolerance with opiate analgesia, and it can be appropriately titrated to provide anesthesia without interruption of motor or autonomic function.

An anesthetic approach to manage diffuse pain is intermittent inhalation therapy with nitrous oxide. It is administered in oxygen through a non-rebreathing face mask with concentration ranging from 25 to 75 per cent.

NEUROSURGICAL PROCEDURES (Table 26–6). Pharmacologic procedures requiring neurosurgery include placement of intraventricular, epidural, or intrathecal catheters and implanted reservoirs or pumps to infuse agents used to manage selected patients with pain and cancer in whom systemic drugs are either ineffective or associated with excessive side effects. These approaches are not useful in managing non-cancer-related chronic pain problems.

Neurostimulatory procedures are performed by implanting electrodes in or on the desired portion of the nervous system and leading the electrodes to an implanted conductive receiver attached to an external transmitter. The technique allows the patient to control the timing and intensity of the stimulation. Electrical stimulation of the dorsal columns of cervical or thoracic spinal cord sometimes controls bilateral or midline neuropathic pain. Unfortunately, tolerance to the analgesic effect alters long-term usefulness of this procedure. Electrodes are usually placed in the epidural space over the dorsal column rather than directly on the spinal cord, thus reducing the risk of cord damage. Electrical stimulation of the periventricular gray matter of the brain stem also has been used for chronic neuropathic pain, especially if dorsal column stimulation or neurolytic blocks fail. Stimulation is delivered for no longer than 20 to 25 minutes at a time, three or four times a day. Tolerance develops more rapidly with increased use of the stimulator. Both animal studies and observations of human beings indicate that periventricular stimulation is associated with total body analgesia but without a decrease in sensory or motor function. This procedure is available in only a few specialized centers.

Medial thalamic stimulation is used to manage chronic but unilateral intractable pain. Electrodes are placed stereotactically in medial thalamus contralateral to the pain. Stimulation results in localized analgesia. This procedure is used to manage the thalamic pain syndrome, phantom limb pain, and peripheral nerve injury pain, particularly when pain involves the head or neck. About 50 per cent of patients with localized neuropathic pain respond to thalamic stimulation.

In addition to neurostimulatory procedures, portions of the nervous system from peripheral nerves to the cerebral cortex can be lesioned to relieve pain. The most commonly used procedure is cordotomy. Other procedures have had only limited success and are marked by significant neurologic morbidity. Cordotomy is the most useful neurosurgical procedure for relief of chronic somatic pain and the most commonly used procedure for the management of patients with localized cancer pain. Cordotomy can be performed as a percutaneous stereotactic radiofrequency procedure or as an open surgical ablation. Because the spinothalamic tract is selectively interrupted, only pain and temperature sensation are lost (on the contralateral side of the body). Cutaneous sensation and motor power remain intact, although some ipsilateral weakness or ataxia occurs transiently in about 20 per cent of patients. Cordotomy is most useful to manage unilateral pain below the neck. Initial pain relief occurs in 90 per cent of patients. This figure drops to 50 per cent at 6 months and about 40 per cent at the end of 1 year. One to 2 per cent of postcordotomy patients develop burning dysesthesias (anesthesia dolorosa), which are often as distressing as the original pain. Because of both the limited duration of its effectiveness and the risk of producing neuropathic pain, cordotomy is not indicated for management of chronic nonmalignant pain. Bilateral cordotomy can be performed to manage midline or perineal pain associated with cancer. If performed in the cervical area, bilateral cordotomy risks producing sleep-induced apnea. The second risk of bilateral cordotomy is bladder dysfunction. With unilateral cordotomy, 7 to 10 per cent of patients develop mirror pain on the opposite side of the body even when the original pain is relieved. Mirror pain can occur in the absence of a definable lesion in the affected area, and its pathogenesis is unknown. Other neuroablative procedures are rarely used.

Management of Cancer Pain

Figure 26–1 provides an algorithm for the management of cancer pain. It attempts to integrate assessment techniques, drug therapy, and anesthetic, neurosurgical, and behavioral approaches and stresses continuity of care. Treatment of cancer pain must begin with a careful diagnostic assessment that ad-

dresses not only the medical nature of pain but also its psychological and social components. At the time of assessment, a plan is developed to treat both the cancer, if possible, and the pain itself. If the anticancer treatment is effective, pain relief usually occurs, and the drugs used for analgesia can be discontinued without difficulty. Pain relief begins with analgesic drugs. Incorporated in Figure 26–1 is the World Health Organization's Cancer Pain Relief Program. It proposes an analgesic drug ladder moving from nonopioid drugs alone or in combination with adjuvant drugs through weak opioids to strong opioids. If pain relief is achieved with this program, no further therapy is necessary. In patients with severe, persistent pain not responsive to analgesic drugs or in whom the side effects of the drugs are not tolerated, physicians should first try switching to alternate analgesics or changing the route or timing of drug administration. For example, intrathecal opioids are indicated for relief of pain in patients in whom systemic analgesics produce confusion or excessive sedation.

If the pain is unresponsive to analgesic drugs and is localized (e.g., intercostal pain from tumor infiltration of the chest wall), neurolytic blocks are indicated. If the pain is unilateral and below the waist, cordotomy should be considered. For more diffuse pain unresponsive to analgesics, neurostimulatory procedures, including nitrous oxide inhalation and chemical hypophysectomy, may be considered. Behavioral approaches, which include relaxation techniques, breathing exercises, and cognitive control of pain, serve as adjuvants and should be integrated into the management of patients with chronic pain.

As the algorithm indicates, whatever the techniques of pain management used in patients with cancer, the physician is responsible for delivering continuing care, constantly reassessing both the diagnosis and the treatment to achieve optimum relief of pain and suffering for both patient and family.

Bonica JJ (ed): The Management of Pain. 2nd ed. Philadelphia, Lea & Febiger, 1989. *This two-volume text provides detailed descriptions of acute and chronic pain syndromes with excellent anatomic graphics.*

Cousins M, Bridenbaugh P (eds.): Neural blockade. *In* Clinical Anesthesia and Management of Pain. 2nd ed. Philadelphia, J.B. Lippincott Co, 1988. *This text describes the commonly used anesthetic procedures in acute and chronic pain management.*

International Association for the Study of Pain: Classification of chronic pain, descriptions of chronic pain syndromes and definitions of pain terms. Pain (Suppl) 3:S1–S225, 1986. *This useful volume contains descriptions of chronic pain syndromes and definitions of pain terms.*

Payne R, Foley KM (eds.): Current Therapy in Pain. Philadelphia, B.C. Decker, 1987. *This paperback pocket book provides short, well-summarized practical management approaches for common pain disorders.*

Loeser JD, Egan KJ (eds.): Managing the Chronic Pain Patient. New York, Raven Press, 1989. *This concise book provides practical guidelines for the evaluation and treatment of patients with chronic pain.*

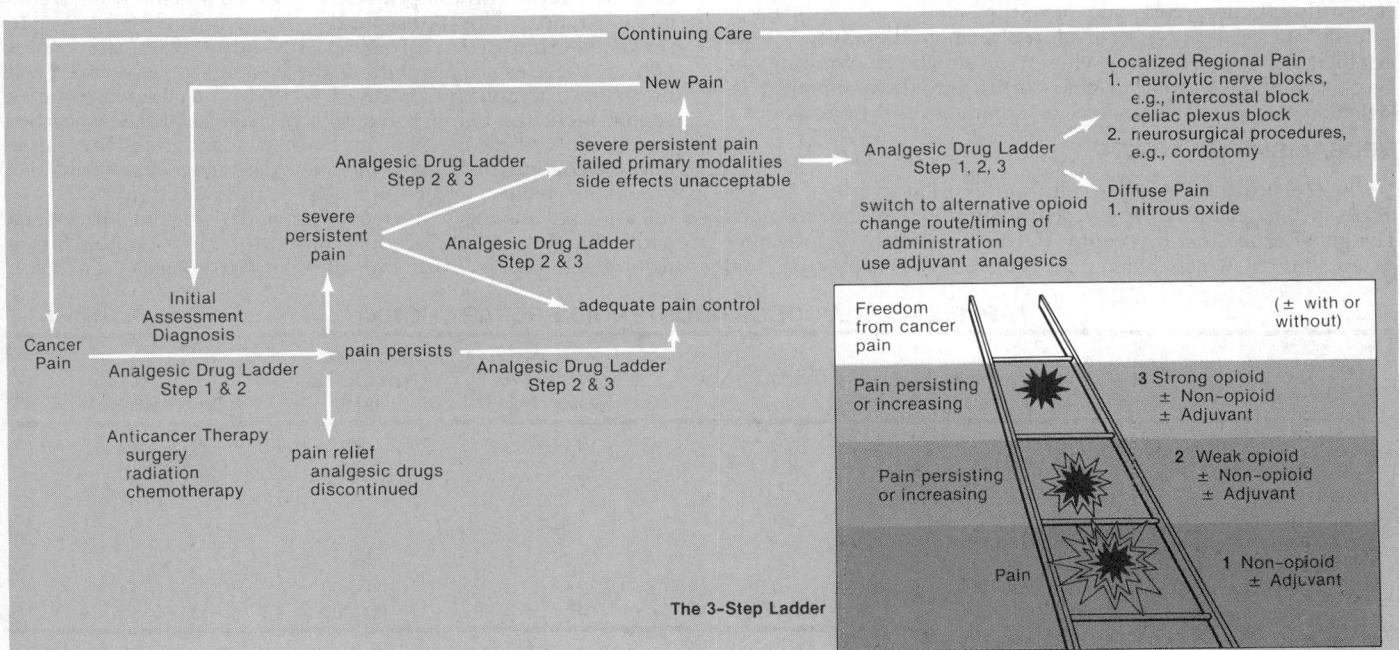

FIGURE 26–1. Algorithm for the management of cancer pain.

27 Glucocorticosteroid Therapy

Barton F. Haynes

In 1949, demonstration that the symptoms of rheumatoid arthritis could be treated with adrenal glucocorticosteroids ushered in a new era of therapy for immune-mediated diseases. With the introduction of glucocorticosteroids into clinical medicine has come the ability to cure adrenal insufficiency (Addison's disease) and to treat a wide spectrum of previously untreatable inflammatory conditions. However, glucocorticosteroid therapy is a double-edged sword with serious and often devastating side effects associated with its use. Understanding the mechanisms of action as well as the advantages and disadvantages of different glucocorticosteroids and their treatment regimens is essential for the physician to use appropriate clinical judgment in glucocorticosteroid administration.

BIOCHEMISTRY AND PHARMACOLOGY

Glucocorticosteroids are one of the three classes of steroids, the others being mineralocorticosteroids and the sex hormones, that are synthesized by the adrenal cortex. Glucocorticosteroids are endogenously synthesized from cholesterol to cortisol (hydrocortisone) via pregnenolone and progesterone. Cortisol is the principal circulating glucocorticosteroid in humans. The existence of glucocorticosteroid activity depends on the presence of a hydroxyl group at carbon 11 of the steroid molecule. Cortisol and prednisone are 11-ketocorticosteroids and therfore lack glucocorticosteroid activity until converted in the liver to the corresponding 11-beta-hydroxyl compounds, cortisol and prednisolone. All glucocorticosteroid preparations marketed for topical or local use are 11-beta-hydroxyl steroids, which do not require bioconversion for activity. Hydrocortisone has an approximate plasma half-life of 90 minutes (Table 27–1) and is metabolized in a number of tissues, particularly the liver. Glucocorticosteroids are irreversibly reduced and conjugated with glucuronic acid in the liver, thus enhancing excretion by the kidney. Ninety-five per cent of circulating endogenous cortisol is bound to plasma proteins—the majority to corticosteroid-binding globulin (transcortin). Adrenal cortisol production is regulated by hypothalamic production of corticotropin-releasing hormone that induces anterior pituitary production of ACTH (see Ch. 217).

The common synthetic glucocorticoids used clinically are listed in Table 27–1. These drugs differ in their plasma half-life, relative anti-inflammatory potency, and salt-retaining potency. Cortisone and cortisol (hydroxycortisone) have the highest sodium-retaining potency and are used especially as replacement therapy in adrenal insufficiency but are rarely chosen in situations requiring the long-term administration of glucocorticosteroids in supraphysiologic doses as anti-inflammatory or immunosuppressive agents.

MECHANISMS OF ACTION

Glucocorticosteroids enter cells via diffusion and bind to hormone-specific cytoplasmic glucocorticosteroid protein receptors. The glucocorticosteroid receptor (GR) is a member of a receptor superfamily to which belong the vitamin D receptor, thyroid hormone receptor, and retinoic acid receptor. Intracellular GR is present in an inactivated form in the cytosol of most mammals. Upon interaction of the GR with corticosteroids, a binding region for DNA is exposed on the GR. The activated GR is translocated to the nucleus, binds to glucocorticosteroid-response elements on DNA and, in doing so, induces subsequent transcription of specific mRNA's.

FACTORS THAT AFFECT RESPONSES TO GLUCOCORTICOSTEROIDS. In general, the potency of a steroid (Table 27–1) is correlated with the binding affinity of the molecule for intracellular GR. In addition, plasma protein concentrations influence glucocorticosteroid bioavailability; when patients with hypoalbuminemia are treated with glucocorticosteroids, they have an increased incidence of steroid side effects. In patients with severe liver disease, the conversion of glucocorticosteroids to the 11-beta-hydroxyl (active) form may not be efficiently made. Another factor that affects bioavailability of steroids is the rate of steroid metabolic degradation. For example, concomitant administration of phenobarbital or phenytoin enhances the rate of glucocorticosteroid clearance by the liver by increasing the activity of liver microsomal enzymes.

Two mechanisms of resistance to glucocorticosteroid effects have been described. First, certain leukemias and tumors have been shown to be resistant to steroid lytic effects owing to lack of or decreased numbers of GR. Second, one study has suggested that the presence of autoantibodies to lipocortins (a family of steroid-inducible proteins) can be responsible for poor responses to glucocorticosteroids in patients with autoimmune diseases.

ANTI-INFLAMMATORY EFFECTS. The effects of glucocorticosteroids following receptor binding are complex and can be manifested at both the molecular and cellular levels. One family of proteins that mediates anti-inflammatory activities of glucocorticosteroids is the lipocortins. Lipocortins inhibit synthesis of the inflammatory molecules (leukotrienes, thromboxanes, prostaglandins, and platelet-activating factor) by inhibition of the activity of phospholipase A_2. In general, glucocorticosteroids act via suppression of the production and/or function of many mediators of the inflammatory response (Table 27–2).

EFFECTS ON CELLS THAT MEDIATE INFLAMMATORY AND IMMUNE RESPONSES. Glucocorticosteroids exert profound effects on neutrophil differentiation, migration, and function (Table 27–2). Administration of glucocorticosteroids in vivo causes a redistribution of bone marrow neutrophils as well as increased production of neutrophils resulting in a peripheral neutrophilia, preventing ingress of neutrophils to areas of inflammation. Glucocorticosteroids inhibit neutrophil adherence to endothelium, neutrophil chemotaxis, neutrophil plasminogen activator production, and neutrophil superoxide generation.

Glucocorticosteroids redistribute monocytes out of the peripheral circulation with the peak effect 4 to 6 hours following steroid administration. This redistribution of mononuclear phagocytes prevents extravasation of monocytes into inflammatory sites. Glucocorticosteroids also inhibit the clearance of opsonized cells by tissue macrophages by interferring with macrophage Fc receptor–mediated binding to antibody-coated cells. Glucocorticosteroids inhibit all mechanisms necessary for granuloma formation, including monocyte chemotaxis, monocyte giant cell formation, monocyte plasminogen activator and interleukin 1 release, and monocyte phagocytosis and killing of intracellular pathogens. The ability of glucocorticosteroids to inhibit inflammatory mediator release by both the lipoxygenase and cyclo-

TABLE 27–1. GLUCOCORTICOSTEROID PREPARATIONS

	Anti-inflammatory Potency	Equivalent Dose (mg)	Sodium-retaining Potency	Approximate Plasma Half-life (min)	Biologic Half-life (hr)
Hydrocortisone	1	20	2+	90	8–12
Cortisone	0.8	25	2+	30	8–12
Prednisone	4	5	1+	60	12–36
Prednisolone	4	5	1+	200	12–36
Methylprednisolone	5	4	0	180	12–36
Triamcinolone	5	4	0	300	12–36
Betamethasone	20–30	0.6	0	100–300	36–54
Dexamethasone	20–30	0.75	0	100–300	36–54

From Garber EK, Targoff C, Paulus HE: *In* Paulus HE, Furst DE, Droomgoole SH (eds.): Drugs for Rheumatic Diseases. New York, Churchill Livingstone, 1987, pp 446; with permission.

TABLE 27–2. GLUCOCORTICOSTEROID EFFECTS ON IMMUNE CELLS AND HUMORAL FACTORS

Glucocorticoid effects on leukocyte movement

Lymphocytes
- Circulating lymphocytopenia 4–6 hours following drug administration secondary to redistribution of cells to other lymphoid compartments
- Depletes recirculating lymphocytes
- Selectively depletes T lymphocytes (especially CD4 subset) more than B lymphocytes and natural killer cells

Monocyte-Macrophages
- Circulating monocytopenia 4–6 hours following drug administration, probably secondary to redistribution
- Inhibits accumulation of monocyte-macrophages at inflammatory sites

Neutrophils
- Circulating neutrophilia
- Accelerated release of neutrophils from the bone marrow
- Blocks accumulation of neutrophils at inflammatory sites, probably secondary to reduced adherence

Eosinophils
- Circulating eosinopenia, probably secondary to redistribution
- Decreased migration of eosinophils into immediate hypersensitivity skin test sites

Glucocorticoid effects on leukocyte function

Lymphocytes
- Delayed hypersensitivity skin testing suppressed by inhibition of recruitment of monocyte-macrophages
- Lymphocyte proliferation to antigens suppressed more easily than proliferation to mitogens
- Mixed leukocyte reaction proliferation suppressed
- High concentrations in vitro suppress T lymphocyte–mediated cytotoxicity
- Antibody-dependent cell-mediated cytotoxicity not depressed
- Natural killer cell cytotoxicity suppressed
- Regulatory effects on helper and suppressor cell populations
- Decrease in T cell interleukin 2, gamma interferon, and colony stimulation factor production
- Lysis of cortical thymocytes and activated peripheral T cells

Monocyte-Macrophages
- Cutaneous delayed hypersensitivity suppressed by inhibition of lymphocyte effect on the macrophage
- Probable blockade of Fc receptor binding and function
- Depressed bactericidal activity
- Possible decrease in monocyte chemotaxis
- Decrease in monocyte interleukin 1 release

Neutrophil
- Probably no effect of phagocytic and bactericidal capability
- Antibody-dependent cellular cytotoxicity increased
- Probably decreased lysosomal release but little effect on lysosomal membrane stabilization at pharmacologic concentrations
- Chemotaxis inhibited only by suprapharmacologic concentrations

Glucocorticoid effects on humoral factors
- Mild decrease in immunoglobulin levels but no decrease in specific antibody production
- Complement metabolism probably unaffected
- Decreased reticuloendothelial clearance of antibody-coated cells
- Effects on kinins and prostaglandins
- Inhibits plasminogen activator release
- Potentiates the actions of catecholamines
- Possibly antagonizes histamine-induced vasodilatation

Adapted, with permission, from the Annual Review of Pharmacology and Toxicology, Vol. 19, © 1979 by Annual Reviews, Inc.

oxygenase pathways leads to decreased production of prostaglandin E_2, thromboxane B_2, and leukotriene B_4 by tissue macrophages.

Eosinophils and basophils, like monocytes, are redistributed out of the circulation following glucocorticosteroid administration in vivo. Eosinophil adherence, chemotaxis, and killing are inhibited by glucocorticosteroids, correlating with the observed efficacy of corticosteroid therapy in clinical syndromes characterized by tissue or peripheral eosinophilia such as *idiopathic hypereosinophilic syndrome* (see Ch. 150) and *eosinophilic fasciitis* (see Ch. 262). Basophil histamine and leukotriene release is also inhibited by glucocorticosteroids.

As with other immune cell types, glucocorticosteroids exert profound effects on both lymphocyte traffic and lymphocyte cell function. Glucocorticosteroid administration in vivo induces a rapid redistribution of T cells out of the circulation with CD4+ T cells preferentially decreased over CD8+ T cells. B cells are only minimally redistributed out of the circulation, whereas natural killer cells are spared the lymphopenic effect and remain in the circulation following glucocorticosteroid administration in vivo. Although glucocorticosteroids do not lyse normal circulating T cells, they do lyse cortical thymocytes and activated mature T cells.

Functionally, corticosteroids administered in vivo (high divided-dose therapy) result in suppression of B cell immunoglobulin production after 2 to 4 weeks of therapy. Similarly, while natural killer cells (CD16+ large granular lymphocytes bearing Fc receptors for IgG) are not depleted from the circulation, glucocorticosteroids markedly inhibit the ability of natural killer cells to kill other cell types. In general, most of the recognized lymphocyte functions—proliferation, mediator production, response to mediators, and cytotoxic effector function—have been shown to be decreased by corticosteroids. However, among immune cells, some lymphocyte functions are more resistant to corticosteroids than others (Table 27–2).

Both T cells and monocytes participate in granuloma formation. Thus, granulomatous hypersensitivity diseases such as *sarcoidosis* are generally responsive to steroid therapy. By contrast, infectious diseases such as *tuberculosis* that are held in check by granulomatous inflammation are prone to exacerbation or relapse during high-dose glucocorticosteroid therapy, owing to glucocorticosteroid-induced inhibition of granuloma formation.

EFFECTS ON CONNECTIVE TISSUE. Glucocorticosteroids reduce bone formation and increase bone resorption rates as well. Parathyroid hormone levels are elevated by glucocorticosteroid administration, most likely reflecting glucocorticosteroid-mediated inhibition of calcium absorption from the gastrointestinal tract. Glucocorticosteroids inhibit wound healing by suppressing prostaglandin synthesis and fibroblast collagen synthesis. Glucocorticosteroids inhibit connective tissue glycoaminoglycan biosynthesis and promote abnormal small blood vessel formation. During chronic administration of corticosteroids, these effects can lead to osteopenia, loss of connective tissue in skin and tendons, skin striae, and telangiectasia.

PRINCIPLES OF THERAPY

The modern principles of clinical use of glucocorticosteroids were established in 1966 by George Thorn, who emphasized that the following considerations were necessary. Prior to use of glucocorticosteroids as pharmacologic agents, the physician should ask: How serious is the underlying disorder? How long will therapy be required? What is the anticipated effective steroid dose? Is the patient predisposed to any of the known hazards of glucocorticosteroid therapy (such as glucose intolerance, osteoporosis, peptic ulcer disease, tuberculosis, hypertension, or psychiatric difficulties)? Which glucocorticosteroid preparations should be used? Can other modes of therapy be used to minimize either steroid dosage or steroid side effects? Is an alternate-day glucocorticosteroid regimen indicated?

INDICATIONS FOR USE. Glucocorticosteroids are most often used for their anti-inflammatory and immunosuppressive effects and for replacement therapy in adrenal insufficiency (see Ch. 217). The use of glucocorticosteroids as antitumor agents is described in Ch. 164. Steroids have been used to stabilize the cardiovascular system in hypotensive states such as septic shock, although recent large clinical trials have not demonstrated any efficacy for glucocorticosteroids in decreasing mortality in septic shock. Glucocorticosteroids are administered in the treatment of brain and spinal edema, particularly in the setting of primary tumors or metastases to the brain or spinal cord. Steroids have been postulated to work in brain edema by decreasing sodium in edema fluid, by stabilizing vascular permeability, and by decreasing production of CSF. In some cases, an antitumor effect by high-dose steroids may occur. Glucocorticosteroids are given for hypercalcemia associated with sarcoidosis or certain tumors. In this setting the therapeutic effect is related to an increase in renal excretion of calcium and a decrease in calcium absorption from the gastrointestinal tract.

Steroid effects on monocytes, neutrophils, lymphocytes, eosinophils, and basophils (Table 27–2) make glucocorticosteroids effective anti-inflammatory and immunosuppressive agents in many rheumatic diseases. For instance, glucocorticosteroids are the mainstay of therapy for *polymyalgia rheumatica, temporal arteritis* (see Ch. 267), and severe manifestations of *systemic lupus erythematosus* (see Ch. 261).

Immunosuppressive regimens that include glucocorticosteroids have been used to inhibit T cell– and monocyte-mediated allograft rejection such as occurs in heart and renal transplantation. Although many antibody- and immune complex–mediated diseases are treated with glucocorticosteroids, antibody-forming cells (B lymphocytes and plasma cells) are relatively resistant to the suppressive effects of steroids such that very high doses of steroids are needed to suppress B cell immunoglobulin production. Thus, the beneficial effects of glucocorticosteroids in immune complex–mediated diseases are likely mediated by the immune system subsequent to immune complex formation. It has been suggested, for example, that glucocorticosteroids are effective in autoimmune hemolytic anemias and other cytopenias by inhibiting the binding of antibody-coated cells to Fc receptors of macrophages in the reticuloendothelial system, thus preventing cell clearance and destruction.

Glucocorticosteroids are extensively used in the treatment of asthma and immediate hypersensitivity allergic conditions. Although the precise mechanisms of action are undefined, steroids are thought to work in asthma and other allergic reactions by inhibition of prostaglandin and leukotriene formation, by suppression of expression of lymphocyte surface receptors for IgE, and by depletion of intracellular histamine. Other specific actions of glucocorticosteroids relevant to asthma include prevention and reversal of late-phase reactants, reduction in mucus secretion, and augmentation in beta-adrenergic responsiveness.

Other clinical situations in which glucocorticosteroids have been used include a wide range of dermatologic and ophthalmologic conditions and prevention of reactions to intravenous contrast material.

LOCAL CORTICOSTEROID ADMINISTRATION. In some situations, local glucocorticosteroid therapy that delivers a concentrated dose of drug only to the affected site is preferable to systemic therapy. Examples of effective local therapy include topical glucocorticosteroid cream for contact dermatitis, administration of glucocorticosteroids for various ocular inflammatory conditions, and injection of microcrystalline preparations of corticosteroids intra-articularly or in bursae to control local joint or bursal inflammation. In each of these situations, if sufficient topical therapy is administered for a long enough time, systemic absorption of steroids occurs and predisposes the patient to systemic side effects and toxicities of glucocorticosteroids. An important advance in the treatment of asthma and severe allergic rhinitis has been the use of inhaled (for asthma) or intranasal (for rhinitis) glucocorticosteroids (see Ch. 57 and 246).

SYSTEMIC THERAPY. Several factors should be considered in the choice of a particular glucocorticosteroid preparation. For anti-inflammatory and immunosuppressive regimens, a steroid drug that possesses little or no mineralocorticosteroid activity is preferred to minimize salt retention and hypertension (see Table 27–1). Cortisol (hydrocortisone) has the greatest degree of mineralocorticosteroid activity, and this preparation is frequently used as replacement therapy in adrenocortical insufficiency (see Ch. 217.6).

There is a direct correlation between plasma and biologic half-life, potency, and toxic side effects of glucocorticosteroid preparations (see Table 27–1). Dexamethasone, betamethasone, and triamcinolone are longer acting, more potent, and associated with more deleterious side effects than the shorter-acting prednisone and methylprednisolone. Thus, prednisone is used more commonly in daily and alternate-day regimens, whereas dexamethasone is routinely used only when continuous glucocorticosteroid effects are needed, e.g., to control brain edema. The shorter-acting glucocorticosteroids such as prednisone are essential for constructing regimens for patients to ensure that the shortest duration of steroid effect needed to control the immune process being treated is used.

DAILY GLUCOCORTICOSTEROID THERAPY. For most of the immunologic diseases that require glucocorticosteroid therapy, the most common regimen is administration of prednisone orally in a single daily morning dose or in divided doses throughout the day. Divided-dose therapy is more potent therapeutically than daily or alternate-day glucocorticosteroids, and likewise, divided-dose therapy is more toxic than either daily or alternate-day regimens, particularly with regard to predisposition to infections and suppression of the hypothalamic-pituitary-adrenal (HPA) axis. Thus, for immune-mediated diseases, the shorter-acting prednisone is generally used in a manner that closely mimics the normal diurnal cortisol cycle. Prednisone is optimally given early in the morning (6 to 8 A.M.) such that exogenously administered steroid levels peak early in the day and then fall later in the evening to allow endogenous ACTH secretion to occur. Given that the diseases for which steroids are used are heterogeneous in etiology, treatment response, and severity, no single set of strict guidelines is available for glucocorticosteroid use. Nonetheless, general guidelines exist that pertain to most situations.

Once the decision has been made that glucocorticosteroid therapy is appropriate (such as for severe manifestations of *systemic lupus erythematosus* or in combination therapy with cyclophosphamide for *systemic necrotizing vasculitis*), glucocorticosteroid therapy should be initiated with prednisone, 1 to 2 mg per kilogram body weight in three to four divided doses (Fig. 27–1). Since divided-dose therapy is a potentially toxic regimen as well as the most anti-inflammatory and anti-immunosuppressive, divided-dose therapy should be tapered to single-dose daily therapy once clinical remission has been achieved. To change from divided-dose daily therapy to single-dose daily therapy, the divided dose (e.g., 20 mg prednisone three times a day) is consolidated to one dose orally in the morning with the same total (e.g., 60 mg prednisone once a day). The single daily dose can then be gradually tapered until the lowest single daily dose that can control the disease is reached or glucocorticosteroid

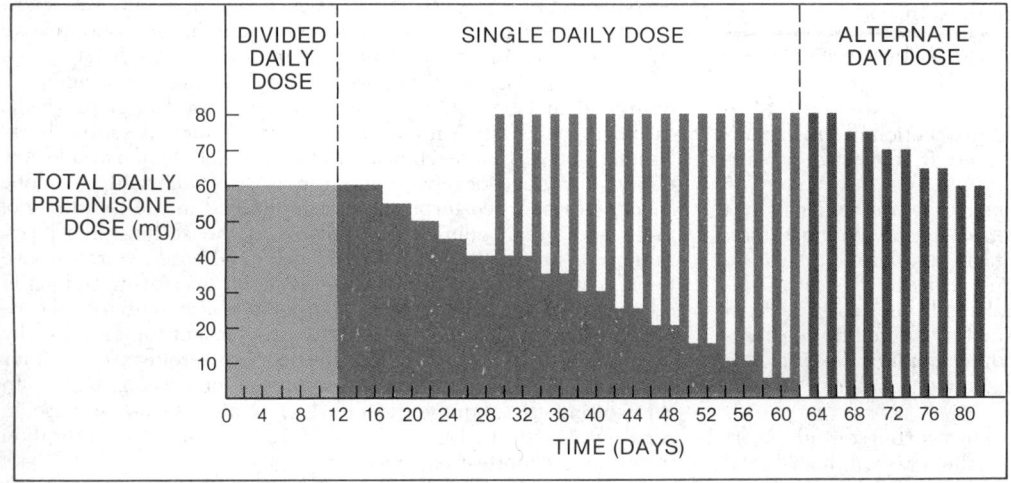

FIGURE 27–1. Schematic method of tapering oral glucocorticosteroids from divided-dose therapy to daily single dose to an alternate-day dose regimen.

TABLE 27–3. TOXIC SIDE EFFECTS OF GLUCOCORTICOSTEROID ADMINISTRATION

Cardiovascular and fluid balance
Hypertension
Sodium and fluid retention
Hypokalemic alkalosis
Dermatologic
Vascular fragility
Inhibition of fibroblast collagen synthesis, striae, impaired wound healing
Endocrine-metabolic
Suppression of HPA axis
Negative balance of nitrogen, potassium, calcium
Hyperglycemia
Hyperlipoproteinemia
Nonketotic hyperosmolar states
Suppression of growth in children
Secondary amenorrhea, acne, virilization
Truncal obesity, moon facies, mediastinal and spinal canal lipomatosis
Fatty infiltration of the liver
Gastrointestinal
Peptic ulcer disease
Pancreatitis
Intestinal perforation
Immunologic
Alteration of immune cell number and function
Opportunistic infections
Suppression of delayed hypersensitivity skin tests
Rare hypersensitivity reactions
Musculoskeletal
Osteopenia, osteoporosis, bone fractures
Aseptic necrosis of bone, bone pain
Myopathy
Neuropsychiatric
Pseudotumor cerebri
Psychiatric symptoms (psychosis, personality changes)
Psychological dependence on glucocorticoids
Ophthalmic
Glaucoma
Posterior subcapsular cataracts

therapy can be stopped altogether. Adjunctive nonsteroidal therapy for the disease in question, such as nonsteroidal anti-inflammatory agents for connective tissue diseases, is important for facilitating the ease of steroid tapering. Single-dose daily therapy (particularly the lower doses, less than 40 mg daily) provides for some normal HPA function in some individuals and also provides for periods of normal immune cell function to prevent opportunistic infections. After initiating glucocorticosteroid therapy, since most inflammatory diseases often are self-remitting illnesses, one should always seek to taper and, if possible, discontinue corticosteroids to prevent or limit toxic side effects.

The decision to reduce the daily steroid dosage is reached when (a) the disease activity is controlled, (b) other steroid-sparing drugs are added to the patient's regimen and the disease is controlled, or (c) the side effects due to glucocorticosteroids are so severe that dose reduction is mandatory. Collapsed vertebral bodies due to severe osteoporosis and opportunistic infections are two consequences of glucocorticosteroid therapy which dictate a reduction in steroid dosage as soon as possible.

ALTERNATE-DAY GLUCOCORTICOSTEROID THERAPY. One effective regimen for tapering glucocorticosteroid therapy is to convert the regimen from a daily divided dose to a single daily dose and then to a single dose on alternate days. The eventual goal in most disease states is to taper off therapy altogether if possible. In many inflammatory diseases such as *polyarteritis nodosa, Wegener's granulomatosis,* and *sarcoidosis,* it is relatively easy to taper glucocorticosteroid therapy to an alternate-day regimen; in others, such as *temporal arteritis* and *systemic lupus erythematosus,* it is more difficult. Nonetheless, if the patient can be tapered to an alternate-day regimen, a considerable service is done for the patient, as the level of unwanted side effects on alternate-day steroids is markedly reduced compared with equivalent-dose daily regimens.

Figure 27–1 illustrates one method of tapering corticosteroids when they are used to induce remission in a steroid-sensitive immune-mediated disease. This is a stylized example, and the tempo and increments of drug tapering need to be modified according to the clinical setting and the severity and degree of response of each individual patient. In this example, therapy is begun to induce remission of clinical symptoms at a dose of prednisone of 20 mg orally three times daily. After 2 weeks, the divided dose is consolidated to one 60-mg daily oral dose. After tapering the single daily dose of prednisone to 30 mg daily, and if the disease remains in remission, a conversion to alternate-day therapy can be attempted. The rationale for alternate-day glucocorticosteroid therapy is to administer a dose of a short-acting steroid at regular 48-hour intervals which will maintain suppression of disease activity while avoiding the toxic side effects associated with daily regimens. There are many ways to convert from a daily to an alternate-day glucocorticosteroid regimen. It is important to go slowly to prevent disease relapse and to make the patient as comfortable as possible with nonsteroidal anti-inflammatory drug supplements on the days off prednisone.

Another common pitfall is to give too little glucocorticosteroid on the "on" day. One effective way to convert to alternate-day therapy is initially to double one of the daily doses of steroids and to maintain the other prednisone dose on the second day (Fig. 27–1). The daily dose of 30 mg is doubled to 60 mg and kept there while the alternate daily dose is gradually tapered to zero and becomes the "off" day. After the dose has been converted to an alternate-day regimen of prednisone 60 mg on the "on" day and 0 mg on the "off" day, the level of the prednisone dose on the "on" day can begin to be tapered. In most instances both the speed and the amount of decrements shown in the example in Figure 27–1 will have to be modified (usually speed decreased and intervals between doses increased) to accommodate each patient's disease severity and clinical course. Specifically, when tapering the "off" day steroid from 20 mg to 0 mg, it frequently is necessary to use 2.5-mg or 1-mg decrements to get to 0 mg. Also, after the "off" day dose has been tapered to 0 mg, it is usual to hold the "on" day at its current level (in the example, 60 mg per day) for 1 to 2 weeks prior to beginning to taper the "on" day to lower doses. Finally, when the "on" day reaches 20 mg, small decrements (1 to 2.5 mg) are usually indicated to reach the lowest allowable dose or to taper off completely.

The regimen shown in Figure 27–1 would be most typical of a 2-month prednisone taper in a patient with uncomplicated *systemic necrotizing vasculitis* who was also being treated with a cytotoxic agent. On the basis of the plasma half-life of prednisone, the highest single dose that one could administer on an alternate-day basis without suppressing the HPA axis on the "off" day is 80 to 120 mg. A short-acting glucocorticosteroid is essential for an alternate-day regimen. For example, using dexamethasone or betamethasone in an alternate-day regimen defeats the purpose of the alternate-day schedule in that these long-acting glucocorticosteroids have biologic half-lives longer than 24 hours.

BURST OR INTERMITTENT-PULSE GLUCOCORTICOSTEROID THERAPY. For some clinical situations, short courses or bursts of corticosteroid therapy, either alone or in combination with other drugs, control the clinical symptoms. Severe poison ivy or poison oak contact dermatitis is an example of a common disease in which "burst" therapy is used. Patients are usually given 60 mg of prednisone or methylprednisolone orally for 2 or 3 days; then the dose is rapidly tapered by 10-mg decrements per day until the drug is completely discontinued. On this type of "burst" regimen, there is little danger of glucocorticosteroid-induced side effects. High-dose "burst" or "pulse" intravenous glucocorticosteroids came into widespread use in the early 1970's for the management of acute renal allograft rejection. Intravenous pulse glucocorticosteroid therapy has been used in progressive rheumatic diseases such as *systemic lupus erythematosus* and in nonrheumatic diseases such as *idiopathic rapidly progressive glomerulonephritis* and in *Goodpasture's syndrome.* Although efficacy in many clinical situations remains controversial, in certain situations such as acute allograft rejection and recent-onset renal failure in *lupus nephritis,* clinical efficacy has been demonstrated.

Methylprednisolone is generally employed for "pulse" regimens because of its high potency and low salt-retaining activity. Intravenous pulse regimens are theoretically desirable in order to obtain a rapid and prolonged therapeutic effect with fewer glucocorticosteroid side effects. While most anti-inflammatory and immunosuppressive effects of glucocorticosteroids that occur with intravenous pulse doses of methylprednisolone also occur at lower doses, certain effects have been seen only at high doses of glucocorticosteroids. These effects include inhibition of granulocyte aggregation, inhibition of T cell interleukin 2 receptor expression, and prolonged suppression of natural killer cell activity. Recently, intravenous pulse methylprednisolone therapy has been suggested to improve monocyte Fc receptor function in patients with *systemic lupus erythematosus*. It is important to administer large doses of intravenous methylprednisolone slowly over 1 hour to avoid abrupt potassium and fluid shifts, which can lead to acute cardiac dysfunction.

A question is frequently asked regarding the use of ACTH versus glucocorticosteroids. There is no convincing evidence that ACTH is superior to glucocorticosteroids in the treatment of any disease. ACTH administration has several drawbacks. ACTH can be given only parenterally, and response to ACTH depends on an induced adrenal glucocorticosteroid response, the magnitude of which is variable.

SIDE EFFECTS OF GLUCOCORTICOSTEROID THERAPY

Suppression of the HPA Axis. Although precise criteria are not available to establish the minimal dose of glucocorticosteroid that can cause suppression of the HPA axis, in some individuals short courses of oral glucocorticosteroid therapy (the equivalent of 30 mg per day for 1 week) can be associated with abnormal HPA function for as long as 12 months. Thus, prophylactic glucocorticosteroids should be considered during times of maximal stress (trauma or major surgical procedures) in the following patients: (a) those with a known diagnosis of primary or secondary adrenal insufficiency, (b) those currently treated with exogenous steroids for chronic diseases, (c) those treated daily with exogenous steroids (prednisone 30 mg daily) for a period exceeding 1 week during the past 12 months, (d) those with signs or symptoms suggestive of hypoadrenalism and an abnormal rapid ACTH stimulation test (see Ch. 217.5), and (e) those scheduled to undergo, or with a history of, bilateral adrenalectomy or hypophysectomy.

If patients who are suspected of HPA axis suppression are to be subjected to severe stress such as a major surgical procedure, they should receive parenteral hydrocortisone in doses of 100 mg every 4 to 6 hours during surgery and for several days thereafter, depending on recovery period (see Ch. 217.6).

To determine suppression of the HPA axis in a person who has recently received glucocorticosteroid therapy, a rapid ACTH stimulation test can be performed (see Ch. 217.5 for procedures). Recovery of HPA function once glucocorticosteroids have been discontinued is a slow process. As yet there are no proven therapies to hasten the process.

OTHER SIDE EFFECTS

Other toxic side effects of glucocorticosteroid administration are listed in Table 27–3. The side effects involve many organ systems and can be devastating. The frequency and severity of toxic side effects in most cases are directly related to the dose and duration of therapy. Unfortunately there are no proven regimens for limiting the complications and side effects of glucocorticosteroid therapy other than treating the patient with the lowest dose of steroid that will control the disease and discontinuing the drug as soon as the disease warrants doing so.

To minimize steroid-induced osteopenia and associated fractures, it has been suggested that the 24-hour urine calcium output be measured after 1 to 3 months of glucocorticosteroid therapy and oral calcium and possibly vitamin D be given based on the level of urinary calcium excretion.

Infections represent the most serious and potentially life-threatening complication of corticosteroid therapy. In patients on long-term daily doses of glucocorticosteroids, the index of suspicion should be high for occult infections. For example, joint inflammation that persists or develops in the rheumatoid arthritis patient on oral corticosteroid therapy should be suspected of

being infectious and the possibility excluded by arthrocentesis. The best method of preventing infectious complications of glucocorticosteroid therapy is always to taper the drug to the lowest possible dose and to attempt either to taper the dose to an alternate-day regimen or to stop steroid therapy completely. One common mistake in the management of glucocorticosteroid therapy is to leave the patient on the dose of the drug that induced remission in the disease instead of tapering the dose to the lowest level possible. During or after tapering of glucocorticosteroids, patients may develop symptoms of glucocorticosteroid withdrawal, such as myalgias and arthralgias, that in some cases may mimic symptoms of the underlying disease.

Camussi G, Tetta C, Bussolino F, Baglioni C: Anti-inflammatory peptides (antiflammins) inhibit synthesis of platelet-activating factor, neutrophil aggregation and chemotaxis, and intradermal inflammatory responses. J Exp Med 171:913–927, 1990. *Recent article describing mechanism of action of lipocortins at a molecular level.*

Flower RJ: Lipocortin and the mechanisms of action of the glucocorticosteroids. Br J Pharmacol 94:987–1015, 1988. *In-depth review of the role that lipocortins play in mediating the anti-inflammatory effects of glucocorticosteroids.*

Garber EK, Targoff C, Paulus HE: Corticosteroids in the rheumatic disease: Chronic low doses, chronic high doses, "pulses," intra-articular. In Paulus HE, Furst DE, Dromgoole SH (eds.): Drugs for Rheumatic Diseases. New York, Churchill Livington, 1987, pp 443–476. *Comprehensive review of steroid use in rheumatic diseases, including intra-articular glucocorticosteroid administration.*

Haynes BF, Fauci AS: The differential effect of in vivo hydrocortisone on the kinetics of subpopulations of human peripheral blood T lymphocytes. J Clin Invest 61:703, 1978. *Original paper describing the effect of glucocorticosteroids on subsets of human T cells, with detailed kinetic studies.*

Kaliner M: Mechanism of glucocorticosteroid action in bronchial asthma. J Allergy Clin Immunol 76:321–329, 1985. *Review article with in-depth analysis of effect of steroids on allergic reactions, including asthma.*

Kerhl J, Fauci AS: The clinical use of corticosteroids. Ann Allergy 50:2, 1983. *An outstanding review article on the theoretical and practical aspects of glucocorticosteroid use.*

Napolitano LM, Chernow B: Guidelines for corticosteroid use in anesthetic and surgical stress. Int Anesthesiol Clin 26:226, 1988. *Excellent review article with guidelines for perioperative treatment with glucocorticosteroids of patients suspected of having HPA suppression.*

Thorn GW: Clinical considerations in the use of corticosteroids. N Engl J Med 274:775, 1966. *The classic paper on clinical use of corticosteroids.*

28 Common Poisonings

William O. Robertson

DEFINITION. Man's chemical environment was recognized as a threat to health long before the birth of Christ. Well-documented outbreaks of occupational mercury and lead "poisonings" had been recorded and preventive measures implemented by 200 B.C. The Middle Ages saw arsenic poisoning employed as a political weapon. More recent times have seen increasing recognition of industrial toxins, "accidental poisoning" in childhood, purposeful overdoses in adults, adverse reactions to drugs, and environmental hazards for us all. The common theme is entrance of an exogenous chemical into an organism and subsequent disruption of its metabolism. The term "poison" has undergone quantitative redefinition so that now such ubiquitous substances as table salt and drinking water are firmly established as being "poisonous." Recall that more than 400 years ago, Paracelsus cautioned "All substances are poisons: There is none that is not a poison. The right dose differentiates a poison and a remedy." Finally, the host-organism itself has contributed to a better comprehension of the word "poison," as genetic variability has been recognized to determine the impact of a given molecule in such hereditary disorders as phenylketonuria, glucose-6-phosphate dehydrogenase deficiency, and others. As man's understanding of life has expanded, the connotation of poisoning has undergone substantial evolution.

ETIOLOGY. Approximately 1.2 million chemical entities had been identified and coded by 1950; the number had risen to more than 4.3 million by 1976. By 1992, the number will exceed 11 million. Although not all of these compounds have been marketed, many new organic compounds have appeared in the home and the workplace. For example, available formulations of pesticides have increased 50-fold over the past 30 years. Moreover, manufacturing processes have released additional compounds into the workplace or the environment with capabilities of serving as poisons. Currently employed methods to determine carcinogenicity, mutagenicity, and teratogenicity indict chemicals as dangerous when simultaneous epidemiologic data from humans fail to support such contentions—e.g., formaldehyde, fluorides, dioxins. Since proving a negative remains so ephemeral, it appears likely that "scare incidents" that eventually prove groundless—e.g., cranberries in the 1960's, sturgeon (Hg) in the 1970's, and Agent Orange (dioxins) in the 1980's—will be even more commonplace.

New chemical techniques have permitted prompt and complete identification of poisonings and have uncovered the causes of such diverse entities as Minamata disease (teratogenesis consequent to methyl mercury), an outbreak of ascending paralysis affecting more than 4000 with more than 400 deaths in Iraq (also caused by methyl mercury), the "gray syndrome" in premature infants (caused by chloramphenicol), mesotheliomas induced by asbestos, and an epidemic of angiosarcoma of the liver among industrial workers (caused by vinyl chloride). Nevertheless, many unknowns remain and justify careful prospective monitoring of industry, of the home, and of the environment. Unfortunately, the combination of more "synthetic chemicals," vastly more precise testing techniques, a press far more devoted to Rachel Carson's *Silent Spring* than to Dupont's "better living through chemistry," and an increasingly litigious society has created an era of "toxic torts" and its consequences, plus a very anxious and concerned public and profession. As a consequence, primary care physicians are bound to be involved in disputes stemming from industrial, occupational, and environmental origins.

INCIDENCE. Over the past 25 years progressively more reliable data have been gathered about deaths from poisonings, the leading agents, and the number of such deaths attributable to each among children less than five years old and among the overall population (Table 28–1). Although concern for infants and toddlers prompted the creation of our nation's Poison Center Network, deaths from poisoning among that group have plummeted over the past 30 years; these children were, fortunately, greatly underrepresented in 1984, accounting for only 2.2 per cent of poisoning deaths despite the fact that their "accidental ingestions" account for 62 per cent of the 1,368,000 human exposures summarized by the National Data Collection System of the American Association of Poison Control Centers in 1988. By 1989, the percentage had fallen still further; viewed over time, some 450 deaths occurred nationwide among children less than 5 years of age in 1962 from accidental poisoning due to household products and prescription items, compared to only 31 in 1989—a remarkable decline in mortality. Among adults precise data are more difficult to retrieve. Incomplete data attest that a minimum of 12,000 deaths occur annually as a result of suicide by poisoning.

EPIDEMIOLOGY. There are significant differences in the epidemiology of poisonings among children under 5 years of age compared with the remainder of the population. With adults, occupational and industrial exposures, suicide gestures or attempts, and homicides depend upon host factors and environmental settings as well as involved chemicals. In contrast, among children under 5, host and environmental factors are less variable. In the United States, occurrences peak at 24 to 32 months of age, and more male than female children are involved; poisonings happen most frequently between 11 A.M. and 12 noon or between 5 and 6 P.M. and in places of easiest exposure—the kitchen, the bedroom, and the bathroom. In addition, illness in the family or "life stress situations" increase the likelihood of accidental ingestion.

PREVENTION. Avoiding exposure to the toxin is the ultimate precaution; among adults, a variety of approaches have been employed—some with obvious effectiveness, others without. For example, the use of mercury in the felting process of hats has been outlawed since 1941; that source of mercury poisoning has disappeared in the hatting industry. Beryllium has been excluded from fluorescent light bulbs, and that source of exposure no longer exists. Similarly, where arsenic has been eliminated from pesticidal preparations and where naphthylamine has been eliminated from the rubber industry, human illness has been avoided. Some of these steps have resulted from legislative processes; others are the result of voluntary activity on the part of industry or an aware public.

Among children some approaches have also proved effective; others are without much evidence of success. For example, efforts directed at altering toddlers' exploratory behaviors in family settings have not proved effective. In contrast, the use of safety caps on medicine bottles had important consequences. For the 10-year period between 1959 and 1969, almost 100 deaths occurred annually from accidental salicylate poisoning in children under 5; in 1988, only one such death was reported. Several variables have been cited as definitely contributory: (1) the manufacturers' voluntary reduction of the number of tablets as well as of the amount of aspirin per bottle; (2) the introduction of a favorable flavor to the "baby aspirin" as an attractive alternative to larger tablets; (3) programs of professional and public education; (4) the appearance of acetaminophen as a rival to aspirin, with its subsequent capture of 30 per cent of the analgesic-antipyretic market, and more recently, their replacement by still newer nonsteroidal anti-inflammatory drugs (NSAID's) attempting to avoid Reye's syndrome; and (5) the mandated use of safety caps or child-resistant containers. All have had an impact, but current professional opinion holds that safety caps have contributed approximately 60 per cent of the variance. As safety caps have subsequently been applied to other prescription products and dangerous household items such as petroleum distillates and caustics, their impact has been felt there also. Unfortunately, safety caps may have a negative effect among the geriatric population, among whom as many as 50 per cent cite them as contributing to their lack of compliance in taking prescribed medications.

Since 1953, more than 500 poison centers have been established across the country to provide professionals and patients with ingredient information, toxic potentials, and treatment alternatives. Initially, the FDA's National Clearinghouse of Poison Control Centers was intended to serve as the coordinating unit; it also provided technical information to centers. In recent years, several microfiche systems—particularly "Poisondex" (Micromedex, Denver) which has evolved to a CD-ROM system—have been developed to catalogue product information and to outline management approaches; they are capable of storing information on more than 400,000 products in a limited space and in an easily retrievable manner. Moreover, such systems avoid filing errors and permit updating of information on a quarterly basis.

Over the years the American Association of Poison Control Centers has served to produce educational material aimed at preventing poisoning, to establish standards for the operation of poison centers, to conduct self-assessment examinations for those staffing poison centers, and to implement a nationwide program aimed at regionalizing the poison center network. More recently, the American Academy of Clinical Toxicology and the American Board of Medical Toxicology have been developed to serve as the specialty society and certifying body, respectively, to further

TABLE 28–1. DEATHS DUE TO "ACCIDENTAL" POISONING IN THE UNITED STATES IN 1985

	All Ages	Under 5 Years	5–44 Years	45 + Years
Total solids and liquids	4091	55	2835	1201
Medications	3612	32	2618	962
Analgesics, antipyretics	1209	4	1016	189
Opiates	867	2	779	86
Sedatives, hypnotics	32	1	22	9
Psychotropic drugs	267	5	160	101
Other CNS drugs	448	6	400	42
Other drugs	1560	11	981	563
Nondrugs	479	23	217	239
Alcohol	305	2	137	166
Paints, solvents, cleaners	85	8	52	25
Pesticides	21	6	5	10
Corrosives, caustics	11	1	1	9
Foods, plants	6	0	2	4
Other	51	6	20	25
Gases and vapors	1079	25	608	446
Carbon monoxide	880	14	518	348

Data from National Safety Council Accident Facts. Chicago, National Center for Health Statistics, 1988.

the academic and professional goals of physicians involved in such programs.

DIAGNOSIS. The diagnosis of an accidental (or a purposeful) poisoning can be made only if considered; this is true for either the adult or child with unexplained signs or symptoms. Once the possibility of poisoning is entertained, a careful search is made for a possible container and its label or for a solid medication form and its drug-identifying imprint; next, the toxic potential of the substance can be verified from existing information or by contacting the nearest poison center. Often the presenting clinical signs and symptoms are so characteristic as to permit diagnosis—e.g., the hyperventilation (following vomiting) of acute salicylism, the extrapyramidal manifestations of phenothiazine reactions. Sometimes diagnostic confirmation can be established by the patient's response to a specific antidote, e.g., naloxone. On other occasions, analysis of specimens of body fluids—blood, urine, vomit, gastric contents, or stool—is necessary for diagnosis. As a generalization, "routine toxic screens" have proved to be of relatively little value in the child and are decried by many experts as inaccurate, confusing, and not helpful in the adult. Where the history or the environment provides a lead to the potential toxins, modern technology is proving increasingly useful. In the absence of such leads, helpful results are admittedly scarce.

Particularly helpful to toxicologists have been the Consumer Product Act of 1970 and the Commission Coordinating Safety Packaging Regulations, which have promulgated adequate labeling of hazardous substances across the country. *The label on the container is the single most useful information in accidental poisonings.* In the absence of a label, generic information about ingredients of household, industrial, and pharmaceutical products is available from a poison center or from a particularly useful textbook: *Clinical Toxicology of Commercial Products*. The information on the prescription bottle, on the package insert, or from the imprint of the solid medication form (such imprints exist on virtually all tablets and capsules) is equally important and ought to be diligently pursued.

Once the ingested poison has been identified, the problem remains to determine its potential for harm in the particular patient. That potential depends upon the amount and form ingested, the toxicity of the agent, the time lapse involved, and a variety of host factors. The amount ingested can sometimes be estimated by observers or by determining the amount of material remaining in the container. The toxicity of a particular poison can be assessed by reference to known data on human experiences, to animal LD_{50}'s, and to derivative "minimal lethal doses." One must be particularly cautious about overinterpreting LD_{50}'s or animal studies; in many instances the results are not transferable to the human. A toxicity rating has proved useful in estimating the degree of risk to the patient (Table 28–2).

In recent years, toxicologic analysis of body fluids has assumed an increasingly significant role in the diagnosis and management of poisoning, but it remains a relatively small one. Technical developments perfecting chemical analysis by mass spectrophotometry, gas-liquid chromatography, and spin resonance now allow toxic screening for a variety of poisons from minuscule amounts of body fluids. Commercial laboratories as well as a number of hospital, public health, and university laboratories provide qualitative and quantitative analyses for sedatives, narcotics, psychotropics, heavy metals, pesticides, and other compounds, all of which enable a speedy and accurate diagnosis. Nevertheless, such determination (i.e., specifying the type and amount of barbiturate in the blood) often does not alter management of the patient. Thus, in instances of barbiturate overdose, measurements of blood gases and pH prove more effective in coping with the clinical problem than does the quantitative determination of barbiturate level. Notable exceptions occur when specific quantification is critical in deciding on therapy—e.g., the use of acetaminophen blood levels and the Matthews-Rumack nomogram in deciding on the use of its antidote (*N*-acetylcysteine) before clinical signs or symptoms of illness appear, or the use of the serum salicylate concentration and the Done nomogram in determining the need for therapy in acute salicylate ingestion; and the value of the serum iron concentration along with clinical signs and symptoms in contemplating chelation therapy with desferrioxamine for iron poisoning. So too, identifying the presence of methyl alcohol or ethylene glycol can be critical in therapeutic management. Regardless of these several exceptions, the point remains that historical and clinical features plus the routinely available laboratory tests are usually paramount. Assisting the physician are a number of texts listed at the end of this chapter.

TREATMENT. Even before the ingested (or inhaled) substance has been identified and its toxic potential determined, first aid measures and supportive care ought to be initiated. Subsequent efforts are directed toward (1) preventing absorption of the substance; (2) curtailing its conversion in the body to its active form or hastening its conversion to an inactive one; (3) neutralizing or counteracting its clinical effect; and (4) enhancing its excretion from the body. In the majority of instances instituting measures to enable the patient to tolerate the temporary impact of the toxin and then to recuperate on his or her own remains the most effective course of action and often prevents subsequent poisonings as a result of overzealous treatment.

Supportive Measures. Prompt attention to supportive measures before a crisis has arisen, is, in fact, usually the single most critical element in managing the overdosed patient. The airway must be maintained, ventilation assured, cardiac output sustained, peripheral vascular collapse avoided, convulsions controlled, and hypertension and increased intracranial pressure lowered. Physical and chemical options ought to be carefully reviewed in advance of the patient's arrival if possible. Life support mechanisms can tide the patient over a period of compromised function as a result of anesthesia, an accidental overdose, or the purposeful induction of "barbiturate coma." But those measures must be carefully planned, carried out by skilled personnel, and monitored in detail if optimal benefit is to be achieved.

Prevention of Absorption. This is best accomplished in the conscious child or adult by *induction of emesis* as opposed to gastric lavage. Although gastric lavage has a tradition in emergency medicine, its yield of ingested material falls short of the returns by emesis. Moreover, despite improved emergency transport systems, there are significant time delays in delivering the patient to a health care facility where lavage can be undertaken. During that time, significant absorption takes place. By contrast, efforts to induce vomiting can be initiated in the home—particularly if syrup of ipecac is available there. If not, it is readily obtained from local pharmacies, 24-hour corner groceries, emergency vehicles, and neighbors. One should administer 15 ml to a child or 15 to 30 ml to an adult together with 200 to 300 ml of any fluids—water, soft drinks, milk, or juices—and wait 10 to 15 minutes with an appropriate receptacle for vomiting to occur. If no vomiting ensues in 20 minutes, one should repeat the initial dose of syrup of ipecac and administer more fluids. If no syrup of ipecac is available, one should try gagging the patient but should be prepared for failure; one should then encourage the patient to drink 30 to 45 ml of liquid dishwashing detergents (anionic or nonionic but *not* cationic detergents) together with 240 ml of fluid. If the patient has already arrived in the emergency room, apomorphine can be used. It proves effective in 4 to 5 minutes but results in a drowsy patient despite use of naloxone. In all circumstances one should avoid table salt as an emetic agent; its use can compound the problem with acute hypernatremia. One should always avoid emesis in the comatose or convulsing patient or in the patient who has ingested a caustic. Syrup of ipecac proves effective in acute phenothiazine ingestions, but not in the face of chronic overdose; any form of emesis is maximally effective in the first 1 to 1.5 hours after ingestion; seldom is it useful after 2 hours' delay.

TABLE 28–2. TOXICITY RATING

Rating	Probable Lethal Dose	
	mg/kg	*For 70-kg Man*
6—Supertoxic	<5	A taste <7 drops
5—Extremely toxic	5–50	7 drops to 1 tsp
4—Very toxic	50–500	1 tsp to 1 oz
3—Moderately toxic	500 mg–5 grams	1 oz to 1 pint
2—Slightly toxic	5–15 grams	1 pint to 1 quart
1—Practically nontoxic	>15 grams	>1 quart

From Gosselin RE, Hodge HC, Smith RP: Clinical Toxicity of Commercial Products. 5th ed. © 1984, The Williams & Wilkins Company, Baltimore.

Gastric lavage, using a large-bore tube and 1000 to 3000 ml of half-strength saline as the rinse, together with terminal instillation of activated charcoal, is the only option for the unconscious patient. In patients over 2 years of age, concomitant use of a cuffed endotracheal tube is indicated to avoid aspiration. Despite the fact that most toxins are absorbed rapidly and thus escape delayed evacuation efforts, on occasion substantial portions of ingested agents have been recovered, especially in suicidal patients who have consumed poisons that delay gastric emptying, slow intestinal motility, or depress overall body function. In those instances attempts at evacuation are recommended but cannot be expected to be effective in more than one of five patients.

Activated charcoal can be used to complement either of the measures discussed above, but not with syrup of ipecac until after emesis has occurred. Since the mid-1980's, increasing numbers of emergency physicians are resorting to exclusive use of activated charcoal in overdose patients who make it to the emergency room, avoiding both induction of emesis and gastric lavage; a substantial data base supports their contention. The large surface area of charcoal permits significant adsorption of the toxin, precluding its absorption from the gut. Given by mouth or via nasogastric tube in amounts of 5 to 15 times the amount of the ingested toxin, activated charcoal has diminished absorption by as much as 50 per cent with significant therapeutic benefits. Recent pharmacologic research supports the contention that absorption may be prevented by early intervention with charcoal but, equally importantly, finds that excretion of those compounds that are recycled via the gastrointestinal tract can be significantly increased by repetitive oral instillation of activated charcoal.

Cathartics, laxatives, enemas, and *colonic irrigations* are "heroic" measures devoid of evidence of effectiveness; in fact, cathartics can increase the rate of absorption of some barbiturates.

Inhibition of metabolism of a potential toxin to its active form or conversion to an inactive form is an option and, when feasible, may prove beneficial. For example, methyl alcohol becomes active only after it is converted to formaldehyde and formic acid; administering ethyl alcohol to the patient takes advantage of substrate competition (it is favored over methyl alcohol by the enzymatic processes involved), permitting significant reduction in the rate of metabolism of methyl alcohol and resulting in diminished formation of formaldehyde and formic acid, which in turn can be more easily scavenged by existent metabolic processes.

In other instances, enhancement of enzymatic activity may *activate* a toxin. For example, pretreatment of the pregnant woman and fetal liver with phenobarbital enhances conjugation of bilirubin, but such pretreatment augments the conversion of carbon tetrachloride to its deleterious metabolite.

Chelating agents also limit the entry of certain toxins into metabolic pathways and augment excretion of the inactivated material. This approach has been particularly useful in poisonings by heavy metals—treatment of arsenic, mercury, and lead with dimercaprol (BAL), D-penicillamine, and edetate (EDTA), respectively. Similarly, desferrioxamine is useful in both acute and chronic iron poisoning.

Specific antidotes to counteract the effects of specific toxins are limited to a few compounds, but when one exists its usefulness is great. Paramount is the example of naloxone, an opiate derivative, which, when administered in adequate amounts (often *considerably more* than the recommended 0.4 mg) to a patient with heroin overdose, results in the patient's sitting up and talking within 20 seconds! Administered to the nonoverdosed patient, naloxone is devoid of any action, thus constituting a unique example of an antagonist drug without any agonist effects. Most other antidotes have agonist as well as antagonist effects. Common examples of such antidotes include atropine for organophosphate and carbamate insecticide poisoning, methylene blue for methemoglobinemia, nitrites plus thiosulfate for cyanide ingestion, N-acetylcysteine for acetaminophen overdoses, pyridoxine for isoniazid toxicity and diphenhydramine for phenothiazine-induced extrapyramidal reactions. In addition, recent advances in immunology have resulted in the use of portions of antibodies ("Fab" fragments) to "neutralize" the clinical effects of overwhelming digoxin poisonings. Introduced as Digibind, this antidote has established itself as a remarkably successful remedy for dangerously moribund overdosed patients, reversing cardiac arrhythmias in minutes. Moreover, monoclonal antibodies to various toxins are being developed for possible clinical use—either via injection into the patient or by being affixed to perfusion columns.

Enhancing elimination of a toxin can be accomplished by several mechanisms. For example, in carbon monoxide poisoning, use of 100 per cent oxygen by ventilatory mask has both theoretical and practical benefit. In instances of phencyclidine ingestion, continuous gastric lavage, taking advantage of "ion trapping" of the recycled phencyclidine via the gastric mucosa, is reported to be effective. Ion trapping is also employed in acute salicylate poisoning via alkalinization of the urine. In the kidney tubule, free salicylate molecules ionize in the presence of an alkaline medium and are not resorbed, thus being "captured" in the urine and excreted into the bladder. In contrast, amphetamine (a weak base) is captured in the kidney tubule by acidifying the urine with ascorbic acid or ammonium chloride. In general, forced osmotic diuresis, particularly chemical diuresis with common diuretics (e.g., furosemide), is of little or no benefit in enhancing the excretory processes.

By contrast, *dialysis* and *hemoperfusion* have proved to be effective therapeutic tools, although not as effective as had been initially believed. For example, a decade ago many patients with barbiturate overdose were subjected to extracorporeal or peritoneal dialysis; today, fewer than 1 in 300 such patients are so treated. If renal shutdown has occurred, as in mercury poisoning, dialysis will prove lifesaving, although it is unlikely to augment excretion of the mercury molecule. Exceptions do exist, as in dialysis for ethylene glycol overdoses. Hemoperfusion and lipid dialysis both serve as effective mechanisms in eliminating specific offending substances from the body, e.g., ethchlorvynol. To be effective, a significant proportion of the total body toxin must be present in the blood and must not be tightly bound to serum protein. For many compounds, such as digoxin, tricyclic antidepressants, and phenothiazines, these conditions are not met, and dialysis and hemoperfusion do little to reduce the total body burden of toxin. Knowledge of the "apparent volume of distribution" of a compound permits prediction of the usefulness of dialysis or hemoperfusion (see Ch. 78.1).

Occasionally, still other techniques, such as *exchange transfusions* in boric acid or iron poisoning, may be useful. So-called *gut lavage*, a virtually continuous through-and-through rinse of the bowel via instillation of large amounts of physiologic fluids into the intestine through a nasogastric tube, has been reported effective in paraquat overdoses when no alternatives exist. Careful consideration of the metabolic pathways of the involved substance combined with empiric evidence of previous outcomes serves as the best guide for management.

Treatment of Specific Common Poisonings. In addition to the general principles of treatment discussed above, a few common poisonings warrant specific mention.

Aspirin (salicylate) poisoning formerly accounted for 20 per cent of ingestions among children under 5 years of age; today, it is responsible for only 1 to 2 per cent. However, it remains a concern for all age groups—particularly because of its widespread use as a potential suicidal agent among the elderly. Acute ingestions in excess of 100 mg per kilogram of body weight deserve induction of emesis; aspirin leads to rapid metabolic acidosis in children under 4 years of age and to initial respiratory alkalosis in the adult. Both groups vomit; this permits early detection and helps in differentiation from acetaminophen ingestion. Alkalinizing the urine proves remarkably effective with the single acute ingestion; one should consult the Done nomogram for prognosis. The administration of intravenous $NaHCO_3$ (3 mEq per kilogram of body weight) to young children usually proves effective in raising urine pH above 7.0. A later second or third dose of approximately one half of that amount may be necessary to sustain alkalinization of the urine and thereby promote ionization and reduce reabsorption of salicylate. The use of acetazolamide to alkalinize the urine should be avoided; its mechanism of action also accelerates transport of salicylate into the central nervous system (CNS). Urinary elimination of the salicylate moiety removes the cause of the acidosis—a far more effective approach to therapy than treatment of the systemic acidosis itself. In the adult, initial blood pH may be elevated; nonetheless, it is the urine pH that is critical to monitor. In general, additional potassium administration is necessary only for the chronically intoxicated patient or later in the course of acute intoxications in adults. Occasionally dialysis may be warranted, but ordinarily general supportive measures prove sufficient. Chronic overdoses are far less responsive to any specific interventions, but supportive treatment can be crucial.

Acetaminophen has captured 30 per cent of today's analgesic-antipyretic market; liquid formulations are being augmented by solid preparation forms, some of which are in "extra strength" dosages. In Britain, acetaminophen has been a particularly popular suicidal substance; management is often complicated by the fact that no significant symptoms may appear until after irreversible liver damage has occurred. If recognized early—preferably less than 8 hours and certainly less than 16 hours after ingestion—determination of the serum level and comparison of it against standards on the Matthews-Rumack nomogram permit an appropriate decision about the possible use of an antidote, either N-acetylcysteine or methionine (both sulfhydryl donors). Both appear to enter into metabolic pathways via glutathione mechanisms and to preclude the formation of an epoxide derivative of acetaminophen that binds covalently to liver macromolecules, resulting in liver cell destruction. An intravenous preparation of the antidote is available that is strongly favored and widely used in Britain; it ought to be available in the United States soon. Currently, only an oral form is available in the United States, and its use presents difficulties because of associated emesis. Of special note is the apparent diminished susceptibility to toxicity in the preadolescent compared with the adult.

Significant overdoses of *anticholinergic substances* in various forms (e.g., tricyclic antidepressants, atropine, antihistamines, phenothiazines, jimson weed) produce fever, flushing, widely dilated pupils, and CNS signs and symptoms varying from somnolence and coma to delirium and seizures. Each of these specific drugs may also produce additional specific symptoms by other mechanisms—e.g., diphenhydramine hydrochloride (Benadryl) occasionally results in extrapyramidal reactions; tricyclic antidepressants cause cardiac arrhythmias. For this class of drugs, physostigmine is available both as a diagnostic agent and as a therapeutic substance; because administration of physostigmine may itself induce seizures in 15 to 20 per cent of treated patients, its use has declined significantly. The dose is 0.5 mg administered slowly intravenously for the child under 5 and 1 to 2 mg for the adult, repeated as often as necessary to control seizures. Today, however, most centers rely on diazepam treatment instead. In all instances atropine should be immediately available during physostigmine infusion, and Valium also ought to be available should a convulsion occur. Tricyclic antidepressant overdoses are now numerically the most serious of prescription medicine hazards. These are best approached by using diazepam (Valium) or phenobarbital to control seizures, by maintaining a blood pH above 7.45 to prevent tachyarrhythmias either by administering $NaHCO_3$ or by controlled ventilation in the obtunded patient, and by use of conventional cardiac drugs should arrhythmias ensue.

Acute petroleum distillates (hydrocarbons) cause their most significant damage as a function of their initial action on the lungs via aspiration; such aspiration occurs at the time of ingestion or inhalation. Both in laboratory animals and in humans, large amounts of various petroleum distillates have been consumed and retained without development of any signs or symptoms save for odoriferous eructations ("smelly burps") and diarrhea. As a general rule, neither lavage nor induction of emesis is indicated in such ingestions unless some additional toxin (e.g., parathion) has been dissolved in the hydrocarbon. When such is the case, induction of emesis has supplanted gastric lavage as the treatment of choice. When pulmonary aspiration has occurred, supportive measures are introduced; antibiotics and steroids are widely used but without much evidence of effectiveness.

Use patterns of anticonvulsants have changed in recent years with the advent of valproic acid and the increased use of carbamazepine (Tegretol). Valproic acid overdoses are similar to those of other sedatives and, in fact, are often less severe. However, valproic acid interacts with other drugs, particularly other sedatives, potentiating their actions. The greatest concerns are hepatic necrosis and a Reye-like syndrome. Valproic acid should be avoided during pregnancy because it is associated with an increase in fetal neural tube defects. Carbamazepine, also a potential teratogen, is noted for its propensity to induce seizures in the overdosed patient, who otherwise appears to be heavily sedated. No specific antidote is available; routine supportive therapy is used. Techniques aimed at enhancing excretion, other than use of repetitive doses of oral activated charcoal, have not been proven satisfactory and are thus not advised.

Carbon monoxide (see Ch. 528) ranks high as a contributor to common poisonings, suicides, and accidental deaths. The mechanism of action involves acute interruption of both oxygen transport and oxygen metabolism, with a rapid cessation of life functions. Prompt recognition of exposure and removal of the patient from the contaminated environment are essential. Hastening of excretion of carbon monoxide by administration of oxygen and consideration of hyperbaric oxygen treatment are currently the hallmarks of management.

Caustic compounds, including acids and alkalis, appear to exert their toxic effects largely via alterations of pH and their consequences on the gastrointestinal tract. Experimental evidence suggests that the damage done by alkalis is complete within 30 seconds after exposure; that done by acids may be somewhat slower to appear. Current recommendations for management are avoidance of major efforts to empty the gastrointestinal tract, neutralization of the offending compound by the administration of a protein-containing substance (such as milk), and careful assessment of the esophagus for the possibility of acute burns. This last point frequently necessitates esophagoscopy because the presence or absence of burns in the mouth proves nonpredictive of the status of the esophagus. In addition to concerns about the acute situation—managed by dilatation, steroids, and antibiotics—much interest now focuses on follow-up for 20 to 40 years because of a significantly increased risk of carcinoma of the esophagus.

Cyanide has gained its deserved reputation for toxicity by its ability to inhibit oxygen utilization at the level of the cell via cytochrome oxidase inhibition; severe metabolic acidosis can occur almost instantaneously. Most exposures are occupational; occasional exposures are the result of homicidal efforts, particularly associated with capsule tampering, and rare consequences are found subsequent to *l*-mandelonitrile-β-glucuronic acid (Laetrile) administration or nitroprusside overdose. As soon as cyanide poisoning is suspected, administration of nitrite—via a 3 per cent solution intravenously or amyl nitrite inhalation—is crucial. It converts hemoglobin to methemoglobin, which selectively binds cyanide. This is followed by administration of sodium thiosulfate to convert cyanide to the less toxic thiocyanate. Recent experience in Europe suggests the use of dicobalt edetate may be even more effective—but avoidance is the goal.

Drugs of abuse haunt the profession, the emergency room, and our society. Were the offending agent easily identified with certainty—e.g., heroin—the immediate remedy would be obvious—naloxone. Such instances are almost nonexistent; more than 90 per cent of what is bought and sold "on the street" is not what it has been represented to be. Even imprinted capsules have been counterfeited in efforts to "con" the buyer. In other instances the basic ingredient has been "cut" with an inert substance or "laced" with some other psychoactive substance. Enormous geographic variations seem to exist across the country, with phencyclidine ("angel dust," PCP) being particularly popular in Los Angeles and Detroit, Ritalin in Seattle, and heroin and cocaine ("crack") in New York.

The laboratory may be helpful in instances of opiate overdose but is of virtually no value for lysergic acid diethylamide (LSD) or PCP (see Ch. 15). As a consequence, symptomatic management predominates; the unconscious or convulsing adult may routinely be approached as a potential heroin addict, an alcoholic, or a hypoglycemic individual; the hyperactive, "spacey" patient prompts consideration of PCP, LSD, and related sympathomimetic agents (amphetamine, phenylpropanolamine, etc.), as well as recreational cocaine or psychosocial decompensation. Supportive measures may include monitoring, restraints, sedatives (diazepam is "customary"), succinylcholine, hydration, and ventilatory and cardiac measures. As a generalization, the acute management proves far more successful than treatment of the underlying problem, but efforts ought to be directed at the latter, as it provides the only true solution to the basic problem.

Ethyl alcohol (see Ch. 14) is mentioned here to stress its ubiquity and the epidemiologic point that it is remarkably prevalent as a cause of admission to hospital for children, with both purposeful and accidental ingestions, as well as a cause of birth defects among newborns. Also, ethyl alcohol augments the potential toxicity of a number of other compounds, such as diazepam.

Halogenated hydrocarbons (including chlorinated insecticides such as chlorophenothane, or DDT) serve as a source of a myriad of occupational, industrial, and pharmacologic exposures. Almost invariably lipid soluble, most are readily absorbable by the gastrointestinal tract, the respiratory epithelium, or the skin. Fortunately, most are metabolically rather stable compounds within the human organism; thus reproduction of still more hazardous metabolites is minimized. Nonetheless, many of the compounds gain access to fat storage deposits or neural tissue and cause both central and peripheral nervous system symptoms. For some (e.g., 2,3,7,8-tetrachlorodibenzodioxin, or dioxin) there are concerns about long-term toxicity and teratogenicity. Treatment modes include elimination of subsequent exposures, attempts to retrieve unabsorbed quantities from the gastrointestinal tract, and general supportive measures in response to symptoms.

Iron salts ($FeSO_4$, Fe gluconate) represent a hazard confined almost exclusively to children who "accidentally" consume prenatal tablets. Recently increasing numbers of iron poisoning have been recognized in adults. While initial reports of a 50 per cent mortality rate were greatly inflated (instead it hovers at approximately 1 per cent), iron poisoning typifies the problem of the "unsuspected toxin" about which parents, parent surrogates, and physicians may be uninformed. When ingestions are known to exceed 50 to 60 mg per kilogram or when serum levels (taken 3 to 6 hours after ingestion) exceed 400 to 500 μg per deciliter, observation and chelation with desferrioxamine ought to be seriously considered, particularly if clinical symptoms such as upper abdominal pain, nausea, and vomiting are present. Management of the acute ingestion calls for prompt gastric emptying and efforts to minimize absorption of the iron salts. More serious overdoses have prompted heroic measures, including surgical extirpation of ingested tablets and attempts at exchange transfusion. To date, studies have documented no serious consequences from ingestion of iron as a component of children's chewable vitamin preparations despite predictions to the contrary.

Methanol and *ethylene glycol* present significant problems of metabolic acidosis in clinically poisoned patients. Diagnosis is often considered following discovery of an unexplained anion gap. These compounds both depend upon alcohol dehydrogenase for their metabolism. The current approach to therapy takes advantage of this situation and provides ethanol (5 to 10 grams per hour intravenously) as a competitive inhibitor of toxin metabolism—thus slowing the formation of toxic metabolites, formaldehyde, and formic acid from methanol, or glycoaldehyde and glycolic, glyoxylic, and oxalic acids from ethylene glycol, to rates of formation permitting these products to be disposed of by ordinary metabolic or excretory pathways. For emphasis, an alternative approach currently employed in Europe involves 4-methyl-pyrazole administered to block alcohol dehydrogenase activity, thus accomplishing the same objective as that sought with ethyl alcohol. It is likely to be available in the United States soon. In the meantime, for large overdoses hemodialysis may be required to eliminate the offending toxin.

Organophosphate and carbamate insecticides can both prove exquisitely toxic in minute amounts. The mechanism of action involves inhibition of acetylcholine metabolism via cessation of cholinesterase function. Prompt recognition of symptoms secondary to acute exposure can prove lifesaving. Detecting symptoms secondary to chronic exposure (e.g., peripheral neuropathy) can serve to eliminate much patient distress and employee unhappiness. In general, acute distress is ushered in via excessive secretions in the upper airway, with respiratory distress, diffuse muscular weakness, nausea, vomiting, and collapse. Treatment requires prompt and repeated administration of large amounts of atropine for both types of poisoning. Pralidoxime (2PAM) is also strongly recommended to assist in the rejuvenation of cholinesterase levels. Introduced in large measure as a "safer" replacement for DDT, these compounds have been responsible for large numbers of acute poisonings but, as far as can be determined, are yet to be implicated in carcinogenicity, teratogenicity, or chronic liver disease.

Paraquat (and its associated congeners) is a particularly popular and effective herbicide. While controversy rages about the consequences of environmental exposures, no controversy exists on the issue of acute, purposeful overdoses; they are devastating. Paraquat is a harsh gastrointestinal irritant that also inhibits renal function; its most destructive impact is on the respiratory tract, where it inhibits superoxide dismutase and kills via "oxygen toxicity." Current approaches to therapy favor such dramatic efforts as "gut lavage," with some suggestion that hemoperfusion might be warranted. However, overdoses are likely to be lethal.

Theophylline and its congeners have been recognized as inducing seizures, cardiac arrhythmias, and occasional deaths in overdose situations. More recently, "therapeutic misadventures" have been recognized; inadvertent overdoses, alterations of theophylline metabolism by viral infections and nutritional variations, and the tendency to use theophylline in large quantities for relatively minor illnesses all increase the likelihood of such occurrences. Beta blockers can be used in managing the clinical symptoms of overdose—particularly the associated anxiety and tachycardia—but should not be used in asthmatic individuals. Children seem more resistant to the serious side effects than do adults, but occasionally both groups may have to be considered for hemoperfusion. Peritoneal and extracorporeal hemodialysis have both been reported to be ineffective.

Although ingestions of *plants and plant elements* constitute the single most frequent reason for telephoning poison centers, the overall problem is best put in perspective by Fraser's analysis of Britain's most recent 20-year experience with poisonings:

> Plants are the most overrated poisons of childhood. In earlier decades there were occasional deaths, most caused by the umbelliferae (particularly hemlock water dropwort) and the solanaceae (various nightshades). From 1958 to 1977 there were three deaths, and in one the role of the ingestion in the child's demise is doubtful. The others were caused by hemlock and by *Amanita phalloides* (death cup), both in children aged five and nine. Laburnum is frequently cited as the most toxic and commonly fatal poisonous plant in both children and adults, but there appears to be no report this century of childhood poisoning death. One adult death in unusual circumstances has been recorded.

Confirming this observation is the fact that the more than 90,000 plant ingestions reported to poison centers in 1988 led to but a single death—of an adult who ate water hemlock.

CONCLUSION. Chemical hazards have always been a way of life. Today their numbers continue to escalate. But modern technology permits both identification and quantification of minuscule amounts of some toxins—uncovering, for example, tamperings with cyanides. At the same time, "media hype" may distort risks—for example, with regard to the purported dangers of methamphetamine laboratories—to such an extent that the prudent physician is overcome with frustration. As a consequence, while the physician is well advised to add possible poisoning to the differential diagnosis for any unexplained collection of signs or symptoms in a patient of any age, unless he or she is confident of the timeliness and completeness of his or her understanding about a specific item, additional consultation is strongly advised.

Arena J, Drew RH: Poisoning: Chemistry, Symptoms and Treatment. 5th ed. Springfield, Ill., Charles C Thomas, 1986. *Derived from years of experience and leadership in the poisoning field, this book is well organized, carefully edited, and readable, with a remarkable collection of cases and common sense.*

Bryson PD. Comprehensive Review in Toxicology. Rockville, Md., Aspen Publishers, 1989. *Authored by an experienced practicing medical toxicologist, this remarkably thorough text clarifies a number of significant clinical concerns.*

Dreisbach RH, Robertson WO: Handbook of Poisoning. 12th ed. Los Altos, Calif., Lange Publishing Company, 1987. *This pocket-sized book is both comprehensive and concise. Up-to-date and always helpful to review for omissions in one's approach, it proves particularly valuable to the primary care physician.*

Ellenhorn MJ, Barceloux DG: Medical Toxicology: Diagnosis and Treatment of Human Poisoning, New York, Elsevier, 1988. *The latest and by far most comprehensive and complete human toxicology text; lucidly written, particularly well indexed, and appropriately clinical in its management recommendations.*

Goldfrank LR, Flomenbaum N, Lewin N, et al.: Toxicologic Emergencies. 4th ed. Norwalk, CT, Appleton-Century-Crofts, 1990. *Probably the most clinically relevant and readable of all the texts available, it summarizes a remarkable amount of experience in readily retrievable form—and in a format aimed at anticipating the reader's needs.*

Gosselin RE, Hodge HC, Smith RP: Clinical Toxicology of Commercial Products.

5th ed. Baltimore, Williams & Wilkins Company, 1984. *Long established as the "bible" of the field, this compendium provides a concise overview of poisoning issues, as well as a thorough and well-edited clinical description of approximately 50 generic poisonings. It has a comprehensive listing of trade-name entities and generic items in household and commercial product fields. Authoritative the world over.*

Haddad LM, Winchester JF: Clinical Management of Poisoning and Drug Overdose. 2nd ed. Philadelphia, W. B. Saunders Company, 1990. *A recent book with contributions chiefly by American experts, this is currently a most comprehensive text for the recognition and clinical management of poisoning.*

Klaassen CD, Amdur MD, Doull J: Toxicology: The Basic Science of Poisons. 3rd ed. New York, Macmillan, 1986. *This text constitutes the "compleat" basic science approach for the toxicologist. With 42 contributors and critical editing, the final product covers the field from salt to water to radiation.*

Journals: Virtually any clinical journal may prove the source of a fascinating case report or a valuable review in the field of poisoning. Lancet, JAMA, N Engl J Med, and the traditional medical and pediatric specialty journals are particularly valuable resources. In the more limited field of clinical toxicology the following are of note: (1) Veterinary and Human Toxicology: The official journal of the American Association of Poison Control Centers and the American Academy of Clinical Toxicology, always updating the clinical field. (2) The American Journal of Emergency Medicine, published by W. B. Saunders Company, whose September issue annually provides nationwide incidence data from the American Association of Poison Control Centers (AAPCC). (3) Clinical Toxicology: A blend of industrial, environmental, and accidental cases appears here, together with results of bench research. (4) Emergency Medicine: A controlled circulation journal particularly noted for "The Toxic Emergency," a periodic contribution of Donald Kunkel. (5) The Annals of Emergency Medicine, focusing on many acute toxic episodes.

29 NSAID's: Aspirin and Aspirin-like Drugs

Gerald Weissmann

HISTORY

Salicylates as Antipyretics and Analgesics

On June 2, 1763, the Royal Society received a communication from Reverend Edmund Stone of Chipping Norton in Oxfordshire. Its opening lines are probably unmatched in clinical pharmacology:

> Among the many useful discoveries which this age has made, there are very few which better deserve the attention of the public than what I am going to lay before your Lordship. There is a bark of an English tree, which I have found by experience to be a powerful astringent and very efficacious in curing aguish and intermittent disorders.

The tree was the willow (*Salix alba*), the astringent bark of which contains salicin, the glycoside of salicylic acid. Stone had discovered that salicylates reduced the fever and aches produced by a variety of acute, shiver-provoking illnesses, or agues.

In 1990, the salicylate most commonly used is acetylsalicylic acid, aspirin. At over-the-counter doses (1 to 3 grams per day) aspirin is *analgesic* and *antipyretic*. In addition, at lower doses (80 to 325 mg per day) aspirin is used to prevent coronary and cerebral thrombosis by virtue of its *antiplatelet* effect. And for 100 years very high doses (4 to 8 grams per day) have been used to reduce the redness and swelling of joints in rheumatic fever, gout, and rheumatoid arthritis.

Salicylates also have a wide variety of other biologic effects, only some of which are related to their current use in clinical medicine. Salicylates can dissolve corns on the toes, a *keratolytic* effect; provoke loss of uric acid from the kidneys, their *uricosuric* property; and kill bacteria in vitro, their *antiseptic* action. Aspirin inhibits the formation of prostaglandins and thereby inhibits the clotting of blood, induces peptic ulcers, and promotes fluid retention by the kidney. Cell biologists use aspirin and salicylates to inhibit anion transport across cell membranes, to interfere with the activation of white cells, and to uncouple oxidative phosphorylation by isolated mitochondria. Botanists use salicylates to induce flowering of *Impatiens;* indeed, the function of salicylates in plants such as the voodoo lily or skunk cabbage is

to induce temperature rises of 12 to 16°C in the course of efflorescence. Salicylates therefore not only reduce fever but also produce it! Finally, molecular biologists use salicylates to activate genes that code for heat-shock proteins in the lampbrush chromosomes of *Drosophila*.

"About six years ago," wrote Stone in his letter to the Royal Society, "I accidentally tasted [the willow bark], and was surprised at its extraordinary bitterness; which immediately raised in me a suspicion of its having the properties of the Peruvian bark." Peruvian bark (*cinchona*) was a venerable remedy for the ague. Stone proceeded to offer a skillful rationale for the use of willow bark in febrile disorders: the traditional doctrine of signatures—i.e., that "many natural maladies carry their cures along with them, or their remedies lie not far from their cause." Since moist shires, like those drained by the Avon or Isis, abound in both fevers and willows, Rev. Stone set out to test whether the former might be cured by the latter. Six years of careful clinical observation and the treatment of 50 patients with willow extracts prepared in water, tea, or beer culminated in his letter to the Royal Society. The eighteenth century had found a predictable remedy for fever.

Hippocrates (fourth century B.C.) had advocated the chewing of willow leaves for relief of the pains of childbirth, and there are references by Pliny (first century) and Galen (second century) to the *analgesic* property of willow, but it remained for Stone to put extract of willow bark into our pharmacopoeia as an effective *antipyretic* agent.

By 1828, at the Pharmacologic Institute of Munich, Buchner isolated a tiny amount of the active glycoside, salicin, in the form of bitter-tasting, yellow, needle-like crystals. Two years later, Leroux in Paris improved on the extraction procedure and obtained 1 ounce of salicin from 3 pounds of the bark. By 1838, Raffaele Pira of Pisa, writing in the *Comtes Rendu de l'Academie de Science*, described how he obtained a pure substance from salicin by hydrolyzing the glycoside in a CrO_3-mediated oxidation via an aldehyde intermediate. He gave it the name by which we know it today: "*l'acide salicylique*," or salicylic acid. Willow bark was not alone in providing a rich natural source of salicylates. Meadowsweet (*Spireae ulmaria*) yielded ample quantities of an ether-soluble oil from which a *Spirsäure* was crystallized in 1835 by the Swiss chemist Karl Jakob Lowig. In 1839 Dumas demonstrated that the *Spirsäure* of Lowig was nothing else than the *acide salicylique* of Piriâ. Another Gallic pharmacologist, Auguste Andre Thomas Cahours (1843), showed that oil of wintergreen—a traditional remedy for aguish disorders—contained the methyl ester of salicylic acid and prepared *acide salicylique* from it.

As was to be the case in much of nineteenth century chemistry, French and British scientists were slightly ahead of the Germans in the study of natural products, whereas Germans held the edge in synthetic know-how. Forced to compete with the French and British dye industries which supplied their textile mills with pigments imported from overseas colonies, the Germans replied by inventing cheap aniline dyes, creating in their train such giant enterprises as I. G. Farben. By 1833, the pharmacist E. Merck of Darmstadt had obtained a clean preparation of salicin which was cheaper by half than the impure willow extracts used as antipyretics, but a cheap, pure, acceptable remedy was not available until 1860, when Kolbe and his students at Marburg succeeded in the first synthesis of salicylic acid and its sodium salt from phenol, CO_2, and sodium. Using industrial variations of the Kolbe synthesis, one of his students, Friedrich von Heyden, established in 1874 the first large factory in Dresden devoted to the production of synthetic salicylates. The availability of cheap salicylic acid spread its clinical use far and wide.

Salicylates as Anti-inflammatory Drugs

The first successful treatment of acute rheumatism was reported in 1876 by Stricker and Ries in the *Berliner Medizinische Wochenschrifft* and by Maclagan writing in *The Lancet*. Stricker and Ries reported the complete cure of acute "polyarthritis rheumatica" by sodium salicylate at doses of 5 to 6 grams per day. Almost simultaneously, Maclagan reported his results with salicylic acid and salicin at similar dosage levels; he paid tribute to the still prevalent doctrine of signatures, pointing out that cases of acute rheumatism were most abundant in moist areas where the willow grows.

Stricker and Ries and Maclagan had demonstrated a clinical property of high-dose salicylates that was not to be tested in the laboratory until the 1930's: They found that salicylates reduce not only fever and pain but also redness and swelling. That anti-inflammatory property was next used to advantage by the Parisian, Germain See, who in 1877 introduced salicylates (both *acid salicylique* and salicin) as effective treatments for gout and "chronic poly-arthritis." See had great success among his well-off clientele with the use of salicylates in acute and chronic gout, so great indeed that the *British Medical Journal*, in an editorial note, called him to task for charging up to 80 pounds sterling to treat a patient with gout by means of 6 to 8 grams of sodium salicylate per day, when the price of the drug was but 5 pence per gram! There the matter rested, with high doses of sodium salicylate more or less accepted as a new treatment in many rheumatic diseases, while lower doses (1.5 to 2.0 grams per day) seemed to relieve aches and pains.

Aspirin

In 1898 a new chapter was written: Felix Hofmann was an aniline dye chemist at the Friedrich Bayer–Eberfeld division of the I. G. Farben cartel when his father complained to him of gastric irritation from the sodium salicylate he was taking for "rheumatism." Hofmann searched the chemical literature for less acidic derivatives and hit upon acetyl derivatives of sodium salicylate first described by G. Von Gilm in 1859 and 10 years later by a certain H. Kraut (sic). Although von Gilm and Kraut had outlined synthesis of the compound, they had no notion of what its biologic effects might be. Hofmann repeated the synthesis (via acetic anhydride) and tried acetylsalicylic acid first on himself and then on his father: It proved more palatable, less irritating to the stomach, and—he claimed—more effective. Hofmann took the material to his supervisor, Heinrich Dreser, head of Bayer's laboratory of pharmacology, who reported that aspirin performed better both in laboratory and in clinic and called the new drug *aspirin*, the a from *acetyl* and the *spirin* from the German *Spirsäure*.

The Aniline Derivatives as Analgesics and Antipyretics

Competitors entered the field as the markets expanded for other drugs that could reduce fever and pain. Based on anecdotal accounts from the Alsace that a product formed from aniline treated with vinegar made a useful febrifuge, Karl Morner in 1889 synthesized the material—acetanilide—and isolated its metabolites. Acetanilide itself, unfortunately, caused bone marrow depression and anemias in a distinct number of patients, so other derivatives were sought. Acetanilide and the widely used phenacetin are metabolized to *N-acetyl-p-aminophenol*, which by various anagramatic combinations yields the generic names *acetaminophen* in the United States and *paracetamol* in the United Kingdom. In 1955 acetaminophen acquired a tradename in the United States that was to make it famous: *Tylenol*—also from ace*tyl*-p-aminoph*enol*.

NSAID's vs. Cortisone

Neither acetanilide nor phenacetin proved as useful as aspirin in the treatment of rheumatic fever or rheumatoid arthritis: They were not anti-inflammatory. For half a century (1900–1950) clinicians appreciated that there was something unique about high-dose salicylates. At levels over 4 grams per day, only salicylates—of all the analgesics—were anti-inflammatory. They also brought under control the erythrocyte sedimentation rate and levels of C-reactive protein in serum. Indeed, when James Reid in 1948 demonstrated an inverse relationship between plasma salicylate levels and signs of rheumatic inflammation, he asked "Does sodium salicylate cure rheumatic fever?" The answer came from well-controlled and definitive studies in the 1950's that were prompted by the discovery of ACTH and cortisone, the most potent anti-inflammatory compounds ever described.

Each of over two dozen studies concluded that neither steroids (cortisone and its derivatives) nor salicylates (aspirin or sodium salicylate) actually cure rheumatic fever or rheumatoid arthritis—and that in the short run both types of agents are equally effective at suppressing acute inflammation. Since the course of acute rheumatic fever is easier to document than that of rheumatoid arthritis, it is worth paying attention today to the back-to-back trials of steroids versus aspirin and sodium salicylate. These were performed by the Medical Research Council of Britain and the American Heart Association (reported in 1955) and the Combined Rheumatic Fever Study Group of the United States (reported in 1961) and showed that salicylates at doses high enough to yield plasma levels of 25 to 35 mg per deciliter (6 to 9 grams per day) were as effective anti-inflammatory agents as cortisone or prednisone in rheumatic fever.

NSAID MODE OF ACTION: INHIBITION OF PROSTAGLANDIN SYNTHESIS

Unfortunately, until 1971 no useful hypothesis had emerged as to how salicylates exert their various effects. Pharmacologists had shown that salicylate analgesia was due to a peripheral effect—as opposed to morphine's central action. In contrast, physiologists maintained that salicylates did not reduce fever by peripheral action but worked directly on the fever centers of the hypothalamus. Renal physiologists found that low doses of salicylates raised uric acid in the blood by blocking tubular secretion by the kidney while, paradoxically, high doses of salicylates lowered uric acid by blocking its tubular absorption. Clinicians found that the latter property explained the utility of salicylates in both acute and chronic gout. It was more difficult to explain how aspirin inhibited platelet function, caused salt and water retention, and provoked severe dyspepsia. And why did some patients develop nasal polyps, with sniffles and wheezes: aspirin "hyper-sensitivity"?

The most important recent contribution to the story of aspirin-like drugs was made by John Vane (now Sir John) at the Royal College of Surgeons in London in 1971. Vane had been impressed that many forms of tissue injury are followed by release of prostaglandins, the oxidation products of arachidonic acid. Prostaglandins E_1 and F_2 had been shown to be associated with acute vasodilation and fever. Vane and his colleagues found that aspirin-like drugs inhibited the biosynthesis of prostaglandins E_2 and $F_2\alpha$ from radiolabeled arachidonic acid in studies in vitro. Moreover, they found that platelets taken from volunteers given aspirin and indomethacin 1 hour before venipuncture failed to make prostaglandins in response to thrombin, and that catecholamine-induced release of prostaglandins from canine spleens could be inhibited by indomethacin—albeit less consistently than by aspirin or sodium salicylate.

All that remained was to show how and when prostaglandins caused redness and swelling with heat and pain and to study the exact means whereby aspirin-like drugs inhibited the enzyme that transformed arachidonic acid to the stable prostaglandins E_1 and E_2, etc. The enzyme has been found to be a 70-kDa homodimer localized to microsomal membranes; it has been cloned and sequenced and was first called "prostaglandin synthase," then "cyclo-oxygenase," and today is known as "prostaglandin H synthase" (Fig. 29–1). This single enzyme catalyzes two reactions: the bis-deoxygenation of arachidonic acid to form prostaglandin H_2 (cyclo-oxygenase activity) and the reduction of hydroperoxides to the corresponding alcohols. This enzyme therefore produces stable prostaglandins of the E and F series via the unstable *endoperoxide* intermediates, PGG_2 and PGH_2. The endoperoxides, which are critical for platelet function, are transformed by platelets to a most potent vasoconstricting and platelet-aggregating substance, thromboxane B_2. Meanwhile, Vane had isolated a potent vasodilator, prostacyclin (prostaglandin I_2), which was also made from arachidonate by the cyclo-oxygenase of endothelial cells. Since platelets make thromboxane B_2, which constricts the smooth muscle of blood vessels, and since blood vessel walls make prostacyclin I_2, which powerfully relaxes blood vessels and inhibits platelet aggregation, the hunt was on for ways of inhibiting the synthesis of thromboxane but not prostacyclin.

Vane and his associates in the 1970's had amassed convincing evidence that the prostaglandin hypothesis of aspirin action was largely correct. They pointed out that almost all aspirin-like drugs (by then generally called "nonsteroidal anti-inflammatory drugs," or NSAID's) inhibited prostaglandin synthetase and that the potency of these drugs (ID_{50}) in this regard pretty much paralleled their clinical potency or their effect in experimental animals; e.g., aspirin was anywhere from one fortieth to one two-hundredth as active as indomethacin and from one fifth to one fiftieth as active as ibuprofen. Indeed, by 1990, over 40 NSAID's had reached the clinic and each of them at one dose or another inhibits the synthetase. It should also be noted, however, that since 1971, inhibition of PG synthetase has been a sine qua non for their introduction! Only NSAID's, but not central analegesics such as morphine or codeine, inhibited PG synthetase, nor did antihistamines, antiserotonin drugs, cortisone, and its analogues. Moreover, concentrations of NSAID's that could be achieved in the circulation (allowing for protein binding) were in excess of those required to inhibit the enzyme in disrupted cell preparations.

Vane and his colleagues argued that stable prostaglandins not only were produced at sites of inflammation, but alone or in concert with other mediators could provoke all the cardinal signs of inflammation. Indeed, prostaglandins E_1 and E_2 *do* induce vasodilation; they promote edema when dilated blood vessels have been made leaky by histamine; they produce fever when injected either into the cerebral ventricles or directly into the anterior hypothalamus; and they sensitize pain receptors of the skin to such other pain-provoking humors as bradykinin and histamine. Sound explanations were offered for a few troubling discrepancies. Acetaminophen was ineffective at inhibiting prostaglandin synthesis by enzyme preparations from a variety of tissues but was effective against the synthetase from brain. And although nonacetylated salicylates were roughly one tenth as potent as aspirin in vitro, studies of urinary prostaglandin metabolites showed that sodium salicylate effectively diminished excretion of these metabolites in man. Sodium salicylate also effectively reduced prostaglandin release in models of experimental inflammation in animals.

NSAID SIDE EFFECTS

Perhaps the most persuasive aspect of the prostaglandin hypothesis was its explanation of the clinical side effects of NSAID's. A major problem with NSAID's at anti-inflammatory doses is that they provoke stomach irritation and sometimes ulceration. Aspirin is the worst offender in this regard. This irritative property is due to the need for endogenous prostaglandins by the gastric mucosa in order to regulate its overproduction of acid and to synthesize the mucous barrier that prevents its self-digestion. But now an *exogenous* prostaglandin E_1 analogue (misoprostol) has been approved for the prevention and treatment of NSAID-induced ulcers.

Moreover, most NSAID's prevent the body from excreting salt and water properly, especially when heart or liver disease compromises renal blood flow. NSAID's block the formation of the vasodilator PGI_2 by kidney cells, and renal blood supply is reduced even further. Another side effect of NSAID's—but not sodium salicylate—is induction of the aspirin sensitivity syndrome in those genetically susceptible: wheezing, sneezing, and polyp formation. Nowadays, thanks to the elucidation of arachidonic acid metabolism, we attribute these consequences to the diversion of arachidonate from blocked PGH synthase to the 5-lipoxygenase pathway which is not inhibited by NSAID's. It is by means of the lipoxygenase pathways that leukotrienes C, D, and E are formed, and these have been implicated in aspirin hypersensitivity.

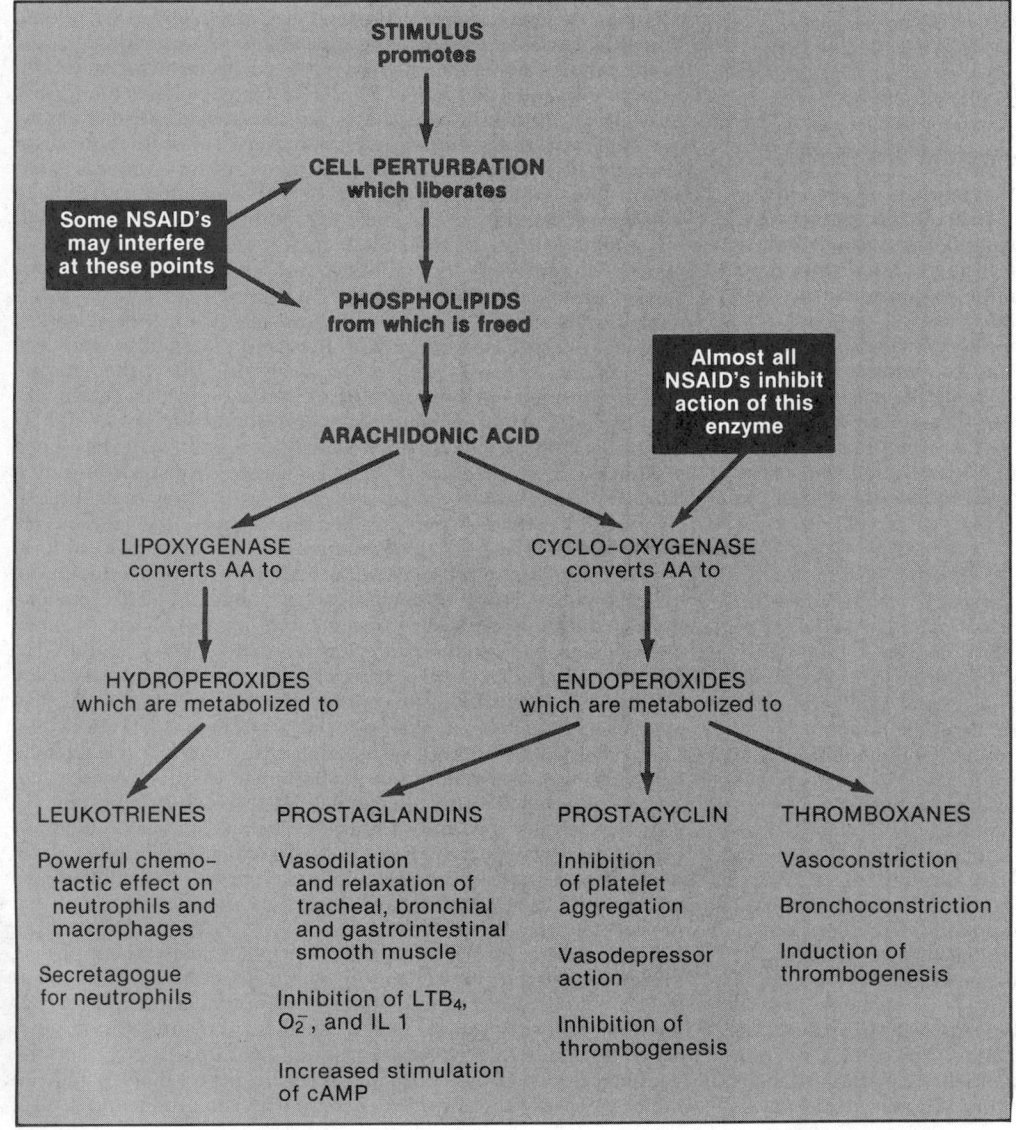

FIGURE 29–1. The inflammatory cascade. LTB_4 = leukotriene B_4; O_2^- = super-oxide anion; IL 1 = interleukin 1; cAMP = cyclic adenosine monophosphate.

Finally, the most common side effect of NSAID's, and especially of aspirin, is their interference with platelet function. Patients on these drugs sometimes suffer from untoward bleeding after tooth extraction, minor surgery, or trauma. Weiss and Aledort in 1967 showed that aspirin inhibits normal platelet aggregation both in vitro and in vivo. All NSAID's that inhibit PGH synthase—again with the exception of sodium salicylate—inhibit platelet function by blocking formation of endoperoxides and thromboxane A_2, which are intermediates in platelet stimulus-response coupling.

INHIBITION OF PGH$_2$ SYNTHASE

The interaction of NSAID's with the PGH synthase has been studied in detail at the molecular and physiologic levels. Lands and Kulmacz have shown that aspirin and indomethacin interact in a complex, biphasic fashion with the enzyme, whereas other NSAID's such as ibuprofen, naproxen, and meclofenamate simply interfere with binding of arachidonate to its oxidation site. Aspirin and indomethacin bind rapidly, in a reversible, competitive manner to the arachidonate-binding site, and then go on to inactivate the synthase irreversibly. Aspirin, moreover, acetylates serine residue 506 of the enzyme. When the PGH synthase is that of the platelet, it remains inactivated for the life of the cell, and thromboxane cannot be made. However, in endothelial cells, which can synthesize new enzyme, prostacylin synthesis is inhibited no more than a few days. Indeed, Fitzgerald has showed that low oral doses of aspirin (less than 325 mg per day) can irreversibly block the PGH synthase activity of a pool of platelets in the portal circulation *before* salicylate appears in the general circulation. These two observations explain why it is possible, by means of low-dose aspirin, to inhibit formation of the endoperoxides (PGG$_2$, PGH$_2$) and thromboxane A_2—all of which promote clotting and vasoconstriction—without inhibiting synthesis of prostacyclin (PGI$_2$), which inhibits platelet function and dilates blood vessels.

NSAID ACTIONS NOT DEPENDENT ON PROSTAGLANDINS

The hypothesis that the local production of prostaglandins leads to *inflammation* has been only partly substantiated. Whereas Vane's proposal that all NSAID's inhibit the transformation of arachidonic acid to stable prostaglandins (i.e., PGE$_2$ and PGI$_2$) has turned out to be largely correct, we lack sufficient evidence to generalize this proposition to all products of the arachidonic acid cascade and to all NSAID's at all dosages. The three major antipyretic, analgesic drugs exert diverse effects on prostaglandin biosynthesis. When used to treat rheumatic diseases in dosages of 4 to 8 grams, aspirin has antipyretic, anti-inflammatory, and analgesic effects and can inhibit the synthesis of prostaglandins in disrupted cell preparations. At the intermediate dosage indicated for analgesia (650 mg every 3 to 4 hours), aspirin has antipyretic and analgesic but not anti-inflammatory activity. And at its lowest clinical dosage (80 to 325 mg per day), aspirin exerts only its antiplatelet effect. Levels of salicylate in the plasma of individuals given intermediate, analgesic doses of aspirin are sufficient to inhibit prostaglandin biosynthesis in vivo by kidneys, platelets, and vascular endothelium, whereas the low levels of aspirin given to prevent thrombosis affect only prostaglandin synthesis by platelets. By contrast, rheumatologists have known since the 1950's that higher plasma concentrations (18 to 30 mg per deciliter) are required to achieve an anti-inflammatory effect. Those observations suggest two possibilities: Either the PGH synthase of cells that provoke inflammation is relatively insensitive to aspirin or aspirin at higher concentrations has a mode of action beyond its capacity to inhibit prostaglandin biosynthesis to which it owes its anti-inflammatory property.

Further evidence that aspirin-like drugs exert clinical effects that do not depend on inhibiting prostaglandin biosynthesis can be drawn from the properties of sodium salicylate and acetaminophen. Although sodium salicylate shares many of the properties of aspirin, it fails to inhibit prostaglandin biosynthesis in disrupted cell preparations at concentrations that may be achieved in plasma (approximately 5 mM). Moreover, clinical studies show that since nonacetylated salicylates do not inhibit platelet function in vitro or ex vivo, they do not cause bleeding. Indeed, acetaminophen, which also fails to inhibit prostaglandin biosynthesis, does not affect platelet aggregation, nor is it by any means anti-inflammatory. We must therefore conclude that pain and fever can effectively be reduced without inhibiting the synthesis of prostaglandins at all (Table 29–1).

PRO- AND ANTI-INFLAMMATORY PROPERTIES OF PROSTAGLANDINS

The Vane hypothesis is further weakened by findings from many laboratories, including our own, that stable prostaglandins (PGE$_1$, PGE$_2$, PGI$_2$) possess not only proinflammatory but also anti-inflammatory properties. It has been well appreciated that these compounds produce vasodilation, act in synergy with complement component C5a or leukotriene B4 to produce edema, mediate fever and myalgia in response to interleukin 1, and act in synergy with bradykinin to provoke pain. They also inhibit the function of T-suppressor cells. All of these are *proinflammatory* effects of prostaglandins.

On the other hand, Zurier and others had shown that high doses of these stable prostaglandins inhibit inflammation in animal models of arthritis, and much lower doses inhibit inflammation induced by local skin irritants. Since the early 1970's we have known that PGI$_2$ and stable prostaglandins of the E type inhibit the activation in vitro of neutrophils, platelets, and mononuclear phagocytes by interfering with their stimulus-response coupling. NSAID's increase cellular cAMP in these cells, levels of which are regulated via prostaglandin receptors. The relevance in vivo of these data obtained in vitro is supported by the observation that one can reduce experimental arthritis or glomerulonephritis in rats by treatment with systemic PGE$_1$. These are *anti-inflammatory* effects of prostaglandins.

As a class, NSAID's are planar, organic anions that partition across the lipid bilayers of plasma membranes in accordance with the Nernst equation. The more acidic the pH (as at inflammatory sites) the greater the lipophilicity of NSAID's, which subsequently interfere with cell function, including assembly of a superoxide anion–generating system by a cell-free, membrane-rich preparation from neutrophils, the activity of phospholipase C in mononuclear cells, the 12-hydroperoxyeicosatetraneonic acid peroxidase in platelets, and signal transduction in neutrophils and lymphocytes.

The first effect of aspirin-like drugs on cell metabolism was found to be the uncoupling of oxidative phosphorylation by isolated mitochondria; until Vane's work in 1971 this was held to be their major mode of action! More recent studies have shown that aspirin (but not acetaminophen) alters the uptake of precursor arachidonate and its insertion into the membranes of cultured human monocytes and macrophages. Salicylates also inhibit anion transport across a variety of cell membranes, including those of

TABLE 29–1. EFFECTS OF COMMONLY USED ANALGESIC AND ANTIPYRETIC AGENTS

	Acetylsalicylic Acid					
	Low Dose*	Intermediate Dose*	High Dose*	Sodium Salicylate	Newer NSAID's†	Acetaminophen
Antipyretic	0	+	+	+	+	+
Analgesic	0	+	+	+	+	+
Anti-inflammatory	0	0	+	+	+	+
Inhibit PG synthesis of platelets	+	+	+	0	+	0
Inhibit PG synthesis systemically	0	+	+	±	+	0

*Low dose, 80 to 325 mg per day; intermediate dose, 650 mg to 3 grams per day; high dose, >3 grams per day.
†Includes indomethacin, ibuprofen, naproxen, diclofenac, piroxicam.

the mammalian red cell and rabbit choroid plexus and renal tubular epithelium. Again, the capacity of salicylates to inhibit anion movements is not shared by acetaminophen. Finally, NSAID's inhibit synthesis of cartilage proteoglycan and bone metabolism (both in vitro and in vivo) by mechanisms that do not depend on the inhibition of the PGH synthase. It is a matter of clinical concern that some classes of NSAID's (e.g., salicylates), but not all (e.g., piroxicam), inhibit proteoglycan synthesis, thereby promoting loss of cartilage matrix.

NSAID's INTERFERE WITH NEUTROPHIL FUNCTIONS

Recent work has shown that aspirin-like drugs affect stimulus-response coupling in the most abundant cells of acute inflammation: neutrophils. Neutrophils injure tissues by releasing proteases, inflammatory peptides, reactive oxygen species such as O_2^- and H_2O_2, and lipid irritants such as platelet-activating factor and leukotriene B_4. Activation of the neutrophil in response to soluble stimuli (chemoattractants) or to immune complexes follows general pathways of stimulus-response coupling of secretory cells and is inhibited by all NSAID's studied so far.

NSAID's—indomethacin, piroxicam, diclofenac, and ibuprofen (at micromolar concentrations)—inhibit the cell-cell aggregation of human neutrophils induced by chemoattractants and mediated by the cell surface adhesion molecule CD11b/CD18. Although *all* NSAID's inhibit aggregation, only some inhibit enzyme release and/or O_2^- generation. Millimolar concentrations of sodium salicylate and aspirin alike (levels achieved in the treatment of rheumatoid arthritis or rheumatic fever) are required to inhibit the aggregation of neutrophils. However, at these concentrations sodium salicylate *does not* interfere with the activation of platelets or synthesis of thromboxane A_2. In contrast, aspirin at one tenth to one hundredth of these concentrations inhibits platelet aggregation and completely inhibits thromboxane biosynthesis via its effect on PGH synthase. It is therefore likely that the shared anti-inflammatory effects of aspirin and sodium salicylate are related to their common inhibition of neutrophil activation rather than to their divergent actions on prostaglandin biosynthesis. In contrast to aspirin and sodium salicylate, acetaminophen has no effect on neutrophil aggregation.

Inhibitory effects of NSAID's on neutrophil activation in vitro can also be demonstrated in the clinic. Indeed, neutrophils derived from the synovial fluid of patients with rheumatoid arthritis produced less superoxide anion following 10 days of therapy with piroxicam, whereas cells from normal volunteers given ibuprofen or piroxicam for 3 days failed to aggregate normally in response to chemoattractants. Sodium salicylate, an ineffective inhibitor of PGH synthase in vitro, is as effective as aspirin at inhibiting neutrophil activation.

It is somewhat paradoxical that both NSAID's and prostaglandins of the E series have similar *inhibitory* effects on the activation of such inflammatory cells as the neutrophil or platelet. Addition of PGE_1 or PGE_2 to human neutrophils at nanomolar to micromolar concentrations fails to override the inhibition by piroxicam of superoxide generation induced by chemoattractants. In the presence of piroxicam, superoxide anion generation was diminished by a factor of approximately 10 to 40 nmoles per liter of cytochrome c reduced per 10^6 cells. Recent studies, with the clinically useful PGE_1 derivative misoprostol, also show additive or synergistic rather than antagonistic effects between NSAID's and prostaglandins.

At anti-inflammatory concentrations, NSAID's appear to uncouple receptors with their effector molecules in the plasmalemma, including those regulated by at least one guanine nucleotide–binding (G) protein. Pertussis toxin, via its capacity for ADP-ribosylation of the alpha subunit of some plasma membrane G proteins, interferes with signal transduction in a variety of cells, including the neutrophil. Compared to pertussis toxin, sodium salicylate alone inhibits only modestly the production of superoxide induced by chemoattractants while inhibiting aggregation to a far greater extent. However, sodium salicylate blocks the inhibitory effect of pertussis toxin on neutrophils: Cells coincubated with both pertussis toxin and sodium salicylate regained their pertussis toxin–inhibited capacity to generate superoxide anion. This paradoxical effect of salicylate suggests that salicylates interfere with the action of pertussis toxin near the site of its interaction with the alpha subunit of the G protein. NSAID's (salicylate, piroxicam, and indomethacin) block the pertussis toxin–dependent ADP-ribosylation of the G protein in purified neutrophil membranes, and salicylates and piroxicam inhibit, in part, the pertussis toxin–sensitive formation of diacylglycerol that follows cell activation.

THE PHYLOGENY OF NSAID STUDIES

A final blow to the generality of the prostaglandin hypothesis comes from the sea. The cell biology of marine sponges, such as *Microciona prolifera*, was first examined by Robert Hooke, who in 1685 suggested in *Microcosmographica* that all living creatures contained a commonality of substructure that under the microscope resembled the "cells of monks." We may recall that the name "cell" derives from Hooke's studies of onion root tips and sponges. *M. prolifera*, which is both the most primitive and most ancient of animal creatures (10^9 years in ancestry), offers a unique model for investigating the anti-inflammatory effects of NSAID's. The activation of sponge cells in the course of cell-cell aggregation is not influenced by stable prostaglandins, nor do sponge cells contain cyclo-oxygenase activity. Nevertheless, aggregation of marine sponge cells is inhibited by NSAID's—either by aspirin or sodium salicylate and by 12 other NSAID's tested, but not by acetaminophen. After dispersion of the cells by treatment with EDTA and removal of the chelator with calcium, cell-cell aggregation of the *M. prolifera* cells is rapidly induced by phorbol esters or by addition of an inophore that raises cytosolic calcium. They are also aggregated by a species-specific aggregation factor called MAF, a 20×10^6 MW proteoglycan, and by arachidonic acid. Both aspirin and sodium salicylate—at millimolar concentrations—inhibit aggregation of these cells in response to MAF. Ibuprofen, piroxicam, and diclofenac—at micromolar concentrations—but not acetaminophen, also inhibit aggregation of these primitive cells. Since the concentrations of NSAID's that inhibit aggregation of marine sponges are the same as those that inhibit neutrophil aggregation, and since marine sponges *cannot* make prostaglandins, we may conclude that these effects—like those of NSAID's on insects (*Drosophila* chromosomes) or plants (voodoo lilies) or human cells (neutrophils)—are unlikely to result from their inhibition of prostaglandin synthesis.

Abramson S, Weissmann G: The mechanisms of action of nonsteroidal antiinflammatory drugs. Arthritis Rheum 32:1–9, 1989. *The physicochemical properties of NSAID's may alter the fluidity of the plasma membrane and thereby disrupt molecular interactions required for normal signal transduction across the lipid bilayer. The alternative hypothesis to J.R. Vane's.*

Clinch D: Why not have definitive trials of gastrointestinal safety for non-steroidal anti-inflammatory drugs? Proc R Soc Med 81:158–160, 1988. *A discussion of gastric inflammation and ulceration associated with NSAID's, which also shows that 74 per cent of NSAID-associated ulcers occur within 6 months of treatment.*

Ferreira SH, Vane JR: New aspects of the mode of action of nonsteroid antiinflammatory drugs. Ann Rev Pharm 14:57–73, 1974. *This review surveys work between 1973 and 1974 on the possible mode of action and on the clinical effects of that group of drugs variously known as non-narcotic analgesics, nonsteroidal anti-inflammatory drugs, aspirin-like drugs, or antiphlogistic acids.*

Graham GG: Pharmacokinetics and metabolism of nonsteroidal antiinflammatory drugs. Med J Aust 147:597–602, 1987. *This review of the few controlled studies shows that plasma levels of NSAID's, when in the therapeutic range, correlate with response.*

Hennekens CH, et al.: Final report on the aspirin component of the ongoing physicians' health study. N Eng J Med 321:129–135, 1989. *Aspirin at low doses prevents myocardial infarction.*

Kulmacz RJ: Topography of prostaglandin H synthase. Antiinflammatory agents and the protease-sensitive arginine 253 region. J Biol Chem 264:14136–14142, 1989. *The best recent review of how NSAID's work on inhibition of the enzyme.*

Pedersen AK, FitzGerald GA: Dose-related kinetics of aspirin: Presystemic acetylation of platelet cyclooxygenase. N Eng J Med 311:1206–1210, 1984. *How aspirin affects platelets in vivo.*

Raskin I, Ehmann A, Melander WR, Meeuse BJ: Salicylic acid: A natural inducer of heat production in arum lilies. Science 237:1601–1602, 1987. *How salicylates work in plants.*

Ritossa F: A new puffing pattern induced by temperature shock and DNP in Drosophila. Exp XII:571–573, 1962. *Sodium salicylate induces heat shock proteins in Drosophila.*

Rodnan GP, Benedek TG: The early history of antirheumatic drugs. Arthritis Rheum 13:145–165, 1970. *A superb review of NSAID's before the days of prostaglandins.*

Tainter ML, Ferris AJ: Aspirin in Modern Therapy. New York, Bayer Company Division of Sterling Drug, Inc., 1969. *A review of NSAID history, with a discussion of their mode of action before the prostaglandin hypothesis.*

Vane JR: Inhibition of prostaglandin synthesis as a mechanism of action for aspirin-like drugs. Nature (London) New Biol 231:232–235, 1971. *The classic.*

PART V
PRINCIPLES OF HUMAN GENETICS

30 Human Heredity

James B. Wyngaarden

The appreciation of genetic factors as arbiters of human disease is a relatively recent development in medical history. Scattered references to inheritance of biologic characteristics may be found in the records of several millenia, including the frequently cited Talmudic exemption from circumcision of males born into families of bleeders, but discernible patterns of hereditary transmission were recognized first in the eighteenth and nineteenth centuries. In the 1750's Maupertuis described the autosomal dominant inheritance of polydactyly. The essential features of X-linked inheritance of hemophilia were described in the early 1800's by several writers and the pattern was formally outlined by Nasse in 1820. The pattern of inheritance now recognized as autosomal recessive was described by Adams in 1814, and the biologic consequences of consanguinity first reported by Bemiss in 1857. In 1876, Galton introduced the twin method of separating effects of heredity from those of environment; later he initiated quantitative studies of polygenic inheritance.

Genetics as an experimental science owes its origins to Gregor Mendel and his cross-breeding of garden peas, tall and short, yellow seed and green seed, round seed and wrinkled seed. From these studies Mendel derived concepts of dominant and recessive traits, hereditary factors (which we now call *genes*), alternative factors (*alleles*), true breeding plants with two identical factors (*homozygotes*), and non–true breeding plants with alternative factors (*heterozygotes*). His experiments led to the formulation of laws of *unit inheritance* (that "factors" retain their identity from generation to generation and do not blend in the hybrid), of *segregation* (that two members [alleles] of a single pair of factors [genes] are never found in the same gamete but always segregate), and of *independent assortment* (that members of different pairs of genes [nonalleles] assort to gametes independent of one another). These laws, formulated in 1865, had almost no immediate impact on biologic thought, but they are now cornerstones of genetics. They were rediscovered about 1900 by several workers independently and first applied to human disease by Sir Archibald Garrod in his concept of "inborn errors of metabolism" in 1908.

DNA AS GENETIC MATERIAL

In 1944 Avery and his associates at the Rockefeller Institute established that the hereditary information in the transforming principle of pneumococci resided in its deoxyribonucleic acid (DNA). From that date onward DNA has been considered the basic material of the gene. In 1953 Watson and Crick proposed a molecular model for the structure of DNA, consisting of two polynucleotide strands twisted together in a double helix with the purine and pyrimidine bases facing inward and attached to each other, binding the two chains. This model offered a rational structure for replication of DNA and for storage of hereditary information within sequences of purine and pyrimidine bases. This structure has since been established by x-ray crystallography. The genetic code, namely the precise triplet sequences of purine and pyrimidine bases in the structural gene that specify the individual amino acids of a polypeptide chain, was discovered by Nirenberg in 1961.

The amount of DNA in each human cell is sufficient to code for approximately 1 million polypeptides of average length. Estimates of the number of structural genes in humans range from 50,000 to 100,000; large amounts of DNA constitute noncoding sequences whose function is as yet obscure. Only a small number of structural genes has been identified. In the most recent update of his catalogue of *Mendelian Inheritance in Man*, McKusick lists phenotypic variations or diseases of 2656 established genetic loci, plus of an additional 2281 loci not yet fully validated, thus implying that at least 4937 genes have undergone mutation so as to cause human disease or polymorphism. In humans, hereditary information is distributed in 23 pairs of chromosomes—22 pairs of autosomes and one pair of sex chromosomes (X + Y, male; X + X, female)—plus the unpaired "mitochondrial chromosome" (see below).

THE GENE AND PROTEIN SYNTHESIS

In specifying the amino acid sequence of a polypeptide, a structural gene first transfers its information to a complementary strand of messenger RNA (mRNA), which in turn governs the order of amino acids in a polypeptide. The transfer of information from DNA to RNA involves no change of language (nucleotide → nucleotide) and is called *transcription;* the transfer of information from RNA to polypeptide involves a new language (nucleotide → amino acid) and is called *translation*. Almost all protein synthesis takes place in ribosomes, cytoplasmic bodies composed of another type of RNA (ribosomal RNA) and protein. An exception is a small amount of specific protein synthesis that takes place in mitochondria.

MUTATION

Broadly defined, a mutation is a stable, heritable alteration in the structure of DNA which can be passed from cell to progeny. From the standpoint of evolution, mutations are essential for the generation of sufficient genetic diversity to permit species to adapt to their environment through the mechanism of natural selection

Mutations may involve millions of base pairs in the structure of a chromosome, as in duplications, deletions, and translocations of a portion of one chromosome to another. Mutations can involve an entire human genome of 3 billion base pairs, as in triploidy, in which a third copy of the entire chromosomal apparatus occurs. At the other extreme, a mutation can be minute and involve a small deletion or insertion, or a replacement of only a single base pair *(point mutation)*. If deletions or insertions occur in a coding region, they give rise to *frame-shift* mutations because they alter the reading frame distal to the mutation. Thus frame-shift mutations alter the protein sequence and frequently result in peptide chain termination through generation of a stop codon.

Point mutations, replacement of one base by another in a coding region, may be of three types: (1) a *synonymous* mutation (about 23 per cent of random base substitutions in coding regions), in which the base replacement does not lead to a change in the amino acid but only to a different codon for the same amino acid; (2) a *missense* mutation (about 73 per cent of base substitutions in coding regions), in which the base change results in substitution of one amino acid for another; and (3) a *nonsense* mutation (about

119

4 per cent of base substitutions in coding regions), in which the base change generates one of the termination codons.

Large deletions may interrupt a coding region and cause an absence of a protein product. Or, if the deletion removes a bridge between two coding regions, the result may be a fusion or hybrid protein containing the initial sequence of one protein and the terminal portion of the other. Such deletions may result from unequal crossing over between homologous genes. In addition, there are complex mutations involving transcriptional, splicing, and RNA processing mutations.

THE GENETIC DIVERSITY OF MAN

The cause of genetic heterogenicity, i.e., of differences between members of homologous gene pairs, is *mutation* of gene structure. Variations of chromosome content are introduced by *recombination*, a process in which genetic material is exchanged between homologous chromosomes during the pairing that takes place in meiosis, and by *translation*, a process in which chromosomal breakage and reunion result in the insertion of whole segments of chromosomes in new locations within the same or another chromosome. Additional variations in genetic constitution, or genotype, result from the *random distribution* ("independent assortment") of one member of each paired chromosome into daughter cells during reductive division of the germ cells. The interplay of all these forces provides each human being except monovular twins with a unique inheritance.

POLYMORPHISM

Many proteins exist in two or more forms in the normal population. These multiple forms are due to the presence in the population of multiple genes (alleles) at the same genetic locus coding for the same protein. If the most common allele at a given locus accounts for fewer than 99 per cent of the alleles in the population, *polymorphism* is said to occur. By definition, when polymorphism exists at a genetic locus, at least 2 per cent of the population must be heterozygous at that locus. Table 30–1 lists selected proteins for which polymorphism has been demonstrated electrophoretically. Most of these genetically determined variations in protein structure are unassociated with clinical disease.

As many as 28 per cent of human genetic loci show multiple alleles in the population. Moreover, the average individual is detectably heterozygous at 7 per cent of his or her loci. Since most detection methods require a change in the charge of the protein, they can detect only about one third of the actual base changes that are possible, because only one third of point mutations result in a substitution of an amino acid with a different charge. Thus, all individuals may actually be heterozygous at as many as 20 per cent of their loci.

At most genetic loci (e.g., the gene for β-globin) one standard allele accounts for the vast majority of alleles in the population, and alternative alleles are rare. At other loci, no single allele occurs with sufficient frequency to be designated standard or normal. The α-chain of haptoglobin, a plasma protein, represents one such extreme example of genetic polymorphism. In this instance all polymorphic forms of haptoglobin appear to function equally in hemoglobin binding. Polymorphisms represent conspicuous examples of human biochemical diversity.

THE HUMAN GENE MAP

About 2500 autosomal loci are known and another 2100 are strongly indicated on the basis mainly of characteristic patterns of inheritance of alternative forms of a given trait. At least 3000 of these are associated with a disease phenotype. This implies that at least 3 to 6 per cent of the 50,000 to 100,000 human genes have undergone mutation so as to cause human disease. The chromosomal locations are known for over 2100 of these loci. In addition, over 160 loci have been assigned to the X-chromosome.

HUMAN GENETIC DISEASE

Genetics is concerned with the study of hereditary variations. When variations are extreme and impair the health, fitness, or reproductive capacity of the individual, we consider them diseases. These extreme variations are of three principal types: (1) chromosomal aberrations, (2) single-gene differences that exhibit

TABLE 30–1. SOME PLASMA PROTEINS AND CELLULAR ENZYMES THAT EXHIBIT ELECTROPHORETICALLY DETECTABLE POLYMORPHISMS

Protein	Locus Name
Plasma proteins	
Haptoglobin (α-chain)	Hp α
Transferrin	Tf
Vitamin-D binding protein	Gc (for group-specific component)
Ceruloplasmin	Cp
α-1-Antitrypsin	Pi (for protease inhibitor)
α-1-Acid glycoprotein	Oro (for orosomucoid)
β-2-Glycoprotein I	—
Properdin factor B	Bf
Complement	
Second component	C2
Third component	C3
Fourth component	C4
Sixth component	C6
Enzymes	
Pancreatic amylase	AMY_2
Cholinesterase	E_2
Red blood cell enzyme	
Acid phosphatase 1	ACP_1
Adenosine deaminase	ADA
Adenylate kinase	AK_1
Carbonic anhydrase 2	CA_2
Diaphorase (NADPH-dependent)	DIA_2
Esterase D	ESD
Galactose-1-uridyltransferase	GALT
Glucose-6-phosphate dehydrogenase	Gd
Glutamic pyruvic transaminase	GPT
Glutathione peroxidase	GPX
Glutathione reductase	GSR
Glyoxalase I	GLO
Peptidase A	PEPA
Peptidase C	PEPC
Peptidase D	PEPD
Phosphoglucomutase 1	PGM_1
Phosphoglucomutase 2	PGM_2
Phosphogluconate dehydrogenase	PGD
Uridine monophosphate kinase	UMPK
White blood cell enzymes	
Aconitase (soluble)	$ACON_S$
Cytidine deaminase	CDA
α-L-Fucosidase	αFUC
α-Glucosidase	αGLUC
Glutamic-oxaloacetic transaminase (mitochondrial)	GOT_M
Hexokinase 3	HK_3
Malic enzyme (mitochondrial)	ME_M
Phosphoglucomutase 3	PGM_3

mendelian patterns of inheritance, and (3) polygenic disorders, in which two or more, often multiple, genes each contribute to the characteristic in question. Examples of the first two categories are relatively easy to recognize. They are discussed in Ch. 31 and 33. Many genetic diseases are dependent upon environmental factors for their expression, e.g., phenylalanine ingestion in phenylketonuria or milk ingestion in galactosemia. Other hereditary diseases are kept in abeyance by specific environmental factors: Scurvy is an inborn error of metabolism (absence of the hepatic enzyme that converts L-gulonolactone to L-ascorbic acid in man, monkey, and guinea pig) kept in remission by vitamin C; metabolic cretinism is foiled in its expression by the administration of thyroid hormone. The greatest difficulty in sorting out the relative importance of genetic and environmental influences is encountered with common diseases. In disorders such as rheumatoid arthritis, essential hypertension, and coronary artery disease, genetic influences are important but hard to identify in specific biochemical terms. In most polygenic disorders, genetic factors are multiple and still beyond definition.

The pace of genetic advance across the full spectrum of molecular biology to human heredity is currently very rapid. The revolution in biology of the past three decades is increasingly molding medical science and practice. New insights into the genetic control of the immune response (see Ch. 250) are explaining disease susceptibilities and facilitating organ and tissue transplantation. Susceptibility to cancer is being explained by the interplay between oncogenes, anti-oncogenes, and environmental exposures (see Ch. 157). As additional genetic mechanisms are disclosed, they will illuminate more and more human diseases and from time to time suggest new avenues of therapy.

THE FAMILY HISTORY. A careful family history is indispensable in the assessment and understanding of hereditary disease. The interviewer should ascertain whether anyone in the family has had a condition similar to that of the patient, and whether this condition or any other "runs in the family." Particularly in the case of rare disorders one should inquire whether the parents are related, and, if this is not known, whether they or their families came from the same village or community and whether their forebears may have intermarried. Since some disorders are more common in certain ethnic groups than in others, the ethnic origin of the parents should also be elicited.

The rarer the recessive disorder in a specific population, the greater is the likelihood of parental consanguinity. Tay-Sachs disease is relatively rare in non-Jews, in whom the gene frequency is low, but a high proportion of non-Jewish parents of Tay-Sachs children are consanguineous. By contrast, Tay-Sachs disease is relatively common in Jews of eastern European origin, in whom the gene frequency is relatively high. In parents of Jewish children with Tay-Sachs disease in the United States the frequency of consanguinity is only slightly higher than in the general population.

Certain ethnic backgrounds increase the likelihood of certain diagnostic possibilities while decreasing that of others. Thalassemia is chiefly a disorder of people of the Mediterranean region and of Southeast Asia, familial Mediterranean fever is a disorder of Armenians and Sephardic Jews, acatalasia is a disease of Japanese and Koreans, and gout is very common among the Maori. By contrast, cystic fibrosis is rare in blacks, phenylketonuria is uncommon in Jews, and sickle cell anemia does not occur in Caucasians.

PEDIGREE ANALYSIS. The chief method of study of an inherited disease in humans is the observation of its pattern of distribution in kindreds, i.e., of its pedigree pattern. The construction of a pedigree pattern begins with the individual first detected, who is referred to as the proband, index case, or propositus (female = proposita). The pedigree pattern allows one to judge whether the distribution conforms to mendelian principles of segregation and assortment and thus represents single-factor inheritance. Patterns that do not conform to mendelian principles may represent polygenic traits in which a number of genes each contributes a minor effect. Valid pedigrees depend on accurate and extensive information about the kindred. This information is likely to be more reliable when based on observer detection than when based on memory.

MONOGENIC DISORDERS. Disorders caused by single mutant genes show one of four simple (mendelian) patterns of inheritance: (1) autosomal dominant, (2) autosomal recessive, (3) X-linked dominant, or (4) X-linked recessive. Dominant traits are those expressed in the heterozygote (as well as in the homozygote or hemizygote). Recessive traits are those expressed in the homozygotes (or hemizygotes) but silent in the heterozygote. The terms *dominant* and *recessive* refer to the phenotypic expression of the trait, not to the expression of the gene. Thus it is incorrect to speak of a dominant or recessive gene. A gene is either expressed or not expressed. Whether the trait is considered dominant or recessive often depends upon the level of observation. Sickle cell anemia is a recessive trait; i.e., it requires a double dose of the abnormal gene for expression at the clinical level. Nevertheless, the sickle gene is expressed in single dose as well, giving rise to carriers with SA hemoglobin. Recessive traits are *codominant* when viewed biochemically at the level of the gene product.

With few exceptions, each of the approximately 5000 mendelian diseases is rare. The overall population frequency of monogenic disorders is about 10 per 1000 live births, comprising about 7 per 1000 dominants, about 2.5 per 1000 recessives, and about 0.4 per 1000 X-linked conditions (see Table 30–2).

If a particular disease shows a mendelian pattern of inheritance, its pathogenesis, no matter how complex, must be due to a single abnormal protein molecule. For example, in sickle cell disease, such seemingly unrelated disturbances as hemolytic anemia,

TABLE 30–2. PREVALENCE OF SELECTED MONOGENIC DISORDERS AMONG LIVEBORN INFANTS*

Disorder	Estimated Prevalence
Autosomal Dominant	
Familial hypercholesterolemia	1 in 500
Polycystic kidney disease	1 in 1250
Huntington disease	1 in 2500
Hereditary spherocytosis	1 in 5000
Marfan syndrome	1 in 20,000
Autosomal Recessive	
Sickle cell anemia	1 in 625 (U.S. blacks)
Cystic fibrosis	1 in 2000 (Caucasians)
Tay-Sachs disease	1 in 3000 (U.S. Jews)
Cystinuria	1 in 7000
Phenylketonuria	1 in 12,000
Mucopolysaccharidoses (all types)	1 in 25,000
Glycogen storage disease (all types)	1 in 50,000
Galactosemia	1 in 57,000
Homocystinuria	1 in 200,000
X-linked	
Duchenne muscular dystrophy	1 in 7000
Hemophilia	1 in 10,000

*Data assembled from Galjaard, Carter, and Motulsky.

painful crises, nephropathy, vascular occlusions, and *Salmonella* osteomyelitis are all physiologic consequences of a single missense mutation, resulting in a single amino acid substitution in the β-globin chain. When two or more phenotypic characters are controlled by a single gene, that gene is said to have *pleiotropic* effects.

AUTOSOMAL DOMINANT TRAITS. Autosomal genes are those genes situated on chromosomes other than the X or Y. When there are two alleles, A and a, at a locus, three possible genotypes exist: AA, Aa, and aa. Genotypes AA and aa are *homozygotes;* Aa is a *heterozygote.*

Dominant traits are fully manifest in the presence of a gene in the heterozygous state, i.e., when only one abnormal gene (*mutant allele*) is present and the corresponding partner allele on the homologous chromosome is normal. Figure 30–1 shows a typical pedigree of transmission of an autosomal dominant trait. The following features are characteristic: (1) Each affected individual has an affected parent (unless the condition arose by a new mutation in a germ cell that formed the individual); (2) an affected individual will bear, on average, an equal number of affected and unaffected offspring; (3) males and females will be affected in equal numbers; (4) each sex can transmit the trait to male and female offspring (i.e., male-to-male transmission is possible); (5) normal children of an affected individual will have only normal

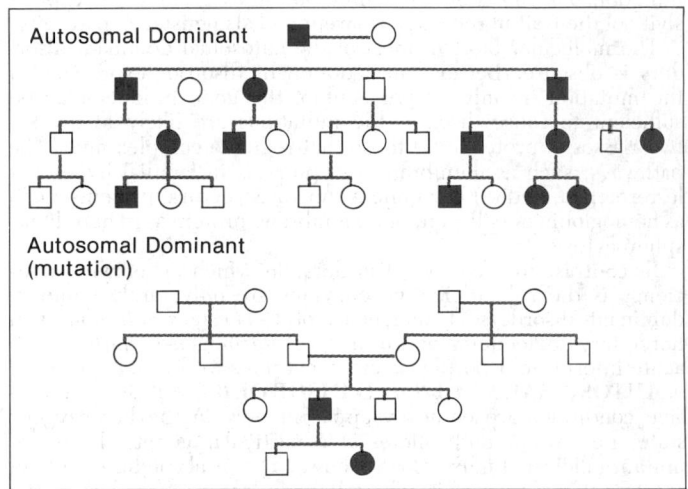

FIGURE 30–1. Pedigrees of autosomal dominant traits. In the lower pedigree the normal parents of the affected individual suggest the possibility of a new mutation. Solid symbols indicate those affected. (For details see text.)

offspring; and (6) when the trait does not impair viability or reproductive capacity, there will be *vertical* transmission of the trait through successive generations.

Most autosomal dominant disorders show two additional characteristics that are not seen in recessive disorders: (1) marked variability in severity, or *expressivity,* and (2) delayed age of onset. Dominant traits in humans often exert only mild effects. Occasionally the expression of the abnormal gene is so weak that a generation appears to be skipped because the carrier of the abnormal gene is clinically normal. When this is the case, the trait is said to be *nonpenetrant.* When a gene of a dominant trait exists in the homozygous state, the effect may be very severe, perhaps lethal. Examples are common in animals in which experimental matings can be constructed, but rare in humans, because matings of two affected heterozygotes are exceptional. One example is homozygous familial hypercholesterolemia. Others possibly include achondroplasia and Osler-Weber-Rendu syndrome. Delayed age of onset is seen in Huntington's disease and adult polycystic kidney disease. These disorders do not become manifest clinically until adult life, even though the mutant gene has been present since conception.

In every autosomal dominant disease some affected persons owe their disorder to a new mutation rather than to an inherited allele. Since a reasonable estimate of the frequency of mutation is of the order of 5×10^{-6} mutations per gene per generation, and since a dominant trait requires a mutation in only one of the parental gametes, one would expect that about 1 in 100,000 newborn persons would possess a new mutation at any given genetic locus. Many mutations will be silent or will involve a recessive function and not be manifest in a single gene dose. However, others will cause a defective gene product that gives rise to a dominant trait.

The percentage of patients with dominant disorders that represents a new mutation is inversely proportional to the effect of the disease upon *biologic fitness,* i.e., survival to adult life, and reproductive capacity. If a dominant mutation produces early death or absolute infertility, genetic transmission is impossible, and all cases represent new mutations. In tuberous sclerosis, the severe mental retardation reduces biologic fitness to about 20 per cent of normal, and the proportion of cases due to new mutations is about 80 per cent. In dominant conditions such as familial hypercholesterolemia, in which there is no reduction in biologic fitness, virtually all cases have a family pedigree showing classic vertical transmission

New mutations appear to be more frequent in the germ cells of fathers of relatively advanced age. Both Marfan syndrome and achondroplastic dwarfism display such "paternal age effect." Fathers of sporadic cases of both conditions are an average of 5 to 7 years older than the general population of fathers or than fathers who transmit these syndromes because of an inherited mutation. Diagnosis of a new mutation must exclude low expressivity of the trait in the carrier parent and also mistaken paternity.

The molecular basis of most of the autosomal dominant disorders is obscure. Because in a dominant disorder expression of the mutation in only 50 per cent of the gene product may be sufficient to cause disease, the mutations are likely to involve two classes of proteins: (1) those that regulate complex metabolic pathways, such as membrane receptors as in familial hypercholesterolemia, and (2) key nonenzymic or structural proteins, such as hemoglobin or collagen, or a membrane protein as in hereditary spherocytosis.

In contrast to recessive disorders, in which an enzyme deficiency is the rule, defective enzymes are only rarely found in dominant disorders. Deficiencies of *C-1–esterase inhibitor* in hereditary angioedema and of *uroporphyrinogen-1 synthetase* in acute intermittent porphyria are exceptions to this general rule.

AUTOSOMAL RECESSIVE DISORDERS. Autosomal recessive conditions are clinically apparent only in the homozygous state, i.e., when both alleles at a particular genetic locus are mutant alleles. Figure 30–2 shows a typical pedigree of an autosomal recessive trait. The following features are characteristic: (1) The parents are clinically normal; (2) only siblings are affected; (3) males and females are affected in equal proportions; (4) if an affected individual marries a homozygous normal person, none of the children will be affected but all will be heterozygous

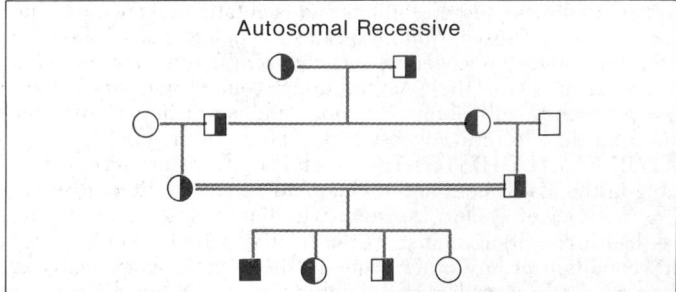

FIGURE 30–2. Pedigree of autosomal recessive trait. Note that both parents are heterozygous. One sib is affected, two are carriers, and one is normal. Double line (═══) indicates that parents are related by descent (first cousins).

carriers; (5) if an affected individual marries a heterozygous carrier, one half of the children will be affected, and the pedigree pattern will superficially suggest a dominant trait; (6) if two individuals who are homozygous for the same mutant gene marry, all of their children will be affected; (7) if both parents are heterozygous at the same genetic locus, one fourth of their children will be homozygous affected, one fourth will be homozygous normal, and one half will be heterozygous carriers of the same mutant gene; and (8) the less frequent the mutant gene is in the population, the greater is the likelihood that the affected individual is the product of consanguine parents.

In actual practice, unless the kinship is very large, the ratio of affected to unaffected sibs is frequently greater than one in four. Inclusion of probands in the enumeration loads the results in favor of the trait. In a sibship of 100 or even 10 the loading factor is not pronounced. However, in all ascertainable one-child sibships the involvement is 100 per cent, in two-child sibships it is 67 per cent (when the fundamental probability is 50 per cent), in three-child sibships it is 57 per cent, and so on. In small sibships a correction must be made for *bias of ascertainment.* The simplest method is to exclude the proband from the calculation and to determine the proportion of affected children among the remaining sibs.

In most autosomal recessive conditions the clinical presentation tends to be more uniform than in dominant diseases, and the onset is often early in life. Recessive disorders are commonly diagnosed in childhood. Approximately 630 well-established recessive traits have been recognized in humans, and in over 300 of these the mutant enzyme or other protein has been identified.

A *completely* recessive disease is one in which the heterozygote is clinically normal. When some features of the disease are detectable in the heterozygote, the disease is sometimes said to show *intermediate inheritance,* or to be *incompletely recessive* or *incompletely dominant.* The ambiguity of these terms from classic genetic studies of phenotypes is further emphasized by results of different methods of detection of gene effects. In many instances of completely recessive inheritance, refined biochemical observations enable the recognition of the trait in the clinically normal heterozygote. An example is Tay-Sachs disease, in which clinically normal parents and some sibs can be shown to be heterozygotes by assay of hexosaminidase A in leukocytes. Because of its importance in genetic counseling, the detection of healthy heterozygous carriers of genes that in the homozygous state cause overt disease is one of the most significant aspects of medical genetics. Since by definition a dominant trait is one that is detectable in the heterozygous state, Tay-Sachs disease (and many others) is recessive when the clinical phenotype is considered and dominant when the biochemical phenotype is determined.

In pure form a recessive disease requires the inheritance of identical mutant genes from both parents. When the mutant genes are rare, the likelihood that any two unrelated parents are carriers for the same defect is small. Inheritance of two different mutant genes derived from the same locus gives rise to *heterollelic compounds.* Individuals with Hb SC disease are genetic compounds who have inherited a different abnormal β-globin gene from each parent. Genetic compounds are also known in cystinuria, phenylketonuria, certain of the mucopolysaccharidoses, "homozygous" familial hypercholesterolemia, and several other disorders.

If the parents of a child with a recessive disorder have a common ancestor who carried a mutant gene, then the likelihood that two of the descendants would each have inherited the gene becomes relatively great. The less frequent the gene, the stronger is the likelihood that an affected individual has resulted from a consanguine mating. First cousins share, on the average, one eighth of their genes. When two first cousins marry, an offspring has, on the average, one sixteenth of the loci homozygous for a gene derived from a common ancestor. In general, offspring of first-cousin mating are slightly more likely to have congenital malformations, as well as mental defects and metabolic diseases, than are children born to unrelated parents.

Increased frequency of consanguinity is not observed if the recessive disease is common. Sickle cell anemia, phenylketonuria, cystic fibrosis, and Tay-Sachs disease are examples in which the carrier (heterozygote) state is frequent in certain populations and in which consanguinity is usually not present in the parents. Increase in consanguinity would also not be expected in dominant or X-linked traits or genetic compounds.

A high percentage of recessive disorders involves abnormalities of enzyme proteins. In most reactions the normal maximal enzyme activity is greatly in excess of catalytic requirements; i.e., the concentration of a substrate is usually maintained at a point well below saturation for the enzyme that metabolizes it. Hence a reduction to 50 per cent of normal activity in a heterozygote does not impair the health of the carrier, whereas a total or nearly total deficiency may result in a serious inborn error of metabolism. These conditions are discussed in Ch. 31.

X-LINKED INHERITANCE. Diseases or traits that result from genes located on the X chromosome are termed X-linked. Since the female has two X chromosomes, she may be either heterozygous or homozygous for the mutant gene, and the trait may exhibit recessive or dominant expression. The male has only one X chromosome and therefore is *hemizygous* for X-linked traits. Males can be expected to express X-linked traits regardless of their recessive or dominant behavior in the female. Thus, the terms X-linked dominant or X-linked recessive refer only to expression of the trait in females.

Since males transmit their X chromosome only to daughters, an important feature of X-linked inheritance is the absence of male-to-male transmission. Affected males transmit the trait to all of their daughters and none of their sons.

Since the female carries two X chromosomes in each cell, it might be expected that the concentrations of proteins determined by genes on the X chromosome would be twice that of males who carry only one X chromosome per cell. This is not the case, and the explanation is provided by the process of X-inactivation first proposed by Mary Lyon, and often termed the *Lyon hypothesis*. In all adult female cells only one of the X chromosomes is genetically active. Early in differentiation one of the X chromosomes becomes inactive and forms the *Barr body*. Inactivation is random so that for each cell there is an equal probability that the paternally or maternally derived X chromosome will be inactivated. Once one of the two X chromosomes is inactivated, the same X chromosome remains inactive throughout all subsequent cell divisions. Thus, on the average one half of the cells of a female will express the X chromosome of her father, and one half of her mother: In this respect the normal female is a mosaic. If one of the X chromosomes carries a mutant gene, the probability is that the mutant phenotype will be expressed in one half of her cells. However, this statistical probability may be disturbed in at least two ways: (1) Since inactivation of one of the X chromosomes occurs early in development and is random, some females may by chance have many more cells that carry an active X chromosome derived from one parent than from the other; and (2) if one of the X chromosomes carries a mutant gene that confers a metabolic disadvantage upon cells with that mutation, these cells may survive less frequently during development, and the female offspring may have cells that carry predominantly or exclusively the active X chromosome without the mutation.

Over 160 loci have been identified on the human X chromosome, and many have been mapped to specific regions on the long or the short arm of the chromosome.

X-Linked Dominant Traits. This mode of inheritance (Fig. 30-3) is uncommon. Its characteristic features are as follows: (1)

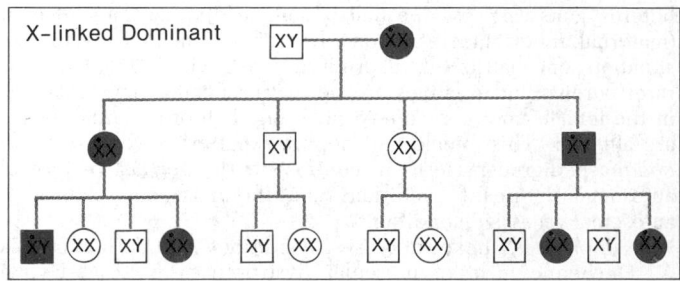

FIGURE 30–3. Pedigree of dominant X-linked trait. The X chromosome bearing the abnormal gene is designated by a small dot.

Females are affected about twice as often as males, (2) heterozygous females transmit the trait to both sexes with a frequency of 50 per cent, (3) hemizygous affected males transmit the trait to all of their daughters and none of their sons, and (4) the expression is more variable and generally less severe in heterozygous females than in hemizygous affected males. Examples of X-linked dominant inheritance include the Xg(a$^+$) blood group, vitamin D-resistant (hypophosphatemic) rickets, and pseudohypoparathyroidism.

Some rare X-linked dominant disorders occur only in the heterozygous female, because the condition is lethal in the hemizygous affected male. Additional characteristics of this form of inheritance are as follows: (1) An affected mother transmits the trait to one half of her daughters (heterozygotes), and (2) an increased frequency of abortions occurs in affected women, the abortions representing affected male fetuses. Examples of disorders that appear to fit this mode of inheritance include incontinentia pigmenti, focal dermal hypoplasia, orofaciodigital syndrome, and hyperammonemia caused by ornithine transcarbamylase deficiency.

X-Linked Recessive Traits. This mode of inheritance (Fig. 30-4) is relatively common. Its characteristic features are as follows: (1) The disorder is fully expressed only in the hemizygous affected male. (2) Heterozygous females are usually normal; occasionally they may exhibit mild features of the disorder; rarely they may be almost as severely affected as the hemizygous affected male (this variability is attributed to the probability that a disproportionate percentage of *normal* X chromosomes of the heterozygous female may have been inactivated early in development [see "Lyon hypothesis," above]). (3) On average, a heterozygous female transmits the trait to one half of her sons (hemizygous affected), but the other half are normal. (4) On average, one half of daughters of a heterozygous female are carriers and one half are normal. (5) All daughters of an affected male married to a normal female are carriers, and no sons of such a union are affected (no father-to-son transmission). (6) In the rare event of the union of an affected male and a heterozygous female, one half of daughters are homozygous affected and one half are

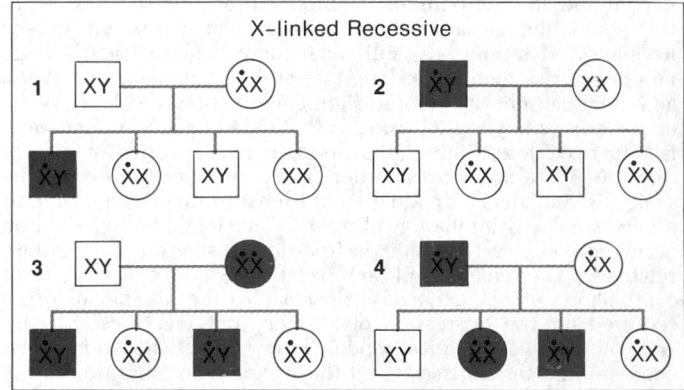

FIGURE 30–4. Pedigrees of X-linked recessive trait. The X chromosome bearing the abnormal gene is designated by a small dot. Affected individuals are indicated by solid squares (males) and circles (females). Pedigree 1 is commonly observed; pedigree 4 is rare.

heterozygous carriers; one half of sons are hemizygous affected (maternal inheritance) and one half are normal. Thus in this situation, one half of all offspring are affected. (7) If the trait is rare, parents and relatives are normal except for male relatives in the female line; e.g., on average, one half of maternal uncles are affected. This "uncle and nephew" pattern gives rise to an *oblique* pedigree pattern, in contrast to the vertical pattern of autosomal dominant conditions and the horizontal pattern of autosomal recessive conditions.

Examples of X-linked recessive conditions include hemophilia A, Duchenne form of muscular dystrophy, the Lesch-Nyhan syndrome, glucose-6-phosphate dehydrogenase deficiency, and Fabry's disease. In several of these, e.g., Duchenne muscular dystrophy and Fabry's disease, heterozygous females may exhibit mild or even moderately severe forms of the disease. Color blindness is also an X-linked inherited trait, but it is sufficiently frequent (occurring in about 8 per cent of Caucasian males) that the occurrence of homozygous color-blind females is not rare.

It is important to distinguish between X-linked inheritance and *sex-influenced autosomal dominant inheritance*. Baldness and hemochromatosis are examples of autosomal dominant traits that are sex influenced. Heterozygous females express the gene for baldness only when a source of testosterone becomes available (e.g., a masculinizing tumor of the ovary). Heterozygous females rarely develop clinical hemochromatosis because menstruation and pregnancy mitigate the accumulation of iron.

Y-LINKED INHERITANCE. A gene on the Y chromosome is transmitted through the father to all of his sons and none of his daughters. The only genes currently known to be located on the Y chromosome are those that determine "maleness" and an antigen that influences graft rejection. The maleness gene (testes determining factor) has been cloned.

POLYGENIC INHERITANCE. Most phenotypic traits are determined by the collaboration of many genes at different loci rather than by single gene effects. Polygenic inheritance is suggested for traits that show continuous variation in the form of a normal distribution curve. Height and intelligence are examples of polygenic traits in which the extremes of the distribution are not necessarily considered abnormal. Parents and offspring, and on average siblings also, have 50 per cent of their genes in common. Second-degree relatives share on average one fourth of all genes $(\frac{1}{2})^2$, and third-degree relatives (cousins) share one eighth $(\frac{1}{2})^3$. Thus as the degree of relation becomes more distant, the probability of inheriting the same combination of genes is reduced, and the degree of resemblance is likely to be less.

Many of the common chronic diseases of adults (such as essential hypertension, diabetes mellitus, hyperuricemia, hypercholesterolemia, coronary artery disease, and schizophrenia) and the common birth defects of children (such as cleft palate and lip and congenital heart disease) that tend to run in families fit best into the category of *multifactorial genetic disease*. This category should be suspected when the pedigree of a disease does not support inheritance in a simple dominant or recessive manner. In multifactorial genetic disease there is both a polygenic component and an environmental component of causative factors. In the population at large there are *risk* genes present in low frequency. If in any one individual there is a particularly large number of risk genes, the latent disorder becomes overt. When an individual inherits just the right combination of risk genes, he or she passes beyond a "risk threshold" at which environmental factors may determine the expression and severity of disease (Fig. 30–5). In order for another family member to develop the same disease, that individual would have to inherit the same or a very similar combination of genes. The likelihood of such an occurrence is clearly greater in first-degree than in more distant relatives. The chances of any relative's inheriting the right combination of risk genes also decrease as the number of genes required for the expression of a given trait increases. Elegant and complex mathematical models have been advanced for polygenic-multifactorial disease, but these should not obscure the fact that each of the risk genes must express itself, like any other gene, by way of a specific biochemical product. Eventually the vague concept of genetic susceptibility of polygenic inheritance must yield to the basic premise that genes control the synthesis of specific proteins with specific functions. We may anticipate

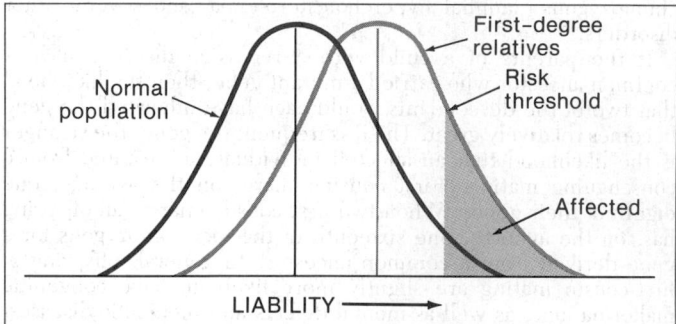

FIGURE 30–5. Diseases that conform to a polygenic multifactorial model of inheritance lead to an increased prevalence of disease among the relatives of affected individuals. This increased prevalence is most evident among first-degree relatives.

that risk genes will be identified in the future using restriction fragment length polymorphism (RFLP) and complex linkage analysis models.

To date the genetic loci most prominently associated with disease susceptibility are those composing the major histocompatibility (MHC) locus or human leukocyte antigen (HLA) system. There are seven internationally recognized, highly polymorphic components of the human MHC: HLA-A, -B, and -C, collectively known as class I antigens, are formed on most nucleated cells; HLA-DR, -DQ, and -DP, collectively known as class II antigens, are restricted primarily to B lymphocytes, monocytes, macrophages, activated T cells, and endothelial cells; and HLA-D, a functional activity recognized through the complex proliferative responses to allogeneic cells in mixed lymphocyte cultures. The products of these genes are proteins that are found on the surface of body cells and that enable an individual's immune system to distinguish its own cells (self) from those of someone else (nonself). Each HLA locus in the population consists of multiple alleles, each of which produces an immunologically distinct protein. HLA-A has at least 24 alleles, HLA-B has at least 52, C has at least 11, D has at least 26, DR has at least 20, DQ has at least 9, and DP has at least 6. The inheritance of certain alleles predisposes to the development of certain diseases, in some instances when the individual is exposed to a particular environmental challenge. For example, the frequency of B27 allele in the white population is approximately 8 per cent. In patients with ankylosing spondylitis the frequency of B27 is over 90 per cent. In Australian aborigines and black Africans the B27 antigen is virtually absent and the frequency of ankylosing spondylitis is sharply reduced. A Caucasian with the B27 antigen is approximately 120 times more likely to develop ankylosing spondylitis than one who does not posses the antigen; the increased liability among Japanese with the B27 antigen is 300 times. Reiter's syndrome may follow an infection of the bowel or urinary tract with *Shigella, Salmonella,* or *Yersinia* organisms. No less than 20 per cent of B27-positive individuals with *Shigella* infections develop Reiter's syndrome. Other examples include the association of HLA-DR and -DQ with type 1 insulin-dependent diabetes mellitus, HLA-DR3 with endocrine disorders, HLA-DR2 with narcolepsy, and HLA-A3 with hemochromatosis.

Multifactorial or polygenic inheritance must not be confused with *genetic heterogeneity*. Hypercholesterolemia and hyperuricemia behave as multifactorial traits when viewed at the population level. At the family level, however, it is sometimes possible to identify a single locus that is mainly responsible for the disease in that family. Examples include familial hypercholesterolemia, an autosomal dominant trait present in about 5 per cent of subjects with premature myocardial infarctions, which in single-gene dosage produces atherosclerosis in the absence of any extraordinary environmental factor; or hypoxanthine-guanine phosphoribosyltransferase deficiency, an X-linked recessive trait present in about 0.5 per cent of subjects with gout, which in the hemizygous state produces marked purine overproduction without any relationship to obesity or alcohol consumption.

MITOCHONDRIAL INHERITANCE. Each mitochondrion contains several circular chromosomes that code for certain ribosomal and transfer ribonucleic acids (RNA's) and for 13 polypeptides involved in oxidative phosphorylation, the chief function of the mitochondrion. The mitochondrial code differs from that of nuclear DNA and that of any contemporary prokaryote; it is similar to that of bacteria. Mitochondrial inheritance is exclusively matrilineal. Diseases that are thought to involve mitochondrial mutations include Leber hereditary optic atrophy, infantile bilateral striatal necrosis, and myoclonic epilepsy with "ragged red fibers."

GENE FREQUENCY. The distribution of a mutant gene in the general population may be calculated on the basis of the Hardy-Weinberg equation. If the frequency of a particular gene A is p, then that of its alternative allele is $(1 - p) = q$. There will be three genotypes in the population: Those who are homozygous AA, those who are heterozygous Aa, and those who are homozygous aa. In a randomly mating population the frequencies of these genotypes will be in the proportion $p^2(AA)$, $2pg(Aa)$, and $q^2(aa)$. An important consequence of this distribution is that irrespective of the initial frequency of the genes A and a in the population, the proportion of the three genotypes will tend to remain constant in succeeding generations, provided that there is no difference in biologic fitness of any of the genotypes. If there is unequal viability or fertility among the three genotypes, or if mating is not random, the frequency calculations require considerable correction, and in small populations major changes in gene frequency can occur on the basis of chance alone.

If the frequency of a recessive disease in a particular population is known, the frequency of heterozygous carriers and of the abnormal gene can be calculated. Thus for a recessively inherited disease aa (q^2) with a frequency of 1 per 10,000 (e.g., albinism), the frequency of the gene a (q) will be 1 per 100, and that of heterozygous carriers will be $2 \times p \times q = 2 \times 99/100 \times 1/100$ = approximately 1 in 50. Thus, in this particular example there will be 200 clinically unaffected carriers of the abnormal gene for every affected individual. Table 30–2 lists the frequency of several inherited diseases. Cystic fibrosis, a recessively inherited disease, has a prevalence in the white population of about 1 per 2500 (q^2); thus the frequency of the gene (q) is 1 in 50 and of heterozygous carriers is approximately 1 in 25, or 4 per cent of the white population. A similar calculation with respect to sickle cell anemia among United States blacks ($q^2 = 1/625$) yields a frequency of heterozygous carriers of 1 in 12.5, or 8 per cent of the United States black population.

The frequency of most genes in the population is relatively stable. When a gene is rare and severely disadvantageous, the rate of its introduction into a population by spontaneous mutation is balanced by the rate of elimination of the disadvantageous gene by natural selection. The frequency of the disadvantageous gene, however, can be stabilized at a high level if the heterozygotes are slightly favored (increased biologic fitness) and leave a greater number of progeny than either homozygote. When a rare form of a species is present at a frequency that cannot be maintained by recurrent mutation alone, a *balanced polymorphism* is said to exist. Usually this means that the rarer of two allelic forms occurs with a frequency of at least 1 per cent of the population. When this is found, *heterozygote advantage* should be suspected. An example of such a balanced polymorphism is the increased resistance of individuals heterozygous for the sickle cell trait to falciparum malaria. Although persons with sickle cell disease (homozygotes, SS hemoglobin) often die before they can reproduce, and thus remove the sickle cell gene from the population, the prevalence of heterozygotes (SA hemoglobin) may nevertheless reach 40 per cent in certain West African populations. Death from falciparum malaria is much less frequent in carriers of the sickle cell trait than in noncarriers, and thus the heterozygote does have an advantage. Whether the extraordinary frequency of heterozygotes for the sickle cell gene in West Africa is due entirely to differential mortality or in part to differential fertility is uncertain, but this example suffices to illustrate that the effects of genes can be assessed only in relation to a particular environment. In most instances, however, a distinct advantage for the heterozygote of a polymorphic trait (of which there are many; see Ch. 31) cannot be demonstrated, and the possibility exists that certain polymorphic traits are genetically neutral.

The term *genetic load* has been used to describe the total genetic disability of a population. It comprises both a *mutational load*, based on recurrent mutation of a normal gene to a lethal or sublethal gene, and a *segregational load*, resulting from segregation of the harmful gene from advantaged heterozygotes, as in the example of sickle cell heterozygotes discussed above. Each individual has been estimated to have three to eight genes, which, if homozygous instead of heterozygous, would be lethal. The relative contribution of the segregational and mutational loads to the total genetic load is uncertain.

Beaudet AL, Scriver CR, Sly WS, et al.: Introduction to Human Biochemical and Molecular Genetics. New York, McGraw-Hill Book Company, 1990. *A concise, historical perspective and summation of what we know about basic principles of human genetics, which emphasizes causes (mutations), pathogenesis, and therapy.*

Cavalli-Sforza LL, Bodmer WF: The Genetics of Human Populations. 2nd ed. San Francisco, W.H. Freeman and Company, 1978. *An authoritative textbook of human genetics.*

Galjaard H: Genetic Metabolic Diseases. Early Diagnosis and Prenatal Analysis. Amsterdam, Elsevier/North Holland Biomedical Press, 1980. *An 850-page book on hereditary disorders, about one third of which is devoted to methods and results of prenatal diagnosis.*

McKusick VA: Mendelian Inheritance in Man. 9th ed. Baltimore, Johns Hopkins University Press, 1990. *A catalogue of autosomal dominant, autosomal recessive, and X-linked phenotypes, with brief descriptions and literature references for each.*

Scriver CR, Beaudet AL, Sly WS, et al.: The Metabolic Basis of Inherited Disease. 6th ed. New York, McGraw-Hill Book Company, 1989. *Authoritative discussions of all inborn errors of metabolism for which there is a substantial body of metabolic or biochemical information.*

Vogel F, Motulsky AG: Human Genetics: Problems and Approaches. 2nd ed. Berlin, Springer-Verlag, 1986. *A superb and up-to-date treatment of human genetics.*

31 Inborn Errors of Metabolism

James B. Wyngaarden

The inspired concept of inborn errors of metabolism, developed by Archibald Garrod in the first decade of this century, marks the birth of biochemical genetics. Garrod's studies of alcaptonuria, pentosuria, albinism, and cystinuria led to the proposal of a new category of diseases in which a block in a metabolic pathway arises from an inherited deficiency of a specific enzyme. This concept was proved in 1948 when Gibson found a deficiency of NADH-dependent methemoglobin reductase in recessive methemoglobinemia. This was soon followed by the discovery in 1952 by Cori and Cori of a deficiency of glucose-6-phosphatase in von Gierke's disease, in 1953 by Jervis of phenylalanine hydroxylase deficiency in phenylketonuria, and in 1956 by LaDu of homogentisic acid oxidase deficiency in alcaptonuria as originally predicted by Garrod. By 1990 deficiencies of over 300 different enzymes have been associated with hereditary disease. Of even greater importance in the history of genetics was the remarkable insight in Garrod's hypothesis that the primary action of a gene is to control the synthesis of a specific enzyme. Decades later Beadle (1945) independently proposed the one gene–one enzyme hypothesis anticipated by Garrod.

In 1949 Pauling, Itano, and associates observed that sickle cell hemoglobin exhibited abnormal electrophoretic behavior and introduced the concept of *molecular disease*, in which a structural alteration in a macromolecule accounted for a specific functional change that was responsible for a disease state. In 1953 Ingram demonstrated the substitution of a single amino acid residue in the β-chain of sickle cell hemoglobin, confirming the concept of molecular disease and initiating an ever-lengthening series of findings of structural alterations in macromolecules that result from gene mutations. For a time "missing" enzyme diseases and hemoglobinopathies were thought to represent distinct categories of disease, perhaps representing defects of control and structural genes, respectively. More sensitive techniques have disclosed low levels of residual activity of the deficient enzyme in many inborn errors of metabolism. In some cases the mutation has affected a critical portion of the enzyme, radically reducing its catalytic activity; in others the mutation has rendered the enzyme highly unstable. In the case of erythrocytes that lack a nucleus and cannot continue to synthesize new protein, enzyme lability results in low enzyme activity values in the older cells. In several instances amino acid sequence studies of enzymes have disclosed single amino acid substitutions analogous to the defect in sickle hemoglobin. Thus many inborn errors of metabolism are molecular diseases in which the *primary* defect lies in the genetic specification of the protein.

INBORN ERRORS AND MUTANT PROTEINS

Although most of the well-defined inborn errors of metabolism are inherited as recessive conditions, in principle any human phenotype showing mendelian genetics must be based on a specific variant or missing protein. Thus not only autosomal and X-linked recessive but also autosomal and X-linked dominant conditions may be expressed through abnormal proteins. Examples in which a mutant protein has been identified include autosomal recessive, alcaptonuria (homogentistic acid oxidase); X-linked recessive, Lesch-Nyhan syndrome (hypoxanthine-guanine phosphoribosyltransferase); autosomal dominant, acute intermittent porphyria (uroporphyrinogen I synthetase). No example of an X-linked dominant condition in which the mutant protein has been identified can be cited as yet. In one condition of this category, X-linked familial hypophosphatemic rickets, a defect in Na-dependent phosphate transport is suspected but the membrane carrier has not been identified. The concept of inborn errors of metabolism has broadened considerably since first propounded by Garrod. A reasonable definition would include any condition of clinical significance that shows a mendelian mode of inheritance, but in practice the term is restricted to conditions that have recognizable biochemical manifestations.

A mutant protein that cannot be detected by functional assay may nevertheless retain immunologic reactivity. However, in some instances no protein can be detected by functional or immunologic means. In the terminology of microbial genetics, the former class of mutants is frequently called CRM(+) ("krim" positive) and the latter CRM(−). The presence of CRM(−) material suggests that the genetic defect is due to a missense mutation with a consequent amino acid substitution that destroys the activity but not the antigenicity of the mutant enzyme. In most cases in which mutant enzymes have been studied, cross-reactive material has been detected. However, in the Lesch-Nyhan syndrome only 1 CRM(+) mutant has been found among 14 studied. At the pseudocholinesterase locus, 17 CRM(+) mutants and 18 CRM(−) mutants have been recognized. A CRM(−) reaction does not prove that no protein is present; the protein may be so altered that both enzyme function and immunologic reactivity have been lost.

Mutation does not necessarily result in loss of enzyme activity. Several examples of increased activity are known. The best examples are three types of phosphoribosylpyrophosphate synthetase overactivity associated with purine overproduction and gout. In one there is a 2.5-fold increase in enzyme activity per molecule; in another, excessive activity is a reflection of diminished affinity for normal intracellular nucleotide inhibitors; in a third, the overactivity results from an increased affinity for ribose 5-phosphate, a substrate of the reaction. All of these changes reflect alterations of enzyme structure. Some of the clinical conditions in which an abnormality of a specific protein has been observed are listed in Tables 31–1 and 31–2. Others include deficiencies of peptide hormones, abnormalities of binding proteins (receptor diseases) and of epidermal proteins, and defects in transmembrane transport (e.g., cystinuria). Chromosome mapping data exist for many inborn errors.

GENETIC HETEROGENEITY

When two or more mutations produce identical or closely similar clinical syndromes, *genetic heterogeneity* is said to exist. In some instances the mutations may be at different loci (*nonallelic* genes), whereas in others they may occur in different portions of the same locus (*allelic* genes). Hemophilia can be caused by a mutation at either of two distinct loci on the X-chromosome, one leading to a deficiency of Factor VIII (classic hemophilia) and the other to a deficiency of Factor IX (Christmas disease). By contrast, the multiple variants of G6PD, over 315 as of 1990, represent different structural gene mutations at a single locus. A striking example of both allelic and nonallelic heterogeneity is hereditary methemoglobinemia, which can be produced by at least ten different mutations at three distinct loci: two at the locus for the α-chain of hemoglobin, three at the locus for the β-chain, and at least five at the locus for NADH methemoglobin reductase.

One of the most stunning developments of the last decade is the recognition that many genetic diseases present in many variant forms, and that the same disease entity can be caused by an array of mutations affecting the structural gene in different potentially large series of allelic variations. Duchenne muscular dystrophy can result from deletions, translocations, duplications, and point mutations of the dystrophin gene, all resulting in apparent absence of dystrophin in skeletal muscle. In the allelic but milder condition, Becker muscular dystrophy, dystrophin is present but is of altered size or quantity.

In view of the multiple alleles that occur at many genetic loci (genetic polymorphism, see Ch. 30), persons who appear to be homozygous for a genetic trait may actually have inherited different abnormal alleles from each parent. Such individuals are said to be *genetic compounds*. The clinical syndrome in a genetic compound may be intermediate in severity and manifestations between the syndromes produced by homozygosity for either allele. A classic example is hemoglobin SC disease, which results when an offspring inherits a Hb S gene (beta-6$^{glu \rightarrow val}$) from one parent and a Hb C gene (beta-6$^{glu \rightarrow lys}$) from the other. Another is the mucopolysaccharide storage disease resulting from inheritance of one gene for Hurler's disease (severe) and one for Scheie's disease (mild). In both these examples the severity is intermediate between the diseases associated with the respective homozygous states. Table 31–3 lists selected inherited diseases for which genetic compounds have been demonstrated.

ETIOLOGY. The etiology of an inborn error of metabolism is a mutant gene. If the amino acid sequence of the mutant protein is known, it is possible to deduce the nature of the mutation from the genetic code. For example, the human variant of glucose-6-phosphate dehydrogenase, G6PD Hektoen, differs from normal G6PD in a single amino acid substitution, HIS→TYR. This substitution corresponds to a mutation from GTA(or G) to ATA(or G) in a codon in the structural gene for G6PD. The G6PD locus emerges as the locus of the human genome with the greatest apparent extent of genetic polymorphism. Nevertheless, extensive tests carried out with numerous endonuclease probes within the gene and flanking regions of the gene, covering over 300 restriction sites, have surprisingly revealed only one restriction fragment length polymorphism (RFLP). Most of the amino acid sequence information of human mutant proteins has been obtained from studies of red blood cell proteins, such as hemoglobin and G6PD. At least four types of mutations can be discerned by this approach: deletions, duplications, missense mutations, and frame-shift mutations.

Another type of mutation, the nonsense mutation, has also been demonstrated in humans, using DNA restriction enzyme analysis and DNA sequencing techniques. The partial nucleotide sequence of β-globin mRNA isolated from a unique patient with homozygous β°-thalassemia disclosed a replacement of an adenine by a uracil in the codon for position 17. This changed the RNA codon from AAG to AUG, a termination codon. As a result a nonfunctional partial β-chain, only 16 amino acids long, was synthesized. Hb McKees-Rock represents another example of mutation of an amino acid codon to a terminator codon, but in this case the β-globin is shortened by only two amino acids and is functional.

DNA cloning techniques permit direct study of the altered DNA sequence in many human mutations, even those that involve genes that code for quantitatively minor proteins, such as most enzymes. The new technique of polymerase chain reaction (PCR) permits amplification of very minute quantities of DNA and, together with use of suitable restriction enzymes and gene probes, enables investigators to produce quantities of DNA adequate for sequence analysis in situations in which this would previously have been impossible. These techniques are greatly accelerating the precise definition of genetic errors at the DNA level.

In addition, the discovery of an array of restriction endonucleases, enzymes capable of cleaving DNA at precise sites characterized by specific short recognition sequences, has permitted identification of RFLP's as genetic markers of human disease.

TABLE 31–1. DISORDERS IN WHICH DEFICIENT ACTIVITY OF A SPECIFIC ENZYME HAS BEEN DEMONSTRATED IN HUMAN BEINGS*

Condition	Enzyme with Deficient Activity	Condition	Enzyme with Deficient Activity
Acatalasia	Catalase	Gout, primary	PP-ribose-P synthetase (increased)
Acid phosphatase deficiency	Acid phosphatase	Granulomatous disease, X-linked	NADPH oxidase
Acyl CoA dehydrogenase deficiency	Acyl CoA decarboxylase	Hemolytic anemia	Adenosine deaminase
Adrenal hyperplasia	Cholesterol desmolase	Hemolytic anemia	Aldolase A
Adrenal hyperplasia	3-β-Hydroxysteroid dehydrogenase	Hemolytic anemia	Diphosphoglycerate mutase
Adrenal hyperplasia	21-Hydroxylase	Hemolytic anemia	γ-Glutamylcysteine synthetase
Adrenal hyperplasia	11-β-Hydroxylase	Hemolytic anemia	Glucose phosphate isomerase
Adrenal hyperplasia	17-α-Hydroxylase	Hemolytic anemia	Glutathione peroxidase
Albinism	Tyrosinase	Hemolytic anemia	Glutathione reductase
Alcaptonuria	Homogentisic acid oxidase	Hemolytic anemia	Glutathione synthetase
Aldosterone deficiency I	18-Hydroxylase (corticosterone methyl oxidase I)	Hemolytic anemia	Hexokinase
		Hemolytic anemia	Phosphofructokinase, muscle M.
Aldosterone deficiency II	18-OH-Dehydrogenase	Hemolytic anemia	Phosphoglycerate kinase
Alpha-methylacetoaceticaciduria	β-Ketothiolase	Hemolytic anemia	Pyrimidine 5′-nucleotidase
Anemia, megaloblastic	Dihydrofolate reductase	Hemolytic anemia	Pyruvate kinase
Apnea, drug-induced	Pseudocholinesterase	Hemolytic anemia	Triosephosphate isomerase
Argininemia	Arginase	Histidinemia	Histidine:ammonia lyase
Argininosuccinic aciduria	Argininosuccinate lyase	HMG-CoA lyase deficiency	3-Hydroxy-3-methylglutarate-CoA lyase
Aspartylglycosaminuria	Aspartyl glycosaminidase		
Ataxia, intermittent	Pyruvate decarboxylase	Homocystinuria I	Cystathionine beta-synthase
Cerebrotendinous xanthomatosis	Mitochondrial 26-hydroxylase	Homocystinuria II	N(5,10)-Methylenetetrahydrofolate reductase
Cholesteryl ester deficiency (Norum-Gjone disease)	Lecithin cholesterol acyltransferase (LCAT)	4-Hydroxybutyricaciduria	Succinic semialdehyde dehydrogenase
Citrullinemia	Argininosuccinate synthetase		
Coproporphyria	Coproporphyrinogen III oxidase	3-Hydroxy-3-methylglutaryl-CoA lyase deficiency	3-Hydroxy-3-methylglutaryl-CoA lyase
Crigler-Najjar syndrome	Glucuronyl transferase	Hydroxyprolinemia	Hydroxyproline oxidase
Cystathioninuria	γ-Cystathionase	Hyperalaninemia	β-Alanine-α-ketoglutarate aminotransferase
2,8-Dihydroxyadenine nephrolithiasis	Adenine phosphoribosyl transferase		
Disaccharide intolerance I	Invertase	Hyperammonemia I	Ornithine transcarbamylase
Disaccharide intolerance II	Invertase, maltase	Hyperammonemia II	Carbamyl phosphate synthetase
Disaccharide intolerance III	Lactase	Hyperammonemia III	N-Acetylglutamate synthetase
Ehlers-Danlos syndrome, type VI	Collagen lysyl hydroxylase	Hyperglycerolemia	ATP:glycerol phosphotransferase
Ehlers-Danlos syndrome, type VII	Procollagen peptidase	Hyperglycinemia, ketotic I	Propionyl CoA carboxylase, α subunit
Epidermolysis bullosa	Collagenase		
Ethanolaminosis	Ethanolamine kinase	Hyperglycinemia, ketotic II	Propionyl CoA carboxylase, β subunit
Fabry's disease	α-Galactosidase A		
Farber's lipogranulomatosis	Ceramidase	Hyperglycinemia, nonketotic form	Glycine forminimotransferase
Formiminotransferase deficiency	Forminimotransferase	Hyperlysinemia	Lysine-α-ketoglutarate reductase
Fructose intolerance	Fructose-1-phosphate aldolase "B"	Hyperphenylalaninemia: DHPR-deficient form	Dihydropteridine reductase (DHPR)
Fructose-1,6-diphosphatase deficiency	Fructose-1,6-diphosphatase	Hyperphenylalaninemia: GTP-CH-deficient form	Guanosine-triphosphate cyclohydrolase (GTP-CH)
Fructosuria	Hepatic fructokinase	Hyperphenylalaninemia: 6-PTS-deficient form	6-Pyruvoyl tetrahydropterin synthase (6-PTS)
Fucosidosis	α-L-Fucosidase	Hyperprolinemia I	Proline oxidase
Galactokinase deficiency	Galactokinase	Hyperprolinemia II	δ-1-Pyrroline-5-carboxylate dehydrogenase
Galactose epimerase deficiency	Galactose epimerase		
Galactosemia	Galactose-1-phosphate uridyl transferase	Hypoglycemia	Glycogen synthase
		Hypophosphatasia	Alkaline phosphatase
Gangliosidosis, G_{M1}	β-Galactosidase A,B	I-cell disease	UDP-N-acetylglucosamine: lysosomal enzyme N-acetyl glucosaminyl-1-phosphotransferase
Gangliosidosis, G_{M2} (Tay-Sachs disease)	β-Hexosaminidase A		
Gangliosidosis, G_{M2}	β-Hexosaminidase A	Ichthyosis, X-linked	3-β-Hydroxy steroid sulfatase
Gangliosidosis, G_{M2} (Sandhoff's disease)	β-Hexosaminidase B	Immunodeficiency disease	Adenosine deaminase
		Immunodeficiency disease	Purine nucleoside phosphorylase
Gangliosidosis, G_{M3}	UDP-N-acetyl-galactosaminyl transferase	Immunodeficiency disease	Uridine monophosphate kinase
		Intestinal lactase deficiency (adult)	Lactase
Gaucher's disease	Glucocerebrosidase	Isovaleric acidemia	Isovaleryl CoA dehydrogenase
G6PD deficiency (favism, primaquine sensitivity, etc.)	Glucose-6-phosphate dehydrogenase	Ketoacidosis, infantile	Succinyl CoA:3-ketoacid CoA-transferase
Glutaric aciduria I	Glutaryl-CoA dehydrogenase	Krabbe's disease	Galactocerebroside β-galactosidase
Glutaric aciduria II	Acyl-CoA dehydrogenase, multiple	Lactic acidosis, congenital	Dihydrolipoyl dehydrogenase
Glutathionemia	γ-Glutamyl transferase	Lactosyl ceramidosis	Neutral β-galactosidase
Glycogen storage disease Ia	Glucose-6-phosphatase	Leigh's necrotizing encephalomyelopathy	Pyruvate carboxylase
Glycogen storage disease Ib	Glucose-6-phosphate translocase		
Glycogen storage disease II	α-1,4-Glucosidase	Lesch-Nyhan syndrome	Hypoxanthine-guanine phosphoribosyl transferase
Glycogen storage disease III	Amylo-1, 6-glucosidase		
Glycogen storage disease IV	Amylo-(1,4 to 1,6)-transglucosidase	Lipase deficiency, congenital	Lipase (pancreatic)
Glycogen storage disease V	Muscle phosphorylase	Lipoprotein lipase deficiency (type I hyperlipoproteinemia)	Lipoprotein lipase
Glycogen storage disease VI	Liver phosphorylase or phosphorylase kinase		
Glycogen storage disease VII	Muscle phosphofructokinase	Lysine intolerance	L-Lysine:NAD-oxidoreductase
Gout, primary	Hypoxanthine-guanine phosphoribosyl transferase	Male pseudohermaphroditism	Testicular 17,20-desmolase

Table continued on following page

TABLE 31–1. DISORDERS IN WHICH DEFICIENT ACTIVITY OF A SPECIFIC ENZYME HAS BEEN DEMONSTRATED IN HUMAN BEINGS* Continued

Condition	Enzyme with Deficient Activity	Condition	Enzyme with Deficient Activity
Male pseudohermaphroditism	Testicular 17-ketosteroid dehydrogenase	Myopathy	Myoadenylate deaminase
Male pseudohermaphroditism	Steroid 5α-reductase	Myopathy, lipid	Carnitine palmitoyl transferase I or II
Mannosidosis	α-Acid-mannosidase	Niemann-Pick disease	Sphingomyelinase
Maple sugar urine disease	Branched-chain keto acid decarboxylase	Ornithinemia with gyrate atrophy	Ornithine-δ-aminotransferase
Metachromatic leukodystrophy I	Arylsulfase A (cerebroside sulfatase)	Orotic aciduria I	Orotate phosphoribonyl transferase and orotidine-5′ phosphate decarboxylase
Methemoglobinemia	Cytochrome b_5 reductase		
Methionine adenosyl transferase deficiency (hypermethioninemia)	Methionine adenosyl transferase	Orotic aciduria II	Orotidylic decarboxylase
2-Methylacetoacetyl-CoA thiolase deficiency	2-Methylacetoacetyl-CoA thiolase	Oxalosis I (glycolic aciduria)	Alanine: glyoxylate aminotransferase
		Oxalosis II (glyceric aciduria)	D-Glyceric dehydrogenase
β-Methyl crotonyl glycinuria I	β-Methyl crotonyl-CoA carboxylase	5-Oxoprolinuria (pyroglutamic aciduria)	Glutathione synthetase
Methylene tetrahydrofolate reductase deficiency	Methylene tetrahydrofolate reductase	Pentosuria	L-Xylulose reductase
Methylmalonic aciduria I (vitamin B_{12}-unresponsive)	Methylmalonic CoA mutase	Phenylketonuria	Phenylalanine hydroxylase
		Phosphoglycerate mutase deficiency	P-glycerate mutase
Methylmalonic aciduria II (vitamin B_{12}-responsive)	ATP: cobalamine adenosyl transferase	Porphyria, acute hepatic	Porphobilinogen synthetase
		Porphyria, acute intermittent	Uroporphyrinogen I synthetase
Mevalonic aciduria	Mevalonate kinase	Porphyria, congenital erythropoietic	Uroporphyrinogen III cosynthase
Mitochondrial myopathy	NADH-CoA reductase	Porphyria cutanea tarda	Uroporphyrinogen decarboxylase
Mucolipidoses II and III	N-Acetylglucosamine-1-phosphotransferase	Porphyria variegata	Protoporphyrinogen oxidase
		Prolidase deficiency	Prolidase (Peptidase D)
Mucolipidosis IV	Ganglioside neuramindase	Propionic aciduria	Propionyl-CoA carboxylase
Mucopolysaccharidosis IH (Hurler's)	α-L-Iduronidase	Protoporphyria	Heme synthetase (ferrochelatase)
		Pulmonary emphysema, or cirrhosis	α-1-Antitrypsin
Mucopolysaccharidosis IS (Scheie's)	α-L-Iduronidase	Pyridoxine-dependent infantile convulsions	Glutamic acid decarboxylase
Mucopolysaccharidosis II (Hunter's)	Iduronate sulfatase		
Mucopolysaccharidosis IIIA (Sanfilippo's)	Heparan sulfate sulfatase	Pyrimidinemia	Dihydropyrimidine dehydrogenase
		Pyruvate carboxylase deficiency	Pyruvate carboxylase
Mucopolysaccharidosis IIIB (Sanfilippo's)	N-Acetyl-α-D-glucosaminidase	Refsum's disease	Phytanic acid α-hydroxidase
		Renal tubular acidosis with deafness	Carbonic anhydrase B
Mucopolysaccharidosis IIIC	Acetyl-CoA:alpha glucosaminide N-transferase	Rickets, vitamin D dependent	25-Hydroxycholecalciferol 1-hydroxylase
Mucopolysaccharidosis IIID	N-Acetyltransglucosamine-6-sulfate sulfatase	Saccharopinuria	Saccharopine dehydrogenase
		Sarcosinemia	Sarcosine dehydrogenase complex
Mucopolysaccharidosis IVA (Morquio's)	Galactose-6-sulfatase	Sialidosis	α-Neuraminidase
		Sulfite oxidase deficiency	Sulfite oxidase
Mucopolysaccharidosis IVB	β-Galactosidase	Sulfite oxidase and xanthine dehydrogenase deficiency	Molybdenum cofactor
Mucopolysaccharidosis VI (Maroteaux-Lamy)	Arylsulfatase B		
		Trypsinogen deficiency	Trypsinogen
Mucopolysaccharidosis VII	β-Glucuronidase	Tyrosinemia A	Fumarylacetoacetate hydrolase
Multiple carboxylase deficiency, late-onset	Biotinase	Tyrosinemia II (Richner-Hanhart syndrome)	Tyrosine transaminase
Multiple carboxylase deficiency (several forms)	Holocarboxylase synthetase	Urocanic acidemia	Urocanase
		Valinemia	Valine transaminase
Muscle lactate dehydrogenase deficiency	Muscle-specific subunit of LDH	Wolman's disease	Acid lipase
		Xanthinuria	Xanthine oxidase
Myeloperoxidase deficiency with disseminated candidiasis	Myeloperoxidase	Xanthurenic aciduria	Kynureninase
		Xylosidase deficiency	Xylosidase

*Based upon McKusick VA: In Scriver CR, Beaudet AL, Sly WS, et al. (eds.): The Metabolic Basis of Inherited Disease. 6th ed. New York, McGraw-Hill, 1989, with modifications.

Polymorphisms result from mutational events that either alter an existing or create a new recognition site, thus generating fragments of either greater or lesser lengths than are found in the case of normal individuals. Linkage maps of the human genome are made possible by the RFLP technique, and genetic linkage analysis can identify DNA markers close to human disease loci. This in turn permits the strategy of mapping and cloning genes prior to the identification of their products, a process called "reverse genetics." This approach has led to cloning of the genes for chronic granulomatous disease, Duchenne muscular dystrophy, and hereditary retinoblastoma and to mapping of the genes for Huntington disease, adult polycystic kidney disease, neurofibromatosis, von Hippel–Lindau disease, polyposis of the colon, and cystic fibrosis to specific sites in the human genome. Members of the last group of genes are likely to be cloned in the foreseeable future. The cloned gene can be inserted into an organism or cell in which it can be expressed, and the synthesized protein can then be identified. These approaches have led to the identification of dystrophin, the protein absent in Duchenne muscular dystrophy, as the prototype of reverse genetics. Duchenne muscular dystrophy is the first disorder in which the sequence of analysis proceeding from mapping of the gene, through identification and characterization of mRNA and cDNA, to the recognition of the protein, has run its full course. These recent developments are discussed in Ch. 32.

PATHOGENESIS OF GENETIC DISEASE. The consequence of a mutation depends on the function normally served by the product of the gene. Mutations in genes for rRNA or tRNA would very likely affect protein synthesis generally and might be incompatible with life. No such mutations have been identified in mammalian systems, although they are known in bacteria.

Defects involving nonenzymic proteins undoubtedly account for a large number of genetic diseases, but relatively few have been defined biochemically. The hemoglobinopathies are an exception. Over 580 hemoglobin variants are now known. Many additional examples exist of mutations affecting nonenzymic proteins, and more are being discovered with increasing frequency.

TABLE 31–2. SOME DISORDERS IN WHICH A DEFICIENCY OF A PLASMA PROTEIN HAS BEEN DEMONSTRATED IN HUMAN BEINGS

Condition	Plasma Protein
Afibrinogenemia	Fibrinogen
Agammaglobulinemia, X-linked	IgA, IgG
Agammaglobulinemia, selective IgA	IgA
Agammaglobulinemia, selective IgG	IgG
Analbuminemia	Albumin
Atransferrinemia	Transferrin
Complement deficiency states, selective C1q, C1r, C1s, C2, C3, C4, C5, C6, C7, C8	C1q, C1r, C1s, C2, C3, C4, C5, C6, C7, C8
Factor VII deficiency	Factor VII
Factor X (Stuart factor) deficiency	Factor X
Fibrin-stabilizing factor deficiency	Factor XIII
Hageman trait	Factor XII
Hemophilia A	Factor VIII
Hemophilia B	Factor IX
Hereditary angioedema	C1-inhibitor
Hypoprothrombinemia	Factor II
Parahemophilia	Factor V
PTA deficiency	Factor XI

PTA = plasma thromboplastin antecedent.

In one of these, the ZZ variant of α-1-antitrypsin deficiency, two amino acid substitutions (missense mutations) in α-1-antitrypsin lead to the production of a modified protein that is not susceptible to normal post-translational processing. As a consequence carbohydrate residues are not added to the protein in the normal manner, and the defective glycoprotein accumulates in liver cells, possibly because the altered molecule cannot be secreted. Other examples in which a specific mutant protein has been identified include various lipoproteins, the abnormal plasma membrane receptor in familial hypercholesterolemia, the abnormal cytoplasmic androgen receptor in the complete form of testicular feminization, an abnormal insulin in familial hyperproinsulinemia, and an abnormal protein called dynein in the microtubules of cilia in Kartagener's syndrome.

The largest number of known inborn errors of metabolism involves deficiencies of enzymes that catalyze discrete steps in biosynthetic or catabolic sequences. The consequences of metabolic blocks depend upon the function of the affected sequence and the properties of the affected substrates. In some conditions the disease is manifested by the inability to form a specific product, as in the failure of melanin production in one form of albinism. In others, accumulation of the precursor of a blocked reaction results in toxicity or in a storage disease. In phenylketonuria the block in phenylalanine hydroxylase results in accumulation of phenylalanine and overproduction of toxic phenylketone products. Deficiencies of various catabolic enzymes explain the progressive tissue accumulations in the mucopolysaccharidoses and sphingolipidoses. In some enzyme deficiencies,

TABLE 31–3. INHERITED METABOLIC DISEASES FOR WHICH GENETIC COMPOUNDS HAVE BEEN DEMONSTRATED

α-1-Antitrypsin deficiency
Cystinosis
Cystinuria
"Homozygous" familial hypercholesterolemia (LDL receptor-internalization defect)
Galactosemia (galactose-1-phosphate uridyltransferase deficiency)
Gaucher's disease (glucocerebrosidase deficiency)
Glucosephosphate isomerase deficiency
Hemoglobin α-chain variants
Hemoglobin β-chain variants
Hurler-Scheie syndrome (α-L-iduronidase deficiency)
Iminoglycinuria
Metachromatic leukodystrophy (cerebroside sulfatase deficiency)
Hereditary methemoglobinemia (NADH dehydrogenase deficiency)
Phenylketonuria (phenylalanine hydroxylase deficiency)
Pseudocholinesterase deficiency
Pyruvate kinase deficiency

LDL = low density lipoprotein; NADH = reduced form of nicotinamide adenine dinucleotide.

disease results from failure to modify another protein. For example, in some types of Ehlers-Danlos syndrome collagen polypeptide synthesis is normal but enzymes essential in cross-linking are deficient, with the result that fragile collagen is produced.

TREATMENT OF INBORN ERRORS OF METABOLISM. Treatment of the patient with an inherited disorder depends upon accurate diagnosis and an understanding of the pathophysiology of the disease, including an appreciation of the interaction of genetic and environmental factors. Well-known examples are phenylketonuria, which predisposes to toxic reactions to dietary phenylalanine, and G6PD deficiency, which predisposes to hemolysis following ingestion of fava beans, during the course of acute viral hepatitis and infectious mononucleosis, or after administration of certain drugs, including aspirin and phenacetin. In such instances control of environmental factors may mitigate or neutralize the effect of the genetic change.

The balance of this chapter is devoted to a discussion of forms of treatment of value in specific hereditary disorders.

Treatment at the Metabolite Level. This approach usually involves nutritional or pharmacologic measures, or both.

Dietary Restriction of Substrate. Dietary restriction often reduces the excessive substrate that accumulates behind a metabolic block. A general reduction in protein intake prevents brain damage in disorders of the urea cycle associated with ammonia intoxication, including argininosuccinicaciduria and citrullinemia. A diet low in phenylalanine is effective in preventing growth and mental retardation in phenylketonuria, if started soon after birth. A fructose-free diet controls the symptoms of hereditary fructose intolerance resulting from deficiency of fructose-1-phosphate aldolase. Similarly, a diet that is virtually galactose free averts brain damage and cataract formation in children with galactokinase or galactose-1-phosphate uridyl transferase deficiency.

Replacement of the Deficient End-Product. A metabolic block may also result in a critical shortage in the product of the reaction or later products of the sequence. Replacement may alleviate the deficiency state. Goiter resulting from a block in thyroxine production can be treated and cretinism prevented by replacement of thyroid hormone. In the adrenogenital syndromes, corticosteroid administration supplies the missing hormone, corrects the disordered steroidal secretory pattern, and leads to remission of the clinical manifestations. In orotic aciduria, administration of uridine supplies the pyrimidines needed for hematopoietic functions and corrects the macrocytic anemia, and also suppresses orotic acid synthesis and urolithiasis.

Depletion of Storage Substances. In some hereditary disorders the clinical consequences result from accumulation of stored materials in the tissues, and removal of the excess material may ameliorate the effects of the genetic lesion. Removal of stored copper in Wilson's disease by penicillamine and of excess iron in hemochromatosis by frequent phlebotomy illustrates this approach. Use of uricosuric agents to deplete the body of uric acid in tophaceous gout and of cholestyramine to reduce serum cholesterol levels in familial hypercholesterolemia are additional examples. The use of cysteamine to help eliminate cystine in cystinosis is a recently introduced example.

Use of Metabolic Inhibitors. When a toxic metabolite accumulates because of a metabolic error, it may be possible to control its production by use of an appropriate metabolic inhibitor. Allopurinol inhibits xanthine oxidase and controls uric acid production in gout and 2,8-dioxyadenine production and renal stone formation in patients with homozygous adenine phosphoribosyl-transferase deficiency. Clofibrate, which inhibits synthesis or release of glyceride from the liver, reduces blood lipid levels to normal in type III hyperlipoproteinemia. Use of mevinolin, a potent inhibitor of 3-hydroxy-3-methylglutaryl-CoA reductase, in patients with hypercholesterolemia who are heterozygous for mutations at the LDL receptor locus, is a recent example. This drug reduces the rate of synthesis of cholesterol.

Treatment at the Level of the Dysfunctional Protein
Amplification of Enzyme Activity. Many enzyme proteins require cofactors for biologic activity. In some inborn errors the mutation affects the ability of the apoenzyme to combine with its cofactor. In other genetic disorders there is a metabolic defect in the conversion of a precursor vitamin to its active cofactor form.

In both situations administration of the appropriate cofactor may increase the catalytic activity of the apoenzyme. Pyridoxine (vitamin B$_6$) is a cofactor for cystathionine synthetase. In more than one half of patients with homocystinuria caused by deficient synthetase activity, administration of large doses of pyridoxine partially overcomes the block in homocysteine metabolism. Similarly the ketoacidosis of some patients with methylmalonicaciduria is corrected by treatment with pharmacologic doses of vitamin B$_{12}$, and the clinical and hematologic abnormalities of patients with hereditary dihydrofolate reductase deficiency are corrected by administration of small doses of 5-formyltetrahydrofolate, which bypasses the metabolic block (replacement of deficient end-product).

Phenobarbital and certain other drugs increase production of smooth endoplasmic reticulum and of certain of its enzymes, including NADPH-cytochrome C reductase, cytochrome P-450, and several drug-hydroxylating enzymes. Administration of phenobarbital to patients with unconjugated hyperbilirubinemia in a variant of the Crigler-Najjar syndrome or with Gilbert's syndrome may reduce plasma bilirubin levels following induction of hepatic glucuronyl-transferase.

Replacement of Mutant Protein. Direct replacement of the missing protein is an attractive approach to the treatment of recessively inherited diseases. Greater success has been achieved in deficiencies of nonenzymic than of enzymic proteins. Examples include replacement of gamma globulin in agammaglobulinemia, of albumin in analbuminemia, and of Factor VIII in hemophilia. In each of these cases, the deficient gene product is a plasma protein. The metabolic and immunologic defects of patients with adenosine deaminase deficiency are transiently corrected by infusion of irradiated erythrocytes containing normal levels of adenosine deaminase.

Much less success has attended efforts to replace missing enzymes that normally function within cells. Enzyme infusions have been attempted in the mucopolysaccharidoses, Gaucher's disease, Tay-Sachs disease, and Pompe's disease, but therapeutic benefits are unproved. The lysosomal storage diseases are perhaps the best candidates for treatment by administration of exogenous enzyme, for cells have highly specific mechanisms for taking up exogenous proteins and delivering them to lysosomes. However, the exogenous protein must bind to a specific recognition site on the plasma membrane of the target cell so that it can be selectively internalized. Enzymes have been coupled covalently to other molecules for which tissues contain receptors, on the theory that in this manner the enzyme might be conveyed to the lysosomes along with the primary ligand. Recently bovine adenosine deaminase cross-linked to polyethylene glycol (PEG) has been administered by intravenous infusion to patients with adenosine deaminase deficiency and severe combined immunodeficiency disease. PEG treatment of the enzyme confers both stability and immunologic neutrality to the enzyme. Weekly injections have resulted in sustained blood adenosine deaminase levels and gradual improvement in immunologic function over several months.

Modifying the Mutant Protein. Many proteins can be modified by the addition of subgroups. For example, sickle cell hemoglobin can be carbamylated by cyanate at the valine in position 1 of the β-chain, which then blocks the hydrophobic bonding of the normal val-1 to the mutant val-6 of β-globin of Hb S, thereby preventing sickling in vitro. Severe toxic reactions, such as peripheral neuropathy, sharply limit the clinical usefulness of cyanate therapy in patients with sickle cell disease. Nevertheless, this approach holds promise for the future.

Organ Transplantation. Allotransplantation of organs has been attempted in a variety of inherited diseases. In some instances, transplantation is done strictly to supply the recipient with a tissue that can replace a missing protein; in others, the transplant also (or only) replaces a damaged organ. Examples of the former include bone marrow transplants for a number of immunodeficiency states, such as lymphopenic hypogammaglobulinemia, (Swiss type), Wiskott-Aldrich syndrome, and severe combined immunodeficiency disease, as well as for lysosomal storage diseases and β-thalassemia; and liver transplants for type I glycogen storage disease, ornithine transcarbamylase deficiency, and homozygous familial hypercholesterolemia. Examples of the latter

include liver transplants for hepatic failure from Wilson's disease, α-1-antitrypsin deficiency, and hepatorenal tyrosinosis; and heart transplants for hereditary cardiomyopathy. The greatest experience has involved renal transplantation, which has been performed in Alport's syndrome, renal amyloidosis, cystinosis, Fabry's disease, Gaucher's disease, oxalosis, and some other conditions. The results in most instances have paralleled those of renal transplantation for other forms of end-stage renal disease. There has been no evidence of reactivation of the renal lesion in patients with Alport's syndrome, or of development of cystinosis or Fabry's disease in the transplanted kidneys. Amyloidosis has recurred in the graft on rare occasions. By contrast severe recurrent oxalosis has developed in a number of transplanted kidneys. Patients with Fabry's disease have developed measurable levels of the missing enzyme, ceramide trihexosidase, in plasma following renal transplantation, and there have been a few long-term survivals. Nevertheless, renal transplantation in patients with inborn errors of metabolism should be limited to replacement of failed kidneys. Results do not warrant use of renal transplantation primarily for enzyme replacement.

Other Surgical Procedures. Surgical removals also play a role in certain hereditary disorders. Examples include splenectomy in hereditary spherocytosis and colectomy in preventing neoplastic transformation in polyposis of the colon. Also, surgery offers a quick and permanent cure for polydactyly as well as for certain other dominantly inherited defects.

Genetic Engineering. The use of recombinant DNA technology in the diagnosis and treatment of inborn errors is discussed in Ch. 32.

McKusick VA: Phenotypic diversity of human diseases resulting from allelic series. Am J Hum Genet 25:446, 1973. *An analytical review of different disorders that can result from series of mutations involving the same gene.*

Scriver CR, Beaudet AL, Sly WS, et al. (eds.): The Metabolic Basis of Inherited Disease. 6th ed. New York, McGraw-Hill Book Company, 1989. *Authoritative discussions of all inborn errors of metabolism for which there is a substantial body of metabolic or biochemical information.*

32 Expectations from Recombinant DNA Research

W. French Anderson

Over the past 15 years, a revolution has occurred in DNA research, variously referred to as recombinant DNA technology, genetic engineering, molecular cloning, gene splicing, or biotechnology. The new DNA research is making a major impact on clinical medicine in four areas: (1) understanding of the molecular basis of human (particularly genetic) diseases, (2) prenatal diagnosis, (3) production of human biologic products, and (4) gene therapy. Categories 1 to 3 are already a reality, and human gene therapy is fast approaching that status.

THE MOLECULAR BASIS OF HUMAN DISEASES

Although the human diseases studied by recombinant DNA techniques at present are the genetic diseases, the power of this technology is beginning to be felt in many other areas of human physiology and pathophysiology. All living processes are ultimately controlled by genes. Therefore, as genes are "cloned" (i.e., isolated) and as their products (which can be obtained in large amounts once the gene is cloned; see below) are studied both in vitro and in vivo, more is learned about the reactions that the genes govern. The result is that the normal physiology of a process becomes better understood. An example is the regulation of the hematopoietic system. As the genes for various growth factors and cytokines are obtained and their products made available for study (e.g., granulocyte-macrophage colony-stimulating factor [GM-CSF], erythropoietin, interleukin 2 [IL2], and so forth), a much clearer understanding is emerging on how proliferation and differentiation are controlled in the bone marrow. Another example is the immune system, in which the genes for the various cell surface receptors (e.g., IL2 receptor, T cell receptor, and so on) are being cloned and analyzed.

It is the genetic diseases, however, that have primarily bene-fited from the recombinant DNA revolution. Most studied are the thalassemias and hemoglobinopathies (see Ch. 136). A dozen years ago the genetics of β-thalassemia was extremely confusing. There were various clinical classifications to account for the range of severity seen. It was assumed that there must be different genotypes and that many patients were probably genetic com-pounds. Now, most of the genes that can produce β-thalassemia have been sequenced, and the mechanisms underlying the var-ious β-zero and β-plus thalassemias have been elucidated (see Ch. 136). Not only has this information led to a better compre-hension of the thalassemia syndromes, but also it has made prenatal diagnosis and genetic counseling much more accurate. Similar progress in the understanding of a number of other genetic diseases is under way.

PRENATAL DIAGNOSIS

Prenatal diagnosis can be used for the detection of a number of genetic diseases; see, for example, Ch. 36, and also the discussion in the chapter on sickle cell anemia (Ch. 136). Recom-binant DNA technology has greatly expanded the accuracy, range, and safety of this procedure. Previously, it was necessary to obtain the gene product in sufficient amounts to be detectable by biochemical methods. For example, in the prenatal diagnosis of β-thalassemia, fetal blood would be sampled at around 18 weeks of gestation (either by fetoscopy or placental aspiration), with a 5 per cent fetal mortality rate. Globin chains would then be fractionated. Analysis of fetal DNA, on the other hand, can be carried out on a small number of amniotic cells (with a fetal mortality rate of only 0.3 per cent) or from chorionic villi (with a fetal loss of 4 per cent but with the distinct advantage of making a diagnosis as early as 9 to 10 weeks of gestation).

There are a number of techniques that can be used to analyze fetal DNA for single-gene disorders. First is the straightforward method of restriction endonuclease mapping. A restriction en-zyme cuts DNA at a specific short (4- to 6-nucleotide) sequence. If a genetic disorder alters the sequence recognized by a restric-tion enzyme, digestion of the fetal DNA with that enzyme provides an immediate diagnosis. Unfortunately, there are only a few situations in which this technique is applicable (e.g., sickle cell anemia). A second procedure is to make a linkage analysis with a restriction fragment length polymorphism (known as RFLP) (see Ch. 31). This approach has become increasingly valuable as sufficient RFLP's have been located to make a roadmap of the entire human genome. Finally, a procedure that promises to be extremely valuable is the use of oligonucleotide probes that are specific for individual mutations. In theory, every genetic disease could be detected directly by hybridizing a normal and "mutant" oligonucleotide probe to a sample of fetal DNA.

It is clear that the new technology will revolutionize prenatal diagnosis. What is uncertain is how long it will take to transfer these sophisticated procedures from research laboratories to routine clinical use.

HUMAN BIOLOGICS PRODUCED BY BIOTECHNOLOGY

Genetic engineering is currently being used by biotechnology companies to produce large quantities of previously unavailable human biologics (usually peptides or proteins). What products are being made? Why these products? How are they being made? How good are they?

A number of human proteins produced by the new technology are now used clinically. Insulin, growth hormone (GH), and α and β interferon were the first ones licensed by the United States Food and Drug Administration (FDA). Examples of other biolog-ics made by recombinant DNA technology are gamma interferon, interleukin 2 (IL2), tumor necrosis factor (TNF), erythropoietin, and hepatitis B vaccine. In each case, the biologic was chosen because of the importance of the protein in treating specific human disease states (either established: insulin, GH; or postu-lated), the commercial market expected for the compound, and the ability to apply recombinant DNA techniques to synthesize large quantities of the human protein in bacteria (or in yeast or other cells) inexpensively.

The Technology

A gene is a sequence of nucleotides in DNA which codes for a product. In order to get a bacterium (the most common biologic

"factory" in use at present) to produce a human protein, it is necessary to obtain a DNA copy of the protein—in other words, to obtain a piece of double-stranded DNA that carries the precise sequence of nucleotides that codes for the protein. This DNA is then inserted into a bacterial plasmid—a circle of naturally occurring nonchromosomal DNA that replicates freely in the cytoplasm of a bacterium. Any gene (bacterial, plant, animal, or human) that is inserted into the plasmid with the correct control signals can, in theory, be transcribed and translated into protein within the bacterium. The synthesized protein can then be purified from the bacterial cells.

There are a number of ways to acquire a human gene suitable for engineered protein production in bacteria. One procedure is to sequence a portion of the human protein of interest and then, by using the genetic code, determine the DNA sequence that would give the known amino acid sequence. Then a segment of DNA one and one half to several dozen nucleotides long is chemically synthesized so as to be exactly complementary to a portion of the expected sequence of the messenger RNA (mRNA). "Exactly complementary" means that the DNA "probe" has T (thymine) where the mRNA has an A (adenine), a C (cytosine) where the mRNA has a G (guanine), and so forth. This DNA probe can be tagged with radioactivity and then used to find (by hybridization) the desired mRNA in extracts of the appropriate human cells. The mRNA is isolated, purified, and shown to be capable of being translated in vitro to give the predicted human protein. This mRNA is then transcribed into full-length comple-mentary (or copy) DNA, called cDNA, by the enzyme reverse transcriptase. The resulting DNA is an exact code of the mRNA for the human protein. It can now be made double stranded (by the action of other enzymes) and inserted into a bacterial plasmid along with the appropriate control signals.

Several requirements must be met in order to obtain large quantities of human proteins in bacteria. The human gene must be attached within the plasmid to a bacterial control signal that will be switched on at a high level. Several such "promoter" regions are used, including those from the lactose operon, from the bacteriophage lambda, and so on. Second, other regulatory signals (for example, a binding site so that the transcribed RNA will attach to and be translated by ribosomes) must be present adjacent to the human gene. Third, any hard-to-handle portion of DNA (for example, nucleotides producing a leader sequence of amino acids or an intervening sequence) should be removed, since bacteria are not equipped to carry out many of the post-transcriptional and post-translational modifications that eukaryotic cells can perform. Fourth, the human protein must be protected from proteinases within the bacterium.

How good are these biologically engineered human proteins? They should be perfectly acceptable for administration to patients. In most cases, they should be pure and contain no infectious contaminants or animal antigenic material. However, unless purified extensively, they might contain clinically relevant amounts of bacterial antigenic substances. In addition, since some products isolated directly from the body have a number of biologic compounds bound to them, the clinical effect of a "pure" engi-neered product (e.g., albumin) might be somewhat different from that of the natural product.

The Next Products

What human biologics are now under development? Those being prepared for human trials fall into four broad categories: vaccines, blood components, neurohormones, and diagnostics.

VACCINES. The first recombinant DNA vaccine approved by the FDA (July 1986) for clinical use was that for hepatitis B. Specific vaccines for influenza and malaria are in clinical trials. Potential vaccines for a number of other diseases are currently in preparation, e.g., leprosy, tuberculosis, typhoid, acquired immunodeficiency syndrome (AIDS), and so forth. This new generation of vaccines should be superior to those in use today. A precise portion of the antigenic surface of a virus or a parasite can be selected and the DNA complement to this moiety pre-pared. Since a bacterial control signal will transcribe any sequence of DNA attached to it, the DNA coding for just the antigenic site desired can be inserted into bacteria for large-scale production of material. Or the DNA could be inserted into, for example, vaccinia in order to take advantage of a well-characterized vaccination agent. It appears to be possible to prepare highly specific vaccines by this approach.

BLOOD COMPONENTS. Several different types of blood components are being prepared for clinical trials.

Clotting Factors. The genes for factor VIII, von Willebrand's factor, and factor IX have been obtained. Human protein C has also been cloned.

Albumin. The great demand for albumin as a plasma expander has resulted in a major effort to produce human albumin by genetic engineering techniques. The advantage of engineered albumin (besides increased availability and decreased cost) should be that there will be no risk of hepatitis, AIDS, or other infectious contamination.

Thrombolytic Agents. Blood clots are a major cause of death and disabling diseases in the United States. Consequently, readily available clot-specific thrombolytic agents would be clinically useful. Biotechnology is being employed to isolate the genes for, and to engineer the production of, tissue-type and urokinase-type plasminogen activators. These proteins should be superior to the currently available agents, urokinase and streptokinase. Tissue plasminogen activator is now in clinical use.

Biologic Response Modifiers. The family of interferons, the family of interleukins, several colony-stimulating factors (GM-CSF, G-CSF, M-CSF), TNF, and other molecules are under active clinical investigation. Considerable effort is being expended to identify other factors, particularly a molecule that would stimulate the earliest pluripotent stem cell. Major advances in clinical manipulation of the immune system are expected when the genes of the major histocompatibility complex and the immunoglobulin gene families are more fully understood.

NEUROHORMONES. This complex group includes a large number of hormones, various neuropeptides, and the neurotransmitters with their receptors. Insulin and growth hormone are already used clinically.

DIAGNOSTICS. Since viruses consist of sequences of DNA or RNA with a coat, diagnostic techniques that would rapidly and accurately identify the presence of specific viruses in body tissues or fluids by using DNA probes are being developed. Polymerase chain reaction (PCR) is a new technology that greatly enhances the sensitivity of these diagnostic tests.

OTHER AREAS. Finally, two other areas need to be mentioned. A further understanding of oncogenes, tumor suppressor genes, and antimetastasis genes and their roles in cancer should lead to the development of drugs or antibodies that could be used to inhibit specific steps in the pathway leading from a normal to a malignant cell. Second, the tremendous potential of recombinant DNA research to produce useful new agricultural plants and improved farm animals should have a large effect on the food supply of the world.

GENE THERAPY

By gene therapy is meant the insertion of a normal gene into the appropriate cells of a patient in such a way that the exogenous gene produces a product that will cure, or at least ameliorate, the genetic defect. For some genetic conditions (specifically those caused by a single gene mutation that produces a defective product that can be isolated), gene therapy should be a beneficial therapeutic procedure in the future.

The Technology of Gene Therapy

It is now possible by the use of recombinant DNA technology to isolate specific normal genes from the DNA of human tissue. A gene can be isolated if it can be recognized, and it can be recognized if the protein product that it makes can be isolated. The defective product in many genetic diseases is a protein (e.g., an enzyme in many of the inborn errors of metabolism; β-globin in sickle cell anemia or Cooley's anemia). In a manner similar to that described above in the section on human biologics, a DNA probe can be synthesized. With this probe it is possible to locate the gene in human DNA, isolate (i.e., clone) it, and purify it. Any gene can be cloned once a probe for the gene exists.

The cloned gene can be inserted into cells in any one of a number of ways. The three most commonly used techniques are (1) microinjecting directly into a cell's nucleus, (2) forming a calcium phosphate precipitate of the DNA and then incubating tissue culture cells with this precipitate, and (3) inserting the gene into a nonpathogenic virus and infecting cells with this recombinant virus. All three procedures have been used successfully to insert cloned genes into cells growing in tissue culture. By far, the most efficient procedure at present is the use of retrovirus-based vectors carrying exogenous genes.

Vectors derived from retroviruses possess several advantages as a gene delivery system. First, up to 100 per cent of cells can be infected and can express the integrated viral (and exogenous) genes. Second, as many cells as desired can be infected simultaneously. Third, under appropriate conditions, the DNA can integrate as a single copy at a single, albeit random, site. Finally, the infection and long-term harboring of a retroviral vector usually do not harm cells. Several retroviral vector systems have been developed; those projected for human use are constructed from the Moloney murine leukemia virus. Evidence obtained from studies with experimental animals and in tissue culture indicates that retroviruses can be used as a reasonably efficient delivery system.

The next question is, what target cell to use? At present, the only human cells that can be used effectively for gene transfer are blood cells. No other cells (except, perhaps, skin cells) can be extracted from the body, grown in culture to allow insertion of exogenous genes, and then successfully reimplanted into the patient from whom the tissue was taken. In the future, as more is learned about how to package the DNA and to make it tissue specific, the intravenous route would be the simplest and most desirable. However, attempting to give a foreign gene by injection directly into the bloodstream is not advisable with our present state of knowledge, since the procedure would be enormously inefficient and there would be little control over the DNA's fate.

Ethics

The ethics of gene therapy in humans has been discussed for many years. Essentially all observers have stated that they believe that it would be ethical to insert genetic material into a human being for the sole purpose of medically correcting a severe genetic disorder in that patient—in other words, somatic cell gene therapy. Attempts to correct a patient's reproductive cells (i.e., germ line gene therapy) or to alter or improve a "normal" person by gene manipulation (i.e., enhancement or eugenic genetic engineering) are controversial areas. However, somatic cell gene therapy for a patient suffering a serious genetic disorder would be ethically acceptable if carried out under the same strict criteria that cover other new experimental medical procedures. The techniques now being developed by clinical investigators for human application are for somatic cell, not germ line, gene therapy.

What criteria should be satisfied prior to the time that somatic cell gene therapy is tested in a clinical trial? Three general requirements are that it should be shown in animal studies that (1) the new gene can be put into the correct target cells and will remain there long enough to be effective; (2) the new gene will be expressed in the cells at an appropriate level; and (3) the new gene will not harm the cell or, by extension, the recipient. These criteria are very similar to those required prior to the use of any new drug, therapeutic procedure, or surgical operation. The requirements simply state that the new treatment should get to the area of disease, correct it, and do more good than harm.

Although retroviruses have many advantages for gene transfer, they also have disadvantages, which leads to questions about safety. One problem is that they can rearrange their own structure, as well as exchange sequences with other retroviruses. There is a built-in safety feature with the mouse retroviral vectors now in use, however; these mouse structures have a very different sequence from known primate retroviruses, and there appears to be little or no homology between the two. Therefore, it has been possible to build a relatively safe retroviral vector.

Even with a "safe" vector, however, the problem of insertional mutagenesis remains. Since a retroviral vector incorporates into the genome randomly, it may inactivate an important gene or, worse, activate an oncogene. It is uncertain how great a danger this problem poses but it is thought to be small. As with any new clinical protocol, the total expected benefit for the patient must be weighed against potential risks. Ultimately, local institutional review boards and the National Institutes of Health Recombinant DNA Advisory Committee (RAC) together with its Human Gene Therapy Subcommittee, as well as the FDA, must decide if a given protocol is ready for human application.

Present Capabilities

The first human gene transfer clinical protocol was approved by the NIH and the FDA on January 19, 1989, after several months of extensive public review. The protocol was as follows:

A retroviral vector was built that carried a bacterial marker gene. The vector, called N2, was constructed from the Moloney murine leukemia retrovirus. The marker gene was NeoR (standing for resistance to neomycin), a bacterial gene that makes an enzyme (neomycin phosphotransferase) that inactivates one subclass of neomycin-like antibiotics. The objective was to use the marker gene as a means of acquiring information about a new form of cancer therapy called TIL adoptive immunotherapy.

Tumor-infiltrating lymphocytes (TIL) are cells from tumor suspensions cultured in IL2 that can mediate cancer regression when adoptively transferred back into the patient. About 40 per cent of patients with malignant melanoma or renal cell carcinoma have an objective response. The mechanism of this anticancer action is not known. It was postulated that if the TIL could be marked by the N2 vector, then the survival and traffic of these cells in vivo could be monitored. To accomplish this objective an aliquot of TIL from each patient received the NeoR gene via retrovirus-mediated gene transfer ex vivo. The gene-modified cells were then grown in parallel with the nontransduced TIL. Both populations were returned to the patient, and the marked cells were monitored by analyzing blood and tumor biopsies over time.

Five patients with advanced malignant melanoma were each given a single infusion of autologous gene-marked TIL between May 22 and July 21, 1989. The data from these patients demonstrated that TIL can be identified in the bloodstream for 3 weeks in all patients, and then in occasional blood samples at very low levels at later times. Marked TIL could be isolated from tumor specimens, in one patient at 2 months after infusion. No side effects or other problems resulted from the administration of the gene-modified TIL in the five patients.

The success of the human gene transfer clinical protocol has opened the door for attempts at gene therapy itself. A human gene therapy clinical protocol was approved by the NIH RAC on July 31, 1990, and the first patient was treated on September 14, 1990. The protocol calls for inserting a normal human adenosine deaminase (ADA) gene into autologous T lymphocytes of children suffering from ADA deficiency and returning these gene-corrected T cells to the patient. ADA deficiency is one cause of severe combined immunodeficiency (SCID), a rare genetic disease that often is fatal in the first years of life. The primary defect is in the T lymphocytes, so the correction of the patient's T cells should be beneficial.

Clinical protocols are being prepared which are designed to treat other genetic diseases (e.g., hemophilia, thalassemia, Gaucher's disease), cancer (e.g., insertion of cytokines that possess antitumor activity into TIL), viral diseases (e.g., insertion of a soluble CD4 gene into autologous cells of AIDS patients), and cardiovascular diseases (e.g., insertion of the tissue plasminogen activator gene into vascular endothelial cells seeded onto vascular grafts in order to attempt to reduce clot formation).

Overview

It now appears that effective delivery-expression systems are available that will allow reasonable attempts at somatic cell gene therapy. The first clinical trials have begun.

Gene therapy is a procedure with enormous potential. It should, in the future, provide a treatment for many types of serious diseases. Some claims made about the potential of genetic engineering in humans are highly unlikely. Patients with multigenic diseases, in which the genes as well as the intracellular products involved are unknown, will not be candidates for gene therapy for a long time to come, if ever. Likewise, characteristics such as personality and intelligence are probably outside the realm of this technique's potential. Only traits produced by identifiable single genes can be approached by genetic engineering.

The power to cure a genetic defect is an awesome one. But the goal of biomedical research is, and has always been, to alleviate human suffering. Gene therapy, with proper safeguards imposed by society, is a logical part of that effort.

Eglitis MA, Anderson WF: Retroviral vectors for introduction of genes into mammalian cells. BioTechniques 6:608, 1988. *This review explains the technology of retrovirus-mediated gene transfer.*

Friedmann T: Progress toward human gene therapy. Science 244:1275, 1989. *This recent review covers the whole field of human gene therapy.*

33 Chromosomes and Their Disorders

John L. Hamerton

Cytogenetics is the study of the chromosomes and their behavior as it relates to transmission of the genetic material from parent to offspring. Errors in chromosome behavior and structure are the cause of a wide range of clinical syndromes.

Humans have 46 chromosomes, which consist of 22 pairs of homologous chromosomes (identical in regard to morphology and constituent gene loci) and one pair of sex chromosomes (X and Y), one partner of each pair being derived from the mother and one from the father. The genes are arranged along the chromosomes in linear order, each gene having a precise position or *locus*. Genes that have their loci on the same chromosome are said to be *linked*, or more precisely, to be *syntenic*. Alternate forms of a gene that occupy the same locus are called *alleles*. Any one chromosome bears only a single allele at a given locus, although in the population as a whole there may be multiple alleles, any one of which can occupy that specific locus.

CELL DIVISION

The number of chromosomes found in somatic cells is constant and is termed the diploid (2n) number. Each gamete, however, has only half the *diploid* number and is said to be *haploid* (n). In order to maintain this regularity two types of cell division occur: *mitosis*, which is the cell division occurring in somatic tissues during growth and repair, and *meiosis*, which is the specialized form of cell division occurring during the formation of the gametes.

MITOSIS. The function of mitosis is the distribution and maintenance of the continuity of the genetic material in every cell of the body. This process consists of a number of different phases, which results in an equal distribution of the chromosomes to the two daughter cells. The cell cycle has four stages: mitosis or M, G_1, S, and G_2. The G_1 phase follows mitosis, during which RNA and protein synthesis occurs. S is the period during which DNA replication takes place and the DNA content of the cell doubles, and G_2 is the period during which energy requirements for cell division are built up and any repair of errors in DNA synthesis takes place.

MEIOSIS (Fig. 33–1). This process occurs only during the formation of the gametes and results in four daughter cells, each with the haploid number of chromosomes. In males each primary spermatocyte forms four functional spermatids that develop into sperm, while in females each oocyte forms only one ovum, the remaining products of meiosis being nonfunctional polar bodies.

The first division of meiosis consists of an extremely long and complex *prophase* during which DNA replication occurs. This is divided into a number of stages during which crossing over and reassortment of genetic material occur. Initially the chromosomes are apparently single threads that begin to shorten and thicken. This is followed by the commencement of pairing of homologous chromosomes (*synapsis*). After pairing is completed, the chromosomes continue to shorten and are now known as *bivalents*, which are held together only at specific points (*chiasmata*). At this stage of prophase each homologous chromosome can be seen to be visibly doubled (two chromatids) so that each bivalent, which continues to shorten and thicken, consists of four chromatids.

The end of prophase is marked by the disappearance of the nuclear membrane and the formation of a spindle, heralding entry into *metaphase* of the first meiotic division. The bivalents are arranged on the equatorial plate of the spindle as a result of a series of complex chromosome movements. The homologous centromeres are undivided at this point and lie opposite each other on the equatorial plate (co-orientation). As soon as this process is complete, the paired homologues separate and move to opposite poles (*anaphase*). The cell then proceeds to the second meiotic division. This is essentially a mitotic division in which the chromosomes have already doubled so that there is no need for DNA synthesis. In addition, the genetic material has undergone exchange at meiosis I so that the sister chromatids are not genetically identical.

The major consequences of meiosis are threefold: (1) the halving of the chromosome number; (2) the co-orientation of the bivalents on the metaphase plate, which ensures the regular distribution of the chromosomes to the daughter cells; and (3) the independent assortment of genetic material that results both from genetic crossing over and from the random assortment of the maternal and paternal homologues to the two daughter cells in meiosis I.

Two processes are fundamental to meiosis: chromosome pairing, which results in formation of the bivalents, and chiasma formation. Chiasmata have two main functions: They are the points on the chromosomes at which genetic crossing over takes place, and they serve to maintain bivalent association throughout the prophase and metaphase. Meiosis thus ensures genetic variability as a result of random segregation of the parental homologous chromosomes and the exchange of genetic material by crossing over between nonsister chromatids.

METHODS FOR THE PREPARATION OF CHROMOSOMES

Since nondividing chromosomes cannot be analyzed, dividing cells are required for chromosome analysis. The cell type most commonly used is the mitogenically stimulated peripheral blood lymphocyte. Skin fibroblasts, bone marrow cells, amniotic fluid cells, and chorion villus cells are also used for special tests. Dividing cells are accumulated at metaphase. In order to accomplish this, colcemid, a drug that destroys the mitotic spindle, is added to the culture medium toward the end of the culture period. The cells are then subjected to hypotonic treatment, followed by fixation and spreading on microscope slides. The slides are then stained.

Staining techniques may result in either a nonbanded or a banded appearance of the chromosomes. Most laboratories today use one of several banding techniques, since this results in a great deal of additional information. These methods provide a means for the precise identification of an extra or missing chromosome and the precise localization of breakpoints in chromosome rearrangements (Fig. 33–2).

Recent developments have resulted in the expansion of the number of visible bands from between 200 and 300 to between 1000 and 2000. This allows the recognition of small deletions and duplications. Most laboratories today work with chromosomes in which between 400 and 800 bands can be recognized.

HUMAN CHROMOSOME NOMENCLATURE

The 46 human chromosomes consist of three types designated by the position of the centromere or primary constriction. These are metacentric, submetacentric, and acrocentric, depending upon whether the position of the centromere is median, submedian, or terminal. Now that each individual chromosome pair can

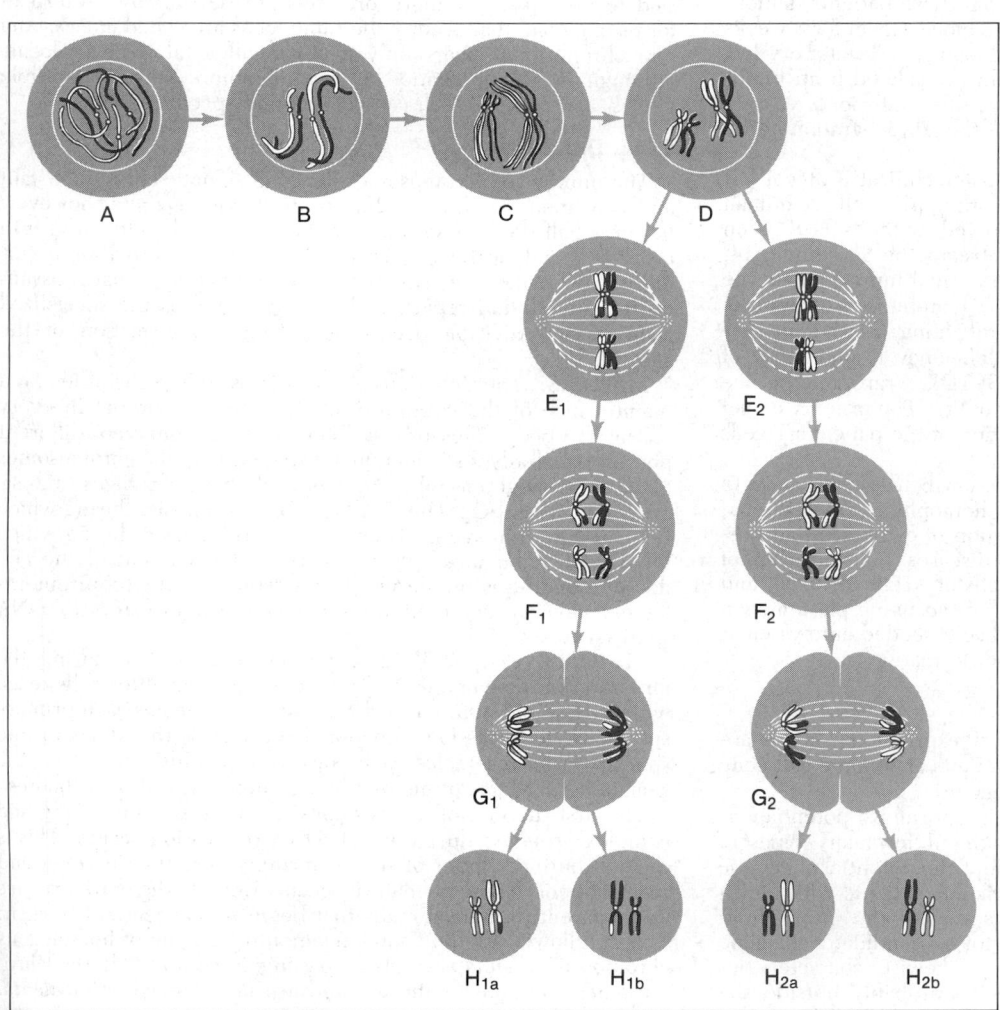

FIGURE 33–1. The stages of the first division of meiosis. Paternal and maternal chromosomes are shown in red and white, respectively. A to D, Stages of prophase. E to G, Metaphase 1 to anaphase 1. H_1 to H_2, Daughter cells with haploid number of chromosomes prior to entering the second division of meiosis. Note the chromosome exchanges that have taken place.

be recognized, the chromosomes are numbered from 1 to 22 in descending order of length. In the female the two sex chromosomes, designated X chromosomes, are identical, while in the male the two sex chromosomes, designated X and Y, are morphologically different.

Chromosome Variants

This term refers to consistent minor chromosome changes often involving the short arms of the acrocentric chromosomes, the long arm of the Y chromosome, or the constitutive heterochromatin near the centromere of chromosomes 1, 9, and 16. These have little obvious clinical significance but may be useful as genetic markers. They occur much more frequently in the population than do major chromosome abnormalities, and they often segregate in families in a mendelian manner. Recent studies suggest that about 70 per cent of newborn infants carry one or more variant chromosomes.

Nomenclature

The nomenclature used to describe the chromosomes, chromosome bands, chromosome variants, and chromosome rearrangements is given in detail in an International System of Human Cytogenetic Nomenclature (ISCN) (1985). A shorthand notation is used to describe the chromosome complement of an individual. In this notation the number of chromosomes is specified first, followed by the listing of the sex chromosomes. Thus a normal female karyotype is designated 46,XX and a normal male karyotype 46,XY. Any deviations from a normal karyotype are written after the sex chromosomes. An individual autosome is referred to by its number, its short arm by the letter "p," and its long arm by the letter "q." A "+" or "−" sign written after the p or q indicates an increase (+) or decrease (−) in the length of the arm. When written before a designated chromosome the sign indicates that the chromosome is extra (+) or missing (−).

Examples: 46,XY,18q− describes a male with 46 chromosomes, including one chromosome 18 whose long arm is diminished in length.

47,XX,+21 describes a female with 47 chromosomes, including an extra chromosome 21 in addition to the 46 chromosomes of the normal karyotype.

A diagrammatic representation of the human chromosome 1 showing differing degrees of chromosome banding is given in Figure 33–3.

CHROMOSOME ABNORMALITIES

Chromosome abnormalities can be divided into two classes: abnormalities of number and of structure.

Abnormalities of Chromosome Number. These arise from nondisjunction, that is, from *the failure of two homologous chromosomes in the first division of meiosis or of two sister chromatids in mitosis or the second division of meiosis to pass to opposite poles of the cell* (Fig. 33–4). Nondisjunction results in cells with abnormal chromosome numbers. If these cells are gametes, fertilization will result in a zygote with an abnormal chromosome number. If nondisjunction occurs during an early cleavage division of a zygote, then a chromosome mosaic may result. This is an individual with two or more cell lines differing in chromosome complement. Table 33–1 gives examples of chromosome abnormalities resulting from nondisjunction.

Abnormalities of Chromosome Structure. These result from chromosome breakage and reunion. When a chromosome breaks it can rejoin in its old form (restitution) or it can rejoin with another broken chromosome (reunion). Reunion leads to a structural rearrangement that can be *balanced* or *unbalanced*. If it is balanced the amount of genetic material is presumed to be identical to that found in a normal cell, and there is a simple rearrangement of the distribution of this material. Types of balanced rearrangements include the balanced reciprocal translocation, robertsonian translocations, and inversions. Balanced chromosome rearrangements do not usually lead to any clinical change. If the rearrangement is unbalanced this indicates loss or gain of chromosome material. Loss includes a deficiency or a deletion. Gain includes a duplication. Such unbalanced rearrangements usually result in changes in the clinical phenotype.

CHROMOSOME DELETION. Deletion is the loss of a chromosome segment following chromosome breakage. Deletions may be terminal or interstitial or result in ring chromosomes (Fig. 33–5A, B, and E).

INVERSIONS (Fig. 33–5C and D). These result from two chromosome breaks and inversion of the intervening segment and can be detected only by chromosome banding studies that show a changed banding sequence. Inversions result in disturbances in chromosome pairing and in the formation of unbalanced as well as balanced gametes.

BALANCED RECIPROCAL TRANSLOCATION (Fig. 33–6). This results from exchange of chromosome segments between

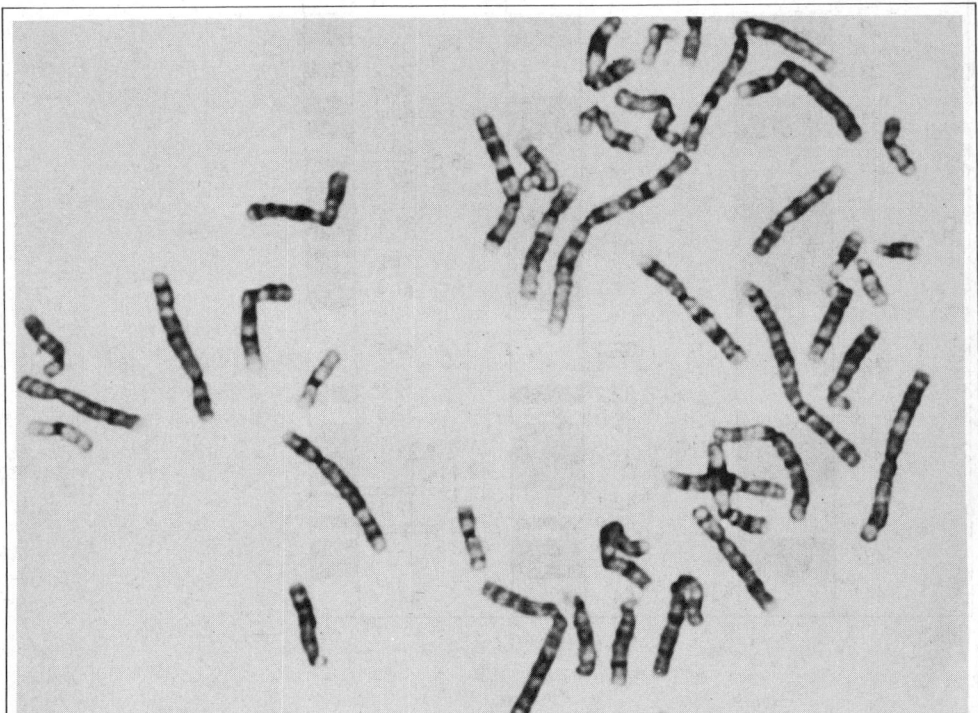

FIGURE 33–2. Human chromosomes at mitotic metaphase. G-banding, approximately 550-band stage. (Courtesy of Dr. H. S. Wang.)

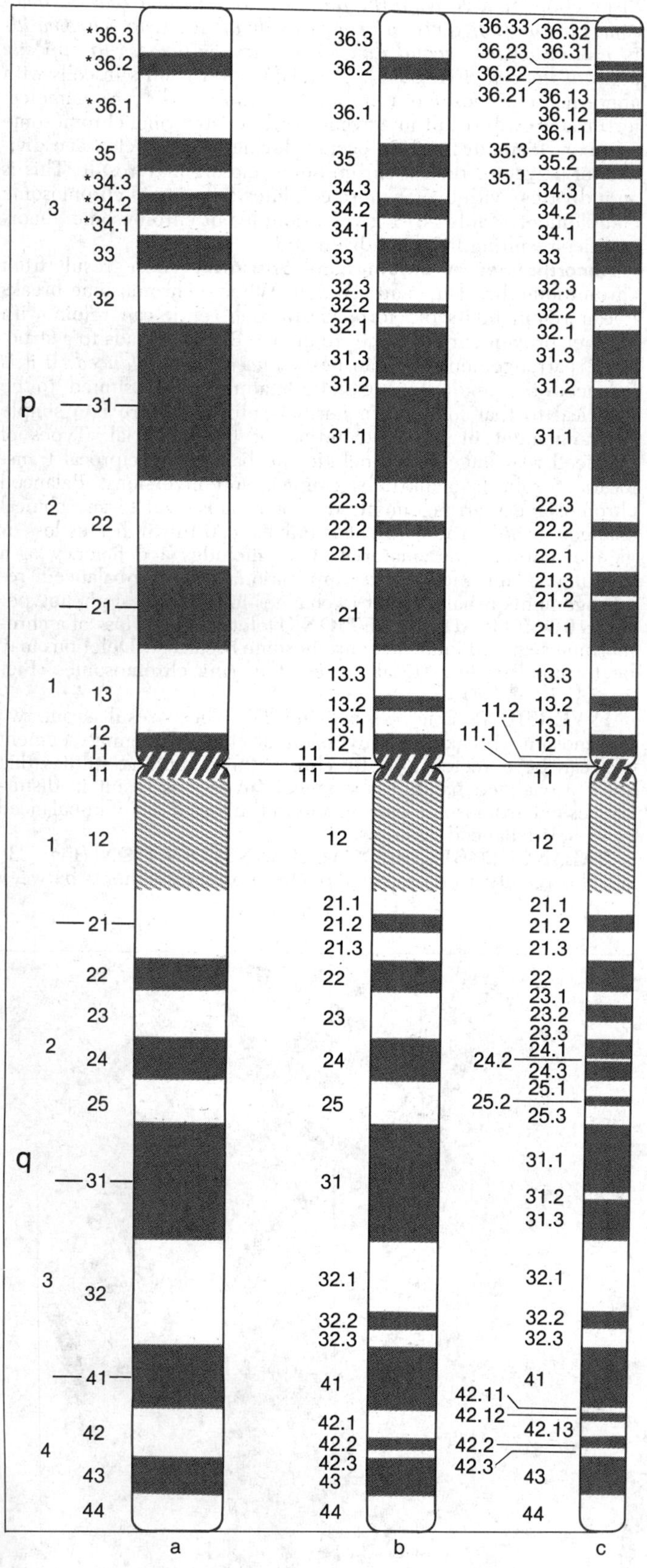

FIGURE 33–3. Human chromosome 1. Idiogram showing chromosome bands at different resolutions. *a*, Approximately 400 bands; *b*, 550 bands; *c*, 850 bands. The band nomenclature and subdivision are according to the internationally agreed upon system (ISCN 1985).

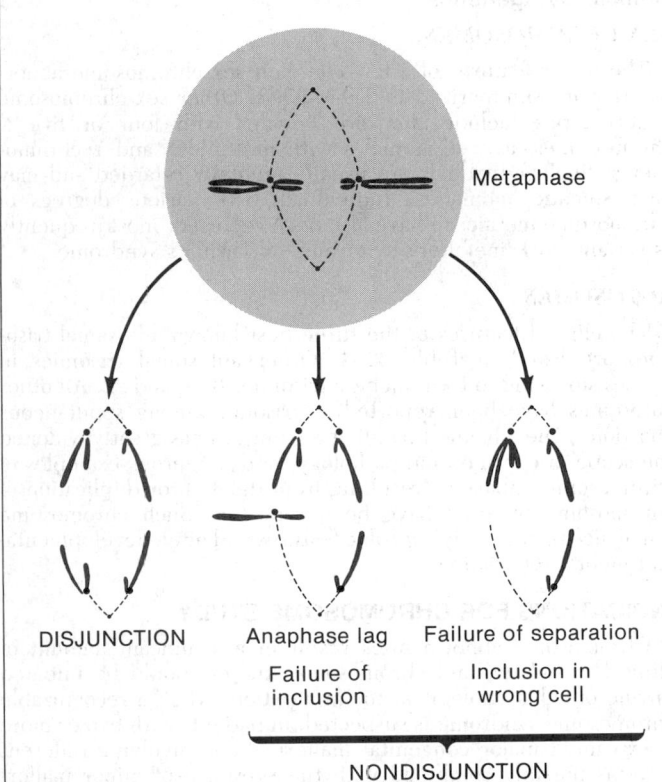

FIGURE 33–4. Diagram illustrating chromosome disjunction and two types of nondisjunction—anaphase lagging and failure of separation. (From Hamerton JL: Human Cytogenetics. Vol 1. New York, Academic Press, 1971.)

nonhomologous chromosomes. An individual carrying such a rearrangement has a higher frequency of abnormal gametes as the result of a disturbance in chromosome pairing at meiosis. Such individuals themselves have a balanced chromosome complement and are clinically normal, but they may have a high risk of having congenitally malformed children and/or spontaneous abortions. Normal children may also be born, and such persons require careful genetic counseling.

ROBERTSONIAN TRANSLOCATION. This is a specific type of unequal reciprocal translocation that occurs between acrocentric chromosomes, resulting in the formation of a new metacentric chromosome from two acrocentric chromosomes. Such rearrangements may be important in the transmission of Down's syndrome when one of the chromosomes involved is chromosome 21, the other usually being chromosome 14.

POPULATION CYTOGENETICS

Chromosome abnormalities form a significant component of the deleterious genetic load carried by the human population.

TABLE 33–1. EXAMPLES OF CHROMOSOME ABNORMALITIES DUE TO NONDISJUNCTION IN HUMANS

Sex Chromosomes	Autosomes†
47,XXY (Klinefelter's syndrome) *46,XY/47,XXY	21-trisomy (47,XX or XY, +21)
47,XYY	13-trisomy (47,XX or XY, +13)
47,XXX	18-trisomy (47,XX or XY, +18)
45,X (Turner's syndrome) *45,X/46,XX (ovarian dysgenesis)	21-monosomy (45,XX or XY, −21)

*Examples of chromosome mosaics due to nondisjunction or chromosome loss during an early cleavage division.
†In describing a chromosome abnormality the words "trisomy" and "monosomy" refer simply to an additional or missing chromosome.

About 6 per 1000 newborn babies have a major chromosome abnormality that may result in some degree of morbidity or mortality at some time during life. The frequency of the different types of chromosome abnormalities found when large numbers of newborn infants are screened is shown in Table 33–2.

Chromosome abnormalities found among infants at birth are, however, only a very small proportion of the total load of chromosome abnormalities seen at conception. The majority of these are lethal or sublethal and are lost during gestation as either very early abortions or failures of implantation (monosomies, and so on), or as recognized abortions and perinatal deaths. This group includes most trisomies, triploids (3n), and tetraploids (4n). A significant proportion of infants dying in the perinatal and neonatal periods have been shown to have a major chromosome abnormality. About 50 per cent of all embryos and fetuses spontaneously aborted have a chromosome abnormality, and about 6 per cent of stillborn infants and those dying in the perinatal period have abnormal chromosomes.

In addition to the large number of data on newborn babies and spontaneous abortions, there are now data on large numbers of mothers who have received amniocentesis because of a maternal age of 35 and over. A recent study of over 50,000 amniocenteses shows that, overall, about 2 per cent of the fetuses in midtrimester pregnancies in mothers aged 35 and above have a chromosome abnormality.

X CHROMOSOME INACTIVATION

In 1961 Mary Lyon proposed an hypothesis to account for dosage compensation for X-linked genes between males and females in humans and mammals. She based her hypothesis on observations of the mosaic patterns created by X-linked coat color genes in female mice and the observation by Barr and Bertram of a condensed chromatin mass in neurons of female cats. These observations have subsequently been extended to other tissues and species, including humans. The Lyon hypothesis states that

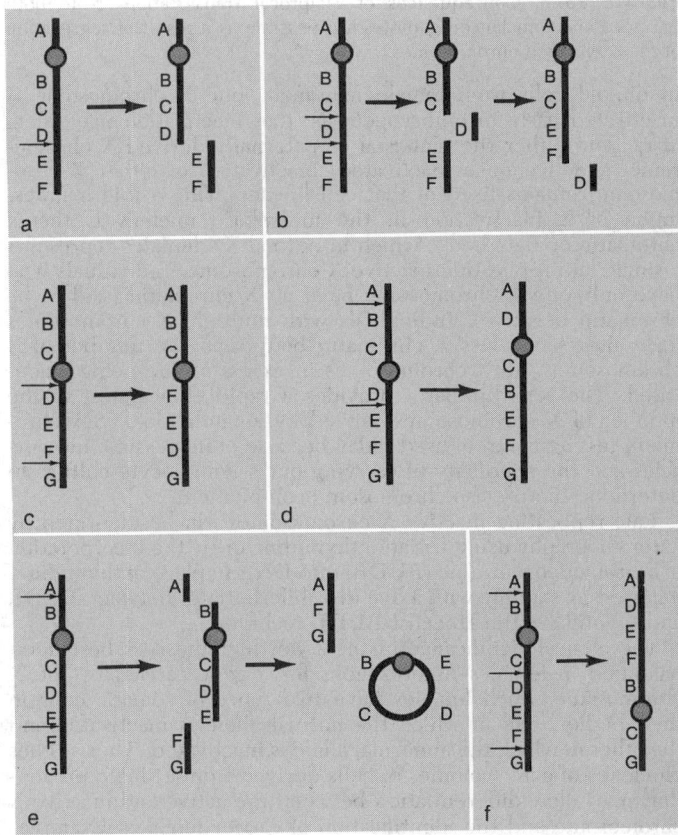

FIGURE 33–5. Types of chromosome rearrangement: *a*, terminal deletion; *b*, interstitial deletion; *c*, paracentric inversion; *d*, pericentric inversion; *e*, ring chromosome; *f*, segmental shift. (From Hamerton JL: Human Cytogenetics. Vol 1. New York, Academic Press, 1971.)

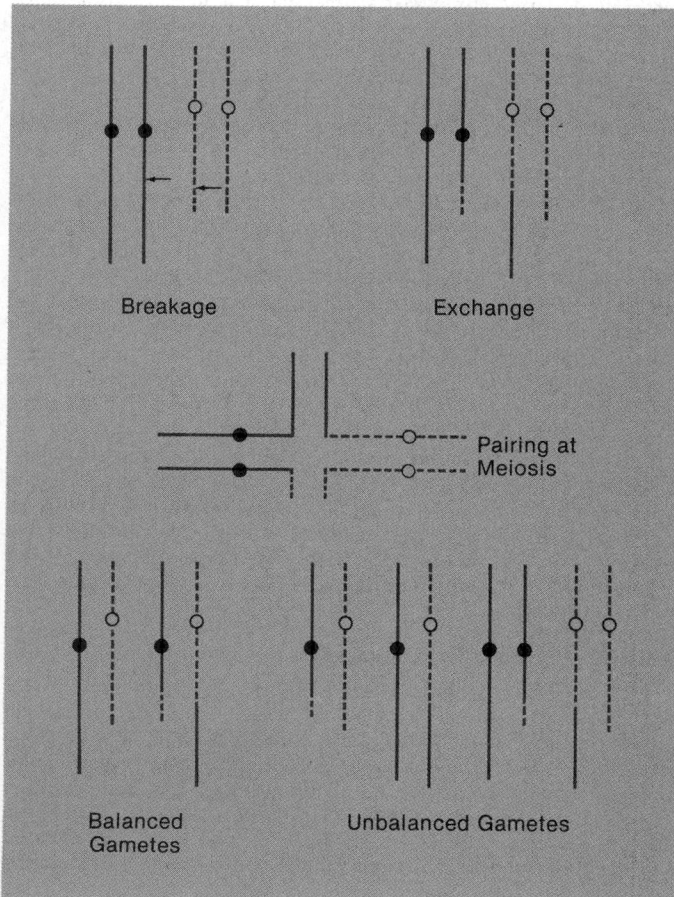

FIGURE 33–6. Consequences of reciprocal translocation. Note both balanced and unbalanced gametes are possible as a result of segregation of the exchanged chromosomes.

in diploid cells from female mammals, one X chromosome is inactivated early in embryogenesis; that inactivation may affect at random either the maternal or paternally derived X chromosome; and that once inactivated, inactivation of either X chromosome remains fixed in that cell lineage. The visible manifestation of X inactivation in the interphase nucleus is the X chromatin or Barr body, which in normal XX females represents a single late replicating inactive X chromosome. Individuals who have only one X chromosome have no X chromatin (said to be chromatin negative). Individuals with multiple X chromosomes have always one less X chromatin body than the number of X chromosomes, all X chromosomes in excess of one being inactivated. The sex chromatin provides a rapid clinical test of the number of X chromosomes carried by an individual. Sex chromatin testing is rarely used today because of its possible inaccuracies and the simplicity of carrying out a lymphocyte culture to determine the precise chromosome complement.

Late-replicating inactive X chromosomes can be identified by autoradiography using tritiated thymidine or by the incorporation of 5-bromodeoxyuridine (BUDR) into DNA in place of thymidine, followed by staining with a dye that differentiates between BUDR and thymidine (the Hoechst-BUDR technique).

The clinical significance of the Lyon hypothesis is best demonstrated in females heterozygous for a gene carried by the X chromosome. Such females have two types of somatic cells in their bodies, one in which the normal allele is inactivated and the other in which the abnormal allele is inactivated. Thus studies on clones of cells (colonies of cells derived from a single progenitor) may allow differentiation between the active and inactive X chromosome and the identification of carrier females. Examples of diseases in which carrier detection has been based on this phenomenon include the Lesch-Nyhan syndrome, Fabry's disease, testicular feminization syndrome, and mucopolysaccharidosis type II (Hunter's syndrome).

Clinical Cytogenetics

SEX CHROMOSOMES

The major features of a few common sex chromosome abnormalities are summarized in Table 33–3. Other sex chromosome abnormalities include the rare females with four or five X chromosomes, as well as males with multiple X and Y chromosomes. Such individuals are usually mentally retarded and may have somatic anomalies. Individuals with various degrees of chromosome mosaicism have also been reported, most frequently as variants in Klinefelter's syndrome or Turner's syndrome.

AUTOSOMES

The clinical features of the three best known autosomal trisomies are listed in Table 33–4. Other autosomal trisomies in fetuses surviving to term include trisomies 8, 9, and 22. All other autosomes have been reported as trisomic among spontaneous abortions. The advent of banding techniques has greatly widened the scope of chromosome pathology, and numerous examples of chromosome imbalance resulting from deletion or duplication of chromosome material have been reported. Such chromosome imbalance results in dysmorphic features and often developmental and mental retardation.

INDICATIONS FOR CHROMOSOME STUDY

Chromosome abnormalities result in a significant amount of clinical pathology, and chromosome studies should be initiated to rule out this etiologic factor in a patient when a recognizable chromosome syndrome is suspected; in patients with two or more unexplained major congenital malformations involving different systems possibly combined with the presence of minor malformations; and in patients with unexplained developmental or mental retardation. Certain cases of abnormal sexual development, leukemia, and certain solid tumors associated with congenital malformations and known to be associated with specific chromosome abnormalities (aniridia, Wilms' tumor, retinoblastoma) require chromosome studies. Chromosome banding is mandatory to identify the chromosome involved as well as to rule out possible structural changes not detectable by other means.

Chromosome Breakage Syndromes

Three diseases are commonly associated with unrepaired chromosome breaks. These are Fanconi's anemia (FA), ataxia-telangiectasia (AT), and Bloom's syndrome (BS). These are so characterized because in addition to their typical clinical features they share the propensity to chromosome breakage that can be seen in cultured cells and that commonly occurs with several times the frequency observed in normal individuals. Each of these diseases is inherited as an autosomal recessive condition. Two of these conditions are associated with congenital malformations (BS and FA), and all three have an increased frequency of malignancy.

TABLE 33–2. FREQUENCY OF CHROMOSOME ABNORMALITIES AMONG LIVE BIRTHS*

Sex Chromosomes	Frequency
Male	
47,XYY	1:1022
47,XXY	1:1022
Other	1:1277
Female	
45,X	1:9586
47,XXX	1:958
Other	1:2739
Autosomal trisomics	
+D	1:18984
+E	1:8136
+G	1:802
Balanced structural	1:517
Unbalanced structural	1:1675
Total	1:167

*Based on 54,952 babies: 35,779 males, 19,173 females.

TABLE 33–3. COMMON SEX CHROMOSOME ABNORMALITIES

Chromosome Complement	Eponym	X Chromatin	Frequency (live birth)	Phenotype
Males 47,XXY	Klinefelter's syndrome	Positive	1:1000	Often tall, eunuchoid males with hypogonadism, feminine distribution of hair, gynecomastia, testicular atrophy after puberty with hyalinized tubules, Leydig cell hyperplasia, often low IQ. May have psychosocial difficulties (see Ch. 222).
47,XYY	None	Negative	1:1000	Often no phenotype abnormalities; usually tall to very tall. May have psychosocial problems.
Females 45,X and other variants of the X chromosome and mosaics	Turner's syndrome or ovarian dysgenesis	Negative or positive	1:10,000	These patients have ovarian dysgenesis with webbing of neck, short stature (< 153 cm). Often congenital heart disease, skeletal defects, and renal anomalies. This is Turner's syndrome. Other patients may have ovarian dysgenesis without webbing of the neck and with much less frequent somatic anomalies. Invariably they are of short stature (< 153 cm) (see Ch. 224).
47,XXX	None	Double	1:1000	This is extremely variable. Often no phenotypic abnormalities but may be mentally retarded or may have psychosocial problems. Often fertile although may be infertile.

TABLE 33–4. THREE BEST-KNOWN AUTOSOMAL TRISOMIES

Chromosome Complement	Eponym	Frequency (live birth)	Phenotype
21-Trisomy (47,XX, +21 47,XY, +21)	Down's syndrome Mongolism	1:700	Typical facial appearance, epicanthic folds, upslanting palpebral fissures, broad bridge of the nose, protruding tongue, open mouth, hypoplastic superior helices, flattened facial profile. Invariable mental retardation, muscular hypotonia, and often congenital heart disease (Fig. 33–7).
18-Trisomy (47,XX, +18 47,XY, +18)	Edwards' syndrome	1:8000	Full-term infants of low birth weight with severe mental and motor retardation. Usually have a prominent occiput and frequently occurring facial abnormalities, including micrognathia, a Grecian nose, low-set and malformed ears, cleft lip and palate. The facial appearance is disproportionately small for the size of the cranium, which itself is small. Flexion deformities of fingers are often severe. Mental retardation is often severe. Congenital heart defect is common. Survival for more than a few months is rare.
13-Trisomy (47,XX, +13 47,XY, +13)	Patau's syndrome	1:20,000	Usually low birth weight infants of full-term gestation with a typical facial appearance, including a broad nose, hypertelorism, microphthalmia, anophthalmia, often with coloboma, and micrognathia. They are usually microcephalic, ears are low-set and malformed, and there is a large broad and bulbous nose. There are often flexion deformities and frequent polydactyly and syndactyly. Survival is usually very short.

TABLE 33–5. PHENOTYPES ASSOCIATED WITH SMALL CHROMOSOME ABNORMALITIES AND THEIR INHERITANCE

Phenotype	Chromosome Abnormality	Origin
Cri du chat	5pter–p15 (del)	Paternal
Aniridia/Wilms tumor (*WAGR*)	11p13 (del)	Maternal in sporadic cases
Retinoblastoma (*RB1*)	13q14.2 (del)	?
Prader-Willi syndrome (*PWCR*)	15q11.2–13 (del or dup)	Paternal
Angelmann syndrome (*ANCR*)	15q11.2–13 (del)	Maternal
Cat-eye syndrome	22pter–q11 (dup)	Maternal
DiGeorge malformation complex	22pter–q11 (del)	Maternal
Trichorhinophalangeal syndrome II	8q13–22 (del)	Maternal; maternally transmitted when inherited
Miller-Dieker syndrome	17p13 (del)	Paternal
Beckwith-Wiedemann syndrome	11p15.5 (dup)	Paternal

Data primarily from Hall, 1990.

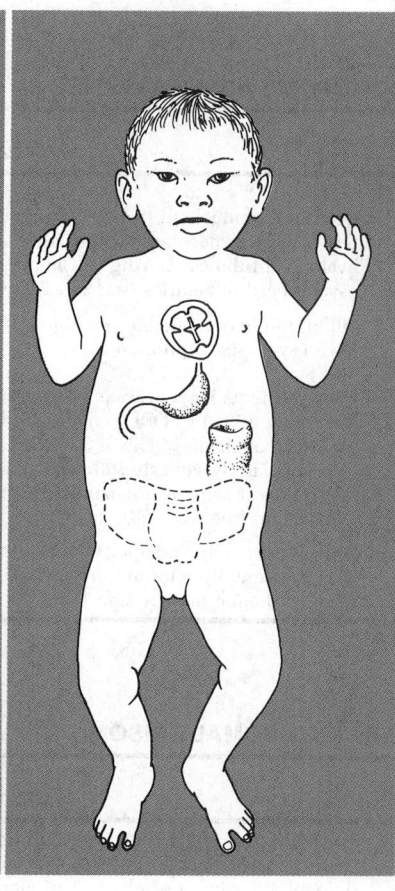

Growth failure

Mental retardation

Flat occiput

Dysplastic ears

Many "loops" on finger tips

Simian crease

Medial axial triradius

Unilateral or bilateral absence of one rib

Intestinal stenosis

Umbilical hernia

Dysplastic pelvis

Hypotonic muscles

Big toes widely spaced

Broad flat face

Slanting eyes

Epicanthus

Short nose

Small and arched palate

Big wrinkled tongue

Dental anomalies

Short and broad hands (clinodactyly)

Congenital heart disease

Megacolon

FIGURE 33–7. Clinical findings in trisomy 21. (From Vogel F, Motulsky AG: Human Genetics: Problems and Approaches. Berlin, Springer-Verlag, 1986.)

This may be the consequence of alterations in DNA repair process.

Sister chromatids can be differentially stained by a modification of the Hoechst-BUDR technique. This permits the identification of exchanges between sister chromatids. Such sister chromatid exchanges (SCE) occur with an increased frequency in BS and in normal individuals may be increased as the result of exposure to chromosome-damaging agents.

New Chromosomal Syndromes—Microcytogenetics

The advent of high-resolution chromosome banding has allowed a much greater definition of banding patterns and has thus allowed the recognition of smaller deletions and duplications of chromosome material. This has led to the development of "microcytogenetics" and the observation that several hereditary syndromes of uncertain etiology and involving multiple systems have been shown to be associated with small chromosome deletions (Table 33–5). Particularly interesting is the observation that both the Prader-Willi and Angelmann syndromes are apparently caused by very similar small chromosome deletions involving 15q11.2–13. In the case of the Prader-Willi syndrome the deleted chromosome is invariably inherited from the father, whereas in the Angelmann syndrome the abnormal chromosome is inherited from the mother. It has been suggested that the differences between these two conditions are due to the imprinting of the abnormal chromosome, which varies with its origin. The nature of such imprinting is at present unknown, but it has been suggested that DNA methylation may play a role. Recently it has been suggested that both chromosome 15's are maternal in origin (maternal isodisomy or heterodisomy) and that there is no paternal contribution in some cases of Prader-Willi syndrome in which there is no evidence of a chromosome abnormality. Other studies have shown that this observation does not apply to all such families lacking a detectable abnormality, and the final determination of the nature of the defect in Prader-Willi syndrome must await further molecular studies.

Heritable Fragile Sites

Chromosome breakage is usually random; however, some individuals may exhibit breakage or a nonstaining chromosome region (chromosome gap) at a specific site in a significant proportion of metaphases. In many cases such sites may be induced by the use of folate-deficient culture medium, although a few sites are folate insensitive. These specific sites, known as fragile sites, may represent alterations in the DNA and are often heritable. While most fragile sites are not associated with disease or other clinical problems, the fragile site at Xq28 is known to be associated with one common form of X-linked mental retardation among males.

PRENATAL DIAGNOSIS

The diagnosis of chromosome abnormalities at midtrimester gestation is now a routine procedure for certain pregnancies. It involves the aspiration of a small sample of amniotic fluid (amniocentesis), culturing of the fetal cells contained in the fluid, and determination of the karyotype of these cells and thus of the fetus. The major indications for the use of this technique for the detection of chromosome abnormalities are (1) maternal age—usually offered to all mothers over the age of 35 at the time of delivery; (2) presence of a parental chromosome abnormality—if one parent is a balanced translocation carrier and particularly if the translocation was detected as the result of the previous birth of a clinically abnormal infant; (3) previous trisomy—those cases in which the mother has previously had a trisomic infant or possibly in which she is known to have had a previous instance of spontaneous abortion in which the abortus was karyotyped and shown to be trisomic; and (4) abnormal levels (high or low) of α-fetoprotein.

The safety and reliability of amniocentesis as a diagnostic technique have now been well established by numerous studies, and it is generally accepted that amniocentesis increases the risk of miscarriage by 0.5 to 1 per cent above the inherent risk for that individual without intervention. Other risks of the test, including fetal and maternal morbidity, are negligible. In competent hands the test has been shown to have nearly 100 per cent reliability for the detection of chromosome abnormalities.

Recently, direct transcervical and transabdominal aspiration of the chorionic villus (chorionic villus sampling, or CVS) has been used both for the prenatal diagnosis of chromosome abnormalities and for the isolation of DNA for the diagnosis of several different genetic diseases. Clinical trials have shown that CVS results in only a slightly higher risk to the fetus than genetic amniocentesis (GA). Because of the nature of the tissue obtained by CVS, the frequency of confined mosaicism is greater in cells obtained by CVS than in cultured amniocytes derived directly from the fetus. This may present greater interpretive problems to the cytogenetic laboratory. With improved ultrasonographic resolution it may be possible to perform GA earlier in pregnancy, at around the thirteenth week of gestation. Clinical trials of early GA are needed to determine its safety and accuracy.

These newer techniques hold promise of being able to perform a genetic diagnosis at the end of the first or early in the second trimester of pregnancy.

DeGrouchy J, Turleau C: Clinical Atlas of Human Chromosomes. 2nd ed. New York. John Wiley & Sons, 1984. *A review of chromosomal syndromes with numerous illustrations and references.*

Evans JA, Hamerton JL: Chromosomal anomalies. *In* Clarke AM, Clarke ADB, Berg JM (eds.): Mental Deficiency, The Changing Outlook. 4th ed. London, Methuen, 1985. *A review of chromosome abnormalities and their relationship to mental retardation.*

Hall JG: Genomic imprinting: Review and relevance to human diseases. Am J Hum Genet 46:857–873, 1990. *A review of a possible new mechanism of genetic regulation and its relationship to human disease.*

Hamerton JL: Population cytogenetics: A perspective. *In* Adonolfi M, Baron P, Giarnelli F, et al. (eds.): Pediatric Research: A Genetic Approach. London, Heineman Medical Books, 1982. *Deals with frequency of chromosome abnormalities in populations.*

ISCN: An International System of Human Cytogenetic Nomenclature. Birth Defects Original Article Series 21:1–116. New York, March of Dimes, 1985. *The basic handbook of nomenclature rules for human chromosomes including high-resolution banding.*

Vogel F, Motulsky AG: Human Genetics: Problems and Approaches. 2nd ed. Berlin, Springer-Verlag, 1986. *A detailed treatise on human genetics from both a basic and a clinical viewpoint. Numerous references. Chapter 2 deals extensively with human cytogenetics.*

34 Congenital Malformations

Lewis B. Holmes

INCIDENCE

Two per cent of newborn infants have serious malformations, most of which are compatible with survival. Many additional malformations, such as genitourinary, vertebral, and heart defects, are identified during childhood and the teenage years. Many adults with congenital malformations are unaware of the significance of these problems for their health or the potential significance for their unborn children.

ETIOLOGIES

The recognized causes of malformations include genetic abnormalities, environmental factors, and the combined effects of mutant genes and environmental factors, i.e., multifactorial inheritance (Table 34–1). Multifactorial inheritance is the most common of these etiologies. However, the cause of at least 40 per cent of all malformations is not known. One example of a cause that is neither environmental nor genetic is a vascular abnormality. Occlusion of blood vessels during development has been postulated to cause intestinal atresia and hydranencephaly; absence of vessels and abnormal persistence of vessels have been observed in absence of the radius and absence of the tibia.

A few hereditary malformations have been shown to be due to biochemical abnormalities, such as a deficiency of 5α-reductase in individuals with pseudovaginal perineoscrotal hypospadias, an autosomal recessive disorder characterized by ambiguous genitals. An abnormal α-2 chain in type I collagen has been identified in skin fibroblasts from a woman with type I osteogenesis imperfecta, a skeletal dysplasia inherited as an autosomal dominant trait (see Ch. 189).

In multifactorial inheritance, clinical studies of human and

TABLE 34–1. RECOGNIZED ETIOLOGIES OF MALFORMATIONS PRESENT IN ADULTS

	Examples
1. Genetic abnormalities	
a. Single mutant gene	
i. Autosomal dominant trait	Polycystic kidney disease, adult type Polysyndactyly
ii. Autosomal recessive trait	Mohr's syndrome (oro-facial-digital syndrome, type II)
iii. X-linked dominant trait	Telecanthus-hypospadias (BBB) syndrome
iv. X-linked recessive trait	Metacarpal 4-5 fusion
b. Chromosome abnormalities	
i. Trisomy of autosomes	Down's syndrome
ii. Interstitial deletion	Aniridia-Wilms' tumor
iii. Sex chromosome abnormalities	45,X (Turner's syndrome); 47,XXY (Klinefelter's syndrome)
2. Environmental factors	
a. Uterine facts	Amniotic band syndrome
b. Intrauterine infection	Congenital rubella syndrome
c. Drugs	Fetal hydantoin syndrome
3. Genetic plus environmental factors (multifactorial inheritance)	Heart defects Cleft lip and/or palate Hypospadias Pyloric stenosis Hirschsprung's disease

laboratory examples have shown that several genes (including major genes) are involved, as well as environmental factors such as maternal influences, uterine factors, the season of the year, and socioeconomic class. Most individuals with a malformation attributed to multifactorial inheritance are the only affected members of their families. However, affected individuals have an increased risk of having affected sibs or affected children. The recurrence risk is usually between 1 and 10 per cent, which is 10 to 40 times greater than the incidence of the malformation in the general population.

About 0.6 per cent of newborn infants have a major chromosome abnormality, but many do not survive to the adult years. Down's syndrome results from the most common trisomy, and survival of most affected newborns to the adult years is now expected. Down syndrome is due to trisomy 21 in 95 per cent of cases, with the other 5 per cent due to translocation or other unusual chromosome abnormalities. In trisomy 21, the extra chromosome comes from the mother 75 per cent of the time. Since women over age 35 now are having a smaller portion of all pregnancies, 80 per cent of the infants with Down's syndrome are being born to women of less than 35 years.

Common sex chromosome abnormalities, such as 47,XYY and 47,XXX, are usually not associated with any congenital malformations. Boys with 47,XXY (Klinefelter's syndrome) may have abnormal physical features that are evident in the teenage years. Girls with the 45,X (Turner's) syndrome are usually recognized in infancy because of associated lymphedema, webbed neck, heart defects, and short stature or in the teenage years because of failure of puberty to occur spontaneously.

CLINICAL RELEVANCE

The following examples illustrate the potential significance of a malformation to the affected adult and his or her children.

Relevance to the Health of the Affected Person

CONGENITAL ABSENCE OF ONE KIDNEY. About 1 in 700 infants has unilateral renal agenesis. Most affected individuals are asymptomatic. However, they have an increased risk of structural malformations of the ureter, such as ureteropelvic junction stricture, and associated infections, hypertension, and so forth. The affected female may have a bicornuate uterus or absence of the half of the uterus on the same side as the renal aplasia. Affected males may have absence of the vas deferens on the same side. Parents with unilateral renal agenesis have an increased risk of having infants with either the same malformation or bilateral renal agenesis, which is fatal.

BRACHYDACTYLY, TYPE E. Owing to premature closure

of epiphyses, persons with this autosomal dominant disorder have short hands and feet with a variable pattern of shortening of the first, fourth, and fifth metacarpals and metatarsals and distal phalanges of the thumb and great toe. They also have a mild-to-moderate degree of shortness of stature. Severe hypertension is often a problem in the affected teenager and young adult. The cause of the hypertension has not been determined.

BRANCHIO-OTO-RENAL SYNDROME. The person with this autosomal dominant disorder has a pattern of malformations that includes malformed ears, preauricular tags, preauricular sinus, and branchial cleft sinus. The mildly affected adult is often not diagnosed until a more severely affected child is born. The affected adult may have significant hearing loss or renal hypoplasia.

KLIPPEL-FEIL SYNDROME. The person with fusion or hemivertebrae of one or more cervical vertebrae usually has a short neck, limited rotation of the head, a low hairline, and a webbed neck. Common associated problems include hearing loss, heart defects, Sprengel's deformity, and genitourinary anomalies, such as aplasia of müllerian structures.

POLYCYSTIC KIDNEY DISEASE. The affected individual with the adult form has an increased risk of having cerebral aneurysms and pancreatic cysts. Prenatal diagnosis using DNA probes is now possible in some families; recent studies show at least two genes can cause this type of polycystic kidney disease (see Ch. 89).

Relevance to Increased Risk of Having Affected Children

MULTIFACTORIAL INHERITANCE. The adult with one of the common malformations attributed to this process has an increased risk of having an affected child. For malformations that show an altered sex ratio, the sex of the affected parent is important in determining the risk of having an affected child (Table 34–2). In general, the parent of the less frequently affected sex has a greater risk of having affected children. For example, *intestinal aganglionosis* (Hirschsprung's disease) is much more common in males than females, but the affected female has a much greater risk of having affected children (Table 34–2).

With early surgical closure and better treatment of the associated hydrocephalus and urinary tract infections, males and females with *spina bifida* (myelomeningocele) are surviving to adult years and usually have normal intelligence. Both affected males and affected females may be fertile. The affected adult has an increased risk of about 3 per cent that each child will have a neural tube defect.

HYPERTELORISM. The mother who has a broad bridge of the nose and hypertelorism* has an increased risk of having severely malformed sons. For example, the female who carries the X-linked gene for the telecanthus-hypospadias (BBB) syndrome shows only hypertelorism, but sons who inherit this gene have a severe malformation syndrome that may include hypertelorism, broad nasal bridge, cleft lip and palate, heart defects, imperforate anus, hypospadias, and mental deficiency. Mothers with the autosomal dominant disorder known as the Opitz-Frias (or G) syndrome also have hypertelorism and a broad bridge of the nose. Their affected sons and daughters have at birth aspiration due to a laryngotracheoesophageal cleft, stridor, and associated malformations such as cleft lip, heart defects, hypospadias (males), and imperforate anus. Unfortunately, the physical features of broad nasal bridge and hypertelorism are nonspecific, and the risk for the woman with no affected children cannot be determined.

MENTAL RETARDATION. There are many causes of mental retardation. The mildly retarded woman without striking physical abnormalities may be a carrier of significant and relatively common genetic abnormalities that give her an increased risk of having severely affected sons. Two examples are the fragile-X syndrome and the Coffin-Lowry syndrome. The fragile-X syndrome is a common cause of mental retardation, mild facial abnormalities, and sometimes macro-orchidism in males. The

*Hypertelorism can be determined most precisely from an anteroposterior radiograph that shows an increased bony interorbital distance.

TABLE 34–2. RISK OF AFFECTED CHILDREN FOR PARENT WITH MALFORMATION ATTRIBUTED TO MULTIFACTORIAL INHERITANCE

Malformation	Risk of Affected Child (per cent)	Prevalence of Condition in General Population (per cent)
1. Intestinal aganglionosis (Hirschsprung's disease)	2.0	0.02
2. Hypospadias	6.0	0.8
3. Club foot	1.4	0.13
4. Congenital hip dislocation	4.3	0.8
5. Ventricular septal defect	4.0	0.2
6. Pyloric stenosis	4 (affected father) 13 (affected mother)	
7. Cleft palate	6.2	0.3
8. Spina bifida (meningomyelocele)	2.0	0.14

affected female may show mosaicism for the marker X chromosome, an abnormality of the distal portion of the long arm of the X chromosome that can be identified in cytogenetic studies only if special media and processing are used. The woman who has the X-linked gene for the Coffin-Lowry syndrome shows only mild mental retardation, short stature, short and hyperextensible hands, and tufted distal phalanges. The affected male is much more severely affected, with severe mental deficiency, short stature, stiff joints, coarse facial features, pectus carinatum, and large, soft hands.

PRENATAL DIAGNOSIS

The techniques used most often for diagnosing malformations in the fetus are cell culture of amniocytes removed at 16 to 18 weeks of gestation, assay for α-fetoprotein (AFP) in the amniotic fluid and maternal serum, and ultrasound imaging. Early amniocentesis is now offered at 12 to 14 weeks of pregnancy at some medical centers. Parents who have previously had a child with trisomy 21 have a 1 per cent risk of having a second child with trisomy 21 regardless of the mother's age. For the woman who has previously had a child with anencephaly or spina bifida, prenatal diagnosis includes amniocentesis to measure the level of AFP and ultrasound imaging for hydrocephalus, the cranial defect in anencephaly, and the spinal defect in meningomyelocele. A neural tube defect is confirmed by an increase in the level of AFP and acetylcholinesterase in the amniotic fluid. Both the amniocytes removed at amniocentesis and the chorionic villi removed transcervically at 9 to 11 weeks of gestation can be used to identify chromosome abnormalities, hemoglobinopathies, and metabolic disorders in the fetus. Limb malformations, diaphragm defects, ventral abdominal wall defects, hydrocephalus, and renal agenesis can be investigated with ultrasound imaging. However, the accuracy of prenatal diagnosis varies with the quality of the equipment used and the experience of the sonographer.

Prenatal screening for neural tube defects and chromosome trisomies is now available as an option in prenatal care. Serum AFP is measured in the mother at 15 to 17 weeks of pregnancy. Errors in diagnosis result from incorrect gestational age and alterations in the range of normal values in obese women with diabetes mellitus. The pregnant woman with an elevated serum level of AFP should have ultrasound imaging and if no abnormality is seen, amniocentesis for AFP and acetylcholinesterase. Elevations in AFP also occur in twin pregnancies, intrauterine death, and other malformations such as esophageal atresia, omphalocele, and hereditary nephrosis. A skin-covered neural tube defect, such as a lumbar meningocele, will be missed in prenatal screening with serum AFP. Measuring maternal serum levels of AFP, estriol, and hCG identifies 60 per cent of the infants with trisomy 21 (low AFP and estriol and high hCG). In general, prenatal AFP screening is most effective if carried out by individuals who are experienced in identifying the causes of false-positive and false-negative values and who educate the parents initially about the steps involved and the benefits and accuracy of the testing.

FETAL SURGERY

Catheters have been introduced to relieve malformations that cause obstruction of the flow of urine or of cerebrospinal fluid.

This approach is experimental. One major problem is to identify an abnormality early enough to permit intervention before the fetus has suffered irreversible lung hypoplasia, the usual cause of death in infants with oligohydramnios from urinary tract obstruction. Another problem is that the fetus in whom only hydrocephalus or urinary tract obstruction is visible by ultrasonography may have multiple malformations that become apparent only after birth.

PREVENTION OF MALFORMATION

Pregnant women with several different medical diseases or exposures have an increased risk of having children with birth defects. If the patient is informed of this risk before conception or soon after conception, these risks can be either lessened or eliminated. These efforts at prevention require special efforts in education, as most women receive routine prenatal care too late to benefit from counseling. Specific opportunities in prevention include the following:

CHRONIC ALCOHOLISM. Exposure of the fetus to high maternal levels of alcohol causes growth retardation before and after birth, microcephaly, brain malformations, mental deficiency, and a characteristic pattern of craniofacial features (fetal alcohol syndrome). The lower the level of exposure, the less the risk of damage to the fetus. If the pregnant woman decreases her alcohol consumption at any time in pregnancy, it is beneficial to the fetus, although a decrease before or soon after conception is the most beneficial.

DIABETES MELLITUS. The woman with insulin-dependent diabetes mellitus is two to three times more likely to have a child with serious malformations than the nondiabetic woman. The malformations include spina bifida, anencephaly, heart defects, vertebral and genitourinary malformations, and multiple malformations. The risk of having a malformed infant correlates inversely with the quality of control of her disease, glucose metabolism in particular, very early in pregnancy. The lower the level of glycosylated hemoglobin before or soon after conception, the lower her risk of having a malformed child.

MATERNAL PHENYLKETONURIA (PKU). Children with PKU identified at birth through neonatal screening for metabolic diseases will have normal development and intelligence if the dietary treatment (low phenylalanine, low protein) is begun soon after birth. The diet is usually discontinued in the early school years. However, successfully treated females with PKU who are no longer on the diet have a risk of over 90 per cent that any pregnancy will either end in a spontaneous abortion or result in a child with microcephaly and mental deficiency, and often heart defects as well. The risk of damage to the fetus correlates with the blood level of phenylalanine in the mother. If the woman with PKU resumes the low-phenylalanine diet before conception she has her best chance of having a normal child. If the diet is resumed in the first trimester, as soon as she knows she is pregnant, the child is less severely damaged than if no dietary treatment is used during pregnancy. Unfortunately, many young women with PKU are not aware of their risk of having children with serious birth defects.

Ardinger HH, Buetow KH, Bell GI, et al.: Association of genetic variation of the transforming growth factor-alpha gene with cleft lip and palate. Am J Hum Genet 45:348, 1989. *A new finding that shows how DNA technology may help clarify the genetic aspects of multifocal inheritance.*

Hanley WB, Clark JTR, Schoonheyt W: Maternal phenylketonuria (PKU)—a review. Clin Biochem 20:149, 1987. *A thorough review of the teratogenic effects of PKU in the pregnant woman and efforts at preventing these effects.*

Jones KL: Smith's Recognizable Patterns of Human Malformation. 4th ed. Philadelphia, W. B. Saunders Company, 1988. *A thorough tabulation of recognized malformation syndromes.*

Kimberling WJ, Fain PR, Kenyon JB, et al.: Linkage heterogeneity of autosomal dominant polycystic kidney disease. N Engl J Med 319:913, 1988. *Shows that more than one gene causes this type of polycystic kidney disease.*

Nelson K, Holmes LB: Malformations due to presumed spontaneous mutations in newborn infants. N Engl J Med 320:19, 1989. *The first clinical assessment of the apparent etiology of all congenital malformations in a large, unselected population of newborn infants.*

Roodhooft AM, Birnholz JC, Holmes LB: Familial nature of congenital absence and severe dysgenesis of both kidneys. N Engl J Med 310:1341, 1984. *Shows the potential genetic significance of unilateral renal agenesis in an adult.*

Shepard TH: Catalog of Teratogenic Agents. 6th ed. Baltimore, The Johns Hopkins University Press, 1989. *A summary of experimental and clinical intervention on the potential teratogenic effects of common drug and other environmental exposures.*

Wald NJ, Cuckle HS, Densem JW, et al.: Maternal serum unconjugated oestriol

as an antenatal screening test for Down's syndrome. Br J Obstet Gynecol 95:344, 1988. *Shows the basis for expanded prenatal screening with three maternal serum constituents: α-fetoprotein, hCG, and estriol.*

35 Genetic Counseling

Margretta R. Seashore

Genetic counseling can be defined as a process in which an individual or family obtains information about a genetic condition that may affect them. The purpose of genetic counseling is to enable individuals and families to make important decisions about marriage, reproduction, and health management based on the facts of the genetic situation for which a risk is perceived. This process is part of a thorough genetic evaluation in which the diagnosis is made or confirmed, the genetic model is developed, the information is communicated, the options are discussed, and psychosocial support is offered. Any breakdown in this progression may lead to information being misunderstood, misinterpreted, or misused.

DIAGNOSIS

The first step in genetic counseling is to confirm the diagnosis. The worst error that can be made is to provide an elegant and sophisticated analysis for the wrong disorder. The importance of this step cannot be overemphasized. Many persons have been given general diagnoses, such as mental retardation, for which there can be a multitude of genetic as well as nongenetic explanations. The increasing definition of the molecular pathology of many disorders has heightened the importance of recognizing genetic heterogeneity. For example, at least 20 different forms of muscular dystrophy have been identified which are clinically similar. Both X-linked and autosomal recessive forms are known. At least two, Becker and Duchenne dystrophy, are X-linked conditions that are allelic but clinically quite distinct. Differentiations of this kind must be made with as much accuracy as possible if the patient and family are to be given the most precise answers.

The confirmation of the diagnosis uses five medical tools, four of which are very familiar to all clinicians. These are medical records, medical history, physical examination, conventional laboratory tests, and molecular genetic analysis. The importance of reviewing medical records seems obvious, yet it can be a difficult task to accomplish completely. Validation of the rate of progression of symptoms and signs, the development of the present physical findings, and the results of prior laboratory tests are all best determined from the medical records. In addition, the status of family members can sometimes be assessed from examination of their medical records. Often the medical geneticist has been told of a relative who "had the same problem" only to learn from that individual's medical records that the relative's problem was entirely different.

The medical history provides clues to the beginnings and progression of symptoms and signs which may provide valuable hints to diagnosis. The pattern of progression in the degenerative neurologic disorders provides important diagnostic information. A history of more than two spontaneous miscarriages may suggest a chromosomal translocation in one parent. Early death of infants in the pedigree may suggest an inborn error of intermediary metabolism.

The physical examination again provides the opportunity to consider genetic heterogeneity. For example, there are many genetic causes of short stature. The details of the physical examination may provide the information on which the correct genetic diagnosis depends. Precise measurement of anthropometric features can be compared with values in the literature and the diagnostic considerations narrowed.

Conventional laboratory tests often provide helpful diagnostic information to complete the genetic diagnosis. Radiographic appearance of bones is often the critical information in diagnosing

TABLE 35–1. MOLECULAR DIAGNOSTIC TOOLS IN GENETIC COUNSELING: CONDITIONS FOR WHICH DNA-BASED DIAGNOSIS HAS BEEN ACCOMPLISHED

Adult polycystic kidney disease
Duchenne muscular dystrophy
Cystic fibrosis
Fragile-X syndrome
Hemophilia A
Huntington disease
Multiple endocrine neoplasia
Myotonic dystrophy
Neurofibromatosis type 1
Neurofibromatosis type 2
Ornithine transcarbamoylase deficiency
Phenylketonuria
Tay-Sachs disease
Thalassemias
Sickle cell anemia
Wiskott-Aldrich syndrome

the chondrodystrophies, for example. Measurement of proteins, such as α_1-antitrypsin, can demonstrate the most important feature of a condition.

The development of molecular diagnostic tools that can provide precise definition of the mutation or utilize linkage to a specific genetic marker has revolutionized genetic counseling. In the past, the chromosomal location of specific genes was inferred from pedigree information for the X chromosome and linkage to specific protein markers for autosomes. Now the chromosomal location of many more genes is known, linkage to specific DNA markers has been established, and many genes of clinical importance have been cloned and sequenced. It is likely that within the next two decades, the entire human genome will be mapped and entirely sequenced. More than 1500 genes have now been mapped to specific locations in the human genome. Many of these comprise specific genes or linkage markers for some of the 2000 single-gene conditions that appear in the McKusick catalog of mendelian phenotypes. The number of conditions that show linkage to known genetic markers or to anonymous DNA probes grows daily. These new tools can be used to enhance the precision of genetic diagnosis and counseling (see Ch. 32 for molecular methods). Table 35–1 lists examples of many of the genetic conditions that can be diagnosed using these molecular tools. This list is being expanded at a rapid rate and should not be taken to be complete. At least one disease has been mapped to each chromosome (Table 35–2). Any condition mapped to a specific chromosomal location can theoretically be diagnosed

TABLE 35–2. EXAMPLES OF ONE CONDITION MAPPED TO EACH CHROMOSOME

Genetic Condition	Map Location
Charcot-Marie-Tooth neuropathy 1	1q
von Hippel–Lindau syndrome	3p
Huntington disease	4pter–p16
Familial polyposis of the colon	5q21–p22
Congenital adrenal hyperplasia	6p21.3
Cystic fibrosis	7q31–q32
Langer-Gideon syndrome	8q24
Friedreich ataxia	9q13–q21
Multiple endocrine neoplasia IIB	10pter–q11
Wilms' tumor–aniridia syndrome	11p13
Stickler syndrome	12q14
Wilson disease	13q14–q21
Variegate porphyria	14q
Xeroderma pigmentosum (comp group F)	15
Adult-type polycystic kidney disease	16p13
Neurofibromatosis	17q11.2
Kidd blood group	18q11–q12
Myotonic dystrophy	19q13.3–q13.3
Alagille syndrome	20p12–p11
Alzheimer disease 1	21pter–q21
NF2 (bilateral acoustic neuroma)	22q11–q13.1
Duchenne muscular dystrophy	Xp21.3–p21.1

using molecular methods, given the appropriate molecular probes and informative family members.

THE GENETIC MODEL

The next essential step to be taken before the genetic counseling visit with the patient and family can take place is the development of the genetic model. The patient has come with the question "what is it and is it inherited?" Arrival at a diagnosis leads to the answer to the first part of the question. The second part is crucial to the process of genetic counseling. The development of the genetic model requires use of the family history, the precise diagnosis, and knowledge of the possible genetic mechanisms. The diagraming of the pedigree from the family history may fit such an obvious genetic model that further analysis is simple. When the physical examination and laboratory studies are typical of a recognized genetic condition such as Duchenne muscular dystrophy and the pedigree demonstrates a clear pattern of X-linked inheritance, the development of the genetic model is straightforward. More often, however, the pedigree is less clear. Where there is familial aggregation without an obvious mendelian pattern or the individual is the only affected member of the family at present, all possible genetic mechanisms must be considered and excluded or confirmed. The genetic model must then be used to identify those at risk for the condition.

Three general genetic mechanisms must be considered: chromosomal, mendelian, and multifactorial. The chromosomal disorders should be considered as a possible explanation for multiple anomalies, mental retardation, recurrent miscarriages, and unexplained stillbirths. These are considered in detail in Ch. 33. Empiric figures must be used to predict the recurrence of chromosomal abnormalities in a family. These range between 1 and 10 per cent, and the literature must be consulted with reference to the specific situation.

When a clear mendelian pattern is seen and the disorder is a recognized mendelian condition, counseling is based on that pattern. When the family history fails to demonstrate a mendelian pattern, the diagnosis is reviewed and the medical literature consulted to determine the inheritance pattern for the specific disorder. With autosomal recessive conditions the birth of an affected child may be the first signal that a set of parents is heterozygous for a rare recessive condition. Here the genetic model depends on the correct diagnosis and the known inheritance pattern for that disorder. For X-linked conditions, the decision must be made whether the affected individual represents a new mutation or inheritance from a heterozygous mother who by chance has no affected relatives. In the past, Bayesian calculations based on the pedigree have been the mainstay of this kind of analysis. Today, however, molecular diagnostic tools have refined the ability to determine heterozygosity in this situation. For dominantly inherited conditions, the literature must be consulted to determine the proportion of patients who represent new mutations, a figure that can approach 50 per cent. When a new mutation is the explanation, others in the family are not at risk, but each offspring of the affected individual has a 50 per cent risk of inheriting the gene. Variability in expression can confound the analysis of a family demonstrating an autosomal dominant condition. The possibility of gonadal mosaicism, although rare, can never be eliminated. In general, however, the absence of the condition in any other family member makes the likelihood high that the patient represents a new mutation. Frequently no mendelian hypothesis can be sustained, yet there is familial aggregation of the disorder. Many conditions, such as neural tube defects and cleft lip and palate, appear to be multifactorial in origin with both genetic and environmental components. Genetic counseling for these conditions must rely on empiric figures for the specific condition.

THE COUNSELING PROCESS

Once the genetic model has been established, the process of communicating this information to the patient and family must begin.

The process of genetic counseling itself has the following components: transferring information about the genetic risks, putting the risks in perspective, providing a summary of the disorder, and discussing the options. It must begin with the individual who brought the original question. An explanation of the genetic risks requires imparting factual information using scientific concepts that are not familiar to everyone. It is important that the facts which form the basis of the development of the genetic model be clearly explained. However, it is neither possible nor desirable to present an entire course in medical genetics to the anxious patient and family. Therefore, the relevant facts must be carefully culled from the counselor's knowledge store and communicated clearly. It is important to remember that persons may be very anxious and find it difficult to absorb complex material, especially if they are fearful about the implications of the information. The strategy of first presenting a brief summary of the conclusions and their implications, stating that the evidence for this conclusion will presently be discussed, can allay some fears and relieve some of the distraction that prevents families from hearing this kind of information.

If the condition is a chromosome disorder, the structure and ways of identifying chromosomes must be mentioned and the specific disorder illustrated. Using teaching aids such as diagrams and photographs of chromosomes is helpful, the normal situation providing a frame of reference. When the condition is a mendelian disorder, the basic concepts of single-gene inheritance must be discussed briefly, but the discussion should center on the mode of inheritance involved in the particular family and not be clouded with a great deal of extraneous material about other modes of inheritance. Families without a prior family history of the disorder may have difficulty with the fact that the disorder has never been seen in their family. An explanation of heterozygosity may help clarify autosomal recessive inheritance. Autosomal dominant inheritance is easy to understand when there are affected individuals and the pedigree demonstrates a clear vertical pattern. Of more difficulty to the family is the new mutation. Careful examination of other family members must be performed before the presence of the condition can be excluded. As with the chromosome disorders, the use of such teaching aids as gene diagrams, sample pedigrees, and other models may be extremely valuable.

A second important component of genetic counseling is putting the risk in perspective. Many workers in the field (see Hsia) have noted that perception of risk may be of more importance in family decision making than the actual numerical value of the risk. This perception depends on at least two factors: risk compared to background risk, and overall burden, a combination of risk and severity. A risk of 1 in 4 of recurrence in a second child, in the case of PKU for example, is very much greater than a risk of 1/10,000 in the general population. Conversely, a risk of 1/10,000 may sound high to a couple who believe that the chances of something being wrong with an unborn child is 1 in a million. The presentation of such risk figures can change the perception of that risk. For example, a 1 in 4 chance of recurrence of PKU is also a 3 to 1 chance against recurrence. The judgment of burden, first put forth by C.O. Carter, is a very personal one. Physical handicap may be a severe burden for one family, whereas another may find that tolerable but mental handicap unacceptable. Helping families to think about risks in these ways is an important component of genetic counseling.

Genetic counseling also includes a description of the disorder. Many persons go to their local library in an attempt to find literature about the disorder or ask medical friends to do so. Often this results in misinformation or information that is out of date. Providing written material about the disorder is often helpful. Many genetic counseling clinics have pamphlets, booklets, and other literature to provide. The family should also be furnished with a written report of the counseling summarizing the important points.

REPRODUCTIVE OPTIONS AND PRENATAL DIAGNOSIS

If risk to future unborn children is at issue, as it so often is, the family in whom a risk for genetic disease has been identified must be told about the reproductive options available to them. Aside from refraining from having children at all, the options can enhance the chances of having healthy children for the family at risk. Adoption should be discussed. Reproductive technologies such as in vitro fertilization with a donor egg or artificial insemination by donor should be addressed. The risk of the same genotype in a donor must be excluded. Appropriate referral to experts in those areas of alternative reproductive options must be made.

Prenatal diagnosis is an important reproductive option for families that are at high risk for the birth of a child with a genetic disorder. Indications for prenatal diagnosis are summarized in Table 35–3.

Prenatal diagnosis is also used to address pregnancies at risk because of maternal disease or maternal exposure to a potential teratogen. The concern is not necessarily genetic, but there is a risk for a condition that can be diagnosed during fetal life.

The methods in prenatal diagnosis depend on the following: imaging the fetus; examination of DNA in cells of fetal origin; analysis of chromosomes in fetal cells; examination of proteins from cells of fetal origin; examination of proteins, metabolites, and other small molecules of fetal origin; and direct visualization of the fetus.

Imaging of the fetus is largely performed using ultrasonography. Estimation of fetal age and assessment of fetal growth can be readily performed. Fetal anatomy and organ function can be evaluated. Anatomic abnormalities such as spina bifida, anencephaly, hydrocephalus, limb malformations, cardiac malformations, and renal anomalies can be visualized.

The genetic material of the fetus, both chromosomes and specific DNA segments, can be analyzed using cells of fetal origin obtained either at amniocentesis or by chorionic villus sampling (CVS). The major autosomal and sex chromosomal aneuploidies can be diagnosed in this way, along with chromosomal rearrangements, deletions, insertions, and the like. Any DNA-based diagnosis that can be performed on cells can be performed on fetal cells. Cells of fetal origin obtained either at amniocentesis or by CVS can also be used to measure enzyme activity, characterize proteins, look for stored material, or perform other biochemical studies specific to the disorder being diagnosed. In most cases, such studies will have been preceded by family studies that have characterized the disorder and demonstrated the informativeness of the methods to be used.

Enzymes, proteins, and other chemicals of biologic importance can be measured in amniotic fluid. Such analyses include measurement of α-fetoprotein and acetylcholinesterase in the evaluation of neural tube defects and 17-OH progesterone in congenital adrenal hyperplasia.

No risk to the unborn fetus has been recognized as a complication of ultrasonography. Midtrimester amniocentesis (15 to 20 weeks' gestation) is associated with a less than 0.5 per cent risk of miscarriage incident to the procedure. Direct trauma to the fetus is very rare in experienced hands, and other risks such as respiratory difficulties, hip dislocation, and club foot are controversial. CVS (9 to 11 weeks' gestation) has a slightly higher risk than amniocentesis, estimated at about 2 per cent or less. Both the transcervical and the transabdominal approaches are being used, and the procedures continue to be critically evaluated. The timing of both amniocentesis and CVS is also being studied, with later CVS and earlier amniocentesis as possibilities.

Fetoscopy is infrequently performed and normally is done only when other diagnostic avenues have failed. It can be used to visualize fetal anatomy and to obtain fetal blood samples, for example to confirm a chromosomal or biochemical diagnosis. Occasionally biopsy of fetal tissues such as liver or skin can be performed to look for a specific condition.

Prenatal diagnosis performed for a pregnancy determined to

TABLE 35–3. INDICATIONS FOR PRENATAL DIAGNOSIS

Advanced parental age (usually maternal)
Family history of inherited disease
Risk of chromosome disorder
   Previous child with chromosomal abnormality
   Parent with known chromosomal translocation
Heterozygote screening based on ethnicity
   Tay-Sachs (Ashkenazi Jews; French Canadians)
   Thalassemias (Mediterraneans, Arabs, Indo-Pakistanis)
   Sickle cell anemia (Blacks, Mediterraneans, Arabs, Indo-Pakistanis, Turks, Southeast Asians)
Pregnancy screening
   Maternal serum α-fetoprotein

TABLE 35–4. CONDITIONS THAT HAVE BEEN DIAGNOSED PRENATALLY*

Disorder	Diagnostic Method
All defined chromosomal disorders	Cytogenetic analysis
Adrenoleukodystrophy	DNA and long-chain fatty acid
Cystinosis	Cystine uptake
Cystic fibrosis	DNA analysis
Duchenne muscular dystrophy	DNA analysis
Ectodermal dysplasia	Fetoscopy, skin biopsy
Fabry disease	α-Galactosidase A
Gaucher disease	β-Glucosidase
GM$_2$-gangliosidosis I (Tay-Sachs)	Hexosaminidase A
Hemoglobinopathies	DNA analysis
Hemophilia A	DNA analysis
Metachromatic leukodystrophy	Aryl-sulfatase A
Mucopolysaccharidosis I (Hurler)	α-L-Iduronidase
Neural tube defects	α-Fetoprotein, ultrasonography, amniotic fluid acetylcholinesterase
Omphalocele	α-Fetoprotein, ultrasonography
Osteogenesis imperfecta	Ultrasonography
Phenylketonuria	DNA analysis

*See Milunsky for more information.

be at risk following heterozygote or pregnancy screening tests is specific to the disorder being sought. Tay-Sachs disease and the hemoglobinopathies are the major examples of heterozygote states being identified in at-risk populations. Since the gene for cystic fibrosis has been mapped and the mutation associated with about 70 per cent of the cases identified, there has been much discussion of population screening for that gene. At present, the limitations in identifying the other mutations have made population screening difficult. However, in a family that already has an individual affected with cystic fibrosis, prenatal diagnosis can be done using DNA-based analysis of fetal cells. Table 35–4 lists some conditions that can be diagnosed prenatally.

Pregnancy screening, usually done by measuring α-fetoprotein in maternal serum, identifies fetuses at risk for open body wall defects, including spina bifida, anencephaly, omphalocele, and gastroschisis. More specific diagnosis is usually attempted using fetal imaging and measurement of proteins such as α-fetoprotein and acetylcholinesterase in amniotic fluid. Recent studies have suggested that maternal serum α-fetoprotein concentration is low in a percentage of pregnancies in which the fetus has trisomy 21. The biologic explanation for this observation is lacking, but the association has allowed refinement of the risk assessment for fetal aneuploidy based on maternal age and maternal serum α-fetoprotein concentration, and amniocentesis can be offered to the woman whose new risk assessment warrants it.

It is of utmost importance that the pregnant woman for whom prenatal diagnosis is performed be given extremely clear counseling. Spelling out the expectations and limitations of the testing prior to any procedures is critical. The diagnoses that are being sought must be explained. It is very easy for the woman to conclude that a normal test result shows that the baby will be "normal," when in fact only a short list of pathologic conditions has been excluded. Normalcy is never completely assured. It is helpful to point out that a condition or conditions have been sought for which the patient had a risk higher than that of the general population. The result after these conditions have been excluded is that the pregnancy stands at the same risk for many other potential problems as others in the general population.

Much more difficult is the situation in which the result of the test is not normal. Although it is best that this possibility be discussed beforehand and the options considered, it is no longer considered necessary that the woman make a decision prior to learning the test results. The implications of the diagnosis must be reviewed with care, sensitivity, and accuracy. The options for the woman are to terminate the pregnancy or to carry it to term. The decision to terminate must be made in collaboration with the obstetrician who will perform the procedure so that the process can be described and possible complications reviewed. The choice of procedure depends on the stage of pregnancy, and the complications are specific to the particular procedure. In general, a second-trimester termination is a more complicated procedure than a first-trimester termination. Psychosocial support after the procedure is crucial. Most families who elect to terminate a pregnancy go through a period of grieving for the loss of the hoped-for normal child. Many such pregnancies were planned and wanted. The family should be offered the chance to visit with the genetic counselor to discuss their normal feelings of sadness and loss and to join a support group if one is available. There is no evidence for long-term psychological sequelae of genetic pregnancy termination.

Thoughtful genetic counseling challenges the skills of the physician in diagnosis, analysis, communication, and support. Rarely is it the province of only one person, but rather it requires the collaborative efforts of an experienced team. From the initial evaluation through the development of the genetic model and identification of those at risk to the completion of the transfer of information, the use of these skills serves to enable patients and their families to make intelligent, informed, and reasoned decisions for their futures.

Collins FS, Gelehrter TD: Principles of Medical Genetics. Baltimore, Williams & Wilkins, 1989. *A new and good general human genetics textbook, up-to-date in molecular material.*

Frets P, Duivenvoorden H, et al.: Factors influencing the reproductive decision after genetic counseling. Am J Med Genet 35:496–502, 503–509, 1990. *Others in the series of articles on the psychodynamics of genetic counseling.*

Hsia YE, Silverberg R, et al.: Counseling in Genetics. New York, Alan R. Liss, 1979. *Thorough discussion of all aspects of genetic counseling by several very experienced geneticists and counselors.*

Lippman-Hand A, Fraser F-C: Genetic counseling—the post-counseling period. II. Making reproductive choices. Am J Med Genet 4:73, 1979. *The third in a series of articles on the psychodynamics of genetic counseling.*

McKusick V: Mendelian Inheritance in Man. 9th ed. Baltimore, Johns Hopkins University Press, 1990. *Exhaustive catalog of mendelian phenotypes.*

Milunsky A: Genetic Disorders and the Fetus: Diagnosis, Prevention and Treatment. 2nd ed. New York, Plenum Press, 1986. *Extensive textbook on prenatal diagnosis.*

Weatherall DG: The New Genetics and Clinical Practice. Oxford, Oxford University Press, 1985. *Details about modern methods of molecular diagnosis of genetic disorders.*

36 Approach to the Patient with Cardiovascular Disease

Thomas W. Smith

Common to the care of all patients with cardiovascular disease is a data base on which sound diagnostic and therapeutic decisions can be made. This chapter outlines an approach to cardiovascular data collection that emphasizes general principles and strategies and is intended to complement the more specific consideration of disease entities in the chapters that follow. One of the endlessly fascinating aspects of medicine is that each patient presents to the physician a unique story of his or her past history and present illness. Textbook descriptions of disease therefore convey at best a set of findings that the author regards as typical but that never quite fit in detail the findings present in any one individual patient. Hence, an open mind is essential during the evaluation of each patient so that diagnostic possibilities are not overlooked or prematurely discarded.

A dazzling array of diagnostic tests is now available for the evaluation of patients with evident or suspected cardiovascular disease. Sensitivity and specificity are known, or can be estimated, for each method under a given set of clinical circumstances. Redundancy must be avoided to achieve a favorable cost:benefit ratio (e.g., radionuclide ventriculography often yields information regarding ventricular function that can be obtained from a two-dimensional echocardiogram, and both methods may be superfluous if the patient undergoes left ventriculography as part of a cardiac catheterization procedure). The emerging discipline of decision analysis (see Ch. 20), with emphasis on the proper application of Bayes' theorem, should help in formulating strategies for the development of an adequate cardiovascular data base.

Although accurate diagnosis is a key element in patient care, prognosis is also vitally important to the patient and often to the physician, who must formulate a program of treatment. Information over and above that needed to establish a diagnosis is typically required to allow an accurate prediction of outcome. This exercise in probability statistics is challenging and deserves careful attention as an essential component of the comprehensive care of the patient.

COMPONENTS OF THE CARDIOVASCULAR WORKUP

The three essential components of the clinical data base are the history, physical examination, and laboratory studies. Although this sequence of data acquisition is typically followed, the value of returning to the bedside (often repeatedly) to refine the assessment of historical information and physical findings as the workup progresses cannot be overstated.

History

The cardinal symptoms of cardiovascular disease are listed in Table 36–1. *Dyspnea* (an abnormally uncomfortable awareness of breathing) and the related items in the first line are discussed in detail in Ch. 40. Historical information is particularly important in distinguishing among heart failure, pulmonary disease (including pulmonary emboli), metabolic disturbances producing aci-

dosis, and anxiety as factors causing dyspnea. The nature of onset and duration of symptoms, relation to position, and precipitating and alleviating factors all provide important clues to the underlying pathophysiologic process.

Fatigue and *weakness* are common to many physical and emotional disease states and are nonspecific; nevertheless, it is important to record quantitative information in the history (e.g., flights of stairs or distance on level ground that the patient can manage) for current and future reference. *Cough*, initially dry and irritative, is a common early manifestation of elevated left-heart filling (and hence pulmonary venous) pressures. *Hemoptysis* should be characterized in regard to color and nature of admixture of blood and sputum to help distinguish between pulmonary (e.g., bronchitis, pulmonary infarction) and cardiac causes (e.g., pulmonary edema, hemorrhage from loss of bronchial vein integrity, as in mitral stenosis). *Cyanosis* is discussed in Ch. 40.

Chest pain or discomfort should be characterized in terms of location, quality, course of onset and offset, duration, and precipitating and alleviating factors. Pain due to ischemic heart disease is considered in Ch. 48, but one should remember that the original meaning of the term angina is *choking* rather than pain, and it is often described by the patient with words such as "pressure" or "squeezing" discomfort. Pericardial pain is more likely to be left sided, sharp in character, and related to breathing and position. Pleuritic pain also tends to be localized and sharp and is related to breathing or coughing. Chest wall pain is often long lasting and associated with tenderness to pressure applied at the trigger area.

Palpitation refers to an awareness of the heart beat, usually occurring in response to a change in cardiac rhythm or rate or by increased contractile force. It is a common anxiety-related symptom in patients without heart disease. Awareness of irregularity of the heart beat is more closely correlated with cardiac rhythm disturbances. *Dizziness* and *syncope* are frequent manifestations of cardiac arrhythmias and demand careful evaluation, often with 24-hour electrocardiographic (ECG) monitoring. These symptoms also occur as a consequence of orthostatic hypotension due to reduced blood volume, vasodilator drugs, or autonomic dysfunction. Obstruction to venous return from any cause also predisposes to these symptoms. *Claudication* refers to pain or an uncomfortable sensation of tiredness, usually in calf and/or thigh muscles, that occurs in response to exertion and is relieved by rest. This common symptom of peripheral arterial insufficiency is further discussed in Ch. 54.

TABLE 36–1. CARDINAL SYMPTOMS OF CARDIOVASCULAR DISEASE

Dyspnea, orthopnea, paroxysmal nocturnal dyspnea, wheezing
Fatigue, weakness
Cough, hemoptysis
Cyanosis
Chest pain or discomfort
Palpitations, dizziness, syncope
Edema
Pain in extremities with exertion (claudication)

Edema refers to swelling, usually of a dependent part of the body, due to retention of excess fluid. It is typically maximal in the feet at the end of the day and resolves, at least partially, by morning. Local factors such as deep venous disease predispose to unilateral edema. Patients confined to bed usually accumulate fluid in the sacral area.

The Physical Examination

Five elements constitute the cardiovascular physical examination. These are

1. Physical appearance
2. Venous pressure and pulse contours
3. Arterial pressure and pulse contours
4. Movement of the heart
5. Auscultation

PHYSICAL APPEARANCE. This is important in assessing the nature and severity of heart disease and also in providing clues to systemic diseases that affect the heart. Important cardiac problems are frequently encountered in patients with Marfan's syndrome, Turner's syndrome, Down's syndrome, the pickwickian syndrome, scleroderma, and thyroid disease, all of which are often recognizable on the basis of careful inspection of the patient's appearance. The funduscopic examination yields important information with regard to hypertension, diabetes mellitus, and sometimes infective endocarditis (Roth's spots). Cheyne-Stokes respirations are often seen in patients with advanced heart failure. Sometimes a highly specific cardiac diagnosis can be made on the basis of the physical appearance, such as the association of atrial septal defect with the bony abnormalities of the upper extremity that constitute the Holt-Oram syndrome. Cyanosis and clubbing of the fingertips indicate right-to-left shunting in patients with congenital heart disease.

VENOUS PRESSURE AND PULSE. Both external and internal jugular veins require careful inspection: external for estimation of mean right atrial pressure and internal for wave form as well as pressure. Figure 36–1 illustrates the typical features of the normal jugular venous pulse and indicates the terminology applied to the various aspects of this wave form. The A wave reflects right atrial contraction and occurs immediately prior to the carotid arterial pulse and first heart sound. The X descent occurs with right atrial relaxation and continues with early right ventricular contraction. The C wave, often superimposed on the beginning of the A wave, coincides with the carotid pulse itself.

The V wave in the normal jugular venous pulse represents passive right atrial filling behind a closed and competent tricuspid valve. The Y descent reflects sudden termination of the V wave with right ventricular relaxation and opening of the tricuspid valve. The X descent is normally the more evident of the two declining phases of the jugular venous pulse. These phenomena are best noted with the patient so positioned that the top of the venous column can be observed throughout the cardiac cycle. Estimation of the central venous pressure is accomplished by estimating its height in centimeters above the sternal angle of Louis, adding 5 cm to allow for the normal relation of the right atrium to the external chest wall. Normal venous pressure varies from 5 to 10 cm of H_2O. The A wave tends to be accentuated in disease states characterized by reduced right ventricular compliance, tricuspid stenosis, or rhythm disturbances in which the atrium contracts against a closed tricuspid valve ("cannon" A waves). Tricuspid insufficiency produces systolic or regurgitant waves that obliterate the normal jugular venous V waves. Abnormalities associated with pericardial disease are discussed in Ch. 51.

ARTERIAL PRESSURE AND PULSE. Examination of the arterial pulse yields critically important information regarding the cardiovascular system. Arterial pressure should always be measured in both arms because of the unexpected discrepancies that are encountered in disease states or that are occasionally due to congenital anomalies. Use of a cuff of appropriate size is essential, and the arterial blood pressure should be recorded in both supine and standing position to assess volume status and the adequacy of reflex vasoconstrictor responses. Pulsus paradoxus refers to a decrease in systolic blood pressure of greater than 10 mm Hg on inspiration and is a typical feature of pericardial tamponade.

The carotid arteries provide the most direct reflection of cardiac activity because of their central location in proximity to the left ventricle and aorta. The amplitude of the carotid pulse is typically increased under circumstances associated with higher cardiac output, including fever, anemia, hyperthyroidism, and arteriovenous fistulas. The regularity (or lack thereof) indicates disturbances of rhythm or hemodynamics as in pulsus alternans. The wave form of the arterial pulse yields clues regarding runoff from the aorta, as in aortic insufficiency or arteriovenous fistula; a bisferious quality is often present in aortic insufficiency and should be distinguished from the spike-and-dome contour encountered in patients with hypertrophic cardiomyopathy with obstruction (i.e., hypertrophic subaortic stenosis). The volume of the carotid pulse is typically reduced in heart failure and in mitral or aortic stenosis. Peripheral arterial pulses other than the carotid pulses should be felt and compared, with particular attention to a pulse delay at the femoral artery as a manifestation of coarctation of the aorta. Patients with claudication should have their lower extremity pulses examined both at rest and with exercise, since the latter maneuver often accentuates asymmetries.

MOVEMENT OF THE HEART. Observation, palpation, and percussion are the traditional means for physical examination of cardiac movements. Inspection of the precordium reveals asymmetries that serve as clues to chronic cardiac hypertrophy, particularly in congenital disease. The partial left lateral decubitus position is optimal for observation as well as palpation of the left ventricle in most patients. Diffuse left parasternal cardiac movement is often best appreciated with the heel of the palm, whereas higher frequency events (S_1, ejection clicks, S_2, opening snap, and thrills) are best felt with firm pressure and the tactile use of the fingertips. Precordial movements should be described at the apex, left parasternal area, and the right and left second intercostal spaces. The normal tapping impulse of the left ventricular apex is replaced by a more diffuse and sometimes dyskinetic impulse in patients with cardiac enlargement from a variety of causes. Displacement of the left ventricle is typically downward and to the left with cardiomegaly. Systolic overload with concentric hypertrophy increases the duration of the apex impulse and can be distinguished from the hyperdynamic impulse accompanying volume overload lesions, such as mitral or aortic insufficiency. Right ventricular enlargement produces a left parasternal systolic lift that is occasionally mimicked by the anterior motion of the heart with systolic expansion of the left atrium in the presence of severe mitral insufficiency. Pulmonary hypertension may be accompanied by a palpable pulmonary artery segment in the second left interspace and by a palpable pulmonic component

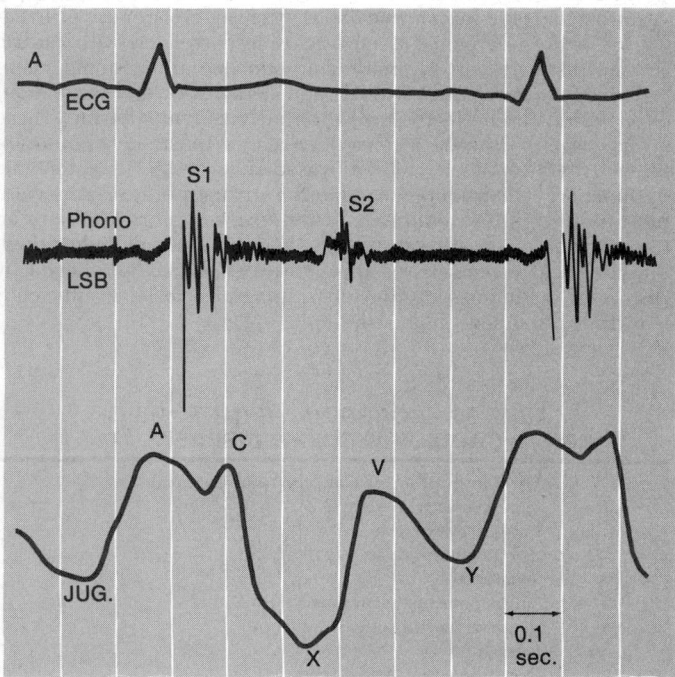

FIGURE 36–1. Normal jugular venous pulse.

of the second sound (P_2). Prominent third or fourth heart sounds can often be palpated as well as heard.

Thus, with the data gleaned from physical appearance, the venous and arterial pulse characteristics, and cardiac motion properties, the experienced clinician is armed with substantial information about cardiac anatomy and physiology before employing the stethoscope.

AUSCULTATION. Satisfactory cardiac auscultation requires a stethoscope that fits the ears snugly but comfortably and has the shortest tubing consistent with convenient use. The examination should be carried out in a quiet area, which sometimes requires moving the patient to a more suitable place when ambient noise levels are excessive. A systematic approach, as in all facets of physical examination, is important. Apart from the most obvious and dramatic auscultatory events, one generally hears only what one listens for. Beginning at the apex, the timing and nature of the first and second heart sounds are determined. Separable components of these events should be carefully noted. If the first sound has more that one component, S_4, asynchronous closure of mitral and tricuspid valves, and ejection clicks must be distinguished. Higher frequency transient systolic and diastolic sounds are listed in Table 36–2 and should be listened for explicitly. Murmurs should be identified and characterized, using the diaphragm to distinguish high-frequency events and the bell for lower frequency sounds. The examination should include listening with the patient sitting and leaning forward, supine, and in the left lateral decubitus position. Position may have a particularly marked effect on the character and loudness of pericardial friction rubs. Standing, exercising, isometric handgrip, and the Valsalva maneuver are important in specific circumstances, as outlined in the chapters that follow.

The plethora of sophisticated laboratory examinations now available should refine, rather than render obsolete, physical diagnostic skills. Every opportunity should be taken to review physical findings with the additional insights provided by noninvasive and invasive laboratory studies.

Laboratory Studies

Laboratory studies of patients with cardiovascular disease run the gamut from routine examinations (chest radiograph, electrocardiogram) that should be performed on virtually every patient being evaluated to highly sophisticated techniques that would be appropriate for specific individual subsets of patients. Remarkable progress in the past decade in noninvasive techniques now permits adequate evaluation of many patients without need for cardiac catheterization. Nevertheless, catheterization and angiography are essential components of the cardiovascular workup in most patients with advanced valvular or coronary artery disease.

ELECTROCARDIOGRAM. The standard 12-lead electrocardiogram remains a cornerstone of the clinical cardiologic evaluation. Although vectorcardiography and other more sophisticated approaches have their proponents, the standard 12-lead ECG remains a highly cost-effective screening test. It is reviewed in detail in Ch. 39.4. Detailed clinicopathologic correlations accumulated over more than two generations provide a wealth of background information. The most important applications are in assessment of cardiac arrhythmias, in which analysis of the P wave and the QRS complex, and their temporal relation to each other, forms the basis for the definition and clinical diagnosis of rhythm disturbances. Existence and location of myocardial ischemia and infarction represent other important components of the information inherent in the ECG. Right and left ventricular hypertrophy patterns, as well as right and left atrial abnormalities, are well described. Characteristic electrocardiographic findings are frequently important in the assessment of congenital heart disease.

The 12-lead electrocardiogram augmented with a standard exercise protocol is important in the assessment of ischemic heart disease (see Ch. 48.1). Both establishment of coronary artery obstructive disease and useful prognostic information are available from this study. Risk stratification in patients who have had myocardial infarctions is heavily dependent upon the exercise ECG. The predictive accuracy of the exercise ECG examination for coronary artery disease in specific patient subsets is well defined. It is important not only to classify ST-segment depression but also to assess duration of exercise, maximum heart rate achieved, blood pressure response, time of onset of ST-segment depression, and time of resolution. A decrease in blood pressure during exercise correlates closely with advanced three-vessel or left main coronary artery obstructive disease. As in all such examinations, the diagnostic and predictive accuracy is dependent on the population of patients studied, and false-positive exercise ECG results are relatively commonly encountered in women, especially from populations with a low predicted incidence of obstructive coronary artery disease.

Assessment of symptoms of palpitations, dizziness, and syncope now rests heavily on the 24-hour (Holter) ECG. This approach is essential in the evaluation of cardiac arrhythmias and of response to antiarrhythmic drug regimens. Recent technical advances permit the assessment of transient ST-segment and T-wave changes reflecting myocardial ischemia, findings of particular value in the assessment of patients with variable threshold or "silent" ischemia.

CHEST RADIOGRAPHY. Posteroanterior and lateral views are a component of virtually every cardiovascular evaluation. Important findings are reviewed in Ch. 39.1. Chest radiography always supplements, rather than replaces, physical examination, since the two approaches yield complementary information. Echocardiography yields more accurate and specific information regarding individual chamber sizes. Evidence of calcification of cardiac structures should be sought on the chest radiograph, although fluoroscopic examination and echocardiography both tend to be more sensitive for this purpose.

ECHOCARDIOGRAPHY. This noninvasive technique uses high-frequency sound waves that reflect from cardiac structures, permitting the imaging of cardiac anatomy and motion. The technique is considered in detail in Ch. 39.3. Two-dimensional echocardiography has largely replaced the M-mode display, although the latter provides superior quantitative details regarding wall thickness and chamber dimensions. This examination is now standard in the assessment of ventricular function and valvular abnormalities.

The Doppler method is the standard technique for assessment of intracardiac blood flow, shunts, and valvular stenosis and regurgitation. In selected patients, echocardiographic information, together with full clinical assessment, permits valvular surgery without prior cardiac catheterization. Echocardiography is diagnostic in cases of left atrial myxoma, mitral valve prolapse, and hypertrophic cardiomyopathy. It is frequently useful for visualization of vegetations on heart valves in patients with infective endocarditis. Pericardial fluid and tamponade are routinely assessed by echocardiography, which is also useful in guiding pericardiocentesis.

Transesophageal echocardiography is available in most referral centers and gives particularly high-resolution images of the heart and proximal great vessels.

TABLE 36–2. SYSTOLIC AND DIASTOLIC SOUNDS

Systolic
  Early
    Ejection sounds (aortic, pulmonary)
    Systolic ejection clicks (mitral apparatus)
    Opening click of aortic valve mechanical prosthesis
  Mid to late
    Mitral valve clicks (prolapse)

Diastolic
  Early
    Opening snaps
    Early third sound of pericardial constriction or mitral regurgitation
    Opening click of mitral valve mechanical prosthesis
    "Tumor plop" of atrial myxoma
  Mid
    Third heart sound or gallop (S_3)
    Summation gallop ($S_3 + S_4$)
    Pericardial knock
  Late (presystolic)
    Fourth heart sound (S_4)

High-resolution B-mode ultrasonography with color Doppler imaging is of substantial value in the noninvasive diagnosis of both peripheral arterial (including carotid) and venous disease.

RADIONUCLIDE STUDIES. These tests involve injection of radioisotopes into the circulation with detection by special instrumentation. One of the most useful of these techniques is radionuclide ventriculography, also referred to as gated blood pool scanning. Technetium 99m (^{99m}Tc) bound to albumin stays in the blood pool and permits imaging of the size and contractile function of cardiac chambers. Special applications include detection of intracardiac shunts by "first pass" methods. Most commonly, the technique is used to assess left and right ventricular function by measurement of end-systolic and end-diastolic dimensions, permitting evaluation of regional wall motion and the derivation of values for right and left ventricular ejection fractions.

Scanning with radioactive thallium (^{201}Tl) permits assessment of myocardial perfusion. The radioisotope is injected at maximum exercise and localizes in cardiac muscle as a function of coronary flow; areas of diminished myocardial perfusion are visualized as "cold" spots on the myocardial image. Viable but ischemic myocardium subsequently fills in with more homogeneous ^{201}Tl distribution, whereas previous infarction produces a persistent cold spot.

Scanning with ^{99m}Tc pyrophosphate can be used to visualize areas of myocardial necrosis and is occasionally useful in evaluation of patients with suspected myocardial infarction when other studies are equivocal.

CLINICAL APPLICATION. The safety of noninvasive techniques tempts the clinician to overutilize them, since no physical harm is likely to result and some incremental information is often obtained. Cost-effectiveness considerations must be kept in mind, however, and the use of these tests must be orchestrated so that the essential clinical decisions can be made without unnecessary cost and inconvenience to the patient. Some elements of noninvasive test information are superfluous if the patient is destined to undergo complete evaluation by cardiac catheterization and angiography. Newer noninvasive techniques including fast computed tomographic (CT) scanning and magnetic resonance imaging (MRI) need to be incorporated into cost-effective diagnostic strategies as these methods become more widely available.

CARDIAC CATHETERIZATION. This invasive approach provides information on intracardiac and vascular pressures and flows. Gradients across stenotic valves and great vessels can be measured and systemic and pulmonary blood flows quantified. Contrast agents can be injected selectively to define the anatomy of cardiac chambers, coronary vessels, and pulmonary and peripheral vessels. The technique of cardiac catheterization and angiography is considered in detail in Ch. 39.5. This diagnostic approach is usually employed when a cardiac surgical or catheter-based interventional procedure is under consideration.

Other applications of cardiac catheterization include electrophysiologic studies with pacing and mapping procedures to evoke and localize the source of cardiac rhythm disturbances. Endomyocardial biopsy is a standard technique for the assessment of transplant rejection, unexplained cardiomyopathy, suspected myocarditis, suspected infiltrative diseases such as cardiac amyloidosis, or doxorubicin cardiotoxicity.

Cardiac catheterization procedures form the basis for therapeutic interventions, including percutaneous transluminal coronary angioplasty, or ablative procedures, such as those for the management of patients with Wolff-Parkinson-White syndrome refractory to drug therapy.

Although cardiac catheterization involves substantial expense and a small but finite risk of morbidity and mortality, this approach remains indispensable in the assessment of a wide array of cardiac problems that remain unsolved after complete noninvasive assessment. A frequent problem is the adult patient with a chest pain syndrome consistent with angina pectoris but with a negative or equivocal exercise electrocardiogram. Such patients may be severely disabled by these symptoms and attendant anxiety. Even though coronary artery surgery may not loom as a likely therapeutic approach, coronary arteriography can be of substantial value, especially when normal coronary anatomy is found, directing the diagnostic evaluation in more productive directions and restoring a previously incapacitated patient to full activity.

TABLE 36–3. A COMPARISON OF THREE METHODS OF ASSESSING CARDIOVASCULAR DISABILITY

Class	New York Heart Association Functional Classification	Canadian Cardiovascular Society Functional Classification	Specific Activity Scale
I	Patients with cardiac disease but without resulting limitations of physical activity. Ordinary physical activity does not cause undue fatigue, palpitation, dyspnea, or anginal pain.	Ordinary physical activity, such as walking and climbing stairs, does not cause angina. Angina with strenuous or rapid or prolonged exertion at work or recreation.	Patients can perform to completion any activity requiring ≥7 metabolic equivalents, e.g., can carry 24 lb up eight steps; carry objects that weigh 80 lb; do outdoor work (shovel snow, spade soil); do recreational activities (skiing, basketball, squash, handball, jog/walk 5 mph).
II	Patients with cardiac disease resulting in slight limitation of physical activity. They are comfortable at rest. Ordinary physical activity results in fatigue, palpitation, dyspnea, or anginal pain.	Slight limitation of ordinary activity. Walking or climbing stairs rapidly, walking uphill, walking or stair climbing after meals, in cold, in wind, or when under emotional stress, or only during the few hours after awakening. Walking more than two blocks on the level and climbing more than one flight of ordinary stairs at a normal pace and in normal conditions.	Patient can perform to completion any activity requiring ≥5 metabolic equivalents but cannot and does not perform to completion activities requiring ≥7 metabolic equivalents, e.g., have sexual intercourse without stopping, garden, rake, weed, roller skate, dance fox trot, walk at 4 mph on level ground.
III	Patients with cardiac disease resulting in marked limitation of physical activity. They are comfortable at rest. Less than ordinary physical activity causes fatigue, palpitation, dyspnea, or anginal pain.	Marked limitation of ordinary physical activity. Walking one to two blocks on the level and climbing more than one flight in normal conditions.	Patient can perform to completion any activity requiring ≥2 metabolic equivalents but cannot and does not perform to completion any activities requiring ≥5 metabolic equivalents, e.g., shower without stopping, strip and make bed, clean windows, walk 2.5 mph, bowl, play golf, dress without stopping.
IV	Patient with cardiac disease resulting in inability to carry on any physical activity without discomfort. Symptoms of cardiac insufficiency or of the anginal syndrome may be present even at rest. If any physical activity is undertaken, discomfort is increased.	Inability to carry on any physical activity without discomfort—anginal syndrome *may be* present at rest.	Patient cannot or does not perform to completion activities requiring ≥2 metabolic equivalents. *Cannot* carry out activities listed above (Specific Activity Scale, Class III).

Reproduced by permission of the American Heart Association, Inc., from Goldman L, et al.: Comparative reproducibility and validity of systems for assessing cardiovascular functional class: Advantages of a new specific activity scale. Circulation 64:1227, 1981.

ELEMENTS OF A COMPLETE CARDIOVASCULAR DIAGNOSIS

Coordinated use of the history, physical examination, and laboratory studies permits a full diagnosis to be established in nearly all patients, including the following five elements:

1. Etiology of the cardiovascular problem
2. Anatomic abnormalities, including quantification to the extent possible
3. Physiologic status, including pressures, flows, and relevant gradients
4. Functional capacity (see Table 36–3)
5. Prognosis

Diagnostic Strategies

The most appropriate approach to a patient with suspected cardiovascular disease depends on the age and clinical presentation of the patient. A systolic ejection murmur at the base in a healthy teenager with an otherwise normal clinical evaluation, including ECG and chest radiograph, should ordinarily constitute adequate grounds for reassurance and avoidance of more elaborate studies. In an elderly patient with a systolic ejection murmur at the base, slow-rising carotid arterial pulses, and symptoms suggesting possible aortic stenosis, however, the chest radiograph, electrocardiogram, and echocardiogram with Doppler study are necessary, at a minimum, to determine whether further and more aggressive evaluation is warranted.

Since prevention is a highly desirable goal in cardiovascular medicine, certain diagnostic tests may be warranted in individual patients even in the absence of specific symptoms. In addition to careful history and physical examination, serum cholesterol measurements are appropriate in most patients, especially those with a family history of coronary artery disease, to assess risk and to guide therapeutic intervention. Use of exercise electrocardiography in sedentary, middle-aged individuals who are contemplating an exercise program remains controversial; many physicians would advocate this procedure, especially if the patient has risk factors for coronary artery disease.

There is no simple formula for defining the data base that is adequate for clearance of patients for noncardiac surgery. A simple, informal stress test of walking up one or more flights of stairs to observe the presence or absence of dyspnea or chest discomfort often obviates the need for more expensive and elaborate formal exercise testing. When extensive procedures such as peripheral vascular surgery or abdominal aortic aneurysm resection are contemplated in older patients with known or suspected coronary artery disease, aggressive diagnostic workup, sometimes including cardiac catheterization and coronary arteriography, may be necessary because of limitations imposed by vascular disease on exercise electrocardiography or other approaches to assessment of cardiac reserve requiring exercise stress.

Perloff JK: Physical Examination of the Heart and Circulation. 2nd ed. Philadelphia, W. B. Saunders Company, 1990. *A pocket-sized compendium of up-to-date information, well illustrated and referenced.*

37 Epidemiology of Cardiovascular Disease

William T. Friedewald

Cardiovascular diseases have been the major health problem and the leading cause of death in the United States for several decades. The various statistics defining the magnitude of the problem are staggering. Estimates suggest that over 60 million people have some form of cardiovascular disease. In 1987, 977,000 people died of cardiovascular disease, which accounted for 46.0 per cent of all deaths. This problem also ranks as the leading reason for social security disability, limitation in physical activity, and hospital bed use, accounting for 46 million bed days in 1984. In 1986 it was estimated that cardiovascular diseases carried a direct health expenditure cost of $62 billion and additional indirect costs of $65 billion.

COMPONENTS OF CARDIOVASCULAR DISEASE

Cardiovascular disease is a general diagnostic category consisting of several separate diseases. One component, congenital heart disease, occurs at a rate of approximately 7 per 1000 live births, leading in 1986 to 5800 deaths, 3300 of which occurred before the age of 1 year. Another component, rheumatic heart disease, has had a dramatic 90 per cent decline over the last 40 years in the age-adjusted death rate (Table 37–1). Although 1.9 million people still have the disease, with approximately 6300 deaths in 1987, it has become a minor contributor to the overall cardiovascular disease problem. Coronary heart disease and cerebrovascular disease continue to be the major components of cardiovascular disease. Each year an estimated 1.25 million heart attacks occur (of which 800,000 are first attacks), leading to 512,000 deaths in 1987. Eight and one-half per cent of men and 3.7 per cent of women aged 45 to 64 years have overt coronary heart disease, and over the age of 65, these percentages increase to 17.8 in men and 12.0 in women. Cerebrovascular disease is found in 2.0 per cent of men (1.8 per cent of women) between the ages of 45 and 64 and 6.3 per cent of men (5.5 per cent of women) aged 65 and older, with 150,000 deaths due to this cause in 1987.

CARDIOVASCULAR DISEASE MORTALITY

These diseases have not always been the major health problem of the United States. In 1900 the five leading causes of death were (1) pneumonia and influenza combined, (2) tuberculosis, (3) diarrhea, enteritis, and ulceration of the intestines, (4) diseases of the heart, and (5) intracranial lesions of vascular origin. These categories all had rates greater than 100 per 100,000 population. By 1940, only two disease categories still had rates greater than 100 per 100,000: diseases of the heart and cancer and other malignant tumors. The infectious diseases had, to a large extent, been controlled, and their mortality rates have continued to fall. The "epidemic" of cardiovascular disease, especially coronary heart disease, had begun. By 1963, the mortality rate from coronary heart disease reached a peak; there has been a progressive and steady decline since then (Fig. 37–1). Despite the continued magnitude of the coronary heart disease problem, the focus recently has been on this dramatic reversal. Not only is the percentage of decline large, but also the impact on the total number of deaths in the United States is large and has led to an increase in life expectancy. In fact, the recent rate of improvement in life expectancy compares with that seen in the 1940's,

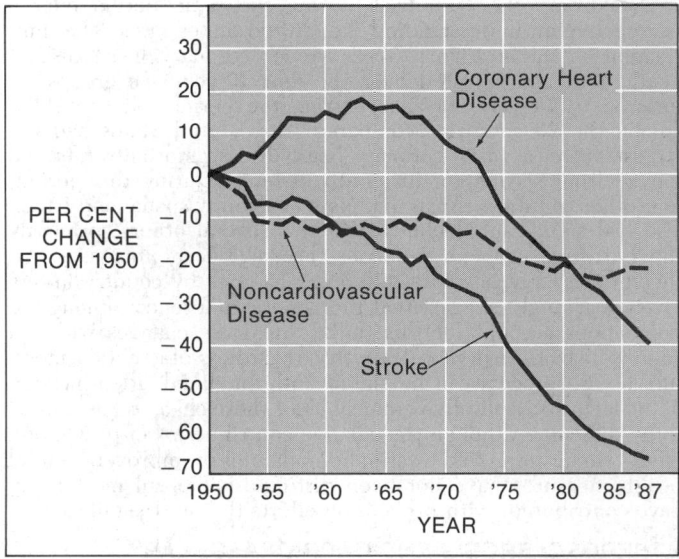

FIGURE 37–1. Per cent change in age-adjusted death rates in the United States, 1950 to 1987. (Source: Vital Statistics of the United States, National Center for Health Statistics.)

TABLE 37–1. AGE-ADJUSTED DEATH RATES* FOR MAJOR CARDIOVASCULAR DISEASES AND ALL OTHER CAUSES OF DEATH COMBINED IN THE UNITED STATES, 1905 TO 1987

Year	All Causes	All Causes Except Cardiovascular Diseases	Cardiovascular Diseases			
			Total	Coronary Heart Disease	Cerebrovascular Disease	Rheumatic Heart Disease
1905	1673.5	1315.9	357.6	NA	134.4	NA
1915	1443.4	1072.6	370.8	NA	123.3	NA
1925	1299.9	920.5	379.4	NA	114.2	NA
1935	1165.8	777.9	387.9	NA	94.4	NA
1945	947.4	556.9	390.5	NA	85.4	18.4
1955	764.6	368.5	396.1	200.0	83.0	11.2
1960	760.9	367.4	393.5	214.6	79.7	9.6
1965	739.0	364.8	374.2	215.8	72.7	7.4
1970	714.3	368.0	346.3	200.4†	66.3	6.3
1975	630.4	337.0	293.4	170.1†	53.7	4.8
1980	585.8	325.4	260.4	149.8	40.8	2.6
1985	546.1	318.5	227.6	125.5	32.3	1.9
1987	536.2	321.8	214.4	114.0	30.1	1.7

*Rate per 100,000 population age adjusted to the United States population, 1940.
†Comparability ratio applied to convert rate to level comparable to rates for 1980 and 1987.
NA = Not available.

when tuberculosis and other infectious diseases were being controlled. In 1987 a 45-year-old person could, on the average, expect to live 3.3 years longer than would have been expected in 1965. Estimates suggest that 45 per cent of this declining total mortality rate is due to the decline in coronary heart disease. The decline in death due to cerebrovascular disease, although even more impressive with a 66 per cent decrease since 1950, has been less of a contributing factor because cerebrovascular disease is less prevalent.

Declines in coronary heart disease mortality have been greater in young adults, but there has been a remarkable uniformity among blacks and whites and among men and women. Despite some early doubts when the reversal in rates was beginning, this decline in coronary mortality is real and not artifactual. It cannot be explained by (1) problems in trend measurement, such as a shift in classifying deaths as due to some other disease, (2) the waning of periodic respiratory epidemics that can contribute to the deaths of many patients with coronary heart disease, or (3) the depletion of the pool due to other causes of death in people expected to be susceptible to coronary heart disease. In addition, the decline has been too steep and long lasting to be reasonably explained by a simple random, temporary downturn. Determining precisely when the true decline began is complicated by these factors, but the increasing rate most likely changed to a decline in the mid 1960's, perhaps somewhat earlier in women.

Data from other countries during the same period offer a perspective on understanding the United States rates. The multinational data in Figure 37–2 are for coronary heart disease death rates age adjusted over the four 10-year age groups for men 35 to 74 years of age. During the period 1969 to 1985, among the 29 countries compared, the United States had the largest decrease in its coronary heart disease mortality rate and moved from second to thirteenth in rank. During this period, four other countries (Australia, New Zealand, Canada, and Israel) also had significant declines, whereas several others, primarily the Eastern European countries, had significant increases. Although the large absolute difference in rates by country in any given year might suggest that the genetic differences among the populations account for this range, the large changes within a country over time demonstrate that regardless of genetic factors, the disease process can be significantly modified. Identification of the factors specifically responsible for these changes has proved to be difficult. Although the relative contributions of prevention efforts versus improved treatment modalities or improved general health measures have not been distinguishable, all most likely have contributed, with prevention efforts the most significant.

ATHEROSCLEROSIS AND CARDIOVASCULAR DISEASE

The major pathologic process leading to disease of the heart and blood vessels is atherosclerosis, with hypertension either a contributing or a primary problem. Atherosclerosis in its most malignant and rare form begins in early childhood and becomes rapidly manifest as clinical coronary heart disease or sudden death in adolescence. The more common and highly prevalent form begins to develop in adolescence and slowly progresses over several decades, gradually occluding the arterial lumen and eventually manifesting clinically as a stroke, angina pectoris, claudication, myocardial infarction, or, most devastatingly, sudden death. Although the factors that may lead to an acute clinical event, such as arterial spasm, acute thrombosis, or embolism, are not completely understood, the underlying, if not immediate, problem is predominantly atherosclerosis.

Laboratory and clinical research efforts continue in the search for the underlying cause or causes of atherosclerosis, examining those factors that may initiate the process as well as those that may cause the milder, highly prevalent, presumed early forms of the disease (i.e., fatty streaks on the arterial surface) to progress in many individuals to the more serious, complicated, and obstructing form of the disease. Other research efforts are concentrating on the later, but still preclinical, stages of the process, searching for improved and more quantitative diagnostic techniques. Meanwhile, epidemiologic research efforts have made and continue to make major contributions to both prevention and treatment approaches to the cardiovascular disease problem through identification of personal and environmental characteristics that markedly increase an individual's probability of developing specific cardiovascular diseases.

RESEARCH IN CARDIOVASCULAR DISEASE

The research approach that has been repeatedly used in several large observational studies of cardiovascular disease is exemplified by the Framingham Heart Study, begun in 1948 in a relatively small town in Massachusetts. A sample (5209 men and women aged 30 to 62) of the total population agreed to be part of this study, undergoing thorough examinations every 2 years, with intense follow-up for the development of both fatal and nonfatal diseases. This population has remained under close scrutiny continuously since originally recruited and examined over the 2-year period from 1948 to 1950. Similar studies have been performed in other groups in the United States, as well as around the world. In Tecumseh, Michigan, 8624 men and women; in Evans County, Georgia, 3102 men and women; in Albany, New York, 1913 male civil servants; and in Chicago, Illionis, 1264 male gas company employees and 1983 male employees of the Western Electric Company were recruited and observed over several years. The critical elements of these studies have been the (1) inclusion of relatively large numbers of people to allow for important and sufficiently powerful subsample analyses, (2) enrollment of participants by methods that would make them reasonably representative of the total population from which they were recruited, (3) careful determination of all the variables (such

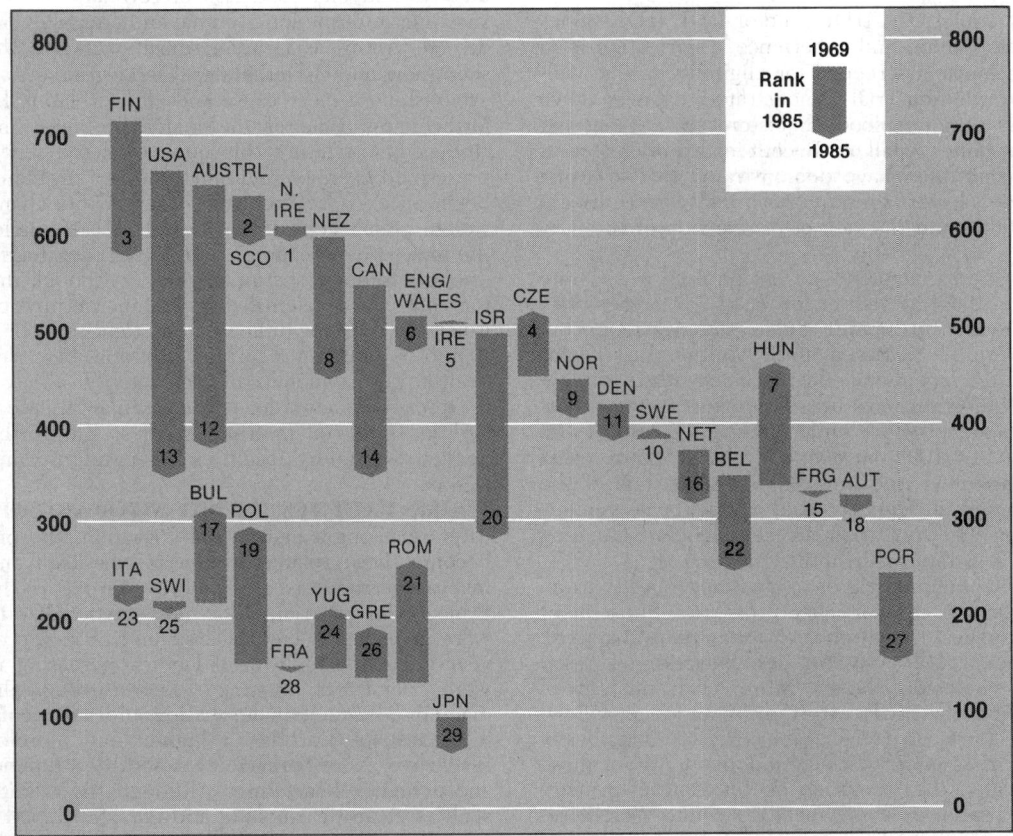

FIGURE 37–2. Age-adjusted coronary heart disease mortality rates per 100,000 population for men, ages 35 to 74, by country, 1969 to 1985. (Source: World Health Organization, World Health Statistics Annual.)

as height, blood pressure, smoking and dietary histories, and blood chemical determinations) in a standardized, reproducible manner, and (4) meticulous follow-up of all the participants for the development of fatal and nonfatal events recorded and defined in a predetermined and standardized fashion.

RISK FACTORS IN CARDIOVASCULAR DISEASE

From these United States studies and others worldwide, a consistent list of so-called risk factors for subsequent cardiovascular disease has been identified. These risk factors can be grouped into two broad categories: *unmodifiable* (such as older age, male gender, and family history of premature heart disease) and potentially *modifiable* (such as cigarette smoking, high blood pressure, high blood cholesterol level, diabetes, and the less prognostic factors of overweight, physical inactivity, and psychological factors). These factors can be used to identify clearly those in the population who are at especially high risk of developing cardiovascular disease.

CIGARETTE SMOKING. Cigarette smoking is established as a risk factor not only for lung cancer, emphysema, and bronchitis but also for coronary, cerebral, and peripheral vascular disease. This association has been seen in many countries, among widely diverse ethnic groups, in both sexes, and across various adult age groups. In addition, the risk increases with heavier cigarette use and the longer one has smoked. Equally important has been the observation that this increased risk falls rapidly over time when people quit smoking. For coronary heart disease, approximately 40 per cent of the increased risk is removed within 5 years of quitting, although it takes several more years of nonsmoking to achieve the level associated with someone who has never smoked.

HIGH BLOOD PRESSURE. High blood pressure is a powerful risk factor for cerebrovascular disease as well as for coronary heart disease and the atherosclerotic process directly. An estimated 58 million people have high blood pressure, defined as a level equal to or greater than 140 mm Hg systolic or 90 mm Hg

diastolic or as being on a regimen of antihypertensive medication. An important result of the epidemiologic studies was the observation that the relationship between blood pressure and cardiovascular risk was not only a positive one (a higher blood pressure resulted in a higher disease rate) but also a smooth one (there was no sharp breakpoint in the curve such that below a certain blood pressure level the risk remained constant or became nonexistent) Thus, the lower the blood pressure, within reasonable physiologic limits, the lower the level of risk. These observations prompted several important intervention trials, which have now clearly established the value of aggressively treating elevated blood pressure.

BLOOD CHOLESTEROL LEVELS. A clear and positive relationship between cholesterol levels and subsequent coronary heart disease has repeatedly been demonstrated. Later information refined the nature of this association but did not weaken it. Cholesterol in the plasma is transported by the lipoproteins. The cholesterol level associated with the low density lipoprotein (LDL) fraction was seen to be positively correlated with coronary heart disease, whereas the cholesterol associated with the high density lipoprotein (HDL) was negatively correlated (the higher the level, the lower the risk). These initial observations have been verified in several different populations and have been shown to be independent of each other, as well as of other known risk factors. As with blood pressure and cardiovascular disease risk, for both LDL cholesterol and HDL cholesterol, the curve is smooth (in the populations studied, there was no breakpoint in the curve observed). The evidence regarding HDL, although more recent than that for LDL, supports a powerful role for HDL in coronary heart disease risk and may explain some of the difference in risk between men and women, with women having higher average levels of HDL than do men. This ratio of LDL to HDL, an efficient method of combining the information from the two separate measures, has been shown to be more predictive than either measure alone. The appropriate clinical use of the mix of LDL, HDL, and/or LDL:HDL values must await more information and experience. Information from over 350,000 American men screened for eligibility in the Multiple Risk Factor Intervention Trial demonstrated that even down to and below levels of total blood cholesterol of 182 mg per deciliter, the risk continues to fall off. Recent intervention studies in hypercholesterolemic men have demonstrated that lowering blood cholesterol levels lowers subsequent coronary heart disease morbidity and mortality and the rate of progression of coronary atherosclerosis.

Each of these three risk factors alone can be used to separate groups of people into those at high or low risk. But as these risk factors occur simultaneously in individuals, the risk range becomes even larger (Fig. 37–3). Based on the Multiple Risk Factor Intervention Trial screenee data, the coronary heart disease mortality rate (1.6/1000 screenees) for nonsmokers in the lowest tertile of diastolic blood pressure and cholesterol is nine times lower than the rate (14.6/1000) for the highest risk group, using only these three variables. Age uniformly remains one of the most powerful factors at all levels of risk, as does male gender, with women realizing a 10- to 20-year differential before attaining the same level of risk as men with similar risk factors.

OBESITY. Initial epidemiologic data identified obesity as an important risk factor for coronary heart disease. Subsequent analyses, however, suggested that obesity was not a primary risk factor but rather acted indirectly through elevation of blood pressure and blood cholesterol levels. More recent analyses of the data from the Framingham Heart Study, with longer follow-up of people in the cohort, have once again suggested that obesity is indeed a primary risk factor that acts independently of these other factors. Clinically, the resolution of this issue of primary versus secondary causation is somewhat irrelevant. Weight reduction should lower the risk of coronary heart disease, whether it acts through a lowered blood pressure and/or cholesterol level or as a lowered risk factor itself.

DIABETES. Diabetes is a powerful and independent risk factor for cardiovascular disease, which remains the major cause of death in diabetic persons. An important remaining issue is whether an elevated blood glucose level is responsible for the observed higher rate of cardiovascular disease and, if it is, whether lowering or, preferably normalizing the glucose level will lower the risk. Regardless of the answers, for the present the important observation is that diabetic individuals are at higher risk of cardiovascular disease, and thus careful attention should be paid not just to the blood glucose level and its control but also to the other risk factors that may coexist in a given patient and additionally elevate the risk.

PHYSICAL INACTIVITY. An association between a less active lifestyle and increased risk of coronary heart disease has been shown in multiple longitudinal and cross-sectional studies in such diverse groups as London transit workers, United States longshoremen, and United States college graduates. However, studies establishing a clear cause-and-effect relationship have not been forthcoming. One of the major problems in the randomized studies investigating this question has been adherence to the prescribed exercise regimen. Another problem is that as people begin an exercise program, other factors change as well. Overweight people tend to lose weight, HDL cholesterol levels rise, the diet tends to change, and those individuals who are cigarette smokers frequently stop smoking. Although these covarying factors make the scientific evaluation of physical exercise as an isolated risk factor difficult, they tend to favor the recommendation of a prudent exercise program because of the multiple healthful consequences of such activity.

Other risk factors for cardiovascular disease have been identified in single or multiple studies, but further information is needed to establish them as independent, important prognostic factors.

RISK FACTORS AFTER MYOCARDIAL INFARCTION. After surviving a myocardial infarction, the primary risk factors become those related to the infarct itself and the damage to myocardial tissue (see Ch. 48.2). As part of the Coronary Drug Project clinical trial, 2789 post–myocardial infarction patients were given usual medical care and observed over a period of 5 years. The most powerful factors increasing risk in this group were persistent resting electrocardiographic abnormalities (namely ST segment depression and ventricular conduction defects), use of diuretics, a higher (and therefore more activity-restrictive) New York Heart Association functional classification, and a higher heart rate. Although the traditional risk factors, such as cigarette smoking and elevated blood cholesterol levels and blood pressure, remained prognostic, they were weaker factors overshadowed now by primary damage to the myocardium. In addition, with sudden death as the initial clinical presentation of cardiovascular disease in approximately one quarter of patients, it is obviously important to establish effective prevention modalities before the onset of clinical disease. Much current myocardial infarction research is focusing on therapeutic approaches that seek to minimize the extent of myocardial damage or even prevent the development of the infarct entirely. Nonetheless, the greatest potential for continuing and accelerating the decline in cardiovascular disease rates rests with prevention or treatment of the factors that lead to clinical presentation of disease and more profoundly of the factors that lead to or accelerate the atherosclerotic process.

CHANGES IN RISK FACTORS. Significant changes have

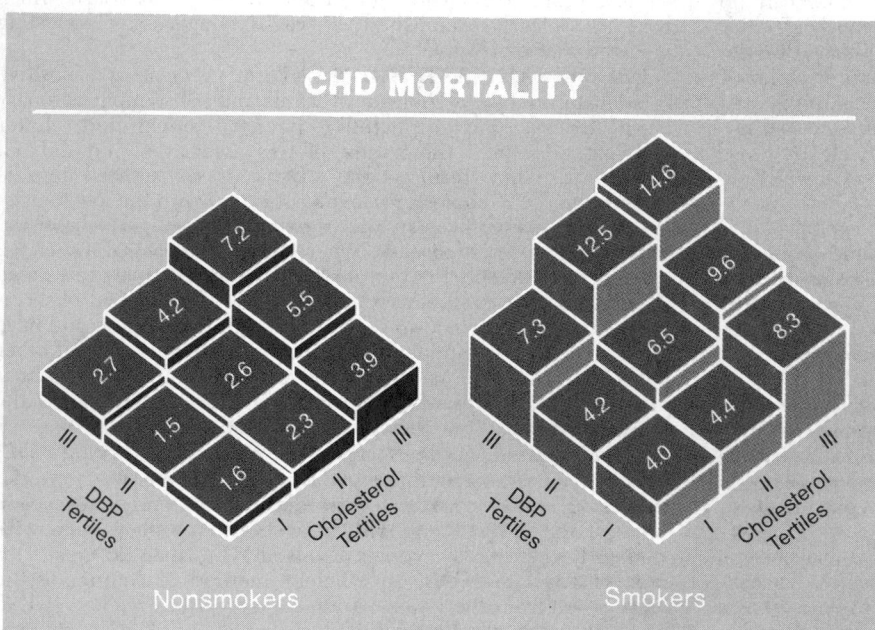

FIGURE 37–3. Age-adjusted CHD mortality rates per 1000 screenees for the Multiple Risk Factor Intervention Trial among smokers and nonsmokers for cholesterol tertiles (I = ≤ 196, II = 197–228, III = ≥ 229) and diastolic blood pressure (DBP) tertiles (I = ≤ 79, II = 80–87, III = ≥ 88).

occurred nationally in the major modifiable risk factors. In 1965, 50 per cent of men aged 20 or greater were cigarette smokers. In 1987 that figure had dropped to 32 per cent. For women the change has been modest, falling from 32 per cent in 1965 to 27 per cent in 1987. From 1965 to 1983, consumption of tobacco fell from 11.5 to 6.6 pounds per capita. In 1971 and 1972 only 16.5 per cent of people with high blood pressure (defined as a level equal to or greater than 160 mm Hg systolic or 95 mm Hg diastolic or as being on a regimen of antihypertensive medication) were effectively controlled. By the late 1970's, this figure had increased to 34 per cent nationally, and by the mid 1980's to 57 per cent in a sample from seven states. During this same period, visits to a physician for high blood pressure increased by 58 per cent. In addition, salt sales fell from 2.2 pounds per capita in 1972 to 1.4 in 1985. Average blood cholesterol levels in men fell from 217 mg per deciliter in the period between 1960 and 1966 to 211 in the late 1970's. Additional decline is suspected, but later national blood levels are not available. Annual food availability surveys, which serve as estimates of actual food consumption data (which are not routinely collected), show some dramatic changes between 1965–67 and 1983–85. The annual per capita availability in pounds of whole milk fell from 240 to 125, of eggs from 40 to 33, of meat from 124 to 121, and of animal fats and oils from 17 to 13. The availability in pounds of low-fat milk rose from 42 to 111, of poultry from 31 to 48, of fresh fruits from 79 to 88, and of vegetable fats and oils from 35 to 51. These impressive changes clearly demonstrate that the United States public can and will modify lifestyle behavior and suggest that additional gains in the prevention of the cardiovascular diseases can be made.

Goldman L, Cook EF: The decline in ischemic heart disease mortality rates: An analysis of the comparative effects of medical interventions and changes in lifestyle. Ann Intern Med 101:825, 1984. *An interesting attempt at quantification of the relative contribution of lifestyle and treatment factors to the decline in coronary heart disease mortality.*

Gordon T, Garcia-Palmieri MR, Kagan A, et al.: Differences in coronary heart disease in Framingham, Honolulu and Puerto Rico. J Chronic Dis 27:329, 1974. *A valuable comparison of the relationship between risk factors and subsequent coronary heart disease in three geographically and ethnically diverse populations.*

Health, United States, 1990. U.S. Department of Health and Human Services, Public Health Service, National Center for Health Statistics. DHHS Publication No. (PHS) 89–1232, March, 1989. *A frequently updated report presenting national data on morbidity and mortality, health delivery costs, and prevention programs with detailed tables.*

The Joint National Committee on Detection, Evaluation, and Treatment of High Blood Pressure: The 1984 Report of the Joint National Committee on Detection, Evaluation, and Treatment of High Blood Pressure. Arch Intern Med 144:1045, 1984. *A succinct and still authoritative review of the major clinical issues involving high blood pressure with a list of key references.*

Proceedings of the Conference on the Decline in Coronary Heart Disease Mortality. U.S. Department of Health, Education, and Welfare, Public Health Service. DHEW Publication No. (NIH) 79–1610, 1979. *A careful review of the issues bearing on the decline, with a useful appendix.*

Report of the Expert Panel on Detection, Evaluation, and Treatment of High Blood Cholesterol in Adults. U.S. Department of Health and Human Services, Public Health Services, National Institutes of Health. NIH Publication No. 89–2925, January, 1989. *A concise review of the major issues involving blood cholesterol and health risks, with a list of key references.*

The Surgeon General's Report on Nutrition and Health, 1988. U.S. Department of Health and Human Services, Public Health Service. DHHS (PHS) Publication No. 88–50210, 1988. *A remarkably complete and reasonably concise summary of the relationship between major nutrients and disease.*

World Health Statistics Annual 1970–1990. World Health Organization. *International vital statistics and population data in tabular form by country.*

38 Cardiac Function and Circulatory Control

John Ross, Jr.

FUNCTIONAL ANATOMY OF THE HEART

The right ventricle is thin walled (3 to 4 mm) and somewhat irregular in shape, with the interventricular septum being largely formed by the left ventricle. The right ventricle is more compliant than the left, the upper limit of normal for right ventricular end-

diastolic pressure being 6 mm Hg (Table 38–1). The left ventricle has a thicker wall (8 to 9 mm), and the upper limit of normal for the left ventricular end-diastolic pressure is higher (12 mm Hg, Table 38–1). The left ventricle has an ellipsoidal shape, shortens more in its short axis, and normally empties about two thirds of its contents during ejection (see "ejection fraction," Table 38–1, average normal ejection fraction 65 per cent).

In addition to its four muscular chambers with accompanying valves, the heart has an electrical activation and conduction system, an autonomic neural supply, and a coronary circulation. The three main coronary arteries divide into lesser branches and eventually send small, penetrating vessels directly into the myocardium to supply a very dense capillary network. During coronary vasodilation, approximately one capillary per muscle cell provides a rich blood supply to the heavily working myocardium.

The electrical subsystem includes the sinoatrial (SA) node, comprising special pacemaker cells with continuous phase 4 depolarization, and the atrioventricular (AV) node, which exhibits delayed or decremental conduction, allowing atrial depolarization to precede ventricular depolarization by approximately 140 msec and atrial contraction thereby to serve as a "booster pump" for filling the ventricles. From the AV junction (or node) the electrical impulse rapidly spreads through the specialized His-Purkinje conduction system in approximately 40 msec to reach the ventricles, which contract slightly out of phase (left before right), left ventricular contraction beginning about 50 msec after the onset of the QRS complex.

The nervous subsystem supplying the heart consists of sympathetic and parasympathetic divisions. There is a rich network of sympathetic nerve terminals containing norepinephrine distributed throughout the atria and ventricles, which allows reflex regulation of the contractility of the myocardium via β-adrenergic receptors on the myocardial cells, which also are accessible to circulating catecholamines. Sympathetic nerves also innervate the coronary arteries. The sympathetic nerves also heavily innervate the SA node and AV junction, where increases in sympathetic tone increase the heart rate (enhanced rate of phase 4 depolari-

TABLE 38–1. PRESSURES AND VOLUMES IN THE NORMAL HEART

Pressures
Left sided
  1. Left atrial pressure (normal mean pressure ≤ 12 mm Hg)
  2. Left ventricular pressure
    a. Peak systolic pressure (same as aorta)
    b. Maximum dP/dt (1200–3500 mm Hg/sec)
    c. Left ventricular end-diastolic pressure (normal ≤ 12 mm Hg)
  3. Aorta
    a. Systolic pressure (wide normal range, usually 100–150 mm Hg in adults)
    b. Diastolic pressure (wide normal range, usually 60–90 mm Hg in adults)
Right sided
  1. Right atrial pressure (normal mean pressure ≤ 6 mm Hg)
  2. Right ventricular pressure
    a. Peak systolic pressure (normal 15–30 mm Hg)
    b. Right ventricular end-diastolic pressure (normal ≤ 6 mm Hg)
  3. Pulmonary artery
    a. Systolic pressure (normal 15–30 mm Hg)
    b. Diastolic pressure (normal 4–12 mm Hg)

Volumes
Left sided (at rest)
  1. Left ventricular end-diastolic volume (normal 70–100 ml/m²)
  2. Left ventricular end-systolic volume (normal 25–35 ml/m²)
  3. Stroke volume (wide normal range, usually 40–70 ml/m²)
  4. Ejection fraction (stroke volume divided by end-diastolic volume [normal 0.55–0.80])

Time-related measurements
  1. Heart rate (wide normal range, usually 60–100 beats/minute)
  2. Cardiac index (2.5–4.2 liters/min/m²)

Resistances
  1. Systemic vascular resistance (770–1500 dynes sec cm⁻⁵)
  2. Pulmonary vascular resistance (20–120 dynes sec cm⁻⁵)

zation), improve conduction velocity through the AV junction, and enhance synchronicity of the ventricular muscle. Enhanced strength of muscle contraction and increased velocity of both muscle contraction and relaxation accompany the increased heart rate during sympathetic stimulation, as with excitement or exercise. Parasympathetic fibers from the vagus nerves containing acetylcholine provide heavy innervation to the right and left atria, the SA node, and the AV junction, but there are few parasympathetic nerve terminals in the ventricles or the conduction system below the AV junction. Activation of the parasympathetic system has a slowing effect on the SA node (reduced rate of phase 4 polarization) and slows conduction through the AV junction, providing reciprocal neural control with the sympathetic nervous system. The contractility of atrial muscle is depressed by parasympathetic stimulation, but there is minimal effect on the ventricles because of their sparse innervation by vagal fibers.

Unlike skeletal muscle, cardiac muscle can regulate its contractility, or inotropic state. The force of cardiac muscle contraction, as well as its velocity, is normally regulated to a large degree by the amount of free calcium (Ca^{++}). Ca^{++} enters the cell when the calcium "gate" is open during phase 2 of the action potential (Fig. 38–1). This provides some of the activating Ca^{++}, but the action potential (and the increasing Ca^{++} itself) triggers much more Ca^{++} release from the sarcoplasmic reticulum (Fig. 38–1). Ca^{++} then binds to a subunit of troponin on the actin filament, causing a conformational change that uncovers the active site, and allows a tension-generating bond to occur between actin and myosin. More Ca^{++} allows more sites to bind. *Between* contractions, the sarcoplasmic reticulum rapidly and actively sequesters Ca^{++} (Fig. 38–1), so that the level at the myofilaments falls below that required for the actin-myosin interaction. Ca^{++} is also extruded more slowly against an electrical and chemical gradient. One important mechanism is a 3:1 sodium for calcium exchange across the sarcolemma (Fig. 38–1), which is driven mainly by the sodium gradient generated by the sodium/potassium ATPase membrane pump. Myocardial contractility is normally increased by catecholamines, which stimulate the β receptors and augment intracellular cyclic adenosine monophosphate (AMP), which leads to phosphorylation of the calcium channel and increased Ca^{++} influx during the action potential. Increasing extracellular calcium also augments myocardial contractility. Increased rate of Ca^{++} reuptake by the sarcoplasmic reticulum also occurs, leading to more rapid relaxation.

A variety of other mechanisms stimulate myocardial contractility in the normal and failing heart. Digitalis, by inhibiting membrane sodium/potassium ATPase, causes an increase of in-

tracellular sodium, which decreases the sodium gradient, thereby leading to increased intracellular Ca^{++} and enhanced contractility (Fig. 38–1). β-Adrenergic agonist drugs such as dobutamine are used to treat the acutely failing heart as well. Some newer positive inotropic agents (e.g., amrinone and milrinone) act largely by inhibiting phosphodiesterase, leading to increased intracellular cyclic AMP, and other new drugs are under study that may increase the sensitivity of the myofilaments to Ca^{++}.

DIASTOLIC PROPERTIES OF THE HEART. A major feature of relaxed cardiac muscle is its intrinsic stiffness while at rest. Skeletal muscle, when isolated from its bony supports, can be overstretched easily, but cardiac muscle at first stretches readily but then, when stretched further, reaches an elastic limit, giving a much steeper relation between length and resting tension at long muscle lengths. Thus, within the walls of the ventricles, particularly the left ventricle, there is an extracellular network of collagen fibers which prevent overdistention with sudden changes in the venous return to the heart.

This property of heart muscle results in a nearly exponential relation between cardiac volume and pressure wherein small changes in volume produce large pressure changes as the ventricle is further filled beyond the upper limit of normal for left ventricular end-diastolic pressure (Fig. 38–2). Thus, the slope of this relation or chamber stiffness ($\Delta P/\Delta V$) increases as the ventricle is filled, and compliance ($\Delta V/\Delta P$) falls. Of course, when an abnormal chamber, such as a hypertrophied left ventricle, is compared with a normal chamber at the same cardiac volume, the entire diastolic pressure-volume relationship is shifted upward and steepened (Fig. 38–2), and the abnormal chamber is said to be stiffer or less compliant than normal. Even in chronically dilated hearts (as in the normal heart), it does not appear possible to stretch sarcomere lengths much beyond 2.2 μm, the optimum sarcomere length, so that the heart never appears to operate on a descending limb of the relation between resting sarcomere length and the active tension developed after muscle stimulation.

A thick, hypertrophied ventricle with decreased compliance causes increased resistance to filling, which can lead to diastolic cardiac dysfunction even when systolic function is maintained. In this setting atrial dilation and hypertrophy occur in order to maintain the atrial contribution to ventricular filling. The importance of this contribution is apparent in patients with severe hypertrophy caused, for example, by aortic stenosis or hypertrophic obstructive cardiomyopathy. Loss of an appropriately timed atrial contraction often results in marked exacerbation of dyspnea and left heart failure. In these patients, during sinus rhythm the left ventricular end-diastolic pressure is markedly elevated owing to a large A wave, whereas mean diastolic pressure, which is reflected back through the pulmonary veins

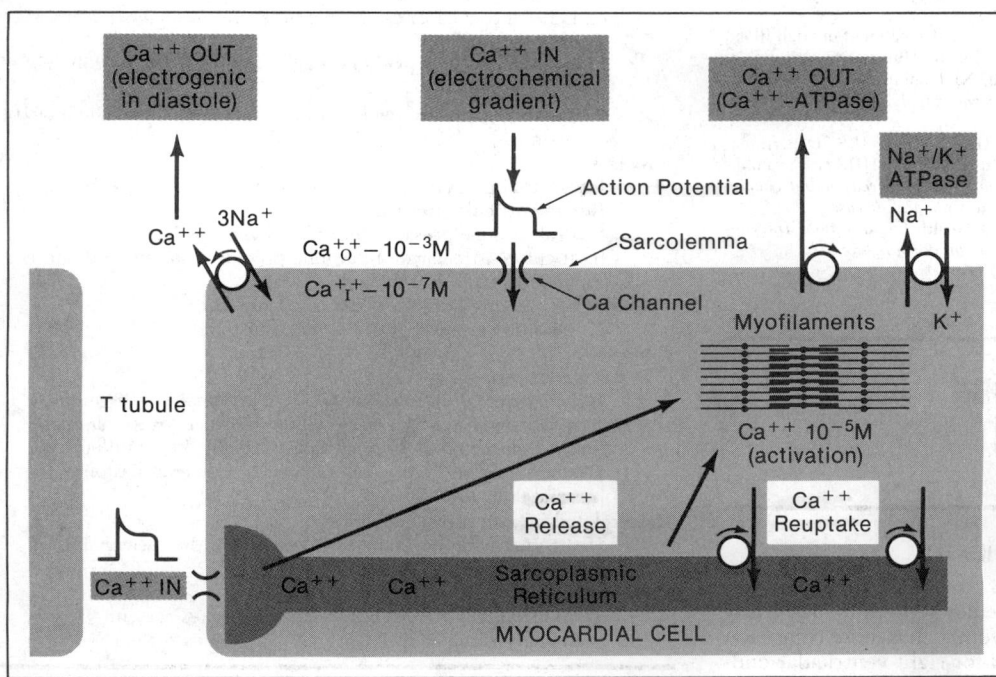

FIGURE 38–1. Movements of Ca^{++} during the cardiac cycle in a myocardial cell. Inward movement occurs across the sarcolemma during the action potential and also triggers Ca^{++} release from the sarcoplasmic reticulum. Free Ca^{++} is rapidly removed from the cytoplasm by the sarcoplasmic reticulum and slower extrusion across the sarcolemma occurs by Na^+-Ca^{++} exchange and by an active Ca^{++} pump (Ca^{++}-ATPase). (Adapted from West JB (ed.): Best and Taylor's Physiological Basis of Medical Practice. 11th ed. © 1985, the Williams & Wilkins Co., Baltimore.)

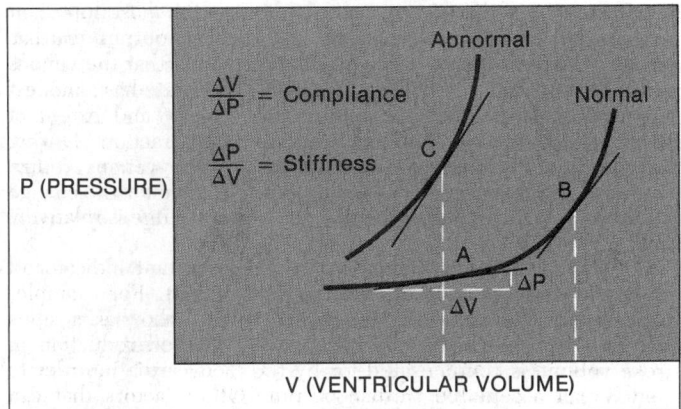

FIGURE 38–2. Diastolic pressure-volume curves of left ventricle under normal conditions and in the presence of severe ventricular hypertrophy (abnormal). Note the nearly exponential shape of the curves. The stiffness at any point on the normal curve ($\Delta P/\Delta V$) is shown by a tangent. Notice that ventricular stiffness increases (tangent A to tangent B) with ventricular filling to a larger ventricular volume. The stiffness of two ventricular chambers can be compared at a common volume, and comparison of the stiffness of the normal with that of the abnormal (hypertrophied) ventricle shows that the latter is markedly increased (tangent A versus tangent C). Compliance is the inverse slope ($\Delta V/\Delta P$) of the curve, and therefore the abnormal ventricle has a markedly reduced compliance. (Adapted from West JB (ed.): Best and Taylor's Physiological Basis of Medical Practice. 11th ed. © 1985, the Williams & Wilkins Co., Baltimore.)

into the lungs, is maintained at a lower level. When atrial contraction and the A wave "kick" are lost, as in atrial fibrillation, there is an increase in mean left atrial pressure in an attempt to maintain the same level of end-diastolic pressure and cardiac output.

CARDIAC CONTRACTION AND ITS REGULATION

DETERMINANTS OF CARDIAC PERFORMANCE. There are four major determinants of the performance of both ventricles. These factors are interrelated but considered separately for convenience.

1. Preload
2. Afterload
3. Contractility
4. Heart rate

The Preload. This refers to the loading condition on the heart at the end of diastole, which is primarily set by the venous return to the heart. In isolated heart muscle, it is defined as the force stretching the resting muscle to a given length prior to contraction. In the intact heart, it is less easily defined. Estimates of preload include measurements of the ventricular end-diastolic volume or the end-diastolic pressure (although the two are not linearly related, Fig. 38–2), and in acutely ill patients, it may be convenient to measure the ventricular "filling pressure" (the mean right or left atrial pressure, or the pulmonary artery wedge pressure) as an index of the preload. Within limits, as the preload increases, there is an increase in cardiac performance manifested by an increase in systolic pressure development or the volume of blood ejected. This represents the ascending limb of the familiar Frank-Starling relationship.

This overall relationship is often referred to as a ventricular function curve (Fig. 38–3). Some measure of cardiac performance, such as the stroke volume or stroke work (stroke volume × arterial pressure), is plotted as a function of some measure of the preload, such as the filling pressure or the end-diastolic pressure. The concept of the ventricular function curve is important, since it allows an objective assessment of the contractility of the ventricles. For example, the normal ventricle has a steep function curve, relatively small changes in end-diastolic pressure producing large changes in performance, whereas the failing ventricle has a downwardly displaced and flattened curve (Fig. 38–3). Such curves can permit a comparison between subjective signs or symptoms and objective measurements. Since the failing left ventricle operates near the peak of its ventricular function curve, the combination of a high filling pressure and low cardiac output

(Fig. 38–3, point D) explains the clinical picture of dyspnea and fatigue (see Ch. 40).

An important distinction must be made between the right atrial pressure, which represents the filling pressure of the right ventricle and can be estimated from the jugular veins, and the left atrial pressure, which is the filling pressure of the left ventricle. The mean left atrial pressure can be assessed from the mean pulmonary artery (or "capillary") wedge pressure, often measured by a flow-directed balloon catheter. In manipulating the volume status of the acutely ill patient, except in cases of isolated right ventricular failure, it is preferable to measure the left ventricular filling pressure, because the failing left ventricle usually has a more important role in determining arterial pressure and the forward cardiac output.

The Afterload. Afterload refers to the load against which the ventricle must contract when it ejects blood. In isolated heart muscle, it can be accurately defined as the load (or force) resisting shortening after the muscle is stimulated to contract and lift a load. In the intact heart, afterload is often estimated as the systolic arterial pressure. A better measure of the afterload is the systolic wall stress, which can be related to the systolic pressure, heart size, and wall thickness through the simplified Laplace relation:

$$\sigma = \frac{PR}{2h}$$

in which σ = wall stress or force/cross-sectional area, P = intraventricular pressure, R = radius of chamber (radius of curvature of the wall), and h = wall thickness.

The effect of afterload on performance is relatively straightforward. As arterial pressure is increased, the stroke volume tends to fall because the ventricle has greater difficulty in ejecting blood against a higher load. Such an effect is seen most clearly in experimental preparations when the preload is held constant (and cannot compensate for changes in afterload), and an inverse relation between the afterload (or systolic ventricular pressure) and the stroke volume is observed. In the intact circulation, changes in preload and afterload are closely related. For example, as the arterial pressure is increased in the normal heart, the left ventricle has greater difficulty in ejecting blood, which results in larger end-systolic and end-diastolic volumes, and the increasing preload then tends to restore the stroke volume.

Another way of representing ventricular function is the pressure-volume loop and the end-systolic pressure-volume relation (Fig. 38–4). (The slope of the latter relation has been used as a

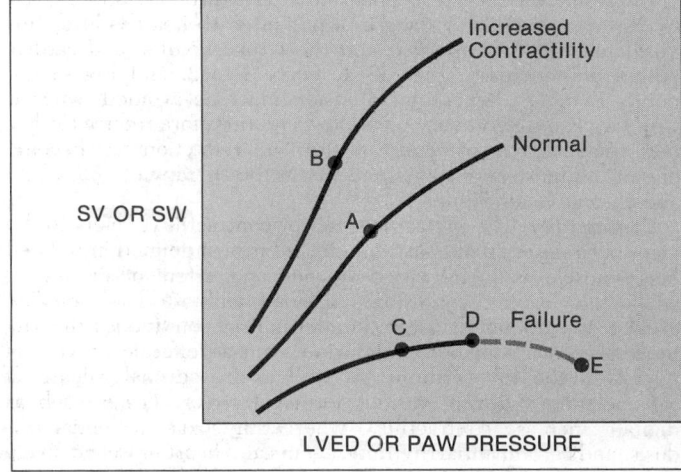

FIGURE 38–3. Left ventricular function curves relating the left ventricular filling pressure to ventricular performance expressed as stroke volume (SV) or stroke work (SW). The filling pressure can be expressed as either the left ventricular end-diastolic (LVED) pressure or the pulmonary artery wedge (PAW) pressure. Curves indicate normal, increased, or depressed ventricular contractility. Points A and B show the effects of a positive inotropic drug, which increases ventricular performance while reducing the filling pressure. See text for further discussion.

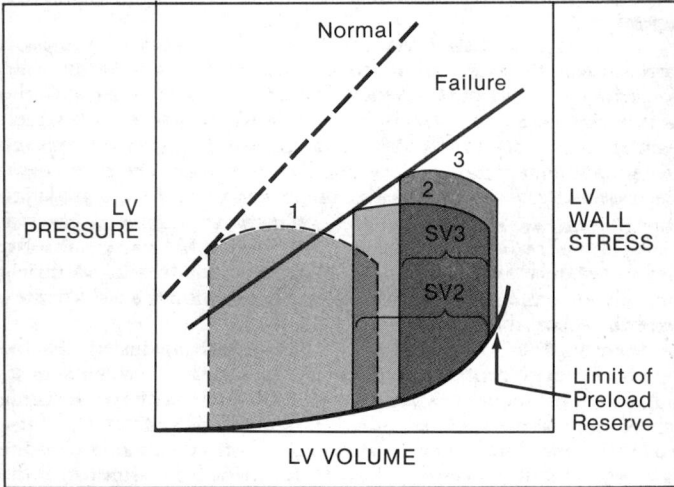

FIGURE 38–4. Left ventricular (LV) diastolic and end-systolic pressure-volume relations together with pressure-volume loops under normal conditions (*dashed lines*) and during heart failure when the linear end-systolic pressure-volume relation is shifted downward and to the right (failure). Beat 2 to beat 3 shows the effect of acutely increasing the left ventricular systolic pressure with a pure vasoconstrictor when there is little or no preload reserve; the stroke volume drops (SV2 to SV3). In chronic heart failure, the dilated left ventricle may be operating under basal conditions similar to beat 3, and left ventricular wall stress (right-hand ordinate) may be elevated despite a normal left ventricular systolic pressure. Under these circumstances use of a vasodilator drug may relieve this "afterload mismatch" and allow the ventricle to improve the stroke volume by lowering the wall stress (beat 3 to beat 2). (Adapted from West JB (ed.): Best and Taylor's Physiological Basis of Medical Practice. 11th ed. © 1985, the Williams & Wilkins Co., Baltimore.)

load-independent measure of contractility.) The end-systolic pressure-volume relation is shifted upward by enhanced contractility and downward by depressed contractility on heart failure (Fig. 38–4). The failing left ventricle exhibits enhanced sensitivity to afterload (decreased slope of the end-systolic pressure-volume relation), and when it reaches the limit of its preload reserve, any further increase in afterload (expressed as pressure or wall stress in Figure 38–4), such as by increased systemic vascular resistance and/or progressive heart failure, causes the stroke volume to fall (Fig. 38–4, beat 2 to beat 3, and Fig. 38–3, point E). This condition has been termed "afterload mismatch."

If systemic vascular resistance and arterial pressure are reduced by use of a vasodilator drug in a patient with heart failure, this mismatch will be improved and the stroke volume and cardiac output will increase (Fig. 38–4, beats 3 to 2, and Fig. 38–3, points E to D). Severe hypotension must be avoided, since it will compromise coronary blood flow and therefore reduce cardiac performance. The principle of afterload reduction has become one of the most important concepts in the therapy of both acute and chronic heart failure.

Contractility. The inotropic state, or contractility, refers to the vigor of contraction of heart muscle and is best defined in isolated heart muscle as an increased velocity and extent of shortening when the loading conditions (preload and afterload) do not change. Contractility is altered under normal conditions primarily by reflex release of norepinephrine from adrenergic nerve terminals in the myocardium, as well as by adrenal release of catecholamines during various forms of stress. Drugs such as digitalis increase contractility, whereas hypoxia, ischemia, acidosis, and certain antiarrhythmic agents and heart muscle damage reduce contractility. In terms of ventricular function curves, drugs that increase contractility shift the curve upward and to the left, increasing stroke volume or stroke work at a given end-diastolic pressure (Fig. 38–3, points A to B). With depression of contractility, the ventricular function curve shifts down and to the right, with a reduction in stroke volume at a given left ventricular end-diastolic pressure (Fig. 38–3).

Heart Rate. The frequency of contraction is an important determinant of cardiac performance and one of the most important mechanisms available to increase the cardiac output (cardiac output = stroke volume × heart rate), provided that the venous return is increased (see below). Increased heart rate has a modest positive inotropic effect, increasing the velocity and extent of shortening while reducing the duration of contraction. During the response to moderate exercise, when the venous return increases, a higher heart rate is mainly responsible for the change in cardiac output, since the increase in stroke volume is relatively small.

The level of the heart rate may be an important indicator of the cardiovascular status of an individual patient. For example, in a patient with acute severe heart failure who has a sinus tachycardia of 140 beats per minute, the marked reduction in stroke volume is compensated for by the tachycardia in order to maintain an acceptable cardiac output. Other factors that can raise the resting heart rate must also be considered, including fever, anemia, thyrotoxicosis, and anxiety.

ASSESSMENT OF CARDIAC PERFORMANCE. Quantitative indices of cardiac performance can be measured in the cardiac catheterization laboratory or in critical care units. For reference, normal pressures, cardiac volumes, cardiac output, and vascular resistance are listed in Table 38–1. Volume measurements are normalized to allow interpatient comparison by dividing by the body surface area (square meters), obtained from a standard table based on height and weight. The maximum value of the first derivative of left ventricular pressure during isovolumetric systole (dP/dt) is sometimes used as a measure of contractility. One very useful index of ventricular function is the ejection fraction, which is the stroke volume divided by the end-diastolic volume. A normal ejection fraction of the left ventricle is 0.55 or greater, and in severe heart failure the ejection fraction may be reduced to less than 0.20.

As discussed above, *ventricular function curves* (Fig. 38–3) are often employed to demonstrate changes in inotropic state, whereas changes in preload move the ventricle up and down on a *single* curve. Experimentally, they are produced by progressive infusions of fluid, whereas in the clinical setting often only two points on a curve are available, before and after an intervention.

When two ventricular function curves are compared, they generally are compared at the same level of mean arterial pressure, since, as discussed above, the stroke volume of the ventricle is changed by altered afterload. Hence, decreased afterload would shift the relation between stroke volume and filling pressure upward, and increased afterload would shift the relation downward. In heart failure, such an effect is sometimes represented as an apparent "descending limb" of function. As discussed earlier, in such a setting, the preload reserve is exhausted and lowering the afterload would improve the stroke volume and cardiac performance (Figs. 38–3 and 38–4).

Venous return and cardiac output curves can be used to represent cardiocirculatory responses under experimental conditions, and although venous return curves cannot be performed in humans, they allow insight into the highly important role of the venous return. The heart behaves as a demand pump, ejecting whatever blood is returned to it under normal conditions, and only in heart failure or when filling is impaired (as in constrictive pericarditis) does the heart itself become the limiting factor for cardiac output. Therefore, the return of blood to the heart (the venous return), which is regulated by a number of mechanical, neural, and humoral factors, through its influence on preload is a key determinant of cardiac performance under normal conditions.

In A.C. Guyton's analysis, cardiac function is represented by a cardiac output curve that intersects a venous return curve at any given-state condition (Fig. 38–5). Noncardiac factors that influence the venous return include the volume of blood in the vascular bed (transfusion shifts the venous return curve upward, whereas bleeding shifts it downward). The position of the venous return curve is also affected by neurohumoral factors, increased sympathetic tone shifting the venous return curve upward and to the right and vice versa; venoconstriction produced by increased sympathetic tone also displaces blood from the peripheral circulation toward the central (cardiopulmonary) circulation, whereas decreased tone to the veins causes pooling of blood in the peripheral circulation. With this framework, changes in *both*

1. Basal oxygen requirements
2. Systolic pressure (or wall stress)
3. Heart rate
4. Myocardial contractility (inotropic state)
5. Wall shortening against a load (related to cardiac work)

Systolic pressure, *heart rate*, and *contractility* are the major determinants of MVo_2, whereas shortening of the wall utilizes relatively less oxygen. There is a nearly linear relation between systolic pressure development by the left ventricle and MVo_2, and with the Laplace equation, this relation can also be expressed as systolic wall stress versus MVo_2. Thus, as systolic pressure doubles, the MVo_2 of the left ventricle approximately doubles. There is also a nearly linear relationship between heart rate and the MVo_2 and, again, an approximate doubling of the MVo_2 occurs as the heart rate increases twofold. If the heart rate and systolic pressure are held constant and a positive inotropic agent is administered, a rather marked increase in MVo_2 can be demonstrated, associated with a pronounced increase in the velocity of shortening and some increase in the extent of myocardial fiber shortening. It is possible that this extra energy expenditure is related, at least in part, to increased oxygen use by the calcium sequestration mechanism of the sarcoplasmic reticulum. Decreased contractility of the myocardium has been shown to cause a reduction of MVo_2.

The oxygen cost of myocardial fiber shortening against a load is relatively low. This is exemplified by experiments in which the systolic arterial pressure was elevated while the cardiac output and heart rate were held constant, and a marked stimulation of MVo_2 was produced, whereas if the cardiac output was increased over a wide range while the arterial pressure and heart rate were constant, only small changes in MVo_2 occurred. These findings indicate a high oxygen cost of "pressure work" and a relatively low oxygen cost of "volume work." The importance of heart rate and systolic pressure has resulted in the use of simplified indices of MVo_2, such as the heart rate × blood pressure (the "double product"). In clinical studies, this provides a means of estimating the effect of an antianginal drug (such as a beta blocker) on cardiac oxygen requirements during exercise.

The fact that myocardial energy expenditure, expressed as MVo_2, is closely linked to mechanical cardiac performance carries important implications in various disease states. For example, in valvular heart disease, chronic mitral regurgitation places a large volume overload on the heart due to the low impedance backward leak into the left atrium. In this condition, the systolic left ventricular pressure is not elevated, and since the left ventricle is performing extra "volume work," the MVo_2 of the left ventricle is not significantly increased. Therefore, in the absence of coronary artery disease, oxygen supply-demand imbalance and angina pectoris are rarely seen in chronic mitral regurgitation. In contrast, in patients with aortic stenosis, the high left ventricular systolic pressure with elevated MVo_2 of the entire chamber can lead to reduction of coronary vasodilator reserve. Therefore, subendocardial ischemia with angina pectoris is quite common in aortic stenosis, particularly during exercise or when left ventricular failure is beginning to occur, even in the absence of coronary artery disease. Of course, in chronic coronary artery disease, during exercise virtually all of the major determinants of MVo_2 are augmented, and in the presence of a stenosed coronary artery with impaired vasodilator reserve, coronary blood flow cannot keep pace with enhanced oxygen demands, and regional myocardial ischemia with angina pectoris occurs (see Ch. 48.1).

REGULATION OF CORONARY BLOOD FLOW

In keeping with the high energy requirements of the normal myocardium, coronary blood flow is relatively high, averaging 60 to 90 ml per minute per 100 grams in the normal human left ventricle when an individual is at rest. Extraction of oxygen by the heart is the highest of any organ, so that little additional oxygen extraction can occur during stress. This means that changes in oxygen demand of the heart are met chiefly by alterations in oxygen supply through changes in coronary blood flow, reflected by a nearly linear positive relation between the MVo_2 and the coronary blood flow. Although cardiac metabolism

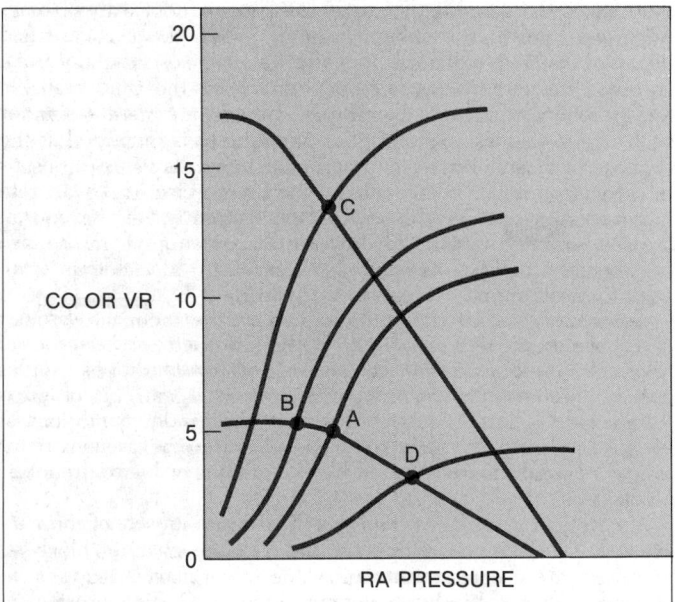

FIGURE 38–5. Relationship between the filling pressure of the heart, expressed as the right atrial (RA) pressure, and either cardiac output (CO) or venous return (VR). Venous return curves are represented as an inverse relation between the cardiac output or venous return and the right atrial pressure; the lower curve represents normal conditions and the upper curve shows the effect of marked sympathetic stimulation during exercise. The series of cardiac output curves shows a positive relation between right atrial pressure and cardiac function. Any steady-state condition is represented by the intersection of these two curves. Shown are normal conditions (A), electrical pacing of the heart (B), severe exercise (C), and heart failure (D). See text for further discussion.

cardiac performance and peripheral circulatory regulation (venous return) can be represented as they influence the cardiac output. Positive inotropic interventions, decreased afterload, and other factors shift the cardiac output curve upward, and opposite effects, including heart failure, shift it downward (Fig. 38–5).

The importance of venous return can be illustrated by the response to electrical cardiac pacing to increase the heart rate, a response in which myocardial contractility is increased. Since no significant effects on the peripheral circulation occur, no change in the cardiac output is observed. This response occurs because the normal heart operates near the flat portion of the normal venous return curve (near the point of venous collapse), and therefore even though the cardiac output curve is shifted upward, the venous return curve is unchanged, and there can be no alteration of the cardiac output (Fig. 38–5, points A to B). The response to exercise using this diagram is discussed subsequently under integrated responses.

REGULATION OF MYOCARDIAL OXYGEN CONSUMPTION

The heart is almost entirely supplied with energy from ATP and creatine phosphate produced by aerobic metabolism, and for practical purposes, the total energy expenditure of the normal heart can be equated with its oxygen consumption. The myocardial oxygen consumption (MVo_2) of the left ventricle can be determined using the Fick principle as the product of its coronary blood flow and the arteriovenous oxygen difference, calculated using blood samples from an artery and from the coronary sinus. Since the heart is a continuously active organ, its oxygen consumption is high relative to other organs, and the MVo_2 of the normal human left ventricle at rest is approximately 6 to 8 ml per minute per 100 grams.

The determinants of the MVo_2 of the heart (most of which is used by the left ventricle) consist of the basal oxygen consumption, which supplies energy for cell maintenance processes including the calcium and sodium pumps, protein synthesis, and so on. The remainder of the oxygen expenditure is controlled by the type of activity that the heart is called upon to perform. The determinants of MVo_2 are is the main determinant of coronary blood flow, several additional factors can be of importance:

1. MVo₂
2. Coronary perfusion pressure
3. Systolic compression
4. Alpha-adrenergic tone to the coronary arteries (or exogenous vasoconstrictors)
5. Vasodilators (epinephrine, exogenous vasodilator substances)

Since the MVo_2 is influenced by each of the major determinants of cardiac performance, coronary blood flow is altered in the appropriate direction. There is evidence that release of the ATP metabolite adenosine, a potent coronary vasodilator, is involved in some of the responses of the coronary blood flow to altered cardiac performance and metabolism, although a number of other stimuli to vasodilation (such as decreased Po₂, decreased pH, and increased K⁺ during enhanced metabolic activity) may also be important.

Under normal conditions, the mean coronary perfusion pressure is not a major determinant of coronary blood flow, except as it affects the systolic arterial pressure and therefore the MVo_2. Of course, on a moment-to-moment basis, the phasic pattern of coronary blood flow to the left ventricle shows a slow fall during diastole as the aortic pressure falls, as well as a sharp drop during systole as the squeezing action of the left ventricular wall compresses the intramural vessels and shuts down coronary blood flow, particularly to the subendocardial layers. However, the mean flow has been shown to be independent of the mean coronary perfusion pressure within certain limits, a phenomenon termed "autoregulation." Studies in which the coronary arteries are perfused *separately* from the aorta show that between mean coronary perfusion pressures of about 60 and 150 mm Hg coronary blood flow is maintained constant, provided that the MVo_2 of the heart does not change (Fig. 38–6). When the coronary perfusion pressure drops below 60 mm Hg, the coronary bed reaches the limit of autoregulation and tends to become fully dilated; at that point, perfusion pressure becomes the major determinant of coronary blood flow, and flow drops as pressure falls below that value with an exponential relation between pressure and flow typical of a passive blood vessel (Fig. 38–6). Obviously, in coronary artery disease the coronary perfusion pressure can become extremely important, since the perfusion pressure beyond an area of stenosis may be relatively low.

Systolic compression of coronary vessels in the inner (subendocardial) left ventricular wall almost entirely shuts off coronary blood flow during systole, but this does not occur in the outer wall (subepicardium). During diastole, flow to the subendocardium becomes slightly higher than in the outer wall, in order to compensate for the loss of flow during systole, a phenomenon that makes the vasodilator reserve in the subendocardium somewhat *less* than in the subepicardium. When the coronary bed becomes maximally dilated, this effect also makes subendocardial coronary blood flow highly dependent upon the time available for diastolic perfusion. For example, if heart rate increases under such circumstances, systolic time per minute is increased at the expense of diastolic time, and coronary flow falls. This can occur in coronary artery disease, when, during exercise, the heart rate increases and coronary blood flow consequently falls beyond an area of coronary stenosis (decreased oxygen supply), in the face of increased oxygen demands. β-adrenergic blockade is often used to treat angina pectoris in this setting (Ch. 48.1).

α-Adrenergic constrictor influences on the coronary vascular bed have been demonstrated. Although such an effect is of relatively minor significance under normal conditions, under certain circumstances of reflex activation it can be of great significance. There is recent evidence that under conditions of exercise-induced ischemia, α-adrenergic coronary vasoconstrictor tone exists and can be reduced by vasodilators or by α-adrenergic blockade.

A variety of substances can relax the smooth muscle of coronary arteries, including nitroglycerin and calcium channel blockers, and these are used to treat angina due to coronary artery spasm, as well as exercise-induced angina pectoris. Certain prostaglandins and agents such as vasopressin and ergonovine are coronary vasoconstrictors, and ergonovine is used as a diagnostic test to evoke coronary spasm in patients with variant angina.

Recently, endothelium-derived relaxing factor (EDRF) has been established as an important endogenous mediator of large artery dilation in response to increased flow, and its release also is responsible for the coronary vasodilator properties of several substances, including acetylcholine and bradykinin. The absence of the endothelium (as in certain coronary atherosclerotic lesions) can alter the vascular responses to such stimuli.

REGULATION OF THE PERIPHERAL CIRCULATION

The heart pumps blood sequentially through the pulmonary and systemic circulations. Throughout the circulation, the small arterioles provide the main site for vascular resistance regulation. There is a wide variability in cardiac output distribution and in oxygen extraction by various organs; for example, the kidneys have a high blood flow (20 per cent of the cardiac output) and a low oxygen extraction, whereas the coronary circulation has a lower flow but a much higher oxygen extraction. The large conduit arteries have a high velocity of blood flow (aorta = 31 cm per second), whereas in the capillaries, the enormous total cross-sectional area results in marked slowing of blood flow (0.05 cm per second), allowing exchange of metabolites. The veins contain 75 to 80 per cent of the total blood volume in the circulation and serve a capacitance function, i.e., as a blood volume reservoir.

The general organization of the systemic circulation is such

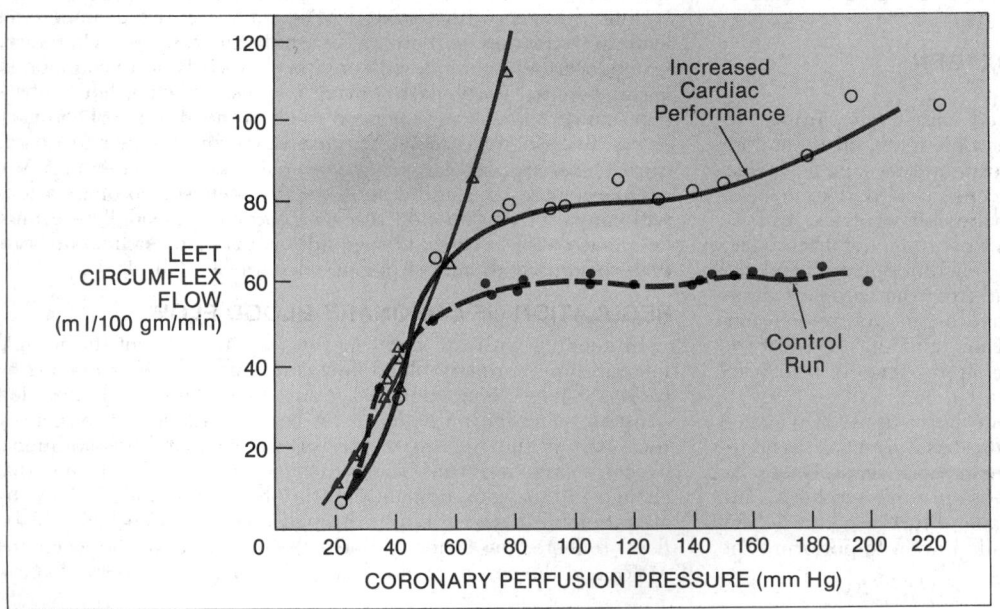

FIGURE 38–6. Autoregulation in the coronary circulation. When the left ventricular work is held constant and the coronary perfusion pressure is altered (coronary artery separately perfused from a controlled pressure source), coronary blood flow remains relatively constant over a wide range (*closed circles,* control run). At a coronary perfusion pressure below approximately 60 mm Hg, the limit of vasodilator reserve is reached, autoregulation is lost, and coronary flow is directly determined by the coronary perfusion pressure. The pressure-flow relation then falls on a curve of maximum vasodilation (passive pressure-flow curve of a distensible blood vessel, *open triangles*). Coronary blood flow is regulated at a higher level when cardiac performance and hence MVo_2 are increased (*open circles,* increased cardiac performance). (Adapted from West JB (ed.): Best and Taylor's Physiological Basis of Medical Practice. 11th ed. © 1985, the Williams & Wilkins Co., Baltimore.)

that the arterial bed serves as a pressure reservoir from which the circulations to the various organs operate in parallel. Thus, each organ takes the blood supply that it requires by regulating its *local* vascular resistance primarily on the basis of metabolic needs (autoregulation, as discussed earlier for the coronary circulation), whereas the *total* peripheral vascular resistance (TPVR) is primarily controlled by cardiovascular reflexes and maintains the pressure in the arteries. Thus, blood pressure = cardiac output × TPVR, and it is protected by the reflexes. For example, during tilting or standing abruptly, venous return and cardiac output fall (venous pooling), but a reflex increase in TPVR prevents a marked drop in the blood pressure.

REFLEX NEURAL CONTROL. The autonomic nervous system and certain neurohumoral factors maintain circulatory homeostasis through regulation of the heart rate, myocardial contractility, vascular tone in the arterioles and small veins, and the blood volume.

The high-pressure baroreceptors, which sense stretch in the walls of arteries, are located in the carotid sinuses and aortic arch. They increase their afferent impulse traffic when the blood pressure rises, and vice versa, and these nerve impulses affect the cardiovascular regulatory centers in the medulla. For example, as arterial pressure is increased, the enhanced impulse traffic stimulates the vagus to slow the heart rate and simultaneously inhibits the cardioaccelerator center. Simultaneously, the vasoconstrictor center is also inhibited, reducing sympathetic tone to the peripheral arterioles and also lowering venous tone. Thus, the reduced peripheral vascular resistance and venous return, together with the slowed heart rate, lower the increased blood pressure toward its previous level. With a decrease in blood pressure, as with moderate bleeding, opposite effects would occur, tending to restore the lowered blood pressure. With a significant drop in blood pressure, reflex release of catecholamines from the adrenal glands also occurs.

Reflex control of the heart and circulation is also under the influence of higher brain centers, as when marked emotional stress activates the sympathetic nervous system. Such central stimulation, as well as reflex activation of the sympathetic nervous system via receptors in the exercising skeletal muscle, produce the marked sympathetic stimulation of exercise. At rest, there appears to be little sympathetic tone affecting heart rate or myocardial contractility, and the heart rate is primarily under the control of parasympathetic influences.

Low-pressure baroreceptors (stretch receptors) are also located in the heart, particularly in the atria and the pulmonary veins, with fewer in the ventricles (see also blood volume regulation). Increased stretch of the atrial receptors can induce tachycardia (the Bainbridge reflex). More marked stretch of these low-pressure receptors produces a depressor reflex, with withdrawal of sympathetic tone and a fall in peripheral vascular resistance, which contributes to high-pressure baroreceptor regulation of the blood pressure. Syncope in some patients with aortic stenosis and high intracardiac pressure may be due to sudden activation of these intracardiac receptors.

REGULATION OF BLOOD VOLUME. The magnitude of blood volume is an important factor affecting cardiovascular function, and it is important in long-term regulation of the blood pressure. Loss of fluid volume occurs primarily through the kidneys, whereas sweating, respiratory, and gastrointestinal losses are less important (except during extreme conditions). Since approximately 20 per cent of the resting cardiac output passes through the kidneys, they provide an ideal location for regulating sodium and water balance. In addition, the hypothalamic osmoreceptors that regulate thirst and antidiuretic hormone (ADH) secretion are of great importance. Since these subjects are discussed in detail in Ch. 75, only selected cardiovascular factors are mentioned here.

An increase in blood volume, as might occur by increased intake of salt and water, would increase the diastolic volume of the cardiac chambers and the cardiac output. Atrial receptors sensitive to stretch activate vasodilating reflexes to the kidneys, increasing renal blood flow, and atrial receptors also reflexly stimulate the central nervous system to diminish the secretion of ADH. These factors would tend to increase the output of urine and sodium excretion, restoring the blood volume toward normal. A decrease in effective blood volume would have opposite effects.

Also, a peptide called atrial natriuretic factor (ANF) has been isolated which causes renal sodium loss and is also a vasodilator. It is released by the atria upon stretch, and ANF levels rise with acute and chronic circulatory congestion.

An additional highly important control mechanism for the regulation of arterial pressure and blood volume is the renin-angiotensin system (see Ch. 44). Reduction in renal perfusion (reduced pressure and flow) is sensed by the juxtaglomerular apparatus, which releases renin, whereas increased effective blood volume shuts off the stimulus for renin release. Renin enzymatically promotes the formation of angiotensin I from a precursor in the bloodstream, which is then converted to angiotensin II by the converting enzyme. Angiotensin II is a powerful vasoconstrictor, but small subpressor doses of angiotensin II also increase aldosterone secretion. Aldosterone, in turn, acts on the kidney to promote retention of salt and water, thereby counteracting the original stimulus of decreased effective blood volume.

With congestive heart failure, there is increased retention of salt and water, which leads to edema formation and increased blood volume. There may be increased aldosterone levels in severe heart failure secondary to reduced renal perfusion and activation of the renin-angiotensin system. Diuretics are used in this setting, and in severe heart failure with hyponatremia that is unresponsive to diuretics, use of an angiotensin-converting enzyme inhibitor may reverse this process by lowering angiotensin II and aldosterone levels, as well as by lowering vascular resistance and afterload on the left ventricle.

INTEGRATED CARDIOVASCULAR RESPONSES

It is important to emphasize the significance of interactions between the peripheral circulation and the heart in considering integrated responses. Certain peripheral circulatory factors, including the total peripheral vascular resistance and the venous capacitance, affect two important mechanical determinants of cardiac performance, the preload and the afterload. Venous return, of course, primarily determines the cardiac output. In addition, feedback control by neurohumoral reflex mechanisms simultaneously regulates both the heart and the peripheral circulation.

CHANGES IN VENOUS RETURN. Venous return to the right heart varies with normal respiration. It increases during inspiration as intrathoracic pressure falls (thereby increasing the pressure gradient for right heart filling), and moment-to-moment operation of the Frank-Starling mechanism in both ventricles to vary the stroke volume keeps the output per minute of the two sides of the heart in equilibrium.

A more marked stimulus, the Valsalva maneuver, which is useful in the physical diagnosis of heart murmurs, causes a marked decrease in the venous return to the heart because of the abrupt elevation of intrathoracic pressure, and after 15 to 20 seconds the associated drop in blood pressure produces reflex tachycardia and increased myocardial contractility. During this phase of the maneuver, cardiac murmurs associated with blood flow across a narrowed valve, such as that of aortic stenosis, diminish in intensity because of the reduced cardiac output, whereas the murmur associated with hypertrophic cardiomyopathy increases owing to the effect of reduced heart size and increased contractility to narrow the left ventricular outflow tract.

Vasodilator drugs that have a considerable venodilating effect, such as nitroglycerin, nitroprusside, and captopril, can have different effects on the cardiac output in the normal circulation and in congestive heart failure. Thus, in the normal circulation the cardiac output falls with nitroprusside, since the venous return curve is shifted downward as blood volume is displaced from the central circulation and pooled in the peripheral veins (decreased effective blood volume), whereas during cardiac failure, the associated unloading of the left ventricle by the arteriole-dilating action of this drug releases blood from the central circulation, which counterbalances the drug's venodilator effect; therefore, the venous return curve is not shifted downward, and the marked shift upward of the cardiac output curve due to reduced afterload results in an increased cardiac output (Fig. 38–5, points D to A).

It is also important to note that certain chronic cardiac conditions can limit the venous return to the heart because of impaired cardiac filling. These include chronic constrictive pericarditis and restrictive cardiomyopathy.

CHANGES IN HEART RATE. The lack of effect on cardiac output of changing heart rate by electrical pacing over a wide range has been previously discussed. But the usual increases in heart rate that occur as a component of cardiocirculatory reflex responses are ordinarily accompanied by increased myocardial contractility, venoconstriction, and an increased cardiac output. Below a certain level of heart rate, as in complete heart block with a ventricular rate of 40 beats per minute, the resting cardiac output may not be maintained, since the stroke volume is maximal (preload reserve fully utilized) and the ventricular output becomes rate limited. In addition, with marked resting tachycardia (approaching 200 beats per minute or more), as in paroxysmal atrial or ventricular arrhythmias, the available diastolic filling time is shortened because of the increased number of contractions per minute, and inadequate ventricular filling leads to a fall in the cardiac output. The loss of an appropriately timed atrial contraction in some dysrhythmias may further contribute to inadequate cardiac filling.

EXERCISE. Many mechanisms can come into play to cause the increased cardiac output that accompanies normal exercise. In nonsedentary individuals during low levels of exercise, increased stroke volume, combined with a mild increase in heart rate, augments the cardiac output. With marked exercise, as sympathetic stimulation and circulating catecholamine levels increase, the increased venous return causes further utilization of the Frank-Starling mechanism, and the stroke volume is further enhanced as increased myocardial contractility augments the ejection fraction. However, the stroke volume reserve is relatively small. The most important cardiac mechanism allowing a very high cardiac output during intense exercise in such individuals is augmented heart rate, which may reach 180 beats per minute or higher. Increased myocardial contractility also combines with decreased total peripheral vascular resistance (caused by marked vasodilation in the exercising muscles) to shift the cardiac output curve upward. In addition, increased sympathetic tone shifts the venous return curve upward (decreased venous capacitance), and it is steepened by decreased venous and arteriolar resistance. Therefore, the intersection of the venous return and cardiac output curves occurs at a markedly increased cardiac output, with only a mild elevation of the right atrial pressure (Fig. 38–5, points A to C). Thus, *both* peripheral and circulatory adaptations are involved in the exercise response.

Braunwald E (ed.): Heart Disease: A Textbook of Cardiovascular Medicine. 3rd ed. Philadelphia, W.B. Saunders Company, 1988, pp 383–425. *Up-to-date review of cardiac performance from the cellular level to the intact heart. Also includes the pathophysiology of heart failure.*

Ross J Jr: Assessment of cardiac function and myocardial contractility. *In* Hearst JW (ed.): The Heart. New York, McGraw-Hill Book Company, 1986, pp 265–298. *Current concepts concerning left ventricular function under normal and abnormal loading conditions, including heart failure and valvular heart disease.*

West JB (ed.): Best and Taylor's Physiological Basis of Medical Practice. 11th ed. Baltimore, Williams & Wilkins Company, 1985, pp 207–262, 284–307. *Basic physiology text that assumes little advanced knowledge. Pathophysiologic examples are concerned with cardiac function, circulatory control, myocardial oxygen consumption, coronary circulation, and heart failure.*

39 Specialized Diagnostic Procedures

39.1 RADIOLOGY OF THE HEART

Murray G. Baron

The heart casts a homogeneous shadow on the chest film. No internal detail can be seen within its contours because the radiodensities of blood, myocardium, and other cardiac tissues are so similar that one cannot be distinguished from the others. Only the two borders of the silhouette, where the heart contacts the radiolucent, air-containing lung, can be clearly discerned in any one projection. Changes in the size and/or shape of the cardiac chambers and great vessels usually alter the shape of the heart and its contours. However, because the heart is a three-dimensional structure and all of the cardiac chambers do not form borders in any one projection, multiple views are required to accurately evaluate its image. With the advent of echocardiography, the routine need for this "cardiac series" has disappeared. However, a remarkable amount of information regarding the heart can be gleaned from the standard frontal and lateral projections. As they are a part of most routine medical examinations, they are a useful screening tool for the detection of heart disease as well as for evaluating the severity of known disease, documenting the natural history of the disease, and assessing the efficacy of treatment.

ROENTGEN ANATOMY (Fig. 39–1)

Radiographic examination of the chest consists of at least a posteroanterior film. The right cardiac border in this projection has two components: a straight, vertical upper half formed by the superior vena cava and a gently convex lower half representing the lateral wall of the right atrium. Some patients are able to lower their diaphragms sufficiently during inspiration to uncover a small, straight segment of the inferior vena cava between the diaphragm and the right atrium.

The left cardiac border is composed of four distinct curves. The uppermost bulge represents the aortic knob. This is formed by the most distal portion of the aortic arch, beyond the left subclavian artery, where it turns downward to become the descending aorta. The prominence below the knob is formed by the main pulmonary artery and the subvalvular portion of the outflow tract of the right ventricle. The lowermost third of this border represents the anterolateral wall of the left ventricle. Between this and the outflow tract of the right ventricle is a short, flat or slightly concave segment where the left atrial appendage reaches the border of the heart.

In the lateral view (Fig. 39–1C), the anterior border of the cardiac silhouette is formed by the body and outflow tract of the right ventricle. The heart lies in the anterior portion of the chest, and the right ventricle abuts on the lower third of the sternum. The outflow tract and pulmonary artery slope posteriorly, and air-containing lung is interposed between the heart and the anterior chest wall, forming the "retrosternal clear space." The upper half of the posterior border of the cardiac silhouette, beginning at the carina and extending downward, is formed by the posterior wall of the left atrium and the lower half by the posterior wall of the left ventricle. The left atrial contour is usually not well visualized because it blends with the shadows of the posterior mediastinum. The shadow of the inferior vena cava can usually be seen extending obliquely and anteriorly from the diaphragm. The lowermost portion of normal left ventricular margin crosses the shadow of the cava about 2 cm above the left leaf of the diaphragm.

Alterations in the contour of the heart usually reflect dilatation and/or hypertrophy of the chambers, changes secondary to some underlying lesion. Many times, the pattern of these changes together with the appearance of the pulmonary vasculature points to the specific primary abnormality. Chest films are not sensitive or accurate as a detector of cardiac hypertrophy because the thickened myocardium often encroaches more on the chamber lumen rather than extending outward and enlarging the heart (Fig. 39–2). With severe hypertrophy, as in hypertrophic cardiomyopathy, the heart enlarges to the left and the apex becomes blunted and rounder than usual. However, this is not a pathognomonic appearance. On the other hand, dilatation of one or more chambers tends to alter the cardiac silhouette in a characteristic and recognizable manner.

HEART SIZE

A normal cardiac silhouette is no guarantee that the heart is normal. Angina, for example, no matter how severe, does not affect heart size unless there is also decompensation of the left ventricle. Similarly, the patient with restrictive cardiomyopathy may be in severe congestive failure with a normal-appearing

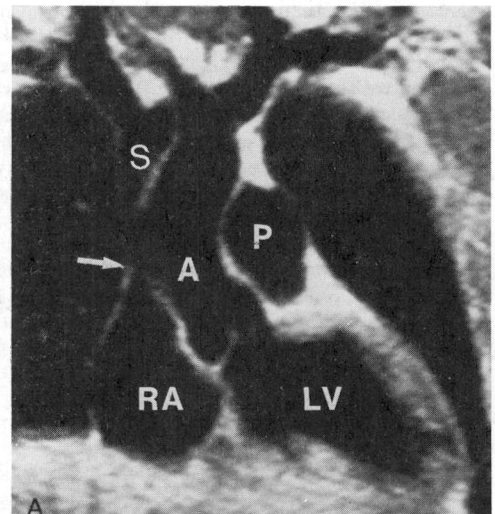

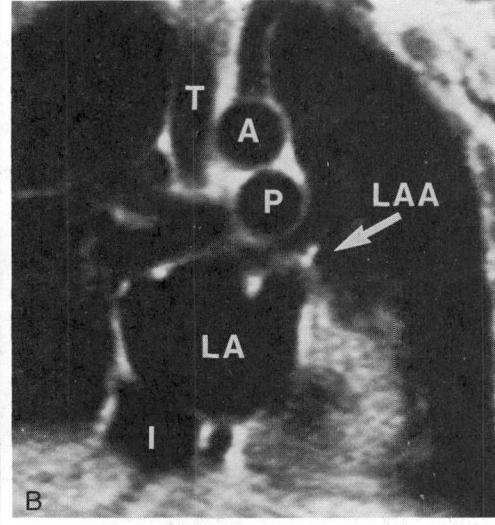

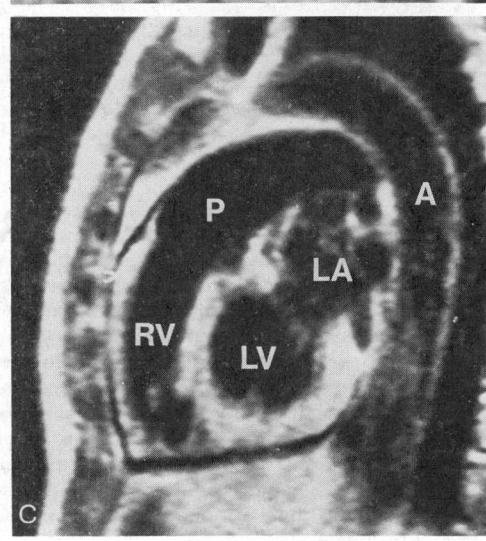

FIGURE 39–1. Normal roentgen anatomy. Magnetic resonance images. *A,* Coronal section at level of aortic valve. The right border of the cardiac silhouette is formed by the superior vena cava (S) and the right atrium (RA). The arrow indicates the caval-atrial junction. The lower portion of the left cardiac border is formed by the left ventricle (LV). A = Ascending aorta; P = main pulmonary artery. *B,* Coronal section at level of left atrium. The upper portion of the left cardiac border is formed by the aorta (A), main pulmonary artery (P), and left atrial appendage (LAA). LA = Left atrium; I = inferior vena cava; T = trachea. *C,* Sagittal section near midline. The right ventricle (RV) forms the anterior surface of the heart, abutting the sternum. The pulmonary artery (P) extends upward and posteriorly from the ventricle. The posterior border of the heart is formed by the left atrium (LA) and left ventricle (LV).

heart. Conversely, enlargement of the heart always indicates the presence of cardiac or pericardial disease. Therefore, accurate evaluation of heart size is important.

Over the years, various measurements have been proposed as objective means for assessing heart size. The simplest of these is the transverse cardiac diameter. This has proved to be of little value because the normal range is so great and its size varies with the age, sex, and body habitus of the patient. However, when the transverse cardiac diameter is considered together with the patient's body surface area, a satisfactory distinction can be made between normal and abnormal. This is not a practical solution, as the data needed to calculate body surface area are usually not available when reviewing chest films. An approximation of body habitus can be gained from the size of the patient's chest. The cardiothoracic ratio is measured by dropping a vertical line through the heart and measuring the greatest distance to the right and left cardiac borders (Fig. 39–2). The sum of the two is the transverse cardiac diameter. The transverse thoracic diameter is the greatest width of the chest, measured from inner surfaces of the ribs. Dividing this into the transverse cardiac diameter gives the cardiothoracic ratio. A ratio of less than 0.6 can be considered within the limits of normal. Setting this value at 0.5, as is often done, produces many false-positive results.

In most cases, accurate measurements of the cardiac silhouette are not necessary, and a reasonably experienced observer can achieve a similar degree of accuracy by visually estimating heart size. Regardless of the method used, several cautions must be observed if overreading of abnormality is to be avoided. The single factor having the greatest effect on apparent cardiac size is the degree of inspiration. The volume of the heart is essentially constant throughout the cardiac cycle. With expiration, as the diaphragm moves up, the vertical diameter of the heart is

shortened and there is a compensatory increase in its transverse diameter. Because of the increase in width, the heart appears larger on expiratory films. The degree of inspiration can be gauged from the relationship of the diaphragm to the ribs. On a properly positioned frontal chest film, a reasonable degree of inspiration is indicated if the diaphragm is pulled down below the posterior portion of the ninth rib.

When the anteroposterior diameter of the chest is small, the heart may be compressed between the sternum and the spine so that it splays to one or both sides. For this reason, the heart often appears enlarged in patients with a straight back syndrome or with a pectus excavatum deformity of the sternum. An epicardial fat pad (actually it is truly extrapleural fat, outside of the pericardium) can occur in one or both cardiophrenic angles and makes the heart appear larger than it actually is. However, the fat often causes the cardiophrenic angle to appear abnormally obtuse or makes the cardiac apex indistinct. In addition, on a properly exposed film, the slightly more radiolucent image of the fat can usually be distinguished from the greater density of the heart.

A change in the size of the cardiac silhouette can also occur between systole and diastole. This is important because chest films are exposed at random with reference to the phase of the cardiac cycle and so may be misleading when comparing the heart size on two films of the same patient made at different times. This usually does not create a problem, as in the majority of cases the difference in the transverse cardiac diameter between the two phases is small, measuring no more than several millimeters. However, in younger patients, especially the more athletic ones, with a slow heart rate and large stroke volume, phasic change in the cardiac diameter can be as much as 2 cm.

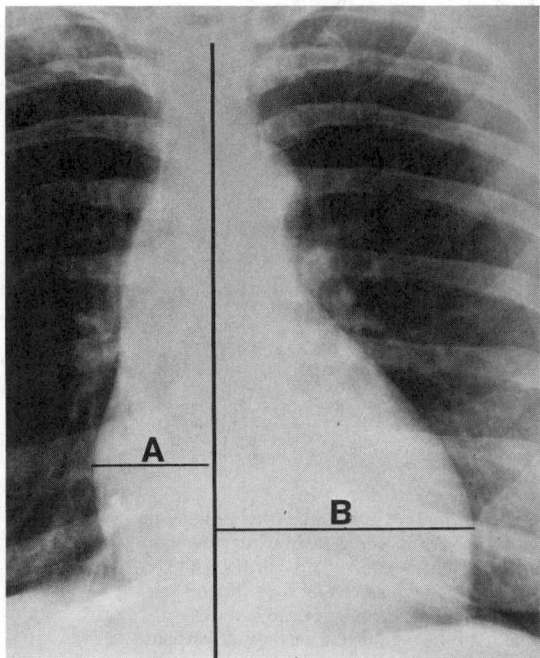

FIGURE 39–2. Measurement of the transverse cardiac diameter. Severe aortic stenosis with a 95-mm systolic gradient across the valve. The heart, although considerably hypertrophied, is normal in size and configuration. A vertical line is drawn through the heart. The greatest distance to the right cardiac border (A) and to the left cardiac border (B) are then measured. Transverse cardiac diameter = A + B.

CHAMBER ENLARGEMENT

Left Atrium

Dilatation of the left atrium alone, in the absence of a left-to-right shunt, is most often due to disease of the mitral valve, although it can also result simply from atrial fibrillation. The two "popular" roentgen signs of left atrial enlargement, a double contour within the right cardiac border and elevation of the left main bronchus, are both accurate when present but are insensi-

tive and not seen in about half of the cases of significant mitral valve disease. In order to produce a discernible margin within the cardiac silhouette, the thickness of the heart must increase sharply at some point. This occurs in mitral valve disease when the left atrium enlarges and protrudes posteriorly from the back of the heart. The right border of the left atrium is then silhouetted against the lung, and its contour is seen within the right side of the cardiac silhouette (Fig. 39–3A). This is not apparent with lesser degrees of left atrial enlargement. When the right atrium enlarges, as is common in longstanding mitral disease, it blends in with the enlarged left atrium and the double contour is lost. Thus, the double contour is not present with mild left atrial enlargement or in severe cases of mitral disease. Furthermore, the radiologic technique used for chest films is chosen to provide optimal images of the lungs. If the heart is enlarged, it will be underexposed and a double contour may not be seen within its opaque silhouette. For the same reason, the position of the left main bronchus often cannot be clearly visualized through the mediastinal shadow.

The most sensitive sign of left atrial enlargement in the frontal chest film is a convexity of the left atrial appendage segment on the left border of the heart (Fig. 39–3). The left atrial appendage extends anteriorly along the left border of the heart. When the appendage dilates, it forms a bulge on the left cardiac contour immediately below the main pulmonary artery segment. As the left atrium enlarges, it extends to the right and can form a portion of the right border of the cardiac silhouette (Fig. 39–3B).

Left Ventricle

The appearance of the dilated left ventricle depends to a large extent on the underlying cause. When it is due to insufficiency of the aortic or mitral valve, the ventricle elongates and its apex is displaced downward, to the left and posteriorly (Fig. 39–4). When the dilatation is due to coronary artery disease or primary myocardial disease, the ventricle tends to assume a more globular shape; thus, the apex is still displaced to the left. In the lateral view, the downward extension of the enlarged left ventricle covers more of the inferior vena caval shadow than normally. Thus, the crossing of the left ventricular margin with that of the cava occurs nearer to the diaphragm. Unfortunately, the practical usefulness of this sign is limited because a factitious appearance often results if the patient is rotated only slightly from a true lateral projection.

Enlargement of the left ventricle produces a smoothly curved dilatation of the lower left portion of the cardiac silhouette. A localized bulge in this contour most often represents a ventricular aneurysm (Fig. 39–5). Dilatation of the left ventricle is usually

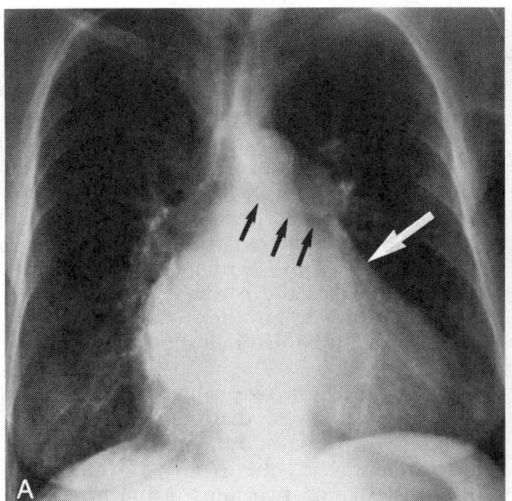
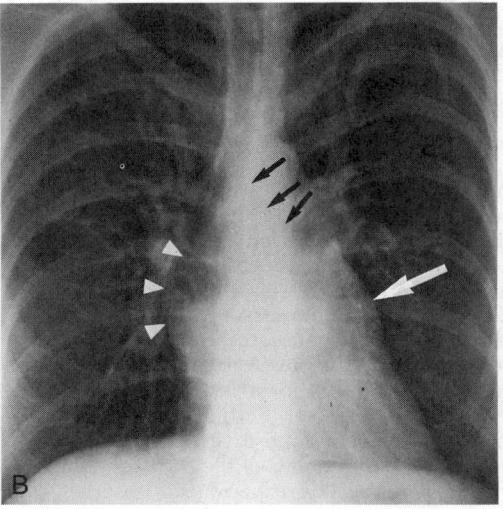

FIGURE 39–3. Left atrial enlargement in mitral valve disease. *A*, Patient 1: The enlarged left atrium causes the central portion of the cardiac silhouette to be abnormally dense. The right border of the atrium is seen within the right side of the cardiac silhouette. The left main bronchus (*small arrows*) is elevated. The region of the left atrial appendage (*white arrow*) is slightly concave because this structure was resected at the time of previous mitral commissurotomy. *B*, Patient 2: The enlarged left atrial appendage bulges from the left side of the heart (*white arrow*) while the body of the atrium (*arrowheads*) extends beyond the right atrium to form a part of the right heart border. There is no double density seen within the heart, and the left main bronchus (*small arrows*) is not elevated.

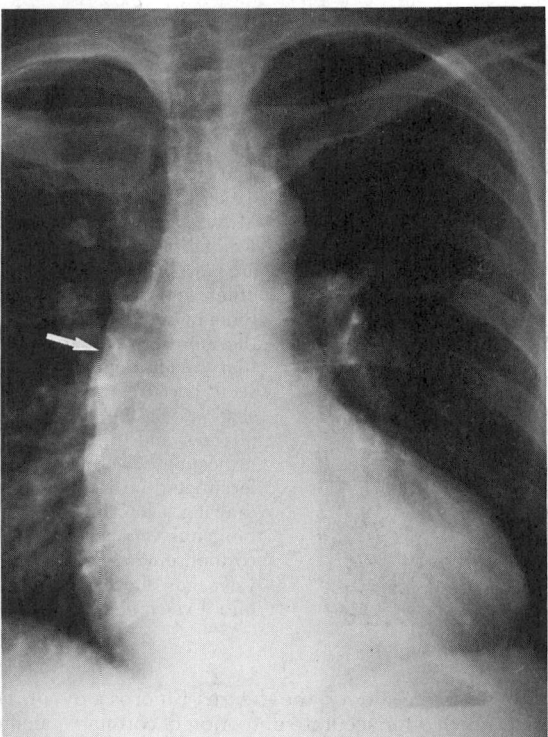

FIGURE 39–4. Left ventricular dilatation, aortic insufficiency. The apex of the heart is displaced downward and to the left. The ascending aorta (*arrow*) is diffusely dilated. The pulmonary vasculature is normal.

associated with elevation of left ventricular end-diastolic pressure. This increases the resistance to left atrial emptying and can result in dilatation of the atrium. Thus, left atrial enlargement in the presence of a large left ventricle does not necessarily indicate the presence of mitral valve disease.

Right Atrium

Enlargement of the right chambers of the heart alone is uncommon in adults. When seen, it is usually due to subacute bacterial endocarditis of the tricuspid and/or pulmonic valves, most often in drug addicts. Cardiac lesions involving the right

side of the heart also occur with the carcinoid syndrome. Dilatation of the right atrium causes an accentuation and outward bowing of its curvature on the lower half of the right cardiac contour. With greater degrees of dilatation, the cardiac silhouette enlarges to the right (Fig. 39–6).

Right Ventricle

The right ventricle is the most difficult of the four cardiac chambers to evaluate on chest films. Except for a small area in the subpulmonic region, the chamber does not form a border in the frontal projection. Even moderate right ventricular enlargement may produce no abnormality in this view other than some elevation of the main pulmonary artery. As right ventricular size increases, the transverse diameter of the heart enlarges to the left, and the cardiac apex may become elevated (Fig. 39–6). Thus, enlargement of either or both ventricles displaces the apex of the heart to the left. It is often not possible to distinguish between biventricular enlargement or dilatation of one or the other of the ventricles.

As the right ventricle enlarges, its area of contact with the sternum, seen in the lateral projection, extends upward and tends to obliterate the retrosternal clear space. This is a nonspecific sign, as it depends on the shape of the chest and the size of the left ventricle as well as the size of the right ventricle.

CALCIFICATION

Calcium deposits, because they have a greater radiodensity than the cardiac soft tissues, can be seen within the cardiac silhouette. Valvular calcification most often involves the mitral and aortic valves, and is consistent with significant stenosis. This is particularly true of the mitral valve. The calcium is deposited in irregular clumps, near the valve commissures. The two valves insert on a common fibrous tendon and are in contact with each other. They lie within the midportion of the cardiac silhouette in the frontal projection, just to the left of the spine (Fig. 39–7A). Determination of which valve is calcified may be difficult. They can be separated on fluoroscopy because the motion of the aortic valve approaches the vertical, whereas the orbit of mitral motion is oriented nearer to the horizontal. The distinction can also be made on films in the lateral view. If a line is drawn from the left main bronchus (seen as a circular shadow superimposed on the

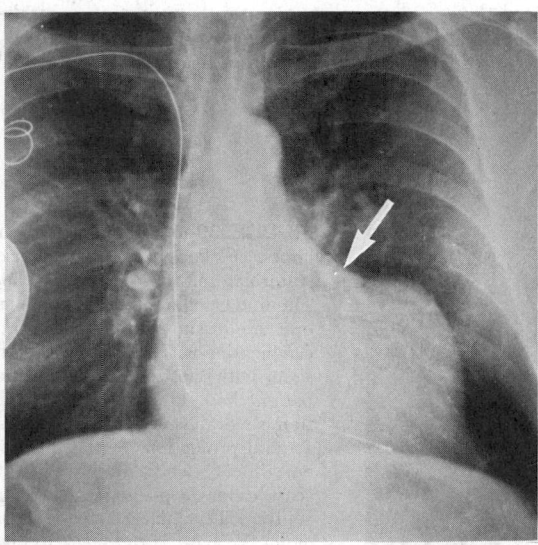

FIGURE 39–5. Left ventricular aneurysm. A bulge on the lower portion of the left cardiac border, formed by the anterolateral wall of the left ventricle, represents a ventricular aneurysm. The patient had suffered a myocardial infarct 1 year previously. The left atrial appendage segment (*arrow*) is normal. A transvenous pacemaker has been inserted through the right subclavian vein. The electrode tip is situated in the apex of the right ventricle.

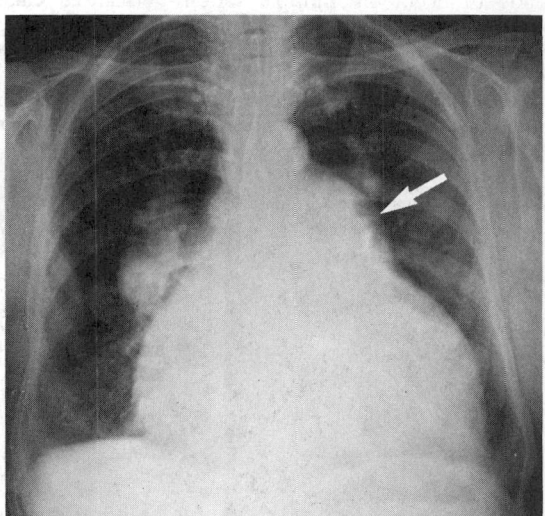

FIGURE 39–6. Right ventricular enlargement. Resistive pulmonary hypertension, secondary to atrial septal defect. The main pulmonary artery (*arrow*) and the right pulmonary artery are markedly dilated. The left pulmonary artery was also dilated but is hidden by the heart in this view. There is a sudden "cutoff" of the vascular shadows just beyond the hila. This is characteristic of resistive pulmonary hypertension. The right ventricle is enlarged, elevating the cardiac apex and displacing it to the left. The accentuation of the curvature of the lower right cardiac border and enlargement of the cardiac silhouette to the right are caused by dilatation of the right atrium.

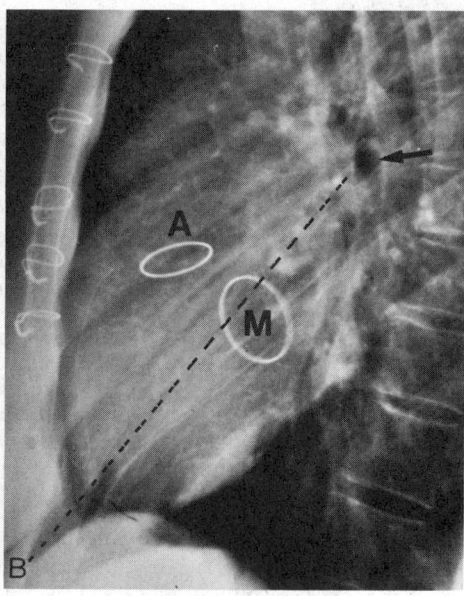

FIGURE 39–7. Location of the mitral and aortic valves. Both mitral and aortic valves have been replaced by porcine heterografts. The circular stents indicate the location and tilt of each valve. M = Mitral valve; A = aortic valve. *A*, Frontal projection. The two valves are normally in contact with each other, and it is difficult to separate them in the frontal projection. Furthermore, on a routinely exposed film, calcific deposits are not easily seen because of the overlapping shadows of the descending aorta (*arrows*) and the spine. *B*, Lateral projection. The valves can be differentiated on the lateral view by drawing a line from the left main bronchus (*arrow*) to the anterior costophrenic sulcus. The aortic valve lies above this line and the mitral valve below it.

lowermost part of the trachea) to the anterior costophrenic angle, the mitral valve is below this line and the aortic valve is above it (Fig. 39–7B).

Calcification of the mitral annulus, most often occurring in elderly females, can be distinguished from valvular calcification because it forms a heavy, relatively smooth curvilinear shadow in the form of an O or a C. Calcification of the wall of the left atrium, although rare, is virtually pathognomonic of rheumatic heart disease. It appears as fine, linear calcific shadows seen through the cardiac silhouette outlining the contour of the left atrium.

Calcification of the myocardium in coronary artery disease indicates a previous transmural infarct and frequently a ventricular aneurysm. The calcified scar is visualized as a fine, curvilinear density, most often on the anterolateral aspect of the heart, seen best in the frontal view (Fig. 39–8A), or in the lower portion of the interventricular septum, seen best in the lateral projection (Fig. 39–8B). Calcification of the pericardium is usually coarser and tends to occur in clumps. Often pericardial calcium is distributed in the interventricular sulcus and the atrioventricular grooves but when extensive, the deposits may coalesce and completely surround the heart (Fig. 39–9).

It is uncommon to see calcification of the coronary arteries on chest films because the deposits are thin and their shadows are blurred by the motion of the heart. Fluoroscopy or fast CT scanning is needed for accurate detection of coronary calcification. Although a high percentage of patients with significant coronary stenosis show coronary artery calcification, in individual patient assessment this is not a particularly meaningful statistic. Most of these data come from cardiac catheterization laboratories and are based on a highly selected patient population. The incidence of coronary artery calcification without significant accompanying stenosis increases with age, and calcification in asymptomatic individuals over 75 is of questionable significance. On the other hand, its occurrence below the age of 55 is highly significant. A search for coronary calcification is indicated in those younger patients with atypical symptoms that, in themselves, are not sufficient to justify coronary arteriography.

PERICARDIAL EFFUSION

The pericardium is a serosal lined sac containing a small amount of fluid. It completely invests the heart, except for a small area on its posterior surface between the entrances of the pulmonary veins and the superior and inferior venae cavae. When fluid accumulates in the pericardium, the sac distends smoothly, enlarging the cardiac silhouette and giving it a flask-shaped appearance. This shape can also be seen with a dilated, failing heart. Differentiation of the two conditions is readily made from

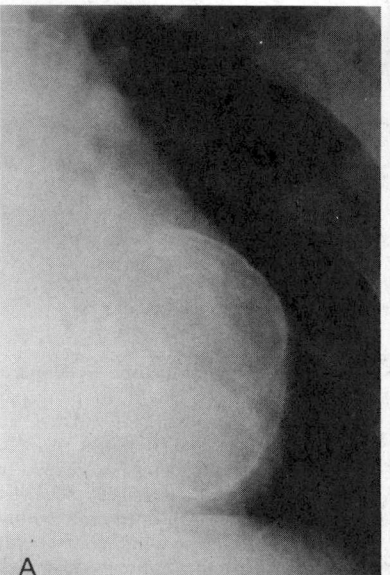
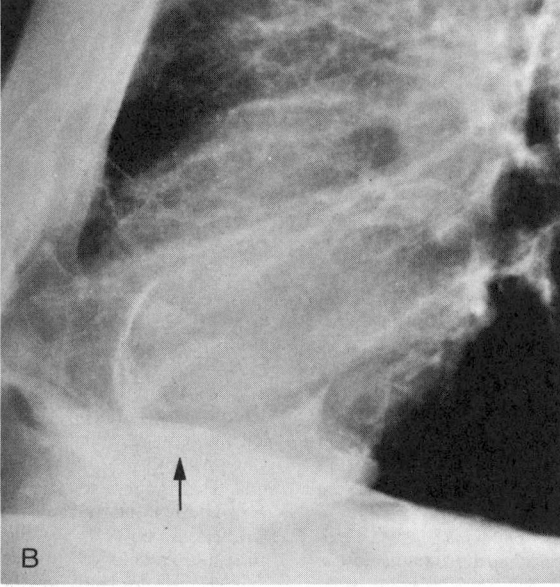

FIGURE 39–8. Calcified myocardial infarcts. *A*, Patient 1: Frontal projection. Anterolateral left ventricular aneurysm. The fine calcific line outlines an anterolateral aneurysm of the left ventricle. The calcific deposit is much finer than that seen with pericardial calcification. The patient had suffered a myocardial infarction several years earlier. *B*, Patient 2: Lateral projection. Septal infarction. The curvilinear calcific deposit is within the scarred lower portion of the ventricular septum. The infarct extended posteriorly along the base of the heart to involve the diaphragmatic wall of the left ventricle (*arrow*).

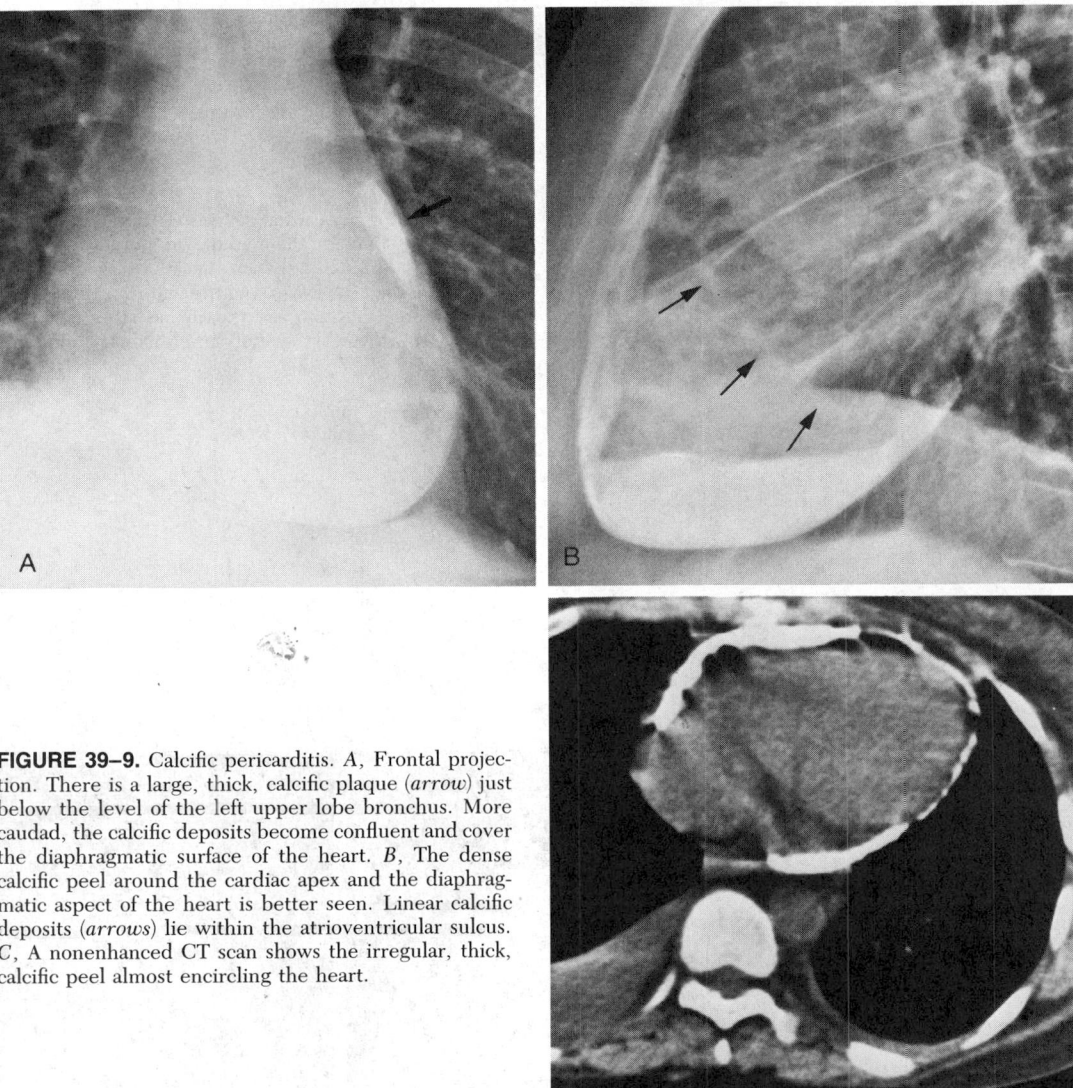

FIGURE 39–9. Calcific pericarditis. *A*, Frontal projection. There is a large, thick, calcific plaque (*arrow*) just below the level of the left upper lobe bronchus. More caudad, the calcific deposits become confluent and cover the diaphragmatic surface of the heart. *B*, The dense calcific peel around the cardiac apex and the diaphragmatic aspect of the heart is better seen. Linear calcific deposits (*arrows*) lie within the atrioventricular sulcus. *C*, A nonenhanced CT scan shows the irregular, thick, calcific peel almost encircling the heart.

the appearance of the pulmonary hila on the chest film and usually is apparent by echocardiography.

The pericardial sac extends onto the great vessels reaching to, or slightly above, the level of the bifurcation of the main pulmonary artery (Fig. 39–10). As the sac distends it tends to overlap and obscure the hilar vessels. On the other hand, as the heart fails, the vessels become congested and appear more prominent than normal (Fig. 39–11).

Posterior displacement of the epicardial fat line provides a second reliable sign of pericardial effusion. In adults, fat is often insinuated between the myocardium and the visceral pericardium (the epicardium). This is sometimes seen in the lateral projection as a curvilinear, radiolucent shadow outlining the anterior aspect of the heart. The outer surface of the parietal pericardium borders on the mediastinal fat behind the sternum. The soft tissue density between these two fat lines, therefore, represents the pericardium, the epicardium, and the fluid between them. When normal, this stripe is no more than 1 to 2 mm thick. As fluid accumulates in the pericardial sac, the epicardial fat line is displaced posteriorly and the pericardial stripe widens (Fig. 39–12).

PULMONARY VASCULATURE

Almost all of the linear shadows in the lung are cast by the pulmonary arteries and veins. The terminal branches of the vessels are too small to be visualized as individual structures. The same is true of the interstitial tissues that support the alveoli and form the primary and secondary interlobular septae. However, the summation of their shadows does give the pulmonary field an overall grayish cast. The large vessels are seen because they are set off against the surrounding air-containing alveoli.

INTRACARDIAC SHUNTS

The caliber of the pulmonary vessels reflects the volume of blood flow into the lungs. When this volume is diminished because of a right-to-left shunt, the pulmonary vessels become smaller and, as a result, the lungs appear more radiolucent. This occurs only when blood from the right side of the heart can bypass the lungs. Thus, even in severe isolated pulmonary vascular stenosis, the pulmonary vascularity is within normal limits. Increased size and prominence of the pulmonary vessels, both central and peripheral, usually reflect the increased pulmonary blood flow secondary to a left-to-right shunt (Fig. 39–13A). The vessels in the lower as well as the upper lung fields are dilated. Although the pulmonary arteries and veins become abnormally prominent when there is congestive failure, there are usually additional signs of pulmonary venous hypertension or interstitial edema which distinguish the appearance from that of shunt vasculature.

The vessels to the lower lobes carry about 60 to 70 per cent of

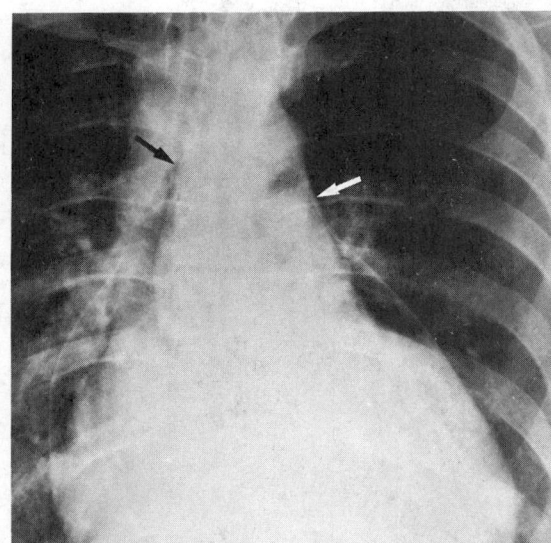

FIGURE 39–10. The superior pericardial reflection. Pericardial effusion following tap. During pericardiocentesis, some of the withdrawn fluid was replaced with air. The normal pericardium is now outlined between the intrapericardial air and the air in the lungs and is seen as a thin linear shadow along the outer border of the cardiac silhouette. The film is made in the erect position and the air has risen to the highest point of the pericardial cavity (*arrows*), above the level of the pulmonary hila and almost reaching to the aortic arch.

FIGURE 39–11. Hilum overlay sign. *A*, Pericardial effusion. The heart is diffusely enlarged. Its silhouette extends outward and obscures the hilar shadows in each lung. *B*, Dilated cardiomyopathy. The heart is diffusely enlarged. The failing left ventricle has caused congestion of the hilar vessels and they are more prominent than normal.

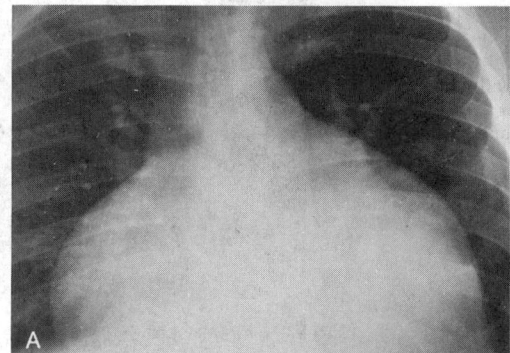
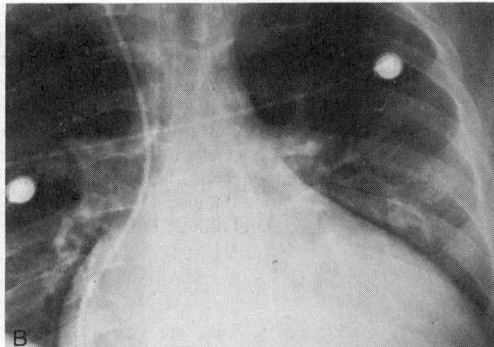

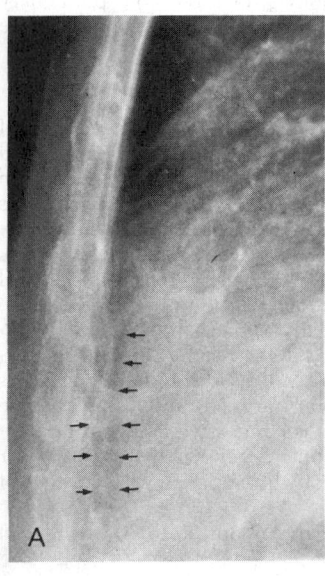
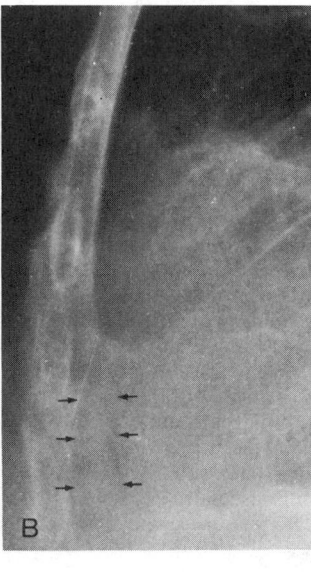

FIGURE 39–12. Pericardial effusion. Posterior displacement of epicardial fat line. The two lines of arrows point to the substernal fat and the subepicardial fat layers. *A*, Normal. The fine line of soft tissue density between the fat layers represents the epicardium, the pericardium, and the fluid between them. *B*, Same patient with a pericardial effusion. The epicardial fat line is displaced posteriorly, and the pericardial stripe is abnormally wide.

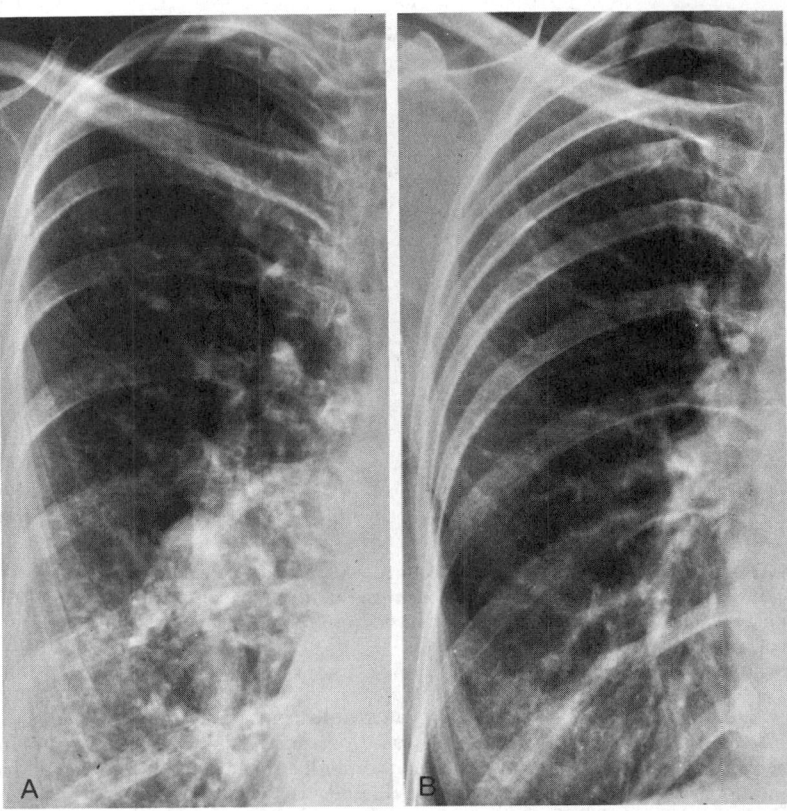

FIGURE 39–13. Pulmonary vasculature. *A*, Atrial septal defect, left-to-right shunt. All pulmonary vessels, to the lower lobes as well as the upper lobes, are dilated, indicating increased blood flow. *B*, Mitral stenosis, pulmonary venous hypertension with redistribution of the pulmonary vasculature. The lower lobe vessels are constricted and the upper vessels, which now carry more blood, are of greater caliber.

the pulmonary blood flow and normally are of greater caliber than the vessels to the upper lobes. As pulmonary venous pressure increases, the lower lobe vessels tend to constrict. This increases resistance to blood flow, resulting in blood being shunted to the upper lungs and dilatation of the upper lobe vessels. This redistribution of pulmonary vasculature is a reliable sign of pulmonary venous hypertension (Fig. 39–13*B*). With sufficient further increase in the venous pressure, interstitial pulmonary edema develops.

PULMONARY EDEMA

Normally, there is a constant circulation of fluid from the capillaries through the interstitium and back to the bloodstream by way of the lymphatics. As pulmonary venous pressure increases, more and more fluid leaks from the capillary bed, the capacity of the lymphatics is exceeded, and the interstitium becomes waterlogged. Because the interlobular septae at the outer bases of the lungs are oriented parallel to the x-ray beam on an erect film, when thickened, they can be seen as parallel, short, horizontal lines in the lung, above the costophrenic sulci (Kerley B lines). Kerley A lines also represent interlobular septae that are longer and usually are seen in the upper lung fields. They are within the depth of the lung and usually do not reach the pleural surface. Most of the other septae, although thickened, cannot be identified as individual structures, but their summation pattern creates random "noise" on the film that tends to obscure the shadows of the pulmonary vessels (Fig. 39–14). Edema of the bronchial walls and the peribronchial connective tissues causes the shadows of the bronchial walls to become thickened and less distinct. This "peribronchial cuffing" is most often seen in the superior portion of the pulmonary hilum, where the anterior segmental bronchus of the upper lobe is viewed on end. When the interstitium can no longer accommodate the excess fluid, it spills into the alveoli (Fig. 39–15). At this point, the typical auscultatory findings of pulmonary edema appear.

FIGURE 39–14. Interstitial pulmonary edema. *A*, Close-up of the right upper lobe. Portable film of a patient with acute myocardial infarct. The pulmonary vessels are well outlined. *B*, Two days later, the patient became tachypneic. There were no abnormal auscultatory findings in the lungs. Radiographically, the lung fields are noisy, with numerous, random shadows obscuring the outline of the pulmonary vessels. The appearance and the time sequence of the changes are characteristic of interstitial pulmonary edema.

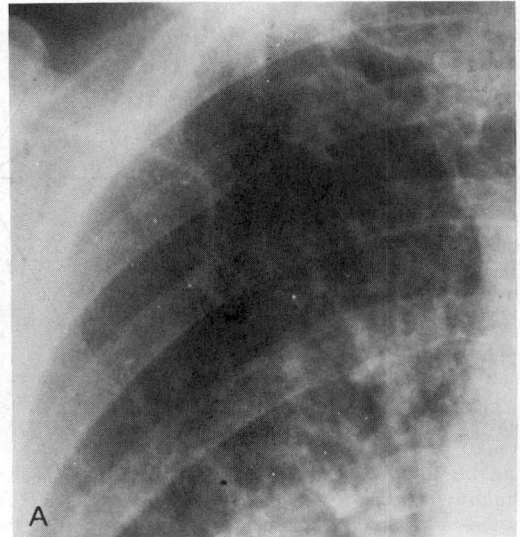
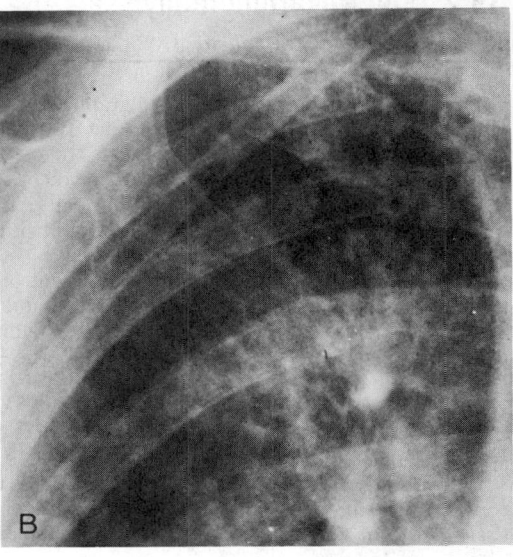

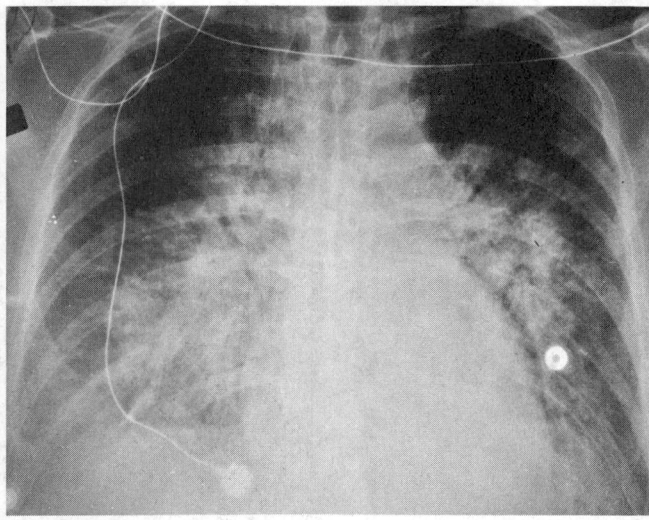

FIGURE 39–15. Alveolar pulmonary edema, acute myocardial infarction. There are patchy areas of consolidation in the perihilar regions of both lungs. Dilatation of the heart after a massive myocardial infarction may not be seen for the first 24 to 48 hours.

Pulmonary arterial hypertension can result from a left-to-right intracardiac shunt, mitral valve disease, or extracardiac disease such as repeated episodes of pulmonary embolization. The central pulmonary arteries become grossly dilated. Instead of gradual tapering as they bifurcate, there is a sudden, sharp change in the caliber of the vessels. The size and number of the smaller arterial branches decrease, creating an appearance that has been likened to a "pruned tree" (Fig. 39–6). With severe pulmonary hypertension, the right heart chambers may dilate. Once this picture of resistive pulmonary hypertension develops, it is difficult to determine whether the original cause was cardiac or extracardiac. The radiographic appearance of pulmonary hypertension is relatively specific but not sensitive. Clinically significant hypertension can be present with a normal-appearing pulmonary vascular bed.

Baron MG: Radiology and Angiocardiography. *In* Onkman FFY (ed.): The Ciba Collection of Medical Illustrations. Vol. 5: The Heart. Summit, N.J., CIBA Publications Department, 1969.
Chen JT: The plain radiograph in the diagnosis of cardiovascular disease. Radiol Clin North Am 21:609, 1983.
Felson B: The mediastinum. Semin Roentgenol 4:41, 1969.
Lane EJ Jr, Carsky EW: Epicardial fat: Lateral plain film analysis in normals and in pericardial effusion. Radiology 91:1, 1968.
Meszaros WT: Lung changes in left heart failure. Circulation 47:859, 1973.

39.2 Electrocardiography

Joseph C. Greenfield, Jr.

The electrocardiogram (ECG) is a graphic representation of the electrical activity generated by the heart during the cardiac cycle and is recorded from the body surface. In 1903, Wilhelm Einthoven used a string galvanometer to record the first EKG (Elektrokardiogramm, Ger.) Shortly thereafter, a clinically useful instrument was manufactured by the Cambridge Scientific Instrument Company. Following the pioneering work of Frank N. Wilson and his associates in the development of lead systems in the 1930's, the ECG became standardized and now consists of 12 leads. The recorders currently in use obtain at least three leads simultaneously, and many use digital processing to improve recording characteristics. At present, the ECG is the most commonly employed noninvasive diagnostic tool in cardiology. Approximately 90 million ECG's are recorded each year in the United States alone.

ELECTROPHYSIOLOGY. Cardiac muscle may be divided conveniently into specialized conducting tissue and myocardial tissue for contraction. Some cells of the specialized conducting

TABLE 39–1. POSITION OF CHEST LEADS

V_1	Fourth intercostal space (ICS) at the right sternal border
V_2	Fourth ICS at the left sternal border
V_3	Halfway between V_2 and V_4
V_4	Fifth ICS at the left midclavicular line
V_5	Fifth ICS at the left anterior axillary line
V_6	Fifth ICS at the left axillary line

When several sequential ECG's are to be obtained, e.g., in the coronary care unit, it is important to mark the location of the chest electrodes to minimize changes in the waveform resulting from variation in electrode placement.

A similar configuration on the right chest can aid in the diagnosis of right ventricular infarction.

tissue possess the potential for spontaneous depolarization, a process termed automaticity. The electrical activity of all myocardial cells is made possible by the presence of ionic gradients maintained across the membranes of individual cells.

Myocardial activation normally begins with the spontaneous calcium-dependent depolarization of cells within the sinoatrial (SA) node located at the junction of the right atrium and superior vena cava. The impulse propagates in a wavelike fashion through the atrial myocardium to the atrioventricular (AV) node located in the lower portion of the interatrial septum. Conduction through the AV node primarily involves the calcium-dependent process of depolarization and is delayed owing to membrane properties of nodal cells. The membrane properties in the proximal and distal segments of the AV node vary such that conduction in the proximal segment is slow and may occur with decrement, whereas conduction in the distal segment is more rapid.

The impulse is rapidly transmitted through the bundle of His, which bifurcates into the narrow right bundle branch (RBB) and the fibers that become the left bundle branch (LBB). The LBB divides further into two main collections of fibers forming the anterior (superior) and posterior (inferior) fascicles. The distal portion of the specialized conducting system is a network of smaller fibers, the Purkinje system, which delivers the propagated impulse to the remaining ventricular tissue, resulting in a synchronized myocardial contraction.

LEAD SYSTEMS. Ten electrodes are used in the standard ECG lead system. One is placed on each of the four limbs and six at different locations on the anterior chest wall (Table 39–1). The right leg electrode functions as a ground lead. In recording the standard frontal plane limb leads, I, II, and III, the right arm, left arm, and left leg are used as follows: Lead I measures the potential difference between the right arm ($-$) and the left

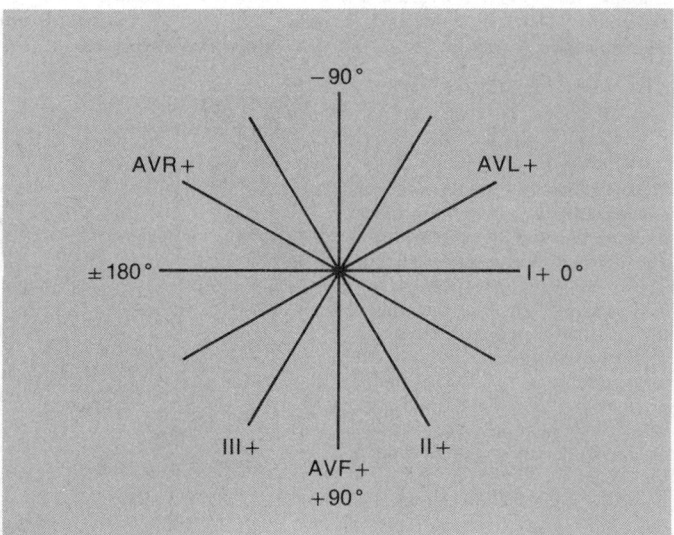

FIGURE 39–16. The limb leads are used to form a hexaxial reference system for the frontal plane. The axis of each lead is separated by approximately 30 degrees from the axes of the two adjacent leads.

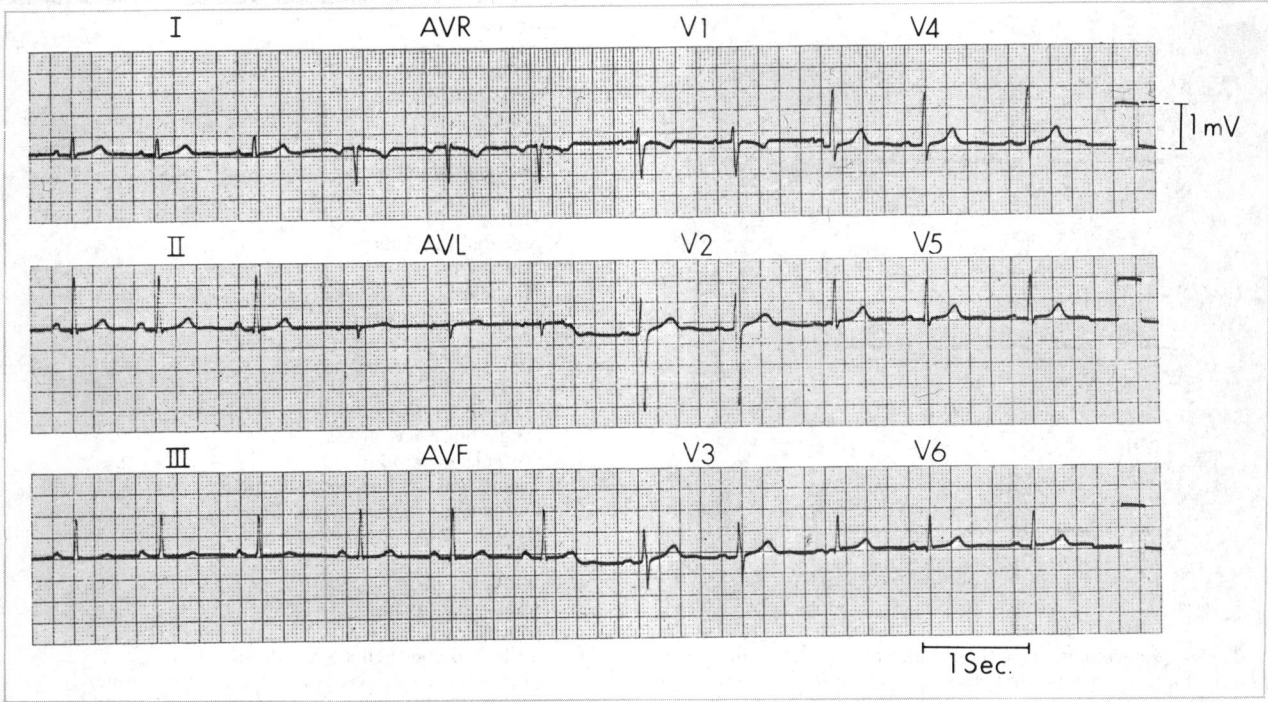

FIGURE 39–17. Normal electrocardiogram; the three leads in each column or lead set are recorded simultaneously.

arm (+). Lead II measures the potential difference between the right arm (−) and the left leg (+). Lead III measures the potential difference between the left arm (−) and the left leg (+). This is the original bipolar lead configuration designed by Einthoven. The other three frontal plane leads—aV$_R$, aV$_L$, aV$_F$—are constructed using a modified central terminal of Wilson, which augments the voltage output, hence the prefix aV. The exploring electrode, placed on the right arm (aV$_R$), left arm (aV$_L$), and left leg (aV$_F$), functions as a positive unipolar lead. The relationship among the six frontal plane leads is shown in Figure 39–16. The six chest leads also function as positive unipolar leads, using the central terminal as the reference point. The ECG leads are displayed in sequence, beginning with lead I, II, and III, followed by aV$_R$, aV$_L$, and aV$_F$, and then the chest leads from V$_1$ through V$_6$. A normal ECG recorded in this manner is illustrated in Figure 39–17.

Normally the ECG is recorded on a graph, using a standard paper speed of 25 mm per second. The paper is marked with a light vertical line every millimeter (0.04 second) and a heavy vertical line every 5 mm (0.20 second). The paper also has horizontal lines separated by 1 mm and a dark horizontal line every 5 mm. Vertical deflection is calibrated in terms of voltage, so that 10 mm equals 1.0 mV.

WAVEFORMS. The waveforms and intervals of the ECG are shown in Figure 39–18. The P wave reflects the electrical activity recorded during atrial depolarization and, in the normal ECG, precedes ventricular depolarization. The QRS complex occurs during ventricular depolarization. The Q wave is the initial downward deflection, the R wave is the initial upward deflection, and the S wave is the second downward deflection. A second upward deflection or a third downward deflection is defined as R' or S', respectively. A Q, R, and S may not be present in each lead; e.g., if the entire lead is negative, it is termed a QS wave. The time from the onset of the P wave to the beginning of QRS is the PR interval; normally the range is 0.12 to 0.20 second. The QRS duration normally is less than 0.10 second. The T wave is inscribed during the period of ventricular repolarization. The electrical activity during atrial repolarization usually is masked by the QRS complex. The interval from the end of QRS to the beginning of the T wave is termed the ST segment. The interval from the onset of QRS to the end of the T wave is the QT interval and is a function of rate. A small deflection following the T wave is the U wave; the precise origin of this waveform is unknown.

LEARNING ELECTROCARDIOGRAPHY. There are two general approaches to learning electrocardiography: (1) the pattern recognition method and (2) the spatial vector approach. In the former, the student memorizes the multiple normal and abnormal waveforms for each lead and gains the necessary expertise through experience in interpreting a large number of ECG's with clinical correlation. This technique is used by all experienced electrocardiographers, and illustrations of this approach are provided in the legends of Figures 39–21 to 39–25. In the spatial vector approach, popularized by R. P. Grant, the waveform is reduced to a vector representing the magnitude and direction of the mean electrical forces of P, QRS, and T. Using this technique, the student can quickly learn to define the normal ECG and the major abnormalities. This approach is based on the fact that the magnitude of a wave in any lead is a function of the relationship between the electrical axis of the heart and that lead (Fig. 39–19). From the hexaxial reference system of the six frontal plane leads illustrated in Figure 39–16, the spatial vector approach can be used to obtain the mean frontal plane axis for the normal electrocardiogram (Fig. 39–17). The QRS complex is

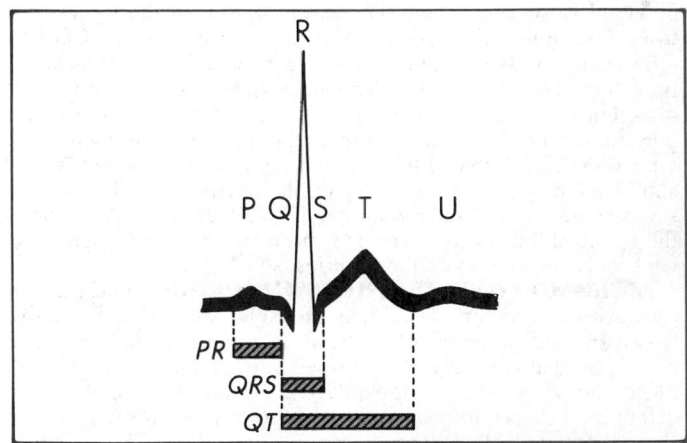

FIGURE 39–18. The ECG waveforms and intervals (horizontal bars) are illustrated. For description, see text.

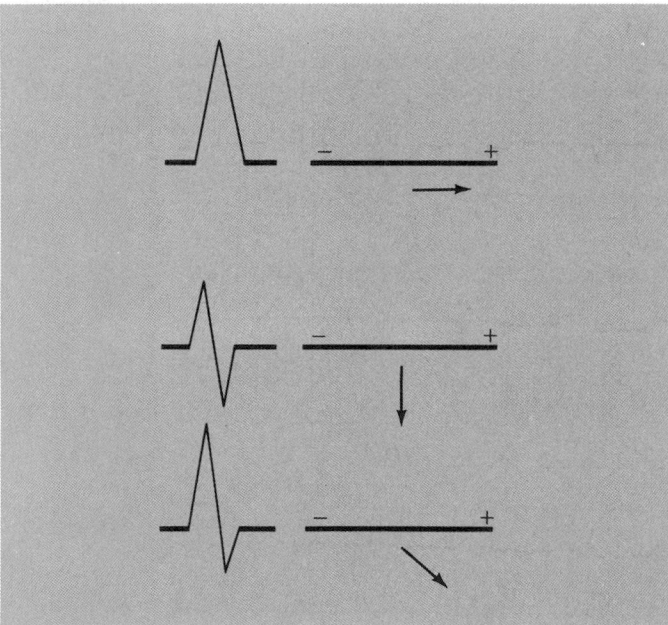

FIGURE 39–19. Determination of the relationship between the mean electrical axis of a wave and the waveform in a given lead. The top row depicts an entirely positive waveform; thus, the axis is parallel to the lead. In the second row the waveform is biphasic and the summation of the positive and negative parts is zero. In this instance, the mean electrical axis of the wave is perpendicular to the lead. (Note that the arrow could be drawn in the opposite direction and still be perpendicular to the lead.) In the third row, a biphasic waveform is shown in which the majority of the area is positive. The mean electrical axis is roughly at a 45-degree angle to the lead.

upright (positive) in lead I; thus the mean axis must be between +90 degrees and −90 degrees, i.e., on the positive side of a line perpendicular to lead I. Since the QRS complex is also positive in leads II and III, the axis must be between +30 and +90 degrees. Since the mean QRS complex is slightly negative in lead aV_L, the mean QRS vector is approximately +70 degrees. A similar determination then can be made for P and T waves. In the frontal plane, the mean P vector should be between 0 and +80 degrees, and the mean QRS and T vectors should lie between −30 and +90 degrees. A mean QRS vector more negative than −30 degrees is considered left-axis deviation and more positive than +100 degrees is defined as right-axis deviation. The angle between the mean QRS and T vectors in the frontal plane should be less than 80 degrees. Application of the spatial vector technique to the transverse plane is somewhat more difficult, since the six percordial leads do not define a precise reference system. An estimate of the vector can be obtained by noting when the waveforms make their transition from a negative to a positive deflection. In a normal ECG, the QRS transition is between V_2 and V_5, and the T wave makes its transition before the QRS. The next step is to determine the direction of the initial 0.04-second vector of the QRS. It is this portion of the QRS that defines the presence of myocardial infarction. The initial 0.04-second vector should lie between 0 and +90 degrees in the frontal plane; outside this range it suggests myocardial infarction (see Fig. 39–22). The direction of the terminal 0.04-second vector is used to aid in the diagnosis of ventricular conduction abnormalities (see Fig. 39–24).

APPROACH TO INTERPRETING AN ECG. The diagnostic categories in which an ECG may be useful are outlined in Table 39–2. In interpreting an ECG, it is important to develop a routine so that each aspect of the recording is carefully analyzed. Since the waveforms of the ECG are influenced to a certain extent by the age and body habitus of the patient, this information should be available to the electrocardiographer. The following eight sequential steps are useful for proper ECG interpretation.

1. *Quality of the ECG recording.* This includes proper stan-

TABLE 39–2. DIAGNOSTIC CATEGORIES IN WHICH AN ECG IS USEFUL

Arrhythmias	+ +
Electronic pacemaker function	+ +
Intraventricular conduction disturbances	+ +
Chamber enlargement	
Left and right atrial enlargement	+
Left and right ventricular hypertrophy	+
Myocardial infarction	
Old	+
Acute	+
Myocardial ischemia	+
Pericardial disease	
Pericarditis	±
Pericardial tamponade	±
Electrolyte disturbances	
Hypo- and hyperkalemia	+
Hypo- and hypercalcemia	+
Miscellaneous disorders	
Congenital heart disease	±
Muscular dystrophy	±
Emphysema and/or cor pulmonale	±
Pulmonary emboli	±
Hypothermia	±
Myxedema	±
Drug effects	
Antidysrhythmic drugs (e.g., quinidine)	±
Digitalis	±
Antineoplastic agents (e.g., doxorubicin)	±
Phenothiazine derivatives (e.g., chlorpromazine)	±
Antidepressant drugs (e.g., amitriptyline)	±
Antiparasitic compounds (e.g., emetine)	±

The symbols indicate the necessity for ECG to establish diagnosis:
  + + ECG is essential for diagnosis.
    + ECG is important for diagnosis.
    ± ECG may be useful for diagnosis.

dardization (Fig. 39–20), lead placement (Fig. 39–21), and identification of significant artifacts. The student must learn to evaluate the quality of the recording. Serious misdiagnosis can result if the quality of the ECG is ignored.

2. *Measurements.* The heart rate can be estimated adequately by employing the method outlined in Table 39–3. The amplitude, duration, and intervals of the various waveforms are measured in the standard frontal plane limb leads. Abnormality of the QRS duration, PR interval, and QT interval also is determined in these leads. Proper measurement of the waveforms is enhanced by simultaneous recording of three leads, since the interrelationships between the waveforms can be easily seen. The QT interval must be corrected for heart rate. The corrected QT interval (QT_c) is given by Bazet's formula:

$$QT_c = \frac{QT}{\sqrt{RR \text{ interval (seconds)}}}$$

and should be between 0.33 and 0.47 second.

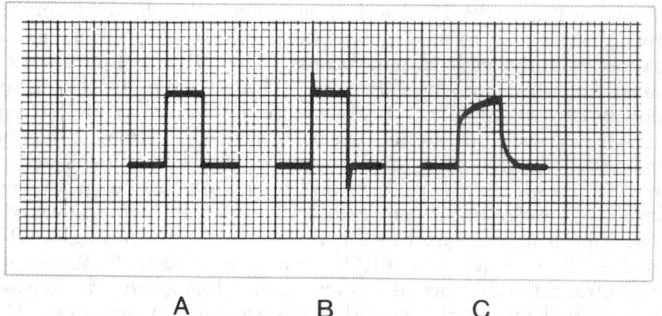

    A   B   C

FIGURE 39–20. In *A*, a correct standardization having a true square wave response is illustrated. *B* represents a standardization obtained from an instrument in which the response is underdamped; the amplitude of the waves will be spuriously enhanced. In *C*, the recorder is overdamped, resulting in both a spuriously decreased amplitude and an increased width of the waveform.

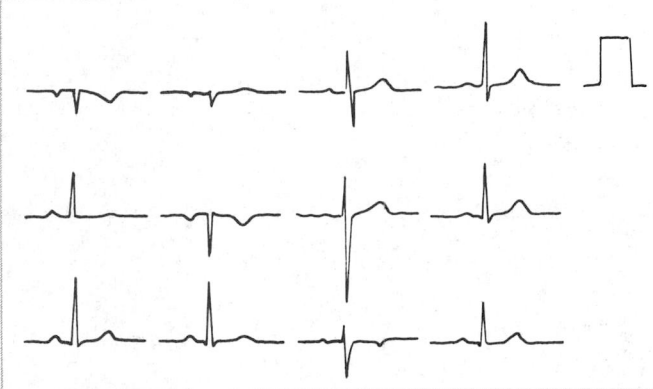

FIGURE 39–21. Two examples of incorrect lead placement from the same patient illustrated in Figure 39–17. Both the left and right arm leads and chest leads V1, 2, 3 are reversed. Reversal of the arm lead results in a mirror image recording of lead I and is easily recognized, since the P wave is negative. If missed, a spurious diagnosis of lateral wall infarction may be made. Reversal of the right precordial leads may result in an incorrect diagnosis of either right ventricular hypertrophy or posterior wall infarction.

3. *Determination of rhythm.*

4. *Examination of P wave.* Determine if atrial enlargement (see Fig. 39–23) or intra-atrial block is present.

5. *Examination of QRS.* Determine if myocardial infarction (Fig. 39–22), ventricular hypertrophy (Fig. 39–23), or ventricular conduction defect (Fig. 39–24) is present.

6. *Examination of ST segment.* Determine if abnormal displacement of the ST segment is present; depression is termed subendocardial (Fig. 39–25) and elevation subepicardial (Fig. 39–22) injury. The ST segment is shortened in hypercalcemia and prolonged in hypocalcemia.

7. *Examination of T wave.* Defining the significance of T-wave abnormalities is the most difficult aspect of electrocardiography. In general, marked T-wave abnormalities that occur either without other ECG abnormalities or with myocardial infarction are defined as ischemic or primary T-wave changes (Fig. 39–22). T-wave abnormalities that occur with conduction defects or ventricular hypertrophy are spoken of as secondary (Fig. 39–23). The T waves also are important in the diagnosis of drug effects and electrolyte abnormalities.

8. *Comparison with patient's previous ECG's.* It is extremely important to compare a new tracing with a previous electrocardiogram for two reasons: (1) Although the ECG may still be within the normal range, significant changes may have occurred; and (2) a comparison allows the electrocardiographer to date specific abnormalities that may have important therapeutic implications.

COMPUTER INTERPRETATION OF THE ECG. The development of algorithms to process and interpret ECG's has progressed to the point that, at present, there are several acceptable programs available for routine clinical use. Although these programs are important in decreasing processing time and enhancing storage, they must be viewed as an assist device to the electrocardiographer and not as a replacement.

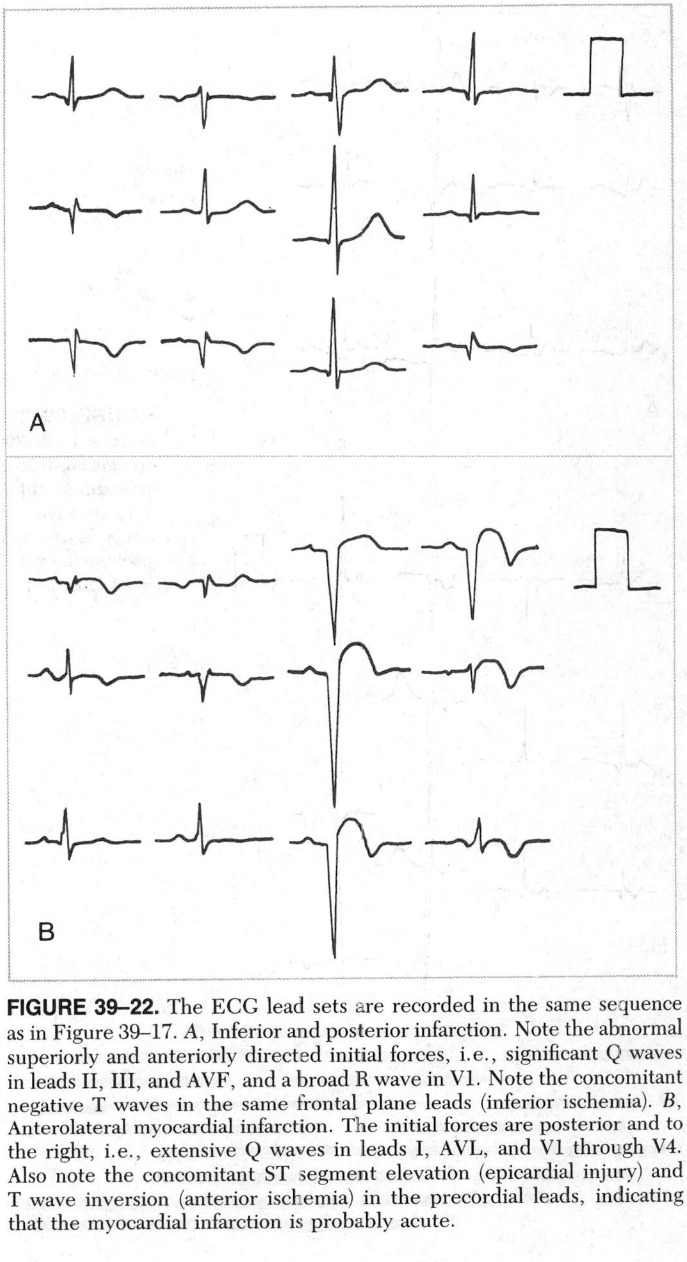

FIGURE 39–22. The ECG lead sets are recorded in the same sequence as in Figure 39–17. *A,* Inferior and posterior infarction. Note the abnormal superiorly and anteriorly directed initial forces, i.e., significant Q waves in leads II, III, and AVF, and a broad R wave in V1. Note the concomitant negative T waves in the same frontal plane leads (inferior ischemia). *B,* Anterolateral myocardial infarction. The initial forces are posterior and to the right, i.e., extensive Q waves in leads I, AVL, and V1 through V4. Also note the concomitant ST segment elevation (epicardial injury) and T wave inversion (anterior ischemia) in the precordial leads, indicating that the myocardial infarction is probably acute.

OTHER RECORDING TECHNIQUES. Several of the other ECG recording techniques and uses are described in Table 39–4.

The vectorcardiogram (VCG) is used to obtain a true orthogonal lead system (XYZ leads) so that the cardiac dipole is in the center of the chest. Since it is time consuming to record a VCG properly, it is not generally used. The VCG is primarily beneficial in

TABLE 39–3. DETERMINATION OF HEART RATE

Interval in Large Boxes Between Two Complexes	Heart Rate (beats/min)
1	300
2	150
3	100
4	75
5	60
6	50

The ECG recording paper is marked vertically by light lines; every fifth line is heavily marked. The time increment separating two heavy lines (one large box) is 0.02 second. To determine the rate rapidly, note the interval between two complexes and estimate the rate from this table.

TABLE 39–4. DIAGNOSTIC USES OF OTHER ECG RECORDING TECHNIQUES

Vectorcardiograms: old myocardial infarction, ventricular hypertrophy, ventricular conduction abnormalities
Body surface mapping: precise definition of instantaneous depolarization and repolarization—primarily experimental at present
Signal-averaged ECG: prediction of serious ventricular arrhythmias
Exercise electrocardiography: transient subendocardial or transmural injury
Ambulatory monitoring: arrhythmias, transient subendocardial injury
Transtelephone monitoring: arrhythmias, pacemaker function
His bundle recordings: arrhythmias and conduction defects
Esophageal leads: arrhythmias

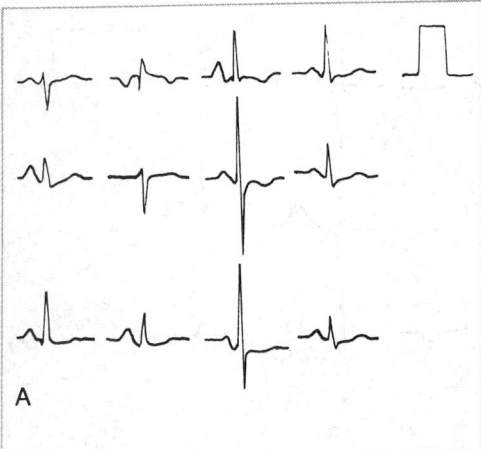

A

B

FIGURE 39–23. *A*, Right ventricular hypertrophy. The mean frontal plane axis is to the right, and there is excessive voltage in the right precordial leads. Also note the tall symmetrical P wave in lead II, indicating right atrial enlargement. *B*, Left ventricular hypertrophy. Note the excessive voltage in the lateral precordial leads and the inverted T waves in the same leads, indicating abnormal repolarization. The wide (greater than 0.12 second) biphasic P wave in lead V_1 is indicative of left atrial enlargement.

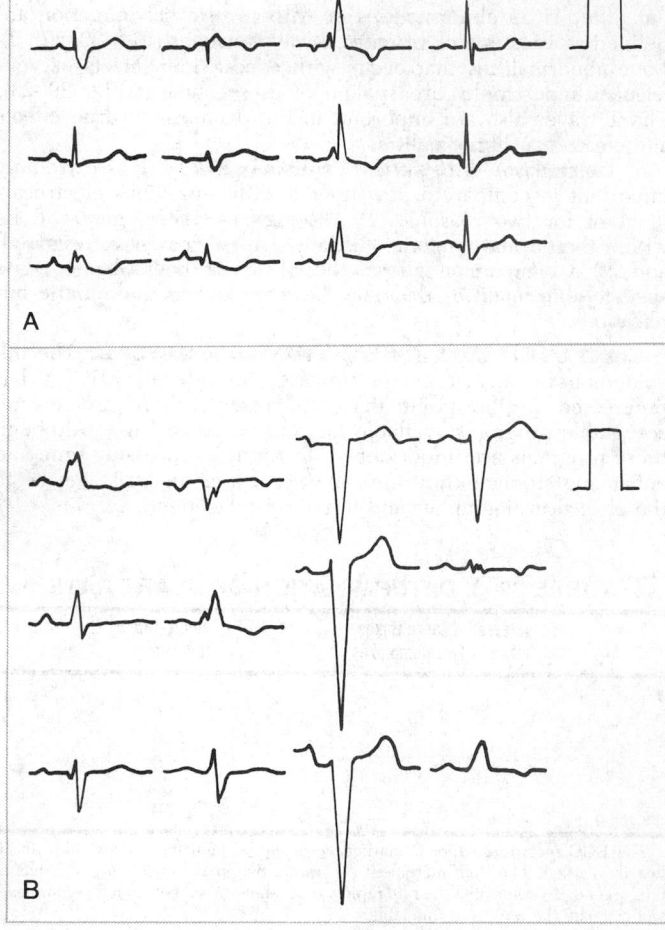

A

B

FIGURE 39–24. *A*, Right bundle branch block. The QRS duration is greater than 0.12 second, and the axis of the terminal 0.04 second of the QRS is to the right and anterior. *B*, Left bundle branch block. The QRS duration is greater than 0.12 second, and the terminal 0.04 second of the QRS is to the left and posterior. Note the secondary T wave changes in leads I and V_6.

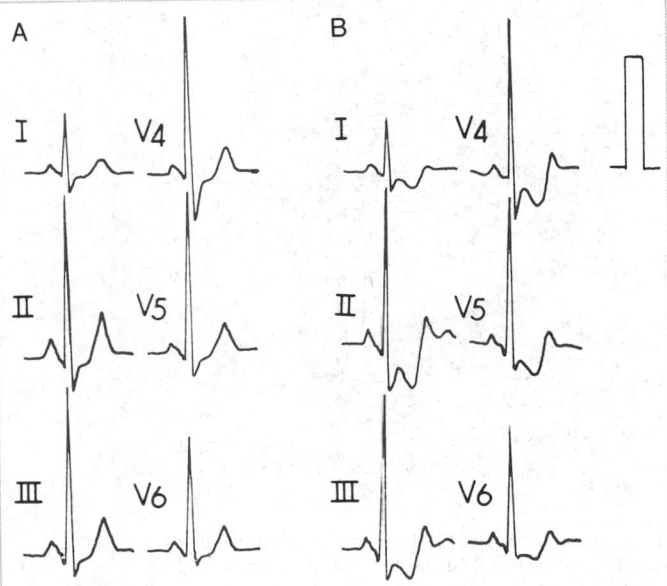

FIGURE 39–25. Recording obtained (*A*) prior to and (*B*) during an exercise test. Note the depression and downward sloping of the S-T segment wave during exercise. This is a typical pattern of subendocardial injury.

teaching electrocardiography and in enhancing the diagnosis of myocardial infarction, conduction defects, and ventricular hypertrophy.

A further refinement is body surface mapping, in which multiple precordial leads are obtained and a computer is utilized to generate a continuous body surface map of the change in electrical potential during depolarization and repolarization.

These techniques are still in the experimental stage, but ultimately may prove to be important in obtaining maximal information on the electrical activity of the heart. Low amplitude signals from the terminal part of QRS and the ST segment can be detected by signal averaging techniques and represent fractional conduction in infarcted regions. Current data suggest that the signal-averaged ECG may be useful in predicting patients with a high likelihood of having serious ventricular arrhythmias.

The ECG stress test is a widely used technique designed to assess the ability of the coronary circulation to deliver oxygen at a rate commensurate with the metabolic needs of the myocardium. Because myocardial metabolism is almost entirely aerobic, an inadequate increase in coronary flow quickly results in ischemia of the inner layers of the heart. The characteristic ST segment response is flat (square wave) or downward sloping. An abnormal ST segment is 0.1 mV or greater, measured 0.08 second after the end of the QRS complex (Fig. 39–25).

Chou TC, Helm RA: Clinical Vectorcardiography. 2nd ed. New York, Grune & Stratton, 1974. *Complete coverage of vectorcardiography.*

Lipman, BS, Massie E, Kleiger RE: Clinical Scalar Electrocardiography. 7th ed. Chicago, Year Book Medical Publishers, 1984. *Excellent general text covering all phases of electrocardiography.*

Marriott HJL: Practical Electrocardiography. 8th ed. Baltimore, Williams & Wilkins Company, 1983. *A comprehensive description of electrocardiography.*

39.3 Echocardiography

Richard L. Popp

PULSED REFLECTED ULTRASOUND

Echocardiography includes a family of diagnostic procedures that use ultrahigh-frequency sound waves to record the structure of the heart, and the blood flow velocities within the heart, throughout the cardiac cycle. Sound frequencies in the range of 1 to 10 million cycles per second, or megaHertz (MHz), are transmitted from a piezoelectric crystal along a carefully defined path within the thorax. A transducer is placed on the chest wall,

and a short burst of ultrasound is transmitted through the chest and into the underlying cardiac structures. The transducer then acts as a sound receiver until the next pulse. At each interface of materials with differing acoustic impedance, part of the sound is reflected or refracted and the remaining sound energy is further transmitted for subsequent acoustic reflection. The acoustic reflecting interfaces oriented perpendicular to the path of sound travel produce reflected sound that is received by the transducer on the chest wall as an "echo" of the transmitted sound. The location of each reflecting surface relative to the transducer can be calculated from the known velocity of sound in tissue and the elapsed time between sound transmission and reception of the echo. This series of depth readings is displayed on an oscilloscope for each pulse of sound, as shown in Figure 39–26. The strength of each echo is indicated by the brightness of the signal on the display device. Blood within the heart chambers usually gives signals of low amplitude that are not displayed. This "brightness-modulated" (B-mode) record of the reflecting interfaces is the building block for both two-dimensional (2D) and time-motion (M-mode) echocardiography.

One thousand pulses per second are created with typical instruments used clinically. A high sampling rate facilitates tracking motion of cardiac structures, yet there is usually enough time for the sound to return from even the most distant reflectors before the next pulse. Sequentially directing the sound beam along a given path, usually a pie-shaped sector of a circular plane, for each successive pulse produces a two-dimensional map of the structures underlying the transducer, called a 2D echocardiogram (Fig. 39–26). Clinical instruments sweep the sound beam through an arc of 60 to 90 degrees, by electronic or mechanical means, to create an imaging plane for visualizing a cross-section of the heart. Thus each 2D ultrasonic image is made up of multiple individual lines of sound reflection information. Depending on the basic pulse repetition rate, the time required for a single sound pulse to travel round trip through the thorax, and the number of such pulses per 2D image, 15 to 60 individual 2D image frames per second are available for interpretation. The images usually are presented on a digital scan converter that interpolates data between the scan lines and gives the impression of watching the heart in motion. The standardized examination provides multiple 2D cross-sectional planes through all parts of the heart using specific transducer locations, as shown in Figure 39–27. The dynamic three-dimensional structure of the heart can be understood by mentally assembling these multiple slices. An electrocardiogram is included as a reference signal in these studies.

A single direction of the sound beam, within the 2D image, may be selected for special attention and very high sampling rate. In this case, a given sound beam direction is repeatedly sampled, and the motion along the path of the sound beam is displayed with respect to time. The usual display is on an oscilloscope or strip chart recorder and is called a time-motion, T-M, or M-mode echocardiogram (right panel, Fig. 39–26). This method of recording is especially useful for identifying precise timing of motion of cardiac structures, such as valves, with respect to the electrocardiogram, phonocardiogram, or Doppler echocardiogram (to be described below). Historically, the M-mode echocardiogram was the first to be used.

Normal or abnormal patterns of cardiac chamber size and connection, wall thickness, wall motion, valve structure, and valve motion all are well assessed by echocardiographic study (Figs. 39–28 and 39–29). It is the method of choice for visualizing many abnormal structures, such as vegetations of infective endocarditis, intracardiac tumors, mural thrombi, and pericardial fluid.

During acute and chronic ventricular ischemia and acute infarction, the echocardiographic images accurately show the extent of myocardial thinning and segmental akinesis or dyskinesis. Exercise-induced segmental abnormalities may be observed as well. The acute complications of myocardial infarction that may be detected by imaging and Doppler echocardiography include pericardial effusion with or without cardiac tamponade, flail mitral leaflet (ruptured papillary muscle), acute mitral regurgitation of papillary muscle dysfunction, acute ventricular septal

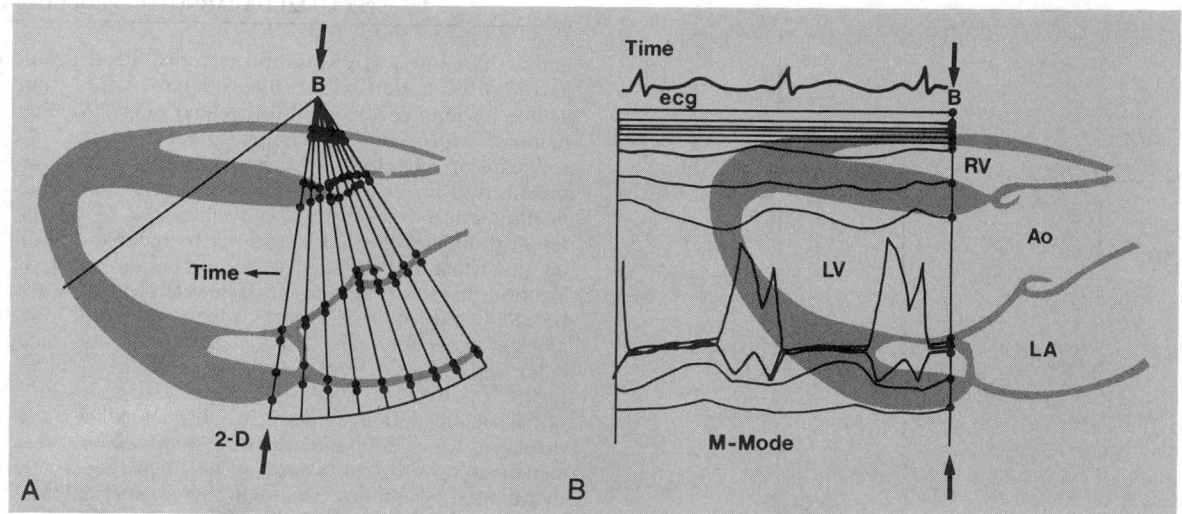

FIGURE 39–26. *A,* A schematic two-dimensional (2D) image of a cross-section of the heart oriented as displayed by echocardiography. The sound transducer is located on the anterior chest wall to the left of the sternum, at B. Sequential sound pulses and the returning echoes from reflecting interfaces are displayed as individual lines (*large arrows*), with dots of light defining the loci of reflectors. B = Brightness-modulated display. Many such lines, accumulated over 1/60 to 1/15 second, make up a single 2D image. *B,* A schematic time-motion (M-mode) echocardiogram produced by tracing out the location of structures moving during the cardiac cycle under a stationary sound transducer. As in *A,* the transducer on the chest wall creates a B-mode (B, *arrows*) display of sequential pulses and traces the motion pattern of each echo-producing interface. The M- and W-shaped patterns represent the anterior and posterior mitral valve leaflets, respectively. Ao = Aorta; ecg = electrocardiogram; LA = left atrium; LV = left ventricle; RV = right ventricle. (Modified from Popp RL, Rubenson DS, Tucker CR, et al.: Echocardiography: M-mode and two-dimensional methods. Ann Intern Med 93:844, 1980.)

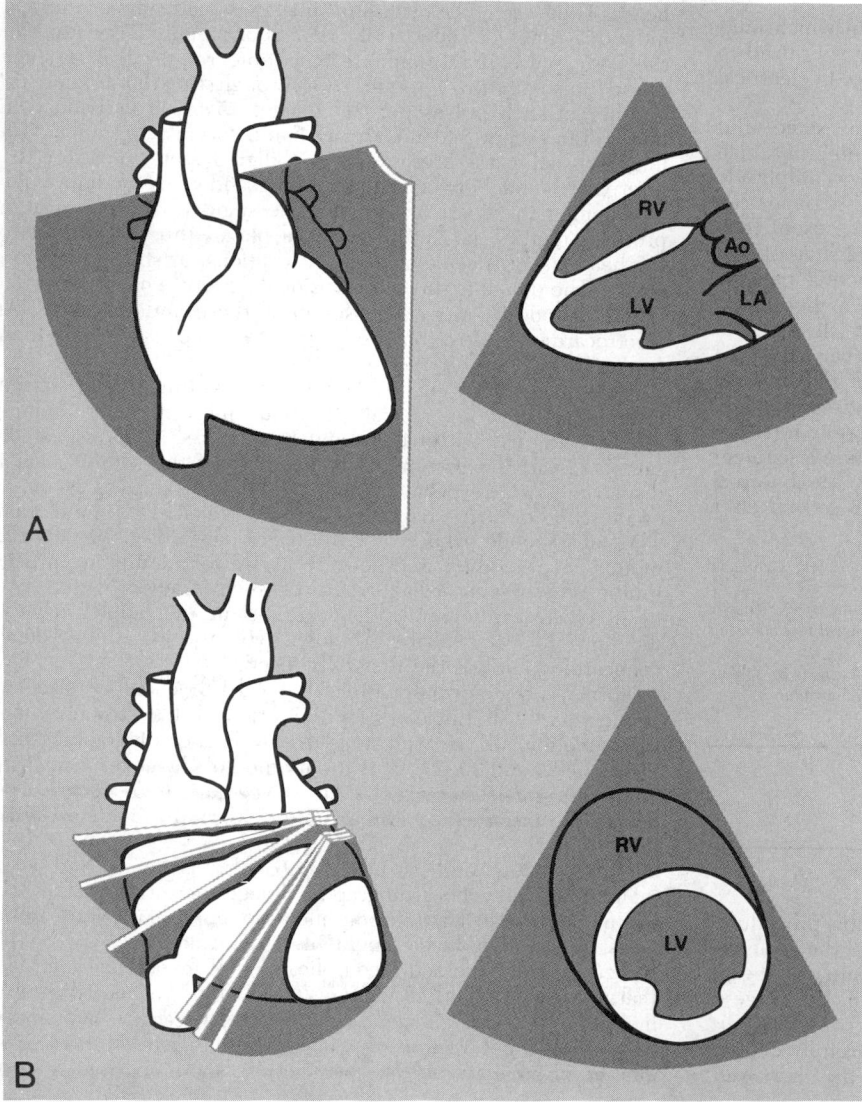

FIGURE 39–27. Schematic illustration of some standard 2D imaging planes used for clinical cardiac studies. *A,* Parasternal transducer position, with the imaging plane oriented parallel to the long axis of the left ventricle (LV) and intersecting a portion of the right ventricular outflow tract (RV), aortic root (Ao), and left atrium (LA). *B,* Transducer position as in *A,* but the imaging planes (six illustrated) are oriented parallel to the left ventricular short axis.

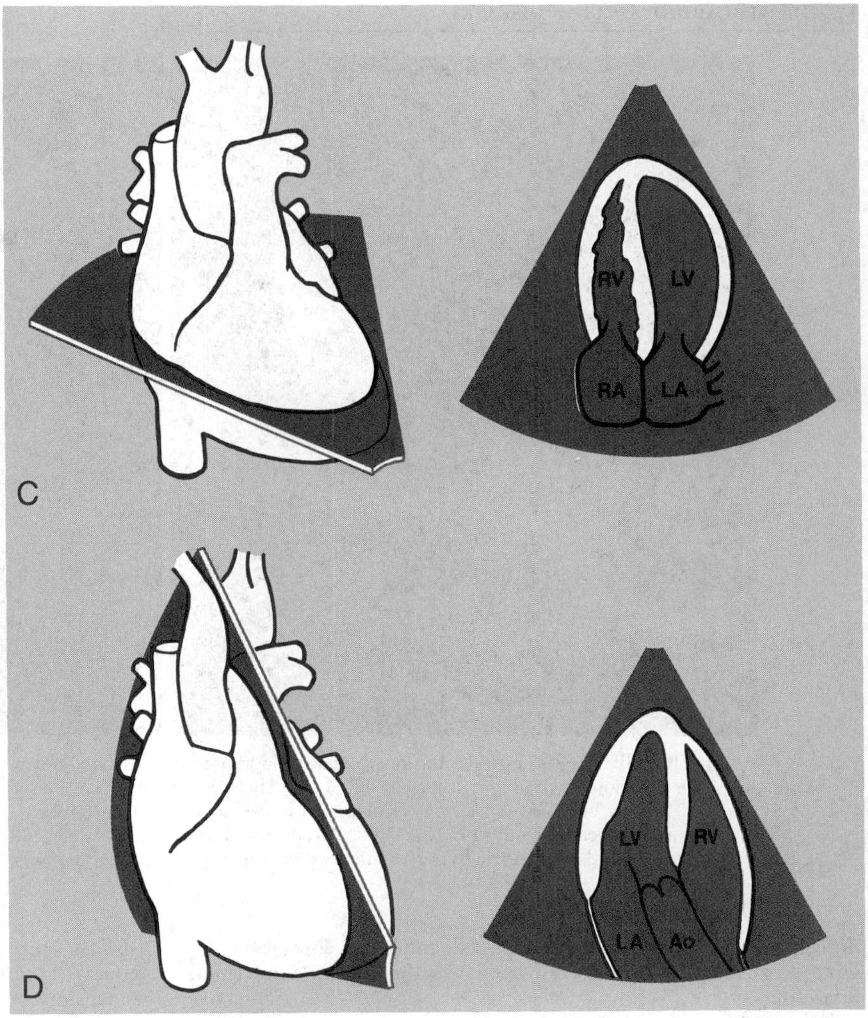

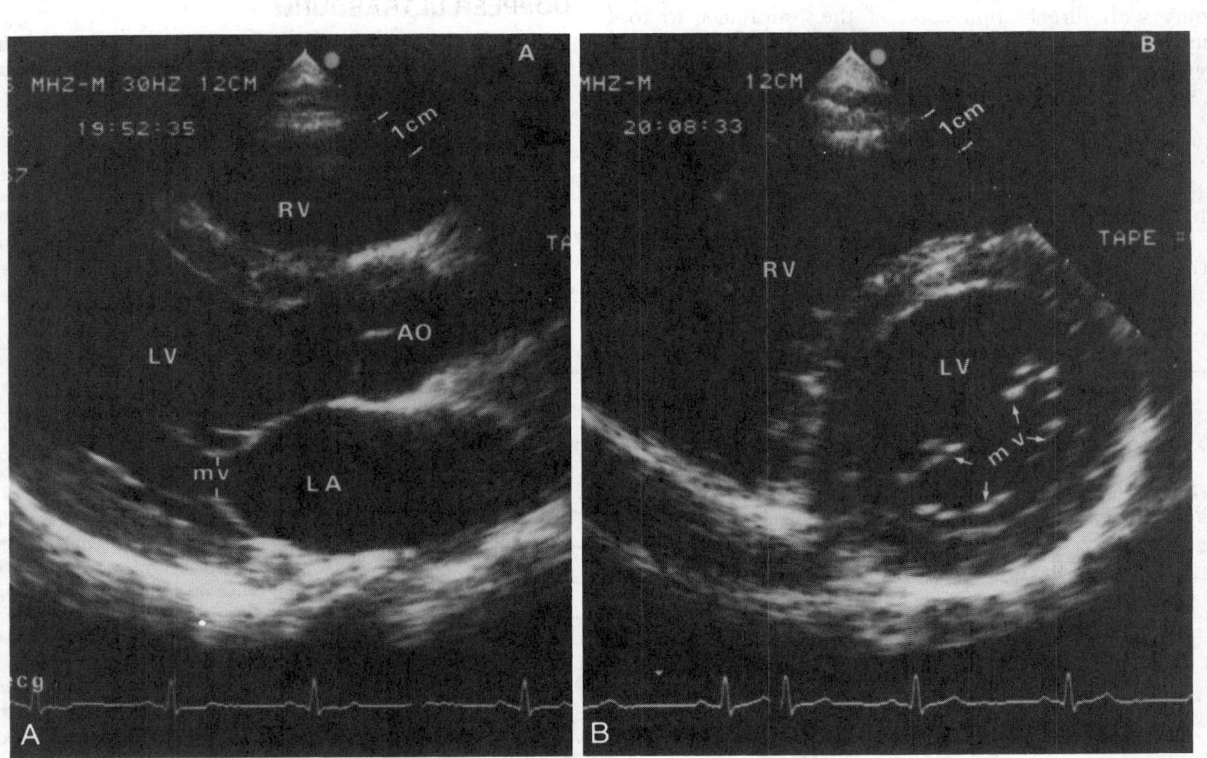

FIGURE 39–27 *Continued C,* Apical transducer position, with the imaging plane oriented to show the four main chambers of the heart (4-chamber view). The 2D image is displayed relative to the transducer so that the cardiac apex is shown near the transducer. RA = right atrium. *D,* Transducer position as in *C,* but the imaging plane is oriented parallel to the left ventricular long axis, as in panel *A.* (Redrawn from Popp RL, Fowles RE, Coltart DJ, et al.: Cardiac anatomy viewed systematically with two-dimensional echocardiography. Chest 75:579, 1979.)

FIGURE 39–28. Two-dimensional echocardiographic images of a normal heart. Panels *A* and *B* were obtained with transducer positions and imaging plane orientations as shown in Figure 39–27*A* and *B,* respectively. Abbreviations as in Figure 39–27. mv = Mitral valve leaflets. (Note depth calibration scale at 1-cm intervals along right margin of each image.) The electrocardiograms (ecg) at the bottom of the panels are interrupted to indicate the timing of each image frame (late diastole in *A,* early diastole in *B*).

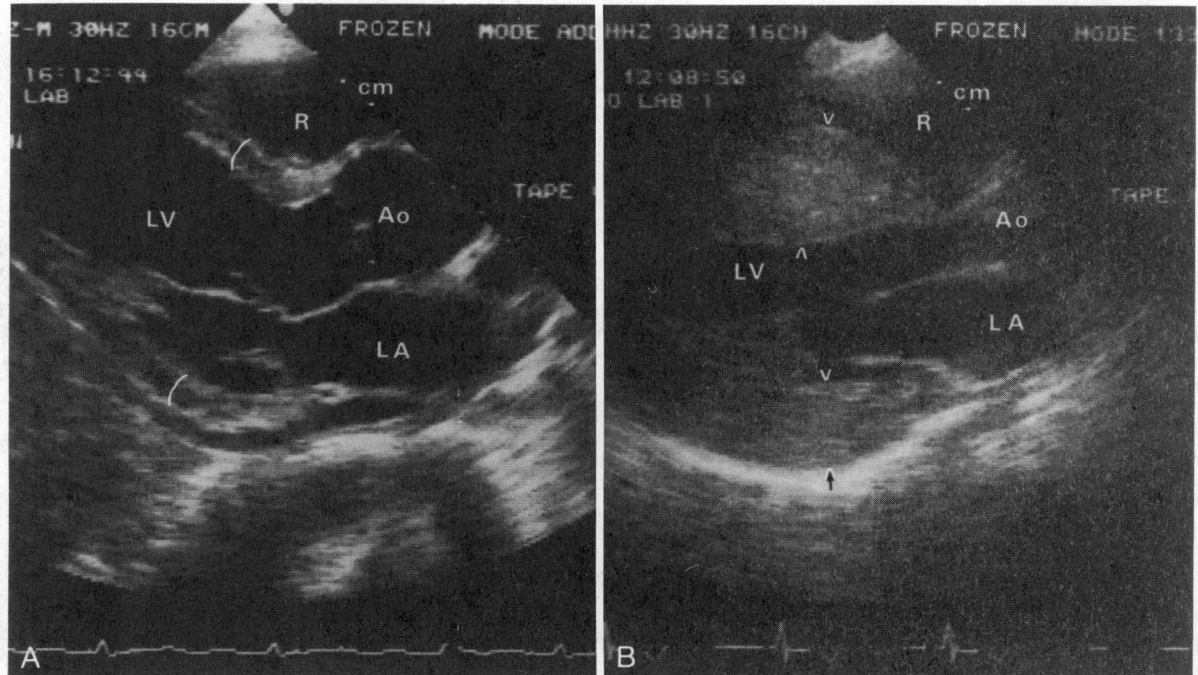

FIGURE 39–29. Two-dimensional echocardiographic images obtained with transducer position and image plane orientation as shown in Figure 39–27A. *A,* The left ventricle (LV) has normal wall thickness (white brackets). A relatively echo-free space posterior to the lower bracket, and extending toward the left atrium (LA), represents a small pericardial effusion. *B,* The LV cavity is small and the walls (*arrowheads*) are massively thickened in a patient with concentric hypertrophic cardiomyopathy. Ao = Aorta; cm = centimeter scale; R = right ventricle.

defect, myocardial rupture with pseudoaneurysm formation, infarct expansion producing true aneurysm, and right ventricular infarction.

Echocardiographic imaging also may be performed "invasively," as when transesophageal transducers are used or during thoracotomy with direct application of the transducer to the epicardium. These approaches produce superb images owing both to lack of sound scattering in the thorax and to the feasibility of using very high-frequency (5 to 10 MHz) ultrasound, which has high physical resolution but poor soft tissue penetration. Intravenous injections of many fluids, such as physiologic saline solution, contain myriad microbubbles of gas, which may be visualized by echocardiography as they travel through the right side of the heart. The gas does not pass through the pulmonary capillary bed, so if microbubble echoes are seen immediately in the left side of the heart, one may assume an intracardiac shunt is present, and a delayed appearance implies an intrapulmonary

shunt. Direct intra-aortic or intracoronary injection of various contrast agents has been used in attempts to visualize coronary perfusion areas of the left ventricle and experimentally to assess washout rates with altered coronary flow.

DOPPLER ULTRASOUND

Sound energy is transmitted as a series of compression-rarefaction waves with a given periodicity or wave frequency. Sound reflected from stationary surfaces has the same basic frequency as the transmitted sound, as shown in Figure 39–30. However, if the reflector or reflectors are moving relative to the direction of sound transmissions, the sequential interaction of the compression-rarefaction waves with the reflector results in a change in the frequency of the sound, as shown in Figure 39–30. This frequency shift is the Doppler effect, and it enables calculation of the velocity of the reflector if one knows the originally transmitted frequency, the received frequency, the speed of

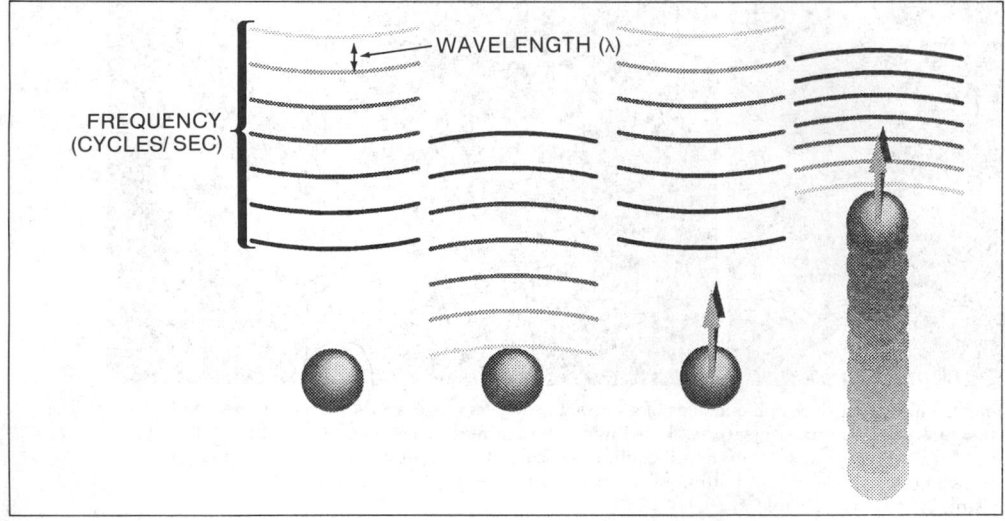

FIGURE 39–30. Schematic diagram of the Doppler principle as applied in echocardiography. From left to right: Sound waves of a given frequency (cycles/sec) and wave length (λ) are transmitted into the chest. Sound reflected from a stationary target has the same frequency as that transmitted. Sound directed toward a moving target interacts with the reflector and alters the frequency of the returning sound by a factor related to the speed of the moving target, the original sound frequency, and the angle of interception of the two.

sound in the medium (soft tissues), and the angle between the sound beam and the direction of the moving reflectors. The moving column of blood, with its cells and fluctuations in spatial distribution of cells, is the source of the Doppler frequency shift measured by echocardiography. An indicator of the beam direction undergoing Doppler frequency analysis is superimposed on the 2D image to help orientation and facilitate placing the beam in the general direction of flow. Fortunately, the change in frequency obtained with clinical instruments is in the audible range, so one may optimally match the direction of the sound beam with the direction of the blood flow by adjusting the transducer while listening to the signal. A beam-to-flow angle of zero degrees is desirable, since the calculated velocity is a function of the cosine of this angle (cos $0° = 1$), but an angle of up to 20 degrees produces underestimation of velocities of up to only 6 per cent.

Blood flow toward or away from the transducer produces an increase or decrease in sound frequency, respectively, so both the velocity and the direction of the blood are measurable. These signals are usually displayed with velocities calculated from received Doppler shifted frequencies plotted versus time. The velocity spectrum is arranged above or below a baseline to convey information on flow direction, as shown in Figures 39–31 and 39–32.

Pulsed wave (PW) Doppler echocardiography is performed with pulses of ultrasound as described above, and frequency analysis is possible for sound returning from any given distance from the transducer. Thus, a signal received during systole from the left atrium and indicating high-velocity flow directed into the atrium from the ventricle signifies mitral regurgitation. This technique has proved especially valuable in locating intracardiac shunts, such as atrial or ventricular septal defects (Fig. 39–31) and patent ductus arteriosus. Since the product of the mean flow velocity (centimeters per second) and cross-sectional flow area (square centimeters) is volumetric flow (cubic centimeters per second), flow within the pulmonary artery or left ventricular outflow tract, or across the tricuspid or mitral valves, can be estimated. Comparison of flows across the pulmonary artery and aorta gives an estimate of shunt flow across the septal defects, for example. Measurement of cardiac output by this method is useful clinically; however, the procedure is technically demanding.

PW methods provide spatial resolution but have limited velocity resolution because of the physical-mathematical constraints of sampling periodically. This trade-off is the opposite of that with continuous wave (CW) Doppler echocardiography, which uses one transducer to transmit, and another to receive, reflected sound continuously. CW Doppler methods have no spatial resolution within the path of the beam but can display frequency shifts corresponding to very high flow velocities. A major series of applications of Doppler echocardiography derives from the relationship of measured velocities to corresponding drops in pressure within the heart or vascular system. A cardiac valve stenosis presents an obstacle to flowing blood, which results in an increased velocity through the area of obstruction. This convective acceleration is the major factor producing a drop in pressure (ΔP, or pressure gradient) across the stenosis. The pressure difference can be accurately estimated instantaneously by CW Doppler echocardiography from the maximum flow velocity (V) achieved ($\Delta P = 4V^2$), as first shown by Holen and co-workers (1976). The ability to obtain intracardiac and intravascular pressure information noninvasively has been a significant advance in the capabilities of echocardiography. Many patients with aortic or mitral stenosis or both now have adequate preoperative hemodynamic assessment on the basis of clinical features and echocardiography only. The method for calculating instantaneous and mean pressure drops across a stenotic aortic valve is shown in Figure 39–32.

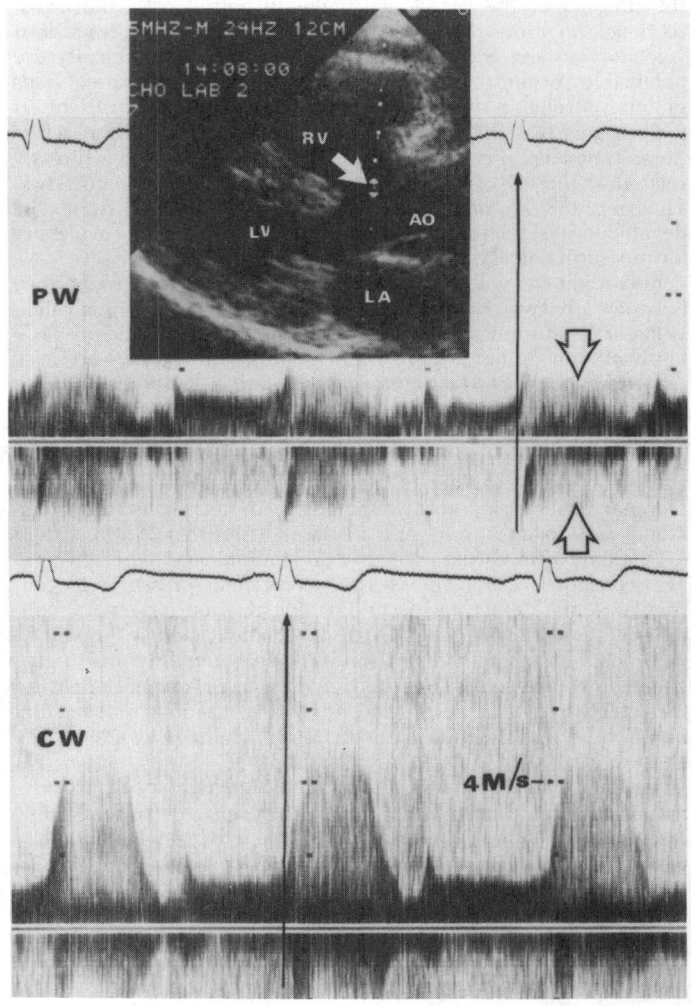

FIGURE 39–31. Methods of displaying a Doppler echocardiographic study in a patient with ventricular septal defect. The black panel above is a 2D image taken with transducer position and image plane orientation as in Figure 39–27A. The white arrow points to the sample volume indicator for pulsed-wave (PW) Doppler ultrasound analysis. This illustration is from a patient with a large defect of the septum between the right ventricle (RV) and left ventricle (LV). The white panels below are spectral displays of the Doppler ultrasound signals in a patient with a small ventricular septal defect. The PW record indicates a frequency shift (*open arrows*) from the area of the sample volume (above), which occurs in systole after the onset of the electrocardiographic QRS (*long arrow*). The continuous-wave (CW) record indicates high-velocity (>4 M/s) flow somewhere along the dotted line shown above. The systolic pressure difference between the right and left ventricles can be calculated from the CW signal as shown in Figure 39–32. The location of the signal origin is defined by PW, while the CW signal defines high-flow velocity quantitatively but is ambiguous regarding signal locus. Other abbreviations as in Figure 39–26.

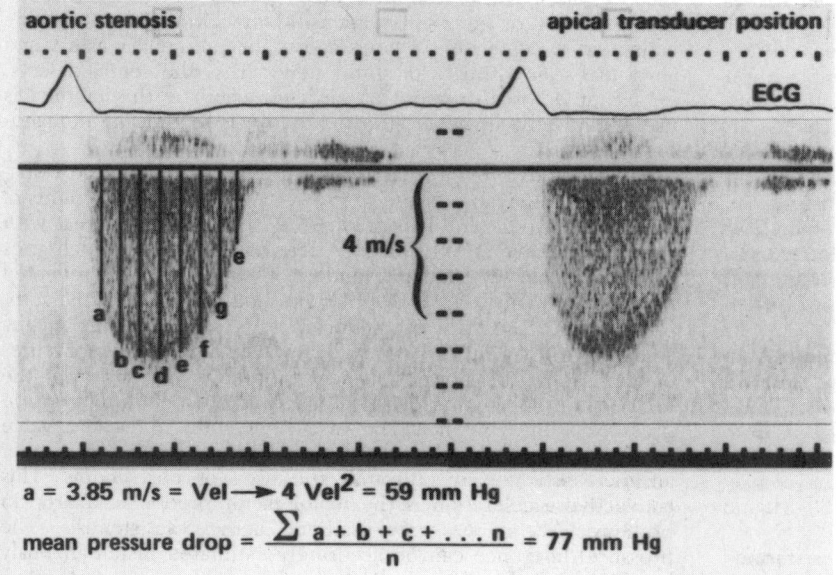

aortic stenosis — **apical transducer position**

ECG

4 m/s

$$a = 3.85 \text{ m/s} = \text{Vel} \longrightarrow 4 \text{ Vel}^2 = 59 \text{ mm Hg}$$

$$\text{mean pressure drop} = \frac{\sum a + b + c + \ldots n}{n} = 77 \text{ mm Hg}$$

FIGURE 39–32. Continuous-wave Doppler ultrasound recording of aortic outflow velocities from a patient with aortic stenosis. The transducer is at the apex, so flow toward the aorta is registered below the baseline in this spectral display of velocity (M/s) versus time. The systolic signal occurs after each QRS of the electrocardiogram (ECG). Instantaneous (vertical lines a through e) maximum velocities (Vel) are assumed to occur in the most narrow part of the stenosis and to correspond to instantaneous pressure drops across the stenosis. The formulae for calculating the instantaneous and mean pressure drops in mm Hg are given below. n = Number of samples.

The pressure drop across a stenotic valve is dependent on both the valve area and the blood volume crossing the valve per unit of time. Aortic valve area is accurately estimated by applying the Gorlin formula (see Ch. 39.5) using Doppler ultrasound–derived values for ejection time, stroke volume, and pressure gradient. Alternatively, one may calculate the flow per beat (see above) from the mean flow velocity and cross-sectional area of the left ventricular outflow tract immediately below the stenotic valve and assume that this same flow is represented by the product of the mean flow velocity within, and the cross-sectional area of, the stenotic valve. The outflow tract flow velocity, outflow tract area, and aortic valve flow velocity are obtainable, permitting calculation of the aortic valve area. This method is reliable even when aortic regurgitation is present. It is fortuitous that the time required for the pressure drop across the mitral valve to reach one half of the maximum level is directly related to the valve area at virtually all clinically relevant flows. Thus mitral valve area may be accurately calculated from data developed by Holen and colleagues (1977) without the necessity for measuring stroke volume.

Recording the velocity of blood flowing across a narrow orifice between any two chambers or cardiovascular loci permits calculation of the absolute pressure level in one chamber if the pressure in the other chamber is known. For example, the systolic pressure difference between the right ventricle and right atrium can be calculated from the velocities recorded from tricuspid regurgitant flow. The sum of jugular venous or right atrial pressure and the atrioventricular pressure difference is the right ventricular systolic pressure. The prevalence of tricuspid regurgitation detectable by Doppler echocardiography sufficient to perform this calculation ranges from over 70 per cent (in normal subjects) to 80 per cent (in patients with cardiomyopathy and pulmonary hypertension). This concept is useful in assessing ventricular pressures in ventricular septal defect and is under investigation for several conditions. Quantitating the pressure gradient across prosthetic valves and assessing the central or perivalvular origin of regurgitant prosthesis leaks noninvasively are major advances because the alternative of catheter placement to get similar information may require trans-septal catheterization of the left side of the heart or direct left ventricular puncture.

Advancing microprocessor technology for high-speed processing of ultrasonic echoes has permitted superposition of flow direction and velocity information, obtained from Doppler frequency shift analysis throughout the imaging field, upon the 2D image itself. The velocity data are coded in color and shade for direction and velocity, respectively, and are presented as a color velocity map within the cardiac chambers of the 2D image at frame rates of 12 to 30 per second. This flow velocity tomographic image is similar to angiographic projectional images in that it gives the appearance of blood moving normally or abnormally across the valves and within the chambers (see Color Plate 4A and B). Clinical instruments generally provide standard 2D, M-mode, PW, and CW Doppler audio and spectral displays as well as the color flow velocity images.

Echocardiography has some advantages over competing imaging technologies. These include no risk from ionizing radiation, portability of equipment, noninvasive imaging, high imaging rate, no requirement for contrast injection, and generally low cost for the study. Its disadvantages include poor-quality images in 5 to 20 per cent of various patient groups and lack of complete quantitative data from most clinical laboratories.

Feigenbaum H: Echocardiography. 3rd ed. Philadelphia, Lea & Febiger, 1986. *This encyclopedic text is useful for the neophyte as well as the advanced student. Its strength in discussion of M-mode and 2D methods is not quite matched in areas discussing Doppler ultrasonography.*

Hatle L, Angelsen B: Doppler Ultrasound in Cardiology. 2nd ed. Philadelphia, Lea & Febiger, 1985. *The most authoritative text on this subject. The chapters on the physics of blood flow and Doppler analysis are excellent. The comprehensive illustrations of pathologic and normal flow velocity patterns are superb. Much of the information included is not published elsewhere.*

Holen J, Aaslid R, Landmark K, et al.: Determination of pressure gradient in mitral stenosis with a non-invasive ultrasound Doppler technique. Acta Med Scand 199:455, 1976. *The classic work describing the clinical use of the relationship between maximum blood velocity detected by Doppler ultrasonography and pressure gradient calculated from the velocity.*

Holen J, Aaslid R, Landmark K, et al.: Determination of effective orifice area in mitral stenosis from non-invasive ultrasound Doppler data and mitral flow rate. Acta Med Scand 201:83, 1977. *Original description of the pressure half-time method for estimation of mitral orifice area using Doppler ultrasonography.*

Popp RL: Echocardiography (Part 1). N Engl J Med 323:101, 1990. Echocardiography (Part 2). N Eng J Med 323:165, 1990. *A recent review of the clinically accepted uses of echocardiography.*

Popp RL, Macovski A: Ultrasonic diagnostic instruments. Science 210:268, 1980. *A more detailed discussion of the instrumentation for producing ultrasonic images than given in this chapter.*

39.4 Nuclear Cardiology

Barry L. Zaret

Nuclear cardiology is based upon the ability of externally placed instruments to detect, define, and quantify radiation emanating from cardiac structures following injection of a radioisotope. The utility of nuclear procedures for defining pathophysiologic, prognostic, and diagnostic phenomena in cardiac patients has been established. The procedures can be safely repeated and are suitable for both imaging and biodistribution studies. Changes in cardiac function, ventricular volume, myocardial perfusion, viability, and metabolism can be evaluated in appropriate clinical circumstances.

At present, a major clinical application of nuclear cardiology is in the assessment of global and regional cardiac performance. This is achieved with radionuclides that remain within the intravascular space during the period of study. Computer technology is critical for such measurement. Cardiac performance can be assessed in two general ways: during the first pass of the isotope through the central circulation or following its equilibration in the cardiac blood pool. First-pass radionuclide angiocardiography is completed within 30 seconds following intravenous injection of a technetium–99m (^{99m}Tc) compound. There is temporal and anatomic segregation of the radioactive bolus during its first transit through the central circulation. Thus it is possible to make concomitant measurements of right and left ventricular function without concern that radioactivity present in one ventricle is interfering with the analysis of the other. Analysis of time-activity curves generated from the respective ventricular regions allows determination of ventricular ejection fraction (Fig. 39–33). Count rates emanating from a cardiac chamber are proportional to the volume of the chamber. In addition to analysis of ejection fraction, rates of ventricular filling and emptying, and ventricular volumes, quantitative and qualitative assessments of regional wall motion can be made from the same data.

The alternative and much more widely used approach to assessing cardiac performance involves equilibration radionuclide studies. Physiologic signals are introduced that convert the conventional static imaging procedure into a dynamic assessment of cardiac function. To obtain this goal, ^{99m}Tc is bound to the patient's own erythrocytes. The ^{99m}Tc label remains evenly distributed throughout the intravascular blood volume for several hours. With the use of the electrocardiogram, nuclear data are segregated according to the time of their occurrence within the cardiac cycle. Data are summed over several hundred cardiac cycles, and composite data are quantified and displayed as sequential 10- to 50-msec points, which together define a representative cardiac cycle. The ventricular volume curve derived from these data is suitable for direct measurement of ejection fraction, rates of filling and ejection, and ventricular volumes. The data are also displayed as a series of images that, when projected in cinematic format, provide a direct visual assessment of the regional contraction patterns of the heart (Fig. 39–34). Computer techniques, particularly regional ejection fraction, now make it possible also to quantify regional function motion accurately. With the regional ejection fraction technique, the left ventricular blood pool in the left anterior oblique position is divided into five discrete areas corresponding to septal, apical, and lateral regions. Individual time-activity curves are obtained from each of these regions, thereby providing quantitative regional analysis.

Both first-pass and equilibrium techniques can be employed to study cardiac performance under conditions of rest and exercise. Data may be accumulated during supine, semisupine, or upright bicycle exercise. Often critical data emerge only when the patient is evaluated during stress. The normal response to exercise involves an augmentation in the pump function of both ventricles, generally defined as an increase in ejection fraction of at least 5 per cent (in absolute ejection fraction units) and the presence of normal regional wall motion. Abnormal exercise ventricular reserve may be encountered in a variety of pathophysiologic conditions involving coronary artery disease and intrinsic myocardial, valvular, and congenital heart disease.

The study of cardiac performance employing nuclear techniques has been particularly useful in coronary artery disease. The ejection fraction is the single best clinical indicator of global ventricular pump performance. The index is of major prognostic importance in patients with coronary artery disease, either immediately following myocardial infarction or in the chronic or subacute phases of disease. Analysis of the ventricular ejection fraction is based upon radioactivity counts. It is not dependent upon geometric assumptions concerning ventricular shape or ventricular volume. In coronary artery disease, particularly following myocardial infarction, asymmetric contraction patterns are common. In these ischemic ventricles, cavitary shapes frequently cannot be approximated by idealized geometric models. Consequently, in coronary artery disease, ejection fraction is measured most accurately by the nuclear approach. Using portable equipment, it is possible to study cardiac performance at the bedside of the acutely ill. Such studies have demonstrated substantial abnormalities in the functioning of the ischemic left ventricle during the acute phase of myocardial infarction. Right ventricular infarction occuring in the course of inferior wall infarction has been identified and further defined. The important negative prognostic impact of functional left ventricular aneurysm formation during acute anterior infarction has been defined. Assessment of regional and global function also is an important means of evaluating the effect of thrombolytic therapy for acute infarction.

Abnormalities of ventricular performance are found in approximately 85 per cent of patients with coronary artery disease studied during exercise stress. Myocardial ischemia is reflected in abnormal ventricular reserve. Abnormal responses of the ejection fraction may be encountered in a variety of conditions, but the development of new regional abnormalities of wall motion is quite specific for coronary artery disease. Abnormal exercise performance has important prognostic implications, particularly following infarction.

In addition, recent technical advances now make it possible to

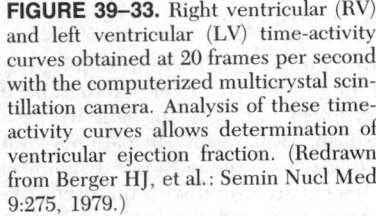

FIGURE 39–33. Right ventricular (RV) and left ventricular (LV) time-activity curves obtained at 20 frames per second with the computerized multicrystal scintillation camera. Analysis of these time-activity curves allows determination of ventricular ejection fraction. (Redrawn from Berger HJ, et al.: Semin Nucl Med 9:275, 1979.)

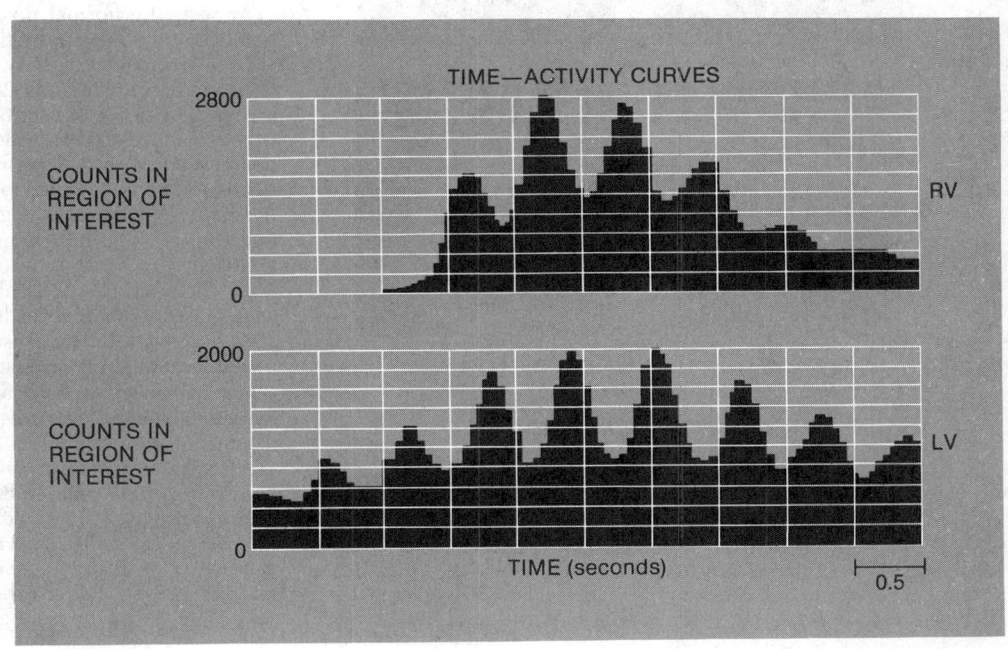

monitor ventricular function in ambulatory patients using a miniaturized detector system employing the principles of equilibrium radionuclide angiocardiography. With this approach, abnormalities of ventricular performance have been noted during routine activities in patients with coronary disease. This new technique, still under active investigation, offers promise for the study of silent myocardial ischemia.

Radionuclide assessment of ventricular performance may also be employed in the evaluation of patients with valvular disease at rest or exercise. Resting measurement of cardiac function provides important preoperative prognostic data and may also be of value in defining the physiologic significance of valvular lesions such as mitral regurgitation. For example, normal left ventricular function in a patient with severe mitral regurgitation would imply a primary valvular problem, whereas severe ventricular dysfunction would suggest secondary mitral regurgitation resulting from diffuse myocardial disease. Assessment of performance under hemodynamic stress may help define the advent of irreversible damage in valvular heart disease. This is particularly important in aortic regurgitation, in which irremediable change in left ventricular function is frequently present by the time valve surgery is considered.

Assessment of ventricular performance and ventricular volumes is critical to the understanding and treatment of congestive heart failure. Knowledge of the degree of impairment in ventricular performance has prognostic and therapeutic relevance. In addi-tion, an important group of patients with primary diastolic dysfunction (normal systolic function and impaired measures of diastolic filling) has been defined well with nuclear techniques. This group may involve as much as 20 to 40 per cent of patients presenting for evaluation of clinical congestive heart failure. It is highly important to define such patients, since routine heart failure therapy is not effective. These patients appear to respond to calcium channel blocking agents.

Radionuclide studies also have been employed in the evaluation of myocardial function in patients with lung disease in which the major hemodynamic burden falls on the right ventricle. Right ventricular performance can probably be evaluated best with the first-pass technique. Abnormalities in right ventricular performance have been noted at rest and during exercise in patients with chronic obstructive pulmonary disease. Pharmacologic interventions may modify abnormal right ventricular performance.

These techniques also have been utilized for long-term studies assessing cardiac therapy. A prototype example has been the application of radionuclide angiocardiography for the serial assessment of ventricular function in patients receiving the antineoplastic agent doxorubicin. Use of this agent has been limited by the frequent development of a drug-induced cardiomyopathy. Serial measurement of cardiac ejection fraction during the course of therapy has led to a set of dosage guidelines that help avert cardiotoxicity.

MYOCARDIAL PERFUSION IMAGING

Myocardial perfusion imaging utilizes radionuclides that traverse the myocardial capillary system and enter the myocardial cell. The radionuclide currently employed for these studies is thallium-201 (^{201}Tl). This tracer is considered a potassium analogue, since its distribution generally mirrors that of intracellular potassium. Thallium-201 is produced in the cyclotron and has a physical half-life of approximately 72 hours. After intravenous injection it is rapidly extracted and distributed within the myocardium according to regional myocardial blood flow and regional cellular viability. Recently, a new group of ^{99m}Tc perfusion tracers, the isonitriles, has been developed. These radiopharmaceuticals, although currently still experimental, should be in the clinical arena shortly. They offer several potential advantages over ^{201}Tl. These include better imaging characteristics, ability to administer a higher dose, better suitability for tomographic studies, and biologic properties that involve lack of major washout following administration. This latter property allows for delayed imaging following administration, particularly in the acute situation, thereby allowing definition of risk zones in acute ischemic syndromes. The ability to administer a ^{99m}Tc bolus intravenously allows for measurement of ejection fraction prior to perfusion imaging. The isonitrile images may also be ECG gated, allowing for better image resolution as well as potential quantification of regional function.

At rest, the normal myocardial perfusion image demonstrates homogeneous uptake in the left ventricular wall with a central area of decreased activity corresponding to the left ventricular cavity. In approximately 20 per cent of normal persons, there is a region of decreased uptake at the cardiac apex corresponding to a normal relative apical thinning. Abnormal image patterns of decreased myocardial perfusion demonstrate a region of relatively decreased radionuclide uptake. Images are obtained in multiple positions. The normal right ventricle is not visualized at rest because of its smaller mass compared with that of the left ventricle.

In the resting state, abnormalities usually represent either acute or remote myocardial infarction. However, studies have also demonstrated perfusion defects at rest in patients with unstable angina or coronary spasm and, rarely, in patients with severe obstructive coronary disease in the absence of clinical evidence of acute ischemia. Defects are noted with high sensitivity during the early hours of acute myocardial infarction. Within the first 6 hours, virtually all infarcts may be identified. After 24 hours, sensitivity falls to 80 to 90 per cent.

In most patients with coronary artery disease without previous infarction, myocardial perfusion patterns appear normal at rest. This is to be expected, since coronary blood flow is relatively uniform at rest, even in the presence of severe coronary obstruction. The major physiologic abnormality in coronary disease is

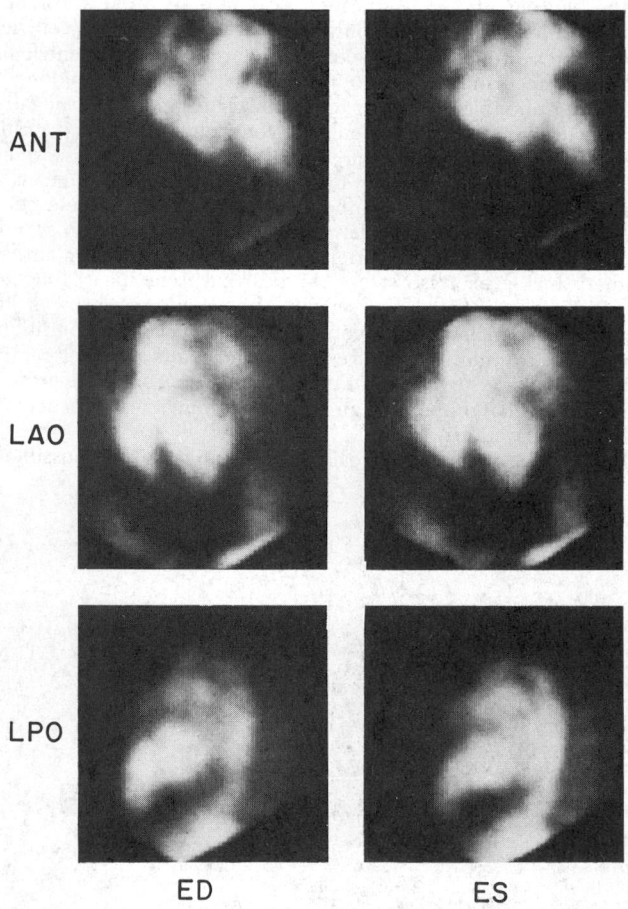

ANT

LAO

LPO

ED   ES

FIGURE 39–34. Gated cardiac blood pool studies obtained in the anterior (ANT), 45-degree left anterior oblique (LAO), and left posterior oblique (LPO) positions. End-diastolic images (ED) are shown on the left and end-systolic (ES) on the right. Note that radioactivity is present throughout the entire cardiac blood pool. A large anteroapical left ventricular aneurysm is appreciated in all three positions. Note that in the LAO position image the left ventricle is the posterior cardiac structure and the right ventricle the anterior structure. These are separated by the interventricular septum, which is displayed as an area devoid of radioactivity. (Reproduced from Berger HJ, et al.: Radiol Clin North Am 18:441, 1980.)

diminished coronary vascular reserve. Therefore, to detect perfusion abnormalities in coronary disease it is necessary to study patients under conditions of increased myocardial blood flow. Most work has employed exercise as an appropriate stress. Thallium-201 is injected at peak exercise, and imaging is begun within 10 minutes after injection. Since thallium is rapidly extracted by myocardium, it can be injected during the period of maximal heterogeneity of regional myocardial blood flow, and its distribution reflects this heterogeneity. Comparison of images obtained immediately following exercise with those obtained following a redistribution phase 2 to 4 hours after exercise allows definition of transiently ischemic zones (Fig. 39–35). Defects present on exercise but not at redistribution are most consistent with transient ischemia; defects that are unchanged are most consistent with previous infarction and scar; and defects that are present at redistribution but are markedly increased during exercise are most consistent with transient ischemia superimposed upon the scar. Recently, it has been recognized that delayed imaging may be important for detecting viable yet ischemic myocardium that appears as a fixed defect on the initial stress and redistribution images. For this purpose 24-hour imaging studies, with or without a second injection of radioisotope, have been employed. In this manner, up to 40 per cent of fixed defects have been demonstrated to have some reversibility. The overall sensitivity of this technique for detecting significant ischemic disease is approximately 80 per cent. The specificity of the technique is excellent. This technique is of greatest value diagnostically in patients with equivocal exercise electrocardiograms, abnormal baseline electrocardiograms, or suspected false-positive or false-negative conventional exercise tests. Both imaging with the patient at rest and exercise/redistribution studies have been of value in evaluating thrombolysis and reperfusion. Exercise studies also are of major value in assessing prognosis following infarction in stable coronary disease and in evaluating patients after coronary angioplasty. In addition to the magnitude of the perfusion defect, increased lung uptake has been demonstrated to be a potent prognostic index in coronary disease patients.

An alternative means of stress perfusion imaging involves use of the coronary vasodilator, dipyridamole. Thallium myocardial distributions following dipyridamole provide data comparable to those noted with exercise. However, with pharmacologic stress, evaluation is based upon differences in flow without implying ischemia, whereas with exercise, evaluation is based upon heterogeneity of flow, generally associated with ischemia. Dipyridamole studies are of particular value in patients unable to exercise.

This type of study has been of particular value in identifying myocardial ischemia in peripheral vascular disease patients undergoing preoperative cardiac evaluation.

Thallium planar imaging is now increasingly quantitative. Computer techniques provide objective definition of the presence and extent of defects as well as quantification of regional tracer washout kinetics. Contemporary evaluation of thallium imaging data should include quantitative interpretation of visual data.

Single photon emission computed tomography (SPECT) thallium studies are currently employed widely. In comparative studies with planar imaging, SPECT has been shown to have similar diagnostic accuracy. A major current use involves definition of multiple vascular bed involvement in coronary disease. Although its clinical role has not been completely defined, it is anticipated that SPECT studies involving the isonitriles will prove to be a significant diagnostic advance.

INFARCT-AVID IMAGING

An additional radionuclide approach involves definition of acute myocardial infarction and regions of acute myocardial necrosis. This is performed with "infarct-avid" radiotracers, which bind selectively to regions of acute infarction. The current agent for this procedure is ^{99m}Tc stannous pyrophosphate. Acute infarcts are visualized as regions of increased radionuclide uptake. The mechanism of abnormal pyrophosphate accumulation appears to be related to regional calcium deposition, as well as binding to denatured proteins. Pyrophosphate uptake also is dependent upon sufficient residual blood flow to allow entry of the radioactive tracer.

The infarct zone can be visualized within 24 to 48 hours of the onset of infarction. Maximal visualization generally occurs from 48 to 72 hours after the infarct. Images usually are not positive within the first 24 hours unless thrombolysis has occurred. Images generally are no longer positive 7 to 10 days after the infarct. Pyrophosphate infarct imaging is most valuable in patients presenting several days after infarction when other studies are equivocal or nondiagnostic.

Radiolabeled antimyosin antibody has recently been proposed as an alternative means of infarct-avid imaging. Initial trials with this agent have been quite promising with respect to infarct definition and prognostic impact. In addition, antimyosin imaging studies have been employed for defining acute myocarditis in patients with heart failure and for defining cardiac transplant rejection.

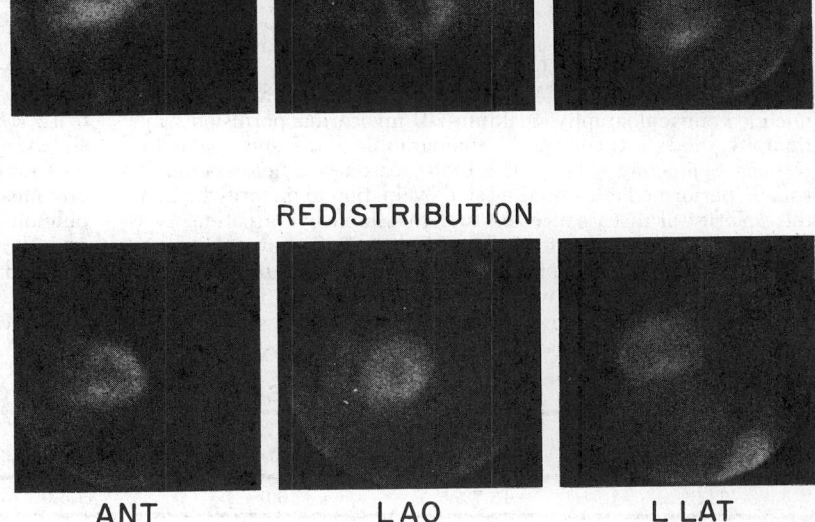

EXERCISE

REDISTRIBUTION

ANT   LAO   L LAT

FIGURE 39–35. Exercise (upper panels) and redistribution (lower panels) thallium-201 myocardial perfusion images in a patient with significant coronary artery disease. Anterior position (ANT) images are shown in the left panels, left anterior oblique (LAO) images in the middle panels, and left lateral (L LAT) images in the right panels. Note a significant perfusion defect present in the anteroseptal wall seen in the LAO image and in the anteroapical wall seen in the L LAT image during exercise, with substantial redistribution and filling in of the perfusion defect on the redistribution images. This study is consistent with transient myocardial ischemia and coronary artery disease involving at least the left anterior descending coronary artery.

POSITRON TOMOGRAPHY (PET)

This technique involves imaging and quantification of the intracardiac distribution of positron-emitting radionuclides. By virtue of the types of radionuclides available and the instrumentation employed, this technique has provided new insight into metabolism and coronary flow. Since carbon–11 is a positron emitter, a variety of biologically active compounds can be radiolabeled and used for imaging. These include fatty acids, metabolites, receptor ligands, and neurotransmitters.

There has been great interest recently in PET studies of myocardial metabolism and perfusion. Of most immediate clinical impact has been the demonstration that increased regional glucose accumulation in areas that are hypoperfused represents viable tissue with a substantial likelihood of improved function with revascularization. This has been demonstrated using fluorodeoxyglucose as the radiopharmaceutical. This "glucose-perfusion mismatch" offers major opportunities for evaluating stunned and hibernating myocardium in ischemic heart disease as well as ischemic cardiomyopathy. Recent additional comparative studies have also involved radiolabeled acetate, palmitate, and glucose. Finally, tomographic perfusion imaging involving positron-emitting rubidium, water, and nitrogen-labeled ammonia has also shown promise, although experience is currently somewhat limited.

Gerson MC: Cardiac Nuclear Medicine. New York, McGraw-Hill Book Company, 1987. *This multiauthored text contains 11 chapters devoted to nuclear cardiology and provides an excellent overview of technical aspects of the field as well as appropriate clinical applications.*

Wackers FJ: Myocardial perfusion imaging. *In* Gottschalk A, Hoffer PB, Pochen EJ (eds.): Diagnostic Nuclear Medicine. Baltimore, Williams & Wilkins Company, 1988, pp 291–354. *An excellent overview of myocardial perfusion imaging. This review contains 218 references.*

Zaret BL, Berger HJ: Nuclear cardiology. *In* Hurst JW (ed.): The Heart. 7th ed. New York, McGraw-Hill Book Company, 1990, pp 1899–1950. *A comprehensive review of all aspects of nuclear cardiology, with 309 individual references cited.*

39.5 Cardiac Catheterization and Angiography

William H. Barry

Cardiac catheterization provides a unique, comprehensive, and quantitative assessment of cardiac structure and function and is frequently utilized in the diagnosis and management of patients with heart disease. With the further application of this procedure for bedside hemodynamic monitoring, intracardiac electrophysiologic testing, endomyocardial biopsy, percutaneous transluminal coronary angioplasty, and percutaneous balloon valvotomy, it has become increasingly important for the internist to understand the indications, capabilities, and risks of cardiac catheterization.

INDICATIONS FOR CARDIAC CATHETERIZATION AND ANGIOGRAPHY

The accuracy of noninvasive evaluation has increased remarkably recently, because of the greatly improved sensitivity and specificity of two-dimensional Doppler echocardiography, radionuclide ventriculography, thallium-201 myocardial perfusion scintigraphy, and fast computed tomographic (CT) and magnetic resonance imaging (MRI). Therefore, cardiac catheterization is usually performed after noninvasive evaluation to quantify further the severity of disease present and to establish if a patient is a candidate for surgical intervention. Table 39–5 shows the diagnoses of a typical series of patients referred for cardiac catheterization. The vast majority of patients undergoing this procedure have coronary artery disease, with valvular disease a distant

second. Table 39–6 lists the usual indications for cardiac catheterization and coronary angiography in patients with coronary artery disease or valvular heart disease.

TECHNIQUES AND THEIR HAZARDS

ARTERIAL AND VENOUS ACCESS. Two basic approaches are used for insertion of catheters into arteries and veins. The first involves incision of the skin overlying the vessel, dissection of the vessel free of surrounding tissue, and incision of the vessel with direct insertion of the catheter. The advantage of this method, usually reserved for the brachial artery or antecubital vein, is that it provides direct access to the vessels, so that they may either be tied off (vein) or repaired (brachial artery) after completion of the catheterization procedure, decreasing the likelihood of hematoma formation. The disadvantages of the technique are that an incision is required in the skin, increasing the patient's discomfort in the postcatheterization period; and there is a significant (2 to 3 per cent) incidence of thrombosis of the brachial artery. However, this approach is usually preferred in patients with severe atherosclerotic disease of the aorta or iliofemoral arteries.

In the Seldinger technique, an artery or vein is punctured percutaneously with a needle, and by means of a thin, flexible guide wire, an arterial or venous sheath or a catheter is inserted into the vessel. The percutaneous technique is employed most frequently for the femoral artery and vein, the axillary artery, or the subclavian or internal jugular vein. This technique is relatively simple, and no sutures are required. The disadvantage is that one does not have direct control of the vessels after withdrawal of the catheters or sheaths, and control of postcatheterization bleeding may be more difficult than with the direct approach. Patients must therefore be relatively immobile for at least 4 to 6 hours. At present, the percutaneous femoral approach in which the femoral artery and femoral vein are punctured is most commonly utilized for cardiac catheterization and coronary angiography.

Catheterization and angiography can cause stroke or myocardial infarction due to vessel occlusion by clot from the tip of the catheter, dislodgment of atherosclerotic material, or dissection of the vessel wall, although the incidence of these complications is low (Table 39–7). Catheterization of the left side of the heart generally carries a much higher risk than that of the right because of the ability of the lung vascular bed to filter out thrombi. To decrease the risk of thrombosis and embolization, heparin is usually administered prior to catheterization of the left side of the heart. The anticoagulant effect of heparin is usually reversed with protamine at the termination of the procedure, before the final withdrawal of the sheath or catheter. Angiography carries a higher risk than simple pressure measurements of the left side of the heart because of the additional catheter manipulation, selective placement of the catheters within the coronary arteries, and use of angiographic contrast solution, especially in patients with more severe cardiac diseases. In addition, risk is increased in patients over 60 years of age, in patients with severe heart failure, and in patients with significant valvular heart disease.

PRESSURE MEASUREMENTS. Measurement of intracardiac pressures, by attaching the end of the fluid-filled catheter to an external pressure transducer, is an essential part of the cardiac catheterization procedure. Phasic pressure waveforms up to 12 Hz may be recorded with this technique (Fig. 39–36), and all the pressures within the cardiac chambers are routinely measured, with the exception of the left atrial pressure. The pulmonary capillary "wedge" pressure, in which a segment of the pulmonary arterial tree is occluded either with the catheter tip or with a small balloon attached to the end of a catheter (a flow-directed Swan-Ganz type of catheter), is recorded to approximate the true left atrial pressure (Fig. 39–36). The normal values for intracardiac pressures are given in Ch. 38.

TABLE 39–5. DIAGNOSES OF 562 PATIENTS CONSECUTIVELY STUDIED

Coronary Artery Disease (CAD)	Valvular Disease	CAD and Valvular Disease	Cardiomyopathy	Normal Persons	Congenital Heart Disease	Miscellaneous
62.6%	16.7%	6.0%	5.9%	6.4%	1.4%	0.9%

Adapted from Barry WH, et al.: Cathet Cardiovasc Diagn 8:401, 1979.

TABLE 39–6. POSSIBLE INDICATIONS FOR CARDIAC CATHETERIZATION AND ANGIOGRAPHY

Suspected Coronary Artery Disease	Suspected Valvular Disease
1. Angina, especially if: unstable refractory to treatment strongly positive treadmill ECG young person with positive family history	1. Aortic stenosis if: angina syncope CHF
2. After acute myocardial infarction (including patients who have received thrombolytic therapy) if: angina positive treadmill ECG	2. Aortic regurgitation if: CHF angina progressive cardiac enlargement
3. In selected patients suspected to have "silent" ischemia: occupational hazards strong family history of infarction/sudden death	3. Mitral stenosis* if: CHF refractory to digitalis and diuretics recurrent emboli with atrial fibrillation
4. Patients with ischemic cardiomyopathy and congestive heart failure (CHF)	4. Mitral regurgitation if: CHF progressive cardiac enlargement
5. In patients with high risk (age, diabetes, lipid disorder) prior to major noncardiac surgery; in patients at risk for coronary artery disease in whom cardiac surgery is planned	
Additional Miscellaneous Indications: Congenital heart disease Pericardial disease Percutaneous transluminal coronary angioplasty Electrophysiologic study Biopsy Hemodynamic monitoring Balloon valvotomy	

*Operation may be performed without catheterization if diagnosis is certain.

The shape as well as the magnitude of the intracardiac pressure waveforms contains diagnostic information. For example, in mitral regurgitation there is a large v wave in the left atrial or pulmonary artery wedge pressure recording (Fig. 39–37). A large v wave in the right atrial pressure tracing indicates tricuspid insufficiency. Simultaneous pressures are usually measured in the pulmonary wedge position and left ventricle to quantitate mitral valve function. A pressure gradient in diastole between the pulmonary wedge pressure and left ventricular diastolic pressure is seen, for example, in mitral stenosis (Fig. 39–38). Left ventricular and aortic pressures are measured simultaneously to assess aortic valve function.

Comparison of pressures in different chambers can also be very

TABLE 39–7. COMPLICATIONS OF CARDIAC CATHETERIZATION AND ANGIOGRAPHY*

	Per Cent Incidence in	
Complication	Patients with CAD†	Patients with Valvular‡ Heart Disease
Death	0.10	0.1
Myocardial infarction	0.06	0.2
Cerebrovascular accident	0.07	0.4
Arrhythmia	0.47	2.0
Vascular complications	0.46	1.7
Other	0.58	2.4
TOTAL	1.74	6.8

*Adapted from The Registry of Society for Cardiac Angiography and Interventions. Cathet Cardiovasc Diagn 17:5–21, 1989.
†Data on 222,553 patients.
‡Data on 1483 patients.

useful. In patients with pericardial constriction, there is equalization of the right atrial and pulmonary artery wedge pressures, and the mean right atrial pressure is greater than one third of the right ventricular systolic pressure. Measurement of intracardiac pressures during exercise or pacing stress may provide useful information as well. For example, patients with mitral stenosis or mitral insufficiency may have relatively normal resting pressures but abnormally high pulmonary artery wedge pressures with exercise. Patients with coronary artery disease may have normal left ventricular diastolic pressures at rest, which elevate markedly during angina produced by pacing tachycardia, reflecting ischemic left ventricular dysfunction.

MEASUREMENT OF CARDIAC OUTPUT. The most accurate way to measure cardiac output is by the Fick method, in which oxygen consumption is measured by determining the oxygen content in expired air collected over a 3-minute period. This allows determination of oxygen consumption in milliliters per minute. Collection of samples from the pulmonary artery (mixed venous sample) and a systemic artery allows determination of the arteriovenous (AV) oxygen difference. If the value for hemoglobin concentration in the blood is known, this allows calculation of the milliliters of blood that had to flow through the lungs to acquire the amount of oxygen consumed.

$$\text{Cardiac output (liters/min)} = \frac{\text{oxygen consumption (ml } O_2/\text{min)}}{\text{A-V } O_2 \text{ difference (ml } O_2/\text{liter blood)}}$$

$$\text{A-V } O_2 \text{ difference (ml } O_2/\text{liter blood)} = 13.9 \times \text{hemoglobin (gm/dl)} \times (\% \text{ sat A} - \% \text{ sat V})$$

Cardiac output may be normalized by dividing by body surface area (m^2) and expressed as cardiac index. In patients with intracardiac shunts, correction for the shunt must be made. This occurs most commonly in adult patients with atrial septal defects or ventricular septal defects with a left-to-right shunt. The pulmonary artery saturation in these conditions is elevated relative to the true mixed venous saturation, which is most closely approximated by the superior vena cava saturation. Standard methods exist for quantification of left-to-right and right-to-left intracardiac shunts.

Another method commonly used for measurement of cardiac output is dye dilution, in which indocyanine green dye is injected into a peripheral vein, with continuous sampling of the dye concentration in blood drawn from a peripheral artery.

The cardiac output is calculated as $\dfrac{i}{c \times t}$ where i is the quantity of indicator injected, c is the average arterial concentration of the indicator during its first pass, and t is the total duration of the dye concentration curve. The product of c and t is easily determined by planimetry of the area under the first-pass curve. Cardiac output determined by dye dilution may be inaccurate in patients with extremely low outputs or with mitral or aortic regurgitation. The dye curve is also distorted by the presence of intracardiac shunts and in fact may be used in certain circumstances to diagnose the presence and direction of an intracardiac shunt.

With the "thermodilution" method the indicator is not dye, but cold saline injected into the right atrium. Temperature changes are detected with a thermistor in the pulmonary artery. The advantages of the thermodilution method are that it is relatively unaffected by mitral and aortic regurgitation and it may be repeated frequently to measure serial outputs. It is influenced by respiration, by the presence of shunts that increase pulmonary flow, and by the presence of tricuspid regurgitation. At the present time, the Fick method is most commonly employed in the cardiac catheterization laboratory, and the thermodilution method is most commonly utilized in intensive care unit settings where patients are being monitored with catheters in the right side of the heart.

From measurements of cardiac output and pressure gradients across vascular beds, the systemic and pulmonary vascular resistances may be calculated. Elevations in systemic vascular resis-

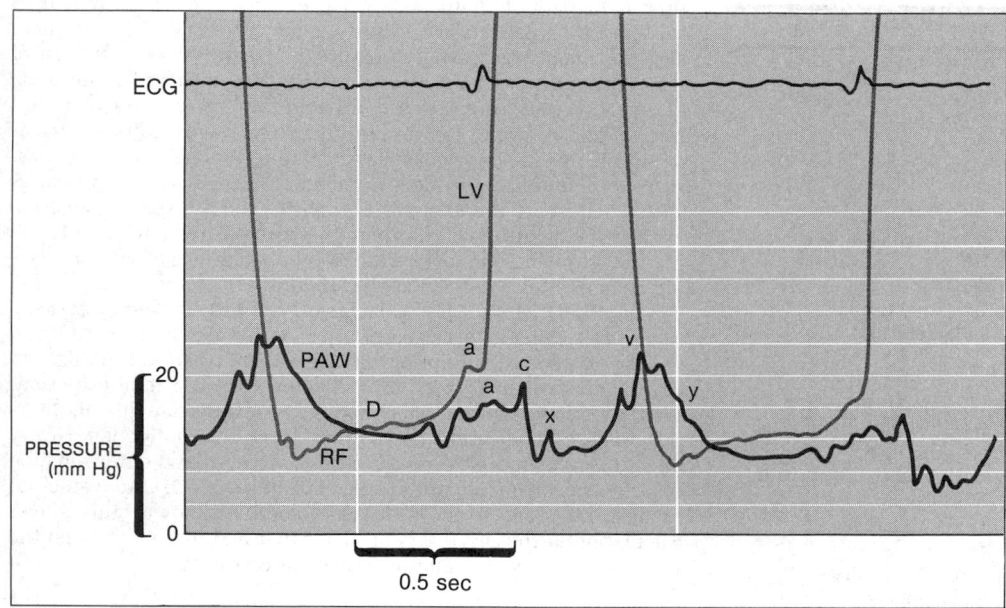

FIGURE 39–36. Simultaneous pulmonary artery wedge (PAW) pressure and left ventricular pressure (LV) in a normal patient. RF = Rapid LV filling; D = diastasis of LV filling; a = atrial contraction pressure wave. Note the delay of the PAW pressure relative to LV pressure.

tance are important in patients with chronic congestive heart failure and may identify those patients who will respond favorably to vasodilator therapy. Pulmonary vascular resistance is frequently elevated in patients with severe left ventricular failure and elevated pulmonary venous pressures, in patients with mitral valve disease, in patients with left-to-right shunts, and always in patients with primary pulmonary hypertension. Measurement of changes in pulmonary and systemic vascular resistances and in cardiac outputs and pressures before and after administration of vasodilator drugs may be helpful in guiding treatment of patients with specific disorders and is frequently employed in the catheterization laboratory setting.

Determination of cardiac output simultaneous with measurement of pressure gradients across the aortic, mitral, tricuspid, or pulmonic valve allows estimation of valve area by use of the Gorlin formula (see Fig. 39–38). The calculated valve area may differ significantly from the true valve area, particularly in the presence of very low cardiac output or valvular insufficiency. Nevertheless, this measurement is often useful in guiding surgical interventions.

ANGIOGRAPHY. During routine cardiac catheterization, left ventriculography and coronary angiography are commonly per-

formed. For left ventriculography, contrast material is injected into the left ventricular chamber and cineangiographic filming is performed at 30 to 60 frames per second. Ejection fraction is determined as the fraction of end-diastolic ventricular volume ejected each systole. In patients with mitral regurgitation, the degree of regurgitation is usually graded on a simple 1+ to 4+ scale. In patients with coronary artery disease, segmental contraction abnormalities are frequently present, and these may be quantified by a variety of regional indices of left ventricular performance.

Injection of dye into the aortic root allows assessment of the degree of aortic insufficiency, and right ventricular contrast injection allows assessment of the tricuspid valve. Pulmonary angiography may also be performed to assess the pulmonary vasculature and to detect presence of pulmonary emboli.

Adverse effects of cardiac angiography include a negative inotropic effect due to calcium binding by the contrast agent and an intravascular volume-expanding effect due to hyperosmolality of the contrast material. The myocardial depressant effects of contrast agents are usually not a problem unless ventricular function is severely compromised. In these patients, the risks of left ventriculography may be reduced by using newer nonionic,

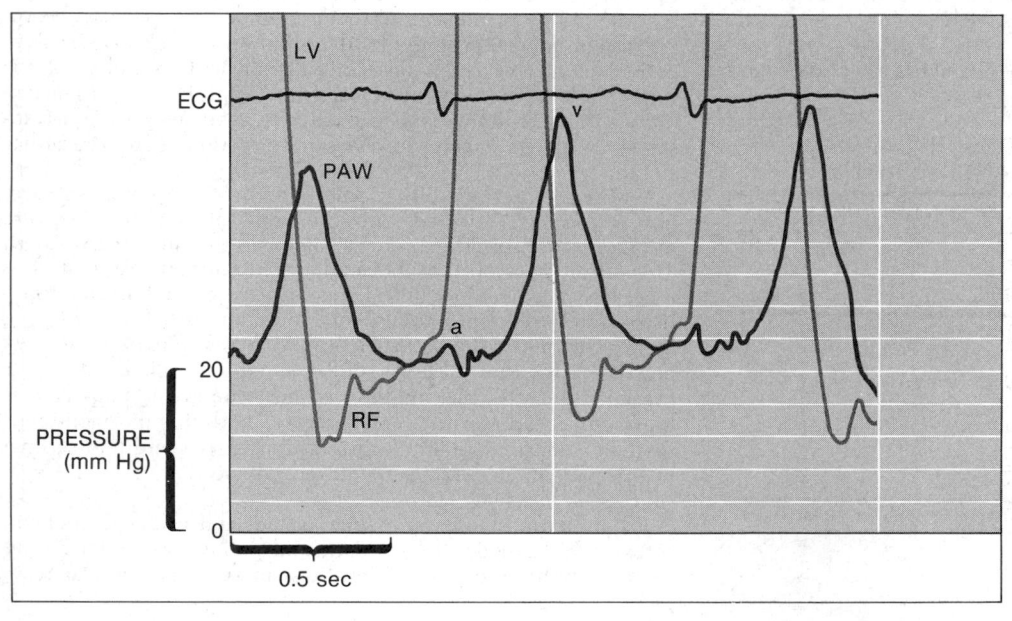

FIGURE 39–37. Simultaneous PAW and LV pressures in a patient with severe mitral regurgitation. Note large v wave with rapid y descent.

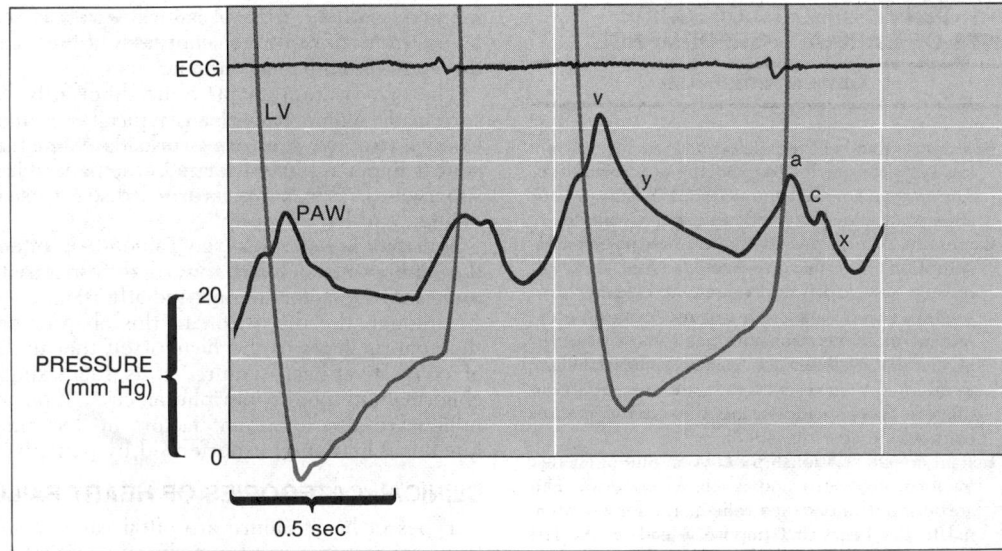

FIGURE 39–38. Simultaneous PAW and LV pressures in a patient with mitral stenosis. Note the slow y descent and the large gradient throughout diastole between PAW and LV diastolic pressures. The actual mitral valve area (M.V.A.) may be estimated as:

$$M.V.A. = \frac{\text{diastolic mitral flow (ml/sec)}}{38 \sqrt{\text{diastolic pressure gradient}}}$$

Thus, for a given M.V.A., the pressure gradient across the valve goes up as the *square* of mitral valve flow. This explains why the PAW pressure rises so markedly with increased cardiac output and hence increased mitral valve flow. Increased heart rate shortens diastolic time, and hence increases the mitral valve flow rate per unit of diastolic time at any given cardiac output.

non–calcium-binding contrast agents or digital image enhancement techniques that permit use of a small volume of contrast material.

Coronary cineangiography is performed by injecting a contrast agent selectively into the right or left main coronary ostia and filming at 30 frames per second. The degree of coronary artery obstruction in multiple views is assessed by measuring the percentage of narrowing of the artery at the site or sites of obstruction or by determining the percentage of area of stenosis by video-densitometric measurements. The presence and location of collateral vessels in relationship to partially or totally occluded coronary artery narrowings are also determined. In patients with no or only minor coronary artery narrowings, but with a suggestive history of chest pain, ergonovine may be infused intravenously to precipitate coronary artery spasm, which then can be documented angiographically.

Descriptions of the indications, techniques, and risks of newer procedures that also involve cardiac catheterization and angiography, such as coronary angioplasty, endomyocardial biopsy, balloon valvotomy, and electrophysiologic study, are beyond the scope of this brief summary but may be found in the selected references included.

Detre K, Holubkov R, Kelsey S, et al.: One year follow-up results of the 1985–1986 National Heart, Lung, and Blood Institute's percutaneous transluminal coronary angioplasty registry. Circulation 80:421–428, 1989. *Representative report of current success rate and complications.*

Grossman W: Cardiac Catheterization and Angiography. 3rd ed. Philadelphia, Lea & Febiger, 1986. *Excellent comprehensive text on catheterization and angiography.*

Latac B, Cribier A, Koning R, Lefelsure E: Aortic stenosis in elderly patients aged 80 or older: Treatment by percutaneous balloon valvuloplasty in a series of 92 cases. Circulation 80:1514–1520, 1989. *Summary of results of percutaneous balloon aortic valvotomy.*

Mason JW, O'Connell JB: Clinical merit of endomyocardial biopsy. Circulation 75:972–980, 1989. *Summary of indications for endomyocardial biopsy.*

Palacios I, Block PC, Wilkins GT, Weyman AE: Follow-up of patients undergoing percutaneous mitral balloon valvotomy. Circulation 79:573–579, 1989. *Summary of current results of percutaneous balloon mitral valvotomy.*

Registry Committee of the Society for Cardiac Angiography and Interventions: Complications of cardiac catheterization. Cath Cardiovasc Diagn 17:5–21, 1989. *Excellent current description of type and incidence of complications associated with cardiac catheterization and coronary angiography.*

40 Heart Failure

Thomas W. Smith

The heart generates the motive force to satisfy the metabolic needs of tissues by delivery of blood containing oxygen and nutrients. The minute-to-minute adjustments in the distribution of the cardiac output according to physiologic priorities (e.g., muscular exercise, heat loss, and digestion) require a complex regulatory system that must also serve to protect vital organs such as the heart and brain when cardiac output is compromised.

The normal or failing heart, in terms of its structure and function, may be examined as a pump, as a muscle, or as a component of the circulatory system. This chapter addresses aspects of heart failure common to the various disease entities discussed in subsequent chapters.

GENERAL ASPECTS

Textbooks commonly define heart failure as a condition in which the heart cannot pump an adequate supply of blood at normal filling pressures to meet the metabolic needs of the body. Clinicians and clinical investigators, however, define heart failure operationally as a syndrome in which ventricular dysfunction is accompanied by reduced exercise capacity. Table 40–1 provides explanations of terms commonly used to describe determinants of cardiac performance.

Heart failure is encountered with increasing frequency, the number of hospital discharges in the United States with this diagnosis having more than doubled in the period from 1973 to 1986. Most of this increase is attributable to an aging population with a high incidence of cardiovascular disease; heart failure is now the most common DRG throughout the United States for patients aged 65 and above.

Despite advances in the medical and surgical management of cardiovascular disease, the prognosis for patients with overt heart failure remains quite limited. About half of patients die within 4 years after this diagnosis; among the group with advanced heart

TABLE 40–1. TERMS USED TO DESCRIBE DETERMINANTS OF CARDIAC PERFORMANCE

Term	Relation to Cardiac Function
Afterload	Resistance that the ventricle must overcome during systole in order to eject the stroke volume. The two major determinants are aortic impedance (see below) and left ventricular volume.
Energetics	Generally determined as myocardial oxygen consumption. For any contractile state, the wall tension developed and maintained during contraction represents the major mechanical determinant of oxygen consumption. An increase in myocardial wall tension occurs in heart failure as filling pressure increases and the ventricle dilates, thereby increasing the energy cost of contraction (see Fig. 40–3).
Impedance (during ejection)	Instantaneous relationship between rate of change in aortic pressure and aortic blood flow. The aortic input impedance reflects the forces external to the heart that impose a load on the left ventricle, including stiffness of aortic wall. Determined primarily, but not exclusively, by total peripheral vascular resistance to runoff from the arterial tree. Normal peripheral resistance is approximately 1500 dynes • sec/cm^{-5} or 15 peripheral resistance units (also known as Wood's units).
Inotropic state	A measure of contractility.
Preload	Rigorously, stretch of myocardial fibers at end-diastole; commonly used as a synonym for venous return to the heart or end-diastolic volume.

failure, 50 per cent or more die within 1 year. Several factors have been shown to be independent predictors of survival in patients with heart failure. The extent of impairment of ventricular function, usually judged by left or right ventricular ejection fraction, is correlated with prognosis, as are reduced cardiac index and elevated ventricular filling pressures. Exercise capacity, as well as peak O$_2$ consumption and New York Heart Association functional class, are valid predictors of survival. Neurohumoral activation as evidenced by elevated plasma norepinephrine levels, basal plasma renin activity, or plasma atrial natriuretic factor has adverse prognostic significance, as does hyponatremia. The occurrence of either ventricular or supraventricular arrhythmias is predictive of shorter survival. Of note, about 40 to 50 per cent of deaths among heart failure patients occur suddenly and are thought to be due in large part to ventricular arrhythmias, occurring at times when patients are relatively compensated and out of hospital. Antiarrhythmic drug therapy has not yet been shown to alter this situation, but the automatic implantable cardioverter/defibrillator shows promise.

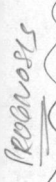

Given the limited outlook despite application of all available treatment modalities for patients with heart failure, the clinician must do everything possible to *prevent* progression of heart disease to the point where cardiac reserve and compensatory mechanisms are exhausted and the syndrome of overt congestive heart failure supervenes.

The term *heart failure* is often used as a synonym for myocardial failure, emphasizing the impaired performance of the heart as a muscle and as a pump. It also provides a rationale for medical treatment. Subsequent chapters deal with syndromes in which the cause of circulatory compromise lies elsewhere, such as in abnormalities of the heart valves or pericardium or inappropriate heart rates.

Imbalance between circulatory demands and cardiac response sets the stage for the syndrome of heart failure. Volume overload is generally tolerated better than pressure overload. Aortic or mitral insufficiency produces *volume* overload that may be tolerated for years without overt heart failure; *pressure* overload from aortic stenosis, in contrast, usually results in earlier onset and more rapid progression of heart failure. Gradually developing

overloads are accommodated better than acute overloads. Thus, gradually developing chronic mitral regurgitation is often present for years without signs of failure, whereas acute mitral regurgitation from a ruptured chorda tendinea can precipitate life-threatening pulmonary edema.

The myocardium adapts quite differently to volume and pressure loads. Volume overloads typically produce dilation followed by hypertrophy; pressure overloads characteristically elicit concentric hypertrophy until late in the natural history when dilation supervenes. Primary myocardial disease usually results in both dilation and hypertrophy.

Precipitating stresses (see Table 40–2) often tip the balance of the compromised heart toward decompensation and constitute important items for therapeutic attention.

Although the discussion in this chapter deals primarily with the abnormalities of the heart itself that underlie the syndrome of congestive heart failure, it is increasingly recognized that abnormalities of the peripheral circulation and neurohormonal milieu are also important factors in determining the degree of functional limitation experienced by patients with heart failure.

CLINICAL CATEGORIES OF HEART FAILURE

Types of heart failure are often categorized according to five features: duration (acute or chronic), initiating mechanisms, the ventricle primarily affected, the clinical syndrome, and the underlying physiologic derangements.

Acute Versus Chronic Heart Failure

The clinical manifestations of heart failure often begin insidiously and progress gradually into a chronic state. Alternatively, onset may be abrupt, as after acute myocardial infarction or chorda tendinea rupture.

Compensatory mechanisms in both acute and chronic heart failure include increased systemic vascular resistance and redistribution of blood flow. However, these adaptive mechanisms in acute and chronic heart failure differ quantitatively and sometimes also in direction. For example, *acute* distention of the left atrium generally promotes a sodium-poor diuresis, whereas *chronic* distention of the left atrium elicits salt and water retention.

Initiating Mechanisms

Each initiating mechanism has its own distinctive characteristics. For example, the symptoms and signs that evolve in rheumatic heart disease differ from those of hypertensive heart

TABLE 40–2. PRECIPITATING OR EXACERBATING FACTORS IN CONGESTIVE HEART FAILURE

Increased demand:
  Anemia
  Fever
  Infection
  Fluid overload
  Increased dietary salt intake
  High environmental temperature
  Renal failure
  Hepatic failure
  Thyrotoxicosis
  Arteriovenous (AV) shunt (Paget's disease of bone)
  Respiratory insufficiency
  Emotional stress
  Pregnancy
  Obesity
Arrhythmias
Pulmonary embolism
Ethanol ingestion
Thiamine deficiency
Uncontrolled hypertension
Poor compliance with therapeutic regimen
Drugs
  Beta-adrenergic blockers
  Antiarrhythmic drugs (e.g., disopyramide)
  Salt-retaining drugs
    Steroids
    Nonsteroidal anti-inflammatory agents

disease, whereas both have a different natural history from that of cor pulmonale. Even a single etiology, arteriosclerosis, may have distinctly different consequences, depending on the size and location of affected vessels. Progressive narrowing and gradual occlusion of distal branches of the coronary arteries may be so covert that shortness of breath and fatigue may be misinterpreted as the general physical decline of advancing age. In contrast, abrupt closure of a major coronary artery may result in myocardial necrosis followed by an acute low output state or by progressive chronic heart failure.

Left Versus Right Heart Failure

One ventricle bears the brunt of many disease processes and fails before the other. Because of the prevalence of cardiac disorders that overload or damage the left ventricle, heart failure most often begins with that ventricle. Breathlessness is the most common presenting symptom and is a direct consequence of elevated left ventricular filling pressure and pulmonary congestion. When the right ventricle fails, systemic venous congestion and peripheral edema predominate. Left ventricular failure is the most common cause of right ventricular failure, and breathlessness may improve as right ventricular output falls and pulmonary congestion diminishes.

The mechanism by which left ventricular failure causes the right ventricle to fail is not clear. Pulmonary hypertension secondary to left ventricular failure may contribute, but the degree of pulmonary hypertension is often insufficient to constitute a formidable burden on the right ventricle. Interdependence of the two ventricles, with failure of shared muscle in the ventricular septum, may also contribute. Right ventricular failure is an uncommon cause of left ventricular failure, but there is a relatively high frequency of independent left ventricular disease in elderly patients with right ventricular failure.

The combination of left and right ventricular (biventricular) failure, with elevated filling pressures of both ventricles causing pulmonary and systemic venous hypertension, results in the syndrome known as "congestive heart failure." This term implies reduced effort tolerance, breathlessness, distended neck veins, hepatic engorgement, and peripheral edema.

Backward Versus Forward Heart Failure

"Backward failure" refers to elevated cardiac filling pressures and attributes to the consequent venous congestion a critical role in the evolution of the syndrome of heart failure. "Forward failure" refers to decreased cardiac output and inadequate perfusion of organs. This distinction has limited clinical usefulness and has largely been replaced by more specific consideration of ventricular filling pressures and cardiac output.

High Versus Low Output Failure

The separation into "high" and "low" output failure distinguishes certain clinical manifestations, rather than causes, of myocardial failure. It serves (1) to distinguish a type of myocardial failure ("high output failure") in which the circulation remains brisk and the extremities tend to remain warm despite elevated venous pressures and a lower cardiac output than existed prior to the onset of heart failure; (2) to emphasize that the cardiac output and the circulatory adjustments during heart failure are conditioned by the state that existed prior to heart failure; and (3) to relate etiology to typical clinical features of heart failure. In regard to this last point, the more common causes—arteriosclerosis, myocardial disease, valvular disease, hypertension, and pericardial disease—tend to produce low output states; other, less common causes, including hyperthyroidism, Paget's disease of bone, anemia, beriberi, and arteriovenous fistula, tend to be associated with high output states. The essence of cardiac failure, however, remains the inability of the heart to increase its output appropriately in relation to demand.

Congestive Failure Versus Congested State

Elevated volume of the circulation, with preserved ventricular function, characterizes the "congested state." It is commonly encountered in intensive care facilities, where vigorous volume infusions are often used to combat systemic hypotension. It is encountered on a chronic basis in severe anemia and chronic renal insufficiency and less often in Paget's disease or beriberi.

In these situations, venous hypertension results from expanded intravascular volume, rather than from impaired myocardial contractile state.

In time, myocardial failure may supervene, with an inadequate increase in cardiac output for the increment in oxygen uptake during exercise. Correction of inciting factors and administration of diuretics are effective in both the "congested state" and in "congestive heart failure."

Systolic Versus Diastolic Failure

Recent studies indicate that up to one third of patients evaluated for symptoms and signs of heart failure have normal or nearly normal left ventricular ejection fractions, but because of the low compliance of the chamber they require substantially elevated filling pressures to maintain an adequate forward stroke output. These patients with diastolic dysfunction usually suffer from one (or more) of three underlying problems: (1) left ventricular hypertrophy (e.g., due to hypertension, aortic stenosis, or hypertrophic cardiomyopathy); (2) myocardial ischemia, which impairs ventricular relaxation; and (3) infiltrative disease (most commonly amyloidosis). Much of the discussion that follows focuses on the "classic" syndrome of congestive heart failure that accompanies a dilated heart with impaired systolic function. It is essential to distinguish these patients from those with predominant diastolic dysfunction, who require a distinctly different therapeutic approach (see below). Echo-Doppler study usually provides definitive information distinguishing these patient subsets, as does radionuclide ventriculography.

SUBCELLULAR BASIS FOR CONTRACTION

Cardiac contraction is initiated by depolarization of the sarcolemmal membrane, which activates slow calcium channels that undergo a transient increase in calcium permeability. The resulting calcium influx triggers the release of a much larger amount of calcium from the sarcoplasmic reticulum with consequent sarcomere shortening; the sarcoplasmic reticulum then resequesters calcium to turn off myofilament interaction, permitting myocardial relaxation.

Contractile force in heart muscle is generated by interactions among contractile proteins in repeating units (sarcomeres) that compose the individual muscle fibers (myofibrils). Within each sarcomere, the contractile proteins are arranged in thick filaments consisting of myosin and thin filaments consisting of actin and the modulator proteins troponin and tropomyosin. Interaction of calcium with one of three proteins composing troponin initiates the contractile process by removing a troponin-tropomyosin–induced inhibition of thick and thin filament interaction.

Changes in the length of heart muscle during contraction and relaxation are explained by the sliding filament hypothesis. During contraction, the thin actin filaments are propelled past the myosin thick filaments by force generated by ATP-dependent movement of cross-bridges consisting of the head portion of the myosin molecule. As the muscle shortens, the cross-bridges disengage and then engage other sites with a ratchet-like action. Depending on the number of cross-bridges that interact at a given time, different tensions are developed. Energy-dependent uptake of cytosolic calcium by the sarcoplasmic reticulum allows cross-bridge disengagement and relaxation to occur. Abundant mitochondria generate energy for the contractile machinery by oxidative phosphorylation fueled by free fatty acids and, to a lesser extent, glucose.

For the sarcomere, as for the whole heart (see Preload, below, and Table 40–1), the tension developed during contraction is directly related to its end-diastolic length. Stretching to permit optimal thick and thin filament overlap increases the ability of individual contractile elements to develop force. There are still many uncertainties regarding molecular details of the contractile process, and much is still to be learned about cardiac "success" as an essential background against which to examine basic mechanisms in cardiac "failure."

PATHOPHYSIOLOGIC INTERPLAY

Because of their location, structure, and function, the heart and lungs operate as a functional unit. The continuity of the muscle that surrounds the ventricular chambers, the shared ventricular septum, and the encasing pericardium ensure coordinate function, yet each ventricle functions as a separate muscular pump with its own atrial booster pump. In the normal heart, at least 50 per cent of the ventricular end-diastolic volume is ejected with each beat. Although many properties of ejection are inherent in the architecture and physiology of cardiac muscle, adaptability to changing metabolic needs is provided by a superimposed set of neurohumoral adjustments that modulate cardiac rate, loading, and contractility.

Each ventricle has its own capacity to withstand and repair the stresses imposed by normal and abnormal function. The two ventricles also have different designs in keeping with their different physiologic functions. Before birth, both ventricles bear similar pressure loads. After birth, the right ventricular workload decreases as pulmonary arterial pressure falls. The greater workload of the mature left ventricle, together with the greater prevalence of diseases that compromise the left side of the heart and its blood supply, result in the preponderance of left over right ventricular dysfunction in groups of patients in whom ischemic disease and hypertension are common.

ASSESSMENT OF CARDIAC PERFORMANCE

In terms of its performance, the heart may be assessed as a pump, as a muscle, or as a component of the circulatory system. Hemodynamic pressure and flow measurements characterize its behavior as a pump. Principles of muscle mechanics are used to describe its behavior as a muscle. Its adequacy as a component of the circulatory system is reflected in the consequences of reduced cardiac output, redistribution of blood flow, organ hypoperfusion, and pulmonary or systemic venous congestion.

Heart as a Pump: Hemodynamics

By the time overt heart failure is apparent, the large functional reserve of the normal heart is compromised and a variety of mechanisms operate to compensate for its diminished performance. Despite an inappropriately low cardiac output, the blood pressure at rest tends to remain normal or even increases, albeit with frequent reduction in pulse pressure.

CARDIAC OUTPUT. In response to peripheral demands, a complex set of control mechanisms modulates heart rate and the extent of stretch and shortening of myocardial fibers and, hence, the stroke volume and the cardiac output (stroke volume times heart rate). Three principal variables determine the stroke volume (Table 40–1): preload, afterload (resistance to ventricular emptying during systole), and the contractile state of the heart. For practical purposes, three of the principal determinants of cardiac output—preload, afterload, and heart rate—are readily measured. Contractile (inotropic) state remains difficult to assess in formal quantitative terms, but noninvasive (echo-Doppler) and minimally invasive (radionuclide ventriculography) methods yield the requisite data for most clinical decision making. Ejection fraction is commonly used as a clinically useful index (albeit impure) of contractile state, and the maximum rate of pressure rise during the isovolumetric phase of systole (dP/dt) is a useful measure in invasive hemodynamic investigations.

Relationships among these determinants vary with the state of the heart and circulation. Thus when contractility is impaired, stroke output and cardiac output tend to be maintained by ventricular dilation (Frank-Starling mechanism), limiting the value of cardiac output as a measure of inotropic state to experimental circumstances in which preload, afterload, and heart rate can be held constant.

Indicator-dilution techniques can be used in the ICU or cardiac catheterization laboratory for determination of cardiac output. In resting adults, the normal range is between 2.5 and 3.6 liters per minute per square meter of body surface area. Decreased cardiac output at rest occurs only in advanced stages of cardiac impairment. A blunted cardiac output response to exercise occurs much earlier. Supine exercise in normal subjects should increase the cardiac output by at least 600 ml per minute for each 100-ml increment in oxygen consumption; lower values indicate reduced cardiac performance. In heart failure the arteriovenous oxygen difference is abnormally wide, resulting chiefly from the low oxygen content of venous blood returning to the heart. Oxygenation of blood in the lungs remains nearly normal until pulmonary vascular congestion becomes sufficiently severe to create ventilation-perfusion mismatch with effective shunting, or abnormal diffusion barriers to oxygen transport.

During exercise, cardiac output normally increases as a linear function of oxygen consumption, although for any level of exercise the cardiac output tends to be lower in the upright position. Increases in cardiac output in the upright posture are accomplished principally by increases in heart rate rather than in stroke volume. In heart failure, cardiac output is particularly dependent on heart rate, both at rest and during exercise.

VENTRICULAR END-DIASTOLIC PRESSURE AND VOLUME. Impaired systolic ventricular emptying leads to an increase in the end-systolic residual volume of blood in the ventricle, predisposing to an increase in end-diastolic volume. Since this is inconvenient to measure or monitor, ventricular end-diastolic pressure is customarily followed for clinical purposes on the premise that a change in pressure is effected by a change in ventricular volume. Exceptions occur, however, including structural changes in the myocardium (fibrosis, edema, and hypertrophy) and pericardial constriction that cause disproportionate rises in end-diastolic pressure relative to volume. Acute ischemia also produces transient reduction in left ventricular compliance. Conversely, in some states of chronic volume overload, compliance increases so that increased volumes are accommodated at end-diastole with relatively modest pressure increases.

A left ventricular end-diastolic pressure greater than 12 to 15 mm Hg is abnormal. The corresponding upper limit for the right ventricle is 6 to 10 mm Hg. It is straightforward to estimate the right ventricular end-diastolic pressure by measuring the central venous pressure. In the absence of mitral obstruction or increased pulmonary vascular resistance, pulmonary arterial diastolic pressure approximates left ventricular end-diastolic pressure. Pulmonary capillary wedge pressure or diastolic pressure measured with a Swan-Ganz catheter is widely used in ICU settings to monitor left ventricular filling pressures.

To summarize, the performance of heart muscle depends on two essential components: fiber length (Frank-Starling mechanism) and inherent contractility (inotropic state). The normal heart autoregulates to maintain cardiac output. The variables involved are preload, afterload, contractility, and heart rate. With chronic overloading, the heart undergoes dilation, hypertrophy, or both.

PRELOAD. According to the Frank-Starling mechanism, an increase in end-diastolic volume (preload) results in more forceful contraction with enhancement of ventricular emptying and stroke volume. A unique ventricular function curve exists for each state of contractility (Fig. 40–1). The curve for a failing ventricle is shifted downward and flattened such that stroke volumes are reduced despite abnormally high end-diastolic volumes or pressures. The elevated filling pressures are responsible for congestion and edema in the venous beds leading to the failing ventricle.

In the normal heart, the Frank-Starling mechanism serves to match the stroke outputs of the two ventricles. In heart failure, this mechanism plays the additional role of helping to support the cardiac output.

AFTERLOAD. Afterload refers to the resistance that the ventricle must overcome during systole in order to eject the stroke volume. It incorporates all factors that oppose shortening of the ventricular fibers. In practice, it is estimated for the left heart either from the arterial blood pressure or from calculation of systemic vascular resistance (ratio of blood pressure to flow, expressed in units of dynes · sec/cm^{-5} or in peripheral resistance units). Right ventricular afterload (pulmonary artery pressure) can be estimated satisfactorily in most patients by echo-Doppler measurements.

In the assessment of patients, the relationship of blood pressure to cardiac output and peripheral resistance (P/Flow = R) is quite useful. Interventions that cause an increase in cardiac output without changing systemic blood pressure must cause vasodilation, thereby decreasing peripheral vascular resistance or afterload. Improved emptying of the left ventricle is usually accompanied by a decrease in its filling pressure (pulmonary capillary wedge or pulmonary artery diastolic pressure).

If preload and contractility remain constant, increasing after-

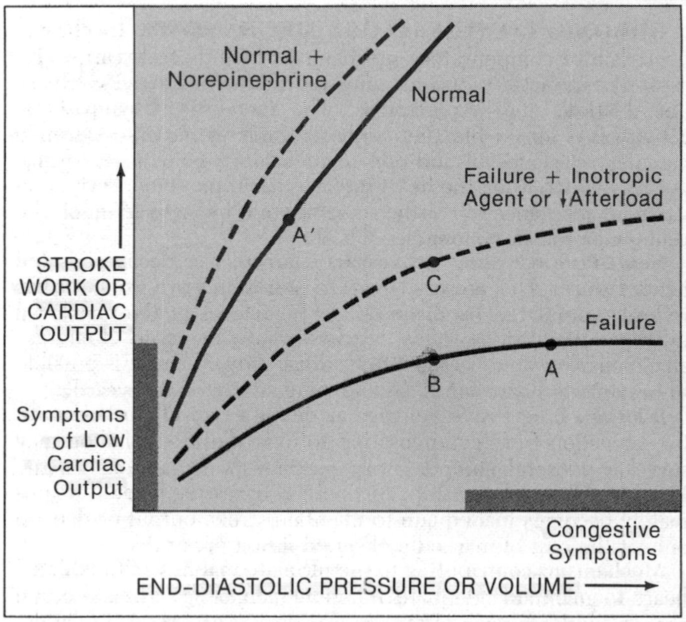

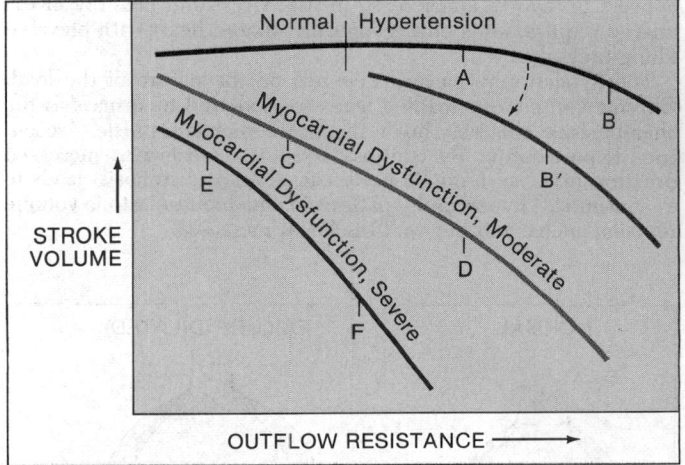

FIGURE 40–1. Schematic diagram demonstrating the relationship between ventricular end-diastolic pressure or volume and cardiac index in a normal and a failing heart. The normal left ventricle increases its stroke output as preload (often measured clinically as pulmonary capillary wedge pressure) increases, moving up the ascending limb of the curve until reserve is exhausted. In heart failure, the ventricular function curve is displaced downward and to the right. An increase in contractility, as after administration of norepinephrine or digitalis, displaces the curve to the left; i.e., a larger stroke output is accomplished at any given filling pressure. A and A' represent the operating points at rest of a hypothetical patient with heart failure and of a normal person, respectively. Reduction of physical activity allows the failing heart to meet the demands of the metabolizing tissues. Treatment of heart failure by a reduction in preload (e.g., with a diuretic or a vasodilator acting predominantly on the venous bed) causes a shift from point A to B on the same ventricular function curve. Administration of a positive inotropic agent or a vasodilator producing afterload reduction shifts the curve as shown, resulting in improvement of the circulatory state in the direction shown by a shift from point A to C.

load in the normal heart tends to decrease both the extent and the speed of contraction to a minor extent. Reduction in afterload has the opposite effects. Within broad physiologic limits, the normal ventricle maintains a relatively constant stroke volume as afterload is increased (Fig. 40–2). The impaired ventricle responds quite differently, with progressive diminution in its ability to eject blood against a given afterload as the severity of myocardial dysfunction advances. Figure 40–2 illustrates the rationale for afterload reduction in the management of heart failure.

CONTRACTILITY (INOTROPIC STATE). Modulation of sympathetic nervous activity provides the major component of short-term adjustment of contractile state in the normal heart and also mediates increases in heart rate and venous tone. Unlike the Frank-Starling mechanism, the increase in force and velocity of contraction is accomplished without any increase in fiber length (end-diastolic volume). Contractility does not limit the output of the normal heart. By contrast, the failing heart is limited in its myocardial performance, indicated by displacement of the ventricular function curve as shown in Figure 40–1.

An objective index of myocardial contractility that could be measured independent of myocardial fiber length would be useful (1) to assess the effects on the myocardium of interventions such as the administration of digitalis or other inotropic agents; (2) to determine serial changes in inotropic state in an individual during the evolution of heart failure and in response to treatment; and (3) to compare the inotropic state in different individuals. However, distinction between the effects of loading conditions and intrinsic contractility is difficult because of the strong influence of loading on hemodynamic measurements. Changes in preload or afterload can modify ventricular performance greatly without affecting intrinsic inotropic state. Since conventional hemodynamic measurements do not take heart size into account, comparisons of contractility in hearts of different size are difficult to interpret.

Ejection Fraction. This term denotes the fraction of the right or left ventricular end-diastolic volume ejected per beat. It is useful as an integrative measure of contractility and is determined by contrast ventriculography, by gated blood pool radionuclide imaging, or by echocardiography. The normal left ventricular ejection fraction ranges from 0.56 to 0.78. A reduced ejection fraction in a patient with normal valves and a dilated ventricle strongly suggests decreased contractility, particularly in the absence of increased afterload. Abnormalities of regional myocardial function are often evident in the pattern of ventricular contraction demonstrated by these techniques and suggest focal ischemic disease, but may also be observed in primary cardiomyopathic disorders.

Other Techniques. Simultaneous graphic recording of the electrocardiogram, phonocardiogram, and carotid arterial pulse contour provides another noninvasive means of assessing cardiac function but has been almost entirely supplanted by the more clinically useful echo-Doppler assessment. Accurate measurement of ventricular dP/dt can be accomplished at cardiac catheterization and provides a measure of contractile state less subject to the influence of loading conditions than most other approaches; its use is largely confined to research applications.

FIGURE 40–2. Relation of left ventricular stroke volume to systemic outflow resistance in normal and diseased hearts. A family of curves may be described, depending on the severity of the myocardial disease. If cardiac function is normal, a rise in resistance results in hypertension, since cardiac output remains fairly constant. Heart failure in a hypertensive patient could be shown by a move to either point B, a high resistance with normal function, or point B', which represents a shift to a slightly depressed ventricular function curve. When myocardial dysfunction is more severe, as shown by the lower two curves, blood pressure is no longer directly determined by resistance, since stroke volume and resistance are inversely related. Consequently, arterial pressure may be similar at points E and F despite marked differences in cardiac output and resistance. It is also apparent that a reduction in outflow resistance does not affect significantly the stroke volume of the normal ventricle. However, it can produce a marked increase in the stroke volume of the failing ventricle (F→E). (Adapted from Cohn JN, Franciosa JA: Vasodilator therapy of cardiac failure. N Engl J Med 297:27, 1977. By permission of the New England Journal of Medicine.)

CHRONIC COMPENSATORY MECHANISMS. In chronic heart failure compensatory mechanisms include tachycardia, increased contractility due to sympathetic nervous activity, chamber dilation, and hypertrophy. The increase in sympathetic activity is a mixed blessing, since it tends to increase systemic vascular resistance in addition to its salutory effects on cardiac output by increasing the heart rate and inotropic state. Peripheral vascular resistance is further augmented by activation of the renin-angiotensin system (see Ch. 44).

Heart Rate. Chronic tachycardia characterizes decompensated heart failure. The increase in rate stems in part from cardiac reflexes stimulated by distention of structures at the venoatrial junctions (Bainbridge reflex). Tachycardia is, in terms of energy, an expensive way to support the cardiac output, and it is possible to precipitate heart failure by inducing sustained tachycardia.

Dilation. Progressive ventricular dilation typically occurs with the transition from compensation to overt failure. Dilation may serve as a useful compensatory mechanism for a time via the Frank-Starling relationship, but with progressive disease it ultimately becomes inadequate to maintain stroke output or does so only at the cost of markedly elevated filling pressures.

Mechanisms contributing to the ultimate inability of the dilated heart to maintain adequate function include (1) ultrastructural changes with slippage of sarcomeres during progressive dilation; as a result, they are not stretched to generate optimal contractility; and (2) increased wall tension (law of Laplace, Fig. 40–3) resulting in increased myocardial oxygen consumption; a corollary is that in contrast to the normal heart, in which the wall tension decreases in the course of systole, wall tension tends to remain high throughout contraction in the dilated heart. Thus chronic dilation has important limitations as a compensatory mechanism in cardiac failure.

Hypertrophy. Sustained abnormal pressure or volume loads lead to an increase in ventricular mass. This involves changes in gene expression and increased protein synthesis. Decreased protein degradation rates may occur as well in response to mechanical overload or dilation. The stimulus for hypertrophy appears to involve an increase in wall stress and possibly in the energy requirements of a chronically dilated heart with elevated filling pressures.

The hypertrophy pattern depends on the nature of the load. Chronic volume overloading leads to increased total mass as the chamber size enlarges, but wall thickness changes little ("eccentric" hypertrophy). By contrast, chronic exposure to increased pressure (e.g., systemic hypertension or aortic stenosis) leads to a "concentric" hypertrophy pattern in which end-diastolic volume remains unchanged but wall thickness increases.

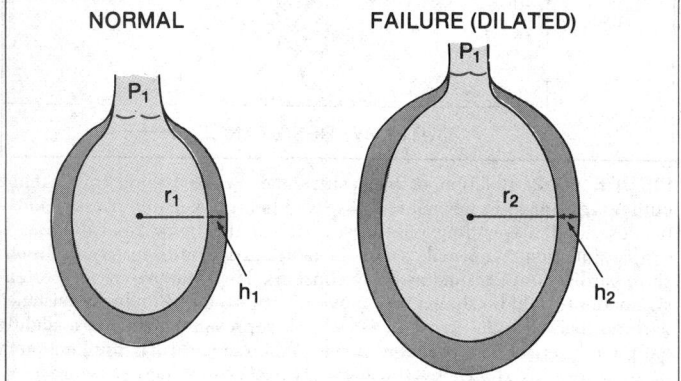

FIGURE 40–3. Laplace relationship applied to the dilated heart. The tension developed in the wall of the heart during systole (T) is a directional force that is proportional to the product of the mean pressure that the wall is supporting (P) and the mean radius (r). To a first approximation, $T = \dfrac{Pr}{2}$. Dilation of the heart $(r_2 > r_1)$ at the same pressure $(P_1 = P_2)$ increases wall tension $(T_2 > T_1)$. Should the wall become thinner during dilatation, the wall stress would increase as the cross-sectional area of myocardium (h) decreased.

Abnormal electrical conduction patterns can interfere with the normal, smoothly coordinated contraction pattern of the normal heart, as can myocyte loss with focal or diffuse fibrosis. Ischemic myocardial damage tends to cause hypertrophy and remodeling of residual muscle because the geometry of the abnormal ventricle causes it to operate at a mechanical disadvantage and also because normal muscle must work, and expend energy, in moving and stretching adjacent damaged muscle or scar.

In early or mild hypertrophy, muscle mass and capillary vessels increase proportionately, preserving the nutritive and contractile properties of the myocardium. With progressive hypertrophy (in the absence of ventricular dilation), additional sarcomeres are laid down, wall thickness increases, and ventricular wall stress tends to be maintained at a normal level despite increased cavity pressure, as indicated in Figure 40–3. This process ultimately exacts a price, however, since increased wall thickness often leads to increased wall stiffness (reduced compliance), thus necessitating a disproportionate rise in filling pressure to maintain adequate end-diastolic ventricular volume. The increasingly recognized syndrome of diastolic ventricular dysfunction, which occurs relatively commonly in the presence of a preserved ventricular ejection fraction, leads to elevated pulmonary or systemic venous pressures, which contribute to symptoms of dyspnea or peripheral edema. In addition, beyond a certain point, coronary flow reserve diminishes and contractile function declines. Thus, once unremitting hypertrophy begins, the myocardium has embarked on the road to overt failure.

Despite the depressed contractile state associated with later stages of hypertrophy, circulatory function is maintained for a time by the combination of increased muscles mass, dilation, and augmented sympathetic drive. With continuing loss of myocardial contractility, or loss of muscle cells (e.g., from ischemic or inflammatory processes), circulatory compensation can no longer be maintained. The typical clinical and hemodynamic manifestations of congestive heart failure then emerge as cardiac output fails to meet demands and filling pressures increase.

Heart as a Muscle

Consideration of the ventricular performance of the failing heart usually centers on the contraction phase. Events during diastole, however, influence ventricular compliance and hence filling pressures, as well as the subsequent contraction and the energy supply for contraction and relaxation.

RELAXATION AND DISTENSIBILITY. Diastolic filling of the ventricle depends on the time available (a function of heart rate), the timing and properties of atrial systole, and the diastolic properties of the ventricle. Relaxation of cardiac muscle is an energy-requiring process (see above) that is quite vulnerable to adenosine triphosphate (ATP) depletion caused by ischemia. Although heart failure per se does not necessarily impair ventricular relaxation, associated processes of hypertrophy, fibrosis, and ischemia often reduce chamber distensibility and further increase filling pressures to levels producing pulmonary edema. This problem can be particularly severe in hypertrophic cardiomyopathy and in diseases such as amyloidosis that markedly reduce left ventricular diastolic compliance. Elderly patients with hypertension and diabetes mellitus seem especially prone to diastolic ventricular dysfunction. Management of the subset of patients with predominant diastolic dysfunction is discussed below.

ENERGETICS. The heart depends on aerobic metabolism for its supply of energy, the bulk of which is spent to support contraction. The major determinants of oxygen consumption of the heart include the interrelated components of rate, ventricular pressure, volume, work, wall tension, and contractile state. The time integral of systolic tension relates closely to myocardial oxygen consumption, whereas fiber shortening has a minor effect on myocardial oxygen consumption.

The cellular and biochemical basis for heart failure remains unsettled. It is generally agreed that there are no consistent defects in energy metabolism or in protein synthesis and turnover. Current investigation is centered on excitation-contraction coupling and mechanisms that control calcium homeostasis.

Compensatory mechanisms in advanced heart failure tend to increase myocardial oxygen requirements by several mechanisms, including increased preload due to salt and water retention and enhanced sympathetic drive with consequently increased after-load, contractility, and heart rate. Increased preload and afterload are also the result of activation of the renin-angiotensin-aldosterone system.

Heart as Component of the Circulatory System

With loss of cardiac reserve and onset of overt heart failure, peripheral mechanisms are called upon to sustain blood pressure and to distribute the limited cardiac output to vital beds.

VENOUS HYPERTENSION. As the ejection fraction falls and the ventricle fails to empty properly during systole, the volume of unexpelled blood increases with an accompanying increase in diastolic pressure in the ventricles and in the atria and proximal veins. Other elements that contribute to the venous hypertension include (1) increased tone in venous capacitance vessels; (2) blood volume expansion as a consequence of renal sodium and water retention; and, on occasion, (3) incompetence of mitral or tricuspid valves with regurgitation of blood from ventricle to atrium as the valve becomes incompetent from intrinsic valvular disease, papillary muscle dysfunction, ventricular dilation, or inadequate closure during an arrhythmia.

PERIPHERAL MECHANISMS TO SUSTAIN BLOOD PRESSURE AND CARDIAC OUTPUT. To sustain and distribute the cardiac output, and to maintain systemic arterial pressure, important peripheral mechanisms are activated.

In the normal circulation, the cardiac output doubles in response to a four- or fivefold increase in total body oxygen consumption. When functional impairment is such that the cardiac output cannot keep pace with peripheral demands, blood flow is redistributed to defend vital areas such as the brain and heart. The autonomic nervous system participates in this modulation of the circulation and contributes also to activation of mechanisms that mediate the retention of sodium and water.

Peripheral vasoconstriction and tachycardia characterize the common forms of heart failure. However, despite a generalized increase in sympathetic nervous activity, norepinephrine stores in the heart muscle are depleted because of its enhanced turnover rate. Pharmacologic agents such as reserpine or guanethidine further deplete cardiac catecholamine stores and can aggravate heart failure, as can β-adrenergic antagonists such as propranolol and the many other drugs of this class.

The contribution of the parasympathetic nervous system to the control of heart rate and baroreceptor activity is impaired in heart failure, but therapeutic implications of these phenomena are not yet clear.

Peripheral Vasoconstriction. Peripheral arteriolar and venous constriction, mediated in large part by increased sympathetic nervous and renin-angiotensin system activity, is an important compensatory mechanism in heart failure that has both positive and negative consequences, as noted earlier. The extent to which accumulation of sodium and water in the arteriolar wall contributes to increased arteriolar resistance is as yet unclear.

Venoconstriction augments venous return by facilitating the return of blood to the central veins, increasing central venous pressure and hence preload. The principal determinant of elevated filling pressures, however, is the inability of the failing ventricle to eject the venous return.

Redistribution. Maintenance of oxygen and substrate delivery to brain and myocardium during states of limited cardiac output requires diversion of flow from skin, kidneys, splanchnic viscera, and skeletal muscle. This redistribution of blood flow initially occurs during activity or stress as cardiac output fails to increase sufficiently to meet the increment in metabolism; in severe heart failure, redistribution operates also at rest. The redistribution of blood flow to essential beds depends on the balance among sympathetic and renin-angiotensin system activities and local metabolism. The vasculature of skin, kidney, splanchnic beds, and skeletal muscle is richly innervated. Furthermore, these tissues have relatively low metabolic rates at rest, permitting sympathetic nervous and angiotensin II–mediated vasoconstriction to override local vasodilator effects of metabolites. By contrast, the circulations to brain and myocardium are less subject to α-adrenergically mediated vasoconstrictor influences because these organs, with their high oxygen consumption, produce metabolic dilator substances that offset increased sympathetic tone.

Under normal physiologic circumstances, exercise with the attendant need for heat dissipation induces an increase in cutaneous blood flow. Patients in heart failure, by contrast, fail to increase cutaneous flow despite this increased need for heat loss. Thus the patient in heart failure preserves systemic arterial pressure and flow to vital organs by suffering the consequences of impaired heat loss as well as limitation of blood flow to exercising muscle groups.

THE VALSALVA MANEUVER. An abnormal response to the Valsalva maneuver, in which intrathoracic pressure is maintained at approximately 40 mm Hg for 10 to 12 seconds, is characteristic of left ventricular failure. In normal subjects there is a characteristic decrease in blood pressure and pulse pressure and increase in heart rate; at cessation of straining, the blood pressure, pulse pressure, and bradycardia tend to overshoot. By contrast, in the presence of left ventricular failure there is a "square wave" response in which normal reflex responses are blunted. Hence blood pressure increases at the onset of straining, stays elevated throughout the maneuver, and decreases abruptly to baseline after the maneuver with no overshoot; tachycardia is absent.

SALT AND WATER RETENTION. As overt heart failure develops, there is typically a decrease in renal blood flow and glomerular filtration rate, with an associated redistribution of renal blood flow. These changes contribute to the sodium and water retention that characterizes heart failure, but the nature and extent of the response differ according to the severity of heart failure, as discussed subsequently under diuretics. Hemodynamic abnormalities are undoubtedly involved in activating the renin-angiotensin-aldosterone system both via direct effects on the kidney and via indirect effects stemming from activation of mechanoreceptors in the distended left atrium. Recognition of the role of hyperaldosteronism in the genesis of sodium and water retention has resulted in the development of aldosterone antagonists as useful adjuncts in the therapy of heart failure.

Sweat and saliva are sodium poor in patients with decompensated heart failure. Antidiuretic hormone (arginine vasopressin) levels tend to be elevated in heart failure and may contribute to elevated systemic vascular resistance, but probably are not important in salt or water retention.

An increase of about 10 to 20 per cent in circulating blood volume contributes to maintenance of cardiac output and perfusion of vital organs in moderate-to-severe heart failure, augmenting ventricular end-diastolic volume and thereby tending to improve pump performance. The resulting elevation of filling pressure, however, promotes edema formation by raising venous and capillary pressures proximal to the failing ventricle. By the time the circulating blood volume has increased by 20 per cent, the extravascular fluid volume may well have increased by a factor of two.

Exercise Testing

Graded treadmill or bicycle exercise testing has been used investigatively to determine maximum total body oxygen uptake (aerobic capacity). The endpoint of fatigue generally coincides with the point at which aerobic metabolism can no longer meet tissue demands and lactate production begins (anaerobic threshold). This approach has also been used to assess quantitatively the effects of therapeutic interventions for the treatment of heart failure.

CLINICAL MANIFESTATIONS OF HEART FAILURE

The signs and symptoms of heart failure depend on which ventricle has failed and the severity and duration of failure. The clinical picture in left ventricular failure is dominated by *symptoms* of pulmonary congestion and edema. By contrast, right ventricular failure is dominated by *signs* of systemic venous congestion and peripheral edema. Weakness, fatigue, and effort intolerance are common to right or left ventricular failure as well as biventricular failure.

Left Ventricular Failure

The symptom of breathlessness predominates in patients with left ventricular failure and varies with position and activity. Noteworthy physical signs are most evident in the heart, lungs, or respiratory control mechanisms.

DYSPNEA. Dyspnea (breathlessness) during limited exertion is typically the earliest symptom of left heart failure and is usually associated with an increased rate of breathing (tachypnea). Although many details of the physiologic basis for the sensation of dyspnea remain unclear, some aspects of the etiology of respiratory symptoms from pulmonary congestion deserve consideration. Since the bronchial capillaries drain for the most part via the pulmonary veins, congestion tends to develop in alveolar and bronchial vascular networks simultaneously. Interstitial edema surrounding pulmonary capillaries appears to stimulate juxtacapillary receptors known as J-receptors, which in turn elicits a reflexly mediated pattern of rapid and shallow breathing. At the same time, bronchial congestion stimulates mucus production, and the distended bronchial capillaries may rupture, with resulting cough and hemoptysis. Bronchial mucosal edema causes increased resistance in small airways, producing wheezing and respiratory distress known as cardiac asthma. The increased work of moving fluid-laden, noncompliant lungs must be accomplished in the face of decreased blood flow to respiratory muscles and also increased diffusion barriers to oxygen exchange across the alveolar-capillary interface, contributing to respiratory muscle fatigue and the sensation of dyspnea.

Thus, the symptom of dyspnea in left heart failure clearly relates to the increase in blood volume and interstitial fluid content of the lungs at the expense of air. Ventilation increases, and the awareness of dyspnea becomes more severe as minute ventilation approaches the maximal ventilatory capacity.

ORTHOPNEA. Dyspnea that occurs soon after lying flat (and is relieved by sitting up) is known as orthopnea. The pathophysiologic basis for orthopnea is the increase in venous return from the lower extremities and splanchnic bed to the lungs in the recumbent position, together with the reabsorption of peripheral edema that accumulates during the day. Orthopnea is a relatively reliable marker for left ventricular failure, whereas the dyspnea associated with chronic lung disease or musculoskeletal disorders is typically less aggravated by lying flat. Patients usually learn to avoid dyspnea of this sort by sleeping with the head and thorax on two or more pillows. In advanced heart failure, orthopnea may be so severe as to cause the patient to sleep upright in a chair. An orthopneic cough has the same significance as orthopnea and is presumably the consequence of venous congestion and edema. Patients with left heart failure may also complain of precordial distress in the supine position that is difficult to distinguish from symptoms caused by myocardial ischemia.

NOCTURIA. In early heart failure, limitation of renal blood flow with upright activity during the day gives way to more normal renal perfusion and diuresis while supine at night. This causes nocturia, a common early symptom of incipient heart failure.

PAROXYSMAL NOCTURNAL DYSPNEA. Severe respiratory distress may arouse the patient from sleep. Relief is urgently sought by sitting up and often by finding an open window. In addition to exacerbation of pulmonary vascular congestion and edema during supine sleep, blunting of the respiratory center response to sensory input from the lungs during sleep, together with increased venous return, allows pulmonary venous congestion and edema to accumulate and trigger the alarming episode of breathlessness.

ACUTE PULMONARY EDEMA. In an episode of acute left ventricular failure, pulmonary venous and capillary pressure can increase abruptly to levels exceeding plasma oncotic pressure, with consequent rapid accumulation of edema fluid in the interstitial spaces and alveoli. Interstitial pulmonary edema leads to an increase in respiratory rate (see foregoing discussion) and tends to produce alveolar hyperventilation and respiratory alkalosis. However, when free fluid enters the alveoli and bronchioles, respiratory acidosis may occur owing to an intolerable increase in the work of breathing. Hypoxemia also occurs commonly because of imbalances between alveolar ventilation and alveolar blood flow (ventilation-perfusion mismatch or "shunting").

Symptoms of pulmonary edema may begin with a nonproductive cough, with wheezing, or with frank dyspnea. Apart from tachypnea and possibly evidence of underlying heart disease on physical examination, few physical signs may be present initially. Later, as free fluid accumulates in distal airways, rales become audible at the lung bases and extend upward accompanied by rhonchi as the episode progresses. In severe acute pulmonary edema, the patient is typically pale, sweating, cyanotic, gasping for breath, and sometimes producing pink or blood-tinged frothy sputum.

HEMOPTYSIS. Rust-colored sputum containing heart failure cells (alveolar macrophages containing hemosiderin) sometimes occurs in severe chronic left heart failure and is seen with particular frequency in patients with advanced mitral stenosis. Frankly bloody sputum should suggest the possibility of pulmonary infarction, but expectoration of substantial quantities of blood can also occur as a consequence of rupture of engorged bronchial capillaries in patients with chronic left heart failure, including that caused by uncorrected mitral stenosis.

CHEYNE-STOKES RESPIRATION. Advanced heart failure may be accompanied by periodic breathing with alternate periods of apnea and hyperventilation. Because of slowing of the circulation time from lungs to brain, the arterial Po_2 reaches its peak and the arterial Pco_2 its nadir during apnea. At this time alveolar gas tensions are exactly opposite. During hyperpnea the alveolar Po_2 reaches its peak and the alveolar Pco_2 its nadir. Thus, changes in arterial blood gases are responsible for the cyclic ventilation, which in turn causes the changes in alveolar gas tensions. As would be expected from this delay of the normal negative feedback loop, the longer the circulation time, the longer are the cycles of hyperventilation and apnea. The neurologic changes of advanced age predispose to Cheyne-Stokes breathing, as does cerebrovascular disease.

Physical and Laboratory Signs of Left Heart Failure

The patient with decompensated left heart failure is generally tachypneic, pale, dusky, and sweaty. The handshake is cold because of peripheral vasoconstriction, and tachycardia is present. The pulse pressure is usually narrow, often with a modest increase in diastolic pressure. The neck veins are not distended if the left ventricle alone has failed.

THE HEART. Cardiac enlargement is often evident upon inspection, percussion, and palpation of the apical impulse and is confirmed by radiographic and echocardiographic examination. This finding is more typical of valvular or primary myocardial disease than of ischemic heart disease. With increased left heart filling pressure, pulmonary venous pressure increases and the pulmonary arterial pressure must also increase. The pulmonic component of the second heart sound (P_2) therefore tends to increase in intensity. In the presence of left ventricular dilation, papillary muscle dysfunction, or both, the mitral valve leaflets may fail to appose properly, resulting in mitral incompetence.

Gallop Rhythm. The presence of a protodiastolic third heart sound (S_3 gallop) in an adult with heart disease usually signifies the presence of ventricular failure. The timing of the normal first and second sounds and the abnormal third sound, in conjunction with an increased heart rate, results in the characteristic cadence of the gallop rhythm. The third heart sound occurs in early diastole coincident with rapid ventricular filling. The S_3 gallop appears to be produced by vibrations of the ventricular walls as the rapidly inflowing blood is abruptly arrested. A third heart sound is a normal finding in children and in young adults.

Presystolic gallop rhythms result from the atrial contribution to ventricular filling. The atrial or S_4 gallop is characteristic of decreased ventricular compliance and typically results from left ventricular hypertrophy or ischemia rather than from myocardial dysfunction or failure, although an S_4 gallop is typically present in patients with symptoms and signs of heart failure due predominantly to diastolic dysfunction. When a patient with an audible fourth heart sound develops overt heart failure, a third sound may appear, causing a quadruple rhythm. If the heart rate is sufficiently rapid or the PR interval is prolonged, S_3 and S_4 may merge, producing a summation gallop. The presence of a summation gallop has the same clinical implication as other protodiastolic (S_3) gallop rhythms.

Pulsus Alternans. The presence of alternating strong and weak beats (the fundamental rhythm remaining regular) usually signifies advanced heart failure. Pulsus alternans can be detected by palpation or by sphygmomanometry and often follows an atrial or ventricular premature beat for several cycles. Mechanical alternans of this sort is only rarely associated with electrical alternans. Pulsus alternans has been attributed to a severe disturbance of excitation-contraction coupling, the detailed pathophysiology of which is unclear.

THE LUNGS. The sequence of pulmonary findings with advancing left heart failure has been described in the foregoing section on acute pulmonary edema.

THE ELECTROCARDIOGRAM. Electrocardiographic abnormalities result from underlying cardiac disease, therapeutic agents (e.g., digitalis), or both and yield little information regarding the functional status of the heart.

RADIOLOGIC ASPECTS. The chest radiograph is usually quite helpful in the diagnosis and assessment of left ventricular failure (see Ch. 39.1). The cardiac silhouette is typically, but not invariably, enlarged and may assume telltale configurations that are determined by the underlying disease process. In contrast to normal, the pulmonary vasculature is prominent in the upper lung zones, reflecting pulmonary venous hypertension and redistribution of blood flow because of encroachment upon the lower lung vessels by edema and possibly fibrosis. Enlarged hilar shadows and prominent septal lines, particularly near the costophrenic angles (Kerley's B lines), are typical findings. Alveolar edema results in a generalized clouding of the lung fields but can occur in focal or patchy distributions that are difficult to distinguish from pneumonia. Pleural effusions sometimes occur in predominantly left-sided heart failure but are more characteristic of biventricular failure. Interstitial and alveolar edema may lessen or disappear with onset of right ventricular failure. A widened superior vena cava shadow suggests right ventricular failure and systemic venous congestion.

NONINVASIVE ASSESSMENT. Echocardiographic study constitutes a cost-effective approach to the evaluation of patients with heart failure, and together with Doppler study in most instances is advisable at an early stage in the workup of this group of patients (see Ch. 39.3). Valuable information can be obtained in every etiologic class of patients, including those with ischemic disease, cardiomyopathy, valvular disease, hypertensive disease, congenital disease, and cor pulmonale. Echo study is of particular value in making the important distinction between predominant systolic and diastolic ventricular dysfunction.

CARDIAC CATHETERIZATION. Invasive evaluation is usually appropriate in patients who are candidates for cardiac surgery or catheter-based interventional procedures such as coronary angioplasty or valvuloplasty, as discussed in Ch. 39.5. Right ventricular endomyocardial biopsy is valuable in patients suspected of having inflammatory or infiltrative disease and for assessment of myopathic effects of certain antineoplastic drugs (e.g., doxorubicin). Endomyocardial biopsy is routinely done using a percutaneous jugular approach at intervals following cardiac transplantation for assessment of the adequacy of immunosuppressive therapy.

PULMONARY FUNCTION TESTS. The course of left ventricular failure, including the response to treatment, can be followed by consecutive determinations of vital capacity, although this practice has been largely supplanted by other approaches in recent years. With interstitial pulmonary edema, expiratory flow rates at low lung volumes are reduced and distal airways tend to close prematurely during expiration, trapping gas within the lungs and disturbing the normal relation of ventilation to perfusion. This produces a widening of the alveolar-arterial P_{O_2} difference and a decrease in arterial P_{O_2} due to venous admixture. Arterial oxygen saturation is typically nearly normal, however, unless intrinsic lung disease is present. The arteriovenous oxygen content difference increases with decreasing cardiac outputs as tissue extraction of oxygen becomes more complete. Systemic arterial P_{CO_2} remains normal or low unless ventilation is compromised in the course of pulmonary edema. Endotracheal intubation and assisted ventilation may be indicated if progressive carbon dioxide retention is documented by serial blood gas measurements.

Right Ventricular and Biventricular Failure

CLINICAL MANIFESTATIONS. Isolated right ventricular failure is uncommon in adults and is usually a consequence of cor pulmonale secondary to intrinsic lung disease or, on occasion, chronic volume overload from a congenital intracardiac left-to-right shunt (e.g., atrial septal defect). Right ventricular failure is encountered most often as a complication of left ventricular failure. In the presence of elevated right heart filling pressures, neck veins are distended and fill from below. Hepatic enlargement and tenderness to gentle palpation result from passive congestion, and manual compression over the liver causes further distention of the neck veins (hepatojugular reflux). In the presence of biventricular failure, signs of right ventricular failure may dominate, but the presence of dyspnea and rales should suggest additional left ventricular failure. Accompanying low cardiac output results in signs of increased sympathetic nervous activity and of organ hypoperfusion. It should be remembered that a critically lowered cardiac output from any cause sufficient to produce metabolic acidosis occasions hyperventilation in defense of acid-base balance, and this must be distinguished from the tachypnea of left heart failure. Advanced right-sided or biventricular failure may be associated with anorexia, weight loss, and malnutrition ("cardiac cachexia").

Cyanosis. Cyanosis is caused by 5 or more grams per 100 ml of unoxygenated hemoglobin in the subpapillary venous plexus of the skin. This occurs in right heart failure because the congested venules contain blood from which considerable oxygen has been extracted because of the slow flow. This is typically accompanied by relatively normal arterial P_{O_2} values unless intrinsic lung disease or intracardiac shunting is present. Cyanosis is usually absent in left heart failure unless caused by a complication (e.g., pneumonia) or by pulmonary edema.

Abnormal Heart and Lungs. Although dyspnea accompanying left ventricular failure may be partially relieved by onset of right ventricular failure, some dyspnea usually persists, together with tachypnea and basal rales. Tricuspid valvular insufficiency commonly accompanies severe right ventricular dilation and failure and contributes to systemic venous engorgement. The murmur of tricuspid insufficiency is distinguished from that of mitral insufficiency by its location (lower left border of sternum), by its tendency to increase during inspiration, and by associated physical signs, such as hepatic pulsation and systolic waves in the jugular venous pulse. Doppler echocardiography greatly assists in the assessment of this problem. Pleural effusion, often unilateral, is more common in right-sided or biventricular than in isolated left ventricular failure.

Systemic Venous Congestion. Elevation of systemic venous pressure is a sine qua non of right heart failure. Responsible mechanisms include (1) the inability of the failing ventricle to eject the venous return without abnormally high filling pressures, causing (2) an increase in the volume of blood in the large systemic veins; and (3) increased venomotor tone resulting from increased sympathetic nervous system activity. Increased systemic venous pressure is responsible for the hepatomegaly, occasional splenomegaly, and peripheral edema that characterize decompensated right ventricular failure. Usually less apparent are the associated congestion and edema of the gastrointestinal tract.

Pressure in the jugular venous system, a useful index of right atrial pressure, may be estimated from the height of the column of blood distending the cervical veins. The cervical veins are normally flat in the upright posture in the absence of raised intrathoracic pressure, whereas in right heart failure they are prominent and distended. The wave form of venous pulsation is usually best appreciated from inspection of the right internal jugular vein, adjusting the angle of the patient's upper body to bring out the top of the venous pressure column. Tricuspid insufficiency distorts the normal venous pulse by producing a systolic or C-V wave that has no counterpart in the normal jugular venous pulse. Occasionally, compression over the liver is necessary to display the increased blood volume in the venous system, but the examiner must avoid being misled by venous distention from involuntary expiration against a closed glottis (the Valsalva maneuver).

Liver. The liver is typically enlarged and tender in right heart failure. If the onset is acute, right upper quadrant pain may result from constraint of the swollen liver by its tight capsule. Splenomegaly is uncommon except in prolonged passive congestion of the liver, and pain or tenderness of the spleen should raise the question of superimposed systemic embolization and splenic infarction.

Early congestion of the liver may cause modest increases in the concentrations of hepatic enzymes such as alkaline phosphatase in serum, and increases in serum bilirubin may occur. Hyperbilirubinemia from this cause usually consists of a combination of conjugated and unconjugated bilirubin. Frank jaundice is uncommon unless hepatic congestion is associated with long-standing pulmonary congestion or pulmonary infarction.

Hypoglycemia may occur if cardiac output is severely compromised and hepatic congestion is marked and protracted. This is attributed to depletion of liver glycogen stores and increased formation of lactic acid from glucose induced by hypoxia.

Repeated and prolonged episodes of right heart failure with reduced hepatic blood flow and elevated venous pressures can cause atrophy and centrilobular necrosis of liver cells and can lead to extensive fibrosis ("cardiac cirrhosis") that is difficult to distinguish from posthepatitic cirrhosis. Hepatic failure with precoma or coma is a rare, preterminal complication of this sequence of events.

Extracellular Fluid Compartments. The fluid compartments of the body are normally maintained constant by neurohormonally mediated interplay among intake (governed by thirst and appetite), exchanges of fluid and electrolytes (governed by passive and active transport mechanisms), and excretion (regulated primarily by the kidneys). In heart failure, excessive retention of sodium and water by the kidneys results in an isosmotic expansion of extracellular fluid, including the circulating blood volume. In mild heart failure, retention of sodium and water may serve to expand the blood volume to sustain venous return and the forward output of the failing heart through the Frank-Starling mechanism. However, retention of salt and water only exacerbates pulmonary and systemic congestion and edema when the myocardium can no longer respond positively to increased filling pressure and volumes.

The distribution of excess extracellular ("third space") fluid varies among patients. Under the influence of gravity, edema accumulates in the feet and ankles of ambulatory patients but shifts to the sacral region in the bedridden patient. Localization occurs in areas of low tissue pressure, such as the back of the ankle. Colloid osmotic pressure and the integrity of the lymphatic system also influence extracellular fluid distribution.

Peripheral Edema. Dependent edema developing over the course of the day and subsiding by morning is a characteristic feature of right heart failure. It is a direct consequence of elevated systemic venous pressure and is typically preceded by a gain in weight. Persistent edema is accompanied relatively frequently by complications such as low-grade cellulitis, and the combination of edema and sluggish venous flow predisposes to deep venous thrombosis and pulmonary embolism.

Pleural Effusion. The infrequency of hydrothorax in isolated right ventricular failure dictates that the association of pleural effusion and cor pulmonale should lead one to search for another cause, such as pulmonary infarction. It is, however, common in biventricular failure. Hydrothorax results from impaired removal of isotonic fluid from the pleural space because of elevated venous pressures in both the pulmonary and the systemic circulations, compromising transcapillary exchange of water at the pleural surface and also impeding lymphatic drainage. Hydrothorax contributes to dyspnea reflexly, probably by stimuli from lungs and chest wall, as well as by displacing ventilated lung tissue from the relatively fixed volume of the thoracic space. Pulmonary embolism and infarction may contribute to pleural effusion in two ways: by transit of fluid from the infarcted area of the lung to the pleural space or by aggravation of heart failure.

Ascites. The presence of free fluid in the abdominal cavity is a late manifestation of right heart failure, usually associated with systemic venous hypertension, peripheral edema, and hydrothorax. It is commonly encountered in the setting of tricuspid valve disease or chronic constrictive pericarditis. Elevated pressures in portal and hepatic veins and in the systemic veins draining the peritoneum contribute to the formation of ascites, but renal retention of sodium and water is a prerequisite. It may

contribute to anorexia and can cause abdominal discomfort or pain in patients with severe right ventricular failure.

Pericardial Effusion. Patients with chronic heart failure commonly have increased amounts of fluid in the pericardial sac that can be demonstrated echocardiographically. Only rarely, however, does it accumulate to an extent that produces further hemodynamic compromise (tamponade).

Anasarca. Advanced and protracted right ventricular failure without adequate treatment can cause edema fluid to accumulate throughout the body, most conspicuously in subcutaneous tissues as well as abdominal and thoracic cavities. Face and arms are typically spared until the preterminal stages of failure. This clinical picture occurs rarely in the present era of potent diuretics.

Gastrointestinal Tract. Systemic venous hypertension leads to edema of the bowel wall. These changes interfere with absorption of drugs or foods only when heart failure is severe, but reduced bioavailability of furosemide and perhaps other drugs can occur under these circumstances. In severe congestive heart failure, anorexia, nausea, and vomiting may occur from reflex, central, local, or drug-induced causes. Protein-losing enteropathy can occur in the setting of severe right heart failure.

Brain. Nonspecific complaints, including headache and insomnia, are common in heart failure and are usually attributable to some diminution of cerebral blood flow and triggering mechanisms such as dyspnea that contribute to insomnia. Neurologic or behavioral aberrations are more frequent when the burdens of a limited cardiac output are superimposed on antecedent neurologic disease (e.g., cerebrovascular disease or prior stroke) or on personality disorder. Irritability, restlessness, and limited attention span are associated with severe congestive heart failure. Stupor and coma supervene when cardiac output is critically reduced.

Kidney. Oliguria occurs with decompensation in isolated right or left heart failure but is more prominent in the latter or in biventricular failure. The urine is sodium poor but has a relatively high specific gravity (1.020 to 1.030). Prerenal azotemia is common, particularly in the presence of intrinsic renal disease or after vigorous diuresis. Azotemia with high urine specific gravity is characteristic of heart failure (and dehydration) and stands in contrast to the low specific gravity expected with renal insufficiency due to intrinsic renal disease. Blood urea nitrogen is typically elevated out of proportion to serum creatinine. Proteinuria is common but does not usually exceed 1 gram per day.

Other Manifestations. In chronic severe congestive heart failure, weakness and gradual loss of tissue mass are frequent concomitants and may progress to cachexia. At this late stage, the patient is usually suffering from anorexia and often gastrointestinal symptoms and electrolyte disturbances as well. Although organ hypoperfusion and congestion play an important part in this syndrome, the physician must maintain vigilance to avoid additional contributions from overvigorous use of digitalis and diuretics.

Anxiety. This is a common feature of cardiac disease by the time the heart fails. Manifestations of anxiety may be difficult to distinguish from symptoms of the underlying cardiac disorder because of the nonspecific nature of complaints such as breathlessness. Symptoms related to hyperventilation as well as palpitations may contribute to the patient's anxiety by reinforcing the impression that organic heart disease is present. The physician must proceed with the separate assessment of organic and psychosomatic aspects of the disease process, recognizing that a careful history and physical examination, together with judicious use of noninvasive diagnostic methods, help to establish the extent to which organic heart disease is responsible for the patient's symptoms.

CLINICAL MANAGEMENT OF HEART FAILURE
General Approaches

The management of congestive heart failure includes three general types of approaches. The first is removal of the underlying cause. This deserves top priority in all cases and includes measures such as surgical correction of valvular lesions or congenital malformation. It also includes medical treatment of hypertension or infective endocarditis when present.

The second approach consists of removal of precipitating causes of heart failure. Frequently the initial development or exacerba-

TABLE 40–3. MEASURES IN THE MANAGEMENT OF CONGESTIVE HEART FAILURE

A. Improve pump performance of the failing ventricle
 1. Cardiac glycosides (digoxin)
 2. Sympathomimetic drugs (dopamine, dobutamine)
 3. Other positive inotropic drugs (amrinone)
 4. Pacemaker for bradycardia or loss of atrioventricular synchrony
B. Reduction of cardiac work load
 1. Rest (physical and emotional)
 2. Correction of obesity
 3. Vasodilator drugs
 4. Assisted circulation (e.g., intra-aortic balloon counterpulsation)
C. Control salt and water retention
 1. Limit dietary sodium intake
 2. Diuretics
 3. Mechanical removal of fluid
  a. Thoracentesis
  b. Paracentesis
  c. Dialysis
  d. Phlebotomy

tion of heart failure is related not to worsening of the underlying cardiac condition but rather to a superimposed stress. Typical factors that can precipitate overt congestive heart failure, apart from changes in the status of the heart itself, are listed in Table 40–2.

The third set of measures, treatment of clinical manifestations of heart failure, occupies the remainder of this chapter. This approach may in turn be divided into three categories, as summarized in Table 40–3:

1. Measures to improve the contractile performance of the heart.
2. Measures to reduce cardiac work.
3. Measures to control excessive retention of salt and water.

As listed in Table 40–3, several therapeutic entities are available in each category. Cardiac glycosides and sympathomimetic agents constitute the principal drugs that enhance the pumping performance of the failing heart. In addition, placement of a pacemaker may improve pumping performance either by supporting a more appropriate heart rate or by restoring atrial augmentation of ventricular filling if synchronous atrioventricular contraction can be achieved (see Ch. 42).

Reduction of the work load of the failing heart can be accomplished by physical and emotional rest, by appropriate treatment of obesity, and by vasodilator therapy. Under specific circumstances, assisted circulation with the intra-aortic balloon pump can usefully contribute to this goal.

Finally, control of the excessive retention of salt and water is approached by instituting a low-sodium diet and the use of diuretic drugs. Under some circumstances, mechanical removal of fluid is of value.

These measures are customarily applied in a stepwise fashion, as outlined in detail in Table 40–4.

Strategy of Heart Failure Management

The many etiologies and degrees of severity of heart failure demand an individualized approach to each patient. Nevertheless, certain general principles apply to the management of various subsets of patients. The comments that follow are relevant to patients with *systolic* ventricular dysfunction (i.e., reduced ejection fraction). In the past, it has not been considered appropriate to institute specific therapeutic measures until symptoms of overt heart failure occur—that is, until the patient makes the transition from functional class I to class II. This recommendation could change, depending on the outcome of current therapeutic trials of vasodilator administration to patients with ventricular dysfunction but without overt heart failure. The first approach (see Table 40–4) in all instances includes judicious limitation of activity, advising the patient to avoid physical exertion that produces undue dyspnea or exhaustion. The degree of restriction should be tailored to the severity of heart failure. It is important not to limit activity so severely that skeletal muscle deconditioning, rather than the underlying cardiac problem, becomes the limiting factor in the patient's activity. Physical activity should, however, be markedly restricted in the setting of acute decompensation of chronic heart failure, a situation in which hospitalization is generally advisable.

PHARMACOTHERAPY. A diuretic, a vasodilator (usually an angiotensin converting enzyme inhibitor), or a cardiac glycoside may be added in early class II, with the choice of one or more based on the balance between risk and expected benefit. In many cases, modest doses of a mild diuretic such as a thiazide restore the patient to an essentially asymptomatic state. A vasodilator such as captopril or enalapril should be used if there is evidence of elevated peripheral vascular resistance (systemic hypertension) and no contraindications exist (e.g., postural hypotension or renal impairment, especially in the presence of bilateral renal artery stenosis). Dietary sodium restriction may be limited to avoidance of heavily salted foods and the use of the salt shaker at the table.

TABLE 40–4. STEPS IN THE MANAGEMENT OF CHRONIC CONGESTIVE HEART FAILURE

| Steps | Functional Class | | |
	II	III	IV
A	*Restrict physical activity:* Limit competitive sports and heavy labor	Reduce work schedule; rest periods during day	Limit to house and finally to bed and chair
B	*Dietary sodium restriction:* Eliminate salt shaker and heavily salted foods	Eliminate salt in cooking and at table (Na intake ~ 1.2 to 1.8 grams)	As in III, plus low-sodium foods (Na intake <1 gram)
C	*Diuretics:* Thiazide or low-dose loop diuretic	Loop diuretic (progressive doses); consider adding distally acting (K-sparing) diuretic	Loop diuretic with distally acting (K-sparing) and/or thiazide diuretic
D	*Vasodilators:* Hydralazine and isosorbide dinitrate *or* an ACE inhibitor (captopril or enalapril) ——————————————————————→		Intravenous nitroprusside
E	*Digitalis glycosides:* Conventional maintenance doses ——————————————————————→		Dose to maintain serum level in 1.5 ng/ml range
F			*Other inotropic drugs (intravenous):* Dopamine, dobutamine, amrinone
G			*Consider cardiac transplantation* *Thoracentesis, paracentesis* *Hemodialysis; extracorporeal ultrafiltration* *Assisted circulation (e.g., intra-aortic balloon pump)*

Special low-sodium foods are expensive and can be so unpalatable as to impair nutrition.

When symptoms persist or evolve on the simple regimen outlined above, combination therapy with diuretics, vasodilators, and cardiac glycosides should be considered. Intensification of the diuretic regimen is often necessary. Problems such as mitral regurgitation are particularly amenable to treatment with vasodilators, as discussed below.

As the severity of heart failure advances, increased restriction of physical activity is usually necessary, and patients often require rest periods during the day as class III symptoms evolve. When patients remain symptomatic during ordinary activity on a program that includes loop diuretics, digitalis, and vasodilators, detailed evaluation is advisable to search for precipitating causes and to consider the possibility of more aggressive approaches. In patients who have progressed to functional class IV, hospitalization is often advisable and the use of intravenous sympathomimetic agents can be considered, in addition to optimization of the vasodilator, diuretic, and cardiac glycoside regimens. In patients who meet appropriate criteria, cardiac transplantation should also be considered at this time if not earlier.

During episodes of decompensation, the hazards of deep venous thrombosis and pulmonary embolism must be guarded against, and the use of minidose heparin (see Ch. 54) is a relatively safe and effective approach during hospitalization. At these times, emotional as well as physical rest is important, and anxiety-provoking situations should be carefully avoided. Marked anxiety or insomnia may be treated with benzodiazepines such as diazepam or the shorter-acting agent triazolam.

DIET. Rigid salt restriction can usually be avoided until diuretics are no longer capable of controlling the accumulation of salt and water. Water intake does not, in general, require specific restriction unless dilutional hyponatremia supervenes.

OXYGEN. Patients with hypoxia, and certainly those with pulmonary edema, benefit from oxygen inhalation, conveniently given by nasal prongs at 4 to 6 liters per minute. In general, supplemental oxygen is worthwhile whenever the arterial oxygen saturation falls below 90 per cent. This is a particularly effective way of reducing right ventricular afterload, since oxygen is a potent pulmonary arteriolar vasodilator.

PHYSICAL REMOVAL OF FLUID. The availability of potent diuretics limits the need for thoracentesis or paracentesis, but these procedures may be important diagnostically when the accumulation of fluid in serous cavities is not readily explained on the basis of heart failure alone. Pulmonary embolism, for example, is a relatively common cause of pleural effusion, and a diagnostic thoracentesis often provides critically important information leading to this diagnosis. Drainage of pleural or ascitic fluid should be carried out slowly, at a rate of not more than about 1500 ml per hour, and the total quantity of fluid removed on any single occasion should not exceed about 1500 ml because of the risk of fluid shifts from the vascular to the extravascular compartment, with consequently inadequate ventricular filling pressures. Particular caution is required in patients (such as those with aortic stenosis or hypertrophic cardiomyopathy) who have reduced ventricular compliance and require high ventricular filling pressures to maintain adequate stroke volume.

Acute Pulmonary Edema

Acute pulmonary edema is a medical emergency in which the immediate therapeutic goals are to (1) improve oxygenation; (2) reduce venous return (preload); (3) reduce anxiety; and (4) treat causal and precipitating factors. Placement of flow-directed pulmonary artery (Swan-Ganz) and arterial lines for monitoring of pressures and arterial blood gases is often advisable. The patient is placed in a trunk-up, legs-down posture and given humidified 100 per cent oxygen, by positive pressure mask if possible. Vital signs are monitored frequently, and an intravenous cannula is inserted for secure intravenous access. Arterial blood gas, blood urea nitrogen (BUN) or creatinine, electrolyte, and complete blood count measurements are obtained at once. An electrocardiogram and chest radiograph (taken with a portable machine if necessary) should also be obtained, and electrical conversion of supraventricular or ventricular tachyarrhythmias should be con-

sidered if present and if not due to digitalis excess. Ultrasound (echocardiographic) study is indicated at the earliest opportunity if the nature and extent of underlying cardiac disease are not entirely clear.

Morphine given intravenously (2 to 10 mg, repeated every 10 to 15 minutes) reduces venous return and allays anxiety; naloxone should be available in case of respiratory depression. Nitroglycerin given sublingually or intravenously further reduces venous return; nitroprusside given intravenously may be used if the blood pressure is adequately maintained and afterload reduction is desirable. Furosemide should be given intravenously in a 20- to 40-mg dose and repeated in increasing doses as necessary to achieve a diuresis. Aminophylline, 250 to 500 mg given slowly intravenously (5.6 mg per kilogram), may be useful to relieve bronchospasm and promote diuresis but can exacerbate sinus or ectopic tachycardias.

If severe respiratory distress persists, tourniquets applied to three of four extremities and rotated every 15 to 20 minutes may be of value. If respiratory acidosis (pH of 7.10 or less) or severe hypoxemia ($PO_2 < 50$ mm Hg) persists, endotracheal intubation and controlled positive-pressure ventilation should usually be instituted. Phlebotomy and hemodialysis deserve consideration in refractory cases. Digitalis has a secondary role in this clinical setting, except occasionally in the management of supraventricular tachyarrhythmias. Superimposed hypotension and low cardiac output states are considered in Ch. 41. Concurrently, vigorous attention should be directed to the identification and management of precipitating factors (see Table 40–2).

Diuretics

Salt and water retention with consequent expansion of the intravascular and interstitial compartments is a sine qua non of chronic congestive heart failure and accounts for many of the common signs and symptoms. Elimination of excess salt and water is an essential goal in management of heart failure.

Two stages characterize diuretic use: first, the elimination of accumulated excess fluid; and second, maintenance of optimal "dry" weight. Care of patients in the hospital typically focuses on elimination of excess fluid, which is facilitated by the controlled salt intake and limited activity of hospitalized patients. Maintenance of optimal fluid balance out of hospital requires adjustments in the context of the individual patient's diet and activity. A sound approach is the use of the mildest diuretic program that is consistent with maintenance of appropriate fluid balance and a salt intake that promotes a nutritious diet. Severe sodium restriction is usually unnecessary except in very severe congestive heart failure. Overly rigorous restriction of sodium intake, together with use of potent diuretics, is a well-known formula for impaired renal function, oliguria, and prerenal azotemia, particularly in the elderly.

CONTROL OF SODIUM BALANCE. The key role of diuretics in management of heart failure relates to the central role of the kidney as a target of many of the neurohumoral and hemodynamic changes that occur in heart failure. Reduced cardiac output causes activation of the renin-angiotensin system in the kidney, with consequent reduction in renal blood flow and increased glomerular filtration fraction, leading to increased resorption of salt and water by the proximal tubule. Elevated plasma angiotensin II levels contribute to increased systemic vascular resistance and increase aldosterone release from the adrenal. Increased renal sympathetic nerve activity also tends to reduce renal blood flow and to release renin from the macula densa, as well as directly augmenting sodium resorption along other segments of the nephron. Intrarenal blood flow redistribution contributes to the formation of relatively concentrated urine (Fig. 40–4). Plasma vasopressin levels are frequently elevated in patients with heart failure, causing further limitation of free water clearance. Together with the increase in thirst of patients with advanced heart failure, this leads to a hyponatremic state that is a particularly ominous prognostic sign in heart failure.

Diuretics intervene in the pathophysiology of heart failure by reducing the reabsorption of sodium and its accompanying anions, as well as water, by the renal tubule. The four major classes of diuretics in current clinical use are summarized in Table 40–5. Each of these agents affects renal tubular function in a distinct way, and each tends to produce a characteristic set of abnormal-

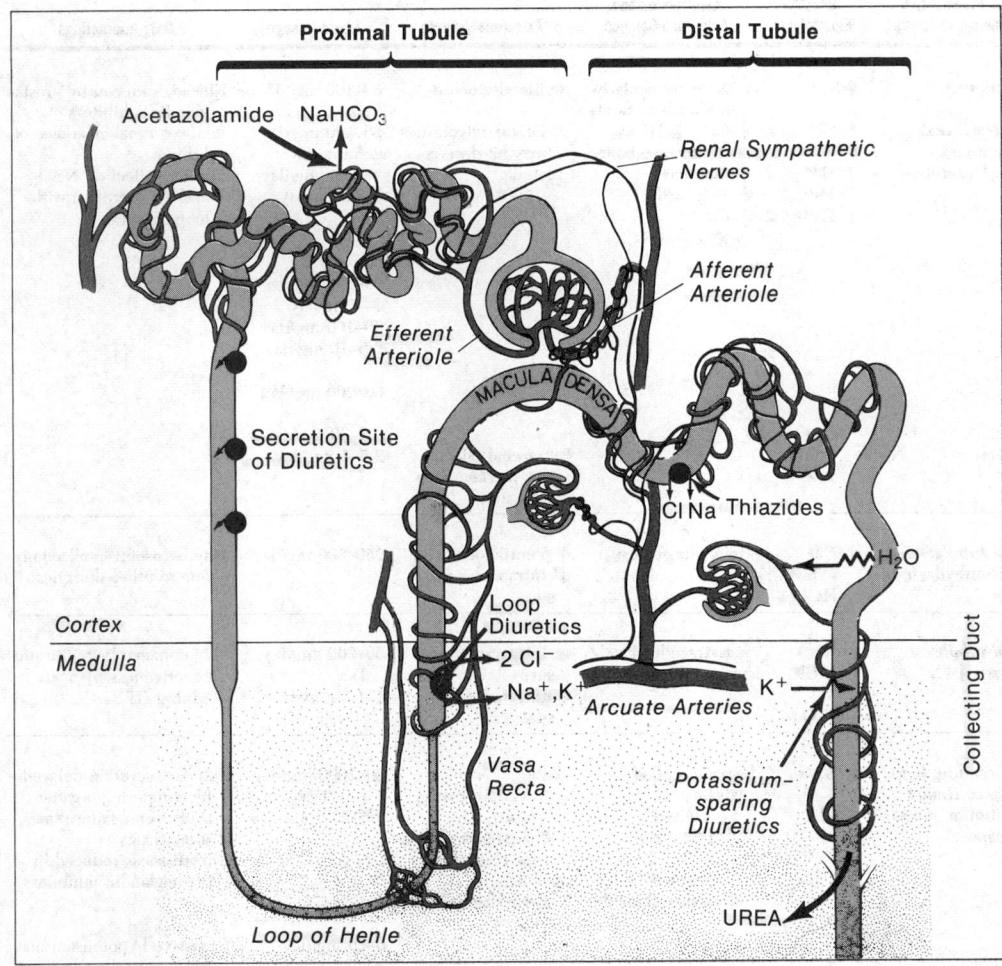

Proximal Tubule   **Distal Tubule**

Acetazolamide   NaHCO₃

Renal Sympathetic Nerves

Afferent Arteriole

Efferent Arteriole

MACULA DENSA

Secretion Site of Diuretics

Cl Na Thiazides

H₂O

Cortex

Medulla

Loop Diuretics

2 Cl⁻

Na⁺, K⁺   Arcuate Arteries   K⁺

Collecting Duct

Vasa Recta

Potassium-sparing Diuretics

UREA

Loop of Henle

FIGURE 40–4. Sites of diuretic action in the mammalian nephron. Fluid resorption across the proximal tubule accounts for approximately two thirds of the resorption of filtered sodium and H₂O. Neuronal, hormonal, and hemodynamic factors, both extrinsic and intrinsic to the kidney, affect the volume and content of urine formation by altering the rate of formation of glomerular filtrate, thereby altering the balance of Starling forces between the proximal tubule and postglomerular peritubular capillaries. Agents that alter the rate of formation of glomerular filtrate, such as ACE inhibitors, may enhance the delivery of solute and water to more distal segments of the nephron that are sensitive to diuretics. Nonsteroidal anti-inflammatory drugs may diminish the glomerular filtration rate, thus reducing the flow of urine to distal diuretic-sensitive portions of the nephron. A reduction in systemic blood pressure, or in renal artery pressure distal to the stenotic arterial lesion, below that necessary for formation of glomerular filtrate renders the kidney refractory to any diuretic. With the exception of the osmotic diuretics that are freely filtered at the glomerulus, most diuretics reach their site of action along the nephron after being secreted into the tubular lumen by the organic anion secretory transport system of the straight proximal tubule (pars recta).

About one third of the glomerular filtrate arrives at the descending limb of Henle's loop; no active transport of solute occurs here, although the tubular epithelium is highly permeable to water, which leaves the nephron for the increasingly hyperosmotic medullary interstitium. Most of the solute transport responsible for maintaining the hypertonicity of the medullary interstitium occurs in the water-impermeable thick ascending limb of Henle's loop. Here, a NaK cotransport system in the luminal membrane is coupled to the uptake of two chloride ions, a process dependent upon the electrochemical driving force for sodium generated by the NaK-ATPase on the basolateral membrane of these cells. This Na/K/2 Cl cotransport system on the luminal membrane of the tubular cells is the site of action for the loop diuretics (furosemide, bumetanide, and ethacrynic acid). Inhibition of cation transport by loop diuretics prevents the normal generation of the hypertonic medullary interstitium, thus reducing the osmotic gradient for free water clearance of ADH-sensitive tubular cells in the collecting duct, and also delivers large amounts of solute and water to the distal nephron, thus overwhelming distal Na⁺ and Cl⁻ resorption sites.

The thick ascending limb approaches its own glomerulus as it re-enters the cortex and passes between the afferent and efferent arterioles to form the juxtaglomerular apparatus (JGA), the tubular contribution to which is termed the macula densa. Loop diuretics may directly stimulate the release of renin by the JGA, an action that may contribute to the extrarenal vascular effects of these drugs. The distal convoluted tubule begins beyond the macula densa. Na⁺ and Cl⁻, as well as other ions (e.g., Ca⁺⁺), are resorbed in this segment. The thiazide diuretics and related drugs inhibit NaCl resorption in this segment, although the mechanism is unknown; they also enhance Ca⁺⁺ resorption by tubular cells in this segment. Salt resorption by this distal, water-impermeable portion of the nephron allows the formation of a dilute urine, hence the term "cortical diluting segment." Thiazide-induced inhibition of NaCl resorption in this segment therefore may lead to hyponatremia, particularly when accompanied by elevated ADH levels and increased thirst.

The cortical collecting duct actively resorbs NaCl via an aldosterone-sensitive mechanism. This leads to increased net resorption of Na⁺ into cells and hence to a lumen negative potential difference that favors the secretion of K⁺ and H⁺ ions. This is why increased Na⁺ concentrations and high flow rates in the cortical collecting duct, as after loop or thiazide diuretic administration, lead to enhanced passive K⁺ secretion. Anti-aldosterone drugs, such as spironolactone, competitively inhibit aldosterone's binding to its receptor, thereby limiting Na⁺ permeability by the apical membrane and reducing K⁺ secretion.

As illustrated, the blood supply to each nephron is derived from several sources. The afferent arteriole that enters the glomerulus is richly innervated with sympathetic nerve endings, particularly as it enters the glomerulus at its vascular pole within the juxtaglomerular apparatus. Increased sympathetic discharge to the kidney results in increased net NaCl resorption even in the absence of changes in glomerular hemodynamics. Elevated efferent sympathetic activity, as is often seen in decompensated congestive heart failure, would be expected to result in avid retention of solute due to reduced renal perfusion, increased renin release, and enhanced tubular resorption of solute. Dopamine is a potent renal vasodilator and may directly affect tubular epithelia to reduce NaCl resorption, thus acting as a natriuretic agent. Exogenously administered dopamine, particularly when infused at rates of 2 to 3 μg per minute, may be a useful adjunct to diuretic therapy in selected with advanced CHF.

TABLE 40–5. DIURETICS: ACTION, DOSAGE, AND DRUG INTERACTIONS

Diuretic	Brand Name	Principal Site and Mechanism of Action	Effects on Urinary Electrolytes	Effects on Blood Electrolytes and Acid-Base Balance	Extrarenal Effects	Usual Dosage*	Drug Interactions
Thiazides and Related Compounds							
Chlorothiazide	Diuril	*Distal tubule:*	$\uparrow Na^+$	$\downarrow Na^+$, particularly in elderly patients	$\uparrow$ Blood glucose	50–100 mg, IV or p.o.	Efficacy reduced by prostaglandin inhibitors
Hydrochlorothiazide	Hydro-Diuril	Inhibit NaCl reabsorption and	$\uparrow Cl^-$	$\downarrow Cl^-$, $\uparrow HCO_3^-$	$\uparrow$ LDL/triglycerides (may be dose related)	25–100 mg/day	Reduces renal clearance of lithium
Trichlormethiazide	Metahydrin	$\uparrow Ca^{2+}$ excretion	$\uparrow K^+$	—mild metabolic alkalosis		2–8 mg/day	
Chlorthalidone	Hygroton		$\uparrow H^+$	$\uparrow$ Uric acid		25–100 mg/day	Additive effect on NaCl and K$^+$ excretion with loop diuretics
Metolazone	Zaroxolyn		$\uparrow Mg^{2+}$ $\downarrow Ca^{2+}$	$\uparrow Ca^{++}$ $\downarrow K^+$, $\downarrow Mg^{2+}$		5–10 mg/day	
Cyclothiazide	Anhydron					2–6 mg/day	
Hydroflumethizide	Diucardin					25–200 mg/day	
Polythiazide	Renese					1–4 mg/day	
Quinethazone	Hydromox					50–100 mg/day	
Methyclothiazide	Enduron Aquatensen					2.5–10 mg/day	
Benzthiazide	Aquatag Exna					50–200 mg/day	
Bendroflumethiazide	Naturetin					2.5–30 mg/day	
Indapamide	Lozol	Vasodilator			Extrarenal effects less marked with indapamide	2.5–5 mg/day	
Carbonic Anhydrase Inhibitor							
Acetazolamide	Diamox	*Proximal tubule:* Carbonic anhydrase inhibitor	$\uparrow Na^+$, $\uparrow K^+$ $\uparrow HCO_3^-$	Metabolic acidosis	$\uparrow$ Ventilatory drive $\downarrow$ Intraocular pressure	250–500 mg/day	May be useful in alkalemia due to other diuretics
Osmotic Diuretics							
Mannitol	Osmitrol	*Proximal tubule* (primarily)	$\uparrow Na^+$, $\uparrow Cl^-$	$\uparrow$ Extracellular volume transiently	$\downarrow$ Intracranial pressure	50–200 gm/day, IV	May enhance loop diuretic effectiveness by maintaining GFR
Glycerol	Glyrol		$\uparrow H_2O$		$\downarrow$ Intraocular pressure	1–1.5 gm/kg	
Loop Diuretics							
Furosemide	Lasix	*Thick ascending limb of loop of Henle:* Inhibition of Na/K/Cl cotransport	$\uparrow\uparrow Na^+$	Hypochloremic alkalosis ($\uparrow HCO_3^-$)	Acute: $\uparrow$ Venous capacitance	20–1000 mg/day, p.o./IV	Tubular secretion delayed by competing organic acids (renal failure) and some drugs
Bumetanide	Bumex		$\uparrow\uparrow Cl^-$	$\downarrow K^+$, $\downarrow Na^+$ $\downarrow Cl^-$, $\downarrow Mg^{2+}$ $\uparrow$ Uric acid (less than thiazide)	$\uparrow$ Systemic vascular resistance Chronic: $\downarrow$ Cardiac preload	0.5–20.0 mg/day	Effectiveness reduced by prostaglandin inhibitors
Piretanide†	Arelix Diumax Tauliz					6–20 mg/day	Excessive hypotension may occur in patients treated chronically with a loop diuretic when begun on an ACE inhibitor
Ethacrynic acid	Edecrin				Ototoxicity	50–200 mg/day, IV	Additive ototoxicity with aminoglycosides
Mefruside†	Baycaron Mefiusal	Similar to thiazides				25–50 mg/day	Longer duration of action than furosemide
Muzolamine† Torasemide†		Less K$^+$ wasting				2.5–5 mg/day	
Potassium-Sparing Diuretics							
Spironolactone	Aldactone	*Collecting duct:* Aldosterone antagonist	$\downarrow K^+$ $\uparrow Na^+$ $\uparrow Cl^-$	$\uparrow K^+$, particularly in patients with $\downarrow$ GFR; metabolic acidosis	Gynecomastia	25–100 mg/day	Useful adjunct to therapy with K$^+$-wasting diuretics; triamterene with indomethacin may cause abrupt $\downarrow$ GFR
Canrenoate† (potassium)							
Triamterene	Dyrenium	Inhibit apical membrane Na$^+$ conductance	$\uparrow HCO_3^-$			100–300 mg/day	
Amiloride	Midamor					5–10 mg/day	

*Route of administration is p.o. except as noted.
†Not yet licensed for use in the United States.
GFR = glomerular filtration rate; LDL = low density lipoproteins; ACE = angiotensin-converting enzyme.

ities in electrolyte patterns, fluid balance, and acid-base homeostasis. The more potent the diuretic, the greater the potential risk for severe and sometimes life-threatening disturbances of electrolyte and acid-base balance.

THIAZIDES. Because of their effectiveness by oral administration, their predictable effects, and their relative freedom from toxicity, thiazide diuretics are very commonly used in the management of heart failure. The thiazide diuretics include several agents with chemical and pharmacologic similarities. The prototype is chlorothiazide. Chlorthalidone and metolazone are heterocyclic compounds that share the basic benzothiadiazine nu-

cleus. All of these drugs inhibit sodium chloride reabsorption in the distal tubule. This effect is not dependent upon the weak carbonic anhydrase inhibitory activities common to most of these drugs. By inhibiting sodium chloride transport in the distal tubule, dilution of tubular fluid is prevented and delivery of solute and water to the hydrogen- and potassium-secreting sites in the collecting duct is enhanced. Calcium reabsorption is also promoted by the thiazides, probably by enhancement of calcium entry into epithelial cells of the distal tubule and perhaps by mild volume depletion as well.

The thiazides are useful in the initial management of mild to moderate congestive heart failure. Their utility is limited, however, by avid solute reabsorption in the more proximal nephron segments. Thiazides are largely ineffective when the glomerular filtration rate is less than 30 ml per minute. They are often useful in the treatment of refractory edema in combination with loop diuretics, as discussed subsequently.

Potentially troublesome side effects include potassium depletion, hyperuricemia, glucose intolerance, and plasma lipid elevations, as discussed below. Care must be taken to avoid gastric and small bowel irritation from the potassium chloride supplements that are often required in conjunction with thiazide diuretics.

CARBONIC ANHYDRASE INHIBITORS. Related to the thiazides are the carbonic anhydrase inhibitors, of which acetazolamide is the only agent currently available. This drug results in urinary sodium and bicarbonate losses until the plasma bicarbonate level falls to the point at which renal tubular bicarbonate reabsorption (both proximal and distal) exceeds the filtered load of bicarbonate. Thus, these agents tend to have a transient effect. The sodium and potassium loss accompanying bicarbonate excretion is moderate, but acetazolamide may be of value in patients with high serum bicarbonate levels, as may occur in cor pulmonale or metabolic alkalosis. The presence of metabolic acidosis, e.g., from renal failure or hepatic failure, constitutes a contraindication to its use.

LOOP DIURETICS. These agents are the most potent diuretics in common clinical use and are capable of inducing a natriuresis of up to 20 per cent of the filtered load of sodium for limited periods. They are of particular value in three situations: in acute pulmonary edema, used intravenously; in severe or refractory heart failure; or when renal function is impaired. Ethacrynic acid is chemically different from furosemide and its analogues but appears to share a similar set of pharmacologic properties. These diuretics act to inhibit the Na/K/2 Cl transport system that is responsible for solute reabsorption in the thick ascending limb of the loop of Henle. Each of these drugs is secreted into the tubular lumen by the organic acid secretory pathway, and their effects may therefore be delayed or decreased by exogenous (e.g., probenecid) or endogenous (organic anion accumulation in uremia) competitive inhibitors of the transporter.

Gastrointestinal absorption of furosemide, the most commonly used of the loop diuretics, is variable, with an average bioavailability of 60 per cent. This is substantially diminished when the drug is given with meals. Congestive heart failure can decrease absorption rates of both furosemide and bumetanide. The nonsteroidal anti-inflammatory drugs, including aspirin, tend to blunt the natriuretic response to all of the loop diuretics.

The loop diuretics in general produce systemic hemodynamic changes that precede and are presumably unrelated to the degree and extent of diuresis they induce. Acute administration of furosemide causes a rapid increase in venous capacitance, with a consequent decline in cardiac filling pressures. This effect is accompanied by an increase in plasma renin activity that can produce an appreciable rise in systemic vascular resistance. These effects on the peripheral vasculature tend to plateau in the lower dose range at about a 20-mg intravenous dose of furosemide. Although the loop diuretics are potent inhibitors of Na/K/2 Cl cotransport, this process is not clinically important outside the kidney, except in the cochlea, where it is thought to account for the eighth nerve toxicity that is seen with loop diuretics, particularly ethacrynic acid. The ototoxicity of loop diuretics is synergistic with that of aminoglycoside antibiotics.

Bumetanide and piretanide tend to have higher bioavailability and greater potency than furosemide and may be slightly less ototoxic. Other differences among these closely related compounds appear to be small and probably clinically unimportant.

An important advantage of the loop diuretics is their rapid onset of action, with a diuretic response typically appearing within a few minutes of intravenous administration.

POTASSIUM-SPARING DIURETICS. Two groups of drugs fall into this class: (1) the aldosterone antagonist and (2) the direct inhibitors of sodium permeability in the collecting duct. The aldosterone antagonist most frequently used is spironolactone, although canrenoate and canrenone have essentially identical effects. The aldosterone antagonists compete with the native hormone for cytoplasmic receptors in responsive cells, ultimately reducing sodium reabsorption. Therapeutic efficacy of these agents is limited when used alone, but they are often useful in combination with other potent diuretics.

Amiloride and triamterene are structurally related compounds that inhibit sodium uptake in collecting duct epithelial cells by inhibiting sodium conductance. A principal effect of these drugs is to reduce renal potassium secretion, which may be useful in concert with the action of potassium-wasting compounds such as the thiazides and loop diuretics but which may lead to clinically important hyperkalemia, particularly in patients with renal failure. The potassium-sparing diuretics tend to cause a mild metabolic acidosis. In patients with chronic obstructive pulmonary disease, these agents may be preferred to diuretics that enhance renal hydrogen losses and secondarily reduce ventilatory drive. Apart from causing hyperkalemia, these drugs are relatively benign. Spironolactone can cause troublesome gynecomastia.

OSMOTIC DIURETICS. These agents are rarely of use in the management of heart failure, but it should be remembered that radiographic contrast dyes are filtered by the glomerulus and act as osmotic diuretics, increasing urinary loss of salt and water. This volume-contracting effect can be important in fragile patients, such as those with severe aortic stenosis. An important characteristic of osmotic diuresis is its ability to maintain urine flow even at very low glomerular filtration rates, as occur in hypotension or dehydration.

COMBINED DIURETIC REGIMENS. Combined use of diuretics in patients with heart failure is usually considered for two main reasons: to avoid electrolyte disturbances that occur with the isolated use of a powerful agent such as a loop diuretic, especially in chronic therapy, and to augment salt and water excretion in the face of refractory edema. A third possible indication is the avoidance of ototoxicity from large doses of loop diuretics.

Combined use of potassium-sparing diuretics with a more proximally acting agent such as a thiazide or a loop diuretic constitutes a common practice. The potassium-sparing diuretics limit potassium and hydrogen ion loss induced by diuretics that act more proximally.

The combination of a loop diuretic with a thiazide or metolazone often results in a synergistic augmentation of salt and water excretion. This combination of agents is capable of producing marked intravascular volume depletion and electrolyte disturbances. Potassium wasting can be severe, and serum potassium levels require close monitoring. In general, this combination of diuretics should be initiated in a hospital setting, with careful regulation of the regimen on an outpatient basis with weight measurements taken daily and frequent checks of serum electrolyte and creatinine levels.

COMPLICATIONS OF DIURETIC THERAPY. Problems complicating diuretic therapy include intravascular volume depletion and hypotension from overly vigorous diuresis; hyponatremia, often due to prolonged diuretic therapy with inadequate sodium intake and often with excessive water intake; hypokalemia from the use of thiazides or loop diuretics, or both, with inadequate potassium supplementation, predisposing to cardiac arrhythmias with or without concomitant digitalis excess; hyperkalemia from potassium-sparing diuretic administration and potassium supplements; metabolic alkalosis with or without potassium depletion; hyperuricemia secondary to thiazide or loop diuretic administration; magnesium depletion, often occurring in parallel with potassium losses; and increased serum low density lipoprotein and triglyceride levels in patients receiving thiazides.

As a final comment, many patients treated for congestive heart failure spend a period of weeks developing the excessive fluid accumulation that characterizes this disease state; there is little virtue and much potential harm in attempting to correct this problem in an unduly short period of time. In general, in the absence of acute pulmonary edema, a reasonable goal (even in the era of DRG's) is about 1 kg of fluid loss per day.

Digitalis Glycosides

Cardiac glycosides have been used in the management of heart failure for more than 200 years and remain the only drugs currently available for long-term ambulatory use that have a positive inotropic effect. The relatively narrow therapeutic-toxic ratio of cardiac glycosides renders them particularly difficult to use, and the clinician should have a detailed understanding of the actions and pharmacokinetics of one drug of this class, such as digoxin. Because digoxin has supplanted almost entirely the use of other cardiac glycosides in the United States, the discussion focuses on this agent.

BASIC MECHANISM OF CARDIAC GLYCOSIDE ACTION. A consensus exists that the sequence of events leading to the positive inotropic effect of digitalis on both normal and failing cardiac muscle is as summarized in Figure 40–5. The digitalis glycosides bind to a site on the extracellular facing aspect of NaK-ATPase, the enzyme constituting the "sodium pump" that moves sodium and potassium across cell membranes against their respective concentration gradients. The complete amino acid sequences of the alpha and beta subunits of the enzyme are known. When a cardiac glycoside binds to the alpha subunit, that individual sodium pump unit is completely inhibited. When a fraction of NaK-ATPase sites on a cardiac myocyte are occupied, intracellular sodium concentration tends to rise. Through the mechanism of sodium-calcium exchange, this leads in turn to augmentation of the intracellular calcium content. Since calcium constitutes the trigger that leads to the contractile event, the increase of intracellular calcium stores (up to a point) enhances the contractile state of both normal and failing myocardium.

The electrophysiologic toxicity commonly observed with excessive doses of digitalis is probably due to the same fundamental mechanism of sodium pump inhibition. At higher doses and myocardial concentrations of the drug, impairment of sodium and potassium transport leads to characteristic disturbances of impulse formation and conduction, as discussed below. It is likely that intracellular calcium overload contributes to the cardiotoxicity of the digitalis glycosides, at least under circumstances that have been studied experimentally.

ELECTROPHYSIOLOGIC EFFECTS. Most of the antiarrhythmic effects of digitalis are the results of its actions at the level of the atria and atrioventricular junction. Conduction velocity is increased by cardiac glycosides in atrial and ventricular myocardium, but it is decreased in the AV conduction system and His-Purkinje system. Similarly, the effective refractory period is shortened in atrial and ventricular myocardium but tends to be lengthened in specialized conduction tissues. These effects are largely mediated by increased vagal tone, rather than by direct effects of cardiac glycosides, although the latter can be documented at the upper end of the dose range. Of particular importance in the management of supraventricular tachyarrhythmias is the tendency of digitalis to lengthen the refractory period and to slow conduction in the atrioventricular node. At toxic doses and blood levels, digitalis enhances sympathetic nerve traffic to the heart, thus increasing the propensity to ectopic impulse formation at atrial, atrioventricular junctional, and ventricular levels.

HEMODYNAMIC EFFECTS. The positive inotropic action is a direct effect of digitalis on cardiac myocytes. Endogenous norepinephrine stores are not necessary to permit expression of this effect. A useful way to appreciate the effect of digitalis on the intact circulation is by consideration of the ventricular function curves shown in Figure 40–1. In contrast to diuretics, which reduce preload and shift the circulatory state to the left along a given ventricular function curve, a positive inotropic agent shifts the entire curve upward and to the left toward the normal curve. Since contractility does not limit cardiac output in the normal circulation, digitalis would not be expected to change output in normal subjects. This is the case. As soon as the contractile state becomes limiting, however, digitalis increases cardiac output and lowers filling pressures of both the right and the left ventricles. Thus, cardiac glycosides are of clinical value in patients with congestive heart failure in the presence or absence of supraventricular tachyarrhythmias such as atrial fibrillation or atrial flutter. Although opinion is less uniform regarding patients in sinus rhythm, recent studies have documented benefit in the majority of patients who have dilated, failing ventricles with poor systolic function. These patients must be carefully distinguished from those with predominant diastolic dysfunction (noncompliant ventricles and elevated filling pressures but normal ejection fractions) who are unlikely to benefit. Thus, patients who are most likely to benefit are those having cardiomegaly with impaired systolic contraction, often accompanied by S_3 gallops. There is no convincing evidence of desensitization or tolerance to the cardiac effects of digitalis, and the positive inotropic effects are sustained over periods of months and years in patients with congestive heart failure.

To summarize, as pathologic processes such as ischemia, volume or pressure loads, or primary myocardial disease lead to reduced contractility, compensatory mechanisms emerge. Elevated end-diastolic pressure and volume augment ventricular performance through the Frank-Starling mechanism. Sympathetic tone tends to increase, thus enhancing contractile state, and the process of ventricular hypertrophy generates additional contractile elements. Each of these mechanisms, however, exacts a price. Excessive elevation of filling pressures results in pulmonary or peripheral edema. Excessive sympathetic tone results in tachycardia and, together with elevated renin-angiotensin system activity, in increased peripheral vascular resistance as well as increased myocardial oxygen consumption. With the progression of underlying cardiac disease, the compensatory mechanisms ultimately fail, or the consequences of these mechanisms become limiting (for example, with emergence of pulmonary edema). Administration of cardiac glycosides under these circumstances enhances myocardial contractility, decreasing the dependence of the circulation on compensatory mechanisms and providing improved cardiac reserve. Improved ventricular function yields a higher cardiac output at any given ventricular filling pressure. With the alternative therapeutic modalities now available, there is little virtue in giving cardiac glycosides to the brink of toxicity. Rather, conventional doses (see below) resulting in serum digoxin concentrations not exceeding 1.5 to 1.7 ng per milliliter appear to yield the best risk-benefit ratio.

PHARMACOKINETICS, BIOAVAILABILITY, AND DOSAGE CONSIDERATIONS. Summarized in Table 40–6 are the important pharmacokinetic variables and dosage ranges for cardiac glycosides in current clinical use. The values cited are averages, and individual variation is to be expected.

Digoxin. This is the most widely used preparation, particularly in hospitalized patients. Its virtues include flexibility of route of administration and intermediate duration of action. Digoxin is excreted exponentially (i.e., first-order kinetics) with a half-life of about 36 hours in young, healthy, normal subjects. In older patients with cardiac disease but without elevated BUN or serum creatinine levels, a half-life of 48 hours represents a more appropriate first approximation. Such patients excrete approximately one third of body stores daily, for the most part in unchanged form, although about 10 per cent of patients excrete substantial quantities of the inactive metabolite dihydrodigoxin, which arises through bacterial biotransformation in the gut lumen. The excretion of digoxin by the kidney is directly proportional to glomerular filtration rate (and hence creatinine clearance) and is relatively independent of the rate of urine flow in patients with intact renal function. Clearance may decrease somewhat in patients with prerenal azotemia. There is also evidence for some secretion of the drug at the renal tubular level.

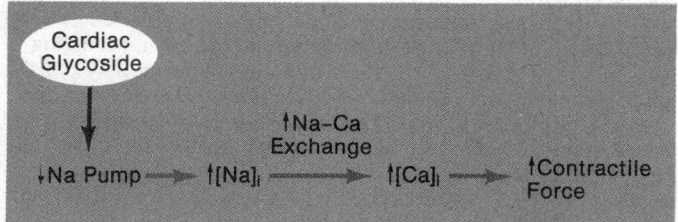

FIGURE 40–5. Schematic representation of the mechanism of inotropic action of cardiac glycosides. Binding of digitalis to NaK-ATPase inhibits this enzyme and hence the active outward transport of Na^+ across the myocardial cell membrane. Na^+ pump inhibition leads to increased intracellular Na^+ ($[Na]_i$) content and activity, which in turn alters Na-Ca exchange with consequent increase in Ca influx, decrease of Ca efflux, or both. The resulting increase in intracellular Ca ($[Ca]_i$) is presumed to mediate the observed increase in myocardial contractile force.

TABLE 40–6. PHARMACOLOGY OF CARDIAC GLYCOSIDES

Agent	Gastrointestinal Absorption	Onset of Action* (minutes)	Peak Effect (hours)	Average Half-Life†	Principal Metabolic Route (Excretory Pathway)	Average Digitalizing Dose		Usual Daily Oral Maintenance Dose‖
						Oral‡	Intravenous§	
Digoxin	55%–75%¶ (Lanoxicaps 90%–100%)	15–30	1½–5	36–48 hours	Renal; some gastrointestinal excretion	1.25–1.50 mg	0.75–1.00 mg	0.25–0.50 mg**
Digitoxin	90%–100%	25–120	4–12	4–6 days	Hepatic#; renal excretion of metabolites	0.70–1.20 mg	1.00 mg	0.10 mg

Modified from Smith TW: Drug therapy: Digitalis glycosides. N Engl J Med 288:719, 1973. By permission of the New England Journal of Medicine.

*For intravenous dose.

†For normal subjects (prolonged by renal impairment with digoxin and probably by severe hepatic disease with digitoxin).

‡Divided doses over 12 to 24 hours at intervals of 6 to 8 hours.

§Given in increments for initial subcomplete digitalization, to be supplemented by further small increments as necessary.

‖Average for adult patients without renal or hepatic impairment; varies widely among individual patients and requires close medical supervision.

¶For tablet form of administration (may be less in malabsorption syndromes and in formulations with poor bioavailability).

#Enterohepatic cycle exists.

**Approximately 20 per cent lower maintenance doses are required if gel solution in capsules (Lanoxicaps) is used. Maintenance dose must be reduced in patients with renal impairment (see text).

Therapy can be instituted in patients without urgent indications by starting the daily maintenance dose without a loading dose. This results in stable plateau concentrations of the drug in four to five excretory half-lives, or about 1 week. In patients with severe renal impairment, the half-life of the drug is prolonged to as much as 4 to 5 days, and steady-state levels are reached on a daily maintenance regimen only after 3 to 4 weeks.

Digoxin is extensively bound to tissues (large volume of distribution), and the drug is consequently not effectively removed from the body by hemodialysis. Lean body mass should be used for purposes of dosage calculation. Infants and children absorb and excrete digoxin much as do adults, although secretion at the renal tubular level may be somewhat more important in prepubertal patients.

An important interaction between digoxin and quinidine has been described, leading to a substantial increase in steady-state serum digoxin levels (averaging about twofold) when conventional quinidine doses are added to a maintenance digoxin regimen. Increases in the serum digoxin level are also observed when verapamil or amiodarone is given concurrently.

Bioavailability of digoxin in the standard tablet formulation is 55 to 75 per cent. The higher estimate is usually used in converting oral to intravenous doses. A preparation in which digoxin is dissolved in an encapsulated gel gives higher bioavailability, requiring a slight adjustment in the standard maintenance doses, as noted in Table 40–6. Previously marketed preparations with poor bioavailability properties are no longer available in the United States, thanks to action by regulatory agencies.

The maintenance digoxin dose required to replace daily losses varies from about 37 per cent of the body content in patients with normal renal function to 14 per cent in patients with essentially no renal function. The latter figure is an average, however, and some patients require substantially more or less than the maintenance dose that would be predicted by the 14 per cent figure. A useful approximation of daily per cent of loss of digoxin from the body is given by the following expression:

$$\text{Per cent daily loss} = 14 + \frac{C_{Cr} \text{ in ml/min}}{5}$$

Useful nomograms have been developed for loading and maintenance doses of digoxin, but it is important that these be used only as first approximations and that the patient be followed closely until a stable steady state is reached. Adjustments subsequently are required with changes in renal function, related either to intrinsic renal disease or to altered renal perfusion due to cardiac disease.

Digitoxin. This cardiac glycoside is the least polar and the most slowly excreted of the cardiac glycosides in current use. It is the principal constituent of the whole leaf of the digitalis plant. Gastrointestinal absorption of digitoxin is virtually complete. The drug binds avidly to serum albumin, and only about 3 per cent

of the drug circulates in the free, pharmacologically active state at conventional doses and serum levels. It thus differs substantially from digoxin, which is only about 23 per cent bound to plasma proteins at usual doses. Because of the high degree of serum protein binding, renal clearance of digitoxin is minimal and the drug is metabolized to a variety of poorly defined derivatives, presumably in the liver. Some enterohepatic cycling occurs in the case of digitoxin but is not important for digoxin. The half-time for digitoxin excretion averages about 5 to 6 days and is not appreciably affected by altered renal function.

Standard pharmacology texts give details of pharmacokinetics of other glycosides such as deslanoside and ouabain, which are rarely if ever used clinically at present in the United States.

DIGITALIS USE IN CONGESTIVE HEART FAILURE. The therapeutic use of digitalis in patients with normal sinus rhythm is complicated by the lack of any easily measurable therapeutic endpoint, such as that provided by the ventricular rate in patients with atrial fibrillation. Digitalis is of value in patients with symptoms and signs of heart failure due to ischemic cardiomyopathy, valvular disease, hypertensive heart disease, many types of congenital heart disease, and dilated cardiomyopathies and in some patients with cor pulmonale and overt right ventricular failure. The drug is of no demonstrated benefit in isolated mitral stenosis with normal sinus rhythm unless right ventricular failure is present. Similarly, little benefit can be expected in patients with pericardial tamponade or constrictive pericarditis. The latter disease states are all characterized by mechanical limitations to cardiac function, rather than by impairment of myocardial contractility. In hypertrophic cardiomyopathy with an obstructive element, digitalis may in fact be deleterious if left ventricular contractility increases and produces greater outflow obstruction. As noted previously, patients with symptoms of dyspnea on exertion due to high diastolic filling pressure from decreased ventricular compliance, but with well-preserved ejection fractions, are unlikely to benefit from digitalis if sinus rhythm is present.

The prophylactic use of digitalis in patients with diminished cardiac reserve who are expected to undergo a major stress such as surgery remains controversial. Many clinicians prefer to withhold digitalis until a specific indication arises.

The use of digitalis in the management of supraventricular rhythm disturbances is considered in Ch. 42. The drug is potentially dangerous in patients with Wolff-Parkinson-White syndrome.

INDIVIDUAL SENSITIVITY TO DIGITALIS. Table 40–7 lists factors that influence the sensitivity of individual patients to digitalis. These are factors intrinsic to the patient, rather than factors that influence *apparent* sensitivity, such as alterations in drug bioavailability or in the excretion pattern of the drug.

Electrolyte and Acid-Base Disturbances. Potassium depletion increases the likelihood that patients will develop digitalis toxic-

TABLE 40–7. FACTORS INFLUENCING INDIVIDUAL SENSITIVITY TO DIGITALIS

Type and severity of underlying cardiac disease
Serum electrolyte derangement
    Hypokalemia or hyperkalemia
    Hypomagnesemia
    Hypercalcemia
    Hyponatremia
Acid-base imbalance
Concomitant drug administration
    Anesthetics
    Catecholamines and sympathomimetics
    Antiarrhythmic agents
Thyroid status
Renal function
Autonomic nervous system tone
Respiratory disease

ity. Hypokalemia has a primary arrhythmogenic effect of its own and also tends to increase cellular binding of digitalis glycosides. Potassium depletion must be guarded against carefully in patients on potassium-wasting diuretics. Magnesium depletion also predisposes to digitalis toxicity and is a common concomitant of diuretic therapy. Elevated serum calcium levels may enhance ventricular automaticity and may also predispose to digitalis toxicity.

Acid-base disturbances appear to exert their effects largely through shifts in serum potassium concentration, and the acid-base disturbances per se usually have little effect within the range commonly encountered clinically.

Drug Interactions. Several drugs, including cholestyramine, colestipol, and neomycin, decrease absorption of orally administered digoxin, as do nonabsorbable antacids and Kaopectate. Quinidine, verapamil, and amiodarone all increase steady-state serum digoxin levels.

Type and Severity of Underlying Heart Disease. The most important factor influencing individual digitalis sensitivity is the type and severity of underlying heart disease. Otherwise healthy subjects are remarkably tolerant of large doses of digitalis, and toxicity typically manifests itself as disturbances of atrioventricular conduction rather than life-threatening tachyarrhythmias. In patients with advanced heart failure or severe focal ischemia, however, the therapeutic ratio of digitalis is remarkably low, and these patients may experience potentially life-threatening toxicity at doses and serum levels no more than twice the optimal amount.

Digitalis and Ischemic Heart Disease. The effects of digitalis on myocardial oxygen consumption, and therefore its use in patients with ischemic heart disease, depend primarily on the prior state of the ventricle. In the normal-size ventricle, the enhanced contractile state may modestly increase oxygen consumption. If failure and ventricular dilation are present, however, digitalis administration tends to reduce cardiac dimensions and thereby reduces wall tension (Laplace's relation) such that myocardial oxygen consumption may not increase or may even be reduced. It is important, therefore, to assess carefully the state of ventricular function prior to instituting digitalis therapy in patients with ischemic disease.

The role of digitalis therapy in acute myocardial infarction is limited. Other measures are generally preferable in the management of mild congestive heart failure in this setting. When symptoms and signs of overt left ventricular failure persist despite optimal use of diuretics and vasodilators, digitalis may be added at about 75 per cent of the usual loading dose. The loading dose should be given over a period of 18 to 24 hours with close monitoring of cardiac rhythm. It is customary to use digoxin in the presence of atrial fibrillation, which is typically a manifestation of heart failure in patients with acute myocardial infarction.

Some evidence suggests that patients may experience excess mortality when maintained on digitalis long-term following acute myocardial infarction, but most studies indicate that the mortality trends are accounted for by baseline variables such as greater severity of heart failure, rather than a deleterious effect of conventional doses of digoxin.

Advanced Age. It is unlikely that advanced age per se has an independent adverse effect on digitalis tolerance, but the reduced renal and pulmonary functions that attend advanced age require appropriate consideration.

Renal Failure. Factors influencing digitalis absorption and elimination, as well as rapid shifts in electrolytes with hemodialysis, predispose to digitalis toxicity. It is wise to leave an extra margin of safety in digitalis doses in managing these patients.

Thyroid Disease. Hyperthyroidism tends to reduce the response of patients to digitalis, whereas hypothyroidism increases the likelihood of digitalis toxicity. The failure of a patient with atrial fibrillation to respond to standard doses of digoxin with appropriate slowing of the heart rate should raise the question of occult thyrotoxicosis.

Pulmonary Disease. It is generally agreed that patients with chronic pulmonary disease, and especially with acute respiratory insufficiency, experience an increased frequency of digitalis intoxication. This may be related both to the underlying lung disease and hypoxia and to the sympathomimetic drugs that these patients often receive. It should be assumed that patients with a variety of pulmonary diseases may be sensitive to the arrhythmogenic effects of conventional doses and serum levels of cardiac glycosides.

SERUM DIGITALIS CONCENTRATIONS. Assay of serum digoxin concentration is routinely performed in most clinical laboratories, usually with the radioimmunoassay technique. There is a relatively constant ratio of serum or plasma to myocardial digoxin concentration, and thus the clinical effect of digoxin is directly related to the serum level. Nevertheless, there is considerable overlap in serum levels between patients with and without evidence of toxicity. Thus, serum concentration data must always be interpreted in the overall clinical context. Mean serum digoxin concentrations in groups of patients without evidence of toxicity, and with an expected therapeutic effect, average 1.4 ng per milliliter. Doubling the digoxin dose in a patient on a steady-state regimen can be expected to double the serum concentration when a new steady state is reached.

Serum digitoxin concentrations average about 10-fold higher than those of digoxin because of the binding of digitoxin to serum proteins.

The upper limit of the "therapeutic" range for digoxin is usually taken as about 2.0 ng per milliliter, but patients with supraventricular tachyarrhythmias, including atrial fibrillation and atrial flutter, may require appreciably higher levels to gain adequate control of the ventricular response and may tolerate these higher levels with no evidence of toxicity. Conversely, unusually sensitive patients may experience toxicity at serum levels as low as 1.0 ng per milliliter. It is not necessary to monitor serum digoxin levels routinely in patients who are doing well on standard maintenance doses of the drug. Serum levels may be of use, however, in the assessment of unexpected responses to therapy, including lack of the expected therapeutic response (Is the patient taking the drug?) or in situations in which digitalis toxicity is suspected (for example, multifocal ventricular premature beats in a patient with overt congestive heart failure who is taking digoxin).

DIGITALIS TOXICITY. At the cellular level, exposure to excessive levels of cardiac glycosides causes increased automaticity and decreased conduction. These abnormalities are reflected in a broad array of rhythm disturbances that are often difficult to distinguish from those caused by underlying heart disease. Commonly encountered rhythm disturbances, in decreasing order of incidence, include ventricular ectopic rhythms, AV block, atrial arrhythmias, sinoatrial arrhythmias, AV dissociation, and accelerated AV junctional rhythms.

Sinus Node and Atrium. Slowing of the sinus rate in patients with congestive heart failure is largely mediated by improved cardiac function and withdrawal of elevated sympathetic tone. Sinus rate is not a very useful indicator of digitalis effect, since it tends to remain rapid in the presence of fever, infection, anemia, thyrotoxicosis, or a variety of other conditions that predispose to sinus tachycardia. At high toxic doses, digitalis can cause direct depression of sinus node automaticity, or more likely sinoatrial exit block, which produce bradyarrhythmias.

Atrioventricular Node. The effective refractory period of the atrioventricular (AV) node is prolonged by digitalis, chiefly through increased vagal activity. In addition, the conduction velocity through the AV junction is reduced. As digoxin doses are increased, first-degree block (PR interval > 0.20 second) may appear, followed by second-degree AV block of the Mobitz type I or Wenckebach variety (see Ch. 42). With still higher doses, complete AV dissociation and third-degree block can occur. A typical manifestation of digitalis toxicity in the presence of atrial fibrillation is AV dissociation, often accompanied by increased automaticity of pacemakers in the AV junction. This causes regularization of a previously irregular ventricular rate.

His-Purkinje System. Digitalis-induced increase in the automaticity of cells in the His-Purkinje system is a relatively common manifestation of digitalis excess and is responsible for rhythm disturbances, including ventricular premature beats, ventricular bigeminy, and ventricular tachycardia.

Clinical Manifestations of Digitalis Toxicity. Gastrointestinal Symptoms. Anorexia, nausea, and vomiting are common consequences of digitalis toxicity. Unfortunately, these are present prior to the onset of rhythm disturbances in only about 50 per cent of cases.

Neurologic Symptoms. Headache, fatigue, malaise, disorientation, confusion, delirium, and seizures can occur, and visual symptoms, including disturbances of color vision, are well known. In fact, the gastrointestinal symptoms actually arise from the effects of digitalis on the chemoreceptor trigger zone in the medulla rather than as a result of direct irritation of the gastrointestinal system.

Massive Cardiac Glycoside Overdose. Suicidal or accidental digitalis overdose can produce the entire array of typical cardiac arrhythmias, including refractory ventricular fibrillation. In addition, hyperkalemia is sometimes encountered owing to interference with sodium and potassium transport across cell membranes throughout the body. This must be taken into account in considering the use of potassium supplements in cases in which massive toxicity may occur.

Treatment of Digitalis Intoxication. The most important element of successful treatment is early recognition that a cardiac rhythm disturbance is due to digitalis toxicity. For many of the most common manifestations, such as occasional ventricular premature beats, first-degree AV block, or atrial fibrillation with a slow ventricular response, temporary withdrawal of the drug with electrocardiographic monitoring (if indicated) until the arrhythmia has disappeared constitutes adequate management. The maintenance dose should then be adjusted to prevent recurrence. Arrhythmias that impair cardiac function because of rates that are too rapid or too slow, or those that suggest the possibility of progression to more malignant arrhythmias, require more aggressive management. Ventricular tachycardia due to digitalis toxicity requires immediate vigorous treatment. Bradyarrhythmias, including sinus bradycardia, sinoatrial arrest, or exit block, and atrioventricular block of second or third degree can sometimes be treated effectively with atropine, 0.5 to 1.0 mg given intravenously. Pervenous electrical pacing should be instituted if atropine is not rapidly effective.

Potassium. Potassium repletion is useful in the treatment of ectopic tachyarrhythmias when hypokalemia is present or when the serum potassium level is in the low normal range. Potassium must be given with caution in other circumstances because of the risks of hyperkalemia, particularly in the presence of renal impairment or of conduction disturbances.

Lidocaine and Phenytoin. These are the most useful drugs in the treatment of ectopic rhythm disturbances caused by digitalis. They tend to have minimal adverse effect on sinoatrial or AV conduction. Lidocaine is given intravenously in 100-mg bolus doses every 3 to 5 minutes, followed by a maintenance intravenous infusion of 15 to 20 µg per kilogram of body weight per minute, as required to maintain control of the rhythm disturbance and to avoid neurologic signs and symptoms. Phenytoin* is given in a dose of 100 mg by slow intravenous infusion, repeated every 5 minutes until onset of toxicity or control of the arrhythmia, followed by an oral maintenance dose of 400 to 600 mg per day if control of the rhythm disturbance is achieved.

*This use is not listed in the manufacturer's directive.

Beta-Adrenergic Blocking Drugs. Beta blockade has been useful in the treatment of some arrhythmias caused by digitalis excess but tends to decrease conduction as well as myocardial contractility and therefore is not widely used in this setting.

Quinidine and Procainamide. These drugs carry a risk of depression of sinoatrial and atrioventricular node function and can also depress myocardial contractility. Other agents are usually preferable for use in digitalis toxicity.

Direct Current (DC) Countershock (also see Ch. 42). This is generally inadvisable in the presence of digitalis intoxication because it may evoke severe arrhythmias in this setting. However, it must occasionally be used when other methods have been ineffective in the presence of a life-threatening arrhythmia. Risk is decreased when lower energy levels are employed, and careful titration is essential. Cardioversion is generally a benign procedure in patients without digitalis-induced rhythm disturbances.

Steroid-Binding Resins, Hemodialysis, and Hemoperfusion. These techniques have not been demonstrated to be effective in the management of advanced digitalis intoxication and are not recommended. Hemodialysis may be of value in controlling the serum potassium level in patients with refractory hyperkalemia.

Digoxin-Specific Antibodies. Purified Fab fragments of digoxin-specific antibodies are available for treatment of advanced digitalis toxicity of sufficient severity to be potentially life threatening. More than 2000 patients have now been treated, with a high degree of efficacy and with adverse side effects largely limited to those expected from withdrawal of digitalis effects. This approach is recommended for patients in whom conventional measures are not rapidly effective.

Vasodilators

Cardiac loading has a strong dependence on the resistance and capacitance properties of the peripheral vascular bed. Thus, vasodilator therapy in heart failure is designed to reduce the preload or afterload, or both, of a failing ventricle by relaxing vascular smooth muscle in the periphery. Vasodilators have been shown to improve survival in patients with continuing symptoms of heart failure who are taking digitalis and diuretics.

PRINCIPLES OF VASODILATOR THERAPY. As summarized in Figure 40–2, the normal ventricle is able to respond to increased afterload with an increase in the force of contraction such that there is little, if any, change in stroke volume until extreme elevations in afterload are encountered. As the ventricle fails, the relationship between afterload and stroke volume shifts downward and to the left so that a relatively modest change in outflow resistance causes a substantial alteration in stroke volume. This constitutes both a pathophysiologic problem and a therapeutic opportunity. The opportunity follows from the uniform increase in peripheral vascular resistance observed in untreated patients with decompensated congestive heart failure. Activation of the sympathetic nervous system and of the renin-angiotensin system accounts for most of the increase in peripheral resistance. These responses of the peripheral vascular system to a perceived decrease in cardiac output have survival value under conditions of hemorrhage or dehydration by redirecting the cardiac output to essential beds, including the brain and coronary circulation. Since congestive heart failure was presumably not an evolutionary pressure, it is not surprising that these primitive mechanisms for the defense of blood flow to vital organs prove maladaptive in the patient with chronic congestive heart failure.

As illustrated in Figure 40–1, the failing heart responds to a reduction in afterload by shifting its ventricular function curve toward normal, although the inotropic state remains unchanged. An attractive feature of afterload reduction is the ability to increase cardiac output without increasing preload or myocardial oxygen consumption.

VASODILATOR AGENTS. In the following discussion, primary consideration is given to vasodilator therapy for left ventricular failure, although the failing right ventricle also benefits from reduced pulmonary vascular resistance. The most potent afterload-reducing agent in the pulmonary circulation is oxygen; there is, as yet, no drug that reliably exerts a preferential afterload-reducing effect in the pulmonary circulation.

The action of vasodilator drugs is described in terms of effects on the venous bed (preload) or the arteriolar bed (afterload). Table 40–8 summarizes data on the vasodilators in current clinical use in the management of heart failure.

Venous Dilators. These reduce the vascular smooth muscle tone in the systemic venous bed, increasing its capacitance and shifting blood volume from the arterial to the venous side of the circulation. Thus, patients with pulmonary vascular congestion and edema due to high left heart filling pressures obtain symptomatic relief, limited only by the necessity to maintain a level of preload that results in an adequate forward cardiac output. The most selective agents for this purpose are the nitrates, including nitroglycerin and the longer-acting orally administered compounds such as isosorbide dinitrate. Many investigators believe that much or most of the clinical benefit of vasodilator use derives from the venous dilator component. In chronic congestive heart failure, administration of agents that preferentially dilate the arteriolar bed without a preload-reducing component, such as minoxidil and hydralazine, fails to show sustained benefit.

Arteriolar Dilators. These reduce left ventricular afterload and tend to redistribute blood flow among organ beds in ways that are, unfortunately, not always predictable. The improvement in blood flow to exercising skeletal muscle is relatively limited. Nevertheless, the forward stroke output of the left ventricle is delivered with a lower wall tension, such that myocardial oxygen consumption is favorably affected. The most selective agent routinely used in obtaining an afterload-reducing effect is hydralazine.

Balanced Vasodilators. The balanced vasodilators exert an effect on both preload and afterload through a generalized relaxing effect on vascular smooth muscle. The prototype short-acting agent of this kind is nitroprusside. This agent has found widespread application in the management of acute heart failure states, including acute pulmonary edema. Used with care, it can also improve the circulatory state of patients with combined hypotension and low forward output, provided that adequate arterial pressure can be maintained by the use of volume loading or inotropic drugs or both. The tendency of nitroprusside to reduce systemic arterial pressure is offset to a considerable extent by the increased stroke output. The unloading effect of nitroprusside is most helpful when the left ventricular filling pressures are maintained in the vicinity of 15 mm Hg, which may require administration of intravenous fluids. An important advantage of nitroprusside in intensive care unit settings is its short duration of action, permitting minute-to-minute titration of the circulatory state.

A regimen yielding a balanced vasodilator effect is hydralazine and nitrates, the latter often given as the long-acting oral preparation isosorbide dinitrate. In an important multicenter study (Cohn, 1986), the protocol randomly assigned patients taking digitalis and diuretics to hydralazine with isosorbide dinitrate, to prazosin, or to placebo. The group treated with hydralazine and nitrates showed a 38 per cent mean reduction in mortality during the initial year of treatment, and the improved survival was sustained to the 3-year point. The prazosin-treated group showed no significant difference from the placebo group. An analogous, albeit smaller, study in Scandinavia in class IV patients demonstrated a similar improvement in survival in patients on diuretics and digoxin randomized to receive in addition the ACE inhibitor enalapril. The hydralazine-nitrate combination is now being compared to enalapril in a multicenter randomized trial (VHeFT-II) with survival as the primary endpoint.

The ACE inhibitors captopril and enalapril are available as balanced vasodilators for the management of patients with heart failure. Multicenter trials have demonstrated sustained improvement in symptoms and exercise tolerance, and large-scale therapeutic trials with survival endpoints are currently in progress in several subsets of patients. Many clinicians find that captopril and enalapril provide a relatively simple and controllable approach to vasodilator therapy, and hence constitute vasodilators of choice in many centers. Special caution and the use of very small initial doses of these drugs, which can produce severe hypotension and renal failure, are required. An irritating, persistent dry cough is a class effect of ACE inhibitor drugs that occurs in up to 10 per cent of patients.

Not all patients who appear to be reasonable candidates for vasodilator use in advanced heart failure can tolerate the drugs initially, and not all of the group that initially tolerates the regimen still show demonstrable benefit at the end of 3 months. Although results can be optimized by careful selection of patients and judicious use of available agents, the fact remains that some patients with advanced heart failure are unable to tolerate vasodilators, chiefly because of postural hypotension.

Combined Drug Therapy

Although patients with mild heart failure (early class II symptoms) can often be managed with a single class of drugs, accumulating evidence indicates that combination therapy with all

TABLE 40–8. MAJOR VASODILATOR DRUGS*

Drug	Mechanism of Action	Venous Dilating Effect (Preload Reduction)	Arteriolar Dilating Effect (Afterload Reduction)	Usual Dosage	Comments
Nitroglycerin	Direct	+++	+	10–100 µg/min, IV 5–20 mg, transdermal 0.4 mg, s.l.	Tolerance may be a problem with sustained continuous use. May be used sublingually to control acute increases in left atrial pressure.
Isosorbide dinitrate	Direct	+++	+	5–20 mg q. 2 hr, s.l. 10–60 mg q. 4 hr, p.o.	Improved survival shown in chronic CHF when used with hydralazine.
Nitroprusside	Direct	+++	+++	5–150 µg/kg/min IV; usual dose, 50–75 µg/kg/min	Used IV only. Drug is light sensitive. Hazard of thiocyanate or cyanide toxicity with prolonged high doses.
Hydralazine	Direct	0	+++	10–75 mg q. 6 hr p.o.	Sustained benefit in heart failure not shown when used as sole vasodilator.
Prazosin†	Alpha-adrenergic blockade (alpha₁ selective)	+++	++	1–5 mg q. 6 hr p.o.	Extra caution required with initial doses. Tolerance requires dosage adjustments and complicates use in heart failure.
Captopril	Angiotensin converting enzyme (ACE) inhibitor	+++	++	6.25–25.0 mg q. 6–8 hr, p.o.	Approved by F.D.A. for use in chronic CHF. Acute renal failure can occur with initial doses; initiate use with extra caution. Avoid potassium-sparing diuretics.
Enalapril	ACE inhibitor	+++	++	2.5–10 mg q. 12 hr p.o.	

*All of these agents may cause severe hypotension, and special caution is required with initial use, particularly in patients with severe congestive heart failure. Heart rate changes with all agents listed are usually minor unless a hypotensive response elicits reflex tachycardia; prazosin can cause bradycardia with initial use. Calcium channel blocking drugs (verapamil, diltiazem, and dihydropyridines including nifedipine) are effective vasodilators but are not recommended for management of heart failure with systolic dysfunction because of their potential negative inotropic effects on the heart.

†Prazosin was not found to improve survival compared to placebo when added to diuretics and digoxin in patients with class II and III chronic heart failure (Cohn, 1986). CHF = congestive heart failure; F.D.A. = Food and Drug Administration.

three major classes of drugs tends to keep heart size and wall stress as well as symptoms at a minimum while allowing the patient maximal effort tolerance within the limits imposed by the underlying cardiac problem. Implicit in the scheme outlined in Table 40–4 is the working hypothesis that in patients with compromised contractile function, combination therapy with a diuretic, vasodilator, and digitalis yields optimal benefit while allowing each drug to be used at a dose level as far as possible from its toxicity threshold. There is substantial evidence documenting the additive beneficial hemodynamic effects of a vasodilator and a positively inotropic drug such as digoxin, as well as additive effects of combined use of digoxin and an ACE inhibitor on exercise tolerance. The experienced clinician usually elects to add these classes of agents to the regimen one at a time to permit assessment of the incremental response at each step, but in most cases evaluates the response to combined treatment with all three classes in patients who remain symptomatic at levels of activity they wish to maintain.

Treatment of Diastolic Ventricular Dysfunction

The elements of therapy in patients with predominant diastolic dysfunction differ in certain important ways from those in patients with "classic" congestive heart failure accompanying a dilated ventricle with impaired systolic function. Pulmonary congestion is appropriately treated in both subsets of patients with diuretics and other means of preload reduction, including venodilators. Nitroglycerin taken sublingually can be used effectively by patients to forestall or slow the progression of episodes of elevated left ventricular filling pressures that might otherwise progress to frank pulmonary edema. It is important to avoid excessive preload reduction in the predominant diastolic dysfunction patient, however, in order to avoid symptoms and signs of low cardiac output. Anti-ischemic and antihypertensive treatment should be pursued aggressively when these disorders and their attendant pathophysiology underlie diastolic ventricular dysfunction, with removal of ischemia and regression of hypertrophy as the goals of therapy. Atrial augmentation of ventricular systole is particularly important in these patients, and every effort should be made to maintain or restore normal sinus rhythm or pacemaker-induced AV synchrony. Calcium channel blocking drugs may be of benefit in some patients with predominant diastolic dysfunction but are generally to be avoided in the presence of severe systolic dysfunction because of their potential negative inotropic effects. Finally, positively inotropic agents such as digoxin have no established role in the management of patients with predominant diastolic dysfunction and are contraindicated in patients with hypertrophic cardiomyopathy and dynamic outflow tract obstruction.

Refractory Heart Failure

Therapeutic advances have left in their wake a subset of patients with marked impairment of ventricular function (often with left ventricular ejection fractions in the 10 to 20 per cent range) who survive but are severely symptomatic on maximal tolerated doses of diuretics, digitalis, and vasodilators. Those who meet additional relevant criteria (including preserved function of other organ systems, no elevation of pulmonary vascular resistance, no active infection) may be referred for consideration of heart transplantation after detailed explanation of the potential risks and benefits of this procedure. This procedure now has relatively widespread application since the advent of cyclosporine for immunosuppression, and more than 150 centers in the United States now have active programs. Survival exceeds 60 per cent in transplanted patients at 5 years in larger series, compared with an expected mortality well in excess of 50 per cent at 12 months in patients treated by conventional means, and functional recovery is often gratifying. Expectations must be tempered by the very limited availability of donor hearts, however, which has recently plateaued in the 1500 to 2000 per year range in the United States.

Treatment of acute decompensation using intravenous β-adrenergic or dopaminergic agonists, or the phosphodiesterase inhibitor amrinone, is covered in Ch. 41. Longer-term use of orally active β-adrenergic agonist drugs has proved disappointing, in part because of rapid development of tolerance, and cannot be recommended. Several phosphodiesterase inhibitor drugs are under continuing clinical study, including amrinone, milrinone,* and enoximone.* These agents have both vasodilator and positive inotropic properties related to enhancement of cyclic adenosine monophosphate levels in vascular smooth muscle and myocardium. Although symptoms appear to be improved in some patients treated chronically with these investigational agents, statistically compelling evidence of sustained efficacy or improved survival is lacking. The artificial heart has been developed sufficiently for placement in several patients, but results to date have been disappointing because of unsolved thromboembolic problems, and mechanical assist devices are in current investigational use mainly to provide a bridge to heart transplantation in potentially suitable candidates.

*Investigational drug.

ACKNOWLEDGMENT: Ralph A. Kelly, M.D., has made major contributions to the coverage of diuretics, including Figure 40–4.

Berger BE, Warnock DG: Clinical uses and mechanisms of action of diuretic agents. In Brenner BM, Rector FC (eds.): The Kidney. Philadelphia, W. B. Saunders Company, 1986, pp 433–455. *A compact summary of clinically relevant information as stated in the title.*

Captopril Multicenter Research Group: A placebo-controlled trial of captopril in refractory congestive heart failure. J Am Coll Cardiol 2:755, 1983. *A well-designed controlled trial demonstrating improved clinical state and effort tolerance among 92 patients with heart failure refractory to digitalis and diuretics randomized to additional treatment with placebo or the ACE inhibitor captopril, which was subsequently approved by the United States Food and Drug Administration for the indication of congestive heart failure. Results are typical of a number of similar clinical trials with ACE inhibitors.*

Cohn JN, et al.: Effect of vasodilator therapy on mortality in chronic congestive heart failure: Results of a VA cooperative study. N Engl J Med 314:1547, 1986.

CONSENSUS Trial Study Group: Effects of enalapril on mortality in severe congestive heart failure. Results of the Cooperative North Scandinavian Enalapril Survival Study. N Engl J Med 316:1429–1435, 1987. *The above two studies establish the role of balanced vasodilator therapy in improving survival when added to diuretics and digoxin (which were continued) in patients with chronic congestive heart failure. At a mean follow-up of 2.3 years, the study of Cohn et al showed improved survival (risk reduction of 34 per cent) among patients treated with hydralazine and nitrates. Mortality in the prazosin-treated group was indistinguishable from that in the group receiving placebo. Overall mortality, as expected, was high (36 to 47 per cent at 3 years) and was higher still in the CONSENSUS trial, which enrolled class IV heart failure patients. Mortality was reduced by 31 per cent at 1 year by addition of enalapril to the regimen in the CONSENSUS trial.*

Packer M (ed.): Physiologic determinants of survival in congestive heart failure. Circulation 75:IV-1–IV-111, 1987. *This supplement to Circulation contains 14 papers reviewing the various factors influencing prognosis in heart failure and current aspects of vasodilator, inotropic, and antiarrhythmic therapy and their potential impact on survival.*

Pouleur H (ed.): Diastolic function in heart failure: Clinical approaches to its understanding and treatment. Circulation 81:III-1–III-158, 1990. *This supplement to Circulation contains 21 papers covering virtually all clinically relevant aspects of diastolic dysfunction, including pathophysiology, role in heart failure, and therapeutic implications.*

Smith TW (ed.): Digitalis Glycosides. Orlando, Fla., Grune & Stratton, 1986. *This 348-page book summarizes available information on all aspects of the basic and clinical pharmacology, clinical use, and toxicity problems related to the cardiac glycosides.*

Smith TW, Braunwald E, Kelly RA: The management of heart failure. In Braunwald E (ed.): Heart Diseases. 4th ed. Philadelphia, W. B. Saunders Company, 1991. *A detailed consideration of general and specific aspects of congestive heart failure management with more than 500 references.*

41 Shock

David W. Ferguson

Shock—a rude unhinging of the machinery of life.
SAMUEL GROSS, 1972

Rather than a specific disease, shock is a complex clinical syndrome, the successful treatment of which requires vigilant medical attention, precise hemodynamic monitoring, and a thorough understanding of the basic principles of circulatory physiology and the pharmacology of cardiac and vasoactive medications. This chapter reviews the basic principles of circulatory control as they relate to the shock syndrome, the systemic and cellular mechanisms involved in the pathogenesis of the shock state, the differential diagnosis of shock, and the clinical characteristics of specific shock syndromes and provides general and specific recommendations pertaining to current therapy of this disorder.

DEFINITION. The term "shock" (Fr. *choc*), first used by the French physician LeDran in 1773 to describe the clinical characteristics of patients after severe gunshot trauma, is a nonspecific term now used to describe complex pathophysiologic syndrome(s) arising from any of a multitude of etiologies. Common to all of these syndromes of shock is a failure of the circulatory system to maintain cellular perfusion and function. Shock usually results from a critical impairment of blood flow to vital organs and tissues and/or the inability of those tissues to utilize essential nutrients. The common denominator in all forms of shock is microcirculatory insufficiency, which may arise from a wide variety of causes. Nevertheless, the end result of irreversible shock is cellular membrane dysfunction, abnormal cellular metabolism, and eventually cellular death. Shock is inferred from clinical evidence of major organ hypoperfusion in the setting of hemodynamic instability usually associated with relative or absolute hypotension. An understanding of the pathophysiology and treatment of shock requires a firm foundation in normal circulatory control mechanisms.

MECHANISMS OF CIRCULATORY CONTROL— NORMAL AND DURING SHOCK

The basic underlying abnormality in all forms of shock is a state of disordered cellular metabolic support. Shock of any etiology is associated with reduced or insufficient cellular oxygen consumption. Since all cellular functions depend upon adequate tissue perfusion, an understanding of the pathophysiology of shock requires an understanding of the normal determinants of tissue perfusion.

Major Determinants of Tissue Perfusion

The basic functions of the circulation are the delivery of oxygen and essential nutrients to peripheral tissues and the removal of metabolic wastes from those tissues. In most cases of shock, there is either insufficient delivery or inappropriate distribution of oxygen and nutrients. These disorders account to a large extent for the impairment of tissue metabolic consumption that characterizes the shock syndrome.

The major determinants of normal tissue perfusion are listed in Table 41–1. Perfusion of peripheral tissues depends upon cardiac, vascular, and microcirculatory factors. Perfusion of any organ depends upon systemic arterial pressure (the driving force for blood flow through the organs), the resistance offered by the vasculature of that organ, and the patency of nutritional capillaries within the organ.

Systemic arterial pressure is determined by cardiac output and the resistance of the total vascular tree:

$$\text{Arterial Pressure} = \text{Cardiac Output} \times \text{Total Vascular Resistance}$$

Vascular resistance is predominantly a function of the radius or caliber of blood vessels, which is influenced by neurogenic, humoral, and myogenic factors that regulate the tone of vascular smooth muscle. Thus, blood flow to any one organ depends on cardiac function, vascular muscle tone, and the caliber of resistance beds both in the systemic arterial tree and within the organ itself. The determinant of exchange of substrates and metabolites within the tissue is the microcirculation. A patent nutritional capillary network is the critical interface between the circulation and the cell. The following discussion reviews the critical cardiac, vascular, and microcirculatory determinants of tissue perfusion which are important in understanding the pathophysiology and treatment of shock.

CARDIAC FACTORS. *Cardiac Output.* Cardiac output is the product of heart rate and stroke volume. When averaged over time, the cardiac output of the right ventricle equals that of the left ventricle.

$$\text{Cardiac Output} = \text{Heart Rate} \times \text{Stroke Volume}$$

In normal resting adults, a heart rate of 70 beats per minute and a stroke volume of 70 to 75 ml per beat produce a cardiac output

TABLE 41–1. MAJOR HEMODYNAMIC DETERMINANTS OF TISSUE PERFUSION

I. **Systemic arterial pressure**
  A. Total vascular resistance
    1. Total arteriolar resistance, vascular muscle tone
      a. Tissue metabolites
      b. Neurohumoral factors
      c. Toxins
    2. Blood viscosity
  B. Cardiac output
    1. Heart rate: Bradyarrhythmias and tachyarrhythmias
    2. Stroke volume
      a. Preload (cardiac filling pressure and volume)
        1) Total circulating blood volume
          a) External loss
          b) Internal loss or sequestration
          c) Red blood cell mass
          d) Capillary hydrostatic pressure
          e) Capillary permeability
          f) Oncotic pressure
        2) Distribution of blood volume
          a) Body position (gravity)
          b) Intrapericardial pressure
          c) Intrathoracic pressure
          d) Venous tone
          e) Skeletal muscle pump
        3) Atrial contraction
          a) Contractile state
          b) Timing (AV synchrony)
        4) Diastolic filling time (heart rate)
      b. Inotropic state
        1) Total functioning ventricular muscle mass
        2) Intrinsic (myocardial) control mechanisms
          a) Adrenergic receptors
          b) Excitation-contraction coupling
         3) Extrinsic (noncardiac) neurocirculatory control mechanisms
          a) Circulating catecholamines
          b) Autonomic nervous system
          c) Myocardial depression
         4) Myocardial perfusion (oxygen supply)
          a) Aortic diastolic pressure
          b) Fixed and nonfixed coronary obstructions
          c) Metabolic coronary vasodilation
          d) Neurogenic control mechanisms
         5) Myocardial oxygen demand
          a) Heart rate
          b) Cardiac size
          c) Afterload
          d) Contractility
          e) Pharmacologic agents
        6) Physiologic depressants
          a) Acidosis
          b) Hypoxemia
          c) Alkalosis (severe)
        7) Pharmacologic depressants
        8) Humoral agents
          a) Catecholamines
          b) Myocardial depressant factors
      c. Afterload
        1) Aortic diastolic pressure
          a) Systemic vascular resistance
          b) Arterial viscoelasticity
          c) Aortic root blood volume
        2) Ventricular size (law of Laplace)
        3) Impedance

II. **Organ vascular resistance**
  A. Occlusive vascular disease
  B. Local arteriolar and venular resistance
    1) Neurogenic factors
    2) Humoral factors
    3) Local autoregulation
  C. Blood viscosity

III. **Nutritional microcirculatory patency**
  A. Precapillary sphincter tone
  B. Postcapillary venular tone
  C. Intracapillary aggregation of blood components
  D. Capillary endothelial integrity

of approximately 5 liters per minute. A decrease in cardiac output to less than 2 liters per minute per square meter of body surface area (cardiac index) may result in severe shock, particularly if imposed over a short time interval.

Heart Rate. Normal individuals tolerate a wide range of heart rates, from approximately 30 to 180 beats per minute, assuming underlying normal cardiac function. An increase in heart rate is one of the earliest physiologic responses to a fall in arterial pressure and is modulated by the autonomic nervous system. Physiologic ranges of tachycardia usually increase cardiac output, but marked increases in heart rate may limit cardiac diastolic filling time and thereby result in a low cardiac output and a fall in arterial blood pressure. The tolerable limits for heart rate decrease with underlying cardiovascular impairment. For example, ventricular tachycardia or rapid atrial fibrillation in a patient with recent myocardial infarction produces a reduction in cardiac output and arterial pressure that, if uncorrected, may result in cardiogenic shock. Immediate treatment to restore normal cardiac rate and rhythm is essential in such a patient.

However, management of the patient in shock who is noted to be tachycardic requires an appreciation of the differential diagnosis of the tachycardia. In the setting of sinus tachycardia, the clinician needs to realize that a "compensatory tachycardia" is often seen in patients with fever, anemia, sepsis, hemorrhage, or severe hypovolemia. In these settings, sinus tachycardia is an appropriate reflex circulatory adjustment to maintain cardiac output. It would therefore be deleterious to attempt to treat the tachycardia alone (e.g., with β-adrenergic or calcium channel blocking agents) without determining the underlying etiology of the tachycardia (e.g., hypovolemia) and correcting the primary defect rather than its physiologic compensatory response.

Marked bradycardia may also cause a reduction in cardiac output and result in hypotension. In many situations, bradycardia is vagally mediated and responds to anticholinergic maneuvers (e.g., atropine). Many commonly utilized medications (e.g., β-adrenergic and calcium channel blockers) may aggravate bradycardia in patients with acute circulatory insults or may attenuate normal sympathetically mediated tachycardic responses. Sinus bradycardia and atrioventricular (AV) block are often seen immediately following myocardial infarction and should be reversed if they contribute to hypotension.

Stroke Volume. Stroke volume is the amount of blood ejected by the ventricle with each cardiac contraction and is determined by cardiac preload, inotropic state, and afterload. A decrease in stroke volume may be caused by (1) a decrease in cardiac filling (preload), (2) a decrease in myocardial contractility (inotropic state), or (3) an increase in cardiac afterload (Figs. 41–1 and 41–2).

Preload is defined as the stretch or tension on an individual sarcomere just prior to the onset of fiber shortening. Clinically, preload refers to the volume of blood filling the ventricle at the end of diastole (presystole). Ventricular preload regulates the subsequent force of cardiac contraction as described by Starling's law of the heart. Preload is often assessed clinically as ventricular filling pressure rather than volume. The clinician must remember that it is the *compliance* (distensibility) of the ventricle that determines the relationship between pressure and volume:

Compliance = Change in Volume / Change in Pressure

Thus, the "optimal" preload (as assessed by filling pressure) for an individual patient may vary significantly with alterations in the compliance of the ventricle.

The most important determinant of cardiac preload is the total circulating blood volume. A reduction in blood volume may be either absolute or relative to the capacity of the vascular tree. Absolute reduction in blood volume is apparent when blood or fluids are lost, causing a hypovolemic state leading to hypovolemic shock, as seen in such clinical disorders as hemorrhage (internal or external), excessive vomiting, diarrhea, burns, renal loss of fluid (diabetes mellitus or diabetes insipidus), excessive diuresis, and excessive perspiration without fluid replacement. Internal losses of fluid occur with disorders such as peritonitis, pancreatitis, intestinal obstruction with extravasation of fluid, splanchnic ischemia with bowel necrosis and gangrene, fractures with extensive muscle trauma, hemothorax, and hemoperitoneum.

However, total blood volume must be not only adequate but also appropriately distributed for preload to be sufficient to maintain stroke volume. The chief determinants of the distribution of preload include body position (gravity), venous tone, intrathoracic and intrapericardial pressure, and the skeletal muscle pump. Compression of the heart may prevent its filling, as in pericardial tamponade or tension pneumothorax. Mechanical obstruction to blood flow may cause hypotension and shock in patients with atrial myxoma, a ball-valve thrombus, or pulmonary embolism. Positive-pressure ventilation may also decrease venous return and cardiac filling. Relative decreases in blood volume occur when there is loss of vascular tone because of the administration of anesthetics or ganglionic blockers, after spinal cord injury or surgery, and in patients with neuropathy or autonomic insufficiency. Pooling of blood thus results in a decrease in cardiac filling pressure.

Another important determinant of ventricular preload is atrial contraction and the rate of diastolic filling of the ventricle. Although atrial contraction in a normal heart may determine only 5 to 10 per cent of the subsequent ventricular stroke volume, in a diseased heart the contribution of atrial contraction to the subsequent ventricular stroke volume may be as great as 40 to 50 per cent. This is the primary reason that patients with hypertrophic cardiomyopathy, critical aortic stenosis, or acute myocardial infarction undergo rapid hemodynamic decompensation with the onset of atrial fibrillation and loss of an organized atrial component to ventricular preload.

Inotropic state refers physiologically to the magnitude and rate of myocardial fiber contraction under a given set of loading conditions. From the clinical standpoint, inotropic state refers to the contractile strength of the heart and is determined by a number of factors. These include the total mass of functioning

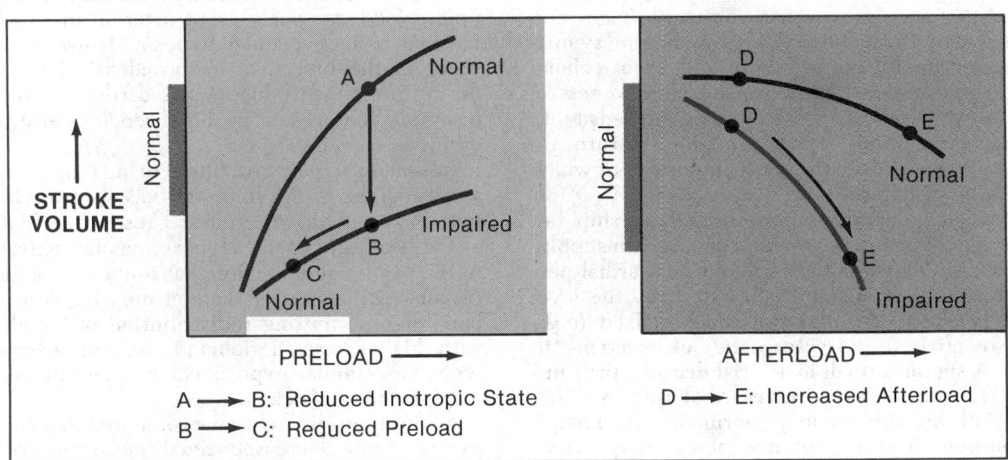

FIGURE 41–1. Effects on stroke volume of alterations in preload, afterload, and contractility.

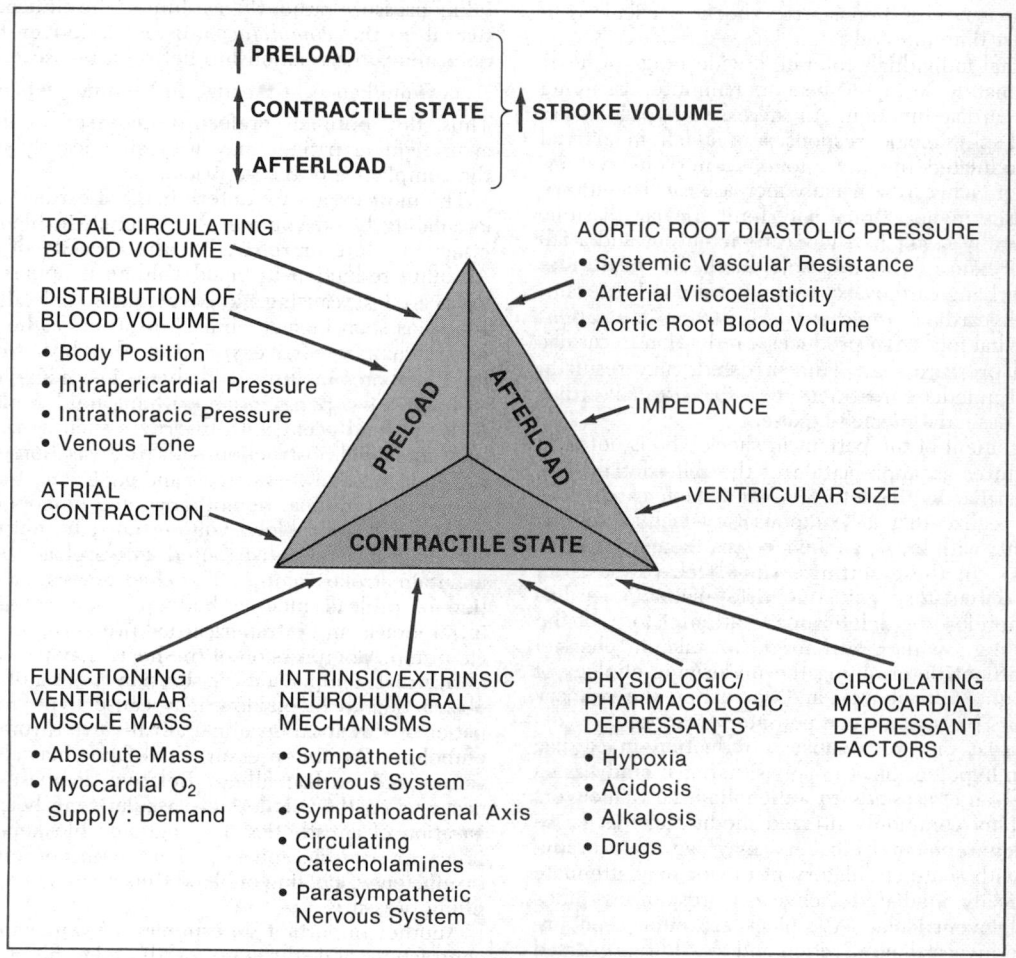

FIGURE 41–2. Determinants of stroke volume.

ventricular muscle, myocardial perfusion, intrinsic and extrinsic neurocirculatory control mechanisms, and the presence or absence of physiologic and pharmacologic stimulants or depressants. In addition, certain shock states may be associated with circulating "myocardial depressant factors" that impair cardiac performance.

Detailed autopsy studies in patients dying of cardiogenic shock following myocardial infarction have demonstrated that loss of greater than 30 to 35 per cent of functioning left ventricular muscle mass results in marked impairment of cardiac inotropic performance to a degree that is usually incompatible with maintenance of an effective cardiac output.

An important determinant of cardiac contractile performance is the sympathetic nervous system via activation of β-adrenoreceptors in the heart that increase cardiac contractile vigor and heart rate. These effects are mediated both by efferent sympathetic nerves impinging on the myocardium and by catecholamines released from the adrenal medulla. The effectiveness of such cardiac stimulants depends upon the number and sensitivity of cardiac β-adrenergic receptors. These receptors in turn are modified by various disease states, the most important of which is underlying chronic heart failure.

Myocardial performance depends upon the relationship between myocardial oxygen demand and myocardial oxygen supply. Myocardial oxygen supply depends primarily on myocardial perfusion, which is determined to a significant extent by the level of arterial diastolic pressure and the presence of fixed (e.g., atherosclerotic) or reactive (e.g., vasospastic) obstructions to coronary blood flow. A significant fall in arterial diastolic pressure (e.g., to <60 mm Hg) may produce myocardial ischemia that further impairs overall hemodynamic performance by further reducing cardiac output. In the presence of coronary artery disease, resistance to flow is due largely to structural changes in the coronary vessel wall, and maximal vasodilation tends to occur distal to the site of coronary stenosis because of excessive accumulation of vasodilator metabolites. In this setting, arterial pressure becomes the determinant of perfusion to the ischemic segment through collateral vessels or across a coronary narrowing.

Among the pathophysiologic depressants common in shock are *hypoxia* and *acidosis*. Tissue hypoxia is a cellular diagnosis that is clinically inferred by evidence of organ dysfunction in the setting of cardiovascular abnormalities known to be associated with impairment of tissue perfusion. Hypoxemia, on the other hand, is a laboratory diagnosis based upon an arterial blood gas determination of reduced oxygen tension (Po_2) and/or increased alveolar-arterial oxygen tension gradient. The clinician often relies upon blood gas analyses of arterial and mixed venous oxygen tensions to infer cellular hypoxia. However, tissue hypoxia may occur in the presence of normal arterial oxygen tension (e.g., during profound reductions of cardiac output), and cellular hypoxia may be present in the absence of arterial hypoxemia (e.g., cyanide poisoning).

In shock, hypoxemia often results from ventilation-perfusion abnormalities in the lung and has several effects on the circulation. A direct vascular effect causes vasodilation in organs such as the heart and brain. Hypoxemia also activates chemoreceptors in the carotid sinus region, causing a sympathetic vasoconstrictor response in vessels of skeletal muscle, skin, and the splanchnic bed, thus permitting redistribution of blood to the vital organs with higher oxygen demand. Severe arterial hypoxemia with secondary cellular hypoxia is a cause of myocardial depression in many forms of shock.

Acidosis results from anaerobic metabolism with the release of lactate, from decreased renal perfusion with accumulation of organic acids, and from hypoventilation with secondary respiratory acidosis. Acidosis reduces myocardial contractility and the vasoconstrictor response to various endogenous and exogenous neurohumoral agents.

Finally, a number of pharmacologic agents utilized in the treatment of critically ill patients have direct or indirect depressant effects on the myocardium and should be avoided if at all possible. These include sedative hypnotic agents, anesthetic agents, antiarrhythmic agents, β-adrenergic blocking agents, and calcium channel antagonists.

Afterload is best understood as the sum of forces that the ventricle must overcome in order to eject blood. Afterload is determined primarily by the diastolic arterial pressure at the root of the aorta, ventricular size (law of Laplace), and vascular impedance. The diastolic pressure at the root of the aorta is determined primarily by total systemic vascular resistance, arterial viscoelasticity, and the volume of blood present in the root of the aorta at the onset of ventricular contraction. Impedance is the sum of factors opposing blood flow from the ventricle and is determined by inertial, viscous, resistance, and compliance components. Impedance relates to the dynamic relation of changes in pressure and flow. In general, clinicians cannot accurately measure impedance and therefore rely upon a *calculated resistance*, derived from measurement of the ratio of pressure gradient to flow across a circulation, for assessment of afterload (i.e., calculated systemic vascular resistance = [mean arterial pressure − mean right atrial pressure] / [systemic cardiac output]).

VASCULAR FACTORS. These determine the resistance to blood flow and the transcapillary exchange of gases and nutrients within tissue beds. Resistance to flow of blood through an organ bed is determined by the viscosity of the blood and by the length and cross-sectional area of the blood vessels perfusing that organ. The cross-sectional area is the most important component, as vascular resistance is inversely proportional to the fourth power of the radius of the vessel. The radius is in turn determined by the tone of vascular smooth muscle in the wall of the vessel. Vascular smooth muscle tone is modulated by neurogenic influences mediated primarily through the sympathoadrenal system and by circulating humoral and local metabolic factors.

Neurogenic Control. Sympathoadrenal discharge to the circulatory system is regulated by medullary neurons in the vasomotor centers of the brain stem. Activity of these neurons is modulated by afferent neural impulses originating in various peripheral sensory receptors located in strategic areas throughout the body. Important among these receptors are the arterial (sinoaortic) and cardiopulmonary baroreceptors, chemoreceptors, and somatic receptors in skeletal muscle. Activities originating in higher portions of the central nervous system also impinge upon the brain stem vasomotor centers and thereby centrally modulate sympathetic and parasympathetic output.

The heart functions both as a muscle pump and as a peripheral sensory and endocrine organ. *Cardiopulmonary baroreceptors,* located primarily in the posterior wall of the left ventricle, are tonically active mechanoreceptors that are activated by expansion and stretch of the myocardium. When activated by an increase in cardiac preload, these "low pressure" receptors exert an afferent inhibitory influence on brain stem cardiovascular centers and thereby decrease efferent sympathetic outflow from these centers. Conversely, reduction in the stretch of these ventricular receptors, as during hypovolemia or assumption of upright posture, results in a lessening of their tonic afferent inhibition on brain stem centers and releases efferent sympathetic activity to cause reflex vasoconstriction, tachycardia, and the release of renin.

The *arterial baroreceptors,* located in the carotid sinus and aortic arch regions, are "high-pressure" mechanoreceptors that are activated by an increase in arterial pressure. When activated, these receptors exert an afferent inhibition on the brain stem vasomotor centers, thereby decreasing efferent sympathetic drive and resulting in vasodilation and bradycardia. Conversely, when deactivated by a fall in arterial pressure, the afferent inhibitory arterial baroreceptor input to the brain stem is decreased, resulting in an increase in sympathetic efferent tone with compensatory vasoconstriction and tachycardia.

In addition to inhibitory receptors such as the cardiac and arterial baroreceptors, peripheral excitatory afferent mechanisms also exist which contribute importantly to reflex control of the

circulation. Severe hypoxia, often found in association with shock, activates excitatory *chemoreceptors* located in the carotid sinus region. This exerts an excitatory afferent influence on the brain stem centers, resulting in an increase in efferent sympathetic tone and vasoconstriction. *Somatic receptors* are metabolic receptors in exercising muscle that are activated by metabolic products of exercise and produce an afferent excitatory influence on the brain stem cardiovascular centers. This effect results in an increase in efferent sympathetic discharge to nonexercising muscles, with resultant vasoconstriction and increase in blood pressure to compensate for metabolic vasodilation occurring in exercising muscle beds.

During circulatory perturbations, synergistic and/or antagonistic activation of these multiple reflex pathways may occur. The net effect on cardiovascular homeostatic mechanisms depends upon the relative influence of these various regulatory pathways, along with a number of other neurohumoral responses not discussed here. For example, during moderate acute hemorrhage, the reduction of central cardiopulmonary blood volume and decrease in blood pressure simultaneously deactivate the cardiopulmonary baroreceptors and the arterial baroreceptors. These two baroreflex pathways synergistically produce an increase in sympathetic efferent outflow from the brain stem vasomotor centers. Similarly, in certain shock states, the combined deactivation of arterial baroreceptors by hypotension and the activation of the chemoreceptor reflex by hypoxia results in a significant synergistic effect on the ventilatory response as well as the circulatory sympathetic drive.

Conversely, there may be situations in which reflex responses have competing effects. This may occur, for example, when cardiac receptors are activated following acute myocardial infarction by the dyskinetic bulge of the left ventricle, while the arterial baroreceptors are deactivated because of hypotension. In the experimental preparation, the inhibitory influence of the bulging left ventricular wall on the sympathetic outflow predominates and overrides the arterial baroreflex, preventing vasoconstriction and thus causing a decrease in the afterload on the damaged left ventricle. Teleologically, this effect may be beneficial, as it tends to decrease left ventricular work following such an acute myocardial insult.

HUMORAL FACTORS. A number of circulating humoral agents play important roles in cardiovascular homeostasis. The release of hormones such as renin, vasopressin, adrenal steroids, prostaglandins, kinins, atrial natriuretic factor, and catecholamines is partially mediated through the autonomic nervous system and partly through direct and indirect cellular effects of toxins, ischemia, and antigens in various organs. These hormones have direct cardiovascular and renal effects and indirect effects on central and/or peripheral adrenergic transmission.

Renin-Angiotensin. The release of renin, synthesized primarily in the juxtaglomerular apparatus of the kidney, is regulated by various stimuli, including renal afferent arteriolar pressure, sodium concentration within the macula densa, stimulation of renal sympathetic nerves, circulating angiotensin II, and electrolyte concentration in circulating plasma. A fall in arterial blood pressure or an increase in sympathoadrenal discharge to the kidney results in the release of renin. Renin functions as a proteolytic enzyme, resulting in the conversion of inactive angiotensinogen to angiotensin I, which is further converted to angiotensin II by angiotensin-converting enzyme, primarily in the lung. Angiotensin II is a very potent direct-acting vasoconstrictor that also facilitates the release of norepinephrine from sympathetic nerve terminals. The net result is peripheral vasoconstriction in an attempt to maintain arterial pressure. In addition, the increase in angiotensin II causes an increase in release of aldosterone with consequent retention of sodium and water.

Vasopressin. This important osmolality-regulating and vasoconstrictor hormone is released from the posterior pituitary primarily in response to increases in osmolality as well as in response to hypovolemia. Vasopressin appears to play a role in the circulatory control response to shock, both through its antidiuretic effect and through its vasoconstrictor action. In addition, vasopressin stimulates release of ACTH and cortisol. Release of vasopressin is reduced by stretch of left atrial receptors during hypervolemia and by stretch of the arterial baroreceptors during hypertension; conversely, during hemorrhage and systemic hypotension, or when patients are on cardiopulmonary bypass, blood levels of vasopressin increase significantly. Vasopressin may be released by as little as a 10 per cent reduction in blood volume. Thirst and the release of vasopressin may be induced by a central nervous system action of angiotensin. From the standpoint of managing the shock patient, it is important to realize that vasopressin secretion is stimulated by nausea, morphine, and hypoxia and may be inhibited by catecholamines and alcohol.

Kinins. A variety of potent vasodilator polypeptides are formed by the action of certain proteolytic enzymes on plasma protein precursors. Bradykinin serves as the prototype for this class of endogenous peptides. Their major physiologic role may be the local regulation of blood flow and function of such organs as the salivary gland, pancreas, and kidney. In pathophysiologic states, kinins are believed to play a part in the hyperemia associated with inflammation and as vasodilators in hypotension produced by anaphylactic reactions. Renal kinins may cause diuresis and natriuresis.

Serotonin and Histamine. Serotonin released from platelets and histamine released from mast cells during anaphylaxis or during complement activation in shock may play an important role in regulating local vascular tone and capillary permeability.

Prostacyclin and Thromboxane A$_2$. Prostaglandins may be released in various organs during ischemia and may contribute to reactive hyperemia and vasodilation. The prostaglandin endoperoxides formed in platelets and in blood vessels are pivotal in the synthesis of two potent substances with opposing effects on the formation of thrombi. Prostacyclin, a powerful vasodilator and inhibitor of platelet aggregation, is synthesized in the vascular wall, mostly in the endothelial layer, from endoperoxides. In the platelets, however, endoperoxides are converted to thromboxane A$_2$, which causes vasoconstriction and platelet aggregation. In shock, damage to endothelial cells may inhibit synthesis of prostacyclin; in addition, platelets may release thromboxane A$_2$, causing intravascular platelet aggregation, clumping, and vasoconstriction.

Neuropeptides. Recent experimental and clinical studies in shock have emphasized the potentially important role of certain neuropeptides in regulating cardiovascular adjustments to shock and trauma. Among these important mediators are endogenous opioids (e.g., β-endorphin), thyrotropin-releasing hormone (TRF), and adrenocorticotropin (ACTH). β-Endorphin and adrenocorticotropin are stored in the pituitary gland and secreted concomitantly under stress. These agents appear to modulate autonomic function through central nervous system action, and they may play a role in the peripheral integration of autonomic nervous system activity. The β-endorphins, in particular, may play an important role in the pathophysiology of certain types of shock, most notably hemorrhagic, endotoxic (septic), and spinal shock. β-Endorphins may contribute directly or indirectly to myocardial depression during shock states. Experimental and limited clinical studies have suggested that pharmacologic blockade of the action of such endogenous opiates, by the use of specific antagonists such as naloxone, may improve cardiovascular stability in certain shock states. However, the precise role of these agents and such therapy remains to be defined (see Management).

Thyrotropin-releasing hormone (TRF) is a neuropeptide with potent central cardiovascular actions. Although frequently thought of primarily as a hypothalamic hormone with specific endocrinologic actions (e.g., stimulating release of thyroid-stimulating hormone from the pituitary), a major fraction of TRF is found outside of the hypothalamus in the brain and spinal cord. Experimental studies have suggested that exogenously administered TRF improves cardiorespiratory function in certain shock states, possibly through antagonism of adverse physiologic effects of endogenous opioids. The clinical importance of TRF in shock states in humans remains to be defined.

Atrial Natriuretic Factors. These biologically active peptides are released from specific granules in atrial myocytes and to a lesser extent from ventricular myocytes. These peptides bind to specific high-affinity receptors located in adrenal, renal, and vascular beds. These peptides produce direct vasorelaxant effects on vascular smooth muscle and natriuretic effects in the kidney. In addition, atrial natriuretic factor inhibits the action of renin and the production of aldosterone. Animal studies have suggested that these agents may alter the sensitivity of baroreceptors. While atrial natriuretic factor has been found to be elevated in pathophysiologic states such as severe heart failure, the exact role of these peptides in severe hemodynamic disorders such as shock remains unclear.

Catecholamines. The catecholamines norepinephrine and epinephrine are potent modulators of cardiovascular homeostasis. Released primarily from sympathetic nerve terminals, norepinephrine increases myocardial contractility and heart rate through activation of β-adrenoceptors and therefore increases cardiac output. In addition, norepinephrine has potent α-adrenergic actions and produces vasoconstriction, although the magnitude of this effect varies from tissue to tissue. Norepinephrine is a potent vasoconstrictor in skin, muscle, and splanchnic beds, whereas it may produce vasodilation in coronary vascular beds through a β$_2$-adrenergic mechanism. Epinephrine is released primarily from the adrenal glands, where the ratio of its release to that of norepinephrine is 10:1. Epinephrine has α, β$_1$, and β$_2$ effects and produces a modest increase in cardiac output through β$_1$ effects. However, epinephrine redistributes cardiac output away from the kidney and splanchnic circulation toward skeletal muscle, where its β$_2$ effect predominates with vasodilation. In other beds, epinephrine has significant α-vasoconstricting effects. Epinephrine may also effect release of norepinephrine from adrenergic nerve terminals through a prejunctional action.

Local Autoregulatory Mechanisms. Blood vessels have an intrinsic ability to autoregulate vascular tone and thereby maintain blood flow over a wide range of perfusion pressures. This property is independent of systemic neurogenic influences or humoral factors. Different vascular beds vary with respect to their ability to maintain blood flow. The cerebral, coronary, and renal circulations have the most developed autoregulatory mechanisms. Thus, during a fall in arterial pressure, vasodilation in these vascular beds maintains blood flow and oxygen delivery to the brain and heart and helps to preserve sodium and water balance. Although a myogenic response intrinsic to the smooth muscle may partially explain the phenomenon, accumulation of tissue metabolites following a transient period of ischemia may also cause vasodilation and restore blood flow. The specific mediator of metabolic vasodilation is not known, but it is likely that a combination of changes in oxygen, carbon dioxide, hydrogen ions, and other cations, in osmolality, in the amount of adenosine compounds, and in Krebs cycle intermediates and other metabolites released in the immediate environment of blood vessels contributes to adjustments in vascular tone.

Finally, apart from neural and humoral influences, the presence of occlusive vascular disease may play an important role in determining resistance to flow through regional circulations. This effect depends upon both fixed physical obstruction to the cross-sectional area of the perfusion bed and abnormalities in vascular reactivity induced by atherosclerotic changes in the vascular endothelium.

MICROCIRCULATION AND TRANSCAPILLARY EXCHANGE. The most critical aspect of the pathogenesis of shock takes place at the level of the microcirculation. In essence, all shock can be considered a form of microcirculatory failure. Delivery of a significant amount of blood to an organ does not guarantee that all the segments of that organ and all capillaries are perfused appropriate to the regional metabolic demand.

Intraorgan Blood Flow Distribution. Adequate tissue perfusion depends upon blood flow through vascular channels in which diffusion between the blood and tissues can occur. These channels are referred to as nutritional capillaries, as contrasted to nonnutritional vessels that do not permit capillary exchange. The latter are referred to as arteriovenous shunts. An example of the importance of the intraorgan redistribution of blood flow is observed in myocardial infarction, in which an increase in coronary blood flow may not increase perfusion to the infarcted segment. Under some circumstances, a coronary vasodilator may redistribute flow away from ischemic into nonischemic regions (e.g., administration of a potent intravenous vasodilator to a patient with severe fixed coronary obstruction with consequent induction of a coronary steal phenomenon). Similarly, the pattern of intraorgan blood flow may be critical in the kidney. Acute tubular necrosis associated with shock may reflect a reduction in glomerular filtration in the outer cortex because of a localized increase in vascular resistance in this region and a selective reduction in blood flow. Interventions that alter total renal blood flow can produce significant redistribution of flow within the kidney; for example, renal vasoconstriction following adrenergic discharge tends to shunt blood away from the outer cortex, whereas renal vasodilators (including the loop diuretic furosemide) shunt blood toward the outer cortical nephrons.

Pre- and Postcapillary Resistance. The precapillary sphincters regulate the patency of nutritional or "exchange" capillaries. The tone of these sphincters may be modulated by neurohumoral factors that contribute to the circulatory adjustments in shock. The metabolic products at the local tissue level are important determinants of the tone of these sphincters, which regulate the total functional capillary surface area and in turn determine the potential capillary area available for intravascular-to-extracellular fluid and solute exchange. The capillary hydrostatic force driving fluid out of the capillaries into the extracellular space depends on the ratio of post- to precapillary resistances. In hypovolemic or hemorrhagic shock, the fall in arterial pressure causes activation of the sympathoadrenal system, constriction of precapillary resistance vessels, and a fall in capillary hydrostatic pressure, facilitating movement of fluids from the extracellular to the intravascular space. This partially restores intravascular volume. Hematocrit, viscosity of blood, and plasma oncotic pressure fall. With persistent hypotension and ischemia, the vasoconstrictor response of precapillary resistance vessels becomes less pronounced because of tissue acidosis while resistance of postcapillary vessels (venules) increases. This creates a situation in which more fluid is lost from the vascular to the interstitial space. Thus, venular resistance and the reactivity of venules to the various vasoactive agents involved in shock become important. Venules may even be relatively more reactive than precapillary resistance vessels to catecholamines, which activate α-vasoconstrictor receptors. This differential effect in favor of postcapillary vasoconstriction also further increases hydrostatic pressure and intravascular fluid loss.

Capillary Permeability and Oncotic Pressure. Colloid osmotic pressure is a major determinant of intravascular volume. Albumin is the main osmotically active protein in plasma. The balance between colloid osmotic pressure and capillary hydrostatic pressure determines the balance between intravascular and extracellular fluid spaces. A significant degree of hypovolemia and hemoconcentration may take place either because of excessive capillary hydrostatic pressure from an increase in the ratio of post- to precapillary resistance or because of a reduction in plasma protein and consequent reduction of plasma oncotic pressure. Reduction of circulating plasma proteins may occur as a result of increased capillary permeability and loss of plasma proteins from the intravascular to the extracellular space. The balance between oncotic and hydrostatic pressures is also an important determinant of the level of pulmonary edema and is critical in the management of the shock lung syndrome. An appreciation of the important interplay between hydrostatic and colloid pressures is crucial to the selection of appropriate intravenous volume replacement in the therapy of many types of shock. Similarly, nutritional support of the critically ill patient is important in the effort to maintain adequate production of albumin.

Shock resulting from increased vascular permeability, as in anaphylactic shock or snake venom poisoning, is characterized by a dramatic reduction of plasma volume. Hematocrit rises sharply and oncotic pressure drops. This increase in capillary permeability may be partly related to release of histamine, metabolites, or humoral factors that alter endothelial permeability.

Intravascular Hemagglutination and "Blood Sludging." Erythrocytes, leukocytes, and platelets undergo agglutination to a variable degree in association with the shock syndromes in thermal burn, sepsis, trauma, and perhaps even hemorrhage. These aggregates may cause obstruction of nutritional capillaries as well as arterioles. The precipitating events are numerous. They may include platelet aggregation by catecholamines; damage to endothelial lining of small blood vessels and capillaries with subsequent fibrin deposition and accumulation of microthrombi; hypoxia increasing the rigidity of red blood cells; oxygen free radicals generated by endothelial cells or neutrophils; and release of vasoactive peptides and anaphylatoxins as a result of complement activation. These may cause additional damage to endothelial cells and increase the tone of precapillary sphincters, leading to further reduction in tissue perfusion and cellular injury.

PATHOPHYSIOLOGY AND STAGES OF SHOCK

From a conceptual standpoint, shock can be considered to progress through stages of lesser to greater severity and from reversible to irreversible derangements of metabolic processes. This conceptual framework involves stages of compensated, decompensated, and irreversible shock as summarized in Figure 41–3 and Table 41–2.

STAGE I—COMPENSATED SHOCK. In early shock, hypotension may arise from either a fall in cardiac output or peripheral vasodilation. The fall in cardiac output and arterial pressure

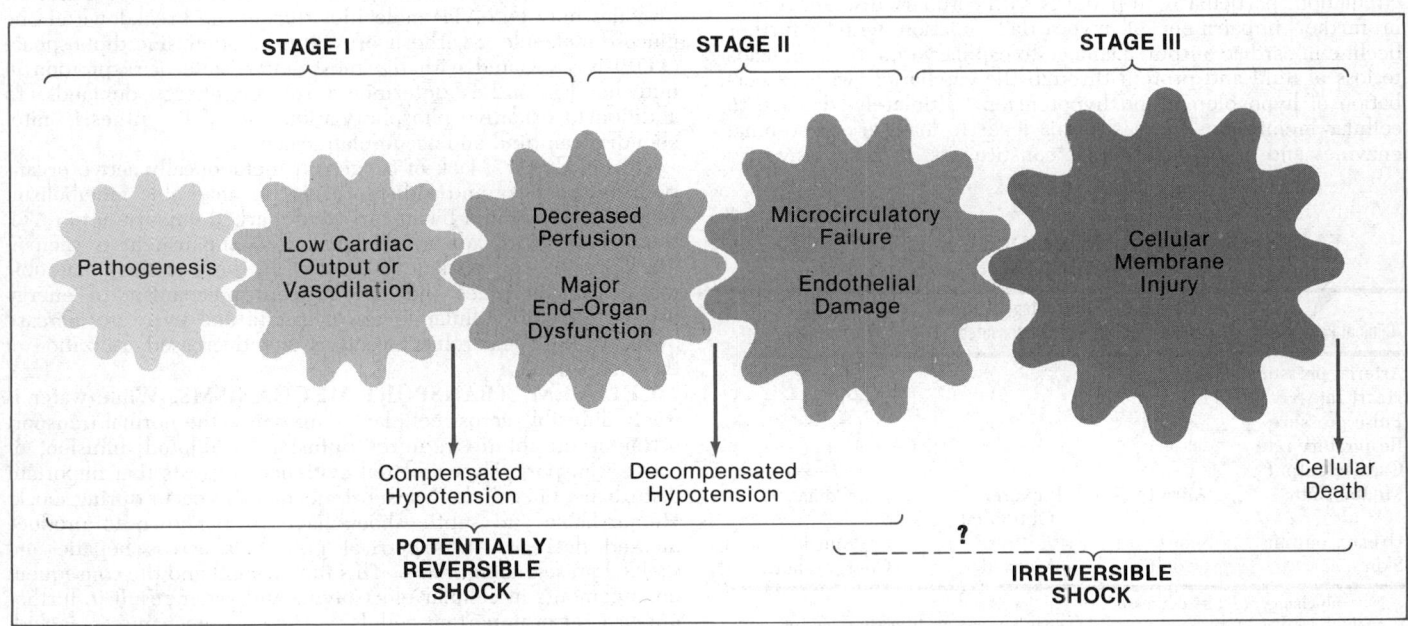

FIGURE 41–3. Pathophysiology of shock.

triggers compensatory mechanisms, which attempt to restore arterial pressure and blood flow to vital organs such as the brain and heart. At this stage, symptoms and signs of hemodynamic impairment are often subtle, and a high degree of clinical suspicion is required to identify early signs of hemodynamic compromise. Arterial pressure is usually maintained or mildly reduced; there is an increase in heart rate and a narrowing of pulse pressure; and there may be mild anxiety and early peripheral vasoconstriction. If shock is identified and vigorously treated at this stage, the syndrome may be successfully reversed in many cases.

STAGE II—DECOMPENSATED SHOCK. At this stage in the progression of shock, the compensatory mechanisms invoked during stage I to maintain perfusion of vital organs are insufficient to compensate for the hemodynamic insult. Patients may demonstrate impairment of major organ perfusion as manifested by altered mental state (impaired cerebral perfusion), reduced urine output (renal hypoperfusion), and myocardial ischemia (coronary flow impairment). The patient in this stage demonstrates the classic clinical picture of shock with hypotension, tachycardia, tachypnea, and narrowed pulse pressure (rapid, weak, and thready pulse). The external appearance of the patient reflects excessive sympathetic drive with acrocyanosis, peripheral vasoconstriction, and diaphoresis (cold and clammy extremities). Rapid aggressive intervention is required to restore cardiac output and perfusion of the tissues in this stage, prior to the onset of irreversible shock.

STAGE III—IRREVERSIBLE SHOCK. Excessive and prolonged reduction of tissue perfusion leads to significant alterations in cellular membrane function, aggregation of blood cells in the microcirculation, and "sludging" in the capillaries. The vasoconstriction that has taken place in the less vital organs in order to maintain blood pressure is now excessive and has reduced perfusion to such a point that cellular damage occurs. In this stage of shock, arterial pressure continues to fall progressively to a critical level at which vital organ perfusion is reduced and a vicious circle of further impairment ensues. Critical impairment of renal perfusion leads to acute tubular necrosis. Ischemia of the gastrointestinal tract leads to necrotic damage of the mucosa with a breakdown of this natural barrier and the subsequent absorption into the circulation of bacteria and their toxins with secondary detrimental effects on other organs. A generalized endothelial damage and disseminated intravascular coagulation may occur. Bacterial toxins may react with neutrophils and cause the release of vasodilator polypeptides that contribute to the fall in arterial pressure. Severe acidosis results from anaerobic metabolism as peripheral organs fail to receive nutrients sufficient to maintain aerobic metabolic pathways. Decreased perfusion of the coronary circulation, particularly in patients with coronary disease, results in further impairment of myocardial function with a further decline in cardiac output. Damage to capillary endothelium leads to loss of fluid and protein through the capillaries, with exacerbation of hypovolemia and hypotension. Ultimately, damage to cellular membranes from ischemia leads to leakage of lysosomal enzymes and other intracellular constituents, to progressive reduction in high-energy phosphate levels, and to cellular destruction. This terminal stage of shock is characterized by irreversible impairment of subcellular machinery, as discussed in the following section.

CELLULAR AND BIOCHEMICAL FACTORS IN SHOCK

MITOCHONDRIAL FUNCTION. Mitochondrial electron transport–linked mechanisms provide greater than 95 per cent of the body's energy needs under normal resting conditions. To do this, mitochondria utilize more than 90 per cent of the available cellular oxygen. The delivery of this essential oxygen depends upon maintenance of adequate tissue perfusion and the integrity of the capillary-interstitial-cellular interface. Shock of many diverse etiologies has been shown to result in progressive defects in mitochondrial metabolism.

Hypoxia alone may reduce the rate of adenosine triphosphate (ATP) synthesis by mitochondria, but it does not cause significant damage to mitochondrial membrane functions unless it is severe, sustained, or associated with ischemia, which also reduces the availability of other substrates. In fact, adaptation to hypoxia appears to take place such that when mitochondria are isolated from animal tissues after the animals have been exposed to brief periods of hypoxia, their capacity to respire and synthesize ATP in vitro is enhanced. During ischemia or shock, mitochondria cannot respond to increased energy needs by normal increases in oxidative phosphorylation.

Possible mechanisms involved in mitochondrial abnormalities during shock include structural changes (e.g., swelling), alterations of enzyme systems secondary to loss of critical cofactors, decreases in mitochondrial magnesium levels, increases in mitochondrial calcium concentration, alterations in mitochondrial sodium and potassium content, inhibition of mitochondrial function by agents such as free fatty acids, and free radical oxidation of phospholipids in the mitochondrial membranes.

It is unclear whether the degree of mitochondrial damage is a uniform feature in all tissues of the patient with shock or is manifested to a greater degree in some organs than in others. In experimental models, hepatic mitochondrial damage appears to dominate, whereas cerebral mitochondrial function appears to be preserved until very late in the experimental shock state. Experimental studies suggest that mitochondrial dysfunction may be reversed by interventions in the very early stages of shock, but the limits of this critical period of reversibility are unknown at present.

METABOLIC ALTERATIONS. Survival of aerobic cells depends on the availability of substrates and oxygen to the mitochondria, which provide most of the high-energy phosphate needs of the cell and utilize most of the available oxygen in the process. During oxidative phosphorylation, 36 moles of ATP are produced per mole of glucose, whereas in the anaerobic state, glycolysis provides only two ATP molecules during the breakdown of one glucose molecule. Synthesis of ATP from adenosine diphosphate (ADP) is associated with the most active state of respiration in mitochondria and is determined by cell energy demands. In addition to oxidative phosphorylation and ATP synthesis, mitochondria can bind and accumulate calcium.

During shock, a lack of oxygen in metabolically active organs such as the liver and kidney results in anaerobic metabolism. This is demonstrated by an early and marked impairment in ATP production. With advanced shock, this impairment is seen in other organs such as skeletal muscle. In these organs, anaerobic metabolism becomes the predominant mechanism of energy production, and cellular levels of lactate and pyruvate increase owing to both anaerobic glycolysis and decreased utilization of these substrates.

CELLULAR TRANSPORT MECHANISMS. While water is freely diffusible across cellular membranes, the normal transport of important solutes requires diffusion, facilitated diffusion, or active transport. Experimental evidence suggests that important disturbances in cellular transport mechanisms occur during shock. Hemorrhagic and septic shock have been shown to produce marked decreases in electrical potentials across hepatic and skeletal muscle membranes. This impairment and the consequent derangements in cellular electrolytes and water result in further impairment of important cellular enzymatic mechanisms, including glycolytic and gluconeogenic pathways.

TABLE 41–2. PATHOPHYSIOLOGIC STAGES OF SHOCK—CLINICAL SIGNS

Clinical Parameters	Stage I (Compensated)	Stage II (Decompensated)	Stage III (Irreversible)
Arterial pressure	N or (−)	(− −)	(− − −)
Heart rate	(+)	(+ +)	(+ + +) to (− − −)
Pulse pressure	(−)	(− −)	(− − −)
Respiratory rate	N	(+ +)	(+ + +) to (− − −)
Cardiac output	(−)*	(− −)	(− − −)
Mental status	Anxiety	Impaired/Obtunded	Coma
Urinary output	N or (−)	(− −)	Anuric
Skin	Cool*	Mottled	Cold, cyanotic

N = no change; (−) = decreased; (+) = increased.

*A high cardiac output and warm skin may be present in early stages of septic shock.

RETICULOENDOTHELIAL DYSFUNCTION. The reticuloendothelial system functions to remove foreign protein and particulate matter from the circulation. An important relationship between reticuloendothelial integrity and function, phagocytic activity, and survival has been suggested in experimental models of shock. Shock results in depression of this system, probably due to impairment of perfusion of the liver and spleen. While the precise abnormalities in reticuloendothelial function in shock remain to be defined, evidence suggests that at least part of the abnormality is due to impairment of opsonization activity resulting in impaired phagocytosis. This may result in the accumulation of toxic substances such as endotoxin, cellular aggregates, and immunologic complexes.

INSULIN RESISTANCE. Circulatory failure and shock are associated with hyperglycemia and abnormal glucose tolerance. While insulin levels often increase in shock, tissue response to insulin appear to be impaired, although the mechanism(s) responsible for this abnormality are not well defined.

OXYGEN-HEMOGLOBIN AFFINITY. Delivery of oxygen to the tissues depends upon the cardiac output and the oxygen carrying capacity of blood:

$$O_2 \text{ Delivery} = \text{Cardiac Output} \times \text{Blood } O_2\text{-Carrying Capacity}$$

Over 98 per cent of oxygen in the circulating blood is bound to hemoglobin. The oxygen-carrying capacity of blood is thus critically dependent upon the amount of hemoglobin and the saturation of the hemoglobin with oxygen. Normal hemoglobin, when 100 per cent saturated, carries 1.38 ml of oxygen per gram of hemoglobin. Thus, 100 ml of arterial blood with normal hemoglobin content (e.g., 15 grams), which is 96 to 98 per cent saturated (e.g., $Po_2 = 95$ to 100 mm Hg), carries 20 ml of oxygen to the tissues. Mixed venous blood returning to the right heart has an oxygen saturation of 75 per cent at a Po_2 of 40 mm Hg and contains 15 ml of oxygen per deciliter. The normal arteriovenous (AV) oxygen content difference is therefore 5 ml per deciliter of blood. The extraction of oxygen from hemoglobin by the tissues is not complete and depends to a large extent on the affinity of hemoglobin for oxygen, i.e., the shape of the oxygen-hemoglobin dissociation curve.

Hydrogen ions (Bohr effect), carbon dioxide, and 2,3-diphosphoglyceric acid (2,3-DPG) cause greater dissociation of oxygen from hemoglobin because of their preferential affinity for reduced hemoglobin. The concentration of 2,3-DPG in red cells results from a side reaction of glycolysis and increases during anemia, hypoxia, and acidosis. A drop in hemoglobin, hypoxemia, and acidosis may thus be partly compensated for by a shift of the oxygen dissociation curve to the right, favoring greater delivery of oxygen to the tissues at the same Po_2. This compensatory mechanism, in addition to the increase in cardiac output, provides for better oxygenation as extraction of oxygen increases at the expense of the oxygen reserve in venous blood. In certain tissues, however, such as the myocardium, extraction of oxygen at rest is already large, and any additional oxygen demand or a decrease in oxygen-hemoglobin dissociation such as in alkalosis requires greater delivery of oxygen, i.e., higher coronary blood flow.

In shock, the pH, carbon dioxide, and 2,3-DPG levels are changing, and one cannot calculate oxygen extraction from values of arterial Po_2 because the shape of the oxyhemoglobin dissociation curve cannot be predicted accurately. It is preferable to measure oxygen content or saturation of venous and arterial blood; if saturation is lower than predicted from values of Po_2, one can deduce that there is a shift of the dissociation curve to the right, and vice versa. Overzealous correction of acidosis with bicarbonate may, through the Bohr effect on hemoglobin affinity for oxygen, actually reduce oxygen delivery to the tissues. Hypophosphatemia (reported during hyperalimentation) may decrease 2,3-DPG and oxygen delivery.

LYSOSOMAL ABNORMALITIES. While present in most tissues, the higher concentrations of lysosomes in the body are found in the liver, kidney, and spleen. Lysosomes are cytoplasmic vesicles that contain a variety of potent hydrolytic enzymes bound in a latent form. These enzymes are capable of hydrolyzing a wide variety of intra- and extracellular macromolecules. When released from organelles as a consequence of certain forms of cellular injury, these enzymes may contribute to the pathogenesis or the propagation and perpetuation of shock. They are most active at an acid pH, which makes them potentially more destructive in the setting of hypoxia and shock.

Numerous morphologic and biochemical observations implicate the lysosomal enzymes in the perpetuation of shock, but at this time the evidence for their primary involvement is unclear. In organs such as the liver, spleen, and intestine, the lysosomes enlarge during the early phases of shock. This is associated with a decrease in the total activity of lysosomal hydrolases in tissues and a corresponding increase in activity in the soluble fraction of the tissue homogenate. This indicates a loss of lysosomal membrane integrity in vivo. The lysosomes obtained from animals in shock demonstrate an enhanced release of enzymes in vitro. A reduction in lysosomal membrane integrity has also been observed in animals after administration of endotoxin. In several animal studies, the levels of hydrolases found in blood, lymph, or serum seem to correlate with severity of shock.

MYOCARDIAL DEPRESSANT FACTOR(S). Initially described in 1966 in the plasma of cats following hemorrhagic shock, myocardial depressant factor (MDF) is an incompletely understood factor associated with almost all forms of shock. Experimental and clinical studies have described elevated plasma levels of MDF in cases of hemorrhagic, septic, cardiogenic, traumatic, and burn shock. An apparent common denominator in these various shock states that is related to the plasma level of MDF is the degree of splanchnic hypoperfusion that occurs. A critical component appears to be marked impairment of pancreatic perfusion, which is believed to result in pancreatic ischemia and acidosis leading to lysosomal disruption. The release of lysosomal enzymes and activation of zymogenic enzymes (e.g., conversion of trypsinogen to trypsin and chymotrypsinogen to chymotrypsin) appear to be related to the formation of MDF. MDF is believed to be released from leaky acinar cells in the pancreas and carried to peripheral sites of the circulation. MDF has been demonstrated in both intact animals and isolated tissue preparations to exert a potent negative inotropic action. The resulting impairment in cardiac output leads to further pancreatic hypoperfusion, and a positive feedback loop is believed to result in further release of this agent. In addition to the cardiodepression, MDF appears to produce vasoconstriction in splanchnic resistance vessels and impairs function of the reticuloendothelial system.

A number of agents have been demonstrated to be effective in preventing the formation of MDF in various shock states. These include the synthetic glucocorticoids, the protease inhibitor aprotinin, angiotensin-converting enzyme (ACE) inhibitors, angiotensin receptor antagonists, thromboxane antagonists, thromboxane synthetase inhibitors, lipoxygenase inhibitors, opiate receptor antagonists, and vasodilator prostaglandins. In addition, agents that have been shown to significantly counteract the negative inotropic actions of MDF include digitalis glycosides, glucagon, isoproterenol, dopamine, amrinone, and calcium ion. The precise role played by MDF in the pathogenesis of clinical shock syndromes remains to be defined.

COMPLEMENT ACTIVATION. The complement system consists of a series of discrete plasma proteins that are present as inactive precursors until they are activated by highly specific biochemical reactions. Activation of the complement system results in the cleavage of several low molecular weight vasoactive peptides from the complement molecules. These peptides in turn have a wide variety of significant biologic effects. For example, during the activation of C2, a cleavage product occurs that has kinin-like activity, which then can significantly influence capillary permeability. Two other activation peptides, C3a and C5a, release histamine from mast cells, have chemotactic activity, and constrict vascular smooth muscle. Another fragment, C3B, acts as an opsonin and facilitates phagocytosis. Polymorphonuclear leukocytes may be attracted chemotactically through activation of esterases on their surface and may release their lysosomal enzymes if the concentration of the complement reaction product C5a is large enough. Platelets may have an increase in their procoagulant activity. In addition to the direct and indirect effects of the fragments of activated complement on cells, their aggregation as complexes on the surface of cell membranes causes cellular destruction. The expressions of all these effects are increased capillary permeability, increased leukocyte accumulation and infiltration, release of lysosomal enzymes, and activation of intravascular coagulation factors. Clinically, these result in such entities as glomerulitis, necrotizing vasculitis, the Schwartzmann reaction, thrombocytopenia, and other manifestations of microcirculatory collapse and intravascular plugging seen in prolonged shock and endotoxemia.

Although the side effects of complement activation in shock are detrimental, leading to cellular death, the fundamental biologic activities of the complement components are beneficial in enhancing phagocytosis and mediating the inflammatory response to local infection or irritation, in the neutralizing of viruses, and, finally, in modulating the immune response.

EICOSANOIDS. These lipid substances, derived from arachidonic acid (eicosatetraenoic acid), have recently been implicated as important mediators of ischemic and circulatory shock. During ischemic and shock states, a variety of these substances are produced, the most important of which are the vasoconstrictor prostaglandins (PG), thromboxanes (TX), and leukotrienes (LT).

PGF_2-α has been found to be increased in animals with hemorrhagic, endotoxic, cardiogenic, and burn shock and has been identified as a potent vasoconstrictor of coronary, mesenteric, and renal vessels and is believed to play some role in the pathogenesis of circulatory shock. TXA_2 is believed to play three important roles in shock: (1) induction of vasoconstriction, (2) aggregation of circulating platelets, and (3) induction of leakage in lysosomal membranes. It is believed to play a role in myocardial ischemia, sudden death, and circulatory shock. Recent experimental evidence suggests that thromboxane synthetase inhibitors may play a protective role in certain types of myocardial ischemia, trauma, and endotoxic shock.

Leukotrienes (LTs) are the major biologically active products of the lipoxygenase pathway of arachidonic acid metabolism and are produced by pulmonary parenchymal cells, macrophages, mast cells, white blood cells, and connective tissue cells. These agents appear to be potent vasoconstrictors and bronchoconstrictors. The exact role, if any, that these agents play in the pathogenesis of shock remains to be defined experimentally.

OXYGEN FREE RADICALS. Oxygen free radicals may be generated in tissues during shock states. The unpaired electron in these radicals may react with any cellular component, but particularly with unsaturated fatty acids and sulfhydryl amino acids, and cause cellular damage. The clinical documentation of the relative importance of these factors and the effectiveness of their elimination awaits further experimentation in humans.

TUMOR NECROSIS FACTOR. Tumor necrosis factor (TNF, cachectin) is a recently recognized endogenous mediator of shock and inflammation. TNF is derived from mononuclear phagocytes on exposure to lipopolysaccharide endotoxin, and TNF appears to be responsible for many of the deleterious effects of endotoxin. TNF appears to be one of the primary mediators of experimental septic shock, with many of the lethal cytotoxic effects of endotoxin being due to host cell effects mediated by this agent. Biologic effects attributed experimentally to TNF include the suppression of lipoprotein lipase biosynthesis by adipocytes, induction of antigenic determinants on fibroblasts and endothelial cells, stimulation of products of prostaglandin E_2 and collagenase, and activation of neutrophils. This latter effect appears responsible for many of the inflammatory changes seen in sepsis that lead to tissue damage. TNF also exerts a catabolic effect on bone and cartilage and is an endogenous pyrogen. TNF appears to share many of the same bioactivities of other inflammatory cytokines such as interleukin-1. The precise role of TNF in clinical shock is under active investigation.

ETIOLOGY OF SHOCK—CLASSIFICATION

While the end result of most shock syndromes involves irreversible deterioration of cellular and subcellular metabolic processes and structural integrity, it is clinically useful to consider the differential diagnosis of shock from a functional standpoint. This classification scheme emphasizes potential initiating pathogenic mechanisms. Most cases of shock can be considered to arise from one of four basic abnormalities: (1) hypovolemia, (2) cardiac functional impairment, (3) obstruction of major vascular conduits, and (4) inappropriate distribution of cardiac output

secondary to abnormal vasodilation. These functional etiologies of shock are outlined in Table 41–3. Common clinical syndromes representative of the functional types of shock are discussed below.

HYPOVOLEMIC SHOCK. Perfusion of major organs and peripheral tissues depends upon the integrity of a vascular pump (heart), a capacitance vascular tree, and an intravascular blood volume. Hypovolemic shock is the most common type of shock seen clinically and is due to an absolute and often sudden reduction in circulating blood volume relative to the capacity of the vascular system. The classic hemodynamic features of this type of shock include tachycardia, hypotension, reduced cardiac filling pressures, and peripheral vasoconstriction (see Table 41–2). An important aspect of this type of shock is the *rapidity* with which hypovolemia occurs. A sudden reduction in circulating blood volume of 10 per cent in previously healthy individuals results in mild reduction in arterial pressure and moderate reduction in cardiac output. A sudden reduction in blood volume of 20 per cent produces moderate hypotension and moderately severe reductions in cardiac output. The loss of 40 per cent of circulating blood volume produces profound reductions in arterial pressure and cardiac output. These hemodynamic consequences are accentuated in patients with pre-existing cardiovascular,

TABLE 41–3. ETIOLOGIC CATEGORIES OF SHOCK

I. **Hypovolemic shock**
  A. Hemorrhagic (e.g., trauma, gastrointestinal hemorrhage)
  B. Hypovolemic, nonhemorrhagic
    1. External fluid loss (e.g., vomiting, diarrhea, polyuria, burns)
    2. Internal extravascular sequestration (e.g., peritonitis, pancreatitis)

II. **Cardiogenic shock**
  A. Acute myocardial infarction
    1. Loss of critical muscle mass (e.g., large anterior wall infarction)
    2. Acute mechanical lesion (e.g., ventricular septal rupture, mitral insufficiency)
    3. Acute right ventricular infarction
    4. Left ventricular free wall rupture
    5. Left ventricular aneurysm
  B. Valvular heart disease
    1. Critical valvular stenosis (e.g., aortic or mitral stenosis)
    2. Severe valvular insufficiency (e.g., acute aortic or mitral insufficiency)
  C. Nonvalvular obstructive cardiac lesions
    1. Atrial myxoma or ball-valve thrombus
    2. Cardiac tamponade
    3. Restrictive cardiomyopathy (e.g., amyloid)
    4. Constrictive pericardial disorder
  D. Nonischemic myopathic processes
    1. Fulminant myocarditis
    2. Physiologic depressants (e.g., acidosis, hypoxia)
    3. Pharmacologic depressants (e.g., calcium channel blockers)
    4. Pathophysiologic depressants (e.g., myocardial depressant factor)
  E. Dysrhythmias
    1. Severe bradyarrhythmias (e.g., high-degree AV block)
    2. Tachyarrhythmias
      a. Ventricular (e.g., ventricular tachycardia)
      b. Supraventricular (e.g., atrial fibrillation or flutter with rapid ventricular response)

III. **Vascular obstructive shock**
  A. Massive pulmonary embolism
  B. Tension pneumothorax
  C. Excessive positive-pressure ventilation
  D. Aortic dissection

IV. **Distributive shock and miscellaneous**
    1. Sepsis
    2. Anaphylaxis
    3. Massive tissue injury (e.g., crush)
    4. Prolonged ischemia/hypoxia
    5. Neurogenic shock
    6. Endocrine disorders
      a. Addisonian crisis
      b. Profound hypothyroidism
    7. Drug or toxin induced

pulmonary, renal, or cerebrovascular disorders. In contrast, a similar degree of volume loss occurring over a longer period of time (days to weeks) may not be accompanied by the same magnitude of hemodynamic impairment.

Hypovolemia may occur as a result of loss of blood volume secondary to hemorrhage (internal or external) or may arise as a result of the loss of fluid and electrolytes. This latter form of hypovolemia may occur following severe loss of gastrointestinal fluids (e.g., diarrhea, vomiting), renal losses (e.g., polyuria), external losses of fluids secondary to impairment of surface tissue integrity (e.g., burns), or internal losses of fluids without a change in total body water (e.g., third-space sequestration of fluids).

As previously noted, hypovolemia usually results in the induction of neurohumoral compensatory mechanisms that produce the characteristic features of shock (e.g., tachycardia, tachypnea, and peripheral vasoconstriction). However, it has been known for some time, although poorly appreciated by clinicians, that profound exsanguinating hemorrhage may present as paradoxical bradycardia (or absence of tachycardia) due to activation of cardiac mechanoreceptors in the setting of vigorous contraction of a "volume-depleted" ventricle. Recent observations in normal humans have demonstrated that abrupt decreases in cardiac filling pressures can result in sympathetic inhibition with profound hypotension and bradycardia. This afferent inhibition from ventricular receptors may override the hypotension-induced deactivation of arterial baroreceptors. Thus, the presentation of a patient with obvious hypovolemic hypotension in the absence of tachycardia should alert the clinician to the possibility of massive volume loss and the need for vigorous volume resuscitation.

CARDIOGENIC SHOCK. Cardiogenic shock may arise from a number of underlying etiologies, the usual common denominator of which is inadequate stroke volume. A strict hemodynamic operational definition, based upon invasive hemodynamic monitoring, is necessary to differentiate cardiogenic from hypovolemic shock.

Cardiogenic shock most commonly presents as an acute deterioration of cardiac function, although this may be superimposed on chronic impairment. The most common etiology of cardiogenic shock is acute myocardial infarction. Cardiogenic shock in this setting carries a mortality of 50 to 90 per cent, varying according to the mechanism of the hemodynamic insult and the aggressiveness of treatment. Shock following myocardial infarction is more common in the setting of anterior infarctions than inferior infarctions. However, large inferoposterior infarctions or inferior infarctions with significant right ventricular involvement may produce cardiogenic shock. Detailed anatomic studies of patients succumbing to cardiogenic shock following acute infarction, in the absence of mechanical lesions, have demonstrated that impairment of 30 to 35 per cent or more of functioning ventricular muscle usually accompanies this syndrome.

In addition to large losses of functioning ventricular muscle mass, cardiogenic shock may arise from the development of intracardiac mechanical defects. These include acute ventricular septal rupture, acute mitral insufficiency (papillary muscle dysfunction or rupture), and left ventricular free wall rupture. The frequency of shock due to acute mitral insufficiency and ventricular septal rupture is evenly divided between anterior and inferior infarctions.

Non–infarct-related etiologies of cardiogenic shock include critical valvular heart disease, disorders of pericardial restraint, obstructive myopathic cardiac disorders, acute cardiomyopathies of diverse etiologies, and marked disorders of cardiac rate and rhythm. In addition, an element of myocardial depression may be a significant factor in the pathogenesis of shock from sepsis and severe hemorrhage. These noninfarction etiologies are outlined in Table 41–3.

VASCULAR OBSTRUCTIVE SHOCK. The most common example of shock secondary to acute obstruction of the vascular tree is acute cardiac tamponade with resultant impairment of diastolic ventricular filling. This may arise as a result of trauma, infection, neoplasm, or cardiac rupture. It is the rapidity of accumulation of pericardial volume, rather than the absolute volume, that is the critical determinant of the hemodynamic impairment in cardiac tamponade. Rapid accumulations of as little as 100 to 200 ml of blood in the pericardium may produce tamponade. Similarly, therapeutic removal of small amounts of

fluid (e.g., 50 to 100 ml) may be all that is required to relieve tamponade and allow diastolic ventricular filling to resume and cardiac output to rise.

Other examples of obstructive shock include massive pulmonary embolism with obstruction of the right ventricular outflow or main pulmonary artery, tension pneumothorax, and abrupt aortic occlusion due to dissection or massive thromboembolism.

DISTRIBUTIVE SHOCK. This functional classification involves shock syndromes manifested by decreased vascular resistance that is not adequately compensated for by alterations in cardiac output. The classic example of distributive shock is endotoxin sepsis.

The incidence of septic shock in the hospital setting appears to have increased over the past several decades, probably as a consequence of multiple medical advances in other areas. It is estimated that 1 per cent of hospital admissions are complicated by gram-negative sepsis, and the mortality from septic shock ranges from 30 to 80 per cent. Rather than a primary community-acquired phenomenon, septic shock more commonly arises in hospitalized patients and is one of the most common causes of mortality in intensive care unit patients.

Septic shock is most commonly associated with gram-negative infections, and approximately 40 per cent of gram-negative bacteremias are complicated by shock. Gram-negative septic shock is most often an example of an opportunistic infection. The most common gram-negative organisms associated with septic shock include Escherichia coli, Klebsiella, Enterobacter, and Pseudomonas species. The most common sources for these infectious agents are the genitourinary and gastrointestinal tracts, followed by respiratory tract, wounds, and sites of indwelling vascular access. Important non–gram-negative organs associated with septic shock include some gram-positive Staphylococcus and Streptococcus species and fungal organisms such as Candida.

Host factors important in the propensity for development of septic shock include advanced age, diabetes, debilitation and malnutrition, chronic alcohol or intravenous drug use, neoplastic diseases, immunocompromised state (especially granulocytopenia), and multiple organ failure.

Septic shock often follows a trimodal pattern of hemodynamic presentation: "warm" shock, "cold" shock, and multisystem organ failure. Early sepsis is often associated with a decrease in systemic vascular resistance, due most likely to the release of vasodilatory mediators such as bradykinin and histamine, and an increase in cardiac output ("warm" shock). The early stages of sepsis are characterized hemodynamically by low cardiac filling pressures, increased cardiac output, tachycardia, fever, and decreased whole-body oxygen consumption. This latter effect is likely due to impaired mitochondrial oxygen utilization and deficient oxygen delivery to cells despite an increase in overall cardiac output (maldistribution of cardiac output). Late in the sequence of septic shock, there is a decline in cardiac output and profound hypotension with severe acidosis, hypoxemia, and hypoxia ("cold" shock). Recent evidence suggests that the initial increase in cardiac output is often followed by a decrease in ventricular ejection fraction, possibly due to a myocardial depressant factor, myocardial edema, or altered responsiveness to adrenergic stimuli.

Lipopolysaccharide endotoxin appears to be a common etiologic factor in septic shock, as previously reviewed in this chapter (Cellular and Biochemical Factors in Shock). The end stages of septic shock are often associated with multiple organ system failure with profound derangements in cardiovascular, pulmonary, and renal systems. The adult respiratory distress syndrome is a common complication of septic shock and is discussed below.

COMMON COMPLICATIONS OF SHOCK

DISSEMINATED INTRAVASCULAR COAGULATION. Disseminated intravascular coagulation (DIC) is a syndrome often seen in shock, particularly that due to gram-negative septicemia, and is associated with a high mortality rate. The clinical hallmark of DIC is the simultaneous occurrence of intravascular clotting and fibrinolysis, although bleeding dominates the clinical picture in most cases. The syndrome causes renal cortical necrosis, generalized ischemic damage of multiple organs, consumption of coagulation factors, and bleeding and may also contribute to the pathogenesis of shock lung.

ADULT RESPIRATORY DISTRESS SYNDROME. The adult respiratory distress syndrome (ARDS), previously known as "shock lung," is a common complication of various shock syndromes and emphasizes the disastrous complications of microcirculatory failure. ARDS is defined physiologically as the presence of severe hypoxemia ($PaO_2/F_{IO_2} < 150$ torr), chest roentgenographic evidence of generalized pulmonary infiltrates, reduced lung compliance, absence of significant elevations of pulmonary venous pressures as confirmed by invasive hemodynamic monitoring (e.g., pulmonary capillary wedge pressure < 18 mm Hg), and absence of alternative explanations for the clinical presentation.

ARDS is most commonly seen in association with sepsis but may also complicate major trauma, aspiration of gastric contents, multiple blood transfusions, drug overdose, and primary pneumonic infections. The onset of ARDS may be extremely rapid (e.g., within 1 to 2 hours) but more often follows the initiating event by 24 to 48 hours. In most series, the mortality associated with ARDS is greater than 50 per cent and as great as 90 per cent in patients with combined ARDS and sepsis. The presence of other shock-associated disorders, such as multiple organ failure or severe infections, increases the mortality.

Three pathologic phases of ARDS have been described. An early exudative phase (24 to 96 hours) is characterized by death of alveolar type I cells, regional microatelectasis, and accumulation of protein-rich edema and fibrin with endothelial cell swelling. Complement-mediated neutrophil activation is a prominent early feature and likely contributes to endothelial damage. A second proliferative phase is characterized by the formation of hyaline membranes and rapid proliferation of type II alveolar cells. A chronic or late proliferative phase is characterized by widespread fibrosis. ARDS appears to produce inhomogeneous lesions in the lung, with the dependent portions being affected to a greater extent.

The physiologic consequences of ARDS include severe hypoxemia, reduced lung compliance, reduced functional residual lung capacity, increased dead space ventilation, pulmonary hypertension, and a nidus for superimposed pulmonary infection. The cause of death in patients who develop ARDS in the setting of shock is usually not respiratory failure. Early deaths are usually due to the underlying illness, and late deaths are related to complications of the treatment of this type of patient. Secondary lung infection is a common complication of ARDS. In those patients surviving ARDS, approximately one third have persistent pulmonary symptoms.

ACUTE RENAL FAILURE. Acute renal failure is a common complication of shock, regardless of primary etiology, and is responsible for considerable morbidity and mortality in this syndrome. Current mortality rates for acute renal failure developing in all hospitalized patients average 40 to 60 per cent. The most common causes of acute renal failure in hospitalized patients include decreased renal perfusion (of particular concern in the shock patient), administration of radiographic contrast agents, and administration of nephrotoxic drugs, particularly the aminoglycoside antibiotics.

The most common mechanism of acute renal failure in the setting of shock is probably acute tubular necrosis, otherwise known as vasomotor nephropathy. The pathogenesis of this disorder usually involves severe reductions in renal cortical blood flow due to marked preglomerular vasoconstriction. Vasomotor nephropathy is usually manifested by oliguria but can occasionally present as total anuria, persists for 1 to 3 weeks, and can be followed by a recovery phase associated with marked diuresis. In most patients, the serum creatinine rises 1 to 4 mg per deciliter per day, and the mortality increases with total increases of 3 mg per deciliter or more.

In the management of the shock patient, close attention needs to be paid to monitoring urine output and ensuring that cardiac preload and cardiac output are adequate to maintain renal perfusion. The onset of anuria requires that postrenal obstructive etiologies be excluded rapidly. In the case of trauma, consideration must be given to vascular insults (renal artery or renal vein occlusion) and to rhabdomyolysis as possible etiologies of renal failure.

CLINICAL PRESENTATION

The classic clinical presentation of shock is a patient who is hypotensive (systolic arterial pressure less than 90 mm Hg or more than 60 mm Hg less than baseline); has a tachycardia with a weak and thready pulse; is hyperventilating; has cold, clammy, cyanotic skin; and has a dulled sensorium ranging from agitation to stupor or coma. The patient is frequently oliguric (urine output less than 30 ml per hour) or anuric.

This classic shock pattern of presentation is not always present, and the recognition of the subtle or early presentation of shock may be crucial. For example, a patient may have a "normal" blood pressure (e.g., 110/70), but this may actually represent "relative hypotension" if the patient has a history of severe hypertension. Early shock may be indicated only by unexplained agitation or tachycardia in the absence of cardiovascular collapse. Some patients with septic or neurogenic shock may present with peripheral vasodilation and warm hyperperfused extremities (socalled warm shock).

Finally, the clinical manifestations of the patient may be altered by pre-existing disease or by chronic pharmacologic agents. If possible, rapid assessment of medical history and medication regimens should be obtained during the initial assessment of the patient.

Assessment of the Shock Patient

GENERAL PRINCIPLES. There are five major goals in the management of the patient in shock: (1) rapid recognition of the shock state; (2) correction of the initial insult, (3) correction of the secondary consequences of the shock state, (4) maintenance of the function of vital organs, and (5) identification and correction of aggravating factors. All five goals are approached simultaneously in an organized and methodical way so as to ensure optimal therapy (Fig. 41–4). The prognosis of a patient in shock is determined in part by the etiology of the shock state (e.g.,

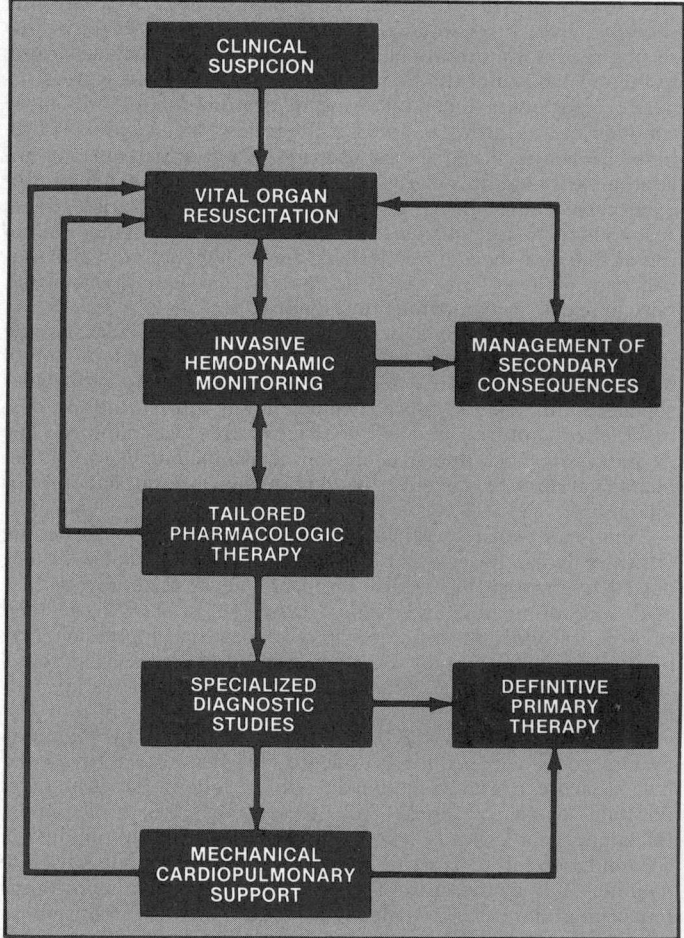

FIGURE 41–4. Strategy for management of the shock patient.

hypovolemic traumatic shock in a young, healthy adult carries a mortality of less than 20 per cent in many centers, whereas cardiogenic shock due to massive anterior wall myocardial infarction carries a mortality of greater than 70 per cent even in the most aggressive medical center). Prognosis is also affected by the duration of shock and consequent secondary organ dysfunction and by the speed of recognition and appropriateness of medical intervention. Finally, the prognosis of the patient in shock is also affected by the preshock status of the patient with respect to pre-existing medical conditions.

CRITICAL CARE TEAM. Successful and sophisticated management of a patient in shock requires an integrated team approach that begins to function upon initial contact with the patient and extends through periods of resuscitation, early stabilization, diagnostic evaluation, definitive therapy, and recovery phases of treatment. In addition to a primary physician knowledgeable in critical care who is responsible for the overall coordination of patient-care efforts, the management of these patients requires a number of other highly motivated, well-trained, and objective but empathetic professionals. Such a team includes critical care nurses, respiratory therapists, hemodynamic monitoring technicians, special procedure and diagnostic technicians, nutrition/dietetic consultants, and physical therapists. Finally, the immediate availability of multiple surgical and medical subspecialty consultants is essential for the care of these complexly and critically ill patients.

MEDICAL HISTORY AND PHYSICAL EXAMINATION. A rapid but thorough medical history and a complete but directed physical examination should be performed during the initial assessment and early management of the shock patient. Particular attention should be directed to the recent medical history and the details of the present illness in an effort to rapidly identify precipitating or causative factors of shock. Pertinent medical history should be obtained with emphasis placed on pre-existing cardiopulmonary, renal, hepatic, neurologic, and hematologic disorders. A complete listing of current medications and known allergies should be obtained from the patient, medical record, or closest relative.

A systematic and complete "head-to-toe" physical examination should be performed, consistent with the patient's clinical condition. During the examination, particular attention should be directed to assessment of the patient's airway, ventilation, circulation, and neurologic status. In the case of trauma, the patient's axial skeleton should be appropriately splinted until critical injuries to the head, spine, pelvis, and extremities have been excluded.

Sinus tachycardia is one of the earliest compensatory mechanisms for a fall in arterial pressure or cardiac output, and the differential diagnosis of this increase in heart rate includes the seven H's of hypovolemia, hypotension, heart failure, hypoxemia, hyperthermia, hyperthyroidism, and reflex hyperadrenergic state (e.g., reflex tachycardia seen in some cases of anterior wall myocardial infarction). Other important possible causes of tachycardia include anxiety and pulmonary embolism. The clinician must remember that unexplained tachycardia may be one of the earliest indications of impending cardiovascular collapse and therefore must not be ignored or inappropriately treated until the differential diagnosis is appropriately addressed.

The most important initial assessment of the patient should be directed to the patency and adequacy of the airway. If the patient is unable to ventilate or cannot adequately protect the airway, endotracheal intubation is indicated. Initial assessment of circulatory reserve can be obtained by palpation of central arteries (e.g., femoral) and by sphygmomanometric measurement of blood pressure. Particular attention should be focused on the pulse pressure, as a narrow pulse pressure suggests marked impairment of stroke volume.

INTRAVENOUS ACCESS. At least two large-bore intravenous catheters (16 gauge or larger) should be inserted in peripheral extremities, and at least one central venous sheath (8 Fr or greater) should be inserted under optimal sterile conditions as rapidly as possible. During placement of these venous access catheters, blood can be obtained for essential hematologic and chemical studies and for blood typing and cross-matching. In most circumstances, isotonic fluids (e.g., normal saline or Ringer's lactate) should be infused through these catheters pending further assessment of the patient.

INITIAL HEMATOLOGIC/BIOCHEMICAL DETERMINATIONS. Essential initial laboratory determinations should include those that may alter immediate therapy. These include complete blood count, serum electrolytes (sodium, potassium, calcium, magnesium), and arterial blood gases. Additional laboratory parameters should be obtained as indicated by the patient's presentation and the most likely etiologies for the shock state (e.g., blood culture; toxicology screen; cardiac enzyme panels).

A key element in the therapy of a patient in shock is hemodynamic monitoring.

Patient Monitoring

Management of the patient in shock requires accurate and serial measurements of heart rate and rhythm, respiratory rate and adequacy of gas exchange, systemic arterial pressure and cardiac filling pressures, tissue perfusion, and end-organ function. A reference for normal hemodynamic parameters in adults is provided in Table 41–4.

ELECTROCARDIOGRAPHIC MONITORING. Continuous electrocardiographic monitoring permits assessment of cardiac rate and rhythm and allows prompt detection of serious cardiac arrhythmias such as ventricular tachyarrhythmias, atrial fibrillation, high-degree AV block, and marked sinus bradycardia. The use of a monitoring lead, or preferably several leads, that provides adequate assessment of atrial as well as ventricular rhythms (e.g., MCL_1) is essential. Serial standard 12-lead electrocardiograms permit indirect assessment of myocardial ischemia and may be required for analysis of complex rhythm disorders.

ARTERIAL PRESSURE MONITORING. An indwelling arterial catheter is essential for continuous on-line assessment of arterial pressure and also provides a convenient access for obtaining blood samples. Assessment of arterial pressure by sphygmomanometry is not adequate for most patients with shock, is often an unreliable indicator of true core blood pressure in the hypotensive patient, and fails to provide continuous on-line assessment of blood pressure in patients with rapidly changing cardiovascular states. The choice of insertion site for arterial line placement depends upon the status of the patient being monitored, the presence and severity of peripheral vascular disease, and the expertise of the critical care team. In general, the more severe the shock state, the more central should the arterial catheter be placed in order to assess core blood pressure. In contrast, the

TABLE 41–4. NORMAL RESTING ADULT HEMODYNAMIC PARAMETERS

Parameter	Wave	Range (mm Hg)
Hydrostatic pressures		
Systemic arterial pressure		
Systemic arterial	Systolic	100–140
	Diastolic	60–90
	Mean	70–105
Right heart pressures		
Right atrial	"a"	2–10
	"v"	2–10
	Mean	2–8
Right ventricular	Systolic	15–30
	Diastolic	2–8
Pulmonary arterial	Systolic	15–30
	Diastolic	4–12
	Mean	9–18
Pulmonary capillary wedge	"a"	3–15
	"v"	3–15
	Mean	2–10
Cardiac output determinations		
Cardiac index (L/min/m²)		2.6–4.2
Arterial–mixed venous oxygen content difference (ml/dl)		3.0–5.0

From Grossman W: Cardiac Catheterization and Angiography. 3rd ed. Philadelphia, Lea and Febiger, 1986.

more central the placement, the higher the complication rate with long-term use of these catheters. The clinician must therefore assess the risk-benefit ratio of arterial cannulation sites in each individual patient. In patients with intense endogenous adrenergically medicated vasoconstriction or under the influence of potent vasoconstricting drugs, monitoring of pressure in small peripheral arteries such as the radial may be inadequate owing to vessel constriction. In the most severely ill patient, rapid insertion of a femoral arterial catheter under optimal sterile conditions provides the most accurate means of monitoring blood pressure. This catheter can always be removed and replaced with a more distal one as the patient's hemodynamic status improves. Alternative sites for arterial pressure monitoring include the radial, brachial, axillary, and dorsalis pedis arteries.

Complications associated with arterial pressure monitoring include bleeding, arterial thrombosis, vasospasm, infection, aneurysm or pseudoaneurysm formation, embolization (distal and proximal), limb ischemia, and pain. Appropriate care must be taken to ensure adequate collateral circulation prior to insertion of the arterial line, if possible, and to follow the patient closely for early signs of ischemia, infection, or embolization at or distal to the insertion site. These catheters should be changed to a new site, under sterile conditions, at least every 72 hours.

CARDIAC FILLING PRESSURE ASSESSMENT. Cardiac preload may need to be assessed invasively in patients with shock, as the physical examination is often not sensitive enough to determine accurately the state of cardiac filling, much less to monitor rapidly changing trends in this important determinant of cardiac output and blood pressure. The relative risk-benefit ratio of invasive hemodynamic monitoring must be assessed in each individual patient. In those patients requiring invasive monitoring, the assessment of central venous pressure (e.g., superior vena caval pressure) alone is inadequate for most patients in shock, as this pressure reflects only diastolic filling of the right ventricle. Central venous pressure monitoring alone may be adequate for the young patient who clearly has no underlying cardiac or pulmonary impairment, is not on a mechanical ventilator, and suffers only from clearly identified hypovolemic shock secondary to trauma. In the critically ill shock patient, the use of a flow-directed pulmonary artery catheter with cardiac output capability is often required for optimal management.

A flow-directed pulmonary artery balloon catheter (Swan-Ganz catheter) is an essential component of the monitoring of most patients in shock. This catheter can be inserted either peripherally from a median antecubital vein or through more central venous access sites such as the percutaneous internal jugular, external jugular, subclavian, or femoral venous approach. Such a catheter can be inserted "blindly" by pressure waveform analysis or under fluoroscopic guidance. During initial catheter insertion, measurements should be obtained of right atrial, right ventricular, pulmonary arterial, and pulmonary capillary wedge pressures during held end-expiration without a Valsalva maneuver. These measurements provide assessment of the preload of the right ventricle (right atrial and right ventricular end-diastolic pressures) and of the left ventricle (pulmonary arterial diastolic and pulmonary capillary wedge pressures). In the absence of significant vascular obstruction between the pulmonary artery and the left ventricle (e.g., severe fixed pulmonary arteriolar hypertension, pulmonary venous occlusive disease, mitral stenosis), the pulmonary capillary wedge pressure should reflect left ventricular end-diastolic pressure and thereby provide an index of left ventricular preload. In the presence of very rapid heart rates or acute severe aortic insufficiency, the pulmonary capillary wedge pressure may not reflect true left ventricular filling pressure.

The clinician must remember, however, that the left ventricular volume is the critical determinant of preload, and the relation between this volume and the left heart filling pressure depends upon the compliance (distensibility) of the ventricle. At the bedside, the clinician can determine in vivo Starling curves in the individual patient by assessing cardiac output at various levels of cardiac filling pressure during incremental volume loading. This also allows an assessment of the compliance of the ventricle by relating the volume infused to the resulting filling pressure. By obtaining measurements of heart rate, blood pressure, cardiac

output, pulmonary capillary wedge pressure, and arterial oxygen tension, the optimal preload in an individual patient can be determined which provides adequate perfusion without compromising ventilation.

In selected patients, a series of oximetry blood samples should be obtained during the initial insertion of the pulmonary artery catheter. This is most important in the patient with presumed cardiogenic shock in the setting of a new systolic murmur in whom the differential diagnosis includes ventricular septal rupture (diagnosed by step-up in oxygen saturation from the right atrium to the pulmonary artery) versus mitral insufficiency. It is essential to obtain blood samples from the superior vena cava, right atrium, pulmonary artery, and systemic artery to perform an adequate oximetry series. As a rule of thumb, there should be no greater than a 7 per cent step-up in oxygen saturation from the superior vena cava to the pulmonary artery in the absence of a left-to-right intracardiac shunt.

In general, only right heart catheters that have the added capability for assessment of cardiac output should be utilized in the monitoring of the shock patient. A proximal lumen for right atrial injection, coupled with an in-line thermistor for assessment of temperature at the tip of the catheter in the pulmonary artery, permits bedside assessment of cardiac output by the thermodilution technique. This indicator-dilution technique utilizes injection of cold saline into the right atrium and the time-dependent appearance of the "cold" indicator in the pulmonary artery to construct an indicator-dilution curve for assessment of cardiac output.

In addition, the Swan-Ganz catheter provides a distal monitoring port in the pulmonary artery which can be utilized for drawing pulmonary artery blood samples for chemical determinations. Important among these is the assessment of mixed venous oxygen saturation and content. Simultaneously obtaining arterial and mixed venous (pulmonary arterial blood in the absence of a left-to-right intracardiac shunt) blood samples permits assessment of arterial–mixed venous oxygen content difference, where O_2 content difference (ml/dl) = hemoglobin (grams) × saturation difference × 1.38 (ml O_2 per gram hemoglobin that is 100 per cent saturated). This provides an inverse assessment of cardiac output by the Fick principle and is complementary to the thermodilution technique for measurement of cardiac output. As cardiac output increases, arterial–mixed venous oxygen content difference should narrow, and vice versa, assuming constant hemoglobin content and oxygen consumption. The normal arterial–mixed venous oxygen content difference is 3.0 to 5.0 ml per deciliter and is a clinically useful reflection of oxygen extraction as well as an indicator of the adequacy of cardiac output in relation to systemic metabolic demand.

Newer modifications of the pulmonary artery catheter with an in-line fiberoptic system permit continuous assessment of pulmonary artery saturation (mixed venous saturation), based upon reflectance spectrophotometry. The mixed venous oxygen saturation is determined by the relationship between oxygen delivery and oxygen consumption in the systemic circulation and can be considered a reflection of "oxygen reserve." In general, mixed venous oxygen saturations greater than 65 per cent represent adequate reserves, whereas those less than 35 per cent indicate severe impairment of tissue oxygenation (assuming an arterial $F_{I_{O_2}} = 0.21$, room air).

Continuous monitoring of mixed venous oxygen saturation with fiberoptic catheters provides another complementary continuous assessment of a patient's hemodynamic status. A reduction in mixed venous oxygen saturation may be produced by a decrease in cardiac output, decrease in arterial oxygen saturation, decrease in hemoglobin, or increase in oxygen consumption (e.g., hyperthermia, pain, seizures). Conversely, an increase in mixed venous oxygen saturation may indicate an increase in cardiac output, an increase in inspired oxygen concentration, a decrease in oxygen consumption (e.g., hypothermia, pharmacologic paralysis, anesthesia), a decrease in peripheral tissue oxygen extraction (e.g., sepsis), a left-to-right shunt, or an artifactual increase in mixed venous saturation due to a wedged catheter.

A reduction of mixed venous oxygen saturation to less than 50 per cent is frequently associated with the development of anaerobic metabolism. An important exception to this generalization is sepsis, in which a decrease in tissue oxygenation is associated with an increase in mixed venous oxygen saturation, probably due at least in part to peripheral AV shunting.

Finally, the assessment of pulmonary arterial blood gases permits analysis of pH, P_{CO_2}, and P_{O_2} in the systemic venous return and may have important applications for monitoring the success of cardiopulmonary resuscitation in certain patients.

Further modifications of the Swan-Ganz catheter have permitted monitoring of intracardiac electrocardiograms and the passage of temporary pacing wires into the right ventricle for external electrical pacing of patients with hemodynamically significant bradyarrhythmias.

The clinician must remember that the Swan-Ganz catheter is expensive to insert and monitor, and complications such as arrhythmias, infection, and pulmonary infarction may accompany its use. Rigorous attention to detail and expertise in the use of this catheter are essential to ensure an optimal risk-benefit ratio during its use. These catheters should be inserted only by physicians adequately trained in the use of these devices who possess extensive knowledge pertaining to indications, potential complications, and analysis of the information they provide. The patient with indwelling Swan-Ganz and arterial catheters requires continuous monitoring of pressure waveforms to detect catheter migration or occlusion. Rigorous attention to sterile technique should be employed in the care of the patient with such catheters.

URINARY CATHETER. An indwelling bladder catheter permits hourly assessment of urinary output, a reflection of effective renal perfusion. A decline in urinary output to less than 20 ml per hour is often an indication of inadequate renal perfusion. The most frequent cause of oliguria in the setting of shock is hypovolemia. Fluid deficits are often underestimated, particularly in the presence of sepsis. If oliguria persists despite adequate administration of volume expanders, as confirmed by left heart filling pressures, then additional therapies such as dopamine may be required. The diagnosis of anuria should be made only once it is confirmed that the bladder catheter is patent and there is no obstruction from the renal pelvis to the catheter.

PHYSIOLOGIC SCORING SYSTEMS. Potentially beneficial prospective data acquisition and management systems for evaluating patients requiring admission to critical care environments for shock and other conditions have been under development for over 10 years. These systems have utilized commonly obtained clinical and laboratory data to formulate a prognostic score soon after a patient's admission and thereby attempt to predict a "seriousness-of-illness" index and projected mortality. The goal behind such systems is to guide appropriateness of therapy and utilization of intensive care resources. These attempts to define the extent of physiologic derangements at the time of patient presentation may provide important information relative to management of patients with shock. At present, however, no universally accepted scoring system has been developed.

SPECIALIZED DIAGNOSTIC STUDIES

In addition to the standard diagnostic studies (e.g., electrocardiogram, chest roentgenogram, hematologic and biochemical blood studies) employed in the management of shock patients, certain auxiliary specialized studies may be of benefit in the management of these patients.

ECHOCARDIOGRAPHY. Two-dimensional echocardiography with Doppler capability provides a rapid, noninvasive, and sensitive bedside tool for the evaluation of the patient with unexplained shock. The echocardiogram is particularly useful for providing the following: (1) rapid assessment of generalized and regional myocardial systolic function, (2) evaluation for intrapericardial fluid accumulation and echocardiographic suggestion of tamponade physiology (diastolic right ventricular collapse), (3) assessment of cardiac valves for stenosis, regurgitation, and vegetations, (4) evaluation for intracardiac shunts (e.g., ventricular septal rupture) and left ventricular aneurysm, (5) assessment of prosthetic valve function, and (6) assessment for aortic dissection (transesophageal echocardiography). Noncardiac ultrasound examinations are invaluable for assessment of certain intra-abdominal, pelvic, retroperitoneal, intrathoracic, and other deep masses and fluid accumulations. Identification of abdominal aortic aneurysms, deep venous thromboses, and fetal-uterine abnormalities is an additional feature of ultrasonography that may play an important role in the management of the shock patient.

NUCLEAR MEDICINE STUDIES. A variety of isotope imaging studies may be of benefit in the management of the shock patient. Ventilation-perfusion lung scans may be useful in the diagnosis or exclusion of massive pulmonary emboli. Renal perfusion studies may be of benefit in the differential diagnosis of acute renal failure. First-pass radionuclide ventriculograms provide important information about systolic and diastolic function of the right and left ventricles. Labeled red cell and white cell scans may be of benefit in identifying localized sites of bleeding or abscesses, respectively. Brain flow studies may be of benefit in assessing neurologic status in the shock patient and may help in identifying potential central nervous system pathology.

COMPUTED TOMOGRAPHY AND NUCLEAR MAGNETIC RESONANCE IMAGING. These techniques provide noninvasive anatomic detail of most major regions of the body and can often be very useful in the evaluation of selected patients in shock (e.g., suspected aortic dissection, retroperitoneal hemorrhage, brain stem stroke).

INTERVENTIONAL CARDIOVASCULAR RADIOLOGY STUDIES. Cardiac catheterization is an essential component in the initial evaluation and management of the patient with cardiogenic shock. In addition to providing necessary anatomic diagnosis as a guide to definitive surgical therapy in some patients, cardiac catheterization may provide the route for definitive nonsurgical therapy in certain forms of cardiogenic shock. This includes the use of percutaneous transluminal balloon coronary angioplasty for reperfusion therapy in cardiogenic shock following myocardial infarction, and balloon valvuloplasty as therapy for cardiogenic shock in high surgical risk patients with critical aortic stenosis. Other noncardiac vascular diagnostic procedures are often required for localization of vascular trauma (e.g., aortic dissection), confirmation of suspected massive pulmonary embolism, and definitive therapy in certain cases (e.g., percutaneous insertion of inferior vena cava filter in survivors of submassive pulmonary emboli despite adequate anticoagulation).

Techniques under development for further specialized monitoring of shock patients include transcutaneous monitoring of arterial oxygen and carbon dioxide tensions, tissue electrodes for direct measurement of tissue oxygenation, measurement of respiratory muscle strength by assessment of maximum airway pressures, assessment of respiratory muscle fatigue by measuring tension-time index of the diaphragm, continuous monitoring of end-tidal P_{CO_2} by capnography for assessment of arterial P_{CO_2}, thermal dye techniques for measurement of extravascular lung water, and double-indicator dilution techniques for evaluation of pulmonary endothelial integrity.

THERAPEUTIC GUIDELINES IN SHOCK MANAGEMENT

Management of the patient in shock consists of primary therapy directed at the underlying insult and secondary therapy directed at the consequences of the shock state. Primary therapy depends upon identification of the etiology of the shock state. Examples of primary therapy are surgical repair of a ruptured abdominal aortic aneurysm, pericardiocentesis for cardiac tamponade, and antibiotic therapy for sepsis. Major efforts in the initial management of patients with shock are simultaneously directed at identification and reversal of the primary etiology while at the same time managing the secondary consequences of the shock state (Fig. 41–4). Selected aspects of this management are reviewed.

PAIN CONTROL. Patients in shock are often in pain and may be frightened or agitated. Care must be taken to avoid approaches to these problems that can worsen the underlying hemodynamic instability of the patient. Essentially all pharmacologic measures for pain control or anxiolysis produce some degree of hemodynamic compromise and must therefore be carefully titrated with close observation of the patient's hemodynamic and ventilatory status. In the setting of shock, all medications must be administered via the intravenous route, as absorption of intramuscular or subcutaneous medication is unpredictable and therefore unreliable.

In general, severe pain can be most easily managed by judicious administration of a reversible narcotic such as morphine sulfate (2 to 4 mg IV increments). Potential side effects following morphine include vasodilation with hypotension (mediated by histamine release, direct vasodilation, and neurogenic mechanisms), vagally mediated bradyarrhythmias, respiratory depression, nausea and vomiting, and biliary spasm. The primary route of morphine metabolism is hepatic glucuronic acid conjugation. Patients with hepatic dysfunction, common in shock states, may be very sensitive to the effects of morphine, as may be the elderly. An advantage of morphine and similar opioid agonists is the capacity for rapid pharmacologic antagonism with agents such as naloxone, should adverse effects follow their administration. Naloxone may have additional benefits in shock, as discussed below.

OXYGEN ADMINISTRATION. Oxygen is a drug, and its use should be guided by considerations applicable to the use of other drugs in the treatment of shock. In general, oxygen should be administered initially to most patients in shock, in view of the likelihood of impaired peripheral oxygen delivery. However, the administration should be performed via a high-flow system (one that delivers the entire inspired oxygen atmosphere), so that the fraction of inspired oxygen administered to the patient (FI_{O_2}) is controlled. This permits bedside assessment of the degree of arterial hypoxemia (defined by the alveolar-arterial oxygen gradient), as the calculation of alveolar P_{O_2} depends upon a known FI_{O_2}. Clinically useful high-flow systems include Venturi masks in the nonintubated patient and ventilators in the intubated patient. An attempt should be made to provide sufficient oxygen to achieve an arterial oxygen saturation of 90 per cent or higher. In the patient requiring positive-pressure ventilation, an attempt should be made to achieve this with an FI_{O_2} of 0.60 or less, in order to reduce the incidence of pulmonary oxygen toxicity. This may be facilitated by the judicious use of positive end-expiratory pressure (PEEP). Continuous assessment of arterial oxygen saturation can be guided by the use of pulse oximetry, but significant alterations in management must be based upon direct assessment of arterial blood gases.

Mechanical ventilation is indicated in the management of the shock patient for the following: (1) apnea or ventilatory failure (acute respiratory acidosis), (2) failure to adequately oxygenate with high-flow system, (3) mechanical splinting of the flail chest wall, (4) relief of the metabolic stress of the work of breathing in selected patients, and (5) adjunctive therapy for other interventions. During mechanical ventilation, careful attention must be paid to the hemodynamic effects of positive intrathoracic pressure. This requires an indwelling pulmonary artery catheter and close assessment of cardiac filling pressure, cardiac output, and arterial blood gases.

CORRECTION OF HYPOVOLEMIA. Hypovolemia is the most common cause of shock seen clinically and may occur in any type of shock, whether or not it is associated with external signs of blood or fluid loss. If there is no evidence of actual fluid or blood loss, there may be significant volume shifts from the intravascular to extracellular spaces because of increased capillary permeability and endothelial damage. This may occur in any vascular bed but is most common in the splanchnic and pulmonary beds. In any shock syndrome associated with decreased tissue perfusion, fluid may also shift intracellularly because of changes in cellular membrane permeability.

The effective and sustained maintenance of cardiac output is critically dependent upon an adequate preload (ventricular filling pressure). The administration of potent inotropic and vasopressor agents in the presence of hypovolemia may be ineffective and often aggravates the clinical condition rather than improves it. As previously discussed, the accurate assessment of cardiac filling pressures often requires the use of invasive hemodynamic monitoring with an indwelling Swan-Ganz catheter. Attempts should be made to provide adequate left heart filling pressures, based upon assessment of the pulmonary capillary wedge pressure and cardiac output. This usually requires maintaining the true (e.g., pulmonary capillary wedge–intrathoracic pressures) filling pressures at or above 10 to 12 mm Hg, but even higher filling pressures (e.g., 18 to 20 mm Hg) may be required in the presence of a noncompliant left ventricle (e.g., acute myocardial infarction shock). These concerns must be balanced by the relative risk of

pulmonary hydrostatic toxicity in some patients with high filling pressures, particularly in the setting of ARDS.

In most cases of shock presenting as profound hypotension and in the absence of obvious acute pulmonary edema, initial management includes positioning the patient in reverse Trendelenburg position (unless head or chest injury contraindicates this position) to permit gravitational return of lower limb blood volume to the central circulation. This should be followed by rapid insertion of large-bore intravenous catheters and the initiation of volume resuscitation with warmed crystalloid solutions. Intravenous infusion volumes of up to 200 ml per minute may be required in some patients and usually require pressurized volume infusion systems. Initial assessment of the adequacy of volume resuscitation can be based upon examination of neck veins, blood pressure, state of consciousness, and clinical signs of tissue perfusion such as color, warmth, capillary refill, and urine volume. In those patients who fail to respond to rapid volume resuscitation, consideration should be given to instituting assessment of cardiac filling pressures with invasive hemodynamic monitoring.

If the patient has cardiogenic shock or signs of pulmonary edema, one should insert a Swan-Ganz catheter prior to administration of volume expanders. If, as frequently happens, the physical examination is misleading and the patient's pulmonary artery diastolic or capillary wedge pressures are less than 12 to 15 mm Hg, one should administer 250 to 500 ml of a crystalloid to the patient every 10 to 15 minutes until achieving a steady left heart filling pressure of 15 to 20 mm Hg. If perfusion of tissues fails to improve or worsens and filling pressures remain above 15 to 20 mm Hg or if true pulmonary edema supervenes, then volume infusion should be stopped and inotropic therapy initiated.

PNEUMATIC ANTI-SHOCK GARMENTS. Lower body external compression garments may be of benefit in certain cases of hypovolemic shock, particularly those involving major trauma. The prototype device is the military anti-shock trouser (MAST) garment. Although controversial, the MAST garment appears to offer potential beneficial effects in certain patients. The MAST suit has been found to increase arterial pressure in hypovolemic shock patients, control certain forms of hemorrhage (e.g., lower abdominal or pelvic), improve carotid and upper body blood flow, and improve the ability of prehospital personnel to start intravenous lines. The mechanisms of action of the garment remain controversial but probably involve decreasing radius of blood vessels compressed by the suit, decreasing the volume of compressed compartments, and increasing venous return. However, potential adverse effects of this device have been identified. These include restriction of blood flow to compressed extremities with increased ischemia, restriction of ventilation, profound hypotension following excessively rapid deflation, renovascular insufficiency, lower extremity compartmental syndromes, arterial thrombosis, and increased bleeding from some vascular injuries. The MAST garment may be of limited short-term benefit for out-of-hospital resuscitation of the traumatic shock patient but should be used only by personnel experienced in the differential diagnosis of shock and familiar with the complications of this device. Prophylactic placement of a noninflated MAST garment should be considered in certain shock patients prior to transport from the scene of trauma to a medical facility, or between medical facilities, especially when the mode of transport (e.g., helicopter) may limit resuscitation techniques.

VOLUME-EXPANDING AGENTS. Debate continues regarding the ideal agent for intravascular volume repletion. In general, this depends upon the etiology of the hypovolemia. Crystalloids are usually the initial agents used for volume resuscitation. Proposed advantages of crystalloids include the argument that the key problem in shock is often shrinkage of the extracellular fluid compartment, which is more appropriately repleted with crystalloid; excessive increases in pulmonary vascular pressures are less likely with crystalloids than colloids; crystalloids are free of the potential for anaphylaxis seen with some colloids; crystalloids can provide safe and effective restoration of circulating blood volume for short periods of time; crystalloids improve microcirculatory flow by reducing blood viscosity; and crystalloids are generally less expensive than colloids.

Selected patients may benefit from colloid administration. Potential advantages of colloids include the finding that smaller volumes of colloids are required to achieve volume repletion because these agents remain in the circulation because of their higher oncotic pressure; greater maintenance of plasma oncotic pressure with colloid than with crystalloid repletion; and the potential metabolic advantages of certain colloid preparations. Obviously, loss of massive amounts of blood in the setting of major trauma should be managed with administration of blood products in combination with crystalloids.

Commonly utilized crystalloids include isotonic normal saline and Ringer's lactate solution. Normal saline contains 140 mEq of sodium and 140 mEq of chloride, whereas Ringer's lactate solution contains 130 mEq of sodium, 4 mEq of potassium, 108 mEq of chloride, and 28 mEq of lactate. When large volumes of fluid are administered, isotonic saline can produce a dilutional acidosis, which can be avoided if Ringer's lactate is used. In contrast, large infusions of Ringer's lactate may produce hyperkalemia in the renal failure patient, and some patients with severe shock may have difficulty metabolizing lactate. In general, initial crystalloid resuscitation of the hypovolemic trauma patient should be given at a ratio of 3:1 per unit of estimated whole blood loss. Crystalloid infusions should be delivered through large-bore catheters with pressure infusion bags if needed, and every effort should be made to infuse solutions previously warmed to normal core body temperature.

Commonly utilized colloids in the management of shock include whole blood, plasma, serum albumin, gelatin preparations, and plasma substitutes such as dextran and hydroxyethyl starch (Hetastarch). Whole blood requires cross-matching and carries the potential risk of disease transmission. However, in cases of massive hemorrhage, whole blood is the preferred agent for volume repletion. Alternative procedures include the administration of packed red blood cells together with crystalloid or colloid volume expanders. Considerations for the use of colloid volume expanders such as albumin or hydroxyethyl starch include major volume resuscitations in which the patient is estimated to have circulating blood volume deficits of 30 per cent or more. In these patients, additional blood component therapy is dictated by the coagulation profile, hemoglobin concentration, and platelet count.

Fresh frozen plasma is a readily available source of biologically active coagulation factors and may therefore be appropriate in some cases of shock. However, other volume expanders may be as effective. In addition, fresh frozen plasma should be considered as an important reserve of coagulation factors and administered when needed for these functions.

Albumin is available as purified albumin, salt-poor purified albumin, and plasma protein fraction albumin. Although it is true that albumin remains in the intravascular space for a longer period than do crystalloids, this is a time-dependent phenomenon and the plasma half-life of exogenously administered albumin is approximately 16 hours. Albumin is clinically available as 5 per cent and 25 per cent solutions in isotonic saline. Potential disadvantages of albumin include potential for lowering serum ionized calcium levels, risk of anaphylaxis, the potential for exacerbating interstitial edema in shock conditions associated with capillary leak (e.g., sepsis, ARDS, intestinal obstruction), and the cost of these preparations. Albumin preparations should not be used indiscriminately.

Dextran is a large polymer of glucose and is commercially available as preparations with average molecular weights of 40,000 and 70,000 (dextran-40 and dextran-70). Both dextran preparations remain in the intravascular space for a significant period of time, longer for dextran-70 (up to 24 hours) than for dextran-40 (several to 12 hours). These agents are eliminated by renal clearance. Theoretically, dextran is an ideal volume expander because of its long "dwell time" in the intravascular space and its biodegradability. Dextran increases plasma volume to a degree equal to or greater than that infused, although this effect is limited by the induced diuresis. The effective volume expansion of dextran-40 is significantly greater than that achieved with 5 per cent albumin and much less expensive. However, the potential advantages of dextran are significantly counterbalanced by serious side effects. The side effects associated with dextran include platelet dysfunction and coagulation abnormalities, anaphylactic reactions, and renal failure. In addition, obligate diuresis occurs following dextran infusion, and therefore urine output cannot be used as an indicator of the sufficiency of volume repletion. Finally, dextran may interfere with cross-matching of blood, can falsely elevate some determinations of blood glucose levels, and may interfere temporarily with the immune function of the reticuloendothelial system.

A newer synthetic colloid used in volume expansion is hydroxyethyl starch (Hetastarch), which resembles glycogen. This agent is available in a 6 per cent solution with average molecular weight of particles being 69,000. Hetastarch has a long half-life in the plasma of greater than 2 weeks. The blood volume expansion achieved with Hetastarch is equal to or greater than that achieved with dextran or albumin, and the side effects appear less. Minor alterations in laboratory coagulation parameters are seen with Hetastarch infusion, but clinical bleeding is rare in doses of less than 1500 ml per day. Hetastarch is not immunogenic, does not produce histamine release, and has a very low incidence of anaphylactic reactions. Serum amylase levels are increased following Hetastarch administration, but no clinical evidence of pancreatic dysfunction is noted.

Hetastarch, as well as the other volume expanders discussed, does not carry oxygen and therefore must be administered in association with blood in patients with massive hemorrhage. During the use of all volume expanders, patients must be carefully monitored for signs of volume overload, especially pulmonary edema.

Limited experimental and clinical trials are currently investigating the potential role of red blood cell substitutes for resuscitation of patients with severe hemorrhagic shock. The use of fluorocarbon red blood cell substitutes, capable of transporting small quantities of oxygen, appears interesting and of potential benefit in selected patients. However, the dilutional effect of these agents and the need for high levels of oxygen administration in such patients may limit the efficacy of this therapy.

CORRECTION OF ACIDOSIS. A significant secondary complication in shock of any etiology is the development of metabolic acidosis as a consequence of tissue ischemia. Severe acidosis impairs metabolic processes, impedes normal neurovascular interactions, and may prevent effective pharmacologic actions of various vasopressor and inotropic agents administered to the shock patient.

The differential diagnosis of metabolic acidosis is aided by calculation of the anion gap, where the anion gap = $[Na^+] - ([Cl^-] + [HCO_3^-])$ and should be approximately 12 to 16 mEq per liter. Increases in the anion gap are due to increased endogenous acid production (e.g., lactic acidosis, diabetic ketoacidosis, alcoholic ketoacidosis, starvation), increased exogenous acids (e.g., aspirin toxicity, methanol, ethylene glycol, paraldehyde), or decreased acid excretion (e.g., renal failure). A metabolic acidosis with normal anion gap is usually due to gastrointestinal or renal loss of bicarbonate or may be a complication of parenteral hyperalimentation.

If arterial pH is less than 7.00 and respiratory acidosis has been excluded as the etiology, intravenous sodium bicarbonate should be administered and titrated to maintain a pH in the range of 7.30 or higher. Care must be taken to avoid overcorrection and the induction of metabolic alkalosis, as this may also impair cardiac function and decrease oxygen delivery to the tissues by shifting the oxyhemoglobin dissociation curve to the left. In addition, inappropriate administration of sodium bicarbonate may produce sodium and water overload, can induce hypokalemia, and may worsen central nervous system acidosis.

TREATMENT OF ARRHYTHMIAS. In general, the physician managing the patient in shock should treat disturbances of cardiac electrical activity only if these disturbances produce hemodynamic instability (e.g., hypotension, heart failure, myocardial ischemia) or if the specific rhythm is of clear prognostic significance (e.g., high-degree AV block in the setting of an anterior wall myocardial infarction). It must be remembered that all of the currently available antiarrhythmic agents possess known adverse side effects, and many of them have negative inotropic properties to some degree. Thus, an attempt to "abolish" the appearance of premature ventricular complexes on the monitor in an otherwise electrically stable patient is not appropriate. It is the patient and not the monitor which must be evaluated and treated.

Ventricular fibrillation is managed with nonsynchronized electrical countershock, delivered as rapidly as possible. Standard cardiopulmonary resuscitation may be required until a shock can be delivered or during intervening periods between defibrillation attempts.

Sustained ventricular tachycardia with profound hemodynamic instability should be treated with synchronized electrical countershock. An initial electrical dose of 100 joules should be applied, and repeated if necessary, prior to increasing energy dose. If the ventricular tachycardia is sustained and causes severe hemodynamic compromise, the patient may be treated with intravenous lidocaine, with an initial bolus of 1.0 to 1.5 mg per kilogram, followed by initiation of a continuous infusion at 2 mg per minute and a repeat bolus of 0.5 to 0.75 mg per kilogram 10 to 15 minutes later. Patients who are prone to serious complications following lidocaine are those 65 years of age or older, those in severe heart failure, and those with compromised hepatic function. These are important factors to consider in the management of the shock patient. In particular, care must be taken to follow plasma drug levels in those patients who require sustained infusions. Every effort should be made to discontinue these drugs as soon as possible once the patient has been stabilized, in order to avoid drug-related toxicity. Alternative agents for management of sustained ventricular tachycardia include bretylium and procainamide.

Accelerated idioventricular rhythm is seen frequently in patients with acute myocardial infarction. This is usually a benign rhythm that does not require treatment.

Sinus tachycardia is often an initial autonomically mediated compensatory response to a fall in arterial pressure and cardiac output. Particularly in the young patient, rapid rates of sinus tachycardia must be distinguished from other forms of supraventricular tachycardia in order to avoid inappropriate attempts at conversion of this rhythm. Sinus tachycardia should be considered a diagnostic sign rather than a dysrhythmia.

Supraventricular tachyarrhythmias (atrial tachycardias, atrial flutter, atrial fibrillation) that are associated with marked hemodynamic compromise are best treated with synchronized electrical cardioversion. Atrial flutter may respond to energies as low as 10 to 20 joules, whereas atrial fibrillation may require 100 to 200 or more joules. Medical therapy of these arrhythmias includes the use of digitalis glycosides, calcium channel blockers, and/or β-adrenergic blockers. However, these latter two classes of drugs are relatively contraindicated in the shock patient. Inappropriate administration of potent intravenous calcium channel blockers for treatment of supraventricular tachycardias in patients with underlying shock has been associated with adverse outcomes, including death.

Sinus bradycardia may be a manifestation of rapid, profound, exsanguinating hemorrhage as previously discussed. Other mechanisms of sinus bradycardia include vagally mediated responses to local (e.g., cardiac receptor) or generalized (e.g., pain) noxious stimuli. Sinus bradycardia is commonly seen following inferior wall myocardial infarction, owing to activation of cardiac afferents and inhibitory cardiac reflexes. Sinus bradycardia usually responds to atropine (0.6 to 1.0 mg IV). Care must be taken to avoid too small a dose of atropine (e.g., ≤0.4 mg), as this may induce a centrally mediated vagal response that paradoxically worsens the bradycardia. An adult patient should not be considered "atropine-resistant" until he or she has received a total intravenous dose of 3.0 mg atropine.

Conduction disturbances such as AV block carry a variable prognosis, and the approach to therapy depends on the underlying mechanism and clinical state. In the setting of acute inferior wall myocardial infarction, AV block is usually neurogenically mediated by afferent inhibitory cardiac reflexes, responds to atropine, and has a good prognosis. In contrast, AV block in the setting of anterior wall infarction is usually due to ischemic impairment of the AV node or His bundle, frequently does not respond to atropine, and has a poor prognosis, as it reflects a large infarction. If atropine fails to counteract and reverse the hemodynamic compromise of AV block, external (transthoracic)

or internal (transvenous) electrical pacing can be employed. In general, it is preferred to re-establish organized AV synchrony, with associated atrial loading of ventricular preload, rather than to rely on ventricular pacing alone. This may occasionally require the use of combined atrial and ventricular synchronized electrical pacing modalities.

CORTICOSTEROIDS. The potential beneficial effect of steroids has been suggested to relate primarily to their action on cellular membranes, with stabilization of lysosomal membranes thought to be a primary focus of their effect. Steroids may also prevent the release of β-endorphin, which can cause myocardial depression. The use of steroids in clinical shock remains controversial. At present, there are no well-controlled trials supporting the routine use of steroids in most forms of shock, and several trials have shown no benefit of steroids in the management of septic shock. One of the most controversial areas in critical care medicine is the role of supraphysiologic doses of corticosteroids in the management of septic shock and ARDS. Despite initial enthusiasm for the use of steroids in septic shock in the 1970's, no conclusive data in humans are currently available to support the widespread use of corticosteroids in septic shock. This applies to other nonendocrine forms of shock as well. Similarly, there are no well-accepted data to support the routine use of corticosteroids in patients with ARDS, regardless of the underlying etiology. This applies to ARDS following aspiration and drowning as well as to that occurring in the setting of sepsis. While controversial, recent data from multicenter sepsis studies suggest that steroids may actually worsen the prognosis of patients with sepsis-related ARDS.

The one clear indication for corticosteroid administration in human shock is acute adrenal crisis with cardiovascular collapse. In this setting, prompt therapy with steroids is lifesaving. In addition to steroids, these patients also require vigorous volume repletion and careful monitoring and repletion of serum glucose.

OPIOID ANTAGONISTS. As previously discussed, shock of various etiologies has been associated with an increase in circulating levels of endogenous opioid substances, the most common of which appears to be β-endorphin. Experimental studies in animals with septic shock have suggested that this agent plays an important role in mediating the hypotensive and cardiodepressant effects of sepsis. Experimental studies of hypovolemic and septic shock in animals have suggested that acute antagonism of endogenous opiates with naloxone may produce beneficial hemodynamic effects.

Limited clinical trials since 1981 have suggested that pharmacologic antagonism of these opioids by the administration of the narcotic antagonist naloxone may produce beneficial hemodynamic effects in patients with septic shock. However, these studies have not been conclusive, and contradictory reports of no benefit have been published. A major area of potential concern relates to the most appropriate dose of naloxone to be administered, and in what types of shock this agent might be beneficial. At the present time, this appears to be an area of intense interest, but detailed prospective trials in large numbers of patients need to be performed to resolve the question of benefit. Reports of potential adverse effects following naloxone administration to patients with shock include reversal of opiate analgesia, pulmonary edema, ventricular arrhythmias, and unexpected hypotension.

SYMPATHOMIMETIC AMINES. These drugs are used to increase cardiac output through their inotropic action and to redistribute blood flow to vital organs by their selective vasoconstricting action. The net desired effect of these agents is therefore an increase in arterial pressure and/or cardiac output with improved perfusion of ischemic regions. Unfortunately, no single agent appears to produce the effects desired in all forms of shock, which is not surprising in view of the various mechanisms of the shock state. There are also two potential problems associated with the use of these types of agents. If arterial pressure is elevated significantly, the hypertension can cause a detrimental increase in cardiac afterload and increase myocardial oxygen demand (see Fig. 41–1). Thus, judicious elevation of arterial pressure to levels adequate for peripheral perfusion is the goal, while avoiding excessive hypertension. The blood pressure range needed to meet these criteria varies with each patient. Reasonable guidelines are to achieve a systolic arterial pressure of 110 to 130 mm Hg and to maintain diastolic arterial pressure in the 60- to 80-mm Hg range. The second and related potential problem associated with these agents is their vasoconstricting effect. While some degree of vasoconstriction is desired in nonessential organ beds, it should be avoided in critical organs. Thus, the proper use of sympathomimetic amines requires a thorough knowledge of their cardiovascular effects. These effects depend primarily upon the affinity of the individual agent for various types of adrenergic receptors.

ADRENERGIC RECEPTORS. The adrenergic receptors are classified as α or β receptors with respect to their cardiac and vascular actions. Over the past 10 years, both prejunctional and postjunctional adrenergic receptors have been identified, and various subtypes of receptors have been characterized. Several have been cloned and their primary structure has been defined. However, from a practical clinical standpoint, the catecholamines utilized to treat shock can be understood by considering three specific types of postsynaptic adrenergic receptors. The α receptors are located primarily in blood vessels and mediate vasoconstriction. The β receptors are present in the blood vessels as well as the myocardium. Activation of β_1 receptors in the heart produces an increase in myocardial contractility and heart rate. Activation of β_2 receptors in blood vessels produces vasodilation. The same catecholamine may activate both α and β receptors, depending on the dose and the organ in which it is acting. The net effect depends to a large extent on the relative distribution of the various receptor subtypes in the organ. The sympathomimetic amines that are commonly used clinically in the management of the patient in shock include dopamine, dobutamine, epinephrine, norepinephrine, and isoproterenol. The relative actions and potencies of these agents are summarized in Table 41–5.

Administration of each of these catecholamines to patients carries the potential for adverse side effects. Common to all of these agents are the potential complications of cardiac arrhythmias, nausea, vomiting, ischemia of major organs with prolonged infusions of potent vasoconstrictors, and localized skin necrosis with inadvertent extravasation of these agents.

INOTROPIC AND VASOPRESSOR AGENTS. _Norepinephrine._ Norepinephrine is the primary neurotransmitter of the sympathetic nervous system. It increases myocardial contractility by activating β_1 receptors and thus may increase cardiac output. In blood vessels, it activates primarily α receptors, thereby producing vasoconstriction. The magnitude of its effect on blood vessels varies from one organ to another. Norepinephrine is a very potent vasoconstrictor in skin, muscle, and splanchnic beds, whereas in the coronary vessels it activates the β_2 receptors as well as the α receptors. Because there is a paucity of α receptors in the coronary vessels (in contrast to other vascular beds), norepinephrine causes vasodilation of the coronary arteries.

Norepinephrine offers several distinct advantages in the treatment of shock. It increases cardiac output and redistributes blood flow away from the extremities and toward the heart and brain and increases arterial pressure. This in turn increases coronary blood flow to ischemic myocardium. Because it is a potent peripheral vasoconstrictor, norepinephrine may be particularly useful in septic shock, a condition associated with significant peripheral vasodilation and resultant hypotension.

Norepinephrine should be administered intravenously through a secure catheter, preferably a centrally placed one, in order to diminish the risk of extravasation, which can result in severe

tissue necrosis. Norepinephrine should be initiated at a dose of approximately 0.050 μg per kilogram per minute and the infusion titrated to achieve the desired hemodynamic effect. Upper recommended limits of infusion are approximately 1.0 μg per kilogram per minute. Norepinephrine is rapidly cleared from the circulation with a half-life of 2 to 3 minutes, although this is variable. It is enzymatically degraded in the liver and kidney and is also cleared by regional reuptake into sympathetic nerve terminals.

If hypoxia, hypovolemia, and acidosis have been corrected, the lack of a response to norepinephrine is probably an indication of significant myocardial damage. Prolonged infusions of norepinephrine, or infusions of large doses, are associated with major end-organ (e.g., liver and kidney) ischemic necrosis. It is a potent vasoconstrictor of the pulmonary circulation and should be used with caution in patients with pulmonary hypertension.

Dopamine. This is one of the most commonly utilized drugs in the treatment of shock, probably related to its unique dose-dependent pharmacologic effects. Dopamine is the naturally occurring precursor of norepinephrine. When administered in low doses (1 to 3 μg per kilogram per minute), dopamine activates dopaminergic (DA) vasodilatory receptors in the renal, mesenteric, cerebral, and coronary circulations. DA-1 receptors are located on postsynaptic membranes and mediate vasodilation, and presynaptic DA-2 receptors prevent the release of endogenous norepinephrine, thereby potentiating the vasodilating effects in these circulations. In infusion ranges of 3 to 10 μg per kilogram per minute, dopamine activates β_1-adrenergic receptors and increases heart rate, myocardial contractility, and cardiac output. In doses greater than 20 μg per kilogram per minute, dopamine produces vasoconstriction through activation of α-adrenergic receptors in the arteries and veins of most vascular beds. Thus, at the upper infusion ranges, dopamine may distribute blood flow away from the extremities and toward the kidney, gut, heart, and brain. However, it is necessary to administer moderate to large doses to maintain arterial pressure and coronary blood flow, particularly following myocardial infarction. These larger doses oppose the dopaminergically mediated vasodilation in some vascular beds.

Epinephrine. Epinephrine is an endogenous catecholamine that is produced and released primarily from the adrenal medulla. Epinephrine activates myocardial β_1 receptors and vasoconstrictor α receptors in most vessels except in skeletal muscle and coronary vessels, where it activates β_2 receptors when administered in low doses. It increases cardiac output but redistributes blood flow away from the kidney and splanchnic circulations toward skeletal muscle. At low doses (0.005 to 0.02 μg per kilogram per minute in adults), epinephrine primarily stimulates β-adrenergic receptors and produces peripheral vasodilation and increases in heart rate and contractility. As the infusion rate is increased, α-vasoconstrictor effects become more prominent. Epinephrine also has important respiratory effects, with β_2 receptor–mediated bronchodilation and inhibition of mast cell degranulation. Epinephrine is a potent renal artery vasoconstricting agent in humans, even at low doses, and this limits its clinical utility.

Epinephrine is rapidly cleared from the circulation by the liver and kidney and has a half-life of approximately 2 minutes. Metabolism is via the enzymes catechol-O-methyl transferase and monoamine oxidase. Epinephrine is also well absorbed from the tracheobronchial tree, and this agent may be administered via injection through an endotracheal tube during initial resuscitation of patients in cardiac arrest or those in whom venous access is not yet available.

Isoproterenol. Isoproterenol is a synthetic nonselective β-adrenergic agonist that activates primarily vascular β_2 receptors, resulting in vasodilation, and myocardial β_1 receptors, resulting in an increase in heart rate, contractility, and cardiac output. The magnitude of the vasodilator effect of isoproterenol varies in different vascular beds, depending on the density of β_2 receptors and the affinity of the drug for them. The major vasodilator action of isoproterenol is in skeletal muscle beds.

Isoproterenol is _not_ recommended for either cardiogenic or septic shock. In cardiogenic shock, it significantly increases myocardial oxygen demands, and despite the increase in coronary

TABLE 41–5. INITIAL HEMODYNAMIC EFFECTS OF CATECHOLAMINES

Catecholamine	Heart Rate	Arterial Pressure	Cardiac Output	Systemic Resistance
Norepinephrine	(+)	(+ +)	(+)/NC	(+ +)
Epinephrine	(+)	(+)	(+)	(+)/NC
Dopamine	(+)	(+)	(+)	(+)/NC
Isoproterenol	(+)	(−)/NC	(+ +)	(−)
Dobutamine	NC/(+)	NC	(+)	NC/(−)

Note: There may be marked regional variations in reactions of different vascular beds to these agents. (+) = increase; (−) = decrease; NC = no change.

blood flow, the ischemic region of the myocardium may be hypoperfused as indicated by increased lactate production. The use of isoproterenol for shock should probably be limited to the temporary treatment of hemodynamically significant, atropine-resistant high-grade AV block until a temporary pacemaker can be inserted. Even in this condition, the potential for inducing vasodilatory hypotension and increasing ventricular arrhythmias must be recognized. In addition, by overcoming hypoxia-induced pulmonary vasoconstriction in some patients, isoproterenol may increase intrapulmonary shunting of blood and result in a worsening of arterial oxygenation.

Dobutamine. This synthetic sympathomimetic amine has predominant β_1 activity. In contrast to dopamine, dobutamine has much less α-vasoconstricting activity but equal positive inotropic effects. Thus, in equal inotropic doses, dobutamine tends to lower the pulmonary capillary wedge pressure while dopamine tends to increase it. Dobutamine is reported to have a lower incidence of cardiac arrhythmias. In experimental models of myocardial infarction, the administration of dobutamine resulted in significantly smaller infarcts than did dopamine, possibly owing to the intracardiac release of norepinephrine produced by dopamine. Thus, especially in the setting of acute myocardial infarction with pump failure but without significant hypotension, dobutamine may be a preferred agent over dopamine for improving cardiac output.

Dobutamine is usually initiated at an infusion rate of 2 to 5 μg per kilogram per minute and titrated to desired hemodynamic effect. The usual infusion rate is 5 to 15 μg per kilogram per minute. The plasma half-life of dobutamine is approximately 2 to 3 minutes in patients with heart failure, with clearance achieved via catechol-O-methyl transferase.

Amrinone. Amrinone is a bipyridine that differs from the sympathomimetic amines and digitalis glycosides with respect to its mechanism of action. Amrinone has phosphodiesterase-inhibiting action that is thought to be (at least in part) the mechanism of its inotropic effect. It possesses positive inotropic and, to a lesser extent, chronotropic actions and is a potent vasodilator. In patients with heart failure, amrinone augments cardiac dP/dt without significant increases in heart rate or blood pressure and reduces left heart filling pressures as well as systemic vascular resistance. There is, however, wide variability in responses of individual patients to amrinone, which makes dosing guidelines difficult to apply.

The recommended dosage for amrinone is an initial intravenous loading dose of 0.75 mg per kilogram over 3 to 5 minutes, followed by a continuous infusion of 5 to 10 μg per kilogram per minute, and a second loading dose of equal magnitude 30 minutes after the initial load. The total daily dose of amrinone should not exceed 10 mg per kilogram.

Amrinone has a relatively long half-life. It is not approved for use in children. Intravenous amrinone has been associated with thrombocytopenia in approximately 4 per cent of patients, and elevation of liver enzymes is reported with long-term infusion. This agent may be considered as an alternative to dobutamine in patients with severe cardiogenic low output syndromes. In addition, the combined use of amrinone and dobutamine or dopamine may be considered in some patients who fail to respond to one agent alone.

Digitalis Glycosides. In general, digitalis glycosides are not indicated as inotropic agents in the management of shock. This is related to the narrow therapeutic-to-toxic ratio and the difficulty in titrating the dose. In addition, the vasoconstrictor actions of digitalis may exacerbate splanchnic ischemic in the shock patient. The one possible role of digitalis in the management of the shock patient may be heart rate control in patients with atrial fibrillation who cannot be successfully electrically cardioverted. However, even in this condition, digitalis must be given very carefully and the patient monitored closely for adverse effects, particularly if there is superimposed renal impairment.

VASODILATOR AGENTS IN SHOCK. While at first glance the administration of vasodilator agents to patients in shock may seem contradictory, the clinical utility of these agents in certain disorders of low cardiac output emphasizes the critical relationship between the contractile state of the ventricle and the afterload against which it must contract. In general, the beneficial effects of vasodilators are to (1) decrease myocardial metabolic demands by decreasing cardiac preload and cardiac size, (2) to decrease ventricular afterload and increase cardiac output without adversely affecting mean perfusion pressure, and (3) to dilate microcirculatory vessels. An important point that must be stressed is that the beneficial effects of vasodilator agents in the therapy of severe heart failure and/or shock depend upon the presence of adequate (e.g., not reduced) cardiac filling pressures and the ability of the ventricle to respond to changes in preload or afterload (e.g., absence of fixed obstructions to cardiac flow, such as is seen with critical aortic stenosis).

Reduction in Preload. Patients in cardiogenic shock may require a high preload and filling pressure to maintain an adequate stroke volume. However, an excessive elevation of filling pressure is detrimental because of pulmonary congestion and increased myocardial oxygen demand. A reduction in myocardial oxygen demand without a significant reduction in stroke volume can be achieved by decreasing ventricular volume and size in patients who have abnormally elevated cardiac filling pressures (e.g., pulmonary capillary wedge pressures of 18 mm Hg or greater) and evidence of pulmonary congestion. Reduction in cardiac size decreases myocardial wall tension, which is a major determinant of myocardial oxygen requirements. Preload may be reduced by the use of diuretic agents or venodilating drugs. The goal of venodilator therapy is to decrease cardiac preload and cardiac size without altering arterial blood pressure. As previously noted, the efficacy of such an approach depends upon the compliance of the ventricle. A reduction in excessively high cardiac preload may be of benefit not only in reducing myocardial oxygen demands, but also in relieving pulmonary venous congestion and pulmonary edema. In some patients with marked increases in preload, in association with marked impairment of contractile performance and borderline hypotension, it may be desirable and necessary to combine a vasodilator agent with an inotropic agent so as to maintain mean arterial pressure within acceptable bounds.

Reduction in Afterload. It is possible to reduce afterload on a failing ventricle without adversely altering mean arterial pressure, by nature of the increase in cardiac output that usually follows the reduction in afterload. However, such an approach requires close hemodynamic monitoring, and systemic hypotension is always a potentially catastrophic side effect of afterload reduction in patients with severely compromised hemodynamic status. During administration of afterload-reducing vasodilators, the systolic arterial pressure should not fall more than 10 mm Hg (unless the patient is being treated for hypertension), and the diastolic arterial pressure (coronary perfusion pressure) should be maintained at or above 60 to 65 mm Hg in most patients. Reduction in ventricular afterload is ideal in the patient with severe heart failure, marked pulmonary venous hypertension with pulmonary edema, and impaired cardiac output but without systemic arterial hypotension of significant degree.

Arteriolar vasodilators are particularly effective in the management of shock due to acute intracardiac left-to-right shunts or regurgitant lesions. Examples of these conditions include acute ventricular septal rupture, acute mitral insufficiency due to papillary muscle rupture, and acute aortic insufficiency due to flail aortic valve leaflet complicating bacterial endocarditis. By acutely reducing impedance to ventricular ejection, nitroprusside may limit the degree of left-to-right shunt in the setting of a septal defect or the degree of mitral insufficiency or aortic insufficiency by reducing resistance to ventricular ejection. However, this effect is frequently achieved at the expense of an increase in heart rate due to unloading of arterial baroreceptors by this agent.

Microcirculatory Vasodilation. In some patients, despite prolonged administration of dopamine or norepinephrine, tissue perfusion is not improved. The reason may be that extensive myocardial damage has occurred. It is also possible that constriction of microcirculatory vessels may prevent perfusion of exchange capillaries.

Nitroprusside. Nitroprusside is a cyanide-containing, direct-acting, smooth muscle–vasodilating agent that causes relaxation of both arteries and veins. It is the classic "balanced" vasodilator, with effects on both capacitance and resistance vessels. The mode of action of nitroprusside is believed to involve activation of soluble guanylate cyclase with consequent elevation of cGMP in vascular smooth muscle cells, leading to activation of cGMP-dependent protein kinase activity. It does not depend upon the sympathetic nervous system or adrenergic receptors. Its onset of action is within seconds of administration, and its duration of effect is 1 to 3 minutes. Nitroprusside can be initiated as an intravenous infusion at approximately 10 μg per minute, with the rate increased every 5 to 10 minutes by 10 μg per minute increments until the desired hemodynamic effect is achieved.

In the setting of power failure following myocardial infarction, nitroprusside should be administered only to patients who are instrumented with indwelling systemic and pulmonary arterial catheters, as the clinician needs to follow arterial and cardiac filling pressures closely during infusion of this very potent vasodilator.

The principal complications associated with nitroprusside infusion include the possibility of hypotension, thiocyanate/cyanide toxicity with prolonged (≥72 hour) infusions of high doses, and a reduction in arterial oxygen tension due to pulmonary vascular vasodilating effects and consequent increase in ventilation-perfusion mismatching.

Nitroglycerin. This is also a very effective vasodilator with predominant effects on the venous capacitance vessels and lesser effects on arteriolar resistance vessels. When therapy is initiated, nitroglycerin can be started as an intravenous infusion of 10 μg per minute, then titrated upward in 10 μg per minute increments every 3 to 5 minutes as indicated by hemodynamics. Nitroglycerin is particularly effective in the management of acute pulmonary edema complicating myocardial infarction. Adverse side effects include headache, hypotension, and occasional nausea and vomiting.

MECHANICAL AND ARTIFICIAL CARDIOPULMONARY ASSISTANCE IN SHOCK. Recent advances have made available various mechanical support devices for the temporary management of patients with medically refractory shock of various etiologies. While clinical experience is limited and controlled clinical trials often are not available, consideration of such devices is appropriate in certain subgroups of patients.

Intra-aortic Balloon Counterpulsation. The intra-aortic balloon pump (IABP) has been used for 15 years in the management of certain types of cardiogenic shock. Currently, the device can be inserted percutaneously through a femoral artery and advanced under fluoroscopic guidance to the thoracic aorta just distal to the left subclavian artery. The balloon is mechanically inflated with carbon dioxide or helium during diastole and rapidly deflated at the onset of ventricular systole. The primary effects of the balloon are therefore (1) an increase in diastolic aortic root (coronary perfusion) pressure, and (2) a mechanical reduction in aortic root blood pressure and volume (impedance) at the onset of systole. The desired hemodynamic effects of the intra-aortic balloon pump are an increase in coronary perfusion pressure, a reduction in ventricular afterload, an increase in forward cardiac ejection fraction, and a reduction in left-to-right or backward cardiac flow.

The IABP is most useful in the management of patients with cardiogenic shock due to acute ventricular septal rupture or acute papillary muscle rupture or dysfunction with mitral insufficiency. In contrast to similar afterload-reducing effects achieved with nitroprusside, the IABP can reduce impedance to ventricular ejection without causing an increase in heart rate (myocardial oxygen demand). At the same time, the mechanical increase in peak augmented diastolic arterial pressure provides an increase in myocardial oxygen supply. The IABP may also be of temporary benefit in patients with ischemia-induced ventricular depression in the setting of high-grade coronary artery lesions, until revascularization can be achieved (i.e., coronary angioplasty or coronary artery bypass surgery) or following cardiopulmonary bypass.

The IABP should be considered only a temporary support device and should be used only in patients who have a correctable cardiac lesion or reasonable likelihood of recovery from an acute cardiac insult. Despite optimal technique, a major complication rate of approximately 10 to 30 per cent is reported with the device, most notably secondary to distal limb ischemia, vascular damage, or infection. The IABP is contraindicated in patients with aortic insufficiency, severe peripheral vascular disease, or inability to tolerate systemic anticoagulation. The IABP may be a useful support device for patients undergoing major surgery (cardiac or otherwise) in the presence of severe impairment of cardiac function.

Cardiac Assist Devices and Artificial Heart. Significant progress has been made over the past 33 years since the first heart-lung machine was used in 1957 to support a patient with cardiogenic shock following acute myocardial infarction. In selected patients with refractory cardiogenic shock, external left and/or right cardiac assist devices have been used to "bridge" patients to cardiac transplant or permit patient survival for a long enough period to allow recovery of intrinsic myocardial function (e.g., in certain patients with severe inflammatory myocarditis). These assist devices require surgical thoracotomy for insertion of large vascular conduits involving the great vessels or the atria and ventricles themselves. Major complications including infection, bleeding, and thrombosis with systemic embolization have been reported with these devices. However, they have been successfully used as a bridge to successful cardiac transplantation in selected patients.

Implantable mechanical heart devices have been reported in a small number of patients, but no long-term success has been achieved and major complications are associated with these devices. Implantable artificial hearts have been utilized for up to 243 days in patients awaiting cardiac transplantation.

Extracorporeal Membrane Oxygenator and Bedside Cardiopulmonary Bypass. Additional recent experience has been reported with emergent bedside initiation of full cardiopulmonary bypass via percutaneous femoral arterial and venous approaches, utilizing a portable cardiopulmonary bypass machine with membrane oxygenator. Limited experience has been reported with this technique in patients with refractory shock or cardiac arrest.

NUTRITIONAL SUPPORT OF THE SHOCK PATIENT

A frequently overlooked but extremely important aspect of the care of the shock patient is nutritional support. In many cases, wound healing, tissue repair, weaning from ventilator support, and therefore long-term survival may be adversely influenced by failure to appreciate the metabolic stresses of the shock state and to provide adequate nutritional support during the early as well as later phases of treatment. Time is a crucial element in the nutritional support of the shock patient. The physician must not allow his or her attention to other traditional details of management to prevent or delay attention to this important aspect of the patient's care. In general, most patients developing shock have suffered major metabolic insults and can rapidly develop catabolic states. This is particularly true of the intubated patient or the patient maintained NPO for extended periods of time following resuscitation. In the case of intubation, the placement of an endotracheal tube should routinely be followed by the placement of a nasogastric tube for initial gastric decompression and then conversion to a gastric feeding tube. Potential contraindications to nasogastric tube placement include midline craniofacial and head trauma, suspected or potential esophageal perforation, and known obstruction of the esophagus.

As soon as possible, patients should begin receiving nutritional support via enteral or parenteral routes. Close monitoring should be performed on a routine basis with daily determinations of calorie intake and biweekly determinations of serum albumin, electrolytes, total lymphocyte count, transferrin level, liver function studies, and prothrombin time. Estimations of carbohydrate, protein, and fat requirements should be based upon the patient's nitrogen balance, nature of insult, and associated medical problems. Continuing assessment of vitamin and essential trace metal levels is important in the long-term care of these patients.

Abboud FM, Heistad DD, Mark AL, Schmid PG: Reflex control of the peripheral circulation. Prog Cardiovasc Dis 18:371–403, 1976. *Review of the major factors of autonomic circulatory control operative in both healthy human subjects and under various disease states.*

Altura BM, Lefer AM, Schumer W: Historical perspective of shock. *In* Altura BM, Lefer AM, Schumer W (eds.): Handbook of Shock and Trauma. New York, Raven Press, 1983. *Provides historical review of the development of understanding of pathophysiology and treatment of shock.*

Bernton EW, Long JB, Holaday JW: Opioids and neuropeptides: Mechanisms in circulatory shock. Fed Proc 44:290–299, 1985. *Reviews potential roles of endogenous opioids, thyrotropin-releasing hormone, and other neuropeptides in central cardiovascular regulatory mechanisms during shock.*

Beutler B, Cerami A: Cachectin/tumor necrosis factor: An endogenous mediator of shock and inflammation. Immunol Res 5:281–293, 1986. *Provides a perspective on the biologic role of tumor necrosis factor as a mediator of the cellular toxicity associated with endotoxic shock.*

Bone RC, Fisher CJ, Clemmer TP, et al. and the Methylprednisolone Severe Sepsis Study Group: A controlled clinical trial of high-dose methylprednisolone in the treatment of severe sepsis and septic shock. N Engl J Med 317:653–658, 1987. *Report of a large, prospective, double-blind, placebo-controlled trial of methylprednisolone in management of patients with sepsis and septic shock, showing no benefit of this steroid and an increase in secondary infections in the steroid-treated patients.*

Chaudry IH: Cellular alteration in shock and ischemia and their correction. Physiologist 28:109–117, 1985. *Presents an overview of cellular and subcellular events in shock in a well-organized manner.*

Ellrodt AG: Sepsis and septic shock. Emerg Med Clin North Am 4:809–840, 1986. *Provides well-referenced overview of most important areas in etiology, pathophysiology, and treatment of septic shock.*

Goldberg LI, Rajfer SI: Dopamine receptors: Applications in clinical cardiology. Circulation 72:245–248, 1985. *Reviews the cardiovascular and renal actions of dopamine and emphasizes the unique effects of this agent on dopaminergic receptors.*

Lefer AM: Eicosanoids as mediators of ischemia and shock. Fed Proc 44:275–280, 1985. *Provides an overview of the variety and role of eicosanoids identified in ischemic and circulatory shock and discusses potential pharmacologic modulation of these mediators.*

Lefer AM: Interaction between myocardial depressant factor and vasoactive mediators with ischemia and shock. Am J Physiol 252 (Regulatory Integrative Comp. Physiol. 21):R193–R205, 1987. *This excellent review discusses a variety of vasoactive mediators produced in ischemia and shock states, with particular emphasis on myocardial depressant factor, and reviews new pharmacologic approaches to the blockade of these mediators.*

McSwain NE Jr.: Pneumatic anti-shock garment: State of the art 1988. Ann Emerg Med 17:506–525, 1988. *Provides exhaustive experimental and clinical information on the use of external pneumatic pressure trousers (MAST suit) in the management of hypotension and shock.*

Parrillo JE, Burch C, Shelhamer JH, et al: A circulating myocardial depressant substance in humans with septic shock. J Clin Invest 76:1539–1553, 1985. *Study of the cardiodepressant effect of serum extract from patients with septic shock and myocardial depression.*

Sanders JS, Ferguson DW: Profound sympathoinhibition complicating hypovolemia in humans. Ann Intern Med 111:439–441, 1989. *Reviews the potential mechanisms responsible for paradoxic autonomic response to acute hypovolemic hypotension in humans.*

Shapiro BA, Cane RD: Blood gas monitoring: Yesterday, today, and tomorrow. Crit Care Med 17:573–581, 1989. *Reviews the history of blood gas determination and provides an up-to-date assessment of new monitoring techniques.*

Suffredini AF, Fromm RE, Parker MM, et al.: The cardiovascular response of normal humans to the administration of endotoxin. N Engl J Med 321:280–287, 1989. *Report of careful hemodynamic measurements obtained in normal human subjects following administration of bacterial endotoxin, demonstrating left ventricular systolic depression independent of changes in ventricular volume or systemic vascular resistance.*

Tobin MJ: Respiratory monitoring in the intensive care unit. Am Rev Resp Dis 138:1625–1642, 1988. *Extensive review of recent advances in monitoring ventilation/respiration parameters in the intensive care environment.*

Zimmerman JJ, Dietrich KA: Current perspectives on septic shock. Pediatr Clin North Am 34:131–163, 1987. *Comprehensive overview of pathophysiology of septic shock.*

42 Cardiac Arrhythmias

J. Thomas Bigger, Jr.

Optimal management of cardiac arrhythmias requires knowledge of their (1) mechanism, etiology, and natural history and (2) effect on the hemodynamic state. Before selecting therapy, the physician should thoroughly assess the patient's physical, psychological, and biochemical state. The chosen treatment—whether drugs, devices, or surgery—must be monitored closely for its initial and continued effectiveness and for adverse effects. This chapter discusses mechanisms, electrocardiographic (ECG) recognition, and management of cardiac arrhythmias.

ANATOMIC CONSIDERATIONS

Normal Specialized Impulse-Generating and Conducting System

SINUS NODE. The sinus node is situated at the junction between the superior vena cava and the right atrium. The node surrounds a large central artery arising from the right (55 per cent) or left (45 per cent) circumflex coronary artery. Two types of special muscle fibers are found in the node: P (pacemaker) and T (transitional) cells. P cells are small (diameter of 5 to 10 μ) ovoid or stellate cells that have a low density of mitochondria, sarcoplasmic reticulum, and myofibrils, suggesting a lack of contractile function. P cells occur in tight clusters and attach only to other P cells or T cells; intercellular attachments are sparse, correlating with the slow conduction in the sinus node.

T cells are intermediate in size, structure, and cellular organization between P cells and ordinary atrial myocardium. T cells may attach either to P cells or to working myocardial cells. T cells surround the sinus node and presumably serve both to organize impulses leaving the node and to hinder access of premature ectopic atrial impulses.

INTERNODAL TRACTS. Three internodal tracts connecting the sinus node to the atrioventricular (AV) node have been described: anterior, middle, and posterior. The *anterior internodal tract* also connects to the left atrium via the interatrial bundle of Bachmann. The three internodal tracts are widely separated in the interatrial septum but converge above and behind the AV node.

Internodal tracts contain working atrial cells interspersed with large cells that resemble ventricular Purkinje cells. Because internodal pathways are difficult to trace by serial microscopic sections, some doubt their presence or functional significance. Internodal tracts continue to function in high extracellular K^+ concentrations, a property that has been used to demonstrate their functional continuity and preferential internodal conductivity.

ATRIOVENTRICULAR NODE. The AV node lies beneath the endocardium of the right atrium near the septal leaflet of the tricuspid valve and immediately anterior to the ostium of the coronary sinus. The AV nodal artery usually arises from the right coronary artery. In the central portion of the AV node, the myocytes form tangled swirls with ample interconnections. Ultrastructurally, cells in the mid-AV node resemble the sinus node T cells. Toward the distal end of the AV node, myocytes pallisade into linear arrays as they form the bundle of His.

The region between the ostium of the coronary sinus and the posterior margin of the AV node is richly supplied by cholinergic ganglia. Retronodal chemoreceptors may trigger vagal reflexes during ischemia of the posterior wall of the heart. These reflexes can produce marked bradycardia, peripheral vasodilatation, nausea, sweating, and salivation.

HIS-PURKINJE SYSTEM. The AV bundle (bundle of His) is a thick, cable-like structure about 15 mm in length that emerges from the anterior, inferior border of the AV node (Fig. 42–1). The bundle of His penetrates the central fibrous body and courses to the crest of the muscular interventricular septum, where it divides into left and right bundle branches. The His bundle is the only normal route for AV conduction. Damage to the AV bundle can cause AV conduction delay or block. The His bundle is generously supplied with arterial blood from the anterior and posterior descending coronary arteries; therefore, extensive coronary disease is required to produce ischemic damage.

The left bundle branch is a broad sheet of fibers that cascade under the noncoronary cusp of the aortic valve and down the left side of the interventricular septum. The left bundle branch connects first with myocardium in the septum and near the papillary muscles, causing early activation of these regions.

The right bundle branch emerges from the bundle of His and courses down the right side of the interventricular septum to make its first connections with ventricular myocardium near the base of the anterior papillary muscle. From here, peripheral branches spread up the interventricular septum and the free wall of the right ventricle.

The terminal Purkinje fibers form extensive interconnected lacy networks on the endocardium of both ventricles. In human hearts, no Purkinje fibers are found in the outer two thirds of the ventricular walls. Purkinje cells are large—15 to 30 mm in diameter and 20 to 100 mm in length—with a round, centrally located nucleus in the cell. Purkinje fibers contain fewer myofibrils and mitochondria than working ventricular muscle. External to the sarcolemmal basement membrane is a thick surface coat of negatively charged glycoproteins that function in Ca^{2+} binding

FIGURE 42–1. The anatomy and characteristic action potentials of the specialized impulse-generating and conducting system of the heart. *A*, A diagram of the conduction system of the heart. SAN = Sinoatrial node; AVN = atrioventricular node; HB = bundle of His; RBB = right bundle branch; LBB = left bundle branch; PF = Purkinje fiber. *B*, Typical action potentials from the sinus node (SN), atrium (AT), atrioventricular node (AVN), Purkinje fiber (PF), and ventricular muscle (VM). *C*, Relationship of deflections in the His bundle (HB) electrogram to depolarization of the sites shown in *B* and to the electrocardiographic deflections. Depolarization of the lower atrial septum (A), bundle of His (H), and ventricular septum (V) is recorded in the bipolar His bundle electrogram. The H deflection partitions the PR interval into two subintervals: the AH interval, representing atrioventricular nodal conduction, and the HV interval, which measures conduction to the His-Purkinje system. (From Braunwald E: Heart Disease: A Textbook of Cardiovascular Medicine. Philadelphia, W. B. Saunders Company, 1980.)

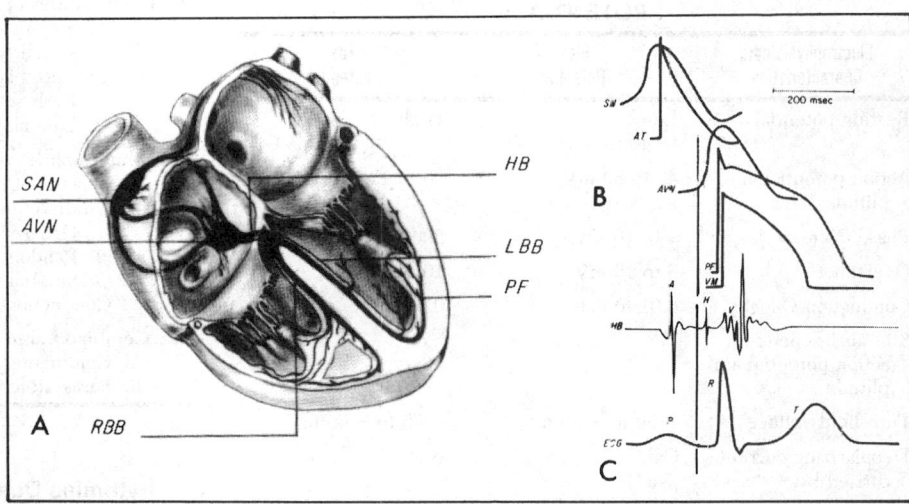

and exchange. Intercalated disks are well developed in Purkinje fibers and provide low-resistance pathways for current flow and for diffusion of ions and small molecules.

Function of the Specialized Impulse-Generating and Conducting System

The normal heartbeat begins in the sinus node and spreads slowly through perinodal fibers to reach specialized atrial tracts and ordinary atrial muscle (Fig. 42–1). Specialized atrial tracts transmit the cardiac impulse rapidly from the sinus node to the AV node and to the left atrium. The cardiac impulse slows dramatically in the AV node, accounting for most of the PR interval in the ECG. Conduction accelerates tremendously in the His bundle, and excitation of the bundle branches and peripheral Purkinje fibers occurs with blazing speed. The great mass of ordinary ventricular muscle is activated almost simultaneously over much of its endocardial surface. Then activation spreads to the epicardium to complete the cardiac excitation cycle.

BRIEF REVIEW OF CARDIAC CELLULAR ELECTROPHYSIOLOGY

RESTING POTENTIAL. The sarcolemma of cardiac cells is a hydrophobic phospholipid bilayer. Protein molecules that cross the entire width of the membrane provide hydrophilic channels and permit hydrated cations or anions to cross the sarcolemma. Ion-selective channels and energy-dependent ion pumping establish transmembrane gradients of Na^+ and K^+ that determine the resting voltage difference of about -80 to -90 mV across the sarcolemma, the *resting transmembrane voltage* (Vm).

ACTION POTENTIALS. When cardiac cells activate, a complex sequence of voltage changes occurs as a function of time and membrane ionic currents. Figure 42–2 diagrams the four phases of a Purkinje fiber *action potential*. Sinus and AV nodal cells have a slowly rising phase 0 and lack distinct phases 1, 2, and 3 (see Fig. 42–1). During phase 4, many cells have a steady transmembrane voltage, but automatic fibers in the sinus node and His-Purkinje system spontaneously depolarize and can initiate impulses that propagate to the rest of the heart.

OVERDRIVE SUPPRESSION. In the normal heart, P cells in the sinus node depolarize and overdrive subsidiary pacemaker cells in the atrial specialized tracts, coronary sinus region, or His-Purkinje system. The faster subsidiary pacemakers are overdriven, the more Na^+ centers the cell per unit of time. As the $[Na]_i$ increases, the activity of the Na^+/K^+ exchange pump becomes more electrogenic; i.e., the ratio of Na^+ out to K^+ in increases, hyperpolarizing the cell and counteracting pacemaker activity. If the dominant pacemaker stops, there is a pause in rhythm. However, as the $[Na]_i$ is pumped out, outward pump current declines until spontaneous depolarization resumes. As the pump

current declines, the firing rate in the subsidiary pacemaker increases gradually—the "warm-up" phenomenon.

FAST AND SLOW RESPONSES. Cardiac action potentials are classified as *fast* or *slow* responses (Table 42–1). The *fast response* (Fig. 42–3) is generated by intense inward i_{Na}, has a large, fast-rising phase 0, propagates rapidly, and has a large safety factor for conduction. Working myocardial cells in the atria, ventricles, and Purkinje fibers have fast responses. The *slow response* has a slowly rising phase 0, propagates slowly, and has a low safety factor for conduction (Fig. 42–3). Cells in the sinus node, pectinate muscles, AV node, and AV rings have slow responses. Depolarization in slow response fibers is due to slow inward current (i_{si}) carried by Ca^{2+} and, to a lesser extent, Na^+ ions.

REFRACTORINESS. Refractoriness is involved in the pathogenesis of many arrhythmias and in the action of antiarrhythmic drugs. The effective refractory period (ERP), the minimum interval between two propagating responses, is closely linked to

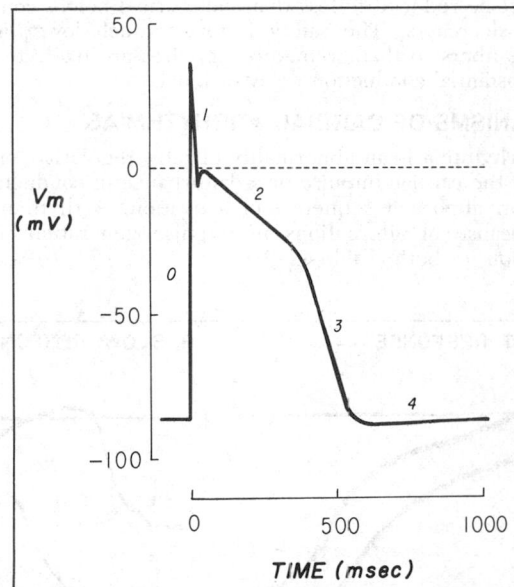

FIGURE 42–2. The cardiac action potential of a Purkinje fiber has five distinct phases: rapid depolarization (0), early repolarization (1), plateau (2), rapid repolarization (3), and diastole (4). (From Braunwald E: Heart Disease: A Textbook of Cardiovascular Medicine. Philadelphia, W. B. Saunders Company, 1980.)

TABLE 42–1. COMPARISON OF SLOW AND FAST ACTION POTENTIALS

Electrophysiologic Characteristics	Slow Potential	Fast Potential
Resting potential	Low (−40 to −70 mV)	High (−75 to −90 mV)
Action potential amplitude	40 to 80 mV	90 to 120 mV
Phase 0 Vmax	1 to 10 V/sec	200 to 800 V/sec
Overshoot	0 to 15 mV	10 to 30 mV
Conduction velocity	0.01 to 0.1 m/sec	0.5 to 3.0 m/sec
Stimulus-dependent action potential amplitude	Yes	No
Threshold voltage	−50 to −30 mV	−75 to −65 mV
Depolarizing current carried by	Ca^{2+} (Na^+)	Na^+
Ionic current activates	Slow (0.5 msec)	Fast (10 to 20 msec)
Ionic current inactivates	Slow (0.5 msec)	Fast (50 to 100 msec)
Channel blocked by	Mn^{2+}, LA^{3+}, verapamil diltiazem, nifedipine	Tetrodotoxin, class 1 antiarrhythmics

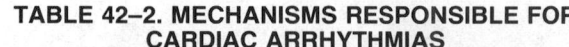

TABLE 42–2. MECHANISMS RESPONSIBLE FOR CARDIAC ARRHYTHMIAS

I. **Abnormalities of impulse generation**
   A. Alterations of normal automaticity
   B. Abnormal automaticity
   C. Triggered activity
      1. Early afterdepolarizations
      2. Late afterdepolarizations

II. **Abnormalities of impulse conduction**
   A. Slowing of conduction and block
   B. Unidirectional block and reentry
      1. Ordered reentry
      2. Random reentry
      3. Summation and inhibition
   C. Conduction block, electrotonus, and reflection

III. **Combined abnormalities of impulse generation and conduction**
   A. Conduction showed by phase 4 depolarization
   B. Parasystole

action potential duration (APD) in fast-response fibers because recovery from inactivation in the Na^+ channel closely parallels repolarization. However, in sinus and AV nodal cells (slow responses), refractoriness can outlast full repolarization so that the ERP is much longer than the APD.

RESPONSIVENESS AND CONDUCTION. The term *membrane responsiveness* applies to the response of a cardiac fiber to a stimulus. Changes in the maximum rate of depolarization during phase 0 (max) provide an index of changes in availability of the Na^+ current. In cardiac Purkinje fibers and other fast-response fibers, $\dot{V}_{max}$ is strongly dependent on Vm at the instant of excitation; as soon as the fiber is fully repolarized, it is fully responsive. In slow-response fibers, responsiveness does not return until well after repolarization is complete. There is a considerable safety factor for conduction in fast-response fibers; $\dot{V}_{max}$ must be reduced to less than half normal before conduction velocity decreases. The safety factor is much lower in slow-response fibers so that premature impulses are likely to experience substantial conduction delay or block.

MECHANISMS OF CARDIAC ARRHYTHMIAS

An arrhythmia is an abnormality of rate, regularity, or site of origin of the cardiac impulse or a disturbance in conduction that causes an abnormal sequence of activation. Arrhythmias may arise because of alternations in impulse generation, impulse conduction, or both (Table 42–2).

Arrhythmias Due to Abnormalities of Impulse Generation

Many arrhythmias arise because of either depressed or enhanced normal automaticity. Abnormal automaticity and triggered activity also are important mechanisms for arrhythmogenesis.

ALTERED NORMAL AUTOMATICITY. Only a few cardiac cell types develop normal automaticity: sinus node, internodal tracts, fibers near the ostium of the coronary sinus, distal AV node, and the His-Purkinje system.

Sinus Node. The rate of firing in the sinus node can be altered by autonomic activity or intrinsic disease. Increased vagal activity can slow or stop sinus node pacemakers by increasing membrane K^+ conductance of P cells. Increased sympathetic nerve traffic to the sinus node causes sinus tachycardia.

Purkinje Fibers. Augmented automaticity due to increased sympathetic nerve activity in the His-Purkinje system is a common cause of human arrhythmias. AV junctional pacemakers can fire faster than a normal sinus node because of selective traffic on sympathetic nerves, local release of catecholamines, or enhanced responsiveness of β-adrenergic receptors. Also, vagal and sympathetic activity can increase together; the vagus slows the sinus rate and AV conduction while sympathetic activity increases the firing rate in the His-Purkinje system.

In diseased hearts, automaticity in the His-Purkinje system may become reduced. In the sick sinus syndrome, it is typical for the ventricular escape pacemakers to be depressed, producing long pauses when the sinus node pacemaker fails. In AV block due to bundle branch disease, ventricular pacemakers also may be abnormally slow.

Abnormal Impulse Generation

Abnormal automaticity or triggered activity can generate impulses even in fibers that are incapable of normal automaticity, e.g., ordinary atrial or ventricular muscle cells.

ABNORMAL AUTOMATICITY. Abnormal automaticity refers to spontaneous diastolic depolarization in depolarized cells. Pur-

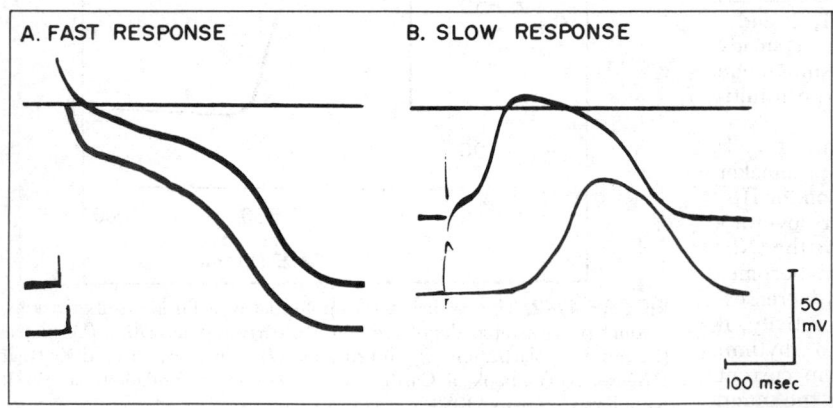

A. FAST RESPONSE   B. SLOW RESPONSE

50 mV

100 msec

FIGURE 42–3. Two types of cardiac action potentials: (*A*) fast action potential, (*B*) slow action potential. (From Wit AL, Rosen MR, Hoffman BF: Electrophysiology and pharmacology of cardiac arrhythmias. II. Relationship of normal and abnormal electrical activity of cardiac fibers to the genesis of arrhythmias. Am Heart J 88:515–524, 1974. With permission of the publisher.)

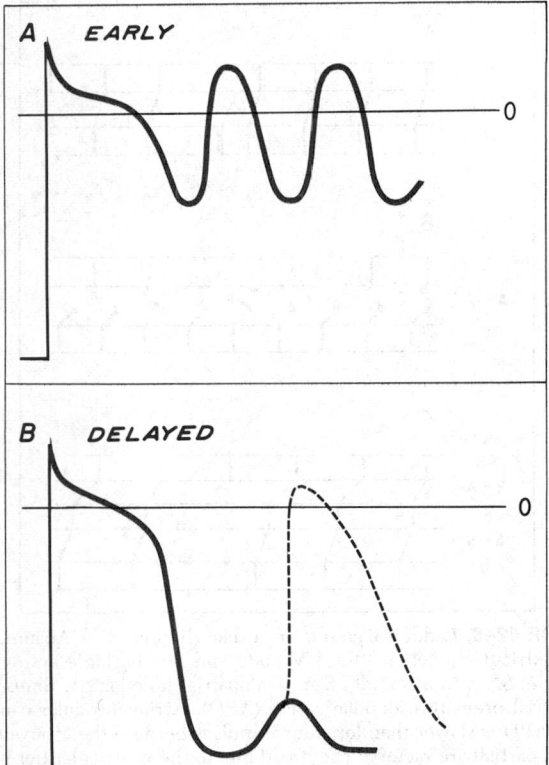

FIGURE 42–4. Afterdepolarizations and triggered activity. *A*, Early afterdepolarization. Repolarization of the Purkinje fiber is interrupted by two secondary depolarizations, which can activate adjacent fibers and cause arrhythmias, e.g., torsades de pointes. *B*, Delayed afterdepolarizations. After full repolarization, the Purkinje fiber depolarizes. If the afterdepolarization reaches threshold voltage, a propagating response can occur. (From Bigger JT: Electrophysiology for the clinician. Eur Heart J 5(Suppl B):1–9, 1984.)

kinje fibers, atrial cells, and ventricular cells can show spontaneous diastolic depolarization and repetitive automatic firing when their resting Vm is reduced to −60 mV or below. Abnormal automaticity is seen in Purkinje fibers depolarized by acute myocardial infarction. Abnormal automaticity and repetitive firing can be evoked in normal atrial or ventricular cells by applying depolarizing current. Abnormal automaticity is not readily suppressed by overdrive pacing.

TRIGGERED ACTIVITY. Repetitive firing in heart muscle can be caused by triggered activity. Triggered activity is *not* a form of automaticity but is capable of producing a sustained tachyarrhythmia. Two primary mechanisms can initiate triggered activity: early afterdepolarizations and delayed afterdepolarizations (Fig. 42–4).

Early Afterdepolarizations. Early afterdepolarizations are secondary depolarizations that occur before repolarization is complete, often from the action potential plateau (Fig. 42–4). Experimentally, early afterdepolarizations have been produced in cardiac Purkinje fibers by stretching or crushing, hypoxia, cooling, low [K]$_o$, high [Ca]$_o$, catecholamines, and chemicals and drugs (such as veratrine, aconitine, quinidine, sotalol, or N-acetyl procainamide). Torsades de pointes in humans is thought to be the counterpart of triggered activity due to early afterdepolarizations.

Delayed Afterdepolarizations. A delayed afterdepolarization is a secondary depolarization occurring after full repolarization has been achieved which is dependent on the previous action potential (Fig. 42–4). Delayed afterdepolarizations can reach threshold and cause a single premature depolarization or trigger a series of impulses. Delayed afterdepolarizations can be induced by digitalis, easily in the His-Purkinje system and with more difficulty in specialized atrial or ordinary ventricular cells. Some of the digitalis-induced ventricular tachycardias in humans behave like triggered activity produced by digitalis in isolated tissue preparations. In the atria, coronary sinus, and mitral valve, delayed

afterdepolarizations and triggered activity can be caused by catecholamines.

Arrhythmias Caused by Abnormalities of Impulse Conduction

Reentry seems to be a common cause of cardiac arrhythmias in humans, e.g., paroxysmal supraventricular tachycardia and constantly coupled ventricular premature complexes. Reentrant arrhythmias usually are started by an initiating premature complex; i.e., they are self-sustained but are not self-initiated. To start reentry, one-way conduction block must occur and there must be an anatomic or functional "barrier" that forms a circuit (Fig. 42–5). Also, the path length of the reentrant circuit must be greater than the wavelength of the cardiac impulse (wavelength = conduction velocity × refractory period). For reentry to occur, conduction must be very slow, refractoriness very short, or both. Reentry has been demonstrated in anatomic loops (e.g., rings of Purkinje fibers) or anatomic obstacles (e.g., scars). Reentry occurring in unbranched bundles or sheets of cardiac muscle has been given specialized names, e.g., reflection or leading-edge reentry.

Reentry can be subdivided into random and ordered forms. In random reentry, the cardiac impulse conducts over circuits that change their location and size as a function of time, e.g., atrial and ventricular fibrillation. In ordered reentry, the circuit for reentrant activity is relatively constant.

LEADING-EDGE REENTRY. Reentrant excitation can be initiated in vitro by premature stimulation in small, thin pieces of normal atrium that contain no anatomic obstacles or loops of tissue. Conduction is slowed because activation occurs when the tissue is partially refractory. Block occurs in some regions because of local differences in refractory periods. The pathway for reentrant activity can stabilize and be sustained.

Cranefield PF: The Conduction of the Cardiac Impulse. Mount Kisco, N.Y., Futura Publishing Company, 1975. *A monograph that reviews the concepts of fast and slow action potentials and their role in the genesis of reentrant cardiac arrhythmias.*

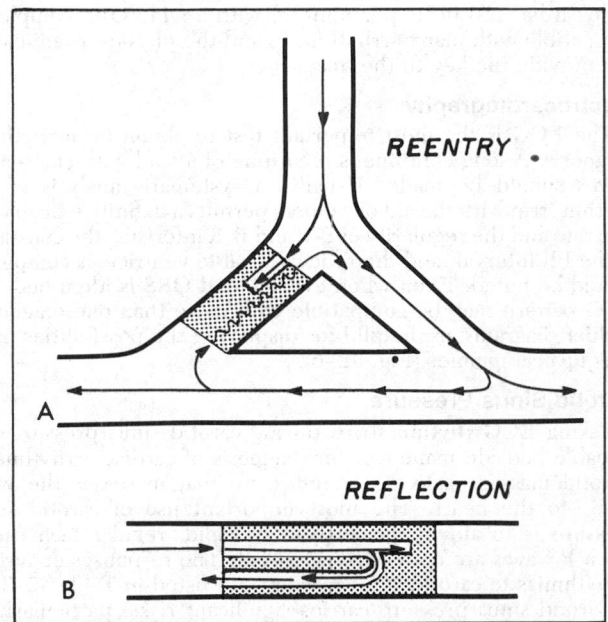

FIGURE 42–5. Two models of reentry according to Schmitt and Erlanger. *A*, Diagram showing a loop of cardiac fibers that could represent either a terminal branch of a Purkinje fiber ending on ventricular muscle or a loop of the Purkinje syncytium. In this case, one-way block and slow conduction permit reentry. *B*, A linear strand of cardiac muscle showing a depolarized zone in a portion of its cross-section. One-way block occurs in the depolarized zone, permitting the propagating impulse to reflect back in the direction from which it came. (From Braunwald E: Heart Disease: A Textbook of Cardiovascular Medicine. Philadelphia, W. B. Saunders Company, 1980.)

Fozzard HA, Haber E, Jennings RB, et al. (eds.): The Heart and Cardiovascular System, Scientific Foundations. New York, Raven Press, 1986. *The section of cardiac electrophysiology and arrhythmias contains detailed reviews of current knowledge and thought on the electrophysiology of the heart, the genesis of cardiac arrhythmias, and the epidemiology of human arrhythmias. Other sections contain excellent reviews of the embryology, anatomy, and pathology of the heart. Profusely illustrated and exhaustively referenced.*

Hackel DB: Anatomy and pathology of the cardiac conducting system. *In* Edwards JE, Lev M, Abell MA (eds.): The Heart. Baltimore, Williams & Wilkins Company, 1974, pp 232–247. *A concise description of the normal anatomy and pathology of the conduction system.*

Noble D: The Initiation of the Heartbeat. London, Oxford University Press, 1979. *An account of cardiac electrophysiology for medical students and clinicians who are unfamiliar with electronics and mathematics. Even the most difficult concepts of cardiac excitation are explained clearly and concisely. Selective references to the classic papers in electrophysiology.*

Noble D: The surprising heart: A review of recent progress in cardiac electrophysiology. J Physiol 353:1–50, 1984. *A detailed review of cellular electrophysiology of the heart. Amply referenced.*

DIAGNOSTIC APPROACHES TO CARDIAC ARRHYTHMIAS

The history, physical examination, 12-lead electrocardiogram, 24-hour continuous electrocardiographic recordings, exercise tests, intermittent electrocardiographic recordings, and clinical electrophysiologic studies are the primary tools used in the diagnosis of cardiac arrhythmias. Decisions about treatment may require other laboratory studies to define better the etiology of heart disease, other aspects of the functional status of the heart, e.g., left ventricular function or perfusion, or function of other organ systems.

History and Physical Examination

The primary purposes of the history are (1) to formulate a hypothesis about the presence and type of arrhythmia, (2) to detect factors that trigger the onset of the arrhythmia or intensify arrhythmic symptoms, (3) to establish the frequency and pattern of occurrence of the arrhythmia, and (4) to establish the functional consequences of the arrhythmia.

The physical examination provides information about the presence and type of heart disease and the degree of cardiac impairment. The physical examination in conjunction with the ECG can aid in the differential diagnosis of arrhythmias. A regular tachycardia, 150 beats per minute, with a wide QRS complex is compatible with many arrhythmias, and the physical examination can provide the key to the diagnosis.

Electrocardiography

The ECG is the most important test to obtain for arrhythmia diagnosis. A long continuous recording of a lead with clear-cut P waves should be made. Usually, a systematic analysis of the rhythm strip with the aid of calipers permits a definitive diagnosis. The rate and the regularity of P-P and R-R intervals, the constancy of the PR interval, and the ratio of atrial to ventricular complexes should be noted. Even when every P and QRS is identified, the ECG pattern may be compatible with more than one diagnosis. Ladder diagrams are helpful for displaying the possibilities in an unequivocal manner (Fig. 42–6).

Carotid Sinus Pressure

Taking ECG rhythm strips during carotid sinus pressure is a valuable bedside maneuver for diagnosis of cardiac arrhythmias. Carotid massage activates a reflex arc that increases the vagal traffic to the heart. The most important use of carotid sinus pressure is to aid in the analysis of rapid, regular tachycardia when P waves are not clearly apparent. The responses of various arrhythmias to carotid sinus massage are listed in Table 42–3.

Carotid sinus pressure carries significant risks, particularly in older patients, i.e., syncope, convulsions, stroke, prolonged asystole, or ventricular tachyarrhythmias. In patients with digitalis toxicity, carotid sinus pressure may provoke malignant ventricular arrhythmias.

Special Procedures to Detect Atrial Activation

All of the P waves must be identified to make rhythm analysis reliable. P waves can be detected using special lead placement, e.g., the Lewis lead, esophageal electrograms, or transvenous bipolar catheter electrodes.

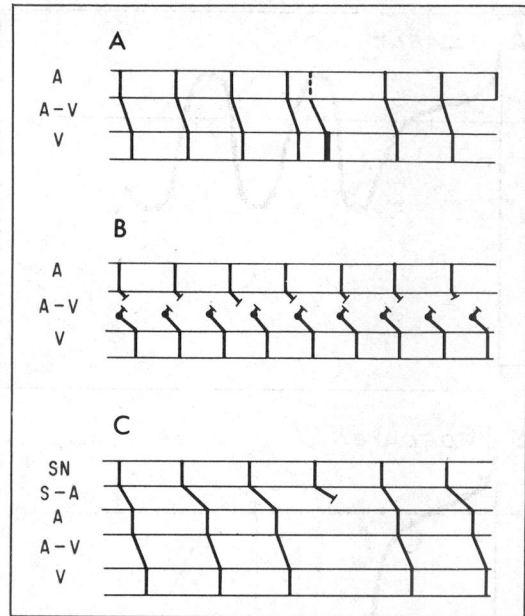

FIGURE 42–6. Ladder diagrams of cardiac rhythm. A = Atrium; A-V = atrioventricular junction (the A-V node and His-Purkinje system); V = ventricle; SN = sinus node; S-A = sinoatrial junction. *A,* Sinus rhythm with atrial premature depolarization (APD). Atrioventricular conduction of the APD is slower than for sinus impulses because the atrioventricular node is partially refractory. The broad line in the ventricular tier indicates aberrant ventricular conduction of the APD, which occurs because the premature impulse arrives during the relative refractory period of the His-Purkinje system. *B,* Atrioventricular junctional rhythm. The A-V junctional automatic rhythm captures the ventricles but shows retrograde block. The sinus node controls the atria, but the sinus impulse finds the A-V node refractory and is blocked; i.e., there is interference between the sinus and junctional rhythm. *C,* Type I (Wenckebach) sinoatrial block. The sinus impulse travels through the perinodal junctional tissues with increasing delay until block finally occurs. (From Braunwald E: Heart Disease: A Textbook of Cardiovascular Medicine. Philadelphia, W. B. Saunders Company, 1980.)

Ambulatory ECG Recording

In 1961, Holter described the technique of ambulatory ECG recording. A light, portable tape recorder continuously records the ECG for 24 hours while the patient performs his or her usual daily activities and records the activities and symptoms in a diary. The primary indications for ambulatory ECG recordings are listed in Table 42–4.

INTERMITTENT RECORDERS. When symptoms occur only occasionally, intermittent recorders permit monitoring lasting from a few days to many weeks even though the ECG recordings are brief (seconds to minutes). These recorders may be attached to patients continuously or intermittently.

Hard-wired Recorders. Intermittent recorders of the hard-wired type are continuously attached to the patient by electrodes and cables. Patients activate these recorders by pressing a switch. Some units have 40 to 100 seconds of electronic memory and sample the ECG continuously, replacing old data with new. When activated, 30 to 60 seconds of ECG prior to patient activation are recorded. Data are retrieved from hard-wired systems either by direct playback or by telephonic transmission.

Intermittently Attached Recorders, Telephonic Transmission. These devices are typically about the size and shape of a radio-paging unit. The patient applies ECG leads when symptoms occur. Units with memory can store one to three ECG samples for subsequent telephone transmission. Commercial services provide immediate evaluation of the ECG transmission. Transmissions are acted on in accordance with the instructions of the patient's physician.

Intracardiac Recording and Stimulation *(Endocardial Electrical Stimulation)*

Over the past 25 years, intracardiac recording and stimulation have developed as a diagnostic and therapeutic tool for the

TABLE 42–3. EFFECT OF CAROTID SINUS PRESSURE ON TACHYARRHYTHMIAS

Arrhythmia	Response to Carotid Sinus Pressure
Sinus tachycardia	1. Gradual slowing during massage, gradual speeding after massage
Paroxysmal supraventricular tachycardia (AV nodal)	1. No effect, or 2. Abrupt conversion to sinus rhythm, or 3. Slight slowing
Paroxysmal supraventricular tachycardia (anomalous AV connection)	1. No effect, or 2. Abrupt conversion to sinus rhythm, or 3. Slight slowing
Nonparoxysmal supraventricular tachycardia	1. No effect, or 2. AV block, slowed ventricular rate, or 3. Gradual slowing of ventricular rate
Atrial flutter	1. AV, slowed ventricular rate, or 2. No effect, or 3. Atrial fibrillation
Atrial fibrillation	1. AV block, slowed ventricular rate, or 2. No effect
Ventricular tachycardia	1. No effect, or 2. AV dissociation

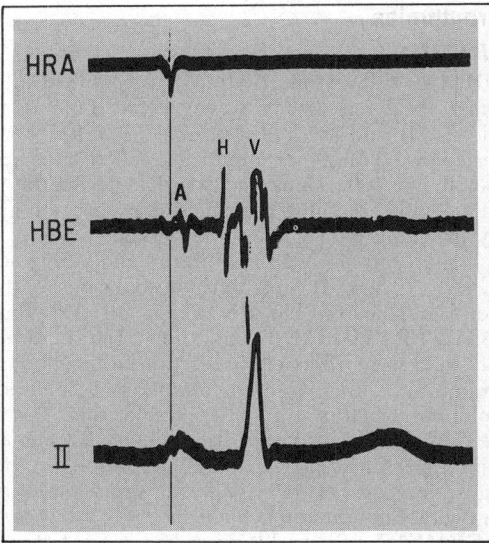

FIGURE 42–7. Intracardiac recordings. A high right atrial bipolar electrogram (HRA), His bundle bipolar electrogram (HBE), and tracing from lead II of the electrocardiogram. A = Atrial depolarization; H = depolarization of the His bundle; V = depolarization of the upper ventricular septum. The PA interval represents intra-atrial conduction time (upper to lower atrium); AH represents atrioventricular nodal conduction; and HV represents the His-Purkinje conduction time. The thin vertical line correlates the onset of atrial activation in the three recordings. (From Braunwald E: Heart Disease: A Textbook of Cardiovascular Medicine. Philadelphia, W. B. Saunders Company, 1980.)

management of human cardiac arrhythmias. Local electrical activity can be recorded from the portions of the heart that are electrically silent on the body surface ECG, e.g., sinus node, His bundle, right bundle branch, left bundle branch, selected sites in the right or left ventricle. The sequence and time of activation of atria and ventricles can be mapped, and AV conduction can be partitioned into AV nodal and His-Purkinje components (Fig. 42–7). Recordings from selected sites are used with pacing and programmed stimulation sequences to evaluate automaticity, conduction, refractoriness, and the causes of arrhythmias

TABLE 42–4. INDICATIONS FOR LONG-TERM CONTINUOUS ECG RECORDINGS

I. Detect and quantify arrhythmias or conduction defects in patients with symptoms (e.g., syncope or other central nervous system symptoms, palpitations, or angina pectoris)

II. Quantify arrhythmias, conduction defects, or ischemia in patients with predisposing conditions
  A. Sick sinus syndrome
  B. Pre-excitation syndromes
  C. AV conduction defects
  D. Pacemaker malfunction
  E. Mitral value prolapse
  F. Long QT syndrome
  G. After myocardial infarction
  H. Angina pectoris
  I. Hypertrophic or dilated cardiomyopathy
  J. Heart failure

III. Evaluate activity
  A. To detect exercise-related arrhythmias or conduction defects
  B. To detect ischemia during activity

IV. Evaluate therapy
  A. Antiarrhythmic drug treatment
  B. Fad diets
  C. Drugs with cardiac adverse effects
  D. Pacemakers
  E. Automatic implantable cardioverter/defibrillator
  F. Surgery
    1. Ischemia or arrhythmias after coronary artery bypass graft surgery
    2. Pre-excitation after division of anomalous AV connection
    3. AV conduction after surgical division or catheter ablation of the His bundle

in intact man. These techniques not only have enhanced our understanding of arrhythmias and conduction defects but also have improved our ability to select and evaluate therapy. Some of the major clinical uses of electrophysiologic studies are listed in Table 42–5.

Bigger JT Jr, Reiffel JA, Coromilas J: Ambulatory Electrocardiography. In Platia EV (ed.): Nonpharmacologic Management of Cardiac Arrhythmias. Philadelphia, J.B. Lippincott Company, 1986, pp 36–61. *A comprehensive review of the technology, indications, and clinical uses of ambulatory electrocardiography. Liberally illustrated and referenced.*

Horowitz LN, Josephson ME, Kastor JA: Intracardiac electrophysiologic studies as a method for the optimization of drug therapy in chronic ventricular arrhythmias. Prog Cardiovasc Dis 23:81, 1980. *Gives the details of electrophysiologic methods for evaluating drug therapy of malignant ventricular arrhythmias.*

Josephson ME, Seides SF: Clinical Cardiac Electrophysiology: Techniques and Interpretations. Philadelphia, Lea & Febiger, 1979. *A detailed description of the techniques of clinical electrophysiology and the interpretation of the findings. Intended for the internist and clinical cardiologist without an extensive background in cardiac electrophysiology.*

Morganroth J: Ambulatory Holter electrocardiography: Choice of technologies and clinical uses. Ann Intern Med 102:73, 1985. *A concise review of the current status of ambulatory electrocardiography.*

Wenger NK, Mock MB, Ringqvist I (eds.): Ambulatory Electrocardiographic Recording. Chicago, Year Book Medical Publishers, Inc., 1981. *Manuscripts from a workshop held at the National Heart, Lung, and Blood Institute. The topics of methodology, recording and analysis systems, quality control, and clinical, epidemiologic, and research applications are discussed thoroughly.*

SPECIFIC CARDIAC ARRHYTHMIAS

Clinically, cardiac arrhythmias are classified by their presumed site of origin, i.e., atrial, AV junctional, or ventricular, and as premature complexes, bradycardia, or tachycardia. It would be desirable to use the precise mechanism to classify clinical arrhythmias, but this is impossible because we do not know the precise mechanism of many cardiac arrhythmias. For some arrhythmias, e.g., the ventricular arrhythmias, prognostic significance can be assigned with reasonable precision. When this is the case, a prognostic classification is useful for guiding decisions about management. In this section, we use a classification based on the site of origin and rate as the framework within which to discuss the definition, pathophysiology, ECG diagnosis, significance, and management of each arrhythmia. The emergency and chronic treatments of cardiac arrhythmias are outlined in Tables 42–6 and 42–7.

Atrial Arrhythmias

SINUS RHYTHM

ECG DIAGNOSIS. Sinus rhythm is recognized in the ECG by a normal atrial rate and P wave vector, i.e., an upright P wave in leads III and aV_f and a normal PR interval. In adults, sinus rates below 60 or 50 per minute are called sinus bradycardia and those above 100, sinus tachycardia. Heart rate changes synchronized with breathing are called sinus arrhythmia and are caused by changing parasympathetic nervous activity. Sinus arrhythmia is more pronounced in children and young adults than in the elderly. Marked sinus arrhythmia can be difficult to distinguish from sinoatrial block or ectopic atrial rhythms.

CLINICAL FEATURES. Resting heart rate in sinus rhythm varies with age: from 130 to 160 per minute in infants to 50 to 100 per minute in adults. Gender, temperature, emotion, effort, and neurohumoral factors also influence sinus rate. The maximum heart rate during exercise varies from almost 200 per minute in healthy young persons to less than 140 per minute in the elderly. Many drugs increase or decrease the sinus rate, usually by interacting with autonomic mechanisms.

MANAGEMENT. Sinus bradycardia is treated only when symptomatic. When acute and symptomatic sinus bradycardia is due to increased vagus nerve activity, heart rate can be increased by intravenous (IV) atropine injection. Rarely, IV isoproterenol infusion may be needed. Chronic symptomatic sinus bradycardia is an indication for an electronic pacemaker. Treatment of sinus tachycardia is based on the cause, usually extracardiac.

ATRIAL PREMATURE COMPLEXES

Atrial premature complexes (APC's) arise in the atria outside the sinus node. APC's occur in normal and diseased hearts. In heart disease, APC's herald sustained atrial arrhythmias such as flutter, fibrillation, or paroxysmal supraventricular tachycardia.

ECG DIAGNOSIS. APC's typically have premature P waves, abnormal P wave morphology, and a prolonged PR interval. Early APC's can be difficult to see because the P wave is superimposed on the T wave. Also, APC's can block in the AV node to produce pauses that can be misinterpreted as a sinus pause or sinoatrial block. Usually, APC's reset the sinus node so that the sum of the pre- and postextrasystolic P-P intervals is less than two sinus cycles (Fig. 42–8). If sinus reset does not occur because the APC occurs late or the perinodal refractory period is long, a compensatory pause occurs. An APC can conduct aberrantly, causing the QRS to be wide and bizarre like a VPC (Fig. 42–9). Aberrant conduction occurs when APC's activate one of the bundle branches, usually the right, during its relative refractory period. Left bundle branch block aberrancy implies an abnormality in the left bundle branch (Fig. 42–9).

MANAGEMENT. The objective of treating APC's is to control symptoms or prevent sustained symptomatic arrhythmias. In

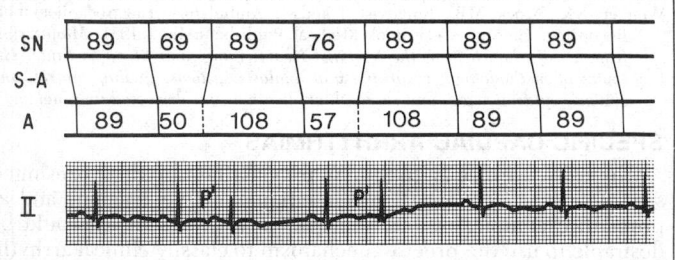

FIGURE 42–8. Atrial premature depolarization (APD). The ladder diagram correlates with the events in the lead II electrocardiographic strip below. SN = Sinus node; S-A = junctional tissues between sinus node and atrium; A = atrium. The time intervals in the ladder diagram are given in msec $\times$ 10^{-1} (e.g., 89 represents 890 msec). The third and fifth P waves are APD's (P'). These P' waves are premature and inverted. The P'R interval is prolonged, and QRS duration is normal. The APD's capture the sinus node and reset it; therefore, the pause following APD's is less than compensatory. (From Braunwald E: Heart Disease: A Textbook of Cardiovascular Medicine. Philadelphia, W. B. Saunders Company, 1980.)

TABLE 42–5. INDICATIONS FOR CLINICAL ELECTROPHYSIOLOGIC STUDIES—ENDOCARDIAL ELECTRICAL STIMULATION

I. To evaluate mechanism, site, and extent of arrhythmia and/or conduction defect
  A. Sick sinus syndrome
  B. Pre-excitation syndrome
  C. Supraventricular tachycardia
  D. Distinguish between supraventricular arrhythmias with aberration and ventricular arrhythmias
  E. Type I AV block with bundle branch block
  F. Type II AV block with normal QRS
  G. Bifascicular block occurring in acute myocardial infarction

II. To search for a cause for syncope
  A. Evaluate sinus node function
  B. Evaluate AV node function
  C. Evaluate function of His-Purkinje system
  D. Evaluate functional characteristics of anomalous AV connections
  E. Provoke arrhythmias
    1. Supraventricular tachycardia
    2. Atrial flutter or fibrillation
    3. Ventricular tachycardia

III. To evaluate therapy
  A. Drug therapy
    1. Prevent inducible arrhythmias
    2. Measure conduction and refractoriness in anomalous AV connections
    3. Evaluate adverse effects
      a. Sinus node function
      b. AV node function
      c. His-Purkinje system
      d. Effect on device function
  B. Surgical therapy
    1. Preoperative endocardial catheter mapping
      a. Location of anomalous AV connections
      b. Location of VT circuit
      c. Need for concomitant pacemaker implantation
    2. Postoperative evaluation
      a. Presence of anomalous AV connections
      b. Arrhythmia inducible
  C. AICD therapy
    1. Preoperative evaluation
      a. Determine that VT or VF is inducible
      b. Determine that VT or VF is drug resistant
      c. Determine need for concomitant pacemaker implantation
    2. Intraoperative evaluation
      a. Determine quality of rate-sensing electrograms
      b. Determine quality of patch electrograms
      c. Determine defibrillation thresholds
      d. Induce clinical arrhythmia to test sensing and termination of ventricular arrhythmias by the AICD
    3. Postoperative evaluation
      a. Induce VT or VF to test the performance of the AICD
      b. Acquaint the patient with the sensation of AICD discharge
  D. Pacemaker therapy
    1. Evaluate condition for suitability for pacemaker therapy
      a. Supraventricular tachycardia due to reciprocation in the AV node
      b. Supraventricular tachycardia due to reciprocation in anomalous AV connections
      c. Reentrant ventricular tachycardia
    2. Determine the information needed to select pacemaker type and parameters

IV. To apply ablation therapy
  A. Posterior septal anomalous AV connections (experimental)
  B. AV node or bundle of His
  C. Ventricular tachycardia (experimental)

AICD = Automatic implantable cardioverter defibrillator; VT = ventricular tachycardia; VF = ventricular fibrillation.

patients with normal hearts, treatment should be focused on general hygienic measures; rest and reducing the use of tobacco, alcohol, or caffeine often reduce the frequency of APC's. In some patients with intermittent, sustained atrial arrhythmias, APC's should be treated with digitalis or class I, II, or IV antiarrhythmic drugs to prevent sustained arrhythmias.

TABLE 42–6. EMERGENCY TREATMENT OF CARDIAC ARRHYTHMIAS

Arrhythmia	Usual First Treatment	Other Effective Treatments	Comments
Atrial fibrillation	Digitalis	Cardioversion; propranolol; acebutolol; verapamil	If hypotensive due to rapid ventricular rate, cardiovert. Avoid propranolol or verapamil in patients with heart failure or hypotension. Avoid digitalis or verapamil in Wolff-Parkinson-White syndrome.
Atrial flutter	Cardioversion	Digitalis; verapamil; propranolol; acebutolol; rapid atrial pacing	Very large doses of digitalis, e.g., 4–6 mg, often are required to achieve AV block in atrial flutter.
Paroxysmal supraventricular tachycardia (AV nodal)	Vagal maneuvers; adenosine; verapamil	Digitalis; propranolol; acebutolol; procainamide	Do not treat wide QRS complex tachycardia with verapamil unless the diagnosis of PSVT is certain. Use cardioversion for PSVT with hypotension.
Paroxysmal supraventricular tachycardia (anomalous AV connection)	Vagal maneuvers; adenosine; verapamil	Cardioversion	If the RP interval suggests anomalous AV connection, an electrophysiologic study should be considered.
Sick sinus syndrome	Pacemaker	Digitalis; pacemaker plus drug with class I antiarrhythmic action	Digitalis usually improves atrial tachyarrhythmias without aggravating sinus bradycardia or AV block.
Nonparoxysmal AV junctional tachycardia	Stop digitalis	Potassium; observation	If the arrhythmia is caused by digitalis toxicity and serum K^+ is low, digitalis should be stopped and potassium should be given.
Sustained ventricular tachycardia	Cardioversion	Lidocaine; procainamide	If VT is well tolerated, intravenous lidocaine or procainamide can be tried.
Ventricular fibrillation	Cardioversion	—	Lidocaine, bretylium tosylate, or propranolol may be helpful when ventricular fibrillation recurs several times immediately after cardioversion.
Digitalis-toxic atrial tachycardia with block or ventricular tachycardia	Lidocaine; phenytoin	Potassium	Avoid cardioversion or bretylium tosylate, which may precipitate ventricular fibrillation.
Digitalis-toxic asystole or AV block	Pacemaker	Fab fragments of digoxin-specific antibodies; dialysis	If associated with malignant hyperkalemia, these rhythms are always fatal unless treated promptly with Fab fragments of digoxin-specific antibodies.

TABLE 42–7. CHRONIC TREATMENT OF CARDIAC ARRHYTHMIAS

Arrhythmia	Usual First Treatment	Other Effective Treatments	Comments
Atrial fibrillation	Digitalis	Drug with class I antiarrhythmic action and digitalis; digitalis and propranolol; digitalis and verapamil	Drugs with class I antiarrhythmic action are used to maintain sinus rhythm; propranolol, acebutolol, or verapamil is used as adjunct to control ventricular rate in atrial fibrillation.
Atrial flutter	Drug with class I antiarrhythmic action	Digitalis; propranolol; verapamil	
Paroxysmal supraventricular tachycardia (AV nodal)	Digitalis	Drug with class IC antiarrhythmic action; propranolol	
Paroxysmal supraventricular tachycardia (anomalous AV connection)	Drug with class IC antiarrhythmic action	Drug with class IA antiarrhythmic action	Surgical ablation is preferable if patient also has atrial fibrillation with rapid ventricular response, if the anomalous AV connection has a short refractory period, or if the patient is noncompliant or has adverse effects from drugs.
Sick sinus syndrome	Pacemaker	Pacemaker and digitalis; pacemaker and drug with class I antiarrhythmic action	With the arrhythmias effectively treated, prognosis is determined by the severity of associated heart disease.
High-grade AV block	Pacemaker	—	No drugs are needed.
Symptomatic ventricular premature complexes or unsustained VT	β blocker	Drug with class I antiarrhythmic action	For benign and potentially malignant ventricular arrhythmias, β blockers are safest and often control symptoms. When heart failure is present, disopyramide and flecainide are relatively contraindicated.
Sustained ventricular tachycardia	Drug with class I antiarrhythmic action	Drug with class III antiarrhythmic action	Treatment must be guided by a method with high predictive accuracy, e.g., endocardial electrical stimulation. A common sequence of drugs is: class IA → class IA + class IB → class IC → class III. If drugs fail or are not evaluable, an implantable cardioverter/defibrillator usually is the best treatment. In selected cases, surgical excision of the arrhythmogenic tissue is the best choice.

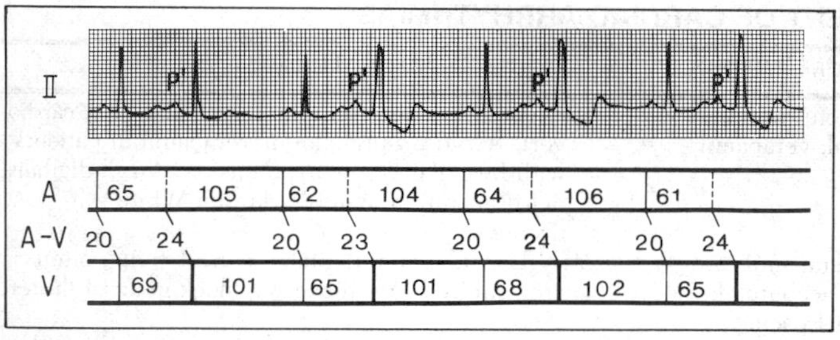

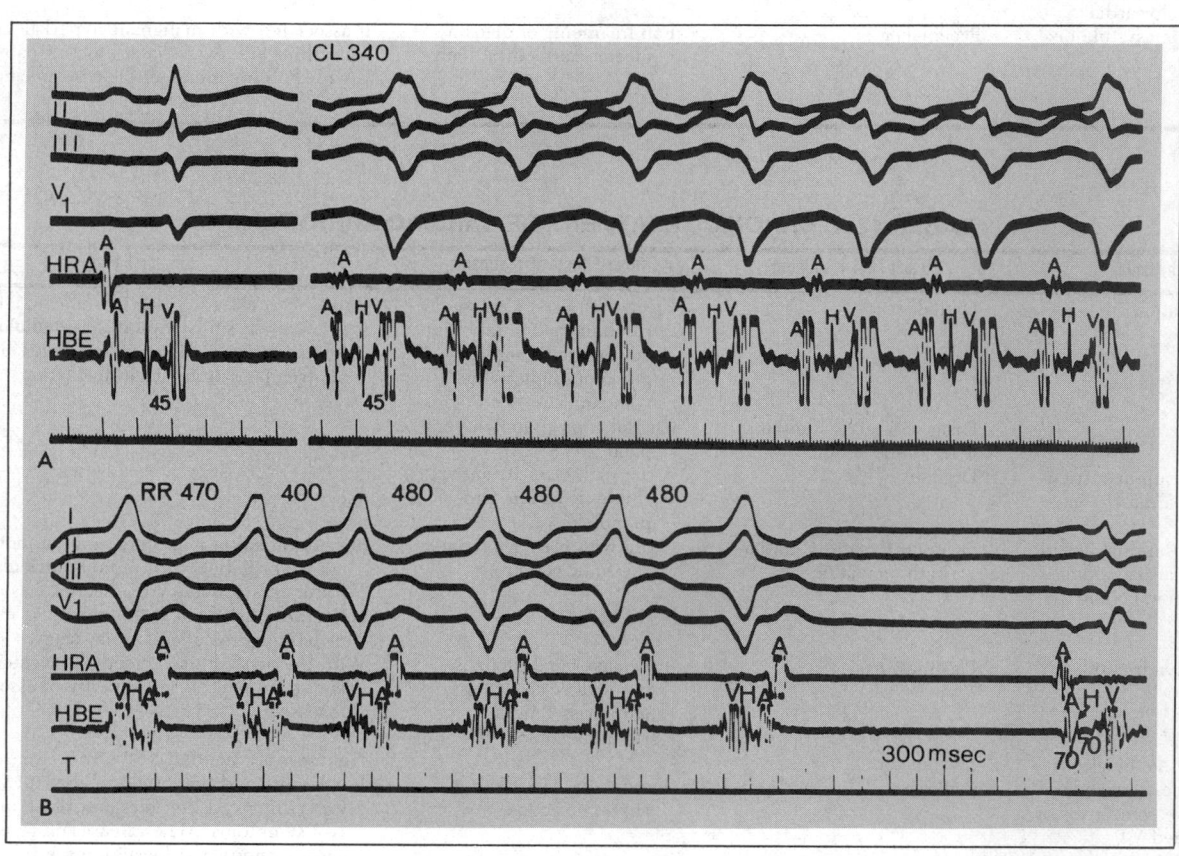

FIGURE 42–9. Atrial premature depolarizations (APD's) with aberrant conduction. The ladder diagram depicts the events in the lead II electrocardiographic strip above. A = Atrium; A-V = atrioventricular node and His-Purkinje system; V = ventricle. Time intervals are in msec × 10⁻¹ (65 represents 650 msec). APD's are represented by dashed lines in the atrial tier; the wide QRS complexes are represented by a wide bar in the ventricular tier. APD's occur in a bigeminal pattern. The even (ectopic) P waves (P') are premature and have configurations slightly different from the odd P waves. Although the P-P' interval is relatively long (>600 msec), the P'-R interval is also prolonged, and the QRS complex following each P' is aberrant (left bundle branch block configuration)—a pattern of aberration suggesting bundle branch disease. Note that the QRS complex after the longest P-P' interval (second QRS) is least aberrant. (From Braunwald E: Heart Disease: A Textbook of Cardiovascular Medicine. Philadelphia, W. B. Saunders Company, 1980.)

ECG DIAGNOSIS. Typically, paroxysmal supraventricular tachycardia (PSVT), also known as paroxysmal atrial or nodal tachycardia and reciprocating AV nodal tachycardia, has the following electrocardiographic features: a regular, rapid rate of 150 to 230 per minute; QRS duration less than 100 msec; and an abnormal P wave in a fixed relationship to each QRS. The P wave often is superimposed on the T wave or the QRS complex. PSVT starts abruptly, usually initiated by an APC or VPC. Often, the atrial rate in PSVT is about 185 per minute. The rate of PSVT often is faster in infants and children, in the Wolff-Parkinson-White (WPW) syndrome, and in thyrotoxicosis. The rate of PSVT is likely to be slower when AV node disease or certain drugs are present. The R-R intervals in typical PSVT are extremely regular except for the first or last few cycles of an episode. Carotid sinus massage either has no effect on PSVT or terminates it. In the presence of AV nodal disease or drugs that depress nodal conduction, e.g., digitalis or verapamil, fixed 2:1 AV block or AV Wenckebach can occur during PSVT.

The QRS complexes may be wide, resembling ventricular tachycardia, due either to a pre-existing wide QRS or to aberrant conduction of the rapid atrial rhythm. If AV dissociation can be documented, the rhythm originates in a subatrial location and is not PSVT. His bundle recording can differentiate between PSVT and ventricular tachycardia (Fig. 42–10).

The mechanism of PSVT is often AV nodal reentry initiated by an APC. The PSVT in the WPW syndrome is reentrant using

FIGURE 42–10. His bundle recording in regular tachycardia with a wide QRS complex. *A,* Supraventricular tachycardia. The left panel is a record taken during sinus rhythm; the QRS is normal. The right panel is a record taken during tachycardia; a left bundle branch block pattern is present. The normal HV interval in the His bundle electrogram (HBE) indicates that the rhythm is supraventricular tachycardia with aberrant conduction. *B,* Ventricular tachycardia. The last six depolarizations of a tachycardia and the first of sinus rhythm are shown. A left bundle branch block pattern is present during the tachycardia. In the His bundle electrogram, the ventricles depolarize (V) before the bundle of His (H), indicating that the rhythm is ventricular tachycardia. Ventriculoatrial conduction shows a stable 1:1 pattern. (From Caracta AR, Damato AN: Significance of His bundle electrocardiography. *In* Fowler NO (ed.): Cardiac Diagnosis and Treatment. 2nd ed. New York, Harper and Row, 1976, pp 979–1008.)

the anomalous AV connection in the retrograde direction and the AV node in the antegrade direction (Fig. 42–11).

Nonparoxysmal atrial tachycardia probably is due to ectopic automaticity or triggered activity in the atrium. Atrial tachycardia with AV block suggests digitalis toxicity, particularly if the atrial rate is slow, e.g., 140 beats per minute.

CLINICAL FEATURES. PSVT occurs in normal as well as diseased hearts. Attacks of PSVT begin abruptly, cause palpitations, and may also end abruptly. The patient may learn maneuvers that are likely to stop the tachycardia, e.g., cough, Valsalva maneuver, or facial immersion. The hemodynamic effects of PSVT vary tremendously and depend on rate and the severity of heart disease. When PSVT is rapid, e.g., 180 to 220 beats per minute, systemic arterial pressure often falls and diastolic pressure rises in both ventricles, even in persons without heart disease. Prolonged and rapid supraventricular tachycardia can cause marked salt and water retention.

MANAGEMENT. Vagal maneuvers (e.g., Valsalva maneuver or carotid sinus massage), adenosine, or verapamil is effective in about 90 per cent of the episodes. When PSVT causes hypotension or heart failure, DC cardioversion should be used. For prevention of recurrences of PSVT due to AV nodal reentry, digitalis usually is tried first. If digitalis fails, potent drugs with class I antiarrhythmic action are quite effective. Surgery may be preferred to drugs in the WPW syndrome with recurrent symptomatic tachyarrhythmias.

ATRIAL FLUTTER

ECG DIAGNOSIS. Typically, atrial flutter has the following ECG features: rapid atrial rate, 250 to 350 beats per minute, narrow QRS, and ventricular rate of 125 to 175 per minute, i.e., 2:1 AV conduction ratio (Fig. 42–12). In atrial flutter, the baseline of the ECG has a characteristic saw-toothed or undulating appearance best seen in leads II, III, and aV_F. Quinidine and other drugs with class I action can slow atrial flutter rate dramatically. In persons with a normal AV node, the AV conduction ratio usually is 2:1. Higher ratios suggest AV node disease or drug effect. Rarely, atrial flutter conducts to the ventricles with a 1:1 ratio, resulting in a ventricular rate of about 300 and hemodynamic collapse. The QRS complex usually is normal during atrial flutter but may be wide owing to pre-existing bundle branch block.

CLINICAL FEATURES. Atrial flutter usually signifies either intrinsic heart disease or adverse extrinsic influences on the heart. Atrial flutter is associated with scarred atria due to rheumatic heart disease, coronary heart disease, or primary myocardial disease. Also, atrial flutter is associated with atrial enlargement, e.g., interatrial septal defect, mitral or tricuspid stenosis/regurgitation, or chronic ventricular failure. Atrial flutter occurs in toxic or metabolic conditions that affect the heart, e.g., thyrotoxicosis, alcoholism, or beri-beri, or when the pericardium is inflamed or infiltrated, e.g., with pneumonia or bronchogenic carcinoma. In all these conditions, atrial flutter is much less common than atrial fibrillation. Atrial flutter tends to be unstable, either reverting to sinus rhythm or converting to atrial fibrillation. Probably because the atria contract vigorously in atrial flutter, systemic emboli are less common during atrial flutter than during atrial fibrillation.

MANAGEMENT. The best choice for the acute treatment of symptomatic atrial flutter is atrial pacing or DC cardioversion because digitalis usually fails to slow the ventricular rate and digitalis, verapamil, or drugs with class I antiarrhythmic action usually fail to convert atrial flutter to sinus rhythm. IV verapamil or β blockers can be useful temporizing measures to control heart rate while arrangements are made for DC cardioversion. A drug with class I antiarrhythmic action alone or with digitalis is the usual treatment to prevent recurrence of atrial flutter.

ATRIAL FIBRILLATION

ECG DIAGNOSIS. Atrial fibrillation has the following features: absence of P waves; irregular atrial activity at a rate of 350 to 600 per minute; and rapid, irregularly irregular ventricular rhythm (150 to 200 per minute). The cardinal feature is the presence of fibrillatory waves best seen in ECG leads II, III, aV_F, or V_1 and at slow ventricular rates. Conditions or drugs that shorten the AV nodal refractory period, e.g., exercise, fever, hyperthyroidism, or catecholamines, increase the ventricular rate. Conversely, factors that prolong AV nodal refractoriness slow ventricular rate.

FIGURE 42–11. Mechanism of supraventricular tachycardia utilizing an accessory pathway. The upper panel demonstrates an electrocardiogram recorded in a patient with Wolff-Parkinson-White syndrome during straight atrial pacing and the introduction of a premature atrial beat. The first five beats are preceded by a stimulus artifact (S); a short PR interval and a wide QRS complex indicate the presence of pre-excitation. Following the introduction of a premature beat, a narrow QRS tachycardia is initiated. The events underlying this supraventricular tachycardia are diagrammatically shown in the lower panels. During sinus rhythm (A), fusion is present owing to conduction over the AV node (AVN) and the accessory pathway (AP). In B, an atrial premature depolarization blocks the accessory pathway and conducts with delay over the AV node, thus dissociating the activity of the normal and accessory pathways. In C, the impulse conducting through the ventricle travels retrograde over the accessory pathway and reenters the atrium, establishing a tachycardia. D demonstrates schematically the reentry circuit underlying supraventricular tachycardia resulting from reentry confined to the AV node.

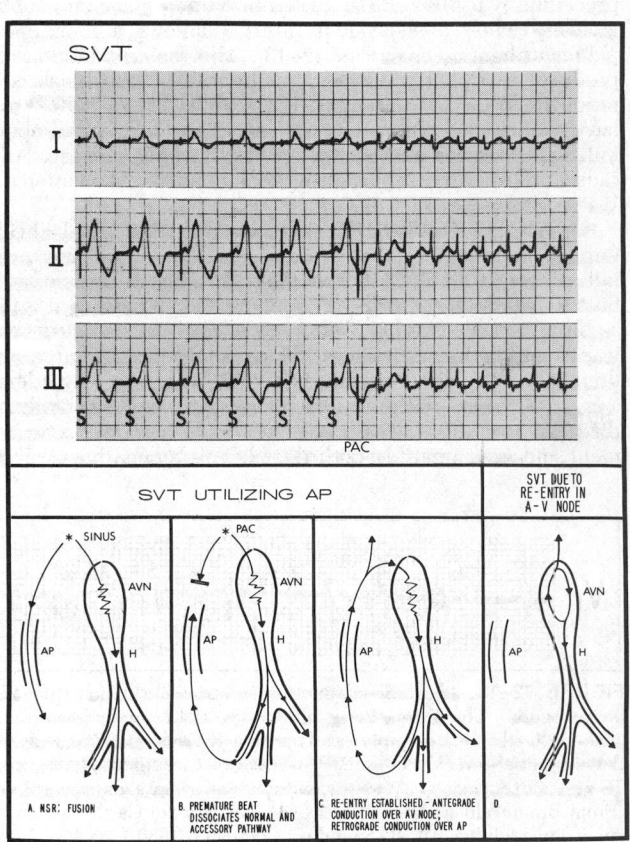

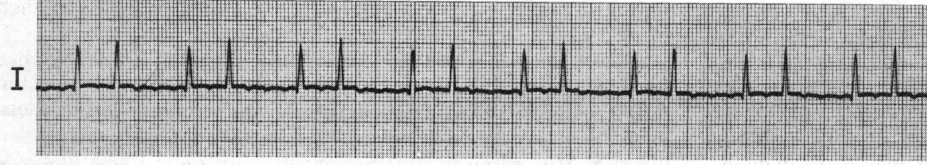

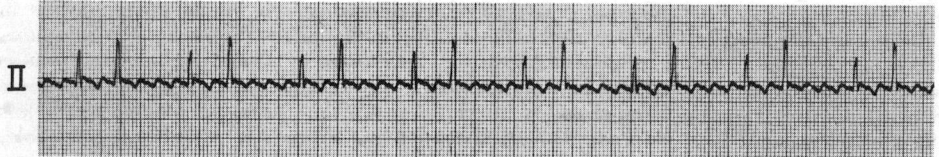

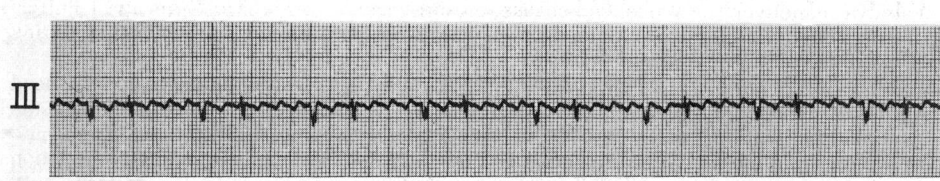

FIGURE 42–12. Atrial flutter with varying AV block. This electrocardiogram, recorded during a period of varying AV block induced by a vagal maneuver, demonstrates the characteristic "saw-toothed" appearance of P waves during atrial flutter.

Because atrial fibrillation is so common, this diagnosis should be entertained for any rapid rhythm that has irregularly irregular R-R intervals. Patients with the WPW syndrome may develop extremely rapid ventricular rates during atrial fibrillation.

Atrial fibrillation coexists with many other arrhythmias and conduction defects; two occur frequently and are critically important to diagnose correctly. The first is AV junctional arrhythmia caused by digitalis toxicity. As digitalis slows the ventricular rate, AV junctional automaticity increases. First, junctional escape complexes terminate long R-R intervals or the ventricular rate becomes regular at a slow rate. Then the junctional focus accelerates to produce nonparoxysmal AV junctional tachycardia. The second is aberrant conduction of supraventricular impulses that must be distinguished from VPC's. The duration of refractoriness in the His-Purkinje system is directly proportional to the preceding R-R interval. In atrial fibrillation, aberrant conduction is likely when a short R-R interval follows a long one—the Ashman phenomenon (Fig. 42–13). Aberrant conduction usually produces a triphasic (RSR') right bundle branch block configuration in lead V$_1$ and normal initial QRS forces. VPC's usually have a mono- or biphasic QRS pattern in lead V$_1$ and abnormal initial QRS forces and are followed by a longer pause. Another cause of repetitive aberrant QRS's in atrial fibrillation is the WPW syndrome (Fig. 42–14).

CLINICAL FEATURES. Like atrial flutter, atrial fibrillation implies myocardial or pericardial disease or adverse extrinsic influences. Atrial fibrillation is about 20 times as common as atrial flutter. Although atrial fibrillation may be paroxysmal, it is usually a chronic, stable rhythm. When atrial fibrillation occurs abruptly in patients with serious heart disease, the consequences may be dramatic, e.g., disconcerting palpitations, pulmonary edema, or angina pectoris. If the ventricular rate is well controlled with digitalis, atrial fibrillation may cause little hemodynamic impairment and is compatible with decades of uneventful survival. As with atrial flutter, atrial fibrillation occurs in many etiologic forms of heart disease. Chronic atrial inflammation and lack of effective atrial contraction promote left atrial thrombi and increased risk for systemic emboli. Atrial fibrillation may occur as an isolated arrhythmia in patients without heart disease or any other systemic illness. This condition has been called "lone atrial fibrillation."

MANAGEMENT. The objective of treating acute atrial fibrillation is to slow the rate. For symptomatic hypotension, immediate cardioversion is indicated. Usually, rate is controlled with IV digoxin (see Table 42–11). Verapamil or β-blocking drugs are useful adjuncts for achieving rate control but can aggravate heart failure or cause hypotension. Digitalis and verapamil are best avoided in patients with WPW because they can increase the ventricular rate and trigger ventricular fibrillation. The objectives of chronic treatment of atrial fibrillation are to (1) control ventricular rate, (2) prevent thromboemboli, and (3) maintain sinus rhythm.

MULTIFOCAL ATRIAL TACHYCARDIA

ECG DIAGNOSIS. The ECG features of multifocal atrial tachycardia are frequent APC's, often occurring in runs that have dramatically different P wave morphology and marked variability in P-P interval.

CLINICAL FEATURES. This rhythm occurs in patients with decompensated or overtreated chronic obstructive pulmonary disease. These patients often have severe derangement of arterial blood gases and electrolytes and are being treated aggressively with theophylline and/or catecholamines.

MANAGEMENT. Multifocal atrial tachycardia is resistant to digitalis therapy. Therapy is directed at improving ventilation and eradicating infection to improve arterial blood gases. The dose of bronchodilators may need to be reduced as well. Verapamil can be used to control the arrhythmia while adjusting the other medications.

SINOATRIAL BLOCK

ECG DIAGNOSIS. Impulses generated in the sinus node may conduct slowly or block in the junction between the sinus node and atrium. First-degree SA block, i.e., a delay in conduction from sinus node to the atrium, cannot be recognized in the standard ECG but can be identified by electrophysiologic studies. Second-degree SA block can be diagnosed electrocardiographically. Type I second-degree SA block is recognized by Wenckebach periodicity of the P-P intervals (Fig. 42–15). In type II second-degree SA block, the P-P interval suddenly lengthens to a value almost precisely twice the usual P-P interval. Third-degree SA block causes atrial arrest.

CLINICAL FEATURES. SA block indicates intrinsic sinus node disease, electrolyte disturbance, or an adverse drug effect,

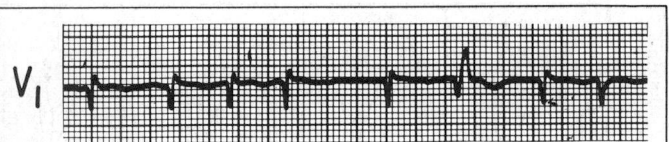

FIGURE 42–13. Aberrant conduction in atrial fibrillation (the Ashman phenomenon). The sixth QRS complex has a right bundle branch appearance. Note that this complex ends a long R-R–short R-R sequence and that its initial forces are similar to those of the other QRS complexes. These features suggest aberrant conduction of a supraventricular impulse. (From Braunwald E: Heart Disease: A Textbook of Cardiovascular Medicine. Philadelphia, W. B. Saunders Company, 1980.)

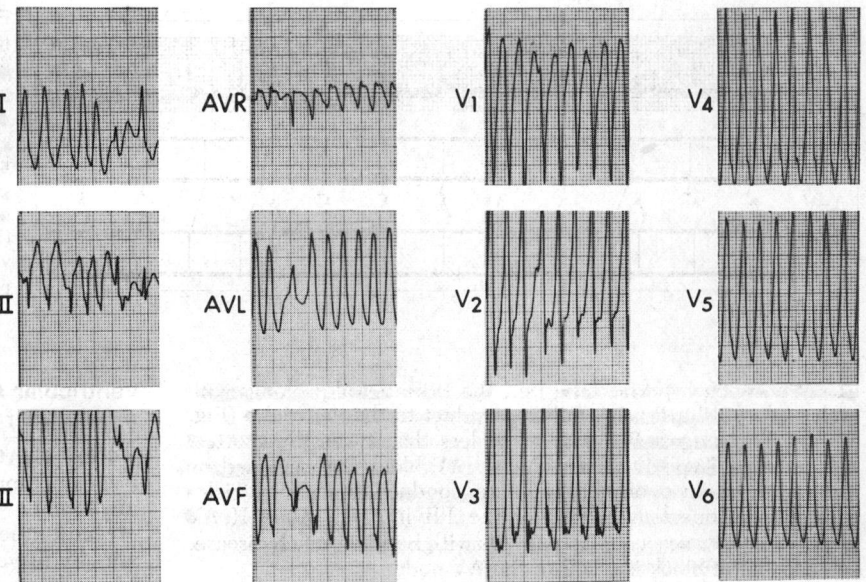

FIGURE 42–14. Atrial fibrillation in the Wolff-Parkinson-White syndrome. The electrocardiogram demonstrates the irregularly irregular response associated with anomalous-appearing QRS complexes resulting from atrial fibrillation with rapid conduction over the accessory pathway to the ventricle.

TG M79212

most often digitalis. Drugs with class I antiarrhythmic action can cause SA block in patients with pre-existing sinus node dysfunction.

Sick Sinus Syndrome. The sick sinus syndrome is characterized by intrinsic inadequacy of sinus node pacemaking and/or conduction failure between the sinus node and the rest of the atrium. In the bradycardia-tachycardia syndrome, recurrent supraventricular tachyarrhythmias alternate with sinus bradycardia and/or subatrial bradyarrhythmias. Conduction disturbances are common in the atria, AV node, bundle branches, and ventricles, but ventricular ectopic activity is rare.

Symptoms in sick sinus syndrome may be intermittent, varied, and difficult to correlate with ECG changes. Syncope, dizziness, and palpitations are common, probably because these symptoms are used for case finding and diagnosis. Congestive heart failure or angina can be aggravated. Cerebral thromboembolism is common in the bradycardia-tachycardia syndrome.

MANAGEMENT. Persistent, symptomatic sinus bradycardia is an indication for pacemaker therapy. Digitalis can be used to control the atrial tachyarrhythmis and, contrary to expectation, usually does not aggravate coexistent bradyarrhythmias. After pacemaker implantation, drugs with class I antiarrhythmic action can be used to control tachyarrhythmias. Symptoms can be improved with pacemaker therapy in the bradycardia-tachycardia syndrome, but cerebral thromboembolism continues. The prognosis of effectively treated sick sinus syndrome is determined by associated heart disease. Treatment of atrial fibrillation in the

sick sinus syndrome can cause severe bradycardia. A temporary ventricular pacemaker should be used when attempting to convert atrial fibrillation with slow ventricular rate to sinus rhythm.

AV Junctional Arrhythmias

AV JUNCTIONAL PREMATURE COMPLEXES

ECG DIAGNOSIS. AV junctional premature complexes are much less common than either APC's or VPC's. Typical ECG features are an abnormally premature or absent P wave and a premature QRS complex with a normal configuration. The position of the premature P wave (P′) is critical to the diagnosis. The P′ may occur 0.10 second or less before, during, or 0.20 second or less after the premature QRS. P′ is inverted in leads II, III, and aV$_F$. The clinical significance of AV junctional premature complexes is similar to that of nonparoxysmal AV junctional tachycardia (see below).

NONPAROXYSMAL AV JUNCTIONAL TACHYCARDIA

ECG DIAGNOSIS. Nonparoxysmal AV junctional tachycardia is caused by enhanced automaticity in the AV junction. The junctional focus fires 70 to 130 per minute (Fig. 42–16). The QRS complex usually is normal or slightly aberrant. If the AV junctional focus captures the atria, the retrograde P may be positioned 0.10 second or less in front of the QRS, simultaneous with the QRS, or 0.20 second or less after the QRS. This arrhythmia often is associated with AV nodal conduction impairment and AV dissociation. The atrial rhythm may intermittently capture the junctional focus and ventricle (see Fig. 42–19).

CLINICAL FEATURES. Nonparoxysmal AV junctional tachycardia has great significance because it is associated with acute inferior myocardial infarction, digitalis toxicity, acute carditis (e.g., viral myocarditis or acute rheumatic fever), or surgical trauma.

MANAGEMENT. Treatment should be focused on the underlying condition, e.g., myocarditis or digitalis toxicity. In acute inferior myocardial infarction and after open heart surgery, nonparoxysmal AV junctional tachycardia is usually transient and requires no therapy. In digitalis toxicity, this arrhythmia should prompt intensive management of toxicity.

AV BLOCK

ECG DIAGNOSIS. AV block is classified as first-, second-, and third-degree. First-degree AV block, i.e., a prolonged PR interval, is caused by conduction delay in the AV node. Second-degree AV block is subdivided into type I (AV nodal) and type II (His-Purkinje). Type I second-degree AV block has character-

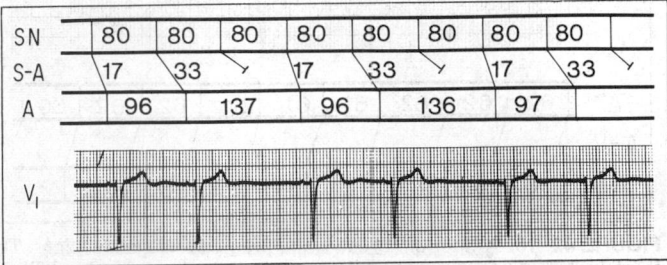

FIGURE 42–15. Second-degree sinoatrial block, type I (Wenckebach). The ECG shows periodicity of the P waves and QRS complex. The PR is constant. This pattern is consistent with a constant sinus node rate of 75 per minute (sinus cycle length = 800 msec) with 3:2 sinoatrial shock. The sinoatrial conduction times are assumed. (From Braunwald E: Heart Disease: A Textbook of Cardiovascular Medicine. Philadelphia, W. B. Saunders Company, 1980.)

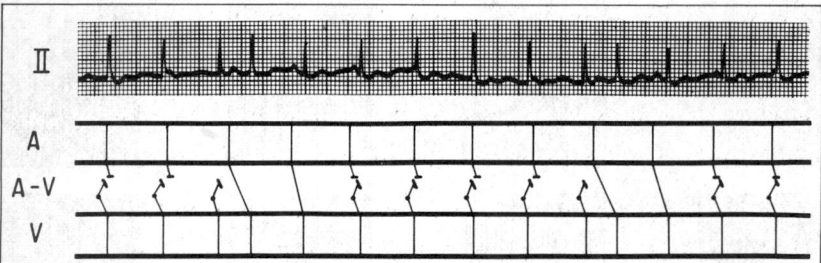

FIGURE 42–16. Nonparoxysmal atrioventricular junctional tachycardia with atrial capture of the ventricles. Two independent rhythms coexist: sinus tachycardia at 107 beats per minute and atrioventricular junctional tachycardia at 115 beats per minute. Sinus rhythm always controls the atria. The ventricles are usually controlled by the AV junctional focus, because its rate is faster. When time relationships are appropriate, atrial depolarizations propagate through the AV junction and capture the ventricles. (From Braunwald E: Heart Disease: A Textbook of Cardiovascular Medicine. Philadelphia, W. B. Saunders Company, 1980.)

istic Wenckebach periodicity; i.e., the PR interval prolongs with each cycle until a P wave fails to conduct to the ventricles (Fig. 42–17). The longest R-R interval is less than twice the shortest R-R interval. Type II second-degree AV block is recognized by the sudden failure of a P wave to conduct to the ventricles without previous lengthening of the PR interval. Type II AV block nearly always occurs in patients with bundle branch disease, and the site of block is distal to the AV node.

In third-degree AV block, sinus or some other atrial rhythm controls the atria while the ventricles are controlled by an independent AV junctional or ventricular pacemaker. The QRS usually is prolonged, and the ventricular rate is between 35 and 50.

CLINICAL FEATURES. First-degree AV block causes no symptoms but may cause the first heart sound to be soft because the AV valves almost close before ventricular contraction. Second-degree AV block usually causes no symptoms unless the ventricular rate becomes very slow. It may be possible to discern second-degree AV block by characteristic pulse intervals, intermittent prominent A waves, and changing intensity of the first heart sound. In complete heart block with sinus rhythm, the pulse is slow, full, and regular; intermittent cannon A waves occur in the jugular venous pulse; and the first heart sound varies markedly in intensity.

MANAGEMENT. First-degree AV block requires no treatment. Type I second-degree AV block usually resolves without the need for a temporary pacemaker. When type I block is caused by a chronic AV junctional disease, block can progress slowly to complete AV block. Type II second-degree AV block usually results from chronic bundle branch disease and often progresses to complete heart block. Chronic, symptomatic second- or third-degree AV block should be treated with an implanted pacemaker.

Ventricular Arrhythmias
VENTRICULAR PREMATURE COMPLEXES (VPC's)

ECG DIAGNOSIS. The QRS is premature, wide, and often bizarre in appearance; the ST segment and T wave are opposite in direction to the QRS complex; and no premature P wave precedes the premature QRS complex (Fig. 42–18). As the impulse leaves its ectopic site of origin, it activates the ventricle in an abnormal sequence, accounting for the striking QRS-T abnormalities. Typically, a VPC is followed by a fully compensatory pause, i.e., the RV interval plus the VR interval is equal to two R-R intervals in sinus rhythm (Fig. 42–18). VPC's may be *interpolated* between two successive sinus complexes. "Concealed" retrograde conduction of the interpolated VPC into the AV node causes the PR interval of the subsequent sinus complex to prolong. Certain patterns of VPC's have special names. When every other QRS is a VPC, the pattern is termed *bigeminy;* a VPC every third QRS is termed *trigeminy;* and two successive VPC's are termed a *pair* or a *couplet.*

CLINICAL FEATURES. Infrequent VPC's are commonly found even in young persons, and VPC frequency increases with age. While sporadic VPC's in persons with normal hearts do not seem to affect outcome adversely, VPC's confer significant risk of subsequent cardiac death in heart disease. When VPC's are caused by drug toxicity, e.g., digitalis, quinidine, or tricyclic antidepressants, lethal rhythm disturbances may ensue unless the drug is discontinued. A strong association exists between myocardial infarct size and the frequency of VPC's in acute myocardial infarction and a weak association between poor left ventricular function and frequency of VPC's during recovery.

MANAGEMENT. The most important issue in the treatment of VPC is the selection of patients for treatment. In general, only very symptomatic VPC's need treatment, and drugs with class II antiarrhythmic action (β-adrenergic blockade) are the first choices for treatment of benign and potentially malignant ventricular

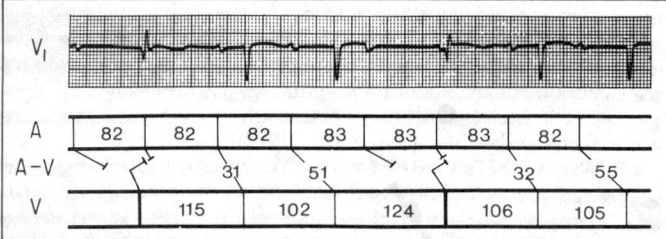

FIGURE 42–17. Sinus rhythm with type I second-degree atrioventricular block (Wenckebach) and junctional escape complexes. Sinus rhythm is regular at a rate of 73 beats per minute. The third P wave from the left begins a 3:2 Wenckebach cycle. The first PR interval of the cycle is quite long (0.31 sec), and the PR increment in the second cycle is large (an additional 0.20 sec). The third P wave of the cycle is blocked in the A-V node. The PR interval following the pause is short (0.10 sec), and the QRS complex is aberrant; this is a junctional escape complex. The tracing demonstrates both impaired conduction and enhanced automaticity in the A-V junction. Type I A-V block nearly always occurs in the A-V node, and A-V junctional escape complexes are presumed to arise in the bundle of His or the most proximal portions of the bundle branches. (From Braunwald E: Heart Disease: A Textbook of Cardiovascular Medicine. Philadelphia, W. B. Saunders Company, 1980.)

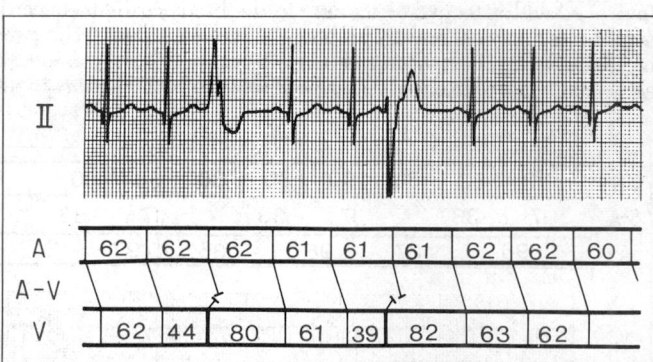

FIGURE 42–18. Multiformed ventricular premature depolarizations. The third and sixth QRS complexes are VPD's with strikingly different configurations. Also, the coupling interval of the two VPD's differs by 50 msec. Such a difference in configuration may be due either to a different site of origin or to a difference in the sequence of ventricular activation from the same site of origin. (From Braunwald E: Heart Disease: A Textbook of Cardiovascular Medicine. Philadelphia, W. B. Saunders Company, 1980.)

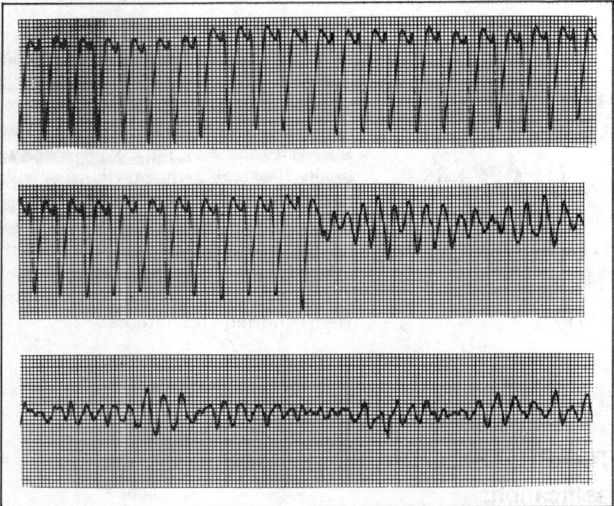

FIGURE 42–19. Ventricular tachycardia and ventricular fibrillation. Three continuous strips from lead V₄ of a Holter electrocardiograph. The top strip shows ventricular tachycardia at 214 cycles per minute—an unusually rapid rate for ventricular tachycardia. Ventricular fibrillation begins in the middle strip and continues on the bottom strip. Note the irregularity in amplitude and period of deflections recorded during ventricular fibrillation. (From Braunwald E: Heart Disease: A Textbook of Cardiovascular Medicine. Philadelphia, W. B. Saunders Company, 1980.)

arrhythmias. IV lidocaine or procainamide is usually used to treat VPC's occurring immediately after myocardial infarction or cardiac surgery.

VENTRICULAR TACHYCARDIA (VT)

ECG DIAGNOSIS. The most prevalent definition of ventricular tachycardia is three or more VPC's in succession at a rate of 100 per minute or greater. Ventricular tachycardia may be unsustained, i.e., last less than 15 to 30 seconds, or sustained (Fig. 42–19). In a tachycardia with wide QRS complexes, two findings strongly suggest VT: *ventricular captures* and *fusion complexes*. Sinus impulses may capture the ventricle during VT, producing either a normal QRS (ventricular capture) or a QRS intermediate in contour between normal and the QRS of ventricular tachycardia (fusion complex). Sustained VT can be difficult to distinguish from supraventricular arrhythmias with a wide QRS complex. A His bundle recording can easily distinguish between these two possibilities (see Fig. 42–10).

CLINICAL FEATURES. Unsustained VT nearly always occurs in patients with heart disease, most often in those with coronary heart disease. Two weeks after myocardial infarction, about 10 per cent of patients have VT detected by a single 24-hour continuous ECG recording. Patients with class III or IV heart failure have a 40 to 50 per cent prevalence of VT in a 24-hour ECG. Most episodes of VT in either setting are brief, i.e., three to five consecutive VPC's, and asymptomatic, yet increase the risk of dying two- to fourfold. Sustained VT is rare and has a poor prognosis. As with other tachyarrhythmias, the severity of symptoms in sustained VT is related primarily to the rate of the tachycardia and left ventricular function. Blood pressure and mental status are not useful for distinguishing between VT and PSVT with aberrant conduction. Sustained VT is prone to deteriorate into ventricular fibrillation.

MANAGEMENT. The management of symptomatic, unsustained VT is the same as that described above for VPC's. Sustained VT in chronic heart disease is treated acutely with IV lidocaine or procainamide, if the patient is hemodynamically stable, or by DC cardioversion if unstable (Fig. 42–19). Baseline studies should include 48 hours of continuous ECG recording, exercise testing, endocardial electrical stimulation, and cardiac catheterization with coronary angiography. The drug/dose finding and long-term management of these patients should be guided by rigorous methods with high predictive accuracy. The standard method is endocardial electrical stimulation. A programmatic noninvasive approach using 24-hour continuous ECG recordings

and exercise tests also can be used. The usual sequence for drug testing is class IA (e.g., quinidine or procainamide), IA plus IB (e.g., quinidine and mexiletine), and III (amiodarone), or an unapproved drug (e.g., dl-sotalol). If an effective drug is not found, an implantable defibrillator is usually the best treatment. In selected cases, surgery is the best choice.

ACCELERATED IDIOVENTRICULAR RHYTHM (AIVR)

ECG DIAGNOSIS. Accelerated idioventricular rhythm is defined as three or more consecutive QRS complexes of ventricular origin with a rate between 50 and 100 (Fig. 42–20). Fusion QRS complexes often begin or end an episode of AIVR.

CLINICAL FEATURES. AIVR occurs in about 30 per cent of patients with acute myocardial infarction, equally commonly in inferior or anterior infarcts. AIVR frequently follows coronary reperfusion. AIVR is usually asymptomatic and therefore needs no treatment. The incidence of ventricular fibrillation and hospital mortality is not increased in patients who have AIVR.

VENTRICULAR PARASYSTOLE

ECG DIAGNOSIS. Ventricular parasystole is an automatic rhythm in the His-Purkinje system that competes with sinus rhythm. Parasystole has two cardinal features: variable coupling of VPC's and a common denominator for interectopic intervals. Entrance block removes the parasystolic focus from the suppressant influence of the sinus impulses, permitting a stable automatic rhythm to emerge; the ectopic focus activates the ventricle every time it fires unless the ventricle is refractory (Fig. 42–20).

CLINICAL FEATURES. Parasystole often is resistant to antiarrhythmic drug therapy, and untreated patients seem to have a good prognosis.

VENTRICULAR FLUTTER AND FIBRILLATION

ECG DIAGNOSIS. The diagnosis of ventricular flutter is made when the ventricular tachyarrhythmia has large sinusoidal or zigzag QRS's and the rate is between 240 and 280 per minute. Multiform VT or torsades de pointes is recognized by the periodic twisting of the points of the QRS complexes (Fig. 42–21). Ventricular fibrillation is recognized in the ECG by the absence of QRS complexes and T waves and the presence of low-amplitude baseline undulations that are variable in both amplitude and periodicity (Fig. 42–19).

CLINICAL FEATURES. Ventricular flutter is rarely recorded because it is unstable and tends to convert to sinus rhythm or, more often, to ventricular fibrillation. Ventricular flutter or fibrillation is catastrophic. Cardiac pumping ceases instantly, the patient loses consciousness, and, if cardiopulmonary resuscitation is not started within a few minutes, the patient dies. Identifiable causes are acute myocardial ischemia or infarction; marked electrolyte disturbances, e.g., hypokalemia; marked hypothermia; electrocution; and drug toxicity. Most victims of ventricular fibrillation who are resuscitated do *not* have one of these condi-

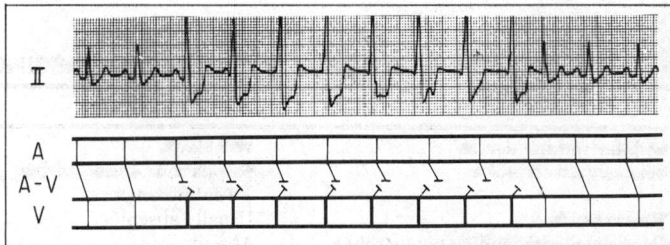

FIGURE 42–20. Accelerated idioventricular rhythm. Sinus rhythm at 88 cycles per minute is interrupted by a rhythm with wide QRS complexes at 95 cycles per minute. Note that the PR interval progressively shortens at the onset of the ventricular rhythm and that sinus rhythm continues unperturbed by the ventricular rhythm (atrioventricular dissociation). After eight QRS complexes of ventricular rhythm, sinus rhythm resumes. (From Braunwald E: Heart Disease: A Textbook of Cardiovascular Medicine. Philadelphia, W. B. Saunders Company, 1980.)

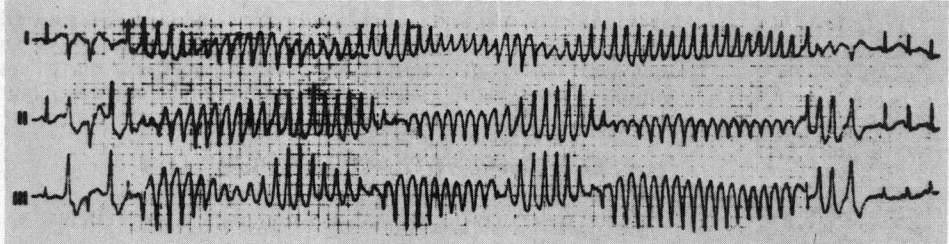

FIGURE 42–21. Torsades de pointes. Sinus rhythm associated with a long QT interval is present at the beginning and at the end of this rhythm strip. Sinus rhythm is interrupted by a rapid wide QRS tachycardia. Note that during the tachycardia, the direction of the points of the QRS complex appears to revolve around an imaginary isoelectric line. (From Krikler DM, Curry DVL: Br Heart J 38:118, 1976. With permission of the British Heart Journal and authors.)

tions but do have advanced coronary atherosclerosis and poor ventricular function.

MANAGEMENT. The only effective treatment for ventricular fibrillation is prompt defibrillation. In most cases, ventricular fibrillation does not recur after defibrillation. When it does, lidocaine, bretylium, or propranolol may help to stabilize the rhythm. When no transient or reversible cause for ventricular fibrillation is found (e.g., myocardial infarction, electrolyte abnormality, or drug toxicity), the process for evaluating long-term treatment is much the same as described above for sustained VT. Unfortunately, a smaller fraction of patients, about 60 to 70 per cent, have VT induced by programmed ventricular stimulation. Nevertheless, the uninducible patients have a high recurrence rate for ventricular fibrillation.

The management of multiform VT (torsades de pointes) is based on its pathophysiology: toxic drug effects, hypokalemia and/or hypomagnesemia, and slow heart rates. Treatment may include avoidance of drugs with class I antiarrhythmic action, ventricular pacing, reducing the level of the culprit drug, repletion of electrolytes, treatment with IV Mg^{2+}, or catecholamine infusion.

PROGNOSTIC CLASSIFICATION OF VENTRICULAR ARRHYTHMIAS. Table 42–8 outlines the classification of ventricular arrhythmias as determined by the presence of heart disease, left ventricular function, and arrhythmia characteristics. Prognosis is an important basis for deciding whom to treat and how to sequence the treatment choices.

Bigger JT Jr, Reiffel JA: Sick sinus syndrome. Ann Rev Med 30:91, 1979. *A comprehensive review of the human sinus node dysfunction. Liberally referenced.*

Marriott HJL: Practical Electrocardiography. 8th ed. Baltimore, Williams & Wilkins Company, 1988. *A textbook designed to emphasize the simplicities of the ECG, provide only those concepts that make everyday ECG interpretation more intelligible, and provide illustrations and discussion of all important ECG patterns. Excellent for learning or reviewing the ECG patterns of arrhythmias.*

Zipes DP: Specific arrhythmias: Diagnosis and treatment. *In* Braunwald E (ed.): Heart Disease. A Textbook of Cardiovascular Medicine. 3rd ed. Philadelphia, W. B. Saunders Company, 1988, pp 658–716. *Detailed description of the clinical features, electrocardiographic recognition, and treatment of cardiac arrhythmias. Contains 52 figures and 372 references.*

ANTIARRHYTHMIC DRUGS

Classification

Antiarrhythmic drugs have been classified according to their mechanisms of action into four classes (Table 42–9). One could think of digitalis as having class V drug action, i.e., a strong cholinergic action that can repolarize stretched or damaged atrial cells and thereby speed conduction. Digitalis glycosides slow conduction in the AV node, tending to slow or abolish reentrant rhythms that use the AV node.

Use-Dependent Block of Ionic Channels

Many antiarrhythmic drugs act on ionic channels in the sarcolemma. Drugs with class I antiarrhythmic action block the Na^+ channel so that ionic conductance falls to zero until the drug dissociates from the channel. Most drugs with class I antiarrhythmic action bind to open or inactivated channels; drug-associated channels have slow or incomplete reactivation. Drug binding and Na^+ channel blockade increase with rate, producing *use-dependent block*. If the association and dissociation of drug from the Na^+ channel both are rapid, use-dependent block attains a steady state after a few action potentials and, if the interval between action potentials is reasonably long, little block persists at the time of the next action potential upstroke. If dissociation is slow, use-dependent block requires many action potentials to develop fully as the degree of block increases with each depolarization.

Specific Antiarrhythmic Drugs

This section gives a brief summary of the pharmacology and indications for each antiarrhythmic drug. This information is supplemented by information given in tables; Table 42–10 gives pharmacokinetic data for the drugs and Table 42–11 gives information on contraindications, precautions, and adverse effects.

DRUGS WITH CLASS IB ANTIARRHYTHMIC ACTION

LIDOCAINE. Lidocaine is a local anesthetic used frequently to treat ventricular arrhythmias in intensive care units. It has

TABLE 42–8. PROGNOSTIC CLASSIFICATION OF VENTRICULAR ARRHYTHMIAS*

	Benign	Potentially Malignant	Malignant
Risk for sudden death	Very low	Low to moderate	High
Clinical presentation	Palpitations; detected by routine exam	Palpitations; detected by routine exam or screening	Palpitations; syncope; cardiac arrest
Heart disease	Usually absent	Present	Present
Cardiac scarring and/or hypertrophy	Absent	Present	Present
VPC frequency	Low to moderate	Moderate to high	Moderate to high
Paired VPC and/or unsustained VT	Absent	Common	Common
Sustained VT	Absent	Absent	Present
Hemodynamic effects of arrhythmia	Absent	Absent to mild	Moderate to severe

VPC = Ventricular premature complex(s); VT = ventricular tachycardia.
*The characteristics listed in this table are typical but do not represent the full range of observations. For example, benign ventricular arrhythmias can be frequent and occasionally repetitive. For potentially malignant or malignant ventricular arrhythmias, the risk within a class depends strongly on left ventricular ejection fraction.

TABLE 42–9. CLASSIFICATION OF ANTIARRHYTHMIC DRUGS ACCORDING TO THEIR MECHANISM OF ACTION

Class	Action	Drugs
I	**Sodium channel blockade**	
B	Minimal phase 0 depression	Lidocaine, mexiletine, tocainide
	Slow conduction 0 to 1+	
	Shorten repolarization	
A	Moderate phase 0 depression	Disopyramide, moricizine, procainamide, quinidine
	Slow conduction 2+	
	Prolong repolarization*	
C	Marked phase 0 depression	Encainide, flecainide, indecainide, propafenone
	Slow conduction 4+	
	Little effect on repolarization	
II	**β-Adrenergic blockade**	Acebutolol, propranolol
II	**Prolong repolarization**	Amiodarone, bretylium, sotalol
IV	**Calcium channel blockade**	Diltiazem, verapamil

*Moricizine does not prolong repolarization.

two major advantages: It reaches a steady state rapidly after starting or changing the dose, and it lacks significant adverse hemodynamic effects.

Pharmacology. Lidocaine prevents reentrant rhythms, decreases automaticity in Purkinje fibers, and increases the ventricular fibrillation threshold. Lidocaine has an intense depressant action on depolarized tissues but almost none on normal cardiac cells. Lidocaine has a negligible effect on the ECG. Lidocaine shortens the ERP of the His-Purkinje system. Lidocaine has no significant effect on the autonomic nervous system.

Indications. Lidocaine is used only for ventricular arrhythmias, particularly those caused by acute myocardial infarction, open heart surgery, and digitalis intoxication. Lidocaine is relatively ineffective for ventricular arrhythmias in chronic coronary heart disease or cardiomyopathy.

Pharmacokinetics. Lidocaine is administered intravenously and, rarely, intramuscularly. Steady-state plasma lidocaine concentration depends strongly on hepatic blood flow. About 70 per cent of plasma lidocaine is bound to α_1 acid glycoprotein, an acute phase reactant. At a given total plasma concentration, the free concentration falls as the α_1 acid glycoprotein increases in the first few days after infarction or surgery.

MEXILETINE. Mexiletine is an orally active local anesthetic, available in the United States since 1986, that is similar to lidocaine chemically and electrophysiologically.

Pharmacology. Mexiletine has an antiautomatic effect on Purkinje fibers and depresses phase 0 of fast action potentials more than lidocaine. It shortens the action potential duration and ERP of Purkinje fibers and ventricular muscle. Mexiletine has little effect on the ECG.

Indications. Like lidocaine, this drug is not indicated for atrial arrhythmias. In chronic coronary heart disease or cardiomyopathy, the drug is about 60 per cent effective in controlling symptomatic, unsustained ventricular arrhythmias, less than drugs with class IA or IC antiarrhythmic action.

PHENYTOIN. Phenytoin is an anticonvulsant that has been used as an antiarrhythmic since the 1960's. Phenytoin is electrophysiologically similar to lidocaine and has no significant effect on the ECG. Phenytoin has complex central autonomic actions that decrease efferent traffic on cardiac sympathetic nerves during digitalis toxicity. Phenytoin has no peripheral cholinergic or β-adrenergic blocking activity.

Indications. Phenytoin is used to treat paroxysmal atrial flutter or fibrillation, supraventricular arrhythmias, and ventricular arrhythmias caused by digitalis but is ineffective for the common atrial arrhythmias, e.g., atrial flutter, atrial fibrillation, and PSVT. Phenytoin is effective against ventricular arrhythmias after acute myocardial infarction or open heart surgery, but lidocaine is easier to use. Plasma concentrations above 10 μg per milliliter are effective for reducing ventricular arrhythmias in the year after myocardial infarction. Phenytoin, like other drugs with class I antiarrhythmic action, is relatively ineffective against recurrent, sustained VT in patients with chronic coronary heart disease.

Pharmacokinetics. The enzymes that metabolize phenytoin can saturate at antiarrhythmic plasma concentrations, causing plasma concentration to rise sharply to toxic levels. Phenytoin should not be infused because its alkaline pH causes severe phlebitis.

TOCAINIDE. Tocainide is an orally effective analogue of lidocaine that was approved in 1984 for use in the United States. Tocainide has cardiac electrophysiologic effects almost identical

TABLE 42–10. PHARMACOKINETIC PROPERTIES OF ANTIARRHYTHMIC DRUGS

Drug	Volume of Distribution (L/kg)	Half-time of Elimination (Hours)	Bioavailability	Major Route of Elimination	Protein Binding (%)	Effective Plasma Concentration (μg/ml)
Digoxin	10.0	24–72	50–80	Kidney	25	>0.0008
Lidocaine	1.0	1–3	—	Liver	70	1–5
Mexiletine	9.5	8–14	80–90	Liver	60	0.7–2.0
Phenytoin	0.7	18–30	60–80	Liver	90	8–20
Tocainide	3.0	10–14	80–90	Kidney, liver	10	6–15
Disopyramide	0.8	7–9	75–90	Kidney	Dose-dependent	2–5
Moricizine	4.5	3–5	35–45	Liver	>90	—
Procainamide	2.0	3–6	75–85	Kidney, liver	15	4–20
Quinidine	2.5	5–9	70–80	Liver	90	2–6
Encainide	4.0	1–3	20–40	Liver	80	—
Flecainide	10	13–30	>90	Kidney, liver	40	0.2–1.0
Indecainide	5.0	7–9	>90	Kidney	50	0.4–1.0
Propafenone	3.5	3–10	3–40	Liver	95	—
Acebutolol	1.2	2–4	35–45	Kidney, liver	25	—
Propranolol	4.0	3–6	20–50	Liver	>90	0.04–0.9
Amiodarone	60.0	500–1000	30–40	Liver	>95	0.5–2.5
Bretylium	6.0	8–12	20–30	Kidney	5	—
dl-Sotalol	2.0	7–15	>90	Kidney	0	1.0–4.0
Diltiazem	5.5	2–6	40–50	Liver	75	0.5–2.0
Verapamil	4.0	4–10	10–35	Liver	90	0.1–0.2

TABLE 42–11. ADVERSE EFFECTS OF ANTIARRHYTHMIC DRUGS

	Contraindications	Precautions	Adverse Effects
Digoxin	Hypersensitivity to the drug	Reduce dose in renal insufficiency; hypokalemia, hypomagnesemia, and hypercalcemia predispose to digitalis toxicity; may accelerate the ventricular response to atrial flutter or fibrillation in Wolff-Parkinson-White syndrome; may worsen outflow obstruction in hypertrophic obstructive cardiomyopathy; serum digoxin concentration increased by quinidine and verapamil; absorption may be increased by some antibiotics; use cautiously with β blockers or calcium channel antagonists in atrial fibrillation	Ventricular arrhythmias, including ventricular tachycardia; accelerated junctional rhythms; atrial tachycardia with AV block; AV dissociation; progression of AV block Anorexia; nausea, vomiting; visual disturbances; weakness
Lidocaine	Known hypersensitivity to local anesthetics of the amide type; patients with Stokes-Adams syndrome, or with severe degrees of SA, AV, or intraventricular block in the absence of a pacemaker	Accumulation in heart failure or hepatic insufficiency or after prolonged infusions; reduce dosage in children and elderly patients; safety in malignant hyperthermia not established; cimetidine and propranolol increase plasma lidocaine concentration	Bradycardia, hypotension, and cardiovascular collapse Drowsiness, confusion, dizziness, respiratory depression, and arrest; vomiting; visual disturbances; convulsions; twitching; unconsciousness; allergic reactions secondary to lidocaine sensitivity
Mexiletine	Cardiogenic shock; pre-existing second- or third-degree AV block in the absence of a pacemaker	Patients with first-degree AV block, sinus node dysfunction, intraventricular conduction abnormalities; may worsen arrhythmias; mexiletine levels increased by cimetidine; use cautiously in patients with a history of seizures, hypotension, heart failure, or liver disease	GI distress, lightheadedness, tremor, coordination difficulties, diplopia, paresthesia, confusion
Phenytoin	History of hypersensitivity to hydantoin products; sinus bradycardia, SA block, second- or third-degree AV block; Stokes-Adams syndrome	Use cautiously in presence of hypotension and myocardial depression; may worsen arrhythmias; discontinue if skin rash develops; may cause hypoglycemia; multiple drug interactions; may be associated with congenital malformations	Hypotension and bradycardia with rapid IV injection Nystagmus, ataxia, slurred speech; Stevens-Johnson syndrome; sensory neuropathy; lymphadenopathy; pancytopenia; megaloblastic anemia, gingival hyperplasia, hyperglycemia, hypocalcemia
Tocainide	Hypersensitivity to this drug or to local anesthetics of the amide type; second- or third-degree AV block in the absence of a pacemaker	May cause blood dyscrasias, pulmonary fibrosis, pneumonitis; may aggravate heart failure or worsen ventricular arrhythmias; may accelerate the ventricular response in atrial fibrillation; accumulates in severe renal or hepatic insufficiency	Nausea, vomiting, lightheadedness, dizziness, tremor, diplopia, paresthesia, confusion, *agranulocytosis*, thrombocytopenia, hypoplastic anemia
Disopyramide	Cardiogenic shock; pre-existing second- or third-degree AV block in the absence of a pacemaker; congenital QT prolongation; known hypersensitivity to the drug	*Use cautiously with left ventricular dysfunction,* sick sinus syndrome, bundle branch block, or AV block; prior digitalization suggested for atrial flutter or fibrillation to prevent increase in ventricular rate. May precipitate myasthenic crisis, glaucoma, or urinary retention; may cause hypoglycemia; serum level may be lowered by phenytoin	*Heart failure;* worsening of arrhythmias; AV block; hypotension; may cause significant prolongation of QRS and QT intervals *Urinary retention;* dry mouth; constipation; blurred vision; impotence; cholestatic jaundice; fever; thrombocytopenia; granulocytopenia; gynecomastia
Procainamide HCl	Second- or third-degree AV block unless a pacemaker is present; torsades de pointes; lupus-like syndrome; hypersensitivity to the drug	Reduce dosage in renal insufficiency; may accelerate the ventricular response in atrial fibrillation or atrial flutter; may exacerbate myasthenia gravis	Hypotension; worsening of ventricular arrhythmias; myocardial depression; AV block *Lupus-like syndrome;* GI distress; *agranulocytosis;* hemolytic anemia; fever; thrombocytopenia; rash; myalgia; hallucinations; psychosis
Quinidine sulfate	Hypersensitivity to quinidine; complete AV block; complete bundle branch block or other severe intraventricular conduction defects exhibiting marked QRS widening; myasthenia gravis; arrhythmias due to digitalis toxicity	May accelerate the ventricular response to atrial flutter or atrial fibrillation; *concurrent use with digoxin increases plasma digoxin levels;* drugs that increase hepatic drug-metabolizing enzymes decrease the plasma concentration of quinidine; may worsen heart failure; test dose recommended because of idiosyncratic response; may require change in oral anticoagulant dose	Hypotension; worsening of ventricular arrhythmias; asystole; may increase AV or bundle branch block; may cause significant prolongation of QRS and QT intervals; *syncope; torsades de pointes* *Diarrhea;* nausea; *thrombocytopenia;* hemolytic anemia; granulocytopenia; fever; visual disturbances; hypersensitivity reaction; cinchonism; rash

TABLE 42–11. ADVERSE EFFECTS OF ANTIARRHYTHMIC DRUGS *Continued*

	Contraindications	Precautions	Adverse Effects
Encainide	Second- or third-degree AV block or right bundle branch block with associated hemiblock unless a pacemaker is in place; cardiogenic shock; known hypersensitivity; asymptomatic ventricular arrhythmias after myocardial infarction	May worsen sinus node dysfunction; increases pacing thresholds; may suppress ventricular escape rhythms; reduce dose with renal insufficiency; cimetidine increases encainide serum concentration	*New or worsened ventricular tachycardia or ventricular fibrillation;* second- or third-degree AV block; increases mortality when used to treat potentially malignant ventricular arrhythmias after myocardial infarction Dizziness; visual disturbances; headache; vertigo; leg cramps
Flecainide	Second- or third-degree AV block or right bundle branch block with associated hemiblock unless a pacemaker is in place; cardiogenic shock; known hypersensitivity to the drug; asymptomatic ventricular arrhythmias after myocardial infarction	May worsen sinus node dysfunction; increases pacing thresholds; may suppress ventricular escape rhythms; avoid concurrent administration of disopyramide or verapamil	*New or worsened ventricular tachycardia or ventricular fibrillation* in patients with sustained ventricular arrhythmias; *heart failure,* second- or third-degree AV block Dizziness; *visual disturbances;* dyspnea; hepatic dysfunction; blood dyscrasias
Propafenone	Uncontrolled congestive heart failure or cardiogenic shock; sinoatrial or AV block in the absence of an electronic pacemaker; bradycardia; bronchospastic disorders; manifest electrolyte disorders; and known hypersensitivity to the drug	Reduce dose in hepatic or renal dysfunction; may worsen arrhythmias; increases plasma digoxin or warfarin concentrations; decreases the clearance of some β blockers; quinidine or cimetidine increases plasma concentrations; use cautiously with β-blockers or calcium entry blockers	New or worsened ventricular arrhythmias in patients with sustained ventricular arrhythmias; safety unknown when used to treat potentially malignant ventricular arrhythmias after myocardial infarction; aggravates asthma or chronic bronchitis; aggravates congestive heart failure; dizziness, taste disturbances, blurred vision; anorexia, nausea, and vomiting; agranulocytosis
Acebutolol	Severe sinus bradycardia; second- and third-degree AV block; overt cardiac failure; cardiogenic shock	Myocardial infarction or exacerbation of angina may occur following abrupt withdrawal; may mask symptoms of hypoglycemia or hyperthyroidism; cautious use in renal insufficiency or with concurrent α-adrenergic or catecholamine-depleting drugs	Congestive heart failure; bradycardia; hypotension; increase in AV block Fatigue; headache; dizziness; arterial insufficiency; bronchospasm; impotence
Propranolol	Cardiogenic shock; sinus bradycardia; second- or third-degree AV block; asthma; congestive heart failure	Exacerbation of angina or myocardial infarction may occur following abrupt withdrawal; may mask symptoms of hypoglycemia or hyperthyroidism; may cause severe sinus bradycardia following termination of tachycardia; may worsen hypertension in pheochromocytoma unless used with an α-adrenergic blocking drug	Congestive heart failure; bradycardia; increase in degree of AV block; hypotension Bronchospasm; arterial insufficiency; Raynaud's phenomenon; mental depression; sleep disturbances; weakness; impotence; disorientation; memory loss; blood dyscrasias
Amiodarone	Severe sinus node dysfunction; marked sinus bradycardia; second- or third-degree AV block; history of syncope due to bradycardia unless a pacemaker is in place	Raises serum digoxin concentration; potentiates the effect of oral anticoagulants; increases levels of quinidine, procainamide, phenytoin; may potentiate bradycardia or AV block when used with β blockers or calcium antagonists; may worsen arrhythmias	Sinus bradycardia *Pulmonary fibrosis;* interstitial pneumonitis; corneal microdeposits; photosensitivity; blue-gray pigmentation; hypo- or hyperthyroidism; *hepatic injury;* nausea; vomiting; anorexia; constipation; tremor; malaise; gait disturbance; *peripheral myopathy or neuropathy*
Bretylium tosylate	*Severe hypotension may occur in patients with fixed cardiac output;* may aggravate digitalis toxicity; reduce dosage in renal insufficiency	*Hypotension, especially postural hypotension;* transient hypertension and increased frequency of ventricular arrhythmias Nausea and vomiting, usually with rapid IV infusion; increases sensitivity to catecholamines	
Dilitiazem	Sick sinus syndrome; second- or third-degree AV block in absence of a ventricular pacemaker; systolic BP <90 mm Hg	Cautious use in renal or hepatic insufficiency; additive effects on AV conduction when used with digitalis or β blockers	Bradycardia; hypotension; AV block Edema; headache; nausea; dizziness; rash; abnormal hepatic enzymes
Verapamil	*Severe left ventricular dysfunction; hypotension or cardiogenic shock;* sick sinus syndrome (except with a pacemaker); second- or third-degree AV block; concurrent intravenous β blockers and intravenous verapamil; known hypersensitivity to verapamil	Reduce oral dose with hepatic dysfunction; avoid use with disopyramide; use cautiously with renal insufficiency, β blockers, quinidine, or severe hypertrophic obstructive cardiomyopathy; raises serum digoxin level; *may accelerate ventricular response in atrial flutter or fibrillation in the presence of the Wolff-Parkinson-White syndrome;* may potentiate activity of neuromuscular blocking agents	Hypotension; AV block; heart failure; bradycardia; asystole (with IV use); *severe hypotension or ventricular fibrillation when given IV to patients with ventricular tachycardia* Peripheral edema; headache; elevation of liver function tests; constipation

to those of lidocaine and has almost no effect on the ECG. Also, it is well tolerated hemodynamically.

Indications. Tocainide is indicated for the oral treatment of sustained or symptomatic unsustained ventricular arrhythmias. The drug is similar to mexiletine in its efficacy; i.e., it controls about 60 per cent of the chronic unsustained ventricular arrhythmias. There is good concordance between the effect of IV lidocaine and oral tocainide on ventricular arrhythmias.

DRUGS WITH CLASS IA ANTIARRHYTHMIC ACTION

DISOPYRAMIDE. Disopyramide has been available in the United States for the oral treatment of ventricular arrhythmias since 1978. Disopyramide suppresses normal automaticity in Purkinje fibers and depresses phase 0 of fast action potentials and slows conduction. Disopyramide appears more potent than quinidine in increasing atrial or ventricular refractoriness but seems less potent in the His-Purkinje system. Therapeutic concentrations cause little change in heart rate or PR or QT intervals and increase the QRS duration by about 25 per cent. It increases the ERP of the atrium and ventricle but not the AV node or His-Purkinje system. Disopyramide has a prominent anticholinergic action that counteracts its direct effects on the sinus and AV nodes.

Indications. Disopyramide is indicated for the treatment of symptomatic, unsustained ventricular arrhythmias. It also terminates attacks of PSVT and decreases the frequency of recurrences. It is about as effective as quinidine for preventing recurrence of atrial fibrillation after cardioversion. Disopyramide prolongs the ERP of anomalous AV connections and can control arrhythmias in the WPW syndrome.

PROCAINAMIDE. Procainamide has been used since the 1950's for the treatment of atrial and ventricular arrhythmias. The cardiac electrophysiologic effects of procainamide are similar to those of disopyramide and quinidine. It suppresses automaticity in cardiac Purkinje fibers, slows the phase 0 depolarization in fibers with fast action potentials, and delays repolarization and increases refractoriness in the atrium, His-Purkinje system, and ventricle. Procainamide produces a small increase in the PR and QT intervals in the ECG and produces a 20 to 30 per cent increase in the QRS duration at therapeutic plasma concentrations. Also, procainamide increases slightly the ERP of the atrium, has little effect on the refractoriness of the AV node, and prolongs the conduction time and ERP of the His-Purkinje system slightly in humans. Procainamide has no significant anticholinergic or α-adrenergic blocking properties.

Indications. Procainamide is indicated for the treatment of atrial fibrillation, atrial flutter, PSVT, symptomatic, unsustained ventricular arrhythmias that do not respond to β blockers, and sustained VT. It can suppress digitalis-toxic ventricular arrhythmias, but lidocaine or phenytoin is a better choice.

Pharmacokinetics. Procainamide is biotransformed in the liver to N-acetyl procainamide (NAPA), and steady-state plasma concentrations can equal or exceed those of procainamide. NAPA is qualitatively different electrophysiologically from procainamide; it has little class I action but a pronounced class III antiarrhythmic action. NAPA is eliminated by the kidney and can accumulate to toxic levels when renal or congestive heart failure is present. Procainamide's adverse effects often preclude chronic therapy.

QUINIDINE. Quinidine, an alkaloid derived from the bark of the cinchona tree, has been used for the treatment of atrial and ventricular arrhythmias since the 1920's.

Pharmacology. Quinidine has powerful direct effects on most types of cardiac cells and has significant anticholinergic and α-adrenergic blocking activity. Quinidine has little effect on normal sinus nodes, but can markedly depress abnormal ones. Quinidine substantially decreases normal automaticity in cardiac Purkinje fibers but has little effect on abnormal automaticity. Quinidine increases atrial and ventricular pacing and fibrillation thresholds. Quinidine depresses phase 0 of atrial, ventricular, and Purkinje cells. Quinidine delays repolarization and increases the effective refractory period of atrial, ventricular, and Purkinje cells. In humans, quinidine causes a small increase in heart rate and in the PR, QRS, and QT intervals in the ECG, and usually prolongs the HV interval slightly.

Indications. Quinidine is indicated for the chronic treatment of atrial flutter or fibrillation, PSVT, and symptomatic ventricular arrhythmias. For symptomatic benign or potentially malignant ventricular arrhythmias that do not respond to β blockers, quinidine can be used if the benefits outweigh the risks. Quinidine is selected for malignant arrhythmias if it renders them uninducible by programmed ventricular stimulation or if it abolishes unsustained VT from Holter recordings.

DRUGS WITH CLASS IC ANTIARRHYTHMIC ACTION

Four drugs with class IC antiarrhythmic action were approved for use in the United States: flecainide in 1986, encainide in 1987, and indecainide and propafenone in 1989. Propafenone has class II action (β blockade) as well. These four drugs have little effect on the normal sinus node but can depress abnormal sinus nodes. They decrease spontaneous phase 4 depolarization in Purkinje fibers and markedly depress phase 0 in fast-response cardiac cells. They slow conduction substantially and shorten the ERP in atrium, ventricle, and His-Purkinje system. In humans, chronic oral doses prolong the refractory periods of the atrium, ventricle, and anomalous AV connections. They increase the AH and HV intervals and the PR, QRS, and QT intervals in the ECG much more than drugs with class IA action. Encainide and propafenone have important active metabolites.

Indications. At the present time, drugs with class IC antiarrhythmic action are indicated only for the treatment of life-threatening, sustained ventricular arrhythmias when other drugs have failed. Treatment should be initiated in hospital. However, encainide and flecainide are extremely effective against PSVT in the WPW syndrome, AV nodal PSVT, and paroxysmal atrial fibrillation and have been recommended for treatment of these arrhythmias in patients without structural heart disease. Encainide and flecainide *increased* the mortality rate in the Cardiac Arrhythmia Suppression Trial, a controlled study that enrolled patients with left ventricular dysfunction and asymptomatic or minimally symptomatic ventricular arrhythmias after myocardial infarction. It is prudent to assume that other drugs with class IC action and perhaps drugs with class IA or IB antiarrhythmic action have the same effect on mortality rate.

DRUGS WITH CLASS II ANTIARRHYTHMIC ACTION

Propranolol, the first β blocker in the United States, was approved more than 20 years ago. Of the many β-adrenergic blocking drugs now available, only acebutolol and propranolol are approved for the treatment of chronic atrial or ventricular arrhythmias; atenolol and metroprolol are indicated to reduce mortality in acute myocardial infarction (when started within hours of symptom onset); and propranolol and timolol are indicated to reduce cardiovascular mortality in patients who have survived the acute phase of infarction. Timolol also reduces nonfatal reinfarction. When there are no contraindications, drugs with class II antiarrhythmic action are the preferred treatment for potentially malignant ventricular arrhythmias. There are many significant differences among the β-adrenergic blocking agents that govern the choice for an individual patient, e.g., cardioselectivity, intrinsic sympathomimetic action, electrophysiologic effects, and pharmacokinetics.

Pharmacology. Beta blockers decrease automaticity in the sinus node and His-Purkinje system when it is enhanced by sympathetic influences but have little effect when catecholamines are absent. Propranolol has little effect on phase 0 depolarization of cardiac fibers at low concentrations. At high concentrations, i.e., 1000 to 3000 ng per milliliter, phase 0 depolarization is depressed. Propranolol shortens while other β blockers can prolong action potential duration in atrial, ventricular, and particularly His-Purkinje cells; these effects are unrelated to β-blocking activity. In humans, propranolol and other β blockers increase the ERP of the AV node, a major antiarrhythmic effect, but have little effect on atrial or ventricular refractoriness.

Indications. Propranolol is indicated for supraventricular arrhythmias, particularly those induced by catecholamines and those associated with the WPW syndrome or thyrotoxicosis, for symptomatic APC's, and to control the ventricular rate in atrial flutter or fibrillation. It is also indicated for ventricular arrhythmias caused by catecholamines. Propranolol, acebutolol, or another β blocker is the first choice for the treatment of symptomatic but benign or potentially malignant VPC's.

DRUGS WITH CLASS III ANTIARRHYTHMIC ACTION

AMIODARONE. Amiodarone is a benzofuran derivative, 37 per cent iodine by weight, originally developed as a smooth muscle relaxant and coronary vasodilator to treat angina pectoris. In 1986, amiodarone was approved by the United States Food and Drug Administration as a last resort treatment for malignant ventricular arrhythmias. There have been no controlled studies of its efficacy.

Pharmacology. Amiodarone substantially prolongs action potential duration and ERP in atrium, ventricle, and Purkinje fibers (a class III action). Amiodarone slows sinus rate by a direct effect. Under laboratory conditions, amiodarone can have a substantial class I antiarrhythmic effect. In man, amiodarone slows the sinus rate and increases the PR and QT intervals in the ECG with less effect on the QRS. Also, it increases the atrial, AV nodal, and ventricular refractory periods and prolongs the HV interval (a class I action).

Indications. Amiodarone is indicated only for treatment of recurrent ventricular fibrillation or recurrent, hemodynamically unstable sustained VT that has not responded to other antiarrhythmic drugs or when other drugs cannot be tolerated. Treatment must be assessed by a method with high predictive accuracy. Endocardial electrical stimulation is the method of choice. About 20 per cent of patients with inducible VT can be rendered uninducible, and these patients do well. In another 40 to 50 per cent, the VT rate slows enough to control symptoms during sustained VT. In this group, recurrences of VT are not reduced much but usually are not fatal. Patients who have inducible symptomatic, sustained VT after being loaded with amiodarone should be considered for some alternate treatment. Because of the serious nature of the arrhythmias for which amiodarone is indicated and the unpredictable time course of effect, amiodarone should be started in a hospital setting.

BRETYLIUM TOSYLATE. Bretylium is a postganglionic adrenergic neuron blocker that was approved in the United States in 1978 for intramuscular or intravenous use as an antiarrhythmic drug.

Pharmacology. Bretylium causes marked lengthening of the action potential duration and ERP of ventricular muscle and Purkinje fibers (class III action). It is selectively taken up in peripheral adrenergic nerves and causes the acute release of norepinephrine; later, it produces chemical sympathectomy, preventing the norepinephrine release during nerve action potentials. Bretylium has no significant effect on phase 0 depolarization or conduction (i.e., it has no class I action), but it does increase the ventricular fibrillation threshold. Bretylium does not depress myocardial performance but can cause severe postural hypotension by interfering with the efferent limb of the baroreceptor reflex arc.

Indications. Bretylium is indicated for the therapy and prophylaxis of ventricular fibrillation and for the treatment of life-threatening ventricular arrhythmias, e.g., sustained VT, that have failed to respond to first-line antiarrhythmic drugs, e.g., lidocaine. Use of bretylium should be restricted to intensive care units. It is interesting that ventricular fibrillation usually responds within minutes while the full effect on unsustained VT and VPC's takes hours.

dl-SOTALOL. dl-Sotalol is an experimental drug being proposed for treatment of malignant or symptomatic, potentially malignant ventricular arrhythmias. It has class III action as well as substantial class II action. It is more effective than amiodarone at rendering sustained VT uninducible and is much safer.

DRUGS WITH CLASS IV ANTIARRHYTHMIC ACTION

VERAPAMIL. Verapamil is a papavarine derivative that has been used since 1962 as a coronary vasodilator. Later, its calcium channel blocking properties were discovered and, in 1981, it was approved for use in the United States for the treatment of angina pectoris and supraventricular arrhythmias.

Pharmacology. Verapamil slows spontaneous firing in isolated sinus node preparations; the effect is less marked in vivo because of reflex sympathetic nervous activity caused by peripheral vaso-

dilation. Verapamil decreases normal automaticity in Purkinje fibers and abolishes delayed afterdepolarizations and triggered activity in experimental digitalis toxicity. Verapamil prolongs refractoriness and conduction in the AV node by blocking Ca^{2+} channels. This action accounts for the ability of verapamil to terminate and prevent PSVT. Verapamil can abolish experimental VT due to slow potentials. Also, verapamil can delay ischemic injury and prevent arrhythmogenic electrophysiologic effects caused by transient ischemia. Verapamil also has α-adrenergic blocking properties. In humans, verapamil slows heart rate and increases the PR interval without any change in the QRS and QTc.

Indications. Intravenous verapamil is about 80 per cent effective for a rapid conversion (45 to 60 seconds) of PSVT to sinus rhythm (Table 42–11). Verapamil should not be given IV to patients with heart failure or those with wide QRS tachycardias until the rhythm is *proven* to be PSVT.

Verapamil can provide temporary control of rapid ventricular rate in atrial fibrillation. A 5- to 10-mg IV dose of verapamil slows the ventricular rate about 20 per cent for 15 to 30 minutes while a more permanent treatment is being established. Verapamil can be used orally to prevent PSVT or to help control the ventricular rate in atrial flutter or fibrillation.

Diltiazem shows promise for the acute and chronic treatment of PSVT.

DRUGS WITH MISCELLANEOUS ANTIARRHYTHMIC ACTION

ADENOSINE. Adenosine became available for use in the United States in 1990. It depresses automaticity in sinus node and conduction in the AV node; these are direct effects not blocked by atropine. A 10- to 20-mg dose of this drug terminates PSVT within 20 seconds in more than 90 per cent of cases by blocking conduction in the AV node in AV reciprocating tachycardia or in the slow antegrade AV nodal pathway in AV nodal tachycardia. It is not effective for terminating intra-atrial reentry and therefore is ineffective for atrial tachycardia, atrial flutter, or atrial fibrillation. It has less adverse hemodynamic effect than verapamil but frequently causes transient, minor adverse effects.

Bigger JT Jr, Hoffman BF: Antiarrhythmic Drugs. *In* Gilman AG, Goodman LS, Rall TW, Murad F (eds.): The Pharmacological Basis of Therapeutics, 8th ed. New York, MacMillan Publishing Company, 1990, pp 840–873. *A concise summary of the pharmacology and clinical use of antiarrhythmic drugs. Selectively referenced.*

Siddoway LA, Roden DM, Woosley RL: Clinical pharmacology of old and new antiarrhythmic drugs. Cadiovasc Clin 15:199, 1985. *A discussion of the pharmacodynamics, pharmacokinetics, drug interactions, and clinical use of antiarrhythmic drugs. Extensively referenced.*

The Physicians Desk Reference. Oradell, N.J., Medical Economics Company, Inc. *A yearly publication that gives accurate full prescribing information for all drugs.*

ELECTRICAL MODALITIES IN THE MANAGEMENT OF CARDIAC ARRHYTHMIAS

Temporary or permanent cardiac pacemakers and DC cardioversion or external defibrillation are well-established forms of electrical therapy. In 1985, an automatic implantable cardioverter/defibrillator was approved by the FDA.

Cardiac Pacemakers

Permanent pacemakers were first implanted in the 1960's, and over the ensuing 25 years the pacemaker industry has matured, providing highly sophisticated and diverse products for management of bradyarrhythmias and, to a lesser extent, tachyarrhythmias. About 100,000 pulse generators are implanted each year in the United States, about half of the world's pacemaker implants. There are approximately 500,000 patients with pacemakers living in the United States.

INDICATIONS FOR CARDIAC PACING. The joint report of the American College of Cardiology and American Heart Association divided indications into three classes: I, definitely indicated; II, possibly indicated; and III, not indicated (Table 42–12). Pacing is indicated for bradycardia with complete heart block or advanced second-degree AV block with symptoms such as transient dizziness, lightheadedness, near syncope or syncope,

TABLE 42–12. DEFINITE INDICATIONS FOR IMPLANTED PACEMAKER

A. Complete heart block, permanent or intermittent with any one of the following complications:
1. Symptomatic bradycardia
2. Congestive heart failure
3. Conditions that require treatment with drugs that suppress ventricular escape rhythms
4. Asystole $\geq$ 3 seconds or ventricular rate <40 per minute
5. Mental confusion that clears with temporary pacing

B. Complete heart block or advanced second-degree AV block that occurs during myocardial infarction and persists

C. Chronic bi- or trifascicular block with one of the following:
1. Intermittent complete heart block
2. Type II second-degree AV block associated with symptomatic bradycardia

D. Sinus node dysfunction with documented symptomatic bradycardia

E. Hypersensitive carotid sinus syndrome with recurrent syncope and asystole >3 seconds provoked by minimal carotid sinus pressure

F. Symptomatic supraventricular tachycardia that does not respond to medical treatment

TABLE 42–13. CODE FOR PACEMAKER MODES

Chamber Paced	Chamber Sensed	Response to Sensing
V = Ventricle	V = Ventricle	I = Inhibited
A = Atrium	A = Atrium	T = Triggered
D = Double (atrium and ventricle)	D = Double (atrium and ventricle)	D = Double (atrium triggered and ventricle inhibited)
	O = None	O = None

Inter-Society Commission for Heart Disease Resources. Table 42–13 shows the first three letter codes. The three letters indicate the chamber paced, the chamber sensed, and the response to sensing. The fourth and fifth positions describe programmable and antitachycardia features and are used less frequently.

SELECTION OF THE PACEMAKER MODE. Selection of the appropriate pacemaker has become more complex as options have become more diverse. Table 42–14 summarizes common selections, considering the atrial rhythm and status of AV and VA conduction.

COMPLICATIONS. Transvenous implants are associated with cardiac perforation, arrhythmias, infection, thrombosis, emboli, and lead fracture or displacement. Thoracotomy carries the risk of general anesthesia, bleeding, infection, postoperative respiratory compromise, and late threshold increases. With either route of implantation, the pulse generator may erode through the skin. Pacemakers can be inhibited by intense magnetic fields such as large telephone transformers, microwave devices, diathermy, cautery, antitheft devices, and certain types of motors, e.g., electric razors. Unipolar pacemakers may be inhibited by local myopotentials. The "pacemaker syndrome" was first defined as lightheadedness or syncope related to long cycles of AV asynchrony that occurred during VOO or VVI pacing. The definition also includes (1) episodic weakness or syncope associated with alternating AV synchrony and asynchrony, (2) inadequate cardiac output associated with continued absence of AV synchrony or with fixed asynchrony (persistent VA conduction), and (3) patient awareness of beat-to-beat variation in vascular pulsation.

PACEMAKER FOLLOW-UP. Implanted pacing devices require careful follow-up. Regular transtelephonic monitoring permits early detection of battery depletion. At the present time, the principal problem in pacemaker follow-up is the diversity of pacemaker models and methods for interrogating pacemaker function.

marked exercise intolerance, and congestive heart failure. Asymptomatic conditions that are definite indications are permanent high-grade AV block after myocardial infarction or surgical repair of congenital heart disease, or complete heart block with a ventricular rate less than 40 per minute.

LEAD PLACEMENT. More than 90 per cent of permanent pacing leads are placed via cephalic, subclavian, or external jugular veins. Most transvenous leads are stainless steel, multifilament helical coil wires insulated with polyurethane or silicone rubber. These leads are small, steerable, and fracture resistant. Leads are anchored by tines or a screw-in arrangement at their tips. Both unipolar and bipolar electrodes are commonly used. For simple ventricular pacing, one lead is placed in the right ventricular apex. For dual chamber pacing, a second lead is placed in the right atrium.

PULSE GENERATORS. Modern pacemaker generators weigh 40 to 50 grams, are powered by lithium batteries that last 7 to 10 years, and have circuitry for sensing intracardiac electrograms. Pacemakers can be interrogated to evaluate the pulse generator or reprogrammed to meet changing requirements. Multiprogrammability provides flexibility in obtaining diagnostic information and individualizing the pacemaker prescription.

MODES OF CARDIAC PACING. Pacemaker modes are expressed in the three- or five-letter notation proposed by the

TABLE 42–14. INDICATIONS FOR PACING MODES

AV Conduction	Atrial Rhythm		
	Normal	*Bradycardia*	*Bradycardia-Tachycardia*
Normal	None indicated	AAI	AAI
AV block; normal VA conduction time	VDD, DDD	DDD, DVI	DVI, VVI
AV block; prolonged VA conduction time	DVI	DVI	DVI

AAI: Fixed-rate atrial pacing occurs unless inhibited by sensed atrial complexes. This mode can be used for patients with symptomatic sinus node dysfunction and normal AV conduction.

VDD: Ventricular pulses are delivered when atrial complex is sensed and inhibited when ventricular complex is sensed. The VDD mode is used when adequate atrial rates and sensing are present, along with high-grade AV block and normal VA conduction. VDD pacing provides atrial augmentation of ventricular filling and avoids the pacemaker syndrome but is contraindicated for patients with supraventricular tachyarrhythmias.

DVI: Both chambers are paced at a preselected rate and AV interval. Pacing is inhibited by ventricular but not atrial activity. The DVI mode is used when synchronous AV contraction is needed in patients with symptomatic atrial bradycardia. The pacing rate does not increase during exercise. DVI pacing is contraindicated in patients who have supraventricular tachyarrhythmias.

DDD: Both atria and ventricles are paced and sensed. The atrial or ventricular pacemaker pulses are inhibited when either atrial or ventricular premature activity is detected. When atrial activity is sensed, a ventricular pulse is provided. This mode of pacing provides synchronous AV contraction over a wide range of heart rates. DDD pacemakers are adaptive: totally inhibited in sinus rhythm with normal AV conduction; AAI pacing during sinus bradycardia with normal AV conduction; VDD pacing during sinus rhythm with impaired AV conduction; DVI pacing during sinus bradycardia with impaired AV conduction. DDD pacemakers are contraindicated in patients with persistent or frequently occurring atrial tachyarrhythmias and those with long VA conduction times who can develop pacemaker-mediated reciprocating tachycardia.

VVI: This mode can be used for any symptomatic bradyarrhythmia. The VVI mode is contraindicated in patients who have had the pacemaker syndrome, those with congestive heart failure, and those who need rate-responsive pacing.

Rate-Responsive Pacing (VVIR): Many patients who need increased heart rate during exercise have relative contraindications for DDD pacing, e.g., inadequate sinus node function or atrial fibrillation. Rate-responsive pacing is provided by sensing the activity level and increasing the pacing rate. Heart rate can be increased by as much as 90 per minute, i.e., from 60 at rest to 150 during exercise, providing an increase in cardiac output and exercise capability.

DC Cardioversion

DC cardioversion was introduced in 1962, and has become a mainstay in the management of cardiac arrhythmias. Cardioversion depolarizes all or most of the heart, interrupts reentrant circuits, and terminates arrhythmias. It is effective for atrial fibrillation, atrial flutter, PSVT, ventricular tachycardia, or ventricular fibrillation. Drug-resistant arrhythmias, e.g., atrial flutter, may respond readily to DC cardioversion. Because of its speed, cardioversion is preferable to drug therapy for arrhythmias that adversely affect hemodynamics, such as rapid atrial arrhythmias, sustained ventricular tachycardia, or ventricular fibrillation. Elective cardioversion is indicated for atrial fibrillation of recent onset (<6 months) to control symptoms and hemodynamic abnormalities and lower the risk of systemic embolism.

LIMITATIONS AND CONTRAINDICATIONS. Chronic atrial fibrillation, i.e., greater than 6 to 12 months in duration, is so likely to recur after cardioversion that digitalis therapy may be preferred. Contributing causes (e.g., hyperthyroidism, pericardial inflammation, pulmonary thromboembolism, chronic obstructive pulmonary disease, or alcohol abuse) should be controlled before cardioversion; otherwise, atrial fibrillation is likely to recur. Sinus rhythm is difficult to maintain after cardioversion of atrial fibrillation in patients with heart failure or large left atria (>45 mm in diameter by echocardiography). In the bradycardia-tachycardia syndrome, cardioversion often produces inadequate rhythms, and atrial fibrillation usually resumes within a few hours. Cardioversion is contraindicated for arrhythmias caused by digitalis intoxication because it can precipitate ventricular fibrillation.

ANTICOAGULATION. Despite the lack of a controlled evaluation, a standard anticoagulation practice has evolved for patients with atrial fibrillation. Most patients who have been fibrillating for more than 3 weeks are anticoagulated, particularly those with (1) a history of embolization, (2) a prosthetic mitral valve, (3) an enlarged left atrium, or (4) congestive heart failure. The prothrombin time is kept at 1.5 to 2.0 times the normal value with warfarin for 3 or more weeks before and a week after cardioversion.

RESULTS. The immediate results of cardioversion are excellent (Table 42–15). The main long-term problem following cardioversion is reversion to atrial fibrillation. Class I antiarrhythmic drugs decrease the chance of recurrence of atrial fibrillation 1 year after cardioversion from about 75 to 50 per cent.

COMPLICATIONS. Few complications attend technically excellent cardioversion. Occasionally, transient SA or AV block or ventricular arrhythmias occur immediately after DC shock, especially with excessive digitalis. In the sick sinus syndrome, the sinus may fail to resume control of cardiac rhythm after cardioversion. Atropine, isoproterenol, and/or external pacing usually maintain the patient until a temporary transvenous pacemaker can be inserted. Occasionally, worsening heart failure or frank pulmonary edema occurs within a few hours after cardioversion. The cause of this syndrome is unknown. Elevation of myocardial creatine kinase after DC cardioversion is rare.

Automatic Implantable Cardioverter/Defibrillator

The first automatic implantable defibrillator (AID), a device that responded only to ventricular fibrillation, was implanted in 1980. The first automatic implantable cardioverter/defibrillator (AICD) was implanted in 1982. This unit detected and cardioverted ventricular tachycardia as well as providing defibrillation. Antitachycardia pacing was added to AICD units in the 1990's.

INDICATIONS. The AICD currently is recommended for patients who have had a documented episode of life-threatening ventricular tachyarrhythmia or cardiac arrest not associated with the acute phase of myocardial infarction. Also, patients should have inducible ventricular tachycardia or ventricular fibrillation unsuitable for drug or surgical therapy. These initial indications are being extended.

IMPLANTATION. The electrode systems are implanted via a thoracotomy. The 292-gram power unit is implanted subcutaneously in an abdominal pocket. During implantation, defibrillation thresholds and detection of ventricular tachycardia/fibrillation are tested extensively to ensure proper function. The AICD usually lasts about 5 years.

The device monitors the ECG continuously. When ventricular tachycardia or fibrillation is detected and verified, the AICD charges its capacitors and delivers a 20- to 30-joule pulse.

FOLLOW-UP. The AICD is a complex device that requires careful follow-up. Potential problems with the device include (1) depletion of the battery, (2) lead breakage or migration, (3) inappropriate discharges, (4) infection, and (5) skin erosion. After implantation, a magnet test should be performed every 2 months to evaluate the device and reform the capacitors. The rate cut-off and other features are programmable to meet changing needs during follow-up.

Between 1980 and the end of 1990 more than 10,000 AID or AICD units were implanted. Follow-up reveals a 1-year cardiovascular mortality of about 10 per cent and a sudden death rate of about 2 per cent. Although the device is complex and expensive, it is highly effective for selected patients with malignant ventricular arrhythmias.

DeSilva RA, Graboys TB, Podrid PJ, Lown B: Cardioversion and defibrillation. Am Heart J 100:881–895, 1980. *A thorough review of the history, theory, and practice of cardioversion and defibrillation.*

Frye RL, Collins JJ, DeSanctis RW, et al.: Guidelines for permanent cardiac pacemaker implantation, May 1984. J Am Coll Cardiol 4:434, 1984. *A report of a task force to review cardiac pacing. The report defines indications for cardiac pacing and makes recommendations about the selection of devices for treatment of specific clinical problems. This report is used as a standard by the medical profession, regulatory agencies, and reimbursement sources.*

Mirowski M: The automatic implantable cardioverter-defibrillator: An overview. J Am Coll Cardiol 6:461, 1985. *A review of the concepts, evolution, clinical use, and follow-up of the automatic implantable cardioverter defibrillator by the originator of the device.*

Parsonnet V, Bernstein AD: Pacing in perspective: Concepts and controversies. Circulation 73:1087, 1986. *A perspective on cardiac pacing. Provides a concise view of the history, development, practice, and future directions in cardiac pacing.*

Winkle RA, Mead RH, Ruder MA, et al: Long-term outcome with the automatic implantable cardioverter-defibrillator. J Am Coll Cardiol 13:1353–1361, 1989. *The clinical events and outcome in 270 patients with AICD implants. Provides an excellent perspective on the current use of the device.*

SURGICAL TREATMENT OF CARDIAC ARRHYTHMIAS

The objective of arrhythmia surgery may be (1) to remove the arrhythmic focus, (2) to interrupt a reentrant pathway, or (3) to prevent the ventricles from responding to supraventricular tachyarrhythmias (Table 42–16). For surgery to be seriously considered, the arrhythmia must pose significant risk to life or interfere substantially with the quality of life.

Supraventricular Arrhythmias

INTERRUPTION OF THE BUNDLE OF HIS. Atrial flutter and fibrillation can be palliated by interruption of the His bundle

---

TABLE 42–15. ENERGY FOR CARDIOVERSION/DEFIBRILLATION

Arrhythmia	Recommended Initial Energy* (joules)	Comments
Atrial flutter	50	100% conversion; most convert with about 25 joules.
Atrial fibrillation	200	85–95% conversion; a few patients may require 300- to 400-joule DC shocks to cardiovert.
Paroxysmal supraventricular tachycardia	100	100% conversion
Ventricular tachycardia	50	90–95% conversion; 80% convert with <10 joules; a few need 100 joules or more.
Ventricular fibrillation	300–400	90–95% defibrillation; many convert at 200 joules or below but time is of the essence in successful defibrillation.

*An energy level with a high probability of converting the arrhythmia.

TABLE 42–16. SURGERY FOR CARDIAC ARRHYTHMIAS

Arrhythmia	Operative Approach
Atrial fibrillation	Ablation of AV node and implantation of a pacemaker
	Left atrial exclusion (highly experimental)
Ectopic atrial focus	Excision of the focus after accurate mapping
PSVT (Pre-excitation)	Surgical division of anomalous AV connection
PSVT (AV nodal)	Partial catheter ablation of AV node
	Retronodal surgical resection
	Division of His bundle, implantation of pacemaker
Ventricular tachycardia (coronary heart disease)	Endocardial resection guided by mapping
Ventricular tachycardia (arrhythmogenic right ventricular dysplasia)	Simple ventriculotomy; isolation of arrhythmic site
Ventricular tachycardia (after repair of tetralogy of Fallot)	Resection of infundibulectomy scar
Multiform ventricular tachycardia (long QT syndrome)	Left stellate ganglionectomy

and implantation of a ventricular pacemaker when drug therapy cannot control ventricular rate. The need for such surgery has diminished with the advent of β-adrenergic blockers, verapamil, and catheter ablation.

Catheter Ablation. A catheter technique for His bundle ablation has been found to be safe and effective. Using fluoroscopy, a multielectrode catheter is placed so as to record the bundle of His depolarization. Then one or more large energy shocks are delivered to the electrode that records the largest His bundle depolarization. Shocks can be repeated until AV conduction is interrupted.

EXCISION OF AUTOMATIC FOCI. Rhythms originating in automatic or tiny reentrant ectopic foci can be removed or ablated. The key to removal or ablation is accurate localization by epicardial and/or endocardial activation mapping.

INTERRUPTION OF REENTRANT PATHWAYS. Surgery is very effective for PSVT that uses an anomalous AV connection as an essential portion of the circuit or for atrial fibrillation with rapid ventricular response in the WPW syndrome. Preoperative electrophysiologic studies are used to delineate the mechanism of PSVT, the site of the accessory AV connection, and the route of cardiac excitation during PSVT. During operation, the anomalous AV connection(s) is located precisely using cardiac stimulation and epi- or endocardial mapping during sinus rhythm, ventricular pacing, and PSVT. Traditionally, division of anomalous AV connections is done on cardiopulmonary bypass with the atrium open. More recently, dissection and cryoablation have been used successfully without cardiopulmonary bypass. Centers with major programs obtain cure rates greater than 85 per cent, with surgical mortalities less than 1 per cent. These results usually make surgery a better choice than drug treatment.

Sustained Ventricular Tachycardia

VENTRICULAR ANEURYSMS. The largest surgical experience has been gathered in patients with recurrent, sustained VT and coronary heart disease; most of these patients have left ventricular aneurysms, two- or three-vessel disease, and severely impaired left ventricular function. The rate of VT tends to be slow and easily induced and can be mapped during electrophysiologic studies. Accurate preoperative endocardial maps are critical because adequate endocardial maps are often impossible to obtain at surgery. At surgery, the arrhythmogenic tissue is removed or ablated with a cryoprobe. Map-guided excision, isolation, or cryoablation is about 80 per cent effective in controlling sustained VT during 1 to 3 years of follow-up. However, the perioperative mortality is about 15 to 20 per cent owing primarily to the advanced coronary disease and severity of left

ventricular dysfunction. Selection of ideal cases lowers the mortality rate to about 8 to 12 per cent.

ARRHYTHMOGENIC RIGHT VENTRICULAR DYSPLASIA. Patients who have VT due to right ventricular arrhythmogenic dysplasia usually can be cured by an incision across the dysplastic area that shows the latest activation in sinus rhythm and earliest activation during VT. Small areas of dysplasia can be excised and large areas can be isolated if simple incision is not successful.

TETRALOGY OF FALLOT. VT occurs rarely in patients who have had total repair of tetralogy of Fallot. Epicardial excitation mapping at surgery shows that VT arises in the right ventricular infundibular scar, and scar resection effects a cure.

LONG QT SYNDROME. Patients with the congenital form of the long QT syndrome can have recurrent attacks of malignant, multiform VT of the torsades de pointes type. These rhythms are associated with cardiac arrest and sudden cardiac death. Unequal sympathetic nerve traffic to the heart is part of the explanation for the heterogeneous electrophysiologic condition of the ventricles. Excision of the left stellate ganglion markedly reduces the mortality rate in high-risk patients with the congenital long QT syndrome.

Cox JL: The status of surgery for cardiac arrhythmias. Circulation 71:413–417, 1985. *A perspective on surgery for both supraventricular and ventricular arrhythmias.*

Cox JL: Patient selection criteria and results of surgery for refractory ischemic ventricular tachycardia. Circulation 79:163–177, 1989. *An update on selection of patients in the era of the automatic implantable cardioverter defibrillator.*

Cox JL, Gallagher JJ, Cain MM: Experience with 118 consecutive patients undergoing operation for the Wolff-Parkinson-White syndrome. J Thorac Cardiovasc Surg 90:490–501, 1985. *A review of a large, successful experience with surgery for anomalous AV connections.*

Guiraudon GM, Klein GJ, Sharma AD, Yee R: Surgical alternatives for supraventricular tachycardias. Am J Cardiol 64:92J–96J, 1989. *A review of the operative treatment of a wide range of supraventricular tachycardias.*

Klein GJ, Guiraudon GM: Surgical therapy of cardiac arrhythmias. Cardiol Clin 1:323–340, 1983. *A summary of concepts that form the basis for surgical treatment of cardiac arrhythmias.*

43 Sudden Cardiac Death
Douglas P. Zipes

DEFINITION AND INCIDENCE

Sudden cardiac death is unexpected natural death from cardiac causes. The cardiac cause results in a disturbance in cardiac function which produces abrupt loss of cerebral blood flow. Death occurs within 1 hour of the onset of acute symptoms. In 25 per cent of patients who die from coronary heart disease, sudden cardiac death may be the first sign of trouble. Although some patients at risk for sudden cardiac death may be symptomatic prior to the event, their complaints are often too nonspecific to be helpful. An estimated 350,000 sudden cardiac deaths occur annually in the United States, or about one every 90 seconds. This represents almost half of all cardiovascular deaths and almost one fourth of all deaths. The incidence of sudden cardiac death due to coronary heart disease is declining along with the overall decrease in coronary heart disease mortality. These decreases may relate to more frequent and effective treatment of hypertension, angina, and myocardial infarction and attention to additional risk factors.

The incidence of sudden cardiac death peaks between 0 and 6 months and between 45 and 75 years of age. Risk factors for sudden cardiac death parallel those for coronary heart disease and include male sex, cardiac enlargement, obesity, cigarette smoking, glucose intolerance, hypertension, social isolation, stress, and excess alcohol consumption. The presence of coronary heart disease and past myocardial infarction add additional risks. Following myocardial infarction, more than five to ten premature ventricular complexes (PVC's) per hour, three or more repetitive PVC's, late potentials recorded on signal-averaged electrocardiograms, and left ventricular dysfunction are variables identifying patients at increased risk of sudden cardiac death. Angiographic or hemodynamic characteristics are not significantly different between patients who have coronary artery disease and suffer sudden cardiac death and those who do not die suddenly.

Sudden cardiac death, stroke, and myocardial infarction all occur more frequently in the morning hours upon rising, from 6:00 A.M. to noon, at a time when a hypercoagulable state with increased platelet aggregability or coronary vasoconstriction exists. Autonomic mechanisms may also be important in modulating this hypercoagulable state and in triggering sudden cardiac death.

CAUSES

Substrate

Ventricular myocardial abnormalities such as hypertrophy, dilated cardiomyopathy, inflammatory changes, diseases of the heart valves, and primary electrophysiologic abnormalities (Table 43–1) are responsible for about 25 per cent of sudden cardiac deaths, with the remaining 75 per cent due to coronary artery disease. Occasionally, patients without structural heart disease suffer ventricular fibrillation. The long QT syndrome is one of several electrophysiologic abnormalities that can predispose to sudden cardiac death (Table 43–1). It may be acquired by exposure to several antiarrhythmic drugs such as quinidine, phenothiazines, and tricyclic antidepressants or may result from electrolyte disturbances such as hypokalemia or hypomagnesemia. It may also be congenital, with (Jervell-Lange-Nielsen syndrome) and without (Romano-Ward syndrome) neural deafness. Preliminary information suggests that a specific electrophysiologic mechanism is responsible, called early afterdepolarizations.

At autopsy, 90 per cent or greater narrowing of at least one coronary artery is noted in three quarters of patients dying with sudden cardiac death, and almost two thirds have three vessels with 75 per cent or more stenosis. Old myocardial infarction is found in about two thirds of autopsies. No specific high-risk coronary artery or lesion site, proximal versus distal, has been identified. Acute thrombotic occlusion is noted in 60 to 75 per cent, usually at the site of a fissured plaque, providing clues about mechanisms of sudden cardiac death. For example, in sudden cardiac death, as in unstable angina, plaque rupture with thrombus formation may result in myocardial ischemia and precipitate fatal ventricular arrhythmias. Also, platelet microthrombi from ulcerated arterial plaques may produce multiple areas of myocardial necrosis that can cause electrical instability and ventricular fibrillation. It is likely that a non–flow-limiting intimal plaque serves as a nidus for acute formation of a lumen-occluding thrombus in a significant number of patients with sudden cardiac death. Certainly coronary artery spasm or other factors that reduce myocardial blood flow without an increase in demand, as well as an increase in myocardial oxygen demand with a fixed supply, may be critical.

Prostacyclin (PGI_2), a potent inhibitor of platelet activation and a vasodilator, may be important. In dogs, PGI_2 given intravenously reduces the incidence of ventricular fibrillation after circumflex coronary artery occlusion, as do specific thromboxane synthase inhibitors. The latter presumably work by blocking conversion of prostaglandin endoperoxide PGH_2 to thromboxane A_2, causing PGH_2 accumulation, which then can be converted to prostacyclin. Prostacyclin also modulates sympathetic activity to the heart at presynaptic sites and can reduce the incidence of ventricular fibrillation by reducing sympathetic effects. Local release of serotonin in atherosclerotic vessels may also be important by reducing coronary blood flow, increasing platelet aggregation, and causing the development of an occlusive thrombus and electrical instability.

Other biochemical clues are being investigated. For example, inhibition of carnitine acyltransferase, which reduces the accumulation of long-chain acylcarnitines in the sarcolemma and the initial electrophysiologic derangements associated with hypoxia and also the accumulation of lysophosphatidylcholine, lowers the early occurrence of ventricular tachycardia or ventricular fibrillation in cats subjected to coronary artery occlusion.

Of great interest is the observation that only 20 per cent of those patients who are successfully resuscitated from ventricular fibrillation evolve an acute myocardial infarction. This means that if thrombosis of a coronary artery causes the ischemia responsible for the ventricular fibrillation, it is transient because flow must be restored to prevent infarction. Ventricular fibrillation recurs in 30 per cent within 1 year and 45 per cent by 2 years in those survivors who do not, versus only about 2 per cent in those who do, evolve a transmural myocardial infarction after resuscitation. Therefore, patients without infarction are at increased risk for another episode of sudden cardiac death.

Ischemia responsible for the biochemical changes noted above is conducive to arrhythmia development. Myocardial ischemia results in loss of membrane integrity with cellular efflux of potassium and influx of calcium, development of acidosis, reduction of transmembrane resting potentials, and enhanced automaticity in some tissues. Reperfusion causes continued influx of calcium that may result in triggered arrhythmias. The electrophysiologic changes following myocardial ischemia can create areas of slow conduction and unidirectional block, changes necessary for reentry to occur, as well as areas of abnormal automaticity and triggered activity. These factors can lead to ventricular tachycardia/fibrillation. Tissue healed after previous injury appears more susceptible to the electrical destabilizing effects of acute ischemia. The combination of a triggering event such as a premature ventricular complex and a susceptible myocardium may be the fundamental combination for development of a lethal arrhythmia. Triggering events and a susceptible myocardium may be dissociated from each other so that in the absence of a susceptible myocardium, triggering events may occur innocuously. Similarly, the presence of a susceptible myocardium without a triggering event may not give rise to arrhythmias.

TABLE 43–1. CAUSES AND CONTRIBUTING FACTORS IN SUDDEN CARDIAC DEATH

Coronary artery abnormalities
  Coronary atherosclerosis
  Congenital abnormalities of coronary arteries
  Coronary artery embolism
  Coronary arteritis
  Miscellaneous mechanical obstructions of coronary arteries
  Functional obstruction of coronary arteries
Hypertrophy of ventricular myocardium
  Left ventricular hypertrophy associated with coronary atherosclerosis
  Hypersensitive heart disease without significant coronary atherosclerosis
  Hypertrophic myocardium secondary to valvular heart disease
  Hypertrophic cardiomyopathy
  Primary or secondary pulmonary hypertension
Myocardial diseases and heart failure
  Chronic congestive heart failure
  Acute cardiac failure
Inflammatory, infiltrative, neoplastic, and degenerative processes
Diseases of the cardiac valves
Congenital heart disease
Electrophysiologic abnormalities
  Abnormalities of the conducting system
  Prolonged QT interval syndrome
  Idiopathic ventricular fibrillation
Electrical instability related to neurohumoral and central nervous system influences
  Catecholamine-dependent lethal arrhythmias
  Central nervous system related
Sudden infant death syndrome and sudden death in children
Miscellaneous
  Sudden death during extreme physical activity
  Mechanical interference with venous return
  Dissecting aneurysm of the aorta
  Toxic/metabolic disturbances
  Mimics of sudden cardiac death

Modified from Myerburg RJ, Castellanos A: Cardiac arrest and sudden cardiac death. *In* Braunwald EB (ed.): Heart Disease: A Textbook of Cardiovascular Medicine, 3rd ed. Philadelphia, W. B. Saunders Company, 1988, pp 742–777; with permission.

Arrhythmias

More than 90 per cent of sudden cardiac deaths are due to a lethal cardiac rhythm disturbance, approximately 80 per cent to

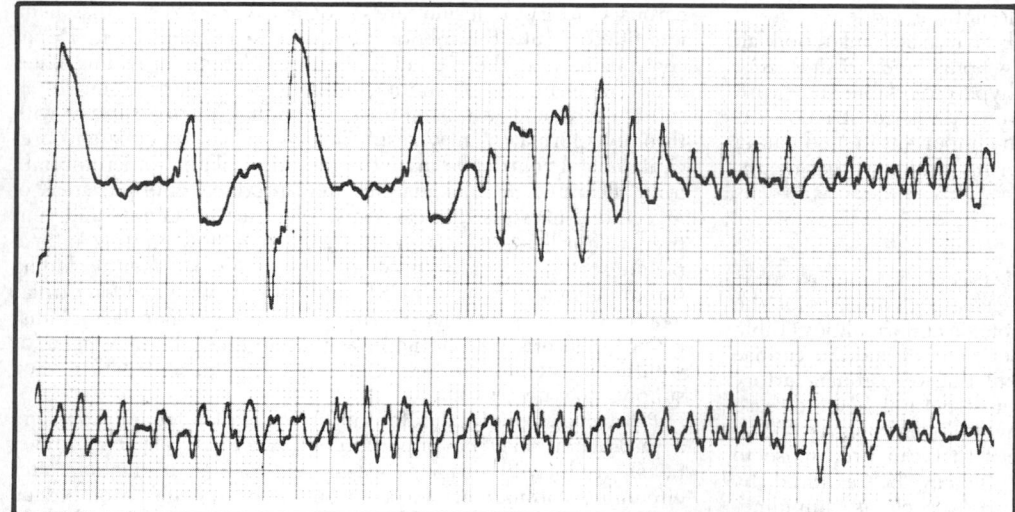

FIGURE 43–1. Ventricular tachycardia fibrillation. Several multiform premature ventricular complexes initiate a run of ventricular tachycardia that progresses to ventricular fibrillation. Monitor lead. Continuous recording.

ventricular tachycardia/fibrillation (Fig. 43–1), and 20 per cent to a severe bradyarrhythmia or ventricular asystole (Fig. 43–2). Ventricular tachycardia leading to ventricular fibrillation is often preceded by increases in sinus rate, advancing grades of ventricular ectopy, and loss of sinus arrhythmia (suggesting a decrease in vagal tone). Only a small percentage of patients have ischemic ST changes. Bradycardia and ventricular asystole occur more commonly in a severely diseased heart and may represent diffuse involvement of subendocardial Purkinje fibers by the ischemic process. Atrioventricular block occurs less often than asystole. Less frequent nonarrhythmic mechanisms of sudden cardiac death include electromechanical dissociation, ventricular rupture, cardiac tamponade, acute mechanical obstruction to flow, and acute dissection of a major blood vessel.

THERAPY AND OUTCOME

Untreated ventricular fibrillation produces irreversible brain damage within 3 to 5 minutes and death shortly thereafter. Although some patients may be resuscitated after longer periods of sustaining a ventricular tachyarrhythmia, the probability of a favorable outcome deteriorates rapidly in proportion to the duration of the unattended cardiac arrest, with older patients doing more poorly than younger. Some patients may have ventricular tachycardia with an output inadequate to maintain consciousness but sufficient to maintain brain viability, permitting a longer time interval between the onset of loss of consciousness and irreversible brain damage or death.

Therapy for a patient suffering cardiac arrest begins initially with establishing the diagnosis of the cardiac arrest, delivering a blow to the chest to attempt "thumpversion" of ventricular tachycardia, and clearing the airway. Basic life support activities including mouth-to-mouth ventilation, and chest compression should be started and continued until advanced life support activities begin. These include initially electrical cardioversion/ defibrillation for treatment of ventricular tachycardia/fibrillation, pacing for bradyarrhythmia/asystole, and drug administration. After successful resuscitation, the patient is admitted to a monitoring unit where treatment goals are to provide hemodynamic support, prevent a second cardiac arrest, and evaluate causes of the first.

Early ventricular defibrillation is the most important factor influencing survival. In the hospital, no time should be wasted in instituting electrical cardioversion or defibrillation. Out of hospital, prompt cardiopulmonary resuscitation (CPR) by bystander laypersons awaiting the arrival of emergency rescue personnel significantly improves the percentage of patients subsequently discharged alive from the hospital. Presumably this difference is due to CPR-related protection of the central nervous system.

Elements required to achieve the highest survival rates from out-of-hospital cardiac arrest include witnessed arrest, rapid telephone notification of the emergency medical service, early initiation of cardiopulmonary resuscitation, rapid arrival of emergency personnel equipped with a defibrillator, early advanced airway management, and prompt intravenous drug therapy. Significant risk factors for death after cardiopulmonary resuscitation include hypotension and pneumonia prior to arrest, time for restoration of normal rhythm exceeding 15 minutes, need for intubation, the presence of hypotension, and, after resuscitation, a need for vasopressors.

The rhythm disturbance responsible for the cardiac arrest influences outcome dramatically. Patients who have ventricular tachycardia have the best prognosis but constitute the smallest group of only about 10 per cent of all cardiac arrests. It is possible that many more cardiac arrests begin as sustained ventricular tachycardia and progress to ventricular fibrillation and that patients found with ventricular tachycardia do better because their arrest is treated earlier. Forty to 60 per cent of patients who

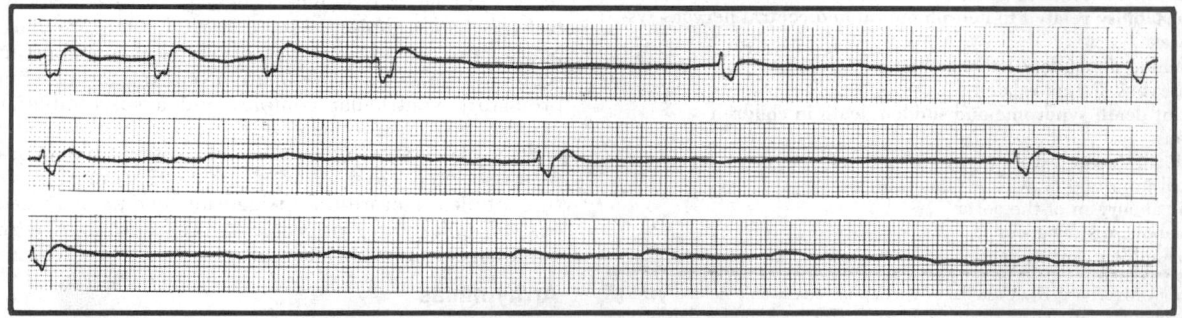

FIGURE 43–2. Sudden cardiac death due to asystole. A ventricular escape rhythm progressively slows, terminating in complete asystole. Monitor lead. Continuous recording.

have ventricular fibrillation are successfully resuscitated and admitted to the hospital alive, and about half of those are ultimately discharged alive. Patients who have bradyarrhythmia or asystole as the initiating event or at initial contact have the worst prognosis, with only about 10 per cent admitted to hospital alive and few if any subsequently surviving. Similarly, patients whose rhythm following defibrillation is a bradyarrhythmia of less than 60 beats per minute also have a poor prognosis, with 95 per cent dying prior to or during hospitalization.

Long-term therapy for prevention of ventricular tachyarrhythmias includes pharmacologic, electrical, and surgical options (see Ch. 42). In patients with ventricular tachycardia/fibrillation inducible by programmed electrical stimulation, serial electrophysiologic testing can identify drug regimens that prevent arrhythmia recurrence in approximately 20 to 40 per cent of patients. In an additional 20 per cent of patients, drugs can slow the ventricular tachycardia and reduce arrhythmia-related mortality to less than 3 per cent per year. For patients in whom ventricular tachycardia/fibrillation cannot be prevented or significantly slowed, medical antiarrhythmic therapy is generally unsuccessful and the sudden death mortality is 20 to 40 per cent per year. In these patients, surgical resection of the arrhythmogenic substrate or implantation of a pacemaker/cardioverter/defibrillator may be indicated. Both subendocardial resection and defibrillator implantation are highly effective in preventing sudden cardiac death. The choice of procedure depends on the arrhythmia diagnosis and the nature of the cardiac disease. Operative mortality is 10 to 15 per cent for surgical resection versus 3 per cent for device implantation, with left ventricular function being the most important predictor of risk. Arrhythmic mortality following device implantation is less than 2 per cent per year.

Bayes-deLuna A, Coumel P, Leclercq JF: Ambulatory sudden cardiac death: Mechanisms of production of fatal arrhythmia on the basis of data from 157 cases. Am Heart J 117:151–159, 1989. *An original study on ECG recordings of patients at the time of sudden cardiac death.*

Epstein SE, Quyyumi AA, Bonow RO: Sudden cardiac death without warning. N Engl J Med 321:320–324, 1989. *Suggestions on the coronary mechanisms responsible for sudden cardiac death.*

Kremers MS, Black WH, Wells PJ: Sudden cardiac death: Etiologies, pathogenesis and management. DM 35:381–445, 1989. *A thorough review of sudden cardiac death.*

Muller JE, Tofler GH, Stone PH: Circadian variation and triggers of onset of acute cardiovascular disease. Circulation 79:733–743, 1989. *A review of some of the triggers of sudden cardiac death.*

Winkle RA, Mead RH, Ruder MA, et al.: Long-term outcome with the automatic implantable cardioverter-defibrillator. J Am Coll Cardiol 13:1353–1361, 1989. *An original study on the largest single series of patients receiving the implantable defibrillator.*

44 Arterial Hypertension

Suzanne Oparil

Systemic hypertension is the most prevalent cardiovascular disorder in the United States, affecting over 60 million Americans. Almost 40 per cent of all black adults and more than half of the entire population over age 60 have hypertension. In spite of increasing public awareness and a rapidly expanding array of antihypertensive medications, hypertension remains one of the leading causes of cardiovascular morbidity and mortality. Efforts to prevent, diagnose, and treat hypertension remain an important concern of national health care. Advances in the diagnosis and treatment of hypertension are likely responsible for the decline in cardiovascular mortality which has occurred in the last 20 years. However, the adverse metabolic effects of some classes of antihypertensive drugs and the disappointing results of antihypertensive treatment in coronary disease prevention have raised questions that challenge traditional approaches to the management of the hypertensive patient. Antihypertensive treatment should be undertaken in the context of overall management of cardiovascular disease risk factors, and its ultimate goal should be reduction of overall cardiovascular risk.

TABLE 44–1. CLASSIFICATION OF BP IN ADULTS AGED 18 YEARS OR OLDER*

BP Range (mm Hg)	Category†
DBP	
<85	Normal BP
85–89	High-normal BP
90–104	Mild hypertension
105–114	Moderate hypertension
≥115	Severe hypertension
SBP, when DBP	
<90 mm Hg	
<140	Normal BP
140–159	Borderline isolated systolic hypertension
≥160	Isolated systolic hypertension

*Classification based on the average of two or more readings on two or more occasions. BP indicates blood pressure; DBP, diastolic blood pressure; and SBP, systolic blood pressure.

†A classification of borderline isolated systolic hypertension (SBP, 140 to 159 mm Hg) or isolated systolic hypertension (SBP, ≥160 mm Hg) takes precedence over high-normal BP (DBP, 85 to 89 mm Hg) when both occur in the same person. High-normal BP (DBP, 85 to 89 mm Hg) takes precedence over a classification of normal BP (SBP, <140 mm Hg) when both occur in the same person.

Reprinted with permission from The 1988 Report of the Joint National Committee on Detection, Evaluation, and Treatment of High Blood Pressure. Arch Intern Med 148:1023, 1988.

DEFINITION

Arterial hypertension is defined as elevated arterial blood pressure (BP). Since BP in the general population falls on a gaussian curve of normal distribution, it is impossible to define with precision the limits of "normal" BP. In addition, the BP of a given individual varies widely over time, depending on many variables, including sympathetic nervous system activity, posture, state of hydration, and skeletal muscle tone. Accordingly, any definition of hypertension must be arbitrary. The Joint National Committee on Detection, Evaluation and Treatment of High Blood Pressure recommends the scheme shown in Table 44–1 for the diagnosis of hypertension in individuals aged 18 years or older. The diagnosis of hypertension in adults is made when the average of two or more diastolic BP measurements on at least two subsequent visits is 90 mm Hg or higher or when the average of multiple systolic BP readings on two or more subsequent visits is consistently greater than 140 mm Hg (Table 44–2). The patient should be clearly informed that a single elevated reading does not constitute a diagnosis of hypertension but is a sign that further observation is required.

Essential, primary, or **idiopathic hypertension** is arterial hypertension of unknown cause. Over 95 per cent of all cases of arterial hypertension are in this category.

Secondary hypertension is arterial hypertension of known

TABLE 44–2. FOLLOW-UP CRITERIA FOR INITIAL BP MEASUREMENT FOR ADULTS AGED 18 YEARS OR OLDER*

BP Range (mm Hg)	Recommended Follow-up
DBP	
<85	Recheck within 2 years
85–89	Recheck within 1 year
90–104	Confirm within 2 months
105–114	Evaluate or refer promptly to source of care within 2 weeks
≥115	Evaluate or refer immediately to source of care
SBP, when DBP	
<90 mm Hg	
<140	Recheck within 2 years
140–199	Confirm within 2 months
≥200	Evaluate or refer promptly to source of care within 2 weeks

*BP indicates blood pressure; DBP, diastolic blood pressure; and SBP, systolic blood pressure. If recommendations for follow-up of DBP and SBP are different, the shorter recommended time for recheck and referral should take precedence.

Reprinted with permission from The 1988 Report of the Joint National Committee on Detection, Evaluation, and Treatment of High Blood Pressure. Arch Intern Med 148:1023, 1988.

cause. Fewer than 5 per cent of all cases of systemic hypertension are in this category. The importance of identifying patients with secondary hypertension is that they sometimes can be cured by surgery or can be easily controlled by specific medical treatment. Thus the morbidity and mortality of potentially ineffective empiric medical therapy can be avoided and the cumulative cost of medical treatment reduced. The most common causes of secondary hypertension are summarized in Table 44–3.

Malignant hypertension is the syndrome of markedly elevated BP (diastolic BP usually greater than 140 mm Hg) associated with papilledema. **Accelerated hypertension** is the syndrome of markedly elevated BP associated with hemorrhages and exudates (grade 3 Kimmelstiel-Wilson [K-W] retinopathy). If untreated, accelerated hypertension presumably progresses to a malignant phase. Both accelerated and malignant hypertension are associated with widespread degenerative changes in the walls of resistance vessels. These syndromes are characterized by extreme BP elevations, sudden onset, fulminant course, and evidence of severe, generalized vascular damage, including grade 3 or 4 K-W retinopathy, hypertensive encephalopathy, hematuria, and renal dysfunction. Malignant hypertension is usually fatal unless treated promptly and vigorously. If BP can be controlled, prognosis depends on the state of renal function.

Complicated hypertension is the descriptive term for arterial hypertension of any etiology in which there is evidence of cardiovascular damage related to the BP elevation. Hypertensive complications commonly include stroke, congestive heart failure, renal failure, myocardial infarction, and arterial aneurysm.

Borderline hypertension is intermittent hypertension in which some BP measurements are elevated and some are normal in the untreated patient. Patients with borderline hypertension tend to maintain pressures that are above average for the general population and are at greater risk of cardiovascular morbidity and mortality than the general population. As a group, these patients manifest increased cardiac output, more rapid heart rate, and higher left ventricular ejection rate than either the normotensive population or the population of patients with stable hypertension.

White coat or **office hypertension** refers to the elevation in BP manifested by some patients due to the stress and anxiety of an office visit. Studies using ambulatory monitoring have suggested that as many as 30 per cent of patients diagnosed as hypertensive by standard office measurements are actually normotensive. However, the true incidence and significance of this phenomenon remain controversial.

INCIDENCE AND PREVALENCE

Approximately 60 million persons in the United States have hypertension. The prevalence of hypertension increases with age in all groups: blacks, whites, men, and women (Fig. 44–1). Diastolic hypertension is roughly twice as common among 50-year-olds as among 30-year-olds, and systolic hypertension increases greatly in prevalence after age 45, probably reflecting age-regulated reductions in compliance of the large conduit vessels. Hypertension is an extremely common health problem in the geriatric population, afflicting approximately 65 per cent of the population in the 65- to 74-year-old group. Data from the 1976 to 1980 National Health and Nutrition Examination Survey (NHANES II) indicate that blacks have a higher prevalence of hypertension than whites (38 per cent versus 29 per cent). The reason for the increased prevalence of hypertension among blacks is unclear, but it has been attributed to heredity, greater salt intake, and greater environmental stress. Men have a higher overall prevalence of hypertension than women (33 per cent versus 27 per cent). Hypertension is more common in men than in women up to approximately age 50; after that time, hypertension is more common in women. The increased prevalence of hypertension in postmenopausal women is related to a combination of weight gain and hormonal alterations.

Data from NHANES II indicate that most hypertensive patients have small elevations in BP (Fig. 44–2). Approximately 50 per cent of all hypertensives in the 18- to 74-year age group, or 15 per cent of the entire adult population of the United States, have mild hypertension (see Table 44–1). These figures reflect the preponderance of white hypertensives sampled by NHANES II. Blacks tend to have more severe hypertension than whites. Five per cent of hypertensives, most of whom are elderly, have isolated systolic hypertension.

ETIOLOGY AND PATHOGENESIS OF ESSENTIAL HYPERTENSION

The cause of elevated BP cannot be identified in more than 95 per cent of cases; these individuals are said to have essential hypertension. Essential hypertension tends to cluster in families and represents a collection of genetically based diseases and/or syndromes with a number of underlying inherited biochemical abnormalities. Of the numerous pathologic features of essential hypertension, many undoubtedly represent compensatory mechanisms that offset the primary abnormality. Pathophysiologic factors that have been implicated in the genesis of essential hypertension include increased sympathetic nervous system activity, overproduction of an unidentified sodium-retaining hormone, chronic high sodium intake, inadequate dietary intakes of potassium and calcium, increased or "inappropriate" renin secretion, deficiencies of vasodilators such as prostaglandins, congenital abnormalities of the resistance vessels, diabetes mellitus, insulin resistance, obesity, increased activity of vascular growth factors, and altered cellular ion transport. The tools of molecular biology provide, for the first time, the means of defining the genetic basis of the hypertensive diseases and for designing rational preventive and therapeutic strategies. To date, no specific set of

TABLE 44–3. CAUSES OF SECONDARY HYPERTENSION

Systolic and diastolic hypertension
  Renal
    Renal parenchymal disease
      Chronic nephritis
      Polycystic disease
      Collagen vascular disease
      Diabetic nephropathy
      Hydronephrosis
      Acute glomerulonephritis
    Renal vascular disease
    Renal transplantation
    Renin-secreting tumors
  Endocrine
    Adrenal
      Primary aldosteronism
      Overproduction of 11-deoxycorticosterone (DOC), 18-OH-DOC, and other mineralocorticoids
      Congenital adrenal hyperplasia
      Cushing's syndrome
      Pheochromocytoma
    Extra-adrenal chromaffin tumors
    Hyperparathyroidism
    Acromegaly
  Pregnancy-induced hypertension
  Coarctation of the aorta
  Neurologic disorders
    Dysautonomia
    Increased intracranial pressure
    Quadriplegia
    Lead poisoning
    Guillain-Barré syndrome
  Postoperative
  Drugs and chemicals
    Cyclosporine
    Oral contraceptives
    Glucocorticoids
    Mineralocorticoids, including licorice and carbenoxolone
    Sympathomimetics
    Tyramine and MAO inhibitors

Isolated systolic hypertension
  Aging, with associated aortic rigidity
  Increased cardiac output
    Thyrotoxicosis
    Anemia
    Aortic valvular insufficiency
  Decreased peripheral vascular resistance
    Arteriovenous shunts
    Paget's disease of bone
    Beriberi

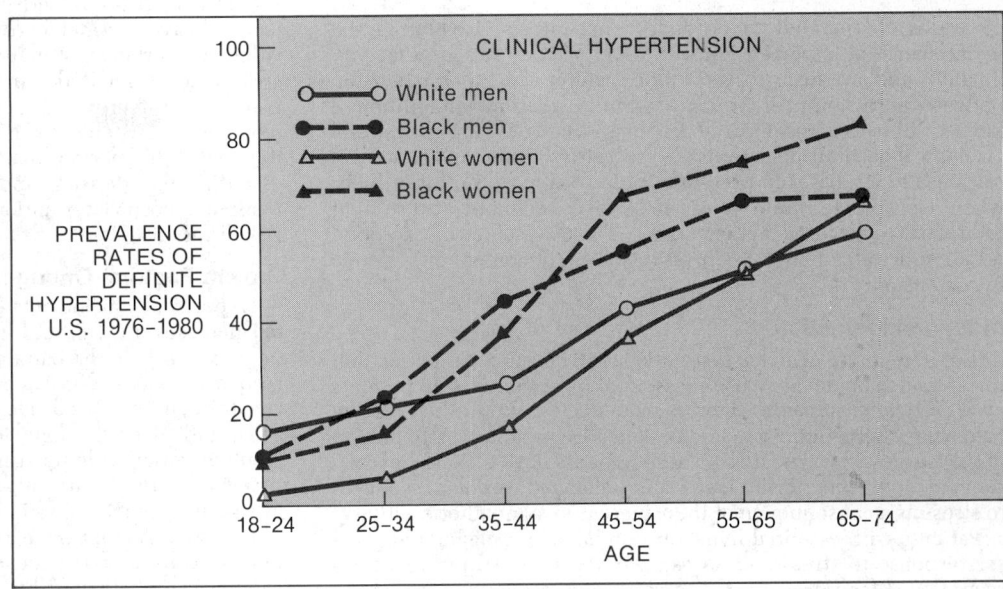

FIGURE 44–1. The prevalence of hypertension in the United States defined as the average of three blood pressure measurements of 140/90 mm Hg or higher on a single occasion or reported taking of antihypertensive medications. (Prepared using data from the 1976–1980 National Health and Nutrition Examination Survey. Modified from Hypertension Prevalence and the Status of Awareness, Treatment and Control in the United States: Final Report of the Subcommittee on Definition and Prevalence of the 1984 Joint National Committee. Hypertension 7:457–468, 1985; by permission of the American Heart Association.)

BP-regulating genes has been identified, nor have genetic markers that permit early detection of individuals at risk for developing hypertension been characterized.

Genetic Factors

The mechanisms by which BP is genetically controlled are diverse, interrelated, and incompletely understood. Studies in normotensive first-degree relatives of essential hypertensives have demonstrated differences in electrolyte excretion and circulating renin levels that may make this group susceptible to the development of hypertension. Thus, inherited abnormalities in the renin-angiotensin-aldosterone system, perhaps including alterations in sympathetic nervous drive to renin release and/or an intrinsic defect in the ability of the kidney to handle volume overload, may contribute to the pathogenesis of essential hypertension.

Specific molecular defects in cell membrane transport systems, such as pumps or cotransport, have been described in hypertensive subjects and related to the pathogenesis of hypertension. Several abnormalities in Na^+ handling, including increased passive entry of Na^+, increased maximal rate of Na^+/Li^+ exchange, and decreased apparent affinity of the Na^+-K^+ pump for internal Na^+, have been found in red blood cells of human hypertensives. An important consequence of these alterations in cellular handling of Na^+ is an increase in intracellular Na^+ concentration, which results in an increased intracellular free Ca^{2+} concentration. A positive correlation between platelet Ca^{2+} and BP has been reported. The membrane defects observed in blood cells of human essential hypertensives could be shared by other cell types, such as vascular smooth muscle cells, sympathetic neurons, and renal tubule cells, which are involved in the maintenance of vascular tone and volume homeostasis and in the pathogenesis of hypertension. Thus, the abnormalities in membrane Na^+ and Ca^{2+} handling described in human hypertensives could account for the circulatory alterations that lead to systemic hypertension. Further study is needed to determine which genes are responsible for these abnormalities and to establish more precisely the mechanisms by which their expression leads to the development of genetically mediated hypertension in humans.

Renal Sodium Handling

A defect in the excretion of salt and water may be central to the pathogenesis of hypertension. The normal kidney plays an important role in maintaining intravascular volume and BP. It responds to increments in perfusion pressure by increasing sodium and water excretion, thus reducing intravascular volume and restoring BP to normal levels. Hemodynamic, neural, and humoral factors participate in the control of volume and BP homeostasis by regulating renal sodium handling. In hypertensive subjects, this relationship is perturbed, such that higher perfusion

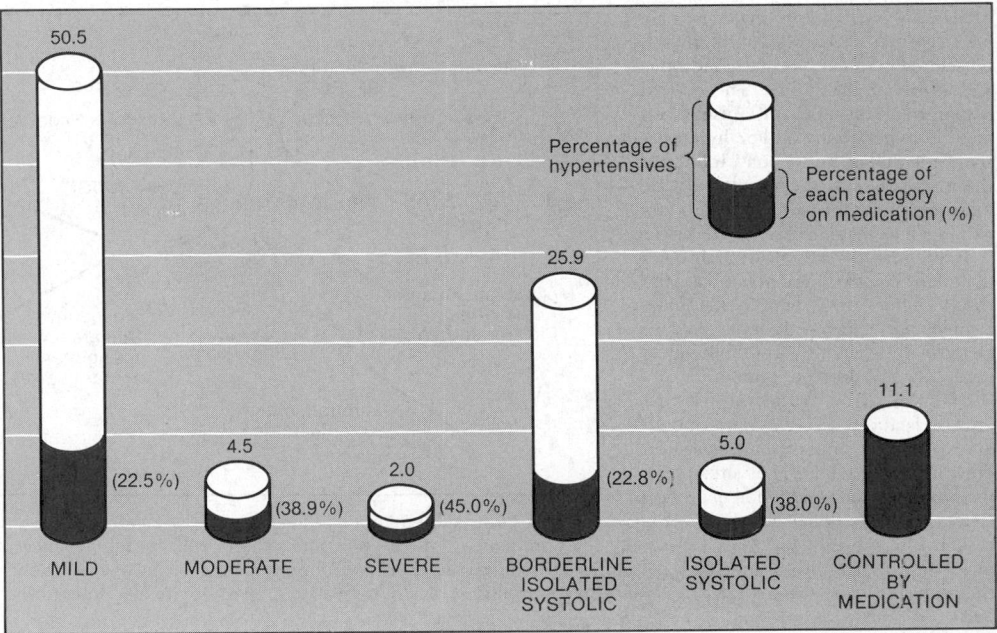

FIGURE 44–2. Percentage of civilian, noninstitutionalized population, 18 to 74 years of age, with hypertension categorized by blood pressure (BP) *(figure over column)* and percentage of each category receiving medication *(dark column)*. Hypertension is defined as BP, 140/90 mm Hg or above or use of antihypertensive medication. (Prepared using data from the 1976–1980 National Health and Nutritional Examination Survey. From Hypertension Prevalence and the Status of Awareness, Treatment and Control in the United States: Final Report of the Subcommittee on Definition and Prevalence of the 1984 Joint National Committee. Hypertension 7:457–468, 1985; by permission of the American Heart Association.)

pressures are needed to produce a natriuresis, facilitating the maintenance of hypertension. A variety of neurohumoral factors, intrinsic and extrinsic to the kidney, influence the relationship between perfusion pressure and sodium excretion. In addition, a kidney subjected to elevated BP over time develops structural changes that limit its ability to excrete sodium and water in response to increases in pressure. Kidneys altered in this fashion, when transplanted into a normotensive recipient, cause that individual to become hypertensive. Thus, a defect in excretion of salt and water may be central to the pathogenesis of systemic hypertension.

Autonomic Function

The autonomic nervous system is involved in the initiation and maintenance of elevated BP in essential hypertension. In patients with early hypertension, there is evidence for diminished resting parasympathetic inhibition and enhanced sympathetic stimulation of the cardiovascular system. These patients have elevated plasma renin and norepinephrine levels and enhanced vascular responses to stress as a consequence of their increased sympathetic activity.

Patients with essential hypertension have an exaggerated pressor response to stress and an exaggerated depressor response to relaxation. Blood pressure falls during meditation and other states of relaxation and rises during isometric exercise and the stress of mental arithmetic in these patients to a greater extent than in normotensive control subjects. The impressive fall in BP that is frequently seen when a hypertensive patient is removed from his home environment and brought into the hospital suggests that environmental stress exacerbates hypertension. The increased prevalence of hypertension in urban populations compared to rural groups and the occurrence of age-related rises in BP in societies with changing value systems but not in those with a stable social structure give evidence for a psychogenic contribution to essential hypertension. Stress presumably mediates its pressor effect through the sympathetic nervous system.

Hemodynamics

Cardiac output is elevated early in the course of essential hypertension and may cause secondary increases in peripheral vascular resistance which are responsible for maintaining the hypertension. This concept of total body autoregulation has been used to explain the adaptation of resistance vessels to increases in cardiac output. According to the theory of total body autoregulation, systemic resistance vessels respond to an increased cardiac output and increased intravascular volume by constricting in order to reduce tissue blood flow to normal. Patients with essential hypertension of recent onset generally show a pattern of increased cardiac output (about 15 per cent greater than normotensive control levels), tachycardia, and venoconstriction, with normal or even low peripheral vascular resistance at rest. In contrast, patients with longstanding established hypertension usually have normal cardiac output and increased peripheral vascular resistance. Longitudinal studies of untreated hypertensive patients have documented a fall in cardiac output, due mainly to a decrease in stroke volume, and an increase in total peripheral resistance over time. These observations are compatible with the notion that increases in cardiac output initiate essential hypertension and that changes in peripheral vascular resistance occur later and are more important in maintaining the BP elevation.

Growth Factors, Oncogenes, and Vascular Hypertrophy

Hypertrophy of blood vessels, whether primary or secondary to increases in BP and hence vessel wall tension, plays an important role in the pathogenesis of hypertension. The myogenic response to elevations in BP and flow is characterized by vasoconstriction, increased calcium influx into vascular smooth muscle cells, and, over the long term, increased myocyte growth. The resultant vascular hypertrophy tends to reduce blood flow to the tissues and to elevate intravascular pressure. Stimuli to growth of vascular smooth muscle cells are summarized in Figure 44–3. The growth factors have contractile effects on vascular smooth muscle cells and trigger many of the same cellular signaling events as are activated by vasoconstrictor agents such as norepinephrine and angiotensin II. Conversely, many of the endogenous vasoconstrictors stimulate vascular smooth muscle cell growth via receptor-mediated mechanisms. Of the endogenous vasoconstrictors, angiotensin II is a particularly important autocrine and paracrine regulator of vascular hypertrophy. Blood vessel walls contain an active renin-angiotensin system, and inhibition of vascular angiotensin II production with angiotensin-converting enzyme (ACE) inhibitors prevents or reverses vascular hypertrophy more effectively than treatment with other classes of antihypertensive agents that have equipotent blood pressure–lowering effects. Further, recent evidence suggests that captopril may prevent restenosis following angioplasty, suggesting that angiotensin II may participate in the vascular remodeling characteristic of the atherosclerotic process.

Contractile agonists and many growth factors share cellular signaling effects that are related to the vascular growth response. These agents activate phospholipase C, which hydrolyzes phosphatidylinositol bisphosphate to generate inositol trisphosphate and diacylglycerol. The former mobilizes Ca^{2+} from intracellular stores; the latter modulates Ca^{2+}-sensitive protein kinase C, which activates Na^+/H^+ exchange and alkalinizes the cell. Cellular alkalinization is associated with both vasoconstriction and growth and/or division. Alternate signaling events, including cyclic AMP production, have been described with some growth factors.

Proto-oncogenes, including c-fos, c-myc, and c-jun, that are induced in association with these signaling events render the

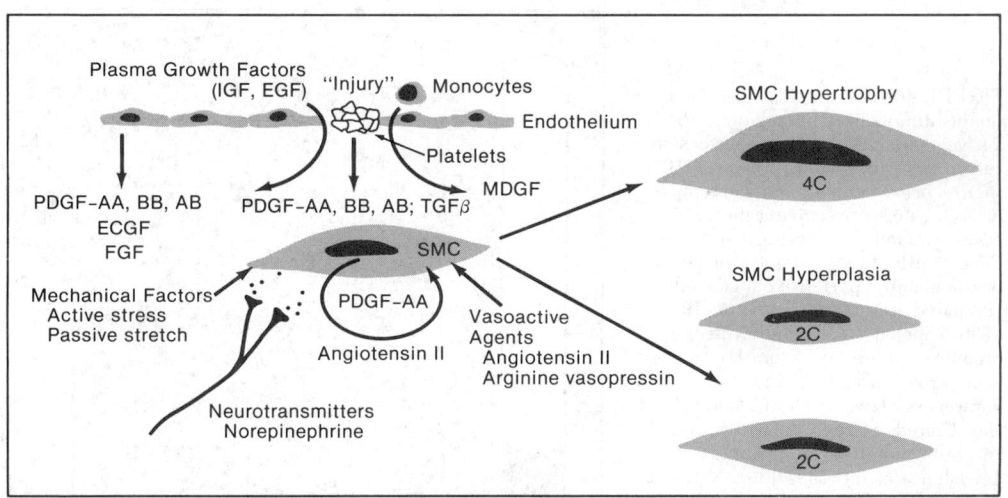

FIGURE 44–3. Factors that may play a role in growth regulation of smooth muscle cells under normal conditions and after vascular injury. The growth response of the smooth muscle cell may be hypertrophy and/or hyperplasia. Endothelial injury may influence the growth of smooth muscle cells by increased influx of plasma growth factors, such as insulin-like growth factor I (IGF), into the vessel wall through denuded vessel segments or as the result of increased endothelial macromolecular permeability; release of growth factors from platelets (e.g., platelet-derived growth factors [PDGF-AA, BB, AB]; transforming growth factor β [TGF β]) or monocytes (e.g., macrophage-derived growth factor [MDGF]) at sites of injury; or increased production of growth factors by endothelial cells (e.g., PDGF-AA, BB, and AB; endothelial-derived growth factor [ECGF]) or of smooth muscle cells themselves as a response to the injury. Other factors that may influence growth of smooth muscle cells in the absence of vessel injury include norepinephrine and other neurotransmitters, mechanical factors, and contractile agonists from circulating blood or endothelial cells or generated by smooth muscle cells themselves. (From Owens GK: Control of hypertrophic versus hyperplastic growth of vascular smooth muscle cells. Am J Physiol 257:H1755–H1765, 1989; with permission.)

cells competent to replicate their DNA in response to growth factors. Whether the protein products of these competence genes are responsible for vascular growth is uncertain. The regulation of vascular growth in hypertension is an area of active investigation and may give rise to new approaches, including gene therapy, to antihypertensive treatment.

Insulin Resistance

Peripheral resistance to insulin has been described in essential hypertension. The level of insulin resistance and the defect in whole-body glucose utilization are positively correlated with the severity of the hypertension. Insulin resistance in hypertension appears to be independent of both obesity and glucose tolerance as measured by standard glucose tolerance tests. Whole-body insulin-induced glucose uptake and nonoxidative glucose disposal (glycogen synthesis and glycolysis) are markedly reduced and plasma insulin levels are elevated, presumably as a compensatory mechanism, in insulin-resistant subjects. Several mechanisms have been hypothesized to explain the relationship between hyperinsulinemia and BP elevation (Fig. 44–4): (1) Hyperinsulinemia could elevate BP by increasing sodium reabsorption in the distal nephron and possibly in the proximal tubule as well, thus expanding plasma and extracellular fluid volume. (2) Hyperinsulinemia in the presence of normal blood glucose levels increases sympathetic nervous system activity, which can, in turn, elevate BP. (3) Insulin is a potent stimulus for receptor-mediated growth of vascular endothelial and smooth muscle cells, thus leading to increased peripheral vascular resistance and BP. (4) Insulin, by altering plasma free fatty acid levels, modulates Na^+-K^+-ATPase activity, thus altering cellular cation transport in a manner that could increase peripheral vascular tone and BP. Interventions that reduce insulin resistance, such as weight loss, diets low in carbohydrates and high in unsaturated fats, and aerobic exercise, reduce both BP and insulin resistance, supporting the concept that essential hypertension is an insulin-resistant state. Further study is needed to elucidate the relationships among hypertension, insulin resistance, and two related syndromes—obesity and diabetes mellitus.

DIAGNOSIS

Initial Evaluation

The initial evaluation of the hypertensive patient should determine baseline arterial BP, assess the degree of end-organ damage, screen for secondary causes of hypertension, identify other cardiovascular risk factors, and characterize the patient (sex, race, age, lifestyle, concomitant illnesses) to facilitate choice of therapy, drug selection in particular.

BP MEASUREMENT. The accurate and reproducible measurement of BP by the cuff technique is the most critical part of the diagnostic evaluation. On the initial visit, the BP should be taken after the patient has been seated comfortably for at least 5 minutes with his or her arm bared. Constriction of the upper arm by a rolled sleeve should be avoided, as it distorts the BP measurement. Two or three measurements should be taken at each visit, and at least 2 minutes should be allowed between readings. Proper cuff size is critical to accurate BP measurement. The cuff bladder should be long enough to encircle at least two thirds of the arm. Falsely elevated readings can be obtained when the bladder is too short, and the error is magnified if the cuff is also too narrow. Mercury manometers are preferred, but aneroid manometers can be used if they are standardized frequently against a mercury manometer.

To obtain an accurate systolic pressure, the cuff should be inflated rapidly to at least 30 mm Hg above the systolic pressure, as determined by palpation of the radial artery. This inflation is necessary to avoid underestimating the pressure because of the auscultatory gap, an unexplained disappearance of Korotkoff's sounds for some interval between systole and diastole. The systolic reading is taken as the level of pressure at which clear Korotkoff's sounds are heard with each heart beat. The diastolic reading is taken at the level when sounds become muffled (Korotkoff phase IV) and when sounds disappear (phase V). Both readings should be recorded. It is not known whether the level of muffling or of disappearance is a more accurate reflection of the intra-arterial diastolic pressure, so selection of one over the other as the clinical measurement of diastolic pressure is a matter of convenience and reproducibility. Baseline BP should be calculated from the average of two separate measurements determined at least 2 weeks apart. However, patients with diastolic BP greater than 115 mm Hg or elevated BP with evidence of ongoing end-organ damage should be started on therapy immediately.

The use of home BP recordings by either the patient or another person in the household or of 24-hour ambulatory BP recordings or both are useful, particularly in monitoring patients with labile hypertension, anxious patients whose BP readings tend to be falsely elevated in the doctor's office, and patients whose doses of antihypertensive medications need to be adjusted frequently. Home recordings should be taken at various times of day, in various positions, and during periods of both stress and relaxation in order to assess the effects of diurnal variations in hormones, posture, and emotional state on BP. Not only do home BP measurements provide additional information on the patient's true BP profile, but involving the patient in his or her care and informing him or her of therapeutic goals may provide incentive for nonpharmacologic therapies, such as weight loss, and may also enhance medication compliance. Standard sphygmomanometers and stethoscopes are appropriate for this purpose and are preferred over automated indirect BP measuring devices, which are often inaccurate. The patient's skill at BP measurement should be tested at frequent intervals by a professional.

Studies using ambulatory BP monitoring suggest that traditional office BP measurements overdiagnose hypertension by 20 to 30 per cent. In addition, these studies suggest that mean ambulatory pressures may better assess end-organ risk than do serial office measurements. These findings are controversial because of potential selection biases, uncertainty over the risks of stress-related hypertension, and the argument that office visits are no more stressful than many work and home environments. Current ambulatory monitoring systems are too cumbersome and

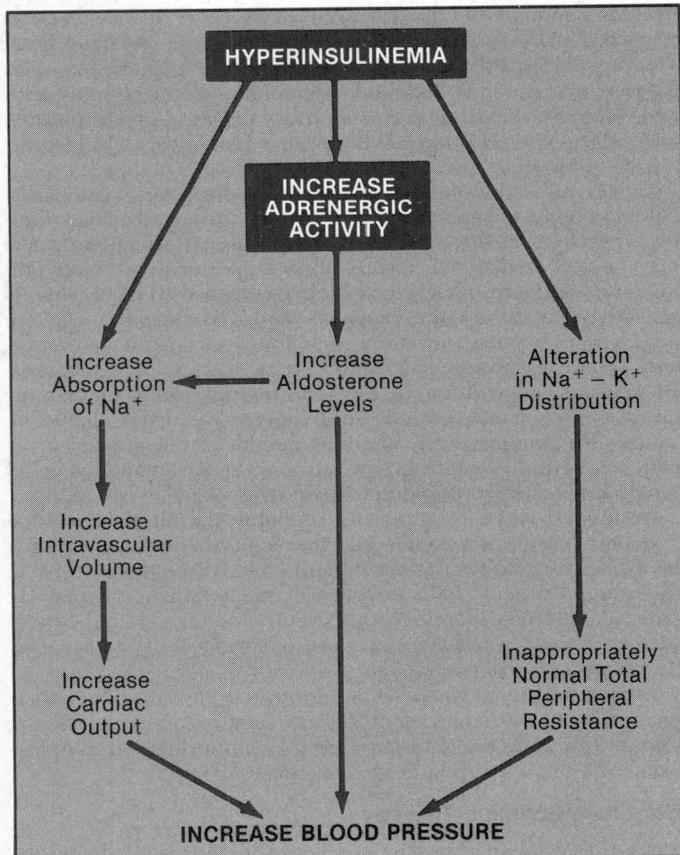

FIGURE 44–4. Physiologic mechanisms involved in insulin resistance–related hypertension. (From Reisin E: Sodium and obesity in the pathogenesis of hypertension. Am J Hypertension 3(2):164–167, 1990; with permission.)

expensive for routine assessment of BP. The controversy they have generated, however, does emphasize the value of home BP measurements made by the patient and/or the patient's family.

Accurate BP determination can be particularly difficult in elderly patients because of stiffening of arterial walls. The loss of arterial wall compliance can result in falsely elevated BP measurements by use of a standard sphygmomanometer, so-called pseudohypertension. Such an occurrence should be suspected in elderly patients diagnosed as having hypertension but lacking evidence of end-organ damage. Use of the Osler maneuver can sometimes identify this phenomenon. During the Osler maneuver, the BP cuff is inflated above the level of systolic BP. If the pulseless radial or brachial artery remains palpable, there may be sufficient stiffening of the artery to falsely elevate the BP measurement. Intra-arterial BP determinations may be necessary for the accurate diagnosis of hypertension in this setting.

Selection of Patients for Evaluation for Secondary Hypertension

Once a diagnosis of stable hypertension has been established, the need for antihypertensive treatment should be assessed, and, where indicated, diagnostic evaluation for secondary causes of hypertension should be undertaken. In view of the rarity of secondary causes of hypertension and the high cost and risk of elaborate diagnostic studies, the routine pretreatment workup should be limited to defining the severity of the hypertension and identifying its complications and associated cardiovascular risk factors. All of the secondary causes combined account for less than 5 per cent of the adult hypertensive population, but since some patients with secondary hypertension are potentially curable, diagnostic evaluation is warranted in selected patients. These include the following:

1. Those in whom routine history, physical examination, or routine laboratory data suggest a specific secondary cause
2. Those who are younger than 30 years of age, since they have the greatest prevalence of correctable secondary hypertension
3. Those in whom drug therapy is inadequate or unsatisfactory
4. Those whose hypertension has suddenly worsened
5. Older patients who develop new-onset hypertension

MEDICAL HISTORY. A careful, complete history should be obtained and a physical examination performed in all hypertensive patients before therapy is started. The medical history should include any previous history of hypertension, including prior and current antihypertensive treatment; a history of factors regarded as predisposing to hypertension, including excessive salt intake, the use of drugs that are known to elevate BP (Table 44–3), stressful occupation, and a family history of hypertension and its complications; evidence of hypertensive complications, including congestive heart failure, coronary artery disease, renal dysfunction, and stroke; and a history of other cardiovascular risk factors, including diabetes, obesity, cigarette smoking, and lipid abnormalities. Discussion of family history should include mention of familial diseases associated with secondary hypertension, including familial renal disease, polycystic kidney disease, medullary thyroid cancer, pheochromocytoma, and hyperparathyroidism. Discussion of the patient's personal habits should include exercise habits, ethanol consumption, and any unusual dietary practices. All current medications should be considered, particularly agents such as corticosteroids, nonsteroidal anti-inflammatory agents, antihistamines, sympathomimetics, appetite suppressants, phenothiazines, tricyclic antidepressants, and monoamine oxidase inhibitors that may exacerbate existing hypertension or antagonize or adversely interact with drug therapy. The physician should also begin assessing the patient's understanding of his or her illness and willingness to alter lifestyle if necessary. A history of weakness, muscle cramps, and polyuria suggests hypokalemia and the possibility of hyperaldosteronism; a history of headaches, palpitations, or hyperhidrosis suggests pheochromocytoma.

PHYSICAL EXAMINATION. The physical examination should include two or more BP measurements, at least one of which is obtained in the standing position; funduscopic examination for hypertensive retinopathy; careful examination of the cardiovascular system for evidence of congestive heart failure, cardiomegaly, myocardial dysfunction, and peripheral vascular disease; examination of the abdomen for bruits; auscultation over all scars for evidence of arteriovenous fistulas, and a careful neurologic examination for the stigmata of stroke. Since poor prognosis has been correlated with severity of retinopathy, presence of left ventricular hypertrophy, and coexisting atherosclerotic disease, physical findings related to these complications should be well documented.

LABORATORY EVALUATION. Pretreatment laboratory tests can be restricted to those generally performed as part of a routine medical checkup: hematocrit, urinalysis to exclude proteinuria and hematuria suggestive of renal disease, creatinine or blood urea nitrogen levels to assess renal function, serum potassium levels, chest film to assess heart size and rule out aortic coarctation, and electrocardiogram. Other tests that can be obtained as part of most automated blood chemistry batteries, such as the blood glucose, serum cholesterol, triglyceride, and uric acid levels, are helpful in assessing other cardiovascular risk factors and can be used as a baseline for monitoring the effects of antihypertensive treatment. Serial electrocardiograms and echocardiograms may be useful in assessing the effects of hypertension and antihypertensive treatment on the heart.

TREATMENT

The goal of antihypertensive therapy is to reduce overall cardiovascular risk. In any given patient, the decision to initiate therapy is governed by the extent of the BP elevation and the presence or absence of cardiovascular complications or additional cardiovascular risk factors, or both. Antihypertensive treatment is indicated in patients with diastolic BP measurements of 95 mm Hg or higher and in those with lesser elevations (90 to 94 mm Hg) who are at high risk of developing cardiovascular morbidity or mortality. The high-risk group includes patients with target-organ damage, diabetes mellitus, and/or other major risk factors for coronary artery disease. The initial goal of therapy is to lower diastolic BP to levels below 90 mm Hg with minimal adverse effects. Excessive BP reduction (diastolic BP below 80 mm Hg and systolic BP below 130 mm Hg) should be avoided, particularly in elderly patients and those with coronary artery disease, because it may actually increase the risk of death from ischemic heart disease, presumably secondary to coronary hypoperfusion. This J-curve phenomenon has been demonstrated in patients with and without pre-existing coronary artery disease. An effort should be made to correct other cardiovascular risk factors in all hypertensive patients.

In patients with moderate to severe hypertension, even partial BP reduction has been shown to decrease cardiovascular morbidity. Therefore, in these patients, a more limited therapeutic goal may be accepted if side effects of antihypertensive therapy are intolerable at doses necessary to achieve normal BP. For patients with diastolic BP in the range of 90 to 94 mm Hg who are otherwise at low risk, an initial trial of nonpharmacologic therapy with careful BP monitoring should be carried out. If the diastolic BP remains above 90 mm Hg despite nonpharmacologic therapy for a 3- to 6-month period, antihypertensive drugs should be added. Nonpharmacologic therapy should be encouraged in all patients with hypertension, as it may reduce the dosage of medication required for adequate BP control.

Antihypertensive treatment is probably indicated in isolated systolic hypertension, since pharmacologic therapy has recently been shown to be well tolerated and effective in lowering BP in this group. Patients with systolic BP greater than 160 mm Hg are generally considered to deserve treatment. The efficacy of such treatment in reducing cardiovascular morbidity and mortality has yet to be demonstrated.

Pharmacologic treatment is not indicated in borderline hypertension in the absence of other risk factors for cardiovascular disease or end-organ damage. Careful monitoring and nonpharmacologic therapy are indicated for these patients.

Nonpharmacologic Therapy

Since the nonpharmacologic interventions useful in hypertensive persons are not costly and are generally beneficial in promoting good health, their gradual introduction should be attempted in all hypertensive patients. Although permanent modifications in diet and lifestyle are difficult to achieve, in motivated patients, they may obviate the need for drug treatment or reduce the dosage requirements of antihypertensive drugs for adequate BP control.

WEIGHT REDUCTION. There is a clear, direct relationship between body weight and resting BP. Epidemiologic studies have consistently shown that overweight individuals have an increased risk of hypertension and increased cardiovascular risk. Weight loss is closely correlated with reduction in BP and is potentially the most efficacious of all nonpharmacologic measures in the treatment of hypertension. This effect is independent of dietary sodium restriction and is seen in both obese and nonobese hypertensive individuals. In addition to reducing BP, weight loss independently reduces cardiovascular risk and tends to improve the patient's self-image and sense of well-being. Patients should avoid appetite suppressants, which contain sympathomimetics such as phenylpropanolamine that can elevate BP. However, significant weight loss is difficult to achieve and even more difficult to maintain. Most patients regain the lost weight within 1 year. Nevertheless, all overweight hypertensive patients should be encouraged to lose weight.

ALCOHOL RESTRICTION. Alcohol consumption elevates BP, both acutely and chronically, and cross-sectional studies have demonstrated an association between increased BP and increased levels of alcohol consumption. The regular ingestion of 1 ounce of alcohol per day (two drinks) is estimated to raise systolic BP by 2 to 6 mm Hg. Therefore, abstinence or moderation of alcohol consumption (restriction of intake to 1 ounce of ethanol, corresponding to 2 ounces of 100 proof distilled liquor, 4 ounces of wine, or 24 ounces of beer daily) should be encouraged.

EXERCISE. Both cross-sectional and longitudinal studies have demonstrated a lower prevalence of hypertension in physically active people. Regular isotonic exercise, such as jogging, bicycling, or swimming, produces modest reductions in BP in persons with mild to moderate hypertension. Exercise also reduces cardiovascular risk independent of weight loss while promoting a sense of well-being. Therefore, all hypertensive patients should be encouraged to participate in regular isotonic or aerobic exercise. Current recommendations for BP reduction and reduction of overall cardiovascular risk include aerobic exercise maintaining 70 to 80 per cent of maximal heart rate (maximal heart rate calculated by subtracting age from 220) for 20 to 30 minutes three times a week. Patients should work gradually toward this goal.

DIETARY SODIUM RESTRICTION. Although dietary sodium restriction is commonly recommended by physicians to hypertensive patients, studies evaluating the antihypertensive efficacy of sodium restriction in unselected patients with essential hypertension have not demonstrated a clear benefit. A recent meta-analysis of published studies of dietary sodium restriction in hypertensive patients found only a small reduction in BP and concluded that there is little evidence that reduction of sodium intake has a beneficial effect on BP control. Further, BP increases have been observed in some hypertensive patients when dietary sodium intake is reduced. The observed heterogeneity in BP response to dietary sodium restriction has given rise to attempts to classify hypertensive patients as salt sensitive or salt resistant and to develop biochemical indices of salt sensitivity. Patients with low renin activity, frequently encountered in elderly and black patients, are more likely to respond to sodium restriction with a decrease in BP. Further, sodium restriction can minimize diuretic-induced hypokalemia and may enhance the ease of BP control with diuretic therapy and should be encouraged in patients who are receiving diuretics. Moderate sodium restriction (4 to 6 grams of salt per day) can be generally recommended to hypertensive patients, realizing that only a subset of patients will benefit. This can be effected by the simple and tolerable measures of not adding salt to food during preparation or at the table and avoiding processed foods containing salt as the preservative. Salt substitutes in which sodium is replaced with potassium are useful in hypertensive patients who do not have renal dysfunction. Patients should be instructed to avoid concomitant decreases in calcium and potassium intake.

DIETARY CALCIUM SUPPLEMENTATION. Epidemiologic studies have suggested an inverse relationship between dietary calcium intake and BP: Hypertensive persons, according to their dietary recalls, ingest less calcium than normotensive persons. Clinical studies of the BP-lowering effects of calcium supplementation have produced mixed results. Only a fraction of the hypertensive patients given oral calcium supplementation (1 gram of elemental calcium per day) show significant reductions in BP. Patients with salt-sensitive essential hypertension who are ingesting a high salt diet appear to be sensitive to the BP-lowering effects of dietary calcium, whereas patients with salt-resistant hypertension are not. This issue requires more study, but early data suggest that patients with salt-sensitive essential hypertension may benefit from oral calcium supplementation. Maintenance of oral calcium intake at levels of 1 gram per day or greater may also be beneficial for other reasons, such as the prevention of osteoporosis and gastrointestinal malignancy.

DIETARY POTASSIUM SUPPLEMENTATION. Epidemiologic studies have demonstrated an inverse relationship between dietary potassium intake and BP, and several recent controlled studies have demonstrated a small but significant reduction in BP with dietary potassium supplementation. The antihypertensive effect of potassium supplementation appears to be related to concomitant sodium intake, in that the higher the sodium intake, the more effective potassium supplementation is in reducing BP. Hypertensive patients should maintain adequate potassium intake ($\sim$ 100 mEq per day) by adequate ingestion of fresh fruits and vegetables and, if necessary, by use of potassium supplements. Potassium supplementation should be avoided or used only with extreme caution in patients with renal insufficiency, in diabetics, and in patients receiving potassium-sparing diuretics. Hypokalemia, whether due to diuretic use or to poor dietary intake, should be treated. Hypokalemia should particularly be avoided in patients receiving digoxin and in those with known coronary artery disease, as it predisposes to arrhythmia. Use of potassium-sparing diuretics should be considered in patients who are hypokalemic prior to initiation of diuretic therapy or who develop hypokalemia while receiving a nonpotassium-sparing diuretic.

SPECIAL DIETS. Dietary manipulations, such as changing to a vegetarian diet, increasing total fiber intake, decreasing total fat intake while increasing polyunsaturated fats relative to saturated fats, or increasing ingestion of fish oils, have been shown in preliminary studies to lower BP. They may, in addition, lower other cardiovascular risk factors. The mechanisms of antihypertensive action of these diets are unknown. Further studies are necessary to evaluate the role of these special diets in BP lowering, and it is premature to recommend them to patients with essential hypertension who lack other cardiovascular risk factors.

SMOKING CESSATION AND CAFFEINE RESTRICTION. Caffeine and nicotine raise BP acutely, but neither cigarette smokers nor coffee drinkers have an increased incidence of sustained hypertension, and there is no evidence that quitting smoking or caffeine products benefits BP control. Accordingly, patients should be advised to avoid cigarettes and coffee or tea immediately prior to having their BP checked. Because of the high incidence of associated malignancy and accelerated cardiovascular disease, smoking cessation should be strongly urged in all patients. Further, moderation in consumption of caffeine-containing beverages is advisable, in part because coronary disease risk may be increased in heavy coffee drinkers.

RELAXATION/STRESS REDUCTION. Relaxation and stress management produce only modest BP lowering even in highly motivated patients. Therefore, although these techniques may have beneficial side effects, including decreased anxiety and an improved sense of well-being, they have limited clinical application in the treatment of hypertension.

OVERALL RECOMMENDATIONS FOR NONPHARMACOLOGIC TREATMENT OF ESSENTIAL HYPERTENSION. Nonpharmacologic antihypertensive therapy should be used in all hypertensive patients, either as definitive treatment or as an adjunct to drug therapy. Therapy should be tailored to the individual characteristics of each patient—for example, weight reduction and exercise for the overweight patient and moderation in alcohol consumption for the heavy drinker. A reasonable generalized approach for all patients includes (1) reduction of dietary sodium and increases in dietary calcium and potassium, (2) weight loss for the overweight patient, (3) regular exercise, (4) moderation of alcohol consumption, and (5) smoking cessation. Such an approach has been shown to produce significant sustained reductions in BP while reducing overall cardiovascular risk.

Pharmacologic Therapy

THERAPEUTIC BENEFIT

Epidemiologic studies, including the Framingham Study, have clearly demonstrated that elevated BP is correlated with an increased incidence of cardiovascular disease, including stroke, renal failure, congestive heart failure, and myocardial infarction. The risk of cardiovascular complications is proportional to the degree of BP elevation. Clinical trials have shown that treatment of moderate to severe hypertension (diastolic BP > 105 mm Hg) reduces overall cardiovascular mortality. In the Veterans Administration Cooperative Study Group Trial, pharmacologic treatment of severe hypertension (diastolic BP 115 to 120 mm Hg) reduced morbidity and mortality by 90 per cent; treatment of moderate hypertension (diastolic BP 105 to 114 mm Hg) reduced overall cardiovascular complications by 50 per cent; treatment of patients with mild hypertension (diastolic BP 90 to 104 mm Hg) did not produce a significant reduction in cardiovascular morbidity and mortality overall. Only those individuals with mild hypertension who were above 50 years of age or had pre-existing cardiovascular or renal disease benefitted from therapy. Other studies, in contrast, have demonstrated clear benefits of pharmacologic treatment of patients with mild hypertension. The Hypertension Detection Follow-Up Program Study demonstrated a 20 per cent reduction in overall mortality in patients with mild hypertension (diastolic BP 90 to 104 mm Hg) who had aggressive treatment of their hypertension. Importantly, in those patients with the mildest degrees of hypertension (diastolic BP 90 to 94 mm Hg), survival was the most significantly improved. The European Working Party Trial demonstrated improved survival in elderly patients (60 to 80 years) being treated for mild hypertension. Clearly, treatment of moderate or severe hypertension significantly reduces overall cardiovascular morbidity and mortality. Although less conclusive, there is also sufficient evidence to recommend pharmacologic treatment of mild hypertension.

Most clinical trials of antihypertensive drugs have shown reductions in the incidence of congestive heart failure, renal failure, and stroke but have demonstrated less impressive reductions in morbidity and mortality from coronary artery disease. A new meta-analysis of clinical trials of antihypertensive drugs (chiefly diuretics and β blockers), in which mean reductions in diastolic BP of 5 to 6 mm Hg were achieved, showed a 42 per cent reduction in incidence of stroke and a 14 per cent reduction in coronary artery disease (Collins et al.). Diuretics and β blockers, the most commonly used medications in these large clinical trials, have metabolic side effects that increase coronary risk. Newer antihypertensive agents with fewer metabolic side effects and with neutral or even positive effects on coronary risk may reduce coronary morbidity and mortality further. Large clinical trials employing the newer agents are needed to assess their overall benefit.

GENERAL CONSIDERATIONS

The increasing number and variety of drugs available for use in hypertension, coupled with our rapidly expanding knowledge of the pathophysiology of hypertension and of the adverse effects of these drugs in individual patient groups, make it increasingly possible to individualize antihypertensive treatment. When used as monotherapy, most agents effectively control hypertension in over 50 per cent of patients with mild or moderate disease. Thus, it is possible to use a single agent to provide effective BP control with minimal side effects in many patients. Therapy should be initiated with the agent best tolerated and most likely to be effective in lowering BP in a given patient. If the initial agent is ineffective at maximal recommended doses or has undue side effects, an alternative agent from another class should be tried. When monotherapy is unsuccessful, a second agent, usually of a different class, should be added. Additional agents should be added or substituted as necessary to provide effective and well-tolerated BP control (Fig. 44–5).

Prescription of antihypertensive therapy should take into consideration the physiologic, economic, and social characteristics of each patient in order to provide effective BP control as simply and as inexpensively as possible. Expensive, complicated, and

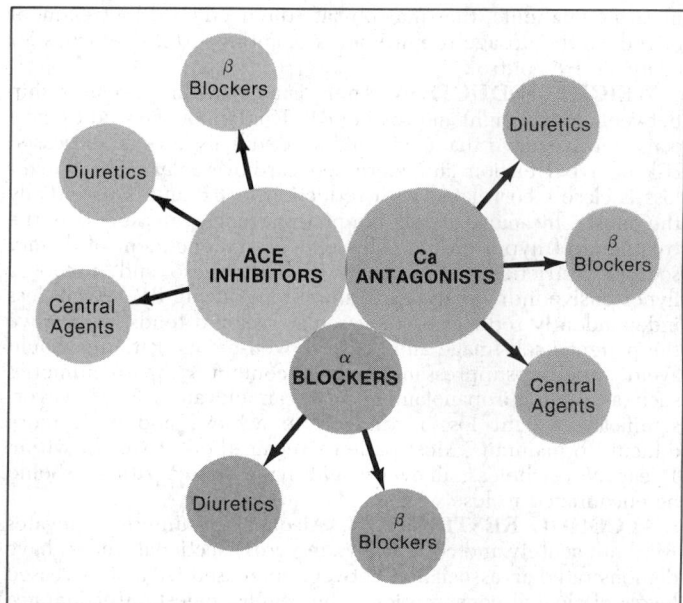

FIGURE 44–5. Proposed program for individualized antihypertensive therapy. Initial treatment should be with an angiotensin-converting enzyme (ACE) inhibitor, Ca antagonist, or α blocker. If this is unsuccessful in controlling blood pressure, an agent from another class should be substituted or a second agent should be added, as indicated in the diagram. Agents can then be added or substituted as necessary to provide effective and well-tolerated blood pressure control. (Modified from Zanchetti A: Angiotensin-converting enzyme inhibitors in essential hypertension. J Cardiovasc Pharmacol 9(Suppl 3):S2–S5, 1987; with permission.)

inconvenient regimens promote poor compliance. Patient involvement in his or her own care should be encouraged. Keeping patients informed of their illness and having patients measure and record their own BP's have been shown to improve BP control.

After initiating therapy, patients should be seen once every 1 to 4 weeks (depending on the severity of hypertension) for titration of antihypertensive drug dosage and once every 3 to 4 months once BP control is achieved. This allows for frequent assessment of treatment effectiveness and side effects and also emphasizes the physician's interest in the patient. Recommended dose ranges for individual drugs are listed with each agent in Tables 44–4 and 44–5, and for combination agents in Table 44–6. Common adverse effects are summarized in Table 44–7.

Once a patient's BP is controlled on a particular regimen, fixed combination tablets may be substituted in order to simplify the regimen and reduce medication costs (Table 44–6). However, such fixed combinations preclude individualized dosage titration, and therefore physicians may need to return to multiple tablet regimens as the patient's dose requirements change.

Step-down therapy, or withdrawal of antihypertensive medication under close monitoring, should be attempted in patients with mild or moderate hypertension whose BP has been adequately controlled for 1 year or more. Dosages should be titrated slowly downward and medications discontinued one at a time, if possible. Therapy should not be discontinued abruptly. Step-down therapy is generally most effective in patients who are also receiving nonpharmacologic treatment for their hypertension. Regular follow-up is crucial for all patients who have antihypertensive therapy discontinued, because BP can rise again to hypertensive levels, even after years of normal BP off therapy.

SPECIFIC DRUGS

DIURETICS. Thiazide diuretics were the principal agents used in most of the major trials of antihypertensive therapy that demonstrated significant reductions in overall cardiovascular morbidity and mortality, including significant reductions in congestive heart failure, stroke, and renal failure. These trials did not show significant reductions in mortality related to coronary artery disease, however. This failure to reduce the incidence of myocardial infarction, considered in conjunction with their adverse metabolic side effects, has led to growing concern about the effects of diuretics on overall cardiovascular risk, particularly in patients with mild hypertension.

Thiazide diuretics are effective in lowering BP in all patient groups, particularly in blacks and the elderly. They are inexpensive and generally well tolerated and consequently are widely used. Diuretics have been used safely in combination with all other classes of antihypertensive agents and generally provide additional BP reduction; therefore, they are a logical second agent when combination therapy is needed.

Thiazide diuretics are associated with a number of metabolic alterations, including kaliuresis, with an average fall in serum potassium of 0.6 mEq per liter, although profound hypokalemia can occur. The clinical significance of this decrease in serum potassium is controversial, but it may be arrhythmogenic in some patients. This interpretation was supported by the finding from the Multiple Risk Factor Intervention Trial (MRFIT) that patients with resting ECG abnormalities receiving thiazide diuretics had an increased incidence of sudden death. Although this finding has not been substantiated by other clinical trials, the potential arrhythmogenic effect of diuretic-induced hypokalemia remains worrisome, particularly in light of the failure of diuretics to improve coronary disease–related mortality. Hypokalemia should especially be avoided in patients at increased risk for arrhythmia, including those receiving digoxin, diabetics, and patients with known coronary artery disease.

Thiazide diuretics cause increases in total cholesterol, LDL cholesterol, and triglyceride levels. These increases tend to diminish with time, but well-controlled studies indicate that significant elevations in lipids persist with long-term thiazide treatment. Although the clinical significance of these alterations in lipid levels is not known, they may have a deleterious effect on overall cardiovascular risk.

Other metabolic side effects of thiazide diuretics include glucose intolerance, elevations in serum uric acid and calcium levels, and decreases in serum magnesium levels. These effects tend to be small but may become problematic in patients with related disorders. Therefore, thiazide diuretics should be used cautiously in diabetics and in patients with a history of gout or hypercalcemia. Other less common thiazide-induced metabolic alterations include hyponatremia and metabolic alkalosis. The most common subjective adverse effects of thiazide use are impotence, decreased libido, muscle cramps, and fatigue.

Recent studies have shown that adequate BP reduction can be achieved with much lower doses of thiazide diuretics than were traditionally used. Metabolic adverse effects tend to be minimized with the lower doses of thiazides. A starting dose of thiazide diuretic is the equivalent of 12.5 mg of hydrochlorothiazide in the general hypertensive population and 6.25 mg of hydrochlorothiazide in the elderly hypertensive patient. Because of their adverse metabolic side effects, their deleterious effects on cardiovascular risk factors, and their failure to reduce coronary morbidity and mortality, it seems prudent, when economically feasible, not to use thiazide diuretics as first-line therapy in patients with mild to moderate hypertension but to reserve them for use in combination with other classes of agents in patients with moderate to severe disease.

Loop diuretics such as furosemide and bumetanide are indicated in hypertensive patients with congestive heart failure or other edematous states or with renal insufficiency. **Potassium-sparing diuretics** are appropriate treatment for patients who are hypokalemic prior to initiation of diuretic therapy or who develop hypokalemia with the use of a non–potassium-sparing diuretic. Potassium-sparing diuretics are also magnesium sparing and may prevent the hypomagnesemia common in thiazide diuretic use. Diabetics, patients with renal insufficiency, and patients receiving ACE inhibitors, β-adrenergic blocking drugs, oral potassium

TABLE 44–4. DIURETICS FOR AMBULATORY TREATMENT OF HYPERTENSION

Generic Name	Trade Name (Manufacturer)	Adult Dosage (mg/day)	Duration (hr)	Dispensing Unit (mg)
Benzothiadiazine diuretics				
Thiazides				
Chlorothiazide	Diuril (MSD)*	250–500	6–12	250, 500
Hydrochlorothiazide	Esidrix (CIBA)	12.5–50	12–18	25
	HydroDIURIL (MSD)			50
	Oretic (Abbott)			
Bendroflumethiazide	Naturetin (Squibb)	5–20	18–36	2.5, 5.0
Benzthiazide	Aquatag (Tutag)	25–50	12–18	10
				50
	Diucen (Central)			
	Edemex (Savage)			
	Exna (Robins)			
	Lemazide (Lemmon)			
Cyclothiazide	Anhydron (Lilly)	1–2	18–24	2
Hydroflumethiazide	Saluron (Bristol)	25–50	18–24	50
Methyclothiazide	Aquatensen (Wallace)	2.5–10.0	24–48	5.0, 2.5
	Enduron (Abbott)			
Polythiazide	Renese (Pfizer)	2–4	24–48	1, 2, 4
Trichlormethiazide	Methahydrin (Merrell Dow)	2–4	24–48	2
	Naqua (Schering)			4
Indapamide	Lozol (USV Pharmaceutical)	2.5–5.0	18–24	2.5
Phthalimidines	Hygroton (USV Pharmaceutical)	12.5–50	24–72	25, 50, 100
Chlorthalidone	Chlorthalidone (Parke-Davis)			25, 50
	Thalitone (Boehringer-Ingelheim)			
Metolazone	Zaroxolyn (Pennwalt)	2.5–5.0	12–24	2.5, 5.0, 10.0
	Diulo (Searle)			2.5, 5.0, 10.0
Quinazolines	Hydromox (Lederle)	50–100	18–24	50
Quinethazone				
Loop diuretics				
Furosemide	Lasix (Hoechst-Roussel)	20–1,000	3–6	20, 40, 80
Ethacrynic acid	Edecrin (MSD)	50–400	3–6	25, 50
Bumetanide	Bumex (Roche)	0.5–2.0	1–4	0.5, 1.0
Potassium-sparing diuretics				
Spironolactone	Aldactone (Searle)	50–100	3–6	25, 50, 100
	Spironolactone (Parke-Davis)			25
Triamterene	Dyrenium (SKF)*	50–100	3–6	50, 10
Amiloride	Midamor (MSD)	5–10	24	5

*MSD = Merck Sharp & Dohme; SKF = Smith Kline & French.

supplementation, or salt substitutes high in potassium chloride are prone to hyperkalemia. Potassium-sparing diuretics should be used with caution in these patients. Dosing information for the currently available diuretics is summarized in Table 44–4.

BETA-ADRENERGIC RECEPTOR BLOCKING AGENTS. Beta-blockers are used extensively in the treatment of hypertension. They are available as nonselective agents that block β_1- and β_2-adrenergic receptors equally, cardioselective agents that have higher affinity for β_1 receptors, and agents with intrinsic sympathomimetic activity (ISA). Labetalol has both α_1-adrenergic antagonist and nonselective β antagonist activity. The antihypertensive effect of β blockers is attributed to their negative inotropic and chronotropic properties, which tend to decrease cardiac output. In addition, β blockers inhibit renin release and produce a delayed vasodilator effect of uncertain mechanism. Beta blockers have been used effectively and safely in combination with all other classes of antihypertensive agents. They must be used cautiously in combination with calcium channel blockers that have significant negative inotropic and chronotropic activity, as these effects of the two classes of agents may be additive. Beta blockers are routinely used in combination with vasodilators to blunt reflex tachycardia.

Beta blockers are more effective in lowering BP in younger patients than in the elderly and in whites than in blacks. Since β blockers are effective in the treatment of angina and in the secondary prevention of myocardial infarction, they are the drugs of choice in hypertensive patients with known coronary artery disease. Recent evidence, uncorroborated by large clinical trials, has suggested that β blockers may also be effective in the primary prevention of myocardial infarction in hypertensive patients. Beta blockers are very effective in younger patients and are the drugs of choice in hypertensive patients with sympathetic hyperactivity, as evidenced by a fast resting heart rate and a wide pulse pressure.

The most common adverse effects of β blockers are related to

TABLE 44–5. ANTIHYPERTENSIVE DRUGS IN AMBULATORY TREATMENT OF HYPERTENSION

Generic Name	Trade Name (Manufacturer)	Adult Maintenance Dose (mg/day)	Frequency of Administration (times/day)	Duration of Action (hr)
Sympatholytic agents				
Centrally acting agents				
Methyldopa	Aldomet (MSD)	250–2000	2	6–12
Clonidine	Catapres (Boehringer-Ingelheim)	0.2–0.8	2	6–12
Clonidine patch	Catapres-TTS (Boehringer-Ingelheim)	1 patch (0.1,0.2,0.3 mg)	weekly	7 days
Guanfacine	Tenex (Robins)	1–3	1	12–24
Guanabenz	Wytensin (Wyeth)	8–64	2	8–12
Reserpine and rauwolfia alkaloids	Serpasil (CIBA)	0.1–0.25	1	24
Beta-adrenergic blocking agents				
Propranolol	Inderal (Ayerst)	40–640	2	6–12
Metoprolol	Lopressor (CIBA)	100–450	2	12
Atenolol	Tenormin (ICI)	50–100	1	24
Nadolol	Corgard (Squibb)	40–320	1	24
Timolol	Blocadren (MSD)	20–60	2	6–12
Pindolol	Visken (Sandoz)	10–60	2	6–12
Acebutolol	Sectral (Wyeth)	400–1200	1 or 2	12–24
Penbutolol	Levatol (Reed & Carnrick)	20	1	24
Alpha-adrenergic blocking agents				
Prazosin	Minipress (Pfizer)	2.5–20	2 or 3	3–6
Prazosin sustained release	Minipress XL (Pfizer)	2.5–20	1	24
Terazosin	Hytrin (Abbott)	1–20	1	24
Doxazosin	Cardura (Roerig)	2–8	1	24
Mixed alpha- and beta-adrenergic blocking agent				
Labetalol	Normodyne (Schering) Trandate (Glaxo)	200–800	2	3–6
Ganglion-blocking agent				
Mecamylamine	Inversine (MSD)	2.5	2	12–24
Peripherally acting sympatholytic agent				
Guanethidine	Ismelin (CIBA)	10–300	1	24
Angiotensin-converting enzyme inhibitors				
Captopril	Capoten (Squibb)	75–450	3	4–8
Enalapril	Vasotec (MSD)	5–40	1 or 2	12–24
Lisinopril	Prinivil (MSD) Zestril (Stuart)	10–40	1	24
Quinapril*	Accupril (Parke-Davis)	5–40	1 or 2	12–24
Cilazaril*	Inhibace (Roche)	1.25–5	1	24
Calcium channel blocking agents				
Nifedipine	Procardia (Pfizer)	30–120	3 or 4	6–8
Nifedipine sustained release	Procardia XL (Pfizer)	30–90	1	24
Diltiazem	Cardizem (Marion)	90–240	3 or 4	6–8
Diltiazem sustained release	Cardizem SR (Marion)	120–240	2	12
Verapamil	Isoptin (Knoll) Calan (Searle)	240–480	3 or 4	6–8
Verapamil sustained release	Isoptin SR (Knoll) Calan SR (Searle)	120–480	1 or 2	12–24
Nicardipine	Cardene (Syntex)	30–90	3	6–8
Nitrendipine*	Baypress (Miles)	10–80	1 or 2	12–24
Isradipine*	DynaCirc (Sandoz/Glaxo)	2.5–20	2	12
Direct vasodilators				
Hydralazine	Apresoline (CIBA)	20–300	2 or 3	6
Minoxidil	Loniten (Upjohn)	5–10	1 or 2	Up to 72
Pinacidil	Pindac (Lilly)	25–50	2 or 3	3–6

*These agents have not been approved by the FDA for the treatment of hypertension.

their mechanism of action. The negative chronotropic and inotropic effects of β blockers may precipitate severe bradycardia, AV block, and congestive heart failure in susceptible patients and therefore should be avoided in patients with a history of bradycardia, cardiac conduction abnormalities, or heart failure. Beta blockers should be used with caution in patients with chronic obstructive pulmonary disease or peripheral vascular disease, since β₂ blockade may exacerbate bronchospasm, peripheral vascular constriction, and Raynaud's phenomenon. Cardioselec-

tive agents have a theoretical advantage in such patients because of their lower affinity for β₂ receptors, but this selectivity diminishes with increasing dose and is probably trivial at usual clinical doses. Central nervous system side effects such as fatigue, impotence, and decreased mental acuity can occur with β blockers, particularly in the elderly. These can be minimized with the use of less lipophilic agents, such as atenolol, acebutolol, nadolol,

TABLE 44–6. COMBINATION AGENTS FOR TREATMENT OF HYPERTENSION

Generic Name	Trade Name (Manufacturer)	Daily Dose (pills/day)	Pill Content (mg/mg)
Combination diuretics			
HCTZ/spironolactone	Aldactazide (Searle)	1–2	25/25
HCTZ/triamterene	Maxzide (Lederle)	1–2	25/75,50/75
HCTZ/triamterene	Dyazide (SKF)	1–4	25/50
HCTZ/amiloride	Modurectic (MSD)	1–2	50/15
ACE inhibitors and diuretics			
Captopril/HCTZ	Capozide (Squibb)	2–4	25/15,25/25 50/15,50/25
Enalapril/HCTZ	Vaseretic (MSD)	1–2	10/25
Beta-blocking agents and diuretics			
Propranolol/HCTZ	Inderide (Wyeth-Ayerst)	2–4	40/25,80/25
Propranolol LA/HCTZ	Inderide LA (Wyeth-Ayerst)	1	80/50 120/50 160/50
Atenolol/chlorthalidone	Tenoretic (ICI)	1	50/25 100/25
Timolol/HCTZ	Timolide (MSD)	1–2	10/25
Nadolol/bendroflumethiazide	Corzide (Princeton)	1	40/5,80/5
Labetalol/HCTZ	Normozide (Schering)	2	100/25 200/25 300/25
Vasodilators and diuretics			
Hydralazine/HCTZ	Apresazide (CIBA)	2–4	25/25,50/50 50/25
Hydralazine/HCTZ	Apresoline-Exidrix (CIBA)	2–4	25/15
Prazosin/polythiazide	Minizide (Pfizer)	2–4	1/0.5,2/0.5 3/0.5
Centrally acting agents and diuretics			
Methyldopa/chlorothiazide	Aldoclor (MSD)	2–8	250/150 250/250
Methyldopa/HCTZ	Aldoril (MSD)	2–4	250/15 250/25 500/30 500/50
Clonidine/chlorthalidone	Combipres (Boehringer-Ingelheim)	2–3	0.1/25 0.2/25 0.3/25
Reserpine/chlorothiazide	Diupres (MSD)	1–2	0.125/250 0.125/500
Reserpine/methychlothiazide	Diutensen-R (Wallace)	1–4	0.1/2.5
Reserpine/quinethazone	Hydromox (Lederele)	1–2	0.125/50
Reserpine/HCTZ	Hydropres (MSD)	1–2	0.125/25 0.125/50
Reserpine/trichlormethiazide	Naquival (Schering)	1–2	0.1/4
Reserpine/polythiazide	Renese-R (Pfizer)	0.5–2	0.25/2
Reserpine/hydroflumethiazide	Salutensin-Demi Salutensin (Bristol)	1–2	0.125/25 0.125/50
Reserpine/HCTZ	Serpasil-Esidrix (CIBA)	1–2	0.1/25 0.1/50
Reserpine/chlorthalidone	Demi-Regroton Regroton (Rorer)	1	0.25/25 0.25/50
Deserpidine/methychlothiazide	Enduronyl Enduronyl-Forte (Abbott)	0.5–2	0.25/50 0.5/5
Deserpidine/HCTZ	Oreticyl Oreticyl-Forte (Abbott)	2–4	0.125/25 0.125/50 0.250/25
Guanethidine/HCTZ	Esimil (CIBA)	1–4	10/25
Rauwolfia/bendroflumethiazide	Rauzide (Princeton)	1–4	50/4
Other combinations			
Reserpine/hydralazine	Serpasil-Apresoline (CIBA)	2–4	0.1/25 0.2/25
Reserpine/hydralazine/HCTZ	Ser-Ap-Es (CIBA)	3–6	0.1/25/15

HCTZ = Hydrochlorothiazide.

labetalol, and timolol, which are less likely to enter the brain. Beta blockers should be used with caution in insulin-dependent diabetics, as they mask symptoms and delay recovery from hypoglycemia. Beta blockers adversely effect the serum lipid profile by reducing HDL cholesterol and increasing triglycerides.

Labetalol has both α and β antagonist properties; its most prominent pharmacologic effect is α_1 adrenergic receptor antagonist activity, similar to prazosin. Labetalol is particularly effective in lowering BP in blacks and in the elderly. It has no significant effect on serum lipid levels and has been used safely in patients with chronic obstructive pulmonary disease and peripheral vascular disease. The most common side effects of labetalol include fatigue, dizziness, headache, and gastrointestinal complaints. There is a low incidence of orthostatic hypotension with labetalol.

Because of their frequent adverse effects and their negative effect on the lipid profile, traditional β-blocking agents are not recommended for initial antihypertensive therapy in the general population. They remain useful in patients with established coronary artery disease. The newer mixed adrenergic blocking agents, such as labetalol, which are generally better tolerated and have a neutral to positive effect on serum lipid levels, are recommended for initial antihypertensive therapy in the general population. Dosing information for the currently available β blockers is summarized in Table 44–5.

CALCIUM CHANNEL BLOCKERS. The calcium channel blockers inhibit vascular smooth muscle contraction by blocking the influx of calcium into the cell. Their predominant antihypertensive effect is a decrease in peripheral vascular resistance. The calcium channel blockers are effective in reducing BP in a majority of unselected hypertensive patients, but like diuretics, they are particularly efficacious in blacks and the elderly. Calcium channel blockers are useful in the treatment of angina, so they are a logical choice for the treatment of hypertension in patients with coronary artery disease. Recent evidence suggests that calcium channel blockers, like β blockers, reduce the incidence of reinfarction. The antivasospastic property of calcium channel blockers may benefit patients with Raynaud's phenomenon, esophagospasm, and irritable bowel syndrome. The calcium channel blockers have been used safely and successfully in combination with all other classes of antihypertensive agents, but they (particularly verapamil) should be used cautiously in combination with β blockers, because of common negative inotropic and chronotropic properties.

The calcium channel blockers are well tolerated and convenient now that sustained-release formulations are available. They are

TABLE 44–7. COMMON ADVERSE EFFECTS OF ANTIHYPERTENSIVE DRUGS

Drugs	Side Effects	Precautions and Special Considerations
Diuretics		
Thiazides and related sulfonamides	Hypokalemia, hyperuricemia, glucose intolerance, hypercholesterolemia, hypertriglyceridemia, sexual dysfunction	May be ineffective in renal failure; hypokalemia increases digitalis toxicity; and hyperuricemia may precipitate acute gout.
Loop diuretics	Same as for thiazides	Effective in chronic renal failure; cautions regarding hypokalemia and hyperuricemia same as above; hyponatremia may be found, especially in the elderly.
Potassium-sparing agents	Hyperkalemia	Danger of hyperkalemia in patients with renal failure or diabetes or those receiving ACE inhibitors.
Amiloride hydrochloride	Sexual dysfunction	—
Spironolactone	Gynecomastia, mastodynia, sexual dysfunction	—
Adrenergic antagonists		
Beta-adrenergic blockers	Bradycardia, fatigue, insomnia, bizarre dreams, sexual dysfunction, hypertriglyceridemia, decreased HDL cholesterol	Should not be used in patients with asthma, chronic obstructive pulmonary disease, congestive heart failure, heart block (> first degree), and sick sinus syndrome. Use with caution in patients with diabetes and peripheral vascular disease. Sudden withdrawal of these drugs may be hazardous in patients with abrupt discontinuance.
Centrally acting agents Methyldopa	Drowsiness, dry mouth, fatigue, —	Rebound hypertension may occur with abrupt discontinuance. May cause liver damage and positive direct Coombs' test (rare hemolytic anemia).
Reserpine	Sexual dysfunction, nasal congestion, lethargy	Contraindicated in patients with a history of depression; use with caution in patients with a history of peptic ulcer.
Alpha₁-adrenergic blockers	"First-dose" syncope, orthostatic hypotension, weakness, palpitations, dizziness, headache, fluid retention	Use cautiously in elderly patients.
Combined α- and β-adrenergic blockers	Nausea, fatigue, dizziness, headache, orthostatic hypotension	Use with caution in patients with cardiac failure, chronic obstructive pulmonary disease, sick sinus syndrome, heart block (> first degree), diabetes.
Vasodilators		
Vasodilators	Headache, tachycardia, fluid retention	May precipitate angina in patients with coronary heart disease.
Hydralazine hydrochloride	Positive antinuclear antibody (without other changes)	Lupus syndrome may occur (rare at recommended doses).
Minoxidil	Hypertrichosis, ascites (rare)	May cause or aggravate pleural and pericardial effusions.
Angiotensin-converting enzyme inhibitors		
Angiotensin-converting enzyme inhibitors	Cough	Can cause reversible acute renal failure in patients with bilateral renal artery stenosis; neutropenia may occur in patients with autoimmune collagen disorders; proteinuria may occur (rare at recommended doses).
Calcium channel blocking agents		
Calcium channel blocking agents	Headache, hypotension, dizziness	
Verapamil hydrochloride	Constipation, bradycardia	Use with caution in patients with congestive heart failure or heart block.

free of significant metabolic adverse effects, including alterations in lipid levels. Negative inotropic effects are seen with all calcium channel blockers but are most pronounced with verapamil and can cause significant suppression of myocardial contractility. Therefore, verapamil should be avoided in patients with left ventricular dysfunction. Verapamil also has a significant negative chronotropic effect and should be used cautiously in patients with conduction abnormalities. Verapamil is indicated for the treatment for certain tachyarrhythmias and is the drug of choice in hypertensive patients who have such arrhythmias. All of the calcium channel blockers can cause constipation, but this effect is most problematic with verapamil. The most common adverse effects of the dihydropyridine derivatives (nifedipine, nitrendipine, nicardipine, isradipine) are related to their vasodilator action. These include lightheadedness, flushing, tachycardia, and periorbital and pedal edema. These adverse effects are less common with sustained-release preparations. Calcium channel blockers generally are free of central nervous system side effects, including sexual dysfunction. They are metabolized by the liver and may require dosage adjustment in patients with hepatic disease but can be used safely in patients with renal disease. All of the calcium channel blockers can increase serum digoxin levels. This is a particular problem with verapamil. Dosing information for the currently available calcium channel blockers is summarized in Table 44–5.

ANGIOTENSIN-CONVERTING ENZYME (ACE) INHIBITORS. ACE inhibitors inhibit the enzymatic conversion of angiotensin I to angiotensin II with consequent reductions in peripheral vascular resistance, sympathetic nervous system activity, and renal sodium and water retention. They effectively lower BP in all of the major subgroups of hypertensive patients, including the elderly. Blacks are generally less sensitive to the antihypertensive effects of ACE inhibition than are whites, but increasing the dose of ACE inhibitor or adding a diuretic abolishes the racial difference. ACE inhibitors reduce afterload and are the drugs of choice in patients with hypertension and congestive failure. The combination of an ACE inhibitor, diuretic, and digoxin prolongs survival in patients with severe congestive failure (New York Heart Association class IV). ACE inhibitors are particularly useful in hypertensive patients with diabetes, since they decrease proteinuria and stabilize renal function in patients with diabetic nephropathy. They are also particularly effective in the control of hypertension secondary to renal vascular disease. However, in patients with renal artery stenosis in a solitary kidney, bilateral renal artery stenosis, or transplant renal artery stenosis, ACE inhibition may precipitate acute renal failure. Renal function should be monitored closely if ACE inhibitors are used in this setting. Further, ACE inhibitors have been reported to minimize the adverse metabolic effects of diuretic therapy. Therefore, the ACE inhibitor–diuretic combination is appealing. ACE inhibitors are well tolerated and generally free of adverse effects on the CNS, sexual function, and metabolism. Specifically, they do not adversely affect lipid levels, glucose tolerance, or uric acid levels.

Class-specific adverse effects of ACE inhibitors include hypotension, hyperkalemia, acute renal failure, angioedema, and cough, which tends to be nonproductive and worse at night. Cough is the most common adverse effect of the ACE inhibitors, with an incidence that approaches 25 per cent. Hypotension is generally a first-dose phenomenon in patients who are in a high renin state, such as those on a low-salt diet or receiving diuretic therapy. It can be minimized by starting with a very low dose of ACE inhibitor and, if possible, withholding diuretics prior to initiation of ACE inhibition. Hyperkalemia rarely occurs in patients with normal renal function. However, in patients with diabetes or renal dysfunction or those receiving potassium-sparing diuretics, potassium supplements, or nonsteroidal anti-inflammatory agents, clinically significant hyperkalemia may be precipitated by ACE inhibitor therapy. Angioedema is a rare but potentially catastrophic side effect of ACE inhibitors.

Side effects of ACE inhibitors thought to be related to the sulfhydryl group (currently found in captopril only) include proteinuria, rash, taste disturbances, and bone marrow suppression. The incidence of these side effects is related to the dose of the ACE inhibitor or to the presence of renal insufficiency. When the captopril dose is limited to less than 150 mg per day in a person with normal renal function, these side effects are infrequent. The risk of neutropenia is highest in patients with connective tissue disease and related renal dysfunction. Rash, taste disturbances, and proteinuria tend to be self-limited and to resolve with cessation of captopril therapy. These side effects have also been reported with nonsulfhydryl-containing ACE inhibitors, but much less frequently.

Captopril should be taken prior to eating, as food may decrease its absorption. The other ACE inhibitors are well absorbed even in the presence of food. Captopril is the shortest acting of the ACE inhibitors and generally requires at least twice-daily dosing for effective BP reduction. The other ACE inhibitors have longer half-lives and are generally effective when administered once a day. All of the ACE inhibitors are excreted by the kidney and require dosage adjustment in patients with renal impairment. Dosing information for the currently available ACE inhibitors is summarized in Table 44–5.

CENTRALLY ACTING AGENTS. The traditional centrally acting antihypertensive agents—clonidine, methyldopa, and guanabenz—have been a mainstay of antihypertensive therapy for several decades. However, in recent years their use has been limited by a high incidence of side effects and the need for frequent dosing. The recent release of transdermal clonidine and long-acting guanfacine, both of which allow for more convenient dosing with fewer side effects, expands the role of centrally acting agents in the treatment of hypertension.

The centrally acting agents are predominantly α_2 adrenoceptor agonists, stimulating adrenoceptors in the brain stem and hypothalamus, thereby inhibiting sympathetic outflow from the central nervous system and decreasing BP, heart rate, and peripheral vascular resistance. These agents are as effective as the other major classes of antihypertensive agents in lowering BP. They have no significant effects on glucose regulation, serum lipid levels, or renal function.

The most common side effects of the centrally acting agents are dry mouth, drowsiness, and fatigue. These occur initially in as many as 30 per cent of patients receiving the traditional centrally acting agents but tend to diminish with continued therapy. Less frequent side effects include orthostatic hypotension, sexual dysfunction, and decreased mental acuity. Transdermal clonidine and guanfacine are better tolerated and have a significantly lower incidence of side effects than the traditional agents. Abrupt discontinuation of the traditional agents, particularly clonidine, has been associated with a withdrawal syndrome characterized by headache, nausea, anxiety, vomiting, and rebound hypertension that may require emergent therapy. BP in this setting can be reduced and symptoms alleviated with reinitiation of previous therapy. The withdrawal syndrome has not been associated with transdermal clonidine or guanfacine. Approximately 10 to 20 per cent of patients receiving methyldopa develop a positive direct Coombs' reaction, but only a very small percentage (< 1 per cent develop hemolytic anemia. Drug-induced hepatitis and/or fever is rarely associated with methyldopa use. Transdermal clonidine is associated with a local rash in 10 to 15 per cent of patients. The rash is generally a mild, localized erythema, but vesicular eruptions have been reported. It disappears with discontinuation of therapy.

The centrally acting agents are effective in all the major subgroups of hypertensive patients but should be used cautiously in the elderly because of their adverse effects on baroreflex and central nervous system function. The more convenient dosing of guanfacine and transdermal clonidine makes these agents more acceptable to patients than the traditional oral centrally acting agents. Transdermal clonidine with its once-weekly dosing is well suited for patients who are forgetful, who do not like to be reminded daily of their illness, or who have their medicines administered to them by family or friends. The centrally acting agents have been used safely and successfully in combination with all of the major classes of antihypertensive agents, including diuretics. Dosing information for the currently available centrally acting agents is summarized in Table 44–5.

ALPHA-ADRENERGIC RECEPTOR BLOCKERS. The α-adrenergic antagonists lower BP by reducing peripheral vascular resistance, principally by inhibiting norepinephrine-induced vasoconstriction in vascular smooth muscle. The hypotensive effect is not accompanied by significant alterations in heart rate, cardiac output, glomerular filtration rate, or renal plasma flow. The α antagonists are effective in all major subgroups of hypertensive patients and have been used safely in combination with all of the major classes of antihypertensive agents, including diuretics and β blockers. Contrary to common clinical perception, long-term trials have not demonstrated the development of tolerance to the antihypertensive effects of the α antagonists.

The α antagonists have no significant adverse metabolic effects and, in fact, have a beneficial effect on the serum lipid profile. They decrease total cholesterol and/or LDL cholesterol and increase HDL cholesterol. Thus, the α antagonists provide a dual benefit in lowering cardiovascular risk.

The major side effects of the α antagonists include headache, dizziness, weakness, and mild fluid retention. Orthostatic hypotension, which is usually most prominent with the initial dose, can occur with all the α antagonists but is best documented with prazosin. The effect can be minimized by initiating therapy with a small dose at bedtime. The α antagonists are generally free of central nervous system–mediated side effects, such as dry mouth, fatigue, and sexual dysfunction. The development of longer-acting α antagonists with minimal side effects and positive effects on serum lipid levels expands the role of these agents as initial antihypertensive therapy, particularly in patients with underlying diseases such as chronic obstructive pulmonary disease, peripheral vascular disease, diabetes, and hyperlipidemia. Dosing information for the currently available α-adrenergic antagonists is summarized in Table 44–5.

VASODILATORS. The direct vasodilators relax arterial smooth muscle with little effect on venous capacitance vessels. BP is reduced secondary to a decrease in peripheral resistance in association with reflex-mediated increases in heart rate, stroke volume, and cardiac output, as well as expansion of the plasma and extracellular fluid volumes.

Common side effects include tachycardia, fluid retention, palpitations, headache, nasal congestion, and, in patients with underlying coronary artery disease, myocardial ischemia. It is generally necessary to administer hydralazine or minoxidil in combination with a diuretic and β blocker to minimize fluid retention and block reflex-mediated increases in heart rate and cardiac output. Long-term administration of hydralazine, particularly in doses greater than 300 mg per day, may induce systemic lupus erythematosus. The lupus reaction generally resolves following discontinuation of hydralazine therapy but occasionally may require several years for complete resolution. Side effects of minoxidil include hirsutism, which makes minoxidil unacceptable to female patients, nausea, fatigue, and skin rash. Minoxidil use has been associated with unexplained pericardial effusion, occasionally with tamponade.

The direct vasodilators are generally reserved for adjunctive therapy in patients with severe refractory hypertension. Minoxidil has been safely and effectively used in patients with severe hypertension complicated by renal insufficiency. The combination of a vasodilator and diuretic with a β blocker (triple therapy) is effective in treating patients with severe, refractory essential or renal hypertension. Dosing information for the currently available vasodilators is summarized in Table 44–5.

Special Patient Groups

THE ELDERLY. Approximately two thirds of persons between the ages of 65 and 74 years have hypertension. Both diastolic hypertension and isolated systolic hypertension in the elderly are associated with a two- to three-fold increased risk of cardiovascular mortality. Multiple clinical trials have demonstrated reduced cardiovascular morbidity and mortality with treatment of diastolic hypertension in the elderly. Whether treating isolated systolic hypertension in the elderly has a similar effect on prognosis is a topic of current study.

The drugs used in the treatment of diastolic or isolated systolic hypertension in the elderly are the same as those used in the nonelderly. Because older persons are particularly sensitive to pharmacologic intervention, antihypertensive medications should be prescribed cautiously at lower than the recommended starting dose for the general population of hypertensives and adjustments made slowly (6- to 8-week intervals). Elderly persons are more prone to orthostatic hypotension because of decreased sensitivity of their baroreceptors. Accordingly, supine and standing BP should be checked regularly in order to avoid orthostasis. Agents particularly prone to cause severe orthostatic hypotension (guanethidine, prazosin, and guanadrel) should be avoided in the elderly. All of the major classes of antihypertensive drugs have been shown to be effective in elderly patients, although the β blockers may be slightly less effective in this group.

DIABETICS. Hypertension is twice as common in diabetics as in the general population. Diabetics with hypertension have a greatly increased risk of developing cerebral vascular disease, coronary artery disease, and renal disease compared to normotensive diabetics. Nonpharmacologic approaches, including weight loss, exercise, and decreased alcohol consumption, benefit both glucose and BP control. Because of their proven effectiveness and lack of significant adverse effects, recommended first-line agents for BP control in diabetics include calcium channel blockers, ACE inhibitors, and α-adrenergic blockers. The ACE inhibitors are gaining favor in the treatment of hypertension in diabetic patients because of recent evidence that they reduce the proteinuria and slow the rate of deterioration in renal function due to diabetic nephropathy. Alpha blockers are favored as antihypertensive treatment in diabetics because of their positive effects on the serum lipid profile. Diuretics are effective in lowering BP in hypertensive diabetics, but their effects on serum potassium, lipid levels, and glucose tolerance are particularly worrisome in this group. Similarly, β blockers are effective but should be used with caution in insulin-dependent diabetics because they tend to mask the symptoms of hypoglycemia and inhibit recovery of glucose levels. Potassium supplements and potassium-sparing diuretics should be used with caution in diabetics because of the frequent occurrence of hyporeninemic hypoaldosteronism in patients with diabetic nephropathy.

BLACKS. Hypertension tends to be more common, earlier in onset, and more severe in blacks than in whites. Organ damage secondary to hypertension also occurs more frequently in blacks than in whites. However, hypertension in blacks can be treated as successfully as hypertension in whites.

Pharmacologic therapy is generally the same for blacks and whites, with only subtle differences in responsiveness to various treatment regimens. Diuretics and calcium channel blockers are very effective in the treatment of black patients. Beta blockers and ACE inhibitors provide less reduction of BP in blacks than in whites at equivalent doses, but at higher doses or in combination with diuretics, racial differences are obliterated. Centrally acting agents and vasodilators are equally effective in whites and blacks.

SECONDARY HYPERTENSION
Renal

RENOVASCULAR HYPERTENSION. Renovascular disease is the most common (1 to 2 per cent) cause of curable hypertension. Lesions of the renal vessels produce a fixed obstruction to perfusion, stimulating the intrarenal baroreceptor and perhaps the macula densa to augment renin secretion. Angiotensin and aldosterone are increased secondarily, resulting in sodium and water retention. Elevated circulating angiotensin II and aldosterone levels are primarily responsible for BP elevation early in the course of renovascular hypertension, and increased sodium and water retention and enhanced sympathetic nervous system activity play dominant roles in the chronic phase of the syndrome. Deficiencies of antihypertensive factors, such as prostaglandins and renomedullary neutral lipid, may also contribute to the pathogenesis of renovascular hypertension.

Any lesion that obstructs either large or small renal arteries can cause renovascular hypertension. The most common and clinically important of these are intrinsic lesions of the large vessels, because they can be physically removed and the hypertension either cured or ameliorated. Atherosclerotic disease is found in two thirds of patients with renovascular hypertension, fibrous or fibromuscular disease in one third. Patients with atherosclerotic renal artery lesions tend to be older and to have higher systolic BP and more frequent extrarenal arterial disease than patients with essential hypertension and are more likely to develop target-organ damage. Patients with fibromuscular disease tend to be younger and predominantly female and are less likely to develop cardiovascular complications. Prognosis is generally worse in atherosclerotic disease than in fibromuscular disease.

Patients most likely to have renovascular hypertension include those with hypertension of abrupt onset, especially in the young or in late middle age or old age; those with malignant hypertension or sudden acceleration of benign hypertension; and those who fail to respond to medical therapy. Generally, these patients have moderately severe to severe fixed diastolic hypertension. The presence of an upper abdominal bruit, particularly one that is systolic-diastolic or continuous in timing, is high pitched, and radiates laterally from the midepigastrium, is strongly suggestive of functionally significant renal artery stenosis. Such bruits have been described in one half to two thirds of patients with surgically proven renovascular hypertension. Because of the high cost of the diagnostic evaluation for renovascular hypertension, diagnostic study should be reserved for patients with one or more of the characteristics discussed above.

Screening tests for renovascular hypertension include abdominal ultrasonography, the captopril renogram, and pharmacologic screening with an ACE inhibitor. **Abdominal ultrasonography** provides an inexpensive, noninvasive means of assessing renal size and ureteral anatomy and does not require administration of radioactive isotopes. It is useful in evaluating patients in whom renal parenchymal disease and obstructive uropathy are part of the differential diagnosis. The **captopril renogram** provides an indirect index of glomerular filtration rate or estimated renal plasma flow and its dependence on intrarenal angiotensin II by measuring renal uptake of radiolabeled diethylene triamine pentaacetic acid (DTPA) or Hippuran before and after ACE inhibition with captopril. It has replaced the rapid-sequence or hypertensive intravenous pyelogram as the most commonly used screening test for renovascular hypertension. A positive captopril renogram indicates that a stenotic lesion is both hemodynamically and functionally significant and predicts a good result from renal revascularization; renal revascularization corrects the abnormalities in the captopril renogram. The sensitivity and specificity of the captopril renogram as a screening test in a large population with a low probability of disease have not yet been tested, however. **Pharmacologic screening** with an ACE inhibitor is a sensitive but not highly specific means of evaluating patients for renovascular hypertension. Administration of a single oral dose of ACE inhibitor leads to increases in plasma renin activity and decreases in BP that are exaggerated in patients with renovascular hypertension. Responses to this pharmacologic screening test reflect the angiotensin dependence of the patient's BP and thus are critically dependent on volume and sodium status. False-positive results are seen in patients who are volume depleted or are being treated with antihypertensive therapy, patients with malignant hypertension, and some patients with high- and normal-renin essential hypertension.

Diagnosis of functionally significant renal artery stenosis has traditionally been made by a combination of selective renal angiography and differential renal vein renin measurement. Renal angiography defines the anatomy of the stenotic renal artery, information needed to plan the approach to revascularization. With the advent of safe and highly effective percutaneous techniques for renal revascularization, many angiographers now elect not to perform renal vein renin determinations in patients with typical lesions but to proceed immediately to angioplasty and use the BP response as a test of the functional significance of the lesion. In some centers, the captopril renogram has replaced renal vein renin determinations as a functional test in patients with documented renal artery stenosis.

In general, the therapeutic approach to patients with renovascular hypertension is to attempt revascularization with percutaneous transluminal angioplasty at the time of diagnosis in those with anatomically favorable lesions. If angioplasty is unsuccessful or if restenosis occurs after successful dilatation, the procedure can be repeated. If repeat angioplasty is unsuccessful, surgical revascularization should be attempted in patients with favorable lesions who can tolerate the procedure, particularly if BP is uncontrolled on medical treatment or renal function is deteriorating. Only patients with anatomically unfavorable lesions and those who are not surgical candidates should receive medical treatment at the time of diagnosis without a prior attempt at revascularization. Medical therapy is used more often in older patients who have atherosclerotic renal artery disease and overt

extrarenal vascular disease than in younger patients with fibromuscular disease.

ACE inhibitors, given alone or in combination with a diuretic, are generally effective in controlling BP while sparing renal function and maintaining negative sodium balance in patients with hypertension due to unilateral renal artery stenosis. These simple regimens are well tolerated and represent the medical treatment of choice in most patients with renovascular hypertension. The ACE inhibitors induce acute, reversible renal failure in a subset of patients with renovascular hypertension: those with bilateral renal artery stenosis or renal artery stenosis in a solitary kidney, whether native or allograft, or with unilateral renal artery stenosis and severe parenchymal disease in the contralateral kidney. This form of reversible renal insufficiency results from impairment in the autoregulation of glomerular filtration secondary to blockade of the intrarenal renin-angiotensin system in the presence of reduced renal artery perfusion pressure. Normal autoregulation of glomerular filtration rate, which is dependent on an intact intrarenal renin-angiotensin system, is lost when an ACE inhibitor is administered.

Renal size and function must be carefully monitored in patients being treated medically for renovascular hypertension, even if BP is satisfactorily controlled. Renal function can deteriorate and renal mass can be lost very rapidly in patients with atherosclerotic disease who are treated medically. Progressive loss of renal mass, presumably related to parenchymal ischemia due to progression of the renal artery lesion, is common in medically treated patients with renovascular hypertension and is unrelated to BP control. Significant reduction in renal length is the most sensitive index of loss of renal mass. Serial (every 3 to 6 months) estimates of renal size are important in the follow-up of patients who are receiving medical treatment for renovascular hypertension.

Adrenal

Primary aldosteronism and pheochromocytoma are relatively rare causes of hypertension which are clinically important because the associated hypertension can usually be cured with appropriate surgical or targeted drug therapy. These syndromes are discussed in detail in Ch. 217.8 and 229, respectively.

ORAL CONTRACEPTIVE–INDUCED HYPERTENSION. A small percentage of women who use oral contraceptives experience the onset of hypertension that resolves with withdrawal of oral contraceptive therapy. Genetic characteristics, such as family history of hypertension and black race, as well as environmental characteristics, such as pre-existing and occult renal disease, obesity, and middle age (> 40 years), increase susceptibility to oral contraceptive–induced hypertension. The diagnosis of oral contraceptive–induced hypertension can be made by documenting the onset of hypertension de novo during contraceptive therapy and the resolution of the hypertension on drug withdrawal. This form of hypertension usually begins during the first year of oral contraceptive administration.

Oral contraceptive–induced hypertension can, in part, be prevented by avoiding the use of these agents in women who are at high risk. Evidence of thromboembolic disease or chronic hypertension of any cause is a contraindication to use of oral contraceptive. A family history of hypertension and a personal history of pre-existing or occult renal disease or of pregnancy complicated by hypertension are relative contraindications to oral contraceptive use. Women over 35 years of age, particularly if obese, should be cautioned about the increased risk of developing hypertension while ingesting oral contraceptives. Such patients should be followed closely: BP measurement and a funduscopic examination should be performed and an interval history obtained on several occasions during the first year of treatment and at yearly intervals thereafter.

The prevalence of oral contraceptive–induced hypertension is not related to the formulation or dose of estrogen, but since the incidence of thromboembolic complications is related to the dose of estrogen in the contraceptive, it is preferable to use preparations of relatively low estrogen content.

HYPERTENSIVE CRISIS

Hypertensive crises are subclassified as hypertensive urgencies or emergencies, depending on evidence of ongoing end-organ

TABLE 44–8. ANTIHYPERTENSIVE DRUGS FOR MANAGEMENT OF HYPERTENSIVE CRISIS

Drugs	Intramuscular (mg*)	Single Dose (mg*)	Continuous Infusion (μg/kg/min)	Onset of Action	Adverse Effects
Oral agents					
Clonidine (Catapres)†	—	0.2 p.o. initially, then 0.1 at 1-hr intervals as needed up to total dose of 0.7	—	30–60 min	Hypotension, headache, nausea, dizziness
Nifedipine (Procardia)†	—	10–20 sublingually or buccally initially, then at 30-min intervals as needed × 3	—	5–10 min	Hypotension, flushing, headache, tachycardia, nausea, coronary ischemia (rare)
Parenteral agents					
Direct vasodilators					
Sodium nitroprusside (Nipride)	—	—	0.5–10	Immediate	Nausea, vomiting, muscle twitching, apprehension, sweating, thiocyanate intoxication
Diazoxide (Hyperstat)	—	50–100 at 5–10-min intervals until satisfactory BP is achieved	Rarely used	3–5 min	Tachycardia, palpitations, flushing, headache, nausea, vomiting, aggravation of angina or congestive heart failure or both, hyperglycemia, hyperuricemia, hypotension
Hydralazine (Apresoline)	10–40 at 30-min intervals until satisfactory response is achieved	10–20 at 30-min intervals until satisfactory BP is achieved	Rarely used	Intramuscularly 30 min; intravenously 5–10 min	Tachycardia, palpitations, flushing, headache, vomiting, aggravation of angina or congestive heart failure or both
Sympathetic blocking drugs					
Ganglion-blocking agent					
Trimethaphan camsylate (Arfonad)	—	—	4–90	5–10 min	Urinary retention, paralytic ileus, paralysis of pupillary reflex and accommodation of eye, dry mouth, orthostatic hypotension
Central nervous system–active agent					
Methyldopa hydrochloride (Aldomet ester)	—	250–500; may be repeated at 6-hr intervals	—	2–3 hr	Drowsiness
Alpha-adrenergic receptor blocking agents					
Phentolamine (Regitine)	5–15	5–15 (rapid injection essential)	—	Instantaneous	Tachycardia, flushing
Labetalol	—	20 initially over 2 min, then 40–80 at 10-min intervals as needed up to 300 total	2/min to a total dose of 300	Instantaneous	Postural dizziness with or without postural hypotension; paradoxical pressor responses have been reported; nausea, vomiting, scalp tingling, burning in throat and groin
Calcium channel blocking agent					
Nicardipine (Cardene)†	—	5/h initially, titrated upward by 1–2.5/h every 15 min as needed up to 15/h		1–5 min	Hypotension, flushing, headache, diaphoresis, dizziness, nausea, tachycardia

*Start with the smallest dose shown. Subsequent doses and intervals of administration should be adjusted according to the BP response.

Start infusion slowly and adjust rate according to response to BP. Constant surveillance is mandatory. Concentration of solution can be adjusted according to patient's fluid requirements.

The total dose should be contained in a volume of at least 20 ml, and the solution should be administered from a 20- or 50-ml syringe. BP should be monitored continuously during injection. Rate of injection should not exceed 0.5 ml per minute. To avoid hypotension, the injection should be stopped frequently when the BP is falling.

Diluted up to 100 ml and injected during a 30- to 60-minute period.

†Not approved by FDA for this indication.

damage. In the absence of neurologic, cardiovascular, or renal deterioration and funduscopic abnormalities, patients with severely elevated BP (> 200/120 mm Hg) require urgent treatment, but usually not hospital admission. However, in the presence of evidence of ongoing end-organ damage, patients with severely elevated BP should be treated emergently with parenteral medications in an intensive care unit. The distinction between the need for urgent versus emergent intervention is based not on the absolute BP, but instead on the effect of the BP elevation on target organs. A BP of 190/130 mm Hg may be well tolerated in a patient with chronic hypertension, whereas that BP reading in another patient may precipitate acute renal insufficiency, left ventricular failure, cerebral edema, or other vascular crisis, thereby creating a medical emergency. The triggering mechanism for the arteriolar lesion responsible for the development of accelerated or malignant hypertension is unknown but has been related to the absolute level or rate of rise of arterial pressure, the presence of disseminated intravascular clotting, or activation of the renin-angiotensin system. The syndrome is perpetuated by the deposition of fibrin in arteriolar walls, which leads to retinopathy, renal damage, and increased renin release. Usually the etiology of any particular hypertensive crisis is not known, and therapy must be generalized. However, when the etiology is known, specific treatment should be instituted whenever possible.

Symptoms of hypertensive crisis include headache, malaise, dizziness, blurred vision, chest pain, palpitations, and shortness of breath. Clinical and laboratory signs of hypertensive crisis include funduscopic changes (arteriolar narrowing, arteriovenous nicking, hemorrhages, exudates, papilledema); changes related to renal insufficiency; microangiopathic hemolytic anemia; signs of left ventricular dysfunction (gallops, jugular venous distention, cardiomegaly, tachycardia, pulmonary edema); and evidence of increased intracranial pressure (confusion, somnolence, stupor, neurologic deficits, seizures). Patients with hypertensive emergencies may present with stroke, subarachnoid hemorrhage, intracranial hemorrhage, aortic dissection, left ventricular failure, or myocardial ischemia. Importantly, however, severely elevated BP is often discovered coincidentally without any related signs or symptoms.

Evaluation of a patient with hypertensive crisis includes a pertinent history, with a special attempt to elicit symptoms relating to the etiology or consequences of the severely elevated BP. Physical examination includes determination of supine, sitting, and standing BP, neurologic evaluation, funduscopic examination, cardiac auscultation with evaluation of left ventricular size and function, and palpation of distal pulses. Chest radiography, electrocardiography, complete blood cell count with blood smear, and renal chemistries and urinalysis should be performed. If by history, physical examination, or laboratory data the patient has evidence of ongoing (new or worsening) end-organ damage, the patient should be considered to be having a medical emergency.

The goal in treating hypertensive crisis is a prompt but gradual reduction in BP to just above normotensive levels. Precipitous or excessive reductions in BP may impair the body's ability to regulate blood flow, causing end-organ hypoperfusion. Ideally, BP should be reduced to 150 to 160/100 to 110 mm Hg and maintained at that level for a few days. Then, with initiation or reinitiation of long-term therapy, BP levels can slowly be returned to the normotensive range.

Hypertensive urgencies are best treated with oral agents that allow effective titration of BP over a short period of time. Both clonidine and nifedipine are especially well suited to this purpose. Recommended dose schedules for these agents in the setting of hypertensive urgency are listed in Table 44-8. If clonidine loading successfully reduces a patient's BP, chronic clonidine therapy should be initiated. Approximately 80 per cent of the oral loading dose given daily on an every-12-hour schedule generally maintains BP adequately and serves as a good starting point for outpatient dose titration. Patients who respond acutely to nifedipine should be started on long-term calcium channel blocker therapy. All patients presenting with hypertensive urgency and treated with oral therapy should be monitored for at least 6 hours to document persistent BP reduction and should be seen in outpatient follow-up within 1 week.

Patients presenting with hypertensive emergencies require parenteral antihypertensive therapy administered in an intensive care setting. Table 44-8 lists the antihypertensive drugs most commonly used in the management of hypertensive emergencies, with recommended doses and common adverse effects. As above, the goal of therapy is to effect an immediate but gradual decline in BP to approximately 160/100 mm Hg. Most patients presenting with critically elevated BP are volume depleted, and consequently the indiscriminate administration of diuretics may exacerbate their hypertension. All patients presenting with severe hypertension should have supine and standing BP checked, and if they have orthostatic changes in BP, diuretics should be withheld. However, in patients with clinical evidence of volume overload, diuresis is indicated, both to improve left ventricular filling pressure and to reduce BP.

Calhoun DA, Oparil S: Treatment of hypertensive crisis. N Engl J Med 323:1177, 1990. *An up-to-date review of the emergency treatment of hypertension.*

Collins R, Peto R, MacMahon S, et al.: Blood pressure, stroke, and coronary heart disease. Part 2, short-term reductions in blood pressure: Overview of randomised drug trials in their epidemiological context. Lancet 335:827, 1990. *A new meta-analysis of 14 randomized trials of antihypertensive drugs, including 37,000 individuals treated for a mean of 5 years, shows significant treatment-related reduction in stroke and coronary artery disease.*

The Joint National Committee on Detection, Evaluation, and Treatment of High Blood Pressure: The 1988 Report of the Joint National Committee on Detection, Evaluation, and Treatment of High Blood Pressure. Arch Intern Med 148:1023, 1988. *Detailed recommendations for the diagnosis and pharmacologic and nonpharmacologic treatment of systemic hypertension.*

Veterans Administration Cooperative Study Group on Antihypertensive Agents: Effects of treatment on morbidity in hypertension: I. Results in patients with diastolic blood pressures averaging 115 through 129 mm Hg. JAMA 202:1028, 1967. *Demonstration that male hypertensive patients with diastolic blood pressure averaging 115 mm Hg or above represent a high-risk group in which hypertensive therapy exerts a significant beneficial effect.*

Veterans Administration Cooperative Study Group on Antihypertensive Agents: Effects of treatment on morbidity in hypertension: II. Results in patients with diastolic blood pressure averaging 90 through 114 mm Hg. JAMA 213:1143, 1970. *Demonstration that treatment of male patients with mildly elevated blood pressure is more effective in preventing congestive heart failure and stroke than in preventing the complications of coronary artery disease and that the degree of benefit of treatment is related to the level of prerandomization blood pressure.*

Working Group on Management of Patients with Hypertension and High Blood Cholesterol: National education programs working group report on the management of patients with hypertension and high blood cholesterol. Ann Intern Med 114:224, 1991. *Detailed recommendations for the management of patients with hypertension and hypercholesterolemia with or without concomitant atherosclerotic disease.*

45 Pulmonary Hypertension
Alfred P. Fishman

The normal pulmonary circulation is not prone to develop pulmonary hypertension. On the one hand, it is endowed with a large capacity, great distensibility, and low resistance to blood flow; on the other, it contains no baroregulatory mechanisms comparable to those in the systemic circulation that can go awry or overshoot. Amputation of more than half of the normal pulmonary circulation, as by pneumonectomy, or doubling of the pulmonary blood flow through normal lungs, as during exercise, elicits a barely perceptible increase in pulmonary arterial pressure. In contrast, when widespread disease or disturbed ventilation-perfusion relationships increase pulmonary vascular resistance and limit distensibility, modest increments in pulmonary blood flow generally elicit considerable increments in pulmonary arterial pressure.

Definitions

The term "pulmonary hypertension" refers to pulmonary *arterial* hypertension unless otherwise specified. Criteria for pulmonary hypertension depend on the altitude: In the resting individual at sea level, a mean pulmonary arterial pressure greater than 19 to 20 mm Hg establishes the diagnosis; the corresponding limit at altitude is higher—at about 15,000 feet, a mean pulmonary arterial pressure greater than 25 mm Hg signifies pulmonary hypertension.

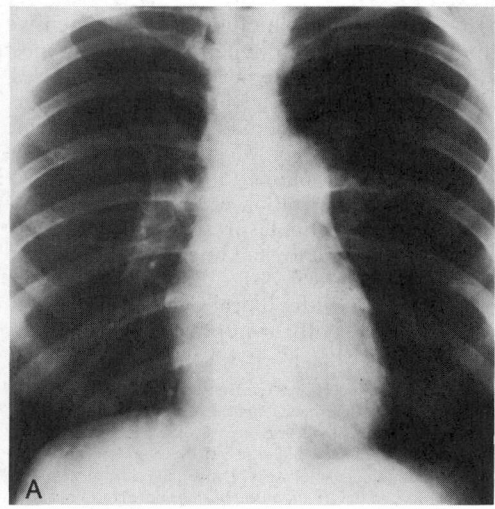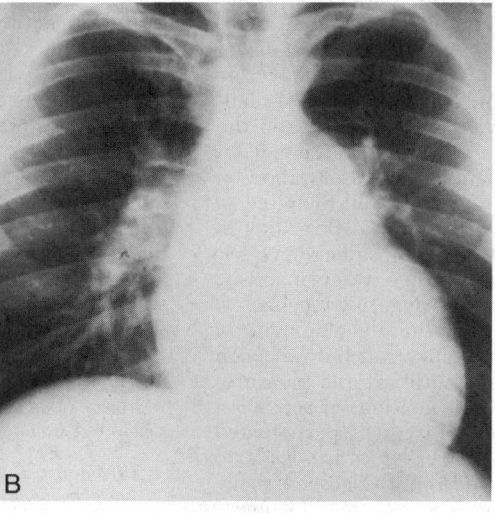

FIGURE 45–1. Pulmonary hypertension, cor pulmonale, and right ventricular failure in two patients with primary pulmonary hypertension. *A*, Pulmonary hypertension and cor pulmonale. *B*, Pulmonary hypertension, cor pulmonale, and right ventricular failure (systemic venous congestion).

Pulmonary *venous* hypertension is a different entity with respect to etiology, pathogenesis, clinical manifestations, and management. It is said to exist when pulmonary venous or left atrial pressure exceeds 12 mm Hg; this limit applies at altitude as well as at sea level. In the normal pulmonary circulation, an acute increase in pulmonary venous pressure to the range of 20 to 30 mm Hg runs the risk of causing pulmonary edema. The sample levels are less threatening when sustained chronically, as in mitral valve disease, presumably because of thickening of alveolar-capillary walls.

Cor pulmonale is a consequence of pulmonary hypertension. It is defined as enlargement of the right ventricle, i.e., hypertrophy, dilatation, or both, as a consequence of disease of the respiratory apparatus. In chronic cor pulmonale resulting from sustained pulmonary hypertension, hypertrophy usually dominates the course of the illness until the later stages when the right ventricle fails; at this juncture, dilatation generally predominates (Fig. 45–1).

THE NORMAL PULMONARY CIRCULATION

In the normal adult, the small muscular arteries and arterioles constitute the "resistance" vessels. In the adult at sea level, these vessels are thin walled and sparsely equipped with muscle; in the fetus and in the native resident at altitude, the muscle is thicker and more extensive.

Hemodynamics

Because of the low resistance and high distensibility of the pulmonary vascular bed and the pulsatile nature of pulmonary blood pressure, the large pulmonary blood flow is accomplished by only a small drop in mean pressure between the pulmonary artery and the left atrium (Table 45–1). The mean pressure difference at rest is ordinarily about 5 to 10 mm Hg.

TABLE 45–1. REPRESENTATIVE VALUES AT REST FOR THE NORMAL PULMONARY CIRCULATION AT SEA LEVEL AND AT ALTITUDE

	Sea Level	14,900 ft
Pulmonary arterial pressure (mm Hg, systolic/diastolic, mean)	20/12, 15	38/14, 25
Cardiac output (liters/min)	6.0	6.0
Cardiac index (liters min/m², body surface area)	3.1	3.1
Left atrial pressure (mm Hg)	5.0	5.0
Pulmonary vascular resistance (R units*)	0.1†	0.2

*R units express calculated resistance in terms of $\frac{mm\ Hg}{ml/sec}$. To convert to C.G.S. units (dynes · sec · cm⁻⁵), the value in R units is multiplied by 1328.

†Based on the data in this table, at sea level, $R = \frac{15-5}{6000/60} = 0.1$ R units.

The normal pulmonary hemodynamics of adults residing at sea level and at altitude are indicated in Table 45–1. Because of the passive nature of the pulmonary vascular bed, the pulmonary arterial pressure—particularly in hypertensive states—must be assessed with respect to the pulmonary blood flow (cardiac output). At the same levels of cardiac output, the pulmonary arterial pressure is consistently higher at altitude than at sea level because of the increase in pulmonary vascular tone elicited by hypoxia.

Calculation of pulmonary vascular resistance (Table 45–1) has become a popular expedient for depicting the state of the pulmonary resistance vessels (small muscular arteries and arterioles) and for inferring whether a change in the tone of these vessels occurs after an intervention, e.g., the administration of a vasodilator agent. However, in pursuing the goal of detecting *active* change, due regard is not always paid to the possible obscuring effects of passive change. Also, for practical reasons—especially in human studies—outflow pressures (left atrium) are often ignored or assumed. In order to minimize shortcomings inherent in applying the resistance formula to a distensible system for which it was not intended, two precautions have proved useful in providing interpretable values for resistance: (1) accurate assessment should be made not only of pulmonary arterial pressure and pulmonary blood flow but also of left atrial (pulmonary wedge) pressure, and (2) if resistances before and after an intervention are to be compared, comparisons should be made at the same level of either the pressure drop across the lungs (the numerator of the resistance equation) or the pulmonary blood flow (the denominator). In this way, passive changes in the pulmonary circulation do not cloud the search for vasomotor activity. Fortunately, the second criterion becomes less stringent in states of severe pulmonary hypertension in which disease has curtailed the extent and distensibility of the pulmonary circulation.

Regulation by Local Chemical Stimuli

It was noted above that the pulmonary circulation is devoid of a baroregulatory apparatus comparable to the carotid sinus apparatus in the systemic circulation. Indeed, local stimuli dominate the control of the pulmonary circulation. Of the local stimuli, hypoxia is the most powerful. Acidosis per se is a fairly weak stimulus, except in reinforcing the pressor effect of hypoxia. Hypercapnia is also a modest pressor agent that acts, presumably, by way of the local acidosis that it generates.

SECONDARY PULMONARY HYPERTENSION

Of the two subsets of pulmonary arterial hypertension, the secondary form (Table 45–2) is by far the more prevalent. As a rule, the clinical manifestations of secondary pulmonary hypertension are dominated by signs and symptoms of the underlying disease, generally cardiac or respiratory. Pulmonary hypertension of mild to moderate degree, as in normal native residents at high altitude, is generally asymptomatic for a lifetime. In contrast,

TABLE 45–2. CLASSIFICATION OF CHRONIC PULMONARY (ARTERIAL) HYPERTENSION

Secondary
  Cardiac disease
    Acquired disorders of the left side of the heart causing
      pulmonary venous hypertension
      Left ventricular failure
      Mitral valve disease
      Left atrial myxoma
      Decrease in left ventricular compliance
    Congenital heart disease
      Pre-tricuspid
      Post-tricuspid
  Respiratory diseases
    Obstructive airways disease
    Diseases of the lung parenchyma
      Alveolar
      Interstitial
    Pulmonary vascular disease
      Collagen vascular disease
      Thromboembolic disease
    Neuromuscular disorders
      Abnormal chest bellows
      Disordered respiratory control mechanisms
Primary pulmonary (arterial) hypertension
Pulmonary veno-occlusive disease

severe pulmonary hypertension, as occurs in chronic mountain sickness or in primary pulmonary hypertension, can be accompanied by evidences of right heart failure and a tendency to easy fatiguability, syncope, arrhythmias (especially in hypoxic states), and sudden death.

The most common causes of pulmonary (arterial) hypertension are heart disease and lung disease (Table 45–2). Regardless of the root cause of the pulmonary arterial hypertension, sooner or later the resistance (precapillary) vessels of the lungs undergo anatomic change that contributes to the pulmonary hypertension. However, the initiating mechanisms are generally dissimilar in heart disease and lung disease: As a rule, pulmonary arterial hypertension secondary to acquired heart disease begins with a disorder of the left ventricle that leads to pulmonary venous hypertension followed by pulmonary arterial hypertension; rarely does an increase in pulmonary blood flow per se cause pulmonary hypertension. In contrast, an increase in pulmonary blood flow not infrequently triggers pulmonary arterial hypertension in congenital heart disease and, as during exercise, aggravates preexisting pulmonary hypertension in both acquired and congenital heart disease.

Cardiac Disease

Acquired disorders of the left side of the heart and certain types of congenital heart disease often lead to pulmonary hypertension.

ACQUIRED DISORDERS. Left ventricular failure is the predominant cause of pulmonary hypertension and of right ventricular failure. Myocardial disorders and lesions of the mitral and aortic valves are the most common left ventricular disorders leading to pulmonary hypertension. Left ventricular disorders increase pulmonary venous pressure, which, in turn, evokes an increase in pulmonary arterial pressure that suffices to maintain antegrade flow; this automatic adjustment is presumably reflex. But, in time, three types of morphologic changes appear as a consequence of the pulmonary venous hypertension: (1) occlusive intimal and medial changes in pulmonary precapillary vessels as well as in pulmonary venules and veins; (2) perivascular interstitial edema, which not only contributes directly to the increase in resistance to blood flow but also stimulates perivascular fibrosis; under the influence of gravity, the vascular and perivascular changes are most marked in the dependent portions of the lungs; and (3) occlusion of small pulmonary vessels by emboli or thrombi; especially in states of slowed systemic blood flow, emboli are much more apt to arise from thrombi in the veins of the extremities than from the right side of the heart. Depending on the reversibility of the vascular and perivascular lesions, relief of the pulmonary venous hypertension, as by mitral valve commissurotomy or replacement for mitral valvular disease, generally reduces the pulmonary arterial pressure.

CONGENITAL HEART DISEASE. Congenital defects that produce left to right shunting of blood within the heart or between the great vessels are commonly associated with pulmonary arterial hypertension. As a rule, this shunting interferes with the normal transition from the thick-walled fetal pulmonary circulation to the thin-walled adult state. Moreover, arterial hypoxemia is often part of the congenital heart syndrome. The net effect of the interplay between the hemodynamic abnormalities, arterial hypoxemia, and the persistent fetal pulmonary circulation is to promote intimal proliferation and medial hypertrophy, which, in time, may dominate in sustaining the pulmonary hypertension and in determining its reversibility. Heart-lung transplantation has been used in small series of patients with Eisenmenger's complex. The results to date have been encouraging, i.e., about 50 per cent alive at 4 years. Deaths were due primarily to infection and, in a few instances, to bronchiolitis obliterans and cerebral embolism.

Respiratory Disease

Failure of any major component of the respiratory apparatus can lead to pulmonary hypertension. For convenience, the components can be sorted into the airways, lung parenchyma, chest bellows, and respiratory control mechanisms. In turn, pulmonary hypertension often taxes the right heart to the point of enlargement (cor pulmonale) by way of dilatation and hypertrophy.

OBSTRUCTIVE AIRWAYS DISEASE. Chronic bronchitis and emphysema (chronic obstructive lung disease, or COPD) is the most common cause of pulmonary hypertension and cor pulmonale. Even though chronic bronchitis and emphysema generally coexist, the chronic bronchitis is predominantly responsible for the alveolar hypoxia and the low Po_2, high Pco_2, and resultant low pH that lead to pulmonary hypertension. In patients with obstructive airways disease, "blue bloaters" are chronically hypoxemic and pulmonary hypertensive whereas "pink puffers" develop transient pulmonary hypertension in the course of an acute respiratory infection that leads to arterial hypoxemia. A key clinical sign of pulmonary hypertension is right ventricular enlargement (cor pulmonale). However, right ventricular enlargement may be difficult to prove in a particular patient with obstructive airways disease until right ventricular failure supervenes. The onset of right ventricular failure is often heralded by striking cyanosis, unexplained drowsiness, inappropriate behavior, systemic venous congestion, and hepatomegaly. Right ventricular gallops (S_3 and S_4) are generally present, and the murmur of tricuspid insufficiency can often be elicited. Arterial blood gas analysis reveals that the Po_2 is low ($Po_2 < 40$ to 50 torr), the Pco_2 is high ($Pco_2 > 50$ torr), and respiratory acidosis is present.

Electrocardiographic evidence of right ventricular enlargement is often equivocal in patients with bronchitis and emphysema because of rotation and displacement of the heart, widened distances between electrodes and the cardiac surface, and acute cardiac dilatation. As a rule, consecutive changes in the electrocardiogram are more useful than a single electrocardiogram in detecting that the right ventricle has been overloaded acutely by pulmonary hypertension: T waves in the right precordial leads (V_1 to V_3) flatten and become inverted, the mean electrical axis of the QRS complex shifts to the right, ST segments become depressed in leads II, III, and aV_F, and right bundle branch block (generally incomplete) often appears; these changes reverse as arterial hypoxemia is relieved and pulmonary blood pressures decrease.

Echocardiography is widely used as a noninvasive approach to estimating pulmonary arterial pressure. Three separate techniques are available: M-mode for determining right ventricular and atrial dimensions, two-dimensional for analysis of the motions of the right ventricular, atrial, and septal walls and of the pulmonic and tricuspid valves, and Doppler (pulse wave, continuous wave, and color flow imaging) for determining velocities of blood flow across the pulmonic and tricuspid valves. In practice, these techniques are generally applied as a package. They are costly, complex, and often inaccurate, except when pulmonary hypertension is severe enough to cause considerable tricuspid insufficiency. Consequently, cardiac catheterization is usually resorted to soon after pulmonary hypertension is suspected, with two goals in mind: (1) to determine directly the pulmonary arterial and wedge pressures and the cardiac output for the calculation of pulmonary vascular resistance; and (2) if pulmonary hypertension does exist, to assess the contribution of congenital and acquired cardiac lesions to its pathogenesis. Echocardiography can be useful in following the course of pulmonary hypertension and cor pulmonale, and the effects of pulmonary vasodilators, if it is performed serially, before and after cardiac catheterization.

Treatment of the patient with obstructive airways disease in whom pulmonary hypertension either develops or intensifies because of a bout of bronchitis or pneumonia is directed at maintaining tolerable levels of arterial oxygenation (e.g., arterial $Po_2 > 50$ mm Hg) while treating the upper respiratory infection. Because of persistent arterial hypoxemia, continuing oxygen administration may be necessary even after maximal recovery from the upper respiratory infection. This need is often met by delivering oxygen at low flow rates via a nasal cannula. It has been shown that continued, prolonged oxygen therapy can slow the progression of pulmonary hypertension and its sequelae. Pulmonary vasodilators have little role in treating pulmonary hypertension associated with obstructive airways disease if oxygen and antibiotic therapy are properly administered.

Heart-lung transplantation has been successfully applied to patients with obstructive airways disease, notably cystic fibrosis. Lung transplantation is also being tested for patients with intractable, end-stage bronchitis and emphysema (COPD), as well as for widespread pulmonary fibrosis and primary pulmonary hypertension (see below).

DISEASES OF THE LUNG PARENCHYMA. These diseases may be further subdivided into alveolar, interstitial, and vascular.

Alveolar. Pulmonary hypertension is a frequent concomitant of alveolar disorders, such as pulmonary edema and the respiratory distress syndromes. In the respiratory distress syndromes, pulmonary hypertension is quite common, occasionally in conjunction with pulmonary venous hypertension secondary to fluid overload but more often as a consequence of mechanical influences exerted by pulmonary edema and atelectasis operating in conjunction with respiratory acidosis. This concomitant disorder requires no special treatment, since it follows the course of the illness, decreasing spontaneously as the patient recovers. The pathogenesis and management of these disorders are considered elsewhere.

Interstitial. A wide variety of inflammatory processes, such as sarcoidosis, asbestosis, and "idiopathic fibrosing alveolitis," can affect the interstitium of the lungs. Early on, the major consequence is a diffusion defect in association with a restrictive ventilatory defect that is characterized by concentric reduction in lung volumes and a low diffusing capacity without evidence of airways obstruction. In time, ventilation-perfusion balances become upset and arterial hypoxemia intensifies as fibrosis progresses. At this juncture, the initial hypocapnia resulting from the reflex stimulation of intrapulmonary receptors is succeeded by eucapnia and then hypercapnia. The small muscular arteries and arterioles are caught up in the inflammatory process, and pulmonary hypertension gradually sets in as a consequence of increasing pulmonary vascular resistance due to mechanical vascular obstruction and arterial hypoxemia. The stage is then set for cor pulmonale and right heart failure.

Supplemental oxygen, especially during exercise and sleep, helps to minimize the hypoxic contribution to the pulmonary hypertension. Corticosteroids are the mainstay of therapy but are apt to be least effective when marked fibrosis and pulmonary distortion, reflected in honeycombing, dominate the condition. Lung transplantation, primarily of a single lung, has been used as a last resort in patients with widespread pulmonary fibrosis. The results reported from a few clinics in this country and abroad have been gratifying, but long-term observations are not yet available.

DISEASES OF THE PULMONARY VESSELS. In this category, the most common cause of pulmonary hypertension is thromboembolic disease. At the opposite extreme is obliterative capillary disorder of unknown etiology known as "pulmonary capillary angiomatosis." Among the more uncommon disorders is primary pulmonary hypertension (see below), which has attracted considerable attention because of its implications for the diagnosis

and treatment of other types of pulmonary hypertension. Between these extremes of incidence is a variety of pulmonary vascular diseases that cause pulmonary hypertension as part of systemic disorders, e.g., scleroderma, lupus erythematosus. The latter are often included in the category of interstitial lung disease because the interstitium as well as the vessels is often directly affected by the inflammatory process.

Collagen Vascular Disease. The incidence of pulmonary hypertension and right heart failure in systemic lupus erythematosus (SLE) is high (Fig. 45–2). The incidence of this complication of SLE is much higher in females than in males. Raynaud's phenomenon is a common occurrence in women with SLE who develop pulmonary hypertension. As a rule, the parenchyma of the lungs as well as the pulmonary blood vessels is involved in the inflammatory process leading to pulmonary hypertension.

On rare occasions, scleroderma of the lungs may affect only the microvasculature. Much more usual for progressive systemic sclerosis (scleroderma) and its variants (CREST and overlap syndromes) is for pulmonary hypertension to be a consequence of combined interstitial and vascular disease. Pulmonary hypertension is quite common in patients with progressive systemic sclerosis or the CREST syndrome but is often overlooked until manifestations of heart failure ensue.

Thromboembolic Disease. Pulmonary hypertension and cor pulmonale can occur acutely or chronically as a result of pulmonary thromboembolic disease. The acute form is caused by massive obstruction of major pulmonary arteries that generally leads to death unless the large clots either attenuate spontaneously or by thrombolytic agents or heroic surgery. Chronic pulmonary thromboembolic disease is a much more prevalent and manageable problem.

Three categories of pulmonary thromboembolic disease leading to chronic pulmonary hypertension can be identified depending on the size of the affected pulmonary arteries. This classification is useful as long as it is recognized that some degree of overlap among categories is almost inevitable. It should also be kept in mind that most instances of nonfatal pulmonary thromboembolism—a common clinical occurrence—are not associated with pulmonary hypertension because of the localized nature of the one or more embolic lesions.

Chronic pulmonary thromboembolism accompanied by pulmonary hypertension is manifested by dyspnea on exertion, easy fatiguability, and occasionally angina-like pain in the chest. Three different syndromes have been identified according to the pulmonary vessels primarily affected.

Small Pulmonary Arteries and Arterioles (Resistance Vessels). This rare syndrome can be indistinguishable in onset and progression from that of primary pulmonary hypertension (Fig. 45–3A). Indeed, not long ago, textbooks referred to it as a syndrome of "multiple pulmonary emboli." However, it now seems likely that the syndrome is caused by widespread in situ thrombi in the distal arterial tree rather than by emboli. The etiology of the widespread in situ thrombosis is speculative.

Neither angiography nor ventilation-perfusion scans are capable of identifying microvascular thrombosis as the cause of the pulmonary hypertension, but scans can exclude thromboembolic disease of larger proximal arteries. Biopsy or autopsy reveals the thrombotic nature of the occlusive vascular disease.

Treatment generally consists of long-term anticoagulation using warfarin-type agents and/or antiplatelet agents. Since the microvascular clots are organized, this antithrombotic therapy probably does more to prevent the formation of new clots than to treat the existing clots. In principle, vasodilator therapy holds as much promise in this disorder (which mimics primary pulmonary hypertension) as it does in primary pulmonary hypertension per se. However, no trials of this hypothesis are as yet available.

Intermediate Pulmonary Arteries. Moderate-sized emboli may lodge in intermediate arteries directly or after fragmentation or lysis of larger clots in major vessels. These lesions are demonstrable both by ventilation-perfusion scans and by angiography.

Once chronic pulmonary hypertension is established in patients with this type of pulmonary vascular occlusive disease, it is generally irreversible except when associated with large organized proximal clots that can be removed surgically (see next section). Attention is therefore directed at preventive measures, particularly at eliminating sources of emboli. Symptomatic relief of breathlessness, enhanced cerebration, and relief of arterial hy-

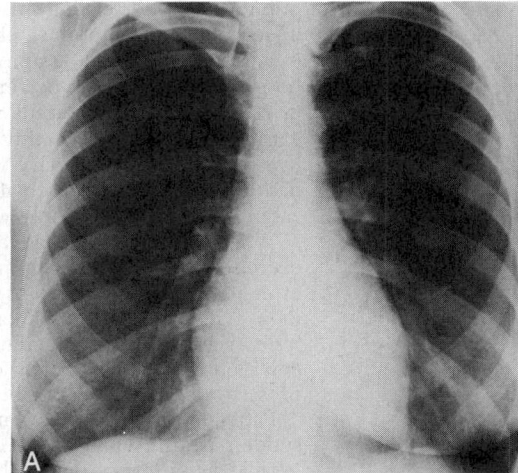
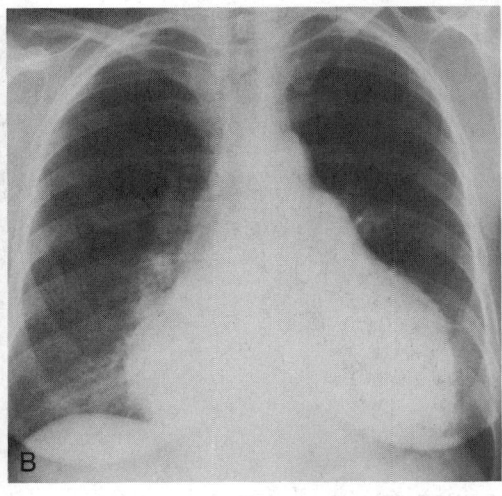

FIGURE 45–2. Pulmonary hypertension in a young woman with systemic lupus erythematosus. *A,* 1974. Pulmonary hypertension and cor pulmonale. *B,* 1981. Cor pulmonale and right ventricular failure.

poxemia can be accomplished by supplemental oxygen. Anticoagulation and/or antiplatelet therapy is routine, as described elsewhere for thromboembolic disease.

Major Pulmonary Arteries. This syndrome results from one or more large clots of long standing in the proximal pulmonary arterial tree which have been incorporated into the vessel wall and cause obstruction and pulmonary hypertension. The clot presumably originates as a large undetected embolus to the lungs. Propagation of the clot proximally and distally, followed by organization, culminates in severe pulmonary hypertension due to obstruction to pulmonary blood flow by poorly compliant proximal pulmonary vessels (Fig. 45–3*B*).

This disorder is amenable to surgery. All patients with unexplained (primary) pulmonary hypertension should be given ventilation-perfusion scans to exclude this possibility. A perfusion defect that is segmental or larger calls for selective pulmonary angiography to localize the site of the organized clot and its proximal extent.

Surgical treatment consists of thromboendarterectomy. It is indicated when clot in the proximal pulmonary arterial tree persists after prolonged anticoagulation, i.e., warfarin sodium for more than 6 months. Presurgical delineation of the extent and boundaries of the obstructive vascular lesions can be helped by combining angiography with magnetic resonance imaging and/or fiberoptic angioscopy. Surgery is formidable, entailing cardiopulmonary bypass during hypothermia punctuated by periods of circulatory arrest. Successful surgery is often followed by a bout of pulmonary edema confined to the large area of lung that was hypoperfused preoperatively. However, successful surgery is gratifying: It is followed by dramatic relief of the pulmonary hypertension and alleviation of symptoms. Lifetime anticoagulation using warfarin sodium is instituted after the surgical procedure.

NEUROMUSCULAR DISORDERS. Disorders of respiratory control mechanisms, of the chest bellows, or of a combination of the two can cause hypertension in lungs that are normal or nearly normal. These disorders, of diverse etiologies that range from kyphoscoliosis to poliomyelitis, have alveolar hypoventilation as the common denominator. Just as in the case of obstructive airways disease, the pulmonary hypertension is associated with alveolar hypoxia and arterial hypoxemia, hypercapnia, and respiratory acidosis. Because of the predominant role of alveolar hypoxia in the syndrome of alveolar hypoventilation, patients are often initially seen because of right heart failure. However, in contrast to obstructive airways disease, the abnormal alveolar and arterial blood gases are due to *global* alveolar hypoventilation rather than to ventilation-perfusion abnormalities; e.g., the alveolar-arterial P_{O_2} gradient is normal or nearly normal in the syndrome of alveolar hypoventilation, whereas it is characteristically large in obstructive airways disease.

Chest Bellows. This category includes skeletal deformity of the chest as well as muscular disorders and extreme obesity (Fig. 45–4). Severe kyphoscoliosis accompanied by dwarfing of the thorax is the prototype of chest deformities that can lead to alveolar hypoventilation. Mutilating operations on the thorax can have the same effect. The predominan mechanism is an inordinate increase in the work of breathing.

Respiratory Control Mechanisms. The Guillain-Barré syndrome or a stroke can impair the central drive to breathe sufficiently to cause alveolar hypoventilation. As indicated elsewhere, certain of the sleep apnea syndromes are also associated with alveolar hypoventilation.

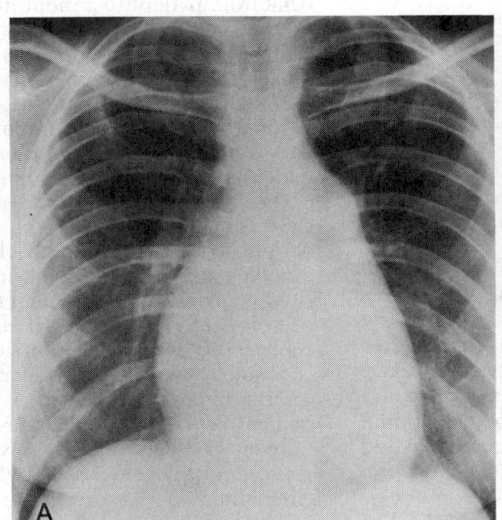
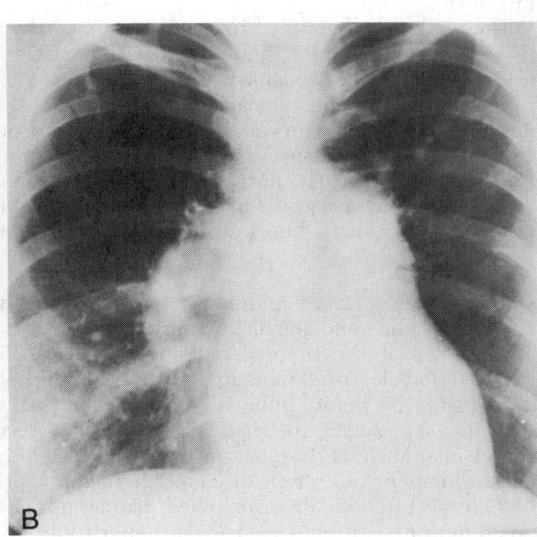

FIGURE 45–3. Pulmonary hypertension due to thromboembolic disease. *A,* A 33-year-old woman with clinical diagnosis of primary pulmonary hypertension. Autopsy showed widespread organized clots in resistance vessels (small muscular arteries and arterioles) throughout the lungs. *B,* A 35-year-old woman with organized clots in major pulmonary arteries. Note hypoperfused upper lobes. Thromboendarterectomy restored blood flow to the right upper lobe and relieved the pulmonary hypertension.

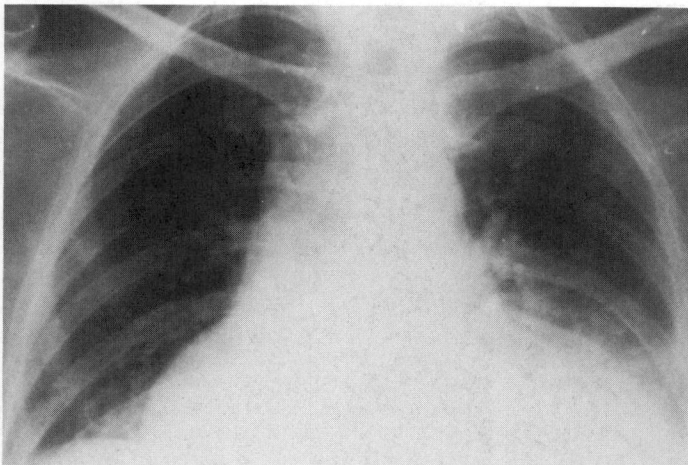

FIGURE 45–4. Cor pulmonale and severe right ventricular failure in global alveolar hypoventilation due to extreme obesity.

Chest Bellows and Respiratory Control Mechanisms. These are the true neuromuscular disorders, as exemplified by central nervous system and paralytic poliomyelitis. In these disorders, both the ventilatory drive and the respiratory muscles per se are directly affected. Alveolar hypoventilation may become manifested years after the acute infection as the ventilation finally fails to keep pace with the metabolic demand, e.g., during stress, fever, or further respiratory infection.

The treatment of alveolar hypoventilation in patients with normal lungs is ideally one of restoring ventilation toward normal or at least improving oxygenation. The practicality of these goals depends on the etiology. In kyphoscoliosis and the muscular dystrophies, ventilation can be supported at night, thereby resting the respiratory muscles, using a body cuirass. This approach is generally less feasible in extreme obesity, in which right ventricular failure that begins with alveolar hypoxia and pulmonary hypertension is accompanied by left ventricular failure due to systemic causes. When assisted ventilation is impractical, supplemental oxygen is useful in minimizing arterial hypoxemia.

PRIMARY PULMONARY HYPERTENSION

Primary pulmonary hypertension is a synonym for "unexplained" pulmonary *arterial* hypertension. The diagnosis is made by exclusion. It is an uncommon disorder that accounts for about 1 per cent of all causes of cor pulmonale encountered at autopsy. Until recently, virtually all reports of primary pulmonary hypertension dealt with sporadic cases. During the past few years, about 25 families have been identified in which the disease seems to be hereditary. Whether more painstaking family histories would show that some sporadic cases are actually familial is unknown.

The clinical hallmarks of primary pulmonary hypertension are (1) clinical, radiographic, and electrocardiographic manifestations of pulmonary hypertension; (2) demonstration by right-heart catheterization of the typical hemodynamic constellation of abnormally high pulmonary arterial pressures and pulmonary vascular resistance in association with a normal pulmonary wedge pressure and a nearly normal or low cardiac output; and (3) inability to find a cause for the pulmonary hypertension in a disorder of the heart, lungs, or systemic circulation.

Clinical Picture

Instances of primary pulmonary hypertension have been reported in males and females of virtually all ages, although the average age at the time of diagnosis is 30 to 36 years. After puberty, females predominate, most strikingly between 10 and 40 years of age. Before puberty, no sex differential is discernible.

In its early stages, the disease is difficult to recognize. Initial complaints, such as dyspnea on exertion, easy fatigability, and chest discomfort are often discounted. In the sporadic case, the first clue is often an abnormal chest radiograph or electrocardiograph indicative of right ventricular hypertrophy (Fig. 45–5). But

these are late manifestations. In many clinics, echocardiography (all three modes) is used to buttress the clinical suspicion of pulmonary hypertension raised by the combination of otherwise unaccountable symptoms, physical examination, chest radiography, and electrocardiography. Echocardiography serves no purpose if pulmonary hypertension 'can be excluded on clinical grounds. Nor is it helpful in blatant pulmonary hypertension except for following noninvasively the response of pulmonary hypertension to pulmonary vasodilator therapy. Direct determination of pulmonary circulatory pressures by cardiac catheterization is currently the only way to prove the diagnosis.

When the disease is advanced, dyspnea, particularly during exercise, is common. Many patients are tachypneic and complain of nondescript chest pain as well as breathlessness. Other common symptoms are weakness, fatigue, and effort syncope. In time, right-sided heart failure develops. On rare occasion, an enlarged pulmonary artery causes hoarseness because of compression of the left recurrent laryngeal nerve.

Patients with severe pulmonary hypertension seem prone to sudden death. Thus, death has occurred unexpectedly during normal activities, cardiac catheterization, and surgical procedures and after the administration of barbiturates or anesthetic agents. The mechanisms for sudden death are not clear, although in a few instances bradycardia and atrioventricular dissociation were seen to culminate in cardiac arrest and death.

On physical examination, the jugular venous pulse usually shows a prominent "a" wave. Right ventricular hypertrophy causes a cardiac thrust along the left sternal border, and a distinct impulse is typically palpable over the region of the main pulmonary artery. The pulmonic component of the second sound is markedly accentuated, the second heart sound is narrowly split, and an ejection click is heard in the pulmonic area. Often a fourth heart sound emanating from the hypertrophied left ventricle is heard at the lower left sternal border. In some patients an ejection murmur is audible at the pulmonic area; as pulmonary arterial pressures approximate systemic arterial levels, the murmur of pulmonary valvular insufficiency (Graham-Steell) often appears.

Right ventricular failure is accompanied by jugular venous distention and an RV gallop (S_3); inspiration intensifies the gallop. The liver becomes enlarged and tender and hepatojugular reflux can be elicited; in time dilation of the failing right ventricle leads to tricuspid insufficiency manifested by a holosystolic murmur, best heard in the fourth interspace to the left of the sternum, which increases in intensity during inspiration. The liver develops expansile pulsations synchronous with the heart beat. Hydrothorax and ascites are uncommon even in the face of hepatomegaly and peripheral edema.

RADIOGRAPHY. In the early stage, the chest radiograph is generally normal. Later it shows cardiac enlargement in association with enlargement of the pulmonary trunk, while the peripheral pulmonary arterial branches are attenuated; the lung fields are free of widespread interstitial disease and may appear oligemic. Although fullness of the central pulmonary arterial trunks and peripheral "pruning" are distinctive, appearances vary somewhat from patient to patient in accord with the level and duration of the pulmonary hypertension and the age of the patient. Radiographic evidence of right ventricular enlargement (cor pulmonale) usually becomes overt only late in the course of the pulmonary hypertension (see Fig. 45–1).

Lung scans and angiography help to exclude multiple pulmonary emboli. Rarely do these procedures prove to be more enlightening than the standard chest radiograph.

Other Laboratory Tests. The electrocardiogram almost always shows some evidence of right ventricular enlargement and usually of right atrial enlargement. Echocardiography, as indicated above, can then provide additional information about the nature of the right ventricular enlargement (hypertrophy and/or dilatation), the presence of right-sided valvular insufficiencies, and myocardial contractility. Pulmonary function tests are generally normal except for a low diffusing capacity, often in association with mild arterial hypoxemia at rest. A high incidence of antinuclear antibodies has recently been described in patients with "primary" pulmonary hypertension, raising the possibility that some may represent collagen vascular disease confined to the pulmonary circulation.

The results of cardiac catheterization are consistent with diffuse

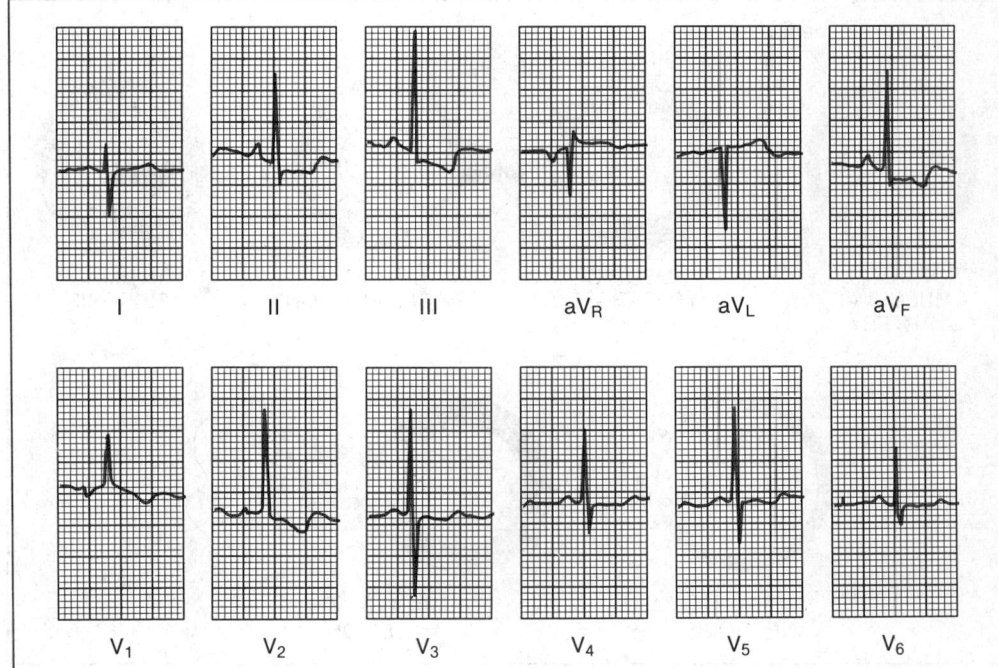

FIGURE 45–5. Unsuspected primary pulmonary hypertension. Routine electrocardiogram in an asymptomatic 32-year-old man was the first clue to the presence of primary pulmonary hypertension.

obliterative disease of the pulmonary precapillary vessels: Pulmonary arterial hypertension is associated with a normal pulmonary wedge pressure and a normal, or nearly normal, cardiac output (see Pathophysiology). Cardiac catheterization is most valuable in excluding cardiac causes of pulmonary arterial hypertension and in screening the response of the pulmonary circulation to vasodilator agents.

Pathology

With respect to corroborating the clinical diagnosis, pathology is generally most helpful in two respects: (1) excluding secondary pulmonary hypertension, and (2) demonstrating occlusive vascular disease of the small pulmonary (muscular) arteries and arterioles. For a long while, pathologists touted the "plexiform" lesion as pathognomonic of primary pulmonary hypertension. However, biopsy and autopsy have shown that the vascular lesions of primary pulmonary hypertension are quite heterogeneous (Fig. 45–6) and that plexiform lesions can also occur in instances of secondary pulmonary hypertension, e.g., Eisenmenger's complex. The heterogeneity of the pulmonary vascular lesions in primary pulmonary hypertension has been underscored by recent experience with the familial form of the disease. As things stand now, primary pulmonary hypertension seems to be the final common pathway for diverse unknown etiologies (Table 45–3), and plexiform lesions probably represent a healed pulmonary arteritis that occurred sometime in the evolution of the occlusive vascular disease.

The seat of the disease is the small pulmonary arteries (between 40 and 100 μ in diameter) and arterioles. The obliterative lesions are diverse, affecting one or more layers of the small muscular arteries and arterioles. The full-blown "classic" picture of concentric intimal fibrosis, medial hypertrophy, necrotizing arteritis, and plexiform lesions is common, but often one or more ingredients are missing. Thrombi are commonly found at autopsy in primary pulmonary hypertension but are generally assigned a subsidiary role in pathogenesis, i.e., preterminal slowing of the circulation in damaged, partially obstructed vessels, rather than a primary role.

Pulmonary capillary angiomatosis is an extraordinary cause of primary pulmonary hypertension. Proliferative lesions of the pulmonary capillary bed lead to high resistance to blood flow in a segment of the pulmonary circulation that is generally unaffected in more conventional types of primary pulmonary hypertension.

TABLE 45–3. SUGGESTED ETIOLOGIES FOR PRIMARY PULMONARY HYPERTENSION

Etiology	Comment
Autoimmune mechanisms	Especially in young women, associated with Raynaud's phenomenon and collagen diseases, such as disseminated lupus erythematosus, rheumatoid arthritis, progressive systemic sclerosis, polyarteritis nodosa, and dermatomyositis.
Persistence of fetal pulmonary vascular bed	A distinct syndrome in neonatal life that is questionably related to the adult syndrome.
Dietary pulmonary hypertension	Suggested by an outbreak of primary pulmonary hypertension related to an anorectic agent, aminorex. Only 2% of those who ingested the drug developed pulmonary hypertension, suggesting individual predisposition. Pulmonary hypertension (with different vascular lesions) also produced experimentally by ingesting seeds of leguminous plant *Crotalaria spectabilis*.
Sustained vasoconstriction	A classic suggestion that is difficult to accept as initiating mechanism; more likely a contributing factor.
Combined portal and pulmonary hypertension	Common denominator suggested by occurrence of pulmonary hypertension in some patients with hepatic cirrhosis. Also related to mechanism of dietary pulmonary hypertension.
Multiple pulmonary emboli	Once considered to be the major cause of primary pulmonary hypertension. May still be difficult to distinguish on clinical grounds but can almost always be distinguished morphologically.
Familial pulmonary hypertension	Although familial instances do occur, and individual susceptibility has been demonstrated in some instances, the connecting links between inherited defect or predisposition and clinical disease are unclear.

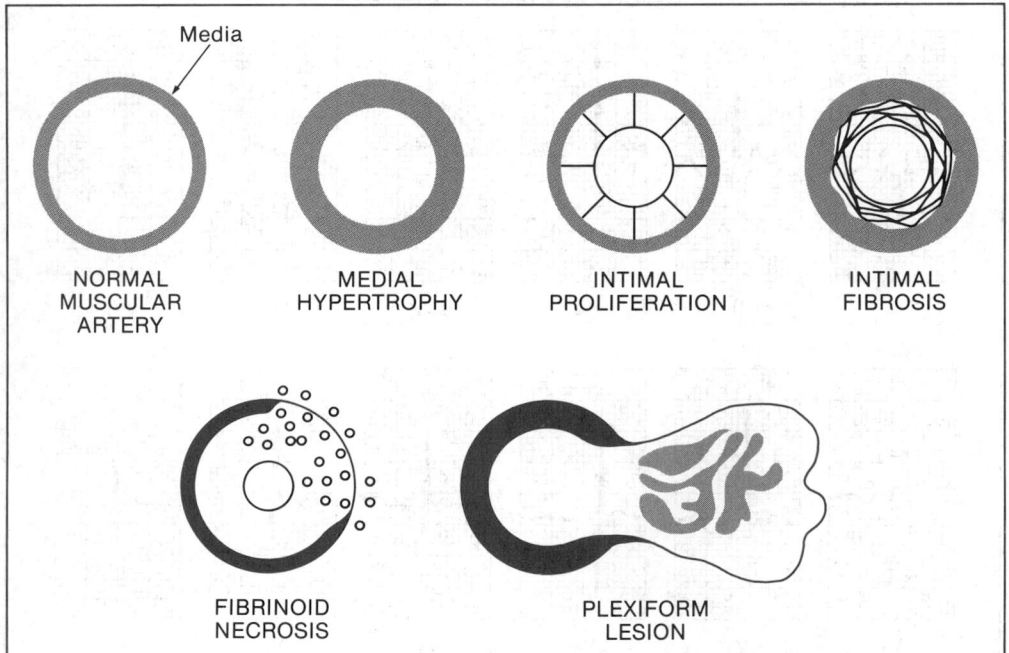

FIGURE 45–6. The heterogeneity of pulmonary vascular lesions in primary pulmonary hypertension. (Modified after Wagenvoort CN, Wagenvoort N: Pathology of Pulmonary Hypertension. Copyright © 1977. By permission of John Wiley & Sons, Inc.)

Pathophysiology

The hemodynamic hallmarks of primary pulmonary hypertension studies at rest are well known: a high pulmonary arterial pressure in association with a nearly normal cardiac output and a normal left atrial (pulmonary wedge) pressure. As a result of this constellation, calculated pulmonary vascular resistance is high, generally leading to the logical conclusion that the resistance vessels, i.e., the small muscular arteries and arterioles, are the predominant sites of vascular obstruction. During exercise, as cardiac output increases, pulmonary arterial pressures increase; the increments in pressure in the pulmonary hypertensive circuit are generally much more striking than in the normotensive pulmonary circulation.

Diagnosis

The diagnosis of primary pulmonary hypertension rests on two pillars: (1) the detection of pulmonary hypertension, and (2) exclusion of known causes of high pulmonary arterial pressure. The history is of utmost importance. For example, the occurrence of Raynaud's syndrome directs attention to the possibility of disseminated sclerosis (scleroderma). Pulmonary function tests are useful in excluding diffuse pulmonary disorders, particularly interstitial fibrosis and granuloma. Serologic testing, especially in young women, may direct attention to covert connective tissue disorders, such as lupus erythematosus. The value of cardiac catheterization in eliminating acquired or congenital heart disease has been indicated above. Even after these procedures, distinction is often not possible, particularly between primary pulmonary hypertension and pulmonary arterial hypertension secondary to pulmonary emboli. This distinction has recently come into prominence because of the increasing awareness that proximal pulmonary organized clots, i.e., in major pulmonary arteries, can be removed surgically. Evidence, as by angiography, of more recent pulmonary emboli calls for anticoagulant therapy. Finally, once the diagnosis of primary pulmonary hypertension is established, the use of vasodilators has to be weighed.

Treatment

The aim of treatment in primary pulmonary hypertension is to decrease pulmonary arterial pressure, preferably in conjunction with an increase in cardiac output. By this combination, the afterload on the right ventricle decreases and organ blood flow improves. In recent years, attempts have been made to identify pulmonary vasodilators that, by decreasing pulmonary vascular resistance, provide symptomatic relief and prolong life.

THE NATIONAL REGISTRY. To help in pursuing this goal, the National Heart, Lung, and Blood Institute has established a national registry by which experiences with the disease and with the use of pharmacologic agents can be shared. To date, about 194 patients have satisfied the criteria for inclusion in the registry and 102 have died (Dr. Carol Vreim, personal communication). Although the data have not yet been thoroughly analyzed, enough information is already on hand to underscore the difficulties in evaluating therapy: (1) The natural history of primary pulmonary hypertension is inconsistent, probably in keeping with the diverse etiologies that can elicit pulmonary hypertension. (2) Instances are being reported of long-term survival without vasodilator therapy. (3) Unless documented by morphologic studies, i.e., lung biopsy or autopsy, secondary pulmonary hypertension—notably pulmonary emboli and less often vasculitis—can masquerade clinically as primary pulmonary hypertension. (4) All vasodilators, except those destroyed during a single pulmonary circulatory transit (currently acetylcholine and prostacyclin), cannot be administered so that they act solely on the pulmonary circulation; as a corollary, all run the risk of troublesome side effects on the heart and systemic circulation. (5) For both acute and chronic administration, optimal therapeutic doses are difficult to establish. (6) Criteria for efficacy in acute studies are inconsistent; many rely almost entirely on a drop in calculated pulmonary vascular resistance even though pulmonary arterial pressure usually remains unchanged and the work of the right ventricle increases. (7) Symptomatic improvement after the acute administration of a presumed pulmonary vasodilator is most closely related to an increase in cardiac output. (8) The acute response to a pulmonary vasodilator is not a reliable predictor of the chronic response. Because of these reservations, optimism for the use of pulmonary vasodilators in primary pulmonary hypertension remains cautious. The ideal would still be prevention (as in thromboembolic disease) or treatment according to etiology (e.g., corticosteroids for interstitial granulomas due to sarcoidosis).

PULMONARY VASODILATORS. Most protocols designed to test pulmonary vasodilators acutely currently center on the response to rest and exercise. Several clinical and hemodynamic changes are sought as desirable endpoints:

1. Improvement in exercise tolerance. This increase in physical capacity is usually accompanied by an increase in cardiac output and presumably improved distribution of blood flow to peripheral organs and tissues.

2. A decrease in the level of pulmonary arterial hypertension, both at rest and during exercise.

3. A decrease in calculated pulmonary vascular resistance. Although this goal is often attained in acute experiments, its

TABLE 45–4. SOME VASODILATOR DRUGS CURRENTLY USED IN THE MANAGEMENT OF PRIMARY PULMONARY HYPERTENSION*

	Mechanism of Action	Acute Testing	Usual Maintenance Therapy	Major Side Effects; Comments
Nitroprusside	Directly on vascular smooth muscle; relaxes both systemic arteries and veins.	10 µg/min IV, increasing by 10 µg/min every 4 min until systemic systolic < 95 torr or PA† systolic > 10 torr over control (max 60 µg/min).	Hydralazine 10 mg every 6 h, increasing up to 50 mg every 6 h, + isosorbide dinitrate 10 mg every 6 h, increasing up to 50 mg every 6 h.	Systemic vasodilation and hypotension, cyanide toxicity at high concentrations. Half-life of a few minutes.
Hydralazine	Directly on vascular smooth muscle, presumably via prostacyclin production; greater dilator effect on arterioles than on veins; myocardial stimulant.	10 mg IV repeated once after 10 min. Resting hemodynamics followed by exercise 20 min later.	Hydralazine, start with 10 mg every 6 h, increase to 50–75 mg every 6 h.	Flushing, nasal congestion, conjunctivitis, CNS† stimulation, drug fever, muscle cramps. Lupus-like syndrome at doses of 200–400 mg/day. Side effects lessened by gradual increase in dosage. Surprisingly few side effects reported as yet in treating primary pulmonary hypertension.
Isoproterenol	Beta-adrenergic agonist; relaxes vascular smooth muscle when tone is high; increases venous return to heart; positive inotropic and chronotropic effects.	1 µg/min IV and increasing by 1 µg/min until heart rate > 120/min or PA systolic > 10 torr over control, up to maximum dose of 5 µg/min.	Isoproterenol (sublingual) 10 mg every 4 h, increasing up to 20 mg every 3 h. Terbutaline 5 mg tid.	Palpitation, tachycardia, flushing, cardiac arrhythmias exceedingly common.
Phentolamine	Alpha-adrenergic blocker; dilates both systemic arterioles and large veins; positive inotropic effect.	0.5 mg/min IV to a maximum of 10 mg.	Phentolamine 25 mg every 6 h, increasing to 50 mg every 3 h while awake. Phenoxybenzamine 10 mg daily, increasing by 10 mg every 4 days to a maximum of 40 mg daily. Prazosin 2 mg tid, increasing up to 5 mg tid.	Tachycardia, cardiac arrhythmias, angina, gastrointestinal stimulation.
Nifedipine‡§	Interferes with calcium fluxes in vascular smooth muscle.	10 mg sublingually repeated once after 15 min. Exercise 15 min later.	Nifedipine 50 mg bid.	Systemic vasodilation and hypotension; flushing, rhythm disturbances; dysesthesias, peripheral edema; currently the most popular vasodilator agent for empiric trial (without hemodynamic testing).

*Based on a table developed by a working group as part of suggested protocols for use by centers for primary pulmonary hypertension, recently established by the National Heart, Lung, and Blood Institute. Members of this working group were Drs. Edward H. Bergofsky (chairman), Michael Beaven, Alfred P. Fishman, Michael Heymann, John T. Reeves, Lynne M. Reid, and Marvin A. Sackner. (From Fishman AP [ed.]: Update: Pulmonary Diseases and Disorders. Copyright © 1982 by McGraw-Hill, Inc. Used by permission of McGraw-Hill Book Company.)

†PA = pulmonary arterial; CNS = central nervous system.

‡Some clinics prefer the calcium channel blocker diltiazem, up to 30 mg three times daily, for oral maintenance therapy.

§This use of nifedipine is not listed in the manufacturer's directive.

clinical value is doubtful unless an increase in cardiac output (with minimal increase in heart rate) occurs in conjunction with a decrease in pulmonary arterial pressure.

It should be kept in mind that agents given to relax the pulmonary vessels cause systemic vasodilation if they gain access to the systemic circulation; in turn, systemic vasodilation unloads the left ventricle. As far as the pulmonary circulation is concerned, this unloading is a passive mechanism for decreasing pulmonary arterial pressure. Instead of causing pulmonary vasodilation, pulmonary arterial pressure falls passively as blood is shifted from the pulmonary circulation to the systemic circulation. It seems likely that effective pulmonary vasodilators currently in use exert both active and passive effects.

Criteria for acute pulmonary vasodilation in response to a potential vasodilator vary from clinic to clinic. As a result, some reports using more rigid criteria, e.g., a 30 per cent drop in pulmonary vascular resistance accompanied by a drop in pulmonary arterial pressure and an increase in cardiac output, conclude

that about one third of patients with primary pulmonary hypertension respond to pulmonary vasodilators. Others, using less rigid criteria, are more sanguine about the prospects for eliciting vasodilation. Clearly, because of its effects on the work of the heart, the greater the drop in pulmonary arterial pressure, the brighter the prospects for sustained clinical improvement. Evidence is accumulating that successful pulmonary vasodilation promotes long-term survival. This likelihood, plus the fact that an increase in cardiac output is almost invariably accompanied by symptomatic relief, is encouraging the search for effective pulmonary vasodilators that can be taken chronically by mouth or via the skin in dosages that do not evoke deleterious systemic side effects.

A battery of drugs was used until recently in acute testing for the capability of the hypertensive pulmonary circulation to vasodilate. These included agents that acted directly on pulmonary resistance vessels (nitroprusside and hydralazine) and others that acted on adrenergic receptors (isoproterenol, phentolamine, and the quinazoline derivative, prazosin) (Table 45–4). However,

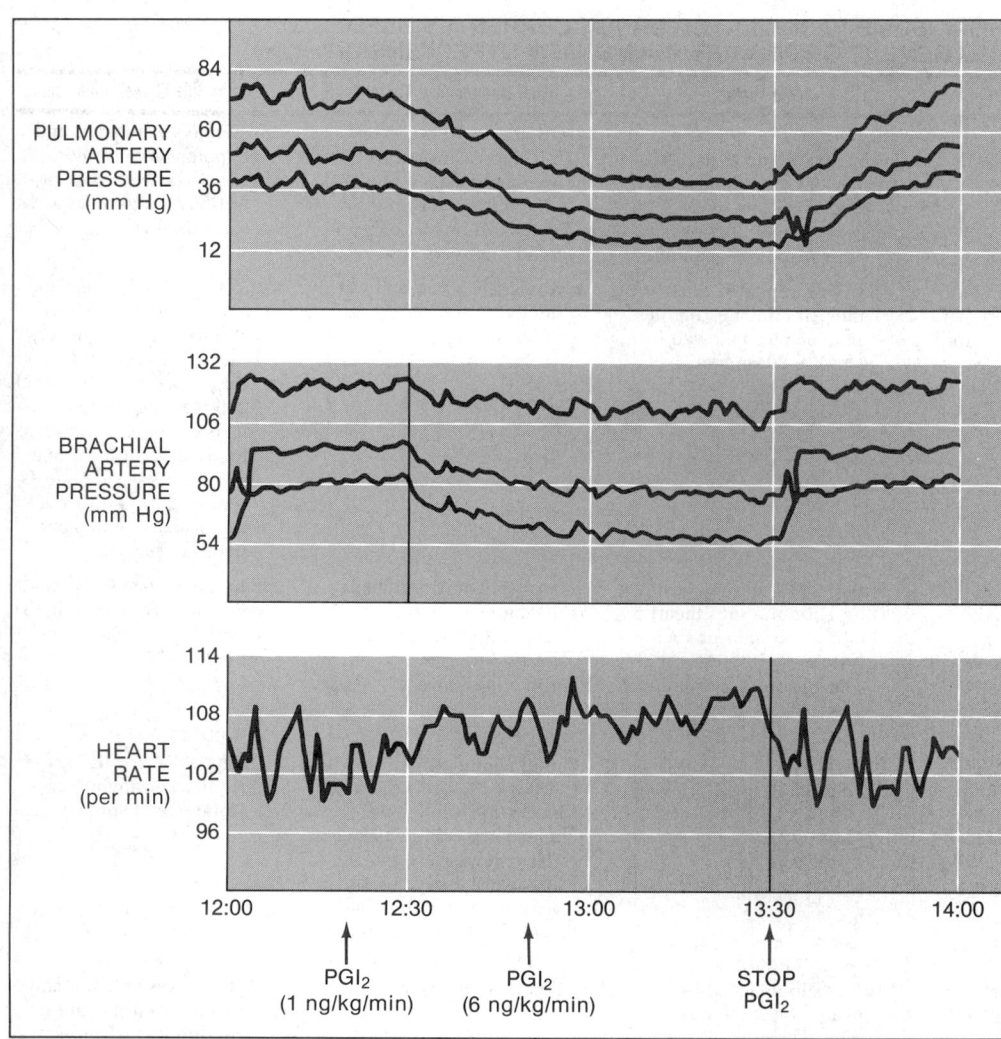

FIGURE 45–7. Prostacyclin administered intravenously to a patient with primary pulmonary hypertension. An abrupt drop in pulmonary arterial pressure occurs at the start of the infusion (with little effect on systemic arterial pressure or heart rate) (*first arrow*). Cessation of the infusion (about 1 hour later) is followed by a prompt return of pulmonary arterial pressure to high levels. (Courtesy of Dr. Harold Palevsky.)

these have been superseded during the last few years by prostacyclin and calcium channel blockers, i.e., nifedipine or diltiazem.

Prostacyclin. Enthusiasm remains high about the effectiveness of prostacyclin (PGI_2) in screening for pulmonary vasomotor responsiveness (vasodilation) in patients with primary pulmonary hypertension (Fig. 45–7). Indeed, it has come to be regarded as "the gold standard." This agent seems to have several attractive features: (1) It is a powerful relaxant of increased pulmonary vascular tone; i.e., it is a potent vasodilator; (2) it reduces pulmonary vascular resistance in a dose-dependent way so that dosage can be titrated to achieve maximal pulmonary vasodilation without undue systemic side effects, e.g., headache, nausea, flushing, and vomiting; (3) adverse effects stop when the infusion stops; and (4) it seems to indicate whether there is a vasoconstrictive element to the pulmonary hypertension that other pulmonary vasodilators might affect. Unfortunately, it is still an investigational drug available only for intravenous use.

Calcium-Blocking Agents. The designation "calcium channel blocker" or "calcium antagonist" is applied to a heterogeneous group of agents of different structural, pharmacologic, and electrophysiologic properties. The agents currently receiving the most clinical attention as potential pulmonary vasodilators are nifedipine and diltiazem. Both are administered orally for both acute testing and chronic therapy. As a rule, the agent is pushed to the limit of tolerance in attempting to achieve the optimal chronic pulmonary vasodilator effect. But severe side effects, e.g., systemic hypotension, often limit the maximum dosage. Of the two, nifedipine is the more popular. Verapamil, once used extensively, has fallen into disuse, largely because of its undesirable negative inotropic effect.

Nifedipine is a synthetic agent that is one of a large family of dihydropyridine compounds unrelated to other vasoactive or cardiotonic drugs. It is available in capsule form. The usual dose is 10 mg three or four times a day, but in some clinics higher dosages are tried until systemic side effects ensue. It is a potent systemic vasodilator used for the treatment of angina pectoris and is thought to be particularly useful when an element of coronary vasospasm is present. The latter use is not listed in the manufacturer's directive. Myocardial depressant effects are typically evident only in patients with severe ventricular dysfunction. It is now the agent of choice when acute trials using prostacyclin or nifedipine show that pulmonary vasodilation can be elicited, or it may be used empirically when preliminary hemodynamic trials of the various pulmonary vasodilators are not feasible.

HEART-LUNG TRANSPLANTATION. Technical and immunosuppressive considerations, as well as a shortage of organ donors, have exerted a large influence on the choice of transplant procedures. Currently, heart-lung transplantation is the preferred choice for primary pulmonary hypertension and certain congenital cardiac disorders affecting the heart and lungs, e.g., Eisenmenger's complex. Bilateral lung transplantation is preferred for chronic bronchitis and emphysema on the one hand and for sepsis, e.g., cystic fibrosis, on the other. Single lung transplantation is used predominantly for patients with end-stage widespread fibrosis (in whom the level of pulmonary hypertension is generally modest).

In patients with primary pulmonary hypertension, heart-lung transplantation is generally reserved for patients with limited life expectancy, e.g., 12 to 18 months, pursuing a downhill course with evident cor pulmonale, often in right ventricular failure; bouts of syncope lend urgency to surgical intervention. Many patients accepted for transplantation die while awaiting the procedure. In some patients, the prolonged infusion of prostacyclin (for 2 months to 2 years) has made it possible to sustain candidates for the operation. The results of heart-lung transplantation have been encouraging with respect to both the quality of life, e.g., improved exercise tolerance, and mortality. About 75 per cent of patients are alive after 1 year, about two thirds after the second year, and almost 50 per cent after the third year. Among the serious complications of heart-lung transplantation have been bronchiolitis obliterans and infections, both presumably related to the postoperative lifelong immunosuppression.

Prognosis

The diagnosis of primary pulmonary hypertension carries with it a poor prognosis. Although death usually occurs within a few years after the onset of symptoms, instances of long-term survival do occur. Exceptions to the rule of a short and fatal course have also been reported. Epidemics of primary pulmonary hypertension have been attributed to the ingestion of aminorex; in many patients in whom the drug was stopped, the pulmonary hypertension subsided. At present, there is no specific treatment for primary pulmonary hypertension. Pulmonary vasodilators have, in some patients, improved exercise tolerance and the quality of life but have not yet been shown to prolong life. Neither anticoagulants nor corticosteroids have been of value. The cause of death is generally right ventricular failure. In some patients, sudden death terminates the illness.

PULMONARY VENO-OCCLUSIVE DISEASE

Pulmonary venous hypertension is usually secondary to lesions of the left side of the heart (mitral valvular disease, left heart failure, left atrial myxoma) but also occurs after obstruction of large pulmonary veins (metastatic carcinoma, tuberculosis, or histoplasmosis), massively enlarged lymph nodes (sarcoidosis), or fibrosing mediastinitis of unknown cause.

However, there are also a small number of patients in whom unexplained progressive obliteration of small pulmonary veins and venules leads to pulmonary venous and then pulmonary arterial hypertension. The entity has been called pulmonary veno-occlusive disease. Despite its name, evidence of vascular injury, possibly viral, occurs not only on the pulmonary venous side but also on the pulmonary arterial side, leaving the pulmonary capillaries unaffected.

CLINICAL PICTURE. Predominantly children and young adults are affected, but the age range has been from infancy to 48 years. There seems to be no sex difference. Although hints exist of possibly related familial cardiac disorders, the patients are too few to do more than raise suspicion of a familial or common environmental cause.

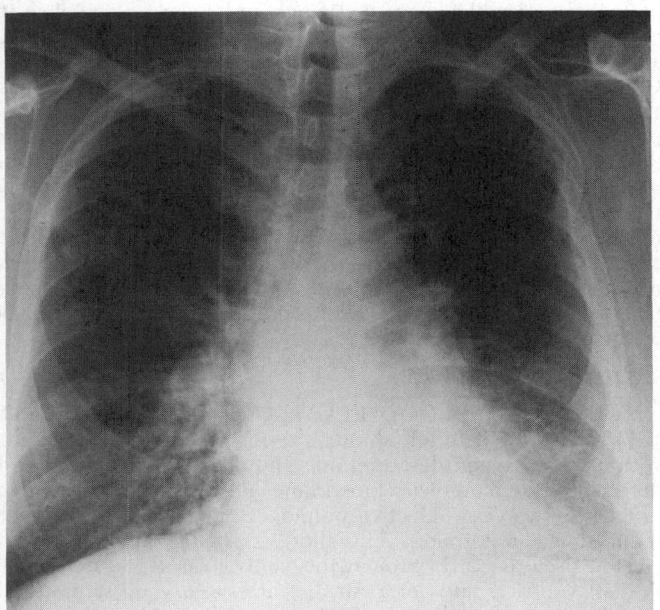

FIGURE 45–8. Pulmonary veno-occlusive disease. Severe pulmonary hypertension in association with pulmonary congestion and edema. Diagnosis was established by lung biopsy.

There is generally little clinical or hemodynamic basis for distinguishing between primary arterial pulmonary hypertension and pulmonary veno-occlusive disease. Even the pulmonary wedge pressure is usually normal in both. However, in some instances, in a patient who proves to have a normal mitral valve and left ventricle, evidence appears of pulmonary venous congestion and edema (bibasal crackles, Kerley B lines, increased vascular markings on the chest radiograph). Another clue is the occurrence of pleural effusions in a patient who otherwise seems to have primary (arterial) pulmonary hypertension. With these few exceptions, the patients are generally diagnosed as having primary (arterial) pulmonary hypertension until autopsy discloses distinctive lesions affecting primarily the small pulmonary veins and venules (see below).

LABORATORY TESTS. Cardiac catheterization discloses a high pulmonary arterial pressure, usually with a normal pulmonary wedge pressure. The low wedge pressure has been attributed to the interruption of blood flow by the occluding catheter into a venous bed in which widespread vascular occlusions preclude inflow from tributaries to the occluding catheter. In a few patients, lung biopsies have established the diagnosis during life.

PATHOLOGY. Both lungs are involved, but the venous lesions may be more marked in one region than in another (Fig. 45–8). As a rule, the pulmonary arteries as well as the pulmonary veins are affected, but the lesions are different. Most striking are the morphologic changes in the pulmonary veins and venules, which are narrowed or occluded by fibrous tissue; up to 95 per cent of the veins and venules may be affected, but complete occlusion is uncommon. Bronchial veins and bronchopulmonary anastomoses share in the occlusive process. Hypertrophy in the walls of the pulmonary arteries may also be quite striking, whereas the pulmonary capillary bed is generally unaffected. Thrombi in the pulmonary arteries are common. The lungs show congestion, edema, and focal fibrosis, which may become extensive.

Treatment has been disappointing, since the lesions are generally irreversible. Often, either anticoagulants or platelet-inhibiting agents are administered. Pulmonary vasodilators have been tried empirically with some anecdotal descriptions of effectiveness. The usual duration of life after the patient is found to have pulmonary hypertension ranges from a few weeks in infants to several years in adults, with 7 years the maximum.

Eysmann SB, Palevsky HI, Reichek N, et al.: Two-dimensional and Doppler-echocardiographic and cardiac catheterization correlates of survival in primary pulmonary hypertension. Circulation 80:353–360, 1989. *Echocardiography can be used as a guide to prognosis in primary pulmonary hypertension once the diagnosis has been made and repeat cardiac catheterization is inadvisable.*

Fishman AP: Pulmonary circulation. *In* Fishman AP, Fisher A (eds.): Handbook of Physiology: The Respiratory System, Vol. I. Bethesda, MD, American Physiological Society, 1986, pp 93–165. *A comprehensive survey of the regulation of the pulmonary circulation, particularly useful as a background for considering pathogenesis of clinical pulmonary hypertension. Emphasis is placed on the concept of pulmonary vascular resistance, the interpretation of pulmonary wedge pressures, and the identification of pulmonary vasomotor activity.*

Fishman AP (ed.): The Pulmonary Circulation: Normal and Abnormal. Philadelphia, University of Pennsylvania Press, 1990. *A survey of current understanding of mechanisms, management (medical and surgical), and treatment of pulmonary hypertension, including both secondary and primary. A feature of the volume is a summary of findings of the National Registry on Primary Pulmonary Hypertension, which began in 1981 and involved 35 medical centers.*

Higenbottam T, Wheeldon D, Wells F, et al.: Long-term treatment of primary pulmonary hypertension with continuous intravenous epoprostenal (prostacyclin). Lancet 1:1046, 1984. *This paper describes the first of seven patients, unmanageable by oral vasodilators, who were treated by continuous infusion of prostacyclin for months up to 2 years. After 1 year of continuous self-administration of prostacyclin intravenously, the patient remained greatly improved.*

Lloyd JE, Atkinson JB, Pietra GG, et al.: Heterogeneity of pathologic lesions in familial primary pulmonary hypertension. Am Rev Respir Dis 138:952–957, 1988. *The heterogeneity of the pulmonary vascular lesions in familial primary pulmonary hypertension argues against the idea of a unique anatomic change in pulmonary resistance vessels as the hallmark of the disease.*

Long WA, Groves BM, Rubin LJ, et al.: Acute hemodynamic effects of prostacyclin in 100 primary pulmonary hypertension patients. Ann Intern Med, in press. *A report of an interinstitutional study of prostacyclin as a vasodilator agent in primary pulmonary hypertension. This agent is now the "gold standard" for acute testing of pulmonary vasodilators.*

Loscalzo J: An overview of thrombolytic agents. Chest 97:117S–123S, 1990. *A review of the mechanisms by which thrombi develop, the pharmacologic agents to lyse thrombi, and the mechanisms of action of these agents.*

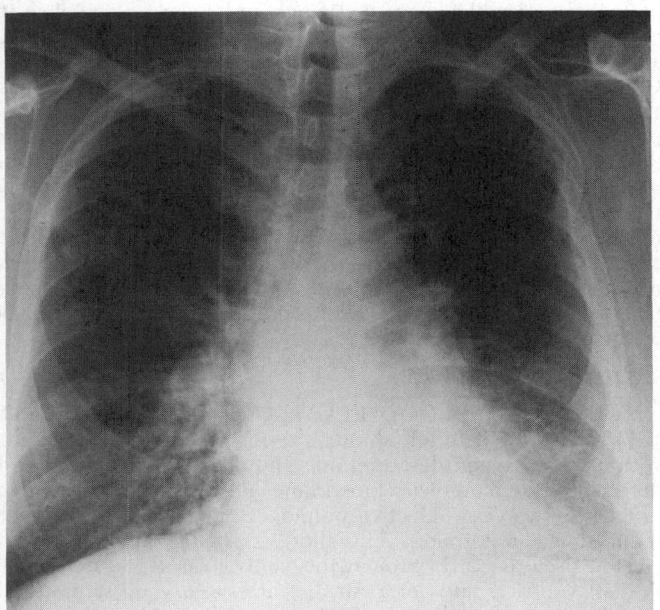

FIGURE 45–8. Pulmonary veno-occlusive disease. Severe pulmonary hypertension in association with pulmonary congestion and edema. Diagnosis was established by lung biopsy.

Palevsky HI, Schloo BL, Pietra GG, et al.: Primary pulmonary hypertension: Vascular structure, morphometry, and responsiveness to vasodilator agents. Circulation 80:1207–1221, 1989. *Correlation of histologic structure (obtained either by biopsy or at autopsy) with vasodilator responsiveness. An appreciably thickened intima correlated with poor pulmonary vasodilation.*

46 Congenital Heart Disease

Samuel Kaplan

Congenital diseases of the heart occur in about 8 to 10 of 1000 live births. The spectrum of severity varies widely. One fourth to one third are symptomatic in the first year of life, frequently as neonates. In others, such as in patients with a functionally normal bicuspid aortic valve, the lesion may remain silent throughout life. With the development of palliative or radical surgical treatment, another large group has evolved that was treated during infancy or childhood and has reached adult life. Accordingly, adults with congenital heart disease fall into several groups: Some have anomalies with a natural history for long survival, others have had successful palliative or "curative" surgery in childhood, and still others have had lesions that were mild in childhood but have increased in severity in adult life (e.g., aortic stenosis).

Etiology

The cause is usually unknown in individual patients. The etiology of congenital heart disease is thought to be multifactorial, primarily due to an interaction between genetic predisposition and intrauterine environmental factors. It is estimated that congenital heart disease is associated with chromosomal abnormalities in 5 per cent of cases and with single mutant genes and environmental factors in 3 per cent each. Among *chromosomal abnormalities* the prevalence of congenital heart disease is about 50 per cent in trisomy 21 (Down's syndrome), 95 per cent in trisomy 18, 90 per cent in trisomy 13, and 35 per cent in Turner's (XO) syndrome. Among *single mutant gene* disorders (autosomal dominant or recessive or X-linked phenotypes), the more frequent syndromes in which the heart is involved are hypertrophic cardiomyopathy and the syndromes of Noonan and Holt-Oram. Numerous *environmental factors* have been implicated. Women who contract rubella during the first trimester of pregnancy may give birth to infants with pulmonic stenosis (especially pulmonary artery branch stenosis), persistent patent ductus arteriosus, and less often other defects. Other viruses have also been implicated, but the evidence that they produce congenital heart disease is not so strong. These include cytomegalovirus, coxsackievirus, and herpesvirus. Among drugs implicated in congenital heart disease are the anticonvulsants, especially phenytoin and trimethadione, and lithium salts (with an apparent predilection for atrioventricular [AV] valve disease, especially Ebstein's malformation of the tricuspid valve), progesterone, warfarin, and amphetamines. The offspring of diabetic women are at greater risk for a variety of congenital heart diseases. Patent ductus arteriosus is more frequent in children born at high altitudes. It is estimated that about one half of the offspring of alcoholic mothers have congenital heart disease, usually left to right shunts.

Counseling

Parents of children with congenital heart disease are concerned about the cause and the possibility of recurrence in future pregnancies. This concern is greatest when the child is first born or the baby succumbs during the neonatal period. An explanation should be offered about the known causes of congenital heart disease and guilt feelings allayed. The prevalence of congenital heart disease in a second infant is 1 to 4 per cent. Although this figure is higher than in the general population, it is still quite low, and parents should be supported if they decide to have another child. When congenital heart disease has recurred in two siblings, the prevalence is higher in a third pregnancy (estimated to be 3 to 12 per cent). Many women with congenital heart disease who had corrective surgery during childhood have reached childbearing age. The prevalence of congenital heart disease in their children ranges from 3 to 16 per cent and is highest in left ventricular obstructive lesions. Recurrence risks are low in the offspring of fathers with congenital heart disease (1 to 3 per cent).

Circulatory Shunts

PATHOPHYSIOLOGY

MAGNITUDE AND DIRECTION. Factors that determine the magnitude and direction of intra- and extracardiac shunts are the size of the defect, pressure differences between the cardiac chambers or vessels, and resistance to ejection produced by outflow obstruction, as well as the ratio of systemic to pulmonary vascular resistance. Since normal systemic vascular pressures and resistances greatly exceed those in the pulmonary circuit, flow across small defects (such as ventricular septal defects) is from left to right but is limited in magnitude by the small opening. When the defect is large and nonrestrictive, peak systolic pressures in the ventricles are virtually identical, so that the direction and magnitude of flow are regulated by outflow resistance. If systemic vascular resistance significantly exceeds that in the pulmonary circuit with large defects (in the absence of pulmonic stenosis), torrential left to right shunts are present. The magnitude of the shunt is decreased as pulmonary vascular resistance approaches that in the systemic circuit, and it is bidirectional or right to left with continued increase of pulmonary resistance. When severe pulmonic stenosis is present, resistance to right ventricular ejection virtually equalizes peak systolic pressures in both ventricles so that flow across ventricular defects is right to left or bidirectional. A major determinant of direction and magnitude of shunting at the atrial level is the diastolic distensibility of the ventricles. Flow, frequently torrential, is from left to right, since the thin-walled right ventricle is easily filled even though atrial pressures are equal and low.

PULMONARY HYPERTENSION. This complication (see Ch. 45), common in congenital heart disease, results from increased pulmonary blood flow and/or resistance. Torrential pulmonary blood flow (as in secundum atrial septal defects) can be accommodated by the pulmonary circulation without increase in pressure. Pulmonary hypertension develops frequently in the presence of large defects at the ventricular level or communications between the aorta and pulmonary arteries. In infants and small children with these defects, "hyperkinetic" pulmonary hypertension is present. This term refers to a vasoactive pulmonary bed that undergoes vasodilation in response to oxygen or tolazoline. These agents reduce the level of pulmonary arterial pressure by pulmonary vasodilation even though pulmonary blood flow increases. Hyperkinetic pulmonary hypertension is uncommon in adults but is seen in some with secundum atrial septal defects. Generally, pulmonary vascular disease is present in adults, so that pulmonary vascular resistance is greatly increased even when pulmonary blood flow is not excessive (see Eisenmenger's Syndrome below). The status of the pulmonary vascular bed determines the clinical picture, prognosis, and feasibility of surgical treatment of intra- and extracardiac shunts. The goal of management is to prevent the development of severe pulmonary vascular changes by surgical ablation of the shunt. This implies serial measurements of pulmonary and systemic pressures and resistances, especially in infants and toddlers with large ventricular or aortopulmonary defects.

RIGHT TO LEFT SHUNTS

PULMONARY BLOOD FLOW AND SYSTEMIC DESATURATION. Right to left shunts are characteristically associated with arterial oxygen desaturation. The degree of desaturation is determined by pulmonary blood flow and the magnitude of right to left shunt. When effective pulmonary blood flow is markedly reduced (as in tetralogy of Fallot), systemic venous blood is ejected preferentially through the ventricular septal defect into the left ventricle and aorta, so that arterial oxygen saturation is severely reduced and cyanosis is obvious. On the other hand, right to left shunts may be associated with markedly increased pulmonary blood flow (as in transposition of the great arteries). In this situation pulmonary venous blood is almost fully saturated so that systemic arterial saturation is only moderately decreased. Cyanosis is not as intense in the latter group of patients, but they suffer from volume loading and failure of the left ventricle.

ARTERIAL HYPOXEMIA. *Cyanosis*, a dusky purple color of the skin but especially the mucous membranes and nail beds, is due to reduced hemoglobin in the arterial blood from right to left shunts. Clinical cyanosis may not be evident until the arterial oxygen saturation is below 85 per cent (normal is 94 to 98 per cent). *Clubbing* of fingers and toes is common, especially when arterial hypoxemia is marked. This sign may appear in childhood (beyond the age of 1 year) and is progressive. When arterial oxygen saturation returns to normal (at rest and during exercise), as occurs after surgical correction, clubbing regresses and even severe forms disappear within 2 to 3 years after operation.

When the hematocrit exceeds 65 to 70 per cent, symptoms of hyperviscosity appear and include excruciating headaches, fatigue, paresthesias, faintness, dizziness, visual disturbances, myalgias, and arthralgias. In adults these symptoms are alleviated with cautious venesection of 500 ml with immediate fluid replacement. Within 48 hours a second venesection of 500 ml can be undertaken if symptoms of hyperviscosity persist. The only indication for venesection is symptomatic hyperviscosity. A high hematocrit (65 to 75 per cent) in an asymptomatic patient is not an indication for venesection because the incidence of intravascular thrombosis (including cerebral vascular accidents) is not increased. However, repeated venesections to lower the hematocrit are not well tolerated and frequently result in iron deficiency with hypochromic and microcytic red blood cells. Furthermore, microcytosis aggravates hyperviscosity, resulting in extreme fatigue, headaches, faintness, paresthesias, dizziness, and decreased effort tolerance. These patients are treated for 1 week with small doses of oral iron (325 mg ferrous sulfate daily) because the hematocrit may rise rapidly on therapy. This treatment may be repeated for 1 to 4 weeks until iron stores are replenished and symptoms disappear. Another important cause of an elevated hematocrit is dehydration, which is treated with fluid replacement. Patients with erythrocytosis and hyperviscosity may have a bleeding diathesis due to a combination of thrombocytopenia, accelerated fibrinolysis, hypofibrinogenemia, prolonged prothrombin time, and prolonged partial thromboplastin time. These coagulation abnormalities may be improved by cautious venesection, which is used to prepare patients for elective noncardiac surgery. Patients with erythrocytosis may have hyperuricemia due to low fractional excretion (not to urate overproduction). Arthralgias are common, although acute gouty arthritis is less frequent.

BRAIN ABSCESS AND PARADOXICAL EMBOLUS. Brain abscess occurs in older children and adults. Predisposing factors include previous occlusive microcirculatory disease from thrombosis or emboli. Clinical recognition may be difficult because the onset is insidious, symptoms are vague, and fever is low grade. In others, the onset is more acute, with headache, seizures, and localized neurologic signs that are dependent on the size and site of the abscess and the presence of increased intracranial pressure. The diagnosis is established with computed tomography or magnetic resonance imaging or both. Treatment is with antibiotics, generally followed by surgical drainage. In patients with right to left shunts, venous blood bypasses the lungs so that emboli arising from systemic veins enter the systemic circulation directly to occlude an artery anywhere in the body, especially the brain. This complication is rare.

SHUNT LESIONS
Atrial Septal Defect

Atrial septal defects occur more frequently in females and are designated according to their site in the septum. The most common are in the region of the fossa ovalis (*ostium secundum defect*) and are among the most prevalent congenital cardiac anomalies in adults. A less frequent variety (*sinus venosus defect*) occupies the upper part of the atrial septum and is closely related to the entry of the superior vena cava. This structure receives one or more anomalously draining pulmonary veins, usually from the right lung. (The *ostium primum defect* is discussed under Endocardial Cushion Defect, below).

The principal factors that determine the magnitude of the left to right shunt are the size of the defect, the relative compliance of the cardiac chambers, and the vascular resistances in the pulmonary and systemic circulations. If the defect is moderate or large (>2 cm in diameter in an adult), the greater distensibility of the right atrium and ventricle and the low pulmonary vascular resistance allow an abundant left-to-right shunt. On the other hand, in infancy the relatively thick and less compliant right ventricle limits the magnitude of left to right shunts. Large defects with torrential left to right shunts produce right atrial and ventricular enlargement, which encroaches on the left-sided chambers. Pulmonary pressures and resistances are generally normal. In the unusual instances in which they are elevated, the pulmonary circulation remains vasoactive, so that pressures and resistances return to normal after surgical ablation of the shunt. Those with severe pulmonary vascular disease are described under Eisenmenger's Syndrome.

DIAGNOSIS. Although symptoms are trivial and physical signs subtle, the diagnosis is usually made during childhood. However, many escape detection in the first decade of life and are recognized in later years only because of effort dyspnea and fatigue. Superimposed coronary artery disease or systemic hypertension can cause the left ventricle to be less distensible, favoring the development or worsening of these symptoms because of a further increase in left to right shunt and right volume overload. In some instances the presence of the defect is first appreciated when pulmonary hypertension develops with persistence of a torrential left to right shunt. The advent of atrial arrhythmias, fibrillation, flutter, or paroxysms of supraventricular tachycardia is not well tolerated. These events increase in frequency beyond the fourth decade. Some patients with an uncomplicated atrial septal defect are recognized for the first time because of an abnormal "routine" chest roentgenogram.

In children failure to gain weight is common but by no means the rule. The characteristic physical appearance is that of a thin child with nearly normal height and a gracile habitus. Generally, adults have a normal physical appearance, but again some are thin and gracile. The jugular venous pulse shows "a" and "v" waves of equal heights reflecting the normal left atrial pulse because the atria are in free communication. Dominant "a" waves suggest the presence of pulmonary hypertension, and dominant "v" waves are associated with tricuspid regurgitation. Right ventricular volume overload results in an easily palpable left parasternal lift. The importance of this sign cannot be overemphasized, and in some the dilated pulmonary artery is palpated in the second left interspace. The soft mid-systolic murmur, seldom accompanied by a thrill, is best heard at the upper left sternal edge and is produced by increased blood flow into the pulmonary artery. A loud murmur is widely transmitted to the chest anteriorly and posteriorly, especially in slightly built patients. The murmur is preceded by an accentuated first heart sound and sometimes by a pulmonic ejection sound. The auscultatory hallmark is the easily audible, widely split second heart sound. This split is virtually fixed in all phases of respiration and during the Valsalva maneuver. When the defect is large, a mid-diastolic murmur is audible at the lower left sternal edge and is produced by extravagant flow across the tricuspid valve. An early diastolic murmur of pulmonary regurgitation may accompany pulmonary hypertension, but this is rare.

The *electrocardiogram* shows right-axis deviation and right ventricular hypertrophy (generally rsR¹ in right precordial leads). This pattern is due to terminal depolarization of the hypertrophied right ventricular outflow tract. Less frequent findings include tall P waves (because of right atrial enlargement), complete right bundle branch block, a prolonged PR interval, and Wolff-Parkinson-White syndrome. Supraventricular arrhythmias may be detected in untreated adults or many years after surgical closure of the defect. These consist of atrial fibrillation or flutter, paroxysmal atrial tachycardia, and multiple premature atrial contractions. Left-axis deviation usually denotes the presence of an ostium primum atrial defect but is seen occasionally in secundum defects. Another rare finding is a normal electrocardiogram.

The *chest roentgenogram* is often distinctive, especially in adults. Varying degrees of cardiac enlargement are due to dilatation of the right atrium and ventricle, which displaces the normal or relatively small left-sided chambers posteriorly. The large pulmonary trunk contrasts with the smaller aortic knob, which is especially notable on the posteroanterior view. The primary branches of the pulmonary artery are enlarged and the vascularity is increased toward the periphery of both lung fields.

Echocardiography not only is diagnostic but also is useful in excluding other suspected anomalies. In uncomplicated secundum atrial defects the right ventricular end-diastolic dimension is increased and the ventricular septal motion is flat or paradoxical. Real-time two-dimensional echocardiograms define the location and size of the defect and also confirm the significant enlargement of the right atrium. The deformity of the ventricular septum resulting from right ventricular volume overload is recognized, and its encroachment into the left ventricular cavity is visualized. Flow disturbance across the interatrial septum can be detected by measurements based on the Doppler principle. The pulmonary and aortic flows can be estimated by two-dimensional echo and Doppler techniques, and the difference between these flows represents the shunt volume. *Mitral valve prolapse* may be associated with secundum atrial septal defects and in many instances the suspicion is raised by the echocardiogram. Since various criteria are used for the echo diagnosis of mitral valve prolapse, caution should be exercised in the diagnosis of combined atrial septal defect and mitral valve prolapse. It is probable that the association has been overestimated.

There is an ongoing debate about whether *cardiac catheterization* is indicated in all patients. Physical examination supplemented by the electrocardiogram and chest roentgenogram usually suggests the diagnosis. This can be confirmed by visualizing the site of the defect and pulmonary venous connection by echocardiography, which also estimates the pulmonary-systemic flow ratio as well as the pulmonary arterial pressure. However, cardiac catheterization should be undertaken in the adult in whom pulmonary hypertension or coexisting coronary artery disease is suspected.

NATURAL HISTORY. The vast majority of secundum atrial septal defects are recognized and treated surgically during childhood or adolescence. Spontaneous closure does occur, but this is usually prior to the age of about 3 years. Although life expectancy is shortened, adult survival is the rule and some live to an advanced age. Pregnancy is usually well tolerated, especially in women who were asymptomatic prior to pregnancy.

COMPLICATIONS. After the age of 40 years complications are frequent, and most patients who survive beyond the age of 60 years show symptoms of effort dyspnea and fatigue. Death may be unrelated to the defect, but when a relationship exists cardiac failure is the most common cause. Heart failure may be due to right ventricular failure alone or may be intensified by a dilated tricuspid valve ring with resultant incompetence. The prevalence of atrial arrhythmias increases after the fourth decade and may precipitate heart failure, especially when the ventricular response is rapid in the presence of a large shunt. Coronary artery disease or systemic hypertension may result in a less distensible left ventricle, which favors an increase in left to right shunting. Pulmonary hypertension may be due to the high pulmonary blood flow or may progress to a state in which pulmonary and systemic vascular resistances are virtually identical and the shunt is abolished or reversed (see Eisenmenger's Syndrome). Infective endocarditis is rare in isolated lesions.

TREATMENT. Treatment is surgical ablation of the shunt, especially when the pulmonary systemic flow ratio exceeds 2:1. Devices inserted through a percutaneous cardiac catheter have been developed to close secundum atrial septal defects. These devices are undergoing clinical trial and if successful would obviate the need for open heart surgery. At this time surgery is advised and is preferably accomplished between the ages of about 3 and 4 years, when the surgical risk is minimal. In these young patients the right ventricular dimension returns to normal. Surgical treatment in older children and adolescents usually improves the size of the right-sided chambers, but they may not return to normal. When the operation is performed in adults, patchy fibrosis of the chronically volume-loaded right ventricle persists, as does some degree of right ventricular dilatation. These residua may explain the blunted chronotropic response during exercise, with resultant decreased cardiac output and decreased working capacity. Nevertheless, patients in the fifth, sixth, or even seventh decade with high pulmonary blood flow and low resistance benefit

from surgical repair, which can be done with a comparatively low risk. Defects in older patients can be closed surgically despite moderate pulmonary hypertension and cardiac failure, provided there is still a significant left to right shunt. Operation is contraindicated when pulmonary vascular resistance is greatly elevated so that the shunt is abolished or reversed. Late-onset arrhythmias occur in fewer than 5 per cent, 10 to 20 years after surgery. The most common are atrial flutter, atrial fibrillation, paroxysmal supraventricular tachycardia, and frequent premature atrial contractions. Less frequent arrhythmias are sick sinus syndrome, junctional tachycardia, and complete heart block.

LUTEMBACHER'S SYNDROME

This condition consists of a secundum atrial septal defect with acquired mitral stenosis. Obstruction to left ventricular inflow aggravates the left to right shunt across the atrial septum. Atrial fibrillation is common. A prominent jugular "a" wave is visible because left atrial pressure is transmitted to the right atrium and the systemic venous return. Physical findings resemble those described under secundum atrial septal defects. Auscultatory findings of mitral stenosis are present but may not be obvious. The echocardiogram is diagnostic in that signs of mitral stenosis are superimposed on right ventricular volume overload. Patients with this condition experience great symptomatic relief after intracardiac repair.

ENDOCARDIAL CUSHION DEFECT

The embryonic endocardial cushions contribute to the development of the mitral and tricuspid valves and to the growth and convergence of the atrial and ventricular septa. Maldevelopment during this stage of cardiac morphogenesis results in varying degrees of complex malformations involving the AV valves and the atrial and ventricular septa. The *ostium primum defect* is situated in the lower portion of the atrial septum overlying both the mitral and tricuspid valves. A cleft in the anterior leaflet to the mitral valve is usual, and the tricuspid valve is frequently thickened but otherwise normal. The ventricular septum is intact functionally. *Common AV canal* (complete endocardial cushion defect) consists of a common defect of both the intra-atrial and intraventricular septa with a single AV valve. This valve, common to both ventricles, has an anterior and posterior leaflet with a lateral leaflet in each ventricle. This anomaly is relatively common in patients with Down's syndrome. *Transitional forms* are intermediate between AV canal and ostium primum defects.

OSTIUM PRIMUM DEFECTS. Ostium primum defects may be associated with recurrent lower respiratory tract infections with or without congestive heart failure during infancy and early childhood. However, the majority are asymptomatic and are recognized because of the murmur of mitral incompetence. In others, the degree of mitral regurgitation is trivial. The physical signs resemble those of ostium secundum defects with superimposed mitral regurgitation. The electrocardiogram is distinctive in that there is a superior counterclockwise frontal plane axis (left-axis deviation), varying degrees of right ventricular hypertrophy (rsR^1 is common), and sometimes voltage criteria for left ventricular hypertrophy because of mitral regurgitation. The chest radiograph simulates an ostium secundum atrial septal defect. The echocardiogram is also characteristic, showing enlargement of both right ventricle and right atrium, a low lying atrial septal defect, and a cleft in the anterior mitral leaflet. The mitral valve apparatus is displaced so that the anterior mitral leaflet encroaches upon the left ventricular outflow. Cardiac catheterization demonstrates the left to right atrial shunt, the level of pulmonary arterial pressure, and the degree of mitral valve incompetence. Left ventriculography shows the characteristic "goose-neck" deformity produced by the abnormal position of the mitral valve. Surgical treatment is advised during infancy or childhood with the purpose of obliterating the left to right shunt and alleviating mitral valve incompetence. In adult life, many years after surgery, atrial arrhythmias may occur as described under secundum atrial septal defect. In addition, a small number of patients have progressive mitral valve incompetence that may require mitral valve replacement.

COMPLETE AV CANAL. Congestive cardiac failure, significant elevation of pulmonary artery pressures and resistances, and intercurrent pulmonary infections are common during infancy.

At that time surgical treatment is undertaken to attempt to prevent progression of these complications. Without treatment, survival of these patients to adolescence and adult life is usually associated with the development of severe pulmonary vascular disease (see Eisenmenger's Syndrome) or congenital obstruction to right ventricular outflow, which limits pulmonary blood flow.

Ventricular Septal Defect

The most common form of congenital heart disease is an isolated ventricular septal defect. Perimembranous defects are the most frequent (Fig. 46–1). The magnitude of the shunt depends on the size of the defect and status of the pulmonary vascular bed. A small defect limits the size of the left to right shunt so that cardiac chambers are normal in size and pulmonary arterial pressures and resistances remain within normal limits. Large defects are associated with a marked increase in pulmonary blood flow, as well as varying degrees of elevation of pulmonary arterial pressures and resistance. In these instances pulmonary vascular disease may be progressive, so that systemic and pulmonary vascular resistances are virtually equal (Eisenmenger's syndrome) (see Ch. 39.5).

SMALL VENTRICULAR SEPTAL DEFECTS. Spontaneous closure of the defect is frequent, especially in the first year of life, and is estimated to occur in more than one half of instances. If the defect does not close spontaneously within the first 3 years of life, the clinical condition is likely to remain unchanged. These patients are generally asymptomatic and have a normal heart size. A systolic thrill may be palpable at the lower left sternal edge and is accompanied by a harsh, loud pansystolic murmur that is widely distributed but loudest at the site of the thrill. The electrocardiogram and chest roentgenogram are normal. These defects may be visualized by two-dimensional echocardiography if they are greater than 2 mm in diameter. However, Doppler interrogation of the right ventricular septum identifies turbulence

at the site of the defect, and color flow imaging confirms the site of left to right shunting. It is now believed that spontaneous closure of a small ventricular septal defect may also occur in early adult life. This notion is based on the fact that congenital ventricular septal defects are seldom found in older adults. Sometimes the development of an ejection click heralds a course that in a few years is associated with complete disappearance of all abnormal auscultatory findings when the defect is completely closed. Uncomplicated small ventricular septal defects do not require surgical closure, and the only treatment is prophylaxis against infective endocarditis.

LARGE VENTRICULAR SEPTAL DEFECTS. Large defects with unrestricted flow from the left to the right ventricle and into the pulmonary vascular bed are common in early life and rare in adults. These defects are associated with increased pulmonary vascular pressure and resistance. Furthermore, volume loading of the left heart may lead to superimposed left ventricular failure. Symptoms are present during infancy, especially between the ages of 2 and 6 months, and are produced by congestive cardiac failure, poor physical development, and recurrent pulmonary infections. These infants may respond to anticongestive measures. If this improvement is maintained, especially beyond the age of 1 year, the defect frequently decreases in size, with continuing clinical improvement. However, in a significant number, response to therapy is not maintained, physical development remains poor, and signs of pulmonary hypertension persist. In these instances surgical closure of the defect is indicated, since the mortality rate from surgery is acceptably low and soon after operation there is a growth spurt when heart failure and pulmonary hypertension regress.

Clinical improvement in some babies with a large ventricular septal defect may be due to the development of *acquired pulmonic stenosis*, which limits pulmonary blood flow. Generally, right ventricular outflow tract obstruction is due to infundibular hypertrophy and is progressive. During infancy or early childhood the clinical course changes in that signs of heart failure improve and heart size decreases because pulmonary blood flow is limited by the pulmonic stenosis. Right ventricular pressure rises to approximate that of the left ventricle, with resultant right to left shunting and cyanosis. The clinical picture resembles that of tetralogy of Fallot (see below).

VENTRICULAR SEPTAL DEFECT WITH AORTIC REGURGITATION. The ventricular septal defect is usually small or moderate in size and its presence is known from infancy. During childhood or adolescence aortic valve regurgitation occurs because of prolapse of the right or, at times, the noncoronary cusp. The clinical picture is extremely variable, from the asymptomatic child with a small left to right shunt and trivial aortic regurgitation to the symptomatic young adult with congestive cardiac failure, angina pectoris, massive cardiomegaly, and florid aortic regurgitation. The latter patient requires surgical closure of the defect and relief of aortic regurgitation; this generally requires aortic valve replacement. The asymptomatic patient with mild regurgitation needs to be observed closely. Some believe that closure of the ventricular defect prevents further prolapse of the aortic valve. Others recommend simultaneous aortic valvuloplasty prior to the development of significant valvular regurgitation and left ventricular dysfunction.

VENTRICULAR SEPTAL DEFECT WITH LEFT VENTRICULAR–RIGHT ATRIAL SHUNT. The AV septum is divided by the insertions of the tricuspid valve and the mitral valve. The insertion of the tricuspid valve is below that of the mitral. Thus, this area is common to the right atrium and left ventricle, and a defect in this area allows shunting from the left ventricle directly into the right atrium. In others the defect is below the tricuspid valve and is associated with an abnormal tricuspid septal leaflet. The physical signs simulate those of an isolated small to moderate ventricular septal defect, but color flow imaging identifies the shunt from left ventricle to right atrium. This condition should be treated surgically.

OTHER DEFECTS ASSOCIATED WITH VENTRICULAR SEPTAL DEFECTS. *Patent Ductus Arteriosus.* In some instances the murmurs of both lesions are audible, so that a continuous murmur is present at the upper left sternal edge and a holosystolic murmur is heard at the lower left sternal edge.

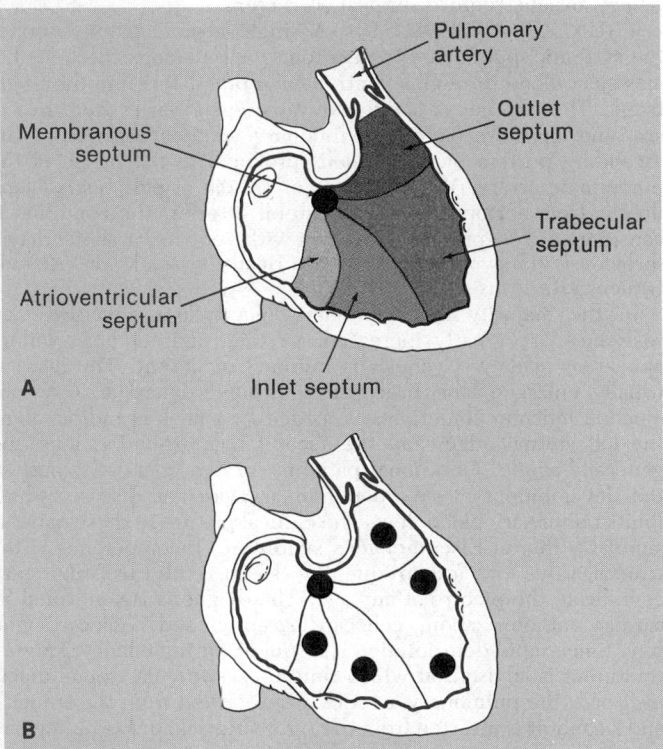

FIGURE 46–1. Diagrams of the right side of the ventricular septum. Anterior portions of the right ventricle and atrium have been removed, as has the tricuspid valve. *A,* Subdivisions of the ventricular septum. *B,* Locations of ventricular septal defects (VSD). 1. Perimembranous VSD (most common type). 2. Subpulmonic VSD (also known as infundibular, conal, or outlet VSD). 3. Atrioventricular canal VSD. 4, 5, and 6. Muscular VSD's in various parts of the septum; defects may be single or multiple. VSD's may extend to adjacent parts of the septum so that perimembranous VSD's may involve the inlet, trabecular, or outlet septum. The tricuspid valve may straddle the defect (rare in isolated VSD).

However, in many patients the physical findings are dominated by either the ventricular defect or the patent ductus arteriosus. Echocardiography combined with Doppler interrogation and color flow imaging is helpful in the diagnosis, disclosing shunting at the ventricular level as well as a patent ductus arteriosus.

Secundum Atrial Septal Defect. In patients with a ventricular septal defect and an ostium secundum atrial septal defect, the clinical picture is usually dominated by the ventricular defect. This combination of defects is more likely to be present during infancy and may result in torrential pulmonary blood flow, pulmonary hypertension, and congestive heart failure. The defects are recognized by echocardiography and, if uncontrolled by medical measures, are both treated surgically during the same procedure.

Coarctation of the Aorta. Signs of coarctation of the aorta usually dominate, and sometimes the signs of ventricular septal defect are erroneously attributed to the collateral circulation associated with coarctation.

Communications Between the Aorta and Pulmonary Arteries

PATENT DUCTUS ARTERIOSUS. Persistent patency of the ductus arteriosus is more frequent in females, in premature babies, in infants born at high altitude, and in infants whose first trimester of intrauterine life is complicated by maternal rubella. The aortic end of the ductus is opposite the origin of the left subclavian artery, and the vessel enters the pulmonary artery, usually at its bifurcation.

The hemodynamic effects of a patent ductus arteriosus depend on the size of the communication, the length of the ductus, and the resistance relationships between the systemic and pulmonary circulations. Generally, the flow through the ductus is small to moderate so that pulmonary arterial pressures and resistances remain normal. These patients usually are asymptomatic, and the only abnormal physical sign is a typical continuous murmur. This murmur, sometimes accompanied by a thrill, is heard best at the upper left sternal edge, rises to a peak in late systole, continues without interruption through the second sound, and wanes during the course of diastole. Larger shunts with a significant aortic runoff result in a wide pulse pressure and a "waterhammer" or bounding arterial pulse. The left atrium and ventricle enlarge to accommodate the increased pulmonary blood flow, and this is recognized by a lateral and downward displacement of the apical impulse, which is lifting in character. The typical continuous murmur is still present, but in addition an apical mid-diastolic murmur may be audible because of increased flow across the mitral valve. When pulmonary arterial pressure and resistance rise to systemic levels, flow across the ductus is limited. In patients with pulmonary hypertension, effort dyspnea is common, the wide pulse pressure disappears, and right ventricular enlargement is prominent. The auscultatory findings are dominated by those produced by pulmonary hypertension in that the typical continuous murmur disappears and is replaced by a short systolic murmur frequently preceded by an ejection click, a booming second heart sound due to loud pulmonic valve closure, and sometimes an early diastolic murmur of pulmonic valve incompetence. Occasionally the shunt through the ductus is reversed so that the descending aorta is perfused with desaturated pulmonary arterial blood. This results in cyanotic lower extremities with clubbing of the toes and normal color and shape of the fingers and fingernails.

The *electrocardiographic findings* are normal when the ductus is small. Moderate or large flows result in left ventricular hypertrophy. In the presence of severe pulmonary hypertension right ventricular hypertrophy dominates. The *chest roentgenogram* is normal if the flow is small. With larger flows the heart is enlarged because of left atrial and left ventricular prominence, the pulmonary arterial trunk and aorta are enlarged, and there is pulmonary plethora. With the development of severe pulmonary hypertension, heart size decreases, there is prominence of the right ventricle and especially the main pulmonary artery, and the size of the aorta may not be increased. In older patients the ductus may calcify. The *echocardiogram* defines and identifies the degree of chamber enlargement and visualizes the ductus.

Evidence of continuous flow is recorded using Doppler interrogation of the ductus arteriosus and the major pulmonary arteries.

Surgical correction is advisable by division of the ductus. In the adult with a large left to right shunt and normal pulmonary vascular resistance, surgery is also advised. Extensive calcification of the ductus increases the surgical risk, but surgery should still be advised if the shunt is large. Occasionally, an adult is seen with a small, hemodynamically insignificant patent ductus. The decision of surgical treatment for these patients must take into account that they are at risk for infective endocarditis, but on the other hand they may remain asymptomatic and some may experience spontaneous closure of the defect. Thus individual judgment is required in these patients. Devices inserted through a cardiac catheter have been developed to close a patent ductus arteriosus. These devices are undergoing clinical trial and if successful would obviate the need for thoracotomy.

AORTIC-PULMONARY SEPTAL DEFECT. This rare anomaly consists of a communication between the ascending aorta and the pulmonary arterial trunk. The defect is generally large and associated with a torrential pulmonary blood flow and pulmonary hypertension. Congestive cardiac failure is common during infancy and childhood. In the absence of severe pulmonary hypertension the signs are dominated by a wide pulse pressure, cardiomegaly, a systolic murmur at the left and right upper sternal edges, and occasionally a continuous murmur. The electrocardiogram generally shows biventricular hypertrophy, although isolated left or right dominance may be present. Roentgenographic examination of the chest defines the degree of cardiomegaly and shows prominence of the pulmonary artery and ascending aorta, as well as pulmonary plethora. The echocardiogram is helpful in defining the presence of two semilunar valves (which excludes the diagnosis of truncus arteriosus) and shows a normal relationship of a large aorta and pulmonary artery. The diagnosis is confirmed by aortography. The hemodynamic effects are measured at the same time by cardiac catheterization. These defects usually require surgical correction.

TRUNCUS ARTERIOSUS. A single arterial trunk supplies the systemic, pulmonary, and coronary circulations. Both ventricles eject blood through a ventricular septal defect into the single trunk. The number of semilunar valve cusps varies from two to six, and in most patients pulmonary arteries arise from the ascending portion of the truncus proximal to the origin of the innominate artery. When the major source of pulmonary blood flow is from aortopulmonary collateral arteries, the condition is considered to be pulmonary atresia with ventricular septal defect (previously known as truncus arteriosus type IV or pseudo–truncus arteriosus).

In the majority the pulmonary blood flow, pressure, and resistance are greatly increased, so that signs of heart failure appear in infancy. Cyanosis is minimal or absent. The heart is usually enlarged, the precordium is hyperdynamic, a systolic ejection murmur sometimes preceded by a click is audible along the left sternal edge, and the second heart sound is loud and generally single. Occasional patients survive infancy because of the development of severe pulmonary vascular disease, which limits pulmonary blood flow. The clinical picture in these patients simulates that of Eisenmenger's syndrome. Incompetence of the truncal valve or, less frequently, stenosis of this valve may complicate the picture at any age. The diagnosis is confirmed by cardiac catheterization, echocardiography, and angiocardiography. Since rapid deterioration is frequent during infancy, surgical treatment is advised, at which time the ventricular septal defect is closed, the pulmonary arteries are detached from the truncus, and a conduit is inserted from the right ventricle to the pulmonary arteries.

Communication Shunts Between the Aortic Root and the Right Heart

CORONARY ARTERIAL FISTULA. A fistulous branch, most frequently from the right coronary artery, enters the right atrium or right ventricle and occasionally the pulmonary trunk. The right coronary artery becomes massively dilated. Although the volume of shunt from the coronary artery to the right heart is variable, it is usually small. The diagnosis is suspected when an atypically located continuous precordial murmur is heard. The electrocardiogram and chest roentgenogram are normal. Studies using the Doppler technique demonstrate the site of entry of the fistula. The diagnosis is confirmed with an aortic root injection of contrast material that demonstrates the large, tortuous right coronary artery and its site of entry into the right heart. Surgical treatment is advised.

CONGENITAL ANEURYSMS OF THE SINUSES OF VALSALVA. The usual aneurysm involves the right or noncoronary sinus, which begins as a blind pouch or diverticulum. The aneurysms may remain as unruptured diverticula but usually enter the right ventricle or right atrium. Patients with these aneurysms are generally asymptomatic and the left to right shunt is small. The diagnosis is suspected because of an atypically located continuous murmur and confirmed by echocardiography and ascending aortography. Surgical treatment is advisable even in asymptomatic patients. Acute rupture of a large aneurysm in a previously healthy young adult produces a dramatic clinical picture. This is characterized by sudden onset of dyspnea, chest pain, brisk arterial pulses, and a loud continuous murmur. Cardiac failure with pulmonary edema supervenes rapidly. The electrocardiogram shows left or combined ventricular hypertrophy. The chest roentgenogram shows cardiomegaly with prominent vascular markings due to pulmonary arterial overcirculation and prominent pulmonary veins and signs of pulmonary edema. The diagnosis is confirmed by two-dimensional echocardiography and Doppler methods, supplemented by cardiac catheterization and aortography. Surgical correction is urgently indicated in acute rupture.

ANOMALOUS ORIGIN OF THE LEFT CORONARY ARTERY FROM THE PULMONARY TRUNK. The right coronary artery originates normally from the aorta, and the left coronary artery receives blood from intercoronary anastomoses so that blood flow in the left coronary artery drains *into* the pulmonary trunk. Thus left ventricular myocardial perfusion is significantly compromised. Generally symptoms are present within the first few months of life because of myocardial infarction, congestive cardiac failure, and mitral valve incompetence due to papillary muscle dysfunction. About 15 per cent of patients with this anomaly reach adult life because of exuberant intercoronary anastomoses, which may produce a continuous murmur. The electrocardiogram is important because signs of anterior and anterolateral myocardial infarction are present in a relatively young person. The chest roentgenogram shows cardiomegaly with dominance of the left ventricle. The origin of the left coronary artery from the aorta cannot be demonstrated by echocardiography. The diagnosis is confirmed by selective right coronary arteriography, which demonstrates the dilated right coronary artery, the intercoronary anastomoses, and opacification of the left coronary artery from these anastomoses as it enters the pulmonary artery. Reconstitution of normal coronary flow from the aorta to the left coronary artery is advised, although in many instances fibrosis of the left ventricle has resulted in permanent damage to ventricular function.

Pulmonary Arteriovenous Fistula

Fistulous communications between the pulmonary arteries and pulmonary veins may be multiple, small, and diffuse in both lungs or large and relatively localized. Hereditary hemorrhagic telangiectasia (Rendu-Osler-Weber syndrome) with angiomas of the buccal and nasal mucous membranes, gastrointestinal tract, and liver is present in about one half of patients or other members of their family. Desaturated pulmonary arterial blood flows through the fistula and enters the pulmonary vein without oxygenation. When total flow across the fistulous communications is significant, left atrial and left ventricular blood is desaturated, resulting in cyanosis and digital clubbing. Pulmonary arterial pressure remains normal because the flow across the fistula is at low pressure and resistance; cardiomegaly is unusual and heart failure uncommon. Hemoptysis may occur and is sometimes massive. Recurrent epistaxes and gastrointestinal bleeding are features of hereditary hemorrhagic telangiectasia. Transitory central nervous symptoms, including dizziness, vertigo, speech disturbances, visual aberrations, motor weakness, and convulsions, may result from paradoxical emboli, cerebral thromboses, or abscess. Findings on auscultation of the chest may be normal; in others soft systolic or continuous murmurs are audible anywhere

in the chest. The electrocardiogram is usually normal. Roentgenographic examination of the chest shows the presence of large fistulas only. Selective pulmonary arteriography is diagnostic and visualizes the site, extent, and distribution of the fistulas. Large localized fistulous communications are treated surgically by lobectomy or wedge resection. Smaller communications may be obliterated by embolization; these emboli are introduced selectively through a strategically placed catheter in the branch of the pulmonary artery that feeds the fistula. Successful treatment is usually followed by disappearance of symptoms, although in some there is postoperative growth of small previously unrecognized fistulas and recurrence of symptoms.

OBSTRUCTIVE LESIONS WITH OR WITHOUT SHUNTS

Tetralogy of Fallot

Fallot originally described a combination of four defects consisting of pulmonic stenosis, ventricular septal defect, overriding aorta, and right ventricular hypertrophy. The important lesions are pulmonic stenosis and ventricular septal defect. In the normally developing ventricular septum, the infundibular septum above is aligned with the muscular septum below. In Fallot's tetralogy the infundibular septum deviates anteriorly, resulting in malalignment with a ventricular septal defect at the site of malalignment. The anteriorly placed hypoplastic infundibular septum encroaches on the right ventricular outflow tract with a reciprocal increase in aortic root size so that the aorta overrides the ventricular septum. Right ventricular hypertrophy is obligatory because right ventricular pressure is systemic as a result of outflow obstruction and ejection against systemic resistance. Right ventricular outflow obstruction is usually a combination of infundibular and valvular pulmonic stenosis, but the pulmonary trunk may be small and pulmonary artery branch stenosis may be present (Fig. 46–2).

The severity of right ventricular outflow tract obstruction determines the hemodynamics and therefore the clinical picture. Severe obstruction is common, pulmonary blood flow is decreased, and blood is shunted from the right ventricle across the ventricular defect into the aorta. This right to left shunt results in systemic hypoxemia manifested as marked cyanosis, digital clubbing, and erythrocytosis. When obstruction to right ventricular outflow and a ventricular septal defect coexist without right to left shunting, the condition is known as acyanotic tetralogy of Fallot.

In severe cases, *cyanosis* is present from birth. In others, this finding develops in infancy, generally before the first birthday.

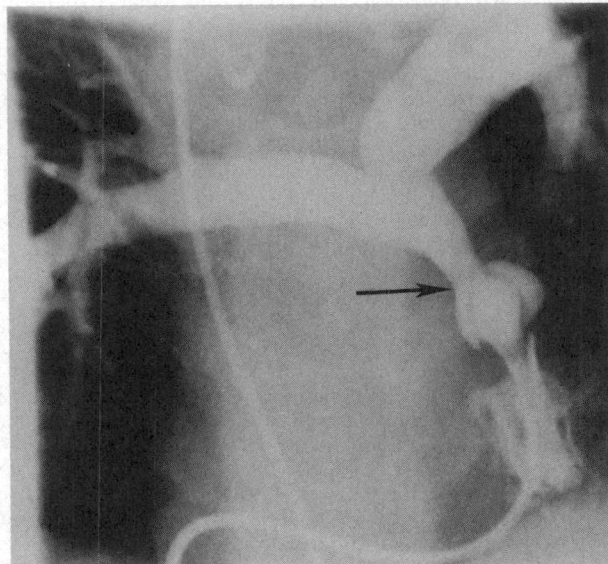

FIGURE 46–2. Cineangiograms in tetralogy of Fallot. Contrast injected in outflow of the right ventricle showing subvalvular obstruction, pulmonary valve stenosis with small annulus (*arrow*), and supravalvular stenosis with short pulmonary arterial trunk.

The absence of cyanosis in the neonatal period is related to maintenance of pulmonary blood flow via a patent ductus arteriosus, which closes spontaneously in the first few months of life. Cyanosis increases in intensity progressively during the first years and is associated with poor physical development. *Dyspnea* with exertion is usual.

Hypoxic ("blue") spells occur primarily in infants with hypoxemia. These spells consist of a sudden onset of dyspnea, restlessness, increased cyanosis, gasping respirations, and syncope. They are associated with a further decrease of arterial Po$_2$ and a reduction of an already compromised pulmonary blood flow. These frightening episodes are treated by placing the child in a knee-chest position and by administering oxygen and intravenous bicarbonate if acidemia develops. The frequency and severity of these episodes can be reduced by oral propranolol. However, surgical treatment is generally indicated to increase pulmonary blood flow and thus relieve the hypoxemia.

Squatting is common in children with hypoxemia, who may assume this position to relieve dyspnea associated with exertion. Physical activity is usually resumed within a few minutes. Squatting decreases the magnitude of right to left shunt by increasing systemic vascular resistance and pulmonary blood flow. Adults seldom squat because they know the limitation of their exercise tolerance and discontinue physical activity before arterial Po$_2$ is significantly decreased.

Physical examination confirms the presence of delayed growth and development, cyanosis, and clubbing. Characteristically, the heart size is normal but the apical impulse is tapping owing to right ventricular hypertrophy. The systolic murmur, sometimes accompanied by a thrill, is produced by the right ventricular outflow tract obstruction. Auscultatory findings are variable; the systolic murmur, which is loudest at the upper left sternal edge but is widely transmitted, may be mid- or pansystolic. The murmur is less intense when the obstruction is severe. Aortic blood flow is increased, and this may result in an early ejection click. The second heart sound is single, produced by aortic valve closure, and pulmonic valve closure is generally inaudible. In rare instances a systolic and diastolic murmur may be audible in any part of the chest, anteriorly or posteriorly, and is produced by bronchial collateral flow to the lung or rarely by a patent ductus arteriosus. This auscultatory finding is frequent with pulmonary atresia.

Roentgenographically the heart size is normal, with a rounded, elevated cardiac apex likened to a wooden shoe (coeur en sabot). There is a concavity in the region of the main pulmonary artery, and the pulmonary vasculature is diminished. The aorta is large and arches to the right in 20 per cent. The *electrocardiogram* shows right-axis deviation and right ventricular hypertrophy. Sometimes the P wave is tall and peaked. *Echocardiography* demonstrates the major intracardiac abnormalities. Echocardiographic examinations show the large ventricular septal defect, the degree of aortic override, and thick right ventricle; the right ventricular outflow tract obstruction may be visualized or inferred from Doppler turbulence in this area. The echocardiogram also helps to distinguish tetralogy of Fallot from other anomalies that may closely simulate this condition, namely, double outlet right ventricle with pulmonic stenosis, arterial transposition with pulmonic stenosis and ventricular septal defect, and a group of complex cardiac malformations consisting primarily of single ventricle and pulmonic stenosis.

These abnormalities are also excluded by *cardiac catheterization and angiocardiography*. Cardiac catheterization confirms that the peak systolic pressures in both ventricles are virtually identical and that there is a significant gradient across the right ventricular outflow. The degree and direction of shunting at the ventricular level are also demonstrated. Arterial oxygen saturation is decreased and at rest is usually between 75 and 85 per cent. Selective right ventriculography identifies the site or sites of right ventricular outflow tract obstruction, the narrowed pulmonic valve ring, the presence of abnormalities of the pulmonary arterial trunk, and any stenoses of the pulmonary arterial branches (Fig. 46–2). In patients with pulmonary atresia, the anatomy of pulmonary blood flow is complex. Although there may not be filling of the main pulmonary artery, a central confluence of left and right intrapulmonary arteries may be present. Left ventriculog-

raphy shows the position and size of the ventricular septal defect and the presence of an overriding aorta. In a few instances, a large coronary artery courses over the right ventricular outflow; preservation of this artery during surgical repair is essential. *Surgical treatment* is usually advised during infancy or childhood. The type of surgical procedure and its timing are still controversial. Infants with severe anoxemia in the first few months of life are frequently treated with a systemic to pulmonary arterial shunt to augment pulmonary arterial blood flow. Beyond the age of 1 to 2 years correction of the defect is advised, at which time any previous systemic to pulmonary shunt is taken down. Older children should have surgical correction of the anomaly because they are generally symptomatic. In all groups surgical correction is more difficult when there is severe deformity of the right ventricular outflow, including a small pulmonic valve ring. The surgical procedure consists of closure of the ventricular septal defect and relief of obstruction by infundibular resection and/or pulmonic valvotomy. Right ventricular outflow may need to be enlarged.

Ebstein's Anomaly of the Tricuspid Valve

This abnormality consists of an abnormal tricuspid valve that is displaced into the right ventricular cavity so that portions of the valve leaflet are attached to the right ventricular wall rather than to the AV ring. The portion of the right ventricle proximal to the tricuspid valve is thin, functions as an extension of the right atrium, and is known as an "atrialized right ventricle." Leaflets of the tricuspid valve are generally redundant and frequently incompetent. The right atrium is large and an atrial septal defect or patent foramen ovale may be present. Increased right atrial pressure, as from tricuspid regurgitation, results in a right to left shunt across the atrial septum and cyanosis of varying degrees. Pulmonary blood flow is decreased.

Ebstein's anomaly in adults varies considerably in severity, so that many patients have active and productive lives, but survival beyond age 50 years is unusual. Symptoms vary in intensity, and with mild anomalies the only complaint is fatigue. Cardiac arrhythmias are frequent and generally supraventricular, the most common being attacks of paroxysmal atrial tachycardia. The precordium is quiet to palpation. Auscultation reveals a systolic murmur, sometimes accompanied by a thrill over most of the anterior left chest, and third and fourth heart sounds are audible, resulting in triple or quadruple rhythms. A diastolic murmur is frequent, appears to be superficial, and may mimic a pericardial friction rub. Other auscultatory findings include multiple systolic ejection clicks and an opening snap of the tricuspid valve. The *electrocardiogram* shows right bundle branch block, tall and/or broad P waves, and a prolonged PR interval. Wolff-Parkinson-White syndrome (usually type B) is present in some. *Roentgenographic examination* shows a variable heart size; in extreme instances massive cardiomegaly is present because of great enlargement of the right atrium (Fig. 46–3). The outflow portion of the right ventricle is sometimes visible in the region usually occupied by the pulmonary artery in the posteroanterior view. The pulmonary vasculature is normal to decreased, and the aorta is small. The *echocardiogram* shows significant delay in tricuspid valve closure and an increased amplitude of motion of the tricuspid valve. The large right atrium and the displaced tricuspid valve can also be visualized. Surgical treatment should be advised in symptomatic patients, especially those with progressive cyanosis. Therapy consists of tricuspid valvuloplasty or valve replacement and ablation of the anomalous pathways between the atrium and ventricle in patients with Wolff-Parkinson-White syndrome and supraventricular tachycardia.

Tricuspid Atresia

In this condition there is no communication between the right atrium and right ventricle so that the entire systemic venous return enters the left heart through a defect in the intra-atrial septum. The left ventricle ejects blood into the normally related aorta and through a ventricular septal defect into the pulmonary arteries. If these vessels are transposed, the aorta arises from a hypoplastic right ventricle that fills from a ventricular septal defect. These patients have a marked increase in pulmonary blood flow and pressure so that heart failure and minimal cyanosis are common in infancy. Survival usually depends upon pulmonary arterial banding to limit pulmonary arterial flow. When the great arteries are normally related, the right ventricle can be minute and associated with marked pulmonic stenosis or atresia. In these patients pulmonary blood flow is derived from a patent ductus arteriosus or collateral bronchial flow. In other instances the left ventricle ejects its blood through a ventricular septal defect into a small right ventricle and then into the pulmonary artery.

Symptoms are usual during infancy and with decreased pulmonary blood flow consist of cyanosis, anoxemia, and poor physical development. Minimal cardiac enlargement is present, and the mid-systolic murmur along the left sternal edge is nonspecific. Left-axis deviation with left ventricular hypertrophy is usual, and these *electrocardiographic findings* in the presence of cyanosis suggest the diagnosis. *Roentgenograms* of the chest show pulmonary undercirculation but are otherwise nonspecific. The *echocardiogram* confirms absence of the tricuspid valve, delineates the size of the small right ventricle, confirms the presence of a large left ventricle, and identifies the presence or absence of transposition of the great arteries. Most infants with decreased pulmonary blood flow require enlargement of the intra-atrial septal defect to ensure easy communication between the two atria as well as a systemic to pulmonary shunt. In later years more radical surgery is undertaken with anastomosis of the right atrium to the pulmonary artery and closure of the intra-atrial septal defect. This procedure effectively separates pulmonary and systemic blood flows, abolishes cyanosis, and improves exercise tolerance. A similar procedure is also used in patients who had pulmonary arterial banding during infancy.

Single Ventricle

Atrial blood empties through two separate AV valves or a common valve into a single ventricle from which the aorta and pulmonary artery arise. Associated cardiac abnormalities are present, but their nature varies considerably. The most frequent ones are transposition of the great arteries, pulmonic stenosis, and aortic origin from a rudimentary outlet chamber. The clinical picture depends on the nature of the associated anomalies. If pulmonic stenosis is severe, cyanosis and anoxemia dominate. In the absence of pulmonic stenosis, pulmonary blood flow and vascular resistance are increased. The clinical picture is then dominated by congestive heart failure. Although these malformations are complex, surgical palliation is undertaken. In the presence of pulmonic stenosis the blood flow is increased with a systemic pulmonary shunt. On the other hand, high pulmonary blood flow is treated with a pulmonary arterial band. In later years, a surgical connection is established between the right atrium and pulmonary artery, and the atria are partitioned so that systemic venous return flows into the pulmonary artery and pulmonary venous return is ejected from the single ventricle into the aorta. When the aorta arises from a rudimentary chamber, systemic flow depends on an unobstructed communication between the single ventricle and the rudimentary chamber. This communication (the bulboventricular foramen) may narrow, resulting in a variable but often significant subaortic gradient. This complication may occur at any time, even postoperatively, and produces cardiomegaly and heart failure.

Inflow Obstruction to the Left Ventricle

Conditions of inflow obstruction are grouped together because they result in high pulmonary venous pressure with potential pulmonary edema. The lesions may occur anywhere from the insertion of the pulmonary veins into the left atrium to the area of the mitral valve. They are extremely rare abnormalities. *Pulmonary vein stenoses* at their site of entry into the left atrium are difficult to treat surgically or by balloon angioplasty. *Cor triatriatum* consists of a diaphragmatic partition of the left atrium. The upper portion receives the pulmonary veins, and the distal portion communicates with the mitral valve or through an atrial septal defect into the right atrium. The opening in the diaphragm is generally small so that symptoms are present in early life. The condition is surgically correctable by excision of the diaphragm and closure of associated atrial septal defects. A *supravalvular ring* above the mitral valve produces a similar clinical picture. *Congenital mitral stenosis* may be due to marked abnormality of the mitral valve apparatus, which includes fused, thickened mitral valve leaflets with short chordae, or the valve may have a parachute deformity in which the leaflets are also abnormal but the chordae converge and insert into a single papillary muscle.

Hypoplastic Left Heart Syndrome

Varying degrees of underdevelopment of the left side of the heart coexist, including marked underdevelopment of the left ventricle and atrium, and stenosis or atresia of the aortic and mitral orifices with hypoplasia of the ascending aorta. This complex malformation is a significant cause of cardiovascular death in the neonatal period. Attempts at surgical management have not been standardized.

OBSTRUCTIVE AND REGURGITANT LESIONS
Pulmonic Stenosis with Intact Ventricular Septum

Obstruction to right ventricular outflow can be valvular, subvalvular, supravalvular, or a combination of obstructions at these sites. Valvular obstruction, the most common variety, results from varying degrees of commissural fusion so that the deformed valve appears domelike. Dysplastic thick valve leaflets are less common and may accompany Noonan's syndrome. Subvalvular obstruction usually accompanies severe valvular stenosis, is due to infundibular hypertrophy, and occasionally is seen as an isolated abnormality with a normal pulmonic valve. Pulmonary arterial branch stenosis may be isolated or may occur at multiple sites and may be associated with supravalvular stenosis. These peripheral lesions are a feature of congenital rubella.

The hemodynamic consequences of valvular pulmonic stenosis are produced by the severity of obstruction. When the right ventricular outflow gradient is between 50 and 80 mm Hg the obstruction is considered to be moderate; pressures below and above that range are considered mild and severe, respectively. Pulmonary arterial pressure is normal or low. The arterial oxygen saturation is normal except when the obstruction is severe (sometimes with suprasystemic right ventricular pressure). Poor right ventricular compliance with or without an increase in right

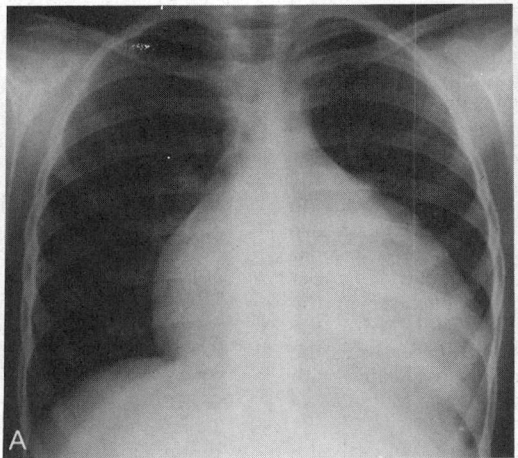
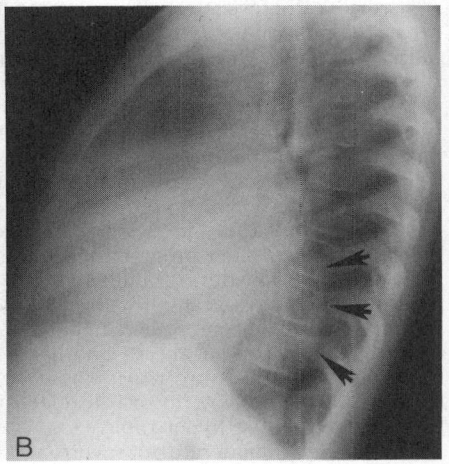

FIGURE 46–3. Chest roentgenograms in Ebstein's anomaly of the tricuspid valve. *A,* Posteroanterior view showing globular cardiac silhouette with narrow waist simulating pericardial effusion. *B,* Left anterior oblique view showing marked cardiomegaly due to massive right atrial enlargement, which extends posteriorly (*arrows*) and also encroaches on the anterior clear space.

ventricular end-diastolic pressure increases right atrial pressure and may result in right to left shunting across the intra-atrial septum.

Symptoms are usually absent when the obstruction is mild or moderate, but when it is severe, effort dyspnea may be present. The physique is frequently normal, and some patients appear robust. When the stenosis is *mild*, the venous pressure is normal and the heart is not enlarged. A systolic murmur of varying intensity with mid-systolic peaking is heard best at the upper left sternal edge and is preceded by a pulmonic ejection click. The second heart sound may be normal, but the pulmonic component is frequently delayed and of normal intensity. The electrocardiogram is normal or shows signs of minimal right ventricular hypertrophy. The chest *roentgenogram* shows prominence of the pulmonary arterial trunk because of poststenotic dilatation, but the heart size and pulmonary vasculature are normal. Echocardiography shows the domed stenotic valve. When pulmonic stenosis is *moderate*, the venous pressure may be normal or slightly elevated, with a prominent "a" wave in the jugular pulse. A right ventricular parasternal lift is palpable and may be accompanied by a systolic thrill at the upper left sternal edge. The systolic murmur, frequently preceded by an ejection sound, is accentuated in late systole. The second heart sound is split with a delayed and diminished pulmonic component. Electrocardiographic evidence of right ventricular hypertrophy is usual, sometimes with a prominent spiked P wave. The chest roentgenogram shows a normal or mildly enlarged heart, prominence of the pulmonary arterial trunk, and normal pulmonary vasculature. The abnormal valve is visualized by echocardiograms.

In *severe* pulmonic stenosis cyanosis may be present, owing to a small cardiac output or a right to left shunt across the intra-atrial septum. A large presystolic "a" wave is usual in the jugular venous pulse and the increased venous pressure may be transmitted to the liver, resulting in a presystolic pulsation. The heart is moderately or greatly enlarged, with a conspicuous parasternal right ventricular lift. The systolic ejection murmur is usually loud, frequently accompanied by a thrill, and audible maximally at the upper left sternal edge, but it may radiate widely over the entire precordium and into the neck and back. The murmur is accentuated in late systole, frequently encompasses the aortic component of the second heart sound, and may be preceded by an ejection sound. The pulmonic component of the second heart sound is either inaudible or soft and very late. The electrocardiogram shows gross right ventricular hypertrophy with tall P waves attributed to right atrial enlargement. The chest roentgenogram confirms the cardiac enlargement, prominence of the right ventricle and atrium, poststenotic dilatation of the pulmonary artery, and pulmonary vasculature that is either normal or decreased. The echocardiogram demonstrates systolic doming of the stenotic leaflets into the dilated pulmonary arterial trunk. In the presence of significant obstruction, the right ventricular wall is thick, the right atrium is enlarged, and the intra-atrial septum bows toward the left. The degree of obstruction is quantified with Doppler techniques by applying a modified Bernoulli equation using peak velocity of flow ($P = 4v^2$, where P = pressure gradient and v = peak flow velocity).

Cardiac catheterization demonstrates the pressure gradient across the pulmonic valve and determines the degree of severity. Selective right ventriculography visualizes the site and nature of the obstruction. During ventricular systole contrast material is seen as a jet through the domed stenotic valve. Subvalvular hypertrophy, which may intensify the obstruction, is also demonstrated by this method.

The clinical course of patients with mild obstruction is usually good, and progression of the disease is unusual, especially in adolescence and adult life. Many with moderate obstruction also do well, although their progress needs to be evaluated at regular intervals, especially during childhood. Progression of the obstruction is detected clinically by the change in character of the murmur, which becomes accentuated in late systole. Also, the width of the splitting of the second heart sound increases as the right ventricular pressure rises. These signs are associated with an increase in the severity of the electrocardiographic signs of the right ventricular hypertrophy.

Treatment of moderate to severe obstruction is by valvulo-

plasty, accomplished by a balloon catheter inserted percutaneously. Rapid inflation and deflation of the balloon placed across the valve annulus significantly increases the size of the valve orifice. This results in an immediate decrease in right ventricular pressure which is maintained for years, and recurrence of obstruction is unusual. Postvalvuloplasty pulmonary valve regurgitation is infrequent and when present is mild. The results in adults with severe obstruction may not be as good. Right ventricular dysfunction may persist despite relief of gradient, and this has been attributed to a poorly compliant ventricle because of persistent hypertrophy and fibrosis. Surgery is reserved for patients with dysplastic pulmonary valve leaflets.

Bicuspid Aortic Valve

This condition is said to occur in about 2 per cent of the population. The valve consists of two commissures and two cusps, one of which is generally larger. The bicuspid aortic valve may have normal function so that there is no systolic gradient across the valve and during diastole the valve remains competent. This normal function may continue throughout life, and the bicuspid valve may be found only incidentally at necropsy. In others, abnormality of the aortic valve can be suspected during examination of teenagers or young adults. These findings relate to minor degrees of valvular obstruction and/or incompetence. The auscultatory findings consist of short, soft systolic murmurs heard at the upper right sternal edge. An early aortic ejection click, which precedes the murmur, excludes an innocent murmur. In others, the systolic murmur may be followed by a short, high-pitched early diastolic murmur of aortic incompetence. The diagnosis may be confirmed by echocardiography, which demonstrates only two aortic leaflets (Fig. 46–4).

The natural course of bicuspid aortic valves is variable. In some, the valve may function normally for many decades and produce no abnormal clinical signs. In others the valve leaflets become thickened, fibrotic, and calcified, so that clear signs of aortic stenosis of varying severity develop during early or mid-adult life. In others, there is eversion or prolapse of one of the aortic cusps, resulting in progressive aortic regurgitation that can become severe. A bicuspid aortic valve is particularly susceptible to infective endocarditis, which may convert a benign lesion into one associated with acute severe aortic regurgitation.

Congenital Valvular Aortic Stenosis

See Ch. 49 for a discussion of this lesion.

Subvalvular Aortic Stenosis (Discrete)

Obstruction to left ventricular outflow is produced by a fibrous membrane situated just below the aortic valve. The membrane is a collar-like structure extending from the intraventricular septum and involving the anterior mitral leaflet. The high-velocity jet of blood flowing through the obstructed area during ventricular systole impinges on the aortic valve, which results in fibrous thickening and incompetence of the valve. The clinical picture simulates that of valvular aortic stenosis with important exceptions. An aortic ejection sound is usually absent, and the murmur occupies the whole of systole. This condition is frequently mistaken for a ventricular septal defect or mitral incompetence. Mild forms of obstruction may coexist with other lesions, especially a ventricular septal defect. This obstruction may be unrecognized

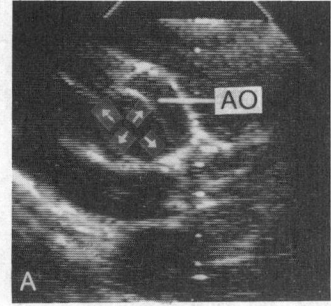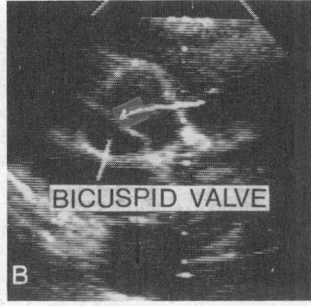

FIGURE 46–4. Short axis echocardiogram of bicuspid aortic valve (AO). *A*, Open valve orifice during systole (*arrows*). *B*, Competent bicuspid valve during diastole. Arrow points to line of apposition of valve leaflets.

at the time of surgical closure of the ventricular septal defect, and the obstruction may progress over the ensuing years. A useful differential sign is the presence of an early diastolic murmur of aortic valve incompetence, which is a common finding when the obstruction is moderate or severe. Laboratory findings simulate those described under valvular aortic stenosis. However, the echocardiogram is diagnostic in that the discrete membrane is visualized. Cardiac catheterization and angiocardiography measure the severity of obstruction and outline the membrane by left ventriculography or aortography if the aortic valve is incompetent. Indications for surgery are liberalized, since continued damage to the aortic valve should be prevented. Excision of the membrane gives immediate good results, but complications include damage to the anterior mitral leaflet with resultant regurgitation or conduction abnormalities, including complete heart block from trauma to the intraventricular septum. Furthermore, there may be recurrence of obstruction from regrowth of the membrane.

A rarer form of subaortic stenosis is a long, narrow fibromuscular channel frequently associated with hypoplasia of the aortic ring. This disease is more frequent in childhood and is difficult to treat surgically because relief of obstruction may require enlargement of the aortic valve ring. In extreme cases a valve-bearing conduit is inserted between the left ventricle and the aorta.

Hypertrophic Cardiomyopathy

See Ch. 50.

Supravalvular Aortic Stenosis

The obstruction may be localized to a segmental hourglass-shaped narrowing immediately above the aortic sinuses. Beyond the area of obstruction the aorta may be normal in diameter or show varying degrees of tubular hypoplasia, frequently involving the ascending aorta but occasionally extending for a varying length along the course of the aorta, even to its bifurcation. Aortic valve leaflets may be thickened, with resultant mild aortic regurgitation. During systole the aortic valve leaflets may impinge upon the orifices of the coronary arteries so that coronary flow is impaired; this may be further aggravated by the coronary arteries themselves, which can be enlarged and tortuous but have a narrow lumen. Supravalvular aortic stenosis is frequently associated with the *Williams syndrome*, consisting of typical facies (broad, prominent forehead, flattened bridge of the nose, epicanthal folds, and long upper lip), mild mental retardation, and low-pitched voice; children with this syndrome are particularly friendly and converse easily. In the absence of the Williams syndrome, supravalvular aortic stenosis occurs sporadically and is sometimes familial. Pulmonary arterial branch stenosis may coexist. Carotid and brachial arterial pulses may be asymmetric, with more conspicuous pulses on the right side. This finding has been attributed to preferential flow into the innominate artery. Other components of the clinical picture simulate those described under valvular aortic stenosis. Echocardiography visualizes the ascending aorta, identifies the area and severity of obstruction, and defines the degree of aortic hypoplasia. Cardiac catheterization and angiocardiography confirm the severity of the obstruction, visualize the anatomy of the aorta and the obstruction, and demonstrate severity of pulmonary arterial branch stenosis, if present. Surgical treatment to relieve the obstruction is advised when the gradient is severe. However, surgical treatment is complicated, especially when the transverse and thoracic aortae are markedly hypoplastic.

Coarctation of the Aorta

Narrowing of the aortic lumen may occur at isolated or multiple sites in the aorta. By far the most common site of discrete obstruction is just distal to the origin of the left subclavian artery. The lesion is more frequent in males and is also seen in patients with Turner's (XO) syndrome. Associated cardiac malformations are frequent, the most common being a bicuspid aortic valve, congenital aortic stenosis with or without incompetence, ventricular septal defect, and lesions of the mitral valve with or without valvular regurgitation. Extensive collateralization usually develops, especially from branches of the subclavian, internal mammary, superior intercostal, and axillary arteries. These vessels join the intercostal arteries of the descending aorta and inferior epigastric branches of the femoral arteries, which allow channels for arterial blood to bypass the area of coarctation. These collateral vessels can become enormously enlarged and tortuous by early adult life.

Children and young adults are generally asymptomatic. However, hypertension may develop in the arteries above the coarctation and may be associated with epistaxis and throbbing headaches. Other symptoms include leg fatigue, complaints of cold extremities, and occasionally intermittent claudication. Beyond the second decade coarctation may be discovered by the finding of brachial arterial hypertension during routine physical examination. The methods of presentation in adults include infective endocarditis, usually involving the aortic valve, and rupture of the aorta or dissecting aneurysm may occur, especially in the 20's and 30's. The site of rupture is either in the proximal aorta or in an aneurysm in the area of coarctation. Cerebral vascular disease with resultant cerebral hemorrhage or infarction may result from complications of hypertension or from the rupture of an aneurysm, usually of the circle of Willis. Hypertension and associated atherosclerosis of the coronary circulation may result in congestive cardiac failure, sometimes preceded by acute myocardial infarction. Pregnancy is usually well tolerated, especially if hypertension is controlled. However, the risk of aortic rupture is increased, especially toward the end of the third trimester.

Classic signs of aortic coarctation are the disparity in pulsations and blood pressures of the arms and legs. The bounding pulses of the arms and carotid vessels contrast with the weak, delayed, or absent femoral and/or distal arterial pulses in the legs. Also, the blood pressure in the arms exceeds that in the legs. This applies especially to the systolic reading, and there is a further rise of systolic blood pressure in response to exercise. If the systolic arterial pressure in the right arm exceeds that of the left arm by more than 30 mm Hg, the left subclavian artery is involved in the coarctation. Collateral arterial circulation may be visible but is usually palpable, especially in the back, at the angles of the scapulae and in the axillae. Murmurs are variable in location, quality, and intensity. The usual is a precordial midsystolic murmur heard best at the left sternal edge, but it may be loudest in the back between the scapulae. Additional systolic or sometimes continuous murmurs are audible over the anterior or posterior chest and are produced by flow through the large, tortuous collateral arteries. The *electrocardiogram* is usually normal during childhood and adolescence. In adults, varying degrees of left ventricular hypertrophy are present. *Roentgenographic* examinations during childhood may not be striking. However, prominence of the left ventricle occurs thereafter and during adult life. The heart may be moderately enlarged. Notching of the inferior border of the ribs from collateral vessels is common. This may be unilateral if one of the subclavian arteries arises below the area of coarctation. Poststenotic dilatation of the descending aorta is usual and is demonstrated by a barium esophagram, and the prominent left subclavian artery produces a shadow in the left mediastinum. *Echocardiography* visualizes the area of coarctation, the large left subclavian artery, poststenotic dilatation of the descending aorta, and associated intracardiac anomalies, especially those of the aortic valve. The site of obstruction, localized aortic aneurysms, and the aortic size are well visualized by magnetic resonance imaging. Two options are now available for therapy and consist of surgical resection or angioplasty. Successful surgical coarctectomy has been undertaken for more than four decades with a low operative mortality. Experience with angioplasty is more recent and follow-up relatively short. There is also debate as to whether angioplasty should be reserved for recoarctation, but successful angioplasty of native coarctation has also been accomplished. Long-term follow-up after surgical coarctectomy in childhood indicates that complications are frequent when patients reach adult life. These consist of recurrence of coarctation, hypertension, atherosclerotic coronary artery disease, aneurysm at the site of coarctectomy, and progressive aortic stenosis and/or regurgitation. It is therefore imperative that patients be followed regularly and treatment instituted (especially for hypertension) prior to onset of complications.

Pulmonic Valvular Regurgitation

Isolated congenital pulmonic valve regurgitation is rare and seldom produces symptoms; an early diastolic murmur at the upper left sternal edge is the only abnormal sign. However, pulmonic valvular regurgitation may accompany other conditions such as those associated with severe pulmonary hypertension or after surgical transection of the pulmonic valve ring for the treatment of severe obstruction of the right ventricular outflow.

Absence of Pulmonic Valve

Absence of the pulmonic valve is a congenital anomaly in which pulmonic valve leaflets are virtually absent. Although the lesion may be isolated it is usually associated with other defects, especially tetralogy of Fallot or isolated ventricular septal defect.

Vascular Rings and Other Aortic Arch Anomalies

The more common anomalies are double aortic arch, right aortic arch with left ligamentum arteriosum, origin of the right subclavian artery from the thoracic aorta distal to the left subclavian artery, anomalous origin of the innominate or left carotid arteries, and anomalous left pulmonary artery, which arises from the elongated pulmonary trunk and courses between the trachea and the esophagus. The clinical picture is extremely variable, and in many instances there are no symptoms. Tracheal compression, especially during infancy, produces respiratory distress with wheezing and a brassy cough. Dysphagia may occur in older patients. Surgery is advised in symptomatic patients to relieve the tracheal and esophageal compression.

THE TRANSPOSITIONS

Transposition of the Great Arteries

In this condition the aorta arises from the right ventricle and the pulmonary artery from the left ventricle. Systemic venous return is to the right atrium, and pulmonary venous return is to the left atrium. Systemic venous blood flows through the tricuspid valve into the right ventricle and is ejected into the aorta. Pulmonary venous blood flows from the left atrium through the mitral valve into the left ventricle and is ejected into the pulmonary artery. Thus, the circulations are parallel. Survival is dependent on mixture of blood through the foramen ovale, a ventricular septal defect, or patency of the ductus arteriosus. This condition is a common malformation that occurs predominantly in males, with symptoms in the neonatal period or soon thereafter.

ISOLATED "SIMPLE" TRANSPOSITION OF THE GREAT ARTERIES. In this malformation the ventricular septum is intact. Mixing of systemic and pulmonary blood occurs primarily from bidirectional shunting across the foramen ovale. This condition produces symptoms and signs of anoxemia in the neonate, is suspected in an otherwise normal neonate who is cyanotic and tachypneic, and is verified by echocardiography, which demonstrates the abnormal origin of the great arteries, as well as the fact that the aorta is usually anterior to the pulmonary artery. Emergency balloon atrial septostomy that ruptures the foramen ovale allows greater mixing at the atrial level and decompresses the left atrium. The arterial switch operation is the treatment of choice in the neonate whereby the origins of the great arteries are transected and the pulmonary artery is connected to the stump of the vessel arising from the right ventricle and the aorta to the left ventricle with implantation of the coronary arteries into the new aorta. This procedure is preferred over intra-atrial redirection of venous return because many years after the latter operation supraventricular tachy- or bradyarrhythmias or systemic (right) ventricular failure occurs.

TRANSPOSITION OF THE GREAT ARTERIES WITH VENTRICULAR SEPTAL DEFECT. When the septal defect is small, the clinical picture is similar to that of simple transposition, and many of these small defects close spontaneously. If the ventricular septal defect is large and nonrestrictive, significant mixing of blood occurs and symptoms are frequently delayed. The clinical picture is dominated by signs of congestive cardiac failure with minimal cyanosis. In the untreated state there is progressive pulmonary hypertension with severe pulmonary vascular disease. Surgical treatment is required during infancy, and the preferred procedure is the arterial switch and closure of the ventricular septal defect. Another option is pulmonary arterial banding during infancy to restrict pulmonary blood flow and prevent the onset of pulmonary vascular disease. In later years, usually during childhood, the second stage is undertaken, in which the pulmonary artery is debanded and transected, the ventricular septal defect is closed so that the left ventricle ejects blood into the aorta, and a conduit is placed from the right ventricle to the transected pulmonary artery (*Rastelli procedure*).

TRANSPOSITION OF THE GREAT ARTERIES WITH PULMONIC STENOSIS. The importance of this condition is that it may closely simulate the clinical picture produced by tetralogy of Fallot. The condition generally requires an aortic pulmonary shunt during infancy to increase pulmonary blood flow and relieve the symptoms of anoxemia. In later years the Rastelli procedure is undertaken.

Double Outlet Right Ventricle

In this malformation both the pulmonary artery and the aorta arise from the right ventricle, and the only outlet from the left ventricle is a ventricular septal defect. The clinical picture simulates a large, uncomplicated ventricular septal defect with pulmonary hypertension. The echocardiogram is diagnostic in that there is discontinuity between the anterior mitral leaflet and the aorta, since the latter structure arises from the right ventricle. Uncontrollable heart failure and pulmonary hypertension are frequent during infancy so that pulmonary arterial banding is usually required. In later years, generally during childhood, the Rastelli operation is advised. Another option is the arterial switch operation. Double outlet right ventricle may be complicated by pulmonic stenosis when the condition simulates that described under Tetralogy of Fallot.

Corrected Transposition (L Transposition of the Great Arteries)

This condition consists of *ventricular inversion* and transposition of the great arteries. Systemic venous blood enters a normal right atrium, flows through a mitral valve into the left ventricle, and is ejected into the pulmonary artery. Pulmonary venous blood flows from the left atrium through a tricuspid valve into the right ventricle and is ejected into the aorta. If the condition is uncomplicated, blood flow and hemodynamics are normal. However, associated anomalies are usual, such as ventricular septal defect, pulmonic stenosis, left AV valve (tricuspid) anomalies, including an Ebstein-like malformation of this valve, and AV conduction abnormalities—frequently complete AV block. The clinical picture is dominated by the associated lesions. The chest roentgenogram may suggest the abnormal origin of the great arteries in that the ascending aorta occupies the upper left border of the cardiac silhouette in the posteroanterior view. Since ventricular inversion is present, the electrocardiogram may show absence of q waves in leads I and V_6, initial q waves in III, aVF, and V_1, and prominent T waves in the right precordial leads. During surgical treatment the bundle of His may be injured because it is located abnormally, so that complete heart block may occur. In others, significant regurgitations via the Ebstein-like tricuspid valve requires valve replacement.

Anomalous Pulmonary Venous Connection

The anomalous pulmonary venous return may be partial or total. *Partial anomalous pulmonary venous return* simulates the clinical picture produced by a secundum atrial septal defect. In fact, one of these forms is the sinus venosus defect.

TOTAL ANOMALOUS PULMONARY VENOUS CONNECTION. The site of entry of the pulmonary veins may be supradiaphragmatic (into a left superior vena cava or vertical vein, coronary sinus, right superior vena cava, or right atrium) or infradiaphragmatic (portal vein, hepatic veins, or inferior vena cava). Thus, there is no connection between the pulmonary vein and the left atrium. Generally the pulmonary veins converge to form a single trunk, which then enters the systemic venous circulation. Varying degrees of pulmonary venous obstruction are present and depend on the length of the common pulmonary venous trunk before its entry into the systemic vein as well as localized areas of obstruction.

The clinical picture is variable. In some instances, especially those of infradiaphragmatic connection, pulmonary edema and cyanosis are present in the neonatal period or soon thereafter. When there is a large intra-atrial communication and obstruction to pulmonary venous return is moderate, symptoms occur in later infancy and the clinical picture is dominated by congestive cardiac failure. When pulmonary venous obstruction is absent and there is a large communication between the right and left atria, symptoms may be delayed until early childhood and very occasionally adolescence. The clinical picture of these patients simulates that produced by a large left to right shunt at the atrial level.

The *electrocardiogram* reflects the hemodynamic state so that symptomatic infants have marked right ventricular hypertrophy with prominent P waves. Chest *roentgenograms* in neonates with pulmonary venous obstruction are characterized by pulmonary edema with a normal heart size. In older infants the heart is large and pulmonary overcirculation evident. In older children with pulmonary venous connection to the left superior vena cava, the cardiac silhouette has the appearance of a snowman or figure 8. The supracardiac shadow is produced by marked dilatation of the left superior vena cava, innominate vein, and right superior vena cava. The *echocardiogram* shows signs of right volume overload, and color flow imaging identifies the site of entry of pulmonary veins. *Cardiac catheterization* demonstrates the severity of pulmonary hypertension, and pulmonary arteriograms show return of contrast material to the pulmonary veins and their anomalous site of insertion into the systemic venous circulation. Surgical treatment is indicated when the common pulmonary venous trunk is anastomosed to the left atrium, the atrial septal defect closed, and the anomalous connection to the systemic venous system obliterated. Results of surgical treatment have been good, with greatest risk in symptomatic neonates.

CARDIAC MALPOSITION

Knowledge of the position of the heart as well as the location (situs) of abdominal viscera aids in defining the nature of these anomalies. Roentgenography of the abdomen helps identify abdominal situs by localizing the position of the stomach bubble and other abdominal structures, but many viscera cannot be visualized by this method alone. Generally, atrial and visceral situs are related; if the viscera are normally located, the atria have a normal position. In abdominal situs inversus, the left atrium is usually to the right and the right atrium to the left. Location of the atria is further and more accurately assessed by evaluation of the tracheobronchial air column on chest roentgenogram. A normal tracheobronchial tree with an epiarterial bronchus on the right indicates normal atrial situs, and this finding is independent of the position of the heart.

Dextrocardia

The heart is in the right chest, and the cardiac apex points to the right. Associated abdominal situs inversus (mirror-image dextrocardia) in adults is usually associated with a normally functioning heart. However, poorly motile cilia may result in sinusitis and bronchiectasis (Kartagener's syndrome). Dextrocardia may be discovered by physical examination when the heart sounds are more clear in the right chest or accidentally on a routine chest film. The electrocardiogram demonstrates the mirror image, so that the P, QRS, and T are inverted in lead I; aV$_R$ and aV$_L$ are the reverse of normal, and the right precordial leads resemble those usually recorded from the left chest. *Isolated dextrocardia* with abdominal viscera in normal position (situs solitus) is invariably associated with various combinations of severe cardiac malformations, the most common being ventricular inversion, single ventricle, pulmonic stenosis, abnormalities of the AV valves, and anomalies of systemic and pulmonary venous return.

Isolated Levocardia

Isolated levocardia is accompanied by varying degrees of anomalous position of abdominal viscera (heterotaxia) so that situs inversus is partial or complete. Severe cardiac malformations are usual, including various combinations of anomalies of systemic and pulmonary venous return, common AV canal, pulmonic stenosis or atresia, defects of the atrial and ventricular septa, and single ventricle.

Mesocardia

Mesocardia is the term used when the heart is centrally located in the chest or the cardiac silhouette on roentgenogram is toward the right chest. The cardiac anatomy is normal with normal relationships of the cardiac chambers, venous return, and origin of the great arteries. Cardiac malformations are usually absent.

Asplenia Syndrome

This condition is characterized by absence of the spleen, undefinable situs of the abdominal viscera (situs ambiguus), bilateral *right-sidedness*, and complex, severe cardiac malformations. Bilateral right-sidedness is identified by bilateral trilobed lungs with bilateral epiarterial bronchi. In the majority the liver is located centrally so that the liver edge is palpable across the entire upper abdomen. The stomach is located on the right in about half the patients, and varying degrees of malrotation of the small bowel are present. Both atria have the morphologic characteristics of the right atrium. Common cardiovascular anomalies include total anomalous pulmonary venous connection, transposition of the great arteries, pulmonic stenosis or atresia, complete AV canal, single ventricle, and dextrocardia. The condition is suspected in a deeply cyanotic male infant with dextrocardia and a centrally placed liver. Howell-Jolly and Heinz bodies in the peripheral red blood cells are suggestive of asplenia, but these findings are not conclusive. Infants with asplenia are susceptible to severe intercurrent infections so that continued antibiotic prophylaxis has been suggested as a preventive measure. Aortopulmonary shunts during infancy are indicated when severe anoxemia is present owing to pulmonic stenosis, and right atrial-pulmonary shunts (Fontan) are advised in later years.

Polysplenia Syndrome

The features of this condition are multiple splenic masses (two or more), ambiguous abdominal situs, and *bilateral left-sidedness*; while cardiovascular abnormalities are frequent, they are generally not as complex as in the asplenia syndrome. The lungs are bilobed and epiarterial bronchi are absent. The liver is frequently located centrally in the upper abdomen, and the stomach is right- or left-sided. Malrotation of the bowel is common. Both atria have the morphologic features of the left atrium. The hepatic segment of the inferior vena cava is frequently absent so that systemic venous return is by way of the azygos vein. The cardiac apex points to the left in the majority. Pulmonary venous return may be normal, arterial transposition is present in only a minority, and pulmonic stenosis is unusual. The cardiac malformations are generally associated with left to right shunts at atrial or ventricular levels.

THE ADULT WITH "UNCURED" CONGENITAL HEART DISEASE

Strategies of management of symptomatic patients with congenital heart disease have changed recently so that the majority are treated during infancy or early childhood. Many adolescents and adults now exist who have trivial lesions, have remained asymptomatic, and have lived a normal lifestyle. Other patients have anomalies that are silent until adult life. Palliative surgery may have been undertaken in another group who have remained relatively well and have now approached adult life. Another cohort of patients who may not have had surgical treatment during early life develop progressive pulmonary hypertension during childhood, and in adult life their lesions are associated with severe pulmonary vascular disease. This section discusses these groups of patients.

VENTRICULAR SEPTAL DEFECTS. A significant number of patients seen in pediatric cardiac clinics have trivial shunts across a small ventricular septal defect. They remain asymptomatic throughout the growing years, and as adults the only abnormal physical sign is a long, harsh systolic murmur, which may be accompanied by a thrill and is heard best at the lower left sternal edge. It is unusual to see such patients beyond the age of 40 years so that it has been assumed that many of these defects close spontaneously. While the defect remains, these patients are at risk to develop infective endocarditis and occasionally aortic regurgitation or discrete subaortic stenosis.

VALVULAR PULMONIC STENOSIS. Generally, asymptomatic children with mild pulmonic stenosis (resting peak right ventricular pressure less than one half of systolic systemic pressure) do not require surgical treatment. There is no consensus about the course of untreated mild to moderate pulmonic stenosis. The generally held belief, however, is that progressive increase in severity is unusual, especially if the patient is beyond the age of 12 years. This optimistic view also applies to those who had a valvotomy during childhood, which relieved the obstruction. Restriction of physical activity is not required, pregnancy is well tolerated, and, although infective endocarditis of the pulmonic valve is not common, prophylaxis is advisable at the time of risk for this complication.

CONGENITAL COMPLETE HEART BLOCK. Fetal echocardiography may be prompted by the recognition of intrauterine bradycardia, and this test unmasks the presence of complete atrioventricular (AV) block. This study is especially important during pregnancy of mothers with connective tissue disease, such as systemic lupus erythematosus, since the offspring are at greater risk for complete AV block. It is suggested that antinuclear antibodies of the IgG category cross the placenta and damage the fetal conduction system. This occurs in mothers whose disease is active but also when there are no overt clinical manifestations and only positive serologic evidence is present. In about 70 per cent of children with complete AV block the lesion is isolated, and the remainder have associated complex cardiac malformations, such as ventricular inversion or single ventricle. Familial complete AV block is well recognized. Adolescents and adults with isolated congenital complete AV block are usually asymptomatic, but it is not possible to predict episodes of syncope. The pulse rate is inappropriately slow for age. The large stroke volume and vasodilatation produce jerky pulses, systolic hypertension, and cardiomegaly. Cannon waves may be visible in the jugular venous pulse. The first heart sound varies in intensity and may be followed by a nonspecific mid-systolic ejection murmur. The diagnosis is confirmed by the electrocardiogram, in which there is no constant relationship between the P waves and QRS complexes. Usually the QRS is of normal duration, which suggests that the site of the lesion is above the bundle of His. Marked ventricular slowing may be recorded by continuous, 24-hour electrocardiographic monitoring, especially during sleep. It is not known whether there is any relationship between the slow ventricular rates during sleep and the prognosis. Since patients with congenital complete AV block have been observed in late adult life, there is a generally held view that the prognosis is good. However, the lesion is not benign, in that complications may occur at any time and are not predictable. Syncope is an indication for implantation of a permanent pacemaker. Decisions about treatment in asymptomatic patients are more difficult. The demonstration of ventricular tachycardia or fibrillation during continuous electrocardiographic monitoring or graded exercise testing is an indication for pacemaker implantation. There remains a group of asymptomatic patients in whom treatment is not standardized, including those with premature ventricular contractions during and after exercise, extreme nocturnal bradycardia, and ventricular depolarization initiated from a focus low in the bundle of His.

EISENMENGER'S SYNDROME. This syndrome is associated with marked elevation of pulmonary vascular resistance with reversed or bidirectional shunt, which is intracardiac or between the aorta and pulmonary arteries. Thus, pulmonary vascular disease is the hallmark of this syndrome, and the site of the shunt is incidental. Medial hypertrophy of pulmonary arteries and arterioles is present and is associated with cellular, fibrotic, and fibroelastic intimal reactions, and in more severe forms plexiform lesions encroach into the lumen of the vessel. These changes in the pulmonary vascular bed are directly related to pulmonary arterial pressure. Extension of muscle into the peripheral arteries occurs when pulmonary hypertension is still associated with increased pulmonary blood flow. With progressive vascular disease, a reduction in the number of small arteries may precede obliterative pulmonary vascular disease.

Historically these patients are frequently symptomatic during infancy and early childhood because of congestive cardiac failure, poor physical development, and recurrent lower respiratory tract infections. As pulmonary vascular resistance rises, the left to right shunt decreases so that symptoms improve. These children may lead nearly normal lives, but their stamina is limited and mild exertional cyanosis is evident. In early adult life there is progressive anoxemia with intensification of cyanosis, digital clubbing may be extreme, and, erythrocytosis increases. Progressive decrease in effort tolerance develops over many years, culminating in congestive cardiac failure in early or mid-adult life. Other symptoms are produced by hyperviscosity, a bleeding diathesis, or hyperuricemia. Angina pectoris attributed to right ventricular ischemia, syncope, and palpitations from premature atrial or ventricular contractions may be present. Jugular venous pressure is increased, with a prominent "v" wave in the presence of complicating tricuspid valve regurgitation. Hepatomegaly and marked dependent edema with ascites are usual with heart failure. The heart size is increased to a variable extent, greatest when there are shunts at the atrial level and when there is complicating tricuspid and/or pulmonic valve incompetence. The precordium is active with a right ventricular heave along the left sternal edge. Pulmonary arterial pulsations and the second heart sound may be palpable at the upper left sternal edge. The systolic murmur varies in intensity and is frequently initiated by a pulmonic ejection click. The second heart sound is booming, single, or narrowly split in ventricular shunts, but wide, fixed splitting may be audible in isolated atrial shunts. Signs of pulmonary and/or tricuspid valve regurgitation are superimposed when there is dilatation of these valve rings secondary to pulmonary hypertension or right ventricular failure. The *electrocardiogram* shows marked right ventricular or biventricular hypertrophy with prominent P waves. Complete right bundle branch block may be present, especially when the shunt is at the atrial level. In others the electrocardiogram is influenced by the underlying anomaly (e.g., single ventricle, ventricular inversion, etc.). The *chest roentgenogram* confirms the degree of cardiomegaly. The pulmonary trunk is enlarged with prominence of the primary divisions, which diminish in caliber in the peripheral branches. The *echocardiogram* helps to identify the anatomy of the underlying intracardiac or extracardiac malformation. *Cardiac catheterization* is undertaken when the diagnosis cannot be established by clinical findings and noninvasive studies. One of the purposes of catheterization is to determine whether the pulmonary vascular bed is vasoactive, as indicated by a fall in pulmonary artery pressure and resistance during the breathing of 100 per cent oxygen. Another major indication is to exclude the presence of left ventricular inflow lesions, which result in elevation of pulmonary venous pressure and secondary pulmonary hypertension. Angiocardiography carries a small increased risk because the contrast medium may produce a fall in systemic vascular resistance and increased right to left shunting with a further fall in systemic arterial saturation.

Symptomatic *erythrocytosis* is treated with cautious venesection, and repeated phlebotomies are avoided because of the risk of iron deficiency. *Hemoptysis* occurs from coagulopathies, from rupture of pulmonary vessels, or from pulmonary arterial thrombosis or embolism. This symptom is usually limited to adult life, blood loss is not excessive, and symptomatic treatment is all that is needed. However, hemoptysis can be life threatening if associated with hypotension, an increase in the degree of hypoxemia, and the development of acidemia. Long-term anticoagulation is not indicated. *Syncope* and *sudden death* cannot be predicted, but patients with Eisenmenger's syndrome between the ages of about 20 and 40 years are at risk. The mechanism is not clear but has been attributed to arrhythmias, probably ventricular tachyarrhythmias, which result in hypotension and an increase in right to left shunting. *Pregnancy* is not well tolerated, and sudden death has been reported during the third trimester or in the postpartum period.

Treatment. Surgical treatment of the cardiac anomaly is contraindicated because these patients succumb to the effects of pulmonary vascular disease. Palliation has been successful in the presence of transposition of the great arteries, ventricular septal defect, and severe pulmonary vascular disease; the procedure involves redirection of the venous return but the ventricular defect is not closed. The experience with transplantation of the heart and lungs is still small and follow-up is short, but this therapy is being watched with interest because patients with progressive symptoms are at great risk of dying. Drugs have been used to attempt to manipulate pulmonary and systemic vascular resistance to reduce the right to left shunt; generally the results have been disappointing.

COMPLEX CARDIAC MALFORMATIONS. When pulmonic stenosis is an important part of the anomaly, surgical aortopulmonary shunting is undertaken during infancy or childhood to alleviate hypoxemia. In others with torrential pulmonary blood flow and pulmonary hypertension, pulmonary arterial banding is undertaken in infancy to prevent progressive pulmonary vascular disease. Many have now reached adolescence or adult life with normal or low pulmonary vascular resistance. These patients are candidates for operation using the Fontan principle (caval or right atrial anastomosis to the pulmonary artery).

THE ADULT WITH SURGICALLY "CURED" CONGENITAL HEART DISEASE

Surgical treatment for extracardiac anomalies has been undertaken for over four decades, and 35 years have elapsed since the introduction of surgical procedures for intracardiac congenital malformations. Immediate results after operation continue to be excellent, even dramatic, but it is now recognized that complications may develop many years after surgery.

INTRA-ATRIAL SURGERY. Many anomalies may be treated by an approach through the right atrium. These include atrial septal defects of all types, endocardial cushion defects, transposition of the great arteries, and total anomalous pulmonary venous connection. Frequently, isolated ventricular septal defects are closed surgically transatrially, and the defect (especially the more common perimembranous defect) is approached through the tricuspid valve and the shunt obliterated. Persistent *conduction disturbances* may occur immediately after operation or appear for the first time many years later. These consist of supraventricular arrhythmias (atrial flutter or fibrillation, paroxysmal supraventricular tachycardia, and junctional rhythm), sick sinus syndrome, or varying degrees of AV block. These rhythm disturbances occur even when there is complete anatomic correction of the abnormality. The treatment of these abnormalities in conduction is similar to the treatment of these arrhythmias of any cause. The *function of the right ventricle* and competence of the tricuspid valve have also been of concern, especially in transposition of the great arteries.

INTRAVENTRICULAR SURGERY. Right ventriculotomy is the approach used in most patients who require intraventricular surgery. The more common lesions treated this way include some forms of ventricular septal defect, tetralogy of Fallot with or without pulmonary atresia, and various forms of transposition of the great arteries. Some of these complications may be reduced in future years, since earlier operation is being advised, especially in some patients with tetralogy of Fallot.

Conduction Disturbances. Permanent complete heart block from intraoperative trauma to the conduction system has decreased to a point where it is no longer a major problem soon after operation. *Bifascicular block* (left anterior hemiblock with complete right bundle branch block) may occur from intraoperative trauma to the bundle of His and its branches. These patients usually remain well for many years after operation, but the conduction abnormality may progress to complete AV block. Bifascicular block does not require treatment. *Sudden unexpected cardiac arrest* may occur many years after operation. While this catastrophe may occasionally occur from complete AV block, more frequent mechanisms are ventricular tachyarrhythmias and deterioration into ventricular fibrillation. The risk of ventricular tachycardia is higher in patients who have multiple unifocal or multifocal premature ventricular contractions at rest. Bursts of ventricular tachyarrhythmia may be recorded during 24-hour electrocardiographic recording or unmasked during or immediately after graded exercise testing. While these arrhythmias may occur in patients who have had adequate relief of right ventricular outflow tract obstruction and in whom the ventricular defect is closed, there appears to be greater risk when residual defects are present, such as severe pulmonic stenosis, persistent large shunts across the ventricular septum, and right ventricular aneurysms. Significant residual defects should be treated by reoperation, and the ventricular arrhythmia may be abolished by excision of arrhythmogenic right ventricular aneurysms. Medical treatment of the ventricular tachycardia is indicated and although there is a choice of many drugs, phenytoin (Dilantin) has been used with particular success.

Reconstruction of the Right Ventricular Outflow Tract. Treatment of extreme forms of tetralogy of Fallot, especially pulmonary atresia, and many forms of transposition of the great arteries with pulmonic stenosis or previous arterial banding requires a prosthesis to establish continuity between the right ventricle and the pulmonary artery. During the last decade the most frequently used prosthesis consisted of a Dacron tube with an aortic valve bearing a porcine heterograft. The durability of this prosthesis is unpredictable, since recurrence of obstruction may occur anywhere along its length from narrowing of the anastomotic sites or from development of an exuberant neointima that encroaches on the lumen of the Dacron tube. Because of these complications, a human valve bearing aortic or pulmonary homografts is being used with greater frequency.

Congenital Aortic Stenosis. See above.
Valvular Pulmonic Stenosis. See above.
Coarctation of the Aorta. See above.

Adams FH, Emmanouilides GC, Riemenschneider TA: Moss' Heart Disease in Infants, Children and Adolescents. 4th ed. Baltimore, Williams and Wilkins, 1989. *The standard comprehensive text on all aspects of congenital heart disease.*

Cohen M, Fuster V, Steele PM, et al.: Coarctation of the aorta. Long-term follow-up and prediction of outcome after surgical correction. Circulation 80:840, 1989.

Garson A, Nihill MR, McNamara DG, et al.: Status of the adult and adolescent after repair of tetralogy of Fallot. Circulation 59:1232, 1979. *Long-term results are evaluated with emphasis on complications in the adult.*

Girod DA, Fontan F, Deville C, et al.: Long-term results after the Fontan operation for tricuspid atresia. Circulation 75:605, 1987. *These principles are also applicable to other complex cardiac malformations with inadequate pulmonary blood flow.*

Giuliani ER, Fuster V, Brandenberg RO, et al.: Ebstein's anomaly. Mayo Clin Proc 54:163, 1979. *Clinical features and natural history are reviewed in a lucid manner.*

Kirklin JW, Barratt-Boyes BG: Cardiac Surgery. New York, John Wiley and Sons, 1986. *Comprehensive analyses of combined clinical experiences from two respected pioneers in all aspects of cardiac surgery, especially congenital heart disease.*

Kopecky SL, Gersh BJ, McGoon MD, et al.: Long-term outcome of patients undergoing surgical repair of isolated pulmonary valve stenosis. Follow-up at 20 to 30 years. Circulation 78:1150, 1988. *These long-term results set the standard against which the results of valvuloplasty will be compared.*

Mullins CE: Pediatric and congenital therapeutic cardiac catheterization. Circulation 79:1153, 1989. *A description of the present status of catheter interventional procedures for congenital heart disease.*

Perloff JK: The Clinical Recognition of Congenital Heart Disease. 3rd ed. Philadelphia, W.B. Saunders Company, 1986. *A book that focuses on the anatomic and physiologic derangements in congenital heart disease, setting the stage for an understanding of the history, physical signs, electrocardiogram, chest roentgenogram, and echocardiogram. All age groups are dealt with.*

Perloff JK, Child JS: Congenital Heart Disease in Adults. Philadelphia, W.B. Saunders Company, 1991. *All major aspects of diagnosis and management are discussed in a sophisticated and authoritative manner.*

Wernovsy G, Hougen TJ, Walsh EP, et al.: Midterm results after the arterial switch operation for transposition of the great arteries with intact ventricular septum: Clinical, hemodynamic, electrocardiographic, and electrophysiologic data. Circulation 77:1333, 1988.

47 Atherosclerosis

Russell Ross

Atherosclerosis is responsible for the majority of cases of myocardial and cerebral infarction and thus represents the principal cause of death in the United States and western Europe. Atherosclerosis is the descriptive term for thickened and hardened lesions of the medium and large muscular and elastic arteries. It is a lipid-rich lesion, in contrast with arteriosclerosis, which is the generic term used for thickened and stiffened arteries of all sizes. Other forms of arteriosclerosis include focal calcific arteriosclerosis (Mönckeberg's arteriosclerosis) and arteriolosclerosis, a disease of small vessels.

The lesions of atherosclerosis occur within the innermost layer of the artery, the intima, and are largely confined to this region of the vessel. The lesions are generally eccentric and, if they become sufficiently large, can occlude the artery and thus the vascular supply to a tissue or organ, resulting in ischemia or necrosis. If this occurs, it often leads to the characteristic clinical sequelae of myocardial infarction, cerebral infarction, gangrene of the extremities, or sudden cardiac death.

THE NORMAL ARTERY

The normal artery consists essentially of a tube lined on its luminal aspect by a continuous layer of endothelium and on its outer aspect by loose connective tissue containing fibroblasts and smooth muscle cells, which package an intermediate layer of pure smooth muscle cells that are bound together in such a manner that, by working with the elastic laminae and the collagen and proteoglycans that surround the cells, the smooth muscle cells contract and maintain the tonus of the artery wall as the blood flows through with each systole and diastole.

The lining cells of the artery, the endothelium, represent the interface with the cells of the blood. It is at this interface that different blood cell types can interact with the endothelium and, under appropriate circumstances, lead to the development of lesions of atherosclerosis. These cells are the platelet, the monocyte, and the lymphocyte. Their potential roles in atherogenesis are discussed below.

THE LESIONS OF ATHEROSCLEROSIS

The two principal forms of atherosclerosis are the early lesion, or fatty streak, and the advanced lesion, or fibrous plaque, which can become an advanced complicated lesion.

The Fatty Streak

The fatty streak is the most common and ubiquitous lesion of atherosclerosis. It occurs at all ages and in Western society is present at birth in some infants and is common in young children. The lesions of atherosclerosis are confined principally to the intima. Initially, the fatty streak appears to contain two cell types: foam cells that consist of macrophages filled with lipids (principally in the form of cholesteryl esters) and T lymphocytes (principally CD-8+ with some CD-4+ cells). The macrophages are derived from blood-borne monocytes that are chemotactically attracted into the artery wall, where they develop into foam cells. As the fatty streak enlarges, it does so by continuing attachment and migration of monocytes into the intima with their consequent development into macrophages. Subsequently, smooth muscle cells appear to migrate into the intima from the media and also begin to accumulate lipid and take on the appearance of foam cells. As the fatty streak becomes larger and more advanced, it contains varying numbers of smooth muscle cells mixed together with lymphocytes and the predominant lipid-filled macrophages. Fatty streaks can be found in young individuals at the same anatomic sites that are later occupied by advanced lesions, as well as at sites where they may either regress and disappear or remain as fatty streaks throughout life.

The Fibrous Plaque

The fibrous plaque is also located in the intima and characteristically leads to the eccentric thickening of the artery that often results in occlusion of the lumen. The fibrous plaque is typically covered at its luminal aspect by a thickened cap of dense connective tissue containing a special form of flattened, pancake-shaped smooth muscle cell that has formed the dense collagenous matrix in which it is embedded. Beneath this cap, the lesion is highly cellular and contains large numbers of smooth muscle cells, some of which may be full of lipid droplets. It also contains numerous macrophages, many of which take the form of foam cells, together with variable numbers of T lymphocytes. These collections of cells usually overlie a deeper area of necrotic foam cells and debris. This necrotic area sometimes becomes calcified and often may contain cholesterol crystals. (Figure 47–1 details the cellular composition of a fibrous plaque.)

The Complicated Lesion

The complicated lesion is a fibrous plaque that has undergone extensive degeneration and often calcification. It may contain

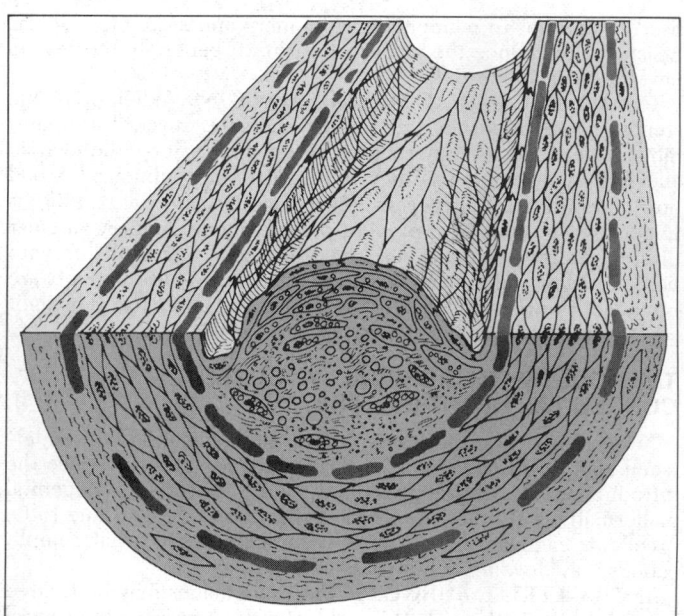

FIGURE 47–1. The *fibrous plaque*, which characteristically consists of numerous proliferated smooth muscle cells together with macrophages and variable numbers of lymphocytes. In this diagram, the fibrous plaque is covered by an intact endothelial monolayer and contains a fibrous cap of smooth muscle cells. These smooth muscle cells lie in a dense connective tissue matrix that covers a deeper collection of smooth muscle cells and macrophages, both of which may contain numerous lipid droplets and take the form of foam cells mixed together with variable numbers of lymphocytes. These collections of cells lie in a mixture of connective tissue matrix and free extracellular deposits of lipid. The fibrous plaque usually intrudes into the lumen owing to its proliferative nature. This diagram represents only in general terms the relative appearance of such a lesion.

ulcerations, cracks, and fissures, which serve as sites for platelet adherence, aggregation and thrombosis, and subsequent organization. When this occurs, thrombosis may result in sudden occlusion of the artery.

Morbid Anatomy of the Lesions

Fatty streaks are flat lesions that often appear as yellow discolorations on the surface of the artery but seldom intrude into the lumen and thus cause no clinical sequelae. The fibrous plaques and complicated lesions are raised lesions that are often pearly gray in appearance but may be discolored when associated with erythrocytes and thrombi.

Localization of the Lesions

The arteries most commonly involved with atherosclerosis are the aorta; the femoral, popliteal, and tibial arteries; the coronary arteries; the internal and external carotid arteries; and the cerebral arteries.

In the aorta, the abdominal portion is commonly involved with lesions of atherosclerosis at an earlier age, and, as in the thoracic aorta, lesions most commonly form around orifices of branches and bifurcations of the artery. There is a greater incidence of atherosclerotic lesions in the leg arteries, whereas they are relatively rare in the vessels of the upper limbs. Atherosclerosis of the smaller arteries, particularly those of the legs and the coronary arteries, is more common in cigarette smokers or in individuals who have glucose intolerance.

Coronary atherosclerosis is most prominent in the main stems of the coronary arteries, particularly in the segments closest to the ostia of the coronary vessel. The degree of luminal narrowing in the coronary arteries can be variable; however, atherosclerosis is generally present in the epicardial segment of the vessels, whereas the intramural coronary arteries are generally spared. Typically, after coronary bypass surgery, the perianastomotic site of the bypass is often (30 per cent of the time) involved in the development of a new lesion of atherosclerosis, which is probably related to mural thrombi that readily form at these sites.

The carotid and cerebral arteries generally have a patchy

distribution of the lesions of atherosclerosis, which often first appear at the base of the brain in the carotid, basilar, and vertebral arteries.

The pulmonary arteries are generally spared of lesions of atherosclerosis, except in association with pulmonary hypertension.

RISK FACTORS

The risk factor concept evolved from epidemiologic studies of the incidence of coronary artery disease conducted in the United States and in Europe. Prospective studies demonstrated a consistent association of characteristics observed in apparently healthy individuals with the subsequent incidence of coronary artery disease in the same individuals. These studies demonstrated an association between an increase in the concentration of plasma lipoproteins, principally low density lipoprotein (LDL) and thus plasma cholesterol (see Ch. 172), and the rate of occurrence of new events of coronary artery disease. Also observed was an increased incidence of the disease in relation to cigarette smoking, hypertension, clinical diabetes, age, male sex, obesity, stress and particular personality characteristics (denoted as type A), and genetic factors. Because of these associations, each of these characteristics was termed a risk factor for atherosclerosis (see Ch. 37). At least three independent predictors of risk for individuals within a population are valuable in anticipating increased incidence of atherosclerosis. These are hyperlipidemia, cigarette smoking, and hypertension.

Hyperlipidemia

There is a clear association between chronic hypercholesterolemia and increase in incidence of ischemic heart disease. The Framingham Study demonstrated this association, particularly in men between the ages of 20 and 40. When the plasma cholesterol levels are greater than 220 mg per deciliter, there is a marked increase in the relative incidence of myocardial infarction, which is most easily demonstrated in individuals with familial hypercholesterolemia. The range of normality is not entirely clear in defining cholesterol and triglyceride levels for a given population as they relate to increased risk of ischemic heart disease. However, in the United States, 200 mg per deciliter is considered to be the upper limit of normal for the plasma cholesterol level, which increases from birth through young adulthood until the age of approximately 50 in men and to somewhat older ages in women. Similarly, there is an age-related increase in plasma triglyceride levels. Triglyceride is associated with increases in very low density lipoproteins (VLDL), whereas elevation in plasma cholesterol level is generally associated with increase in LDL.

Abnormal accumulation of lipoproteins in the plasma can occur from overproduction, from deficient removal, or from a combination of these abnormalities. There are numerous forms of genetically derived hyperlipoproteinemias that are either monogenic or polygenic. Perhaps more common are forms of hyperlipoproteinemia that are secondary to other disease, such as diabetes, renal disease, alcoholism, hypothyroidism, and the dysglobulinemias, or to treatment with corticosteroids or estrogens (see Ch. 172).

HOMOZYGOUS FAMILIAL HYPERCHOLESTEROLEMIA. Patients with homozygous familial hypercholesterolemia (FH disease) represent one of the best demonstrations of the capacity of hypercholesterolemia to induce the cellular changes that lead to atherogenesis. Although FH disease is much rarer than the secondary hyperlipoproteinemias or other forms of genetic hyperlipidemia, we know a great deal about its course in humans and in an animal model, the Watanabe heritable hyperlipidemic rabbit, as well as diet-induced hypercholesterolemia in the nonhuman primate. In the case of genetic hyperlipidemia, the plasma cholesterol and LDL levels are inordinately high owing to faulty or missing LDL receptors. When LDL is bound to its normal receptor, it suppresses the activity of the rate-limiting enzyme for cholesterol synthesis, HMG-CoA-reductase. In individuals with FH disease, the liver and peripheral cells continue to synthesize large amounts of cholesterol because absent or faulty receptors fail to generate a feedback inhibitory signal and cholesterol synthesis goes on unabated. Under these conditions, plasma cholesterol levels reach 500 to 1000 mg per

deciliter or higher, and rampant atherosclerosis develops, with advanced occlusive lesions. This can occur at very young ages, and myocardial infarcts have been described in young children with this disease.

TREATMENT OF HYPERCHOLESTEROLEMIA. The Lipid Research Clinic Trials have demonstrated that it is beneficial to lower plasma levels in patients with chronic elevations of LDL. These studies showed that the decrease in plasma cholesterol levels can be correlated with a reduction in the incidence of myocardial infarction and thus atherosclerosis. Premature ischemic heart disease is usually associated with hypercholesterolemia, particularly when levels of plasma cholesterol are greater than 240 mg per deciliter. When this occurs, the incidence of atherosclerotic disease can be as high as fivefold greater than for individuals with plasma cholesterol levels below 200 mg per deciliter.

Hypertriglyceridemia is usually associated with increases in VLDL in the plasma, which may be complicated by increases in cholesterol as well. Patients with increased VLDL levels who come from families with familial combined hyperlipidemia are at increased risk for atherosclerosis, whereas those with elevated VLDL levels from families with monogenic familial hypertriglyceridemia are not at increased risk. Increased VLDL levels can increase the risk of atherosclerosis if it accompanies other risk factors, such as diabetes mellitus or cigarette smoking.

It is important to examine all patients over the age of 20 for hyperlipidemia, particularly if they have a family history of premature ischemic heart disease. This is best done by measuring the concentrations of cholesterol and triglyceride in plasma after an overnight fast. Cholesterol levels above 200 mg per deciliter or triglyceride levels above 250 mg per deciliter, or both, are indicative of hyperlipidemia, requiring attention and therapy, the first step of which should be dietary intervention. Such patients should be brought to normal weight if this is excessive and maintained on a diet low in saturated fat and cholesterol. Those with hypertriglyceridemia should limit or eliminate intake of alcohol. In general, reduction of intake of calories, cholesterol, and saturated fat is the best approach to begin with in most patients. Severe hyperlipidemia with cholesterol levels in excess of 350 mg per deciliter or triglyceride levels in excess of 400 mg per deciliter, or both, is usually representative of a genetic disorder and often first manifests with xanthomas. Such patients' families, particularly first-degree relatives, should also be examined.

If dietary approaches are unsuccessful, then regimens including bile acid–binding resins or one of the more recently developed lipid-lowering drugs should be considered (see Ch. 172). Use of such agents is dependent not only on their efficaciousness, but on their long-term effects as well. Their use before puberty and during pregnancy is currently not recommended.

High Density Lipoprotein (HDL)

In epidemiologic studies, elevations of high density lipoprotein particles in the plasma are inversely related to the incidence of atherosclerosis and its sequelae. Elevation of the HDL cholesterol level is "protective" against ischemic heart disease; conversely, the individuals with abnormally low levels of HDL are at increased risk.

HDL has been postulated to participate in transfer of cholesterol out of cells. Women generally have elevated HDL levels prior to menopause. If their HDL level is decreased in association with diabetes or obesity, they are at increased risk for ischemic heart disease. Regular strenuous exercise, decreased cigarette smoking, and diet rich in some fish oils (eicosapentaenoic acid) are associated with increased HDL levels, although the basis for the increase is poorly understood.

Cigarette Smoking

Cigarette smoking is one of the most common risk factors associated with increased incidence of atherosclerosis, and when it is reduced or eliminated, the risk of developing the disease decreases. Stroke, myocardial infarction, and intermittent claudication are common in male cigarette smokers, who, together with female smokers, show an increased incidence of symptoms associated with atherosclerosis. In addition to atherosclerosis of the large coronary arteries, cigarette smokers characteristically have occlusive disease of the leg arteries. There is a mean increase of approximately 70 per cent in the death rate and a three- to fivefold increase in the risk of ischemic heart disease in males who smoke more than one pack of cigarettes per day, compared with nonsmokers.

Sudden death is frequently associated with cigarette smoking, and of particular importance is the observation that cessation of cigarette smoking leads within a year to reduction of the risk of the sequelae of atherosclerosis to levels of that of nonsmokers. The basis for atherosclerosis in cigarette smokers is not well understood.

Glucose Intolerance and Diabetes Mellitus

Both insulin-dependent and non–insulin-dependent diabetics show at least a twofold increase in the incidence of myocardial infarction, compared with nondiabetics. Younger diabetics have a marked increase in the risk of atherosclerosis and thus of ischemic heart disease, and diabetic women appear to be even more prone than diabetic men. Gangrene of the lower extremities is one of the principal sequelae of atherosclerosis in diabetics. It is not clear what factors are responsible for the increased incidence of atherosclerosis in diabetes.

Hypertension

Elevation in blood pressure is an important risk factor associated with increased incidence of atherosclerosis and is of particular importance since this is a factor that is easily diagnosed and highly treatable. The risk of atherosclerosis and its sequelae increases progressively with increase in blood pressure, and when the blood pressure exceeds 160 mm Hg systolic and 95 mm Hg diastolic in middle-aged men the risk is five times greater than in normotensive men with blood pressure of 140 mm Hg systolic and 90 mm Hg diastolic or less. The increase in diastolic pressure may be more important than that in systolic pressure in both hypertensive men and women. After the age of 50, hypertension may be more important as a risk factor in predicting increased incidence of atherosclerosis than hypercholesterolemia. Recent intervention studies of individuals with hypertension have demonstrated that a reduction of diastolic pressure levels below 105 mm Hg can significantly reduce the incidence of symptomatic cerebrovascular disease, ischemic heart disease, and congestive heart failure in men (see Ch. 44). When multiple risk factors are present, including hypertension, it is particularly important to treat the hypertension, since it is the most easily accessible and treatable aspect of this disease process.

Obesity

When body weight is greater than 20 per cent above the norm, there is an increased risk of ischemic heart disease. Obesity may particularly accelerate atherosclerosis in individuals below the age of 50. Obesity is generally associated with hypertriglyceridemia, hypercholesterolemia, glucose intolerance, and hypertension.

Physical Activity

There are many studies related to the value of increased physical activity in reducing the incidence of ischemic heart disease. The Framingham Studies suggest that sedentary individuals are more susceptible to atherosclerosis and to sudden death than individuals who maintain an active lifestyle. It has been suggested that increased physical activity may elevate the level of HDL. Appropriately supervised physical training can improve exercise performance in patients with angina due to ischemic heart disease.

Genetic Factors

Clearly, genetic factors are critical in atherosclerosis. The best example of this is the increased incidence of atherosclerosis in individuals with homozygous familial hypercholesterolemia and familial combined hyperlipidemia. Other risk factors, such as hypertension and diabetes mellitus, can also be inherited, and it is possible that protective factors, such as increased HDL, may

also be inherited, although the latter is not well understood. As a consequence, family history must be included in assessing the risk for a given individual.

THE PATHOGENESIS OF THE LESIONS OF ATHEROSCLEROSIS

The lesions of atherosclerosis as they occur in the intima of the artery essentially consist of three biologic entities. First and foremost of these is an increase in the number of intimal smooth muscle cells, together with an accumulation of macrophages and variable numbers of lymphocytes. The increased number of smooth muscle cells is responsible for the second entity, the formation of large amounts of connective tissue matrix containing collagen, elastic fibers, and proteoglycans. The third entity, lipid, accumulates in hyperlipidemic individuals within the smooth muscle cells and the macrophages and in many instances causes them to develop into foam cells. Lipid also accumulates within the surrounding connective tissue matrix but may be absent from lesions of patients that are normocholesterolemic, subject to other risk factors. Thus the advanced lesions of atherosclerosis represent the culmination of a usually longstanding proliferative disease process in which it becomes important to understand the basis for the proliferation of smooth muscle, accumulation of macrophages, formation of new connective tissue, and accumulation of lipid.

The Response to Injury Hypothesis of Atherosclerosis

During the past 15 years, it has been possible to develop a hypothesis that takes into account most of what is known concerning risk factors, the biology of the artery wall, the cells involved, and the biologic processes that result in the lesions of atherosclerosis.

The response to injury hypothesis of atherosclerosis suggests that some form of "injury" affects the lining endothelial cells. The injury may alter the functional characteristics of the endothelium, leaving the endothelium morphologically intact. Thus endothelial injury could alter the permeability of the endothelium, its nonthrombogenic character, its ability to form vasoactive substances and growth factors, and its capacity to regenerate. At the other extreme, endothelial injury may lead to endothelial cell-cell disjunction and endothelial retraction, exposing the underlying connective tissue or accumulated foam cells, such as macrophages, that form the first and ubiquitous lesion of atherosclerosis, the fatty streak.

In hypercholesterolemic animals, including nonhuman primates, swine, rabbits, and rats, the first change that occurs in the artery wall is a chemotactic attraction of circulating monocytes and lymphocytes, which increasingly adhere to the surface of the endothelial cells in clusters located throughout the arterial tree. The adherent monocytes migrate on the surface of the endothelium, penetrate between endothelial junctions, localize subendothelially, accumulate lipid, and become intimal foam cells. The accumulation of these intimal lymphocytes and monocytes that become converted to lipid-laden macrophages represents the initial lesion of atherosclerosis, the fatty streak. These fatty streaks expand by continued attraction and accumulation of lymphocytes and monocytes in the artery. They also expand by migration of some smooth muscle cells from the underlying media into the intima, where they localize beneath the accumulated macrophages and also accumulate lipid.

With increasing time, level, and duration of hypercholesterolemia, endothelial cell-cell junctions separate and endothelial cells retract, permitting lipid-laden macrophages to enter the circulation and home to the spleen and lymph nodes. This occurs particularly at branches and bifurcations of the artery. Sometimes the exposed macrophages or connective tissue, or both, can be thrombogenic and induce platelets to adhere at these sites. Sites where mural thrombi have formed become loci of increased migration and proliferation of smooth muscle cells that accumulate and form large amounts of connective tissue matrix. Thus sites of platelet adherence and aggregation subsequently may become sites of intimal smooth muscle proliferation.

At other anatomic sites, the endothelium may remain intact, but the fatty streak expands by the continued attraction and accumulation of monocytes. Many of the macrophages in the lesions also synthesize DNA and replicate, further aggravating the proliferative component of the lesions.

Numerous investigations have attempted to determine what factors are responsible for the migration and proliferation of smooth muscle cells in the intima. Growth factors able to induce smooth muscle cell migration and proliferation can be formed and secreted by several cells. Of particular importance is the capacity of platelets to release growth factors and of activated macrophages to release the same as well as other types of growth factors. The growth factors that may play a critical role in atherogenesis include platelet-derived growth factor (PDGF), a potent growth factor for mesenchymal connective tissue cells such as fibroblasts and smooth muscle, and transforming growth factor beta (TGF-β), a factor that may act in an inhibitory fashion and can induce formation of large amounts of connective tissue.

PDGF is a potent mitogen that, at nanogram and picogram levels, can induce cells such as smooth muscle to multiply, and TGF-β can induce them to form new connective tissue. PDGF and TGF-β can be derived from platelets, from activated macrophages which are probably the principal cellular source of PDGF, and from appropriately stimulated or "injured" endothelial cells. Thus, if endothelial injury occurs, appropriate opportunities may be present for the release of mitogens such as PDGF

from all three cells. Such growth factor release may be related to increased incidence of atherogenesis in experimental animals. There is also evidence that smooth muscle cells, once they have been induced to proliferate in the artery wall, may in themselves be capable of expressing the gene for PDGF and of secreting this growth factor so that they may, in effect, stimulate themselves in an autocrine fashion to continue the proliferative response.

The response to injury hypothesis of atherogenesis suggests that the "injury" to the endothelium results in cellular changes that lead to a modified form of inflammation in which monocytes and lymphocytes enter the artery wall and the monocytes become macrophages that can secrete growth factors, act as scavenger cells, and accumulate lipid and become foam cells. The fatty streak then becomes converted into a smooth muscle proliferative lesion, or fibrous plaque, and probably does so by local release within the artery of growth factors derived from activated macrophages, injured endothelium, and/or platelets that may interact with the artery wall at sites where the protective cover of the endothelium may be altered. These changes are diagrammatically shown in Figure 47–2, which suggests how the lesions of atherosclerosis may form.

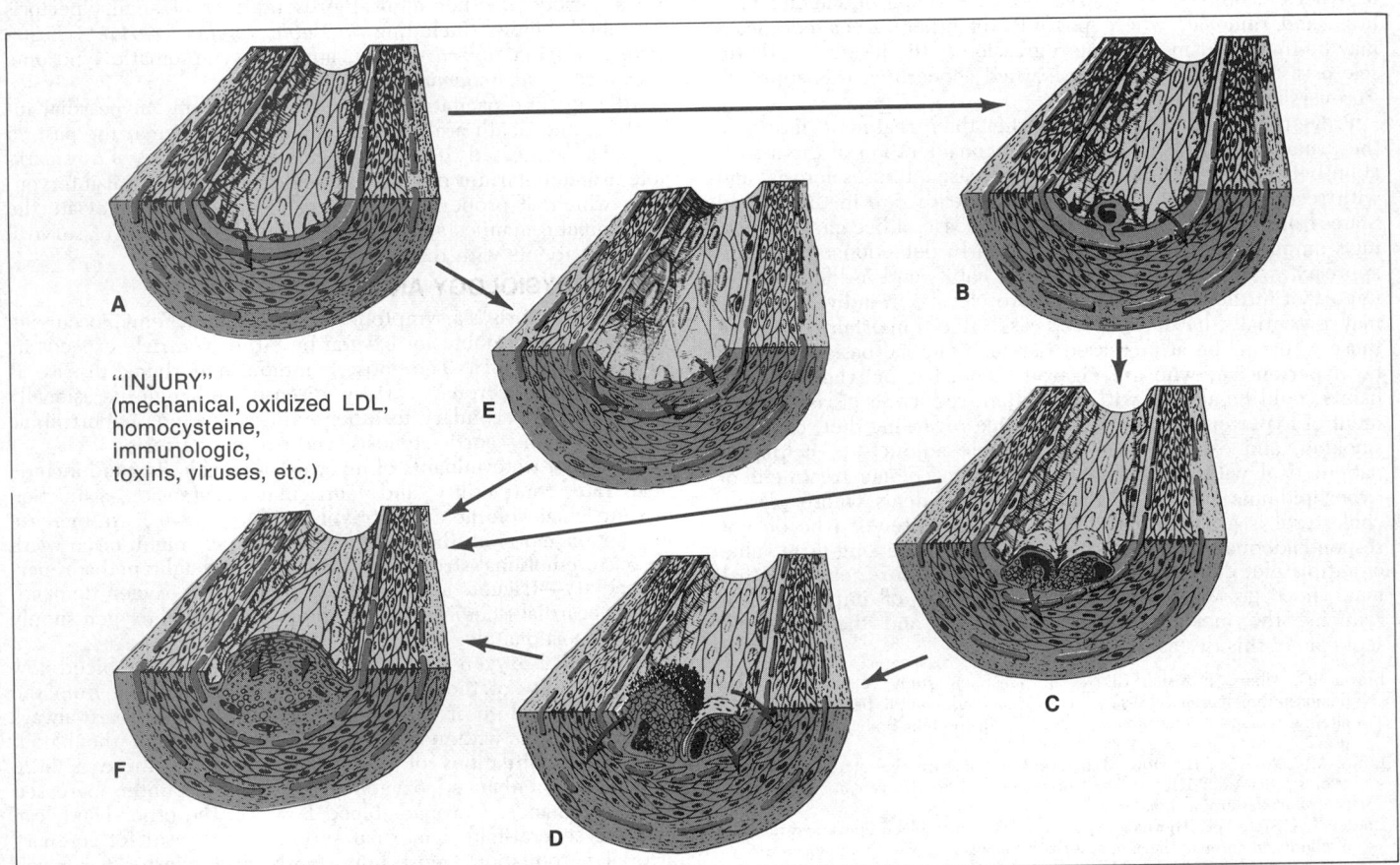

FIGURE 47–2. Endothelial injury: The response to injury hypothesis. Advanced intimal proliferative lesions of atherosclerosis may occur by at least two pathways. The pathway demonstrated by the clockwise (*long*) arrows to the right has been observed in experimentally induced hypercholesterolemia. Injury to the endothelium (*A*) may induce growth factor secretion (*short arrow*). Monocytes attach to endothelium (*B*), which may continue to secrete growth factors (*short arrow*). Subendothelial migration of monocytes (*C*) may lead to fatty streak formation and release of growth factors such as platelet-derived growth factor (PDGF) (*short arrow*). Fatty streaks may become directly converted to fibrous plaques (*long arrow* from *C* to *F*) through release of growth factors from macrophages or endothelial cells or both. Macrophages may also stimulate and/or injure the overlying endothelium. In some cases, macrophages may lose their endothelial cover and platelet attachment may occur (*D*), providing three possible sources of growth factors—platelets, macrophages, and endothelium (*short arrows*). Some of the smooth muscle cells in the proliferative lesion itself (*F*) may form and secrete growth factors such as PDGF (*short arrows*).

An alternative pathway for development of advanced lesions of atherosclerosis is shown by the arrows from *A* to *E* to *F*. In this case, the endothelium may be injured but remain intact. Increased endothelial turnover may result in growth factor formation by endothelial cells (*A*). This may stimulate migration of smooth muscle cells from the media into the intima, accompanied by endogenous production of PDGF by smooth muscle as well as growth factor secretion from the "injured" endothelial cells (*E*). These interactions could then lead to fibrous plaque formation and further lesion progression (*F*). (From Ross R: The pathogenesis of atherosclerosis—an update. N Engl J Med 314:496, 1986. Reprinted by permission of the New England Journal of Medicine.)

The response to injury hypothesis also offers an opportunity to consider means of preventing and intervening in the formation of the lesions of atherosclerosis. Clearly, alteration in lifestyle habits, including changes in dietary habits and alteration of risk factors associated with increased incidence of atherosclerosis, could be potentially important in preventing these cellular changes from occurring and possibly in inducing lesion regression.

Regression of Atherosclerosis

In experimental animals the fatty streak is clearly capable of regressing and disappearing entirely if hypercholesterolemic animals are placed on a normocholesterolemic regimen for a sufficient period of time. There is evidence to suggest that fatty streaks can also regress in humans, based upon examination of individuals who decreased their dietary intake of lipids and atherogenic foods. Fibrous plaques or complicated lesions in humans may also be partially reversible, based upon angiographic studies. It is not yet clear how far a lesion must progress before it becomes irreversible. Cessation of cigarette smoking is associated with decreased risk, and this in combination with treatment of hypertension, dietary intervention, treatment of diabetes mellitus, and removal, where possible, of other associated causes may be important in inducing regression of the lesions of atherosclerosis. More remains to be learned concerning this approach to reversing the disease process.

Prevention of atherosclerosis, rather than treatment, has to be the principal goal for all patients. In consideration of the association between hyperlipidemia and increased atherosclerosis, and with recognition of the decline in the death rate in the United States from premature ischemic heart disease, it becomes increasingly important to understand that early detection of risk and approaches toward change in dietary habits and in lifestyles are important in the prevention of atherosclerosis in individuals who may potentially be at increased risk. It is important to detect those who may be at increased risk on a familial basis, who may be hypertensive, who are cigarette smokers, or whose dietary habits could be altered with a resultant reduction in risk. Treatment of hypertension, as well as advice regarding diet, cigarette smoking, and exercise, can be valuable adjuncts to helping a patient deal with these problems. Pharmacologic treatment of hyperlipidemia should be limited to individuals whose plasma cholesterol is greater than 240 mg per deciliter or who do not respond adequately to dietary management. The long-term value of antiplatelet drugs and, potentially in the future, of drugs that may affect growth factor activity could be of importance in reducing the incidence of atherosclerosis and the long-term sequelae of this disease process.

Brown BG, Albers JJ, Fisher LD, et al.: Treatment study: A randomized trial demonstrating coronary disease regression and clinical benefit from lipid altering therapy among men with high apolipoprotein B. N Engl J Med, in press.

Brown MS, Goldstein JL: How LDL receptors influence cholesterol and atherosclerosis. Sci Am 251:158, 1984. *A discussion of how LDL receptor interactions control cholesterol metabolism.*

Gordon T, Castelli WP, Hjortland MC, et al.: Diabetes, blood lipids, and the role of obesity in coronary heart disease risk for women. The Framingham Study. Ann Intern Med 87:393, 1977.

Gordon T, Castelli WP, Hjortland MC, et al.: High density lipoprotein as a protective factor against coronary heart disease. The Framingham Study. Am J Med 62:707, 1977. *These two papers represent epidemiologic studies that relate the role of several of the principal risk factors on atherosclerosis and indicate the potential protective effect of HDL in atherosclerosis.*

Report of the Working Group on Arteriosclerosis of the National Heart, Lung, and Blood Institute. Vol. 2. Department of Health, Education and Welfare (National Institutes of Health) Publication No. 82–2035. Washington, D.C., Government Printing Office, 1981. *This represents an overview of a large number of individuals who have examined both the epidemiology and the nature of the lesions of atherosclerosis.*

Ross R: The pathogenesis of atherosclerosis—an update. N Engl J Med 314:488, 1986.

Ross R, Glomset JA: The pathogenesis of atherosclerosis. N Engl J Med 295:369, 1976. *These two papers review the anatomic structure of the artery wall, lesions of atherosclerosis, and the potential roles of the cells in atherosclerosis. They provide a hypothesis for how atherogenesis may come about.*

Steinberg D: Metabolism of lipoproteins and their role in the pathogenesis of atherosclerosis. Atherosclerosis Rev 18:1, 1988.

48 Disorders of the Coronary Arteries

48.1 ANGINA PECTORIS

William J. Rogers

Angina pectoris, a common clinical manifestation of coronary artery disease, afflicts over 3 million persons in the United States. The term "angina pectoris," derived from the Greek *ankhein* (to choke), was coined by William Heberden in 1768 to describe a clinical syndrome of exertional chest discomfort, but the cardiac origin of the syndrome was not fully appreciated until Caleb Parry proposed in 1799 that angina was due to insufficient delivery of blood to the heart muscle, particularly during exercise.

Today angina pectoris is generally defined as a discomfort within or adjacent to the chest, typically provoked by exertion or anxiety, usually lasting for several minutes, alleviated by rest, and not resulting in myocardial necrosis. Besides this common syndrome of what is often termed *classic exertional angina*, there are a variety of other clinical presentations of angina pectoris described below, including *unstable angina, variant (Prinzmetal's) angina, mixed angina,* and an asymptomatic syndrome known as *silent ischemia.*

Although incapacitating recurrent chest pain, myocardial infarction, and death are potential sequelae of angina, the past 25 years has witnessed the emergence and refinement of a remarkable armamentarium of pharmacologic and mechanical interventions which, if properly utilized, can considerably alleviate the symptomatic manifestations and extend the duration of survival of most patients with this common condition.

PATHOPHYSIOLOGY AND CLASSIFICATION

Angina pectoris is a symptom of myocardial ischemia, occurring when the requirement for oxygen by either ventricle exceeds its supply (Fig. 48–1). The most common underlying disease is atherosclerotic coronary artery disease, although occasionally angina occurs secondary to other entities, such as hypertrophic cardiomyopathy, aortic stenosis, and coronary arteritis.

The major determinants of myocardial oxygen demand include heart rate, contractility, and ventricular wall tension, a function of ventricular volume and intraventricular pressure. An increase in one or more of these determinants—as might occur with exercise, emotional stress, or other states of heightened adrenergic activity—triggers an increase in myocardial oxygen demand, and myocardial ischemia results unless myocardial oxygen supply rises proportionately.

Myocardial oxygen supply is governed by coronary blood flow and the ability of the myocardium to extract oxygen from the blood delivered to it. Unlike other organs, the heart always extracts oxygen with near maximal efficiency from the blood, even under situations of minimal demand, so there is little potential for enhanced oxygen extraction to counter increased oxygen demands. Coronary blood flow, on the other hand, can increase several-fold in normal subjects as a result of coronary arterial vasodilation, most importantly at the arteriolar level, triggered by the local build-up of lactate, adenosine, and other vasoactive substances as myocardial oxygen demands increase.

In the presence of obstructive coronary artery disease, myocardial ischemia may result when the coronary arterial stenosis prevents autoregulatory vasodilation so that coronary blood flow can no longer increase proportional to rising oxygen demands. In other situations, myocardial ischemia may occur when oxygen demands are constant but there is a *primary decrease in coronary blood flow* mediated via (1) coronary artery spasm, (2) rapid evolution of the underlying atherosclerotic plaque (plaque disruption) leading to a reduced coronary arterial lumen caliber, and/or (3) intermittent microvascular plugging by platelet aggregates.

In some patients with *exertional angina,* ischemia is primarily a manifestation of increased oxygen demands in the face of fixed coronary blood flow, whereas in patients with primary *vasospastic angina,* ischemia results when coronary artery spasm causes blood flow to diminish in the face of stable oxygen demands. However,

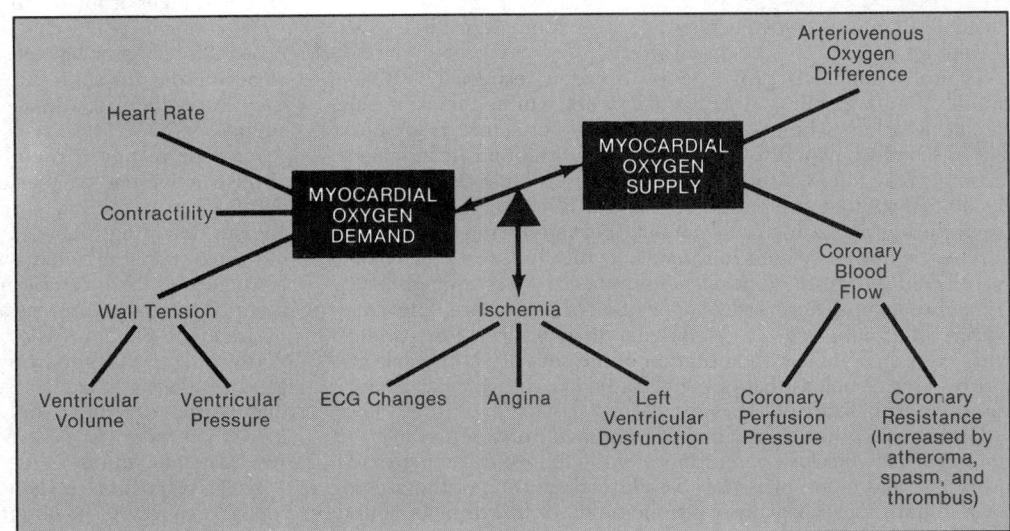

FIGURE 48–1. Ischemia occurs when oxygen demand exceeds supply.

many, if not most, patients fall between these two extremes, experiencing angina as a result of both heightened oxygen demands and diminished supply, and are said to have *mixed angina.*

As shown in Figure 48–1, angina is but one manifestation of myocardial ischemia. Ischemia typically begins in the subendocardium, where wall tension is high and compressive forces limit coronary microvascular flow, and then spreads like a wavefront toward the epicardium. The electrocardiogram often depicts ST-segment depression or T-wave inversion as manifestations of subendocardial ischemia but may show ST-segment elevation (injury current) if ischemia is prolonged and extends transmurally. These electrocardiographic changes may occur without typical anginal symptoms, a condition termed *silent ischemia.*

Segmental left ventricular contraction abnormalities occur in the region of the myocardium served by the coronary arterial branches distal to the stenosis responsible for the ischemia (the culprit lesion), and, if about 10 per cent or more of the myocardium is rendered ischemic, a reduction in global function of the left ventricle may be detectable. In addition to abnormal systolic function during ischemia, increased diastolic stiffness of the left ventricle manifests by a rising left ventricular end-diastolic pressure and rising pulmonary venous pressure. Consequently, transient clinical evidence of left ventricular failure may occur during episodic ischemia and may explain why many patients describe their angina not as pain but as a feeling of "breathlessness" or "chest tightness."

It is prognostically and clinically useful to classify anginal syndromes into stable and unstable categories. *Unstable angina* refers to angina of recent onset (within 2 months) or angina that has begun to intensify or to occur at rest or with a lower level of exertion within the previous 2 months. *Stable angina,* as the name implies, describes a relatively constant pattern of pain with regard to its severity and precipitating factors within the recent months. Some authorities classify angina of recent onset as "stable angina" if it is precipitated by moderate or severe levels of exertion and maintains a constant threshold over time, because "stable angina" has to begin at some point in time.

Of patients with unstable angina, up to 20 per cent progress to acute myocardial infarction within the next 3 months. Coronary angiography and angioscopy reveal that more than 50 per cent of patients with unstable angina have multivessel disease with eccentric, irregular, or ulcerated atherosclerotic lesions associated with endothelial disruption and adherent thrombus. Left main coronary artery disease occurs in about 10 per cent of patients with unstable angina. It is likely that unstable angina represents a point on a continuum between stable exertional angina and acute myocardial infarction.

Variant angina, originally described by Printzmetal, is characterized by rest pain accompanied by transient ST-segment changes (often ST elevation resembling acute myocardial infarction, although ST depression can also occur) and ventricular arrhythmias. Variant angina is a form of unstable angina caused by coronary arterial spasm, usually within a coronary artery

narrowed by plaque, but occasionally within an angiographically normal appearing artery.

HISTORY AND PHYSICAL EXAMINATION

The diagnosis of angina pectoris often requires considerable clinical skill because there is no totally specific symptom, physical finding, or laboratory examination to confirm its presence. The history is probably the most powerful tool for diagnosing angina and provides the skilled interviewer an assessment of both the stability (or instability) of the syndrome as well as its severity (Table 48–1). The patient should be instructed to describe the chest discomfort according to its character, location, radiation, duration, precipitating and alleviating factors, accompanying symptoms, and change in pattern over the past few weeks or days.

As indicated above, the typical *history* is that of exertional chest discomfort of several minutes duration alleviated by rest. The discomfort typically involves the region of the sternum (substernal or, more properly, retrosternal location) but may instead manifest itself in any region between the jaw and epigastrium. Commonly the discomfort radiates to the shoulders or arms, especially the left, to the neck or jaw, and less commonly to the back or epigastrium. Most patients perceive angina as a deep or visceral (rather than superficial) sensation and describe it as a "tightness," "heaviness," or "choking sensation" rather than as a definite pain. The discomfort is usually of several minutes duration; discomfort of less than 1 minute's duration is rarely angina, and discomfort at full intensity exceeding 20 minutes in duration should arouse suspicion of myocardial infarction or discomfort unrelated to myocardial ischemia. The pain of

TABLE 48–1. CANADIAN CARDIOVASCULAR CLASSIFICATION OF ANGINA SEVERITY*

Class	Signs
I	"Ordinary physical activity does not cause . . . angina, such as walking and climbing stairs. Angina with strenuous or rapid or prolonged exertion at work or recreation."
II	"Slight limitation of ordinary activity. Walking or climbing stairs rapidly, walking uphill, walking or stair climbing after meals, or in cold, or in wind, or under emotional stress, or only during the few hours after awakening. Walking more than two blocks on the level and climbing more than one flight of ordinary stairs at a normal pace and in normal conditions."
III	"Marked limitation of ordinary physical activity. Walking one to two blocks on the level and climbing one flight of stairs in normal conditions and at normal pace."
IV	"Inability to carry on any physical activity without discomfort—anginal syndrome *may be* present at rest."

*From Campeau L: Grading of angina pectoris. Circulation 54:522, 1976. Reproduced by permission of the American Heart Association, Inc.

unstable angina, however, may wax and wane repeatedly over several hours.

Typically angina is provoked by exertion, especially walking uphill, climbing stairs, vigorous arm work, coitus, or exercising in cold weather (when peripheral vascular resistance is greater). The discomfort may also be provoked by emotion (fear, anger, anxiety), may follow a meal, or may occur on lying down (angina decubitus) owing to increased ventricular filling pressure, or may occur during sleep (nocturnal angina), perhaps owing to increased adrenergic output related to dreams. Typically, exertional angina is relieved promptly (within 5 minutes) by rest; emotionally triggered angina may last longer; both usually are alleviated within 3 to 5 minutes with sublingual nitroglycerin. For patients with exertional angina, quantitation of the severity of the discomfort by a scale such as that of the Canadian Cardiovascular Society can be useful (Table 48–1).

During an episode of angina, *the physical examination* may be normal or may disclose one or more of the following: an increased heart rate and blood pressure; paradoxical splitting of the second heart sound; a precordial presystolic bulge or fourth heart sound (S_4), both due to enhanced atrial contraction into a ventricle rendered stiff by ischemia; a systolic bulge due to left ventricular dyskinesis; a diastolic bulge or S_3 gallop as evidence of significant left ventricular failure; a mid- to late-systolic murmur of mitral regurgitation related to ischemia-induced mitral papillary muscle dysfunction; or transient rales or other evidence of pulmonary venous congestion.

Other conditions that should be considered in the *differential diagnosis* of angina include the following: gastrointestinal disease—especially disordered esophageal motility, gastroesophageal reflux, peptic ulcer disease, and cholecystitis; exertional bronchospasm related to asthmatic bronchitis; chest wall discomfort related to costochondritis, muscle spasm, herpes zoster, or anxiety states, the last often presenting as submammary sharp pain of a few seconds' duration; and other cardiac and vascular diseases such as pericarditis, myocardial infarction, aortic dissection, or pulmonary embolism. These should be readily distinguished from angina in most cases by a detailed history, physical examination, and appropriate laboratory tests.

LABORATORY EVALUATION

Certain laboratory studies may help to establish a diagnosis of angina pectoris by confirming the presence and extent of underlying coronary artery disease.

ELECTROCARDIOGRAM. Although often normal at baseline, the electrocardiogram (ECG) *during* an episode of spontaneous or provoked angina may demonstrate horizontal or downsloping depression of the ST segment, T-wave peaking or inversion, and, rarely, transient ST-segment elevation. Such ECG changes, when transitory and accompanied by typical anginal discomfort, make the diagnosis of myocardial ischemia with a high degree of confidence. However, taken alone, and occurring on the resting ECG, such ST and T-wave changes are regarded as nonspecific because they accompany many other conditions including hyperventilation, electrolyte abnormalities, left ventricular hypertrophy, pericarditis, myocarditis, and the administration of digitalis and other drugs.

EXERCISE ECG. The exercise ECG or graded exercise test is a widely used clinical provocative test for myocardial ischemia in which the patient is required to exercise, usually on a treadmill or bicycle, at gradually increasing workloads until ischemic electrocardiographic changes, angina, or other limiting symptoms occur. With the increasing workload of progressive exercise, heart rate and systolic blood pressure should rise. The product of heart rate and systolic blood pressure (the double product) correlates with myocardial oxygen demand and defines an anginal threshold for a given subject. During exercise a clinically positive response is the occurrence of typical anginal chest discomfort, whereas an electrocardiographically positive response is the occurrence of 0.1 mV horizontal or downsloping ST depression at 0.08 second after the J point of the ECG.

The sensitivity of the graded exercise test for diagnosing coronary artery disease ranges from 54 to 94 per cent and is greatest in patients with the most extensive coronary artery disease. The specificity (negative test when coronary disease is absent) ranges from 67 to 97 per cent. False-positive tests are *more common* when the test is utilized in patients with a low probability of coronary disease (as for example, with the screening of asymptomatic subjects), and false-positive exercise tests are *least common* in patients with a history of typical exertional angina.

Exercise testing is useful not only for diagnosing the presence of obstructive coronary artery disease, but also for following the natural course of the disease in patients with chronic stable angina, detecting high-risk coronary artery disease, and estimating prognosis. Left main or multivessel coronary artery disease is suggested by exercise-induced hypotension, by 3.0-mm or more ST-segment depression, by downsloping ST segments, and by ischemic ST depression occurring within the first 3 minutes of exercise and/or persisting 5 or more minutes after exercise. A good prognosis is suggested by a negative exercise test or one that becomes positive only after the patient has exercised for more than three stages (> 9 minutes), or to a heart rate exceeding 160 beats per minute.

Exercise testing is generally safe; experienced laboratories report a mortality of about 1 per 10,000 tests and a morbidity requiring hospitalization of 2.4 per 10,000. Exercise testing should not be performed in patients with significant aortic stenosis, hypertension, congestive heart failure, or unstable angina, and, when exercise testing is performed, resuscitative equipment should be immediately available.

RADIONUCLIDE STUDIES. Two radionuclide-enhanced accompaniments to exercise testing are commonly utilized: myocardial perfusion imaging and radionuclide ventriculography. These tests may localize the ischemic myocardial zone and are not influenced by factors that alter interpretation of the baseline ECG such as ST-T wave changes.

Exercise myocardial perfusion imaging utilizes a radionuclide (commonly, the potassium analogue, thallium-201) that, after intravenous injection during peak treadmill exercise, distributes to the myocardium via the coronary arterial circulation and is taken up rapidly by viable myocardium in proportion to coronary blood flow. Immediate imaging discloses perfusion defects (cold spots) in zones of myocardial ischemia or prior infarction (scar). Regions of myocardial perfusion deficit correlate with severe stenosis of the coronary artery supplying the region: i.e., septum—left anterior descending coronary artery; inferior wall—right coronary artery; posterolateral wall—left circumflex coronary artery. Repeat imaging 3 to 4 hours later (more reliably, 24 hours later) shows uptake of the radionuclide by previously ischemic zones, but not by zones of prior infarction, allowing differentiation of the two. For patients unable to exercise, a dipyridamole thallium examination (investigational) may be performed; patients are administered intravenous dipyridamole, which produces vasodilation of normal or minimally atherosclerotic coronary arteries, often stealing coronary blood flow from stenotic vessels and creating regional myocardial ischemia. Thallium-201 is then injected, and imaging is performed and interpreted in a manner analogous to that for exercise thallium-201 studies.

Exercise radionuclide ventriculography consists of imaging the left ventricular blood pool first at rest and then with exercise. Imaging is performed by either the "first-pass technique," in which there is injection of a large bolus of radionuclide (commonly, technetium-99m) and assessment of cardiac blood pool activity over the next few beats as the tracer is cleared, or by the multigated equilibrium technique (MUGA), in which the red blood cells are labeled with a radionuclide and composite left ventricular function is estimated from all beats occurring during the next several minutes' observation. In most normal subjects, systolic function of the left ventricle increases during exercise, and ejection fraction (ratio of stroke volume to end-diastolic volume) rises by 0.05 or greater. Myocardial ischemia is suggested if the ejection fraction with exercise fails to rise by 0.05, if it falls, or if segmental left ventricular wall motion abnormalities appear during exercise.

In general, the radionuclide enhancements to exercise testing are expensive and are not routinely required. Perfusion scintigraphy or radionuclide ventriculography can, however, be useful in interpreting the physiologic significance of angiographically proven coronary lesions, in assessing equivocal or suspected false-positive conventional exercise tests, in evaluating patients with chest pain following coronary revascularization surgery or angioplasty, in screening for residual ischemia in patients following myocardial infarction, and in assessing patients with abnormal ECG findings (e.g., left bundle branch block). Echocardiographic imaging of regional ventricular wall motion has been used in a manner analogous to radionuclide ventriculography.

CORONARY ARTERIOGRAPHY. Coronary arteriography, the selective visualization of the major epicardial coronary arteries by radiographic contrast material, is the most precise means currently available to document the presence and extent of obstructive coronary artery disease. The results of coronary arteriography coupled with assessment of left ventricular systolic function (ejection fraction) provide powerful prognostic information concerning the natural history of coronary artery disease and, along with the clinical evaluation, can suggest the need for coronary artery revascularization by angioplasty or bypass graft surgery.

Coronary arteriography is indicated in patients with angina whose symptoms are severe (class III to IV) or unstable, in patients with angina or other evidence of myocardial ischemia following myocardial infarction, and in many patients with recurrent chest pain of uncertain etiology. Coronary arteriography is also often performed in certain categories of patients in whom angina may or may not be present, for example, those over age 40 about to undergo cardiac valve replacement or other noncoronary cardiac surgery, those with refractory ventricular arrhythmias, survivors of out-of-hospital cardiac arrest, those with heart failure thought secondary to coronary artery disease, and those with convincing electrocardiographic evidence of extensive ischemia, either during exercise testing or during electrocardiographic monitoring at rest or during normal daily activities.

Coronary artery stenoses of 70 per cent or greater diameter narrowing are generally considered flow limiting and thus clinically significant; however, coronary stenoses may be considerably underestimated on arteriography. If the coronary arteriograms are normal, the smooth muscle constrictor, ergonovine maleate, may be carefully administered intravenously in an attempt to evoke angiographic and electrocardiographic evidence of localized coronary arterial spasm in patients suspected of having coronary vasospasm.

The risks of coronary arteriography are low and are related to the skill and experience of the operator and to the severity of the patient's cardiac disease; complications are increased in patients with severe left main coronary artery disease and in those with severe left ventricular dysfunction. Experienced operators report procedural mortality in 0.2 per cent, myocardial infarction in 0.25 per cent, embolization in 0.1 per cent, and severe vascular complication at the entry site in 0.7 per cent.

GENERAL MANAGEMENT

Patients diagnosed with angina pectoris should be counseled concerning the potential serious and unpredictable nature of the condition but also advised that powerful new pharmacologic and mechanical interventions are available that may ameliorate symptoms and, in many cases, extend survival. Patients with unstable angina should undergo hospital admission to rule out myocardial infarction, to receive intensive pharmacologic therapy, and, in most cases, to undergo coronary arteriography. All patients with angina should be thoroughly instructed in risk factor modification, particularly dietary management of cholesterol and saturated fat intake, smoking cessation, and blood pressure control. A search should be made for potentially correctable conditions such as aortic stenosis, severe anemia, thyrotoxicosis, and tachyarrhythmias that might be contributing to the myocardial oxygen supply/demand imbalance causing angina.

PHARMACOLOGIC THERAPY

The goals of pharmacologic therapy of angina pectoris are to restore the imbalance between myocardial oxygen demand and supply by reducing oxygen demands, increasing coronary blood flow, or both. The most important categories of antianginal drugs are the nitrates, β blockers, and calcium channel blockers. Additionally, patients with unstable angina benefit from heparin and aspirin.

NITRATES. Nitrates alleviate angina predominantly by reducing oxygen demands, but they may improve coronary blood flow as well. Nitrates reduce oxygen demands by relaxing vascular smooth muscle, producing venodilation at low dosages but arterial and arteriolar dilation as well at higher dosages. Their major effect at usual dosages is peripheral venous pooling, which diminishes systemic venous return, thus reducing left ventricular end-diastolic pressure and volume, left ventricular wall tension, and myocardial oxygen demands. To a lesser extent, the diminished peripheral arteriolar resistance lessens myocardial oxygen demands by reducing systemic blood pressure and left ventricular wall tension. Unfortunately, the fall in systemic blood pressure may trigger a slight rise in heart rate, which augments oxygen demands. Nitrates may also improve coronary blood flow by dilating coronary vessels, reversing or preventing coronary spasm, and enhancing collateral blood flow. Furthermore, the effect on lowering left ventricular end-diastolic pressure, noted above, may allow better perfusion of subendocardial tissue.

The most commonly used nitrate preparations are nitroglycerin and isosorbide dinitrate. Nitroglycerin is available in a variety of formulations: intravenous, topical, buccal, oral, sublingual, and lingual aerosol (Table 48–2), each with different onset and duration of action. For an acute anginal attack, one of the rapidly acting preparations such as sublingual nitroglycerin is preferable, whereas for chronic prophylaxis of angina a longer-acting nitroglycerin formulation such as isosorbide dinitrate is helpful. Failure to respond to long-acting nitrates may occur if inadequate doses are utilized; however, to minimize adverse reactions, these preparations should be initiated at low doses and then titrated upward until the desired clinical response or limiting side effects occur. Topical nitroglycerin paste can be an effective formulation but, for optimal absorption, it should be spread over a wide area of skin rather than concentrated beneath the applicator paper. Intravenous nitroglycerin is useful in the treatment of unstable angina in hospitalized patients. The drug is usually begun at doses of 10 to 20 μg per minute and titrated upward by dosage increments of 10 to 20 μg at intervals of 10 to 15 minutes until chest pain is controlled or until limiting side effects, such as hypotension, occur. Once pain is stabilized with intravenous nitroglycerin, substitution of one of the long-acting preparations can usually be accomplished.

Adverse reactions to nitrate administration include cutaneous flushing, headaches, postural dizziness, nausea, and vomiting. Attenuation or resolution of these side effects usually occurs with continued administration of the drug. Nitrate tolerance or hyporesponsiveness has been noted with preparations providing constant plasma levels over many hours. It is believed that nitrate tolerance can be prevented by using the smallest effective dose of nitrate, by using less frequent dosing, and by allowing a nitrate-free interval of 8 to 12 hours daily. For example, sustained release isosorbide dinitrate produces less tolerance when administered at 8:00 AM and 2:00 PM than when given at 8:00 AM and 8:00 PM; furthermore, nitroglycerin patches are more apt to retain effectiveness if there is an overnight patch-free interval.

BETA BLOCKERS. Beta-adrenergic blockers alleviate angina predominantly by reducing oxygen demand. These drugs competitively inhibit the action of catecholamines on β receptors throughout the body. By blocking the β_1 or cardiac β receptor, these agents lower heart rate, blood pressure, and myocardial contractility, three major determinants of myocardial oxygen utilization, and thus attenuate the rise in oxygen consumption normally occurring during exercise. By slowing the heart rate, β blockers also prolong diastole, allowing more time for diastolic coronary perfusion to occur, thus indirectly augmenting coronary flow.

Many β blockers are currently available (Table 48–3) in the United States, and each has the potential to diminish angina, although not all of them are currently approved for the treatment of angina. The available agents differ according to various pharmacologic properties, and these differences may favor the use of one agent over another in certain clinical situations.

For example, cardioselectivity, a feature of some β blockers, permits selective blockade of the cardiac β_1 receptor and is potentially advantageous in patients with reactive airways disease

TABLE 48–2. AVAILABLE DOSAGE FORMS OF NITROGLYCERIN AND ISOSORBIDE DINITRATE

Medication	Dosage Form	Recommended Dosage	Onset of Action (min)	Antianginal Duration
Nitroglycerin	Intravenous	Start at 10–20 μg/min	Immediate	Transient
	Aerosol spray	0.4 mg	2	10–30 min
	Sublingual	0.3–0.8 mg	2–5	10–30 min
	Transmucosal (buccal)	1–3 mg	2–5	30–300 min
	Oral sustained release	6.5–19.5 mg	15–45	2–6 h
	Topical ointment, 2%	1.2–5.0 cm	15–60	3–8 h
	Transdermal disc or patch	10–30 mg/24 h	30–60	Up to 24 h
Isosorbide dinitrate	Sublingual	2.5–10 mg	5–20	45–120 min
	Oral	20–60 mg	15–45	2–6 h
	Oral sustained release	40 mg	15–45	Up to 8 h

*Modified from Abrams J: Am J Med 74(Suppl 6B):85–94, 1983; with permission.

who are dependent upon chronic β_2 stimulation. Selectivity is lost, however, as the dose of the cardioselective β blockers is increased; furthermore, patients with true asthma rarely tolerate β blockade, regardless of the agent used. Beta blockers with longer half-life allow once-daily dosing and, theoretically, promote better patient compliance. The ultrashort-acting intravenous β blocker esmolol may be useful in patients, including those with unstable angina, in whom rapid onset of action is desired and in whom rapid reversal would be advantageous should adverse hemodynamic effects occur. Finally, agents with partial agonist activity (intrinsic sympathomimetic activity [ISA]) activate the β receptor minimally at rest, when adrenergic tone is low, but predominantly block the β receptor under situations of heightened adrenergic tone, such as exercise or anxiety. These agents are less apt to slow the resting heart rate than non-ISA β blockers, but might prove less useful in patients with unstable or rest angina because of their weak agonist activity. Unlike other β blockers, ISA β blockers have not uniformly shown potential for improving survival in patients following myocardial infarction.

For the treatment of angina, β blockers are generally administered orally in small doses and titrated upward at 1- to 2-day intervals until clinical benefit is observed, an adverse reaction occurs, or some physiologic marker of β blockade is noted, such as a slowing of the resting heart rate to 50 to 60 beats per minute. Side effects include bradycardia, hypotension, atrioventricular (AV) block, heart failure, and central nervous system complaints (fatigue, depression, nightmares). Beta blockers are, of course, contraindicated in patients already having any of those findings. Beta blockers may contribute to lack of recognition of hypoglycemia and are thus relatively contraindicated in patients with brittle diabetes. Discontinuation of β blocker therapy should be done by gradual tapering because rebound unstable angina and myocardial infarction may occur with sudden cessation.

CALCIUM CHANNEL BLOCKERS. Calcium channel blockers alleviate angina by reducing myocardial oxygen demands as well as by increasing coronary blood flow. Calcium channel blockers limit the uptake of calcium by vascular smooth muscle and cardiac muscle required for excitation-contraction coupling, and thereby produce systemic arteriolar dilation, systemic venodilation, and reduced inotropism, all of which reduce myocardial oxygen demands. Furthermore, coronary arteries are dilated and spasm is opposed, thus enhancing myocardial oxygen delivery.

The available calcium channel blockers have considerable dissimilarity in chemical structure and adverse clinical actions (Table 48–4). Two of the agents, verapamil and diltiazem, reduce sinus node automaticity, decrease AV conduction, and thus often slow the resting heart rate. Nicardipine and nifedipine, on the other hand, are potent arterial dilators, often causing mild hypotension and reflex sinus tachycardia. All of the calcium channel blockers should be used with caution in patients with significant impairment of systolic left ventricular function (ejection fraction less than 30 per cent) and discontinued if heart failure worsens. Mild peripheral edema is common with nicardipine and nifedipine, constipation is common with verapamil, and AV block may occur in response to verapamil or diltiazem, especially with concomitant β blocker use and in patients with baseline conduction abnormalities. Serum digoxin levels may also rise upon institution of a calcium channel blocker, especially verapamil.

Calcium channel blockers are of particular benefit in patients with vasospastic or mixed angina but are also effective in those having exertional angina. Therapy is generally begun with the doses shown in Table 48–4 and gradually advanced over 2- to 3-day intervals until symptoms or other evidence of ischemia improves or until a limiting adverse reaction occurs.

COMBINATION THERAPY AND CHOICE OF AGENT. The antianginal therapy preferred in a given clinical situation may be dictated by the type of anginal presentation and by concomitant medical conditions (Table 48–5). Therapy is usually begun with sublingual nitroglycerin for treatment of acute anginal attacks and a sustained release nitrate preparation for anginal prophylaxis, owing to the relatively low cost and reasonably low side effect profile of these agents. In most patients, angina is incompletely controlled with nitrates alone, necessitating the use of a second drug. For patients having exertional angina, β blockers

TABLE 48–3. BETA BLOCKERS AVAILABLE IN THE UNITED STATES*

Medication	Approved for Angina	Cardioselective	ISA	Primary Clearance	Half-Life (hrs)	Usual Dosage[1]
Acebutolol	No	Yes	Yes	Renal	3–4	400 mg qd
Atenolol	No	Yes	No	Renal	6–9	50 mg qd
Carteolol	No	No	Yes	Renal	5–6	2.5 mg qd
Esmolol	No	Yes	No	N/A	0.15	50 μg/kg/min[3]
Labetalol[2]	No	No	No	Hepatic	6–8	200 mg bid
Metoprolol	Yes	Yes	No	Hepatic	3–7	100 mg qd
Nadolol	Yes	No	No	Renal	20–24	40 mg qd
Penbutolol	No	No	Yes	Renal	5	20 mg qd
Pindolol	No	No	Yes	Both	3–4	10 mg bid
Propranolol	Yes	No	No	Hepatic	4	60 mg bid
Timolol	No	No	No	Both	4–5	10 mg bid

*Modified from The Medical Letter 31:71, 1989; with permission.
[1]Listed, except for esmolol, are the lowest maintenance doses for control of hypertension.
[2]Labetalol also has α_1 selectivity.
[3]Lowest dose for control of supraventricular tachycardia.

TABLE 48–4. CALCIUM CHANNEL BLOCKERS AVAILABLE IN THE UNITED STATES*

Medication	Initial Dosage	Resting Heart Rate	AV Block	Edema	Constipation
Diltiazem	30 mg qid	Decreased	+ +	+	No
Sustained release	60–120 mg bid[1]				
Nicardipine	20 mg tid	Increased	No	+ + +	No
Nifedipine	10 mg tid	Increased	No	+ + +	No
Sustained release	30 mg qd				
Verapamil	80 mg tid	Decreased	+ + +	+	Yes
Sustained release	240 mg qd[1]				

Under "Unique Adverse Reactions[2]" spanning AV Block, Edema, Constipation.

*Modified from The Medical Letter 31:41–42, 1989; with permission.
[1]Initial dosage recommended for treatment of hypertension.
[2]All calcium channel blockers can cause hypotension and exacerbate heart failure.

may be combined with nitrates and often prove synergistic; i.e., β blockers prevent the nitrate-induced reflex tachycardia while the vasodilating action of nitrates reduces the tendency of β blockers to precipitate heart failure. For patients suspected of having vasospastic or mixed angina, a combination of nitrates and a calcium channel blocker is often effective. For patients having recurrent angina despite two-drug therapy, addition of the third drug (triple therapy) is often employed. For patients with persistent systems, attention should be directed toward maximizing the dose of each agent while considering the feasibility of mechanical revascularization.

ANTIPLATELET AND ANTITHROMBIN THERAPY. With the recognition that intracoronary thrombosis is often present in patients with unstable angina has come the demonstration that both aspirin and heparin may be protective against adverse events, including progression to myocardial infarction and death in patients with unstable angina. Unless there are contraindications, therefore, all patients with unstable angina should receive aspirin 325 mg daily. Hospitalized unstable angina patients should be treated with intravenous heparin with or without concomitant aspirin. The role of thrombolytic therapy for unstable angina is speculative and the subject of ongoing clinical trials. Once unstable angina stabilizes with medical therapy, angioplasty, or bypass surgery, daily aspirin therapy should be maintained for 1 year or longer.

CORONARY REVASCULARIZATION

Pharmacologic therapy, when used aggressively, can control the symptoms of angina in many patients and return them to a normal or nearly normal lifestyle. However, many physicians and patients elect to proceed with mechanical interventions for improving coronary blood flow—coronary artery bypass surgery or percutaneous transluminal coronary angioplasty. These procedures are each being performed in more than 200,000 patients annually in the United States.

TABLE 48–5. CHOICE OF ANTIANGINAL THERAPY

Situation	Choice of Therapy[1]
Type of anginal presentation	
Stable exertional angina	N, BB, CaB
Unstable angina[2]	N, CaB, BB
Vasospastic angina	N, CaB
Concomitant conditions in patient with angina	
Hypertension	BB, CaB
Diabetes	N, CaB
Heart failure	N, BB,[3] CaB[3]
AV block	N, nicardipine, or nifedipine
COPD, peripheral vascular disease	N, CaB, cardioselective BB[3]
Bradyarrhythmias	N, nicardipine, or nifedipine
Tachyarrhythmias	BB, diltiazem, or verapamil
Recent myocardial infarction	BB, ASA

[1]Drug of first choice for monotherapy is listed first. Combination therapy may also be used in most instances.
[2]Aspirin and intravenous heparin are also useful in unstable angina.
[3]Use with caution in this situation.
Abbreviations: BB = β blocker; CaB = calcium channel blocker; N = nitrate.

Coronary artery bypass surgery, popularized as a treatment for ischemic heart disease approximately 20 years ago, consists of anastomosing a reversed segment of saphenous vein between the ascending aorta and one or more stenotic coronary arteries. The procedure carries an operative mortality of approximately 1 to 3 per cent, higher in patients with disease of the left main coronary artery, with significant left ventricular dysfunction and with age greater than 65 years. Perioperative myocardial infarction occurs in 2.5 to 10 per cent of the patients. About 10 per cent of the grafts occlude within the first year postoperatively, 2 per cent occlude per year during the next 6 years, and 5 per cent occlude per year over the next 5 years. Owing to graft occlusion and progression of coronary artery disease in native vessels, angina recurs in 2 to 4 per cent of patients each year postoperatively. Recently, following the demonstration of lower rates of graft occlusion (1 per cent per year or less), internal mammary arteries rather than free saphenous vein grafts have been utilized as conduits, especially for left anterior descending artery revascularization.

Percutaneous transluminal coronary angioplasty was introduced by Gruentzig in 1979, primarily as a treatment for isolated, discrete, noncalcified, proximal stenoses in patients with single-vessel disease. As equipment has improved and operator experience has grown, the range of coronary artery lesions approachable by balloon angioplasty has expanded to encompass almost the entire spectrum formerly managed by bypass surgery. Currently, the only categories of patients having coronary artery disease in whom angioplasty is contraindicated are those with minimal coronary narrowing (no lesion of 60 per cent or greater diameter stenosis), left main stenoses, and severe diffuse multivessel disease. Angioplasty should not be performed unless in-hospital cardiovascular surgery backup is available.

Elective angioplasty is successful initially in approximately 90 per cent of patients; failures are due primarily to inability to cross the lesion with the balloon catheter or to abrupt reclosure of the vessel by dissection or thrombus following dilation. Procedure-related complications of elective angioplasty are as follows: death, 1 per cent; myocardial infarction, 4 to 5 per cent; emergency bypass surgery, 4 to 5 per cent. Complications are higher with emergency procedures, with multivessel disease, or when angioplasty is performed on complex (eccentric, angulated, or long) atherosclerotic lesions. A major limitation of coronary angioplasty is restenosis of the dilated artery in 25 to 30 per cent of patients, usually occurring within the first 6 months following angioplasty and usually amenable to repeat angioplasty.

Patients having balloon angioplasty have much shorter hospitalizations than those undergoing bypass surgery and are probably more likely to return to gainful employment. However, the long-term role of angioplasty compared to bypass surgery is unknown, particularly for patients having multivessel disease. The direct comparison of these two revascularization modalities in such patients is the subject of ongoing randomized clinical trials.

Revascularization with either angioplasty or bypass surgery is unequivocally indicated under two circumstances: (1) to alleviate incapacitating angina when medications have failed, and (2) to improve survival in certain patient subsets. Bypass surgery has been shown to improve longevity compared to continued medical therapy in patients with greater than 50 per cent stenosis of the left main coronary artery, in those with three-vessel coronary artery disease and abnormal ventricular function (ejection fraction between about 30 and 50 per cent), in those with multivessel disease with proximal left anterior descending artery involvement, and in those with residual ischemia (spontaneous or exercise-provoked) following myocardial infarction. Continued medical therapy rather than mechanical revascularization is recommended for patients with minimally obstructive (< 60 per cent diameter stenosis) coronary artery disease, especially if coronary artery spasm is suspected; for patients with chest pain atypical for angina and lacking confirmation of ischemia by objective testing; for patients without left main disease who have normal ejection fraction and good symptomatic response to antianginal therapy; for patients with left main coronary artery stenoses less than 50 per cent; for patients with prior bypass surgery and chest pain but without objective evidence of ischemia; for patients with severe left ventricular dysfunction (ejection fraction less than 20 per cent) whose primary limitation is heart failure rather than myocardial ischemia; and for elderly patients (>75 years) who have coronary disease but lack disabling angina.

Conti CR, Hill JA, Mayfield WR: Unstable angina pectoris: Pathogenesis and management. Curr Probl Cardiol 14:551–623, 1989. *A comprehensive summary of recent clinical experience in managing unstable angina with pharmacologic therapy, angioplasty, and bypass surgery.*

Frye RL, Fisher L, Schaff HV, et al.: Randomized trials in coronary artery bypass surgery. Prog Cardiovasc Dis 30:1, 1987. *A survey of the important randomized clinical trials comparing bypass surgery with continued medical therapy for patients with coronary artery disease.*

Hill JA, Pepine CJ: Silent myocardial ischemia. Annu Rev Med 39:213–219, 1988. *Most myocardial ischemia is asymptomatic, occurs during normal daily activities, and has prognosis, in general, similar to that of painful ischemia.*

Julian DG (ed.): Angina Pectoris. New York, Churchill Livingstone, 1985. *An exhaustive discussion of the historical background, epidemiology, prognosis, hemodynamics, clinical classification, physical examination, laboratory findings, and medical and surgical management of angina pectoris.*

Weiner DA, Frishman WH (eds.): Therapy of Angina Pectoris. A Comprehensive Guide for the Clinician. New York, Marcel Dekker, Inc., 1985. *An extensive description of the pathophysiology, clinical evaluation, and pharmacologic and mechanical therapy of angina pectoris.*

Willerson JT: Selection of patients for coronary arteriography. Circulation 72 (Suppl V):V3–V22, 1985. *A discussion of the various categories of patients commonly undergoing coronary arteriography and the rationale for each.*

48.2 ACUTE MYOCARDIAL INFARCTION

Burton E. Sobel

DEFINITIONS AND HISTORICAL CONSIDERATIONS. Literally, acute myocardial infarction is a focus of necrosis resulting from inadequate perfusion of the tissue. What is generally implied by the term, however, is the clinical syndrome resulting from such ischemia and manifested by sudden cardiac death; "typical" signs and symptoms of infarction such as crushing chest pain and diaphoresis, malignant ventricular arrhythmia, and congestive heart failure or shock; or atypical presentations that can be clinically silent or subtle with new-onset or accelerated angina, atypical chest pain mimicking "indigestion," impaired cerebral perfusion with syncope, or signs simulating those of a cerebrovascular accident or psychosis. Coronary thrombosis was recognized as a potential cause as early as 1910 in Obrastzow and Straschesko's report of coronary thrombosis with "status anginous" and respiratory embarrassment, and in 1912 by Herrick, who described clinical features typical of sudden coronary occlusion. Although diminution of perfusion has not been questioned, the contribution of thrombotic occlusion at sites of severe atherosclerosis as a primary phenomenon rather than as an epiphenomenon was resolved only recently. Its pivotal role was established unequivocally by early angiographic study of afflicted patients. Early catastrophic complications of infarction include ventricular fibrillation, rupture of the ventricular free wall, ventricular septal rupture (with shock and left to right shunting), or papillary muscle rupture (with profound mitral or tricuspid regurgitation). Later complications include ventricular mural thrombus with peripheral embolization and cerebrovascular accident, congestive heart failure with or without ventricular true or pseudoaneurysm, ventricular dilatation and infarct expansion, and sudden cardiac death. Progression of underlying coronary artery disease in survivors of acute myocardial infarction may result in unstable angina pectoris, "silent ischemia" (with electrocardiographic [ECG] changes without symptoms), recurrent infarction, or sudden death.

INCIDENCE AND ETIOLOGY

INCIDENCE. Heart disease, the leading cause of death in the United States, accounts for more than 30 per cent of total death, most of which is attributable to acute myocardial infarction. Age-adjusted death rates for infarction have declined dramatically, however, since 1950 (from more than 300 per 100,000 population to slightly less than 200). Nevertheless, because of population growth, the total number of infarct-related deaths in the United States has not declined, and heart disease remains responsible for more years of potential life lost before age 65, regardless of gender or race, than any other illness.

Infarction accounts for 750,000 hospital admissions in the United States annually. Diagnosed coronary disease is present in as many as 7 million Americans and kills 514,000 annually. Sudden death, precluding hospitalization, occurs in more than 350,000. Even among those who die after the prehospital phase, death is most often sudden. The impressive decline in age-adjusted death rates attributable to acute myocardial infarction over the past 25 years, a decrease of as much as 47 per cent according to some estimates, probably reflects a decreased incidence and severity of coronary atherosclerosis antedating the recent intense interest in diet, fitness, and smoking cessation. It may reflect in part early and aggressive treatment of predisposing conditions such as hypertension, widespread use of β-adrenergic blockers in patients with angina, the benefits of community-based CPR and defibrillation programs, the impact of coronary care units, and consequences of aggressive revascularization.

ETIOLOGY. Although most infarcts result from thrombotic occlusion superimposed on severe coronary atherosclerosis, severe atherosclerotic disease may exist for years with no change in severity of effort-induced angina. Occurrence of angina with progressively less effort or at rest, protracted angina simulating the pain of infarction, and acceleration of angina despite intense medical management and the absence of exacerbating factors such as anemia, arrhythmia, hypertension, congestive heart failure, thyrotoxicosis, or obesity often reflect dynamic changes in obstructing plaques with consequent intermittent thrombosis. Q-wave infarcts (previously called transmural) appear to result when occlusive thrombi persist, as documented angiographically in more than 90 per cent of patients with infarction. Non–Q-wave infarcts (previously called subendocardial) result often from incomplete or spontaneously recanalized thrombotic occlusions after ischemia sufficiently persistent to elicit necrosis. Reocclusion with early recurrent infarction is common. A common denominator of all acute coronary syndromes (sudden cardiac dath, new-onset angina, unstable angina, acute myocardial infarction) appears to be instability of atherosclerotic plaques with intramural hemorrhage, fissuring, and plaque rupture, all of which may precipitate acute thrombotic occlusion.

Risk factors for infarction parallel those for atherosclerosis in general. Diabetes mellitus, hypertension, truncal obesity, smoking, increased concentrations of low density lipoprotein (LDL) cholesterol and decreased concentrations of high density lipoprotein (HDL) cholesterol in plasma, increased concentrations of lipoprotein (a), elevated plasma homocysteine, and genetic predisposition to atherosclerosis manifested by a strong family history apply to both, as discussed in Ch. 47. Changes such as hyperglycemia and elevation of triglycerides in plasma early after infarction may be inappropriately interpreted as indicative of diabetes or hyperlipidemia when in fact they reflect transiently impaired insulin release because of reduced pancreatic blood flow, augmented glycogenolysis secondary to catecholamines, increased gluconeogenesis secondary to 17-OH corticosteroids, increased concentrations of plasma free fatty acids, and augmented hepatic synthesis of triglycerides. Conversely, plasma cholesterol may be diminished because of hepatic dysfunction and may be misinterpreted as the absence of hypercholesterolemia that would otherwise be evident. The fall in HDL cholesterol is greater than that of total cholesterol and may persist for 6 to 8 weeks.

TABLE 48–6. CONDITIONS OTHER THAN CORONARY ATHEROSCLEROSIS THAT MAY CAUSE ACUTE MYOCARDIAL INFARCTION

Coronary emboli	Causes include aortic or mitral valve lesions, left atrial or ventricular thrombi, prosthetic valves, fat emboli, intracardiac neoplasms, infective endocarditis, and paradoxical emboli.
Thrombotic coronary artery disease	May occur with oral contraceptive use, sickle cell anemia and other hemoglobinopathies, polycythemia vera, thrombocytosis, thrombotic thrombocytopenic purpura, disseminated intravascular coagulation, antithrombin III deficiency and other hypercoagulable states, macroglobulinemia and other hyperviscosity states, multiple myeloma, leukemia, malaria, and fibrinolytic system shutdown secondary to impaired plasminogen activation or excessive inhibition.
Coronary vasculitis	Seen with Takayasu's disease, Kawasaki's disease, polyarteritis nodosa, lupus erythematosus, scleroderma, rheumatoid arthritis, and immune-mediated vascular degeneration in cardiac allografts.
Coronary vasospasm	May be associated with variant angina, nitrate withdrawal, cocaine or amphetamine abuse, and angina with "normal" coronary arteries.
Infiltrative and degenerative coronary vascular disease	May result from amyloidosis, connective tissue disorders such as pseudoxanthoma elasticum, lipid storage disorders and mucopolysaccharidoses, homocystinuria, diabetes mellitus, collagen vascular disease, muscular dystrophies, and Friedreich's ataxia.
Coronary ostial occlusion	Associated with aortic dissection, luetic aortitis, aortic stenosis, and ankylosing spondylitis syndromes.
Congenital coronary anomalies	Including Bland-White-Garland syndrome of anomalous origin of the left coronary artery from the pulmonary artery, left coronary artery origin from the anterior sinus of Valsalva, coronary arteriovenous fistula or aneurysms, and myocardial bridging with secondary vascular degeneration.
Trauma	Associated with and responsible for coronary dissection, laceration, or thrombosis (with endothelial cell injury secondary to trauma such as angioplasty); radiation; and cardiac contusion.
Augmented myocardial oxygen requirements exceeding oxygen delivery	Encountered with aortic stenosis, aortic insufficiency, hypertension with severe left ventricular hypertrophy, pheochromocytoma, thyrotoxicosis, methemoglobinemia, carbon monoxide poisoning, shock, and hyperviscosity syndromes.

Several causes of acute myocardial infarction (Table 48–6) other than atherosclerosis merit particular consideration. Embolization of coronary arteries secondary to infective or marantic endocarditis (associated with drug abuse or collagen vascular disease), calcium deposits or thrombi from prosthetic or calcified valves, ventricular mural thrombi, or atrial thrombi or myxomas may be responsible. Coronary thrombosis caused by trauma or by oral contraceptives in women, perhaps attributable to diminished antithrombin III or increased plasminogen activator inhibitor type 1 (PAI-1) in plasma; vasculitis; vasospasm (idiopathic or associated with cocaine or amphetamine abuse); coronary vascular degeneration (including accelerated atherosclerosis) after cardiac transplantation; or inflammatory small vessel coronary disease (0.1- to 1.0-mm diameter vessels) associated with diabetes, collagen vascular diseases, or disorders affecting extracellular matrix may be implicated.

Occasionally, acute myocardial infarction may occur in association with syndrome X (angina with "normal" coronary arteries) or variant angina. Diminished elaboration of endothelial cell–derived relaxing factor or release of vasoconstrictors such as endothelin may contribute.

PATHOLOGY AND PATHOPHYSIOLOGY

PATHOLOGY. Coronary atherosclerosis is particularly prominent at branch points of vessels. Atherosclerotic lesions appear initially as "fatty streaks"—i.e., lipid-laden cells, presumably monocytes or macrophages, adhering to the endothelial surface and ultimately penetrating the intima. More advanced fibrous plaques comprise not only lipid-laden cells but also connective tissue and proliferating smooth muscle cells. The most advanced lesions, called complicated plaques, exhibit fibrocalcific degeneration with intra- and extracellular lipid, calcium, fibrous tissue, necrotic debris, extravasated blood, and a fibrous tissue cap. Platelet-rich mural thrombi are often associated with the surface. Atherogenesis may reflect endothelial injury; permeation of atherogenic lipoproteins such as oxidized LDL; platelet and monocyte mitogens; and impaired reverse cholesterol transport attributable to low HDL. It is undoubtedly linked intimately to thrombosis. For example, platelet-derived growth factors may contribute to atherogenesis, impaired endothelial cell function caused by early atherosclerosis may predispose to platelet adhe-

sion and activation, diminished endothelial elaboration of activators of fibrinolysis or augmented release of inhibitors may predispose to thrombosis, and vasospasm in atherosclerotic vascular segments may potentiate platelet activation through augmentation of sheer forces.

The spectrum of injury manifest in myocardium depends not only on the intensity of impairment of myocardial perfusion but also on its duration. Accordingly, no conventional microscopic or gross changes may be evident in hearts of patients who die suddenly as a result of an acute coronary event. Typical infarction is manifest by coagulation necrosis followed ultimately by fibrosis. Contraction-band necrosis occurs when ischemia is followed by reperfusion or accompanied by massive adrenergic stimulation, often with myocytolysis.

In patients who succumb with a history of preceding unstable angina, morphologic manifestations of frank infarction may be lacking. However, platelet microemboli and vascular mural thrombosis of diverse ages are seen, indicative of the underlying pathophysiology involving repetitive thrombotic phenomena initiated by dynamic changes in complicated atherosclerotic plaques. In victims of infarction reflected by evolutionary ECG changes, the classic differentiation of transmural from nontransmural infarction based on ECG criteria (the presence or absence of Q waves after complete evolution of the insult) serves only as a crude generalization in view of bidirectional overlap of morphologic lesions associated with each ECG pattern.

PATHOPHYSIOLOGY. The right and left coronary arteries arise independently from individual ostia associated with right and left aortic valve cusps. The left anterior descending (LAD) and circumflex coronary arteries arise as the left main coronary artery bifurcation and supply the anterior left ventricle, the bulk of the interventricular septum, and the lateral and posterior left ventricular walls. The apex, lateral wall, and posterior wall may be supplied by the right posterior descending coronary artery, diagonals from the LAD, and the posterior left ventricular branch of the right coronary artery, respectively. When the posterior descending coronary artery that supplies the posterior interventricular septum arises from the left circumflex, the circulation is called left dominant. More often, the posterior descending artery arises from the terminal portion of the right coronary artery (right dominant circulation). The posterior left ventricular branch of the right coronary artery supplies the atrioventricular (AV) node in 90 per cent of subjects. Another branch (in 55 per cent of subjects) supplies the sinus node. The right ventricle is supplied by the right coronary artery. Although the posterior division of the left bundle branch has a dual blood supply (from both the left and right coronary arteries), the anterior fascicle of the left bundle and the right bundle are each supplied primarily by branches of the left anterior descending coronary artery.

In view of anatomic considerations it is not surprising that right coronary artery occlusion is manifested frequently by sinus bradycardia, AV block, right ventricular infarction, or left ventricular infarction of modest extent. Conversely, markedly impaired left ventricular function with pulmonary congestion or edema indicative of extensive injury and intraventricular conduction defects such as hemiblock are more typical of left coronary artery occlusion.

Acute insults are generally attributable to thrombosis initiated by hemorrhage or rupture of complicated atheromatous plaques with deprivation of blood flow to myocardium as a final common denominator. Even if recanalization is induced relatively promptly (spontaneously, mechanically, or with fibrinolytic drugs), regional myocardial perfusion may not be sustained (the "no reflow" phenomenon) because of endothelial cell swelling, platelet and leukocyte plugs, or complement-mediated microvascular inflammation. In addition to hypoxia, decreased removal of noxious metabolites, including potassium, calcium, amphiphilic lipids, and oxygen-centered free radicals, impairs ventricular performance and may evoke lethal arrhythmias. Inflammation of endocardial surfaces and stasis associated with dyskinesis can lead to ventricular mural thrombi. Epicardial inflammation may initiate the pericardial involvement seen with as many as 20 per cent of Q-wave infarcts.

Systolic Function. Even transitory deprivation of oxygen and accumulation of metabolites are manifest promptly by diminished regional systolic contractile function and wall thickening detectable by echocardiography, abnormal wall motion detectable by radionuclide ventriculography, diminished cardiac cycle–dependent variation of backscattered ultrasound detectable by tissue characterization, and, if extensive, diminished stroke volume. Restoration of perfusion may promptly restore function of depressed myocardium even after prolonged intervals ("hibernating" myocardium). Often, however, impairment of function persists even if blood flow is restored early ("stunning")—when injury is not yet irreversible. In general, hypokinesis and dyskinesis reflect the locus and extent of myocardial injury. Expansion of infarction and ventricular dilatation begin as early as 24 hours after the onset of infarction with thinning of the infarct zone and realignment of layers of tissue within and adjacent to it. Rupture, seen in 20 per cent of fatal infarcts, may result, particularly when cardiogenic shock, malignant arrhythmia, or antecedent ventricular hypertrophy is present. Rupture may occur also with small infarcts because the well-preserved ventricular function increases wall stress.

Ventricular aneurysms are seen with early cardiac imaging in as many as 20 per cent of patients with Q-wave infarction. Clinically, they may be recognized only late, manifested by congestive heart failure, recurrent ventricular arrhythmia, or recurrent emboli. They may be accompanied by persistent ST-segment elevation in electrocardiograms obtained 6 or more weeks after infarction.

Because coronary artery disease is usually generalized, ischemia "at a distance" may be evident. As left ventricular end-diastolic volume and pressure increase because of impaired regional pump function, intramural diastolic ventricular pressure increases and myocardial perfusion declines. Peripheral arterial vasoconstriction and systemic venous constriction can no longer compensate for diminished stroke volume, and blood pressure falls. With decline of cardiac output and acceleration of heart rate, coronary flow declines further. Ischemia at a distance may be manifest simply as an ECG derangement or may result in a vicious circle in which stuttering infarction ultimately leads to profound left ventricular failure and cardiogenic shock.

Normally perfused zones may initially exhibit compensatory hyperfunction with excessive wall thickening in systole. However,

as the heart dilates over 24 to 48 hours, hyperfunction regresses.

Diastolic Function. Early after the onset of infarction, distensibility of ischemic myocardium first increases and then decreases. Effective ventricular filling can be maintained only with an increase in left ventricular end-diastolic volume and pressure (LVEDP). The increased LVEDP results in elevated pulmonary venous pressure, decreased pulmonary compliance, interstitial and ultimately alveolar pulmonary edema, hypoxemia, and exacerbation of myocardial ischemic injury. As the infarct thins and shrinks and if infarct expansion does not predominate, ventricular dilatation may regress, and diastolic cardiac and pulmonary pressures may return toward normal.

Right Ventricular Function. Impaired right ventricular function was recognized initially in the extreme, when right coronary artery occlusion led to gross right ventricular infarction. However, similar manifestations can occur when inferior left ventricular infarction and right coronary or left circumflex occlusion exist in the presence of a left dominant circulation. Right ventricular dysfunction diminishes cardiac output disproportionately to left ventricular injury. High-grade bradyarrhythmias are common, including those resulting from third-degree heart block, occasional profound arterial oxygen desaturation because of augmented right atrial pressure and right to left shunting through a patent foramen ovale, and exacerbation or extension of left ventricular infarction because of hypotension and diminished cardiac output.

Compensatory Mechanisms. Reflexly augmented sympathoadrenal and vagal discharge may give rise to tachycardia, ventricular arrhythmia, and bradycardia (sinus node depression or heart block), as well as pallor, cutaneous vasoconstriction, and diaphoresis. Initially, compromised cardiac output is maintained by the combination of increased heart rate and ventricular dilatation with recruitment of the Frank-Starling mechanism. Right ventricular infarction impairs hemodynamics most dramatically early in its course. As healing progresses and the right ventricle becomes less complaint, its conduit function is restored, permitting maintenance of cardiac output at the expense of augmentation of right ventricular filling pressure.

Effects of Myocardial Infarction on Organs Other Than the Heart. Augmentation of pulmonary venous pressure may cause diminished pulmonary compliance, dyspnea, pulmonary vascular redistribution detectable radiographically, interstitial and alveolar pulmonary edema, respiratory decompensation, and hypoxemia.

Cerebral hypoperfusion may result in restlessness or, rarely, psychosis. Coupled with dyspnea in the elderly, it may be manifest only by confusion and combativeness. Increased sympathoadrenal tone reflected by markedly elevated plasma catecholamines and adrenocortical stimulation may be prominent as well. Plasma concentrations of atrial natriuretic peptide decrease initially but then increase, perhaps because of heart failure and atrial stretch. Elevated plasma concentrations of vasopressin, angiotensin (with β-adrenergic stimulation of renin release), and aldosterone contribute to fluid retention and hyponatremia. Impaired pancreatic blood flow inhibits insulin secretion.

In addition to the typical increase in erythrocyte sedimentation rate and leukocytosis, a modest increase in plasma fibrinogen and an augmentation of circulating PAI-1 occur as part of the acute phase reaction to infarction. Impairment of fibrinolysis and augmentation of platelet activation by circulating catecholamines may predispose to continuing coronary and ventricular mural thrombosis. Plasma viscosity increases because of increased fibrinogen, α_2 globulins, and hemoconcentration several days after the onset of infarction, most markedly when left ventricular failure or shock supervenes.

Determinants of Prognosis. Immediate survival depends primarily on whether or not ventricular fibrillation occurs, and if so, whether it can be treated instantly. Community-based emergency systems with defibrillation capability, the use of defibrillators by appropriately trained lay personnel, and rapid hospitalization of patients with suspected evolving infarction have improved early survival. Even among hospitalized patients, fatality is generally attributable to ventricular fibrillation, which can, of course, often be interrupted by immediate defibrillation.

Judging from ambulatory electrocardiograms and recordings obtained in coronary care units, mortality associated with acute myocardial infarction is attributable to primary ventricular fibrillation in 85 per cent or more of instances. Only rarely is electrical asystole responsible. The association between primary ventricular fibrillation and "warning arrhythmias" (high-grade ventricular ectopy and R-on-T phenomena) is not strong, although ectopy as well as fibrillation may reflect intermittent or severe ischemia with compromise of ventricular performance exacerbating ischemia, thereby predisposing to fibrillation. Ventricular premature complexes activating the ventricle during its vulnerable period can, of course, trigger fibrillation. Nevertheless, pharmacologic suppression of ventricular ectopy per se does not necessarily protect the heart against fibrillation. In fact, suppression with type IA or IC agents, β blockers, calcium channel blockers, or type III agents may increase the incidence of asystole in patients being treated with lidocaine.

In some instances mortality may result from fibrillation secondary to cardiac decompensation accompanying profound congestive heart failure, hypotension, or shock (secondary ventricular fibrillation). Accordingly, determinants of late mortality include "infarct size" measured enzymatically or by other means at the time of the index infarct (Fig. 48–2). Diminution of left ventricular ejection fraction is a powerful descriptor.

Late mortality is determined also by the likelihood of recurrent infarction and the frequency and severity of episodic ischemia. Both may reflect progression of underlying atherosclerotic coronary artery disease and thrombosis. Complex ventricular ectopy after hospital discharge predicts subsequent mortality as well. Most late cardiac death is sudden, arrhythmic death (Fig. 48–3).

The Status of the Infarct-related Artery. Coronary thrombolysis and mechanical revascularization have revolutionized primary treatment of acute myocardial infarction largely because they salvage myocardium when implemented early after the onset of ischemia. In addition, however, prognostic benefit of an open infarct-related artery is evident even when recanalization can be induced only 6 hours or more after onset of symptoms, when salvage of substantial amounts of jeopardized ischemic myocardium is no longer likely. An open infarct-related artery is reflected ultimately by improved ventricular function, improved collateral blood flow from the infarct-related artery, decreased infarct expansion, decreased ventricular aneurysm formation, improved ventricular remodeling, diminished left ventricular dilatation, decreased late arrhythmia associated with ventricular aneurysms, decreased late potentials on the signal-averaged electrocardiogram, and decreased mortality.

SIGNS AND SYMPTOMS

"Typical" Q-wave infarction is manifested by prodromal symptoms of fatigue, chest discomfort, or malaise in the days preceding the event. Onset of infarction occurs often in the early morning

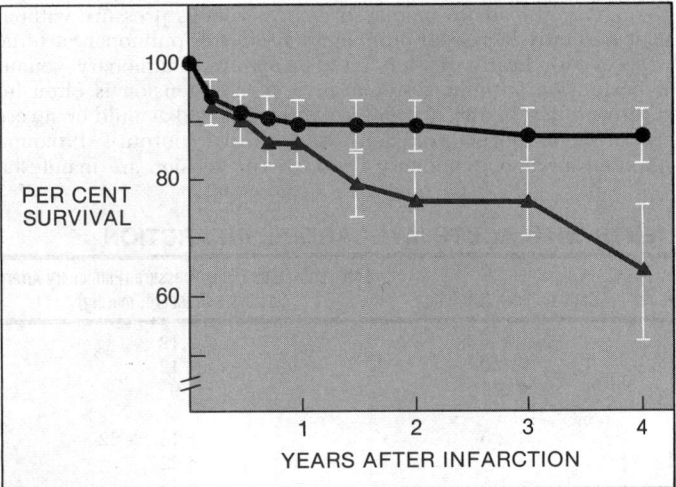

FIGURE 48–2. The influence of the extent of an initial infarct on survival. Infarct size index was estimated enzymatically and expressed as CK-g-equivalents per square meter of body surface area in 173 patients who survived for at least 24 hours. Survival was greater for those with small (< 15 CK-g-eq) *(circles)* compared with large (≥ 15 CK-g-eq) *(triangles)* infarcts. (From Geltman EM, et al.: Circulation 60:805, 1979. Reproduced by permission of the American Heart Association, Inc.)

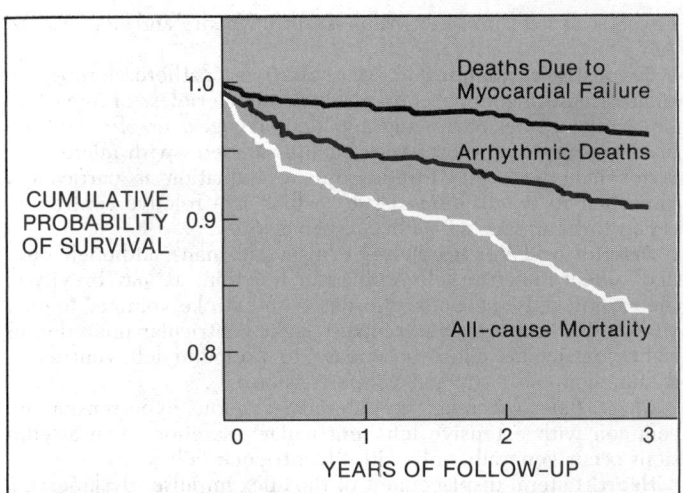

FIGURE 48–3. The large contribution of arrhythmia (sudden cardiac death) to overall mortality throughout the follow-up interval in victims of acute myocardial infarction. The ordinate shows survival from the time of hospital discharge after acute myocardial infarction. The number of patients alive and in follow-up were 0 years, 867; 1 year, 777; 2 years, 704; and 3 years, 314. (Adapted from Marcus F, et al.: Am J Cardiol 61:8, 1988; with permission.)

hours, presumably in part because of the increased catecholamine-induced platelet aggregation and diminished plasma concentrations of PAI-1 after awakening. Onset is generally not directly associated with severe exertion.

Typical pain is intense, severe, unremitting for 30 to 60 minutes, crushing or squeezing in nature, retrosternal, and often radiating down the ulnar aspect of the left arm and into the neck, teeth, or jaw. Occasionally the pain is epigastric. Diaphoresis, weakness, a sense of impending doom, profound restlessness, confusion, presyncope, hiccuping (presumably reflecting irritation of the diaphragm), nausea and vomiting, and palpitations are common. Decreased systolic ventricular performance accounts for impaired perfusion of vital organs and reflexly mediated compensatory responses to hypotension such as restlessness and impaired mentation, pallor, cutaneous vasoconstriction and sweating, tachycardia, and prerenal failure. Impaired left ventricular diastolic function leads to pulmonary vascular congestion with shortness of breath and tachypnea and pulmonary edema with orthopnea. Impaired right ventricular diastolic function leads to systemic venous hypertension, edema, hepatomegaly, and further compromise of left ventricular cardiac output.

Myocardial infarction may be clinically silent (in as many as 1 per cent of patients), with the diagnosis established only retrospectively by ECG criteria. The patient may recall only an episode of "indigestion" or nothing. Stoicism, an unusually high pain threshold, disorders impairing function of the nervous system such as diabetes mellitus, or obtundation caused by medications or impaired cerebral perfusion may prevent recognition of typical chest pain.

PHYSICAL FINDINGS TYPICAL OF ACUTE MYOCARDIAL INFARCTION. Typical clinical findings can be summarized as follows:

General Appearance. Pallor, diaphoresis, and restlessness are present.

Vital Signs. Heart rate is often increased secondary to sympathoadrenal discharge, ventricular ectopy, accelerated idioventricular rhythm, ventricular tachycardia, atrial fibrillation or flutter, or other supraventricular arrhythmias, especially when atrial infarction or heart failure is present. Bradyarrhythmias attributable to impaired sinus node function, AV nodal block, or infranodal block may be evident. The blood pressure is generally elevated initially with arterial vasoconstriction, in contrast to the case with acute pulmonary embolism, in which initial hypotension is frequent. However, with right ventricular infarction or severe left ventricular dysfunction, hypotension occurs. The respiratory rate is usually increased in response to pulmonary congestion. Coughing, wheezing, and production of frothy sputum may occur.

Fever is usually present within 24 to 48 hours and may exceed 39°C.

Funduscopic Examination. Manifestations of atherosclerotic vascular disease including copper wiring of arterioles, of hypertension with arterial narrowing and hemorrhages, or of conditions predisposing to atherosclerosis such as diabetes with microaneurysms may be seen. Funduscopic examination is particularly important to detect hemorrhage, which is a relative contraindication to treatment with fibrinolytic agents.

Arterial and Venous Pulses. Pulsus alternans, although rare, may reflect impaired left ventricular function, as may brevity of the carotid pulse secondary to decreased stroke volume. Jugular venous distention may accompany right ventricular infarction or right ventricular failure secondary to profound left ventricular dysfunction and pulmonary hypertension.

Chest. Rales secondary to pulmonary venous hypertension are common with extensive left ventricular infarction; pleural effusions occur generally only with biventricular failure.

Heart. Lateral displacement of the apex impulse, dyskinesis, a palpable S_4, and a soft S_1 may be indicative of diminished contractility of the compromised left ventricle; paradoxical splitting of S_2 may reflect left bundle branch block or prolongation of the pre-ejection period with delayed aortic valve closure despite decreased stroke volume; accentuated S_4 and S_3 may reflect diminished left ventricular compliance; a mitral regurgitation murmur indicative of either papillary muscle dysfunction or rupture or annulus dilatation may be audible even if cardiac output is diminished markedly; a pericardial friction rub may be evident. Premature ventricular beats, brief runs of ventricular tachycardia, or accelerated idioventricular rhythm are common.

Abdomen. Hepatojugular reflux may be elicited even when hepatomegaly is not marked.

Extremities. Peripheral cyanosis, edema, and pallor may indicate vasoconstriction, and diminished cardiac output may reflect right ventricular dysfunction or failure.

Neurologic Findings. Patients with acute myocardial infarction are prone to frank cerebrovascular insults as a result of ventricular mural thrombi and consequent embolization (with an incidence of approximately 1 per cent). Recrudescence of signs or symptoms of a prior cerebrovascular accident may occur secondary to diminished cerebral perfusion. In contrast, the incidence of myocardial infarction in patients with cerebrovascular accidents is substantial.

The incidence of myocardial infarction appears to be greater and its prognosis worse in patients with depression. Infarction may precipitate reactive depression whether or not β-adrenergic blocking agents or other central nervous system (CNS)–active agents are administered.

HEMODYNAMIC MANIFESTATIONS. Hemodynamic observations are of inestimable value in guiding therapy. A categorization of hemodynamic subsets of patients is shown in Table 48–7.

Patients Requiring Invasive Monitoring. Not all patients with infarction require hemodynamic monitoring with right heart catheterization and/or invasive arterial pressure monitoring.

Those who are hemodynamically stable without apparent complications such as tachycardia, refractory arrhythmia, respiratory compromise, impairment of cerebral, hepatic, or renal function, or persistent or recurrent pain indicative of recurrent or refractory ischemia, pericarditis, or incipient cardiac rupture can generally be managed without invasive hemodynamic monitoring. Effective management may be facilitated by balloon flotation right heart catheter hemodynamic monitoring in patients with pulmonary congestion indicative of pulmonary venous hypertension reflected by physical findings or chest roentgenographic abnormalities, but many patients with mild complications can be managed conservatively. Patients with peripheral hypoperfusion despite initial administration of fluids to replete or expand vascular volume and those with severe, refractory, or progressive congestive heart failure, potentially catastrophic complications of acute infarction refractory arrhythmias, persistent pain, or hemodynamic instability should be evaluated by balloon flotation right heart catheter hemodynamic monitoring.

Monitoring catheters should generally be introduced through compressible sites, particularly because of the high likelihood that thrombolytic agents will be used early in the treatment of infarction. They should remain in place for no more than 72 hours to avoid the risk of infection and can often be removed much more promptly. Sometimes ascertainment of systemic and pulmonary venous pressure, cardiac output, and peripheral vascular resistance is sufficient for subsequent management without the need for continuous monitoring. In other instances the effects of vasodilators, diuretics, agents with positive inotropic effects, and therapeutic alterations of vascular volume should be monitored over the ensuing 48 to 72 hours.

Hemodynamic Subsets. Patients are categorized with respect to cardiac output (increased, normal, or diminished), systemic arterial blood pressure (increased, normal, or diminished with or without increased or decreased systemic vascular resistance), and the presence or absence of pulmonary venous hypertension (augmented pulmonary arterial wedge pressure) (Table 48–7).

Patients without diminished systemic arterial blood pressure or pulmonary venous hypertension may have normal or hyperdynamic hemodynamics (the latter reflected by a high cardiac output with or without hypertension caused by sympathoadrenal stimulation). Systemic arterial hypotension may be attributable to relative or absolute hypovolemia or to right ventricular infarction (generally reflected by augmented systemic venous pressure). Rarely, it reflects decreased peripheral vascular resistance caused by vagotonia or sepsis. The noncompliant left ventricle requires augmented filling pressure to sustain cardiac output. Accordingly, relative hypovolemia may exist despite moderately elevated left ventricular filling pressure. Central venous pressure cannot be relied upon for assessment of vascular volume.

Right ventricular failure with or without concomitant tricuspid regurgitation leads to increased central venous pressure without concomitantly increased pulmonary venous or pulmonary arterial occlusive (indicative of left atrial) pressure. Pulmonary venous hypertension without systemic arterial hypotension is often indicative of left ventricular failure (differentiated as mild or severe in terms of normal or depressed cardiac output). Profound hypotension and pulmonary venous hypertension are manifesta-

TABLE 48–7. HEMODYNAMIC SUBSETS AMONG PATIENTS WITH ACUTE MYOCARDIAL INFARCTION

Hemodynamic Subset		Systemic Arterial Blood Pressure	Cardiac Index (L/m²/min)	Left Ventricular Filling Pressure (Pulmonary Artery Occlusive Pressure; mm Hg)
I	Normal hemodynamics	Normal	2.7 ± 0.5	≤ 12
II	Hyperdynamic state	Increased	> 3.0	< 12
III	Hypovolemia*	Decreased	≤ 2.7	≤ 9
IV	Left ventricular failure			
	A. Mild	Normal	≤ 2.5	> 18, ≤ 22
	B. Severe	Normal or decreased	≤ 1.8	≥ 22
V	Cardiogenic shock	Decreased	≤ 1.8	≥ 18
VI	Shock attributable to right ventricular infarction†	Decreased	≤ 1.8	≤ 18

Adapted from Forrester JS, et al.: Medical therapy of acute myocardial infarction by application of hemodynamic subsets. N Engl J Med 295:1404, 1976. By permission of the New England Journal of Medicine.

*Relative hypovolemia may result in hypertension even if pulmonary artery pressure is moderately elevated (≤ 18) if left ventricular compliance is decreased associated with infarction or failure.

†Central venous (systemic venous) pressure is often markedly elevated (upper limit of normal = 6 mm Hg).

tions of cardiogenic shock. The vicious circle of cardiogenic shock—progressive infarction with declining cardiac output, further compromise of perfusion, and ultimately extensive necrosis with profound failure and shock—is generally irreversible without prompt mechanical support of the circulation and coronary revascularization with thrombolytic drugs, angioplasty, or surgery.

In general, hemodynamic status reflects the extent of left ventricular infarction. However, an infarct of modest extent superimposed on a previous infarct can profoundly compromise hemodynamics. Initial impairment of ventricular performance may exceed that attributable to irreversible injury because of myocardial stunning early after the onset of infarction. Right ventricular involvement may compromise cardiac output more than anticipated from the extent of left ventricular injury alone.

LABORATORY DETERMINATIONS

The objectives of acquiring laboratory data include determination of the presence or absence of infarction (diagnosis and differential diagnosis); characterization of the locus, nature (Q or non-Q), and extent of infarction (estimation of infarct size); detection of recurrent ischemia or infarction (extension of infarction); detection of early and late complications of infarction; and estimation of prognosis.

The complete blood count and platelet count (which may decrease after heparin) are useful not only diagnostically but in assessing suitability for treatment with thrombolytic drugs. The leukocyte count may be normal initially but generally increases within 2 hours and peaks in 2 to 4 days with predominance of polymorphonuclear leukocytes and a shift to the left. Elevations generally persist for 1 to 2 weeks. Other components of the acute phase reaction contribute to elevations of the erythrocyte sedimentation rate (ESR) within 48 hours with subsequent changes paralleling those in the leukocyte count. Because of increased pulmonary and sometimes systemic venous pressure, contraction of plasma volume is common after acute myocardial infarction, manifested not only by hemoconcentration but also by prerenal failure with elevation of plasma creatinine and blood urea nitrogen. Arterial blood gases should be assayed if necessary to evaluate hypoxemia resulting from pulmonary congestion, atelectasis, or ventilatory impairment secondary to complications of infarction or excessive sedation or analgesia. Fingertip oximetry may be adequate and can obviate the need for arterial puncture and bleeding in patients treated with thrombolytic drugs. The chest radiograph is particularly useful in determining the presence or absence of cardiomegaly (often correlated with the presence or absence of increased LVEDP or left atrial pressure, and of pulmonary venous hypertension), pulmonary edema, pleural effusions, Kerley B lines, and other criteria of congestive heart failure. A small cardiac silhouette and clear lung fields in a patient with systemic hypotension may be indicative of relative or absolute hypovolemia. A large cardiac silhouette with similar hemodynamics may reflect hemopericardium and tamponade or right ventricular infarction compromising cardiac output. Chest radiographic findings indicative of pulmonary venous hypertension may occur later and persist longer because of delay in fluid shifts between vascular, interstitial, and alveolar spaces.

Sequential ECG findings remain hallmarks of diagnosis despite the occasional occurrence of infarction without any acute changes and the nonspecific nature of some of the ECG changes that may be seen. The diagnosis can be established with certainty when typical ST elevation persists for hours and is followed by T-wave inversion within the first few days and Q waves subsequently. However, initial ST depression or T-wave inversion is difficult to differentiate from that seen with ischemia without infarction or in unrelated conditions (Table 48–8). ST-segment depression followed by T-wave inversion without evolution of Q waves can result from non–Q-wave infarction or subendocardial ischemia without infarction. Q-wave infarction cannot be differentiated from non–Q-wave infarction initially if ST elevation is lacking and Q waves have not yet developed. Infarction is often associated with nonspecific ECG changes including intraventricular conduction delays; ventricular and supraventricular arrhythmias; signs of atrial infarction, such as changes in P-wave morphology, elevation or depression of the PQ segment, atrial flutter or fibrillation, or a wandering atrial pacemaker; and signs of right ventricular infarction such as ST elevation or Q waves detectable

TABLE 48–8. CONDITIONS ASSOCIATED WITH ELECTROCARDIOGRAPHIC CHANGES THAT MAY OBSCURE OR SIMULATE THOSE INDICATIVE OF ACUTE MYOCARDIAL INFARCTION

Abnormality	Examples
Intraventricular conduction abnormalities	Left bundle branch block, left anterior superior fascicular block, infranodal arborization block, right ventricular transvenous or epicardial pacing
Electrolyte disturbances	Hypo- or hyperkalemia, hypocalcemia
Pre-excitation	Wolff-Parkinson-White syndrome
Early repolarization	
Cerebrovascular accident	
Myocarditis	Inflammatory, infiltrative, viral, collagen vascular disorders, pheochromocytoma, cardiac allograph rejection, neuromuscular disorders such as muscular dystrophy and Friedreich's ataxia
Left ventricular hypertrophy	Hypertrophic cardiomyopathy, dilated cardiomyopathy, valvular heart disease, hypertension
Right ventricular hypertrophy	Cor pulmonale, acute pulmonary embolus, pneumothorax
Cardiac tumors	
Pericarditis	

in right-sided precordial leads. The appearance of abnormalities in a large number of ECG leads is often indicative of extensive injury or concomitant pericarditis. Anterior and anterolateral infarcts tend to involve more left ventricular myocardium than inferior or true posterior infarcts.

MACROMOLECULAR MARKERS OF INFARCTION. Detection of elevated concentrations in plasma of macromolecules released from irreversibly injured myocardium has become the definitive diagnostic criterion of infarction. Enzymes, including creatine kinase (CK), aspartate serum transaminase (AST), and lactate dehydrogenase (LDH); myoglobin; and myosin light chains, among numerous other constituents, egress from irreversibly injured ischemic myocardium within several hours after the onset of the insult. Their elevated concentrations in plasma constitute sensitive diagnostic findings. Specificity is limited, however, because of their ubiquitous distribution in skeletal muscle and other tissues. Assay of activity in plasma of the MB isoenzyme of CK (MB CK) is the cornerstone of diagnosis because of the marked abundance of this isoenzyme in myocardium and virtual absence from most other tissues, and its consequent sensitivity (detection of necrosis of less than 100 mg of myocardium). Characteristic sequential changes of plasma MB CK include elevations above normal within 4 hours, a two- to 10-fold peak in 16 to 24 hours, and a return to baseline within 3 to 4 days. The magnitude and persistence of elevations are useful in estimating the extent of infarction.

Initially normal enzyme values are seen often when patients present very early after the onset of infarction. Thus, discharge from an emergency room of a patient with a history consistent with myocardial infarction should not occur without several hours of observation and repeat determinations. If infarction has occurred more than 24 hours before admission, is of very modest magnitude, or is stuttering in nature, enzyme elevations may be lacking because of the predominance of clearance over rates of release into the circulation. Assay of myosin light chains or the $LDH_1:LDH_2$ isoenzyme ratio, which remains elevated for several days after infarction because of the slow clearance of LDH, may be helpful. Late detection of infarction is sometimes facilitated by myocardial infarct scintigraphy with technetium-99m (^{99m}Tc)-pyrophosphate or radiolabeled antimyosin antibodies (investigational).

Generally, MB CK is assayed at the time of admission and at 12- to 24-hour intervals until the diagnosis is established. Determination of total CK is less specific and is redundant. Recently, assays detecting post-translational conversion of individual iso-enzymes of CK to isoforms have been shown to permit even earlier diagnosis (within 2 to 3 hours of infarction). Recanalization is reflected by sudden washout of the tissue isoform into plasma. Isoform analysis is likely to become useful for monitoring interventions such as coronary thrombolysis. Determination of plasma concentrations of myoglobin, a protein with a short half-life in the circulation, offers similar promise, but results may be distorted by changes in renal function with prerenal failure.

IMAGING. Several noninvasive modalities permit detection of regional wall motion and hypokinesis or dyskinesis, as well as estimation of overall ventricular performance (Fig. 48–4). These include two-dimensional and color flow Doppler echocardiography, radionuclide ventriculography, ultrafast (cine) computed tomography, and gated magnetic resonance imaging. Because of cost considerations and convenience, only the first two are used widely. Sensitivity and specificity of abnormal wall motion as criteria of acute myocardial infarction exceed 90 per cent, particularly in patients without previous infarction. Assessment of segmental function and overall left ventricular performance has prognostic implications and is essential when infarction is extensive (elevations of MB CK exceeding 150 IU per liter) or complicated by shock or profound heart failure, in part to identify potentially surgically correctable complications and to detect ventricular true or false aneurysms and thrombi (Fig. 48–5) that can be treated with anticoagulants or fibrinolytic drugs. Imaging is useful also to detect pericardial effusion, concomitant valvular or congenital heart disease, and marked depression of ventricular function that may interdict treatment with calcium antagonists or β-adrenergic blockers. Doppler echocardiography is particularly useful in estimating the severity of mitral or tricuspid regurgitation, detecting ventricular septal defects secondary to rupture, assessing diastolic function, and monitoring cardiac output calculated from flow velocity and aortic valve area. When right ventricular infarction is suspected or when infarction is superimposed on a previous insult or associated with ECG phenomena such as left bundle branch block that obscure diagnosis, assessment of right ventricular function and delineation of regional wall motion may be particularly helpful.

Infarct-avid agents such as ^{99m}Tc-pyrophosphate and radiolabeled antimyosin antibodies (investigational) can sensitively detect infarction and define its locus. However, positive results with infarct scintigraphy cannot be obtained generally until 24

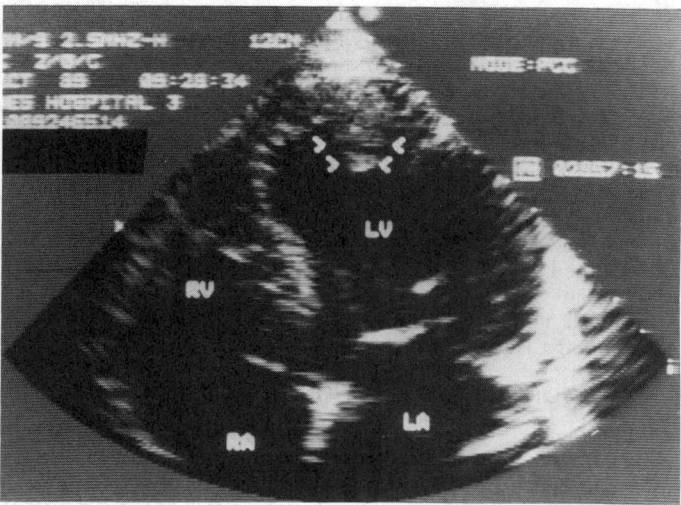

FIGURE 48–5. An apical four-chamber two-dimensional echocardiographic still frame demonstrating thrombus in the apex of the left ventricle (*arrows*) associated with acute myocardial infarction. LV = Left ventricle; RV = right ventricular; RA = right atrium; LA = left atrium. (Courtesy of Dr. J. E. Perez, Washington University School of Medicine, St. Louis, MO.)

hours or more after the onset of infarction and may be simulated by accumulation of tracer in temporally remote infarcts. Perfusion scintigraphy with tracers such as thallium-201 or ^{99m}Tc-isonitrile is sometimes useful when the diagnosis is obscure.

Positron emission tomography with tracers of intermediary metabolism (Fig. 48–6), perfusion (Fig. 48–7), or oxidative metabolism (Fig. 48–7) permits quantitative assessment of the distribution and extent of impairment of myocardial oxidative metabolism and regional myocardial perfusion (Fig. 48–8). It has been particularly useful in defining the efficacy of therapeutic interventions designed to salvage myocardium and has been used diagnostically to differentiate reversible from irreversible injury in hypoperfused zones.

DIFFERENTIAL DIAGNOSIS

When the history of acute myocardial infarction is typical, the initial electrocardiogram abnormal and followed by definitive sequential changes, and MB CK elevated in the initial or subsequent plasma samples with typical sequential changes, the diagnosis is straightforward. A presumptive diagnosis can be made when any two of these criteria are present. Unfortunately, however, the diagnosis may be obscure in patients seen very early after the onset of infarction and in those with ECG manifestations of prior ischemic or other types of heart disease, electrocardiographically silent infarcts, or atypical presentations. Differentiation from ischemia without infarction (unstable angina, aortic stenosis in the elderly, ischemia attributable to right ventricular overload, new-onset angina, or inadequate myocardial perfusion in markedly hypertrophied left ventricles or in association with marked aortic insufficiency) and from pericarditis with pain simulating that of infarction may be difficult without the aid of laboratory tests and cardiac imaging. A critical differential diagnostic consideration is aortic dissection. It should be suspected whenever pain is atypical or not associated with ECG changes typical of infarction.

Pleurodynia, pulmonary embolism or infarction, pneumothorax, pneumonitis, musculoskeletal pain associated with bursitis, the shoulder/hand syndrome, pectoral lymphadenopathy, herpes zoster before eruption of the typical vesicles, myalgia, and costochondritis may simulate infarction superficially but can usually be differentiated easily on the basis of physical findings, results of laboratory tests, and chest radiography. Pain of abdominal origin that may masquerade as infarction includes that caused by cholecystitis or cholelithiasis, pancreatitis, duodenal or gastric ulcer, gastritis, esophagitis, esophageal spasm, or esophageal reflux associated with a hiatal hernia.

CARE OF THE PATIENT

The focus of treatment differs in the prehospital, hospital (coronary care unit and step-down unit), and convalescent phases

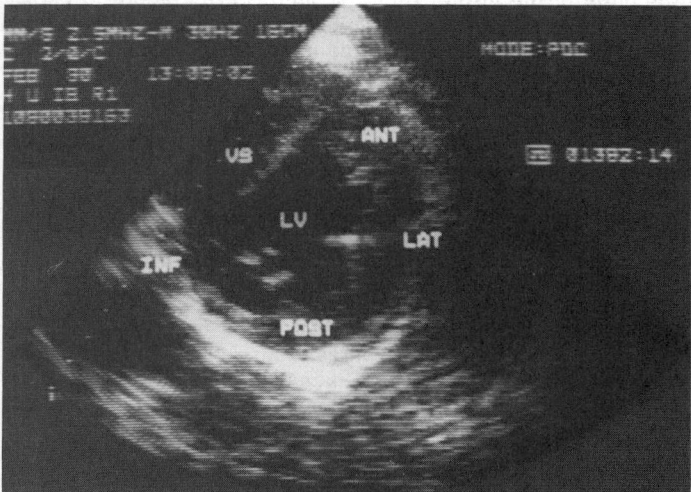

FIGURE 48–4. A still-frame short-access two-dimensional echocardiogram illustrating an inferoposterior left ventricular aneurysm after acute myocardial infarction evident as an outpocketing of the thinned left ventricular wall on the perimeter of the left ventricular cavity in the region corresponding to 6 to 9 o'clock, with the center of the clock face envisioned as central. The echo densities within the left ventricular cavity posteriorly and laterally are caused by papillary muscles. ANT = Anterior; LAT = lateral; POST = posterior; INF = inferior; VS = ventricular septum; LV = left ventricular cavity. (Courtesy of Dr. J. E. Perez, Washington University School of Medicine, St. Louis, MO.)

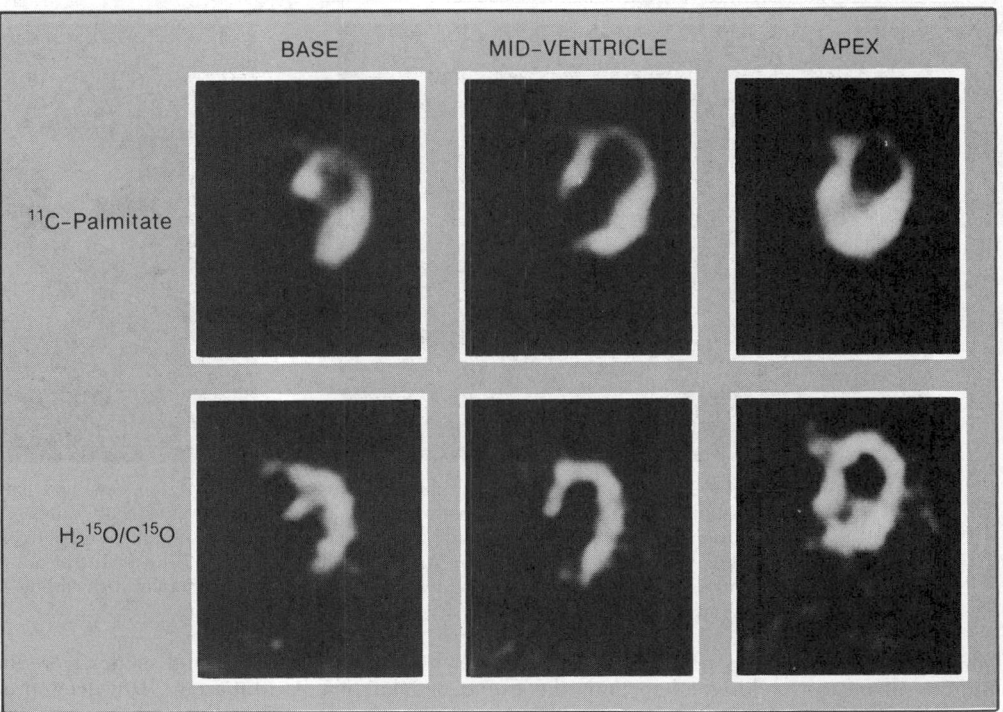

FIGURE 48–6. Positron emission tomograms at three levels of the left ventricle obtained from a subject with myocardial infarction after late spontaneous coronary recanalization. Anterior myocardium is at the top right, the left ventricular free wall at the bottom right, and posterior myocardium at the bottom left. Reconstructions acquired after intravenous administration of ^{11}C-palmitate show the persistent anterior defect despite homogeneous myocardial perfusion imaged with $H_2^{15}O$ and blood pool subtraction with $C^{15}O$. The discontinuity posteriorly in some tomographic sections is attributable to the mitral valve apparatus. (From Bergmann SR, et al.: Prog Cardiovasc Dis 28:165, 1985; with permission.)

despite considerable overlap of objectives in each. Most death caused by infarction occurs early and is attributable to primary ventricular fibrillation. Thus, initial objectives are immediate ECG monitoring and reversal of ventricular fibrillation should it occur.

TREATMENT IN THE PREHOSPITAL PHASE. Community-based systems in Belfast, Ireland; Columbus, Ohio; Los Angeles, California; and Seattle, Washington, have conclusively documented the effectiveness of rapidly responding rescuers such as police and firefighters trained in defibrillation. Approximately 65 per cent of deaths caused by infarction occur in the first hour. More than 60 per cent (39 per cent of those who would succumb) can be saved by defibrillation initiated by a bystander or first-responding rescuer. Additional objectives of prehospital care by paramedical and emergency room personnel include adequate analgesia (generally with morphine), reduction of excessive sympathoadrenal and vagal stimulation pharmacologically, prophylaxis and treatment of malignant ventricular arrhythmias (generally with lidocaine), and support of cardiac output, systemic blood pressure, and respiration. Atropine (0.5 mg IV at 5-minute

intervals to a maximum of 2 to 4 mg) is particularly useful in counteracting excessive vagal tone often underlying bradyarrhythmias and hypotension. It is indicated when heart rate is disproportionately diminished with respect to blood pressure, when hypotension (sometimes secondary to morphine) is refractory despite augmentation of left ventricular filling pressure, or when impaired AV nodal conduction with Wenckebach block is evident. If bradycardia persists, pacing may be required.

The advent of coronary thrombolysis as primary therapy for Q-wave infarction has already revolutionized management of patients in the hospital. Prehospital phase coronary thrombolysis initiated by paramedical personnel under medical supervision appears likely to become important as well because of its promise for salvaging more myocardium because of earlier interruption of ischemia.

TREATMENT IN THE HOSPITAL PHASE. Cardiac care units (CCU's) have reduced early mortality attributable to acute myocardial infarction by approximately 50 per cent, largely by immediate implementation of defibrillation. They have proven to be optimal facilities for continuous ECG monitoring, invasive

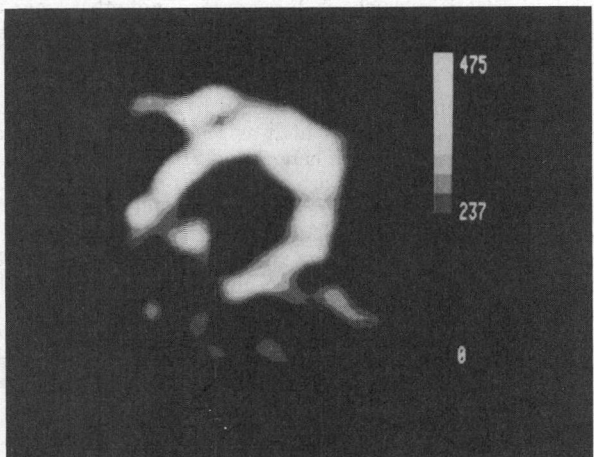
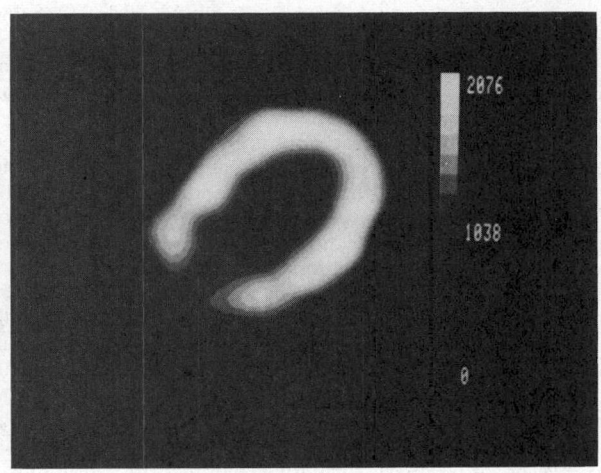

FIGURE 48–7. A single midventricular positron emission tomographic reconstruction obtained from a normal subject. Perfusion (*left*) assessed with $H_2^{15}O$ and myocardial oxidative metabolism (*right*) assessed with ^{11}C-acetate are homogeneous. The scales indicate counts per pixel. Orientation is the same as in Figure 48–6. (Courtesy of Dr. S. R. Bergmann, Washington University School of Medicine, St. Louis, MO.)

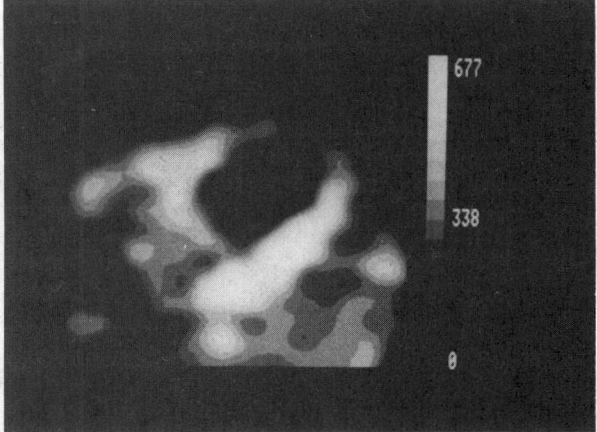 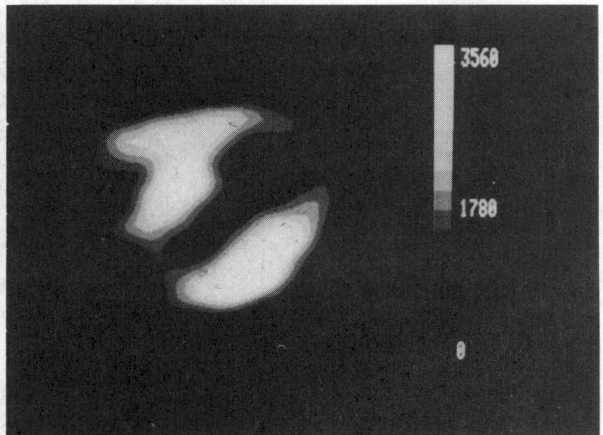

FIGURE 48–8. Midventricular tomographic reconstructions of perfusion (*left*) and oxidative metabolism (*right*) obtained after intravenous administration of $H_2{}^{15}O$ and ${}^{11}C$-acetate after acute anterior myocardial infarction. A large perfusion deficit is evident anteriorly with a concordant decrease in myocardial oxygen consumption reflected by decreased ${}^{11}C$-acetate uptake. (From Walsh MN, Geltman EM, Brown MA, et al.: Noninvasive estimation of regional myocardial oxygen consumption by positron emission tomography with carbon-11 acetate in patients with myocardial infarction. J Nucl Med 30:1798, 1989; with permission.)

hemodynamic monitoring when indicated, implementation and titration of measures designed to limit the extent of infarction and salvage jeopardized ischemic myocardium, and induction of recanalization of infarct-related arteries pharmacologically.

Care in the CCU. In addition to continuous ECG monitoring, several general measures should be implemented. Diet should include liquid only during the first 24 hours because of the risk of aspiration with the frequent nausea and vomiting, and possible cardiac arrest. Stool softeners are helpful to avoid constipation, straining, and consequent circulatory derangements. Patients with uncomplicated infarction need be confined to bed for only 1 day. Physical activity should be limited (bed-chair regimen) throughout the 2- to 3-day CCU stay, with gradual and carefully monitored resumption of ambulatory activity in the late hospital phase. Sedative, anxiolytic, and hypnotic drugs at night may be helpful but cannot replace optimal communication by compassionate physicians and nurses and the reassurance it provides. Oxygen should be given to avoid hypoxemia. High doses may be counterproductive because of vasoconstriction and lack of augmentation of myocardial oxygen delivery in normoxemic patients.

Refractory or severe pain should be treated with intravenous morphine, meperidine, or pentazocine. Repeated intravenous doses of 4 to 8 mg of morphine at intervals of 5 to 15 minutes can be given with relative impunity until the pain is relieved or toxicity is manifest by hypotension, vomiting, or depression of respiration. Prodigious quantities are sometimes required (2 to 3 mg per kilogram). Should toxicity occur, a morphine antagonist such as naloxone can reverse it. Morphine-induced hypotension in a patient without incipient or overt pulmonary edema can be minimized by maintenance of the patient in a supine position, elevation of the legs, administration of fluids, and administration of atropine if heart rate is not increased.

Continuing chest pain indicative of ischemia should be treated with agents diminishing myocardial oxygen requirements and potentiating myocardial perfusion. Intravenous nitroglycerin titrated (10 to 200 µg per minute) to avoid hypotension reduces peripheral arterial resistance and ventricular afterload. Higher doses diminish systemic venous tone, blood pressure, and ischemic zone perfusion. Favorable effects are probably mediated by diminished afterload and preload and decreased LVEDP facilitating myocardial perfusion. Although coronary vasodilation in intramural vessels is often already maximal as a result of accumulation of vasodilator metabolites locally, nitrates may dilate epicardial vessels and reduce vasospasm, thereby reducing shear forces otherwise contributing to platelet activation and potentiating propagation of coronary thrombi. Tolerance to continuously administered intravenous nitrates occurs rapidly, often within hours.

Oral calcium channel blockers such as nifedipine and diltiazem are often useful because they reduce ventricular afterload (nifed-

ipine) and modestly reduce heart rate and contractility as well (diltiazem). However, prognosis appears to be affected adversely in patients with congestive heart failure or impaired left ventricular function that persists after myocardial infarction by treatment with diltiazem and possibly other calcium channel blockers as well. Oral or intravenous conventional or ultra–short-acting β-adrenergic blockers such as esmolol may ameliorate ischemia and pain by lowering heart rate and hence myocardial oxygen requirements. Theoretically, calcium antagonists and β-adrenergic blockers may exert anti-injury effects as well by diminishing inward calcium flux in cardiac myocytes.

Despite the use of effective analgesia with nitrous oxide given by inhalation in concentrations of 20 to 50 per cent combined with oxygen in Europe and elsewhere, this agent is not used widely in the United States. Its effects on ventricular afterload are favorable, and it is generally well tolerated for intervals as long as 24 to 48 hours when used intermittently.

Limitation of Infarct Size. Because the evolution of infarction is dynamic and determined in part by the imbalance between myocardial oxygen requirements and oxygen supply, early treatment focuses not only on prompt recanalization of the infarct-related artery but also on diminution of myocardial oxygen requirements without compromise of perfusion of vital organs. Myocardial protection can be enhanced with β-adrenergic blockers to reduce heart rate; arterial vasodilators such as nifedipine, nitrates, or angiotensin-converting enzyme (ACE) inhibitors to reduce ventricular afterload; and diuretics with pulmonary venous dilating properties such as furosemide and ethacrynic acid to reduce left ventricular preload. Beta-adrenergic blockers are likely to be useful in most patients without specific contraindications such as heart failure, bradycardia, or bronchial constriction. Other agents should be titrated to optimize left ventricular filling pressure (often to as high as 18 to 22 mm Hg because of decreased ventricular compliance) and cardiac output while maintaining adequate systemic arterial blood pressure (Table 48–9).

Coronary Thrombolysis. The potential value of coronary thrombolysis has been recognized for more than 30 years. Its emergence as primary therapy was delayed, however, until the pivotal role of thrombosis in causing Q-wave infarction had been established unequivocally by coronary arteriography, the impact of extensive infarction on mortality had been established, and salvage of myocardium by decreasing oxygen requirements had been found to be limited. The "modern" era of coronary thrombolysis began in the late 1970's with the demonstration that intracoronary administration of plasminogen activators recanalized occluded arteries and immediately relieved pain. Recanalization was soon documented in 70 to 75 per cent of patients given intracoronary streptokinase. However, intracoronary dosing entailed serious disadvantages including risk and delay associated with the obligatory cardiac catheterization. Intravenous administration was soon

TABLE 48–9. THERAPEUTIC INTERVENTIONS TAILORED TO SPECIFIC HEMODYNAMIC SUBSETS

Hemodynamic Subset		Intervention	Remarks
I	Normal hemodynamics	None required	
II	Hyperdynamic state	Beta-adrenergic blockade	Analgesics and anxiolytic drugs may be helpful.
III	Hypovolemia	Intravenous fluids to augment effective vascular volume	Marked increases in pulmonary artery occlusive pressure reflecting pulmonary venous hypertension and increased left ventricular filling pressure may occur if heart failure is unmasked or exacerbated; manifestations may include dyspnea, hypoxemia, bronchospasm and rales, and pulmonary congestion evident radiographically.
IV	Left ventricular failure		
	A. Mild	Systemic arterial vasodilators	Diuretics may be useful if failure is refractory.
	B. Severe	Systemic arterial vasodilators and diuretics	Cardiotonic agents may be helpful if hypotension supervenes, but their use can exacerbate the imbalance between myocardial oxygen requirements and supply; sympathomimetic and dopaminergic agents may be helpful, but their benefit on hemodynamics is usually only transitory and may exacerbate ischemic injury.
V	Cardiogenic shock	Coronary recanalization and circulatory support	
VI	Shock attributable to right ventricular infarction	Augmentation of vascular volume and cardiotonic agents	

Adapted from Forrester JS, et al.: Medical therapy of acute myocardial infarction by application of hemodynamic subsets. N Engl J Med 295:1404, 1976. By permission of the New England Journal of Medicine.

shown to be effective in recanalizing approximately 50 per cent of infarct-related arteries when streptokinase was used and 75 to 80 per cent (comparable to the optimal recanalization rates with any agent by any route of administration) when tissue-type plasminogen activator (t-PA) was used (Fig. 48–9). The superiority of intravenously administered second- compared with first-generation plasminogen activators in recanalizing coronary arteries may reflect (1) more modest plasminemia with its consequent procoagulant and platelet-activating effects counteracting thrombolysis; (2) a lack of "plasminogen steal" with consequent maintenance of high concentrations of clot-associated plasminogen available for activation to plasmin induction of lysis; and (3) the feasibility of safe administration of high concentrations of activator with less degradation of hemostatic proteins.

Induction of coronary thrombolysis with intravenously administered activators of plasminogen improves ventricular function

and decreases mortality both early and late after infarction, particularly when initiated within a few hours after the onset of ischemia. Even when initiated only 6 hours or more after the onset of infarction, restoration of patency of the infarct-related artery appears to confer benefits reflected by improved collateral blood flow, improved ventricular remodeling, decreased infarct expansion, decreased late potentials manifest in signal-averaged electrocardiograms potentially indicative of arrhythmogenicity, improved late ventricular function, decreased ventricular aneurysm formation, decreased late arrhythmia associated with those aneurysms that do develop, and decreased mortality.

It is convenient and useful to consider two generations of fibrinolytic drugs. The first, typified by streptokinase, urokinase, and APSAC (acetylated plasminogen streptokinase activator complex) induces activation of free plasminogen and clot-associated plasminogen indiscriminately. First-generation drugs invariably

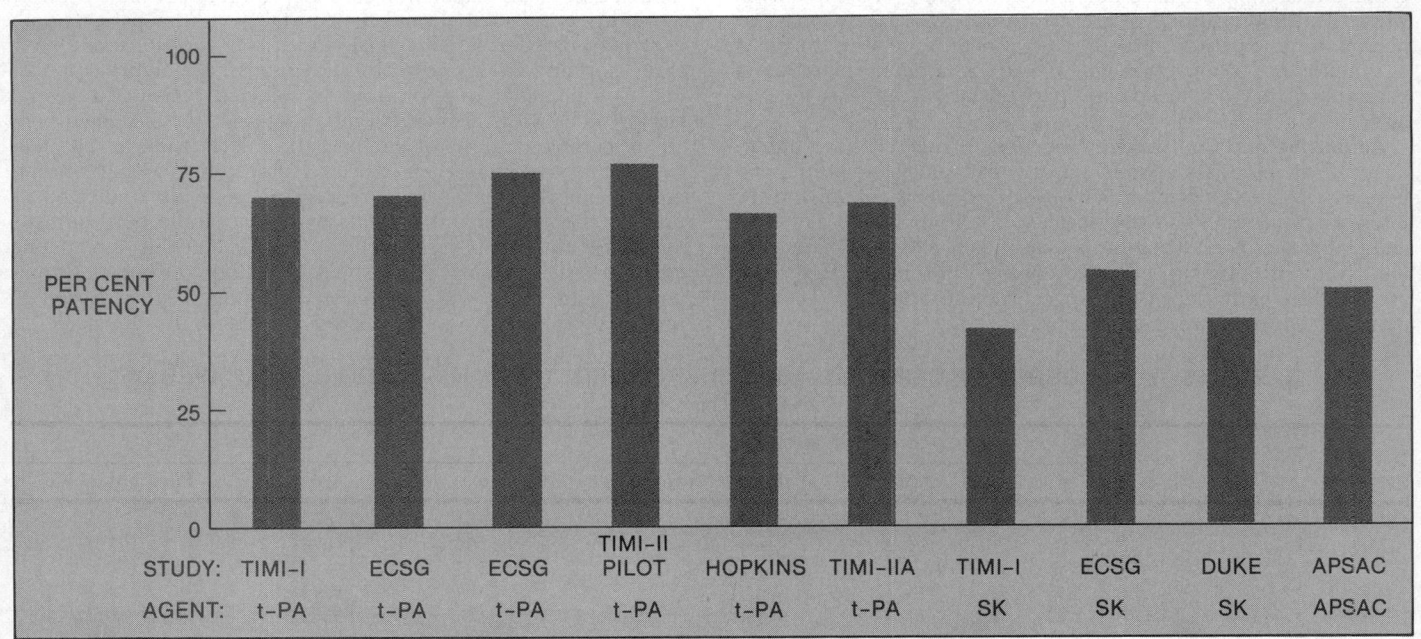

FIGURE 48–9. Angiographically defined patency of infarct-related arteries 90 minutes after treatment within 4 to 8 hours after onset of symptoms with streptokinase (SK), tissue-type plasminogen activator (t-PA), or acetylated plasminogen streptokinase activator complex (APSAC) reported in 10 large studies involving 1654 patients. TIMI = Thrombolysis in Myocardial Infarction; ECSG = European Cooperative Study Group. (From Tiefenbrunn AJ, Sobel BE: Fibrinolysis 3:1, 1988; with permission of Churchill Livingstone.)

elicit a systemic lytic state characterized by depletion of circulating fibrinogen, plasminogen, and hemostatic proteins and by marked elevation of concentrations of fibrinogen degradation products in plasma. Their lack of clot selectivity is therefore associated with an increased risk of bleeding and possible protection against early reocclusion in inadequately anticoagulated patients.

Second-generation drugs, typified by t-PA and single-chain urokinase plasminogen activator, activate plasminogen in the fibrin domain preferentially compared with free plasminogen in the circulation. Thus they exhibit relative clot selectivity. In optimal dosage they induce clot lysis without inducing a systemic lytic state. They are less prone to predispose to hemorrhage requiring transfusion.

Recanalization is more frequent and more rapid with second- than with first-generation agents, perhaps in part because of clot selectivity and lack of induction of plasminemia, which may induce procoagulant effects that attenuate fibrinolysis and plasminogen steal and diminish the intensity of fibrinolysis.

The risks of coronary thrombolysis with plasminogen activators include bleeding, most of which is confined to sites of vascular access. Marked depletion of fibrinogen indicative of a systemic lytic state may be a marker of pharmacologic effects that can lead also to bleeding. Marked prolongation of bleeding time may reflect bleeding risk somewhat more specifically. Although intracranial hemorrhage had been feared, the incidence of cerebrovascular accidents in patients treated with thrombolytic agents is no greater than that seen with conservative treatment without fibrinolytic drugs (Table 48–10). The incidence of hemorrhagic stroke is somewhat greater and that of thrombotic or embolic stroke somewhat less, but the disparity is not reflected by an increased incidence of fatal cerebrovascular accidents and is more than offset by the favorable impact of fibrinolytic agents on survival after infarction.

Plasminogen activators should not be given to patients with active internal bleeding or a bleeding diathesis, suspected aortic dissection, hemorrhagic retinopathy, recent trauma (including surgery or prolonged and traumatic cardiopulmonary resuscitation), intracranial neoplasm, or hypertensive crisis. Relative contraindications include peptic ulcer disease, remote cerebrovascular accident, and hepatic failure. Safety has not been established for pregnant women. In general, thrombolytic agents should be used in patients 75 years of age or less who present with suspected Q-wave infarction within 6 hours after the onset of symptoms in whom contraindications are not present. Treatment may be helpful in some patients first seen 6 hours or more after the onset of symptoms. Its impact on non–Q-wave infarction, infarction in patients of very advanced age, and unstable angina is not yet clear.

Adjunctive and Conjunctive Measures. Clinical efficacy of coronary thrombolysis depends on the frequency, rapidity, and persistence of recanalization, all of which depend not only on the intensity of fibrinolysis but also on the inhibition of coagulation and platelet-induced thrombosis that undoubtedly occur concomitantly. Even optimally effective coronary thrombolysis is compromised by early thrombotic reocclusion in 6 to 20 per cent of patients with initial recanalization.

Calcium antagonists have potential value as anti-injury agents in the setting of reperfusion, as antiplatelet agents, and as coronary vasodilators, effects that may minimize activation of platelets in the vicinity of lysed thrombi by reducing shear forces. Nitrates may diminish excessive coronary reactivity and hence ischemia. Reperfusion arrhythmias, if they compromise hemodynamics or threaten to degenerate into ventricular fibrillation, can often be suppressed with lidocaine. Alpha-adrenergic blocking agents are attractive theoretical alternatives. Accelerated idioventricular arrhythmia often does not require pharmacologic intervention. Perhaps of most importance are conjunctive anticoagulation with a powerful antithrombin such as heparin or hirudin (currently investigational) and conjunctive use of antiplatelet agents such as aspirin or antibodies and antagonists to the platelet glycoprotein IIb/IIIa receptor, prostacyclin and PGE_2 analogues, thromboxane receptor antagonists and synthetase inhibitors, and serotonin antagonists (all investigational at present).

Contrary to initial expectations, not all patients treated with thrombolytic drugs should be subjected to obligatory early cardiac catheterization and angioplasty. A strategy comprising arteriography and angioplasty in only those patients who exhibit recurrent or persistent symptoms and signs of ischemia appears to be safer (Table 48–11) and as effective as obligatory angiography for all patients in preserving ventricular function and reducing mortality. The value of rescue angioplasty, i.e., angioplasty performed when occlusion has proven to be refractory to recanalization with fibrinolytic drugs, has not been established.

Mechanical Revascularization. Compared with pharmacologic thrombolysis, mechanical recanalization (angioplasty or surgery) may enhance flow more markedly or more rapidly in patients who sustain infarction while in a cardiac catheterization laboratory. However, except in such rare instances or in centers dedicated to immediate angioplasty as primary therapy, it has not yet proven to be superior. Immediate angioplasty or surgery cannot be provided universally because of contention for facilities, the need for large teams of highly trained personnel on a 24-hour per day basis, and other logistic constraints. Risks of primary angioplasty exceed those of elective angioplasty for coronary artery disease with angina. Surgical facilities and personnel should be readily available in view of the 10 per cent incidence of life-threatening complications encountered. Restenosis rates after balloon angioplasty or other investigational approaches such as laser or mechanical atherectomy exceed 30 per cent within 6 months despite vigorous use of anticoagulants, antiplatelet drugs, calcium antagonists, vasodilators, and intracoronary stents. Although restenosis rates after coronary surgery are much lower, morbidity is substantial, and the mortality risk for patients with evolving infarction is not trivial. In view of the remarkably low early mortality attainable with intravenous fibrinolytics (approximately 5 per cent in appropriately selected patients in several large studies with second-generation agents), the sustained benefit of coronary thrombolysis, and the effectiveness of late mechanical intervention when indicated after initial coronary thrombolysis, mechanical revascularization is generally indicated as primary therapy only for patients with contraindications to pharmacologic thrombolysis, those with immediate life-threatening conditions such as cardiogenic shock refractory to coronary thrombolysis, and those with infarction resulting from occlusion of previously placed coronary artery bypass grafts amenable to

TABLE 48–10. INCIDENCE OF CEREBROVASCULAR ACCIDENT (CVA) IN CONTROLLED STUDIES OF CORONARY THROMBOLYSIS

Study	Thrombolytic Agent			Control Group		
	n	Agent	Per Cent with CVA	n	Agent	Per Cent with CVA
GISSI	5860	SK	1.1	5852	Placebo	0.9
AIMS	502	APSAC	0.4	502	Placebo	1.0
ISIS-2	8592	SK	0.7	8595	Placebo	0.8
ASSET	2516	t-PA	1.1	2495	Placebo	1.0
ECSG*	722	t-PA	1.1	366	Placebo	0.5
TOTAL	18,192		0.9	17,810		0.9

Adapted from Tiefenbrunn AJ, et al.: Coronary thrombolysis—it's worth the risk. JAMA 261:2107, 1989. Copyright 1989, American Medical Association.

*Two studies, one with placebo, one with t-PA with and without angioplasty.

GISSI = Gruppo Italiano per lo Studio della Streptochinasi nell'Infarto Miocardico; AIMS = APSAC Intervention Mortality Study; ISIS-2 = International Study of Infarct Survival; ASSET = Anglo-Scandinavian Study of Early Thrombolysis; ECSG = European Cooperative Study Group.

SK = Streptokinase; APSAC = anisoylated plasminogen streptokinase activator complex; t-PA = tissue-type plasminogen activator.

TABLE 48–11. OUTCOME AFTER INVASIVE COMPARED WITH CONSERVATIVE MANAGEMENT*

Event	Management Strategy after Thrombolysis		
	Invasive	*Conservative*	*P Value*
Death	5.2%	4.7%	0.49
Death or reinfarction	10.9%	9.7%	0.25
Coronary artery bypass grafting	11.9%	10.5%	0.18
Intracranial hemorrhage	0.9%	0.7%	0.70
Any adverse endpoint†	13.0%	10.6%	0.04

Adapted from the TIMI Group: Comparison of invasive and conservative strategies after treatment with intravenous tissue plasminogen activator in acute myocardial infarction: Results of the thrombolysis in myocardial infarction (TIMI) phase II trial. N Engl J Med 295:1404, 1976. By permission of the New England Journal of Medicine. Inclusion and exclusion criteria are delineated in the referenced article.

*The percentages of adverse clinical events during the initial 42 days of follow-up are shown in these results from a study of 3262 patients with Q-wave infarction randomized to treatment with (invasive strategy) or without (conservative strategy) obligatory angiography and angioplasty early after acute myocardial infarction treated initially with tissue-type plasminogen activator. The invasive strategy was not superior.

†Death, nonfatal reinfarction, intracranial hemorrhage, or coronary bypass grafting after angioplasty.

angioplasty. The role of salvage angioplasty for occlusions refractory to fibrinolysis remains to be established, in part because candidates are likely to have already sustained extensive irreversible injury by the time failure of thrombolysis can first be established.

PROPHYLAXIS AND TREATMENT OF ARRHYTHMIA. Continuous ECG monitoring is essential for 72 hours after the onset of infarction and optimally throughout hospitalization by telemetry to immediately detect ventricular fibrillation and numerous arrhythmias that may occur. Some degenerate into ventricular fibrillation because of augmentation of myocardial oxygen requirements, impaired ventricular performance with consequent exacerbation of ischemia, or both.

Both primary and secondary (to hemodynamic decompensation, hypoxemia, electrolyte disturbances, or progressive cardiac or pulmonary failure) ventricular fibrillation should be treated by immediate electrical countershock. Fibrillation may be confused with electrical asystole when the vector of fibrillation is perpendicular to the axis of the recording lead used for monitoring. True asystole requires confirmation with multiple leads and differentiation from fine ventricular fibrillation. If the distinction between ventricular fibrillation and asystole cannot be made with certainty, fibrillation should be assumed to be present. Other established components of cardiopulmonary resuscitation and advanced cardiac life support are invaluable, but the primacy of immediate restoration of effective cardiac rhythm cannot be overemphasized. Electrical countershock should be implemented immediately rather than deferred until after endotracheal intubation and other emergency measures. If true electrical asystole is documented, immediate external, transvenous, or transthoracic cardiac pacing is essential, although prognosis in this situation is grim.

When ventricular fibrillation accompanies acute myocardial infarction, lidocaine is the drug of choice for prevention of immediate recurrence. Prophylactic administration remains somewhat controversial because adverse effects (central nervous system depression, seizures, proarrhythmic, asystolic, and cardiodepressant effects) may offset potential benefit. Repeat bolus injections of 0.5 to 1.0 mg per kilogram body weight every 5 minutes to a total of 4 mg per kilogram, followed by maintenance infusions of 1 to 2 mg per minute are used for this purpose in younger patients without prior cardiac disease who can be treated within the first few hours after the onset of infarction when the risk of primary ventricular fibrillation is greatest. After successful resuscitation when ventricular fibrillation has occurred, lidocaine should be administered by continuous infusion (20 to 50 μg per kilogram of body weight per minute), particularly if frequent, closely coupled, multiform, or repetitive ventricular premature complexes or ventricular tachycardia occurs. Blood levels should be maintained in the range of 2 to 5 μg per milliliter. Recurrent ventricular fibrillation, refractory to lidocaine, may be suppressed after a considerable lag period by intravenous bretylium given in 5- to 10-mg per kilogram doses or by amiodarone (0.75 μg per kilogram loading dose followed by infusion of 5 to 10 μg per minute [still investigational in the United States]). Other promising antifibrillatory drugs are currently investigational in the United States.

High-grade ventricular ectopy or bursts of ventricular tachycardia should be treated with lidocaine. If they persist for more than a few hours after hospitalization, their management is similar to that applicable in other circumstances. Procainamide and quinidine are generally the drugs of choice. Torsades de pointes may respond to overdrive pacing or intravenous magnesium sulfate. Accelerated idioventricular rhythm should not be treated unless hemodynamic decompensation occurs, in which case sequential or atrial overdrive pacing or atropine may be effective.

Supraventricular Arrhythmias. Treatment of these arrhythmias is the same as when they occur under other circumstances and is indicated when they impair hemodynamics or compromise myocardial viability by augmenting oxygen requirements. Sinus tachycardia is usually secondary to excessive sympathoadrenal tone associated with extensive infarction and impaired ventricular performance, pericardial inflammation and irritation of the sinus node, relative or absolute hypovolemia, hypoxemia secondary to pulmonary venous congestion and respiratory impairment, congestive heart failure, or other potentially remediable factors. Atrial fibrillation or atrial flutter may be indicative of failure or atrial infarction. In the absence of the Wolff-Parkinson-White syndrome, these conditions should be treated with calcium channel blockers such as verapamil, digitalis glycosides, or a short-acting β-adrenergic blocker such as esmolol to control ventricular rate. Procainamide (intravenous or oral) or quinidine (oral) is often effective in restoring and maintaining sinus rhythm. When decompensation is evident, rapid atrial pacing (to terminate atrial flutter) or electrical cardioversion (to terminate either atrial fibrillation or flutter) should be used. When hemodynamics are compromised or myocardial viability is threatened, paroxysmal supraventricular tachycardias should be managed initially by augmentation of vagal tone with carotid sinus compression or the Valsalva maneuver, calcium channel blockers, intravenous adenosine, or electrical cardioversion. The safety of adenosine in patients with infarction has not yet been established unequivocally.

Bradyarrhythmias. Sinus bradycardia occurs often, particularly in patients with inferior myocardial infarction. If refractory to atropine, it may require temporary transvenous pacing. A wandering atrial pacemaker or first-degree AV block rarely requires specific treatment. Higher degrees of AV block or AV block associated with hypotension refractory to atropine may require sequential pacing to sustain adequate hemodynamics.

Long-term pacing is needed only when heart block persists throughout the hospital phase, sinus node function is markedly impaired, Mobitz II second- or third-degree block occurs intermittently, or block is associated with newly acquired bundle branch block or other criteria of conduction system impairment. It is difficult to prove that long-term pacing improves survival after myocardial infarction because mortality is so high, with the extensive infarction frequently responsible. Nevertheless, temporary transvenous pacing may stabilize hemodynamics, and long-term pacing may be justified prophylactically in patients at high risk.

TREATMENT TAILORED TO HEMODYNAMICS. Invasive hemodynamic monitoring is of inestimable value in patients with clinically complicated acute myocardial infarction. It permits rapid delineation of left ventricular filling pressure, effective vascular volume, the presence or absence of mitral regurgitation and its severity, ventricular septal rupture (with oximetry), right ventricular systolic and diastolic pressure and function, and cardiac output and peripheral vascular resistance. Selection of therapy based on hemodynamics is delineated in Table 48–9 and is predicated on the following considerations:

1. Hypertensive patients with increased cardiac output and normal pulmonary artery wedge pressure may benefit from infusions of β-adrenergic blockers such as esmolol to reduce myocardial oxygen requirements.

2. Hypotension associated with relative or absolute hypovole-

mia reflected by lack of substantial elevation (above 18 mm Hg) of left ventricular filling pressure generally responds to augmentation of vascular volume with intravenous fluids. Pulmonary artery wedge pressure should be monitored to preclude excesses leading to pulmonary edema. Hypotension with markedly elevated right ventricular diastolic, right atrial, and central venous pressures may implicate right ventricular infarction, which responds often to augmentation of vascular volume and stimulation of the heart with cardiotonic agents such as dobutamine, dopamine, or β-adrenergic agonists. Systemic arteriolar vasodilators secondarily decrease impedance of right ventricular outflow if they ameliorate left heart failure and can be used when systemic arterial diastolic pressure is adequate.

3. Sudden and profound hypotension may reflect a catastrophic insult such as pulmonary embolism (manifested by pulmonary arterial hypertension and hypoxemia) or rupture of the ventricular septum (detectable by augmented right ventricular and pulmonary artery pressure associated with an oxygen step-up in the right ventricle). Alternatively, it may reflect left ventricular papillary muscle rupture with mitral regurgitation manifested by large V waves in the pulmonary artery wedge pressure recording. When caused by free wall rupture with hemopericardium, hemodynamic manifestations of pericardial tamponade are apparent, with a diastolic pressure plateau in all four cardiac chambers, impairment of right ventricular filling, and confirmatory echocardiographic findings of pericardial fluid and diastolic right atrial and right ventricular collapse. Mechanical insults should be treated by immediate surgery if hemodynamic stability can be maintained with only pharmacologic and circulatory support. Surgery can be delayed for 1 to 2 weeks if stability can be maintained without such measures and the patient can be monitored meticulously.

4. Hypotension associated with markedly elevated pulmonary artery wedge pressure is generally indicative of severely impaired left ventricular performance and cardiogenic shock. Supportive measures and cardiotonic agents are generally ineffective unless the ischemia responsible can be relieved by coronary thrombolysis, angioplasty, or surgery. Mechanical circulatory support may be necessary to permit acquisition of definitive diagnostic information pertinent to potentially remediable insults such as septal or free wall rupture, mitral regurgitation, or coronary reocclusion. Intra-aortic balloon counterpulsation or circulatory support with a left ventricular assist device may be particularly useful as a temporizing measure or as a bridge to cardiac transplantation.

5. Pulmonary venous hypertension with normal systemic arterial pressure is indicative of relative or absolute excess of vascular volume and left heart failure that should be treated with vasodilators to reduce both ventricular preload and afterload, diminish the commonly associated mitral regurgitation accompanying left ventricular failure, and diminish left atrial and pulmonary venous hypertension. Intravenous nitroprusside, nitroglycerin, or parenteral or oral ACE inhibitors may be effective. Caution must be exercised to avoid marked changes in concentrations of electrolytes in plasma. If pulmonary congestion is severe or pulmonary edema is present but cardiac output is reasonably well maintained and associated with an adequate systemic arterial blood pressure, contraction of vascular volume by removal of fluid (phlebotomy with reinfusion of blood cell elements, slow continuous ultrafiltration, and rarely peritoneal dialysis) may be effective. If pulmonary congestion persists or if cardiac output and systemic arterial pressure are low, loop diuretics (having the advantage also of pulmonary venodilation) may be helpful. Hemodialysis is dangerous because of the risk of precipitous changes in filling pressures and cardiac performance. Cardiotonic agents (dobutamine or dopamine, digitalis, and phosphodiesterase inhibitors such as amrinone or milrinone [investigational]), previously a mainstay of therapy for congestive heart failure with diminished cardiac output and hypotension, may be necessary but entail the risk of exacerbating imbalance between myocardial oxygen supply and demand and are generally not dramatically effective alone.

6. Hypotension with or without pulmonary venous hypertension indicative of left heart failure is generally associated with increased peripheral vascular resistance in patients with infarc-

tion. In rare instances it may be decreased, in which case vasoconstrictors (such as dopamine in relatively high doses, epinephrine particularly if cardiac rate is not accelerated, and rarely, although usually fruitlessly, norepinephrine) may be indicated. The decrease of resistance is often caused by other factors, such as occult sepsis, which must of course be recognized. In patients with profound ventricular failure, circulatory support with intra-aortic balloon counterpulsation or left ventricular assist devices may permit performance of diagnostic catheterization and identification and treatment of surgically remediable lesions.

Care in the Step-down Unit. Patients with uncomplicated myocardial infarction require CCU care generally for no more than 72 hours. Subsequent care is facilitated in a step-down unit equipped with telemetry for continuous ECG monitoring. Therapeutic objectives include immediate recognition and treatment of ventricular tachycardia, ventricular fibrillation, and bradycardia caused by sinus node dysfunction or AV block; daily clinical and appropriate laboratory monitoring for prompt detection and treatment of complications, including deep venous thrombosis (sometimes manifest–by fever and Homans' sign), pulmonary emboli, post–myocardial infarction pericarditis with a friction rub, tachycardia, and fever (generally managed with aspirin to avoid impaired infarct healing that may occur with nonsteroidal anti-inflammatory agents or corticosteroids), ventricular thrombi, ventricular true or false aneurysm, or catastrophic mechanical complications including cardiac rupture; treatment to minimize the risk of recurrent infarction; assessment of prognosis based on evaluation of left ventricular function, exercise tolerance, and the severity of spontaneous or inducible ischemia; and gradual and judicious progressive ambulation followed by a rehabilitation program after discharge.

In patients who have been treated with thrombolytic agents, heparin can be discontinued after 5 to 7 days, and secondary prevention of thrombosis can be continued with daily aspirin. For those with ventricular mural thrombus or extensive hypokinesis, congestive heart failure, or ventricular aneurysm predisposing to mural thrombus, anticoagulation with warfarin is appropriate for 6 months. Patients with non–Q-wave infarction without congestive heart failure should be treated with calcium channel blockers to prevent recurrence. Those with Q-wave infarction without failure or other contraindications should be treated for 6 months or more with β-adrenergic blockers devoid of intrinsic sympathomimetic activity to reduce the incidence of reinfarction and enhance survival.

Complications detected by telemetry (episodic ischemia with ST-segment deviation, arrhythmia, heart block, new-onset bundle branch block, tachycardia with minimal exertion), physical findings suggestive of congestive heart failure, markedly impaired ventricular performance documented echocardiographically or by radionuclide ventriculography, or manifestations of recurrent coronary occlusion such as recurrent pain, unexplained tachycardia, exacerbation or appearance of heart failure, hypotension, or impaired ventricular performance justify consideration of coronary arteriography before discharge from the hospital, with mechanical revascularization if indicated. In patients without such complications and particularly those treated initially with thrombolytic drugs, submaximal (7 to 10 days) or symptom-limited (predischarge) exercise testing should be performed to determine whether arteriography is indicated. Exercise-induced ischemia manifested by ST-segment depression of 1 mm or more, reversible thallium perfusion defects, a hypotensive response to modest workloads, ventricular arrhythmias, diminution of ejection fraction, or induction of wall motion abnormalities with or without angina pectoris is an indication for coronary arteriography. Marked impairment of ventricular performance (resting ejection fraction less than 40 per cent) or anticipated stringent physical occupational requirements are relative indications. Thallium scintigraphy or exercise echocardiography may be useful when baseline ECG abnormalities obscure interpretation]. Dipyridamole thallium scintigraphy or dobutamine stress echocardiography (currently investigational in the United States) may substitute for exercise testing in patients unable to exercise for noncardiac reasons. Risk for development of sustained ventricular tachycardia or ventricular fibrillation can be estimated by high-resolution electrocardiography with frequency- or time-domain analysis of signal-averaged recordings, which provides criteria independent

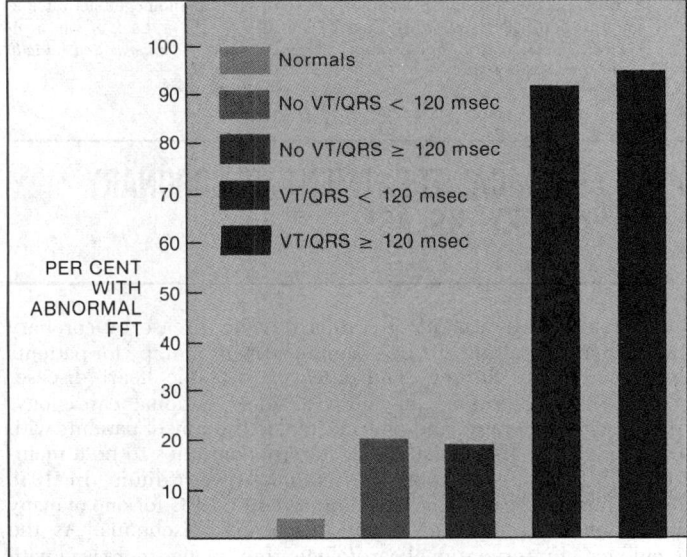

FIGURE 48–10. The predictive value for risk of sustained ventricular tachycardia (VT) of abnormalities detectable by high-resolution electrocardiography performed by fast-Fourier transform (FFT) frequency-domain analysis in 169 subjects with and without coronary artery disease and myocardial infarction categorized with respect to the presence or absence of QRS complex prolongation indicative of left bundle branch block or other intraventricular conduction delays. High-resolution ECG abnormalities correlated closely with the likelihood of occurrence of sustained VT whether or not conduction disturbances were present. (From Lindsay BD, et al.: Circulation 77:122, 1988. Reproduced by permission of the American Heart Association, Inc.)

of left ventricular dysfunction (Fig. 48–10). Ambulatory continuous ECG monitoring is often used, but the occurrence of the complex ventricular ectopy targeted for detection is generally concordant with severe left ventricular dysfunction after infarction.

CONVALESCENCE

Most patients can be discharged within 1 to 2 weeks. Complications at any time may require a longer hospital stay. Objectives of management during convalescence include (1) prevention of recurrent infarction (continued use of β-adrenergic blockers after Q-wave infarction, calcium channel blockers after non–Q-wave infarction with preserved left ventricular function, and aspirin); (2) prevention of late complications of infarction such as peripheral or cerebral embolus from ventricular mural thrombus with continued anticoagulation for 3 to 6 months in patients at high risk of harboring mural thrombi; (3) risk factor modification including

cessation of smoking, treatment of hypertension, diabetes, and hyperlipidemia, and implementation of a carefully monitored exercise rehabilitation program under supervision or for appropriately motivated patients at home; (4) prompt detection and evaluation of potential progression of underlying coronary artery disease manifested by signs or symptoms of ischemia including angina pectoris; and (5) prevention of sudden cardiac death with β-adrenergic blockers in patients without specific contraindications. Indiscriminate use of antiarrhythmic agents, particularly type I_c drugs, to suppress asymptomatic ventricular ectopy should be avoided because of the risk of increasing mortality (Fig. 48–11).

Patients with non–Q-wave infarctions require special consideration. This syndrome appears often to be a manifestation of incomplete or nonsustained thrombotic coronary occlusion. Early prognosis is good compared with prognosis for patients with Q-wave infarction. However, mortality late after infarction may exceed that after Q-wave infarction because of reocclusion, reinfarction, or sudden cardiac death reflecting recurrent ischemia. Survivors of non-Q infarction in whom ventricular function is well maintained benefit from treatment with calcium channel blockers. Beta-blockers are more likely to improve survival after Q-wave infarction; aspirin is indicated in both groups.

THE OUTLOOK

Early mortality associated with acute myocardial infarction has declined dramatically over the past three decades. Before the advent of CCU's, hospital mortality was approximately 30 per cent. Aggressive defibrillation reduced it by half. Protection of jeopardized ischemic myocardium and early pharmacologic coronary recanalization followed by mechanical revascularization when indicated have lowered mortality even further, to 5 per cent or less among patients 75 years of age or less with no contraindications to thrombolysis in whom treatment can be initiated within several hours after the onset of symptoms. Consolidation of these gains requires continued surveillance and management of patients throughout convalescence to allow recognition and prevention of recurrent ischemia; retardation of progression of coronary artery disease; prompt recognition of its occurrence; and vigorous medical, mechanical, and surgical intervention when required.

Bergmann SR: Positron emission tomography. *In* Gerson M (ed.): Cardiac Nuclear Medicine. New York, McGraw-Hill Book Company, 1990. *A comprehensive and elegant review addressing technology, instrumentation, applications in research, and utility in diagnosis.*

Braunwald E: Thirty-five years of progress in cardiovascular research. Circulation (Suppl III) 70:III-8, 1984. *Lucid and thorough articulation of the major conceptual themes and paradigms underlying treatment of acute myocardial infarction and their evolution during the modern era.*

The Cardiac Arrhythmia Suppression Trial Investigators: Preliminary report: Effect of encainide and flecainide on mortality in a randomized trial of arrhythmia suppression after myocardial infarction. N Engl J Med 321:406, 1989. *A noteworthy report of the unexpected adverse influences of type I_c antiarrhythmic agents when utilized in the treatment of ventricular ectopy in asymptomatic patients who have sustained acute myocardial infarction.*

Collen D, Topol EJ, Tiefenbrunn AJ, et al.: Coronary thrombolysis with recombinant human tissue–type plasminogen activator: A prospective, randomized, placebo-controlled trial. Circulation 70:1012, 1984. *The initial study demonstrating effective coronary thrombolysis with sparing of fibrinogen in patients with acute myocardial infarction treated with tissue-type plasminogen activator produced by recombinant DNA technology.*

Davies MJ, Woolf N, Robertson WB: Pathology of acute myocardial infarction with particular reference to occlusive coronary thrombi. Br Heart J 38:659, 1976. *A seminal study demonstrating the pathophysiologic connections between complex atherosclerotic plaques and sudden cardiac death.*

DeWood MA, Spores J, Notske R, et al.: Prevalence of total coronary occlusion during the early hours of transmural myocardial infarction. N Engl J Med 303:897, 1980. *Demonstration of the high incidence of occlusive coronary thrombi in patients studied angiographically soon after the onset of chest pain who have sustained acute Q-wave infarctions.*

Ellis AK, Little T, Masud Z, et al.: Early noninvasive detection of successful reperfusion in patients with acute myocardial infarction. Circulation 78:1352, 1988. *A recent report demonstrating the value of macromolecular markers such as myoglobin in the detection of recanalization.*

Forrester JS, Litvack F, Grundfest W, et al.: A perspective of coronary disease seen through the arteries of living man. Circulation 75:505, 1987. *Angioscopic illustrations supporting the hypothesis that acute coronary syndromes are attributable to dynamic changes in complex atherosclerotic plaques with characteristic durations of thrombosis accounting for differences between the syndromes.*

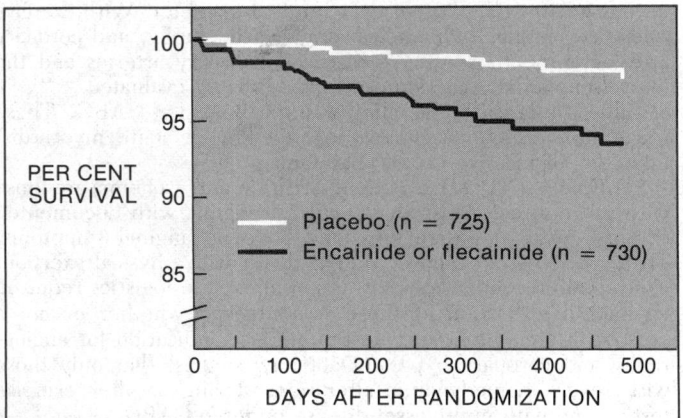

FIGURE 48–11. Survival among 1455 patients randomly assigned to treatment with encainide or flecainide compared with those assigned to placebo calculated with respect to death attributable to arrhythmia or cardiac arrest. (Adapted from Cardiac Arrhythmia Suppression Trial Investigators: N Engl J Med 321:406, 1989. By permission of the New England Journal of Medicine.)

Fry ETA, Sobel BE: Coronary thrombolysis. *In* Zipes DP, Rowlands DJ (eds.): Progress in Cardiology. Philadelphia, Lea & Febiger, 1990, pp 199–239. *A recent review of the impact of coronary thrombolysis on acute myocardial infarction with extensive reference to clinical trials performed with diverse plasminogen activators.*

Geltman EM, Ehsani AA, Campbell MK, et al.: The influence of location and extent of myocardial infarction on long-term ventricular dysrhythmia and mortality. Circulation 60:805, 1979. *An investigation establishing the association between the extent of myocardial injury sustained and long-term morbidity and mortality after acute myocardial infarction.*

Gruppo Italiano per lo Studio Della Streptochinasi nell'Infarto Miocardico (GISSI): Long-term effects of intravenous thrombolysis in acute myocardial infarction: Final report of the GISSI study. Lancet 2:871, 1987. *The pivotal report demonstrating improved survival after coronary thrombolysis in patients with acute myocardial infarction.*

Gunnar RM, Bourdillon PDV, Dixon DW, et al.: Guidelines for the early management of patients with acute myocardial infarction. A report of the American College of Cardiology/American Heart Association Task Force on Assessment of Diagnostic and Therapeutic Cardiovascular Procedures (Subcommittee to Develop Guidelines for the Early Management of Patients With Acute Myocardial Infarction). J Am Coll Cardiol 16:249, 1990. *This task force report summarizes the rationale and accepted approaches to treatment of all aspects of acute myocardial infarction based on full understanding of pertinent pathophysiologic principles.*

Jaffe AS, Serota H, Grace A, et al.: Diagnostic changes in plasma creatine kinase isoforms early after the onset of acute myocardial infarction. Circulation 74:105, 1986. *Observations indicating the value of analysis of isoforms of creatine kinase in plasma for prompt detection of acute myocardial infarction.*

Kanovsky MS, Falcone RA, Dresden CA, et al.: Identification of patients with ventricular tachycardia after myocardial infarction: Signal-averaged electrocardiogram, Holter monitoring, and cardiac catheterization. Circulation 70:264, 1984. *Delineation of the relationship between changes evident by high-resolution electrocardiography and the risk of ventricular tachycardia after acute myocardial infarction.*

Kennedy JW, Martin GV, Davis KB, et al.: The Western Washington intravenous streptokinase in acute myocardial infarction randomized trial. Circulation 77:345, 1988. *Report of a major clinical trial supporting the hypothesis that an open infarct-related coronary artery is beneficial even if recanalization cannot be induced very early after the onset of symptoms.*

Lindsay BD, Markham J, Schechtman KB, et al.: Identification of patients with sustained ventricular tachycardia by frequency analysis of signal-averaged electrocardiograms despite the presence of bundle branch block. Circulation 77:122, 1988. *Observations indicating that frequency-domain analysis of signal-averaged electrocardiograms provides information predictive of risk of sustained ventricular tachycardia even when intraventricular conduction abnormalities are present.*

Marcus FI, Cobb LA, Edwards JE, et al.: Mechanism of death and prevalence of myocardial ischemic symptoms in the terminal event after acute myocardial infarction. Am J Cardiol 61:8, 1988. *The prominence of arrhythmia as a cause of death late after acute myocardial infarction is underscored by these findings from a longitudinal study of survivors of acute myocardial infarction.*

Maroko PR, Kjekshus JK, Sobel BE, et al.: Factors influencing infarct size following experimental coronary artery occlusions. Circulation 43:67, 1971. *Laboratory observations demonstrating that myocardial infarction is a dynamic process amenable to favorable modification by reduction of myocardial oxygen requirements.*

Puleo PR, Perryman B, Bresser MA, et al.: Creatine kinase isoform analysis in the detection and assessment of thrombolysis in man. Circulation 75:1162, 1987. *The value of assay of creatine kinase isoforms in plasma for early detection of recanalization induced by fibrinolytic agents is demonstrated.*

Roberts R, Croft C, Gold HK, et al.: Effect of propranolol on myocardial infarct size in a randomized blinded multicenter trial. N Engl J Med 311:218, 1984. *Despite favorable effects in experimental animals, reduction of myocardial oxygen requirements in victims of acute myocardial infarction does not appear to reduce the extent of necrosis judging from results of this large-scale randomized multicenter study.*

Seacord LM, Abendschein DR, Nohara R, et al.: Detection of reperfusion within 1 hour after coronary recanalization by analysis of isoforms of the MM creatine kinase isoenzyme in plasma. Fibrinolysis 2:151, 1988. *A report demonstrating that serial assay of plasma creatine kinase isoforms permits very prompt detection of coronary recanalization.*

Sobel BE (ed.): Coronary thrombolysis. Review in depth. Coronary Artery Dis 1:1, 1990. *A review with components from Collen and Lijnen, Sheehan, Ohman and Califf, Guerci, and Muller and Topol addressing features of first- and second-generation fibrinolytic drugs, similarities and differences between the two, and mechanisms responsible for both.*

Tiefenbrunn AJ, Sobel BE: The impact of coronary thrombolysis on myocardial infarction. Fibrinolysis 3:1, 1989. *A review of pathophysiologic mechanisms, principles underlying treatment with plasminogen activators, and benefits resulting from early coronary thrombolysis.*

The TIMI Study Group: Comparison of invasive and conservative strategies after treatment with intravenous tissue plasminogen activator in acute myocardial infarction: Results of the thrombolysis in myocardial infarction (TIMI) phase II trial. N Engl J Med 320:618, 1989. *A definitive report from a large number of centers comparing survival after coronary thrombolysis with that following obligatory early angiography and demonstrating the advantages of a conservative strategy focusing on thrombolysis alone.*

Topol EJ, Califf RM, George BS, et al.: A randomized trial of immediate versus delayed elective angioplasty after intravenous tissue plasminogen activator in acute myocardial infarction. N Engl J Med 317:581, 1987. *Lack of benefit of immediate angioplasty after coronary thrombolysis was demonstrated initially in this important trial.*

48.3 SURGICAL TREATMENT OF CORONARY ARTERY DISEASE

Lawrence H. Cohen

The surgical treatment of coronary heart disease by coronary artery bypass grafting (CABG) is an important therapy for patients with acute and chronic syndromes of ischemic heart disease. Despite the enormous advances in interventional cardiology, thrombolytic therapy, and pharmacologic therapy of patients with coronary heart disease, surgical therapy continues to be a mainstay of direct reperfusion of ischemic myocardium. In 1988 approximately 240,000 patients underwent CABG for one of many indications of acute and chronic myocardial ischemia. As the incidence of interventional cardiologic therapy has increased with percutaneous transluminal coronary angioplasty (PTCA), the indications for CABG have changed and evolved so that the two procedures are now considered complementary to each other. PTCA is generally indicated for the less severe anatomic manifestations of obstructive coronary lesions, namely single-vessel disease, whereas CABG continues to be the treatment of choice for multivessel coronary disease.

The selection of patients for CABG has evolved strikingly since the advent of this procedure on a large scale in 1967 by the Cleveland Clinic Foundation, although a few individual cases had been done earlier by Sabiston and DeBakey. At the outset of surgical therapy, the patients who were operated upon were the younger, healthier patients with relatively few coronary lesions and good ventricular function. The patients most often considered for CABG today are those on the other end of the spectrum who tend to be older and sicker and have more advanced arterial disease, oftentimes with the ravages of coronary heart disease manifested by severe left ventricular dysfunction. In addition, there are numbers of patients with acute myocardial ischemia requiring operation who were seldom considered candidates for surgery when the operation was introduced. CABG has thus evolved into a procedure with a wide spectrum of indications requiring a considerable amount of ingenuity, new uses of conduits, better myocardial protection, and advanced techniques for life support.

INDICATIONS FOR CORONARY BYPASS SURGERY

In general, the patients selected for CABG should be those who have failed intensive medical therapy for the treatment of chronic angina or acute myocardial ischemia and who, by demonstration on coronary arteriography, have one or more significant lesions greater than 70 per cent luminal diameter. With exercise tolerance testing, radionuclear angiocardiography, and coronary arteriography, the patient's diseased coronary arteries and the impact on cardiac function can be completely evaluated.

Table 48–12 lists the clinical indications for CABG. These range from "silent" ischemia to an evolving acute myocardial infarction or massive myocardial damage.

SILENT ISCHEMIA. Patients with "silent" ischemia are those with exercise and ECG evidence of ischemia with documented coronary arterial obstruction who have no anginal symptoms. These patients often have sudden death with physical exertion. Considerable controversy has arisen about the logistics required for the identification of these patients and whether or not a positive exercise tolerance test should be indication for angiography and coronary bypass. Data now suggest that only those with severe hemodynamic alterations during or after exercise testing and with multivessel disease undergo CABG.

CHRONIC STABLE ANGINA. This is the largest group of patients who are considered for coronary bypass surgery. These patients, predominantly male and predominantly in their sixth decade of life, have effort angina or stress-related angina that is more or less controlled by medical therapy but with considerable reduction in lifestyle. These patients require β blockade, calcium

TABLE 48–12. INDICATIONS FOR CORONARY ARTERY BYPASS SURGERY

Chronic ischemia
  "Silent" ischemia
  Chronic stable angina
Acute myocardial ischemia
  Unstable angina
  Subendocardial infarction
  Postinfarction angina
  Acute evolving myocardial infarction
  Myocardial infarction with shock
With other cardiac operations
  Valve surgery
  Mechanical sequelae of myocardial infarction
    Ventricular septal defect
    Ruptured septal defect
    Left ventricular aneurysm

channel blockers, vasodilators, and antiplatelet aggregation agents, which may produce a considerable number of untoward effects. Arteriography of patients in this category shows at least two and usually three or more significant obstructions in their coronary arteries. They may have normal but often have reduced left ventricular function, especially as measured by the left ventricular ejection fraction, due to prior myocardial infarction(s). Occasionally, CABG may be considered for a patient with single-vessel disease who is symptomatic despite medical treatment, who is not a candidate for or who has failed angioplasty, and whose single diseased artery is unusually large and dominant.

UNSTABLE ANGINA. Unstable angina refers to a condition of accelerated anginal patterns not controllable by the usual medical therapy; it may manifest as rest angina, nocturnal angina, or almost continuous chest pain with ECG abnormalities indicating ischemia but not infarction, and it often requires the most intensive of therapies in the Coronary Care Unit. Patients with unstable angina should be stabilized, if possible, and treated with intravenous vasodilators such as nitroglycerin; they may occasionally even require the use of intra-aortic balloon support pump for the stabilization of hemodynamics, anginal symptoms, and ECG abnormalities. A cooperative national prospective study in the 1970's showed that stabilization of patients prior to bypass surgery is far preferable to operating on patients emergently when they are truly unstable. By decreasing left ventricular myocardial oxygen consumption, intensive β blockade and other pharmacologic agents actually decrease operative mortality when patients with this syndrome are operated upon.

SUBENDOCARDIAL INFARCTION. The patient with a subendocardial myocardial infarction has a small leak of myocardial enzymes not associated with a Q-wave type infarction pattern on ECG. Clinically, these patients are very similar in presentation to patients with unstable angina and may have severe angina. Their angiographic patterns of obstructive disease are the same as those with unstable angina, and they are considered for operation with the same degree of aggressiveness as are patients with unstable angina, provided that they are otherwise good candidates for surgery.

EVOLVING MYOCARDIAL INFARCTION. Those with evolving myocardial infarction present in the throes of a myocardial infarction, usually from occlusion of the anterior descending artery or posterior circulation, are considered for operation when they may be operated upon within approximately 6 hours of the onset of chest pain. A number of cardiac centers with excellent logistical set-ups have performed large numbers of operations in these patients with excellent results and ultimate reduction of myocardial necrosis. These large studies evolved from earlier studies which showed that patients who had sustained an acute occlusion in the cardiac catheterization laboratory, for example, could be taken to the operating room, undergo a rapid CABG procedure, generally survive, and usually abort a major myocardial infarction. These patients usually have triple-vessel coronary disease, since those with single-vessel disease are excellent candidates for thrombolytic therapy and/or PTCA. Patients with acute evolving infarction with triple-vessel disease may also be candidates for thrombolytic therapy, but if this is not successful they should be considered for expeditious operation.

POSTINFARCTION ANGINA. Postinfarction angina is an important clinical syndrome that occurs in patients who have had a myocardial infarction which was thought to be complete but is now threatening to extend either in the area of the prior infarction or in a new area of ischemia. This syndrome, left untreated, usually results in extension of the myocardial infarction and oftentimes severe mechanical sequelae of myocardial infarction. A major advance in the surgical therapy of coronary heart disease has been the aggressive treatment by CABG of this syndrome, which may occur within hours to days of the completed myocardial infarction. Untreated, it is a harbinger of further difficulty and a high mortality. Results of surgery for this syndrome are similar to those for unstable angina, provided that the patient is not in shock preoperatively.

MYOCARDIAL INFARCTION WITH SHOCK. This relatively small group of patients requiring CABG have suffered occlusion of a coronary artery which has produced massive destruction of the left ventricle, usually in excess of 40 per cent of the volume of the left ventricle. This syndrome often leads to immediate sudden death, but in some instances, by support with appropriate pharmacologic and mechanical devices, the patients are stabilized enough in the intensive care unit to be considered for emergency CABG. Careful evaluation of the residual left ventricular function in nonischemic areas and the anatomy of the distal coronary vessels is extremely critical in these patients, since patients with poor residual myocardial function or poor distal vessels are not usually candidates for conventional CABG. This treatment should be considered only in patients otherwise in good health and generally in the younger age group. Operative mortality in the best of centers averages 25 to 40 per cent.

CORONARY BYPASS WITH OTHER CARDIAC OPERATIONS. For sequelae of myocardial infarction when there is a mechanical abnormality associated with a myocardial infarction, coronary bypass is often done. These include infarction ventricular septal defect, ruptured or dysfunctional papillary muscle producing mitral regurgitation and left ventricular aneurysm, pseudoaneurysm, or left ventricular rupture. These are all sequelae of a transmural myocardial infarction and may occur from days to weeks following the original infarction and are often associated with multiple-vessel coronary disease. Coronary bypass should be done as an adjunctive procedure during simultaneous repair of these defects.

In cardiac valve disease, a very high percentage of patients in the adult population have coexistent coronary artery lesions. These patients require a concomitant coronary bypass operation if valve surgery is to be done because of the added reduction in coronary blood flow to the left ventricular myocardium imposed on the hemodynamic burden produced by the valve lesion itself. In some series of patients operated upon for valve disease, fully 30 to 40 per cent of the patients require concomitant CABG. The long-term outlook for patients with valve disease and coronary disease, despite the fact that the coronary disease may be grafted completely, is not as satisfactory as for those who have valve disease without concomitant coronary artery disease. In the workup of any adult for valvular heart surgery over the age of 40, coronary arteriography is generally indicated.

ANATOMIC INDICATIONS FOR CORONARY ARTERY BYPASS GRAFTING. Finally, there are some anatomic indications for CABG regardless of symptomatology. Severe occlusive lesion of the left main coronary artery of greater than 70 per cent diameter is indication for immediate surgery, regardless of the severity of the patient's clinical symptoms. Similarly, acute failure of a coronary angioplasty may often require emergency CABG, either because of failure to improve the lesion over subsequent dilations or because a failed angioplasty usually results in an acute myocardial infarction from coronary occlusion.

BASIS OF SURGICAL TREATMENT OF CORONARY ARTERY DISEASE

The basis of the surgical attack on coronary arteries is the bypass principle, one that has been in use for many years in regard to ischemic problems in many arterial beds throughout the body: the aortoiliofemoral arteries, the renal arteries, and the cerebral arteries. In a coronary bypass a conduit is sutured distal to the obstructing lesion and connected proximally to either the aorta or some other systemic artery, much as a detour in a road is used to get to a destination beyond a highway blockage. CABG utilizes autogenous conduits, since artificial grafts, which need to be sutured to coronary vessels that measure 1 to 2 mm, at the present time have poor long-term patency. A reversed saphenous vein was first used as the conduit for CABG. It is readily available and allows considerable flexibility. Other readily available conduits used since the early days of coronary surgery are the left and right internal mammary arteries. These arteries run under the chest wall bilaterally, supplying blood to the chest wall and breast, and can be dissected off the chest wall, dropped down, and used as a conduit to a coronary artery beyond the blockage. The advantages of this conduit are that it is an autogenous artery with a better size match to the coronary artery vessel and it has a natural proximal long-term patency rate better than that of the saphenous vein. The size match is better, the arterial wall is more consistent with that of coronary artery, and a number of other physiologic observations suggest that it is the bypass graft of choice for coronary arteries, particularly the left anterior descending. More recently, the gastroepiploic artery, which must be brought through the diaphragm, has also been considered for CABG.

Operations are performed on cardiopulmonary bypass with moderate systemic hypothermia and cardioplegic solutions to render the heart totally flaccid and motionless without expending energy stores and allowing for the performance of very small anastomoses. Hemodilution and the avoidance of blood transfusions are desirable and obtainable with a variety of extracorporeal perfusion techniques. Over the quarter century that CABG has been performed, complete revascularization of the patient—that is, the placement of a graft beyond every major stenosis—yields significantly better long-term survival and prevents cardiac events better than incomplete revascularization. In the average multivessel patient undergoing CABG, at least three or four bypass grafts are the rule in the modern era. The safety of the operation is unquestionably improved because of myocardial protection with various forms of cardioplegic solutions and the availability of intra-aortic balloon pumping.

The surgical mortality after coronary bypass surgery varies with the acuity of the presenting symptoms, the state of left ventricular function, and other patient risk factors. There is no statistical difference in mortality among varying numbers of grafts, but mortality is clearly dependent upon the function of the left ventricle prior to surgery. The operative mortality for coronary bypass in the multivessel younger age group with good left ventricular function is about 1 per cent. In the acutely ischemic

syndromes, operative mortality may vary from 2 to 25 per cent, depending upon whether it is postinfarction angina or acute myocardial infarction with shock. The effect of age is to perhaps double the operative mortality in patients over 70, particularly those with acute ischemic events. Increased ventilator dependency, stroke rate, etc., are also clearly more frequent in the older age group undergoing CABG.

Postoperative care consists of management of all organ subsystems, including renal, pulmonary, cerebral, and general metabolic function. Low cardiac output following cardiac surgery is treated by monitoring devices to measure cardiac output, pulmonary vascular resistance, and left and right ventricular filling pressures. Optimization of these filling pressures determines which type of pharmacologic agent or mechanical assist device to use in the management of this complication. Cardiac arrhythmias are extremely common and occur in about 30 per cent of patients, most often atrial fibrillation. Perioperative myocardial infarction (Q wave) occurs much less frequently than in previous decades, and it is now estimated to be around 2 to 5 per cent. Hypertension is often an accompanying feature and must be vigorously controlled with the use of vasodilating drugs such as nitroprusside or nitroglycerin to limit myocardial oxygen consumption in this critical postoperative period. It is of interest that unless there is severe associated hemodynamic instability, a postoperative perioperative infarction apparently has little or no effect on long-term survival and little effect on the hospital course. Mediastinitis may occur in a small percentage of cases, usually about 1 to 2 per cent in most large centers, which may be increased with the use of bilateral internal mammary arteries, particularly in diabetic patients. Postoperative management of this complication includes open drainage and irrigation and then closure with antibiotic irrigation tubes and occasionally in some instances the placement of a pectoral muscle flap to improve the healing.

Postoperative management now includes the routine use of antiplatelet therapy with daily aspirin. It has been demonstrated in randomized prospective trials that the addition of one aspirin tablet per day is effective in improving graft patency, presumably by the prevention of platelet "stickiness" in the grafts.

REOPERATIONS

Coronary bypass surgery is palliative surgery and unless the disease is totally controlled biochemically with extensive rehabilitation of patients undergoing this operation, symptoms may recur as a result of progression of disease in previously ungrafted normal vessels, or new disease may occur involving the bypass grafts themselves. Thus, reoperation is a necessity in some patients and increases with the length of time from surgery unless internal mammary artery bypass grafts are used exclusively. The indications for reoperative CABG are similar to the primary

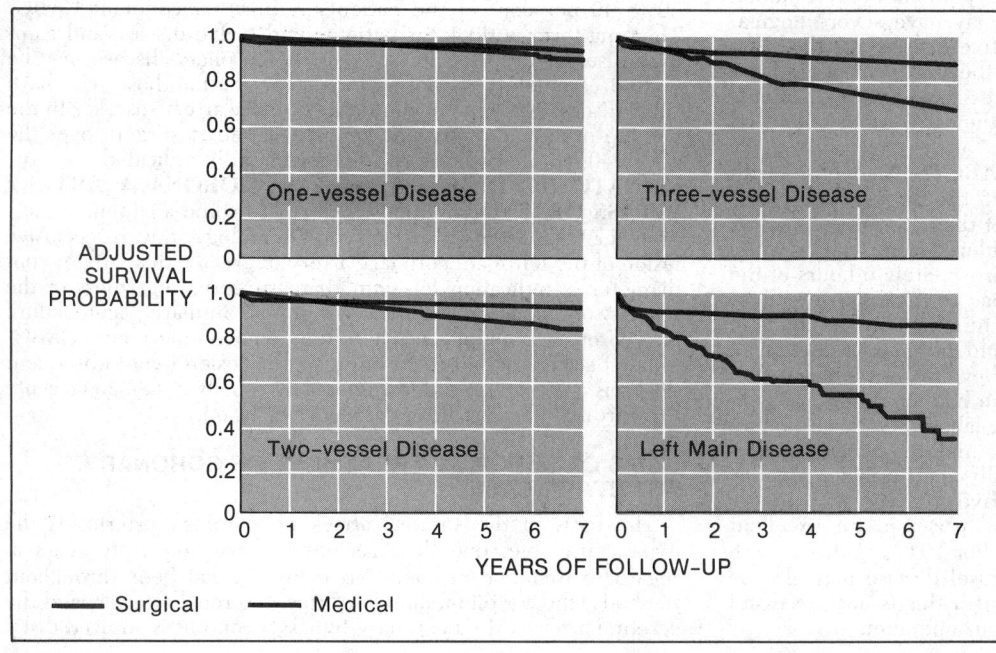

FIGURE 48–12. Survival treated medically or surgically with one-vessel, two-vessel, three-vessel, and left main coronary artery disease. (From Califf RM, et al.: JAMA 261:2077, 1989. Copyright 1989, American Medical Association.)

operation indications, but the patient must be aware that the risk is somewhat higher (5 to 10 per cent) and the benefits to be gained are somewhat lower than in the previous operation. This is because of the inherent difficulty with reoperative surgery due to the extensive adhesions around the heart, the possibility of myocardial ischemia due to manipulation of partially obstructed grafts filled with atheromatous material, and increased risk of bleeding. The risk of reoperative coronary bypass varies considerably with the experience of the team and the approach to myocardial protection.

LATE RESULTS OF CORONARY BYPASS SURGERY

The current operative mortality has stabilized at 2 to 5 per cent despite the increased number of aged patients, complexity of disease, numbers of reoperations, left ventricular dysfunction, and extension to almost all forms of acute myocardial ischemia. The probability of long-term survival and prevention of late cardiac events is related to the function of the left ventricle, complete revascularization, type of conduits used (internal mammary arteries versus saphenous veins), and patient rehabilitation. In general, the 5-year late survival of patients with multivessel disease completely revascularized is 90 to 95 per cent and the 10-year survival is 85 to 90 per cent (Figs. 48–12 and 48–13). The long-term graft patency is clearly better with an internal mammary artery than with a saphenous vein graft, 95 per cent versus 75 per cent at 5 years and 50 per cent at 10 years. It is apparent that if one considers every major clinical risk factor, the outcome with use of the internal mammary artery is statistically significantly better than that with the saphenous vein. In the long term, it is apparent that patients with left main coronary stenosis or with multivessel disease have improved survival and protection from cardiac events over similar medical patients in both prospective randomized studies and retrospective studies. Effects on ventricular function are less easy to document, but it is apparent that the ischemic or stunned myocardium may show significant improvements in left ventricular function after CABG

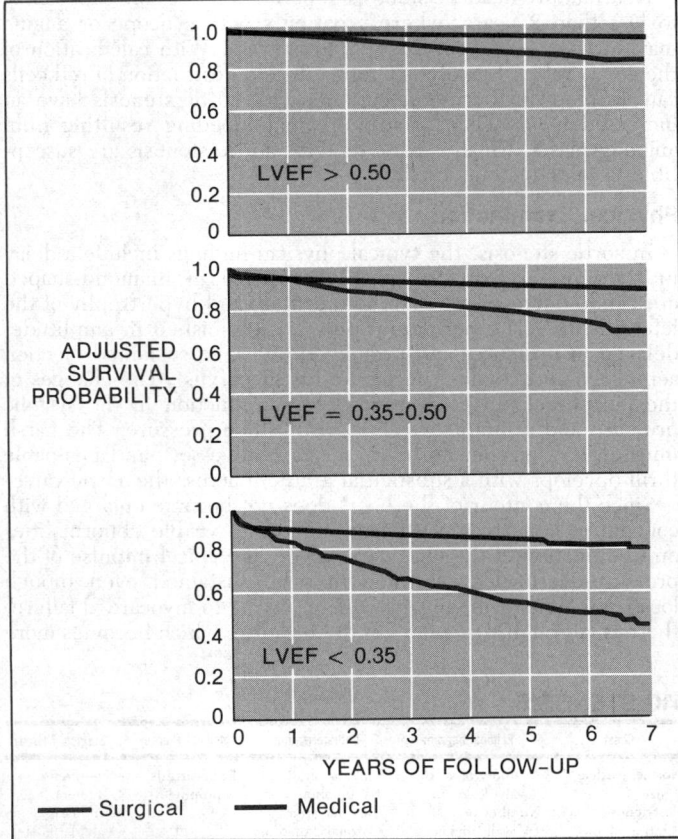

FIGURE 48–13. Projected survival of patients treated medically or surgically with a left ventricular ejection fraction (LVEF) greater than 0.50, between 0.35 and 0.50, and less than 0.35. (From Califf RM, et al.: JAMA 261:2077, 1989. Copyright 1989, American Medical Association.)

and that CABG may prevent further deterioration of function in the severely dysfunctional left ventricle.

Califf RM, Harrell FE, Lee KL, et al.: The evolution of medical and surgical therapy for coronary artery disease. JAMA 261:2077, 1989. *A 15-year perspective on the evolution of medical and surgical treatment, indicating that the surgical treatment, particularly in the last decade, has improved markedly so that not only the early but the late survival is improved over that with medical therapy because of newer revascularization techniques and better myocardial protection.*

Cohn LH: Surgical treatment of acute myocardial infarction. Cardiology 76:167, 1989. *This paper is a review of the various acute ischemic syndromes related to coronary occlusion and the results of both pure bypass surgery and surgery associated with the mechanical sequelae of myocardial infarction.*

Loop FD, Bruce WL, Cosgrove DM, et al.: Influence of the internal-mammary-artery graft on 10-year survival and other cardiac events. N Engl J Med 314:1, 1986. *This is a long-term follow-up of patients treated with internal mammary arteries versus those treated with only saphenous vein grafts for anterior descending coronary bypass. This large, well followed-up series (including angiography) shows conclusively that the internal mammary is the preferable conduit for coronary bypass surgery.*

Naunheim KS, Fiore AC, Wadley JF, et al.: The changing mortality of myocardial revascularization: Coronary artery bypass and angioplasty. Ann Thorac Surg 46:666, 1988. *This paper analyzes risk factors and outcomes for patients operated on in different eras and shows the marked change in the demography of patients operated upon in the late 1980's compared with the late 1970's.*

49 Valvular Heart Disease
Charles E. Rackley

The clinical manifestations of valvular heart disease result from either stenosis or incompetence of cardiac valves, or both. These mechanical disturbances lead to either pressure or volume overload on the affected chambers. The most frequently involved cardiac chamber in valvular heart disease is the left ventricle, which compensates for chronic volume or pressure overload with dilatation and hypertrophy. Myocardial oxygen requirements are related to the increased mechanical work and hypertrophy of the myocardium. In the advanced stage of valvular heart disease, myocardial decompensation, a reduction in cardiac output, and decreased coronary perfusion can impair oxygen delivery despite increased myocardial oxygen demands.

Although rheumatic heart disease remains prevalent in the temperate climates of the world, control of streptococcal infections in the United States has reduced the incidence of rheumatic fever and subsequent rheumatic heart disease. Today mitral valve prolapse is the most common valvular abnormality. A bicuspid aortic valve is the most common cause of aortic stenosis, but degeneration and calcification of the aortic valve are recognized with increasing frequency in the aging adult.

Recognition of a heart murmur on physical examination is the usual means of initially diagnosing valvular heart disease. Thus, the clinical examination remains important for detection of valvular heart disease, recognition of cardiac deterioration, and assessment of follow-up status. The noninvasive technologies of electrocardiography, chest radiography, echocardiography, radionuclide angiography, and stress testing play an important role in assessing the impact of valvular heart disease on cardiac function and determining the timing of operative intervention. Cardiac catheterization continues to be important in the accurate measurement of gradients across stenotic valves, evaluation of left ventricular function, and recognition of concomitant coronary artery disease. In recent years advances in echocardiography have resulted in more accurate assessment of valvular orifice size, and catheterization is reserved to confirm impressions and to identify underlying coronary artery disease.

GENERAL APPROACH TO THE PATIENT WITH VALVULAR HEART DISEASE
History

The patient with valvular heart disease usually recalls a history of a heart murmur, and therefore the first recognition of the murmur may be helpful in establishing the etiology. Although cardiac murmurs are frequent in healthy, physicially active children and adolescents, congenital valvular etiologies are often recognized at birth. Detection of a heart murmur in early adulthood often suggests a congenital or rheumatic basis, whereas development of the murmur in later years is often due to the degenerative changes in valvular structure. In addition to ascertaining the earliest detection of the heart murmur, the physician should carefully assess the patient's physical activities and note the initial onset of dyspnea or fatigue. The physician's interpretation of the patient's symptoms dictates the appropriate timing of noninvasive and invasive cardiac studies as well as the decision for surgical correction.

Physical Examination

The physical examination of the patient with valvular heart disease should be performed in the standard manner. Particular attention should be paid to the vital signs. Fever should raise the possibility of infective endocarditis. Palpation of the peripheral pulse may indicate stenosis or incompetence of the aortic valve. The habitus can suggest Marfan's syndrome as well as other heritable disorders of connective tissue. Funduscopic examination can demonstrate subtleties in arterial pulsations in aortic incompetence or the characteristic hemorrhages or Roth's spots in infective endocarditis. Careful attention to the vessels in the neck can reveal abnormalities in venous pulsation, reflecting right ventricular failure or tricuspid stenosis or incompetence. Carotid arteries reveal pulsatile abnormalities and transmitted bruits from the aortic valve.

Cardiac examination must include inspection, palpation, percussion, and auscultation. These maneuvers should be performed with the patient both in the sitting and in the recumbent positions. Auscultation at the apex, left sternal border, and pulmonic and aortic areas should be performed with the patient in the sitting, recumbent, and left lateral decubitus positions as well as after mild exercise. The remainder of the examination consists of documenting fluid retention, such as hepatic enlargement, ascites, and peripheral edema.

AORTIC STENOSIS
Etiology and Pathology

Aortic stenosis (Table 49–1) can result from a congenital abnormality, rheumatic fever, or degeneration with calcification in the aging patient. A bicuspid valve is the most common congenital abnormality, and invariably there is a raphe in one of the cusps that indicates failure of the commissure to develop. Rarely, a unicuspid valve can be present at birth. Although the bicuspid valve may not be initially stenotic, fibrosis and thickening lead to eventual reduction of the orifice size with calcification. Rheumatic fever produces scarring of the leaflet margins, and there is eventual fusion of the commissures with calcification. More than 50 per cent of adults with aortic stenosis will be found to have a bicuspid valve, but fibrosis and calcification may make it difficult to determine whether the valve is bicuspid or tricuspid. In the aging patient with degenerative aortic stenosis, calcium deposits usually develop in the sinuses and annulus, whereas the margins of the leaflets remain free.

In any of the conditions producing hemodynamic stenosis of the aortic valve, the systolic hypertension in the ventricular chamber is compensated by concentric hypertrophy of the myocardial wall. As myocardial failure develops from depression of the contractile state, dilatation of the ventricle will occur. Fibrosis

of the myocardium also occurs. Myocardial oxygen consumption remains high owing to the elevation of systolic pressure within the left ventricle and the increase in left ventricular mass. Thus, significant aortic stenosis creates conditions in which high myocardial oxygen demands are inadequately supported by reduced oxygen supply, which leads to subendocardial ischemia. Eventually, with a decline in the inotropic state of the myocardium, the ventricle dilates and the ejection fraction is decreased below the normal range. Further elevation of the left ventricular end-diastolic pressure results in pulmonary venous hypertension. The increased myocardial oxygen demands in aortic stenosis with the underperfused subendocardial myocardium can produce arrhythmias, chest pain, and even sudden death. In adults there may be coexistent coronary artery disease, which further contributes to myocardial ischemia.

Clinical Features

Chest pain, syncope, and heart failure are the characteristic symptoms of aortic stenosis, even though a gradient across the valve can exist for years before the patient develops symptoms. Children with a severe gradient can suddenly develop symptoms, whereas in adults the increase in mortality occurs later in the course of the disease.

The chest discomfort is exertional and indistinguishable from that of ischemic heart disease. Approximately 50 per cent of patients with aortic stenosis above the age of 40 years have underlying coronary artery disease whether exertional chest pain is present or not. Syncope can be an initial symptom of aortic stenosis and is probably related to the same mechanism as the chest pain, that is, critical reduction in myocardial oxygen supply with increased demands. Orthostatic syncope can result from the inability of the cardiac output to increase with abrupt assumption of the upright position, whereas exertional syncope is further aggravated by peripheral vasodilatation unaccompanied by an increase in cardiac output. Arrhythmias due to myocardial ischemia can also contribute to syncope and sudden death. When aortic stenosis is found at autopsy, approximately 15 per cent of the patients will have died suddenly without previous symptoms.

Heart failure in aortic stenosis generally reduces life expectancy to less than 2 years, whereas patients with syncope or angina may survive, on the average, 2 to 5 years. With calcification of the aortic valve, hemolytic anemia due to destruction of red cells can develop; furthermore, patients with aortic stenosis have an increased incidence of gastrointestinal bleeding resulting from angiodysplasia. Finally, patients with aortic stenosis are susceptible to infective endocarditis.

Physical Examination

In aortic stenosis, the typical physical findings include a delay in the upstroke of the peripheral pulse, a diamond-shaped crescendo-decrescendo systolic murmur, and hypertrophy of the left ventricle. The peripheral pulse is diminished in amplitude, delayed in upstroke, and prolonged owing to sustained ejection across the aortic valve (pulsus tardus et parvus). The changes in the peripheral pulse are caused by a reduction in the systolic pressure and a gradual decline in diastolic pressure. The harsh murmur is often transmitted to the carotid vessels, and a palpable thrill develops with a substantial gradient across the aortic valve.

Since the contour of the heart does not become enlarged with concentric hypertrophy, there may be no visible abnormalities on examination of the chest. However, the apical impulse of the pressure-overloaded ventricle may be sustained even though localized. When the ventricle dilates owing to myocardial failure, there is lateral displacement of the impulse, which becomes more

TABLE 49–1. AORTIC STENOSIS

Etiology	Physiology	Symptoms	Physical Examination	Electrocardiogram	Chest	Echocardiogram	Catheterization	Medical Therapy	Surgical Therapy
Congenital Rheumatic Degenerative	LV* pressure overload LV hypertrophy Decreased LV compliance	Chest pain Syncope Heart failure	Delayed arterial pulse wave Aortic thrill Diamond-shaped aortic area, left sternal border and apex	LV hypertrophy	Normal cardiac size Poststenotic dilatation of ascending aorta	Anatomy of aortic valve/calcium Number of cusps LV wall thickness Echo Doppler estimate of valvular gradient Valvular area	Valvular gradient LV function Valvular area Coronary anatomy Mitral lesions	Endocarditis prophylaxis	Symptoms Gradient >50 mm Hg Valvular area <0.8 cm²

*LV = left ventricular.

diffuse. Detection of palpable systolic vibrations over the primary aortic area, with the patient in the sitting position during full expiration, often correlates with a gradient across the aortic valve of more than 40 mm Hg. An atrial (S_4) gallop is usually audible, and an ejection click may be heard along the left sternal border. The aortic second sound becomes diminished, except in calcific stenosis of the elderly, in which the margins of the leaflets usually maintain their mobility. Fibrosis and fusion of the aortic leaflets may result in a single S_2 at the base. Mechanical or electrical prolongation of left ventricular systole can create reverse splitting of S_2. The diamond-shaped ejection murmur develops after the first sound, peaks in mid- and late systole, and disappears before the second heart sound. There is a tendency toward late peaking of the murmur with increasing severity of the stenosis. If an ejection click is present, the murmur develops immediately after the click and can sometimes be erroneously identified as a holosystolic murmur. The murmur is most intense over the aortic area and along the left sternal border, but in the elderly patient, the musical quality of the murmur can sometimes be loudest at the apex. The intensity in the apical area can be confusing and may make it difficult to distinguish this murmur from that of mitral regurgitation. A faint diastolic blow is often audible along the left sternal border, since the severely stenotic valve may have a mild degree of incompetence.

Laboratory Studies

ELECTROCARDIOGRAM. Left ventricular hypertrophy is the most common finding on the electrocardiogram, with an increase in QRS amplitude and ST-T changes of a strain pattern. Left-axis deviation can develop as well as conduction disturbances and left bundle branch block. As the left ventricle becomes noncompliant, there may be enlargement of the left atrium with a negative P wave in lead V_1. Because of myocardial fibrosis, Q waves can develop in the precordial leads, but these as well as the ST-T wave abnormalities are indistinguishable from underlying coronary artery disease.

CHEST RADIOGRAPH. Cardiac size remains unchanged in the early phase of aortic stenosis, since hypertrophy does not increase the cardiothoracic ratio. Poststenotic dilatation and prominence of the ascending aorta may be present. Calcification is often present but may require fluoroscopy for confirmation. Development of heart failure will enlarge the left ventricle and cause pulmonary congestion. Since a bicuspid aortic valve is sometimes associated with coarctation of the aorta, rib notching should always be sought on the chest film.

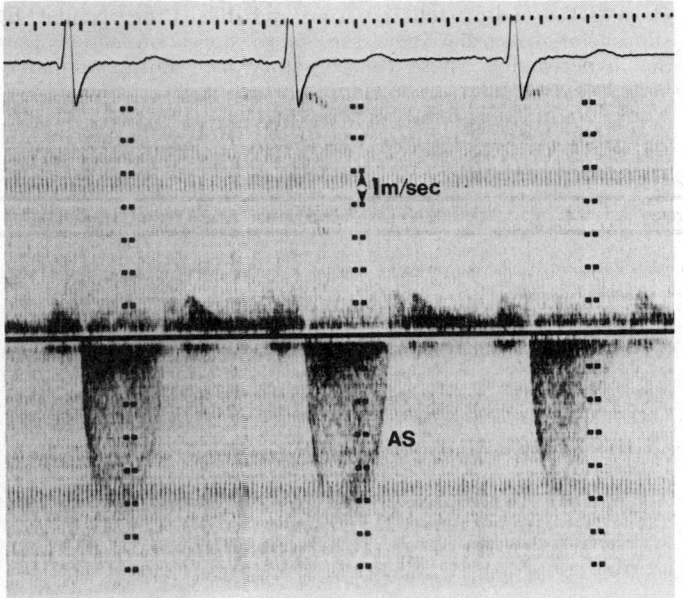

FIGURE 49–1. Continuous wave Doppler recording from the ascending aorta in a patient with severe aortic stenosis. The peak velocity is approximately 5 m/sec. Utilizing the modified Bernoulli equation, a peak instantaneous gradient across the aortic valve of 100 mm Hg can be calculated. Peak-to-peak gradient at catheterization was 80 mm Hg.

ECHOCARDIOGRAM. The echocardiogram can demonstrate thickening of the aortic leaflets, determine the number of leaflets, detect calcification of the valves, and estimate left ventricular wall thickness and function. Two-dimensional echocardiography can give an estimated size of the aortic orifice, and the Doppler technique can assess accurately the systolic pressure gradient across the valve. Thus, available echocardiographic techniques can provide accurate detection and assessment of aortic stenosis (Fig. 49–1).

CARDIAC CATHETERIZATION. The pressure gradient across the aortic valve can be accurately measured with simultaneous measurements of left ventricular and aortic pressures. A decline in cardiac output is associated with a reduced pressure gradient across the valve, and the valvular area tends to be overestimated when the cardiac output is reduced and only the pressure gradient is analyzed.

The size of the normal aortic orifice is 2.5 to 3 cm², and mild stenosis develops when the orifice is reduced to 0.75 to 1.5 cm². Moderate stenosis is present when the valvular size is less than 0.75 cm² and severe stenosis when the valvular area is less than 0.5 cm². Surgery is usually advised when the aortic valve gradient is greater than 50 mm Hg or the valve area is less than 0.8 cm². Left ventricular angiography is helpful in determining the presence of mitral regurgitation. With the information available from echocardiography, cardiac catheterization may be primarily indicated for coronary arteriography, since 50 per cent of patients over the age of 40 years will have underlying coronary artery disease.

Differential Diagnosis

In children, valvular aortic stenosis has to be differentiated from congenital forms of both supra- and infravalvular lesions. In hypertrophic cardiomyopathy with obstruction, the systolic ejection murmur is similar to that of valvular aortic stenosis, but the peripheral pulse is hyperdynamic with a rapid upstroke and a double-notch or bisferious contour compared with the delayed upstroke observed in valvular stenosis. With rupture of the chordae or papillary muscle, acute mitral regurgitation may produce a harsh systolic murmur. This murmur can be transmitted to the left atrial wall and aorta, resulting in a palpable and audible "aortic" murmur. However, the murmur of acute mitral regurgitation transmitted into the aortic area is holosystolic rather than midsystolic. A systolic ejection murmur accompanies significant aortic regurgitation and is generally caused by turbulence of the large stroke volume across the aortic valve.

Medical Therapy

Prophylaxis with antibiotics is indicated for dental, genitourinary, and gastrointestinal procedures in the asymptomatic patient to reduce the likelihood of infective endocarditis. Prophylaxis should be routine throughout life in a patient with a stenotic or prosthetic valve (Table 49–2). Prosthetic valves require intramuscular or intravenous antibiotics for prophylaxis. If the patient with aortic stenosis develops a supraventricular tachycardia, digitalis and an antiarrhythmic drug may be necessary to slow the ventricular response. Development of chest pain warrants catheterization to evaluate underlying coronary artery disease, but the use of nitrates should be undertaken with great caution, since arterial pressure may fall and further reduce coronary blood flow. Since life expectancy is reduced when aortic stenosis becomes symptomatic, chest pain, syncope, or heart failure warrants appropriate studies and consideration for surgery. Aysmptomatic patients with hemodynamically significant aortic stenosis are at significant risk for cardiac events within 2 years and should be followed closely.

Surgical Therapy

In children with aortic stenosis, surgery may be considered before the development of symptoms. If the pressure gradient is high, valvuloplasty can sometimes be performed before calcification has developed. The operative mortality for aortic valve replacement is 2 to 3 per cent and is less than 5 per cent if coronary bypass surgery is also performed. Even if heart failure has developed, surgery with prosthetic valve replacement can improve ventricular function. A mechanical valve will require

TABLE 49–2. ANTIBIOTIC PROPHYLAXIS IN AORTIC STENOSIS

Category	Drug	Dose and Route of Administration
Dental procedures and surgery of the upper respiratory tract		
Most patients	Penicillin	2 grams penicillin V orally 1 hour prior to procedure and 1 gram 6 hours later
Allergic to penicillin	Erythromycin	1 gram orally 1 hour prior to procedure and 500 mg 6 hours later
Prosthetic valves, not allergic to penicillin	Ampicillin and gentamicin	Ampicillin 1–2 grams plus gentamicin 1.5 mg/kg IM or IV 30 min before procedure; no repeat dose necessary
Prosthetic valves, allergic to penicillin	Vancomycin	Vancomycin 1 gram IV over 60 min, begun 60 min before procedure; no repeat dose necessary
Gastrointestinal and genitourinary tract surgery and instrumentation		
Most patients	Ampicillin and gentamicin	Ampicillin 2 grams plus gentamicin 1.5 mg/kg IM or IV 30 min before procedure; may repeat once 8 hours later
Allergic to penicillin	Vancomycin and gentamicin	Vancomycin 1 gram IV plus gentamicin 1.5 mg/kg IM or IV over 60 min before procedure; may be repeated once 8–12 hours later
Minor or repetitive procedures	Amoxicillin	Amoxicillin 3 grams orally 1 hour before procedure and 1.5 grams 6 hours later

long-term coagulation, but the porcine valve can be utilized in older patients or in those in whom anticoagulation is contraindicated. Currently, the porcine valve usually lasts 10 years or longer before deterioration in adults, but it is not recommended in children or adolescents. If indicated, coronary bypass surgery should also be performed at the time of valve replacement. The 10-year survival of combined aortic valve replacement and coronary revascularization approaches 55 per cent. Late cardiac events occur at a rate of approximately 6 per cent per year and include thromboembolic neurologic insults, myocardial infarction, congestive heart failure, endocarditis, bleeding, peripheral thromboembolism, and reoperation. Valvuloplasty is an option in severely ill or elderly patients, but the restenosis rate remains high. Octogenarians are those most likely to benefit from percutaneous valvuloplasty, since operative mortality may be as high as 30 per cent. Hospital mortality for the procedure in patients 80 years old or older has been reported at 6.5 per cent, with 1-year survival at 70 per cent. Surviving patients describe marked symptomatic improvement.

AORTIC REGURGITATION

Etiology and Pathology

Aortic regurgitation (Table 49–3) can be caused by disease conditions that render the aortic leaflets incompetent or affect the ascending aorta with dilatation of the annulus of the aortic valve. Rheumatic fever produces scarring and fibrosis of the valvular margins. Myxomatous degeneration of the aortic cusp can lead to incompetence. Hypertension, as well as arteriosclerosis, can be associated with scarring of the aortic valve and mild incompetence. Congenital lesions, such as bicuspid aortic valve, are predominantly stenotic, but scarring and calcification can result in associated incompetence as well. An aneurysm of the sinus of Valsalva may be associated with a ventricular septal defect as well as aortic regurgitation.

Conditions that affect the ascending aorta and produce valvular incompetence include syphilis, heritable disorders of connective tissue, arthritic diseases, and cystic medial necrosis of the aorta. In syphilis, the granulomatous process can result in calcification of the aorta, extreme dilatation, and ostial narrowing of the coronary arteries. Myxomatous degeneration of the aortic valve occurs in Marfan's syndrome. Ankylosing spondylitis, rheumatoid arthritis, and Reiter's syndrome are arthritic conditions that can cause aortic root dilatation and aortic cusp thickening. Cystic medial necrosis and aortic ectasia can produce extreme dilatation of the aorta with secondary aortic regurgitation. Acute aortic regurgitation can result from dissection of the aorta, perforation of the valve with infective endocarditis, rupture of a sinus of Valsalva, and mechanical complications of a prosthetic aortic valve.

Physiology

Aortic regurgitation imposes a volume overload on the left ventricle. Although the end-diastolic pressure may be normal or slightly elevated in the early phases, progressive regurgitation elevates the end-diastolic pressure and dilates the chamber by slippage of myocardial fibers, sarcomere replication, and myocardial hypertrophy. These compensatory mechanisms support a large left ventricular stroke volume, which is often achieved with an ejection fraction above 50 per cent.

TABLE 49–3. AORTIC REGURGITATION

Etiology	Physiology	Symptoms	Physical Examination	Electrocardiogram	Chest	Echocardiogram	Catheterization	Medical Therapy	Surgical Therapy
Chronic									
Rheumatic fever	Chronic volume overload	Fatigue	Wide arterial pulse pressure	LV hypertrophy and strain	Enlarged LV	Valvular anatomy	Contrast from aorta to LV	Preload and afterload reduction	LV systolic echo dimension >55 mm
Connective tissue disorders		Dyspnea	Enlarged LV		Dilated aorta	Aortic root size	LV function		
Hypertension, atherosclerosis	LV* dilatation	Edema	Diastolic aortic murmur			Enlarged LV		Diuretics	Ejection fraction <50%
Syphilis	LV hypertrophy		Systolic ejection murmur			Mitral valve fluttering		Digitalis	
Cystic medial necrosis			Third sound			LV function			
Aortic ectasia			Apical diastolic rumble						
Congenital heart disease									
Acute									
Endocarditis	Acute LV diastolic pressure and volume overload	Pulmonary edema	Loud diastolic musical murmur	LV strain	Pulmonary edema	Valvular anatomy	Contrast from aorta to LV	Preload and afterload reduction	Urgent surgery
Aortic dissection			Right and left sternal border radiation with thrill		Normal heart size	Aortic size and intimal flap	Aortic and intimal flap		
Ruptured sinus of Valsalva			Soft S$_1$ and third sound						
Prosthetic valve			Continuous murmur if rupture into right side of heart						

*LV = left ventricle, ventricular.

The systolic ejection of a large stroke volume into the high-impedance area of the systemic circulation increases the systolic pressure. Systolic wall stress or afterload can be maintained within the normal range by hypertrophy of the myocardium, but myocardial oxygen demand is significantly increased. A progressive decline in aortic diastolic pressure due to regurgitation of blood into the left ventricle can reduce coronary blood flow and thus create conditions for subendocardial ischemia in severe chronic aortic regurgitation.

The gradual volume overload of chronic aortic regurgitation can be tolerated for years before the inotropic state of the myocardium deteriorates. Eventually, the declining ejection fraction and inotropic state, along with limits to the dilatation hypertrophy mechanism, cause marked elevation of the left ventricular filling pressure with pulmonary venous capillary congestion.

Left ventricular hemodynamics in acute aortic regurgitation, compared with those in chronic aortic regurgitation, are immediately disturbed, since the regurgitant volume may be imposed on a normal end-diastolic volume. Under such circumstances, sudden incompetence of the aortic valve can severely elevate the left ventricular filling pressure, since the acute dilatation of the left ventricle is limited. With such rapid regurgitation through the aortic valve, the mitral valve may close prematurely, and the aortic diastolic murmur may persist beyond the diminished first heart sound.

Clinical Course

Since the chronic volume overload of aortic regurgitation is well tolerated, patients may remain asymptomatic for long periods of time. The patient may be aware of prominent precordial activity as well as exaggerated pulsation of the carotid arteries. Diffuse sweating patterns and vague abdominal discomfort are less frequent symptoms. The accelerated development of angina, heart failure, or sudden death within several years has been observed in patients with a pulse pressure greater than 140/40 mm Hg and left ventricular enlargement demonstrated on electrocardiography or chest radiograph. Dyspnea, orthopnea, and paroxysmal nocturnal dyspnea result from impaired left ventricular contractility in pulmonary venous hypertension. Although tachycardia may impair ventricular function, the shortened diastolic filling period can be beneficial in reducing the duration of the aortic regurgitation. Chest pain and syncope are infrequent symptoms. Chest pain is often associated with underlying coronary artery disease, and syncope is usually attended by arrhythmias.

With acute aortic regurgitation, pulmonary edema is often the presenting manifestation. Severe chest pain suggests aortic dissection when acute aortic incompetence develops.

Physical Examination

In aortic regurgitation, the physical findings reflect the large left ventricular stroke volume into the systemic circulation and the rapid diastolic run-off into the left ventricle. The peripheral pulse is characteristically bounding, and additional manifestations of the wide pulse pressure include head bobbing, pulsation of the retinal arterioles, bounding carotid pulse, pistol shot sounds over the femoral arteries, a to-and-fro murmur elicited from the femoral artery with slight compression of the stethoscope, and capillary pulsations in the nail beds. With connective tissue and arthritic diseases that produce aortic regurgitation, there may be characteristic changes in habitus, such as the musculoskeletal type in Marfan's syndrome and kyphosis of the thoracic spine in ankylosing spondylitis.

The precordium is hyperdynamic with a laterally displaced apical impulse. The auscultatory hallmark is the high-pitched, blowing, decrescendo diastolic murmur heard best along the left sternal border while the patient is in the sitting position during full expiration. As the regurgitation becomes more severe, a diastolic rumble or Austin Flint murmur due to vibration of the anterior leaflet of the mitral valve in the regurgitant jet may be audible at the apex. If the ascending aorta is dilated, the diastolic murmur may be heard along the right sternal border as well. With extreme left ventricular dilatation, mitral regurgitation can produce an apical systolic murmur, and heart failure is attended by a ventricular gallop at the apex.

With acute aortic regurgitation due to disruption of an aortic leaflet or dissection dilating the aortic annulus, the diastolic murmur may be harsh with palpable vibrations along the left sternal border. A perforated or prolapsed aortic leaflet, as well as the detached aortic intima from dissection, can generate prominent musical qualities in the diastolic murmur.

Laboratory Studies

ELECTROCARDIOGRAM. The electrocardiogram typically reveals left ventricular hypertrophy with increased QRS voltage amplitude and ST-T wave changes of the strain pattern. With acute aortic regurgitation, the hypertrophy may be absent, and the ST-T wave changes can indicate myocardial ischemia.

CHEST RADIOGRAPHY. Significant cardiomegaly usually attends chronic aortic regurgitation, with the increase in size due to dilatation of the left ventricle. The ascending aorta is often prominent. Calcium in the aortic valve or annulus is best appreciated by fluoroscopy, but calcification of the ascending aorta caused by syphilis can be detected on the chest film. Left ventricular failure will be accompanied by pulmonary congestion and venous prominence.

ECHOCARDIOGRAM. Echocardiography has become the most useful noninvasive tool to recognize anatomic abnormalities of the aortic valve and to assess dimensions of the annulus and ascending aorta. The intensity of the regurgitant flow can be appreciated by the vibrations of the anterior mitral leaflet, and the echo Doppler and color techniques can estimate the severity of the regurgitation. Left ventricular chamber dimensions and wall thickness permit calculation of end-diastolic volume and hypertrophy. Finally, an end-systolic dimension of 55 mm has been proposed by several investigators to represent the limit of surgically reversible dilatation of the left ventricle so that aortic valve replacement should be performed before this chamber size is exceeded. Additional clinical experience has challenged the validity of the 55-mm systolic limit, since postoperative reduction in chamber size remains variable. Thus, echocardiographic studies of left ventricular dimensions and function are important in evaluation, follow-up, and timing for aortic valve replacement in aortic regurgitation.

EXERCISE TESTING. Although exercise capacity can be measured and followed periodically in patients with aortic regurgitation, exercise testing is best clinically used in combination with radionuclide angiography. A reduction in exercise ejection fraction by 5 per cent or more is considered by some an indication for surgery even in the absence of symptoms.

CARDIAC CATHETERIZATION. Cardiac catheterization can confirm the presence of aortic incompetence when contrast material injected into the aorta regurgitates into the left ventricle. The primary clinical indications for catheterization are to recognize coexisting lesions, such as mitral regurgitation, and to detect coronary artery disease. Dimensions of the aortic annulus and the ascending aorta are useful for the choice of a prosthetic device in the operative procedure.

Differential Diagnosis

In the evaluation of a diastolic murmur along the left sternal border, aortic insufficiency is far more common than pulmonic insufficiency. The pulsatile characteristics of the peripheral circulation can be helpful in differentiating an aortic from a pulmonic origin of the diastolic murmur. In systemic hypertension, accentuated tambour qualities of the second heart sound can sometimes suggest mild aortic regurgitation, but the level of the diastolic blood pressure can be helpful in distinguishing incompetence from reverberations of the second sound. Any condition that causes aortic stenosis through immobility of the valve leaflets is often accompanied by some degree of aortic regurgitation.

Medical Therapy

Antibiotic prophylaxis is indicated for the prevention of endocarditis. When symptoms of heart failure develop, vasodilating agents such as hydralazine, prazocin, or nifedipine may be beneficial, but benefits are rarely maintained. Thus, the use of digitalis, diuretics, and afterload-reducing agents is primarily of short-term benefit in aortic regurgitation.

Surgical Therapy

A major clinical decision in aortic regurgitation is the timing of aortic valve replacement before irreversible dilatation of the left ventricle has developed. The echocardiographic dimensions and evidence of reduced left ventricular function are now being utilized to advise valve replacement before symptoms of heart failure are manifested. Even after heart failure has developed, patients still improve clinically after aortic valve replacement. Valve replacement can be undertaken with a mortality of less than 3 to 5 per cent. The type of prosthetic valve will depend on the patient's age and the ability to be anticoagulated. In aortic dissection, there may also be replacement of the ascending aorta, since acute regurgitation requires intervention.

MITRAL STENOSIS

Etiology and Pathology

Rheumatic fever remains the predominant cause for mitral stenosis (Table 49–4). Calcification of the mitral valve annulus in the elderly patient can occasionally cause hemodynamic obstruction. Space-occupying lesions, such as left atrial myxoma, or thrombus formation can rarely obstruct the mitral valve. The characteristic pathologic change in rheumatic fever is fibrosis and scarring, particularly at the margins of the valve. This process can also extend into the chordae, with shortening and fusion. Eventually, fibrotic and destructive changes lead to calcification of the valve, and pulmonary venous hypertension causes thickening of the pulmonary veins and capillaries with eventual intimal and medial proliferation of the pulmonary arteries. With longstanding mitral stenosis and pulmonary hypertension, right ventricular hypertrophy and fibrosis develop.

Physiology

The hemodynamic abnormalities in mitral stenosis result from obstruction of diastolic blood flow into the left ventricle. The normal cross-sectional area of the mitral valve ranges from 4 to 6 cm^2, and turbulence of diastolic flow occurs when the valvular orifice is reduced below 2 cm^2. Increased demands for cardiac output, such as in exercise or fever, may be necessary to produce the diastolic murmur when the mitral valve orifice is reduced to 1.5 to 2 cm^2. In the second stage of progressive reduction in the mitral orifice size, a diastolic gradient develops between the left atrium and left ventricle under resting conditions when the valvular area is 1.5 to 1 cm^2. In the advanced stage, mitral orifice size is less than 1 cm^2, and left atrial and pulmonary hypertension becomes significant. The pulmonary capillary pressure often exceeds 20 to 25 mm Hg, and this leads to significant pulmonary arterial hypertension, pressure overload on the right ventricle, and compensatory hypertrophy of the right ventricle. Although the cardiac output can be maintained until the late stage of severe mitral stenosis, exercise will not produce a normal increase in cardiac output owing to impaired diastolic filling. Another hemodynamic complication in chronic mitral stenosis is atrial fibrillation due to left atrial enlargement. Atrial fibrillation and the increased ventricular response can aggravate hemodynamic abnormalities by reducing the diastolic filling period and leading to further elevation of pressure in the lungs.

Clinical Features

The average age at which rheumatic fever occurs is 10 to 12 years, and generally there is a 10-year period before the murmur of mitral stenosis can be detected. Mitral stenosis affects females more than males, and symptoms usually develop between the ages of 25 and 30 years. In temperate zones, mitral stenosis can accelerate in childhood, with severe hemodynamic impairment by the age of 10 to 12 years. Dyspnea is the most common symptom secondary to pulmonary venous hypertension and can be precipitated by any circumstance that increases cardiac output, such as exercise or febrile conditions. Paroxysmal atrial fibrillation can precipitate symptoms by increasing the ventricular rate. As the stenosis progresses, patients experience symptoms with minimal effort or at rest. With longstanding mitral stenosis and chronic pulmonary hypertension, the compensatory thickening of the pulmonary capillaries can protect the lungs from extravasation of fluid despite severe elevations of pulmonary pressure.

Systemic embolization resulting from underlying atrial fibrillation and left atrial thrombus development can also be a manifestation of mitral stenosis. Females can become symptomatic in the second trimester of pregnancy, when the blood volume increases significantly and elevates pulmonary pressures. As the blood volume diminishes late in the third trimester, the symptoms may slightly improve. With severe enlargement of the left atrium and infringement on the mainstem bronchus, persistent cough may develop. Hemoptysis can result from rupture of small vessels in the bronchi due to longstanding venous hypertension. Infective endocarditis can complicate mitral stenosis at any stage, but this generally occurs when mitral regurgitation is present as well.

Physical Examination

The classic physical findings of mitral stenosis are an accentuated first sound at the apex, an opening snap, and a diastolic rumble. If the condition is severe, the diminished peripheral pulse and blood pressure reflect a reduced left ventricular stroke volume. Patients may display typical "mitral facies" with florid congestion of the cheeks. The distended neck veins indicate right ventricular failure with secondary tricuspid regurgitation. If tricuspid stenosis coexists with mitral stenosis, a prominent a wave may be observed in the jugular vein.

Inspection of the precordium may reveal activity along the left sternal border, indicating right ventricular enlargement and pulmonary hypertension. On palpation, the accentuated first sound, the opening snap (OS), and the diastolic rumble can sometimes be felt at the apex. With significant right ventricular dilatation, the left ventricular apical impulse may be displaced laterally, and the right cardiac border may be percussed to the right of the sternum. The opening snap can vary from 0.04 to 0.10 second after the second sound at the apex. The higher the left atrial pressure, the closer the opening snap to the second heart sound (S$_2$), and thus the S$_2$-OS interval indicates the severity of the mitral stenosis. The opening snap is a high-pitched sound and is heard best with the patient in the left lateral decubitus position. The opening snap can sometimes be appreciated at the base of the heart but must be differentiated from a split pulmonic second sound. The diastolic rumble at the apex is a low-pitched murmur following the opening snap. If sinus rhythm is present, there will be presystolic accentuation due to atrial contraction. Since the murmur of mitral stenosis may be faint in the early stages, to complete the physical examination, the patient should exercise by performing sit-ups or hopping on one foot to increase the heart rate. With the increased flow across the mitral valve, the diastolic rumble may be more easily detected.

The diastolic murmur of pulmonic insufficiency should be sought along the left sternal border, but this can be difficult to distinguish from aortic regurgitation. A widened systemic pulse pressure favors aortic over pulmonic insufficiency with mitral stenosis. Rarely, tricuspid stenosis can simultaneously occur with

TABLE 49–4. MITRAL STENOSIS

Etiology	Physiology	Symptoms	Physical Examination	Electrocardiogram	Chest	Echocardiogram	Catheterization	Medical Therapy	Surgical Therapy
Rheumatic	Pressure overload	Dyspnea	Loud S$_1$	Broad, notched	Enlarged LA	Square wave of	Elevated PA*	Dental	Symptoms
Myxoma	LA* and	Fatigue	Opening snap	P wave in	Prominent	EF slope of	wedge	prophylaxis	Valvular area
Calcification	pulmonary	Palpitations	Diastolic rumble	lead II	pulmonary	mitral valve	pressure	Digitalis for	<1.0 cm^2
Congenital	veins	Hemoptysis	Signs of pulmonary		veins	Estimation of	and normal	atrial fibrilla-	
			hypertension:			gradient and	LV diastolic	tion	
			RVH*			orifice size	pressure	Warfarin	
			↑ P$_2$					(Coumadin)	
			Diastolic blow						

*LA = left atrium; RVH = right ventricular hypertrophy; PA = pulmonary arterial.

the mitral stenosis. The murmur of tricuspid stenosis is heard along the lower left sternal border and is greatly accentuated with inspiration. Finally, some degree of mitral incompetence often accompanies mitral stenosis and produces an apical systolic murmur of varying intensity.

Laboratory Studies

ELECTROCARDIOGRAM. The electrocardiographic changes of mitral stenosis include left atrial enlargement and right ventricular hypertrophy due to pulmonary hypertension. Characteristic notching and prolongation of the P wave are most prominent in leads II, III, and aV_F. The terminal portion of the P wave is usually negative in lead V_1. Right-axis deviation and an increased amplitude of the R wave in V_1 are evidence of right ventricular hypertrophy.

CHEST RADIOGRAPH. Radiographic evidence of mitral stenosis includes left atrial enlargement, pulmonary venous hypertension, and right ventricular prominence. The enlarged left atrium produces a double contour along the right cardiac silhouette, as well as straightening of the left cardiac border due to the large left atrial appendage. This change produces elevation of the left mainstem bronchus. The pulmonary venous hypertension redistributes the blood flow to the apices of the lungs, with a reduction in blood volume of the lower lung. Pulmonary arterial hypertension renders the hilar arteries more prominent. Kerley's B lines due to fibrosis and lymphatic engorgement appear as transverse linear densities at the lung bases above the diaphragm.

ECHOCARDIOGRAM. The echocardiogram is the most accurate noninvasive technique for detection of mitral valve stenosis (Fig. 49–2), which is recognized by the characteristic square wave motion of the E to F slope of the valve during diastole. The concordant movement of anterior and posterior mitral valve leaflets is one of the cardinal echocardiographic findings in mitral stenosis. Calcification produces additional echoes from the stenotic valve. The two-dimensional echo can accurately measure the diastolic area of the mitral valve, and the echo Doppler technique can estimate the pressure gradient across the valve, as well as left atrial and left ventricular dimensions, and provide an assessment of left ventricular function. Thrombus or a myxoma in the left atrium produces multiple echoes during diastolic filling.

EXERCISE TESTING. Treadmill or bicycle exercise testing can establish aerobic capacity and the degree of exercise impairment. These observations can be useful in following the young patient with mitral stenosis during the early stages of the disease. The response of the heart rate to exertion and early symptoms of fatigue or dyspnea can be documented with an exercise test.

CARDIAC CATHETERIZATION. Hemodynamic confirmation of mitral stenosis requires measurement of the diastolic pressure gradient across the mitral valve. Left atrial pressure can be obtained directly through trans-septal puncture or as reflected in the pulmonary capillary wedge pressure and recorded simultaneously with the left ventricular pressure. The Gorlin formula (see Ch. 39.5) permits calculation of the mitral orifice size based on the diastolic flow derived from the forward cardiac output and the simultaneous pressure gradient across the valve. The mitral valve gradient can vary from 5 to 25 mm Hg. In an individual without symptoms, mitral valve area can range from 1.5 to 2.0 cm^2. In those exhibiting symptoms with usual activity, valvular size may be 1.5 cm^2 or less, and patients with marked limitations usually have an orifice size less than 1.0 cm^2. Sometimes, a minimal mitral valve gradient is obtained under resting circumstances, but exercise can markedly increase pulmonary pressures to the level of heart failure. At the time of catheterization, associated valve lesions should be assessed, such as mitral regurgitation, aortic stenosis, and aortic regurgitation. If the patient is above 40 years of age, coronary arteriography should also be performed.

Differential Diagnosis

Several cardiac conditions can be confused with the symptoms and physical findings of mitral stenosis. A left atrial myxoma can produce dyspnea or syncope with an opening snap and a diastolic rumble. Primary pulmonary hypertension in young women can be associated with dyspnea and an accentuated pulmonic second sound, but other auscultatory findings are lacking. An atrial septal defect can mimic mitral stenosis with an accentuated first sound, opening snap, and diastolic rumble. However, the accentuated first sound is due to tricuspid valve closure, the opening snap is a split pulmonic second sound, and the diastolic rumble is created by flow across the tricuspid valve.

Medical Therapy

Medical therapy is directed at reducing the incidence of rheumatic fever, prophylaxis for infective endocarditis, control of atrial fibrillation with a rapid ventricular response, and anticoagulation for thromboembolic phenomena. The patient should continue on rheumatic fever prophylaxis until he or she is 30 years of age.

Since atrial fibrillation can aggravate and precipitate symptoms of pulmonary congestion, digitalis should be administered to control ventricular response. Anticoagulation on a chronic basis should be considered in all patients with mitral stenosis and atrial fibrillation. If the patient develops pulmonary edema with atrial fibrillation, cardioversion should be attempted. Ideally, the patient should be anticoagulated 2 weeks prior to elective cardioversion for atrial fibrillation. Quinidine should be started 2 days before the elective procedure, and if digitalis has been administered, this may be discontinued 1 day prior to the cardioversion. If cardioversion is successful, the patient should remain on long-term anticoagulation and quinidine therapy. For thromboembolic phenomena from the left atrium, anticoagulation is indicated. For acute embolism to the extremities or abdomen, surgical embolectomy may be beneficial.

Valvuloplasty via catheter is being performed in selected patients with mitral stenosis, particularly in children, in young women desiring to become pregnant at a later date, and in the elderly at high surgical risk.

Surgical Therapy

The decision for surgery is based on the development of symptoms of pulmonary congestion during activity or at rest. In addition to pulmonary congestion, recurrent atrial fibrillation with aggravation of pulmonary congestion, thromboembolic phenomena, and hemoptysis can be indications for surgery. Mitral commissurotomy remains the procedure of choice with a pliable mitral valve without calcification or mitral regurgitation and carries an operative mortality of less than 1 per cent. This procedure should be considered particularly for the young female who has a desire for pregnancy. Sometimes commissurotomy can be performed before the development of significant symptoms. Patients may benefit for 5 to 20 years after commissurotomy, but if symptoms occur at a later time, mitral valve replacement may be required. Mitral valve replacement carries an operative mor-

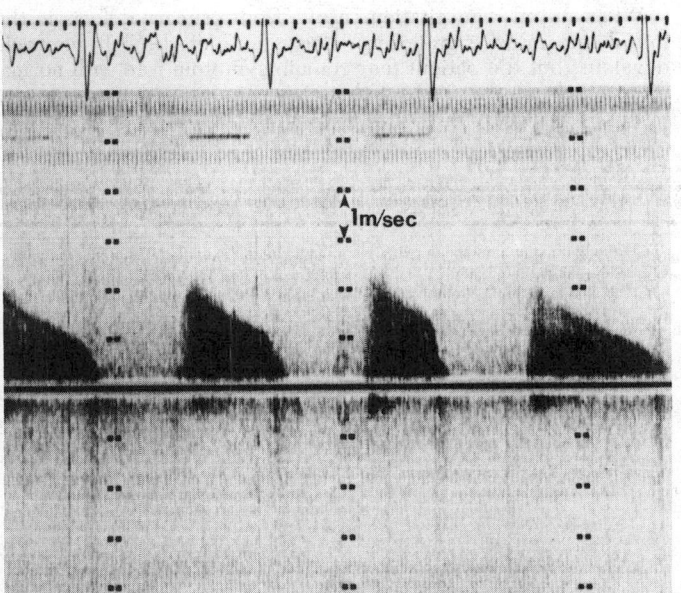

FIGURE 49–2. Continuous wave Doppler echocardiogram of mitral valve flow in a patient with mitral stenosis and atrial fibrillation.

1m/sec

tality of 2 to 3 per cent. The type of mitral valve depends on the age of the patient as well as the circumstances for anticoagulation in a young female. The porcine valve can be inserted without the need for chronic anticoagulation but may require replacement after 10 years. If the valve is calcified or if the patient has had a previous commissurotomy, a prosthetic device is preferred. When there is a contraindication to anticoagulation, as in the aging patient, the porcine valve can be inserted.

Anticoagulation and antibiotic prophylaxis are required in patients with a prosthetic valve. Should atrial fibrillation persist with a rapid ventricular response, digitalis will still have to be administered. Long-term complications of prosthetic mitral valves, such as thrombus formation, infection, and mechanical dysfunction, are estimated to occur at a rate of 1 to 2 per cent per year. Thromboembolism occurs at a rate of 3 per cent per year with a mechanical mitral valve, whereas with the porcine valve, the incidence is 1 to 2 per cent per year.

MITRAL REGURGITATION
Etiology and Pathology

Mitral valve prolapse has now become the leading cause of mitral regurgitation (see next section), although rheumatic heart disease remains an important cause of mitral regurgitation (Table 49–5). Connective tissue disorders, coronary artery disease, annular calcification, and any condition producing left ventricular dilatation can create incompetence of the mitral valve. Several congenital cardiac conditions, such as partial atrioventricular (AV) canal, corrected transposition of the great arteries, and isolated cleft of the mitral valve seen with the ostium primum atrial septal defect, can be associated with mitral valve regurgitation.

Acute mitral regurgitation can result from sudden disruption of the normal function of the mitral valve apparatus. Ruptured mitral valve chordae from endocarditis, myxomatous degeneration of the valve, or trauma can produce sudden mitral regurgitation. Acute myocardial infarction can rupture the papillary muscle, and infective endocarditis can perforate the mitral valve leaflet or the chordae. Mechanical disturbances with a prosthetic mitral valve can lead to mitral incompetence.

Physiology

Incompetence of the mitral valve apparatus during systolic ejection permits regurgitation into the left atrium and pulmonary veins. The extent of the hemodynamic abnormalities imposed on the left ventricle and the left atrium is influenced by the chronic or acute nature of the valvular disturbance as well as the pre-existing functional state of the left ventricle. In chronic mitral regurgitation, a volume overload is imposed on the left ventricle, and the size of the regurgitant volume determines the increase in the end-diastolic volume. Systolic regurgitation into the left atrium produces a prominent v wave, which accentuates the normal filling of the left ventricle from the pulmonary venous inflow. With chronic mitral regurgitation, distensibility of the left atrium and pulmonary veins and increased compliant properties of the left ventricle permit rapid ventricular diastolic filling. As a result of the increased atrial and ventricular compliance, mean left atrial pressure and left ventricular end-diastolic pressure often remain within the normal range in chronic mitral regurgitation.

In *chronic mitral regurgitation,* the large total left ventricular stroke volume maintains the forward stroke volume despite the regurgitant volume into the left atrium. Total left ventricular output may reach six times the normal forward cardiac output. Left ventricular hypertrophy accompanies the increased left ventricular end-diastolic volume. Eventually, the contractile properties of the left ventricular myocardium decline, and the end-systolic volume is abnormally increased. The ejection fraction declines, even though the value may remain near the normal range in the early stage of left ventricular decompensation. An increase in the end-systolic volume elevates the pressure and wall stress values beyond those that can be attributed solely to changes in wall thickness or hypertrophy. This occurrence has been designated as a mismatch in afterload and preload. Even though the deterioration of the contractile state of the left ventricle may gradually elevate the left ventricular end-diastolic pressure, in rare instances the left atrium enlarges to such dimensions that ventricular end-diastolic and left atrial pressures remain normal, as encountered in the giant left atrium syndrome.

In coronary artery disease, mitral regurgitation results from abnormalities of posterior wall motion and papillary muscle function. Ischemia of the papillary muscle has been proposed as a mechanism, and disturbances in posterior wall motion are usually present with mitral regurgitation. When the residual scar after myocardial infarction exceeds 20 per cent of the total surface area of the ventricle, compensatory dilatation of the left ventricle is often attended by some degree of mitral regurgitation.

Severe dilatation of the left ventricle from either a primary volume overload or secondary myocardial decompensation eventually results in mitral regurgitation. Dilatation of the left ventricular chamber displaces the papillary muscles so that coaptation of the leaflets is impaired during systolic ejection. Conditions producing ventricular dilatation are further aggravated by depression of the contractile state, and the left ventricular hemodynamic abnormalities primarily reflect myocardial failure with an additional overload on the ventricle.

In *acute mitral regurgitation,* a sudden pressure overload is imposed on the left atrium and pulmonary veins from the left ventricular regurgitant volume. This pressure overload is intensified by the inability of the left atrium and left ventricle to dilate suddenly. The v wave in the left atrium may be as high as 60 to 70 mm Hg, resulting in acute pulmonary edema.

Clinical Features

When mitral regurgitation results from primary defects in the mitral apparatus, significant enlargement of the left ventricle develops, but the patient may remain symptom free with normal exercise tolerance. Since pulmonary venous hypertension and

TABLE 49–5. MITRAL REGURGITATION

Etiology	Physiology	Symptoms	Physical Examination	Electrocardiogram	Chest	Echocardiogram	Catheterization	Medical Therapy	Surgical Therapy
Chronic									
Prolapse	LV volume overload	Initially asymptomatic	Holosystolic apical murmur	LV hypertrophy	Enlarged LV Enlarged LA	Enlarged LV and LA	Contrast from LV to LA	Afterload reduction	Symptoms LV echo
Rheumatic	LV dilatation and hypertrophy	Fatigue	Decreased S₁			Mitral valve anatomy	LA v wave	Diuretics	Diastolic dimension
Coronary artery disease	LA* enlargement	Dyspnea	Third sound					Digitalis	>60 mm†
Annular calcification									
Connective tissue disorder									
LV* dilatation									
Prosthetic valve									
Acute									
Ruptured chordae	Pressure overload LA and pulmonary veins	Acute pulmonary edema	Harsh holosystolic murmur radiating into back	No change Acute myocardial infarction	Normal LV and LA dimension	Abnormal mitral valve apparatus	Massive LA regurgitation	Preload and afterload reduction	Surgery may be urgently required
Ruptured papillary muscle	No change in LV dimension		Third sound		Pulmonary edema		Large v wave		
Perforation of leaflet							Normal-sized LA		
Prosthetic valve									

*LV = left ventricle or ventricular; LA = left atrium or atrial.
†Proposed.

congestion are not early features of mitral regurgitation, fatigue due to reduced forward cardiac output is a more frequent symptom than dyspnea. Gradual impairment of the contractile state is attended by further enlargement of end-systolic and end-diastolic volumes and elevation of the left ventricular end-diastolic and left atrial pressures. Atrial fibrillation commonly develops when the left atrium enlarges and further aggravates heart failure.

In coronary artery disease, significant mitral regurgitation is usually accompanied by symptoms of impaired left ventricular function, such as dyspnea, fatigue, and orthopnea. This condition is sometimes designated the *ischemic cardiomyopathy syndrome*. In acute syndromes of mitral regurgitation, pulmonary edema is often the initial presentation because of the suddenly imposed pressure and volume overload on the left atrium and pulmonary venous system.

Physical Examination

The typical physical finding of mitral regurgitation is the apical holosystolic murmur, but the intensity, variation during the ejection phase, and radiation over the precordium are influenced by the underlying mechanism. The peripheral pulse can sometimes be rapid in upstroke with a short duration because of the abbreviated systolic ejection time, since a large volume of blood is regurgitated into the left atrium. The precordium may reveal a diffusely hyperdynamic impulse, and the first heart sound at the apex is diminished. The characteristic holosystolic murmur radiates into the axilla and often to the left sternal border. A protodiastolic or ventricular gallop sound is frequently audible and may be followed by an early diastolic rumble due to the large inflow of blood from the left atrium. When mitral regurgitation is caused by left ventricular dilatation and depression of the contractile state, the systolic murmur may be mid-, late, or holosystolic. Under these circumstances, the systolic murmur is usually grade II/VI or less and is accompanied by a left ventricular (S_3) gallop sound.

In acute mitral regurgitation due to rupture of the mitral valve apparatus, the murmur is harsh, grade III or IV/VI, and accompanied by a palpable thrill at the apex.

Laboratory Studies

ELECTROCARDIOGRAM. In chronic mitral regurgitation, the electrocardiogram will show evidence of left ventricular dilatation and hypertrophy with increased QRS voltage and ST-T wave changes in the lateral precordial leads. Left atrial enlargement will produce a negative P wave in lead V_1, but atrial fibrillation often develops in the late stages. When coronary artery disease is the etiology of mitral regurgitation, there is often evidence of an inferior or posterior wall myocardial infarction.

CHEST RADIOGRAPH. Left ventricular enlargement due to the volume overload can be appreciated from the standard chest film. Left atrial enlargement will cause a prominence along the right sternal border, but the pulmonary venous pattern may show no abnormalities until heart failure and venous congestion have developed.

ECHOCARDIOGRAM. The echocardiogram can define the anatomy of the mitral valve apparatus as well as left atrial and left ventricular chamber dimensions and function. Calcification of the valve leaflets and the annulus can be recognized. Depression of left ventricular ejection fraction and increases in end-diastolic and end-systolic dimensions are observed in secondary causes of mitral regurgitation with heart failure. With acute mitral regurgitation, a flail leaflet, ruptured chordae, or nidus of infection with infective endocarditis can sometimes be identified by the echocardiogram. The echo Doppler and color techniques can assess the intensity of the regurgitant jet into the left atrium. Finally, left ventricular end-diastolic and end-systolic dimensions have been used to identify the optimal time for mitral valve replacement before significant and irreversible myocardial deterioration has taken place.

EXERCISE TESTING. The standard exercise tests and radionuclide angiography can quantify functional capacity and document early deterioration in patients with mitral regurgitation.

CARDIAC CATHETERIZATION. Left ventriculography confirms mitral regurgitation by demonstrating systolic regurgitation of contrast material into the left atrium. Although the magnitude of the regurgitation can be quantified, the mechanism is not always apparent from left ventriculography. Left ventricular end-diastolic and end-systolic dimensions can be utilized to calculate ejection fraction, left ventricular mass, wall stress, and regurgitant volume per beat into the left atrium. The difference between the angiographic left ventricular stroke volume—that is, the end-diastolic volume minus the end-systolic volume on left ventriculography—and the forward stroke volume, calculated from the Fick or thermodilution methods, yields the regurgitant stroke volume per beat across the mitral valve. Coronary artery disease and the wall motion abnormalities contributing to disturbance in mitral valve function can also be confirmed at catheterization. The prominent v wave of mitral regurgitation can be recorded in the left atrium or the pulmonary capillary wedge pressure tracing. In acute mitral regurgitation, dimensions of the left ventricle and left atrium may be normal, but the regurgitant v wave can rise to 60 to 70 mm Hg. Cardiac catheterization can also detect coexistent lesions in the aortic valve. Since the left ventricular ejection fraction may be maintained in the normal range despite deterioration of the contractile state, additional assessment of the contractile state is important in all causes of mitral regurgitation. Calculation of end-systolic wall stress from pressure, volume, and wall thickness dimensions has proved useful in recognizing early deterioration of the contractile state in mitral regurgitation.

Differential Diagnosis

A holosystolic murmur identifies mitral regurgitation, even though the mechanism may not be apparent. Tricuspid regurgitation can cause a holosystolic murmur at the lower left sternal border, but inspiration accentuates the murmur more than in mitral regurgitation. If the murmur is not holosystolic, conditions such as aortic stenosis could be considered, along with papillary muscle dysfunction and mitral valve prolapse. In calcific aortic stenosis of the elderly patient, the murmur may sometimes be more prominent in the apex and may be confused with that of mitral regurgitation. A ventricular septal defect also causes a harsh holosystolic murmur at the lower left sternal border, but this generally radiates to the right of the sternum, compared with the axillary radiation of the murmur in mitral regurgitation.

Medical Therapy

In the early phase of mitral regurgitation without symptoms, only antibiotic prophylaxis is warranted. The same antibiotic program as described for mitral stenosis should be administered to these patients. When atrial fibrillation develops, digitalis is indicated to slow the ventricular response. Afterload-reducing agents, such as nitrates and antihypertensive drugs, have been found useful in maintaining the forward stroke volume in mitral regurgitation. Once heart failure develops, diuretics and inotropic agents are required, but major consideration should be given to surgery.

Surgical Therapy

The operative mortality of mitral valve replacement in mitral regurgitation has remained higher than the 2 to 3 per cent in mitral stenosis and for the symptomatic patient may range from 5 to 10 per cent. In the past, surgery has been delayed until patients develop symptoms, but the advanced symptomatic stage and depressed left ventricular function contribute to high operative mortality rates. When the ejection fraction falls below 20 per cent, operative mortality for mitral valve replacement may be as high as 25 per cent. Therefore, surgery should be considered before the patient becomes extremely symptomatic. An echocardiographic diastolic dimension greater than 60 mm has been proposed as a predictor for mitral valve replacement. In the selection of the optimal prosthetic device, the patient's age, underlying condition, and circumstances for anticoagulation must be considered. When technically feasible, valvular reconstruction is employed in order to preserve the anatomy. The mechanical prosthetic valve in the mitral position is more likely to develop thrombotic material than in other locations, so anticoagulation must be maintained. Any contraindication to anticoagulation warrants consideration of a porcine valve. Thromboembolism in patients with mechanical valves who are on anticoagulation occurs at a rate of 3 per cent per year, and for preoperative functional classes I through III, there is a yearly mortality rate of 3 per cent over a 10-year follow-up period. With a porcine valve, the rate of thromboembolism is lower but may reach 1.5 per cent per year.

MITRAL VALVE PROLAPSE

Etiology and Pathology

Although an isolated systolic click has been regarded as benign for decades, echocardiography has identified prolapse of the mitral valve in as many as 5 per cent of the adult population. A variety of synonyms include the midsystolic click–late systolic murmur, click murmur syndrome, and Barlow's syndrome. Pathologic findings include myxomatous degeneration of the valve and redundancy of the valve leaflets. These changes can also involve the chordae as well as the mitral valve. Although the underlying mechanism is still incompletely understood, these changes in the mitral valve are seen with several connective tissue diseases, including Marfan's syndrome and osteogenesis imperfecta, and sometimes with coronary artery disease. The syndrome occurs most frequently in women in early adulthood and can also be found in families.

Physiology

The abnormalities of mitral valve prolapse can affect both anterior and posterior leaflets, but the posterior leaflet is most frequently involved. With the onset of ventricular systole, normal closure of the mitral valve takes place, but redundancy of the leaflets results in further upward motion of the valve into the left atrium. Sudden cessation of the valvular motion is thought to generate the click, and the lack of proper positioning of the two leaflets results in the systolic regurgitant murmur in mid- and late systole. Occasionally, both the anterior and posterior leaflets prolapse, and in extreme conditions, there can be extensive prolapse of both leaflets in the absence of a click or murmur. In a small number of patients, progressive degenerative changes in the valve or rupture of the chordae or both can produce severe mitral regurgitation.

Clinical Features

The majority of patients with mitral valve prolapse remain asymptomatic, but a spectrum of symptoms can be encountered. Symptoms include palpitations, fatigue, chest pain, orthostatic changes, and psychological aberrations. Frequently, symptoms fail to correlate with the prominence of the physical findings and the extent of mitral regurgitation. Circulatory studies on changes in tilting, along with heart rate and blood pressure response, have led to the designation of dysautonomia in certain of these patients. In 10 to 15 per cent of affected individuals, palpitations may become frequent, and in a smaller number there may be progressive mitral regurgitation. Infective endocarditis occurs with a slightly higher incidence than in the normal population. Sudden deaths associated with this syndrome have been sporadically reported.

Physical Findings

Patients are often female, with a thin habitus and a narrow anteroposterior chest diameter. The principal findings are the early to midsystolic click and a mid- or late systolic murmur. The timing of the click as well as the characteristics of the murmur can vary widely. Often the murmur is crescendo and decrescendo, but it can be sustained in its frequency. The click or the murmur may be present alone, and not infrequently, both click and murmur are absent. The click and the murmur are influenced by the dimensions of the ventricle, and maneuvers that decrease ventricular filling, such as standing and the Valsalva maneuver, will result in movement of the click closer to the first sound, followed by early onset of the murmur. Conditions that increase filling of the ventricle, such as the squatting maneuver, can delay the onset of the click and the murmur.

Laboratory Studies

ELECTROCARDIOGRAM. The electrocardiogram may reveal a variety of T wave and ST-segment changes, along with atrial or ventricular ectopic beats. Most commonly, the T wave is slightly inverted in the inferior and lateral precordial leads, and occasionally there is associated ST-segment depression. Rarely, QT prolongation with deep coving of the T wave is seen in the precordial leads. Runs of premature beats, both from the atrium and the ventricle, can be recorded by Holter monitoring. Symptoms may not correlate with the frequency and occurrence of cardiac ectopic activity.

CHEST RADIOGRAPH. The habitus is asthenic; the chest has a narrow anteroposterior diameter, and the cardiac silhouette is elongated.

ECHOCARDIOGRAPHY. The echocardiogram is the diagnostic technique of choice for mitral valve prolapse (Fig. 49–3). In one form, late systolic prolapse of the posterior leaflet resembles an inverted question mark. In the second form, there may be prolapse of the posterior leaflet throughout the systolic ejection phase with a hammock type of configuration. The echocardiographic findings of prolapse can be recognized in the absence of the click and the murmur. At other times, the click and murmur are not attended by echocardiographically evident prolapse of the leaflet. The standard for diagnosis of mitral valve prolapse is the two-dimensional echo, which can define the plane of the mitral annulus and demonstrate extension of the mitral valve leaflets beyond the annulus into the left atrium. Color Doppler can display the amount of mitral regurgitation.

EXERCISE TESTING. Stress testing can aggravate or precipitate cardiac irritability in these patients. Furthermore, the exercise test can document the patient's fatigue and musculoskeletal symptoms, which often are at variance with the echocardiographic findings.

CARDIAC CATHETERIZATION. Although left ventriculography has been the standard invasive method for documenting redundancy and prolapse of the mitral leaflets, the precision of echocardiography has obviated the necessity of catheterization in the majority of patients with prolapse. Atypical chest discomfort sometimes requires coronary arteriography to exclude coronary artery disease. Wall motion abnormalities have been recognized on the ventriculogram, but these do not correlate with coexisting abnormalities in the coronary arteries. Prolapse of the tricuspid valve can also occur. With mitral valve prolapse in connective tissue disorders, there may be associated aortic regurgitation.

Differential Diagnosis

The mid- and late systolic murmur, as well as the crescendo-decrescendo qualities of mitral valve prolapse, can be similar to the murmur of regurgitation in papillary muscle dysfunction. In coronary artery disease or hypertrophic cardiomyopathy with

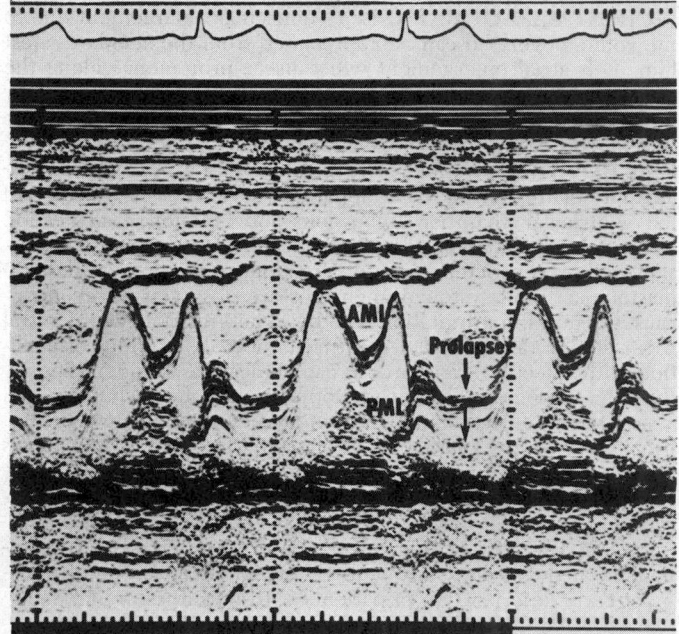

FIGURE 49–3. M-Mode echocardiogram of a patient with mitral valve prolapse. Note the systolic posterior motion of the anterior (AML) and posterior (PML) mitral valve leaflets.

obstruction, the crescendo-decrescendo murmur may be similar to that of mitral valve prolapse. However, the harsh intensity of the murmur is much louder with the hyperdynamic contraction of hypertrophic cardiomyopathy. Maneuvers that increase the murmur of mitral valve prolapse intensify the murmur of cardiomyopathy with obstruction even more. However, in the latter condition, the murmur is often holosystolic. If ventricular irritability is present, the intensity of the murmur of hypertrophic cardiomyopathy with obstruction will be much louder in the post-extrasystolic beat.

Treatment

The majority of patients with mitral valve prolapse require no treatment. Ventricular ectopy and symptoms of palpitations can be effectively managed with β-blocking drugs. However, fatigue in these patients can sometimes be aggravated with β blockade. With a prolonged QT interval or syncope, treatment with an antiarrhythmic is warranted. Infrequently, control of ectopy may be difficult despite the use of standard antiarrhythmic agents.

Infective endocarditis is a potential problem in these patients. Originally, all patients were advised to have antibiotic prophylaxis. Statistical studies now suggest that only those patients with an audible click and murmur should be treated with antibiotic prophylaxis. Patients with prolapse demonstrated on echocardiography without a click or murmur may be at no greater risk than the normal population. When mitral regurgitation becomes progressive with chamber enlargement or with ruptured chordae, mitral valve replacement may be necessary. Mitral valve reconstruction and mitral valve annuloplasty are preferred by some surgeons to total valve replacement. Fortunately, for the majority of patients, reassurance and conservative follow-up constitute the best treatment.

TRICUSPID STENOSIS

The most common cause of stenosis of the tricuspid valve remains rheumatic fever, but this condition is invariably associated with involvement of left-sided valves by the same rheumatic process. Rare conditions such as carcinoid tumor, endocardial fibroelastosis, and right atrial myxoma can create stenosis or obstruction of the tricuspid valve. Tricuspid stenosis causes right atrial hypertension and elevated systemic venous pressure. Stenosis of the tricuspid valve may serve as a protective mechanism for the pulmonary vascular bed in patients with mitral stenosis. Symptoms of tricuspid stenosis are dyspnea and fatigue, but the pulmonary manifestations of mitral stenosis can diminish with the development of significant stenosis of the tricuspid valve. Pulsations in the neck veins and peripheral edema develop.

Physical examination reveals a prominent, often giant, a wave in the neck veins caused by the vigorous atrial contraction against the stenotic valve. The diastolic murmur is heard best along the left lower sternal border and is presystolic if sinus rhythm is present or midsystolic with atrial fibrillation. The murmur increases prominently with inspiration, but an opening snap is rarely heard. Since mitral stenosis is usually concurrent, the auscultatory maneuvers must specifically locate the tricuspid stenosis murmur. If tricuspid stenosis is the dominant hemodynamic lesion, pulmonary hypertension and right ventricular hypertrophy will not be detected on the physical examination.

The electrocardiographic finding is a tall, tented P wave in leads II, III, and aV$_F$ with absence of right ventricular hypertrophy. The chest radiograph should reveal a large right atrium without prominence of the pulmonary arteries. The echo Doppler technique may detect and assess the gradient across the tricuspid valve. If cardiac catheterization is performed, simultaneous catheters must be placed in the right atrium and the right ventricle for accurate detection of the pressure gradient. Respiratory variations will introduce inaccuracies in a pull-back tracing across the tricuspid valve. Treatment consists of antibiotic coverage. If surgery is performed for lesions in the left side of the heart, correction of the tricuspid lesion can also be undertaken.

TRICUSPID INSUFFICIENCY

Tricuspid insufficiency is, most commonly, secondary to right ventricular dilatation and hypertrophy. Tricuspid regurgitation can rarely result from infective endocarditis, myocardial infarction, trauma, prolapse, or congenital heart disease such as atrial septal defect or Ebstein's anomaly. Symptoms of tricuspid regurgitation are those of hepatic congestion or peripheral edema.

On physical examination, atrial fibrillation is commonly present and large cv waves can be detected in the jugular veins. The murmur is holosystolic along the left sternal border and increases with inspiration. The electrocardiogram often reveals atrial fibrillation without other significant features. The chest film demonstrates a prominent right atrium and ventricle. The echocardiogram can document prolapse of the tricuspid leaflets as well as a nidus of infection or disruption of a chorda. Contrast-echo and echo Doppler techniques can accurately detect and assess the amount of tricuspid regurgitation. Therapy usually consists of treatment of conditions leading to right ventricular failure. Should surgery be performed for left-sided lesions, the tricuspid valve can be inspected. Often the leaflets are anatomically normal, and annuloplasty is indicated rather than valve replacement. If the tricuspid valve is replaced, along with insertion of mitral and aortic prostheses, mortality remains high at 20 per cent.

PULMONIC REGURGITATION

Regurgitation of the pulmonic valve is most commonly secondary to severe pulmonary hypertension, which can be caused by mitral stenosis, chronic lung disease, or pulmonary emboli. Inflammatory diseases and endocarditis can sometimes render the pulmonic valve incompetent, and previous surgery for congenital heart disease may create pulmonic regurgitation. The murmur (Graham Steell) is typically a high-pitched diastolic blow along the left sternal border similar to that in aortic regurgitation. No characteristic electrocardiographic changes are found, but the chest radiograph often demonstrates a prominent pulmonary artery echo. The color Doppler technique easily detects regurgitation in the pulmonary outflow tract. Cardiac catheterization is useful only to exclude aortic regurgitation as a cause of the diastolic murmur. Treatment consists of management of pulmonary hypertension with medical agents or occasionally with mitral valve surgery.

PULMONIC STENOSIS

Stenotic lesions of the pulmonic valve are almost always caused by congenital malformations (see Ch. 46). Rarely, hypertrophic cardiomyopathy can involve the right side of the heart with obstruction of the right ventricular outflow tract.

Aortic Valve Disease

Letac B, Cribier A, Koning R, et al.: Aortic stenosis in elderly patients aged 80 or older: Treatment by percutaneous balloon valvuloplasty in a series of 92 cases. Circulation 80:1514, 1989. *A review by the founders of this procedure for a common valvular condition in aging patients.*

Pellikka PA, Nishimure RA, Bailey KR, et al.: The natural history of adults with asymptomatic hemodynamically significant aortic stenosis. J Am Coll Cardiol 15:1012, 1990. *Clinical guidelines for the asymptomatic patient.*

Mitral Valve Disease

Duren DR, Recker AE, Dunning AJ: Long-term follow-up of idiopathic mitral valve prolapse in 300 patients: A prospective study. J Am Coll Cardiol 11:42, 1988. *Clinical events in the most common abnormality of cardiac valves.*

Rackley CE, Edwards JE, Karp RB: Mitral valve disease. *In* Hurst JW (ed.): The Heart. 7th ed. New York, McGraw-Hill Book Company, 1989, p 820.

Rappaport E: Natural history of aortic and mitral valve disease. Am J Cardiol 36:221, 1975. *A 10-year follow-up of the stenotic and regurgitant lesions of the aortic and mitral valves.*

Valve Surgery

Chavez AM, Copgrove DM, Lyth BW, et al.: Applicability of mitral valvuloplasty techniques in a North American population. Am J Cardiol 62:253, 1988. *Alternatives to surgical replacement of the mitral apparatus.*

Lindblom D, Lindblom U, Quist J, et al.: Long-term survival rates after heart valve replacement. J Am Coll Cardiol 15:566, 1990. *Analysis of risk, benefits, and complications in long-term follow-up of prosthetic valves.*

Rackley CE, Katz NM, Wallace RB: Artificial valve disease. *In* Hurst JW (ed.): The Heart. 7th ed. New York, McGraw-Hill Book Company, 1989, p 871.

50 Diseases of the Myocardium

Joseph K. Perloff

"Cardiomyopathy" means heart (cardio) muscle disease (myopathy). The term is appropriately applied to disorders characterized by *primary* involvement of ventricular myocardium. Because these disorders of cardiac muscle are primary, they are by definition not in response to coexisting or pre-existing disease of the heart or circulation. The cardiomyopathies are best classified according to their anatomic and pathophysiologic types as dilated, hypertrophic, or restrictive (Table 50–1, Fig. 50–1). In each category, the cause or causes may or may not be known.

DILATED CARDIOMYOPATHY

DEFINITION AND GENERAL DESCRIPTION OF FINDINGS. Dilated cardiomyopathy is characterized by an increase in left ventricular or biventricular internal dimensions without a proportional increase in septal and free wall thicknesses. The principal physiologic impairment is in systolic function (depressed contractility).

Certain *general pathophysiologic principles* apply. Injured myocytes do not regenerate but are replaced by connective tissue. Hypertrophy of remaining cells does not adequately compensate for the loss of contractile elements. Ventricular volumes increase, cardiac output falls, and left ventricular filling pressure rises. Stroke volume is initially maintained despite depressed ejection fraction. This state of compensated systolic dysfunction is ultimately replaced by decompensated heart failure in which cardiac output is critically limited. The development of mitral and tricuspid regurgitation adds to the hemodynamic burden and further depresses cardiac output. Hypervolemia and peripheral vasoconstriction contribute additionally to net ventricular overload.

Three major threats confront the patient with chronic dilated cardiomyopathy, namely, progressive hemodynamic deterioration, systemic embolization, and sudden death. An insidious decrease in exercise tolerance is followed by frank exertional dyspnea, orthopnea, and paroxysmal nocturnal dyspnea. Both ventricles are usually involved, but the clinical manifestations of left ventricular failure generally predominate. The mechanisms of sudden death are diverse and include ventricular tachycardia or fibrillation, severe bradycardia, electromechanical dissociation, systemic embolization of mural thrombi from the dilated left ventricle (Fig. 50–2), and pulmonary embolization from venous thromboses.

On *physical examination*, the arterial pulse exhibits a relatively narrow pulse pressure and pulsus alternans. A "proportional pulse pressure" (calculated as the difference between systolic and diastolic blood pressures divided by the systolic pressure) of 25 per cent or less identifies approximately 90 per cent of patients with cardiac indices of 2.2 liters per minute per square meter or less. The jugular venous pulse exhibits elevated a and v waves with preserved x and y descents until tricuspid regurgitation increases the v wave and blunts the x descent. Precordial palpation identifies a displaced, hypodynamic left ventricular impulse. Auscultation detects third and fourth heart sounds. Systolic murmurs originate from mitral and tricuspid regurgitation. Occasional patients have disproportionate right ventricular failure (peripheral edema, ascites, and hepatic congestion). Im-

TABLE 50–1. PATHOPHYSIOLOGIC CLASSIFICATION OF THE CARDIOMYOPATHIES

1. Dilated
2. Hypertrophic
   a. Asymmetric (eccentric)
   b. Symmetric (concentric)
3. Restrictive (nondilated, nonhypertrophic)
   a. Increased septal/wall thickness
   b. Normal septal/wall thickness

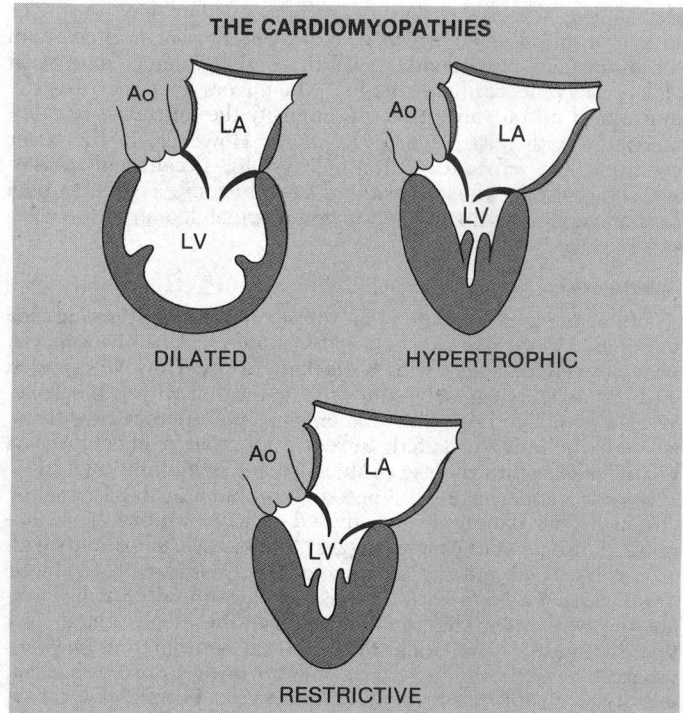

FIGURE 50–1. Schematic illustrations of dilated, hypertrophic, and restrictive cardiomyopathies. (Modified from Roberts WC, Ferrans VJ: Pathologic anatomy of the cardiomyopathies. Human Pathol 6:287, 1975. Reprinted with permission from W. B. Saunders Co.)

portantly, rales are typically absent despite elevated left ventricular filling pressure because chronic exudation of fluid is associated with an increase in lymphatic drainage so that the alveoli remain relatively dry.

The *electrocardiogram* may show nothing more than nonspecific ST-T wave abnormalities, but occasionally Q wave "infarct patterns" are present and are believed to reflect myonecrosis. Left bundle branch block is relatively frequent in chronic idiopathic dilated cardiomyopathy, but Chagas' disease is most commonly associated with right bundle branch block.

The *chest roentgenogram* reveals varying degrees of cardiomegaly. The increase in heart size principally reflects dilatation of the ventricles, although the atria are enlarged as well. Elevated left ventricular filling pressure is reflected chiefly in prominent central (hilar) pulmonary veins and in upper lobe vascular redistribution, rather than by radiologic evidence of pulmonary edema. Increased lymphatic drainage is the reason (see above).

Two-dimensional echocardiography identifies increased internal dimensions of the ventricles at end-diastole, normal or reduced septal and free wall thicknesses, and depressed ventricular function (Fig. 50–3). Although global hypokinesis is the rule, regional wall motion abnormalities occur and are believed to reflect zones of myonecrotic injury. Doppler echocardiography with color flow imaging establishes the presence and degree of atrioventricular (AV) valve regurgitation. Two-dimensional echocardiography and technetium-99m radionuclide imaging shed light on abnormal ventricular function and wall motion. Magnetic resonance imaging provides refined morphologic information and, together with two-dimensional echocardiography, serves to identify left ventricular endocardial thrombi (see Fig. 50–2).

INCIDENCE. It has been estimated that in 1989 there were approximately 140,000 patients with idiopathic dilated cardiomyopathy in the United States. Each year, approximately 20,000 new patients come to attention, and about 10,000 die.

ETIOLOGY, PATHOGENESIS, AND PATHOLOGY. The dilated cardiomyopathies are caused by myocardial injury that results in depressed systolic function and progressive ventricular dilatation. Table 50–2 lists most of the etiologic categories. Pathogenetic mechanisms—clinical and experimental—include myocarditis (infectious or noninfectious), immune or autoimmune processes, genetic factors (immune-response genes), hormonal

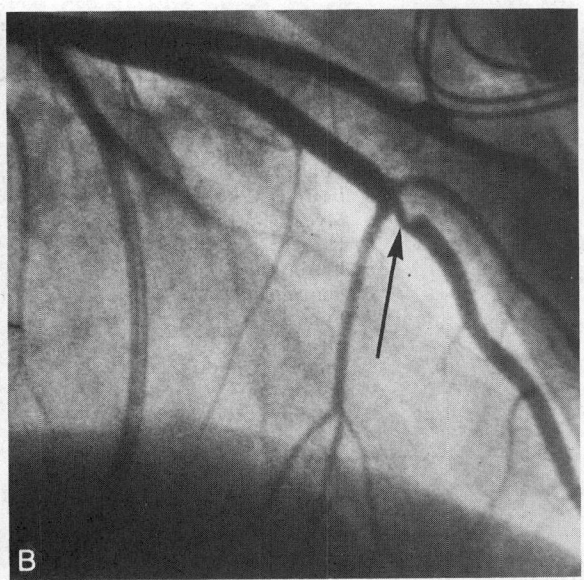

FIGURE 50–2. *A,* Two-dimensional echocardiogram showing an endocardial thrombus *(arrowheads)* in the apex of the left ventricle (LV) of a patient with dilated cardiomyopathy. *B,* Coronary arterial embolus *(arrow)* to the left anterior descending artery in another patient with idiopathic dilated cardiomyopathy.

imbalances, free radicals, calcium overload, and altered blood supply (abnormal coronary microvasculature).

The majority of cases of dilated cardiomyopathy are believed to represent sequelae of myocarditis, generally infectious. The histologic diagnosis of myocarditis is now on firmer ground because of the Dallas criteria established by a group of experienced pathologists (Fig. 50–4). Every major type of infectious agent has been implicated as causative (Table 50–2), although with widely divergent incidence. In western Europe and the United States, infectious myocarditis is most commonly due to viruses, especially enteroviruses.

The most convincingly documented cause of human myocarditis is coxsackievirus group B infection. Experimental murine coxsackievirus B3 results in an initial phase of active intramyocardial viral replication and cell necrosis during which physical exercise or immunosuppressive agents enhance replication of the virus and reinforce tissue injury. In the next phase, virus is not detectable in the myocardium. Defects in immunoregulation are believed to result in an inability to attenuate the stimulus for autoimmune responses (suppressor cell defect), ineffective viral clearance (natural killer cell deficiency), and prolonged antigenic stimulation that may trigger the immune responses. The net result is immunopathic myonecrosis. Reduction of the offending lymphocyte population appears to coincide with a decrease in late myocyte injury. Infected animals may recover, die, or progress to a late third stage in which the dilated heart contains little or no inflammation but, instead, large areas of fibrosis.

The histologic features of dilated cardiomyopathy on endomyocardial biopsy do not necessarily correspond to the symptomatic or hemodynamic status. It is likely, therefore, that many cases of primary myocarditis initially escape clinical detection. In the late phase of the natural history, active inflammatory cell infiltration is absent or nearly so. Chronic dilated cardiomyopathy is then characterized by the presence of areas of fibrosis interwoven among shrunken or hypertrophied myocytes (Fig. 50–4). At this stage, the designation *idiopathic dilated cardiomyopathy* is commonly applied because thorough clinical evaluation fails to identify a specific cause in more than 80 per cent of patients. The association in human subjects between myocardial inflammation initiated by cardiotropic viruses and the subsequent development of dilated cardiomyopathy is persuasive but not conclusive.

In South America, up to 15 per cent of the rural population have primary myocardial injury due to infection by *Trypanosoma cruzi* (Chagas' disease). Chagas' cardiomyopathy is characterized by an acute tissue invasive phase followed by a chronic phase of extensive myocardial fibrosis believed to be the result of a lymphocyte- or an antibody-mediated autoimmune reaction. Chronic chagasic injury not only affects myocytes (with a peculiar propensity to cause apical left ventricular aneurysm) but also has a predilection for specialized tissues (right bundle branch block) and for cardiac parasympathetic ganglia (denervation).

Noninfectious inflammation of the myocardium occurs with systemic diseases of connective tissues (autoimmune disorders). Systemic lupus erythematosus is an example. Of the *toxic agents* that directly injure ventricular myocardium, ethyl alcohol (ethanol) is the most common, and has been implicated in at least 10 per cent of patients with dilated cardiomyopathy. The undesirable acute myocardial effects of ethyl alcohol are masked by

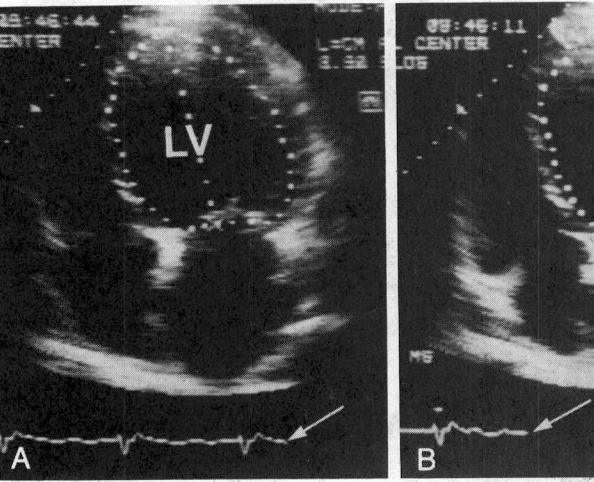

FIGURE 50–3. Two-dimensional echocardiograms with endocardial markers *(A)* during systole and *(B)* during diastole in a patient with dilated cardiomyopathy. The minimal change in dimensions indicates a markedly reduced left ventricular (LV) ejection fraction.

TABLE 50–2. ETIOLOGIC CLASSIFICATION OF THE DILATED CARDIOMYOPATHIES

I. Idiopathic
II. Inflammatory
  A. Infectious
    1. Viral
    2. Bacterial
    3. Mycobacterial
    4. Parasitic
    5. Rickettsial
    6. Spirochetal
    7. Fungal
  B. Noninfectious
    1. Autoimmune disease
    2. Peripartum
    3. Hypersensitivity reactions
    4. Transplantation rejection
III. Toxic
  A. Ethyl alcohol
  B. Chemotherapeutic agents
  C. Elemental compounds
  D. Catecholamines
IV. Metabolic
  A. Nutritional
  B. Endocrinologic
  C. Electrolyte abnormalities
V. Familial cardiomyopathy
  A. Neuromyopathic
    1. Progressive muscular dystrophy
    2. Myotonic muscular dystrophy
    3. Friedreich's ataxia
  B. Hereditary dilated cardiomyopathy
VI. Abnormal coronary microvasculature

the beneficial effects of peripheral vasodilatation and the positive inotropic response to catecholamines, but in the autonomic blockaded heart, ethanol causes a significant decrease in contractility. Both ethanol and acetaldehyde (its first metabolite) adversely affect myocardial metabolism. Alcoholic cardiomyopathy is attributed to the toxicity of ethanol and acetaldehyde on the myocardial cell. In addition to the effects of ethyl alcohol and its metabolites, constituents of the brew may also depress contractility. Cobalt added to beer to stabilize foam is a case in point. In the beriberi heart disease of chronic alcoholics, high-output heart failure of thiamine deficiency is imposed upon the depressed myocardium of alcoholic cardiomyopathy. There is a positive epidemiologic association between excessive alcohol ingestion

and systemic hypertension. An important clinical aspect of alcoholic cardiomyopathy is its reversibility, at least initially. However, pathologic studies late in the natural history reveal myocardial cell necrosis with replacement fibrosis.

A host of other toxic substances and drugs reportedly cause myocardial injury either as a result of excessive exposure or as idiosyncratic responses. Catecholamine excess may cause myonecrosis. Doxorubicin (Adriamycin) and other anthracycline chemotherapeutic agents are additional examples. The structural changes in response to anthracycline antitumor agents are dose related. Doxorubicin rarely results in acute heart failure and only occasionally produces arrhythmias or conduction disturbances. About 2 to 5 per cent of patients receiving 500 mg of the drug per square meter slowly develop overt heart failure, but over one half of patients have abnormal responses to exercise and exhibit histologic changes on endomyocardial biopsy. The microscopic pattern of doxorubicin-induced myocardial injury is characterized by the gradual appearance of vacuolar degeneration, myofibrillar loss, and juxtaposition of disrupted cells among normal cells.

The distinct clustering of *peripartum cardiomyopathy* in the last month of gestation and especially in the first 3 postpartum months supports the contention that the disorder is uniquely coupled to pregnancy. Incidence has been estimated from 1 in 3000 to 1 in 15,000 confinements. Myocardial inflammation is sufficiently frequent to warrant the designation "myocarditis," but the inflammation is not infectious. Despite diligent search, no role of cardiotropic viruses has been established. The peripartum myocardial injury is believed to result from an autoimmune mechanism triggered by release of myocyte antigens from the late-term pregnant uterus.

Metabolic derangements that adversely affect systolic function and result in dilated cardiomyopathy include endocrinopathies, trace element deficiencies, and electrolyte abnormalities. In diabetes mellitus, there is convincing evidence of a cardiopathy (myocardial injury) separate from extramural coronary artery disease. The relative roles of microvascular disease, interstitial PAS-positive material, and fibrosis remain unsettled. Dilated heart failure in hyperthyroidism principally reflects pre-existing impairment of contractile reserve made clinically overt by the hypermetabolic state. An analogy is the high-output state of beriberi (vitamin B_1 deficiency) in chronic alcoholics. In classic Asian beriberi, however, dilated heart failure is due to thiamine deficiency per se in individuals without myocardial depression from other causes. Teenagers who excessively consume processed foods deficient in thiamine may suffer from heart failure provoked by strenuous exercise. The principal initial physiologic effect of thiamine deficiency is on the peripheral circulation, but persistent deficiency may lead to dilated cardiomyopathy. Abnormal regu-

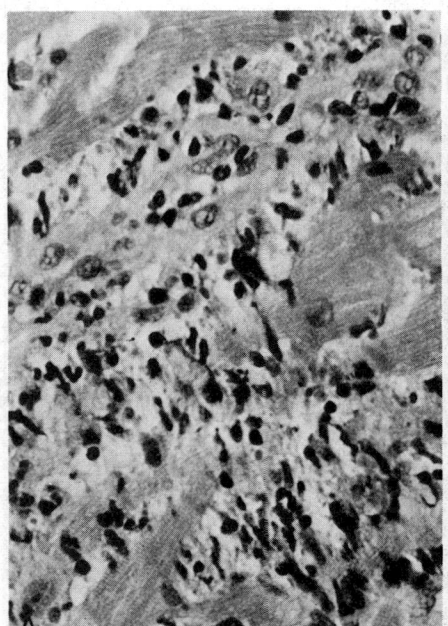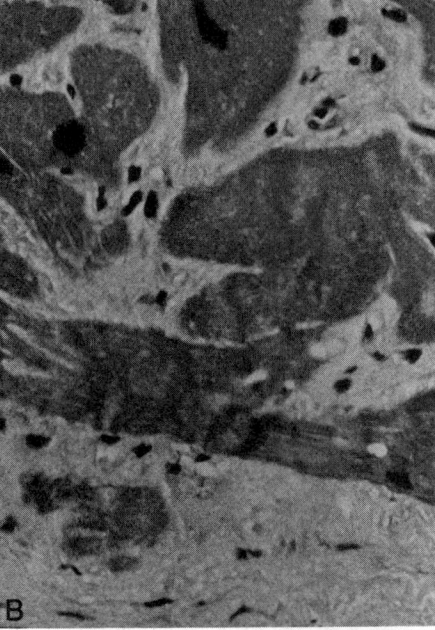

FIGURE 50–4. Endomyocardial biopsies from two patients. *A*, Early stages showing the inflammatory cells and myocyte damage of myocarditis. *B*, Late stage showing extensive replacement of myocardium by fibrous tissue.

lation of carnitine, a naturally occurring amino acid required for mitochondrial oxidation of long chain fatty acids, has also been associated with dilated heart failure.

Electrolyte disorders that adversely affect cardiac contractility include deficiencies of calcium, phosphate, magnesium, and potassium. If the availability of calcium is inadequate, ejection fraction falls, as in patients receiving large transfusions of blood preserved with citrate. which chelates calcium, or in patients with hypoparathyroidism. Hypophosphatemia leads to inadequate stores of high-energy phosphate compounds, as in alcoholism, diabetes, and hyperalimentation. Magnesium, a cofactor for thiamine-dependent reactions and for sodium-potassium adenosine triphosphatase (ATPase), may be depleted by impaired gastrointestinal absorption or increased renal excretion (diuretics).

A number of heredofamilial *neuromyopathic disorders* are associated wtih dilated cardiomyopathy. Examples include X-linked, slowly progressive muscular dystrophy (Becker dystrophy), certain patients in the late stages of Duchenne dystrophy, Friedreich's ataxia, and the childhood form (but not the adult form) of myotonic muscular dystrophy.

DIAGNOSIS. Dilated cardiomyopathy should be suspected in relatively young patients who present with cardiac enlargement, cardiac failure, systemic emboli, and ventricular arrhythmias. Chest pain indistinguishable from myocardial infarction (myonecrosis caused by the cardiotropic virus) sometimes accompanies acute myocarditis. The diagnosis of dilated cardiomyopathy hinges on firm exclusion of pre-existing or coexisting heart or vascular disease. Cardiac catheterization has given way to noninvasive diagnostic procedures, especially two-dimensional echocardiography (see Fig. 50–3), except for the exclusion of ischemic cardiomyopathy (coronary artery disease) in older patients, especially males.

If dilated cardiomyopathy presents early in its course, throat and stool cultures and viral titers should be secured and serially compared. Up to 50 per cent of patients with clinical myocarditis have evidence of recent coxsackievirus B infection, especially types 1 to 5. Myocardial inflammation has been identified by gallium-67 scintigraphy, but more specifically by endomyocardial biopsy from the right ventricular septum (Fig. 50–4). Twenty-four hour Holter monitors are used to detect ventricular arrhythmias.

TREATMENT AND PROGNOSIS. Dilated cardiomyopathy entails four major therapeutic concerns: the potential presence of ongoing myocardial injury, the hemodynamic state of the dilated heart, the threat of systemic emboli, and the risk of ventricular arrhythmias.

During the tissue-invasive stage of acute infectious myocarditis, immunosuppressive agents provoke viral replication and are therefore proscribed. The majority of patients who present with active infectious myocardial inflammation do so after the acute tissue-invasive stage. Attempts at pharmacologic suppression of persistent myocarditis require documentation of the presence of inflammation. Although immunosuppression for biopsy-proven myocarditis in human subjects remains controversial, experience with cardiac transplant patients teaches us that immunosuppressive therapy can be lifesaving. Many patients with virus-induced myocarditis improve during treatment with prednisone and azathioprine, and relapses have occurred after discontinuing immunosuppression. Whether or not immunosuppression is used, clinical status improves in up to one half of patients with biopsy-proven myocarditis. Not surprisingly, even patients who clinically improve may have persistent abnormalities of ventricular systolic function. The grim prognosis of peripartum cardiomyopathy, coupled with evidence of noninfectious myocardial inflammation, argues for treatment with immunosuppressive agents, but the relatively high incidence of spontaneous improvement is a confounding variable. Mortality rates in the acute and subacute stages of peripartum cardiomyopathy range from 30 to 60 per cent. Improvement in symptoms, heart size, and ventricular function, when it occurs, does so early, generally within 1 month of presentation. The severity of early compromise in left ventricular function does not predict long-term outcome, but if normalization of function is not achieved by 6 months, the outlook is poor. The risk of recurrences during subsequent pregnancies is related to ventricular function. Alcoholic cardiomyopathy often responds dramatically to abstention even after patients have

become significantly symptomatic. Continued ethanol consumption is associated with an inexorable deterioration and a 3-year mortality of up to 80 per cent. Abstention should be undertaken in hospital so that compliance can be assured, diet monitored, and arrhythmias controlled.

Doxorubicin (Adriamycin) cardiotoxicity is generally irreversible and is the cause of death in over 60 per cent of patients so afflicted. Careful monitoring during doxorubicin therapy minimizes the risk. Potential cardiomyopathy in response to doxorubicin can be identified by radionuclide angiography, two-dimensional echocardiography, or endomyocardial biopsy. Patients without additional cardiac risks are best studied after 450 mg per square meter of drug administration. Although a decline in ejection fraction at rest or with exercise arouses legitimate concern of myocyte damage, the frequency of false positivity mandates that damage be confirmed by endomyocardial biopsy before therapy is withdrawn. Cardiotoxicity of doxorubicin is related not only to peak levels but also to cumulative dose. Toxicity is reduced by slow infusion rates.

The treatment of dilated ventricles with depressed systolic function and elevated filling pressure requires an awareness of the complex interplay among a host of variables, including neurohormonal interactions and adaptations, and the relationship between central hemodynamics and regional blood flow. The chief pharmacologic agents employed are vasodilators (afterload reduction) and diuretics. The role, if any, of digitalis glycosides remains open to question. Vasodilator therapy and diuretics are initially employed empirically, but refined adjustments require a flotation catheter for hemodynamic monitoring in order to achieve an optimal balance between a reduction in left ventricular filling pressure and maintenance of a satisfactory cardiac output. Reductions in ventricular filling pressure and systemic vascular resistance can result in a decrease in *total* stroke volume but an increase in *forward* stroke volume, apparently due to attenuation of mitral regurgitation and a decrease in left ventricular volume.

The use of β blockade in chronic dilated cardiomyopathy is seemingly contradictory and at present controversial. There is a contrasting effect between short- and long-term administration of the β-adrenergic blocker metoprolol. Short-term administration results in acute depression of systolic function, whereas long-term administration results in improved systolic function. The following mechanisms have been proposed to account for improvement after long-term (3 to 12 months) metoprolol therapy. Chronically elevated levels of circulating catecholamines and a high local release of norepinephrine tend to worsen heart failure. There is down-regulation of β receptor density in severe heart failure. Long-term treatment with metoprolol results in moderate receptor up-regulation, which may facilitate a more normal response to sympathetic stimulation.

The risk of systemic emboli in dilated cardiomyopathy argues for the use of long-term anticoagulants, which are obligatory if a thrombus announces itself as a systemic embolus or if an endocardial thrombus is found during noninvasive imaging. Systemic emboli generally arise from a thrombus attached to the left ventricular endocardium (see Fig. 50–2). A second predisposing cause of embolization is atrial fibrillation. Pulmonary emboli are not uncommon and originate from peripheral venous thromboses rather than from right ventricular endocardium.

Sudden, unexpected cardiac arrest accounts for approximately half of all deaths in patients with dilated cardiomyopathy. The conventional wisdom attributes sudden death to ventricular tachyarrhythmias, but Holter monitoring does not reliably identify patients at risk of dying suddenly from ventricular tachycardia or fibrillation. This is so because the mechanisms of unexpected cardiac arrest in advanced heart failure are diverse. A significant majority of patients experience severe bradycardia or electromechanical dissociation at the time of arrest, with ventricular tachycardia or fibrillation occurring in the minority.

Cardiac transplantation has been a major step forward in the treatment of patients with advanced heart failure, over half of whom have primary dilated cardiomyopathy. Impressive improvements in post-transplantation survival are due chiefly to advances in immunosuppression. However, because of the substantial disparity between donor availability and patient need, every attempt should be made to stabilize candidates so that transplantation can be done electively. Patients referred for urgent transplantation cannot be considered refractory to medical therapy until vasodilators and diuretics are systematically administered during continuous hemodynamic monitoring. When that is done, oral vasodilator and diuretic therapy is possible in 80 per cent of "refractory" patients, with a 6-month actuarial survival of 75 per cent despite an initial ejection fraction of 0.15 per cent ± 0.04.

Aretz HT, Billingham ME, Edwards WD, et al.: Myocarditis: A histopathologic definition and classification. Am J Cardiovasc Pathol 1:3, 1986. *The biopsy diagnosis of myocarditis hinges on the identification of inflammatory cells and evidence of subsequent damage as defined by the Dallas criteria established in this report.*

Dec GW, Palacios IF, Fallon JT, et al.: Active myocarditis in the spectrum of acute dilated cardiomyopathies: Clinical features, histologic correlates, and clinical outcome. N Engl J Med 312:885, 1985. *A series of 27 patients with dilated cardiomyopathy of recent onset in which biopsy-proven myocarditis and subsequent improvement were frequent, whether or not immunosuppressive drugs were given.*

Luu M, Stevenson WA, Stevenson LW, et al.: Diverse mechanisms of unexpected cardiac arrest in advanced heart failure. Circulation 80:675, 1989. *This report deals with the multifactorial mechanisms of sudden death in advanced heart failure, calling attention to severe bradycardia and electromechanical dissociation in the majority of patients at the time of cardiac arrest.*

O'Connell JB, Costanzo-Nordin MR, Subramanian R, et al.: Peripartum cardiomyopathy: Clinical, hemodynamic, histologic, prognostic characteristics. J Am Coll Cardiol 8:52, 1986. *Characterization and prognosis of 14 patients who developed peripartum cardiomyopathy despite good general health and prenatal care. The relatively high incidence of myocarditis is documented and discussed.*

O'Connell JB, Mason JW: Immunosuppressive therapy in experimental and clinical myocarditis. Pathol Immunopathol Res 7:292, 1988. *This review summarizes the studies of immunosuppression in active myocarditis and describes a multicenter trial designed to resolve the issue of efficacy.*

Perloff JK (ed.): The Cardiomyopathies. Cardiology Clinics. Philadelphia. W. B. Saunders Company, 1988. *This concise volume surveys the clinical and experimental aspects of the three major categories of cardiomyopathies, covering etiology, clinical manifestations, diagnosis, and treatment.*

Regan TJ: Alcoholic cardiomyopathy. Prog Cardiovasc Dis 27:141, 1984. *A comprehensive review of the pathogenesis, preclinical course, and prognosis of alcoholic cardiomyopathy.*

THE HYPERTROPHIC CARDIOMYOPATHIES

DEFINITION. This category of cardiomyopathies is represented grossly by asymmetric (eccentric) or symmetric (concentric) hypertrophy of the left ventricle in the absence of another cardiac or systemic disease capable of producing an increase in ventricular mass (see Table 50–1). In the asymmetric variety, the septum is disproportionately thick relative to the left ventricular free wall beneath the mitral annulus (see Fig. 50–1). In the symmetric variety, the septum and left ventricular free wall are of equal thickness. Ventricular cavity size is normal or reduced in both types.

ETIOLOGY. Hypertrophic cardiomyopathy occurs in both familial and sporadic forms. Autosomal dominance is the usual mode of inheritance in the genetically transmitted form of the disease. Sporadic occurrences may represent new mutations, reduced penetrance in first-degree relatives, autosomal recessive transmission, or nongenetic occurrence. Biochemical determinants in the pathogenesis are not firmly established but have focused on two interrelated hypotheses—the proposed intrauterine links between myocyte development and norepinephrine stimulation and/or excess intracellular calcium. Studies of regional myocardial blood flow and metabolism using positron emission tomography suggest a metabolic abnormality in the disproportionately thick septum.

PATHOLOGY. Genetic hypertrophic cardiomyopathy is characterized by two gross morphologic and two histologic features. The gross morphologic features are asymmetric septal hypertrophy and a catenoid ventricular septal configuration. Asymmetric hypertrophy may involve the entire septum (base to apex, Fig. 50–5), or much less commonly the hypertrophy is principally if not exclusively apical or midventricular, at the level of the papillary muscles. The most typical histologic feature—cellular disarray—is significantly more common and quantitatively considerably more extensive in hypertrophic cardiomyopathy than in other cardiac disorders or in normal subjects. In its proper clinical and pathologic context, extensive septal cellular disarray remains an important marker of genetic hypertrophic cardiomy-

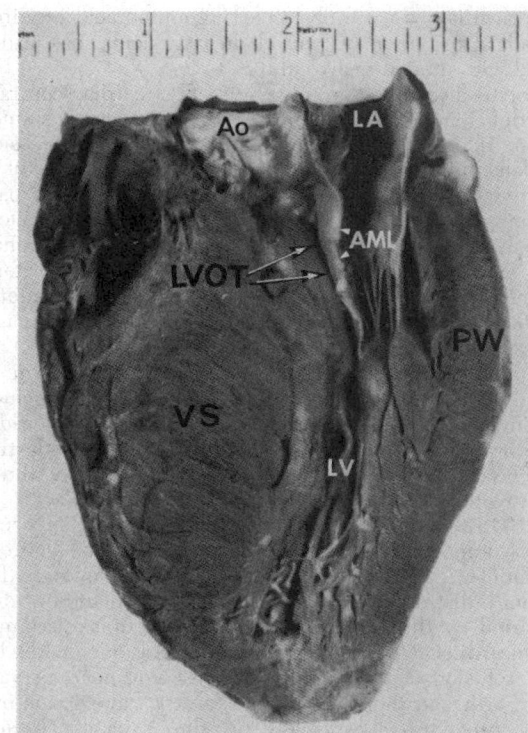

FIGURE 50–5. One of Teare's original cases of "asymmetrical hypertrophy of the heart." The ventricular septum (VS) is substantially thicker than the left ventricular posterior wall (PW). The cavity of the left ventricle (LV) is much reduced. The base of the ventricular septum bulges into the left ventricular outflow tract (LVOT) adjacent to the anterior mitral leaflet (AML). Ao = Aorta; LA = left atrium. (From Teare D: Asymmetrical hypertrophy of the heart in young adults. Br Heart J 20:1, 1958, with permission. Labels superimposed.)

opathy. The second histologic feature—thick-walled intramural coronary arteries with narrow lumens—occurs in more than three fourths of patients with genetic hypertrophic cardiomyopathy, especially in the ventricular septum. The pathogenetic and clinical significance of the thickened intramural coronary arteries is unresolved.

PHYSIOLOGY. Characterization of the physiologic derangements in genetic hypertrophic cardiomyopathy forms the basis for an understanding of the clinical manifestations, diagnosis, and treatment. The principal physiologic features include a hypercontractile left ventricular free wall (enhanced systolic function) (Fig. 50–6A), hypocontractile ventricular septum, left ventricular cavity obliteration (Fig. 50–6A), and impaired diastolic function. In the normal heart, ventricular contraction consists of an isovolumetric phase that occupies about 10 per cent of systole and an ejection phase with fiber shortening that occupies 80 to 90 per cent of systole. In genetic hypertrophic cardiomyopathy, a third phase is added. High-velocity ejection is completed in the first 60 to 80 per cent of systole, following which the cavity obliterates and the ventricle contracts isometrically. Thus, hypertrophic cardiomyopathy is characterized by enhanced systolic function, a prolonged and abnormally powerful isometric contraction phase followed by impaired relaxation and increased chamber stiffness during diastole.

Classic genetic hypertrophic cardiomyopathy is accompanied by a singular physiologic feature that continues to generate lively interest—the left ventricular to aortic dynamic pressure gradient. Entrapment of the catheter tip during cavity obliteration spuriously elevates the recorded systolic pressure within the left ventricle. However, echocardiography with Doppler interrogation and color flow imaging has provided convincing evidence of a true obstructive pressure gradient. Anterior mitral leaflet-septal contact is believed to be the cause of the gradient, and the Venturi effect is regarded as the responsible pathogenetic mechanism.

The gradient is "dynamic," a term that calls attention to its lability and its response to certain physical and pharmacologic

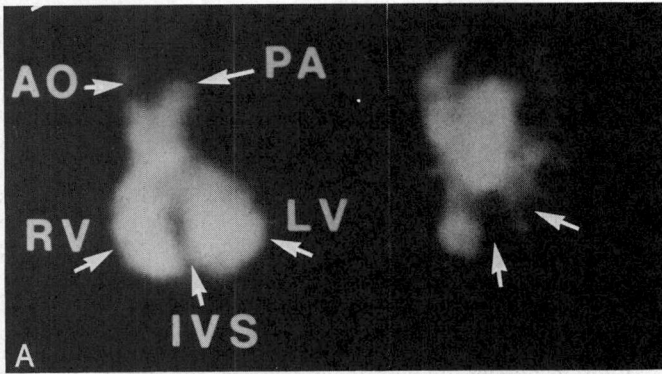

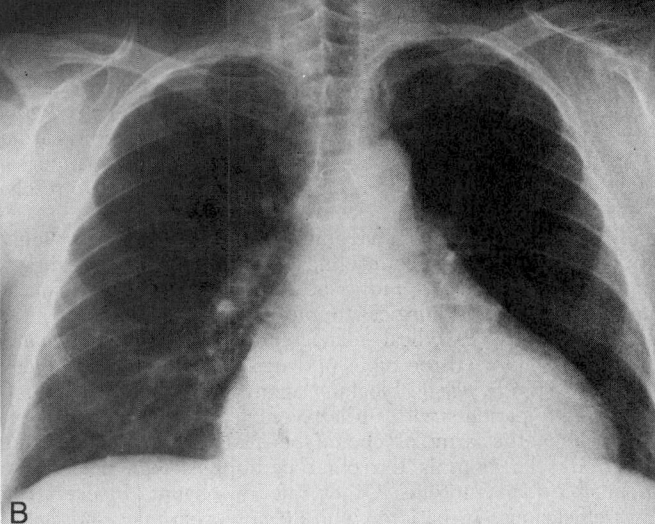

FIGURE 50–6. *A*, Technetium-99m gated radionuclide angiography in genetic hypertrophic cardiomyopathy (diastolic and systolic images). During systole, the left ventricular (LV) cavity obliterates, and the thick interventricular septum (IVS) becomes evident. RV = Right ventricle; Ao = aorta; PA = pulmonary artery. *B*, Left ventricular dilatation and failure 20 years after ventriculomyomectomy in a patient with genetic hypertrophic cardiomyopathy.

interventions. Interventions that reduce left ventricular cavity size intensify the gradient and vice versa. The gradient increases during the straining phase of the Valsalva maneuver; during prompt standing from the squatting position; following the compensatory pause initiated by a premature beat; and in response to isotonic exercise, tachycardia, digitalis, isoproterenol, amyl nitrite, and nitroglycerin. The gradient decreases during the overshoot phase of the Valsalva maneuver, during the Müller maneuver, upon squatting, in response to isometric exercise (handgrip), and in response to β-adrenergic blockade or α-adrenergic stimulation. In patients with significant gradients, administration of inotropic drugs or volume-depleting diuretics can be accompanied by sudden and serious deterioration.

CLINICAL MANIFESTATIONS. The clinical picture ranges from asymptomatic patients who are incidentally found to have hypertrophic cardiomyopathy to severely ill patients with incapacitating symptoms. The widespread use of echocardiography has allowed detection of asymptomatic patients who come to attention because of an abnormal physical examination or electrocardiogram, or because of a first-degree relative with hypertrophic cardiomyopathy. The symptomatically overt disease typically becomes manifest in relatively young adults (third to fifth decades), but it is not uncommon for patients to present after 60 years of age. In infants, the disorder presents as a murmur and marked congestive failure, with the majority of afflicted babies dying before their first birthday. In adults, it is not uncommon for the disease to declare itself dramatically as syncope or sudden death in previously healthy young persons engaged in strenuous exertion. The most common symptoms are dyspnea, fatigue, chest pain (similar to, if not identical with, angina pectoris), and syncope. The most prevalent symptom is dyspnea, which is

intensified by exertion and which is believed to be chiefly related to high end-diastolic pressures (left ventricular diastolic dysfunction). Clinical deterioration in adults is typically slow with two major exceptions—sudden death or the onset of atrial fibrillation. Loss of coordinated atrial contraction in the face of impaired left ventricular diastolic function results in acute dyspnea (sudden increase in end-diastolic and pulmonary venous pressures).

In older subjects, chest pain coupled with electrocardiographic Q waves (see later) prompts a diagnosis of atherosclerotic coronary artery disease, which may coexist. However, symptoms resembling angina pectoris occur in relatively young patients without extramural coronary artery disease, and have been attributed to small vessel (intramural) coronary disease, decreased capillary to fiber ratio of hypertrophy, and impaired diastolic function which impedes coronary blood flow. Observations based upon positron emission tomography have not detected ischemia at rest in mildly symptomatic patients.

Cerebral symptoms vary from lightheadedness to frank syncope. Patients sometimes feel pain in the upright position (promptly corrected by lying down) or in response to physical exercise. Occasional patients report such a history for years without apparent clinical deterioration. Syncope or presyncope has been attributed to disturbances in rhythm or conduction (see below), to an inability to increase cardiac output because of impaired diastolic function or obstruction to left ventricular outflow, or to stimulation of intraventricular baroreceptors that impairs peripheral vasoregulation.

The *physical examination* in asymptomatic patients without systolic gradients is unimpressive except for a relatively prominent left ventricular impulse and a fourth heart sound. The jugular venous pulse may exhibit a prominent A wave (increased force of right atrial contraction) that does not reflect pulmonary hypertension, but instead is a response to reduced distensibility of the right ventricular cavity caused by massive thickening of the ventricular septum (see Fig. 50–5). The increase in velocity of left ventricular ejection causes a brisk rate of rise of the systemic arterial pulse while the pulse pressure remains normal (small waterhammer pulse). Twin peaking of the arterial pulse coincides with a mid- to late-systolic trough, a feature better recorded than palpated. Precordial palpation sometimes detects a *triple* apical impulse composed of double systolic movement coupled with presystolic distention. A systolic thrill may be present at the apex and toward the lower left sternal edge in patients with left ventricular outflow gradients, but the thrill is related more closely to mitral regurgitation than to the outflow gradient. Auscultation detects a prominent apical fourth heart sound, a normal first sound, and at the left base a second sound that is usually normally split, sometimes narrowly split or single, and occasionally paradoxically split. Despite the increased velocity of left ventricular contraction, aortic ejection sounds are exceptional. Systolic murmurs in patients with left ventricular outflow gradients represent combinations of midsystolic murmurs caused by increased velocity of ejection and longer, if not holosystolic, apical murmurs caused by mitral regurgitation. The murmur is typically loudest at the apex, with radiation into the axilla or to the left lower sternal edge, less prominently to the base, and seldom into the neck. The systolic murmur is less important because of its presence than because of the diagnostic significance of its response to physical and pharmacologic interventions (Table 50–3). Third heart sounds occur in the presence of mitral regurgitation and are occasionally followed by brief after-

TABLE 50–3. EFFECTS OF BEDSIDE PHYSICAL INTERVENTIONS ON THE SYSTOLIC MURMUR OF HYPERTROPHIC OBSTRUCTIVE CARDIOMYOPATHY

Increased Intensity of Murmur
  Dynamic exercise
  Straining phase of Valsalva maneuver
  Prompt standing after squatting
Decreased Intensity of Murmur
  Release (overshoot) phase of Valsalva maneuver
  Squatting
  Isometric exercise (handgrip)

vibrations that create the auscultatory impression of short mid-diastolic murmurs. A high-frequency early diastolic murmur of aortic regurgitation makes the diagnosis of hypertrophic cardiomyopathy doubtful.

Electrocardiograms are normal in a minority of asymptomatic patients but are almost invariably abnormal in symptomatic patients with left ventricular outflow gradients. P-wave morphology generally shows a left atrial abnormality alone, but occasionally a right atrial configuration coexists. The PR interval is often short but only rarely associated with pre-excitation, even when the short PR interval is accompanied by initial force slurring reminiscent of a delta wave. Atrial fibrillation, the most common sustained supraventricular rhythm disturbance, is not accompanied by accelerated AV conduction. Ventricular arrhythmias are relatively common (see below). Arrhythmic syncope is ominous and heralds sudden death that is attributed to ventricular tachycardia or fibrillation. The propensity for ventricular arrhythmias has been attributed, at least in part, to electrical instability inherent in the cellular disarray (nonuniform anisotropy) and to the disparity between the duration of mechanical systole and electrical activation. The potentially malignant ventricular arrhythmias that prevail in genetic hypertrophic cardiomyopathy are essentially unknown in the hypertrophic cardiomyopathy of Friedreich's ataxia, whether asymmetric or concentric, and cellular disarray has not been found at necropsy in Friedreich's disease.

Prominent Q waves occur in upward of 50 per cent of cases. The Q waves tend to be abnormal because of their depth rather than their duration. The Q waves have been ascribed to abnormal electrophysiologic properties in areas of cellular disarray. Electrocardiographic evidence of left ventricular hypertrophy is common but not invariable and is reflected in the increased voltage and ST-segment and T-wave abnormalities. Distinctive giant T-wave inversions in mid to left precordial leads imply *apical* hypertrophic cardiomyopathy (Fig. 50–7).

In the *chest roentgenogram,* enlargement of the left atrium is relatively common, especially when significant mitral regurgitation coexists with atrial fibrillation. Left ventricular size and contour range from normal to a convex silhouette projecting to the left, inferior and posterior. The aortic root is inconspicuous.

The echocardiogram is the mainstay of the *laboratory diagnosis* of hypertrophic cardiomyopathy, providing virtually all necessary clinical diagnostic information. The cardinal echocardiographic features of genetic hypertrophic cardiomyopathy are disproportionate thickness of the ventricular septum (at least 15 mm measured at the minor axis level), with a septal/posterior wall ration of 1.5:1 or more, a small left ventricular cavity, exaggerated contractility of the left ventricular free wall, and a relatively hypocontractile ventricular septum. Two-dimensional echocardiography establishes the location and extent of disproportionate septal thickness (Fig. 50–7A) and occasionally shows a ground-glass appearance of the septum believed to be related to cellular disarray. High-velocity ejection through a left ventricular outflow tract that is narrowed by the disproportionately thick septum causes systolic anterior motion of the mitral leaflets (Venturi effect). Doppler interrogation with color flow imaging establishes the left ventricular outflow dynamics and the presence and degree of mitral regurgitation. Pulsed Doppler echocardiography (sample volume slightly on the ventricular side of the mitral annulus) has been a major step forward in characterizing the abnormalities of left ventricular diastolic function.

Technetium-99m gated radionuclide ventriculography identifies the thickness of the ventricular septum, the relative motions of septum and free wall, and the left ventricular cavity size in diastole and systole (Fig. 50–6A). Magnetic resonance imaging, with its capability of recording in multiple planes, offers refined morphologic information on the septum and free walls.

Prior to noninvasive imaging, *cardiac catheterization* provided the standards for the clinical diagnosis of hypertrophic cardiomyopathy. Catheterization is now reserved for older patients in whom coronary angiography is employed in an attempt to resolve the cause of chest pain.

TREATMENT. The management of hypertrophic cardiomyopathy includes genetic counseling, medical therapy according to hemodynamic subgroup and associated symptoms, the management of arrhythmias, surgical therapy, and prophylaxis for infective endocarditis. Medical management of the hemodynamic subgroups employs three types of drugs—calcium channel blocking agents, β-adrenergic blocking agents, and disopyramide. In symptomatic patients with no left ventricular to aortic gradient, verapamil is the drug of choice because diastolic dysfunction (impaired relaxation) is the chief pathophysiologic mechanism responsible for symptoms. Other calcium channel blockers may be as efficacious. In patients who do not experience satisfactory symptomatic improvement on verapamil alone, β blockers are added to reduce the heart rate and prolong the diastolic filling period.

Treatment of symptomatic patients with latent (provokable) left ventricular outflow gradients primarily employs β-adrenergic blockers. Calcium channel blockers might serve a useful purpose as negative inotropic agents, but drug-induced peripheral vasodilatation can augment left ventricular outflow obstruction. The negative inotropic effect of disopyramide does not run this risk (see below).

Symptomatic patients with resting left ventricular to aortic gradients are first treated with disopyramide, provided that intravenous administration appreciably reduces or abolishes the gradient. If subsequent oral administration relieves both the

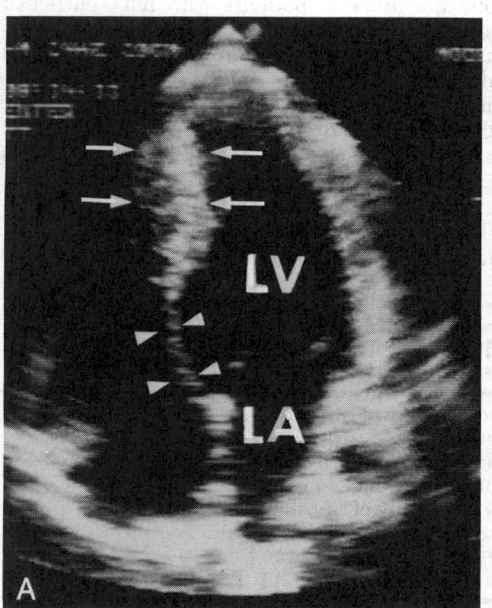

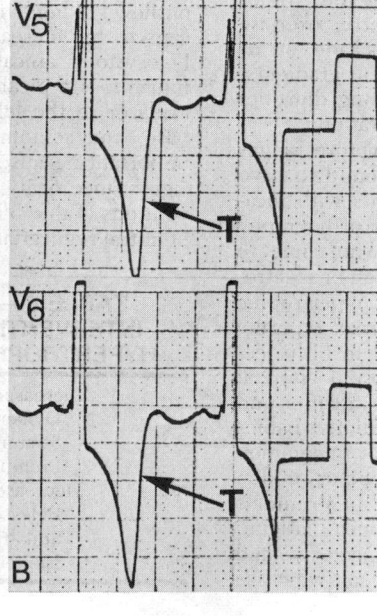

FIGURE 50–7. *A,* Two-dimensional echocardiogram showing hypertrophic cardiomyopathy involving the apical half of the ventricular septum *(arrows).* The basal septum *(arrowheads)* is not thickened. *B,* Typical electrocardiogram in apical hypertrophic cardiomyopathy showing giant T-wave negativity *(arrows)* in leads V_5 and V_6.

symptoms and the gradient, the drug is continued. If not, a β blocker can be added. Calcium channel blockers are used cautiously if at all because their vasodilating effect can appreciably augment the gradient and provoke symptoms.

The management of arrhythmias focuses on ventricular arrhythmias and atrial fibrillation. The recommended method of screening patients for ventricular arrhythmias is 48- to 72-hour ambulatory electrocardiographic monitoring. Sudden death occurs about eight times more frequently in patients with asymptomatic ventricular tachycardia recorded on this type of ambulatory monitoring than in those without ventricular tachycardia so recorded. The highest yield for asymptomatic ventricular tachycardia is in patients with resting gradients, extensive hypertrophy, syncope, or a family history of sudden death. Clinical trials have not yet shown that antiarrhythmic therapy reduces the risk of sudden death, but treatment is recommended for patients with frequent repetitive firing of three or more ventricular beats, and in the rare patient with prolonged episodes of asymptomatic ventricular tachycardia. Quinidine, procainamide, or disopyramide are initially used, with dose levels adjusted according to blood levels and according to efficacy by repeated ambulatory monitoring. Amiodarone is effective in abolishing the ventricular arrhythmias, but there are significant side effects, and recent data suggest that abolition of ventricular tachycardia on ambulatory monitoring does not prevent sudden death. The drug is best confined to high-risk patients in whom more conventional antiarrhythmic therapy has failed.

Atrial fibrillation requires treatment because of its adverse effect on diastolic filling (removal of the booster pump benefit of atrial systole and shortening of the diastolic filling period because of the increased heart rate). Every effort should be made to restore sinus rhythm. If the need is urgent, digoxin, verapamil, or a β blocker are used to slow the ventricular response while prompt cardioversion is arranged. If cardioversion is not considered urgent, the patient should be anticoagulated and treated with digoxin or β blockers, together with quinidine, procainamide, or disopyramide. If sinus rhythm is not restored, cardioversion is then required. If patients cannot be maintained in sinus rhythm, amiodarone should be considered because it may be efficacious in relatively low doses.

Surgery in hypertrophic cardiomyopathy consists of excision of a portion of the basal septum (ventriculomyomectomy). The objective is to enlarge the outflow tract, abolish the gradient, and reduce if not eliminate mitral regurgitation by reducing the Venturi effect on the mitral leaflets. Although a success rate in excess of 90 per cent has been reported in symptomatic patients with resting gradients, ventriculomyomectomy is recommended only for patients with resting gradients in whom medical therapy has failed. In patients with resting gradients and either recurrent or chronic atrial fibrillation, surgery should be considered when sinus rhythm cannot be maintained. The efficacy of successful ventriculomyomectomy in reducing the risk of sudden death remains open to question.

Susceptibility to infective endocarditis is confined to patients with resting left ventricular outflow obstruction because of the coexisting mitral regurgitation and anterior mitral leaflet/septal contact. Prophylaxis is recommended only in this subgroup.

PROGNOSIS. Except for the infant with clinically overt hypertrophic cardiomyopathy in the first year of life, the natural history is usually characterized by slow progression. The most ominous threat is sudden death, which often occurs during exercise in younger patients who were previously clinically well. Sudden death accounts for an appreciable proportion of the annual mortality, which is about 4 per cent. The advent of atrial fibrillation can rapidly and significantly accelerate clinical deterioration, and the risk of systemic embolization is relatively high. A small proportion of patients develop progressive left ventricular dilatation and failure late in the natural course of their disease or many years after ventriculomyomectomy (see Fig. 50–6B). The dilated left ventricle is extensively replaced with fibrous tissue.

Maron BJ, Nichols PF, Pickle LW, et al.: Patterns of inheritance in hypertrophic cardiomyopathy: Assessment by M-mode and two-dimensional echocardiography. Am J Cardiol 53:1087, 1984. *This important paper focuses on the mode of inheritance of hypertrophic cardiomyopathy in 367 relatives from 70 families.*
Perloff JK: Pathogenesis of hypertrophic cardiomyopathy. *In* Goodwin JF (ed.): Heart Muscle Disease. Lancaster, England, MTP Press Ltd., 1985, pp 7–22.

Pathogenesis is dealt with in light of anatomic, physiologic, and clinical features of hypertrophic cardiomyopathy. The catecholamine hypothesis is elaborated.
Rosing DR, Idanpaan-Heikkila U, Maron BJ, et al.: Use of calcium channel blocking drugs in hypertrophic cardiomyopathy. Am J Cardiol 55:185B, 1985. *An important long-term drug study dealing with 227 patients treated with verapamil. A policy regarding drug administration is recommended, and the beneficial and adverse effects are reviewed.*
Sasson Z, Rakowski H, Wigle ED: Hypertrophic cardiomyopathy. *In* Perloff JK (ed.): The Cardiomyopathies. Philadelphia, W. B. Saunders Company, 1988. *A comprehensive critical review of all of the major aspects of hypertrophic cardiomyopathy.*
Takenaka K, Dabestani A, Gardin JM, et al.: Left ventricular filling in hypertrophic cardiomyopathy: A pulsed Doppler echocardiography study. J Am Coll Cardiol 7:1263, 1986. *Left ventricular diastolic filling characteristics were studied by pulsed Doppler echocardiography in patients with and without systolic anterior motion of the mitral leaflets.*

THE RESTRICTIVE CARDIOMYOPATHIES

DEFINITION. The restrictive cardiomyopathies, the least common of the three major categories of cardiomyopathic disorders (see Table 50–1), are characterized by a *primary* abnormality of *diastolic* function (impaired filling) with normal or nearly normal systolic function (contraction). The term "restrictive cardiomyopathy" is not appropriately applied when the primary derangement is one of systolic function that precedes and is variably associated with diastolic impairment (late-stage dilated cardiomyopathy, for example) or when impaired diastolic function is secondary to cardiac hypertrophy. The restrictive cardiomyopathies show little or no increase in end-diastolic or end-systolic dimension of either the right or left ventricle—hence the designation "nondilated, nonhypertrophic cardiomyopathy."

Ventricular filling is not a passive event in which inflow merely distends a compliant recipient chamber, but instead is a complex, active, energy-dependent process. The abnormality of diastolic filling in the restrictive cardiomyopathies results in a higher filling pressure for a given increment in volume. Ventricular filling is completed in early diastole with little or no filling in late diastole, functionally analogous to constrictive pericarditis. The differential diagnosis can be difficult, but information from echocardiography, computed tomography, and magnetic resonance imaging generally permits restrictive cardiomyopathy to be distinguished from constrictive pericarditis.

Impaired diastolic function in the restrictive cardiomyopathies can be idiopathic, i.e., in the absence of morphologically detectable myocardial or endomyocardial disease, or can occur because of interstitial deposition of abnormal substances (infiltrative), because of intracellular accumulation of abnormal substances (storage diseases), or because of endomyocardial diseases (Table 50–4).

Noninfiltrative Restrictive Cardiomyopathies

IDIOPATHIC RESTRICTIVE CARDIOMYOPATHY. This term applies to the clinical and hemodynamic findings of restric-

TABLE 50–4. CLASSIFICATION OF THE RESTRICTIVE CARDIOMYOPATHIES

Myocardial
A. Noninfiltrative
   Idiopathic
   Scleroderma
B. Infiltrative
   Amyloid
   Sarcoid
   Gaucher's disease
   Hurler's disease
C. Storage diseases
   Hemochromatosis
   Fabry's disease
   Glycogen storage diseases

Endomyocardial
   Endomyocardial fibrosis
   Hypereosinophilic syndrome
   Carcinoid
   Metastatic malignancies
   Radiation
   Anthracycline toxicity

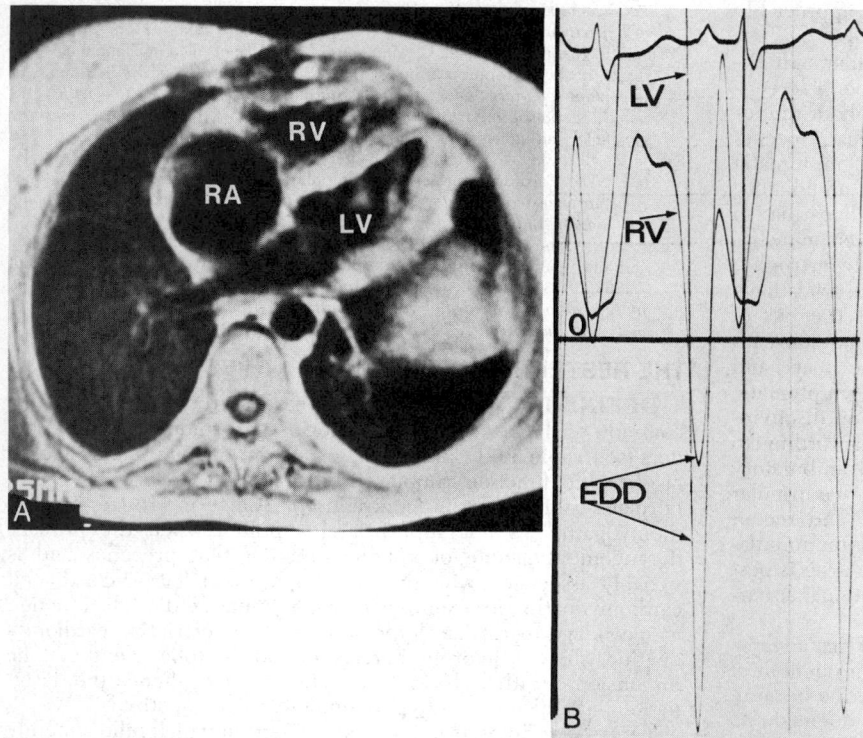

FIGURE 50–8. *A*, Magnetic resonance image in a patient with idiopathic restrictive cardiomyopathy. The right ventricle (RV) and left ventricle (LV) are normal in size, and the septum, pericardium, and ventricular free walls are of normal thicknesses. The right atrium (RA) is enlarged. The left atrium is not well shown in this view, but was also enlarged. *B*, The right ventricular (RV) and left ventricular (LV) pressure pulses show marked early diastolic dips (EDD), but the diastolic configurations differ.

tive heart disease in the absence of discernible morphologic cause. Ventricular cavity sizes and ventricular septal and free wall thicknesses are normal or nearly so. Microscopic examination including histochemical stains may show nothing more than mild interstitial fibrosis. Idiopathic restrictive cardiomyopathy is sometimes familial and is believed to be a biochemical abnormality of the energy-dependent rapid filling phase of ventricular relaxation. The decline in cytosolic calcium required for myocardial relaxation is probably mediated by sarcolemmal Na^+-Ca^{2+} exchange. The fault in idiopathic restrictive cardiomyopathy may reside in a failure of an appropriate decline in cytosolic calcium needed for relaxation.

Patients with idiopathic restrictive cardiomyopathy present with clinical signs and symptoms of high systemic and pulmonary venous pressures. The jugular venous pulse resembles that of constrictive pericarditis, and peripheral edema and ascites reinforce the impression. Atrial fibrillation is not uncommon. Auscultation detects a prominent third heart sound (right or left ventricular in origin), and murmurs of AV valve regurgitation are common. Chest roentgenograms show pulmonary venous congestion and pleural effusions. The cardiac silhouette reflects biatrial enlargement without ventricular dilatation.

Two-dimensional echocardiography with Doppler interrogation and color flow imaging discloses normal or nearly normal systolic ventricular function, impaired diastolic function, relatively normal ventricular cavity sizes, and marked biatrial dilatation in response to reduced ventricular distensibility and AV valve regurgitation. Magnetic resonance imaging is efficacious in confirming the absence of pericardial thickening (Fig. 50–8A). Intraventricular pressure pulses reveal an early diastolic dip followed by a diastolic plateau, but the configurations of the diastolic portions of the pressure pulses differ because the myocardial restriction is not uniform in the two ventricles (Fig. 50–8B).

The clinical course of idiopathic restrictive cardiomyopathy can be protracted even in the presence of chronic atrial fibrillation. High-degree heart block is relatively common and may require a permanent pacemaker. Digitalis glycosides are useful in controlling the ventricular response to atrial fibrillation but otherwise have little to offer because ventricular systolic function is normal or nearly so. The biochemical fault in idiopathic restrictive cardiomyopathy may lie in failure of the decline in cytosolic calcium required for ventricular relaxation, so calcium channel

antagonists theoretically may have a therapeutic role in improving diastolic relaxation, although their efficacy is unproven.

SCLERODERMA. Scleroderma heart disease is primarily the result of insidious fibrosis involving myocardial interstitium as well as pericardium and AV conduction. Echocardiographic studies occasionally disclose patterns of restrictive or dilated cardiomyopathy.

Infiltrative Restrictive Cardiomyopathies

AMYLOIDOSIS. Amyloid heart disease is the paradigm of the infiltrative restrictive cardiomyopathies. Amyloid causes tissue injury chiefly because interstitial deposits replace normal contractile elements of the myocardium. When amyloid fibrils consist mainly of light chains, deposition tends to involve the heart, tongue, gastrointestinal tract, nerves, and skin. When the fibrils are chiefly protein, amyloid tends to involve the liver, kidney, and spleen. The differences between these two varieties of amyloid are, however, less than categoric.

Histologically, cardiac amyloidosis is characterized by interstitial deposition in all four cardiac chambers and also in cardiac valves (especially the AV valves) in the walls of intramural coronary arteries and arterioles, in the pericardium, and in the impulse and conduction system. Deposition of amyloid in myocardial interstitium impairs diastolic ventricular function, leaving systolic function normal or nearly so, at least initially. As amyloid insidiously and progressively replaces contractile elements, systolic function suffers but may remain well preserved despite advanced amyloid infiltration.

The clinical manifestations of cardiac amyloidosis reflect the anatomic and physiologic derangements described above. Biventricular circulatory congestion is the most common feature, but right-sided congestion often dominates the clinical picture, with peripheral edema and ascites outweighing orthopnea and nocturnal dyspnea. Angina pectoris occurs in approximately one third of patients and is believed to be caused by amyloid involvement of the coronary arteries. Impairment of sinus node function and of AV conduction occurs in about 35 per cent of cases. Atrial fibrillation is a less frequent occurrence. Upwards of one third of patients experience orthostatic hypotension, lightheadedness, or frank syncope (amyloid autonomic neuropathy). Sudden death is comparatively common.

On physical examination, the arterial pulse is normal or small.

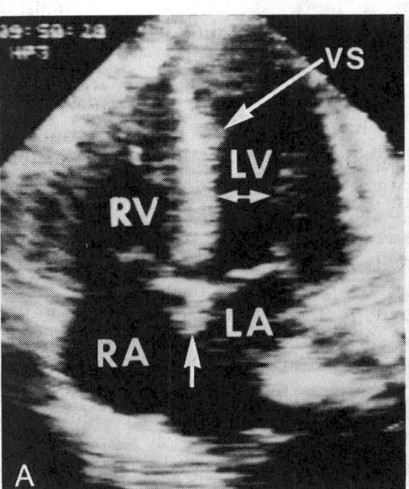
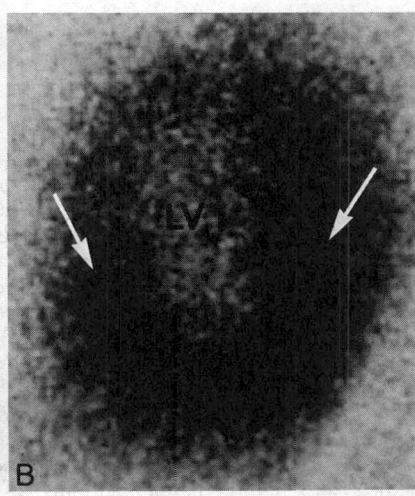

FIGURE 50–9. *A*, Two-dimensional echocardiogram in a patient with amyloid heart disease (restrictive cardiomyopathy). There is thickening of the ventricular septum (VS) and of the walls of both ventricles. The left ventricular (LV) cavity is small. There is echo dropout in the atrial septum, the inferior portion of which (*vertical arrow*) is thickened. RV = Right ventricle; RA, LA = right and left atria. *B*, Technetium-99m pyrophosphate scan (left anterior oblique view) from a patient with amyloid heart disease. The isotope accumulated in the thick ventricular septum and left ventricular free wall (*arrows*). The left ventricular (LV) cavity is small.

The jugular venous pulse is often visible even when the patient sits bolt upright, with wave forms that resemble those of constrictive pericarditis. Auscultation detects a soft first heart sound (PR interval prolongation), no murmur or soft systolic murmurs of AV valve regurgitation, and third heart sounds but not fourth heart sounds. Peripheral edema, hepatomegaly, and ascites are common, even in the absence of pulmonary rales and orthopnea.

The electrocardiogram shows left or right atrial P-wave abnormalities and varying degrees of AV block. QRS voltage is characteristically low. Poor R-wave progression or QS deformities in right precordial leads are believed to reflect myocardial replacement with amyloid.

Echocardiography has been a major step forward in the clinical diagnosis of cardiac amyloidosis. Two-dimensional imaging discloses a symmetric increase in thickness of the ventricular septum and left ventricular free wall, with an increase in right ventricular wall thickness, but normal to small ventricular cavity sizes (Fig. 50–9A). Two-dimensional imaging also serves to identify thickening of the interatrial septum (Fig. 50–9A), and of the AV valves. Real-time imaging often discloses a distinctive "granular/sparkling" appearance of the thickened ventricular myocardium. Rarely, the ventricular septum is thicker than the posterior wall, prompting a mistaken diagnosis of asymmetric hypertrophy. Pulsed Doppler diastolic filling patterns reflect the presence and degree of amyloid infiltration of the myocardium. Early, intermediate, and advanced stages have been identified. Advanced cardiac amyloidosis is characterized on pulsed Doppler inflow interrogation by a typical "restrictive pattern" (increased early diastolic ventricular inflow velocities with shortened deceleration times, decreased "a" velocities, and normal isovolumic relaxation time). Color flow imaging frequently reveals mitral and tricuspid regurgitation, much less commonly aortic and pulmonic regurgitation, all usually mild. Technetium-99m pyrophosphate cardiac scans are useful diagnostic adjuncts in the diagnosis of advanced cardiac amyloidosis (Fig. 50–9B). The mechanism of intense uptake of the tracer is unclear, but accumulation is biventricular and relates to the thickness of ventricular myocardium. Based upon the above clinical and diagnostic assessments, the diagnosis of cardiac amyloidosis can generally be made without recourse to histochemical tissue confirmation from endomyocardial biopsy.

The prognosis and clinical course of cardiac amyloidosis depend upon where in the spectrum of cardiac involvement a given patient lies. Progressive congestive heart failure and atrial fibrillation are generally reserved for patients with marked ventricular wall thicknesses, granular/sparkling tissue texture, decreased systolic function, and atrial enlargement. Amyloid involvement of major epicardial coronary arteries can cause ischemia and infarction.

Treatment of cardiac amyloidosis is supportive, usually ineffective, and occasionally inadvertently harmful. Progression cannot currently be arrested, and regression is unknown. Overzealous use of diuretics may reduce ventricular filling pressures and relieve symptoms of circulatory congestion, but at the expense of an undesirable fall in cardiac output. Digitalis glycosides are potentially proarrhythmic and have adverse effects on already depressed sinus node and AV node function. Should cardioversion be attempted for atrial fibrillation, the abnormal sinus node may fail as an effective pacemaker. An artificial ventricular pacemaker is required for high-degree heart block, but the thresholds may be abnormally high because of amyloid deposits at the site of electrode implantation. Treatment of angina pectoris with nitroglycerin may provoke hypotension owing to decreased ventricular filling and may reinforce the tendency to orthostatic hypotension.

SARCOIDOSIS. Myocardial involvement at necropsy has been identified in up to 25 per cent of patients with generalized sarcoidosis. However, only about 5 per cent of patients with proven sarcoidosis have clinically overt involvement of the heart. Physiologic derangements initially reflect interstitial infiltration that causes impaired diastolic function with normal or nearly normal systolic function. Subsequent injury to contractile elements with fibrous replacement results in impaired systolic function.

The sites most frequently involved in myocardial sarcoidosis are the left ventricular free wall, the basal aspect of the ventricular septum, the right ventricular free wall, and the walls of the atria. The basic lesion is a noncaseating granuloma, which may be accompanied by lymphocytic infiltration and patchy fibrosis. The peculiar affinity for involvement of the cephalad portion of the ventricular septum may result in complete heart block. Accordingly, cardiac sarcoidosis may dramatically announce itself as a Stokes-Adams episode or sudden death. Relevant to this discussion is the restrictive phase of sarcoid cardiomyopathy, although pulmonary hypertension, high-degree heart block, and papillary muscle dysfunction are important clinical associations.

Echocardiography and imaging with technetium-99m pyrophosphate, gallium, and thallium-201 may be useful in detecting myocardial sarcoid. Endomyocardial biopsy is seldom efficacious because the biotome is not likely to sample one of the common sites of cardiac sarcoidosis.

Prognosis is determined not only by the restrictive cardiomyopathy but also by the risks of high-degree heart block, ventricular arrhythmias, and pulmonary hypertension. Steroid treatment has been advocated for biopsy-proven myocardial sarcoidosis. Sarcoid granulomas in the heart are supposedly more responsive to steroids than granulomas in other organs. Myocardial granulomas may be replaced by connective tissue with aneurysmal thinning of the ventricular wall.

GAUCHER'S DISEASE. This is an inherited disorder of glucocerebroside metabolism. The cerebroside accumulates in the reticuloendothelial system as well as in brain and myocardium. Infiltration of the myocardium by Gaucher cells can cause decreased ventricular compliance.

HURLER'S DISEASE. This autosomal recessive disorder is the prototype of the mucopolysaccharidoses. Hurler cells laden with mucopolysaccharide moieties infiltrate the myocardial interstitium and are accompanied by increased interstitial fibrous tissue. The result is reduced diastolic distensibility (restriction). Although as many as one third of deaths in the Hurler syndrome result from congestive heart failure, it is difficult clinically to isolate myocardial involvement per se from the hemodynamic effects of infiltration of mitral and aortic valves, the ischemic effects of infiltration of coronary arteries, and the coexisting effect of systemic hypertension.

Storage Diseases

HEMOCHROMATOSIS. Primary hemochromatosis is a recessive inborn error of metabolism characterized by multiple organ parenchymal intracellular deposition (storage) of iron. Deposition of iron in reticuloendothelial cells is relatively innocuous, but parenchymal cell deposits are potentially harmful. The initial myocardial iron deposits are in the subepicardium, subendocardium, and papillary muscles, with subsequent deposition in the ventricular free walls and septum. Myocardial cell disruption is followed by fibrous replacement. The AV conduction system may be involved, but the sinus node is usually spared. Approximately one third of untreated patients with histologically proven primary hemochromatosis die of congestive heart failure. A phase of restrictive cardiomyopathy has been confirmed. Patients with clinical and hemodynamic evidence of cardiac restriction may also have decreased systolic function with normal left ventricular cavity size. Dilated heart failure is the most common ultimate sequela.

Progressive diastolic dysfunction with rising ventricular filling pressures is symptomatically expressed as effort dyspnea, but right-sided failure may dominate the clinical picture. When systolic dysfunction supervenes, the physical signs resemble those of dilated cardiomyopathy. In either case, hepatic enlargement may be due to the hemochromatosis per se rather than to passive congestion.

Symptomatic cardiac hemochromatosis is usually associated with electrocardiographic abnormalities, chiefly ST-T changes or supraventricular arrhythmias. Despite histologic involvement of ventricular muscle and atrioventricular conduction system, ventricular arrhythmias and conduction disturbances are uncommon.

Because cardiac hemochromatosis is the most common cause of death in these patients, and because phlebotomy is an effective therapy if begun early enough, accurate diagnosis is of considerable practical importance. A significant minority of patients die within a short time after the diagnosis is made. The echocardiogram initially shows a nondilated, concentrically thick left ventricle with evidence of diastolic dysfunction but normal or nearly normal ejection fraction. Suspected cardiac involvement has been confirmed by endomyocardial biopsy, although myocardial iron can be focal and variable in location. Multiple biopsy sites are necessary to minimize the chance of sampling error.

Heart failure may respond to iron depletion therapy if initiated when cardiac muscle cells are viable and before there is significant myocardial fibrosis. The corollary to this observation is that prevention of myocardial fibrosis can be achieved when early recognition of myocardial infiltration with iron is effectively treated by phlebotomy.

FABRY'S DISEASE. This is an X-linked recessive disorder of glycosphingolipid metabolism due to a specific enzyme deficiency. The result is intracellular glycolipid accumulation in vascular endothelial lysozymes as well as in heart muscle and valves (particularly mitral), skin, cornea, kidneys, gastrointestinal tract, and central nervous system. The disease is fully expressed in the male and incompletely expressed in the female (X-linked). Males usually die by the fourth or fifth decade from cardiac failure, renal failure, hypertension, or cerebrovascular disease.

Accumulation (storage) of glycolipid in cardiac muscle can result in an increase in mass and myocardial restriction. Echocardiography in the typical male with Fabry's disease reveals increased septal and free wall thicknesses (presumably a consequence of glycolipid storage) with normal left ventricular internal dimensions. Lysosomal accumulation of glycolipids in mitral leaflets does not correlate with clinical severity of disease, but left ventricular mass does.

GLYCOGEN STORAGE DISEASES. These disorders result from a deficiency of one or more of the enzymes involved in the biosynthesis and degradation of glycogen. Most cases of glycogen storage disease causing restrictive cardiomyopathy belong to type II, that is, Pompe's disease. The glycogen that is stored in cardiac muscle cells, skeletal muscle cells, and liver is biochemically normal but present in excessive amounts.

Pompe's disease is always fatal, usually within the first 2 to 3 years of life. The combination of marked cardiomegaly (increased free wall and septal thicknesses) with skeletal muscle weakness (flaccidity) in infants who appear normal at birth is diagnostically distinctive. The characteristic echocardiographic findings in Pompe's disease are dramatic thickening of ventricular septum and of right and left ventricular free walls with reduced cavity sizes. The electrocardiogram is distinctive, exhibiting a remarkable increase in QRS amplitude with a short PR interval.

Restrictive Cardiomyopathies Due to Endomyocardial Disease

ENDOMYOCARDIAL FIBROSIS. This is a common form of cardiomyopathy in tropical and subtropical Africa, is encountered less often in South America and Asia, and more recently has been reported in Western Europe and the United States in patients who have never been in the tropics. Endomyocardial fibrosis accounts for 15 to 25 per cent of deaths due to heart disease in equatorial Africa. The disease involves both the right and left ventricles in about 50 per cent of cases but is isolated to the left ventricle in approximately 40 per cent and to the right ventricle in 10 per cent. Dense endomyocardial thickening of the inflow tracts of the ventricles includes the AV valves, so that mitral and tricuspid regurgitation are important features. The ventricular outflow tracts are not involved. Functional derangements consist of impaired diastolic filling and AV valve regurgitation with relatively well-preserved systolic function. In the presence of intractable biventricular failure and AV valve regurgitation, surgical resection of the fibrous endocardium with valve replacement has been advocated as a therapeutic option.

HYPEREOSINOPHILIC SYNDROME. This syndrome is defined as (1) persistent eosinophilia of 1500 per cubic millimeter for at least 6 months, or death before 6 months; (2) lack of evidence of recognized causes of eosinophilia despite careful evaluation; and (3) signs and symptoms of organ system involvement, especially the heart and nervous system. The capability of the eosinophil and its contents to cause tissue damage (the "Gordon phenomenon") has been known for over 50 years and is held responsible for initial damage to the endocardium. Platelet thrombi form over the denuded endocardium with a morphologic evolution that ultimately results in pathologic findings indistinguishable from those described above in endomyocardial fibrosis. It has been argued persuasively that idiopathic hypereosinophilic syndrome and endomyocardial fibrosis are the same disease at different stages of development. Conversely, it has been proposed that geochemical factors (thorium excess together with magnesium deficiency) might cause tropical endomyocardial fibrosis.

Endomyocardial biopsies lend support to the hypothesis that endocardial endothelial cells and the microvasculature are the primary targets, whereas thrombosis is secondary. In any event, endocardial fibrosis and restrictive cardiomyopathy ensue. Because of the endocardial thrombi, peripheral emboli are common. Involvement of the posterior mitral leaflet and the septal and posterior tricuspid leaflets result in mitral and tricuspid regurgitation, as in endomyocardial fibrosis described above.

Echocardiography is useful in the noninvasive diagnosis. The combination of small ventricles and large atria is typical although not diagnostic, but together with apical obliteration, the diagnosis is reasonably secure.

Treatment is limited. The surgical option is as mentioned earlier for endomyocardial fibrosis.

CARCINOID ENDOCARDIAL DISEASE. The carcinoid syndrome results in cardiac involvement as a late complication in 50 per cent of cases. Endocardial abnormalities may cause a restrictive cardiomyopathy, although the principal overt cardiac manifestations reflect involvement of the pulmonic and tricuspid valves with stenosis and regurgitation. In the presence of significant pulmonic or tricuspid valve disease, detection of coexisting restriction is difficult even with current techniques of pulsed Doppler inflow interrogation.

MALIGNANT ENDOMYOCARDIAL DISEASE. Cardiac metastases are present in over 60 per cent of patients with malignant melanoma, and there is a relatively high incidence of involvement of the heart in bronchogenic carcinoma, carcinoma of the breast, lymphoma, and leukemia. Restriction of ventricular filling caused by endomyocardial infiltration is rare and is more commonly due to pericardial tumor or radiation.

RADIATION HEART DISEASE. Radiation-induced endocardial and myocardial fibrosis can cause restrictive cardiomyopathy, sometimes with disproportionate involvement of the more exposed anterior right ventricle. Functional abnormalities due to interstitial fibrosis demonstrated by echocardiography and radionuclide angiography occur up to 15 years after radiation. Importantly, the pericardium is the most frequent cardiovascular site of radiation heart disease, and the differential diagnosis between radiation-restrictive cardiomyopathy and radiation injury to pericardium is difficult.

ANTHRACYCLINE CARDIOMYOPATHY. There is convincing evidence that doxorubicin and other anthracycline antitumor agents can cause dilated cardiomyopathy as well as restrictive cardiomyopathy due to endomyocardial fibrosis. Light microscopy of biopsy specimens has disclosed fibrous thickening of the endocardium. Hemodynamic studies may record a restrictive diastolic "dip-and-plateau" in the left and/or right ventricle. The risk of myocardial injury is dose-related, although cardiotoxicity sometimes occurs at lower doses in individuals with prior mediastinal (and cardiac) radiation.

Child JS, Perloff JK: *In* Perloff JK (ed.): The Cardiomyopathies. Philadelphia, W. B. Saunders Co., 1988. *A comprehensive review of the various types of myocardial and endomyocardial restrictive cardiomyopathies.*

Cueto-Garcia L, Tajik AJ, Kyle RA, et al.: Serial echocardiographic observations in patients with primary systemic amyloidosis; Smith TJ, Kyle RA, Lie JT: Clinical significance of histopathologic patterns of cardiac amyloidosis. Mayo Clin Proc 59:547, 589, 1984. *Two comprehensive articles that deal with the pathology and serial echocardiographic diagnoses of cardiac amyloidosis.*

Dabestani A, Child JS, Henze E, et al.: Primary hemochromatosis: Anatomic and physiologic studies characteristic of the cardiac ventricles and their responses to phlebotomy. Am J Cardiol 54:153, 1984. *Clinically occult cardiac involvement was identified by echocardiography and equilibrium blood pool imaging. Therapeutic phlebotomy ameliorated or reversed the deleterious effects of cardiac iron deposition if initiated prior to irreversible connective tissue replacement.*

Fauci AS, Harley JB, Roberts WC, et al.: The hypereosinophilic syndrome. Ann Intern Med 97:78, 1982. *This comprehensive National Institutes of Health conference deals with clinical, pathophysiologic, and therapeutic considerations in the hypereosinophilic syndrome and with the relationship of the disorder to endomyocardial fibrosis.*

Siegel RJ, Shah PK, Fishbein MC: Idiopathic restrictive cardiomyopathy. Circulation 70:165, 1984. *This form of cardiomyopathy is characterized chiefly by elevated left and right ventricular filling pressures, normal global ventricular systolic function, and normal or nearly normal ventricular septal and wall thicknesses and internal dimensions in the absence of specific infiltrative disorders or of diseases of pericardium or coronary arteries.*

Stewart JR, Fajardo LF: Radiation-induced heart disease: An update. Prog Cardiovasc Dis 27:173, 1984. *An informative review of the pathology, physiology, pathogenesis, diagnosis, treatment, and prevention of radiation-induced heart disease.*

51 Diseases of the Pericardium

Ralph Shabetai

Diseases of the pericardium typically present in one or more of three clinical forms: acute pericarditis, pericardial effusion, and pericardial constriction. Pericardial involvement may progress from inflammation to effusion and then constriction, or it may present as effusion or constriction without clinical evidence of preceding inflammation.

ETIOLOGY

The pericardium may be involved in a large number and variety of diseases. The most important are listed in Table 51–1. Pericardial disease may be asymptomatic but may also cause dramatic symptoms and signs.

The clinical syndromes of pericardial disease are listed in Table 51–2.

INFECTIONS WITH LIVING AGENTS. *Virus Infection.* Many viruses may cause pericarditis; the common offenders are listed in Table 51–1. The number of cases of idiopathic pericarditis that are caused by preceding viral infection is unknown.

TABLE 51–1. MAJOR CAUSES OF PERICARDIAL DISEASE

1. Inflammation	
Virus	
Coxsackie (usually B)	(E)
Echo	(E)
Other	
Bacterial	
Pneumococcus	(E)
Staphylococcus	(E,C)
Meningococcus	(E,C)
Mycobacterium tuberculosis	(E,C)
Haemophilus influenzae	(C)
Other	
Fungus	
Histoplasma capsulatum	(E,C)
Other	
Other living organisms	
Parasites	(E)
Protozoa	(E)
Nonliving agents	
Trauma	(E,C)
Radiation	(E,C)
Chemical	
Chemotherapeutic agents	
2. Idiopathic	
(Many may be viral, but unproven)	(E,C)
3. Neoplastic	
Secondary to carcinoma of	
Lung	(E,C)
Breast	(E,C)
Other	
Lymphoma	(E)
Primary	
Mesothelioma	(E)
Other	
4. Metabolic	
Chronic renal disease	
Associated with dialysis	(E)
End-stage uremia	(E)
Myxedema	(E)
Chylopericardium	(E)
Hypoalbuminemia	(E)
5. Myocardial injury	
Myocardial infarction	
Acute	
Dressler's syndrome	(E)
Congestive heart failure	(E)
6. Trauma	(E,C)
Postpericardiotomy syndrome	(E)
Postoperative	(C)
7. Connective tissue disorders and hypersensitivity	
Acute rheumatic fever	
Rheumatoid arthritis	(C)
Systemic sclerosis	
Lupus erythematosus	
Drugs	
Procainamide	
Others	
8. Congenital	
Absence of left pericardium	
Partial	
Complete	
Cyst	
Other	

(E) = effusion common; (C) = constrictive pericarditis common.

Bacterial Infection. Bacterial pericarditis is still important, although the spectrum has altered. Pneumococcal pericarditis, once a frequent complication of pneumonia, is now rare, whereas infection by staphylococci, fungi, and exotic organisms is more common, especially in persons at either extreme of age and in the immunologically compromised host. Meningococcal pericarditis may be a manifestation of either direct infection or hypersensitivity.

TABLE 51-2. CLINICAL SYNDROMES OF PERICARDIAL DISEASE

Dry, fibrinous pericarditis
  Usually acute (R)
Lax pericardial effusion
  Chronic effusive
Cardiac tamponade (R)
Constrictive pericarditis
  Subacute
  Chronic
Effusive-constrictive pericarditis

(R) = Relapse or recurrence common.

Tuberculosis. Tuberculous pericarditis is less common now that tuberculosis is better controlled and treated. Pulmonary tuberculosis may be present, but often pericardial effusion is an isolated manifestation. *Mycobacterium tuberculosis* can be recovered from only one third of effusions. Even pericardial biopsy findings are not uniformly positive. Commonly, the diagnosis is presumptive and based on circumstantial evidence, such as a positive skin test result or a history of recent contact.

Haemophilus influenzae infection is an important cause of constrictive pericarditis in children.

Fungal Infection. In an otherwise normal population fungal pericarditis is uncommon, but infection with *Histoplasma capsulatum* should be considered in patients who reside in the Ohio Valley. Similarly, coccidioidomycosis should be considered in patients who have been in the San Joaquin Valley of California.

PERICARDIAL INFLAMMATION CAUSED BY NONLIVING AGENTS. *Trauma.* Blunt and sharp trauma is an important cause of pericarditis and may lead to pericardial effusion with or without tamponade and ultimately to constrictive pericarditis. Common examples of acute trauma include gunshot and knife wounds. Impact against a steering wheel, explosions, and crushing are the major causes of blunt injuries.

Radiation. The pericardium may be exposed to considerable injury when radiotherapy is employed to treat neoplasia, for example, Hodgkin's disease and lung or breast neoplasms. The latent period between radiation and clinical pericardial disease may extend for many years.

PERICARDIAL DISEASE IN METABOLIC DISORDERS. *Renal Disease.* Pericardial disease continues to be one of the more frequent major complications of chronic dialysis and may cause cardiac tamponade. Fortunately, constrictive pericarditis is rare. The etiology is not understood: It may be a manifestation of end-stage renal disease, but the process of dialysis itself may be responsible in whole or in part.

Myxedema. Pericardial effusion may occur and accounts in part for apparent cardiomegaly on chest radiograph; it may also contribute to the low voltage and T-wave inversion that, in addition to sinus bradycardia, characterize the electrocardiogram. Pericardial effusion may contain cholesterol crystals.

CHYLOPERICARDIUM. Chylopericardium, a pericardial collection of fluid bearing a large quantity of chyle, may be idiopathic but often follows surgical or other trauma of the thoracic duct.

MYOCARDIAL INFARCTION. Acute dry, fibrinous pericarditis can be detected in about one third of patients with acute myocardial infarction. Autopsy evidence is more common. Acute pericarditis early in the course is often a contiguous inflammation over the infarction but may also represent reaction to myocardial injury. Rupture of an infarction, aneurysm, or pseudoaneurysm creates greater or lesser degrees of hemopericardium, the former usually ending fatally.

In some patients, pericarditis (often accompanied by effusion) occurs in the weeks or months following acute myocardial infarction. This syndrome (Dressler's) is thought to be a delayed autoimmune reaction and is often recurrent.

CONNECTIVE TISSUE DISORDERS. Pericardial reaction may occur in virtually all of these disorders. Acute pericarditis is a constituent of rheumatic pancarditis but does not progress to constriction. On the other hand, subacute constrictive pericarditis can occur in rheumatoid arthritis. Pericarditis is an important

manifestation of lupus erythematosus, both spontaneous and induced by drugs such as procainamide, and can cause tamponade.

HEART FAILURE. In patients with fluid retention, small pericardial effusion may be seen by echocardiography.

CONGENITAL LESIONS AND CYSTS. Partial absence of the pericardium produces a striking abnormality on the chest radiograph. Pericardial cysts are more frequent. They are filled with clear fluid and most often occupy the right cardiophrenic angle, although they may occupy atypical locations. They are benign and usually produce no symptoms.

ACUTE (FIBRINOUS) VIRAL OR IDIOPATHIC PERICARDITIS

SYMPTOMS. Findings are often preceded by generalized malaise and fever. The chief symptom is chest pain, which may be either sharp or crushing. Frequently, the pain is precordial but may shift to the left side, simulating pleurisy. Characteristically, the pain is relieved by sitting up and exacerbated by deep inspiration. Thus, pericardial pain has features that may suggest either myocardial ischemia or pleural inflammation. Referral of pain to the right trapezius ridge is a specific but uncommon sign of its pericardial origin.

CLINICAL FINDINGS. *Pericardial Friction Rub: The Pathognomonic Sign of Pericardial Inflammation.* Classically, the rub has components accompanying atrial systole, ventricular systole, and ventricular diastole (see LMSB line, Fig. 51–1). Commonly, the rub is biphasic and must be distinguished from to-and-fro murmurs. When it is monophasic, it must be differentiated from systolic murmurs. It is typically superficial and scratchy, and although it may be widely distributed over the precordium, it is usually most apparent at the left sternal edge. Appreciation is enhanced by firm pressure with the diaphragm of the stethoscope. Changes in posture and the respiratory cycle may alter the intensity. Pericardial friction rubs are often transient and should be sought frequently when pericarditis is suspected. They must be distinguished not only from cardiac murmurs but also from mediastinal crunch due to air in the mediastinum, crepitations from surgical emphysema, and artifacts produced by movement of the skin against the stethoscope.

LABORATORY FINDINGS. *Electrocardiogram.* The typical findings of pericarditis are shown in Figure 51–2. ST-segment elevation, although common, is not invariably present, depression of the ST segment being usual in leads aV_R and V_1. Depression of the PR segment, although highly specific, is less common than ST-segment elevation.

On a single tracing and without clinical information, ST-segment elevation cannot always be distinguished from the early repolarization normal variant or from the early stage of acute myocardial infarction. In the latter, evolution of the pattern in serial tracings is helpful. In acute pericarditis, the ST segment returns to baseline without inversion of the T wave (which may occur later if pericarditis becomes chronic), whereas in acute myocardial infarction, T-wave inversion typically occurs before the ST segment becomes isoelectric.

Other Laboratory Findings. The erythrocyte sedimentation rate is elevated and there is variable leukocytosis. Viral titers may confirm the origin of the illness but are seldom performed in clinical practice. Gallium radioisotope scanning may display the epicardium, but this expensive test is required only in exceptional cases. Plasma levels of cardiac enzymes may be elevated, but this determination need not be made routinely.

DIAGNOSIS. The diagnosis can usually be made reliably from symptoms and signs. When any of the conditions listed in Table 51–1 is suspected, the symptoms and signs of pericarditis should be specifically sought and the diagnosis confirmed by electrocardiography. When the pain simulates that of pleurisy, pneumonia or pulmonary infarction must be considered. When it is retrosternal and crushing, myocardial infarction must be ruled out. On occasion, other major causes of chest discomfort, such as acute pulmonary embolism or dissection of the aorta, need to be considered.

CLINICAL COURSE, PROGNOSIS, AND MANAGEMENT. Commonly, this is a self-limiting disease. However, its natural history is seldom observed, as it usually responds rapidly to treatment with nonsteroidal anti-inflammatory agents such as

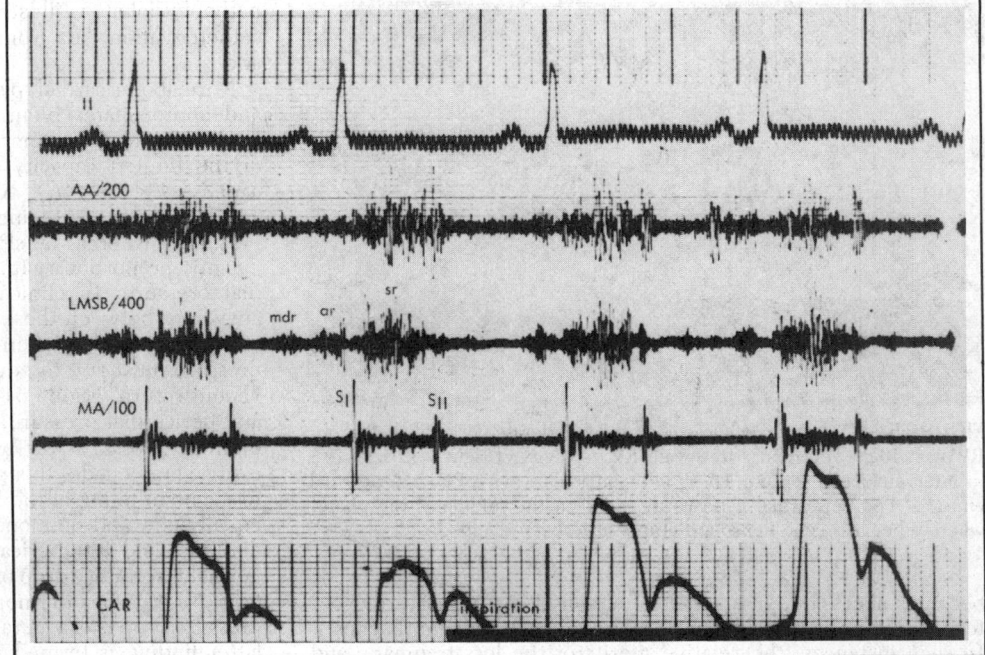

FIGURE 51–1. Phonocardiography of pericardial friction rub. AA = Aortic area; LMSB = left mid-sternal border; MA = mitral area. Note the three-component rub heard along the left mid-sternal border. Numbers refer to filter settings. (Reproduced by permission from Spodick DH: Am Heart J 81:114, 1971.)

indomethacin (25 to 50 mg three to four times a day) or ibuprofen. Even aspirin is often satisfactory. Resistant cases may require steroid treatment—for instance, prednisone, starting with 75 mg a day and rapidly tapering to the minimum dose that suppresses symptoms and signs.

Detectable pericardial effusion occurs in a small proportion of cases and may progress to cardiac tamponade. Similarly, acute pericarditis may rarely lead to chronic constrictive pericarditis.

Recurrent Pericarditis. Perhaps the most troublesome of all complications is frequent recurrence over a period of years. The patient is greatly disturbed by the frequent occurrence of disabling pain, and when steroidal agents must be used for resistant cases, their side effects may become significant.

PERICARDIAL EFFUSION

LAX PERICARDIAL EFFUSION. Pericardial effusions that do not raise intrapericardial pressure more than 3 or 4 mm Hg do not cause symptoms. The physical findings are variable and frequently do not provide valuable clinical clues. Pericardial effusion should be strongly suspected in the setting of acute pericarditis if the cardiopericardial silhouette is enlarged on the chest radiograph. A previous radiograph showing a normal-sized silhouette is particularly helpful. The diagnosis can be made with certainty by echocardiography (Fig. 51–3).

PERICARDIAL EFFUSION COMPLICATING ACUTE PERICARDITIS. When echocardiograms are performed rou-

tinely in acute pericarditis, effusion is found in a considerable proportion of cases. However, in clinical practice, echocardiography is not required if the heart size remains normal, there is no evidence of cardiac tamponade or myocarditis, and the findings subside within 48 to 72 hours after beginning treatment. Myocarditis should be suspected when depolarization changes, such as left or right bundle branch block, or conduction abnormalities develop and when a third heart sound is audible. In such cases, echocardiography is often useful in distinguishing cardiac chamber enlargement from pericardial effusion.

ETIOLOGY OF PERICARDIAL EFFUSION. The causes of pericardial effusion are indicated in Table 51–1. Pericardial effusion must always be considered in patients who have or are likely to have one of these disorders, but especially when there is or has been evidence of acute pericarditis or when there is circulatory compromise. When the patient has a possible cause of cardiac tamponade or constrictive pericarditis, pericardial disease must be ruled out before attributing circulatory abnormalities to heart disease.

PERICARDIOCENTESIS. When the venous pressure is normal, systemic arterial hypotension is absent, and the etiology of pericardial effusion has been established with reasonable certainty, pericardiocentesis is seldom needed. On the other hand, if the clinician suspects or diagnoses purulent effusion, or cardiac tamponade that is not responding satisfactorily to medical treatment, removal of pericardial fluid via a needle or open drainage

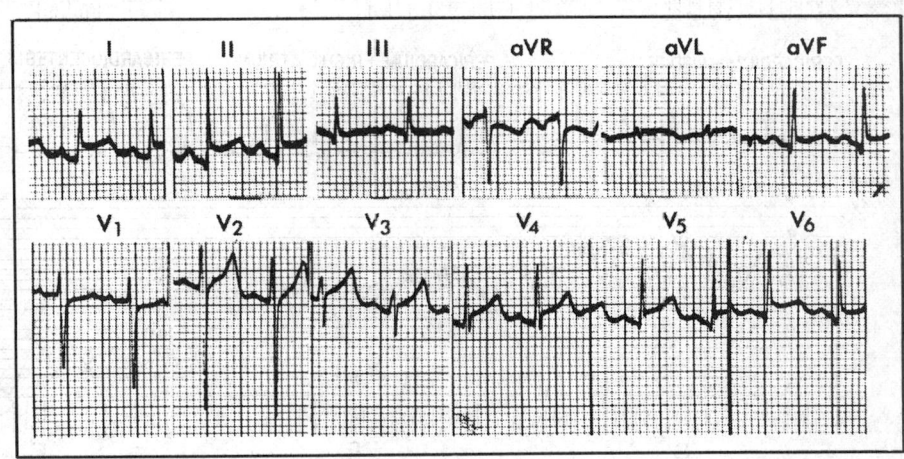

FIGURE 51–2. ECG from a case of acute pericarditis. Note the ST-segment elevation in leads I, II, aV$_F$ and V$_4$ to V$_6$ and ST segment in leads aV$_R$ and V$_1$. (From Shabetai R: The Pericardium. New York, Grune & Stratton, 1980.)

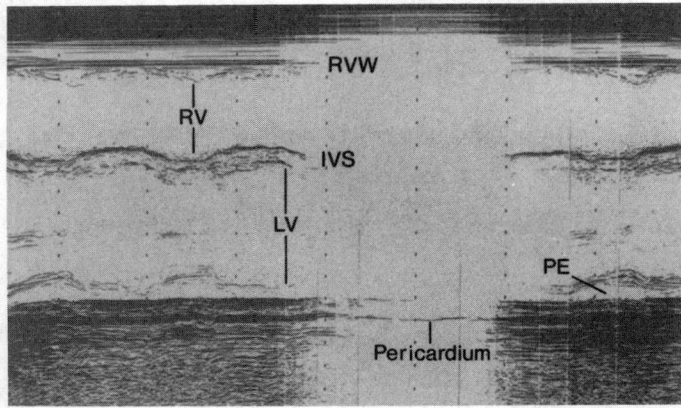

FIGURE 51–3. M-mode echocardiogram of moderate pericardial effusion. RVW = Right ventricular free wall; RV = cavity of right ventricle; IVS = interventricular septum; LV = left ventricular cavity; PE = pericardial effusion. The pericardial echo is identified in the middle of the photo, where other less echo-dense structures have been damped.

becomes necessary. In a smaller fraction of cases, pericardiocentesis is required to establish a tissue or bacteriologic diagnosis. In such instances, the relative merits of the less traumatic and less expensive pericardiocentesis, versus surgical drainage, must be weighed against local experience and preference and the relative importance of pericardial biopsy in establishing the diagnosis.

Lax pericardial effusions have minimal hemodynamic effects, but when large and chronic, as, for example, in idiopathic chronic effusive pericarditis, a number of clinicians recommend surgical drainage.

CARDIAC TAMPONADE

ETIOLOGY AND PATHOPHYSIOLOGY. Pericarditis of virtually any cause may be associated with pericardial effusion, and virtually any pericardial effusion can progress to cardiac tamponade. The important causes are indicated in Table 51–1. The pathophysiology is illustrated in Figure 51–4, taken from cardiac catheterization data from a patient with severe cardiac tamponade.

Normal pericardial pressure is subatmospheric (Fig. 51–4F) and approximates pleural pressure. When pericardial effusion rapidly accumulates, pericardial pressure rises abruptly because of the limited capacity of the parietal pericardium to stretch acutely (Fig. 51–4D). A few hundred milliliters accumulating rapidly can generate intrapericardial pressures in excess of 20 mm Hg, whereas a slowly developing effusion may assume gigantic proportions with only minimal elevation of intrapericardial pressure. In clinical practice, cases may be encountered anywhere between these two ends of the spectrum.

If effective circulation is to be maintained, systemic venous pressure must rise to equal intrapericardial pressure to maintain venous return. Figure 51–4E indicates equilibration of right atrial and pericardial pressure. Unless the pre-existing left ventricular diastolic pressure was higher than pericardial pressure during cardiac tamponade, this pressure also must rise to the same level to maintain filling of the left ventricle. Figure 51–4 A to E shows equally elevated pulmonary wedge, right atrial, right ventricular diastolic, and intrapericardial pressures. During inspiration the normal inspiratory drop of systemic venous pressure is maintained (Fig. 51–4A), but the normal systemic arterial systolic and pulse pressure drop is exaggerated during inspiration (Fig. 51–4C). The latter finding is termed pulsus paradoxus. Systemic arterial hypotension is absent (Fig. 51–4C) in mild-to-moderate cardiac tamponade. Surgical causes such as trauma or rupture of the heart or the aorta into the pericardium are usually associated with profound hypotension. In medical cases, cardiac output is often reduced to the range shown in Figure 51–4, but in surgical cases still lower cardiac outputs are often observed.

CLINICAL FINDINGS. The chief component in recognizing tamponade is thinking of it. Cardiac tamponade must be considered whenever evidence suggesting heart disease or heart failure develops in a patient who may reasonably be suspected of a disorder listed in Table 51–1. In extreme cases consciousness may be impaired, and arterial blood pressure may drop to shock

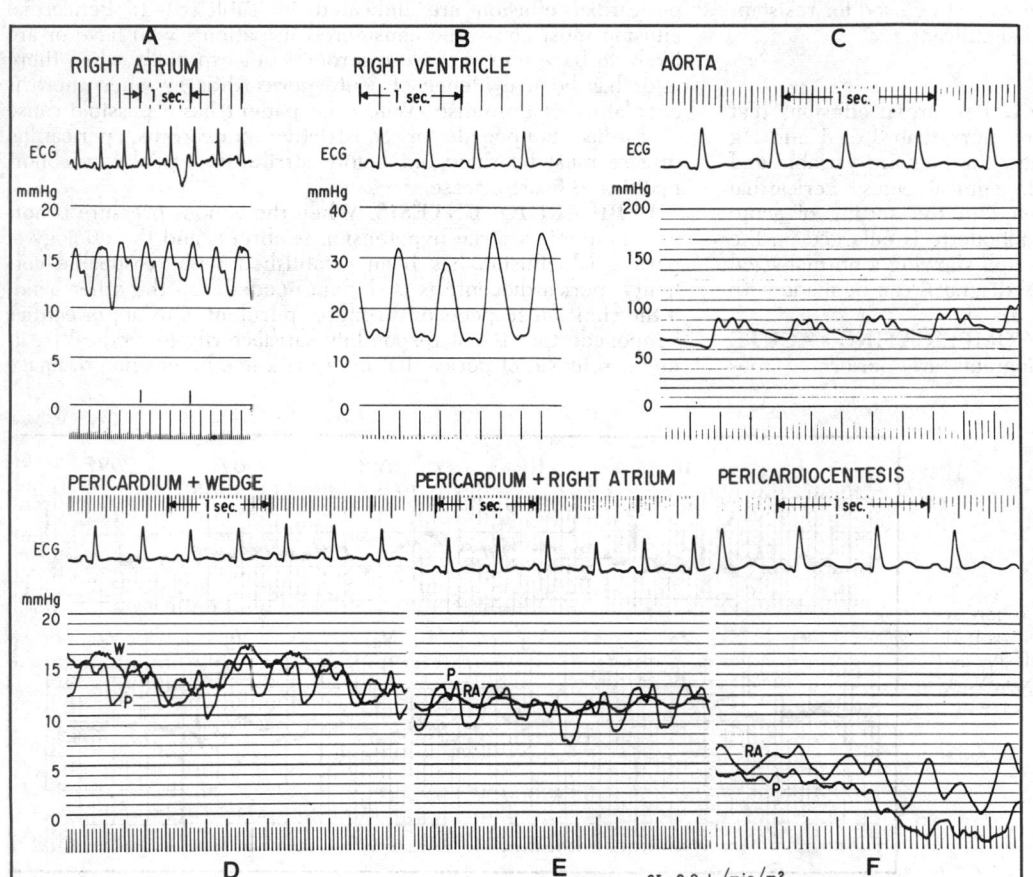

FIGURE 51–4. Hemodynamic data from a patient with cardiac tamponade. See text for discussion.

levels. Frequently there is oliguria, because cardiac tamponade, with the resulting drop in cardiac output and blood pressure, is a powerful stimulus for sodium retention by the kidney. Pericardial pain may or may not be present; often there is a sensation of fullness of the chest and sometimes frank dyspnea.

Venous Pressure. Important evidence of cardiac tamponade includes abnormal jugular venous pulses. The venous pressure is elevated, usually considerably so, unless there is concomitant acute blood loss or severe dehydration. The right atrial (and therefore the jugular) pulse is monophasic, the normal inspiratory drop is maintained, and the predominant wave is the x descent, occurring when the ventricle ejects (Fig. 51–4A). The prominent x descent is detected as a sharp inward movement of the internal jugular pulse synchronous with the carotid pulse. The y descent is reduced or abolished because of the attenuated early diastolic dip of ventricular pressure (Fig. 51–4B).

Pulsus Paradoxus. Severe pulsus paradoxus may be detectable by palpation of any arterial pulse. When extreme, the pulse disappears during inspiration; when less extreme, it diminishes but can still be palpated. In the presence of severe hypotension, pulsus paradoxus may be difficult to detect but then is usually more evident in large arteries. Pulsus paradoxus is quantified with a sphygmomanometer. As the cuff is deflated, pulsus paradoxus is estimated as the difference between pressure occurring when the first blood pressure sound can be heard only during expiration and that occurring when the sound is heard throughout the respiratory cycle. More accurate measurement requires direct monitoring of systemic arterial pressure. In clinical practice this intervention is necessary only when monitoring of arterial blood pressure is essential.

Friction Rub. In some cases of cardiac tamponade, a pericardial friction rub is present; otherwise, precordial examination tends not to be helpful.

LABORATORY FINDINGS. The echocardiogram is definitive. The chest radiograph usually shows cardiac enlargement, but in acute cases the volume of pericardial effusion may be too small to increase the cardiothoracic ratio. The electrocardiogram is often not helpful, but when pericardial effusion is large, especially in cardiac tamponade secondary to neoplasm, electrical alternans may occur. Alternation is usually confined to the QRS complex; more specific for pericardial effusion, but less common, is alternation of P, QRS, and T waves.

TREATMENT. Unless tamponade is mild or moderate and rapidly improves following medical treatment of the cause, prompt removal of pericardial fluid is mandatory. In acute cases only a small portion of the fluid need be removed, because of the steep pressure-volume curve of the pericardium. In experienced hands, pericardiocentesis has an acceptable risk. When experience is limited, tamponade is recurrent, or biopsy is needed, subxiphoid surgical drainage is preferred.

CONSTRICTIVE PERICARDITIS

DEFINITION AND ETIOLOGY. Constrictive pericarditis produces thickening, fibrosis, and often calcification of the pericardium with restriction of the diastolic filling of the ventricles. The most common causes are listed in Table 51–1. In the United States and western Europe, constrictive pericarditis most often is idiopathic, secondary to neoplasm or radiation, post-traumatic, or due to connective tissue disease. Tuberculosis and pyogenic infection are less common causes than they used to be. More subacute and fewer chronic cases are therefore seen, and heavy calcification of the pericardium is less frequent.

PATHOPHYSIOLOGY. The pathophysiology and hemodynamics are shown in Figure 51–5 from the study of a stock car driver with post-traumatic pericarditis. Panel A shows pressures recorded simultaneously from both ventricles. In early diastole there is a prominent dip of pressure, and in mid and late diastole the pressure forms a plateau. The two plateaus are elevated and equal. During early diastole, ventricular filling is faster than normal, signified by the early diastolic dip, at the end of which cardiac volume reaches the limit set by the rigid pericardium. The ventricular diastolic pressures are then elevated but do not rise through the remainder of diastole, signifying absence of further ventricular filling. Elevation of left ventricular diastolic pressure to approximately 20 mm Hg causes elevation of right ventricular systolic pressure.

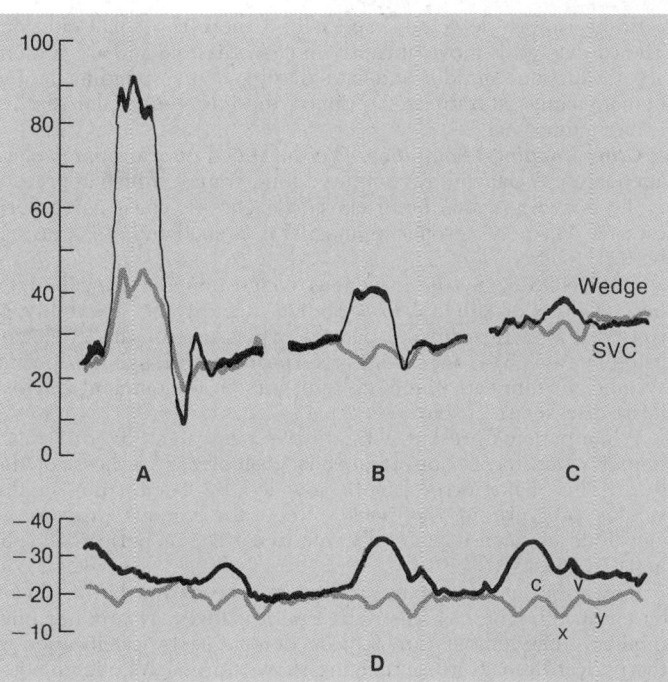

FIGURE 51–5. Hemodynamic data from a case of constrictive pericarditis. See text for details. (From Shabetai R: Profiles of constrictive pericarditis, restrictive cardiomyopathy and cardiac tamponade. *In* Grossman W [ed.]: Cardiac Catheterization and Angiography. 2nd ed. Philadelphia, Lea & Febiger, 1980.)

Panel B shows simultaneous pressure records from the right ventricle and right atrium. In contradistinction to cardiac tamponade, right atrial pressure is biphasic, showing a prominent x descent with ventricular ejection and prominent y descent coincident with the early diastolic dip of ventricular pressure. The y descent can be recognized at the bedside as a sharp inward movement of the jugular pulsation out of phase with the carotid pulse. Respiratory variation is absent. Panel C shows simultaneous pulmonary wedge and superior vena cava pressures, confirming equilibration of filling pressures on the two sides of the heart. Panel D shows pressures simultaneously recorded from the pulmonary artery and the pulmonary wedge position. In late diastole all cardiac pressures equilibrate around 20 mm Hg.

CLINICAL FINDINGS. Elevation of the filling pressure of the left side of the heart causes dyspnea and pulmonary congestion, which in severe cases is evident on the chest radiograph. Elevated filling pressure of the right side of the heart causes peripheral edema; hepatic enlargement, congestion, and dysfunction; and frequently ascites.

When ventricular filling is suddenly checked at the end of the early diastolic pressure dip, a loud third heart sound ("pericardial knock") is frequently audible. The apex beat may not be palpable, or there may be systolic retraction. Ascites is often prominent in relation to peripheral edema. The liver is usually enlarged and pulsatile. When present, palmar erythema, spider angiomas, and mild jaundice testify to severe, chronic hepatic congestion.

The abnormally small ventricular end-diastolic volume reduces stroke volume even when systolic function is well maintained, as it usually is.

LABORATORY FINDINGS. By chest radiography, the heart is normal in size to moderately enlarged. In chronic cases, particularly those associated with tuberculosis, calcification may be seen in the pericardium. The electrocardiogram usually shows T-wave inversions and frequently a wide, notched P wave due to chronic elevation of left atrial pressure. In longstanding cases, atrial fibrillation often supervenes. Liver function test results are abnormal, and hypoalbuminemia may be compounded by protein-losing enteropathy.

Echocardiography. The echocardiogram is less helpful than in pericardial effusion. Sometimes increased thickness of the pericardium can be detected, especially if there is a small effusion. The cardiac walls move abruptly in early diastole and are stationary throughout middle and late diastole, corresponding to the hemodynamic alterations. Motion of the interventricular septum is often abnormal.

Other Imaging Techniques. The thickened pericardium is more adequately visualized by computed tomography, which at present is the imaging technique of choice for chronic constrictive pericarditis. Magnetic resonance imaging is as good and, on occasion, better.

DIAGNOSIS. Systemic venous congestion not explained by heart failure or other causes should suggest the possibility of constrictive pericarditis, especially when one of the etiologies listed in Table 51–1 is present or suspected. Although nonspecific systolic murmurs are common, murmurs of predominant valvular heart disease are absent.

When patients present with massive edema and liver dysfunction, the most common erroneous diagnosis is cirrhosis of the liver. This major error can be avoided by examination of the venous pressure in the neck. When the venous pressure is elevated, anasarca is generally due to cardiac or pericardial, not hepatic, causes.

Pericardial effusion may produce a large "water-bottle" heart on chest radiograph. Constrictive pericarditis may produce only minimal enlargement but may be detectable by calcification of the pericardium. Cardiac imaging shows normal systolic function and normal cardiac valves. The ventricles are often small and fill rapidly in early diastole but not at all for the remainder of diastole. This finding, together with increased thickness of the pericardium, establishes the diagnosis.

Restrictive cardiomyopathy is a disease of heart muscle (see Ch. 50) that mimics constrictive pericarditis. Characteristically, however, left ventricular diastolic pressure exceeds that on the right. In some cases, endomyocardial biopsy and occasionally exploratory thoracotomy are needed to establish the correct diagnosis.

TREATMENT. For the vast majority of patients, the treatment of choice is pericardiectomy. The patient may be prepared by modest diuresis. With modern techniques of cardiopulmonary bypass, especially in cases that are not too far advanced, the operation yields gratifying clinical improvement, although full benefit may not be evident for about 6 months.

Engel PH: Echocardiographic findings in pericardial disease. *In* Fowler NO (ed.): The Pericardium in Health and Disease. Mt. Kisco, NY, Futura Publishing Company, 1985. *An up-to-date, well-written discussion.*

Klopfenstein HS, Schuchard G, Wann LS, et al.: The relative merits of pulsus paradoxus and right ventricular diastolic collapse in the early detection of cardiac tamponade. An experimental echocardiographic study. Circulation 71:829, 1985. *Describes the correlation between hemodynamics and echocardiographic abnormalities in cardiac tamponade.*

Shabetai R: The Pericardium. New York, Grune & Stratton, 1980. *A comprehensive monograph dealing with the normal pericardium and pericardial diseases.*

Shabetai R, Fowler NO, Fenton JC, et al.: Pulsus paradoxus. J Clin Invest 44:1882, 1965. *An experimental study of the mechanisms of pulsus paradoxus.*

Spodick DH: Pathogenesis and clinical correlations of the electrocardiographic abnormalities of pericardial disease. Cardiovasc Clin 8:201, 1977. *A well-illustrated and complete account of theory and clinical application.*

52 Miscellaneous Conditions of the Heart: Tumor, Trauma, and Systemic Disease

Bernadine P. Healy

CARDIAC TUMORS

Tumors of the heart and pericardium are uncommon, and as a cause of clinical cardiac disease they are especially rare. Consecutive autopsy studies suggest that primary tumors of the heart are seen in only 1 in 2000 postmortem examinations; tumors secondary to metastases are roughly 20 times more frequent than primary lesions. A number of factors have made cardiac tumors a more visible current medical problem. With improved medical diagnostic technology, we are more apt to recognize both primary and secondary cardiac tumors; and with better therapy, patients with metastatic neoplasms live longer, increasing the likelihood for the heart to develop secondary cancers.

In part because of their relative rarity as a cause of clinical heart disease, cardiac tumors often go unrecognized. A general awareness of the pathophysiology of the heart afflicted with tumor and the ways in which it so often mimics more common forms of heart disease is essential to diagnosis and recognition of options for therapeutic intervention.

Primary Tumors of the Heart

Primary tumors of the heart are almost always benign and are considerably less common than tumors secondary to metastatic disease. The myxoma, of endocardial origin, is overwhelmingly the most common and best known of the primary cardiac tumors. Less common is the rhabdomyoma, a benign congenital tumor of myocardium most often seen in children. The sarcoma is the predominant malignant form of primary heart tumor and includes a variety of types, such as rhabdomyosarcoma, angiosarcoma, and fibrosarcoma. Among these tumor types, the myxoma is of greatest clinical importance in terms of relative frequency, tendency to produce symptoms, and ease of diagnosis and therapy.

The cardiac myxoma has been recognized as a pathologic entity for several hundred years, occurring with an incidence of about 0.03 per cent at autopsy. Myxomas are typically solitary, smooth-surfaced, globular tumors, which vary in size from 1 to 8 cm (average 5 cm), and most are pedunculated. In about 90 per cent of cases they occur in the left atrium; most of the rest occur in the right atrium. They are attached to the interatrial septum in the region of the fossa ovalis. Clinical presentation is related to location of the tumor, as well as to the presence of a pedicle. Larger myxomas, generally over 3 cm in diameter, are more apt to be symptomatic. The presence of a pedicle, allowing the myxomas to move about in the cardiac chambers, also correlates with symptomatology.

Myxomas occur most frequently (75 per cent) in women and usually manifest with symptoms in persons between the ages of 35 and 60 years. Because myxomas are most commonly located in the left atrium, signs and symptoms of cardiac dysfunction are usually referable to left-sided cardiac disease. The most common clinical cardiac problem is congestive heart failure, present in roughly half of patients, and often the heart failure is paroxysmal and precipitated by positional change, such as lying down. Other signs include chest pain, murmurs of mitral stenosis or regurgitation or both, syncope, and arrhythmias (including atrial fibrillation, often paroxysmal in nature). Other, noncardiac manifestations of atrial myxomas include systemic or pulmonary embolism, fever, malaise, arthralgias, and hematologic abnormalities suggestive of chronic infection. With these clinical manifestations, it is not surprising that atrial myxomas often have been misdiagnosed as rheumatic mitral valve disease, infective endocarditis, fever of unknown origin, or connective tissue disease. Indeed, cardiac myxomas may be viewed as the "great simulators"; their correct clinical diagnosis is among the most challenging in internal medicine.

Some of the challenge and error in the clinical recognition of cardiac myxomas have been diminished by the advent of improved noninvasive techniques. Echocardiography, particularly two-dimensional study, readily identifies atrial tumors and has virtually eliminated the need for invasive contrast angiography. Radionuclide ventriculography (gated blood cardiac scan) will also identify a moving filling defect within the cardiac chambers and can be used in making the diagnosis of intracavitary tumor. Once the diagnosis of cardiac myxoma has been made, the only treatment is surgical excision. Undiagnosed atrial myxomas are often fatal, but when considered, are readily detected and, once detected, straightforwardly treated and virtually always cured.

Secondary Tumors of the Heart

The heart may be a target for secondary tumor invasion. Cancer has been reported to involve the heart in anywhere from 5 to 20 per cent of patients with metastatic malignant disease, with an apparent increase in reported involvement of the heart in recent years. Almost any type of primary neoplasm may involve the heart. Malignant melanomas are among the most common solid tumors that spread to the heart. Cardiac lesions occur in 40 to 50 per cent of patients with metastatic disease, and as a group, melanomas constitute approximately 3 per cent of all cardiac metastases. Leukemias frequently infiltrate the heart, with microscopic invasion evident in approximately half of patients. Other tumors that frequently metastasize to the heart include carcinomas of the lung, breast, and thyroid, the lymphomas, and the sarcomas, including Kaposi's sarcoma. Carcinomas of the lung and breast, because of their relative frequency among malignancies, together account for approximately 50 per cent of the secondary tumors of the heart.

What is most striking about cardiac invasion by metastatic tumor is that it is so often clinically silent, despite what may be extensive disease. The clinical manifestations of cardiac metastases are myriad and generally reflect the anatomic site of invasion. Congestive heart failure, cardiac arrhythmias, and signs of pericardial constriction are among the most common clinical manifestations of cardiac metastases. Myocardial ischemia and infarction may also result from coronary compression or invasion. Although most cardiac metastases are diagnosed post mortem, they may be clinically detected by a variety of means. When a malignant pericardial effusion is present, cytologic examination of pericardial fluid readily provides diagnosis. Identification of a mass in one or more cardiac chambers or of an irregularity in chamber contour or wall thickness may be accomplished by cross-sectional cardiac echocardiography, radionuclide ventriculography, or invasive contrast angiography. Pathologic examination is necessary, however, to identify tumor type. Unlike treatment for myxomas, surgery for primary or secondary malignancies of the heart is generally ineffective. The major role for cardiac surgery is to obtain tissue for pathologic diagnosis or to alleviate mechanical obstruction. Radiotherapy and chemotherapy are utilized, depending on tumor type.

CARDIAC DISEASE SECONDARY TO CANCER THERAPY. Cardiac disease or dysfunction may also occur as a consequence of chemotherapy and radiotherapy and may obscure even further the diagnosis of metastatic tumors of the heart. Many of the antineoplastic drugs, particularly doxorubicin (Adriamycin), produce a dose-dependent toxicity that leads to a dilated congestive cardiomyopathy. Doxorubicin causes a characteristic degeneration of the myocyte that can be detected by myocardial biopsy. Radiotherapy may also produce dose-dependent cardiac damage to all three layers of the heart. Pericarditis and pericardial effusions are most common, but fibrosis of the myocardium and of mural and valvular endocardium may occur. Prevention is the best therapy for radiation- and drug-induced cardiac damage, which is generally irreversible.

CARDIAC TRAUMA

Trauma is a major cause of morbidity and mortality in our society, and tragically it often affects those who are otherwise healthy. Cardiac trauma results from either a penetrating object or a nonpenetrating blunt assault on the thorax. Death may immediately occur as a result of asystole, ventricular fibrillation, or exsanguination. Those who survive long enough for transport to a hospital pose immediate diagnostic and therapeutic challenges.

Penetrating wounds of the heart are believed to be fatal in over 90 per cent of instances, with most patients never reaching medical attention. Stab and gunshot wounds may lacerate any portion of the heart. Pericardial laceration with cardiac tamponade or exsanguination is most common, usually in conjunction with rupture of some portion of the myocardium. Because of their anterior location, the right ventricle and pulmonary outflow tract are particularly susceptible. Valve lacerations leading to incompetence and coronary injuries leading to ischemia or infarction, or both, are of particular importance for survivors, who may be left with residual lesions.

The diagnosis of cardiac trauma in the setting of a penetrating wound of the thoracic cavity is not always straightforward. Patients usually present acutely with hypotension due either to cardiac tamponade or to hemorrhage. The diagnosis is assumed when profound hypotension is present in the setting of a penetrating mediastinal wound with or without an object in or near the cardiac silhouette. In this setting, emergency thoracotomy, preferably in an operating room, is virtually always necessary for both diagnosis and therapy. The wisdom of performing a diagnostic pericardiocentesis has been challenged, as false-negative readings may result from local clot formation. Pericardiocentesis may be necessary, however, to stabilize a patient with cardiac tamponade prior to emergency thoracotomy. Once the diagnosis of trauma has been made and cardiac surgical repair initiated, the survival rate may be as high as 70 per cent.

Nonpenetrating trauma to the chest cavity may also cause a similar range of cardiac injuries requiring emergency thoracotomy. Unlike penetrating wounds, however, physical evidence of trauma to the chest wall may be minimal or even absent, and the severity of chest wall trauma does not correlate with likelihood or extent of cardiac injury. Among the most common causes of cardiac trauma are steering wheel injuries to the sternum. Others include sports activities, industrial accidents, and personal assaults. The myocardium is the major site of injuries, which may range in severity from mild myocardial contusion to rupture of the ventricle or interventricular septum. Pericardial laceration, valve disruption, coronary artery thrombosis, or great vessel rupture, particularly of the ascending aorta, may also occur.

Diagnosis is difficult, since symptoms are often absent or misleading. Symptoms of chest pain similar to that associated with myocardial infarction are the most frequent. Cardiac arrhythmias and hypotension may also signal cardiac injury in the proper setting. Survivors of myocardial injury may develop false aneurysms with their usual complications. Early and late cardiac arrhythmias (atrial or ventricular) may be caused by myocardial contusions, and the electrocardiographic abnormalities may include those of myocardial infarction or acute pericarditis. Serum enzyme assays (creatine kinase, MB fraction) and echocardiography are helpful in making the diagnosis, and if coronary compromise is suggested, cardiac catheterization with coronary angiography would be appropriate. Treatment depends on the extent of cardiovascular compromise. Pain and arrhythmias alone are treated similarly to those of acute myocardial infarction, except that anticoagulants should be strictly avoided. Thoracotomy is necessary if there are signs of myocardial rupture or pericardial tamponade. Late complications, such as valvular or interventricular septal rupture or false aneurysms of the heart or aorta, require surgical correction.

CARDIAC MANIFESTATIONS OF SYSTEMIC DISEASE

The heart may be afflicted secondarily by a variety of systemic conditions and diseases. The most frequent cardiac manifestations of systemic disease are those common disorders that primarily involve the vascular system and produce cardiac dysfunction by virtue of increased volume or pressure load on the heart or interruption in blood flow to the myocardium. Systemic hypertension, whether essential, renal, or endocrine in cause, often leads to cardiac hypertrophy and heart failure. Atherosclerosis is a systemic vascular disease with the heart as a prime target. Less common are the anemias, which produce a volume load and at times hypoxic insult to the heart, leading to congestive heart failure. In addition to these widely recognized disorders, there are several systemic diseases that secondarily involve the heart in a distinctive fashion. Examples of these disorders include the connective tissue diseases (e.g., systemic lupus erythematosus [SLE], progressive systemic sclerosis, and polyarteritis nodosa); endocrine-humoral disorders (thyroid disease, pheochromocytoma, and metastatic carcinoid); and systemic infiltrative disease (amyloidosis).

CONNECTIVE TISSUE DISEASES. Although the connective tissue diseases may affect the heart only secondarily, the cardiac disorder may dominate the clinical course. In systemic lupus erythematosus, the endocardium, myocardium, and pericardium all are potential targets. A fibrinous pericarditis is a common cardiac lesion and frequently produces clinical symptoms. Fibrofibrinous thrombotic lesions may develop on the surface of the cardiac valves (a condition termed Libman-Sacks endocarditis) and are usually clinically silent. On occasion this endocarditis may lead to significant mitral or aortic valve dysfunction. Myocarditis may occur but is an infrequent result of SLE. Coronary arteritis and thromboembolism may also develop, and in patients with corticosteroid-treated lupus, in particular, there may be accelerated coronary atherosclerosis.

Progressive systemic sclerosis (PSS) or scleroderma may produce cardiac dysfunction by means of its effect on the myocardium. Focal fibrosis and necrosis of myocardium may lead to a picture of dilated congestive cardiomyopathy. Morphologic and clinical evidence now suggests that the etiology of the myocardial disease in PSS is small vessel coronary spasm, causing ischemia, i.e., a Raynaud's phenomenon of the coronary arteries. Polyarteritis nodosa may cause a focal or a diffuse coronary arteritis, with formation of coronary thrombosis or aneurysm or both. The latter may lead to myocardial ischemia or infarction and, combined with systemic hypertension, to congestive heart failure. Cardiac manifestations of the connective tissue diseases are diagnosed and treated with the standard technology and methods used for valvular, myocardial, pericardial, or coronary disease. Therapy also includes the immunosuppressive drugs used for treatment of the systemic diseases.

ENDOCRINE-HUMORAL DISORDERS. Thyroid disease has long been known to target the heart. Thyroid hormone increases oxygen consumption and metabolic rate, has a direct inotropic and chronotropic effect on the heart, and has been shown to have a direct trophic effect on the myocardium, inducing a physiologic pattern of hypertrophy. The major clinical manifestation of thyroid hormone excess is a hyperkinetic heart and circulation. Other symptoms include a variety of arrhythmias (atrial fibrillation, in particular), and, with severe disease, congestive heart failure may develop. Although less common, hypothyroidism may produce an idiopathic dilated cardiomyopathy, but its etiology is obscure. More often, hypothyroidism causes bradycardia and pericardial effusions. The latter may contain cholesterol crystals, a finding believed to be characteristic of a myxedema-associated effusion. Identification of the basis for these cardiac disorders is confirmed by abnormal serum thyroxine levels. Thyroid hormone levels should be obtained routinely in patients with idiopathic atrial fibrillation and in those with heart failure of obscure etiology.

Pheochromocytomas, which are chromaffin cell tumors, produce norepinephrine and, to a varying degree, epinephrine, which may cause systemic hypertension as well as induce direct myocardial toxicity. Autopsy studies have shown focal myocardial contraction band necrosis and fibrosis in as many as 50 per cent of patients with this tumor. Similar lesions may be produced in experimental animals with catecholamine infusions and are believed to relate to norepinephrine-induced calcium overload. Although this tumor may cause cardiomyopathy, it is exceedingly rare.

CARDIAC AMYLOIDOSIS. This disorder may be primary but occurs most often secondary to systemic conditions, including multiple myeloma, systemic amyloidosis, familial Mediterranean fever, and aging. Amyloid may infiltrate myocardium and coronary arteries, and less often the cardiac valves, and typically causes increased myocardial mass and focal fibrosis. The latter leads to decreased myocardial compliance and ultimately congestive heart failure—a picture that may simulate hypertrophic or restrictive cardiomyopathy. Cardiac amyloid deposits may also affect the conduction system of the heart, causing a variety of arrhythmias. The diagnosis of cardiac amyloid is confirmed by myocardial biopsy. Therapy for the cardiac dysfunction of amyloidosis is the standard treatment for arrhythmias or heart failure or both. A proclivity to digitalis toxicity, possibly related to conduction system infiltration by amyloid, should be considered when treating heart failure in these patients.

Doherty NE, Siegel RJ: Cardiovascular manifestations of systemic lupus erythematosus. Am Heart J 110:1257, 1985. *A review article summarizing present information on the clinical and morphologic aspects of the heart in systemic lupus erythematosus.*

Follansbee WP, Curtiss EI, Medsger TA, et al.: Physiologic abnormalities of cardiac function in progressive systemic sclerosis with diffuse scleroderma. N Engl J Med 310:142, 1984. *Description of cardiac dysfunction in patients with PSS, showing by noninvasive techniques the relationship of circulatory disturbances to ventricular dysfunction.*

Frazee RC, Mucha P Jr, Farnell MB, et al.: Objective evaluation of blunt cardiac trauma. J Trauma 26:510, 1986. *A review of the cardiovascular consequences of blunt chest trauma, describing CK-MB elevations, arrhythmias, and ven-*

tricular dysfunction as assessed by echocardiography in a wide range of cardiac injuries.

McDonnell PJ, Mann RB, Bulkley BH: Involvement of the heart by malignant lymphoma: A clinicopathologic study. Cancer 49:944, 1982. *A clinicopathologic study of the cardiovascular manifestations of lymphomatous involvement of the heart and a general review of the range of malignant tumors of the heart and how they cause cardiac dysfunction.*

Morkin E, Flink IL, Goldman S: Biochemical and physiologic effects of thyroid hormone on cardiac performance. Prog Cardiovasc Dis 25:435, 1983. *An in-depth and current review of the effect of thyroid hormone on the normal heart and its role in disease.*

Salcedo EE, Adams KV, Lever HM, et al.: Echocardiographic findings in 25 patients with left atrial myxoma. J Am Coll Cardiol 1:1162, 1983. *Describes the use of echocardiography to diagnose myxomas noninvasively.*

Schrader ML, Hochman JS, Bulkley BH: The heart in polyarteritis nodosa: A clinicopathologic study. Am Heart J 109:1353, 1985. *A clinicopathologic study of the heart in polyarteritis nodosa and a review of the literature.*

Skhvatsabaja LV: Secondary malignant lesions of the heart and pericardium in neoplastic disease. Oncology 43:103, 1986. *A review of clinical and laboratory data in 240 patients with metastatic tumors of the heart and pericardium, focusing on clinical symptoms and diagnosis.*

53 Diseases of the Aorta

Lawrence S. Cohen

The aorta is vital to the proper functioning of every organ system in the body. The coronary arteries are the first arteries to arise from the aorta, followed by vessels of the head and central nervous system and then the gastrointestinal, renal, and genitourinary arteries. Disease in any segment of the aorta, therefore, can have profound consequences upon bodily function. The aorta is susceptible to four major disease processes: *aneurysm, dissection, arteriosclerotic occlusive disease,* and *aortitis.*

At its origin the aorta is approximately 3 cm in diameter. The ascending aorta is approximately 5 cm in length, coursing in a left-to-right direction in the same ejection axis as the left ventricle. The aortic arch is also approximately 5 cm in length and takes an upward, posterior, and leftward direction, terminating along the left border of the thoracic vertebrae. The aortic arch lies entirely within the superior mediastinum. The descending thoracic aorta is contained in the posterior mediastinum. It is a bit narrower than the ascending aorta and is approximately 20 cm in length. It runs to the diaphragm at the level of the twelfth thoracic vertebra and supplies the arteries to the spinal cord. The abdominal aorta is the continuation of the thoracic aorta, ending at the level of the fourth lumbar vertebra. The average length is 15 cm, with an average diameter of 2 cm at its origin and a slightly smaller diameter at its lower end.

ANEURYSM

Definition

An aneurysm is a widening of a vessel involving the stretching of fibrous tissue within the media of the vessel. A true aneurysm is a widening of the vessel, whereas a false aneurysm represents a localized rupture of the artery with sealing over by clot or adjacent structures. The natural history of aneurysms is to enlarge. Not only does the etiologic process tend to continue and progress but also the law of Laplace is a factor. As described by Laplace, the tension in the wall of a spherical chamber enclosing a fluid under pressure is related to the pressure under which the fluid is kept and the radius of curvature of the containing vessel. As the radius increases so does wall tension. Hence, enlargement of the vessel begets more enlargement.

It is convenient to classify aneurysms according to etiology, morphology, and location. Arteriosclerosis is the most common cause of aneurysms. Other causes are cystic medial necrosis, trauma, and infection, including syphilis. Rarer causes are rheumatic aortitis, Takayasu's syndrome, temporal arteritis, and relapsing polychondritis. Marfan's syndrome is characterized by cystic medial necrosis (Ch. 187). In some forms of Ehlers-Danlos syndrome, rupture of blood vessels, including the aorta, may occur. Aneurysms can be classified into three morphologic types: (1) fusiform, in which the aneurysm encompasses the entire circumference of the aorta and assumes a spindle shape; (2)

saccular, in which only a portion of the circumference is involved and in which there is a neck and an asymmetric outpouching of the aneurysm; and (3) dissecting, in which an intimal tear permits a column of blood to dissect along the media of the vessel. This is often called a dissecting hematoma. Location is a further way to classify aneurysms. Aneurysms involve (1) the ascending aorta, including the sinuses of Valsalva; (2) the aortic arch; (3) the descending thoracic aorta, originating just distal to the left subclavian artery; and (4) the abdomen, most commonly distal to the renal arteries.

The most proximal portion of the ascending aorta comprises the sinuses of Valsalva. Aneurysms in this location are usually congenital in origin. Most involve either the right sinus or the right portion of the noncoronary sinus. Aneurysms of the sinus of Valsalva are often silent until they rupture into the right side of the heart, usually the right ventricle or right atrium. This event may occur spontaneously or may be a consequence of infective endocarditis. Other causes of aortic sinus aneurysm are Marfan's syndrome, syphilis, and infective endocarditis. Aneurysms of the ascending aorta may be arteriosclerotic, but cystic medial necrosis with or without other features of Marfan's syndrome is more common. Syphilis was once a common cause of ascending aortic aneurysm but has all but disappeared as an etiology. The more distal the aortic location of the aneurysm, the more likely it is to be arteriosclerotic.

Clinical Manifestations

Clinical manifestations of aneurysms of the thoracic aorta (other than rupture) are due to compression, distortion, or erosion of surrounding structures. Pain is the most common symptom. Pain in a gradually enlarging aneurysm is insidious and may be described as boring and deep. Increasing intensity of pain is an ominous sign and may presage impending rupture.

Aortic valve regurgitation may be associated with aneurysms of the ascending aorta. Distortion of the aortic annulus and separation of the aortic valve cusps accounts for the regurgitation. If regurgitation occurs rapidly, the clinical consequences can be dramatic, with the patient developing acute pulmonary edema. Many patients develop a murmur of aortic regurgitation gradually and may be relatively asymptomatic. Aneurysms of the transverse aortic arch are less common than are aneurysms in other sites. The consequences of such aneurysms are often formidable, since the innominate and carotid arteries arise from the transverse aortic arch. In addition, the arch is contiguous with other vital structures such as the superior vena cava, pulmonary artery, trachea, bronchi, lung, and left recurrent laryngeal nerve. Symptoms may include dyspnea, stridor, hoarseness, hemoptysis, cough, or chest pain.

The most common site of an aneurysm of the descending thoracic aorta is between the origin of the left subclavian artery and the diaphragm. Arteriosclerosis is the most common cause, with age, hypertension, and probably smoking contributing as risk factors. One factor in the pathogenesis of aneurysms of the descending aorta may be the immobility of the aorta at this site and the unique stresses imposed on the aorta immediately distal to the left subclavian artery. Distortion of the architecture in this area may result in sufficient turbulence to cause elastic tissue degeneration, accelerated arteriosclerosis, and localized dilatation.

Pain from descending thoracic aortic aneurysm is often intrascapular but can vary considerably. Hoarseness may occur from stretching of the left recurrent laryngeal nerve. Hemoptysis may occur owing to leakage into the left lung. Thoracic aortic aneurysms, like those of the abdominal aorta, threaten life by potential rupture. They are rarely complicated by thrombosis or embolism. Thoracoabdominal aneurysms involve the celiac, superior mesenteric, and renal arteries. Fortunately, they are not common, for they represent a great challenge to the vascular surgeon. Although some are caused by cystic medial necrosis, most are of arteriosclerotic origin and occur in older men.

The most common form of aneurysm is the abdominal aortic aneurysm. The prevalence of this aneurysm at autopsy is in the 1 to 3 per cent range but is even more common in men over 60. Its frequency in men outnumbers that in women by 6:1. Almost all of these aneurysms are below the renal arteries. Most are of arteriosclerotic origin, but trauma, infection (including syphilis),

and arteritis make up a small fraction. A fortunate feature of these aneurysms is their accessibility on physical examination. Rupture of an abdominal aneurysm is the greatest threat and may lead to a rapid demise because of shock and hypotension. Other less acute symptoms may also occur. Pain in the lower back is a sign of enlargement of the aneurysm and at times is a warning of impending rupture. Almost all abdominal aortic aneurysms are lined with clot or have ulcerated plaques. Embolization of atherothrombotic material may lead to a variety of symptoms, ranging from digital infarction to anuria from a shower of emboli to the kidneys.

The likelihood of rupture increases with increasing aortic aneurysm size. Sixty to 80 per cent of patients with lesions 7 cm or larger die of rupture, and 95 per cent of patients with lesions over 10 cm die of aneurysm rupture. The risk of rupture in aneurysms 5 cm or less is considerably lower. Given these data, general guidelines about surgical repair have emerged. Aneurysms associated with aortic thrombosis or distal embolic events should be repaired promptly. Aneurysms suspected of rupture or acute expansion should be treated surgically immediately. Although there are differences of opinion concerning when elective repair of asymptomatic aneurysms should be undertaken, once the aneurysm exceeds 5 cm in diameter, the prognosis on continued medical management becomes increasingly guarded.

Diagnosis

Palpation is usually the first step in diagnosing abdominal aneurysms. Ultrasound imaging is an excellent technique to confirm the diagnosis, as it is noninvasive, inexpensive, and accurate to within 2 to 3 mm of aneurysm size when compared with the findings at surgery. Computed tomography (CT) scanning utilizing contrast material is equal in effectiveness to ultrasound in the detection and sizing of abdominal aortic aneurysms. Often lumbar spine x-ray films clearly outline the walls of an abdominal aortic aneurysm if there is calcium in the walls. Aortography, either arterial or venous with digital subtraction, may not reflect the true size of the aneurysm; an extensive laminated clot may reduce the lumen.

Joyce JW: Aneurysmal disease. *In* Spittell JA Jr (ed.): Clinical Vascular Disease. Philadelphia, F. A. Davis Company, 1983, pp 89–101. *A concise summary of aneurysmal disease, including management guidelines for aneurysms in all aortic locations.*

Spittell JA Jr: Abdominal aortic aneurysms. Hosp Pract 21:105, 1986. *This is a short, well-illustrated practical management update. Modern diagnostic tools are discussed, and management strategies are reviewed.*

DISSECTING ANEURYSM OF THE AORTA

The incidence of aortic dissections is not known exactly, but it is estimated that approximately 2000 acute cases occur in the United States each year.

Classification of aortic dissection is based upon duration and anatomic location of the dissection. Dissection is considered acute if it occurred within 2 weeks, and chronic if it occurred more than 2 weeks, prior to the institution of therapy.

Aortic dissection is more commonly classified by site of the intimal tear and extent of dissecting hematoma. In type I and type II dissections, the intimal tear is in the ascending aorta, usually within a few centimeters of the aortic valve. In type I aneurysms, the dissecting hematoma extends and involves at least the aortic arch and often the descending aorta as well. Type II aneurysms involve the ascending aorta only. Type III aneurysms are characterized by an intimal tear in the descending aorta, usually immediately distal to the left subclavian artery. The dissecting hematoma usually propagates distally but at times may extend in a retrograde manner to the aortic arch (Fig. 53–1).

Etiology

The most consistent etiologic factor in aortic disection is hypertension. Other conditions are associated with dissection in the absence of hypertension. Marfan's syndrome has been discussed. There is a peculiar association between pregnancy and dissection. It is postulated that hormonal changes during pregnancy may alter the composition of the aorta and make it more susceptible to rupture. Stresses and strains of labor may also be a factor.

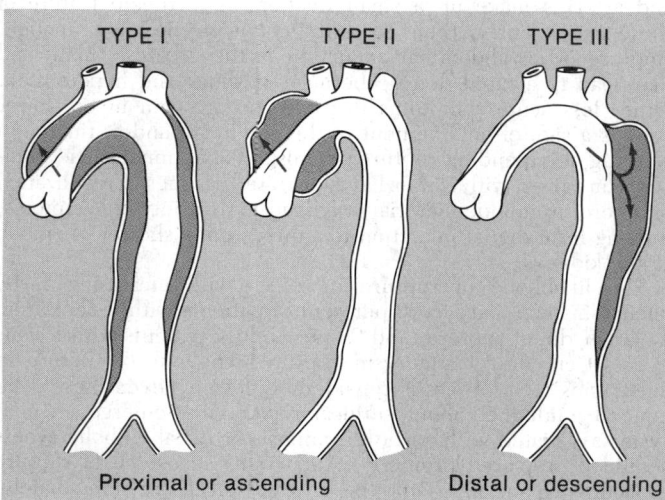

FIGURE 53–1. Classification of dissecting aneurysms of the aorta. (Modified from DeBakey.)

TYPE I   TYPE II   TYPE III

Proximal or ascending   Distal or descending

Valvular aortic stenosis, particularly that due to a bicuspid valve, is associated with dissection. Turbulence established beyond the stenotic valve increases lateral forces, thereby enhancing the likelihood of an intimal tear and development of a dissection. The association between coarctation of the aorta and dissection is well known. The years of proximal aortic hypertension prior to repair of the coarctation may establish the conditions that ultimately lead to aortic dissection. In addition, there is a high incidence of bicuspid aortic valves in patients with coarctation of the aorta. Before the advent of antimicrobial agents, syphilitic aortitis was the most common cause of aortic dissection. It is now unusual. Trauma may be a cause of dissecting aneurysm. Other unusual etiologies are the Ehlers-Danlos syndrome and relapsing polychondritis.

Pathogenesis

Aortic dissection begins most frequently in an intimal tear in the ascending aorta a short distance above the aortic valve. The primary tear is often referred to as the *entry intimal tear*. The *re-entry* or *secondary tear* occurs more distally. The basic pathologic condition resides in the underlying media, the chief supporting layer of the aorta. Most tears are transverse or circumferential, reflecting the direction of the muscular fibers of the media.

The two key ingredients of aortic dissection are arterial hypertension and medial degeneration. In any given patient, one or the other of these abnormalities may be the more important. Many patients with Marfan's syndrome or the Ehlers-Danlos syndrome develop dissecting aneurysms without ever developing hypertension. Alternatively, individuals with longstanding hypertension may develop dissection without any apparent specific weakness of the aortic medial wall. Additional factors in the pathogenesis of aortic dissections are the anatomy and motion of the heart and great vessels themselves. The heart beats an average of 70 times per minute, over 80,000 times per day, and over 35 million times per year. The heart is not absolutely fixed in place but is limited in its anterior-posterior movement by the sternum and vertebral column, respectively. Its motion is both side to side and twisting as it ejects blood into the ascending aorta. This produces a flexing stress in the ascending aorta and contributes to the frequency of ascending aortic dissections. The descending aorta becomes fixed distal to the left subclavian artery, accounting for the alternative predilection for dissection to occur at that site. Once an intimal tear occurs, the dissecting hematoma is propagated through the weakened medial wall. The forces that continue the propagation are the arterial pressure and the pulse wave properties (dp/dt) of left ventricular ejection. Some dissecting hematomas rupture back into the aortic lumen at a distal site. Rupture may also occur externally into the pericardial or pleural space.

Clinical Manifestations

Pain is often excruciating and may occur primarily in the anterior chest. It may migrate to the back as the dissecting hematoma works it way down the aorta. Patients sometimes describe an accentuation of the pain with each heart beat, suggesting the driving force of the pulse wave. Pain may occur in the neck, jaw, or teeth if the aortic arch is involved. Less common symptoms are syncope, stroke, paraplegia, or loss of pulses in any of the extremities. Rarely, a dissection may be clinically silent and be suggested only by an abnormal roentgenogram. If aortic regurgitation occurs owing to the dissection, patients may develop congestive heart failure. A diastolic murmur is usually present in these circumstances, although the duration of the murmur may be relatively short if the filling pressure in the left ventricle rises rapidly because of the acute nature of the regurgitation. Such murmurs may be heard commonly along the right sternal border.

The clinical presentation and physical findings in patients with aortic dissection are determined by the course taken by the dissecting hematoma. (1) Loss of any pulse can occur as the circulation to any major artery arising from the aorta may be compromised. (2) Aortic regurgitation may result from disruption of the supporting structures of the aortic valve. (3) Neurologic symptoms may occur if the head and neck vessels are compromised by the dissection. Paraplegia may occur owing to loss of blood supply to the spinal cord. A number of other physical findings may be seen in patients with aortic dissection. These include Horner's syndrome due to compression of the superior cervical ganglion, vocal cord paralysis and hoarseness due to pressure against the recurrent laryngeal nerve, superior vena cava syndrome, pulsating neck masses, dyspnea due to tracheal or bronchial compression, hemorrhagic pleural effusion, myocardial infarction if the hematoma dissects retrograde across a coronary ostium, and symptoms and signs of mesenteric infarction. Persistent fever has also been described.

Diagnosis

Time is often of utmost importance in management. Once the patient is stabilized, aortography should not be delayed. Routine laboratory tests do not generally add much to the diagnosis. Leukocytosis is a common but nonspecific finding. A chest roentgenogram may be normal but will often show widening of the aortic shadow (Fig. 53–2). Aortic angiography is the definitive procedure, yielding precise information necessary for proper management. The extent of the dissection, the entry and reentry

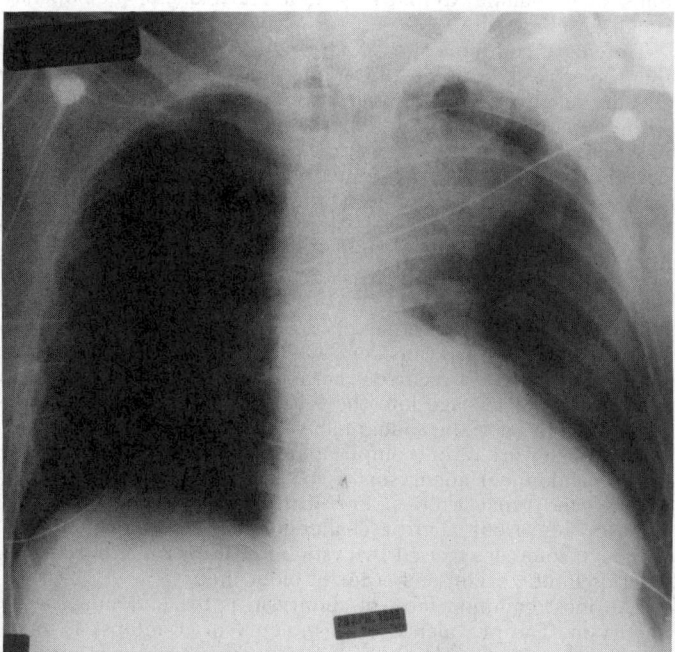

FIGURE 53–2. Chest roentgenogram of a patient with a dissecting aneurysm demonstrating marked enlargement of the aortic arch and descending aorta.

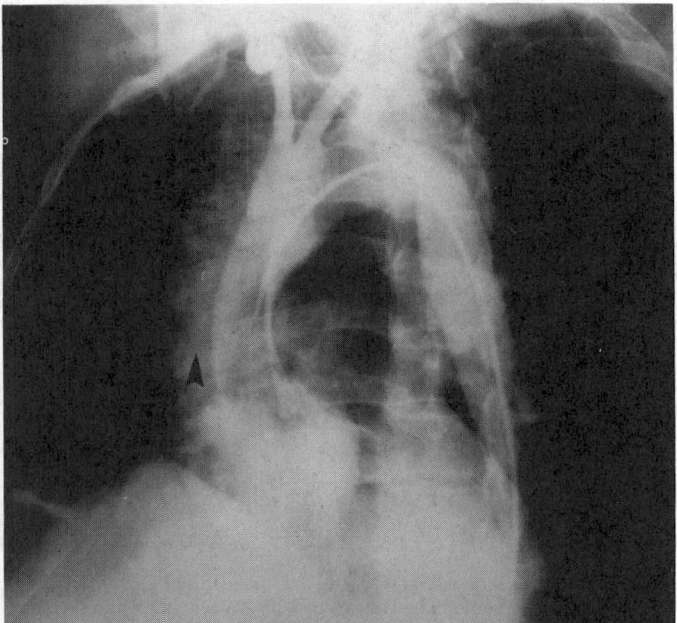

FIGURE 53–3. Aortic root angiogram in the left anterior oblique projection. The black arrowhead demonstrates the false lumen caused by the aortic dissection.

sites, the competence or degree of regurgitation of the aortic valve, and aortic branch vessel involvement can all be ascertained (Fig. 53–3).

The differential diagnosis of a patient with chest or back pain, pulmonary edema with a new murmur of aortic regurgitation, any acute neurologic syndrome, or sudden loss of pulse in an extremity should include aortic dissection.

Computed tomography with the use of contrast material is also highly accurate in demonstrating aortic dissection, although it is not always possible to perform this examination rapidly. Two-dimensional echocardiography does not necessitate the use of contrast agents or ionizing radiation and is easily performed. False-negative and false-positive diagnoses remain a problem with this procedure, but it is nevertheless useful (Fig. 53–4). Transesophageal echocardiography is a powerful new diagnostic tool, as the majority of the aorta can be imaged well from the transducer placed in the esophagus (Fig. 53–5). Magnetic resonance imaging is also capable of diagnosing aortic dissection and does not require the use of contrast agents for vascular imaging.

Prognosis

In untreated aortic dissection, the prognosis is poor. Approximately 20 per cent of patients die in 24 hours, 60 per cent in 2 weeks, and 90 per cent in 3 months. The principal cause of death is not the initial intimal tear but is related to the effects of propagation of the dissecting hematoma. Progressive aortic regurgitation may occur if the hematoma dissects in a retrograde direction. Rupture into the pericardial or pleural space is often a fatal complication.

Treatment

Prompt diagnosis and institution of therapy are critical to the success of treatment. Since the most important known factors in the propagation of the dissecting hematoma are hypertension and the rate of rise of the aortic pressure pulse (dp/dt), efforts must be undertaken to alter both of these. An intravenous drip of sodium nitroprusside is started, and the infusion is titrated to reduce the systolic blood pressure to 100 to 120 mm Hg. The infusion rate can usually be started at 1 µg per kilogram per minute. Simultaneously, propranolol should be given in intermittent intravenous boluses of 0.5 to 1.0 mg until the heart rate is in the range of 60 beats per minute. When possible, an intra-arterial line to measure blood pressure accurately and a central venous line or Swan-Ganz catheter should be utilized. Once the patient's blood pressure and other hemodynamic and clinical features are stable, aortography should be performed. Computed tomographic scanning or echocardiography may be of some diagnostic aid at this stage while awaiting aortography.

Operative intervention is usually indicated if the dissection involves the ascending aorta, as in types I and II aneurysms. These aneurysms are unstable and pose the threat of retrograde dissection, rupture, severe aortic regurgitation, or fatal pericardial tamponade. This type of acute dissection can be corrected surgically with a mortality rate in the range of 20 per cent. Type III aneurysms that involve the distal or descending aorta can generally be treated medically. If the patient's condition stabilizes, drug therapy can be continued into the chronic phase. Surgical intervention for the patient with a type III aneurysm is indicated if there is evidence of increasing size of the dissecting hematoma, impending rupture, inability to control pain, or bleeding into the pleural space.

The operative approach must be flexible and individualized. For patients with ascending aortic dissection and involvement of the annulus or root, it is often necessary to replace the entire

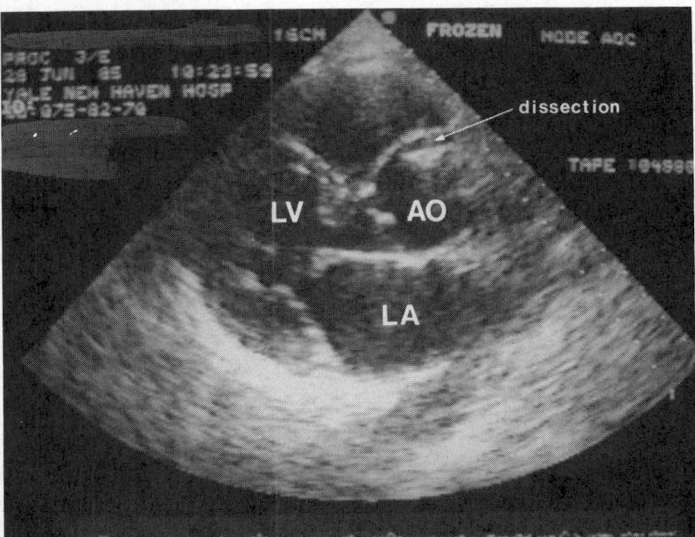

FIGURE 53–4. Echocardiogram, long-axis parasternal view of a patient with dissecting aneurysm. The dissection arises in the proximal aortic root. LV = Left ventricle; AO = aortic root; LA = left atrium.

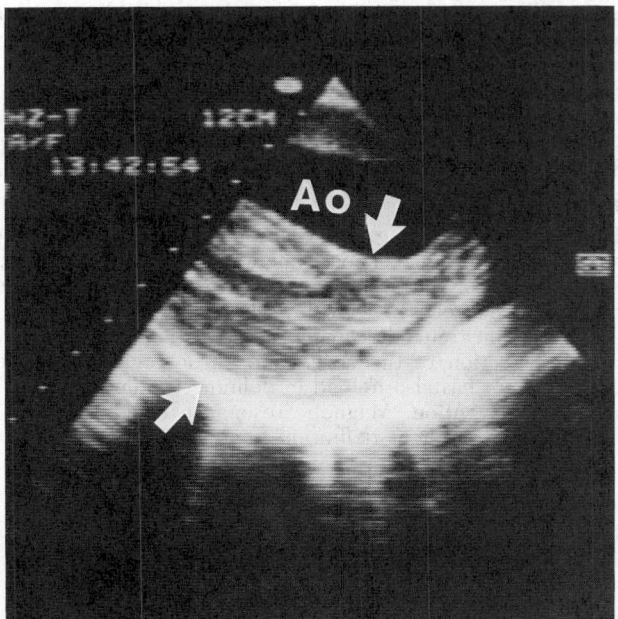

FIGURE 53–5. Transesophageal echocardiogram demonstrating an ascending aortic dissection. The top arrow points to an intraluminal clot. The bottom arrow points to the outer aortic wall.

aortic root and aortic valve with a composite conduit, which is attached proximally to the aortic annulus and distally to the aorta after obliteration of the false lumen. The coronary ostia are then reimplanted into the tubular graft. If the ascending aorta is involved but the sinuses of Valsalva are spared, operative repair consists of resection of the aneurysmal portion with replacement by a synthetic tubular graft. This same technique applies for descending aortic dissections. In all cases, the false lumen is obliterated. Management and follow-up of patients initially treated either surgically or medically is the same. Continued meticulous control of blood pressure and administration of β blockers to control dp/dt are warranted. The systolic blood pressure should be kept below 130 mm Hg at rest and the heart rate below 72 beats per minute at rest.

Cooke JP, Safford RE: Progress in the diagnosis and management of aortic dissection. Mayo Clin Proc 61:147, 1986. *This excellent short article concentrates on the available diagnostic studies in patients with aortic dissection.*

Eagle KA, Quertermous T, Kritzer GA, et al.: Spectrum of conditions initially suggesting acute aortic dissection but with negative aortograms. Am J Cardiol 57:322, 1986. *This study defines the differential diagnosis of aortic dissection, discusses the frequency of false-negative aortographic findings, and contrasts the clinical features of patients with and without dissection.*

Roberts WC: Aortic dissection: Anatomy, consequences, and causes. Am Heart J 101:195, 1981. *A well-illustrated review of aortic dissection with emphasis on pathologic findings.*

Slater EE, DeSanctis RW: The clinical recognition of dissecting aortic aneurysm. Am J Med 60:625, 1976. *The clinical, roentgenologic, and laboratory findings in 124 patients with dissecting aneurysm of the aorta are discussed. Patients with dissections of the proximal aorta were younger and had a higher incidence of Marfan's syndrome, cystic medial necrosis, anterior chest pain, pulse deficits, neurologic compromise, aortic regurgitation, and congestive heart failure. Back pain, hypertension, and atherosclerosis characterized patients with distal dissection.*

Wheat MW Jr: Acute dissecting aneurysms of the aorta: Diagnosis and treatment—1979. Am Heart J 99:373, 1980. *The author, a surgeon, presents arguments for vigorous medical therapy in order to control hypertension and rate of pressure development in the aorta.*

MARFAN'S SYNDROME

Patients with Marfan's syndrome (see Ch. 187) develop both aortic aneurysm and aortic dissection. Myxomatous degeneration of valve leaflets may also occur. The mitral valve cusps may be involved. The chordae tendineae may elongate or rupture, predisposing to mitral valve prolapse, or flail mitral valve with mitral regurgitation. Regurgitation at either the mitral or the tricuspid valve may be the most prominent finding in certain patients. However, the most commonly affected tissue is the aorta. The aorta enlarges, beginning with the sinuses of Valsalva. The enlargement most often extends to the innominate artery, although at times the entire aorta may be involved in what has been referred to as annuloaortic ectasia. Aortic dilation may begin as early as the fifth year of life or as late as the sixth decade.

Aortic regurgitation may occur secondary to participation of the aortic root in the development of an aortic aneurysm. Dissection of the aortic root may lead to acute aortic regurgitation. Dilation of the pulmonary artery is common.

Diagnosis

Dilation of the aortic root is easily measured by echocardiography. Two-dimensional echocardiography shows the classic flask-shaped dilation of the aorta extending from the aortic valve to the innominate artery (Fig. 53–6). Echocardiography may also be used to demonstrate the major complications of aortic root dilation, dissection of the aorta, and aortic regurgitation. The echocardiogram has also helped in defining the optimal time for operative intervention. Magnetic resonance imaging is also capable of giving excellent definition to abnormalities of the aorta (Fig. 53–7).

Therapy

It is now generally agreed, although not absolutely proven, that β blockade may inhibit the pace of aortic dilation. Therefore, it is appropriate to obtain serial echocardiograms in patients thought to have Marfan's syndrome. When incipient dilation of the aorta is recognized, institution of a β blocker may be warranted. By diminishing the velocity with which the left ventricle ejects blood, the forces on the weakened aortic wall may be lessened.

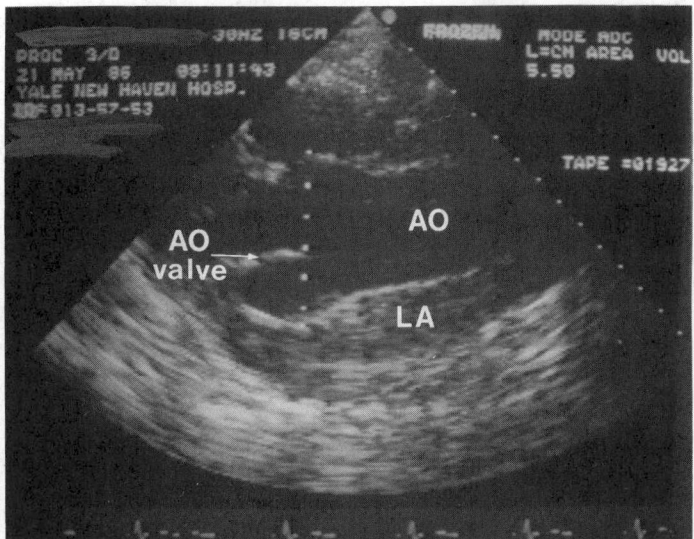

FIGURE 53–6. Echocardiogram, long-axis parasternal view of a patient with Marfan's syndrome. The sinuses of Valsalva are flared and the aortic root is dilated.

Complications of aneurysms in the ascending aorta account for more than 90 per cent of deaths from Marfan's syndrome. The likelihood of both aortic dissection and aortic regurgitation increases as the size of the aortic root increases. Operation in the face of an acute dissection is fraught with considerable hazard. Therefore, prophylactic operation is recommended if the aortic root enlarges to 6 cm on echocardiography. The operation most commonly utilized for patients with Marfan's syndrome is replacement of the ascending aortic aneurysm with a composite tube graft that includes a prosthetic valve at its proximal end. The coronaries are anastomosed to the sides of the tube graft. The aneurysm is wrapped around the tube graft to help establish hemostasis. The overall hospital mortality of the procedure is 2 per cent (Gott and colleagues). Although it may seem radical to recommend aortic replacement to a patient who may be asymptomatic, the adverse prognosis of the patient with Marfan's syndrome whose aorta dilates to greater than 6 cm in diameter probably warrants this recommendation.

Gott VL, Pyeritz RE, Magovern GJ Jr, et al.: Surgical treatment of aneurysms of the ascending aorta in the Marfan syndrome. N Engl J Med 314:1070, 1986. *The results of ascending aorta replacement with a composite graft in 50 consecutive patients with Marfan's syndrome are reported. Because of the unfavorable natural history of Marfan's syndrome, the authors recommend prophylactic repair when the aneurysm reaches a diameter of 6 cm.*

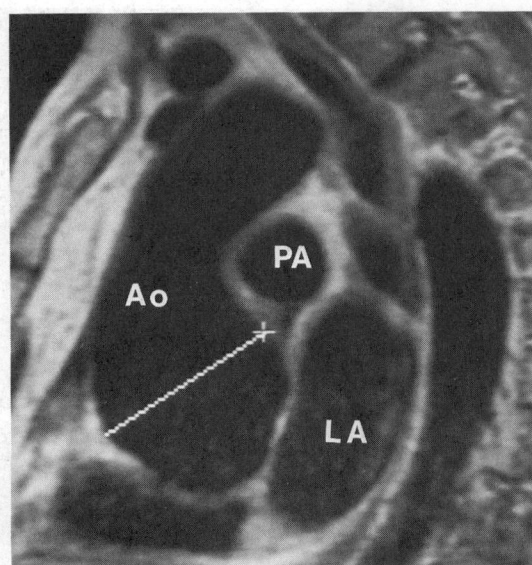

FIGURE 53–7. Magnetic resonance image, sagittal view, showing an aneurysm of the ascending aorta in a patient with Marfan's syndrome.

Halpern BL, Char F, Murdoch JL, et al.: A prospectus on the prevention of aortic rupture in the Marfan syndrome with data on survivorship without treatment. Johns Hopkins Med J 129 123, 1971. *This is one of the first articles to advocate the prophylactic use of β blockers in patients with the Marfan's syndrome in order to prevent further dilation and dissecting aneurysm.*

MISCELLANEOUS FORMS OF AORTITIS AND THE AORTIC ARCH SYNDROME

Arteritis

A number of inflammatory processes can involve the aortic arch and its major branches. Aortic arteritis, no matter what the etiology, may cause narrowing or occlusion of the major arch vessels. Blood supply to the areas supplied by the innominate artery, the left common carotid artery, and the left subclavian artery may be impaired. Symptoms may include transient ischemic attacks, syncope, disorders of vision or speech, claudication of the upper extremities or of the muscles of the jaw, decreased pulses in the neck and upper extremities, or symptoms of basilar artery insufficiency. As a group, these entities are called the aortic arch syndrome. They include aortitis due to syphilis, tuberculosis, giant cell arteritis, polyarteritis nodosa, Takayasu's syndrome, or dissecting aneurysm. Kawasaki's mucocutaneous lymph node syndrome may cause an aortitis, but the coronary arteries are the principal vessels involved. Giant cell arteritis may cause the aortic arch syndrome in addition to temporal and ophthalmic artery disease.

Takayasu's arteritis may be a more specific form of aortitis. Initially it was thought that the arteritic process was limited to the aortic arch and its branches. Subsequent studies have demonstrated that the arteritis is not confined to these areas. Three varieties are now recognized. In one type, the involvement is localized to the aortic arch and its branches. The second type involves the descending thoracic aorta and abdominal aorta without the arch. The third type contains features of both. There is a preponderance of females with "pulseless disease." Although early reports were more common in Japan, increasing numbers of patients are being recognized in the United States. The presence of hypertension with absent pulses in the upper extremities has caused this syndrome to be called reversed coarctation.

Lupi-Herrera E, Sanchez-Torres G, Marcushamer J, et al.: Takayasu's arteritis: Clinical study of 107 cases. Am Heart J 93:94, 1977. *A review of Takayasu's arteritis involving 107 patients. This entity is not limited to Asian patients. It is a nonspecific inflammatory process affecting the aorta and its main branches.*

TRAUMATIC AORTIC DISEASE

The most common form of trauma to the aorta is due to deceleration injuries, often seen in automobile accidents. Since the descending aorta is relatively immobile, deceleration injuries characteristically affect the portion of the aorta immediately distal to the left subclavian artery. Nonpenetrating aortic injury may cause internal bleeding with no external evidence of chest injury. Hypotension or shock, left hemothorax, absence of femoral pulses, and pale lower extremities round out the clinical picture. A chest roentgenogram may show mediastinal widening. Prompt surgical intervention may be life saving.

54 Vascular Diseases of the Limbs

Hermes A. Kontos

VASCULAR DISEASES OF THE LIMBS CAUSED BY ABNORMAL RESPONSES OF VASCULAR SMOOTH MUSCLE

Raynaud's Phenomenon and Disease

DEFINITION. Raynaud's phenomenon is a syndrome manifested by attacks of pallor and cyanosis of the digits in response to cold or to emotion. As the attack abates, these color changes are replaced by redness. When the disorder is primary, it is called Raynaud's disease; when it is secondary to another disease or cause, it is called Raynaud's phenomenon.

ETIOLOGY AND INCIDENCE. Raynaud's disease is the most common cause of Raynaud's phenomenon, accounting for 60 per cent of patients with this disorder. The cause of Raynaud's disease is unknown. Although it can begin at any age, it becomes clinically manifest most commonly between the ages of 20 and 40 years. Raynaud's disease is much more common in women than in men. Two theories have been advanced to explain its occurrence. Raynaud believed that it is caused by increased sympathetic nerve activity. However, measurements of the sympathetic nerve traffic in the median nerve failed to show differences between patients with Raynaud's disease and normal individuals. Lewis discovered that attacks of Raynaud's phenomenon could be induced after interruption of the sympathetic nerves. He concluded that the cause of the disorder was a fault in the arterial wall that rendered the vessels hyperresponsive to the vasoconstrictive effects of cold. He ascribed the vasospastic attacks to spasm of the digital arteries as a result of this hypersensitivity. Little is known about the defect in the vessel wall, which renders the vessel hypersensitive to cold. The circulation of the digits of patients with Raynaud's disease is not hypersensitive to infused norepinephrine. Also, determination of the arteriovenous concentration differences of norepinephrine and epinephrine across the hand showed that there was no excessive release of catecholamines from the hands of patients with Raynaud's disease. More recently, accelerated destruction of platelets and release of agents such as serotonin or thromboxane A_2 have been proposed as causing vasoconstriction in some patients with Raynaud's phenomenon. It is not known whether platelet destruction is the cause of spasm in such patients or a consequence of it.

In a recent study, 26 per cent of patients with the variant type of angina pectoris were found to have migraine, and 24 per cent were found to have Raynaud's phenomenon. This suggested that some patients with Raynaud's phenomenon may have a generalized defect that predisposes arteries in many regions to vasospasm. An association of Raynaud's phenomenon with idiopathic pulmonary hypertension has also been reported. This association may reflect a very high level of peripheral vascular tone secondary to the severe reduction in cardiac output.

Secondary Raynaud's phenomenon is observed frequently as a manifestation of the diseases listed in Table 54–1.

In the presence of arterial obstruction, vasoconstrictive stimuli that normally do not cause clinical manifestations result in more

TABLE 54–1. CAUSES OF SECONDARY RAYNAUD'S PHENOMENON

1. Occlusive arterial disease
   a. Arteriosclerosis obliterans
   b. Buerger's disease
   c. Arterial embolism
   d. Vasculitis
   e. Arterial thrombosis
2. Connective tissue diseases
   a. Scleroderma
   b. Rheumatoid arthritis
   c. Systemic lupus erythematosus
3. Vascular injury
   a. Repetitive minor occupational trauma, as in pneumatic hammer operators, pianists, typists, or users of hand-held vibrating tools
   b. Frostbite
4. Neurogenic causes
   a. Thoracic outlet compression by cervical rib, by scalenus anticus muscle, or in hyperabduction syndrome
   b. Carpal tunnel syndrome
   c. Sympathetic causalgia
   d. Spinal cord diseases
5. Drugs or exposure to chemicals
   a. Ergotamine
   b. Ergotism
   c. Methysergide
   d. Polyvinyl chloride
   e. Beta-adrenergic receptor blockers
   f. Antimetabolite drugs (cisplatin, vinblastine, bleomycin)
6. Intravascular coagulation or aggregation
   a. Cryoglobulinemia
   b. Cold agglutinins

severe reduction in blood flow and may cause Raynaud's phenomenon.

Raynaud's phenomenon is very often associated with connective tissue diseases; it is particularly frequent in scleroderma. Almost all patients with scleroderma develop Raynaud's phenomenon at some time during the course of their illness. A distinctive syndrome consisting of calcinosis, Raynaud's phenomenon, abnormal esophageal motility, sclerodactyly, and telangiectasia (CREST syndrome) is recognized. Raynaud's phenomenon may be the presenting manifestation in connective tissue diseases and may precede the appearance of other manifestations by several years. The presence of abnormal nail fold capillaries in patients with Raynaud's phenomenon has predictive value for the future development of scleroderma. Structural changes in the vessel wall that limit flow and increase the sensitivity to vasoconstrictive influences appear to account for the frequent occurrence of Raynaud's phenomenon in these diseases. Vascular injury may also result from repetitive minor occupational trauma or from a severe exposure to cold, as in frostbite. Consequent hypersensitivity to cold causes Raynaud's phenomenon. Occupationally induced Raynaud's phenomenon is frequently secondary to exposure to a source of vibration. It is referred to as vibration white finger. It usually develops after several years of using hand-held vibrating power tools.

Neurogenic lesions cause Raynaud's phenomenon because of irritation of sympathetic nerves and consequent vasoconstriction. Intense or sustained vasoconstriction caused by drugs may also result in Raynaud's phenomenon, as in 3 to 6 per cent of patients taking β-adrenergic receptor–blocking drugs. Propranolol is the main offender. These drugs block a β-adrenergic vasodilative mechanism in the digits and may also enhance the vasoconstrictive effects of norepinephrine. A high incidence of Raynaud's phenomenon was described during administration of certain antimetabolite drugs, such as cisplatin, vinblastine, and bleomycin. Raynaud's phenomenon was associated with hypomagnesemia, which might have been responsible for vasoconstriction.

Intravascular aggregation or coagulation of blood elements may obstruct the vessels and cause ischemia and Raynaud's phenomenon.

PATHOPHYSIOLOGY. The pallor during the attack of Raynaud's phenomenon is explained by intense vasoconstriction or spasm of the digital arteries. This results in severe reduction in blood flow. In a later stage of the attack, the vasoconstriction becomes less severe, and the capillaries and veins are partially filled with blood whose hemoglobin becomes markedly deoxygenated. This accounts for the cyanosis. Upon rewarming, cyanosis is replaced by an intense red color associated with reactive hyperemia. Between attacks, blood flow to the digits is usually reduced, especially in patients who have trophic changes, but may be normal in some patients. In those patients without trophic changes, blood flow to the hand during maximum vasodilation is the same as in normal individuals, but it is severely reduced in those with trophic changes, a reflection of structural changes in the blood vessels.

PATHOLOGY. In the early stages of the disease, the digital blood vessels are histologically normal. In longstanding cases, the intima becomes thickened, and the media may be hypertrophied. In severe progressive cases, complete obstruction from thrombosis may occur, and gangrene of the tips of the digits may ensue.

CLINICAL MANIFESTATIONS. The onset of Raynaud's disease is usually gradual. The patient notices an occasional mild and short-lasting attack during winter. Over succeeding years, the severity and duration of the attacks may increase. A wide variation in severity is present. Most commonly, the attacks are provoked by exposure to cold. In some patients, attacks are also precipitated by emotion. The attacks may be terminated by rewarming, or they may abate spontaneously. Between attacks, in a warm environment, the patient is asymptomatic, and physical examination shows no abnormalities. Some patients, however, complain of chronically cold hands and feet, and they may have cold fingers with cyanosis on examination. In a typical attack of Raynaud's phenomenon, the digits become pale. Usually, all digits are affected symmetrically. The pallor is sharply demarcated at the level of the metacarpophalangeal joints, a reflection of spasm of the digital arteries. At a later stage during the attack, the

pallor is replaced by cyanosis. The patient may have feelings of coldness, numbness, and occasionally pain. Upon rewarming, the cyanosis is replaced by intense redness, and the patient may feel tingling or throbbing. Most commonly, only the hands are affected. Frequently, both hands and feet are affected. Rarely, the nose, cheeks, ears, and chin are affected also.

Atypical attacks are not infrequent. In these, the involvement of the digits may be asymmetric, with only one or two digits being affected. In some cases, only a portion of the digit is affected. In these instances, the most severely affected portion of the digit is the most distal one. Thus, one may see pallor of the fingertip or of the terminal phalanx of one digit. In other cases, more than one phalanx may be involved.

In severe, progressive cases, trophic changes may occur after a few years of involvement. The hair may disappear from the dorsal aspect of the digits. The nails grow more slowly and become brittle and deformed. The skin becomes atrophic, thin, and tight (sclerodactyly). Ulcerations may develop at the fingertips or around the nail bed. These heal slowly and may become infected. They are extremely painful, especially at night. When they heal, they leave characteristic small, pitted scars.

DIAGNOSIS. The diagnosis of Raynaud's phenomenon can usually be made on the basis of the history of vasospastic attacks in the digits, precipitated by cold and relieved by warming. In atypical cases or when the patient's description of the attack is not clear, provocation of an attack may be helpful. This may be done by immersing the hands in water at a temperature of 10 to 15°C. Whole-body exposure to cold is more successful in provoking attacks. A negative result does not exclude Raynaud's phenomenon.

In typical cases, Raynaud's phenomenon is easily distinguished from acrocyanosis, but when involvement is atypical, the differentiation may be more difficult. Distinguishing features include the following: The color changes in Raynaud's phenomenon are episodic, whereas in acrocyanosis they are sustained. Pallor is not a prominent feature of acrocyanosis. Cyanosis is the more typical color change, whereas in Raynaud's disease digital pallor is characteristic. In Raynaud's disease, only the digits are involved, whereas in acrocyanosis the color changes usually involve the whole hand or foot and sometimes even more proximal portions of the limbs. In Raynaud's disease the skin of the palms is usually dry, whereas in acrocyanosis it is wet and clammy with sweat. Finally, acrocyanosis rarely causes trophic changes and ulcerations.

Obstruction of major arteries from arteriosclerosis, angiitis, embolism, or thrombosis may lead to color changes in the digits that simulate Raynaud's phenomenon. The distinction is made by the demonstration of changes in arterial pulses and by the fact that the color changes in these disorders are likely to be confined to one limb rather than symmetric. Arteriography, which demonstrates the arterial lesion, is helpful. However, secondary Raynaud's phenonenon may be superimposed upon any of these diseases. In Raynaud's phenomenon, Doppler velocity studies show patent arteries and sharply peaked blood flow velocity patterns in the digits. Arteriography shows normal major arteries and diffuse spasm of the digital arteries.

The distinction of Raynaud's disease from secondary Raynaud's phenomenon is based mainly on the exclusion of disorders known to cause secondary Raynaud's phenomenon. The exclusion of obstructive arterial disease is discussed above. Connective tissue disorders, particularly scleroderma, are excluded by the absence of arthralgias or arthritis, alterations of esophageal motility, and the absence of a pulmonary oxygen diffusion defect. The presence of a normal sedimentation rate and the absence of circulating autoantibodies, such as antinuclear antibodies, provide additional reassurance. A careful occupational history is necessary to exclude Raynaud's phenomenon secondary to minor repetitive trauma. A history of drug ingestion or exposure to chemicals is helpful in identifying drug-induced Raynaud's phenomenon. Neurologic disorders can be recognized by their somatic neurologic manifestations. Thoracic outlet compression syndromes can be excluded by the appropriate maneuvers. The presence of intravascular agglutination or coagulation of the blood elements may be suspected if, in the presence of cyanosis, the blood cannot be expelled from vessels by pressure, and when there are isolated areas of redness as the attack abates during rewarming. Confirmation is obtained by demonstrating the cold agglutinins or cryoglobulins in the patient's blood.

TABLE 54–2. TREATMENT OF RAYNAUD'S PHENOMENON

Frequency and Severity of Vasospastic Attacks	Suggested Treatment
1. Rare or mild attacks	Protective measures, cessation of smoking, and no drug therapy
2. Frequent or severe attacks without trophic changes	Protective measures and calcium antagonists
3. Frequent attacks with trophic changes but no open ulcers	Protective measures plus calcium antagonists or oral reserpine plus liothyronine
4. Frequent attacks with active, painful ulcers	Intravenous PGE$_1$, intra-arterial reserpine followed by calcium antagonists; or reserpine plus liothyronine; or oral misoprostol

TABLE 54–3. SOME DRUGS USEFUL IN THE TREATMENT OF RAYNAUD'S PHENOMENON

1. Calcium antagonists
   a. Nifedipine*
   b. Diltiazem*
2. Alpha-adrenergic receptor blockers
   a. Phenoxybenzamine*
   b. Tolazoline
   c. Prazosin*
3. Drugs that interfere with sympathetic nerve activity
   a. Reserpine*
   b. Guanethidine*
   c. Alpha-methyldopa*
4. Vasodilators
   a. PGE$_1$*
   b. PGE$_2$*
   c. PGI$_2$*
   d. Iloprost
   e. Misoprostol*
5. Miscellaneous
   a. Liothyronine*

*Investigational drug for this purpose.

PROGNOSIS. The prognosis of patients with Raynaud's disease is good. There is no mortality associated with the disease and morbidity is low; it is generally limited to loss of portions of digits as a result of ulcerations. In approximately 50 per cent of patients with Raynaud's disease, the disorder improves and may disappear completely after several years. In only a fraction of 1 per cent of patients is amputation necessary. Approximately 15 per cent of patients with Raynaud's phenomenon eventually develop a connective tissue disorder, particularly scleroderma.

The prognosis in secondary Raynaud's phenomenon depends on the course of the primary disorder. In scleroderma, the prognosis is unsatisfactory, particularly when the disease has caused digital ulcerations.

TREATMENT. Management of patients with Raynaud's phenomenon must be tailored to the individual needs of the patient, taking into consideration the frequency and severity of the attacks (Table 54–2). All patients benefit from reassurance and protective measures against exposure to cold. The patients should limit the duration of exposure to cold to the greatest extent possible. They should wear heavy clothing, protecting not only the hands and feet but also the face and trunk, especially when there is a cold wind; this is important because exposure to cold of other portions of the body may reflexly induce vasoconstriction in the digits and precipitate Raynaud's phenomenon. When prolonged exposure to cold is unavoidable, the use of electrically powered or solid fuel–powered hand and foot warmers is advisable. These patients should be taught to recognize and terminate attacks by returning promptly to a warm environment, placing their hands in warm water, or using a warm-air hairblower to warm their hands rapidly. Smoking causes cutaneous vasoconstriction; therefore, tobacco smoking is contraindicated in Raynaud's phenomenon. The use of induced vasodilation by placing the hands in warm water (43°C) has been reported to raise skin temperature and minimize the severity of attacks of Raynaud's phenomenon. Biofeedback to teach patients to raise skin temperature voluntarily has been shown to limit the duration and frequency of vasospastic attacks, but its effect is nonspecific because it is also seen in control patients who received no such treatment and in those in whom biofeedback is used to teach relaxation. In patients with Raynaud's phenomenon secondary to vibration, the use of vibrating tools must cease. However, termination of exposure to vibration does not always eliminate Raynaud's phenomenon.

The simple measures outlined above usually suffice for patients with infrequent or mild attacks. When Raynaud's phenomenon is more frequent or more severe, and especially when it has resulted in trophic changes or ulcerations, these measures need to be supplemented by drugs. The aim of drug therapy is to induce vascular smooth muscle relaxation, thereby relieving spasm, raising resting blood flow, and limiting the degree of ischemia during attacks. The drugs most frequently used in treating patients with Raynaud's phenomenon are shown in Table 54–3. For most patients, the drug of choice is a calcium antagonist. Nifedipine* has been found to be effective in several well-controlled, double-blind studies. The drug is administered at a dose of 10 to 20 mg three or four times daily. Diltiazem,* at a dose of 60 mg three or four times daily, may be substituted, if nifedipine is not well tolerated or if it causes side effects. In one study of very severely affected patients, verapamil was found not to be effective. The angiotensin-converting enzyme inhibitors enalapril and captopril are also effective in reducing the frequency and decreasing the severity of Raynaud's phenomenon. They have been less extensively studied than calcium antagonists, although they appear equally effective. Enalapril is administered by mouth in a dose of 10 to 20 mg once daily, and captopril in a dose of 25 to 50 mg two to three times daily.

Reserpine* is the best-studied drug among the group that interferes with the function of the adrenergic nervous system. It is administered by mouth in doses of 0.1 to 0.5 mg daily. In cases in which ulcerations have developed, it may be given intra-arterially in a dose of 0.5 to 1 mg, dissolved in saline and administered into the brachial or radial artery by slow infusion over several minutes. The drugs in this group may also be administered by means of tourniquet-controlled intravenous injection (Bier's block). The administration by the last two routes gives a much higher local concentration and largely avoids systemic side effects.

In controlled trials, nitroglycerin* ointment or topical prostaglandin E$_2$* (PGE$_2$) has been found effective in Raynaud's phenomenon. The topical application of these drugs is advantageous because their local relaxant action is not counteracted by reflex vasoconstriction secondary to changes in blood pressure that may occur when they are given systemically.

Prostaglandin E$_1$* (PGE$_1$) or prostacyclin* (PGI$_2$) administered intravenously has a beneficial effect in patients with Raynaud's phenomenon. These drugs can be given by constant intravenous infusion in a dose of 6 to 10 ng per kilogram per minute for a few hours or up to 3 days. Iloprost is an experimental stable analogue of PGI$_2$. It is administered intravenously in a dose of 0.5 to 2 ng per kilogram per minute for several hours. Misoprostol* is an analogue of PGE$_1$. It is administered by mouth in a dose of 0.2 mg three or four times daily. It is reported that the beneficial effect outlasts this therapy by several weeks. All these drugs act by inducing vasodilation and also by inhibiting platelet aggregation.

A novel but effective way of inducing vasodilation in the digits is via the iatrogenic induction of hyperthyroidism by the administration of sodium liothyronine* (triiodothyronine), 75 μg daily. The resultant hypermetabolism elicits thermoregulatory reflex cutaneous vasodilation. The combination of triiodothyronine and reserpine has been found to be most effective.

Preganglionic sympathectomy to eliminate vasoconstrictor tone may have a beneficial immediate result, but the long-term results are disappointing. The duration of benefit is limited by regeneration of the nerves. If sympathectomy is contemplated, it is advisable to try sympathetic blockade with local anesthetics to verify a beneficial result. A recently devised technique that

*Investigational drug for this purpose.

involves surgical stripping of the palmar and digital arteries to bring about a local sympathectomy may also be tried, but its results have not been fully evaluated.

Coffman JD, Davis WT: Vasospastic diseases: A review. Prog Cardiovasc Dis 18:123, 1975. *A comprehensive, well-referenced review of vasospastic diseases.*

Cohen RA, Coffman JD: β-Adrenergic vasodilator mechanism in the finger. Circ Res 49:1196, 1981. *Demonstration of a β-adrenergic, humorally activated, vasodilative mechanism in the arteriovenous anastomoses of the human finger. Blockade of this mechanism may explain the occurrence of Raynaud's phenomenon in patients taking β-adrenergic receptor–blocking drugs.*

Fagius J, Blumberg H: Sympathetic outflow to the hand in patients with Raynaud's phenomenon. Cardiovasc Res 19:249, 1985. *Demonstration that sympathetic nerve activity in patients with Raynaud's phenomenon under baseline conditions and during maneuvers that increase sympathetic nerve traffic does not differ from that in normal controls. The results do not support the theory that Raynaud's disease is caused by increased sympathetic nerve activity.*

Harper FE, Maricq HR, Turner RE, et al.: A prospective study of Raynaud's phenomenon and early connective tissue disease. Am J Med 72:883, 1982. *This study of capillaries of the nail fold shows that the presence of capillary abnormalities in patients with Raynaud's phenomenon may have predictive value for the future development of scleroderma.*

Janini SD, Scott JS, Coppock PAB, et al.: Enalapril in Raynaud's phenomenon. J Clin Pharmacol Ther 13:145, 1988. *Report of a prospective double-blind crossover trial showing that enalapril is effective in reducing the frequency and severity of attacks of Raynaud's phenomenon.*

Kontos HA, Wasserman AJ: Effect of reserpine in Raynaud's phenomenon. Circulation 39:259, 1969. *An analysis of the effects of reserpine given intra-arterially and orally on hand blood flow in patients with Raynaud's disease. It also contains evidence against the hypothesis that defective catecholamine metabolism may account for Raynaud's disease. Beneficial results from oral administration of reserpine are also presented.*

Miller D, Waters DD, Warnica W, et al.: Is variant angina the coronary manifestation of a generalized vasospastic disorder? N Engl J Med 304:763, 1981. *Provocative study showing high incidence of migraine and Raynaud's phenomenon in patients with variant angina, suggesting the possibility that we may be dealing with a generalized vasospastic disorder.*

Roath S: Management of Raynaud's phenomenon: Focus on newer treatments. Drugs 37:700, 1989. *Comprehensive consideration of drug therapy in Raynaud's phenomenon.*

Smith CR, Rodeheffer RJ: Treatment of Raynaud's phenomenon with calcium channel blockers. Am J Med 78 (Suppl 2B):39, 1985. *Concise consideration of the pathophysiology of Raynaud's phenomenon and review of available evidence concerning the effectiveness of treatment with calcium antagonists.*

Acrocyanosis

DEFINITION. Acrocyanosis is a rare disorder characterized by persistent cyanosis of the skin of the hands and, less commonly, of the feet associated with reduced skin temperature.

ETIOLOGY. Acrocyanosis is a primary disorder of unknown cause. It is much more common in women than in men. The onset of the disease is usually in young adults or middle-aged persons. The high incidence of the disease among patients with psychiatric disorders is of unknown significance.

PATHOPHYSIOLOGY. The smaller precapillary vessels (arterioles) are abnormally constricted, causing reduction in blood flow and accounting for cyanosis and reduced skin temperature. The veins are secondarily dilated. Constriction of the arterioles occurs under normal environmental conditions and becomes more pronounced on exposure to cold because of increased sensitivity of these vessels to the effects of cold. An important feature of acrocyanosis is the reduced venous tone. No venous obstruction is present. These features can be demonstrated by elevating the involved limb and eliminating the blue color or intensifying the blue color by placing the limb in a dependent position and overfilling the veins.

CLINICAL MANIFESTATIONS. Patients with acrocyanosis have persistent blue discoloration of the hands. Less commonly, the feet are also involved. In some cases, the blue color extends to more proximal portions of the limbs. The skin is cold, and the palms are wet and clammy from sweat. No pallor is usually present. In some cases, there may be spots of pallor surrounded by confluent cyanosis. The blue color is intensified by exposure to cold, and it is converted into purplish or red color by exposure to heat. There are few accompanying symptoms. The patient has feelings of coldness and, occasionally, numbness. Ulcerations and other trophic changes are distinctly unusual. Patients with acrocyanosis seek medical advice either because they are frightened or because the cyanosis is cosmetically unappealing.

DIAGNOSIS. The distinction between acrocyanosis and Raynaud's phenomenon is discussed above in the section on Raynaud's phenomenon. Differentiation from cyanosis secondary to arterial obstruction can be made on the basis of normal pulses, by the bilateral and symmetric occurrence of acrocyanosis, and, if necessary, by the angiographic verification of absence of obstruction. The limitation of the cyanosis to the hands and feet, the improvement in a warm environment, and the absence of reduced arterial blood saturation distinguish acrocyanosis from generalized, systemic cyanosis.

TREATMENT. Since acrocyanosis is a benign disease, no drug therapy is usually required. Reassurance and protection from cold usually suffice. In some cases, cosmetic considerations or unusually severe symptoms may necessitate drug therapy. In these cases, the same drugs that are useful in Raynaud's phenomenon may be tried.

Lewis T, Landis EM: Observations upon the vascular mechanism in acrocyanosis. Heart 15:229, 1930. *Classic description of the clinical features of acrocyanosis. Evidence is presented showing that the disease is the result of an abnormal responsiveness of the smaller blood vessels.*

Livedo Reticularis

DEFINITION. Livedo reticularis is a reticular, bluish discoloration of the skin of the extremities that produces a lacy, irregular appearance outlining central areas of normal-appearing skin. The etiology is not known. The disorder usually begins in young individuals before age 20 to 30 years. It is equally common in men and women but more often symptomatic in women.

PATHOLOGY. Proliferative lesions of the arterioles of the skin with perivascular infiltration have been described. In some cases, there may be thrombosis of arterioles leading to cutaneous infarction and ulceration. Similar changes are seen in the veins.

PATHOPHYSIOLOGY. The mechanism of livedo reticularis is presumed to be similar to that of acrocyanosis, namely, constriction of arterioles followed by stasis and dilation of capillaries and veins. The latter are filled with desaturated blood. The reticular appearance of livedo reticularis reflects the anatomic arrangement of the affected vessels. It is believed that the bluish areas represent the arborizations of peripheral capillaries from central penetrating arterioles. Blood flow is faster in the central regions closer to the penetrating arteriole, whereas the more distant areas have lower flow, with consequent stasis and cyanosis.

CLINICAL MANIFESTATIONS. Patients seek medical attention for cosmetic reasons or because they are frightened by the bluish discoloration. The lower extremities are involved more often than the upper extremities. The patient usually has no symptoms. In some cases, there may be paresthesias or a feeling of coldness. The bluish discoloration becomes more intense on exposure to cold and may disappear in a warm environment. Ulcerations occur rarely; when they do, they appear in winter and heal in summer.

TREATMENT. In most cases no treatment is required. Protection from cold and abstinence from tobacco are useful. In severe cases, drugs useful in the treatment of Raynaud's phenomenon, such as nifedipine and reserpine, may be tried.

Feldaker M, Hines EA, Kierland RR: Livedo reticularis with ulcerations. Circulation 13:196, 1956. *Report of the clinical and pathologic features of 18 patients with livedo reticularis with ulcerations. A brief review of the earlier literature is included.*

Erythromelalgia (Erythermalgia)

DEFINITION. Erythromelalgia is a disorder manifested by episodes of erythema accompanied by increased skin temperature and by pain involving the feet and, less commonly, the hands. It may be primary or secondary to other disorders. Erythromelalgia is considered further in Ch. 280.

PATHOPHYSIOLOGY. The symptoms of erythromelalgia are dependent on skin temperature. Rise in skin temperature above a certain level causes the manifestations. In each person this critical point is fairly constant. Vasodilation and consequent hyperemia are the usual causes of the rise in skin temperature. However, an increased blood flow is not essential, since once symptoms have been induced by heat, they may continue even though blood flow is reduced to zero with a cuff inflated above the systolic pressure levels. These features suggest that the cause of the disorder is abnormal sensitivity of the cutaneous pain fibers to heat or tension from the dilated blood vessels.

CLINICAL MANIFESTATIONS. The onset of the disease is

gradual. With progression, the frequency and duration of the attacks become more pronounced. Eventually, symptoms may become almost continuous and cause total disability. During an attack the patient complains of burning pain, usually in the feet and, less commonly, in the hands. The pain is usually located in the balls of the feet and in the tips of the toes and in the corresponding parts of the hands. Pain is aggravated by dependency and ameliorated by elevation of the limbs. Exposure to heat aggravates the disorder, whereas cold provides relief. Trophic changes, ulcerations, and gangrene are rare.

DIAGNOSIS. Peripheral neuropathy may cause burning pain simulating erythromelalgia. The pain may be accompanied by cutaneous vasodilation. The detection of the associated sensory and motor manifestations of peripheral neuropathy should help distinguish this condition from erythromelalgia. Arteriosclerosis obliterans or thromboangiitis obliterans may also produce localized burning pain and redness. The alterations in the arterial pulses and the absence of high skin temperature distinguish these conditions from erythromelalgia. Vascular damage from prolonged exposure to cold, as after frostbite, may simulate erythromelalgia. In these cases, the condition is more persistent, and the history of cold exposure should help make the distinction possible.

TREATMENT. Avoidance of exposure to heat, particularly dry heat, prevents attacks of erythromelalgia. Elevation of the extremity and application of cold may terminate an attack. Aspirin, 0.5 gram orally, relieves the pain in many cases. The response is sometimes so striking that it is of diagnostic value. Vasoconstrictive agents, such as methysergide or epinephrine, or β-adrenergic blocking agents, such as propranolol, have been reported to be effective in some patients. In secondary cases, treatment of the primary disorder may alleviate the attacks.

Babb RR, Alarçon-Segovia D, Fairbairn JF: Erythermalgia: Review of 51 cases. Circulation 29:136, 1964. *Description of the features of primary and secondary erythromelalgia based on a study of a large number of patients.*

Lewis T: Clinical observations and experiments relating to burning pain in the extremities, and to so-called "erythromelalgia" in particular. Clin Sci 1:175, 1933. *A classic paper with detailed clinical descriptions of the manifestations of erythromelalgia. The paper also presents clinical investigations pertinent to the pathogenesis of the disease.*

VASCULAR DISEASES OF THE LIMBS CAUSED BY DAMAGE FROM COLD

Immersion Foot (Trench Foot)

DEFINITION AND ETIOLOGY. Immersion foot is characterized by vascular damage resulting from prolonged exposure of the extremities to cold by wearing wet socks or wet footwear. Usually, the exposure is for several days at about 0°C. Dependency of limbs and immobility, as well as conditions that lead to general debility (lack of sleep and starvation), are contributory factors. The condition occurs primarily in soldiers at war.

Immersion foot has been described in survivors of shipwrecks, who were immobilized in crowded small craft for prolonged periods of time and exposed to wetness and cold. Maceration of the skin with sea water and secondary infection also contribute.

PATHOPHYSIOLOGY. This condition results from vascular injury. The initial effect of cold is to cause vasoconstriction. Loss of heat is facilitated by moisture. The resultant ischemia causes tissue and vascular injury with increased endothelial permeability. There is extensive extravasation of protein and fluid. As a result, there may be increased hematocrit, sludging, and further aggravation of ischemia.

PATHOLOGY. Little is known about the earliest pathologic change in the blood vessels in immersion foot. Most of the available information has been obtained from advanced cases with extensive vascular injury and gangrene. In these cases, the small arteries exhibit periarterial fibrosis and thickening and may be occluded. The veins show perivenous fibrosis, inflammatory reaction, and hemorrhage. The nerves may also be affected. In cases of immersion foot at relatively high temperatures, hyperhydration of the plantar stratum corneum may be the only finding.

CLINICAL MANIFESTATIONS. Three successive stages, each with distinct clinical manifestations, are recognized. During exposure to the wet, cold environment, there is vasoconstriction. The involved extremity becomes pale and cool, and the patient has paresthesias and a feeling of coldness. A second hyperemic stage follows. Patients are observed most commonly during this stage, because this is when they seek attention. The involved

extremity is red, hot, and edematous. There may be pain or paresthesias. The swelling may be aggravated by heat and by placing the limb in a dependent position. Subsequently, blebs appear, filled with serous or hemorrhagic fluid. Hemorrhages may occur into the skin and subcutaneous tissue. This stage may persist for several days. In severe cases, gangrene may supervene. The condition may be complicated by lymphangitis, cellulitis, and thrombophlebitis. Mild cases or those treated early may recover after this second hyperemic phase. In other cases, a third late vasospastic phase occurs in which there is increased sensitivity to cold and typical secondary Raynaud's phenomenon, with excessive sweating, pain, and paresthesias of the lower extremities. This phase may persist for years.

TREATMENT. If the patient is seen in the initial vasoconstrictive phase, bed rest with the extremity in the horizontal position and a warm environment are necessary. During the hyperemic phase, the extremity should be placed at heart level and kept cool to diminish edema. Local care to keep the foot dry and clean should be instituted to avoid infection. Control of pain may require analgesics or narcotics. Sympathectomy may be helpful in the hyperemic stage and also in preventing the late vasospastic phenomena.

Abramson DI, Lerner D, Shumacker HB, et al.: Clinical picture and treatment of the later stage of trench foot. Am Heart J 32:52, 1946. *Clinical report based on the study of 633 patients with trench foot. Emphasis is placed on the late sequelae of the disorder.*

Frostbite

DEFINITION AND ETIOLOGY. Frostbite results from freezing of the tissues and consequent vascular injury. In most cases, frostbite occurs during prolonged exposure to temperatures below 0°C. Other environmental factors also play a role, such as high wind and humidity. Predisposing factors include vascular disease, inadequate clothing, lack of acclimatization, and general debility.

PATHOPHYSIOLOGY. Tissue damage results from cold-influenced vasoconstriction. Freezing causes water crystal formation in cells and dehydration. Endothelial damage with increased permeability to protein ensues, causes edema, and further contributes to stasis and eventual thrombosis.

PATHOLOGY. The vessels show endothelial swelling and vacuolization and proliferative changes. Subsequently, there are inflammatory reactions and atrophic changes in the skin.

CLINICAL MANIFESTATIONS. Initially, the patient notices a prickling sensation followed by numbness. The skin becomes bloodless and appears white and cold. This is followed by redness, swelling, and increased temperature. Blisters may form 24 to 48 hours after thawing. They are filled with either serous yellow or hemorrhagic fluid. There may be hemorrhages under the nail beds. Necrosis and gangrene may supervene. The subsequent course may be similar to that of sudden arterial occlusion, including ischemia and gangrene. Spontaneous amputation may require several weeks or months. After an attack of frostbite, the affected extremities may remain sensitive to cold for a period of time or permanently, and secondary Raynaud's phenomenon may occur.

TREATMENT. Frostbite should be treated with immediate rewarming. If frostbite affects deep tissues, rewarming should be done with water at 40 to 44°C. Muscular exercise of the involved limb and massage should be avoided, because they tend to increase edema and pain. If pain is severe, it should be treated with analgesics or narcotics. After the tissues have thawed, the exposed parts should remain at room temperatures. Vesicles should be left untouched, and the limb should be left exposed, without dressings. Antibiotic therapy should be used if infection is present. Sympathectomy has been reported to be beneficial in the initial stages as well as in preventing the delayed sequelae of frostbite.

Washburn B: Frostbite. N Engl J Med 266:974, 1962. *Comprehensive consideration of the clinical features, pathology, diagnosis, prevention, and treatment of frostbite.*

Chilblain (Pernio)

DEFINITION. Chilblain is an inflammatory condition of the skin of the extremities induced by cold and characterized by erythema, itching, and ulceration. The cause is unknown. It is more common in cold, damp climates, as in England, than in the United States. Women are affected more commonly than men. In most patients, the disease begins before the age of 20 years.

PATHOLOGY. In chronic cases, the lesions consist of angiitis with intimal proliferation, thickening of the arterial wall, and perivascular infiltration with lymphocytes and polymorphonuclear leukocytes. There may be necrosis of the adipose tissue and chronic inflammatory infiltrates in the subcutaneous tissue.

CLINICAL MANIFESTATIONS. Both acute and chronic forms of the disease are recognized. The typical patient is a young woman who, in the winter, notices bluish-red discoloration and edema of the skin of the lower limbs associated with burning and warmth. The lesions are persistent and are associated with itching. They generally last from 7 to 10 days and then clear up, sometimes leaving residual pigmentation of the skin. In severe cases, the lesions may become hemorrhagic, or blebs may appear. Infection may supervene.

With repeated exposure to cold, susceptible persons may develop chronic lesions. These are erythematous, ulcerative, and hemorrhagic lesions that begin as raised, red areas 0.5 to 1 cm in diameter. These lesions are then transformed into blebs and finally ulcerate. Healing occurs in the summer, leaving a permanently pigmented region.

DIAGNOSIS. Acute chilblain is distinguished from other forms of dermatitis by its characteristic distribution and by its relationship to cold. Chronic chilblain needs to be distinguished from erythema induratum and erythema nodosum. Erythema induratum of Bazin is caused by *Mycobacterium tuberculosis*. If the infection is active, the differential diagnosis may be made by the microscopic demonstration or culture of bacteria. Erythema induratum affects the upper part of the legs more frequently than the lower part. The lesions are more nodular, deeper, and infiltrative. They are also more permanent, whereas those of chronic chilblain clear up in the summer. Erythema nodosum is a more acute process, and it is usually associated with a systemic reaction, consisting of fever, malaise, and arthralgias. There is no seasonal association.

TREATMENT. In mild cases, protection from cold, local application of anti-inflammatory ointments, avoidance of scratching, and cessation of smoking are usually sufficient. In more severe cases, drugs that have been found useful in the treatment of Raynaud's phenomenon, such as reserpine or nifedipine, may be effective.

Eskell J: Reserpine in the treatment of chilblains. Practitioner 189:792, 1962. *Report of a controlled clinical trial of reserpine in patients with chilblain showing excellent benefit.*

Lynn RB: Chilblains. Surg Gynecol Obstet 99:720, 1954. *Concise description of the clinical and pathologic features of chilblain.*

Rustin MHA, Newton JA, Smith NP, et al.: The treatment of chilblain with nifedipine: The results of a pilot study, a double-blind placebo-controlled randomized study and a long-term open trial. Br J Dermatol 120:267, 1989. *Report of a controlled trial showing that nifedipine accelerated the clearance of chilblain and prevented the development of new lesions. It also caused symptomatic relief and resolution of edema and perivascular infiltration.*

VASCULAR DISEASES OF THE LIMBS CAUSED BY ORGANIC ARTERIAL OBSTRUCTION

Arteriosclerosis Obliterans

DEFINITION. Arteriosclerosis obliterans consists of segmental arteriosclerotic narrowing or obstruction of the lumen in the arteries supplying the limbs.

ETIOLOGY AND INCIDENCE. The etiology of arteriosclerosis in general is discussed in another chapter (see Ch. 47).

Arteriosclerosis obliterans is the most common cause of arterial obstructive disease of the extremities. The disease becomes clinically manifest usually between the ages of 50 and 70. It is unusual in individuals younger than 30 years of age. Men are affected more often than women. The lower limbs are involved much more frequently than the upper limbs. The most commonly affected vessel is the superficial femoral artery. The distal aorta and its bifurcation into the two iliac arteries and the popliteal artery are the next most frequent sites of involvement. The presence of diabetes mellitus influences arteriosclerosis obliterans in a number of important ways. In diabetics, arteriosclerosis

obliterans is likely to be more progressive. This is reflected in a much higher incidence of intermittent claudication in diabetics. The disease affects arterial vessels of smaller caliber and more distally located vessels more frequently than in nondiabetics. The incidence of involvement of vessels below the knee with arteriosclerosis obliterans in diabetics is considerably higher than in nondiabetics.

PATHOLOGY. The lesions of arteriosclerosis obliterans are typical atheromatous plaques involving the intima of the arteries. As a rule, there is superimposed thrombus formation. The media of the vessels shows degenerative changes. Calcification of the media is frequent and may take the form of a ringlike arrangement, as in Mönckeberg's sclerosis. Medial calcification is twice as frequent in diabetics as in nondiabetics. These arteriosclerotic lesions are segmental, and they are typically multiple. Weakening of the media may give rise to aneurysmal dilation of the involved artery. Such arteriosclerotic aneurysms are most common in the popliteal fossa or in the femoral artery below the inguinal ligament. They may be filled with thrombi.

PATHOPHYSIOLOGY. The arterial obstruction or narrowing causes reduction in blood flow during exercise or at rest. Clinical symptoms are caused by the consequent ischemia. The most important feature of the stenosis in determining ischemia is the cross-sectional area of the stenotic segment. Because the vascular bed of the extremities generally has a high resting vascular tone and, therefore, a large capacity for vasodilation, a moderate degree of stenosis can be compensated fully by downstream dilation. Stenoses that decrease the cross-sectional area of the vessel by less than 75 per cent do not usually affect resting blood flow. When the prevailing flow rates are high, as in exercise, decreases of 60 per cent or more in cross-sectional area are required before a reduction in flow occurs. Vasodilation in response to ischemia is the result of the action of local mechanisms. These include myogenic mechanisms related to reduction in intravascular pressure or metabolic mechanisms due to release of vasodilative metabolites from the ischemic tissues. These local mechanisms compete with neurogenic mechanisms that, when activated, cause vasoconstriction. Increased sympathetic activity, as from exposure to cold, may, therefore, induce ischemia in the presence of an arterial obstructing lesion.

The presence or absence of ischemia in the face of severe arterial stenosis or obstruction is frequently determined by the degree of development of collateral circulation. Some collateral vessels are present in the normal limb but are not used until obstruction takes place. They open up immediately after an acute arterial occlusion. Others take several weeks or months to become fully developed. Little is known about the responsiveness of collateral vessels. They are subject to neurogenic vasoconstriction from the action of adrenergic nerves. They dilate in response to increased blood pressure, resulting in improved collateral blood flow.

CLINICAL MANIFESTATIONS. The symptoms of arteriosclerosis obliterans are intermittent claudication, pain at rest, and trophic changes in the involved limb. Intermittent claudication denotes pain that develops in a limb on exercise and disappears when the patient rests. The pain is usually described as a cramp or a tightness or as severe fatigue of the exercising muscles. The amount of exercise necessary to induce the pain is usually constant for any given patient. The pain is usually bilateral. In some patients, the pain disappears by slowing the pace of walking without complete cessation of exercise. The location of the pain is distal to the arterial obstruction. The most frequently affected muscles are those of the calf, because of the high frequency with which the femoral artery is involved. The muscles of the lower part of the back, the buttocks, the thigh, and the foot may also be affected.

Pain at rest occurs when a pronounced reduction in resting blood flow is present. It is a sign of severe disease. The pain may be localized to one or more toes, or it may have a stocking-type distribution. The character of the pain is usually burning or gnawing. It is generally worse at night. It is improved by placing the limb in a dependent position and by cooling. There may be associated coldness and numbness, together with cyanosis or pallor of the extremity.

Examination discloses reduced or absent arterial pulses distal to the obstruction. There may be bruits audible over the aorta or its branches. These may be systolic, or they may be continuous.

In advanced cases, examination may reveal signs of ischemia. The skin temperature may be abnormally low, or there may be pallor or cyanosis. Ischemic damage may cause persistent reddish or reddish-blue discoloration. There may be trophic changes, including a dry, scaly, and shiny skin. The hair may disappear, and the toenails may become brittle, ridged, and deformed. There may be ulcerations or gangrene. The ischemic ulcers are usually at pressure points and may be inflamed and painful.

Leriche's syndrome refers to isolated aortoiliac disease, which produces a fairly characteristic clinical picture. There is intermittent claudication of the low back, buttocks, and thigh or calf muscles. There is atrophy of the limbs and pallor of the skin of the feet and legs. Impotence may also be present. Arterial pulses in the legs are absent; they may be present but weak in the femoral arteries. Systolic bruits may be audible over the femoral arteries and lower abdomen.

Arteriosclerotic aneurysms may occur, and present as pulsatile, expansible masses in the popliteal fossa or in the femoral artery below the inguinal ligament. These may cause symptoms by pressure on adjacent structures, and, occasionally, by embolism of peripheral vessels or by hemorrhage into the tissues.

DIAGNOSIS. The diagnostic approach to the patient with arteriosclerosis obliterans should be directed at establishing the site of the arterial obstruction, its severity, the degree of ischemia, and the adequacy of the collateral circulation. Palpation of the arterial pulses and auscultation of bruits usually suffice to determine the presence and site of arterial obstruction. Trophic changes and alterations in skin color and temperature indicate ischemia. The latter, as well as the adequacy of the collateral circulation, can be further ascertained by determining the blood pressure at the ankle at rest and during exercise. Several tests may be helpful. With the patient in a warm environment, so that vasoconstrictor tone is low, the leg is raised to a 45-degree angle while the patient is supine. The color of the plantar surface of the foot is observed. Pallor during this test is indicative of severe arterial insufficiency. Venous and capillary filling times can be measured when the patient shifts from the recumbent to the sitting position. Ordinarily, delay in flushing by more than 20 to 30 seconds indicates inadequate collateral circulation. The systolic blood pressure in the dorsalis pedis or posterior tibial arteries can be determined with the use of a Doppler velocitometer at rest as well as during exercise. Ordinarily, this pressure should not be lower than 90 per cent of the level of systolic pressure in the brachial artery. In the presence of severe ischemia, pressures may fall to very low levels. As a rule, pressures less than 30 mm Hg indicate ischemia of sufficient severity to cause gangrene.

The confirmation of arterial obstruction is carried out by arteriography, which is essential to establish the exact anatomy of the arterial vessels and to determine the advisability of surgery.

Arterial embolism is usually distinguishable from arteriosclerosis obliterans because of the sudden onset of the ischemic manifestations and the usually unilateral involvement. Intermittent claudication may occur in severe anemia, in venous disease, and in muscle phosphorylase deficiency (McArdle's syndrome). These conditions are distinguished from arteriosclerosis obliterans by the presence of normal pulses. Ergotamine or methysergide toxicity may cause severe vasospasm, which may affect the large arteries and diminish pulses. The history of drug ingestion may help distinguish these from arteriosclerosis obliterans. In difficult cases, angiography shows the generalized vasospasm and absence of segmental obstructions. A number of conditions of nonvascular nature, such as arthritis and lumbar disc disorders, may cause pain in the limbs and may be confused with intermittent claudication. The presence of normal pulses and other manifestations of these diseases distinguishes them from arteriosclerosis obliterans. In diabetics, ulcerations may be present as a result of diabetic neuropathy. The cause of these ulcers may be difficult to ascertain in the presence of arteriosclerosis obliterans.

TREATMENT. Patients with arteriosclerosis obliterans without evidence of ischemia should be treated medically. Limitation of physical activity, avoidance of tobacco smoking (which causes vasoconstriction), and a regular exercise program are advisable. The treatment of hyperlipidemia, if present, may prevent development of new arteriosclerotic lesions. The control of diabetes, if present, is required. Patients should maintain the skin of the affected limbs clean, dry, and soft and protect it from cold and trauma. Infections and trauma should be attended to promptly.

There is no evidence that vasodilative drugs are effective in the treatment of arteriosclerosis obliterans. In fact, they may be harmful under certain circumstances by lowering arterial blood pressure and reducing collateral blood flow or by diverting blood to proximal healthy areas, thereby reducing the perfusion pressure in the more distal portions of the limb. Pentoxifylline, 400 mg administered orally three times daily, has been shown in controlled trials to prolong the duration of exercise and the distance the patient is able to walk prior to the onset of claudication. The drug acts by increasing red cell membrane deformability, thereby reducing effective blood viscosity.

Surgical treatment is advisable when ischemia is present or if intermittent claudication seriously interferes with the patient's activities. Surgery involves either endarterectomy of the stenotic artery or a bypass operation. Bypass can be performed with either a vein graft or synthetic material. Vein grafts are preferred because of the lower incidence of thrombosis. It is essential that the presence of patent vessels below the obstruction be ascertained before the grafting procedure is carried out. Axillofemoral or femorofemoral grafts for aortoiliac disease have been successful. The larger the size of the vessels grafted, the higher the rate of successful restoration of blood flow.

Percutaneous transluminal angioplasty offers an attractive alternative to surgery in the treatment of arteriosclerosis obliterans. It is simple, has low morbidity, and is less costly than surgery. In this technique, the segmental stenosis or obstruction is dilated by suddenly inflating at the site of the lesion a balloon introduced into the artery by percutaneous catheterization. High success rates and good long-term rates of patency of the dilated vessels have been reported. Angioplasty is more successful in larger vessels, when the stenotic segment is relatively short and when the vessel is not completely occluded. Restenosis of lesions dilated by angioplasty occurs in 20 to 30 per cent of the patients within a year. It may be due to thrombosis or, more commonly, to intimal and medial proliferation.

Atherectomy is a newly introduced alternative to balloon angioplasty. In this technique, the obstructing lesion is eliminated by shaving off successive layers with a special atherectomy catheter equipped with a rotary cutting device. The technique may be advantageous when used for repeat angioplasty following restenosis.

If the anatomy of the disease makes surgery impossible and ischemic manifestations are present, bed rest is essential. The affected extremity should be kept in a slightly dependent position at 20 to 30 degrees below horizontal, and direct application of heat should be avoided. The limb is best kept warm by placing it under a cradle, under which the temperature is regulated below 38°C. Analgesics or narcotics may be required to control pain. Ulcers should be kept clean with warm saline soaks and debrided. Appropriate antibiotics should be used if infection is present. Intra-arterial administration of PGE_1* may be beneficial in patients with gangrene or ulceration in whom surgery is not possible. Amputation may be necessary to arrest advancing gangrene. The level of amputation is chosen by the presence of warm, viable tissue having normal color.

Long-term anticoagulants are of questionable value. Fibrinolytic therapy with intravenous streptokinase is reported to be helpful in a few patients with recent onset of the disease.

Preganglionic lumbar sympathectomy may be performed as an acute intervention to treat ischemic manifestations of arteriosclerosis obliterans. Before surgery, it must be demonstrated that the interruption of sympathetic nerves is likely to cause improvement in the circulation of the limb. This is done by inducing temporary sympathetic blockade with local anesthetics. This is essential, especially in diabetics in whom peripheral neuropathy may have already produced spontaneous sympathectomy. Sympathectomy does not influence the long-term prognosis of intermittent claudication.

PROGNOSIS. Arteriosclerosis obliterans in the absence of diabetes is a slowly progressive disease. No significant deterioration may be detected for several years. In the presence of diabetes, the disease tends to progress more rapidly, and the

---

*Investigational drug for this purpose.

prognosis is less satisfactory. The location of obstructing lesions also influences the prognosis. When the lesions are in larger arteries, the probability of successful surgical intervention or percutaneous angioplasty is higher, and the prognosis is better. Frequently arteriosclerosis obliterans is only one of the manifestations of a generalized arteriosclerotic process. Mortality results from arteriosclerotic involvement of other vascular beds, such as the coronary or the cerebral circulation, with death from myocardial infarction or stroke.

Coffman JD: Intermittent claudication and rest pain. Physiologic concepts and therapeutic approaches. Prog Cardiovasc Dis 22:53, 1979. *A comprehensive, well-referenced consideration of the clinical features, diagnosis, and treatment of arteriosclerosis obliterans.*

Freiman DB, Spence R, Gatenby R, et al.: Transluminal angioplasty of the iliac and femoral arteries: Follow-up results with anticoagulation. Radiology 141:347, 1981. *Transluminal angioplasty for the treatment of obstructive disease of the iliac and femoral arteries. Excellent results are reported in 192 patients.*

Porter JM, Culter BS, Lee BY, et al.: Pentoxifylline efficacy in the treatment of intermittent claudication: Multicenter controlled double-blind trial with objective assessment of chronic occlusive arterial disease patients. Am Heart J 104:66, 1982. *A controlled trial of pentoxifylline in patients with intermittent claudication demonstrating objectively improved exercise tolerance.*

Schadt DC, Hines EA, Juergens JL, et al.: Chronic atherosclerotic occlusion of the femoral artery. JAMA 175 937, 1961. *A long-term follow-up study showing slow progression of arteriosclerosis obliterans.*

Thromboangiitis Obliterans (Buerger's Disease)

DEFINITION. Thromboangiitis obliterans is an obstructive arterial disease caused by segmental inflammatory and proliferative lesions of the medium and small arteries and veins of the limbs.

ETIOLOGY. The cause of thromboangiitis obliterans is unknown. Almost all patients with this disease are moderate or heavy smokers, particularly of cigarettes. Many show cutaneous hypersensitivity to intradermally injected tobacco products. There is a high prevalence of HLA-A9 and HLA-B5 antigens in affected persons. An autoimmune mechanism is suggested by a study of cellular and humoral immune responses of 39 patients with thromboangiitis obliterans. Lymphocytes from 77 per cent of these patients exhibited cellular sensitivity to human type I and type III collagen, both of which are constituents of the vascular wall. In addition, approximately 50 per cent had significant levels of anticollagen antibodies in their blood. By contrast, normal controls and patients with arteriosclerosis obliterans had considerably lower levels of cellular sensitivity to collagen and no circulating anticollagen antibodies.

INCIDENCE. Thromboangiitis obliterans is a disease mostly of young males. The disease begins most frequently between the ages of 20 and 40 years, and the ratio of men to women affected varies from 9:1 to as high as 75:1. There is a high prevalence of the disorder in Israel, the Orient, and in India as compared with the United States and Western Europe, suggesting the possibility of a genetic predisposition. The disease has been occasionally reported to occur in familial form.

PATHOLOGY. The disease affects small and medium-sized arteries and veins in segmental fashion. Acute lesions are manifested by proliferation of the intima and thrombosis. There is inflammatory infiltration with polymorphonuclear leukocytes, lymphocytes, and giant cells of all coats of the artery or vein, extending into the thrombus. The media remains intact. Calcium or cholesterol deposition does not occur. These lesions are distinguished from those of arteriosclerosis obliterans because of the more cellular thrombus, the preservation of the media, and the inflammatory infiltration of all coats of the vessel. Older lesions become less cellular, and eventually they may be transformed into a dense scar. Typically, in any one vessel, lesions of varying ages are seen.

CLINICAL MANIFESTATIONS. The typical patient with thromboangiitis obliterans is a young man who smokes cigarettes heavily, has manifestations of ischemia of the extremities, and has a history or evidence of superficial thrombophlebitis. Common presenting complaints are Raynaud's phenomenon with digital ulcerations or pain from ischemia. Pain in thromboangiitis obliterans may be of several types. The most frequent is pain at rest in one or more digits. This pain may be accompanied by manifestations of ischemia, such as color or temperature changes

of the skin. This type of pain may be a forerunner of ulceration or gangrene. In the presence of these trophic lesions, there may be localized pain that is aching in character and more severe at night. Another type of pain may occur along the course of the inflamed blood vessels. Ischemic neuropathy may result and cause a paroxysmal, shocklike pain, which may follow the distribution of sensory nerves. Paresthesias may accompany this type of pain. Typical intermittent claudication occurs commonly in the lower extremities. It most often occurs in the arch of the foot because of involvement of the vessels of the leg and sparing of the femoral and iliac arteries. Some patients have intermittent claudication of the forearm or hand. Sensitivity to cold with paresthesias and the development of secondary Raynaud's phenomenon are common. Migratory superficial thrombophlebitis is manifested by the development of inflamed, tender, red segments of the superficial veins, which subside over a period of several weeks.

Physical examination discloses impaired arterial pulsations in the more distal portions of the limbs, such as the radial, ulnar, dorsalis pedis, and posterior tibial arteries. The more proximal arteries are normal, a finding that contrasts with arteriosclerosis obliterans. There may be cyanosis or pallor or persistent redness in the digits, and associated changes in temperature may be noted. Postural changes in color are also common. Gangrene or ulcerations of the digits may be present in both upper and lower extremities. Edema of the foot is common. Occasional patients have involvement of visceral arteries with stenosis or occlusion of mesenteric, coronary, cerebral, or renal arteries and manifestations of ischemia of these organs.

DIAGNOSIS. The diagnosis of thromboangiitis obliterans should be entertained when there is evidence of ischemia of the extremities from arterial occlusive disease in association with migratory superficial thrombophlebitis. The age and sex of the individual and the involvement of the upper extremities are additional helpful characteristics. Arteriography may be helpful in disclosing segmental multiple occlusions of the medium-sized and small arteries associated with collateral vessel visualization. The larger arteries are generally spared, a finding that also helps distinguish the disorder from arteriosclerosis obliterans. Final confirmation may be obtained only from biopsy material of an early lesion and histologic demonstration of the characteristic inflammatory and proliferative lesion of the disease.

PROGNOSIS. Thromboangiitis obliterans is not usually life threatening except in rare individuals in whom the visceral arteries are involved. The disease, however, results in disability and amputation of the extremities in a high percentage of cases. It is generally more rapidly progressive than arteriosclerosis obliterans, especially in individuals who refuse to stop smoking.

TREATMENT. Cessation of tobacco smoking is essential. Continuation of smoking results in a progressive course. If the patient stops smoking, new lesions do not develop or they develop more rarely. The approach to the patient with thromboangiitis obliterans is generally the same as that to patients with advanced arteriosclerosis obliterans. It consists of conservative measures, including protection from cold, local care in the event of ulceration or gangrene, and eventually amputation, if these lesions occur. Sympathectomy is tried frequently and may be effective, at least temporarily, if vasospasm is a prominent feature. Vasodilative drug therapy can be tried in cases of Raynaud's phenomenon with ulcerations, but its effectiveness is questionable.

Adar R, Papa MZ, Halpern Z, et al.: Cellular sensitivity to collagen in thromboangiitis obliterans. N Engl J Med 308:1113, 1983. *An important study showing high incidence of cellular sensitivity to collagen and the presence of circulating anticollagen antibodies in patients with thromboangiitis obliterans. The results have profound implications concerning the etiology of the disease and offer possible means of differentiating it from arteriosclerosis obliterans.*

McKusick VA, Harris WS, Ottesen OE, et al.: Buerger's disease: A distinct clinical and pathologic entity. JAMA 181:5, 1962. *A concise and thoughtful consideration of the clinical features, arteriographic findings, and histopathology of 30 cases with Buerger's disease.*

Sudden Arterial Occlusion

DEFINITION. Sudden arterial occlusion may result from obstruction of an artery of the extremity by embolism or by thrombosis in situ. The clinical manifestations are the result of the consequent ischemia.

ETIOLOGY. The major cause of sudden arterial occlusion is arterial embolism. The heart is the most frequent source of emboli in this syndrome. Emboli may arise from thrombi in the left atrium in the presence of atrial fibrillation or mitral valve disease, usually mitral stenosis. Emboli may also arise from mural thrombi from a myocardial infarction or in the presence of a cardiomyopathy. Septic emboli may arise from vegetations from the mitral or aortic valves in the presence of bacterial endocarditis. Less commonly, emboli may arise from an arteriosclerotic plaque in more proximal parts of the arterial tree or from aneurysms. In rare cases, the embolus may arise from the venous side and enter the arterial tree via a patent foramen ovale (paradoxical embolism). More rarely, the embolus consists of calcium fragments from a calcified valve leaflet, cholesterol crystals from an arteriosclerotic plaque, or foreign materials such as a bullet.

Sudden arterial thrombosis occurs in about 10 per cent of the cases of arteriosclerosis obliterans. The condition is rare in thromboangiitis obliterans or in polyarteritis nodosa. Acute arterial thrombosis may occur in conditions in which the coagulability of the blood is increased in the presence of normal vessels, such as in polycythemia vera or in cryoglobulinemia. Rarely, arterial thrombosis may occur in the presence of normal vessels in infections such as septicemia, pneumonia, peritonitis, tuberculosis, ulcerative colitis, and other debilitating diseases. Trauma from penetrating wounds, as from arterial puncture or catheterization, may cause arterial occlusion.

PATHOLOGY. The structure of emboli that arise from thrombi in the heart or from aneurysms is the same as that of the parent thrombi. Emboli lodge in an artery and obstruct the vessel. There may be extension of the thrombus distally by further clotting of the blood. The fate of the embolus varies. In some cases it may become organized and finally be recanalized, and in other cases it may become fragmented and the fragments may lodge in more distal vessels.

PATHOPHYSIOLOGY. The sudden arterial occlusion causes reduction of blood flow to the more distal portions of the limb and consequent ischemia. There have been suggestions that vasoactive agents released from the emboli, such as serotonin from platelets, may cause contraction of vascular smooth muscle in more distal portions of the vascular tree and result in vasospasm that further aggravates ischemia. The severity and extent of ischemia depend on the size of the vessel occluded and on the extent of collateral circulation. The larger the occluded vessel, the more likely it is that severe ischemia would result.

CLINICAL MANIFESTATIONS. Sudden arterial occlusion causes the abrupt onset of severe pain accompanied by manifestations of ischemia in about half the patients. In the remainder, the onset is gradual with either mild pain or numbness and paresthesias. Pain is present in about 75 per cent of the cases. There may be muscular weakness or outright paralysis. A saddle embolus of the aortic bifurcation causes abdominal pain, nausea, and vomiting and may result in a shocklike state.

Examination of the patient discloses diminished or absent pulses distal to the occlusion. Evidence of ischemia is present with low skin temperature and pallor or cyanosis or a combination of the two. If the occluded artery is superficial, the site of lodgment of the embolus may be identified as a tender region. The subsequent course depends on the adequacy of the collateral circulation. If this is adequate, gradual improvement occurs. Otherwise, gangrene supervenes.

DIAGNOSIS. The diagnosis of sudden arterial occlusion is usually relatively easy in the patient who has the acute onset of pain and ischemia of an extremity. If the cause is an embolus, its source may be evident. Rarely, patients with acute thrombophlebitis of the iliac and femoral veins may have feeble or absent arterial pulses and show manifestations resembling those of ischemia from an arterial embolus. In these cases, the demonstration of the feeble pulse and the presence of distended veins and pronounced edema help make the differentiation possible.

PROGNOSIS. The outcome of acute arterial obstruction depends on the size of the vessel affected, the age of the patient, the extent of the collateral circulation, and the timing of therapeutic intervention. When a large artery is occluded, the prognosis is poor without surgical treatment. In older patients with pre-existing arterial occlusive disease, the prognosis is poor because of obstruction of multiple vessels, including collateral vessels.

TREATMENT. The goal of therapeutic intervention is the removal or dissolution of the thrombus and re-establishment of patency of the occluded artery. This goal can be achieved by surgical embolectomy or by thrombolytic therapy. Urgent embolectomy is the preferred method of treatment when a large artery is occluded, such as with a saddle embolus of the bifurcation of the aorta. When smaller vessels are occluded and the thrombus is not easily accessible or when the patient's general condition does not permit surgical intervention, intravenous or intra-arterial streptokinase or urokinase may be given, if there are no contraindications for their use. Streptokinase is given intravenously as a bolus of 250,000 IU, followed by an infusion of 100,000 IU per hour. The infusion is continued for 72 hours. Intra-arterial administration can be used instead, in a dose of about one tenth of the intravenous dose; it can be coupled with angioplasty. Thrombolytic therapy is followed by conventional anticoagulants. The success rate of thrombolytic therapy is critically dependent on how early it is administered after the onset of symptoms. It is more effective for thrombotic lesions than embolic ones. Streptokinase or urokinase cannot be safely followed by surgery because of the danger of bleeding from the arteriotomy. The choice of therapy, therefore, must be carefully considered.

If neither therapeutic approach can be used, the patient should be treated conservatively. The patient should be placed at rest. The limb should be placed in a slightly dependent position under a cradle whose temperature is controlled at 30 to 35°C. Anticoagulation with heparin should be started as soon as possible to prevent extension of the thrombus and to prevent formation of additional emboli. If vasospasm is prominent, lumbar sympathectomy may be tried to reduce vasomotor tone and improve blood flow to the limb.

When a patient is treated by conservative medical measures, he or she should be followed closely for evidence of deterioration. If this occurs, immediate surgical intervention and embolectomy should be attempted. The results of embolectomy depend, to a large extent, on the timing of intervention. Therefore, surgery should not be delayed longer than a few hours. If therapy fails, gangrene may supervene, and amputation may become necessary.

Haimovici H: Peripheral arterial embolism. Angiology 1:20, 1950. *Detailed consideration of the clinical features of the arteries of the limbs based on study of 330 cases.*

Hargrove WC, Barker CF, Berkowitz HD, et al.: Treatment of acute peripheral arterial and graft thromboses with low-dose streptokinase. Surgery 92:981, 1982. *A report of good results from the use of intra-arterial streptokinase for the treatment of acute arterial thrombosis.*

Hinton RC, Kistler JP, Fallon JT, et al.: Influence of etiology of atrial fibrillation on incidence of systemic embolism. Am J Cardiol 40:509, 1977. *A study of the pathology of arterial embolism in 333 patients with atrial fibrillation. The paper emphasizes that the risk of embolism is independent of the cause of atrial fibrillation.*

VASCULAR DISEASES OF THE LIMBS CAUSED BY ABNORMAL COMMUNICATION BETWEEN ARTERIES AND VEINS

Arteriovenous Fistula

DEFINITION. Arteriovenous fistula is an abnormal direct communication between an artery and a vein.

ETIOLOGY. Arteriovenous fistulas in the limbs may be congenital or acquired. Congenital fistulas are usually multiple; acquired ones are usually single. The most common type is iatrogenic, created to carry out renal dialysis. Acquired arteriovenous fistulas may also result from trauma caused by penetrating wounds or surgical procedures.

PATHOPHYSIOLOGY. The low resistance of the direct communication between artery and vein results in a high arterial inflow into the vein, with a resultant increase in venous pressure. The elevated venous pressure causes engorgement of the vein and distention and may lead to the production of varicose veins. In the region of the fistula, blood flow is high, whereas more distal portions are deprived of capillary blood flow and may show ischemia and trophic changes.

Large fistulas cause a reduction in systemic vascular resistance and impose a burden on the heart because of the associated increase in cardiac output. Total blood volume may be increased. Left ventricular failure may eventually result.

PATHOLOGY. In the region of the fistula the veins become thickened, whereas the artery undergoes thinning and loss of elastic and muscular fibers in the media.

CLINICAL MANIFESTATIONS. The patient may be totally asymptomatic, and the discovery of the fistula may be accidental. In other cases, there may be pain in the location of the fistula, edema, varicosities, and asymmetry in the size of the limbs. In some cases, the presenting symptoms may be those of cardiac decompensation with dyspnea on exertion, palpitations, and orthopnea. Examination of the involved limb reveals tortuous, dilated superficial veins and venous pulsation at the site of the fistula. The temperature of the skin may be high, and distal portions of the limb may show ischemic changes. A bruit or a thrill may be heard over the fistula during systole. At other times, a continuous bruit may be present. The extremity may be swollen, or the girth of the limb may be increased because of hypertrophy of the soft tissues. Temporary compression of the artery proximal to the fistula causes immediate increase in systemic vascular resistance and leads to reflex decrease in heart rate (Branham's sign), a change that may be helpful diagnostically.

DIAGNOSIS. When the fistula is superficial and large, the diagnosis can be made easily. If this is not possible from the physical examination, arteriography should be attempted for a definitive diagnosis. The oxygen saturation of the venous blood from the involved limb is higher than that of its contralateral part, and this comparison may be helpful in making the diagnosis.

TREATMENT. The treatment of choice is surgical intervention with closure of the fistula and re-establishment of the continuity of the involved artery and vein. If such restoration is not possible, ligation of the artery or vein or both may be necessary, but this may lead to arterial or venous insufficiency of the limb. In some cases, the fistula involves an anomalous artery. In this case, the ligation of the artery and the obstruction of the veins by the injection of sclerosing solutions may give a satisfactory result. It may not be practical to treat surgically patients with multiple fistulas. In these cases, conservative measures consisting of local care, relief of pain, and wearing elastic bandages may be helpful. If the fistula is inoperable and cardiac decompensation is present or threatened, amputation may be necessary.

Nickerson JL, Elkin DC, Warren JV: The effect of temporary occlusion of arteriovenous fistulas on heart rate, stroke volume, and cardiac output. J Clin Invest 30:215, 1951. *A classic study of the systemic hemodynamic effects of arteriovenous fistulas in a large number of patients.*

Rossi P, Carillo FJ, Alfidi RJ, et al.: Iatrogenic arteriovenous fistulas. Radiology 111:47, 1974. *A comprehensive review of 154 cases of iatrogenic arteriovenous fistulas. The paper provides a good review of the literature.*

Glomus Tumor (Glomangioma)

DEFINITION. Glomangioma, or glomus tumor, is a benign tumor of the glomus body.

PATHOLOGY. The glomus tumor is an encapsulated structure consisting of a hypertrophied arteriovenous anastomosis. The tumor varies in size from 0.5 to 2.5 cm in diameter. It can be found in various parts of the upper and lower extremities but is most frequently located in the nail beds.

CLINICAL MANIFESTATIONS. The most common symptom is severe burning pain in the location of the tumor. The pain may precede the appearance of the tumor. Pain may occur spontaneously, or it may be precipitated by exposure to heat or cold. Occasionally, the tumor is exquisitely sensitive to touch, and even the slightest pressure from contact with clothing may cause severe pain. Severe disability and atrophy of the limb from disuse may occur secondary to fear of pain. Examination of the involved area shows a reddish, purplish, or bluish mass that is sharply demarcated. At times, the tumor may not be easily visible or palpable. In this case, pressure with the head of a pin may help identify the location of the tumor. When it is located under the nail bed, the nail and the phalanx may be visibly deformed, thereby giving a clue to the location of the tumor. Ultrasonography or magnetic resonance imaging is useful in the diagnosis of small glomus tumors.

TREATMENT. The glomus tumor is a benign tumor. Surgical excision results in complete relief without recurrence.

Cooke SAR: Misleading features in the clinical diagnosis of the peripheral glomus tumour. Br J Surg 58:602, 1971. *The clinical manifestations of glomus tumor are described based on the study of 24 cases.*

Fornage BD: Glomus tumors in the fingers: Diagnosis with US. Radiology 167:183, 1988. *This report shows that ultrasonography is useful in the diagnosis of small glomus tumors.*

DISEASES OF THE VEINS OF THE LIMBS

Thrombophlebitis and Deep-Vein Thrombosis

DEFINITION. Thrombophlebitis refers to venous thrombosis with accompanying inflammation of the venous wall. For important practical reasons, superficial thrombophlebitis is distinguished from deep-vein thrombosis. Superficial thrombophlebitis does not cause embolic complications, but deep-vein thrombosis is a frequent cause of pulmonary embolism.

PATHOLOGY. Thrombi in veins consist mostly of red cells with a few platelets held together with fibrin. They propagate in the direction of the bloodstream by extension of the thrombotic process. They attach to the wall of the vein at one end, while the more proximal end floats freely into the lumen of the vessel. This is the portion that is commonly broken off and travels to the lungs. Varying degrees of inflammatory reaction of the venous wall may be present. Venous thrombosis may exist in the absence of inflammation, as is the case in some patients with malignancy. This is referred to as "phlebothrombosis." In most cases, however, inflammation and thrombosis coexist. The disorder may start as a pure thrombotic process, and inflammation usually occurs secondary to the presence of the thrombus.

INCIDENCE. Deep-vein thrombosis is a common disorder. It is more common in women than in men. All races seem to be affected equally, at least in developed countries. The incidence of the disease increases with advancing age. The disease is very common in hospitalized patients. Approximately one third of the patients over age 40 who have undergone major surgery or have had an acute myocardial infarction develop deep-vein thrombosis. The incidence is even higher after certain operations such as repair of hip fractures or prostatectomy. Patients with thrombotic strokes have an equally high incidence of deep-vein thrombosis. This occurs almost exclusively in the paralyzed limb.

Superficial thrombophlebitis occurs most commonly in patients with varicose veins, possibly as a result of minor trauma. It is also frequent after pregnancy. A migratory type of superficial thrombophlebitis also occurs in patients with thromboangiitis obliterans.

PATHOGENESIS. Venous stasis, injury to the venous wall, and a hypercoagulable state are the three main factors that lead to venous thrombosis. In most cases, more than one of these factors are present, and their effect may be cumulative. The combination of venous stasis and changes in the clotting mechanism of the blood accounts for the increased incidence of deep-vein thrombosis in pregnancy and during administration of oral contraceptives. Venous stasis is the major factor in the development of venous thrombosis in patients with heart disease, in paralyzed patients, in patients undergoing major surgery, in those who have varicose veins, and in healthy individuals after long trips. Increased viscosity, leading to stasis, and alterations in the clotting factors of the blood account for the high incidence of polycythemia vera. Patients with familial deficiencies of certain anticlotting factors are susceptible to recurrent thrombophlebitis. These include deficiencies of antithrombin III, protein S, protein C, and heparin cofactor II. Injury to the venous wall may result from administration of certain vasoconstrictive or chemotherapeutic agents, or it may result from infectious agents. Patients with malignancies may have migrating thrombophlebitis, which has been attributed to low-grade activation of intravascular coagulation.

CLINICAL MANIFESTATIONS. The presence of superficial thrombophlebitis is usually easily ascertained by finding the inflamed vein. This may be apparent as a red, tender cord. By contrast, deep-vein thrombosis frequently causes few distinctive clinical features; about one half of patients with deep-vein thrombosis are asymptomatic. The first manifestation of deep-vein thrombosis may be the occurrence of pulmonary embolism. Pain in the region of the thrombosed veins at rest or only during exercise and edema distal to the obstructed veins are the usual symptoms of deep-vein thrombosis. Examination of the patient may disclose several helpful manifestations. Edema or pitting of the malleolar fossa may be present and may cause loss of the normal concavity of that portion of the leg. There may be a difference between the two legs in the circumference of the calf. A difference in maximal circumference in excess of 1.4 cm in men and 1.2 cm in women is highly suspicious. The temperature of the skin may be increased as a result of the inflammatory reaction, and palpation may disclose the thrombosed veins in the calf or in the popliteal fossa. There may be tenderness to palpation. Increased resistance or pain on voluntary dorsiflexion of the foot (Homans' sign) may be present. A useful sign is the presence of tenderness on inflation of a blood pressure cuff around the calf. Most normal individuals tolerate this without pain up to pressures of 160 to 180 mm Hg.

Thrombosis of the iliac and femoral veins usually presents with a characteristic clinical picture consisting of rapidly advancing swelling of the entire limb. The thrombosed vein may be tender if it extends below the inguinal ligament. Collateral distended veins may be present in the upper thigh. In some cases, secondary ischemia may occur as a result of the very high venous pressure that impedes arterial inflow. Cyanosis of the toes and even gangrene may occur under these circumstances.

Thrombosis of the subclavian vein may result in swelling of the upper extremity, and collateral veins may be present. In axillary thrombosis, a similar clinical picture occurs; the thrombosed vein may be felt in the axilla. A history of walking on crutches or sleeping in a sitting position on a bench with the arms behind the backrest may be helpful. Thrombosis of the superior vena cava causes increased venous pressure in the neck and face with distention of the neck veins in the upper part of the chest.

In septic thrombophlebitis, there may also be systemic manifestations of infection, such as fever, chills, and leukocytosis. In cases in which septic phlebitis begins from infected needles or catheters, an inflamed, tender cord may appear at the site of the venipuncture.

DIAGNOSIS. Iliofemoral thrombophlebitis is usually easily recognized by the rapid swelling of the entire limb, engorged collateral veins in the thigh, and signs of inflammation, such as increased skin temperature.

By contrast, in the majority of cases of deep-vein thrombosis involving the calf, popliteal area, and thigh, the clinical picture is not sufficiently distinctive to allow diagnosis with a high degree of confidence. Confirmation of the diagnosis must be provided by resorting to one or more of a number of diagnostic tests. The most commonly employed tests are the following:

X-ray Venography. Venography is one of the most accurate means of making the diagnosis of deep-vein thrombosis. The test involves the injection of a contrast medium into the venous system, which has been previously emptied of blood by gravity. The test relies on finding a filling defect or a sharp cutoff, indicating the presence of occluding thrombus in the vein. The test may result in inflammatory reaction followed by thrombosis in a few cases. It is sensitive and highly specific; for these reasons, venography is considered the "gold standard" in the diagnosis of deep-vein thrombosis.

Radionuclide Venography. This test is similar to x-ray venography except that instead of contrast medium, a radioisotope, such as ^{99m}Tc-macroaggregated albumin, is injected in a foot vein. External scanning detects venous obstruction and the presence of collateral circulation. In another variation of the technique, ^{99m}Tc-labeled red cells from the patient's own blood are injected intravenously, and a blood pool scan is obtained. The sensitivity and specificity of the technique are somewhat less than those of x-ray venography. The technique is probably better in detecting venous thrombosis in the thigh than in the calf.

Radioisotope-labeled Fibrinogen. This test consists of intravenous administration of fibrinogen labeled with ^{125}I and the subsequent incorporation of the radioactive material into the thrombus. The accumulation of radioactivity is detected by external counting. This test detects an active thrombophlebitis; it may be negative in cases in which the active process has stopped but thrombi exist in the veins. The reliability of the test depends on the location of the thrombus. It is of little use in detecting pelvic thrombi because of the high background due to the bladder and iliac arteries. It is most useful in detecting thrombosis of the calf. Another disadvantage is that it requires 1 or 2 days for sufficient counts to build into the thrombosed vein for detection. This test is, therefore, most useful in longitudinal screening of high-risk populations.

Liquid Crystal Thermography. This test relies on the detection of small increases in skin temperature as a result of the venous inflammation. The test is easy to perform. It has high sensitivity but relatively low specificity. It can be a useful adjunct to ultrasonography or impedance plethysmography for monitoring patients at risk.

Ultrasonography. This test utilizes the Doppler principle to detect venous obstruction. Thus, during various maneuvers that alter venous flow, such as deep inspiration, the Valsalva maneuver, or leg compression, the ultrasonogram may detect the presence of obstructed veins. The disadvantages of the technique are that a high degree of stenosis is necessary for the test result to be abnormal and that it does not distinguish between occlusion from external pressure and occlusion by thrombus. Also, the result may be negative if an effective collateral circulation has developed. The test is most sensitive for thrombosis of the veins above the knee.

"Duplex" Ultrasonography. This technique makes use of simultaneous real-time ultrasound imaging, combined with pulsed gated Doppler evaluation of blood flow. The technique allows direct visualization of the major vascular channels together with evaluation of the blood flow. Modern instruments display the Doppler signal in the form of a colored real-time image (color-flow Doppler). This technique has excellent specificity and sensitivity for deep-vein thrombosis above the knee. It is less reliable in detecting small calf thrombi. Its reliability is so high for thrombosis in the thigh that it can be used as a substitute for venography.

Impedance Plethysmography. This test detects alterations in blood volume of the extremities by detecting changes in the electrical impedance of the tissues. The test is carried out during respiratory maneuvers or during alterations in blood flow by occluding the limb with a pneumatic pressure cuff. Like ultrasonography, this test requires significant proximal obstruction for positive results. The reported sensitivity and specificity of the last two tests are high (over 90 per cent).

Choice of Tests. The choice of tests to be performed depends to a large extent on their availability. If all are available, it is preferable to use duplex ultrasonography. Because this technique does not detect small thrombi in the calf with consistency, it is necessary to repeat the test after a few days to eliminate the possibilty of extension into the thigh of existing deep vein thrombosis in the calf. If duplex ultrasonography is not available, it is preferable to use conventional ultrasonography or impedance plethysmography and to resort to venography if the results of these tests are inconclusive. The radioactive fibrinogen test and thermography should be reserved for screening of patients at high risk.

DIFFERENTIAL DIAGNOSIS. A number of conditions that cause localized pain or edema in the lower extremities may be confused with deep-vein thrombosis. A ruptured popliteal synovial membrane or cyst (Baker's cyst) may simulate most of the manifestations of venous thrombosis. The diagnosis can be suspected if there is a history or physical findings of arthritis of the knee joint. The diagnosis may be confirmed by an arthrogram revealing the entry of dye from the joint into the calf muscles. Rupture of the calf muscles may cause pain, tenderness, and edema and may simulate thrombophlebitis. The diagnosis can be made from the history of strenuous or unusual exercise, the presence of ecchymosis from extravasated blood, and the palpation of a hematoma. Sometimes the patient reports an audible snap during the activity when the pain first occurred. The differential diagnosis is important because anticoagulants are contraindicated in this condition. A severe muscle cramp may cause pain and swelling for a considerable period of time. Other manifestations of thrombophlebitis are, however, lacking in this situation. The pain of a lumbar disc may be localized in the calf. There are no other manifestations of venous thrombosis, however, and there may be neurologic findings to identify the cause of the pain. Lymphedema is recognized by its slower and gradual onset and the absence of signs of inflammation and of collateral veins. Finally, cellulitis may be confused with superficial thrombophlebitis.

COMPLICATIONS. Pulmonary embolism is a frequent and serious complication of deep-vein thrombosis. About 80 to 90 per cent of pulmonary emboli arise in the deep veins of the lower limbs. Although deep-vein thrombosis may begin frequently in the veins of the calf, it is only when the thrombosis extends above the knee that serious pulmonary embolism occurs.

About 5 per cent of patients with deep-vein thrombosis develop venous insufficiency with stasis dermatitis (postphlebitic syndrome). This is more likely to occur in those with more proximal venous obstruction. A rare complication of iliofemoral thrombophlebitis is venous claudication, in which the patient develops pain on exercise which is relieved by rest, as in arterial occlusive disease.

PROPHYLAXIS. Prophylactic therapy against deep-vein thrombosis should be attempted in high-risk patients (Table 54–4). The exact regimen used must take into consideration the risk of deep-vein thrombosis and consequent pulmonary embolism and the potential risk of hemorrhagic complications from the prophylactic therapy. Low-dose heparin is currently the most commonly used prophylactic technique. For surgical patients, this consists of administration of 5000 units of heparin subcutaneously 2 hours before surgery and then every 8 or 12 hours until the patient is ambulatory. This method is effective in reducing the incidence of deep-vein thrombosis and pulmonary embolism in patients subjected to a variety of surgical procedures. It is also effective in reducing the incidence of deep-vein thrombosis in patients following acute myocardial infarction, but it is not known whether there is a reduction in the incidence of pulmonary embolism. Low-dose heparin has been shown to be ineffective in patients undergoing surgery for hip fracture and hip replacement, and its effectiveness has not been established in urologic procedures. Higher dose heparin adjusted to give an activated partial thromboplastin time (APTT) in the upper limits of the therapeutic range has been reported to be more effective than low-dose heparin. In addition, the administration of dihydroergotamine mesylate, 0.5 mg subcutaneously, together with low-dose heparin, is more effective in preventing deep-vein thrombosis than heparin alone in surgical patients. Ergotamine acts by inducing venoconstriction and also by altering the coagulability of the blood. Warfarin and other similar drugs are also effective in protecting patients from thromboembolism during a variety of surgical techniques. Low molecular weight dextran given on the day of surgery and at suitable intervals thereafter has been reported in most cases to give favorable results. There is a risk of fluid overload, and, to a lesser extent, hemorrhagic complications. This method can be used in instances in which there is a high risk of bleeding from anticoagulants. Drugs that interfere with platelet aggregation, such as aspirin and other nonsteroidal anti-inflammatory agents, have not been shown convincingly to be effective as prophylactic agents. In patients in whom anticoagulation is contraindicated, such as patients with neurosurgical procedures, it is prudent to use conservative means of prophylaxis. These include early ambulation, elastic stockings, and external periodic calf compression. The external compression devices have been reported to be effective. There are no risks associated with their use; the only negative aspect is low patient acceptance during prolonged use, because they are uncomfortable or cumbersome.

TREATMENT. Anticoagulation is not necessary for the treatment of superficial thrombophlebitis. Local measures, sometimes coupled with administration of anti-inflammatory drugs, such as indomethacin, suffice to bring about healing and relief of symptoms.

Full anticoagulation is the preferred treatment for deep-vein thrombosis. Heparin is preferred for initiation of treatment because of its immediate action, whereas warfarin-type drugs may not become fully effective for a considerable period of time. Heparin inhibits coagulation by binding and activating antithrombin III, an inhibitor of activated Factor X. Heparin is best administered by constant infusion. Initially a bolus of 5000 units is given intravenously, followed by constant infusion of 750 to 1000 units per hour. The dose is adjusted by monitoring the APTT so that a level about two times the normal control is achieved. APTT is checked 4 to 6 hours after the initial bolus and once a day thereafter. An alternative method is intermittent intravenous administration of 5,000 to 10,000 units every 4 to 6 hours. If no suitable veins are found, heparin may be administered subcutaneously in a dose of 15,000 to 30,000 units every 12 hours. After 5 days of heparin therapy, oral warfarin at a dose of 10 to 15 mg daily is given until the one-stage prothrombin time (PT) is 1.2 to 1.5 times the normal level. Subsequently, a daily maintenance dose is administered to maintain the PT at the desired level. Warfarin brings about anticoagulation by decreasing the level of Factors II, VII, IX, and X. Many drugs interact with warfarin. Some of them potentiate its action and others inhibit it. If the patient requires other drug therapy while on warfarin, each drug should be carefully screened for potential interaction. If bleeding occurs in the course of heparin therapy, its effect can be counteracted by administration of 1 mg of protamine per 100 units of heparin. If bleeding develops in the course of warfarin treatment, the patient should receive vitamin K_1 intramuscularly to reduce PT to the therapeutic range (0.25 to 1.0 mg usually suffices). If bleeding is serious, blood or fresh frozen plasma may be necessary.

Thrombolysis with fibrinolytic agents, such as streptokinase or urokinase, administered intravenously in patients with deep-vein thrombosis has been shown to achieve more complete dissolution of the thrombus and better preservation of the venous architecture than conventional anticoagulants. These drugs act by causing activation of plasminogen to plasmin, thereby causing dissolution of the thrombus. Streptokinase is administered intravenously as an initial bolus of 250,000 to 500,000 IU, followed by an infusion of 100,000 IU per hour for 24 to 72 hours. The effectiveness of the drug diminishes after the first 24 hours. Urokinase is less likely to cause anaphylactic reactions, but it is more expensive. It is given in a dose of 4400 IU per kilogram as a bolus, followed by an infusion of 4400 IU per kilogram per hour for the same duration as streptokinase. Human recombinant tissue-type plasminogen activator is also capable of dissolving venous thrombi and pulmonary emboli. A controlled trial of this agent in deep-vein thrombosis is now in progress. Thrombolytic therapy is the preferred method of treatment of patients with iliofemoral or subclavian-axillary vein thrombosis. In patients with more distal deep-vein thrombosis, the high effectiveness of heparin and its lower rate of hemorrhagic complications render this the preferred method of treatment.

TABLE 54–4. PREVENTION OF VENOUS THROMBOEMBOLISM

Representative patient groups	1. Medical patients without predisposing factors on short bed rest 2. Young patients without predisposing factors undergoing brief (<1 hr) general surgical procedure	1. Medical patients with predisposing factors or on prolonged bed rest 2. Middle-aged or old patients without predisposing factors undergoing general surgical procedure longer than 1 hr	1. Patients with hip fracture 2. Patients undergoing extensive orthopedic or pelvic surgery 3. Middle-aged or old patients with predisposing factors or with previous venous thrombosis undergoing general surgical procedure longer than 1 hr
Approximate incidence of venous thrombosis	5%	20–40%	50–70%
Approximate incidence of pulmonary embolism	Almost zero	5%	10%
Suggested prophylaxis	None	Low-dose heparin or intermittent pneumatic compression	Warfarin, low-dose heparin plus either intermittent pneumatic compression or dihydroergotamine; or higher dose heparin

In patients in whom anticoagulation is contraindicated, simple measures—elevation of the extremity and local heat—should be used. When the risk of pulmonary embolism is low, as in the case of deep-vein thrombosis limited to the calf, these measures suffice. In patients with deep-vein thrombosis extending above the knee, in whom the risk of pulmonary embolism is high, implantation of an inferior vena caval filter or ligation of the inferior vena cava may also be considered. This form of therapy should also be used when anticoagulation needs to be terminated because of complications, when recurrent thromboembolism occurs in the presence of adequate anticoagulation, and when septic thromboembolic disease not controlled by antibiotics is present.

Bed rest should be continued until local signs of inflammation, including tenderness and edema, subside. After 7 to 15 days the patient is allowed to walk wearing elastic stockings. If no discomfort occurs, resumption of full activity is allowed 1 to 2 weeks later. Anticoagulation for 3 months is usually sufficient to prevent recurrence of deep-vein thrombosis.

Beisaw NE, Comerota AJ, Groth HE, et al.: Dihydroergotamine/heparin in the prevention of deep-vein thrombosis after total hip replacement. J Bone Joint Surg 70A:2, 1988. *Report of a controlled, randomized multicenter trial showing greater effectiveness of the combination of dihydroergotamine plus heparin than either drug alone in the prophylaxis of deep-vein thrombosis in patients undergoing total hip replacement.*

Grassi CJ, Goldhaber SZ: Interruption of the inferior vena cava for prevention of pulmonary embolism: Transvenous filter devices. Herz 14:182, 1989. *A consideration of the uses of inferior vena cava filters for the prevention of pulmonary embolism.*

Hirsh J, Hull RD: Treatment of venous thromboembolism. Chest 89:426S, 1986. *A thoughtful consideration of various aspects of the use of anticoagulants in the treatment of venous thromboembolism.*

Hull RD, Raskob GE, Hirsh J: Prophylaxis of venous thromboembolism: An overview. Chest 89:374S, 1986. *A concise and thoughtful analysis of the methods for preventing deep-vein thrombosis.*

Mudge M, Hughes LE: The long term sequelae of deep vein thrombosis. J Surg 65:692, 1978. *A report of long-term follow-up of patients who had evidence of venous thrombosis after surgery. The sequelae of venous thrombosis are described.*

Peterson CE, Kwaan HC: Current concepts of warfarin therapy. Arch Intern Med 146:581, 1986. *A concise consideration of the pharmacology and use of warfarin in the treatment of thrombotic disease.*

Shafer KE, Jaffe AS: Thrombolytic therapy: Current and potential uses. Drug Ther 13:95, 1983. *A concise consideration of the uses of thrombolytic agents.*

Sharma GVRK, Cella G, Parisi AF, et al.: Thrombolytic therapy. N Engl J Med 306:1268, 1982. *Detailed consideration of the use of streptokinase and urokinase in vascular thrombosis.*

White RH, McGahan JP, Daschbach MM, et al.: Diagnosis of deep-vein thrombosis using duplex ultrasound. Ann Intern Med 111:297, 1989. *A review of the use of duplex ultrasonography in the diagnosis of deep-vein thrombosis.*

Varicose Veins

DEFINITION. Varicose veins are prominent, abnormally distended, and tortuous veins.

INCIDENCE. Approximately 20 per cent of adults develop varicose veins. A familial history is present in 15 per cent of patients. They are more common in women than in men by a factor of 5 to 1. Most women date the onset of varicose veins from the time of pregnancy. The veins of the lower extremities are most frequently affected because of the effects of gravity on venous pressure.

ETIOLOGY. Congenitally absent or defective valves are a recognized cause of varicose veins in early life. Varicose veins may develop secondary to sustained elevations of venous pressure from obstruction of the veins. The cause of the obstruction may be thrombosis secondary to thrombophlebitis or external pressure, as is the case in pregnancy, ascites, and tumors. However, in most affected individuals, no clearly identifiable cause or precipitating factor can be found. The possibility of a genetically determined structural defect in the venous wall has been suggested. Individuals with varicose veins in the lower extremities have been found to have increased venous distensibility and reduced amounts of collagen and hexosamine in the wall of unaffected veins. In the face of such a generalized defect, a sustained elevation in venous pressure from the effects of gravity in the lower extremities or from other factors may lead to stretching of the walls and, finally, to incompetence of the valves and overdistention of the veins. An association of varicose veins with hemorrhoids and diverticulosis of the bowel suggests the possibility that increased intra-abdominal pressure during bowel movements may play a role in their pathogenesis.

CLINICAL MANIFESTATIONS. Most patients are asymptomatic, especially in the early stages of the disease. They may seek attention because the dilated, tortuous varicosities are cosmetically unappealing. In some cases, aching in the lower extremities and edema, especially after prolonged standing or exercise, may be present. The edema usually subsides overnight. When the communicating veins are incompetent, symptoms are more common. Prolonged venous insufficiency leads to the postphlebitic syndrome, with sustained edema, induration, and fibrosis. Eventually, trophic changes with brownish discoloration of the skin and ulceration may result. Ulcers usually occur above the medial malleolus. An incompetent communicating vein may be identified in the vicinity of the ulcer. The arterial pulses are normal, and no evidence of ischemia is present.

DIAGNOSIS. Clinical inspection suffices to make the diagnosis. The Trendelenburg test can identify the presence of defective valves and incompetent communicating veins. With the patient recumbent, the leg is elevated to empty the veins, and a tourniquet is then applied to occlude the superficial veins. The patient is instructed to resume the erect position, and the tourniquet is released. If the venous valves are incompetent, the veins immediately become distended as a result of the backflow. If two tourniquets are applied, the distention of the veins in the intervening portion of the limb identifies the presence of incompetent communicating veins. The patency of the deep venous system can be examined by venography. It is prudent to exclude other causes of edema, such as congestive heart failure and renal disease.

PROGNOSIS. The prognosis of uncomplicated superficial varicose veins is excellent. The postphlebitic syndrome, once established, is usually progressive and resistant to treatment.

TREATMENT. Simple measures usually suffice to treat uncomplicated varicose veins. These consist of frequent periods of rest with elevation of the limbs, external pressure with elastic stockings or bandages, and avoidance of obstruction of the veins by garments such as girdles. In more severe or advanced cases, ligation and stripping of the saphenous veins or injection of sclerosing solutions may become necessary to prevent the postphlebitic syndrome. An injection/compression technique in which the sclerosing solution is injected into a vein emptied of blood, followed by compression by external pressure, is simple, cheap, and effective. It is widely used in Europe. When stasis ulcers are present, local care with warm, wet dressings is necessary. If infection is present, local and systemic antibiotics may be administered. If considerable fibrosis is present, it may be necessary to excise the entire area and carry out skin grafting to eliminate ulceration.

Beresford SSA, Chant ADB, Jones HO, et al.: Varicose veins: A comparison of surgery and injection/compression sclerotherapy. Lancet 1:921, 1978. *A 5-year follow-up comparing the effects of surgery and injection/compression sclerotherapy for varicose veins.*

Hobbs JT: The Treatment of Venous Disorders: A Comprehensive Review of Current Practice in the Management of Varicose Veins and Post-thrombotic Syndrome. Philadelphia, J. B. Lippincott Company, 1977. *A well-written, comprehensive consideration of the clinical features, diagnosis, and treatment of varicose veins and post-thrombotic syndromes.*

DISEASES OF THE LYMPHATIC VESSELS OF THE LIMBS

Lymphangitis

DEFINITION. Lymphangitis is an inflammation of the lymphatic vessels. It is usually of bacterial origin.

ETIOLOGY. In most cases the responsible infective agent is the hemolytic streptococcus or *Staphylococcus aureus*, coagulase-positive. The bacteria gain access to the lymphatics via local trauma or from ulcerations. In many instances no identifiable portal of entry can be found. Infection spreads from the lymphatics to the regional lymph nodes.

PATHOLOGY. Various stages of inflammation are found in the subcutaneous tissue and regional lymph nodes.

CLINICAL MANIFESTATIONS. The local manifestation of lymphangitis consists of a red streak that appears at the site of initial entry of the infective organism and extends to the regional lymph nodes. The latter are swollen and tender. There may be a surrounding area of cellulitis. Systemic accompaniments of infection may constitute the presenting manifestations.

DIAGNOSIS. The local manifestations of lymphangitis and the accompanying systemic reaction are usually sufficient to make the diagnosis. Leukocytosis with predominance of polymorphonuclear leukocytes may be present. Confirmation is obtained by culturing the organism from the portal of entry or from the subcutaneous tissues. Acute lymphangitis may be difficult to distinguish from a generalized cellulitis or from thrombophlebitis.

PROGNOSIS. With treatment the prognosis is good when one is dealing with an initial attack in an otherwise normal limb. In the case of recurrent attacks, lymphedema may develop and residual increase in the girth of the limb may occur.

TREATMENT. This consists of systemic administration of the appropriate antibiotics. In addition, surgical drainage of the focus of infection is important. Supportive measures, including rest and elevation of the infected limb and local warm, wet dressings, are also helpful. The use of elastic support hose may be necessary for a period of several weeks to prevent lymphedema. In recurrent cases, the causes of secondary lymphedema should be sought.

Schinger A, Martin WJ, Spittell JA: Acute lymphangitis and cellulitis. Minn Med 48:191, 1965. *Concise consideration of the clinical features, diagnosis, and treatment of lymphangitis*

Lymphedema

DEFINITION. Lymphedema refers to edema from accumulation of lymph secondary to obstruction to its flow.

ETIOLOGY AND INCIDENCE. Lymphedema can be primary or secondary. The most frequent type of primary lymphedema is simple congenital lymphedema, which is not familial and is present at birth. A congenital familial form (Milroy's disease) is inherited as an autosomal dominant trait. Another hereditary form is associated with Noonan's syndrome in about 15 per cent of cases. Lymphedema praecox becomes manifest in puberty and is associated with congenital hypoplasia of the lymphatics. A late form may become manifest in middle age.

Primary lymphedema is more common in women. Most cases are manifest at birth or become apparent before age 40. A syndrome characterized by yellow nails, recurrent pleural effusion, and lymphedema is believed to be secondary to multiple lymphatic abnormalities in the areas involved. A familial syndrome consisting of recurrent intrahepatic cholestasis and lymphedema is probably due to defective hepatic lymphatic vessels as well as those in the extremity.

Secondary lymphedema results most commonly from trauma. It commonly results from surgical removal of lymph nodes and from fibrosis secondary to radiation following surgery for cancer. Lymphoma or metastatic carcinoma involving the lymph nodes may also cause obstruction to the flow of lymph and lymphedema. Filarial infection in the tropics is a cause of secondary lymphedema.

PATHOLOGY. In cases of congenital lymphedema there is absence or hypoplasia of the lymphatic vessels. In secondary lymphedema there are numerous small, irregular lymphatics, together with tortuous and sometimes greatly enlarged varicose lymphatic vessels.

CLINICAL MANIFESTATIONS. Typically, lymphedema begins gradually with an enlargement of the involved limb without other manifestations. The swollen extremity is soft and pitting. The edema subsides at night. With time, the skin becomes thickened and cannot be raised into a fold, and the edema becomes more persistent. The lower extremities are involved most often. In about half the patients the edema is unilateral. Superimposed lymphangitis and cellulitis may occur, and in longstanding cases lymphangiosarcoma may develop.

DIAGNOSIS. The diagnosis of lymphedema may be confirmed with a radioisotope lymphogram. ^{99m}Tc-labeled rhenium sulfur colloid, ^{99m}Tc-labeled antimony trisulfide colloid, or ^{99m}Tc-labeled human serum albumin microcolloid is injected in the web spaces of the foot. The ilioinguinal region is scanned 30 and 60 minutes later. In lymphedema, the uptake of isotope by the lymph nodes is reduced, whereas in edema due to venous obstruction it is greater than normal owing to increased lymph flow. The precise diagnosis of the type of lymphedema is made by lymphangiography. Contrast medium is injected directly into a lymphatic vessel in the foot, or a water-soluble contrast agent is injected intracutaneously and taken up by the lymphatics. By this technique, a distinction can be made between absence or hypoplasia of the lymphatic vessels, on the one hand, which characterizes congenital lymphedema, and the hyperplasia and numerous small lymphatics, which characterize secondary lymphedema, on the other.

PROGNOSIS. Primary lymphedema is usually a slowly progressive disorder, not easily amenable to treatment. The prognosis of secondary lymphedema depends on the cause. In cases in which it results from infection, it can be effectively managed by treatment with antibiotics.

TREATMENT. In primary lymphedema this is aimed at keeping the limb as free of edema as possible to prevent fibrosis and secondary infection. Frequent elevation of the limb, the use of elastic stockings, and the administration of diuretics may be useful. In cases not controlled by these simple measures, benzopyrones have been reported to be useful. These drugs break down protein by activating macrophages; hence, they reduce viscosity and facilitate the flow of lymph. Surgery may be tried in advanced cases to remove subcutaneous tissue and to induce new lymph vessel formation. Anastomosis of small lymphatic vessels with veins by microsurgery has been reported to give good results in some cases.

Allen EV, Ghormley RK: Lymphedema of the extremities: Etiology, classification and treatment; report of 300 cases. Ann Intern Med 9:516, 1935. *Comprehensive consideration of the clinical features of primary and secondary lymphedema in a large series of cases.*

Browse NL: The diagnosis and management of primary lymphedema. J Vasc Surg 3:181, 1986. *A concise account of the diagnosis and management of primary lymphedema.*

Browse NL, Stewart G: Lymphoedema: Pathophysiology and classification. J Cardiovasc Surg 26:91, 1985. *An up-to-date description of the pathophysiology and classification of lymphedema.*

Gloviczki P, Calcagno D, Schirger A, et al.: Noninvasive evaluation of the swollen extremity: Experiences with 190 lymphoscintigraphic examinations. J Vasc Surg 9:683, 1989. *Report of the use of lymphoscintigraphy with ^{99m}Tc-labeled antimony trisulfide in the diagnosis of lymphedema.*

Partsch H, Wenzel-Hora BI, Urbanek A: Differential diagnosis of lymphedema after indirect lymphography with iotasul. Lymphology 16:12, 1983. *Description of the usefulness of indirect lymphangiography using a water-soluble contrast medium for the differential diagnosis of lymphedema.*

Pillar NB: Lymphoedema, macrophages and benzopyrones. Lymphology 13: 109, 1980. *Discussion of the role of macrophages in lymphedema. The effectiveness of benzopyrones in this disease is ascribed to activation of macrophages.*

Weissleder H, Weissleder R: Lymphedema: Evaluation of qualitative and quantitative lymphoscintigraphy in 238 patients. Radiology 168:729, 1988. *Report of the application of lymphoscintigraphy using ^{99m}Tc-labeled human serum albumin microcolloid in the diagnosis of lymphedema.*

PART VII
RESPIRATORY DISEASES

55 Introduction

John F. Murray

Respiration includes all the processes that contribute to O_2 uptake and CO_2 elimination. The lungs are the major organs of gas exchange, but the nose, oropharynx, extrapulmonary airways, brain, spinal cord, nerves, thoracic cage, respiratory muscles, lymph nodes and vessels, and cardiovascular system are also involved. Thus respiratory diseases, literally interpreted, include a large variety of abnormalities arising in all the different structures concerned with gas exchange. In general, a more limited definition applies, and respiratory diseases are considered to include disturbances of the air passages, lungs, pleura, chest wall, muscles of respiration, and mediastinum (excluding the heart, systemic vessels, and esophagus).

Acute respiratory diseases are probably the most common afflictions of humankind and are responsible for more absences from school and work than any other type of illness. Chronic respiratory diseases, particularly emphysema and bronchitis, are second only to cardiovascular diseases as causes of disability payments. Cancer of the lung kills more persons each year than any other kind of malignancy. Because of the extremely high incidence of these and other respiratory diseases, it is important that all physicians, not just internists and chest specialists, be well versed in the clinical manifestations and methods of diagnosis, treatment, and prevention of the most common disorders. The material concerned with respiratory diseases here and elsewhere in the book is intended as a primer of necessary knowledge with which to recognize and to treat the major respiratory diseases; additional information is available in the references cited at the end of each chapter.

Patients with respiratory disease often seek medical attention because they have at least one of three cardinal manifestations: *cough* (including its derivative hemoptysis), *chest pain*, and *dyspnea*. These are nonspecific and sometimes trivial abnormalities, but the frequency with which they are associated with serious underlying thoracic disease means that the complaints must always be considered carefully and often become the focus of diagnostic evaluations. Because of the clinical importance of cough, chest pain, and dyspnea, the mechanisms, special features, and diagnostic approach to each symptom are briefly reviewed in the following pages. Further information can be found under the headings of the specific diseases in which these symptoms occur.

COUGH

Healthy persons seldom cough; their scant bronchial secretions, although constantly being produced, are imperceptibly carried up the tracheobronchial system by the action of cilia and, after reaching the pharynx, swallowed. Coughing is an essential defense mechanism that protects the airways from the adverse effects of inhaled noxious substances and also serves to clear them of retained secretions. Patients recognize that coughing indicates an abnormality, and this symptom is the second most common reason given for seeking medical advice.

MECHANISM. Coughing may be produced voluntarily, but more often it results from reflex stimulation. Extrathoracic cough receptors are located in the nose, oropharynx, larynx, and upper trachea. Intrathoracic rapidly adapting irritant receptors, which cause cough, are located in the epithelium of the lower trachea and large central bronchi, which are the air passages from which coughing effectively clears secretions or removes foreign material.

Depending on which cough receptors are activated, afferent stimuli travel to the brain via the trigeminal, glossopharyngeal, superior laryngeal, or vagus nerve. Efferent pathways include the recurrent laryngeal nerves, to cause closure of the glottis, and the corticospinal tract and peripheral nerves, to cause contraction of the thoracic and abdominal musculature. The cough reflex begins with a deep breath followed by glottic closure, relaxation of the diaphragm, and contraction of the expiratory muscles. Collectively, these acts generate a positive pressure of 100 to 300 mm Hg within the thorax, which is suddenly released when the glottis opens. During cough, the *volume* rate of flow out of the lungs (liters per second) is only slightly greater than or the same as it is during a forced expiratory maneuver, a fact that is not always appreciated. However, because the positive pressure in the pleural space is higher than the luminal pressure in the trachea and central bronchi, a pressure difference is created that causes the posterior membranous portion of the airway walls to fold inward and nearly to obliterate the lumen. By this means, the *linear* velocity of airflow through the narrowed channels (centimeters per second) is markedly increased, and a shearing force is created that dislodges secretions and particles from the mucosal surface.

PRODUCTIVE COUGH. The daily quantity of bronchial secretions produced by a normal person is not known, but it is sufficiently small to be removed by mucociliary action alone, and coughing and expectoration are not required. Secretions can accumulate in the tracheobronchial system in the presence of one or more of the following abnormalities: excessive production, altered physical properties, and deficient clearance. Thus, productive cough, which clears retained secretions from the airways, is an important defense mechanism and one of the hallmarks of acute and chronic inflammatory conditions of the lungs and airways. Patients who are unconscious or intubated or who, for other reasons, cannot cough must have their tracheobronchial secretions removed by suctioning to prevent the complications of atelectasis and/or bronchopulmonary infection.

NONPRODUCTIVE COUGH. In addition to the cough that serves an expectoration function, another type of cough—an irritative phenomenon—is encountered frequently. The stimulus may be mechanical, chemical, thermal, or inflammatory, including reactions from infection. There is increasing evidence that alteration of the surface epithelium of the major airways, into which the terminal filaments of irritant receptors are inserted, exposes the receptors more directly or somehow sensitizes them to the effects of stimulants; the cough reflex thus becomes hyperreactive, and coughing occurs in response to ordinarily innocuous stimuli. When the causes of chronic cough are analyzed, asthma often heads the list. Indeed, chronic nonproductive cough, especially at night, may be the sole presenting complaint of patients who subsequently prove to have bronchial asthma. An intractable, dry cough is now recognized as an important side effect of angiotensin-converting enzyme inhibitors.

COMPLICATIONS. Coughing seems to provoke more coughing. Paroxysms of coughing, as in pertussis, may terminate in vomiting, which seems to break the cycle. Paroxysmal attacks may also terminate in syncope. The mechanism of *cough syncope* is uncertain, but the effects of increased intrathoracic pressure on venous return, cardiac output, and blood flow to the brain are believed to play a role. At times, severe coughing attacks have continued to the point of utter exhaustion. The muscular force developed during coughing may be sufficient to cause occasional fractures of ribs (*cough fractures*) and even compression fractures of vertebral bodies.

DIAGNOSTIC APPROACH. It is difficult to generalize about a condition as common but as varied as coughing. Obviously, many episodes of coughing are innocent and transient. The essential first step in evaluating a patient complaining of cough is to obtain a thorough history with particular attention to the following aspects: (1) acute or chronic, (2) productive or nonproductive, (3) character, (4) time relationships, (5) type and quantity of sputum, and (6) associated features. A specific diagnosis of the cause of chronic intractable cough can be made by history alone in the majority (80 per cent) of patients.

An acute cough is usually associated with viral laryngotracheobronchitis but may signify other bronchopulmonary infections. Less commonly, acute episodes of coughing may be the chief manifestation of the inhalation of various immunologic or irritative substances. A chronic cough is the diagnostic hallmark of chronic bronchitis but also occurs in asthma, tuberculosis, bronchiectasis, and bronchogenic carcinoma. The frequency with which chronic bronchitis and bronchogenic carcinoma coexist, both being a complication of cigarette smoking, has led to the important axiom that *any change in the character or pattern of a chronic cough warrants immediate diagnostic evaluation, with special attention directed toward the detection of bronchogenic carcinoma.*

A productive cough usually implies an underlying inflammatory process, often infectious, but in many conditions in which secretions would be anticipated, the cough is described as nonproductive. The cough may be characterized as "brassy," from major airways involvement, or "barking" or "croupy," from laryngeal disease. Paroxysmal coughing with "whoops" is characteristic of pertussis. A cough that occurs mainly at night may accompany congestive cardiac failure; one occurring at meals suggests esophagogastric disease, such as hiatal hernia or diverticulum; and the cough of severe bronchitis or bronchiectasis is often worse upon awakening because of pooling of secretions during sleep. Each of these patterns tends to recur repeatedly under similar circumstances.

A description of the secretions produced in association with cough is diagnostically useful. Foul-smelling sputum indicates anaerobic infection, as in lung abscess or necrotizing pneumonia. Abundant frothy, saliva-like sputum is a well-known but rare symptom of bronchoalveolar carcinoma. Pink, foamy sputum, which is often voluminous, indicates pulmonary edema. In pneumococcal pneumonia, the classic rust-colored or "prune juice"–colored sputum may be observed. The chronic production of copious purulent sputum with intermittent blood streaking, especially on change of postures, is an important clue to bronchiectasis.

The associated features of coughing episodes are of considerable clinical importance: wheezing—a disorder with obstruction to airflow, such as asthma; stridor—involvement of the pharynx–larynx–extrathoracic trachea; fever and chills—acute infection; weakness and weight loss—tuberculosis or other chronic infection or malignancy; and recurrent pneumonias—bronchiectasis, foreign body, or obstructing tumor. In view of the importance of cigarette smoking in the pathogenesis of cough, a careful smoking history is crucial to the evaluation of cough.

Physical examination may reveal signs of pulmonary involvement that provide clues to the specific diagnosis. Regardless of the presence or absence of physical findings, evaluation of significant cough entails roentgenographic examination of the chest. When indicated, simple pulmonary function tests will demonstrate abnormalities of airflow and/or lung volumes. In patients whose routine spirometric tests are normal, bronchial provocation studies are indicated. Appropriate studies of sputum, especially culture and cytology, are often the easiest and most direct way of establishing a diagnosis. Fiberoptic bronchoscopy or other special diagnostic tests are sometimes needed.

TREATMENT. The ideal treatment of cough is elimination of its underlying cause. This is possible in most kinds of bronchopulmonary infections by suitable antimicrobial treatment of the responsible microorganism. Cessation of cigarette smoking nearly always eliminates the cough of chronic bronchitis. Disabling, irritative, nonproductive cough may be suppressed by an antitussive drug such as codeine, 15 mg every 6 hours. In contrast, productive cough should not be suppressed because retention of secretions impairs the distribution of inspired air, which worsens gas exchange, and promotes the development of atelectasis and secondary infection. Adequate hydration, not overhydration, is traditionally recommended, although its effect on pulmonary secretions is difficult to substantiate. Expectorants and ultrasonic aerosols have not been shown to be beneficial. When secretions are difficult to raise because of their physical properties and/or ineffective coughing, respiratory physical therapy with postural drainage and percussion may be helpful, and a trial is warranted.

HEMOPTYSIS

Regardless of whether the sputum is grossly bloody or merely blood streaked, the expectoration of any blood whatsoever denotes hemoptysis. Patients with chronic bronchitis may produce faintly blood-tinged sputum from time to time, but apart from this exception every patient with hemoptysis deserves a thorough diagnostic workup. A substantial proportion of all patients who expectorate bloody sputum have a serious disease, although the causes have changed in recent decades: Tuberculosis has become less common and bronchogenic carcinoma has become more common; bronchitis-bronchiectasis remains important. Other conditions that may manifest with hemoptysis include pulmonary embolism, mitral stenosis, pulmonary arteriovenous fistula, and Goodpasture's syndrome. All series include an appreciable number (5 to 15 per cent) of undiagnosed cases despite complete investigation.

Diagnostic Approach

The amount of expectorated blood may vary widely, from slight streaking of sputum to massive exsanguinating hemorrhage. The patient may not be aware of the pulmonary origin of the bleeding and often states that the blood "welled up" in his or her throat. For this reason, patients with true hemoptysis may seek the services of an otolaryngologist. Although it is always wise to examine the nasopharynx thoroughly, it is rare that hemoptysis is due to lesions in the upper respiratory tract.

Bleeding of esophageal, gastric, or duodenal origin may be confused with bleeding from the respiratory tract. Hematemesis can usually be differentiated from hemoptysis by the presence of symptoms of gastrointestinal involvement, such as nausea and vomiting, a history of peptic ulcer disease or alcoholism, or signs of cirrhosis. Prompt endoscopy will settle the issue in doubtful cases.

The history and physical examination may provide clues to the underlying cause of hemoptysis but are seldom diagnostic. Chest roentgenograms, which should be obtained in all patients complaining of hemoptysis, may reveal evidence of old or new inflammatory lesions, probable malignancies, or vascular abnormalities. At times, the underlying lesion may be obscured by the densities caused by the presence of blood itself. Once the bleeding has stopped, however, intra-alveolar blood usually clears within a week, so that delayed roentgenographic examinations are often helpful. Routine laboratory evaluation should include a complete blood count and tests to exclude a coagulopathy. It is useful to collect and measure the quantity of blood coughed up, but much may be swallowed or retained in the lungs and airways.

Virtually every patient with significant hemoptysis should undergo bronchoscopy to determine the site of bleeding and its cause, but the timing of the procedure is controversial. It is always desirable to determine from which bronchus the blood is coming; this is absolutely necessary in patients bleeding massively who are being considered for surgery, but it is also extremely difficult because the tracheobronchial system contains so much blood that it is frequently impossible to identify a bleeding point. The fiberoptic bronchoscope is often used in patients with hemoptysis, but many experts prefer the rigid scope because its larger lumen permits easier aspiration of blood and, when necessary, control of bleeding by packing.

TREATMENT. Fortunately, intrapulmonary bleeding usually stops spontaneously, and massive or life-threatening hemoptysis is unusual (fewer than 1.5 per cent of all cases). When bleeding is brisk, the patient should be hospitalized and kept with the affected lung, from which the bleeding is occurring, in the dependent position; the airways should be kept free of blood—coughing may suffice, but suction may be necessary; and strong sedatives, which abolish cough, should be avoided, but mild sedatives, to relieve anxiety, are often advisable. A thoracic surgeon should be notified about the problem, and an endotracheal tube and suction apparatus must be ready at the bedside.

If massive bleeding suddenly occurs, the tube can be inserted blindly into the right main bronchus and the balloon inflated to separate the two lungs and keep the blood confined to one of them. If circumstances permit, it is even better to put a balloon catheter, under bronchoscopic guidance, into a lobar or segmental bronchus to isolate the blood to as small a region of the lung as possible. Blood transfusions are given according to the usual clinical guidelines of quantity of blood lost, hematocrit, blood pressure, pulse rate, and urine output.

After the bleeding stops, the patient should be examined as outlined to determine the cause of the hemorrhage as well as the extent and severity of the underlying disease or diseases. Then, in consultation with a thoracic surgeon, a rational decision can be made concerning the need for and likelihood of success of an operation. Ordinarily, localized lesions (e.g., bronchial adenoma or sequestration) are resected, and generalized lesions (e.g., widespread bronchiectasis or multiple fistulas) are left alone. However, there is considerable clinical ground between these two extremes, and each patient must be considered individually.

The accepted treatment for "massive" hemoptysis has been rapid identification of the site of bleeding and, when possible, its surgical removal, usually by lobectomy but occasionally by pneumonectomy. However, the overall benefits of this approach have never been convincingly validated, and there is increasing emphasis on medical treatment followed by elective lung resection of carefully selected patients. Nonsurgical management of persistent severe hemoptysis includes bronchial artery embolism, which stops the bleeding, at least temporarily, in virtually all patients.

CHEST PAIN

Various types of chest pain are extremely common. Chest pain is one of the most frequent symptoms that cause the sufferer to seek medical attention. Because there is no clear relationship between the intensity of the discomfort and the importance of its underlying cause, all complaints of chest pain must be considered carefully. Pain that is virtually diagnostic because of its typical pattern of onset, location, and relation to effort and to respiratory movements is found in pleurisy, intercostal neuritis, costochondral disease, and disorders of the chest wall. The location and character of pain from myocardial ischemia are also characteristic but may be simulated by the pain of acute and chronic pulmonary hypertension. Occasionally, chest pain is elusive and difficult to diagnose, but it must always be taken seriously. A *meticulous history* is essential in evaluating chest pain. From the patient's story alone, a differential diagnosis can be formulated that serves as the basis for subsequent examinations.

MECHANISM. The anatomy, physiology, and biochemistry of pain in the body are reviewed in Ch. 26. Chest pain is no different from other types in that receptors and afferent pathways transmit a stimulus to the central nervous system, where that stimulus is perceived as pain. However, the capacity of various intrathoracic structures to serve as a source of pain differs. The lung parenchyma and the visceral pleura covering it are insensitive to ordinarily painful stimuli. In contrast, pain often accompanies involvement of the parietal pleura, the major airways, the chest wall, the diaphragm, or the mediastinal structures, including the heart. The mechanism of pain in myocardial ischemia is unknown, but the actuating event is clearly an imbalance between myocardial oxygen supply and demand. The pain of pericarditis may be in part related to involvement of the adjacent pleura, thus accounting for the striking respiratory component of what is primarily a cardiac disease. Pain in the esophagus is provoked by stimulation of receptors from acid reflux or muscle spasm.

PLEURAL PAIN. Pleurisy, or acute inflammation of the pleural surfaces, usually causes chest pain that has several distinctive features. The pain is restricted in distribution rather than diffuse, is nearly always on one side or the other, and tends to be distributed along the intercostal nerve zones. Pain from diaphragmatic pleurisy is often referred to the shoulder and side of the neck. The most striking and important characteristic of pleural pain is its clear relationship to respiratory movements. The pain may be variously described as "achy," "sharp," "burning," or simply a "catch," but whatever its designation, it is typically worsened by taking a deep breath, and coughing or sneezing causes intense distress. Patients with pleurisy frequently also complain of dyspnea because the aggravation of their pain during inspiration makes them conscious of every breath. Movement of the trunk, including bending, stooping, or even turning in bed, increases pleural pain, and patients usually find and remain in the position in which movements of the affected region are most restricted.

The rapidity of development of pleural pain provides a clue to its cause. An immediate onset attends pulmonary embolism or spontaneous pneumothorax; a slower but still acute onset over a few hours, especially with fever and cough, accompanies pneumonia; finally, a gradual onset over days or even weeks, often associated with features of chronic illness, such as weakness and weight loss, suggests tuberculosis or malignancy.

INTERCOSTAL NEURITIS. The distribution and superficial and knifelike quality of the pain of intercostal neuritis may resemble pleural pain and sometimes may even be mistaken for myocardial ischemia. Usually, the pain of intercostal neuritis is worsened by vigorous respiratory movements such as coughing, sneezing, and straining but, unlike pleurisy, not by ordinary breathing. A neuritic origin may be suggested by the presence of lancinating or electrical shock sensations unrelated to movements, and hyperalgesia or anesthesia over the distribution of the affected intercostal nerve provides further confirmatory evidence.

COSTOCHONDRAL DISEASE. Pain localized to the costosternal cartilaginous junctions may be confused with other, more serious causes of chest pain. The discomfort is usually described as dull with a gnawing, aching quality; there is little, if any, relationship to respiratory or other movements, although the pain may be most noticeable when the patient is lying in bed at night. The diagnostic key lies in the fact that there is tenderness to palpation that is clearly localized to one or more of the costal cartilages. Redness, swelling, and enlargement of the costal bridges (*Tietze's syndrome*) may be present, but the frequency of these is overemphasized. The most common sites of costosternal perichondritis are the second, third, and fourth cartilages, but any part of the large and complex cartilaginous shield along the central and lower portions of the anterior thoracic cage may be involved.

DISORDERS OF THE CHEST WALL. The system of joints, muscles, and fasciae involved in movements of the thoracic wall is complex. Because these structures are in constant motion throughout a person's life, it is surprising that "rheumatic" pains of the chest do not occur more frequently than they do. Fibrositis of the muscle-bone attachments may simultaneously involve the chest wall and other parts of the skeleton. Similarly, spondylitis of the thoracic spine may have its rib cage component, and many less definable skeletal disorders may produce discomfort in the chest. Localized pain in the thoracic cage may be related to unusually severe exercise or motion of the involved area. At times, the abnormality appears to be spontaneous, although even in these cases it is possible that pain was delayed in onset after either injury to the muscles of the chest wall or fractures of ribs during minor trauma or an unnoticed episode of coughing.

PULMONARY HYPERTENSION. The pain of pulmonary hypertension may simulate the pain of myocardial ischemia in its substernal location, its pattern of radiation, and its crushing or constricting quality. This type of pain may occur in patients with acute pulmonary hypertension, especially from multiple and/or massive pulmonary emboli. A similar pain has been noted in patients with chronic pulmonary hypertension from vasculitis or mitral stenosis, but the relationship is controversial. The mechanism of the pain is unknown, but it is believed to differ in the acute and chronic varieties. In the former it is related to sudden distention of the main pulmonary artery and stimulation of mechanoreceptors, and in the latter to an imbalance between the oxygen supplied to and utilized by the pressure-overloaded right ventricle. Although substernal pain related to the sudden onset of pulmonary hypertension is a well-recognized complication of pulmonary embolism, more commonly emboli cause pain in the lateral part of the chest that is typically pleuritic in character whether or not they produce pulmonary infarction.

MYOCARDIAL ISCHEMIA. Among the most important types of chest pain is that of myocardial ischemia, which is usually caused by coronary artery atherosclerosis (see Ch. 47). These attacks are provoked by an imbalance, which may be transient or permanent, between the supply of and demand for oxygen by the ventricular myocardium. Ischemic pain spans a continuum of severity from angina pectoris on the one hand to myocardial infarction on the other. Typical anginal pain is induced by exercise, heavy meals, and emotional upsets; the pain is usually described as a substernal "pressure," "constriction," or "squeezing" that, when intense, may radiate to the neck or down the ulnar aspect of one or both arms. Variant or Prinzmetal's anginal pain is similar in location and quality to typical angina pectoris but occurs in cycles at rest rather than during stressful episodes. Both typical and variant types of angina pectoris are relieved by coronary vasodilator drugs such as nitroglycerin. Typical angina also decreases with rest or removing the inciting stress. In contrast, the pain of myocardial infarction, although similar in location and character to anginal pain, is usually of greater intensity and duration, is not alleviated by rest or by nitroglycerin, may require large doses of opiates, and is often accompanied by diaphoresis, nausea, hypotension, and arrhythmias. Although patients are often short of breath during attacks of myocardial ischemia, and myocardial infarction may induce severe pulmonary edema, the pain itself is neither related to breathing nor affected by respiratory movements.

OTHER SOURCES. Pericarditis causes pain that is usually pleuritic in nature but may be steady and substernal; typically, the pain is worse while the patient is recumbent or lying on the left side. Dissecting aneurysm of the aorta is associated with severe, unremitting anterior chest pain that often radiates through to the back or into the abdomen. A deep substernal pain may result from esophageal reflux or spasm or from spontaneous mediastinal emphysema. Finally, psychogenic disorders may be associated with various forms of chest pain, the most common of which is a substernal tightness or aching sensation that may last from 30 minutes to several days. The pain may vary somewhat in intensity from time to time, and the ancillary features of myocardial infarction and a respiratory component are absent.

DIAGNOSTIC APPROACH. The approach to the general problem of the diagnosis of chest pain varies according to how seriously ill the patient is when first seen. Patients with acute chest pain who are gravely ill, as evidenced by hypotension, intense dyspnea, profuse diaphoresis, agitation, and restlessness, are usually evaluated first in the emergency room. The chief diagnostic considerations in this common clinical complex are myocardial infarction, pulmonary embolism, and dissecting aneurysm; less likely possibilities are tension pneumothorax, pericardial tamponade, and ruptured esophagus. An initial tentative diagnosis can usually be made from the results of a careful history and physical examination, supplemented by an electrocardiogram and chest roentgenograms. Except when the electrocardiogram reveals clear evidence of acute myocardial ischemia, definitive diagnosis depends on the results of later studies, such as ventilation-perfusion lung scans, pulmonary angiography, aortography, serial enzyme determinations, and coronary artery catheterization.

Patients with less severe chest pain may present during an episode of pain or afterward. Again, a detailed history of the character and behavior of the pain provides the best guide for the selection of subsequent diagnostic studies. Most patients will require an electrocardiogram, ideally taken during an episode of pain, and chest roentgenograms; then, on the basis of the results of these examinations, diagnostic evaluation proceeds as needed for the particular entities under consideration.

TREATMENT. The treatment of chest pain depends on its cause. Anginal pain responds to coronary artery vasodilator drugs, whereas myocardial infarction usually requires opiates, often in large doses. Pleural pain responds to analgesics, given as required. However, pleurisy in association with pneumonia may be alleviated by anti-inflammatory drugs such as indomethacin; in refractory cases, intercostal nerve block is needed. For costochondral and other types of chest wall pain, mild analgesia, reassurance, and time usually suffice; rapid relief can be obtained, when necessary, by injection of local anesthetic agents into the involved area.

DYSPNEA

When healthy persons undertake a steadily increasing amount of physical activity, they will eventually become aware of their breathing; the exercise required to provoke this sensation depends on their physical fitness. If they increase the level of activity even further, the awareness will increase as the sensation becomes progressively more unpleasant; if they stop exercising, the feeling will quickly disappear. The sensation experienced by normal subjects during physical exertion is aptly described as "shortness of breath" but not as dyspnea. The term dyspnea implies that the awareness is disproportionate to the stimulus and, moreover, that the sensation is abnormally uncomfortable. Many patients will describe their breathing discomfort as "breathlessness," but many others will complain only of "tightness," "choking," "inability to take a deep breath," "suffocating," and simply "can't get enough air." Thus dyspnea is difficult to define and quantify precisely, although various rating scales are in use. As with the evaluation of chest pain, a thorough history is required to explore all the vagaries of this elusive symptom.

MECHANISM. It is impossible to find a common mechanism for what appears to be the same or similar sensation of difficulty in breathing that may occur in respiratory, cardiac, erythropoietic, metabolic, and psychogenic disorders. Dyspnea in patients with respiratory diseases is believed to have a reflex origin and thus must begin with stimulation of receptors in one or more of the organs concerned with breathing. There are three types of intrapulmonary receptors (stretch, irritant, and C-fibers, which include the J- and probably other receptors), each of which has its afferent pathway to the central nervous system in the vagus nerve. There are also receptors in the muscles and tendons that participate in breathing, and chemoreceptors are situated in systemic arteries and the brain. The theory of "length-tension inappropriateness" postulates that misalignment of muscle spindles in the respiratory musculature serves as the genesis of dyspnea. An attractive explanation is that dyspnea is the subjective perception of the intensity of the stimuli that are generated by *all* the receptors activated during or in association with the act of breathing. Another theory proposes that the presence and intensity of dyspnea depend on the level of motor output to the respiratory muscles, but it is not certain how this activity is sensed.

PATTERNS. Dyspnea occurs with many underlying conditions and in several different patterns. Some of these are sufficiently characteristic to warrant separate designations. Episodes of breathlessness that wake patients from a sound sleep are called *paroxysmal nocturnal dyspnea;* these are most often observed in patients with chronic left ventricular failure but may also occur in patients with chronic pulmonary diseases because of pooling of secretions, gravity-induced decreases in lung volumes, or sleep-induced increases in airflow resistance. *Orthopnea,* or the onset or worsening of dyspnea on assuming the supine position, like paroxysmal nocturnal dyspnea, is found in patients with heart disease and occasionally in patients with chronic lung disease. The inability to assume the supine position (instant orthopnea) is particularly characteristic of the rare condition of paralysis of both hemidiaphragms. *Platypnea* denotes dyspnea that occurs in the upright position and *trepopnea* the even rarer form of dyspnea that develops in either the right or the left lateral decubitus position. Both the terms *hyperpnea,* an increase in minute volume, and *hyperventilation,* an increase in alveolar ventilation in excess of carbon dioxide production, indicate that ventilation is increased above normal. However, neither term carries any implication about the presence or absence of dyspnea.

DIAGNOSTIC APPROACH. The differential diagnosis of the dyspneic patient begins with a careful history. In patients with chronic respiratory or cardiac disease, dyspnea initially develops only during physical activity, and the amount of exertion required to provoke the symptom relates in a general way to the severity of the underlying condition. Sudden episodes of dyspnea, unrelated to physical activity, typically occur with pulmonary embolism, spontaneous pneumothorax, and anxiety; the acute attacks in each of these disorders characteristically remit, but bouts of breathlessness may recur with varying severity.

The results of the history and physical examination, routine blood tests, electrocardiography, and chest roentgenography nearly always indicate whether the dyspneic patient is suffering from a respiratory, cardiac, hematologic, renal, or hepatic abnormality. Special diagnostic studies are often then required to determine what specific kind of disease is present. Measurements of lung volumes, expiratory flow rates, and diffusing capacity, studies during exercise, and noninvasive tests of cardiac function are particularly valuable in three difficult clinical situations: (1) differentiating between dyspnea of cardiac and pulmonary origin and, if abnormalities of both systems coexist, as is often the case, estimating the severity of each; (2) identifying the presence of either pulmonary vascular obstructive disease or diffuse pulmonary infiltrative disorders in dyspneic patients whose routine studies, including chest roentgenograms, are normal; and (3) helping to establish, by ruling out significant cardiorespiratory abnormalities, that dyspnea in a given patient is psychogenic in origin (a diagnosis that is always tenuous).

TREATMENT. Unlike cough, for which there are effective antitussives, and pain, for which there are powerful analgesics, there is no category of medications for relief of dyspnea. Cure or alleviation of dyspnea depends on recognizing its origin and treating the basic abnormality. In acute reversible conditions, the dyspnea subsides along with improvement of its underlying cause. In chronic cardiac and pulmonary disorders, sufficient physical exertion will continue to provoke dyspnea, but even in these conditions rehabilitation programs can be used to enable patients to increase their physical activity up to the maximum of the limits imposed by their disease.

CONCLUSION

This introduction to the three most common and important symptoms of *all* diseases of the respiratory system is meant to supplement the material presented not only in the remainder of Part VII but also elsewhere in the book. Acute infections of the upper and lower respiratory tract caused by viruses, bacteria, fungi, protozoa, and helminths are discussed in Parts XX, XXI, and XXII. Systemic diseases in which the lungs may be involved are also discussed elsewhere: Wegener's granulomatosis (Ch. 266), eosinophilic syndromes (Ch. 150), and the "collagen diseases" (Ch. 258 to 268). Various abnormalities of the pulmonary circulation, exclusive of pulmonary embolism, and pulmonary edema, an important disorder (not disease) of the lungs, are discussed chiefly in Part VI.

Simon PM, Schwartzstein RM, Weiss JW, et al.: Distinguishable types of dyspnea in patients with shortness of breath. Am Rev Respir Dis 142:1009, 1990. *A partially successful effort to subdivide various types of dyspnea that supports the belief that different mechanisms are involved in each.*

Jones DK, Davies RJ: Massive haemoptysis. Medical management will usually arrest the bleeding. Br Med J 300:889, 1990. *Short review that supports the recent trend from surgical to medical management.*

Schneider RR, Seckler SG: Evaluation of acute chest pain. Med Clin North Am 65:53, 1981. *Comprehensive description of pain arising from different organs within the thorax; 75 references.*

Stulbarg M: Evaluating and treating intractable cough. Medical Staff Conference, University of California, San Francisco. West J Med 143:223, 1985. *Excellent review of the pathophysiology, causes, diagnosis, and management of intractable cough; 49 references.*

56 Respiratory Structure and Function

John F. Murray

Respiration can be defined as "those processes concerned with gas exchange between an organism and its environment." This definition, which emphasizes that the chief function of the respiratory system is *gas exchange*, is sufficiently comprehensive to apply to all animals, ranging from simple one-celled protozoa to infinitely more complex mammals. In human beings, the basic processes leading to gas exchange, or the uptake of O_2 and the elimination of CO_2, are usually divided into four functional subdivisions:

1. *Ventilation*—the movement of air from outside to inside the body and the distribution of air within the tracheobronchial system to the gas exchange units of the lungs.

2. *Diffusion*—the movement of O_2 and CO_2 across the alveolar-capillary membrane between the gas in alveolar spaces and the blood in pulmonary capillaries.

3. *Perfusion*—the flow of mixed venous blood through the pulmonary arterial circulation, distribution of the blood to the capillaries of the gas exchange units, and removal of the blood from the lungs through pulmonary veins.

4. *Control of breathing*—the regulation of ventilation, usually in accordance with changing metabolic demands.

VENTILATION

Air moves from outside the body into the gas exchange units of the lungs because contraction of the muscles of respiration normally generates sufficient force to expand the lungs and chest wall and to overcome the resistance and inertia in the system. This condition creates a negative pressure within the alveolar spaces that causes ambient air to flow into the lungs. The volume of gas that reaches the individual gas exchange units is determined by the mechanical properties of the lung parenchyma, airways, and chest wall, and by the force provided by the muscles of respiration (or by a mechanical ventilator).

The amount of air that enters the lung with each breath is called the *tidal volume*. When the lungs are fully expanded, the amount of gas they contain is called the *total lung capacity*. The maximal volume of gas that a person can exhale from total lung capacity is called the *vital capacity*, and the amount of gas remaining in the lungs at the end of maximal expiration is called the *residual volume*. Another important static lung volume is the *functional residual capacity*, which is the volume of gas in the lungs at the end of a normal breath. The relationships among these different lung volumes, which vary in different disorders and which will be frequently referred to, are shown in Figure 56-1.

Static Properties

Both the lungs and the chest wall are elastic structures. This means that they can be distended, and when the distending force is removed, they recoil back to their resting volumes. Although the lungs and chest wall are similar in this respect, they differ considerably in their respective resting volumes when there is no expanding force.

The elastic properties of isolated lungs are shown by the dashed line in Figure 56-1. The slope of the line, or the change in volume (ΔV) for a given change in pressure (ΔP), is known as the compliance of the lungs. This curve demonstrates that (1) the lungs collapse almost completely when there is no distending pressure; (2) the slope of the volume-pressure curve is relatively steep at low lung volumes (i.e., as the lungs are beginning to inflate, their compliance is high); and (3) at high lung volumes, the curve flattens (compliance decreases), so that little increase in volume results from a large increase in pressure. The elastic forces of the lungs originate within the tissues that are being stretched, particularly those containing elastin and collagen, and from the surface tension of the film of *surfactant* that lines the air-liquid interface of alveolar spaces. The static properties of the isolated chest wall (including the diaphragm and abdominal contents that must be displaced during breathing) are shown by the solid light red line in Figure 56-1. The chest wall is a compressible and distensible structure that contains an appreciable volume in its resting state. To decrease the volume of the thorax, a force must be applied to overcome the tendency of the chest wall to resist compression and recoil back to its resting position. Conversely, to increase the volume of the thorax, the applied force must overcome the elastic forces in the chest wall that also cause it to recoil back to its resting position.

It is useful conceptually to consider the behavior of the lungs and chest wall separately, but obviously they function together. Because their action is coupled by the pleural pressure that keeps each lung expanded against the chest wall, the lungs and chest wall ordinarily change their volumes by exactly the same amount. Thus the pressures required to change the volume of the respiratory system are obtained by simply adding the separate pressures necessary to inflate the lungs and chest wall to a given volume. The solid dark red line in Figure 56-1 indicates the pressure that must be produced by contraction of the respiratory muscles, or by a mechanical ventilator, to inflate or deflate both the lungs and the chest wall. Figure 56–1 also shows that functional residual capacity is the volume at which the inward recoil force of the lungs is equal and opposite to the outward recoil force of the chest wall; in other words, functional residual capacity is that volume at which the net force of the respiratory system is zero.

During inspiration, the force developed by the contracting muscles of inspiration meets progressively increasing (inward) recoil forces from the combined expansion of the lungs and chest wall. Furthermore, because shortening muscle fibers generate progressively less force, inspiration finally ceases at that volume (total lung capacity) at which the weakening inspiratory muscle forces can no longer overcome the increasing forces required to expand the lungs and chest wall further. Similarly, during expiration, the net force developed by the contracting muscles of expiration meets progressively increasing (outward) recoil forces from the chest wall. In children and young adults, expiration ceases at that volume (residual volume) at which the decreasing expiratory muscle forces can no longer overcome the increasing forces required to compress the chest wall further. In older persons, residual volume is governed mainly by factors that regulate the caliber and patency of peripheral airways; thus even though the expiratory muscles are capable of further compression of the thorax, emptying is prevented by airway closure and trapping of gas in the lungs.

Vital capacity, or the volume between total lung capacity and residual volume, is determined by the factors that influence maximum inspiration and expiration, i.e., the balance of forces generated by the muscles of respiration and by the mechanical properties of the lungs and chest wall combined. Changes in these variables explain the characteristic abnormalities in lung volumes that occur in patients with the respiratory disorders discussed in subsequent chapters.

Lung volumes also vary among healthy persons according to their age, sex, and physical structure (especially height). Because body build varies slightly from one ethnic group to another, it is important to have normal data that pertain to the population being studied. Measured volumes are usually expressed as both the observed value and the percentage of the predicted mean value for a normal subject of the same age, sex, and height. Measured values should not be considered abnormal unless they are clearly outside the range of values likely to be found in normal persons (100 per cent ± 20 per cent for vital capacity and 100 per cent ± 25 per cent for total lung capacity, residual volume, and functional residual capacity).

Routine tests of pulmonary function customarily include measurements by a spirometer or one of a variety of commercially available recording systems of vital capacity and of rates of expiratory airflow (see Dynamic Properties, below). These methods, however, do not measure total lung capacity, functional residual capacity, or residual volume.

To measure *all* the gas in the lungs at any of these volumes, one of two basically different methods must be used: either dilution or washout of an inert gas or whole-body plethysmography. Functional residual capacity is usually determined because it is the normal end-expiratory lung volume and thus is an easy volume for subjects to maintain during the breathing test. During the measurement of functional residual capacity, the subject exhales completely so that this volume, expiratory reserve volume, can be subtracted from the functional residual capacity to obtain the residual volume; total lung capacity is obtained by adding vital capacity to the residual volume.

Gas dilution or *washout* involves measurement of the volume and concentration of an inert gas, such as nitrogen (N_2), neon (Ne), or helium (He). These methods measure the amount of gas that communicates freely with the airways during the breathing maneuver; dilution or washout techniques do not detect gas trapped beyond closed (or very narrowed) airways and in poorly communicating regions, like bullae.

Body plethysmography involves placing the subject in the plethysmograph, a large airtight box resembling a telephone booth, and having him or her breathe through a mouthpiece in which a shutter can be closed to stop the flow of air. When the subject attempts to pant against the closed shutter, the volume of the thorax and gas in the lungs expands and contracts, which changes the pressure measured inside the mouthpiece. Movement of the thorax also changes the pressure in the box by compressing and expanding the gas surrounding the subject. From application of Boyle's law, which states that the pressure times the volume of a gas is constant if temperature remains the same, the volume of gas in the thorax can be calculated. The body plethysmograph measures all the gas present during the breathing maneuver, including that in freely communicating air spaces *and* any that may be trapped behind poorly communicating airways or in closed spaces (e.g., pneumothorax).

In normal subjects, measurements of functional residual capacity by dilution (or washout) and plethysmographic techniques are virtually identical. In contrast, in patients with airways obstruction or bullous disease, the communicating volume may be considerably less than the plethysmographic volume, and the difference is a measure of the noncommunicating (sometimes called "trapped") volume.

Dynamic Properties

To cause air to flow from outside the body into the gas exchange units, a muscular (or other mechanical) force must be exerted to overcome not only the elastic recoil properties of the lungs and chest wall but also their resistive and inertial properties. In contrast to distensibility, which is not affected by the rate of movement, the forces required to offset resistance and inertia

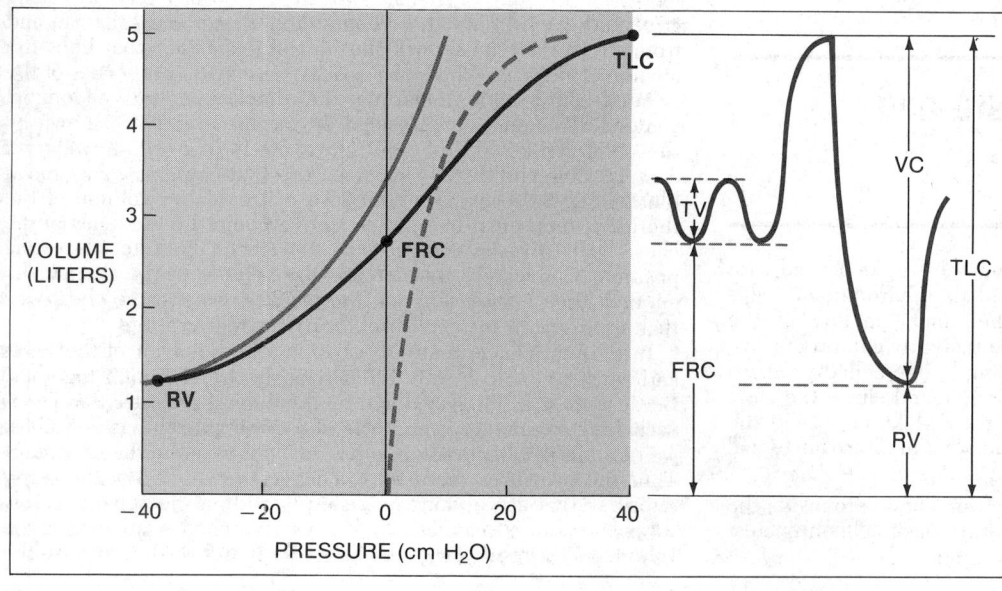

FIGURE 56–1. Schematic representation of the volume-pressure relationships of the chest wall (*solid light red line*), lungs (*dashed light red line*), and chest wall and lungs combined (*solid dark red line*). Total lung capacity (TLC) occurs when the lungs are fully expanded, and residual volume (RV) is the amount of gas remaining in the lungs at the end of a maximal expiration. Functional residual capacity (FRC) occurs at that volume at which the recoil pressures of the chest wall and lung are equal and opposite (i.e., the distending pressure = 0 cm H_2O). On the right is a spirometric tracing (volume-time) of the breathing maneuvers of the person whose pressure-volume curves are on the left. TV = tidal volume; VC = vital capacity.

are markedly influenced by the velocity of airflow. Inertial forces are ordinarily small and usually ignored, although new tests show they may be important in advanced lung diseases.

Resistance to airflow is affected chiefly by the caliber of the air passages. Although the diameter of each successive generation of airways decreases, the combined total cross-sectional area at any level increases steadily throughout the tracheobronchial tree, from the main bronchi to the peripheral airways. This means that airways resistance progressively decreases and that most of the resistance of the human tracheobronchial tree resides in large airways: Direct measurements reveal that between 50 and 80 per cent of total resistance to airflow originates in airways *greater than* 2 mm in diameter. A corollary of this observation is that substantial changes can occur in the caliber of the small peripheral airways without having much effect on total airways resistance. Hence, small airways have been called the lung's "quiet zone," and because they are frequently involved early in the evolution of clinically important lung disease, special tests have been devised to examine their functional behavior.

Changes in the cross-sectional area of airways can also result from changes in lung volume and diseases of the lung parenchyma or the airways themselves. During inflation of the lungs from functional residual capacity, airways are pulled open so that resistance to airflow decreases; during deflation, airways narrow and their resistance increases. Airway caliber changes during inflation and deflation because of the combined effects of the tethering action of the attachments between the lung parenchyma and small bronchioles and the distending effect of pleural pressure on larger airways. Elastic recoil of the lung, which governs the pull of the attachments and the magnitude of pleural pressure, affects the size of all airways, and this, in turn, affects overall resistance to airflow.

Airway narrowing may result from bronchospasm, edema of the mucosal lining, and secretions within the lumen. In addition, changes in the viscosity and density of the inspired gas affect airways resistance, and gas mixtures of different densities are sometimes used to study the dynamic properties of the tracheobronchial system.

Resistance to airflow can be measured in a body plethysmograph; however, this procedure has limited clinical usefulness. Fortunately, the important dynamic properties of the respiratory system can be assessed by several readily available tests of airways function. The simplest and most widely used of these is the forced expiratory volume in 1 second (FEV_1), expressed as a ratio of the forced vital capacity (FVC), or FEV_1/FVC (Fig. 56–2). To perform the FVC maneuver, the subject inhales fully and then exhales as rapidly and completely as possible. In normal persons, the FVC equals the vital capacity from a slow or nonexpulsive maneuver, but in patients with airways obstruction, vigorous expiration may cause airways to narrow and close prematurely, so that the FVC may be less than the vital capacity; the magnitude of the difference between the two values is an indication of the amount of air trapped behind compressed airways. The FEV_1/FVC decreases with age in normal persons after reaching adulthood and is usually higher in women than in men at all ages.

Additional measurements of airways behavior besides the FEV_1 can be obtained from the FVC maneuver (Fig. 56–2): several derivatives of time, such as the $FEV_{0.5}$ and FEV_3 (the subscript denoting the number of seconds after beginning expiration at which the expired volume is measured), the maximal expiratory flow rate (MEFR or often $MEFR_{200-1200 \, ml}$, indicating that the flow rate was measured between expired volumes of 200 and 1200 ml), and the maximal mid-expiratory flow rate (MMFR or often $MMFR_{25-75\%}$, indicating that the rate was measured between expired volumes of 25 and 75 per cent of the FVC). None of these has any particular advantage over the FEV_1 except that the MMFR is less dependent on the effort exerted by the subject than are the other variables and reflects the flow properties of small as well as large airways.

Another way of examining the events during an FVC maneuver is by recording flow against volume instead of volume against time, which provides a maximal expiratory flow-volume curve (Fig. 56–3). From these records, maximal flow rates at any given fraction of the expired vital capacity, usually 50 per cent ($Vmax_{50}$) or 75 per cent ($Vmax_{75}$), can be determined and reported as the percentage of the predicted values for a subject

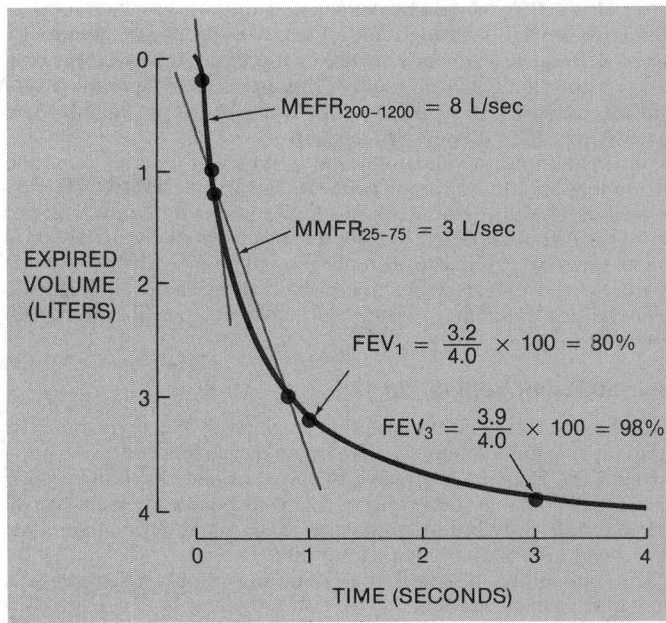

FIGURE 56–2. Schematic representation of a normal forced vital capacity (FVC) maneuver (expired volume against time, *heavy red line*) and the derivation of several variables commonly used to evaluate airways obstruction. $MEFR_{200-1200}$ = maximal expiratory flow rate, measured between expired volumes of 200 and 1200 ml; $MMER_{25-75}$ = maximal mid-expiratory flow rate, measured between 25 and 75 per cent of the total FVC; FEV_1 = forced expiratory volume in 1 second, expressed as percentage of total FVC; FEV_3 = forced expiratory volume in 3 seconds, expressed as percentage of total FVC.

of the same age, sex, and body size. The early portion of the maximal expiratory flow-volume curve, which includes peak flow, is determined by the effort exerted by the subject and is thus called the effort-*dependent* segment; the later portion is less influenced by effort and is called the effort-*independent* segment, or that part of the curve during which expiratory airflow limitation occurs. Additional effort does not increase expiratory airflow (i.e., maximal velocity is limited), because "choke points" develop in

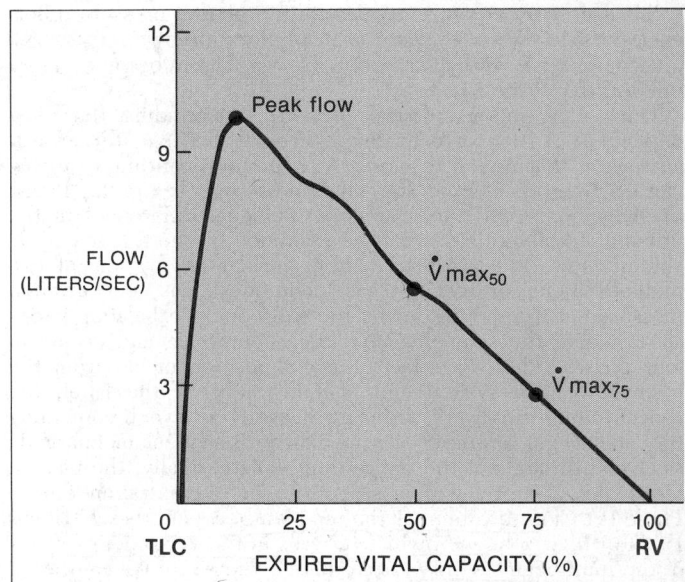

FIGURE 56–3. Typical forced expiratory flow-volume tracing of a normal adult man showing points of peak flow, maximal flow at 50 per cent expired vital capacity ($Vmax_{50}$), and maximal flow at 75 per cent expired vital capacity ($Vmax_{75}$). TLC = total lung capacity; RV = residual volume. (From Smith LH, Thier SO: Pathophysiology: The Biological Principles of Disease. Philadelphia, W. B. Saunders Company, 1981.)

those airways in which the velocity of airflow has increased to equal the speed at which pressures will propagate along the airways. Because events recorded in the effort-independent portion of the flow-volume curve require less cooperation and understanding by the subject, they are more reproducible than those in the effort-dependent portion.

Maximal expiratory flow-volume curves can also be recorded after a few breaths of 79 per cent He and 21 per cent O_2 (He-O_2) as well as after breathing room air (79 per cent N_2 and 21 per cent O_2). Although much has been learned about the behavior of the airways by comparing the curves obtained with the two gas mixtures, these tests have not proved as reliable as originally believed in detecting disease localized to peripheral (small) airways.

Distribution of Ventilation

During the movement of air from outside the body into the lungs during inhalation, the airstream is partitioned as it flows through the branching airways to the terminal respiratory units where gas exchange takes place. Even in healthy persons ventilation is not distributed uniformly, and marked derangements may develop in patients with lung disease.

The unevenness of ventilation found in normal subjects results from the vertical gradient of pleural pressure between the uppermost and lowermost parts of the lungs. The origins of the vertical gradient in different mammals are complex and include the weight of the lungs, their attachments at the hilum, and the shape and effects of the chest wall and abdominal contents; in humans, the weight of the lungs is the most important determinant. Because of the gradient in the pressure surrounding the lungs, alveoli are larger at the top than at the bottom, and there are regional differences in the distribution of inspired ventilation.

When breathing slowly from functional residual capacity, more inspired air is distributed to the dependent regions of the lungs than to the superior regions because the differences in pleural pressure cause the two regions to function on different segments of the same volume-pressure curve. Because the *change* in intrapleural pressure during quiet breathing is the same throughout the pleural space, the lower regions, which are operating on a steeper part of the curve and thus receive more volume for the same pressure change, inflate more than the upper regions. When inspiration continues to total lung capacity, alveoli at the top and bottom of the lungs inflate to nearly the same size because both regions are functioning on the flat portion of the volume-pressure curve, even though the pleural pressure difference persists. When the rate of inspiratory airflow increases, as during exercise, the distribution of ventilation becomes more uniform than it is at rest.

During expiration, pleural pressure surrounding the most dependent portion of each lung becomes positive; this causes airways in that region to close. As expiration continues, airway closure progresses from the lowermost regions up the lungs, involving more and more airways. Regional differences in the distribution of ventilation can be examined by the test of closing volume (Fig. 56–4). After labeling alveolar gas by one of two methods (bolus or resident gas techniques), gas concentration measured at the mouth during the subsequent exhalation varies according to the sequence of regional emptying and occurs in four phases. Phase I reflects the composition of gas from the tracheobronchial system and contains none of the label; the concentration rapidly rises during Phase II as alveoli containing the label begin to empty; a near-plateau is evident in Phase III as alveoli throughout the entire lung deflate; finally, the plateau terminates abruptly with a steep rise in concentration during Phase IV. Closing volume is the junction between Phases III and IV and is that volume at which airways in the dependent regions of the lung begin to close; accordingly, the rising concentration of the label in the subsequent expirate indicates the progressively increasing contributions from the preferentially labeled alveoli in the upper regions of the lung.

Because an increase in closing volume reflects premature closure or narrowing of airways, an increase in closing volume occurs in patients with lung disorders in which the caliber of peripheral airways is decreased from either decreased elastic

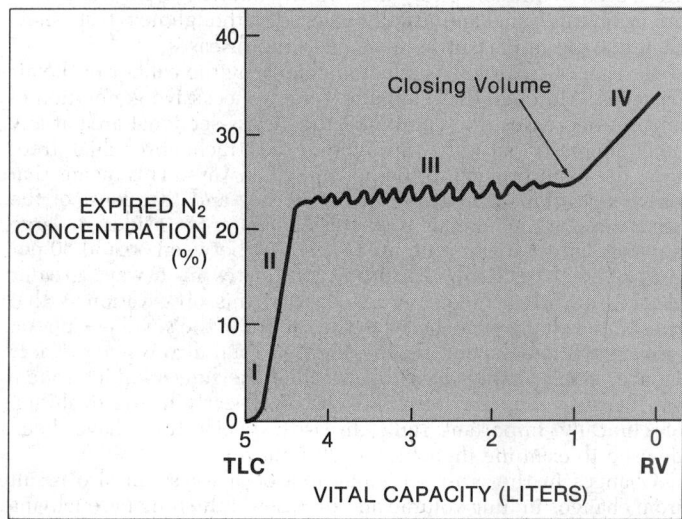

FIGURE 56–4. Representative tracing of expired nitrogen (N_2) concentration after taking a single breath of 100 per cent oxygen. An explanation of the four numbered phases (I, II, III, IV) is provided in the text. TLC = total lung capacity; RV = residual volume. (From Smith LH, Thier SO: Pathophysiology: The Biological Principles of Disease. Philadelphia, W. B. Saunders Company, 1981.)

recoil (e.g., in emphysema) or abnormalities of the airways themselves (e.g., in bronchitis or asthma). Furthermore, increases in closing volume have been detected in asymptomatic patients, usually smokers, and may be an early manifestation of lung disease. In addition, examination of the slope of Phase III is useful because it provides a sensitive measure of the adequacy of the distribution of ventilation. Well-ventilated units fill and empty more completely and rapidly than poorly ventilated units; this means that the concentration of the label will be lower in the better-ventilated regions that empty early during exhalation than in the poorly ventilated regions. Thus, the more uneven the distribution of ventilation within the lung, the steeper the slope of Phase III.

Other tests of the distribution of ventilation utilize the gamma ray–emitting properties of certain radioactive gases, chiefly ^{133}Xe, which are nontoxic and can be detected by external counters after inhalation in low concentrations. The distribution of ventilation can be assessed during a breath hold at end-inspiration after a single breath of ^{133}Xe or at intervals during its elimination by normal breathing after the lung has been labeled uniformly by rebreathing ^{133}Xe from a closed system.

Abnormalities of Ventilation

Lung diseases that cause abnormalities of ventilation are usually divided into two different categories: restrictive and obstructive ventilatory disorders. This classification is not completely satisfactory because it ignores the fact that disturbances of the distribution of ventilation are the earliest and by far the most common abnormality of ventilation and can occur in the absence of manifestations of coexisting obstructive or restrictive disorders.

DISTURBANCES OF DISTRIBUTION. Whenever a disease process involves the lung parenchyma or airways unevenly, abnormalities in the distribution of ventilation are likely to occur because more inspired gas will reach the normal regions of the lung compared with the regions distal to the sites of bronchial narrowing, or the regions in which the distensibility is impaired. Whether these functional changes can be detected depends on the extent and severity of the disease and the sensitivity of the test being used. The slope of Phase III of the closing volume maneuver is the most commonly used test for detecting early abnormalities in the distribution of ventilation. Frequency dependence of compliance is an extremely sensitive test for distribution of ventilation but is seldom used owing to its technical complexities.

RESTRICTIVE VENTILATORY DISORDERS. The term *restrictive ventilatory disorder* denotes a pattern of abnormalities in lung function. The word "restrictive" is employed to indicate a restriction of or limitation to the amount of gas within the lungs. Thus restrictive ventilatory disorders are characterized by reductions in lung volumes (Table 56–1). The hallmark of restriction is a decreased vital capacity, but because this change also occurs in obstructive ventilatory disorders, it is important to exclude the presence of airways obstruction (see Obstructive Ventilatory Disorders, below) or to demonstrate the presence of reductions in other lung volumes, particularly total lung capacity.

Many components of the lungs, chest wall, and respiratory control system determine the amount of gas that can be breathed into the lungs. Accordingly, restrictive ventilatory disorders can develop in diseases that (1) affect the chest wall or respiratory muscles (kyphoscoliosis, myasthenia gravis), (2) cause infiltrations in the lung parenchyma or air spaces (diffuse interstitial fibrosis, pulmonary edema), (3) involve the pleura (pleural thickening), (4) occupy space within the thorax (tumors, effusions, cardiac enlargement), and (5) occur after lung resection (pneumonectomy).

OBSTRUCTIVE VENTILATORY DISORDERS. The term *obstructive ventilatory disorder* denotes the constellation of abnormalities that results from limitation of expiratory airflow, regardless of its cause. Because the functional disturbances depend on the presence of increased airways resistance, obstructive ventilatory disorders are detected mainly by tests of the behavior of the respiratory system under dynamic conditions (Table 56–1). Of the available tests, the FEV_1/FVC is the most widely used, and other tests provide little additional information.

Obstructive ventilatory disorders are found in patients with asthma, bronchitis, emphysema, advanced bronchiectasis, or other diseases that cause narrowing of the tracheobronchial system. When the term "obstructive" was originally employed, it was not possible to differentiate among these various entities, so they were lumped together in the nonspecific category of chronic obstructive pulmonary disease. Now, however, it is possible by means of specialized tests of lung function to sort out the various diseases that cause airways obstruction, even when they coexist; the characteristic features of asthma, chronic bronchitis, and emphysema are described in subsequent chapters.

DIFFUSION

Diffusion can be defined as the movement of molecules from a region of higher to one of lower concentration; accordingly, diffusion tends to eliminate differences in concentration within the various regions accessible to the molecules. Diffusion is a passive process that results from the kinetic motion of the molecules, and no extra energy is required. In the lungs, O_2 moves by diffusion from alveolar gas into pulmonary capillary blood; similarly, in the peripheral tissues, O_2 moves by diffusion from capillary blood into neighboring cells. Carbon dioxide also moves by diffusion but usually in the direction opposite to that of O_2. Both O_2 and CO_2 undergo chemical reactions in the bloodstream at the start and finish of their journeys between the lungs and the peripheral tissues; O_2 reacts solely with hemoglobin, and CO_2 reacts in part with hemoglobin and in part to form bicarbonate.

Diffusing Capacity

The diffusing capacity of the lungs for any gas indicates the quantity of that gas that diffuses across the alveolar-capillary membrane per unit of time in response to the difference in mean pressures of the gas within the alveolus and pulmonary capillary. Most inert gases (e.g., N_2) diffuse across the air-blood barrier so rapidly that the amount taken up by the lungs is not detectably limited by the diffusibility of the gas and the properties of the lungs and blood but is determined solely by the solubility of the gas and the volume of tissue and blood into which it can dissolve. This phenomenon enables the use of highly soluble gases like acetylene, dimethyl ether, or nitrous oxide to measure lung tissue volume and pulmonary capillary blood flow.

The only two gases that can be used to measure the diffusing capacity of the lungs are O_2 and CO. Because of their unique ability to combine with hemoglobin, both have to diffuse across the alveolar-capillary membrane in large quantities to saturate the available hemoglobin at the gas pressure prevailing in the alveoli. Thus it may not be possible for complete equilibrium to occur before the hemoglobin-containing red blood cells leave the pulmonary capillaries and gas transfer ceases. Of the two gases, CO is much more widely used for the measurement of diffusing capacity than O_2 because of the ease and convenience of applying the various CO tests and because CO uptake is always diffusion limited. In contrast, O_2 uptake is not limited by diffusion (i.e., is not a test of diffusing capacity) in normal subjects except during heavy exercise or while breathing low concentrations of O_2.

Two general types of tests using CO are available that involve either a breath-holding maneuver (single-breath method) or continuous rebreathing (steady-state methods). These two methods yield systematically different results, largely because neither technique summarizes accurately the events taking place in the 100,000 gas exchange units of the lung, in each of which P_{CO} varies according to the ventilation and blood flow to the unit. Despite this shortcoming, measurements of pulmonary diffusing capacity have provided useful empiric information concerning the function of the lungs in healthy persons and patients with lung diseases.

The quantity of CO that will diffuse in a known period of time from alveolar gas into capillary blood and combine with hemoglobin in response to a given pressure difference between gas and blood depends on (1) the solubility and diffusibility of CO in each layer of the air-blood barrier, (2) the surface area and thickness of the barrier, and (3) the rate of the chemical reaction between CO and hemoglobin within red blood cells. Because the solubility and diffusibility of CO are physical characteristics that presumably do not change under ordinary circumstances, the two chief components of diffusing capacity are the area and thickness of the alveolar-capillary membrane available for diffusion (D_M) and the pulmonary capillary blood volume (V_C), both of which can be derived by performing several measurements of diffusing capacity (DL_{CO}) with the subject breathing gas mixtures of different concentrations of CO and O_2.

Normal values for CO-diffusing capacity depend chiefly on the person's lung volume and therefore closely correlate with body size, especially height. Less than half the total resistance to diffusion of CO from alveolar gas to capillary blood is attributable to the membrane component, and the greater fraction resides in the chemical reaction that takes place in the pulmonary capillary blood volume. Accordingly, changes in the hemoglobin concentration have a calculable effect on total CO diffusion that should be taken into account when establishing the predicted "normal" value for a patient with anemia or polycythemia.

Diffusing capacity is normally higher when a person is in the supine position than when he or she is in the erect posture because position changes the volume of blood in pulmonary capillaries, and at high compared with low lung volumes because inflation recruits alveolar-capillary surface. When blood flow to the lung increases, as in muscular exercise, capillary blood volume also increases owing to recruitment of previously nonperfused capillaries and dilation of others; these phenomena account for the progressive increase in DL_{CO} during increasingly strenuous levels of exercise. Similarly, the elevated pulmonary arterial pressures encountered in persons who live at high altitudes also recruit capillaries, increase capillary blood volume, and cause an increase in "normal" DL_{CO}. For unexplained reasons (possibly genetic), natives of high altitudes have higher DL_{CO} values than sojourners fully acclimatized to the same altitude.

TABLE 56–1. CHARACTERISTIC CHANGES IN LUNG VOLUMES AND TESTS OF AIRWAYS RESISTANCE IN PATIENTS WITH RESTRICTIVE AND OBSTRUCTIVE VENTILATORY DISORDERS*

Test	Restrictive	Obstructive
Vital capacity	Decreased	Decreased or normal
Residual volume	Decreased or normal	Increased
Total lung capacity	Decreased	Normal or increased
RV/TLC	Normal or slightly increased	Markedly increased
FEV_1/FVC	Normal or increased	Decreased
MMFR	Normal or decreased	Decreased
Slope of phase III	Normal or increased	Increased

*Abbreviations: RV/TLC = ratio of residual volume to total lung capacity; FEV_1/FVC = ratio of forced expiratory volume in 1 second to forced vital capacity; MMFR = maximum mid-expiratory flow rate.

Abnormalities of CO-Diffusing Capacity

On the basis of the physiologic principles that govern the diffusion of CO, it can be inferred that DL_{CO} may increase or decrease in patients with various cardiopulmonary disorders that affect the membrane, the capillary blood volume, or both. When tests of diffusing capacity were first used to study patients with various forms of lung disease, it was assumed that abnormalities of gas transfer would result from thickening of the air-blood barrier by a pathologic process that lengthened the pathway for diffusion of gases; this concept led to the formulation of what became widely known as the *alveolar-capillary block syndrome*. The "block" meant that the distance CO molecules had to travel from gas to blood was increased and, in turn, that extra time was required for diffusion to reach equilibrium across the air-blood barrier. Now it is known that most abnormalities of diffusion are caused by decreased capillary blood volume and that a true alveolar-capillary block is unusual.

Pulmonary vascular disorders, such as pulmonary emboli and pulmonary vasculitis, that affect (directly or indirectly) the pulmonary capillary bed decrease DL by decreasing capillary blood volume. Similarly, DL_{CO} is reduced in patients with infiltrative disorders of the interalveolar septum that obliterate or destroy capillaries. This is the usual mechanism underlying reduction of DL_{CO} in patients with sarcoidosis, diffuse interstitial fibrosis, berylliosis, or collagen diseases of the lung.

Changes in the characteristics of the membrane account for a decreased DL_{CO} in patients with diseases in which some form of intra-alveolar filling process has occurred and the air-to-blood diffusion pathway is actually lengthened: pneumonia, pulmonary edema, and alveolar proteinosis. A decrease in both membrane and blood volume components produces a low DL_{CO} in patients with disorders associated with removal or destruction of lung tissue, such as resectional surgery or emphysema.

An increase in DL_{CO} results occasionally from an increase in capillary blood volume secondary to hemodynamic changes in the pulmonary circulation: an increase in pulmonary arterial or left atrial pressures, as in congestive heart failure, or an increase in pulmonary blood flow, as in atrial septal defect. The DL_{CO} is sometimes increased in patients with bronchial asthma during an attack, but the cause of this change is not known.

PERFUSION

The pulmonary circulation delivers blood in a thin film to the gas exchange units so that O_2 uptake and CO_2 elimination can occur. The physiologic determinants of pulmonary blood flow are analogous to those of ventilation in that the total volumes of ventilation and blood flow must be adequate to meet metabolic needs, and the distribution of both must be such that proportionate amounts of inspired fresh air and incoming mixed venous blood are delivered to individual gas exchange units. Ventilatory volume is controlled by the factors that regulate breathing (see below), whereas the volume of blood flowing through the lungs is determined mainly by the extrapulmonary mechanisms that govern cardiac output.

Distribution of Pulmonary Blood Flow

Pulmonary blood flow is not distributed uniformly throughout the lungs but is normally greatest in the dependent regions, where pulmonary arterial pressure is highest, and, conversely, is least in the superior regions, where pulmonary arterial pressure is lowest. In the upright subject under resting conditions, the apices of the lungs are poorly perfused, and considerably more blood flows, even allowing for differences in the amount of lung tissue, to the basilar regions. The presence of nonuniform blood flow, which is not matched by comparable changes in ventilation, leads to important differences between regions of the lung in their defense capabilities and efficiency of gas exchange.

Regional blood flow is also governed by local factors, the most important of which is vasoconstriction secondary to alveolar hypoxia. As a consequence, blood flow is redistributed away from poorly ventilated gas exchange units, and the matching of ventilation and perfusion is preserved.

Distribution of pulmonary blood flow can readily be measured by injecting radioactive substances, such as ^{125}I-albumin aggre-gates or ^{133}Xe dissolved in saline, and then detecting their location in the lung with an external counter system. Abnormalities in the volume and distribution of pulmonary blood flow may result from diseases that involve the blood vessels themselves (emboli, vasculitis, emphysema), from compression of blood vessels (tumors, cysts), or from vasoconstriction of blood vessels (alveolar hypoxia secondary to local abnormality of ventilation).

Other Functions

The pulmonary circulation has important functions besides providing blood flow for continuous gas exchange: (1) It acts as a filter of virtually the entire venous drainage; (2) it supplies substrates for the nutrition and metabolic needs of the lung, including the synthesis of surfactant; (3) it serves as a reservoir of blood for the left ventricle; (4) it affects endocrine function by modifying the pharmacologic properties of a variety of circulating substances; and (5) it provides a large surface area for the absorption and filtration of liquids and solutes.

CONTROL OF BREATHING

The respiratory system must maintain gas exchange during periods of stress, such as exercise and other forms of increased metabolic needs. The O_2 consumption may increase more than 10-fold from rest to strenuous exercise; over this range, arterial Po_2 remains remarkably constant. The correspondence between the volume of ventilation and the demands for O_2 uptake and CO_2 elimination results from the responsiveness of three reasonably well characterized receptor systems that interact to regulate breathing in normal persons and patients with a variety of disease states: (1) receptors in the airways and lung parenchyma, (2) peripheral chemoreceptors, and (3) central chemoreceptors. Nerve impulse traffic from these receptors is integrated and modulated in the medulla with impulses arising from higher centers in the brain. The medulla can be viewed as the main headquarters for initiating, processing, and relaying messages concerning breathing to other parts of the body via nervous pathways. Some of the resulting medullary neural activity may reach the cerebral cortex and evoke conscious perception of breathing (i.e., the symptom of dyspnea); other impulses may travel through efferent pathways in the autonomic nervous system to the lungs and other organs; still other impulses may descend in the spinal cord to be processed with afferent impulses from peripheral nerves at different cord segments before finally being transmitted to the muscles of respiration and other effectors.

Abnormalities of Control of Breathing

Variations, usually increases, in the rate and depth of breathing occur in patients with many common clinical disturbances such as fever, metabolic diseases, or psychiatric disorders. Several frequently used drugs (e.g., aspirin, antidepressants, and alcohol) also affect ventilation. *Hyperventilation* occurs when ventilation increases out of proportion to CO_2 production and arterial Pco_2 decreases; *hypoventilation* is the converse. *Hyperpnea* signifies an increase in the rate and depth of breathing, such as occurs during exercise, but carries no implication concerning arterial Pco_2 values. It should be emphasized that a decrease in the O_2 pressure (Po_2) of arterial blood has several causes. In contrast, the pressure of CO_2 (Pco_2) is governed simply by the relationship between CO_2 production ($\dot{V}co_2$) and CO_2 elimination by alveolar ventilation (Valv):

$$Pco_2 = k\dot{V}co_2/\dot{V}alv$$

Because alveolar ventilation normally changes to keep pace wth CO_2 production, for practical purposes abnormal arterial Pco_2 values can always be interpreted as indicating hyperventilation or hypoventilation.

Abnormalities of the control of breathing can result from excitation of intrapulmonary receptors (pulmonary embolism, pneumonia, asthma), depression of peripheral chemoreceptors (natives of high altitudes, sedative drugs, severe chronic bronchitis), stimulation of peripheral chemoreceptors (drugs such as doxapram), depression of central chemoreceptors (sedative drugs, obesity, myxedema, neurologic disorders), and stimulation of central chemoreceptors (drugs such as aspirin, irritative neurologic lesions). Special tests of the ventilatory response to breathing gas mixtures with increased CO_2 or decreased O_2 and a test that determines the pressure developed during the first 0.1 second of breathing against a closed mouthpiece ($P_{0.1}$) help define the physiologic derangements in these disorders.

GAS EXCHANGE

The end-product of respiration is gas exchange, which in human beings consists of maintaining the values for PO_2 and PCO_2 in arterial blood within normal limits. As stated previously, respiration consists of ventilation, including the distribution of inspired air throughout the tracheobronchial system, diffusion, blood flow, including the distribution of mixed venous blood throughout pulmonary capillaries, and the control of breathing. Each of these contributes in a unique way to gas exchange such that an impairment in one process cannot be compensated for by improvement in another.

Ambient air consists primarily of N_2 and O_2, with varying amounts of water vapor. As air is inhaled, it is warmed to body temperature and fully saturated with water vapor (PH_2O 37°C = 47 mm Hg); the addition of water vapor has the effect of diluting the inspired mixture of N_2 and O_2 and reduces their respective pressures proportionally. During gas exchange in the alveoli, more O_2 is removed than CO_2 is added; this causes the volume of each respiratory unit to decrease slightly and raises the concentration and pressure of N_2 slightly. When ventilation and perfusion are each uniformly distributed to various units (Fig. 56–5), "ideal" conditions for gas exchange exist, and there is no difference between the PO_2 values in (mean) alveolar gas and arterial blood. The alveolar-arterial PO_2 difference is an important measure of the uniformity of matching of ventilation and perfusion. The difference is derived from a direct measurement of the arterial PO_2, which is subtracted from alveolar PO_2 (PA_{O_2}, calculated according to the following equation

$$PA_{O_2} = PI_{O_2} - PA_{CO_2} \left[FI_{O_2} + \frac{1 - FI_{O_2}}{R} \right]$$

where PI_{O_2} = PO_2 of inspired gas, PA_{CO_2} = alveolar PCO_2 (usually assumed to equal arterial PCO_2), FI_{O_2} = fractional concentration of O_2 in inspired gas, and R = respiratory exchange ratio (often assumed to equal 0.8).

However, gas exchange in healthy lungs is not perfect because there is a small (5 to 10 mm Hg) alveolar-arterial PO_2 difference, which occurs because of the normal presence of a slight nonuniformity in the distribution of ventilation with respect to perfusion and a small right-to-left shunt. It is also noteworthy that the sum of the pressures of the individual gases in mixed venous blood is less than the total atmospheric pressure. Because the tissues and spaces of the body are in approximate equilibrium with venous blood, these structures are also subatmospheric. The "suction" serves to keep the lung expanded against the chest wall and to cause the reabsorption of gas from tissue spaces (e.g., a pneumothorax).

Abnormal Gas Exchange

Measurements of arterial PO_2 and PCO_2 and calculations of the alveolar-arterial PO_2 difference are reliable guides to the overall adequacy of respiration. In determining whether or not an abnormality is present, it must be remembered that normal values for PO_2, but not PCO_2, vary with age and that both PO_2

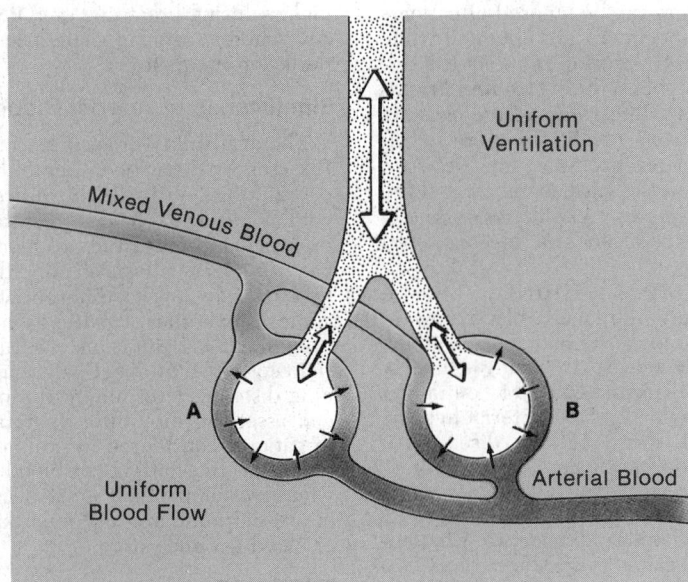

FIGURE 56–5. Schematic representation of gas exchange in an idealized two-compartment model of the lung in which there is uniform distribution of ventilation and blood flow. (Adapted with permission from Comroe JH Jr, et al.: The Lung: Clinical Physiology and Pulmonary Function Tests. 2nd ed. Chicago, Year Book Medical Publishers, 1962. Copyright © 1962, Year Book Medical Publishers, Inc.)

	A	B	A + B	Units
Alveolar ventilation	2.4	2.4	4.8	L/min
Pulmonary blood flow	3.0	3.0	6.0	L/min
Ventilation-perfusion ratio	0.8	0.8	0.8	
Mixed venous PO_2	40	40	40	mm Hg
Mixed venous SO_2	75	75	75	per cent
Mixed venous PCO_2	46	46	46	mm Hg
Alveolar PO_2	101	101	101	mm Hg
Arterial PO_2	101	101	101	mm Hg
Arterial SO_2	97.5	97.5	97.5	per cent
Arterial PCO_2	40	40	40	mm Hg
Alveolar-arterial PO_2 difference	0	0	0	mm Hg

and P_{CO_2} are influenced by the altitude at which the subject is living. There are five physiologic mechanisms known to cause arterial hypoxia, defined as a decrease below normal of arterial P_{O_2}: (1) hypoventilation, (2) decreased diffusion, (3) ventilation-perfusion imbalance, (4) right-to-left shunting of blood, and (5) breathing air (or a gas mixture) with a low P_{O_2}. Except for a few uncommon clinical examples, such as breathing air with its P_{O_2} reduced by combustion of O_2 and addition of smoke or suffocation, item 5 can be ignored. Items 1 to 4 can be distinguished, at least for practical clinical purposes, by analyzing the values from a given blood specimen and a few easy tests.

HYPOVENTILATION. The simplest disturbance of gas exchange occurs when not enough fresh air is breathed into alveolar spaces to raise pulmonary capillary P_{O_2} to normal levels and to allow CO_2 to leave the bloodsteam. Although arterial P_{CO_2} may theoretically increase in patients with other disturbances of gas exchange (ventilation-perfusion abnormalities and right-to-left shunts), for clinical purposes an elevated value should be interpreted as indicating alveolar hypoventilation.

Pure hypoventilation is a relatively uncommon clinical event. When it is found, depression of the central nervous system resulting from anesthetic agents or other sedative drugs is the usual cause. More commonly, hypoventilation occurs in association with other disturbances of oxygenation. When these coexist, they can be recognized by the fact that the decrease in arterial P_{O_2} is more than can be accounted for by the increase in arterial P_{CO_2}.

IMPAIRED DIFFUSION. Decreased diffusion, from either loss of pulmonary capillaries or thickening of the air-blood barrier, does not usually cause important alveolar-arterial P_{O_2} differences *at rest*. Thus abnormalities of diffusion can be ignored in patients with arterial hypoxia whose blood specimens are obtained while they are resting. In contrast, impaired diffusion is one of the two major causes of severely worsening hypoxia during exercise (right-to-left shunting of blood is the other). Regardless of the cause of the diffusing impairment, under resting conditions there is sufficient time to allow gas transfer to reach equilibrium between gas and blood. However, during exercise, cardiac output and the velocity of blood flow through pulmonary capillaries increase; thus the time for gas transfer is reduced and alveolar–end-capillary P_{O_2} differences may occur.

VENTILATION-PERFUSION MISMATCHING. Because the distributions of inspired air and pulmonary blood flow in normal lungs are neither uniform nor proportionate to each other, a slight ventilation-perfusion imbalance exists in healthy persons. Moreover, increased (above normal) mismatching of ventilation and perfusion is by far the most common cause of arterial hypoxia encountered clinically. Virtually all forms of lung disease are associated with a detectable ventilation-perfusion abnormality.

When a unit is underventilated relative to its perfusion (i.e., has a low ventilation-perfusion ratio), O_2 uptake by that unit must decrease so that the P_{O_2} of its end-capillary blood is lower than normal; P_{CO_2} tends to increase but cannot rise above the value in mixed venous blood (Fig. 56–5). Thus the process affects values for P_{O_2} more than P_{CO_2}. Furthermore, in those units that are overventilated owing to a redistribution of inspired air, the high ventilation-perfusion ratio causes P_{O_2} to increase and P_{CO_2} to decrease. But there is an important difference in the effects of these changes in pressures on the actual quantities (contents) of O_2 and CO_2 in the capillary blood leaving units with high ventilation-perfusion ratios. Given the shapes of the respective dissociation curves, O_2 content is not appreciably increased but CO_2 content is decreased. Thus increasing ventilation with respect to perfusion in some regions corrects the tendency to CO_2 retention that would otherwise exist but does not correct the hypoxia caused by low ventilation-perfusion relationships in other units. Another invariable consequence of a ventilation-perfusion abnormality is an increase in the alveolar-arterial P_{O_2} difference.

RIGHT-TO-LEFT SHUNTING. A small right-to-left shunt of blood is found in normal persons, and shunts of considerable magnitude may occur in patients with pulmonary disease. A right-to-left shunt may be visualized as a pathway (or pathways) through which mixed venous blood flows from the right to the left side of the heart without having perfused functioning gas exchange units along the way. Thus there is a continuous admix-

ture of venous blood that has flowed through the abnormal pathway with arterialized blood from normal pathways in the lungs. Arterial hypoxia and an increased alveolar-arterial P_{O_2} difference occur that vary in severity with the magnitude of the shunt and its O_2 content. Right-to-left shunts may occur through intracardiac communications in patients with congenital heart disease. In patients with lung disease, although shunts may be extremely large, they seldom occur through abnormal vascular channels such as pulmonary arteriovenous fistulas; instead, they are caused by blood perfusing normal vessels in regions of the lung that are atelectatic or in which alveoli are filled with edema fluid, pus, or blood; in either case, because gas transfer is impossible, a shunt occurs.

The consequences of a right-to-left shunt are similar to those of a ventilation-perfusion imbalance owing to basic similarities between the two disturbances. A shunt can be viewed as an extreme ventilation-perfusion abnormality in which there is perfusion but *no* ventilation at all. It is impossible to differentiate between a ventilation-perfusion disturbance and a right-to-left shunt while the subject is breathing ambient air; therefore the effects of both are combined and designated venous admixture or a "shuntlike" effect. The two causes of hypoxia can be differentiated by giving the patient 100 per cent O_2 to breathe and measuring arterial P_{O_2} after all the N_2 has been washed out of the lungs. When a ventilation-perfusion abnormality exists, the N_2 is replaced by O_2 and all the blood perfusing the lungs equilibrates at a high P_{O_2} (approximately 600 mm Hg); in this way 100 per cent O_2 is said to "correct" a ventilation-perfusion disturbance. In contrast, in the presence of a right-to-left shunt, the admixture of mixed venous blood continues despite breathing 100 per cent O_2, and arterial hypoxia persists. In fact, the alveolar-arterial P_{O_2} difference in patients with a right-to-left shunt is higher during breathing of 100 per cent O_2 compared with room air, whereas the opposite occurs in patients with ventilation-perfusion inequalities.

Significance of Arterial Blood Gas Values

The availability of accurate rapid analyzers for measuring P_{O_2}, P_{CO_2}, and pH has been one of the major clinical advances of the past 25 years. Virtually the entire therapeutic approach to patients with acute and chronic respiratory failure is dictated by the presence and magnitude of blood gas and pH abnormalities (see Ch. 70). Every physician should know the mechanisms of arterial hypoxia and how to differentiate them, because it is important clinically whether a patient's hypoxia results from hypoventilation, impaired diffusion, ventilation-perfusion mismatching, or right-to-left shunting. Evaluating the course and prognosis of the lung disease, determining the need for and outcome of therapy, and assessing disability, operability, and the limits of resection in patients considered for pulmonary surgery all depend to some extent on the findings of blood gas analysis. Thus all physicians who care for patients must become familiar with the technique of arterial puncture and must know how to interpret the results of blood gas analysis.

EXERCISE

Tests of pulmonary function are customarily performed with the subject seated at rest. The results of these studies provide useful information about the functional abnormalities that characterize common and important pulmonary diseases. Occasionally, the results of routine tests are perfectly normal in symptomatic patients, usually those with exertional dyspnea. In these circumstances, tests during exercise may reveal severe functional disturbances that lead to further evaluation and a diagnosis of either pulmonary vascular or parenchymal infiltrative diseases. Exercise tests are also essential to document the presence of and mechanisms underlying disability.

Chang HK, Paiva M (eds.): Respiratory Physiology. New York, Marcel Dekker, Inc., 1989. *Detailed and authoritative review for advanced students.*

Murray JF: The Normal Lung: The Basis for Diagnosis and Treatment of Pulmonary Disease. 2nd ed. Philadelphia, W. B. Saunders Company, 1986. *Review of normal anatomy, pulmonary physiology, and structure-function correlations.*

Roussos C, Macklem PT (eds.): The Thorax, Parts A and B. New York, Marcel Dekker, Inc., 1983. *Extremely thorough, authoritative discussion of the interrelationships among the thorax, lungs, and respiratory muscles in health and disease.*

Taylor AE, Rehder K, Hyatt RE, et al.: Clinical Respiratory Physiology. Philadelphia, W.B. Saunders Company, 1989. *Useful introduction to pulmonary physiology and its many clinical applications.*

Wagner PD, Rodriguez-Roisin R: State of the art. Clinical advances in pulmonary gas exchange. Am Rev Respir Dis 14:883, 1991. *A summary of the pathophysiologic insights gained from studies of pulmonary gas exchange in various common clinical diseases.*

Wasserman K, Hansen JE, Sue DY, et al.: Principles of Exercise Testing and Interpretation. Philadelphia, Lea and Febiger, 1987. *An instructive and practical book for all persons interested in exercise physiology.*

Wilson AF (ed.): Pulmonary Function Testing: Indications and Interpretations. Orlando, Fla., Grune & Stratton, 1985. *Good summary of pulmonary function testing; well referenced.*

57 Asthma

Jeffrey M. Drazen

DEFINITION

Asthma is a clinical syndrome characterized by recurrent episodes of airway obstruction that resolve spontaneously or as a result of treatment. The etiology of asthma remains unknown. The resolution of the airway obstruction in asthma is a critical feature that distinguishes it from forms of chronic obstructive lung disease. Asthma is also associated with hyperresponsiveness of the airways to a variety of inhaled stimuli; this condition is manifested as an exaggerated bronchoconstrictor response to stimuli that have little or no effect in normal subjects. Current evidence, outlined in Pathogenesis and Pathology below, suggests that asthma may comprise a number of distinct disease entities.

EPIDEMIOLOGY AND STATISTICS

Asthma is an extremely common disorder affecting men and women equally; approximately 4 per cent of the population of the United States has signs and symptoms consistent with a diagnosis of asthma. Although most cases of asthma begin before the age of 25, asthma may begin anytime throughout life. Asthma is a common reason to seek medical treatment. In the United States in 1988, there were 15 million outpatient visits to physicians for asthma and nearly 2 million inpatient hospital days of treatment. More than 4 billion dollars per year are spent on asthma care.

PATHOGENESIS AND PATHOLOGY

Despite the high prevalence of asthma, its cause remains unknown. It is established that the episodic airway narrowing that constitutes an asthma attack results from obstruction of the airway lumen to airflow. Three distinct pathobiologic processes account for this obstruction: (1) constriction of airway smooth muscle, (2) thickening of the airway epithelium, and (3) the presence of liquids within the confines of the airway lumen. Among these mechanisms, the first has received the greatest attention. In this regard, constriction of airway smooth muscle due to the local release of bioactive mediators or neurotransmitters is the most widely accepted reason for airway obstruction in asthma. The sources and mechanisms of release of such molecules in human asthma are still speculative, but potential sources have been identified from experimental studies in lower animals and in isolated human tissues. The cellular sources and mediators thought to be of importance in asthma are summarized below.

HISTAMINE. Histamine, or beta-imidazolylethylamine, was identified as a potent endogenous bronchoactive agent more than 80 years ago. Mast cells, which are prominent in airway tissues, constitute the major pulmonary source of histamine. Recent studies with novel potent antihistamines indicate a role for histamine as one of the mediators of bronchospasm in asthma.

ACETYLCHOLINE. Acetylcholine released from intrapulmonary motor nerves that are branches of the vagi effects constriction of airway smooth muscle through direct stimulation of muscarinic receptors. In the airways these receptors are predominantly of the M_3 subtype. The utility of atropine (and its congeners) in the treatment of asthma provides the major evidence for the importance of acetylcholine in the pathogenesis of asthma.

KININS. Bradykinin and related molecules are cleaved from plasma precursors by the actions of enzymes known as kallikreins. Although there are many sources of kallikreins, at least one type is released from mast cells after appropriate activation. Although no bradykinin synthesis inhibitors or receptor antagonists are in clinical study or use, the potential importance of bradykinin derives from its potency and from the release of kinin-forming enzymes from a cell of potential importance in asthma, the mast cell.

ADENOSINE. Adenosine is a purine nucleoside that is formed during the rapid extracellular metabolism of adenosine triphosphate (ATP). A possible role of adenosine in asthma was first suggested based on the observation that theophylline at therapeutic levels effectively antagonizes the activity of adenosine at the receptor level. Both oral and inhaled forms of theophylline have also been shown to inhibit the adenosine-induced bronchoconstriction in human asthmatics. This evidence for the importance of adenosine in asthma lost some of its strength when enprofylline, a xanthine with a poor adenosine-antagonist effect, was documented to be a more potent antiasthmatic drug than theophylline.

LEUKOTRIENES. The sulfidopeptide leukotrienes—LTC_4, LTD_4, and LTE_4—constitute the material previously known as slow-reacting substances of anaphylaxis, or SRS-A. These molecules and LTB_4 are derived by the sequential lipoxygenation of arachidonic acid, which is released from cell membrane phospholipids during cellular activation. Mast cells, eosinophils, and alveolar macrophages have the enzymatic capability required to produce sulfidopeptide leukotrienes from membrane phospholipids. Two enzyme systems, 5-lipoxygenase and LTC_4 synthase, and a cytosolic protein known as 5-lipoxygenase-activating protein are required to produce the sulfidopeptide leukotriene LTC_4. This molecule is transported out of the cell where it is synthesized and processed extracellularly to LTD_4 and LTE_4. LTC_4 and LTD_4 are about 3000 times more potent than histamine as contractile agonists, while LTE_4 is about 300 times more potent than histamine. Preliminary clinical studies with leukotriene receptor antagonists or synthesis inhibitors have shown efficacy in the treatment of asthma.

PLATELET-ACTIVATING FACTOR (PAF). PAF is a phospholipid with an ether rather than an ester link to a long-chain (C_{16}–C_{20}) fatty acid in the sn–1 position, an acetyl moiety in the sn–2 position, and phosphatidylcholine in the sn–3 position. It is derived from lyso-PAF by the action of specific acetyltransferases and is produced by a variety of inflammatory cells, including mast cells and eosinophils. PAF, through action at specific receptors, is a moderately potent airway contractile agonist, but since the receptors mediating this constriction are rapidly tachyphylactic, it is unlikely that PAF has a major direct role in asthmatic bronchoconstriction. PAF has the ability to induce a state of prolonged airway hyperresponsiveness (see below), which is characteristic of the asthmatic condition.

TACHYKININS. Tachykinins are a series of small peptides, on the order of 10 residues in length, which share a common carboxy terminal sequence—Phe-X-Gly-Leu-Met-NH2. Three tachykinins—substance P, neurokinin A (substance K), and neurokinin B—are found in the terminal axon dendrites of certain sensory nerves. When these nerves are stimulated by appropriate sensory stimuli, the peptides are released into the airway microenvironment, where they can induce airway smooth muscle constriction as well as mucus secretion through action at specific receptors. As these sensory signals pass the terminal ramifications of the axon on their way to the central nervous system, antidromic conduction occurs. Conduction of the antidromic signal to the sensory nerve endings is accompanied by further local release of tachykinins. This process has been termed as "axon reflex." Ordinarily, the peptides released from the nerves are rapidly degraded by specific peptidases located at or near the site of their action or release; inhibition of the function of these peptidases enhances the biologic effects of released peptides. These small peptides have been implicated in asthmatic responses because many stimuli known to cause their release in lower animals have been shown to induce asthma attacks in humans.

Each of these putative mediators of asthma has the potential to effect airway obstruction; their action in concert may induce severe bronchospasm. It is not unreasonable to speculate that there are a variety of asthmatic diatheses that differ in the profile of mediators released, elaborated, or left unchecked at or near their site of action on airway smooth muscle. Elucidation of these pathways may fragment the syndrome we now know as asthma into many diseases.

Pathology of the Asthmatic Response

The pathology of mild asthma, as derived from bronchoscopic and biopsy studies, is characterized by edema and hyperemia of the mucosa and by infiltration of the mucosa with mast cells, eosinophils, and lymphocytes bearing the CD4 phenotype. The lamina propria is thickened, with deposition of types III and V collagen (Fig. 57–1). In cases of more severe asthma, there is thickening of the airway wall due to hypertrophy and hyperplasia of the airway glands and secretory cells, hyperplasia of airway smooth muscle, as well as further deposition of submucosal collagen. Airway epithelium may be shed, leading to a denuded airway. These changes occur in a patchy fashion in mild asthma and become more widespread as the disease becomes more severe. Morphometric studies of airways from asthmatic subjects have demonstrated airway wall thickening of sufficient magnitude to increase airflow resistance and enhance airway responsiveness. In severe asthma, the airway wall is thickened markedly, and there is patchy airway occlusion by a mixture of hyperviscous mucus and shed airway epithelium.

Physiologic Changes in Asthma

The consequence of the airway obstruction induced by smooth muscle constriction, thickening of the mucosa, or free liquid within the airway lumen is an increased resistance to airflow. This condition is manifested by increased airway resistance (R_{aw}) and decreased flow rates throughout the vital capacity. At the onset of an asthma attack, obstruction occurs at all airway levels; during the resolution of the attack, changes reverse first in the large airways (i.e., mainstem, lobar, segmental, and subsegmental bronchi) and then in the more peripheral airways. This anatomic sequence of onset and reversal is reflected in the physiologic changes monitored during an asthmatic episode (Fig. 57–2). As an asthma attack resolves, flow rates first normalize high in the vital capacity, and only later do they resolve low in the vital capacity. Because asthma is an airway disease, there are no primary changes in the static pressure-volume curve of the lungs. However, during an acute attack of asthma, airway narrowing may be so severe as to result in airway closure. Individual lung units tend to close at a volume that is near their maximal volume; this tendency produces a change in the pressure-volume curve such that for a given contained gas volume within the thorax there will be decreased elastic recoil. The decreased elastic recoil at a given overall lung volume further depresses expiratory airflow rates.

Additional factors influence the mechanical behavior of the lungs in the course of an acute attack of asthma. During inspiration, the pleural pressure drops far below the 4 to 6 cm H_2O

below atmospheric pressure usually required for tidal airflow. The expiratory phase of respiration also becomes active as the patient tries to force air from the lungs. As a consequence, peak pleural pressures during expiration, which normally are only a few centimeters of water above atmospheric pressure, may be as high as 20 to 30 cm H_2O. The low pleural pressures during inspiration tend to dilate airways, while the high pleural pressures during expiration tend to narrow airways. During an asthma attack, the net effect is to increase airflow resistance during expiration much more than during inspiration.

The respiratory rate is usually rapid during an acute asthma attack. The tachypnea is not driven by abnormalities in arterial blood gas composition, but rather by stimulation of intrapulmonary receptors, with subsequent effects on the respiratory centers. A consequence of airway narrowing combined with the rapid airflow rates is that there is a heightened mechanical load on the ventilatory pump. During a severe asthma attack, the load can increase the work of breathing by a factor of 10 or more and can predispose to fatigue of the ventilatory muscles.

The patchy nature of the asthmatic airway narrowing results in a maldistribution of ventilation (V̇) relative to pulmonary perfusion(Q̇). There is a shift from the normal situation, in which V̇/Q̇ units with a ratio of near unity are preponderant, to a distribution involving a large number of alveolar-capillary units with a V̇/Q̇ ratio less than unity. The net effect is to induce arterial hypoxemia. In addition, the hyperpnea of asthma is reflected as hyperventilation with a low arterial P_{CO_2}.

CLINICAL PRESENTATION

History

During an asthma attack, patients seek medical attention for shortness of breath accompanied by cough, wheezing, and anxiety. The degree of breathlessness experienced by the patient is not closely related to the degree of airflow obstruction but is often influenced by the acuteness of the attack. Dyspnea may occur only with exercise, so-called *exercise-induced asthma;* may occur after exposure to a specific known allergen, referred to as *extrinsic asthma;* or may occur for no identifiable reason, so-called *intrinsic asthma.* There are variants of asthma in which cough, hoarseness, or inability to sleep throughout the night are the only symptoms. Identification, through careful questioning, of a provoking stimulus both helps to establish the diagnosis of asthma and may help in therapy if the stimulus can be avoided. Most patients with asthma will complain of shortness of breath when exposed to rapid changes in the temperature and humidity of inspired air. For example, in less temperate climates during the winter months, this commonly occurs when the patient leaves a heated house. Airway narrowing induced by breathing cold, dry air forms the basis of one of the diagnostic tests for asthma (see below).

Physical Examination

VITAL SIGNS. A rapid respiratory rate, often 25 to 40 breaths per minute, is common during an acute asthma attack. Tachycardia is also common, as is the presence of pulsus paradoxus, an

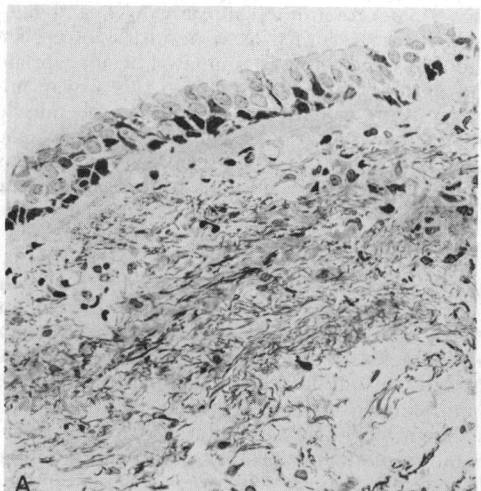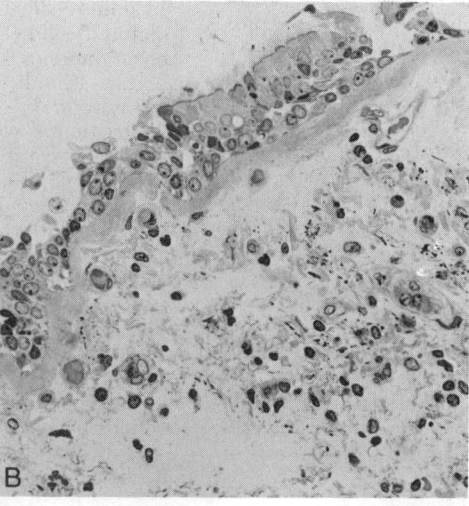

FIGURE 57–1. Photomicrographs of endobronchial biopsy specimens from a normal (*A*) and a mildly allergic asthmatic subject (*B*). The airway biopsy from the asthmatic individual demonstrates the characteristic subepithelial fibrosis, edema, and inflammatory cell infiltration not seen in the normal subject. (Photomicrograph courtesy of W.R. Roche, University of Southampton, United Kingdom.)

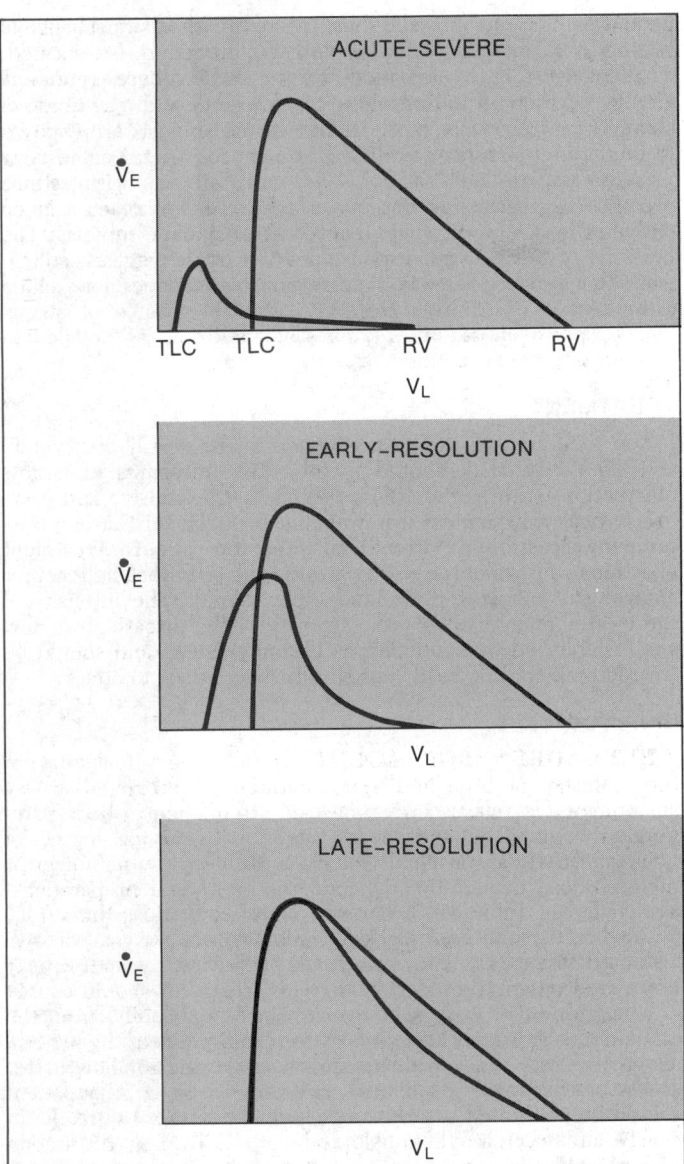

FIGURE 57–2. Schematic flow-volume curves in various stages of asthma; in each figure the colored line depicts the normal flow-volume curve. Predicted and observed total lung capacity (TLC) and residual volume (RV) are shown in the top panel. Note that TLC and RV decrease as flow rates increase with attack resolution. $\dot{V}_E$ = expiratory flow rate; V_L = lung volume.

exaggerated inspiratory fall in the systolic pressure. The magnitude of the pulsus paradoxus is related to the severity of the attack.

THORACIC EXAMINATION. Inspection will reveal that the patient is using the accessory muscles during inspiration; the skin over the thorax may be retracted into the intercostal spaces during inspiration. The chest is usually hyperinflated, and the expiratory phase is prolonged relative to the inspiratory phase. Percussion of the thorax demonstrates hyperresonance with loss of the normal variation in dullness due to diaphragmatic movement. Auscultation reveals wheezing, the cardinal physical finding in asthma; the presence of wheezing does not, however, establish asthma as the diagnosis (Table 57–1). Wheezing is commonly heard during both inspiration and expiration, although it is louder during the latter phase of respiration. The wheezing is characterized as polyphonic in that more than one pitch may be heard at a given time. There may be other accompanying adventitious sounds, including rhonchi, suggestive of free secretions in the airway lumen, or rales, indicative of localized infection or cardiac failure. The loss of intensity or absence of breath sounds in a patient with asthma is an indication of severe airflow obstruction.

TABLE 57–1. DIFFERENTIAL DIAGNOSIS OF WHEEZING OTHER THAN ASTHMA

Common
Acute bronchiolitis (infectious, chemical)
Aspiration (foreign body)
Bronchial stenosis
Cardiac failure
Chronic bronchitis
Cystic fibrosis
Eosinophilic pneumonia

Uncommon
Airway obstruction due to masses
  External compression
    Central thoracic tumors, superior vena cava (SVC) syndrome, substernal thyroid
  Intrinsic airway
    Primary lung cancer, metastatic breast cancer
Carcinoid syndrome
Endobronchial sarcoid
Pulmonary emboli
Systemic mastocytosis
Systemic vasculitis (polyarteritis nodosa)

Laboratory Findings

PULMONARY FUNCTION FINDINGS. A decrease in airflow rates throughout the vital capacity is the cardinal pulmonary function abnormality in asthma. Although essential for the diagnosis of asthma, it is not specific, as other obstructive diseases share this feature. The peak expiratory flow rate (PEFR), forced expiratory volume in the first second (FEV_1), and maximal midexpiratory flow rate (MMEFR) are all decreased in asthma. In very severe asthma, the dyspnea may be so severe as to prevent the patient from performing a complete spirogram. In this case, if 1 second of forced expiration can be recorded, useful values for the PEFR and FEV_1 can be obtained. Gradation of attack severity *must* be assessed by objective measures of airflow; there are no other methods that can do this in an accurate and reproducible fashion. Table 57–2 relates the severity of the attack to the relative depressions of airflow rates. As the attack resolves, PEFR and FEV_1 increase in concert while the MMEFR remains substantially depressed. Further resolution of obstruction is indicated by a normalization of both the FEV_1 and the PEFR while the MMEFR remains depressed. Even when the attack is resolved clinically, it is not uncommon to observe residual depression of the MMEFR, which may resolve over a prolonged course of treatment. Representative schematic flow-volume curves during an asthma attack are shown in Figure 57–2. If the patient is able to cooperate fully, measurements of lung volumes will show increases in total lung capacity (TLC) and residual volume (RV) during the acute attack that resolve with treatment.

ARTERIAL BLOOD GASES. Blood gas analysis need not be done in individuals with mild asthma. If, however, the asthma is of sufficient severity to merit prolonged observation, blood gas analysis is indicated; in such cases, hypoxemia and hypocarbia are the rule. With the subject breathing room air, the Pa_{O_2} is usually between 55 and 70 torr, and the Pa_{CO_2} is usually between 25 and 35 torr. At the onset of the attack, there will be an appropriate pure respiratory alkalemia, while with attacks of prolonged duration, the pH will normalize owing to compensatory metabolic acidemia. The presence of a normal Pa_{CO_2} in a patient with moderate to severe airflow obstruction is reason for concern, as it may indicate that the mechanical load on the respiratory system is greater than what can be sustained by the ventilatory muscles and that respiratory failure is imminent. When the Pa_{CO_2} rises in such settings, the pH will fall quickly because the bicarbonate stores will have been depleted as a result of renal compensation for the prolonged preceding respiratory alkalemia. Since this chain of events can occur rapidly, close observation is indicated for asthmatics with "normal" P_{CO_2} levels and moderate to severe airflow obstruction.

OTHER BLOOD FINDINGS. Asthmatic subjects are commonly atopic; thus blood eosinophilia is common. In addition, elevated serum immunoglobulin E (IgE) levels are common;

TABLE 57–2. RELATIVE SEVERITY OF AN ASTHMATIC ATTACK AS INDICATED BY PEFR, FEV₁, AND MMEFR

Test	Per Cent of Predicted	Asthma Severity
PEFR	80% or greater	
FEV₁	80% or greater	No spirometric abnormalities
MMEFR	80% or greater	
PEFR	80% or greater	
FEV₁	70% or greater	Mild asthma
MMEFR	55%–75%	
PEFR	60% or greater	
FEV₁	45%–70%	Moderate asthma
MMEFR	30%–50%	
PEFR	Less than 50%	
FEV₁	Less than 50%	Severe asthma
MMEFR	10%–30%	

PEFR = peak expiratory flow rate; MMEFR = maximal mid-expiratory flow rate; FEV₁ = forced expiratory volume in the first second.

epidemiologic studies indicate that asthma is unusual in subjects with low IgE levels. If indicated by the patient's history, specific radioallergosorbent (RAST) assays for IgE directed against likely offending antigens can be obtained. Although unusual, asthma alone can result in elevated levels of serum transaminases, lactate dehydrogenases, muscle creatine phosphokinase, ornithine transcarbamylase, and antidiuretic hormone.

RADIOGRAPHIC FINDINGS. The chest radiograph is often normal in subjects with asthma. Severe asthma is associated with hyperinflation, as indicated by depression of the diaphragm and abnormally lucent lung fields. Complications of severe asthma, including pneumomediastinum or pneumothorax, may be detected radiographically. In mild to moderate cases of asthma without adventitious sounds other than wheezing, a chest radiograph need not be obtained; if the asthma is of sufficient severity to merit hospital admission, a chest radiograph is advised.

ELECTROCARDIOGRAPHIC FINDINGS. The electrocardiogram is usually normal, save for a sinus tachycardia, in acute asthma. However, right-axis deviation, right bundle branch block, "P pulmonale," or even ST segment and T wave abnormalities may arise from severe asthma and resolve as the attack subsides.

SPUTUM FINDINGS. The sputum of the asthmatic patient may be clear or opaque with a green or yellow tinge. The presence of color does not invariably indicate infection, and examination of a Gram-stained and Wright-stained sputum smear is necessary. Often the sputum will contain eosinophils, Charcot-Leyden crystals (crystallized eosinophil proteins), Curschmann's spirals (bronchiolar casts composed of mucus and cells), or Creola's bodies (clusters of airway epithelial cells with identifiable cilia).

Differential Diagnosis

Asthma is easy to recognize in a younger patient without comorbid medical conditions who has exacerbating and remitting airway obstruction accompanied by blood eosinophilia. The rapid response to bronchodilator treatment (see below) is usually all that is needed to establish the diagnosis firmly. However, in the patient with cryptic episodic shortness of breath, airway challenge testing by a laboratory familiar with this procedure is indicated. Challenge testing is performed at a time when there is minimal airway obstruction, to determine the presence and magnitude of airway hyperresponsiveness. In such tests, subjects are exposed to increasing amounts of inhaled bronchoconstrictor agonists or breathe graded levels of cold, dry air. Subjects with asthma usually require smaller amounts of a stimulus to reach a given endpoint in airway response than do nonasthmatic subjects. The presence of airway hyperresponsiveness strongly suggests asthma, while the absence of airway hyperresponsiveness does not exclude asthma as a possibility. However, in the absence of airway hyperresponsiveness, other causes of wheezing, as detailed in Table 57–1, should be investigated.

TREATMENT

The treatment of asthma is directed at the airway obstruction and should be documented by objective measures of airflow obstruction, such as the FEV₁ or PEFR. Inexpensive and easy-to-use peak flow meters are available to make this latter measurement accessible to virtually all asthmatic patients. Treatment of asthma consists of the use of bronchodilators, specific receptor antagonists, corticosteroids, and other agents. The intensity of the treatment depends on the severity of the disease. It is now well established that asthma is a chronic disease and should be treated on a chronic basis, not simply from attack to attack.

Bronchodilators

BETA-ADRENERGIC AGENTS. Beta-adrenergic agents are the mainstay of bronchodilator treatment. Constricted airway smooth muscle relaxes in response to stimulation of beta₂-adrenergic receptors. Beta-adrenergic agents with varying degrees of beta₂ selectivity are available for use in inhaled (by nebulizer or metered-dose inhaler [MDI]), oral, or parenteral preparations, as detailed in Table 57–3. Patients with very mild asthma (i.e., fewer than three or four attacks of mild severity per year) or with asthma that occurs in known settings, such as with exercise, may be treated on an as-needed basis. This treatment should consist of a long-duration beta₂-selective inhaler. Two "puffs" from the inhaler at 3- to 5-minute intervals are recommended; the interval allows the first "puff" to dilate narrowed airways to allow better access of the agent to affected areas of the lung. The patient should be instructed to exhale to residual volume, to breathe in slowly, and to actuate the inhaler as he or she inspires. Inspiration to near TLC is recommended, followed by a period of breath holding on the order of 5 seconds, to allow smaller aerosol particles to deposit in more peripheral airways. Aerosol "spacers" are available from many manufacturers for the patient who has difficulty coordinating inspiration and inhaler actuation. Patients with mild to moderate disease should use their inhalers on a regular, daily basis (at 6- to 8-hour intervals) rather than only when they become symptomatic. Depending on the specific type of inhaled beta agent employed, use of the inhaler is possible between scheduled intervals if symptoms of airflow obstruction occur. Patients with moderate to severe asthma may benefit from the addition of an oral beta₂ agent used as indicated by the manufacturer.

The routine use of parenteral beta agonists in adults is not encouraged, as careful studies have shown that inhaled agents

TABLE 57–3. BETA AGONISTS FOR ASTHMA TREATMENT*

Drug	Beta₂ Selective	Form Available for Administration			Comments
		Inhaled	Oral	Parenteral	
Albuterol	Yes	Yes	Yes	No	Available as an MDI or for nebulization
Ethylnorepinephrine	No	No	No	Yes	Fewer central nervous system effects than with epinephrine
Epinephrine	No	Yes	No	Yes	MDI available without prescription
Isoetharine	Yes	Yes	No	No	Available as an MDI or for nebulization
Isoproterenol	No	Yes	No	Yes	Parenteral form is for intravenous use only
Metaproterenol	Yes	Yes	Yes	No	Available as an MDI or for nebulization
Perbuterol	Yes	Yes	No	No	Available as an MDI
Terbutaline	Yes	Yes	Yes	Yes	Although beta₂ is selective in animals, clinical studies do not show selectivity when given subcutaneously

*Based on market drugs in the United States as of February 1, 1990.
MDI = metered-dose inhaler.

have equal efficacy, without the systemic side effects that accompany the use of parenteral agents.

THEOPHYLLINE. Theophylline and aminophylline are bronchodilators of moderate potency used in both inpatient and outpatient management of asthma. The mechanism of action of their effect is not established with certainty but likely is related either to the inhibition of the breakdown of cyclic adenosine monophosphate (AMP) by phosphodiesterase or to the inhibition of adenosine receptors. The utility of theophylline is limited by its toxicity and by the wide variations in the rate of its metabolism both in a single individual over time and among individuals in a population. As a result of this wide variability, monitoring of plasma theophylline levels is indicated to be sure that patients are appropriately treated. Acceptable plasma levels for therapeutic effects are between 10 and 20 μg per milliliter; higher levels are associated with gastrointestinal, cardiac, and central nervous system toxicity, including anxiety, headache, nausea, vomiting, diarrhea, cardiac arrhythmias, and seizures. The last two, catastrophic complications of toxicity may occur when plasma levels exceed 20 μg per milliliter without antecedent mild side effects. Because of these potentially life-threatening complications from treatment, plasma levels need to be monitored with great frequency in hospitalized patients receiving intravenous aminophylline and with less frequency in stable patients receiving, on an outpatient basis, one of the long-acting theophylline preparations. The use of theophylline preparations in patients with mild to moderate asthma managed with other medications has been recently questioned.

Receptor Antagonists

ANTIHISTAMINES. When antihistamines were first developed in the 1940's and 1950's, they were used in asthmatic subjects with unremarkable effect and major soporific side effects. In the past decade, newer, more potent H_1 receptor antagonists, such as terfenadine and astemizole, have emerged, with fewer central nervous system side effects. Although these compounds have not yet come into widespread use for the treatment of asthma, data from clinical trials indicate that they produce bronchodilation and alleviate asthmatic symptoms. It is likely that H_1 receptor antagonists will soon be used more frequently in asthma.

ANTICHOLINERGICS. Atropine has been known to be beneficial in the treatment of asthma for more than a century. Its mechanism of action is thought to be inhibition of the effects of acetylcholine released from intrapulmonary motor nerves that run in the vagus and innervate airway smooth muscle. The central nervous system side effects of atropine, which limited its utility, have been overcome with the development of ipratropium bromide, which is available as a metered-dose inhaler. Although ipratropium bromide has a salutary effect on cough in asthma and is useful in conjunction with a beta$_2$ inhaler in chronic stable asthma, it is not effective treatment for acute bronchospasm.

OTHER RECEPTOR ANTAGONISTS. Antagonists active at the putative receptors for LTD_4 and PAF are being clinically tested for use in the treatment of asthma. Initial trials in both laboratory-induced and spontaneously occurring asthma have shown efficacy, but there are currently no marketed drugs with this mechanism of action available for use in treating asthma.

Anti-inflammatory Agents

SYSTEMIC CORTICOSTEROIDS. Corticosteroids are a widely used and effective treatment for patients with moderate to severe asthma. Their mechanism of action in asthma is not established with certainty but has been linked to the diminished phlogistic potential of the cells resident within the airway as well as a reduction in the number of inflammatory cells within the airway. There is no consensus on the specific type, dose, or duration of dose of corticosteroid to be used in the treatment of asthma. In nonhospitalized patients refractory to standard antiasthma therapy, initial dosages on the order of 40 to 60 mg of prednisone per day tapered over 7 to 14 days are recommended. It has been clearly shown that in patients who cannot stop taking steroids without recurrent uncontrolled bronchospasm, the use of alternate-day oral steroids is preferable to daily treatment. In the patient who requires hospital treatment of his or her asthma, but who is not considered to have life-threatening asthma, an initial intravenous bolus of 2 mg per kilogram of hydrocortisone, followed by continuous infusion of 0.5 mg per kilogram per hour, has been shown to be effective therapy, with beneficial effects observable within 12 hours of starting treatment. In attacks of asthma that are considered life threatening, the use of intravenous methylprednisolone, 125 mg every 6 hours, has been advocated. In each case as the patient improves, oral steroids are substituted for intravenous steroids, and the dose is tapered over 1 to 3 weeks; as outlined below, the addition of inhaled steroids to tapering oral steroids is recommended.

INHALED CORTICOSTEROIDS. Inhaled corticosteroids, which have minimal systemic and side effects, have been shown to be an effective adjunctive therapy to bronchodilators for moderate to severe asthma. Their mechanism of action is presumed to be secondary to the reduction of intraluminal and airway mucosal inflammation. A number of studies have shown that at the recommended doses it is possible to withdraw oral steroids from steroid-dependent asthmatic patients; recent studies have suggested that the use of two to four times the recommended dose of inhaled steroid (i.e., four to six inhalations four to six times per day) results in further improvement in indices of airflow obstruction and asthmatic symptoms. The addition of inhaled steroids to the regimen of any asthmatic who has required a course of oral steroids is strongly advised. The major side effect from inhaled steroids is oral thrush; the risk and severity of this complication can be reduced through the use of aerosol spacers and good oropharyngeal hygiene.

OTHER ANTI-INFLAMMATORY DRUGS. The use of systemic gold (as is used in rheumatoid arthritis) or oral methotrexate has been suggested as adjunctive treatment for patients with severe chronic asthma who cannot be removed from high-dose corticosteroid treatment. These treatments are experimental, and their routine use is not advocated.

Disodium Cromoglycate

Disodium Cromoglycate is a mast cell membrane–stabilizing agent that is of value in the prophylactic treatment of asthma. It is most useful in patients with identifiable stimuli eliciting an asthmatic response, such as exercise or allergen exposure.

Specific Treatment Scenarios

ASTHMA IN THE EMERGENCY ROOM. When a patient with asthma presents for acute emergency care, objective measures of the severity of the attack, including quantification of pulsus paradoxus and measurement of airflow rates (PEFR or FEV_1), should be obtained in addition to the usual vital signs. If the PEFR or FEV_1 is less than 40 per cent of the predicted value, but the attack does not appear to be clinically life threatening, inhaled beta$_2$ agents and intravenous aminophylline (dose to be determined by the patient's previous treatment status) should be given. If the attack is prolonged and has failed to respond to treatment with bronchodilators, intravenous steroids (40 to 60 mg of methylprednisolone) should be administered. Inhaled treatments should be repeated at 20- to 30-minute intervals until the PEFR or FEV_1 improves to greater than 40 per cent of the predicted value. If this improvement fails to occur within 2 hours, admission to the hospital for further treatment is strongly advocated. In the patient whose PEFR and FEV_1 are greater than 60 per cent of predicted values on admission to the emergency room, treatment with inhaled beta$_2$ agonists alone is likely to result in an objective improvement in airflow rates. If a significant improvement occurs, such patients can usually be treated on an outpatient basis with the use of inhaled beta$_2$ agonists; the addition of oral theophylline or of oral or inhaled corticosteroids may be of value, depending on the severity of the attack and the rapidity of its response to treatment. For the patients whose PEFR and FEV_1 are between 40 and 60 per cent of predicted values at the time they are initially evaluated in the emergency care setting, a treatment plan varying in intensity between the two cited above is indicated. It is important to realize that failure to achieve an objective response to treatment, as recorded by measurements of PEFR or FEV_1, is an indication for more intense therapy.

STATUS ASTHMATICUS. The asthmatic subject in whom

the PEFR or FEV$_1$ does not increase above 40 per cent of the predicted value with treatment, who develops an increasing Pa$_{CO2}$ without an improvement in the indices of airflow obstruction, or who develops major complications, such as pneumothorax or pneumomediastinum, should be admitted to the hospital in a care environment where he or she can be closely monitored. Frequent treatments with inhaled beta agonists, intravenous aminophylline to achieve maximal plasma levels, and high-dose intravenous steroids are indicated. Oxygen should be administered by face mask or nasal cannula. If there is objective evidence of infection, it should be treated. If the patient's condition fails to improve with treatment and respiratory failure appears imminent, bronchodilator treatment should be intensified to the maximum tolerated by the patient. If indicated, intubation of the trachea and mechanical ventilation can be instituted; in this case the goal should be to provide ventilation just adequate to sustain life and *not to normalize* arterial blood gases. For example, a Pa$_{CO2}$ of 50 to 60 torr is acceptable for a patient in status asthmaticus.

THE PREGNANT ASTHMATIC. Asthma may be exacerbated, remain unchanged, or remit during pregnancy. There need not be substantial departures from the ordinary management of an asthmatic during pregnancy; however, unnecessary medications should be avoided. Systemic steroids should be used sparingly to avoid fetal complications, and certain drugs should be avoided. These include tetracycline as a treatment for intercurrent infection; atropine and atropine-like drugs, since they may cause fetal tachycardia; terbutaline during active labor because of its tocolytic effects; and iodine-containing mucolytics, such as saturated solution of potassium iodine (SSKI). The use of prostaglandin F$_{2\alpha}$ as an abortifacient should be avoided in asthmatics.

Barnes PJ: A new approach to the treatment of asthma. N Engl J Med 321:1517, 1989. *A good summary of current approaches to the treatment of asthma.*

Beasley R, Roche WR, Roberts JA, et al.: Cellular events in the bronchi in mild asthma and after bronchial provocation. Am Rev Respir Dis 139:806, 1989. *A review of the cellular physiology involved in bronchospastic responses.*

Jeffrey PK, Wardlaw AJ, Nelson FC, et al.: Bronchial biopsies in asthma. An ultrastructural, quantitative study and correlation with hyperreactivity. Am Rev Respir Dis 140:1745, 1989. *A good discussion of the pathology and tissue changes in asthma.*

Rossing TH: Methylxanthines in 1989. Ann Intern Med 110:502, 1989. *A good discussion of the pharmacology of methylxanthine.*

58 Chronic Airways Diseases

Richard A. Matthay

CHRONIC BRONCHITIS AND EMPHYSEMA

Chronic generalized airway disorders that are not the direct result of a "specific" bronchopulmonary disease are discussed in this chapter. Common to most of these diseases is chronic airways obstruction, caused most frequently by a diffuse involvement of peripheral (small) airways or, more rarely, by localized obstruction of central (large) airways. The designation *chronic obstructive pulmonary disease* (COPD) is an imperfect, although widely utilized, term, since it includes several specific disorders with different clinical manifestations, pathologic findings, therapy requirements, and prognoses.

Four *diffuse* airway disorders are examined in this chapter: simple chronic bronchitis, asthmatic bronchitis, chronic obstructive bronchitis, and emphysema. Some classifications include all of these entities in the broad term COPD. Moreover, various combinations of these disorders coexist; for instance, patients often have chronic obstructive bronchitis as well as emphysema. Localized airways obstruction, above and below the tracheal bifurcation, is discussed in a separate section of this chapter.

DEFINITIONS OF TERMS. Unfortunately, *chronic bronchitis* has been used variably to refer to a simple smoker's cough or, as in the British literature, to severe COPD. To reduce ambi-

guity, in this discussion, chronic bronchitis is considered "simple," "obstructive," or "asthmatic," and thus these three terms are applied. It is useful clinically to differentiate between the extremely common simple chronic bronchitis and the less common but often devastating form, chronic obstructive bronchitis. These two entities are therefore described in separate sections.

Simple chronic bronchitis, a syndrome characterized primarily by a chronic productive cough, is the result of low-grade exposure to bronchial irritants in an individual without hyperreactive airways. This syndrome is associated with enhanced mucus secretion, reduced ciliary activity, and impaired resistance to bronchial infection. Simple chronic bronchitis is defined in clinical terms: (1) excessive production of mucus; (2) presence of symptoms, largely cough, on most days for at least 3 months annually during 2 or more successive years; and (3) exclusion of bronchiectasis, tuberculosis, or other causes of these symptoms. The term does not describe the underlying process, which may vary widely. The patient population ranges from those who are asymptomatic except for a morning "cigarette cough" productive of mucus in small amounts *(simple chronic bronchitis)* to patients with a severe, disabling condition manifested by increased resistance to airflow, hypoxia, and often hypercapnia *(chronic obstructive bronchitis).* Chronic obstructive bronchitis, which develops in a relatively small proportion of individuals with simple chronic bronchitis, results in irreversible narrowing of airways. Because the obstruction is in bronchioles and bronchi 2 mm or less in diameter, the term *small airways disease* has been used.

Exposure to bronchial irritants in individuals with hyperreactive, or "twitchy," airways can lead to bronchospasm (i.e., bronchial smooth muscle constriction), frequently accompanied by excessive mucus production and edema of bronchial walls. Recurrent episodes of symptomatic bronchospasm are called *asthma* (discussed in Ch. 57). The present discussion must consider bronchospasm, since a degree of reversible airways obstruction often accompanies other reactions to inhaled noxious agents. In fact, episodic airways obstruction is common in individuals with chronic bronchitis. This combination, called *asthmatic bronchitis,* may closely resemble classic asthma. The term *chronic asthmatic bronchitis* is applied in patients with persistent airways obstruction, a chronic productive cough, and a major problem of episodic bronchospasm.

Emphysema, another lung response to noxious stimuli, is characterized by abnormal, permanent enlargement of air spaces distal to the terminal bronchioles, accompanied by destruction of their walls, and without obvious fibrosis. The alterations in emphysema cause reduction in lung elastic recoil, which permits excessive airway collapse upon expiration and leads to irreversible airflow obstruction.

These definitions are not mutually exclusive; there is considerable crossover between the emphysematous (type A) and bronchial (type B) findings listed in Table 58–1. For example, most individuals with emphysema also have a chronic productive cough. It may be difficult to determine the relative importance of emphysema and chronic obstructive bronchitis, with obliteration of small airways. Accordingly, general terms such as *chronic obstructive pulmonary disease (COPD)* have been used to describe this clinical syndrome.

PATHOPHYSIOLOGY OF AIRWAYS OBSTRUCTION. Airways obstruction denotes slowing of forced expiration. As outlined in Ch. 56, the speed of forced expiration is determined primarily by three factors: intrinsic resistance of the airways, compressibility of the airways, and lung elastic recoil. Reduced maximal expiratory flow (Vmax) results from high airways resistance, reduced lung recoil, and/or excessive airways collapsibility.

In general, a low FEV$_1$/FVC* ratio is indicative of airflow obstruction; the amount of reduction in FEV$_1$ itself establishes the severity of the obstruction (Fig. 58–1). Some prefer to use FEF$_{25-75\%}$, the average flow over the middle half of a forced expiration.

Actual Vmax values have been measured, commonly at 50 per cent or 75 per cent of the forced expired volume (Vmax$_{50\%}$ or

---

*Fev$_1$ = forced expiratory volume in 1 second; FVC = forced vital capacity; FEF = forced expiratory flow.

TABLE 58–1. FEATURES OF THE EMPHYSEMATOUS AND BRONCHIAL TYPES OF COPD

	Emphysematous (Type A)	Bronchial (Type B)
Clinical features		
Dyspnea	Insidious onset, slowly progressive	Often noted first only during chest infections
Sputum	Usually scant and mucoid	Often copious and purulent
Weight loss	Often marked	Usually slight or absent
Chronic cor pulmonale with heart failure	Infrequent until terminal stages of the disease	Common
Chest examination	Quiet chest (except slight wheeze at end expiration), marked hyperinflation	Noisy chest, slight hyperinflation
Chest radiograph	Hyperlucent, overinflated lung; often regional attenuation of vessels	Often evidence of old inflammatory disease
Physiologic tests		
Total lung capacity	Increased	Normal or slightly decreased
Residual volume	Markedly increased	Moderately increased
Lung compliance, static	Increased	Near normal
Lung compliance, dynamic	Normal or slightly low	Very low
Lung recoil	Markedly reduced	Variable
Inspiratory airways resistance	Normal	Increased
Diffusing capacity	Markedly reduced	Variable
Arterial P_{O_2}	Slight reduction at rest; usually falls with exertion	Often very low at rest; variable change with exertion
Arterial P_{CO_2}	Usually normal or low	Often chronically elevated
Resting pulmonary artery pressure	Normal or slightly elevated at rest; increases with exertion	Often markedly elevated at rest
Cardiac output	Often low	Usually near normal

$\dot{V}max_{75\%}$, respectively*). $\dot{V}max_{75\%}$ has become popular in epidemiologic studies because it appears to be more sensitive than the FEV_1.

In clinical practice, FEV_1 is used more widely because it is easy to measure, is quite reproducible, has a relatively narrow normal range, and tends to reflect the clinical severity of disease.

A variety of physiologic abnormalities are associated with obstructive airways disorders (also discussed in Ch. 56). Increased venous admixture and hypoxemia develop owing to ventilation-perfusion mismatching. Unless there is an increase in overall ventilation, this mismatching may also lead to increased physiologic dead space and hypercapnia. Carbon dioxide retention is likely when airways obstruction is severe, respiratory muscle fatigue occurs, and the drive to breathe is depressed. Air trapping and an increase in residual volume develop because obstructed airways tend to close prematurely during a maximal exhalation. In emphysema, total lung capacity may be enhanced as well. The pulmonary diffusing capacity measurement is usually reduced in emphysema owing to loss of functioning alveolar-capillary membrane surface area.

Because of the large total cross-sectional diameter of the small airways, marked alterations are required to produce discernible changes in the FEV_1 values. Several potentially more sensitive tests have been proposed to detect mild abnormalities of the small airways: closing volume, helium response of the maximal expiratory flow volume (MEFV) curve, and frequency dependence of compliance. Although these tests are not used routinely, they may prove useful in research studies for detecting subclinical disease.

Burrows B: Airways obstructive diseases: Pathogenetic mechanisms and natural histories of the disorders. An overview of obstructive lung disease. Med Clin North Am 74:547, 1990. *This is the lead article of an 18-chapter symposium on obstructive lung diseases. The entire symposium is recommended reading and an excellent source of original references.*

Fishman AP: The spectrum of chronic obstructive disease of the airways. *In* Fishman AP (ed.): Pulmonary Diseases and Disorders. 2nd ed. New York, McGraw-Hill Book Company, 1988, p 1159. *A concise, clearly written description of the different types of airways obstructive disorders and how they overlap.*

Snider GL, Kleinerman J, Thurlbeck WM, et al.: The definition of emphysema. Am Rev Respir Dis 132:182, 1985. *Succinct statement of the definition, anatomic subtypes, and clinical diagnosis of emphysema.*

Thurlbeck WM: Pathophysiology of chronic obstructive pulmonary disease. Clin Chest Med 11:389, 1990. *Overview of pathophysiology associated with airways obstruction.*

Simple Chronic Bronchitis and Asthmatic Bronchitis

PREVALENCE AND PATHOGENESIS. "Simple chronic bronchitis" refers to a productive cough for at least 3 months of the year for 2 consecutive years. It affects 10 to 25 per cent of the adult population. Cough with sputum production is more common in men than in women and more common in persons over the age of 40 than in younger individuals. All forms of chronic bronchitis are strongly linked to cigarette smoking. Thus, a large proportion of cigarette smokers, particularly those over age 45, fit the diagnostic criteria for simple chronic bronchitis. Some occupations (e.g., those involving dust, handling grain, and mining) are associated with an abnormally high incidence of chronic bronchitis, even after statistics are corrected for smoking habits. Few individuals with simple chronic bronchitis consult a physician, and then the visit is usually prompted by acute or recurrent respiratory tract infections or wheezing in addition to chronic cough. *Chronic asthmatic bronchitis* tends to develop in elderly individuals; most commonly, they are smokers.

Three direct effects of inhaling bronchial irritants cause chronic bronchitis: (1) stimulation of mucus secretion in the airways, (2) impaired mucus clearance due in part to interference with ciliary activity, and (3) lowered resistance to bronchopulmonary infection because of disturbed alveolar macrophage function. Cough develops owing to accumulation of secretions. As a result of bacterial colonization by organisms usually found in the nasopharynx, normally sterile bronchi now harbor organisms.

Although cigarette smoking is the most important of the identifiable causal factors, not all smokers experience mucus hypersecretion, and no more than 15 to 20 per cent develop airflow obstruction. Little is known about the reasons for the variable susceptibility to hypersecretion and airflow obstruction in smokers or why reversible airways obstruction develops in many patients with chronic bronchitis. Retention of secretions may be a major factor in some instances. Immunologic factors and other mediators of bronchoconstriction may play a role, since some patients have subacute or chronic bronchospasm resembling classic asthma.

PATHOLOGY. Enlargement of mucous glands in the large airways, the most characteristic abnormality, is primarily due to increased numbers of their constituent cells (hyperplasia) rather than to enlargement of cells (hypertrophy). Retained bronchial secretions and variable degrees of inflammatory changes in the bronchial walls are also identified. Narrowing or obliteration of some small airways, increased mucus in these airways, and

---

*Because use of these symbols has caused confusion, it has been suggested that $\dot{V}max_{50\%}$ and $\dot{V}max_{75\%}$ be expressed as $FEF_{50\%}$ and $FEF_{75\%}$, respectively. Moreover, $\dot{V}max_{75\%}$ as defined herein has sometimes been reported as $\dot{V}max_{25\%}$, the 25% referring to the portion of the FVC remaining when the flow measurement is made.

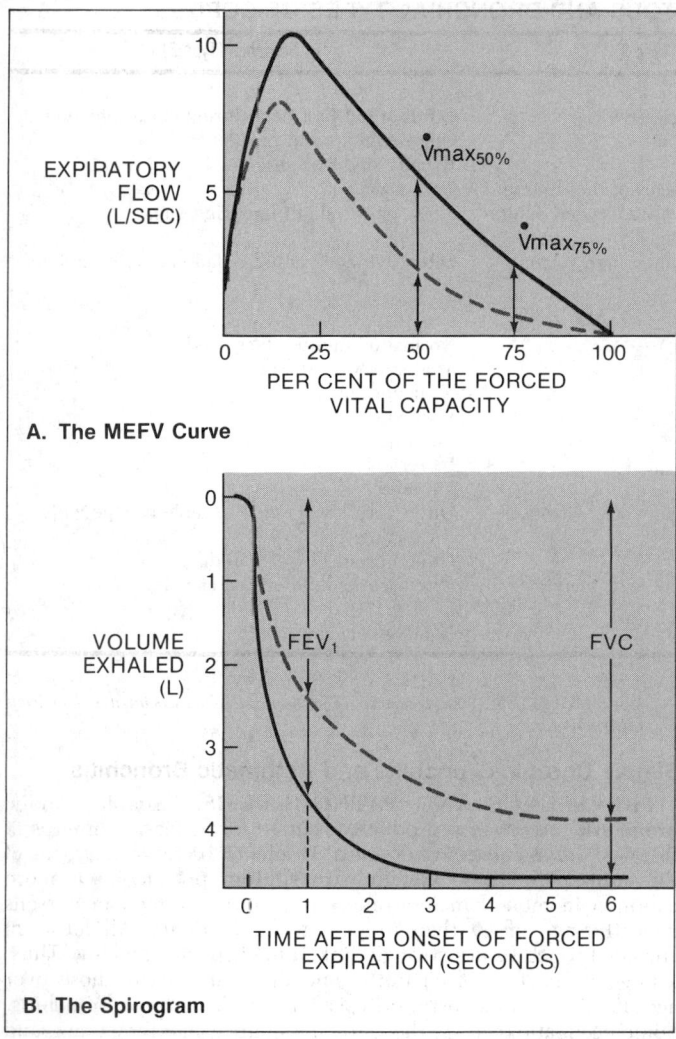

EXPIRATORY FLOW (L/SEC)

$\dot{V}max_{50\%}$

$\dot{V}max_{75\%}$

PER CENT OF THE FORCED VITAL CAPACITY

A. The MEFV Curve

VOLUME EXHALED (L)

FEV_1

FVC

TIME AFTER ONSET OF FORCED EXPIRATION (SECONDS)

B. The Spirogram

FIGURE 58–1. Solid lines are used to show a normal maximal expiratory flow-volume (MEFV) in *A* and a normal spirogram in *B*. Broken lines indicate typical curves for a patient with mild airways obstruction. Measurements of the forced vital capacity (FVC), the forced expiratory volume at 1 second (FEV_1), and forced flow rates at 50 per cent and 75 per cent of the FVC ($\dot{V}max_{50\%}$ and $\dot{V}max_{75\%}$) are depicted as vertical lines. (Adapted from Burrows B: Chronic airways disease. *In* Wyngaarden JM, Smith LH Jr (eds.): Cecil Textbook of Medicine. 17th ed. Philadelphia, W. B. Saunders Company. 1988, p 412).

scattered centrilobular emphysema may be found, even though clinically significant obstruction is absent. Since asymptomatic smokers may have similar small airways and emphysematous changes, it is unclear whether these alterations are related to simple chronic bronchitis, except through a common association with cigarette smoking.

CLINICAL MANIFESTATIONS. When the disease is mild, *cough* occurs when the patient arises or usually after he or she smokes the first cigarette of the day. The cough is productive of a small amount of mucoid sputum and occurs most regularly in the winter months. As the severity increases, the patient coughs throughout the day, symptoms are present throughout the year, sputum volume increases, and episodes of severe coughing develop. Near the end of a severe paroxysm of coughing, wheezing may occur, probably owing to cough-induced bronchospasm. Lying down may induce wheezing, which is probably caused by retained secretions, for cough often provides relief.

Symptoms associated with purulent sputum, suggesting overgrowth of bacteria, may reappear after a viral respiratory infection. *Hemophilus influenzae* and *Streptococcus pneumoniae* may be present, but sputum cultures usually show normal nasopharyngeal flora.

Bacterial organisms probably represent secondary pathogens

rather than being the primary cause of these exacerbations of symptoms. During exacerbations, various degrees of bronchospasm may also develop, blurring the distinction between such episodes and asthma. Whereas *blood-streaked sputum* is noted occasionally, severe or repeated hemoptysis may indicate a more serious entity, such as a pulmonary neoplasm.

The sputum may become chronically purulent as the disorder progresses, and the term *mucopurulent bronchitis* may be applied at this stage of the disease. Rarely, drug-resistant organisms (e.g., *Pseudomonas aeruginosa*) are identified on sputum cultures, especially if the patient has received multiple antibiotics.

In mild disease, the physical examination may be normal. As the disease advances, variable coarse crackles, which may clear or change location with coughing, and scattered wheezes are heard. A forced expiratory maneuver often induces a wheeze or a paroxysm of coughing.

If reversible airways obstruction is present, the patient may resemble the typical asthmatic person, with wheezing and slowing of forced expiration as prominent features.

LABORATORY FINDINGS. The chest radiograph, blood counts, and the differential smear are all normal in the uncomplicated case. Leukocytes and a mixed flora of organisms are noted on sputum examination. Although spirometry often shows some slowing of forced expiration, flow rates may be normal in simple bronchitis. Individuals with *chronic asthmatic bronchitis* may have severe airways obstruction even between acute attacks. During episodes of bronchospasm in patients with asthmatic bronchitis, functional abnormalities are more severe, and both blood and sputum eosinophilia may be present.

COURSE AND PROGNOSIS. In patients with simple chronic bronchitis, symptoms may fluctuate widely. Increased cigarette use, inclement weather, and acute respiratory infections all tend to enhance cough and sputum production. Cessation of smoking in mild cases usually leads to disappearance of symptoms. A slight reduction in ventilatory function is common in simple chronic bronchitis, but progressive respiratory insufficiency does not necessarily develop.

The long-term outcome of patients with asthmatic bronchitis has not been studied extensively. Some patients may become asymptomatic for years after an initial excellent response to therapy, while others require progressively more medication to control bronchospasm. Progress to irreversible airways obstruction occurs in at least a few patients despite good medical management.

DIFFERENTIAL DIAGNOSIS. A persistent, productive cough not attributable to an upper respiratory tract disorder, an allergic reaction of the airways, a specific endobronchial disease, or parenchymal lung disease justifies the diagnosis of chronic bronchitis. Exclusion of a parenchymal lesion requires a chest radiograph. Moreover, a careful upper airway examination should be done, and physical findings, such as a persistent, localized wheeze, must be sought to identify a localized airways disorder. Cystic fibrosis must be excluded in children and in young adults who have severe symptoms of chronic bronchitis (see Ch. 64). In addition, in individuals with one of the immotile cilia syndromes, symptoms of chronic bronchitis may be noted (see Ch. 64).

When there is no identifiable source of chronic bronchial irritation, the diagnosis of simple chronic bronchitis should be made with caution. Sputum and blood eosinophilia should be sought in a nonsmoking patient whose symptoms are associated with exposure to allergens or in a patient with episodes of combined wheezing and dyspnea. Asthmatic bronchitis, which may respond to bronchodilators or corticosteroids, is suggested by high eosinophil levels.

Bronchoscopy and even bronchography or a computed tomography (CT) scan of the chest may be indicated to rule out an endobronchial lesion or localized bronchiectasis in patients with severe or repeated hemoptysis or with physical findings suggesting localized disease. In the routine case, these procedures are not indicated.

Severe mucopurulent bronchitis may be difficult to distinguish from bronchiectasis. In fact, in persons with severe bronchitis, the bronchi may show mild, diffuse, cylindrical dilatation. Saccular bronchiectasis is suggested by (1) repeated pneumonias in the same lung zone, (2) honeycombed areas on the chest radiograph, and (3) recurrent hemoptysis. Bronchography provides an accurate diagnosis, but this invasive procedure is usually indicated only if resection of the bronchiectatic area or areas is considered. Otherwise there is little difference between the therapy for mucopurulent bronchitis and that for bronchiectasis. CT of the chest has been used successfully to diagnose localized and diffuse bronchiectasis.

TREATMENT. Cigarette smoking should stop, and any other bronchial irritants should be removed initially, since this step alone may relieve the symptoms. If the symptoms persist after the maximal effort to avoid provoking factors, the following measures are applied.

Antibiotic Therapy. Infection is considered present when the patient is producing a noneosinophilic, purulent sputum. A 7- to 10-day course of tetracycline or ampicillin (1 gram daily in divided doses) or double-strength sulfamethoxazole-trimethoprim (one tablet twice daily) should be administered. Failure of this antibiotic therapy to clear the sputum warrants a sputum culture and sensitivity test. Successive doses of different antibiotics should be avoided, since this may lead to resistant flora. Therapeutic failure generally is due to inadequate drainage of the airways more often than to an improper choice of antibacterial drugs.

The antibiotic may have to be changed on the basis of drug susceptibility studies when resistant organisms are cultured from the sputum. (For severe, purulent exacerbations, penicillin has proved to be inadequate therapy.)

Bronchodilators. The bronchodilator agents are the mainstays for managing bronchospasm associated with simple chronic bronchitis and for control of any reversible component of COPD. They are also useful in conjunction with bronchial hygiene therapy, described below. Both of the main classes of bronchodilators, the methylxanthines and the beta-adrenergic agonists, help to relieve bronchospasm and to prevent recurrent attacks. The inhaled route of administering beta-adrenergic drugs is usually more effective and rapid in relieving bronchospasm than the oral route. Patients must be carefully instructed, however, in the proper technique for utilizing inhalers. Inhaled atropine may exhibit a combined beneficial effect of reducing copious amounts of sputum and partially relieving bronchospasm in the person with severe bronchitis. The principles and details for therapeutic application of these agents are described in Ch. 57.

Corticosteroids. When significant airways obstruction persists or recurs in the patient with asthmatic bronchitis in spite of maximal therapy with bronchodilators, corticosteroids are indicated. If the patient is ambulatory, modest dosages (e.g., 20 to 40 mg of prednisone per day) are administered for several days and then tapered to the lowest dose that will sustain improvement. Often, improvement is rapid, and the drug can be discontinued in 7 to 10 days. Thereafter, a short "burst" of corticosteroids is used to treat occasional relapses. In some patients, tapering corticosteroids leads to recurrence of symptoms. In these individuals, the dose should be maintained as low as possible to relieve bronchospasm and to prevent recurrent attacks. Alternate-day single-dose corticosteroids should be used for maintenance if possible.

Once bronchospasm has been relieved and a maintenance dose of corticosteroid achieved, an inhaled, poorly absorbed preparation such as beclomethasone should be added. This medication is inhaled from a pressurized container, two to four puffs (100 to 200 g) two to four times daily, depending upon the preparation. The inhaled agent may permit reduction in the maintenance dose of corticosteroid without recurrence of bronchospasm. When significant bronchospasm is present, inhaled corticosteroid agents should be avoided, since this medication may aggravate bronchoconstriction and fail to reach the distal airways. For some patients, premedication with an inhaled bronchodilator (e.g., a beta-adrenergic agent) may relieve airway irritation and permit successful use of inhaled corticosteroids. In general, inhaled corticosteroids replace 7.5 to 10 mg per day of oral prednisone.

After the addition of an inhaled agent, the dose of oral prednisone should be reduced slowly (over several months) to avoid adrenal insufficiency in a corticosteroid-dependent patient who has received months or years of systemic medication. In up to 30 per cent of patients, oropharyngeal candidiasis occurs because of inhaled corticosteroids. This condition responds, however, to specific therapy and rarely requires discontinuation of the inhaled preparation. Nasal symptoms, previously controlled by oral prednisone, may recur, requiring reinstitution of oral agents.

Bronchial Hygiene. These measures are designed to clear retained bronchial secretions. Deep breathing followed by deliberate coughing is the most important maneuver. Sputum production may be more effective if the most involved lung regions are in the superior position (postural drainage) and chest percussion and vibration are applied.

Bronchial hygiene measures may be better tolerated and more effective if the patient is premedicated with an inhaled bronchodilator and then inhales a bland mist to loosen secretions. Although some patients are convinced of its efficacy, objective benefits of bland mist therapy have been difficult to establish. Because patients' reactions to this therapy vary, only measures that prove effective should be continued, since the full program is uncomfortable and time consuming.

To avoid inspissation of secretions, patients should be encouraged to keep well hydrated. Intravenous fluids may be required for acute exacerbations. Although the efficacy of expectorant medications has not been established, some authorities recommend 10 to 12 drops of a saturated solution of potassium iodide three times daily. This program is associated with a high rate of side effects, some severe; yet it does seem beneficial in some patients. Cough syrups and lozenges have little effect on the viscosity of bronchial secretions, but they may relieve a "tickle" in the throat of many persons with bronchitis. Cough sedatives should be used only for acute episodes of a severe, nonproductive cough and are otherwise contraindicated.

Treatment of Severe Exacerbations. Severe exacerbations of asthmatic bronchitis can be life threatening, particularly when associated with severe airways obstruction. The approach to status asthmaticus outlined in Ch. 57 is appropriate, although the patient with asthmatic bronchitis may require more attention to bronchial hygiene measures to clear secretions than does the person with asthma.

Anthonisen NR, Manfreda J, Warren CPW, et al.: Antibiotic therapy in exacerbations of chronic obstructive pulmonary disease. Ann Intern Med 106:196, 1987. *Double-blind placebo controlled trial that reports significant benefit from antimicrobial therapy during exacerbations of chronic bronchitis.*

Burrows B: Irreversible airways obstruction and asthma. Pract Cardiol 8:69, 1982. *This article presents in more detail views concerning the overlap of reversible and irreversible airways obstructive diseases.*

Burrows B, Lebowitz MD, Barbee RA, et al.: Interactions of smoking and immunological factors in relationship to airways obstruction. Chest 84:657, 1983. *This paper presents evidence that chronic asthmatic bronchitis may result from an interaction of the irritant effects of smoking and immunologic factors.*

Iafrate RP, Massey KL, Hendeles L: Current concepts in clinical therapeutics: Asthma. Clin Pharm 5:206, 1986. *A quality review of the use of bronchodilators and corticosteroids in reversible airways diseases.*

IPPB Trial Group: Intermittent positive pressure breathing therapy of chronic obstructive pulmonary disease. Ann Intern Med 99:612, 1983. *This study establishes that there is no significant benefit in positive-pressure breathing over other modalities of delivering bronchodilators.*

Sachs FL: Chronic bronchitis. *In* Pennington JE (ed.): Respiratory Infections: Diagnosis and Management. New York, Raven Press, 1983, p 113. *Comprehensive review of the etiologic role and need for treatment of respiratory infection during exacerbations of chronic bronchitis.*

Stoller JK, Wiedemann HP: Chronic obstructive lung diseases: Asthma, emphysema, chronic bronchitis, bronchiectasis, and related conditions. *In* George RB, Light RW, Matthay MA, Matthay RA (eds.): Chest Medicine. 2nd ed. Baltimore, Williams and Wilkins, 1990. *Comprehensive discussion of the various obstructive lung diseases and their management.*

Chronic Obstructive Bronchitis and Emphysema

PREVALENCE AND PATHOGENESIS. As a major cause of chronic disability in older individuals, chronic obstructive bronchitis and emphysema (COPD) rank behind only heart disease and schizophrenia in the United States. Trends over the past two decades suggest a 60 per cent increase in the prevalence of COPD. This disease is the fifth leading cause of death in the United States, and there has been a 22 per cent increase in the death rate from this condition over the past 20 years. Approximately 75,000 individuals per year die of COPD in the United States, one-half the number of persons dying annually of lung cancer.

Emphysema is common and increases with age. It is present at autopsy in approximately 65 per cent of adult men and 15 per cent of adult women. The prevalence of emphysema is strongly related to cigarette smoking.

Chronic obstructive pulmonary disease is usually diagnosed in those between the ages of 55 and 65. The greater incidence in men than in women most likely reflects the lower incidence of smoking in women in earlier decades. Recent trends, however, show that more teenage girls than boys are starting to smoke. Thus, in several decades COPD may be as common, or more common, in women.

Smoking. Patients with COPD have some combination of chronic obstructive bronchitis and pulmonary emphysema, both of which are closely associated with cigarette smoking. Longitudinal studies confirm a dose-response relationship between cigarette smoking and the rate of pulmonary function decline in patients with COPD. The chronic, progressive destruction of the alveolar structures characteristic of emphysema is thought to occur because of an imbalance between the proteases (proteolytic enzymes) and antiproteases in the lower respiratory tract. According to this concept, proteases, particularly polymorphonuclear neutrophil (PMN) elastase and possibly elastases in pulmonary alveolar macrophages (PAM's), work unimpeded to destroy alveolar structures and their elastin network. Cigarette smokers have increased numbers of PAM's, and PMN's are recruited into their lungs, so that increased numbers of both cell types are recoverable on bronchoalveolar lavage. Recruitment of PMN's into the lungs may occur as a result of the elaboration of chemotactic factors by PAM's stimulated by cigarette smoke. Moreover, smoke components can cause elastase to be released by PMN's by inducing cytotoxic reactions and by stimulating secretion from viable cells. Macrophages exposed to cigarette smoke in vitro or in vivo increase secretion of an elastase-like enzyme. This potential for a greatly increased protease (primarily elastase) burden must be counteracted by the antiprotease defense system of the lungs.

The protease-antiprotease theory of the pathogenesis of emphysema has received further support from the recognition that patients with severe (homozygous phenotype) alpha₁-antitrypsin deficiency have markedly reduced levels of serum alpha₁-antitrypsin and progressive panacinar emphysema. As might be expected, when studied by bronchoalveolar lavage, patients with severe alpha₁-antitrypsin deficiency have little or no alpha₁-antitrypsin in their lower respiratory tracts. Nor do they have alternate antiprotease protection against neutrophil elastase.

Compared with nonsmokers, cigarette smokers without alpha₁-antitrypsin deficiency also show reduced elastase inhibitory capacity because of inactivation of alpha₁-proteinase inhibitor (alpha₁-PI). Chemical oxidation of alpha₁-PI by material in cigarette smoke is postulated as a major cause of the observed decrease in elastase inhibitory capacity. Smoking may interfere with elastin repair mechanisms, as documented by studies both in vivo and in vitro.

Severe genetic deficiency of serum alpha₁-antitrypsin occurs in 0.5 to 2 per cent of patients with COPD. Typically, in such individuals, emphysema is likely to develop by age 40 in smokers and by age 60 in nonsmokers. Presumably, prolonged exposure to irritants, primarily cigarette smoke, further reduces lung antiprotease defenses and induces low-grade inflammation and destructive changes in the parenchyma of the lungs.

The protease-antiprotease hypothesis of the pathogenesis of emphysema does not readily explain all of the observations in experimental and human emphysema. For instance, experimental enzyme-induced emphysema is panacinar rather than centrilobular, the more common type in humans with chronic airflow obstruction. Further, it does not explain the predominant localization of centrilobular emphysema to the upper lung zones or of panacinar emphysema to the lung bases or of paraseptal emphysema to the regions beneath the pleura and adjacent to fibrous septa. There is a close relationship between slowing of forced exhalation and cigarette smoking. The average heavy smoker has a 40- to 45-ml per year decline in FEV₁, whereas the average nonsmoking adult shows a decline of only 20 to 25 ml per year. Nonsmokers with alpha₁-antitrypsin deficiency have approximately an 80-ml per year decline in FEV₁; cigarette smokers with this deficiency have approximately a 150-ml per year decline. When individuals with alpha₁-antitrypsin deficiency stop smoking, this excess rate of decline in FEV₁ ceases. Nevertheless, the average effect of cigarette smoking alone does not explain the more severe reduction in FEV₁ noted in patients with COPD.

Moreover, why is it that only a minority of smokers develop clinically significant COPD? Some individuals may be particularly susceptible for various reasons: respiratory disorders in childhood, intercurrent respiratory infections, and genetic factors, for example.

Can COPD be detected early by screening lung function in young to middle-aged adults? Longitudinal studies are attempting to identify susceptible cigarette-smoking individuals with an excessive rate of decline in pulmonary function throughout adult life. The hypothesis is that the individual who will develop COPD later in life should be identifiable by age 40 because he or she will show at least a mild ventilatory abnormality by then. There is no direct evidence yet, however, that any physiologic test applied early in life detects the individual who will develop disabling COPD.

Alpha₁-Antitrypsin Deficiency. A deficiency in serum antiproteolytic activity associated with a susceptibility to COPD has been noted in several families. The protease inhibitor, or "Pi," phenotype of the subject determines the serum's trypsin inhibitory capacity. Two M genes (Pi MM phenotype) are present in normal individuals. When only Z genes are present (Pi ZZ phenotype), serum alpha₁-antitrypsin levels are severely reduced (<50 mg per deciliter), and the alpha₁-antitrypsin that is present in plasma is less effective in inhibiting neutrophil elastase than the alpha₁-antitrypsin in individuals with the Pi MM phenotype. Deficiency of alpha₁-antitrypsin is transmitted as an autosomal recessive trait. This antiproteolytic deficiency, present in approximately 1 in 4000 of the population, is associated with hepatitis in infancy and the development of emphysema in the third, fourth, and fifth decades. Present in 3 to 5 per cent of the population, the heterozygotic state (Pi MZ phenotype) is associated with a moderately reduced serum antiproteolytic activity, but no predilection for developing an excess of respiratory disorders. Several other Pi genes have been identified (of which S is the most common), but only the Z gene clearly leads to COPD. In Ch. 121 the hepatic manifestations of alpha₁-antitrypsin deficiency are discussed.

PATHOLOGY. Alveolar wall destruction with a nonuniform pattern of air space enlargement is the basic abnormality in emphysema. The orderly appearance of the acinus and its components is disturbed and may be lost, as air spaces are fewer in number but enlarged. In centrilobular emphysema, the process is most severe in the central portion of the lobule, whereas in panacinar emphysema, the defect occurs uniformly throughout the acinus. Both centrilobular and panacinar emphysema may be noted in the same lung. In severe centrilobular emphysema, the entire acinus may ultimately become involved. Centrilobular emphysema generally is the most common form of emphysema in patients with chronic airflow obstruction.

In large airways, inflammation is noted in and around air passages, with narrowing of the lumina, impaction of mucus, and obliterative changes. Abnormalities of the small airways are usually not obvious on cursory examination and require careful morphometric studies.

CLINICAL MANIFESTATIONS. Dyspnea is usually the predominant complaint, but some patients consult a physician initially because of cough, wheezing, recurrent respiratory infections, or, occasionally, weakness or weight loss. Patients may date the onset of chronic symptoms to an acute respiratory infection. In some, shortness of breath is present only during acute exacerbations.

A productive cough is usually present, associated with a thick or "sticky" sputum varying widely in quantity. Copious amounts of purulent sputum, coupled with a severe cough, are noted by some patients.

The physical examination may yield normal findings relatively early in the illness (FEV₁ > 1.0 liter). Auscultation of the chest may reveal rhonchi, or the chest may be quiet, particularly in patients with extensive emphysema. Wheezing, which may be absent on quiet breathing, can often be heard on forced exhalation. As the disease progresses, marked hyperinflation with low diaphragm and a reduced area of cardiac dullness are common. Labored breathing, at times through pursed lips, may be noted after minimal exertion or even at rest. Patients tend to lean forward on their elbows when sitting, assuming a stooped posture, while using accessory muscles of respiration. Cyanosis and dependent edema may be noted.

Occasionally, patients first seek medical attention when signs of right ventricular failure due to cor pulmonale appear. In such cases, the FEV_1 is likely to be below 1 liter and the arterial Po_2 below 45 mm Hg. The pulmonary hypertension in these patients with COPD and cor pulmonale is most closely related to the severity of hypoxemia.

Table 58–1 shows features of relatively distinctive COPD clinical syndromes and their associated underlying pathologic conditions. These two clinical types of COPD, emphysematous (type A) and bronchial (type B), represent extremes of presentation; most individuals, if followed chronically, develop a mixture of findings from the type A and type B groups. Type A patients, described as "pink puffers," often hyperventilate, maintaining normal or nearly normal arterial O_2 and CO_2 tensions. In contrast, type B patients, "blue bloaters," often have a low arterial O_2 tension, high CO_2 tension, cyanosis, and right-sided congestive heart failure. The "blue bloater" syndrome may also result from disordered breathing during sleep, a common problem in patients with COPD.

LABORATORY FINDINGS. The routine blood count and differential study are normal except for erythrocytosis in some COPD patients with hypoxemia. When eosinophilia is found, a reversible (asthmatic-bronchitic) component of the disease should be suspected.

Early in the disease, the chest radiograph may be normal; however, in severe emphysema, lung hyperinflation and an increased retrosternal air space, with flattening of the diaphragm and regional attenuation of blood vessels, are usually noted. Frank bullae outlined by hairline margins are present in some cases. The chest radiograph should not be the sole basis for the diagnosis of COPD, for individuals with perfectly normal lung function may have radiographic findings typical of the disease. Chest CT has frequently been used to determine with accuracy the presence of emphysema and to quantify its severity.

Persistent reduction in FEF rates is the most typical finding in COPD. Two lung volume measurements, the residual volume and the ratio of residual volume to total lung capacity, are elevated. Ventilation-perfusion mismatch and nonuniformity of ventilation are also typical findings, whereas arterial hypoxemia and physiologic shunting vary among patients. When the diffusing capacity is very depressed and the total lung capacity is clearly increased, emphysema is likely to be extensive.

Ventilation-perfusion lung scans should be interpreted cautiously when pulmonary emboli are suspected. These scans reveal the uneven ventilation and perfusion typical of COPD. Areas of diminished perfusion may be mistaken for pulmonary emboli. Accordingly, when pulmonary embolism is suspected in a patient with COPD, a pulmonary angiogram is often required for definitive diagnosis.

The electrocardiogram tends to be normal, particularly early in the course of the disease. Later, the axis is shifted to the right, and there are early R waves in the precordial leads V_1 and V_2 and net negative electrical forces in leads V_5 and V_6. Especially during exacerbations, peaked P waves ("P pulmonale") are present. Unfortunately, these changes do not correlate well with pulmonary artery hypertension and cor pulmonale. The presence of R waves over the right precordium is the most reliable indication of cor pulmonale.

COURSE AND PROGNOSIS. Initially, the response to bronchodilator therapy is variable, dependent upon the degree of bronchospasm. Thereafter, the disease progresses slowly, with an annual average decrement in FEV_1 of 50 to 75 ml. Because the variability in FEV_1 may be greater than the true annual decline, a follow-up of several years is required to determine the rate of loss of lung function. If the patient stops smoking, cough and sputum production may cease. However, most other symptoms progress gradually.

In terms of absolute FEV_1, patients are dyspneic upon moderate exertion when the value is 1.2 to 1.5 liters; they are forced to be relatively sedentary at 1.0 liter; and they are often invalids when the FEV_1 is 500 ml or less. As the FEV_1 drops below 1 liter, severe arterial hypoxemia, hypercapnia, and cor pulmonale are often evident.

Median survival varies considerably. Despite initially very low FEV_1 values, some individuals live 12 to 15 years. Generally, however, when the FEV_1 is more than 1.2 liters, patients survive about 10 years; when the FEV_1 is 1.0 liter, survival is approximately 5 years; and when the FEV_1 is less than 700 ml, survival is about 2 years. Signs of a poor prognosis include a resting tachycardia, severe arterial hypoxemia or hypercapnia or both, and evidence of cor pulmonale. If a patient resides at altitudes higher than 3500 feet, longevity is reduced.

Increased cough and dyspnea are hallmarks of periodic worsening of the disease. Symptoms characteristically occur after an acute respiratory infection and may be accompanied by bronchospasm. Such exacerbations in patients with severe COPD may be life threatening and may lead to acute respiratory failure as well as right ventricular failure. The latter occurs secondary to pronounced increases in pulmonary artery pressure and pulmonary vascular resistance, which, in turn, are due primarily to hypoxic pulmonary vasoconstriction.

DIFFERENTIAL DIAGNOSIS. Three criteria are required to diagnose COPD: (1) The FEV_1 must be reduced, and this reduction must be proportionately more than any lowering in the FVC (i.e., both the predicted percentage of FEV_1 and the FEV_1/FVC ratio must be depressed); (2) in spite of intensive, prolonged medical treatment, this slowing of forced expiration must persist; and (3) other bronchopulmonary disease that might explain the observed physiologic abnormalities must be excluded. Sufficient evidence for the last criterion generally includes absence of extensive parenchymal abnormalities on the chest radiograph and absence of any signs of upper airways obstruction, such as neck mass, stridor, or narrowing of the upper airway seen on the chest radiograph. Irreversibility of the obstructive ventilatory defect may be more difficult to establish. This factor is discussed further in the treatment section.

Assessing the relative contribution of emphysema and intrinsic airway changes can also be difficult. Emphysema is usually severe when the diffusing capacity is very depressed and the chest radiograph shows hyperlucent lungs with attenuation of the vascular markings. In contrast, if the diffusing capacity is normal or nearly normal, extensive emphysema is unlikely. Esophageal balloon measurements, which are required to assess lung elastic recoil (the best guide to the severity of emphysema), are seldom justified as part of the clinical evaluation.

If there is a family history of emphysema or emphysema-type COPD develops at an early age, a homozygous alpha$_1$-antitrypsin deficiency should be considered. Suspicion is heightened when the patient is a nonsmoker or a woman or when the chest radiograph shows a bibasilar distribution of emphysematous changes. Laboratory confirmation is provided by almost complete absence of alpha$_1$ globulin, by a markedly reduced serum trypsin inhibitory capacity, and, most specifically, by demonstration of a pattern of a pure Z phenotype on crossed immunoelectrophoresis of the serum.

TREATMENT. The following are therapeutic goals in patients with COPD: (1) to relieve the portion of airway obstruction that is reversible; (2) to control cough and sputum production; (3) to eliminate and prevent airway infections; (4) to increase exercise tolerance to the maximum allowable at the individual's level of physiologic deficit; (5) to control remedial disease complications, such as arterial hypoxemia and cardiovascular problems; (6) to avoid smoking and other airway irritants, narcotics and sedatives, and noncritical surgery, all of which aggravate the disease; and (7) to relieve the anxiety and depression that are often present in the patient with COPD.

In spite of treatment, most patients with severe COPD show progressive ventilatory deterioration; yet therapy should not be withheld. A comprehensive therapeutic program can reduce symptoms, decrease the frequency of hospital admissions, prevent premature death, and permit patients to lead a more active and satisfying life.

A formal rehabilitation program using a team approach is effective. Nevertheless, good results can also be obtained by a dedicated individual physician, assisted, perhaps, by an office nurse who can help patients with physical therapy and bronchial hygiene measures.

Initial Treatment. During the initial visit, it is impossible to predict with certainty the degree of reversibility of airways obstruction in a patient with COPD. Therefore, all patients should be considered as having potentially reversible disease. Bronchodilators should be administered according to tolerance, as outlined in the therapy for asthmatic bronchitis and asthma. Smoking should be discontinued and other bronchial irritants avoided. As mentioned in the therapy for simple chronic bronchitis, bronchial hygiene measures and, when indicated by purulent mucus production, antibiotics should be used. Diuretics should be given when heart failure is present. In addition, the Pneumovax vaccine and yearly administration of the influenza vaccine are indicated.

The effects of this initial therapy both on symptoms and on pulmonary function test results should be determined and adjustments made in medication to minimize side effects. Apparently ineffective measures (e.g., postural drainage that leads to no symptom relief or sputum production) should be discontinued. Next, if further reversibility of the disease is considered possible, a 3- to 4-week trial of corticosteroids can be initiated. If the acute inhalation of bronchodilator produces a 20 per cent improvement in FEV_1 or if there is a similar increase in FEV_1 several days or weeks after intensive bronchodilator therapy, corticosteroids are likely to be beneficial. Several other findings suggest that corticosteroids may help: (1) a noisy chest or wheeze upon auscultation, (2) sputum or blood eosinophilia, (3) evidence of atopy (e.g., history of hay fever, an elevated serum immunoglobulin E [IgE] level, positive results of allergy skin tests), or (4) associated nasal polyps or vasomotor rhinitis.

Generally, 20 to 40 mg of prednisone daily is given for 3 to 4 weeks, and spirometry tests are used to assess the efficacy of this medication. Other bronchodilators are continued at full doses. When improvement is noted, the corticosteroid dose should be tapered to the lowest maintenance dose possible, as outlined for asthmatic bronchitis. If there is no significant improvement in FEV_1 (e.g., >20 per cent), corticosteroids should be tapered slowly and discontinued.

Maintenance Therapy. Frequently, objective improvement (i.e., increase in FEV_1) cannot be demonstrated with bronchodilator therapy. Yet oral theophylline, combined with an inhaled beta-adrenergic agent, is recommended to prevent superimposed bronchospasm. In COPD, theophylline can (1) enhance respiratory muscle function, in both the fatigued and the nonfatigued state; (2) augment right and left ventricular systolic pump function while decreasing pulmonary artery pressures and pulmonary vascular resistance (potentially helpful in patients with cor pulmonale); and (3) in some patients, reduce dyspnea. The beta-adrenergic agents also improve biventricular systolic pump performance and decrease pulmonary vascular resistance. Whether any of these potentially salutary effects are additive or synergistic when oral theophylline is administered in conjunction with beta-adrenergic agents has not been established.

Aerosolized adrenergic agents are also used (1) to relieve acute attacks of dyspnea; (2) prior to exposure to known bronchial irritants, such as cold air; or (3) as a regular part of a bronchial hygiene program.

If a patient with COPD shows improvement in airflow rates (particularly FEV_1) with bronchodilators or adrenocortical hormones, these agents should be maintained, as in asthmatic bronchitis. Those with a productive cough, retained secretions, or repeated episodes of bronchopulmonary infection should be treated with the same measures as described for simple chronic bronchitis. In addition, some other forms of treatment are uniquely applicable to patients with COPD.

Physical Therapy. Exercise has not been shown to improve lung function, but it may enhance cardiovascular fitness and train skeletal muscles to function more efficiently, thus increasing exercise tolerance. Accordingly, unless contraindicated by an underlying cardiac abnormality, progressively increasing exercise (usually walking) should be prescribed. In most cases, the program can be recommended directly by the physician, but if the patient is severely disabled, a trained physical therapist can initiate an appropriate exercise program. Arterial blood gas levels should be obtained when the patient is at rest and after exercise, prior to instituting a vigorous exercise program, particularly if the FEV_1 is less than 1 liter. Supplemental oxygen should be used during exercise if the patient becomes severely hypoxemic.

Although breathing exercises probably do not alter the usual breathing pattern of COPD, occasionally they are recommended to encourage diaphragmatic breathing. Perhaps it is more useful and more realistic to teach patients slow, deep breathing as a quicker, more effective method for relieving dyspnea than rapid, shallow "panic" breathing. Breath holding should be avoided during exertion. Many authorities now recommend inspiratory muscle training by breathing against a graded resistor, but mechanical devices, intermediate positive-pressure breathing (IPPB) machines, and emphysema belts are of unproven value.

Oxygen Therapy. In some individuals with COPD, there are clear indications for home oxygen therapy. One indication is development of severe exertional hypoxemia (PaO_2 < 40 mm Hg) in patients who respond to supplemental oxygen therapy with an increase in exercise tolerance. A second indication is found in patients with severe, persistent arterial hypoxemia at rest (PaO_2 < 55 mm Hg), accompanied by secondary signs of hypoxemia, after all other therapeutic measures have been exhausted and the patient has completely recovered from exacerbation of the disease. Both continuous oxygen therapy and that spanning 12 to 15 hours per day prolong survival, but continuous therapy (i.e., 10 to 24 hours per day) is associated with longer survival. To raise the PaO_2 to the necessary 60 to 80 mm Hg usually requires 1 to 3 liters of oxygen per minute via nasal prongs.

Since patients may become habituated to this therapy and thus increase their invalidism, oxygen should not be prescribed solely for episodes of dyspnea.

Environmental Control. All patients with severe COPD should be cautioned to avoid high altitudes, and supplemental oxygen may be required for those with severe hypoxemia when they travel by air. Moreover, COPD patients with severe hypoxemia should reside at altitudes below 4000 feet. A change in residence may be indicated in patients who live in areas with heavy air pollution.

Cold winter climates are avoided by some patients who find relief in either warm desert climates or warm, humid regions. No specific climate has been shown to alter the overall course of the disease. Accordingly, the economic and social hardships of a move should be weighed carefully against the potential symptomatic benefit provided by relocation to a more agreeable climate. Before moving, the patient should spend a trial period in the new climate to assess symptomatic benefit.

Treatment of Edema and Cor Pulmonale. Even in the absence of frank right-sided congestive heart failure, pedal edema is common, and control is usually obtained with small doses of diuretics. Ankle edema associated with cor pulmonale is more difficult to control, but oxygen combined with diuretics often suffices. Digitalis is useful for enhancing right ventricular function only if there is concomitant left ventricular failure; accordingly, digitalis should be reserved for combined right and left ventricular failure. Phlebotomy is not required in most oxygen-treated patients but may transiently relieve central nervous system symptoms, especially when the hematocrit is above 60 per cent.

Treatment of Hypercapnia. Chronic hypercapnia is common in late stages of COPD, but it requires no therapy. However, during exacerbations, blood gases must be monitored closely for severe respiratory acidosis, and all narcotics, sedatives, and tranquilizers should be avoided. In patients with stable chronic hypercapnia, mechanically assisted ventilation and respiratory stimulants are unnecessary.

Surgical Therapy. In the absence of significant emphysema (e.g., that manifested by a moderate to severe reduction in diffusing capacity), bullectomy may benefit patients with large bullae compressing normal or nearly normal lung. Careful, detailed preoperative evaluation is required to select suitable candidates for operation.

Supportive Measures. Careful, detailed education of the patient regarding the nature of the disease is essential. The significance of symptoms such as purulent sputum production, potential side effects of medication, and therapeutic goals should be explained. A prompt, prearranged treatment plan for intercurrent exacerbations should be discussed with the patient.

Above all, within the limits of respiratory impairment and within the constraints of therapy, these patients should be encouraged to have an active lifestyle with daily exercise. Some patients benefit from vocational rehabilitation and occupational therapy.

Replacement Therapy in Severe Alpha₁-Antitrypsin Deficiency Emphysema. Chronic, weekly replacement or monthly therapy with intravenous alpha₁-antitrypsin concentrate of normal plasma has been undertaken at the National Heart, Lung and Blood Institute in individuals with severe alpha₁-antitrypsin deficiency. Serum alpha₁-antitrypsin was elevated to levels that are probably required for effective antielastase protection of the lungs (average posttherapy level achieved, 130 mg per deciliter; average pretherapy level, 31 mg per deciliter). Alpha₁-antitrypsin levels after bronchoalveolar lavage increased in these individuals to about 60 per cent of normal, associated with an equivalent restoration of functional antineutrophil elastase activity. Moreover, the incidence of adverse reactions was limited to a transient postinfusion fever in fewer than 1 per cent of the patients.

Recently, recombinant DNA methodology has been used to produce alpha₁-antitrypsin molecules. The future may bring widespread clinical application of this potentially less expensive material administered by intravenous infusion or by inhalation to patients with the PiZZ phenotype. When only mild airways disease is present, this therapy will re-establish the lung antineutrophil elastase defenses and protect the alveolar walls from elastolytic attack.

Treatment of Exacerbations. Antibiotics, increased bronchodilator medications, and even corticosteroids are often indicated for acute exacerbations. Immediate hospitalization is required for severe hypoxemia, increasing carbon dioxide tension, or congestive heart failure. Ch. 40 and 70 outline the management of decompensated cor pulmonale and acute respiratory failure, respectively. The same management utilized in patients with status asthmaticus is indicated in COPD patients with superimposed refractory bronchospasm.

Anthonisen NR: Hypoxemia and O₂ therapy. Am Rev Respir Dis 126:729, 1982. *A succinct review of the British and American studies establishing that oxygen therapy prolongs life in patients with hypoxemic COPD.*

De Marco FJ Jr, Wynne JW, Block AJ, et al.: Oxygen desaturation during sleep as a determinant of the "blue and bloated" syndrome. Chest 79:621, 1981. *One of several papers by this group of investigators proposing that sleep-related breathing disorders are important in COPD patients.*

Gadek JE (ed.): Alpha–1-antitrypsin deficiency. Am J Med 84 (suppl 6A):1, 1988. *Extensive monograph detailing the pathogenesis and potential treatment modalities for lung disease associated with alpha₁-antitrypsin deficiency.*

Higgins MW, Keller JB: Estimating your patients' risk of COPD. J Respir Dis 4:97, 1983. *This paper discusses the use of routine spirometric testing to detect subjects who are at high risk of developing clinically significant airways obstructive disease.*

Hubbard RC, Brantly ML, Sellers S, et al.: Anti-neutrophil-elastase defenses of the lower respiratory tract in alpha₁-antitrypsin deficiency directly augmented with an aerosol of alpha₁-antitrypsin. Ann Intern Med 111:206, 1989. *Establishes that inhaled alpha₁-antitrypsin restores epithelial lining fluid levels of alpha₁-antitrypsin and antineutrophil-elastase activity in patients with severe alpha₁-antitrypsin deficiency.*

Janoff A: Elastases and emphysema. Current assessment of the protease-antiprotease hypothesis. Am Rev Respir Dis 132:417, 1985. *Reviews 10 years of progress in elucidating the pathogenesis of emphysema.*

Petty TL (ed.): Chronic obstructive pulmonary disease. 2nd ed. New York, Marcel Dekker, 1985. *Comprehensive text on all aspects of COPD.*

Snider GL: Pulmonary disease in alpha₁-antitrypsin deficiency. Ann Intern Med 111:957, 1989. *Succinct, up-to-date statement on the pathogenesis and therapy of lung disease in patients with alpha₁-antitrypsin deficiency.*

LOCALIZED AIRWAYS OBSTRUCTION

Extrinsic compression of airways, intraluminal obstruction, and diseases of the airways themselves all can cause localized airways obstruction. Signs and symptoms depend upon the location of the obstruction and upon whether it is partial or complete, variable or fixed. The discussion of localized lesions is divided into obstructions above and below the bifurcation of the trachea.

Obstruction Above the Tracheal Bifurcation

PARTIAL OBSTRUCTION. Stridor, frequently accompanied by inspiratory retraction of the intercostal spaces, is the principal finding in partial obstruction above the main (tracheal) carina. On both forced inspiration and forced expiration, airflow rates are reduced, and there may be a characteristic appearance to the MEFV curve. As shown in Figure 58–2, the site and nature of the obstruction determine the findings on spirometry. When the obstruction is severe, hypoxemia and hypercapnia may result owing to reduced overall ventilation.

Among the intrinsic airways diseases that can cause partial airways obstruction are (1) tonsil and adenoid enlargement, especially in young children; (2) stenosing lesions secondary to trauma; (3) neoplams or granulomatous processes (e.g., sarcoidosis, fungi) involving the hypopharynx, larynx, vocal cords, or

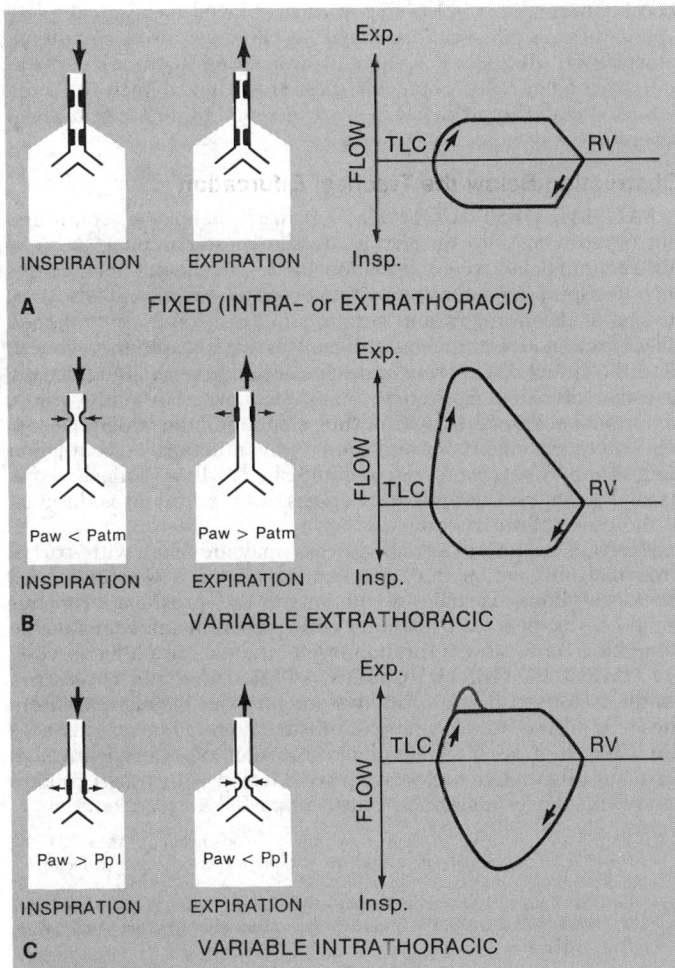

FIGURE 58–2. Airways obstruction above the carina may produce characteristic flow-volume abnormalities, depending on the type and site of obstruction. *A,* If the obstruction is fixed, both inspiratory and expiratory flows will be decreased whether the obstruction is intrathoracic or extrathoracic (for purposes of illustration, obstruction is shown in both locations). Note that this pattern is usually seen when the obstruction is at the level of the thoracic inlet. *B,* When a variable obstruction is extrathoracic in location, the airway narrows during inspiration when airway pressure (P_{aw}) is less than atmospheric pressure (P_{atm}) and inspiratory flow is diminished. Expiratory flows are often limited, but to a lesser extent. *C,* When a variable obstruction is intrathoracic in location, airway pressure is less than pleural pressure (Ppl) during expiration, and expiratory flow is diminished. Inspiratory flows are often limited, but to a much lesser extent. (Reproduced with permission from Burrows B, et al: Respiratory Disorders—A Pathophysiologic Approach. 2nd ed. Copyright © 1983 by Year Book Medical Publishers, Inc., Chicago.)

trachea; (4) bilateral paralysis of the vocal cords; (5) spasm or edema of the larynx; or (6) inflammation in several locations—the pharynx (e.g., peritonsillar abscess), the larynx (e.g., croup), or the trachea (e.g., diphtheria). An enlarged thyroid, a paratracheal neoplasm, or a mediastinal infection can cause extrinsic compression of the airways. An artificial airway, tracheostomy, or surgical repair is indicated when the primary cause of the obstruction cannot be eliminated.

COMPLETE OBSTRUCTION. Rapid asphyxiation results unless complete obstruction above the main carina is relieved promptly. There is a pathognomonic presentation, with absent airflow at the mouth in spite of both inspiratory efforts and inspiratory retraction of the intercostal muscles. Aspiration of poorly chewed food (so-called "café coronary") is the most common cause of acute obstruction. If a sharp blow to the back fails to dislodge the obstructing material, forced pressure is applied to the epigastrium—the *Heimlich maneuver.*

When the glossopharyngeal structures fall back in some obese individuals, complete obstruction of the upper airway occurs.

Local abnormalities in the hypopharynx may also cause complete upper airways obstruction, resulting in disordered breathing, especially during sleep. Frequent awakening, a troubled sleep, and somnolence are characteristic. This clinical picture, often confused with the pickwickian syndrome and other forms of sleep disorders, is discussed in Ch. 203.

Obstruction Below the Tracheal Bifurcation

PARTIAL OBSTRUCTION. A primary neoplasm, compressing or growing into an airway, is the most common cause of obstruction below the bifurcation of the trachea. Other causes include aspiration of foreign bodies, acute or chronic inflammatory lesions of the bronchi, and compression of bronchi by enlarged hilar lymph nodes or mucous plugs. A localized expiratory wheeze over the site of obstruction and hyperinflation of the lung distally are characteristic. Spirometry may be normal or only mildly abnormal because airflow from the remaining lung is unimpaired; yet other tests show nonuniformity of ventilation. A ventilation lung scan may reveal an area of diminished airflow. Bronchoscopy usually provides a definitive diagnosis, and treatment is directed at the cause of obstruction.

Infection and perhaps an abscess may develop with partial bronchial obstruction due to impaired secretion clearance from the distal lung. Partial obstruction of the proximal bronchus should be suspected in patients with recurrent infections in the same lung zone, slow resolution of pneumonia, or a lung abscess.

COMPLETE OBSTRUCTION. "Obstructive atelectasis" is a condition caused by absorption of air into the bloodstream from the lung distal to a complete obstruction. This condition is discussed in Ch. 59. Complete occlusion of a bronchus and resultant obstructive atelectasis may develop with progression of any of the above-mentioned causes of partial obstruction.

Heimlich HJ: A life-saving maneuver to prevent food-choking. JAMA 234:398, 1975. *The original report on a standard method to remove aspirated food from the airways.*

Loughlin GM, Taussig LM: Upper airway obstruction. Semin Respir Med 1:131, 1979. *This is an excellent review of upper airways obstructive disorders in infants and children.*

Miller RD: Obstructing lesions of the larynx and trachea: Clinical and pathophysiologic aspects. *In* Fishman AP (ed.): Pulmonary Diseases and Disorders. 2nd ed. New York, McGraw-Hill Book Company, 1988, p 1173. *An excellent review of the causes, consequences, and treatment of tracheolaryngeal obstruction.*

59 Abnormalities of Lung Aeration

Richard A. Matthay

LOCALIZED HYPOAERATION (ATELECTASIS)

Atelectasis, or reduced aeration of the lung, is present in many bronchopulmonary disorders and assumes a variety of forms. A total loss of ventilation to a lung region (i.e., with total airway collapse) leads to a shunt wherein blood traversing this region fails to participate in gas exchange and behaves as if it were moving directly from the right to the left side of the heart. Accordingly, total atelectasis causes an "absolute" shunt. In contrast to the shuntlike effect of increased venous admixture present in most bronchopulmonary diseases, the absolute shunt is not fully corrected by inhalation of 100 per cent oxygen.

TYPES OF ATELECTASIS AND THEIR PATHOGENESIS. *Obstructive atelectasis* is a condition of alveolar collapse that develops within a few hours after obstruction of an airway distal to the tracheal bifurcation. The collapse occurs because gas in the lung behind the obstruction is slowly absorbed into the bloodstream. If the lung is filled with oxygen-rich gas rather than ambient air, the alveoli collapse more rapidly. Nitrogen in ambient air is poorly soluble, whereas oxygen is rapidly absorbed into the bloodstream. As a result, high inspired oxygen tensions encourage the development of atelectasis behind obstructing mucous plugs.

Contraction atelectasis occurs when fibrotic changes in a local area of the lung increase its recoil. Contraction, or shrinkage, of the involved lung, rather than complete airlessness, results.

Patchy atelectasis develops throughout the lung owing to alveolar instability in adult and infant (newborn) respiratory distress syndromes.

A large pneumothorax, pleural effusion, or other space-occupying lesion in the thorax can increase intrapleural pressure, causing a portion of the lung to decrease in volume. This *compression atelectasis* is more appropriately called *relaxation atelectasis* because the atelectasis results from the tendency of the lung to recoil when the distending forces are relaxed. As small airways close in the affected region because of marked relaxation atelectasis, any air remaining distally is absorbed into the bloodstream.

Although its pathologic significance is unclear, *platelike atelectasis* may be visible on the chest radiograph. This condition is characterized by horizontal radiopaque streaks, usually in the lung bases. Commonly associated with poor lung aeration, these streaks are seen when the patient has been unable to breathe deeply for a sustained period or when the diaphragm is elevated, such as after intra-abdominal surgery.

CLINICAL MANIFESTATIONS. The chronicity and extent of the process determine the physiologic and clinical consequences of atelectasis. When the obstruction evolves slowly, typical of bronchial neoplasms, usually few or no symptoms develop and hypoxemia is minimal. In contrast, profound dyspnea and severe hypoxemia often develop after the acute collapse of a large section of the lung. As blood flow through the nonventilated lung diminishes over several hours, symptoms and hypoxemia lessen. The acute situation typically involves obstructive atelectasis due to aspiration of a foreign body or to retention of secretions (which may develop in the postoperative period).

The type of atelectasis determines the physical findings. In obstructive or contraction atelectasis, the physical findings depend upon the amount of lung involved. In major atelectasis, the trachea and mediastinum shift to the affected side, the diaphragm is elevated, and the involved hemithorax is smaller and shows less respiratory motion than does the unaffected side. Patchy atelectasis is associated with findings like those of the respiratory distress syndrome reviewed in Ch. 70. The underlying condition (e.g., pleural effusion, pneumothorax, space-occupying lesion) determines the findings in relaxation atelectasis. Platelike atelectasis is primarily diagnosed on the basis of a chest radiograph and presents no distinctive abnormalities on physical examination.

DIAGNOSIS, TREATMENT, AND OUTCOME. The chest radiograph confirms the presence of atelectasis. When obstructive atelectasis is suspected, bronchoscopy is required to establish the cause; it may be possible to remove the occluding material through the bronchoscope. However, a bronchogenic neoplasm should always be considered when obstructive atelectasis is present and the patient is not severely ill.

Treatment is directed at the underlying disorder in nonobstructive forms of atelectasis.

When relaxation atelectasis is relieved (e.g., by insertion of a chest tube for a large pneumothorax), the lung usually returns to normal. However, obstructive atelectasis often is accompanied by secondary complications, such as infection, which lead to abscess formation, localized bronchiectasis, and fibrosis. Moreover, after prolonged collapse, the affected lung may fail to reexpand after the obstruction is removed. The *middle lobe syndrome* exhibits a typical sequence of events. In this syndrome, the middle lobe bronchus in the right lung has usually been compressed by large hilar lymph nodes in tuberculosis or other granulomatous lung diseases. Even after the lymph nodes finally decrease in size, the affected lung fails to expand fully, there are often bronchiectatic changes, and the lobe may be a site of recurrent or chronic infection. Although less common, the same sequence of events may occur in other lung regions. The involved lung may have to be resected if recurrent pneumonia, chronic suppuration, or repeated episodes of hemoptysis develop.

LOCALIZED HYPERAERATION

BLEBS AND BULLAE. Blebs are small collections of gas that are entirely enclosed within the visceral pleura. The gas resides between the multiple leaves of the visceral pleura rather than within the lung itself. Blebs are the uncommon result of dissection of air from the lung interstitium into the lung septa and thence into and between the layers of visceral pleura. Blebs are not clinically important except on the rare occasions that they rupture and cause a spontaneous pneumothorax. Sometimes blebs are visible on the plain chest radiograph, particularly in the lung apex; they are more easily seen when there is a pneumothorax and partial collapse of normal surrounding lung.

Bullae are larger air spaces in the parenchyma of the lung (> than 1 cm in diameter) that are associated with destruction. A bulla denotes severe, localized emphysema causing the formation of a large air space. Bullae may occur with several different types of emphysema and are common in patients with chronic obstructive bronchitis and emphysema. Individuals without any generalized obstructive airways disorder and without diffuse emphysema may also develop bullae.

Bullae are commonly located in the apices of the lungs and are often multiple. A lack of an endothelial lining distinguishes bullae from cysts. Moreover, on the chest radiograph, bullae have "hairline" (thin) margins and, unlike cysts, are usually irregularly shaped, are frequently trabeculated, and rarely contain fluid.

When they become large enough to compromise the function of the remaining normal lung and cause shortness of breath, bullae are clinically important. However, like blebs, when small, they are of little significance, unless they rupture and lead to a pneumothorax.

A difficult clinical problem may be to ascertain whether dyspnea is secondary to diffuse emphysema of the lungs or to bullae (observed on the chest radiograph). Surgery may be indicated in the latter case, but it is contraindicated in the former. Ventilation-perfusion radionuclide lung scans, computed tomography (CT) scans, and pulmonary angiograms may be necessary to make this distinction and to evaluate the state of the remaining lung. As a rule, unless associated generalized obstructive airways disease is present, bullae that occupy less than half a hemithorax do not cause severe dyspnea and significant functional impairment. Moreover, when diffuse disease is present, severe slowing of expiratory airflow is unusual, even with very large bullae. An ideal surgical candidate has moderate to severe dyspnea, bullae that fill most of a hemithorax, only mild slowing of flow rates on forced expiration, good perfusion of normal remaining lung on lung scan and pulmonary angiogram, and no evidence of significant emphysema (e.g., the diffusing capacity measurement is normal or only moderately reduced, and lung compliance studies are normal).

The diagnosis is usually made on the basis of the chest radiograph; however, on physical examination, a tympanitic percussion sound and reduced breath sounds may be noted over very large bullae. The radiolucency of a very large bulla on the chest film may be mistaken for a pneumothorax.

BRONCHOGENIC CYSTS. Bronchogenic cysts may occur in the mediastinum or within the lung parenchyma. These congenital malformations can be differentiated from bullae by their epithelial lining. On the chest radiograph, mediastinal cysts are seen as masses in the hilar, the paraesophageal or paratracheal, and, most commonly, the subcarinal region. In the parenchyma, these cysts are most often found in the lower lobes and are usually filled with a proteinaceous material, unless they become infected and communicate with the bronchial tree. They may have thin, even paper-thin, walls. During early development, acquired lung cysts often have relatively thick walls; later even those resulting from lung abscesses may have very thin walls that simulate those of bullae.

Large cysts may cause respiratory symptoms in young children, but adults with these large lesions are usually asymptomatic, and the abnormality tends to be an incidental finding on the chest radiograph. In the differential diagnosis, mediastinal cysts must be distinguished from other mediastinal masses. Lung cysts must be differentiated from acute lung abscesses, cavitated carcinomas, and cystic bronchiectasis. Frequently, thoracotomy and resection of the lesion are required to obtain a specific diagnosis, although chest CT combined with needle aspiration has been useful for diagnosis and drainage.

Only when they have a bronchial connection (communication) do bronchogenic cysts manifest as abnormalities in lung aeration. Although often partially filled with fluid, they may appear as air spaces when there is a bronchial communication. Infection in

fluid-filled cysts is unusual, but if it occurs and does not resolve after a course of antibiotics, the cysts may have to be removed surgically. Cysts containing air can often be distinguished from bullae by their regular outline, lack of trabeculation, and the presence of a fluid level. Distinguishing bronchogenic cysts in the lung from thin-walled cavities secondary to granulomatous infections, prior abscesses, previous pulmonary infarcts, and squamous cell carcinomas may be more difficult.

BRONCHOPULMONARY SEQUESTRATION. In *bronchopulmonary sequestrations* of the intralobular type, cystic lesions may be identified. This sequestration is caused by abnormal budding in the tracheobronchial tree of the early embryo. The involved area is found most often in the bases of the lungs posteriorly, and the affected lung region is nonfunctional. On the chest radiograph, involved areas are opaque.

Only when there is a bronchial communication do air-containing cysts develop, and in such situations secondary infection is the prime concern. These lesions are asymptomatic and are incidental findings on the chest radiograph unless infection develops. An aortogram that shows an abnormal vascular supply distinguishes a sequestration from a simple cyst. The arterial supply to some sequestrations arises at least partially from below the diaphragm. Surgical excision is the only treatment.

THE UNILATERAL HYPERLUCENT LUNG. Swyer-James (also called Macleod's) syndrome, a rare disorder, is generally discovered on the chest radiograph. Increased translucency of one hemithorax is noted because of diminished vascular markings in the lung on that side. On the inspiration chest radiograph, the affected lung is usually not hyperinflated. However, air trapping has been described, and an expiration chest radiograph may show hyperinflation of the affected lung relative to the other uninvolved lung and shift of the mediastinum to the unaffected side. Extensive bronchitis and bronchiolitis are usually noted on biopsy. These abnormalities likely date from childhood. In fact, in some children the condition develops 6 months to 5 years after viral bronchiolitis, and there is a history of some such occurrence in more than half of the patients. Dyspnea, a productive cough, and occasionally hemoptysis may occur.

At bronchoscopy, no obstruction of the main bronchi can be observed. But bronchography shows irregular dilatation of the bronchi to the fifth order, with failure to fill the peripheral airways, and an appearance characteristic of bronchiolar obliteration. Patency of the pulmonary artery on the angiogram differentiates Swyer-James syndrome from pulmonary artery stenosis or atresia. On the affected side, the lung scan shows reduced ventilation and perfusion. Pulmonary function test findings are variable and usually include some evidence of airways obstruction and an increase in residual volume, suggesting air trapping. Severe expiratory obstruction of airflow is uncommon.

Resection is not indicated, and treatment is usually limited to managing infection.

Allison RS, Chirnside AM: Pulmonary sequestration: A review of 12 cases. NZ Med J 596:381, 1983. *Well-written, complete coverage of the types, presentation, and management of pulmonary sequestration.*

Fraser RG, Paré JAP, Paré PD, et al.: Bullous disease of the lung. In Diagnosis of Diseases of the Chest. Vol. III. 3rd ed. Philadelphia, W. B. Saunders Company, 1990, p 2166. *In-depth review of blebs, bullae, and cysts, as well as the unilateral hyperlucent lung.*

Fraser RG, Paré JAP, Paré PD, et al.: Roentgenologic signs in the diagnosis of chest disease. In Diagnosis of Diseases of the Chest. Vol. I. 3rd ed. Philadelphia, W. B. Saunders Company, 1988, p 472. *Excellent overview of atelectasis.*

Murphy DMF, Fishman AP: Bullous disease of the lung. In Fishman AP (ed.): Pulmonary Diseases and Disorders. Vol. 2. 2nd ed. New York, McGraw-Hill Book Company, 1988, p 1219. *Detailed review of blebs, bullae, and cysts of the lung.*

Primrose WR: Spontaneous pneumothorax: A retrospective review of etiology, pathogenesis, and management. Scott Med J 29:15, 1984. *Succinct, up-to-date review of spontaneous pneumothorax.*

Proto AV, Tocino I.: Radiographic manifestations of lobar collapse. Semin Roentgenol 15:117, 1980. *A comprehensive, superb review of chest radiographic features of lobar collapse.*

Rodgers BM, Harman PK, Johnson AM: Bronchopulmonary foregut malformations—the spectrum of anomalies. Ann Surg 203:517, 1986. *A review of the various foregut malformations, including both bronchogenic cysts and sequestration, complete with ultrasound and CT images and a quality bibliography.*

Wagner RB, Johnston MR: Middle lobe syndrome. Ann Thorac Surg 35:679, 1983. *The etiology, pathophysiology, and therapy of this syndrome are up to date.*

60 Interstitial Lung Disease

Ronald G. Crystal

General Description

The interstitial lung diseases (ILD) are a heterogeneous group of diffuse inflammatory disorders of the lower respiratory tract. The term "interstitial lung disease" refers to the fact that the interstitium of the alveolar walls is thickened, usually by fibrosis. While this is true, the ILD are also characterized by derangements of the epithelial and endothelial cells of the alveolar walls and, in many cases, of the small airways and/or blood vessels of the lung parenchyma.

There are many disorders associated with ILD. In some, the ILD is the only manifestation; in others it is a part of a systemic disorder. The natural history of many of the ILD is one of slowly progressive loss of the functional alveolar-capillary units, often eventuating in respiratory insufficiency and death. Because of their insidious nature and the nonspecificity of the accompanying symptoms, such as dyspnea on exertion or a nonproductive cough, the ILD may go undiagnosed and untreated until large numbers of alveolar-capillary units become scarred and irrevocably lost.

These disorders are inflammatory diseases; the bulk of the damage to the lung parenchyma is caused by activated inflammatory cells that have accumulated in the alveolar structures. The diagnosis, staging, and treatment of the ILD require defining the character and intensity of the inflammation in the lung and the derangements of the alveolar structures caused by the inflammation.

Anatomy

The lower respiratory tract is composed of alveoli, grapelike units branching off the terminal bronchioles, and the vascular network of pulmonary arterioles, capillaries, and venules that bring blood to and from the lung (Fig. 60–1). The walls of the alveoli are lined by a single layer of epithelial cells resting on a thin, continuous basement membrane. Ninety-five per cent of the alveolar surface is covered by type I epithelial cells, with the remainder by type II epithelial cells, the cell that produces surfactant, the material that prevents alveolar collapse. Underneath the epithelial basement membrane is the alveolar interstitium, a region containing mesenchymal cells and supporting connective tissue matrix composed of collagen, elastic fibers, proteoglycans, and various glycoproteins. The pulmonary capillaries form a branching network of tubes lined by a single layer of endothelial cells resting on their own basement membrane. The capillaries weave through the interstitium in such a way that the capillary basement membrane often abuts the epithelial basement membrane beneath the type I epithelial cells. It is at these sites that air and blood are in closest approximation and where gas exchange takes place.

The normal alveolar wall is thin (5 to 10 μm wide) compared with the space occupied by air (200 to 300 μm). In the ILD, the walls are thickened several-fold and the space for air is correspondingly less. The derangements that accompany the thickening of the alveolar walls in the ILD can be conceptualized in two groups (Fig. 60–2). In the distortion form of derangement, typified by sarcoidosis and the early phases of hypersensitivity pneumonitis, the alveolar walls are deformed by the accumulation of inflammatory cells in the interstitium, altering the normal architecture. Because there is little injury to the normal structures, this form of derangement is often reversible if the process causing the distortion is eliminated. In the fibrosis form of derangement, typified by idiopathic pulmonary fibrosis and the inorganic dust disorders, the epithelial surface is often altered: Type I epithelial cells are lost, and the surface is repopulated with cuboidal cells derived from proliferating type II cells and bronchiolar cells migrating down from the terminal airways. Alveolar capillary endothelial cells are injured and lost. The interstitium is thickened with edema and proliferation of mesenchymal cells and accumulation of connective tissue products secreted by these cells, particularly collagen. The interstitium is scarred and fibrotic—hence the term "fibrotic lung disease" is also used to refer to these ILD. In the more aggressive forms of fibrosis-type derangements, there are breaks in the epithelial basement membrane through which the interstitial contents protrude; this condition often expands into intra-alveolar fibrotic masses called "intra-alveolar buds" that are eventually incorporated into the alveolar wall, expanding its mass. As the fibrotic form of ILD progresses, the alveolar-capillary units become less distinguishable, and the lung parenchyma takes on the appearance of "end-stage lung" characterized by masses of fibrotic tissue interspaced with cystic areas representing the remnants of alveoli and dilated terminal bronchioles.

Epidemiology

The epidemiology for most of the ILD is not carefully defined, but it is estimated that in the United States their prevalence is approximately 20 to 40 per 100,000 of the population. Conven-

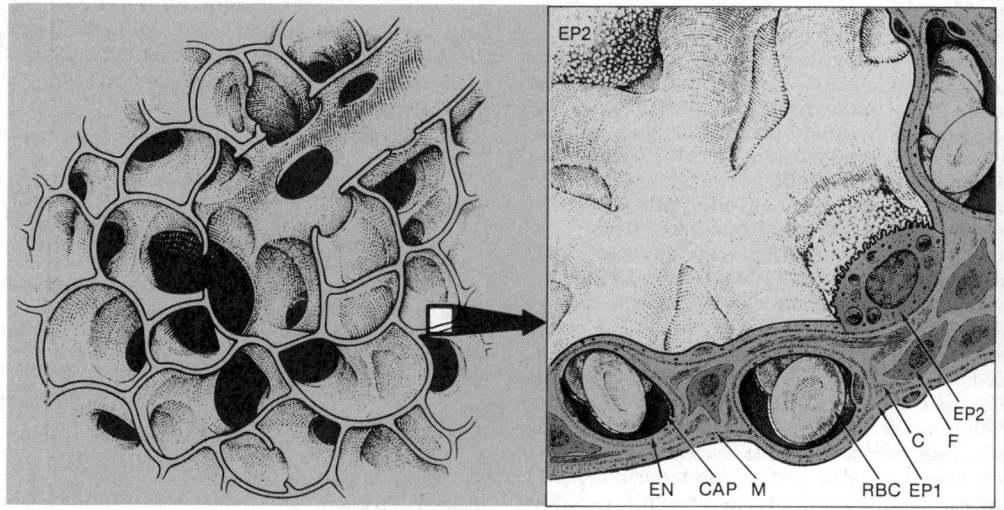

FIGURE 60–1. Structure of the normal lower respiratory tract. *Left,* Representation of a low-power view of the distal lung; the terminal bronchiole is shown but the pulmonary artery and vein are omitted. *Right,* Representation of a high-power view of an alveolus; the cut surface demonstrates the type I (EP1) and type II (EP2) epithelial cells, endothelial cells (EN), basement membranes (M), red blood cells (RBC) in the capillaries (CAP), fibroblasts (F; the most common form of mesenchymal cell in the interstitium), and connective tissue (C). Inflammatory cells are not shown. (From Crystal RG, Bitterman PB, Rennard SI, et al.: Interstitial lung diseases of unknown cause: Disorders characterized by chronic inflammation of the lower respiratory tract. N Engl J Med 310:154, 1984. Reprinted with permission of the New England Journal of Medicine.)

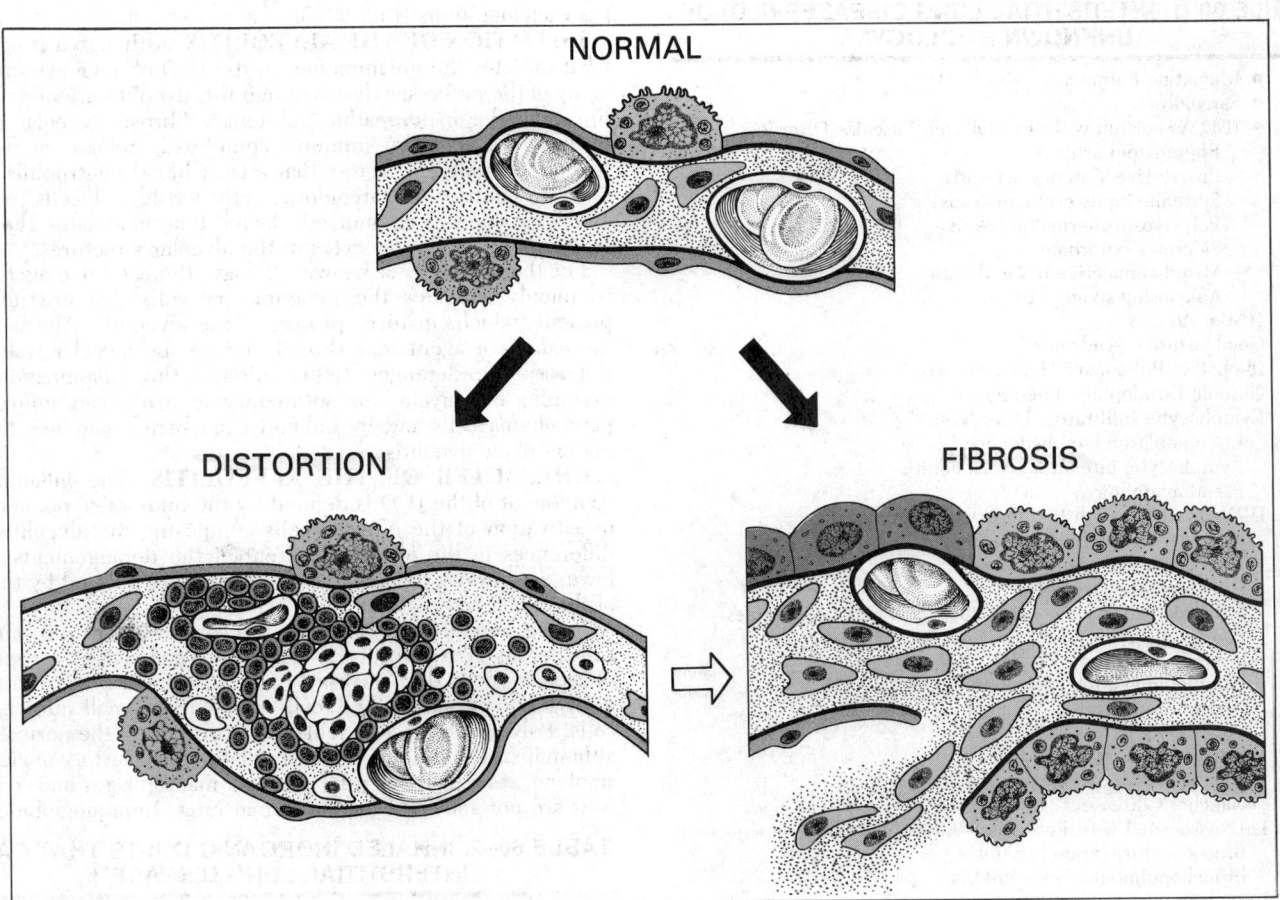

FIGURE 60–2. Typical forms of derangement of alveolar structures in the interstitial lung disorders. *Top,* Schematic of a cut surface of the normal alveolar wall. Shown are the type I and II epithelial cells, endothelial cells lining the capillaries, basement membranes, mesenchymal cells, and interstitial connective tissue. The few inflammatory cells normally present are not shown. *Lower left,* Schematic of a similar view of the alveolar wall deranged by the distortion caused by the accumulations of inflammatory cells. The example used is that of sarcoidosis, in which T cells (primarily CD4+ cells) (pale red) macrophages (white), and granulomas (massed accumulation of macrophages) distort the normal alveolar walls. *Lower right,* Schematic of a similar view of the alveolar wall deranged by fibrosis. The example used is that of idiopathic pulmonary fibrosis. In contrast to the distortion type of derangement, in which there is little damage and change in the lung parenchyma, in the fibrotic form of derangement the type I cells are injured, leaving denuded basement membrane. In some areas, the interstitial contents protrude into the air space, causing intra-alveolar fibrosis. Note that some of the injured type I cells have been replaced by the type II cells and bronchiolar cells that have migrated down from the airways. Capillaries are injured; the basement membranes are thickened; there are expanded numbers of mesenchymal cells; and the density of connective tissue is increased. In the fibrotic type of derangement, there are also large numbers of inflammatory cells distorting the alveolar wall (not shown). In some cases of the distortion kind of derangement, there is sufficient damage to the parenchymal components that the derangements shift into a more fibrotic-type situation.

tionally, the ILD are categorized as those of unknown and known etiology. ILD of known etiology have more subcategories than do ILD of unknown etiology; however, in terms of total numbers of patients, the ILD of unknown etiology predominate. The most common ILD of unknown etiology (Table 60–1) are idiopathic pulmonary fibrosis (IPF), chronic ILD associated with the collagen vascular disorders, and sarcoidosis. Much less common are histiocytosis X, Goodpasture's syndrome, chronic eosinophilic pneumonia, idiopathic pulmonary hemosiderosis, and the ILD associated with the pulmonary vasculitides. The other ILD of unknown etiology are very rare, with fewer than 1000 cases of each reported in the world literature.

The ILD of known etiology are most commonly due to the inhalation of inorganic dusts, particularly crystalline silica, asbestos, and coal dust (Table 60–2), the hypersensitivity pneumonitides (diseases caused by the repeated inhalation of organic dust; Table 60–3), and the drug-induced ILD (Table 60–4). Much less frequent are the ILD resulting from paraquat, radiation, the sequelae of known infectious agents, and the inhalation of gases, aerosols, chemical dusts, fumes, and vapors (Table 60–5). Occasionally, however, large populations develop ILD when exposed to a single agent at one time, such as occurred in Bhopal, India, in 1984 when methyl isocyanate was released into a crowded urban area.

Differential Diagnosis

The initial problem in assessing ILD is to differentiate it from other disorders that may also present with symptoms of respiratory deficiency and diffuse infiltrates on the chest radiograph (Table 60–6). In general, pulmonary edema, high-flow states, hemorrhage, and aspiration pneumonitis can be easily differentiated from the ILD by history and physical examination. The major problem is in ensuring that the patient does not have an infection or malignancy, diagnoses that require an appropriate evaluation of specimens from the lower respiratory tract for the presence of infectious agents or malignant cells, respectively. In some cases, such as opportunistic organisms associated with human immunodeficiency virus (HIV) infection or with filarial infestation, serologic studies are also necessary.

The diagnosis of a specific ILD is made by a combination of historical, physical examination, blood, urine, roentgenographic, physiologic, scintigraphic, and bronchoscopic criteria. In addi-

TABLE 60–1. INTERSTITIAL LUNG DISEASES (ILD) OF UNKNOWN ETIOLOGY*

- Idiopathic Pulmonary Fibrosis (IPF)
- Sarcoidosis
- ILD Associated with the Collagen Vascular Disorders
  Rheumatoid arthritis
  Progressive systemic sclerosis
  Systemic lupus erythematosus
  Polymyositis/dermatomyositis
  Sjögren's syndrome
  Mixed connective tissue disease
  Ankylosing spondylitis

Histiocytosis X
Goodpasture's Syndrome
Idiopathic Pulmonary Hemosiderosis
Chronic Eosinophilic Pneumonia
Lymphocytic Infiltrative Disorders
  Immunoblastic lymphadenopathy
  Lymphocytic interstitial pneumonitis
  Pseudolymphoma
ILD Associated with Pulmonary Vasculitides
  Wegener's granulomatosis
  Lymphomatoid granulomatosis
  Churg-Strauss syndrome
  Systemic necrotizing vasculitides ("overlap" vasculitides)
  Hypersensitivity vasculitis
Inherited Disorders
  Familial idiopathic pulmonary fibrosis
  Neurofibromatosis
  Tuberous sclerosis
  Hermansky-Pudlak syndrome
  Niemann-Pick disease
  Gaucher's disease
ILD Associated with Pulmonary Airway Disease
  Bronchocentric granulomatosis
  Bronchopulmonary aspergillosis
Lymphangioleiomyomatosis
Alveolar Proteinosis
ILD Associated with Liver Disease
  Chronic active hepatitis
  Primary biliary cirrhosis
ILD Associated with Bowel Disease
  Whipple's disease
  Ulcerative colitis
  Crohn's disease
Weber-Christian Disease
Amyloidosis
Hypereosinophilic Syndrome
Pulmonary Veno-occlusive Disease
ILD Caused by Failure of Other Organs
  Chronic left ventricular failure
  Chronic left-to-right intracardiac shunt
  Chronic renal disease with uremia
Graft-vs.-Host Disease
Recovery Phase of Adult Respiratory
  Distress Syndrome

*Disorders indicated with "●" are the most common ILD of unknown etiology.

tion, unless an agent of known etiology is apparent (e.g., long-term asbestos exposure), it is mandatory to evaluate the disease by morphologic means, usually by open lung biopsy. The only exception to this rule is when the ILD is in clear association with a systemic disorder (e.g., a collagen vascular disease, Goodpasture's syndrome) in which the diagnosis can be made by evaluation of organs other than the lung.

Pathogenesis

The ILD are inflammatory disorders in which most of the derangements of the alveolar walls, including the fibrosis, are mediated by inflammatory/immune cells that have accumulated in the lung parenchyma. The inflammation, usually referred to as the "alveolitis" of the disease, not only involves the alveoli but often involves the walls of small airways and sometimes the pulmonary blood vessels. The critical importance of the alveolitis is simply stated: Although dysfunction of the alveolar-capillary units causes the symptoms and impairment of the patient, it is the alveolitis that causes the derangements of the alveolar-capillary units, resulting in their dysfunction and eventual loss as gas exchange units (Fig. 60–3).

INITIATION OF THE ALVEOLITIS. Although it is not clear what initiates the inflammation in the ILD of unknown etiology, many of the processes that maintain the alveolitis are understood. For example, in idiopathic pulmonary fibrosis, alveolar macrophages, activated by immune complexes, release neutrophil-specific chemotactic factors that attract blood neutrophils to the lung. In contrast, in sarcoidosis, activated lung T cells release a monocyte-specific chemotactic factor that modulates the accumulation of blood monocytes in the alveolar structures.

For the disorders of known etiology, the causative agent most commonly activates the inflammatory cells that are normally present, which, in turn, propagate the alveolitis. Alternatively, the causative agent may directly injure the alveolar walls, and the resulting deranged tissue initiates the inflammation. For example, bleomycin, an antineoplastic drug, can injure lung parenchyma cells and by unknown mechanisms induce the formation of an alveolitis.

CHARACTER OF THE ALVEOLITIS. The inflammatory component of the ILD is defined by the number, type, and state of activation of the effector cells composing the alveolitis. The differences in the form and extent of the derangements to the lower respiratory tract in these disorders are defined by the sum of these characteristics.

In the normal lung there are approximately 80 inflammatory cells per alveolus. Most (>80 per cent) are alveolar macrophages, phagocytic cells derived from blood monocytes. The remainder are lymphocytes, mostly T cells, but with a small number of B cells. Polymorphonuclear leukocytes are rare in the normal lung, although small numbers do accumulate with a history of cigarette smoking. As a general rule, alveolar macrophages and T and B cells are not activated in the normal lung. Immunoglobulins are

TABLE 60–2. INHALED INORGANIC DUSTS THAT CAUSE INTERSTITIAL LUNG DISEASE*†

Silica (variants of SiO_2)
- Crystalline silica ("silicosis")
  Amorphous
Silicates
- Asbestos ("asbestosis")
  Talc (hydrated Mg silicates; "talcosis")
  Kaolin (china clay, hydrated aluminum silicate)
  Diatomaceous earth (Fuller's earth, aluminum silicate with Fe and Mg)
  Nepheline (hard rock containing mixed silicates)
  Aluminum silicates (sericite, sillimanite, zeolite)
  Portland cement
  Mica (principally K and Mg aluminum silicates)
Carbon (with or without crystalline silica)
- Coal dust ("coal worker's pneumoconiosis")
  Graphite ("carbon pneumoconiosis")
Metals
  Beryllium ("berylliosis" or "chronic beryllium disease")
  Aluminum ("aluminosis")
    Powdered aluminum ("aluminum lung")
    Bauxite (aluminum oxide; "Shaver's disease")
  Barium (powder of baryte or $BaSO_4$; "baritosis")
  Iron ("siderosis")
  Tin ("stannosis")
  Antimony (oxides and alloys)
  Mixed dusts
    Hematite (mixed dusts of iron oxide, silica, and silicates; "siderosilicosis")
    Mixed dusts of silver and iron oxide ("argyrosiderosis")
  Hard metals
    Titanium oxide
    Tungsten, titanium, hafnium, niobium, cobalt, and vanadium carbides
    Cadmium
Rare earths (cerium, scandium, yttrium, lanthanum)
$CuSO_4$ neutralized with hydrated lime (Bordeaux mixture; "vineyard sprayer's lung")

*The most common inorganic dust–induced interstitial lung diseases are indicated with "●."
†Disorders given a specific name are indicated in quotes in parentheses; others are referred as "(name of the dust) pneumoconiosis."

TABLE 60–3. INHALED ORGANIC DUSTS THAT CAUSE INTERSTITIAL LUNG DISEASE*

Disorder	Causative Agent†
● Farmer's lung	*M. faeni, T. vulgaris, A. fumigatus, T. candidus*
● Humidifier lung, air conditioner lung	*T. vulgaris, T. candidus*, thermotolerant bacteria, protozoa, *Penicillium* species, *Naegleria gruberi*
● Bird breeder's disease‡	Avian proteins, feathers
Maple bark stripper's lung	*Cryptostroma corticale*
Cheese worker's lung	*A. clavatus, Penicillium caseii*
Malt worker's lung	*A. clavatus, A. fumigatus*
Sequoiosis	*Aureobasidium pullulans, Graphium* species
Paprika splitter's lung	*Mucor stolonifer*
Wheat weevil disease	*Sitophilus granarius*
Suberosis	*Penicillium frequentans*
Bagassosis	*T. sacchari*
Mushroom worker's lung	*M. faeni, T. vulgaris*
Pituitary snuff lung	Porcine and bovine proteins
Wood-pulp worker's disease	*Alternaria* species
Sauna-taker's disease	*Aureobasidium* species
Detergent worker's lung	*Bacillus subtilis*
Lycoperdonosis	*Lycoperdon bovista*
Rodent handler's disease	Serum and urine constituents
Dry rot disease	*Merulius lacrymans*
Wood-dust worker's lung	Unknown
Furrier's lung	Unknown
New Guinea lung	*Saccharomonospora irridis*
Coptic disease (mummy unwrapper's disease)	Antigens associated with mummy wrappings
"Summer-type" disease	*Cryptococcus neoformans*
	Cephalosporium species§
	Streptomyces albus§
	Bacillus subtilis§

*The most common interstitial lung disorders caused by inhaled organic antigens are indicated with "●."
†M. = *Micropolyspora*; T. = *Thermoactinomyces*; A. = *Aspergillus*.
‡Includes pigeons, parakeets, budgerigars, turkeys, chickens, and ducks.
§Hypersensitivity pneumonitis has been described in association with these agents, in circumstances in which no common name has been given to the disorder.

present in the normal lower respiratory tract (IgG > IgA >> IgM), as are some complement components. Macromolecules that defend against inflammatory injury, including antiproteases and antioxidants, are also present.

Active, untreated ILD are generally characterized by a marked increase in the number of inflammatory cells in the alveolar walls and on the alveolar epithelial surface. Commonly, this increase in numbers of effector cells is also characterized by a shift in

TABLE 60–4. DRUGS THAT CAUSE INTERSTITIAL LUNG DISEASE

Antineoplastic Agents
Azathioprine
Bleomycin
Cyclophosphamide
Methotrexate
Nitrosoureas
  Carmustine (BCNU)
  Lomustine (CCNU)
  Semustine (methyl-CCNU)
  Chlorozotocin (DCNU)
Melphalan
Busulfan
Chlorambucil
6-Mercaptopurine
6-Thioguanine
Mitomycin C
Procarbazine
Uracil mustard
Zinostatin

Antibiotics
Nitrofurantoin
Penicillins
Sulfonamides
Erythromycin
Tetracycline
Isoniazid
para-Aminosalicylic acid
Niridazole

Cardiovascular Drugs
Hydralazine
Procainamide
Beta blockers (propranolol, practolol, pindolol, acebutolol)
Tocainide
Amiodarone
Reserpine

Central Nervous System Drugs
Phenytoin
Carbamazepine
Chlorpromazine
Imipramine
Amitriptyline
Methylphenidate
Dantrolene
Mephenesin

Ganglionic Blocking Agents
Mecamylamine
Hexamethonium
Pentolinium

Anti-Inflammatory Agents
Gold salts
Phenylbutazone
Beclomethasone
Naproxen

Oral Hypoglycemic Agents
Chlorpropamide
Tolbutamide
Tolazamide

Miscellaneous
Penicillamine
Allopurinol
Cromolyn sodium
Hydrochlorothiazide
Mineral oil
Intravenous drugs containing particulate material
Silicone used for tissue augmentation

TABLE 60–5. OTHER AGENTS KNOWN TO CAUSE INTERSTITIAL LUNG DISEASE

Paraquat
Radiation
Sequelae of Known Infectious Agents
  Bacteria   *Mycoplasma*
  Mycobacteria   *Legionella pneumophila*
  Fungi   Parasites
  Viruses
Inhaled Agents Other Than Inorganic or Organic Dusts
  Gases
    Oxygen   Sulfur dioxide
    Oxides of nitrogen   Methyl isocyanate
    Chlorine gas
  Aerosols
    Aspiration pneumonia   Pyrethrum (a natural
    Fats   insecticide)
    Oils   Toluene diisocyanate
  Chemical dusts
    Synthetic fibers (Orlon, polyesters, nylon, acrylic)
    Bakelite
    Vinyl chloride, polyvinyl chloride powder
  Fumes
    Oxides of Zn, Cu, Mn, Cd, Fe, Mg, Ni, Se, Sn, Sb, V, and brass
    Diphenylmethane diisocyanate
    Trimellitic anhydride
  Vapors
    Hydrocarbons
    Mercury
    Thermosetting resins

their relative proportions. Different patterns of alveolitis are generally referred to by the cell types that are most abundant. For example, when the inflammation is dominated by neutrophils and macrophages, it is referred to as a neutrophil-macrophage alveolitis. The alveolitis patterns most frequently observed in ILD are a macrophage-dominant alveolitis, a lymphocyte-macrophage alveolitis, and a neutrophil-macrophage alveolitis. Eosinophils play a role in the alveolitis of many ILD but rarely dominate it. Subcategories of the common alveolitis patterns have also been described. For example, the granulomatous lung disorders, sarcoidosis and berylliosis, are characterized by a CD4+ T-helper cell–macrophage alveolitis, while chronic hypersensitivity pneumonitis is usually characterized by a CD8+ T-suppressor/cytotoxic cell–macrophage alveolitis, sometimes including neutrophils.

In addition to the numbers and types of inflammatory cells

TABLE 60–6. DISORDERS INVOLVING THE LOWER RESPIRATORY TRACT THAT CAN BE CONFUSED WITH INTERSTITIAL LUNG DISEASE*

Pulmonary Edema
Neoplasms
  ● Leukemic infiltration
  ● Lymphoma
  ● Lymphangitic spread of carcinoma
  Multiple metastases
  Primary pulmonary malignancy
Infections
  ● Viruses†
  Fungi
  Bacteria‡
  ● Mycobacteria
  ● Parasites§
  ● *Mycoplasma*
  Psittacosis
  Q fever
  ● *Pneumocystis carinii*
Pulmonary Hemorrhage
Aspiration

*Disorders frequently confused with the ILD are indicated with "●."
†Of the viruses known to involve the lung—influenza, cytomegalovirus (CMV), varicella zoster, measles, and HIV are most commonly confused with ILD.
‡Particularly *Legionella*.
§*Pneumocystis* and filarial disease are commonly mistaken for ILD.

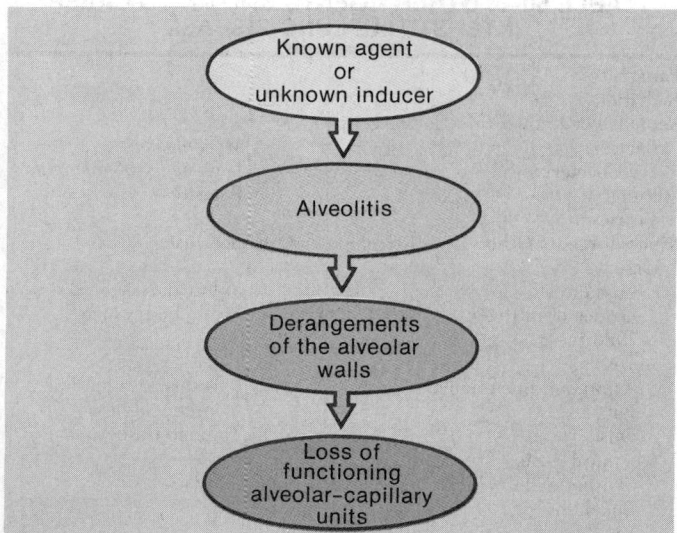

FIGURE 60–3. Pathogenesis of the interstitial lung diseases of unknown and known etiology. In both groups, the inflammation (alveolitis) is responsible for the bulk of the derangements of the alveolar walls. In some disorders, the deranged wall components may accelerate the alveolitis by recruiting additional inflammatory cells. In the disorders of known etiology, the causative agent may directly damage the alveolar structures, which, in turn. initiates and/or accelerates the alveolitis.

present, the consequences of the alveolitis critically depend on the state of activation of these cells. The simple presence of the inflammatory cells in the alveolar structures distorts the alveolar walls but usually is not damaging. When activated, however, some inflammatory cells can injure the alveolar walls, particularly sensitive type I epithelial cells and capillary endothelial cells. If the alveolitis is self-limiting, or if it is suppressed by therapy before the injury becomes too severe, the architecture of the lower respiratory tract can be re-established and normal lung function restored. If, however, the injury is extensive, with mesenchymal cell proliferation and collagen deposition, the normal architecture of the affected alveolar-capillary units can never be fully re-established. Therapeutic success in treating ILD means suppression of the alveolitis and thus prevention of further loss of alveolar-capillary units.

DISTORTION AND FIBROSIS. Whether the derangements of the alveolar walls take the form of distortion and/or fibrosis is dictated by the characteristics of the alveolitis. It is important to recognize that while the distortion type of derangement is usually reversible if the inflammation is suppressed, the consequences of the fibrosis form of derangement are commonly sufficient to prevent a return to the normal architecture.

Accumulation of sufficient numbers of any type of inflammatory cells results in some distortion of the tissue. However, this form of derangement is most significant when the inflammation involves lymphocytes and macrophages, such as when there is an accumulation of activated CD4+ T-helper cells that direct the formation of granuloma. Together, the T cells and masses of macrophages distort the normal architecture but usually do not cause permanent damage.

The fibrosis form of derangement is characterized by injury to parenchymal components, together with the accumulation of mesenchymal cells and their secreted connective tissue products. The neutrophil is the most damaging of all inflammatory cells by virtue of its highly reactive oxygen metabolites that are toxic to the parenchymal cells and its connective tissue–specific proteases that can damage the interstitial collagens and basement membranes. Injury to the epithelial basement membrane has profound consequences because the epithelial cells no longer have a surface upon which to migrate, making it impossible to reconstruct a normal alveolar surface. The eosinophil can also injure lung parenchymal cells and connective tissue, but on a per cell basis it is less potent than the neutrophil. Activated human alveolar macrophages release toxic oxidants and thus can be cytotoxic to

normal lung parenchymal cells. The macrophage also mediates the accumulation of mesenchymal cells and the connective tissue that characterizes the fibrosis type of derangement of the alveolar walls. The fundamental problem is the accumulation of mesenchymal cells in the alveolar walls. Since mesenchymal cells are major producers of collagen, the consequence of an increase in mesenchymal cell numbers is an accumulation of collagen in the alveolar interstitium. As a result, the alveolar wall is thickened and scarred and has decreased compliance. The macrophage mediates the accumulation of mesenchymal cells by releasing exaggerated amounts of at least three mediators, platelet-derived growth factor, fibronectin, and a form of insulin-like growth factor 1 (also called "alveolar macrophage–derived growth factor"). Platelet-derived growth factor, a product of the *c-sis* oncogene, attracts mesenchymal cells and is a potent stimulus for mesenchymal cells to begin traversing the cell cycle. Fibronectin, a 440,000-dalton glycoprotein, attracts mesenchymal cells, attaches them to the extracellular matrix, and stimulates them to enter the cell cycle. The alveolar macrophage form of insulin-like growth factor 1, an 18,000-dalton protein, induces the platelet-derived growth factor or fibronectin-primed mesenchymal cells to continue through the cell cycle and proliferate.

Clinical Features

HISTORY. Occasional patients are detected as having ILD because a routine chest radiograph is noted to be abnormal, but most come to medical attention because of symptoms related to the chest. All ILD are characterized by abnormalities in the transfer of oxygen from air to blood secondary to slowly progressive derangement of the lower respiratory tract. The initial symptoms are those of insufficient oxygen transfer, such as *fatigue* and *breathlessness with exertion*. These symptoms are often initially denied by the patient or are attributed to being "out of shape" or "overweight" or to a prior chest infection, usually a viral syndrome. As the disease progresses, the dyspnea becomes more apparent and eventually is felt when the patient is at rest. In contrast to cardiac-induced dyspnea, paroxysmal nocturnal dyspnea and orthopnea are rare, as are platypnea and trepopnea. Nonproductive cough, pleuritic pain, and hemoptysis are less common presenting complaints. Early in the disease, chest pain is rare, although later, when pulmonary hypertension develops, substernal discomfort may be noted.

The history also plays an important role in the diagnosis of the type of interstitial disease. Since a large number of agents cause ILD, a careful exposure history is essential to determine not only the agents to which the patient has been exposed but also the circumstances, intensity, and duration of exposure. Exposure to agents that cause ILD may be found in nonclassic situations. For example, silicosis has been described in workers involved in the manufacture of pencils, furniture, and tombstones; talcosis in the manufacture of rubber condoms; and hypersensitivity pneumonitis in office buildings where the offending organic antigen was located in the air conditioning system.

The lack of a history of exposure to a known agent that causes interstitial disease is very important in diagnosing the ILD of unknown etiology. For example, pulmonary sarcoidosis is very difficult to distinguish from berylliosis unless there is a negative history of beryllium exposure. Similarly, idiopathic pulmonary fibrosis is difficult to diagnose if an exposure history is unavailable or if there is a clear history of sufficient exposure to one or more agents that cause ILD. Some ILD of unknown etiology are associated with diseases that often involve other organs, such as the collagen vascular disorders, primary biliary cirrhosis, and Wegener's granulomatosis, which may be suspected from the history.

PHYSICAL EXAMINATION. The chest expansion is typically reduced, reflecting the reduced total lung capacity of individuals with ILD. Most have fine, crackling inspiratory and expiratory rales, heard best at the posterior lung bases. These rales have a characteristic sound, described as "Velcro-like" (i.e., the sound of unwrapping a blood pressure cuff) or like the sound of rubbing hair together. Coarse rales, wheezing, and rhonchi are occasionally heard. As the disease progresses, these patients may be tachypneic at rest, but unlike individuals with emphysema, they do not use the accessory muscles of respiration and do not assume the posture of placing their hands on their thighs to "fix" the upper body to assist in respiration.

Early in the disease, examination of the heart is normal. Later, an accentuated P_2 reflects mild pulmonary hypertension. Eventually, obvious evidence of pulmonary hypertension is noted, including a right ventricular heave. Patients with ILD rarely develop frank right-sided failure with liver enlargement and peripheral edema, presumably because they die of the complications of insufficient oxygen delivery before the right ventricle deteriorates.

Clubbing of the fingers and sometimes the toes is common in ILD, particularly in idiopathic pulmonary fibrosis and asbestosis. Cyanosis occurs, but usually very late in the disease. Other physical findings in ILD are those associated with problems with oxygen transport (e.g., left ventricular failure, central nervous system signs) and those characteristic of associated diseases (e.g., the rash of systemic lupus erythematosus, the skin changes of scleroderma).

LABORATORY STUDIES. No blood test is diagnostic for one ILD, and the intensity and character of the alveolitis are not reflected in the blood. The hemoglobin and hematocrit are usually normal despite associated hypoxemia, and the white blood cell count and differential usually bear no relationship to the alveolitis. In most ILD, the sedimentation rate is elevated.

A patient with suspected ILD should have routine blood screening tests for hematologic, liver, renal, and muscle abnormalities and collagen vascular disorders. Screening for HIV infection is mandatory, as some opportunistic infections associated with the HIV-positive state can mimic ILD, and the pulmonary inflammation associated with HIV infection can cause ILD. Other blood tests directed toward specific diseases may be ordered as the workup proceeds and the specific disease is suspected. For example, serologic tests for antibodies against organic antigens are ordered only in the context of suspected hypersensitivity pneumonitis and anti–basement membrane antibodies only when Goodpasture's syndrome is suspected.

Rheumatoid factor and antinuclear antibodies are occasionally present in low titer and do not necessarily indicate the presence of an underlying collagen vascular disorder. Plasma immunoglobulins may be elevated, but this finding is usually nonspecific. Except in those circumstances in which the disease is systemic (e.g., sarcoidosis, a collagen vascular disorder), other screening blood studies are generally normal.

The electrocardiogram (ECG) is usually normal in ILD except for evidence of pulmonary hypertension. As the loss of alveolar-capillary units progresses, the ECG demonstrates a pattern of right atrial and ventricular strain. The hypoxemia of ILD may exacerbate coexisting coronary heart disease, evoking arrhythmias and evidence of coronary insufficiency, particularly with exercise.

RADIOGRAPHIC STUDIES. The posteroanterior and lateral chest films have a major role in establishing the diagnosis of ILD, although 5 to 10 per cent of patients with biopsy-proven disease have a normal chest film. A ground-glass pattern may be seen early in the disease. More typically, the chest radiograph demonstrates a diffuse, finely nodular, reticular, or reticulonodular pattern usually more prominent at the bases (Fig. 60–4). As the disease evolves, the pattern becomes coarser, with cystic areas appearing and, finally, a honeycomb pattern. Initially the pulmonary arteries appear normal, but in the later stages of ILD, evidence of pulmonary hypertension may be present.

A definitive diagnosis of a specific ILD can never be made by the chest radiograph alone. However, certain radiographic patterns are typical of specific diseases or groups of diseases and thus are very helpful in establishing a diagnosis. For example, some ILD are also characterized by hilar and/or paratracheal lymph node enlargement, while others manifest pleural disease.

Except for rare circumstances, radiographic studies other than the routine chest film have little use in the evaluation of ILD. Oblique films, tomography, bronchography, and angiography are occasionally used to evaluate localized lesions on a background of ILD but usually are difficult to interpret. Computed tomographic (CT) scans of the chest are routinely used in the evaluation of those patients in whom questionable hilar or pleural lesions are being evaluated. CT scans are being evaluated for use in assessing the extent of parenchymal changes, but standard criteria for abnormalities are not yet established.

PULMONARY FUNCTION TESTS. The classic physiologic alterations in ILD include reduced lung volumes (vital capacity, total lung capacity), reduced diffusing capacity, and a normal or

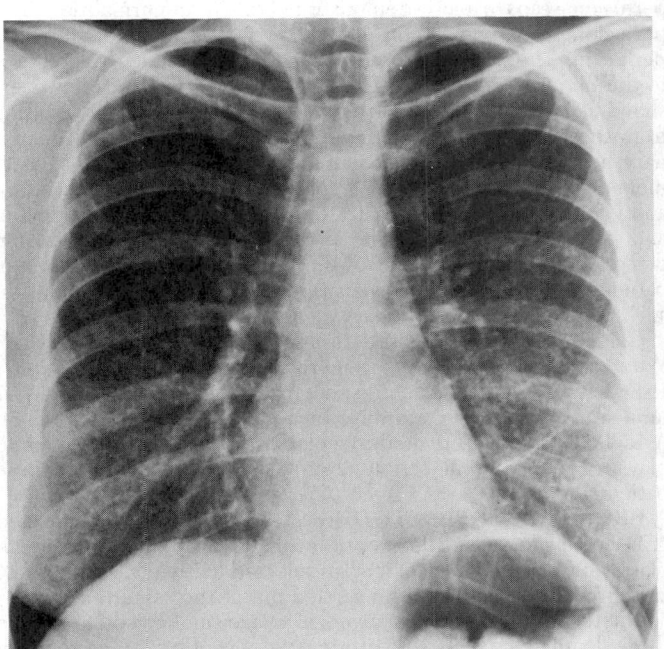

FIGURE 60–4. Chest radiograph of a patient with idiopathic pulmonary fibrosis, typical of the radiographic findings of many interstitial lung diseases. There is a diffuse reticulonodular infiltrate throughout the lung fields, most prominent at the bases. The heart and pleura are normal.

supranormal ratio of forced expiratory volume in 1 second to forced vital capacity. In some ILD, sensitive tests such as flow-volume curves and maximal flow-static recoil curves can detect mild limitation of airflow. Measurement of static lung compliance demonstrates decreased lung volumes for a given transpulmonary pressure, and an increased maximal transpulmonary pressure, i.e., very high negative pressures (relative to the atmosphere), must be generated to open the fibrotic alveoli.

Arterial blood gases typically show mild hypoxemia; carbon dioxide retention is rare, even late in the course of the disease. Patients with ILD tend to hyperventilate and have a reduced PCO_2 and compensated respiratory alkalosis, mostly as a result of an increase in respiratory rate. The drive to hyperventilate is not due to hypoxemia or abnormalities in acid-base status but rather to the subjective sense of dyspnea or to an increased stimulation of the respiratory center from neural signals arising in the deranged lung parenchyma. With exercise, the arterial PO_2 drops, while the PCO_2 remains constant. The loss of alveolar-capillary bed in ILD and hence the limitation of cardiac output seriously impair oxygen delivery and thereby markedly limit the exercise tolerance of these patients. This leads to their propensity to suffer hypoxic damage to vital organs. The arterial pH is usually normal in ILD, but it can fall with exercise as a consequence of oxygen deprivation of muscles, which then resort to anaerobic metabolism.

At rest, the hypoxemia of ILD results from abnormal matching of pulmonary ventilation and perfusion. With exercise, however, an apparent "diffusion block" also contributes. It was originally thought that this block resulted from a limited oxygen diffusion through the thickened alveolar walls, but it is now recognized to be due to red blood cells passing through the functioning pulmonary capillaries too rapidly to permit full saturation of hemoglobin. In rare instances, some of the hypoxemia of ILD results from shunts, either in the lung parenchyma or through a patent foramen ovale in the setting of pulmonary hypertension.

The loss of pulmonary capillary bed in ILD is associated with pulmonary hypertension, first with exercise only and later at rest. The pulmonary hypertension is thought to result from mechanical reasons (e.g., the loss of pulmonary capillary bed) and not from hypoxia-induced vasoconstriction or from local mediators. Right ventricular end-diastolic pressure rises late in the disease, but this rarely leads to frank right-sided failure.

SCINTIGRAPHIC STUDIES. Conventional ventilation and

perfusion scans usually demonstrate diffuse abnormalities. The perfusion scans show multiple subsegmental areas of impaired perfusion. The normal, upright individual has limited blood flow to the upper lobes at rest. The perfusion scan in ILD, however, shows a redistribution of perfusion to the upper lobes, resulting from the loss of pulmonary capillary bed and developing pulmonary hypertension. The ventilation scan shows multiple subsegmental areas of reduced ventilation. Comparison of the perfusion and ventilation scans demonstrates numerous areas of ventilation and perfusion mismatch. The presence of numerous perfusion defects limits the usefulness of these techniques in evaluation of patients with ILD who have suspected pulmonary emboli. In such circumstances, pulmonary angiography is mandatory.

Gallium-67 scans are used to evaluate the alveolitis of ILD. Whereas the normal lung parenchyma takes up little gallium-67, ILD with an active alveolitis demonstrate positive gallium-67 lung scans with either a diffuse or a patchy pattern (Fig. 60–5). A high density of activated alveolar macrophages is thought to play a major role in the lung uptake of gallium-67 in these patients.

BRONCHOSCOPIC STUDIES. Most patients with suspected ILD are evaluated by fiberoptic bronchoscopy to rule out neoplastic or infectious disease. In selected patients (see below), transbronchial biopsy can be carried out at the same time.

The technique of bronchoalveolar lavage can be used to sample the inflammatory cells constituting the alveolitis. To accomplish this, the bronchoscope is wedged into a distal bronchus, and aliquots of sterile saline are used to recover the inflammatory cells and epithelial lining fluid of the lower respiratory tract. In

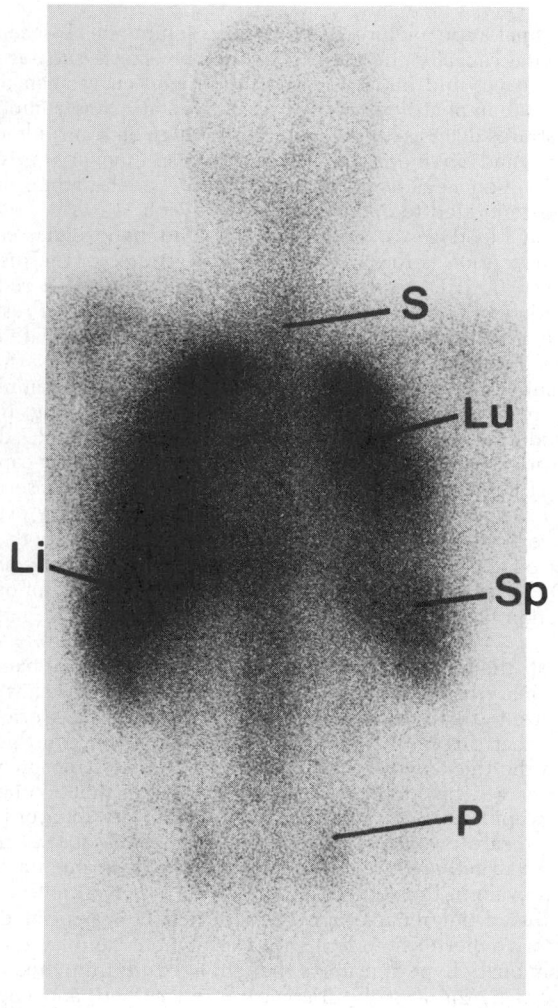

FIGURE 60–5. Gallium-67 scan of a patient with sarcoidosis. There is diffuse uptake of the isotope throughout the lung parenchyma (Lu). Structures that normally take up gallium-67 are also seen, including the spine (S), liver (Li), spleen (Sp), and pelvis (P).

normal individuals, 80 per cent or more of the recovered cells demonstrate alveolar macrophages, with the remainder being lymphocytes (almost all T cells). Polymorphonuclear leukocytes are normally rare. In patients with ILD, the pattern of alveolitis is reflected by the cells recovered by lavage. For example, in pulmonary sarcoidosis, the proportions of T cells may be 30 to 60 per cent, while in idiopathic pulmonary fibrosis, the proportion of neutrophils is often greater than 10 per cent. The diagnostic usefulness of bronchoalveolar lavage has not been established, but it can help to orient the clinician to the category of alveolitis that is present. Furthermore, because alveolar macrophages are phagocytic and ingest foreign materials present in the lung parenchyma, bronchoalveolar lavage can also be used to help diagnose specific agents that cause ILD, including inorganic dust diseases.

BIOPSY. The diagnosis of many ILD depends upon pathologic studies of lung parenchyma. The method of choice is the open lung biopsy, usually performed in the right middle lobe or lingula in an area of "average" disease as judged by the chest film. Transbronchial biopsy through the fiberoptic bronchoscope is useful for diagnosing sarcoidosis, but for most other ILD the samples are too small for a definitive diagnosis to be made.

Staging and Therapy

A patient with ILD should be evaluated to assess the contribution of the disease to functional impairment. The activity of the disease process should be independently assessed. Once both are known, rational decisions can be made concerning prognosis and therapy.

ASSESSMENT OF IMPAIRMENT. The consequences of ILD are assessed by history, chest radiograph, and lung function testing. A careful history of the patient's sensation of breathlessness, combined with an estimate of exercise tolerance, allows a rough estimate of lung derangement. The chest radiograph is somewhat more objective, and comparison with prior films helps to determine if the disease has become more extensive. Pulmonary function tests are the most accurate means to assess impairment. Of the tests routinely available, vital capacity, total lung capacity, diffusing capacity, and arterial Po_2 most accurately gauge the loss of functioning alveolar-capillary units. Measurements of the changes in Po_2 with exercise and of static compliance are more sensitive indicators of the extent of the impairment, but these tests are more difficult to perform and are not widely available.

ASSESSMENT OF ACTIVITY. Alveolitis is confined to the lower respiratory tract, so that its character or extent is difficult to measure directly. Circulating immune complexes and angiotensin-converting enzyme have been suggested as measures of the alveolitis in idiopathic pulmonary fibrosis and sarcoidosis, respectively, but neither test is very sensitive or specific. Similarly, attempts to correlate the chest radiograph or lung function tests with morphologic evidence of the alveolitis have been disappointing, and thus neither can be used to evaluate the alveolitis accurately.

Open lung biopsy, bronchoalveolar lavage, and *gallium-67 scanning* are the best present methods to stage alveolitis. Open biopsy is the most accurate method but is very rarely performed more than once in the course of the disease. Bronchoalveolar lavage and gallium-67 scanning are both sensitive to and specific for the alveolitis, but neither has been fully validated for routine clinical use. At this time, bronchoalveolar lavage is most useful for evaluating the intensity of the neutrophil, eosinophil, and lymphocyte components of the alveolitis and gallium-67 scanning for the macrophage component.

THERAPY. The principal aim of therapy in ILD is to suppress the alveolitis. For the ILD of unknown etiology, the conventional approach is to treat with oral corticosteroids, usually prednisone. Relatively high doses are used (1 mg per kilogram daily) for 1 to 2 months, followed by tapering doses over 2 to 3 months to maintenance levels (0.25 mg per kilogram per day), which are continued for varying periods. The corticosteroids are generally given once daily; it is not known if alternate-day regimens are equally effective. There has never been a large controlled trial of corticosteroids in any ILD, but some patients with ILD respond to corticosteroids in a fashion that cannot be explained by spontaneous remission. "Successful" therapy does not necessarily mean improvement in pulmonary function, chest radiograph, or subjective symptoms, since severely damaged alveoli are lost forever. In this context, successful suppression of the alveolitis usually means no further loss of alveoli. If improvement does occur, it likely results from suppression of the contribution of the inflammation itself to the derangements of the alveolar structures.

If the disease stabilizes, the corticosteroids are usually tapered. If the deterioration begins again after a period of quiescence, corticosteroids are often restarted, but their efficacy under these circumstances is limited. A variety of cytotoxic and other anti-inflammatory drugs have also been used in the treatment of the ILD of unknown etiology, but there has been no controlled series to demonstrate their efficacy.

For the ILD of known etiology, the initial treatment is to remove exposure to the causative agent. If the inflammation persists for months after removal from the known agent, patients are usually treated in a fashion similar to that used for ILD of unknown etiology. The exception to this rule is most of the pneumoconioses, for which no therapy is used.

In all ILD, attention should be given to prompt treatment of lung infections. Bronchodilators are sometimes used in mid to late course in these diseases to help mobilize secretions. Oxygen therapy, particularly with exercise, is often used as the patient reaches the late stage of ILD, but its efficacy in increasing the lifespan of these patients is unproved.

INTERSTITIAL LUNG DISEASES OF UNKNOWN ETIOLOGY

The ILD of unknown etiology represent the majority of all cases of ILD. Although of unknown etiology, each represents a specific entity with distinct features (see Table 60–1). The best understood ILD of unknown etiology are idiopathic pulmonary fibrosis and sarcoidosis.

Idiopathic Pulmonary Fibrosis (IPF)

CLINICAL MANIFESTATIONS. IPF, the "classic" fibrotic lung disease, is characterized by a neutrophil–alveolar macrophage alveolitis and progressive scarring of alveolar-capillary units. In the past IPF was sometimes called the Hamman-Rich syndrome, but this designation is not generally used now. Typically, IPF first manifests in middle age, but all age groups can be affected. The sex distribution is equal. Patients present with dyspnea on exertion and/or a dry cough, often following a viral illness. Fever is rare. Physical examination demonstrates dry, bibasilar rales, often associated with clubbing of the fingers and sometimes of the toes. The chest radiograph typically shows a diffuse reticulonodular infiltrate most prominent at the bases without hilar or pleural abnormalities. Some patients have various "autoimmune" abnormalities that likely represent nonspecific epiphenomena. Circulating immune complexes are common. Pulmonary function tests yield typical findings for ILD, i.e., reduced volumes and diffusing capacity. Routine tests of airflow are normal, but sensitive tests reveal mild airflow limitation, an observation that correlates with morphologic evidence of narrowing of small airways. Patients with IPF have mild resting hypoxemia that drops significantly with physical activity. Typically, a resting Po_2 of 80 torr will fall to 50 torr with the exercise equivalent to walking up one flight of stairs. Ventilation and perfusion studies reveal diffuse, patchy abnormalities with mismatching of air and blood. The gallium-67 scan usually shows a diffuse uptake of isotope throughout the lung parenchyma, and bronchoalveolar lavage reveals an alveolitis pattern dominated by neutrophils and macrophages, with fewer numbers of lymphocytes and eosinophils. The epithelial lining fluid of the lower respiratory tract contains elevated levels of immunoglobulin G (IgG), immune complexes, and neutrophil products, including collagenase and myeloperoxidase. Open lung biopsy shows a diffuse alveolitis that is patchy in its intensity. There is marked derangement of the alveolar walls with a fibrosis-type pattern, including denudation of the epithelial basement membranes; replacement of the type I epithelial cells by type II epithelial cells and bronchiolar cells; loss of capillaries; and expansion of the interstitium with edema, increased numbers of mesenchymal cells, and masses of deranged collagen fibers. The epithelial basement membranes have holes through which the interstitial fibrosis extends into the air spaces.

The clinical course of IPF is characterized by progressive loss of alveolar-capillary units, with eventual respiratory failure and death occurring an average of 5 years after the onset of symptoms. Occasional patients have a rapidly progressive course; others may live for 10 or more years. IPF is associated with a higher than expected incidence of myocardial infarction and pulmonary embolism and, in association with cigarette smoking, a high incidence of lung carcinoma.

DIFFERENTIAL DIAGNOSIS. Although the term "IPF" suggests that the diagnosis is one of exclusion, its features are so characteristic that the diagnosis is usually not difficult. Most confusion arises in distinguishing IPF from ILD associated with the collagen vascular disorders; however, the latter are systemic diseases, whereas IPF is compartmentalized to the lung. To exclude the ILD of known etiology that can mimic IPF, it is mandatory to take a careful history of past exposures to agents that can cause ILD. An open lung biopsy is necessary for diagnosis, but IPF cannot be diagnosed using morphologic criteria alone. While the biopsy features of IPF fit the morphologic categories of "usual interstitial pneumonitis (UIP)," "desquamative interstitial pneumonitis (DIP)," or, more commonly, a mixture of UIP and DIP, these features are not specific for IPF and can be found in other ILD of both known and unknown etiology.

PATHOGENESIS. IPF likely results from uncontrolled inflammatory processes that ensue after any of a variety of insults to the lower respiratory tract of susceptible individuals. The susceptibility to this disease is probably inherited but links to a specific gene locus have not been made. The neutrophil-macrophage–dominated alveolitis, the first known manifestation of IPF, may be driven by immune complexes of unknown origin formed within the lower respiratory tract. The immune complexes are probably associated with enhanced lung B cell immunoglobin production, with at least some of the immunoglobulins directed against local self-antigens. These immune complexes activate alveolar macrophages to release neutrophil-specific chemotactic factors that recruit neutrophils to the alveolar structures. The neutrophils damage the alveolar walls by releasing toxic oxygen radicals and proteases. IPF macrophages spontaneously release exaggerated amounts of platelet-derived growth factor, fibronectin, and the alveolar macrophage form of insulin-like growth factor 1 and thus expand the numbers of mesenchymal cells, resulting in fibrosis of the alveolar walls.

STAGING AND THERAPY. The degree of lung damage in IPF is determined by history, chest radiograph, and pulmonary function testing. The intensity of the alveolitis of IPF can be gauged by gallium-67 scanning and bronchoalveolar lavage, with particular emphasis placed on the intensity of the neutrophil component of the alveolitis. The use of corticosteroids, usually lifelong, is the conventional therapy. Approximately 10 to 20 per cent of patients with IPF improve with corticosteroids, particularly if the disease is detected early, before the alveolitis causes significant abnormalities. The second line of therapy is either the addition of massive doses of methylprednisolone sodium succinate (Solu-Medrol) (2 grams given intravenously [IV] once weekly) or oral cyclophosphamide (1.5 mg per kilogram per day). Either approach helps suppress the alveolitis, but the long-term efficacy is unknown.

Sarcoidosis

Sarcoidosis (Ch. 67) is a multisystem granulomatous disease of unknown etiology characterized in affected organs by a CD4+ T-helper cell–mononuclear phagocyte inflammatory process, noncaseating granulomas, and derangement of normal tissue architecture. While most organs can be affected by sarcoidosis, the lower respiratory tract is the site that most commonly causes morbidity and mortality. Pulmonary sarcoidosis is characterized by sharply circumscribed granulomas in the alveolar, bronchial, and vascular walls, composed of tightly packed cells derived from the mononuclear phagocyte system. In some cases, the alveolar walls are deranged in a fashion similar to that seen in IPF, but much less so. Significant interstitial fibrosis occurs in 20 to 25 per cent of patients. Sarcoidosis is described in detail in Ch. 67 and will not be discussed further here.

ILD Associated with the Collagen Vascular Disorders

All collagen vascular disorders are associated with ILD. In most cases the collagen vascular disorder is apparent before lung involvement is noted, but occasionally the ILD develops first and the other characteristic systemic signs and symptoms appear later. In either case, these disorders are frequently confused with IPF.

RHEUMATOID ARTHRITIS (Ch. 258). The ILD associated with rheumatoid arthritis include (1) an IPF-like disorder, (2) Caplan's syndrome (rheumatoid arthritis associated with coal worker's pneumoconiosis), (3) pulmonary parenchymal rheumatoid nodules, (4) pulmonary arteritis, and (5) apical fibrobullous disease. A few patients with rheumatoid arthritis have been described with dyspnea, severe irreversible airway obstruction with hyperinflation, and morphologic evidence of obliterative bronchiolitis. While some of this terminal airway disease may be related to penicillamine therapy, it may represent another manifestation of rheumatoid arthritis in the lung parenchyma.

The IPF-like disorder is by far the most common pulmonary manifestation of rheumatoid arthritis. Approximately 25 per cent of chest radiographs of patients with rheumatoid arthritis show interstitial changes, and the diffusing capacity is reduced in 50 per cent of all patients. In most cases the lung disease is much milder than IPF. The pathogenesis of the ILD is unknown but assumed to be the consequence of the same processes that affect the joints. The alveolitis is similar to IPF, but the neutrophil component is much less evident. There is no relationship between the extent of disease and the titer of the rheumatoid factor. Most cases of ILD associated with rheumatoid arthritis do not need to be treated. If treatment is instituted, guidelines similar to those for IPF are used. Gold salts, a common therapy for rheumatoid arthritis, can also induce ILD. There is no way to distinguish between gold salt- and rheumatoid arthritis–induced ILD, except that the gold-induced disease may reverse when the drug is discontinued.

PROGRESSIVE SYSTEMIC SCLEROSIS (PSS) (Ch. 262). The most common form of ILD associated with PSS is similar to IPF. The incidence of ILD among patients with PSS is very high; at autopsy, morphologic changes are found in 90 per cent and radiographic evidence of ILD is found in 30 to 40 per cent of patients. PSS patients with the CREST syndrome (calcinosis, Raynaud's phenomenon, esophageal involvement, sclerodactyly, and telangiectasia) rarely develop ILD. The ILD associated with PSS is generally indolent, but if it becomes symptomatic, the 4-year survival rate is about 50 per cent. Although PSS is considered a connective tissue disorder with fibrosis as its main feature, patients with the ILD associated with PSS have an alveolitis, albeit milder than that of IPF. Gallium-67 scans are often positive. For most patients, the alveolitis is dominated by macrophages, but neutrophils and sometimes lymphocytes play a role. The ILD linked with PSS is associated with a higher than normal incidence of bronchogenic carcinoma, particularly bronchoalveolar cell carcinoma.

Occasional patients with PSS develop an ILD characterized by pulmonary hypertension, with relatively less disease of the alveolar-capillary units. Morphologically, there is thickening of the pulmonary arteries with fibrosis and some inflammation. Many of these patients develop rapidly progressive respiratory failure.

The pathogenesis of the ILD associated with PSS is unknown. The therapeutic guidelines are unclear, although patients with progressive disease usually are treated in a similar fashion to those with IPF. Penicillamine has been suggested as an alternative therapy, but its efficacy is unproved.

SYSTEMIC LUPUS ERYTHEMATOSUS (SLE) (Ch. 261). The common manifestations of SLE in the lung include pleurisy with or without effusion, atelectasis, and acute pneumonitis. Less frequently, SLE manifests as uremic pulmonary edema, diaphragmatic dysfunction, parenchymal hemorrhage, or chronic ILD. Most cases of chronic ILD have pulmonary features similar to those of IPF, together with the systemic findings of SLE. Rarely, ILD associated with SLE can also manifest with a lymphocytic alveolitis similar to Sjögren's syndrome, a disorder similar to idiopathic pulmonary hemosiderosis, or a hypersensitivity vasculitis–like condition. Together, the incidence of acute and chronic pulmonary involvement in SLE is fewer than 20 per cent of all cases of SLE, and chronic ILD occurs in fewer than 5 per cent. Chronic ILD can appear insidiously or follow the acute pneumonitis of SLE, a severe illness characterized by fever, tachypnea, radiographic evidence of patchy or diffuse infiltrates, and hypoxemia. The pathogenesis of the ILD associated with SLE is thought to result from the deposition of circulating immune complexes in the alveolar walls. Therapy is usually with corticosteroids, but specific treatment guidelines have not been established. SLE can be associated with pulmonary infection, and this must be distinguished from ILD before corticosteroid therapy is started.

POLYMYOSITIS/DERMATOMYOSITIS (Ch. 268). The incidence of ILD in polymyositis/dermatomyositis is 5 to 10 per cent. The proportion of patients who develop ILD before the extrapulmonary manifestations is higher in polymyositis/dermatomyositis than in any other collagen vascular disorder. The ILD is similar to IPF, but its pathogenesis is unclear. Patients are usually treated with corticosteroids, but methotrexate has been suggested as alternative therapy.

SJÖGREN'S SYNDROME (Ch. 263). Approximately 3 per cent of patients with Sjögren's syndrome develop ILD that manifests as either a mild IPF-like disease or, more commonly, a disorder with a lymphocyte-dominant alveolitis, similar to the lymphocytic infiltration of other organs in these patients. This lymphocytic form of ILD can be mild to severe and can undergo transformation to a lymphocytic malignancy, an event that is invariably fatal. Therapy of either ILD associated with Sjögren's syndrome is controversial; corticosteroids, immunosuppressive agents, and no therapy have all been advocated.

MIXED CONNECTIVE TISSUE DISEASE (Ch. 262). Up to 80 per cent of patients with this systemic disorder have ILD. The lung disease is usually like IPF. Pulmonary hypertension is common and can occur without significant parenchymal involvement. Therapy is usually with corticosteroids, with or without cytotoxic agents.

ANKYLOSING SPONDYLITIS (Ch. 259). Lung disease, manifested as chest wall restriction and upper lobe fibrobullous disease, occurs in about 1 per cent of patients with ankylosing spondylitis. Most patients are asymptomatic, but colonization with organisms such as *Aspergillus* or atypical mycobacteria is common, and hemoptysis and pneumothorax occur in the late stages of the disease. While HLA-B27 (HLA = human leukocyte antigen) is strongly associated with ankylosing spondylitis, it is not common in those patients with the associated ILD. The morphology of the ILD is like that of IPF, together with localized destruction of alveolar walls and bullae. There is no known therapy.

Histiocytosis X

Histiocytosis X (HX) (Ch. 149), also called "pulmonary Langerhans' cell granulomatosis," "primary pulmonary histiocytosis," and "eosinophilic granuloma," is a fibrotic-destructive disorder of the lower respiratory tract associated with an intense mononuclear phagocyte–dominant alveolitis. HX is grouped with the other proliferative disorders of the mononuclear phagocyte system, such as Letterer-Siwe and Hand-Schüller-Christian disease. In adults, HX is primarily a lung disease, although bone, skin, and central nervous system manifestations do occur. At least 50 per cent of all patients have chronic symptoms, and the disease can be fatal. More than 1000 cases have been reported; most new patients are 20 to 40 years of age, and there is an equal sex distribution. Almost all patients with HX have been cigarette smokers.

The patient with HX presents with a nonproductive cough, dyspnea on exertion, or chest pain. Spontaneous pneumothorax occurs in 10 per cent of cases; fever, weight loss, hemoptysis, and wheezing are occasionally noted. Bone involvement is present in a minority of patients. Posterior pituitary involvement with diabetes insipidus is unusual, as are skin lesions. Physical examination commonly reveals decreased breath sounds and rales. The chest radiograph shows upper and midzone small, irregular nodules superimposed on a delicate cystic pattern. The costophrenic angles are usually clear, and the pleura and hila are normal. Pulmonary function tests show a mixed restrictive-obstructive pattern with reduced lung volumes, reduced diffusing capacity, airflow limitation, and hypoxemia that worsens with exercise.

Definitive diagnosis is made by open lung biopsy. The disease is focal but poorly demarcated. There are sites of intense alveolitis dominated by alveolar macrophages and Langerhans' cells. Gallium-67 scans are negative or only mildly positive. Bronchoalveolar lavage reveals a macrophage-dominant alveolitis, and Langerhans' cells can be detected in lavage by ultrastructure and the T6 monoclonal antibody. The pathogenesis of this rare entity is discussed in Ch. 149. The lung disease in adults is considered untreatable.

Goodpasture's Syndrome

Goodpasture's syndrome (Ch. 79) is characterized by diffuse pulmonary hemorrhage, ILD, glomerulonephritis, and circulating anti–glomerular basement membrane (anti-GBM) and anti–alveolar basement membrane (anti-ABM) antibodies. It is assumed that the anti-GBM and anti-ABM antibodies are identical and cross-react with identical components in the kidney and lung basement membranes. Goodpasture's syndrome can be mimicked by SLE, Wegener's granulomatosis, and the systemic necrotizing vasculitides. In the appropriate clinical setting, the diagnosis of Goodpasture's syndrome is straightforward but does require (1) demonstration of the circulating antibodies, (2) characteristic linear deposits of immunoglobulin along the glomerular basement membrane, and (3) demonstration that the antibodies (either those circulating or those eluted from the kidney) are specific. It is usually not necessary to obtain lung tissue to make the diagnosis, but the diagnosis can be confirmed by histologic and immunofluorescence study of lung tissue obtained by transbronchial biopsy.

Almost all of the anti–basement membrane antibodies in Goodpasture's syndrome are IgG, but immunoglobulin A (IgA) anti-GBM and anti-ABM antibodies have been described in the setting of pulmonary hemorrhage and glomerulonephritis. The basement membrane antigen (or antigens) against which the antibodies are directed is thought to be a portion of type IV (basement membrane) collagen that is somehow unmasked in the kidney and lung.

Goodpasture's syndrome occurs mostly in young men. In most cases, evidence of alveolar hemorrhage precedes the clinical evidence of renal disease. Hemoptysis occurs in almost all cases, tends to be recurrent, and occasionally is massive and life threatening. In such cases, death is from asphyxiation. Anemia is almost always present. The chest radiograph reveals interstitial and alveolar infiltrates. The patchy infiltrates due to the hemorrhage often clear, but the interstitial markings, reflecting chronic ILD, often remain. Histologic findings include alveolar hemorrhage, hemosiderin-laden macrophages, focal areas of alveolitis, and interstitial fibrosis. Linear deposits of IgG can be detected in the alveolar walls.

Spontaneous remissions of Goodpasture's syndrome can occur but are rare. Therapy generally consists of corticosteroids, cytotoxic agents, and plasmapheresis.

Idiopathic Pulmonary Hemosiderosis (IPH)

IPH is a rare disorder of unknown cause characterized by alveolar hemorrhage, iron deficiency anemia, transient parenchymal infiltrates on the chest radiograph, and ILD. The disease is most common in individuals less than 20 years of age, but adult cases are seen. The disease is occasionally found in families, but a genetic basis has not been proved. IPH is compartmentalized in the lung and must be distinguished from Goodpasture's syndrome, Wegener's granulomatosis, SLE, and the vasculitides.

The patient with IPH presents with repetitive acute episodes of dyspnea, cough with hemoptysis, and fever. Iron deficiency anemia is common. The chest radiographs associated with these acute episodes reveal transient infiltrates, a miliary pattern, or massive confluent shadows. On this background of intermittent episodes, a chronic ILD develops, with increasing dyspnea, rales, clubbing, and pulmonary hypertension. While the childhood form of the disease is aggressive, with a mean survival of about 3 years, adult IPH tends to be more insidious. Lung function tests are typical for ILD, but the diffusing capacity may be falsely high owing to increased uptake of the carbon monoxide (used as the test gas) by free hemoglobin in the lung parenchyma. Hemosiderin-laden macrophages in sputum or lavage fluid suggest prior parenchymal hemorrhage. In the appropriate clinical setting, when there are no detectable anti-GBM antibodies, a definitive diagnosis of IPH can be made with an open lung biopsy revealing focal hemorrhage, a macrophage-dominant alveolitis with hemosiderin-positive macrophages, and typical findings of ILD. The pathogenesis of this disorder is unknown. Corticosteroids are generally used to treat the acute episodes and the chronic ILD, but there is no evidence regarding their efficacy.

Chronic Eosinophilic Pneumonia (CEP)

CEP is a chronic ILD characterized by cough, dyspnea, malaise, fever, night sweats, weight loss, variable degrees of blood eosinophilia, and a chest film revealing peripheral, nonsegmental, nonmigratory infiltrates. Rarely, acute cases can result in the rapid development of respiratory failure. Hilar adenopathy rarely occurs. Asthma accompanies CEP in 50 to 60 per cent of cases. High proportions of eosinophils are sometimes recovered in sputum or by lavage. A very high sedimentation rate is common, and elevated levels of immunoglobulin E (IgE) during acute episodes have been described. The histologic findings of CEP include a diffuse alveolitis dominated by eosinophils and macrophages with fewer numbers of neutrophils and lymphocytes. Eosinophilic abscesses, multinucleated giant cells, angiitis of small pulmonary vessels, and interstitial fibrosis are common.

Although the stimulus to the accumulation of the eosinophils in the lung is unknown, the eosinophil can damage the cells and matrix of the alveolar walls through its release of toxic oxygen radicals, collagenase, and major basic protein, a highly charged polypeptide associated with the eosinophil granules.

An open lung biopsy is required to make a definitive diagnosis. However, because CEP usually responds dramatically to corticosteroids, a tentative diagnosis is often made on clinical grounds only, without biopsy confirmation, and corticosteroid therapy is instituted. In some patients, the disease is only partly suppressed by corticosteroids, and long-term treatment is required.

Lymphocytic Infiltrative Disorders

This is a group of rare, diffuse ILD characterized by infiltration of the alveolar structures by cells of the lymphocyte series. Most patients present with cough and dyspnea, occasionally with fever. All of the lymphocyte infiltrative disorders of lung can progress to frank lymphoma.

Immunoblastic lymphadenopathy (also called angioimmunoblastic lymphadenopathy) is a systemic disorder, usually of elderly individuals, characterized by generalized lymphadenopathy, hepatosplenomegaly, and variable amounts of ILD. The disease has no known etiology, but associations with drugs have been reported, including antibiotics and phenytoin. A skin rash is observed in one third of cases; there may be a coexistent collagen vascular disorder or hemolytic anemia. There are polyclonal increases in serum immunoglobulins. The alveolar structures exhibit a pleomorphic alveolitis representing all levels of lymphocyte differentiation. Diagnosis is usually made by lymph node biopsy. The disease can remit spontaneously, but patients die of progressive respiratory failure, infection, or malignancy. The response to therapy with corticosteroids and/or cytotoxic agents is variable.

Lymphocytic interstitial pneumonitis is limited to the lung. The signs and symptoms are typical for an insidious, slowly progressive ILD. It is most common in women in their 40's, but it is observed in males and all age groups. The chest radiograph characteristically shows diffuse reticulonodular infiltrates. Most patients have dysproteinemias. Some cases, particularly in the pediatric population, are associated with HIV infection. Hypergammaglobulinemia and hypogammaglobulinemia have been described, and an association with Sjögren's syndrome is common. The diagnosis is made by an open lung biopsy revealing diffuse parenchymal infiltration with mature lymphocytes, plasma cells, and immunoblasts. Granulomas are sometimes observed. Because the infiltrating cells may form germinal centers, the disease is sometimes called "pseudolymphoma." The prognosis of lymphocytic interstitial pneumonitis is variable, and some patients progress to end-stage lung disease or lymphoma. Treatment is with corticosteroids and/or immunosuppressive agents.

ILD Associated with Pulmonary Vasculitis

Many of the systemic vasculitides result in ILD as a consequence of a pulmonary vasculitis causing a secondary alveolitis and derangements of the alveolar structures.

Wegener's granulomatosis is a granulomatous vasculitis of the upper and lower respiratory tracts and kidney (Ch. 266). There is a limited form of the disease without clinically apparent renal disease. All patients have pulmonary involvement, but only one third have symptoms related to the lungs. Airway involvement is common. The parenchymal lung disease can appear as discrete nodules and/or diffuse ILD; either can undergo necrosis and cavity formation. Hemoptysis, cough, sputum production, dyspnea, and pleuritic pain are common. Lung function tests reveal a mixed restrictive-obstructive pattern. Diagnosis is usually made by open lung biopsy. Untreated disease is usually fatal, but with cyclophosphamide therapy long-term survival is the rule.

Lymphomatoid granulomatosis is a systemic vasculitis involving the lung, skin, central nervous system, and kidneys. The lung is always affected, but involvement of other organs is variable. In the lung, the walls of the blood vessels are infiltrated with typical and atypical lymphocytes, together with some granulomas, and there is associated ILD. A mild form of lymphomatoid granulomatosis has been described ("benign lymphocytic angiitis and granulomatosis"). The disease is most common in middle age. Multiple, fleeting nodular densities are seen on the chest film; occasionally there are diffuse infiltrates. Death is usually due to parenchymal destruction with sepsis and occasionally to massive hemoptysis. The diagnosis is usually established by biopsy of the lung or skin. The lung disease often responds to corticosteroids and cyclophosphamide, but the central nervous system lesions do not. Lymphoma occurs in about 10 per cent of cases.

The *Churg-Strauss syndrome* (allergic angiitis and granulomatosis) (Ch. 264) is a form of systemic necrotizing vasculitis that almost always involves the lung, unlike classic polyarteritis nodosa, which rarely does. The pulmonary manifestations, consisting of asthma and diffuse infiltrates, often precede systemic involvement by 1 or 2 years. A history of allergy is common. An elevated sedimentation rate and total eosinophil count are common. The systemic vasculitis involves skin, heart, and gastrointestinal tract. Diagnosis is made by open lung biopsy, which shows a granulomatous vasculitis with eosinophilic infiltration, a secondary diffuse alveolitis, interstitial granulomas, and fibrosis. Treatment is the same as for the other pulmonary vasculitides.

Hypersensitivity vasculitis represents a heterogeneous group of vasculitides whose development is thought to be related to sensitization to antigens such as drugs or serum proteins. Skin involvement is most common; most cases do not involve the lung. When they do, there is a small-vessel polymorphonuclear leukocyte vasculitis with fibrinoid necrosis and secondary ILD. Diagnosis is usually made by skin biopsy, and the disorder is often self-limiting. A similar disorder can occur in association with mixed cryoglobulinemia or Henoch-Schönlein purpura.

Inherited Disorders

There is a small group of rare ILD that are clearly inherited. Almost all are autosomal dominant disorders, although the autosomal recessive disorders Hermansky-Pudlak syndrome, Niemann-Pick disease, and Gaucher's disease may rarely be associated with ILD.

FAMILIAL IDIOPATHIC PULMONARY FIBROSIS. This is a chronic, usually fatal autosomal dominant disorder identical to IPF. Symptoms usually begin in the fifth or sixth decade, but the disease can be manifested earlier. Some of the asymptomatic children of affected family members have evidence of a mild alveolitis yet with normal lung function, suggesting that the disease begins with an alveolitis.

NEUROFIBROMATOSIS (Ch. 467). Von Recklinghausen's disease is an autosomal dominant disorder characterized by pigmented skin lesions and neurofibromas of the peripheral and central nervous systems. In 10 to 20 per cent of adult cases there is a coexisting ILD and/or bullous lung disease. The ILD has histologic features similar to those of IPF, but it is not known whether it responds to similar therapies.

TUBEROUS SCLEROSIS (Ch. 467). This is a hamartomatous autosomal dominant disorder involving the central nervous system, skin, kidneys, eyes, bones, heart, and, in 1 per cent of patients, the lungs. Although the hamartomatous "tumors" are composed of various cell types in most affected organs, in the

lung they are composed only of smooth muscle cells. The accumulation of smooth muscle cells in the alveolar interstitium causes ILD, together with parenchymal destruction. Unlike most ILD, there is little alveolitis. The chest radiograph shows diffuse infiltrates and honeycombing, and lung function tests show a mixed pattern with a dominant obstructive pattern. Pneumothorax is common. There is no known therapy.

ILD Associated with Pulmonary Airway Disease

This term refers to disorders in which the ILD is likely secondary to a primary airway disease. It is unclear if there are many such diseases or only one. The characteristic lesions are necrotic granulomas in the bronchial walls, with the bronchiolar lumina filled with palisading epithelioid cells, cellular debris, and polymorphonuclear leukocytes. A diffuse alveolitis and nongranulomatous fibrosis-type derangements of the alveolar walls are usually present. Approximately one third of patients have asthma, blood eosinophilia, mucus plugging, fungal hyphae identifiable in the airways, and positive sputum cultures for *Aspergillus* organisms. These patients are usually referred to as having *bronchopulmonary aspergillosis* (see Ch. 406). It is unclear, however, whether the fungus is a primary cause of the disease or represents a secondary process.

The remaining two thirds of patients, referred to as having *bronchocentric granulomatosis*, do not have asthma, microscopic evidence of fungi, or blood eosinophilia. The disease can present in an insidious manner or as an acute febrile illness. The chest film usually shows nodular or mass lesions; diffuse infiltrates are seen in about 20 per cent of cases. Lung function tests demonstrate a mixed obstructive-restrictive pattern. Corticosteroids are usually the therapy of choice.

Lymphangioleiomyomatosis

This is a rare disease of women, almost always of childbearing age, characterized by the proliferation of benign but atypical smooth muscle cells in walls of the lymphatics of the lower respiratory tract, pleura, mediastinum, and retroperitoneum. Although it is an ILD characterized by thickening and derangements of the alveolar walls, very little inflammation is present. Eventual destruction of the alveolar walls is common. The clinical findings include dyspnea, recurrent unilateral or bilateral chylous pleural effusions, pneumothorax, hemoptysis, and occasionally peritoneal chylous effusions. The chest radiograph has a characteristic reticulonodular pattern on a background of diffuse cystic changes, similar to that seen in HX. Lung function tests reveal a mixed obstructive-restrictive pattern. An open lung biopsy is required to make the diagnosis. It has been theorized that the disease results from an abnormal response to estrogens, and thus oophorectomy, progesterone, and tamoxifen therapy have all been tried in these patients. There is no proven efficacy of such therapies, and the disease is almost always fatal, usually within 10 years of diagnosis.

Alveolar Proteinosis

In this disorder the alveoli are filled with a periodic acid–Schiff (PAS)–positive lipid and protein-rich granular material. There may be an accompanying mononuclear cell alveolitis and fibrosis-type derangements of the alveolar walls. Although of unknown etiology, alveolar proteinosis can be associated with silicosis, hematologic malignancies, bronchogenic cyst, and mycobacterial and fungal diseases of the lung. Why this material accumulates in the alveoli is unknown but is speculated to result from the breakdown of cells in the lower respiratory tract, from the overproduction of substances normally secreted into the alveolar spaces (e.g., surfactant), from increased transudation of plasma proteins, or from decreased alveolar clearance mechanisms.

The disease usually begins insidiously with dyspnea as the initial symptom. The chest radiograph has a characteristic diffuse, finely nodular alveolar filling pattern. Lung function tests show decreased lung volumes and diffusing capacity. There is usually hypoxemia secondary to pulmonary blood shunting by filled alveoli. Open lung biopsy is ordinarily required for the diagnosis. However, in the appropriate clinical setting, bronchoalveolar lavage recovery of the typical material, together with transbronchial biopsy evidence of alveoli filled with PAS-positive material, is usually diagnostic. Alveolar proteinosis can be fatal but can also spontaneously resolve. The recommended therapy is massive whole-lung lavage with the patient under general anesthesia. Corticosteroid therapy has no proven use and may lead to the development of opportunistic infections.

Miscellaneous Other ILD of Unknown Etiology

There are several ILD of unknown etiology that are reasonably well defined but so rare that there is little information available concerning their pathogenesis and no apparent guidelines relating to their staging and therapy. These are included by list in Table 60–1 but will not be discussed individually here.

INTERSTITIAL LUNG DISEASE OF KNOWN ETIOLOGY

Approximately 135 agents are known to cause ILD, but together they are responsible for only one third of all cases of ILD. In terms of numbers of patients that come to medical attention, the most important agents are crystalline silica, asbestos, coal dust, organic dusts of the *Micropolyspora* and *Thermoactinomyces* genera and those derived from avian proteins, some antineoplastic drugs, nitrofurantoin, and hyperoxia.

Inhaled Inorganic Dusts

ILD resulting from the chronic inhalation of an inorganic dust is called a "pneumoconiosis" (see Table 60–2). The most common are silicosis, asbestosis, and coal worker's pneumoconiosis. The common pneumoconioses are all characterized by fibrosis-type derangements of the lower respiratory tract.

There are several important principles relevant to understanding the pneumoconioses. (1) The dusts themselves cause little damage to the lung parenchyma; it is the inflammatory response to the dusts that causes the loss of functional alveolar-capillary units. (2) A number of defense mechanisms prevent such dusts from reaching the alveoli, and others remove most dusts that might reach the lower respiratory tract. Just because an individual has been exposed to an inorganic dust does not mean that the dust has necessarily caused ILD. (3) Abnormalities on a chest radiograph consistent with exposure to an inorganic dust do not prove that the individual has a functionally significant ILD. (4) These chronic disorders result from the inhalation of high concentrations of inorganic dusts over many years; i.e., history of a brief exposure sometime in the past is not sufficient evidence to implicate a particular dust. (5) No known therapy has proven efficacy for any pneumoconiosis; current "treatment" for all pneumoconioses is permanent removal from inhalation of the causative agent. (6) Many individuals exposed to inorganic dusts also have a history of chronic cigarette smoking; this must be taken into account when evaluating these patients. (7) Physical evidence of the inorganic dust in the lung is useful but not critical in making the diagnosis of a common pneumoconiosis (silicosis, asbestosis, coal worker's pneumoconiosis) as long as the chronic exposure history is very clear and unambiguous. For the other inorganic dusts, however, biopsy evidence is required to make a definitive diagnosis. (8) While the miners and millers who work around these inorganic dusts represent the "classic" exposure situations, inorganic dust materials are widely used in manufacturing. A careful occupational history is required, or the exposure history may be missed. *Coal worker's pneumoconiosis, silicosis, asbestosis,* and *berylliosis* are described in Ch. 527, Occupational Pulmonary Disorders.

Inhaled Organic Dusts

The repeated inhalation of certain organic dusts (see also Ch. 527) causes a granulomatous ILD called *hypersensitivity pneumonitis* or *extrinsic allergic alveolitis.* The term "hypersensitivity pneumonitis" is reserved for those ILD caused by organic dusts derived from living sources. A large number of organic dusts have been implicated (see Table 60–3), but the most common are the thermophilic organisms of the *Micropolyspora* and *Thermoactinomyces* groups and those derived from avian proteins.

The nomenclature relating to hypersensitivity pneumonitis is confusing because the name of the disease usually refers to the situation of exposure (e.g., "maple bark stripper's disease," "humidifier lung"), even though the organic dusts causing different diseases may be identical. For example, *Thermoactinomyces vulgaris* can cause "farmer's lung," "humidifier lung," and "mushroom worker's lung." The most common exposure situations are farmers exposed to moldy hay, individuals exposed to organic antigens growing in humidifiers and air conditioners, and bird breeders, particularly those raising pigeons. The other exposure situations are varied, and the list is ever expanding (see Table 60–3).

Classically, 4 to 6 hours after inhalation of the antigen, a sensitized individual develops acute symptoms of hypersensitivity pneumonitis, including fever, cough, dyspnea, and malaise. The chest film at this time shows diffuse parenchymal infiltrates, and lung function tests demonstrate decreased lung volumes, decreased diffusing capacity, mild airflow limitation, and hypoxemia. If the individual is removed from the antigen exposure, there is gradual improvement in symptoms, the chest film, and lung function tests over a 24-hour period. If the exposures are few, there are few sequelae other than the acute episodes. However, in some individuals, for unknown reasons, repetitive exposure leads to a chronic ILD characterized by lymphocyte-macrophage alveolitis occasionally mixed with neutrophils. Initially, the derangements are of the distortion type, with lymphocytes and granulomas in the alveolar walls. Later, however, there are fibrotic changes, including intra-alveolar fibrosis. Rarely, the chronic form develops in an insidious manner without the acute episodes.

The diagnosis of hypersensitivity pneumonitis is made in the context of a history of exposure to a known causative antigen, the presence of ILD, the presence of antigen-specific antibodies in the blood, and an open lung biopsy demonstrating the characteristic morphology. The gallium-67 scan is usually positive, and bronchoalveolar lavage shows a lymphocyte-macrophage alveolitis, mixed with neutrophils when the exposure has been recent. When the history is typical, a biopsy is not necessary to make the diagnosis, but there must be a clear demonstration of the acute symptoms 4 to 6 hours after inhalation of the antigen.

The mechanisms by which sensitization to these organic dusts causes either the acute or the chronic disease are unknown. T cells, the majority of which have suppressor/cytotoxic (CD8+) surface markers, dominate the alveolitis. The T cells in the lung and blood are sensitized to the offending antigen. Besides the circulating antigen-specific immunoglobulins, levels of IgG and immunoglobulin M (IgM) are increased in the lower respiratory tract. However, there is no evidence that the immunoglobulins play a role in the pathogenesis of the disease, and immune complexes have not been convincingly demonstrated in the lower respiratory tract. One of the confusing aspects of this disease is that although many exposed individuals become sensitized to the organic antigen (as manifested by the presence of antigen-specific antibodies in the blood), only a very small proportion will develop either the acute or the chronic symptoms of hypersensitivity pneumonitis.

The prognosis of chronic hypersensitivity pneumonitis is not clear. In those with farmer's lung, there is a 10 per cent mortality over 6 years, with an additional 30 per cent having significant functional impairment. Management of hypersensitivity pneumonitis is directed toward removing the patient from the source of the antigen and suppressing the alveolitis, usually with corticosteroids.

Drug-Induced ILD

Drug-induced ILD are disorders in which the lower respiratory tract is structurally and/or functionally deranged as a result of a pharmacologic agent. The list of drugs reported to cause ILD is large (see Table 60–4) and includes those producing acute, subacute, and chronic ILD. Drug-induced ILD can be serious and sometimes fatal, but they are usually effectively treated simply by recognizing the disorder and discontinuing the responsible drug.

It is generally assumed that many of the drug-induced ILD are "hypersensitivity" reactions, but proof of an immune basis for these diseases is circumstantial at best. In many cases, it is thought that the drug injures the lung parenchyma in some fashion to initiate an alveolitis that propagates the injury.

Typically, the acute and subacute forms of drug-induced ILD present with respiratory decompensation following a prodrome of fever and cough. At this time there are usually increased heart and respiratory rates, dry rales, and, occasionally, cyanosis. The chest radiograph shows a patchy or diffuse reticulonodular infiltrate that can be confused with pulmonary edema. Pleural effusions are common. Blood studies often show eosinophilia and arterial hypoxemia and hypocarbia. Lung function tests are typical for ILD, and the gallium-67 scan is often positive. Open lung biopsy demonstrates parenchymal cell injury, edema of the alveolar wall, fibrin in the air spaces, and a patchy lymphocyte-macrophage alveolitis, sometimes mixed with neutrophils and/or eosinophils. In some cases, the course is rapidly downhill, requiring mechanical ventilation and oxygen administration. The disease is usually reversible if the drug is discontinued but can be fatal if this is not done early in the course.

One major area of confusion in conceptualizing and categorizing the drug-induced ILD disorders has resulted from the use of the term "pulmonary infiltration with eosinophilia (PIE) syndrome" to describe patients receiving drugs who develop an acute or subacute disorder characterized by blood eosinophilia and parenchymal infiltrates on the chest film. However, the PIE syndrome is far from diagnostic as a drug-induced ILD. Many non–drug-associated ILD of both known (e.g., acute beryllium-induced disease) and unknown etiology (e.g., IPF, sarcoidosis) can be associated with blood eosinophilia, and tropical pulmonary eosinophilia caused by filarial infestation presents in an identical manner. In addition, there is no evidence that the blood eosinophilia has any relevance to the pathogenesis of the disease in the lung. Thus, most clinicians have abandoned the concept of the PIE syndrome and simply think of these disorders as part of the spectrum of ILD in which the presence of blood eosinophilia is a helpful, but not definitive, clue to the diagnosis.

The chronic form of drug-induced ILD is much more insidious and difficult to associate with a drug as the etiologic agent. Fever is less common, and patients usually present with typical ILD. Occasionally there is blood eosinophilia. Because of the insidious nature of the chronic form of drug-induced ILD, many clinicians use lung function tests, particularly the diffusing capacity, to follow patients on drugs commonly associated with the development of ILD. The gallium-67 scan is usually positive. Open lung biopsy usually shows a lymphocyte-macrophage alveolitis with mixed numbers of polymorphonuclear leukocytes. The derangements are of the fibrosis type, often with intra-alveolar fibrosis. Unlike the acute and subacute forms of the drug-induced ILD, the chronic form often persists after the drug is discontinued. The reasons why this occurs are not clear, but it is likely that the injury to the parenchyma has been sufficient to establish a chronic alveolitis that propagates the disorder in the absence of the initial stimulus. In such cases, therapeutic strategies are directed toward suppressing the alveolitis, usually with corticosteroids.

ANTINEOPLASTIC AGENTS. *Bleomycin*-induced disease is common; up to 10 per cent of patients receiving bleomycin develop some ILD, and 1 per cent die of the ILD. Toxicity from this agent occurs in both acute and chronic forms and is potentiated by concomitant therapy with oxygen or irradiation. *Busulfan* lung disease occurs in 2 to 3 per cent of those receiving the drug. The disease is chronic, usually takes at least 1 year of therapy before it appears, and usually does not respond to withdrawal of the drug or to corticosteroids. *Methotrexate*-induced ILD can appear in acute or chronic form. Leucovorin or corticosteroids are not protective, but recovery is common once the drug is stopped. There are increasing numbers of reports of ILD induced by the *nitrosoureas*. The incidence of toxicity is about 1 per cent and occurs 2 months to 3 years after initiation of therapy. *Procarbazine* causes an acute ILD with pleural effusions, peripheral eosinophilia, and an eosinophilic alveolitis. Although *cyclophosphamide* is used to treat many ILD of unknown etiology, it can rarely cause acute or chronic ILD. Several other antineoplastic agents are reported to cause ILD, but very rarely.

ANTIBIOTICS. ILD induced by *nitrofurantoin* is a common adverse drug reaction, occurring in both acute and chronic forms. The acute form, 5 to 10 times more frequent than the chronic form, occurs in sensitized individuals within 1 month of reinstituting treatment. The disease almost always clears when the drug is discontinued. The chronic disease occurs following 6 to 12 months of therapy. Approximately 60 per cent have positive

antinuclear antibodies. The prognosis is good once the drug is stopped, but permanent loss of lung function is common, and approximately 10 per cent die of the disease. The ILD caused by other antibiotics are also mostly acute disorders and are very rare.

CARDIOVASCULAR DRUGS. *Hydralazine* and *procainamide* induce an acute ILD similar to that associated with SLE. In contrast to spontaneously occurring SLE, which is common in blacks and women, the ILD produced by both of these drugs occurs more commonly in whites and affects a significant number of men. Most affected individuals have serum antinuclear antibodies. The disease usually disappears when the drug is stopped. Other drugs that can cause a similar syndrome include isoniazid, phenytoin, and allopurinol. Increasingly, ILD has been observed in association with amiodarone, a useful antiarrhythmic agent. The ILD is usually dose dependent and self-limiting but can be chronic even after the drug has been discontinued. The beta blockers can cause chronic ILD, but rarely. The disease is insidious and like IPF but is often associated with fibrosis elsewhere in the body.

OTHER DRUGS. *Gold salts* can induce ILD after 1 to 6 months of therapy; this form of ILD can be difficult to distinguish from the ILD associated with rheumatoid arthritis. The disease is thought to represent a hypersensitivity reaction. *Mineral oil*–induced ILD, sometimes called "lipoid pneumonia," results from the aspiration of mineral oil used as nose drops or ingested as a laxative. The open lung biopsy demonstrates a typical picture of lymphoid cells, lipid-laden macrophages, and fibrosis. With an appropriate history, however, the diagnosis can be made by recovering lipid-laden macrophages by bronchoalveolar lavage. The intravenous use of drugs meant for oral use can cause ILD by virtue of the presence of particulate material in the drugs, including talc, starch, maltose, or quinine. The disease is usually chronic and characterized by foreign body granulomatous reactions affecting pulmonary capillaries.

Many other drugs are known to cause acute and/or chronic ILD, and the list is ever expanding. Because these disorders are all potentially curable if the drug is stopped, it is critical to have a high index of suspicion of drug-induced disease whenever confronted by a patient with ILD.

Other Agents Known to Cause ILD

Beyond inorganic dusts, organic dusts, and drugs, the most important known causes of ILD are paraquat, radiation, the sequelae of prior infectious processes, hyperoxia, and chronic aspiration pneumonia. The others are very rare and mostly represent anecdotal case reports (see Table 60–5).

PARAQUAT. Poisoning with the herbicide paraquat can occur with oral, parenteral, aerosol, or dermal exposure. Paraquat is available in granules, aerosols, and liquid concentrates; ingestion of the liquid either by accident or by suicidal intent is the most common means of paraquat poisoning. Paraquat is an extremely potent cause of parenchymal derangement and fibrosis and consequent respiratory insufficiency. As little as 1 teaspoon of the concentrate can be fatal. The disease is usually acute, but chronic cases have been described. In acute cases, dyspnea, fever, fatigue, and gastrointestinal complaints occur 1 to 5 days after poisoning. Mouth, pharyngeal, and esophageal ulcerations are common following oral ingestion. Diffuse radiographic changes of ILD are quickly followed by rapidly progressive respiratory failure, usually requiring ventilatory support. Open lung biopsy reveals a neutrophil-macrophage alveolitis and alveolar wall derangements typical of ILD, but very severe. In addition to interstitial fibrosis, intra-alveolar fibrosis is common. In these acute cases, there is a rough correlation between plasma levels of paraquat and survival. If the plasma paraquat concentration 8 hours after ingestion is greater than 1200 µg per liter, death is inevitable. In addition to these acute cases, intermittent low-dose skin exposure may be hazardous and may lead to a chronic ILD.

Paraquat causes ILD by virtue of its propensity to be taken up by parenchymal cells of the lower respiratory tract, where it generates toxic oxygen radicals sufficient to damage the normal parenchymal components severely. There is a secondary alveolitis that further injures the parenchyma and mediates the development of fibrosis-type derangements. Treatment of paraquat poisoning is mostly supportive. Attempts should be made to remove the paraquat (gastric lavage with bentonite, Fuller's earth, or charcoal, followed by charcoal hemoperfusion). Since hyperoxia accelerates paraquat-induced injury, oxygen concentrations should be kept as low as possible. Antioxidant therapy (e.g., vitamin E) has been suggested, but its efficacy is unknown. In chronic cases, corticosteroids are usually used to suppress the alveolitis.

RADIATION. ILD resulting from thoracic irradiation is a common sequela of radiotherapy of breast, lung, or esophageal carcinoma and lymphoma and is potentiated by the concomitant use of antineoplastic drugs known to cause ILD. Radiation-induced lung disease is described in Ch. 530.

SEQUELAE OF KNOWN INFECTIOUS AGENTS. All types of infections of the lower respiratory tract may occasionally result in significant injury and fibrosis. Usually, the ILD remains localized to the site of infection and does not progress after eradication of the infectious agent. A typical example is the localized upper lobe scars left by mycobacterial infection. ILD has been described following *Mycoplasma* infection as well as *Legionella* pneumonia, and there are scattered reports of viral infections causing a progressive ILD. A significant number of individuals with HIV infection develop mild ILD. In some cases, this results from the inflammation associated with opportunistic infections, but in others, it is likely that the inflammation with resulting ILD is secondary to the local HIV infection. Tropical pulmonary eosinophilia due to chronic microfilarial infestation is a subacute ILD (see Ch. 437.3) and can evolve into a chronic ILD.

INHALED AGENTS OTHER THAN INORGANIC OR ORGANIC DUSTS. These agents include gases, aerosols, chemical dusts, fumes, and vapors. Most are rare causes of ILD, and there is little information available concerning pathogenesis, clinical course, staging, or therapy. Most are acute disorders that reverse when the agent is removed unless significant injury to the parenchyma has occurred.

The most common gas causing ILD is *oxygen*. The inhalation of high concentrations of oxygen over several days often causes parenchymal lung damage, particularly in the setting of acute respiratory failure in the intensive care situation (see Ch. 70). Oxygen toxicity can also be chronic. In contrast, the inhalation of gases such as the oxides of nitrogen, chlorine gas, and sulfur dioxide almost always cause only acute injury; if the patient survives the initial insult and respiratory failure, there are rarely any sequelae. In contrast, many of the survivors of methyl isocyanate exposure develop chronic fibrosis-type ILD.

Aerosols are particles of liquid suspended in a gas. The most common examples of ILD due to aerosol inhalation are the acute and chronic ILD resulting from aspiration of gastric contents (see Ch. 528) and the aspiration of mineral oil. Exposure to aerosols of cooking oils, pyrethrum (a neutral insecticide used in commercial and household products), and toluene diisocyanate has also been implicated as a cause of ILD.

ILD due to the inhalation of chemical dusts such as synthetic fibers, Bakelite, and vinyl chloride and polyvinyl chloride powder are probably hypersensitivity-type disorders similar to those associated with the repeated inhalation of organic dusts from living sources. Little is known about the clinical course of these disorders. ILD have also followed the inhalation of various fumes and vapors (see Table 60–5).

Cooper JAD, Jr (ed.): Drug-induced pulmonary disease. Clin Chest Med 2:1, 1990. *Details the pathogenesis and clinical findings in all of the drug-induced interstitial lung disorders.*

Crystal RG, Ferrans VJ: Reactions of the interstitial space to injury. *In* Fishman AP: Pulmonary Diseases and Disorders. New York, McGraw-Hill, 1988, pp 711–738. *General concepts of the processes that derange the alveolar walls.*

Crystal RG, Bitterman PB, Rennard SI, et al.: Interstitial lung diseases of unknown cause: Disorders characterized by chronic inflammation of the lower respiratory tract. N Engl J Med 310:154, 235, 1984. *A general review of the interstitial lung disorders of unknown etiology.*

Crystal RG, Ferrans VJ, Basset F: Biologic basis of pulmonary fibrosis. *In* Crystal RG, West JB (eds.): The Lung. Scientific Foundations. New York, Raven Press, 1991, pp 2031–2046. *Overview of the concepts underlying the development of fibrosis in the interstitial lung disorders.*

Crystal RG, Gadek JE, Ferrans VJ, et al.: Interstitial lung disease: Current concepts of pathogenesis, staging, and therapy. Am J Med 70:542, 1981. *Overviews the concepts of the pathogenesis of the interstitial lung disorders and emphasizes the approaches to staging and therapy.*

Davis WB, Crystal RG: Chronic interstitial lung disease. *In* Simmons DH (ed.): Current Pulmonology. Vol. V. New York, John Wiley and Sons, 1984, pp 347–473. *Reviews each of the interstitial lung disorders.*

DuBois R, Saltini C, Holroyd K, et al.: Granulomatous processes. *In* Crystal RG, West JB (eds.): The Lung. Scientific Foundations. New York, Raven Press, 1991, pp 1925–1938. *General concepts of granulomatous disorders of the lung.*

Keogh BA, Crystal RG: Alveolitis: The key to the interstitial lung disorders. Thorax 37:1, 1982. *Summarizes the importance of alveolitis in the interstitial disorders.*

Morgan WKC, Seaton A: Occupational Lung Diseases. 2nd ed. Philadelphia, W. B. Saunders Company, 1984. *Overall summary of the interstitial lung disorders resulting from the inhalation of inorganic dusts.*

Rom R, Crystal RG: Consequences of chronic particulate exposure. *In* Crystal RG, West JB (eds.): The Lung. Scientific Foundations. New York, Raven Press, 1991, pp 1885–1898. *Recent review of the pathogenesis of the common pneumoconioses.*

Schwarz MI, King TE (eds.): Interstitial Lung Disease. Toronto, B. C. Decker, 1988. *General review of interstitial lung disease.*

61 Introduction to Pneumonia

Waldemar G. Johanson, Jr.

Pneumonia is a term used to indicate inflammation of the distal lung—terminal airways, alveolar spaces, and interstitium. To improve the precision of communication, the term "pneumonia" is usually further qualified with words that imply an etiology, mechanism, anatomic site, or clinical course. Thus, descriptors such as "viral bronchopneumonia," "aspiration pneumonia," "chronic interstitial pneumonia," or "acute bacterial pneumonia" serve to identify patients with clinical illnesses characterized by signs and symptoms of lung inflammation in a variety of clinical situations. This chapter will provide the background for the chapters that deal with specific forms of bacterial pneumonia (see Part XIX).

PATHOPHYSIOLOGY. Bacterial pneumonia can be simply defined as a condition that results when host defense mechanisms are insufficient to meet a bacterial challenge presented to the lungs. This definition emphasizes the two key aspects of bacterial pneumonia—host defenses and the type and route of bacterial challenge.

Bacterial Challenges to the Lungs. Bacteria may be introduced into the lungs by any of four routes (Table 61–1). The most common routes are aspiration of contaminated oropharyngeal secretions and inhalation of airborne bacteria. Organisms arriving in the lungs via the bloodstream may produce pneumonia, but the originating site of infection and the severe systemic effects of sepsis usually outweigh the importance of the resulting pneumonia. Direct extension from a focus of infection adjacent to the lungs is uncommon, and the initial site of infection is always more important.

Aspiration of contaminated oropharyngeal secretions is by far the most common route of lung inoculation leading to pneumonia. Organisms transmitted from person to person are usually deposited in the nose or mouth by one means or another, including the inhalation of large droplets generated by cough, sneeze, or even talking. These organisms initially establish themselves in the nasopharynx or oropharynx, where they join the plethora of organisms already present and multiply to achieve high local concentrations. They gain entry into the lungs in a bolus of secretions in the company of other organisms. Aspiration of large amounts of oropharyngeal secretions occurs regularly in individuals with impaired levels of consciousness, but aspiration of small volumes of secretions occurs regularly, at least during sleep, in normal people as well. The concentration of aerobic bacteria in upper respiratory tract secretions is about 10^8 organisms per

TABLE 61–1. ROUTES OF BACTERIAL INOCULATION OF THE LUNGS

Aspiration of contaminated oropharyngeal secretions
Inhalation of airborne bacteria
Bacteremia
Direct extension into the lungs

milliliter, while that of anaerobic organisms is about 10 times greater. Thus, aspiration of even small quantities of oropharyngeal secretions causes inoculation of the lung with an enormous bacterial challenge.

The number of bacteria present in ambient air is small, although some are available for inhalation with each breath. The organisms present are highly selected by environmental conditions, as they must have survived aerosolization, drying, temperature changes, and ultraviolet irradiation. Further, since only a few bacteria will be inhaled with each breath, those that arrive in the lungs must be capable of causing infection with a very small inoculum; this is not true for most pathogenic bacteria. In fact, the inability of investigators in the early twentieth century to produce pneumonia in experimental animals by exposing them to massive numbers of aerosolized bacteria nearly halted research on the airborne transmission of disease. Subsequently it was learned that a few organisms meet all of the criteria listed above and are often transmitted by the airborne route. *Mycobacterium tuberculosis* was one of the first to be identified. The infective dose may be as low as a single organism, most often resulting in only a positive skin test as the evidence of infection. Many viruses are transmitted by this route as well. However, the list of bacteria capable of transmission by this route is short and includes only organisms that are unusually invasive, such as the plague bacillus, and organisms particularly adapted to certain environments, such as *Legionella*, so that they are present in large numbers in the air in confined spaces, such as buildings served by contaminated air conditioning systems. Organisms capable of airborne transmission often produce outbreaks of infection when groups of susceptible people are exposed, a striking characteristic of *Legionella* infections, for example.

Host Defenses. A variety of mechanisms defend the host against bacterial invasion of the respiratory tract. Some of them should be evident from the discussion above. The anatomy of the upper air passages is an important aspect of defense against inhaled particulates, including bacteria. Droplets that exceed 10 μ in diameter are deposited by inertial impaction in the upper airways, a process that is promoted by the angulations of these structures. About 90 per cent of particles 5 to 10 μ in diameter are deposited along the tracheobronchial tree, while only those particles that are 0.5 to 3 μ in diameter tend to be deposited in the alveoli. Smaller particles tend to behave like gas molecules and are exhaled to a large extent. "Droplet nuclei" is the term applied to particles about 1 to 3 μ in diameter containing a single bacterium, the likely infecting unit for organisms transmitted by the airborne route.

Organisms that are deposited in the upper air passages are immediately exposed to local secretions. The antibacterial capacity of normal respiratory secretions has been investigated for many years without a firm conclusion. There is little doubt that an antibacterial effect can be demonstrated under various experimental conditions or in vitro. These effects have been attributed to a variety of factors, including lysozyme, complement, immunoglobulins, and products of resident bacteria. The biologic significance of these factors remains uncertain, however. Of much greater significance is the process of physical removal effected by the movement of secretions toward the esophagus and ultimate swallowing.

To avoid physical removal, newly arrived bacteria must persist in the upper air passages. This is facilitated by adherence of bacteria to the regional epithelium. Normal mucosal cells of the upper respiratory tract contain cell-surface receptors for a variety of bacteria. The chemical nature of receptors for different species of bacteria is highly variable, and the site of the receptor may be either an integral part of the cell surface or contained in proteins attached to the cell. For example, *Streptococcus pyogenes* binds to fibronectin, a protein that is not an integral constituent of the cell membrane but is acquired normally by respiratory mucosal cells following exposure to respiratory secretions. By contrast, gram-negative bacilli such as *Escherichia coli* or *Pseudomonas aeruginosa* adhere in large numbers to respiratory cells only after the surface fibronectin is removed. While many details of bacteria–host cell adherence remain to be defined, it is clear that this phenomenon is a major determinant of the composition of the normal bacterial flora of the oropharynx and that changes in

adherence are important in promoting or inhibiting colonization of this region by exogenous bacteria.

Under ideal conditions aspiration of oropharyngeal secretions is prevented by the normal swallowing mechanisms and the presence of reflexes that close the vocal cords when foreign materials enter the larynx. The latter are highly effective in preventing the aspiration of large volumes of fluid in normal persons but apparently do not prevent the aspiration of small volumes, at least during sleep. In view of the high concentration of bacteria in oropharyngeal secretions, aspiration of even 0.0001 ml may be important in initiating pneumonia, depending upon the nature of the bacteria aspirated and the state of lung defenses. Aspiration of such volumes may be an everyday occurrence in normal people and the infrequence of pneumonia may be due principally to lung defenses.

The first line of defense against bacteria that have gained entry into the lungs is physical removal from the airways. This is accomplished by the mucociliary escalator, an integrated multifaceted system consisting of the ciliated cells lining the airways, the secretory cells (goblet cells and submucosal glands), and the secretions. Propulsion of secretions toward the mouth is provided by cilia beating at the incredible rate of 1200 times per minute. However, the effectiveness of this activity depends on the perpendicular depth and the viscosity of secretions. The perpendicular depth of secretions within the airways appears to be relatively constant. This is somewhat puzzling when one considers the total cross-sectional area of the airways, which becomes markedly smaller as the numerous peripheral airways converge on the fewer central bronchi and ultimately on the trachea alone. Mucus moves twice as rapidly in the trachea as in small bronchi, but the difference in area is much greater, a finding that has led to speculation that fluid in secretions must be resorbed in proximal airways to maintain the perpendicular depth of the mucous layer in a range compatible with the length of the cilia. Obviously, processes that impair ciliary movement, cause excessive secretion of respiratory mucus, or change the viscosity of secretions may each hinder the effectiveness of this transport system.

Bacteria that penetrate to the distal airways or alveoli are killed in situ prior to physical transport out of the lung. The principal mechanism of bacterial killing is ingestion and killing by phagocytic cells. The quantitative aspects of this phenomenon have been extensively investigated in experimental animals, using a variety of bacterial species. The initial experiments were performed with relatively nonpathogenic staphylococci, and the results indicated that the antibacterial capacity of the lung is enormous and that phagocytosis and killing are accomplished almost solely by resident alveolar macrophages. This finding fits nicely with the concept that the lung is normally sterile and that polymorphonuclear leukocytes constitute a very small proportion of the total phagocytic cells on the alveolar surface. Further, these experiments indicated that neither antibody nor other humoral components are required for phagocytosis of bacteria on the alveolar surface. Subsequent experiments with more highly pathogenic bacteria showed that the situation is more complicated; some species cause a prompt recruitment of neutrophils, and in fact, bacterial killing appears to depend much more upon the availability of neutrophils than on the presence of alveolar macrophages. Further, clearance of viable bacteria from the lung is enhanced by the presence of specific antibody and is delayed in the absence of complement, findings that indicate an important role for circulating factors.

In general, bacterial killing is more efficient following aerosol deposition than following deposition of a fluid bolus containing equal numbers of bacteria. The reasons for this difference are not entirely clear but probably have to do with the local concentration of bacteria; changes induced in the organisms by the process of aerosolization, e.g., loss of capsular material; and the antiphagocytic effects of the fluid bolus in which the bacteria are suspended.

If bacteria on the alveolar surface are not promptly engulfed and killed, an inflammatory response swiftly develops that is characterized by interstitial and alveolar edema and an influx of neutrophils from the vascular space. The chemoattractants responsible for the latter may include bacterial products, activation of complement proteins that are present in small concentration in alveolar lining fluid, and the elaboration of neutrophil chemotactic factors by alveolar macrophages. In any case, once alveolar edema and inflammation are initiated, the process of bacterial ingestion and killing is remarkably retarded. As neutrophils and bacteria accumulate, the local milieu becomes acidic and hypoxic, since ventilation is impaired by alveolar filling. These conditions further impair phagocyte function, so that a population of viable organisms persists, albeit with a reduced rate of multiplication.

In the preantibiotic era, patients with pneumonia often improved dramatically on about the seventh day of illness with a sudden loss of fever, a process that was termed the "crisis" or "breaking of the fever." This event correlated with the development of antibody, which interrupted the standoff between bacteria and phagocytes in the consolidated regions of lung. This clinical phenomenon rarely occurs with antibiotic treatment because the drugs assist in bacterial killing. However, many antibiotics penetrate lung tissue poorly, and treatment must be relatively prolonged.

Community-acquired pneumonias are usually due to a single organism, an observation that appears to contradict the aspiration mechanism that necessarily includes multiple species. The susceptibility of individual bacterial species to lung defenses varies widely. While mucociliary transport is presumably equally effective for all bacteria, phagocytosis by the resident alveolar macrophages clearly is not. Further, previous exposure or immunization may have led to the development of antibody against some species, a factor that promotes phagocytosis and killing by neutrophils. The result of these differences is that the lung's defenses select the organism (or organisms) that will go on to cause pneumonia—the species most capable of evading phagocytosis and killing.

A number of conditions are clinically associated with an increased risk of bacterial pneumonia. Many of these have been confirmed in studies of experimental animals in attempts to relate susceptibility to pneumonia to specific defects in one or another of the lung's defenses (Table 61–2).

CLINICAL MANIFESTATIONS. The signs and symptoms associated with bacterial pneumonia vary widely, depending on several factors, most importantly the nature of the offending pathogen and the state of the host. Extremes in presentation can be easily described, although most patients will fall somewhere between. At one extreme is the previously healthy person with pneumococcal pneumonia. Such patients complain of a brief prodromal upper respiratory illness followed by fever, a single shaking chill, pleuritic chest pain, and a cough productive of purulent or "rusty" sputum. Physical examination reveals signs of consolidation, which are readily confirmed by chest radiography. Gram's stain of the sputum reveals numerous neutrophils and abundant pneumococci. In such a patient there is no doubt that a lower respiratory tract infection is present, and the stain of the sputum strongly suggests the etiology. At the other extreme might be an elderly, confused patient who presents only with deterioration in mental function. Physical examination reveals only rhonchi without signs of consolidation, and the chest radiograph shows only bilateral lower lobe interstitial infiltrates that might represent acute or chronic changes. Gram's stain of the sputum (obtained with difficulty) shows many squamous epithelial cells, a few neutrophils, and a pleomorphic bacterial flora that includes both gram-positive and gram-negative organisms. In such patients it may not be clear whether or not the patient has pneumonia, and the information at hand offers few clues regarding etiology.

The history-taker should explore the presence of risk factors, including chronic illnesses, recent acute illnesses, illness in family

members, use of alcohol or other drugs, and possible exposures to infectious agents. A thorough physical examination, postero-anterior and lateral chest radiographs, and blood leukocyte count with differential should be performed. On the basis of the data available from these steps, it is usually possible to conclude that pneumonia is present. The remaining task is to determine its etiology.

Controversy exists over the proper microbiologic evaluation of the patient with pneumonia because of questions of sensitivity, specificity, cost, and benefit. These problems are created basically by the presence of abundant organisms in the upper tract and the resultant contamination of expectorated specimens. Further, since most patients with pneumonia respond satisfactorily to simple, relatively nontoxic antibiotic regimens, the need to document the etiology of the process is uncertain. It is impossible to define rules that apply to all patients, and knowledgeable physicians will differ in their approach to an individual patient.

There is little disagreement that sputum should be examined microscopically. The portion chosen should be purulent and contain fewer than 10 squamous cells and more than 25 leukocytes per low-power field. A well-done Gram stain will disclose whether or not one species of organism predominates. Often, such specimens contain a vast preponderance of a single species, and if these are encapsulated gram-positive diplococci (pneumococci), clumps of large gram-positive cocci (staphylococci), or small pleomorphic gram-negative coccobacilli (*Haemophilus*), a presumptive diagnosis can be made. Problems arise when a predominant organism is less apparent, when enteric gram-negative bacilli are present, or when an adequate specimen cannot be obtained. Special stains for acid-fast organisms, fungi, *Legionella*, *Pneumocystis carinii*, and others should be used selectively when the clinical situation suggests infection with one of these organisms.

Aerobic culture of expectorated sputum suffers from a lack of sensitivity (organisms causing pneumonia are not detected) and specificity (organisms are present that are not the cause of pneumonia); both have been estimated to occur in up to 50 per cent of cases. The results may be improved by microscopic screening of the specimen prior to culture. Other approaches have included washing the specimen repeatedly to remove contamination by oral secretions and using quantitative culture techniques on the assumption that the organism causing pneumonia will be present in the greatest concentration. While both of these techniques have merit, the time and effort required to perform them preclude their use as a routine part of the evaluation of a sputum specimen.

Contamination of sputum by oral secretions may be avoided by collecting the specimen proximal to the mouth. The most direct approach involves puncture of the trachea with a large-bore needle and insertion of a plastic cannula into the trachea, a technique called transtracheal aspiration. If secretions cannot be harvested by suction, a small amount of sterile saline is injected through the cannula and suction is reapplied. In the hands of experienced operators, this technique provides better results than sputum examination in some situations. It is most useful in documenting the absence of bacteria in the secretions of individuals with nonbacterial (e.g., viral, mycoplasmal, and so on) pneumonias, but these pneumonias can usually be strongly suspected on clinical grounds alone. In patients in whom an accurate bacteriologic diagnosis is urgently required, such as elderly or immunocompromised patients, contamination of tracheal secretions by aspirated oropharyngeal secretions renders the technique of less value. Absolute contraindications to transtracheal aspiration include abnormal bleeding or clotting values and an uncooperative patient. The major complications are bleeding and the occurrence of barotrauma, usually manifested as subcutaneous emphysema in the neck only. Because of the risk of bleeding, the procedure should not be performed in patients with a small trachea (children) or in those with a markedly impaired cough who may not be able to expectorate blood effectively. Transtracheal aspiration remains an excellent method for identifying anaerobic bacteria as responsible for pleuropulmonary infections, if this diagnosis cannot be made by other means.

Another method for bypassing the mouth in the collection of

TABLE 61–2. CONDITIONS ASSOCIATED WITH INCREASED RISK OF BACTERIAL PNEUMONIA

Condition	Impaired Defense Mechanism
Chronic airway obstruction	Reduced mucociliary transport
	Alveolar hypoxia
Pulmonary edema	Reduced phagocyte function
Unconsciousness	Increased aspiration
Immunoglobulin deficiency	Impaired phagocytosis
Neutropenia	Impaired phagocytosis
Viral infection	Altered mucosal adherence
	Reduced mucociliary transport
	Impaired phagocytosis

specimens is to aspirate directly from the area of lung consolidation, using either physical findings or fluoroscopy to guide the approach. This technique, called transthoracic lung aspiration, has proved to be an excellent technique in children with complicated pneumonias, since sputum samples may be impossible to obtain. In adults, especially those with underlying lung disease, the rate of complications, particularly pneumothorax and bleeding, limits its usefulness. This direct approach is further compromised by the fact that the false-negative rate may be as high as 30 per cent.

Fiberoptic bronchoscopy provides a relatively safe way to collect specimens from the periphery of the lung. Specially designed protected brushes are available that permit the operator to obtain endobronchial specimens that have not been contaminated by proximal airway secretions, even though the instrument has traversed the upper airways. Complications of the procedure are infrequent, and the major limiting factors are expense and time. In addition to the small specimens collected by brushing of the peripheral airways, sterile fluid can be instilled and aspirated to obtain material from a larger area of the lung (bronchoalveolar lavage).

Immunologic techniques, such as immunofluorescence, enzyme-linked immunoassay, and DNA hybridization, hold great promise for determining the cause of pneumonia. However, compared with conventional cultures, these techniques are expensive and relatively insensitive. They detect the presence of only a narrow spectrum of related organisms. Because of this specificity, they have a limited role in the evaluation of patients with pneumonia and should be considered only when specific organisms are strongly suspected on clinical grounds.

Last, it must be remembered that cultures of the blood and pleural fluid, if positive, provide results that are highly specific. However, only about 30 per cent of patients with bacterial pneumonia are bacteremic. About the same percentage of pleural fluid aspirates are positive in the absence of antibiotic therapy, but since only 10 to 15 per cent of patients with pneumonia have a pleural effusion, the applicability of this approach is limited. Nevertheless, blood cultures should be obtained in patients with serious illness due to pneumonia, and a diagnostic thoracentesis should be performed in patients with effusions large enough to be aspirated safely.

Proper utilization of these techniques must be individually determined for each patient with pneumonia. In many patients, the history, physical examination, radiographic studies, and evaluation of the sputum by Gram's stain provide all the data that might be reasonably required. Additional procedures should be reserved for those patients in whom a delay in making an accurate diagnosis will have serious consequences or those in whom the diagnosis cannot be reasonably suspected on the basis of simpler approaches.

RADIOGRAPHIC PATTERNS. Careful examination of posteroanterior (PA) and lateral chest radiographs is an invaluable adjunct in the diagnosis of pneumonia and should be part of the evaluation of every patient in whom significant respiratory infection is suspected. While a specific microbiologic diagnosis is seldom, if ever, possible on the basis of radiographic data alone, important clues to the etiology of pneumonia and its distribution and severity may be gained by this technique. Pathogens frequently associated with particular radiographic patterns are summarized in Table 61–3.

The presence of shadows corresponding to pulmonary lobes or segments (lobar or segmental infiltrates) should strongly suggest a bacterial etiology for pneumonia. Such lobar pneumonia is most commonly caused by one of the aerobic pathogens, such as *Streptococcus pneumoniae*, *H. influenzae*, or *Klebsiella pneumoniae*. These infections may be confined to a single lobe or segment or may involve multiple areas of the lung. Radiographically, the infiltrates are usually dense and homogeneous, frequently with obscuration of the borders between adjacent structures (e.g., heart borders or diaphragm). This obliteration of mutual radiographic borders is often termed the "silhouette sign" and is very useful in the localization of densities within the lung parenchyma.

Less well defined and inhomogeneous radiographic densities, often described as "patchy" or "streaky" infiltrates, are commonly observed in bronchopneumonia, a pattern of infection involving

TABLE 61–3. COMMON RADIOGRAPHIC PATTERNS OF PNEUMONIA AND ASSOCIATED PATHOGENS

Pattern	Pathogen
Lobar or segmental infiltrates	*Streptococcus pneumoniae*, *Haemophilus influenzae*, *Klebsiella pneumoniae*, *Escherichia coli*, *Legionella* species
Inhomogeneous infiltrates (patchy or streaky opacities)	*Mycoplasma pneumoniae*, viruses, mixed aerobic/anaerobic organisms (e.g., aspiration), *Legionella* species
Diffuse homogeneous infiltrates	*Legionella* species, viruses, *Pneumocystis carinii*
Nodular opacities	Mycobacterial species, *Aspergillus*, *Candida*, organisms involved in hematogenous spread of infection
Cavitary infiltrates	*Staphylococcus aureus*, gram-negative organisms, anaerobes, *Mycobacterium tuberculosis*, *Aspergillus*

airways rather than lobes and segments. This radiographic pattern may be seen in infections caused by a wide variety of organisms, including bacteria and viruses, and may occur in virtually any clinical setting, including aspiration of oropharyngeal contents by debilitated individuals and the relatively mild pneumonia caused by *Mycoplasma pneumoniae* in otherwise healthy, ambulatory adults.

Diffuse pulmonary infiltrates are less commonly caused by the typical aerobic or anaerobic pathogens associated with lobar pneumonia or bronchopneumonia. This pattern may be indicative of infection with viruses (such as cytomegalovirus or influenza), *Legionella pneumophila*, or opportunistic pathogens such as *P. carinii*. In addition to infection, diffuse homogeneous infiltrates may also be due to pulmonary edema, lung hemorrhage, interstitial lung disease, or the lung injury associated with the adult respiratory distress syndrome (ARDS), making the differential diagnosis of this radiographic pattern particularly complicated. For this reason, the detection of infection superimposed on other forms of lung pathology may be especially difficult and often requires the use of specialized diagnostic techniques, such as bronchoscopy or open lung biopsy.

Important information can be derived not only from the size and shape of the radiographic density but also from its character. In this regard, cavitary shadows generally suggest the presence of a necrotizing infection, with associated destruction of lung tissue. Organisms that frequently produce this radiographic picture include *Staphylococcus aureus*, gram-negative bacteria, mixed anaerobic organisms (such as those associated with aspiration of oropharyngeal contents), *Aspergillus* species, and *Mycobacterium tuberculosis*. Less commonly, nonnecrotizing infection occurring in an area of lung containing cysts or bullae may have a cavitary appearance on the radiograph in the absence of frank lung destruction.

Pulmonary infection may be associated with the appearance of nodular lesions on the chest radiograph. These nodular shadows can range widely in size, from the miliary (<2 mm) lesions of tuberculosis to the large cavitating lesions of septic embolization to the lung. In general, however, disseminated nodular lesions suggest the presence of infection borne to the lung from another source via the bloodstream. Consideration must be given to primary sites of infection, such as endocarditis of the valves of the right side of the heart and septic thrombophlebitis. In patients with unexplained fever despite prolonged courses of antibiotics, fungal infection (e.g., *Candida albicans*) should be considered.

The chest radiograph may also yield valuable information about infectious involvement of structures outside the parenchyma of the lung, including the pleural surface and thoracic lymph nodes. Pleural effusions occur in a wide variety of respiratory infections, including bacterial, viral, fungal, and mycobacterial illnesses. Lateral decubitus radiographs are helpful in documenting the presence of free pleural fluid, and thoracentesis is frequently necessary to distinguish transudative and uncomplicated parapneumonic effusions from complicated parapneumonic effusions or empyema, which may require drainage (see Ch. 62 and 69). Needle pleural biopsy may be useful in the diagnosis of granulomatous infections involving the pleura.

Enlargement of mediastinal and hilar lymph nodes is uncommon in acute bacterial infection of the lung. When present in association with pneumonia, this finding should suggest infection by fungal pathogens or mycobacteria, or an underlying malignancy.

Loss of volume of a pulmonary segment or lobe (partial or complete atelectasis) should raise suspicion regarding an endobronchial lesion obstructing a large airway, with associated infection in the obstructed segment. Such lesions may include bronchogenic carcinoma, foreign body, or mucous plug.

Green GM, Jakab GJ, Low RB, et al.: Defense mechanisms of the respiratory membrane. Am Rev Respir Dis 115:479, 1977. *Still the best, most comprehensive review of lung defense mechanisms.*

Onofrio JM, Toews GB, Lipscomb MF, et al.: Granulocyte-alveolar-macrophage interaction in the pulmonary clearance of *Staphylococcus aureus*. Am Rev Respir Dis 127:335, 1983. *Illustrates how the lung defenses vary in response to differing bacterial challenges.*

Palmer DL, Jones CC: Diagnosis of pneumococcal pneumonia. Semin Respir Infect 3:131, 1988. *A thoughtful review of the usefulness of immunologic studies in diagnosing pneumococcal infections.*

Van Uffelen R, van Saene HKF, Fidler V, et al.: Oropharyngeal flora as a source of bacteria colonizing the lower airways in patients on artificial ventilation. Intensive Care Med 10:233, 1984. *Demonstrates the progression from oropharyngeal colonization to colonization of distal airways to bacterial pneumonia.*

Wanner A: Clinical aspects of mucociliary transport. Am Rev Respir Dis 116:78, 1977. *An excellent, complete review of the mucociliary system.*

62 Lung Abscess

John G. Bartlett

DEFINITION. Lung abscess literally means a collection of pus within a destroyed portion of the lung; thus there are numerous possible causes of such a lesion (Table 62–1). As used clinically, however, the term "lung abscess" refers to a pulmonary infection with parenchymal necrosis, generally caused by bacteria other than mycobacteria. Lung abscesses are usually solitary, but occasionally multiple discrete lesions are observed. Numerous small abscesses confined to a given region of the lung are sometimes referred to as "necrotizing pneumonia." Because they share a common pathogenesis, there is considerable overlap among aspiration pneumonia, lung abscess, and necrotizing pneumonia, and each of these may lead to and coexist with an empyema (a collection of pus within the pleural space).

ETIOLOGY. As indicated in Table 62–1, many different underlying processes can lead to the formation of a lung abscess. By far the most important are necrotizing pulmonary infections, and, of these, anaerobic bacteria are responsible for the majority.

TABLE 62–1. DIFFERENTIAL DIAGNOSIS OF A CAVITARY LESION IN THE LUNG

Necrotizing infections
  Bacteria: Anaerobic bacteria, *Staphylococcus aureus*, enteric gram-negative bacteria, *Pseudomonas aeruginosa*, *Legionella*, *Streptococcus pyogenes*, *Hemophilus influenzae*, *Pseudomonas pseudomallei*, *Actinomyces*, *Nocardia*, *Streptococcus pneumoniae* (?)
  Mycobacteria: *Mycobacterium tuberculosis*, *M. kansasii*, *M. avium-intracellulare*
  Fungi: *Coccidioides immitis*, *Histoplasma capsulatum*, *Blastomyces hominis*, *Cryptococcus neoformans*, *Aspergillus*, *Phycomycetes* (*Mucor*)
  Parasites: *Entamoeba histolytica*, *Paragonimus westermani*
  Septic embolism: *S. aureus*, anaerobes, and so on

Cavitary infarction
  Bland infarction (with or without superimposed infection)
  Vasculitis: Wegener's granulomatosis, periarteritis

Neoplasms
  Bronchogenic carcinoma, metastatic carcinoma, lymphoma (with or without superimposed infection)

Miscellaneous lesions
  Cysts or bullae with fluid collections, sequestration

These organisms account for essentially all "putrid" lung abscesses and nearly all that have been classified as "nonspecific" or "primary." Most of these infections involve multiple bacterial species, which may include aerobic organisms. The dominant bacteria are *Fusobacterium nucleatum*, *Bacteroides melaninogenicus*, *B. intermedius*, peptostreptococcus, aerobic streptococci, and microaerophilic streptococci.

Pneumonia, particularly cases caused by *Staphylococcus aureus* and *Klebsiella pneumoniae*, may also be complicated by abscess formation. Less frequent but well-documented agents of lung abscess include *Streptococcus pyogenes* (group A beta-hemolytic streptococci), *Streptococcus pneumoniae* (especially type 3), *Streptococcus milleri*, *Haemophilus influenzae* (type B), *Pseudomonas aeruginosa*, *Pseudomonas pseudomallei* (melioidosis), *Actinomyces* (actinomycosis), *Legionella*, *Nocardia*, *Paragonimus westermani* (lung fluke), and *Entamoeba histolytica* (amebiasis). Enteric gram-negative bacilli other than *K. pneumoniae* may cause lung abscess, but this occurs almost exclusively in debilitated patients with severe associated medical-surgical conditions. Necrotizing alveolitis is a separate entity diagnosed by microscopic examination and usually caused by *P. aeruginosa*; sometimes these microabscesses coalesce to form radiographically detectable cavities.

INCIDENCE AND PREVALENCE. The incidence of primary lung abscess has decreased substantially since the prechemotherapeutic era. Nevertheless, most large academic centers encounter 10 to 30 cases annually.

EPIDEMIOLOGY. Most lung abscesses, and nearly all involving anaerobic bacteria, involve the normal flora of the oropharynx. Abscesses involving *S. aureus* or gram-negative bacilli are more likely to be nosocomial in origin. Amebic lung abscess results from the direct extension of an hepatic abscess through the diaphragm into the lung. *Nocardia* causes lung abscess almost exclusively in immunocompromised hosts, especially in recipients of corticosteroids. Septic pulmonary emboli commonly lead to multiple solitary abscesses in noncontiguous sites and are usually caused by *S. aureus*, anaerobic bacteria, or *P. aeruginosa*; hematogenous abscesses are most often found in intravenous drug abusers with tricuspid valve endocarditis and patients with septic thrombophlebitis. Lung abscesses due to *P. westermani* and melioidosis are usually acquired in the Far East or Indonesia.

PATHOGENESIS. The formation of an anaerobic lung abscess nearly always involves two coexisting abnormalities: (1) periodontal infection, such as gingivitis or pyorrhea, which provides the inoculum; and (2) aspiration, which provides access to the lung parenchyma. The usual causes for aspiration are those that compromise consciousness and the gag reflex, such as alcoholism, drug addiction, general anesthesia, seizure disorder, sedative use, or neurologic disorders. Other factors predisposing to aspiration include dysphagia resulting from esophageal disorders or neurologic deficits; disruption of the usual mechanical barriers, as with nasogastric intubation, tracheostomy, or nasogastric feeding tubes; or pharyngeal anesthesia, as seen with dental procedures or surgery involving the upper airway. Most healthy persons periodically aspirate small inocula from the upper airways, but these are readily cleared by the normal cough reflex and other pulmonary defense mechanisms without deleterious consequences. Patients who develop aspiration pneumonia and lung abscesses presumably do so because of the relatively large inocula of bacteria and failure of the usual protective mechanisms.

The initial lesion is pneumonitis, or "aspiration pneumonia," which typically involves dependent pulmonary segments, e.g., those favored by gravitational flow. The dependent pulmonary segments in patients who aspirate in the recumbent position are the superior segments of the lower lobes or posterior segments of the upper lobes. Aspiration in the upright or semi-upright position favors involvement of the basilar segments of the lower lobes. Patients who have a defined period of known or probable aspiration demonstrate with sequential radiographs that 7 to 14 days are usually required for the appearance of a typical air-fluid level on chest radiograph.

CLINICAL MANIFESTATIONS. Patients with anaerobic abscesses tend to have indolent symptomatology with medical complaints dating for 2 or more weeks before presentation. The usual symptoms are fever, malaise, cough, sputum production, and pleuritic pain. The frequent observation of weight loss and anemia provides testimony to the chronicity of the infection. There may be "chilliness," but frank rigors are rare, and their presence suggests organisms other than anaerobes. The cough often becomes more productive at the time of cavitation, and it is at this time that the patient is most likely to note the onset of putrid sputum, which is considered diagnostic of anaerobic infection. Putrid sputum is found in 60 per cent of patients with a confirmed anaerobic etiology. Many patients will also note that the sputum has an unusually noxious taste. Most patients have a history of compromised consciousness or other risk factors for aspiration, and many have periodontal infection. Nevertheless, about 10 per cent of patients with anaerobic lung abscesses have no identifiable predisposing condition. Occasional patients with anaerobic lung abscesses are edentulous; the incidence of underlying bronchogenic neoplasms seems particularly high in this group. Patients with lung abscesses due to S. aureus, gram-negative bacilli, and amebae usually have a more fulminant course, with the precipitous onset of symptoms. Other features that may be noted in this group include chills, the lack of putrid discharge, and the absence of the usual associated findings. The physical findings in the early phases of disease are those of pneumonia, with or without a pleural effusion. At a later stage there may be amphoric or cavernous breath sounds, pleural effusions are common, and approximately 25 per cent of patients have an associated empyema.

DIAGNOSIS. The diagnosis of lung abscess is usually established on the basis of a chest radiograph showing a parenchymal infiltrate with a cavity containing an air-fluid level (Fig. 62–1). The differential diagnosis of this roentgenographic finding is included in Table 62–1. Certain roentgenographic features may provide clues to the presence of an infected cyst, bulla, or sequestration. Massive pulmonary fibrosis with necrosis from occupational exposure is usually distinctive. A loculated empyema with an air-fluid level may be differentiated from lung abscess with computed tomography.

Studies for an etiologic agent are often hampered by the limitations of bacteriologic analysis of expectorated sputum. These specimens are useful in detecting mycobacteria, pathogenic fungi, and parasites, and they may be used for cytologic studies. However, routine aerobic cultures often give erroneous results, and they are not valid for meaningful anaerobic culture owing to the universal presence in oral secretions of anaerobes that con-

taminate the specimen during passage through the upper airways. Blood cultures are useful, primarily for patients with infections involving S. aureus or gram-negative bacilli, but most patients with anaerobic abscesses do not have bacteremia. Pleural fluid is a valuable culture source for both aerobic and anaerobic bacteria in any patient with an empyema, so that thoracentesis should be performed before treatment is begun. For most patients with anaerobic pulmonary infections restricted to the pulmonary parenchyma, the preferred specimen source is from a transtracheal aspiration, from a transthoracic needle aspirate, or from a fiberoptic bronchoscopy utilizing a double-lumen catheter with a distal occluding plug, combined with quantitative cultures. Specimen collection prior to institution of antibiotic therapy is preferred. In most cases of anaerobic abscesses, the etiologic agents will not be defined, and the therapeutic regimen will be selected empirically. Bronchoscopy, which used to be performed routinely in patients with lung abscesses, is now usually restricted to patients who fail to respond to antibiotic treatment or who have an atypical clinical presentation. Major concerns are a cavitating neoplasm, an obstructing tumor, or a foreign body.

TREATMENT. The most important facets of the treatment are the administration of appropriate antibiotics and adequate drainage of any associated empyema. Physiotherapy with postural drainage should be utilized when possible; however, this must be done with considerable caution in patients with large lung abscesses because of the possibility of spillage of purulent contents, with extensive involvement of other lobes.

The drugs of choice for the treatment of abscesses caused by aerobic pyogenic microorganisms, Mycobacterium tuberculosis, fungi, and Entamoeba histolytica are reviewed in detail elsewhere in this volume. For aspiration-related lung abscess involving anaerobic bacteria, the three antimicrobial regimens recommended are penicillin, clindamycin, or penicillin plus metronidazole. Penicillin has traditionally been regarded as the favored drug on the basis of its long, well-established track record. There is considerable variation in the dosage recommendations, but most authorities recommend doses of 10 to 20 million units given intravenously per day. This is continued until the patient is afebrile and clinically improved, at which time treatment is changed to intramuscular or oral penicillin using penicillin G, penicillin V, ampicillin, or amoxicillin in doses of 500 to 750 mg three or four times daily. Some authorities suggest an arbitrarily selected total duration of treatment of 3 to 6 weeks, whereas others continue treatment until the chest radiograph changes have cleared or there is only a small, stable residual lesion. The

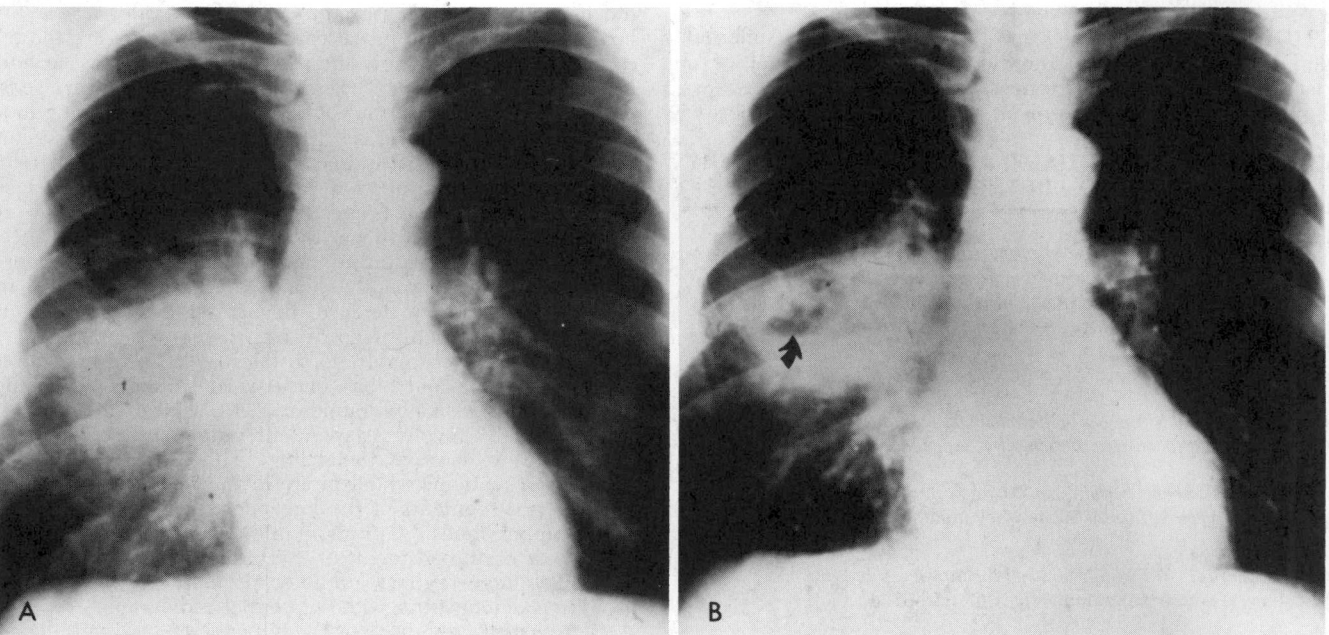

FIGURE 62–1. Chest radiographs of a 55-year-old alcoholic man. The first film (A) shows pneumonitis involving the superior segment of the right lower lobe, a common segment for aspiration pneumonia. The second radiograph (B), taken 1 week later, shows cavitation with an air-fluid level as indicated by the arrow. A transtracheal aspirate yielded F. nucleatum, B. melaninogenicus, and anaerobic streptococci. The final diagnosis was aspiration pneumonia with progression to lung abscess due to anaerobic bacteria.

latter criterion commonly requires 2 to 4 months or longer but may be necessary to prevent relapses.

Clindamycin is active against most penicillin-resistant anaerobes that are found in 20 to 25 per cent of cases, including many or most strains of *B. melaninogenicus*, *B. fragilis*, *B. ruminicola*, and *B. ureolyticus*. Some regard clindamycin as the preferred agent for all lung abscesses due to anaerobic bacteria; others advocate it only for patients who fail to respond to penicillin, have a contraindication to penicillin, or have a serious infection with a fulminant course. The usual regimen is 600 mg given intravenously every 6 to 8 hours until the patient is afebrile and clinically improved, followed by 300 mg orally four times daily. An alternative regimen is penicillin G (above doses) combined with metronidazole (2 gm orally per day in two to four divided doses). Metronidazole is active against nearly all clinically important anaerobes, but penicillin must be added owing to the probable importance of aerobic and microaerophilic streptococci.

The necessity to treat the aerobic components of mixed aerobic-anaerobic infections is controversial, but this is generally advocated for patients who are seriously ill or fail to respond to clindamycin. In such cases, most penicillins are considered equally effective against oral anaerobes, including penicillin G, penicillin V, ampicillin, amoxicillin, ticarcillin, and piperacillin. However, antistaphylococcal penicillins, such as nafcillin or oxacillin, are considered inferior and unacceptable. Cephalosporins are considered nearly equivalent to penicillins in terms of in vitro activity, although the clinical experience is limited. Imipenem and any combination of a betalactam–betalactamase inhibitor are considered almost universally active against clinically important anaerobes. The activity of tetracyclines and erythromycin is variable. Quinolones and trimethoprim-sulfamethoxazole are unacceptable for infections caused by anaerobic bacteria.

Patients with lung abscesses involving *S. aureus* should be treated with a penicillinase-resistant penicillin or a first-generation cephalosporin. Vancomycin is the preferred agent for methicillin-resistant strains of *S. aureus*. This agent or clindamycin may be used for patients with a contraindication to beta-lactam antibiotics. Penicillin G is the preferred agent for infections involving group A beta-hemolytic streptococcal infection. Antibiotic selection for infections involving gram-negative bacilli requires in vitro sensitivity data. This usually consists of an aminoglycoside combined with an expanded-spectrum penicillin, such as ticarcillin for *P. aeruginosa* or a cephalosporin for Enterobacteriaceae. Sulfonamides are preferred agents for *Nocardia* infections.

The expected response to antimicrobial agents is subjective improvement with decreased fever within 3 to 7 days and elimination of fever within 7 to 14 days. The putrid odor of the sputum, when initially present, usually resolves in 3 to 10 days. Delayed response may indicate large cavity size, poor host status, obstruction, erroneous antimicrobial selection, a wrong diagnosis, drug fever, a complicating empyema requiring drainage, or an abscess that requires drainage by physiotherapy, bronchoscopy, or surgery. Radiographic response is delayed; in fact, there is often extension of the infiltrate and increased cavity size or new cavity formation during the first week. Chest radiographs should be followed at 2- to 3-week intervals with the expectation that infiltrates will clear or there will be a small residual scar or a thin-walled cyst.

Bronchoscopy is indicated in patients with an atypical presentation and in those who fail to respond to recommended antimicrobial regimens. The major purpose of the procedure is to differentiate cavitating neoplasms and to detect underlying lesions, such as bronchogenic neoplasms, bronchostenosis, or a foreign body. It may also be used to facilitate drainage.

The major indications for surgery are an uncontrollable or life-threatening hemorrhage, a bronchogenic neoplasm, a bronchial obstruction, or a lung abscess that proves absolutely refractory to medical treatment. Medical failures are rare but are most common in patients with an obstructed bronchus, those with extremely large abscesses, those with abscesses that have been present for an extended period before the institution of treatment, and those with infections involving certain bacteria such as gram-negative bacilli. The usual surgical procedure is lobectomy. Patients with prohibitive operative risks may benefit from percutaneous drainage, but care must be taken to avoid contamination of the pleural space.

PROGNOSIS. The natural course of lung abscesses was best studied in the prechemotherapeutic era. Treatment at that time was nearly equally divided between conservative management using postural drainage and supportive care, and surgery. The mortality rate was about 33 per cent in both groups, and another third of patients developed a chronic debilitating disease or suffered recurrent symptoms. The availability of the Jackson bronchoscope to facilitate drainage had no important bearing on outcome. The technique of resectional surgery was developed at about the time penicillin became available, and the relative merits of these two approaches as the primary therapeutic modality were widely debated. During the past two decades, however, the majority of patients have been treated with antibiotics alone, including those with "delayed closure" (i.e., the persistence of a cavity demonstrated by a chest radiograph at 4 to 6 weeks after the initiation of antibiotic therapy), because most of these cavities eventually resolve if the antibiotics are continued long enough. The mortality rate for aspiration-related lung abscess is currently reported at 5 to 6 per cent. Findings that herald a relatively poor prognosis include (1) large cavity size, particularly cavities greater than 6 cm in diameter; (2) prolonged symptoms prior to presentation, especially symptoms for more than 6 weeks; (3) necrotizing pneumonia characterized by multiple small abscesses in contiguous segments; (4) patients who are elderly, debilitated, or immunologically compromised; (5) abscesses associated with bronchial obstruction; and (6) abscess due to aerobic bacteria, including *S. aureus* and gram-negative bacilli.

PREVENTION. The major preventive measures are factors used to reduce the incidence or magnitude of aspiration, appropriate care of periodontal disease, early treatment of pneumonia, and adequate courses of antimicrobials to prevent relapses.

Bartlett JG: Anaerobic bacterial infections of the lung. Chest 91:6, 1987. *A review of anaerobic pleuropulmonary infections, including 83 cases of lung abscesses with bacteriology, clinical features, and management guidelines.*

Hagan JL, Hardy LD: Lung abscess revisited. A survey of 184 cases. Ann Surg 197:755, 1983. *Update on the surgical point of view concerning lung abscess; 11 per cent were operated on.*

Landay MJ, Christensen EE, Bynum LJ, et al.: Anaerobic pleural and pulmonary infections. AJR 134:233, 1980. *The authors review the roentgenographic features of anaerobic pleuropulmonary infections, including response to antibiotic treatment.*

Levison ME, Mangura CT, Lorber B, et al.: Clindamycin compared to penicillin for the treatment of anaerobic lung abscess. Ann Intern Med 98:466, 1983. *The authors show the superiority of clindamycin versus intravenous penicillin in terms of response rates, relapse rates, and time to defervescence.*

Snow N, Lucas A, Horrigan TP: Utility of pneumonotomy in the treatment of cavitary lung disease. Chest 87:731, 1985. *A description of the procedure and results with percutaneous drainage.*

63 Bronchiectasis

Roger Bone

DEFINITION

The definition of bronchiectasis is primarily an anatomic one, expressed as the *irreversible* dilation of one or more proximal and medium-sized bronchi due to destruction of the muscular and elastic supporting tissues of the bronchial walls. Destruction is generally the result of recurrent or chronic inflammation and intermittent healing with fibrosis. Chronic cough and copious sputum production are nearly universal; dyspnea and orthopnea occur in severe cases.

HISTORICAL PERSPECTIVE AND CURRENT ETIOLOGIES

Before the advent of antibiotics and vaccines, bronchiectasis was a much more significant contributor to patient morbidity and mortality than it is today. Measles, pertussis, tuberculosis, and a variety of childhood respiratory infections commonly set the stage for the development of bronchiectasis. Immunization and aggressive antibiotic therapies have rendered these diseases much less significant precursors to bronchiectasis in the United States; in the developing countries, however, these diseases remain common antecedents.

With immunization and antibiotics also comes the declining absolute incidence of bronchiectasis. Although infection remains a major component in the disease, those cases that do occur are often in patients with one or more predisposing conditions (Table 63–1).

Bronchial Obstruction

Aspiration of foreign bodies (most notably in children), tumors, and occasionally mucus impaction can lead to infection, dilation of bronchi, and subsequent destructive changes. These are generally focal rather than diffuse processes. Bronchiectasis may develop years after aspiration of foreign bodies or inhalational injury. Obstruction, per se, does not appear to cause bronchiectasis but facilitates the condition by interfering with bronchial clearance and thereby encouraging infection.

Congenital or Hereditary Conditions

The cilia of individuals with the immotile cilia syndrome exhibit structural alterations (dynein arms are absent or aberrant) that render them immotile or dyskinetic. The syndrome is probably transmitted as an autosomal recessive trait. Lack of ciliary motility is apparent in several body systems. Men with the condition are infertile, owing to immotile sperm; women have decreased fertility as well. Such patients are prone to the recurrent infections characteristic of bronchiectasis because cilia of the respiratory tract are unable to beat or because they have functional alterations. Mucociliary clearance of bacteria and phagocytic debris is inhibited; chronic sinusitis and bronchiectasis may result.

Patients with Kartagener's syndrome, a subset of the immotile cilia syndrome, may, in addition to bronchiectasis and sinusitis, exhibit situs inversus. It is presumed that situs inversus represents the chance result of embryonic migration of viscera, rather than the normally cilia-dependent placement of internal organs.

Bronchiectasis in patients with cystic fibrosis is a reflection of defects in exocrine gland secretion. In this country, nearly half of the cases of bronchiectasis in children or young adults are attributable to cystic fibrosis. Copious amounts of thickened

TABLE 63–1. PREDISPOSING FACTORS FOR BRONCHIECTASIS

Bronchopulmonary infections	Pertussis, measles; *Staphylococcus aureus*, *Klebsiella*, *Mycobacterium tuberculosis*, *Hæmophilus influenzae*; adenovirus, influenza, herpes simplex; viral bronchiolitis; mycotic (histoplasmosis) or mycoplasmal (?) infection
Bronchial obstruction	Foreign body aspiration; neoplasm; hilar adenopathy (tuberculosis, sarcoidosis); mucoid impaction; chronic obstructive pulmonary disease (COPD; chronic bronchitis, asthma); acquired tracheobronchial disease; amyloidosis
Congenital anatomic defects	Bronchomalacia, bronchial cysts, cartilage deficiency, tracheobronchomegaly, ectopic bronchus, endobronchial teratoma, tracheoesophageal fistula; pulmonary sequestration, pulmonary artery aneurysm; yellow-nail syndrome
Immunodeficiency states	Congenital agammaglobulinemia; acquired immune globulin deficiency; chronic granulomatous disease
Hereditary defects	Ciliary defects (immotile cilia syndrome, ciliary dyskinesia, Kartagener's syndrome); alpha₁-antitrypsin deficiency; cystic fibrosis
Miscellaneous	Young's syndrome; recurrent aspiration pneumonias (alcoholism, neurologic disorders, lipoid pneumonia); irritant inhalation (ammonia, nitrogen dioxide, smoke, talc, silicates, detergents); after heart/lung transplantation (associated with obliterative bronchiolitis)

Adapted from Swartz MN: Bronchiectasis. *In* Fishman AP (ed.): Pulmonary Diseases and Disorders. 2nd ed. New York, McGraw-Hill Book Company, 1988, p 1559; with permission of McGraw-Hill, Inc.

secretions promote the development of infection (for more information, see Ch. 64).

Intralobar sequestration of the lung is a congenital malformation that consists of a detached segment of pulmonary tissue that has a systemic arterial blood supply and that is attached to normal lung and covered by the same pleura. In adults, pneumonia in the sequestered segment may occur. In general, the detached segment has no bronchial attachment to the rest of the lung and, therefore, is not filled with air. With infection, however, connections may become established, allowing progression to bronchiectasis.

Bronchiectasis is also associated with immunodeficiency states; defects in humoral immunity more frequently lead to the disorder than do defects in cellular immunity. Panhypogammaglobulinemia, especially, may lead to bronchiectasis. Such patients have a greatly increased susceptibility to repeated bacterial infections and therefore are at increased risk.

Other Causes

Although no longer common in the United States, bronchiectasis can follow necrotizing pneumonias caused by the tubercle bacillus or staphylococci. Previously, necrotizing pneumonia was not uncommon secondary to measles, pertussis, and influenza. In addition, one third to two thirds of patients with Young's syndrome, a combination of obstructive azospermia and chronic sinopulmonary infections, will develop bronchiectasis. Central bronchiectasis is a finding associated with allergic bronchopulmonary aspergillosis. Brief mention should also be made of the very rare "yellow-nail syndrome"—a combination of lymphedema of the lower extremities, recurrent pneumonia, bronchiectasis, and yellow discoloration of the nails.

PATHOGENESIS AND PATHOLOGY

It is likely that infection and at least some degree of obstruction are necessary for the development of bronchiectasis. Bronchiectatic changes may become irreversible if obstruction persists or if infection produces further bronchial inflammation, destruction, and dilation.

Current views on the pathogenesis of bronchiectasis describe the following scenario. An inhalational or parenteral injury occurs (e.g., corrosive chemical, infectious agent, particulate agent). If the precipitating event is a respiratory infection, it is not necessarily a serious one. Obstruction and stasis occur because secretions, epithelial injury, or a relatively minor obstruction inhibit drainage and clearance and allow infection to continue. The process may be exacerbated in a vulnerable host (one with immunodeficiency, ciliary dysfunction, or reactive airways). Often, the initial insult is unknown; it may be that in the susceptible host repeated cycles of bacterial infection with increasing airway obstruction and destruction develop.

Bronchial dilation predominantly involves medium-sized bronchi but may extend to more distal regions. Bronchi may be dilated to greater than four times their normal size and are often filled with purulent secretions. Peripheral airways in involved regions are often obstructed. In addition, viscous secretions slow mucociliary clearance, and the proteolytic activity of polymorphonuclear leukocytes (of the inflammatory process) contributes to tissue destruction. There is also evidence that purulent secretions themselves are rich in proteases (elastase, collagenase, and cathepsin G) and may be at least partially contributory. The mucosal surface is swollen, inflamed, frequently ulcerated, and sometimes necrotic. Formation of granulation tissue may lead to alterations in the bronchial epithelial lining. This condition is often described as being "polypoid" in appearance—ciliated columnar epithelium is replaced by cuboidal cells or fibrous tissue.

The lower lobes are most frequently involved, the left much more often than the right, presumably because of anatomic differences in drainage attributable to the angle and diameter of more proximal segments. In left lower lobe bronchiectasis, the posterior basal segment is almost always involved, and the apical segment is usually spared.

The radiologic appearance of bronchiectasis can be classified into three types, increasing in severity. In *cylindrical* or *fusiform* bronchiectasis, bronchi are relatively straight and not greatly increased in diameter. Bronchi in *varicose* bronchiectasis are typically dilated and irregular and exhibit bulbous, distorted terminations. The bronchial lumen may be totally obliterated by fibrous tissue; distal portions may become epithelium lined and fluid filled. *Saccular* or *cystic* bronchiectatic segments are dilated, ballooning into pus-filled cavities called saccules as they approach the periphery. These saccules represent totally destroyed and fibrosed segments of the bronchial tree. Larger, more proximal segments may remain relatively unchanged, except for marked inflammation in the bronchial walls and polyposis of bronchial epithelium. The morphology of saccular bronchiectasis is probably attributable to extension of the inflammatory process of the bronchial walls to supporting structures and surrounding lung parenchymal tissue, which are destroyed or fibrosed. Polyposis of bronchial mucosa partially obstructs bronchi proximal to saccular regions, preventing drainage. As a result, these more proximal regions become distended with pus. Squamous metaplasia is common in saccular bronchiectasis but is uncommon in the other types.

Clinical Manifestations and Clinical Course

Today, most clinically significant bronchiectasis originates in early childhood but may not become apparent until much later. Predisposing factors, such as cystic fibrosis, the immotile cilia syndrome, or immunodeficiency states, are usually present.

Cough (sometimes paroxysmal) and sputum production (frequently purulent)—often more severe upon awakening—are observed in 90 per cent of patients. In the preantibiotic era, sputum volumes of as much as 600 ml per day were seen in those with advanced, untreated disease. Fetid sputum and foul breath were also common. Today, these extreme presentations are unlikely; antibiotics and postural drainage have greatly reduced the volume of sputum and have prevented the development of secondary growth of anaerobic bacteria that contributes to such purulence.

Recurrent episodes of infection exacerbate established bronchiectasis. Intercurrent infections may be accompanied by fever, cough, sputum production, and dyspnea. Anorexia and weight loss are associated with multiple bronchiectatic episodes, as is wheezing. Hemoptysis was very common in the past but is not as common today, since the infectious aspect of the disease can be treated. Sinusitis sometimes accompanies bronchiectasis, especially in patients with ciliary defects and immunodeficiency states.

Bronchiectatic patients usually show abnormalities on physical examination. Persistent, medium to coarse, "moist crackles" over involved lobes are most significant. The crackles begin early in inspiration, continue to mid-inspiration, and then fade by the end of inspiration. Diffuse rhonchi and prolonged expiratory phases may also be evident. In patients with extensive disease, dullness and decreased breath sounds may be heard over involved regions. Respiratory expansion may be either increased or decreased. Patients with advanced disease or disease complicated by emphysema may show hyperexpansion, but hyperexpansion is more common in children.

In the preantibiotic era, clubbing and cyanosis were common as the disease progressed (40 per cent of cases). Metastatic abscesses, especially in the brain, were well known. At present, these are all unusual. The incidence of cor pulmonale has also declined dramatically in these patients, except in those with cystic fibrosis and considerable lung destruction. Secondary amyloidosis is rare.

DIAGNOSIS

Since the definition of bronchiectasis is an anatomic one, diagnosis of the disease is based upon demonstration of morphologic alterations in the bronchial tree. Generally, radiologic techniques are used. Patients should also be evaluated for the presence of one of the familial causes of bronchiectasis (Table 63–2)—unless there has been an obvious precipitating event. Bronchiectasis should be suspected in any patient presenting with chronic productive cough (especially if sputum is purulent or there is intermittent blood streaking).

Chest Radiographs

Chest radiographs are crucial for documenting regions of increased markings, cavities, and atelectasis. However, routine chest radiographs may appear normal, especially in the early phases of bronchiectasis (7 to 10 per cent of patients). Often, all that may be seen are nonspecific markings in localized segments of lung. Tubular shadows (tram tracks, tram lines), mucoid impactions, or gloved finger shadows are more significant. Tubular shadows reflect the thickening of bronchial walls, peribronchial fibrosis, and alveolar collapse. Mucoid impactions or gloved finger shadows appear when secretions and pus fill airways with radiodense material.

Compensatory hyperinflation of uninvolved lung regions is common, especially in patients with cystic fibrosis.

Bronchography

Bronchography used to be considered the best method of confirming bronchiectasis and evaluating the extent of its progress. However, it is rarely done, since severely compromised patients or those with bronchospasm may have adverse reactions. In addition, bronchographic studies should not be performed in patients with active disease. Bronchography is rarely indicated today and should not be obtained unless the results will be important to a treatment decision. One example would be to document localized bronchiectasis that might be amenable to surgery. If they are needed, bronchograms should be obtained after several months, when reversible damage to airways has had time to resolve.

Computed Tomography (CT)

In almost all instances, CT replaces the need for bronchography. Adequate visualization of bronchiectatic segments is usually possible, and the problems noted above do not occur with this technique.

Bronchoscopy

Though not of use in diagnosing bronchiectasis, bronchoscopy is useful in identifying obstructions or sources of hemoptysis and in removing secretions. Biopsy of bronchial (or nasal) mucosa for

TABLE 63–2. DIAGNOSTIC FEATURES OF FAMILIAL BRONCHIECTASIS

Disorder	Clinical Findings	Laboratory Tests
Cystic fibrosis (see Ch. 64)	Pancreatic insufficiency, mucoid *Pseudomonas* strain, obstructive azospermia, infertility	Sweat chloride
Immotile cilia syndrome	Infertility, sinusitis, otitis media, Kartagener's syndrome (with or without dextrocardia)	Electron microscopy of cilia, absent mucociliary clearance, immotility in living cells (nasal, sperm)
Alpha$_1$-antitrypsin deficiency	Emphysema, cirrhosis	Serum alpha$_1$-antitrypsin, Pi typing
Immunoglobulin G (IgG) deficiency	Recurrent infections	Quantitative Ig, IgG subclass
Immunoglobulin A (IgA) deficiency	Autoimmune phenomena, atopy	Quantitative Ig
Williams-Campbell syndrome	Disease restricted to chest	On bronchography, expiratory collapse of proximal bronchi
Neutrophil deficiencies	Recurrent infections (with or without thrombocytopenia, with or without pancreatic disease)	Blood smear, differential leukocyte count, nitroblue tetrazolium dye test
Complement deficiencies	Recurrent infections	C3 levels, CH50 determination

From Newth CJL: Bronchiectasis. *In* Wyngaarden JB, Smith LH Jr (eds.): Cecil Textbook of Medicine. 18th ed. Philadelphia, W. B. Saunders Company, 1988, p 439; with permission.

electron microscopic evaluation may be used to confirm ciliary dyskinesia.

Sinus Radiographs

Radiographic evaluation may be helpful in identifying patients in whom sinusitis accompanies bronchiectasis (e.g., immotile cilia syndrome, Young's syndrome).

Pulmonary Function

Patients with extensive bronchiectasis have impairments similar to those seen in chronic bronchitis or emphysema. Cough in patients with saccular or varicose bronchiectasis produces premature collapse of large bronchi, leading to obstruction of expiratory airflow and to air trapping. This collapse is probably due to the inflammatory destruction of proximal bronchial walls. Ineffective cough leads to retention of secretions, predisposing patients to further infection.

Disturbances in respiratory function are dependent upon the anatomic type of bronchiectasis and the degree of lung compromise. Pulmonary function tests in patients with diffuse involvement usually reveal airway obstruction. Forced vital capacity (FVC), forced expiratory volume in 1 second (FEV_1), FEV_1/FVC, and forced expiratory flow ($FEF_{25-75\%}$) are all decreased, and residual volume is increased. Decreased ventilation, perfusion, and ventilation-perfusion ratios are found in involved regions. Nitrogen washout studies may show evidence of maldistribution of inspired air. Hypoxemia may occur in severe bronchiectasis; but carbon dioxide retention tends to occur only in those patients with concomitant severe bronchitis or advanced emphysema. Persistent or progressive hypercapnea is an ominous finding, one that reflects advanced disease and cor pulmonale.

Additional Studies

Sputum cultures may yield evidence of *Haemophilus influenzae, Streptococcus pneumoniae, Streptococcus pyogenes, Pseudomonas aeruginosa, Pseudomonas cepacia, Staphylococcus aureus,* or *Aspergillus,* as well as a number of other organisms. Accurate determination of infective organisms has obvious implications for antibiotic therapies.

White blood cell counts and differentials may help to confirm active infection and to distinguish bronchiectasis from lymphoproliferative disorders. Arterial blood gas levels aid in the assessment of severe respiratory compromise. Sweat chloride tests in patients with bronchiectasis may detect previously undiscovered cystic fibrosis. Quantitative immunoglobulin determinations should be obtained if immunodeficiency is suspected. Nasal or bronchial biopsy is indicated when the immotile cilia syndrome is suspected.

Differential Diagnosis

Bronchiectasis represents permanent lung destruction and needs to be distinguished from reversible changes caused by such entities as pneumonia, bronchitis, and atelectasis, as well as from foreign body aspiration, tuberculosis, and lung abscess. In addition, the presence of any of the numerous predisposing conditions needs to be determined.

COMPLICATIONS

Severe complications are relatively uncommon; hemoptysis does occur. An early onset of disease, especially in those with cystic fibrosis or immunodeficiencies, is associated with decreased lifespan. Such complications as lung abscesses, pneumonia, progression of infection through the pleura to produce bronchopleural fistulas, or empyema are more common in this population than in those who acquire bronchiectasis later in adult life.

TREATMENT AND PROGNOSIS

Since anatomic destruction is irreversible, efforts are directed at medical therapies to prevent disease progression and to control symptoms. Antibiotics to combat (or occasionally prevent) infections, postural drainage, chest physical therapy, hydration, discontinuation of smoking, bronchodilators (in patients with bronchospasm), oxygen (for hypoxic patients during acute exacerbations or for those with chronic respiratory insufficiency), and

treatment for sinusitis are used as appropriate. Patients with bronchiectasis should also receive annual influenza vaccines.

The choice of antibiotics should be guided by the results of the sputum culture. However, these cultures often grow "normal flora," so ampicillin is generally chosen for empiric use. Trimethoprim-sulfamethoxazole or tetracycline is appropriate for patients for whom penicillins are contraindicated. One to 3 weeks of antibiotic therapy may be required to achieve the desired therapeutic effects. Long-term antibiotic therapy and courses of inhaled antibiotics have not proved effective.

Progression within involved bronchial segments is common, but extension to normal regions is unusual. Underlying diseases such as cystic fibrosis, asthma, and the immotile cilia syndrome may render the entire bronchial system vulnerable. Appropriate use of antibiotics is effective in controlling symptoms and minimizing dysfunction and disease progression.

Resection may be curative in that small subset of patients with severe localized disease. Patients with advanced bilateral disease are not surgical candidates and may do well with medical therapies alone. Rarely, surgery is indicated for a patient with massive hemoptysis resulting from vascular deformity within a bronchiectatic segment. If the patient is unable to tolerate surgical resection, bronchial artery embolization may be warranted.

Barker AF, Bardana EJ Jr: Bronchiectasis: Update of an orphan disease. Am Rev Respir Dis 137:969, 1988. *A concise review with 214 references, outlining pathology, etiology, host-insult pathogenesis, prognosis, and suggested evaluation.*

Le Roux BT, Mohlala ML, Odell JA, Whitton ID: Suppurative Diseases of the Lung and Pleural Space. Part II: Bronchiectasis. Chicago, Year Book Medical Publishers, 1986, pp 95–159. *Review with exhaustive bibliography and excellent section on historical perspective; focuses primarily on surgical management of bronchiectasis.*

Slutzker AD, Kinn R, Said SI: Bronchiectasis and progressive respiratory failure following smoke inhalation. Chest 95:1349, 1989. *Case presentation of patient who developed bronchiectasis after inhalational injury.*

Swartz MN: Bronchiectasis. *In* Fishman AP (ed.): Pulmonary Diseases and Disorders. 2nd ed. New York, McGraw-Hill Book Company, 1988, pp 1553–1579. *Comprehensive, well-referenced, and well-illustrated examination of the subject.*

64 Cystic Fibrosis
Roger Bone

DEFINITION

Cystic fibrosis (CF) is a heritable disease that follows an autosomal recessive pattern of transmittance. A child born to two heterozygous carriers has a 1:4 risk of having the disease, a 1:2 chance of being a carrier, and a 1:4 chance of neither being a carrier nor having the disease. CF is the most common lethal genetic disease in the United States; the approximate frequency in Caucasians is 1 in 2000. On the basis of this figure, it is estimated that 1 in 20 is a carrier of the defective gene. Blacks and Asians are seldom affected. CF is characterized by abnormal eccrine and exocrine gland function; mucous glands produce viscous secretions, which lead to chronic pulmonary disease, insufficient pancreatic and digestive function, and abnormally concentrated sweat.

HISTORICAL PERSPECTIVE

Although there are numerous historical associations between salty skin and early death, CF was first described as a distinct clinical entity in the late 1930's. It was initially referred to as "cystic fibrosis of the pancreas," to describe the histologic appearance of that organ late in the course of the disease. Only later was it recognized that all exocrine glands were involved.

PATHOLOGY AND PATHOGENESIS

There have been several diverse lines of research into the basic etiology of CF. The more prominent theories included searches for alterations in the physicochemical properties of exocrine secretions (e.g., defective macromolecular secretion), the regulation of exocrine gland secretions, electrolyte transport, and abnormalities in serum.

Though it has been known for the past few years that the gene for CF is located on the long arm of chromosome 7, the gene has only recently been isolated. The encoded protein contains 1480 amino acids, is very similar to other membrane proteins, and may, in fact, be an ion channel. A deletion of three base pairs in the genetic code results in loss of a phenylalanine residue at position 508. It is believed that the defective protein may be at least partially responsible for alterations in cyclic adenosine monophosphate (cAMP)–mediated chloride secretion.

With the isolation, in late 1989, of the genetic defect that presumably leads to CF, a unifying hypothesis is beginning to emerge. In normal individuals, chloride channels are located on the luminal membranes of epithelial cells. When these channels are open, chloride ions move into the airway lumen, producing an osmotic gradient that draws water into the lumen (Fig. 64–1). Abnormalities in sweat electrolytes of CF patients are probably due to chloride impermeability of the sweat duct epithelium. Anomalous mucus of the lungs and other organs may result from inadequate amounts of water on the luminal side of epithelial membranes, secondary to excessive sodium reabsorption or failure to secrete chloride, either of which would favor water movement from secretions into tissues. There is evidence to suggest that several CF mucous secretions contain inadequate amounts of water and that physical properties of mucous secretions are highly dependent on water content. If altered regulatory mechanisms are the source of these water and electrolyte transport abnormalities, it is possible that the secretion of macromolecules by exocrine cells is not properly controlled and that excessive amounts of mucous glycoproteins and other elements are secreted, which would further diminish clearance of secretions. It is now hoped that research in these directions will have a bearing on new therapies or potential cures for CF. Further efforts will most likely focus on epithelial cell regulatory mechanisms.

CLINICAL MANIFESTATIONS AND CLINICAL COURSE

Cystic fibrosis manifests in any number of ways and can mimic other clinical entities (Fig. 64–2). Early gastrointestinal involvement (i.e., meconium ileus, failure to thrive) leads to the diagnosis of more than 10 per cent of CF patients at birth or during infancy. More typical presentations, however, include early onset of respiratory symptoms such as cough and recurrent respiratory infections later in life.

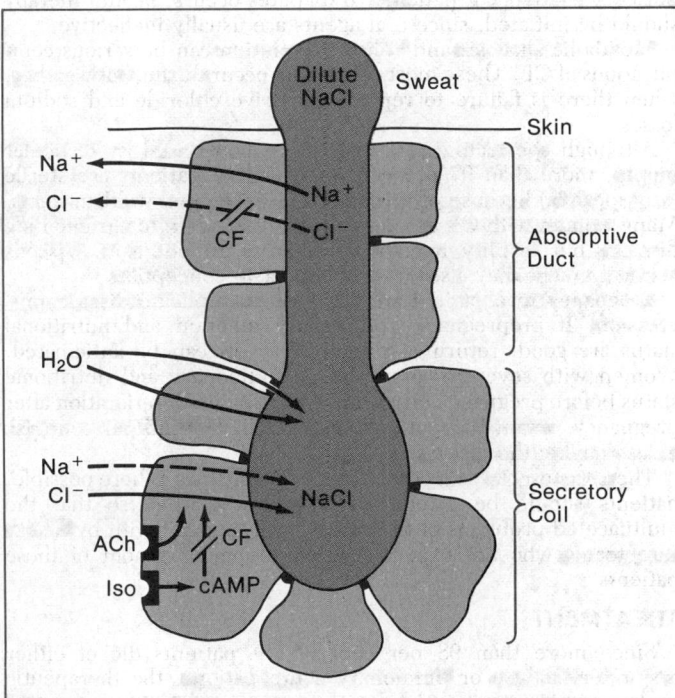

FIGURE 64–1. Electrolyte transport by sweat glands. (From Welsh MJ, Fick RB: Cystic fibrosis. J Clin Invest 80:1523, 1987. Reproduced from *The Journal of Clinical Investigation* by copyright permission of the American Society for Clinical Investigation.)

In many patients, intermittent episodes of acute respiratory infections persist longer than would be expected. Coughing increases and becomes worse at night and upon the patient's awakening. Sputum is viscous and purulent. Disease progression is often marked by a gradual decline in pulmonary function and is punctuated by acute exacerbations. The clinical course of CF is known to change suddenly with the onset of a number of complications. Poor nutritional status (or malnutrition, if present) often correlates with the severity of the pulmonary disease.

DIAGNOSIS
Radiology

Hyperinflation is noted early in the course of CF. As the disease progresses, hyperinflation and evidence of bronchitis increase, and there may be indications of peripheral cuffing, mucus impaction, or bronchiectasis.

Pulmonary Function

It is thought that newborns with CF have normal lung function, but within a short time many children show evidence of decreasing pulmonary function. There is usually demonstrable obstruction of small airways (e.g., decreased maximal mid-expiratory flow rates, reduced expiratory flow rates at low lung volumes, increased residual volume/total lung capacity [RV/TLC] ratios). Spirometry, lung volume measurements, and oxygenation levels are most frequently used to monitor pulmonary function and disease progression. Oxygenation gradually worsens throughout life; when arterial Po_2 values remain below 55 mm Hg, pulmonary hypertension is often present. Significant arterial Pco_2 elevations or forced expiratory volume in 1 second (FEV_1) values less than 30 per cent of those predicted portend end-stage disease; survival then averages 29 months.

Patients with CF often display airway hyperreactivity, which can be demonstrated by exercise testing, histamine challenge, or response to bronchodilators.

Sputum Culture

Although *Staphylococcus aureus, Pseudomonas aeruginosa,* and *Pseudomonas cepacia* are sometimes found in sputum cultures from patients with pulmonary diseases other than CF, their association with this disease is so consistent that attempts to obtain sputum cultures have become an integral part of evaluating any patient suspected of having CF. Sputum cultures may also be useful during exacerbations of the disease.

Pancreatic Function

Ninety to 95 per cent of patients with CF exhibit some degree of exocrine pancreatic dysfunction. Enzyme deficiency leads to maldigestion of protein and fat, which produces bulky, foul-smelling stools. If untreated, these patients fail to gain weight, and growth is inhibited. Poor growth can also be the result of increased energy expenditures associated with the work of breathing in those with severe respiratory symptoms.

Sweat

The discovery that an excessive loss of salt occurs in the sweat of CF patients has been used as the most important diagnostic criterion. Although the sweat glands of patients with CF are histologically normal, they function abnormally—producing secretions that are nearly isotonic, rather than the hypotonic solutions excreted by normal individuals.

Quantitative pilocarpine iontophoresis, performed in laboratories with established expertise, remains the standard for diagnosis of CF. A minimum of 100 mg of sweat needs to be collected, and results should be confirmed by a second test. In children, sodium and chloride concentrations exceeding 60 mEq/per liter are considered diagnostic of CF; in adults the level is 70 mEq per liter.

COMPLICATIONS
Respiratory

The major source of morbidity in patients with CF is pulmonary disease. Atelectasis is not uncommon, and it is usually associated with few symptoms. Evidence of bronchiectasis is common in CF

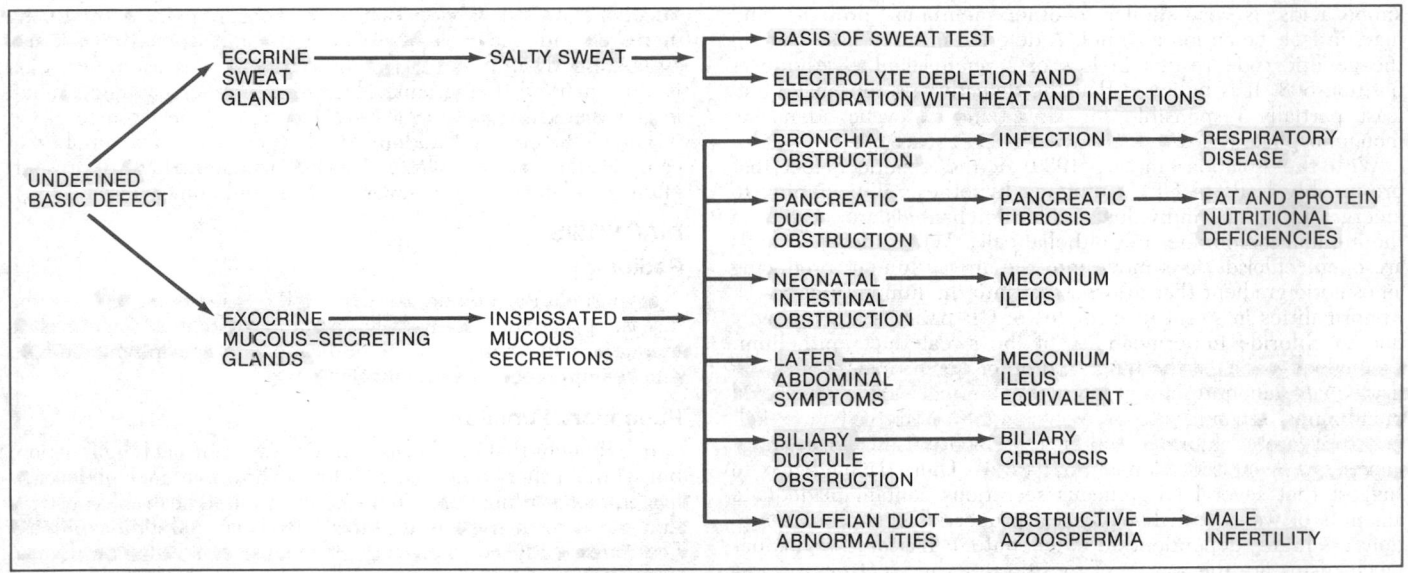

FIGURE 64–2. Clinical manifestations of cystic fibrosis. (From Newth CJL: Cystic fibrosis. *In* Wyngaarden JB, Smith LH Jr (eds.): Cecil Textbook of Medicine. 18th ed. Philadelphia, W. B. Saunders Company, 1988, p 440; with permission.)

patients by 5 to 10 years of age. Chest physiotherapy and antibiotics are often successful in re-expanding atelectatic regions. Surgical resection is only rarely considered, since the bronchiectasis is diffuse.

Pneumothorax is a common complication of CF. Up to one third of older patients experience recurrent episodes of pneumothorax. Because of this high rate, after an initial pneumothorax, attempts are often made to obliterate the pleural space by instillation of sclerosing agents, such as tetracycline. Insertion of a chest tube is usually considered only when the pneumothorax involves more than 10 per cent of a hemithorax.

Hemoptysis may occur if there is an erosion of pulmonary tissue that impinges on a bronchial blood vessel. Small amounts of blood-streaked sputum are common, but expectoration of more significant volumes of blood (>30 ml) often requires hospitalization. Massive hemoptysis is relatively uncommon in patients with CF, but when it occurs, it is life threatening. Bronchoscopy or surgery may be necessary, but radiographically guided bronchial artery embolization is becoming a more frequent treatment maneuver.

Respiratory failure (hypoxemia, hypercarbia) in a patient with CF becomes increasingly difficult to manage. Since CF patients tend to respond poorly to, and experience more complications from, mechanical ventilation than do patients in respiratory failure secondary to other conditions, mechanical ventilation is generally instituted only in the event of acute precipitating events, such as infectious pneumonia or other reversible complications. With disease progression, hypoxemia increases, and pulmonary hypertension and cor pulmonale develop in virtually all CF patients.

Although as many as 50 per cent of patients with CF exhibit antibodies to *Aspergillus fumigatus* in their serum, only a small number develop allergic aspergillosis. Expectoration of rusty brown plugs of sputum is suggestive of this condition.

Digital clubbing occurs in nearly every patient with CF and is often present early in the course of the pulmonary manifestations of this disease. Severity seems to correlate with the degree of pulmonary dysfunction. Hypertrophic pulmonary osteoarthropathy occurs in up to 15 per cent of adolescent and adult CF patients and is often characterized by pain in the joints on ambulation. Symptoms tend to subside when pulmonary symptoms improve.

Other

Intestinal obstruction (caused by meconium ileus or meconium ileus equivalent) can usually be treated medically; intussusception or rectal prolapse usually requires surgical intervention. Patients with CF are often prone to episodes of acute or chronic, crampy, lower right quadrant abdominal pain, reflecting partial intestinal obstruction. These episodes can usually be treated with oral mineral oil and N-acetylcysteine used in conjunction with hyperosmolar enemas that contain agents such as diatrizoate methylglucamine.

Symptomatic biliary cirrhosis occurs in 2 to 5 per cent of CF patients. Patients present with hyperbilirubinemia, ascites, and peripheral edema. Although bleeding esophageal varices are an infrequent complication of CF, they are seen in some patients secondary to hepatic cirrhosis and portal hypertension. Endoscopy is generally used to sclerose the affected vessels.

As fibrosis of the exocrine pancreas continues, hyperglycemia may be encountered in patients with CF, especially in the second and third decades. Diabetes mellitus occurs in approximately 10 per cent of adult CF patients. If diabetes occurs, insulin therapy should be initiated, since oral agents are usually ineffective.

Metabolic alkalosis and volume depletion can be serious complications of CF. These most commonly occur during hot weather, when there is failure to replace excessive chloride and sodium losses.

Although spermatogenesis can be demonstrated by testicular biopsy, more than 97 per cent of male CF patients are sterile (azoospermia) because of incompletely developed wolffian ducts. Many women with CF are anovulatory secondary to chronic lung disease, but fertility may be as high as 20 per cent. Viscous cervical mucus may also prove a barrier to conception.

Pregnancy in a patient with CF can complicate disease progression. If prepregnancy pulmonary function and nutritional status are good, return to pregravid levels can be anticipated. Women with severely compromised pulmonary and nutritional status before pregnancy often show accelerated deterioration after pregnancy. Infants of mothers with CF have a 2.5 per cent risk of also having the disease.

The psychosocial aspects of CF are formidable. Where possible, patients should be cared for in special centers so that the multifaceted problems of the disease can be dealt with by health care teams who are experienced in the management of these patients.

TREATMENT

Since more than 98 per cent of CF patients die of either respiratory failure or pulmonary complications, the therapeutic goals are to prevent and treat the complications of obstruction and infection in the airways, enhance mucus clearance, and improve nutrition. Antibiotics are the key element to increasing survival in this population of patients. Frequent courses of antibiotic therapy are usually necessary; some patients may require them nearly continuously. Antibiotic selection should be guided by sputum culture.

Several species demonstrate great affinity for the respiratory tracts of patients with CF—*Staphylococcus aureus, Pseudomonas aeruginosa*, and, more recently, *Pseudomonas cepacia*. Indeed, their presence is suggestive of CF. Patients with demonstrable infection by *S. aureus* are most often treated with dicloxacillin, cephalexin, the newer cephalosporins, or chloramphenicol. Ciprofloxacin is also being increasingly used but is recommended only for patients older than 10 years of age. Early in the course of the disease, *Pseudomonas* organisms may be sensitive to tetracycline, trimethoprim-sulfamethoxazole, or chloramphenicol, but infection by these organisms is most often treated by using a combination of an intravenously given aminoglycoside and a semisynthetic penicillin (more popular combinations include gentamicin-carbenicillin and tobramycin-ticarcillin). Once found in the sputum, however, *P. aeruginosa* rarely, if ever, is eradicated. Therapeutic benefit therefore seems to be derived from reduction in the microbial load, rather than elimination of the infecting organism. Of late, *P. cepacia* is emerging as a serious problem for CF patients. This species tends to develop resistance to multiple antibiotics and has been associated with severe, frequently fatal pneumonia. *Haemophilus influenzae* infection is most often treated with ampicillin, trimethoprim-sulfamethoxazole, or chloramphenicol.

Chest Physiotherapy

Percussion and postural drainage are mainstays in the treatment of CF. Clearance of pulmonary secretions to prevent the complications that result from plugging of the airways with viscous mucous secretions and the infections that may arise distal to obstruction constitutes a crucial component of therapy.

Bronchodilators

Although positive effects can be demonstrated in the laboratory, long-term benefit from the use of bronchodilators for CF patients has not been established.

Nutrition

Most patients can be maintained on normal diets with pancreatic enzyme supplementation (usually enteric-coated capsules taken with meals). Because defective fat metabolism may lead to deficiencies in the fat-soluble vitamins (i.e., A, D, E, K), supplementation with these is often necessary. Many patients with CF also have higher than normal caloric needs—presumably resulting from the increased workload of breathing and maldigestion.

Exercise and Rehabilitation

Exercise tolerance in patients with CF correlates with the severity of pulmonary obstruction. Although exercise does not improve pulmonary function, it does improve cardiorespiratory fitness, and a program of physical conditioning is recommended. Long-term oxygen therapy can be used for chronic hypoxemia.

PROGNOSIS

Over the past three decades, there can be no question that comprehensive treatment programs have increased the overall survival of patients with CF. In the 1950's, patients lived only a few years; at present, the median survival is to age 24, and significant numbers of patients survive well beyond that. Clinical complexity and individual variability, however, make predictions in any given patient difficult. As mentioned previously, numerous factors are associated with unfavorable prognoses. CF patients who initially present with respiratory symptoms seem to have poorer prognoses. Once lung disease is established, colonization by *Pseudomonas* may indicate a poor prognosis. Males, those who maintain weight, and those in whom pancreatic exocrine function is relatively well preserved seem to do much better than those with severe insufficiency. The most significant determinant of the clinical course is the severity of the pulmonary disease and the rate at which it progresses.

To date, using marker techniques, it has been possible to screen only for carriers of the genetic defect within families of living CF patients. Recent advances in identification of the defective gene promise to have profound effects on our ability to detect heterozygotes, thereby allowing prevention of this devastating disease.

Boat TF: Cystic fibrosis. *In* Murray JF, Nadel JA (eds.): Textbook of Respiratory Medicine. Philadelphia, W. B. Saunders Company, 1988, pp 1126–1152. *Outstanding overview; especially clear review of the clinical manifestations of CF; 207 references.*

Fick RB, Stillwell PC: Controversies in the management of pulmonary disease due to cystic fibrosis. Chest 95:1319, 1989. *Addresses the questions of antibiotic administration (ambulatory, nebulized), corticosteroid use, nutritional support, exercise as a substitute for postural drainage, and surgical resection in this patient population.*

Halley DJJ, Bijman J, deJonge HR, et al.: The cystic fibrosis defect approached from different angles—new perspectives on the gene, the chloride channel, diagnosis and therapy. Eur J Pediatr 149:670, 1990.

O'Loughlin EV: Cystic fibrosis: An inborn error of cellular electrolyte transport? J Paediatr Child Health 26:126, 1990.

Michel BC: Antibacterial therapy in cystic fibrosis: A review of the literature published between 1980 and February 1987. Chest 94(Suppl 2):129S, 1988. *Numerous comparative tables compiled over a 7-year period; 67 references.*

Rubio TT: Infection in patients with cystic fibrosis. Am J Med 81(Suppl 1A):73, 1986. *Compilation and comparison of data from antimicrobial therapy studies over the past 16 years; 40 references.*

Scanlin TF: Cystic fibrosis. *In* Fishman AF (ed.): Pulmonary Diseases and Disorders. 2nd ed. New York, McGraw-Hill, 1988, pp 1273–1294. *An excellent overview, especially regarding the genetics, pathology, evaluation, treatment, natural history, and complications of CF.*

Thomassen MJ, Demko CA, Doershuk CF: Cystic fibrosis: A review of pulmonary infections and interventions. Pediatr Pulmonol 3:334, 1987. *A state-of-the-art review of the topic as of August 1986; 184 references.*

65 Pulmonary Embolism
Robert M. Senior

DEFINITION

Pulmonary embolism is the impaction of material into branches of the pulmonary arterial bed. Although they may completely prevent blood flow, most pulmonary emboli do not produce necrosis of lung parenchyma ("pulmonary infarction") because (1) a dual circulation (bronchial and pulmonary) supports lung parenchymal tissue and (2) exchange of oxygen and carbon dioxide can occur directly between the tissue and alveolar gas. Most pulmonary emboli are blood clots ("thromboemboli"); much more rarely, neoplastic cells, fat droplets (Ch. 66), air bubbles, exogenous materials (such as talc and cornstarch particles in intravenous drug abusers), or pieces of intravenous catheters and catheter introducers occlude pulmonary vessels. The ensuing discussion deals with pulmonary thromboembolism.

PATHOGENESIS

Pulmonary embolism is a complication of venous thrombosis; that is, emboli come from thrombi in peripheral veins, principally the deep veins of the lower extremities and pelvis (Ch. 54), and "travel" through the circulation to the pulmonary artery. In fact, in 70 per cent of patients with pulmonary thromboembolism, coexisting thrombi can be found in the deep veins of the thighs or pelvis. In the remaining cases, it is presumed that the emboli either come from other sites that escape detection or represent the entire thrombus that originated in the lower extremities. Thrombosis of superficial veins of the lower extremities does not lead to pulmonary thromboemboli, and thrombosis confined to deep veins in the leg distal to the popliteal vein infrequently leads to pulmonary thromboemboli. The renal veins can be a source of thromboemboli, particularly in patients with the nephrotic syndrome, but thromboemboli in nephrotic patients do not necessarily arise only from the renal veins. Pulmonary thromboemboli seldom originate in veins of the upper extremities, head, or neck, but they may arise from mural thrombi in the right side of the heart. Venous thromboemboli may be trapped in the right atrium or ventricle, from which they embolize to the lungs intact or fragment in the heart and shower the lungs with emboli at one time or at different times.

Venous thrombosis can be attributed to one or more of the

TABLE 65–1. CLINICAL RISK FACTORS FOR VENOUS THROMBOSIS AND PULMONARY THROMBOEMBOLISM

Common	Uncommon
Surgical and nonsurgical trauma, including burns	Acquired
Congestive heart failure	Lupus anticoagulant
Immobilization (bed rest, stroke, prolonged travel, and so forth)	Nephrotic syndrome
	Inflammatory bowel disease
Malignancy	Persistent thrombocytosis
Previous deep venous thrombosis	Polycythemia vera
Pregnancy, particularly in the puerperium and after cesarean section	Paroxysmal nocturnal hemoglobinuria
	Inherited
Estrogen therapy	Antithrombin III deficiency
Age over 50	Protein C deficiency
Obesity (?)	Protein S deficiency
	Plasminogen activator deficiency
	Elevated plasminogen activator inhibitor
	Homocystinuria

following: stasis of blood, increased tendency for blood to coagulate, and endothelial injury. Many clinical situations have been associated with the risk of proximal deep venous thrombosis (Table 65–1), but practically speaking, most are associated with decreased blood flow in lower extremity veins due to immobilization, elevated systemic venous pressure, extrinsic pressure on pelvic and lower extremity veins, intraluminal venous blockage from previous venous thrombosis, or decreased venous tone.

Pulmonary embolism occurs in 1 to 2 per cent of patients over age 40 following general surgery. The incidence is higher (5 to 10 per cent) with orthopedic surgery of the hip or knee. The risk associated with surgery is increased by advanced age, obesity, a lengthy operative period, underlying malignancy, pre-existent venous disease, prolonged bed rest after surgery, and postoperative infection. Venous stasis due to immobilization is probably a major reason for venous thrombosis associated with surgery, but other factors come into play: increased blood coagulability associated with release of tissue thromboplastin and exposure of subendothelium, postoperative decreased blood fibrinolytic activity, and vessel damage, particularly in surgery of the lower extremities or pelvis.

Cancers of the lung, breast, and abdominal viscera have a strong association with venous thromboembolism, and the thromboembolism may antedate clinical recognition of the malignancy. Factors released from tumors may increase blood coagulability, decrease fibrinolytic activity, and alter endothelial surfaces. Malignancies also predispose to deep venous thrombosis by leading to venous stasis through immobilization and surgical interventions. Some evidence in women with breast cancer points to a thrombogenic effect of anticancer drug therapy. Prolonged bed rest from any cause and paralysis resulting from stroke are also associated with a high incidence of venous thrombosis. Pulmonary embolism is commonly found at autopsy in patients who die of congestive heart failure.

In pregnancy, multiple factors predispose to venous thrombosis: (1) venous stasis induced by compression on pelvic veins, increased intra-abdominal pressure, and hormonal relaxation of vascular smooth muscle; (2) altered blood rheologic properties; and (3) increased concentrations of factors in the coagulation cascade (fibrinogen, Factors VII, VIII, IX, and XII), with concomitant reductions in antithrombin III and fibrinolytic activity. There may be a greater risk of thromboembolism during pregnancy, but there is clearly an increased risk in the puerperal period, particularly after cesarean section. Estrogen therapy has been linked with a higher incidence of venous thrombosis, and the risk appears related to the dose, but the precise degree of increased risk and the mechanisms involved are not certain. Multiple possibilities have been considered, including reduction in antithrombin III concentration, decreased plasminogen activator level, increased platelet aggregability, increased blood viscosity, and increased distensibility of peripheral veins leading to venous stasis.

When pulmonary embolism occurs without an obvious predisposing factor, and particularly when there is a family history of venous thrombosis, one should consider the possibility of a hereditary decrease in an anticoagulant factor (antithrombin III, proteins C and S, or tissue plasminogen activator) or a hereditary increase in plasminogen activator inhibitor (Ch. 155).

INCIDENCE

Pulmonary embolism is a major cause of morbidity and death. The annual incidence in the United States has been estimated at approximately 600,000. About one third of the episodes are fatal, with nearly all of the fatalities either sudden (within 1 hour of onset) or undiagnosed during life. In approximately half of the people who die, there is serious underlying disease apart from venous thrombosis. Autopsy studies have reported pulmonary embolism as a major cause of death (10 to 20 per cent of all deaths occurring in hospitals and 15 per cent of postoperative deaths). The incidence of fatal pulmonary embolism in hospitalized patients may be declining. In one medical center, the incidence of autopsy-documented fatal pulmonary embolism fell from 9.3 per cent to 3.8 per cent over a recent 10-year period. It is interesting that during the same years, there was a concomitant increase, from 4 per cent to approximately 12 per cent, in the percentage of adult patients given anticoagulant therapy.

PATHOPHYSIOLOGY

Pulmonary emboli produce respiratory and hemodynamic responses that reflect the extent of pulmonary vascular obstruction, the time elapsed since embolization, and the presence or absence of pre-existent heart or lung disease.

HYPERPNEA AND ALVEOLAR HYPERVENTILATION. Acute pulmonary embolism stimulates ventilation. The increase in minute ventilation, manifested clinically by increased respiratory rate, usually offsets the increased physiologic dead space produced by obstruction of the pulmonary vascular bed, so that the arterial P_{CO_2} (Pa_{CO_2}) does not rise. On the contrary, the Pa_{CO_2} typically falls below 35 mm Hg, indicating that hyperpnea does not occur solely to preserve a normal Pa_{CO_2}. Similarly, alveolar hyperventilation is not due to hypoxemia, as it occurs even when arterial oxygenation is normal, and it cannot be abolished with supplemental inspired oxygen. The stimulus for alveolar hyperventilation is unknown but presumably involves reflexes initiated from the pulmonary parenchyma in the area of the obstructed vessel. A reduction of Pa_{CO_2} below baseline may occur even among those with chronic hypercapnia. Although a lower than normal Pa_{CO_2} is usual, the Pa_{CO_2} rises in individuals who cannot increase their minute ventilation adequately to compensate for the increased physiologic dead space—for example, in those with neuromuscular disease, those receiving controlled mechanical ventilation, or those with severe pleuritic pain. The Pa_{CO_2} may also rise when there is massive embolization that confines pulmonary blood flow to a severely reduced portion of the pulmonary vascular bed.

HYPOXEMIA. A decrease in arterial oxygen tension (Pa_{CO_2}) is common in acute pulmonary embolism. The mechanisms are complex. Ventilation-perfusion ($\dot{V}a/\dot{Q}$) inequality seems to be the predominant mechanism early in the course of pulmonary embolization, with intrapulmonary shunting as the dominant cause after 48 hours. Regional bronchoconstriction, atelectasis, and pulmonary edema are postulated as the anatomic basis for these physiologic defects. If cardiac output fails to keep up with metabolic demands, as is common with massive pulmonary embolism, mixed venous oxygen saturation falls and accentuates the effects of abnormal $\dot{V}a/\dot{Q}$ and intrapulmonary shunting. If pulmonary hypertension develops and a patent foramen ovale is present, blood may be shunted from the right to left within the heart, another factor causing arterial hypoxemia.

PULMONARY HYPERTENSION AND ACUTE COR PULMONALE. Pulmonary thromboembolism is the most common cause of acute pulmonary hypertension. The rise in pulmonary arterial pressure results primarily from mechanical blockage of the pulmonary vascular bed. Vasoconstrictive reflexes and mediators may also contribute. The rise in mean pulmonary arterial pressure tends to match the extent of blockage of the pulmonary arterial tree, but in patients without pre-existing cardiac or pulmonary disease, mean pulmonary arterial pressure is usually below 20 mm Hg unless pulmonary vascular obstruction exceeds 50 per cent. Pressures of 20 to 40 mm Hg occur only with 50 per cent to 75 per cent obstruction. The pressure seldom rises above 40 mm Hg because the normal right ventricle is incapable of generating higher pressures. A mean pulmonary arterial pressure above 40 mm Hg indicates chronic right ventricular hypertrophy secondary to recurrent pulmonary emboli or other diseases. When a sudden and marked increase in pulmonary vascular resistance causes the mean pulmonary arterial pressure to approach 40 mm Hg, several events occur. Right ventricular diastolic pressure, right atrial pressure, and systemic venous pressure all increase. The cardiac index falls below 2.5 liters per minute per square meter, and systemic hypotension and other clinical signs of hemodynamic distress appear.

PATHOLOGY

Most episodes of acute pulmonary embolism involve multiple emboli. Both lungs are affected about two thirds of the time. Lower lobe vessels are involved more often than upper lobe vessels, and the right lung is affected more often than the left. Emboli in the main branches of the right or left pulmonary arteries are seen in only a small percentage of patients. A large embolus obstructing the main pulmonary artery or straddling the pulmonary artery bifurcation (so-called "saddle embolus") is uncommon even in fatal acute pulmonary embolism. When a thromboembolus is poorly organized, it is apt to fragment in passage through the heart and is thus more likely to impact in smaller vessels than are organized thromboemboli.

The likelihood that emboli will cause pulmonary infarction is determined by the size of the vessels involved, by the extent of obstruction, by the potential for delivery of bronchial arterial blood flow, and by the adequacy of ventilation to the lung tissue supplied by the blocked pulmonary arteries. Occlusions of segmental arterial vessels or smaller branches are more apt to lead to infarction than are emboli lodged in larger vessels. Infarction is also more likely in the setting of elevated pulmonary capillary pressure from any cause—hence the frequency of infarction in patients with congestive heart failure—but otherwise healthy individuals can develop infarcts. Histologically, pulmonary infarction is characterized by intra-alveolar hemorrhage and necrosis of alveolar walls, but little inflammation. Cavitation rarely develops without coexisting pulmonary infection or an infected thrombus.

CLINICAL MANIFESTATIONS

The clinical features of pulmonary embolism can be diverse and confusing and range from no symptoms to sudden death. Occasionally, the principal manifestations are fever, arrhythmias, or refractory congestive heart failure. Usually, however, the presentations are not obscure. Three clinical patterns predominate: (1) sudden dyspnea with no physical findings but tachypnea; (2) sudden pleuritic chest pain and dyspnea accompanied by findings consistent with pleural effusion and pulmonary consolidation; and (3) sudden apprehension, chest discomfort, and dyspnea, with findings of acute cor pulmonale (accentuated pulmonic closure sound in the second left interspace, right ventricular lift, jugular venous distention) and systemic hypotension. It is this last pattern that may culminate in death within a few minutes.

The type of pattern that develops depends upon the extent of pulmonary arterial tree blockage, whether there is pre-existent cardiopulmonary disease, and whether pulmonary infarction occurs. Severe disturbances in pulmonary and systemic hemodynamics seldom occur unless extensive vascular obstruction or pre-existent heart or lung disease is present. Pleuritic pain and signs of pulmonary consolidation and pleural effusion indicate that embolization involves one or more peripheral pulmonary arterial branches. Large discrepancies may exist between the severity of embolization and symptoms. Some patients with massive embolization may appear remarkably comfortable, whereas others with minimal embolization may show great distress.

The most common symptoms of pulmonary embolism are dyspnea and chest pain, each occurring in more than 80 per cent of patients (Table 65-2). Tachypnea is the most common sign. Hemoptysis, on the other hand, often considered typical, is not

TABLE 65-2. SYMPTOMS AND SIGNS IN 327 PATIENTS WITH PULMONARY EMBOLI

Symptoms	Per Cent	Signs	Per Cent
Chest pain	88	Respirations above 16/min	92
Pleuritic	74	Rales	58
Nonpleuritic	14	S_2P* increased	53
Dyspnea	84	Pulse above 100/min	44
Apprehension	59	Temperature above 37.8°C	43
Cough	53	Phlebitis	32
Hemoptysis	30	Gallop	34
Sweats	27	Diaphoresis	36
Syncope	13	Edema	24
		Murmur	23
		Cyanosis	19

*S_2P = intensity of the pulmonic component of the second heart sound.

Apprehension, syncope, increased pulmonic component of the second heart sound, gallop, diaphoresis, murmur, and cyanosis occurred more often with massive emboli (angiographically, at least two lobar arteries obstructed), whereas hemoptysis and pleuritic pain were more often present with submassive emboli.

From Bell WR, Simon TL, DeMets DL: The clinical features of submassive and massive pulmonary emboli. Am J Med 62:355, 1977; with permission.

a usual finding. Its absence, therefore, is not evidence against pulmonary embolism. Similarly, deep venous thrombosis of the lower extremities is seldom clinically apparent. A recent prospective study of adults presenting to the emergency room with pleuritic chest pain found, by pulmonary arteriography, that 21 per cent had pulmonary emboli. Emboli were not found in those under age 40 without risk factors for venous thrombosis; however, among the subjects over 40 without risk factors, 18 per cent had abnormal pulmonary arteriograms.

DIAGNOSIS

Although the history and physical examination may suggest the pulmonary embolism, a diagnosis that rests on clinical grounds alone is often incorrect. The differential diagnosis of pulmonary embolism can encompass many disorders, but principally those leading to acute shortness of breath, substernal or pleuritic chest pain, hemoptysis, and hemodynamic collapse. Thus, at times the possibility of pulmonary embolism must be distinguished from asthma, the hyperventilation syndrome, pneumothorax, pulmonary edema, a fractured rib, herpes zoster before the appearance of vesicles, pleurodynia, pleuritis due to collagen vascular diseases, pneumonia, empyema, bronchiectasis, bronchogenic carcinoma, acute myocardial infarction, pericarditis, dissecting aortic aneurysm, esophageal rupture, and upper abdominal processes such as acute cholecystitis. Several features discount the diagnosis of pulmonary embolism: (1) the absence of a precipitating factor for deep venous thrombosis, (2) recurrent chest pain in the same location, (3) pleuritic chest pain of more than 1 week's duration that is increasing in severity, (4) pleuritic chest pain with normal findings on the chest radiograph, (5) hemoptysis of greater than 5 ml with normal findings on the chest radiograph, (6) pericardial friction rub, (7) purulent sputum, and (8) spiking fever in excess of 39°C lasting more than 1 week.

DIAGNOSTIC STUDIES. When pulmonary embolism is suspected, confirmation of the diagnosis depends upon establishing that there is intravascular obstruction to pulmonary arterial blood flow. The definitive means of making the diagnosis is by pulmonary arteriography; however, a high degree of certainty can also be achieved with ventilation-perfusion scanning. Other approaches to visualizing the pulmonary circulation, such as computed tomography and magnetic resonance imaging, as well as methods of visualizing intrapulmonary thrombi using radioisotopically labeled platelets or monoclonal antibodies to platelet antigens and fibrin, are under development.

Arterial blood gas measurement, the electrocardiogram, the chest radiograph, and thoracentesis may help in the evaluation of patients suspected of having pulmonary embolism, either by favoring or by discounting diagnoses with which pulmonary embolism can be confused, but these studies lack specificity and therefore cannot be used in place of imaging the pulmonary circulation. Many efforts have been made to develop blood tests with specificity for the diagnosis of pulmonary embolism. None has been found useful.

Arterial Blood Gases. Typically in pulmonary embolism, there is a reduction in Pa_{O_2} and a concomitant reduction in Pa_{CO_2}. In patients with arteriographically proven acute pulmonary embolism who do not have previous cardiopulmonary disease, Pa_{O_2} values are less than 50 mm Hg in 13 per cent, 50 to 59 mm Hg in 19 per cent, between 60 and 80 mm Hg in 55 per cent, and greater than 80 mm Hg in 13 per cent. In those with a normal Pa_{O_2}, there is usually an increased alveolar-arterial oxygen difference, reflecting reduced efficiency of alveolar gas exchange, but even a normal alveolar-arterial oxygen difference does not exclude the diagnosis. A Pa_{O_2} less than 50 mm Hg is confined to those with greater than 50 per cent occlusion of major pulmonary arterial branches; however, in individuals with underlying cardiopulmonary disease, less severe degrees of pulmonary vascular obstruction can be associated with severe hypoxemia. Arterial blood gas abnormalities have no specificity for pulmonary embolism (similar abnormalities occur in conditions with which pulmonary embolism is confused).

Electrocardiogram. The main value of the electrocardiogram is to help exclude acute myocardial infarction. The most common finding in pulmonary embolism is sinus tachycardia. With emboli that provoke a substantial rise in pulmonary arterial and right-sided cardiac pressures, patterns of S_1, Q_3, T_3, inverted T waves in leads V_{1-3}, right ventricular strain, right-axis deviation, right bundle branch block, and atrial arrhythmias may occur. These changes, when they occur, are apt to be transient, lasting a few minutes or hours, disappearing as the pulmonary arterial pressure returns toward normal.

Chest Radiograph. A normal chest radiograph is uncommon in acute pulmonary embolism, but the usual radiographic findings are nonspecific: elevation of one of the hemidiaphragms with basilar atelectasis, infiltrates, and unilateral pleural effusion. Cardiac dilatation, dilatation of the main branches of the pulmonary artery, and zones of oligemia may occur with massive embolization. Besides lacking specificity, the chest radiograph shows a poor correlation with pulmonary arteriographic findings. Parenchymal densities tend to be in the lower lung fields, pleural based, and triangular and are ordinarily associated with pleural effusions. These densities usually represent extravascular blood rather than infarcted tissue. In summary, the principal value of the chest radiograph is to help exclude other possible diagnoses.

Thoracentesis. Pleural effusions, usually unilateral, are common with pulmonary embolism. The fluid is most often an exudate and is often hemorrhagic (but has a low hematocrit).

Ventilation-Perfusion Lung Scans. Isotopic scans of pulmonary perfusion (Q scans) provide a sensitive, safe means of assessing regional pulmonary blood flow and therefore have proved to be of great value in the diagnosis of pulmonary embolism. They can be performed alone or in combination with isotopic scans of ventilation (V scan). The combination of scans (V/Q scans) is more specific than the Q scan alone. V/Q lung scanning has become the accepted means of initially assessing the patient suspected of having pulmonary embolism. The strategy of using these scans is summarized in Figure 65–1.

A Q scan requires intravenous administration, with the patient supine, of technetium-99m–labeled particles of macroaggregated albumin, followed by scanning of the thorax with a gamma counter in a minimum of six views (anterior, posterior, right and left lateral, and right and left posterior oblique). The particles, which are slightly larger in diameter than the cross-section of the precapillary vessels of the pulmonary circulation, are injected into a peripheral vein, flow through the peripheral and central venous circulation, the right side of the heart, and the main pulmonary arteries, and finally lodge in precapillary vessels, where they remain for hours. The standard dose of particles blocks less than 0.2 per cent of the pulmonary precapillary vessels in the normal pulmonary vascular bed. For a V scan, the patient usually inhales and then rebreathes air containing radioactive gas, most often xenon-133, or aerosolized radiolabeled particles. Images of the initial breath, equilibration, and washout of the tracer are obtained. Typically, the xenon V scan is performed before the Q scan in the posterior projection with oblique views during washout. The patient is upright if possible. Besides xenon-

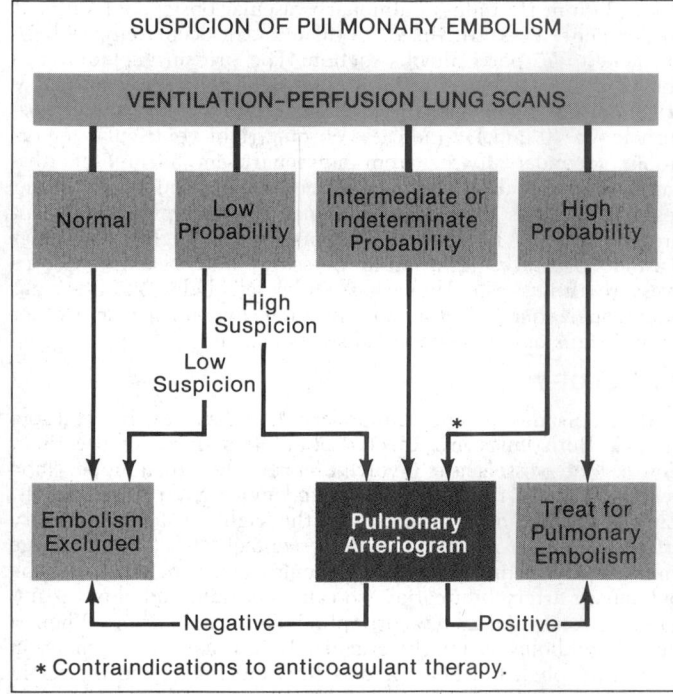

FIGURE 65–1. Ventilation-perfusion lung scanning in the evaluation of the patient suspected of having pulmonary embolism.

133, two other isotopes that are increasingly used for V scanning are krypton-81m– and technetium-99m–labeled particles in aerosols, which have the advantage over xenon-133 of enabling scans to be obtained in the same views as the Q scan with minimal radiation exposure.

A normal Q scan eliminates the diagnosis of pulmonary embolism. A normal scan reveals a homogeneous distribution of activity with an image that conforms to the lungs. In the presence of a pulmonary embolus, the radiolabeled particles are prevented from reaching vessels distal to the embolus, and the scan shows one or more perfusion defects in the image. The sensitivity of the Q lung scan to pulmonary arterial obstruction is excellent, as obstruction of vessels 3 mm in diameter or more leads to defects. Perfusion defects generally show some resolution within 4 to 5 days, but substantial abnormalities commonly persist for several weeks and may be present even a year later.

Defects on Q lung scans are interpreted in conjunction with the chest radiograph. Defects that do not have a corresponding abnormality on the chest radiograph are scored by number and size for the probability of pulmonary embolism. Single defects smaller than segments carry low probability for pulmonary embolism, whereas multiple defects that are segmental or larger carry a substantially higher probability for pulmonary embolism. Perfusion defects that have corresponding abnormalities on the chest radiograph are called "indeterminate," although some evidence indicates that a perfusion defect can be assigned a probability of embolus score based upon its size relative to the radiographic abnormality.

The limitation of the Q scan is nonspecificity. Besides emboli, perfusion defects can be caused by lesions that compress pulmonary vessels, by increased pulmonary vascular resistance, by regional alveolar hypoxia, and by regional loss of pulmonary parenchyma, as in pulmonary emphysema. In practice, obstructive lung disease is the most common clinical condition causing perfusion defects that are not due to pulmonary embolism.

The V lung scans increase the specificity of the Q scans for diagnosing pulmonary emboli because pulmonary emboli do not usually disrupt regional ventilation as much as regional blood flow, unlike other causes of perfusion defects, especially obstructive lung disease (Table 65–3). V scans may indicate the preservation of ventilation when there are perfusion defects ("V/Q mismatches"), the loss of ventilation when there are perfusion defects ("V/Q matches"), and delays of washin or washout indicative of obstructive lung disease. V/Q mismatches establish a higher probability of pulmonary emboli than do perfusion defects alone. With some patterns of V̇/Q̇ mismatch, the diagnosis of pulmonary embolism can be made with virtual certainty (Fig. 65–2). Matched V̇/Q̇ defects are less likely to represent pulmonary embolism, but pulmonary embolism is not excluded.

A multicenter study to evaluate the sensitivity and specificity of V̇/Q̇ scanning in the diagnosis of pulmonary embolism has been completed recently in the United States. This prospective investigation of pulmonary embolism diagnosis (referred to as the PIOPED Study) employed V̇/Q̇ scanning and pulmonary arteriography in a large, randomly selected sample of individuals suspected of having acute pulmonary embolism. The results support the findings of earlier studies (Table 65–3): (1) High-probability scans were confirmed with definitive arteriographic findings of emboli in most cases; (2) normal scans were seldom associated with arteriographic findings of emboli; (3) among low-probability scans the occurrence of embolism was small, particularly when the clinical suspicion for embolism was low; and (4) intermediate or indeterminate scans were of little help in predicting the results of arteriography. Notably, in the majority of instances in which arteriograms were abnormal, scans were abnormal but did not indicate a high probability of embolism.

Pulmonary Arteriography. Pulmonary arteriography is the definitive test for the diagnosis of pulmonary embolism. It involves insertion of a catheter into the pulmonary artery, usually by a percutaneous approach through one of the femoral veins. After the catheter is advanced at least as far as the right or left mainstem branch of the pulmonary artery, or more selectively into lobar or segmental branches, the contrast medium is injected and films are taken in rapid sequence. Radiographic images—anterior, oblique, or lateral views—are examined for filling defects (Fig. 65–3) in branches of the pulmonary artery; these establish the diagnosis of pulmonary embolism. Abrupt terminations ("cutoffs") of pulmonary arterial branches also indicate that diagnosis, although less definitely. The filling defects or cutoffs should be present in vessels of at least 2 to 3 mm in diameter. Other types of abnormalities, including delayed filling and a diminished number of small vessels, are not diagnostic. A normal study has rarely been proved wrong. Arteriography should be done promptly after the onset of symptoms, but it is doubtful that there will be major changes within a few days in most cases.

Pulmonary arteriography is indicated when scans demonstrate an intermediate probability of pulmonary embolism. It is also warranted in the following circumstances: (1) when V̇/Q̇ scans suggest a high probability of pulmonary embolism but there are concerns about using anticoagulation therapy; (2) before using thrombolytic agents; (3) when there are clear-cut contraindications to anticoagulation therapy, so that other forms of treatment will be needed; and (4) when anticoagulation therapy has apparently failed and surgical treatment is being contemplated.

When V̇/Q̇ scans are interpreted as indicating a low probability of pulmonary embolism, it has been considered reasonable to be guided by clinical suspicion about the need for arteriography (see Fig. 65–1). Since approximately 10 per cent of these patients will have an abnormal arteriogram, some clinicians contend that pulmonary arteriography should be done routinely in this situation, irrespective of the level of clinical suspicion. Recent studies, however, cast doubt on whether pulmonary arteriography is necessary in any patients having low-probability scans because long-term follow-up of such individuals indicates that they are unlikely to have clinically apparent pulmonary emboli over the subsequent year without anticoagulant therapy. Assessing the proximal deep veins of the lower extremities may be important in this setting. In a large prospective series, Hull and associates found that an abnormal V̇/Q̇ scan, but not one of high probability, combined with normal results on serial noninvasive tests for thrombosis of proximal veins, carried a very good prognosis without anticoagulant therapy.

Many experts in this field believe that pulmonary arteriography is underutilized because physicians have unwarranted concerns about the safety of the procedure. Pulmonary arteriography for the diagnosis of pulmonary embolism has proved to be very safe. In large series, the risk of a serious complication is 1 to 2 per cent and of death, about 0.25 per cent. The deaths have occurred almost exclusively in people with severe pulmonary hypertension who were given large amounts of contrast media.

THERAPY

Nearly all patients with acute pulmonary embolism who survive long enough to have the diagnosis confirmed will survive the acute episode. Accordingly, the primary goal of therapy is to prevent a recurrence that might be fatal. Additional goals are to reduce the morbidity of the acute episode and to prevent chronic pulmonary hypertension.

The overall therapeutic approach is summarized in Figure 65–4. The cornerstone of therapy is the use of anticoagulant drugs, since most patients with acute pulmonary embolism are hemodynamically stable and do not have a contraindication to anticoagulants. Patients who are treated with therapeutic doses of anticoagulants for an appropriate period seldom have a recurrence of pulmonary embolism, and fatal recurrences are rare indeed. Thrombolytic therapy accelerates restoration of pulmonary blood flow and normal pulmonary hemodynamics and therefore is the initial therapy for massive pulmonary embolism that has produced hemodynamic instability. When anticoagulants and thrombolytic agents are contraindicated or prove ineffective, therapy consists of interruption of the inferior vena cava, combined with pulmonary embolectomy in patients with hemodynamic instability.

Supportive measures can reduce the morbidity of the acute episode and, on occasion, are essential to sustain the patient through a period of hemodynamic crisis. These measures include supplemental oxygen to correct hypoxemia, analgesics for pleuritic pain, and hemodynamic and ventilatory support.

ANTICOAGULANT THERAPY. Anticoagulant therapy guards against future embolization by preventing the formation of new deep venous thrombi and the propagation of residual thrombi in the deep venous system. During anticoagulant ther-

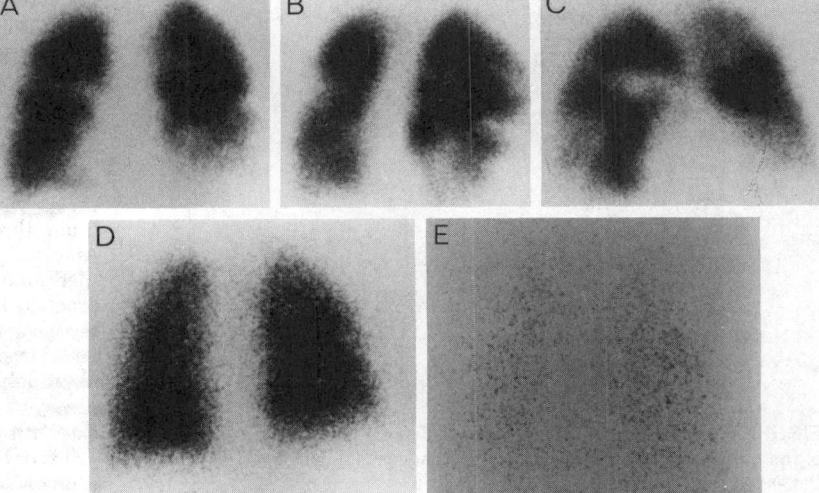

FIGURE 65–2. Selected views of ventilation-perfusion lung scans in a 60-year-old man who experienced sudden, severe shortness of breath 14 days after a suprapubic prostatectomy. The perfusion scans—(A) posterior, (B) right posterior oblique, and (C) left posterior oblique—show multiple segmental defects; the ventilation scans are normal—(D) at equilibrium and (E) at 1 minute of washout. This combination of scan findings indicates a high probability of pulmonary embolism and with the clinical setting is sufficient to make the diagnosis of pulmonary embolism. (Courtesy of Dr. Keith C. Fischer.)

TABLE 65–3. INTERPRETATION OF VENTILATION-PERFUSION (V̇/Q̇) SCINTIGRAMS

Category	Pattern	Approximate Frequency of Pulmonary Embolism Detected by Pulmonary Arteriogram (%)
Normal	No perfusion defects	0
Low probability	Small V̇/Q̇ mismatches	10
	V̇/Q̇ matches without corresponding roentgenographic changes	
	Perfusion defect substantially smaller than roentgenographic density	
Intermediate probability	Severe, diffuse obstructive pulmonary disease with perfusion defects	30
	Perfusion defect of same size as roentgenographic change	
	Single segmental mismatch*	
High probability	Two or more segmental mismatches	90
	Perfusion defect substantially larger than roentgenographic density	

*Controversy exists regarding the important categorization of a single segmental mismatch. This has been considered either of high or intermediate probability. The more conservative interpretation, that is, intermediate probability, has been used in this table.

Adapted from Biello DR: Radiological (scintigraphic) evaluation of patients with suspected pulmonary thromboembolism. JAMA 257:3257, 1987; with permission. Copyright 1987, American Medical Association.

apy, pulmonary emboli and residual deep venous thrombi either organize or undergo dissolution or both. Anticoagulation does not, however, hasten resolution of the thromboemboli within the lungs.

Table 65–4 presents a regimen of anticoagulant agents. Heparin is the initial therapy because its effect is immediate. It may also be a more effective antithrombotic agent than warfarin. Heparin, an acidic glycosaminoglycan obtained from pig intestinal mucosa or beef lung, accelerates the inhibitory effect of antithrombin III upon the coagulation enzymes, thrombin, and Factors IXa, Xa, XIa, and XIIa. In patients who are suspected of having pulmonary embolism, an intravenous bolus of heparin (5000 to 10,000 units) should be given while diagnostic studies are under way, unless there is intracranial bleeding, intracranial lesions predisposed to bleed, or active internal bleeding, all of which are absolute contraindications to heparin.

Heparin is usually administered intravenously by continuous infusion. Intermittent intravenous injection and subcutaneous injection are alternative means of administration, but a higher incidence of bleeding complications may occur with intermittent injection, and it is difficult to establish the correct dose with the subcutaneous route. The risk of recurrent venous thromboembolism is low if the activated partial thromboplastin time is maintained 1.5 to 2 times the control (about 25 seconds beyond the control) at all times. Accordingly, this is the goal of therapy. The usual daily dose is 25,000 to 50,000 units. Heparin therapy should be monitored particularly closely during the first few days

after the thromboembolic event, as the heparin requirements are greatest then.

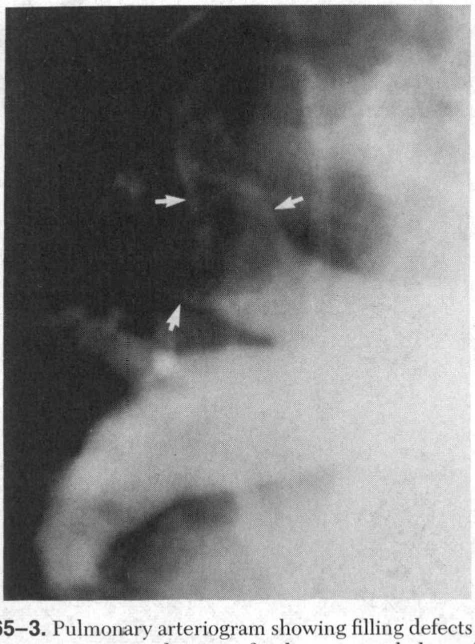

The most common and most serious complication of heparin therapy is bleeding. The risk of bleeding may be more closely related to risk factors, such as trauma, recent surgery, recent invasive procedures, and the inhibition by heparin of platelet function, than to the absolute anticoagulant effect produced by the drug. Thrombocytopenia may also complicate therapy and cause bleeding. Approximately 10 per cent of patients exhibit platelet counts less than 100,000 per cubic millimeter during heparin therapy; there seems to be no correlation between this complication and the type of heparin used. The thrombocytopenia, which appears to have an immunologic basis, seldom occurs until after several days of therapy. A rare complication of heparin-induced thrombocytopenia is thrombosis, mainly of arteries. With long-term administration, heparin can cause accelerated osteoporosis.

After 1 to 2 days of heparin therapy, oral anticoagulation with warfarin is begun. Both agents are continued together for 4 to 5 days, after which the heparin is discontinued. Warfarin acts in the liver to inhibit the gamma-carboxylation of specific glutamic acid residues in several vitamin K–dependent coagulation factors: Factors II, VII, IX, and X (Ch. 155). These gamma-carboxyglutamic acids are required for calcium binding and the expression of functional activity. Since these coagulation cofactors have different half-lives in the circulation, the rates at which they diminish in activity are variable after the start of therapy. The prothrombin time is most sensitive to Factor VII, which has the shortest half-life (4 to 6 hours).

The rationale for overlapping heparin therapy with the first period of warfarin therapy is to ensure a full anticoagulant effect during the time required for depression of the level of all four coagulation cofactors affected by warfarin. It is also done to reduce the risk of thrombosis during the induction of warfarin, since warfarin lowers the concentration of protein C, a vitamin K–dependent protein that has anticoagulant properties because of its capacity to degrade Factors Va and VIIIa proteolytically. Warfarin is not used during pregnancy, since it is teratogenic. In pregnancy, only heparin is used for anticoagulant therapy, and its use has been found safe for the fetus and protective for the mother without producing an incidence of bleeding greater than that expected for the nonpregnant individual.

The dose of warfarin needed for prophylaxis against venous thromboembolism should be adjusted to achieve an increase in the prothrombin time to 1.3 to 1.5 times the control (using rabbit brain thromboplastin for the assay, as is customary in North America). This range is therapeutic and produces less bleeding than amounts aiming for 1.5 to 2 times the control, as was the practice for many years. The optimal duration of anticoagulant therapy is not known. It is generally advised to continue therapy for at least 3 months in all patients, to extend therapy as long as identifiable risk factors are resolving, and to give therapy indefinitely to patients in whom an increased risk for deep venous thrombosis is permanent.

THROMBOLYTIC THERAPY. Thrombolytic agents, by dissolving pulmonary emboli and thrombi in the deep venous

FIGURE 65–3. Pulmonary arteriogram showing filling defects in branches of the pulmonary artery, indicative of pulmonary embolism. (Courtesy of Dr. Noah Susman.)

TABLE 65–4. GUIDELINES FOR ANTICOAGULANT THERAPY WITH HEPARIN AND WARFARIN IN PULMONARY EMBOLISM

Embolism Suspected	Embolism Confirmed
Obtain baseline APTT,* PT, and platelet count and give heparin bolus (5000–10,000 units) IV Order diagnostic test: ventilation-perfusion lung scan or pulmonary arteriogram	Give loading dose of heparin (5000 units) and start constant IV infusion at approximately 1000 units/hr Monitor APTT at 6 hr and thereafter until the APTT is stabilized between 1.5 and 2.0 times control value Monitor platelet count every 3–4 days while administering heparin Start warfarin on day 1 or 2 by instituting the estimated daily maintenance dose (usually 4–10 mg) After at least 5 days of heparin therapy and 4–5 days of joint therapy, stop heparin and check PT 4 hr later Maintain PT off heparin at 1.3 to 1.5 times control or pretreatment value (using rabbit brain thromboplastin) Maintain full-dose anticoagulation for at least 3 mo in patients without continuing risk factors, longer in other patients

*APTT = activated partial thromboplastin time; PT = one-stage prothrombin time (1.3 times control performed with rabbit brain thromboplastin is roughly equal to 2.0 times control with human brain thromboplastin); IV = intravenous.

Adapted from Hyers TM, Hull RD, Weg JG: Antithrombotic therapy for venous thromboembolic disease. Chest 95:37S, 1989; with permission.

system, can alleviate the hemodynamic disturbances caused by pulmonary emboli, eliminate the source of further emboli, and perhaps diminish postphlebitic complications in the lower extremities. Two thrombolytic agents, streptokinase and urokinase, have been used for a number of years. A third, tissue-type plasminogen activator (TPA), generated by recombinant DNA methods, has been used in limited trials, but it is not yet approved by the Food and Drug Administration for the treatment of pulmonary embolism.

Streptokinase and urokinase convert circulating endogenous plasminogen to plasmin, a potent serine protease that dissolves fibrin. Urokinase cleaves plasminogen to plasmin directly, whereas streptokinase forms a complex with plasminogen, allowing expression of plasminogen's normally hidden active site, which then cleaves other plasminogen molecules to plasmin. At equivalent dosage, streptokinase is considerably cheaper than urokinase, but, unlike urokinase, it can produce febrile and allergic reactions. Plasmin formed by either agent lyses the fibrin clot in pulmonary emboli, but unfortunately it also cleaves other molecules in the circulation, including fibrinogen and Factors V and VIII, and it leads to consumption of circulating plasmin inhibitors, in particular, alpha$_2$-antiplasmin. Thus, besides solubilizing pulmonary emboli and deep venous thrombi, these agents can solubilize hemostatic plugs where they are important, such as at incisional sites, and can reduce hemostatic competence generally.

Thrombolytic agents can restore pulmonary arterial pressure and pulmonary parenchymal perfusion toward normal faster than does heparin, but this effect does not appear to result in improved survival rates or pulmonary perfusion when patients are studied a few weeks after the acute episode. Moreover, concerning the rate of recurrence of pulmonary embolism, there is no difference between thrombolytic agents and anticoagulants. With thrombolytic agents, pulmonary capillary blood flow after a year may be more normalized than if only heparin were used, but this is of questionable clinical importance, since pulmonary impairment is rare following pulmonary emboli in either case. One setting in which thrombolytic therapy may offer a clear advantage over heparin is that of angiographically proven massive pulmonary embolism that has produced hemodynamic instability. In this case, the rapid reduction in vascular occlusion that may be achieved with thrombolytic therapy may prove life-saving. Some preliminary evidence has suggested a greater speed of clot resolution with TPA than with other thrombolytic agents, but the studies showing such an effect have not used comparable doses, so these data are difficult to interpret.

The typical thrombolytic regimen involves a loading dose of streptokinase or urokinase, followed by a continuous intravenous infusion for 12 to 24 hours. Other regimens that have been proved effective include single large-bolus infusions of thrombolytic agent into the right atrium over a few minutes and continuous infusions of low-dose thrombolytic agent directly into the

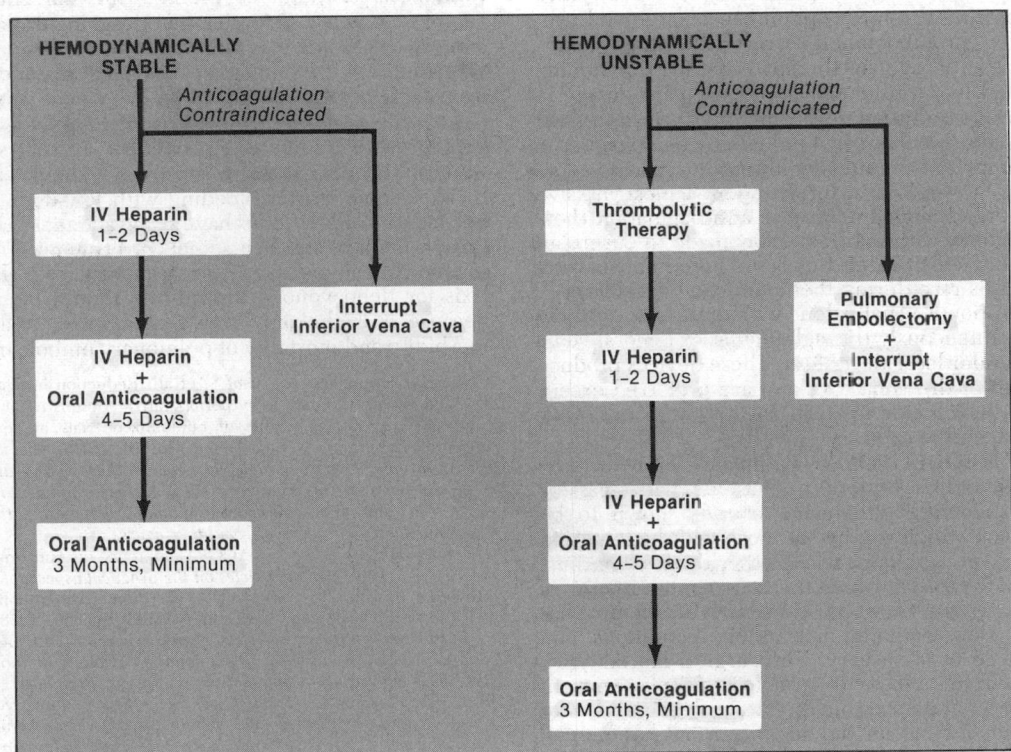

FIGURE 65–4. The therapy of pulmonary embolism.

pulmonary artery at the site of the clot, in combination with systemic heparinization. Whatever thrombolytic regimen is used, it should be followed by anticoagulant therapy (Fig. 65–4).

There is no ideal test for monitoring patients given thrombolytic agents. The usual approach is to document either an anticoagulant effect (lengthening of the prothrombin time, partial thromboplastin time, or thrombin time) or evidence of fibrinogen or fibrin degradation (decreased fibrinogen concentration or increased titers of fibrin degradation products) or both. Because these agents digest substrates besides fibrin in pulmonary emboli, proof that a thrombolytic agent has exerted some effect according to these tests does not, however, prove that it has had an effect upon pulmonary emboli. Nor is it possible to use results from these tests to titrate the dose. On the other hand, clinical effectiveness is usually apparent from improvement in the patient's cardiopulmonary status.

Because thrombolytic agents may start or aggravate bleeding, they are absolutely contraindicated when active internal bleeding is present or within a few months of stroke, neurologic or ophthalmic surgery, or head injury. They are relatively contraindicated within 10 days of major surgical procedures or biopsies of internal organs or arteriographic studies, during pregnancy and the first 10 days post partum, and in a variety of medical states associated with increased risk of bleeding, such as severe hypertension. In the patient who is critically ill from pulmonary emboli, however, the danger of bleeding must be weighed against the potential benefits and the risks of alternate forms of therapy.

VENA CAVAL INTERRUPTION. The principal reasons for interruption of the inferior vena cava are (1) absolute contraindications to anticoagulant therapy (active internal bleeding and recent central nervous system lesions that are bleeding or are predisposed to bleeding), (2) severe internal bleeding that develops during therapeutic anticoagulation, and (3) recurrent emboli despite adequate anticoagulation. Infrequently, vena caval interruption is necessary for septic embolism, after pulmonary embolectomy, or after massive embolization of such severity that further embolization might well be fatal. In the last-noted situation, anticoagulation therapy is used as well.

Like anticoagulation therapy, interruption of the vena cava is only preventive against future emboli. It does not promote resolution of emboli already in the lungs, and it does not correct the hemodynamic effects of emboli. In addition, it may not provide permanent protection against pulmonary embolism, since collateral veins bypassing the interruption can enlarge and provide other routes for thromboemboli to reach the lungs. Since most bleeding during anticoagulant therapy is not life threatening and can be controlled by a reduction in anticoagulant dosage, a conservative approach is advised regarding the interruption of the vena cava. Similarly, recurrence of pulmonary embolism after anticoagulation therapy is begun should not be taken as an automatic indication for vena caval interruption. Unless massive embolism is documented angiographically, anticoagulation therapy should be continued, with maximal effort made to ensure an adequate anticoagulant effect at all times. As noted above, fatal pulmonary embolism is rare during therapeutic anticoagulation.

Vena caval interruption is usually done with umbrellas or filters that are inserted percutaneously through jugular or femoral veins while the patient is under local anesthesia. These devices produce only partial occlusion of the vena cava and are preferred except for septic emboli, in which case ligation or clipping is done with the patient under general anesthesia.

PULMONARY EMBOLECTOMY. Pulmonary embolectomy is rarely performed and is limited to patients with massive pulmonary emboli involving pulmonary arteries shown to be accessible on pulmonary angiography, to those with hypotension and end-organ (brain and kidney) dysfunction despite maximal medical support, and to those in whom there are contraindications to thrombolytic therapy or in whom thrombolytic therapy has proved ineffective. Few patients meet these conditions and survive long enough to have surgery. The surgical mortality for emergency pulmonary embolectomy is at least 25 per cent. In contrast, elective surgery for symptomatic, unresolved pulmonary emboli in large branches of the pulmonary artery has proved effective and reasonably safe. The procedure for chronic emboli, which amounts to an endarterectomy for removal of organized

thromboemboli, can improve functional status, reduce pulmonary arterial pressure, and normalize pulmonary arterial perfusion and arterial oxygenation.

PROGNOSIS

The majority of deaths from pulmonary embolism occur either too quickly for therapy to be given or because the condition is not recognized. If pulmonary embolism goes untreated, survival is only 70 per cent, with death occurring as a result of recurrent thromboembolism within a few weeks of the first episode. In contrast, among those individuals in whom a diagnosis is made and therapy begun, 92 per cent survive and do so without sequelae. Among those few individuals who do not survive despite therapy, two thirds of the deaths are due to associated critical diseases. In those in whom death is caused by pulmonary embolism, systemic hypotension is usually present at the onset of the episode, and pulmonary vascular obstruction is usually greater than 75 per cent. Even when hypotension and acute cor pulmonale are present at the onset of acute pulmonary embolism, however, it does not necessarily mean a fatal outcome. Clinical signs of massive embolization can subside quickly, presumably because vascular obstruction decreases as a result of fragmentation or remodeling of the emboli or because pulmonary vasoconstrictive reflexes and mediators dissipate. The presence of pulmonary infarction has no effect on survival.

In fewer than 1 per cent of those who survive acute pulmonary thromboembolization, the emboli persist and result in a chronic syndrome of exertional dyspnea, pulmonary hypertension, right ventricular enlargement, and right ventricular failure. Individuals presenting with this syndrome usually have a history that contains clues to recurrent episodes of pulmonary embolism and to conditions predisposing to venous thromboembolic disease.

PREVENTION

Several therapeutic regimens reduce the risk of deep venous thrombosis and by doing so decrease the risk of pulmonary thromboembolism. These regimens—which include early ambulation after surgery, low-dose subcutaneous heparin, low-dose warfarin, dextran, external pneumatic calf compression, and gradient elastic stockings—are easy to use, have minimal complications, and require essentially no laboratory monitoring. The most thoroughly proven regimen, low-dose subcutaneous heparin (5000 units twice daily), is effective for (1) general surgery patients with high-risk features (over age 40, obese, previous deep venous thrombosis or pulmonary embolism, current malignancy, and complex surgery), (2) patients undergoing urologic or gynecologic surgery (excluding procedures for gynecologic malignancies), and (3) patients with congestive heart failure and those recovering from acute myocardial infarction. Low-dose subcutaneous heparin is not effective for prophylaxis of deep venous thrombosis in patients with traumatic hip fracture. In that situation, low-dose warfarin or pneumatic compression should be used. Because there is some risk of bleeding with low-dose heparin, it should not be used in patients having intracranial or eye surgery or in those who have suffered spinal cord trauma. For these situations, pneumatic compression is a satisfactory, safe alternative. Prophylaxis for deep venous thrombosis should be used more widely because it is the only way that a substantial reduction in the morbidity and mortality of pulmonary embolism will be achieved.

Collins R, Scrimgeour A, Yusuf S, et al.: Reduction in fatal pulmonary embolism and venous thrombosis by perioperative administration of subcutaneous heparin: Overview of results of randomized trials in general, orthopedic, and urologic surgery. N Engl J Med 318:1162, 1988. *Analysis of randomized trials of prophylactic subcutaneous heparin therapy in various types of surgery indicates that this therapy greatly decreases pulmonary emboli, deep venous thromboses, and deaths due to pulmonary emboli, without causing a concomitant increase in deaths from other causes.*

Dalen JE, Hirsh J (eds.): 2nd ACCP Conference on Antithrombotic Therapy. Chest 95:1S, 1989. *Detailed articles on the practical aspects of anticoagulant therapy.*

Hull RD, Raskob GE, Carter CJ, et al.: Pulmonary embolism in outpatients with pleuritic chest pain. Arch Intern Med 148:838, 1988. *Prospective study of individuals presenting to an emergency room with pleuritic pain showing a substantial occurrence of pulmonary embolism in those over age 40 and in those with predisposing factors for venous thrombosis.*

Hull RD, Raskob GE, Coates G, et al.: A new noninvasive management strategy for patients with suspected pulmonary embolism. Arch Intern Med 149:2549, 1989. *A prospective study with long-term follow-up showing an excellent prognosis without anticoagulant therapy in individuals suspected of having acute pulmonary embolism whose lung scan is not of high probability and whose lower extremity proximal veins do not show thrombosis on serial impedance plethysmography.*

Levine M, Hirsch J, Weitz J, et al.: A randomized trial of a single bolus dosage regimen of recombinant tissue plasminogen activator in patients with acute pulmonary embolism. Chest 98:1473, 1990. *A prospective study of recombinant tissue plasminogen activator (rt-PA) therapy in patients with acute symptomatic pulmonary embolism who were receiving heparin. Patients given a 2-minute infusion of rt-PA at 0.6 mg per kilogram had more resolution of perfusion defects on lung scans 24 hours later than patients given a saline placebo, but at 7 days the resolution of scans was the same in both groups.*

Mitchell JP, Trulock EP: Tissue-plasminogen activator for pulmonary embolism resulting in shock: Two case reports and discussion of the literature. Am J Med 90:260, 1991. *Two patients with relative contraindications to thrombolytic therapy received 100 mg of recombinant tissue plasminogen activator over 2 to 3 hours for pulmonary emboli causing shock. In both patients, there was almost complete restoration of normal hemodynamics within a few hours.*

Moser KM: Venous thromboembolism. Am Rev Respir Dis 141:235, 1990. *Review of deep venous thrombosis and pulmonary thromboembolism, with particular emphasis on the importance of prevention.*

The PIOPED Investigators: Value of the ventilation/perfusion scan in acute pulmonary embolism: Results of the Prospective Investigation of Pulmonary Embolism Diagnosis (PIOPED), JAMA 263:2753, 1990. *A multicenter, prospective study that used pulmonary arteriography to assess the sensitivity and specificity of lung scans in the diagnosis of pulmonary embolism.*

66 Fat Embolism Syndrome

Robert M. Senior

DEFINITION

Fat embolism syndrome refers to the constellation of clinical manifestations that may develop when fat droplets become impacted in the pulmonary microvasculature and other microvascular beds, especially in the brain. The principal clinical features of fat embolism syndrome are respiratory failure, cerebral dysfunction, and petechiae.

CLINICAL SETTING

Fat embolism syndrome occurs almost exclusively as an early complication of traumatic fractures of the pelvis and of long bones, particularly the shaft of the femur. Delays in stabilization of fractures and periods of systemic hypoperfusion after trauma increase the risk of the syndrome. The syndrome develops in 2 to 25 per cent of persons with fresh long bone fractures, depending on criteria for the diagnosis and selection of patients at risk. In contrast, it rarely follows elective orthopedic surgery on long bones, even though fat droplets can be found routinely in the venous blood draining the operative sites. Other forms of trauma that rarely result in fat embolism include massive soft tissue injury, severe burns, and liposuction. Nontraumatic settings occasionally lead to fat embolism. These include conditions associated with fatty liver, prolonged corticosteroid therapy, acute pancreatitis, osteomyelitis, and conditions causing bone infarcts, such as sickle cell hemoglobinopathy.

DIAGNOSIS

There are no laboratory tests that are diagnostic of fat embolism syndrome. Looking for fat droplets in the blood, urine, and sputum is not helpful in making the diagnosis, as droplets may not be present in patients who clearly have fat embolism syndrome but may be found after traumatic fractures in patients without evidence of the syndrome. It is possible, however, that bronchoalveolar lavage and staining the lavage cells with oil red 0 may be helpful. In a recent study, large fat droplets were found in the lavage cells of patients with definite fat embolism syndrome and of patients with possible fat embolism syndrome that was later proved, whereas fat droplets were rare in the lavage cells from normal persons and patients with other causes of respiratory distress. The diagnosis is based on the presence of at least one of the following features within the first 72 hours after traumatic fracture: (1) otherwise unexplained dyspnea, tachypnea, arterial hypoxemia, and diffuse alveolar infiltrates on the chest radiograph; (2) otherwise unexplained confusion or other signs of cerebral dysfunction; and (3) petechiae over the upper half of the body, including the axillae, conjunctivae, and oral mucosa. The diagnosis is definite if all three criteria are present. Further support for the diagnosis is provided by fluffy retinal exudates and hemorrhages and unexplained fever. The diagnosis is unlikely if the signs and symptoms first begin more than 72 hours after the injury. In these situations, more probable causes of respiratory distress are pulmonary edema from massive fluid replacement, aspiration, sepsis, pneumonia, or venous thromboembolism.

PATHOGENESIS

The cellular mechanisms leading to fat embolism syndrome are not fully understood, but it is clear that the syndrome is not simply a consequence of mechanical obstruction of small vessels by fat droplets. An important aspect of the pathogenesis appears to be endothelial injury caused by fatty acids released from impacted fat droplets by lipoprotein lipase, with ensuing increased microvascular permeability and fluid leakage into interstitial spaces.

The fat droplets found in small vessels are from the trauma site. As the first microvascular bed encountered by fat droplets in the venous circulation, the lungs bear the brunt of fat embolization. Presumably, fat emboli in other organs, especially the brain, reach those sites by passing through the pulmonary microvasculature or through right-to-left shunts in the heart.

Although the effects of fatty acids upon endothelium appear to be important in the mechanism of lung injury, the pathogenesis of respiratory failure may be more complex in some cases. Other tissue components besides fat may be liberated from fracture sites, and these as well as the injured pulmonary endothelium may activate the clotting, complement, and contact systems. Thus, the pathogenesis of lung injury may be multifactorial, as in other forms of the adult respiratory distress syndrome, involving thrombi, mediators of inflammation, and products of inflammatory cells.

Hypoxemia explains brain dysfunction in many cases, but not all. In some fatal cases, cerebral symptoms reflect direct brain injury with many fat emboli and associated hemorrhage and necrosis. Moreover, patients with comparable hypoxemia from causes other than fat embolism syndrome seldom have brain dysfunction, and occasional patients with fat embolism syndrome have neurologic features that precede hypoxemia or are disproportionate to the degree of hypoxemia.

The reason for the petechiae is not known, although in some patients thrombocytopenia and disseminated intravascular coagulation may be present. There is also no explanation for the striking localization of the petechiae to the pectoral regions and conjunctivae.

THERAPY

Management of fat embolism syndrome is supportive and consists primarily of ensuring good arterial oxygenation. Supplemental oxygen is given to maintain the arterial oxygen tension in the normal range, 75 to 90 mm Hg. If endotracheal intubation and ventilatory support are necessary, positive end-expiratory pressure may reduce the need for high concentrations of inspired oxygen. Restricting fluid intake and even giving diuretics, if systemic perfusion can be maintained, may minimize fluid accumulation in the lungs. The role of corticosteroids is controversial; there is no clear-cut evidence that they are helpful.

In patients with acute long bone fractures, the risk of fat embolism syndrome is reduced by prompt surgical stabilization of the fractures and by correcting or preventing decreased systemic perfusion. In addition, administration of corticosteroids for a short period (for example, 1.5 mg per kilogram of methylprednisolone intravenously at 8-hour intervals for 2 days) seems to prevent development of the syndrome.

PROGNOSIS

The mortality from fat embolism syndrome is 10 per cent or less and thus is clearly much lower than the 50 per cent or greater mortality for most causes of the adult respiratory distress syndrome. Even severe respiratory failure associated with fat embolism seldom leads to death. In one report of 54 cases, there was not a single fatality from the syndrome, although severe hypoxemia was common during the acute stages.

Chastre J, Fagon J-Y, Soler P, et al.: Bronchoalveolar lavage for rapid diagnosis of the fat embolism syndrome in trauma patients. Ann Intern Med 113:583, 1990. *A report indicating that looking for fat droplets in alveolar macrophages and neutrophils recovered by bronchoalveolar lavage is helpful in making the diagnosis of the fat embolism syndrome.*

Eddy AC, Rice CL, Carrico CJ: Fat embolism syndrome: Monitoring and management. J Crit Ill 2:24, 1987. *Reviews many aspects of posttraumatic fat embolism syndrome.*

Guardia SN, Bilbao JM, Murray D, et al.: Fat embolism in acute pancreatitis. Arch Pathol Lab Med 113:503, 1989. *Describes a patient with fatal fat embolism syndrome that occurred without trauma.*

Peltier LF: Fat embolism: A perspective. Clin Orthop Rel Res 232:263, 1988. *Reviews the progress in understanding the pathogenesis of fat embolism syndrome and its management since the first diagnosis in 1873.*

67 Sarcoidosis

Barry L. Fanburg

DEFINITION

Sarcoidosis, a multisystem granulomatous disease, begins most frequently in people between 20 and 40 years old. The etiology is unknown, but alterations in the immune system are clearly involved in its pathogenesis. Organ involvement is usually asymptomatic, and the disease most frequently regresses spontaneously, but it may progress to a more chronic state of fibrosis with severe functional impairment of various organs. No natural animal models of sarcoidosis have been discovered.

EPIDEMIOLOGY AND GENETICS

Sarcoidosis occurs with similar manifestations world wide, but its incidence differs strikingly, from 0.04 per 100,000 in Spain, for example, to 64 per 100,000 in Sweden. The reported numbers are susceptible to considerable error based upon procedures for evaluation, but large unexplained differences in prevalence clearly exist. The occurrence in blacks has been reported to be more frequent than that in whites. The majority of cases occur during adulthood, but sarcoidosis is also present in the pediatric population.

The disease has been reported to be transmissible in experi-mental animals, but this work still has not been rigorously tested for confirmation. Sarcoidosis is not contagious in humans.

Familial occurrences have been reported in approximately 200 instances, but no specific patterns of parent-child or sibling relationships have emerged. Sarcoidosis has been reported in twins, with a preponderance of monozygotic over dizygotic twins. The disease seems not to be linked with specific human leukocyte antigen (HLA) types.

IMMUNOLOGY

A postulated schema for the immunopathology of sarcoidosis is presented in Figure 67–1. The macrophage most likely initiates the cellular response of sarcoidosis, possibly in response to some unknown presenting antigen. Various factors released by the macrophage, such as interleukin 1, cause accumulation and proliferation of helper T lymphocytes. Factors secreted by the lymphocytes attract and immobilize other inflammatory cells. In addition, B lymphocytes are stimulated to produce increased amounts of immunoglobulins, and fibroblasts are stimulated to proliferate. As the response becomes less active, the number of T lymphocytes decreases, and suppressor T lymphocytes predominate.

As a result of these various immunologic interactions, (1) inflammatory cells proliferate in the affected organ (forming the granuloma), (2) cutaneous delayed hypersensitivity responses to common antigens are depressed, and (3) immune globulins are synthesized and circulate in excess. In addition, circulating immune complexes may be present; high levels of serum antibodies to common environmental antigens such as *Mycoplasma pneumoniae* and various viruses frequently occur; antibody responses to immunization may be exaggerated; and circulating rheumatoid factor, antinuclear antibody, and autoantibodies to T lymphocytes may be present.

Intradermally injected extracts of homogenized tissue of involved organs from patients with sarcoidosis are capable of producing a delayed inflammatory reaction in patients with sarcoidosis. This antigen that causes the so-called *Kveim-Siltzbach reaction* has not been purified, and the basis for its response has not been defined. The reaction differs from a cutaneous delayed hypersensitivity reaction in that it takes 4 to 6 weeks to develop and then persists for several months.

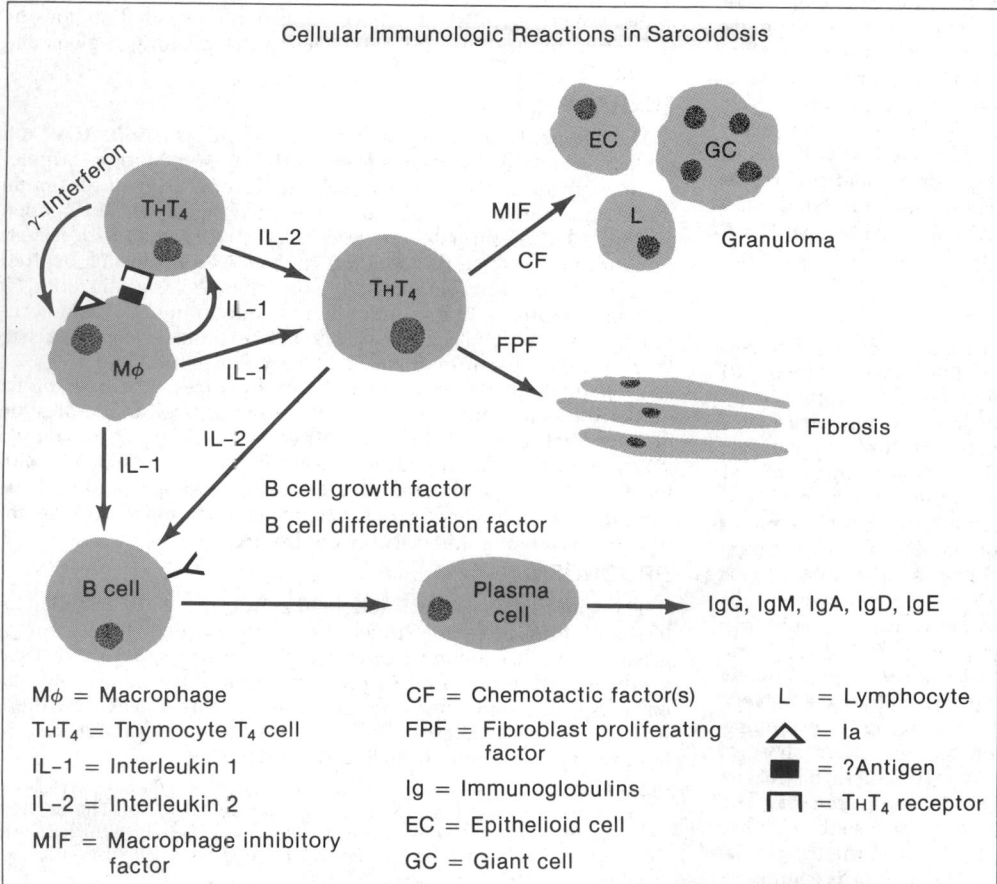

Cellular Immunologic Reactions in Sarcoidosis

Granuloma

Fibrosis

B cell growth factor
B cell differentiation factor

IgG, IgM, IgA, IgD, IgE

Mφ = Macrophage
THT4 = Thymocyte T4 cell
IL–1 = Interleukin 1
IL–2 = Interleukin 2
MIF = Macrophage inhibitory factor

CF = Chemotactic factor(s)
FPF = Fibroblast proliferating factor
Ig = Immunoglobulins
EC = Epithelioid cell
GC = Giant cell

L = Lymphocyte
△ = Ia
■ = ?Antigen
⊓ = THT4 receptor

FIGURE 67–1. Immunologic abnormalities associated with sarcoidosis.

CLINICAL PRESENTATION

Sarcoid lesions may develop in almost any organ system, so that the clinical presentation is quite varied (Fig. 67–2). In fact, "silent" granulomas are frequently present in multiple organs. Most characteristically, the patient is asymptomatic, but the disease is detected by an abnormal chest radiograph, usually showing bilateral symmetric hilar adenopathy often associated with paratracheal adenopathy (Fig. 67–3) and/or reticulonodular parenchymal infiltrates. Patients with sarcoidosis may also present with hilar and paratracheal adenopathy in association with some combination of acute peripheral arthritis, uveitis, and erythema nodosum (the so-called "acute sarcoidosis," or Loeffgren's syndrome). Except for Loeffgren's syndrome, significant constitutional symptoms other than those of fatigue are unusual in sarcoidosis. When anorexia, weight loss, and fever are present, other diseases should be strongly considered.

Lungs

The lungs are the most frequently involved organ, and pulmonary symptoms, when present, include dyspnea on exertion, nonproductive cough, and wheezing. Dyspnea is usually caused by fibrotic or granulomatous pulmonary parenchymal disease, but it may also result from granulomatous obstruction of the upper airways. Granulomas in the nose may cause nasal congestion and in the larynx may result in hoarseness. Hemoptysis is rare in sarcoidosis but may occur from an associated mycetoma in advanced cavitary sarcoidosis. Acute dyspnea secondary to a pneumothorax also occasionally develops in patients with more advanced fibrotic pulmonary disease. Pleural involvement has been reported but is unusual.

Skin

Erythema nodosum may be associated with sarcoidosis as a secondary vasculitic reaction. Sarcoid granulomas also occur directly in the skin to produce a variety of small, asymptomatic macular and papular lesions that are present either superficially or more deeply in the dermis. *Lupus pernio*, consisting of violaceous plaques over the nose, cheeks, and ears, is the most commonly described skin lesion. It may be disfiguring. Granulomas may also occur in scar tissue.

Eyes

Ophthalmologic lesions most commonly consist of inflammation of the uveal tract, but the conjunctiva, retina, and lacrimal glands may also be involved. These lesions may produce nonspecific ocular symptoms of visual impairment and discomfort; chronic lesions may progress to blindness. Anterior uveitis in combination with parotitis and facial nerve palsy has been referred to as *Heerfordt's syndrome*.

Nervous System

Almost any portion of the neurologic system may be affected by sarcoidosis, and the diagnosis may prove difficult. The most common cranial nerve to be involved is the facial nerve, but any cranial nerve may be affected. Disease of the optic nerve may result in papilledema. Palsies of the ninth and tenth cranial nerves manifest as dysphagia, absent gag reflex, and vocal cord paralysis, and disease of the eighth cranial nerve occurs as deafness, tinnitus, and vertigo. Mononeuropathy or polyneuropathy of peripheral nerves causes sensory loss, paresthesias, or motor weakness. Meningitis produced by sarcoidosis is usually insidious in presentation and chronic in its course. Diabetes insipidus results from involvement of the hypothalamus or posterior pituitary gland. Granulomas of the brain may produce a space-occupying lesion and cause headaches, seizures, or focal symptoms. Rarely, personality changes have been observed, and the total constellation of findings resulting from multiple areas of involvement of the nervous system by sarcoidosis may bewilder the diagnostician.

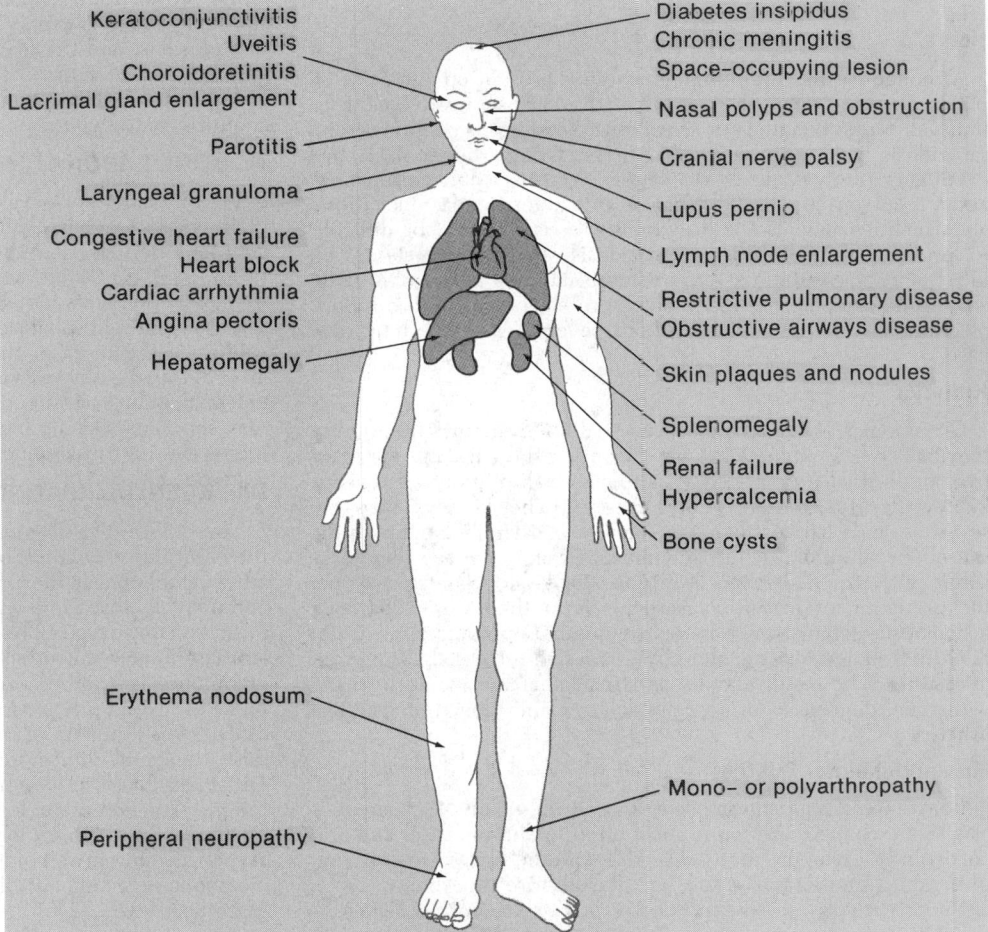

FIGURE 67–2. Organ abnormalities associated with sarcoidosis.

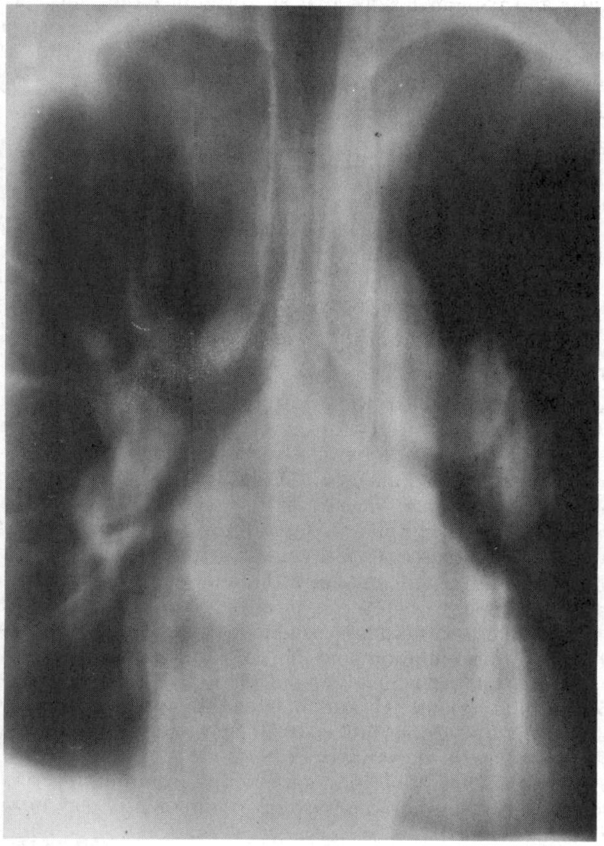

FIGURE 67–3. Tomogram of chest showing hilar and paratracheal adenopathy. (From Murray JF, Nadel J: Textbook of Respiratory Medicine. Philadelphia, W. B. Saunders Company, 1987.)

Heart

Although cardiac granulomas are often present on autopsies of patients with sarcoidosis, symptomatic cardiac involvement is unusual. Granulomatous or fibrotic cardiac lesions resulting from sarcoidosis may cause congestive heart failure, heart block, arrhythmias (often ventricular), angina pectoris, ventricular aneurysm, recurrent pericardial effusion, or sudden death. Since these abnormalities may also be due to other causes, it may be difficult to prove a relationship to sarcoidosis. Cor pulmonale is an infrequent presentation, occurring usually in association with advanced pulmonary fibrosis, but there has been the rare report of pulmonary hypertension without severe restrictive lung disease.

Kidneys

Granulomas of the kidneys are usually infrequent and asymptomatic. When kidney failure occurs, other lesions such as pyelonephritis, nephrocalcinosis, and hyalinization of various kidney structures are usually present. The kidneys may be severely and irreversibly damaged by calcium nephropathy caused by altered calcium metabolism that produces hypercalcemia and hypercalciuria. Symptoms of kidney failure may be the predominant feature of sarcoidosis in these cases. Sarcoid lesions can enzymatically activate vitamin D precursors to 1,25-dihydroxycholecalciferol, thereby increasing intestinal absorption of calcium. The result may be hypercalcemia and hypercalciuria, with renal damage from nephrocalcinosis and recurrent nephrolithiasis.

Musculoskeletal System

Bones, joints, and muscles are frequently involved in sarcoidosis. Bone changes are found most often in chronic cases and are particularly common in blacks with chronic skin disease. The phalanges, metacarpals, and metatarsals are the bones most frequently involved. Osteoporosis, cystic or reticulated changes, and external manifestations of digital deformation and dystrophic

nails may be present. Joints are usually spared destructive changes except in the vicinity of bone lesions.

Arthritic changes may also manifest acutely by monoarthralgias or polyarthralgias or arthritis of the larger joints, such as the ankles, knees, wrists, or elbows. The associated symptoms may be migratory and usually recede with no residual deformities. Although, like the liver, muscles frequently contain asymptomatic granulomas, acute myositis and chronic myopathy with associated muscular enzyme abnormalities are uncommon findings in sarcoidosis. Gout may complicate sarcoidosis, presumably owing to overproduction of purines in widespread granulomas.

Miscellaneous

Although diffuse granulomas may be present, clinical manifestations of liver, gastrointestinal, or pancreatic disease are very unusual. Similarly, clinical evidence for involvement of the endocrine and reproductive systems is rare. As noted earlier, posterior pituitary and hypothalamic involvement may result in diabetes insipidus. Hypopituitarism from anterior pituitary disease occurs very rarely. Alteration in fertility by sarcoidosis has not been described. Peripheral lymph nodes, in contrast to hilar nodes, are seldom more than moderately enlarged and usually go unnoticed by the patient. Although the spleen is moderately enlarged in 5 to 10 per cent of patients, gross enlargement that causes discomfort and predisposes to rupture occurs rarely. Thrombocytopenia is occasionally present and may be associated with hypersplenism. Hypercalcemia may produce nonspecific anorexia and vomiting.

PHYSICAL FINDINGS

Physical findings in the chest in sarcoidosis are often normal despite radiographic abnormalities that may be extensive. Fever is absent, except with Loeffgren's syndrome. Other physical findings usually relate to granulomatous or fibrotic involvement of a specific organ system. Skin lesions may be readily apparent or found only with careful examination. Subcutaneous or muscle nodules may be identified. Slit-lamp examination may be necessary to demonstrate ocular lesions. Lymph nodes are often palpable but usually only moderately enlarged. As noted above, hepatosplenomegaly may be present. Digits may be deformed by bone lesions, and the nails may be dystrophic in cases of chronic disease. Acute arthritic changes may be apparent, in particular in association with erythema nodosum, and must be differentiated from associated gout.

ROUTINE LABORATORY STUDIES

Routine laboratory evaluation may reveal lymphopenia, hyperglobulinemia, hypercalcemia, and/or hypercalciuria. The platelet count is rarely decreased. It is unusual for the sedimentation rate to be significantly elevated, except with Loeffgren's syndrome. Liver function tests may be moderately abnormal, and, in particular, alkaline phosphatase levels may be elevated. With complications of the disease, the expected but nonspecific changes in arterial blood gases and serum chemistries accompany respiratory or renal failure, respectively. Cerebrospinal fluid examination may show nonspecific pleocytosis and increased protein in meningitis caused by sarcoidosis.

DIFFERENTIAL DIAGNOSIS

The differential diagnosis of sarcoidosis depends largely upon the clinical presentation of the patient. With hilar lymphadenopathy, lymphoma is most frequently considered; with pulmonary parenchymal disease, a wide variety of diffuse interstitial diseases must be considered (Ch. 61). Tuberculosis and other granulomatous pulmonary infections must always be ruled out. Eosinophilic granuloma is another diagnostic possibility, particularly when diabetes insipidus is present. Exposure to beryllium may produce disease very similar to sarcoidosis. Pulmonary sarcoid nodules raise the possibility of primary or metastatic tumor. Similarly, sarcoid nodules in the breast or brain may be thought to be tumor. Conglomerate lesions with hilar retraction or eggshell calcification of lymph nodes may be confused with silicosis. Hypercalcemia in sarcoidosis raises the question of a number of metabolic or malignant disorders, especially primary hyperparathyroidism (Ch. 235). Arthritis or arthralgia associated with sarcoidosis may be confused with acute rheumatic fever or gout.

The isolated finding of granulomas on biopsy of various tissues raises the possibilities of foreign body reactions, fungal or tubercular infections, and malignancy associated with granulomatous reactions. Granulomas occurring only in the liver may result in confusion between granulomatous hepatitis and sarcoidosis. The presence of granulomas in the intestinal wall may suggest Crohn's disease. Finally, renal and hepatic impairment or cardiac abnormalities occurring in sarcoidosis may be caused by more common coexisting diseases rather than by sarcoidosis itself.

RADIOLOGIC EVALUATION

Radiologic evaluation of the chest is particularly useful in sarcoidosis, since the disease is so often asymptomatic and so often involves the thorax. Radiologic abnormalities that occur in sarcoidosis have been arbitrarily classified as follows: grade 0—absence of abnormal radiographic findings; grade 1—lymph node enlargement without pulmonary parenchymal abnormalities; grade 2A—combination of lymph node and diffuse pulmonary parenchymal disease; grade 2B—diffuse parenchymal disease without lymph node enlargement; and grade 3—radiographic changes indicating more chronic disease with pulmonary fibrosis ("honeycombing" or hilar retraction). The most frequent parenchymal abnormality is reticulonodularity, consisting of fine linear densities and small, irregular nodules measuring 3 to 5 mm in diameter (Fig. 67–4). Large, conglomerate lesions may be present in association with hilar retraction (Fig. 67–5). Parenchymal infiltrates are at times "fluffy" and have an alveolar pattern. Single or multiple large nodules may occur and may be confused with tumor. Small nodules may cause a miliary pattern suggestive of tuberculosis.

A large variety of other changes may be present on the radiograph. Pleural effusion occurs rarely in sarcoidosis. Mediastinal or hilar lymph nodes may show eggshell calcification. In addition to bullous changes, true cavities may be present that, at times, contain mycetomas. Lobar atelectasis may be caused by intrabronchial granulomas, and postobstructive bronchiectasis may be present. In addition to the more common locations in the short tubular bones of the hands and feet, lytic or sclerotic bone lesions may occur in the ribs.

Computed tomographic (CT) scans can demonstrate lymphadenopathy more clearly and, in particular, can detect anterior mediastinal and subcarinal lymph nodes that have gone undetected on conventional films of the chest (Fig. 67–6). This examination, however, is needed in only a limited number of patients with sarcoidosis.

PHYSIOLOGIC CHANGES

The most common pulmonary physiologic changes occurring in sarcoidosis are decreases in vital capacity and diffusing capacity.

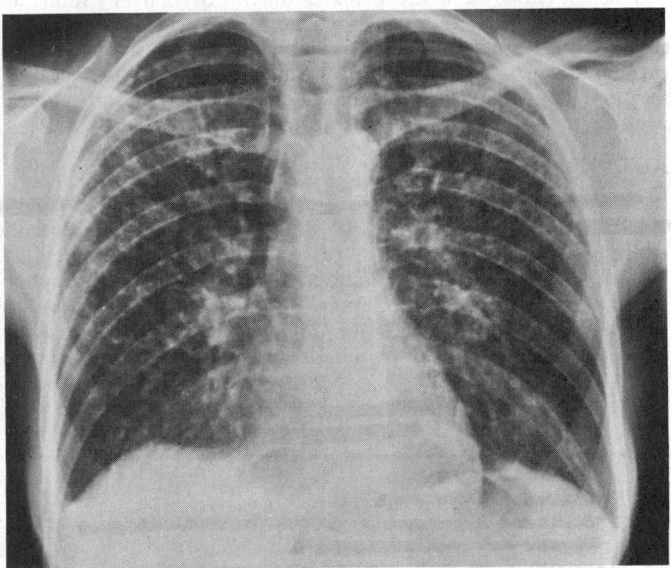

FIGURE 67–4. Chest radiograph showing typical reticulonodular appearance of parenchymal sarcoidosis. (From Murray JF, Nadel J: Textbook of Respiratory Medicine. Philadelphia, W. B. Saunders Company, 1987.)

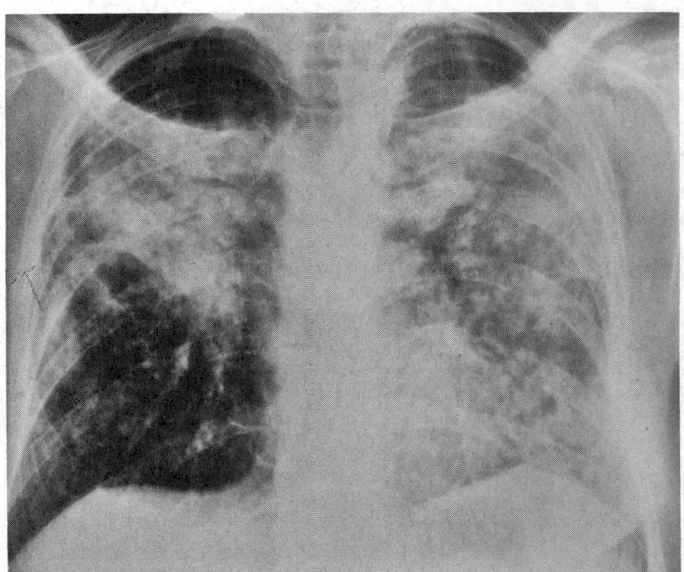

FIGURE 67–5. Chest radiograph showing large conglomerate lesions associated with hilar retraction. (From Murray JF, Nadel J: Textbook of Respiratory Medicine. Philadelphia, W. B. Saunders Company, 1987.)

Although useful in determining the extent of functional impairment at the onset and in following the course of the disease, physiologic changes do not correlate well with symptoms or radiologic abnormalities. At times pulmonary function studies are totally normal despite radiologic evidence of pulmonary disease. Conversely, functional abnormalities, especially of diffusing capacity, may be present when the lung parenchyma appears normal radiographically. Evidence of airway obstruction may also be present, and, at times, this is the predominant feature of sarcoidosis, causing confusion with asthma. An elevation in arterial PCO_2 is unusual, but moderate arterial hypoxemia may be present. As with other interstitial diseases, arterial hypoxemia often worsens with exercise.

APPROACH TO DIAGNOSIS

With a very typical presentation (i.e., bilateral symmetric hilar and paratracheal lymphadenopathy in an asymptomatic patient 20 to 40 years of age or in one with erythema nodosum, uveitis, and arthralgias), the clinical diagnosis of sarcoidosis can be made with a high degree of certainty by physicians familiar with this disease (Table 67–1). In all other cases in which the diagnosis is less clear, further support must be obtained by examination of biopsy material.

Diagnosis by Biopsy

Typical sarcoid granulomas consist of whorls of epithelioid cells surrounding multinucleated giant cells, which may or may not contain inclusion bodies (Fig. 67–7). Mononuclear cells are present at the periphery of the granulomas, and various amounts of fibrosis and/or hyalinization are present throughout the tissue. True caseation is unusual. The histologic appearance, even when typical, is always nonspecific. To strengthen the diagnosis of sarcoidosis, infectious agents and foreign bodies must be excluded by special stains, cultures, and examination under polarized light.

What tissue should be examined by biopsy? In the absence of specific skin lesions, transbronchial biopsy of the lung is usually most specific, since rarely, if ever, will nonspecific granulomas be found (in contrast to liver or lymph nodes). Approximately 60 per cent of patients with sarcoidosis show granulomas on transbronchial lung biopsy even if their chest radiographs are normal; this number increases to 85 to 90 per cent when there is a parenchymal abnormality on chest radiograph. If the transbronchial biopsy yields negative findings but a high suspicion of sarcoidosis exists and there is obvious parenchymal disease on the chest radiograph, a repeat transbronchial biopsy may be justified. Other reasonable approaches at this juncture of evaluation include mediastinoscopy or, at times, open lung biopsy.

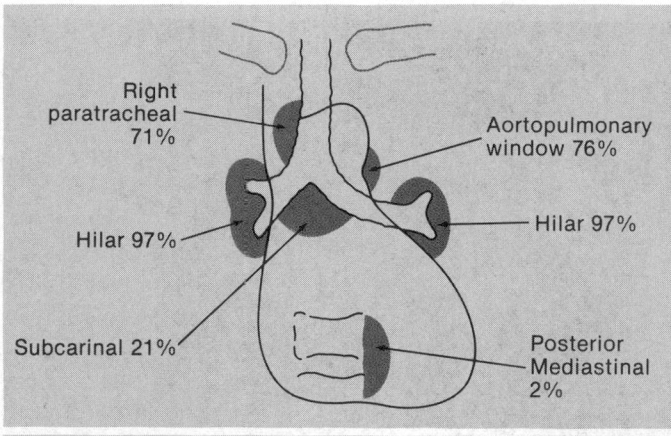

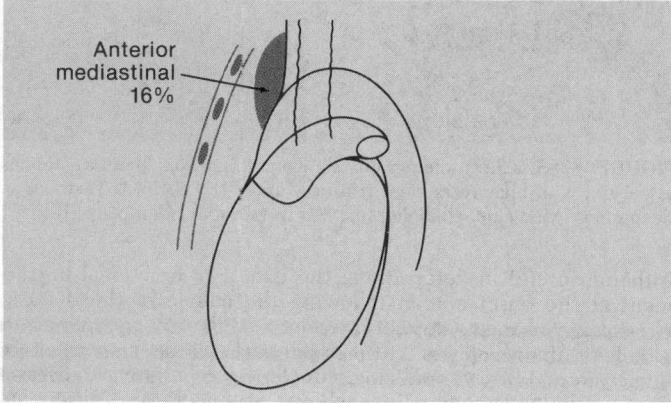

FIGURE 67–6. Schematic representation of CT detection of thoracic lymphadenopathy in sarcoidosis. (Reprinted from Rodan BA, Putman CE: Radiologic alterations in sarcoidosis. *In* Fanburg BL [ed.]: Sarcoidosis and Other Granulomatous Diseases of the Lung. New York, Marcel Dekker, 1983. By courtesy of Marcel Dekker, Inc.)

Blind conjunctival, lacrimal gland, or gingival biopsies are frequently not rewarding in the absence of overt disease at these locations. When these tissues are involved, however, the yield is high. Biopsies of skin lesions are particularly useful, since they may show granuloma and, in association with other findings, may provide an easy diagnosis if foreign body granuloma can be excluded. Biopsy of idenfiable subcutaneous or muscle lesions may also be diagnostic. Biopsy of lesions of erythema nodosum shows a nonspecific panniculitis or vasculitis and therefore is not diagnostic. Other localized lesions, such as those of the pharynx or larynx, require direct biopsy for diagnosis. Diagnosis by biopsy sometimes becomes problematic for neurologic disease caused by sarcoidosis when other tissues do not provide a positive diagnosis, since the involved tissue is often not easily accessible.

Other Available Tests

The Kveim-Siltzbach test lacks precision, and the required antigen is not readily available. It is therefore rarely used. Anergy

TABLE 67–1. FEATURES CONSIDERED IN THE DIAGNOSIS OF SARCOIDOSIS

Primary
1. Clinical and radiologic presentation
2. Biopsy material showing granuloma, but no mycobacterial, fungi, or refractile material

Secondary
1. Anergy to skin tests
2. Positive Kveim-Siltzbach reaction (infrequently performed)
3. Significant elevation of serum angiotensin I–converting enzyme with exclusion of other obvious diseases associated with elevation (e.g., Gaucher's disease, leprosy)

Current Research Modalities
1. Evaluation of cells obtained by bronchial lavage
2. Gallium-67 scanning

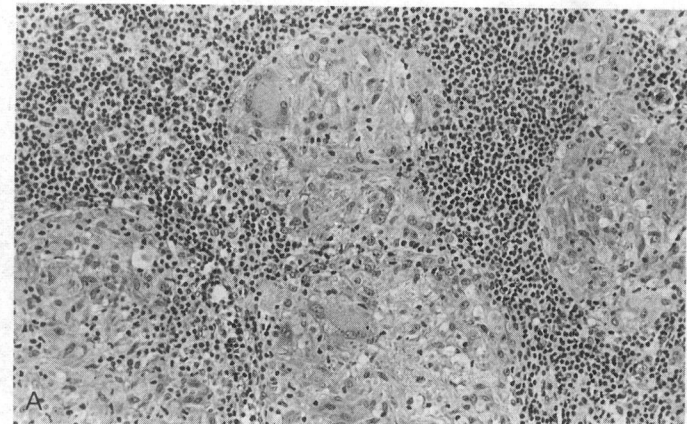

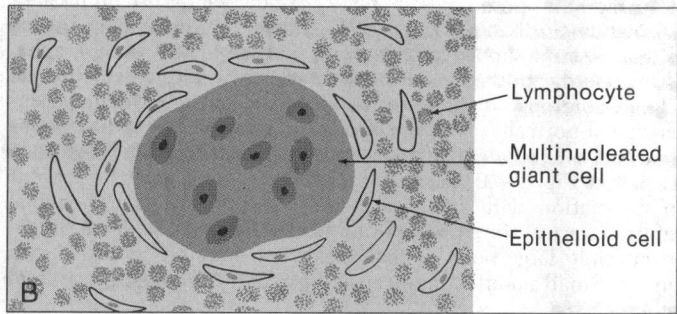

FIGURE 67–7. Typical histologic appearance of the granuloma of sarcoidosis with accompanying schematic representation.

to delayed hypersensitivity skin test antigens is a frequent finding but is obviously not diagnostic of sarcoidosis. Similarly, characterization of cells obtained by bronchial lavage and the use of gallium–67 scanning of the lungs are not in themselves diagnostic of sarcoidosis, although abnormalities consistent with that diagnosis may be found. For this reason, and because of cost and radiation exposure, these last two tests are not routinely justified currently for diagnosis in clinical practice. However, gallium–67 scanning may be useful in detecting unsuspected organ involvement by sarcoidosis, such as that of parotid glands. This observation may support the diagnosis.

Serum angiotensin I–converting enzyme activity is often elevated in sarcoidosis, but a number of other diseases may be similarly associated with its increased activity (e.g., miliary tuberculosis, leprosy, Gaucher's disease). If these diseases can be readily excluded, measurement of this enzyme may be useful. This is the case when the primary diagnostic considerations are lymphoma and sarcoidosis, since angiotensin I–converting enzyme activity is not increased in lymphoma. Elevations of other proteolytic enzymes in serum, such as lysozyme and thermolysin-like metalloendopeptidase, have been evaluated but are not yet commonly used for diagnostic purposes.

ACTIVITY OF DISEASE

Sarcoidosis may remit spontaneously; the concept of "activity of disease" is therefore useful when considering therapeutic strategies (Table 67–2). Activity of disease is very difficult to define, since occult granulomatous lesions may exist throughout many tissues of the body. Clinical findings provide some indication of activity of disease, but often in a nonquantitative and imprecise way, especially when the patient is relatively asymp-

TABLE 67–2. INDICATORS OF "ACTIVITY" OF SARCOIDOSIS

1. Clinical features
2. Worsening of symptoms
3. Worsening of pulmonary function tests/chest radiograph
4. Elevation of serum calcium level
5. Elevation of serum angiotensin I–converting enzyme level
6. Gallium scanning positivity
7. Evidence of alveolitis on bronchial lavage

tomatic. Radiologic and pulmonary function study changes may also be helpful in assessing activity of disease. Bronchoalveolar lavage to measure the percentage of lymphocytes as a reflection of parenchymal inflammation has been advocated. A high percentage of lymphocytes has been referred to as high-intensity alveolitis, denoting a poorer prognosis, but this approach has not gained wide acceptance. Gallium–67 scanning of the lung, which is also thought to reflect inflammation, has been proposed as an indirect method to monitor the intensity of alveolitis; the utility of this assessment of disease activity, similar to that of bronchoalveolar lavage, will need to be determined by more extensive prospective testing. Since elevated activity of serum angiotensin I–converting enzyme in sarcoidosis may be derived from epithelioid cells or granulomas, it has been suggested, without convincing evidence, that serum levels of this enzyme may reflect the granuloma "load" of the body. On the basis of this premise, its measurement is sometimes used to follow disease activity, but there is no assuredly accurate independent assessment of its validity as a guide to therapy or prognosis.

THERAPY

Many patients with sarcoidosis show spontaneous total remission of disease in a period up to 3 years. As many as 80 to 90 per cent of those with hilar and mediastinal lymphadenopathy or Loeffgren's syndrome alone may have remission; fewer patients with parenchymal involvement experience remission spontaneously. Other patients show arrest of the disease with moderate fibrosis, and a small percentage of patients develop progressive fibrosis and organ impairment. Once the disease remits spontaneously, only rarely does it recur. Treatment with corticosteroids causes granulomas to regress but does not appear to affect the natural course of the disease, since granulomas may recur if therapy is stopped. Since the disease may remit spontaneously and since steroids may cause significant side effects, treatment is usually started only if there is an indication of interference with the function of a vital organ (lungs, kidneys, eyes, heart, or central nervous system) or if hypercalcemia is present. All patients with sarcoidosis should be followed carefully so that therapy can be started as soon as deterioration of organ function has been detected.

Prednisone is usually the drug of choice for the treatment of sarcoidosis. The usual starting dosage is 30 to 40 mg per day, but at times a schedule of 50 to 60 mg every other day is used for initial therapy. A response in terms of symptoms or radiologic findings should be seen within 2 to 4 weeks. The steroid dose should be tapered after several weeks, and the eventual maintenance dose should be the lowest one that is effective in maintaining the response that is being followed (see below). Often 10 to 15 mg of prednisone every other day, a dosage that has a low risk of side effects, will suffice. Attempts to stop therapy may be tried after several months, but evidence of disease activity (symptoms, chest radiographic abnormalities, or worsening of pulmonary function) may recur, and prednisone may have to be restarted.

What are the best parameters to follow as indicators of disease activity? As noted earlier, measurements of disease activity are imprecise. Certainly, clinical symptoms should be assessed carefully, and chest radiographic and pulmonary function changes often give indication of disease activity. However, both radiographic abnormalities and pulmonary function changes correlate poorly with clinical parameters. Serum angiotensin I–converting enzyme levels are easily obtained and may provide clues to activity, but tests such as bronchial lavage and gallium–67 scanning are still largely experimental. Failure of response may indicate irreversible fibrosis, a situation in which steroid therapy causes more potential risk than benefit.

All of the usual side effects associated with steroid therapy may occur in patients treated for sarcoidosis (Ch. 27). The dose can usually be reduced sufficiently, however, so that infection with opportunistic organisms occurs rarely. Cosmetic problems of weight gain and fluid accumulation are often the most bothersome side effects. More difficult decisions about steroid therapy arise when there are associated disorders, such as diabetes mellitus, that may be exacerbated by these agents. Since tuberculin skin tests will become positive in patients with sarcoidosis who contract tuberculosis, appropriate prophylaxis or treatment should

be given when the tuberculin skin test is positive or converts to positivity.

Topical steroids have been used for dermatologic and ophthalmologic lesions, and chloroquine and methotrexate have been used for sarcoidosis of the skin. Indomethacin and other nonsteroidal anti-inflammatory agents may be useful for arthritis occurring in Loeffgren's syndrome. Aerosolized steroids approved for use in the United States have not been effective for pulmonary sarcoidosis, but other aerosolized preparations are being tried in Europe. Sarcoidosis that manifests with bronchoconstriction does not respond well to conventional bronchodilator therapy other than steroids. It remains to be determined whether avoidance of sunlight will significantly influence calcium metabolism in sarcoidosis. Dietary calcium restriction may be considered when hypercalcemia is present.

Bascom R, Johns CJ: The natural history and management of sarcoidosis. Adv Intern Med 31:213, 1986. *This is an excellent general review of this controversial area, with 138 references.*

Fanburg BL: Sarcoidosis and Other Granulomatous Diseases of the Lung. New York, Marcel Dekker, 1983. *A comprehensive textbook covering both clinical and experimental aspects of sarcoidosis.*

James DG, Williams WJ: Sarcoidosis and Other Granulomatous Disorders. Philadelphia, W.B. Saunders Company, 1982. *Another good monograph with an extensive review of all phase of sarcoidosis. Excellent clinical descriptions and comprehensive references.*

Roberts WC, McAllister HA Jr, Ferrans VJ: Sarcoidosis of the heart: A clinicopathologic study of 35 necropsy patients (Group I) and review of 78 previously described necropsy patients (Group II). Am J Med 63:86, 1977. *A good compilation of cases of sarcoidosis of the heart.*

Rockoff SD, Ronatagi PK: Unusual manifestations of thoracic sarcoidosis. Am J Radiol 144:513, 1985. *A comprehensive coverage of radiologic features of sarcoidois.*

Stern BJ, Krumholz A, Johns C, et al.: Sarcoidosis and its neurological manifestations. Arch Neurol 42:909, 1985. *A superb review of neurologic manifestations of sarcoidosis.*

Thomas PD, Hunninghake GW: Current concepts of the pathogenesis of sarcoidosis. Am Rev Respir Dis 135:747, 1987. *A current review with emphasis on immunologic features in sarcoidosis.*

Venet A, Hance AJ, Saltini C, et al.: Enhanced alveolar macrophage–mediated antigen-induced T-lymphocyte proliferation in sarcoidosis. J Clin Invest 75:293, 1985. *Further information about immunologic abnormalities in sarcoidosis.*

68 Pulmonary Neoplasms

Charles H. Scoggin

The lung can be affected by a variety of neoplasms (Table 68–1). Bronchogenic carcinoma accounts for more than 90 per cent of all lung tumors. The major management questions of lung cancer are the following: Is the tumor resectable? Is the tumor small cell lung cancer? Other tumors may metastasize to the lung. Benign tumors of the lung are infrequent compared with malignant tumors.

BRONCHOGENIC CARCINOMA

Lung cancer, a primary neoplasm arising within the airways, is a frequent and important neoplasm. In the United States, it is the leading fatal neoplasm of men and women. In 1990, it is estimated that approximately 142,000 will die of lung cancer in the United States. This figure represents 28 per cent of all cancer deaths in the United States. Lung cancer is strongly associated with the use of tobacco products, particularly with cigarettes. Although surgery or radiation therapy may lead to eradication of tumors in a small number of patients, the majority of people with lung cancer will have advanced disease at the time of diagnosis and will die of the disorder within 1 year of its detection. Determining the cell type and the stage of the disease is important in the clinical management of lung cancer, since these factors will affect treatment and prognosis. Four types of tumors account for 95 per cent of all lung malignancies: squamous cell (epidermoid), adenocarcinoma (including alveolar cell), large cell (also known as large cell anaplastic), and small cell lung cancer. Small

TABLE 68–1. WORLD HEALTH ORGANIZATION CLASSIFICATION OF LUNG TUMORS

I. Epithelial tumors
  A. Benign
    1. Papillomas (squamous cell and "transitional")
    2. Adenomas (includes pleomorphic and monomorphic)
  B. Dysplasia, carcinoma in situ
  C. Malignant
    1. Squamous cell carcinoma (epidermoid carcinoma)
    2. Small cell carcinoma
    3. Adenocarcinoma (includes acinar, papillary, bronchiolar, alveolar, and solid with mucus formation)
    4. Large cell carcinoma (giant cell and clear cell)
    5. Adenosquamous carcinoma
    6. Carcinoid tumor
    7. Bronchial gland carcinomas (includes adenoid cystic and mucoepidermoid carcinoma)
    8. Others
II. Soft tissue tumors
III. Mesothelial tumors
  A. Benign mesothelioma
  B. Malignant mesothelioma
IV. Miscellaneous tumors
  A. Benign
  B. Malignant
    1. Carcinosarcoma
    2. Pulmonary blastoma
    3. Malignant melanoma
    4. Malignant lymphoma
    5. Others
V. Secondary tumors
VI. Unclassified tumors
VII. Tumor-like lesions
  A. Hamartoma
  B. Lymphoproliferative lesions
  C. Tumorlet
  D. Eosinophilic granuloma
  E. "Sclerosing hemangioma"
  F. Inflammatory pseudotumor
  G. Others

cell lung cancer is distinguished from other types of lung cancer because it often shows a clinical response to chemotherapy.

Incidence and Prevalence

No population group is exempt from lung cancer. Lung cancer is the leading cause of cancer-related death of men in 28 developed countries of the world. In 1986, lung cancer surpassed breast cancer as the leading cause of death from cancer in women in the United States. The worldwide incidence of lung cancer is anticipated to continue to increase owing to the spread of the use of cigarettes, particularly in the Third World.

Lung cancer, as a major health problem, is a phenomenon of the twentieth century. In 1912, only 374 cases of primary lung neoplasms had been reported in the world's medical literature. There is little doubt that the exposure to cigarette smoke and other carcinogens accounts for the rapid increase in the occurrence of lung cancer.

The exact incidence of each type of lung cancer is difficult to determine. Squamous cell carcinoma is thought to be the most frequent form of the tumor (30 to 35 per cent of all cases), followed by adenocarcinoma, large cell carcinoma, and small cell carcinoma. Adenocarcinoma may be the most frequent lung cancer of women currently, but there is evidence that small cell lung cancer may soon surpass it.

Lung cancer occurs principally in those between the ages of 45 and 75 years. All histologic types of lung cancer in men peak at approximately 70 to 74 years of age. In women, adenocarcinoma peaks at an earlier age than in men (50 to 59 years).

Epidemiology

CIGARETTE SMOKING. About 80 to 90 per cent of all cases of lung cancer are caused by smoking cigarettes (see also Ch. 10 and 158). Cigarette smoking causes cancer in humans and experimental animals in a dose-dependent manner. Consumption of cigarettes is commonly quantitated as number of packs smoked per day and number of years smoked ("pack years"). A person who has smoked 2 packs per day for 20 years (40 pack years) has a 60- to 70-fold increased risk of developing lung cancer compared with a person who has never smoked. Because the duration of smoking is strongly associated with risk of lung cancer, the incidence and death rate from lung cancer are highest in the older age groups. Other factors that are important are depth of inhalation and tar and nicotine content of cigarettes.

Decreased smoking of cigarettes is associated epidemiologically with a declining incidence of lung cancer. A reduction in the prevalence of smoking among men in Sweden, Australia, Canada, and the United States has resulted in a reduction or slowing of deaths from lung cancer in men. A lag phase of about 20 years exists between an increase in cigarette smoking in a particular population and a rise in deaths from lung cancer. This lag is reflected in the current rise in deaths from lung cancer among women of the United States, among whom there was an increase in cigarette consumption in the 1950's. A similar phenomenon is thought to account for the increasing occurrence of lung cancer among Japanese men.

Passive inhalation of cigarette smoke may also be a risk factor for lung cancer. Passive smoke inhalation may cause both lung cancer and breast cancer in women. Sidestream smoke has a higher concentration than mainstream smoke of carcinogens such as nitrosamines, naphthalene, and benzopyrene.

OCCUPATIONAL ASSOCIATIONS. Occupational exposures also increase the incidence of lung cancer: uranium (in miners), haloethers (such as dichloromethyl ether and chloromethyl methyl ether), arsenical fumes, isopropyl oil, nickel, metallic iron, iron oxide, and beryllium. Asbestos exposure in nonsmokers is associated with a four- to fivefold increased incidence of lung cancer. Asbestos and radon gas act as cocarcinogens with cigarette smoke. Smoking increases the risk of bronchogenic cancer 80- to 90-fold in persons also exposed to asbestos. Radon gas exposure may also occur as an environmental pollutant in heavily insulated homes. As many as 12 per cent of homes in the United States may contain unhealthy levels of radon gas. Chronic inflammation of the lung, such as from interstitial fibrosis and areas of scarring, is associated with the occurrence of adenocarcinoma. Certain genetic determinants, such as levels of aryl hydrocarbon hydroxylase, may also be important.

Pathogenesis

CELL OF ORIGIN. The development of lung cancer is a multistep process. The pulmonary endodermal cell seems to be the common stem cell of origin of all lung cancer cell types. Because it demonstrates certain amine precursor uptake and decarboxylation (APUD) properties, small cell lung cancer has been hypothesized to arise from Kulchitsky's cell. There is no direct evidence to support this hypothesis, however.

CIGARETTE SMOKE. Cigarette smoke contains many carcinogens in both the gaseous and the particulate phases. Nitrosamines and other compounds are thought to be important in the gaseous phase. Carcinogens in the particulate phase include benzopyrene and related polycyclic aromatic hydrocarbons, nitrosonornicotine, polonium, and arsenic. Reduction in particulate factors correlates with a decreased incidence of lung cancer.

CELLULAR CHANGES. In the natural history of bronchogenic cancer, bronchial epithelial cells first become cytologically abnormal. At this stage, they are not malignant, nor are they invariably predictive of the eventual development of malignancy. The next step is carcinoma in situ, i.e., carcinomatous changes localized above the basement membrane and productive of no symptoms. The next change is epidermal invasion by tumor cells, followed by metastasis of the tumor. In situ tumors are indolent and slow growing. As malignancy progresses, so too does the rapidity of tumor spread.

CELLULAR EVENTS. Three aspects of the cellular events that attend the transformation of normal bronchial epithelial cells to malignant cells are important: (1) damage to cellular DNA; (2) alteration in cellular oncogene expression; and (3) tumor-derived factors that stimulate cellular division.

Cigarette smoke, ionizing radiation, and chemical carcinogens damage cellular DNA, in part through inducing chromosomal deletions and rearrangements and point mutations. The most

TABLE 68-2. CLINICAL MANIFESTATIONS OF LUNG CARCINOMA

1. Due to primary lesions
Cough	Wheezing
Dyspnea	Weight loss
Hemoptysis	Fever
Sputum	Pneumonia
2. Due to local extension
Chest pain	Dysphagia
Hoarseness	Pericardial effusion
Superior vena cava syndrome	Pleural effusion
Pancoast's syndrome	Diaphragm paralysis
Horner's syndrome	
3. Extrapulmonary manifestations

widely recognized chromosomal abnormality seen in lung cancer is a deletion of genetic material in the 3p14 to 23 region in the malignant, but not the normal, cells of patients with small cell lung cancer. Activation of oncogenes appears to be a common event in bronchogenic carcinoma (Ch. 157). Expression of members of both the *ras* and the *myc* oncogene families has been found in lung tumor cells, in contrast to normal lung cells. Another important factor is the production of so-called "autocrine growth factors" by lung cancer cells. Cultured small cell cancer cells secrete growth factors into their media. This feature is thought to account for their decreased requirement for serum growth factors. One such factor is bombesin/gastrin-related peptide. These growth factors stimulate cell division constantly. They may be of future clinical importance in that monoclonal antibodies to bombesin/gastrin-related peptide inhibit tumor growth of cells in culture and in experimental animals.

Clinical Manifestations

SYMPTOMS OF LUNG CANCER (Table 68-2). Most patients with lung cancer have some symptoms that cause them to seek medical attention. A typical patient will present with pulmonary complaints such as cough, hemoptysis, and weight loss. Only 5 to 15 per cent of patients are asymptomatic when discovered to have bronchogenic carcinoma.

Some Characteristics of Specific Tumors. Squamous cell, or *epidermoid, carcinoma* usually begins as a central lesion that tends to invade locally. The patient often presents with symptoms referable to the airways, such as cough, dyspnea, or hemoptysis. It may also invade the chest wall, diaphragm, or mediastinum. Unlike other primary lung neoplasms, squamous cell tumors may cavitate.

Adenocarcinoma usually begins as a peripheral lesion. It is more aggressive than squamous cell carcinoma. Symptoms at the time of diagnosis often reflect invasion of lymph nodes, pleura, or the other lung or metastasis to other organs, such as the central nervous system or adrenal glands. *Bronchioloalveolar carcinoma*, a special subtype of adenocarcinoma, usually accounts for no more than 1 to 5 per cent of primary lung neoplasms. Bronchioloalveolar carcinoma often manifests as a solitary pulmonary nodule (approximately 60 per cent) but may also appear as a localized infiltrate or area of lobar consolidation mimicking infection. *Large cell carcinoma* usually manifests as a bulky peripheral mass.

Small cell lung cancer should be carefully distinguished from non–small cell lung cancer, from which it differs both in biologic features and in clinical manifestations (Table 68–3). Small cell lung cancer commonly begins as a central tumor, but 70 to 90 per cent of patients have disease outside the original hemithorax at the time of detection. Because of its propensity to metastasize and to produce paraneoplastic syndromes, small cell lung cancer is usually symptomatic for 3 months or less before diagnosis. In contrast, symptoms associated with squamous cell carcinoma appear, on the average, 8 months before the diagnosis is made, and up to 25 per cent of patients with adenocarcinoma are asymptomatic at presentation. The severity of symptoms is also an important prognostic factor, particularly in small cell lung cancer. The more severe the tumor symptoms, the worse the prognosis.

Symptoms Referable to the Chest. Most patients with bronchogenic carcinomas present with symptoms referable to the chest, sometimes reflecting the area of lung involved. Central or endobronchial tumors can manifest as dyspnea, cough, hemoptysis, wheezing, or pneumonitis with fever and purulent sputum. Even small tumors may cause a disproportionately high degree of dyspnea. Hemoptysis, a common complaint, is more frequent in non–small cell lung cancer, since small cell lung cancer is often submucosal in location, without ulceration into the airway itself. Peripheral tumors may manifest as chest pain due to pleural or chest wall involvement.

Spread to thoracic lymph nodes is common in lung cancer, especially in small cell lung cancer. Regional spread to hilar and mediastinal nodes may cause dysphagia due to esophageal compression, hoarseness because of recurrent laryngeal nerve compression, Horner's syndrome due to sympathetic nerve involvement, and elevation of the hemidiaphragm from phrenic nerve compression. Superior sulcus, or Pancoast's, tumor may involve the brachial plexus, resulting in a C7–T2 neuropathy with pain, numbness, and weakness of the arm.

Cardiac involvement is seen at autopsy in 20 to 25 per cent of patients with small cell lung cancer, but less frequently in those with non–small cell lung cancer. Clinical findings of cardiac involvement are arrhythmias, cardiomegaly, and pericardial effusion with pericardial friction rub. Cardiac tamponade may occur.

Systemic Symptoms. Constitutional symptoms of anorexia, weight loss, and generalized weakness are common in lung cancer. Patients may also have fever without obvious infection.

Tumors that obstruct the superior vena cava cause the superior vena cava syndrome: swelling of the head and neck, breast enlargement, and prominence of the superficial veins of the thorax. Bronchogenic carcinoma, particularly small cell lung cancer, may demonstrate extrathoracic spread to other organ systems. Metastasis to the spinal cord causes spinal cord pain and symptoms of cord compression. Pain may precede weakness and sensory changes by days. Metastasis to the liver may cause pain, chemical dysfunction of the liver, and biliary obstruction. Metastasis to the bone may result in pain or bone marrow invasion.

Paraneoplastic Syndromes. Paraneoplastic syndromes are remote effects of tumor. They are described in detail in Ch. 161

TABLE 68-3. COMPARISON BETWEEN NON–SMALL CELL LUNG CANCER AND SMALL CELL LUNG CANCER

	Small Cell Lung Cancer	Non–Small Cell Lung Cancer
Cytopathology	Scant cytoplasm; indistinct nucleoli	Large amount of cytoplasm; prominent nucleoli
Cytogenetics	Deletion of 3p14 → 23	No known specific chromosomal alteration
Biochemistry and hormone production	Multiple enzymes and hormones (neuron-specific enolase, creatinine kinase BB, L-dopa decarboxylase, ACTH, bombesin, ADH, somatostatin, MSH)	Ectopic hormone production rare; paraneoplastic syndromes less common than in small cell lung cancer
Clinical presentation	Hemoptysis rare; most patients symptomatic at presentation; usually metastatic at presentation	Hemoptysis common, symptoms less frequent at time of presentation; dissemination at presentation less common than in small cell carcinoma
Treatment		
Surgery	Seldom, if ever, indicated	Primary hope for cure
Radiation	Limited role; palliation and perhaps prophylaxis of CNS metastasis	Palliation, possible cure
Chemotherapy	Main treatment (up to 80 per cent response)	Effect on survival undetermined

ACTH = adrenocorticotropic hormone; ADH = antidiuretic hormone; MSH = melanocyte-stimulating hormone; CNS = central nervous system.

and 162, to which the reader is referred. They lead to metabolic and neuromuscular disturbances unrelated to the primary tumor, metastases, or treatment. Paraneoplastic syndromes may be the first sign of the tumor or of tumor recurrence. They do not necessarily indicate that a tumor has spread. Paraneoplastic syndromes often respond to treatment of the primary tumor. Osteoarthropathy associated with lung cancer is seen in up to 30 per cent of patients with lung cancer but is rare in patients with small cell lung cancer. Manifestations include digital clubbing and painful periosteal inflammation. Periosteal elevation usually involves the long bones. It may be confused with certain forms of arthritis, including rheumatoid arthritis. Endocrinologic manifestations are well recognized in bronchogenic carcinoma. Up to 10 per cent of epidermoid tumors secrete humoral factors, resulting in hypercalcemia and hypophosphatemia. Metastasis to the adrenal glands may rarely result in adrenal insufficiency. Other endocrinologic manifestations, most common with small cell lung cancer, include Cushing's syndrome due to production of adrenocorticotropic hormone (ACTH), hyperpigmentation from production of melanocyte-stimulating hormone (MSH), and rarely the "somatostatinoma syndrome," which consists of vomiting, abdominal pain, diarrhea, mild diabetes, and cholelithiasis. Patients with lung cancer develop the syndrome of inappropriate antidiuretic hormone secretion (SIADH) in 10 to 15 per cent of cases (Ch. 161). Neuromyopathic manifestations of lung cancer are rare (<5 per cent) but may dominate the clinical picture when they occur (Ch. 162). Such manifestations include the Eaton-Lambert syndrome (seen in small cell lung cancer), polymyositis, subacute cerebellar degeneration, spinocerebellar degeneration, and peripheral neuropathies. Nonbacterial (marantic) endocarditis, migratory thrombophlebitis (Trousseau's syndrome), and disseminated intravascular coagulation as complications of malignancy are described in Ch. 159.

CLINICAL FINDINGS OF LUNG CANCER. Physical examination often does not reflect either the presence of lung cancer or the state of the disease. Digital clubbing may be found in up to 12 per cent of patients and gynecomastia in 5 to 7 per cent of patients (the latter most frequently associated with large cell anaplastic cancer). Acanthosis nigricans may be found with adenocarcinoma, and hyperpigmentation of the palms and soles may be seen with squamous cell carcinoma (Ch. 163). Obstruction of the superior vena cava may cause superior vena cava syndrome. Examination of the head may disclose the presence of Horner's syndrome, i.e., a unilaterally constricted pupil, enophthalmos, narrowed palpebral fissure, and loss of sweating on the same side of the face. Endobronchial obstruction may result in a localized wheeze detected during physical examination of the chest. Lobar collapse may result in an area of decreased breath sounds and dullness to percussion. Decreased movement of a hemidiaphragm may occur as a consequence of phrenic nerve compression. Liver metastasis may cause hepatic enlargement or nodularity. Weakness, altered reflexes, and decreased sensation may be found in patients with tumors metastatic to the central nervous system.

Diagnosis of Bronchogenic Carcinoma

The diagnosis of lung cancer requires detecting the tumor, establishing its cell type, and defining the stage of the malignancy. Determining cell type is important because it guides the approach both to staging and to treatment.

THE CHEST RADIOGRAPH. The presence of lung cancer is usually suggested by abnormalities on the chest radiograph. The most frequent finding is a mass in the lung field. Lesions usually cannot be detected if they are less than 5 to 6 mm. Tumors occur in the right lung more than in the left (3:2) and in the upper lobes more than in the lower lobes. Secondary manifestations seen on the chest radiograph include lobar collapse, pleural effusion, pneumonitis, elevation of the hemidiaphragm, hilar and mediastinal adenopathy, and erosion of ribs or vertebrae due to metastases. Alveolar cell cancer can manifest as a localized infiltrate mimicking pneumonia.

HISTOLOGIC DIAGNOSIS. When lung cancer is suspected, the next step in evaluation after the chest radiograph should be that of obtaining tissue specimens for histologic examination. The diagnostic yield of sputum cytologic evaluation will depend upon the adequacy of the specimen, the expertise of the cytologist, the type of tumor, and the number of specimens examined (three or four specimens are considered adequate). Sputum cytologic study is more likely to be negative in patients with small cell lung cancer than in those with non–small cell lung cancer. A negative sputum study should never be regarded as conclusive evidence for absence of carcinoma.

Bronchoscopy is important both for determining if a tumor is present and for obtaining tissue for histologic diagnosis. The combination of bronchial brushing and forceps biopsy is positive 90 to 93 per cent of the time with tumors located in proximal airways. Bronchial washings are less successful (approximately 80 per cent positive). For lesions that are not proximal enough in the airways for direct visualization, transbronchial biopsy with fluoroscopic guidance may be utilized. Yield of histologic diagnosis is 25 per cent for tumors less than 2 cm in diameter and 65 per cent for larger lesions. Transbronchial needle aspiration can also be employed. Peripheral lesions can be aspirated using a transthoracic needle with guidance by multiplane fluoroscopy or chest computed tomography (CT). Success rates as high as 95 per cent have been reported. Pneumothorax is the major complication. Contraindications to pulmonary biopsy include pulmonary hypertension, hypoxemia with carbon dioxide retention, and a bleeding diathesis.

If a diagnosis is not established by cytologic study of the sputum, bronchoscopy, or needle biopsy, thoracotomy may be necessary. The decision to undertake thoracotomy should be a reasoned one, weighing the importance to the patient of making the diagnosis against other factors such as age or other complicating illness.

In some circumstances, a histologic diagnosis can be made by biopsy of metastatic sites, such as liver, lymph nodes, bone, or bone marrow. When tumor involves the pleural space, combined thoracentesis and pleural biopsy will provide a diagnostic yield of up to 90 per cent.

SCREENING STUDIES. Screening studies for early stages of lung cancer, using chest radiographs alone or in combination with sputum cytology, have been proposed for cigarette smokers who are 45 years of age or older; however, recent trials examining the outcome of screening have failed to demonstrate a benefit. Carcinoembryonic antigen (CEA), neural peptides, and neurogenic enzymes are not currently useful in detecting lung tumor, its metastases, or its recurrence.

Staging of Lung Cancer

Lung cancers are staged first for location (anatomic staging) and then for the patient's ability to withstand various treatments aimed at curing the tumor or increasing life expectancy (physiologic staging). Staging for non–small cell lung cancer differs from that for small cell lung cancer.

NON–SMALL CELL LUNG CANCER. For non–small cell lung cancer, the first and most important decision is whether or not the tumor is operable. Routine staging to exclude inoperable patients has increased the survival of patients undergoing surgical resection of lung cancer. Table 68–4 lists a widely used tumor, node, and metastasis (TNM) system for classifying lung cancer. Patients with stages I and II are considered candidates for surgical resection. Certain patients with stage III cancer may be candidates for surgery with postoperative irradiation of the mediastinum. Surgical resection of N2 disease is controversial. Detection of mediastinal lymph node involvement with cancer is best determined by mediastinoscopy for tumors in the right hemithorax. Tumor assessment of the left hemithorax requires an anterior exploration (a Chamberlain procedure). Transbronchial and percutaneous needle aspiration is sometimes used to evaluate hilar lymph nodes. Size alone cannot be used to judge whether or not mediastinal lymph nodes are involved with metastatic cancer; however, enlarged nodes in the presence of known bronchogenic carcinoma argue strongly for metastatic disease. CT scanning of the chest is useful in excluding the presence of other tumors in the chest. In addition, scanning of the adrenal glands can be useful in determining if adrenal enlargement, possibly due to metastases, is present. Routine bone scan, CT scanning, liver scan, and bone radiographs are not recommended unless the physical examination or history suggests that these organs are involved. Magnetic resonance imaging (MRI) may be helpful in

Primary Tumor (T)

TX: Tumor present as determined by presence of malignant cells in bronchopulmonary secretions, but not radiographically or bronchoscopically visible; no evidence of primary tumor

T0: No evidence of primary tumor

T1S: Carcinoma in situ

T1: Tumor 3 cm or less surrounded by lung or visceral pleura, but without evidence of invasion proximal to lobar bronchus at bronchoscopy

T2: Tumor more than 3 cm or tumor invading visceral pleura or associated with obstructive pneumonitis or atelectasis; involving less than entire lung; at bronchoscopy, proximal extent of visible tumor must be within a lobar bronchus or at least 2 cm distal to carina

T3: Tumor of any size with direct extension into chest wall, diaphragm, or mediastinal pleura or pericardium without involving heart, great vessels, trachea, esophagus, or vertebral body; also includes superior sulcus tumors and tumor in main bronchus within 2 cm of carina but not involving carina

T4: Tumor of any size invading mediastinum or involving heart, great vessels, trachea, esophagus, vertebral body, or carina or presence of malignant pleural effusion

Nodal Involvement

N0: No demonstrable metastasis to regional lymph nodes

N1: Metastasis to peribronchial or the ipsilateral, or both, hilar lymph nodes, including direct extension

N2: Metastasis to ipsilateral mediastinal lymph nodes and subcarinal lymph nodes

N3: Metastasis to contralateral mediastinal lymph nodes, contralateral hilar lymph nodes, ipsilateral or contralateral scalene or supraclavicular lymph nodes

Distant Metastasis (M)

M0: No (known) distant metastasis

M1: Distant metastasis present—specify site(s)

Stage Grouping

Occult carcinoma	TX	N0	M0
Stage 0	T1S	Carcinoma in situ	
Stage I	T1	N0	M0
	T2	N1	M0
Stage II	T1	N1	M0
	T2	N1	M0
Stage IIIa	T3	N0	M0
	T3	N1	M0
	T1–3	N2	M0
Stage IIIb	Any T	N3	M0
	T4	Any N	M0
Stage IV	Any T	Any N	M1

examining adrenal glands, defining hilar masses, and demonstrating chest wall invasion.

SMALL CELL LUNG CANCER. Small cell lung cancer has often metastasized at the time of diagnosis; the TNM system has not proved to be useful. Small cell lung cancer is defined as either limited or extensive (Table 68–5). Limited disease is confined to one hemithorax, with or without involvement of mediastinal lymph nodes. Spread of disease beyond this point is extensive. In addition, performance status is also an important prognostic factor. Survival correlates with degree of symptoms and functional impairment.

Treatment of Bronchogenic Carcinoma

NON–SMALL CELL LUNG CANCER. Both surgery and radiation therapy may benefit patients with non–small cell lung

TABLE 68–5. TWO-STAGE CLASSIFICATION OF SMALL CELL LUNG CANCER

Limited disease (30%)
1. Primary tumor confined to hemithorax
2. Ipsilateral hilar lymph nodes
3. Ipsilateral and contralateral supraclavicular lymph nodes
4. Ipsilateral and contralateral mediastinal lymph nodes
5. Pleural effusion

Extensive disease (70%): more advanced than limited
1. Metastasis in the contralateral lung
2. Distant metastasis (brain, bone, liver, and so on)

cancer, but chemotherapy remains experimental. Newer modalities, such as laser bronchoscopy, may lead to symptomatic improvement by relieving endobronchial obstruction and may have a role in the treatment of carcinoma in situ.

Surgery. Surgical resectability of lung cancer is determined in large measure by the extent of lymph node metastasis. Patients with stage I and stage II non–small cell lung cancer (Table 68–5) should be treated with surgical resection aimed at cure. Patients with stage III disease characterized by ipsilateral intranodal mediastinal lymph node involvement may benefit from surgical resection of the primary and involved lymph nodes. Intranodal disease is defined as tumor completely confined within the capsule of the mediastinal lymph nodes. These patients should also receive postoperative mediastinal irradiation. Patients with superior sulcus tumors that have not metastasized to mediastinal lymph nodes or systemically should be treated with preoperative irradiation and en bloc resection. Irradiation is usually given as 3000 rads in 10 treatments, followed in 3 to 6 weeks by surgical resection. En bloc surgical resection of tumors that have invaded the chest wall, but have not metastasized systemically or to the mediastinal lymph nodes, may benefit. Surgical resection of both superior sulcus and chest wall tumors is associated with increased surgical mortality, compared with other less extensive surgical resections of lung cancer.

Limited resection of tumors yields results comparable to those obtained with more extensive surgical procedures. In general, lobectomy is recommended. Even less extensive procedures, such as lobar segment and wedge resection, are usually reserved for patients with peripheral lesions or limited pulmonary function.

Approximately 40 per cent of patients with non–small cell lung cancer undergo thoracotomy, with an overall 5-year survival from 10 to 35 per cent. At the time of thoracotomy, 75 per cent of patients undergo tumor resection with the aim at cure. The overall survival of patients resected for cure varies according to histopathologic type of tumor: squamous cell carcinoma, 37 per cent; adenocarcinoma, 27 per cent; large cell undifferentiated carcinoma, 27 per cent; and bronchoalveolar carcinoma, 56 per cent. Stage of the tumor is also an important determinant of surgical survival: stage I, 54 per cent; stage II, 35 per cent; and stage III without systemic or mediastinal lymph node metastasis, 19 per cent.

Pulmonary function is another very important factor in the evaluation of patients for surgery. Forced vital capacity greater than 2 liters and a forced expiratory volume in the first second (FEV_1) of greater than 50 per cent of the forced vital capacity predict that a patient can tolerate the consequences of pneumonectomy. Radionuclide scanning has generally replaced differential spirometry as a method of assessing the lung to be resected for its contribution to overall respiration.

Elderly patients should not be excluded from consideration for resection of tumor. The most limiting factor of survival in this age group is not age, but the tumor. Bronchogenic carcinoma is a highly aggressive tumor in the elderly. The average life expectancy of patients with untreated tumor is 8 months. This compares with an average life expectancy in the United States of 11.1 and 14.8 years, respectively, for men and women aged 70 years. Elderly patients carefully selected for surgery have a 5-year survival of 35 to 42 per cent.

Radiation Therapy. Most non–small cell lung cancers are responsive to radiation treatment. Radiation therapy is indicated in patients with stage III disease without metastases or in stage I or stage II patients who refuse surgical treatment. A consistently small but reproducible group of patients with disease in the chest alone benefit from radiation treatment aimed at cure. Patients with operable lung cancer may have a 5-year survival rate with radiation therapy alone of up to 21 per cent. Treatment is generally 5500 to 6000 rads by either split course or continuous fraction irradiation. Acute esophagitis is a common complication. Patients receiving irradiation of a lung for cure of cancer may develop radiation pneumonitis; therefore, patients must have pulmonary function equivalent to that necessary to tolerate pneumonectomy.

Most tumors will respond to irradiation by decreasing in sizes; however, radiation treatment of patients with nonresectable non–small cell lung cancer has been disappointing in prolonging survival.

Postoperative mediastinal irradiation is recommended in patients who have undergone resection and who have intranodal lymph node involvement, but preoperative and postoperative adjuvant radiotherapy for T2 and T3 tumors has not been shown to be beneficial and may even be detrimental. The single exception appears to be superior sulcus, or Pancoast's, tumor.

TREATMENT OF PATIENTS WITH DISSEMINATED NON–SMALL CELL LUNG CARCINOMA. Seventy per cent of patients with non–small cell lung cancer have unresectable disease at the time of diagnosis or thoracotomy. In such patients, irradiation and other forms of palliative treatment are very important.

Radiation Therapy. Irradiation effectively decreases tumor size to reduce endobronchial obstruction and to re-expand the atelectatic lung. Important intrathoracic complications may respond to irradiation: the superior vena cava syndrome, 80 to 90 per cent; hemoptysis, 84 per cent cough, 60 per cent; and atelectasis, 23 per cent. Radiation therapy may also palliate bone pain and cerebral metastases.

Chemotherapy. A response rate of 30 to 40 per cent in non–small cell lung cancer has been achieved with cisplatin regimens, especially in combination with etoposide (VP–16) and/or mitomycin C. This should not be regarded as routine therapy. Substantive improvement in symptoms and survival remains to be proved. Potential benefit to the patient must be weighed against chemotherapy-induced side effects. Peripheral neuropathy, not severe myelosuppression, is usually the main dose-limiting factor. The effectiveness of combined modalities such as chemotherapy plus radiotherapy or chemotherapy plus surgery is still unproved.

SMALL CELL LUNG CANCER. The median survival of patients with untreated small cell lung cancer from the time of diagnosis is 2.8 months. Fewer than 1 per cent of untreated patients will survive 5 years. The treatments of choice for small cell lung cancer are chemotherapy and radiation. Surgical resection has little, if any, role, because at the time of detection the tumor has usually spread beyond the limits of surgical removal. For example, the mean survival with radiation therapy alone (284 days) is statistically greater than the mean survival with surgical treatment (199 days), although it remains very low.

Chemotherapy. Small cell lung cancer is highly responsive to chemotherapy. Moderately intensive therapy with three agents is usually given initially in an attempt to eradicate the tumor. The use of additional drugs beyond three is associated with a disproportionate increase in side effects compared with benefit. Examples of currently employed regimens are cyclophosphamide, methotrexate, and lomustine (CCNU); cyclophosphamide, doxorubicin, and vincristine; and cyclophosphamide, doxorubicin, and etoposide (VP–16). These regimens appear to be approximately equal in producing responses and long-term survival. Objective responses usually occur within 6 to 12 weeks after initiation of treatment. The effective length of treatment is yet to be established. Most protocols involve treatment for 12 months or less. Alternating non–cross-resistant combinations of drugs and using intensive therapy with autologous bone marrow transplantation have not been shown to increase survival. Combined modalities of irradiation and chemotherapy may be of use in limited disease, although this has yet to be conclusively proved.

Most chemotherapy regimens produce a greater than 80 per cent response rate in all patients. Complete response, defined as the absence of any evidence of residual tumor, is seen in greater than 50 per cent of patients with limited disease and in 20 per cent of patients with extensive disease. This results in a median survival of about 14 months in patients with limited disease and 7 months in patients with extensive disease. Twelve to 15 per cent of patients with limited disease will survive 6 to 11 years.

Aggressive chemotherapy produces complications and symptoms in all patients. All experience anemia and leukopenia. Opportunistic infection is an important complication. Approximately 60 per cent of neutropenic patients experience febrile episodes. Herpes zoster occurs in 8 to 12 per cent of patients with small cell lung cancer treated with chemotherapy. Other complications include nausea, vomiting, alopecia, hemorrhagic cystitis, mucositis, electrolyte imbalance, possible cardiotoxicity, and peripheral neuropathy. A long-term complication of chemotherapy for small cell lung cancer is a secondary malignancy: leukemia, lymphoma, and other neoplasms. Risk appears to increase with intensity of drug dosage and the number of drugs utilized. Finally, patients successfully treated for small cell carcinoma are still at risk for non–small cell carcinoma.

Radiation Therapy. Radiation therapy is of proven benefit in controlling bone pain, spinal cord compression, superior vena cava syndrome, and bronchial obstruction. More than 90 per cent of patients have been reported to have palliation of symptoms due to brain metastases. The use of radiation therapy in combination with chemotherapy is controversial and should be reserved for experimental studies.

Prophylactic Cranial Irradiation. Although chemotherapy has increased the survival of patients with small cell lung cancer, this survival has been accompanied by an increased risk of relapse in the central nervous system. The cumulative risk of central nervous system metastases at 2 years may be as high as 80 per cent. This risk is reduced to about 3 to 12 per cent with the use of prophylactic cranial irradiation. Unfortunately, this decreased rate of brain metastasis is not associated with increased survival. Prophylactic cranial irradiation is generally reserved for patients who have achieved a complete response in chemotherapy, but even in these patients, the benefit in terms of increased survival is slight. In all other patients, cranial irradiation should be used when central nervous system metastases are diagnosed. Most patients who survive long term exhibit memory loss, confusion, ataxia, loss of vision, and dysphonia. This encephalopathy is probably a complication of cranial irradiation with a possible contribution by chemotherapy as well.

OTHER CONSIDERATIONS IN THE TREATMENT OF LUNG CANCER

Bone Metastasis. The metastasis of lung cancer to bone most frequently causes pain, but pathologic fracture may also occur. Bone involvement is best detected by bone scan, although large lesions will be visible radiographically. Pain can usually be palliated by radiation to the involved areas.

Hypercalcemia. Hypercalcemia is one of the most important complications of lung cancer. Serum calcium values in excess of 12 mg per deciliter are considered life threatening. Treatment is aimed at lowering the serum calcium level. Treatment of hypercalcemia is discussed in detail in Ch. 235.

Central Nervous System Metastasis. Metastases from lung cancer to the central nervous system usually cause symptoms in proportion to their size and location. Corticosteroids are effective in relieving acute symptoms of increased intracranial pressure in about 75 per cent of patients. Doses of 8 to 12 mg of dexamethasone should be administered on an acute basis. Osmotic agents given to reduce intracranial pressure, such as a 20 per cent solution of mannitol administered intravenously, may be useful in treating cerebral herniation. Acute control of increased pressure should be followed by radiation therapy.

Pleural Effusion. Malignant pleural effusion frequently complicates bronchogenic carcinoma. It is exudative in nature. The diagnosis is made by cytologic examination of the fluid and by pleural biopsy. Effusions complicated by dyspnea or pain should be drained. If the fluid recurs, obliteration of the potential pleural space should be accomplished by introducing a sclerosing agent. This is best performed by insertion of a chest tube to drain the effusion completely, followed by the instillation of 1 gram of tetracycline dissolved in 100 ml of normal saline and 50 ml of 1 per cent lidocaine (Xylocaine) into the chest through the tube. The tube should then be clamped and the patient turned into different positions to distribute the sclerosing fluid along the pleural surface. The tube is then allowed to drain until the amount of fluid over a 12- to 14-hour period is 100 ml or less. Malignant pleural effusions with pH less than 7.0 are associated with a very poor prognosis.

Weakness and Weight Loss. Weight loss, muscle weakness, and difficulty in eating are frequent and distressing manifestations of lung cancer. The pathophysiology of weight loss in lung cancer is poorly understood but can be partially explained by altered carbohydrate and protein metabolism and the release of toxic factors into the circulation. The use of aggressive nutritional support in lung cancer patients in whom traditional forms of treatment have been ineffective is of limited value and may even be adverse.

Cough and Dyspnea. Reversible causes of cough and dyspnea, such as bronchospasm, bronchitis, and pneumonitis, should be excluded. The mainstays of cough control are narcotic cough suppressants. Narcotics and tranquilizers used in low dosage may produce remarkable relief of severe dyspnea. When clearance of large airway secretions becomes difficult, patients may "rattle" when they breathe (so-called "death rattle"). This is particularly distressing to family members. In patients who are terminally ill, scopolamine, 0.4 to 0.6 mg given subcutaneously every 4 hours as necessary, will tend to dry up secretions and relax the smooth muscle of the airways. It is preferred to atropine, since the former is a central nervous system depressant, in contrast to atropine, which is a stimulant.

Pain. The therapeutic goal of managing pain, the most common symptom of advanced lung cancer, should be not only its relief but also its prevention. Narcotics should be taken every 4 hours around the clock to prevent the patient from awakening with pain. There is no single optimal dosage schedule for narcotics. Most patients have their pain controlled with 30 mg of morphine, or its equivalent, given orally on a 4-hour basis. Patients, families, and those caring for the patient should be counseled that tolerance and addiction do not present real clinical problems in patients with advanced lung cancer. The most common adverse side effects of narcotic treatment are constipation and nausea, which must preferably be prevented, but treated aggressively if they appear.

Patients who have been treated for lung cancer with apparent success continue at risk for a second primary lung cancer, or "metachronous" tumor. Such tumors can have a histologic pattern identical with or different from the first primary tumor. Metachronous tumors occur in 1 to 3 per cent of patients with lung cancer. Treatment is determined by the same factors that affect other primary lung tumors; however, the physiologic impact of treatment of the first primary cancer may limit surgical resection or radiation dosage.

Bunn PA (ed.): Lung cancer. Issue dedicated to Mary Jean O'Leary Matthews. Semin Oncol 15:197, 1988. *Very comprehensive review of non–small cell and small cell lung cancer, including biology, pathology, molecular genetics, diagnostic techniques, staging, and treatment.*

Carney DN: The biology of lung cancer. Acta Oncol 28.1, 1989. *Concise review of biology of lung cancer with emphasis on tumor markers.*

Eddy DM: Screening for lung cancer. Ann Intern Med 111:232, 1989. *Excellent review of all recent trials examining screening for lung cancer with lung roentgenography and sputum cytology. Concludes routine screening not recommended because of cost, lack of benefit, and potential harm*

Filderman AE, Shaw C, Matthay RA: Lung cancer part 1: Etiology, pathology, natural manifestations, and diagnostic techniques. Invest Radiol 21:80, 1986. *Particularly good for summarization of roentgenographic manifestations of primary pulmonary malignancies.*

Horton AW: Indoor tobacco smoke pollution. A major risk factor for both breast and lung cancer? Cancer 62:6, 1988. *Reviews risk of involuntary smoke inhalation and risk of lung and breast cancer.*

Iannuzzi MJ, Scoggin CH: Small cell lung cancer: State of the art. Am Rev Respir Dis 134:593, 1986. *Focuses on clinical and investigational aspects of small cell lung cancer.*

Rapp E: Chemotherapy can prolong survival in patients with advanced non–small cell lung cancer—report of a Canadian multicenter randomized trial. J Clin Oncol 6:633, 1988. *Reports on 18-center study sponsored by National Cancer Institute of Canada. In 251 patients studied, survival increased by 7 weeks in treated patients, but with significant toxicity.*

Webb WR: The role of magnetic resonance imaging in the assessment of patients with lung cancer: A comparison with computed tomography. J Thorac Imaging 4:65, 1989. *Reviews role of CT, but also presents the advantages and disadvantages of MRI. MRI has superior ability to discriminate certain tissues and is helpful in demonstrating chest wall invasion, defining mediastinal masses, detecting hilar masses, and distinguishing recurrent tumors from fibrosis in patients with prior irradiation.*

Whang-Peng J, Bun PA, Kao-Shan CS, et al: A nonrandom chromosomal abnormality, del3p(14–23), in human small cell lung cancer (SCLC). Cancer Genet Cytogenet 6:119, 1982. *Description of a chromosomal abnormality found in small cell lung cancer.*

OTHER MALIGNANCIES OF THE LUNG

Carcinoid Tumors

These tumors, sometimes termed "bronchial adenomas," are in fact distinct entities with different clinical courses and histologic manifestations. Three types are recognized: bronchial carcinoids, cylindromas, and mucoepidermoid tumors. Tumors may manifest with endobronchial obstruction or hemoptysis. Carcinoid tumors, including bronchial carcinoids, are considered in Ch. 230.

Scheithauer BW, Carpenter PC, Block B, et al.: Ectopic secretion of a growth hormone–releasing factor: Report of a case of acromegaly with bronchial carcinoid tumor. Am J Med 76:605, 1984. *Reviews different extrapulmonary manifestations of bronchial carcinoid tumors.*

Primary Lymphoma of the Lung

Hodgkin's disease and non-Hodgkin's lymphoma are discussed in Ch. 147 and 148. Such lymphoma may arise in the lymph nodes of the chest or within the lung itself. Patients with tumor involving the lung may present with weight loss, fever, cough, or pleuritic chest pain. Pleural effusion may be an initial or complicating manifestation.

Non-Hodgkin's tumors arising within the parenchyma of the lung are often discrete masses with or without hilar and mediastinal lymph node enlargement. An intrathoracic Hodgkin's tumor mass may cavitate or compress the bronchial tree to cause atelectasis or postobstructive pneumonitis. A common differential diagnosis of hilar adenopathy is that between lymphoma and sarcoidosis (Ch. 67). Enlargement of anterior mediastinal lymph nodes suggests lymphoma, as this is an unusual region of lymphadenopathy in sarcoidosis.

Other lymphoproliferative disorders that involve the lung are pseudolymphoma and lymphocytic interstitial pneumonitis. Pseudolymphoma appears as a nodular lesion, whereas lymphocytic interstitial pneumonitis manifests as a diffuse infiltrate. The diagnosis is made by histologic examination of lung biopsy specimen. Distinguishing between benign disease and true pulmonary lymphoma may be difficult. Some patients who initially present with an apparently benign lymphoproliferative disorder later develop malignant lymphoma. The development of hilar or mediastinal lymphadenopathy suggests the presence of malignancy.

The diagnosis of lymphoproliferative disorders of the lung depends upon histologic examination of tissue obtained by bronchoscopy, transbronchial biopsy, mediastinoscopy, or thoracotomy.

The treatment of Hodgkin's and non-Hodgkin's lymphomas of the lung involves the use of radiation or chemotherapy as would be employed for nonpulmonary lymphoma (Ch. 147 and 148). Pseudolymphoma can be removed by surgical resection. No established treatment for lymphocytic interstitial pneumonitis exists, although chemotherapy has been attempted.

Colby TV, Carrington CB: Pulmonary lymphomas: Current concepts. Pathol Annu 14:884, 1983. *Presents criteria for and classification of pulmonary lymphoid lesions.*

Uncommon Primary Lung Malignancies

Cylindromas are the second most common tumors of the trachea and bronchi. (The most common tumors are bronchogenic carcinomas.) The tumors arise from the mucous glands of the bronchial epithelium. The most common symptoms are airway obstruction and cough. Men and women are equally affected, and the age of occurrence ranges from 30 to 65 years. The diagnosis is made by bronchoscopy and biopsy. Treatment is by surgical resection, although cure may be difficult owing to the tumor's propensity to metastasize.

Mucoepidermoid tumors also arise from the bronchial mucous glands and usually manifest in persons between the ages of 40 and 55. The diagnosis is made by the bronchoscopic finding of a polypoid endobronchial mass, followed by biopsy. Treatment is by surgical resection; the prognosis is better than that with cylindroma. *Carcinosarcoma,* an unusual tumor, contains both malignant epithelial elements and sarcomatous changes. It may occur as a peripheral mass or as an endobronchial lesion; it is treated by surgical resection. *Pulmonary blastomas,* which usually occur in the periphery of the lung, are thought to arise from mesoderm. Surgical resection is the indicated treatment, but the prognosis is poor.

Primary sarcomas of the lung, which are very rare, include fibrosarcomas, leiomyosarcomas, hemangiopericytomas, and osteosarcomas. Treatment is by surgical resection. More recently, Kaposi's sarcoma has been recognized as a cause of pulmonary disease in patients with the acquired immunodeficiency syndrome (AIDS). It may be difficult to distinguish from infection. The diagnosis requires lung biopsy.

Olnibene FP, Steis RG, Macher AM, et al.: Kaposi's sarcoma causing pulmonary infiltrates and respiratory failure in the acquired immunodeficiency syndrome. Ann Intern Med 102:471, 1985. *Description of 66 patients with acquired immunodeficiency syndrome and 30 episodes of pulmonary Kaposi's sarcoma.*

Tumors Metastatic to the Lung

Both hematogenous and lymphatic spread of carcinomas and sarcomas may involve the lung. Patients are often asymptomatic; however, metastatic lesions may cause dyspnea, cough, and chest pain. Diffuse hematogenous tumor spread may cause vascular obstruction, manifested by cor pulmonale with hilar enlargement and clear lung parenchyma.

The radiographic appearance of pulmonary metastases may give some clue to the primary tumor. Solitary nodules are usually associated with cancers from breast, colon, kidney, rectum, cervix, and melanoma. These tumors may also diffusely involve the lung, leading to multiple large nodules or micronodules. In addition, a micronodular pattern is also seen with tumors from the thyroid, trophoblastic tissue, or bone sarcomas. Large, well-defined pulmonary nodules, sometimes with associated hilar enlargement, occur with testicular germinal cell tumors.

Tumors that spread lymphatically include carcinomas from the stomach, pancreas, thyroid, larynx, and lung. These tumors may spread to lung lymphatics through hilar lymph nodes or from parenchymal lymphatics that have been invaded by hematogenous metastases. Enlargement of lung lymphatics is radiographically visible as linear shadows similar to Kerley's lines.

Pleural involvement may appear as a pleural-based mass or as pleural effusion. Metastatic lesions, particularly synovial cell tumors and other bone tumors, may lead to pneumothorax. Certain metastatic lesions may cavitate: metastatic sarcomas, carcinomas of the colon, and epidermoid carcinomas of the head, neck, and the female reproductive system. Osteogenic sarcomas or chondrosarcomas display calcification in metastatic lesions.

The diagnosis of metastatic lesion is confirmed by the histologic examination of tissue obtained by sputum cytology, fiberoptic bronchoscopy, or occasionally thoracotomy. Cytologic findings are positive in as many as 50 per cent of patients. Bronchoscopy and needle biopsy have similar success rates. Decisions on how aggressive to be in seeking confirmation by tissue study of suspected metastatic lesions must be made thoughtfully. The risk to the patient must be weighed against the question of how the confirmation of metastasis will alter the management of the patient.

Treatment of metastases will usually be based upon management of the primary neoplasm. Certain metastatic lesions should be considered for surgical resection, especially those arising from osteogenic sarcomas. On occasion, resection of a solitary metastasis from other primary sources has been reported to be associated with increased survival, but usually without any controlled study. In considering surgical resection of a metastasis, the following criteria should be met: (1) absence of other metastatic lesions within the lung on CT, (2) no evidence of metastasis involving other organs, and (3) sufficient physiologic reserve to tolerate a more extensive resection if simple wedge resection is deemed inadequate.

In general, this means the criteria used for determining tolerance of surgical resection of primary lung cancer should be applied when contemplating resection of metastatic lesions.

In summary, surgical resection of pulmonary metastasis should be considered when the primary tumor is under control, the patient is a good surgical risk, other approaches to treatment are unsatisfactory, and all of the tumor can be resected.

Beattie EJ: Surgical treatment of pulmonary metastases. Cancer 54:2729, 1984. *Brief review of metastatic lesions to the lung that may be appropriate for multiple surgical resections.*

Mountain CF, McMurtrey MJ, Hermes KE: Surgery for pulmonary metastasis: A 20-year experience. Ann Thorac Surg 38:323, 1984. *Report of results of the M.D. Anderson Hospital and Tumor Institute with surgical resection in 443 patients with various tumors metastatic to the lung.*

BENIGN NEOPLASMS OF THE LUNG

Benign neoplasms of the lung are uncommon. They may occur as solitary nodules within lung parenchyma or as endobronchial lesions. Symptoms are nonspecific and include cough, dyspnea, chest pain, and pneumonia.

HAMARTOMAS. Hamartomas, the most common benign tumors of the lung, are usually diagnosed in adults. The tumors consist of unorganized elements, such as fat, fibrous tissue, epithelial tissue, cartilage, and calcification. Calcification leads to the "popcorn" radiographic appearance of the tumor. The majority of hamartomas occur as solitary nodules within lung parenchyma, but about 10 per cent are endobronchial. Hamartomas should be removed because of the potential complications of hemorrhage and bronchial obstruction resulting in atelectasis and pneumonia.

PAPILLOMAS. Papillomas, which arise from the trachea and bronchi, are most commonly found in children. They may be diffuse, leading to repeated pneumonias, bronchiectasis, atelectasis, and chronic infection. Because of diffuse involvement, management may be difficult, and repeated bronchoscopy may be required in an attempt to remove these tumors. Malignant changes may also occur.

OTHER TUMORS. Uncommon benign tumors of the lung include granular cell myoblastomas, lipomas, fibromas, leiomyomas, chondromas, and hemangiomas. They usually first appear as masses radiographically. Complications are similar to those of other benign neoplasms. Surgical removal is the usual treatment.

Arrignoni MG, Woolner LB, Bernatz PE, et al.: Benign tumors of the lung: A ten-year surgical experience. J Thorac Cardiovasc Surg 60:589, 1970. *Excellent review of 130 patients with benign tumors of the lung. Includes clinical, radiographic, and pathologic features.*

SOLITARY PULMONARY NODULE

A solitary pulmonary nodule is a single lesion, regardless of size, surrounded by lung parenchyma on at least two thirds of its circumference, not touching the hilum or mediastinum, and without associated atelectasis or pleural effusion. Important etiologies of solitary pulmonary nodules include neoplasia, infection, and collagen vascular disease. Because of the wide variety of cause and differing treatments, determining the etiology is very important (Table 68–6).

Etiology

Both benign and malignant tumors may manifest as a solitary pulmonary nodule. Approximately 40 per cent of solitary pulmonary nodules are malignant, and of these, 85 to 90 per cent are bronchogenic carcinoma. Bronchogenic carcinomas that are detected as solitary nodules have a much more favorable prognosis (24 per cent 5-year survival) than do those with more complicated presentations (5 to 8 per cent 5-year survival). Patients detected with solitary nodules at stage I of bronchogenic carcinoma have been reported to have almost a 50 per cent 5-year survival. Most benign hamartomas appear as solitary pulmonary nodules. Three to 10 per cent of solitary pulmonary nodules are due to malignancies metastatic to the lung from other organs, especially from renal cell carcinoma, Wilms' tumor, Ewing's sarcoma, choriocarcinoma, bladder carcinoma, rhabdomyosarcoma, osteosarcoma, melanoma, and carcinomas of the breast, colon, testis, head, and neck.

The most common infection that manifests as solitary nodules is that caused by *Coccidioides immitis*. Echinococcal cysts may also appear as a single nodule, as may the lesions of *Histoplasma*

TABLE 68–6. ETIOLOGIES OF SOLITARY PULMONARY NODULES

1. Primary lung malignancies
2. Metastatic malignancies to the lung
3. Benign tumors or tumor-like conditions

Hamartoma	Pseudolymphoma
Herniation of omentum	Herniation of liver
Hemangioma	

4. Pulmonary infections

Fungal	Mycobacterial
Bacterial	Hydatid cyst

5. Foreign body pneumonitis

Lipid pneumonia	Amyloidosis
Pneumoconiosis	Aspiration pneumonia
Talc granulomas	

6. Pulmonary vascular disorders

Pulmonary infarct	Pulmonary hemosiderosis
Pulmonary hemorrhage	

capsulatum and *Blastomyces dermatitidis*. Tuberculosis rarely manifests as a solitary pulmonary nodule.

Certain collagen vascular disorders may present as pulmonary nodules, especially rheumatoid arthritis and Wegener's granulomatosis. Although usually multiple lesions occur, occasionally only a single nodule may be seen. Unusual causes of solitary nodules are pulmonary infarcts and vascular malformations.

Evaluation

The sequence of the approach to a patient with a solitary pulmonary nodule is outlined in Figure 68–1. Evaluation of patients with solitary pulmonary nodules begins with a thorough history and physical examination. Travel to an area endemic for fungal disease such as coccidioidomycosis suggests, but does not prove, this etiology. Weight loss and other constitutional symptoms are consistent with malignancy, although early stages may be asymptomatic. Joint changes may suggest rheumatoid nodules. Age is also an important consideration. Primary lung cancer is uncommon in patients who have never smoked and who are below the age of 30 years. Patients over the age of 50 years with new solitary nodules, particularly if they have smoked, have an increased incidence of malignancy. Geography is also important. Fungal disease is a more common etiology in persons who reside in or have recently visited the American Southwest, whereas malignancy is a more common cause of solitary nodules in individuals living in areas nonendemic for fungal infections such as coccidioidomycosis.

An important step in the evaluation of a solitary pulmonary nodule is a comparison of its radiographic appearance with that of a previous film. A benign etiology is suggested by a lesion that has not enlarged in 2 or more years. On the other hand, if the nodule is new or if there has been progressive enlargement, malignancy or infection is much more likely. Most malignant solitary nodules have a volume doubling time of 60 to 150 days, with a mean of 120 days. In spherical lesions, an increase in diameter of 26 per cent equates to one doubling in volume. Calcification within the node is usually a sign of a benign lesion. Patterns of calcification seen with benign lesions are a dense central nidus of calcium, a concentric or laminated pattern, a diffuse pattern, or a clustered or "popcorn" pattern. Small amounts of calcium may be seen within 1 to 3 per cent of bronchogenic carcinomas or osteosarcomas metastatic to the lung. CT has two important roles in evaluating solitary pulmonary nodules. First, imaging and densitometry can be helpful in detecting calcification. Tomograms of the lung may also serve this purpose. Second, other nodules not seen with standard anteroposterior and lateral chest radiographs may be detected on CT. The use of CT densitometry to identify malignancy by low-density numbers remains experimental.

If a previous radiograph is not available, or if an enlarging lesion is suspected, the ultimate determination of etiology of a solitary nodule is dependent upon either culture confirmation of infection or histologic examination. A lesion can be considered benign only if a specific diagnosis is obtained. Sputum for tuberculosis should be obtained only if tuberculosis is highly suspected. Cytologic findings in sputum are positive in only 10 per cent or fewer of patients with endobronchially invisible bronchogenic carcinomas and 20 per cent of patients with malignancies metastatic to the lungs.

Once the etiology of a solitary nodule is ascertained, treatment will depend upon cause. When a lesion is not obviously benign, percutaneous transthoracic needle aspiration, fiberoptic bronchoscopy, or thoracotomy is indicated. Needle aspiration biopsy yields a specific diagnosis in 85 to 90 per cent of cases. It is helpful to establish a diagnosis of malignancy in patients in whom surgery is not contemplated but in whom a specific diagnosis will help guide management. Fiberoptic bronchoscopy with transbronchial biopsy and bronchial brushing has the advantage over needle aspiration because it is useful in staging lung cancer and has a lower complication rate. Success in obtaining a diagnosis is dependent upon the size of the nodule. Solitary pulmonary nodules less than 2 cm in size or within 2 cm of the hilum are difficult to diagnose with bronchoscopy. Thoracotomy is the most direct means of establishing a diagnosis; however, transthoracic needle biopsy may be used as an alternative to thoracotomy in lesions less than 2 cm in diameter. It also offers the best chance for cure of lung cancer. The possibility of small cell lung cancer is not necessarily a reason for avoiding thoracotomy. Surgical resection of small cell lung cancer presenting as a solitary pulmonary nodule may have a 5-year survival comparable to that with other forms of nodular bronchogenic carcinoma treated with surgical resection (approximately 24 per cent). Indications for thoracotomy include suspicion that the lesion is malignant and resectable and the absence of major surgical risk factors. Contraindications are severe underlying lung disease or heat disease. Mediastinoscopy is indicated only if the chest radiograph shows mediastinal widening, if the solitary nodule is greater than 3 cm in diameter, or if the nodule is centrally located near the hilum of the lung.

Stauffer JL: What to do when you detect a solitary pulmonary nodule. J Respir Dis 7:17, 1986. *Excellent summary of management of solitary pulmonary nodule based upon etiologic consideration and the yield of particular diagnostic approaches. Practical and rational.*

Swensen SJ, Jett JR, Payne WS, et al : An integrated approach to evaluation of the solitary pulmonary nodule. Mayo Clin Proc 65:173, 1990. *Focuses on integrated approach for detection and evaluation of solitary nodule, particularly using CT and transthoracic needle biopsy.*

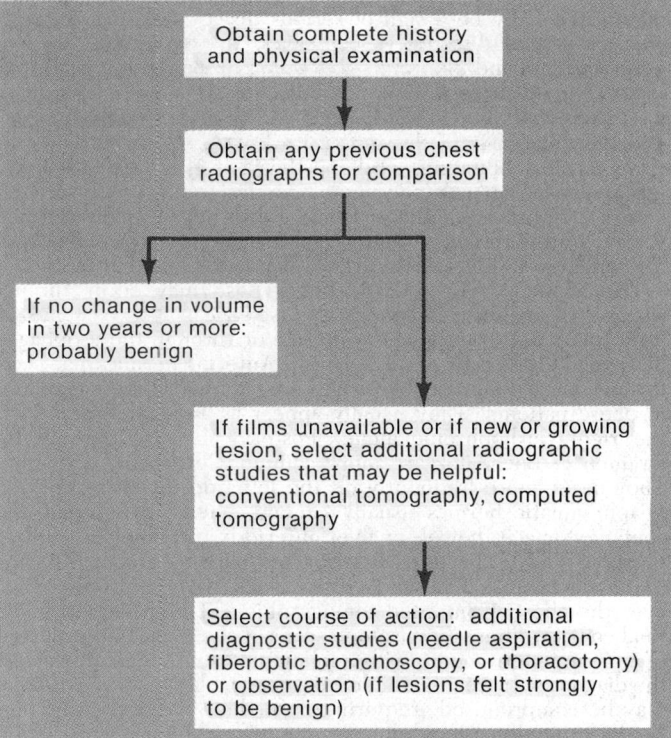

FIGURE 68–1. Approach to the patient with a solitary pulmonary nodule.

69 Diseases of the Diaphragm, Chest Wall, Pleura, and Mediastinum

Bartolome R. Celli

THE DIAPHRAGM

The diaphragm is the most important muscle of respiration. Shaped like a thin dome, it separates the thoracic and abdominal cavities. It has two components: the central noncontractile tendon and the muscle fibers that arise from it and radiate down and outward to insert distally into the circumferential caudal limits of the ribcage. There is a hiatus for each of the structures that pass from the thorax to the abdomen. The diaphragm is neurologically controlled via the phrenic nerve, the motoneurons of which arise in the cervical spinal cord at levels C3–C5. The anatomic arrangement of the diaphragm and its coupling to the ribcage-abdomen account for its mechanical action. Diaphragmatic contraction acts to displace the abdominal contents downward and to raise the ribs up and outward. This action results in the creation of the negative intrapleural pressure of inspiration. Like the heart, the diaphragm, and, to a lesser degree, the other respiratory muscles, must intermittently contract throughout a person's life. Unlike the heart, it has no intrinsic contractile mechanism, and the respiratory cycle is regulated by a complex set of centrally organized neurons and several peripheral feedback mechanisms that synchronizes the diaphragm with many other muscles. This arrangement must be so, since the diaphragm serves other, nonrespiratory functions, such as speech, defecation, and parturition. The blood supply to the diaphragm is very rich and is arranged in such a way as to minimize interruption during contraction. Nevertheless, the muscle itself is highly oxygen dependent.

Disorders of the Diaphragm

DYSFUNCTION AND FATIGUE. The most frequent cause of diaphragmatic dysfunction is lung hyperinflation, either acute, like in asthma, or chronic, like in chronic obstructive pulmonary disease (COPD). Hyperinflation shortens the diaphragmatic fibers and changes the shape of the diaphragm to a flatter state in which the more horizontal fibers do not generate the normally lifting and expanding action of the ribcage but rather produce an inward deforming change in the lower ribcage (Hoover's sign in COPD). These changes, coupled with the increased ventilatory loads secondary to airways resistance and with changes in lung and chest wall compliance, result in greater work by the diaphragm. If the increased demand of energy to perform this work outstrips the energy supply, the diaphragm will fatigue, and ventilation may fail. Diaphragmatic fatigue can be determined by the use of pressure measurements across the diaphragm (transdiaphragmatic pressure, or Pdi) or by the more elaborate power-spectrum analysis of electromyographic signals. Fortunately, both correlate well with simpler clinical signs, such as increased respiratory rate with progressively shallower breathing. As fatigue increases, ventilation is maintained by intermittent expansions of the ribcage and abdomen (respiratory alternans) and then by paradoxical inward motion of the abdomen during inspiration (abdominal paradox). The strategies available to improve diaphragmatic muscle function in patients with impending fatigue are listed in Table 69–1. If the fatigue has resulted in hypercapnia and acidosis, mechanical ventilation must be instituted so that the respiratory muscles can rest. When ventilation is assisted, it should be done for at least 1 to several days, since muscle fatigue of the kind causing ventilatory failure may take that long to abate.

DISORDERS OF DIAPHRAGMATIC MOTION. Diaphragmatic paralysis may be unilateral, which is usually secondary to phrenic nerve involvement by a tumor (bronchogenic carcinoma

TABLE 69–1. THERAPEUTIC MODALITIES TO IMPROVE DIAPHRAGMATIC FUNCTION

Reduce mechanical load
  1. Decrease airways resistance (bronchodilators, treat infection, decrease inflammation)
  2. Reduce hyperinflation
  3. Decrease ventilatory requirements (administer oxygen, control fever, avoid caloric loads)
Improve respiratory muscle contractility and endurance
  1. Oxygen therapy
  2. Improve nutrition
  3. Improve cardiovascular performance
  4. Correct electrolytes (sodium, potassium, calcium, phosphorus)
  5. Administer drugs that improve contractility (theophylline, β_2 agonist, caffeine)
  6. Check for hypothyroidism or drugs that impair contractility (aminoglycosides)
  7. Ventilatory muscle training
Improve respiratory muscle coordination and energy conservation
Rehabilitation
Respiratory muscle resting

being the most frequent). It may result as a complication of neurologic diseases, such as myelitis, encephalitis, poliomyelitis, and herpes zoster. It may result from trauma to the thorax or cervical spine or from compression by benign processes, such as a substernal thyroid, an aortic aneurysm, and infectious collections. With the advent of extensive cardiac surgery, paralysis secondary to cooling of the phrenic nerve has been increasingly noted. Occasionally, the paralysis may be idiopathic. In patients with normal lungs, unilateral paralysis is usually asymptomatic and rarely requires treatment. The diagnosis is suspected when, in the chest roentgenogram, the diaphragmatic leaflet is elevated and is confirmed fluoroscopically by observing paradoxical diaphragmatic motion on sniff and cough. Bilateral paralysis usually results from high cervical trauma (C3–C5) or from myopathies. The myopathy may be generalized (muscular dystrophy, polymyositis, hypothyroidism) or may be limited or may primarily affect the diaphragm (acid maltase deficiency, collagen vascular disorders). In many cases, the etiology remains unknown. The patients may become symptomatic early. The dyspnea is characteristically worsened when the patient assumes the supine position, since abdominal contents displace the diaphragm into the thorax. This situation also results in a significant drop in the vital capacity (>500 ml) and in oxygen saturation. Fluoroscopic observation of diaphragmatic excursions is less reliable in this condition, since the flaccid diaphragm may lag behind the ribcage expansion when accessory muscles contract, thus giving the impression of diaphragmatic contraction. The diagnosis can be suspected by the presence of abdominal paradoxical retraction with inspiration. It can be confirmed by measurement of transdiaphragmatic pressure with and without electromyographic recording. Phrenic nerve conduction time helps establish the diagnosis of neuropathy. The treatment of ventilatory failure secondary to bilateral paralysis consists of intermittent ventilation that has been achieved with different methods (external negative ventilation, nasal positive-pressure ventilation, and rocking beds). In some cases, such as after cardiac surgery, the paralysis will resolve with time, and the ventilation may be discontinued. When used on a permanent basis, but in those with intact muscle function (e.g., in high quadriplegics), diaphragmatic pacing has been life saving.

HICCUP. Hiccup, or singultus, is a common disorder produced by spasm of the diaphragm that is followed by sudden closure of the glottis during an inspiratory effort. Hiccups are usually self-limited but may persist for days or weeks and become very disturbing. In most patients, a cause is never found, but it may occasionally be a sign of serious disease, such as a central nervous system disorder (encephalitis, stroke, tumor), uremia, herpes zoster, and pleural or abdominal processes that invade or irritate the diaphragm. Prolonged hiccups are sometimes psychogenic in origin. In general, hiccups will subside spontaneously or with improvement of the initiating disease. When hiccups are chronic and debilitating, local anesthesia or phrenic nerve crushing may be required (permanent paralysis may occur with the latter). Diaphragmatic flutter is a rare disorder in which rhythmic contractions of the diaphragm occur at a rate of 1 to 8 per second. The etiology and treatment are similar to those of hiccups.

DIAPHRAGMATIC HERNIAS. These may occur through congenitally weak or incompletely fused areas of the diaphragm, from traumatic rupture of the muscle or through the esophageal hiatus (>70 per cent of all hernias). Anterior hernias that occur through the foramina of Morgagni are rare and tend to be found in obese patients. They usually appear as a rounded density in the right cardiophrenic angle. Posterior hernias through the foramen of Bochdalek are more common, especially in infants. They occur more frequently on the left side than on the right. Diaphragmatic hernias usually contain omentum but may also contain stomach, bowel, or liver anteriorly or kidney and spleen posteriorly. The diagnosis is suspected on the basis of the chest roentgenogram and in some cases when there is borborygmus over the chest. Computed tomographic (CT) scans, gastrointestinal contrast films, radioisotope scans of the liver, and induction of a pneumoperitoneum with a follow-up film may help establish the diagnosis. In infants, the hernias may be large, and ventilation may be compromised, requiring immediate surgical correction. In the asymptomatic adult with previous evidence of a hernia, observation is indicated. Surgery may be needed for diagnosis or to relieve strangulation of sac contents. Traumatic diaphragmatic hernias may result from direct penetrating injuries or from abdominal compression. The severity of symptoms depends upon the extension of abdominal contents into the thorax and the presence of strangulation. In other cases, several years may elapse before respiratory and abdominal symptoms recur. The treatment in these cases is surgical. Eventration may resemble a hernia but instead consists of a localized elevation of the diaphragm resulting from impaired muscle development or weakness. It is more frequent in the right anteromedial portion and tends to occur in middle-aged, obese persons. Once differentiated from neoplasm, it rarely requires surgical treatment.

Celi BR: Clinical and physiologic evaluation of respiratory muscle function. Clin Chest Med 10:199, 1989. *Comprehensive, up-to-date review covering the clinical aspects and practical application of respiratory muscle function.*

Newsom-Davis J, Goldman M, Loh L, et al.: Diaphragm function and alveolar hyperventilation. Q J Med 45:87, 1976. *It establishes the role of diaphragmatic dysfunction in generating ventilatory failure. It also introduces intermittent external ventialtion as a therapeutic modality.*

Rochester DF: The diaphragm: Contractile properties and fatigue. J Clin Invest 75:1397, 1985. *Excellent review of the anatomy and physiology of the diaphragm. It covers our understanding of dysfunction and fatigue.*

THE CHEST WALL

The chest wall is an integral part of the pump that moves air in and out of the lungs. It consists of the bony thoracic cage (ribs, sternum, and vertebrae) and the various muscles of respiration. Besides the diaphragm, the intercostal and scalenus muscles are active even during quiet breathing in normal persons. Other muscles, such as the sternocleidomastoid, pectoralis minor and major, serratus anterior, latissimus dorsi, and trapezius, may participate in respiration in cases of increased ventilatory demand. Even the abdominal muscles can take part in ventilation; by contracting in exhalation, they lengthen the inspiratory muscles and place them in an advantageous position for the next inspiratory contraction. The thoracic cage system is a major determinant of ventilation and of static and dynamic lung volumes. Diseases that disrupt the system will alter ventilation and the ventilation-perfusion relationship, thus causing hypoxemia or hypercapnia. Primary disorders of the chest wall may occur from impairments of the neuromuscular apparatus or of the bony thoracic cage. Since alterations in the neuromuscular apparatus are dealt with in different parts of the text, this section discusses primary alterations of the bony thoracic cage.

Disorders of the Chest Wall

The most important diseases of the bony thoracic cage are listed in Table 69–2. They are all linked by a similar pathophysiologic process: (1) alveolar hypoventilation, (2) changes in chest wall compliance, (3) variable lung compression, (4) ventilation-perfusion imbalance, and (5) pulmonary hypertension and cor pulmonale. Clinical symptoms include dyspnea without significant cough, sputum, or pain. The physical examination usually establishes the diagnosis and helps determine the presence of cor pulmonale.

KYPHOSCOLIOSIS. Deformities of the dorsolumbar spine are by far the most common causes of symptomatic derangements of the chest wall. Scoliosis consists of lateral angulation and rotation of the spine and can be categorized as right (most frequent) or left, according to the direction of the convexity of the primary curvature. Kyphosis is less important and consists of anteroposterior angulations of the spine. The severity of scoliosis is quantified by measuring the angle (Cobb's angle) between the upper and lower portions of the spinal curve on a roentgenogram. Only when this angle exceeds 70 degrees is any abnormality of respiratory function detectable. When the angle is greater than

TABLE 69–2. MOST IMPORTANT RIBCAGE DERANGEMENTS

Spine
  Scoliosis (idiopathic, congenital, paralytic)
  Kyphosis
  Ankylosing spondylitis

Sternum, Ribs, or Pleura
  Pectus excavatum
  Thoracoplasty
  Fibrothorax

120 degrees, dyspnea and early respiratory failure are expected. The ribs over the convex side of the deformity are separated and rotated posteriorly, giving rise to the kyphoscoliotic hump. On the concave side, the ribs are crowded and displaced anteriorly. This, combined with decreased thoracic height, results in forward bulging of the anterior wall. Kyphoscoliosis usually begins in childhood and has no specific etiology in most cases. Primary muscle diseases and congenital disorders account for a very small fraction of the total. The patients who have angles greater than 70 degrees may begin to develop symptoms upon exerting effort, and as the angulation increases, respiratory failure and cor pulmonale gradually develop This situation may result in death in the fourth to sixth decade. If the scoliosis is not severe and does not progress, life expectancy may be normal. Static lung volumes are decreased in relation to the severity of the scoliosis. Chest wall and, to a lesser degree, lung compliance are also decreased. The determination of regional lung function shows ventilation-perfusion shifts that result in hypoxemia. When the mechanical load, caused by progressive scoliosis or superimposed infection, is such that the muscles fail, the hypoxemia may be associated with hypercapnia. Hypoventilation and hypoxemia may become worse during sleep, which accounts for the frequent worsening of some patients with otherwise stable kyphoscoliosis.

Several therapeutic approaches are used in kyphoscoliosis and thoracic disorders in general. Surgical correction includes traction, plasters, and attempts to straighten the scoliosis by the use of rods. The effects appear mostly cosmetic (it prevents prgression of the curvature), and the improvement in function is minimal. In patients who are hypoxemic, the addition of oxygen is beneficial. Kyphoscoliosis is one of the few diseases in which the administration of intermittent positive-pressure ventilation results in increases in tidal volume with temporary improvement in lung compliance and lung volumes. In patients with chronic ventilatory failure from scoliosis, nighttime ventilatory assistance either with external devices or with tracheostomy results in reversal of the failure. Efforts must be made to prevent airways disease and to induce the patient to stop smoking. Bronchospasms and respiratory infections must be treated aggressively. If obese, the patient should lose weight.

ANKYLOSING SPONDYLITIS. This inflammatory disease results in the fusion of costotransverse and vertebral joints but also involve sternomanubrial and clavicular joints. With relative fixation of the ribcage in an inspiratory position, most of the ventilatory movement is performed by the diaphragm-abdomen, which is already placed at a mechanical disadvantage, as shown by a normal or greater than normal functional residual capacity. In contrast to kyphoscoliosis, cor pulmonale and ventilatory failure are the exception. Some patients with ankylosing spondylitis may develop upper lobe fibrosis with minimal alterations in gas exchange.

PECTUS EXCAVATUM. This condition is a congenital deformity of the lower portion of the sternum with symmetric bowing of the anterior ribs. In infants it tends to occur with multiple abnormalities and is associated with high mortality. It may also be associated with mitral valve prolapse. When the deformity is severe, the heart and mediastinal structures are laterally displaced. Although some patients may fail to increase cardiac output during exercise in a normal fashion, functional impairment for the most part is limited. Surgical correction is mainly done for cosmetic reasons.

SEQUELAE OF THORACOPLASTY. Thoracoplasty is the general term applied to a series of surgical procedures employed from 1940 to 1950 for the treatment of tuberculosis. The procedures included resection of several ribs with collapse of the lung underneath the resected area. This situation results in paradoxical retraction of that portion of the chest wall. Although it was originally thought to have minimal physiologic consequences, there has been a significant increase in the development of cardiorespiratory failure with cor pulmonale in those patients.

FIBROTHORAX. Fibrothorax resulting from pleural diseases such as intense hemothorax or asbestosis is also considered a primary disease of the chest wall, since the lung itself may not be affected. The disorder may occasionally result in ventilatory and cardiac failure. The treatment of both conditions is similar to that of patients with kyphoscoliosis. Occasional pleurectomy may help patients with fibrothorax secondary to pleural fibrosis.

FLAIL CHEST. This condition is produced by double fractures of three or more adjacent ribs or by combined sternal and rib fractures. The flail segment will paradoxically move inward during inspiration and outward during expiration. The inefficient ventilation increases the work of breathing, which may be even more inefficient if (as is often the case) there is concomitant neuromuscular impairment. Flail chest occurs most frequently with accidental chest trauma, but it also can occur after cardiopulmonary resuscitation. Hypoxemia is very often present as a result of ventilation-perfusion inequality from the flail segment and the frequent underlying lung contusion. It is clear that in most cases artificial ventilation for internal fixation of the flail segment is not necessary. It should be reserved for patients with ventilatory failure. Supportive care with attention to maintaining adequate oxygenation, clear airways, and prevention of infections is the preferred therapy for most patients. When the flail segment is large, operative chest wall fixation may be considered.

Bergofsky EH: Respiratory failure in disorders of the thoracic cage. Am Rev Respir Dis 119:643, 1979. *Still the most comprehensive work on this topic. Easy to read, excellent review.*
Holppner VH, Cockcroft DW, Dosman JH, et al.: Nighttime ventilation improves respiratory failure in secondary kyphoscoliosis. Am Rev Respir Dis 129:240, 1984. *Reviews the use of nighttime ventilation and its effectiveness in reverting ventilatory failure in cases of "pump fatigue."*
Todd TR, Shamji F: Pathophysiology of chest trauma. Thorax 33:979, 1985. *Excellent review of the pathophysiologic changes in respiratory function secondary to chest trauma. Reviews the controversies in treatment.*

THE PLEURA
Anatomy and Physiology

The pleura consists of a layer of variable-sized mesothelial cells and normally has a smooth, glistening, and semitransparent appearance. It is supported by a network of connective and fibroelastic tissue, lymphatics, and vessels. The mesothelial cells are rich in microvilli, and their most important function is to deliver glycoproteins rich in hyaluronic acid, which helps decrease friction between the lung and chest wall. The pleura is defined as "parietal" where it covers the surface of the chest wall, diaphragm, and mediastinum. The parietal pleura is supplied with blood from the systemic circulation, contains sensory nerves, and has cells that are very rich in microvilli. The visceral pleura is that layer covering the entire surface of the lungs, including the interlobar fissures. Its blood supply arises from the low-pressure pulmonary circulation, it has no sensory nerves, and its cells have a lower number of microvilli. Both pleural layers are separated by a cavity and are lubricated by 5 to 10 ml of fluid. This arrangement allows the lung to expand, retract, and deform with ease. It also helps maintain the lung in an inflated state by coupling it with the chest wall. Both functions decrease the work of breathing.

The pleural fluid has a low protein concentration (< 2 grams per deciliter) with a pH and glucose level similar to those of blood. Pleural fluid is formed primarily from the parietal pleura, and part of its turnover is dependent on the same Starling forces that govern vascular and interstitial fluid exchange elsewhere. The parietal pleura has a hydrostatic pressure similar to that of the systemic circulation (30 cm H_2O), while that of the visceral pleura depends on the pulmonary circulation (10 cm H_2O). Oncotic pressure is similar in both (25 cm H_2O), but the pressure within the pleural cavity is affected by the gravity gradient. Thus the pleural space is heterogeneous with a nondependent portion where Starling forces favor outpouring of fluid to the cavity and into parenchymal capillaries. Recent evidence reveals that stomas are present over the parietal surface of the low mediastinum, low chest wall, and diaphragm. These stomas and "lacunae" empty into lymphatics. The current thought is that these subpleural parietal lymphatics represent the major pathway for liquid and solute drainage of the pleural space. Alterations in any of the components of this formation-resorption mechanism frequently lead to the accumulation of pleural fluid. Excessive increases in hydrostatic forces or decreases in oncotic pressures result in low-protein "transudates." Increased outpouring by the capillaries or cells or blocking of lymphatics results in high-protein "exudates." The mechanisms that lead to the accumulation of pleural fluid are shown in Table 69–3.

TABLE 69–3. MECHANISMS THAT LEAD TO ACCUMULATION OF PLEURAL FLUID

1. Increased hydrostatic pressure in microvascular circulation (e.g., congestive heart failure)
2. Decreased oncotic pressure in microvascular circulation (e.g., severe hypoalbuminemia)
3. Decreased pressure in the pleural space (e.g., complete lung collapse)
4. Increased permeability of the microvascular circulation (e.g., pneumonia)
5. Impaired lymphatic drainage from the pleural space (e.g., malignant effusion)
6. Movement of fluid from the peritoneal space (e.g., ascites)

Diagnostic Procedures

HISTORY AND PHYSICAL EXAMINATION. Although a patient's history may suggest pleural disease, it is neither sensitive nor specific. The most frequent symptoms are chest pain, dyspnea, and cough. They may be absent in some large effusions and in critically ill patients. When present, the pain is usually unilateral and sharp and worsens with inspiration, cough, or ribcage movements. It may radiate to shoulder, neck, or abdomen. Dyspnea may result from the compression of lung tissue secondary to the accumulation of fluid, thus creating a ventilation-perfusion mismatch. It may also result from mechanical alterations in diaphragmatic and other respiratory muscles as the amounts of fluid change their length-tension relationship. The degree of dyspnea relates to the volume of fluid, to the intrathoracic pressure it generates, and to its effect on mechanics and gas exchange. Finally, pleural effusions that accumulate in patients with minimal lung compromise are well tolerated, whereas similar effusions in patients with underlying severe lung disease may cause ventilatory failure. The physical examination varies, depending on the severity of the effusion and the underlying lung or systemic disease. Patients breathe shallowly and rapidly, they may have decreased excursions in the affected hemithorax (splinting), and breath sounds are decreased in the affected area. Percussion shows dullness with absent tactile fremitus over the area. Frequently, there are E to A changes (egobronchophony) at the upper border of the fluid.

RADIOLOGIC EXAMINATION. An effusion can be suspected when blunting and medial displacement of the sharp costophrenic angle are present. Accumulation of fluid between the base of the lung and the diaphragm (subpulmonic effusion) is suspected when there is apparent elevation of the hemidiaphragm or widening of the shadow between the gas-containing stomach and the lower margin of the left lung. Up to 300 ml of fluid may fail to be seen in a posteroanterior chest roentgenogram, whereas as little as 150 ml may be seen in a lateral decubitus film. A supine film (frequent in patients in intensive care units) may obscure the diagnosis as the fluid layers posteriorly. A pseudo-tumor occurs when fluid loculates in an interlobar fissure, most commonly in the minor fissure, and gives the radiologic appearance of a tumor. A clue to the diagnosis is the presence of pleural fluid elsewhere and a biconvex lenticular configuration of the mass. When an effusion is suspected, an upright or a lateral decubitus film is usually confirmatory. A collection of pleural air and fluid (hydro-, pyo-, hemopneumothorax) usually produces horizontal and not concave margins. A pneumothorax is identified by noting the contrast between the water density of the visceral pleura centrally and the gas lucency without vascular markings laterally. Small pneumothoraces may be harder to diagnose, but an expiratory film may help outline it. Pleural plaques may be seen when calcified, and if not calcified, they may be detected when the plaques are viewed tangentially but not en face. Other tumors and loculated effusions may be difficult to define. Ultrasonography and CT may provide better definition of pleural and, in many cases, parenchymal abnormalities.

THORACENTESIS AND PLEURAL FLUID ANALYSIS. Thoracentesis may be performed for diagnostic or therapeutic purposes. A thoracentesis is diagnostic in approximately 75 per cent of patients, and even when not diagnostic it helps exclude other important diagnoses, such as empyema. Diagnostic thoracentesis requires a relatively small amount of material (30 to 50 ml), usually obtained with a small-gauge needle. As a rule, newly

TABLE 69–4. CHARACTERISTICS OF PLEURAL FLUID TRANSUDATES

	Absolute Value	Pleural Fluid/ Serum Value
Protein	<3 grams/dl	<0.5
Lactate dehydrogenase (LDH)	<200 units/L	<0.6
Glucose	<60 mg/dl	1.0
White blood cell count	<1000	—

discovered effusions should be tapped. Although there are no absolute contraindications to a diagnostic thoracentesis, relative contraindications include a bleeding diathesis, anticoagulation, a small volume, mechanical ventilation, and low risk-benefit ratio. Therapeutic thoracentesis involves removing larger amounts of fluid. No more than 1000 to 1500 ml should be removed at one time, since pulmonary edema may occur in the re-expanded underlying lung, especially in those cases of tension effusions.

Although the classification of pleural fluid into *transudate* or *exudate* is not absolute, it has proved helpful in directing the clinician to the most useful studies and in suggesting possible diagnoses. To differentiate transudates and exudates, it is cost effective to obtain the following tests on the fluid obtained: total protein, lactate dehydrogenase (LDH), white blood cell count (WBC) with differential, and either glucose level or pH. Table 69–4 shows the characteristics of transudates. Transudates are due to imbalances in hydrostatic and oncotic pressures, such as those seen in congestive heart failure or hypoalbuminemia. They may also result from the peritoneum to the pleural space.

Exudates are defined by the presence of at least one of the following criteria: (1) a pleural fluid/serum protein ratio greater than 0.5; (2) a pleural fluid/serum LDH ratio greater than 0.6; and (3) a pleural fluid LDH greater than two-thirds that of serum. The results obtained from the analysis of exudative effusions suggest some diseases, as shown in Table 69–5. The diagnoses that can be established by thoracentesis include malignancy (malignant cells), empyema (pus), tuberculosis (positive acid-fast bacillus for smear or cultures), fungal infection (positive KOH or culture), lupus pleuritis (LE cells), chylothorax (high triglyceride levels or presence of chylomicrons), urinothorax (a pleural fluid/ serum creatinine ratio of >1), and esophageal rupture (an increased pleural fluid amylase level and pH around 6.0). Since many diagnoses may produce exudative pleural fluid with overlapping values, acid-fast and Gram's stains, aerobic and anaerobic cultures, cell count and differential, and cytologic analysis should be included in the study of these effusions. A predominance of polymorphonuclear leukocytes is most compatible with bacterial infection, while lymphocytes (particularly with a paucity of mesothelial cells) suggest tuberculosis. Lymphocytes are also seen in lymphoma and leukemic effusions. Abundant eosinophils are usually nonspecific and suggest longstanding fluid. When not due to trauma, a bloody effusion is most likely the result of malignancy or pulmonary infarction. A white effusion suggests chyle, choles-

TABLE 69–5. CORRELATION OF PLEURAL FLUID EXUDATE FINDINGS AND CAUSATIVE DISEASE

Tests	Diseases
pH < 7.2	Empyema, malignancy, esophageal rupture, rheumatoid, lupus and tuberculous, pleuritis
Glucose (<60 mg/dl)	Infection, rheumatoid pleurisy, tuberculous and lupus effusions, esophageal rupture
Amylase (>200 units/dl)	Pancreatic disease, esophageal rupture, malignancy, ruptured ectopic pregnancy
Rheumatoid factor, ANA, LE cells	Collagen vascular diseases
Complement (decreased)	Lupus erythematosus, rheumatoid arthritis
Red blood cells (>5000/ml)	Trauma, malignancy, pulmonary embolus
Chylous effusion (triglycerides > 110 mg/dl)	Violation of thoracic duct (trauma, malignancy)
Biopsy (+)	Malignancy, tuberculosis

terol, or lymphoma. A black fluid suggests *Aspergillus* pleural involvement. A yellow-green color may be seen in rheumatoid pleurisy. A putrid odor is diagnostic of anaerobic empyema, while an ammonia odor suggests urinothorax. The value of other diagnostic markers, such as adenosine deaminase (ADA), beta$_2$-microglobulin, and lysozyme, remains to be determined. The complications of thoracentesis include pain, bleeding (local, pleural, or abdominal), pneumothorax, infection, and spleen or liver puncture. With therapeutic thoracentesis, up to 50 per cent of patients experience a temporary fall in PaO_2 of as much as 20 mm Hg.

PERCUTANEOUS PLEURAL BIOPSY. This biopsy is indicated in the evaluation of the patient with undiagnosed exudative effusion (particularly those with lymphocytic predominance), since the most frequently diagnosed diseases are malignancy and tuberculosis. The procedure is performed with the patient under local anesthesia, using a hook-type needle (Cope or Abrams). The contraindications are as follows: a small or loculated pleural effusion; an uncooperative patient; and anticoagulation or bleeding diathesis, including azotemia with abnormal bleeding time. Since pleural seeding may not be uniform, multiple samples are needed. The overall diagnostic yield is around 60 per cent for malignancy and 75 per cent for tuberculosis.

EXPLORATION OF THE PLEURA. In most of the 5 to 10 per cent of cases of patients with pleural effusion in whom a diagnosis cannot be established, the effusion will disappear spontaneously or the cause will become evident. In those patients in whom a diagnosis is considered necessary, a biopsy can be directly obtained through thoracoscopy (introduction of a rigid scope with a cold light source). Besides its high yield, thoracoscopy is useful because it may be performed with the use of local anesthesia and sedatives. In some other cases, it is necessary to perform an open pleural biopsy with the patient under general anesthesia. The main advantage is the possibility of obtaining larger specimens and concomitant lung tissue.

Disorders of the Pleura

TRANSUDATIVE EFFUSIONS

Congestive heart failure is the most common cause of transudative effusions. The evidence indicates that effusions result from biventricular failure with venous hypertension. They are more often bilateral, usually larger on the right, and on the chest roentgenogram, they are associated with vascular congestion and cardiomegaly. In chronic heart failure (months), the total protein level may be greater than 3 grams per deciliter. Thoracentesis is indicated if the patient is febrile, the effusion is very large and unilateral, and there is pleuritic pain or hypoxemia that is disproportionate to the degree of failure. Transudates may also occur in 5 to 10 per cent of patients with cirrhosis of the liver, usually with ascites. This transudate is secondary to movement of ascitic fluid through diaphragmatic defects or lymphatic channels. The effusion is more frequent on the right (70 per cent). If the diagnosis is in doubt, injection of radioactive tracer in the ascitic fluid will show up in the chest within hours of administration. The pleural effusion very often improves as the ascites improves. Occasionally, chemical pleurodesis has been effective in relieving symptomatic recurrent effusions. The transudative effusion seen in up to 20 per cent of patients with the nephrotic syndrome is due to decreased oncotic pressure (hypoalbuminemia) and increased hydrostatic forces. It is frequently bilateral and improves with correction of the protein-losing nephropathy. Peritoneal dialysis and atelectasis may also cause transudative effusions. A rare form of transudate is that seen in obstructions of the urinary system. The effusion (urinothorax) is usually ipsilateral with the obstruction and has the characteristic odor of urine. Relief of the obstruction results in prompt resolution of the effusion.

EXUDATIVE EFFUSIONS

INFECTIONS. Parapneumonic effusion (pleural fluid associated with pneumonias or lung abscess) is the most common cause of exudates. The effusions can be divided into two types: uncomplicated, which resolve spontaneously with antibiotics, or complicated, which require drainage to resolve fully. Complicated effusions are usually rich in white cells (empyema) and/or have a positive Gram stain or cultures. Uncomplicated effusions are usually small, contain moderate amounts of polymorphonuclear neutrophils (PMN's), a glucose level similar to that of blood, a pH higher than 7.3, and an LDH less than 500 units per liter. In contrast, complicated effusions have a large number of PMN's many times over 100,000 per cubic millimeter, a pH less than 7.2, a glucose level lower than 40 grams per deciliter, and an LDH greater than 1000 units per liter. If the effusion is also purulent and contains bacteria, immediate draining is necessary. The more of these features the effusion has, the more likely it is that drainage is needed. Drainage itself is best achieved with a standard chest tube placed in the most dependent portion of the pleural space. If the fever persists over 48 to 72 hours, the pleural space drainage is inadequate (such as when fluid becomes loculated), the antibiotic is inappropriate, or the diagnosis is wrong. If drainage is not effective because of loculation, insertion of an additional tube or instillation of intrapleural streptokinase has been effective. Poorly treated empyemas may result in communications with the bronchial tree (bronchopleural fistulas) or skin (bronchopleurocutaneous fistulas). These require surgical therapy (open drainage with rib resection, decortication, and extensive reconstruction). In some patients whose main problem is uncontrolled pleural sepsis, a thoracotomy with drainage and decortication may be life saving. Pleural involvement by nonbacterial, nontuberculous infection is uncommon and, when present, is usually small. Fungal diseases rarely affect the pleura except for coccidioidomycosis, which may cause a hypersensitivity pleuritis.

OTHER INFECTIVE-INFLAMMATORY DISORDERS. Exudative and frequently infected pleural effusions may result from subdiaphragmatic processes such as upper abdominal abscess, of which a subphrenic site is the most common location. Very frequently postoperative in origin, they may result from hepatic diseases and gastrointestinal perforations. The patients are usually febrile and dyspneic and manifest an elevated hemidiaphragm with ipsilateral decreased motion. Abscesses may also develop in the liver or spleen. Antibiotics alone may not be sufficient, and drainage may be necessary. Pancreatitis and pancreatic pseudocyst can cause pleural effusions, more often on the left side or bilaterally. These exudates may be blood tinged. The amylase level is higher than that in the serum. It tends to normalize as the pancreatic problem improves. Esophageal rupture is an urgent cause of pleural effusion. Close to one half of cases are secondary to endoscopy or esophageal dilatation. It may also be secondary to a foreign body or trauma or may occur spontaneously (Boerhaave's syndrome). Patients complain of chest pain, dyspnea, and dysphagia. Fever is universal, and half will have subcutaneous emphysema. The roentgenogram may confirm the subcutaneous emphysema and may show pneumothorax more frequently on the left side. Pleural effusion occurs in 75 per cent of cases. The fluid findings depend on the time of thoracentesis. Early on, the exudate contains abundant PMN's, to be followed by high concentrations of salivary amylase. Later, anaerobic organisms from the mouth will seed the space, and the pH will rapidly fall and approach a value of 6.0. The diagnosis is established by using barium sulfate or water-soluble water compounds with the patient in the appropriate lateral decubitus position. Early diagnosis and prompt surgical correction result in a greater than 90 per cent survival. If surgical closure is delayed, antibiotics for anaerobes, parenteral nutrition, and mediastinal and pleural drainage are necessary.

TUBERCULOSIS. Pleural effusion occurs in most cases of pulmonary tuberculosis but is frequently inapparent. The effusion may accompany the primary infection, in which case it is serous and results from a hypersensitivity phenomenon. These patients, who are usually febrile, may recover without treatment, but close to two thirds of them will develop active tuberculosis in the following 5 years. A second form occurs when a subpleural focus of *Mycobacterium tuberculosis* ruptures into the pleural space. The immunologic reaction between proteins or the bacterium itself and lymphocytes results in alterations in vascular permeability and an accumulation of cells that characterizes the tuberculous effusion. It is usually rich in protein (>4 grams per deciliter), with a leukocyte count around 5000 cells, of which 90 to 95 per cent are lymphocytes. A predominance of PMNs may occur the first few days after penetration of the bacillus to the pleural space. The glucose level may be low, but rarely lower than 20 mg per deciliter. The pH ranges between 7.0 and 7.3, with a pH over 7.4 virtually excluding tuberculosis. The fluid is characteristically free of mesothelial cells. Recently, the presence of ADA and lysozyme has been found to correlate with tuberculosis. The use of enzyme-linked immunosorbent assay (ELISA) for demonstration of mycobacterial antigen is gaining acceptability. Acid-fast bacilli in a smear are seen in fewer than 10 per cent of cases. Multiple-sample closed pleural biopsy is positive in 50 per cent to 80 per cent of cases, while a culture is positive in 30 per cent to 70 per cent. With all three methods combined, the yield is close to 95 per cent. The clinical presentation may vary, from simulation of an acute pneumonia (60 per cent of cases), with fever, nonproductive cough (80 per cent), and chest pain (75 per cent), to a subacute or more chronic form, with fever being the predominant symptom. The chest roentgenogram shows a normal heart size and small to moderate effusions (4 per cent are actually large). Parenchymal disease is seen in one third of cases. Intermediate-strength purified protein derivative (PPD) is positive in 70 per cent of patients, and if repeated after 6 to 8 weeks, it may become positive in those with a prior negative test. Standard treatment for pulmonary tuberculosis, including isoniazid and rifampin, results in resolution of the fever within 2 weeks, although occasionally the fever may persist for 6 to 3 weeks. The effusion resolves by 6 weeks but may persist for 3 to 4 months. Very ill patients may be helped by short-term corticosteroids. Rarely, surgical drainage of tuberculous empyema or decortication may be necessary.

OTHER INFECTIOUS EFFUSIONS. Actinomycosis, caused by the anaerobic organism *Actinomyces israelii*, may produce purulent pleural effusions. The effusions may bulge the thoracic wall and drain through the chest. Sulfur granules (whitish-yellow or brown interwoven filaments) can be identified in the fluid. Pleural effusions are also common in *Nocardia* infection of the lungs. The effusion is usually purulent with abundant PMN's. Sulfonamides are the treatment of choice. Aspergillosis of the pleura is uncommon, but an inflammatory, thickened pleura is frequently seen in progressive invasive aspergillosis. Pleural effusions due to parasitic diseases are still uncommon but are increasing in frequency, especially among Third World immigrants. Paragonimiasis causes pleural thickening or effusion in up to 48 per cent of patients. This effusion has a triad of characteristic findings: low glucose (<10 grams per deciliter), high LDH (>1000 units per liter), and low pH (<7.1). Complement fixation antibodies higher than 1:64 are diagnostic. Amebiasis and echinococcosis are rare diseases only occasionally seen in most U.S. hospitals.

HEMOTHORAX. Frank blood in the pleural space (hematocrit >20 per cent) is usually the result of trauma, hemothorax, hematologic disorders, or pleural malignancies. Left-sided pneumothorax, particularly with an associated widened mediastinum may indicate rupture or dissection of the aorta. Pleural blood often does not clot and can be readily removed by lymphatics if small. Larger effusions require tube drainage. Persistent bleeding requires surgical correction.

CHYLOTHORAX. Leakage of the lymph from the thoracic duct (chyle) most commonly results from malignancy involving the mediastinum (50 per cent), lymphoma being the most frequent. It may also result from thoracic surgery (20 per cent) or trauma (5 per cent). Since chyle collects within the posterior mediastinum, the chylothorax may not appear for days, until the mediastinal pleura ruptures. The usual milky appearance of the effusion may be confused with a cholesterol effusion or an effusion with many leukocytes. The best diagnostic criterion is the presence of a triglyceride concentration greater than 110 mg per deciliter, with rare instances of values between 50 and 110 mg per deciliter. The major complications of chylothorax are malnutrition and immunologic compromise, as fat, protein, and lymphocytes are depleted with repeated thoracentesis or chest tube drainage. Treatment should include drainage of the pleural space, a decrease in chyle formation by intravenous hyperalimentation, and a decrease in oral intake, with the possible addition of medium-chain triglycerides, which are directly absorbed into the portal circulation. In those cases in which drainage persists, thoracic duct ligation should be considered if the cause is traumatic. If the chylothorax is secondary to tumor, the treatment should address the primary cause. The triad of slow-growing yellow nails, lymphedema, and pleural effusions is termed the "yellow nail syndrome." It is due to either hypoplastic or dilated lymphatics.

IMMUNOLOGIC CAUSES OF PLEURAL EFFUSIONS. Clinical rheumatoid pleurisy occurs in close to 5 per cent of patients with rheumatoid disease, even though autopsy studies suggest up to 50 per cent involvement. It has a striking male predominance, and the effusion appears within 5 years after the onset of the disease; nevertheless, effusions have been known to occur up to 20 years before the onset of articular disease. The fluid is an exudate with a low glucose level (<30 mg per deciliter) and pH and a high LDH level. The complement level in the fluid is usually low, with high titers of rheumatoid factors. The patients may complain of pleuritic chest pain or dyspnea. Fever is not common, in contrast with lupus pleuritis. The effusion does not resolve quickly, but rather over several months; occasionally, it persists for years. The major complication is fibrosis with lung trapping, so that anti-inflammatory agents and careful administration of corticosteroids may be tried. Pleuritic pain or effusion can be the presenting manifestation in 5 per cent of patients with systemic lupus erythematosus (SLE) and can occur at some point in the course of the disease in close to 50 per cent of patients. Pain (86 per cent), cough (64 per cent), dyspnea (50 per cent), pleural friction rub (71 per cent), and fever (57 per cent) are commonly seen. The effusions are exudates, which, in the majority of cases, have normal pH and glucose. The hemolytic complement (especially C–3 and C–4 components) is low, and classic LE cells may be present in the pleural fluid. LE pleuritis is likely if the antinuclear antibody (ANA) titer in the fluid is 1:160. Spontaneous resolution of LE pleuritis is uncommon, but the response to corticosteroids is usually dramatic, with disappearance of the pleuritis within 2 weeks. Sarcoidosis, Wegener's granulomatosis, Sjögren's syndrome, and immunoblastic lymphadenopathy are rare causes of pleural effusions that may involve an immunologic mechanism for their formation.

OTHER CONDITIONS AFFECTING THE PLEURA

ASBESTOSIS. This condition is frequently associated with pleural disease. It may be an effusion, often unilateral, small, and serosanguineous. The cell count is lower than 6000 cells per milliliter with a predominance of either PMN's or mononuclear cells. Eosinophilia of up to 50 per cent of cells has been described. The diagnosis is suspected with known asbestos exposure of variable duration and intensity. The exclusion of malignant mesothelioma when pleural plaques coexist may be difficult and requires follow-up of 2 to 3 years. The effusion tends to resolve in 1 month to a year. When it resolves, it leaves a blunted angle in more than 90 per cent of patients, with 50 per cent showing diffuse pleural thickening. Calcification of the plaques occurs late (20 to 40 years after exposure). Close to 5 per cent of patients may have underlying pulmonary parenchymal asbestosis.

MEIG'S SYNDROME. This syndrome consists of the following triad of features: benign fibroma or other ovarian tumors, ascites, and large effusions (usually on the right side). Most commonly seen shortly after menopause, the symptoms are those of chronic illness, chest pain, and increased abdominal girth. Fluid moves from the abdomen to the thorax through small diaphragmatic defects or lymphatics. The fluid is usually an exudate with a paucity of mononuclear cells. When the condition is suspected, an abdominal CT scan can be done in addition to the pelvic examination and will document the ovarian tumors. Their removal results in resolution of the effusion within 2 to 3 weeks.

UREMIA. Different from the urinothorax and hydrothorax of the nephrotic syndrome, the effusion of uremia accompanies a polyserositis. It is usually an exudate with varying amounts of blood. The effusions will resolve with treatment of the uremia, but repeated thoracentesis may be needed if the patient is very symptomatic (dyspnea, cough, chest pain).

MISCELLANEOUS CAUSES OF INFLAMMATORY EFFUSIONS. Other causes of effusions with an inflammatory component include radiation therapy, esophageal sclerotherapy, enteral feeding misplacement, drug-induced pleural disease (nitrofurantoin, dantrolene, methysergide, methotrexate, procar-

bazine, amiodarone, practolol, mitomycin, bleomycin, and minoxidil). Pleuritis in a lupus-like syndrome has been associated with procainamide, hydralazine, isoniazid, and quinidine. It usually resolves after discontinuation of the medicine and may occasionally require corticosteroids.

MALIGNANCY. Malignant effusions probably are the most common cause of exudate in patients over the age of 60. Direct invasion by carcinoma of the lung is the most frequent cancer, while tertiary spread from liver metastasis or chest wall lymphatic invasion is the most frequent mechanism in breast cancer. Ovarian and gastric cancers represent close to 5 per cent of cases, while 7 per cent of patients may have an unknown primary malignancy at the time of initial diagnosis. The patients may be asymptomatic or may develop cough, pain, and dyspnea; the last-named seems related to changes in chest wall compliance and improves after thoracentesis. The effusion is an exudate with abundant red blood cells (30,000 to 50,000 per milliliter) and mononuclear cells (lymphocytes >50 per cent). Occasionally (5 per cent to 10 per cent), they are transudative, and close to one third may have a pH lower than 7.3 or a glucose level less than 60 mg per deciliter. Pleural fluid cytology is positive in close to 60 per cent of cases, and the biopsy increases the yield only to 70 per cent. Thoracentesis should be repeated if the diagnosis is still suspected. Malignant pleural effusion carries a very poor prognosis, with the exception of breast and small cell carcinoma of the lung, both of which may respond temporarily to therapy. The best method short of pleurectomy or pleural abrasion for control of recurrent malignant effusion is the intrapleural instillation of tetracycline after drainage through a chest tube.

Lymphomas. These may cause exudative effusions, which are frequently diagnostic in the case of non-Hodgkin's lymphoma. Mediastinal invasion with lymphatic blockage and effusion on this basis is suggestive of Hodgkin's lymphoma. Although the prognosis for patients with lymphomatous pleural effusion is poor, they often respond to chemotherapy.

Malignant Mesothelioma. This tumor is related to asbestos exposure in 80 per cent to 90 per cent of cases. Patients usually present with symptoms of dyspnea, cough, weight loss, and pain. Smoking is not a factor. The tumors are diffuse and often encase the underlying lung. The effusion may be massive and often bloody and, in 70 per cent cases, may have a pH lower than 7.3. Cytology is controversial because even when positive it may be difficult to differentiate from metastatic carcinoma. Elevated levels of hyaluronic acid have been documented, and special stains and electron microscopy of biopsy tissue may help in the diagnosis. The prognosis is dismal, with a median survival of 6 to 12 months after diagnosis. Malignant mesotheliomas may be confused with benign mesotheliomas, which have the histologic features of a fibroma. Benign mesotheliomas may reach a large size and may be pedunculated (migrating with position changes). They are often associated with hypertrophic pulmonary osteoarthropathy and clubbing. Treatment involves surgical removal of the mass.

PNEUMOTHORAX. Pneumothorax is defined as an accumulation of gas in the pleural space. It may be caused by (1) perforation of the visceral pleura and entry of gas from the lung; (2) penetration of the chest wall, diaphragm, mediastinum, or esophagus; or (3) gas generated by microorganisms in an empyema. In cases in which gas originates in the lung, the rupture may occur in the absence of known disease (simple pneumothorax) or as a result of parenchymal disease (secondary pneumothorax).

Simple, spontaneous pneumothorax occurs most commonly in previously healthy men 20 to 40 years of age and is due to spontaneous rupture of subpleural blebs at the apex of the lungs. The right lung is more frequently involved than the left, and recurrence is frequent (30 per cent ipsilateral, 10 per cent contralateral). The patients usually present with an acute onset of pain, dyspnea (related to size of pneumothorax), and cough. Physical examination reveals decreased breath sounds and tactile fremitus with increased resonance on the side of the pneumothorax. The chest roentgenogram classically shows the visceral pleural line. As stated before, a small pneumothorax may become evident only with an expiratory or lateral decubitus film. Small amounts of fluid (sometimes blood) are present in 25 per cent of patients. Tension pneumothorax (caused by increased positive pressure through a "ball-value" air leak) can cause mediastinal shift and compromise circulation. Observation may suffice for a small pneumothorax (<20 per cent of the hemithorax) in an asymptomatic patient, since it reabsorbs in 7 to 14 days. Larger pneumothoraces can be treated with air aspiration. In patients with pneumothorax that occupies more than 50 per cent of the hemithorax, in those with tension pneumotherapy, or in those who are very symptomatic, a chest tube should be placed. The tube can be connected to suction or placed under a water seal. The tube should be left 2 to 4 days until the leak seals. After recurrent episodes, chemical pleurodesis or surgical correction is necessary.

Secondary or complicated pneumothorax occurs as a result of trauma or other pulmonary diseases. Widespread emphysema is the most common process causing secondary pneumothorax. It may be caused by rupture of an infected abscess, with spillage of the material into the pleural space (pyopneumothorax). Also seen, but less frequently, are asthma; certain interstitial lung diseases (idiopathic fibrosis, eosinophilic granulomatosis, sarcoidosis, tuberous sclerosis); neoplasms (sarcoma, bronchogenic carcinoma); some rare diseases, such as Marfan's and Ehlers-Danlos syndromes; and endometriosis (catamenial pneumothorax). Iatrogenic injuries (e.g.,) insertion of central lines) and barotrauma are frequently seen in the intensive care unit. The treatment of pneumothorax in patients with underlying lung disease should be aggressive. The patient should be hospitalized and a chest tube inserted, since spontaneous expansion is rare, and because of the decreased pulmonary reserve, even small or moderate pneumothorax may cause significant ventilatory compromise. Surgery must not be regarded lightly since the rate of complications is high, but it may be life saving in some patients. In patients on ventilatory support, a pneumothorax will always be under tension and requires immediate insertion of a chest tube. If a bronchopleural fistula persists, a portion of the minute ventilation will exit through it; hence it is necessary to increase ventilation to compensate for this loss. For severe leak, high-frequency low-pressure ventilation or synchronized chest tube occlusion may be helpful. Frequent complications of chest tube insertion include re-expansion pulmonary edema, lung trauma or infarction, subcutaneous emphysema, bleeding, and infection of a previously sterile pleural space.

Light RW, MacGregor MI, Luchsinger PC, et al.: Pleural effusions: The diagnostic separation of transudates and exudates. Ann Intern Med 77:507, 1972. *Classic paper that divides effusions into transudative or exudative types on the basis of pleural fluid/serum ratios of LDH and protein.*

O'Rourke JP, Yee E. Civilian spontaneous pneumothorax: Treatment options and long-term results. Chest 96:1302, 1989. *Retrospective review of a large number of patients (130) with discussion of therapeutic options.*

Pistolesi M, Miniati M, Giuntini C: Pleural liquid and solute exchange. Am Rev Respir Dis 140:825, 1989. *Reviews the physiology and pathophysiology of pleural liquid. It summarizes the new concepts that have increased the importance of lymphatic drainage for fluid and solute exchange.*

Sahn SA. The pleura: State of the art. Am Rev Respir Dis 138:184, 1988. *Extensive in-depth review of pleural effusions: cause, presentation, and differential diagnosis. With 594 references, the most complete review.*

Wied U, Halkier E, Holier-Madson K, et al.: Tetracycline versus silver nitrate pleurodesis in spontaneous pneumothorax. J Thorac Cardiovasc Surg 86:591, 1983. *Controlled trial that determined the superiority of tetracycline over silver nitrate.*

THE MEDIASTINUM

The mediastinum is the anatomic space that lies in the mid-thorax and separates the two pleural cavities. It is limited by the diaphragm below and the suprasternal thoracic outlet above. The mediastinum contains several vital structures in a small space. Thus, regardless of the cause, mediastinal abnormalities can produce major symptoms. For clinical purposes, it is convenient to divide the mediastinum into anterior, middle, and posterior compartments (Fig. 69–1). The anterior compartment is bounded posteriorly by the pericardium, ascending aorta, and brachial cephalic vessels and anteriorly by the sternum. It contains the thymus, substernal extensions of the thyroid and parathyroid glands, blood vessels, pericardium, and lymph nodes. The middle compartment extends from the posterior limit of the anterior compartment to the posterior pericardial line. It contains the heart, great vessels, trachea, main bronchi, lymph nodes, and

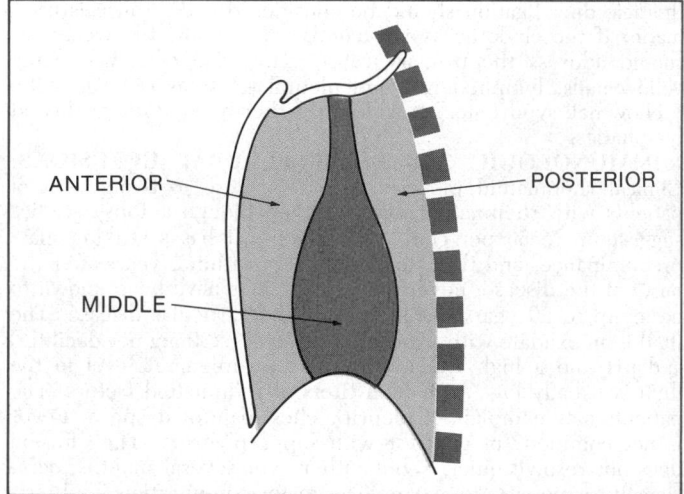

FIGURE 69–1. Anatomic compartments of the mediastinum.

phrenic and vagus nerves. The posterior compartment extends from the posterior pericardial line to the dorsal chest wall. It contains the vertebrae, descending aorta, esophagus, thoracic duct, the azygos and hemiazygos veins, the lower portion of the vagus, the sympathetic chains, and the posterior mediastinal nodes.

Signs and Symptoms of Mediastinal Masses

Most patients with mediastinal masses are asymptomatic, and the finding is incidental on a chest roentgenogram obtained for another reason. The most common symptoms are chest pain, cough, hoarseness, and dyspnea, while stridor, dysphagia, and Horner's syndrome are less frequent. Occasionally, some syndromes are associated with a primary mediastinal lesion. Myasthenia gravis is seen in nearly half of patients with thymoma. Hypoglycemia has been observed in patients with mesotheliomas, fibrosarcomas, and teratomas. Parathyroid tumors may induce hypercalcemia, and neurogenic tumors may press upon the spinal cord, causing neurologic symptoms. The signs on the physical examination are usually minimal and nonspecific. The mass may produce superior vena caval obstruction with typical signs of facial edema, dilated neck veins, and upper extremity edema. The masses may erode the trachea, esophagus, and great vessels, with life-threatening consequences.

Diagnosis of Mediastinal Masses

Most mediastinal masses are detected on a plain chest roentgenogram (Figs. 69–2 and 69–3). CT of the chest should be the initial procedure for evaluating most patients (Fig. 69–4), since it provides good visualization and definition of mediastinal struc-

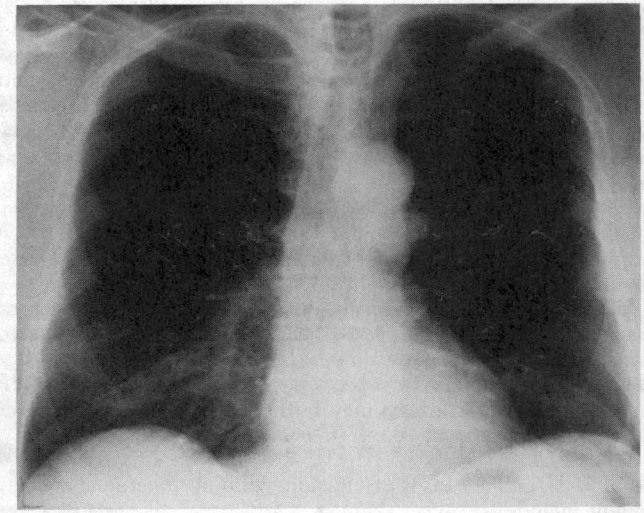

FIGURE 69–2. Posteroanterior roentgenogram of a patient with a mass in the superior portion of the anterior mediastinum.

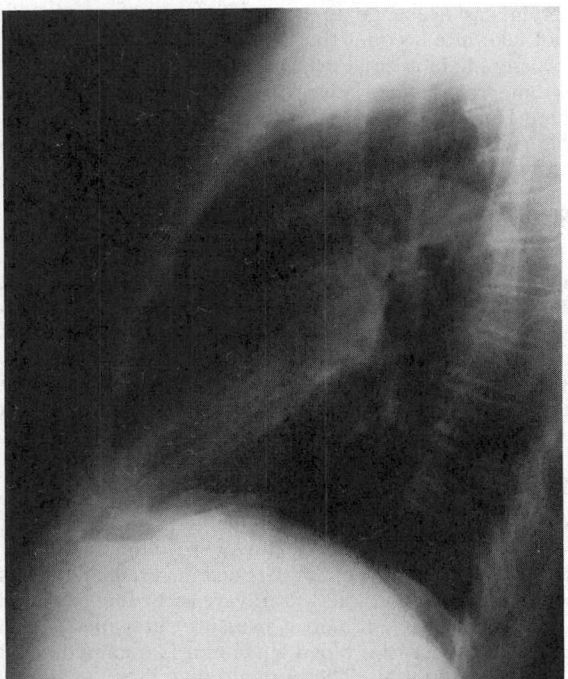

FIGURE 69–3. Lateral chest radiograph of same patient as in Figure 69–2.

tures. If the patient is asymptomatic and if noninvasive information obtained by CT with and without contrast suggests a benign process, conservative management with careful follow-up is justified. The radiologic evaluation may include angiography and barium esophagogram. The role of magnetic resonance imaging (MRI) is currently being investigated, specifically in the evaluation of vessels and blood flow, in which no contrast solution is needed. In patients in whom a specific diagnosis cannot be established with radiologic methods, it may be necessary to obtain tissue for histologic diagnosis. Classically, anterior and middle compartment lesions are reached through mediastinoscopy or mediastinotomy. Thoracotomy may be needed for middle and posterior compartment lesions or when surgery is the treatment of choice for the suspected lesion. Direct sampling, using fluoroscopy or CT-guided needle aspiration, has proved useful, especially in patients whose underlying conditions made thoracotomy or mediastinoscopy a risky procedure.

Disorders of the Mediastinum

TUMORS. The most common cause of a mediastinal mass in older patients is a metastatic carcinoma (most commonly, bronchogenic carcinoma). In young adults, primary mediastinal pathology is more frequent. The common origin of tumors by location is shown in Table 69–6.

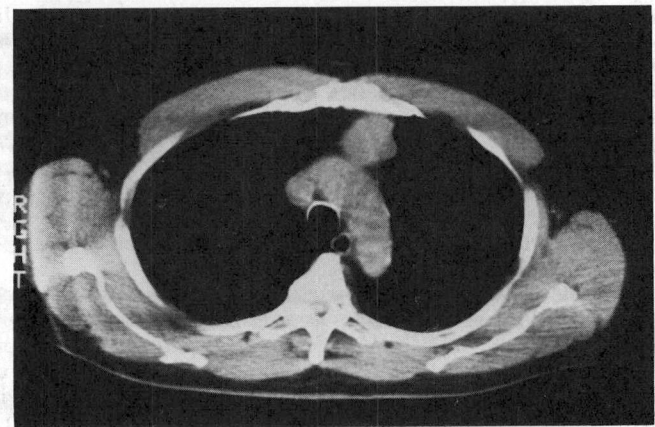

FIGURE 69–4. CT of same patient as in Figures 69–2 and 69–3. The mass proved to be a thymoma. (Courtesy of Elon Gale, M.D., Department of Radiology, Boston Veterans Administration Medical Center.)

TABLE 69–6. MOST FREQUENT CAUSES OF MASSES IN THE MEDIASTINUM

Anterior	Middle	Posterior
Thymoma	Lymphoma	Neurogenic tumors
Lymphoma	Cancer	Enteric cysts
Teratogenic tumors	Cysts	Esophageal lesions
Thyroid	Aneurysms	Aneurysms
Parathyroid	Hernia (foramen of	Diaphragmatic hernias
Aneurysms	Morgagni)	(foramen of Bochdalek)

Neurogenic Tumors. These are the most common primary mediastinal tumors (20 per cent). They are located in the posterior mediastinum. Nonspecific chest pain and nonproductive cough with occasional compression of intercostal nerves and trachea and bronchi are the most frequent symptoms. Most tumors are benign, originating in the nerve sheath (neurilemoma, neurofibroma) or sympathetic ganglion cells (ganglioneuroma). Neuroblastomas (malignant tumors of sympathetic ganglion cell) have a better prognosis than the same tumors occurring as primary malignancies in the adrenals. Neurofibromas may occur in association with von Recklinghausen's disease. Ganglioneuromas and neuroblastomas may secrete hormones that cause flushing, diarrhea, and hypertension. Pheochromocytomas may occasionally arise in the mediastinum. Neurogenic tumors should be resected and postoperative radiation therapy given to neuroblastomas.

Lymphoreticular Tumors. Thymomas account for 20 per cent of mediastinal tumors and are located in the superior portion of the anterior mediastinum. Two thirds of them are malignant. Myasthenia gravis is seen in 40 per cent of cases, and other paraneoplastic syndromes, such as Cushing's syndrome, refractory anemia, and hypogammaglobulinemia, have been reported. All thymomas should be regarded as malignant, and surgical resection should be done, followed by radiation. Lymphatic tumors (17 per cent) also arise in the anterior mediastinum. Hodgkin's lymphoma is the most frequent and carries the best prognosis. Non-Hodgkin's lymphoma, plasmacytomas, and angiomatous lymphoid hamartomas with a similar clinical presentation carry a worse prognosis. Teratomatous tumors constitute 10 per cent of mediastinal tumors. One third of them are malignant at diagnosis. Also located in the anterior compartment, they are embryologically and histologically linked to the thymus. Cystic teratomas are more frequent and may contain squamous cells, hair follicles, sweat glands, cartilage, and linear calcifications. *Intrathoracic goiter* (10 per cent) is usually a benign nodular or follicular enlargement of the thyroid gland. Three quarters of patients present with stridor, cough, and dyspnea. Most frequently located in the anterior mediastinum, it occasionally causes the superior vena cava (SVC) syndrome. Benign cysts are usually asymptomatic and occur as an incidental roentgenographic finding. Bronchogenic cysts develop around the paratracheal area or carina and are seen in the middle and posterior compartments. They are filled with liquid and are lined with respiratory epithelium and cartilage but do not communicate with the tracheobronchial tree. Pericardial cysts occur in the anterior compartment and cardiophrenic angle. They contain clear liquid and are lined by flattened endothelial or mesothelial lining with a bland, fibrous wall. Enteric cysts are located in the posterior mediastinum and are lined by gastric or intestinal epithelium. All developmental cysts are potentially hazardous in that they may become infected, bleed, or rupture into the mediastinum or pleural cavity.

Vascular Tumors. These tumors may have a primary origin in the mediastinum. Vascular hamartoma, lymphangioma, and hemangioma are benign tumors, whereas hemangiopericytoma is malignant. Mesenchymal benign (lipoma) or malignant (liposarcoma, mesothelioma, rhabdomyosarcoma, and mesenchymoma) tumors are rare causes of mediastinal masses.

HERNIAS. Hernias through the diaphragm may also manifest as mediastinal masses. They may be retrosternal through the foramen of Morgagni, posterolateral through the foramen of Bochdalek, or, most commonly, through the esophageal hiatus. When gas is contained in the herniated organ, the presumptive diagnosis is easily made.

PNEUMOMEDIASTINUM. This condition may occur secondary to a tear in the esophagus or tracheobronchial tree or from the dissection of air from ruptured alveoli. Tears in the esophagus and tracheobronchial tree commonly have a traumatic origin, whereas an alveolar rupture may occur spontaneously or as a complication of artificial ventilation. Air may track to the neck and rest of the body, producing subcutaneous emphysema, or into the pleural space and cause pneumothorax. Patients complain of retrosternal pain and dyspnea. There may be subcutaneous emphysema with the classic crepitus. Auscultation may reveal a crunching sound synchronous with the heartbeat (Hamman's sign). Rarely, cardiac function is compromised. A lateral chest roentgenogram is usually diagnostic. Simple, spontaneous pneumomediastinum usually resolves without treatment. When it is severe or results from organ rupture, surgical drainage and repair are required.

SUPERIOR VENA CAVA (SVC) SYNDROME. The SVC syndrome results from the obstruction of blood flow through the superior vena cava. Besides dilatation of the collateral veins of the upper thorax and neck and edema and congestion of the face, patients may have headache, dyspnea, dysphagia, and wheezes. Malignancy is the most frequent cause of SVC syndrome, with bronchogenic carcinoma responsible for more than 70 per cent of cases and lymphoma a distant second. Fibrosing mediastinitis can also occur after granulomatous diseases such as histoplasmosis or in association with the ingestion of methysergide. Aortic aneurysm and retrosternal thyroid are relatively benign causes of SVC syndrome. Because of vessel dilatation, invasive procedures are contraindicated. An effort must be made to obtain tissue elsewhere, and irradiation or chemotherapy must be begun before attempts are made to obtain mediastinal tissue.

Benjamin SP, McCormack LJ, Effler DB, et al.: Primary tumors of the mediastinum. Chest 67:297, 1972. *Excellent experience with 215 patients with mediastinal tumors managed by two surgeons. It establishes the prevalence and localization of primary mediastinal masses.*

Putgatch RD, Faling LJ, Robbins AH, et al.: CT diagnosis of benign mediastinal abnormalities. A J R 135:685, 1980. *Examines the evidence that supports the concept that CT scan of the thorax should be the initial procedure used to evaluate mediastinal masses.*

Weisbrod GL: Percutaneous fine needle aspiration biopsy of the mediastinum. Clin Chest Med 8:27, 1987. *It reviews the experience with fluoroscopy and CT-guided needle aspiration. It reiterates that experience and good cytopathologic interpretation are important to the success of the procedure.*

70 Respiratory Failure

John F. Murray

Adequate respiration consists of the uptake of sufficient amounts of O_2 and the elimination of sufficient amounts of CO_2 to maintain Po_2 and Fco_2 in arterial blood at their respective normal values. It follows that *respiratory failure* is associated with disturbances in the exchange of O_2 and CO_2 between gas in alveoli and blood in pulmonary capillaries and that these abnormalities must be reflected by changes in the Po_2 and Pco_2 in arterial blood. Thus respiratory failure is defined as a condition in which arterial Po_2 is below the normal range (excluding hypoxemia from intracardiac right-to-left shunting of blood) or arterial Pco_2 is above the normal range (excluding respiratory compensation for metabolic alkalosis). This definition, which is physiologically precise as well as clinically applicable, implies that the diagnosis of respiratory failure depends chiefly on laboratory analysis of arterial blood and not on clinical findings.

Respiratory failure is not a disease but a disorder of function that can be caused by a variety of conditions that affect the lungs; in some instances, the lungs are completely normal (e.g., overdose of sedative drugs). Respiratory failure is analogous to heart failure and renal failure, both of which represent the consequences of impaired normal function resulting from numerous disparate diseases.

Respiratory failure is traditionally divided into acute and chronic varieties, depending on the time it takes for the abnor-

malities in gas exchange to occur. This arbitrary classification does not take into account the common clinical occurrence of an acute worsening of arterial Po_2 and Pco_2 in a patient who already has chronic respiratory failure as a result of some underlying disorder. However, the distinction between acute and chronic respiratory failure has important etiologic and therapeutic implications and will be referred to subsequently.

PATHOPHYSIOLOGY OF RESPIRATORY FAILURE

In human beings, respiration has been subdivided into four functional processes: *ventilation, diffusion, perfusion,* and *control of breathing.* Each of these contributes uniquely to the maintenance of normal values of Po_2 and Pco_2 in arterial blood. Therefore, abnormalities in any one of the four processes, if sufficiently severe, will cause respiratory failure; furthermore, in many common respiratory disorders, multiple abnormalities coexist.

Normal Gas Exchange

The physiology of normal gas exchange is described in Ch. 56 and will not be reviewed here. However, understanding what is meant by normal is important, because arterial Po_2 varies with age, and both arterial Po_2 and Pco_2 vary according to the altitude (i.e., the prevailing barometric pressure) at which the person happens to be when the blood specimen is obtained and to the extent of acclimatization. The normal range includes the biologic variabilities among individuals and the analytic variations inherent in the measurements. Because the diagnosis of respiratory failure should be made in the laboratory and not at the bedside, the physician's ability to establish the diagnosis depends on the accuracy of the laboratory tests used to measure Po_2 and Pco_2. Normal mean arterial Po_2 (Pa_{O_2}) values in subjects 20 years of age or older can be calculated from the regression equation $Pa_{O_2} = 100.1 - 0.323$ (age in years). The normal range of variation is ± 5 mm Hg from the mean value. Arterial Pco_2 does not vary with age and is normally within the range of 40 ± 5 mm Hg in healthy persons at sea level. Values of Po_2 *below* or Pco_2 *above* normal limits indicate the presence of respiratory failure.

Abnormal Gas Exchange

The pathophysiology of abnormal gas exchange is also discussed in Ch. 56 and 71. Hypoventilation, impaired diffusion, ventilation-perfusion mismatching, right-to-left shunting of blood, and breathing air with a low Po_2 all cause arterial hypoxia (a decrease below normal of Po_2); in contrast, for practical purposes, only hypoventilation causes arterial hypercapnia (an increase above normal of Pco_2). In view of the therapeutic importance of recognizing the abnormal mechanism (or mechanisms) leading to a patient's respiratory failure, each will be reviewed briefly.

HYPOVENTILATION. Alveolar hypoventilation is present when the arterial Pco_2 is increased. Furthermore, as arterial Pco_2 increases, Po_2 decreases *except* when the patient is breathing gas with an enriched concentration of O_2. Because arterial Po_2 and Pco_2 change in opposite directions by nearly the same amount during hypoventilation, the contribution of hypoventilation to the patient's arterial hypoxia can be readily assessed. (In a 60-year-old person, for example, if $Po_2 = 50$ mm Hg and $Pco_2 = 70$ mm Hg, both have changed from their normal values by the same amount [30 mm Hg] and "pure" hypoventilation is present; in contrast, if $Po_2 = 30$ mm Hg and $Pco_2 = 70$ mm Hg, the change from normal of Pco_2 does not account for the entire change in Po_2; therefore, some other cause in addition to hypoxia from hypoventilation must be present.) Arterial hypoxia from alveolar hypoventilation is not associated with an increased alveolar-arterial Po_2 difference and is "corrected" by breathing 100 per cent O_2.

IMPAIRED DIFFUSION. Abnormalities of diffusion do not cause arterial hypoxia in persons at rest unless they are extremely severe. Although these occur in occasional patients with respiratory failure, for practical purposes the possible contributions of an abnormality of diffusion to a given patient's arterial hypoxia can be ignored except during exercise or at high altitude. This practice is permissible because diffusion disturbances, even when marked, cause only relatively small increases in the patient's alveolar-arterial Po_2 difference, and this abnormality, if it exists, is readily corrected by adding small amounts of O_2 to the inspired air.

VENTILATION-PERFUSION IMBALANCE. When gas exchange units receive more blood flow than ventilation, arterial hypoxia results. Mismatching of ventilation and perfusion is by far the most common cause of arterial hypoxia and can be recognized by giving the patient 100 per cent O_2 to breathe; this causes the alveolar-arterial Po_2 difference from pure mismatching that is present while the patient breathes room air to decrease and arterial Po_2 to increase to normal values (>550 mm Hg). It is important, when performing this test, to use 100 per cent O_2 and to allow enough time for N_2 to be eliminated from the lungs; otherwise, the results are unreliable. Although a "pure" ventilation-perfusion inequality can lead to CO_2 retention, this is an uncommon cause of hypercapnia because as arterial Pco_2 tends to increase, it stimulates peripheral and central chemoreceptors and increases ventilation; this, in turn, reduces Pco_2 back to normal values but, owing to the shape of the oxyhemoglobin dissociation curve, does not correct the hypoxia.

RIGHT-TO-LEFT SHUNTS. Shunts of blood from right to left may occur through abnormal anatomic communications in the lung (e.g., pulmonary arteriovenous fistula) but much more frequently by perfusion of lung units that are completely unventilated because they are either collapsed (atelectasis) or filled with fluid (pulmonary edema, pneumonia, intra-alveolar hemorrhage). Regardless of the cause, an alveolar-arterial Po_2 difference results that increases when the patient breathes 100 per cent O_2 compared with when the patient breathes room air. For reasons similar to those occurring in patients with ventilation-perfusion imbalances, CO_2 retention seldom occurs in patients with right-to-left shunts.

DECREASED INSPIRED Po_2. Expected values of arterial Po_2 are corrected for the influence of decreasing barometric pressure; strictly speaking, therefore, the effects of high altitude on inspired Po_2 and the resulting decreased arterial Po_2 are not an abnormal cause of hypoxia, even though the hypoxia may be severe and dangerous. Occasionally, pathologic hypoxia occurs when ambient Po_2 is reduced because of combustion of O_2 or because of dilution by some other gas, both of which may occur in fires. However, this phenomenon is not of importance when interpreting the results of analysis of arterial blood specimens obtained in the hospital or clinic.

HYPERCAPNIA. In contrast to arterial hypoxia, which may result from five different pathophysiologic derangements, arterial hypercapnia can always be interpreted as signifying alveolar hypoventilation. This is true because arterial Pco_2 (Pa_{CO_2}) is governed by the relationship between CO_2 production (Vco_2) and alveolar ventilation (Va): $Pa_{CO_2} = kVco_2/Va$. Normally, however, even when CO_2 production increases markedly, alveolar ventilation increases proportionately and arterial Pco_2 is maintained within fairly narrow limits. Thus an increase in arterial Pco_2 can always be viewed as respiratory failure in the sense that alveolar ventilation is inadequate to eliminate all the CO_2 being produced at that time. Severe ventilation-perfusion imbalances and right-to-left shunts can produce hypercapnia, but this is uncommon because, as already emphasized, alveolar ventilation usually increases and restores CO_2 to normal values.

An increase or decrease in Pco_2 in the blood has a direct effect on the amount of carbonic acid in the blood and a reciprocal effect on pH. Acute changes in Pco_2 have a more profound effect on pH than chronic changes owing to differences in plasma bicarbonate concentrations. With acute increases or decreases in Pco_2, there is little change in bicarbonate level and a considerable change in pH; after 3 to 5 days of a sustained change in Pco_2, renal compensation has increased plasma bicarbonate in hypercapnia and decreased it in hypocapnia, both tending to restore pH toward normal. Many patients with respiratory failure have mixed respiratory and nonrespiratory acid-base disturbances, which are difficult to define without knowledge of their time course and the level of plasma bicarbonate.

Right-Sided Heart Failure

Acute respiratory failure can cause acute right-sided heart failure (acute cor pulmonale). The normal right ventricle is not a good pressure generator and cannot sustain sudden pressure loads over 40 to 50 mm Hg. Thus acute right-sided heart failure

may develop in any condition in which pulmonary vascular resistance increases abruptly; this happens most commonly in patients with massive pulmonary emboli with obstruction of much of the pulmonary vascular bed (usually >60 per cent). At times, acute cor pulmonale complicates the course of patients with severe bronchial asthma or other forms of marked airways obstruction.

Acute right-sided heart failure may also occur in patients with chronic lung disease during an episode of acute respiratory failure. Most of these patients have right ventricular hypertrophy (chronic cor pulmonale) to begin with, and a subclinical or stable condition is aggravated by the added effects of the superimposed acute lung disease (usually bronchitis or pneumonia). In these patients, right ventricular function is worsened for several reasons: (1) Alveolar hypoxia and acidemia cause pulmonary arterial vasoconstriction; (2) certain lung diseases reduce the cross-sectional area available for perfusion; (3) hyperinflation of the lung increases pulmonary vascular resistance; and (4) arterial hypoxia may depress myocardial contractility. These factors are important to recognize because they are reversible and usually respond well to appropriate treatment of the intercurrent acute disorder.

CAUSES OF RESPIRATORY FAILURE

Because respiratory failure is defined as the presence of arterial hypoxia with or without hypercapnia, two physiologically different types are recognized: failure of ventilation, which is characterized by abnormalities of both O_2 and CO_2, and failure of oxygenation, in which only O_2 is abnormal. For convenience, the multiple causes of respiratory failure can be classified according to which component of the respiratory system is involved, and whether they are either acute or chronic in onset.

Diseases Causing Airways Obstruction

ACUTE. Obstruction may result from acute diseases that involve any portion of the upper and lower airways. The presence of respiratory failure depends on the magnitude and extent of the narrowing. Obstruction of the *extra*thoracic airway (nasopharynx, larynx, extrathoracic portion of the trachea) usually causes stridor, a characteristic alteration of breathing that is associated with harsh, high-pitched respiratory noises that are louder and more pronounced during inspiration than expiration. In contrast, obstruction of the *intra*thoracic airways causes wheezing, an abnormality of breathing in which expiration is louder and longer than inspiration.

Obstruction of the upper airways can result from (1) inflammation-induced swelling of the mucosa secondary to infections, allergic reactions, and, less commonly, thermal or mechanical injuries and (2) impaction of foreign bodies or, occasionally, tumors. Acute obstruction of the upper airways is particularly likely to develop in infants and young children, who have smaller and hence more vulnerable upper passages than do older children and adults.

Acute obstruction of the lower airways is usually caused by swelling of the mucosa, secretions in the lumen, or bronchospasm. Accordingly, bronchial asthma, infections, bronchiolitis, and the inhalation of chemicals (such as nitrogen dioxide in silo-filler's disease) are important causes of acute respiratory failure.

CHRONIC. Diffuse obstruction may result from disorders originating in bronchi (bronchiectasis), bronchioles (bronchiolitis), or the lung parenchyma (emphysema). These abnormalities characteristically progress gradually and lead to chronic respiratory failure. Of considerable importance are the intercurrent episodes of acute disease, usually pneumonia or bronchitis, that complicate the underlying disorder and often worsen the severity of existing respiratory failure.

Diseases Causing Parenchymal Infiltration

ACUTE. The most common cause of acute infiltration of the parenchyma is pneumonia, which usually has an infectious origin but occasionally is caused by inhalation or aspiration of a toxic chemical. Whether acute respiratory failure develops depends on the extent and severity of the disease. Immunologic reactions from drugs, migrating parasites, or leukoagglutinins are uncommon causes of acute respiratory failure but are important because of their special therapeutic requirements.

CHRONIC. More than 100 different conditions can cause chronic diffuse parenchymal infiltration. When severe, any of these can cause chronic respiratory failure. As in patients with chronic airways obstruction, patients with chronic infiltrative diseases may have intercurrent episodes of bronchopulmonary infection that cause acute worsening of their underlying respiratory status.

Diseases Causing Pulmonary Edema

CARDIOGENIC. Pulmonary edema in patients with heart disease may be acute or chronic in onset; both varieties are caused by an increase in the hydrostatic pressure within pulmonary capillaries. Pulmonary edema may follow an acute myocardial infarction or acute left ventricular failure of any cause (hypertensive crises, arrhythmias), or it may be precipitated in patients with valvular or other forms of chronic heart disease by sudden changes in their cardiorespiratory status (from arrhythmias, hypoxemia, or increased systemic blood pressure). Chronic pulmonary edema is found in patients with chronic, usually refractory, heart failure, but even in these patients the amount of edema increases and decreases according to changing hemodynamics and therapy.

INCREASED PERMEABILITY. Acute pulmonary edema can accompany certain conditions that do not involve the heart. The basic pathophysiologic abnormality in most of these disorders appears to be an increased permeability of the pulmonary capillary endothelium and overlying alveolar epithelium. Generalized pulmonary edema with accompanying severe hypoxemia from right-to-left shunting of blood, diffuse infiltrations on chest radiographs, and decreased pulmonary compliance constitute what is known as the *adult respiratory distress syndrome (ARDS)*. This syndrome (not disease) includes the composite manifestations of diffuse injury to the lung parenchyma, which may occur in association with certain usually identifiable clinical disorders (Table 70–1); of these, the sepsis syndrome (infection with systemic complications, such as hypotension and/or metabolic acidosis) is by far the most common. Histologic examination early in the evolution of ARDS reveals prominent injury to the type I alveolar epithelial cells, less severe damage to the capillary endothelium, hyaline membranes, proteinaceous pulmonary edema, and intra-alveolar hemorrhage. Later, the injury may clear or may evolve into a proliferative pattern, with hyperplasia of type II epithelial cells, infiltration by connective tissue cells, and deposition of collagen. Unless the underlying cause of ARDS is rapidly reversible (heroin, air embolism, near-drowning), the clinical course is apt to be prolonged and complicated and is associated with a high mortality (60 to 70 per cent). However, death is much more likely to result from multiple organ failure (see Ch. 71) than from intractable respiratory failure.

TABLE 70–1. PARTIAL LIST OF CONDITIONS THAT HAVE BEEN ASSOCIATED WITH THE ADULT RESPIRATORY DISTRESS SYNDROME

Infections	Inhaled toxins
Sepsis syndrome	O$_2$ (high concentrations)
Pneumonia (any cause)	Smoke
Trauma	Corrosive chemicals (NO$_2$, Cl$_2$,
Fat emboli	NH$_3$, phosgene, cadmium)
Lung contusion	Hematologic disorders
Nonthoracic trauma (including	Intravascular coagulation
head injury)	Massive blood transfusion
Liquid aspiration	Metabolic disorders
Gastric juice	Pancreatitis
Fresh and salt water (drowning)	Uremia
Hydrocarbon fluids	Paraquat ingestion
Drug overdose	Miscellaneous
Heroin and other opiates	Increased intracranial pressure
Salicylates	(including seizures)
Propoxyphene	Eclampsia
Barbiturates	Post cardioversion
	Radiation pneumonitis
	Post cardiopulmonary bypass

Pulmonary Vascular Diseases

ACUTE. Pulmonary embolism is usually accompanied by a decreased arterial Po$_2$ and Pco$_2$, the former from ventilation-perfusion mismatching and the latter reflecting the hyperventilation that nearly always occurs. Pulmonary embolism is also an important cause of worsening respiratory failure in patients with underlying chronic lung disease. Fat emboli and emboli from platelet-fibrin aggregates during disseminated intravascular coagulation are recognized causes of ARDS.

CHRONIC. Pulmonary vasculitis and recurrent thromboembolism are not common conditions and, when present, usually do not cause respiratory failure until the late stages of the disease. Recurrent thromboembolism occurs in intravenous drug abusers and in patients with chronic peripheral venous thrombi, sickle cell anemia, and schistosomiasis. Pulmonary vasculitis occurs in patients with scleroderma, other collagen diseases, and primary pulmonary hypertension.

Diseases of the Chest Wall and Pleura

ACUTE. The most important cause of sudden respiratory failure from acute disorders involving the thoracic cage is injury to the chest wall. Segmental fractures of several ribs or fractures of ribs on both sides of the sternum can result in a flail chest. Besides the impairment of ventilatory function that results from the unstable chest wall, gas exchange abnormalities are often compounded by contusion of the lung underneath the site of injury. Spontaneous or traumatic pneumothorax is an important cause of acute respiratory failure, which may be severe and which often afflicts otherwise healthy persons.

CHRONIC. Severe idiopathic or acquired kyphoscoliosis can cause chronic respiratory failure, which is often associated with cor pulmonale. Patients with massive pleural effusion (or effusions) or with thickened, constrictive pleural layer (or layers) may also have chronic respiratory failure.

Disorders of the Neuromuscular System

Disorders of the neuromuscular system are classified according to which part of the effector system is involved, i.e., the brain, neuronal pathways, or muscles of respiration, rather than into acute and chronic varieties. Patients with these disorders often have perfectly normal lungs; respiratory failure occurs from inability to ventilate normally.

BRAIN DISORDERS. Probably the most common cause of respiratory failure from impaired function of the central nervous system is the use of sedative drugs or anesthetic agents. Suppression of ventilatory drive from opiates, barbiturates, psychic depressants, alcohol, and a variety of sedative drugs results in hypoxia and hypercapnia that may be life threatening. Ventilatory stimuli can also be depressed by many diseases of the central nervous system, including vascular diseases, tumors, and infections.

SPINAL CORD AND PERIPHERAL NERVE DISORDERS. Injuries to the cervical or high thoracic spinal cord may produce immediate respiratory failure from paralysis of the muscles of respiration. Loss of anterior horn cell function in patients with poliomyelitis was an important cause of acute and chronic respiratory failure but is seldom encountered now because of the widespread use of vaccination. Polyneuritis, whether postinfectious (Guillain-Barré syndrome) or toxic, is an uncommon but important cause of respiratory failure in view of its inherent reversibility.

MUSCULAR DISORDERS. The final effectors in the system that controls breathing are the skeletal muscles of respiration. When these muscles are involved by generalized myopathies, such as muscular dystrophy or myasthenia gravis, respiratory failure results. Respiratory failure in patients with myasthenia gravis occurs during myasthenic or cholinergic crises. In contrast, respiratory failure in patients with muscular dystrophy is nearly always chronic and related to an advanced stage in the progression of the disease.

SLEEP APNEA. Brief periods of apnea occur in normal persons during deep sleep. Much more prolonged episodes associated with severe hypoxia have been documented in patients with massive obesity, chronic mountain sickness, enlarged tonsils, and many other disorders. Apnea results from either failure of ventilatory drive or obstruction of the upper airway. Severe sleep apnea can cause chronic respiratory failure, cor pulmonale, psychosis, and pathologic daytime sleepiness, a condition occasionally called the pickwickian syndrome, with somewhat dubious literary authenticity. Sleep apnea is discussed at greater length in Ch. 447.

CLINICAL MANIFESTATIONS

Given the great variety of disorders that can cause respiratory failure, it is obvious that the clinical manifestations in a given patient depend in large part on which underlying disease he or she has; these are dealt with elsewhere in this text. When respiratory failure ensues and if the blood gas disturbances are sufficiently severe, the signs and symptoms of hypoxia, and possibly hypercapnia, become superimposed upon the signs and symptoms of the underlying disease. The clinical manifestations of hypoxia and hypercapnia are nonspecific and usually occur late in the evolution of the clinical problem. This statement underscores the earlier axiom that the diagnosis of respiratory failure is made in the laboratory by blood gas analysis and not at the bedside by clinical examination.

Hypoxia

The signs and symptoms of acute hypoxia are chiefly caused by abnormalities in central nervous system and cardiovascular function. Characteristic features are impaired judgment and motor instability, a clinical picture closely resembling that of acute alcoholism. As hypoxia worsens, the brain stem is affected, and death results from depression of the medullary respiratory centers. The initial cardiovascular effects of acute hypoxia are tachycardia and increased blood pressure; when hypoxia is very severe, bradycardia, myocardial depression, and shock ensue. Recognizable cyanosis of the lips, mucous membranes, and nail beds usually occurs when the concentration of reduced hemoglobin in the capillaries is greater than 5 grams per deciliter. Accordingly, cyanosis can result from decreases in either arterial Po_2 or blood flow. In patients with lung disease, cyanosis cannot be detected by most physicians until arterial Po_2 is less than 50 mm Hg; some observers cannot recognize cyanosis unless arterial Po_2 is less than 40 mm Hg!

In patients with chronic hypoxia, the central nervous system manifestations are drowsiness, inattentiveness, apathy, fatigue, and delayed reaction time. The chronic cardiovascular effects are often minimal, but pulmonary hypertension or even cor pulmonale with signs of right-sided heart failure may be detected on clinical examination. One of the hallmarks of chronic hypoxia is erythrocytosis, which may cause noticeable plethora and changes in the hemoglobin concentration, hematocrit ratio, or red blood cell count.

Hypercapnia

The physiologic consequences of hypercapnia depend not only on the amount of excess CO_2 in the body but also on the rate at which retention develops. Increases in Pco_2 from acute respiratory failure lead to a constellation of progressive disturbances of central nervous system function: apprehension, confusion, drowsiness, coma, and death. The vascular responses represent a mixture of vasoconstriction, from generalized sympathetic activity, and vasodilation, from local accumulation of CO_2; thus the cardiovascular abnormalities are variable and depend on whether vasoconstrictor or vasodilator influences predominate. Tachycardia and sweating are usually present, but blood pressure may be high, low, or normal.

In contrast, if Pco_2 increases slowly, compensation takes place and the clinical consequences may be minimal at values of arterial Pco_2 that would cause death if reached suddenly. There are numerous patients with arterial Pco_2 values over 100 mm Hg who are ambulatory and at times living active lives, although most breathe supplementary O_2 to prevent life-threatening hypoxia. Patients with hypercapnia from chronic respiratory failure frequently complain of headaches and drowsiness; these symptoms are probably attributable to the potent cerebral vasodilating effect of excess CO_2. In addition, patients with chronic hypercapnia may have papilledema, muscular twitching, coarse myoclonic jerky motions, and asterixis. At times, the neurologic findings simulate those of a brain tumor.

TREATMENT OF ACUTE RESPIRATORY FAILURE

The time course of worsening abnormalities varies in patients with acute respiratory failure from almost instantaneous (flail chest, pulmonary embolism) to a gradual crescendo during a period of several hours or even days (respiratory tract infections, bronchial asthma). The demands for treatment and the speed with which it must be provided obviously differ from one patient to another. It is difficult to generalize about such an extremely variable clinical condition, but the principles of treatment of acute respiratory failure are as follows: *first*, establish an airway, administer O_2, and maintain adequate alveolar ventilation; *second*, identify and treat the underlying condition and monitor the patient's progress carefully.

Establish an Airway

The upper airway tends to be occluded in unconscious patients because of relaxation of the oropharyngeal muscles and tongue and the presence of saliva, vomitus, and other secretions. When respiratory arrest occurs away from medical facilities, all material should be cleared from the oropharynx, and the victim should be placed on his or her back with the head tilted backward as far as possible and the jaw extended forward. Sometimes these simple maneuvers are all that is required to enable breathing to resume spontaneously. Further details about the treatment of cardiorespiratory arrest are provided in Ch. 71.

An airway can be established by three different methods: an oropharyngeal tube, an endotracheal tube passed via the nose or mouth, and a tracheostomy. Selection of the procedure depends on available facilities and personnel and on the site and severity of the obstruction.

OROPHARYNGEAL AIRWAY. An oropharyngeal airway is valuable in unconscious patients who are breathing spontaneously (e.g., during recovery from general anesthesia, after a cerebrovascular accident). An oropharyngeal airway is also useful in patients who are apneic during emergency resuscitation but who are receiving some form of assisted ventilation (mouth-to-mouth respiration, bag-mask system). Although an oropharyngeal tube is commonly used in these clinical circumstances, its role must be viewed as temporary, either while the patient is waking up or until an endotracheal tube can be inserted.

ENDOTRACHEAL TUBE. The preferred method of establishing an airway in most emergencies is with an endotracheal tube. Once inserted, the tube is used to remove secretions and to provide ventilation. Endotracheal tubes can usually be passed quickly through the nose or, at times, through the mouth into the trachea by an experienced person; the airway is then sealed by inflating a balloon near the tip of the tube. Endotracheal tubes should be used in nearly all patients with acute respiratory failure severe enough to require control of their airways.

TRACHEOSTOMY. Emergency tracheostomy was formerly the only way of quickly establishing an airway in patients with acute respiratory failure. Now, emergency tracheostomy is contraindicated except in one clinical situation: acute obstruction of upper airways (e.g., from foreign bodies, trauma, or inflammation). Otherwise, intubation with an endotracheal tube is the treatment of choice for control of the airway. Tracheostomy, if needed, can be performed electively at a later time in the operating room under ideal conditions. There is virtually no mortality and very little morbidity with an elective tracheostomy, in contrast to the high incidence of complications associated with emergency tracheostomy performed at the bedside.

The decision to convert a satisfactory endotracheal intubation to a tracheostomy is not an easy one and must be individualized in each case. The availability of tubes of inert plastic with low-pressure cuffs permits endotracheal tubes to be used for weeks rather than days without prohibitive injury; the main mechanical difference between endotracheal and tracheostomy tubes is the trauma to the vocal cords from the former and problems related to the stoma in the latter. The usual reasons for performing a tracheostomy in a patient with a satisfactory endotracheal tube are (1) failure to control secretions (sometimes it is difficult to suction the lungs adequately, especially the left side, through a long endotracheal tube) and (2) the need for prolonged (i.e., several weeks) intubation for assisted ventilation and/or removal of secretions (these circumstances are uncommon but occur particularly in patients with neuromuscular disease and chest wall injuries).

The presence of a tube and its cuff in the airways can cause necrosis of the mucosa of the trachea; at times the entire airway wall may be eroded with penetration of the esophagus (tracheoesophageal fistula) or a neighboring blood vessel (innominate artery), causing severe hemorrhage. Delayed complications after extubation are caused by damage to the trachea or larynx from the tube or cuff; injury to the vocal cords merely impairs phonation, but serious and life-threatening obstruction to airflow can result from stenosis or malacia of the tracheal wall. These complications should be considered and evaluated in any patient who complains of persisting hoarseness or who develops breathlessness or stridor at any time after endotracheal intubation.

HUMIDIFICATION. Insertion of an endotracheal or tracheostomy tube bypasses the normal source of humidification of the inspired air. When this occurs and unhumidified air or gas mixture is breathed, the result is drying of the mucosa and impairment of mucociliary clearance. Thus as long as the upper airway is bypassed, patients must receive air or a mixture of O_2 that is fully saturated with water vapor at their body temperature. This is easily accomplished if the patient is being ventilated, because most commercial ventilators have heated humidifiers in the circuit. If the patient is breathing spontaneously, humidified gas can be delivered through a T-piece connected to the endotracheal or tracheostomy tube. When proper humidification is carried out, remember that there is *no* insensible water loss through the respiratory tract when evaluating the patient's daily fluid balance.

Administer Oxygen

Acute respiratory failure, by definition, includes decreased arterial Po_2. When respiratory failure is severe, death results from the central nervous system or cardiovascular consequences of hypoxia. During emergencies, supplementary O_2 is given without worrying about the concentration being used; in general, the higher the concentration of O_2, the better. After the patient's emergency condition has stabilized, attention is directed to administering O_2 in the lowest possible concentration required to correct the hypoxia. Any more O_2 than required to raise arterial Po_2 to a safe level exposes the patient to the direct toxicity of O_2 on the lung parenchyma and other undesirable effects: suppression of alveolar macrophage function and mucociliary clearance. In patients with chronic obstructive pulmonary disease, especially those with chronic hypercapnia, the administration of O_2 is likely to worsen the CO_2 retention. The further increase in Pco_2 can be explained in part by suppression of preexisting hypoxic ventilatory drive; the remaining increase can be accounted for through the effects of O_2 on the breathing pattern and matching of ventilation-perfusion. In general, the higher the inspired O_2 concentration, the greater the CO_2 retention; this observation underlies the use of "low-flow" O_2 for these patients, as described below under Treatment of Chronic Respiratory Failure.

The usual goal of O_2 therapy in acute respiratory failure is to raise arterial Po_2 to between 60 and 80 mm Hg. Because these values lie on the flat portion of the oxyhemoglobin dissociation curve, most of the available hemoglobin is saturated with O_2; raising arterial Po_2 values even higher adds very little additional O_2 to the blood and may require increases in alveolar Po_2 concentrations to toxic levels. At times, especially when the mechanism of arterial hypoxia is right-to-left shunting of blood, arterial Po_2 may be considerably less than 60 mm Hg even with the patient breathing 100 per cent O_2. When this occurs, other maneuvers, such as addition of end-expiratory pressure, are required to raise arterial Po_2 and to allow a reduction in inspired O_2 concentration.

There are several ways of giving supplementary O_2 to a patient. Which method is chosen depends on the cause and severity of the arterial hypoxia and convenience to the patient. It is important to emphasize that no method can be relied upon to produce a certain increase in arterial Po_2; the response depends on which physiologic mechanism (or mechanisms) is responsible for the

hypoxia. Thus it is always advisable to monitor the effects of O_2 administration by serial analyses of arterial blood.

NASAL CANNULAS OR PRONGS. Nasal cannulas, catheters, or prongs can be used to administer enriched concentrations of O_2. These devices work well even when patients breathe through their mouths. However, because of the drying effects of unhumidified O_2 on the nasal mucous membranes, if more than 5 to 6 liters per minute is needed to achieve satisfactory arterial oxygenation, other methods of administration, such as face masks, are advisable.

RESERVOIR MASKS. When high concentrations of O_2 (40 to 80 per cent) are needed in patients who are not intubated, reservoir masks are used. To ensure optimal efficiency of operation, the masks must be tight fitting to avoid leaks; because this often causes discomfort, it is difficult to deliver high concentrations of O_2 by reservoir masks for long periods.

OTHER METHODS. Virtually all mechanical ventilators have regulators that can be set to deliver an inspired O_2 concentration that ranges from 21 to 100 per cent. The most reliable way of ensuring that patients actually receive high concentrations of O_2 (60 to 100 per cent) when they need it is to use a mechanical ventilator connected to an endotracheal or tracheostomy tube.

Maintain Alveolar Ventilation

Emergency resuscitation after respiratory arrest requires ventilation by mouth-to-mouth respiration or a bag and mask device. As soon as possible thereafter, if the patient does not resume spontaneous breathing, intubation and ventilation by a mechanical ventilator are indicated. Similar considerations apply to patients with acute respiratory failure whose breathing is insufficient to maintain adequate gas exchange. The main indications for mechanical ventilation are ventilatory failure, shown by an elevated or rising Pco_2, or severe refractory hypoxia, shown by a low Po_2 that cannot be corrected without high concentrations of O_2 and often end-expiratory pressure. Special indications include the need to produce alkalosis, as in head injuries and certain drug overdoses; to stabilize the thorax, as in traumatic injuries that result in flail chest; or to aspirate secretions, as in bronchopulmonary infections and failure to cough.

MECHANICAL VENTILATION. The different types of ventilators and modes of ventilation are described in Ch. 71. In general, the settings that are chosen depend on whether or not the patient can initiate each breath and what the underlying disorder is. Patients who cannot synchronize their breathing with the machine frequently become agitated, and their gas exchange deteriorates further. This problem can often be solved by alternate settings of the ventilator; if not, the patient must be sedated or at times paralyzed.

END-EXPIRATORY PRESSURE. Mechanical ventilators ordinarily raise airway pressure during inspiration and allow it to fall to zero (atmospheric) pressure during expiration; this pattern of assisted ventilation is known as intermittent positive-pressure ventilation, or IPPV. At times, it is desirable to add positive pressure to the airway during expiration as well as inspiration to hold the lung at a higher end-expiratory lung volume (functional residual capacity) than it would reach at zero end-expiratory pressure; this pattern of assisted ventilation is known as continuous positive-pressure ventilation, or CPPV. Keeping the lung at a high end-expiratory lung volume prevents closure of alveoli and airways during expiration, redistributes pulmonary edema fluid out of alveoli, and often improves arterial Po_2 considerably. Positive end-expiratory pressure (or PEEP) is particularly useful in patients with the conditions that cause the adult respiratory distress syndrome (Table 70–1).

Although end-expiratory pressure usually results in an improvement in arterial Po_2 and O_2 content, it may also decrease cardiac output by impairing venous return. Accordingly, the actual delivery of O_2 to the tissues of the body may decrease. Thus it is important to monitor both the respiratory and the circulatory responses to end-expiratory pressure to determine the optimal amount of pressure and the need for additional therapeutic interventions. Another common and serious hazard of end-expiratory pressure is its tendency to cause spontaneous pneumothorax and pneumomediastinum.

Identify and Treat the Underlying Condition

Acute respiratory failure always has a precipitating cause. Consequently, the cause of the condition should be identified as soon as possible after emergency measures have been started and the patient's condition has stabilized. Usually, the diagnosis can be established easily by a thorough history and physical examination, analysis of the blood and urine, and chest roentgenogram. Helpful auxiliary tests include those that evaluate central nervous system or cardiac function, those that determine the presence of drugs or poisons in the body, and bacteriologic study of secretions and blood.

Treatment obviously depends on the underlying cause, and the reader is referred to the appropriate chapters of this book for information about therapy for specific pulmonary and other disorders that lead to acute respiratory failure. In all patients with acute respiratory failure, careful attention should be paid to fluid balance. Overhydration is a frequent and serious complication that can usually be avoided by careful attention to fluid replacement and, when needed, monitoring of pulmonary capillary (wedge) pressure.

Many patients cared for in intensive care units are nutritionally depleted at the time of admission or become so soon afterward. Because morbidity and mortality are closely linked to nutritional status, it is important that this be assessed and, when necessary, treated by appropriate enteral or parenteral supplementation.

Monitor the Patient's Progress

The need for monitoring varies from patient to patient according to the response to initial treatment. If the disorder is readily reversible (e.g., bronchial asthma), the patient may respond sufficiently to go home shortly after being seen and treated. Other less rapidly responding conditions causing acute respiratory failure often require hospital care, and seriously ill patients are best treated in special acute care facilities (intensive care units) when available. Intensive care units provide an institutional focus of trained personnel and special equipment for the care of critically ill patients.

All seriously ill patients should have frequent measurements of blood pressure, constant monitoring of heart rate, careful recording of fluid intake and output, and determination of weight daily. Arterial blood gas analysis should be performed as often as needed but usually at least once daily. Special studies include measurement of cardiac output and placement of a Swan-Ganz catheter in the pulmonary artery for determination of pulmonary arterial and wedge pressures and sampling of mixed venous blood; this information is very helpful in guiding fluid replacement and ventilator adjustments, including levels of end-expiratory pressure. In general, wedge pressure values should be maintained in the normal range (5 to 10 mm Hg) and not allowed to increase above 15 mm Hg, especially in patients with ARDS. Less reliance is being placed now, compared with previous years, on values of mixed venous Po_2 as a guide to O_2 delivery, especially in disorders such as sepsis and ARDS. Attention is currently directed at improving O_2 delivery by increasing cardiac output through pharmacologic means or by increasing O_2 content through transfusions of packed red blood cells.

TREATMENT OF CHRONIC RESPIRATORY FAILURE

Patients with chronic lung disease often have sufficient alterations in their daily arterial Po_2 and Pco_2 values that they are said to be in chronic respiratory failure. Therapeutic regimens for these patients, whose disease is relatively stable, are delivered mainly on an outpatient basis and are designed to meet two objectives: (1) preventing or minimizing the number and severity of the intercurrent complications that would otherwise occur and (2) treating maximally all reversible elements of the underlying disorder. Many of the specific remedies are used for both purposes, and the approaches to preventive and maintenance therapy for patients with the most common chronic lung diseases—asthma, bronchitis, and emphysema—are discussed in Ch. 57 and 58.

Despite emphasis on preventing intercurrent complications, these attacks continue to plague the lives of patients with chronic lung disease. Acute episodes of bronchopulmonary infection, pneumothorax, pulmonary embolism, surgical procedures, and misuse of sedatives all add their effects to those of the underlying lung disease and frequently produce serious disturbances of blood gases. These episodes are potentially life threatening, are usually associated with prolonged morbidity, and frequently require hospitalization. The principles of therapy are to maintain oxygen-

ation while treating all new, presumably reversible, elements of the disease in an effort to restore the patient to his or her former level of function.

Oxygen

Patients with chronic obstructive lung disease and superimposed episodes of acute respiratory failure nearly always have severe hypoxia from a combination of hypoventilation and ventilation-perfusion mismatching. Typical arterial blood values are a Po_2 of approximately 30 mm Hg, a Pco_2 of 70 mm Hg, and a pH of 7.30. Neither the hypercapnia nor the acidemia is life threatening, but the hypoxia is potentially fatal. Thus treatment is directed mainly at alleviating the disturbance in oxygenation; the changes in Pco_2 and pH will return to the baseline values for that patient as the acute condition improves. In view of the possibility that O_2 therapy may depress ventilation and cause the Pco_2 to increase further, O_2 is given initially in low concentrations (1 to 3 liters per minute). The goal is to raise Po_2 to satisfactory levels (50 to 60 mm Hg) without depressing ventilation to the extent that unacceptable increases in Pco_2 and decreases in pH (particularly) occur.

The O_2 is usually started at 2 liters per minute, and an arterial blood specimen is analyzed 15 to 30 minutes later to determine the patient's response. Depending on the Po_2 value, the flow of O_2 can be adjusted. If hypoventilation and acidemia result from too much O_2 (e.g., a Po_2 of 80 mm Hg, a Pco_2 of 80 mm Hg, and a pH of 7.25), the supplementary O_2 should not be discontinued, but the flow rate should be decreased. This is necessary because the Po_2 decreases much faster than the stimulus to breathe returns, and cardiac arrest or other serious complications of hypoxia may result.

Intubation-Assisted Ventilation

Low-flow O_2 given in the manner described provides satisfactory relief of hypoxia in most patients with respiratory failure from chronic lung disease. Although the goal of low-flow O_2 is an arterial Po_2 of 50 to 60 mm Hg, at times one has to be satisfied with 40 to 50 mm Hg. When oxygenation cannot be achieved without intolerable hypercapnia and acidemia, the decision whether to intubate and ventilate the patient must be made. Experience with intubation and mechanical ventilation in this group of patients has not been rewarding, particularly because of the prolonged need for assisted ventilation once intubation is performed and the poor prognosis for lengthy survival and return to useful life after recovery from the acute episode. There are no firm guidelines to intubation and assisted ventilation in patients with chronic obstructive pulmonary disease who develop superimposed acute respiratory failure, and it is helpful to have ascertained the wishes of the patient before the event occurs.

Bronchodilators

Most intercurrent episodes of acute respiratory failure in patients with chronic obstructive pulmonary disease are associated with increased airways resistance from the presence of secretions, edema of the mucosa, and bronchospasm. Because it is impossible to discriminate among these, bronchodilator drugs are always included in the treatment regimen to take advantage of the reversibility of whatever element of bronchospasm is present.

When patients seek medical attention for intercurrent attacks, they frequently have already tried—and failed to respond to—oral and aerosolized bronchodilators. In this circumstance, the mainstays of treatment are aerosolized beta$_2$-sympathomimetic drugs, administered at 1- or 2-hour intervals for the first 12 to 24 hours, and intravenous corticosteroids, either methylprednisolone, 60 mg, or hydrocortisone, 100 mg, given intravenously every 6 hours. Much higher doses of corticosteroids (e.g., methylprednisolone, 15 mg per kilogram of body weight per day in divided doses) have been proposed, but there is no evidence to suggest that these are more efficacious in this clinical setting than the lower doses recommended above. Intravenous theophylline, although less popular now than before, and aerosolized anticholinergic drugs are often used as supplementary therapy in patients who are sick enough to warrant hospitalization.

Antimicrobials

Infections are the most frequent and important cause of acute respiratory failure in patients with chronic underlying lung disease. Intercurrent attacks usually begin as a typical cold, with rhinitis, pharyngitis, and headaches. Shortly afterward, lower respiratory involvement appears with increasing cough, sputum production, purulence, wheezing, and breathlessness. These episodes occur several times a year in most patients with chronic obstructive pulmonary disease. (It should be noted that fever, leukocytosis, and new roentgenographic infiltrations are uncommon in this syndrome.) When airway infection is present, the sputum not only is purulent but usually contains numerous microorganisms detectable by Gram's stain of the secretions. Sputum cultures, however, often fail to reveal pathogenic bacteria, although at times *Streptococcus pneumoniae* and/or *Haemophilus influenzae*, may be grown. Regardless of the presence or absence of identifiable pathogens, oral treatment with ampicillin (250 to 500 mg every 6 hours), a combined preparation of trimethoprim-sulfamethoxazole (160 mg and 800 mg, respectively, every 12 hours), or tetracycline (250 to 500 mg every 6 hours) frequently results in decreased volume of sputum, thinning of the secretions, change in sputum appearance from purulent to mucoid, and improvement in blood gases. If parenteral therapy is indicated, second-generation cephalosporins are useful.

When pneumonia is present, signified by the presence of new infiltrations on the chest roentgenogram, Gram's stain of the sputum is likely to show one bacterial species predominating, and the initial selection of antimicrobials should cover this organism. Therapy can be revised, if necessary, when the results of the sputum cultures are available.

Control of Secretions

Many patients complain of thick, tenacious sputum that is troublesome to clear. Although it seems desirable to attempt to alter the character of these secretions to facilitate their removal, there is no clear evidence that it is possible to do so by pharmacologic means. Iodides, enzymes, detergents, and acetylcysteine, administered orally or by aerosol, have been tried extensively, but none has been shown convincingly to be effective. Moreover, each has potential toxic side effects. Similarly, mist tents and ultrasonic nebulizers, once widely used, are seldom employed today. The best way to control secretions is to treat infection with antimicrobials and to ensure adequate (but not excessive) hydration by the administration of intravenous fluids.

Patients with troublesome sputum retention may require intermittent nasotracheal suction to control the volume of secretions. Manual or mechanical percussion serves to loosen secretions and enhances their removal in patients who have retained sputum in their airways. Respiratory physical therapy, especially when carried out by a skilled therapist, may result in an increase in arterial P_{O_2} related to the improvement in the distribution of ventilation from clearance of sputum.

Treatment of Heart Failure

Cor pulmonale is an inevitable complication of severe chronic lung disease. Right ventricular hypertrophy followed by heart failure occurs secondary to the increased work load imposed on the ventricle by the changes in the pulmonary circulation from the effects of lung disease. Resistance to blood flow through the lungs increases when pulmonary blood vessels are destroyed (as in emphysema), obstructed (as in pulmonary thromboembolism), narrowed (from vasoconstriction), or compressed (breathing at high lung volumes), or when the blood is unusually viscous (polycythemia). Patients whose cor pulmonale is well compensated or even inapparent while their chronic lung disease is stable often develop acute right-sided heart failure during intercurrent attacks of acute respiratory failure. Peripheral edema, increased venous pressure, and an enlarged, painful liver are important clues to the presence of acute cardiac decompensation.

Most patients with right-sided heart failure from cor pulmonale, even if severe, have a satisfactory diuresis when they are put to bed, given O_2, and treated appropriately for their underlying lung disease. Diuretics may make patients feel more comfortable by diminishing peripheral edema and hepatic and gastrointestinal congestion faster than spontaneous diuresis; but if used, the drugs should be administered orally in low doses. Intravenous ethacrynic acid or furosemide can cause excessive renal loss of Cl^- that worsens existing acid-base disturbances and depletes intravascular volume sufficiently to decrease cardiac output and blood pressure. A particularly dangerous situation occurs in patients who already have coexisting nonrespiratory (metabolic) alkalosis, often from Cl^--losing diuretics, in addition to their hypercapnia from chronic respiratory failure; when the measures designed to improve ventilation lower arterial P_{CO_2}, the metabolic alkalosis becomes "unmasked," and arterial pH becomes markedly alkaline. When this occurs, the patients can develop cardiac arrhythmias, become comatose, or manifest convulsive seizures or other focal neurologic abnormalities.

If an element of pulmonary edema or pulmonary vascular congestion is present from left-sided heart failure, this may also respond to diuretics. Whether left-sided heart failure can occur secondary to purely right-sided disease is controversial. Of greater importance are coexisting causes of left-sided involvement (e.g., valvular disease, coronary atherosclerosis); furthermore, chronic hypoxia and severe polycythemia may impair left ventricular as well as right ventricular function.

Present evidence indicates that digitalis preparations are not beneficial in patients with cor pulmonale. Also, the use of digitalis is hazardous in patients with chronic respiratory failure owing to the sudden shifts in acid-base balance and electrolyte concentrations that may occur in these patients. Therefore, digitalis drugs should be used only in patients with digitalis-responsive arrhythmias or coexisting left-sided heart failure.

Respiratory Stimulants

With few exceptions, respiratory stimulants are obsolete. Nikethamide, picrotoxin, and ethamivan have been replaced by other less hazardous and more efficient methods of maintaining ventilation. Doxapram, a drug that works by stimulating carotid chemoreceptors rather than neurons in the brain, appears to be much safer than centrally acting stimulants. The chief use of doxapram is to minimize or prevent the depression of ventilation, with consequent increase in P_{CO_2} and decrease in pH, that occurs in some hypoxic patients with hypercapnia who are given O_2 to breathe. Almitrine, another drug that stimulates the carotid chemoreceptors but that can be administered orally, is widely used in Europe to improve arterial P_{O_2} in outpatients with chronic respiratory failure. This drug has not been approved by the Food and Drug Administration for use in the United States.

Sedation

All sedative drugs should be avoided in patients with chronic lung disease and intercurrent acute respiratory failure, including diazepam (Valium) and chlordiazepoxide (Librium), which can suppress ventilation. Exceptions to this cardinal rule are made from time to time, but usually only when the patient is being mechanically ventilated and sedation is required to enable breathing synchronous with the machine.

Postoperative Complications

Patients with chronic respiratory failure are high-risk operative candidates. Moreover, the closer the surgical incision to the thorax, the higher the incidence of postoperative complications. Despite this caveat, it is safe to say that virtually *all* patients who have respiratory failure can safely undergo *nonthoracic* surgery or *nonresectional* thoracic surgery. Postoperative complications can be anticipated and often prevented by attention to the general principles of care outlined in this chapter. Close observation and monitoring are usually required, and these can best be carried out in an intensive care unit.

Derene J-P, Fleury B, Pariente R: Acute respiratory failure of chronic obstructive pulmonary disease. Am Rev Respir Dis 138:1006, 1988. *Recent state-of-the-art review of this common and important complication.*

Johanson WG, Peters JI: Respiratory failure: Pathophysiology and treatment. *In* Murray JF, Nadel JA (eds.): Textbook of Respiratory Medicine. Philadelphia, W.B. Saunders Company, 1988, p 2017. *Detailed discussion of the physiologic abnormalities and therapy directed to improve them.*

Murray JF, Matthay MA, Luce JM, Flick MR. An expanded definition of the adult respiratory distress syndrome. Am Rev Respir Dis 138:720, 1988. *A synthesis of 20 years of studies of this elusive syndrome.*

Pingleton SK: Complications of acute respiratory failure. Am Rev Respir Dis 137:1463, 1988. *A useful compendium of the subject with 420 references.*

PART VIII

CRITICAL CARE MEDICINE

71 Critical Care Medicine

John M. Luce
and Philip C. Hopewell

CHARACTERISTICS OF CRITICAL CARE MEDICINE

Critical care medicine is a body of knowledge that is applied to the management of severely ill patients in critical care units. Many kinds of patients require critical care, but most have dysfunction or failure of one or more organ systems. Circulatory and respiratory failures are the most common kinds of organ system failure dealt with in critical care units. This chapter focuses on their pathophysiology, monitoring, and management.

Critical care medicine is practiced for the most part by internists, anesthesiologists, surgeons, and pediatricians. The parent boards of these disciplines recognize that critical care medicine may become a specialty and now provide certification of special competence in critical care medicine. The American Board of Internal Medicine gave its first critical care certifying examination in 1987. This and subsequent examinations have been taken primarily by pulmonologists, cardiologists, and general internists. These physicians are expected to be familiar with all areas of internal medicine that are relevant to severely ill patients, in addition to ethical issues in critical care.

Consistent with this broad approach, the interdependence of organ systems must be kept in sharp focus in critical care practice. Limited attention to one component of an illness, even if it is predominant, will frequently yield a therapeutic approach that is detrimental to the patient as a whole. For example, treatment directed toward reducing intravascular volume in a patient with the adult respiratory distress syndrome (ARDS) may adversely affect renal and central nervous system function. Conversely, an increase in intravascular volume given to raise cardiac output in a patient with left ventricular infarction may result in noncardiogenic pulmonary edema if parenchymal lung injury pre-exists. Physicians caring for severely ill patients must synthesize an overall management strategy that supports several organ systems and often incorporates the view of numerous consultants. This is one of the major challenges of critical care.

ATTRIBUTES OF CRITICAL CARE UNITS

Critical care units were first developed in the 1950's for patients who required mechanical ventilation because they had poliomyelitis or were recovering from anesthesia. Currently, various kinds of critical care units are found in almost all acute care hospitals in the United States containing more than 200 beds. These units are defined by their ability to provide the environment, facilities, and personnel for the care of severely ill patients. The important features of critical care units are listed in Table 71–1.

Critical care units may have a general orientation, treating all kinds of severely ill patients, or be more specialized, accepting only specific categories of patients as defined by the kind of

TABLE 71–1. FEATURES OF CRITICAL CARE UNITS

High nurse-patient ratio
Ready accessibility of physicians
Ability to provide invasive cardiovascular and respiratory monitoring
Availability of respiratory support techniques
Ability to provide supervised continuous infusion of pharmacologic agents

illness (for example, burn units), organ system involved (coronary and acute neurologic units), specialty service designation (medical and surgical units), or the patient's age (neonatal and pediatric units). In addition to having the basic attributes listed in Table 71–1, specialized units provide medical personnel specifically skilled in the area of care provided by the units and have available particular forms of technology with applications generally limited to the category of patients accepted by them.

Critical care units need administrative policies and procedures that differ from those of other hospital areas. Because of the severity of the illness of their patients, critical care units require clear delineation of administrative and medical lines of authority and responsibility. Critical care units must also have general guidelines for admission and discharge of patients, specifically described roles for nurses and respiratory therapists, standing orders, and programs of continuing staff education and quality assurance. The existence of such policies reduces the apparent ambiguity often inherent in the difficult environment of a critical care unit and enables prompt decision making by health care professionals.

MONITORING OF CARDIOVASCULAR AND RESPIRATORY FUNCTION

The term monitoring refers to the repeated or continuous assessment of patients and their physiologic functions. Critical care units are designed to provide such assessment, particularly as it pertains to specific organ systems. Thus, vital signs, mental status, and urinary output are regularly measured. In addition, a variety of noninvasive and invasive procedures may be performed to measure the cardiovascular and respiratory variables listed in Table 71–2.

Cardiovascular Monitoring

The adequacy of cardiac output ($\dot{Q}T$) and tissue perfusion can be inferred from the strength of peripheral pulses, the warmth and color of the hands or feet, and the time required to refill superficial capillaries after they have been blanched; normally, 2 to 3 seconds is required. Most critical care units also have the capacity to monitor and record heart rate (HR) and heart rhythm electrocardiographically. Manually or mechanically inflatable sphygmomanometers may be used to measure systemic arterial pressure (PsA).

MONITORING OF SYSTEMIC ARTERIAL PRESSURE. Heart rate and PsA may be determined in an on-line fashion with indwelling systemic arterial catheters, which may also be used to obtain samples for systemic arterial blood gas analysis. These catheters are usually placed in the radial or femoral artery. Complications such as local hematoma formation, ischemia distal to the site of insertion, and local infection may be minimized by using pressure dressings, devices that continually flush the catheters with dilute solutions containing heparin, and sterile catheter insertion and maintenance techniques, respectively.

Although HR is easy to measure, stroke volume (SV) is difficult to estimate and requires radionuclide or ultrasonographic studies that cannot routinely be performed at the bedside. Because of this, clinicians commonly must infer SV by estimating preload, one of its three determinants. Preload cannot be measured directly in patients, but it is equivalent to ventricular end-diastolic volume, which itself is similar to—but not always the same as—ventricular end-diastolic pressure.

MONITORING OF CENTRAL VENOUS PRESSURE. Right ventricular end-diastolic pressure may be obtained by passing a catheter into the superior vena cava and measuring mean right atrial pressure ($\overline{P}RA$) when the tricuspid valve is open. Central venous pressure (CVP) monitoring carries the risk of perforating a major vein or the right atrium and providing a nidus for infection, especially if the catheter is inserted in an unsterile fashion or left in place too long. Nevertheless, the pressure measurement provides an approximation of right ventricular preload, if ventricular compliance is normal.

Central venous pressure measurement may also be used to estimate left ventricular end-diastolic pressure and volume if one assumes that right and left ventricular pressures are similar in diastole. The $\overline{P}_{RA}$ is particularly helpful when it is less than its normal level of approximately 5 mm Hg, inasmuch as pressure in the right ventricle is seldom much higher than that in the left. However, the $\overline{P}_{RA}$ may be increased owing to elevated pressure in the pulmonary circulation when left ventricular pressure is normal, just as left ventricular pressure may be elevated when right ventricular pressure is normal. Because of this, it may be preferable to assess left ventricular pressure more directly.

MONITORING OF PULMONARY ARTERY PRESSURE. Left ventricular end-diastolic pressure may be estimated by passing a balloon-tipped catheter into the central venous circulation. With the balloon inflated, the catheter travels with venous blood through the right atrium, right ventricle, and main pulmonary artery; the pressure tracings obtained as the catheter passes through these structures are depicted in Figure 71–1. The catheter then floats into a branch of the pulmonary artery and "wedges" there. Blood flow distal to the balloon ceases, and the "wedge" or pulmonary artery occlusion pressure (P_{PAO}) measured at the catheter tip just distal to the balloon reflects the downstream pressure. This pressure usually is equal to left atrial pressure (P_{LA}), which is the same as left ventricular end-diastolic pressure when the mitral valve is open, assuming that pulmonary venous pressure is not higher. The left ventricular end-diastolic pressure is assumed to be an approximation of left ventricular end-diastolic volume, that is, preload.

In addition to estimating preload, the pulmonary artery catheter with a thermistor incorporated may be used to measure $\dot{Q}_T$. This measurement is done using the indicator dilution technique, in which a bolus of cold liquid, usually dextrose in water, is injected through the proximal port of the catheter that is located in the right ventricle when the distal port is in the pulmonary artery. The cold liquid mixes with venous blood as it flows from the ventricle into the artery, where the temperature decrease is detected by the thermistor. The change in temperature then is used to calculate $\dot{Q}_T$. Although the $\dot{Q}_T$ of the right ventricle is measured, it is assumed to be equivalent to that of the left ventricle.

The indications for pulmonary artery catheterization are listed in Table 71–3. The contraindications include lack of vascular access, untreatable bleeding disorders, and instability of the patient that does not allow time for the procedure. The complications of pulmonary artery catheterization include vascular laceration during insertion and infection, as with central venous catheterization. In addition, because the catheter is passed through the heart, it may cause arrhythmias and heart block. For this reason, pulmonary artery catheterization should be performed under the guidance of electrocardiographic monitoring, with resuscitation equipment and intravenous lidocaine available. A temporary transvenous pacemaker should also be available for patients with pre-existing left bundle branch block, because additional right bundle branch block may develop as the catheter is inserted. The catheter should be passed quickly through the ventricle and should be removed if significant ventricular arrhythmias develop.

Once the catheter is in the pulmonary artery, it may cause vessel rupture or infarction if it migrates into a distal vessel. These complications may be avoided by determining the position of the catheter tip on chest radiographs, monitoring the P_{PA} waveform to be certain that the P_{PAO} tracing is not present when the balloon is deflated, and making sure that a P_{PAO} tracing can be obtained only by inflating the balloon with at least 1 ml of air.

Proper interpretation of measurements made with central venous and pulmonary artery catheters requires that intravascular pressures be referenced to the extravascular pressures around them. Thus, the P_{PAO} will actually be lower than the true ventricular filling pressure if it is measured in a spontaneously breathing patient during inspiration, when pleural pressure may be greatly negative. On the other hand, the P_{PAO} will be higher than the true filling pressure if it is measured in a mechanically

TABLE 71–2. NORMAL VALUES FOR SELECTED CARDIOVASCULAR AND RESPIRATORY VARIABLES

Variables	Symbol	Values Mean	Values Range
Heart rate	HR	70 beats/min	60–80 beats/min
Stroke volume	SV	70 ml/beat	60–80 ml/beat
Cardiac output	$\dot{Q}_T$	5 L/min	4–6 L/min
Mean pulmonary artery pressure	$\overline{P}_{PA}$	15 mm Hg	9–18 mm Hg
Mean left atrial (pulmonary arterial occlusion) pressure	$\overline{P}_{LA}$ ($\overline{P}_{PAO}$)	10 mm Hg	2–14 mm Hg
Pulmonary vascular resistance	PVR	80 dyne • sec • cm^{-5}	70–90 dyne • sec • cm^{-5}
Mean systemic arterial pressure	$\overline{P}_{SA}$	85 mm Hg	70–105 mm Hg
Mean right atrial (central venous) pressure	$\overline{P}_{RA}$ (CVP)	5 mm Hg	0–8 mm Hg
Systemic vascular resistance	SVR	1240 dyne • sec • cm^{-5}	950–1350 dyne • sec • cm^{-5}
Systemic arterial carbon dioxide tension	Pa_{CO_2}	40 mm Hg	35–45 mm Hg
Fraction of inspired oxygen	FI_{O_2}	0.21	
Systemic arterial oxygen tension	Pa_{O_2}	95 mm Hg	90–100 mm Hg
Carbon dioxide production	$\dot{V}_{CO_2}$	200 ml/min	180–220 ml/min
Oxygen consumption	$\dot{V}_{O_2}$	250 ml/min	225–275 ml/min
Minute ventilation	$\dot{V}_E$	6 L/min	5–7 L/min
Dead space ventilation (per breath)	V_D	150 ml	125–175 ml
Tidal volume	V_T	450 ml	400–500 ml
Dead space to tidal volume ratio (per breath)	V_D/V_T	0.32	0.30–0.35
Respiratory rate	F	17/min	12–22/min
pH	pH	7.40	7.38–7.42
Bicarbonate concentration	[HCO_3^-]	24 mEq/dl	22–26 mEq/dl
Hemoglobin	Hb	15 grams/ml	14–16 grams/ml
Systemic arterial oxygen saturation	Sa_{O_2}	98%	96%–100%
Systemic arterial oxygen content	Ca_{O_2}	20 ml/dl	19–21 ml/dl
Mixed venous oxygen tension	$P\bar{v}_{O_2}$	40 mm Hg	38–42 mm Hg
Mixed venous oxygen saturation	$S\bar{v}_{O_2}$	75%	72%–78%
Mixed venous oxygen content	$C\bar{v}_{O_2}$	15 ml/dl	14–16 ml/dl
Arterial–mixed venous oxygen content difference	$C(a - \bar{v})_{O_2}$	5 ml/dl	4–6 ml/dl
Shunt fraction	$\dot{Q}_S/\dot{Q}_T$	<7%	
Maximum inspiratory pressure	MIP	−70 cm H_2O	−60 to −80 cm H_2O
Vital capacity	VC	50 ml/kg	40–60 ml/kg
Forced expiratory volume in 1 second	FEV_1	75% of VC	70%–80% of VC

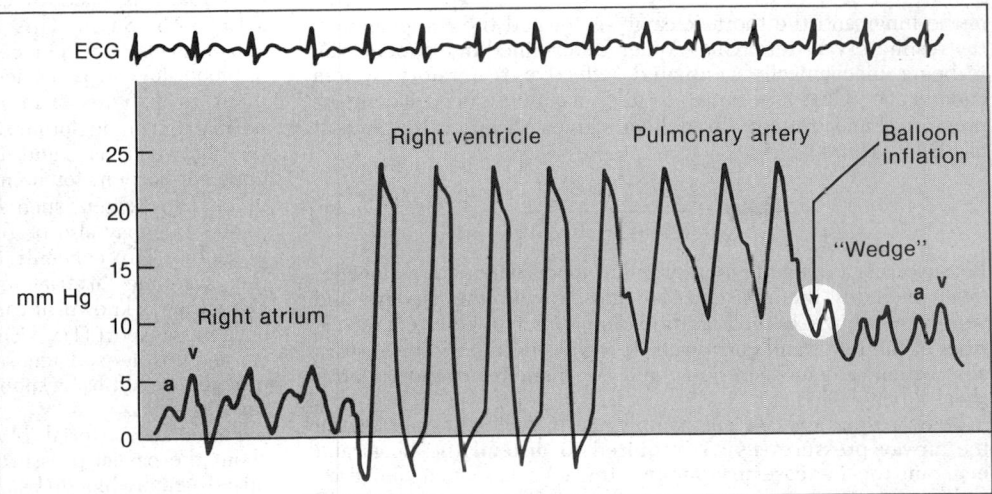

FIGURE 71-1. Tracing of pressures during passage of a pulmonary artery catheter from the internal jugular vein into the pulmonary artery. Pressures and waveform are normal. (From Matthay MA: Invasive hemodynamic monitoring in critically ill patients. Clin Chest Med 4:233, 1983.)

ventilated patient during an inspiration with positive pressure. To avoid erroneous interpretation, the Ppao should be measured in end-expiration. If patients are receiving positive end-expiratory pressure (PEEP) at levels above 10 cm H_2O from the ventilator, approximately one quarter of the PEEP should be subtracted from the measured Ppao to approximate the true Ppao. It is less important to subtract an exact amount than it is to recognize that the Ppao is at best an approximation of left ventricular end-diastolic pressure, which itself is only an approximation of left ventricular end-diastolic volume.

The combination of systemic and pulmonary artery catheterization also facilitates measurement of the pressure across the systemic (Psa minus Pra) and pulmonary (mean pulmonary artery pressure [Ppa] minus Pla or Ppao) circulations. In concert with Qt, these data allow determination of the systemic and pulmonary vascular resistances (SVR, PVR). Pulmonary artery catheterization also provides information about mixed venous blood gas values, as discussed in the next section. Characteristic patterns of cardiovascular and respiratory dysfunction that may be identified by combined systemic and pulmonary artery catheterization are listed in Table 71-4 and are discussed in greater detail later in this chapter.

Respiratory Monitoring

Physical examination may be very helpful in assessing respiratory function. For example, intercostal muscle retraction may reflect respiratory distress. Inward movement of the abdominal wall during inspiration, a sign called abdominal paradox, signifies that the diaphragm is not contracting normally and frequently presages ventilatory failure. In addition, hypoxemia may be suspected if cyanosis of the lips and palate is detected. Nevertheless, cyanosis is an insensitive finding, and respiratory failure can be diagnosed only through systemic arterial blood gas analysis.

ASSESSMENT OF VENTILATION. Samples of systemic arterial blood for measurement of the partial pressures of carbon dioxide (Pa_{CO_2}) and oxygen (Pa_{O_2}), pH, and the bicarbonate concentration ($[HCO_3^-]$) may be obtained from either repeated percutaneous arterial punctures or indwelling arterial catheters. The Pa_{CO_2} is used to assess the adequacy of ventilation and to diagnose hypercapnic respiratory failure, also called ventilatory failure. Similarly, the pH and $[HCO_3^-]$ measurements can be used to determine whether hypercapnia is acute or chronic.

TABLE 71-3. INDICATIONS FOR PULMONARY ARTERIAL PRESSURE MONITORING

To help distinguish cardiogenic from noncardiogenic pulmonary edema
To provide information in the differential diagnosis of shock
To assist in determining the cause of hypoxemia
To characterize the patterns of abnormal cardiovascular function after myocardial infarction
To monitor the effects of various cardiovascular and respiratory therapies

An approximation of Pa_{CO_2} may be made by measuring the end-tidal carbon dioxide tension (PET_{CO_2}) in expired gas. This is most conveniently measured in mechanically ventilated patients. If the PET_{CO_2} is to substitute for the Pa_{CO_2}, the two values should be correlated, using several paired measurements. The PET_{CO_2} usually is slightly less than the Pa_{CO_2}.

Ventilatory variables such as respiratory rate (F) and tidal volume (Vt) and their product, the minute ventilation (Ve), may be accurately measured by a technique called respiratory inductance plethysmography, which uses wire coils embedded in bands that fit around the chest and abdomen to detect movements of these areas. These variables may also be measured by a pneumotachograph or other types of spirometers in patients who are breathing through endotracheal tubes. Neither alveolar ventilation (Va) nor dead space ventilation (Vd) can be directly measured, although the value of Va may be inferred if Ve and Vd are known. The ratio of Vd to Vt per breath can be calculated in patients whose Pa_{CO_2} and PET_{CO_2} are known, using the modified Bohr equation:

$$V_D/V_T = \frac{Pa_{CO_2} - PET_{CO_2}}{Pa_{CO_2}} \quad (1)$$

The Vd/Vt is usually 0.30 to 0.35 in healthy persons breathing spontaneously. In patients with normal lungs being mechanically ventilated, the Vd/Vt is approximately 0.50.

Carbon dioxide production (Vco_2) may be measured by closed systems in patients breathing spontaneously or receiving mechanical ventilation. Once Vco_2 is measured, Vd/Vt is calculated from Equation 1, and Va is inferred, one can determine which abnormality in the alveolar ventilation relationship (Equations 5 and 6) is responsible for ventilatory failure.

Three other variables that reflect ventilatory capability are the maximum inspiratory pressure (MIP), the vital capacity (VC), and the ratio of the forced expiratory volume in 1 second (FEV_1) to the forced VC. In the MIF maneuver, a manometer is used to measure the negative pressure that patients can generate when inspiring from a low lung volume. An MIP that is less negative than -20 cm H_2O suggests the need for ventilatory support, whereas an MIP that is more negative than -20 cm H_2O correlates with successful weaning from mechanical ventilation.

The VC, the greatest amount of gas that can be inhaled or exhaled in a single breath, can be measured with any of a variety of spirometers. The normal VC is approximately 50 ml per kilogram of body weight. A VC of less than 10 ml per kilogram usually indicates the need for institution or continuation of mechanical ventilation. The FEV_1 can also be measured by spirometry. Normally, the FEV_1 is approximately 75 to 80 per cent of the forced VC; reductions in this ratio may occur in patients with airways obstruction due to asthma or chronic obstructive pulmonary disease (COPD).

ASSESSMENT OF RESPIRATORY SYSTEM COMPLIANCE. The amount of pressure required to increase the volume of the lungs and the thoracic cavity is termed the compliance of the respiratory system (CRS). When determined in a patient who is being mechanically ventilated, effective respiratory system compliance (CEFF) is equal to the maximum or peak airway pressure (Pmax) required to deliver a given V_T minus the amount of PEEP. Thus,

$$C_{EFF} = \frac{V_T}{P_{max} - PEEP} \qquad (2)$$

Because it is a dynamic measurement made when gas is flowing, CEFF includes the resistance to gas flow in the airways and ventilator tubing, as well as the volume and pressure characteristics of the lungs and chest wall. It will be influenced by airways obstruction, airway secretions, and the diameter of the endotracheal tube.

Static respiratory system compliance (CSTAT) is a measure of the airway pressure (PSTAT) required to distend the lungs and maintain the increase in volume after a V_T has been delivered and gas is not flowing into or out of lungs. The amount of PEEP should be subtracted in determining this pressure. Thus,

$$C_{STAT} = \frac{V_T}{P_{STAT} - PEEP} \qquad (3)$$

Because it is a static measurement, CSTAT reflects only the compliance of the lungs and chest wall and is not affected by resistance to gas flow. It will be decreased (normal level is 50 to 60 ml per centimeter of water) by conditions, such as ARDS, that decrease lung volume. Weaning from mechanical ventilation is difficult if CSTAT is less than 25 ml per centimeter of water.

ASSESSMENT OF AUTO-PEEP. Another measurement that may be made on mechanically ventilated patients is intrinsic or auto-PEEP. Auto-PEEP occurs in patients with airways obstruction and other disorders who fail to complete expiration either during spontaneous breathing or before they receive the next breath from a mechanical ventilator. This results in air trapping that produces positive pressure at end-expiration. The auto-PEEP effect can reduce cardiac filling pressures and $\dot{Q}_T$ and elevate PPAO readings unless it, like intentionally administered PEEP, is accounted for. Auto-PEEP can be measured in mechanically ventilated patients by stopping airflow at end-expiration just before the next breath, allowing the pressure in the airways and the ventilator tubing to equilibrate, and reading the pressure from the ventilator manometer.

ASSESSMENT OF ARTERIAL OXYGENATION. Just as measurement of Pa_{CO_2} is the means by which ventilatory failure is diagnosed, failure of arterial oxygenation can be diagnosed only by determining the Pa_{O_2}. Introducing the values for Pa_{CO_2} and the partial pressure of oxygen in inspired gas (PI_{O_2}) into the alveolar gas equation (Equation 7) enables determination of the alveolar-arterial oxygen pressure difference, $P(A - a)_{O_2}$, as will be discussed. This information in turn provides insight into the probable cause of hypoxemia in a given patient.

Because systemic arterial blood sampling may be associated with complications, a less invasive approximation of the state of arterial oxygenation often is desirable. This may be accomplished through pulse oximetry, in which the differential absorption of

certain wavelengths of light passed through a finger or other appendage is used to calculate the systemic arterial oxygen saturation (Sa_{O_2}). This technique accurately measures Sa_{O_2} above levels of 80 per cent in patients with adequate peripheral blood flow. It is particularly helpful as a continuous measurement in patients who are relatively stable and in whom a normal oxyhemoglobin saturation curve enables good correlation between Sa_{O_2} and Pa_{O_2}. The Sa_{O_2} measured by oximetry does not account for hemoglobin that is saturated by substances other than oxygen, such as carbon monoxide.

The Sa_{O_2} may also be derived from the Pa_{O_2}. The Sa_{O_2}, the hemoglobin (Hb) concentration, and Pa_{O_2} are the determinants of the systemic arterial oxygen content (Ca_{O_2}) (Equation 9). Once Ca_{O_2} is known, it can be multiplied by the $\dot{Q}_T$ to determine systemic arterial oxygen transport (T_{O_2}) (Equation 8). Thus, systemic arterial blood gas analysis helps diagnose failure of oxygen transport, determine the abnormalities responsible for such failure, and assess its severity.

Pulmonary arterial blood gas analysis provides information about the partial pressure, saturation, and content of oxygen in mixed venous blood ($P\bar{v}_{O_2}$, $S\bar{v}_{O_2}$, $C\bar{v}_{O_2}$). In addition, $S\bar{v}_{O_2}$ may be measured continuously with oximetric pulmonary artery catheters. In combination with values for $\dot{Q}_T$ and Ca_{O_2} obtained by systemic arterial blood gas analysis, the $C\bar{v}_{O_2}$ may be inserted into Equation 10 to calculate the oxygen consumption ($\dot{V}_{O_2}$). Alternatively, $\dot{V}_{O_2}$ may be determined directly by measuring concentrations of oxygen in inspired and expired gas and the inspired and expired volumes. Even if $\dot{V}_{O_2}$ is not calculated or precisely known, the decrease in $P\bar{v}_{O_2}$, $S\bar{v}_{O_2}$, and $C\bar{v}_{O_2}$ and the increase in the arterial–mixed venous content difference, $C(a - \bar{v})_{O_2}$, that characterize inadequate oxygen transport can be assessed by analysis of systemic and pulmonary artery blood samples, as can the increase in $P\bar{v}_{O_2}$, $S\bar{v}_{O_2}$, and $C\bar{v}_{O_2}$ and the decrease in $C(a - \bar{v})_{O_2}$ that characterize inadequate oxygen extraction.

MEASUREMENT OF SHUNT FRACTION. Finally, combined systemic and pulmonary artery blood gas analysis may be used to quantitate the contribution to hypoxemia of right-to-left intrapulmonary shunting of blood. This analysis may be performed in patients receiving 100 per cent oxygen, using the following shunt equation:

$$\frac{\dot{Q}_S}{\dot{Q}_T} = \frac{Cc'_{O_2} - Ca_{O_2}}{Cc'_{O_2} - C\bar{v}_{O_2}} \qquad (4)$$

where $\dot{Q}_S$ is the volume of shunted blood and Cc'_{O_2} is an approximation of end-capillary blood oxygen content, assuming Pc'_{O_2} to be the same as PA_{O_2}, and calculating Cc'_{O_2} on the basis of that assumption. The shunt equation is based on the Fick equation (Equation 10), which will be discussed. A simpler but less precise way of estimating intrapulmonary shunt, which is also based on the Fick equation and assumes a normal $C(a - \bar{v})_{O_2}$ of 5 ml per deciliter of blood, is to divide the $P(A - a)_{O_2}$ by 15 to 20. The normal $\dot{Q}_S$ is 7 per cent or less of $\dot{Q}_T$.

ASSESSMENT OF TISSUE OXYGENATION. As suggested by the previous discussion, the data obtained from combined systemic and pulmonary artery blood gas analysis may be very helpful in managing critically ill patients. Nevertheless, not all

TABLE 71–4. HEMODYNAMIC PATTERNS IN CARDIOVASCULAR AND RESPIRATORY DISORDERS

Situation	PSA	PRA	PPA	PPAO	$C(a - \bar{v})_{O_2}$	$\dot{Q}_T$	PVR	SVR	$P\bar{v}_{O_2}$
Airways obstruction	→↓	→↑	↑	→	→	→↓	↑	→	→
Hypovolemic shock	↓	↓	↓	↓	↑	↓	↑	↑	↓
Pulmonary thromboembolism	↓	↑	↑	→↓	↑	↑↓	↑	↑	↓
Cardiac tamponade	↓	↑	↑	↑	↑	↓	→	↑	↓
Cardiogenic shock	↓	↑	↑	↑	↑	↓	↑	↑	↓
Right ventricular infarction	↓	↑	→	↑	↑	↓	→ ↑	↑	↓
Distributive shock	↓	↓	↓	↓	↓	↑	↓	↓	↑

PSA = systemic arterial pressure; PRA = right atrial or central venous pressure; PPA = pulmonary arterial pressure; PPAO = pulmonary arterial occlusion pressure; $C(a - \bar{v})_{O_2}$ = arterial–mixed venous oxygen content difference; $\dot{Q}_T$ = cardiac output; PVR = pulmonary vascular resistance; SVR = systemic vascular resistance; $P\bar{v}_{O_2}$ = mixed venous oxygen tension.

such patients require such sophisticated monitoring techniques, and the techniques still cannot provide an ideal assessment of oxygenation of a tissue level. The same can be said for serial measurement of serum lactate levels, which some physicians use as a monitoring tool. Despite these and other technologic advances in critical care monitoring, assessment of tissue oxygenation probably is best performed by analyzing individual organ system function by simple biochemical tests, such as renal and hepatic indices, measurement of urine output, and observation of mental status.

PATHOPHYSIOLOGY OF CIRCULATORY AND RESPIRATORY FAILURE

Aerobic metabolism in humans is made possible by four processes that involve the cardiovascular and respiratory systems: (1) *ventilation,* in which oxygen is inhaled from the atmosphere and carbon dioxide is excreted into it; (2) *arterial oxygenation,* in which oxygen is transferred from the alveoli into mixed venous blood in the pulmonary capillaries in exchange for carbon dioxide; (3) *oxygen transport,* in which oxygen is carried in systemic arterial blood to the tissues; and (4) *oxygen extraction and utilization,* in which the tissues take up oxygen from the blood and give up carbon dioxide, which is transported in mixed venous blood to the lungs.

Impairments in any or all of these four processes commonly occur in critically ill patients. As a result, much of critical care monitoring and management involves preventing or correcting the various impairments. In the following section, the four processes are discussed in greater detail, and examples of disorders that cause disturbances in the processes are given (Table 71–5).

Ventilation

The adequacy of ventilation is determined by measurement of the Pa_{CO_2} in systemic arterial blood. At sea level, the normal Pa_{CO_2} is approximately 40 mm Hg. Hypoventilation and hypercapnia exist when the Pa_{CO_2} exceeds this level, and hypercapnic respiratory failure is diagnosed when the Pa_{CO_2} is 50 mm Hg or

TABLE 71–5. KINDS OF CIRCULATORY AND RESPIRATORY FAILURE

Failure	Definition	Abnormality	Examples
Ventilatory failure	Inadequate alveolar ventilation	High Pa_{CO_2}	Narcotic or sedative drug overdose Asthma Chronic obstructive pulmonary disease Neuromuscular diseases
Failure of arterial oxygenation	Inadequate oxygenation of systemic arterial blood	Low Pa_{O_2}	Pneumonia Asthma Chronic obstructive pulmonary disease
Failure of oxygen transport	Inadequate supply of oxygenated blood to tissues	Low Ca_{O_2} or $\dot{Q}T$ or both Low $P\bar{v}_{O_2}$, $S\bar{v}_{O_2}$, $C\bar{v}_{O_2}$ Increased $C(a - \bar{v})_{O_2}$ Lactic acidosis	Anemia Carbon monoxide poisoning Hypovolemic shock Obstructive shock Cardiogenic shock Cardiorespiratory arrest
Failure of oxygen extraction	Inadequate tissue oxygen uptake	Low $\dot{V}_{O_2}$ High $P\bar{v}_{O_2}$, $S\bar{v}_{O_2}$, $C\bar{v}_{O_2}$ Decreased $C(a - \bar{v})_{O_2}$ Lactic acidosis	Cyanide poisoning Distributive shock Adult respiratory distress syndrome Multiple organ system failure

Pa_{CO_2} = systemic arterial carbon dioxide tension; Pa_{O_2} = systemic arterial oxygen tension; Ca_{O_2} = systemic arterial oxygen content; $\dot{Q}T$ = cardiac output; $P\bar{v}_{O_2}$ = mixed venous oxygen tension; $S\bar{v}_{O_2}$ = mixed venous oxygen saturation; $C\bar{v}_{O_2}$ = mixed venous oxygen content; $C(a - \bar{v})_{O_2}$ = arterial–mixed venous oxygen content difference; $\dot{V}_{O_2}$ = oxygen consumption.

greater at sea level, unless this is a compensation for metabolic alkalosis. Hypercapnic respiratory failure is also called ventilatory failure.

The pathophysiology of ventilatory failure is explained by examining the factors that determine the Pa_{CO_2}. The Pa_{CO_2} is directly related to the body's carbon dioxide production per minute ($\dot{V}CO_2$) and inversely proportional to $\dot{V}A$. Thus,

$$Pa_{CO_2} \simeq \frac{\dot{V}CO_2}{\dot{V}A} \tag{5}$$

The normal $\dot{V}CO_2$ of a healthy young person is approximately 200 ml per minute; the $\dot{V}A$ is approximately 5 liters.

Alveolar ventilation is equal to the $\dot{V}E$, which is the amount of gas that enters the upper respiratory tract each minute, minus the $\dot{V}D$, which is the inhaled gas that does not participate in gas exchange, either because it remains in the upper airways or because it enters areas of the lung where blood flow is insufficient for the matching of ventilation and perfusion. The minute ventilation is the product of VT (normally 450 ml) and F (normally 12 to 22 per minute). Thus,

$$Pa_{CO_2} \simeq \frac{\dot{V}CO_2}{(\dot{V}T \times F) - \dot{V}D} \tag{6}$$

From Equations 5 and 6 it follows that hypercapnia can occur (1) if $\dot{V}CO_2$ increases and $\dot{V}A$ does not, (2) if $\dot{V}A$ decreases and $\dot{V}CO_2$ does not, or (3) if $\dot{V}D$ increases out of proportion to $\dot{V}E$. An example of the first situation might be a patient who becomes febrile owing to sepsis syndrome and thereby increases $\dot{V}CO_2$ but cannot increase $\dot{V}A$ because of respiratory muscle weakness. Patients with severe asthma and COPD may have ventilatory failure because $\dot{V}A$ is reduced owing to airways obstruction, especially when $\dot{V}CO_2$ is increased. A primary reduction in $\dot{V}A$ also is seen in narcotic or sedative drug overdose. Diseases such as ARDS, in which $\dot{V}D$ may increase owing to vascular obstruction, can cause ventilatory failure if patients cannot increase $\dot{V}E$ because of, for example, oversedation.

The physiologic consequences of hypercapnia depend largely on the rate of increase in Pa_{CO_2} and the level it reaches. An increased Pa_{CO_2} dilates cerebral blood vessels, increases cerebral blood flow, and may cause headaches and eventually obtundation. More important, every 1 mm Hg rise in Pa_{CO_2} causes the pH in systemic arterial blood to fall by 0.0075 unit. The acute respiratory acidosis that results may depress the function of the heart and other organs until the plasma $[HCO_3^-]$ rises and buffers the fall in pH. Thus, gradual increases in Pa_{CO_2} are compensated for by an increasing $[HCO_3^-]$. Chronic metabolic alkalosis of this sort is of little physiologic consequence. However, as discussed in the next section, an increase in Pa_{CO_2} will result in a reduction of the partial pressure of oxygen in alveolar gas and thus a decrease in the partial pressure of oxygen in systemic arterial blood unless supplemental oxygen is administered.

Arterial Oxygenation

The adequacy of arterial oxygenation is determined by the Pa_{O_2}, which in healthy young persons is approximately 95 mm Hg at sea level. Hypoxemia exists when the Pa_{O_2} is below this value, and hypoxemic respiratory failure is diagnosed if the Pa_{O_2} is less than 50 to 60 mm Hg at sea level. Hypoxemic respiratory failure is also called failure of arterial oxygenation.

The alveolar gas equation states that the partial pressure of oxygen in alveolar gas (PA_{O_2}) is equal to the partial pressure of oxygen in inspired air (PI_{O_2}) minus the partial pressure of carbon dioxide in alveolar gas (PA_{CO_2}), divided by the respiratory quotient (RQ). Thus,

$$PA_{O_2} = PI_{O_2} - \frac{PA_{CO_2}}{RQ} \tag{7}$$

The PI_{O_2} is equal to the fraction of inspired oxygen (FI_{O_2} normally = 0.21) times the barometric pressure corrected for water vapor ($PB - 47$ mm Hg) and is approximately 150 mm Hg at sea level.

The $P_{A_{CO_2}}$ is equal to the Pa_{CO_2} and therefore normally is 40 mm Hg. The RQ is the ratio of $\dot{V}_{CO_2}$ to $\dot{V}_{O_2}$ and usually is assumed to be 0.8. Substituting these values in Equation 7, the $P_{A_{O_2}}$ should equal approximately 100 mm Hg in healthy young persons breathing ambient air at sea level. Normally, with an $F_{I_{O_2}}$ of 0.21, the difference between $P_{A_{O_2}}$ and Pa_{O_2}, the $P_{(A - a)_{O_2}}$, is less than 10 mm Hg.

From Equation 7 and the normal value for $P_{(A - a)_{O_2}}$ just derived, it follows that a fall in the Pa_{O_2} to below 50 to 60 mm Hg can occur if $P_{I_{O_2}}$ decreases, if Pa_{CO_2} increases, or if $P_{(A - a)_{O_2}}$ increases. A marked decrease in $P_{I_{O_2}}$ might occur while breathing air at high altitude where PB is reduced or in a fire that consumes oxygen; in the latter case, $F_{I_{O_2}}$ will be less than 0.21. An increase in Pa_{CO_2} above 40 mm Hg is ventilatory failure by definition; thus, ventilatory failure may cause failure of arterial oxygenation unless the $P_{I_{O_2}}$ is increased by the administration of supplemental oxygen to offset the fall in $P_{A_{O_2}}$. An increased $P_{(A - a)_{O_2}}$ is primarily the result of two processes: ventilation-perfusion mismatching and shunting of mixed venous blood either within the heart or past unventilated areas of the lung, the most extreme form of ventilation-perfusion mismatching. The hypoxemia associated with asthma and COPD is largely attributable to ventilation-perfusion mismatching, whereas the hypoxemia with ARDS is attributable to intrapulmonary shunting.

The physiologic consequences of hypoxemia depend on the rate of decline of Pa_{O_2} and its severity and duration. Some persons who are born at high altitude or who have congenital cyanotic heart disease live normally with a Pa_{O_2} less than 50 mm Hg. However, failure of arterial oxygenation usually leads to some mental impairment and reduced exercise performance regardless of its chronicity, and it is likely to be catastrophic in depressing organ function in patients unaccustomed to hypoxemia.

Oxygen Transport

The amount of oxygen transported to the tissues is the product of the cardiac output $\dot{Q}T$ and the Ca_{O_2}. Thus,

$$\dot{T}_{O_2} = (\dot{Q}T)(Ca_{O_2}) \tag{8}$$

The Ca_{O_2} is the oxygen that is bound to Hb plus the small amount that is dissolved in plasma. This is described by the following equation:

$$Ca_{O_2} = (1.39)(Hb)(Sa_{O_2}) + (0.003)(Pa_{O_2}) \tag{9}$$

where 1.39 is the oxygen-carrying capacity of Hb in milliliters per gram and 0.003 is the solubility of oxygen in plasma at 37°C in milliliters of oxygen per milliliter of blood. If arterial blood has an Hb concentration of 15 grams per milliliter and the Hb is 98 per cent saturated, the Hb carries 19.7 ml of oxygen per deciliter of blood. The amount of oxygen in solution at a Pa_{O_2} of 95 mm Hg is 0.3 ml per deciliter of blood. Thus, the Ca_{O_2} normally is 20 ml of oxygen per deciliter of blood, or 200 ml of oxygen per liter. Multiplying by the normal $\dot{Q}T$ of 5 liters per minute, T_{O_2} is approximately 1 liter per minute.

The relationship between Pa_{O_2}, Sa_{O_2}, and Ca_{O_2} is described by the oxyhemoglobin dissociation curve (Fig. 71–2). Some laboratories use an idealized version of this curve to calculate the Sa_{O_2} and Ca_{O_2} from the measured Pa_{O_2}. However, the idealized curve assumes that Hb and metabolic status are normal. In patients the oxyhemoglobin dissociation curve frequently is shifted to the left owing to alkalosis, Hb with a high affinity for oxygen, or carbon monoxide poisoning (in which Hb also binds carbon monoxide more avidly than oxygen, causing a functional anemia). As a result of this left shift, the Sa_{O_2} is higher at a given Pa_{O_2}, so less oxygen is extracted by the tissues. By contrast, the curve is shifted to the right by acidosis, Hb with a weak affinity for oxygen, and 2,3-diphosphoglycerate, which is produced in increased amounts in response to hypoxia. This right shift results in a lower Sa_{O_2} for a given Pa_{O_2}, so that more oxygen is extracted by the tissues. The true Sa_{O_2} can be known only by oximetric analysis of arterial blood, a fact that is of particular relevance in evaluating patients with carbon monoxide poisoning.

Inspection of the oxyhemoglobin dissociation curve reveals other important aspects of $\dot{T}_{O_2}$. One is that with a normal Hb concentration the Ca_{O_2} remains near 20 ml per deciliter of blood above a Pa_{O_2} of 60 mm Hg and Sa_{O_2} of 90 per cent, but the Ca_{O_2} diminishes rapidly below these levels. Because of this, the physiologic consequences of hypoxemia usually begin to occur at a Pa_{O_2} of approximately 60 mm Hg and can be avoided if the Pa_{O_2} is raised above this level. Note also that the Ca_{O_2} can be increased only slightly by raising the Pa_{O_2} above the normal level of 95 mm Hg. This is because the Hb is fully saturated at this level and only a little more oxygen can be dissolved in blood.

The oxyhemoglobin dissociation curve also gives information regarding the $P\bar{v}_{O_2}$, $S\bar{v}_{O_2}$, and $C\bar{v}_{O_2}$. The relationship between these values and their counterparts in systemic arterial blood is described by the Fick equation, which holds that the oxygen extracted by the tissues, the $\dot{V}_{O_2}$, is the difference between the oxygen transported to the tissues, the $\dot{T}_{O_2}$, and the oxygen returned from the tissues in mixed venous blood to the right side of the heart, which is the product of $\dot{Q}T$ and the $C\bar{v}_{O_2}$. By combining terms, the Fick equation can be expressed as follows:

$$\dot{V}_{O_2} = \dot{Q}T\,(C[a - \bar{v}]_{O_2}) \tag{10}$$

Figure 71–2 shows that the $P\bar{v}_{O_2}$ normally is approximately 40 mm Hg, the $S\bar{v}_{O_2}$ is 75 mm Hg, the $C\bar{v}_{O_2}$ is 15 ml per deciliter of blood, and the $C(a - \bar{v})_{O_2}$ is 5 ml per deciliter blood; given a $\dot{Q}T$ of 5 liters per minute, $\dot{V}_{O_2}$ is approximately 250 ml of oxygen per minute. These values indicate that normally only 25 per cent of the oxygen in systemic arterial blood is extracted by the tissues, leaving a large oxygen reserve. Patients characteristically call upon this reserve when $\dot{V}_{O_2}$ increases or when T_{O_2} decreases owing to a fall in $\dot{Q}T$, Ca_{O_2}, or both. This in turn causes a decrease in the $P\bar{v}_{O_2}$, $S\bar{v}_{O_2}$, and $C\bar{v}_{O_2}$ and an increase in the $C(a - \bar{v})_{O_2}$.

A shift from aerobic to anaerobic metabolism and an increased production of lactic acid may be observed in conditions such as severe anemia; carbon monoxide poisoning; hypovolemic, obstructive, and cardiogenic shock; and cardiorespiratory arrest. These findings are associated with decreases in the $P\bar{v}_{O_2}$ below 30 mm Hg, in the $S\bar{v}_{O_2}$ below 60 per cent, and in the $C\bar{v}_{O_2}$ below 10 ml of oxygen per deciliter of blood, and an increase in the $C(a - \bar{v})_{O_2}$ above 10 ml per deciliter. Such values are indicative of failure of oxygen transport.

From Equation 8, it can be seen that inadequate oxygen transport can result from a decrease either in Ca_{O_2} or in $\dot{Q}T$. Cardiac output itself is the product of HR and SV. Thus,

$$\dot{Q}T = (HR)(SV) \tag{11}$$

Heart rate, which normally averages about 70 beats per minute, is determined by autonomic influences on the intrinsic cardiac pacemakers. Stroke volume, which averages 70 ml per beat, is determined by three factors: (1) preload, the length of cardiac muscle fibers at the start of contraction, which is equal to ventricular end-diastolic volume and is approximated as end-diastolic pressure; (2) afterload, the tension the heart muscle develops during systole, which usually is equated with the blood pressure or the vascular resistance that the ventricle must overcome to pump blood into either the pulmonary or the systemic circulation; and (3) contractility, the inotropic state of the muscle, which may be expressed as the velocity of muscle shortening.

Cardiac output also is equal to the perfusion pressure (Pcirc) across the circulation into which the ventricle is pumping, which is the difference between arterial inflow and venous outflow pressures, divided by the resistance of that circulation (Rcirc). Thus,

$$Rcirc = Pcirc/\dot{Q}T \tag{12}$$

Pulmonary vascular resistance is equal to $P\overline{PA}$ minus $P\overline{LA}$ divided by $\dot{Q}T$. Normally, $P\overline{PA}$ = approximately 15 mm Hg, $P\overline{LA}$ = 10 mm Hg, and $\dot{Q}T$ = 5 liters per minute, so PVR = 1 mm Hg per liter per minute; this usually is multipled by 80 and expressed as 80 dyne · sec · cm^{-5}. On the other hand, SVR is equal to $P\overline{SA}$ minus $P\overline{RA}$, divided by the $\dot{Q}T$. Normally, $P\overline{SA}$ = approximately 85 mm Hg, $P\overline{RA}$ = 5 mm Hg, and $\dot{Q}T$ = 5 liters per minute, so SVR $=$ 16 mm Hg per liter per minute, or 1280 dyne $\cdot$ sec $\cdot$ cm^{-5}.

Oxygen Extraction

Some critically ill patients shift from aerobic to anaerobic metabolism and develop lactic acidosis despite what appears to be a normal or even increased $\dot{Q}T$ and Ca_{O_2}. Such patients have what may be called failure of oxygen extraction. They characteristically have a $P\bar{v}_{O_2}$ of greater than 60 mm Hg, a $S\bar{v}_{O_2}$ of greater than 80 per cent, a $C\bar{v}_{O_2}$ of greater than 18 ml of oxygen per milliliter, and a $C(a - \bar{v})_{O_2}$ of less than 5 ml of oxygen per milliliter of blood. In keeping with Equation 10, failure of oxygen extraction is characterized by a reduction in $\dot{V}_{O_2}$. Such a reduction occurs in cyanide poisoning, in which the cyanide ion interrupts intracellular mitochondrial oxygen transport. More common examples are distributive shock, ARDS, and the syndrome of multiple organ system failure (MOSF).

GENERAL MANAGEMENT OF CIRCULATORY AND RESPIRATORY FAILURE

Abnormalities in ventilation, arterial oxygenation, oxygen transport, and oxygen extraction may exist separately or coexist in critically ill patients. As a result, management of such patients may require therapy to improve these processes either independently or at the same time. The following section provides a general approach to improving ventilation, arterial oxygenation, oxygen transport, and oxygen extraction.

Therapy to Improve Ventilation

The Pa_{CO_2} may be improved by manipulating the variables that affect it: $\dot{V}_{CO_2}$ and $\dot{V}_A$ ($\dot{V}_A$ is equal to $\dot{V}_E - \dot{V}_D$). Manipulation of $\dot{V}_A$ may involve any or all components of the respiratory system. These include the respiratory control centers in the brain stem that regulate $\dot{V}_A$, the nerves that transmit messages from the control centers to the respiratory muscles, the muscles themselves, the chest wall to which the muscles are attached, the pleura that lines the lungs, the lung parenchyma, and the upper and lower airways.

Ventilation may be improved in patients who have overdosed on narcotics by the administration of intravenous naloxone in 0.4-mg doses as required. Antagonists to benzodiazepines and other sedatives are not yet generally available in the United States, although the excretion of some of the drugs that depress ventilation may be enhanced by hemodialysis or charcoal hemoperfusion. At the very least, narcotics and sedatives should be administered cautiously to patients at risk of ventilatory failure. Intravenous doxapram in a bolus of 140 mg and a continuous infusion of 2 mg per minute has been used to overcome drug-induced ventilatory depression and to forestall mechanical ventilation in a variety of patients whose ventilatory failure is thought to be reversible, such as those recovering from anesthesia or having exacerbations of COPD. However, neither this agent nor other ventilatory stimulants can forestall mechanical ventilation indefinitely.

Disorders of the chest wall, such as in massive obesity and kyphoscoliosis, are not usually amenable to specific treatment. This is not true, however, of neuromuscular diseases that cause respiratory muscle weakness or paralysis, as will be discussed. Beyond therapies for neuromuscular diseases, there are few measures that improve respiratory muscle weakness. Theophylline increases ventilatory capacity in some, but not all, patients with COPD. Nutrition also improves respiratory muscle function to a limited extent, but it also increases $\dot{V}_{CO_2}$, which may offset any increase in $\dot{V}_E$.

Pleural and parenchymal diseases limit $\dot{V}_A$ by restricting lung expansion and by increasing $\dot{V}_D$. These disorders also increase the work of breathing, which increases $\dot{V}_{CO_2}$ and may fatigue the respiratory muscles. Evacuation of the pleural space, usually by means of tube thoracostomy, is called for in patients compromised by pneumothorax, hemothorax, or pleural empyema.

Anatomic obstruction of the upper airways should be removed or bypassed when it causes or could cause hypercapnia; this rule applies to excessive soft tissues as well as to aspirated material. Inspissated secretions frequently cause or contribute to ventilatory failure in a variety of patients, including those with neuromuscular diseases, asthma and COPD, and ARDS. Removal of secretions may be facilitated by chest physiotherapy or gentle endotracheal suctioning. In a recent study, iodinated glycerol facilitated secretion clearance in outpatients with COPD, although the effects of this oral mucolytic agent on $\dot{V}_A$ and Pa_{CO_2} were not determined.

The $\dot{V}_{CO_2}$ may be reduced by lowering the metabolic rate and thereby the need for increased ventilation. For example, seizures may respond to phenytoin administration (50 mg per minute given intravenously, up to a loading dose of 1000 mg, followed by 300 mg per day). Shivering may be prevented by chlorpromazine (25 to 75 mg given intramuscularly). Fever may be reduced by the administration of antipyretics, such as aspirin or acetaminophen, which are more effective than cooling blankets or sponge baths in decreasing core temperature.

Unfortunately, the increase in $\dot{V}_D$ caused by obliteration of the pulmonary vasculature due to disorders such as ARDS is rarely amenable to medical measures. Increases in the $\dot{V}_D$ caused by pulmonary thromboembolism may be treated with thrombolytic agents, such as streptokinase.

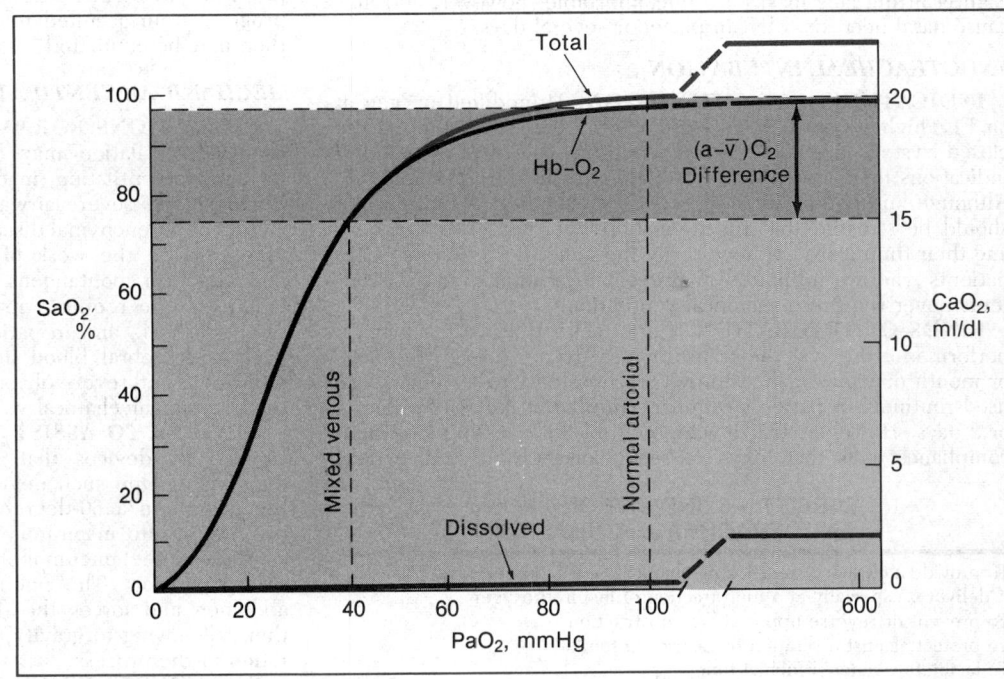

FIGURE 71–2. The oxyhemoglobin dissociation curve, relating the partial pressure of oxygen in systemic arterial blood (Pa_{O_2}), in millimeters of mercury, to systemic arterial oxygen saturation (Sa_{O_2}), in per cent, and to the oxygen content of systemic arterial blood (Ca_{O_2}), in milliliters per deciliter of blood. A normal hemoglobin (Hb) concentration of 15 grams per deciliter of blood is assumed, as is an unshifted dissociation curve. Note that the curve descends steeply below Pa_{O_2} values of 50 to 60 mm Hg, indicating severely reduced oxygen-carrying capacity of Hb below this Pa_{O_2}. The lower line represents oxygen bound to Hb plus oxygen dissolved. Note that dissolved oxygen contributes little to Ca_{O_2} at a Pa_{O_2} in the normal range. (From Luce JM, Tyler ML, Pierson DJ: Intensive Respiratory Care. Philadelphia, W.B. Saunders Company, 1984.)

Therapy to Improve Arterial Oxygenation

The Pa_{O_2} may be improved by manipulating the variables that affect it: Pa_{CO_2}, PI_{O_2}, and $P(A - a)_{O_2}$. Thus, if hypoventilation is the sole cause of hypoxemia, as might be the case in a narcotic overdose, the Pa_{O_2} increases as the Pa_{CO_2} decreases in response to naloxone. Similarly, if the PI_{O_2} is reduced by the combustion of oxygen in a fire or by residence at high altitude, the Pa_{O_2} should improve if the patient breathes atmospheric air with an FI_{O_2} at the same PB as at sea level. Patients whose $P(A - a)_{O_2}$ is increased require therapy for the underlying cause of their hypoxemia as well as supplemental oxygen.

POSITIONING. Alveolar collapse, also called atelectasis, commonly occurs in dependent regions of the lung. Atelectasis is particularly problematic in supine patients whose lung expansion is limited by obesity, pain on deep breathing, or the presence of restricting bandages over the abdomen or chest. Positioning such patients upright from time to time and relieving their pain with narcotics may greatly improve the Pa_{O_2}.

Adults with unilateral parenchymal lung disorders, such as pneumonia, may become more hypoxemic when their diseased lung is dependent. The Pa_{O_2} of these patients may improve when they lie on the side of the nondiseased lung. Pulmonary edema fluid tends to collect in dependent lung regions because the intravascular hydrostatic pressure is greatest there. For this reason, the Pa_{O_2} of patients with pulmonary edema may improve, at least temporarily, if they are moved from the supine to the prone position. Unfortunately, such positioning may complicate nursing care.

OXYGEN DELIVERY SYSTEMS. Hypoxemia usually responds to increasing the FI_{O_2} and thereby the PI_{O_2}. The hypoxemia associated with disorders such as asthma and COPD that are characterized by ventilation-perfusion mismatching but not by intrapulmonary shunt usually is relieved by supplemental oxygen at a low FI_{O_2}. An FI_{O_2} of 0.24 to 0.35 can usually be achieved by delivering oxygen through nasal prongs at flow rates of 5 to 6 liters per minute; higher flow rates dry the nasal mucosa and do not further increase the FI_{O_2} because patients dilute the oxygen with ambient air. Open face masks provide a higher flow of humidified, premixed air and oxygen at an FI_{O_2} of up to 0.5. Such masks can be combined with a Venturi device that allows precise setting of the FI_{O_2} to avoid ventilatory depression in patients who have chronic carbon dioxide retention.

Tightly fitting face masks with a nonrebreathing valve and reservoir bag can be used to provide even higher concentrations of oxygen in patients whose hypoxemia is caused by shunting associated with disorders such as severe pneumonia and ARDS. Tightly fitting face masks are uncomfortable, however, and may cause nasal necrosis if left in place for several days.

ENDOTRACHEAL INTUBATION

INDICATIONS FOR INTUBATION. Humidified oxygen at an FI_{O_2} higher than 0.50 is most reliably delivered through the closed system provided by an endotracheal tube. The other indications for endotracheal intubation are listed in Table 71–6. Although intubation often precedes mechanical ventilation, it should be stressed that the indications for these two therapies and their timing are not necessarily the same. For example, some patients who are intubated to prevent aspiration of gastric contents never require mechanical ventilation.

KINDS OF INTUBATION. Endotracheal intubation may be performed either via the translaryngeal route through the nose or mouth or via a tracheostomy. Tracheostomy tubes once were used routinely in patients requiring intubation for longer than 1 or 2 days. However, the development of low-pressure and high-compliance cuffs that limit tracheal damage from nasal or oral

TABLE 71–6. INDICATIONS FOR ENDOTRACHEAL INTUBATION

To provide a closed system for mechanical ventilation or oxygen delivery, especially at a high fraction of inspired oxygen
To prevent or reverse upper airway obstruction
To protect against aspiration of gastric contents
To facilitate tracheobronchial toilet

tubes, the demonstration that such tubes can be left in place for weeks and even months without severe sequelae, and the documentation of complications after tracheostomy have led to a preference for orotracheal or nasotracheal intubation over tracheostomy in all but a few patients. Such patients include those with laryngeal fractures and those who will require intubation for longer than a month or so. Tracheostomy tubes generally are more comfortable than translaryngeal tubes. Tracheostomy tubes also are easier to suction through, and talking may be made possible by fitting the tubes with a device that directs a stream of air retrograde through the larynx above the cuff site.

Nasal intubation provides good support for the endotracheal tube and often allows patients to swallow their secretions better than when the tube passes orally. Oral intubation may allow passage of a tube with a larger diameter (8 mm or more) than that which the nostril will accommodate and usually is the preferred route during emergency intubations. Whichever route is chosen, the tube diameter should be sufficient to seal the trachea without cuff pressures in excess of 20 to 25 mm Hg. These pressures should be monitored regularly. Tube position should be determined by chest radiograph immediately following insertion and on a regular basis thereafter. Intubation of the right mainstem bronchus, which extends from the trachea at less of an angle than the left mainstem bronchus, should be sought in particular.

COMPLICATIONS OF INTUBATION. In one study, more than half of all patients receiving endotracheal intubation suffered adverse consequences. Excessive cuff pressure requirements (>20 mm Hg), self-extubation, and inability to seal the airway were the most common complications with nasotracheal and orotracheal tubes, occurring in 62 per cent of all endotracheal intubations. Problems associated with tracheostomy, which occurred in 66 per cent of intubations, included stomal hemorrhage, excessive cuff pressure requirements, and subcutaneous emphysema. Follow-up studies of patients receiving intubation and mechanical ventilation revealed a higher incidence of tracheal stenosis after tracheostomy (65 per cent) compared with translaryngeal intubation (19 per cent), although laryngeal complications were more common with nasal and oral tubes.

EXTUBATION. In general, endotracheal tubes may be removed when the original indications for their insertion are no longer present. For example, extubation frequently follows the return of consciousness and an adequate gag reflex in previously comatose patients or the restoration of adequate ventilation and arterial oxygenation in patients with respiratory failure. If an endotracheal tube has been in place only briefly, it may be removed after secretions have been suctioned from above the cuff site and the patient has been seated upright. Depending on physical and mental status, a patient with a tracheostomy may progress from a cuffed to a noncuffed or fenestrated tube and then may be extubated.

MECHANICAL VENTILATION

INDICATIONS FOR MECHANICAL VENTILATION. Mechanical ventilation may be necessary in patients who have inadequate ventilation, inadequate arterial oxygenation, or both. Furthermore, severe airway obstruction caused by asthma and COPD or parenchymal disease caused by disorders such as ARDS may increase the work of breathing to levels that cannot be maintained in spontaneous breathing. Finally, mechanical ventilation may be required in clinically unstable patients, such as those in shock, and in patients who require hyperventilation to decrease cerebral blood flow and intracranial pressure. These indications and severe physiologic abnormalities that may indicate the need for mechanical ventilation are listed in Table 71–7.

DEVICES TO ASSIST VENTILATION. Ventilation can be assisted by devices that substitute for the functions of the diaphragm. One such device is the rocking bed, which swings the patient in a 60-degree arc, forcing the weak or paralyzed diaphragm into inspiratory and expiratory positions by gravity. Another is the pneumobelt, which is used by patients in the sitting position. The pneumobelt intermittently squeezes the abdomen and forces the diaphragm cephalad. The diaphragm then falls owing to gravity, creating a marginally effective inspiration in the process.

NEGATIVE-PRESSURE VENTILATION. Ventilation can

TABLE 71–7. INDICATIONS FOR MECHANICAL VENTILATION

Acute hypercapnia
Minute ventilation greater than 10 L/min
Vital capacity less than 10–15 ml/kg body weight
Maximum inspiratory pressure more positive than −20 cm H_2O
Dead space to tidal volume fraction 0.60 or more
Acute hypoxemia (Pa_{O_2} less than 50–60 mm Hg, especially if inspired oxygen fraction is 0.4 or more, or $P(A − a)_{O_2}$ greater than 300 mm Hg on inspired FI_{O_2} of 1.0)
Clinical instability
Need for hyperventilation therapy

Pa_{CO_2} = systemic arterial carbon dioxide tension; Pa_{O_2} = systemic arterial oxygen tension; $P(A − a)_{O_2}$ = systemic alveolar-arterial oxygen pressure difference; FI_{O_2} = fraction of inspired oxygen.

also be supported by devices that generate a negative pressure around the chest during inspiration to substitute for the negative pleural and airway pressures normally created by contraction of the respiratory muscles. Negative-pressure ventilation can be achieved by enclosing the entire body, except the head and neck, in an "iron lung," by encompassing the thorax in a garment wrap, or by fitting a cuirass to the anterior chest. Like machines that substitute for the diaphragm, negative-pressure ventilators are best suited to stable patients with neuromuscular diseases whose lungs are normal and who do not require endotracheal intubation for delivery of oxygen at a high FI_{O_2}.

POSITIVE-PRESSURE VENTILATION. Because of the limitations of the aforementioned devices, positive-pressure ventilation (PPV) is the kind of mechanical ventilation most widely used today. With PPV, gas is delivered under positive pressure, usually through an endotracheal tube, into the airways and the lungs. In contrast to negative-pressure ventilation, PPV produces a positive airway pressure during inspiration. This pressure inflates the alveoli, providing both ventilation and arterial oxygenation while reducing the work of breathing.

Most positive-pressure ventilators may be used to deliver gas up to either a preset pressure or volume. The first approach allows limits to be established on the Pmax used for lung inflation but allows VT and hence VE to vary, depending on CRS. Alternatively, the ventilators may deliver a preset VT at whatever Pmax is required for lung inflation, which guarantees VE but may increase Pmax and pressure in the alveoli. Cycling of standard ventilators occurs whenever a certain pressure or volume is reached or at preset time intervals. Time-cycled ventilation is used primarily in infants or in adults who are ventilated at a high F that precludes pressure or volume cycling.

Modes of Positive-Pressure Ventilation. Perhaps the simplest mode of PPV is *controlled mechanical ventilation* (CMV), in which the ventilator delivers gas at a preset F and either a preset Pmax or VT (Table 71–8). Volume-cycled CMV most often is used in patients who are unconscious owing to illness or drugs, who are being intentionally hyperventilated, or who are recovering from anesthesia. Patients whose ventilatory drives are intact must often be hyperventilated or given sedatives to diminish their tendency to breathe asynchronously with the ventilator while receiving CMV. As with most other modes of PPV, an inspiratory to expiratory (I/E) ratio of 1:3 or less generally is used with CMV to allow adequate time for expiration and thereby avoid auto-PEEP. Because patients receiving CMV cannot increase their VE voluntarily, their ventilatory status must be followed closely. Thus, the advantage of CMV—complete control of ventilatory function—is also its major limitation.

Assisted mechanical ventilation (AMV) is a PPV mode in which the patient triggers the ventilator to deliver a preset VT. Triggering is accomplished by generating an airway pressure less than that in the ventilator and tubing; if the ventilator is sensitive to this pressure, it will increase F and VE in response to the demands of the patient. The machine will not trigger if it is insensitive, however, and if unduly sensitive it will trigger in response to small fluctuations in airway pressure in addition to attempts to breathe. The latter problem may be circumvented by establishing a proper sensitivity or, if this is not possible, by sedating the patient. Because sedation or neurologic changes may prevent patients from adjusting VE, an obligatory backup (or CMV) rate that will provide to the minimum allowable VE should

be used with AMV. The combination of AMV and CMV, which is called the assist/control mode, offers the great advantage of responding to changes in the patient's status without the close monitoring required of CMV. Traditionally, AMV and CMV have been referred to as intermittent positive-pressure ventilation (IPPV).

A third mode of PPV is *intermittent mandatory ventilation* (IMV), in which the ventilation delivers a preset VT at specific intervals while also providing a flow of gas for spontaneous breathing. The form of IMV most often used today is synchronized IMV (SIMV), in which ventilator breaths are delivered only after the end of a spontaneous expiration, so the patient's lungs are not hyperinflated by receiving spontaneous and machine-delivered inspirations simultaneously. With SIMV, the ventilator F may be set high enough to provide most, if not all, of the patient's VE initially; F then may be lowered as the patient improves. The potential benefits of SIMV include less asynchronous breathing and fewer sedation requirements, reducing mean airway pressure by combining spontaneous and machine breaths, and improving respiratory muscle function by allowing patients to breathe spontaneously. Disadvantages include the lack of a backup to guarantee VE in unstable patients and the possibility of causing respiratory muscle fatigue in patients who receive SIMV at a low ventilator F.

Another PPV mode is *high-frequency ventilation* (HFV), in which gas is delivered to the lungs using either a conventional ventilator with very high internal compressibility, high-pressure jet sources, or an oscillator that entrains ambient air. The ventilator F with HFV is greater than 60 per minute, the I/E ratio is very small, and the VT is either greater than the patient's anatomic VD (convective flow HFV) or less than the VD (nonconvective flow HFV). Although adequate ventilation with a VD/VT in excess of 1.0 would seem to be physiologically impossible, nonconvective flow HFV can achieve adequate carbon dioxide elimination in some patients, probably by enhanced diffusion in the lung. Both convective and nonconvective flow HFV usually produce a Pmax that is less than that with other modes of PPV, although the small I/E ratio usually produces auto-PEEP. The

TABLE 71–8. MODES OF POSITIVE-PRESSURE VENTILATION

Mode	Description	Advantages/Disadvantages
Controlled mechanical ventilation (CMV)	Ventilator F, VT (and thus VE) preset	May be used with sedation or paralysis; ventilator cannot respond to ventilatory needs
Assisted mechanical ventilation (AMV) or assist/control	Ventilator VT preset, but patient can increase F (and thus VE)	Ventilator may respond to ventilatory needs; ventilator may undertrigger or overtrigger, depending on sensitivity
Intermittent mandatory ventilation (IMV)	Ventilator delivers preset VT and F, but patient may also breathe spontaneously	May decrease asynchronous breathing and sedation requirements; ventilator cannot respond to ventilatory needs
Synchronized intermittent mandatory ventilation (SIMV)	Same as IMV, but ventilator breaths delivered only after patient exhales	Same as IMV, plus patient's lungs not overinflated by receiving spontaneous and ventilator breaths at same time
High-frequency ventilation (HFV)	Ventilator F is increased and VT may be smaller than VD	May reduce peak airway pressure; may cause auto-PEEP
Pressure support ventilation (PSV)	Patient breathes at own F; VT determined by inspiratory pressure and respiratory system compliance	Increased comfort and decreased work of breathing; ventilator cannot respond to ventilatory needs
Pressure control ventilation (PCV)	Ventilator peak pressure, F, and inspiratory time preset	Peak inspiratory pressures may be decreased; hypoventilation may occur
Inverse ratio ventilation (IRV)	Inspiratory time exceeds expiratory time	May improve gas exchange by increasing time spent in inspiration; may cause auto-PEEP

F = rate; VT = tidal volume; VD = dead space; VE = minute ventilation; PEEP = positive end-expiratory pressure.

lower Pmax supports the use of HPV in treating patients with bronchopleural fistulas and conditions such as ARDS. However, ventilation and arterial oxygenation may be inadequate with HFV.

Pressure support ventilation (PSV), a fifth mode of PPV, augments spontaneous ventilatory efforts with a level of positive airway pressure that is preset to achieve a desired VT. This mode of ventilation allows patients to set their own F and timing of breaths, which may be more comfortable than other modes of PPV. Pressure support ventilation also is useful in overcoming the work of breathing through an endotracheal tube. Inasmuch as patients must initiate breaths with PSV, it should not be used in unstable patients and is most applicable during weaning.

A sixth PPV mode is *pressure control ventilation* (PCV). With this mode, gas is not delivered at a constant VT. Instead, it is delivered until a preset Pmax is reached, and the patient's V̇E is determined by the preset Pmax, ventilator F, and inspiratory time. In contrast to the square wave gas flow pattern used with CMV and AMV, inspiratory flow with PCV decelerates when the Pmax is reached. Advocates of this mode state that complications are reduced with PCV because Pmax is limited. In addition, the decelerating waveform is thought to provide ventilation of more alveoli. This feature might be particularly helpful in patients with ARDS, although PCV may not provide a V̇E that is sufficient to prevent hypoventilation.

Inverse ratio ventilation (IRV) is the final mode of PPV discussed in this chapter. With IRV, the I/E ratio is increased above the normal level of 1:3 or less to 1:1 or more. The rationale for this approach is that the longer duration of inspiratory positive pressure will open stiff or fluid-filled alveoli and the shorter expiratory time will not allow these alveoli to collapse. Peak airway pressure may also be lower than with other modes of PPV, although the increase in I/E time probably increases auto-PEEP. One drawback to IRV is that this mode often is uncomfortable and requires sedation or paralysis of the patient.

Complications of Positive-Pressure Ventilation. One possible result of PPV is that inflation at high pressure may damage the lung. Such damage has been described traditionally as barotrauma, implying that it is the consequence of pressure changes. However, because alveolar distention occurs as a result of changes in pressure, "volutrauma" may be an equally accurate term. Pneumothorax is a common kind of barotrauma, but subcutaneous and mediastinal emphysema, parenchymal lung cysts, and systemic air embolism may also occur. Some investigators believe that PPV at high pressures and volumes also causes bronchopulmonary dysplasia and diffuse alveolar damage identical to what is found in ARDS and may either cause or perpetuate the syndrome.

In addition to these respiratory effects, PPV may also compromise the cardiovascular system. This is because the positive airway pressure during inspiration reduces venous return to the chest and may depress Q̇T. This effect may be increased if auto-PEEP is produced by PPV. On the other hand, it may be decreased if adequate time is allowed for airway and alveolar pressure to return to ambient levels during exhalation.

An early study reported pneumothorax in 4 per cent of patients receiving PPV in the form of CMV and AMV. Other complications included hyperventilation (11 per cent), hypoventilation (10 per cent), atelectasis (5 per cent), pneumonia (4 per cent), and massive gastric distention with air (1 per cent). Proponents of newer modes of PPV, such as PCV and IRV, claim that complications are limited with their use, but no data support this claim.

Weaning from Positive-Pressure Ventilation. Mechanical ventilatory support generally can be withdrawn when the reasons for its initiation no longer are present. This usually means complete or near-complete resolution of the patient's disease process, whether or not it involves the lungs. Such resolution should be reflected in clinical stability, a return of V̇E to below 10 l per minute, spontaneous VT to between 10 and 15 ml per kilogram, MIP to more negative than -20 cm H_2O, VD/VT to below 0.6, Pa_{O_2} to above 50 to 60 to 100 mm Hg on an FI_{O_2} of 0.4, and $P(A - a)_{O_2}$ to less than 300 mm Hg on an FI_{O_2} of 1.0.

Weaning from AMV and other modes of PPV may be accomplished by connecting the endotracheal tube to a piece of tubing, called a T-piece, that is connected to a source of oxygen that is diluted with air to create the desired FI_{O_2}. The patients then may breathe spontaneously through the T-piece at their own F and

TABLE 71–9. INDICATIONS FOR POSITIVE END-EXPIRATORY PRESSURE

To prevent or reverse atelectasis
To facilitate weaning from mechanical ventilation
To improve arterial oxygenation at a low inspired oxygen fraction

VT until they meet some or all of the weaning criteria just described. Otherwise healthy persons recovering from anesthesia or drug overdoses may be put on a T-piece when they wake up and may be extubated after a brief (15 to 30 minutes) period. Chronically ventilated patients may be put on a T-piece for a few minutes each hour or a few hours each day. When their respiratory muscles are less fatigued and they can tolerate longer periods on a T-piece, discontinuation of the ventilator may be appropriate.

Weaning from SIMV may be accomplished by progressively reducing the ventilator F until the patient can maintain an adequate V̇E by breathing spontaneously. Patients initially receiving AMV or other PPV modes can be weaned with SIMV without ever using a T-piece. Finally, SIMV and PSV may be combined to facilitate weaning. The PSV level is reduced as long as the patient's VT remains adequate; SIMV is begun at an intermediate rate and reduced to an F of 2 or so to inflate the lungs periodically and limit atelectasis.

POSITIVE END-EXPIRATORY PRESSURE

Positive end-expiratory pressure improves arterial oxygenation by increasing lung volume. This has the effect of preventing or reversing atelectasis and redistributing intra-alveolar edema fluid either into a thinner meniscus within the alveoli or out into the interstitium of the lung. The end result is recruitment of alveoli for better oxygen exchange. It should be noted that PEEP does not improve ventilation; in fact, the Pa_{CO_2} may increase because PEEP increases VD/VT by distending the airways and alveoli.

INDICATIONS FOR POSITIVE END-EXPIRATORY PRESSURE. One indication for PEEP is to prevent or reverse atelectasis (Table 71–9). For example, low levels of PEEP, such as 5 cm H_2O, are commonly administered to intubated patients who are supine in bed. Some investigators believe that low levels of PEEP facilitate weaning from mechanical ventilation by maintaining higher lung volumes while patients breathe through an endotracheal tube. They therefore continue PEEP during T-piece trials and when patients are receiving SIMV at a low ventilator F, with or without PSV.

The other major indication for PEEP is to improve arterial oxygenation in patients with diffuse parenchymal lung disorders, such as ARDS. Because their hypoxemia is primarily due to

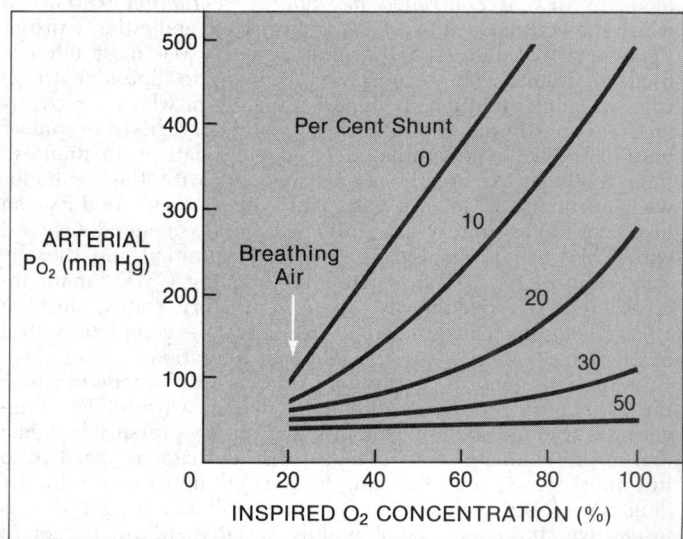

FIGURE 71–3. The relationship of the partial pressure of oxygen in systemic arterial blood (Pa_{O_2}) to the fraction of inspired oxygen (FI_{O_2}) with increasing amounts of shunt. Note that with 30 per cent of the cardiac output being shunted, there is only a slight increase in Pa_{O_2}. (From West JR: Pulmonary Pathophysiology: The Essentials. © 1977, The Williams & Wilkins Co., Baltimore.)

intrapulmonary shunt, such patients often cannot be oxygenated adequately even at an $F_{I_{O_2}}$ of 1.0, as illustrated in Figure 71–3. Administered in levels in excess of 5 cm H_2O, PEEP usually improves the Pa_{O_2} of these patients. It also allows the $F_{I_{O_2}}$ to be reduced to levels of 0.6 or less, thereby minimizing the risk of oxygen toxicity.

MODES OF POSITIVE END-EXPIRATORY PRESSURE. Positive end-expiratory pressure can be administered to spontaneously breathing patients through either a tightly fitting face mask or an endotracheal tube, in which case it is called continuous positive airway pressure (CPAP). It may also be combined with IPPV to create what is called continuous positive-pressure ventilation (CPPV). The improvement in oxygenation that may be produced by these two modes of PEEP depends primarily on the increase in lung volume they achieve, which in turn depends on the increase in airway pressure. As illustrated in Figure 71–4, the increase in airway pressure generally is greater with CPPV than with CPAP. Because of this, patients who merely have atelectasis may often be managed solely with CPAP. However, because they also have edema and because their ventilatory needs are greater, patients with diffuse parenchymal lung disease generally receive CPPV.

COMPLICATIONS OF POSITIVE END-EXPIRATORY PRESSURE. Like its benefits, the complications of PEEP are related to lung volume and airway pressure. The delivery of gas at high pressure to achieve an increase in lung volume throughout the ventilatory cycle is more likely to cause barotrauma (or "volutrauma") than is the delivery of pressurized gas solely during inspiration. It is also more likely to decrease venous return to the chest and thereby depress P_{SA} and $\dot{Q}T$. Although the incidence of complications due to PEEP has not been well studied, it appears to be significant if high levels are used.

WEANING FROM POSITIVE END-EXPIRATORY PRESSURE. Patients who are receiving low levels of PEEP for atelectasis can usually be weaned from PEEP without difficulty. Premature withdrawal or reduction of PEEP in patients with diffuse parenchymal lung disorders can worsen oxygenation, however, and cause clinical deterioration that requires hours or days of therapy to reverse. For this reason, PEEP should be withdrawn slowly, in small (2 to 5 cm H_2O) decrements, with close monitoring of Pa_{O_2} or Sa_{O_2} in such patients. Premature

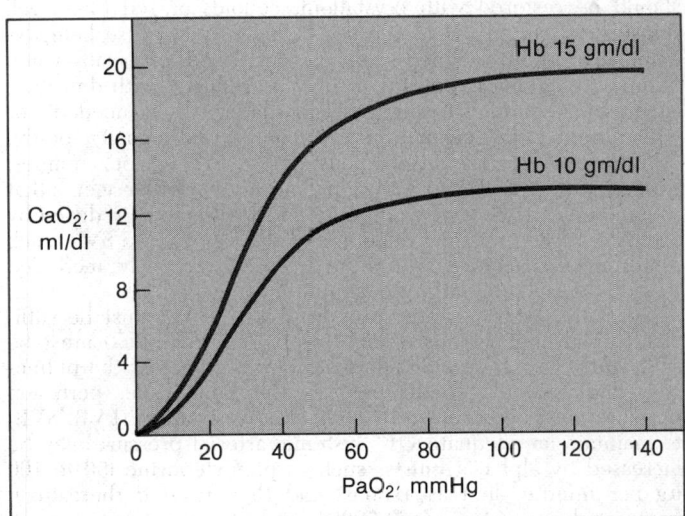

FIGURE 71–5. Importance of blood hemoglobin (Hb) concentration in oxygen transport. At a Pa_{O_2} of 80 mm Hg, arterial blood oxygen content (Ca_{O_2}) can be increased by 50 per cent by raising Hb from 10 to 15 grams per deciliter in an anemic patient. (From Luce JM, Tyler ML, Pierson DJ: Intensive Respiratory Care. Philadelphia, W. B. Saunders Company, 1984.)

reduction of PEEP can be avoided if the disease process for which PEEP was initiated has resolved or is substantially improved, if the Pa_{O_2} is 80 mm Hg or greater on an $F_{I_{O_2}}$ of 0.4 or less, and if these conditions have been present for several hours.

Therapy to Improve Oxygen Transport

Oxygen transport may be improved by manipulating the variables that affect it: Ca_{O_2} and $\dot{Q}T$. The major determinants of Ca_{O_2} are the Hb concentration and Sa_{O_2}. Most physicians are familiar with the need to optimize Sa_{O_2} by the methods discussed earlier, but many forget that T_{O_2} can often be improved by restoring the Hb concentration to normal, as depicted in Figure 71–5.

Carbon monoxide poisoning causes a functional anemia that may impair T_{O_2}. The oxyhemoglobin dissociation curve is also shifted to the left in patients with carbon monoxide poisoning, which results in less oxygen being available to the tissues. Because the Pa_{O_2} is normal, the possibility of carbon monoxide poisoning may be overlooked unless the Sa_{O_2} or the Ca_{O_2} is measured directly. Carbon monoxide poisoning is treated with supplemental oxygen at an $F_{I_{O_2}}$ of 1.0 and occasionally with hyperbaric oxygenation. Both of these maneuvers improve T_{O_2} by dissolving oxygen in plasma and displacing carbon monoxide from Hb.

Manipulation of $\dot{Q}T$ in patients with failure of oxygen transport often involves administration of drugs to alter HR, SV, and vascular pressures and resistances (Table 71–10). Alteration of HR includes measures to reverse bradyarrhythmias or tachyarrhythmias if they are present. In general, sinus bradycardia severe enough to compromise $\dot{Q}T$ and P_{SA} may be treated with parasympatholytic drugs, such as atropine (0.5 to 1.0 mg intravenously); with beta$_1$- and beta$_2$-adrenergic agonists, such as isoproterenol (1 to 2 mg in 500 ml of dextrose and water given at 2 to 20 μg per minute); or with cardiac pacing. Sinus tachycardia may be treated by correcting its underlying causes, which include hypovolemia, pain, and hyperthyroidism.

Supraventricular tachycardia may respond to vagal maneuvers, such as carotid sinus massage; beta$_1$ and beta$_2$ antagonists, such as esmolol (5 grams in 500 ml of dextrose and water given as a loading dose of 500 μg per kilogram over 1 minute, followed by an infusion of 50 μg per minute for 4 minutes); and calcium channel blockers, such as verapamil (5 to 10 mg given intravenously as needed). Ventricular tachycardia is treated with lidocaine or bretylium; ventricular fibrillation is treated with electrical defibrillation. The use of these therapies in cardiopulmonary resuscitation is discussed later.

Manipulation of SV requires alterations of its three determinants: preload, afterload, and contractility. For example, preload

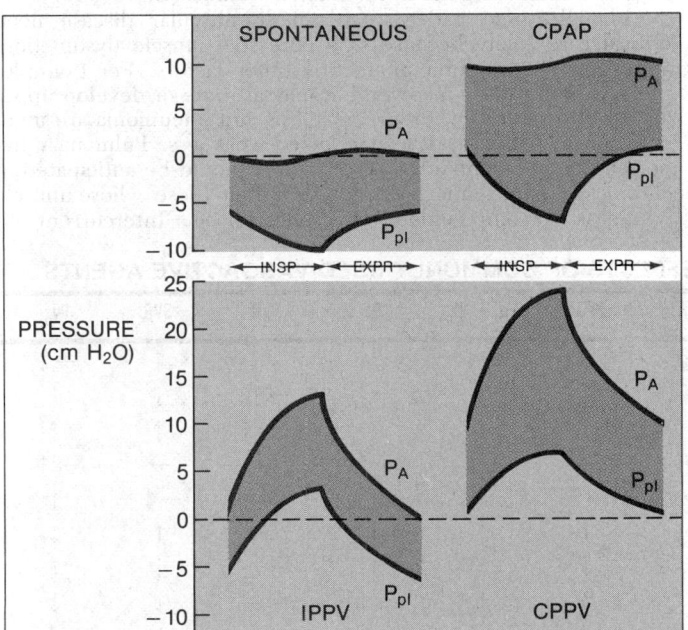

FIGURE 71–4. Schematic representations of airway (P_A) and pleural (P_{pl}) pressures with spontaneous respiration, spontaneous respiration with continuous positive airway pressure (CPAP), intermittent positive-pressure ventilation (IPPV), and continuous positive-pressure ventilation (CPPV). Note that with CPAP and CPPV, the pressure gradient between the airway and the pleural space is increased compared with spontaneous respiration and IPPV, respectively. (From Hinshaw HC, Murray JF [eds.]: Diseases of the Chest. Philadelphia, W.B. Saunders Company, 1980.)

should be restored with crystalloid, colloid, or red blood cell transfusions, when it is decreased sufficiently to cause hemodynamic compromise. When preload is increased, especially when pulmonary edema is present, it may be reduced with diuretics, such as furosemide (40 mg given intravenously as needed), or with nitroglycerin (given transcutaneously, sublingually, orally, or intravenously; the intravenous dose is 10 μg per minute, titrated as high as 200 to 300 μg per minute) or other agents that cause venodilation. Left ventricular afterload may be reduced by agents that cause arterial dilation and thereby reduce SVR, such as nitroprusside (10 μg per minute given intravenously, increased to as high as 300 to 400 μg per minute as needed).

Normally, arterial inflow pressures (PPA, PSA) must be sufficiently high and venous outflow pressures (PLA, PRA) must be sufficiently low to provide adequate perfusion across the pulmonary and systemic circulations. At the same time, perfusion pressure must be balanced by circulatory resistances (PVR, SVR) to maintain an adequate QT. Systemic arterial pressure may be increased by alpha₁ agonists, such as phenylephrine (50 to 100 μg per minute, first as a bolus and then titrated thereafter), norepinephrine (4 to 8 mg in 500 ml of dextrose and water, given at 4 to 12 μg per minute), or high-dose dopamine. Left atrial pressure and PRA may be reduced by nitrates and other agents that decrease preload. Similarly, SVR may be increased by alpha₁ agonists and decreased by drugs such as nitroprusside.

The drugs most commonly used to improve QT in critically ill patients are dopamine and dobutamine. Dopamine may be given in low doses (usually 2.0 to 5.0 μg per minute) to enhance renal and mesenteric perfusion through its dopaminergic effects. Intermediate-dose (5.0 to 10.0 μg per minute) dopamine improves QT through its beta₁ effects, whereas high-dose (>10.0 μg per minute) dopamine increases PSA through its alpha₁ properties. The pharmacologic effects of dopamine are not always predictable in all patients, and the drug must be carefully titrated to achieve its desired effects.

Unlike dopamine, dobutamine does not selectively enhance renal and mesenteric perfusion because it lacks dopaminergic properties. It also does not generally increase PSA or PAO because its alpha₁ properties are balanced by its beta₁ properties; in fact, dobutamine may reduce PSA and PAO in some labile patients when its beta₂ properties predominate. However, dobutamine improves QT through its beta₁ properties. If PSA is reduced, dobutamine may be combined with high-dose dopamine or other alpha₁ agonists. The usual dose of dobutamine is 2.5 to 10 μg per minute, up to a maximum dose of 30 μg per minute.

Therapy to Improve Oxygen Extraction

Oxygen extraction may be improved by increasing $\dot{V}O_2$. In patients with cyanide poisoning, this has traditionally involved administering amyl nitrate by inhalation and sodium nitrite intravenously; these drugs produce methemoglobin, which binds free cyanide ions. Intravenous sodium thiosulfate then is given to enhance conversion of cyanide to thiosulfate, which is less toxic and is readily excreted. Vitamin $B_{12}A$ will soon be available for treating cyanide poisoning in the United States.

Unfortunately, no simple antidote exists for the disturbances in oxygen extraction associated with distributive shock, ARDS, and MOSF. The general approach to these conditions is to improve T_{O_2}, as is discussed further on.

PATHOPHYSIOLOGY, MONITORING, AND MANAGEMENT OF COMMON CAUSES OF CIRCULATORY AND RESPIRATORY FAILURE

Neuromuscular Diseases Causing Respiratory Failure

A wide variety of neuromuscular diseases cause weakness or paralysis that may lead to hypercapnic respiratory failure. These disorders may involve the upper motor neurons (e.g., traumatic quadriplegia), lower motor neurons (e.g., amyotrophic lateral sclerosis), peripheral nerves (e.g., Guillain-Barré syndrome), myoneural junction (e.g., myasthenia gravis, botulism), or the muscles themselves (e.g., muscular dystrophies). The overall approach to patients with these conditions is to diagnose and treat specific neuromuscular disease, if possible, to ascertain precipitating factors prompting critical care unit admission, to evaluate the need for respiratory support, to provide such support on an acute basis, and to consider chronic support when required.

Once weakness or paralysis is appreciated, most neuromuscular diseases causing these symptoms can be differentiated by means of clinical characteristics, cerebrospinal fluid analysis, provocative tests such as the administration of cholinergic drugs, nerve conduction studies and electromyography, and occasionally muscle biopsy. In terms of specific therapy, plasmapheresis is used for patients with the Guillain-Barré syndrome (Ch. 497). Myasthenia gravis is treated with relatively long-acting anticholinesterase agents, such as pyridostigmine, and with plasmapheresis, corticosteroids, and thymectomy (Ch. 509). Specific therapy for botulism involves elimination of malabsorbed neurotoxin from the gut by means of enemas and gastric lavage, administration of trivalent antitoxin, administration of high-dose penicillin, and surgical debridement of contaminated wounds (Ch. 309).

Although some patients with neuromuscular disease need critical care solely because of progressive muscle dysfunction, admission often is precipitated by other factors. For example, patients with bulbar involvement may aspirate or develop upper airway obstruction, whereas atelectasis and pneumonia are more common in patients with generalized weakness. Pulmonary hypertension and right-sided heart failure should be anticipated in chronically hypoxemic patients, including those whose muscle weakness is compounded by kyphoscoliosis. Intercurrent ill-

TABLE 71–10. CARDIOVASCULAR AND RESPIRATORY EFFECTS OF COMMONLY USED VASOACTIVE AGENTS

Agent	HR	PSA	PRA	PPA	PPAO	C(a − v̄)O₂	QT	PVR	SVR	Pv̄O₂
Phenylephrine	→	↑	↑	→↑	↑	→↓	→	→↑	↑	→↓
Norepinephrine	↑	↑	↑	↑	↑	↓	→↑	→↑	↑	↑
Epinephrine	↑	↑	↑	→↑	↑	↓	↑	→	↑	↑
Dopamine, low dose	→	→	→	→	→	→↓	→↑	→	→	→↑
Dopamine, intermediate dose	↑	→	→	→	→↓	↓	↑	→	→↓	↑
Dopamine, high dose	→↑	↑	→	→	↑	↑	↓	→	↑	↓
Dobutamine	↑	↓	↓	→↓	↓	↓	↑	→↓	↓	↑
Isoproterenol	↑	↓	→↓	↓	↓	↑	→↑	→↓	↓	↓
Metaproterenol/albuterol	→↑	→↑	→	→↓	→	→	→↑	→	→	→
Nitroglycerin	→↑	↓	↓	→↓	↓	↓	↓	→↓	↓	↓
Nitroprusside	↑	↓	↓	→↓	↓	↓	↑	→↓	↓	↑
Esmolol	↓	→↓	→	→	→↑	→	↓	→	→	→
Morphine	→↑	→	↓	↓	↓	→	↑	↓	↓	↑

HR = heart rate; PSA = mean systemic arterial pressure; PRA = mean right atrial or central venous pressure; PPA = mean pulmonary arterial pressure; PPAO = mean pulmonary arterial occlusion pressure; C(a − v̄)O₂ = arterial–mixed venous oxygen content difference; QT = cardiac output; PVR = pulmonary vascular resistance; SVR = systemic vascular resistance; Pv̄O₂ = mixed venous oxygen tension.

nesses, such as urinary tract infection and pulmonary thromboembolism, may also occur.

The need for respiratory support in patients with neuromuscular disease can be assessed by the MIP and VC maneuvers. As noted earlier, intubation and mechanical ventilation generally are required if the MIP is less negative than -20 cm H_2O and the VC is approximately 10 ml per kilogram. It should be noted that impaired clearance of secretions may occur at a VC that is less than 30 ml per kilogram and may require intubation but not mechanical ventilation.

Hypoxemic respiratory failure in patients with neuromuscular disease can usually be treated adequately with supplemental oxygen delivered through nasal prongs or a face mask, coupled with frequent repositioning and the delivery of CPAP via a tightly fitting face mask to treat atelectasis. Intubation and mechanical ventilation are usually called for, however, if muscle strength and lung volumes have declined to the level mentioned previously and always are necessary if hypercapnia is acute and severe. Patients with rapidly reversible muscle weakness or paralysis should be intubated by the translaryngeal route in most instances, but tracheostomy is indicated if patients require intubation for longer than a month or so.

No particular kind of ventilatory support has been demonstrated to be superior in patients with neuromuscular disease, although PPV is preferred to negative-pressure ventilation in the critical care unit, especially if admission has been prompted by pneumonia or some other intermittent illness that requires supplemental oxygen at a high FI_{O_2}. The value of various modes of PPV is also open to debate. Nevertheless, because SIMV can be used only in those patients who can generate substantial inspiratory pressures, patients with severe weakness or paralysis are ventilated at least initially with CMV or AMV. In patients who are improving, SIMV may be used if it does not cause fatigue. Weaning by SIMV, T-piece, or PSV should be attempted only when patients demonstrate improvement in the MIP and VC.

Oxygen transport usually is adequate in patients with neuromuscular disease who are not hypoxemic or anemic and who do not have concurrent cardiac disease. Nevertheless, autonomic dysfunction in patients with Guillain-Barré syndrome and other disorders may take the form of either overactivity or underactivity of the sympathetic nervous system. Hypertension, diaphoresis, and tachycardia may be treated with titratable agents, such as esmolol, to prevent overswings in HR and P_{SA}. The hypotension that often accompanies spinal cord injury and other conditions may be treated with intravenous fluids or alpha$_1$ agonists, such as phenylephrine or high-dose dopamine. Bradycardia is treated with atropine. Patients with profound vagal tone in whom bradycardia progresses to asystole may be candidates for cardiac pacing.

Patients with neuromuscular disease also require emotional support. These patients frequently regress psychologically, owing occasionally to central nervous system involvement by their disease and more commonly to their complete dependence on the people caring for them. They and their families usually need frequent reminders that their needs will be met by nurses, physicians, respiratory therapists, and other health care professionals. If their neuromuscular disease can be corrected with time or treatment, they should also be told that their recovery can be expected, in months if not in days.

The difficult question remains of how to help patients who are not expected to recover neuromuscular function. Some patients whose phrenic nerve nuclei are damaged but whose phrenic nerves and diaphragm are intact may be candidates for electrophrenic ventilation, in which the nerves are repetitively stimulated in the lower neck or upper thorax. Others who maintain nearly normal arterial blood gas values only while awake may be ventilated during sleep with rocking beds, pneumobelts, chest cuirasses, and other negative-pressure devices, or by PPV delivered through the mouth or the nose or via a tracheostomy. Unfortunately, however, most patients with chronic severe neuromuscular disease must receive negative- or positive-pressure ventilation around the clock at home or in the hospital. This situation may be unacceptable to the patients and their families.

Asthma and Chronic Obstructive Pulmonary Disease

The primary pathophysiologic abnormalities in asthma and COPD are (1) an increased resistance in airflow resulting from narrowing of the airways by bronchospasm, inflammation, and mucus and (2) loss of airway tethering forces by parenchymal lung destruction. The airflow resistance causes air trapping and an abnormal increase in lung volume. Patients also have hypoxemia caused by mismatching of ventilation and perfusion and hypercapnia caused by the airways obstruction itself plus fatigue of the respiratory muscles.

In patients with asthma and COPD, Pa_{CO_2} usually begins to increase when the FEV_1 is reduced to approximately 750 ml or 25 per cent of the predicted value. This reduction may result from gradually progressive disease but more often occurs in the setting of acute exacerbations of obstruction due, for example, to acute bronchitis. An increase in Pa_{CO_2} without a deterioration in FEV_1 may be the result of decreased ventilatory drive due to narcotic or sedative drugs or the inhalation of oxygen at a high FI_{O_2}. Alternatively, it may result from increased $\dot{V}_{CO_2}$ in a patient with a limited ability to increase $\dot{V}_A$. As previously described, the distinction between acute and chronic respiratory acidosis can be determined by analyzing the relationships between Pa_{CO_2}, pH, and $[HCO_3^-]$. Acute hypoventilation obviously dictates a more prompt response than chronic partially compensated respiratory acidosis, as is also true in patients with neuromuscular disease.

Metabolic acidosis is a more ominous finding than pure respiratory acidosis in the setting of airways obstruction. It implies a failure of oxygen transport to meet the demands imposed by the increased work of breathing. This failure may result from a decrease in Ca_{O_2} due to processes such as hypoxemia or anemia or a decrease in $\dot{Q}_T$ due to concurrent ischemic heart disease, inadequate intravascular volume, or auto-PEEP caused by air trapping. Unless patients with inadequate oxygen transport improve, their condition will rapidly deteriorate.

Patients with asthma and COPD may be treated with beta$_2$-adrenergic agonists, theophylline, anticholinergic agents, and corticosteroids (Ch. 57 and 58). Beta$_2$ agonists, such as metaproterenol and albuterol, relax bronchial smooth muscle through their action on beta$_2$ receptors in the airways and have little effect on beta$_1$ receptors in skeletal muscles, systemic vessels, and the heart. They, therefore, are preferred to agents such as epinephrine and isoproterenol that have mixed beta$_1$ and beta$_2$ properties. The usually mild tachycardia, tremulousness, and other cardiovascular side effects of beta$_2$ agonists can be minimized if the drugs are taken in aerosol form. Average doses of aerosolized metaproterenol and albuterol are 15 mg and 2.5 mg, respectively, given every 2 to 4 hours.

Theophylline has fallen into disfavor because of its limited bronchodilating properties and its potential for toxicity. Theophylline may be administered as aminophylline in a loading dose of 5 to 6 mg per kilogram given intravenously, followed by an infusion of 0.4 to 0.9 mg per kilogram per hour to achieve a mean serum level of approximately 10.0 µg per milliliter. Serum levels should be followed regularly in patients receiving intravenous theophylline.

Aerosolized anticholinergic agents such as ipratropium bromide, which may be given via an inhaler at a dose of 0.04 mg every 2 to 4 hours, are both effective and safe owing to their lack of systemic side effects. Corticosteroids suppress inflammation and increase responsiveness to beta$_2$ stimulation. These agents are available in aerosol, oral, or intravenous forms. In patients critically ill with asthma and COPD, intravenous methylprednisolone is commonly administered in the range of 0.5 to 1.0 mg per kilogram four times per day.

Although hypoxemia invariably is present in patients with severe airways obstruction, the degree of reduction in Pa_{O_2} is generally not sufficient to require respiratory support other than supplemental oxygen delivered with external devices. Hypoxemia should usually be corrected only to a Pa_{O_2} of approximately 60 mm Hg, using as low an FI_{O_2} as possible to avoid ventilatory depression. If a high FI_{O_2} must be used in patients with intercurrent illnesses such as pneumonia, endotracheal intubation and mechanical ventilation may be required.

One cannot definitely state what the criteria are for intubating and ventilating patients with severe airways obstruction. Arterial blood gas and pH values at a single point in time showing marked acute respiratory acidosis with or without metabolic acidosis may be sufficient information on which to base the decision to provide mechanical ventilation. More commonly, however, it is necessary to evaluate the patient during a period while drugs are being administered and to assess the response to therapy. If blood gas values are worsening or not improving in spite of maximal treatment, mechanical ventilation is the next logical step. In addition to the objective evaluation provided by arterial blood gas and pH measurements, subjective assessments are also of value. Patients who are confused, somnolent, or uncooperative may require ventilatory support because their mental status may indicate inadequate oxygen transport and because they cannot cooperate with conservative management.

Severe airways obstruction presents a difficult situation in which to apply PPV. There is need to allow adequate expiratory time to avoid auto-PEEP, but also slow inspiratory flows are desirable to optimize the distribution of ventilation and to minimize the airway pressure required to deliver a preset V_T. To accomplish these goals, at least early in the course of mechanical ventilation, it often is necessary to sedate the patient receiving CMV or AMV in order to provide a slow ventilator F, which allows a small I/E ratio to be used. Some patients will benefit from SIMV in this situation. The V_T should be between 7 and 10 ml per kilogram, and the $F_{I_{O_2}}$ should be adjusted to provide an adequate Pa_{O_2}. The Pa_{CO_2} may rise owing to the relatively low F and V_T, but the pH will not fall precipitously if the rise is gradual. If the Pa_{CO_2} remains elevated, or if the patient already has chronic hypoventilation, it is important not to reduce the Pa_{CO_2} rapidly because doing so will result in uncompensated metabolic alkalosis.

Positive end-expiratory pressure would appear to be contraindicated in patients with asthma and COPD whose lung volumes already are increased above normal. Certainly, high levels of PEEP are potentially dangerous; they also are unnecessary because these patients do not have failure of arterial oxygenation due to diffuse parenchymal lung disease. Nevertheless, PEEP in levels of approximately 5 cm H_2O does not commonly cause hyperinflation in patients with airways obstruction. Indeed, low levels of PEEP may reduce the work or breathing of some obstructed patients by preventing airway collapse during expiration.

The adequacy of oxygen transport in patients with asthma and COPD can generally be assessed by physical examination, measurement of urine output, and monitoring of P_{SA}. Central venous and pulmonary artery catheterization is rarely required but may be helpful in evaluating patients whose Q_T is known or suspected to be depressed and in evaluating their response to fluids and agents such as dopamine or dobutamine. The elevation of P_{PAO} by auto-PEEP should be taken into account when estimating intravascular volume. Serial measurements of C_{eff} in ventilated patients may be useful in assessing the severity of airways obstruction and the response to therapy.

In patients with airways obstruction, weaning from mechanical ventilation may also present difficulties. Patients with asthma may usually be weaned and extubated quickly after they have responded to treatment. Patients with COPD may at best have marginal lung function, however, with persistent retention of carbon dioxide. In general, the arterial blood gas pattern that exists when the patient is "well" should be approximated while mechanical ventilation is still being used. Ideally, weaning with SIMV or a simple T-piece with or without PSV and small amounts of PEEP then can proceed, using previously described criteria.

In some instances, patients with COPD never meet the objective criteria for weaning and extubation. When this occurs, the decisions regarding weaning and extubation are based on subjective criteria, such as level of alertness, cooperation of the patient, and prognosis. These factors obviously cannot be quantitated. Once the patient has demonstrated the ability to maintain a desired V_E spontaneously for 30 to 60 minutes, the endotracheal tube should be removed.

It is important to determine which patients with COPD have a component of reversible respiratory dysfunction and which patients have simply reached the end stage of their disease, as is true of patients with neuromuscular disorders. Although chronic negative- or positive-pressure ventilation may be used to maintain life in a patient with end-stage airways obstruction, the decision

to pursue this course should be carefully considered by the patient and the family, preferably before mechanical ventilation is begun.

Adult Respiratory Distress Syndrome and Multiple Organ System Failure

A constellation of clinical, radiographic, and pathophysiologic findings that result from diffuse injury to the lung parenchyma defines ARDS. The characteristics of this syndrome are (1) severe hypoxemia due to intrapulmonary shunting of blood, (2) decreased C_{RS} due to decreased compliance of the lung, and (3) the presence of diffuse infiltration on the chest radiograph. The common abnormality that accounts for these features is an increase in the permeability of the endothelium of the pulmonary capillary and the epithelium of the alveolar wall. This increased permeability allows fluid to leak from the capillary into the alveolus, even though the hydrostatic pressure within the capillary is normal; hence, noncardiogenic pulmonary edema results.

The adult respiratory distress syndrome is associated with a variety of clinical conditions, the most common of which is sepsis syndrome. A partial list of these conditions is found in Table 71–11. The injury to the lung that occurs in these conditions may be delivered either via the airways or via the circulation. In many instances (e.g., gastric aspiration or diffuse pneumonia), lung injury would appear to be direct. In others (e.g., sepsis syndrome or pancreatitis), the injury presumably is indirect and is mediated by circulating substances.

Regardless of the type or mechanism of injury, the damage to the lungs of patients with ARDS is diffuse, compared with the damage in diseases such as unilateral pneumonia. The damage is nonhomogeneous, however, and some areas of lung parenchyma may be spared. In damaged areas, the lung is atelectatic, edematous, and hemorrhagic. Microscopic examination reveals intra-alveolar collections of proteinaceous fluid, red blood cells, and inflammatory cells. Microthrombi or white cell aggregates may be seen in small vessels. After 24 to 48 hours, hyaline membranes formed by fibrin that has escaped through the capillaries line the alveoli. Subsequently, as repair of the injury occurs, fibrosis may ensue.

Reduction in lung volume is characteristic of ARDS and is caused by a combination of atelectasis, edema fluid, and inflammation and perhaps fibrosis replacing alveolar air. This decrease in lung volume contrasts with the increase in lung volume of patients with airways obstruction. It is largely responsible for the decrease in C_{RS} associated with ARDS, which traditionally has been attributed primarily to lung stiffness. The work of breathing increases considerably because of the decreased C_{RS}.

The major and most frequent gas exchange abnormality in ARDS is hypoxemia caused by the loss of functional alveoli. In severe forms of ARDS, as the process evolves from injury to repair, gas exchange abnormalities also evolve. Lung fibrosis may result in obliteration of capillaries and coalescence of alveoli to produce an increased V_D/V_T. Unless V_E can be increased, which may be difficult, hypercapnia will result.

Some, but not all, patients with ARDS develop dysfunction or failure of one or more organ systems sequentially or simultaneously. By contrast, other patients develop the syndrome of MOSF without having ARDS, although they may have less severe degrees of parenchymal lung injury. Multiple organ system failure is associated with the same clinical conditions as ARDS. Furthermore, as with ARDS, it most commonly is associated with sepsis syndrome. This observation suggests that ARDS is a respiratory manifestation of MOSF, just as distributive shock is

TABLE 71–11. CONDITIONS ASSOCIATED WITH THE ADULT RESPIRATORY DISTRESS SYNDROME AND MULTIPLE ORGAN SYSTEM FAILURE

Sepsis syndrome
Severe trauma
Diffuse pneumonia
Burns and smoke inhalation
Multiple transfusions
Pancreatitis
Anaphylaxis
Drug overdose
Cardiorespiratory arrest

a cardiovascular manifestation. Alternatively, ARDS and MSOF may be aspects of sepsis syndrome. Indeed, some investigators have broadened the use of the term sepsis syndrome to include any generalized inflammatory process that may cause or contribute to widespread organ dysfunction.

This generalized inflammatory process may be mediated by a variety of circulating substances with vasoactive, inflammatory, and tissue-damaging properties. These substances, which may include endotoxin, histamine, arachidonic acid metabolites, complement, myocardial depressant factor, and tumor necrosis factor, may cause systemic vasodilation, microvascular vasoconstriction, altered myocardial contractility, capillary microembolization, and endothelial cell disruption. The end result is increased capillary permeability with intravascular fluid loss, interstitial fluid accumulation, impaired microcirculatory blood flow, and inadequate tissue oxygenation in the lungs and other organs. Patients may die of refractory hypotension, hypoxemia attributable to ARDS, or other manifestations of MOSF, such as disseminated intravascular coagulation.

The diagnoses of ARDS and MOSF are made clinically because there are no reliable markers for the disorders. The diagnoses are supported by documenting the presence of the associated conditions just discussed. Pulmonary artery catheterization, which may aid in management, also suggests the diagnosis of ARDS and MOSF if the characteristic patterns of distributive shock and inadequate oxygen extraction are observed.

It is not clear whether the term sepsis syndrome should be applied to patients with ARDS and MOSF who are not truly infected. Nevertheless, such patients probably should be assumed to be infected unless there is another explanation for their condition. If bacterial infection is suspected or known to exist, broad-spectrum antibiotics, such as ampicillin, metronidazole, and gentamicin, should be given intravenously to cover gram-positive and gram-negative pathogens, and the choice of agent then tailored to culture results. Suspected or documented infections with other organisms should be treated appropriately. In addition, abscesses should be sought by computed tomography (CT) and other techniques when appropriate. If detected, they should be drained percutaneously or at surgery.

The unusual patient with MOSF who does not have severe parenchymal lung disease may benefit from endotracheal intubation and mechanical ventilation merely because he or she is hemodynamically unstable. Vital organ perfusion may also be enhanced if the work of breathing is reduced by mechanical ventilation. Patients with ARDS, however, invariably require both PPV and PEEP to improve arterial oxygenation. The need for such support may be evaluated by monitoring the Pa_{O_2} and $P(A - a)_{O_2}$. Respiratory or metabolic acidosis is ominous in this setting. Because patients with ARDS, MOSF, or both may deteriorate rapidly, it generally is better to provide intubation and mechanical ventilation earlier rather than later.

The use of PPV in patients with ARDS and MOSF varies. Most physicians probably administer CMV, AMV, or IMV with a V_T of 10 to 15 ml/kg, an I/E ratio of 1:3 or greater, and a Pmax as required to deliver a V_T in the aforementioned range. Positive end-expiratory pressure is used at levels necessary to reduce the FI_{O_2} to 0.6 or less. Increasing concern over the possible effects of high alveolar pressures and volumes in causing barotrauma has led some investigators to advocate the use of HFV, PCV, and IRV despite the fact that these newer modes of PPV have not been shown to be superior to older ones. When older modes of PPV are employed, it is argued, V_T should be as low as 5 to 7 ml per kilogram, ventilators should be pressure cycled, and high levels of PEEP should be avoided if possible, even if the FI_{O_2} exceeds 0.6 in the process.

It is not clear that the current concepts of the pathogenesis of lung injury and therapies based upon them will prove superior to concepts and therapies accepted earlier. Nevertheless, it does appear prudent to use all modes of PPV and PEEP carefully. Most patients with ARDS and MOSF probably can be adequately ventilated and oxygenated by CMV, AMV, and IMV at a relatively low V_T and a Pmax of less than 50 cm H_2O. If Pmax exceeds this amount, PCV may be added with or without IRV. Positive end-expiratory pressure should be used at the lowest possible level to achieve an FI_{O_2} of 0.6 or less.

Because barotrauma is such a concern, CSTAT should be monitored frequently in patients receiving PPV and PEEP. In addition, the amount of auto-PEEP should be measured by the method cited previously. Although the auto-PEEP often caused by PCV and IRV has been considered undesirable, auto-PEEP may be just as potentially useful as intentionally administered PEEP in recruiting alveoli. The important point is to include the amount of auto-PEEP in the overall measurement of PEEP so that its effects can be anticipated.

Appropriate use of intravenous fluid is an essential component of the management of ARDS and MOSF. Because pulmonary capillary permeability is increased, administration of fluid, which raises the capillary hydrostatic pressure, tends to increase the amount of lung water. The relationship between capillary hydrostatic pressure and extravascular lung water is shown schematically in Figure 71–6.

On the other hand, adequate pulmonary perfusion may be important in preventing or ameliorating lung damage, and systemic perfusion clearly is essential in maintaining renal, cardiac, and central nervous system function. Thus, the effects of crystalloid, colloid, or red blood cell administration should be carefully monitored with clear endpoints in mind. In addition to measuring PsA and other variables, indices of end-organ perfusion, such as urine output and mental status, should be followed.

Pulmonary artery catheterization may be extremely helpful in assessing hemodynamic status, at least early in the course of ARDS and MOSF. Although the correlation between PPAO and the outcome of these disorders has not been determined, it appears reasonable to maintain the PPAO at a normal or slightly lower than normal level as long as perfusion of vital organs is maintained. If perfusion is inadequate or if QT is depressed by the patient's underlying disease or its treatment, the circulation can be supported with dopamine or dobutamine

Ideally, the combination of specific therapy for associated conditions, such as sepsis syndrome, and appropriate cardiovascular and respiratory system support should improve TO_2 in patients with ARDS and MOSF. It is important to keep this goal in mind for at least three reasons. First, TO_2 and its components (Ca_{O_2} and QT) can be quantified, and therapies that increase one component at the expense of the other may be modified. Second, because there is no specific antidote for the inadequate oxygen extraction that so often characterizes ARDS and MOSF, therapies to improve TO_2 are the only ones available.

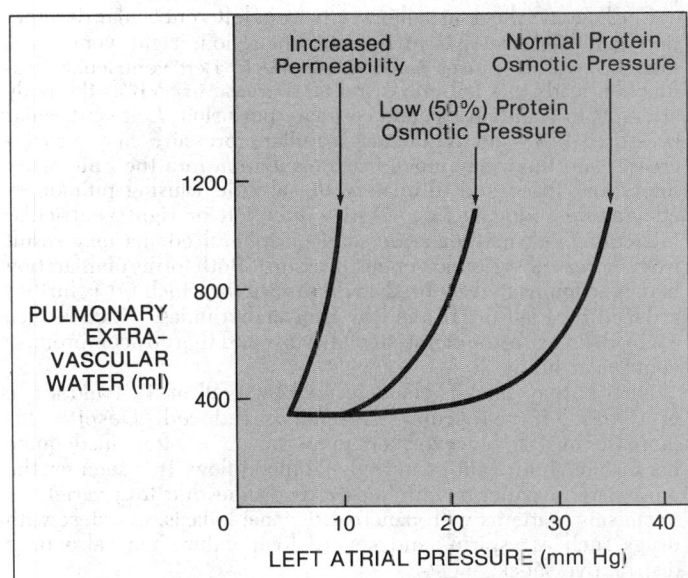

FIGURE 71–6. Schematic representation of the relationship between pulmonary extravascular water volume and left atrial or pulmonary artery occlusion pressure. Right curve represents the relationships when both microvascular permeability and plasma protein osmotic pressures are normal; middle curve represents normal permeability but a reduction in plasma protein osmotic pressure of 50 per cent; left curve shows relationship when permeability of the capillaries is increased (From Hopewell PC, Murray JF: Adult respiratory distress syndrome. *In* Moser KM, Spragg RG [eds.]: Respiratory Emergencies. 2nd ed. St. Louis, The C.V. Mosby Company, 1982; with permission.)

A third reason to improve $\dot{T}o_2$ is that the apparent failure of oxygen extraction in patients with ARDS and MOSF may actually be a complicated form of failure of oxygen transport. This is supported by the demonstration that $\dot{V}o_2$ appears to be dependent upon $\dot{T}o_2$ at some critical level of $\dot{T}o_2$ in these conditions. It is also supported by the finding that some patients with ARDS and MOSF increase $\dot{V}o_2$ and resolve their lactic acidosis with increases in $\dot{T}o_2$. Given this finding, some investigators advocate fluid loading, hypertransfusion with red blood cells, or the administration of dobutamine to patients with ARDS and MOSF to increase Ca_{o_2} and $\dot{Q}_T$ to arbitrarily high levels. The general benefit of this approach has not been determined, however, and it cannot be recommended at the present time.

Large doses of corticosteroids, such as methylprednisolone, have also been given to patients with sepsis syndrome, ARDS, and MOSF and to those at risk of these disorders. These agents have not been shown to improve outcome from the sepsis syndrome, to prevent or ameliorate ARDS, or to influence the development of MOSF, however. Prostaglandin E_1, a pulmonary vasodilator with anti-inflammatory properties, also does not improve survival despite its salutary effect on $\dot{Q}_T$. Broad-spectrum nonabsorbable antibiotics have been given to some patients in the hope that selective decontamination of the gut may reduce a potential source of bacteria and endotoxin, but few data support this strategy. Studies of antiendotoxin antibodies currently are being performed in the hope that these agents will affect the underlying pathogenesis of these conditions. Other experimental therapies designed to neutralize other mediators and cytokines that may be responsible cannot be recommended until they are proved effective in large clinical trials.

Shock (also see Ch. 41)

The concepts contained in Equations 11 and 12 help to explain the various kinds of shock that produce inadequate oxygen transport and oxygen extraction. For example, hypovolemic shock, in which $\dot{Q}_T$ is depressed because SV is inadequate, is associated with either hemorrhage or other intravascular fluid losses. Obstructive shock may result from pulmonary thromboembolism, in which right ventricular output falls because P_{PA} and PVR increase, or from cardiac tamponade, in which an accumulation of pericardial fluid interferes with ventricular filling and SV.

Cardiogenic shock usually results from left ventricular dysfunction following massive myocardial infarction; right ventricular infarction rarely causes cardiogenic shock. Left ventricular dysfunction leads to a fall in SV and an increase in SVR as the body attempts to maintain P_{SA} and coronary perfusion. Left ventricular pressure, P_{LA}, and pulmonary capillary pressure may also increase, and fluid may move via transudation into the pulmonary interstitial space and ultimately the alveoli, causing pulmonary edema and reducing Pa_{o_2}. With either left or right ventricular infarction, P_{RA} may increase, and peripheral edema may result from increased systemic venous pressure. Both forms of infarction may be complicated by bradyarrhythmias, in which $\dot{Q}_T$ is further reduced by a fall in HR, and by tachyarrhythmias, which reduce SV by decreasing the duration of diastole and thereby compromise ventricular filling.

Distributive shock is characterized by a fall in SVR and a rise in $\dot{Q}_T$ as left ventricular afterload is reduced. Despite this increase in $\dot{Q}_T$, however, organ perfusion is often inadequate because of abnormalities in regional blood flow. It is seen for the most part in patients with sepsis syndrome due to a variety of organisms. Patients with pancreatitis, anaphylaxis, overdose with drugs such as aspirin, and severe liver failure may also have distributive shock.

The monitoring of patients with all kinds of shock should involve repeated measurement of vital signs and urine output. Because most patients with shock are hypotensive, they may require systemic arterial catheterization for continuous measurement of P_{SA}. The combination of systemic and pulmonary artery catheterization may also aid in their evaluation and management.

Treatment of the various kinds of shock is based on their underlying pathophysiology. For example, hypovolemic shock is best treated with intravascular fluids, including blood, that restore preload. Alpha$_1$ agonists, such as phenylephrine or high-dose

dopamine, that increase P_{circ} and R_{circ} should be used only temporarily to support P_{SA} because they do not affect the underlying volume loss. Similarly, obstructive shock should be treated with measures that relieve the obstruction. Thus, the abnormal rise in P_{PA} and PVR that accompanies pulmonary thromboembolism may be ameliorated by thrombolytic agents. Oxygen should also be administered to prevent increases in PVR caused by alveolar hypoxia. At the same time, SV may be restored in patients with cardiac tamponade by removing pericardial fluid. The circulation can be supported in patients with these conditions with volume infusion and dobutamine to increase $\dot{Q}_T$, given in concert with alpha$_1$ agonists, if necessary, to maintain P_{SA} and perfusion of the coronary circulation.

The treatment of cardiogenic shock following left ventricular infarction depends on the patient's P_{LA}, as approximated by P_{PAO}. If the P_{PAO} is decreased, $\dot{Q}_T$ may be increased by improving preload. Conversely, if P_{PAO} is increased, it may be decreased by agents that reduce preload, left ventricular afterload, or both variables. Morphine (1 to 10 mg or more given intravenously) is a potent venodilator that reduces preload; this agent also relieves pain and thereby reduces the liberation of endogenous catecholamines that increase SVR during infarction. Nitroglycerin also reduces preload by its effects on the venous circulation and limits ischemia through coronary vasodilation. Nitroprusside is preferred in reducing afterload because its effects are more pronounced on the arterial circulation. It should be noted that decreasing P_{PAO} by reducing preload or afterload will in turn reduce pulmonary capillary pressure and edema formation and also P_{RA}. If right ventricular infarction has occurred, the output of that ventricle may be improved either by volume infusion or by dobutamine. In patients with infarction of either ventricle, P_{SA} may be supported with alpha$_1$ agonists, if necessary, to ensure adequate coronary perfusion.

The general approach to patients with distributive shock is to ensure adequate preload, to add alpha$_1$ agonists to increase P_{SA} and SVR if necessary, and to administer dopamine in low doses to maintain renal and mesenteric blood flow. Dopamine may also be used in beta$_1$- and alpha$_1$-range doses in patients with sepsis syndrome, pancreatitis, and severe liver failure. Epinephrine, which also has alpha$_1$ and both beta$_1$ and beta$_2$ properties, traditionally has been given to patients with anaphylaxis at doses of 0.5 to 1.0 mg (5 to 10 ml of a 1:10,000 solution). Although dobutamine may be useful in increasing $\dot{Q}_T$ in patients with distributive shock, it may cause hypotension and require the simultaneous administration of alpha$_1$ agonists. Isoproterenol probably should be avoided because it is a beta$_1$ and beta$_2$ agonist without alpha$_1$ effects and therefore has unopposed vasodilating properties.

Finally, many patients in shock require mechanical ventilation because of lung disease or to decrease respiratory work. If patients with shock are allowed to breathe spontaneously, a greater portion of the $\dot{Q}_T$ must be diverted to the respiratory muscles. Perfusion of the heart and brain is aided when PPV is provided to experimental animals in shock.

Cardiorespiratory Arrest

Cardiorespiratory arrest is the most profound form of cardiogenic shock and also the most extreme example of failure of oxygen transport. Cessation of effective $\dot{Q}_T$ may be the culmination of a variety of shock states but most commonly is the result of ventricular fibrillation, occurring either primarily or in the course of left ventricular infarction. As $\dot{Q}_T$ abruptly falls, release of catecholamines results in peripheral vasoconstriction in an attempt to preserve blood flow to the brain, heart, and respiratory muscles at the expense of other organs, just as occurs in less severe shock. Lactic acid production increases unless $\dot{Q}_T$ is restored, and the effectiveness of catecholamines is diminished. This in turn results in generalized vasodilation that reduces the distribution of blood flow to vital organs.

Oxygen consumption by the brain is normally about 5 ml of oxygen per minute per 100 grams of brain tissue, and cerebral blood flow averages 50 ml per minute per 100 grams of tissue. Cerebrovascular resistance is minimal during cardiorespiratory arrest because the cerebral circulation cannot autoregulate, so cerebral blood flow is totally dependent on cerebral perfusion pressure, determined by the $\overline{P_{SA}}$ minus intracranial pressure

(ICP), the effective venous outflow pressure of the brain. Central nervous system injury develops when cerebral blood flow is less than approximately 18 ml per minute per 100 grams of tissue. Anaerobic cerebral metabolism is stimulated, but the subsequent increase in lactic acid further induces neuronal damage. Because oxygen utilization is nonuniform within the brain, some areas, such as the frontal and temporal lobes, are more susceptible to ischemia than are areas of lower metabolic activity.

Myocardial $\dot{V}_{O_2}$ is approximately 10 ml of oxygen per minute per 100 grams of tissue in the normally beating heart and 5 ml of oxygen per minute per 100 grams of tissue during ventricular fibrillation. Assuming a normal Ca_{O_2} and an oxygen extraction of 75 per cent, a myocardial blood flow of 60 ml per minute per 100 grams of tissue would be required to meet normal metabolic needs; with ventricular fibrillation this figure would be 25 ml per minute per 100 grams of tissue. Coronary vascular resistance is also likely to be minimal during cardiorespiratory arrest unless coronary vascular disease is present, so myocardial blood flow will be dependent on coronary perfusion pressure, which is the difference between P_{SA} and P_{RA} during diastole. As P_{SA} falls during arrest, myocardial blood flow will fall below the vital levels given earlier, and ischemic injury will result. Myocardial injury will be particularly severe in the presence of coronary artery disease unless metabolic needs are reduced as blood flow is restored.

Cardiorespiratory arrest is treated with cardiopulmonary resuscitation (CPR). This technique is based on the goal of augmenting both Ca_{O_2} and $\dot{Q}T$ by a series of basic life support maneuvers until advanced cardiac life support can be applied (Table 71–12). An important determinant of success in CPR is the provision of adequate $\dot{V}_A$ to normalize Pa_{CO_2} and pH. When cardiac arrest occurs in nonintubated patients, the first step is to open the airway and ensure its patency. The most common cause of obstruction is the tongue. This situation may be corrected simply by tilting the head backward and lifting the chin or lower jaw forward. Mouth-to-mouth ventilation then has to be applied unless a foreign body is obstructing the airway. Two quick breaths sufficient to make the chest wall rise should be given in single-rescuer CPR.

A resuscitator's exhaled air may provide an $F_{I_{O_2}}$ of approximately 0.17 during mouth-to-mouth ventilation, and carbon dioxide will be eliminated because of passive lung deflation. This should alleviate the need for HCO_3^-, which is no longer recommended to reverse metabolic acidosis because it adds carbon dioxide to the body and may cause respiratory acidosis. Commonly, however, oxygen exchange within the lungs is not normal, and significant hypoxemia develops. For this reason, supplemental oxygen should be administered as soon as it is available. Both oxygenation and ventilation can be accomplished via a tightly fitting face mask and ventilation bag, preferably one capable of delivering an $F_{I_{O_2}}$ of 1.0. Endotracheal intubation provides the most reliable closed system for oxygenation and ventilation and also protects the airway against the aspiration of gastric contents.

Closed-chest compression should be administered to patients who do not have a palpable pulse. The patient should be supine and on a firm surface. Sufficient pressure should be applied to the lower half of the sternum to depress it 4 to 5 cm in most adults and 2 cm in children in order to increase P_{SA}. The pressure should be relaxed after each compression, allowing the sternum to return to its relaxed position, which will reduce P_{RA} and enhance coronary perfusion. The recommended compression-relaxation ratio is 1:1, and the rate of compressions should be between 80 and 100 per minute. The adequacy of closed-chest compression should be determined by attempting to palpate a carotid or femoral pulse produced by the compression.

The mechanism by which closed-chest compression causes

TABLE 71–12. BASIC LIFE SUPPORT

Establish unresponsiveness
Call for help
Position victim
Open airway
Check for foreign body in airway
Institute mouth-to-mouth breathing
Check for pulse
Initiate closed-chest compression

blood to circulate is not clear. The original "cardiac pump" theory held that by compressing the chest the heart was squeezed between the sternum and the vertebral column, producing a mechanical systole in which right and left ventricular pressures exceed pulmonary artery and aortic pressures, respectively, causing forward blood flow. Release of the pressure caused diastolic filling of the ventricles because of the gradient between the peripheral venous system and the intrathoracic structures. More recent data suggest that it is the total intrathoracic pressure that causes forward blood flow rather than cardiac compression ("thoracic pump" theory). For example, cough in itself has sustained cardiac output and consciousness in patients with ventricular fibrillation. A variety of experimental studies are consistent with this contention, but "new CPR" based on this model has not proved to be more effective than conventional CPR.

The arrival of persons with additional training or equipment marks the start of advanced cardiac life support. Electrocardiographic monitoring enables proper application of direct-current countershock for defibrillation or conversion of ventricular tachycardia. A current of 200 to 360 joules should be used for ventricular fibrillation. The current given should be increased if there is no response to the initial shock. In patients with ventricular fibrillation, epinephrine should be administered, routinely in doses of 1 mg, or 10 ml of a 1:10,000 dilution, either intravenously (preferably via a central venous catheter) or via an endotracheal tube before countershock is applied. Epinephrine constricts peripheral vessels through its alpha$_1$ effects and enhances myocardial contractility through its beta$_1$ effects; this combination improves cerebral and cardiac perfusion. Intravenous lidocaine in a bolus of 1 mg per kilogram, followed by additional boluses and a continuous infusion of 1 to 4 mg per minute, may also be helpful in treating ventricular ectopy, as may bretylium (initial intravenous bolus of 5 to 10 mg per kilogram, followed by an infusion of 1 to 2 mg per minute). Calcium chloride is no longer recommended in the treatment of cardiorespiratory arrest because it has not been shown to be effective and because it may contribute to ischemic injury.

All patients who have been resuscitated successfully should be transferred as quickly as possible to a critical care unit if they are not there already. At a minimum, electrocardiographic monitoring should be provided. The need for pulmonary artery catheterization depends on the causes and consequences of the cardiorespiratory arrest. Often, at least transiently, it is necessary to provide mechanical ventilation to allow rest and functional recovery of the respiratory muscles and to minimize their oxygen needs.

The major determinant of return of brain function is the adequacy of cerebral perfusion during the period of cardiac arrest. Subsequently, after recovery of cardiac function, all factors that influence oxygen delivery to the brain should be evaluated and made normal when possible. Measures to prevent possible elevations in ICP, such as head elevation, controlling arterial pH and Pa_{CO_2}, and treating seizures and agitation, should be undertaken. Barbiturate loading has not been demonstrated to minimize brain damage; calcium channel blocking agents are being studied at the present time.

ETHICAL ISSUES IN CRITICAL CARE MEDICINE

Critical care units have been utilized in more or less their present form for approximately 25 years, yet their contribution to health care has not been quantified. Studies of patients suspected of having a myocardial infarction have suggested that if there are no early (initial 2 hours in one study, at 24 hours in another) indications of complications, management in a coronary care unit does not offer any advantage over management in a hospital room or at home. Similarly, the outcome of patients with bacteremic pneumococcal pneumonia has not been found to be improved by critical care.

Other diseases commonly encountered in the critical care setting continue to have a poor outcome. One study demonstrated that the in-hospital mortality rate for patients with ARDS who required mechanical ventilation with an $F_{I_{O_2}}$ of 0.5 or greater for more than 24 hours was 66 per cent; patients who required an $F_{I_{O_2}}$ of 1.0 with a PEEP level of 5 cm H_2O or more for 2 hours, or an $F_{I_{O_2}}$ of 0.6 and a PEEP level of 5 cm H_2O or more for 12 hours, had a mortality rate of 92 per cent. The mortality rates of patients with cardiogenic and distributive shock remain between 50 and 75 per cent despite the introduction of pulmonary artery catheterization, a finding that has led to questions regarding the value of this monitoring technique. Cardiopulmonary resuscitation, when performed on hospitalized patients or persons older than 70 years of age out of the hospital, may be successful less than 10 per cent of the time. The survival rate of patients with three or more organ failures after 5 days in a critical care unit approached zero in one large investigation.

Data such as these imply that critical care is of little or no value in several categories of illness. Yet patients in the postoperative period and patients with cardiac arrhythmias, narcotic and sedative drug overdose, reversible neuromuscular diseases, hypovolemic and obstructive shock, and asthma and COPD clearly benefit from critical care. Furthermore, most clinicians treating severely ill patients have hope that the patients will survive, and they thus request that critical care be provided, almost regardless of the published prognosis. One reason for this is that prognostication is difficult in individual patients despite data derived from groups. Another is that patients and their families usually desire critical care if it will prolong life, assuming that self-awareness and social interaction are maintained. A third reason is that physicians may respond to what has been called the technologic imperative: the desire to do everything possible despite the ratio of benefit to cost.

Critical care is extraordinarily expensive. The issue of who should be admitted to critical care units and how aggressively they should be treated is a social, as well as medical, concern. Until this issue is resolved, physicians should base decisions regarding critical care primarily on the wishes of well-informed, mentally capable patients or their surrogates. Patients and surrogates who request critical care should receive it if they can benefit and if space permits. On the other hand, the wishes of mentally capable patients who choose against therapies such as endotracheal intubation and mechanical ventilation should be respected. If the mental capacity to make decisions is not clear, hospital ethics committees may become involved.

Orders not to initiate CPR, which are also called "do not resuscitate," or "DNR," orders, may be written at the request of patients, as just discussed, or may be initiated by physicians, when to the best of their knowledge CPR will not be successful in the broad sense of restoring meaningful life. In most instances, such decisions should be discussed with the patient and, when appropriate, with his or her family. The order should then be written in standard fashion in the order sheet, and a note describing the basis for the order and the decisions that took place should be included in the chart. Such orders clarify the ambiguity that surrounds the decisions concerning critical care for patients with irreversible illnesses and relieve nurses or uninvolved physicians from the responsibility of deciding not to initiate CPR.

Some patients with pre-existing DNR orders may still benefit from critical care. Treating airways obstruction, metabolic abnormalities, or arrhythmias may at least temporarily improve the patient's condition, making the existence of DNR orders a moot point. Nevertheless, DNR orders, when written in a critical care unit, usually represent the start of withholding or withdrawal of life support. Life-sustaining care was withheld or withdrawn from only 5 per cent of the patients in a recent study, but such withdrawal or withholding precipitated about half of the deaths occurring in critical care units. The reason for limiting care was a poor prognosis, including brain death, the complete and irreversible loss of the functions of the cerebral hemisphere and brain stem. Most of the patients from whom life support was withheld or withdrawn were not brain dead, but they nonetheless were not mentally capable of participating in the decision-making process. Only a few had previously expressed their wishes regarding critical care in a "living will" or other format. As a result, family members or other patient surrogates usually had to make decisions limiting treatment on the basis of the physician's recommendations. Developing the prognostic knowledge to make such recommendations on a more rational basis and managing the death of severely ill patients are among the major responsibilities of those who participate in critical care medicine.

Bihari D, Smithies M, Gimson A, et al.: The effects of vasodilation with prostacyclin on oxygen delivery and uptake in critically ill patients. N Engl J Med 317:397, 1987. *Describes the presence of an "oxygen debt" in patients with the adult respiratory distress syndrome and how the "debt" can be repaid with maximization of oxygen transport.*

Danek SJ, Lynch JP, Weg JG, et al.: The dependence of oxygen uptake on oxygen delivery in the adult respiratory distress syndrome. Am Rev Respir Dis 122:387, 1980. *The first clinical study of oxygen supply dependence in patients with the adult respiratory distress syndrome.*

Danis M, Patrick DL, Southerland LI, et al.: Patients' and families' preferences for medical intensive care. JAMA 260:797, 1988. *Through interviews with survivors of critical care and relatives of nonsurvivors, the authors conclude that most patients welcome such care if it prolongs meaningful life.*

Darioli R, Perret C: Mechanical controlled hypoventilation in status asthmaticus. Am Rev Respir Dis 129:385, 1984. *Intentional underventilation of asthmatics to reduce the risk of barotrauma is described.*

Dorinsky PM, Gadek JE: Mechanisms of multiple nonpulmonary organ failure in ARDS. Chest 96:885, 1989. *A recent review of organs other than the lungs that fail in patients with the adult respiratory distress syndrome. Explanations for this phenomenon are offered.*

Gilbert EM, Haupt MT, Mandanas RY, et al.: The effect of fluid loading, blood transfusion, and catecholamine infusion on oxygen delivery and consumption in patients with sepsis. Am Rev Respir Dis 134:873, 1986. *Administering fluids, blood, or catecholamines increased oxygen consumption in patients with septic shock and lactic acidosis.*

Hook EW III, Horton CA, Schaberg DR: Failure of intensive care unit support to influence mortality from pneumococcal bacteremia. JAMA 249:1055, 1983. *This study illustrates that critical care has had no major impact on the outcome of bacteremic pneumococcal pneumonia.*

Kelly MA: Critical care medicine—a new specialty? N Engl J Med 313:24, 1988. *Traces the evolution of critical care medicine.*

Knaus WA, Draper EA, Wagner DP, et al.: An evaluation of outcome from intensive care in major medical centers. Ann Intern Med 104:3, 1986. *Patient outcome was related primarily to the interaction and coordination of critical care unit staff.*

Krischer JP, Fine EG, Weisfeldt ML, et al.: Comparison of prehospital conventional and simultaneous compression-ventilation cardiopulmonary resuscitation. Crit Care Med 17:1263, 1989. *Describes a recent trial of "new" versus conventional CPR; the "new" form was not superior.*

Lain DC, DiBenedetto R, Morris SL, et al.: Pressure control inverse ratio ventilation as a method to reduce peak inspiratory pressure and provide adequate ventilation and oxygenation. Chest 95:1081, 1989. *A clinical study of the effectiveness of pressure control and inverse ratio ventilation as compared with assisted mechanical ventilation.*

Luce JM: Ethical principles in critical care. JAMA 263:696, 1990. *A recent review of the application of ethical principles, such as beneficence, in the critical care unit.*

MacIntyre NR: Respiratory function during pressure support ventilation. Chest 89:677, 1986. *A small trial of pressure support ventilation during weaning.*

Montgomery AB, Stager MA, Cerrico CJ, et al.: Causes of mortality in patients with the adult respiratory distress syndrome. Am Rev Respir Dis 132:485, 1985. *This study demonstrates that most patients with the adult respiratory distress syndrome die of septic complications, including MOSF.*

Norcini JJ, Shea JA, Langdon LO, et al.: First American Board of Internal Medicine critical care examination: Process and results. Crit Care Med 17:7, 1989. *Describes the physicians who took the first ABIM critical care examination and what was expected of them.*

O'Quin RJ, Marini JJ: Pulmonary artery occlusion pressure: Clinical physiology, measurement, and interpretation. Am Rev Respir Dis 128:319, 1983. *A guide to using and interpreting flow-directed pulmonary artery catheters.*

Parillo JE, Burch C, Sheshamer JH, et al.: A circulating myocardial depressant substance in humans with septic shock: Septic shock patients with a reduced ejection fraction have a circulating factor that depresses myocardial cell performance. J Clin Invest 76:1539, 1985. *This investigation provides the best evidence yet for circulating myocardial depressant factor.*

Pepe PE, Marini JJ: Occult positive end-expiratory pressure in mechanically ventilated patients: The auto-PEEP effect. Am Rev Respir Dis 126:166, 1982. *Describes the effects of auto-PEEP and how to measure this parameter in ventilated patients.*

Sahn SA, Lakshiminarayan S, Petty JL: Weaning from mechanical ventilation. JAMA 235:2208, 1976. *Reviews the best overall approach to the task of weaning, although it does not include newer ventilatory modes.*

Shoemaker WC, Kram HB, Appel PL: Therapy of shock based on pathophysiology, monitoring, and outcome prediction. Crit Care Med 18:S19, 1990. *Argues in favor of increasing oxygen transport in patients in shock.*

Smedira NG, Evans BH, Grais LS, et al.: Withholding and withdrawal of life support from the critically ill. N Engl J Med 322:309, 1990. *This recent study documents why, how, and under what circumstances life support was withheld or withdrawn from patients in two critical care units.*

Stauffer JL, Olson DE, Petty TL: Complications and consequences of endotracheal intubation and tracheotomy. Am J Med 70:65, 1981. *The best prospective study of the complications of endotracheal intubation by the translaryngeal route or via tracheostomy.*

Wanzer SH, Federman DD, Adelstein SJ, et al.: The physician's responsibility toward hopelessly ill patients. N Engl J Med 320:844, 1989. *A consensus of ethicists and clinicians reviews how to deal with hopelessly ill patients in critical care units.*

Zwillich WC, Pierson DJ, Creagh CE, et al.: Complications of assisted ventilation: A prospective study of 354 consecutive episodes. Am J Med 57:161, 1974. *A study of complications in patients receiving assisted mechanical ventilation.*

72 Approach to the Patient with Renal Disease

Thomas E. Andreoli

This chapter provides an overview of the cardinal manifestations of diseases of the kidney or urinary tract, together with a relatively simple classification of these disorders. There are four sections. The first section contains a brief consideration of the cardinal functions of the kidney. A more detailed analysis of renal physiology is presented in Ch. 73. The second section enumerates briefly the approach to patients affected with the more common syndromes involving the kidneys and urinary tract. The third section describes the consequences of complete or nearly complete failure of renal function, that is, the uremic syndrome. Finally, the last section considers the relationship between the adaptive response to a reduction in nephron mass and the potential contribution of one of these adaptive responses, renal hyperfiltration, to the pathogenesis of progressive renal disease.

CARDINAL ELEMENTS OF RENAL FUNCTION

URINE FORMATION. The kidneys maintain constancy of the volume and composition of body fluids by forming urine, whose composition is ultimately determined by the dietary intake of solute and water and by the rate and kind of metabolic transformation of endogenous and exogenous carbohydrates, proteins, lipids, and nucleic acids. The kidneys also serve as the major route for the excretion of a large number of drugs. The formation of urine serves two purposes: a *regulatory* function, that is, the maintenance of a constant volume and composition of body fluids; and an *excretory* function, that is, elimination of endogenous and exogenous metabolic end-products.

Urine is formed by a sequence of five events:

1. The glomerulus filters approximately 180 liters of extracellular fluid daily across glomerular capillaries and the visceral epithelium of Bowman's capsule, using as a driving force the mean arterial pressure. The glomerular capillary endothelium and basement membrane and the visceral epithelium of Bowman's capsule are freely permeable to water and solutes of relatively low molecular weight (that is, under 6000 to 8000), moderately permeable to large molecular weight species such as myoglobin (molecular weight, approximately 16,000), and virtually impermeable to macromolecules such as albumin. Filtration is also influenced by molecular charge as well as size. The result is an isotonic, virtually protein-free filtrate whose daily volume is more than 10-fold greater than the volume of extracellular fluid (ECF).

2. The proximal tubule isotonically reabsorbs approximately two thirds of the glomerular filtrate. In the process, certain alterations in the composition of tubular fluid are produced by specialized transport mechanisms: the preferential absorption of sodium with bicarbonate rather than chloride; the virtually complete absorption of organic solutes such as glucose and amino acids; and the absorption of organic acids such as uric acid and other nonamino acids in early segments of the proximal nephron, followed by secretion of these acids into tubular fluid in the late proximal nephron. Thus the volume of tubular fluid delivered to the loop of Henle is approximately one third of the volume of glomerular filtrate, has a sodium concentration equal to that of plasma and a bicarbonate concentration about 10 per cent of that in plasma, and contains little or no glucose or amino acids.

3. The loop of Henle dissociates the absorption of sodium and water. The descending limb of Henle passively abstracts water into the hypertonic medullary interstitium, concentrating the tubular fluid. Conversely, the essentially water-impermeable thick ascending limb of Henle actively absorbs approximately 25 per cent of filtered sodium chloride but little water. As a result, about 18 liters of tubular fluid enter the distal convoluted tubule daily. This fluid, which is approximately 10 per cent of the initial glomerular filtrate, is also maximally dilute, having an osmolality of approximately 50 mOsm per kilogram of H_2O.

4. The distal convoluted tubule primarily absorbs sodium under the influence of aldosterone and secretes protons, ammonia, and potassium.

5. The collecting duct system regulates the osmolality of urine. When antidiuretic hormone (ADH) is present, water is absorbed across the collecting duct and tubular fluid equilibrates osmotically with the hypertonic medullary interstitium; when ADH is absent, the water permeability of collecting ducts is at a minimum and a dilute urine is excreted.

THE KIDNEY AS AN ENDOCRINE RECEPTOR. Among many hormones that regulate renal function, three are of particular importance: parathyroid hormone (PTH), aldosterone, and ADH. PTH enhances the absorption of calcium and magnesium and inhibits the absorption of phosphate and bicarbonate in the proximal tubule by increasing intracellular cyclic 3',5'-adenosine monophosphate (cAMP). PTH also stimulates the renal conversion of 25-hydroxycholecalciferol, the major metabolite of vitamin D_3, to 1,25-dihydroxycholecalciferol, which is the major biologically active form of vitamin D_3 (Ch. 233).

Aldosterone and other mineralocorticoids stimulate the rate of sodium absorption in the distal nephron. Aldosterone also increases the rate of net potassium secretion and net proton secretion (and consequently the rate of bicarbonate regeneration) by the distal nephron.

ADH promotes the formation of a hypertonic urine both by increasing the rate of salt absorption in the thick ascending limb of Henle and by increasing the water permeability of the collecting duct system. Both actions are mediated by ADH-dependent increases in cytosolic cAMP in those renal tubular segments.

THE KIDNEY AS AN ENDOCRINE ORGAN. The kidney plays a major role in prostaglandin production, in the operation of the kallikrein-kinin system, and in the degradation of low molecular weight proteins. The kidney is also the major site for the synthesis of erythropoietin and of renin. Erythropoietin is a glycoprotein produced by renal enzymatic action on a circulating precursor of hepatic origin. The principal action of erythropoietin is to stimulate the rate of red blood cell production by the bone marrow. Synthetic human erythropoietin, produced using recombinant technology, is now available for use in patients with chronic renal failure who are undergoing chronic dialysis.

Renin is secreted by the granular cells of the juxtaglomerular apparatus in response to reductions in renal perfusion pressure or in effective circulating volume. Renin increases the rate of conversion of angiotensinogen to angiotensin I, which in turn is a precursor of angiotensin II. In turn, angiotensin II is a potent vasoconstrictor agent and a strong stimulus to thirst and to aldosterone production. Thus, the kidney, by way of renin production, plays a central role in the volume repletion reaction.

EVALUATION OF PATIENTS WITH RENAL DISEASE

Renal diseases may be intrinsic or may occur as manifestations of systemic disease. Thus the initial history and physical examination are often quite variable in different diseases. The same considerations apply to routine urinalysis, to initial blood chemistry measurements, and to more specialized renal imaging tests, such as renal ultrasonography or intravenous pyelography. Consequently, these findings are considered in the context of the various cardinal renal syndromes.

THE MAJOR RENAL SYNDROMES

Renal disorders are often nonspecific in their manifestations—as hematuria, azotemia, hypertension, or metabolic acidosis, for example. The interpretation of a group of findings obtained by history, physical examination, and routine laboratory studies, however, may be used to describe some of the more common syndromes and disorders affecting the kidneys and urinary tract, which are briefly described below.

THE UNDERPERFUSION SYNDROMES. Table 72–1 lists the major groups of diseases characterized by renal hypoperfusion: (1) renal hypoperfusion secondary to a reduction in effective circulating volume, (2) renal ischemia because of occlusive disease in one or both renal arteries, and (3) reversible renal vasoconstriction secondary to acute transplant rejection or certain drugs.

All three classes of disorders reduce effective renal perfusion and thus are characterized by certain common features. These include (1) a reduced fractional excretion of sodium, (2) hyperreninemia and secondary hyperaldosteronism, and (3) nuclear renal scintiscans indicative of renal underperfusion. When renal underperfusion is severe, oliguria and azotemia also ensue. However, the clinical manifestations of the three groups of disorders differ significantly.

Renal hypoperfusion secondary to a *reduction in effective circulating volume* may occur in association with true volume contraction; an increase in vascular capacitance, as in sepsis; sequestration of fluid in interstitial compartments, as in ascites and the hepatorenal syndrome; or an inability to transfer fluid from the venous to the arterial limbs of the circulation, as in severe congestive heart failure, constrictive pericarditis, or pericardial tamponade. When the effective circulating volume is sufficiently reduced, the kidneys are hypoperfused, the glomerular filtration rate is reduced, and renin is released. This results in oliguria, an elevation in serum blood urea nitrogen (BUN) and creatinine concentrations, and a reduced fractional excretion rate for sodium (that is, generally less than 1 per cent). Although plasma renin levels are elevated, the patients are ordinarily normotensive, presumably because the effective circulating volume is decreased.

Renal ischemia produced by *occlusive disease* of the renal arteries results in renin release from the ischemic kidney without a reduction in effective circulating volume and consequently is manifested primarily as hypertension, since pressor activity is elevated while filling of the arterial tree is normal or only slightly reduced. If the renal arterial occlusive disease is limited to one kidney and the contralateral kidney retains normal function, azotemia is absent. However, if the hypertension results in injury to the unaffected kidney, azotemia may ensue. When both renal arteries are involved, azotemia occurs when renal ischemia is sufficiently severe that renal autoregulatory mechanisms are inadequate to maintain an adequate glomerular filtration rate.

Reversible vasoconstriction of renal microcirculation is a third mechanism for producing renal hypoperfusion, renal salt avidity, and azotemia. This phenomenon occurs in acute renal transplant rejection and in response to certain nephrotoxic agents, particularly cyclosporine and amphotericin B. Restoration of renal perfusion and improvement in renal function generally occur if the

TABLE 72–1. THE UNDERPERFUSION SYNDROMES

Class	Examples
Reduced effective circulating volume	Circulatory collapse
	Congestive heart failure
	Cirrhosis with ascites
Occlusive renal artery disease	Renal artery atherosclerosis
	Fibromuscular hyperplasia
Vasoconstriction of renal micro-vasculature	Acute transplant rejection
	Cyclosporine nephrotoxicity
	Amphotericin B nephrotoxicity

acute rejection episode is treated successfully or when the offending nephrotoxic agent is discontinued.

THE RENAL PARENCHYMAL SYNDROMES. *Acute Glomerular Disorders.* **Glomerulonephritis and the Nephrotic Syndrome** (Ch. 79). Two major types of disorders affect the glomerulus: (1) the *acute nephritic syndrome*, characterized mainly by inflammatory and/or necrotizing lesions within glomeruli, and (2) the *nephrotic syndrome*, a predominantly noninflammatory derangement of the glomeruli characterized by an abnormal "leakiness" of the glomeruli to albumin and other macromolecules.

The etiologic, histologic, and clinical characteristics of the glomerulonephritic and nephrotic syndromes overlap to a considerable degree: (1) A given disease process—for example, systemic lupus erythematosus (SLE)—may produce a mild, focal glomerulonephritis with hematuria, mild proteinuria, but no azotemia; a diffuse proliferative glomerulonephritis with hematuria, proteinuria, and severe renal failure; or membranous nephropathy characterized by a relatively pure nephrotic syndrome. (2) Glomerular lesions may evolve; for example, Goodpasture's syndrome can begin as a mild, focal nephritis and progress to a diffuse, necrotic glomerulonephritis. (3) The extent of glomerular injury, as viewed on renal biopsy, correlates generally but inexactly with the severity of the clinical picture. (4) A given pathogenic mechanism—for example, immune complex disease—may in some instances result in acute glomerulonephritis and in other cases in a pure nephrotic syndrome. (5) In certain disorders such as membranoproliferative nephritis, both a nephritic picture and a nephrotic picture may coexist. (6) The same histologic picture—for example, in nil disease—may occur either as a primary renal disorder or in association with a systemic disorder such as Hodgkin's disease.

These diverse glomerular disorders can be somewhat arbitrarily classified by four major patterns that may be defined by the initial presentation of the patient (Table 72–2). Table 72–3, in turn, lists the most common diseases that present as nephritic, nephrotic, and mixed syndromes. As indicated in Table 72–3, the acute glomerular syndromes may occur as primary renal disorders—for example, postinfectious glomerulonephritis—or in association with a systemic disease—for example, SLE. Accordingly, the clinical findings vary considerably. In primary renal disorders, the antecedent history may reveal nothing except a prior, recent infection and a recent history of hematuria. In Goodpasture's syndrome, pulmonary symptoms may also be present. The physical findings are generally limited to edema and/or hypertension. In glomerular disorders associated with systemic diseases such as vasculitis, gammopathies, or diabetes, the history and physical examination may reveal findings typical of those disorders. Alternatively, a glomerular disorder may commonly be the first manifestation of a systemic disease, as in, for example, SLE.

The Mild Acute Glomerulonephritis Syndromes. In this class of glomerular inflammation, glomerular blood flow is sufficient to

TABLE 72–2. CLASSIFICATION OF MAJOR ACUTE GLOMERULAR SYNDROMES

Class of Disorder	Major Derangement	Major Findings
1. Mild acute glomerulonephritis	Mild glomerular inflammation	Hematuria, proteinuria Absent or mild azotemia Absent or mild edema
2. Severe acute glomerulonephritis	Extensive glomerular inflammation Renal ischemia Primary tubular sodium acquisitiveness	Hematuria, proteinuria Azotemia Plasma volume expansion Hypertension Edema Circulatory overload (if severe)
3. Pure nephrotic syndrome	Glomerular protein leak	Massive proteinuria Reduced plasma oncotic pressure Anasarca Normotensive Sensitive to diuretics
4. Mixed disorders	1 plus 3 or 2 plus 3	Hematuria Massive proteinuria Azotemia (variable) Hypertension (variable) Edema

TABLE 72–3. MAJOR ACUTE GLOMERULAR SYNDROMES

Common Presentation	Primary Renal Disorders	Systemic Disorders
Nephritic syndrome	Postinfectious glomerulonephritis Idiopathic rapidly progressive (crescentic) glomerulonephritis Goodpasture's syndrome Hemolytic-uremic syndrome Hereditary nephritis	Vasculitis: SLE Polyarteritis nodosa Wegener's granulomatosis Henoch-Schönlein purpura
Nephrotic syndrome	Idiopathic nil disease Membranous nephropathy Focal sclerosis	Nil disease in Hodgkin's disease Membranous nephropathy in neoplasia, SLE, and drug toxicity Focal sclerosis in heroin abuse, vesicoureteral reflux, and AIDS Essential cryoglobulinemia Gammopathies Diabetic nephropathy
Nephritic/nephrotic syndrome	Membranoproliferative glomerulonephritis type I type II (dense deposit disease) Mesangioproliferative glomerulonephritis (IgA/IgG nephropathy)	Vasculitides, particularly SLE Diabetic nephropathy

SLE = systemic lupus erythematosus; AIDS = acquired immunodeficiency syndrome; IgA = immunoglobulin A; IgG = immunoglobulin G.

maintain the glomerular filtration at a normal or nearly normal rate. Mild acute glomerulonephritis is characterized by hematuria, red cell casts, modest proteinuria, minimal azotemia, and mild or no edema. Because renal perfusion is not severely compromised, hypertension or salt retention or both are generally absent.

The Diffuse Acute Glomerulonephritis Syndromes. These glomerulonephritic syndromes are usually characterized by diffuse glomerular inflammation and/or necrosis sufficiently severe that hematuria and proteinuria are accompanied by a reduction in filtration rate and, consequently, azotemia of varying degrees. Simultaneously, for reasons that are not well understood, sodium acquisitiveness in acute glomerulonephritis is considerably greater than that expected solely from the reduction in glomerular filtration rate. Plasma albumin is generally normal, so that a significant fraction of retained sodium remains in the vascular compartment and may result in hypertension, plasma volume dilution, circulatory overload, congestive heart failure, and a suppression of plasma renin activity.

Nephrotic Syndrome. In the pure nephrotic syndrome, the glomerular filtration barrier is abnormally permeable to macromolecules, so that massive proteinuria occurs even though the filtration rate may be normal. This large urinary loss of protein contributes to the characteristic hypoalbuminemia in such patients. Hypercholesterolemia also occurs and correlates closely with the degree of hypoalbuminemia.

Nephrotic patients are usually salt acquisitive and edematous. In the nephrotic syndromes the reduced plasma oncotic pressure leads to translocation of fluid to the interstitium, a reduced effective circulating volume, and a secondary sodium acquisitiveness and edema. Patients with the pure nephrotic syndrome often are normotensive, rarely develop circulatory overload, and frequently have elevated plasma renin activities. As further evidence for a reduced effective circulating volume, severely nephrotic patients may have postural hypotension even in the presence of anasarca and may have hemoconcentration and renal hypoperfusion with attendant azotemia following excessive diuretic use.

The Interstitial Nephritis Syndromes (Ch. 80). In the interstitial nephritis syndromes, the primary abnormality is damage to the tubulointerstitial system of the kidney, with secondary glomerular damage. Thus renal tubular function tends to be deranged disproportionately to reductions in glomerular filtration rate.

Generalized tubulointerstitial disorders often damage the juxtaglomerular apparatus and therefore tend to impair renin pro-

duction. As a consequence of hyporeninemia, aldosterone production is curtailed. This combination generally results in hyporeninemia, hypoaldosteronism, modest degrees of salt wasting, hyperkalemia, and hyperchloremic metabolic acidosis. These abnormalities occur even when the glomerular filtration rate is only modestly reduced.

Urinary abnormalities such as hematuria and proteinuria are usually, but not always, relatively modest in patients with tubulointerstitial disease. Three general classes of tubulointerstitial diseases can be defined:

1. *Chronic tubulointerstitial disease* may occur as a consequence of any of a large number of diseases that produce chronic damage to the renal interstitium: chronic hypertension, with progressive ischemia to the renal interstitium; diabetes mellitus, in which microvascular disease within the kidney effects the same end result; occlusive disease of smaller renal vessels, as in sickle cell disease; chronic pyelonephritis; and gout; other causes include exogenous toxins, notably illicit alcohol containing lead, and analgesic abuse, particularly the combination of phenacetin and aspirin. Chronic interstitial disease is generally detected in individuals who have modest degrees of sodium wasting, hyperkalemia, metabolic acidosis, and an acidic urine. These abnormalities may occur even when only mild degrees of azotemia exist. The plasma renin activity is generally reduced, as are rates of aldosterone secretion. Hematuria and massive proteinuria are not common in chronic interstitial disease.

2. *Acute allergic interstitial disease* occurs when patients are treated with antibiotics, notably penicillin and related drugs, or with nonsteroidal anti-inflammatory agents. In addition to producing electrolyte abnormalities similar to those described above for chronic interstitial nephritis, acute allergic interstitial nephritis may severely reduce glomerular filtration and may be associated with marked hematuria and proteinuria and with oliguria.

Oliguria and azotemia associated with acute allergic interstitial nephritis may be difficult to differentiate from those of acute tubular necrosis. In this setting an electrolyte pattern of hyperkalemic, hyperchloremic metabolic acidosis, a reduced plasma renin activity and rates of aldosterone secretion, an elevated fractional excretion rate for sodium, eosinophilia, and the presence of eosinophils in the urine would strongly suggest acute allergic interstitial nephritis.

3. *Acute pyelonephritis*, a form of acute interstitial nephritis due to bacterial invasion of the kidney, usually produces a septic picture with fever, flank pain, leukocytosis, and dysuria (Ch. 84). Factors that predispose to acute pyelonephritis are often present, such as diabetes mellitus, obstructive uropathy, prior instrumentation of the urinary tract, or bacterial endocarditis with septic renal emboli. The most useful clues to the presence of acute pyelonephritis include findings of sepsis, costovertebral angle tenderness, pyuria, leukocyte casts, the presence of bacteria in unspun samples of urine, and positive urine cultures.

Isolated Tubular Defects (Ch. 82). In addition to tubular derangements secondary to diffuse tubulointerstitial disease, there are a number of specific defects of tubular function.

Proximal Tubular Defects. *Renal glycosuria* occurs when the glucose threshold of the proximal nephron is reduced. *Renal phosphate wasting* results when the rate of proximal absorption of phosphate is reduced. Similarly, *aminoaciduria* may result from tubular defects that are either generalized or specific. Finally, the rate of bicarbonate absorption by the proximal nephron may be reduced, resulting in profound bicarbonate wasting, a syndrome entitled *proximal renal tubular acidosis* (Ch. 82).

Renal phosphate wasting, renal glycosuria, renal aminoaciduria, and proximal renal tubular acidosis occurring simultaneously constitute Fanconi's syndrome (Ch. 82). These proximal tubular defects may be congenital or may be found in association with heavy metal poisoning of the proximal nephron, notably by copper in Wilson's disease, following exposure to toxic agents such as maleic acid, and in the gammopathies.

Possible Loop of Henle Defect. The pathogenesis of *Bartter's syndrome* has not been elucidated (Ch. 82). Yet it appears that many of the findings of Bartter's syndrome, including profound salt wasting, potassium wasting, and compensatory hypertrophy of the juxtaglomerular apparatus with hyperreninemia, may be the result of a salt-absorptive defect in the thick ascending limb. A clinical syndrome resembling Bartter's syndrome commonly occurs because of surreptitious ingestion of furosemide or furosemide-like diuretics.

Distal Tubular Defects. *Distal, gradient-limited renal tubular acidosis* represents a specific defect of the distal nephron (Ch. 82). In this disorder the distal nephron is abnormally permeable to protons and cannot therefore maintain an adequately acid urine. In contrast to patients who have tubulointerstitial disease, the classic electrolyte abnormalities in distal, gradient-limited renal tubular acidosis include a tendency to salt wasting, hyperchloremic metabolic acidosis, a urine that is relatively alkaline with respect to arterial pH, and profound hypokalemia. The hypokalemia of distal, gradient-limited renal tubular acidosis is probably a consequence of aldosterone release in response to salt depletion. In contrast to proximal renal tubular acidosis or to the hyperkalemic, hyperchloremic renal tubular acidosis of diffuse tubulointerstitial disease, gradient-limited distal renal tubular acidosis is frequently associated with severe nephrocalcinosis, renal calculi, renal infection, and progressive destruction of renal mass.

Distal, gradient-limited renal tubular acidosis may occur congenitally. The disorder may also occur as a consequence of exposure to exogenous agents, notably amphotericin B and lithium, and in association with the gammopathies.

Collecting Duct Defects. The unique tubular defect of the collecting duct is nephrogenic diabetes insipidus (NDI), in which the collecting duct is refractory to the action of ADH (Ch. 214). Patients with NDI are consistently polyuric, even when large amounts of ADH are administered. The disorder may occur congenitally; in association with certain systemic disorders, such as Sjögren's syndrome and sarcoidosis; and as a result of lithium intoxication or exposure to the antibiotic demethylchlortetracycline.

The Renal Calculus Syndrome. The origin and composition of renal calculi are described in Ch. 88; most renal calculi contain magnesium-ammonium-phosphate, calcium oxalate, uric acid, a combination of calcium oxalate and uric acid, or cystine as their main crystalloids. Of these, all but uric acid stones are radiopaque.

Renal calculi may be asymptomatic and detected only on routine radiographic examination of the kidney, especially isolated calculi that do not move down the urinary tract and staghorn calculi lodged within the renal pelvis. Calculi may obstruct urine flow and consequently lead to pyelonephritis. Therefore, in any patient in whom pyelonephritis is suspected, a careful radiographic and urologic examination for renal calculi is mandatory. *Renal colic* refers to the passage of a renal calculus from the renal pelvis into the ureter characterized by exquisite pain, generally beginning in the flank and radiating into the groin. Patients almost always describe renal colic as the worst pain they have ever experienced. Renal colic is almost invariably accompanied by hematuria, unless the calculus is lodged within a ureter and produces complete unilateral obstruction to urine flow. Under these circumstances, the urine voided by the patient represents red cell–free urine from the unaffected kidney.

Kidney stones are among the more common renal disorders. It is generally prudent, particularly in patients with multiple renal calculi or with a family history of renal calculi, to look for potential underlying causes for stone formation (for example, gout, absorptive hypercalciuria, cystinuria, distal, gradient-limited renal tubular acidosis, or primary hyperparathyroidism). The presence of nephrocalcinosis should alert the physician to the possibility of distal, gradient-limited renal tubular acidosis or to primary hyperparathyroidism.

The patient with renal colic also warrants an evaluation for obstructive uropathy on the affected side and for urinary tract infection. These approaches generally involve culture of the urine, plain films of the abdomen, and, when indicated, ultrasonography of the kidneys, excretory urography, evaluation of parathyroid function, and evaluation for an absorptive hypercalciuric state.

Renal Cystic Disease (Ch. 89). There are three major forms of renal cystic disease: single or multiple cysts, polycystic kidney disease, and microcystic disease of the renal medulla. The clinical characteristics, significance, and clinical presentations of these three kinds of renal cysts vary significantly. There is no evidence that true simple cysts, multiple simple cysts, or polycystic kidney disease progresses to renal neoplasia. However, in more than 30 per cent of patients undergoing chronic hemodialysis therapy for more than 5 years, multiple single cysts develop. These are sometimes termed acquired polycystic kidney disease. About 10 per cent of these cystic transformations subsequently undergo malignant transformation.

Isolated simple cysts, either single or multiple, form sporadically for unknown reasons within the renal parenchyma, generally within the renal cortex. Single cysts in particular usually cause no symptoms; they are generally detected in one of two circumstances: episodes of renal trauma that provoke cyst rupture and hematuria, or on routine excretory urography. The true single, simple cyst (in contrast to the cystic neoplasm; see below) is innocuous and needs no therapy. *Multiple simple cysts* probably represent an extension of the process described above and are also similarly innocuous unless they encroach on renal parenchyma. Multiple simple cysts should be distinguished from polycystic kidney disease, a disorder with a more ominous prognosis. These two forms of multicystic disease can be distinguished by excretory urography; in individuals with multiple simple cysts, the overall size of the kidney is normal and the calyceal system is not elongated and only minimally distorted.

Adult polycystic kidney disease is a form of nephropathy that is generally inherited by autosomal dominance with incomplete penetrance. If a parent has polycystic kidney disease, approximately one half of the progeny will ultimately develop the disorder, although the time at which polycystic kidney disease becomes manifest is highly variable.

Polycystic kidney disease may present with recurrent bouts of hematuria, renal colic, hypertension, or urinary tract infection because of intrarenal obstruction due to cysts. Many patients with polycystic kidney disease develop renal failure, although the rate and extent of development of renal failure depend on the degree of penetrance of the autosomal dominant trait.

Three factors distinguish between patients with polycystic kidney disease and those with multiple simple cysts: (1) a positive family history consistent with an autosomal dominant trait; (2) enlargement of the kidneys, generally detected as a pole-to-pole diameter in excess of 15 to 17 cm and a cortical thickness in excess of 3 cm; and (3) elongation and deformation of the caliceal structure from the progressive enlargement of the parenchymal cysts.

Microcystic kidney disease of the renal medulla, a disorder of children generally inherited as a recessive trait, is characterized by progressive disruption and destruction of the renal medullary architecture by multiple cysts. The disease is generally detected when young children complain of fatigue and are noted to have mild degrees of proteinuria, anemia, and azotemia. The clinical course is characterized by an inordinately high requirement for salt intake in order to maintain blood pressure and an adequate filtration rate and by stunted growth due to chronic illness, to uremia, and to excessive urinary calcium losses. Nephrons are gradually destroyed, usually with progression to end-stage renal disease before the age of 30.

Renal Neoplasia (Ch. 91). Two major classes of renal tumors occur in adults: *renal cell carcinomas* (sometimes called hypernephromas), which originate in the renal cortex, and *transitional cell tumors* of the renal pelvis. Hypernephromas are versatile tumors and are often difficult to diagnose. Many patients present simply with painless hematuria. However, hypernephromas also produce a number of unusual syndromes, including polycythemias, presumably due to excessive erythropoietin production; hypertension, presumably because the neoplasm acts as the equivalent of an arteriovenous fistula and results in renin release by the affected kidney; fever of unknown origin; and hypercalcemia (see Table 91–3).

Transitional cell tumors of the renal pelvis commonly present as hematuria, which may be painless or accompanied by renal colic from the clots that are passed. The systemic manifestations described for hypernephroma are uncommonly found in transitional cell tumors. Examination of urine cytology by a Wright's stain of the urinary sediment may provide a useful diagnostic clue to the presence of these tumors.

Acute Renal Failure (Ch. 76). Acute renal failure refers either to the sudden cessation of urine flow or to sudden oliguria. Acute renal failure caused by acute glomerular disorders is generally evident from the findings described above for the acute glomerulonephritic syndromes. The general approach to the differential diagnosis of acute renal failure, particularly in hospitalized patients, involves the distinction between three major classes of disorders: (1) the underperfusion syndromes indicated in Table 72–1; (2) intrarenal syndromes, especially acute tubular necrosis and acute allergic interstitial nephritis; and (3) postrenal syndromes, that is, oligoanuria resulting from urinary tract obstruction.

The general approach to these patients involves the following cardinal maneuvers: (1) an assessment of circulatory dynamics; (2) a careful history to assess possible antecedent hypotension or exposure to nephrotoxic agents, coupled with a measurement of the fractional excretion of sodium; and (3) renal ultrasonography to exclude the possibility of obstruction of both kidneys, or obstruction of a solitary kidney, as in an individual with renal agenesis or with renal transplantation. These maneuvers are generally helpful in distinguishing between prerenal, intrarenal, and postrenal causes of oliguria. Invasive hemodynamic monitoring, coupled with a fluid challenge, may still be required to exclude rigorously the possibility of oliguria due to a reduced effective circulating volume. A percutaneous renal biopsy may be needed to distinguish between acute tubular necrosis and acute allergic interstitial nephritis. Renal ultrasonography has reduced strikingly the need for retrograde ureteral catheterization as a means for excluding obstructive uropathy.

THE POSTRENAL SYNDROMES (Ch. 81). The postrenal syndromes result from obstruction of urine flow at various loci in the urinary tract from the renal papillae to the urethral meatus. Azotemia and oliguria occur in urinary tract obstruction only when the urinary tract is obstructed bilaterally or when obstruction exists in a sole functioning kidney. The degree of azotemia depends upon the extent of the obstruction; partial obstruction may produce only moderate degrees of azotemia, while complete obstruction of the urinary tract obviously produces anuria. Obstruction of urine flow can irreversibly damage the kidneys. If the obstruction is partial or nearly complete, renal function may be preserved for as long as 4 to 5 weeks following the onset of obstruction. Obstructive uropathy also carries with it the possible complication of urinary tract infection.

Bilateral ureteral obstruction most frequently occurs at three major sites: (1) the *ureteropelvic junction*, where the obstruction is generally due to scar formation or, less commonly, to renal vessels crossing the ureter; (2) the site where the ureters cross the *pelvic brim*—neoplasms are the primary cause of such obstruction, particularly extensive carcinoma of the cervix; and (3) the *ureterovesical junction*, because of either neoplasm or scar formation. Less commonly, other disorders such as *retroperitoneal fibrosis* or disseminated retroperitoneal lymphoma may cause bilateral ureteral obstruction between the ureterovesical junction and where the ureters cross the pelvic brim. The probability of renal calculi causing bilateral ureteral obstruction is small unless one kidney is already nonfunctional and a stone obstructs the outflow of urine from the other kidney. Prostatic enlargement is a common cause of partial or complete obstruction to urine outflow. In contrast to the case in ureteral obstruction, the urinary bladder distends and often results in overflow urinary incontinence. The patient may therefore present with azotemia secondary to a profound reduction in glomerular filtration and yet have significant volumes of urine flow.

Urinary tract obstruction represents a potentially remediable cause of renal failure; every attempt should be made to exclude obstructive uropathy in individuals who are oliguric or anuric. Renal ultrasonography has simplified this task greatly, since it noninvasively detects whether or not the renal calyces are dilated and the ureters are narrowed, as occurs in ureteropelvic junction obstruction; or whether the ureters and renal calyces are both dilated, as occurs in ureterovesical obstruction or urethral obstruction.

RENAL FAILURE: THE UREMIC SYNDROME

The uremic syndrome (Ch. 77) occurs when the functional renal mass is reduced sufficiently that the kidney is no longer able to carry out excretory functions, functions relating to the regulation of the volume and composition of body fluids, functions as an endocrine receptor, and functions as an endocrine organ. The manifestations of *acute* uremia may differ from those of

chronic uremia, but these differences relate more to the rate of development of renal failure than to fundamental differences in pathophysiology.

Uremia is in part a syndrome of "autointoxication." While the chemical agents responsible for this autointoxication have not been clearly identified, uremic syndromes may be ameliorated by dialysis (which generally removes molecules having molecular weights less than 1000 to 2000), and severe protein restriction may minimize the rate of development of the uremic symptoms. Thus it is plausible to presume that the retention of the endproducts of protein metabolism, reflected primarily by the BUN and serum creatinine levels as well as by other factors such as acidosis, is responsible for many of the manifestations of the uremic syndrome.

In early stages, chronic uremia is manifested by relatively nonspecific systemic symptoms, including anorexia, a metallic taste, systemic weakness, and easy fatigability. Hypertension is commonly present, but signs of circulatory volume overload may be absent if dietary solute intake has been curtailed because of anorexia. As uremia progresses, these findings increase in severity and are often accompanied by vomiting, progressively increasing pruritus, marked pallor, and central nervous system symptoms such as lethargy and confusion. In advanced uremia, frank coma and seizure, as well as pericarditis, are common findings. However, advanced central nervous system manifestations of uremia, such as pericarditis or peripheral neuropathy, are relatively infrequent in modern clinical practice because of early intervention with dialysis therapy.

In uremia the major electrolyte alterations include hypocalcemia, presumably due to the inability to form 1,25-dihydroxycholecalciferol as renal mass is reduced and to hyperphosphatemia; hyperphosphatemia, resulting from a reduction in glomerular filtration rate; and metabolic acidosis, which results from a reduction in the renal excretion of "fixed" acids (that is, incompletely combusted organic acids; and sulfate and phosphate, which represent the end-products of protein and nucleic acid metabolism, respectively).

The occurrence of hyperkalemia among uremic individuals is variable and depends on a number of factors, including the rate of potassium intake, the rate of tissue catabolism, and the rate at which renal failure has evolved. In general, patients in whom the uremic syndrome evolves acutely do not develop adaptive mechanisms (either renal or extrarenal) for potassium elimination and are therefore more prone to develop hyperkalemia. In contrast, individuals who approach end-stage renal disease gradually may often be normokalemic even when the glomerular filtration rate is less than 5 per cent of normal. Two factors may account for this phenomenon: (1) The development of renal disease is accompanied by asthenia and anorexia, so that dietary intake of potassium may be minimized; and (2) both renal and extrarenal mechanisms for more efficient potassium excretion are gradually developed.

Uremia, whether acute or chronic, is a catabolic disorder. In individuals with acute renal failure, even extensive hyperalimentation fails to prevent the loss of approximately 0.5 to 1.0 pound daily. In chronic renal failure, weight loss is more gradual and less easily perceived by patients. But in both acute and chronic renal failure, asthenia and loss of lean body mass are inevitable sequelae.

As the functional renal mass is diminished, erythropoietin production is also reduced. Thus within 2 to 3 weeks of the onset of acute renal failure, the combination of diminished erythrocyte production and an accelerated rate of red cell destruction invariably reduces the hematocrit level to the range of 20 to 25 per cent. Similar hematocrits are found in patients with chronic renal failure, particularly prior to dialysis therapy. Polycystic kidney disease represents an exception in that profound reductions of glomerular filtration rate may occur coincident with the maintenance of a hematocrit well in excess of 30 per cent. Presumably, the large renal mass of polycystic kidney disease produces sufficient erythropoietin to maintain an adequate hematocrit.

Individuals with acute renal failure do not develop significant bone disease. In contrast, individuals with chronic, severe reductions in glomerular filtration rate and in functional renal mass often have significant bone disease, termed renal osteodystrophy

(Ch. 237). At least four factors may contribute to the complex bone disorders in uremia: (1) The synthesis of 1,25-hydroxycholecalciferol in the kidney is reduced, with consequent diminished calcium absorption from the gut. (2) The calcium malabsorption leads to secondary hyperparathyroidism, which mobilizes calcium from bone in an attempt to maintain a normal level of serum ionized calcium and in the process produces osteitis fibrosa (Ch. 235). (3) Bone calcium is exchanged for retained protons in buffering the metabolic acidosis of chronic renal failure with partial maintenance of acid-base homeostasis, but at the expense of progressive dissolution of bone. (4) The uremic state impairs protein synthesis in bone and with this the formation of osteoid.

In short, the uremic syndrome results from varying impairment in the ability of the kidney to meet all of its normal metabolic and physiologic obligations: to regulate the volume and composition of body fluids, to excrete the end-products of metabolism, to serve as an endocrine receptor, and to serve as an endocrine organ. Within that framework the particular manifestations of uremia in any given patient will depend largely on the rate at which kidney failure has occurred, the severity of the renal failure (that is, the extent to which residual nephron mass is able to maintain homeostasis), and the homeostatic stresses to which the individual is subjected.

ADAPTATION TO RENAL INJURY AND THE PATHOGENESIS OF PROGRESSIVE RENAL FAILURE

Two additional characteristics of nearly all forms of chronic renal disease warrant particular consideration. First, nephron loss may be accompanied by *adaptive functional changes* in residual nephrons, which tend to minimize the effects of reducing the functional nephron mass on the chemical composition of blood. This argument, generally termed the *intact nephron hypothesis*, considers that in chronic renal disease the function of residual nephrons may be normal or supranormal. Among the cardinal adaptive characteristics described by the intact nephron hypothesis have been an increased glomerular filtration rate per nephron with elevated serum BUN concentrations or increased rates of protein feeding, and an increase in the rate of phosphate excretion per nephron mediated through secondary hyperparathyroidism, such that, in chronic renal failure, serum phosphate levels do not rise until the glomerular filtration rate is reduced to about 30 per cent of normal.

Second, these adaptive responses may ultimately be harmful to the kidney: For example, the maintenance of relatively normal serum calcium and phosphate concentrations in a setting of modest reductions in glomerular filtration rate (that is, to 30 to 40 per cent of normal) by secondary hyperparathyroidism is achieved at the expense of bone dissolution. Likewise, recent observations have provided evidence that increases in protein intake lead to glomerular hyperperfusion and that the elevated glomerular filtration rate produced by this hyperperfusion can result in progressive glomerulosclerosis. Thus, in principle, glomerular hyperperfusion produced by a protein intake that is large in relation to the residual nephron mass could contribute to the progression of chronic renal disease. A corollary to this hypothesis is the possibility that dietary protein restriction early in the course of chronic renal failure might slow the rate of progression of renal disease. A federally sponsored trial assessing the potential benefits of low-protein diets in preserving renal function in various stages of chronic renal failure is currently in progress.

Glassock RJ, Ward H, Adler S: The primary and secondary glomerular diseases. Curr Nephrol 13:1–47, 1990. *A helpful classification of primary glomerular disorders and those secondary to systemic diseases.*

Hricak H: Radiologic assessment of the kidney. *In* Brenner BM, Rector FC (eds.): The Kidney. Philadelphia, W.B. Saunders Company, 1991, pp 969–992. *A discussion of renal imaging studies.*

Klahr S, Schreiner G, Ichikawa I: The progression of renal disease. N Engl J Med 318:1657, 1988. *A detailed analysis of the factors contributing to progressive chronic renal failure.*

Levey AS, Madaio MP, Perrone RD: Laboratory assessment of renal disease: Clearance, urinalysis, and renal biopsy. *In* Brenner BM, Rector FC (eds.): The Kidney. Philadelphia, W.B. Saunders Company, 1991, pp 968–969. *A concise approach to the laboratory evaluation of patients with renal disease.*

Levine E, Grantham JJ, Slusher SL, et al.: A computed tomographic study of acquired cystic disease and renal tumors in long-term dialysis patients. AJR 142:125, 1984.

73 Structure and Function of the Kidneys

Saulo Klahr*

This chapter reviews the structure and function of the normal mammalian kidney as a framework for understanding the derangements that occur with kidney disease.

RENAL STRUCTURE

The kidneys are located retroperitoneally with their upper and lower poles opposite the twelfth thoracic and third lumbar vertebrae, respectively. Because of the presence of the liver, the right kidney is generally lower than the left. Each adult kidney weighs 130 to 170 grams and measures about 12 by 6 by 3 cm. Through the hilus of the kidney pass a renal artery and vein, lymphatics, a nerve plexus, and the *renal pelvis*, which subdivides into the *three major calices* and subsequently into eight or more *minor calices*. A coronal section of the kidney reveals two distinct regions: the medulla and the cortex. The *renal medulla* is composed generally of 12 to 18 conical masses, the *pyramids*. The base of each pyramid is located on the corticomedullary boundary, and the apex extends toward the renal pelvis, forming the *papilla*, which projects into the minor calix. Each papilla is perforated by the distal end of 15 or more *terminal collecting ducts* (of Bellini). The *renal cortex*, about 1 cm in thickness, covers the base of the pyramids and extends medially between the individual pyramids to form the renal columns (of Bertin).

BLOOD SUPPLY

Each kidney is usually supplied by a single artery originating from the aorta at the level of the first lumbar vertebra. This artery generally divides into two branches (anterior and posterior) which enter the renal sinus and give rise to upper, middle, and lower branches *(lobar arteries)*. As these arteries enter the renal parenchyma they form the *interlobar arteries* that course toward the cortex along the lateral borders of the medullary pyramids and then form the *arcuate arteries* at the base of the renal medulla. The *intralobular arteries*, branching at right angles from the arcuate vessels, course through the cortex to the periphery. They give rise to *afferent arterioles*, each of which ends in a fine capillary bed known as a glomerulus. Thus, the glomerulus is supplied by a single afferent arteriole and drained, in turn, by an *efferent arteriole*, which emerges at the glomerular vascular pole and immediately ramifies into numerous peritubular capillaries that surround the tubular segments of the cortex. The *vasa recta*, which extend medially into the medulla, are the capillaries that originate from efferent arterioles of juxtamedullary glomeruli.

The venous system follows the same pattern as the arterial system, with the capillaries forming venules that unite into intralobular, arcuate, lobular, and ultimately renal veins. Each renal vein drains into the inferior vena cava.

THE NEPHRON

The nephron is the functional unit of the kidney. There are approximately 1,200,000 nephrons in each human kidney. Each is composed of a malpighian corpuscle (the *glomerulus* and *Bowman's capsule*) and its attached *tubule*. The tubule contains several distinct anatomic and functional segments: proximal tubule, loop of Henle, distal convoluted tubule, and collecting tubule. The junction of collecting tubules forms the collecting ducts, which traverse the medulla and terminate at the tip of the papilla. There are two distinct populations of nephrons in the human kidney: those with glomeruli located in the outer cortex *(superficial nephrons)* and those with glomeruli situated near the

*The author wishes to thank Dr. David Warnock for assistance in the revision of this chapter.

corticomedullary junction (*juxtamedullary nephrons*). The superficial nephrons, which constitute about 85 per cent of the total nephron population, have short loops of Henle that frequently do not penetrate the medulla. The juxtamedullary nephrons have long loops of Henle that extend into the inner medulla and are in close apposition to the vasa recta.

GLOMERULUS. The glomerulus (Fig. 73–1) is a network of capillaries originating from the afferent arteriole. After dividing into four to eight lobules to form the glomerular tuft, the capillaries rejoin to form the efferent arteriole, which leaves the glomerulus at the vascular pole. The glomerular tuft is surrounded by *Bowman's capsule*, which is an extension of the basement membrane and connective tissue of the proximal tubule. The *urinary* or *Bowman's space* separates the capsule from the glomerular tuft. Bowman's capsule contains a single layer of squamous cells *(parietal epithelial cells)*, which undergo an abrupt transition to taller columnar cells typical of the proximal tubule at the urinary pole of the glomerulus. In the glomerular tuft there are three distinct cell types (endothleial, mesangial, and epithelial), a capillary wall (basement membrane), and an interstitial or supporting region (mesangium).

Capillary Wall. The capillary wall contains endothelial cells, a basement membrane, and epithelial cells (see Fig. 73–1). The *endothelial cells* line the capillary lumen. Fenestrae or pores (approximate diameter of 700 Å) covered by thin diaphragms are present in the attenuated endothelium. The *basement membrane*, a structure with an average thickness in the adult of 3200 Å, contains three distinct areas: a central electron-dense *lamina densa* and, on either side, a *lamina rara externa* and *lamina rara interna* (see Fig. 73–1). The major constituents of the basement membrane are collagen and glycoprotein. Thickening of this structure is seen in a number of glomerular diseases. The *visceral epithelial cells,* or *podocytes,* are the largest of the glomerular cells. Extending from the body of the podocyte are primary processes, from which individual *foot processes,* or *pedicels,* project to come into contact with the lamina rara externa of the basement membrane. Between the foot processes is a space *(filtration slit* or *slit pore)* 250 to 400 Å wide, which is covered by a thin membrane, the *filtration slit diaphragm,* which is located approximately 600 Å from the basement membrane. This slit diaphragm is a zipper-like structure composed of rectangular

pores (40 to 140 Å in a cross-section). The estimated total area of these pores is approximately 3 per cent of the total surface area of the glomerular capillaries. In renal diseases characterized by proteinuria the pedicels of the podocytes are replaced by a continuous band of cytoplasm adjacent to the lamina rara externa (fusion of foot processes).

The Mesangium. The mesangium, the interstitial portion of the glomerular lobules, is composed of *mesangial cells* (axial or intercapillary) and *mesangial matrix.* The latter is a homogeneous fibrillary material containing mucopolysaccharides and glycoprotein. The mesangial cells, which have phagocytic properties, resemble smooth muscle cells, contain myosin, and usually do not communicate directly with the vascular space. The mesangium is unique in that entry of a substance into the space does not require passage through a capillary basement membrane. In human glomerulonephritis, immune deposits are found in the mesangium, often exclusively.

THE TUBULE. The renal tubule is composed of distinct anatomic and functional segments: the *proximal convoluted tubule,* the *pars recta* or *straight portion* of the proximal tubule, the *thin descending* and *ascending limbs of Henle's loop,* the *thick ascending limb of Henle's loop,* the *distal convoluted tubule,* the *cortical collecting tubule,* and the *medullary collecting duct.* These segments differ in their location, length, diameter, characteristics of the lining epithelium, including number and size of mitochondria, appearance of intercellular channels, presence of luminal microvilli (brush border), and complexity of basal infoldings. The functional differences among nephron segments are described below.

JUXTAGLOMERULAR APPARATUS. The juxtaglomerular apparatus is a region near the glomerular vascular pole in which the transition occurs between the *thick ascending limb* and the *distal convoluted tubule* and the *afferent* and *efferent arterioles* come into juxtaposition. Here, the cells of the distal tubule become taller and more numerous *(macula densa),* and cells derived from the afferent arteriole *(juxtaglomerular cells)* are present between the distal tubule and the vascular pole (Fig. 73–1). These cells may be granular (containing renin) or agranular. Adrenergic nerve endings have been demonstrated in the juxta-

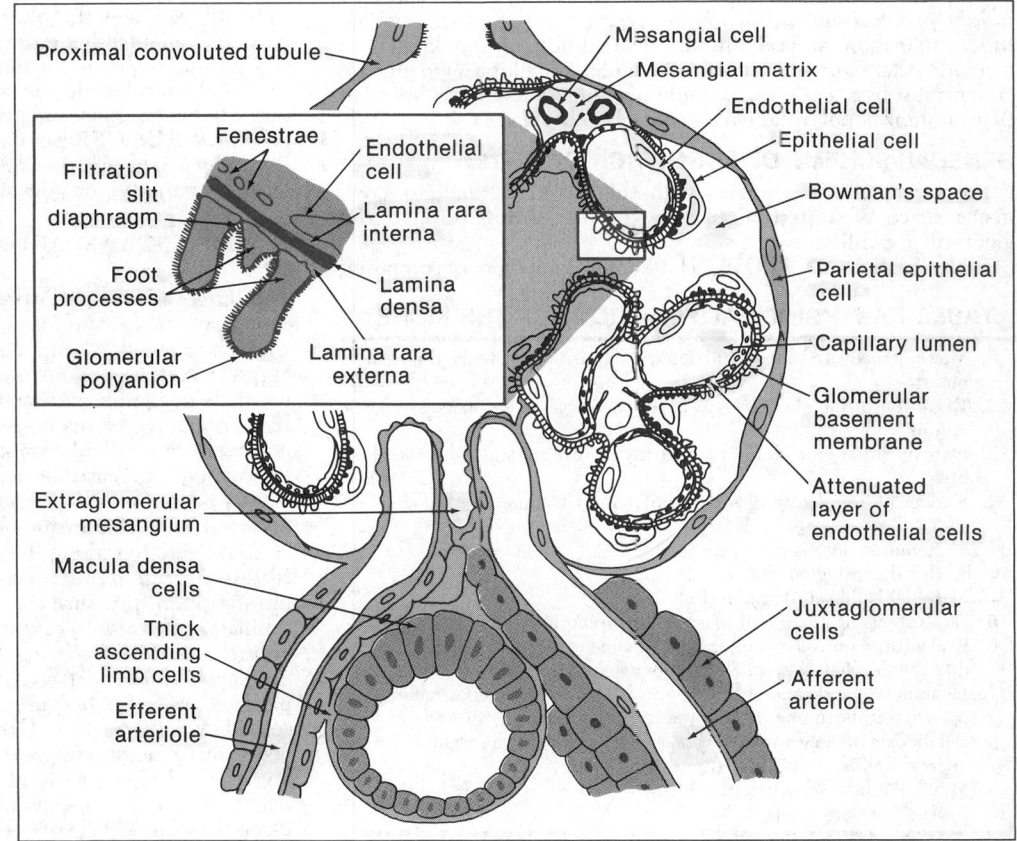

FIGURE 73–1. Schematic representation of the glomerulus, illustrating the three major types of cells (endothelial, epithelial, and mesangial) and the close relationship of the macula densa to afferent and efferent arterioles ("juxtaglomerular apparatus"). Notice that there is no basement membrane interposed between the mesangium and the lumen of the capillaries. The inset shows a magnified view of the capillary wall, illustrating the gaps between the endothelial cells (fenestrae), the three layers of the basement membrane, and the foot processes of the epithelial cells. For more details see text.

Proximal convoluted tubule

Fenestrae

Filtration slit diaphragm

Endothelial cell

Foot processes

Lamina rara interna

Lamina densa

Glomerular polyanion

Lamina rara externa

Mesangial cell

Mesangial matrix

Endothelial cell

Epithelial cell

Bowman's space

Parietal epithelial cell

Capillary lumen

Glomerular basement membrane

Attenuated layer of endothelial cells

Extraglomerular mesangium

Macula densa cells

Thick ascending limb cells

Efferent arteriole

Juxtaglomerular cells

Afferent arteriole

glomerular region. Signals originating from the macula densa can affect glomerular filtration rate (tubuloglomerular feedback).

INTERSTITIUM

The interstitial connective tissue of the kidney is scant and consists primarily of *reticular fibers* and *interstitial cells*. It is more prominent in the medulla than in the cortex. In addition to capillaries, the interstitium contains *lymphatics* and *motor* and *sensory nerves*. This region may be infiltrated by white blood cells and contain increased amounts of connective tissue in a variety of renal diseases.

NORMAL RENAL FUNCTION

The principal functions of the kidney are summarized in Table 73–1. The kidneys play a central role in the *maintenance of volume and ionic composition of body fluids* (homeostasis) by regulating the rate of excretion of water and/or ions. The large changes in urine volume and composition, which occur in response to alterations in the diet, reflect the adaptability of the kidney to the requirements of homeostasis. There is no fixed normal volume or composition of the urine. Normal homeostatic renal function is defined by the capacity of the organ to vary the volume and composition of the urine over a wide range.

The kidney is the main route of excretion of fixed (nonvolatile) metabolic waste products. These substances usually serve no biologic function, and some of them are potentially toxic. Examples include urea (end-product of protein metabolism), uric acid (end-product of nucleic acid metabolism), and creatinine (end-product of creatine metabolism). The kidney also *eliminates exogenous chemicals (drugs, toxins)* and their metabolites.

The kidney participates in endocrine functions as well. In addition to its capacity to *metabolize and excrete certain hormones*, the kidney is the site of *production* of renin, erythropoietin, prostaglandins, 1,25-dihydroxycholecalciferol, and kinins. It is the target organ for several hormones (e.g., parathyroid hormone, atrial peptide, antidiuretic hormone, angiotensin, aldosterone).

The kidney is also involved in the *catabolism of small molecular weight proteins* and in *metabolic interconversions* that regulate the composition of body fluids. The ability of the kidney to convert certain organic acids (lactic, alpha-ketoglutaric) to glucose (a neutral substance) is an example of a metabolic interconversion that minimizes potential changes in plasma pH.

GENERAL SCHEME OF FORMATION OF URINE

Formation of urine begins with the ultrafiltration into Bowman's space of a portion of the plasma flowing through the glomerular capillaries.

RENAL BLOOD FLOW. The renal circulation is composed

TABLE 73–1. PRINCIPAL FUNCTIONS OF THE KIDNEY

1. Maintenance of volume and ionic composition of body fluids (homeostasis)
2. Excretion of metabolic waste products—e.g., urea, uric acid, creatinine
3. Detoxification and elimination of toxins, drugs, and their metabolites
4. Endocrine regulation of extracellular fluid volume and blood pressure
   a. Renin-angiotensin system
   b. Renal prostaglandins
   c. Renal kallikrein-kinin system
5. Control of red blood cell mass: erythropoietin
6. Endocrine control of mineral metabolism: formation of 1,25-dihydroxycholecalciferol and 24,25-dihydroxycholecalciferol
7. Degradation and catabolism of peptide hormones: insulin, glucagon, parathyroid hormone, calcitonin, growth hormone, etc.
8. Catabolism of low molecular weight proteins: light chains, beta$_2$-microglobulin
9. Metabolic interconversions: gluconeogenesis, lipid metabolism
10. Synthesis of growth factors

of two capillary beds in series: the glomerular and the peritubular capillaries. The glomerulus has a high intracapillary hydrostatic pressure because it is interposed between two arterioles, i.e., resistance vessels. Therefore, filtration is favored. The second capillary system (peritubular capillaries in the cortex, vasa recta in the medulla) is a high-flow, low-pressure system that acts as a reservoir for tubular reabsorption and secretion.

The kidneys receive 25 per cent of the cardiac output, or approximately 1.1 liters of blood per minute. In subjects with a physiologic hematocrit of 45 per cent, total renal plasma flow is about 600 ml per minute. Cortical blood flow is about 75 per cent and medullary blood flow 25 per cent of total renal blood flow. Only 1 per cent of the renal blood flow reaches the papilla. As blood flows through the glomerular capillaries, hydrostatic forces drive filtration of 20 per cent of the plasma volume (120 ml per minute) across the capillary wall into Bowman's space (glomerular filtration). The ratio of glomerular filtration rate (GFR) to renal plasma flow is called the *filtration fraction*.

Renal blood flow is maintained relatively constant (*autoregulation*) even in the face of wide variations (80 to 180 mm Hg) in renal arterial perfusion pressure by changes in renal vascular resistance proportional to changes in perfusion pressure. Since the afferent and efferent arterioles determine renal vascular resistance, changes in arteriolar resistance alter renal blood flow. Recent evidence suggests that endothelium-derived relaxing factor (EDRF) and endothelins are major regulators of renal blood flow and vascular resistances. Autoregulation of renal blood flow maintains a constant GFR despite alterations in arterial perfusion pressure. Although the kidneys are innervated by adrenergic nerve fibers, renal sympathetic tone probably does not play a significant role in regulating renal blood flow under basal conditions. Thus, denervation or alpha- or beta-adrenergic blockers does not alter renal blood flow. However, augmented sympathetic activity (e.g., fright, pain, exercise, norepinephrine, congestive heart failure) increases renal vascular resistance and reduces renal blood flow. Both afferent and efferent arterioles contract, but GFR falls less than renal blood flow, suggesting that catecholamines have their major effect at the efferent arteriole. Renal blood flow is increased in infections or by substances inducing fever (pyrogenic reaction), presumably as a consequence of nitric oxide release by macrophages.

GLOMERULAR FILTRATION RATE. The initial step in the formation of urine (ultrafiltration) occurs across the glomerular wall and separates the plasma water and its nonprotein constituents (crystalloids) that enter Bowman's space from the blood cells and protein (colloids), which remain in the capillary lumen. The rate of glomerular ultrafiltration (GFR) is governed by the differences between transcapillary hydrostatic (ΔP) and colloid osmotic pressures ($\Delta \Pi$). GFR is influenced also by the filtration coefficient (K_f), which is a function of both total capillary surface area and the permeability per unit of surface area. Thus:

$$\text{GFR} = K_f(\Delta P - \Delta \Pi) \text{ or GFR} = K_f[(P_{GC} - P_{BS}) - \Pi_{GC}]$$

The difference in hydrostatic pressure (ΔP) between glomerular capillaries (P_{GC}) and Bowman's space (P_{BS}) favors filtration, whereas the colloid osmotic pressure inside the capillaries (Π_{GC}) opposes it. (The colloid osmotic pressure in Bowman's space is normally negligible and can be disregarded.) Hydrostatic pressure (P_{GC}) remains relatively constant along glomerular capillaries; however, the colloid osmotic pressure (Π_{GC}) undergoes a large progressive increase because filtration of "protein-free fluid" results in an increase of protein concentration along the capillary lumen. Hence, the mean effective pressure for ultrafiltration ($\Delta P - \Delta \Pi$) decreases along the glomerular capillary as $\Delta \Pi$ increases. If the rise in glomerular capillary Π is such that effective ultrafiltration pressure becomes zero before the end of the capillary, *filtration pressure equilibrium* ($P_{GC} = \Pi_{GC} + P_{BS}$) occurs, and filtration ceases before the end of the glomerular capillary. Thus, GFR is highly dependent on the glomerular plasma flow rate, because at high flow rates, a slower rise in colloid osmotic pressure (Π_{GC}) occurs. Thus, glomerular filtration takes place across a greater length of the capillary. Hence, increased plasma flow tends to elevate GFR, whereas decreased plasma flow may cause a fall in GFR. As noted previously, renal blood flow and GFR are autoregulated within a wide range of renal arterial pressure. When perfusion pressure falls, the resistance of the afferent arteriole decreases. Thus, glomerular plasma flow and GFR are maintained. Below 80 to 90 mm Hg, renal plasma flow and GFR vary directly with arterial pressure, and the GFR ceases when the pressure falls below 50 mm Hg.

At a physiologic GFR of 120 ml per minute, the filtration rate per nephron (assuming 2,400,000 nephrons in both kidneys) would be 50 nanoliters per minute. However, just as superficial and juxtamedullary nephrons differ anatomically, they also appear to differ functionally. The larger juxtamedullary glomeruli have filtration rates that are about twice as high as the superficial ones. The physiologic implications of this extensive heterogeneity are not clear, although it has been suggested that redistribution of intrarenal blood flow toward deeper nephrons is associated with salt retention and may contribute to edema in hepatic disease and congestive heart failure.

Alterations by disease states of any of the primary determinants discussed above may modify GFR. Thus, GFR can fall as a result of (1) decreased hydrostatic pressure in glomerular capillaries (marked hypotension); (2) increased hydrostatic pressure in Bowman's space (intratubular or urinary tract obstruction); (3) elevated glomerular plasma oncotic pressure as a consequence of increased concentration of proteins in the systemic circulation (dehydration: vomiting, diarrhea); (4) decreased renal plasma flow, which may lead to filtration equilibrium at a more proximal region along the glomerular capillary and hence may decrease the total surface area of capillary available for filtration (e.g., congestive heart failure, hepatic disease); or (5) a decrease in the filtration coefficient (K_f) due to a fall in permeability or to a reduction in total surface area available for filtration (intrinsic renal disease: certain nephrotoxins, acute or chronic glomerulonephritis).

Permselectivity of the Glomerular Capillary Wall. The glomerular capillary wall is highly permeable to small solutes and water. Molecules the size of inulin (molecular weight 5200) or smaller are present in the glomerular filtrate at the same concentration as in plasma water. Constituents with increasing *molecular size* exhibit progressively decreasing concentration in the filtrate.

In addition to molecular size, *molecular configuration*, *deformability*, and *net electrical charge* influence the filtration of macromolecules across the glomerular capillary wall. Negatively charged dextrans, of comparable size to albumin (a polyanion), have a clearance similar to that of albumin (less than 1 per cent that of inulin). By contrast, uncharged (neutral) dextran molecules of the same size as albumin are filtered at a much greater rate (20 per cent the rate of inulin), and filtration of cationic (positively charged) dextrans is even greater. Therefore, at constant molecular size, negative charge of the solute restricts and positive charge accelerates its filtration, suggesting that, phenomenologically, glomerular filtration occurs through pores with negative charges. A negatively charged glycoprotein ("*glomerular polyanion*"), predominantly found lining the foot processes of the epithelial cells, has been identified. Loss of these negative charges, in certain glomerular diseases, may lead to increased filtration of albumin.

HOMEOSTATIC AND EXCRETORY FUNCTIONS OF THE KIDNEY

The formation of urine begins with the elaboration of a protein-free plasma ultrafiltrate across the glomerular capillaries (*glomerular filtration*). As this ultrafiltrate flows through the renal tubule, solutes and water are reabsorbed from lumen to blood (*reabsorption*). Other solutes are secreted into the tubular lumen from the blood (*secretion*). In some cases, both processes (reabsorption and secretion) affect a given substance, permitting flexible regulation of its excretion. Quantitatively, about 170 liters of fluid are ultrafiltered daily, of which less than 1 liter to more than 10 liters may be excreted as urine, depending on the water balance of the individual. Large amounts of filtered sodium, chloride, calcium, magnesium, and phosphate are reabsorbed, with the quantity remaining in the final urine varying according to the dietary intake of each one of these solutes. Substances such as glucose, amino acids, and bicarbonate are almost completely reabsorbed and, under physiologic conditions, do not appear in the urine. The contribution of tubular transport to homeostasis is discussed in more detail below.

TUBULAR TRANSPORT. The renal tubule can be divided functionally into three major segments: (1) the proximal tubule, (2) the loop of Henle, and (3) the distal nephron. Although there are physiologic and morphologic subdivisions of these segments, it is possible to ascribe a general function to each. The proximal tubule reabsorbs, rather nonselectively, a large fraction (two thirds) of the glomerular filtrate. The loop of Henle has unique water and solute transport properties and serves to establish a hyperosmolar medullary interstitium that influences the ultimate concentration or dilution of the urine. The distal nephron is the site of fine regulation of water and electrolyte excretion and appears to be the main target of hormones that control these processes. Since the tubule segments are arranged in series, the function of any segment depends not only on its own intrinsic transport characteristics but also on the volume and composition of the fluid delivered to it from the previous segment.

Proximal Tubule. The proximal tubule reabsorbs sodium, several other solutes, and water at a high rate. Active sodium reabsorption and hydrogen ion secretion are the essential processes to which transport of chloride, several organic solutes, and water is coupled by a variety of mechanisms. Fluid transport is isosmotic, so that concentration gradients of solute across the wall are small. Functionally, the proximal tubule can be divided into three segments:

Initial Portion of the Proximal Tubule. Sodium reabsorption in this portion occurs through cells and intercellular spaces. Transcellular reabsorption of sodium is active, generating a small transtubular electrical potential (1 to 5 mV, lumen negative) (Fig. 73–2). It requires entry of sodium across luminal (brush border) membranes and extrusion of sodium across basolateral membranes. Entry of sodium across luminal membranes is passive and occurs (1) by diffusion, (2) coupled to the transport of other solutes (e.g., glucose, amino acids, phosphate), and (3) in exchange with H^+ secreted from cell to lumen. Sodium extrusion from cells into the intercellular spaces and across the basolateral membrane is an active (energy-requiring) process that is accomplished by the sodium-potassium pump (Na^+-K^+-ATPase). These processes transport solutes out of the lumen and generate slight osmotic gradients which drive water absorption across the permeable proximal tubule.

Preferential reabsorption of bicarbonate from H^+ secretion occurs in this segment, with bicarbonate concentration falling and chloride concentration increasing to an equivalent degree along this segment of the tubule. The reabsorption of glucose and amino acids is active, is coupled to sodium transport, and is nearly complete in this segment. Some permeant solutes, such as urea, are partially reabsorbed by a passive mechanism because of the increase in their luminal concentration as water is absorbed.

Distal Two Thirds of the Proximal Tubule. The luminal fluid of the last two thirds of the proximal tubule is characterized by a low concentration of bicarbonate and by the absence of glucose and amino acids. The tubular fluid remains isosmotic with plasma and has the same concentration of sodium as does the filtrate. The concentration of chloride in the lumen, however, exceeds the concentration of chloride in the peritubular capillary. This concentration gradient for chloride favors its diffusion out of the lumen, generating a lumen-positive potential (which is on the order of 1 to 3 mV). In experiments in vitro in which luminal and peritubular fluids have identical compositions, active sodium transport occurs. Therefore, sodium chloride reabsorption in this segment primarily occurs by active transcellular transport, with a smaller passive flow due to the positive luminal potential and solvent drag.

This segment is the main site of secretion of organic acids (penicillin, uric acid) and other substances such as creatinine. Its rate of sodium and fluid transport is slower, and its capacity for glucose and amino acid reabsorption is modest compared with that of the early segments of the proximal tubule.

Modulation of Reabsorption by the Proximal Tubule. Proximal reabsorption conserves most of the filtered fluid and all of a number of essential solutes. Several factors modulate the transport rate at the proximal tubule and therefore influence the performance of subsequent segments by altering their load.

Transtubular Physical Factors. The hydrostatic pressure (P) in the peritubular capillaries is markedly decreased compared with that in the glomerular capillaries. The colloid osmotic pressure

(Π) is increased owing to filtration of a "protein-free fluid" at the glomeruli. These "Starling forces" thus favor the uptake of fluid by the peritubular capillaries. When Π falls or P rises, the uptake of fluid by peritubular capillaries decreases. This leads to fluid accumulation in the interstitium, increased hydrostatic pressure in this space, and a decrease in net fluid reabsorption.

Glomerular tubular balance refers to a direct relationship between GFR and the prevailing rates of proximal tubular reabsorption and has been ascribed to changes in Π in the peritubular circulation that result from changes in GFR (increases in GFR and hence in filtration fraction lead to a greater protein concentration and increases in Π in the efferent arterioles and peritubular capillaries; a decrease in GFR has the opposite effect). Thus, when GFR increases, a greater amount of fluid is delivered to the proximal tubule; however, the resulting rise in peritubular Π leads to a proportional increase in the reabsorption of fluid in this segment so that the percentage of the filtrate reabsorbed in the proximal tubule remains constant. An alternative mechanism accounting for glomerular tubular balance is a link between fluid reabsorption in the proximal tubule and flow rates of tubular fluid. Increases in GFR, and hence in proximal tubular flow, augment reabsorption; decreases in GFR and in flow decrease reabsorption.

Effects of Hormones on Sodium Reabsorption by the Proximal Tubule. Parathyroid hormone acutely reduces sodium and fluid reabsorption in the proximal tubule; catecholamines may stimulate fluid reabsorption in this segment. Locally generated angiotensin II stimulates sodium reabsorption across the apical membrane of the proximal tubule. Atrial natriuretic peptide antagonizes this effect of angiotensin II on sodium reabsorption.

Loop of Henle. The loop of Henle, which is interposed between the proximal and distal tubules, is a hairpin-shaped structure extending into the renal medulla (Fig. 73–2). Under physiologic conditions it reabsorbs about 25 per cent of the filtered sodium and chloride and 15 per cent of the filtered water. In consequence, the isotonic fluid entering Henle's loop becomes hypotonic to plasma before entering the distal tubule.

The maintenance of water balance requires the excretion of urine of varied tonicity. The formation of a dilute (hypotonic to plasma) or concentrated (hypertonic to plasma) urine takes place by means of a *countercurrent system* that involves not only the loops of Henle but also the distal tubule, the collecting ducts,

and the blood vessels supplying these segments. The excretion of a hypertonic urine involves two basic steps: (1) creation of a hypertonic medullary interstitium and (2) osmotic equilibration of the fluid that enters the medullary collecting duct with the hypertonic interstitium. Antidiuretic hormone (ADH) is required in this latter process. Hypotonic urine is excreted when the fluid that enters the medullary collecting duct does not equilibrate with the hypertonic interstitium owing to low levels or absence of ADH.

In normal human subjects the maximal osmolality of urine that can be achieved is around 1200 mOsm per kilogram. Since the tubular fluid reaches this osmolality by equilibration with the medullary interstitium, it follows that the interstitium must have a similar osmolality. *Countercurrent multiplication* is the process by which the interstitial osmolality is increased from 285 mOsm in the cortex (the same osmolality as plasma) to 1200 mOsm in the papilla. The thin descending and ascending limbs of juxtamedullary nephrons lie in close proximity to each other in the medulla. Flow through them is countercurrent. Fluid obtained from thin ascending limbs has a lower osmolality than fluid obtained from thin descending limbs at comparable levels in the papilla. This is due to functional differences. Whereas the descending limb is highly permeable to water, slightly permeable to urea, and highly impermeable to sodium, the ascending limb is highly permeable to sodium, moderately permeable to urea, and impermeable to water. In normal mammals, the medullary interstitium is hyperosmotic owing to the accumulation of high concentrations of both urea and sodium chloride. The isotonic fluid delivered from the proximal tubule becomes progressively hypertonic as it traverses the thin descending limb owing to net water flow from lumen to interstitium. The highest osmolality of the luminal fluid is achieved at the tip of the loop. This hyperosmolar fluid becomes diluted progressively as it flows up the thin ascending limb, owing to the movement of sodium without water from the lumen to the interstitium. Urea present in the interstitium diffuses inward. However, since the permeability of this segment to sodium chloride is greater than to urea, the net effect is a greater exit of sodium chloride than urea entry, resulting in net addition of solute to the interstitial fluid, and since the thin ascending limb is impermeable to water, the fluid becomes hypotonic with respect to the interstitial fluid at the same level.

The thick ascending limb of the loop actively reabsorbs sodium chloride. The luminal transport step is a furosemide-inhibitable $Na^+/K^+/2Cl^-$ cotransporter. This segment is essentially imperme-

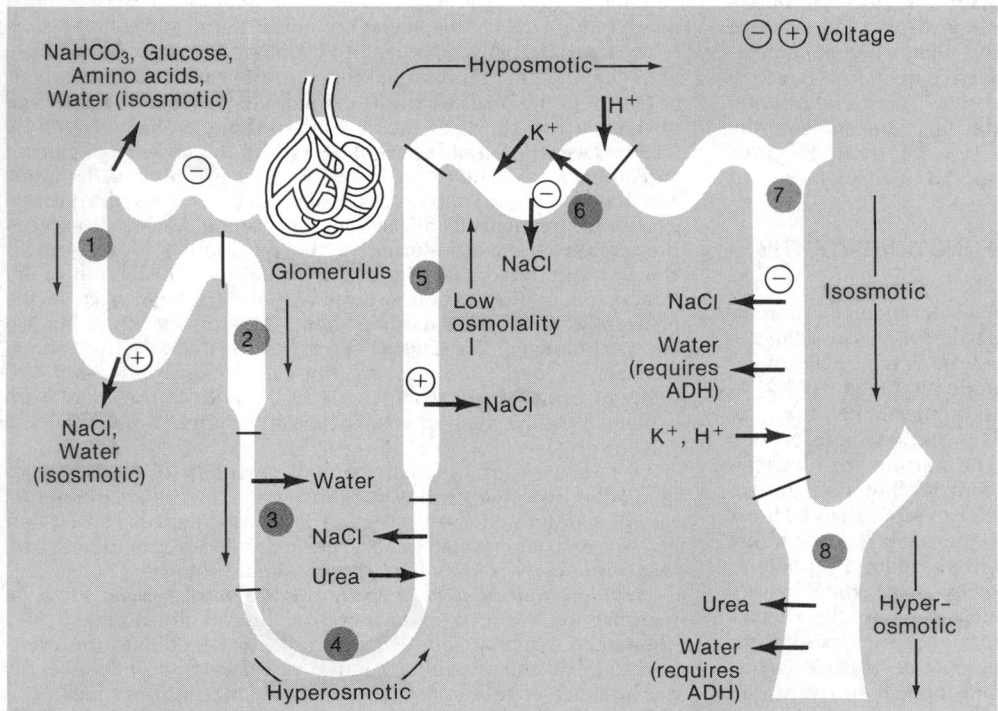

FIGURE 73–2. Schematic representation of the principal processes of transport in the nephron. In the early portion of the proximal tubule (1) salt and water are reabsorbed at high rates, in isotonic proportions. Bulk reabsorption of most of the filtrate (65 to 70 per cent) and virtually complete reabsorption of glucose, amino acids, and bicarbonate take place in this segment. In the pars recta (2) organic acids and bases are secreted and continuous reabsorption of sodium chloride takes place. The loop of Henle comprises three segments; the thin descending (3) and ascending (4) limbs and the thick ascending limb (5). The fluid becomes hyperosmotic, because of water abstraction, as it flows toward the bend of the loop and hyposmotic, because of sodium chloride reabsorption, as it flows toward the distal convoluted tubule (6). Active sodium reabsorption occurs in the distal convoluted tubule and in the cortical collecting tubule (7). This latter segment is water impermeable in the absence of ADH, and the reabsorption of sodium in this segment is increased by aldosterone. The collecting duct (8) allows equilibration of water with the

hyperosmotic interstitium when ADH is present. In the absence of ADH, a large volume of dilute urine is excreted. (Adapted from figure by A Iselin, from Burg MB: Hosp Pract 13:99, 1978. Reproduced with permission.)

able to water, even when ADH is present; therefore, salt transport from lumen to interstitial fluid further decreases the osmolality of the luminal fluid and increases the osmolality of the interstitium, accounting for the countercurrent multiplication that occurs in the renal medulla. The amount of urea present in the fluid of the thick ascending limb is higher than in the fluid entering the thin descending limb. This is due to water abstraction, in excess of urea, out of the latter segment and net urea entry (recycled from the collecting duct) into the thin ascending and descending limbs of Henle's loop.

The fluid emerging from the loop of Henle is virtually always hyposmotic (about 150 mOsm per kilogram) compared with plasma, regardless of the final urine osmolality. With low or absent ADH, the luminal fluid in the collecting system does not equilibrate with the interstitium. Hence, the volume of fluid delivered to the tip of the collecting duct is increased and its osmolality decreased compared with plasma. The osmolality of this fluid can be further decreased to as low as 30 mOsm per kilogram by the reabsorption of solute in excess of water in distal tubule and cortical and medullary collecting ducts.

Since the maximal urine osmolality cannot exceed that in the interstitium, the ability to conserve water by excreting a highly concentrated urine is reduced when the hypertonicity of the medullary interstitium is decreased. This may occur when papillary urea accumulation is reduced, as occurs in protein malnutrition, as a consequence of decreased urea production, or due to reduced interstitial sodium chloride accumulation (use of loop diuretics, hypercalcemia). Reduced levels or absence of ADH (diabetes insipidus) or unresponsiveness of the collecting duct to the action of ADH (nephrogenic diabetes insipidus) may prevent equilibration of the fluid in the collecting duct with the hypertonic interstitium, leading to an impairment in water conservation.

Distal Nephron (Distal Convoluted Tubule, Cortical Collecting Tubule, and Medullary Collecting Duct). The distal nephron accomplishes the final and delicate adjustments in the reabsorption of water, sodium, chloride, phosphate, and calcium in response to aldosterone, ADH, and parathyroid hormone.

The *distal convoluted tubule* is defined anatomically as the segment that extends from the macula densa to the site of transition from homogeneous cells to a mixture of dark and light cells (typical of the collecting duct). The distal convoluted tubule is essentially impermeable to water and unresponsive to ADH. Sodium chloride is reabsorbed at a slower rate than in the proximal tubule or in the loop, but against large concentration gradients. The rate of reabsorption is proportional to the load. The transtubular electrical potential, lumen negative, is related to the reabsorption of sodium and varies from −10 in the initial portion to −45 mV in the distal portion. Most of the reabsorption of sodium chloride occurs transcellularly. Potassium is secreted in this segment from peritubular capillary into the lumen, and there appears to be an active H⁺ transport mechanism located at the luminal membrane, especially at the transition of distal convoluted tubule to cortical collecting tubule.

The *cortical collecting tubule* extends from the end of the distal tubule to the corticomedullary junction. Under basal conditions, water permeability is negligible in this segment. It is increased markedly by ADH. Sodium chloride is actively reabsorbed at this level; therefore, in the absence of ADH the luminal fluid osmolality falls further. When ADH is present the luminal fluid equilibrates with the cortical interstitial fluid and becomes isosmotic with plasma; at the same time, luminal urea concentrations rise (see above). The transtubular electrical potential is about 35 mV, lumen negative; it is related to active reabsorption of sodium and is highly dependent on the levels of mineralocorticoids, which increase sodium reabsorption. Potassium and hydrogen are secreted in this segment. Aldosterone increases sodium reabsorption as well as potassium and H⁺ secretion in this portion of the nephron (Fig. 73–2).

The *medullary collecting duct* starts at the corticomedullary junction and ends on the surface of the papilla. Water and urea permeabilities are low in the absence of ADH. Continuous sodium chloride reabsorption at this level, in the absence of ADH, results in a further drop in urine osmolality. ADH increases water and urea permeability and allows the equilibration of the luminal osmolality with that of the hypertonic interstitium.

To recapitulate, in the proximal tubule salt and water are transported at high rates, in isotonic proportions. Bulk reabsorp-

tion of most of the filtrate (65 to 70 per cent) and virtually complete reabsorption of "metabolically useful" solutes (glucose, amino acids, bicarbonate) take place in this segment. The *loop of Henle* comprises three segments with strikingly different properties of active transport and permeability of water and solute. Because of these properties, the medullary interstitium is made hyperosmolar and acts as the driving force for final water reabsorption. The loop reabsorbs additional sodium chloride (about 25 per cent of that filtered) and water (about 15 per cent of the filtrate) and leaves about 10 per cent of the sodium and 15 per cent of the water to be reabsorbed in the last segments of the tubule.

The distal convoluted tubule and the collecting tubule can establish large sodium gradients between fluid in the lumen and in the peritubular capillary. The collecting ducts, water impermeable in the absence of ADH, become permeable to water in response to the hormone. It is in these segments that the final volume and osmolality of the urine are determined. Salt transport occurs at a slower rate than in the preceding segments but against large concentration gradients. The final regulation of salt excretion takes place in these segments, under the influence of aldosterone. Potassium and H⁺ excretion are regulated also in these segments.

ROLE OF THE KIDNEY IN SODIUM CHLORIDE HOMEOSTASIS. Normally the kidney regulates sodium balance (and hence extracellular fluid volume) in a very efficient manner. The daily intake of sodium varies considerably. In the Western world the average diet contains about 170 mEq per 24 hours. About 98 per cent of this amount is excreted in the urine. However, this represents less than 1 per cent of the amount of sodium filtered (140 mEq per liter × 170 liters = 23,800 mEq) each day. Thus, maintenance of sodium homeostasis is primarily a function of the renal tubule and reabsorption of filtered sodium; changes in GFR appear to be quantitatively less important. Thus, (1) sizable increases in GFR, not accompanied by extracellular fluid (ECF) volume expansion, do not result in a marked natriuresis because of glomerular tubular balance (see above), and (2) the natriuresis of ECF volume expansion occurs under experimental conditions in which GFR is maintained constant or even decreased experimentally. When a normal subject increases the intake of salt, urine sodium excretion increases progressively and reaches a steady-state level equal to intake. During the interval of adjustment, positive sodium balance occurs, with an accompanying retention of water and consequent gain in body weight. When salt intake is suddenly reduced, the opposite effects are observed. Sodium excretion decreases, reaching a level equal to intake within 3 to 5 days with a reduction in total body water and body weight.

Several physiologic mechanisms ordinarily control sodium reabsorption by the kidney to maintain the sodium content of ECF. Changes in sodium mass are not sensed as such, but secondarily as changes in ECF volume. Total ECF volume changes are sensed through their effects on circulatory dynamics ("effective arterial blood volume"). The determinants of effective arterial blood volume are (1) the degree of filling of the arterial tree, which depends in large part on cardiac output, and (2) peripheral vascular resistance, which depends on the compliance of the peripheral vessels and the magnitude of the arterial runoff. Decreases in effective volume (dehydration, hemorrhage, venodilation, venous pooling) lead to renal retention of salt. Increases in effective volume (saline administration, excessive salt intake) lead to a rise in salt excretion by the kidney.

Factors That Influence the Tubular Reabsorption of Sodium. Alterations in effective arterial volume affect handling of sodium by the kidney through the renin-angiotensin-aldosterone system, the sympathetic nervous system, and other less well-defined factors. The last category probably includes changes in intrarenal hydrostatic and oncotic pressures (so-called physical factors), natriuretic (or salt-losing) hormones such as atrial natriuretic peptides, and possibly the distribution of blood flow within the kidneys.

Role of Physical Factors in the Reabsorption of Sodium. A fall in effective arterial blood volume (dehydration, hemorrhage) and the consequent decline in blood pressure decrease renal perfusion. In response to reductions in renal perfusion pressure, glomerular plasma flow decreases more than does glomerular capillary hydrostatic pressure, resulting in a fall in GFR that is proportionally less than the decline in renal plasma flow. This disparity is due to a greater vasoconstriction of efferent compared with afferent arterioles in response to increased levels of catecholamines and angiotensin II. The lesser fall in GFR compared with renal plasma flow increases filtration fraction and hence the concentration of protein in the efferent arterioles and peritubular capillaries. In addition, vasoconstriction of the efferent arteriole results in a fall in hydrostatic pressure (P) in the peritubular capillaries. The increase in Π and the decrease in P in the peritubular capillaries augment sodium and water reabsorption along the proximal segments of the nephron. Thus, in response to contraction of effective arterial volume, the glomerular and peritubular microcirculations act in concert to minimize fluid losses by both lowering GFR and augmenting salt and water reabsorption by the tubules.

Expansion of the ECF volume elicits opposite effects. The increase in renal perfusion pressure leads to not only a rise in GFR but also a proportionally greater rise in renal plasma flow; consequently filtration fraction falls. The net effect is a decrease in peritubular protein concentration and hence in Π, with a decrease in reabsorption of fluid by peritubular capillaries. The importance of such physical factors in the normal control of sodium and water reabsorption is not exactly clear. Since alterations in Π and P in the peritubular capillaries influence fluid reabsorption mainly, if not exclusively, in the proximal tubule, it is likely that changes in physical factors are important only when fluid balance deficits or gains are very large (as, for example, with severe hemorrhage or marked expansion of the ECF volume). Whether significant changes in proximal reabsorption occur in response to more modest alterations in fluid balance (as might result, for example, in response to a diet very low or very high in sodium chloride) remains uncertain.

Redistribution of Blood Flow. Another mechanism potentially altering sodium excretion is redistribution of blood flow. It has been suggested that nephrons with superficially placed glomeruli have less capacity to reabsorb sodium than others. If so, at any given total GFR, the relative amounts of fluid filtered by the two different nephron populations would be an important determinant of sodium excretion. Redistribution of GFR toward the "high reabsorption nephrons" (juxtamedullary nephrons) would be associated with decreased sodium excretion because of the greater capacity of these nephrons to reabsorb sodium. Despite the attractiveness of this theory, evidence favoring it is scant.

Renin-Angiotensin-Aldosterone. Sodium balance is controlled also by *mineralocorticoid hormones, mainly aldosterone.* Only a small but significant fraction (some 2 per cent) of the filtered sodium is under hormonal control. Yet loss or gain of an amount of sodium equivalent to 2 per cent of the filtered load (about 500 mEq per day) has profound effects on sodium balance. Aldosterone increases sodium reabsorption in the distal tubule and collecting duct. Lack of aldosterone leads to loss of sodium in the urine. The factors controlling aldosterone secretion include (1) angiotensin, (2) plasma concentration of potassium, (3) adrenocorticotropic hormone (ACTH), and (4) plasma Na^+ concentration. Circulating levels of angiotensin are increased by hemorrhage, dietary salt restriction, changes in distribution of blood and fluids (venous pooling and edema-forming states), and other states of increased secretion of renin. *Renin* is a proteolytic enzyme secreted by the granular cells of the juxtaglomerular apparatus. The mechanisms controlling its release seem to depend on (1) changes in renal perfusion pressure, (2) factors reflecting the rate of delivery of sodium chloride to the macula densa, and (3) activity of the renal sympathetic nerves. When perfusion pressure or the delivery of sodium falls, or the activity of the sympathetic nerves increases, the release of renin is enhanced. Renin acts on a substrate in plasma, *angiotensinogen,* to form *angiotensin I* (a decapeptide). *Converting enzyme* splits two amino acids from angiotensin I to form *angiotensin II* (an octapeptide). The latter is a potent hormone, central to the regulation of salt and water balance. It produces vasoconstriction and stimulates the secretion of aldosterone, thirst, and the renal reabsorption of sodium. Another split product of angiotensin, *angiotensin III* (a heptapeptide), also increases aldosterone secretion from the zona glomerulosa of the adrenal.

Natriuretic Hormones. A 28-amino acid peptide produced in the cardiac atria (atrial peptide), which has both natriuretic and vasodilating properties, participates in the regulation of extracellular fluid volume and electrolyte balance. Recently an "atrial-like" natriuretic peptide has been shown to be produced in the kidney. Its role is unknown. In addition, a natriuretic substance of hypothalamic origin that inhibits Na^+-K^+-ATPase activity, displaces ouabain that is bound to cellular membranes, and cross-reacts with digoxin antibodies has been described. The roles of these natriuretic substances in the regulation of renal sodium excretion have not been fully defined, but are most apparent during volume expansion.

Other Hormonal Agents. Cortisol, estrogen, growth hormone, and insulin all can enhance sodium reabsorption. Glucagon, progesterone, and parathyroid hormone can decrease it. It is almost certain that when circulating levels of these hormones are elevated (as, for example, estrogen during pregnancy), significant influences occur on sodium reabsorption and thereby excretion. However, there is no evidence that any of them, unlike the factors described previously, are controlled specifically as part of the homeostatic regulation of sodium balance. Of great interest is the possible role played by intrarenally produced substances such as *prostaglandins* and *kinins*. These agents are potent vasodilators and may reduce sodium reabsorption, by altering regional intrarenal vascular resistance or by direct actions on the tubular cells. Their levels change with alterations of sodium balance, but it is not yet clear how extensively they participate in the renal regulation of sodium excretion. In addition, locally generated vasoconstrictors (thromboxanes, endothelins) may affect renal blood flow and tubule function.

Renal Nerves. The renal sympathetic nerves play a prominent role in sodium homeostasis by modulating (1) secretion of aldosterone via the renin-angiotensin system, (2) intrarenal physical factors, (3) the reabsorptive activity of the tubular cells themselves, and (4) GFR. Yet, because of the many other known (and potential) factors involved, a transplanted and, therefore, denervated kidney maintains sodium homeostasis quite well.

RENAL REGULATION OF WATER EXCRETION. The capacity to regulate renal excretion of water, independent of solute excretion, maintains the osmolality of body fluids within narrow limits despite wide variations in intake of water. Roughly 170 liters of water are filtered daily. Of this amount, less than 2 liters, or about 1 per cent of the amount filtered, are excreted. Except for setting an upper limit for the amount of water that can be excreted per unit time, GFR is not involved in the regulation of water excretion. This upper limit assumes importance only when GFR is profoundly reduced as in acute renal failure or advanced chronic renal disease.

The tubule is the major site for renal regulation of water excretion. Net absorption of water occurs all along the nephron and is due to passive diffusion of water down its concentration gradient into a region of higher osmolality. In the proximal tubule, this gradient is established by the active transcellular transport of sodium chloride and other solutes. About two thirds of the filtered water is reabsorbed isosmotically in the proximal tubule. Reabsorption of water in this segment is intimately related to the reabsorption of sodium. Since water reabsorption in the remaining segments of the nephron is to a large extent independent of the reabsorption of solute, the process is referred to frequently as the reabsorption of solute-free water, or simply *free water.*

The reabsorption of free water is dependent largely on interrelationships among four factors: (1) the concentration of solute in the interstitium through which the renal tubule passes, (2) the concentration of solute in the tubular fluid, (3) the permeability of the renal tubule to water and solute, and (4) the circulating levels of ADH. About 15 per cent of the filtered water enters the distal tubule. A variable fraction of this water is reabsorbed by the distal tubules and collecting ducts. Absorption of this final fraction is controlled by antidiuretic hormone (ADH), which serves as the main regulator of the osmolality of body fluids. ADH is synthesized by nerve cells in the hypothalamus and liberated from their terminals in the posterior lobe and pituitary stalk. The major stimulus for the secretion of ADH into the circulation is an increase in plasma osmolality, mediated by osmoreceptors, which are exquisitely sensitive to changes in osmolality. The feedback system they provide helps to maintain the tonicity of plasma within a standard deviation of ± 2 mOsm (a change of less than 1 per cent). Although changes in osmolality are the most sensitive and therefore the primary regulators of ADH release, alterations in ECF volume can modulate ADH release through a baroreceptor pathway, and override the effects of tonicity. However, secretion of ADH is not increased unless volume loss is greater than 10 per cent. Baroreceptor stimulation appears to mediate the increase in ADH secretion resulting from volume contraction. This effect is potentiated by elevated levels of circulating catecholamines, which act directly on these receptors. Angiotensin II, prostaglandins, and nicotine may also affect ADH release through activation of arterial baroreceptors. When a surfeit of body water develops, ADH release is inhibited and a dilute urine is excreted; when a water deficit is present, free water is reabsorbed and the urine becomes concentrated with respect to plasma.

The human kidney can dilute urine 10-fold with respect to plasma (to about 30 mOsm per kilogram) but can concentrate it to a maximum of only fourfold with respect to plasma (to about 1200 mOsm per kilogram). The daily volume of urine depends on the intake of fluid and can be varied from 600 ml to over 24 liters. When a large load of water is ingested, the following events occur: (1) The osmolar concentration (osmolality) of plasma falls; (2) over the next 15 to 20 minutes ADH levels fall, and as a consequence the flow rate of urine increases, reaching a maximum in 45 to 60 minutes. The maximal increase in urine flow occurs when free water excretion is about 15 per cent of GFR.

ROLE OF THE KIDNEY IN THE PRESERVATION OF POTASSIUM BALANCE. The daily intake of potassium ranges from 50 to 150 mEq. Most of the potassium ingested is absorbed (less than 10 mEq is excreted in the stool); thus, maintenance of balance requires the daily excretion of an amount of potassium identical to that absorbed from the gut. Under physiologic conditions, approximately 70 per cent of the potassium filtered is reabsorbed in the proximal tubule. The loop of Henle reabsorbs the remaining 20 to 30 per cent. Distal segments of the nephron can both reabsorb and secrete potassium. The balance between distal reabsorption and secretion determines the net urinary excretion of this cation. On a normal diet (100 mEq per day) the kidneys excrete approximately 90 mEq of potassium per day. The secretion of potassium is influenced by the potassium concentration in renal distal tubular cells, by the magnitude of the electrochemical gradient between cell interior and tubular lumen, and by the luminal flow rate. The factors that regulate potassium excretion in the urine are summarized in Table 73–2. If potassium intake is increased acutely, renal excretion of potassium can rise

TABLE 73–2. FACTORS THAT REGULATE POTASSIUM EXCRETION IN THE URINE

Condition		Effect on K$^+$ Excretion
Dietary K$^+$	High	Increase
	Low	Decrease
Serum levels of K$^+$	High	Increase
	Low	Decrease
Levels of mineralo- or glucocorticoid hormones	High	Increase
	Low	Decrease
Tubular fluid or urine flow rate	Fast	Increase
	Slow	Decrease
Sodium excretion in the urine	High	Increase
	Low	Decrease
Most diuretics		Increase
K$^+$-sparing diuretics (spironolactone, triamterene, amiloride)		Decrease
Inhibitors of renin release or angiotensin II formation (NSAID's, beta blockers, ACE inhibitors)		Decrease
Metabolic alkalosis		Increase
Metabolic acidosis		Decrease
Augmented urine excretion of impermeant anions (sulfate, carbenicillin)		Increase

more than 10-fold. About 50 per cent of the amount administered appears in the urine within 12 hours. The renal response to potassium deprivation is sluggish. Excretion falls to levels of 10 to 15 mEq per 24 hours only after 7 to 14 days of a potassium-free diet. During this interval a deficit of as much as 200 mEq of potassium may be incurred. In adults with increased catabolism (infections, surgery), the renal excretion of potassium may exceed the amount ingested.

Urinary excretion of potassium (Table 73–2) depends on its rate of secretion by the distal tubule. Increased net secretory rates of potassium in this segment could be due to (1) increased active uptake by the peritubular membrane leading to increased cell potassium concentration and increased passive leak across the luminal membrane, (2) increased permeability of the luminal membrane to potassium, (3) decreased active reabsorption of potassium by the luminal membrane, (4) increased lumen-negative electrical potential difference, or (5) increased luminal flow rate.

A high concentration of potassium in distal tubular cells is maintained through the action of a Na$^+$-K$^+$-ATPase located in the peritubular membrane. Potassium uptake via this pump is stimulated by high plasma levels of potassium, alkalosis, aldosterone, and increased sodium reabsorption. All factors that raise cell potassium (increased peritubular pump activity, dehydration) favor its diffusion into the lumen. If the cellular potassium concentration falls (potassium deprivation, acidosis, dilution of body fluids), the rate of potassium translocation into the lumen falls and may be less than the potassium uptake across the luminal membrane. Under these conditions, net reabsorption of potassium may replace net potassium secretion.

The difference in electrical potential across the entire distal tubular cell is established by the active reabsorption of sodium and is about 50 mV (lumen negative to peritubular fluid). The cell interior is negative (-70 mV) in relation to the peritubular capillary. Thus, the luminal membrane potential difference is about 20 mV (cell negative to lumen). This electrical profile favors a greater leak of potassium across the luminal membrane than across the peritubular membrane. Thus, potassium is pumped into distal tubular cells and then leaks across the luminal membrane into the tubular lumen. Such passive translocation of potassium from the cell into the lumen depends not only on the electrical potential difference across the luminal membrane but also on the chemical concentration gradient. An increased lumen-negative electrical potential or factors that increase cellular potassium or lower luminal potassium have been shown to augment potassium secretion.

Augmented sodium reabsorption in the distal tubule increases lumen electro-negativity, which favors potassium secretion from the cell interior into the tubular fluid. Hence, increased distal sodium reabsorption favors potassium excretion. For example, diuretic administration increases sodium delivery distally, which, in turn, increases potassium excretion, particularly in patients with secondary aldosteronism. Hyperkalemia increases potassium excretion by two mechanisms: It stimulates aldosterone secretion directly, and it also enhances renal secretion, presumably via increased cell content of potassium. Alkalosis enhances and acidosis depresses potassium secretion, probably by inducing corresponding changes in renal cell potassium. The rates of *distal tubular flow* also influence potassium excretion, presumably because of the rapid dissipation of the concentration of potassium in the tubular lumen at higher flow rates.

ROLE OF THE KIDNEY IN ACID-BASE BALANCE. The kidney maintains plasma pH in a physiologic range by regulating the concentration of plasma bicarbonate. This is accomplished by the reabsorption of filtered bicarbonate, and the excretion in the urine of 50 to 100 mEq of H$^+$ in the form of ammonium (NH$_4^+$) and titratable acid (the amount of alkali required to titrate the urine to the pH of plasma). Disodium phosphate (Na$_2$HPO$_4$) present in the filtrate is converted to NaH$_2$PO$_4$, which accounts for most of the titratable acid excreted in the urine. Net excretion of acid (titratable acid + ammonium excretion − bicarbonate excretion) equals the daily production of nonvolatile acids under physiologic conditions. Both the *reclamation* of filtered bicarbonate and the *regeneration* of bicarbonate depend on the secretion of H$^+$ from the tubular cells into the lumen. The secreted H$^+$ is generated within the tubular cells by the *carbonic anhydrase–*catalyzed hydration of CO_2 to H_2CO_3, which immediately dissociates into H^+ and HCO_3^-. The H^+ is secreted into the tubular fluid, and the bicarbonate, concomitantly produced intracellularly, enters the peritubular capillary. Thus, H^+ secretion results in addition of bicarbonate to plasma. When the H^+ secreted into the lumen combines with filtered bicarbonate, it forms H_2CO_3, which quickly dissociates to CO_2 and H_2O. As a consequence, a bicarbonate disappears from the lumen, and the net effect is bicarbonate reabsorption (reclamation).

At a physiologic GFR of 170 liters per day and a plasma bicarbonate level of 24 mEq per liter, the reabsorption of over 4000 mEq of bicarbonate requires the secretion of an equivalent amount of H^+, whereas the excretion of net acid requires the secretion of 50 to 100 mEq of H^+ daily (Table 73–3). The process of bicarbonate reclamation operates to reabsorb all the filtered bicarbonate below a critical serum concentration, the *bicarbonate threshold concentration*, which in adult humans is normally about 24 mEq per liter, essentially identical to the concentration of bicarbonate in plasma. When plasma bicarbonate concentration rises and/or GFR is increased, the filtered load of bicarbonate is increased and renal reclamation is incomplete. The excess bicarbonate escapes into the urine, enabling the plasma bicarbonate concentration to return to the threshold level. Under physiologic conditions the virtually complete reabsorption of bicarbonate serves to preserve bicarbonate stores but does not replace the bicarbonate consumed in the buffering of nonvolatile acids. If the secreted H^+ combines with buffers, such as HPO_4^- or NH_3, a new bicarbonate ion (de novo synthesis) is added to the peritubular capillary blood. This results in replacement of the bicarbonate consumed in buffering the daily acid load (Table 73–3).

At times, net acid excretion is absent or has a negative value. This occurs after ingestion of an alkaline load (bicarbonate or substances that can be metabolized to bicarbonate). Ammonium excretion accounts for two thirds and titratable acid for one third of the urinary excretion of acid. When the daily H^+ load increases (e.g., increased catabolism, infection), the rise in acid excretion by the kidney is usually due to increased ammonium excretion. Ammonia (NH_3), produced within the renal proximal tubular cells from glutamine, diffuses into the peritubular capillary or lumen down its concentration gradient. In the lumen it combines with H^+ to form NH_4^+. As noted, each mole of NH_4^+ excreted results in the de novo generation of 1 mole of bicarbonate. Thus, when metabolic acidosis develops and the need for regenerating bicarbonate increases, synthesis of ammonia and NH_4^+ excretion usually increase.

Hydrogen secretion occurs in both proximal and distal segments of the nephron. As the concentration of bicarbonate in the lumen decreases, the concentration of H^+ increases, and as a result a limitation is imposed on the net rate of H^+ secretion. The maximal H^+ gradient achievable between cell and collecting duct lumen is about 800:1 (luminal fluid pH of 4.5).

Factors That Regulate the Renal Secretion of Hydrogen Ions. The major factors that influence the renal secretion of H^+ are (1) *effective circulating volume*, (2) *arterial pH and* P_{CO_2}, (3) *plasma concentration of potassium*, and (4) *mineralocorticoids (aldosterone)*.

Effective Circulating Volume. Hydrogen ion secretion is increased during volume depletion (increased sodium reabsorption) and diminished during ECF volume expansion. Hydrogen secretion is stimulated also when significant amounts of nonreabsorbable anions, i.e., sulfate ions, are present in the distal nephron and when sodium reabsorption is enhanced by any mechanism. Thus, the effective circulating volume of the ECF and the amounts of nonreabsorbable anion accompanying sodium through the distal nephron are important determinants of renal H^+ secretion.

Arterial pH and P_{CO_2}**.** Net acid excretion is increased with acidosis and decreased with alkalosis. Acidosis, resulting from a decrease in the plasma concentration of bicarbonate (metabolic acidosis) or induced by an elevation in P_{CO_2} (respiratory acidosis), augments H^+ excretion and increases the renal synthesis of bicarbonate. Metabolic alkalosis (increased plasma bicarbonate) or respiratory alkalosis (decreased P_{CO_2}) has the opposite effects. The effects of arterial pH on net acid excretion are most likely mediated by changes in renal tubular cell pH. Elevations in arterial P_{CO_2} increase bicarbonate reabsorption, and a fall in arterial P_{CO_2} reduces bicarbonate reabsorption.

Plasma Potassium Concentration. Hypokalemia increases and hyperkalemia decreases H^+ excretion. These effects are due to changes in intracellular H^+ concentration induced by cation shifts between the ICF and the ECF. In hypokalemia, potassium leaves the cell and is replaced by H^+ and sodium. The increase in intracellular H^+ concentration (intracellular acidosis) leads to the enhanced H^+ secretion and bicarbonate reabsorption associated with potassium depletion. In addition, hypokalemia stimulates renal ammonia production. The opposite occurs with hyperkalemia.

Aldosterone. Aldosterone stimulates secretion of both potassium and hydrogen in the distal nephron. Excess of aldosterone may cause metabolic alkalosis, and its deficiency may lead to hyperchloremic metabolic acidosis and hyperkalemia by decreasing H^+ and K^+ excretion.

ROLE OF THE KIDNEY IN MINERAL HOMEOSTASIS. The kidney regulates the homeostasis of minerals not only by modifying the excretion of phosphate, calcium, and magnesium (see below) but also by influencing the metabolism of vitamin D. Vitamin D_3 (cholecalciferol) is metabolized to 25(OH) cholecalciferol in the liver and subsequently to $1,25(OH)_2D_3$ and $24,25(OH)_2D_3$ in the kidney. The $1,25(OH)_2D_3$ is the calcemic hormone produced in the renal cortex in response to hypophosphatemia or elevated levels of parathyroid hormone (when hypocalcemia occurs), and $24,25(OH)_2D_3$ is produced preferentially when the mineral balance is normal. The $1,25(OH)_2D_3$ increases absorption of calcium and phosphate from the gut as well as mineral mobilization from bone. The role of $24,25(OH)_2D_3$ is less well defined; it seems to promote bone mineralization and suppress parathyroid hormone release.

REGULATION OF PHOSPHORUS METABOLISM. The kidneys play a major role in maintaining the serum phosphorus concentration within narrow limits, about 3.0 to 4.5 mg per deciliter in adults. On an average diet, 1 gram of phosphorus is ingested daily, of which 700 mg is absorbed and the rest is excreted in the stool. The kidneys filter about 7 grams of phosphorus daily, of which 6.3 grams (90 per cent) is reabsorbed and 700 mg is excreted in the urine. As serum phosphorus and filtered load of phosphorus rise, the capacity to reabsorb phosphorus increases until a transport maximum (Tm) for phosphorus reabsorption is reached when serum phosphorus concentrations are between 6 and 9 mg per deciliter. Under physiologic conditions, about 70 per cent of the filtered phosphorus is reabsorbed in the proximal tubule and 10 to 15 per cent in the distal tubule and collecting ducts; thus, 5 to 20 per cent of the filtered phosphorus is excreted in the urine. In other words, the tubular reabsorption of phosphate (TRP) ranges normally from 80 to 95 per cent.

Numerous factors (the major ones being dietary phosphorus load and the serum levels of parathyroid hormone) affect the reabsorption of phosphorus. Phosphorus reabsorption approaches 100 per cent in patients fed a very low-phosphorus diet. In contrast, patients ingesting 2 to 3 grams of phosphorus daily can excrete 60 to 70 per cent of this amount in the urine. Changes in phosphorus intake affect phosphorus excretion directly and also by altering the levels of ionized calcium that modify the release of parathyroid hormone. Parathyroid hormone decreases phosphorus reabsorption in both proximal and distal segments of the nephron. An excess of parathyroid hormone may increase fractional excretion of phosphorus from a basal value of 10 per cent to 30 per cent or more. In the absence of parathyroid hormone the tubular capacity to reabsorb phosphorus is increased. Additional factors affect phosphorus reabsorption by the

TABLE 73–3. ROLE OF THE KIDNEY IN ACID-BASE BALANCE

Function	mEq/24 hr
1. Reabsorption of filtered bicarbonate ("reclamation")	≅ 4000
2. Generation of new bicarbonate (net excretion of acid)	50–100
a. Ammonium excretion	35–65
b. Titratable acid excretion	15–35

kidney. Volume expansion of the ECF, calcitonin, glucocorticoids, metabolic acidosis or alkalosis, and glycosuria increase urinary phosphorus excretion. On the other hand, growth hormone, insulin, and respiratory acidosis decrease phosphorus excretion. Vitamin D and its metabolites increase phosphorus reabsorption by the kidney.

RENAL REGULATION OF CALCIUM METABOLISM.

Serum calcium concentrations in humans are maintained between 9 and 10 mg per deciliter despite wide variations in dietary calcium intake. Total serum calcium consists of ultrafilterable calcium (approximately 60 per cent of the total) and calcium bound to protein, primarily albumin. The ultrafilterable fraction includes both the ionized calcium (50 per cent of the total) and calcium complexed to citrate, bicarbonate, and phosphate, which represents 10 per cent of total serum calcium. Serum calcium levels are maintained relatively constant through modification of calcium absorption from the gastrointestinal tract, changes in renal calcium excretion, and mobilization of calcium from bone.

Approximately 1000 mg of calcium is ingested daily in the diet. About 800 mg appears in the stool (from unabsorbed dietary calcium and intestinal secretion) and 200 mg in the urine. The percentage of dietary calcium absorbed from the intestine increases when calcium intake is low and decreases when it is high. Parathyroid hormone and vitamin D participate in these adaptations. Thus, in patients fed a low-calcium diet, the development of mild and transient hypocalcemia increases the release of parathyroid hormone, which augments the renal conversion of $25(OH)D_3$ to $1,25(OH)_2D_3$. This latter compound increases intestinal calcium absorption and mobilizes calcium from bone, synergistically with parathyroid hormone. Thus, serum calcium returns toward normal. On the other hand, in patients fed a high-calcium diet, the mild hypercalcemia that may occur suppresses the release of parathyroid hormone, leading to decreased activity of the renal 1-hydroxylase enzyme and reduced production of $1,25(OH)_2D_3$.

The kidneys filter approximately 10 grams of calcium per day, but usually less than 200 mg appear in the urine. Thus over 98 per cent of the filtered load is reabsorbed. Approximately 55 per cent of the filtered calcium is reabsorbed in the proximal tubule, 20 to 30 per cent in the loop of Henle, 10 to 15 per cent in the distal tubule, and 2 to 8 per cent in the terminal nephron, including the collecting duct. Most maneuvers that decrease sodium and fluid reabsorption in the proximal tubule (infusion of saline, administration of acetazolamide, or mild to moderate hypercalcemia) decrease calcium reabsorption in this segment as well. The reabsorption of calcium in the loop of Henle also parallels sodium reabsorption. It is only distal to the loop of Henle that calcium and sodium are influenced separately and independently.

Parathyroid hormone stimulates the renal absorption of calcium and decreases urinary calcium excretion. Acute parathyroidectomy increases calcium excretion despite a fall in total serum calcium and hence in the filtered load of calcium. However, the degree of calciuria declines when the plasma concentration of calcium falls below 7 mg per deciliter. Pharmacologic doses of vitamin D usually increase intestinal absorption of calcium and bone resorption, leading to increases in serum calcium, the filtered load of calcium, and urinary calcium excretion. Metabolic acidosis or phosphate depletion produces hypercalciuria. Both furosemide and ethacrynic acid inhibit sodium and calcium transport in the thick ascending limb of Henle's loop and increase calcium excretion. Chronic administration of thiazides results in natriuresis and hypocalciuria. This effect may be due to contraction of ECF volume and increased calcium reabsorption in the proximal segments. In addition, thiazides may directly stimulate calcium reabsorption in the distal segment.

RENAL REGULATION OF MAGNESIUM METABOLISM.

Total body magnesium is approximately 2000 mEq (or 25 grams). About 60 per cent of total body magnesium is found in bone. Another 20 per cent is present in muscle. Only a small fraction (about 1 per cent) is present in the ECF. The normal plasma concentration of magnesium in humans is 1.7 to 2.2 mg per deciliter, of which 80 per cent is ultrafilterable and the remainder protein bound. Most of the ultrafilterable magnesium is ionized. Roughly 300 mg or 25 mEq of magnesium is ingested daily in the diet. About two thirds of this amount appears in the stool and one third is eliminated in the urine. The kidney filters about 2 grams of magnesium daily, and approximately 100 mg (5 per cent) appears in the urine; thus, 95 per cent of the filtered magnesium is reabsorbed. Renal excretion of magnesium can be reduced to less than 0.5 per cent of the filtered load during magnesium deprivation. On the other hand, during infusion of magnesium or among patients with advanced chronic renal insufficiency the kidney can excrete 40 to 70 per cent of the filtered magnesium. The proximal tubules reabsorb about 20 to 30 per cent of the filtered magnesium, with 50 to 60 per cent being reabsorbed in the loop of Henle. Expansion of the ECF volume, produced by infusion of saline or chronic administration of mineralocorticoids, reduces the reabsorption of magnesium. A diet deficient in magnesium or the administration of parathyroid hormone enhances the reabsorption of magnesium in the thick ascending limb of Henle's loop. Infusions of calcium, ingestion of alcohol, administration of glucose, diets containing large amounts of magnesium, and diuretics such as furosemide or ethacrynic acid increase the urinary excretion of magnesium. Nephrotoxins, most notably cisplatin and aminoglycosides can cause severe renal Mg^{2+} wasting.

OTHER NONEXCRETORY FUNCTIONS OF THE KIDNEY

In addition to its role in the secretion of renin and the metabolism of vitamin D already discussed, the kidney has several other nonexcretory functions.

REGULATION OF THE RED BLOOD CELL MASS. *Erythropoietin* promotes the differentiation, proliferation, and maturation of red blood cell precursors in the bone marrow. Erythropoietin is produced by interstitial cells and by endothelial cells lining the peritubular capillaries of the cortex and outer medulla of the kidney. The stimulus to increased erythropoietin production by the kidney appears to be decreased renal oxygen tension or decreased renal perfusion (anemia, hypoxia, renal ischemia) or circulatory alterations induced by vasoconstrictors such as norepinephrine, angiotensin, or vasopressin. Increased erythropoietin levels may be seen in association with renal artery stenosis, renal cysts, renal cell carcinoma, and hydronephrosis and after renal transplantation. Production of erythropoietin decreases with hyperoxia, an excess red blood cell volume, and reduced functional renal mass.

RENAL METABOLISM OF PLASMA PROTEINS AND PEPTIDE HORMONES. The kidney is an important catabolic site for low molecular weight proteins (less than 50,000) but not for proteins with a molecular weight exceeding 68,000 (e.g., albumin, immunoglobulins).

Low molecular weight proteins are filterable. In the absence of tubular reabsorption they would be excreted quantitatively in the urine. Reabsorption of proteins or their catabolic products by the kidney prevents their loss in the urine, thereby conserving nutritionally important components. The proteins catabolized by the kidney are broken down to amino acids or polypeptides prior to return into the renal venous blood. The kidney, therefore, contributes to the regulation of their concentrations in plasma and precludes extensive loss of protein components in the urine.

In some patients with abnormalities of renal tubular function, low molecular weight proteins may appear in the urine in the absence of albumin owing to decreased tubular reabsorption. Conversely, in patients with reduced GFR the fractional catabolic rate of low molecular weight proteins (lysozyme, ribonuclease, beta$_2$-microglobulins, insulin, proinsulin, gastrin, glucagon, parathyroid hormone, Bence Jones protein, retinol binding protein, and growth hormone) is decreased and their levels in plasma are elevated.

Insulin, parathyroid hormone, and glucagon are catabolized by the kidney by filtration and subsequent tubular reabsorption as well as by peritubular uptake.

The catabolism of albumin, immunoglobulins, and larger plasma proteins is relatively low, with the kidney accounting for less than 5 per cent of their fractional catabolic rate, unless the nephrotic syndrome is present, in which case albumin catabolism could be significantly increased owing to both urinary losses and increased tubular degradation.

SYNTHESIS OF GROWTH FACTORS. Insulin-like growth factor I (IGF-I) is synthesized in the kidney. IGF-I is localized throughout the collecting ducts in both cortex and medulla. The steady-state levels of IGF-I mRNA in the collecting duct are influenced by the levels of circulating growth hormone. Receptors for IGF-I are present in proximal tubular basolateral membranes but not in membranes from the collecting duct, suggesting that IGF-I produced in the latter site exerts its biologic effect in the proximal tubule (paracrine action). Renal IGF-I is very likely involved in kidney growth or hypertrophy. A role for IGF-I in the regeneration of proximal tubule cells following ischemic injury has also been proposed.

THE KALLIKREIN-KININ SYSTEM. Kallikrein is a peptidase produced in various tissues, including the kidney, which acts on a specific substrate (kininogen) to split off a peptide, kinin. The kinin is destroyed by plasma and tissue peptidases (kininases). Kinins are potent vasodilators. The renal kallikrein-kinin system may constitute a local hormonal mechanism involved in the regulation of renal blood flow and sodium excretion. Renal kallikrein is probably produced by the cortex and excreted into the urine. It acts on a kininogen substrate to produce the potent vasodilator decapeptide (kallidin). Kallikrein excretion is augmented by reduced sodium intake. In contrast, high sodium intake decreases it. Administration of mineralocorticoids increases the excretion of kallikrein, and the increased kallikrein excretion of a low-salt diet is blocked by aldosterone antagonists (spironolactones). However, the role of the renal kallikrein system in sodium homeostasis is not yet established.

RENAL PROSTAGLANDINS. The prostaglandins are 20-carbon unsaturated fatty acids. Both vasodilator prostaglandins (PGE_2, prostacyclin, or PGI_2) and vasoconstrictor substances (thromboxanes) are synthesized in renal cortex (by arteries and glomeruli) and medulla (by interstitial and collecting duct cells) from free arachidonic acid, released from phospholipids. Renal prostaglandins may play a role in control of blood flow and GFR and in sodium and water excretion. They affect renin secretion as well. Prostaglandins may also modulate phosphorus transport and regulate renal ammonia synthesis. Their synthesis is stimulated by bradykinin, angiotensin II, ADH, and catecholamines. The last substances are vasoconstrictors that tend to diminish renal plasma flow. Therefore when constrictor stimuli are operative, renal prostaglandin production may increase, resulting in maintenance of renal blood flow.

Two other pathways of arachidonic acid metabolism have been described in the kidney: (1) an NADPH-dependent mono-oxygenase pathway that leads to the formation of 19- and 20-hydroxyeicosatetranoic acid (19-HETE and 20-HETE), 19-ketoarachidonic acid, and 1,20-dicarboxylic acid; and (2) a calcium-dependent lipoxygenase pathway with synthesis of 15-HETE, 12-HETE, and leukotrienes. The physiologic or pathophysiologic importance of these pathways is unknown, but it should be remembered that the HETE's are potent chemotactic compounds and, therefore, may play a role in inflammatory glomerular disease. Leukotrienes are known to contract vascular and nonvascular smooth muscle and enhance vascular permeability. Thus, they may play a role in the control of renal blood flow and GFR.

Cogan MG: Renal effects of atrial natriuretic factor. Ann Rev Physiol 52:699–708, 1990. *Comprehensive description of the role of atrial natriuretic peptides on glomerular filtration rate and tubular function.*

DuBose TD Jr. (ed.): Acidification mechanisms. Semin Nephrol 10(2):91–180, 1990. *Several contributions in this issue cover different aspects of proton secretion and bicarbonate reabsorption in the nephron.*

Hammerman MR: The growth hormone–insulin-like growth factor axis in kidney. Am J Physiol 257:F503–F514, 1989. *An authoritative editorial on the role of insulin-like growth factors in the kidney.*

Khraibi AA, Knox FG: Renal hemodynamics and sodium chloride excretion. *In* Klahr S, Massry SG (eds.): Contemporary Nephrology. Vol. V. New York, Plenum Publishing Company, 1989, pp 35–79. *A lucid update written by major contributors in the field of renal physiology.*

Norris SH: Renal eicosanoids. Semin Nephrol 10:64–88, 1990. *A detailed review of the role of arachidonic acid metabolites in health and disease.*

Tisher CC, Madsen KM: Anatomy of the kidney. *In* Brenner BM, Rector JC (eds.): The Kidney. 3rd ed. Philadelphia, W. B. Saunders Company, 1986, pp 3–60. *An excellent and clearly written review of kidney structure.*

Vane JR, Angaard EE, Botting RM: Regulatory functions of the vascular endothelium. N Engl J Med 323:27–36, 1990. *An excellent review of the role of vasoconstrictors and vasodilators produced by the vascular endothelium.*

74 Investigations of Renal Function

Vincent W. Dennis

Methods are available to assess the functional integrity of the glomerular ultrafiltration barrier; the presence of urogenital inflammation; the overall rate of glomerular filtration; the ability to dilute, concentrate, or acidify urine; and the ability to conserve or to excrete specific solutes. Measurements of certain values in blood and urine detect abnormalities in renal function and may occasionally point to specific etiologies, but a final diagnosis usually requires direct or indirect visualization of the kidneys and urogenital system or morphologic examination of renal tissue.

PROTEINURIA. Increased urinary excretion of protein is one of the most common and most easily detected signs of renal disease. The normal excretion rate of urinary protein is less than 150 mg per 24 hours for adults, but values as high as 300 mg per 24 hours may occur in apparently healthy adolescents. The normal composition of urinary protein includes about 40 per cent albumin, 40 per cent tissue proteins originating from renal and other urogenital tissues, 15 per cent immunoglobulins and their fragments, and 5 per cent other plasma proteins. Abnormalities may occur in both the quantity and the composition of urinary proteins.

Urinary protein is usually detected by a colorimetric test ("dipstick test"), which depends on the ability of proteins, especially albumin, to alter the color reaction of a pH-sensitive dye. Such qualitative tests may detect protein concentrations as low as 15 mg per deciliter and give a positive test result if a normal amount of protein is present in a concentrated volume of urine. Conversely, abnormal rates of protein excretion may remain undetected in large volumes of dilute urine. It is therefore important to have some estimate of the degree of urine concentration when interpreting a qualitative test for protein. A positive qualitative result for urinary protein usually warrants quantification of the absolute protein excretion rate per 24 hours. Alternatively, the protein-creatinine ratio of a random daytime urine sample correlates well with values from 24-hour collections. Proteinuria usually results from (1) elevated plasma concentration of normal or abnormal proteins, (2) increased glomerular permeability, (3) decreased tubular reabsorption of normally filtered proteins, and (4) alterations in renal hemodynamics (Table 74–1).

Overflow Proteinuria. Changes in plasma protein concentrations may alter the rates of protein excretion by both the normal and the abnormal kidney. This type of proteinuria may occur from the presence in plasma of increased concentrations of proteins not normally present in significant amounts. Examples include light-chain immunoglobulin fragments such as Bence Jones protein associated with plasma cell disorders (see Ch. 151) or myoglobin associated with rhabdomyolysis. The presence of abnormal proteins in either plasma or urine may be confirmed by electrophoresis. Changes in the concentration of normal plasma proteins may also influence passage across the *abnormal* glomerular capillary wall. For example, increases or decreases in the plasma concentration of albumin may increase or decrease its rate of urinary excretion without necessarily indicating improvement or worsening of the renal conditions that led to proteinuria.

Increased Glomerular Permeability. The glomerular capillary wall consists of capillary endothelium, basement membrane, visceral epithelium, and mesangium. Each of these four anatomic components contributes directly or indirectly to the formation and maintenance of the functional ultrafiltration barrier that limits the passage of proteins into the urinary space. The glomerular capillary wall restricts the passage of plasma proteins according to their size (steric hindrance) and surface charge (electrostatic hindrance). At any given molecular size, negative charges on the glomerular capillary basement membrane hinder the passage of negatively charged molecules more than positively charged molecules.

A number of systemic and primary renal diseases may affect one or more glomerular structures and thereby increase the effective permeability of the glomerular capillary wall to proteins. The degree of proteinuria may range from 0.2 to greater than 20 grams per 24 hours. Proteinuria that exceeds about 3 to 5 grams of normal plasma protein per 24 hours provides direct evidence of increased effective permeability of the glomerular capillary wall, since these amounts exceed those that may be filtered by the normal glomerulus and reabsorbed by the renal tubules. Such massive losses of plasma proteins may be responsible for changes in plasma oncotic pressure and thereby set in motion the events that are manifest clinically as the nephrotic syndrome (see Ch. 79).

Because of its low molecular weight and its dominance among plasma proteins, albumin is typically the major urinary protein in this type of proteinuria. However, the relative proportion of albumin in the urine, even if corrected for changes in its proportion in plasma, is lower in some forms of renal diseases than in others. *Selective proteinuria* refers to the ability of the glomerulus to retain higher molecular weight proteins despite increased filtration of low molecular weight proteins. A highly selective proteinuria therefore consists almost exclusively of increased excretion of albumin, whereas a poorly selective proteinuria contains proportionately greater amounts of higher molecular weight proteins and is generally associated with severe disruption of the glomerular capillary wall. This selectivity may be attributed to the glomerulus only if the composition of urinary proteins is not affected significantly by downstream events such as tubular reabsorption. This requirement is presumably met with levels of proteinuria that exceed 3 to 5 grams per 24 hours, but the selectivity pattern of lesser amounts of proteinuria may be significantly influenced by tubular reabsorption. To define glomerular selectivity requires measurements of the relative clearances of specific proteins with increasing molecular weights, such as albumin (69,000), transferrin (90,000), gamma globulin (150,000), and alpha$_2$-glycoprotein (820,000). Although attractive in theory and potentially useful as an index of the severity of glomerular damage, the techniques required to characterize the selectivity of proteinuria are generally too laborious and too imprecise to have achieved widespread clinical applicability. Nevertheless, heavy proteinuria characterized by the dominance of albumin and the absence of higher molecular weight globulins is typical of minimal change or nil lesion (see Ch. 79), whereas the detection of a nonselective pattern is highly suggestive of the presence of some other form of otherwise undefined glomerular disease.

Microalbuminuria refers to increases in albumin excretion that are detectable by sensitive immunoassay but not by current standard clinical techniques. The presence of microalbuminuria in diabetics may predict the development of diabetic nephropathy, whereas its absence may forecast a more favorable prognosis.

Tubular Proteinuria. Many polypeptides and low molecular weight proteins normally present in plasma are filtered freely at the glomerulus and are reabsorbed by the tubules. Examples include polypeptide hormones such as insulin, glucagon, and parathyroid hormone and plasma proteins with a molecular weight smaller than 20,000. Once filtered, these proteins are absorbed by specific endocytic processes that bind and engulf the filtered proteins. The presence of tubular disorders, especially injuries that result from various antibiotics or heavy metals (see Ch. 80), may be associated with increased urinary excretion of low molecular weight proteins and relatively slight increases in the excretion of albumin (*tubular proteinuria*). This pattern is in marked contrast to the predominance of albumin in the urine of patients with glomerular disorders. Patients characterized clinically as having tubulointerstitial rather than glomerular diseases have increased urinary protein excretion (generally less than 2 grams per 24 hours) and increased renal clearance of beta$_2$-microglobu-

lin, especially relative to albumin. Beta$_2$-microglobulinuria is less likely to occur in those disease processes such as diabetes mellitus that cause proteinuria via effects on glomerular permeability. The clinical significance of tubular proteinuria is unclear at this time because there is still insufficient documentation of correlations between tubular proteinuria and detailed functional, biochemical, and morphologic descriptions of the underlying diseases in which it has been observed.

Proteinuria from Altered Renal Hemodynamics. Changes in protein excretion rate may also occur in response to changes in renal hemodynamics. Exercise, major motor seizures, change to the standing position, fever, and vasoactive agents such as renin, angiotensin, and norepinephrine increase urinary protein excretion by mechanisms that seem related to reductions in renal blood flow. Changes in renal blood flow may alter urinary protein excretion in normal subjects as well as in those with abnormal rates of protein excretion. Possible mechanisms include local increases in protein concentration within the glomerular capillary, increased effective permeability of the glomerular capillary wall, increased transglomerular hydrostatic pressure, and increased effective filtration area. Hemodynamic increases in urinary protein excretion are generally transient or additive to other causes of proteinuria.

LEUKOCYTURIA. The urinary leukocyte excretion rate in apparently healthy individuals ranges between 0 and 300,000 leukocytes per hour; rates greater than 400,000 per hour are generally regarded as abnormal. If appropriate cleansing precautions are used, there is no difference in leukocyte excretion rates between apparently healthy males and females or between urine samples obtained from suprapubic puncture and midstream urine.

In practice, leukocyte excretion rates are estimated indirectly by microscopic examination of urinary sediment resuspended after centrifugation of approximately 10 ml of urine. Abnormal leukocyturia probably exists when more than 5 white blood cells occur per high-power field. However, about 20 per cent of urine specimens from patients excreting more than 400,000 white blood cells per hour may demonstrate fewer than 5 leukocytes per high-power field. The indirect method thus underestimates the prevalence of abnormal leukocyturia, although increased numbers of white blood cells per high-power field appear to correspond well to increased rates of leukocyte excretion. Leukocyturia results frequently from urinary tract infection (see Ch. 84) but may also indicate other causes of inflammation, such as tubulointerstitial diseases (see Ch. 80).

HEMATURIA. The detection of hematuria is aided by the widespread use of the multifunctional "dipstick," which includes a section impregnated with orthotolidine. The test is sufficiently sensitive to detect the equivalent of greater than 10,000 red blood cells per milliliter of urine but is negative in normal individuals despite the wide range of red blood cell excretion rates. A positive orthotolidine test occurs in the presence of free hemoglobin or myoglobin in urine. Free hemoglobin in the urine generally results from the lysis of red blood cells in the urine but may also reflect free hemoglobin in the plasma. When indicated, this question can be resolved by direct measurements of plasma hemoglobin and haptoglobin concentrations. Myoglobin in the urine is detected by the differential precipitation of hemoglobin with ammonium sulfate, by spectrophotometry of the ferricyanide derivatives of hemoglobin and myoglobin, by the co-migration on paper electrophoresis of myoglobin with hemoglobin C, or, preferably, by direct immunoassay of myoglobin in plasma or

TABLE 74–1. TYPES OF PROTEINURIA*

Type	Mechanism	Quantity	Molecular Weight	Examples
Overflow	Increased filtration of abnormal plasma proteins across normal glomeruli	Variable (0.2 to >10 grams)	Low (<40,000)	Bence Jones proteinuria, myoglobinuria
Glomerular	Defective glomerular retention of normal plasma proteins	>3–5 grams	High (>68,000)	Glomerulonephritis, nephrotic syndrome
Tubular	Defective reabsorption of normally filtered plasma proteins	<2 grams	Low (<40,000)	Interstitial nephritis, antibiotic injury, heavy metals
Hemodynamic	Increased filtration and possibly decreased reabsorption	<2 grams	Variable (20,000–68,000)	Transient proteinuria, congestive heart failure, fever, seizures, exercise

*Values >150 mg per 24 hours.

urine. Myoglobinuria is usually accompanied by marked increases in plasma concentrations of creatine phosphokinase (CPK).

As with leukocytes, the presence of red blood cells in urine is quantified in terms of red blood cells per high-power field and is normally 0 to 1 in males but may be slightly higher in females. The persistent presence in males or females of even small numbers of red blood cells in urine is cause for concern and may indicate the presence of a coagulopathy, hemoglobinopathy, renal parenchymal disease, tumor, trauma, or inflammation anywhere along the renal and urinary tract (Table 74–2). Hematuria accompanied by proteinuria generally indicates renal parenchymal disease.

GLOMERULAR FILTRATION RATE. Measurements of glomerular filtration rate are used clinically largely as estimates of the mass of functional renal tissue or of the number of functioning nephrons. To be useful in the measure of glomerular filtration rate, a substance should be filtered freely at the glomerulus and not secreted, reabsorbed, catabolized, or synthesized by the kidney. The substance should be harmless, inexpensive, and easy to administer and measure accurately. A number of exogenous substances fulfill some of these requirements, but there is no ideal material of endogenous origin. Overall, however, the most useful indicators of glomerular filtration rate are measurements of the plasma creatinine concentration and creatinine clearance. Creatinine is an end-product of creatine metabolism. Its endogenous production averages about 15 mg per kilogram of body weight per day, correlates with muscle mass, and tends to be constant for a given individual. Creatinine is filtered freely at the glomerulus and is secreted by the proximal tubule to an extent that may increase with elevated plasma concentration. The excretion rate of creatinine thus reflects the combined effects of filtration and secretion, and normally the clearance of creatinine exceeds the glomerular filtration rate. The secretion of creatinine is inhibited by certain drugs, such as cimetidine and trimethoprim, which may increase the plasma creatinine concentration without affecting glomerular filtration rate. Ketonemia may cause spurious increases in measurements of plasma creatinine because acetoacetate interferes with certain automated analytic techniques (Table 74–3).

Figure 74–1 shows the theoretic relationship between plasma creatinine concentration and creatinine clearance and the relationship between creatinine clearance and other measures of glomerular filtration rate, such as inulin clearance. The relationship between plasma creatinine and creatinine clearance is described by a rectangular hyperbola. This reflects the mathematical reality that values on the horizontal axis are determined by the reciprocals of values on the vertical axis, since the formula for creatinine clearance includes the serum creatinine concentration in the denominator. To the extent that creatinine clearance and glomerular filtration rate are equivalent, the same ideal relationship should apply between observed glomerular filtration rate and plasma creatinine concentration, but deviations from this ideal occur.

In the normal range, measurements of plasma creatinine concentration include a significant and variable component of noncreatinine chromogen that is not excreted in the urine. This overestimate offsets in part the error introduced by the renal secretion of creatinine, so that in this range creatinine clearances correlate well with other measures of glomerular filtration rate.

TABLE 74–2. CAUSES OF HEMATURIA ISOLATED FROM OTHER URINE ABNORMALITIES

Urologic
  Urogenital tumor
  Renal cyst or solid tumor
  Nephrolithiasis or urolithiasis (usually painful)
Hematologic
  Coagulopathies, inherited or acquired
  Hemoglobinopathies, especially sickle trait
Nephrologic
  Glomerulopathies, especially immunoglobulin A (IgA) nephropathy
  Benign essential hematuria (attenuated glomerular basement
    membrane)
Menstruation

TABLE 74–3. FACTORS THAT AFFECT PLASMA CREATININE CONCENTRATION WITHOUT CHANGES IN GLOMERULAR FILTRATION RATE

Increase	
Ketonemia	Spurious increase in automated measurements by acetoacetate
Cimetidine, trimethoprim	Inhibition of tubular secretion
Decrease	
Muscle wasting	Reduced creatinine production
Low protein diet	Reduced creatinine ingestion and production

In the presence of renal failure, plasma creatinine concentration rises much more so than that of noncreatinine chromogens, and thus measurements of plasma creatinine concentration approach the true creatinine concentration. Moreover, in the presence of moderate degrees of renal failure, the secretory component of creatinine excretion may increase until the glomerular filtration rate falls below about 10 ml per minute. For these reasons, in the presence of moderate renal failure the clearance of creatinine tends to overestimate the glomerular filtration rate. In advanced renal failure (glomerular filtration rate less than 10 ml per minute), creatinine clearance again approximates the glomerular filtration rate (Fig. 74–1). Despite these shortcomings, measurement of the plasma creatinine concentration is the most useful estimate of filtration rate largely because of the ease with which repeated measurements may be made in individual patients along the course of their disease. In view of the insensitivity in detecting reductions in the glomerular filtration rate to the 50 to 80 ml per minute range, values in the upper range of normal need to be interpreted with special caution and correlated with other clinical data. Patients with chronic renal disease should have at least one and perhaps annual measurements of their 24-hour creatinine excretion to monitor possible changes in creatinine production. Measurements of urinary creatinine are less useful in acute renal failure, since values do not generally reflect a steady state. In the acute setting, about 3 days are required for plasma creatinine concentrations to achieve a steady state, and thus clinically detectable changes may lag behind the time of injury.

The most accurate measures of glomerular filtration rate in humans are obtained with the use of a number of exogenous

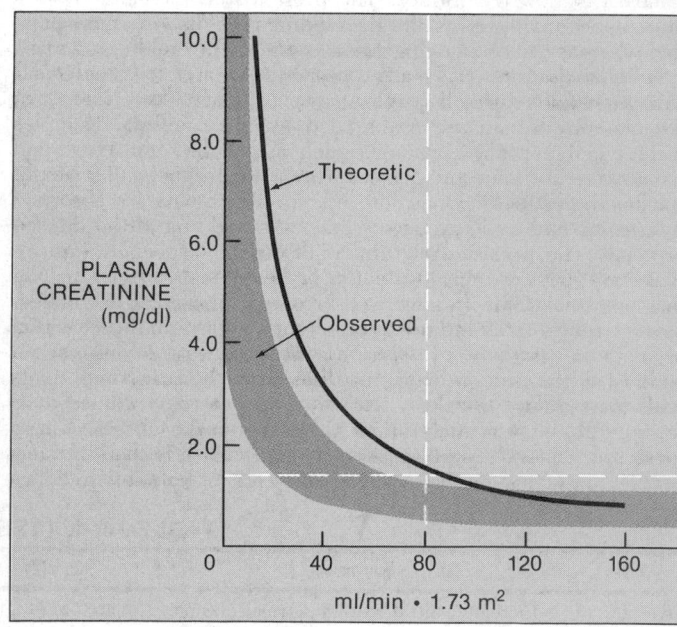

FIGURE 74–1. Relationship between plasma creatinine concentrations and various measures of glomerular filtration rate. The solid line depicts the theoretical relationship between plasma creatinine concentration and creatinine clearance. The color-screened area represents the relationship between plasma creatinine and noncreatinine measures of glomerular filtration rate. The dashed lines denote the limits of normal values. Note the extent to which normal plasma creatinine values may occur in spite of reduced filtration rates.

substances, such as insulin, or a variety of radioisotopically labeled compounds, such as ^{125}I-iothalamate. Standard clearance techniques for these measurements require injection of the compound to a steady-state plasma concentration and then the timed collection of urine.

The blood urea nitrogen (BUN) concentration is an imperfect quantitative indicator of renal filtration despite its frequent use for this purpose. Urea is synthesized by the liver from ammonia derived from the catabolism of proteins and amino acids. Urea production is therefore variable and is influenced by hepatic as well as dietary conditions. At the kidneys, urea is filtered, reabsorbed, and secreted. Reabsorption dominates, but the rate of reabsorption varies with the degree of hydration. Those conditions, such as dehydration, that tend to increase the renal reabsorption of volume also increase the reabsorption of urea. Accordingly, blood urea nitrogen concentration may increase without any abnormality in renal function. Conversely, in the presence of renal excretory failure and reduced filtration rate, the BUN concentration may be influenced significantly by the degree of dietary protein intake. For these reasons, measurement of plasma creatinine concentration provides a more reliable index of renal filtration rate than the BUN. The BUN is used mainly to quantify the balance between the accumulation and excretion of nitrogenous metabolites (i.e., the degree of uremia), especially in the presence of more than moderate reductions in glomerular filtration rate.

RENAL CONCENTRATING AND DILUTING ABILITY.
The total solute concentration of urine is generally assessed clinically by measurement of urinary specific gravity, which relates the weight of a unit volume of urine to an equal volume of water. Because of its simplicity, this technique has persisted despite well-recognized deficiencies. Errors of technique relate primarily to poor calibration of the hygrometer, but even in the absence of faulty technique the specific gravity of urine provides only a rough indication of urinary osmolality. For example, urines that contain high concentrations of urea have lower specific gravities than expected for their osmolality, and urines that contain higher density solutes, such as glucose, iodinated contrast material, or protein, have higher specific gravities relative to their osmolalities. Within these limitations, however, there is a useful correlation between the specific gravity and osmolality of urine such that urinary osmolality in milliosmoles per kilogram of water may be estimated as 40 times the increase in specific gravity of urine above the value of water, which is 1.000. Thus, urine with a specific gravity of 1.007 would have an estimated osmolality of 280 mOsm, similar to that of plasma, and urine with a specific gravity of 1.020 would be distinctly concentrated, with an estimated osmolality of 800 mOsm. Nonetheless, measurements of urinary specific gravity represent only crude estimates of osmolality, and, when indicated, accurate measures of urinary

osmolality may be made easily by measurement of freezing point depression in a cryoscopic osmometer.

Maximal urinary concentrating ability is measured by restricting fluid intake until the patient loses a minimum of 3 per cent or a maximum of 5 per cent of body weight, or until three consecutive urine specimens show no further increase in osmolality. These results are usually achieved within 16 hours of fluid restriction but may occur much earlier in patients with severe inability to conserve water. Once either one of these endpoints is achieved, additional information may be obtained by the subcutaneous administration of 5 units of aqueous vasopressin to determine if any further increase in urinary osmolality can be achieved. Normal subjects achieve maximal urinary osmolality of 1000 ± 200 (SD) mOsm without further change after vasopressin. Patients who have complete or incomplete defects in antidiuretic hormone secretion (ADH), nephrogenic diabetes insipidus, or psychogenic polydipsia will have abnormal and distinctive patterns of response (Fig. 74–2).

Maximal diluting capacity of the kidney is assessed by the rapid administration of 1200 ml of water by mouth to a fasting subject. The osmolality of three hourly urine specimens is measured and should achieve values lower than 80 mOsm or a specific gravity of 1.002. Measurements of the rate or extent of excretion of the administered water are quite variable and are not generally useful. Both maximal diluting and maximal concentrating ability of the kidney may be impaired by diuretics, especially potent loop diuretics such as furosemide and ethacrynic acid, and by diuretic states such as glucosuria.

ACIDIFICATION CAPACITY.
The urine is normally more acidic than body fluids because of the endogenous production and renal excretion of nonvolatile acids derived primarily from sulfate and phosphate contained in dietary protein. Even at low pH, however, the amount of acid excreted as free hydrogen ion is negligible (pH 5.0 equals 0.01 mEq H^+ per liter). Most hydrogen ion is excreted in the form of ammonium or titratable acids. For these reasons, the pH of a random specimen of urine provides only limited information about renal function and essentially no reliable information about the systemic acid-base status.

Assessment of the renal acidification capacity is accomplished by the *ammonium chloride tolerance test*. The basis of this test is to induce mild metabolic acidosis by the administration of ammonium chloride by mouth and to measure the maximal depression in urinary pH, the maximal excretion rate of ammonium and titratable acid, and the percentage of excretion of the administered hydrogen ion equivalent. Because the purpose of the ammonium chloride is to induce metabolic acidosis, its administration is not necessary if acidosis is present spontaneously. Indications for the ammonium chloride test are generally

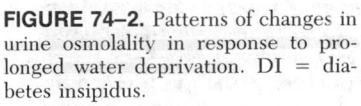

FIGURE 74–2. Patterns of changes in urine osmolality in response to prolonged water deprivation. DI = diabetes insipidus.

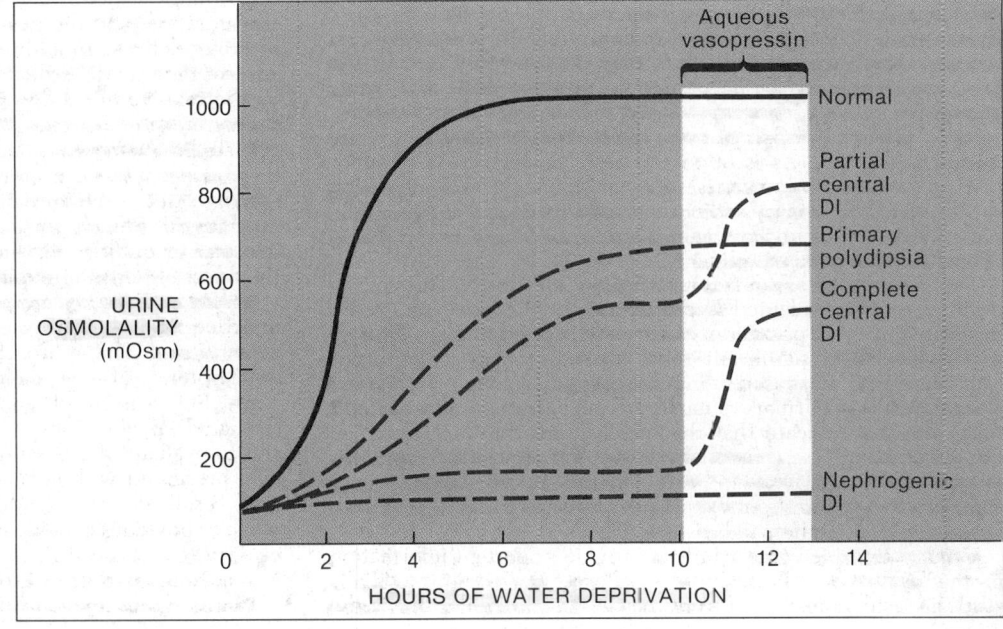

restricted to those conditions, usually suspected abnormalities in distal tubular function, that are associated with only mild reductions in glomerular filtration rate. Ammonium chloride, 0.1 gram per kilogram, is administered by mouth, and urine is collected hourly for 6 to 8 hours. A normal response is to achieve a urinary pH of 5.4 or less and to excrete at least 30 per cent of the administered hydrogen ion equivalent. An abnormal response consists of failure to acidify the urine below pH 5.4 despite a measured reduction in arterial pH. This defines a distal renal tubular acidosis and indicates a defect in maximal acidification capacity. The ammonium chloride tolerance test is not generally performed in patients with renal insufficiency, but, if performed, these patients usually achieve reduction in the urinary pH below 5.4, although there is reduced excretion of ammonium and titratable acid.

URINARY ELECTROLYTES. Measurements of urinary sodium, potassium, and chloride may provide important information but only in a limited set of clinical circumstances. Two types of measurements are made. The absolute daily excretion of sodium, potassium, or chloride (milliequivalents per day) is derived from the electrolyte concentration of a 24-hour collection of urine. Such measurements provide quantification of the daily intake of these electrolytes, provided that two requirements are met. First, total body weight must be constant to indicate balance between intake and output. Second, electrolyte excretion must be limited to the urine, and losses via the gastrointestinal tract or skin must be negligible. Under these conditions, the daily excretion of sodium, potassium, or chloride will reflect the dietary intake, but this information has only limited clinical value.

Measurement of the *concentration* of sodium, potassium, or chloride in a random urine sample may provide information of importance in certain circumstances, such as the evaluation of hyponatremia, acute oliguria, volume depletion, hypokalemia, and metabolic alkalosis. In the evaluation of hyponatremia, a urinary sodium concentration less than 10 mEq per liter indicates the presence of reduced effective extracellular volume with an appropriate increase in mineralocorticoid and ADH activity that leads to the renal retention of sodium and solute-free water. Higher urinary sodium concentrations indicate significant renal losses of sodium such as might occur from diuretics or, less commonly, from mineralocorticoid or glucocorticoid insufficiency or with volume expansion from the inappropriate secretion of ADH. Similarly, in the evaluation of patients with reduced extracellular volume, urinary sodium concentrations greater than 10 to 20 mEq per liter indicate that the kidney is participating in the loss of sodium and volume, perhaps because of diuretics or renal or adrenal insufficiency, whereas urinary sodium concentrations less than 5 to 10 mEq per liter indicate that losses of sodium and volume are occurring via extrarenal routes.

In the setting of acute oliguria, urinary sodium concentration greater than 20 to 40 mEq per liter occurs frequently with acute renal failure or incomplete obstruction, whereas urinary sodium concentrations are generally less than 20 mEq per liter in the presence of severe volume depletion (prerenal azotemia), acute glomerulonephritis, congestive heart failure, coexistent liver disease, or acute renal failure from radiocontrast material or acute rejection (Ch. 76). As is often the case, however, these values may be modified by many factors, including the administration of diuretics, and urinary sodium concentrations are not generally regarded as sufficiently discriminatory to be useful in the differential diagnosis of acute oliguria.

The urinary potassium concentration may be useful in the evaluation of unexplained hypokalemia. In the presence of hypokalemia, urinary potassium concentrations greater than 20 mEq per liter indicate significant renal losses, such as might occur from diuretics, increased mineralocorticoid activity, or magnesium deficiency. Urinary potassium concentrations less than 10 mEq per liter indicate that the hypokalemia may be related to gastrointestinal losses, such as may occur from the surreptitious use of laxatives or may indicate changes in plasma potassium concentration without potassium deficits, such as may occur with hypokalemic periodic paralysis (see Ch. 507).

Urinary chloride concentrations provide important information in the evaluation of metabolic alkalosis. Persistent metabolic alkalosis results most often from the depletion of chloride via the gastrointestinal tract or urine. In the presence of metabolic alkalosis, urinary chloride concentrations greater than 10 mEq per liter suggest the presence of diuretic-induced increases in chloride excretion, severe depletion of potassium, Bartter's syndrome, or increased adrenocortical hormone activity. On the other hand, urinary chloride concentrations less than 10 mEq per liter point to losses of chloride via extrarenal routes, usually vomiting, and indicate further that the metabolic alkalosis is likely to respond to replacement of volume with normal saline.

IMAGING OF THE KIDNEYS AND UROGENITAL TRACT

Imaging techniques of importance in the evaluation of renal abnormalities include roentgenography, ultrasonography, radionuclide studies, and magnetic resonance imaging (MRI). These techniques are used (1) to visualize the number, size, and location of the kidneys; (2) to identify the presence and site of obstruction; (3) to detect and to characterize mass lesions; (4) to visualize renal arteries and veins; and (5) to guide percutaneous diagnostic and therapeutic interventions, such as biopsy and nephrostomy. The choice of a technique is based on its relative simplicity, its safety, its potential to yield results that for a particular suspected disorder are neither falsely positive (lack of specificity) nor falsely negative (lack of sensitivity), and its potential to provide additional information not already available from previous studies.

ROENTGENOGRAPHIC STUDIES. The most simple radiologic study of the kidneys and urogenital system is the plain roentgenogram of the kidneys, ureter, and bladder (KUB), which will often reveal abnormal calcifications and may reveal renal size if the kidneys are not obscured by overlying bowel. If indicated, tomography may be necessary to determine the renal outlines.

Excretory Urogram. The excretory urogram, also known as the intravenous pyelogram, or IVP, is the classic radiologic method to detect anatomic abnormalities of the kidneys and ureters and to evaluate patients with renal abnormalities. The basic excretory urogram is performed by the intravenous injection of iodinated contrast material, which is filtered at the glomerulus and concentrated within the tubular lumina and collecting system by the renal reabsorption of volume. Visualization of the contrast material within the renal parenchyma yields a *nephrogram*, and visualization within the major collecting system yields a *pyelogram*. Each of these phases is dependent on the amount of radiocontrast material that is delivered to the kidneys and filtered and also on the degree of extraction of volume that concentrates the dye within the parenchyma and collecting system. Modern radiocontrast materials are not secreted. Patients with renal insufficiency (e.g., those with plasma creatinine values >3 to 4 mg per deciliter) may not have adequate filtration and concentration of radiocontrast to allow detailed visualization, especially relative to their increased risk for adverse reactions.

A nephrogram normally appears within 1 to 3 minutes after injection of the contrast material. The nephrogram provides an opportunity to determine the number of kidneys, their size and configuration, and the possible presence of inhomogeneous areas or filling defects. In addition, the symmetric and timely appearance of nephrograms bilaterally provides qualitative information on the relative blood flow and filtration rate of each kidney. The pyelogram phase occurs within 5 minutes after the injection of dye as the nephrogram fades. This phase allows visualization of the caliceal system, ureters, and bladder and provides opportunities to detect abnormalities in shape, size, or drainage that might result from intrinsic defects or from extrinsic compression. Vascular or outflow obstructions may result in marked delays in the onset of both the nephrogram and the pyelogram phases.

Retrograde Pyelography. Retrograde pyelography is the direct injection of radiocontrast material into the ureter and upper urinary tract. The approach to this area is achieved via insertion of a ureteral catheter under direct visualization through cystoscopy. Some form of anesthesia may be required. Although retrograde pyelography was used frequently to assess renal size and to evaluate the possibility of ureteral obstruction in patients who presented with advanced renal failure, these questions are now resolved more readily with ultrasonography. Retrograde pyelography does provide more direct and improved visualization of the ureters and calices, and this visualization is useful in the localization and diagnosis of tumors and obstructions.

Percutaneous Pyeloureteral Techniques. The combination of

visualizing techniques such as roentgenographic fluoroscopy or ultrasonography and the availability of percutaneous catheters allows placement of a catheter in the renal pelvis, calices, or perirenal space if these spaces are distended by abnormal collections of fluid. Percutaneous catheter placement allows drainage and irrigation of pyonephrosis, abscesses, and obstructions, as well as placement of temporary nephrostomy catheters.

Renal Arteriography and Venography. The renal vasculature is visualized with radiocontrast material injected via a catheter introduced usually through the femoral vessels. Renal arteriography is performed most often to evaluate possible renal arterial stenosis as a cause or aggravating factor in systemic hypertension and to evaluate renal mass lesions. In general, cystic mass lesions are devoid of vasculature and may stretch and distort normal renal vessels and calices. Solid tumors are frequently vascular with irregular and erratic vessels that fill early as a blush of contrast material.

Renal venography is limited largely to searches for renal vein thrombosis and venous extension of renal cell carcinoma. Because renal venography requires the injection of dye against usually heavy renal venous outflow, turbulence may on occasion distort the distribution of dye and give the appearance of an intravascular filling defect. For this reason, renal venography is sometimes performed with intra-arterial infusion of epinephrine to reduce renal blood flow.

Digital Subtraction Angiography. Digital subtraction angiography uses high-quality image intensifiers and video camera recordings to visualize major arterial vessels following the rapid intravenous injection of radiocontrast material. Standard x-ray sources are used to produce sequential images at rates of about one per second, beginning at the time of injection of radiocontrast material into a central or peripheral artery or vein. Images are intensified electronically, displayed on a video camera, digitized, and stored on magnetic tape in a memory system. Images obtained prior to the arrival of radiocontrast material at a particular vascular region are subtracted electronically from the subsequent images to enhance the contrast between vessels and other tissues. With regard to the detection of renovascular diseases, digital subtraction venous angiography has an overall accuracy of about 70 to 80 per cent, compared with conventional arteriography. Technically successful studies are generally sensitive enough to detect significant renovascular lesions, but false-positive results may be as frequent as 20 to 30 per cent. Because venous angiography does not require an arteriotomy, it can be performed without hospitalization at considerably less cost than direct arteriography.

Computed Tomography. Computed tomography (CT) represents a sophisticated extension of roentgenography and may be performed with or without contrast material. Its usefulness in the evaluation of renal abnormalities consists primarily in its application as a tertiary mode after excretory urograms and ultrasonography to detect and localize mass lesions. Computed tomography may detect cystic masses as small as 0.5 cm in diameter, but the sensitivity is less for noncalcific solid masses (Fig. 74–3). Computed tomography is also useful in detecting and evaluating obstruction and dilatation of the major collecting system in patients allergic to iodinated contrast material or for whom ultrasonography is inconclusive for technical reasons, such as interference by bone, calcifications, or gas.

Adverse Effects of Urography. Two types of adverse effects should be considered in relation to the performance of excretory urograms, angiograms, or CT with intravenous contrast material. First, any exposure to radiation is associated with a finite, statistical risk of permanent alteration in DNA. Depending on the question being asked, alternative modes of visualization, such as ultrasonography, might be considered in certain circumstances, especially those that involve pregnancy or repeated examinations over time.

The second type of adverse effect of excretory urography relates to toxic reactions to the iodinated contrast material. The overall incidence of adverse reactions to intravenous contrast is about 5 per cent for the general population and about 10 per cent for those with any allergies. The most common reactions involve nausea or urticaria; about 10 per cent of reactions will involve life-threatening events, such as hypotension, laryngeal edema, or cardiac arrhythmias.

Radiocontrast urography is a remarkably safe procedure, es-

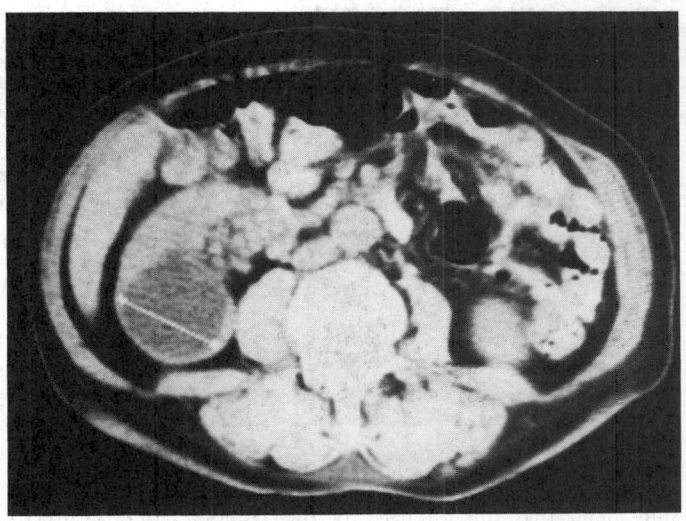

FIGURE 74–3. Computed tomography (CT) of the abdomen. The orientation is looking upward from toes to head. The right kidney is visualized at this level, but only a small portion of the left kidney is shown. There is a large, well-demarcated, homogeneous mass (white diagonal) in the right kidney that has the density of water rather than tissue. This is characteristic of a renal cyst.

pecially when performed in essentially healthy individuals. Not unexpectedly, radiocontrast materials are less safe in individuals who are less healthy. The single most important risk factor for radiocontrast-induced renal injury is the presence of pre-existent renal disease, such as that likely to be present in patients with diabetes mellitus, multiple myeloma, and generalized atherosclerotic disease. Renal function may also deteriorate more frequently following administration of intravenous radiocontrast in patients with advanced age, marked dehydration, hyperuricemia, or proteinuria. Appropriate precautions are indicated: consideration of alternative modes of visualization, attention to optimal hydration, and use of the minimal amount of contrast material consistent with an adequate examination.

ULTRASONOGRAPHY. Ultrasonography represents a major advance in the noninvasive visualization of the kidneys and genitourinary system. The acoustic impedance of a tissue to ultrasonic waves is the product of its density and the velocity of sound in that tissue. Significant differences in acoustic impedance occur among tissues that differ in their content of water, fat, collagen, minerals, and other solids, and interfaces between these tissues will reflect portions of the sound energy back to the transmitting transducer. These reflections are recorded as electrical signals and may be visualized by various display modes. The brightness modulation, or B-mode, displays echoes as bright dots plotted along the vertical and horizontal axes of an oscilloscope at positions corresponding to their point of origin in the area being scanned and in degrees of brightness that correspond to their amplitude. So-called "real-time" imaging, or sonofluoroscopy, produces repetitive scans that give the impression of a continuous image.

Sonography can usually allow delineation of the renal outlines and measurement of the longitudinal and transverse dimensions (Fig. 74–4). Difficulties may arise from overlying ribs that may obscure the upper poles or from similarities in the acoustic impedance of perirenal fat and renal cortex such that the renal margins are poorly defined. The structures within the renal parenchyma are sufficiently similar that few intrarenal echoes are produced except by the vascular and caliceal structures of the renal pelvis. Advanced gray-scale examination of the kidney may permit identification of the cortex, medulla, arcuate vessels, and renal pyramids. The ureters are not normally visualized unless distended.

B-mode ultrasonography has been combined with pulsed Doppler and color Doppler systems to form duplex imaging systems that also provide estimates of the velocity of blood flow in regions or vessels localized precisely by sonography. Doppler techniques depend on the observation that sound waves emanating or

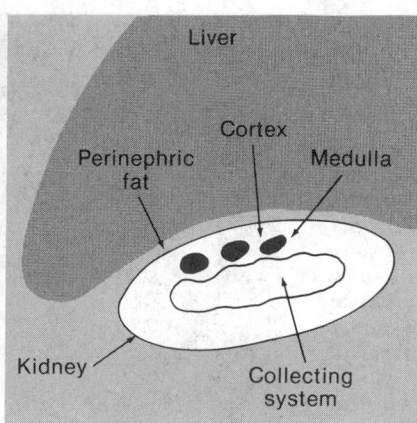

FIGURE 74–4. Ultrasonography *(left)* and schematic *(right)* of a normal right kidney. This was obtained anteriorly by transmission through the liver.

reflected from objects in motion shift their frequency ("Doppler shift") and that the intensity of the Doppler shift is directly proportional to the velocity of the objects in motion, which in the clinical context are red blood cells. Duplex ultrasonography is highly dependent on the skills of the operator but has emerging applications in suspected diseases of the major renal arteries or veins and in acute failure of the transplanted kidney.

The primary applications of ultrasonography to the evaluation of renal abnormalities include assessment of renal size, especially in the presence of severe renal failure, evaluation of mass lesions detected by excretory urography, examination of the perinephric area, and detection and grading of hydronephrosis. Renal ultrasonography may serve as the primary imaging procedure for patients with unexplained acute renal failure, for diabetics and other individuals at higher risk for adverse reactions to contrast material, in the presence of pregnancy, and to diagnose suspected polycystic kidney disease.

Evaluation of Renal Mass Lesions. Ultrasonography is used widely and effectively in the evaluation of renal mass lesions detected by excretory urography. Fluid-filled cysts as small as 1 to 2 cm in diameter may be detected, but reliable detection and evaluation of consistency generally require lesions greater than 2.5 to 3.0 cm. The primary application of ultrasonography is to describe the ultrasonographic characteristics of mass lesions ac-

cording to three patterns: cystic, solid, or complex. Cystic lesions are free of internal echoes, have smooth, sharply defined margins, and cause accentuation of echoes from their far wall. Solid lesions have less distinct margins because of attenuation of the signal by solid tissue and also demonstrate internal echoes related to vessels, connective tissue, or hemorrhage. Complex lesions represent features of both patterns. Because of the inherent limitations of the technique, ultrasonographically defined lesions should be described simply as having the *characteristics* of cysts or solids. Physically solid lesions that may appear on ultrasonography as cysts include melanomas, lymphomas, and certain metastases. Localized areas of hydronephrosis may also appear as cysts.

Renal ultrasonography is most nearly diagnostic in adult polycystic kidney disease and severe hydronephrosis. In other instances, ultrasonography should be regarded as informative rather than diagnostic. In the evaluation of renal mass lesions, combinations of ultrasonography, CT (Fig. 74–3), and arteriography may distinguish between benign cysts and potentially malignant solid tumors with remarkable accuracy. Clinical judgment will still be needed to decide whether even a 90 to 95 per cent level of accuracy is sufficient in an individual instance or whether surgery is indicated to obtain a definite diagnosis.

RADIONUCLIDE SCINTILLATION IMAGING. Radionuclide imaging has not achieved a major role in the evaluation of the kidneys and urinary tract. Two advantages of these techniques, however, make them useful in special circumstances. First, radionuclide imaging does not require the injection of radiocontrast material. Second, radionuclide studies are relatively simple and rapid and may be performed repeatedly at intervals of 24 to 48 hours. For these reasons, radionuclide imaging has perhaps its greatest application in the evaluation of patients at high risk for adverse reaction to radiocontrast material and in the evaluation of patients in the period immediately after renal transplantation. Otherwise, these techniques have few advantages over more direct radiologic and ultrasonographic methods.

With regard to the kidneys, radionuclide imaging techniques involve the intravenous injection of an agent labeled with a radionuclide that emits gamma radiation. Use of a scintillation camera allows the performance of dynamic studies that monitor the passage of a radiopharmaceutical agent through the vascular, renal parenchymal, and urinary tract compartments. Static studies examine the local accumulation of radionuclide activity. At present, radiopharmaceuticals of value in studies of the kidney contain either ^{131}I or ^{99m}Tc (technetium).

Static Imaging. Static imaging of the kidney consists of the administration of a radiopharmaceutical agent, usually ^{99m}Tc-glucoheptonate, that accumulates within the renal parenchyma and persists for several hours. Static imaging provides information on the location, size, and contour of functional renal tissue and may reveal areas of inhomogeneity or filling defects.

Dynamic Imaging. Dynamic scintillation imaging consists of the intravenous injection of a radiopharmaceutical agent and the visualization of its course through the vascular, renal parenchymal, and urinary collecting system by external monitoring of regional radioactivity with a scintillation camera. The time course of the appearance and disappearance of radioactivity is recorded

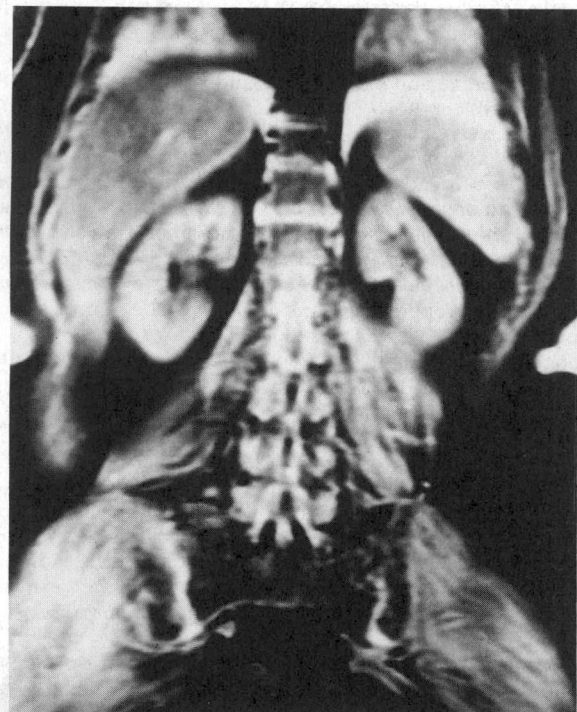

FIGURE 74–5. Magnetic resonance image (MRI) of two normal kidneys in an elderly woman.

in intervals as brief as 1 second. The radiopharmaceuticals used most frequently include ^{131}I-orthoiodohippurate, which is excreted by secretion with only a small component of filtration, and ^{99m}Tc-diethylenetriamine pentacetic acid (DTPA), which is excreted by filtration only.

The time-activity data observed for the passage of either radionuclide generally delineate three discrete phases. The vascular phase is the first 15 to 60 seconds after injection and consists of a rapid increase in radioactivity in the region viewed by the scintillation camera. The second phase occurs over the next 3 to 5 minutes and consists of slower accumulation of regional radioactivity. The third, or excretory, phase refers to the decrease in activity that occurs as the radionuclide is excreted from the region of interest. Unilateral or bilateral disturbances in renal blood flow, renal filtration, renal tubular function, or excretion cause disturbances in the various phases of this renogram. Although some efforts have been made to provide quantification of the various phases, interpretation of renograms still depends for the most part on the recognition of patterns in the scintillation displays. Dynamic imaging is especially useful for comparing excretory function between the right and left kidneys when renal dysfunction is asymmetric, such as may occur with congenital, vascular, or urologic disorders.

MAGNETIC RESONANCE IMAGING. Magnetic resonance imaging represents a new and emerging diagnostic technology that uses high magnetic fields and radiofrequencies to construct images. The method avoids the use of ionizing radiation or the administration of contrast material. Imaging depends instead on the water content and the chemical behavior of hydrogen compounds in the tissues themselves. Magnetic resonance imaging provides images in a tomographic format similar to CT (Fig. 74–5). The technique is very sensitive to blood flow and represents an excellent method for evaluating major vascular structures for patency or tumor involvement.

RENAL BIOPSY

Biopsy of the renal parenchyma by either the percutaneous or the open technique is useful (1) to define the morphologic expression of primary renal diseases, (2) to determine the type and extent of renal involvement by systemic diseases, and (3) to diagnose systemic diseases. The performance of renal biopsy is seldom necessary to *diagnose* systemic diseases. Systemic lupus erythematosus, diabetes mellitus, thrombotic thrombocytopenic purpura, multiple myeloma, Wegener's granulomatosis, and amyloidosis may on occasion display pathognomonic features on renal biopsy, but of these diseases only amyloidosis is likely to require renal biopsy for diagnosis. The others are diagnosed more readily by other means.

Renal biopsy is performed most frequently via the percutaneous technique. The indications for percutaneous biopsy are listed in Table 74–4; the contraindications are the presence of a single kidney, bleeding disorders, and uncontrolled hypertension. In experienced hands, percutaneous renal biopsy is a safe and effective technique that should provide sufficient tissue in more than 90 per cent of the attempts. Complications occur in 5 to 10 per cent of the attempts, and the most frequent complication is gross hematuria that usually resolves uneventfully in 24 to 48 hours. The formation of a perirenal hematoma may on occasion

TABLE 74–4. INDICATIONS FOR RENAL BIOPSY

Presumptive presence of glomerular disease
    Heavy proteinuria (>3 to 5 grams/24 hr)
    Nephrotic syndrome
    Acute nephritic syndrome
Proteinuria with hematuria
Renal involvement by systemic disease
    Connective tissue disease
    Vasculitis
    Amyloidosis
    Suspected Goodpasture's disease
Unexplained acute renal failure
Persistent acute renal failure (beyond 2 to 4 weeks)
Renal transplantation
    Acute rejection
    Chronic rejection
    Recurrence of original disease

require surgical evacuation. Microscopic hematuria occurs very frequently and is not generally considered a complication. Complications that occur less frequently include persistent bleeding, formation of arteriovenous fistula, aggravation of hypertension, and inadvertent biopsy of nonrenal tissue, such as muscle, liver, pancreas, spleen, or small bowel. Although fluoroscopy and ultrasonography may on occasion be useful or even necessary to localize the kidney for biopsy, it is not clear that these added maneuvers diminish the occurrence of complications or notably improve the rate of success. Complications of percutaneous renal biopsy occur more often in younger patients and in those with hypertension or small, diseased kidneys. Because hemorrhagic complications of percutaneous renal biopsy are the most common, the patient should be advised to refrain from strenuous exercises, especially lifting, and from contact sports for at least 2 weeks after biopsy.

The information obtained from a renal biopsy depends on the quality of tissue examination. Tissue should be examined by light microscopy, immunofluorescence microscopy, and, on occasion, electron microscopy. Accurate morphologic definition of possible primary renal disease or of the type and extent of renal involvement by systemic disease is often essential prior to making therapeutic decisions that might involve the use of life-threatening immunosuppressive therapy and to informing the physician and patient about the expected natural history of any renal abnormality. Moreover, for those renal disorders that may be treated ultimately by renal transplantation, knowledge of the nature of the original renal disease is important to predictions of whether that disease is likely to recur in the transplanted kidney.

Dennis V. W., Robinson R. R.: Clinical proteinuria. *In* Stollerman G. H., Harrington W. J., Lamont J. T., et al. (eds.): Advances in Internal Medicine. Chicago, Year Book Medical Publishers, 1986, pp 243–263. *This article provides more detail on the mechanisms and clinical classifications of proteinuria isolated from other renal abnormalities.*

Hertzberg B. S., Carroll B. A.: Ultrasonography of the vascular system. *In* Taveras J. M., Ferrucci J. T. (eds.): Radiology Diagnosis-Imaging-Intervention. Vol 2. Philadelphia, J. B. Lippincott Company, 1990, pp 1–19. *Readable background information on the theory and applications of Doppler imaging.*

Schwab S. J., Hlatky M. A., Pieper K. S., et al.: Contrast nephrotoxicity: A randomized controlled trial of a nonionic and an ionic radiographic contrast agent. N Engl J Med 320:149, 1989. *A recent and extensive study of some of the variables in radiocontrast injury in a general population undergoing angiographic study.*

Walser M.: Progression of chronic renal failure in man. Kidney Int 37:1195, 1990. *A scholarly examination of the methods and results of studies contending that chronic renal failure progresses inexorably and that selected interventions alter that course.*

75 Disorders of Fluid Volume, Electrolyte, and Acid-Base Balance

Thomas E. Andreoli

INTRODUCTION

Electrolyte abnormalities often occur as manifestations of underlying illnesses. In turn, fluid and electrolyte abnormalities, of themselves, produce systemic derangements. This chapter considers four major derangements of fluid and electrolyte balance, namely, volume disturbances, osmolality derangements, abnormalities of potassium balance, and acid-base disorders.

In health, the functional capacities of the mechanisms regulating water and electrolyte balance are so large that one can vary the intake of solutes and water over a wide range without developing perceptible metabolic disturbances. But the limits between which solute and water intake can be varied become narrower as the degree of functional impairment progresses. For example, salt intake in normal individuals can vary from approximately 10 mEq per day to several hundred milliequivalents per day without affecting volume homeostasis. In the presence of chronic renal disease, the minimal requirement rises and the maximal tolerance decreases, so that dietary salt intake must be kept within a much narrower range if volume depletion or volume overload is to be avoided.

75.1 VOLUME DISORDERS

PHYSIOLOGIC CONSIDERATIONS

Protection of extracellular fluid volume is the most fundamental characteristic of fluid and electrolyte homeostasis. It is helpful to use the term *effective circulating volume (ECV)*. The latter cannot be defined in an absolute sense, nor can it be measured explicitly. In operational terms, effective circulating volume may be viewed as adequate filling of the arterial tree, that is, an arterial flow rate sufficient to maintain adequate perfusion of body tissues. The mechanisms regulating volume balance respond primarily to changes in the ECV.

The Body Fluid Compartments

In healthy adults, body water comprises approximately 60 per cent of body weight and exists in two compartments: The intracellular compartment (ICF) contains two thirds of body water, or 40 per cent of body weight; the extracellular compartment (ECF) contains the remaining one third of total body water; and total blood volume, that is, plasma plus formed elements, constitutes one third of the total ECF volume. This "rule of thirds" for the body fluid compartments is useful in the assessment of most clinically encountered fluid and electrolyte disorders. Thus in a healthy 70-kg man, total body water comprises about 40 liters, of which 25 liters is intracellular. The functional extracellular fluid volume is 15 liters, 5 liters of which is blood; and since the normal hematocrit is 40 to 45 per cent, total plasma volume is approximately 2.75 to 3.0 liters.

More than 95 per cent of total body sodium is extracellular, and sodium and its associated anions, primarily chloride and bicarbonate, constitute the principal solutes of the ECF. Albumin and other macromolecules present in plasma are restricted to the vascular bed and constitute 5 per cent of plasma volume, so that plasma is about 95 per cent water. Since capillaries are freely permeable to water and small solutes, interstitial fluid is a protein-poor, but not entirely protein-free, ultrafiltrate of plasma.

Potassium is the principal cation of intracellular fluid, and nearly 98 per cent of total body potassium is intracellular. The principal anions of intracellular fluid vary among different cells. In muscle cells, they include phosphate, sulfate, and negatively charged macromolecules; and in red blood cells, they include the latter anions as well as chloride and bicarbonate.

Regulation of Fluid Transfer Among Compartments

The transfer of fluid between vascular and interstitial compartments occurs at the capillary level and is governed by the balance between hydrostatic pressure gradients and plasma oncotic pressure gradients. This relation may be stated by the familiar Starling equation:

$$J_v = K_f (\Delta P - \Delta \pi)$$

where J_v is rate of fluid transfer between vascular and interstitial compartments, K_f is the water permeability of the capillary bed, ΔP is the hydrostatic pressure difference between capillary and interstitium, and $\Delta \pi$ is the oncotic pressure difference between capillary and interstitial fluids. Under normal circumstances, interstitial tissue pressure is low and the ΔP term in the Starling equation represents the integrated hydrostatic pressure gradient from arteriolar to venular ends of a capillary. Since interstitial fluid is protein poor, the $\Delta \pi$ term in the Starling equation represents the oncotic pressure of plasma proteins, principally albumin; 5 grams of albumin per deciliter of plasma exerts an oncotic pressure of about 15 mm Hg.

Protection of Fluid Balance

As noted earlier, protection of the ECV is the single most fundamental characteristic of body fluid homeostasis. This pri-

TABLE 75–1. THE INTEGRATED VOLUME RESPONSE

	Systemic Hemodynamic Changes	External Salt and Water Balance
Response	Tachycardia ↑ Peripheral resistance ↓ Venous capacitance	Thirst Renal Na$^+$, water retention
Onset	Minutes	Hours
Major activators	Catecholamines ADH Angiotensin II Endothelin 1 Prostaglandin H$_2$ Thromboxane A$_2$	Catecholamines Aldosterone ADH
Major inactivators	Prostaglandin E$_2$ Atriopeptin Nitric acid	Prostaglandin E$_2$ Atriopeptin

ADH = antidiuretic hormone.

macy is underscored by the fact that, in circumstances in which multiple physiologic variables are threatened simultaneously, the homeostatic response invariably protects ECF volume even at the expense of aggravating another electrolyte disorder. For example, a volume-contracted patient who is replenished with water, and not sodium, will retain water and become hyponatremic in an attempt to avoid circulatory collapse. Likewise, the maintenance of metabolic alkalosis in a patient who has vomited and is not repleted with salt depends, in part, on an elevated renal absorptive capacity for sodium bicarbonate. The latter maintains fluid balance at the expense of pH homeostasis.

Two cardinal mechanisms protect extracellular fluid volume: alterations in systemic hemodynamic variables and alterations in external sodium and water balance. Both mechanisms maintain filling of the arterial tree and consequently are activated by external fluid losses; by inability to transfer fluid from the interstitium to the venous system, for example, in ascites; or by impaired fluid transfer from venous to arterial systems, for example, in congestive heart failure, pericardial tamponade, or constrictive pericarditis.

The combination of alterations in systemic hemodynamic variables and alterations in external water and solute balance can be termed the "integrated volume response" (Table 75–1). Increases in pulse rate and blood pressure are modulated not only by ADH, catecholamines, and angiotensin II but also by a series of factors derived from vascular endothelial cells. These factors include endothelin 1, a 21-residue peptide with potent vasoconstrictor properties, and thromboxane A$_2$ and prostaglandin H$_2$, both derived from the cyclo-oxygenase pathway in vascular endothelial cells. The major inactivators of these systemic hemodynamic changes include prostaglandin E$_2$ and atriopeptin, both of which are discussed below, and nitric oxide, an endogenous vasodilator released by vascular endothelial cells.

There are differences in the two response systems, indicated in Table 75–1. Tachycardia, peripheral arteriolar vasoconstriction, and peripheral venoconstriction occur within minutes of external fluid losses, whereas renal salt and water conservation lag behind by 12 to 24 hours. The sensitivities of the two limbs also differ. For example, a 2 to 3 per cent decrease in extracellular fluid volume, which amounts to the loss of 40 to 60 mEq of sodium, results in virtual elimination of sodium from the urine but produces negligible changes in systemic hemodynamic factors, such as heart rate, blood pressure, or systemic vascular resistance. Since there is 2500 to 3000 mEq of exchangeable sodium in the ECF, the system for conserving renal sodium is remarkably sensitive.

Renal Volume Regulation

Figure 75–1 provides a schematic summary of the renal factors regulating volume homeostasis. In general, the system is characterized by a positive limb, activated by volume contraction, and by negative feedback, activated by volume repletion. The separate details of this mechanism are as follows.

SENSING AND EFFECTOR ELEMENTS. Changes in effective ECF volume that exceed acceptable physiologic limits are sensed by baroreceptors located in both the high- and the low-pressure regions of the circulation. The low-pressure barorecep-

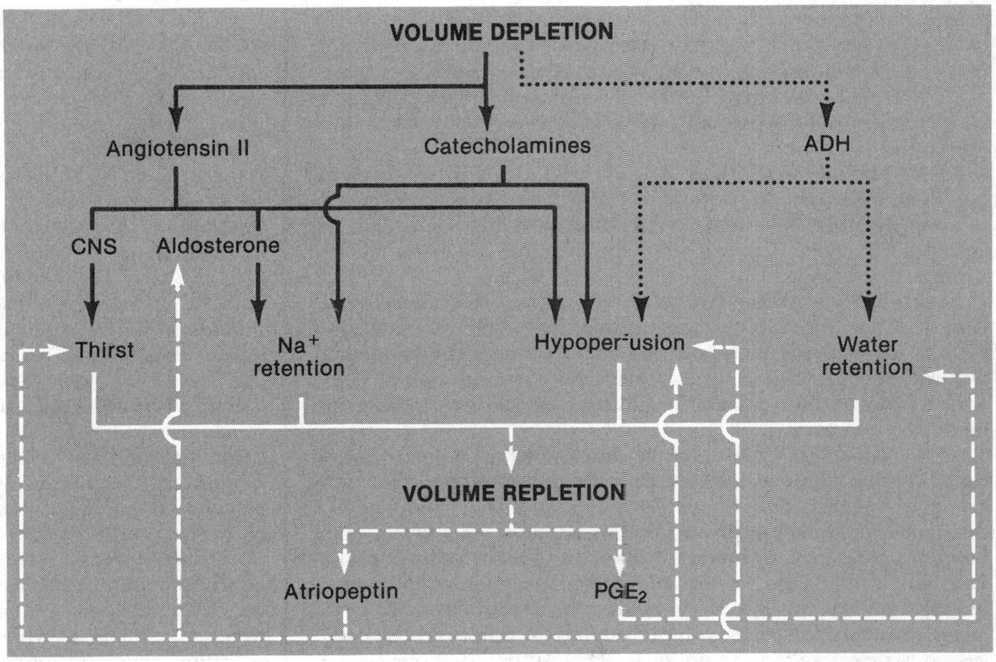

FIGURE 75–1. The volume repletion reaction. The solid and dotted lines originating from "volume depletion" indicate positive mechanisms activated when volume depletion is modest and severe, respectively. The dashed lines originating with "volume repletion" indicate negative feedback mechanisms.

tors are located primarily in the left atrium and in major thoracic veins, whereas the arterial high-pressure baroreceptors are located in the sinus body and aortic arch. Both sets of baroreceptors respond to pressure and stretch stimuli associated with changes in ECV. Activation of these extrarenal baroreceptors by relatively slight reductions in effective circulating volume results in increased sympathetic nerve activity and in rises in plasma catecholamine activity.

This catecholamine response raises blood pressure by increasing arteriolar resistance and heart rate, while simultaneously decreasing venous capacitance. Increases in arteriolar resistance also reduce capillary hydrostatic pressure and therefore promote fluid transfer from interstitial fluid to the vascular compartment. Within the kidney this increase in arteriolar resistance results in renal hypoperfusion. Moreover, adrenergic nerve terminals are in direct contact with proximal renal tubular epithelial cells, and direct stimulation of renal sympathetic nerves increases proximal tubular sodium absorption.

A second effector mechanism activated by stimulation of extrarenal baroreceptors is release of antidiuretic hormone (ADH). When blood volume is isotonically contracted by more than 8 to 10 per cent, afferent stimuli carried by the ninth and tenth cranial nerves result in nonosmotic ADH release by the neurohypophysis. In turn, ADH enhances renal water conservation and, because the hormone also has potent vasoconstrictor activity, reduces renal perfusion.

In addition to these extrarenal baroreceptors, the renal juxtaglomerular apparatus serves as an intrarenal baroreceptor system. Sympathetic nerve stimulation, reductions in afferent arteriolar blood pressure, or reductions in the rates of distal tubular sodium delivery enhance renin release by the juxtaglomerular apparatus. Renal renin release into plasma accelerates the formation of angiotensin II according to the following general scheme:

Renin Substrate
↓ renin
Angiotensin I
↓ pulmonary converting enzyme
Angiotensin II
↓ circulating angiotensinase
Angiotensin III

The octapeptide angiotensin II has three major effects on volume conservation: (1) It is a potent pressor agent; on a molar basis, angiotensin II is a more potent vasoconstrictor than norepinephrine. (2) Angiotensin II is the major stimulus to aldosterone secretion and consequently is a key factor modulating renal sodium conservation. (3) The angiotensin II formed in the central

nervous system is a potent stimulus to thirst. The heptapeptide angiotensin III is also a potent vasoconstrictor but is not as potent a stimulator of aldosterone secretion as is angiotensin II; angiotensin III also stimulates thirst.

Finally, as indicated in Table 75–1, factors produced and released by vascular endothelial cells also play a major role in modulating systemic hemodynamics. The vasoconstricting factors include the potent vasoconstrictor peptide endothelin 1. Moreover, endothelin 1 is also released from the posterior pituitary and may play a role in modulating ADH release. The vasoconstrictor agents derived from the cyclo-oxygenase pathway in vascular endothelial cells include thromboxane A_2 and prostaglandin H_2. Nitric oxide produced by vascular endothelial cells is the major endogenous nitrovasodilator.

RENAL ELEMENTS. The kidneys respond to slight reductions in ECV by increasing the rate of proximal tubular sodium absorption without disturbing either the glomerular filtration rate (GFR) or osmoregulatory mechanisms. In normal circumstances, approximately 70 per cent of filtered sodium is absorbed by the proximal nephron. As long as euvolemia persists, the fractional rate of proximal sodium absorption remains constant when the GRF is varied; this constant relation is referred to as *glomerulotubular balance*.

A number of factors modulate glomerulotubular balance in association with changes in ECV. In empiric terms, this modulation includes a downsetting of glomerulotubular balance in volume-expanded states and an increase in the rate of fractional proximal sodium absorption when filling of the arterial tree is impaired. Among these factors, the hemodynamic regulation of oncotic pressure in peritubular capillaries seems to have a dominant role. At relatively low concentrations, angiotensin II has a vasoconstricting effect on efferent, but not afferent, glomerular arterioles. Therefore this agent, by increasing the glomerular filtration fraction, can increase peritubular capillary oncotic pressure and thereby enhance proximal tubular rates of sodium absorption. At high concentrations, angiotensin II, like norepinephrine, produces afferent glomerular arteriolar constriction, which results in reductions in GFR and in renal ischemia.

The kidney responds to modest sodium depletion by increasing the rate of tubular sodium absorption without altering the GFR. Glomerulotubular balance is reset upward, so that a greater fraction of glomerular filtrate is absorbed in the proximal nephron; both direct stimulation of renal nerves and the effect of angiotensin II on efferent glomerular arterioles contribute in part to this resetting of glomerulotubular balance. Angiotensin II also provides a second mechanism for renal sodium conservation by increasing the rate of aldosterone secretion, which enhances sodium absorption in the terminal regions of the distal tubule.

Finally, increased sodium absorption by more terminal portions of the collecting duct may also be part of the volume repletion reaction. When volume contraction becomes severe, the vasoconstrictive effects of high levels of norepinephrine and angiotensin II tend to reduce both the GFR and the rate of renal sodium excretion.

NEGATIVE FEEDBACK. As indicated in Figure 75–1, atriopeptin and E series prostaglandins (PGE) constitute the principal negative feedback elements of the renal volume regulatory response. The major features of these negative feedback mechanisms are as follows.

Prostaglandins, particularly of the E series, are potent vasodilators. Within the kidney, two cardinal loci of PGE_2 production include renal glomeruli, where angiotensin II activates eicosanoid production and release, and renal medullary interstitial cells, which produce and release PGE_2 in response to increases in medullary osmolality.

As indicated in Figure 75–1, E series prostaglandins suppress renal volume conservation by at least three effects: (1) These agents are natriuretic, although it is not yet established whether the natriuretic effect of prostaglandins is due to changes in renal hemodynamics or to a direct inhibition of tubular sodium absorption. (2) Prostaglandins are potent renal vasodilators and consequently play a major role in protecting the kidneys from ischemia in circumstances such as volume depletion, when levels of the vasoconstrictor agents angiotensin II and norepinephrine are increased. (3) PGE_2 is a direct antagonist of the renal tubular effects of ADH and thus impairs renal water conservation.

An important therapeutic principle follows from a consideration of the renal vasodilatory effects of prostaglandins. Specifically, the use of aspirin and other nonsteroidal anti-inflammatory agents should be avoided in circumstances characterized by a high degree of sodium avidity, that is, by a reduction in ECV. These agents inhibit prostaglandin synthesis and thus reduce the rate of prostaglandin production. Consequently, in sodium-avid states, the use of aspirin or other nonsteroidal anti-inflammatory agents increases the rate of development of renal ischemia and hence azotemia.

Atriopeptin, or atrial natriuretic peptide, is the second negative feedback element in the renal volume regulatory response. This hormone is released from cardiac atrial storage granules in response to atrial distention; immunoreactive atriopeptin has also been identified within the central nervous system. Atriopeptin is discussed in detail in Ch. 211. In the present context, three actions of atriopeptin have particular pertinence: (1) Centrally released atriopeptin suppresses pituitary ADH release and angiotensin II–mediated thirst. (2) Atriopeptin of cardiac origin inhibits aldosterone secretion and hence renal Na$^+$ conservation; atriopeptin may also block terminal nephron Na$^+$ absorption directly. (3) Atriopeptin is a potent vasodilator that increases renal blood flow strikingly. The last-named effect also accounts in part for the natriuretic effects of this peptide.

SUMMARY. When considered in an overall context, two features of the volume repletion reaction illustrated in Figure 75–1 are noteworthy. First, redundant mechanisms protect ECV. Thus, angiotensin II release, catecholamine release, and ADH release all produce overlapping results.

Second, the magnitude of the volume repletion reaction varies, depending on the degree of volume contraction. In modestly volume-contracted states, peripheral vasoconstriction and renal sodium conservation occur, but renal blood flow, GFR, and osmoregulation are unaffected. When volume contraction becomes advanced, nonosmotic ADH release, angiotensin II–mediated thirst, and reductions in the rate of salt delivery to the loop of Henle act in concert to produce hyponatremia. Finally, when catecholamine release and angiotensin II release become sufficiently great that renal blood flow is compromised beyond autoregulatory limits, prerenal azotemia ensues.

VOLUME DEPLETION

DEFINITION. A true hypovolemic state is one in which there is a reduction in total body water, functional ECF volume, and ICF volume; it occurs when the rate of salt and water intake is less than the combined rates of renal plus extrarenal volume losses. In chronic volume-contracted states, input and output may be equal.

ETIOLOGY AND PATHOGENESIS. Three major groups of diseases, occurring individually or in combination, account for most clinically encountered states of true volume contraction. Table 75–2 summarizes these three sets of disorders and the more common specific diseases in each group.

Hormone Deficit. Volume contraction can occur whenever there is loss of ADH or aldosterone. Untreated *diabetes insipidus*, either pituitary or nephrogenic, produces profound volume contraction and hypertonic encephalopathy in patients denied free access to water. The obligatory loss of solute-free water in diabetes insipidus may be as high as 10 to 18 liters daily. Both forms of diabetes insipidus are discussed in Ch. 214.

Addison's disease may impair aldosterone production and hence lead to renal sodium wasting. A second major cause of aldosterone lack occurs in *hyporeninemic hypoaldosteronism*, which may accompany interstitial renal disease. Disorders that damage the renal interstitium, such as hypertension, diabetes mellitus, gout, sickle cell disease, chronic ingestion of lead-containing illicit alcohol, and analgesic abuse, can suppress the ability of the juxtaglomerular apparatus to produce renin. In turn, the low rate of renin secretion results in low rates of aldosterone secretion. Thus hyporeninemic hypoaldosteronism represents a disorder in which impaired aldosterone production results in renal salt wasting, hyperkalemia, and metabolic acidosis. It is not yet known why hyperkalemia, which is a potent stimulus to aldosterone secretion, fails to enhance rates of aldosterone secretion in patients with hyporeninemic hypoaldosteronism.

Renal Deficits. A number of disorders impairing renal tubular sodium or water conservation can lead to volume contraction. For convenience, these derangements may be grouped into three classes.

First, various tubular nephropathies are characterized by specific deficits in salt or water absorption. As mentioned above, nephrogenic diabetes insipidus and interstitial renal disease may produce water and sodium wasting, respectively. Because interstitial renal disease often results in hyperchloremic, hyperkalemic metabolic acidosis, the term "renal tubular acidosis, type IV" is often applied to this disorder. However, the general term "renal tubular acidosis" also includes other sodium-wasting disorders accompanied by hyperchloremic acidosis, such as proximal tubular acidosis, a specific proximal defect in bicarbonate reabsorption, and gradient-limited distal renal tubular acidosis, a specific defect in distal tubular sodium bicarbonate regeneration (Ch. 82).

Alternatively, Bartter's syndrome is a specific tubular nephropathy that results in failure of sodium chloride absorption by distal regions of the nephron; the disorder is accompanied by excessive production of prostaglandins by the renal medullary interstitium and is characterized by sodium chloride wasting, juxtaglomerular hyperplasia, high renin levels, and secondary hyperaldosteronism; the last-named results in hypokalemic metabolic alkalosis.

TABLE 75–2. MAJOR CAUSES OF VOLUME DEPLETION

Renal Losses	Extrarenal Losses
Hormonal Deficit	**Hemorrhage**
Pituitary diabetes insipidus	**Cutaneous Losses**
Aldosterone insufficiency	Sweating
Addison's disease	Burns
Hyporeninemic hypoaldosteronism	
Interstitial nephritis	
Renal Deficits	**Gastrointestinal Losses**
Specific tubular nephropathies:	Vomiting
Renal tubular acidosis	Diarrheal disorders
Proximal	Gastrointestinal fistulas
Distal, gradient-limited	Tube drainage
Bartter's syndrome	
Nephrogenic diabetes insipidus	
Diuretic abuse	
Postobstructive diuresis	
Excessive filtration of	
nonelectrolytes:	
Osmotic diuresis	
Generalized renal disease:	
Chronic renal failure	

Inhibition of tubular sodium absorptive processes due to *chronic diuretic abuse* may also lead to salt wasting, volume contraction, and specific metabolic acid-base abnormalities. These abnormalities are discussed below in connection with Table 75–5 (see below). Diuretics such as furosemide and thiazides produce serum electrolyte changes indistinguishable from those of Bartter's syndrome.

Profound but reversible defects in tubular salt and water absorption may occur during *postobstructive diuresis*, that is, shortly after relief of partial or complete urinary tract obstruction. Salt and water losses may also occur in the *diuretic phase* of acute tubular necrosis. However, profound salt and water losses associated with the diuretic phase of acute tubular necrosis are seen uncommonly if extracellular fluid volume is carefully controlled during oliguric acute tubular necrosis.

Third, glomerular filtration of large amounts of nonelectrolytes may produce volume deficits by overwhelming renal tubular reabsorptive capacity for salt and water; in this instance, water losses predominate, so that hypernatremia generally occurs. This phenomenon, termed *osmotic diuresis* or *solute diuresis*, occurs in diabetic ketoacidosis, hyperglycemic hyperosmolar coma, or hyperalimentation with large glucose loads in chronically debilitated patients; in patients with burns, in whom there are abnormally high rates of urea production; and during mannitol or glycerol administration to patients with central nervous system disorders requiring reductions of intracranial pressure.

Finally, in *chronic renal failure* of any cause, there is an obligatory loss of sodium. The extent of obligatory sodium loss in chronic renal failure is most pronounced in cystic renal diseases, notably medullary cystic disease and polycystic kidney disease (Ch. 89).

Extrarenal Losses. In addition to hemorrhage, two other classes of extrarenal losses account for volume contraction. Simple dehydration may result from increased insensible water loss in *excessive sweating* due to high ambient temperatures or to fever. Because sweat usually contains less than 50 mEq per liter of sodium, the ICF and the ECF share the water loss, and body water osmolality rises while ECF volume loss is modest. *Burns* allow the loss of large amounts of plasma and interstitial fluid through affected areas and therefore can lead rapidly to profound ECF losses.

Finally, gastrointestinal volume losses occur when portions of the 8 to 10 liters of normal gastrointestinal secretions are lost, particularly in secretory diarrheas. Volume depletion is most commonly the consequence of vomiting, gastric drainage, or diarrhea but may occur with any type of bowel fistula. Loss of hydrochloric acid from the stomach may produce metabolic alkalosis, whereas loss of sodium bicarbonate from pancreatic secretions lost through the lower gastrointestinal tract, as in diarrhea, may produce metabolic acidosis.

CLINICAL MANIFESTATIONS. The clinical findings in states of true volume contraction are due both to underfilling of the arterial tree and to the renal and hemodynamic responses to this underfilling. In mild or partially compensated volume contraction, particularly when the latter has occurred gradually, the patient may exhibit nothing more than mild postural giddiness, postural tachycardia, and weakness. In more advanced stages of volume depletion, particularly those occurring acutely, there may be hypotension when the patient is recumbent, tachycardia, and a reduced urine volume. Finally, when volume contraction is severe, the combination of profound fluid loss and increased sympathetic activity produces circulatory collapse characterized by oliguria, a nondetectable blood pressure (except by Doppler studies), tachycardia when the patient is recumbent, and cold extremities. In short, the clinical manifestations of mild to severe volume contraction may range from minimal symptoms to life-threatening circulatory collapse.

The lack of physical findings does not exclude the presence of mild to moderate volume contraction in a given patient. In the postoperative period, 7 to 10 per cent blood volume losses in patients are often accompanied by normal vital signs and by only slight decreases in the central venous pressure or the pulmonary capillary wedge pressure.

Skin turgor and the moistness of mucous membranes are valuable indices to the volume of body water in infants but are unreliable in adults. In young adults, reductions in skin turgor do not occur unless profound volume contraction is present, and normal loss of skin elasticity makes skin turgor difficult to assess in older patients. Similarly, mouth breathing and other factors affect the oral mucosa independently of external volume balances.

The signs and symptoms of volume contraction, regardless of cause, are referable to a reduction in ECV. Consequently, the clinical findings in volume contraction depend primarily on the interplay among four major factors: the magnitude of the volume loss; the rate of volume loss; the nature of the fluid loss, that is, whether the fluid loss is primarily water, a combined sodium plus water loss, or a blood loss; and finally, the responsiveness of the vasculature to volume reduction. Some simple considerations illustrate these relations.

The clinical manifestations of volume contraction are obviously related intimately to the volume and rate of fluid loss. For example, an acute gastrointestinal hemorrhage of 1 liter of blood can easily result in oliguria, coupled with the signs and symptoms of circulatory collapse, while the hematocrit remains constant. In other words, the hemorrhage is sufficiently acute that fluid flux from the interstitial to the vascular bed makes a negligible contribution to expanding the vascular bed. However, the same amount of gastrointestinal blood loss occurring more slowly—for example, over a 1-day period—permits a partial transfer of fluid from the interstitium to the vascular bed and consequently produces a fall in hematocrit; but since the ECV is at least partially restored by this fluid shift, the volume of urine flow and the hemodynamic response to volume contraction may be minimally affected.

Second, the kind of fluid loss significantly affects the clinical findings in volume contraction. Consider, for example, a 1-liter loss of different kinds of body fluids in a 70-kg man having a total body water of 40 liters and a hematocrit of 45 per cent. The acute loss of 1 liter of predominantly solute-free water, as in diabetes insipidus, produces a 2.5 per cent reduction in blood volume; urine flow and systemic hemodynamics are minimally affected. The acute loss of 1 liter of predominantly extracellular fluid produces a 6.6 per cent reduction in blood volume, since sodium is confined to the ECF; in this circumstance, modest oliguria and tachycardia while the patient is recumbent ensue. Last, the acute loss of 1 liter of blood by hemorrhage reduces blood volume by 20 per cent, thus resulting in profound oliguria and near circulatory collapse.

Finally, peripheral vasoconstriction and tachycardia represent important physiologic responses to volume losses. Consequently, the signs and symptoms of volume contraction, even of modest degree, are amplified appreciably in patients with diminished myocardial reserve or reduced sympathetic nervous system function. The former occurs commonly in cardiomyopathies of any cause or in pericardial tamponade or pericardial constriction. The latter occurs commonly in patients subjected to prolonged bed rest, in diabetic patients with autonomic neuropathy, and as a consequence of therapy with certain antihypertensive drugs.

DIAGNOSIS. The pulse, blood pressure, and changes of these variables with position, together with a clinical estimate of the venous pressure and skin temperature, provide an initial assessment of circulatory dynamics. Because these findings may be inconclusive in moderate degrees of volume contraction, a fluid challenge is useful in the evaluation of critically ill patients in whom a volume deficit is thought to be a contributory factor to a reduced cardiac output. A convenient way of achieving this goal is to administer 500 ml of normal saline over 1 to 3 hours.

In patients with a normal cardiac reserve, the effect of a fluid challenge may be monitored safely by evaluating the pulse, blood pressure, and urine flow. In patients with impaired cardiac function, the use of a flow-directed Swan-Ganz catheter for measurement of the pulmonary capillary wedge pressure or cardiac output, as estimated by thermal dilution, provides more precise indicators to early volume overload secondary to a fluid challenge. Because volume contraction is associated with vasoconstriction, both in the venous and the arterial circuits, transient changes in the pulmonary capillary wedge pressure may not accurately reflect the volume status of the patient. During volume expansion, the wedge pressure rises and subsequently falls. The initial pressure elevation is due to fluid infusion into a vasoconstricted, low-capacity vascular bed and should not be misinterpreted to indicate adequacy of volume repletion. The subsequent reduction in wedge pressure coincides with decreases in arterial resistance coupled to increases in venous capacitance. Finally, central venous pressure measurements provide unreliable estimates of pulmonary vascular volume.

The cardinal laboratory findings associated with volume contraction follow directly from the volume repletion mechanism summarized in Figure 75–1. The kidney initially responds to a decrease in effective circulating blood volume by reducing urine volume and sodium excretion. Severe degrees of volume contraction also reduce filtration rate and result in prerenal azotemia.

The urinary sodium concentration and the fraction of filtered sodium excreted in the urine, denoted as Fe_{Na}, are clinically useful indices of renal sodium avidity. The Fe_{Na} is calculated as the urine to plasma sodium concentration ratio divided by the urine to plasma creatinine concentration ratio. In the volume-contracted state, the urinary sodium concentration is generally less than 10 mEq per liter and the Fe_{Na} is less than 1 per cent, whereas in acute tubular necrosis, the urinary sodium concentration is greater than 40 mEq per liter and the Fe_{Na} is greater than 1 per cent. These indices are useful in the differential diagnosis between acute oliguric tubular necrosis and volume contraction associated with prerenal azotemia, with certain notable exceptions.

The urinary sodium indices are not reliable determinants of volume contraction when there is obligatory renal sodium wasting, as in interstitial nephritis. When volume contraction is due to the renal losses listed in Table 75–2 (except for diabetes insipidus), the urinary sodium concentration and the Fe_{Na} may both be elevated even when volume losses are large enough to produce azotemia. The urinary sodium excretion may also be elevated in volume contraction due to upper gastrointestinal losses associated with vomiting or gastric drainage. This occurs during early metabolic alkalosis if the filtered load of bicarbonate exceeds the renal tubular reabsorptive capacity for bicarbonate. During this interval, the urinary chloride concentration is a more reliable index of renal salt avidity. Finally, antecedent diuretic therapy may invalidate Fe_{Na} measurements.

TREATMENT. The major goal of the treatment of volume contraction is to expand the ECV by replacing fluid deficits. The type of fluid, the route and rate of fluid administration, and the total amount of fluid to be given will vary with the particular circumstance. For example, a mild, nonpersisting upper gastrointestinal hemorrhage may be treated appropriately by infusion of normal saline, whereas a major, persisting upper gastrointestinal hemorrhage will generally require replacement with whole blood.

The degree to which a given volume of crystalloid solution expands the ECV depends on solution composition. If glucose metabolism is normal, the infusion of 5 per cent dextrose in water (D_5W) is equivalent to administering solute-free water, which distributes uniformly in total body water. Since less than 10 per cent of total body water is in the intravascular compartment, infusion of 1 liter of D_5W expands the intravascular volume by 75 to 100 ml, that is, by about 2 per cent.

Sodium-free solutions, such as D_5W, are used principally in hypertonic volume-contracted states, such as diabetes insipidus or excessive sweating. If large volumes of glucose-containing solutions are given rapidly, the urine must be monitored for glycosuria, since the osmotic diuresis produced by the latter will cause urinary losses of both sodium and water.

Solutions containing sodium as the principal solute preferentially expand the extracellular fluid volume. Infusion of 1 liter of a normal saline solution increases blood volume by about 300 ml, or about 6 per cent; the remaining portion is distributed in the interstitial compartment. Hypotonic sodium-containing salt solutions expand intravascular volume in a manner intermediate between that of D_5W and normal saline. Sodium-containing crystalloid solutions are indicated primarily in volume-contracted states secondary to renal or gastrointestinal sodium losses (Table 75–2). They are also useful adjuncts to therapy in burns and in hemorrhage.

Colloid-containing solutions, such as iso-oncotic albumin solutions and plasma, preferentially expand the intravascular compartment, since large molecules like albumin are mainly restricted to the intravascular space. This kind of fluid replacement is most helpful in burns, in which cutaneous protein losses are apprecia-

ble, and in circulatory collapse, in which rapid intravascular expansion is critical. In most other instances of volume contraction, the use of colloid-containing solutions is difficult to justify, since the half-life of infused albumin in ill patients is relatively short, only 4 to 6 hours, and the cost of colloid solutions such as iso-oncotic albumin is more than 50 times greater than that of an equal volume of crystalloid solution.

Finally, blood, which contains formed elements, is the most potent expander of the intravascular space. A unit of packed red blood cells will remain entirely in the vascular bed. In most hemorrhagic situations, the combination of packed red blood cells with either normal saline solutions or colloid solutions is adequate for volume replacement. There are few circumstances in modern practice, with the possible exception of massive hemorrhagic shock, in which whole-blood therapy for volume expansion is utilized.

CIRCULATORY COMPROMISE WITHOUT TRUE VOLUME CONTRACTION

DEFINITION. In the previous section, we considered those disorders characterized by inadequate filling of the arterial tree that occur because of fluid losses between the patient and the external environment. Clearly, the cardinal signs and symptoms of these disorders are referable to responses accompanying the integrated volume repletion reaction (Fig. 75–1). There are also disorders in which inadequate arterial filling occurs in the absence of external fluid losses. The signs and symptoms of these disorders mimic closely those that characterize true volume contraction.

ETIOLOGY AND PATHOGENESIS. Table 75–3 lists three commonly encountered classes of derangements that may manifest clinically with tachycardia, acute hypotension, oliguria, azotemia, and a reduced Fe_{Na}. These disorders can be termed "non–volume-contracted circulatory compromise," with the understanding that the term "non–volume-contracted" refers to the absence of body fluid losses between the patient and the external world.

Impaired Cardiac Output. A profound collapse of cardiac output, due to acute myocardial infarction with pump failure (cardiogenic shock) or to acute pericardial tamponade, may clearly result in circulatory collapse. In this instance, failure to fill the arterial tree and to maintain an ECV occurs because the heart fails to translocate blood adequately from venous to arterial beds.

Increased Vascular Capacitance. Circulatory collapse with its attendant signs and symptoms occurs when there is a sudden increase in the capacitance of the vascular bed, most notably in the venous part of the circulation. This kind of increase in ratio of vascular capacitance to vascular volume occurs most commonly in sepsis but may also be seen in circumstances in which peripheral vasodilators, particularly those having a postarteriolar locus of action, are administered injudiciously.

Vascular-Interstitial Fluid Shifts. Profound hypotension, tachycardia, progressive oliguria, and azotemia are also encountered when there is a rapid translocation of fluid from vascular to interstitial compartments, presumably because of a sudden, profound increase in the permeability characteristics of peripheral capillaries. Some common derangements of this type include infarction of the small or large intestine, extensive tissue trauma, acute pancreatitis, and rhabdomyolysis. An analogous mechanism—namely, a marked increase in the permeability of pulmonary capillaries—is also presumed to account for the formation of noncardiogenic pulmonary edema in the adult respiratory distress syndrome.

DIAGNOSIS AND THERAPY. The diagnosis and therapy of

TABLE 75–3. CIRCULATORY COMPROMISE WITHOUT EXTERNAL FLUID LOSSES

I. **Impaired Cardiac Output**
  Acute myocardial infarction
  Pericardial tamponade
II. **Increased Vascular Capacitance**
  Septic shock
III. **Vascular → Interstitial Fluid Shifts**
  Acute pancreatitis
  Bowel infarction
  Rhabdomyolysis
  Noncardiogenic pulmonary edema

acute myocardial infarction with circulatory collapse and of acute pericardial tamponade are considered in detail in Part VI of this book. It is, however, worth citing certain factors particularly germane to the management of fluid therapy in such patients. In individuals affected either by right ventricular infarction or by pericardial tamponade, maintenance of adequate filling of the systemic arterial tree depends critically on providing a relatively high venous preload to the right side of the heart. Attempts at volume contraction in patients with right ventricular infarcts or pericardial tamponade may exacerbate systemic hypotension. Thus treatment of these disorders generally requires concomitant hemodynamic monitoring with a flow-directed Swan-Ganz catheter to avoid excessive preload to the left side of the heart.

In patients with left ventricular infarction and systemic hypotension, particular attention should be directed to excluding the possibility that antecedent true volume depletion—for example, with prolonged diuretic therapy and salt restriction prior to the myocardial infarction—may be a significant contributor to what otherwise might be mistaken for true cardiogenic shock. The findings of acute left ventricular infarction, systemic arterial hypotension, the absence of pulmonary edema on the chest radiograph, a reduced pulmonary capillary wedge pressure, and an antecedent history of prolonged diuretic therapy, when taken together, indicate that improved systemic hemodynamics may be achieved by cautious attempts at volume expansion carried out in combination with serial measurements of the cardiac output and the pulmonary capillary wedge pressure.

The distinction between hypotension due to true volume contraction and that due to an increase in the capacitance-volume ratio of the vascular bed, as occurs in sepsis, is often difficult. This distinction is particularly difficult in individuals who have been in intensive care units for prolonged periods of time and in those at high risk for developing sepsis, such as cancer patients treated with potent chemotherapeutic agents. A useful clue to the presence of septic circulatory collapse is the occurrence of warm extremities coupled with hypotension and oliguria, since true hypovolemia, particularly when advanced, is ordinarily accompanied by profound peripheral vasoconstriction and hence cool and often cyanotic extremities.

True hypovolemia and sepsis may also coexist. In such a circumstance, invasive hemodynamic monitoring may be helpful. Both in true hypovolemia and in sepsis, the pulmonary capillary wedge pressure is reduced; but in septic circulatory collapse, the calculated systemic vascular resistance falls, because of peripheral vasodilation, whereas in true hypovolemia, peripheral vasoconstriction ordinarily raises the systemic vascular resistance. The diagnosis of disorders producing rapid transfer of fluids from the vascular bed to the interstitium, such as trauma, acute pancreatitis, or rhabdomyolysis, is generally evident from clinical appraisal.

The treatment of patients with sepsis and an increased vascular capacitance-volume ratio, as well as those individuals with rapid vascular to interstitial fluid shifts, has as a mainstay the administration of sufficient sodium-containing fluids, generally isotonic saline, to permit adequate filling of the arterial tree. This therapy necessarily expands total body water, particularly in the vascular and interstitial compartments. Consequently, during recovery from the underlying disorder, care must be taken to avoid unnecessary expansion of the vascular bed and consequently the risk of volume-mediated cardiac decompensation.

VOLUME EXCESS

DEFINITION. Volume-expanded states are characterized by an increase in total body water, which is accompanied, in most but not all circumstances, by an increase in total body sodium. Total body salt and water may be increased while the ECV is decreased. In other words, certain volume-expanded states are characterized by dissociation between total body salt and water and the ECV.

ETIOLOGY AND PATHOGENESIS. Volume expansion occurs whenever the rate of salt or water intake exceeds the rate of renal plus extrarenal losses; in chronic volume expansion, the external salt and water balance may be normal. A convenient way of considering volume-expanded states is to view them in the context of three different classes of physiologic explanations (Table 75–4).

TABLE 75–4. DISORDERS OF VOLUME EXCESS

I. Disturbed Starling Forces	II. Primary Hormone Excess
(Reduced effective circulating volume; edema formation)	(Increased effective circulating volume)
Systemic venous pressure increases:	Primary aldosteronism
Right heart failure	Cushing's syndrome
Constrictive pericarditis	SIADH
Local venous pressure increases:	**III. Primary Renal Sodium Retention**
Left heart failure	(Increased effective circulating volume)
Vena cava obstruction	Acute glomerulonephritis
Portal vein obstruction	
Reduced oncotic pressure:	
Nephrotic syndrome	
Combined disorders:	
Cirrhosis	

SIADH = syndrome of inappropriate antidiuretic hormone production.

Disturbances in Starling Forces. The most common diseases encountered in which both volume expansion and edema occur are those in which derangements in the Starling forces regulating fluid transfer between capillaries and interstitium tend to promote expansion of the interstitial compartment at the expense of the ECV. Consequently, renal sodium retention and edema occur. By definition, this group of disorders is characterized by increases in capillary hydrostatic pressure, by decreases in capillary oncotic pressure, or by a combination of these two factors.

Four groups include most edematous states characterized by abnormal Starling forces (Table 75–4). First, the systemic venous pressure may be increased because of primary cardiac disorders, such as right-sided heart failure or constrictive pericarditis. Second, local elevations in pulmonary or systemic venous pressure may occur, as in left-sided heart failure, vena caval obstruction, or portal vein obstruction. Third, a reduction in plasma oncotic pressure, and consequently a net increase in the tendency for fluid to transude from capillaries to interstitium, accounts plausibly for edema formation in the nephrotic syndrome. Finally, a combination of these factors may be responsible for edema formation. For example, both hypoalbuminemia and portal hypertension are major contributory factors to the development of ascites in hepatic cirrhosis.

Plasma renin activity and aldosterone concentrations in these disorders tend to be elevated, although the results also tend to be variable. In advanced cases of disorders characterized by increases in local or systemic venous pressure, most notably in severe congestive heart failure and in cirrhosis, hyponatremia may occur; this finding represents an ominous prognostic sign. Finally, edema formation due to such derangements of Starling forces may result in the "third space" phenomenon, namely, the sequestration of large volumes of interstitial fluid in regions such as the pleural or peritoneal cavities.

Primary Hormonal Excess. These disorders include those disturbances in which there is unregulated production of mineralocorticoids or ADH. The volume expansion that occurs in states of mineralocorticoid excess, such as primary hyperaldosteronism, is due to sodium retention and is accompanied by a primary, preferential expansion of the ECF and consequently by hypertension. The serum sodium level is generally normal. In the syndrome of inappropriate ADH production (SIADH), primary water retention occurs. Consequently, the volume expansion involves both the ICF and ECF; dilutional hyponatremia is the hallmark of SIADH, whereas hypertension is uncommon. Edema is not characteristic in either of these two disorders. Instead, patients with primary aldosteronism or SIADH reach a volume-expanded steady state in which output equals input.

Primary Renal Sodium Retention. The kidneys may also retain sodium abnormally when the ECV is normal and there is no effector excess. For example, in acute glomerulonephritis unidentified renal mechanisms are primarily responsible for edema formation. Patients with acute glomerulonephritis retain salt and water and become hypertensive without reductions in the GFR or in ECV. Furthermore, sodium retention and edema develop when plasma renin activity and aldosterone concentration are normal or reduced and when the serum albumin concentration is normal. Thus, the renal tubule may be abnormally avid for sodium in acute glomerulonephritis. Congestive heart failure may occur as a secondary consequence of the volume expansion.

DIAGNOSIS AND TREATMENT. The recognition and management of volume-expanded states depend on proper identification and treatment of the underlying disorder. Clearly, the cornerstones of therapy in volume-expanded states characterized by sodium excess include salt restriction and diuretics. Table 75–5 provides a summary of some of the major diuretics used commonly and certain of their properties. For convenience, these drugs have been classified according to their sites of action in the nephron.

Proximal Diuretics. The cardinal example of a proximal tubular diuretic is acetazolamide, a carbonic anhydrase inhibitor that blocks proximal reabsorption of sodium bicarbonate. Consequently, prolonged use of acetazolamide may lead to hyperchloremic acidosis, in contrast to all other diuretics, which act at loci prior to the late distal nephron. Metolazone, a congener of the thiazide class of diuretics, blocks sodium chloride absorption in two nephron sites by unknown mechanisms. Specifically, in addition to an action on the early distal tubule, metolazone also inhibits proximal tubular sodium chloride absorption. Since the major locus for phosphate absorption is in the proximal nephron, the phosphaturia accompanying metolazone administration exceeds considerably that observed with other thiazide class diuretics.

Proximal diuretics are rarely used as primary diuretic therapy in modern practice. More commonly, these diuretics, particularly metolazone, are used as supplements to loop diuretics in instances in which loop diuretics alone are ineffective in producing diuresis.

Loop Diuretics. Loop diuretics, such as ethacrynic acid and furosemide, produce diuresis by inhibiting the coupled entry of Na^+, Cl^-, and K^+ across apical plasma membranes in the thick ascending limb of Henle. The latter is responsible for the reabsorption of approximately 25 per cent of filtered sodium. The natriuretic dose-response characteristics of these diuretic agents are considerably more linear than those of all other currently used diuretics. Consequently, the loop diuretics are, for practical purposes, the most potent diuretics currently available; therefore these drugs are commonly referred to as "high-ceiling" diuretics.

Furosemide is the most commonly used loop diuretic. The drug may be administered orally, generally at dosages of 20 to 60 mg every 6 to 8 hours. The onset of action occurs within 1 to 2 hours and is dissipated at 6 hours. Intravenous furosemide, generally in dosages of 20 to 80 mg at 6-hour intervals, is useful in circumstances in which acute diuresis is required, as, for example, in acute pulmonary edema. The onset of action occurs within 10 to 20 minutes, and the effect is dissipated at 3 to 4 hours. Although the dose-response curve with furosemide is more linear than with diuretics of the thiazide class, there is little justification for using intravenous furosemide dosages in excess of 120 to 160 mg. Rather, it is more prudent, in instances of diuretic resistance, to employ combined diuretic therapy—for example, using metolazone together with furosemide.

Early Distal Tubule Diuretics. Early distal tubule diuretics, such as thiazide and metolazone, interfere primarily with sodium chloride absorption in the earliest segments of the distal convoluted tubule. The thiazide diuretics appear to exert their effect by blocking sodium entry from tubular fluid across apical plasma membranes into distal tubular cells.

With the exception of acetazolamide (which impairs bicarbonate absorption), hypokalemia and metabolic alkalosis may complicate the administration of proximal diuretics, loop diuretics, and early distal tubular diuretics. This occurs because the rate of sodium delivery to terminal distal tubular regions, where a significant fraction of potassium and proton secretion occurs, is a major factor promoting these two processes. Consequently, an increased delivery of salt to the late distal nephron, occasioned by inhibition of sodium reabsorption in the proximal tubule, the ascending limb of Henle, or the early distal tubule, leads to accelerated rates of proton and potassium secretion and consequently to hypokalemia and metabolic alkalosis.

In general, early distal tubular diuretics are utilized for the same circumstances as loop diuretics. The major exception to this statement occurs in disorders of calcium metabolism. Loop diuretics are calciuric and therefore are a valuable adjunct to the management of acute hypercalcemia. In contrast, thiazide diuretics promote hypocalciuria and calcium retention and are therefore useful in managing hypercalciuric states, but not hypercalcemia.

Late Distal Nephron Diuretics. Finally, a group of agents inhibit sodium absorption in terminal regions of the distal tubule and concomitantly suppress indirectly potassium secretion and proton secretion. Spironolactone competes with aldosterone; the primary use of this agent is restricted to conditions of aldosterone excess, either primary or secondary. Alternatively, both triamterene and amiloride operate independently of aldosterone. These agents directly block sodium uptake by late distal tubular cells and concomitantly suppress indirectly both potassium and proton secretion. Accordingly, hyperkalemic, hyperchloremic metabolic acidosis may complicate the injudicious use of spironolactone, triamterene, or amiloride. These diuretics are useful especially in managing disorders characterized by secondary hyperaldosteronism, such as cirrhosis with ascites, and in promoting diuresis in hypokalemic patients.

One factor common to the treatment of disorders with reduced ECV's and expanded ECF volumes merits particular consideration. A major factor in edema formation is an increase in the Starling forces promoting fluid translocation from the vascular to interstitial spaces. When potent diuretics are administered to patients with portal hypertension or with hypoalbuminemia, urinary sodium excretion may exceed the rate at which salt and water are transferred from the interstitium to the vascular bed. As a result, vigorous diuretic therapy may result in volume contraction, reduced salt delivery to diluting segments, nonosmotic ADH release, and consequently hyponatremia. In advanced cases of diuretic abuse, hypotension, hemoconcentration, and azotemia also occur.

A like effect occurs in volume-expanded patients, particularly

TABLE 75–5. CHARACTERISTICS OF COMMONLY USED DIURETICS

Diuretic	Primary Effect	Secondary Effect	Complications
I. Proximal Diuretics			
Acetazolamide	↓ Na^+/H^+ exchange	↑ K^+ loss, ↑ HCO_3^- loss	Hypokalemic, hyperchloremic acidosis
Metolazone	↓ Na^+ absorption	↑ K^+ loss, ↑ Cl^- loss	Hypokalemic alkalosis
II. Loop Diuretics			
Furosemide, Ethacrynic acid	↓ Na^+:K^+:2Cl^- absorption	↑ K^+ loss, ↑ H^+ secretion	Hypokalemic alkalosis
III. Early Distal Diuretics			
Thiazide, Metolazone	↓ Na^+ absorption	↑ K^+ loss, ↑ H^+ secretion	Hypokalemic alkalosis
IV. Late Distal Diuretics			
Aldosterone antagonists: Spironolactone. Nonaldosterone antagonists: Triamterene, Amiloride	↓ Na^+ absorption	↓ K^+ loss, ↓ H^+ secretion	Hyperkalemic acidosis

those exhibiting a third space effect and having significant hypo-albuminemia, if relatively large volumes of ascitic fluid are removed by paracentesis. In this circumstance, the transudation of fluid from the vascular space to the interstitial space may result in circulatory collapse.

Johnston CI, Hodsman PG, Kohzuki M, et al.: Interaction between atrial natriuretic peptide and the renin, angiotensin, aldosterone system. Am J Med 87(Suppl 6B):24S, 1989. *A review of the renin-angiotensin system and the interaction with atriopeptin.*

King AJ, Brenner BM, Anderson SH: Endothelin: A potent renal and systemic vasoconstrictor peptide. Am J Physiol 256:F1051, 1989. *A description of the physiology of endothelin.*

Palkovits M, Geiger H, Bahner U, et al.: Atrial natriuretic factor in central nervous system regulatory mechanisms: Effect of experimental alterations in water and salt homeostasis and blood pressure. Miner Electrolyte Metab 16:42, 1990. *A summary of current information about atriopeptin.*

Stein JH, Kunau RT (eds.): Diuretics II Clinical uses. Semin Nephrol 8:317, 1988. *A complete issue of this journal devoted to the clinical application of diuretics.*

Weinman EJ, Andreoli TE (eds.): Diuretics I: Physiology, biochemistry and pharmacology. Semin Nephrol 8:197–314, 1988. *A complete issue of this journal devoted to the physiology of diuretics.*

75.2 OSMOLALITY DISTURBANCES

PHYSIOLOGIC CONSIDERATIONS

In normal individuals, the serum osmolality is virtually constant from day to day, and the serum sodium concentration is an accurate index of body water osmolality. In fact, the normal ranges for serum sodium concentrations or for serum osmolalities in populations of healthy individuals reflect small differences in body water osmolality among individuals, rather than on variations in body water osmolality in a given individual.

It is useful to define "effective ECF osmolality," since the osmoregulatory mechanisms that adjust water balance in normal individuals are determined primarily by changes in cell volume that result from variations in effective ECF osmolality. In dilutional states, the measured and effective ECF osmolalities are approximately equal, since ECF dilution also produces ICF dilution and, at least acutely, cell swelling. Osmoregulatory mechanisms are activated when ECF hypertonicity is due to a solute that is excluded from cells and therefore produces, at least acutely, cell shrinkage; in this case, the measured and effective ECF osmolalities are approximately equal. If the ECF osmolality is increased by solutes such as urea, which penetrate cell membranes readily, acute cell shrinkage does not occur and osmoregulatory mechanisms are not activated. In this case, the measured ECF osmolality is greater than the effective ECF osmolality.

The serum osmolality can be approximated from the following formula:

$$\text{Osmolality} = 2[\text{Na}^+] + \frac{[\text{glucose}]}{18} + \frac{[\text{BUN}]}{2.8}$$

where the glucose and blood urea nitrogen (BUN) concentrations are expressed as milligrams per deciliter and the serum sodium concentration is expressed as milliequivalents per liter. In normal circumstances, glucose contributes 5.5 mOsm per kilogram of H_2O to the serum osmolality. When hyperglycemia occurs, the effective ECF osmolality rises because glucose entry into cells is limited. When azotemia occurs, the effective ECF osmolality does not rise because urea enters cells readily.

Cell Volume Regulation

Starling forces regulate fluid transfer between the ICF and the ECF. Because plasma membranes cannot tolerate even small hydrostatic gradients, the operational Starling forces between ICF and ECF are almost entirely osmotic. Significant changes in cell volume, particularly in the central nervous system, are by themselves potentially lethal. Thus the goals of fluid transport between the ECF and ICF are to maintain constancy of cell volume and to maintain a negligible hydrostatic pressure gradient between cells and the ECF. Since cell membranes are freely permeable to water, these two goals are achieved when the ECF osmolality is normal and intracellular and extracellular osmolalities are identical.

Since cell membranes are partially permeable to sodium and

potassium, there is a tendency for sodium to leak into cells and for potassium to leak out of cells. Because impermeant macromolecules account for a large fraction of intracellular anions, passive sodium and potassium movements tend toward a Donnan distribution, in which total intracellular cations would exceed total interstitial cations, in precise analogy to the way in which total plasma water cations exceed total interstitial cations. If these passive cation movements across cell membranes were unopposed, osmotic water movement into cells would tend to produce cell lysis. Consequently, active transport mechanisms are required to balance intracellular and interstitial cation concentrations.

Specifically, both sodium leakage from the ECF into cells and potassium leakage out of cells into the ECF are counterbalanced exactly by active outward sodium transport coupled to active inward potassium transport. These active transport events maintain the intracellular cation (and therefore osmolar) content equal to that of extracellular fluid and also maintain the predominant extracellular and intracellular distributions of sodium and potassium, respectively. Thus because cellular cation pumps balance cellular cation leaks, cells are *operationally* impermeable to sodium and to potassium. Active sodium efflux coupled to active potassium influx is mediated by membrane-bound $(\text{Na}^+ + \text{K}^+)$–adenosine triphosphatase (ATPase), and the activity of these cellular cation pumps accounts for more than 50 per cent of the basal caloric consumption.

Cation transport mediated by $(\text{Na}^+ + \text{K}^+)$-ATPase is the major factor regulating cell volume when the effective ECF osmolality is normal. When the effective ECF osmolality is increased or decreased, additional processes are required to maintain the constancy of cell volume. These auxiliary mechanisms are of particular importance in minimizing potentially lethal changes in brain volume because of osmotic water shifts into or out of brain cells.

In chronic hypotonic disorders, cell swelling is offset by the loss of potassium chloride from cells. This potassium chloride efflux mechanism appears to be activated by small increases in cell volume produced by ECF dilution. In chronic hypernatremia, brain shrinkage is minimized by the accumulation of additional solutes within brain cells. These latter solutes, often called "idiogenic osmoles," include amino acids and other solutes, including myoinositol, betaine, and urea. As will be discussed in the section on treatment, these auxiliary transport processes affect significantly the therapeutic approach to patients with osmoregulatory failure.

Water Balance

The key elements regulating water balance are summarized in Figure 75–2. The osmoreceptors, both for ADH release and for thirst, respond to small changes in effective ECF osmolality, while baroreceptors respond to changes in ECV. As little as a 2 per cent increase in effective ECF osmolality causes shrinkage of osmoreceptor cells and stimulation of both ADH release from the posterior pituitary and thirst. A second way of stimulating both ADH release and thirst involves volume-mediated stimuli that can operate independently of changes in plasma osmolality. When the ECV volume is reduced by approximately 10 per cent, these volume-dependent mechanisms stimulate ADH release.

Until recently, it was commonly thought that increases in plasma osmolality and in plasma volume directly suppressed water repletion. It now seems likely, however, that suppression of thirst and of ADH release depends on at least two factors, namely, the oropharyngeal reflex (OPR) and release of atrial natriuretic peptide, the latter occurring, in all likelihood, both systemically and in the central nervous system.

SENSORS AND EFFECTORS. Three kinds of *sensor* elements adjust water balance. Two of these, osmoreceptors and the thirst center, respond to small changes in effective ECF osmolality, whereas baroreceptors respond to changes in ECV. The osmoreceptors are situated in the supraoptic and paraventricular nuclei of the hypothalamus, whereas the thirst center is in the organum vasculosum of the anterior hypothalamus. As little as a 2 per cent increase in effective ECF osmolality produced by solutes such as sodium chloride, but not urea, causes shrinkage

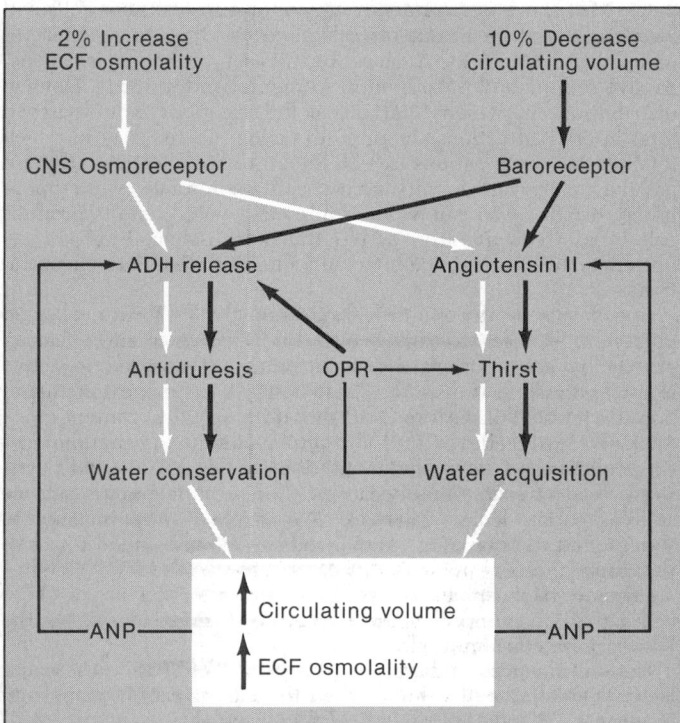

FIGURE 75–2. The water repletion reaction. The white arrows are positive water conservation processes activated by osmolality. The red arrows are water conservation processes that are volume activated. The black arrows indicate negative feedback. (From Reeves WB, Andreoli TE: The posterior pituitary and water metabolism. *In* Wilson JD, Foster DW [eds.]: Williams Textbook of Endocrinology. 8th ed. Philadelphia, W. B. Saunders Company, 1992.)

of osmoreceptor cells and thirst center cells. The osmoreceptors stimulate the release of the *effector* hormone ADH from storage sites in the posterior pituitary gland. The stimulation of thirst by the thirst centers depends on centrally produced angiotensin II.

Endothelin 1 is also released from the posterior pituitary in response to water deprivation. Moreover, administered endothelin 1 increases plasma ADH levels. Thus, endothelin 1 may have a central role in modulating ADH release.

When the ECV is reduced by more than 10 per cent, volume-dependent blood volume produces afferent signals, carried by the ninth and tenth cranial nerves, which result in nonosmotic ADH release. Volume contraction also acts as a potent stimulus to thirst via angiotensin II.

THE ANTIDIURETIC RESPONSE. The cardinal characteristics of the antidiuretic response depend primarily on the integrated activity of two regions of the nephron: the medullary thick ascending limb of Henle, referred to as the diluting segment; and the collecting duct, which may be termed the concentrating segment.

The medullary thick ascending limb absorbs a large amount, possibly as much as 25 per cent, of the filtered load of sodium. Some of this reabsorbed sodium is trapped in the renal medullary interstitium, thus accounting in large part for the hypertonicity of the renal medullary interstitium. However, the medullary thick limb of Henle is also impermeable to water. Consequently, salt abstraction from the thick limb of Henle accounts simultaneously for the development of medullary hypertonicity, thus permitting, in the presence of ADH, maximal antidiuresis, and for the appearance of maximally dilute urine in early distal convolutions, thus permitting, in the absence of ADH, maximal water diuresis.

In normal individuals, approximately 18 liters daily of tubular fluid reaches the early distal tubule; the osmolality of this fluid is quite dilute, approximately 50 mOsm per kilogram of H_2O. Thus in the total absence of ADH and volume contraction, maximal rates of water diuresis include a urinary volume of 18 liters per day having an osmolality of 50 mOsm per kilogram of

H_2O. During antidiuresis, ADH increases the water permeability of collecting ducts (Ch. 214). Tubular fluid equilibrates osmotically with the hypertonic medullary interstitium, reducing urinary volume, concentrating the urine, and conserving body water. When ADH is absent, the water permeability of collecting ducts is low, and absorption of tubular fluid is reduced, so that it escapes unchanged as hypotonic urine.

Finally, since collecting ducts are partially permeable to water in the absence of ADH, a reduced volume of hypotonic fluid reaching collecting ducts equilibrates partially with the medullary interstitium, thereby limiting the ability to dilute urine maximally. In some experimental circumstances, sufficiently significant reductions in the rate of solute excretion result in formation of a hypertonic urine when ADH is absent.

NEGATIVE FEEDBACK. Water repletion activates a negative feedback of water conservation by at least two systems, atriopeptin and OPR (Fig. 75–2). Immunoreactive atriopeptin is released both within the central nervous system and by secretory granules in cardiac atria. The centrally released atriopeptin can suppress ADH release and thirst. Oropharyngeal stimulation by water suppresses ADH release and thirst prior to absorption of water or a fall in plasma osmolality. This mechanism, termed the oropharyngeal reflex, probably depends on neural traffic between the oropharynx and the central nervous system.

Finally, intrarenal PGE_2 suppresses the effects of ADH on nephron segments. PGE_2 is produced by renal interstitial cells in response to increases in medullary osmolality. In turn, PGE_2 impairs water conservation by inhibiting the actions of ADH on nephron segments involved in the antidiuretic response, namely, the medullary thick ascending limb and the collecting duct.

HYPOTONIC DISORDERS

DEFINITION. A hypotonic disorder is one in which the ratio of solutes to water in body fluids is reduced, and the serum osmolality and serum sodium are both reduced in parallel. True hypotonicity must be distinguished from disorders in which the *measured* serum sodium is low while the measured serum osmolality is either normal or increased.

The distinction among these disorders is presented in Table 75–6. The measured serum sodium can be reduced either because there is an increased concentration of small, nonsodium solutes restricted to the ECF or because of a laboratory artifact. In hyperglycemia or excessive mannitol administration, these solutes, which are restricted to the ECF, draw water from the cellular compartment. The serum sodium level is therefore reduced, even though the serum osmolality may be increased. When a small, nonsodium solute is distributed in total body water, as in ethanol intoxication or in azotemia, the serum osmolality rises but the serum sodium concentration remains normal, resulting in an "osmolar gap." The latter is a useful diagnostic aid in intoxication with the different alcohols shown in Table 75–6.

Instances of spurious hyponatremia due to hyperlipemia or hyperproteinemia are becoming less common as more laboratories adopt the use of ion-selective electrodes to measure the serum sodium concentration.

TABLE 75–6. DISTINCTION BETWEEN APPARENT AND REAL HYPOTONICITY

Condition	Measured Serum [Na⁺]	Measured Serum Osmolality
True hypotonicity	↓	↓
Increased nonsodium ECF solutes		
Hyperglycemia	↓	↑
Mannitol administration	↓	↑
Increased nonsodium ECF and ICF solutes		
Ethanol	Normal	↑
Ethylene glycol	Normal	↑
Methanol	Normal	↑
Isopropyl alcohol	Normal	↑
Laboratory artifact		
Hyperlipemia	↓	Normal
Hyperproteinemia	↓	Normal

ETIOLOGY AND PATHOGENESIS. Hyponatremia and simultaneous body water hypotonicity develop whenever water intake exceeds the sum of renal plus extrarenal water losses; in chronic hyponatremia, the net water intake and net water output may be equal. Thus hyponatremia and body fluid hypotonicity occur when there is a primary increase in water ingestion, when the ability of the kidney to dilute urine maximally is limited, or when a combination of these factors is operative.

Dilutional hyponatremia may be the consequence of an absolute increase in water intake that exceeds the ability of a normal kidney to excrete free water, as in *primary polydipsia*, occasionally referred to as psychogenic polydipsia. Patients with this disorder ingest unusually large volumes of water, often in excess of 10 to 15 liters per day, and generally develop mild, clinically asymptomatic hyponatremia.

However, polydipsia may contribute to rather severe hyponatremia in individuals with underlying psychiatric illness. Episodic polydipsia and hyponatremia occur in 3 to 5 per cent of patients in mental hospitals, and polyuria occurs in more than 60 per cent of patients in mental hospitals. This disorder is sometimes described by the acronym PIP syndrome (psychosis, intermittent hyponatremia, and polydipsia). The cause of this syndrome is uncertain. Most patients have, in addition to polydipsia, excessive vasopressin secretion. Carbamazepine, sometimes used to control agitation in psychotic patients, may also contribute to hyponatremia.

More commonly, hyponatremia occurs because the ability of the kidney to excrete a maximally dilute urine is reduced. This inability to dilute urine maximally occurs because of (1) reductions in the rate of salt absorption by the diluting segment, that is, the thick ascending limb of Henle; (2) sustained nonosmotic release of ADH; or (3) a combination of these factors. Table 75–7 summarizes these disorders.

Reduced Sodium Delivery to Diluting Segments. These disorders occur when a reduced sodium intake, without significant sodium depletion or ECF volume contraction, decreases the rate of sodium delivery to the diluting segment and consequently impairs the maximal rate of dilute urine formation, the minimal urinary osmolality, or both. Beer potomania, although an uncommon disorder, illustrates this mechanism for hyponatremia nicely.

Patients with beer potomania derive a substantial part of their caloric intake from the ingestion of large volumes of beer, which contains little salt or protein. Because sodium and urea are the major urinary solutes, dietary restriction of these solutes, particularly sodium, increases the fractional rate of proximal sodium absorption, diminishes the rate of salt delivery to diluting segments, and in turn limits the daily rate of formation of dilute urine. For example, the minimal urinary osmolality is approximately 50 mOsm per kilogram of H_2O; consequently, the excretion of 15 liters of highly dilute urine requires the excretion of 750 mOsm of solute. If the daily urinary solute excretion falls, the maximal amount of dilute urine formed daily is also reduced. Moreover, partial equilibration of reduced volumes of collecting duct fluid with the renal medullary interstitium impairs even further the daily excretion of dilute urine.

Hyponatremia due to reduced solute intake is not restricted to individuals with beer potomania but may occur during starvation,

TABLE 75–7. HYPONATREMIA REFERABLE TO IMPAIRED RENAL EXCRETION OF WATER

I. Reduced Sodium Delivery to the Diluting Segment	III. Mixed Disorders
Starvation	Volume contraction (Addison's disease)
Beer potomania	Edema with deranged Starling forces (congestive heart failure, constrictive pericarditis, and cirrhosis)
? Myxedema	
II. Primary Excess of ADH	
SIADH	
Drug-induced ADH production	
Drug potentiation of ADH action	
Trauma	
Potassium depletion	
? Myxedema	
? Acute intermittent porphyria	

TABLE 75–8. MAJOR CAUSES OF SIADH

Malignant Neoplasia
  Carcinoma: bronchogenic, pancreatic, ureteral, prostatic, bladder
  Lymphoma and leukemia
  Thymoma and mesothelioma
Central Nervous System (CNS) Disorders
  Trauma
  Infection
  Tumors
  Porphyria
Pulmonary Disorders
  Tuberculosis
  Pneumonia
  Ventilators with positive pressure

when intake may be dramatically reduced without parallel reductions in water intake. This form of hyponatremia occurs with increasing frequency in elderly patients in nursing homes who are inadequately supervised.

Patients with beer potomania or starvation are to be distinguished from individuals in whom a reduced ECV accompanied by an increase in total body water or by a reduction in GFR reduces the rate of salt delivery to diluting segments and collecting ducts (see below). In short, beer potomania and starvation are classic examples in which a reduced rate of delivery to the diluting segment, in the absence of ADH release, blunts significantly urinary diluting power in the absence of profound gains or excesses in total body water.

Primary Effector ADH Excess. **The Syndrome of Inappropriate ADH Production (SIADH).** In SIADH, hyponatremia occurs as a result of sustained endogenous production and release of ADH or ADH-like substances; the ECV is normal or increased, and there are no other physiologic or pharmacologic stimuli to ADH release. Table 75–8 lists the major causes of SIADH. A similar process may account in part for the hyponatremia seen in myxedema.

Antidiuretic hormone, or a peptide having comparable biologic activity, is produced by tumors. Increased ADH levels, estimated by either bioassay or radioimmunoassay, have also been noted in patients with cranial disorders such as skull fractures, subdural hematomas, subarachnoid hemorrhage, and brain tumors; in acute intermittent porphyria; and possibly in myxedema. Four different patterns of plasma ADH concentrations have been described in patients with SIADH. Figure 75–3 illustrates three of these patterns; the shaded area in Figure 75–3 illustrates the normal relation between plasma ADH levels and serum osmolality. The pattern denoted "erratic ADH release" in Figure 75–3 accounts for about 37 per cent of patients with SIADH; the hormone is released completely independently of osmotic control. About one third of patients with SIADH have a "reset osmostat"; there is an abnormally low threshold for ADH secretion, but if sufficiently hyponatremic, these patients with SIADH can produce a maximally dilute urine. About 16 per cent of patients with SIADH exhibit the "ADH leak" pattern, namely, sustained ADH production below the osmotic threshold, and normal increases in serum ADH levels with osmotic challenge (Fig. 75–3). Finally, about 14 per cent of patients with SIADH have no detectable abnormality in ADH levels; they fail, for reasons not yet understood, to dilute urine maximally.

The typical features of SIADH are listed in Table 75–9. The cardinal results of the sustained water conservation in SIADH are twofold: hyponatremia and volume expansion. In fact, patients with SIADH who are allowed free access to water generally gain about 3 kg in water weight, or, in other words, nearly 10 per cent of body water. In that respect, patients with SIADH differ from those with hyponatremia secondary to salt depletion, Addison's disease, or diuretic excess, since patients with the latter disorders are volume contracted. However, patients with SIADH, although volume expanded, do not develop edema and thus differ in that respect from patients with congestive heart failure or cirrhosis.

When total body water is expanded by about 10 per cent by water conservation in SIADH, a natriuresis occurs even in the face of hyponatremia. Thus the patient with SIADH reaches a

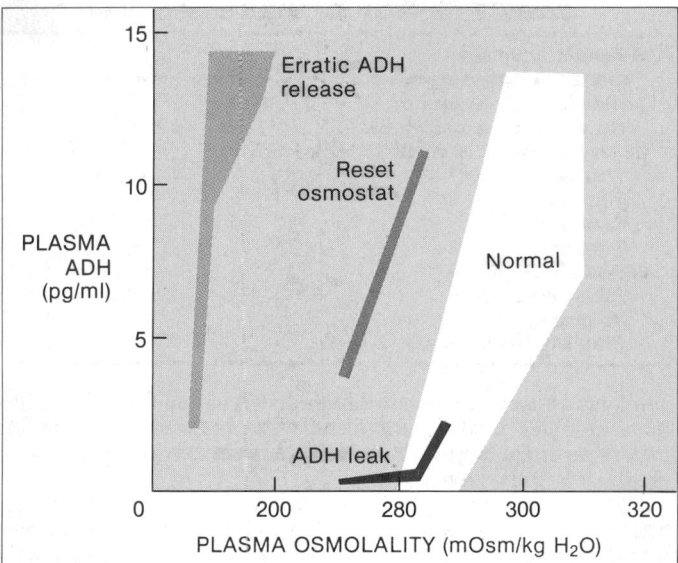

FIGURE 75–3. The patterns of serum ADH abnormalities in SIADH. The shaded areas indicate the normal relation between increases in effective ECF osmolality and ADH levels; the normal osmotic threshold is lower than the normal serum osmolality. The three shaded areas indicate ADH patterns in SIADH. (Adapted from Zerbe R, Strope L, Robertson G: Vasopressin function in the syndrome of inappropriate diuresis. Annu Rev Med 31:315, 1980. With permission from the Annual Review of Medicine, Vol. 31, © 1980 by Annual Reviews, Inc.)

steady state in which body water is expanded by water retention and in which natriuresis, even in the face of hyponatremia, prevents edema formation.

The causes for the natriuresis that is characteristic of SIADH are multiple. First, volume expansion will result in enhanced release of atriopeptin, which enhances urinary sodium wasting both by enhancing glomerular filtration and probably by suppressing tubular sodium absorption. Second, the volume expansion of SIADH also reduces the rate of proximal tubular sodium absorption, as well as the rate of proximal uric acid absorption.

In short, SIADH is a disorder in which hormone-stimulated water conservation results in hyponatremia, volume expansion, and consequently an increased GFR, tubular sodium wasting, and reduced net tubular absorption of creatinine and uric acid, but no edema formation. These characteristics are summarized in Table 75–9. Finally, as indicated in connection with Figure 75–3, the urinary osmolality in patients with SIADH may be either inappropriately high for the level of serum osmolality or maximally dilute.

Other Causes of Excessive ADH Production and/or Release. Table 75–7 lists other circumstances in which an increased level of ADH is the primary factor responsible for hyponatremia. A number of commonly used drugs stimulate ADH release: vincristine, cyclophosphamide, carbamazepine, phenothiazines, morphine, barbiturates, chlorpropamide, amitriptyline, thiothixene, and clofibrate. Chlorpropamide also potentiates the effect of ADH on the water permeability of collecting ducts. The posterior pituitary peptide oxytocin (Pitocin) also has an antidiuretic action, although oxytocin is a much less potent antidiuretic agent than is vasopressin. Thus the administration of intravenous hypotonic solutions containing oxytocin for the purpose of inducing labor may result in profound hyponatremia. Trauma or surgical stress also stimulates ADH release.

Ordinarily, diuretic-induced hyponatremia is related to volume contraction; this kind of body fluid dilution will be discussed below. Chronic severe potassium depletion induced by diuretics can also result in ADH release, although the mechanisms by which potassium depletion stimulates ADH release are unknown.

Mixed Disorders. Hyponatremia occurs commonly in true volume contraction and in edematous states in which filling of the arterial tree is impaired. The former disorders include patients in whom both ECF and total body water are reduced; the latter group comprises those patients with deranged Starling forces,

notably local or systemic increases in venous pressure, which result in inadequate filling of the arterial tree. In both sets of disorders, two factors contribute, individually or in unison, to the pathogenesis of hyponatremia: nonosmotic, volume-mediated ADH release and reductions in the rate of sodium delivery to the diluting segment.

Volume contraction is a potent nonosmotic stimulus to ADH release. Figure 75–4 shows the relations between osmotic and nonosmotic, volume-mediated stimuli and plasma ADH levels in experimental animals; entirely comparable responses occur in humans. Increases in plasma osmolality are related linearly to increases in plasma ADH levels. The relation between blood volume depletion and plasma ADH levels is nonlinear. However, with depletion of more than 7 to 10 per cent blood volume, plasma ADH levels rise sharply and produce an antidiuretic effect even when the plasma osmolality is reduced below normal. In other words, volume-mediated, nonosmotic ADH release occurs primarily when circulatory dynamics are moderately to severely advanced; in that circumstance, volume-mediated stimuli override osmotically mediated ADH release, and hyponatremia ensues.

A second factor that accounts for hyponatremia in volume-contracted states is an inability to dilute urine maximally because the rate of sodium delivery to diluting segments in the thick ascending limb is reduced. This situation occurs because increased rates of proximal tubular sodium absorption are stimulated by reduced sodium intake or by inadequate filling of the arterial tree in conditions with combined ECF volume expansion and reduced arterial tree filling. The significance of volume contraction as a pathogenic factor in this type of hyponatremia can be gauged by noting that hyponatremia occurs during volume contraction in experimental animals with pituitary diabetes insipidus.

Hyponatremia is a common feature of untreated Addison's disease and occurs because of a combination of circumstances. In mineralocorticoid deficiency, the major factors responsible for an inability to handle water loads appear to be ECF volume contraction, glomerular filtration reduction, enhanced proximal tubular salt absorption, and volume-mediated, nonosmotic ADH release. Glucocorticoid deficiency also impairs the ability to handle water loads. One of the factors responsible for water retention in Addison's disease is nonosmotic ADH release, which results from impaired cardiac function.

Hyponatremia occurs commonly in advanced stages of disorders characterized by edema formation and a reduced ECV (Table 75–7), particularly in intractable heart failure and advanced hepatic cirrhosis with ascites. Reduced rates of salt delivery to diluting segments of the renal tubule clearly contribute to the impairment in water excretion in these disorders. In patients with heart failure or severe ascites, the plasma concentrations of ADH tend to be inappropriately high with respect to plasma osmolality, so that nonosmotic ADH release may contribute to the development of hyponatremia in these disorders. Furthermore, since nonosmotic ADH release occurs only with profound reductions in blood volume (Fig. 75–4), the occurrence of hyponatremia in congestive heart failure or cirrhosis indicates profound arterial underfilling. This observation correlates well with the ominous prognosis of hyponatremia in these disorders.

CLINICAL MANIFESTATIONS. The clinical features of hyponatremia are produced by the brain swelling that accompanies acute dilution of total body water and generally become manifest when the serum sodium concentration falls to 120 mEq per liter or less. The early symptoms include lethargy, weakness, and somnolence, which proceed rapidly to seizures, coma, and death as hyponatremia worsens. Untreated acute water intoxication is nearly uniformly fatal and represents a medical emergency. In chronic hyponatremia, central nervous system manifestations are

TABLE 75–9. MAJOR CHARACTERISTICS OF SIADH

Hyponatremia
Volume expansion without edema
Natriuresis
Hypouricemia
Normal or reduced serum creatinine level
Normal thyroid and adrenal function

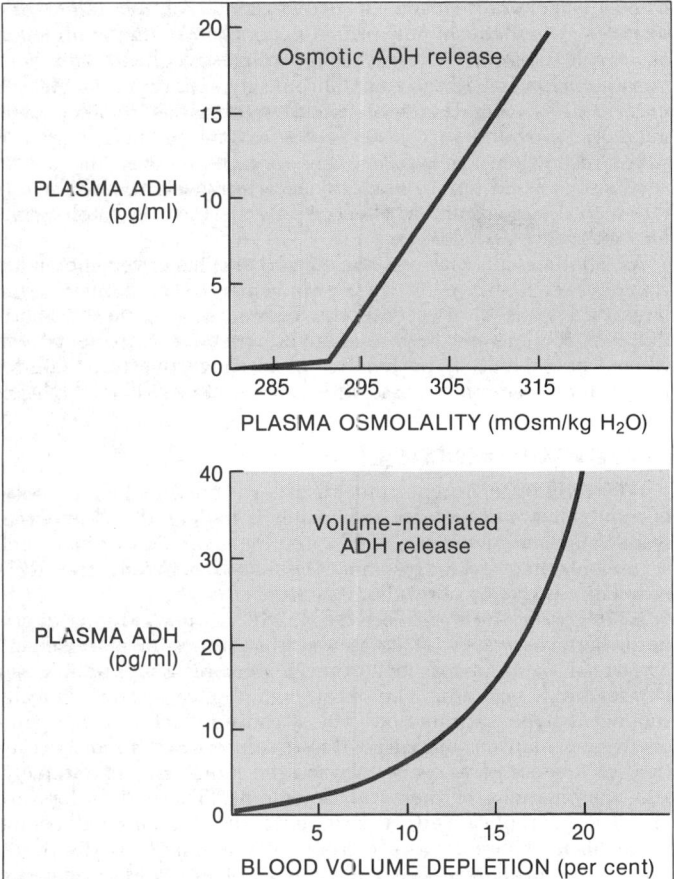

FIGURE 75–4. Relation between plasma ADH concentrations and either effective ECF osmolality (*upper plot*) or the per cent of blood volume depletion (*lower plot*). (Adapted from Dunn FL, Brennan TJ, Nelson AE, et al.: The role of blood osmolality and volume in regulating vasopressin secretion in the rat. J Clin Invest 52:3212, 1973. By copyright permission of the American Society for Clinical Investigation.)

far less common, even when the serum sodium concentration is as low as 100 mEq per liter, because the loss of brain solutes, principally potassium chloride, minimizes brain cell swelling for a given reduction in body water osmolality.

DIAGNOSIS. Hyponatremia should be considered whenever there is a sudden deterioration in central nervous system function, particularly in circumstances such as intractable heart failure, hepatic cirrhosis with ascites, or the administration of large volumes of intravenous fluids. The hyponatremic patient should be evaluated to determine the underlying condition that produced body fluid dilution. This evaluation should include a careful history and physical examination; measurement of the serum creatinine, BUN, and electrolytes; measurement of the urinary sodium concentration, or the Fe_{Na}; measurement of serum and urinary osmolalities; and, when appropriate, evaluation of thyroid and adrenal function.

The history and physical examination are generally adequate for recognizing disorders such as beer potomania or compulsive water ingestion or for noting the ingestion of drugs that stimulate ADH release or enhance ADH action. The presence of edema is characteristic of individuals in whom hyponatremia occurs because of a reduced ECV coupled to ECF volume expansion. In myxedema or Addison's disease, the typical clinical or laboratory findings of these disorders are generally present (Ch. 216 and 217).

The most difficult differential diagnosis among hyponatremic disorders involves the distinction between patients who are modestly volume contracted and those who have SIADH. In both circumstances, the serum sodium and the serum osmolality are reduced, whereas the urinary osmolality is inappropriately high with respect to the reduced serum osmolality. Nonosmotic water conservation in SIADH and in volume contraction is recognized by the presence of a urinary osmolality greater than 120 to 150

mOsm per kilogram of H_2O in association with a reduced serum osmolality. The distinction between the two disorders therefore depends on a clinical and laboratory assessment of ECV.

Patients who are volume contracted may provide a history of volume losses or of diuretic ingestion and may exhibit the signs of ECF volume contraction discussed previously in the section on volume depletion. When the volume losses are due to extrarenal causes, the urinary sodium concentration is less than 10 to 15 mEq per liter and the Fe_{Na} is generally less than 1 per cent. The presence of hyperuricemia may also be a useful clue to the possibility of ECF volume contraction. Prerenal azotemia may occur if the volume contraction is severe. Patients with SIADH are generally normovolemic or slightly volume expanded and therefore exhibit none of the signs of volume contraction. The serum BUN and creatinine levels are normal, and the serum uric acid level is generally reduced. The urinary sodium concentration usually exceeds 30 mEq per liter, and the Fe_{Na} is greater than 1 per cent. Tests of adrenal function yield normal results.

The above studies usually discriminate between SIADH and extrarenal volume contraction. When ECF volume contraction is due to renal salt wasting, urinary sodium losses generally persist unless volume contraction is profound. Moreover, as noted previously (see Volume Depletion), the blood pressure and pulse may be normal in states of modest volume contraction. A useful diagnostic and therapeutic maneuver in this situation is to observe the results of water restriction. When water intake is restricted to 600 to 800 ml daily, patients with SIADH exhibit a highly characteristic response: A 2- to 3-kg weight loss is accompanied by correction of hyponatremia and cessation of salt wasting, usually over a period of 2 to 3 days. If weight loss fails to correct both hyponatremia and urinary sodium wasting simultaneously, the diagnosis of SIADH is doubtful. Rather, renal sodium wasting with ECF volume contraction, due to Addison's disease or the other renal salt-losing disorders listed in Table 75–2, is the more probable diagnosis.

TREATMENT. The goal of treatment in hyponatremia is to correct body water osmolality and therefore restore cell volume to normal by raising the ratio of sodium to water in extracellular fluid. The increase in ECF osmolality draws water from cells and therefore reduces their volume. The choice of therapeutic approach, and whether or not net sodium and water balance is adjusted to be positive or negative during therapy, depends on the serum sodium concentration, the rate at which hyponatremia has developed, the clinical status of the patient, and the underlying disorder.

Acute Hyponatremia. Acute hyponatremia associated with a serum sodium concentration below 120 mEq per liter and with central nervous system manifestations requires immediate therapy. In volume-contracted states, the treatment of choice is to raise the serum sodium level to 125 to 130 mEq per liter over a 6-hour interval by administering hypertonic 3 to 5 per cent saline. As is discussed below, the rapid elevation of serum sodium to values greater than 125 mEq per liter may be hazardous. Since the desired effect is to correct body water osmolality, the amount of sodium administered must be sufficient to raise total body water osmolality to approximately 250 mOsm per kilogram of H_2O, that is, to approximately twice the desired serum sodium concentration. A convenient formula for calculating this sodium requirement is as follows.

$$[125 - \text{measured serum Na}^+] \times 0.6 \text{ body weight} = \text{required mEq of Na}^+$$

The serum sodium level is in milliequivalents per liter, and the body weight is in kilograms. Since 60 per cent of body weight is water, the formula allows an estimate of the amount of sodium required to raise body water osmolality to 250 mOsm per kilogram of H_2O.

The administration of hypertonic saline solutions is hazardous in volume-expanded, salt-retaining states such as congestive heart failure. Furthermore, in SIADH associated with volume expansion and sodium wasting, hypertonic saline alone is ineffective in correcting hyponatremia because the administered salt is excreted promptly in a relatively concentrated urine.

A preferable alternative is to use normal saline in combination with furosemide administration. The diuretic induces urinary salt loss and therefore reduces the risk of ECF volume expansion. Moreover, the diuresis induced by furosemide is characterized by the excretion of urine having a sodium concentration that is appreciably lower than that in plasma. Consequently, the combination of intravenously administered normal saline with a furosemide-induced diuresis of urine that is dilute with respect to plasma provides an effective way of raising the serum sodium level in SIADH or other volume-expanded states. By adjusting the rates of salt administration to be less than urinary salt losses, reductions in ECF volume can be produced simultaneously.

Rate and Magnitude of Correction of Acute Hyponatremia. Since loss of brain solute is a compensatory mechanism for preserving brain cell volume in dilutional states, a serum sodium level of 140 mEq per liter is relatively hypertonic to brain cells that have become partially depleted of solute as a result of hyponatremia. Consequently, raising the serum sodium rapidly to levels greater than 120 to 125 mEq per liter can result in central nervous system damage, such as central pontine myelinolysis. Furthermore, raising the serum sodium concentration to greater than 120 mEq per liter is probably unnecessary.

The major, and still unresolved, controversy surrounding the treatment of hyponatremia concerns the rate at which hyponatremia should be corrected. Mortality rates for severe hyponatremia of 33 to 86 per cent have been cited in support of prompt correction of hyponatremia. These estimates, however, derive largely from single case reports and small series of patients. Thus, these data may overestimate the mortality from hyponatremia. For example, a recent retrospective analysis of all patients with severe hyponatremia (less than 110 mEq per liter) at two university-affiliated hospitals found a mortality rate of only 8 per cent, with most deaths attributed to underlying diseases. Slow or delayed correction of hyponatremia was not associated with higher mortality or with neurologic complications. But the risk of developing neurologic complications was greatest in patients whose serum sodium concentrations were corrected at a rate greater than 0.6 mEq per liter per hour (14 mEq per day).

It has been suggested that rapid correction of hyponatremia may lead to central pontine myelinolysis. This is a demyelinating lesion of the pons, with destruction of myelin sheaths but sparing of the axis cylinders and nerve cells. The majority of patients in whom it has been described have had some form of debilitating disease, such as malnutrition or alcoholism. The clinical characteristics include flaccid quadriplegia or paraplegia, facial weakness, dysphagia, dysarthria, and coma. The possible role of the rate of correction of hyponatremia in the development of central pontine myelinolysis remains uncertain. For example, the incidence of central pontine myelinolysis in hyponatremia is very low, and the rate of correction in patients who develop this condition is no faster than in those who do not. Furthermore, central pontine myelinolysis generally occurs in settings in which additional risk factors, such as alcoholism or malnutrition, could be responsible for the lesion. In experimental animals, the rapid correction of severe hyponatremia to normal sodium levels results in diffuse necrotic brain lesions, whereas rapid correction of mildly hyponatremic levels does not. Thus, the extent of correction and the rate of correction are important factors in the development of neurologic complications.

Given these considerations, it is prudent to correct the serum sodium concentration at a rate of 0.5 mEq per liter per hour until it reaches 120 to 125 mEq per liter. However, young women with acute symptomatic hyponatremia are at greater risk than men for suffering respiratory arrest, severe neurologic sequelae, and death. Thus, it is reasonable to treat these patients with hypertonic saline in an attempt to raise the serum sodium concentration to 125 mEq per liter at a rate of 1.0 to 1.5 mEq per liter per hour. At this point, the patient should be asymptomatic, and the serum sodium level can be gradually returned to normal over several days with water restriction. Overcorrection of the serum sodium concentration (to greater than 130 mEq per liter) is unnecessary and potentially harmful. Even in acutely developing hyponatremia, symptoms and central nervous system signs are uncommon until the serum sodium concentration falls below 120 mEq per liter.

Chronic Hyponatremia. Mild, asymptomatic chronic hyponatremia is generally managed by correction of the underlying disorder, when the hyponatremia occurs in volume contraction or in salt-retaining states, such as congestive heart failure or hepatic cirrhosis with ascites. Chronic hyponatremia in SIADH may be easily corrected by restricting water intake to 800 to 1000 ml daily, provided that patients can adhere to the program of water restriction. An alternative approach involves the use of agents such as lithium or demethylchlortetracycline, which interfere with the renal tubular effects of ADH. However, both agents have other adverse effects.

As another alternative, some workers have recommended reducing renal ability for urinary concentration by administering large oral loads of urea, thereby producing a modest osmotic diuresis. A more palatable maneuver, effective in patients who are not edematous, hypertensive, or in congestive heart failure, is to administer oral furosemide in association with a high-salt diet.

HYPERTONIC DISORDERS

DEFINITION. A hypertonic disorder is one in which the ratio of solutes to water in total body water is increased. All hypernatremic states are hypertonic. In some hypertonic disorders, such as uncontrolled hyperglycemia, the increase in effective ECF osmolality is due to nonsodium solutes.

ETIOLOGY AND PATHOGENESIS. Hypernatremia develops whenever water intake is less than the sum of renal and extrarenal water losses; in chronic hypertonic states, net water balance may be zero. The most common causes of clinically significant hypernatremia occur as a consequence of three pathogenic mechanisms: impaired thirst; solute or osmotic diuresis; excessive losses of water, either via the kidneys or extrarenally; and combinations of these derangements. These disorders are grouped in Table 75–10 according to the primary pathogenic mechanism. There is also a group of miscellaneous disorders, such as hypokalemia, hypercalcemia, and interstitial renal disease, as well as chronic renal failure, which either partially impair renal urinary concentrating ability or partially blunt the responsiveness of collecting ducts to ADH. These disorders rarely cause significant hypernatremia and are not discussed further.

Inadequate Intake of Water. This problem occurs in patients who are comatose or who are otherwise unable to communicate thirst. Because of the exquisite sensitivity of thirst mechanisms to changes in effective body water osmolality, hypernatremia due to inadequate water intake is rare in conscious patients allowed free access to water. Rarely, patients will have a primary thirst deficiency. Patients with Cushing's syndrome or primary hyperaldosteronism commonly have slight elevations in the serum sodium level for unknown reasons.

Finally, "essential hypernatremia" is characterized by a slightly elevated serum sodium level that occurs in the conscious state. The defect in patients with essential hypernatremia appears to be an insensitivity of thirst centers and osmoreceptors to osmotic stimuli. However, both thirst and antidiuresis occur when these patients are volume contracted. Consequently, it has been inferred that volume-mediated stimuli to thirst and ADH release are intact in patients with essential hypernatremia. This disorder may be either congenital or acquired, sometimes in association with histiocytic infiltration of the central nervous system.

Osmotic Diuresis. This is another mechanism for producing renal water losses in excess of sodium losses and therefore

TABLE 75–10. MAJOR CAUSES OF HYPERNATREMIA

I. **Impaired Thirst**
    Coma
    Essential hypernatremia
II. **Solute Diuresis**
    Osmotic diuresis: diabetic ketoacidosis, nonketotic hyperosmolar
      coma, mannitol administration
III. **Excessive Water Losses**
    Renal
      Pituitary diabetes insipidus
      Nephrogenic diabetes insipidus
    Extrarenal
      Sweating
IV. **Combined Disorders**
    Coma plus hypertonic nasogastric feeding

hypertonicity. Osmotic diuresis occurs commonly in uncontrolled glycosuria and may occur during mannitol administration for the treatment of increased intracranial pressure. Since these solutes are restricted to the ECF, the serum sodium level is generally reduced in the early stages of osmotic diuresis, and the effective ECF osmolality is increased primarily by the impermeant non-sodium solute. In prolonged osmotic diuresis, net water losses may be sufficiently great that hypernatremia develops. In this circumstance, the increase in effective ECF osmolality is due to the combined effects of hypernatremia and the nonsodium solute. Hypernatremia due to an osmotic urea diuresis can occur if large amounts of protein and amino acids are administered by nasogastric tube, or if tissue catabolism is great, as in burns. In this circumstance, hypernatremia is entirely responsible for the increased effective ECF osmolality.

Hypernatremia may also occur when large amounts of hypertonic sodium solutions are administered, particularly in patients whose renal function is compromised. Two common examples of this condition include the rapid intravenous administration of multiple ampules of sodium bicarbonate during cardiopulmonary resuscitation and the administration of large amounts of sodium bicarbonate to patients with lactic acidosis.

Hypernatremia may also complicate the administration of normal saline solutions when the endogenous osmolar solute load is high and renal concentrating ability is limited. Patients with diabetic ketoacidosis, who are generally young, have sufficient urinary concentrating ability that hypernatremia does not occur when normal saline solutions are used in the treatment of ketoacidosis. In contrast, the nonketotic hyperglycemic syndrome generally occurs in elderly patients, who can have partial impairment of urinary concentrating power. In this setting, hypernatremia can occur during therapy with normal saline solutions. This complication can be avoided by treating with half-normal saline and thus providing sufficient solute-free water for urinary elimination of the osmolar glucose load.

Excessive Water Losses. Impairment of ADH production, release, or action, as in pituitary or nephrogenic diabetes insipidus, can lead to profound water deficits and to hypernatremia. In such circumstances, the urine volumes are large, the urinary osmolality is low, and the net rate of solute excretion is low, in contrast to individuals undergoing osmotic diuresis, in whom rates of urinary solute excretion are elevated. The diabetes insipidus syndromes are considered in detail in Ch. 214.

Striking water losses may also occur with excessive sweating, particularly during rigorous physical activity by untrained individuals exercising in high humidity. This phenomenon plays a major role in the evolution of heat stroke.

Combined Disorders. Finally, hypertonic dehydration may occur as a combination of these events. A common example in modern clinical practice involves the injudicious administration of large amounts of carbohydrate or amino acids by nasogastric tube, coupled with limited amounts of water, to stroke patients unable to communicate thirst.

CLINICAL MANIFESTATIONS AND DIAGNOSIS. Since two thirds of body water is intracellular, primary water losses tend to have modest effects on circulating volume unless fluid losses are profound. Rather, the clinical manifestations are produced by brain shrinkage that results from increases in effective ECF osmolality. Thus the symptoms of hypertonicity produced either by hypernatremia or by impermeant nonsodium solutes such as glucose are referable to the central nervous system and range from somnolence and confusion to coma, respiratory paralysis, and death. The degree of symptomatology varies with the degree of hypertonicity and with the rate at which hypertonicity develops. In acute hypertonicity, symptoms generally appear when the effective ECF osmolality exceeds 320 to 330 mOsm per kilogram of H_2O, and coma and respiratory arrest may occur when the ECF osmolality exceeds 360 to 380 mOsm per kilogram of H_2O. Chronic hypertonicity generally produces fewer central nervous system manifestations, because brain cells accumulate idiogenic osmoles, which minimize the tendency for brain shrinkage.

TREATMENT. The treatment of acute hypernatremia requires the administration of isotonic dilute saline solutions, generally by an intravenous route. The following factors should be borne in mind when treating acute hypernatremia.

In the highly volume-contracted patient with severe hyperna-tremia, the administration of isotonic saline solutions has two advantages. It provides fluid resuscitation in impending cardiovascular collapse. Moreover, the isotonic salt solution, which is hypotonic with respect to the hypertonic patient, avoids an unnecessary rapid fall in the serum sodium level.

Rapid correction of hypertonicity to a normal serum osmolality is hazardous. Since accumulation of idiogenic osmoles by brain cells is a compensatory mechanism for preserving brain volume in hypertonic disorders, a normal serum osmolality may be relatively hypotonic to brain cells that have accumulated idiogenic solutes. Hence if the serum osmolality is reduced rapidly, central nervous system damage due to brain swelling may occur. A useful guide to circumventing this difficulty is to reduce the serum sodium level by no more than 1 mEq per liter during every 2 hours of the first 2 days of treatment.

Finally, if solutions of D_5W are administered at a rapid rate, hyperglycemia and osmotic diuresis may occur and hence aggravate the hypertonic state. In this circumstance, the use of a 2.5 per cent dextrose solution in one-quarter normal saline is advisable. This solution has been particularly useful in treating hypernatremia associated with volume contraction in children with pituitary or nephrogenic diabetes insipidus.

Ayus JC, Krothapalli RK, Arieff AI: Treatment of symptomatic hyponatremia and its relation to brain damage: A prospective study. N Engl J Med 317:1190, 1987. *A prospective study showing little relation between the rate of correction of hyponatremia and the occurrence of central pontine myelinolysis.*

Berl T: Treating hyponatremia: Damned if we do and damned if we don't. Kidney Int 37:1006, 1990. *A discussion of the relative merits of rapid versus slow correction of hyponatremia.*

Buckalew VM Jr: Hyponatremia: Pathogenesis and management. Hosp Pract 21:49, 1986. *An excellent description of the treatment of hyponatremia.*

Goldman MB, Luchins DJ, Robertson GL: Mechanisms of altered water metabolism in psychotic patients with polydipsia and hyponatremia. N Engl J Med 318:397, 1988. *An account of factors causing hyponatremia in hospitalized patients with affective disorders.*

Reeves WB, Andreoli TE: The posterior pituitary and water metabolism. *In* Wilson JD, Foster DW (eds.): Williams Textbook of Endocrinology. 8th ed. Philadelphia, W. B. Saunders Company, 1992. *A complete analysis of the physiology of water metabolism and osmotic derangements.*

Sterns RH: Severe symptomatic hyponatremia: Treatment and outcome. Ann Intern Med 107:656, 1987. *An extensive retrospective analysis of acute symptomatic hyponatremia that argues that rapid correction of hyponatremia is hazardous.*

Thompson CS, Andreoli TE: Hyponatremia and hypernatremia. *In* Callaham ML (ed.): Decision Making in Emergency Medicine. Philadelphia, B.C. Decker, 1990, pp 172–175. *A practical guide to the diagnosis and treatment of hyponatremia and hypernatremia.*

Zerbe R, Strope L, Robertson G: Vasopressin function in the syndrome of inappropriate diuresis. Annu Rev Med 31:315, 1980. *The patterns of ADH response in SIADH.*

75.3 DISTURBANCES IN POTASSIUM BALANCE

PHYSIOLOGIC CONSIDERATIONS

The body contains approximately 3500 mEq of potassium, of which only 60 mEq, or about 2 per cent, is extracellular. In normal circumstances external potassium balance depends mainly on dietary potassium intake and renal potassium excretion; fecal potassium losses are only about 10 mEq per day unless diarrhea is present. Since 98 per cent of potassium is located intracellularly, primarily in skeletal muscle, regulation of the serum potassium concentration depends not only on external potassium balance but also on potassium exchanges between the intracellular and extracellular compartments.

Transfer Between ICF and ECF

The intracellular compartment acts as a large potassium reservoir in series with the small ECF potassium pool. In potassium-depleted states, a 1 mEq per liter fall in the serum potassium level requires the loss of about 100 to 200 mEq of potassium; hence the bulk of external potassium loss comes from the cellular compartment. Conversely, if large amounts of potassium are administered acutely, the rise in serum potassium level is less than would be expected if the administered potassium were distributed solely in the ECF. In this situation, cellular uptake of potassium obviously occurs and prevents greater increases in the serum potassium concentration. This ability of cells to accumulate potassium can be enhanced strikingly by chronic administration of high-potassium diets.

A number of *effector* mechanisms regulate the partition of potassium between the ICF and ECF. These include active and passive ionic transcellular transport processes.

ACTIVE TRANSPORT PROCESSES. The cardinal transport process regulating K^+ distribution between ICF and ECF is cell membrane–bound $(Na^+ + K^+)$-ATPase, which actively transports potassium into cells and therefore counterbalances the passive leak of potassium from cells into interstitial fluid. Insulin is a second effector that promotes potassium transfer from ECF to ICF. This hormone promotes cellular uptake of potassium independently of cellular glucose uptake by increasing $(Na^+ + K^+)$-ATPase activity. Insulin also reduces sodium permeability; the resultant cellular hyperpolarization of cells produces a passive driving force for potassium accumulation within cells. Furthermore, hyperkalemia augments insulin release. Thus hyperkalemia may be the sensor that stimulates release of insulin, which then serves as an effector for potassium entry into cells. Beta-adrenergic agents, particularly beta$_2$ agonists such as terbutaline, also promote cellular potassium uptake by enhancing $(Na^+ + K^+)$-ATPase activity; it is not yet known whether hyperkalemia can provoke beta agonist release, as it does for insulin release. Finally, mineralocorticoids such as aldosterone, in addition to enhancing renal potassium excretion (see below), also enhance cellular potassium uptake; the mode of aldosterone action in the latter instance is not understood.

PASSIVE TRANSPORT PROCESSES. A number of passive effector mechanisms also regulate the partition of potassium between the ICF and the ECF. First, alterations in the pH of ECF reproducibly shift potassium between the ICF and the ECF: Systemic acidosis, whether metabolic or respiratory, promotes potassium efflux from cells, whereas systemic alkalosis, either metabolic or respiratory, promotes cellular potassium uptake. As a general rule, a reduction in plasma pH of 0.1 unit raises the serum potassium level by 0.6 mEq per liter, whereas a plasma pH increase of 0.1 unit produces a similar reduction in serum potassium. The mechanisms for these pH-induced potassium shifts between ICF and ECF are not understood.

Second, cellular shrinkage produced by increases in effective ECF osmolality raises the intracellular potassium concentration and thereby increases the driving force for passive potassium leakage from the ICF to the ECF. This leakage may result in hyperkalemia when large glucose loads are administered to insulin-deficient diabetic patients who also have hyporeninemic hypoaldosteronism; the insulin lack limits cellular reentry of potassium, and the aldosterone deficiency limits renal potassium excretion. Increases in cellular potassium concentrations produced by cellular shrinkage also contribute significantly to the hyperkalemia of diabetic ketoacidosis, because hyperglycemia raises cellular potassium levels by cell shrinkage and insulin lack prevents accelerated potassium reentry into cells.

Finally, brain cells and renal tubular cells lose potassium when exposed to chronic ECF hypotonicity. However, muscle cells, which are the largest component of ICF potassium, do not appear to participate in this process. Consequently, hypotonic disorders, by themselves, have little effect on the serum potassium level or on external potassium balance.

Renal Handling of Potassium

The kidneys process potassium strikingly differently from the way in which they process sodium. Sodium excretion involves filtration, partial tubular absorption, and appearance of nonabsorbed sodium as urinary sodium excretion. When dietary sodium intake is varied, there is a prompt adjustment in urinary sodium excretion, either in the upward direction, when sodium intake is increased, or in the downward direction, when sodium intake is curtailed.

In contrast, virtually all dietary potassium, ordinarily about 50 to 200 mEq per day, appears in the urine because of tubular secretion of potassium by terminal nephron segments, particularly the late distal convoluted tubule and the cortical collecting duct. These regions of the nephron can increase rates of potassium secretion significantly if dietary potassium intake is augmented; and they carry out net absorption of potassium in kaliopenic states. In other words, these terminal nephron segments regulate external potassium balance by adjusting *renal output* to balance *intake*.

A convenient way of considering distal nephron handling of potassium, and the ways in which effector mechanisms modulate this process, is shown in Figure 75–5. The dashed lines indicate passive processes, and the solid lines denote active transport processes. Basolateral membranes of all terminal nephron segments, including the thick limb of Henle, the distal tubule, and the collecting duct, share two common characteristics: a passive leakage pathway for K^+ efflux and an active $(Na^+ + K^+)$-ATPase for cellular K^+ uptake. The apical membranes of these nephron segments also contain passive potassium leakage pathways, which can be blocked by barium. In the thick ascending limb of Henle, apical membranes contain a furosemide-sensitive coupled entry step that involves electroneutral $Na^+:K^+:2Cl^-$ co-transport, driven by the electrochemical sodium gradient between lumen and cells. In distal tubular and collecting ducts, Na^+ entry into cells involves sodium-specific channels that are blocked by amiloride. Thus in the ascending limb, coupled electroneutral sodium entry into cells does not result in luminal electronegativity (in fact, the lumen in the thick ascending limb is electropositive), whereas in the distal tubule and collecting duct, amiloride-sensitive ionic sodium entry produces luminal electronegativity.

The majority of net K^+ secretion occurs in these latter two segments and is driven indirectly by the rate of sodium entry into cells, which increases luminal electronegativity and increases the activity of basolateral $(Na^+ + K^+)$-ATPase, thus raising cell potassium concentrations. In the loop of Henle, little net potassium secretion occurs, because the lumen is electropositive and because coupled $Na^+:K^+:2Cl^-$ transport from lumen to cells recycles secreted potassium back into cells.

The major elements of the *effector systems* that regulate distal nephron potassium excretion include the rate of distal tubular sodium delivery, dietary potassium intake, plasma pH, aldosterone, impermeant anions, and tubular flow rates. When distal sodium delivery rates are increased, increased sodium entry into cells across apical membranes is accompanied by increased activity of pump $(Na^+ + K^+)$-ATPase, which tends to raise intracellular potassium concentrations. Second, either an increase in

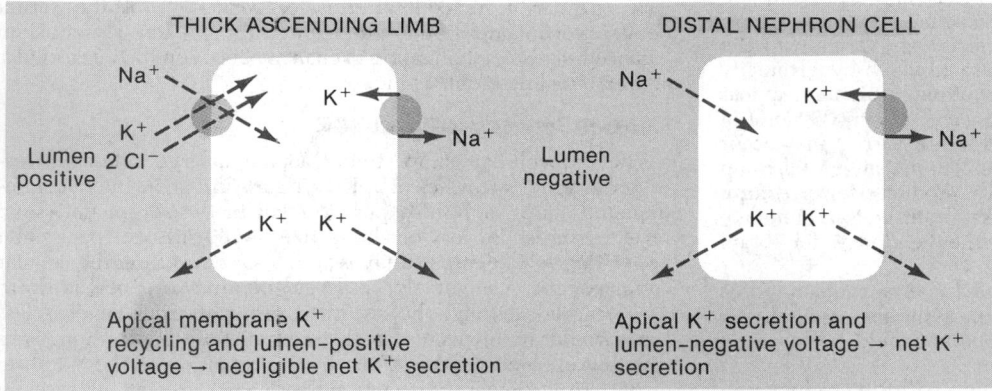

THICK ASCENDING LIMB

Na$^+$

K$^+$

K$^+$ 2 Cl$^-$

Na$^+$

Lumen positive

K$^+$ K$^+$

Apical membrane K$^+$ recycling and lumen-positive voltage → negligible net K$^+$ secretion

DISTAL NEPHRON CELL

Na$^+$

K$^+$

Na$^+$

Lumen negative

K$^+$ K$^+$

Apical K$^+$ secretion and lumen-negative voltage → net K$^+$ secretion

FIGURE 75–5. Handling of potassium in late nephron segments, including the thick ascending limb and the distal nephron. The dashed arrows represent passive transport processes, and the solid arrows represent active transport processes. In the thick ascending limb, K^+ recycling into cells by $Na^+:K^+:2 Cl^-$ co-transport and the lumen-positive voltage reduce the rate of net K^+ secretion. Most urinary K^+ comes from net K^+ secretion by terminal nephron segments, particularly the late distal convoluted tubule and the cortical collecting tubule.

dietary potassium intake or an increase in plasma pH tends, as indicated above, to raise cellular potassium content. Third, urinary excretion of impermeant anions such as sulfate, carbenicillin, or penicillin produces greater luminal electronegativity. Fourth, aldosterone and mineralocorticoids, whose kaliuretic effects may be dissociated from their sodium-sparing effects, increase the permeability of luminal membranes to potassium. These hormones may also augment distal tubular $(Na^+ + K^+)$-ATPase activity. Among these factors, the rate of aldosterone secretion and the rate of distal salt delivery to terminal nephron segments are the cardinal variables.

Each of the above factors modulates one or another portion of a generalized mechanism, namely, an electrochemical gradient favorable to the passive movement of potassium from tubular cells to urine and consequently for net potassium secretion. Conversely, reductions in sodium delivery, potassium restriction, reductions in plasma pH, and mineralocorticoid lack all reduce the magnitude of passive potassium movement from cells to tubular fluid and therefore tend to decrease net potassium secretion. Finally, increases in tubular flow rates, as in osmotic diuresis, also promote potassium secretion, whereas reductions in tubular flow rates decrease potassium secretion. The mechanism responsible for this effect is unknown.

The net rate of urinary potassium excretion in any given circumstance therefore depends on the interplay of these multiple factors in modulating the common effector mechanism for potassium secretion. For example, mineralocorticoid excess in primary aldosteronism commonly leads to severe potassium wasting. This kaliuresis can be curtailed by dietary sodium restriction and accentuated by dietary sodium loading. Conversely, in hyporeninemic hypoaldosteronism, hyperkalemia may be prevented by ensuring a liberal intake of sodium.

The renal adaptation to excess potassium loads occurs over a 24- to 36-hour period. Consequently, hyperkalemia from the ingestion of large oral potassium loads is uncommon in normal individuals. But the renal response to dietary potassium restriction is more sluggish and requires 7 to 10 days for full development. Even under the latter circumstances, urinary potassium losses are rarely less than 20 mEq per day.

Excitable Tissues and the ICF/ECF Potassium Ratio

The clinical consequences of hypokalemia and hyperkalemia are generally due to changes in the excitable characteristics of heart, skeletal muscle, and smooth muscle. Excitable tissues, such as nerve, heart, and skeletal muscle, share certain common properties. At rest excitable tissues are far more permeable to potassium than to sodium. The cell interior is electronegative with respect to extracellular fluid, and this voltage is largely determined by the logarithm of the ratio of intracellular (K_i) to extracellular (K_o) potassium concentrations. When excitable tissues are suddenly depolarized to their threshold voltage, sodium permeability increases profoundly with an accompanying increase in the sodium to potassium permeability ratio. This sodium entry into the cells of excitable tissues occurs through sodium-specific channels having electronegative sites that are activated by sudden depolarization. During depolarization, rapid sodium entry produces the initial spike of the action potential, and the cell interior becomes electropositive.

This voltage-dependent increase in sodium permeability during depolarization to threshold is the most fundamental characteristic of excitable tissues (except in tissues such as the atrioventricular node, where Ca^{2+} influx into cells is responsible for the action potential). If an excitable cell is partially depolarized in the resting state, the rate of rise of action potentials is reduced; the prolonged resting depolarization, by undefined mechanisms, reduces the increase in sodium permeability that accompanies the action potential. This effect of resting depolarization on reducing sodium permeability during action potentials is referred to as inactivation.

Repolarization of excitable cells occurs more slowly than depolarization. During repolarization, potassium permeability rises with respect to sodium permeability, and there is passive potassium efflux from the cell to the ECF. This potassium efflux restores the electronegativity of the cell interior. In nerve and skeletal muscle, potassium efflux occurs almost immediately after the initial spike of the action potential. In cardiac muscle, potassium efflux follows the absolute refractory period and coincides with the relative refractory period (phase 3) of the cardiac action potential.

Hyperkalemia reduces the K_i/K_o ratio and consequently partially depolarizes electrical tissues at rest. Hyperkalemia also increases the potassium permeability of excitable cells. The results of these changes on cardiac excitation are illustrated in the left-hand panel of Figure 75–6. Because partial resting depolarization decreases the rate of sodium entry into cells during excitation, the rate of phase zero depolarization is slower and the peak of phase zero depolarization is markedly reduced. The increased potassium permeability accelerates repolarization and shortens the plateau phase. The net effect of progressive hyperkalemia is therefore to make the heart progressively refractory to excitation.

The effects of hypokalemia on excitable tissues are more complex. Because the K_i/K_o ratio rises in hypokalemia, excitable cells at rest should be hyperpolarized. This occurs initially, but resting depolarization eventually follows, because the high K_i/K_o ratio, by itself, reduces the potassium permeability of excitable cells. The effects of hypokalemia on cardiac muscle fibers are shown in the right-hand panel of Figure 75–6. At rest the cell is partially depolarized because the reduced potassium permeability allows the high extracellular to intracellular sodium ratio to make the cell interior less negative. The initial spike of the action potential is less affected than in hyperkalemia because the reduced potassium permeability offsets the reduced sodium permeability during phase zero depolarization. Since potassium efflux determines the rate of repolarization, the reduced potassium permeability prolongs the relative refractory period. The net effect of these changes in cardiac tissue is to increase the

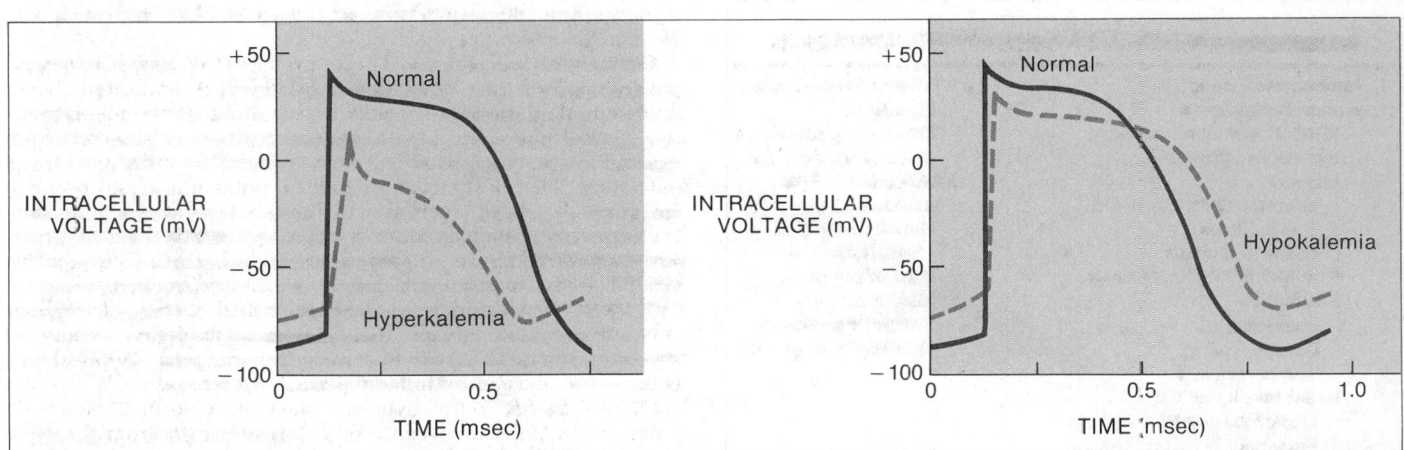

FIGURE 75–6. The effect of increases or decreases in serum potassium on the cardiac action potential. The solid lines represent the normal cardiac action potential; the dashed lines represent the cardiac action potential with either hyperkalemia (*left*) or hypokalemia (*right*).

likelihood of sinus bradycardia and, because of a prolonged relative refractory period, the risk of arrhythmia formation. In skeletal muscle the reduction in membrane permeability to potassium produced by hypokalemia leads, in severe hypokalemia, to generalized paralysis.

HYPOKALEMIA AND POTASSIUM DEPLETION

DEFINITION. Chronic hypokalemia generally reflects a reduction in total body potassium. A 1-mEq reduction in serum potassium level generally implies the net loss of 100 to 200 mEq of potassium from the body. In extreme body potassium depletion, the serum potassium level may be as low as 1.5 to 2.0 mEq per liter. Acute reductions in serum potassium level without parallel reductions in total body potassium occur when potassium is shifted from the ECF to the ICF.

ETIOLOGY AND PATHOGENESIS. Hypokalemia and simultaneous potassium depletion occur whenever renal plus extrarenal potassium losses exceed potassium intake. In advanced body potassium depletion, intake and output of potassium may be equal. The four major causes for hypokalemia are given in Table 75–11.

Inadequate Intake. Reduced potassium intake may result in potassium depletion and hypokalemia because maximal renal conservation of potassium requires, as indicated above, 7 to 10 days. During this interval, the net renal potassium loss may be as much as 150 to 200 mEq.

Excessive Renal Losses. Many of the causes for renal potassium wasting can be analyzed in terms of factors that modulate the common effector system for potassium secretion. *Mineralocorticoid excess* accelerates distal tubular potassium secretion (Fig. 75–5). Consequently, hypokalemia occurs regularly in primary hyperaldosteronism, in Cushing's syndrome, and in secondary hyperaldosteronism. *Chronic licorice ingestion* produces a syndrome that mimics primary hyperaldosteronism, because glycyrrhizinic acid, a component of licorice extract, has physiologic properties similar to those of aldosterone.

In *Bartter's syndrome* sodium chloride wasting and secondary aldosteronism may contribute to potassium depletion (Ch. 82). However, potassium depletion in Bartter's syndrome may also occur either when aldosterone secretion rates are normal or following bilateral adrenalectomy. Consequently, it is believed that a tubular defect in potassium handling also contributes to the hypokalemia of Bartter's syndrome.

Most diuretics having a locus of action prior to the late distal tubule (Table 75–5) increase urinary potassium losses. Enhanced sodium delivery to distal nephron segments is the major factor responsible for the kaliuresis produced by these diuretics, and sodium restriction or volume depletion tends to minimize diuretic-induced potassium losses. Carbonic anhydrase inhibitors such as acetazolamide inhibit proximal bicarbonate absorption and thereby accentuate potassium losses. Distal tubular segments are relatively impermeable to bicarbonate; consequently, increased delivery of bicarbonate to distal nephron regions has an impermeant anion effect that increases luminal electronegativity in these nephron regions.

Osmotic diuresis is commonly associated with increased renal potassium losses, because increased tubular flow rates enhance net potassium secretion. In diabetic ketoacidosis renal potassium losses are common. Yet patients with diabetic ketoacidosis and a reduced total body potassium commonly present with hyperkalemia, because metabolic acidosis tends to promote potassium shifts from the ICF to the ECF. Consequently, profound hypokalemia may develop if body potassium is not replenished concomitantly with insulin therapy and ECF volume expansion (Ch. 218).

Potassium depletion is seen frequently in *chronic metabolic alkalosis*. When the alkalosis is associated with volume contraction, secondary hyperaldosteronism results in renal potassium losses. Potassium depletion in chronic metabolic alkalosis is also enhanced if bicarbonaturia is present, because of the impermeant anion effect produced by bicarbonate delivery to terminal nephron segments. In fact, the hypokalemia associated with upper gastrointestinal fluid losses, as in vomiting or nasogastric suction, is primarily the result of the renal potassium losses produced by secondary hyperaldosteronism or bicarbonaturia or both. The potassium losses from the upper gastrointestinal tract are small, since upper gastrointestinal tract fluid contains only about 10 mEq of potassium per liter.

Hypokalemia may develop during therapy with certain *antibiotics*. Carbenicillin or other penicillin-like antibiotics exist as sodium or potassium salts of impermeant anions and promote kaliuresis because they increase net sodium excretion and because of an impermeant anion effect. Amphotericin B increases the permeability of luminal membranes to potassium and therefore promotes potassium secretion. Gentamicin produces potassium losses by unknown mechanisms.

Hypokalemia and potassium depletion are common findings in *distal, gradient-limited renal tubular acidosis* (Ch. 82). Increased distal sodium delivery and the impermeant anion effect produced by bicarbonate wasting account for most of the potassium losses seen in proximal renal tubular acidosis. Consequently, salt restriction, which enhances the rate of proximal sodium bicarbonate absorption in this disorder, also tends to correct potassium depletion. In gradient-limited distal renal tubular acidosis, hypokalemia may be accentuated by volume losses and secondary hyperaldosteronism. Other factors, not yet understood, also contribute to hypokalemia in this disorder. Hyperkalemia, rather than hypokalemia, commonly accompanies the hyperchloremic acidosis of interstitial disease (type IV acidosis) or of voltage-dependent renal tubular acidosis (see below).

Liddle's syndrome is a rare tubular disorder characterized by hypokalemia, metabolic alkalosis, hypertension, and normal aldosterone secretion rates. Therapy with triamterene, but not with aldosterone antagonists such as spironolactone, ameliorates the disorder. These findings suggest that terminal nephron sodium avidity and potassium secretion independent of aldosterone are major factors in the pathogenesis of Liddle's syndrome. Thus in operational terms, Liddle's syndrome may be described as distal nephron hyperfunction, in regard to Na^+ absorption and H^+ and K^+ secretion.

Gastrointestinal Losses. These provide the major route for potassium depletion, other than the kidney. As indicated above, potassium depletion associated with vomiting is referable primarily to renal potassium losses. Diarrhea produces significant potassium losses, since diarrheal fluid contains 30 mEq per liter of potassium. The most striking diarrheal potassium losses occur in secretory diarrheas, such as with non–beta islet cell tumors of the pancreas, which produce vasoactive intestinal polypeptide, and in laxative abuse. In both secretory diarrheas and chronic laxative abuse, hypokalemia is probably caused by increased rates of K^+ secretion through apical membrane K^+ channels. Villous adenomas of the colon produce potassium depletion because of excessive colonic K^+ secretion from the adenoma. Hypokalemia is uncommonly seen in inflammatory bowel disease.

ECF-ICF Shifts. Acute hypokalemia with a normal total body potassium may occur because of *potassium shifts* from the ECF to the ICF. In *hypokalemic periodic paralysis,* acute shifts of potassium from the ECF to the ICF produce limb and trunk paralysis. The periodic attacks are often precipitated by high-carbohydrate meals. Patients with the disorder can often abort

TABLE 75–11. MAJOR CAUSES OF HYPOKALEMIA

I. Inadequate Intake	III. Gastrointestinal Losses
II. Excess Renal Loss	Vomiting
Mineralocorticoid excess	Diarrhea, particularly
Bartter's syndrome	secretory diarrheas
Diuresis	IV. ECF → ICF Shifts
Diuretics with a pre–late	Acute alkalosis
distal locus	Hypokalemic periodic
Osmotic diuresis	paralysis
Chronic metabolic alkalosis	Barium ingestion
Antibiotics	Insulin therapy
Carbenicillin	Vitamin B_{12} therapy
Gentamicin	Thyrotoxicosis (rarely)
Amphotericin B	
Renal tubular acidosis	
Distal, gradient-limited	
Proximal	
Liddle's syndrome	
Acute leukemia	
Ureterosigmoidostomy	

attacks by exercising affected muscles. The chronic use of acetazolamide can prevent attacks. A condition resembling hypokalemic periodic paralysis occurs with the ingestion of *barium salts* and is endemic in China, where the disorder is referred to as "Pa-Ping." Barium appears to produce hypokalemia by blocking K^+ channels in skeletal muscle and thus blocking efflux of potassium from the ICF to the ECF. *Insulin* therapy and *vitamin B_{12}* therapy also promote potassium shifts from the ECF to the ICF. Hypokalemia can also result rarely from thyrotoxicosis, especially in Asian males, for reasons that are unclear.

CLINICAL MANIFESTATIONS. The clinical effects of potassium deficiency are manifest in one or more organ systems, including skeletal muscle, heart, kidneys, and the gastrointestinal tract. The most serious disturbances are those affecting the neuromuscular system. At serum potassium concentrations in the range of 2.0 to 2.5 mEq per liter, muscular weakness is likely to occur; with more severe hypokalemia, the patient may develop areflexic paralysis, in which case respiratory insufficiency is an immediate threat to survival. The severity of the neuromuscular disturbance tends to be proportional to the speed with which the potassium level has declined.

Losses of large amounts of potassium from skeletal muscle may be accompanied by rhabdomyolysis and myoglobinuria. Hence, rhabdomyolysis sometimes occurs in military recruits subject to severe exercise, sweating, and ECF volume contraction. The secondary hyperaldosteronism that follows excessive salt loss produces urinary potassium wasting and consequently potassium depletion. Potassium depletion secondary to malnutrition and vomiting is also one of the pathogenic mechanisms in alcoholic rhabdomyolysis.

The electrocardiographic abnormalities of potassium depletion, shown in Figure 75–7, affect primarily repolarization segments of the electrocardiogram, in keeping with the effects of hypokalemia on the action potential. The common electrocardiographic manifestations of hypokalemia include sagging of the ST segment, depression of the T wave, and elevation of the U wave. With

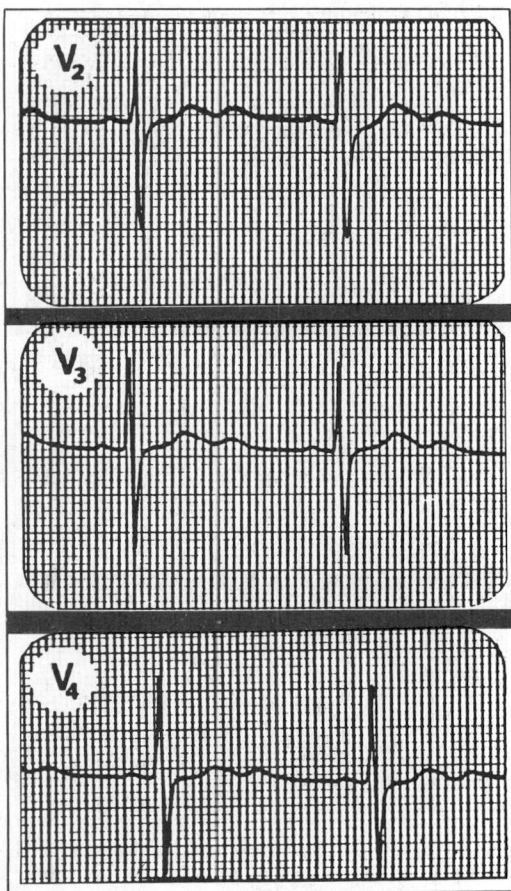

FIGURE 75–7. The electrocardiographic manifestations of hypokalemia. The serum potassium was 2.2 mEq per liter. Note that the ST segment is prolonged, primarily because of a V wave following the T wave, and that the T wave is flattened.

marked hypokalemia, the T wave becomes progressively smaller and the U waves show increasing amplitude. In some cases the merging of a flat or positive T wave with a positive U wave may erroneously be interpreted as a prolonged QT interval. Ordinarily, there are no serious clinical consequences from the abnormalities in cardiac excitation. In patients treated with digitalis, hypokalemia may precipitate serious arrhythmias.

Longstanding potassium depletion may produce renal tubular damage, referred to as hypokalemic nephropathy. Potassium deficiency also affects smooth muscle of the gastrointestinal tract and can result in paralytic ileus.

TREATMENT. The treatment of hypokalemia involves replacement therapy with potassium salts and attempts to correct the underlying disorder. Since diuretic abuse is probably the most common cause for hypokalemia in routine clinical practice, every attempt should be made to identify diuretic ingestion.

Except in extreme circumstances, oral rather than parenteral potassium replacement is prudent. However, when gastrointestinal function is impaired, or when neuromuscular manifestations of hypokalemia are present, parenteral therapy with potassium may be advisable. Since potassium deficits involve both the ICF and the ECF, their correction requires the transfer of administered potassium from the ECF into the ICF. The major problem in parenteral therapy is to avoid intravenous administration of potassium at rates sufficiently great to produce hyperkalemia. A prudent protocol to follow is to add potassium chloride to intravenous solutions at a final concentration of 40 to 60 mEq per liter and to administer no more than 10 to 20 mEq of potassium per hour. Except in unusual circumstances, the total amount of potassium administered daily should not exceed 200 mEq. The serum potassium level should be monitored at appropriate intervals; the frequency of monitoring should be determined by the patient's clinical condition, by the initial serum potassium, by the rate at which the serum potassium changes in a given patient, and by the patient's renal function. Because the electrocardiographic manifestations of hypokalemia are subtle, the electrocardiogram should not be used as a guide to replacement therapy.

Although potassium chloride is the salt of choice for intravenous potassium replacement, oral potassium chloride solutions are not well tolerated because of gastrointestinal irritation. Enteric-coated potassium chloride tablets are to be avoided, because they produce small bowel ulcerations. Oral potassium is administered most conveniently in the form of organic salts such as gluconate or citrate. This form of therapy is, however, not effective in hypokalemic metabolic alkalosis with hypochloremia. In this circumstance, chloride supplementation is required together with potassium replacement and is most easily achieved by administering sodium chloride supplementation.

HYPERKALEMIA AND POTASSIUM EXCESS

DEFINITION. Chronic hyperkalemia can occur with little or no increase in total body potassium. However, acute increases in serum potassium concentrations, produced by potassium shifts from the ICF to the ECF, can occur even when total body potassium is normal or reduced.

ETIOLOGY AND PATHOGENESIS. Hyperkalemia develops whenever the rate of potassium intake or the rate of potassium efflux from cellular to extracellular fluids exceeds the sum of renal plus extrarenal potassium losses. The renal mechanisms for potassium excretion adapt efficiently to increases in the rate of potassium influx to extracellular fluid, particularly from dietary sources. Hence acute or chronic hyperkalemia due to exogenous potassium intake is uncommon, unless renal mechanisms for potassium excretion are compromised. In the latter setting injudicious potassium administration may result in hyperkalemia. This occurs most commonly when intravenous potassium chloride is administered too rapidly; when potassium salts of antibiotics such as pencillin are administered; when transfusions are given with blood that has been stored for long periods; or when salt substitutes containing potassium are used. The occurrence of hyperkalemia in these settings usually requires that renal potassium excretion be impaired.

Acute or chronic hyperkalemia occurs most commonly either

TABLE 75–12. MAJOR CAUSES OF HYPERKALEMIA

I. Diminished Renal Excretion	II. Transcellular Shifts
Reduced GFR	Acidosis
Acute oliguric renal failure	Cell destruction
Chronic renal failure	Trauma, burns
Reduced tubular secretion	Rhabdomyolysis
Addison's disease	Hemolysis
Hyporeninemic hypoaldosteronism	Tumor lysis
Potassium-sparing diuretics	Hyperkalemic periodic paralysis
Voltage-dependent renal tubular acidosis	Diabetic hyperglycemia
	Insulin dependence plus aldosterone lack
	Depolarizing muscle paralysis
	Succinylcholine

GFR = glomerular filtration rate.

because of diminished *renal excretion* or because there is a sudden *transcellular shift* of potassium from the ICF to the ECF. The major causes for hyperkalemia listed in Table 75–12 follow this format.

Diminished Renal Excretion. Hyperkalemia may occur in *acute oliguric renal failure* of any cause. In *chronic renal failure,* hyperkalemia generally does not occur until the GFR has reached markedly low levels. Hyperkalemia may be precipitated in chronic renal failure, however, either by the development of acidosis or, as indicated above, by the injudicious administration of potassium salts. Hyperkalemia also occurs with little or modest reduction in the GFR, if there is impairment of potassium secretion by terminal nephron regions. This occurs in *Addison's disease,* in *hyporeninemic hypoaldosteronism,* and with the injudicious administration of *potassium-sparing diuretics,* such as triamterene or spironolactone. Hyperkalemia in Addison's disease and hyporeninemic hypoaldosteronism may also be exacerbated by the administration of beta-blocking agents or converting enzyme inhibitors.

Hyperkalemia is also a characteristic feature of *voltage-dependent renal tubular acidosis.* The latter is a specific defect in sodium transport of distal nephron segments. This blockade of distal sodium absorption reduces luminal electronegativity and consequently impairs both proton secretion and potassium secretion. Thus, voltage-dependent renal tubular acidosis, like hyporeninemic hypoaldosteronism, is characterized by sodium wasting and hyperkalemia. In hyporeninemic hypoaldosteronism, the urine is acidic, and plasma levels of aldosterone are reduced even during volume contraction, whereas in voltage-dependent renal tubular acidosis, there is impaired urinary acidification but a normal plasma aldosterone response to volume contraction.

Finally, in each of the disorders characterized by diminished renal potassium excretion, hyperkalemia can be aggravated by ECF volume contraction, which reduces sodium delivery to terminal nephron segments, or by acidosis, which promotes cellular potassium efflux.

Transcellular Shifts. The second class of disorders causing acute hyperkalemia includes situations in which there is an abrupt shift of potassium from the ICF to the ECF. This shift occurs in acidosis or in circumstances that result in *cell destruction;* the latter occurs commonly with tissue trauma, burns, rhabdomyolysis, or hemolysis, as well as with lysis of large masses of tumor cells. As indicated previously, hypokalemia predisposes to rhabdomyolysis. Thus the sudden occurrence of hyperkalemia in potassium-depleted patients is a diagnostic clue to the development of rhabdomyolysis.

Hyperkalemic periodic paralysis is an autosomal dominant disorder in which sudden increases in the serum potassium level result in muscle paralysis. The hyperkalemia is often provoked by dietary potassium intake or by exercise. Myotonia occurs commonly in the disorder and appears either between attacks or immediately preceding attacks. The pathogenesis of the disorder is not understood. The acute paralytic attack can be treated by intravenous administration of calcium gluconate or glucose and insulin. Chronic treatment with diuretics such as acetazolamide minimizes the frequency of attacks.

Paradoxical hyperkalemia occurs when *sudden hyperglycemia* develops in insulin-dependent diabetics who also have interstitial renal disease and associated hyporeninemic hypoaldosteronism. The sudden increase in ECF osmolality draws water from cells, raises intracellular potassium concentrations, and therefore promotes passive potassium efflux from cells. The insulin lack minimizes cellular reentry of potassium, and the aldosterone deficiency blunts renal potassium excretion. Insulin therapy promptly corrects the hyperkalemia. Finally, anesthetic agents or other drugs that cause a *depolarizing muscle paralysis,* such as succinylcholine, promote potassium efflux from muscle cells. The loss of cell electronegativity in this situation increases passive potassium efflux from muscle cells.

Pseudohyperkalemia may occur in thrombocytosis or leukocytosis, because clotting of blood promotes potassium release from these cells and may be identified by noting that the *serum* potassium level is elevated while the *plasma* potassium level is normal. This kind of artifact occurs most commonly in patients with myeloproliferative disorders.

CLINICAL MANIFESTATIONS. The most important clinical manifestations of hyperkalemia relate to alterations in cardiac excitability. For this reason the electrocardiogram is the single most important guide in appraising the threat posed by hyperkalemia and in determining how aggressive a therapeutic approach is necessary.

The electrocardiographic manifestations of hyperkalemia, shown in Figure 75–8, follow directly from the effects of hyperkalemia on cardiac action potentials (see Fig. 75–6). The earliest manifestation of hyperkalemia is the development of peaked T waves, which become evident when the serum potassium level exceeds 6.5 mEq per liter. This peaking of the T waves is a manifestation of the accelerated repolarization of the cardiac action potential produced by hyperkalemia. When the potassium concentration exceeds 7 to 8 mEq per liter, diminished cardiac

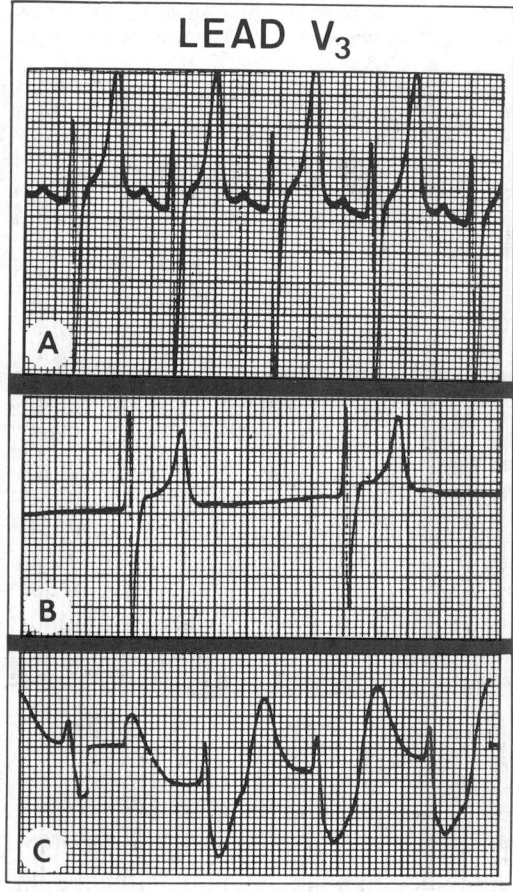

FIGURE 75–8. The effects of progressive hyperkalemia on the electrocardiogram. All of the illustrations are from lead V_3. *A,* Serum K^+ = 6.8 mEq per liter; note the peaked T waves together with normal sinus rhythm. *B,* Serum K^+ = 7.7 mEq per liter; note the peaked T waves and absent P waves. *C,* Serum K^+ = 8.9 mEq per liter; note the classic sine wave with absent P waves, marked prolongation of the QRS complex, and peaked T waves.

excitability results in prolongation of the PR interval, followed by a loss of P waves and widening of the QRS complex. These changes indicate progressive inexcitability of cardiac muscle and are referable to hyperkalemia-induced inactivation of sodium permeability during the initial spike of the action potential. When the serum potassium level exceeds 8 to 10 mEq per liter, the electrocardiogram may develop a sine wave pattern and cardiac standstill can occur.

The correlation between serum potassium concentrations and electrocardiographic abnormalities is approximate at best; in a given patient, progression from peaked T waves to a sine wave pattern may occur rapidly, particularly if the serum potassium concentration rises rapidly. Therefore the development of peaked T waves in conjunction with hyperkalemia should be viewed as a serious disorder; more advanced electrocardiographic manifestations of hyperkalemia should be treated as life-threatening medical emergencies.

TREATMENT. Three kinds of maneuvers are used in the treatment of hyperkalemia: agents such as glucose plus insulin, sodium bicarbonate, or beta agonists, which promote the transfer of potassium from the ECF to the ICF; maneuvers that enhance potassium elimination from the body, such as administration of diuretics or exchange resins or dialysis; and the use of calcium, which does not alter serum potassium concentrations but counteracts the effects of hyperkalemia on cardiac excitability.

Both insulin and sodium bicarbonate promote potassium entry into cells. The administration of 25 grams of glucose, together with 10 units of regular insulin, is an effective way of reducing the serum potassium level rapidly. The glucose may be administered over 30 minutes as a 20 per cent solution, or it may be given as a 50 per cent glucose solution. Insulin promotes potassium entry into cells, and glucose is administered to prevent hypoglycemia. In insulin-dependent diabetic patients in whom sudden hyperglycemia has precipitated the hyperkalemia, insulin administration alone suffices to reduce the serum potassium concentration.

Administering 40 to 150 mEq of sodium bicarbonate intravenously over a 30- to 60-minute interval also promotes potassium entry into cells, particularly if acidosis is also present. This maneuver should be used with caution in patients with compromised renal function because of the risks of hypernatremia and of ECF volume overload.

Potassium shifts from extracellular to intracellular fluids may also be enhanced by the use of aerosolized specific beta$_2$ agonists; albuterol is a commonly used agent of this kind. Agents such as albuterol are most helpful in the management of mild hyperkalemia in chronic disorders such as chronic renal failure and hyperkalemic periodic paralysis.

None of the maneuvers described above removes potassium from the body. Gastrointestinal potassium losses may be produced by the use of cation exchange resins in the sodium cycle, such as sodium polystyrene sulfonate (Kayexalate). Each gram of the resin contains approximately 1 mEq of sodium and exchanges for about 1 mEq of potassium. This stoichiometry is not precise, since the sodium form of the resin also exchanges for other cations in gastrointestinal secretions, including calcium. In chronic hyperkalemia, 20 grams of Kayexalate may be given three or four times a day in a 70 per cent solution of sorbitol. The sorbitol creates an osmotic diarrhea and enhances resin passage through the gastrointestinal tract. In acute circumstances, Kayexalate may also be administered by enema, generally as 100 grams of resin suspended in 200 ml of 20 per cent sorbitol. The use of chronic Kayexalate therapy in patients with chronic renal failure carries with it the risk of sodium overload.

In settings of extreme hyperkalemic cardiotoxicity, when P waves are absent and the QRS complexes are widened, the administration of calcium gluconate, 10 to 30 ml of a 10 per cent solution over a 10- to 20-minute interval, may be life saving. This approach should be undertaken with constant electrocardiographic monitoring and should be used with extreme caution in patients who have received digitalis. In the latter circumstances, calcium administration may unmask digitalis intoxication, especially if other agents are used simultaneously to reduce the serum potassium level. Calcium salts should not be added to bottles of intravenous fluids containing bicarbonate, because water-insoluble calcium salts will form.

The influence of calcium salts in minimizing the cardiotoxic effects of hyperkalemia may be understood by noting, as described under Physiologic Considerations, that depolarization of excitable tissues by elevating serum K^+ concentrations inactivates sodium channels and that the extracellular sides of these sodium channels are electronegative. Divalent cations such as calcium provide a remarkably effective way of screening these electronegative sites. Thus calcium salts raise the voltage gradient across sodium channels by screening electronegative surface charges of these channels on their extracellular fluid sides and consequently restoring the voltage-dependent excitability of these channels.

Finally, acute hemodialysis or peritoneal dialysis provides another mechanism for potassium removal from the body. This approach is particularly advantageous in acute renal failure; when patients are volume expanded and sodium administration may produce congestive heart failure; or when there is a continued efflux of large amounts of potassium from the ICF to the ECF, as in burns or rhabdomyolysis.

Brem AS: Disorders of potassium homeostasis. Pediatr Clin North Am 37:419, 1990. *A concise clinical guide to disorders of potassium balance.*

Brown RS: Extrarenal potassium homeostasis. Kidney Int 30:116, 1986. *An account of extrarenal factors regulating potassium homeostasis.*

Castellino P, Bia M, DeFronzo RA: Adrenergic modulation of potassium metabolism in uremia. Kidney Int 27:793, 1990. *The role of beta-adrenergic agents in regulating potassium homeostasis in uremia.*

Clausen T, Everts ME: Regulation of the Na, K-pump in skeletal muscle. Kidney Int 35:1, 1989. *A description of the ($Na^+ + K^+$-ATPase in skeletal muscle and its regulation by insulin and beta agonists.*

Kurtzman NA, Gonzalez J, DeFronzo R, et al.: A patient with hyperkalemia and metabolic acidosis. Am J Kidney Dis 15:333, 1990. *A concise account of the renal tubular disorders causing hyperkalemia.*

Montoliu J, Almirall J, Ponz E, et al.: Treatment of hyperkalemia with salbutamol inhalation. J Intern Med 228:35, 1990. *A description of the use of beta agonist nebulization in hyperkalemia.*

Tsien RW, Hess P: Excitable tissue—the heart. In Andreoli TE, Hoffman JF, Fanestil DD, et al. (eds.): Physiology of Membrane Disorders. New York, Plenum, 1986, pp 469–490. *A meticulous description of the ionic basis for the cardiac action potential.*

75.4 DISTURBANCES IN ACID-BASE BALANCE

PHYSIOLOGIC CONSIDERATIONS

The pH of arterial blood and interstitial fluid normally ranges between 7.38 and 7.42 despite wide variations in dietary intake of acids or alkali. The arterial pH range over which cardiac function, metabolic activity, and central nervous system function can be maintained is narrow; the widest range of pH values compatible with life is from 6.8 to 7.8, or an interval of one pH unit.

The major buffer system in extracellular fluid is the bicarbonate–carbonic acid pair. The relation between pH, bicarbonate, and carbonic acid concentrations in ECF may be expressed according to the familiar Henderson-Hasselbalch equation:

$$pH = pK + \log \frac{HCO_3^-}{H_2CO_3}$$

where pK is the carbonic acid dissociation constant, HCO_3^- is the plasma bicarbonate concentration, and H_2CO_3 is the plasma carbonic acid concentration. The H_2CO_3 concentration is given by αPa_{CO_2}, where α is the CO_2 solubility constant, and has a value of 0.03, and Pa_{CO_2} is the arterial carbon dioxide tension. Therefore, with a Pa_{CO_2} of 40 mm Hg, the Henderson-Hasselbalch equation becomes the following:

$$7.4 = 6.1 + \log \frac{24 \text{ mM/L}}{1.2 \text{ mM/L}}$$

The arterial pH provides a qualitative, but not quantitative, index to total body water acid-base status because, at any given time, about two thirds of an acid or alkali load is buffered by proton shifts into or out of the ICF, respectively. For this reason, some prefer to use the term "acidemia" for acidosis and "alkalemia" for alkalosis to connote that plasma pH measurements provide quantitative information about the pH status of plasma and interstitial fluid and only qualitative information about total body acid-base balance.

A convenient way to consider the total body buffering capacity is as follows. Bicarbonate is predominantly an extracellular anion, and the total ECF bicarbonate content in a 70-kg man having 15 liters of ECF is (24 mEq per liter × 15 liters), or 360 mEq HCO_3^-. However, about two thirds of a given acid or alkali load is buffered within cells. Consequently, the total body buffering capacity, often referred to as the "bicarbonate space," is calculated as:

$$(\text{Arterial } HCO_3^- \times 0.6 \text{ body weight})$$

that is, using total body water as an index to total buffering capacity. The bicarbonate space is also an index to net acid excess or net base excess. If the arterial HCO_3^- concentration in a 70-kg man is reduced to 15 mEq per liter while the Pa_{CO_2} remains constant, the net acid excess (or net base deficit) is (24 − 15) mEq per liter × 42 liters = 378 mEq. Conversely, if the arterial HCO_3^- concentration rises to 33 mEq per liter while the Pa_{CO_2} remains constant, the net base excess (or acid deficit) is 378 mEq.

Proton shifts between the ECF and ICF stabilize the plasma pH against acute fluctuations. But the ultimate maintenance of pH balance requires that input of acid or base into the body be matched by output of acid or base, so that the HCO_3^-/H_2CO_3 ratio and the total bicarbonate content in the ECF remain constant. The cardinal systems involved in these external processes are the kidneys, for bicarbonate balance, and the lungs, for carbon dioxide balance.

Carbon Dioxide Production and Elimination

VOLATILE ACID INPUT. The largest source of endogenous acid production is from combustion of glucose and fatty acids to carbon dioxide and water or, in other words, to a volatile acid. During aerobic glycolysis, that is, cellular respiration, glucose oxidation involves oxygen utilization and carbon dioxide production according to the following reaction:

$$C_6H_{12}O_6 + 6O_2 \rightarrow 6CO_2 + 6H_2O$$

Since red blood cells contain carbonic anhydrase (c.a.), carbon dioxide hydration in erythrocytes yields the following:

$$CO_2 + H_2O \xrightleftharpoons{\text{c.a.}} H_2CO_3 \rightleftharpoons H^+ + HCO_3^-$$

The protons formed from carbonic acid dissociation are buffered by hemoglobin, whereas bicarbonate leaves red blood cells in exchange for chloride (the familiar chloride shift). In other words, carbon dioxide generation is equivalent to carbonic acid formation, and the bulk of hydrogen ion formed is buffered intracellularly.

A simple way of calculating the daily rate of nonvolatile acid production is to note, from the above reactions, that the production of 1 mole of metabolic water and 1 mole of carbon dioxide represents, through dissociation of carbonic acid, the formation of 1 mole of hydrogen ions.

Since the molecular weight of water is 18, 1 liter of water contains about 55 moles of water. Consequently, the average rate of metabolic water production, about 400 ml daily, yields 22,000 mmol of water and an equal number of carbon dioxide molecules. Thus the rate of volatile acid production amounts to about 22,000 mEq of hydrogen ion daily. The cellular combustion of carbohydrates and fatty acids to carbon dioxide and water is remarkably efficient. Under normal circumstances, organic anions such as lactate and keto acids, which derive from incomplete combustion of carbohydrates and fatty acids, have plasma concentrations of approximately 5 mEq per liter.

VOLATILE ACID OUTPUT. Pulmonary ventilation excretes the carbon dioxide formed by cellular respiration. During blood transit through the lungs, bicarbonate reenters red blood cells and combines with protons to form carbonic acid, which dissociates to carbon dioxide and water. The carbon dioxide so formed diffuses freely through red blood cells and alveolar epithelium, so that the rate of carbon dioxide excretion is governed primarily by the rate of minute ventilation.

MODULATION OF RESPIRATION. The prime factors nor-

mally regulating alterations in the rate of minute ventilation are subtle changes in cerebrospinal fluid (CSF) pH or arterial pH. Sensor chemoreceptors in central medullary centers or in the carotid body are activated by small reductions in CSF pH or arterial pH, respectively; the pH reduction can result either from carbon dioxide accumulation or from nonvolatile acid accumulation, which reduces the plasma bicarbonate concentration. In most circumstances, central medullary chemoreceptors provide the major impetus to altering ventilatory response, and the carotid body chemoreceptors serve as relatively minor stimuli to ventilation. The medullary respiratory centers therefore serve as the major *effector* mechanism for regulating carbon dioxide output by increasing ventilation rate.

The ventilatory response for carbon dioxide removal involves an increase in both tidal volume and respiratory rate. On an average, for every 1 mEq per liter reduction in plasma bicarbonate produced by metabolic acidosis, increased minute ventilation will produce a 1.0 to 1.2 mm Hg fall in the Pa_{CO_2}. In most circumstances, the maximum reduction in Pa_{CO_2} produced by the hyperventilatory response to severe metabolic acidosis is to a Pa_{CO_2} of 12 to 15 mm Hg; hyperventilation to Pa_{CO_2} values less than 10 mm Hg in metabolic acidosis almost never occurs. Conversely, an increase in arterial pH reduces the rate of minute ventilation and therefore results in carbon dioxide retention. For increases in plasma bicarbonate concentrations to 35 mEq per liter, the Pa_{CO_2} usually remains less than 50 mm Hg. When profound metabolic alkalosis occurs, the Pa_{CO_2} may rise further but virtually never exceeds 65 mm Hg.

Renal Bicarbonate Processing

In addition to volatile acid production due to carbon dioxide formation, cellular metabolism also results in the formation of a number of nonvolatile acids. The major source for nonvolatile acid production is the metabolism of sulfur-containing amino acids, such as cysteine and methionine, which results in sulfuric acid formation. Consequently, the daily rate of nonvolatile acid production is closely related to dietary protein intake and to the rate of endogenous protein catabolism. Nonvolatile acids also derive from oxidation of phosphoproteins and phospholipids, which results in phosphoric acid formation; nucleoprotein degradation, which yields uric acid; and incomplete combustion of carbohydrates and fatty acids, which produces lactic acid and the keto acids.

The daily rate of nonvolatile acid production under normal conditions is about 1 mEq per kilogram of body weight. Thus daily nonvolatile acid production would consume the total body fluid buffering capacity in about 2 weeks, were it not for the fact that the kidneys excrete nonvolatile acids and, in so doing, regenerate bicarbonate. Since the minimal urinary pH ordinarily attainable is 5.0 and the amount of nonvolatile acid to be excreted is about 70 mEq per day, renal hydrogen ion excretion, which is equivalent to renal bicarbonate regeneration, occurs mainly as protons trapped in an undissociated form by urinary buffers.

The kidneys also filter large quantities of bicarbonate daily: For a normal plasma bicarbonate concentration of 24 mEq per liter and a glomerular filtration of 180 liters per day, the net amount of bicarbonate filtered daily is approximately 4300 mEq, or about four times the total body buffering capacity. Thus, in addition to generating new bicarbonate, the renal tubules must also absorb filtered bicarbonate.

BICARBONATE REABSORPTION. Virtually all filtered bicarbonate is absorbed, together with sodium, by the proximal tubule. Within renal tubular cells, CO_2 is hydrated to H_2CO_3. Apical membrane Na^+ exchange permits H^+ secretion into urine and Na^+ entry into cells, with subsequent absorption of sodium bicarbonate into blood.

The rate of proximal bicarbonate reabsorption is modulated by the same *effectors* that regulate proximal sodium absorption. Among these, the ECV exerts a central effect. Volume expansion, which resets glomerulotubular balance downward, reduces the fractional rate of proximal bicarbonate reabsorption. Conversely, volume contraction raises the bicarbonate threshold by increasing the fractional rate of proximal tubular sodium bicarbonate reabsorption.

Two other *effectors* regulate, in operational terms, the rate of bicarbonate reabsorption. One of these is the arterial Pa_{CO_2}: High

Pa_{CO_2} values raise the apparent bicarbonate threshold, whereas low Pa_{CO_2} values reduce the rate of the compensatory reabsorption. This factor accounts for the compensatory increase in plasma bicarbonate concentrations in respiratory acidosis. Second, hypokalemia also increases the rate of bicarbonate reabsorption, presumably by raising the intracellular hydrogen ion concentration. This factor accounts for the fact that in hypokalemic, hypochloremic metabolic alkalosis associated with volume contraction, alkalosis can persist after volume deficits are restored. In this circumstance, correction of potassium deficits is required for correction of the alkalosis.

BICARBONATE REGENERATION. The excretion of non-volatile acids and the simultaneous renal regeneration of bicarbonate occur principally in distal nephron segments. Distal renal tubular cells hydrate carbon dioxide to carbonic acid, which dissociates to protons, which are secreted into urine, and bicarbonate anions, which are absorbed into blood. The major mode of proton secretion in terminal nephron segments, particularly collecting tubules, involves an apical membrane proton-ATPase.

The secreted protons titrate urinary buffers, principally phosphate, while sodium is absorbed. Thus the overall reaction is as follows:

$$\underset{(filtered)}{Na_2HPO_4} + H^+ + HCO_3^- \longrightarrow \underset{(excreted)}{NaH_2PO_4} + \underset{(absorbed)}{NaHCO_3}$$

Titratable acid formation normally accounts for about one third of renal acid excretion. The remaining two thirds of acid excretion is accounted for by ammonia (NH_3) secretion by the following sequence:

$$\underset{(filtered)}{NaR} + NH_3 + H^+ + HCO_3^- \longrightarrow \underset{(reabsorbed)}{NaHCO_3} + \underset{(excreted)}{NH_4R}$$

where NaR is the filtered sodium salt of a nonvolatile acid, NH_3 is ammonia produced by renal tubular cells, and the protons and bicarbonate come from carbon dioxide hydration by tubular cells.

Distal acid excretion and bicarbonate absorption are accompanied by sodium absorption. Consequently, *effector* systems that enhance distal sodium absorption, such as aldosterone or increased rates of sodium delivery to terminal nephron segments, also promote terminal nephron hydrogen ion excretion. Three other *effector* mechanisms also increase the rate of hydrogen ion excretion: (1) Delivery of sodium to terminal nephron segments in association with impermeant anions such as sulfate favors proton movement from tubular cells to lumen. (2) Hypokalemia enhances hydrogen ion excretion, particularly in sodium-acquisitive states, presumably because hypokalemia is accompanied by a fall in intracellular pH. (3) Acidosis stimulates ammoniagenesis by renal tubular cells; consequently, in metabolic acidosis, increases in the rate of renal acid excretion are referable primarily to increased rates of ammonium excretion. In other words, these last-named three effector systems enhance renal acid excretion by creating a favorable situation for proton transfer from tubular cells to urine. Conversely, aldosterone deficiency, alkalosis, or reduced rates of salt delivery to terminal nephron segments reduce renal capacity for acid excretion.

pH Disequilibria Between Plasma and CSF

Central rather than arterial chemoreceptors are the prime sensors for pH-mediated changes in respiration. The ventilatory responses to pH changes mediated by respiratory processes and by metabolic processes therefore differ. The blood-brain barrier is freely permeable to carbon dioxide. Consequently, pH changes produced exclusively by hyperventilation or hypoventilation occur almost simultaneously in arterial plasma and in the CSF, and the respiratory response to primary increases or decreases in Pa_{CO_2} occurs almost instantaneously. The blood-brain barrier imposes a lag, however, in the rate at which arterial bicarbonate equilibrates with the CSF. Thus in metabolic acidosis, the arterial pH and bicarbonate concentration fall more rapidly than they do in the CSF; and in metabolic alkalosis, the CSF pH and bicarbonate concentration rise more slowly than they do in arterial plasma. Consequently, in the early stages of acute metabolic acidosis, there may be a 1- to 3-hour delay in the development of a maximal hyperventilatory response. Conversely, when metabolic acidosis is corrected rapidly, hyperventilation may persist for a few hours because of a delay in the rise of cerebrospinal fluid pH.

An unusual situation relating to this effect occurs in diabetic ketoacidosis and in certain other metabolic acidoses associated with impaired central nervous system function. In these situations, carotid body chemoreceptors, rather than central medullary chemoreceptors, provide the major stimulus to respiration driven by a reduced arterial pH. The rapid correction of ECF acidosis by bicarbonate administration reduces the rate at which carotid body chemoreceptors drive ventilation. When this occurs, Pa_{CO_2} levels in plasma and in the CSF rise almost simultaneously; but because of a lag in the rate of bicarbonate entry into the CSF, the CSF bicarbonate/carbonic acid ratio tends to fall. In severe diabetic ketoacidosis, this situation can result in an actual fall in CSF pH simultaneously with a rise in arterial pH produced by intravenous bicarbonate administration.

DEFINITION OF ACID-BASE ABNORMALITIES

The arterial pH is determined by the ratio of the bicarbonate–carbonic acid buffer system, as expressed in the Henderson-Hasselbalch equation. These data also provide an index of total body acid-base balance, because, as indicated in the preceding section, the majority of body buffering occurs within cells. Acid-base disturbance can therefore occur either by altering the serum bicarbonate concentration, referred to as a "metabolic" disorder, or by altering arterial carbon dioxide tension, referred to as a "respiratory" disorder. A convenient way for considering these disturbances is illustrated in Figure 75–9, which illustrates pH isobars (for pH 7.0, 7.4, and 7.8) calculated according to the Henderson-Hasselbalch equation for the bicarbonate concentrations and Pa_{CO_2} values listed on the ordinate and abscissa, respectively.

TYPES OF ACID-BASE ABNORMALITIES. The left-hand panel in Figure 75–9 shows the directional changes in Pa_{CO_2} and bicarbonate concentrations that *initiate* the four basic types of acid-base abnormalities. *Respiratory acidosis* results from hypoventilation and reduces pH by raising the Pa_{CO_2}. *Respiratory alkalosis* results from hyperventilation and raises pH by reducing the Pa_{CO_2}. *Metabolic alkalosis* occurs when increases in the plasma bicarbonate concentration raise pH, and *metabolic acidosis* occurs when reductions in plasma bicarbonate decrease pH.

Any of these initial acid-base disturbances activates *compensatory responses*, illustrated in the right-hand panel of Figure 75–9, that tend to minimize the pH changes produced by the initial acid-base abnormality. By comparing the directional arrows in the left- and right-hand panels of Figure 75–9, it becomes evident that the initial disturbance in any of these four acid-base abnormalities tends to displace the arterial pH away from the pH 7.4 isobar and that the compensatory response partially restores arterial pH values toward the pH 7.4 isobar. The arterial pH, Pa_{CO_2}, and plasma bicarbonate concentrations illustrated in the right-hand panel of Figure 75–9 are the values usually observed clinically in the four primary acid-base disturbances.

The Compensatory Responses. As indicated in Figure 75–9, a compensatory response blunts the effect of the initial insult on pH homeostasis. In *primary respiratory disorders*, the renal response is to change the proximal tubular bicarbonate threshold and consequently the plasma bicarbonate concentration. A good rule of thumb is that for every 1 mm Hg rise or fall in the arterial Pa_{CO_2}, the plasma bicarbonate concentration rises or falls, respectively, by approximately 0.3 to 0.5 mEq per liter. This renal adaptive response is relatively slow, however, and requires 24 to 48 hours for complete expression. Consequently, the renal response to a respiratory acid-base disorder affords relatively little pH compensation in the first 12 to 18 hours in acute respiratory acidosis or alkalosis.

In chronic respiratory acidosis, as, for example, in chronic obstructive pulmonary disease, renal bicarbonate retention provides adequate but not complete compensation for CO_2 retention. Chronic respiratory alkalosis is relatively uncommon in clinical settings. The renal response to chronic respiratory alkalosis is discussed below.

The pulmonary response to primary *metabolic acid-base disorders* involves an alteration in the rate of minute ventilation. In

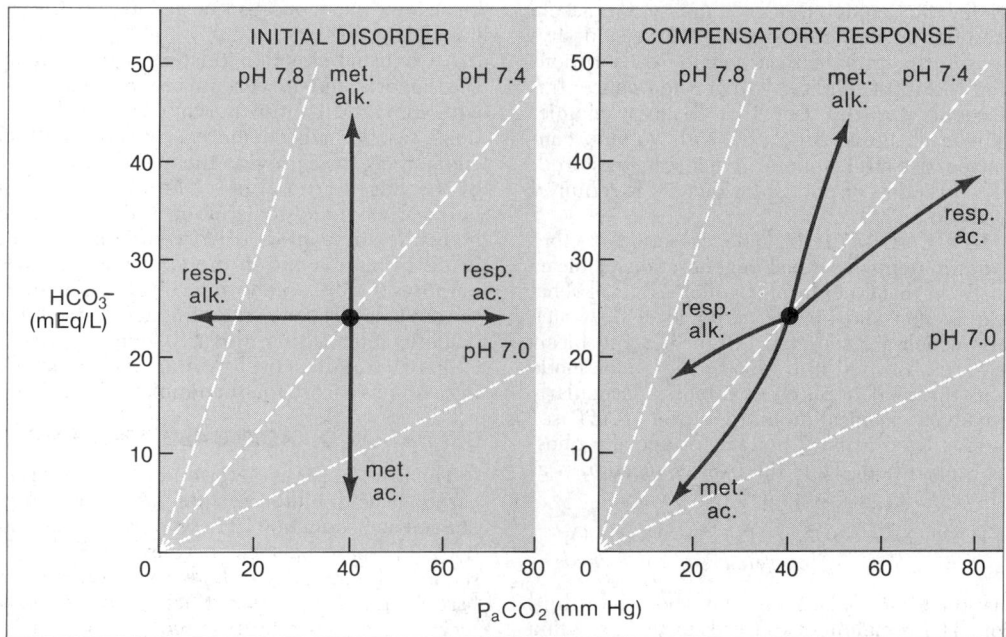

FIGURE 75-9. Schematic frame of reference for considering acid-base disturbances. The dotted lines are the pH isobars for pH values of 7.8, 7.4, and 7.0 computed from the Henderson-Hasselbalch equation for given combinations of arterial bicarbonate values (vertical axes) and arterial carbon dioxide tensions (horizontal axes). The graph on the left shows the initial derangement in HCO_3^- concentrations in metabolic acidosis and metabolic alkalosis and the initial $PaCO_2$ derangement in respiratory acidosis and respiratory alkalosis. Note that each of the four changes in either HCO_3^- or $PaCO_2$ tends to displace the arterial pH from the pH 7.4 isobar. The graph on the right, labeled "Compensatory Response," indicates the general trend of pH, HCO_3^-, and $PaCO_2$ changes actually observed in the four primary acid-base disturbances: respiratory acidosis, respiratory alkalosis, metabolic acidosis, and metabolic alkalosis. Respiratory acidosis and alkalosis are accompanied by compensatory renal bicarbonate retention and loss, respectively. Metabolic acidosis and alkalosis are accompanied by compensatory hyperventilation and hypoventilation, respectively. Note that the compensatory response in each of the four acid-base disorders tends to restore arterial pH values toward the pH 7.4 isobar.

general, a 1 mEq per liter decrease or increase in the plasma bicarbonate concentration produces a 1.0 to 1.2 mm Hg decrease or increase in the arterial Pa_{CO_2}, respectively. This ventilatory response begins within minutes of the onset of the metabolic abnormality. The full expression of the ventilatory response may be delayed for 1 to 3 hours if, as noted above, a pH disequilibrium exists between plasma and CSF.

Three other characteristics of these compensatory responses should be noted. The compensatory responses do not, in general, provide complete compensation for the initial abnormality. Moreover, the magnitude of the compensatory response may vary in individual patients and may be affected by pre-existing conditions. For example, the ventilatory response to sepsis with lactic acidosis is considerably less in patients with chronic obstructive pulmonary disease than in normal individuals. Finally, a near-normal arterial pH may also be due to offsetting metabolic derangements rather than to physiologic compensatory processes. For example, in diabetic ketoacidosis, a fall in arterial pH may be offset by a metabolic alkalosis secondary to vomiting rather than by Kussmaul's ventilation (see below).

THE SERUM ANION GAP. Sodium is the principal cation in extracellular fluids. The sum of plasma chloride plus bicarbonate concentrations is less than the serum sodium concentration; the remaining anions required for electroneutrality, generally not reported with routine serum electrolyte measurements, are referred to as unmeasured anions, or as the serum anion gap. A convenient formula for calculating the serum anion gap is the following:

$$\text{Serum anion gap} = Na^+ - (Cl^- + HCO_3^-)$$

where Na^+, Cl^-, and HCO_3^- are the serum sodium, chloride, and bicarbonate concentrations, respectively. The serum anion gap includes primarily phosphates and sulfates derived from tissue metabolism; lactate and keto acids arising from incomplete combustion of carbohydrates and fatty acids; and negatively charged protein molecules, principally albumin. The normal value for

unmeasured anions, or the serum anion gap, is 10 to 12 mEq per liter; albumin and other proteins normally account for about half of the anion gap.

An *increased* serum anion gap generally indicates the presence of metabolic acidosis. The factors responsible for this kind of metabolic acidosis are discussed in the next section.

A *reduced* serum anion gap provides a clue to the presence of certain other disorders. The anion gap will be reduced if the sodium concentration falls while the chloride plus bicarbonate concentrations are unchanged or, in other words, when the concentration of another cation in serum is increased while the serum osmolality remains normal. This may occur in multiple myeloma of the immunoglobulin G (IgG) variety if the myeloma proteins are cationic at pH 7.4. Hyperviscosity syndromes may also result in a reduced anion gap because of a laboratory artifact: When serum is excessively viscous, automatic pumps deliver decreased volumes of serum to a flame photometer, producing artifactual reductions in sodium concentrations. Rarely, lithium intoxication, hypermagnesemia, and hypercalcemia raise nonsodium cation concentrations sufficiently high to reduce the anion gap.

The serum anion gap will also be decreased if the serum sodium concentration remains normal while the serum chloride plus bicarbonate concentrations are increased. This situation occurs most commonly in hypoalbuminemia. A low serum anion gap also occurs in bromide intoxication, since colorimetric techniques for serum chloride determinations give spuriously high values for chloride plus bromide when bromide is present in relatively high concentrations in serum.

THE URINARY ANION GAP. The urinary anion gap, defined as

$$\text{Urinary anion gap} = (Na^+ + K^+) - Cl^-$$

is a useful measurement in evaluating patients with hyperchloremic acidosis. The test provides an approximate index of urinary NH_4 excretion, as measured by a negative urinary anion gap, that

TABLE 75–13. CHARACTERISTICS OF DISTAL RENAL TUBULAR ACIDOSIS (RTA) SYNDROMES

Condition	Urinary pH	Serum K+	Urinary Anion Gap	Response to Furosemide		Aldosterone Secretion
				Urinary pH	Urinary K+	
Gradient-limited RTA	>5.5	↓	Positive	Unchanged	↑	Normal
Hyporeninemic hypoaldosteronism	<5.5	↑	Positive	↓	↑	Reduced
Voltage-dependent RTA	>5.5	↑	Positive	Unchanged	Unchanged	Normal

is, urinary (Na$^+$ + K$^+$) is less than urinary Cl$^-$. Thus, in hyperchloremic metabolic acidosis, a normal renal response would be a negative urinary anion gap, generally in the range of 30 to 50 mEq per liter. In such an instance, it is likely that the hyperchloremic acidosis is due to gastrointestinal losses rather than a renal lesion. In contrast, a positive urinary anion gap implies a renal tubular disorder, as is discussed below.

URINARY RESPONSE TO ORAL FUROSEMIDE. The urinary response to oral furosemide loading is another useful test for evaluating tubular acidifying capability. The rationale for the test is that in normal individuals blockade of sodium absorption in diluting segments by furosemide increases sodium delivery to distal nephron segments where potassium and protons are secreted (see above) and increases the rate of excretion of the latter two moieties. Consequently, the oral administration of 40 to 80 mg of furosemide should be followed, in a subsequent 4- to 6-hour urinary collection, by an increase in urinary sodium excretion and fractional sodium excretion, an increase in urinary potassium excretion and fractional potassium excretion, and a reduction in urinary pH. In some renal tubular acidosis syndromes, proton and/or potassium excretion is impaired (Table 75–13).

METABOLIC ACIDOSIS

ETIOLOGY AND PATHOGENESIS. A convenient way to consider the metabolic acidoses is to divide them into two groups: normal anion gap and increased anion gap metabolic acidoses (Table 75–14). The pathogeneses of these two groups differ appreciably.

NORMAL ANION GAP METABOLIC ACIDOSIS. The metabolic acidoses having a *normal anion gap* result whenever there are abnormally high net bicarbonate losses. This situation may occur because the kidneys fail to reabsorb or regenerate bicarbonate; because there are extrarenal losses of bicarbonate; or because excessive amounts of substances yielding hydrochloric acid have been administered.

Bicarbonate Losses. Bicarbonate losses occur either when the proximal tubule fails to absorb virtually all filtered bicarbonate, that is, when the apparent bicarbonate threshold is reduced, or when there are losses of bicarbonate from the gastrointestinal tract.

Renal bicarbonate wasting occurs in *proximal renal tubular acidosis*, either alone or as part of Fanconi's syndrome (Ch. 82). The apparent threshold for bicarbonate in this disorder is set below the normal value of 26 mEq of bicarbonate per deciliter of glomerular filtrate and may be as low as 15 to 20 mEq of bicarbonate per deciliter of glomerular filtrate. Consequently, bicarbonate wasting occurs whenever the plasma bicarbonate level is raised above the apparent renal threshold for bicarbonate.

Attempts to correct the acidosis of proximal renal tubular acidosis by bicarbonate administration are generally unrewarding, because increases in the plasma bicarbonate level produced by administering bicarbonate salts are accompanied by corresponding increases in bicarbonaturia. A promising approach to this disorder involves reducing the ECV by sodium restriction. This maneuver exploits the fact that ECF contraction resets glomerulotubular balance upward and consequently increases the fractional rate of sodium, and hence bicarbonate, reabsorption by the proximal tubule.

A converse of this situation is sometimes referred to as *dilutional acidosis*. Individuals who are volume expanded reduce the fractional rate of sodium bicarbonate absorption by the proximal tubule and consequently develop mild reductions in plasma bicarbonate concentrations. *Carbonic anhydrase inhibitors* such as acetazolamide inhibit proximal sodium bicarbonate absorption, resulting in metabolic acidosis. *Primary hyperparathyroidism* also reduces the apparent bicarbonate threshold in the proximal tubule; mild degrees of hyperchloremic acidosis are commonly noted in patients with this disorder.

Gastrointestinal bicarbonate wasting can occur in several circumstances. Both pancreatic and small bowel secretions are rich in bicarbonate; pancreatic fluid, for example, has a pH of approximately 8.0. Hence *diarrheal states* and *ileal drainage* can result in significant bicarbonate losses. *Ureterosigmoidostomy* results in metabolic acidosis because the colon can secrete bicarbonate in exchange for chloride. Thus in patients with this surgical procedure, urine reaching the colon is alkalinized by bicarbonate exchange for chloride, thereby producing a net bicarbonate loss.

Failure of Bicarbonate Regeneration. The second major group of disorders producing hyperchloremic acidosis includes those disorders in which the ability of the distal nephron to regenerate bicarbonate is impaired. Three different tubular disorders account for the majority of cases of renal hyperchloremia encountered clinically. *Classic gradient-limited renal tubular acidosis* is a tubular disorder in which proton secretion may be normal, but because the distal tubule is unable to maintain a steep urine to blood proton concentration gradient, secreted protons are recycled back to blood. The administration of large quantities of phosphate salts permits the excretion of large amounts of titratable acid in this disorder, because the pH of the phosphate buffer system is 6.8, that is, relatively high. Potassium wasting and hypokalemia are common in distal gradient-limited renal tubular acidosis, owing at least in part to secondary hyperaldosteronism stimulated by sodium wasting.

In *hyporeninemic hypoaldosteronism*, which generally occurs in association with interstitial disease, the distal tubular derangements include diminished rates of sodium absorption and diminished rates of proton and potassium secretion. Aldosterone secretion is impaired. Consequently, sodium wasting and hyperkalemic, hyperchloremic acidosis are the hallmarks of this disorder. Diuretics such as *triamterene spironolactone*, and

TABLE 75–14. MAJOR CAUSES OF METABOLIC ACIDOSIS

Normal Anion Gap	Increased Anion Gap
I. Bicarbonate Loss	I. Reduced Excretion of Inorganic Acids
Proximal renal tubular acidosis	Renal failure
Dilutional acidosis	II. Accumulation of Organic Acids
Carbonic anhydrase inhibitors	Lactic acidosis
Primary hyperparathyroidism	Ketoacidosis: alcoholic
Diarrheal states	diabetic
Small bowel drainage	starvation
Ureterosigmoidostomy	Ingestion: salicylates
II. Failure of Bicarbonate Regeneration	paraldehyde
Distal, gradient-limited renal tubular acidosis	methanol
Hyporeninemic hypoaldosteronism	ethylene glycol
Diuretics: triamterene, spironolactone	
III. Acidifying Salts	
Ammonium chloride	
Lysine hydrochloride	
Arginine hydrochloride	
Parenteral hyperalimentation	

amiloride, which interfere with distal tubular sodium absorption, proton secretion, and potassium secretion, also result in hyperkalemic, hyperchloremic metabolic acidosis (Table 75–5).

Finally, *voltage-dependent renal tubular acidosis,* also known as hyperkalemic tubular acidosis, is a disorder characterized by an impaired ability of the distal nephron to absorb sodium and by an inability to secrete either potassium or protons. The latter two secretory deficits appear to be secondary to the defect in sodium absorption, which diminishes the magnitude of the lumen-negative transepithelial voltage in those nephron segments. Aldosterone secretion is normal.

Table 75–13 provides a summary of the distinguishing features of the three renal tubular acidosis syndromes. It should be noted that when hyporeninemic hypoaldosteronism is associated with extensive interstitial disease, the ability to increase urinary potassium excretion or decrease urinary pH in response to furosemide may be blunted.

Acidifying Salts. The third major group of conditions producing hyperchloremic acidosis includes the administration of *acidifying salts,* such as ammonium hydrochloride, lysine hydrochloride, or arginine hydrochloride. In each instance, metabolism of the ammonium or of the amino acids leads to hydrochloric acid formation. *Parenteral hyperalimentation* without the administration of adequate amounts of bicarbonate or bicarbonate-yielding solutes (such as lactate or acetate) can also produce hyperchloremic metabolic acidosis. The acidosis occurs because the synthetic amino acids used in hyperalimentation mixtures contain positively charged amino acids, such as arginine, lysine, and histidine, which yield proton equivalents when metabolized.

INCREASED ANION GAP METABOLIC ACIDOSIS. Metabolic acidoses characterized by an increased anion gap occur either because the kidneys fail to excrete inorganic acids, such as phosphate or sulfate, or because there is net accumulation of organic acids.

Reduced Acid Excretion. Renal failure, either acute or chronic, results in metabolic acidosis with an increased anion gap due to retention of sulfates and phosphates. In chronic renal failure metabolic acidosis occurs because the net amount of ammonium excreted daily falls as functional renal mass diminishes. The plasma bicarbonate concentration in most patients with chronic renal failure ranges between 16 and 20 mEq per liter. Although this degree of acidosis appears relatively modest, the daily acid load is buffered by bone salts; this buffering may contribute to the osteopenia of chronic renal failure (Ch. 237). In acute tubular necrosis, acidosis occurs because of generalized tubular dysfunction, including impaired net acid excretion. The plasma bicarbonate level generally remains above 16 mEq per liter unless sepsis, profound hypoxia, or extensive tissue necrosis complicates the disorder.

Organic Acid Accumulation. Accumulation of organic acids represents the second major cause for metabolic acidosis with an increased anion gap and is the most common cause for acute metabolic acidosis. Normally, the complete combustion of carbohydrates and fatty acids to carbon dioxide and water is highly efficient and results in the production of approximately 22,000 mEq of hydrogen ion per day. Thus, the lungs eliminate, as expired carbon dioxide, more than 300 times as much acid as the 70 mEq of fixed acid excreted daily by the kidneys as titratable acid plus ammonia. Processes that impair cellular respiration, and therefore result in nonvolatile rather than volatile acid production, lead to profound metabolic acidosis. In these circumstances, the interplay of four cardinal factors determines the magnitude of the anion gap acidosis.

The first two of these factors are insulin and glucagon, and the interplay between these two hormones. In disorders such as diabetic ketoacidosis or starvation, insulin lack accelerates lipolysis while aerobic glycolysis is impaired. Concomitantly, glucagon increases augment ketogenesis by the liver.

The third variable is the rate of cellular respiration, which in practical terms is determined by the rate of tissue perfusion with oxygen and the functional state of mitochondria. Lactic acidosis due to hypoperfusion or phenformin therefore is an anion gap acidosis caused by impaired cellular respiration.

The last factor determining the magnitude of the anion gap for such conditions is the extent of renal perfusion, which in turn

regulates the proximal renal tubular threshold for organic acid excretion. Thus in diabetic ketoacidosis, volume expansion with normal saline can convert a large anion gap acidosis to a normal anion gap acidosis, not by correcting the underlying metabolic derangement, which requires insulin, but simply by increasing the rate of renal organic acid excretion.

The syndrome of *lactic acidosis* results from impaired cellular respiration. Lactic acid is produced in muscle, red blood cells, and other tissues as a consequence of anaerobic glycolysis. Lactic acid oxidation involves reduction of nicotine adenine dinucleotide (NAD) by lactic acid dehydrogenase (LDH) according to the following reaction:

$$\text{Lactate} + \text{NAD} \xrightleftharpoons{\text{LDH}} \text{pyruvate} + \text{NADH}$$

Cellular respiration involves mitochondrial oxidation of pyruvate and NADH to carbon dioxide and water. When lactic acidosis occurs because of impaired cellular respiration, the lactate to pyruvate ratio (L/P) rises, as does the NADH/NAD ratio. Thus glycolysis in a setting of impaired cellular respiration results in increased production of nonvolatile lactic acid. Lactic acidosis should not be confused with states in which serum lactate levels are elevated with normal L/P and NADH/NAD ratios, as, for example, in vigorous exercise. Lactic acidosis is also characterized by negative serum nitroprusside (Acetest) reactions, since Acetest tablets react with acetoacetic acid and acetone, but not with lactic acid or beta-hydroxybutyric acid. In lactic acidosis the beta-hydroxybutyric acid/acetoacetic acid ratio is elevated in parallel with the increased NADH/NAD ratio.

Lactic acidosis occurs most commonly in disorders characterized by inadequate oxygen delivery to tissues, such as shock, septicemia, and profound hypoxemia. Drug-induced lactic acidosis may occur with phenformin therapy and isoniazid toxicity; in both circumstances, oxygen utilization by tissues is thought to be impaired. Lactic acidosis also occurs in association with leukemia and diabetes mellitus. A negative serum Acetest reaction in patients with diabetes acidosis is a valuable clue to the coexistence of diabetic ketoacidosis and lactic acidosis. There is also a spontaneous, idiopathic form of lactic acidosis in debilitated patients, which is almost uniformly fatal.

A second group of disorders characterized by an anion gap metabolic acidosis includes those disorders in which cellular respiration may not be impaired, but accelerated rates of organic acid production, particularly from lipolysis, result in an increased anion gap. *Alcoholic ketoacidosis* occurs in patients with chronic alcoholism and a recent history of binge drinking, little or no food intake, and recurrent vomiting. Hypoglycemia may be present. The major pathogenic mechanism for alcoholic ketoacidosis is accelerated lipolysis and hepatic ketoacid production because of relative decreases and increases in the secretion rates for insulin and glucagon, respectively. The Acetest reaction is variably positive, and the beta-hydroxybutyrate/acetoacetate ratio is elevated. Lactate utilization is diminished in this disorder. Patients with alcoholic ketoacidosis have beta-hydroxybutyric acid, rather than lactic acid, as the principal nonvolatile acid. *Diabetic ketoacidosis* is the most common cause of metabolic acidosis with an increased anion gap and occurs because of increased rates of ketogenesis due to insulin lack and inadequate carbohydrate combustion. *Starvation* produces metabolic acidosis by essentially the same mechanism: increased hepatic ketogenesis with reduced caloric intake. Thus in a general sense, alcoholic ketoacidosis, diabetic ketoacidosis, and starvation share at least one common feature: accelerated lipolysis and ketogenesis due to a relative insulin lack coupled with a relative glucagon excess.

Finally, a number of ingested substances result in severe metabolic acidosis with a large anion gap. *Salicylism* produces a complex set of acid-base abnormalities. Salicylates stimulate ventilation through central mechanisms; the decrease in Pa_{CO_2} then results in reductions in plasma bicarbonate concentrations. Since salicylate is a relatively strong acid, the ingestion of large quantities of salicylate can, by itself, contribute to metabolic acidosis and an increased anion gap. Salicylates also interfere with mitochondrial function. As a consequence, a number of as yet unidentified organic acids accumulate in serum and are the major factors responsible for the anion gap acidosis of salicylism.

A number of other agents, including *paraldehyde, methanol,* and *ethylene glycol*, also produce severe metabolic acidosis with organic acid accumulation. In methanol poisoning, formic acid (an end-product of methanol metabolism) accounts in large part for the reduction in serum bicarbonate concentration. In ethylene glycol intoxication, glycolic and lactic acid accumulation accounts for the majority of the reduction in plasma bicarbonate level; however, oxalate deposition in tissues is clearly a major factor in ethylene glycol toxicity. The organic acids responsible for an increased anion gap in paraldehyde intoxication have not been identified.

DIAGNOSIS AND TREATMENT. The diagnosis of metabolic acidosis requires analysis of serum electrolytes and, when indicated, measurement of arterial pH and Pa_{CO_2}. A cardinal clinical manifestation of metabolic acidosis is hyperventilation, which, when severe, is manifest as Kussmaul's respiration. In patients with chronic metabolic acidosis, however, hyperventilation may be difficult to detect clinically.

Severe metabolic acidosis exerts a negative inotropic effect on the heart, which depends, at least in part, on the fact that acidosis diminishes tissue responsiveness to catecholamines. Thus in lactic acidosis, negative inotropy sets the stage for a potentially lethal chain of events: poor tissue perfusion → lactic acidosis → decreased cardiac function → further reduction in tissue perfusion.

Acidosis also affects the delivery of oxygen to tissues. In acidosis, the Bohr effect shifts the oxyhemoglobin dissociation curve to the right. This compensatory mechanism permits the delivery of oxygen to inadequately perfused tissues. However, the protective characteristics of the Bohr effect may be offset by the effect of pH variation on red blood cell 2,3-diphosphoglycerate (2,3-DPG). Increases in red cell 2,3-DPG also shift the oxyhemoglobin dissociation curve to the right. However, acidosis tends to reduce red blood cell 2,3-DPG; this may offset partially the compensatory Bohr effect and therefore aggravate inadequate tissue oxygenation in acidosis.

Since metabolic acidosis is a manifestation of a variety of different diseases, the treatment of metabolic acidosis varies, depending on the underlying process and on the acuteness and severity of the acidosis. Certain general principles serve as useful guidelines for therapy. Those disorders characterized by *failure of bicarbonate regeneration* or *reduced excretion of inorganic acids* represent acidoses in which the kidneys fail to excrete a normal load of nonvolatile acid or, in other words, fail to regenerate approximately 70 mEq of bicarbonate daily. Thus the treatment of these metabolic acidoses requires removal of the offending agent, if patients are receiving triamterene or spironolactone, and the administration of relatively modest amounts of bicarbonate. In chronic renal failure, alkali therapy is generally not required unless the plasma bicarbonate level falls below 16 to 18 mEq per liter. If the acidosis is more severe, bicarbonate supplementation in the form of Shohl's solution (see below) may be instituted. Caution should be exercised to avoid sodium overload or the appearance of tetany, if overalkalinization occurs.

In distal, gradient-limited renal tubular acidosis, the administration of 30 to 60 mEq of bicarbonate daily, either as sodium bicarbonate tablets or as Shohl's solution, usually corrects the acidosis. A 650-mg sodium bicarbonate tablet provides 7.7 mEq of bicarbonate. Shohl's solution is a mixture of sodium citrate and citric acid; 1 ml of Shohl's solution yields the equivalent of 1 mmol of sodium bicarbonate. The cost of sodium bicarbonate, either as tablets or as common baking soda, is considerably less than that of Shohl's solution.

Potassium supplementation is also required in treatment of the disorder. In children with distal renal tubular acidosis, greater quantities of bicarbonate, in the range of 5 to 14 mEq of alkali per kilogram per day, are usually required to avoid growth retardation.

The therapy of patients with metabolic acidosis due to *external bicarbonate loss* varies with the nature of the disorder. As indicated above, sodium restriction, and an attendant rise in the apparent bicarbonate threshold, may be helpful in treating proximal renal tubular acidosis. In acute metabolic acidosis due to gastrointestinal losses, the net bicarbonate deficit may be roughly calculated, as indicated previously, from the reduction in "bicarbonate space," or total body buffering capacity, as follows:

$$(24 \text{ mEq/L} - \text{measured plasma HCO}_3^-) \times 0.6 \text{ body weight (kg)}$$

Bicarbonate therapy should be instituted when the arterial pH falls below 7.1. It is prudent to administer sufficient sodium bicarbonate intravenously to raise the plasma bicarbonate concentration to 16 mEq per liter over a 12- to 24-hour interval, rather than to repair the entire bicarbonate deficit. Calculation of the bicarbonate deficit in this manner is valid only if there are no further bicarbonate losses. If the latter persist, as in cholera or other types of secretory diarrhea, the daily amount of bicarbonate given to maintain the plasma bicarbonate concentration in the range of 16 mEq per liter may actually exceed the calculated bicarbonate space.

The treatment of acidoses due to *accumulation of organic acids* varies with the disorder. In *lactic acidosis*, therapy should be directed toward improving tissue perfusion. Because the disorder results from a failure of conversion of lactic acid and other organic acids to carbon dioxide and water, large amounts of sodium bicarbonate, sometimes in excess of 1000 mEq per 24-hour period, have been used in attempts to avoid lethal acidosis.

The treatment is complicated by the fact that the response to alkali therapy is not predictable. In experimental lactic acidosis, dichloroacetate can raise arterial pH by suppressing endogenous lactic acid production, but bicarbonate therapy worsens the disorder by increasing the rate of splanchnic bed lactate production. Moreover, large amounts of sodium bicarbonate (in the form of ampules containing 44.5 mmol of sodium bicarbonate per 50 ml) can produce cellular shrinkage due to hypertonicity and circulatory overload due to ECF volume expansion. Finally, in controlled clinical trials in patients with lactic acidosis, sodium bicarbonate therapy has failed to improve circulatory dynamics when compared with equimolar sodium chloride therapy.

The treatment of *alcoholic ketoacidosis* generally requires only the administration of saline solutions and glucose. Alkali therapy should not be used unless the metabolic acidosis is in the lethal range. The same considerations apply to starvation ketosis. The insulin release provoked by glucose administration suppresses lipolysis and consequently the overproduction of keto acids.

In *diabetic ketoacidosis*, insulin therapy promotes glucose utilization and, consequently, complete oxidation of keto acids; simultaneously, ketogenesis is reduced. Therefore alkali therapy is ordinarily not required in the disorder. Furthermore, because the hyperventilatory response to acidosis in some diabetic patients is governed by arterial rather than central medullary chemoreceptors, intravenous sodium bicarbonate administration may result in arterial alkalinization, a reduction in the rate of minute ventilation, and a potentially lethal fall in CSF pH. Sodium bicarbonate therapy in diabetic ketoacidosis should therefore be reserved for initial therapy of the disorder when the arterial pH is below 7.0 to 7.1 and cardiac contractility is impaired. Finally, because *salicylates*, *methanol*, and *ethylene glycol* are by themselves tissue toxins, appropriate therapy for ingestion of these toxins includes not only alkalinization but also hemodialysis for removal of the offending agent. Ethanol can be administered to slow the rate of metabolism of methanol to formic acid.

METABOLIC ALKALOSIS

ETIOLOGY AND PATHOGENESIS. The maintenance of the plasma bicarbonate concentration depends on renal bicarbonate reabsorption and renal bicarbonate regeneration (that is, net acid excretion). Consequently, although metabolic alkalosis may be *initiated* by the loss of hydrogen ion from the body—for example, during gastric drainage—the *maintenance* of a sustained metabolic alkalosis requires that the net rate of renal bicarbonate reabsorption or renal bicarbonate generation, or both, be greater than normal. In other words, a steady-state elevation of plasma bicarbonate concentrations to levels greater than 24 mEq per liter requires increased activity of one or more of the effector mechanisms regulating bicarbonate handling by renal tubules. In normal individuals it is therefore difficult to produce metabolic alkalosis by simple alkali loading.

Table 75–15 lists the major clinical causes of metabolic alkalosis. The table includes two disorders in which the apparent threshold for proximal bicarbonate reabsorption is increased, namely, volume contraction and potassium depletion, and disorders that increase net bicarbonate regeneration, including increased rates

TABLE 75–15. MAJOR MECHANISMS FOR METABOLIC ALKALOSIS

ECF volume concentration
Potassium depletion
Increased distal salt delivery
Mineralocorticoid excess
Liddle's syndrome
Bicarbonate loading (posthypercapnic alkalosis)
Delayed conversion of administered organic acids

of distal salt delivery and mineralocorticoid excess, either primary or as a consequence of volume contraction. Table 75–15 also lists Liddle's syndrome, in which the pathogenesis of alkalosis is obscure.

Volume contraction can sustain metabolic alkalosis because of an increase in the apparent rate of bicarbonate reabsorption by the proximal tubule. The most common cause for initiating this kind of alkalosis is hydrochloric acid loss caused by vomiting or gastric suction. In the early stages of gastric fluid losses, there is a modest sodium bicarbonate diuresis, but urinary sodium chloride excretion is reduced. As volume contraction becomes increasingly severe, sodium conservation occurs and potassium bicarbonate is excreted in an attempt to maintain pH homeostasis. Finally, when potassium depletion becomes severe, urinary sodium plus potassium excretion is sharply reduced and paradoxical aciduria occurs: The urine is acidic while the plasma bicarbonate level and pH are both elevated. *Contraction alkalosis* is a frequently misunderstood term; the designation should be reserved for those patients in whom metabolic alkalosis has developed and volume contraction maintains the alkalosis by increasing the apparent proximal tubular threshold for bicarbonate reabsorption. Thus contraction alkalosis is a mirror image of the dilutional acidosis listed in Table 75–14.

Potassium depletion from any cause, when sufficiently severe, can sustain metabolic alkalosis initiated by acid loss, for example, during gastric drainage. Presumably, potassium loss from cells is accompanied by increased hydrogen ion concentrations within cells, including renal tubular cells. Thus potassium depletion, when sufficiently severe, can raise the rate of renal tubular bicarbonate reabsorption and hence maintain a metabolic alkalosis. Consequently, when serum potassium concentrations are reduced to about 2 mEq per liter, metabolic alkalosis due to gastric fluid loss becomes saline resistant but responsive to potassium chloride administration.

Situations in which there occurs *enhanced delivery of sodium chloride* to terminal nephron segments enhance renal acid excretion and therefore lead to metabolic alkalosis by increasing the rate of renal bicarbonate generation. This effect occurs with loop diuretics (Table 75–5), such as furosemide or ethacrynic acid, and with the proximal tubular diuretic metolazone. These diuretics also contribute to the maintenance of metabolic alkalosis by contracting ECF volume and by promoting potassium depletion. Salt wasting is common in *Bartter's syndrome;* metabolic alkalosis due to renal bicarbonate generation is therefore a common feature of the disorder. The administration of large amounts of *impermeant anions* such as carbenicillin also favors distal hydrogen ion secretion. Thus carbenicillin therapy is one of the few circumstances in which an increased anion gap and metabolic alkalosis can be produced simultaneously by the same agent.

Mineralocorticoid excess, either primary or secondary, can also result in metabolic alkalosis because of renal bicarbonate generation. The disorder can occur in volume-expanded patients, as, for example, in primary hyperaldosteronism, in which the alkalosis is unresponsive to sodium chloride loading; and in patients with a reduced ECV and secondary hyperaldosteronism. The alkalosis of mineralocorticoid excess occurs primarily because of increased generation of bicarbonate by terminal nephron segments (or, in other words, by increased renal acid excretion) and is clearly accentuated by potassium depletion. *Liddle's syndrome* is a disorder of unknown cause in which metabolic alkalosis, hypokalemia, and hypertension occur because of an increase in sodium avidity by terminal nephron segments, which can be blocked by triamterene therapy.

When viewed in this context, the disorders listed in Table 75–15, with the exception of posthypercapnic alkalosis, result in metabolic alkalosis by two general kinds of mechanisms. First, metabolic alkalosis may be initiated by a loss of acid from nonrenal sources, for example, gastric fluid loss; and the kidney maintains the metabolic alkalosis by raising the rate of proximal tubular bicarbonate reabsorption. This is the primary mechanism responsible for the alkalosis associated with ECF volume contraction or potassium depletion. Second, the generation of metabolic alkalosis may occur intrarenally, because of increased rates of renal bicarbonate generation (or net acid excretion). This appears to be the major factor responsible for the alkalosis accompanying increased rates of salt delivery to the terminal nephron, mineralocorticoid excess, and Liddle's syndrome. Obviously, there may be considerable degrees of overlap. For example, loop diuretics increase rates of salt delivery to terminal nephron segments and therefore enhance bicarbonate generation. However, these agents also produce hypokalemia and ECF volume contraction and as a consequence raise the apparent threshold for bicarbonate reabsorption. Similarly, in primary aldosteronism, increased distal nephron bicarbonate generation as a cause for alkalosis is accentuated by the effects of hypokalemia on bicarbonate reabsorption.

In normal circumstances it is nearly impossible to produce metabolic alkalosis by increasing dietary alkali intake. In certain situations, however, *bicarbonate loading* can produce either a transient or a steady-state alkalosis. One such circumstance is *posthypercapnic alkalosis.* Patients with chronic hypercapnia develop compensatory increases in plasma bicarbonate concentrations: On an average, chronic hypoventilation results in a 0.3 to 0.5 mEq per liter rise in serum bicarbonate level for each 1.0 mm Hg increase in excess of a Pa_{CO_2} of 40 mm Hg. If ventilatory status is improved acutely, the Pa_{CO_2} will fall quickly but the plasma bicarbonate level will remain elevated, particularly if the patient is salt acquisitive because of congestive heart failure or ECF volume contraction. A common way to accentuate posthypercapnic alkalosis is to maintain patients on ventilators having high positive end-expiratory pressures (PEEP), which causes a central tourniquet effect that reduces cardiac output.

Delayed conversion of *accumulated organic acids* is a second mechanism for producing transient metabolic alkalosis. This may occur after insulin therapy for diabetic ketoacidosis, during the recovery phase of lactic acidosis, and following high-efficiency hemodialysis. In the last-named circumstance, acetate in the dialysis bath is taken up rapidly during dialysis. The accumulated acetate, which represents "potential bicarbonate," is then converted to bicarbonate after dialysis has been completed. Prolonged metabolic alkalosis because of alkali loading is a common feature of the *milk-alkali syndrome.* The alkalosis occurs because of prolonged ingestion of absorbable alkali in patients with impaired renal function due to hypercalcemic nephropathy. Frequent vomiting and attendant ECF volume contraction may also contribute to alkalosis in this disorder.

CLINICAL FEATURES AND DIAGNOSIS. There are no specific signs or symptoms of metabolic alkalosis. Relatively severe metabolic alkalosis can result in cardiac arrhythmias. Severe metabolic alkalosis can also result in severe hypoventilation, especially in patients with reduced renal function. Tetany and increased neuromuscular irritability, which are quite common in acute respiratory alkalosis, are very rare in chronic metabolic alkalosis. Rather, since hypokalemia generally accompanies metabolic alkalosis, muscular weakness and hyporeflexia are often seen in chronic metabolic alkalosis.

The diagnosis is inferred in most cases by routine measurements of serum electrolytes and can be confirmed by arterial blood gas analysis. Hypokalemia is generally present. The finding of an unexplained hypokalemic metabolic alkalosis is suggestive of the presence of Cushing's syndrome due to an extrarenal neoplasm.

The urinary chloride concentration is a useful index for distinguishing metabolic alkalosis due to volume contraction from that due to primary mineralocorticoid excess. In volume-contracted states, the urinary chloride concentration is generally less than 10 mEq per liter. Volume-contracted patients with Bartter's syndrome or volume-contracted patients taking diuretics generally have elevated urinary chloride concentrations. The combination of postural hypotension, hypokalemic metabolic alkalosis, and a urinary chloride concentration greater than 20 mEq per liter is therefore suggestive of diuretic abuse or Bartter's syndrome.

TREATMENT. In metabolic alkalosis associated with hypokalemia and volume contraction, appropriate therapy consists of volume expansion with saline solutions and of potassium replacement (see Disturbances in Potassium Balance). If the metabolic alkalosis is sufficiently severe that significant hypoventilation is present ($Pa_{CO_2} > 60$ mm Hg), the administration of dilute hydrochloric acid or other acidifying salts, such as lysine hydrochloride or arginine hydrochloride, may be required. The use of these amino acid salts carries with it the risk of hyperkalemia that is in excess of that expected simply from the change in arterial pH, presumably because these agents promote potassium efflux from cells. Ammonium chloride, lysine hydrochloride, or arginine hydrochloride should not be used in patients with significant liver disease.

If diuretic abuse can be identified, use of these agents should be discontinued. Indomethacin may partially correct the abnormalities of Bartter's syndrome, although potassium supplementation is almost invariably required. Triamterene is effective in preventing potassium wasting in Liddle's syndrome.

Hypokalemia and metabolic alkalosis due to primary hyperaldosteronism are best treated by potassium chloride supplementation, which tends to correct the metabolic alkalosis partially. Dietary sodium restriction in this disorder also tends to reduce renal potassium wasting. Of course, neither of these maneuvers provides definitive therapy for primary hyperaldosteronism.

MIXED METABOLIC DISORDERS

Mixed metabolic derangements occur commonly. Consequently, the evaluation of metabolic acid-base abnormalities depends on a simultaneous assessment of the anion gap, serum electrolytes, and, when appropriate, arterial blood gases. Electroneutrality requires that the sum of the principal anions in serum ($Cl^- + HCO_3^- +$ anion gap) equals the serum sodium level. Thus unless the serum sodium level changes, a change in the serum concentration of one or more of these principal anions necessitates a reciprocal change in the remaining anions.

Table 75–16 indicates the pattern of serum anion concentrations in single and mixed acid-base disorders. In the single acid-base disturbances, the change in the concentration of one anion is usually balanced by a reciprocal change in one other anion. For example, in hyperchloremic acidosis, the increase in chloride concentration equals the decrease in bicarbonate concentration.

In mixed disorders, the anion patterns are more complex. In a mixed metabolic alkalosis combined with an anion gap acidosis (e.g., diabetic ketoacidosis complicated by vomiting), the identifying pattern is an increased anion gap offset partially or entirely by a reduction in chloride; the serum bicarbonate level is variable. In an anion gap plus hyperchloremic acidosis, the reduction in bicarbonate is offset by increases in both chloride and the anion gap. Finally, in metabolic acidosis combined with hyperchloremic acidosis (e.g., vomiting combined with interstitial nephritis), offsetting changes in serum bicarbonate and chloride concentrations may result in normal anion concentrations.

TABLE 75–16. ANION PATTERNS IN METABOLIC ACID-BASE DISORDERS

Condition	Serum Anion Concentrations		
	HCO_3^-	Cl^-	Anion Gap
Simple Disorders			
Hyperchloremic acidosis	↓	↑	nl
Anion gap acidosis	↓	nl	↑
Metabolic alkalosis	↑	↓	nl
Mixed Disorders			
Metabolic alkalosis + anion gap acidosis	nl, ↑, or ↓	↓	↑
Anion gap acidosis + hyperchloremic acidosis	↓	↑	↑
Metabolic alkalosis + hyperchloremic acidosis	nl	nl	nl

nl = normal.

RESPIRATORY ACIDOSIS

ETIOLOGY AND PATHOGENESIS. Respiratory acidosis occurs whenever there is impairment in the rate of alveolar ventilation. Carbon dioxide elimination involves the following sequence: transfer of carbon dioxide from tissues to the lungs in the form of venous bicarbonate; formation of carbon dioxide within red blood cells by a reversal of the chloride shift, described previously in connection with tissue buffering mechanisms; perfusion of the lungs with systemic venous blood; diffusion of carbon dioxide from pulmonary capillaries to alveoli; and alveolar ventilation. Under normal circumstances, the rate of carbon dioxide hydration within red blood cells and the rate of carbon dioxide diffusion from pulmonary capillaries into alveoli are sufficiently rapid that carbon dioxide accumulation is virtually synonymous with hypoventilation.

Acute respiratory acidosis occurs when there is a sudden depression of the medullary respiratory center, as in narcotic overdose or anesthesia; when there is paralysis of the respiratory muscles, as in profound hypokalemia, neuromuscular disorders (myasthenia gravis), or the administration of agents that impair neuromuscular transmission (aminoglycoside antibiotics); when there is airway obstruction, as in foreign body aspiration or profound bronchospasm; when trauma, such as flail chest, impedes ventilation; and when an acute insult is imposed on a chronic hypercapnic state.

Chronic respiratory acidosis generally occurs in individuals with chronic bronchitis, emphysema, and bullous lung disease; in patients with extreme kyphoscoliosis; and in individuals with extreme obesity (pickwickian syndrome).

The arterial pH and plasma bicarbonate concentrations differ in acute and chronic respiratory acidosis. The compensatory response to carbon dioxide retention is to increase the apparent renal threshold for bicarbonate reabsorption. In general, the plasma bicarbonate concentration rises by approximately 0.3 to 0.5 mEq per liter for every millimeter of Hg increase in the Pa_{CO_2} over 40 mm Hg, until the Pa_{CO_2} reaches 80 mm Hg. This compensatory increase in plasma bicarbonate concentration requires 2 to 3 days for complete expression. Conversely, when chronic hypercapnia is relieved suddenly, there is a 2- to 3-day lag in renal bicarbonate excretion, resulting in posthypercapnic alkalosis.

These concepts are also useful in evaluating the possibility of mixed acid-base disorders occurring in association with respiratory acidosis. For example, since the rate of compensatory bicarbonate retention is delayed in acute respiratory acidosis, the presence of an elevated plasma bicarbonate concentration in a setting of acute carbon dioxide retention should be a clue to the simultaneous occurrence of acute respiratory acidosis and metabolic alkalosis. Similarly, because renal bicarbonate reabsorption is an effective compensatory mechanism for chronic carbon dioxide retention, plasma bicarbonate concentrations below 28 to 30 mEq per liter in patients having chronic Pa_{CO_2} values in excess of 50 mm Hg should alert one to the possible coexistence of acute metabolic acidosis and chronic respiratory acidosis.

Since hypercapnia is synonymous with alveolar hypoventilation, patients with carbon dioxide retention are invariably hypoxemic. A compensatory polycythemia occurs commonly in chronic hypercapnic states.

CLINICAL MANIFESTATIONS. The clinical manifestations of respiratory acidosis vary, depending on the severity of the disorder and on the rate at which carbon dioxide retention has occurred. Acute increases in Pa_{CO_2} values result in somnolence, in confusion, and ultimately in *carbon dioxide narcosis*. Asterixis may also be present. Because carbon dioxide is a cerebral vasodilator, the blood vessels in the optic fundi are often dilated, engorged, and tortuous; in severe hypercapnic states, frank papilledema may occur.

TREATMENT. The only practical treatment for acute respiratory acidosis involves treatment of the underlying disorder and ventilatory support. The possibility of drug abuse should always be considered in otherwise healthy patients who suddenly develop acute respiratory depression; consequently, naloxone (Narcan) therapy should be considered in all comatose patients seen in the emergency room in whom no apparent cause for respiratory depression can be identified.

In patients with chronic hypercapnia who develop sudden increases in Pa_{CO_2} values, attention should be directed toward identifying factors such as pneumonia or pulmonary embolism, which may have aggravated the underlying disorder. It should be emphasized again that oxygen therapy in patients with chronic hypercapnia should be instituted with extreme caution, since hypoxemia may be the primary stimulus to respiration in this setting. Consequently, in such patients, sudden increases in arterial Pa_{CO_2} produced by oxygen administration may result in cessation of respiration. The administration of alkalinizing salts has no place in the management of chronic respiratory acidosis.

RESPIRATORY ALKALOSIS

ETIOLOGY AND PATHOGENESIS. Respiratory alkalosis occurs when hyperventilation reduces the arterial Pa_{CO_2} and consequently increases arterial pH. Acute respiratory alkalosis is most commonly the result of the hyperventilation syndrome in anxiety. Acute hyperventilation may also occur because of damage to the respiratory centers; in acute salicylism; in fever and septic states; and in association with pneumonia, pulmonary emboli, or congestive heart failure. The disorder may also be produced iatrogenically by injudicious mechanical ventilatory support. Chronic hyperventilation occurs in the acclimation response to exposure to high altitudes (a low ambient oxygen tension), in advanced hepatic insufficiency, and in pregnancy.

During acute hyperventilation, plasma bicarbonate concentrations fall by approximately 3 mEq per liter when the Pa_{CO_2} falls to about 25 mm Hg. This fall in plasma bicarbonate level is due largely to proton shifts from the ICF to the ECF and tends to minimize acute changes in arterial pH. In chronic hyperventilation, renal bicarbonate loss provides the compensatory response to the reduction in Pa_{CO_2}. In experimental studies with dogs, approximately 2 to 4 days are required for a maximal renal compensatory response, which involves approximately a 0.4 mEq per liter reduction in plasma bicarbonate concentrations for every 1 mm Hg fall in Pa_{CO_2}.

Hyperventilation and respiratory alkalosis may also occur, as mentioned previously, following the correction of metabolic acidosis and particularly in diabetic ketoacidosis. In all likelihood, hyperventilation persists in this setting because of the lag in the rate at which plasma bicarbonate concentrations rise with respect to ECF bicarbonate concentrations during correction of metabolic acidosis.

CLINICAL MANIFESTATIONS AND TREATMENT. Chronic hyperventilation may be asymptomatic. The acute hyperventilation syndrome is characterized by light-headedness, paresthesias, circumoral numbness, and tingling of the extremities. Tetany occurs in severe cases. Both the acute metabolic alkalosis and the reduction in ionized calcium contribute to the increased neuromuscular excitability.

The treatment of acute respiratory alkalosis involves correction of the underlying disorder. When severe anxiety provokes the hyperventilation syndrome, air rebreathing with a paper bag generally terminates the acute attack. If this maneuver fails, sedation may also be required. If an individual is to be exposed to high altitude, 2 days of pretreatment with acetazolamide, 500 mg daily, will produce a mild metabolic acidosis that will offset the initial respiratory alkalosis on exposure to high altitude and thus minimize symptoms due to hyperventilation on initial exposure to high altitude.

Androgué HJ, Rashad MN, Gorin AB, et al.: Assessing acid-base status in circulatory failure. Differences between arterial and central venous blood. N Engl J Med 320:1312, 1989. *A comparison of arterial blood gases with central venous blood measurements.*

Batlle DC, Hizon M, Cohen E, et al.: The use of the urinary anion gap in the diagnosis of hyperchloremic metabolic acidosis. N Engl J Med 318:594, 1988. *An account of the urinary anion gap in renal tubular disorders. The data in Table 75–13 are adapted in part from this paper.*

Cooper DJ, Walley KR, Wiggs BR, et al.: Bicarbonate does not improve hemodynamics in critically ill patients who have lactic acidosis. Ann Intern Med 112:492, 1990. *This paper compares the effects of sodium chloride and those of sodium bicarbonate on pH balance and hemodynamics in critically ill patients with lactic acidosis.*

Feinstein EI (ed.): Severe metabolic acidosis in an intoxicated patient. Am J Nephrol 8:323, 1988. *An account of the metabolic acid-base derangements in licit and illicit alcohol ingestion*

Kitabchi AE, Murphy MB: Diabetic ketoacidosis and hyperosmolar hyperglycemic nonketotic coma. Med Clin North Am 72:1545, 1988. *A clinical summary of these two disorders.*

Kurtzman NA, Gonzalez J, DeFronzo R, et al.: A patient with hyperkalemia and metabolic acidosis. Am J Kidney Dis 15:333, 1990. *A concise account of the renal tubular disorders causing hyperkalemia and the diagnostic approach to these disorders.*

Madias NE: Lactic acidosis. Kidney Int 29:752, 1986. *A superb discussion of lactic acidosis.*

Norris SH, Kurtzman NA: Does chloride play an independent role in the pathogenesis of metabolic alkalosis? Semin Nephrol 8:101, 1988. *An analysis of the pathophysiology of metabolic alkalosis.*

Stacpoole PW, Lorenz AC, Thomas RG, et al.: Dichloroacetate in the treatment of lactic acidosis. Ann Intern Med 108:58, 1988. *The use of dichloroacetate in the treatment of lactic acidosis.*

Winter SD, Pearson JR, Gabow PA, et al.: The fall of the serum anion gap. Arch Intern Med 150:311, 1990. *A good summary of anion gap acidosis.*

76 Acute Renal Failure

Jared J. Grantham

DEFINITION

Acute renal failure is a syndrome characterized by a relatively rapid decline in renal function that leads to the accumulation of water, crystalloid solutes, and nitrogenous metabolites in the body. Clinically significant acute renal failure is usually associated with a daily increase in the serum creatinine and urea nitrogen levels (azotemia) greater than 0.5 and 10 mg per deciliter, respectively. *Oliguria*, a rate of urine flow less than 400 ml per day, may be observed, but in some cases the urine output may exceed this limit (*nonoliguric* acute renal failure). Complete cessation of urine flow, *anuria*, is relatively uncommon.

ETIOLOGY

Acute renal failure may be seen in a wide variety of clinical settings (Table 76–1). A systematic approach to the causes of acute renal failure facilitates diagnosis in the individual patient. It is important to remember that acute renal failure is a bilateral process, except in patients with only one functioning kidney.

Prerenal

Prerenal causes lead to renal failure by decreasing the effective perfusion of kidney parenchyma. An absolute decrease in blood volume (hypovolemia), the most common prerenal disorder, may be caused by skin, gastrointestinal, and renal losses of water and electrolytes, hemorrhage, and sequestration of fluids in body cavities. In some conditions the kidneys respond as though the blood volume were decreased, when in fact the measured volume is normal or even increased. These oliguric states include congestive heart failure (which may be precipitated by myocardial infarction or dysrhythmia), sepsis, anaphylaxis, and liver failure. Bilateral renal artery occlusion can occur spontaneously owing to emboli from the heart or from an atheromatous aorta. Embolism of atheroma may occur in the course of difficult surgical procedures involving the abdominal aorta.

Postrenal

Although quite rare, *bilateral ureteral obstruction* may be due to calculi, shed papillae in analgesic nephropathy, thrombus, neoplasms, and iatrogenic causes. Commonly in bilateral obstruction one kidney is blocked for several days or weeks before obstruction of the contralateral kidney causes acute renal failure. Acute ureteral obstruction of a solitary kidney is seen occasionally. Acute renal failure can be caused by *urethral obstruction* due to prostatic hypertrophy, prostatitis, bladder and prostate tumors, bladder rupture, calculi, and iatrogenic causes. In hospitalized patients with indwelling urinary catheters, the patency and correct placement of the catheter should always be checked in the evaluation of acute renal failure.

Bilateral renal venous occlusion is rare but may be seen in hypercoagulable states, with intra-abdominal neoplasms, or secondary to surgical procedures.

TABLE 76–1. CAUSES OF ACUTE RENAL FAILURE SYNDROME

Location of Primary Disorder	Clinical Examples
Prerenal	
Absolute decrease in effective blood volume	Hemorrhage, skin losses (burns, sweating), gastrointestinal losses (diarrhea, vomiting), renal losses (diuretics, glycosuria), fluid pooling (peritonitis, burns)
Relative decrease in blood volume (ineffective arterial volume)	Congestive heart failure, dysrhythmias, sepsis, anaphylaxis, liver failure
Arterial occlusion	Bilateral thromboembolism, thromboembolism of solitary kidney, aortic or renal artery aneurysm
Postrenal	
Ureteral obstruction	Bilateral or solitary kidney (calculi, neoplasm, clot, retroperitoneal fibrosis, iatrogenic)
Urethral obstruction	Prostatitis
Venous occlusion	Bilateral or solitary kidney (renal vein thrombosis, neoplasm, iatrogenic)
Intrarenal	
Vascular	Vasculitis, malignant hypertension, vasopressors, eclampsia, microangiopathy, hyperviscosity states, nonsteroidal anti-inflammatory drugs, hypercalcemia, iodinated radiocontrast agents
Glomerulus	Acute glomerulonephritis
Tubular injury	
Ischemia	Profound hypotension, postrenal transplant, vasopressors, microvascular constriction
Intratubular pigments	Hemoglobinuria, myoglobinuria
Intratubular proteins	Myeloma
Intratubular crystals	Uric acid, oxalate, sulfonamides, phenazopyridine hydrochloride
Tubulointerstitial	Interstitial nephritis due to drugs, infection, radiation
Nephrotoxins	Antibiotics (gentamicin, kanamycin, neomycin, amikacin, tobramycin, streptomycin, cephaloridine, amphotericin B); metals (mercury, bismuth, uranium, arsenic, silver, cadmium, iron, antimony); solvents (carbon tetrachloride, glycol, tetrachlorethylene); iodinated contrast agents; streptozotocin, cisplatin

Intrarenal

The renal arterial and arteriolar *blood vessels* may be involved in vasculitis, malignant hypertension, eclampsia, and microangiopathies. Pronounced vasospasm leading to acute renal failure may be seen in scleroderma, during systemic infusions of norepinephrine, secondary to the use of nonsteroidal anti-inflammatory compounds, iodinated radiocontrast agents, or diet pills, or in hypercalcemic states.

Glomerular inflammation (acute glomerulonephritis, Ch. 79) may cause acute renal failure by sharply reducing renal blood flow. *Renal tubules* are susceptible to a number of insults. *Ischemic* injury, sometimes progressing to frank necrosis, may be seen secondary to profound hypotension, especially in elderly persons. The term *acute tubular necrosis* (ATN) is frequently used to describe a clinical syndrome in which there is a simultaneous and progressive deterioration of glomerular and tubular function in the absence of documented glomerular or interstitial nephritis, vascular disease, or obstruction of the collecting system. In the vast majority of patients with ATN, the initiating event is either a decrease in renal plasma flow or exposure to a nephrotoxic agent. In spite of its wide usage, however, the term ATN is not a valid histologic description of the renal injury. In general, the term *acute renal failure* is to be preferred. Rarely, ischemia may be severe enough to cause irreversible necrosis of renal parenchyma. Kidneys transplanted from cadaver sources often undergo oliguric renal failure. The intravenous administration of powerful vasoconstrictors, such as norepinephrine, may

cause acute ischemic tubular injury in certain susceptible patients. Renal tubules are susceptible to injury by high levels of urinary pigments (hemoglobinuria, myoglobinuria), especially in the setting of renal hypoperfusion and ischemia. Several serum proteins are potentially nephrotoxic, including kappa and lambda light chains, which may be abundantly excreted in patients with multiple myeloma. Renal tubules may be occluded by uric acid, oxalate, sulfonamide, or pyridium crystals, leading to acute renal failure.

A wide variety of chemicals are potential tubular toxins. Antibiotics of the aminoglycoside class (one of the most common iatrogenic nephrotoxins), streptomycin, cephaloridine, and amphotericin all injure renal tubules when given in excessive doses. These agents are apparently nephrotoxic even at low therapeutic doses in patients who are oliguric or hypotensive or who have underlying renal disorders. The combined effects of aminoglycosides and certain cephalothin drugs appear to be additive in causing acute renal failure. Heavy metal poisoning is seen rarely but may cause acute tubular necrosis and renal failure. Iodinated radiocontrast agents may directly injure renal tubules in patients with underlying disorders such as diabetes mellitus, systemic lupus erythematosus, and chronic renal insufficiency from nearly any cause. Chemotherapeutic agents such as streptozotocin and cisplatin almost routinely cause acute renal injury that may progress to acute renal failure. Phencyclidine, a psychotropic agent, has caused acute renal failure in a few patients.

INCIDENCE

Acute renal failure is a relatively common syndrome. The incidence in the general outpatient population is not known; in one study about 5 per cent of patients on medical and surgical units in a general hospital experienced an episode of acute renal failure. Approximately 60 per cent of cases are related to surgery or trauma; the remainder have medical or obstetric causes. Overall, about one half of cases of acute renal failure in hospitalized patients may be iatrogenic.

PATHOGENESIS

Ischemia and nephrotoxins are the most common causes of acute renal failure listed in Table 76–1. There are at least three important phases in the acute renal failure syndrome due to ischemia or nephrotoxins. In the first, or *initiation*, phase the kidneys are subjected to an insult that produces parenchymal injury (e.g., temporary cessation of renal blood flow; nephrotoxins or pigments; see Table 76–1 and Fig. 76–1). In some patients who are hypovolemic, the initiation phase can be overridden by plasma volume expansion and the acute renal failure syndrome aborted. More commonly, however, the initiation phase causes profound renal vasoconstriction and an initial decrease in renal blood flow. The initiation phase is followed by the *maintenance* phase, during which renal vasoconstriction may persist, thereby decreasing the formation of glomerular filtrate. The hydraulic permeability of the glomeruli is usually decreased, diminishing further the ability of glomeruli to form filtrate. In addition to factors operating within the glomeruli, injury to renal tubules causes the cells to slough from the basement membranes to form casts that can obstruct urine flow. Moreover, the damaged epithelium of the tubules allows the small amount of glomerular filtrate that is formed to leak back into the peritubular capillaries. These four factors—vasoconstriction, decreased glomerular permeability, intratubular obstruction, and tubular back leak of filtrate (Figs. 76–1 and 76–2)—operate in concert to depress the effective glomerular filtration rate (GFR) in the ischemic and nephrotoxic types of acute renal failure listed in Table 76–1.

In some cases the renal blood flow may return to relatively normal levels 24 to 48 hours after the initiation phase. Despite this, the GFR remains very low owing to the decreased glomerular hydraulic permeability, tubular obstruction, or tubular back leak of filtrate.

The third stage in the pathogenetic sequence is the *recovery* phase. Healing of renal parenchyma and recovery of function may be expected in most types of acute renal failure.

CLINICAL MANIFESTATIONS

The onset of acute renal failure usually follows the initiating event by an interval varying from a few hours to as long as several

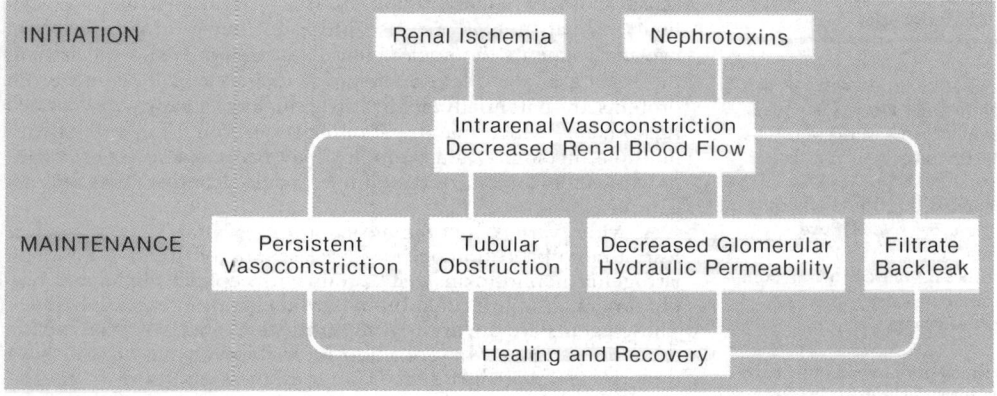

FIGURE 76–1. Pathogenesis of acute renal failure.

days. Patients and physicians usually first notice a reduction in urinary volume in the oliguric types of acute renal failure. Facial edema, tight-fitting rings, and weight gain reflect the retention of water. Rarely, pulmonary edema may be an initial manifestation. Renal pain is uncommon except in association with acute infection, urolithiasis, and tumors. Hematuria is seen in nephritic syndromes and vascular occlusive states but is uncommon in nephrotoxic and transient ischemic states.

The serum creatinine and urea levels rise steadily. In severely oliguric persons of average size, the serum creatinine level rises about 1.5 to 2.0 mg per deciliter per day. When the measured increase in serum creatinine exceeds this range, one should consider hypercatabolic factors; when the measured increase is less, renal clearance of creatinine may be greater than the rate of urine volume flow would suggest. The serum urea nitrogen level usually rises in concert with the creatinine level. However, urea production is altered by food intake, by tissue catabolism, and by blood within the intestines; consequently, the urea levels do not reflect the performance of the kidneys as well as do creatinine levels.

Hyperkalemia due to inadequate renal excretion of potassium may be life threatening early in the course of acute renal failure. Metabolic acidosis due to inadequate renal excretion of hydrogen ions is seen later on. Hyponatremia may be seen in patients who drink unlimited amounts of water or other fluids. Hypocalcemia, hyperphosphatemia, hyperuricemia, and anemia usually develop after several days unless there are mitigating factors, such as rhabdomyolysis and hemolysis. Serum amylase levels may be twice normal in the absence of pancreatitis.

The uremic syndrome develops gradually and, in addition to the features mentioned above, is characterized by the progressive development of anorexia, nausea, vomiting, nervous irritability, hyperreflexia, asterixis, seizures, and coma. Hemorrhagic signs include ecchymoses, gastric and colonic hemorrhage, and pericarditis.

DIAGNOSIS

When renal failure is recognized, it is important to determine the probable cause and remediable factors underlying kidney dysfunction. Table 76–2 lists several key components in the diagnostic approach to renal failure.

The initial objective is to determine whether the renal failure is acute or chronic. The diagnostic evaluation starts at the patient's bedside. With conversant ambulatory patients, the onset of renal dysfunction can usually be determined based on historical changes in urine output (oliguria, polyuria, nocturia), abnormal urine color, and changes in body weight. Chronic renal failure is further indicated by anemia, osteodystrophy, lipiduria, bilateral small kidneys, neuropathy, and a modestly elevated serum level of uric acid.

In the differential diagnosis of acute renal failure, it is important to distinguish among *prerenal, postrenal,* and *intrarenal* factors.

Prerenal Failure

Prerenal failure is suggested by a history of rapid weight loss, flu-like illness, lack of fluid ingestion, bleeding, nasogastric aspiration, diuretic therapy, or orthostatic dizziness. In prerenal failure due to *extracelluar fluid volume contraction,* the physical examination may reveal orthostatic hypotension and tachycardia, poor venous filling and a "thready" pulse, and peripheral vasoconstriction with cool extremities and dry mucous membranes. When prerenal failure occurs in *euvolemic* or *hypervolemic* patients, one usually finds signs of congestive heart failure or liver failure, including distended veins, a third heart sound, pulmonary rales and wheezes, ascites, jaundice, and peripheral edema.

Urinary indices (Table 76–3) show concentrated urine (relatively high specific gravity and osmolality), low fractional excretions of sodium and chloride, and a high urine to plasma creatinine ratio. Diuretics can diminish the diagnostic usefulness of urinary indices and should not be used prior to collecting urine for

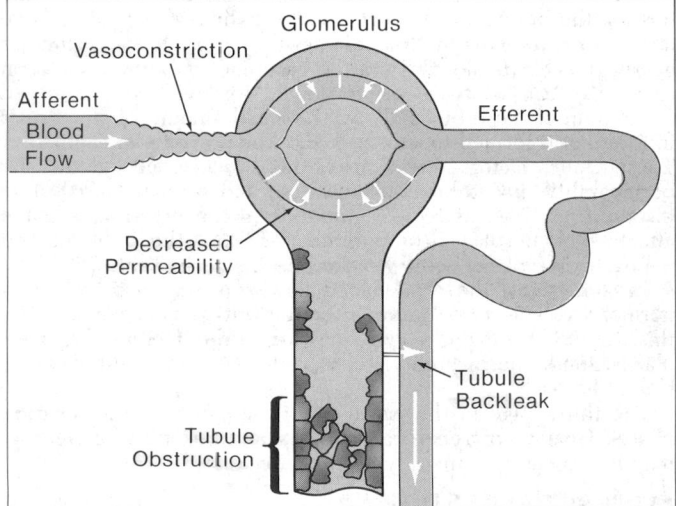

FIGURE 76–2. Possible mechanisms contributing to oliguria in acute renal failure.

TABLE 76–2. DIAGNOSTIC APPROACH TO RENAL FAILURE

1. Review of medical history, clinical setting, medications
2. Physical examination, including evaluation of hemodynamic status
3. Urinalysis, including careful sediment examination
4. Simultaneous chemical analysis of blood and urine. Osmolality, urea, creatinine, sodium, chloride, potassium, uric acid
5. Bladder catheterization
6. Fluid-diuretic challenge
7. Radiologic studies
   Ultrasonography
   Radioisotope scans (pertechnetate ^{99m}Tc, ^{131}I-hippurate)
   CT scan
   Pyeloureterography
     Intravenous pyelography
     Retrograde pyelography
     Antegrade (percutaneous) pyelography
8. Renal biopsy

TABLE 76-3. URINARY INDICES IN ACUTE RENAL FAILURE

Index	Prerenal	Acute Tubular Injury
Urinary osmolality, mOsm/kg H_2O	> 500	< 350
Urinary sodium, mEq/liter	< 20	> 40
Urinary/plasma creatinine	> 40	< 20
Fractional sodium excretion*	< 1	> 1

$$*\frac{Urine/Serum\ [Na]}{Urine/Serum\ [creatinine]} \times 100$$

analysis. Urinalysis and urinary sediment examination are usually unremarkable except for hyaline casts.

When the physical and chemical findings point to prerenal acute azotemia due to a *decrease in extracellular fluid volume*, a fluid challenge of 500 to 1000 ml of isotonic saline may stimulate urine formation in the average adult. In the author's opinion, mannitol and diuretics are contraindicated in volume-depleted patients with prerenal azotemia. In prerenal azotemia associated with an *expanded extracellular fluid volume*, diuretics may be indicated as part of the general plan to improve cardiac function.

Prerenal azotemia due to occlusion of renal arteries is revealed by radioisotope screening tests and arteriography. Urine output generally is scanty. Urinalysis may show hematuria and proteinuria, and urinary indices show an inability to concentrate urinary solutes (Table 76-3).

Postrenal Failure

Obstruction to the flow of urine may be acute or chronic (see Ch. 81). In most cases of acute obstruction of the *upper tract*, the patient notices pain in the flank or lower abdominal regions and fluctuating urine output. *Urethral* obstruction usually causes urinary frequency, dribbling, and lower abdominal fullness. In urinary tract obstruction, infected urine is commonly observed.

The onset of renal failure due to obstruction of the urinary drainage system can be difficult to determine. To cause renal failure, the urinary drainage from both kidneys must be compromised; alternatively, the patient may have only one kidney. Chronic progressive processes, such as retroperitoneal neoplasia, can obstruct the drainage of one ureter weeks or months before the contralateral ureter is obstructed. Obstructive uropathy should be suspected in patients with adenopathy, abdominal scars, palpable bladder, flank tenderness, prostatic enlargement, or pelvic masses with induration.

Urinary findings are nonspecific. The sediment contains leukocytes and erythrocytes in infected patients. The urinary indices are variable. In acute obstruction the indices are identical to those seen in prerenal failure; in obstructions more than 2 days in duration the indices are similar to those seen in intrarenal tubular injury (Tables 76-2 and 76-3).

Bladder catheterization may be diagnostic. With upper tract obstruction, ultrasonography in the hands of an experienced radiologist is the most useful diagnostic test. Rarely, acute obstruction of the urinary tract may occur without dilation of the renal pelvis and cannot be detected by sonography. The ^{131}I-hippurate scan is a noninvasive test that is useful for determining the number and placement of the kidneys and the potential for return of renal function in obstructive uropathy. Bilateral upper tract obstruction is usually nonsynchronous. In such cases the hippurate scan shows asymmetric accumulation of the isotope. The kidney showing the most intense uptake of hippurate is the best candidate for return of function after relief of obstruction. Intravenous pyelography is useful to localize the site of obstruction, but adequate renal function is needed to concentrate the contrast material in the urinary tract. Retrograde pyelography should be reserved for those cases in which the noninvasive methods are not available or those in which equivocal results have been obtained. In some cases the computed tomographic (CT) scan may provide anatomic confirmation of obstruction.

Occlusion of the renal veins is suggested by a history of a hypercoagulable state, pulmonary emboli, hematuria, or proteinuria. Urinary indices are not diagnostic. Radioisotope studies of renal perfusion may be suggestive, but definitive diagnosis depends on renal arteriography or venography.

Intrarenal Failure

Renal failure due to intrinsic dysfunction is suggested by a history of multisystem disease (e.g., systemic lupus erythematosus, vasculitis), fever, malaise, skin rash, hypertension, gross hematuria, hypotensive episode, or exposure to nephrotoxins.

The urinalysis is an invaluable guide in the diagnosis of intrarenal failure. Acute glomerulonephritis is characterized by hematuria, proteinuria, erythrocyte casts, and granular casts. Lipid bodies and broad waxy casts suggest a chronic process. Pus casts indicate acute or chronic interstitial inflammation. Urinary eosinophils are seen in allergic interstitial nephritis. Crystalluria is observed in urate and oxalate disorders. Physicians should be able to recognize these formed elements in the urine and should personally examine a freshly prepared urinary sediment. Acute inflammation of the preglomerular arterioles may or may not be associated with alterations in glomerular capillaries. In the absence of glomerular capillary inflammation, the urinalysis reflects ischemic tubular injury due to reduced renal blood flow. Acute tubular injury does not give specific urinary sediment findings, but celluluria, epithelial cell casts, and coarse granular casts should raise the index of suspicion.

Urinary indices (Table 76-3) are very helpful in differentiating between conditions that cause injury to preglomerular arterioles and glomeruli and those that cause acute tubular injury. In the former the indices show a prerenal pattern, whereas in acute tubular injury the fractional excretion of sodium is increased and the urinary osmolality approaches that of plasma. The conditions that may exhibit low or normal fractional sodium excretion at some point in the course of the acute renal failure syndrome are listed in Table 76-4.

Radiologic tests are relatively nonspecific in the evaluation of intrarenal failure. The ^{131}I-hippurate scan shows accumulation of isotope in both kidneys if some renal perfusion is preserved and viable tubules remain. Renal arteriography may show microaneurysm formation in polyarteritis nodosa. Renal biopsy is usually indicated in the evaluation of glomerulonephritis, vasculitis, or interstitial nephritis but is not commonly used when pyelonephritis or acute tubular injury is suspected.

TREATMENT

There are at least four major objectives in the treatment of acute renal failure: (a) correct the reversible causes, (b) prevent additional injury, (c) convert oliguric to nonoliguric renal failure, and (d) provide general metabolic support during the maintenance and recovery phases of the syndrome.

Correct Reversible Causes

Prerenal and postrenal factors contributing to renal function should be corrected insofar as is possible. Drugs that interfere with renal perfusion or that are directly nephrotoxic should be stopped. In hypotensive patients the blood pressure should be restored by discontinuing antihypertensive drugs and administering isotonic volume-expanding solutions. In elderly patients with longstanding hypertension, a "normal" blood pressure of 110/70 may in fact be inadequate to generate glomerular filtrate. If there is doubt about the status of the plasma volume, an intravenous challenge of isotonic saline (500 to 1000 ml) is warranted. Accident victims with crushed extremities may re-

TABLE 76-4. CONDITIONS ASSOCIATED WITH FRACTIONAL SODIUM EXCRETION LESS THAN 1 PER CENT IN ACUTE RENAL FAILURE SYNDROME

Intense Intrarenal Vasoconstriction
1. Iodinated radiocontrast
2. Acute bilateral ureteral obstruction
3. Severe burns
4. Sepsis
5. Pigment excretion (myoglobin, hemoglobin)
6. Nonsteroidal anti-inflammatory drugs
7. Amphotericin B
8. Norepinephrine, dopamine
9. Liver disease
10. Cardiopulmonary bypass

Vascular Inflammation
1. Acute glomerulonephritis
2. Acute vasculitis
3. Renal transplant rejection

quire several liters of isotonic saline when they are freed from entrapment. In the states listed in Table 76–4 associated with a low fractional sodium excretion due to intrarenal vasoconstriction, a volume challenge combined with 40 to 80 mg of intravenous furosemide may reverse the oliguric state and, in some cases, prevent the maintenance phase of acute renal failure.

Prevention of Additional Injury

Radiocontrast agents are potentially harmful to patients in the maintenance phase of acute renal failure, and alternative diagnostic methods should be used whenever possible. CT scans are often done with contrast enhancement, and physicians are not always aware of this "hidden" source of iodinated radiocontrast material. Nonsteroidal anti-inflammatory drugs and nephrotoxic antibiotics should be avoided if possible. Drug dosages should be adjusted according to guidelines for renal failure, and plasma drug levels should be monitored when possible.

Convert Oliguria to Nonoliguria

Oliguria in and of itself is not harmful, and a normal urinary flow rate does not accelerate the healing process in the acute renal failure syndrome. Nonetheless, the management of patients with acute renal failure is simplified, and the survival rate may be improved by converting oliguria to nonoliguria with diuretics and fluid administration. A trial of furosemide (2 to 10 mg per kilogram given intravenously) is warranted. If urine output exceeding 40 ml per hour is achieved, additional doses of diuretic may be given periodically.

General Support

Conservative management without dialysis may be adequate in many cases. Indwelling urinary catheters should be avoided in uncomplicated cases. Intermittent catheterization using careful sterile technique is usually sufficient in oliguric obtunded patients. In all patients careful attention to fluid status is crucial to successful management. Daily weight measured by a competent assistant or physician is essential in the evaluation of changes in fluid balance. Catabolic patients may be expected to lose about 0.5 kg per day. As a rule of thumb, patients can be allowed to drink a volume of fluid (water, tea, coffee) equal to 500 ml plus the amount of the preceding 24-hour urine output. In febrile patients this fluid limit can be increased. In anorectic patients the fluids are given intravenously.

Sodium, potassium, and chloride are not given to patients in the maintenance phase of acute renal failure, except coincidentally in the food they eat. This may amount to about 1 mEq per kilogram of Na, K, and Cl daily. Protein intake is restricted to 0.7 to 1.0 gram per kilogram of body weight per day and is principally composed of foods high in essential amino acid content. Carbohydrates and fats are given to ensure an adequate caloric intake. In patients who cannot eat, intravenous infusion of essential amino acids and glucose may be necessary, but this regimen contributes a considerable fluid load.

In addition to measurements of daily weight, fluid intake and fluid output, serial determinations of blood pressure (supine and upright), serum electrolytes, creatinine, urea nitrogen, and blood hematocrit are essential for patient management. Hyperkalemia exceeding 6 mEq per liter is a potentially serious complication that can be handled temporarily by ingestion of polystyrene sulfonate exchange resin (25 to 50 grams) in a solution containing sorbitol. Electrocardiographic changes showing widened QRS complexes or atrioventricular (AV) dissociation demand immediate treatment with intravenous sodium bicarbonate (88 mmole), glucose and insulin (25 units regular insulin per liter of 10 per cent glucose), and calcium gluconate (10 per cent solution, 10 to 30 ml). These measures will generally control the serum potassium level until dialysis can be initiated. (See Ch. 75 for a discussion of hyperkalemia.)

Dialysis may be necessary in certain patients in the maintenance phase of acute renal failure. The indications for dialysis include severe hyperkalemia (serum K^+ > 6.5 mEq per liter after treatment), severe metabolic acidosis (serum bicarbonate < 10 mEq per liter after bicarbonate therapy), pulmonary edema due to fluid overload, progressive azotemia (urea nitrogen > 100, creatinine > 10 mg per deciliter), encephalopathy, seizures, bleeding diathesis, pericarditis, and uremic enteropathy.

In uncomplicated cases, peritoneal dialysis may be the most suitable method of treatment. This procedure avoids the wide shifts in blood volume and blood solute composition encountered in hemodialysis, and anticoagulants are not used. Peritoneal dialysis can be used for prolonged treatment if recovery of renal function is slow.

In many cases, one must remove solutes and water from the blood faster than can be achieved by peritoneal dialysis. Also, patients with acute renal failure frequently have pre-existing abdominal injuries. In such cases hemodialysis is the preferred dialytic method. One has rapid access to the circulation by percutaneous catheterization of femoral or subclavian veins. In hemorrhagic states, systemic heparinization is not feasible, and regional anticoagulation with citrate or prostacyclin may be necessary.

PROGNOSIS

The prognosis for recovery must be viewed from at least two perspectives: (1) patient survival and (2) recovery of renal function.

Patient Survival

With the advent of modern dialysis techniques, few if any patients with the acute renal failure syndrome die of uremia. Death is usually a consequence of the underlying disease that caused the acute renal failure or is secondary to trauma and/or sepsis. The mortality rate in traumatized septic patients with acute renal failure is disturbingly high (40 to 80 per cent).

Recovery of Renal Function

The prognosis for recovery of renal function depends on the nature of the underlying disorder that initiated the renal dysfunction. All acute renal failure due to prerenal causes is potentially reversible. In postrenal failure, renal function may be expected to stabilize or improve significantly if the obstruction is relieved.

Acute renal failure due to intrarenal causes has a variable outcome. Glomerulonephritis and vasculitis may respond to immunosuppressive therapy, with complete recovery of renal function. Acute renal failure due to renal tubular injury is usually reversible, provided that the cause of ischemia is removed or nephrotoxins are avoided. Recovery of renal function to near-normal levels is more likely in nonoliguric than in oliguric patients, and in subjects who have strong images on the ^{131}I-hippurate renal scan. The duration of the period of poor renal function is highly variable. Recovery of renal function takes longer in elderly patients than in young persons. Recovery is also prolonged in patients who develop acute renal failure in addition to a chronic renal disorder that compromises baseline function.

The major improvements in renal function usually appear in the first and second weeks after the beginning of the recovery phase. Some mild defects in renal function may persist for months or years after a bout of acute tubular injury.

PREVENTION

The opportunity for major prevention of acute renal failure is in the hands of physicians and surgeons. A few simple measures will diminish the incidence of acute renal failure acquired in the hospital: (1) Patients should be adequately hydrated before receiving iodinated radiocontrast material. (2) Adequate hydration is necessary before certain surgical procedures, specifically repair of abdominal aortic aneurysm and renal transplantation. (3) Adequate hydration is essential before and during chemotherapy using cisplatin and streptozotocin. (4) Pretreatment with allopurinol before chemotherapy of massive tumors will diminish uric acid excretion. (5) Nonsteroidal anti-inflammatory drugs should be avoided in patients with renal diseases. (6) Nephrotoxic antibiotics should be avoided or carefully monitored.

Better, OS, Stein JH: Early Management of shock and prophylaxis of acute renal failure in traumatic rhabdomyolysis. N Engl J Med 322:825, 1990. *Seismic catastrophes entrap victims, leading to rhabdomyolysis and acute renal failure. The critical role of fluid therapy is emphasized in this timely article.*

Brezis M, Rosen S, Epstein FH: Acute renal failure. In Brenner BM, Rector FC Jr (eds.): The Kidney. 3rd ed. Philadelphia, W. B. Saunders Company, 1986, pp 735–799. *This is an exhaustive compendium with 1003 references.*

Harwood TH, Hiesterman DR, Robinson RG, et al.: Prognosis for recovery of function in acute renal failure. Arch Intern Med 136:916, 1976. *A simple noninvasive radioisotope test (^{131}I-hippurate) is shown to be useful in judging the prognosis for recovery of renal function.*

Hou SH, Bushinsky DA, Wish JB, et al.: Hospital-acquired renal insufficiency: A prospective study. Am J Med 74:243, 1983. *A disturbing study that establishes in one hospital the risk for developing acute renal failure.*

Myers BD, Morna SM: Hemodynamically mediated acute renal failure. N Engl J Med 314:97, 1986. *The clinical patterns of acute renal failure are examined systematically in this excellent paper.*

77 Chronic Renal Failure

David G. Warnock

Chronic renal failure (CRF) is a functional diagnosis characterized by a progressive and generally irreversible decline in glomerular filtration rate (GFR). It is caused by a large number of diseases. Nearly 158,000 Americans were treated for end-stage renal disease (ESRD) during 1987. The prevalence in 1977 was only 45,000 patients, so it is apparent that the ESRD programs are expanding. Approximately 12 per cent of the U.S. population was black in 1987, while nearly 28 per cent of the patients in the Medicare ESRD program were black; it is clear that renal failure is much more likely in blacks than in whites. Figure 77–1 summarizes the incidence of CRF for 1987 according to causes (U.S. Renal Data System Report). Diabetes and hypertension are now recognized as the leading causes of CRF in the United States.

This chapter considers the pathophysiology and clinical manifestations of CRF, an approach to the patient with CRF, and principles of management.

PATHOPHYSIOLOGY AND CLINICAL MANIFESTATIONS

The clinical constellation of signs and symptoms of end-stage renal failure is known as the "uremic syndrome" (Table 77–1). In the initial phases of advancing renal failure, most organs function normally, so that the patient often seeks medical attention only when his or her disease has progressed to the uremic stage.

TABLE 77–1. THE UREMIC SYNDROME

1. Electrolyte disorders
   a. Potassium: hyperkalemia, total body depletion
   b. Sodium: salt-losing nephropathy, sodium retention
   c. Acidosis: metabolic acidosis with high "anion gap," type IV renal tubular acidosis (hyporeninemic hypoaldosteronism)
   d. Calcium (see Table 237–1): tendency toward hypocalcemia—phosphate retention and secondary hyperparathyroidism, with vitamin D deficiency
   e. Phosphate: hyperphosphatemia contributes to disorders of calcium metabolism
   f. Magnesium: accumulation due to excessive intake
   g. Aluminum: accumulation due to excessive intake
2. Cardiovascular abnormalities
   a. Accelerated atherosclerosis
   b. Hypertension
   c. Pericarditis
   d. Myocardial dysfunction
3. Hematologic abnormalities
   a. Anemia: erythropoietin deficiency, iron deficiency
   b. Leukocyte dysfunction: infection
   c. Hemorrhagic diathesis: defective platelet function
4. Gastrointestinal disorders
   a. Anorexia, nausea, vomiting, gastroparesis
   b. Gastrointestinal bleeding
   c. Disorders of taste
5. Renal osteodystrophy (see Table 237–1)
   a. Osteomalacia
   b. Osteitis fibrosa (secondary hyperparathyroidism)
   c. Osteosclerosis
   d. Osteoporosis
6. Neurologic abnormalities
   a. Central nervous system: insomnia, fatigue, psychological symptoms, asterixis
   b. Peripheral neuropathy: stocking-glove sensory neuropathy
7. Myopathy: especially of proximal muscles
8. Impaired carbohydrate tolerance: peripheral resistance to insulin, hypoglycemia
9. Endocrine and metabolic disorders
   a. Glucose intolerance: insulin resistance, insulin degradation, hypoglycemia
   b. Other endocrine disorders: fertility, sterility
   c. Hypothermia
10. Hyperuricemia: clinical gout is rare; pseudogout occurs
11. Pruritus, soft tissue calcification, uremic frost

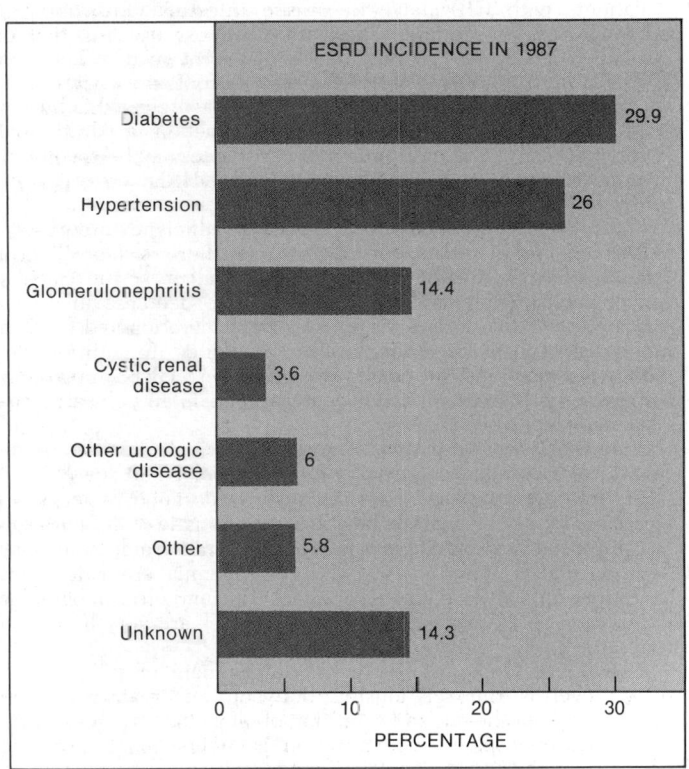

ESRD INCIDENCE IN 1987

Diabetes	29.9
Hypertension	26
Glomerulonephritis	14.4
Cystic renal disease	3.6
Other urologic disease	6
Other	5.8
Unknown	14.3

PERCENTAGE

FIGURE 77–1. Histogram of primary renal diseases leading to end-stage renal disease. (Data based on U.S. Renal Data System, 1988.)

Normally, the adult patient is unaware of advancing renal failure until the GFR has decreased to less than 15 ml per minute. When conservative medical management is no longer adequate, alternative approaches, such as dialysis or transplantation (see Ch. 78), must be considered.

The uremic syndrome results from functional derangements of many organ systems, although the prominence of specific symptoms may vary from patient to patient (Table 77–1). In this chapter, the pathophysiology and clinical manifestations of uremia are discussed by components, even though this is arbitrary and not all of them may be present in the same patient. Azotemia refers to the retention of nitrogenous waste products as renal insufficiency develops. Uremia refers to the final stages of progressive renal insufficiency when the complex, multiorgan system derangements become clinically manifest. A variety of metabolites of proteins and amino acids have been considered possible uremic toxins, but the clinical symptoms of uremia correlate to their blood levels rather poorly. Uremia, in the general sense, results from the accumulation of such metabolites and from the progressive failure of renal catabolic, metabolic, and endocrinologic processes.

WATER, ELECTROLYTE, AND ACID-BASE METABOLISM IN UREMIA. Renal and extrarenal compensatory mechanisms maintain electrolyte and water metabolism in a nearly normal state until the late stages of renal failure. However, characteristic changes develop as renal function declines.

Potassium. The normal human dietary intake of potassium is 1 mEq per kilogram of body weight per day, more than 90 per cent of which is excreted by the kidneys. The potassium excreted in the urine has been largely secreted by distal nephron segments beyond the macula densa. The intracellular concentration of potassium is important in net potassium secretion. The accumulation of potassium in the distal tubular cells is related to the activity of Na-K-ATPase (adenosine triphosphatase) in the basolateral membranes of these cells. The activity of the cell Na-K-ATPase is controlled by diet and mineralocorticoid status. Both normal and uremic subjects adapt to high-potassium diets by increasing potassium excretion per nephron. In addition, the gut can increase its ability to secrete potassium and serves as an important adjunct for potassium adaptation in CRF.

In spite of these adaptive processes, potassium homeostasis in patients with CRF is not normal. In advanced CRF, the serum potassium concentration tends to be higher than normal, even though body stores of potassium may be reduced. Hyperkalemia can be accentuated by trauma, surgery, anesthesia, blood transfusion, acidosis, or increased dietary intake. It can produce serious cardiac abnormalities, but many patients are asymptomatic until cardiac arrest occurs. Occasional patients complain of muscle weakness or paresthesias. The major warning signs are those detected by electrocardiography and include peaked T waves and prolongation of the PR interval and QRS complex.

Sodium. The kidney has a remarkable ability to maintain total body sodium within normal limits until the very end stages of CRF. As renal disease progresses, the remaining nephrons must excrete a proportionately greater quantity of dietary sodium to maintain total body sodium balance. This observation has led to a search for humoral factors that might be responsible for the increased natriuresis per nephron observed in CRF.

Sodium Wasting. Some patients with CRF have salt-losing nephropathy and may lose sodium chloride to the point of extracellular volume contraction and hypotension. These patients will require dietary salt supplementation to prevent their hypotensive symptoms. A variety of renal diseases may be associated with salt wasting, including pyelonephritis, medullary cystic disease, hydronephrosis, interstitial nephritis, and milk-alkali syndrome. The collecting ducts are damaged in these conditions and cannot regulate the final urinary excretion of sodium chloride.

Sodium Retention. Many patients with CRF are unable to increase sodium chloride excretion to appropriate levels with increases in dietary intake. Most come to a new steady state with increased total body weight. When these patients receive an extra salt load, they excrete it promptly and maintain their state of volume expansion. These patients often have the physical findings of expanded extracellular fluid volume: hypertension, peripheral edema, pulmonary vascular congestion, and cardiomegaly. The clinical picture often suggests heart failure, and valvular heart disease or cardiomyopathy may be suspected. Some patients with normal cardiac output may develop relentless sodium retention and require hemofiltration for volume control. These patients tend to be diabetic or have other causes of severe nephrotic syndrome. Volume overload worsens hypertension and thus accelerate all forms of CRF.

Acid-Base Balance. The kidney normally regulates blood pH within narrow limits by reabsorption (proximal tubule) and regeneration (distal tubule) of bicarbonate by secretion of protons into the urinary fluid. When diets high in alkali content are ingested, the kidney excretes less acid, whereas with acid ash diets and endogenous acid production, the kidney reabsorbs and regenerates bicarbonate and secretes hydrogen ion in amounts sufficient to maintain systemic acid-base balance. A maximally acidic urine in the human has a pH of 4.5 to 5.0. The total quantity of acid that can be excreted is a function of the amount of buffer that is excreted and the net rate of proton secretion. The excreted buffers may be filtered or generated; the most important filtered buffer is phosphate, and the most important buffer generated within the kidney is ammonia.

In chronic renal disease, there is a progressive reduction in net ammonia secretion. While the urinary pH may be maximally acid in CRF, the total amount of acid secretion is reduced owing to the limitation on buffer delivery to the distal tubule. In disease processes that disproportionately affect the medulla, the ability to form maximally acidic urine may also be compromised. Metabolic acidosis develops when exogenous intake and endogenous production of acid exceed renal net acid excretion. In chronic metabolic acidosis, extrarenal buffering mechanisms become involved, including bone salts and intracellular buffers. These buffering mechanisms allow for maintenance of relatively stable, but reduced, blood bicarbonate concentrations when the urinary net acid excretion rate cannot keep up with endogenous production of acid. Loss of bone buffer stores contributes to the development of osteomalacia and renal osteodystrophy. As the GFR falls below 10 ml per minute, there is retention of various organic anions and a progressive rise in the "anion gap" [$Na - (Cl + HCO_3)$] to around 20 to 24 mEq per liter, with a reciprocal fall in plasma bicarbonate concentration ("uremic acidosis"). The serum bicarbonate concentration does not usually fall below 12 to 15 mEq per liter. This chronic metabolic acidosis is well tolerated by most patients with CRF, probably reflecting its slow development and respiratory compensation. The overall buffer reserve is limited, however, so that acute acid-base challenges (ketoacidosis, sepsis) can cause severe worsening of the metabolic acidosis.

Another form of renal acidosis, distinct from the uremic acidosis described above, is type IV renal tubular acidosis (RTA), or hyporeninemic hypoaldosteronism with hyperkalemia and hyperchloremic acidosis. This condition can occur in the early stages of CRF when the GFR is only moderately depressed. At this stage the kidney still has the capacity to excrete various organic acids, and therefore patients with type IV RTA, in contrast to those with uremic acidosis, have normal anion gaps. There is a reciprocal fall in plasma bicarbonate levels as chloride concentration increases. Type IV RTA is often seen in all forms of CRF but is most characteristically seen in diabetic patients with progressing renal disease or those with predominantly tubulointerstitial disease. It is described further and compared with other types of RTA in Chapter 82. Potassium retention and overt hyperkalemia are the most significant manifestations of hyporeninemic hypoaldosteronism in CRF.

Calcium. The total serum calcium concentration in patients with CRF is significantly lower than normal, although usually above 7.5 mg per deciliter. Great variability exists, and occasionally the calcium level is very low. Patients with CRF tolerate the hypocalcemia quite well, and rarely is a patient symptomatic from the decreased calcium concentration. Tetany is surprisingly uncommon. It is occasionally precipitated by the infusion of sodium bicarbonate, but the usual muscle twitching and cramping of CRF are primary neuromuscular disorders unrelated to hypocalcemia.

Patients with CRF have decreased intestinal absorption of calcium, and consequently fecal calcium loss exceeds that of normal subjects. Jejunal and ileal malabsorption of calcium in CRF can be corrected by oral administration of active vitamin D analogues. In addition, patients with either acute renal failure or CRF are resistant to the normal calcemic action of parathyroid hormone (PTH). The mechanism of resistance may be secondary to a decreased permissive effect of $1,25\text{-}(OH)_2D_3$ on the bone action of PTH.

Phosphate retention develops as renal insufficiency progresses. With increases in serum phosphate level, there is deposition of calcium phosphate into soft tissues and a fall in serum calcium concentration (both total and ionized). The decrease in serum calcium levels is a potent stimulus to PTH secretion and leads to functional hyperplasia of the parathyroid glands. In addition, the kidney is a major site for catabolism of PTH, so CRF is invariably associated with secondary hyperparathyroidism and elevated circulating levels of PTH.

A subgroup of CRF patients develops hypercalcemia after some months on hemodialysis, usually owing to persistent secretion of PTH from glands that have previously undergone hyperplasia. Occasionally, these patients become symptomatic with bone pain or exhibit signs of metastatic calcification. Parathyroidectomy may be indicated if other causes of hypercalcemia are ruled out. Measurements of serum levels of intact PTH and ultrasonographic localization of hyperplastic glands in the neck are very helpful in this setting.

Phosphate. The most important determinant of serum phosphate level is the relationship between net reabsorption of phosphate from the gut and excretion of phosphate by the kidney. The serum phosphate concentration is higher than normal in patients with a GFR below 20 ml per minute, but actual retention of phosphate can be documented with even less severe declines in GFR.

The retained phosphate is of major pathogenetic importance in the development of secondary hyperparathyroidism in CRF. It is postulated that there are periodic decreases in phosphate excretion as nephrons progressively drop out. The resultant increases in plasma phosphate concentration lead to reciprocal decreases in serum calcium concentration, increased secretion of PTH, and decreased tubular reabsorption of phosphate. This adaptive mechanism will maintain a normal serum phosphate concentration until GFR has fallen to approximately 20 per cent of normal. However, if dietary phosphorus intake is not reduced in patients with advancing renal disease, these adaptive mechanisms cannot compensate fully and hyperphosphatemia ensues. If hyperphosphatemia can be prevented, the expected rise in serum parathyroid hormone will be blunted. In addition to dietary restriction, intestinal absorption of phosphate can be reduced by the use of compounds that bind phosphate in the gut in nonabsorbable form. It appears that calcium carbonate is an effective phosphate binder when taken with meals. Calcium carbonate enhances gut calcium absorption, provides a base equivalent for the treatment of metabolic acidosis, and also effectively binds dietary phosphate. This approach avoids the potentially toxic effects of aluminum (dementia, anemia, bone disease) that can result from the use of aluminum-containing antacids and phosphate binders in patients with CRF.

Magnesium. Patients with CRF tend to have modest elevations in serum magnesium concentration when the GFR has fallen below 20 ml per minute. The urinary excretion of magnesium is diminished, and intestinal magnesium absorption continues normally. Most CRF patients with hypermagnesemia have no associated symptoms or findings. Nevertheless, it is prudent to discontinue magnesium-containing antacids and cathartics in patients with a GFR below 20 ml per minute.

CARDIOVASCULAR ABNORMALITIES. Cardiovascular complications are common in patients with CRF and can be classified into three main categories: atherosclerosis and hyperlipidemia, hypertension, and pericarditis. There may also be a primary myocardial dysfunction in uremia that responds to acute dialysis.

Atherosclerosis. Accelerated atherosclerosis is one of the major factors limiting the longevity of patients with CRF. The most characteristic lipid abnormality is elevated triglyceride concentrations with normal or slightly elevated plasma cholesterol levels (type IV). The incidence of elevated triglyceride concentrations is higher in patients maintained on chronic hemodialysis than in nondialyzed patients. There appears to be a positive relationship between the elevation of plasma triglyceride levels and the increased incidence of occlusive coronary disease. The cause of hypertriglyceridemia in CRF is unknown, but current evidence favors a defect in triglyceride removal rather than an increase in triglyceride production.

Hypertension. Hypertension is common in chronic renal disease, being present in the majority of patients at the onset of maintenance dialysis. At least two factors contribute to its high incidence in CRF: (1) The tendency toward sodium retention and volume expansion is perhaps the most important. Expansion of the extracellular volume is accompanied by an initial rise of cardiac output followed by a rise in peripheral resistance. Patients with volume-sensitive hypertension may have increasing problems with blood pressure control as they progress into renal failure. (2) Alterations of the renin-angiotensin axis are also important contributors to the pathogenesis of hypertension. Angiotensin-converting enzyme inhibitors effectively control hypertension in CRF and can be used as long as hyperkalemia is avoided. A small number of patients with hypertension can be controlled only by bilateral nephrectomy. The vast majority of patients with CRF will have much better control of their hypertension once fluid volume is controlled by dialysis.

Brenner and colleagues have focused their attention on glomerular capillary hypertension rather than systemic arterial pressure. It is known that reduction in renal mass causes functional and structural hypertrophy of the remaining intact nephrons. Increases in glomerular capillary pressures and blood flow may be a central factor in this adaptive hypertrophy. The role of adaptive glomerular hyperfiltration in the progression of chronic renal disease must be viewed as somewhat controversial. This hypothetical framework has provided a therapeutic approach that emphasizes the potential contribution of protein restriction and the use of antihypertensive agents that are effective at the level of the glomerular capillary in the treatment of progressive renal insufficiency

Pericarditis. "Uremic pericarditis" is a term that refers to pericarditis of unknown etiology occurring in association with uremia. Conventionally, pericarditis is classified as "uremic" or "dialysis associated." However, since the pathophysiologic characteristics are similar in both settings, the division into two distinct subtypes appears arbitrary, and therefore the continued use of the term "uremic pericarditis" seems justified. Uremic pericarditis was originally described in nondialyzed patients, whereas currently it is most common in patients who are not dialyzed adequately. Characteristically, the pericardial fluid is hemorrhagic. The onset of pericarditis is usually signaled by pain, often on the left side of the chest with respiratory accentuation. Pain is often severe and frequently associated with a friction rub. The friction rub can be loud, generalized, and even palpable but may also be evanescent. Tamponade can occur with signs of falling blood and pulse pressures, raised jugular venous pressure, and poorly perfused extremities. The hemorrhage is thought to originate from sheared pericardial capillaries that have developed in response to uremic inflammation of the pericardium. It is recognized that in previously nondialyzed patients uremic pericarditis responds to dialysis more rapidly than in patients who develop pericarditis during dialysis. However, the pericarditis in this latter group usually responds to intensification of hemodialysis. Pericarditis should be viewed as potentially lethal, and it may require surgical intervention if tamponade becomes evident. Two-dimensional echocardiography can be very helpful in documenting the magnitude of the pericardial effusion and assessing its functional significance. If "diastolic collapse" can be demonstrated with this technique, then emergent surgical drainage is indicated.

HEMATOLOGIC ABNORMALITIES. Hematologic abnormalities are among the most consistent manifestations of uremia. These abnormalities include anemia, bleeding, and granulocyte and platelet dysfunction.

Anemia. Many patients with CRF have severely reduced hematocrits. Hematocrits in the 15 to 20 per cent range are not uncommon. The manifestations of anemia include pallor, tachycardia, a wide pulse pressure with accentuation by exercise, a systolic ejection murmur best heard over the pulmonary area, and the precipitation of angina pectoris in patients with underlying coronary artery disease.

The primary cause of anemia in CRF is a deficiency of erythropoietin, which is a glycoprotein normally produced in the kidney in response to hypoxia. It is responsible for normal red blood cell differentiation from stem cells. Decreased erythropoietin production results primarily from destruction of renal parenchyma and causes normochromic, normocytic anemia. Circulating inhibitors and protein deprivation that in turn decreases erythropoietin production may also contribute to erythropoietin deficiency.

Other factors may contribute to anemia. Many patients on maintenance hemodialysis are iron deficient. Inadequate iron intake is very common in CRF, and iron deficiency may develop in dialyzed patients because of frequent blood sampling and accidental losses during the course of dialysis. Red blood cell survival is shortened in uremia, probably owing to mechanical factors and changes in the red blood cell membrane composition. In addition, patients with CRF may have additional factors that contribute to anemia, including microangiopathic hemolysis as a result of hypersplenism, and folate and iron deficiency. Erythropoietin therapy has greatly improved the sense of well-being of patients on chronic dialysis. Although difficulties may arise because of iron deficiency, exacerbation of previous hypertension, and seizure disorders, the overall response is gratifying. Although now widely prescribed for the majority of patients on chronic dialysis, the optimal dosing regimens and target hematocrits are still open to debate. The role of erythropoietin therapy in patients with CRF who have not yet become dialysis dependent is being actively investigated. Very careful dose titration is required, since any worsening of hypertension may accelerate the onset of overt renal failure.

Leukocyte Dysfunction. Although the granulocyte count is usually normal, some patients have a tendency toward granulocytopenia or lymphopenia. Moreover, the chemotactic response of granulocytes is subnormal. These factors contribute to impairments in acute inflammatory responses and delayed hypersensitivity and may account for an enhanced susceptibility to infection in CRF.

Hemorrhagic Diathesis. A hemorrhagic tendency, manifested by epistaxis, menorrhagia, or excessive bleeding or bruising after trauma, is common in CRF. Whole-blood clotting time and prothrombin time are usually normal. Bleeding time may be prolonged, perhaps related to the associated abnormalities of platelet function. Platelets are often decreased in number owing to increased peripheral destruction. In addition, there are functional defects, such as decreased adhesiveness and aggregation. These abnormalities are often rapidly corrected by hemodialysis and may be secondary to a dialyzable uremic toxin (e.g., guanidinosuccinic acid). The abnormal bleeding time is not rapidly corrected by dialysis and, as such, may not be a reliable prospective guide to the risk of bleeding complications.

INFECTIONS. Most patients with CRF develop serious infections during the course of their disease. The increased susceptibility to infection could be due to deranged or deficient humoral or cellular immunity, impaired inflammatory reaction, or increased exposure to pathogenic bacteria and viruses. Humoral immunity is, in general, intact. Most patients have normal humoral responses to vaccines, but there may be a requirement for more aggressive immunization, as demonstrated by the difficulty in achieving full responses to hepatitis B vaccine in patients with CRF. Cellular defense mechanisms are often deficient, with impairment of delayed hypersensitivity. Patients with CRF may have low lymphocyte counts, and their lymphocytes do not respond normally to mitogenic stimulation. The neutrophil count is usually normal in CRF, and it rises appropriately in response to infection. However, leukocytes of uremic subjects have a decreased phagocytic function. The chemotactic response of polymorphonuclear leukocytes is also depressed; this function improves with hemodialysis. In addition, patients on hemodialysis are often exposed to bacterial and viral infections. Staphylococcal sepsis is commonly due to cutaneous contamination through the arteriovenous hemodialysis access. Gram-negative sepsis also occurs with greater frequency. Often an infected urinary tract can be implicated as the cause. There is an increase in the frequency of hepatitis in dialysis patients that is related to multiple blood transfusions. The disease is usually asymptomatic, but it can be severe. A significant fraction of patients with CRF who contract hepatitis become chronic carriers. The incidence of hepatitis has been diminished with erythropoietin therapy, effective hepatitis screening, and vaccinations.

GASTROINTESTINAL DISORDERS. Gastrointestinal disorders are common in patients with uremia. Their symptoms have varying presentations and may be quite distressing. The most common early symptom is loss of appetite. Many uremic patients then develop nausea and vomiting, sometimes severe enough to cause loss of salt and water, leading to volume depletion and negative caloric balance, which results in weight loss. The specific cause of these symptoms has not been identified, but they quickly resolve with the institution of dialysis.

Gastrointestinal bleeding is also common in uremic patients. Often it is of minor magnitude and is detected by positive stool guaiac test results, but it can be severe as well. The gastrointestinal bleeding may be the result of scattered petechiae, ulceration, or angiodysplasia. There is also an increased incidence of peptic ulcer disease in CRF. The platelet defects contribute to the increased frequency of gastrointestinal bleeding characteristic of uremic patients, but structural abnormalities must not be overlooked.

OSTEODYSTROPHY. "Renal osteodystrophy" is an all-inclusive term for the skeletal changes in uremia, which include, in decreasing order of frequency, osteitis fibrosa, osteomalacia, osteoporosis, and osteosclerosis (see Ch. 237). Osteitis fibrosa is almost universal in advanced renal failure, the exceptions being those patients with rapidly progressive disease and a short duration of uremia. A number of patients exhibit abnormal radiographs, and some complain of actual bone tenderness or muscle weakness. Renal osteodystrophy becomes a major limi-

tation for patients on long-term dialysis. Spontaneous fractures and bone pain, due to osteitis fibrosa and osteomalacia, can have severe functional consequences. Although vitamin D deficiency plays a major role in osteomalacia, there is a growing realization that aluminum-induced bone disease and iron overload may also contribute to the development and progression of renal osteodystrophy.

NEUROPATHY. Many patients with CRF have abnormalities in central and peripheral nervous system function. Tiredness, insomnia, and psychological symptoms, including agitation, irritability, depression, regression, and rebellion, are common. Patients with secondary hyperparathyroidism have abnormal electroencephalograms (EEG's) characterized by increased frequency of slow wave activity. Patients with secondary hyperparathyroidism caused by CRF may show improvement in their EEG's and psychological symptoms after parathyroidectomy. The mechanism by which PTH exerts these effects on the central nervous system is not known, but a variety of mechanisms may be involved, including changes in brain calcium content, abnormal neuroendocrinologic responses, and alterations in ion transport systems involved in normal neurotransmission.

Peripheral neuropathy is also common in CRF. Clinical manifestations include painful paresthesias of extremities, twitchings, "restless leg syndrome," loss of deep tendon reflexes, muscular weakness, and occasional sensory deficits. Lower extremities are involved much more frequently than upper extremities. Diminished deep tendon reflexes and vibratory sense may be found, but the most common presentation is sensory loss in a stockingglove distribution. Peripheral neuropathy can be drug induced, but its pathophysiology in most patients is unknown. Diabetic patients can develop peripheral neuropathy as part of their underlying disease processes, which only worsens as their CRF progresses.

MYOPATHY. Muscular weakness and wasting develop slowly but are common in patients with end-stage renal failure. Proximal muscles are affected more than distal muscles. There are no distinct histologic features of uremic myopathy, and the precise cause has not been defined. Nutritional factors obviously play a central role in the development and treatment of uremic myopathy. The resting transmembrane potential difference of skeletal muscle cells is abnormally low, and the average mean duration of the action potential is significantly shortened in uremic individuals. The reflexes and results of the sensory examination are normal, and there is no evidence of myositis. In inadequately dialyzed uremic patients, intracellular sodium and chloride contents are elevated, whereas potassium content is reduced. These findings are consistent with either increased permeability of the muscle membrane to these ions or decreased active efflux of sodium. These abnormalities can be corrected by dialysis and have been used as an index of the adequacy of hemodialysis. Polymyositis syndromes with elevated creatinine phosphokinase levels have been observed in patients with CRF, especially in conjunction with various drugs, including colchicine, clofibrate, and lovastatin.

ENDOCRINE AND METABOLIC DISORDERS. Carbohydrate Metabolism. Carbohydrate metabolism is often abnormal in patients with CRF. Fasting blood glucose values are normal or slightly elevated, but glucose tolerance may be abnormal. This state of impaired glucose tolerance is often termed *uremic pseudodiabetes mellitus*. Severe hyperglycemia does not occur unless the patient receives a large load of glucose, e.g., during peritoneal dialysis with hypertonic glucose solutions. Nevertheless, the requirement for exogenous insulin decreases in insulin-dependent diabetics as renal failure progresses. At least two different mechanisms are responsible for the simultaneous coexistence of abnormal glucose tolerance and a decreased requirement for exogenous insulin: (1) enhanced peripheral resistance to insulin and (2) a decreased renal clearance of insulin.

A number of possibilities may explain the insulin resistance in uremia. First, some uremic substances may interfere with the action of insulin, since aggressive hemodialysis decreases exogenous requirements for insulin. Second, potassium deficiency may alter the nature of insulin released from the pancreas. Indeed, proinsulin-insulin ratios rise in nonuremic patients who are potassium deficient. Third, there is decreased binding of insulin to peripheral receptors in CRF. Whatever the reason (or reasons), patients with CRF clearly have some degree of peripheral resistance to insulin.

Insulin is filtered and metabolized by the kidney. With progressing CRF, blood insulin concentrations rise owing to decreased extraction of insulin by renal proximal tubular cells. These observations explain the decrease in insulin requirements of diabetics with progressing CRF, but it is also necessary to postulate a degree of peripheral resistance to insulin to explain the carbohydrate intolerance ("uremic pseudodiabetes") of nondiabetic subjects with CRF. A small number of patients with CRF will not manifest insulin resistance and may in fact develop severe, life-threatening hypoglycemia.

Other Endocrine Disturbances. Pituitary, thyroid, and adrenal function is relatively normal in CRF, although some compromise may be observed in response to stress, infections, and so on. Sexual function is often compromised in CRF, with amenorrhea and infertility occurring in women and impotence and oligospermia occurring in men. Reduced estrogen and testosterone levels can often be observed, and prolactin excess may be of pathogenetic importance.

Hypothermia. Patients with CRF often have reduced basal metabolic rates and abnormalities in temperature regulation. The deficiency or reduced activity of the ubiquitous Na-K-ATPase may play a central role in the reduced rate of metabolism. Overt hypothermia is very common in CRF, with a resetting of the normal temperature from 37°C to as low as 35.5°C. This observation is of practical importance in assessing fever in patients with CRF; a temperature of 37.5°C may denote a serious, acute infection that requires appropriate antibiotic coverage.

Elevation of Uric Acid Level. Approximately two thirds of the total uric acid excretory load is normally removed each day by the kidney. With progression of CRF, hyperuricemia is a consistent finding once GFR has decreased to 20 per cent of normal. However, the correlation between the rise of the serum uric acid level and the severity of CRF is poor. Only rarely does the serum uric acid concentration rise above 10 mg per deciliter unless dehydration is superimposed. Whether or not the elevated serum uric acid levels hasten the development of ESRD is not known. Symptomatic gout does occur in patients with CRF, as well as other forms of arthritis, including "pseudogout" due to crystalline deposits other than uric acid, and deposition of amyloid and beta$_2$-microglobulin.

Pruritus. Generalized pruritus is a frequent symptom of CRF and is occasionally severe and intractable. Usually, there are no dermatologic findings. To date, no single causative factor has been identified. Implicated factors include some dialyzable product of uremia, a high calcium-phosphorus product in extracellular fluid with deposition of calcium salts in the dermal structures, and abnormalities in nerve end-plates. Symptomatic relief has been reported with more frequent dialysis, parathyroidectomy, dietary protein restriction, and exposure to ultraviolet light. Other dermatologic conditions include a sallow, yellow discoloration due to deposition of "urochromes," bronze discoloration due to hemochromatosis, uremic frost due to deposition of urea crystals on the skin surface, and metastatic calcifications.

APPROACH TO THE PATIENT WITH UREMIA

The principles of approach to the uremic patient are based on the general precepts of internal medicine. A detailed clinical history is imperative, with special emphasis on urinary tract symptoms, such as nocturia, hematuria, dysuria, polydipsia, and polyuria. Also of special importance is a complete history of systemic diseases, of exposure to toxins and infections, and of renal diseases in the family. The medical history will often be of diagnostic significance. The physical examination should emphasize the blood pressure, retina, cardiovascular system, renal examination with auscultation for bruits and palpation of size, rectal examination for size of prostate in men, gynecologic examination for pelvic masses in women, extremity examination for edema and nail bed findings, and neuroskeletal examination for evidence of myopathy, neuropathy, and osteodystrophy. Laboratory tests should include a complete blood count and urinalysis.

Additional studies should determine whether a patient has acute reversible renal failure, acute worsening of CRF resulting from aggravating factors, or a chronic progressive disease. Again, the history is important. It is unlikely that a patient with acute renal disease is asymptomatic with elevations of serum creatinine and blood urea nitrogen (BUN) above 10 and 100 mg per deciliter,

respectively. On the other hand, patients with slowly progressing CRF are often asymptomatic with much higher elevations of serum creatinine and BUN. In CRF, the hematocrit tends to be lower, the phosphate concentration is higher, and the urinary sediment is usually benign. However, none of these tests is specific enough to differentiate with certainty between acute renal failure and CRF.

Determination of the kidney size can be helpful in establishing the chronicity of renal disease. Renal sonograms can be used to estimate renal size and identify hydronephrosis or cystic masses. If the kidneys are significantly reduced in size, this almost always indicates chronicity and irreversibility. Normal kidney size tends to favor an acute process, although exceptions exist. Chronic renal processes in which kidney size may be normal or larger than normal include polycystic kidney disease, amyloidosis, scleroderma, and diabetes mellitus. Thus normal renal size does not rule out a chronic process. The sonogram may reveal asymmetric renal size, which may be due to unilateral renal agenesis, or renal arterial disease processes, which would suggest a need for arteriography to assess the renal arteries directly.

It is also important to differentiate between renal and extrarenal causes of azotemia. Extrarenal causes of progressive azotemia may be either prerenal or postrenal. Prerenal causes are those disease processes that decrease the blood flow to the kidneys. This decrease may result from true extracellular fluid volume depletion or from effective volume depletion, as seen with cardiac and liver failure. It is also imperative to rule out postrenal causes of azotemia, including lower or upper urinary tract obstruction. Lower urinary tract obstruction may be diagnosed by having the patient void completely and then measuring the residual urine volume in the bladder via catheterization. By far the most common cause in men is an enlarged prostate. Any time a uremic patient with anuria is seen, it is imperative that lower urinary tract obstruction be ruled out, especially if accompanied by symptoms such as hesitancy in initiating the urinary stream, slow urinary stream, and incontinence. Upper urinary tract obstruction can be established by ruling out residual urine in the bladder and demonstrating dilated renal calices, pelvis, and ureters above the obstruction with sonography. The most common causes of upper urinary tract obstruction include renal stones, congenital obstruction, and bladder cancer. Superimposed volume depletion can limit the usefulness of sonography in diagnosing upper urinary tract obstruction.

Once it has been determined that uremia is secondary to renal parenchymal disease and not due to prerenal or postrenal causes, the physician must ascertain whether a treatable form of parenchymal disease is present. The most common forms of treatable renal disease are listed in Table 77–2. Renal biopsy and arteriography may be helpful and are often considered. In general, although renal arteriography produces excellent visualization of the kidney, it is of limited diagnostic value in patients with uremia. It may be helpful in patients suspected of having polyarteritis nodosa, tumors (although uremia is an uncommon association), and renal disease secondary to severe hypertension. Asymmetry in renal size in the setting of severe hypertension suggests renal artery stenosis and should be evaluated by arteriography.

Renal biopsy may give a definitive histologic diagnosis, provided it is performed before the disease has progressed to such

TABLE 77–2. TREATABLE TYPES OF PARENCHYMAL RENAL DISEASE

Acute hypertensive nephropathy
Analgesic nephropathy
Hemolytic-uremic syndrome
Hypercalcemic nephropathy
Interstitial nephritis
Lupus nephritis
Multiple myeloma
Oxalate nephropathy
Pyelonephritis
Rapidly progressing glomerulonephritis with crescents
Renal vein thrombosis
Wegener's granulomatosis

a degree that the only possible morphologic interpretation is ESRD. Renal biopsy can be performed by a percutaneous route with local anesthesia or as an open biopsy with the patient under general anesthesia. The associated morbidity and mortality are low, but the possibility of complications nevertheless exists. For these reasons, renal biopsy is probably indicated in only a small number of patients with uremia; on the other hand, an argument can be made for an aggressive approach to renal biopsy in those patients who have not yet progressed to end-stage renal failure. Although a consensus does not exist among nephrologists, biopsy should not be done unless the physician has strong feelings that the information to be gained will influence management. In that light, serious consideration of any of the treatable renal diseases listed in Table 77–2 should be pursued with renal biopsy. Contraindications to renal biopsy include uncorrectable bleeding tendencies, severe hypertension, bacteriuria, suspicion of perinephric abscess, hydronephrosis, and extreme obesity. Biopsy is often most useful in patients with normal-sized kidneys and progressive renal disease if they have (or are suspected of having) nephrotic syndrome, collagen vascular disease (especially systemic lupus erythematosus), tubulointerstitial disease, or rapidly progressive glomerular disease.

MANAGEMENT

The management of patients with CRF can be divided conveniently into three separate categories: treatment of aggravating factors, treatment of specific complications of uremia, and consideration of optimal diet and general principles in the long-term follow-up of patients with CRF. We will consider those principles of management that are common to all forms of CRF regardless of etiology.

Aggravating Factors

Patients with CRF are highly susceptible to factors that may cause a deterioration of renal function. These must be sought meticulously and treated immediately so that the underlying renal failure will not be worsened permanently. Table 77–3 lists factors that may rapidly worsen renal function in a patient with previously stable CRF.

VOLUME DEPLETION. One of the most common causes of worsening renal function in a patient with CRF is vascular volume depletion. Vascular volume depletion can be the result of either absolute volume depletion or contraction of the effective arterial blood volume. Common causes of volume depletion include the aggressive use of diuretics coupled with salt and water restriction, and gastrointestinal loss of fluid from either vomiting or diarrhea. Vascular volume depletion can also be "effective" and associated with decreases in renal blood flow. Therefore, aggravating factors that cause decreases in renal blood flow can produce rapid rises in serum creatinine concentrations (Table 77–3). Physical signs of volume depletion should thus be sought. In addition, urinary electrolyte measurements often suggest volume depletion. Patients with CRF may rapidly and irreversibly decrease their GFR with volume depletion, so it is imperative for treatment, either oral or intravenous fluid replacement, to be started as soon as

TABLE 77–3. AGGRAVATING FACTORS FOR PROGRESSION OF RENAL DISEASE

1. Vascular volume depletion
   a. Absolute: aggressive use of diuretics, gastrointestinal fluid losses, dehydration
   b. Effective: low cardiac output, renal hypoperfusion with atheroembolic disease, ascites with liver disease, nephrotic syndrome
2. Drugs: aminoglycosides, prostaglandin synthesis inhibitors in a setting of renal hypoperfusion, diuretics in dosage to cause volume depletion
3. Obstruction
   a. Tubular: uric acid, Bence Jones protein
   b. Posttubular: prostatic hypertrophy, necrotic papillae, ureteral stones
4. Infections: sepsis with hypotension, urinary tract infections
5. Toxins: radiographic contrast material
6. Hypertensive crises
7. Metabolic: hypercalcemia, hyperphosphatemia

feasible. Patients with CRF who are not on chronic dialysis should be hospitalized if there is any doubt that adequate volume repletion can be carried out on an outpatient basis.

DRUGS. Patients with CRF are often treated with a variety of drugs, many of which are nephrotoxic. Table 77–4 lists the nephrotoxic drugs. Of these, the aminoglycoside antibiotics are a common cause of worsening renal failure. In addition, prostaglandin synthesis inhibitors can decrease the creatinine clearance in patients with CRF, especially in a setting of volume depletion. It is prudent to obtain a detailed drug ingestion history whenever a CRF patient with an accelerating rate of renal failure is seen. In addition, drug dosing appropriate to the level of renal function is important to avoid superimposed nephrotoxicity (Table 77–4).

OBSTRUCTION. Acute (less than a day) or subacute (less than a few weeks) obstruction of the urinary tract can occur from multiple causes in patients with CRF. Urinary tract obstruction is conveniently divided into that from tubular causes and that from posttubular causes. The more common etiologies for tubular obstruction include uric acid crystal deposition (as observed with malignancies) and Bence Jones protein deposition (in association with multiple myeloma). More common causes of posttubular obstruction include prostatic hypertrophy and/or prostatism; necrotic papillae, especially in patients with diabetes; and ureteral stones. When the clinical symptoms suggest urinary tract obstruction, it is important that prompt diagnostic and therapeutic measures are undertaken. Rapid in-and-out catheterization rules out bladder obstruction, whereas ultrasonography is useful in ruling out ureteral obstruction. If any doubt persists, then retrograde pyelography should be performed. These measures are simple and safe, and appropriate intervention often prevents progression of azotemia.

INFECTION. Urinary tract infections are significantly worsened when obstruction is present. The rate of infection rises especially after repeated catheterization. Although infection limited to the urinary tract rarely causes progression of renal failure, specific attention should be directed toward evaluating proteinuria, pyuria, and bacteriuria. Increased proteinuria and exaggerated pyuria suggest urinary tract infection. A culture of clean-catch urine should be done under these circumstances. If infection is documented, specific antibiotics are indicated. Care must be exercised to adjust the drug dosage for the degree of renal failure. Uremic patients are also more prone to other infections, such as pneumonia and sepsis, on a de novo basis. These systemic infections, if present, in turn may compromise renal blood flow and result in worsening uremia. The index of suspicion should be high for sepsis in hypotensive CRF patients with urinary tract infection in whom the serum creatinine level is rising.

TOXINS. The list of potential nephrotoxins is long. Therefore, it is important to obtain a good exposure history in patients with CRF. In a hospitalized patient with CRF, when the serum creatinine level starts to rise rapidly, one must consider exposure to radiocontrast materials, nephrotoxic antibiotics, and vasodilators. Volume-depleted patients with CRF, especially diabetics and individuals with multiple myeloma, may experience worsening renal disease because of volume depletion. Fortunately, the prognosis is quite good if the patients are adequately hydrated; it appears that the incidence and severity of contrast dye nephrotoxicity have been reduced with this approach.

HYPERTENSIVE CRISIS. Many patients with CRF are hypertensive. Indeed, hypertension is one of the significant risk factors that may accelerate the rate of progression of renal disease. Thus, strict attention must be paid to adequate control of blood pressure in patients with CRF. Occasionally, patients with CRF develop malignant hypertension with rapidly deteriorating renal function. It is imperative that the blood pressure is quickly controlled in these patients. Even so, the restoration of renal blood flow may be delayed if there are significant vascular abnormalities secondary to accelerated hypertension. This recovery phase can take months, with gradual improvement in the renal function.

METABOLIC FACTORS. Of the metabolic abnormalities that worsen the progression of renal disease, the rises in calcium-phosphorus products are among the most common. The rise in the calcium-phosphorus product not only causes soft tissue calcification but also may be a precipitating factor in the progression of renal disease. This is especially true in patients with multiple

TABLE 77–4. ANTIBIOTIC DOSAGE IN CRF

Major Reduction in Dosage	Moderate Reduction in Dosage	Minor or No Reduction in Dosage	Agents That Should Not Be Used
Flucytosine	Ampicillin	Amphotericin B	Bacitracin
Gentamicin	Carbenicillin	Cefotaxime	Chlortetracycline
Kanamycin	Cefazolin	Cefoperazone	Nitrofurantoin
Oxytetracycline*	Cephaloridine	Chloramphenicol	
Streptomycin	Cephalothin	Clindamycin	
Tetracycline*	Cloxacillin	Doxycycline	
Tobramycin	Co-trimoxazole	Erythromycin	
Vancomycin	(trimethoprim-sulfamethoxazole)	Isoniazid	
	Methicillin	Lincomycin	
	Moxalactam	Nafcillin	
	Oxacillin		
	Penicillin G		
	Ticarcillin		

*Although tetracyclines are not significantly nephrotoxic per se, their dosage should be reduced in CRF because of their hepatotoxicity with increased blood levels (especially with chlortetracycline) and because their antianabolic actions cause an increase in blood urea nitrogen disproportionate to the degree of renal failure. If tetracyclines are indicated in renal failure, doxycycline is the drug of choice because it is cleared by hepatic routes.

myeloma. Vitamin D supplementation and the use of calcium carbonate as a phosphate binder provide reasonable control of the calcium-phosphorus product. Careful monitoring of the serum calcium level and dietary phosphate restriction are also important adjuncts to the care of patients with CRF.

Complications of Uremia

WATER AND ELECTROLYTE ABNORMALITIES. Hyperkalemia. The mean serum potassium concentration is higher than normal, whereas the total body potassium content is lower than normal in CRF. Serum potassium concentrations up to 6 mEq per liter are well tolerated in patients with CRF. However, patients with CRF have difficulty in excreting an acute potassium load. Therefore, potassium concentrations above 6 mEq per liter require treatment. One should initially determine whether the hyperkalemia is a result of some aggravating factor, such as volume depletion, tissue breakdown, transient worsening of acidosis, drugs (spironolactone, amiloride, triamterene, continued oral potassium supplements, converting enzyme inhibitors, nonsteroidal anti-inflammatory agents, beta blockers), fever, or high intake of potassium. If hyperkalemia is of modest degree and due to some aggravating factor, the therapy should be directed toward correcting the source of hyperkalemia. Discontinuation of oral potassium supplements and dietary potassium restriction are rational first steps. However, if hyperkalemia is severe, skeletal muscle weakness and electrocardiographic changes may be present. This situation represents a medical emergency and requires immediate intracellular transfer of potassium and rapid removal of potassium from the body. The treatment of hyperkalemia is described in detail in Ch. 75.

Abnormalities of Sodium Balance. Total body sodium content dictates total extracellular fluid volume. Although the fractional excretion of sodium per nephron increases as renal disease progresses, patients with CRF are nevertheless susceptible to both volume contraction and volume expansion. Since even mild volume depletion may adversely affect renal function in patients with CRF, it is prudent to maintain these patients in a somewhat volume-expanded state. Volume-sensitive hypertension and pulmonary edema are limiting factors, but it is even more hazardous to keep a patient completely free of edema. If a patient should develop orthostatic hypotensive symptoms, salt intake should be liberalized. Ideally, dietary salt intake should be decreased in proportion to the decrease in GFR. Some of the sodium may be given as sodium bicarbonate to correct metabolic acidosis. If the patient is poorly compliant and becomes volume expanded, the use of diuretics, such as furosemide alone or in combination with a thiazide, is indicated, assuming that underlying kidney function is sufficient to permit a satisfactory clinical response to these drugs. If volume expansion causes severe symptoms and does not respond to conventional techniques, acute peritoneal dialysis or hemodialysis is indicated. Hyponatremia and hypernatremia are treated with the same general principles of water restriction or free water administration as in any other patient. Neurologically symptomatic, life-threatening hyponatremia may require the administration of hypertonic sodium chloride, but the resultant volume expansion may then require acute dialysis.

CARDIOVASCULAR ABNORMALITIES. It is important to control the cardiovascular complications of patients with CRF to improve their potential longevity. Hypertriglyceridemia and hypertension are the primary risk factors leading to accelerated atherosclerosis and high cardiovascular mortality. It is not clear whether the course of atherosclerotic vascular disease in patients with CRF can be altered. Even patients who have undergone successful renal transplantation seem to have an increased incidence of cardiovascular deaths. Nevertheless, it seems advisable to adhere to the same dietary principles in patients with hypertriglyceridemia and CRF as in patients without CRF (see Ch. 172). If clofibrate or cholesterol synthesis inhibitors are used, the dose should be decreased proportionately to the degree of renal failure to prevent adverse side effects.

Hypertension is the result of numerous interrelated factors in patients with CRF. It is most commonly volume dependent and volume sensitive. Thus, one of the primary objectives is to decrease intravascular volume, an approach that is sufficient to control hypertension in most patients. If the patient has an adequate urinary volume, the judicious use of diuretics together with a decrease in the dietary intake of salt and water is indicated. Of the available diuretics, furosemide and bumetanide are preferred because of their effectiveness. Excess fluid can also be removed in patients on dialysis by ultrafiltration during the procedure. If volume contraction is not sufficient, then the same general principles apply to the treatment of hypertension in any other patient (see Ch. 44). Additional drugs, such as clonidine, calcium channel blockers, and beta blockers, may be required. Oral inhibitors of angiotensin-converting enzyme have been shown to be particularly useful in some patients. Minoxidil, a direct smooth muscle vasodilator, has also been advocated in patients with otherwise refractory hypertension. There still exists an extremely small number of patients with malignant hypertension that cannot be controlled by any medical regimen. These patients may respond to bilateral nephrectomy.

The diagnosis of uremic pericarditis requires hospitalization and treatment for fear of impending cardiac tamponade. The best initial therapy is daily dialysis for approximately a week. Indomethacin is not effective in uremic pericarditis. If pericarditis remains refractory to increased frequency of dialysis, intrapericardial injection of nonabsorbable steroids may prove therapeutic. Some patients will require partial pericardiectomy if they develop circulatory impairment that does not respond to medical management.

HEMATOLOGIC ABNORMALITIES. The anemia of CRF often improves with maintenance hemodialysis. The rise in hematocrit is not due to stimulation of erythropoietin production but rather to the removal of some circulating factor (or factors) that inhibits the normal response to erythropoietin.

Besides achievement of the best possible metabolic status of the patient with either hemodialysis or transplantation, two general considerations exist for the treatment of anemia: long-term medical management and transfusion. The general aim of medical treatment is to increase the hematocrit to reasonable levels without secondary side effects. Because patients with CRF, especially those on maintenance hemodialysis, are iron deficient, supplemental iron should be given. Iron can be given daily as a ferrous salt or on a periodic basis as intravenous iron dextran. Oral iron supplementation is inexpensive and is associated with very few side effects. Unfortunately, some patients do not absorb iron normally in spite of hemodialysis and require periodic intravenous iron dextran. No consensus on the frequency or dosage exists, and there is the potential for iron overload with hemosiderosis and occasional anaphylactoid reaction to intravenous iron dextran. Most patients with CRF do not have folate deficiency unless they are receiving maintenance dialysis treatment; routine folate supplementation is advisable.

Clinical trials have been recently carried out with recombinant human erythropoietin for the treatment of uncomplicated anemia in patients with ESRD. Gratifying and dose-dependent rises in the hematocrit occurred in response to intravenous erythropoietin administration. The phase III trial confirms that recombinant erythropoietin represents a major breakthrough in treating the anemia of ESRD.

The above findings with erythropoietin have changed the indications for transfusions and androgen therapy in CRF. Many patients with CRF tolerate extraordinarily low hematocrits surprisingly well. This tolerance may be due to increased release of oxygen from hemoglobin during chronic anemia. Substantial increases in overall well-being are observed when the hematocrit is maintained between 25 and 30 per cent. Higher levels are associated with side effects, including hypertension, headaches, and occasionally seizures.

INFECTIONS. Infections are more common in uremic than nonuremic patients. The general approach to the use of antibiotics should be the same in both groups of patients. Ideally, the antibiotic dose should be adjusted by monitoring the serum concentration of the antibiotic. However, this often is not feasible, and therefore after an initial normal loading dose, dosage levels must be adjusted for the degree of renal failure if the antibiotic is excreted by the kidney (Table 77–4). Some antibiotics are more nephrotoxic than others, and nephrotoxicity is potentiated in CRF. If drug sensitivities allow a choice in the treatment of a given infection, the physician should chose the least nephrotoxic antibiotic that is therapeutic.

RENAL OSTEODYSTROPHY. Hyperparathyroidism, decreased amounts of active vitamin D metabolites, and chronic metabolic acidosis all contribute to the development of renal osteodystrophy, as noted above. The goals of treatment are to normalize these abnormalities to the greatest extent possible.

NEUROPATHY. No specific treatment exists for either central or peripheral neuropathy. However, both objective and subjective improvement may occur by prolonging the periods of dialysis and by using dialyzers with a larger surface area. A gratifying improvement in peripheral neuropathy has been noted following successful renal transplantation, even in patients who were well dialyzed before transplantation.

MYOPATHY. No specific therapy exists for myopathy. Patients may improve dramatically with adequate dialysis. Some patients have shown improvement of myopathy following treatment with active vitamin D analogues and aggressive nutritional supplementation. Erythropoietin has a generalized anabolic effect, which may be very useful in this setting. Some patients with secondary hyperparathyroidism may benefit from parathyroidectomy.

CARBOHYDRATE METABOLISM. Abnormalities of carbohydrate metabolism in the nondiabetic patient are of no or minimal clinical significance. In the diabetic patient, insulin dosages must be adjusted to maintain serum glucose values at normal levels. Often, smaller insulin doses will be adequate as CRF progresses. Overt hypoglycemia may develop in a small number of patients with CRF.

URIC ACID. Although uric acid levels are consistently elevated in CRF, they are rarely much above 10 mg per deciliter. There is little evidence to suggest that asymptomatic hyperuricemia should be treated. Elevated uric acid levels in uremic patients should be treated only when there are tophaceous deposits or symptomatic gout. If treatment is elected, allopurinol is the drug of choice, since patients with CRF do not respond to uricosuric agents. Because of potential toxic side effects, the allopurinol dose should be decreased to no more than 100 mg per day in patients with chronic uremia.

PRURITUS. No specific therapy has withstood the test of time in the treatment of pruritus. A few patients get relief following topical application of emulsified oils or the use of oral antihistamine agents. Some patients have benefited from lowering the serum phosphate concentration by more effective dialysis and phosphate restriction. Parathyroidectomy has sometimes relieved intractable pruritus.

Diet

An appropriate diet can be critically important in the management of patients in CRF, for it may provide symptomatic improvement and may also slow the rate of loss of residual renal function. Although nutritional and caloric intake should be individualized for obese and malnourished patients, some general principles are applicable to all patients. In general, the higher the amount of protein in the diet, the higher the serum urea concentration. This occurs because amino acids are metabolized to form urea in addition to all other nitrogenous waste products that have been implicated by factors causing the uremic syndrome. Reducing the amount of protein in the diet lowers the BUN and reduces symptoms. Moreover, the difficulties in controlling serum phosphorus and acidosis are overcome, since a high protein intake is always associated with a high intake of phosphates as well as other inorganic ions. However, if dietary protein intake is too low, protein malnutrition will occur, with loss of strength, body weight, and muscle mass. This condition can be avoided if the protein requirements are met by providing 0.6 gram of protein per kilogram of body weight per day, of which at least 60 per cent contains proteins rich in essential amino acids, e.g., eggs, lean meat, and milk. A high-calorie intake can improve nitrogen utilization at very low nitrogen intakes, so that a diet of adequate calories manifests a protein-sparing (anticatabolic) effect. Providing about 30 kcal per day generally suffices, although this figure may be lowered for obese patients or raised for patients weighing less than their ideal body weight. Accumulated waste products can be reduced even further by lowering the daily protein intake to approximately 20 grams of protein per day, but only if the diet is supplemented with essential amino acids or a mixture of essential amino acids and their alpha-ketoanalogues. Such a regimen will maintain adequate protein nutrition for prolonged periods in patients with advanced renal failure. Alpha-ketoanalogues of essential amino acids are aminated in the body to form essential amino acids and hence body protein. Nitrogen, which otherwise would have accumulated as waste products, is therefore used to build body proteins. Unfortunately, this approach is extremely expensive. Low-protein diets in which daily minimum requirements are met and the very low protein diet supplemented with mixtures of amino acids may slow the rate of loss of residual renal function and possibly postpone the time when therapy with chronic hemodialysis becomes necessary. Compliance in this setting is probably the rate-limiting factor.

Diets should be supplemented with the water-soluble B vitamins plus vitamin C and folic acid; there is no need to supply additional vitamin A or E. Vitamin D should be reserved for treatment of severe renal osteodystrophy. In general, dietary sodium does not need to be severely restricted unless hypertension or edema is present. Most patients with CRF can readily excrete sodium until renal function is markedly impaired (creatinine clearance less than 10 ml per minute), but they cannot rapidly reduce salt excretion when dietary sodium is markedly restricted. For most patients, the diet should contain at least 1.5 to 2.0 grams of sodium per day. As long as the amount of urine excreted is greater than 1 liter per day, it is unusual to have to restrict potassium in the diet. Renal potassium excretion is promoted by increasing the dietary salt content. With use of these guidelines, uremic symptoms and the consequences of renal insufficiency can be controlled for most patients. Once chronic hemodialysis becomes necessary, the diet should be altered to meet the added requirements related to dialysis therapy.

Patients with CRF should be seen at regular intervals to monitor the progress of their disease. The frequency of these visits will depend upon the presence of other diseases, e.g., hypertension and heart failure, and on how rapidly residual renal function is being lost. All patients should be seen at least every 3 months, at which time a medical history is taken and a physical examination is performed. In addition, laboratory values, including hematocrit, white blood cell count, serum urea nitrogen and creatinine concentrations, and electrolyte values, should be obtained. Monitoring the progress of renal insufficiency is generally accomplished by measuring the serum creatinine concentration as an indirect index of the GFR. Alternatively, 24-hour urine collections can be obtained to measure creatinine and urea clearances, as an approximation of the GFR and a general indication of dietary protein intake. For most patients, the loss of residual renal function proceeds at a constant rate; this rate is different for each patient, although generally patients with polycystic kidney disease have a slower rate of loss of renal function than do those with diabetic nephropathy. When the reciprocal of serum creatinine concentration reaches 0.1 or less (a creatinine concentration of 10 mg per deciliter), the patient is close to the time when dialysis becomes necessary. It must be emphasized that the serum creatinine level is a reflection of muscle mass, which decreases as CRF progresses. In addition, creatinine secretion may be relatively well maintained as the GFR falls, so that creatinine clearance and serum creatinine will progressively overestimate the "true" GFR. Therefore, wide variations exist between individual patients with CRF when serum creatinine values are compared with the GFR. These considerations eliminate any absolute relationship between the serum creatinine level and the need for dialysis. Nevertheless, in the individual patient, the serum creatinine concentration provides the most immediately available marker for following the progression of renal insufficiency.

Dubach UC, Rosner B, Sturmer T: An epidemiologic study of abuse of analgesic drugs: Effects of phenacetin and salicylate on mortality and cardiovascular morbidity (1968–1987). N Engl J Med 324:159, 1991. *The authoritative 20-year follow-up on Dr. Dubach's group of 623 Swiss women who were exposed to phenacetin. A classic of epidemiologic research and clinical investigation.*

Eschbach JW, Abdulhadi MH, Browne JK, et al.: Recombinant human erythropoietin in anemic patients with end stage renal disease: Results of a phase III multicenter clinical trial. Ann Intern Med 111:992, 1989. *This is an important report of results from the phase III clinical trial using recombinant human erythropoietin to treat uncomplicated anemia in patients with end-stage renal failure undergoing hemodialysis. The authors demonstrate a remarkable dose-dependent rise in hematocrit in response to intravenous erythropoietin, which eliminates transfusions, reduces iron overload, and improves quality of life.*

Ihle BU, Becker GJ, Whitworth JA, et al.: The effect of protein restriction on the progression of renal insufficiency. N Engl J Med 321:1773, 1989. *A prospective, randomized study of 64 patients with CRF. There was a fourfold increase in ESRD in those patients who ate a regular diet, compared with those on a protein-restricted diet.*

Klahr S, Schreiner G, Ichikawa I: The progression of renal disease. N Engl J Med 318:1657, 1988. *A scholarly review of the physical, hormonal, and metabolic factors that may be involved in the progression of renal disease.*

Kopple JD, Jahn H, Massry SG, et al.: Kidney Int 36(Suppl 27):S1, 1989. *This supplement represents contributions from more than 100 leading interdisciplinary specialists on various aspects of uremia. Clinical symptoms, pathogenesis, and treatment of uremia and its complications are discussed in great detail.*

Meyer TW, Anderson S, Rennke HG, et al.: Reversing glomerular hypertension stabilizes established glomerular injury. Kidney Int 31:752, 1987. *These studies support the view that glomerular hypertension is an essential hemodynamic derangement that is responsible for progressive renal injury in the rat. Reduction of glomerular capillary pressure with converting enzyme inhibition or dietary protein restriction can arrest the progression of renal injury in the remnant rat model even if therapy is delayed until glomerular injury is established.*

Rostand SG, Brown G, Kirk K, et al.: Renal insufficiency in treated essential hypertension. N Engl J Med 320:684, 1989. *Despite acceptable blood pressure control, renal function may continue to deteriorate in approximately 15 per cent of treated patients. Black patients were twice as likely as white patients to have elevations in serum creatinine concentrations, even though diastolic blood pressure was maintained at 90 mm Hg.*

Salusky IB, Foley FN, Nelson P, et al.: Aluminum accumulation during treatment with aluminum hydroxide and dialysis on children and young adults with chronic renal disease. N Engl J Med 324:527, 1991. *A very provocative report that suggests that aluminum accumulation is a serious problem with serious sequelae in ESRD, even at previously accepted "safe" doses.*

Slatopolsky E, Weerts C, Norwood K, et al.: Long-term effects of calcium carbonate and 2.5 mEq/liter calcium dialysate on mineral metabolism. Kidney Int 36:897, 1989. *Calcium carbonate was shown to be an effective phosphate binder in large doses (10.5 grams per day). Hypercalcemia was prevented by lowering dialysate calcium concentration, thus obviating phosphate binders that contain aluminum.*

US Renal Data System: USRDS 1989 Annual Report. The National Institutes of Health, National Institute of Diabetes and Digestive and Kidney Diseases, Bethesda, Md., August 1989.

Warnock, DG: Uremic acidosis. Kidney Int 34:278, 1988. *A review of the renal responses to chronic acidosis, with an emphasis on the adaptations that develop during chronic renal insufficiency. The importance of chronic metabolic acidosis in the development of renal osteodystrophy is emphasized.*

Wollam GL, Tarazi RC, Bravo EL, et al.: Diuretic potency of combined hydrochlorothiazide and furosemide therapy in patients with azotemia. Am J Med 72:929, 1982. *A crossover study that demonstrates the importance of plasma volume expansion in chronic renal disease patients with hypertension. Hydrochlorothiazide caused a diuresis in patients who were resistant to furosemide.*

---

78 Treatment of Irreversible Renal Failure

78.1 DIALYSIS

Robert G. Luke

Each year approximately 1.3 in 10,000 of the United States population develop end-stage renal disease (ESRD) and require one of the various forms of renal replacement therapy: chronic hemodialysis in a center or at home; continuous ambulatory or cycling peritoneal dialysis (CAPD or CCPD); or transplantation from a live-related or cadaveric donor. For almost all of the United States population, most of the costs of such treatment are covered by the Renal Medicare Program, and by the early 1990's approximately 130,000 patients are expected to participate. The number of patients with ESRD continues to increase about 10 per cent per year, but most rapidly in the age group over 65 years. Diabetic glomerulosclerosis and hypertensive nephrosclerosis now contribute equally to cause 60 per cent of all ESRD, with chronic glomerulonephritis (5 per cent), polycystic kidney disease (7 per cent) and chronic interstitial kidney disease (5 per cent) accounting for most of the rest. Overall the program is a success, since it provides ready access to renal replacement therapy for virtually all U.S. residents with ESRD. Cost per patient (approximately $32,000 per year) has fallen, when inflation is considered.

The overall incidence of ESRD is four times greater in blacks than in whites, and all except congenital causes are increased in blacks.

Choice of renal replacement therapy is dictated by the availability of a live-related donor (best results), the age of the patient (transplantation is less frequently performed over the age of 65 years), and the presence of important systemic extrarenal disease (which may preclude surgery or immunosuppression). Preliminary hemodialysis is usually necessary before cadaveric transplantation. Home hemodialysis requires the support of a partner, an adequate home, self-motivation by the patient, and reasonably stable medical circumstances. Such patients have better rehabilitation and survival rates than those on in-center hemodialysis, but this may relate to patient selection factors. The cost of home dialysis is less than that of in-center dialysis. In general, patients are best served when all modalities of treatment for ESRD are readily available and well integrated.

TECHNICAL ASPECTS

As renal excretory function becomes progressively impaired, solutes accumulate in the body and eventually contribute to the uremic syndrome (see Ch. 77) and, ultimately, to death. These solutes, especially those of low molecular weight such as urea, can be removed efficiently from the blood by the process of diffusion across a semipermeable membrane down a chemical concentration gradient (dialysis). Substances higher in concentration in the dialysate than in the plasma, such as bicarbonate, will diffuse into the plasma. The membrane must be nontoxic and compatible with red blood cells, white blood cells, platelets, and plasma proteins. A synthetic membrane is used in extracorporeal hemodialysis; the lining membrane of the peritoneal cavity is used in peritoneal dialysis.

Hemodialysis

Membranes of varying hydraulic conductivity and solute permeability can be used in dialyzers of varying surface area and extracorporeal blood volume (100 to 250 ml in adults) to accommodate patients of different sizes, including infants. To remove accumulated sodium chloride and water, ultrafiltration across artificial membranes is induced by a transmembrane hydrostatic pressure, either positive on the blood side or negative on the dialysate side. The removal of over 1 liter of fluid per hour is feasible and predictable based on the ultrafiltration coefficient of the dialyzer. The essential components of a dialysate delivery and monitoring system of an artificial kidney apparatus are shown in Figure 78–1. Blood flow rates of 200 to 300 ml per minute are usual. Heparin is given intermittently or infused continuously (1000 to 10,000 units in total) to prevent clotting of blood in the dialyzer during the 3- to 6-hour procedure; dosage is controlled by the whole-blood or activated clotting time.

Dialysate contains normal serum levels of sodium and chloride, a variable potassium concentration (0 to 4 mEq per liter) depending on the patient's need for removal of potassium, and acetate (normally metabolized to bicarbonate) or bicarbonate (35 mEq per liter) to correct the metabolic acidosis. Bicarbonate may be preferable to acetate in some patients, either because acetate is not metabolized normally (in which case the normally transient increase in "anion gap" in the plasma will persist) or because it may contribute to hypotension during the hemodialysis procedure. A slight respiratory alkalosis is common during dialysis because of loss of CO_2 across the dialyzer. It persists transiently at the end of the hemodialysis procedure because, although the extracellular base deficit has been corrected, the respiratory center continues to respond transiently to intracellular acidosis. Calcium levels in the dialysate—3.5 mEq per liter—are higher than ionized calcium levels in blood to allow a calcium influx

from the dialysate, since most patients with chronic renal failure are in negative calcium balance. Dialysate flow rates are usually 500 ml per minute and thus the patient's blood "sees" 120 liters of fluid during a standard 4-hour dialysis.

High-flux dialysis now allows selected patients shorter dialysis times (2 to 3 hours) because of newer, more permeable membranes with higher clearances and dialyzers that allow more precise control of the rate of ultrafiltration. Patients must have a vascular access that permits blood flow rates of 300 ml per minute and must avoid high interdialytic intake of sodium chloride and water because of the limited time for fluid removal. Bicarbonate is required in the dialysate.

Peritoneal Dialysis: CAPD and CCPD

In peritoneal dialysis clearances of low molecular weight substances are less than those for hemodialysis (for example, a urea clearance of 20 to 25 ml per minute versus 150 ml per minute for hemodialysis), but clearance of some larger, perhaps also toxic, substances is greater because of the greater permeability of the peritoneal membrane to these larger molecules and the longer duration of treatment. When required, fluid removal is carried out by means of osmotic movement of water using high concentrations of glucose (1500 to 4500 mg per deciliter) in the dialysate. Exchange volumes during peritoneal dialysis are commonly 1 to 3 liters each hour. Several types of automated machines are available that deliver set volumes of fluid into the abdomen and then allow drainage after a set "dwell" time. The most common type now in use is the cycler, which is relatively simple, uses commercially prepared dialysate in bags, and automatically cycles up to 16 liters of dialysate in and out of the abdomen during a period of 8 hours (often overnight). Heparin (no systemic effect) and antibiotics are usually added during treatment of peritonitis, the most common complication of the procedure.

CAPD makes use of the fact that small molecular weight solutes reach complete equilibration with peritoneal fluid in 4 to 6 hours. Thus the patient exchanges 1.5 to 3.0 liters of sterile dialysate containing hypertonic glucose (1.5, 2.5, or 4.25 per cent) and physiologic electrolytes three to five times a day through a Tenckhoff peritoneal dialysis catheter and is able to maintain adequate removal of solutes and water. Since insulin-dependent diabetics have more complications of vascular access because of their vasculopathy and since regular insulin can be given in the dialysate with excellent control of the blood sugar, CAPD offers advantages to patients with diabetic glomerulosclerosis. In infants and children, the higher peritoneal surface area relative to body size also facilitates CAPD. In contrast to poorer dialysis of small molecular weight solutes compared with hemodialysis, dialysis of larger molecules (molecular weight >500) is increased. Many patients have been managed successfully by CAPD for 5 to 10 years, but long-term technique failure rates remain higher than for chronic hemodialysis, mainly because of problems with the peritoneal catheter or recurrent peritonitis.

CCPD is increasingly popular because the number of daily "connects" is reduced from four to two by employing the cycler during sleep and a single prolonged CAPD-type daytime exchange. This method is convenient for working patients or for blind or disabled patients who require helpers with their connections. When patients on CAPD or CCPD are admitted to the hospital and cannot perform exchanges, the cycler is usually employed. Rapid, hourly exchanges with the cycler are also useful for treating peritonitis.

Permanent vascular access is usually obtained by creation of an end-to-side arteriovenous fistula in the forearm or insertion of a prosthetic arteriovenous graft when the vessels themselves are inadequate. The fistula functions longer and, if feasible, is preferable. The permanent indwelling peritoneal catheter is made of radiopaque Silastic, is 25 cm long, and includes an intra-abdominal (located in the pelvis), subcutaneous (with a Dacron felt cuff barrier to bacteria at each end), and external segment.

SELECTION OF TREATMENT MODALITY

There is general agreement that successful renal transplantation offers the best rehabilitation, especially if a compatible related live donor is available (see Ch. 78.2). Unfortunately, the rate of renal transplantation in the United States appears to have reached

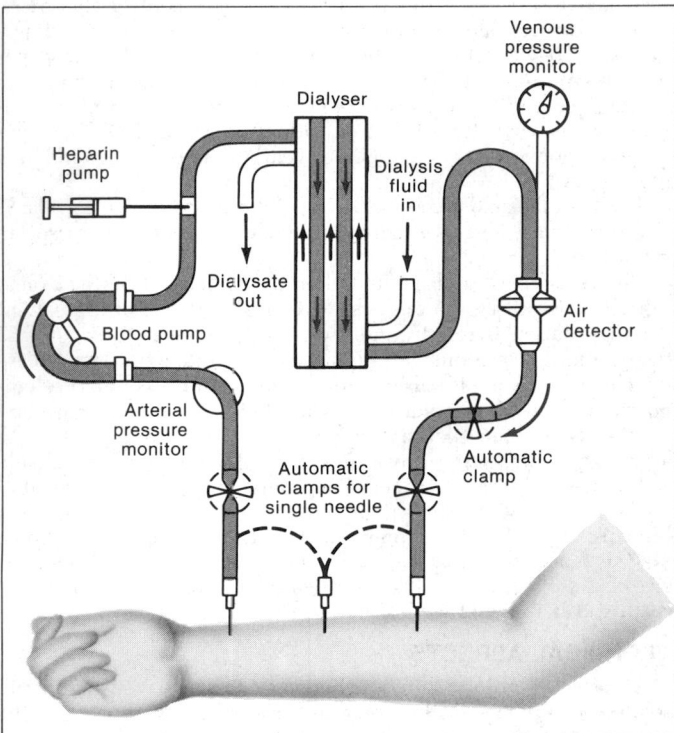

FIGURE 78–1. Essential components of a dialysis delivery system, which, together with the dialyzer, make up an "artificial kidney." In isolated ultrafiltration, no dialysis fluid is used (bypass mode). Also shown is the apparatus for using a single needle for inflow and outflow of blood from the patient. (From Keshaviah PR, Shaldon S: In Drukker W, Parsons FM, Maher JF [eds.]: Replacement of Renal Function by Dialysis. 3rd ed. Boston, Martinus Nijhoff Publishers, 1988.)

a plateau at about 10,000 per year, because of the continued high refusal rates by families of potential cadaveric donors. This means that the vast majority of ESRD patients must continue to rely on some form of dialysis therapy. This situation is influenced by age: Under 25 years of age, 50 per cent of patients with ESRD have a functioning transplant, but over 60 years of age, only 2 per cent have one. Many patients utilize all forms of renal replacement therapy at some stage of their treatment—for example, after loss of function of an allograft or after failure of vascular or peritoneal access.

All patients should have a thorough explanation of, and exposure to, all of the various renal replacement therapies, unless a specific absolute contraindication to one modality exists (e.g., human immunodeficiency virus [HIV] seropositivity for renal transplantation). Relative indications and contraindications are common (Table 78–1). The intermittent nature of clearance in hemodialysis contrasts with its continuity in CCPD or CAPD.

Initiation of Dialysis

Before initiating chronic dialysis, careful discussion with the patient and family should address the issue of whether such treatment is in the patient's best interest. For example, if there is extensive irremediable extrarenal disease, such as severe cerebrovascular disease or a painful malignancy, it may be wiser to continue conservative treatment only. Uniformly brief survival in patients with acquired immunodeficiency syndrome (AIDS) and ESRD has in general discouraged chronic dialysis in such patients. This is not true for patients who are HIV seropositive only.

Dialysis should be initiated when conservative management of chronic renal failure is beginning to be inadequate but before the development of uremic symptoms. In general, dialysis becomes necessary at a creatinine clearance of 4 to 8 ml per minute or a serum creatinine of about 10 mg per deciliter. However, the patient's general clinical state is more important than the level of blood urea nitrogen (BUN) or creatinine. It is especially important to institute therapy before the onset of pericarditis, peripheral neuropathy, or an impaired nutritional state secondary to anorexia or other uremic gastrointestinal symptoms, as subsequent recovery is then quite prolonged and mortality rate increased. A vascular access site should be prepared, if feasible, a few months before dialysis to allow it to mature adequately. If uremia develops abruptly, acute vascular access can be maintained for up to several months by an indwelling subclavian vein catheter or intermittently via the femoral vein. Permanent peritoneal access is prepared 1 to 2 weeks prior to use to prevent fluid leaks, which predispose to peritoneal and subcutaneous infections.

In *diabetic nephropathy* renal failure may accelerate or compound microangiopathic complications—especially retinopathy, gastropathy, and peripheral neuropathy—and many nephrologists therefore prefer to initiate replacement therapy earlier in such patients, perhaps when the serum creatinine level approximates 4 to 8 mg per deciliter. The progression of diabetic glomerulosclerosis to ESRD at that stage tends to be quite rapid.

Hypertension is an important complication in most patients who reach ESRD. Patients surviving for 20 years or more on chronic dialysis uniformly demonstrate good control of blood pressure. Antihypertensive medications can usually be tapered after initiation of dialysis, and blood pressure can be controlled by adjustment of plasma and extracellular fluid volume by ultrafiltration during dialysis and by dietary salt and water restriction. Sympatholytic drugs or drugs that cause postural hypotension are best avoided, since they interfere with the ability to remove fluid adequately by ultrafiltration. A reduction in urinary volume commonly accompanies the onset of dialysis because of lessening of solute osmotic diuresis. The concept of "dry weight" is a clinically important one in a patient on chronic dialysis, regardless of modality of therapy. This is the postdialysis weight at which the patient has an acceptable blood pressure and a plasma volume adequate for avoiding symptoms of diminished cardiac output or of pulmonary congestion. Short-term changes in weight are always due to salt and water deficits or excesses, but careful supervision is required to detect changes in body mass in either direction over longer periods. Interdialytic weight gains should not exceed 2 to 3 kg but unfortunately often do so in patients who are not compliant with dietary salt and fluid restrictions.

Most dialysis patients thus have "volume-dependent" hypertension and require antihypertensive medications only if they are noncompliant with salt and water intake. In perhaps 10 per cent of patients, however, blood pressure is "renin dependent," and hemodialysis is accompanied by persistent rebound hypertension due to rising circulating levels of angiotensin II resulting from ultrafiltration of plasma. Previously bilateral nephrectomy was sometimes employed to control blood pressure in such patients, but the advent of such potent drugs as captopril and minoxidil has virtually eliminated the need for this procedure. Furthermore, it is especially important to avoid bilateral nephrectomy when some recovery of renal function may occur in time, as after an episode of primary or secondary malignant hypertension or after rapidly progressive glomerulonephritis.

Dialysis disequilibrium describes a syndrome in which confusion, headache, and focal neurologic signs develop owing to more rapid dialysis of solutes from the plasma than from the intracellular compartment, especially from the brain. Thus an osmotic gradient can be set up between brain cells and extracellular fluid and lead to cerebral edema. This complication usually occurs in patients with acute or chronic renal failure and uremic symptoms and/or a very high BUN. Short dialysis with a low blood flow usually prevents this problem, which does not occur in patients maintained on chronic dialysis and is extremely rare during initiation of any of the forms of peritoneal dialysis because of their lesser efficiency.

Hepatitis B (Hb_sAg) is carried in the plasma of some patients

TABLE 78–1. SELECTION OF TREATMENT*

Clinical Factor	Preferred Modality	Comment
Insulin-dependent diabetes mellitus	PD	See text
Obesity	HD	Glucose load, hyperlipidemia with PD
Noncompliance	HD	Peritonitis with self-connects, missing exchanges
Work requires travel	PD	Freedom from machine
Severe peripheral vascular disease	PD	Avoids vascular access, ischemia, steal syndromes
Severe angina, congestive heart failure	PD	Less cardiovascular stress and hypotension and smoother control of extracellular fluid and vascular volume
Hernia	HD	PD may exacerbate or cause; repair before PD
Back pain	HD	PD may exacerbate
Ostomy	HD	Infection
Extensive intra-abdominal adhesions	HD	Difficulty with catheter placement, low clearance
Large, muscular build	HD	Better clearance
Small build or child	PD	Relatively good PD clearance
Transplant planned	PD/HD	HHD requires 6 weeks to train vs. 1 week for PD
Transplant not possible or unacceptable in younger patient	HHD	Longer survival of treatment modality than PD; independence
Hypoalbuminemia	HD	Loss of 12 grams/day of protein in PD fluid

*Transplant is not considered here but, if feasible, is generally preferred.
PD = CAPD or CCPD; HD = hemodialysis; HHD = home hemodialysis.

TABLE 78–2. RELATIVE INDICATIONS FOR PERITONEAL DIALYSIS (PD) OR HEMODIALYSIS (HD) FOR MANAGEMENT OF ACUTE RENAL FAILURE

Clinical Circumstance	Comment
1. Recent cerebral surgery, vascular accident or trauma	PD preferred; risk of hemorrhage with heparin and of fluid shifts in brain during HD
2. Hypercatabolic states (e.g., multiple injuries)	HD preferred; PD may not provide adequate clearance of urea, and so on
3. Recent cardiac surgery or myocardial infarction	PD preferred; increased risks of hypotension and arrhythmias with HD
4. Recent abdominal surgery	HD preferred; loss of fluid via incisions during PD; ileus requires surgical placement of PD catheter
5. Acute hemorrhage or severe coagulopathy	PD preferred; but in certain circumstances HD without heparin feasible
6. Complicating severe lung disease	HD preferred; PD may cause atelectasis and impair vital capacity by interfering with movement of diaphragm

with chronic renal failure, who therefore constitute a serious risk to dialysis staff and other patients, since there is repeated exposure to the patient's blood. Separate dialysis facilities and staff are needed for such patients if home dialysis or transplantation is not feasible. Routine monitoring for Hb$_s$Ag is now performed in patients initially testing negative for the antigen, and active immunization is available and indicated for patients and staff. Non-A, non-B hepatitis also remains an epidemiologic problem. Universal precautions (gloves, gown and mask, and special arrangements for disposal of needles) are now routine in dialysis units and offer adequate protection against the less infective HIV. Routine testing of patients and staff and isolation of HIV-seropositive patients are not required.

The Achilles heel of CAPD and CCPD is peritonitis, most often due to gram-positive skin organisms. Fortunately, most episodes can be managed in an outpatient setting with intraperitoneal antibiotics. Fungal peritonitis usually requires catheter removal; recurrent or multiple gram-negative organisms suggest primary intra-abdominal pathology, such as diverticulitis.

Hemodialysis and acute peritoneal dialysis are also employed in the treatment of acute renal failure, the most frequent cause of which is acute tubular necrosis (see Ch. 76). These patients are often quite ill, and survival is aided by frequent "prophylactic" dialysis to maintain a BUN of less than 100 mg per deciliter. The relative merits of hemodialysis and peritoneal dialysis for acute renal failure are outlined in Table 78–2.

Continuous Arteriovenous Hemofiltration

The technique of continuous arteriovenous hemofiltration can be uniquely valuable, especially in patients with acute cardiorenal failure and a low cardiac output. This procedure employs a membrane with a very high ultrafiltration coefficient, which allows fluid and solute removal at low blood perfusion pressures and flow rates. No blood pump or complex monitoring devices are required, and the procedure can be readily performed in an intensive care setting with femoral artery and vein cannulation in very ill, often fluid-overloaded patients in whom hemodialysis or peritoneal dialysis would be very difficult or impossible. Intravenous administration of electrolyte replacement solutions may be necessary with intravenous nutrition if indicated. Heparin is needed.

ROUTINE MANAGEMENT

Patients on chronic hemodialysis usually require a slightly reduced protein intake (0.8 to 1.0 gram per kilogram), but a more stringent control of salt and potassium intake, to maintain satisfactory levels of blood urea nitrogen, potassium, and blood pressure. CAPD patients are encouraged to ingest 1.0 to 1.2

grams per kilogram because of dialysate protein losses. Depending on peritoneal ultrafiltration rates, they may also tolerate a higher intake of salt and water. Hyperkalemia remains a significant cause of death in patients on chronic dialysis, usually due to dietary indiscretion. Monitoring of adequacy of dialysis requires assessment both of clinical well-being, including nutritional state, and of BUN and serum electrolytes, including calcium and phosphorus. The BUN reflects urea production rates and is dependent on protein intake and endogenous protein catabolism as well as on adequacy of urea removal by dialysis. Provided nutrition and protein intake are adequate, a BUN less than 90 mg per deciliter immediately prior to dialysis is usually acceptable. Plasma chemistries are checked monthly in the absence of clinical problems. Because of controlled prospective studies on the amount of dialysis necessary to prevent uremic complications, the increased use of high-flux, shorter time dialysis, and the use of lower dialysis plasma flows (higher hematocrits secondary to erythropoietin treatment), prescription of dialysis treatment is now being more closely individualized in terms of the patient's size and protein intake, duration of dialysis, type of dialyzer, and required clearance and dialysis blood flow rates.

In most patients, supplemental oral base (sodium bicarbonate) is not required; the serum HCO$_3$ should be kept above 20 mEq per liter in the predialysis blood. Dialysis is almost always inadequate to maintain serum phosphorus in an acceptable range (3.5 to 5.0 mg per deciliter) and, as in the conservative management of renal failure, oral phosphate binders are necessary. Aluminum hydroxide contributes to aluminum toxicity (see below), and its use is avoided or minimized by substituting calcium carbonate or acetate, by the prudent use of magnesium-containing antacids, and by avoidance of high-phosphate foods. Because of loss of water-soluble vitamins, including folic acid, from the blood during dialysis, routine administration of supplements of these substances is necessary. Oral iron is also given because there is a chronic small loss of blood that cannot be returned to the patient at the end of each dialysis. Use of recombinant human erythropoietin is now routine for treatment of renal anemia and constitutes the major therapeutic advance since the start of chronic dialysis in the 1960's. The replacement hormone is given intravenously during each dialysis or is administered subcutaneously. Hematocrit is maintained at about 35 per cent; lack of response usually indicates iron deficiency or malignant or chronic inflammatory disease. Hypertension sometimes develops as the hematocrit increases, but it usually responds to reduction of extracellular fluid volume.

COMPLICATIONS OF CHRONIC DIALYSIS

The major clinical complications experienced by patients on chronic dialysis are renal osteodystrophy, vascular access infections and thromboses, pericarditis and ascites, beta$_2$-microglobulin amyloidosis, and acquired renal cystic disease. (Table 78–3). The major cause of death remains cardiovascular disease, but the high incidence of coronary atherosclerosis probably reflects the risk factors of hypertension, smoking, and hyperlipidemia (and perhaps of a high calcium-phosphate product) rather than any specific effects of chronic dialysis per se. Dialysis does cause some cardiovascular stress during the procedure owing to ultra-

TABLE 78–3. COMPLICATIONS IN PATIENTS ON CHRONIC DIALYSIS

Accelerated cardiovascular disease	During dialysis
Hypertension	Hypotension
Renal osteodystrophy	Cramps
Serositis	Bleeding
Pericarditis	Leukopenia with pulmonary
"Dialysis ascites"	sequestration of WBC's
Pleural effusion	Hypoxia
Access infections and thrombosis	Electrolyte disturbances
Dialysis dementia	Dialysis disequilibrium
Pseudogout, tenosynovitis	CAPD
Pruritus	Exacerbation of symptoms of
Poor nutrition	abdominal hernia or back
Hepatitis B (Hb$_s$Ag) carrier state	pain
A$_2$ amyloid	Peritonitis
Acquired renal cystic disease	

WBC's = white blood cells.

filtration and reduction of plasma volume and to a modest reduction of arterial oxygen levels (by 10 to 20 mm Hg). This latter is due to hypocarbia secondary to loss of CO_2 across the dialyzer or to sequestration of blood leukocytes in alveolar capillaries after the activation of complement by the dialyzer membrane; a transient leukopenia is usual during the first hour of dialysis. Episodes of hypotension and hypoxia secondary to those dialysis effects frequently provoke angina in patients with coronary vascular disease.

Renal osteodystrophy is discussed elsewhere from the standpoint of both pathogenesis and treatment (see Ch. 237). Normal serum levels of calcium, phosphate, bicarbonate, and parathormone should be maintained. Calcium supplements, phosphate binders, and 1,25-$(OH)_2$ cholecalciferol (given orally or given intravenously during hemodialysis) may be needed. Rarely, soft tissue calcification, hypercalcemia, and progressive osteitis fibrosa cystica may necessitate subtotal parathyroidectomy. Osteomalacia usually responds to 1,25-$(OH)_2$ cholecalciferol, but one resistant type, in which an excess of aluminum is found on bone biopsy, appears to respond only to diminishing bone aluminum by chelating agents, such as desoxyferamine.

Serositis, manifested by pleural effusion, ascites, or pericarditis, may complicate chronic dialysis. The pathogenesis is not established, although onset often accompanies infection, stress, or protein catabolism. The diagnosis is dependent on elimination of other causes. In general, the abnormal fluid has the characteristics of an exudate and, especially in the case of the pericardial sac, may be hemorrhagic. Patients with pericardial effusion may develop pericardial tamponade, especially during dialysis, when intravascular volume and pressure in the right side of the heart are being reduced. Atrial arrhythmias are also common. If pericardial effusion occurs, dialysis should be carried out daily with very careful control of anticoagulation. If hemodynamic, radiologic, or ultrasonic assessment shows no improvement, surgical treatment by pericardial stripping or medical treatment by pericardiocentesis and insertion of a locally long-acting steroid, such as triamcinolone, is indicated. "Dialysis ascites" can be an intractable management problem. Poor nutrition and fluid overload often contribute, and insertion of a LeVeen shunt (one-way valve with bacterial filter between peritoneum and vena cava) may be necessary. Tuberculosis is an important differential cause of these complications, and diagnosis is dependent on histologic findings and culture, since anergy is common. Pleural effusion is less common and less troublesome than pericarditis and ascites.

Access infections are commonly due to *Staphylococcus aureus* infection, may be associated with bacteremia or septicemia or even bacterial endocarditis, and may require excision of the graft. Nafcillin and vancomycin are commonly used; the latter is convenient, since the absence of renal excretion often permits maintenance of adequate blood levels by weekly intravenous dosage during hemodialysis. Access problems are the most frequent cause of admission to hospital in the dialysis population. These include thrombosis, aneurysms, and infection of the graft. Arteriovenous fistulas last, on the average, longer than synthetic grafts, but each may function for several, even many, years. Steal syndromes may develop with pain in the hand during dialysis, especially in patients with diabetic vascular disease. Very high blood flows through fistulas may contribute to congestive heart failure, but this is quite unusual.

Dialysis dementia is a progressive fatal disease of the central nervous system associated with speech and motor defects, dementia, and seizures. It is now rare because of improved procedures for preparation of dialysate from tap water and reduction in its aluminum content. Past and present use of oral aluminum-containing phosphate-binding agents, however, continues to be associated with aluminum toxicity manifested as microcytic anemia (unresponsive to iron), muscle weakness, and a bone syndrome of pain and pathologic fractures unresponsive to 1, 25-$(OH)_2$ cholecalciferol or parathyroidectomy—indeed, it is made worse by the latter. Diagnosis is by special staining for aluminum of a nondecalcified bone biopsy. Serum aluminum levels, even after desoxyferamine infusion, are not reliable for diagnosis. Treatment involves infusion of desoxyferamine during dialysis, supplemented, as necessary, by a specific cartridge in the dialysis circuit to increase clearance of the aluminum-desoxyferamine complex.

Pseudogout and *tenosynovitis* occur quite frequently in dialysis patients and respond well to drugs such as indomethacin. *Pruritus*

is a troublesome symptom and is sometimes attributable to a high blood calcium-phosphate solubility product or to hyperparathyroidism. In some cases, pruritus, despite correction of the above factors, remains resistant to treatment.

The *dialysis procedure* itself may be complicated by hypotension and muscle cramps; both are related to rates of ultrafiltration and usually respond to injections of small amounts of hypertonic fluids, such as 0.3 M NaCl or 20 per cent mannitol. Contributory causes of hypotension are autonomic insufficiency, diminished cardiac function, and hypotensive drugs. In patients who are prone to ventricular ectopy, it is important to avoid hypoxia by use of supplemental oxygen and rapid changes in serum potassium by modifying dialysate potassium concentration. This is especially true in patients on cardiac glycosides. Other complications of the dialysis procedure are air embolism, bleeding secondary to heparin, loss of blood due to clotting of the dialyzer, and electrolyte disturbances due to errors in the dialysate. Fortunately, these are all now quite unusual. Indeed, death or serious morbidity due to complications of the hemodialysis procedure itself in properly trained or supervised patients is now exceedingly rare.

Two important new syndromes are recognized as complications after 5 or more years of dialysis: beta$_2$-microglobulin (A_2) amyloidosis and acquired renal cystic disease. A_2 amyloidosis results from retention of beta$_2$-microglobulin (molecular weight of 11,800; component of human leukocyte antigen [HLA] proteins on most cell membranes), which accumulates, after polymerization, in bone, joints, and tendons; carpal tunnel syndrome, bone pain, and arthritis are common. There is no specific treatment; prevention may be possible by use of more permeable dialyzer membranes. Intrarenal cysts also develop in patients on dialysis, but not after renal transplantation. Because some of these progress into renal adenocarcinoma, intermittent ultrasound examinations are probably indicated in patients on long-term dialysis.

LIMITATIONS OF DIALYSIS

For chronic dialysis, hemodialysis remains the "gold" standard, and many patients continue to do well even after 10 to 15 years of treatment. The 5-year survival rate for American patients is 40 per cent and ranges from 90 per cent in children to 20 per cent in adults over 64 years. This form of treatment is inherently limited, however, because of low clearances and because the endocrine and regulatory functions of the native kidney are not replaced by the "artificial kidney," (except for erythropoietin and 1, 25-$(OH)_2$-cholecalciferol.) Indeed, life saving though dialysis is, the patient with an endogenous creatinine clearance of even 20 ml per minute is usually better off than one on maintenance chronic dialysis or CAPD.

Especially in elderly patients with multisystem disease who may not improve on chronic dialysis, a "trial of dialysis" for a defined period of a few weeks may be indicated. Withdrawal from chronic dialysis in such circumstances by an informed patient is ethical.

Drukker W, Parsons FM, Maher JF: Replacement of Renal Function by Dialysis. 2nd ed. Boston, Martinus Nijhoff Publishers, 1988. *This is a complete reference work for all technical and clinical aspects of dialysis.*

Fisher JW, Bommer J, Heidelberg JE, et al.: Statement on the clinical use of recombinant erythropoietin in anemia of end-stage renal disease. Am J Kidney Dis 14:163, 1989. *A full discussion of current indications and methods for use of erythropoietin in patients with ESRD.*

Kleinman KS, Coburn W: Amyloid syndromes associated with hemodialysis. Kidney Int 35:567, 1989. *A complete and thoughtful review of the new amyloidosis related to beta$_2$-microglobulin.*

Salusky IB, Foley J, Nelson P, et al.: Aluminum accumulation during treatment with aluminum hydroxide and dialysis in children and young adults with chronic renal disease. N Engl J Med 324:527, 1991. *Aluminum hydroxide is less effective than calcium carbonate as a phosphate-binding agent for the control of hyperphosphatemia and is associated with aluminum retention in patients who are receiving chronic dialysis therapy.*

Sherrard DJ, Andress DL: Aluminum-related osteodystrophy. Ann Intern Med 39:307, 1989. *A concise review of aluminum toxicity and its primary manifestations.*

Twardowski ZJ, Nolph KD, Khanna R: Peritoneal dialysis: New concepts and applications. *In* Stein JH (ed.): Contemporary Issues in Nephrology. Vol 22. New York, Churchill-Livingstone, 1990. *A comprehensive and up-to-date account of clinical status of all aspects of CAPD and CCPD treatment and complications of therapy.*

78.2 RENAL TRANSPLANTATION

John J. Curtis

In the 1920's, Alexis Carrel developed the technique of vascular anastomoses. This momentous surgical breakthrough made possible David Hume's and Joseph Murray's human allograft attempts in the early 1950's. Similarly, Willem Kolff fashioned dialysis techniques and machinery that set the stage for George Thorn's group at Harvard Medical School to advance clinical dialysis to a viable and familiar therapy. Both accomplishments were eventually joined, with synergistic results, to effect truly dramatic changes in the management of chronic renal disease.

Those involved in other forms of organ transplantation envy the advantages produced by the combination of dialysis techniques and allograft transplantation. Because of the combination of these two effective renal replacement therapies, the volume of kidney transplant operations is vastly greater than that of other transplantation procedures. Patients can freely move back and forth between dialysis and transplantation, so that life does not depend on only one form of treatment. Kidney transplantation leads the field of organ replacement therapies by a large and growing margin.

Other advances in knowledge flow from these milestone developments. Peter Medawar's description of second set reactions and his insights into cellular immunology were preeminent advances in thinking. Both ideas are still actively advancing our understanding of human life. The close collaboration of pharmaceutical companies such as Burroughs-Wellcome and clinical researchers such as Roy Calne resulted in the development of azathioprine. Azathioprine made kidney transplantation possible in nonrelated individuals.

Today, several pharmaceutical companies are in the forefront of advancing transplantation. In few areas of endeavor are the accomplishments of academic centers, clinicians, industry, government, and patients themselves so truly beneficial to all concerned. The advance in kidney transplantation is one of medicine's success stories of the 1980's.

IMMUNOLOGIC ASPECTS OF KIDNEY TRANSPLANTATION

In kidney transplantation, the translation of understanding of the human immune system into clear-cut clinical advances is dramatic. Small lymphocytes are central to the problem of kidney allograft rejection. Both T and B lymphocytes are important players in kidney allograft rejection. B lymphocytes make circulating antibodies. The T lymphocyte, however, is critical: Acute rejection is dependent on the presence of T lymphocytes.

T lymphocytes constitute a heterogeneous group: Helper, suppressor, cytotoxic, and natural killer (NK) T lymphocytes are recognized by the presence of characteristic antigens on their cell membranes. The helper T lymphocyte is required for the rejection process. It participates in initial recognition of foreign antigen on transplanted tissue. Foreign antigens stimulate the T helper lymphocyte to release lymphokines that produce both growth and differentiation of other T and B lymphocytes.

Newly developed immunosuppressive agents target T lymphocytes and the lymphokines they produce. These new agents may be both more potent and more specific than those used in the past. Further understanding of the methods by which foreign antigens are presented to lymphocytes and the lymphokine communication network (in which the T helper cell is central) will yield more specific immunosuppression.

In the late 1960's, Daussett advanced the science of immunology with the description of the human lymphocyte antigen (HLA) system. The major histocompatibility complex (MHC), which in humans is on chromosome 6, codes for two classes of antigens (class I [A, B, and C] and class II [D, DR, DQ, DP, and DO]) on cell membranes. Inheritance of these cell antigen markers is co-dominant. Each parent transmits one set of HLA antigens (haplotype) to his or her child. Nearly all cells, except red blood cells, express class I antigens, while B lymphocytes, monocytes, and endothelial cells express class II antigens. These antigens are pivotal in the rejection process.

Transplantation usually succeeds if all known class I and class II antigens between donor and recipient are identical. Unfortunately, from a matching prospective, the MHC is the most polymorphic coding system known in human biology. Most donors and recipients cannot be perfectly matched for MHC coded antigens unless the organ comes from a close family member. Figure 78–2 shows that siblings of a given patient with ESRD may be either two-haplotype matches (25 per cent likelihood), one-haplotype matches (50 per cent likelihood) or zero-haplotype matches (25 per cent likelihood). True parents are usually a one-haplotype match. As noted in the figure, ABO blood groups must also be compatible to ensure successful transplantation.

In animal and human recipients of kidney allografts, matching for both class I and class II antigens correlates with successful graft outcomes. The source of most human kidney transplants, however, is a cadaveric donor (a donor who has died but whose kidneys are still viable). Finding a good HLA match is more difficult from cadavers than from blood relatives. Although retrospective analysis of cadaveric transplantation data shows the benefit of class I and class II matching, the benefit is not as dramatic as for kidneys from relatives.

Transplantation centers in the United States currently follow a policy of mandatory sharing of six-antigen (both class I and class II) matches for cadaveric kidneys. Organ banks consider other factors besides HLA match (e.g., the patient's age and length of time on a waiting list) in the distribution of cadaveric kidneys.

Unquestionably important for both living-related transplantation and cadaveric transplantation is the "crossmatch" test. Tissue typing laboratories perform this test before all kidney transplant operations. Technicians incubate leukocytes from the potential donor (living-related or cadaveric) with serum from the potential recipient and serum complement. If the serum of the recipient destroys the membranes of the leukocyte of the potential donor, the laboratory reports the test as positive.

The surgeon usually cancels the transplant operation if the crossmatch is positive. Such a result signifies circulating antibodies against the HLA antigens. A positive crossmatch predicts nearly immediate and severe ("hyperacute") allograft rejection if the transplant is done. Investigators are testing modifications of the crossmatching procedure to find a more sensitive, yet more specific, test. The current tests, however, have all but eliminated hyperacute rejections. More sensitive tests could decrease other types of early rejection ("accelerated rejections").

Currently, many patients on waiting lists for kidney transplants have developed broad anti-HLA sensitization. Exposure to blood transfusions, failed previous transplants, or pregnancy causes such sensitization to HLA antigens. Nearly one third of patients awaiting transplantation fall into this "highly sensitized," difficult-to-transplant category. Such patients benefit from receiving the best HLA antigen match possible.

Physicians have tried other strategies, such as plasmapheresis and extracorporeal immunoadsorption, to find a suitable method of overcoming the problem of circulating preformed antibodies. These trials offer promise but are not yet established practice. The more common use of erythropoietin in patients awaiting transplantation will reduce the exposure to blood transfusions. The introduction of this new therapy to dialysis promises to decrease the rate of development and degree of circulating antibodies in patients with ESRD.

INDICATIONS FOR KIDNEY TRANSPLANTATION

The most common diseases that result in referral of patients for transplantation are (1) diabetes mellitus with renal failure, (2) hypertensive renal disease, and (3) glomerulonephritis. These three causes of ESRD account for nearly 75 per cent of candidates.

No specific cause of intrinsic and irreversible renal failure is considered a contraindication to kidney transplantation. Nonetheless, all patients should have reversible causes of renal dysfunction excluded (e.g., incomplete obstruction) prior to consideration of renal replacement therapy. Most patients undergo a period of chronic dialysis prior to receiving an allograft. Listed in Table 78–4 are selected diseases that can cause renal failure and need special consideration before renal transplantation is

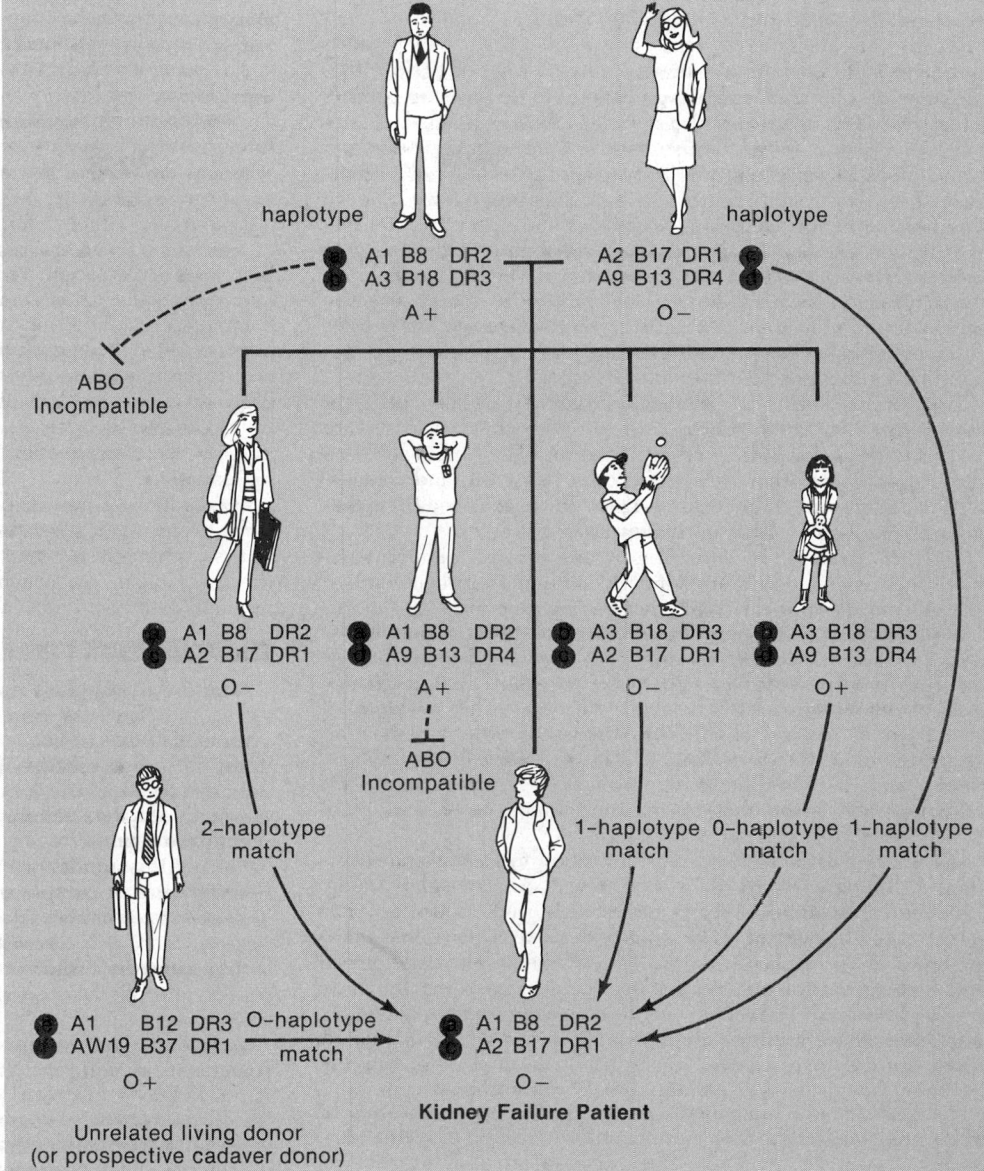

FIGURE 78–2. Family tree of HLA genotypes and unrelated HLA genotype.

chosen as therapy. The listed diseases are not contraindications to transplantation, yet the outcome may be less satisfactory for patients with these diseases compared with other renal diseases.

Patients with renal failure induced by diabetes (Kimmelstiel-Wilson disease) make up the greatest population of patients currently referred for transplantation. A decade ago, such patients

were not routinely considered for kidney transplantation, but today many nephrologists consider this the treatment of choice for diabetic patients. The change in medical practice for this condition has resulted in a major extension of life expectancy of patients whose kidneys fail from diabetes.

The long-term outcome for patients with diabetes is less likely to result in full rehabilitation than for patients with forms of renal disease that do not have other organ involvement. Although allograft replacement restores normal renal function to such patients, kidney transplantation does not correct the diabetes. Long-term complications of diabetes do not reverse, and new complications develop. Eventually, other organ involvement with diabetic disease limits both survival and rehabilitation in diabetic recipients of renal allografts.

Today, living-related transplantation offers patients with diabetic renal failure the highest likelihood of prolonged survival. Most centers perform transplantations earlier in diabetic patients than in those referred with other forms of renal disease. If diabetic patients can undergo transplantation before extensive damage occurs in other organs, such as the eye and heart, rehabilitation will be more satisfactory. Late referral of diabetic patients is not in their best interest. Such patients may develop severe neurologic and cardiovascular disease to a degree that excludes them from transplantation.

Hypertension is better treated than in the past, yet the

TABLE 78–4. FACTORS LIMITING SUCCESS OF RENAL TRANSPLANTATION IN CERTAIN DISEASES

Disease	Comment
Hemolytic uremic syndrome	Disease can recur and cause graft failure rapidly; cyclosporine may increase the risk of recurrence.
Sickle cell disease	Improved hematocrit can result in increased incidence of sickle crises.
Scleroderma	Long-term vascular and gastrointestinal problems of scleroderma can limit rehabilitation.
Oxalosis	Recurrence of stone disease can be severe.
Cystinosis and Fabry's disease	Disease activity continues.
Focal glomerulosclerosis	Graft loss from recurrence is common.

incidence of end-stage renal failure due to hypertension has not decreased. It ranks second only to diabetes as a cause of renal failure in patients sent to renal transplant units. Such patients often have suffered from a malignant phase of hypertension. It is more common for elevated blood pressure to destroy the kidneys of black patients than of white patients. Kidney transplantation in this group of patients often restores normal renal function and normal blood pressure control. The reason the number of patients referred to transplant centers with end-stage failure due to hypertension is not decreasing is unclear and deserves intensive investigation. Black patients tend to have slightly poorer success with renal transplants than do white patients. The high prevalence of hypertension as a cause of renal failure in blacks may be responsible for the poorer outcome. Most investigators believe that immunologic factors, rather than original disease, are responsible for slightly poorer allograft survival.

The various forms of glomerulonephritis usually progress (slowly) to end-stage function. Patients with these diseases are ideal candidates for kidney transplantation. They often have no medical problems other than their kidney disease, and replacement of kidney function restores them to normal health. Rehabilitation can be excellent in this group of patients.

Listed in Table 78–4, however, is one form of glomerulonephritis that causes continuing difficulty in renal transplant centers. Focal glomerulosclerosis (FGS) is an idiopathic form of glomerulonephritis that (like many other forms of glomerulonephritis) can recur in the allograft. Patients with FGS have a rate of graft loss from recurrent disease (20 to 30 per cent) that is greater than in other forms of glomerular disease. The problem of recurrence of disease should be discussed with patients and prospective family kidney donors. The histologic lesion of focal sclerosis can occur in other circumstances (e.g., reflux nephritis), and recurrence in the allograft does not appear to be a problem in such cases.

Age is never an absolute contraindication to kidney transplantation. Although infants have had successful transplantations, most centers maintain infants on dialysis until body size has increased to 10 to 20 kg. Older patients are also becoming more numerous in transplant clinics. Older age (>60 years) never precludes successful transplantation but does increase the risks of complications. Transplant centers usually encourage older patients who have multiple medical problems (rather than isolated kidney failure) to remain on dialysis. On both ends of the age spectrum, however, transplantation is becoming more common.

The presence of malignancy is considered a contraindication to kidney transplantation, as is severe atherosclerotic or pulmonary disease. Patients with active liver disease are also usually excluded. Infection with the HIV virus is a relative contraindication. Anecdotal case reports suggest that such patients may progress more rapidly from carrier status to clinical AIDS when given immunosuppressive therapy. Social circumstances (inability to take medications or arrange follow-up) can also make kidney transplantation an impossibility.

EVALUATION OF THE DONOR AND RECIPIENT OF THE KIDNEY TRANSPLANT

The transplant team that will perform the surgery and follow-up should evaluate the donor (living-related) and potential recipient of the transplant. This evaluation is best done at the center where the transplantation will be done, before the actual transplantation date. The evaluation team usually includes a transplant surgeon, nephrologist, urologist, social worker, and psychiatrist.

Evaluation of the living donor focuses on three issues. Physicians must document that the patient does not have any significant medical problems that would increase the risk of surgery. The donor's motives should be appraised to ensure that the donation is altruistic. Finally, the renal function and the anatomy of the donor's renal arteries need to be defined, usually with a renal arteriogram. This evaluation is best performed in the hospital.

Evaluation of the recipient also has three goals. The physicians should assess the patient's overall medical status, aware that the recipient may face both major surgery and potent immunosuppression in the future. Emphasis should be placed on the recipient's cardiovascular risks and urologic status. The recipient's

original disease often is uncertain, and the transplant center should attempt to define this for the record. Knowledge of the original kidney disease is often important in the posttransplant management of the patient. Finally, the recipient needs to understand the risks and benefits of transplantation surgery.

The patient's social circumstance and ability to arrange follow-up also need evaluation. A discussion that explores the degree of the patient's understanding of the disease process and the planned intervention is part of the evaluation. Both audiovisual aids and personal discussions with nurses, physicians, and other kidney transplant patients are key to the patient's preparation.

Potential recipients found to have correctable cardiovascular or urologic lesions are encouraged to have repair of the lesions before transplantation. Bilateral nephrectomy of native kidneys before transplantation is rarely done. In the past, this was a more common procedure for the control of severe hypertension. A nephrectomy is suggested if the native kidneys are infected in such a fashion that only their removal will protect the patient from serious infections after transplantation. Occasionally, patients excrete such large amounts of protein from diseased native kidneys that nephrectomy is recommended because of protein malnutrition.

Preparation of the recipient with deliberate blood transfusions was a common procedure before the routine use of cyclosporine but is no longer so popular as in the past. An understanding of the mechanism by which such blood transfusions altered the immune response is still a matter of investigation.

THE ADMISSION FOR KIDNEY TRANSPLANTATION

Cadaveric transplant operations can be better "planned" than in the past because improved allograft harvesting and storage techniques have removed some of the urgency from the procedure. It is not elective surgery, however, and is still highly dramatic for the recipient. The pretransplantation evaluation of the recipient should help prepare the patient for the actual day of the transplantation.

During this admission, the transplant surgeon places a kidney allograft into the recipient's iliac fossa. An anastomosis is created between the donor renal artery and the hypogastric artery. The surgeon must also connect the donor renal vein to the iliac vein and implant the ureter into the recipient's bladder. These three connections all have variations, and all need skillful surgical technique.

On return from the operating room, the transplant recipient's first transplant admission has begun. Three issues face the patient. If the kidney is not working immediately ("immediate nonfunction"), the reason (or reasons) need to be identified. If the kidney is working, careful observation for possible rejection is begun. In either case, a new immunosuppressive regimen starts.

Immediate nonfunction of the allograft is becoming less common with improvement of techniques for procurement and storage. It is due, most often, to an acute tubular necrosis (ATN)–like syndrome in which there is reversible ischemic damage to the allograft that will heal, given time. Recent evidence strongly suggests that this phenomenon, while similar to classic ATN, differs in that the immune system plays a major role.

Obstruction, vascular thrombosis, and ureteral compression from hematoma should be considered in cases of primary nonfunction. Renal scans and ultrasound tests, as well as the patience of the managing physician, are indicated. Occasionally, an immediate return to the operating room is required. Most patients with immediate nonfunction, however, have reversible renal impairment that does not require surgical intervention.

Allografts that work immediately after the release of the vascular clamps engender immediate optimism. Observation is key in the postoperative management. It is usually in the first 3 months after transplantation that reversible acute rejections commonly occur. Many of these rejections occur during the initial hospital stay. All patients should have daily assessment of renal function, and when physicians notice impairment, a rapid diagnosis of cause (rejection versus other causes) is in order. Despite pressures to cut costs, early discharge is not in the best interest of the kidney transplant patient, although most feel well within a few days after the transplant operation. The more frequently that patients are observed in the months after transplantation, the better their care and the greater the likelihood that rejections will be reversed. The transplant physician should encourage close observation as a more important goal than early discharge.

During the first hospital stay, patients are given potent immunosuppressive agents. Immunosuppressive regimens remained stable from the 1960's through the early 1980's. Azathioprine and prednisone were the two drugs employed. Physicians became experienced with these two agents and with their predictable complications and eventually settled on the proper dose and schedule.

The Food and Drug Administration (FDA) approved cyclosporine in 1983 for general use in transplantation. Since then, the transplant community has developed a frenzy for new and different immunosuppressive protocols. Transplant centers often change to new protocols before research groups test the older protocols with randomized controlled trials. Nonetheless, as transplant groups have experimented with new and different immunosuppressive agents, results have improved markedly over the results seen with "conventional therapy" (azathioprine and prednisone).

Currently, many centers in the United States use sequential, or "induction," therapy. Four drugs are used. Initially, either antilymphocyte globulin (ATG) or monoclonal antibody (OKT3) is given as the primary immunosuppressive agent. These anti–T lymphocyte agents are continued until the allograft functions well. Then, cyclosporine, azathioprine, and prednisone are added, and ATG or OKT3 is discontinued shortly thereafter. Other groups begin with a regimen of cyclosporine, azathioprine, and prednisone immediately preceding the transplant operation ("triple drug therapy"). Some groups believe that a combination of cyclosporine and prednisone, or cyclosporine alone, is adequate therapy.

Many groups treat recipients of living-related allografts with a different immunosuppressive regimen than that used for recipients of cadaveric kidneys. Living-related donor recipients generally require less immunosuppression. These patients are usually given lower doses of fewer different immunosuppressive agents.

The addition of cyclosporine and the routine use of anti–T lymphocyte agents, while credited with improved allograft success rates, make management more complex. Cyclosporine can cause impairment of renal function that is difficult to distinguish from rejection. OKT3 and ATG can cause febrile reactions and may result in renal dysfunction.

Cyclosporine has revolutionized organ transplantation. Transplant groups have achieved a 10 to 15 per cent improvement in initial and long-term allograft survival rates with cyclosporine. Some investigators believe that the added immunosuppression of this agent overcomes the risks of rejection with poorly matched allografts. Others suggest that preparation of recipients with pretransplant blood transfusions is no longer necessary. Both of the above benefits of cyclosporine remain controversial. Most agree, however, that cyclosporine has improved allograft success rates while allowing a decrease in other immunosuppressive agents. Fewer fungal or bacterial infections occur in transplant recipients despite the decreased use of other immunosuppressants.

Cyclosporine does not affect the immunorecognition or priming of T lymphocytes to express surface receptors. Its mechanism of action is inhibition of synthesis of interleukin 2 and gamma-interferon. This is a more specific and more easily reversed action than that associated with glucocorticoids and antimetabolites. Increasing specificity of immunosuppressive agents is leading to both improved allograft survival and greater safety.

Unfortunately, one of cyclosporine's major side effects is nephrotoxicity. Investigators have shown acute, "reversible," and chronic kidney damage. Cyclosporine also markedly slows recovery from ATN and potentiates nephrotoxicity due to other substances. Cyclosporine is difficult to monitor, and clinical toxicity is common even in experienced hands. Besides nephrotoxicity, cyclosporine commonly causes tremor, palmar and plantar paresthesia, hyperglycemia, hepatotoxicity, hypertrichosis, gingival hypertrophy, and hyperkalemia.

As of this writing, OKT3 is the only monoclonal antibody commercially available. The antibody is directed against the T lymphocyte receptor for antigen and is thus a "pan" T lymphocyte agent. More specific monoclonal antibodies remain in investigational status.

OKT3 is effective in the treatment of acute rejection. Most patients who do not respond to the more traditional acute rejection therapy (bolus methylprednisolone) respond well to OKT3. This antibody is also used as prophylactic immunosuppression in the immediate posttransplant period as part of some sequential protocols. It is one of the most potent agents available for reversal and prevention of T lymphocyte–mediated rejection.

Like cyclosporine, however, OKT3 has several drawbacks. Humans develop antibodies against this murine antibody that eventually limit its effectiveness. After a single course of treatment, many patients do not respond to further therapy. Unfortunately, the reversed rejection episodes sometimes flare or recur. OKT3 that is given intravenously usually produces a "first-dose reaction" that results from cytokine release.

This first-dose reaction varies markedly among patients, from mild to life threatening. Fever, chills, dyspnea, wheezing, tachycardia, hypotension, nausea, and vomiting are common. The fever is of special concern because febrile patients with renal transplant may also be infected and OKT3-induced temperature elevation may mimic fever from other critical causes.

OUTPATIENT FOLLOW-UP

If the transplant admission goes without complication, it is possible for patients to be discharged as early as a week after surgery. Unless arrangements can be made for daily outpatient visits after discharge, however, most centers keep patients in the hospital for longer periods. Complications can lengthen this first admission to months. Geography, financial resources of the patient, facilities of the center, and clinical judgment of the physicians involved result in initial hospital stays that vary markedly in length. The author's opinion is that longer initial in-hospital stays are to the benefit of the patient. Nonetheless, whether patients are in the hospital or are outpatients, the two major problems faced by them in the initial period are infection and rejection.

Two forms of rejection have already been alluded to previously: hyperacute rejection and accelerated rejection. Both, by definition, occur before the end of the first week. Hyperacute rejection is rare with current crossmatch techniques. Accelerated rejections are less well understood and more common. Accelerated rejections often do not respond to therapy and some investigators believe that such rejection episodes also suggest the presence of circulating antibodies. It is possible that more sensitive crossmatch techniques will decrease the frequency of accelerated rejections.

Acute and chronic rejections are more common. Acute rejection episodes occur in most kidney transplant recipients. These episodes usually occur after the first week and can occur at any time, even years after the transplant. Mediated by T lymphocytes, such rejections are often associated with marked cellular infiltration of the allograft with edema. Vascular lesions also occur and suggest a poor prognosis.

Most acute rejection episodes, if diagnosed early, will respond to increased dosages of immunosuppressive agents. Diagnosis is usually made when a sudden impairment in the function of the allograft is noted. Other causes of impaired function must be ruled out. Confirmation of acute rejection can be obtained with renal scans and allograft biopsies. The most common other reason for impaired allograft function is toxicity from cyclosporine.

Chronic rejection is a phenomenon less well understood than acute rejection. Most cadaveric allografts eventually show histologic changes of rejection. These changes are mostly vascular and are similar to the histology of nephrosclerosis. Eventually, the allograft develops fibrosis and glomerular lesions that appear secondary to ischemia. There is neither a good understanding of chronic rejection nor an accepted effective therapy.

Serial "flow sheet" measurements of serum creatinine concentration reveal a gradual trend for slow but progressive impairment of allograft function. The renal scan reveals a more marked loss of renal blood flow than of glomerular filtration rate (GFR), and renal biopsy reveals fibrosis and vascular narrowing. Patients are generally asymptomatic. Recurrence of original kidney disease and cyclosporine toxicity are two other causes of allograft impairment that can mimic chronic rejection.

Despite the fact that the serum creatinine concentration is a somewhat gross measurement of renal function, it is the most commonly used test for clinical follow-up. Other tests are regularly promised in the literature to diagnose rejection earlier and more definitively. None of these laboratory tests, however, has yet replaced the serum creatinine level. Blood urea nitrogen and urinalysis are routinely obtained. It is the sequential measurement of serum creatinine concentration, however, that proves most useful clinically.

Renal scans and isotope measurements of renal blood flow (^{131}I-orthoiodohippurate) and GFR (^{99m}Tc-diethylenetriamine) are employed frequently to provide additional functional assessment of renal function. Ultrasound has proved useful for visualizing the structure of the allograft and to rule out obstruction. It has almost replaced the use of intravenous pyelography (IVP). Arteriography of the transplant renal artery is useful in making the diagnosis of stenosis. Although an invasive procedure, an arteriogram of the allograft can also provide information about the small vessels of the allograft in a more global fashion than renal biopsy. Biopsy of the allograft is also an invasive procedure. Transplant physicians believe that it gives the most useful assessment of the allograft and aids in differentiating the causes of allograft dysfunction. When other clinical assessment leaves considerable doubt in the mind of the managing physician concerning the cause of impaired function, a biopsy is indicated. More recently, the technique of fine-needle biopsy has gained popularity. This technique is considerably safer than the percutaneous core biopsy, yet its sensitivity and specificity remain controversial.

Infections during the first few weeks after transplantation cause fever and can cause impairment of allograft function. They may be confused with rejection. Wound, intravenous line, and catheter-related infections are common and are not usually due to opportunistic organisms when they occur within a few weeks of transplantation.

Opportunistic infections usually occur a month or more after the transplant operation. While *Aspergillus, Nocardia,* and *Toxoplasma* were once somewhat common, newer immunosuppressive protocols have resulted in a change in the spectrum of opportunistic infections. Viral infections, especially cytomegalovirus, have become dominant. Many investigators believe this is a result of the use of more specific anti–T lymphocyte preparations, such as OKT3. Infection with cytomegalovirus can be asymptomatic. It also can be so severe as to cause coma and death. Fortunately, most of these infections after transplantation, characterized by spiking fevers, leukopenia, and general malaise, last only 1 to 2 weeks and then resolve without sequelae.

Immunosuppressed kidney transplant patients believed to be infected should be hospitalized and aggressively managed. Infections in this group are the leading early cause of mortality, and aggressive management can usually reverse the process without need of sacrificing the allograft.

LONG-TERM FOLLOW-UP

Long-term immunosuppression is surprisingly well tolerated by most kidney transplant recipients. Nonetheless, it is this therapy that accounts for most of the posttransplant morbidity and mortality. Vascular disease, infections, malignancy, and chronic liver disease pose the most serious problems for recipients of kidney transplants. Immunosuppressive agents either cause or aggravate these four medical problems. Table 78–5 lists some of the more common medical problems encountered in kidney transplant clinics.

Like the general population, kidney transplant patients are most likely to die of atherosclerotic vascular disease. Kidney transplant patients, however, die of myocardial infarctions and cerebrovascular accidents at an earlier age. The reason for this precocious onset of vascular disease is not entirely understood.

Kidney transplant patients experience a high incidence of hypertension. The hypertension is multifactorial in nature. Some immunosuppressive drugs (cyclosporine and prednisone) can cause hypertension, as does kidney disease. Even if the allograft is normal, the diseased native kidneys can maintain elevated blood pressure. Stenosis of the artery of the transplanted kidney may also be a factor.

TABLE 78–5. MEDICAL COMPLICATIONS AFTER KIDNEY TRANSPLANTATION

Cardiovascular Events
  Myocardial infarction
  Cerebrovascular accident

Hypertension
  Stenosis of transplant renal artery
  Native kidney induced
  Drug induced
  Renal impairment of the allograft

Malignancies
  Skin carcinomas
  Lymphomas

Erythrocytosis
  Induced by native kidneys (?)
  Thromboembolic disease

Bone Disease
  Osteoporosis
  Aseptic necrosis
  Persistent hyperparathyroidism

Infections
  Listeria monocytogenes
  Pneumocystis carinii
  Cryptococcus
  Aspergillus
  Nocardia
  Toxoplasma
  Mycobacteria
  Legionella pneumophila
  Cytomegalovirus (CMV)
  Herpes simplex virus (HSV)
  Varicella zoster virus (VZV)
  Hepatitis viruses
  Papovaviruses
  Human immunodeficiency virus (HIV)
  Epstein-Barr virus (EBV)

Gastrointestinal Problems
  Peptic ulcer
  Pancreatitis
  Diverticulitis
  Hepatitis

Glucocorticoid-Induced Complications
  Obesity
  Cataracts
  Hyperglycemia
  Myopathy

Endocrine and Metabolic Disorders
  Secondary hyperparathyroidism
  Proximal and distal types of renal tubular acidosis
  Asymptomatic hyperuricemia and gout
  Mild hyperkalemia
  Glycosuria without an increased serum glucose concentration
  Hypophosphatemia

Miscellaneous
  Idiopathic polyarthritides
  Hirsutism
  Lymphocele
  Warts
  Psychiatric affective disorders

Kidney transplant patients have abnormal lipid profiles that physicians consider a risk factor for atherosclerotic death. These abnormal lipid patterns are believed to be an effect of the immunosuppressive drugs. Some patients continue to have proteinuria in the nephrotic range after transplantation, which may contribute to the abnormal lipid profile.

Besides hypertension and abnormal lipid profiles, there is convincing evidence that renal transplant patients usually have vascular disease even before the transplant. This vascular disease may relate to their time on dialysis and the hypertension associated with their chronic renal failure.

Most successful recipients of renal transplants enjoy a quality of life that is superior to that achieved on dialysis. Women frequently give birth after transplantation, and men can father children. It is unusual for patients with successful transplants not to return to full-time employment. Many return to a lifestyle similar to that preceding the onset of kidney disease. On the other hand, the experience of chronic disease, frequent hospitalizations, disability financing, and fear of allograft failure with long-term complications of transplant immunosuppression limit full rehabilitation for some patients.

In the United States in 1987, the average 1-year allograft survival rate was 77 per cent for recipients of cadaveric kidneys. It was 90 per cent for recipients of allografts from relatives. This is a remarkable advance compared with survival rates of 50 per cent for cadaveric kidneys just a few years ago. Some individual centers now experience cadaveric allograft survival rates of nearly 90 per cent. Mortality and morbidity continue to decrease as allograft survival rates increase. It seems likely that even these rates of success will improve in the near future.

The long-term use of immunosuppressive agents causes or aggravates most of the complications listed in Table 78–5. Investigators are directing considerable efforts at making such therapy unnecessary. Soon patients may be able to tolerate foreign antigens of the donor kidney but react normally to other foreign antigens. Limited tolerance has been achieved in animal models. If similar types of tolerance can be created in humans, graft survival will improve, and the morbidity and mortality of kidney transplantation will be drastically reduced.

Success can create problems. The number of patients on waiting lists for kidney transplantation is growing faster than the number of transplant operations. In 1988, there were only 4083 cadaveric donors in the United States. About 2000 living-related donor transplants are performed each year, and this number has been relatively stable for the past 5 years. The shortage of donor kidneys is the most consequential limitation of kidney transplantation as we enter the 1990's.

Alexander JW: The cutting edge: A look to the future of transplantation. Transplantation 49:237, 1990. *A review of the growth of kidney transplantation and predictions about future growth.*

1989 Annual Data Report of the United States Renal Data System. Washington, D.C., National Institutes of Health, pp 1–41. *Most recent statistics concerning ESRD treatment in the United States.*

Class FHJ, van Rood JJ: The hyperimmunized patient: From sensitization toward treatment. Transplant Int 1:53, 1988. *The reasons that patients develop antibodies against HLA antigens and current strategies for dealing with this problem are reviewed.*

Combined Report on Regular Dialysis and Transplantation in Europe, XIX, 1988. Nephrol Dialysis Trans 4 (Suppl 4) 5, 1989. *A review of recent trends in immunosuppressive regimens in Europe.*

Kahan BD: Cyclosporine. N Engl J Med 321:1725, 1989. *A detailed description of cyclosporine from pharmacology to future prospects.*

Shapiro ME, Reed MH, Strom TB, et al.: The role of a primate model of renal transplantation in the development of new monoclonal antibodies. Am J Kidney Dis 14 (Suppl 2):58, 1989. *A brief description of testing of new monoclonal antibodies.*

79 Glomerular Disorders

William G. Couser

About 120,000 patients in the United States require hemodialysis or transplantation for chronic renal failure at an annual cost in excess of 2 billion dollars. Two thirds of these have some glomerular disease.

In this chapter, glomerular diseases are classified on a clinical basis into three groups: (1) primary renal diseases that usually present with the abrupt onset of hematuria, red cell casts, proteinuria, and decreased glomerular filtration rate (GFR) (acute nephritic syndrome or glomerulonephritis [GN]); (2) primary renal diseases that usually present with the insidious onset of heavy proteinuria and relatively normal GFR (nephrotic syndrome); and (3) secondary glomerular diseases resulting from renal involvement by a variety of systemic illnesses, which may be either nephritic or nephrotic. This approach has the virtue of simplicity, but it is useful only if its limitations are fully appreciated. Distinguishing between primary and secondary renal diseases is sometimes difficult and arbitrary. For example, immunoglobulin A (IgA) nephropathy is recognized as a primary renal disease, and Henoch-Schönlein purpura is classified as a secondary one, although they probably represent only differing clinical manifestations of the same process and often overlap. Most of the diseases that present as acute GN may cause the nephrotic syndrome, although they do so uncommonly, and some nephrotic glomerular diseases may occasionally exhibit nephritic features.

IMMUNE MECHANISMS AND THE GLOMERULAR RESPONSE TO INJURY

Two immunologic mechanisms of glomerular disease are generally accepted: (1) Rare patients develop GN due to deposition of antibody to glomerular basement membrane (GBM) antigens, which results in a typical uninterrupted linear staining pattern along all glomerular capillary walls when viewed by immunofluorescence microscopy (see Fig. 79–7). (2) Much more commonly, GN is associated with discontinuous, or granular, deposits of immunoglobulin and complement (see Figs. 79–2B, 79–3B, and 79–8). These deposits may occur at three sites: (1) within the glomerular mesangium, as in IgA nephropathy, Henoch-Schönlein purpura, and early lupus nephritis; (2) along the subendothelial surface of the capillary wall between endothelial cells and GBM, as seen in more severe forms of lupus nephritis and type I membranoproliferative glomerulonephritis (MPGN); and (3) on the outer, subepithelial surface of the capillary wall, as in membranous nephropathy and the so-called subepithelial "humps" in poststreptococcal glomerulonephritis (PSGN). Granular, or immune complex, deposits at mesangial and subendothelial sites either can result from the passive glomerular trapping of preformed immune complexes from the circulation or may form in situ owing to initial glomerular localization of free antigens followed by antibody binding to them. Subepithelial immune complex deposits appear to form only on a local basis. Figure 79–1 illustrates schematically how immune deposits at each of these sites are related to normal glomerular structures and some of the morphologic lesions that result.

Several glomerular diseases that are believed to be immunologically mediated do not have immune deposit formation in glomeruli. For example, minimal change nephrotic syndrome (MCNS) exhibits a marked increase in capillary wall permeability without immune deposits or histologic changes; and idiopathic rapidly progressive glomerulonephritis (RPGN) is characterized

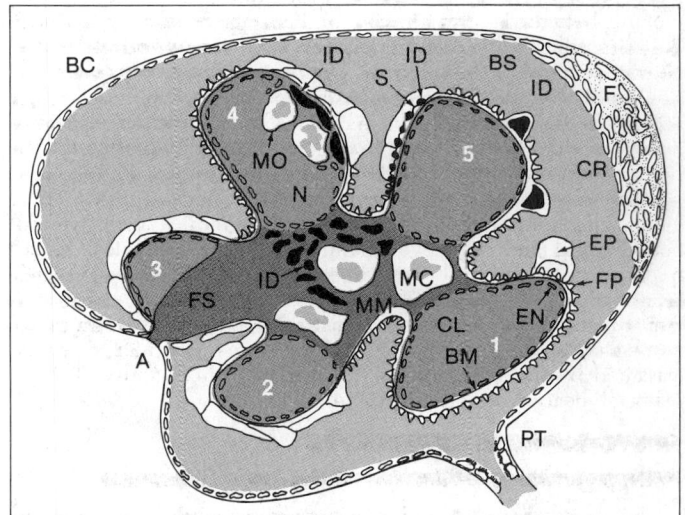

FIGURE 79–1. A highly schematized illustration of a cross-section of a single glomerulus showing normal glomerular architecture and some of the characteristic changes seen in glomerular diseases. One lobule with five capillary loops is illustrated within Bowman's capsule (BC). The capillary loops are supported by the intercapillary mesangium, containing mesangial cells (MC) and mesangial matrix (MM). Note that the normal glomerular capillary wall (loop 1) is composed of three layers: Endothelial cells (EN), basement membrane (BM), and epithelial cells (EP) with epithelial cell foot processes (FP).

TABLE 79–1. SUMMARY OF PRIMARY RENAL DISEASES THAT PRESENT AS ACUTE GLOMERULONEPHRITIS

Diseases	Poststreptococcal Glomerulonephritis (PSGN)	IgA Nephropathy	Goodpasture's Syndrome	Idiopathic Rapidly Progressive Glomerulonephritis (RPGN)
Clinical Manifestations				
Age and sex	All ages, mean 7, 2:1 male	15–35, 2:1 male	15–30, 6:1 male	Mean 58, 2:1 male
Acute nephritic syndrome	90%	50%	90%	90%
Asymptomatic hematuria	Occasionally	50%	Rare	Rare
Nephrotic syndrome	10–20%	Rare	Rare	10–20%
Hypertension	70%	30–50%	Rare	25%
Acute renal failure	50% (transient)	Very rare	50%	60%
Other	Latent period of 1–3 weeks	Follows viral syndromes	Pulmonary hemorrhage; iron deficiency anemia	None
Laboratory Findings	↑ ASO titers (70%) Positive streptozyme (95%) ↓ C3–C9 Normal C1, C4	↑ Serum IgA (50%) IgA in dermal capillaries	Positive anti-GBM antibody	Positive ANCA
Immunogenetics	HLA-B12, D "EN" (9)*	HLA-Bw 35, DR4 (4)*	HLA-DR2 (16)*	None established
Renal Pathology				
Light microscopy	Diffuse proliferation	Focal proliferation	Focal→diffuse proliferation with crescents	Crescentic GN
Immunofluorescence	Granular IgG, C3	Diffuse mesangial IgA	Linear IgG, C3	No immune deposits
Electron microscopy	Subepithelial humps	Mesangial deposits	No deposits	No deposits
Prognosis	95% resolve spontaneously 5% RPGN or slowly progressive	Slow progression in 25–50%	75% stabilize or improve if treated early	75% stabilize or improve if treated early
Treatment	Supportive	None established	Plasma exchange, steroids, cyclophosphamide	Steroid pulse therapy

*Relative risk

by severe glomerular inflammatory changes with crescent formation without detectable immune deposits.

The type and severity of histologic and functional glomerular disease induced by immune deposits in glomeruli depend on many factors, including the quantity, composition, and site of the deposits. Most glomerular antibody deposits contain predominantly immunoglobulin G (IgG), which activates complement via the classic complement pathway. When deposits are in mesangial and subendothelial sites, they are accessible to circulating inflammatory cells. Chemotactic and immune adherence mechanisms recruit participation of neutrophils, macrophages, and platelets and these effector cells cause damage to glomeruli by release of proteolytic enzymes and toxic oxygen metabolites. An inflammatory glomerular lesion results, with clinical manifestations that include hematuria, proteinuria, and loss of renal function. IgA deposits activate complement less well and predominantly by the alternate complement pathway. When immune deposits form at a subepithelial site, as in membranous nephropathy, they are not accessible to circulating cells and the resulting lesion is a noninflammatory one, with the nephrotic syndrome apparently induced by a direct effect of the C5b–9, or membrane attack complex, portion of complement on capillary wall permeability. Thus, glomerular immune complex deposits may induce a spectrum of both clinical and histologic manifestations. The clinical consequences range from the acute nephritic syndrome with acute renal failure, as seen in some cases of PSGN, to idiopathic nephrotic syndrome with normal renal function, as in membranous nephropathy. Table 79–1 lists the glomerular diseases, classified by the mechanisms that produce them and with their major clinical presentations noted.

ACUTE GLOMERULONEPHRITIS

Pathophysiology of the Acute Nephritic Syndrome

The terms *acute GN* and *acute nephritic syndrome,* which are synonymous, refer to the abrupt onset of hematuria and proteinuria, usually associated with some impairment in renal function and often with retention of salt and water, leading to hypertension and edema. Virtually all of these abnormalities are present in patients with PSGN but are less frequently found with other causes of the acute nephritic syndrome. The most common primary renal diseases that produce the acute nephritic syndrome are summarized in Table 79–2, where their major distinguishing clinical and pathologic features are compared. The syndrome may

also result from MPGN, which is discussed under diseases that cause the nephrotic syndrome, and from glomerular involvement in several of the systemic diseases to be discussed subsequently.

HEMATURIA. Hematuria is the hallmark of the acute nephritic syndrome. When hematuria is associated with proteinuria and red blood cell (RBC) casts, it usually reflects an acute glomerular inflammatory process that has the potential for rapid loss of renal function. RBC's probably reach the urine through breaks or "gaps" in the capillary wall and form casts as they become embedded in concentrated tubular fluid with an increased protein concentration. Hematuria and RBC casts may occasionally be seen in other diseases in which capillary wall

TABLE 79–2. CLASSIFICATION OF RAPIDLY PROGRESSIVE (CRESCENTIC) GLOMERULONEPHRITIS

Type of RPGN	Frequency
Anti-GBM Antibody–Mediated RPGN	20%
Goodpasture's syndrome	
Idiopathic anti-GBM nephritis	
Membranous nephropathy with crescents	
RPGN Associated with Granular Immune Deposits	40%
Postinfectious	
Poststreptococcal glomerulonephritis	
Bacterial endocarditis	
"Shunt" nephritis	
Visceral abscesses, other nonstreptococcal infections	
Noninfectious	
Systemic lupus erythematosus	
Henoch-Schönlein syndrome	
Mixed cryoglobulinemia	
Solid tumors	
Primary Renal Disease	
Membranoproliferative glomerulonephritis	
IgA nephropathy	
Idiopathic "immune complex" nephritis	
RPGN Without Glomerular Immune Deposits	40%
Vasculitis	
Polyarteritis	
Hypersensitivity vasculitis	
Wegener's granulomatosis	
Idiopathic RPGN	

disruption occurs, such as malignant hypertension and hereditary nephritis.

PROTEINURIA. In acute GN, proteinuria invariably accompanies hematuria but rarely exceeds 3.5 grams per day and is therefore in the "nonnephrotic" range. Proteinuria in acute GN reflects an increased urinary content of serum proteins due to some combination of three factors: (1) a generalized increase in the permeability characteristics of the glomerular capillary wall itself, (2) altered glomerular hemodynamics, and (3) mechanical disruptions in capillary wall structure. Thus, proteinuria in acute GN is "nonselective" and contains serum globulins as well as albumin. The pathophysiology of glomerular protein excretion is discussed in more detail below under Nephrotic Syndrome.

IMPAIRED RENAL FUNCTION. When glomerular inflammation is severe enough to cause hematuria and proteinuria, the GFR is usually reduced. This may range from a minimal reduction in GFR with normal serum creatinine values to oliguria or anuria requiring dialysis. Multiple factors account for the reduced GFR, including the effects of acute immune injury on glomerular pathophysiology and the development of glomerular intracapillary thromboses, acute tubular necrosis secondary to glomerular ischemia, tubular obstruction by casts, and compression of the glomerular tuft by proliferating epithelial cells forming crescents. The return of renal function to normal depends not only on cessation of the process that initiated the injury but also on the extent of irreversible structural changes that have occurred, such as necrosis, sclerosis, and fibrosis.

HYPERTENSION. Hypertension is a common manifestation of the acute nephritic syndrome in PSGN and may be a presenting sign in older patients. It is largely volume dependent, reflecting impaired renal excretion of sodium and water, with reduced levels of plasma renin and aldosterone. Hypertension can generally be controlled by strict adherence to sodium restriction.

EDEMA. Edema in the acute nephritic syndrome, like hypertension, reflects extracellular fluid volume expansion due to renal retention of salt and water. The mechanisms of renal sodium retention in acute GN are poorly understood but include a reduced filtered sodium load as well as enhanced sodium reabsorption in either the distal nephron or deep juxtamedullary nephrons. Edema and fluid retention are seen in more than 90 per cent of patients with acute PSGN but are less common in other diseases causing the acute nephritic syndrome. Unlike nephrotic edema, in the nephritic syndrome, edema is often present in nondependent areas, such as eyelids, face, and hands. The key to management is effective sodium restriction, since diuretics may not be effective in the acute stage of GN.

Couser WG: Mediation of immune glomerular injury. J Am Soc Nephrol 1:13, 1990. *An in-depth review of the pathogenetic mechanisms that underlie immune glomerular disease.*

Madaio MP, Harrington JT: Medical intelligence. Current concepts: The diagnosis of acute glomerulonephritis. N Engl J Med 309:1299, 1983. *This short review provides a useful outline of the diagnosis and classification of acute glomerulonephritis, emphasizing the distinctive clinical and laboratory features of each of the diseases that cause the acute nephritic syndrome.*

Whitley K, Keane WF, Vernier RL: Acute glomerulonephritis: A clinical overview. Med Clin North Am 68:259, 1984. *This article reviews the pathogenetic mechanisms, clinical presentations, laboratory features, and renal biopsy findings in each of the major disease entities that cause acute glomerulonephritis.*

Isolated Hematuria

The presence of persistent abnormal hematuria (more than five RBC's per high-power field in more than one fresh-voided urine specimen), without systemic disease, RBC casts, significant proteinuria, or impaired renal function, is a common medical problem that may or may not reflect renal parenchymal disease. It is more common in children and adolescents than in adults. A careful medical and urologic evaluation must be performed with appropriate laboratory, radiologic, and urologic procedures to exclude nonglomerular lesions of the urinary tract, such as infection, prostatism, papillary necrosis, polycystic and medullary sponge kidney, renal or urinary tract tumors, arteriovenous malformations, renal stones, blood dyscrasias, and hemoglobinopathies. The presence of dysmorphic RBC's in the urine by phase microscopy suggests a glomerular origin for hematuria. The "loin pain–hematuria syndrome" is a disorder usually seen in young women taking oral contraceptives who develop recurrent episodes of gross hematuria accompanied by loin pain and mild

hypertension in the absence of proteinuria or reduced renal function. The condition appears to be benign and is reversible when oral contraceptives are discontinued.

If no cause of hematuria can be found and no evidence of systemic or renal disease is present, isolated hematuria appears to be a benign entity, and only careful follow-up is indicated. Renal biopsy is performed in such patients only if evidence of progressive renal disease develops or if the patient requires further evaluation for other purposes such as insurance or employment. When such patients do undergo renal biopsy, the results usually reveal a mild, nonprogressive form of glomerular disease, often focal GN with or without mesangial IgA deposits.

Bauer DC: Evaluation of hematuria in adults. West J Med 152:305, 1990. *A concise review of the causes of hematuria in adults and the approach to diagnosis as it should be pursued by a primary care physician.*

Trachtman H, Weiss RA, Bennett B, et al.: Isolated hematuria in children: Indications for a renal biopsy. Kidney Int 25:94, 1984. *This paper reviews the findings in 76 children and adolescents who had biopsies for isolated hematuria and identifies a family history of hematuria and episodes of gross hematuria as the best predictors of significant renal pathology.*

Isolated Proteinuria

A more detailed discussion of proteinuria is given in Ch. 74. Like isolated hematuria, proteinuria in the nonnephrotic range *without* hematuria or decreased renal function may indicate a significant glomerular disease but usually does not. When increased urinary protein excretion is suggested by qualitative analyses such as the dipstick test, it must be confirmed by an accurate measurement of 24-hour protein excretion. Values in excess of 150 mg per day in adults, and 140 mg per square meter per day in children, are regarded as abnormal if an accurate 24-hour urine collection has been obtained. Reliable estimates of proteinuria can also be obtained by measuring protein-creatinine ratios in random daytime urine specimens. Values in excess of 0.2 are abnormal and above 3.5 suggest nephrotic range proteinuria. Abnormal protein excretion may be intermittent or persistent (fixed).

INTERMITTENT PROTEINURIA. The most common causes of intermittent proteinuria are *exercise,* assumption of the *upright position* (postural proteinuria), and *fever.* Up to 10 per cent of patients admitted on a routine medical basis may exhibit transient proteinuria. The basis for proteinuria in most of these conditions is probably hemodynamic, although subtle alterations in glomerular architecture have not been excluded. Total protein excretion is usually less than 2.0 grams per day, renal function is normal, and 20-year follow-up studies have shown resolution of the proteinuria in a majority of cases with no evidence of progressive renal disease.

PERSISTENT PROTEINURIA. Persistent or fixed proteinuria can also occur without glomerular disease. *"Overflow" proteinuria* occurs when excess production of filterable, low molecular weight proteins exceeds the tubular reabsorptive capacity, as occurs with the production of lysozyme (molecular weight 14,000) in myelomonocytic leukemia or L-chains in plasma cell dyscrasias such as multiple myeloma. In some cases up to 5.0 grams of L-chains may be excreted daily. Another nonglomerular cause of proteinuria is renal tubular disease in which normal quantities of proteins such as lysozyme or beta$_2$-microglobulin are filtered but not reabsorbed. This situation can result in urinary excretion of up to 2.0 grams of such proteins daily in a variety of interstitial nephropathies and disorders of tubular function.

Isolated, fixed, nonnephrotic proteinuria of glomerular origin is associated with an increased incidence of hypertension and a somewhat decreased life expectancy in long-term follow-up studies, but progressive renal disease is rare. Renal biopsy in such patients usually reveals some glomerular abnormality. The spectrum of lesions in isolated proteinuria is wide and similar to that discussed above in isolated hematuria. In patients with fixed proteinuria of less than 2.0 grams per day without hematuria, systemic disease, or impaired renal function, renal biopsy is usually not performed unless a change in clinical status occurs or the patient requests a biopsy for other purposes.

Abuelo JG: Proteinuria: Diagnostic principles and procedures. Ann Intern Med 98:186, 1983. *A well-written summary of the different types of proteinuria, their causes and prognosis, with emphasis on the approach to evaluation of patients with mild proteinuria and normal renal function.*

SPECIFIC RENAL DISEASES THAT PRESENT AS ACUTE GLOMERULONEPHRITIS (GN) (see Table 79–1)

The prototype of acute postinfectious GN is PSGN, but glomerular disease may follow infection with a variety of other bacterial and nonbacterial agents: both gram-positive and gram-negative bacteria, viruses, mycoplasma, fungi, protozoa, helminths, and spirochetes. Many of these associations have been noted only in patients with endocarditis or infected ventriculoatrial shunts. It is important to distinguish between specific postinfectious glomerular diseases, such as PSGN, and the nonspecific role of many infections, particularly viral illnesses, in producing "exacerbations" of underlying glomerular disease. These exacerbations are usually characterized by a transient increase in proteinuria and hematuria associated with the infection, usually without an intervening latent period.

Poststreptococcal Glomerulonephritis (PSGN)

Etiology, Incidence, and Epidemiology. GN occurs only following infection with a group A (beta-hemolytic) streptococcus of nephritogenic M type, usually type 12 in the United States. Streptococcal pharyngitis is the most common antecedent event in the North, and PSGN occurs with a frequency of less than 5 per cent after a latent period of 6 to 20 days (average of 10). The disease is often sporadic, occurs in the winter and spring, is more common in males, and is accompanied by serologic evidence of recent streptococcal infection in more than 80 per cent of cases. In the South, streptococcal pyoderma or impetigo is more common, the attack rate is higher (25 to 50 per cent), the latent period is longer (14 to 21 days, average of 20), and the disease affects males and females equally, often occurring in epidemic form in more temperate climates in the summer and fall.

Pathogenesis. Granular immune complex deposits in glomeruli cause the clinical and histologic features of PSGN. The presence of these deposits, hypocomplementemia, and the latent period between infection and the onset of GN suggest that the disease is similar to experimental acute serum sickness, in which acute GN is mediated by formation of glomerular deposits containing antigen and antibody to it 8 to 10 days following a single injection of antigen. The deposits are thought to reflect glomerular trapping of circulating immune complexes, but they may also form on a local basis. Streptococcal antigens have been identified in glomerular deposits early in PSGN in some patients. The presence of C3 in the deposits and the prominent infiltrate of neutrophils and mononuclear cells in the acute stage suggest a lesion that is mediated by complement, neutrophils, and macrophages.

Pathology. Figure 79–2 illustrates the typical findings in acute PSGN by light microscopy, IF, and EM. The histologic lesion in PSGN is a diffuse (all glomeruli involved) proliferative GN with a marked hypercellularity involving glomerular endothelial and mesangial cells, as well as neutrophils and mononuclear cells with narrowing or occlusion of capillary loops (Fig. 79–2A). Proliferation of epithelial cells in Bowman's space results in formation of glomerular "crescents" in severe disease. Extensive crescent formation is seen in about 5 per cent of patients and correlates with a more severe initial disease and reduced likelihood of complete recovery. Coarsely granular deposits of IgG and C3 occur along the glomerular capillary walls and in the mesangium (Fig. 79–2B). By electron microscopy there are discrete electron-dense subepithelial nodules or "humps" (Fig. 79–2C) that persist for about 8 weeks. Subepithelial humps are a highly characteristic feature of PSGN, although they may occasionally be seen in other types of bacterial postinfectious GN and type I MPGN.

Clinical Findings. PSGN is the prototype of the acute nephritic syndrome and causes all of the findings discussed above under Pathophysiology of the Acute Nephritic Syndrome. The disease is most common in children between 3 and 12 years of age, with a mean age of about 7, and is rare in infancy and in adults over 50. The typical presentation of PSGN is the abrupt onset of hematuria (90 per cent), which is usually evident as dark or "smoky" urine, accompanied by *malaise* and sometimes gastrointestinal symptoms, such as abdominal pain, nausea, and vomiting. Central nervous system manifestations may include headaches

and occasionally seizures. *Edema* is an early and frequent sign, often in a periorbital distribution most evident on arising and sometimes progressing to peripheral edema and anasarca. *Hypertension* is present in 60 to 70 per cent of patients and reflects renal retention of salt and water with volume overload. Proteinuria is usually present as well. About 20 per cent of hospitalized patients develop nephrotic range proteinuria, usually transiently and during the recovery phase. Renal function is impaired in about 50 per cent of patients.

Prognosis. Three clinical courses can be defined in PSGN: complete recovery, no recovery, or partial recovery with progressive disease. In more than 90 per cent of cases, complete recovery occurs with spontaneous diuresis in an average of 4 to 7 days. Even patients who require dialysis during the acute phase usually recover spontaneously without specific therapy. Abnormal hematuria and proteinuria may persist for up to 2 years. Progressive renal disease is a very uncommon consequence of PSGN, however, if renal function returns to normal and proteinuria is less than 500 mg per day.

Fewer than 5 per cent of patients with PSGN have oliguria lasting more than 9 days; the prognosis in these patients is worse. Although spontaneous complete recovery has been reported with oliguria or anuria for up to 25 days, this is unusual. Many patients with prolonged oliguria have a crescentic glomerular lesion. About half of these will still recover spontaneously. In the remainder, the disease behaves like RPGN, with no recovery at all or with only partial recovery of renal function, which may be followed by persistent proteinuria and progressive renal disease, leading to renal failure in months to years. Patients with PSGN who have oliguric renal failure lasting more than 1 week, particularly adults, should undergo a renal biopsy. If extensive crescent formation is found, they should be considered for therapy as outlined below under Treatment.

Laboratory Features. Laboratory findings consist of an abnormal urinalysis, elevated antibodies against streptococcal exoenzymes, and reduced serum complement levels. The urinalysis usually reveals signs of glomerular inflammation with proteinuria, RBC's, white blood cells (WBC's), and casts. RBC casts are present in 60 to 85 per cent of cases when a freshly voided urine is examined. The urine is often concentrated and exhibits biochemical characteristics of prerenal azotemia, including a low urinary sodium concentration, indicating severe glomerular disease with good preservation of tubular function.

Beta-hemolytic streptococci are detected by culture in only 25 per cent of untreated patients, but serologic tests generally confirm recent streptococcal infection. The anti–streptolysin O (ASO) titer exceeds 200 Todd units within 1 to 3 weeks and may remain elevated for months. An increase in ASO titer may not be seen if penicillin therapy is initiated early or if the antecedent infection was in the skin. Antibodies to other streptococcal enzymes are usually elevated as well. The streptozyme test utilizes five of these antigens in a single assay and is quite sensitive and specific. More than 90 per cent of patients with PSGN have a reduced level of total hemolytic complement or C3 during the first 2 weeks of illness, with most returning to normal within 8 weeks. The pattern of complement component depression suggests alternate pathway activation, with levels of C1q and C4 usually normal.

Diagnosis. The differential diagnosis of acute GN with hypocomplementemia includes other forms of postinfectious GN, such as subacute bacterial endocarditis (SBE) or shunt nephritis, systemic lupus erythematosus (SLE), and type I MPGN. Only MPGN is difficult to exclude by clinical and laboratory criteria. A similar pattern of alternate complement pathway activation is seen in MPGN, a disease that may also occasionally follow streptococcal infection, and MPGN must be considered when nephrotic range proteinuria and hypocomplementemia persist for longer than 2 months. The diagnosis of PSGN can usually be made by the presence of typical clinical features of the acute nephritic syndrome following a streptococcal infection by an appropriate latent period, and by hypocomplementemia and serologic evidence of recent streptococcal infection. Because patients with PSGN usually recover spontaneously and no specific therapy is indicated, the diagnosis is often made clinically without a renal biopsy. Biopsy is indicated, however, if atypical features are present, such as prolonged oliguria, anuria, persistent hypocomplementemia, the nephrotic syndrome, or clinical or serologic evidence of systemic disease.

Treatment. In most patients with PSGN, there is no need for specific therapy, since spontaneous recovery can be anticipated. Antibiotics should be given if cultures are positive for group A streptococci, but penicillin therapy does not alter the incidence or severity of PSGN. Manifestations of sodium retention, such as hypertension, edema, and congestive heart failure, can usually be managed with careful sodium restriction, but diuretics and antihypertensive agents may be employed if necessary. Dialysis may be required temporarily in some patients, most of whom will still recover normal renal function spontaneously.

There are no data on which to base a recommendation for therapy in patients with prolonged oliguria and a crescentic glomerular lesion on biopsy. Although up to 50 per cent of such patients may recover spontaneously, the prognosis is sufficiently guarded to warrant considering therapy with pulse steroids or plasma exchange, as outlined below under RPGN.

Nissenson AR, moderator: Post-streptococcal acute glomerulonephritis: Fact and controversy. Ann Intern Med 91:76, 1979. *An excellent overview of the microbiology, epidemiology, clinical manifestations, laboratory features, pathogenesis, and sequelae of PSGN, with 128 references.*

Rodriguez-Iturbe B: Epidemic poststreptococcal glomerulonephritis. Kidney Int 25:129, 1984. *An excellent review of the pathogenesis, laboratory findings, clinical features, and long-term prognosis in acute poststreptococcal nephritis, with 65 references.*

Glomerulonephritis in Subacute Bacterial Endocarditis (SBE)

Glomerular disease in SBE ranges in severity from the proteinuria and hematuria seen in 70 per cent of patients, usually with normal renal function, to occasional cases of crescentic GN with acute renal failure. It is more common in chronic cases with right-sided cardiac involvement and negative blood cultures, as may occur in patients who abuse drugs. A wide variety of organisms have been implicated, most commonly *Staphylococcus aureus* and *Streptococcus viridans*. A similar syndrome may be seen in patients with infected ventriculoatrial shunts for hydrocephalus (shunt nephritis), often due to *Staphylococcus albus*. Serologic abnormalities are often present, including hypocomplementemia with activation of both the classic and the alternate complement pathways, cryoglobulinemia, and positive rheumatoid factor. Renal biopsy usually demonstrates a focal proliferative GN, often with necrosis and intracapillary thrombi. Granular deposits of IgG, IgM, and C3 occur in mesangial and subendothelial areas, implicating an immune complex rather than an embolic mechanism in the pathogenesis of the lesion. Renal function usually returns to normal following appropriate antibiotic

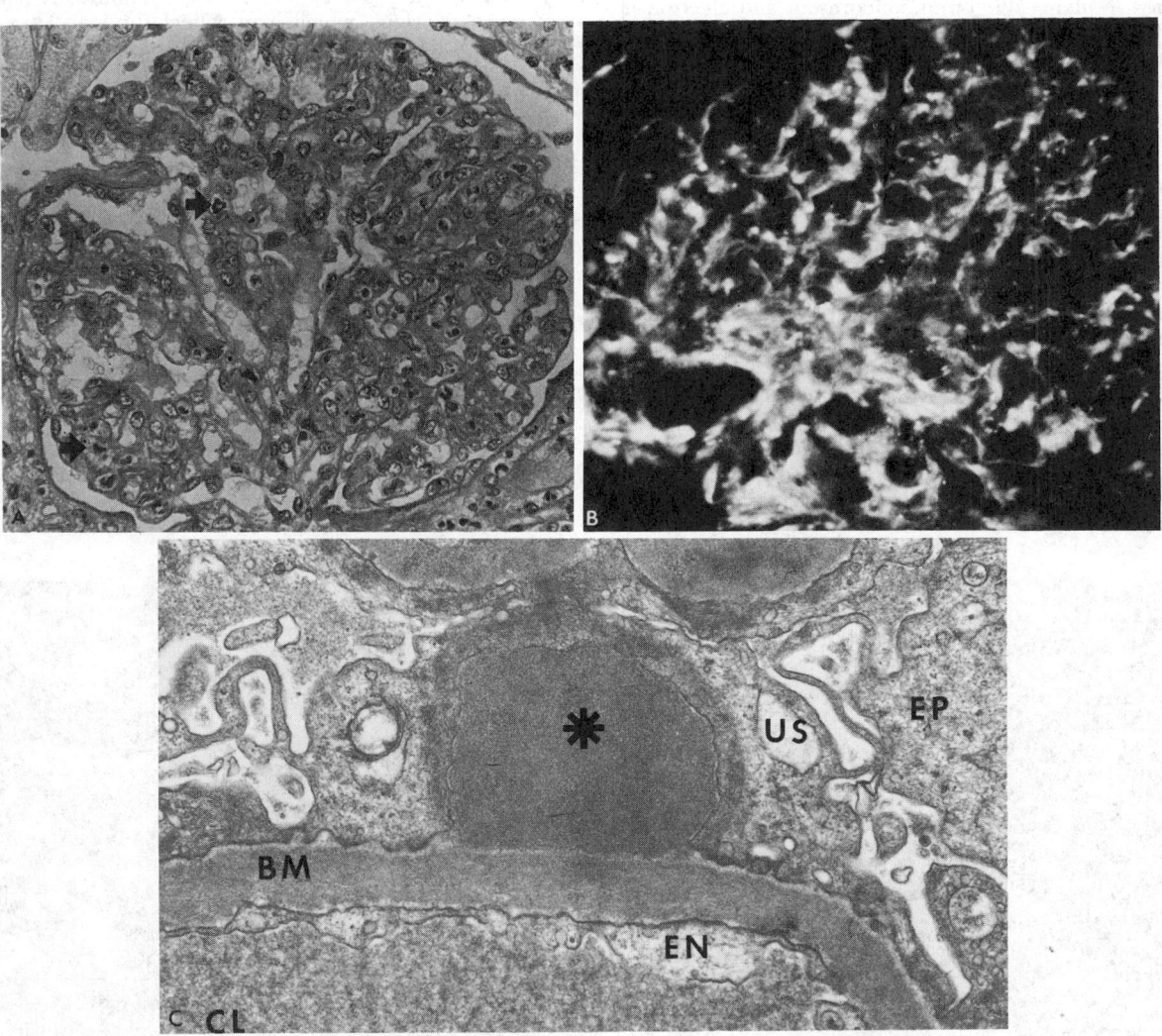

FIGURE 79–2. The renal lesion of poststreptococcal glomerulonephritis (PSGN). *A*, Light microscopic section of a renal biopsy from a patient with acute PSGN showing a marked increase in glomerular cells and infiltration by polymorphonuclear leukocytes (*arrows*) (periodic acid–Schiff stain; ×300). *B*, Immunofluorescent staining for IgG from the same biopsy reveals a coarse, granular pattern of deposits on the capillary walls and in the mesangium (×350). *C*, Electron microscopy in acute PSGN reveals a characteristic electron-dense "hump" on the subepithelial surface (*) with effacement of epithelial foot processes around the deposit. BM = Basement membrane; CL = capillary lumen; EN = endothelial cell; EP = epithelial cell; US = urinary space (×14,400). (Reproduced with permission from Couser WG, Salant DJ, Stilmant MM. *In* Flamenbaum W, Hamburger RJ [eds.]: Nephrology. Philadelphia, J.B. Lippincott Company, 1982, pp 265–301.)

therapy and eradication of the infection. However, recovery may be slow if the lesion is severe or crescents are present.

Feinstein EI, Eknoyan G, Lister BJ, et al.: Renal complications of bacterial endocarditis. Am J Nephrol 5:457, 1985. *This discussion, with 69 references, of endocarditis and glomerulonephritis in a patient who is an intravenous drug abuser presents a comprehensive review of glomerular disease associated with both endocarditis and drug abuse.*

Neugarten J, Gallo GR, Baldwin DS: Glomerulonephritis in bacterial endocarditis. Am J Kidney Dis 3:371, 1984. *This paper reviews 107 patients with endocarditis and notes that 22 per cent had glomerulonephritis with a spectrum of renal lesions and that* Staphylococcus aureus *was the predominant organism. The relationship among renal lesion, therapy, and prognosis is discussed.*

Glomerulonephritis with Visceral Abscesses

The abrupt onset of acute renal failure associated with proteinuria, hematuria, and red cell casts may occur in patients with a pyogenic visceral abscess. Abscesses are most frequently located in the respiratory tract but have been reported at numerous other sites, including the abdomen and uterus. Endocarditis may be present but usually is not, and blood cultures are commonly negative. In contrast to PSGN, SBE, and shunt nephritis, serologic studies, including complement levels, are usually normal. A variety of bacteria have been implicated. The glomerular lesion is usually a proliferative GN with crescents, and monocytes may be prominent in glomeruli. Immunofluoresent and electron microscopic studies do not usually reveal immune deposits, so that the pathogenesis of this lesion is unclear. Recovery of renal function has occurred in about half of the patients reported with acute renal failure who were successfully treated to eradicate the infection, but the overall mortality is quite high.

Beaufils M: Glomerular disease complicating abdominal sepsis. Kidney Int 19:609, 1981. *A detailed review of nonstreptococcal postinfectious glomerulonephritis, including SBE- as well as abscess-related lesions. The frequency with which renal biopsies reveal glomerular disease as a cause of acute renal failure in patients with sepsis is striking, since most such patients would not be so extensively studied in the United States.*

Glomerular Disease in Acquired Immunodeficiency Syndrome (AIDS)

Up to 50 per cent of patients with AIDS have abnormal proteinuria, and 10 per cent develop nephrotic syndrome. A variety of glomerular, tubular, and interstitial lesions have also been noted, presumably induced by infections, drug exposure, and other factors. However, a majority of patients with nephrotic syndrome have focal glomerulosclerosis. A rapid loss of renal function may occur in this subset of patients.

Bourgoignie JJ, Meneses R, Ortiz C, et al.: The clinical spectrum of renal disease associated with human immunodeficiency virus. Am J Kidney Dis 12:131, 1988. *A review of 100 cases of AIDS with renal manifestations that emphasizes the frequency of nephrotic syndrome and focal glomerulosclerosis as well as the poor prognosis of this type of renal lesion.*

Glassock RJ, moderator: Human immunodeficiency virus (HIV) infection and the kidney. Ann Intern Med 112:35, 1990. *This authoritative review covers all aspects of renal involvement in AIDS, including fluid and electrolyte disturbances, AIDS nephropathy, and HIV infection in patients on dialysis or undergoing renal transplantation.*

IgA Nephropathy (Berger's Disease)

Overview and Incidence. IgA nephropathy is the most common cause of primary glomerular disease in Europe, Australia, and the United States. The disease is now regarded as a monosymptomatic form of *Henoch-Schönlein purpura* (HSP), but clinical manifestations are milder than in HSP and are usually confined to the kidney. HSP is discussed later in this chapter and also in Ch. 154.

Pathogenesis. The pathogenesis of the renal lesion in IgA nephropathy and HSP is not known. It appears to be a consequence of mesangial formation of immune deposits composed predominantly of IgA (see Fig. 79–3B). The IgA may represent the antibody component of an immune complex containing a nonrenal antigen. A similar glomerular lesion may develop in liver disease associated with elevated portal pressure. The glomerular IgA deposits appear to be predominantly polymeric and of mucosal origin, which may reflect the association of disease activity with viral infections of the upper respiratory and gastrointestinal tracts.

Pathology. The typical lesion of IgA nephropathy has a focal distribution, meaning that some glomeruli are involved while others are spared, and is also segmental, with lesions in some glomerular tufts but not others (Fig. 79–3A). Mesangial expansion and hypercellularity are common, but the characteristic lesion is focal and segmental proliferative GN. When crescents are present, they are usually small and rarely involve more than 30 per cent of glomeruli. Immune deposits are present diffusely in the mesangium of all glomeruli and contain IgA as the predominant immunoglobulin, accompanied by C3 in 60 per cent and IgG in 30 per cent of cases (Fig. 79–3B). C1q and C4 are usually absent, suggesting alternate complement pathway activation. Some patients have deposits along the subendothelial aspect of the capillary wall or in the subepithelial space and generally have more severe disease and more proteinuria.

Clinical and Laboratory Findings and Diagnosis. IgA nephropathy is two to three times more common in males than in females, and most patients present before the age of 35. The classic

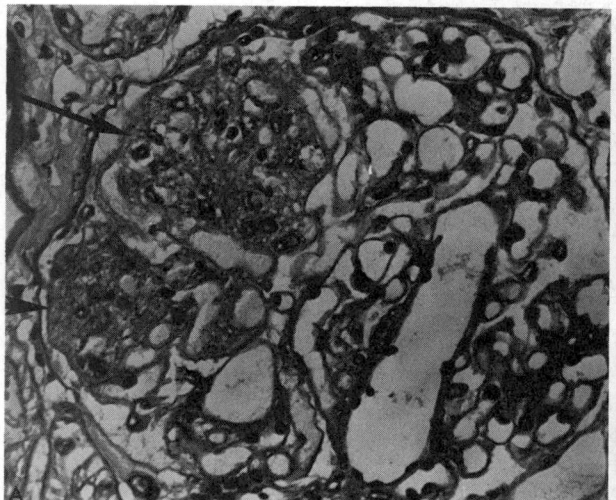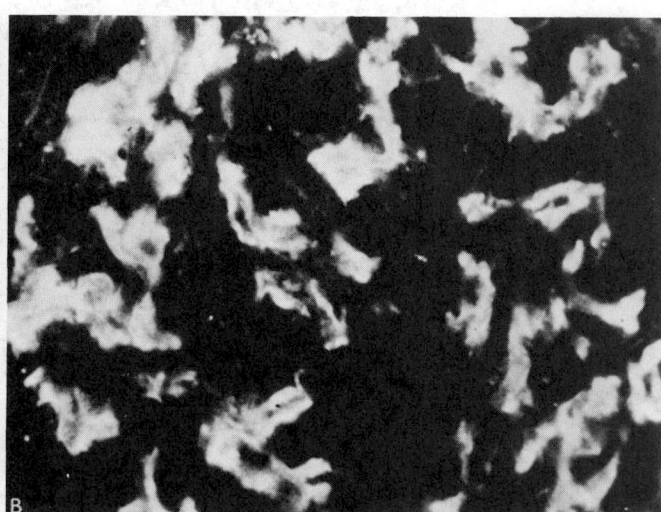

FIGURE 79–3. The renal lesion of IgA nephropathy. *A*, Light microscopic section from a patient with gross hematuria and focal glomerulonephritis due to IgA nephropathy. There is segmental involvement of the glomerulus, which shows mesangial matrix increase and hypercellularity in two lobules (*arrows*). Adjacent lobules are essentially normal (periodic acid–Schiff stain, ×350). *B*, Immunofluorescence microscopy on the same biopsy reveals bright, diffuse staining for IgA in all mesangial areas. No significant capillary wall staining is present. IgG and C3 may be found in a similar pattern but with less intensity (×450). (Reproduced with permission from Couser WG, Salant DJ, Stilmant MM. *In* Flamenbaum W, Hamburger RJ [eds.]: Nephrology. Philadelphia, J.B. Lippincott Company, 1982, pp 265–301.)

presentation is *gross hematuria* that occurs coincident with, or immediately following (24 to 48 hours), a viral upper respiratory infection (50 per cent), flu-like illness (15 per cent), a gastrointestinal syndrome (10 per cent), or other infectious prodrome. Associated findings often include mild fever, malaise, myalgias, dysuria, and loin pain. The remainder of cases are identified during medical evaluation for persistent, asymptomatic hematuria or proteinuria. The absence of a latent period, as well as normal levels of complement and antistreptococcal antibodies, distinguishes this disease clinically from PSGN. Moreover, other features of the acute nephritic syndrome, including edema and hypertension, are seen in fewer than half of the patients. Only about 25 per cent of patients have impaired renal function during active disease, and the serum creatinine level rarely exceeds 3 mg per deciliter. Proteinuria is usually less than 1 gram per day. A subset of patients with steroid-sensitive nephrotic syndrome may have mesangial IgA deposits but are believed to have primary MCNS.

Gross hematuria usually lasts only 2 to 6 days, but microscopic hematuria often persists between attacks. Fifty per cent of patients will have only a single episode of gross hematuria. The remainder have recurring episodes for many years, often preceded by viral infections.

There are no laboratory findings diagnostic of IgA nephropathy. About half of all patients have elevated serum levels of IgA that do not correlate with disease activity. Circulating immune complexes containing IgA are present intermittently, and deposits of IgA, C3, and fibrin may be present in the dermal capillaries of normal skin. The incidence of this disease is greater in persons with HLA-Bw 35 and HLA-DR4 (HLA, human leukocyte antigen) phenotypes.

Course and Prognosis. Progression to renal failure occurs in 15 to 20 per cent of patients within 6 months, and a 50 per cent death or dialysis rate is projected over 20 years. While there are no clinical or pathologic features that permit accurate prediction of progression, patients who tend to do worse are male, have a prolonged clinical course, develop hypertension or proteinuria exceeding 3 grams per day, or have extensive glomerulosclerosis present on biopsy.

Treatment. No specific form of therapy has been shown to alter the long-term clinical course of this disease. Rigorous control of hypertension is important. Mesangial deposits of IgA occur with a high frequency in renal allografts but rarely compromise graft function.

Clarkson AR, Woodroffe AJ, Aarons I, et al.: IgA nephropathy. Ann Rev Med 38:157, 1987. *A very current and detailed summary of IgA nephropathy that includes comments on clinical manifestations, pathology, natural history, and pathogenesis.*
D'Amico G: The commonest glomerulonephritis in the world: IgA nephropathy. Q J Med 64:709, 1987. *An in-depth review of IgA nephropathy with an excellent summary of the rationale for designing treatment options.*
Julian BA, Waldo FB, Rifai A, et al.: IgA nephropathy, the most common glomerulonephritis worldwide. Am J Med 84:129, 1988. *A concise but complete review of the epidemiology, clinical features, immunopathogenesis, and approach to therapy of IgA nephropathy from an experienced clinical center.*

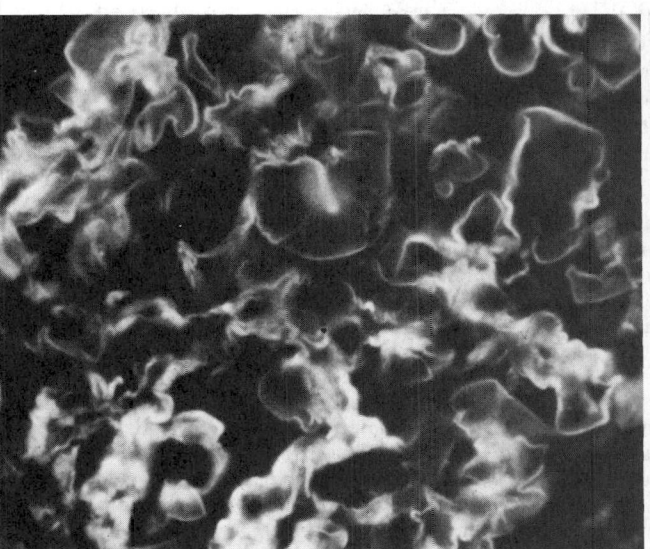

FIGURE 79–5. Immunofluorescence microscopy on a renal biopsy from a patient with Goodpasture's syndrome reveals continuous, uninterrupted, linear deposition of IgG along all capillary walls. This pattern is characteristic of anti-GBM disease (×450). (Reproduced with permission from Couser WG, Salant DJ, Stilmant MM. *In* Flamenbaum W, Hamburger RJ [eds.]: Nephrology. Philadelphia, J.B. Lippincott Company, 1982, pp 265–301.)

Rapidly Progressive Glomerulonephritis (RPGN)

Overview. The term RPGN is applied to any glomerular disease in which rapid loss of renal function occurs in association with extensive crescent formation in many glomeruli, usually more than 50 per cent (Fig. 79–4). RPGN may occur in severe cases of a wide variety of glomerular diseases, which are listed in Table 79–2, or it may occur alone as a primary renal disease. The classification system used here is based on pathogenetic mechanisms. Accurate prognosis and selection of appropriate therapy require that the underlying mechanisms be defined. About 20 per cent of cases of RPGN are mediated by anti-GBM antibody deposition and 40 per cent by glomerular immune complex formation (usually in association with some systemic disease process such as PSGN or SLE), and 40 per cent are primary renal lesions with no significant glomerular immune deposits, which are classified here as idiopathic RPGN (Table 79–2).

RPGN DUE TO ANTI-GBM ANTIBODY. Although much is known of the mediation of immune glomerular injury from studies of experimental anti-GBM nephritis, this mechanism accounts for fewer than 5 per cent of cases of GN seen clinically. Anti-GBM GN is characterized by the abrupt onset of a proliferative GN, usually with crescents, and a characteristic linear deposition of IgG seen along the GBM by immunofluorescence (Fig. 79–5). In about two thirds of cases, pulmonary hemorrhage accompanies GN, and the disease is termed Goodpasture's syndrome. The remaining one third of patients have anti-GBM nephritis without pulmonary involvement.

Goodpasture's Syndrome. Pathogenesis. The events that initiate anti-GBM antibody production are not known. Antibody reactive with GBM and alveolar basement membrane mediates the glomerular disease in anti-GBM nephritis with and without pulmonary hemorrhage. The development of lung hemorrhage appears to require the presence of prior lung damage to allow antibody deposition. Genetic factors are clearly important in this disease. There is a strong association with HLA-DRw2 (relative risk of 15 to 34 times normal). Anti-GBM antibody production is a self-limited event usually lasting several months. Exacerbations

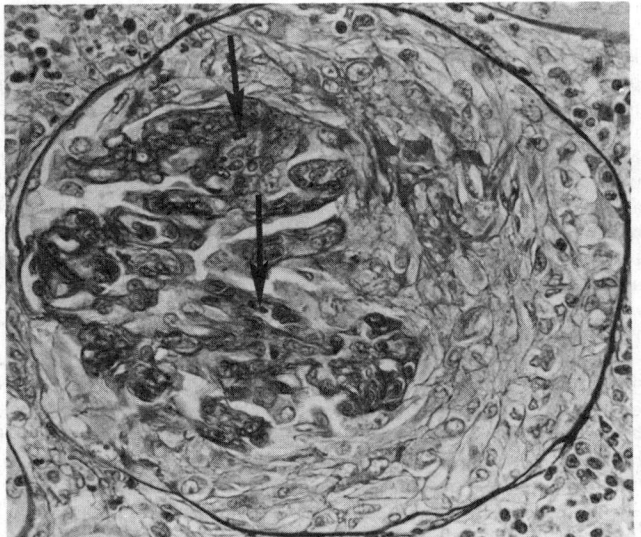

FIGURE 79–4. Light microscopy from a patient with idiopathic RPGN reveals the presence of a large cellular crescent in Bowman's space surrounding and compressing the glomerular capillary. A few polymorphonuclear leukocytes are seen in the glomerulus (*arrows*) (periodic acid–Schiff stain, ×275). (Reproduced with permission from Couser WG, Salant DJ, Stilmant MM. *In* Flamenbaum W, Hamburger RJ [eds.]: Nephrology. Philadelphia, J.B. Lippincott Company, 1982, pp 265–301.)

of disease associated with increased antibody levels may be triggered by infectious complications. Antibody binding to GBM mediates glomerular injury by mechanisms that involve complement activation and participation of both neutrophils and macrophages. Fibrin deposition in Bowman's space is believed to initiate glomerular crescent formation.

Pathology. The early histologic lesion in Goodpasture's syndrome is a focal proliferative and necrotizing GN that progresses to diffuse involvement with crescent formation. Extensive interstitial infiltrates may also be present, perhaps owing to antibody deposition on tubular basement membranes. There is a characteristic, continuous, linear pattern of IgG deposition along the capillary wall, accompanied by C3 in about 70 per cent of cases (Fig. 79–5). Tubular basement membrane deposits may also occur. Electron microscopy is not diagnostic.

Clinical Features. Goodpasture's syndrome is a disease of young males (6:1 male-female ratio) characterized by a triad of *pulmonary hemorrhage, GN, and anti-GBM antibody production*. It usually begins with pulmonary hemorrhage manifested as hemoptysis, pulmonary alveolar infiltrates seen on the radiograph, dyspnea, and iron deficiency anemia. The pulmonary symptoms are followed within days to weeks by the development of hematuria, proteinuria, and rapid loss of renal function. Over half of patients with Goodpasture's syndrome are azotemic when first seen. Hypertension and fluid retention are uncommon. Preceding flu-like illness or exposure to other pulmonary toxins, such as volatile hydrocarbon solvents and cigarettes, is common. Until recently, 80 per cent of cases required treatment for end-stage renal disease within 1 year, although some patients with mild disease recover spontaneously. Up to 30 per cent of patients may die as a consequence of the pulmonary hemorrhage.

Laboratory Findings and Diagnosis. The only laboratory finding specific for anti-GBM nephritis is the demonstration of antibody to GBM in the serum or as linear deposits of IgG in glomeruli. The antibody can be detected quickly in serum by indirect immunofluorescence using normal human kidney substrate in a test that is similar to the fluorescent antinuclear antibody test. The indirect immunofluorescence assay is positive in 80 to 90 per cent of patients with Goodpasture's syndrome. More sensitive enzyme-linked immunosorbent assays (ELISA) are also available and are positive in more than 95 per cent of patients. It is urgent to make a diagnosis and to initiate therapy early in RPGN of all types. An anti-GBM assay, as well as a renal biopsy, should therefore be obtained as soon as possible after the diagnosis of RPGN is suspected. The demonstration of anti-GBM antibody is critical, since a variety of other diseases may result in similar pulmonary and renal manifestations, including SLE, polyarteritis nodosa, Wegener's granulomatosis, and other forms of systemic necrotizing vasculitis.

Treatment. As in all forms of RPGN, the success of treatment is critically dependent upon how quickly it is initiated. The overall survival rate in Goodpasture's syndrome has risen from less than 10 per cent 15 years ago to over 50 per cent today owing to earlier diagnosis and detection of milder cases, better general medical care, and probably some improvements in specific therapy for the disease. There is little evidence that oral steroids or immunosuppressive agents alone significantly alter the course of the renal lesion. The pulmonary hemorrhage commonly responds either to high-dose oral prednisone therapy or to intravenous "pulse" methylprednisolone (see treatment of idiopathic RPGN below). However, steroid pulse therapy does not appear to benefit the renal lesion. Most centers now treat anti-GBM disease with vigorous plasma exchange therapy combined with prednisone, 1 mg per kilogram per day, and cyclophosphamide, 2 to 3 mg per kilogram per day. Plasma exchanges of up to 4 liters per day are performed on a daily or alternate-day basis until anti-GBM antibody is no longer detectable in the circulation and disease progression has halted. Therapy may require several weeks. Replacement is with albumin or, when pulmonary hemorrhage is active, with fresh frozen plasma. Overall survival in anti-GBM nephritis appears to be improved by plasma exchange therapy. However, the response rate in patients who are oliguric on presentation or who have serum creatinine levels exceeding 6 mg per deciliter is very low, again emphasizing the need for early diagnosis. In patients with end-stage renal

disease due to anti-GBM nephritis, renal transplantation appears to be safe if delayed until anti-GBM antibody is no longer detectable in the serum.

Anti-GBM Glomerulonephritis Without Pulmonary Hemorrhage. Some patients have the same anti-GBM antibody–mediated renal disease as seen in Goodpasture's syndrome, but antibody localization does not occur in lungs and pulmonary hemorrhage is therefore absent. The patients are generally older than those with Goodpasture's syndrome (mean age about 50), and males and females are equally affected. In all other respects, the clinical and pathologic findings, course, and treatment are the same as those discussed above for Goodpasture's syndrome. Because such patients present with an idiopathic form of acute RPGN without pulmonary hemorrhage and may respond to plasma exchange therapy, it is important that the possibility of anti-GBM nephritis be considered in all patients who present in this fashion and that circulating anti-GBM antibody studies and renal biopsy be performed early.

Savage COS, Pusey CD, Bowman C, et al.: Antiglomerular basement membrane antibody mediated disease in the British Isles 1980–4. Br Med J 292:301, 1986. *Experience with 71 patients in a single center is reviewed, disclosing two patterns of disease: young women in their twenties with Goodpasture's syndrome and women in their sixties with glomerulonephritis alone. The poor response to plasma exchange in patients with serum creatinine levels exceeding 6 mg per deciliter or in those requiring dialysis is emphasized.*

Walker RG, Scheinkestel C, Becker GJ, et al.: Clinical and morphological aspects of the management of crescentic anti–glomerular basement membrane antibody (anti-GBM) nephritis/Goodpasture's syndrome. Q J Med 543:75, 1985. *This review of 22 patients with anti-GBM nephritis details the clinical features of this disease. Anuria and greater than 80 per cent crescents are identified as poor prognostic signs, and a beneficial effect of plasma exchange is suggested.*

RPGN DUE TO GLOMERULAR IMMUNE COMPLEX FORMATION. Patients with RPGN associated with granular deposits of immunoglobulin and complement in glomeruli account for about 40 per cent of all patients seen with crescentic GN. In most cases the glomerular disease is a manifestation of some well-defined systemic illness, such as SLE, Henoch-Schönlein purpura, or other forms of vasculitis, or of another well-defined primary renal disease, such as PSGN, MPGN, or, rarely, IGA nephropathy. In all of these disorders, the correct diagnosis can usually be made from the associated clinical, laboratory, and pathologic findings. Prognosis depends considerably on the underlying disease. For example, about 50 per cent of patients with RPGN secondary to streptococcal infection will recover spontaneously without specific therapy, while in RPGN due to SLE spontaneous recovery virtually never occurs. Therapy for the glomerular disease per se is the same as that outlined below under treatment for idiopathic RPGN and includes the use of methylprednisolone pulse therapy and/or plasma exchange.

IDIOPATHIC RPGN. Pathogenesis. RPGN as a primary renal disease is usually not associated with significant glomerular deposits of anti-GBM antibody or immune complexes. The disease mechanism in such patients is undefined but probably immune in nature. Whatever the mechanism leading to capillary wall damage, leakage of fibrin into Bowman's space apparently initiates epithelial cell proliferation and crescent formation. Some of the vague prodromal clinical manifestations, the development of crescentic GN without immune deposits, and the frequent presence of anti-neutrophil cytoplasmic antibody (ANCA) are quite similar to findings in several of the vasculitides. This disease is a form of vasculitis, although inflammatory changes are confined primarily to the glomerular capillaries.

Pathology. There is extensive glomerular crescent formation with circumferential cellular crescents usually involving 50 to 100 per cent of glomeruli (see Fig. 79–4). There is a rough correlation between the percentage of glomeruli with crescents, the severity of clinical disease, and the prognosis. Prominent proliferative changes suggest a postinfectious etiology and a better prognosis. Fibrinogen and fibrin polymers are present in the crescents. The glomeruli at most show only focal granular deposits of IgM and C3, which are nonspecific. Electron microscopy may show "gaps" or rupture of the capillary wall but usually does not show immune deposits.

Clinical Manifestations and Diagnosis. Idiopathic RPGN is a disease of older patients (mean age of 58). There is a slight male predominance. Many patients have a prodrome that resembles a viral illness with myalgias; arthralgias; loin, back, and abdominal pain; fever; and malaise. Minor hemoptysis is common, and fleeting pulmonary infiltrates may be seen on the radiograph. No specific inciting events have been identified. RPGN presents as an acute nephritic syndrome, including *hematuria, proteinuria,* and *rapidly decreasing renal function,* often without hypertension or edema. As in anti-GBM nephritis, the progression of renal disease is usually very rapid, with up to 50 per cent of patients oliguric at the time of presentation and half of these sufficiently uremic to require immediate dialysis. The remaining patients may require dialysis within 1 to 3 weeks. At the time of presentation, the disease is often relatively acute and potentially reversible.

The laboratory features of idiopathic RPGN are entirely nonspecific. ASO titers, antinuclear and anti-GBM antibodies, circulating immune complexes, and complement levels are normal or negative. The diagnosis is made by renal biopsy in a patient with deteriorating renal function, evidence of glomerular disease in the urinary sediment, absence of anti-GBM antibody, and lack of clinical or serologic evidence of other systemic diseases, such as SLE.

Treatment and Prognosis. Treatment with oral steroids and/or cytotoxic agents has been of little apparent benefit, and a death or dialysis rate of about 75 per cent in 2 years is reported. Favorable prognostic factors include a young age at the time of onset, a history of a preceding infectious episode, absence of oliguria and hypertension, a serum creatinine level below 6 mg per deciliter at presentation, and fewer than 50 per cent crescents in the renal biopsy. Success rates approaching 75 per cent have been reported in patients treated with either methylprednisolone pulse therapy or plasma exchange. Methylprednisolone, 30 mg per kilogram to a maximum of 3 grams, is given intravenously over 20 minutes on a daily or alternate-day basis three times, followed by oral prednisone, 2 mg per kilogram, which is tapered over several months. About 75 per cent of patients, including some who were oliguric and on dialysis, have shown a dramatic response, with a return of renal function to normal or nearly normal levels. Responses have generally been evident within 5 to 10 days and have continued over 4 to 6 weeks. About 25 per cent will progress to renal failure despite an impressive initial response. Very similar results have been reported in patients treated with intensive plasma exchange (plus prednisone and cyclophosphamide). Neither form of therapy has yet been shown in a prospective, controlled study to improve long-term patient or kidney survival over what might be achieved with more conservative measures. Until such data are available, the author's feeling is that both pulse therapy and plasma exchange probably represent significant advances in the treatment of idiopathic RPGN. Steroid pulse therapy is safer and cheaper and appears to be as effective as plasma exchange. There are no data on the efficacy of cytotoxic drugs in this disease. However, if there is evidence of segmental necrotizing glomerular lesions, ANCA, or systemic manifestations consistent with vasculitis, cyclophosphamide should probably be given concurrently with steroids.

Idiopathic RPGN appears to recur rarely in allografted kidneys.

Couser WG: Rapidly progressive glomerulonephritis: Classification, pathogenetic mechanisms, and therapy (in-depth review) Am J Kidney Dis 11:449, 1988. *A very current and complete review of RPGN with emphasis on pathogenetic mechanisms and therapy, including 195 references.*

Falk RJ, Jennette JC: Anti-neutrophil cytoplasmic autoantibodies with specificity for myeloperoxidase in patients with systemic vasculitis and idiopathic necrotizing and crescentic glomerulonephritis. N Engl J Med 318:1651, 1988. *This paper emphasizes the utility of determining ANCA levels in patients with idiopathic crescentic glomerulonephritis and the overlap between this disease and small vessel vasculitis, including Wegener's granulomatosis.*

Glassock RJ: Natural history and treatment of primary proliferative glomerulonephritis: A review. Kidney Int 28:S136, 1985. *In this review of treatment of several forms of glomerulonephritis, the section on crescentic glomerulonephritis provides a thoughtful and comprehensive review of the literature on treatment of RPGN, with useful guidelines and recommendations.*

NEPHROTIC SYNDROME

The nephrotic syndrome is not a disease; it is a group of signs and symptoms commonly seen in patients with glomerular diseases that are characterized by a marked increase in capillary wall permeability to serum proteins rather than (or sometimes in addition to) glomerular inflammatory changes. The primary abnormality in nephrotic syndrome is the excretion of large amounts (greater than 3.5 grams per day) of protein in the urine. Other manifestations that may occur secondary to *proteinuria* include *hypoalbuminemia, edema, hyperlipidemia,* and *lipiduria.* In contrast to the acute nephritic syndrome, the onset of the nephrotic syndrome is usually insidious, gross hematuria and red cell casts are infrequent, and renal function is often normal at the time of presentation.

The list of diseases that may cause the nephrotic syndrome is extensive and includes virtually every disorder that may affect the glomerulus. About one third of adults and one tenth of children have the nephrotic syndrome as a manifestation of some systemic disease, usually diabetes, SLE, or amyloidosis. In two thirds of adults and most children, the nephrotic syndrome is idiopathic and a manifestation of one of three types of primary glomerular disease: MCNS or its variants, membranous nephropathy, or MPGN. The relative frequencies of these diseases and their identifying characteristics are presented for comparison in Table 79–3. It is important to note that the occurrence of the nephrotic syndrome in patients over 45 may be associated with occult malignancy. The association of Hodgkin's disease with MCNS and of solid tumors of the lung, breast, and gastrointestinal tract with membranous nephropathy is discussed below. All of the diseases discussed in the section on acute GN can also cause the nephrotic syndrome, although they do not commonly do so.

Pathophysiology of the Nephrotic Syndrome

PROTEINURIA. Glomeruli are normally perfused with plasma containing more than 60,000 grams of protein per day, but less than 150 mg of protein is excreted in the final urine. The filtration barrier, which includes the endothelial cells, basement membrane, epithelial cells, and slit diaphragms, restricts the transcapillary passage of proteins on the basis of their size, shape, and electrical charge. The size barrier is primarily at the level of the endothelial cells and GBM. The glomerular filtration barrier is discussed in Ch. 73.

Glomerular hemodynamic factors also alter protein filtration. Thus, in situations of reduced renal perfusion, renal blood flow (RBF) may be reduced while GFR is maintained by adaptive changes in other determinants of GFR, such as intracapillary hydraulic pressure. Under these circumstances the filtration fraction (GFR/RBF) is increased, resulting in a higher than normal protein concentration at the efferent end of the glomerular capillary. This may produce an increased diffusion of protein across the capillary wall, resulting in proteinuria in the absence of glomerular disease in conditions such as congestive heart failure and other states of reduced renal perfusion (see Isolated Proteinuria, above).

Proteinuria, the hallmark of the nephrotic syndrome, exceeds 3.5 grams per day in adults or 40 mg per square meter per hour in children. Fixed nephrotic range proteinuria with the nephrotic syndrome generally occurs only in the presence of diffuse glomerular disease. The immune mechanisms that cause an increase in the permselective properties of the glomerular capillary wall may induce a loss of net negative charge on the capillary wall, as appears to occur in MCNS, leading to a marked increase in urinary albumin excretion without significant change in the excretion of other serum proteins (*selective proteinuria*). Other diseases with extensive capillary wall immune deposits, such as membranous nephropathy, or disorders of basement membrane biochemistry or structure, such as those found in diabetes or hereditary nephritis, are associated with apparent structural defects and increased filtration of all serum proteins (*nonselective proteinuria*). More than 40 grams of protein may be excreted in the urine each day in some patients. It is this loss of protein that leads to the other clinical and biochemical manifestations of the nephrotic syndrome.

HYPOALBUMINEMIA. Serum albumin concentration decreases to less than 3.0 grams per deciliter when the rate of urinary protein loss and renal catabolism of filtered albumin (which may exceed 10 grams per day in the nephrotic syndrome) exceeds the rate of hepatic synthesis. Hepatic albumin synthesis is normally 12 to 14 grams per day in adults and may increase in the nephrotic syndrome but can be limited by various factors, including age, poor nutritional status, and liver disease. Thus, some patients may exhibit significant hypoalbuminemia with proteinuria of less than 10 grams per day, while others excreting larger amounts of protein are better able to maintain serum albumin levels.

EDEMA. Edema in the nephrotic syndrome results in part from a reduction in plasma oncotic pressure such that capillary hydraulic pressure exceeds oncotic pressure in peripheral capillaries and fluid leaves the capillaries. Although the reduction in effective circulating volume that occurs may result in increased renal retention of salt and water through normal compensatory mechanisms, more than 50 per cent of patients with the nephrotic syndrome have normal or increased plasma volume and normal or low levels of plasma renin during sodium retention, suggesting a primary renal contribution to salt retention in the nephrotic syndrome through mechanisms that remain poorly defined.

HYPERLIPIDEMIA. Hyperlipidemia is common in the nephrotic syndrome and is inversely proportional to the serum albumin concentration. Hypercholesterolemia and elevated phospholipids are the most constant abnormalities observed, but increased levels of low and very low density lipoproteins, triglycerides, and chylomicrons are also seen. The primary mechanism appears to be increased hepatic synthesis of cholesterol, triglycerides, and lipoproteins, but reduced catabolism of these compounds has also been demonstrated.

LIPIDURIA. In a nephrotic urinary sediment, lipids are seen as free fat, oval fat bodies (degenerated renal tubular epithelial cells containing cholesterol esters), and fatty casts, all of which exhibit a Maltese cross pattern under polarizing light. Lipiduria parallels the level of urine protein excretion rather than the serum lipid levels.

Complications of the Nephrotic Syndrome

The most clinically important metabolic complications of the nephrotic syndrome are severe protein malnutrition, which may require appropriate nutritional supplementation, hypercoagulability with a tendency to form thrombi in both renal and peripheral veins leading to thromboembolic complications, and acute renal failure.

Hypercoagulability is thought to be a consequence of altered clotting factor levels in the nephrotic syndrome, including reduced levels of factors IX, XI, and XII; elevated levels of factors V and VIII, fibrinogen, beta-thromboglobulin, and platelets; a reduction in levels of antithrombin III and antiplasmin; and increased susceptibility of platelets to aggregation. There is a high incidence (10 to 40 per cent) of thrombus formation in renal, pulmonary, and peripheral veins, and occasionally in arteries, with frequent thromboembolic phenomena. The incidence of renal vein thrombosis appears to be particularly high in patients with the nephrotic syndrome due to membranous nephropathy. Routine anticoagulation is not indicated unless emboli occur.

Acute renal failure in the nephrotic syndrome very rarely occurs owing to rapid progression of the underlying renal disease, since most diseases that cause the nephrotic syndrome progress very slowly. However, acute renal failure does occur as a consequence of several potentially treatable disorders superimposed on nephrotic glomerular disease. These include (1) reduced renal perfusion due to low plasma volume, which can result in acute tubular necrosis, particularly following a surgical procedure or biopsy; (2) interstitial renal edema in patients with MCNS and significant peripheral edema, who may develop intrarenal swelling sufficient to produce increased intrarenal pressure, cessation of filtration, and acute renal failure (this may be reversible with diuretic therapy); (3) drug-induced allergic interstitial nephritis, particularly in patients receiving diuretic therapy; (4) bilateral acute renal vein thrombosis; and (5) reduced glomerular perfusion due to nonsteroidal anti-inflammatory drugs, which inhibit synthesis of vasodilatory prostaglandins and reduce glomerular plasma flow in states of volume contraction or diffuse glomerular disease. Nonsteroidal anti-inflammatory agents may also cause acute allergic interstitial nephritis, which may be accompanied by a reversible nephrotic syndrome with a glomerular lesion like that in MCNS.

Other complications that may also be associated with the nephrotic syndrome include reduced levels of IgG (which may dispose to bacterial infection); proximal tubular dysfunction with signs of Fanconi's syndrome; deficiencies of trace metals such as iron, copper, and zinc; and loss of vitamin D with development of osteomalacia and secondary hyperparathyroidism. Measurements of thyroid function, such as thyroxine (T_4) radioimmunoassay and triiodothyronine (T_3) resin uptake, may falsely suggest reduced function, but free T_4 and thyroid-stimulating hormone (TSH) levels are generally normal.

Bernard DB: Extrarenal complications of the nephrotic syndrome (nephrology forum). Kidney Int 33:1184, 1988. *A detailed and comprehensive review of the pathophysiology and treatment of systemic complications of nephrotic syndrome presented in a lucid and comprehensive fashion, with 153 references.*

TABLE 79–3. SUMMARY OF PRIMARY RENAL DISEASES THAT PRESENT AS IDIOPATHIC NEPHROTIC SYNDROME

	Minimal Change Nephrotic Syndrome (MCNS)	Focal Glomerular Sclerosis (FGS)	Membranous Nephropathy	Membranoproliferative Glomerulonephritis (MPGN)	
				Type I	Type II
Frequency*					
Children	75%	10%	<5%		10%
Adults	15%	15%	50%		10%
Clinical Manifestations					
Age	2–6, some adults	2–6, some adults	40–50	5–15	
Sex	2:1 male	1.3:1 male	2:1 male	male-female	
Nephrotic syndrome	100%	90%	80%	60%	
Asymptomatic proteinuria	0	10%	20%	40%	
Hematuria	20%	60–80%	60%	80%	
Hypertension	10%	20% early	Infrequent	35%	
Rate of progression	Does not progress	10 years	50% in 10–20 years	10–20 years	5–15 years
Associated conditions	Allergy, Hodgkin's disease	None	Renal vein thrombosis, cancer, SLE	None	Partial lipodystrophy
Laboratory Findings	Manifestations of nephrotic syndrome	Manifestations of nephrotic syndrome	Manifestations of nephrotic syndrome	Low C1, C4, C3–C9	Normal C1, C4, low C3–C9 C3 nephritic factor
Immunogenetics	HLA-B8, B12 (3.5)†	Not established	HLA-DRW3 (12–32)†	Not established	
Renal Pathology					
Light microscopy	Normal	Focal sclerotic lesions	Thickened GBM, spikes	Thickened GBM, proliferation, lobulation	
Immunofluorescence	Negative	IgM, C3 in lesions	Fine granular IgG, C3	Granular IgG, C3	C3 only
Electron microscopy	Foot process fusion	Foot process fusion	Subepithelial deposits	Mesangial and subendothelial deposits	Dense deposits
Response to Steroids	90%	15–20%	May be slow progression	Not established	

*Approximate frequency as a cause of idiopathic nephrotic syndrome. About 10 per cent of adult nephrotic syndrome is due to various diseases that usually present with acute glomerulonephritis (Table 79–1).
†Relative risk.

Cameron JS: The nephrotic syndrome and its complications. Am J Kidney Dis 10:157, 1987. *A stimulating and provocative analysis of what is known of the pathophysiology of fluid retention in nephrotic syndrome and including an analysis of the causes and treatment of some of the underlying disorders by an experienced clinician and student of these diseases.*

Kaysen GA, Myers BD, Couser WG, et al.: Biology of disease: Mechanisms and consequences of proteinuria. Lab Invest 54:479, 1986. *An in-depth review that correlates the pathophysiology of glomerular protein filtration with observations in patients with nephrotic syndrome and discusses the mechanisms and the consequences of massive urinary protein loss.*

Primary Renal Diseases That Present as the Nephrotic Syndrome

MINIMAL CHANGE NEPHROTIC SYNDROME (MCNS)

As indicated in Table 79–3, MCNS accounts for about 75 per cent of cases of idiopathic nephrotic syndrome in children and up to 20 per cent of adults. Synonyms include minimal change disease, nephropathy or glomerulopathy, lipoid nephrosis, and nil disease.

Pathogenesis. The pathogenesis of MCNS is not known. The disease is characterized by a loss of net negative charge on the capillary wall and can recur promptly in the transplanted kidney, suggesting the presence of a circulating factor that neutralizes glomerular polyanion, resulting in loss of the charge barrier and a selective type of proteinuria. The association of MCNS with Hodgkin's disease, its responsiveness to steroids and alkylating agents, and the tendency for remission to follow some viral infections, particularly measles, have focused attention on the possibility of an abnormality in T lymphocytes, perhaps involving production of a lymphokine with properties that induce increased glomerular capillary permeability.

Pathology. By definition, the diagnosis of MCNS requires the absence of abnormalities on light microscopy and of immune deposits on immunofluorescence. Diffuse epithelial cell foot process effacement, or "fusion," is the abnormality usually seen on electron microscopy, but some morphologic abnormalities may occur in MCNS, including mild to moderate focal or diffuse proliferation of mesangial cells; mesangial deposits of IgM, IgA, or C3 seen on immunofluorescence; and the presence of focal glomerulosclerosis (FGS) by light microscopy. In the presence of FGS, response to steroids is poor, and progressive loss of renal function is commonly seen. This observation has led several authors to consider FGS a separate disease (see below). However, in some patients the FGS lesion appears to develop late in the course of MCNS and may simply be a histologic marker of a more severe and less responsive form of MCNS mediated by a similar mechanism.

Mesangial proliferation and mesangial IgM deposits may occur together or separately and usually predict a poor (or delayed) response to steroids and an increased possibility of progression. As with FGS, there have been attempts to classify such disorders into separate disease categories (mesangial-proliferative GN, IgM nephropathy). When progression occurs in patients with MCNS and mesangial proliferation and/or IgM deposits, glomeruli develop changes typical of FGS.

Clinical Features. The peak incidence of MCNS is in children 2 to 6 years of age, in whom it virtually always presents as a full-blown nephrotic syndrome. In childhood, boys are affected twice as often as girls. One third of patients have a preceding upper respiratory tract infection or other identifiable antecedent event. In the absence of volume contraction, renal function and blood pressure are normal, but up to one third of patients, when first seen, may have a reduced GFR due to hypovolemia and reduced renal perfusion. Urinary protein excretion may exceed 40 grams per day in severe cases, and the serum albumin level is less than 2.0 grams per deciliter in more than 90 per cent of children. The complications of this disease are discussed above under complications of the nephrotic syndrome in general. In addition, there is an association between MCNS and Hodgkin's disease in which the nephrotic syndrome may be the presenting sign of an occult lymphoma. Allergic reactions to nonsteroidal anti-inflammatory agents may produce nephrotic syndrome and MCNS on biopsy, usually associated with interstitial nephritis and reduced renal function.

Laboratory Findings. The laboratory findings in MCNS are those of the nephrotic syndrome of any etiology. Proteinuria is

"selective" (greater than 90 per cent albumin) in about 85 per cent of cases. Complement levels are usually normal. A consistent finding is a marked reduction in ASO titers (less than 100 Todd units).

Course and Treatment. Before steroids and modern antibiotics were available, the spontaneous remission rate in MCNS was estimated at 25 to 40 per cent. During that era, the mortality rate in children exceeded 50 per cent in 5 years owing to infections or thromboembolic complications. The mortality rate now is about 7 to 12 per cent in nephrotic children and less than 2 per cent in those who respond to steroids. Some of this improvement reflects the development of effective antibiotics and better general medical care. Steroid therapy has never been shown in a controlled study to improve survival in patients with MCNS. However, the usual dramatic resolution of the nephrotic syndrome following steroid administration, as well as the fact that survival has improved since the presteroid era, has led to the widespread belief that such treatment is beneficial.

Conventional doses of oral prednisone are 60 mg per square meter per day in children and 2 mg per kilogram per day in adults, given daily for 4 weeks, followed by alternate-day therapy for 4 more weeks and then a tapering course over 4 to 6 months. Within 4 weeks, 90 per cent of children will have responded, and 90 per cent of adults will respond within about 8 weeks. There is little value in continuing steroid therapy beyond 8 weeks if abnormal levels of proteinuria persist. The 10 per cent of patients who fail to respond generally have FGS (see below).

Of the steroid responders, roughly 50 per cent will remain free of proteinuria or develop infrequent relapses that respond to steroids, eventually entering permanent remission. The remainder will become either "frequent relapsers" (more than twice a year) or steroid dependent, often with a high incidence of steroid side effects. Some can be managed conservatively with salt restriction, diuretics, and a high-protein diet. In children, the clinical manifestations of the nephrotic syndrome are usually more severe, and steroid toxicity may require the use of an additional drug. Both cyclophosphamide, 2 to 3 mg per kilogram per day (75 mg per square meter per day in children), and chlorambucil, 0.2 to 0.3 mg per kilogram per day, given for 8 to 12 weeks, have been shown to increase the frequency and duration of remission in steroid-sensitive MCNS. However, because of their gonadal toxicity, teratogenic potential, and other side effects, these agents should be used only when both the nephrotic syndrome and steroid side effects are severe. About half of such patients treated with a second drug are reported to be in remission 4 years later, suggesting that complete remission can be achieved with drug therapy in almost 90 per cent of patients with MCNS.

Meyrier A, Simon P: Treatment of corticoresistant idiopathic nephrotic syndrome in the adult: Minimal change disease and focal segmental glomerulosclerosis. Adv Nephrol 17:127, 1988. *A comprehensive analysis of therapeutic approaches and responses to therapy as well as prognosis in adult patients with MCNS and FSG. This paper is unique in separating adults from children and emphasizes the indications and complications of cytotoxic drug therapy.*

Nolasco F, Cameron JS, Heywood EF, et al.: Adult-onset minimal change nephrotic syndrome: A long-term follow-up. Kidney Int 29:1215, 1986. *This paper reviews the clinical course and response to therapy in 89 adults with MCNS and documents a higher incidence of complications and slower response to therapy compared with children with this disease.*

FOCAL GLOMERULOSCLEROSIS (FGS)

Overview. FGS is a histologic lesion found in some patients with otherwise typical MCNS, and it correlates well with steroid resistance and progressive renal failure. Controversy exists regarding whether it should be classified as a separate glomerular disease or should be viewed as one end of a spectrum that ranges from pure steroid-responsive MCNS with no morphologic abnormalities to typical FGS. The author favors the views that mesangial proliferation, mesangial IgM deposits, and FGS are part of the MCNS spectrum. However, the clinical features of patients with idiopathic nephrotic syndrome and FGS in early biopsies are sufficiently different from those who do not have these lesions to warrant separate consideration.

Pathogenesis. The etiology and pathogenesis of the lesion of FGS are unknown. Presumably, the basic mechanism underlying the generalized increase in capillary wall permeability may be the same as that in MCNS, and the structural lesion may be the consequence of either the greater severity of this process in such patients or the presence of some additional, as-yet-unidentified factor (or factors). Experimentally, FGS has been attributed to glomerular hypertension and hypertrophy.

Pathology. The diagnosis of FGS is made by renal biopsy in which sclerotic lesions are seen only in some glomeruli (focal) and within an affected glomerulus are present only in some capillary loops (segmental). The presence of sclerosis involving occasional entire glomeruli (global sclerosis) is a common finding that increases with age in all patients and does not have prognostic significance. The FGS lesion itself is an expansion of the mesangial matrix, with wrinkling and collapse of adjacent capillary loops, development of periodic acid–Schiff (PAS)–positive intracapillary hyaline deposits, adhesions to Bowman's capsule, and often foamy cells and focal epithelial cell proliferation (Fig. 79–6). Glomeruli that do not contain the lesion of FGS exhibit changes identical to those of MCNS, indicating that the increase in capillary permeability is a diffuse one not confined to the areas of sclerotic lesions. Interstitial infiltrates and tubular atrophy usually accompany lesions of FGS. IgM and C3 are frequently deposited nonspecifically in sclerotic lesions and may occasionally be seen more diffusely in the mesangium.

Clinical Features. FGS is present in 5 to 15 per cent of patients with idiopathic nephrotic syndrome and is associated with a higher frequency of hematuria (65 per cent), hypertension (10 per cent), and renal insufficiency (10 per cent) on presentation than is seen in MCNS (Table 79–3). Sterile pyuria is also common. Proteinuria is nonselective, presumably reflecting the focal areas of structural damage to the capillary wall associated with lesions of FGS. While most patients have the nephrotic syndrome, a significant minority are detected with asymptomatic proteinuria, a finding that is rarely seen in MCNS. When all of these features accompany the finding of FGS in an early biopsy, only about 20 per cent of such patients will respond to steroid therapy and many of these do not remain steroid responsive. The presence of the nephrotic syndrome, hematuria, hypertension, decreased renal function, and mesangial hypercellularity on biopsy tends to indicate a poor prognosis.

A smaller group of patients appears to have clinically typical MCNS without hematuria or hypertension but shows early lesions of FGS on biopsy. Often such biopsies are obtained later in the course of the disease after several episodes of steroid-responsive nephrotic syndrome, and such patients may remain steroid responsive for many years and progress very slowly or not at all. When all patients with FGS on initial biopsy are studied, only about 40 per cent are in renal failure at the end of 10 years.

Laboratory Features. There are no distinctive laboratory abnormalities, except for the increased incidence of hematuria and presence of nonselective proteinuria, that differentiate patients with FGS from those with pure MCNS.

Course and Treatment. Patients with FGS on initial biopsy, especially if hematuria, hypertension, and nephrotic syndrome are present, are often resistant to steroids and may progress to renal failure in an average of about 10 years. The level of proteinuria is clearly related to prognosis, and 80 per cent of all patients with nonnephrotic proteinuria retain normal renal function for more than 10 years. About 15 to 20 per cent of all patients with FGS and the nephrotic syndrome will show a response to steroids, sometimes months to years after therapy, a phenomenon that justifies a trial of steroid therapy as outlined above for MCNS in such patients. A remission can be induced in up to 40 per cent of adults with combined steroid and cytotoxic drug therapy. If a remission is achieved, the prognosis is considerably better, and such patients may behave like those with MCNS. Alkylating agents such as cyclophosphamide and chlorambucil have been shown to increase the frequency and duration of steroid-induced remission in FGS, as they have in MCNS.

Patients with FGS who progress to renal failure have a high incidence of recurrent disease in renal transplants. Factors that have been correlated with recurrence include mesangial hypercellularity, a rapidly progressive course (less than 3 years), and receipt of a well-matched living-related donor transplant. In four-antigen matches, the recurrence rate may be as high as 80 per cent, although it is less than 50 per cent for all patients with end-stage renal disease due to FGS. With recurrence, patients develop the nephrotic syndrome within a few hours to 1 week, accompanied by lesions of FGS in the transplant and usually a shortened graft survival.

Korbet SM, Schwartz MM, Lewis EJ: The prognosis of focal segmental glomerulosclerosis of adulthood. Medicine 66:304, 1986. *This detailed analysis of 46 patients with idiopathic nephrotic syndrome and focal glomerulosclerosis emphasizes clinical features, prognosis, and therapy.*

Meyrier A, Simon P: Treatment of corticoresistant idiopathic nephrotic syndrome in the adult: Minimal change disease and focal segmental glomerulosclerosis. Adv Nephrol 17:127, 1988. *A comprehensive analysis of therapeutic approaches and responses to therapy as well as prognosis in adult patients with MCNS and FSG. This paper is unique in separating adults from children and emphasizes the indications and complications of cytotoxic drug therapy.*

Pei Y, Cattran D, Delmore T, et al.: Evidence suggesting under-treatment in adults with idiopathic focal segmental glomerulosclerosis. Am J Med 82:938, 1987. *This analysis of 103 cases of FGS from Canada emphasizes the remission rate of up to 40 per cent with appropriate steroid and cytotoxic drug therapy and points out the markedly improved prognosis in adult patients who experience a remission.*

HEROIN NEPHROPATHY. In some centers, up to 25 per cent of new cases of FGS and 10 per cent of all cases of end-stage renal disease occur in young adults with a history of parenteral drug abuse, usually including heroin. Other renal lesions such as GN secondary to bacterial endocarditis, hepatitis B–associated membranous nephropathy, large vessel vasculitis, amyloidosis, and interstitial nephritis related to embolized foreign material are also seen in addicts. However, the entity of nephrotic syndrome with FGS, hypertension, and rapidly progressive renal disease appears to be the most common drug-related lesion. A similar lesion may cause nephrotic syndrome in patients with AIDS (see above), with or without a history of drug abuse. Discontinuation of drug use has resulted in stabilization or improvement in renal function in some patients, but no other form of therapy has proved beneficial. The role of the injected drugs or other foreign substances in the pathogenesis of this lesion is not known.

Dubrow A, Mittman N, Ghali V, et al.: The changing spectrum of heroin-associated nephropathy. Am J Kidney Dis 5:36, 1985. *This study of 35 heroin abusers with nephrotic syndrome confirms the presence of FGS as a common underlying lesion but emphasizes the increasing frequency with which amyloid is seen as the cause of nephrotic syndrome.*

Membranous Nephropathy

Overview. Membranous nephropathy is an uncommon disease in childhood but is the most common cause of idiopathic nephrotic

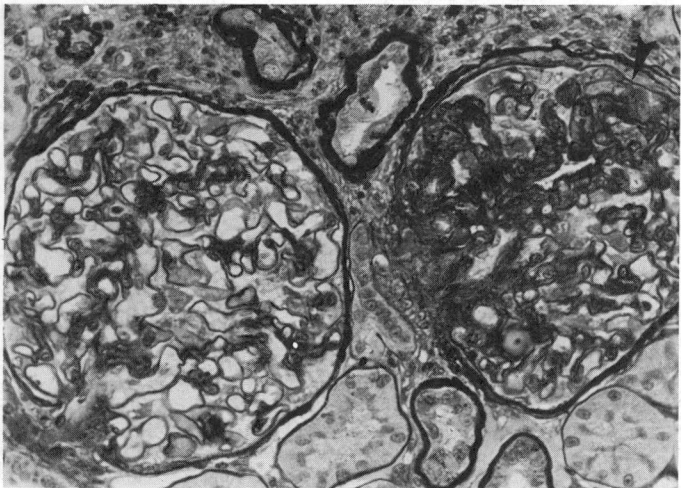

FIGURE 79–6. Renal biopsy from a patient with nephrotic syndrome, FGS, and decreased renal function. By light microscopy the glomerulus on the left appears almost normal with only slight mesangial matrix increase, while the glomerulus on the right is partially sclerotic with an adhesion to Bowman's capsule at one o'clock (*arrowhead*). Two atrophic tubules with thickened basement membranes in the upper part of the field are surrounded by fibrosis and mononuclear cells. (Periodic acid–Schiff stain, ×350.) (Reproduced with permission from Couser WG, Salant DJ, Adler S, et al. *In* Brenner BM, Lazarus JM [eds.]: Acute Renal Failure. Philadelphia, W.B. Saunders Company, 1983, p 403.)

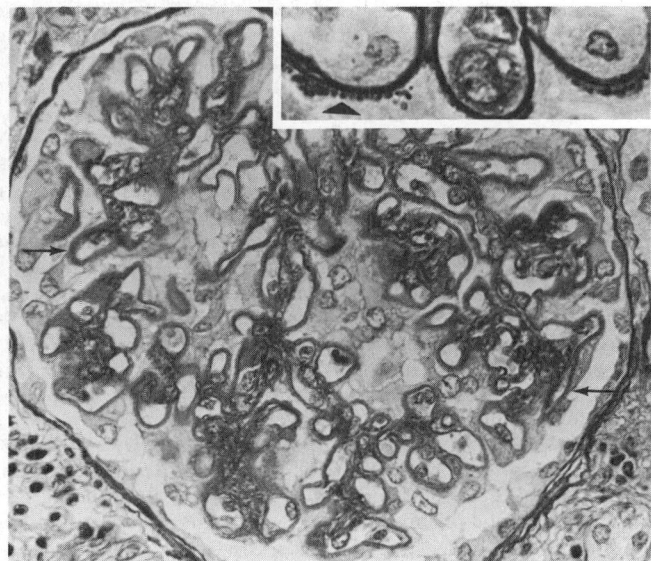

FIGURE 79–7. Light microscopy in early membranous nephropathy shows minimal thickening of the glomerular capillary walls (*arrows*) without any increase in cells or mesangial matrix. In the inset, three capillary loops stained with silver methenamine demonstrate the "spike" of basement membrane between deposits (*arrowheads*) (periodic acid–Schiff stain, ×350; inset: silver methenamine stain, ×900). (Reproduced with permission from Couser WG, Salant DJ, Stilmant MM. *In* Flamenbaum W, Hamburger RJ [eds.]: Nephrology. Philadelphia, J.B. Lippincott Company, 1982, pp 265–301.)

syndrome in adults, in whom it accounts for about 50 per cent of all cases (Table 79–3). As with all other causes of idiopathic nephrotic syndrome, the diagnosis can be made only by renal biopsy.

Pathogenesis. Experimentally, subepithelial immune deposits may result from the binding of antibody to an epithelial cell membrane antigen or to exogenous antigens that become localized at this site, usually on the basis of charge-charge interactions with glomerular anionic structures. In humans, the idiopathic form of membranous nephropathy appears to be an autoimmune disease. Subepithelial immune deposits induce proteinuria by a mechanism that probably involves the C5b–9, or membrane attack, portion of the complement system.

The role played by inciting agents, such as drugs or hepatitis

virus, in initiating this process is unknown. A strong association exists between idiopathic membranous nephropathy and HLA-DRw3 (a relative risk of about 4), an association also noted in patients who develop membranous nephropathy while taking drugs. Although most cases are idiopathic, some develop in association with a variety of other conditions, including *drugs* (penicillamine, gold, captopril), *infectious agents* (hepatitis B, various parasitic infestations), *SLE*, and *malignancy*, particularly solid tumors of the lung, breast, and gastrointestinal tract. The nephrotic syndrome may be the presenting sign of an otherwise occult neoplasm, and older patients with idiopathic membranous nephropathy should be carefully evaluated for malignancy. An identical lesion occurs in about 15 per cent of patients with SLE and may be the presenting sign of this disease when other systemic and serologic manifestations are absent. Young females who present with what appears to be idiopathic membranous nephropathy must be carefully followed for later development of SLE. Other associations, such as those with Sjögren's syndrome, mixed connective tissue disease, diabetes, thyroiditis, syphilis, sarcoidosis, and sickle cell disease, are documented but rare.

Pathology. On light microscopy, glomeruli may appear entirely normal early, but as the disease progresses, a diffuse thickening of capillary walls occurs without any increase in glomerular cellularity (Fig. 79–7). A silver methenamine stain usually demonstrates the spikelike extensions of basement membrane between areas of subepithelial deposits, and the subepithelial deposits themselves may be seen with a PAS stain. A diffuse, very finely granular pattern of immune deposits of IgG and C3 is found along the subepithelial surface of all capillary loops (Fig. 79–8). Electron microscopy demonstrates electron-dense deposits in an exclusively subepithelial distribution with effacement of overlying foot processes (Fig. 79–9).

Clinical Manifestations. The mean age of onset of idiopathic membranous nephropathy in the United States is 40 to 50, and males predominate about 2 to 1. However, the disease has been reported in patients as young as 2 and as old as over 70. More than 80 per cent of patients present with the nephrotic syndrome, but 20 per cent may be seen first with asymptomatic proteinuria. Microscopic hematuria is present in about 60 per cent of cases in adults, but red cell casts are rare. Hypertension is uncommon and renal function is usually normal at the time of presentation. The association of membranous nephropathy with other disease processes has been discussed above under Pathogenesis.

Two complications of this disease are important: (1) Patients may develop a *superimposed anti-GBM nephritis* with crescent formation and a clinical course similar to that of RPGN. This

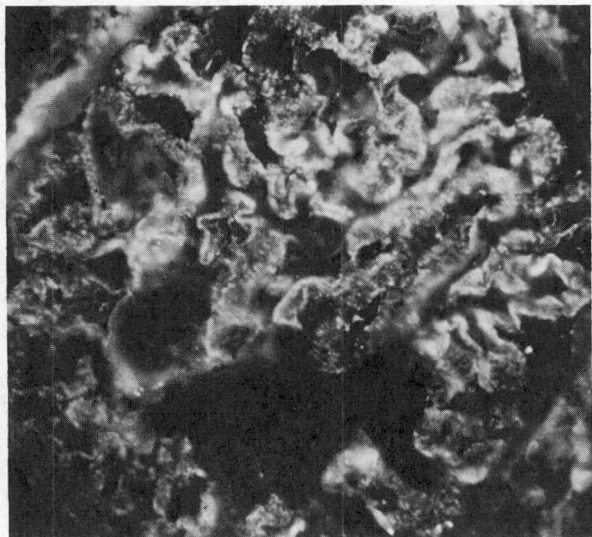

FIGURE 79–8. Immunofluorescence microscopy in membranous nephropathy demonstrates diffuse, finely granular staining of IgG (and C3) on all capillary walls, usually without mesangial deposits (×400). (Reproduced with permission from Couser WG, Salant DJ, Stilmant MM. *In* Flamenbaum W, Hamburger RJ [eds.]: Nephrology. Philadelphia, J.B. Lippincott Company, 1982, pp 265–301.)

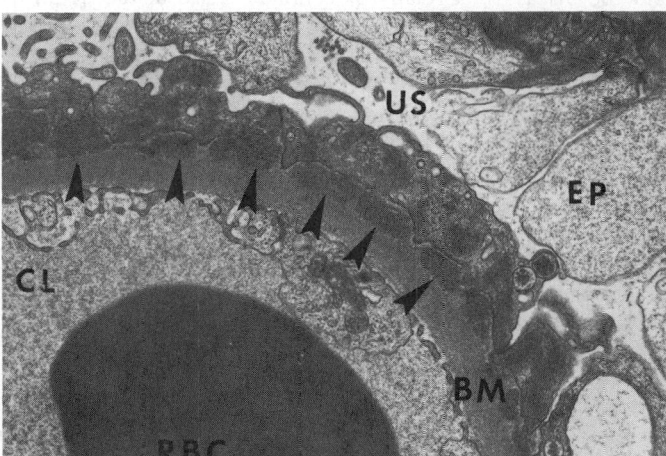

FIGURE 79–9. Electron micrograph of a glomerulus in membranous nephropathy showing many electron-dense subepithelial deposits (*arrowheads*) between the basement membrane and effaced epithelial cell foot processes. A red blood cell is present in the capillary lumen (×15,000). BM = Basement membrane; CL = capillary lumen; EP = epithelial cell; RBC = red blood cell. (Reproduced with permission from Couser WG, Salant DJ, Adler S, et al. *In* Brenner BM, Lazarus JM [eds]: Acute Renal Failure. Philadelphia, W.B. Saunders Company, 1983, p 406.)

possibility must be considered in otherwise stable patients who experience a rapid deterioration in renal function accompanied by a nephritic urine sediment. (2) An incidence of *renal vein thrombosis* as high as 50 per cent has been reported in membranous nephropathy. Any patient in whom a thromboembolism is suspected should be studied for renal vein thrombosis and treated with long-term anticoagulation to reduce thromboembolic complications if a venous thrombosis is demonstrated.

Laboratory Studies. There are no laboratory abnormalities specific for idiopathic membranous nephropathy. Because of the frequency of various associated conditions, the laboratory workup should include determinations of antinuclear and anti-DNA antibody, serum complement levels, rheumatoid factor, cryoglobulins, hepatitis B antigen, VDRL, and tests to exclude diabetes. In older patients, a careful clinical and radiologic search for occult malignancy is justified. If the patient has unusual flank pain, hematuria, or a reason to suspect pulmonary emboli, the renal veins should be studied by venography.

Course and Treatment. The disease has a widely variable clinical course, with substantial fluctuations in proteinuria and an uncertain prognosis. The spontaneous remission rate is about 25 per cent in adults. Another 25 per cent of patients have persistent nephrotic range proteinuria for many years but retain normal renal function. The remaining 50 per cent of adults, and 10 to 15 per cent of children, experience a slowly progressive deterioration of renal function that results in end-stage renal disease in an average of about 15 years, although more rapid progression may be seen. No clinical or pathologic criteria have been identified that will predict the future clinical course in an individual patient.

The variable clinical course in idiopathic membranous nephropathy makes any assessment of benefits from therapy difficult, since large numbers of patients must be followed in a prospective controlled fashion to obtain meaningful data. The results of steroid therapy have been inconsistent and generally not clearly beneficial. Concomitant administration of cyclophosphamide appears to have a definite beneficial effect in reducing proteinuria and slowing disease progression. Since fewer than 50 per cent of patients will develop progressive disease, the author recommends cytotoxic drugs only in males with proteinuria in excess of 10 grams per day and in patients with evidence of progressive loss of renal function.

Recurrent membranous nephropathy in a renal transplant is rare but has been reported in several patients who have progressed to end-stage renal disease in a period of 4 years or less. Recurrence usually has not adversely affected graft survival. Significantly more cases of de novo membranous nephropathy have been reported in renal allografts than cases of recurrence, and the disease is a relatively common cause of the nephrotic syndrome in transplant patients.

Couser WG, Abrass CK: Pathogenesis of membranous nephropathy. Ann Rev Med 39:517, 1988. *A current review of the present understanding of the pathogenetic mechanisms in membranous nephropathy as they relate to treatment and prognosis; with 81 references.*

Ponticelli C, Zucchelli P, Passerini P, et al.: A randomized trial of methylprednisolone and chlorambucil in idiopathic membranous nephropathy. N Engl J Med 320:8, 1989. *The latest results of a large controlled study of therapy in membranous nephropathy comparing steroids and cytotoxic drugs with no treatment document impressive benefits of this therapeutic approach in inducing a remission of nephrotic syndrome and preserving renal function. While the specific agents and protocols used here may be arbitrary, the efficacy of steroid and cytotoxic drug therapy in membranous nephropathy is well established by this study.*

MEMBRANOPROLIFERATIVE GLOMERULONEPHRITIS (MPGN)

Overview. The term membranoproliferative glomerulonephritis refers to a clinicopathologic entity found primarily in young adults and characterized by idiopathic nephrotic syndrome, hypocomplementemia, and a histologic lesion having the lobular appearance of glomeruli with both thickening of the basement membrane and cellular proliferation. These histologic and clinical features are probably common to at least two separate and perhaps unrelated diseases, which are now referred to as type I MPGN (that with subendothelial immune deposits) and type II MPGN (dense deposit disease). Type I MPGN is about twice as common as type II, and the two diseases cause about 10 per cent of cases

of idiopathic nephrotic syndrome in both children and adults (Table 79–3). However, unlike the other glomerular diseases that cause idiopathic nephrotic syndrome, about 20 per cent of patients present with an acute nephritic syndrome, and nephritic features are common in both of these diseases.

Pathogenesis. Type I MPGN. Several features of type I MPGN suggest that it is a chronic immune complex GN: (1) the granular deposits of IgG and C3 in a subendothelial and mesangial distribution, (2) the activation of the classic complement pathway, (3) the frequent presence of cryoglobulins and circulating immune complexes, (4) the presence of similar lesions in patients with some forms of postinfectious GN, including shunt nephritis and nephritis associated with chronic hepatitis B antigenemia, and (5) the production of similar lesions in animals immunized chronically with a foreign serum protein. However, the etiology of the disease, the nature of the antigen (or antigens) involved, and the reasons for the chronicity of the process remain unknown.

Type II MPGN. This disease does not appear to be an immune deposit disease, and the nature of the dense deposits remains unclear. Despite much study of the unique abnormalities in complement metabolism associated with this disease, and the identification of C3 nephritic factor in the serum, the role of the complement abnormalities, if any, in the pathogenesis of the disease remains undefined. There is no animal model of dense deposit disease, and similar lesions have not been described in other renal diseases.

Pathology. Type I MPGN. Light microscopy reveals a diffuse proliferative GN with thickening of the glomerular capillary walls, increase in mesangial cells and matrix, and a lobulated appearance of the glomerulus (Fig. 79–10). The thickened capillary walls are due to subendothelial immune deposits and interposition of mesangial matrix between GBM and endothelium, resulting in a double contour, splitting, or "tram track" appearance of the capillary walls on silver stain. Crescents are present in fewer than 10 per cent of cases. Coarsely granular deposits of C3, and often of IgG, IgM, C4, properdin, and fibrin, occur in the mesangium and in peripheral capillary loops in a pattern much like that seen in diffuse proliferative, or class IV, SLE. By electron microscopy, there are dense subendothelial and mesangial deposits present as well as mesangial matrix interposition with capillary wall thickening and narrowing of the capillary lumen.

Type II MPGN. The histologic findings in type II MPGN are very similar to those in type I disease except that crescents are present in up to 30 per cent of patients and correlate with a worse prognosis. The dense deposits may be seen as PAS-positive, ribbon-like deposits within the capillary wall as well as along

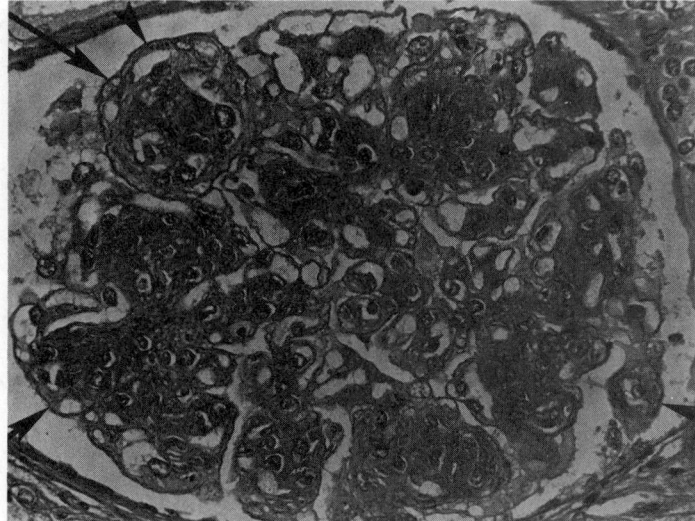

FIGURE 79–10. Light microscopy in membranoproliferative glomerulonephritis shows glomerular hypercellularity, segmental thickening of the basement membrane (*arrowheads*), and lobulation of glomerulus (*arrows*). (Periodic acid–Schiff, ×350.) (Reproduced with permission from Couser WG, Salant DJ, Stilmant MM. *In* Flamenbaum W, Hamburger RJ [eds.]: Nephrology. Philadelphia, J.B. Lippincott Company, 1982, pp 265–301.)

Bowman's capsule and tubular basement membrane. C3 is present along the margins of these deposits. Granular immune deposits of IgG are much less common than in type I disease. Electron microscopy reveals extensive replacement of the lamina densa with homogeneous, dark-staining material that may also be seen in the mesangium, Bowman's capsule, and tubular basement membrane.

Clinical Features. There are only minor differences in the clinical manifestations of types I and II MPGN. What follows is a description of patients with the more common type I disease. The differences observed in type II disease are commented on below. MPGN is a disease of children and young adults, rarely seen before age 5 and relatively uncommon after age 30. Males and females are affected approximately equally. The nephrotic syndrome is the presenting sign in about 50 per cent of patients and develops during the course of the disease in more than 80 per cent. Up to 20 per cent may present with an acute nephritic syndrome (which is more common in type II), and the remainder are detected with asymptomatic hematuria or proteinuria or both. Preceding upper respiratory tract infections have occurred in about half of patients with type I MPGN and may have been streptococcal. Hematuria is a common feature of the disease. Hypertension is present in one third, and 25 per cent have a reduced GRF on initial presentation.

The clinical course is quite variable. One third of patients develop end-stage renal disease within 6 to 10 years, one third have persistent nephrotic syndrome with relatively stable renal function, and one third have persistent nonnephrotic proteinuria or hematuria. Fewer than 5 per cent experience spontaneous remissions. In the long term, at least 50 per cent of patients with type I will reach end-stage renal disease in 15 to 20 years, while type II progresses somewhat more rapidly (6 to 10 years). Poor prognostic signs include a reduced GFR at onset, the presence of the nephrotic syndrome, early hypertension, gross hematuria, and the presence of either crescents or sclerosis on a renal biopsy.

Type I MPGN recurs in about 25 per cent of patients who receive renal transplants but rarely interferes with graft function.

The clinical features of type II disease that differ from those of type I include a higher frequency of both the nephrotic syndrome and acute nephritic episodes, a lower frequency of asymptomatic hematuria and proteinuria, more rapid progression to renal failure (probably due to the greater frequency of nephritic episodes), more frequent and persistent hypocomplementemia (see below), and a higher frequency of recurrence in transplants. Type II disease is also associated with partial lipodystrophy in some patients.

Laboratory Abnormalities. Type I MPGN is characterized by fluctuating levels of complement with depression of both classic (C1q, C4) and alternate pathway components at some time in most patients. In type II disease, hypocomplementemia is more frequent and persistent, and only alternate pathway activation is usually seen with a reduction in C3 and other alternate pathway proteins such as properdin and factor B, while classic pathway components are usually normal. Most type II patients have a circulating IgG autoantibody (C3 nephritic factor, or C3 Nef) directed against the C3 convertase of the alternate complement pathway. The definitive diagnosis of either type I or type II MPGN can be made only by renal biopsy with complete immunofluorescence and electron microscopic studies.

Treatment. Improvement or stabilization in renal function in MPGN has been reported with 2-year courses of alternate-day steroid therapy and with a "cocktail" of drugs including steroids, cytotoxic agents, anticoagulants, and antiplatelet agents. However, side effects of such treatments are significant. There is currently no therapeutic regimen of established safety and efficacy in these diseases.

Bennett WM, Fassett RG, Walker RG, et al.: Mesangiocapillary glomerulonephritis type II (dense-deposit disease): Clinical features of progressive disease. Am J Kidney Dis 13:469, 1989. *This paper reviews 27 patients with dense deposit disease and documents the clinical features as well as the clinical and morphologic correlates of a poor prognosis.*
Cameron JS, Turner DR, Heaton J, et al.: Idiopathic mesangiocapillary glomerulonephritis. Comparison of types I and II in children and adults and long-term prognosis. Am J Med 74:175, 1983. *An excellent clinical review of 104 well-studied patients that discusses the clinical and laboratory findings in types I and II MPGN, the differences between children and adults, and the long-term prognosis and prognostic features.*

GLOMERULAR INVOLVEMENT IN SYSTEMIC DISEASES

The most common systemic diseases resulting in glomerular involvement are the various forms of vasculitis. With the group of diseases referred to as systemic necrotizing vasculitis, a distinction is made between necrotizing vasculitis involving medium-sized and larger vessels (the polyarteritis nodosa group, including classic PAN, allergic granulomatosis, and "overlap" syndromes), and necrotizing vasculitis involving small vessels and capillaries (hypersensitivity vasculitis or microscopic PAN plus several well-defined clinical syndromes, including SLE, HSP, and mixed essential cryoglobulinemia). The only other common vasculitic syndrome with significant renal involvement is Wegener's granulomatosis.

Polyarteritis Nodosa (PAN)

Classic PAN, a disease of older adults sometimes associated with drug abuse (particularly amphetamines) and hepatitis B antigenemia, is described in detail in Ch. 265. Renal involvement, which occurs in 90 per cent of cases, is usually manifest first as hematuria with an active urinary sediment and mild proteinuria. In 70 per cent of cases, the renal lesion is primarily an ischemic one caused by vasculitic involvement of arcuate and interlobular arteries. This involvement is best demonstrated by abdominal angiography and is generally not seen on renal biopsy. Aneurysmal dilatation is present in renal, hepatic, and mesenteric vessels. In 30 per cent of patients, a focal necrotizing GN with crescents may be seen. Both types of glomerular involvement may sometimes occur in the same patient. Immune deposits are generally not found in the glomerulus, and the pathogenesis of the renal disease is uncertain. Renal failure is a major cause of death and may either be a slowly progressive process or develop acutely in association with accelerated hypertension. In patients with PAN who develop hypertension and acute renal failure, renal cortical necrosis is common, and there is little reversibility. More often, the disease is a slowly progressive one in which vigorous control of hypertension, use of oral steroids, and addition of cytotoxic agents, such as cyclophosphamide, have achieved 5-year survival rates of more than 80 per cent of patients in uncontrolled studies.

Milder renal lesions may occur in the other two subgroups of this category. In allergic granulomatosis, allergic symptoms, asthma, pulmonary involvement, and eosinophilia are prominent features of the disease. In the overlap syndromes, both allergic manifestations and small vessel involvement may occur in the presence of the classic large vessel involvement seen in PAN.

Balow JE: Renal vasculitis. Kidney Int 27:954, 1985. *A comprehensive review of the classification, pathogenesis, and clinical features of the various forms of systemic necrotizing vasculitis involving the kidney. The utility of angiography in the diagnosis of PAN and the indications for cytotoxic drug therapy are stressed.*

Wegener's Granulomatosis

Wegener's granulomatosis is a granulomatous and necrotizing vasculitis but also involves large vessels, usually of the upper and lower respiratory tract and kidney (see Ch. 266). The disease presents most frequently in the fourth or fifth decade of life and affects more men than women. Presenting signs usually are respiratory and include purulent rhinorrhea, painful sinusitis, otitis, keratoconjunctivitis, oral ulcerations, and multiple bilateral nodular pulmonary infiltrates. Renal involvement eventually develops in more than 80 per cent of patients and, if left untreated, may result in the death of up to 30 per cent. Early renal involvement is manifest by hematuria, proteinuria, and mild renal impairment with a focal and necrotizing proliferative GN, usually without immune deposits. However, severe diffuse necrotizing and crescentic GN may develop rapidly. Necrotizing granulomatous vasculitis may be seen in biopsies of the respiratory tract but is often not evident in renal biopsies. The presence of granulomas may be the only pathologic finding that distinguishes Wegener's granulomatosis from PAN. Spontaneous improvements in renal disease have not been reported. Antineutrophil cytoplasmic antibody levels are usually elevated in Wegener's granulomatoses and may parallel disease activity. Although the diagnosis can usually be made on clinical grounds, a renal biopsy is generally performed early in the disease to identify potentially severe renal involvement that may be clinically silent and to distinguish Wegener's granulomatosis from other diseases with pulmonary and renal manifestations, such as Goodpasture's syndrome, which would be treated differently. Prognosis and therapy are discussed in Ch. 266.

Sack KE: Wegener's granulomatosis (medical staff conference). West J Med 150:329, 1989. *A current review of the clinical manifestations, diagnosis, approach to cytotoxic drug therapy, and complications of treatment of Wegener's granulomatosis.*

Hypersensitivity Vasculitis (Microscopic PAN, Allergic Vasculitis, Leukocytoclastic Angiitis)

Hypersensitivity vasculitis is a form of systemic necrotizing vasculitis of small vessels in which the clinical manifestations do not fall into a well-recognized syndrome, such as SLE, HSP, or essential mixed cryoglobulinemia (see Ch. 264). The disease is believed to be a manifestation of immune complex formation in small vessels and frequently follows exposure to some offending antigen, such as an infectious agent, drug, or foreign protein, by about a 7- to 10-day latent period. However, about half of patients will not have an identifiable antecedent event. The skin is most commonly involved, with palpable purpura. Other frequent manifestations include microangiopathic hemolytic anemia and pulmonary infiltrates with hemoptysis.

Clinical renal involvement is present in about 50 per cent of cases and is usually manifest initially as asymptomatic proteinuria associated with a segmental necrotizing GN on biopsy. Impairment in renal function is present in 20 to 40 per cent of cases, and up to 10 per cent may develop acute oliguric renal failure. Antineutrophil cytoplasmic antibodies are often positive in these patients. On biopsy, these patients generally have extensive necrotizing glomerular lesions with abundant crescent formation and negative immunofluorescence studies. Treatment considerations are similar to those outlined above for idiopathic RPGN, including high-dose steroid pulse therapy and possibly plasma exchange. There is good evidence to support the use of additional cytotoxic agents, such as cyclophosphamide, in the treatment of RPGN due to vasculitis.

Serra A, Cameron JS, Turner DR, et al.: Vasculitis affecting the kidney: Presentation, histopathology, and long-term outcome. Q J Med 210:181, 1984. *Fifty-three patients with vasculitis involving the kidney are reviewed. The finding of a segmental necrotizing glomerular lesion accompanied by systemic symptoms, such as fever, malaise, or weight loss, was considered diagnostic of a small vessel vasculitis. Clinical features in such patients were identical to those in patients who had histologic evidence outside the kidney. The paper is an excellent review of the wide spectrum of clinical manifestations of vasculitis and the frequency of crescentic glomerulonephritis in such patients as well as the relatively poor prognosis.*

Wilkowski MJ, Velosa JA, Holley KE, et al.: Risk factors in idiopathic renal vasculitis and glomerulonephritis. Kidney Int 36:1133, 1989. *This review from the Mayo Clinic of 170 patients with renal vasculitis and glomerulonephritis provides useful data on clinical manifestations and prognostic features in this disorder.*

Systemic Lupus Erythematosus (SLE)

The current diagnostic criteria and clinical manifestations of SLE are considered in more detail in Ch. 261. This section discusses only renal involvement. About 70 per cent of patients have clinical manifestations of renal disease, ranging from microscopic hematuria and proteinuria to an acute nephritic syndrome with acute renal failure and typical nephrotic syndrome. Renal biopsies reveal some abnormalities in most patients.

CLASSIFICATION. The most common classification system used for renal involvement in SLE is the World Health Organization (WHO) classification based on histopathologic criteria (Table 79–4).

Class I (Normal Kidneys). Only very rarely do patients with diagnostic criteria for SLE have entirely normal kidneys by light microscopy, immunofluorescence, and electron microscopy, and they do not have clinical manifestations of glomerular disease.

Class II (Minimal or Mesangial Lupus Nephritis). This is the earliest and mildest form of renal involvement in SLE and is characterized by mesangial deposits of immunoglobulin and C3 with (class IIB) or without (class IIA) focal proliferative changes seen on light microscopy. Clinical manifestations of proteinuria and hematuria are present in most patients, but the nephrotic syndrome and renal insufficiency are very uncommon and do not develop unless progression to a more severe lesion occurs, as happens in about 20 per cent of patients. Five-year survival is higher than 90 per cent, and no specific therapy is indicated for the renal lesion.

Class III (Focal Proliferative Lupus Nephritis). This is a stage in a continuum between mesangial lesions alone and diffuse proliferative lupus nephritis. Focal proliferative changes are present in fewer than 50 per cent of glomeruli, but all glomeruli contain immune deposits of IgG, IgA, C3, and usually IgM and fibrin-related antigens. Deposits are predominantly mesangial, but occasional subendothelial deposits may be seen. All patients have proteinuria, but the nephrotic syndrome and renal insufficiency occur in fewer than 20 per cent and may remit following steroid therapy. Serologic abnormalities, including hypocomplementemia, are more severe than in class II disease. Long-term prognosis with this lesion is also good (90 per cent 5-year survival). However, there is a relatively high incidence of transformation to class IV disease, resulting in a reduction in 5-year survival to about 70 per cent, with almost half of the deaths occurring from renal failure. The most reliable predictor of progression is probably the presence of subendothelial deposits on electron microscopy.

Class IV (Diffuse Proliferative Lupus Nephritis). This is the severest of the glomerular lesions in lupus, with proliferation seen in more than 50 per cent of glomeruli, frequently with crescent formation and necrosis. Extensive mesangial and subendothelial deposits contain all immunoglobulins, C3, and fibrin. Mesangial and subendothelial deposits are present on electron microscopy, often with subepithelial deposits as well. Proteinuria is seen in all patients, and nephrotic range proteinuria is present in 50 per cent at onset and 90 per cent some time during the course of the disease. Renal function is decreased in 75 per cent at the time of presentation, and serologic evidence of disease activity, including hypocomplementemia, elevated levels of anti-DNA antibody, and circulating immune complexes, is present in most patients. The long-term prognosis for this lesion has improved considerably over the years, with most centers now achieving survival rates of about 75 per cent at 5 years. The best prognosis is in those patients in whom a remission of the nephrotic syndrome and normalization of serologic parameters are achieved within 1 year of starting therapy.

Class V (Membranous Lupus Nephritis). About 15 per cent of patients with SLE develop a glomerular lesion that may be indistinguishable from idiopathic membranous nephropathy, with extensive subepithelial deposits of all immunoglobulins and C3. The nephrotic syndrome and a slowly progressive renal disease are common (see Table 79–3). Patients may have undetectable levels of antinuclear antibody at the time of presentation. The

TABLE 79–4. HISTOLOGIC CLASS, CLINICAL PRESENTATION, AND PROGNOSIS IN SLE NEPHRITIS

Histologic Type	WHO Class	Frequency (%)*	Proteinuria (%)	Nephrotic Syndrome† (%)	Azotemia‡ (%)	Death (%)	Uremic Death (%)
Normal	I	<5					
Mesangial	II	15	68	0	12	18	0
Focal proliferative	III	20	100	15	18	30	11
Diffuse proliferative	IV	50	100	87	75	58	36
Membranous	V	15	100	88	20	38	6

*Per cent of patients with SLE who show this lesion on biopsy.
†Proteinuria exceeding 3.0 grams per 24 hours.
‡Serum creatinine exceeding 1.2 mg per deciliter or BUN exceeding 25 mg per deciliter.

incidence of systemic manifestations of SLE and serologic abnormalities in general is also lower in patients with a membranous lesion. The long-term prognosis for patients with this lesion does not differ significantly from those with class II disease. As in idiopathic membranous nephropathy, there appears to be an increased incidence of renal vein thrombosis. Therapy as discussed under idiopathic membranous nephropathy is usually recommended.

TREATMENT OF LUPUS NEPHRITIS. In patients with active renal disease and a class III or IV lesion, steroids have a beneficial effect in lupus nephritis. High-dose steroid therapy is given for a period of 4 to 6 weeks and subsequently tapered and adjusted according to responses in renal function, serologic parameters, and extrarenal disease. In the presence of crescents and deteriorating renal function, steroid pulse therapy, as discussed above under idiopathic RPGN, may result in more rapid return to maximal renal function. The addition of a cytotoxic agent, such as cyclophosphamide, to oral steroid therapy may result in better preservation of renal function in a subset of patients with evidence of active class III or IV disease and mild chronic changes by biopsy. Thus a renal biopsy appears to be useful as a basis for selecting therapy in patients with active lupus nephritis. Administration of cyclophosphamide as a monthly intravenous pulse provides a therapeutic effect equivalent to a daily oral dose, with fewer side effects.

With development of renal failure, disease activity in SLE usually subsides. Renal transplantation has been carried out in a large number of patients without significant problems.

Balow JE: Lupus as a renal disease. Hosp Pract 23:129, 1988. *An excellent overview of the immune basis for lupus nephritis, the clinical and pathologic features, the classification and approach to therapy, which emphasizes the extensive National Institutes of Health (NIH) experience, and results with steroids and pulse cyclophosphamide.*

Balow JE, moderator: Lupus nephritis. Ann Intern Med 106:79, 1987. *This review from a group with extensive experience in the classification and treatment of lupus nephritis summarizes current understanding of the pathogenesis and treatment of renal disease in SLE.*

Henoch-Schönlein Purpura (HSP)

Henoch-Schönlein syndrome, or anaphylactoid purpura, is another systemic necrotizing vasculitis of small vessels in which systemic manifestations include palpable purpura (100 per cent) on the lower extremities and buttocks due to a leukocytoclastic vasculitis of dermal vessels; arthralgias of large joints, usually the knees and ankles (70 per cent); gastrointestinal involvement with colic and bleeding (25 per cent); and renal involvement, usually with a focal necrotizing GN (see Ch. 154). About 30 per cent of patients have clinical evidence of renal disease in the form of hematuria or acute nephritic syndrome. Except for the systemic manifestations, the disease is very similar in its morphologic and clinical characteristics to IgA nephropathy but is of somewhat greater severity. Typically, the disease presents with an acute nephritic syndrome, usually without edema or hypertension, developing within 3 months of the onset of other systemic manifestations of HSP. Many patients have an infectious episode prior to the onset of renal disease. Up to 25 per cent of adults may develop a severe crescentic lesion with RPGN. The nephrotic syndrome has been reported to develop in over 50 per cent, and progressive renal failure occurs in at least 25 per cent of patients. The renal involvement is much less severe in children. Predictors of progressive disease include presentation with an acute nephritic syndrome, nephrotic syndrome, crescents, and subepithelial deposits or subendothelial "lead-shot" lesions by EM. Most patients have self-limited episodes of renal involvement, usually lasting 1 week or less. However, recurrences are common.

The pathogenesis of HSP is unknown but is presumed to be immunologic and similar to that of IgA nephropathy. Similar immunogenetic associations in the two diseases, as well as the clinical, histologic, and immunopathologic similarities, strongly suggest that a common underlying disease mechanism is involved.

No treatment has been shown to be of benefit in the nephritis of HSP. Short courses of steroids may be useful in controlling systemic manifestations but do not appear to benefit the renal lesion. Patients who develop crescents and a clinical picture of RPGN should be considered for treatment as outlined above under idiopathic RPGN.

Fogazzi GB, Pasquali S, Moriggi M, et al.: Long-term outcome of Schönlein-Henoch nephritis in the adult. Clin Nephrol 31:60, 1989. *This paper describes 16 adult patients with HSP and reviews the literature. The clinical manifestations are well reviewed and the poor prognosis in adults emphasized.*

Meadow AR, Glasgow EF, White RHR, et al.: Schönlein-Henoch nephritis. Q J Med 41:241, 1972. *This older article provides an excellent review of the clinical features in a large series of adult patients with HSP.*

Essential Mixed Cryoglobulinemia (EMC)

Low concentrations of mixed cryoglobulins, usually type III with polyclonal IgG and IgM with rheumatoid factor activity, are seen in a variety of immune glomerular disorders, autoimmune diseases, vasculitides, and neoplastic syndromes, in which they rarely produce symptoms (Ch. 264). Type II mixed cryoglobulins, composed of monoclonal IgM rheumatoid factor and polyclonal IgG, are characteristic of a disorder called essential mixed cryoglobulinemia (EMC), in which dependent vascular purpura, Raynaud's phenomenon, arthralgias, weakness, and GN are the principal clinical manifestations. Cryoprecipitates from these patients often contain hepatitis B antigen. The disease is one of middle age and affects women somewhat more often than men.

Renal involvement is present in about 40 per cent of cases and is usually preceded by purpura and arthralgias. The severity of renal disease ranges from microscopic hematuria and proteinuria to an acute nephritic syndrome with acute renal failure. In contrast to most of the other vasculitic syndromes, the nephrotic syndrome is a rather frequent occurrence, and severe hypertension is common. Laboratory abnormalities include a markedly elevated sedimentation rate, cryoglobulins, rheumatoid factor activity, and sometimes an artifactual decrease in levels of early complement components, with C3 and later components often normal. The glomerular lesion is a diffuse proliferative and exudative GN, sometimes accompanied by vasculitis, with large PAS-positive proteinaceous deposits present in many capillaries. The subendothelial capillary deposits are composed predominantly of IgG and IgM, with lesser amounts of C3 and fibrin. In patients with acute nephritic syndrome and renal failure, the prognosis is poor. However, in all patients with renal disease more than 50 per cent may recover with or without therapy, and the survival rate at 10 years is about 75 per cent. Although steroids and cytotoxic agents alone have not been shown to be of consistent benefit in the renal lesion, plasma exchange therapy may improve the prognosis in patients with severe renal disease.

D'Amico G, Colasanti G, Ferrario F, et al.: Renal involvement in essential mixed cryoglobulinemia: A peculiar type of immune-mediated renal disease. Adv Nephrol 17:219, 1988. *This is an excellent and detailed analysis of the renal disease in essential mixed cryoglobulinemia, with a description of clinical features, pathology, natural history, and response to therapy, including over 50 references.*

Thrombotic Microangiopathy (Hemolytic Uremic Syndrome and Thrombotic Thrombocytopenic Purpura)

Hemolytic uremic syndrome (HUS) and thrombotic thrombocytopenic purpura (TTP) are referred to collectively by some authors as thrombotic microangiopathy. The two disorders can be clinically indistinguishable, may have a common, although poorly understood, pathogenesis, and respond to similar therapy.

HEMOLYTIC UREMIC SYNDROME (HUS). HUS is a syndrome of microangiopathic hemolytic anemia, thrombocytopenia, and renal impairment, which usually occurs abruptly in children about 3 to 10 days following episodes of gastroenteritis or viral upper respiratory tract infection. Gastroenteritis is often associated with verotoxin producing *Escherichia coli* infections. A similar syndrome occurs less commonly in adults, often associated with complications of pregnancy or during the postpartum period (postpartum acute renal failure) or associated with the use of oral contraceptives. HUS also occurs in adults following treatment with a variety of antineoplastic agents. Acute renal failure develops in up to 60 per cent of children but usually resolves spontaneously within about 2 weeks with only supportive therapy. Chronic renal failure occurs in only 10 per cent of patients, usually those who suffer loss of renal function in a gradual, progressive manner, who have oliguria lasting longer than 2 weeks, or who have total anuria. Laboratory features of the disease include microangiopathic hemolytic anemia, thrombocytopenia, increased numbers of reticulocytes, elevated bilirubin levels, reduced haptoglobin levels, and elevated levels of fibrin split products, usually with only minimal laboratory evidence of disseminated intravascular coagulation. In TTP (see below) levels of fibrin split products are less commonly elevated. The glomerular lesion is one of intimal hyperplasia of arterioles and intracapillary fibrin thrombi, sometimes with areas of focal necrosis. The anemia and thrombocytopenia are presumably due to trapping of platelets and destruction of red cells in the areas of capillary thrombosis. The pathogenesis of the syndrome is unknown but probably involves glomerular endothelial cell injury by some as yet unidentified circulating factor, with subsequent fibrin deposition and thrombosis.

In typical HUS in children, only supportive therapy, including early dialysis, is required, since the rate of spontaneous recovery is very high. In adults, the prognosis is considerably worse because renal involvement is more severe and development of bilateral cortical necrosis more common. This is particularly true in cases associated with pregnancy and oral contraceptives. No form of therapy has been determined to be effective in HUS, although aspirin, antiplatelet agents, heparin, fresh frozen plasma infusions, and plasma exchange have all been advocated by some authors. In adults with severe disease, treatment with plasma exchange as described below for TTP, in addition to steroids, antiplatelet agents, and aspirin, is probably indicated.

THROMBOTIC THROMBOCYTOPENIC PURPURA (TTP). TTP is clinically and pathologically very similar to HUS (see Ch. 154). The differences that distinguish this end of the spectrum of thrombotic microangiopathy are (1) a more common occurrence in young adults, (2) fever as a frequent manifestation of the disease, (3) neurologic abnormalities that tend to predominate and cause death, and (4) a lesser degree of renal involvement, with acute renal failure in only about 10 per cent of cases. Hematuria is the most common manifestation of renal disease. Proteinuria, generally less than 5 grams per day, and a serum creatinine level in excess of 2 mg per deciliter occur in about 50 per cent of cases. Histologically, the renal lesion is the same as that in HUS. TTP has a considerably worse prognosis than HUS, with about a 75 per cent mortality within 3 months, and spontaneous recovery is rare.

A wide variety of therapeutic regimens have been employed in TTP. The most promising results have been obtained with plasma exchange, often in combination with fresh plasma, antiplatelet agents, and steroids, a regimen that has produced rather dramatic clinical remissions in several patients with apparently severe and advanced disease. In refractory cases, splenectomy may confer an additional benefit.

Kaplan BS, Proesmans W: The hemolytic uremic syndrome of childhood and its variants. Semin Hematol 24:148, 1987. *This scholarly review by pediatric nephrologists emphasizes the multiple etiologies of HUS and provides an excellent overview of management.*

Remuzzi G: HUS and TTP: Variable expression of a single entity (nephrology forum). Kidney Int 32:292, 1987. *This nephrology forum by an experienced clinical investigator is a lucid review of the classification, clinical features, pathology, pathogenesis, and treatment of HUS/TTP. The review emphasizes the similar features of these two overlapping syndromes, with 191 references.*

80 Tubulointerstitial Diseases and Toxic Nephropathies

T. Dwight McKinney

COMMON FEATURES OF TUBULOINTERSTITIAL DISEASES

Tubulointerstitial disease (tubulointerstitial nephritis or nephropathy, interstitial nephritis) refers to a diverse group of acute and chronic disorders that primarily affect the renal tubules and interstitium. In contrast, in other primary renal diseases, most notably glomerulonephritis, the tubules and interstitium are only secondarily involved. Approximately 30 per cent of all cases of chronic renal insufficiency in the United States result from tubulointerstitial diseases. Usually the cause of tubulointerstitial disease can be identified. Renal function may improve or stabilize with appropriate therapy.

CLINICAL MANIFESTATIONS

In tubulointerstitial diseases, functional renal tubular defects, which are present to some degree in advanced renal insufficiency of any cause, are frequently out of proportion to the degree of renal insufficiency as measured by reduction in glomerular filtration rate (GFR). In fact, the finding of such a disproportional loss of tubular compared with glomerular function should lead one to suspect the diagnosis of tubulointerstitial disease (Table 80–1). Urinary concentration in response to water deprivation or exogenous antidiuretic hormone may be reduced, particularly in chronic interstitial nephritis. This may result in decreased maximal urinary osmolarity, polyuria (generally <3 liters per day), and nocturia. Concentration defect, an acquired form of nephrogenic diabetes insipidus, may result from interference with the action of antidiuretic hormone on the collecting ducts or anatomic damage or disruption of the medullary structures involved in the urinary concentrating mechanism (Ch. 214). Damage to the proximal tubules may result in excessive urinary excretion of substances normally reabsorbed in this location. Bicarbonaturia (proximal renal tubular acidosis), phosphaturia, aminoaciduria, uricosuria, glycosuria, kaliuresis, and low molecular weight proteinuria may occur. These losses may cause low plasma levels of some of these substances, particularly phosphate, bicarbonate, and urate. The presence of multiple proximal tubular defects is referred to as Fanconi's syndrome (Ch. 82). In addition to proximal renal tubular acidosis, failure of the distal nephron to acidify the tubular fluid maximally results in classic distal renal tubular acidosis. Hyperkalemic (type 4) distal renal tubular acidosis may also occur. All of these cause a hyperchloremic (normal anion gap) metabolic acidosis (Ch. 75). Hyperkalemia may result from a primary failure of potassium secretion by the distal nephron but more commonly results from decreased renal production of renin and subsequent secondary hypoaldosteronism. Patients with tubulointerstitial disease may also fail to conserve sodium normally. In some, this is due to the hyporeninemic hypoaldosteronism noted above. Renal sodium wasting may result in signs of extracellular fluid volume depletion when sodium intake is restricted and may cause worsening of renal function. With acute and, to a lesser extent, chronic interstitial nephritis, these tubular defects may be accompanied or, indeed, overshadowed by other signs, symptoms, and laboratory abnormalities of renal failure (Ch. 76 and 77).

DIAGNOSIS

A specific diagnosis of tubulointerstitial renal disease can often be made or inferred from historical information, physical examination, or laboratory tests. Renal biopsy is the most definitive

TABLE 80–1. MANIFESTATIONS OF RENAL TUBULOINTERSTITIAL DISEASES

1. Tubular dysfunction disproportionate to reduction in GFR
2. Tubular abnormalities
   a. Reduced maximal urinary concentrating ability (polyuria, nocturia)
   b. Renal tubular acidosis (hyperchloremic metabolic acidosis)
   c. Partial or complete Fanconi's syndrome

Phosphaturia	Uricosuria
Bicarbonaturia	Glycosuria
Aminoaciduria	

   d. Sodium wasting
   e. Hyperkalemia
3. Renal endocrine deficiencies
   a. Hyporeninemic hypoaldosteronism (hyperkalemia, metabolic acidosis)
   b. Calcitriol deficiency (renal osteodystrophy)
   c. Erythropoietin deficiency (anemia)
4. Urinalysis
   a. May be normal but usually contains cellular elements
   b. Proteinuria is usually modest (<3.5 grams per day) and consists largely of low molecular weight "tubular" proteins, such as lysozyme and beta$_2$-microglobulin

method of diagnosis, but this is not always necessary. Pathologic features are discussed below. Radiographic, ultrasonographic, and radionuclide examinations generally show only evidence of acute or chronic renal insufficiency but may provide a specific diagnosis, such as urinary tract obstruction or polycystic kidney disease.

PROGNOSIS AND TREATMENT

The prognosis usually depends on the specific cause of tubulointerstitial renal disease, as discussed below. General supportive therapy, such as treatment of electrolyte disorders, and management of acute and chronic renal failure are discussed in Ch. 76 and 77.

COMMON FEATURES OF TOXIC NEPHROPATHIES

The term toxic nephropathy refers to those renal disorders resulting directly or indirectly from exposure of the kidneys to exogenous chemicals and physical factors, including both drugs and environmental agents, and abnormal concentrations of substances normally present in the body fluids, such as calcium and uric acid. Drug-related renal disease is the most important cause of toxic nephropathy. Toxic nephropathy often results in tubulointerstitial disease, but it is not synonymous with it.

Several factors predispose the kidneys to toxic injury: (1) The kidneys receive approximately 20 per cent of the resting cardiac output and, therefore, are exposed to more blood-borne materials than any other organ except the lungs. (2) The high metabolic rate of the renal tubules required for active transport processes makes them particularly vulnerable to toxic insults. (3) The large glomerular capillary surface area is a major site for trapping immune complexes or for antigen-antibody reactions in situ. (4) Some substances (e.g., aminoglycosides) are selectively concentrated in the renal cortex because of specific transport processes located in the proximal tubules, whereas others (e.g., phenacetin) are concentrated in the medulla owing to the renal countercurrent system. This selective concentration accounts, in part, for the anatomic distribution of damage by some nephrotoxins. (5) Certain substances are converted to less soluble forms with resultant precipitation (e.g., urate to uric acid) consequent to acidification of tubular fluid in the distal nephron. This may lead to tubular obstruction.

Nephrotoxins injure the kidneys in a variety of ways, both direct and indirect (Fig. 80–1). Indirect injury, for example, may result from immunologic reactions or from secondary effects, such as drug-induced hypotension or hemolysis. These mechanisms, alone or in concert, may cause an array of renal disorders, ranging from isolated functional tubular defects to reversible acute renal failure to progressive end-stage renal disease.

ACUTE INTERSTITIAL NEPHRITIS

PATHOLOGY AND PATHOGENESIS

Characteristically, in acute interstitial nephritis (AISN) mononuclear cells infiltrate the interstitium, particularly in the cortex. Eosinophils, especially in cases of drug-related AISN, and occasionally small numbers of polymorphonuclear leukocytes may also be present. Inflammatory cells may invade the tubule walls and, in severe cases, may be associated with areas of tubular necrosis. The infiltrate may be diffuse or patchy; the extent of the infiltrate corresponds in general to the degree of renal functional impairment. In addition to the cellular infiltrate, the renal tubules are separated by interstitial edema, but no fibrosis is present. With prolonged AISN, interstitial fibrosis may develop, and the pathologic picture may merge into that of chronic interstitial nephritis. In primary AISN the glomeruli are generally normal, although there may be some mesangial prominence. The predominant mononuclear inflammatory cells in infiltrates are T cells. Both helper/inducer and suppressor/cytotoxic T cells are present. These observations suggest that both T cell–mediated delayed hypersensitivity reactions and cytotoxic T cell injury may be involved in AISN. In some cases immunoglobulins and complement components are demonstrable in the interstitium and/or tubular basement membrane by immunofluorescence. Rarely, electron microscopy may reveal electron-dense deposits in these areas, suggestive of immune complexes. Finally, in occasional cases there may be linear deposition of immunoglobulins and complement in the tubular basement membrane, indicative of anti–tubular basement membrane antibodies. There is, therefore, considerable evidence for immune injury mediated by cellular and humoral mechanisms as the cause of AISN. Usually, however,

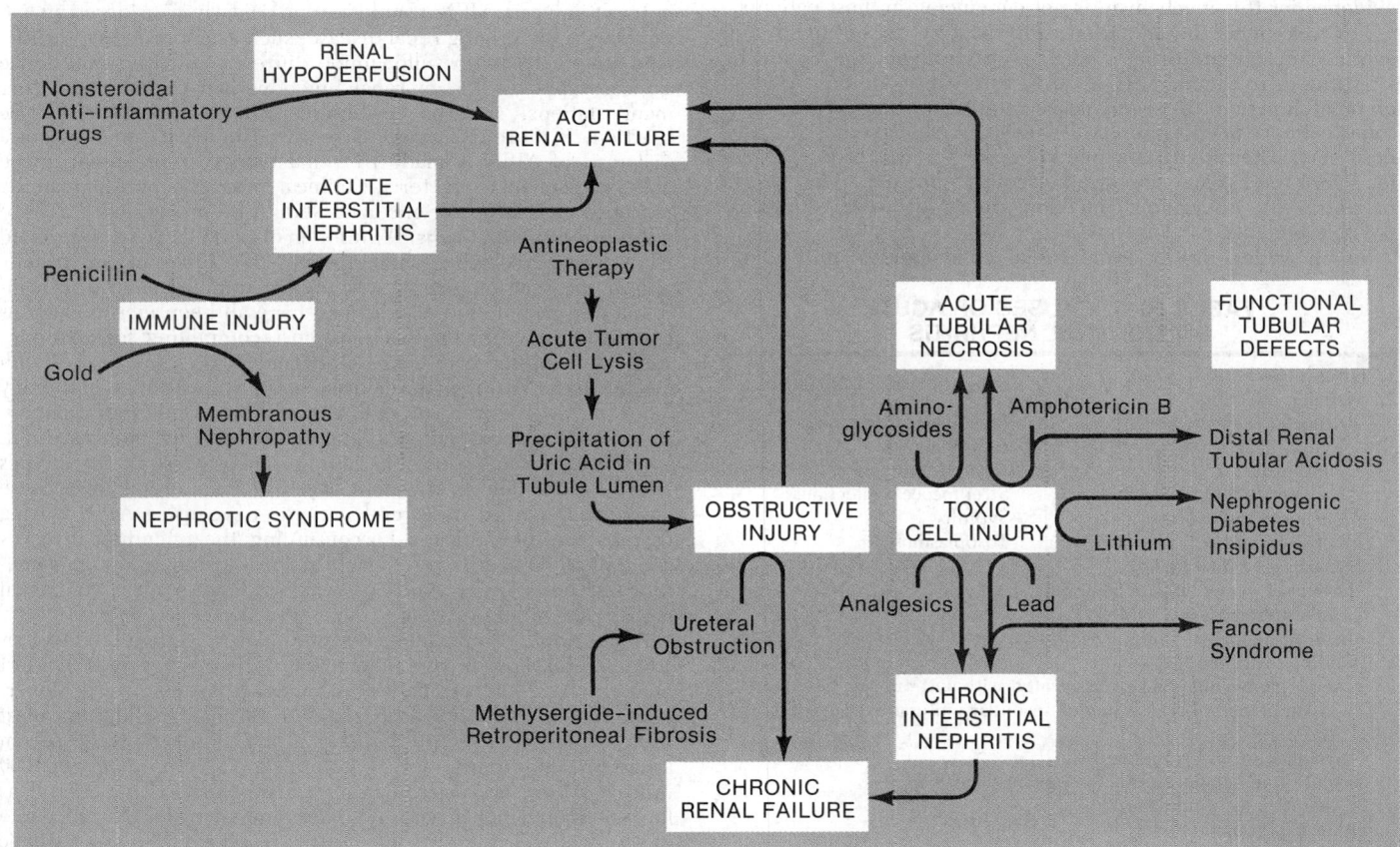

FIGURE 80–1. Types of toxin-induced renal disease.

the immunopathogenetic mechanisms involved in a given case of AISN remain unknown.

ETIOLOGY

Acute interstitial nephritis may result from a variety of causes (Table 80–2). Drug-related AISN is becoming more frequently recognized as an important cause of acute renal insufficiency, probably because of (1) the more widespread use of renal biopsy, (2) the increasing number of drugs being used, and (3) the characteristic clinical presentation.

DRUG-INDUCED ACUTE INTERSTITIAL NEPHRITIS. The list of drugs that have been implicated as etiologic in AISN continues to expand (Table 80–3). AISN is a rare complication of drug therapy, but because of the frequency with which these agents are used, drugs account for a substantial portion of all cases of acute renal failure.

Penicillins. Several penicillin congeners may cause AISN, including amoxicillin, ampicillin, carbenicillin, methicillin, mezlocillin, nafcillin, oxacillin, and penicillin G. Methicillin has been responsible for most reported cases, but the clinical syndrome is similar for the other penicillins. It is reasonable to presume that AISN may occur with any penicillin. Typically, penicillins have been taken for about 2 weeks prior to the onset of signs and symptoms of AISN, but this time interval has varied from 2 days to several weeks. The disorder appears to be more frequent in men and children. There is no correlation between the dosage of the drug administered and subsequent development of AISN. The most frequent manifestations are hematuria (which may be gross and associated rarely with red cell casts in the urinary sediment), proteinuria (usually less than nephrotic range), pyuria (eosinophiluria is frequently present and strongly suggests the diagnosis of AISN), fever eosinophilia (this may be evanescent), azotemia (often associated with oliguria), and skin rash. Serum immunoglobulin E (IgE) levels may be elevated. Renal sodium wasting and hyperchloremic metabolic acidosis with hyperkalemia (hyperkalemic distal renal tubular acidosis) may also occur. The pathogenesis of the disorder is uncertain. Binding of penicillin haptens to renal tubule basement membranes may result in formation of anti–tubular basement membrane antibodies, but evidence for this mechanism is not convincing in most patients.

For treatment, the offending drug must be discontinued, and another appropriate drug for the underlying infection should be substituted. In the majority of cases, this will result in restoration of renal function. Recovery may require several weeks, with some patients needing interval dialysis. A short course of high-dose corticosteroids (1 mg per kilogram per day of prednisone for 1 to 2 weeks) may accelerate recovery, but the added risk in patients with underlying infections must be weighed against possible benefits.

Sulfonamides. Both antimicrobial sulfonamides and sulfon-

TABLE 80–2. CAUSES OF ACUTE INTERSTITIAL NEPHRITIS

1. Drug-related (Table 80–3)
2. Systemic infections

Brucellosis	Mycoplasmal pneumonia
Cytomegalovirus	Polyomavirus
Diphtheria	Rocky Mountain spotted fever
Infectious mononucleosis	Streptococcal infections
Legionnaires' disease	Syphilis
Leptospirosis	Toxoplasmosis

3. Primary renal infections
   Bacterial pyelonephritis (Ch. 84)
   Renal tuberculosis
   Fungal nephritis
4. Immune disorders
   Acute glomerulonephritis associated with anti–tubular basement membrane antibodies and/or secondary interstitial nephritis (Ch. 79)
   Systemic lupus erythematosus
   Acute rejection of a renal transplant (Ch. 78.2)
   Necrotizing vasculitis
5. Other conditions
6. Idiopathic

TABLE 80–3. DRUGS ASSOCIATED WITH ACUTE INTERSTITIAL NEPHRITIS

Antimicrobial Drugs

Cephalosporins	Para-aminosalicylic acid
Chloramphenicol	Penicillins*
Ciprofloxacin	Polymyxin B
Erythromycin	Rifampin*
Ethambutol	Sulfonamides*
Isoniazid	Tetracyclines
	Vancomycin

Nonsteroidal Anti-inflammatory Drugs*

Miscellaneous

Allopurinol*	Methyldopa
Antipyrene	Phenindione
Azathioprine	Phenylpropanolamine
Bismuth	Phenytoin
Captopril	Probenecid
Carbamazepine	Sulfinpyrazone
Cimetidine	Sulfonamide diuretics*
Clofibrate	Triamterene
Gold	

*Most frequent or clinically important.

amide diuretics (thiazides, furosemide, chlorthalidone, acetazolamide) have been implicated in AISN. Although frequently these are prescribed in combination with other drugs (e.g., sulfamethoxazole plus trimethoprim as antimicrobials and hydrochlorothiazide plus triamterene as diuretics), it is most likely that the sulfonamide moiety of these combinations is responsible for AISN. Typically, evidence for AISN develops several days after therapy is begun, but rechallenge of a patient with a past history of sulfonamide-induced AISN may result in signs and symptoms within hours of exposure. The clinical presentation is in many ways similar to that described for the penicillins. Pyuria, hematuria, eosinophilia, and azotemia are frequent. A skin rash is present in a minority of patients. Renal failure may be severe and may require temporary dialysis, but recovery is the rule when the offending drug is discontinued. A brief course of corticosteroids may hasten recovery if no contraindication to their use is present.

Drug-induced AISN should be particularly considered in patients with underlying renal disease, such as nephrotic syndrome, who are treated with sulfonamide diuretics and who experience a more rapid decline in renal function than expected or other manifestations, such as eosinophilia, that suggest an allergic reaction. If diuretic therapy is required in a patient in whom a diagnosis of AISN is made by renal biopsy or presumed to be present based on characteristic clinical findings, a nonsulfonamide diuretic, such as ethacrynic acid, should be prescribed.

Antituberculous Drugs. A number of patients have developed AISN while receiving chemotherapy for tuberculosis, usually with more than one agent. Although rifampin, isoniazid, ethambutol, and para-aminosalicylic acid have all been incriminated as causing AISN, the evidence is most compelling for rifampin. AISN appears to occur more often and to be more severe with intermittent therapy with rifampin or after reinstitution of therapy following a drug-free interval than during continuous therapy. Fever, chills, flank pain, and anuria may develop after readministration of a single dose of rifampin. In contrast to other types of acute renal failure, transient hypercalcemia of unknown cause has been reported in several patients developing AISN during therapy for tuberculosis. Discontinuing the offending drugs is generally followed by recovery of renal function, although sometimes rather slowly. Corticosteroids do not appear to hasten recovery of renal function.

Allopurinol. Allopurinol-associated AISN generally develops after several days of treatment (mean interval of 3 weeks). Most patients have an exfoliative maculopapular skin rash, fever, eosinophilia, and decreased renal function. In addition, most have evidence of acute hepatic injury. Elevations of serum aspartate aminotransferase, sometimes to values in excess of 1000 units per liter, are present in about two thirds of patients. This form of allopurinol toxicity is severe and carries a mortality rate of approximately 20 per cent. Deaths result from severe systemic reactions, sepsis, gastrointestinal bleeding, or acute hepatic or renal failure. The cause of allopurinol toxicity is uncertain. Clinical and laboratory manifestations suggest a severe systemic hypersensitivity reaction. Most reported patients have been treated with conventional doses of the drug (200 to 400 mg per day), but most have had underlying renal insufficiency prior to development of allopurinol toxicity. Serum concentrations of the major metabolite of allopurinol, oxipurinol, are elevated in renal insufficiency. Hypersensitivity to this or another metabolite may be responsible for the syndrome. In addition, about one half of the reported patients were receiving concomitant diuretic therapy. Whether this represents a causal relationship or merely coincidence is uncertain, as allopurinol is commonly prescribed to treat hyperuricemia that develops with diuretic therapy. Treatment of allopurinol toxicity consists of discontinuing the drug and instituting supportive measures, including dialysis, when indicated. Although corticosteroids have been given to many patients, their efficacy is unproved. The incidence of allopurinol toxicity can be reduced by prescribing the drug only for clearly documented indications, such as recurrent gouty arthritis or uric acid nephrolithiasis, and not for asymptomatic hyperuricemia per se (including diuretic-induced hyperuricemia). The dose should be reduced in patients with underlying renal insufficiency.

Other Drugs Associated with AISN. Of the numerous other drugs reported to cause AISN, perhaps the most important are the nonsteroidal anti-inflammatory drugs (see Ch. 29). For the remainder of the agents listed in Table 80–3, AISN appears to be a very rare complication. Nevertheless, when manifestations characteristic of AISN occur in patients receiving these drugs (or other drugs not listed), the diagnosis of AISN should be entertained. In this setting it may be simplest to discontinue the suspected drug and replace it with an alternative agent. On the other hand, in patients for whom no suitable alternative exists, it may be necessary to confirm or exclude the diagnosis of AISN by renal biopsy.

AISN ASSOCIATED WITH INFECTION. Systemic bacterial, viral, rickettsial, mycoplasmal, and parasitic infections have been associated with AISN. Infections with group A beta-hemolytic streptococci are, perhaps, the most frequent, especially in children. The pathogenesis of AISN related to systemic infection is uncertain. Possibly, renal deposition of antigens related to the infectious agent elicits humoral and cell-mediated immune reactions that result in renal injury, as discussed earlier. Many patients with AISN associated with systemic infections have received antibiotic therapy and may have drug-induced AISN (see above). Therapy consists of treatment of the underlying infection and supportive measures. The prognosis for recovery of renal function is usually quite favorable.

Acute bacterial pyelonephritis is a common cause of AISN. The clinical presentation with fever, chills, flank pain, and bacteriuria is characteristic (Ch. 84). Similarly, renal parenchymal fungal and mycobacterial infections may cause acute renal interstitial inflammation. All of these can result in renal scarring but only rarely cause acute renal failure.

AISN ASSOCIATED WITH IMMUNE DISORDERS. Varying degrees of acute and chronic interstitial nephritis may accompany numerous renal or systemic diseases of presumed immune origin. Several types of glomerulonephritis are associated with interstitial inflammation that may be out of proportion to the degree of glomerular injury (Ch. 79). In some, there may be antibodies to the tubular basement membranes. Although glomerulonephritis is generally the primary renal lesion in systemic lupus erythematosus, interstitial nephritis is the predominant finding in some patients (Ch. 79 and 261). Acute and chronic interstitial inflammation is the hallmark of renal transplant rejection (Ch. 78.2). Renal involvement with necrotizing vasculitis is generally manifest as a focal segmental glomerulonephritis, but in some patients, particularly those with Wegener's granulomatosis, there may be prominent interstitial involvement.

OTHER CONDITIONS ASSOCIATED WITH AISN. Sarcoidosis (Ch. 67), may involve the kidneys in a number of ways, including acute (granulomatous) interstitial nephritis, chronic interstitial nephritis (often associated with hypercalcemia and hypercalciuria), and primary glomerulonephritis. Rarely, AISN may cause acute renal failure in sarcoidosis. There have been isolated case reports of AISN following therapy with recombinant leukocyte interferon.

IDIOPATHIC AISN. In occasional patients with AISN, a specific cause cannot be identified. Some of these have evidence, such as eosinophilia, suggesting a hypersensitivity reaction to an unknown antigen. In addition to acute interstitial inflammation, renal biopsies sometimes demonstrate evidence for anti–tubular basement membrane antibodies. Others have granulomatous interstitial nephritis in the absence of an obvious etiology. The course of idiopathic AISN is variable, with some patients recovering spontaneously or in response to corticosteroid therapy and others progressing to renal insufficiency.

CLINICAL MANIFESTATIONS

In AISN the GFR may decline abruptly, often with oliguria. The urinary sediment typically contains numerous leukocytes. In cases of drug-induced AISN, eosinophils are frequently present as well. Hematuria is ordinarily present, and red blood cell casts, although rare, may be observed. Proteinuria is usually present but modest (<3.5 grams per day), except in AISN due to nonsteroidal anti-inflammatory drugs (see below). The fractional excretion of sodium tends to be high, as it is in most cases of acute tubular necrosis (see Ch. 76). A spectrum of renal tubular defects may be present (Table 80–1). In cases of drug-induced AISN (see above), other manifestations of drug allergy, such as fever, skin rash, and eosinophilia, are frequent. In AISN occurring as part of a systemic process, such as systemic lupus erythematosus, clinical and laboratory manifestations of the primary disease may dominate the clinical presentation. The diagnosis of AISN is established by examination of renal tissue obtained by biopsy (or autopsy). In drug-induced AISN, the diagnosis is often inferred from characteristic clinical and laboratory findings. The outcome of AISN depends on the underlying disease process. In drug-induced disease, renal function generally improves once the offending drug is stopped. Corticosteroid therapy may be beneficial, as discussed above. With prolonged and severe AISN, variable degrees of chronic renal insufficiency may result.

CHRONIC INTERSTITIAL NEPHRITIS

PATHOLOGY

Chronic interstitial nephritis (CISN) is characterized pathologically by interstitial fibrosis with atrophy and loss of renal tubules. The glomeruli may be normal but frequently are contracted. There is generally a patchy interstitial infiltrate of chronic inflammatory cells. The renal vasculature may show evidence of associated hypertension. In addition to these general findings, there may be others that suggest a specific disease, such as casts typical of multiple myeloma.

ETIOLOGY (Table 80–4)

CISN may result from persistence or progression of many of the acute forms of interstitial nephritis (Table 80–2) or may evolve without an obvious preceding phase of acute injury. Many of the specific causes of CISN are discussed subsequently; some of the remainder are commented on briefly below.

Urinary tract obstruction (including vesicoureteral reflux), the single most important cause of CISN, is discussed in Ch. 81. Perhaps the second most important group of disorders comprises those caused by nephrotoxins, most of which are discussed later as toxic nephropathies. In addition to exogenous toxins, certain endogenous chemical abnormalities may result in CISN. The major renal complication of *chronic hypokalemia* is nephrogenic (vasopressin-resistant) diabetes insipidus, which results in mild polyuria, but chronic interstitial nephritis with modest renal insufficiency may rarely occur as well. *Hypercalcemia* also produces mild polyuria due to nephrogenic diabetes insipidus. Acute hypercalcemia also acts on the glomeruli and renal vasculature to reduce GFR in a manner largely reversible with correction of hypercalcemia. Chronic hypercalcemia results in nephrocalcinosis and chronic interstitial nephritis with reduced GFR that may be only slowly and incompletely reversible. In addition, nephrocalcinosis may cause distal renal tubular acidosis (Ch. 82). In the absence of urinary tract obstruction, *chronic bacterial pyelonephritis* rarely causes severe renal failure. Renal *tuberculosis* can

TABLE 80–4. CAUSES OF CHRONIC INTERSTITIAL NEPHRITIS

1. Persistence or progression of acute interstitial nephritis (Table 80–2)
2. Chronic urinary tract obstruction (Ch. 81)
3. Nephrotoxins
   Drugs: analgesics, nitrosoureas
   Endogenous substances: hypercalcemia, hypokalemia, oxalate, uric acid
   Metals: cisplatin, copper, lead, lithium, mercury
   Radiation
4. Chronic bacterial pyelonephritis (Ch. 84) or renal tuberculosis (Ch. 332)
5. Immune disorders
   Chronic glomerulonephritis with interstitial nephritis (Ch. 79)
   Chronic rejection of a renal transplant (Ch. 78.2)
   Systemic lupus erythematosus (Ch. 261)
   Sjögren's syndrome (Ch. 263)
6. Associated with neoplasia or paraproteinemias
   Leukemia   Waldenström's macroglobulinemia
   Lymphoma   (Ch. 151)
   Amyloidosis (Ch. 197) Cryoglobulinemia (Ch. 79)
          Multiple myeloma (Ch. 151)
7. Cystic diseases
   Medullary cystic disease
   Polycystic kidney disease (Ch. 89)
8. Miscellaneous
   Diabetes mellitus Advanced renal failure
   Sickle cell   Idiopathic
    hemoglobinopathies
   Vascular diseases

result in acute and chronic tubulointerstitial disease. Tuberculous ureteral strictures may cause hydronephrosis.

A variety of *immune disorders* may be associated with both acute and chronic interstitial nephritis, including several types of glomerulonephritis (Ch. 79), chronic renal transplant rejection (Ch. 78.2), and systemic lupus erythematosus (Ch. 261). Renal involvement in *Sjögren's syndrome* is usually in the form of CISN. The most common functional abnormalities are distal renal tubular acidosis and urinary concentrating defects (Ch. 263).

Neoplastic and *paraproteinemic* disorders may be associated with CISN. In patients with lymphomas and leukemias, particularly acute lymphoblastic leukemia, neoplastic cells may infiltrate the renal interstitium and cause renal enlargement. Adjacent renal tubules may be compressed and destroyed, but renal function is rarely compromised. Renal disease in patients with *amyloidosis* (Ch. 197), *Waldenström's macroglobulinemia* (Ch. 151), and *mixed cryoglobulinemia* (Ch. 79) usually involves the glomeruli, but, rarely, there may be prominent tubulointerstitial involvement. Renal failure is a common cause of death in patients with *multiple myeloma,* especially in those with Bence Jones proteinuria (monoclonal immunoglobulin light chain paraproteins). CISN, often associated with cast nephropathy, is the most important cause of renal failure in multiple myeloma. Large, dense eosinophilic casts occur within the tubule lumina, surrounded by a chronic interstitial infiltrate. Renal failure appears to result both from obstruction of the renal tubules by these casts and/or from direct toxic effects of the Bence Jones proteins. In addition to renal insufficiency, multiple myeloma may cause proximal and distal renal tubular acidosis, Fanconi's syndrome, urinary concentrating defects, and the nephrotic syndrome. The last is usually associated with renal amyloidosis. Recovery from renal failure due to CISN with cast nephropathy is rare in contrast to that occurring from other abnormalities in these individuals, particularly hypercalcemia.

MISCELLANEOUS FACTORS

In *diabetes mellitus* and *sickle cell hemoglobinopathies,* CISN may be accompanied by papillary necrosis. Hyperkalemia and hyperkalemic distal renal tubular acidosis may occur in both. In diabetic patients this is generally due to hyporeninemic hypoaldosteronism. Urinary concentrating defects are particularly common in sickling disorders. Chronic reduction in renal blood flow from a variety of *renovascular disorders* causes atrophy of both

the renal tubules and the glomeruli, along with interstitial fibrosis. *Advanced renal disease* of any etiology results in interstitial fibrosis with mild interstitial inflammation, tubular atrophy, and glomerulosclerosis characteristic of the "end-stage" kidney. Cysts of varying size may also be present. In many cases, these changes are so severe that it is not possible to determine whether the underlying cause of renal failure was tubulointerstitial, glomerular, or vascular in origin. In occasional cases of CISN, sometimes accompanied by granulomas, no recognized cause can be identified.

CLINICAL AND LABORATORY MANIFESTATIONS

The clinical manifestations may be primarily those of renal tubular functional defects (Table 80–1) or may primarily reflect those of advanced renal failure. Sterile pyuria may be seen, but, in contrast to AISN, eosinophilia and eosinophiluria are not. Historical and laboratory findings may suggest a specific diagnosis, e.g., flank pain, and radiographic or ultrasonographic evidence of hydronephrosis suggesting obstructive nephropathy. Clinical presentations unique to certain entities are discussed elsewhere.

TOXIC NEPHROPATHIES (Table 80–5)

Drug-induced acute interstitial nephritis, an important type of nephrotoxic renal injury, is discussed in the preceding section with other causes of acute interstitial nephritis. Other important toxic nephropathies are discussed below.

Analgesic Nephropathy

Chronic interstitial nephritis leading to chronic renal failure may result from excessive consumption of certain analgesic agents. In the United States, 2 to 10 per cent of all cases of end-stage renal disease are thought to be due to analgesic nephropathy (AN). In other countries, AN is an even more important cause of chronic renal failure. For example, about 20 per cent of all cases of end-stage renal disease in Australia result from AN. The drugs most commonly associated with AN are phenacetin or acetaminophen (phenacetin is largely converted to acetaminophen soon after ingestion), usually in combination with aspirin. Generally, the offending agents are taken in the form of proprietary drugs, but sometimes they are obtained by prescriptions from physicians. In many countries the availability of phenacetin in proprietary drugs is now greatly restricted. Acute acetaminophen poisoning may cause acute renal failure due to acute tubular necrosis (Ch. 76).

PATHOGENESIS AND PATHOLOGY

Although phenacetin, acetaminophen, and aspirin may be nephrotoxic when consumed in large quantities over extended periods, there is some debate about which of these may be the most noxious to the kidney. The combination of acetaminophen or phenacetin with aspirin appears to be more nephrotoxic than either drug alone. Prospective epidemiologic studies show a convincing correlation between the amount of phenacetin or acetaminophen consumed and the development of renal disease.

TABLE 80–5. PROMINENT OR COMMON NEPHROTOXINS

Anticonvulsants: paramethadione, phenytoin, trimethadone
Antihypertensive drugs: angiotensin-converting enzyme inhibitors
Antimicrobials: aminoglycosides, amphotericin B, cephalosporins, ethambutol, isoniazid, para-aminosalicylic acid, penicillins, rifampin, sulfonamides, tetracyclines, pentamidine, acyclovir
Antineoplastic agents: cisplatin, methotrexate, mitomycin C, nitrosoureas, radiation
Sulfonamide diuretics: acetazolamide, chlorthalidone, furosemide, thiazides
Endogenous compounds: Bence Jones proteins, calcium, hemoglobin, myoglobin, oxalate, uric acid
Halogenated alkanes, hydrocarbons, and solvents: carbon tetrachloride, ethylene glycol, paraquat, toluene
Iodinated radiographic contrast media
Metals: arsenic, bismuth, cadmium, copper, gold, lead, lithium, mercury
Nonsteroidal anti-inflammatory drugs
Miscellaneous compounds: acetaminophen, allopurinol, amphetamines, azathioprine, cimetidine, cyclosporine, heroin, methoxyflurane, methysergide, D-penicillamine, phenacetin, phenindione, silicon

The generally accepted requirement for the presumptive diagnosis of AN is a cumulative ingestion of 3 kg or more of the above drugs or daily consumption of 1 gram per day for 3 or more years. In most reported cases of AN, consumption has far exceeded these amounts.

The pathogenesis of AN is still uncertain. Both aspirin and acetaminophen are concentrated within the kidney, and for acetaminophen, and perhaps aspirin, a concentration gradient exists within the kidney from the renal cortex to the medulla. Phenacetin and acetaminophen are metabolized to reactive species that covalently bind to proteins and result in oxidative tissue damage by depleting reducing equivalents such as glutathione. Aspirin may exacerbate this toxicity by inhibiting glutathione production. In addition, aspirin is a potent inhibitor of prostaglandin synthesis. This latter action may lead to a reduction in renal medullary blood flow and result in ischemic damage. In addition to aspirin, other nonsteroidal anti-inflammatory drugs that also inhibit prostaglandin synthesis have been associated with papillary necrosis. The ultimate importance of these other drugs as a cause of chronic interstitial nephritis will require long-term observations, as many of them have been only recently used on a wide scale.

In the initial stages of AN, there is patchy necrosis of interstitial cells, loops of Henle, and capillaries in the inner medulla, with calcium deposition and lipid accumulation in the involved areas. With continued exposure to these drugs, the process progressively involves the outer medulla and often results in total papillary necrosis. In advanced stages, the renal cortex is thin, and the renal tubules are atrophic. There is interstitial fibrosis accompanied by a round cell infiltrate. The glomeruli are initially spared, but later they and the arterioles become sclerotic. If AN is complicated by bacterial infection, focal collections of acute inflammatory cells are evident. The necrotic papillae may remain in situ, often with cavities in them, or they may totally detach from the medulla and slough into the renal pelvis.

CLINICAL AND LABORATORY MANIFESTATIONS

AN is usually associated with a characteristic group of signs, symptoms, and laboratory findings. The diagnosis of AN is often overlooked because patients frequently do not admit to taking analgesics or, if they do, will not provide a true estimate of the amount consumed. When the diagnosis is suspected, therefore, the possibility of AN should be vigorously pursued by discussions with family members or physicians who have cared for the patient previously. AN occurs more frequently in women (usually middle age) with a female-male ratio of 3:1 to 6:1. Although patients may consume analgesics for a variety of complaints, especially headaches, more often than not there is no disease that warrants taking large amounts of analgesics. In many patients there is a large psychological component to their clinical presentation. In some patients there is a family history of heavy analgesic use. Anemia is present in most patients and is frequently more severe than can be attributed to their degree of renal insufficiency. In addition to renal insufficiency, anemia may result from hemolysis or gastrointestinal blood loss due to peptic ulcer disease or gastritis, which also occur commonly. Hypertension is present in about one half of patients but generally appears after renal disease is obvious. Malignant hypertension occasionally develops.

Urinalysis frequently reveals pyuria. Urinary tract infections are present in approximately one half of patients at some point and may be associated with leukocyte casts in the urinary sediment. Sloughing of a necrotic papilla into the urinary tract may be associated with gross hematuria, flank pain (ureteral colic), passage of tissue in the urine, and an abrupt decline in renal function. Proteinuria is generally modest (< 2 grams per day), but as the disease progresses, occasional patients develop focal sclerosing glomerulopathy with heavy proteinuria. Generally, progression to end-stage renal failure occurs over a period of several years. Renal tubular abnormalities may be reflected by hyperchloremic metabolic acidosis due to decreased renal acidification, mild polyuria with an inability to concentrate the urine above the osmolality of blood due to nephrogenic diabetes insipidus, and an inability to reduce appropriately urinary sodium excretion with sodium deprivation (renal salt wasting).

Early in the course of the disease, the kidneys may be of normal size and contour when evaluated radiographically or by ultrasonography. In the late stages, the kidneys are small with a thin cortex and an irregular surface. A variety of findings on intravenous urography or retrograde pyelography—including caliceal clubbing, papillary cavities, and caliceal filling defects due to the presence of a sloughed papilla (ring sign)—may suggest papillary necrosis. Demonstration of papillary necrosis in the absence of its more common causes (e.g., diabetes mellitus, urinary tract obstruction, often with infection, or sickle cell disease) should suggest AN. Finally, patients with AN are at increased risk for development of transitional cell carcinoma of the urinary tract, particularly of the renal pelvis. The appearance of hematuria should lead to prompt evaluation to exclude a uroepithelial neoplasm. This evaluation should generally include examination of the urine for neoplastic cells, cystoscopy, and retrograde pyelograms.

PREVENTION AND THERAPY

Obviously, avoidance of drugs implicated as causes of AN will prevent the disorder. Public education about the dangers of excessive analgesic consumption is important. In Canada removal of phenacetin from proprietary analgesic mixtures has been associated with a decline in the incidence of AN. This has not been the case in Australia, however.

The most important factor in treatment of established AN is cessation of analgesic use. For individuals who habitually abuse analgesics, this requires a great deal of education and encouragement. Often psychological counseling is needed. For patients with diseases requiring analgesics—e.g., rheumatoid arthritis—alternative forms of therapy are indicated. With cessation of analgesic use, renal function will generally stabilize or improve. If renal disease is clearly established and drug use continues, renal function inexorably declines, often to the point of end-stage renal disease, over a period of several years. Urinary tract infections, ureteral obstruction from sloughed papillae, hypertension, and dehydration are conditions that may cause a more rapid decline in renal function, and all should be treated promptly.

Nonsteroidal Anti-inflammatory Drugs

During the last decade, several drugs that inhibit production of the various prostaglandins have been marketed. These agents are referred to collectively as nonsteroidal anti-inflammatory drugs (NSAID's) (see Ch. 29). With more widespread use of these drugs, several renal and electrolyte complications have been recognized.

The functions of renal prostaglandins have yet to be completely elucidated. Vasodilator prostaglandins (PGE_2, PGI_2) are important in maintaining renal blood flow in states of sodium depletion or when "effective" arterial blood volume is low. These states are generally associated with elevated levels of circulating angiotensin II and catecholamines. By causing renal vasodilation, prostaglandins preserve renal blood flow while allowing angiotensin II and catecholamines to maintain systemic blood pressure by increasing systemic vascular resistance. Prostaglandins also cause a natriuresis, stimulate renin release, and antagonize the effect of antidiuretic hormone. Many of the renal and electrolyte complications of prostaglandin inhibition by NSAID's (Table 80–6) are predictable, based on these recognized functions of the prostaglandins.

TABLE 80–6. RENAL AND ELECTROLYTE COMPLICATIONS OF NONSTEROIDAL ANTI-INFLAMMATORY DRUGS

1. Renal failure
   a. Hemodynamic (major risk factors are sodium depletion and low "effective" arterial blood volume)
   b. Acute interstitial nephritis with or without the nephrotic syndrome
   c. Glomerulonephritis associated with diffuse vasculitis
   d. Papillary necrosis with chronic interstitial nephritis
2. Sodium and fluid retention
3. Hyperkalemia, metabolic acidosis (occurs more often in patients with renal insufficiency, sodium depletion, or other factors predisposing to hyperkalemia)

HEMODYNAMICALLY MEDIATED ACUTE RENAL FAILURE. This has been reported in several patients receiving NSAID's, most notably indomethacin. This type of renal failure appears to result from renal hypoperfusion and occurs shortly after drug therapy is instituted. Patients at risk are those with sodium depletion (e.g., from diuretic therapy) or low "effective" arterial blood volumes (e.g., nephrotic syndrome, congestive heart failure, and hepatic cirrhosis with ascites), older individuals, and patients with underlying renal disease. Individuals receiving triamterene may be especially at risk. This type of acute renal failure is usually associated with oliguria and low fractional excretion of sodium and thus resembles prerenal azotemia (see Ch. 76). The urinary sediment is generally unremarkable. Renal biopsies have shown evidence of acute tubular necrosis. Azotemia generally resolves promptly after discontinuation of the offending drug. Occasional patients, however, require temporary dialysis.

ACUTE INTERSTITIAL NEPHRITIS (AISN). AISN resulting in acute renal failure has been described in several patients in association with NSAID's, particularly fenoprofen. Heavy proteinuria, often in the nephrotic range, is peculiar to this form of drug-induced AISN. In addition to copious proteinuria, there are other features of AISN due to NSAID's that differ from those associated with other drugs. For example, eosinophilia, eosinophiluria, and skin rashes are uncommon. As with other types of drug-induced AISN, however, urinalysis frequently reveals microscopic hematuria and pyuria. In addition to histopathologic changes of AISN (described earlier), electron microscopy of the glomeruli reveals fusion of podocyte foot processes. Unlike hemodynamically mediated acute renal failure, AISN usually appears only after the offending drug has been administered for several days to several months. The disorder usually resolves with discontinuation of the drug, but recovery may not occur until several months later, and interval dialysis may be required. Corticosteroid therapy is believed by many to hasten recovery, and in the absence of contraindications, it is reasonable to prescribe a short course of high-dose corticosteroids (1 mg per kilogram per day of prednisone) if renal failure is severe and spontaneous recovery does not occur within several days of stopping the drug.

OTHER RENAL COMPLICATIONS OF NSAID's. In addition to the above causes of acute renal insufficiency, *systemic vasculitis* with *glomerulitis* and *papillary necrosis* with chronic interstitial nephritis may occur rarely in association with NSAID's.

RETENTION OF SODIUM (AND FLUID). This is perhaps the most common renal side effect of NSAID's. Although this retention may not present a problem in persons with normal cardiovascular and renal function, it may result in worsening of pre-existing congestive heart failure or hypertension. Finally, inhibition of prostaglandin synthesis may result in *hyperkalemia* and *metabolic acidosis* due to inhibition of renin secretion and secondary hypoaldosteronism. Underlying renal insufficiency, sodium depletion, or concomitant administration of other drugs that predispose to hyperkalemia (e.g., potassium-sparing diuretics) increases the risk for developing the latter electrolyte abnormalities.

Antimicrobial Drugs

Renal damage from penicillin, sulfonamide, and antituberculous antimicrobials usually results from AISN, described earlier. Additional antibiotics may cause renal disease manifested in other ways.

AMINOGLYCOSIDES. The aminoglycosides, excreted primarily by glomerular filtration, accumulate in the renal cortex to levels higher than those in serum. They may cause several renal tubular functional abnormalities, the most clinically relevant of which are potassium and magnesium wasting, which may result in hypokalemia and hypomagnesemia. The most important manifestation of aminoglycoside renal toxicity, however, is acute renal failure. This results from both a direct effect of these drugs on glomerular filtration and tubular toxicity causing acute tubular necrosis. Up to 10 per cent of patients receiving aminoglycosides develop some degree of acute renal failure, accounting for 10 to 15 per cent of all cases of this disorder in the United States. Generally, this failure is manifested by a rise in the serum creatinine level after several days of therapy with one of the aminoglycosides. At times, renal failure may become evident only after the drug has been discontinued. Acute renal failure is usually mild and of the nonoliguric variety. However, oliguria and severe renal failure requiring dialysis may be seen.

The most nephrotoxic aminoglycoside is neomycin, which is, therefore, not administered parenterally. It may rarely cause acute renal failure when given orally or by enema to decrease the bowel flora. The least nephrotoxic is streptomycin. Tobramycin and netilmicin are, perhaps, less nephrotoxic than gentamicin and amikacin. Risk factors for development of aminoglycoside toxicity include the dose of drug administered; the length of therapy; simultaneous administration of other potential nephrotoxins, particularly cephalosporins; renal insufficiency; advanced age; extracellular fluid volume depletion; liver disease; and, possibly, potassium depletion. In older individuals the GFR normally declines, although this is unaccompanied by an elevated serum creatinine level. Failure to consider this variable when calculating the maintenance dose of aminoglycosides is a major (and preventable) factor in production of acute renal failure.

Management of acute renal failure following aminoglycoside administration consists of discontinuing the drug and substituting another appropriate antibiotic if continued treatment is necessary. When no alternative antibiotic can be found, aminoglycosides may be continued in appropriately reduced doses. In this setting, serum aminoglycoside levels should be monitored. Supportive measures are similar to those indicated with acute renal failure of other causes (Ch. 76). The prognosis for recovery of renal function after several days is excellent.

CEPHALOSPORINS. Renal failure due to acute tubular necrosis and acute interstitial nephritis may rarely accompany treatment with the cephalosporins. The combination of a cephalosporin and an aminoglycoside carries a risk higher than for either drug alone, requiring close monitoring of renal function when this combination of agents is used.

TETRACYCLINES. Tetracyclines inhibit protein synthesis and, therefore, shunt amino acids into urea. The enhanced synthesis of urea elevates the blood urea nitrogen (BUN) without a concomitant elevation of serum creatinine or a reduction in GFR. In normal individuals this is of little consequence. In patients with underlying insufficiency, however, the increase in BUN may be dramatic. With the exception of doxycycline and minocycline, which do not accumulate in renal failure and which require only minor dosage adjustments, tetracyclines should be avoided in individuals with significant renal insufficiency. Demeclocycline causes a dose-related nephrogenic diabetes insipidus. This property has been used to treat some hyponatremic patients, particularly those with the syndrome of inappropriate secretion of antidiuretic hormone (Ch. 75). Demeclocycline has been reported to cause acute renal failure, however, when used to treat hyponatremic patients with hepatic cirrhosis. Although the renal failure is reversible, demeclocycline (and other tetracyclines) should be avoided in these patients. Outdated tetracyclines can cause Fanconi's syndrome.

AMPHOTERICIN B. Most patients receiving more than 2 grams of this antifungal agent develop one or more renal abnormalities. Defects in distal nephron function are the first to appear: distal renal tubular acidosis, nephrogenic diabetes insipidus, and renal potassium wasting. These alterations may occur without a reduction in GFR and are generally reversible with discontinuation of the drug. Metabolic acidosis and hypokalemia should be treated with supplemental alkali and potassium salts. Acute renal insufficiency, which may be progressive and incompletely reversible, is a major side effect of amphotericin B. This side effect is dose related and appears to result both from direct renal tubular toxicity and from ischemia due to renal vasoconstriction. Acute renal failure is more likely to occur in patients who are sodium depleted from whatever cause: diuretics, vomiting, and so on, and in patients with underlying renal insufficiency. Sodium repletion may protect against amphotericin B nephrotoxicity. Once moderate azotemia is present (BUN > 50 mg per deciliter), consideration should be given to prescribing the drug on alternate days or to temporarily discontinuing therapy until renal function improves. The risk of renal insufficiency has to be weighed, of course, against the severity of the underlying infection and whether alternative antifungal therapy is available.

Radiographic Contrast Agents

Acute renal failure resulting from acute tubular necrosis is an uncommon, but important, complication of iodinated radiographic contrast agents used, for example, in intravenous urography, arteriography, or contrast-enhanced computed tomography. The incidence of acute renal failure associated with these agents has varied in large series from 0 to 13 per cent but is much higher in certain groups of patients. Risk factors include underlying renal insufficiency, diabetes mellitus, older age, dehydration, history of prior acute renal failure following use of contrast agents, multiple contrast procedures in a short period, concomitant exposure to other nephrotoxins, and, perhaps, multiple myeloma. In addition, acute renal failure is more likely after administration of larger doses of these agents. Clearly, individuals at highest risk are diabetic patients with renal insufficiency. The incidence of acute renal failure following exposure to these agents in this population of patients may be as high as 75 per cent. In the absence of other risk factors, diabetes per se does not appear to pose a major risk.

Pathogenetic factors in radiocontrast-induced acute renal failure may include ischemia resulting from renal arteriolar vasoconstriction due to the hypertonicity of these agents, tubular obstruction due to precipitation of proteins, and direct tubular toxicity. In addition, as with any drug, anaphylaxis with hypotension is a rare cause of acute renal failure. Patients who develop acute renal failure generally have an elevation in serum creatinine level within 24 hours of exposure to radiocontrast agents. The peak in creatinine elevation typically occurs within 7 days. Renal insufficiency is usually moderate and resolves in a few days, but it may be severe and necessitate temporary dialysis. With advanced underlying renal disease, the acute insufficiency may be irreversible. In patients at risk, the serum creatinine concentration should be measured the day after exposure to these agents to determine if nephrotoxicity has occurred. A persistent nephrogram at this time also suggests renal injury.

Prevention of renal failure in patients at high risk includes avoidance of dehydration, minimizing the amount of contrast administered (no more than 0.88 mg of iodine per kilogram of body weight), and using alternative diagnostic methods such as ultrasonography, if possible. Non-ionic agents do not appear to be any less nephrotoxic than ionic ones. Hypertonic mannitol (25 to 50 grams given over 1 hour) immediately following exposure to radiographic contrast agents may reduce the incidence of acute renal failure in high-risk patients. Treatment of acute renal failure due to contrast agents is similar to that resulting from other etiologies (Ch. 76).

Nephropathies Resulting from Antineoplastic Therapy

Several drugs used in the treatment of neoplasia may produce renal toxicity. Some of these may cause isolated abnormalities in renal tubular function, whereas others may produce acute or chronic renal insufficiency. For some of these compounds, renal damage represents the dose-limiting toxicity.

CISPLATIN. Cisplatin and its metabolites are eliminated primarily by urinary excretion. Acute tubular necrosis, which may occur after intravenous administration of the drug, is dose related, being uncommon with single doses less than 50 mg per square meter but occurring in most patients with doses above 100 mg per square meter. The cause of cisplatin toxicity is uncertain, but it appears similar to that produced by other heavy metals (see below). Concomitant administration of cisplatin and other nephrotoxins, such as aminoglycosides, increases the risk of acute renal failure. Generally, azotemia appears a few days after administration of the drug and is usually reversible over a period of 2 to 4 weeks. With severe acute renal failure and/or repeated administration of cisplatin, chronic renal insufficiency due to chronic interstitial nephritis may develop. The incidence of acute renal failure due to cisplatin can be reduced by ensuring adequate hydration and establishing a saline diuresis prior to and during administration of the drug and by continuously infusing the drug slowly over several hours or a few days. Hypomagnesemia due to renal magnesium wasting may occur in as many as 50 per cent of patients treated with cisplatin. Hypomagnesemia may be severe, may develop in the absence of renal insufficiency, and may persist for several weeks following cisplatin therapy. Other renal tubular abnormalities, such as potassium wasting,

decreased urinary concentrating ability, and low molecular weight proteinuria, may also be observed but are generally of little clinical importance.

METHOTREXATE. This folic acid antagonist is eliminated principally by urinary excretion. Nephrotoxicity is rare with low doses (5 to 60 mg per square meter). With high-dose therapy (500 to 7500 mg per square meter), the drug precipitates in the renal tubule lumina and causes acute renal failure from tubular obstruction. Direct tubular toxicity may also play a role. Nephrotoxicity may be reduced by vigorous (intravenous) hydration to maintain a urine flow of greater than 100 ml per hour for several days following high-dose therapy. In addition, the urine pH should be kept above 7 by alkali administration, since methotrexate is more soluble in alkaline solutions. Development of renal insufficiency prolongs the half-life of methotrexate and increases the likelihood of systemic toxicity.

NITROSOUREAS. A number of nitrosoureas used in cancer chemotherapy, including streptozocin, carmustine (BCNU), lomustine (CCNU), and methyl CCNU, may produce several types of renal toxicity. Streptozocin may cause proteinuria, sometimes resulting in nephrotic syndrome, due to glomerular injury; acute tubular necrosis leading to acute renal failure; and a variety of renal tubular abnormalities, including proximal renal tubular acidosis, glycosuria, phosphaturia, and aminoaciduria. Proteinuria is generally the first manifestation of renal toxicity. Should this occur, therapy should be withheld and only cautiously restarted if this resolves. Azotemia developing after streptozocin should lead to permanent discontinuation of the drug. The other nitrosoureas given in multiple courses over several weeks have been associated with a very high incidence of chronic renal insufficiency. In one series the majority of patients receiving at least six courses of therapy developed insidious chronic renal insufficiency, sometimes resulting in uremia, without an antecedent episode of acute renal failure and without abnormalities in the urinary sediment. The principal pathologic findings are chronic interstitial nephritis and glomerulosclerosis. Any nitrosoureas should generally be discontinued at the first sign of an otherwise unexplained decrease in renal function.

MITOMYCIN C. There is a 5 to 40 per cent incidence of nephrotoxicity following mitomycin C therapy. Toxicity is dose related and generally appears after repeated courses and/or a cumulative dose of 60 mg per square meter. Renal injury is manifested by proteinuria (usually mild) and azotemia. Renal insufficiency may develop gradually or abruptly. In the latter instance, the clinical features are similar to those of the hemolytic uremic syndrome (Ch. 79) and include thrombocytopenia, microangiopathic hemolytic anemia, and acute renal failure. Renal pathologic findings consist of glomerular alterations (mesangial fragmentation, capillary thrombi, and hemorrhage) and thrombosis and fibrinoid necrosis of the arterioles. There is no established therapy except for supportive measures for renal failure developing after administration of mitomycin C. Renal function should be monitored closely in patients receiving this drug, and therapy should probably be discontinued if otherwise unexplained azotemia occurs.

MISCELLANEOUS ANTINEOPLASTIC AGENTS. Nephrotoxicity has occasionally been reported with other cancer chemotherapeutic agents, including 5-azacytidine, daunorubicin, doxorubicin, mithramycin, dacarbazine, and recombinant leukocyte A interferon. Administration of recombinant interleukin 2 to patients with advanced cancer is commonly associated with acute renal insufficiency, probably resulting from severe prerenal azotemia. Finally, therapy resulting in massive acute killing of neoplastic cells may cause the tumor lysis syndrome (see below).

RADIATION NEPHRITIS (Also see Ch. 530). Exposure of the kidneys during abdominal irradiation for cancer may subsequently result in damage of varying degree. Manifestations range from mild proteinuria, urinary concentrating defects, and benign hypertension with a reduced GFR to malignant hypertension with end-stage renal failure. Evidence for renal damage occurs several months to years after renal irradiation, and the severity bears a general relationship to the amount of irradiation received. Clinically evident renal injury is uncommon with less than 1000 to 2000 cGy but develops in approximately 50 per cent of patients receiving doses higher than this. In the early stage of radiation nephritis, tubular necrosis, medial and intimal thickening of the small renal arteries, and damage to the glomerular endothelium are present. Later, glomerulosclerosis, collagenous thickening of the small renal arteries, and interstitial fibrosis are prominent. The incidence of radiation nephritis can be minimized by limiting the total dose of abdominal irradiation in a single course to 2000 cGy over 2 weeks and by shielding the kidneys as much as possible. Malignant hypertension resulting from unilateral radiation nephritis can be cured by nephrectomy.

URIC ACID AND THE TUMOR LYSIS SYNDROME. Patients with certain hematologic malignancies, particularly acute lymphoblastic leukemia and poorly differentiated lymphomas, may rarely develop spontaneous acute renal failure from obstruction of the renal tubules by uric acid. More frequently, this complication follows aggressive chemotherapy or radiation therapy, which kills cells and releases massive amounts of purine uric acid precursors. The resulting hyperuricemia greatly increases the filtered load of urate. Its solubility is exceeded in acidified tubular urine, and uric acid precipitation occurs in the renal tubules, often resulting in acute obstructive renal failure. A ratio of urinary uric acid/creatinine concentrations greater than 1:1 suggests the diagnosis of acute uric acid nephropathy. During massive cell lysis, phosphate is also released in large amounts, and hyperphosphaturia with intrarenal precipitation of calcium phosphate may contribute to the renal failure. Hyperkalemia due to release of intracellular potassium may also be observed. Prevention of acute renal failure secondary to massive tumor cell killing includes establishing a urinary output of 3 or more liters per 24 hours and treatment with high-dose allopurinol (300 to 400 mg per square meter per day) prior to institution of cytotoxic therapy. The role of urinary alkalinization is uncertain. Although this will increase the solubility of uric acid, a high urinary pH will favor precipitation of phosphate salts in the renal tubules. If renal failure occurs despite the foregoing precautions, hemodialysis is indicated for supportive therapy and for removing uric acid and other cellular products. This practice allows renal function to recover, generally in a few days. Chronic interstitial nephritis (gouty nephropathy), a complication of chronic hyperuricemia and gout, is discussed in Ch. 183.

Metal Nephropathies

The diagnosis and treatment of intoxication with trace metals are discussed in detail in Ch. 533. Only certain aspects of this subject related to the kidney are discussed below. Acute intoxication with some metals may cause both acute renal injury with a reduction in GFR and renal tubular dysfunction. With chronic intoxication, the most common form of injury is chronic interstitial nephritis manifested by renal tubular abnormalities with or without reduction in GFR. In certain instances glomerular injury may also occur. Metal intoxication is often treated by chelation therapy. Unfortunately, some of the drugs used for this purpose, e.g., penicillamine, may also be nephrotoxic, as discussed below.

LITHIUM. Lithium carbonate, used in the treatment of affective disorders, causes a variety of renal abnormalities. The most frequent is a form of vasopressin-resistant nephrogenic diabetes insipidus. This is of little consequence in most patients. Polyuria (urine volumes > 3000 ml per day) may result but usually abates when lithium therapy is stopped. The diuretic amiloride may significantly reduce the polyuria associated with lithium. Incomplete distal renal tubular acidosis and mild renal sodium wasting may also result from lithium therapy. Chronic interstitial nephritis occurs in some lithium-treated patients. However, since CISN is more frequent in individuals with affective disorders than in the general population, the importance of lithium is debated. However, a history of acute lithium intoxication may predispose to development of chronic renal insufficiency.

LEAD. Lead poisoning may result from acute exposure, such as from ingestion of lead-containing paint, but more often from chronic exposure, such as in foundry and battery workers or from consumption of illicit alcoholic beverages ("moonshine"). Acute intoxication, more common in children, is manifested primarily by abdominal colic, hemolytic anemia, and encephalopathy. Acute interstitial nephritis with eosinophilic inclusions in the proximal tubular cells, tubular necrosis with a reduction in GFR,

and Fanconi's syndrome may also occur. Whether acute lead intoxication without further exposure results in chronic renal disease in later years is unclear. Chronic lead intoxication causes interstitial nephritis with variable reductions in GFR and renal tubular dysfunction. Some patients develop gout and hypertension as a result of chronic lead intoxication ("saturnine gout"). Chronic lead intoxication should be considered in individuals with the triad of gout, hypertension, and chronic renal insufficiency. A history of exposure to lead should be sought and a $CaNa_2$–ethylenediaminetetra-acetic acid (EDTA) infusion carried out to evaluate lead stores (Ch. 533). Treatment of acute lead intoxication consists of preventing further exposure to the metal, supportive care, and chelation with dimercaptopropanol (BAL) or $CaNa_2$-EDTA. Chronic renal insufficiency resulting from lead may sometimes improve during chelation therapy but may also progress despite this therapy.

MERCURY. Acute intoxication with mercurial salts may cause tubular necrosis and severe renal failure. The strong affinity of mercury for sulfhydryl groups, along with the hypotension that frequently accompanies acute intoxication, probably accounts for the acute renal injury. Acute exposure may occur rarely in industrial settings or with intentional ingestion of mercurial salts. Treatment of acute poisoning from mercurial salts consists of chelation therapy with dimercaptopropanol or penicillamine and supportive care (Ch. 533). Chronic exposure to organomercurials may result in subtle renal damage manifested by increased urinary excretion of low molecular weight proteins and renal tubular enzymes (tubular proteinuria). Chelation therapy is ineffective in removing organomercurials. Chronic exposure to mercurial compounds may also cause the nephrotic syndrome as a result of glomerular damage, most commonly from membranous nephropathy. The pathogenesis of this disorder is uncertain, as mercury is not demonstrable in the glomeruli.

GOLD. Proteinuria may complicate the treatment of rheumatoid arthritis with gold salts, more frequently with parenteral than with oral administration. Proteinuria may develop at any time, but usually after several months of therapy. Rarely, it may be severe enough to result in the nephrotic syndrome associated with membranous nephropathy. It is unlikely that gold per se is directly responsible for the glomerular injury, since the metal can be demonstrated in the renal tubules, but not in the glomeruli. Gold may in some way modify an intrinsic protein so that it becomes antigenic and elicits the immune reactions that produce membranous nephropathy. Membranous nephropathy may also occur in patients with rheumatoid arthritis who have not been treated with gold. The appearance of proteinuria in a patient receiving gold should prompt discontinuation of the drug. This practice generally results in disappearance of the proteinuria, but this disappearance may occur only several months later.

ARSENIC. Arsenic is used in a number of industrial applications and is present in several commercial products, such as insecticides. In addition, illicit alcohol may be contaminated with the metal. Gastrointestinal symptoms and peripheral neuropathy are the most prominent manifestations of acute arsenic poisoning but acute tubular necrosis may also occur. Like mercury, arsenic has a high affinity for sulfhydryl groups of proteins. Cellular damage resulting from this interaction and from hypotension are the most likely causes of acute renal damage. Treatment of arsenic poisoning includes supportive measures and chelation therapy with dimercaptopropanol. Arsine gas may cause acute renal failure secondary to hemoglobinuria from acute hemolysis and from hypotension.

CADMIUM. With chronic low-level exposure—for example, in alkaline battery workers—cadmium accumulates in the renal cortex. This may result in mild proteinuria, of both glomerular and tubular origin, and in early renal insufficiency. The incidence of proteinuria increases with the length of exposure.

MISCELLANEOUS METALS. *Bismuth* has been reported to cause both acute tubular necrosis and the nephrotic syndrome. Acute *copper* poisoning may produce acute tubular necrosis, most likely resulting from hemolysis with hemoglobinuria and from hypotension. Chronic copper accumulation in Wilson's disease (Ch. 192) may be associated with proximal renal tubular acidosis and other components of Fanconi's syndrome and mild renal insufficiency. In rare instances, renal injury has been reported with *antimony, thallium,* and *uranium* intoxication. *Platinum* nephrotoxicity is discussed under cisplatin.

Oxalate

End-stage renal failure from chronic interstitial nephritis and from recurrent nephrolithiasis is the major complication of primary hyperoxaluria and may rarely occur in enteric hyperoxaluria as well (Ch. 171).

Acute intoxication with ethylene glycol is the major cause of acute renal failure due to oxalate. Ethylene glycol is the principal component of antifreeze and is usually ingested by desperate alcoholics, by children accidentally, or in a suicide attempt. Ethylene glycol is metabolized to several toxic substances, one of which is oxalic acid. Intoxication with ethylene glycol causes acute renal failure, profound metabolic acidosis of the anion gap variety (Ch. 75), and acute central nervous system and pulmonary dysfunction. Renal failure results from massive deposition of oxalate within the renal tubules. This is usually accompanied by large numbers of calcium oxalate crystals in the urinary sediment. Ethylene glycol intoxication is managed by (1) administration of ethyl alcohol to slow the metabolism of ethylene glycol by competing for alcohol dehydrogenase; (2) hemodialysis to remove the parent compound, to allow treatment with sodium bicarbonate therapy, which may be required in amounts that would otherwise result in pulmonary edema and hypernatremia, and to treat acute renal failure; and (3) administration of pyridoxine and thiamine to help shunt ethylene glycol into other metabolic pathways that result in less toxic metabolites. If patients survive acute intoxication, chances for recovery of renal function are good, but many will require temporary dialysis for several days prior to functional renal recovery.

Angiotensin-Converting Enzyme (ACE) Inhibitors

Acute renal failure has been reported in patients with bilateral renal artery stenosis or stenosis of the renal artery supplying a solitary kidney following treatment with ACE inhibitors. Usually, ACE inhibitor–associated acute renal failure is thought to be hemodynamic in origin, resulting from loss of autoregulation of renal blood flow and GFR. Sometimes, however, acute renal failure following captopril therapy has been accompanied by skin rash, eosinophilia, and eosinophiluria, a constellation of findings strongly suggesting allergic interstitial nephritis. Acute renal failure in both the above settings generally resolves with discontinuation of the ACE inhibitor but may recur upon rechallenge with the drug. Membranous nephropathy with the nephrotic syndrome may also occur in association with captopril therapy. This complication may resolve slowly after discontinuation of the drug. Membranous nephropathy occurring during therapy with captopril and penicillamine (see below) may possibly be related to the active sulfhydryl group that they contain.

D-Penicillamine

Therapy with this drug for metal chelation, rheumatoid arthritis, scleroderma, or cystinuria is complicated by proteinuria in 4 to 7 per cent of patients, often sufficiently severe to result in the nephrotic syndrome. Proteinuria, which may be associated with mild azotemia, usually results from membranous nephropathy (Ch. 79). Rarely, rapidly progressive glomerulonephritis accompanied by pulmonary hemorrhage occurs. Proteinuria generally resolves or decreases when D-penicillamine therapy is discontinued, but usually only after several months.

Methoxyflurane

This fluorinated anesthetic agent may cause a dose-related postoperative nephrogenic diabetes insipidus and acute renal failure. Similar complications have rarely been reported with enflurane. The initial polyuric acute renal failure may progress to oliguria in severe cases. Renal function may recover after several days, but persistent renal failure, which has required long-term dialysis, may develop. The pathogenesis of methoxyflurane-induced acute renal failure is uncertain. The drug is metabolized to fluoride and oxalate. Although oxalate is nephrotoxic (see above), it is believed that the major toxic product is fluoride, since nephrotoxicity correlates with blood levels of this ion and fluoride produces nephrotoxicity in experimental animals. Volume depletion due to the urinary concentrating defect may also contribute to acute renal failure.

Miscellaneous Nephrotoxins

Exposure to *hydrocarbons*, frequently in the form of paint or glue sniffing, has been associated with a variety of (generally) reversible abnormalities, including azotemia, renal tubular acidosis, Fanconi's syndrome, proteinuria, hematuria, and pyuria. Similar findings may result from exposure to halogenated alkane solvents, such as *carbon tetrachloride*, and insecticides, such as *paraquat*. *Silicon* exposure—for example, in sandblasters—has been implicated in a connective tissue–like disease with multiple serologic abnormalities and progressive renal failure associated with both glomerular and renal tubular pathologic changes that appear to be immune mediated.

Heroin abuse is associated with a variety of glomerular lesions, including amyloidosis, and glomerulonephritis due to bacterial endocarditis or hepatitis B infection. In some patients, however, these etiologies cannot be implicated. Most commonly, focal sclerosing glomerulopathy is found, often resulting in the nephrotic syndrome. Recently, it has been found that many of these patients have human immunodeficiency virus (HIV) infections with or without full-blown acquired immunodeficiency syndrome (AIDS) (Part XXI). Heroin-associated nephropathy generally results in progressive renal failure unless abuse of the drug is stopped.

The nephrotic syndrome may occur as a rare complication of *trimethadione* and *methimazole*. *Sulfonamides* and intravenous *amphetamines* may cause systemic vasculitis that results in renal damage from segmental renal infarction or glomerulonephritis (Ch. 79 and 264). Acute renal insufficiency is a major complication of cyclosporine A therapy of organ transplantation (Ch. 78.2). Administration of cyclosporine A for several months may be associated with occlusion of renal arterioles, CISN, and a reduced GFR. The antiviral drug acyclovir may cause acute renal failure because of precipitation of the agent in the tubular lumina with resultant intrarenal obstruction. A similar process may occur in patients treated with high-dose sulfadiazine. Pentamidine used to treat *Pneumocystis carinii* and other protozoal diseases results in acute renal insufficiency in approximately 25 per cent of cases. *Nifedipine*, like many other drugs, may cause prerenal azotemia because of hypotension but, in addition, may also rarely cause reversible acute renal failure in the absence of a fall in blood pressure and without abnormalities in the urinary sediment.

Retroperitoneal fibrosis as a complication of long-term treatment of migraine headaches with *methysergide* may obstruct the ureters. *Anticoagulant therapy* may cause ureteral obstruction from intraluminal blood clots or from ureteral compression by a retroperitoneal hematoma.

Acute and Chronic Interstitial Nephritis

Adler SG, Cohen AH, Border WA: Hypersensitivity phenomena and the kidney: Role of drugs and environmental agents. Am J Kidney Dis 5:75, 1985. *An excellent review of the various types of immune-mediated renal injury that may result from numerous pharmacologic agents.*

Benabe JE, Martinez-Maldonado M: Tubulo-interstitial nephritis associated with systemic disease and electrolyte abnormalities. Semin Nephrol 8:29, 1988. *This paper provides a concise review of interstitial diseases associated with hypokalemia, hypercalcemia, hyperuricemia, multiple myeloma, sarcoidosis, Sjögren's syndrome, systemic lupus erythematosus, and tuberculosis (136 references).*

Boucher A, Droz D, Adafer E, et al.: Characterization of mononuclear cell subsets in renal cellular interstitial infiltrates. Kidney Int 29:1043, 1986. *Using monoclonal antibodies, the authors found that the predominant mononuclear cells in interstitial cellular infiltrates of 33 renal biopsies, including 11 with AISN or CISN, were T cells. However, the relative proportions of the different T cells subsets varied among the biopsies.*

Cameron JS: Allergic interstitial nephritis: Clinical features and pathogenesis. Q J Med 66:97, 1988. *A very good review of this topic, with an emphasis on drug-induced AISN and pathogenetic factors (165 references).*

Cotran RS, Rubin RH, Tolkoff-Rubin NE: Tubulo-interstitial diseases. *In* Brenner BM, Rector FC Jr (eds.): The Kidney. 3rd ed. Philadelphia, W. B. Saunders Company, 1986. *An excellent review of this topic (353 references).*

Eknoyan G: Chronic tubulointerstitial nephropathies. *In* Schrier RW, Gottschalk CW (eds.): Diseases of the Kidney. 4th ed. Boston, Little, Brown and Company, 1988. *A detailed review of this topic (337 references).*

Hande KR, Noone RM, Stone WJ: Severe allopurinol toxicity. Am J Med 76:47, 1984. *This report describes 7 patients with allopurinol toxicity treated by the authors and reviews another 78 cases from the literature. Dosage guidelines for allopurinol for patients with varying degrees of renal insufficiency are proposed.*

Hostetter TH, Hostetter MK: Infection-related chronic interstitial nephropathy.

Semin Nephrol 8:11, 1988. *This paper provides an excellent discussion of the pathogenetic factors responsible for the renal damage that may accompany renal infections.*

Toto RD: Review: Acute tubulointerstitial nephritis. Am J Med Sci 299:392, 1990. *A recent review of the pathogenesis, pathophysiology, differential diagnosis, and treatment of this disorder (114 references).*

Toxic Nephropathy (General References)

Humes HD, Weinberg JM: Toxic nephropathies. *In* Brenner BM, Rector FC Jr (eds.): The Kidney. 3rd ed. Philadelphia, W. B. Saunders Company, 1986. *An extensive, and well-written review with 579 references.*

Roxe DM, Krumlovsky FA: Toxic interstitial nephropathy from metals, metabolites and radiation. Semin Nephrol 8:72, 1988. *This paper contains a succinct review of nephrotoxicity resulting from cadmium, mercury, uranium, lead, oxalate, and radiation (102 references).*

Walker RJ, Duggin GG: Drug nephrotoxicity. Ann Rev Pharmacol Toxicol 28:331, 1988. *A concise review of the pathophysiologic mechanisms involved in aminoglycoside, amphotericin B, cephalosporin, acetaminophen, and cyclosporine A nephrotoxicity (74 references).*

Weinberg JM: The cellular basis of nephrotoxicity. *In* Schrier RW, Gottschalk CW (eds.): Diseases of the Kidney. 4th ed. Boston, Little, Brown and Company, 1988. *This chapter provides an exhaustive review of the pathophysiology of nephrotoxic renal injury (581 references).*

Analgesic Nephropathy

Buckalew VM Jr, Schey HM: Renal disease from habitual antipyretic analgesic consumption: An assessment of the epidemiologic evidence. Medicine 65:291, 1986. *This paper reviews the worldwide evidence that indicates that habitual analgesic use is an important cause of renal diseases (74 references).*

Eknoyan G, Qunibi WY, Grissom RT, et al.: Renal papillary necrosis: An update. Medicine 61:55, 1982. *A comprehensive review of the various causes of papillary necrosis, including analgesic nephropathy.*

Kincaid-Smith P, Nanra RS: Lithium-induced and analgesia-induced renal diseases. *In* Schrier RW, Gottschalk CW (eds.): Diseases of the Kidney. 4th ed. Boston, Little, Brown and Company, 1988. *This recent chapter contains a thorough review of these disorders (298 references).*

Sandler DP, Smith JC, Weinberg CR, et al.: Analgesic use and chronic renal disease. N Engl J Med 320:1238, 1989. *This paper describes the results of a multicenter case-control study of 554 adults with recently diagnosed kidney disease. The risk of developing renal disease was markedly increased in individuals who used phenacetin or its major metabolite acetaminophen on a daily basis.*

Nonsteroidal Anti-inflammatory Drugs

Dunn MJ, Patrono C (eds.): Renal effects of nonsteroidal anti-inflammatory drugs. Am J Med 81(Suppl 2B):1, 1986. *The several papers from the proceedings of this symposium deal with most aspects of this topic (1068 references).*

Henrich WL: Nephrotoxicity of nonsteroidal antiinflammatory agents. *In* Schrier RW, Gottschalk CW (eds.): Diseases of the Kidney. 4th ed. Boston, Little, Brown and Company, 1988. *This chapter contains a thorough discussion of the renal, fluid, and electrolyte complications of NSAID's (159 references).*

Porile JL, Bakris GL, Garella S: Acute interstitial nephritis with glomerulopathy due to nonsteroidal anti-inflammatory agents: A review of its clinical spectrum and effects of steroid therapy. J Clin Pharmacol 30:468, 1990. *This paper reviews 43 reported cases of acute renal failure and/or nephrotic range proteinuria occurring after treatment with NSAID's. The disorder was more frequent in women and the elderly and had a good prognosis for resolution with discontinuation of the NSAID. The authors believe the evidence suggests that steroids do not alter the course of this disorder.*

Antimicrobial Drugs

Branch RA: Prevention of amphotericin B–induced renal impairment: A review on the use of sodium supplementation. Arch Intern Med 148:2389, 1988. *This paper reviews the evidence that suggests that sodium loading may ameliorate amphotericin B nephrotoxicity.*

Fisher MA, Talbot GH, Maislin G, et al.: Risk factors for amphotericin B nephrotoxicity. Am J Med 87:547, 1989. *This report indicates that risk factors for amphotericin B nephrotoxicity include drug dose, diuretic use, and abnormal baseline renal function.*

Humes HD, O'Connor RP Jr: Aminoglycoside nephrotoxicity. *In* Schrier RW, Gottschalk CW (eds): Diseases of the Kidney. 4th ed. Boston, Little, Brown and Company, 1988. *An up-to-date comprehensive review of this disorder (265 references).*

Perez-Ayuso RM, Arroyo V, Camps J, et al.: Effect of demeclocycline on renal function and urinary prostaglandin E$_2$ and kallikrein in hyponatremic cirrhotics. Nephron 36:30, 1984. *In this report, five of eight hyponatremic cirrhotic patients given demeclocycline developed acute reversible renal insufficiency with a reduction in GFR from an average of 72 to 31 ml per minute.*

Sawyer MH, Webb DE, Balow JE, et al.: Acyclovir-induced renal failure. Am J Med 84:1067, 1988. *This report describes four patients with intrarenal obstruction and crystalluria resulting from acyclovir.*

Radiographic Contrast–Induced Nephrotoxicity

Berkseth RO, Kjellstrand CM: Radiologic contrast–induced nephropathy. Med Clin North Am 68:1, 1984. *A comprehensive review of this topic (101 references).*

Cronin RE: Southwestern Internal Medicine Conference: Renal failure following radiologic procedures. Am J Med Sci 298:342, 1989. *A recent and excellent review of this topic (148 references).*

Schwabe SJ, Hlathy MA, Pieper KS, et al.: Contrast nephropathy: A randomized controlled trial of a nonionic and an ionic radiographic contrast agent. N Engl J Med 320:149, 1989. *In this study, 443 patients were randomized to undergo cardiac catheterization with either an ionic or a nonionic contrast agent. There was no difference in the nephrotoxicity of the two agents in patients at low or high risk of developing acute renal failure.*

Nephrotoxicity Associated with Antineoplastic Therapy

Belldegrun A, Webb DE, Austin HA III, et al.: Renal toxicity of interleukin-2 administration in patients with metastatic renal cell cancer: Effect of pretherapy nephrectomy. J Urol 141:499, 1989. *In this study of 135 patients with advanced cancer, including 52 with renal cell carcinoma, posttherapy depression of renal function was more severe in patients whose pretherapy serum creatinine concentration was elevated to 1.5 mg per deciliter or higher.*

Narins RG, Carley M, Bloom EJ, et al.: The nephrotoxicity of chemotherapeutic agents. Semin Nephrol 10:556, 1990. *This paper provides succinct reviews of the nephrotoxicity associated with several contemporary chemotherapeutic agents (89 references).*

Hainsworth JD, Johnson DH, Porter LL: Nephrotoxicity associated with antineoplastic therapy. *In* McKinney TD (ed.): Renal Complications of Neoplasia. New York, Praeger, 1986. *A thorough review of this topic with a particularly extensive discussion of cisplatin nephrotoxicity (174 references).*

Hande KR: Hyperuricemia, uric acid nephropathy and the tumor lysis syndrome. *In* McKinney TD (ed.): Renal Complications of Neoplasia. New York, Praeger, 1986. *A comprehensive review of this topic (86 references).*

Jorkasky DK, Singer I: Drug-induced tubulo-interstitial nephritis: Special cases. Semin Nephrol 8:62, 1988. *This paper provides a concise review of the nephrotoxicity associated with several drugs, including methotrexate, cisplatin, and the nitrosoureas (118 references).*

Rieselbach RE, Garnick MB: Renal diseases induced by antineoplastic agents. *In* Schrier RW, Gottschalk CW (eds.): Diseases of the Kidney. 4th ed. Boston, Little, Brown and Company, 1988. *This chapter provides a thorough review of this topic (179 references).*

Metal Nephropathies

Cullen MR, Robins JM, Eskenazi B: Adult inorganic lead intoxication: Presentation of 31 new cases and a review of recent advances in the literature. Medicine 62:221, 1983. *This article describes clinical characteristics in 31 patients with lead intoxication resulting from industrial exposure, along with a review of the topic (207 references).*

Falck FY Jr, Keren DF, Fine LJ, et al.: Protein excretion patterns in cadmium exposed individuals. High resolution electrophoresis. Arch Environ Health 39:69, 1984. *In this study, 7 of 39 men chronically exposed to industrial sources of cadmium had mild proteinuria, and 5 had mild elevations of serum creatinine concentrations.*

Katz WA, Blodgett RC Jr, Pietrusko RG: Proteinuria in gold-treated rheumatoid arthritis. Ann Intern Med 101:176, 1984. *In this report, 41 of 1283 (3 per cent) patients receiving oral gold treatments for rheumatoid arthritis developed proteinuria. In 9 this was in the nephrotic range. The results suggest that oral gold is less nephrotoxic than parenteral gold therapy.*

Tubbs RR, Gephardt GN, McMahon JT, et al.: Membranous glomerulonephritis associated with industrial mercury exposure. Am J Clin Pathol 77:409, 1982. *This report describes two patients with industrial exposure to mercury who developed biopsy-proven membranous nephropathy with heavy proteinuria. In one case proteinuria resolved after cessation of exposure to mercury, and this correlated with a decline in urinary mercury excretion from high to normal values.*

Wedeen RP: Heavy metals. *In* Schrier RW, Gottschalk CW (eds.): Diseases of the Kidney. 4th ed. Boston, Little, Brown and Company, 1988. *This chapter reviews the renal complications that may accompany intoxication with several heavy metals (161 references).*

Toxic Nephropathy (Miscellaneous References)

Baldwin DS, Gallo GR, Neugarten J: Drug abuse with narcotics, amphetamines and other agents. *In* Schrier RW, Gottschalk CW (eds.): Diseases of the Kidney. 4th ed. Boston, Little, Brown and Company, 1988. *This chapter provides a good discussion of the several renal complications that may result from drug abuse, along with representative photographs of histopathologic findings (118 references).*

Diamond JC, Cheung JY, Fang LST: Nifedipine-induced renal dysfunction. Am J Med 77:905, 1984. *This paper describes four patients with underlying renal insufficiency who had reversible acute declines in renal function during nifedipine therapy in the absence of hypotension.*

Gabow PA, Clay K, Sullivan JB, et al.: Organic acids in ethylene glycol intoxication. Ann Intern Med 105:16, 1986. *This paper describes three patients with ethylene glycol intoxication, acute renal failure, and metabolic acidosis successfully treated by a combination of ethanol infusion and hemodialysis.*

Hricik DE, Dunn MJ: Angiotensin-converting enzyme inhibitor induced renal failure: Causes, consequences, and diagnostic uses. J Am Soc Nephrol 1:845, 1990. *This is a comprehensive review of this topic. Emphasis is placed both on the renal failure that may accompany administration of this class of drugs in individuals with renovascular disease and the potential use of these agents for diagnosing renovascular disease.*

Krochak RJ, Baker DG: Radiation nephritis: Clinical manifestations and pathophysiologic mechanisms. Urology 27:389, 1986. *A succinct review of this topic.*

Myers BD, Sibley R, Newton L, et al.: The long-term course of cyclosporine-associated chronic nephropathy. Kidney Int 33:590, 1988. *This paper describes the progressive decrease in renal function and the histologic changes occurring in a group of 37 cardiac transplant recipients treated with cyclosporine A. Compared with a group of 24 other patients with other types of immunosuppression treated for the same length of time (24 months), patients treated with cyclosporine A had a higher incidence of hypertension and proteinuria and a lower GFR.*

Ntoso KA, Tomaszewski JE, Jimenez SA, et al.: Penicillamine-induced rapidly progressive glomerulonephritis in patients with progressive systemic sclerosis: Successful treatment of two patients and a review of the literature. Am J Kidney Dis 8:159, 1986. *Two cases of crescentic glomerulonephritis due to penicillamine are described along with a brief review of types of renal disorders that may complicate therapy with this drug.*

Streicher HZ, Gabow PA, Moss AH, et al.: Syndromes of toluene sniffing in adults. Ann Intern Med 94:758, 1981. *Clinical features of 25 cases of toluene sniffing are reported. The most prominent renal-electrolyte manifestation was hyperchloremic metabolic acidosis.*

81 Obstructive Uropathy

Saulo Klahr

Obstructive uropathy refers to the structural or functional changes in the urinary tract that impede the normal flow of urine. It occurs in a wide variety of settings and is a relatively common cause of impaired renal function (obstructive nephropathy). Obstructive uropathy may also cause dilatation of the urinary tract (hydronephrosis). Since the consequences of obstructive uropathy are potentially reversible, prompt diagnosis and appropriate treatment are important to prevent permanent loss of renal function, which is directly related to the degree and duration of the obstruction.

INCIDENCE

Obstructive uropathy, a relatively common disorder, is seen in all age groups. Hydronephrosis has been found at autopsy in 3.5 to 3.8 per cent of adults and in 2 per cent of children, mostly as a consequence of congenital abnormalities of the urinary tract. Urolithiasis occurs predominantly in young adults (ages 25 to 45) and is three times more common in men than in women. In patients older than 60 years, obstructive uropathy is seen more frequently in men than in women owing to benign prostatic hyperplasia and prostatic carcinoma. In 1985, approximately 166 patients per 100,000 population were hospitalized with a presumptive diagnosis of obstruction, and 387 patient visits per 100,000 population were related to obstructive uropathy. Approximately 450,000 surgical procedures for benign prostatic hyperplasia are performed annually in the United States.

ETIOLOGY

Obstruction can occur anywhere in the urinary tract from the renal tubules (uric acid nephropathy) to the urethral meatus (phimosis) (Table 81–1). Clinically, it is helpful to divide the causes of obstruction into *upper urinary tract* (lesions located above the ureterovesical junction) and *lower urinary tract* (below the ureterovesical junction) factors. The causes of upper urinary tract obstruction can be divided into *intrinsic* (intraluminal or intramural) and *extrinsic* (Table 81–1). Intraluminal obstruction is due to stones, clots, or sloughed papillary tissue. Intramural causes are either anatomic (tumors, strictures) or functional (defects in peristalsis: pyeloureteral or vesicoureteral junctions). Extrinsic causes of obstruction can be classified based on the system of origin of the obstructing lesion (Table 81–1).

Clinically, the age and sex of the patient are helpful in narrowing the differential diagnosis. In children, congenital causes of obstructive uropathy are common (stenosis at the ureteropelvic or ureterovesical junction, urethral valves, and so on). In the middle-aged woman, cervical cancer is a common cause of extrinsic ureteral or ureterovesical junction obstruction. In elderly men, benign prostatic hyperplasia and prostatic carcinoma are frequent causes of obstruction.

PATHOLOGY AND PATHOPHYSIOLOGY

The effects of urinary tract obstruction on renal function are due to several factors with complex interactions. Following the

TABLE 81–1. CAUSES OF URINARY TRACT OBSTRUCTION

Upper Urinary Tract	Lower Urinary Tract
A. Intrinsic Causes 1. Intraluminal a. Intratubular deposition of crystals (uric acid, acyclovir) b. Ureter: stones, clots, renal papillae 2. Intramural a. Ureteropelvic or uretero-vesical junction dysfunction b. Ureteral valve, polyp, stricture, or tumor **B. Extrinsic Causes** 1. Vascular system a. Aneurysm: abdominal aorta, iliac vessels b. Aberrant vessels: ureteropelvic junction c. Venous: retrocaval ureter 2. Reproductive system a. Uterus: pregnancy, prolapse, tumors, endometriosis b. Ovary: abscess, tumors, ovarian remnants c. Gartner's duct cyst, tubo-ovarian abscess 3. Gastrointestinal tract: Crohn's disease, diverticulitis, appendiceal abscess, tumors, pancreatic tumor, abscess, or cyst 4. Retroperitoneal disease: a. Retroperitoneal fibrosis (idiopathic, radiation, drugs) b. Inflammatory: tuberculosis, sarcoidosis c. Hematomas d. Primary tumors (lymphoma, sarcoma, and so on) e. Metastatic tumors: cervix, bladder, colon, prostate, and so on) f. Lymphocele g. Pelvic lipomatosis	1. Phimosis, meatal stenosis, paraphimosis 2. Urethra: strictures, stones, diverticulum, posterior or anterior urethral valves, periurethral abscess, urethral surgery 3. Prostate: benign hyperplasia, abscess, carcinoma 4. Bladder a. Neurogenic bladder: spinal cord defect or trauma, diabetes, multiple sclerosis, cerebrovascular accidents, Parkinson's disease b. Bladder neck dysfunction c. Bladder calculus d. Bladder cancer 5. Trauma a. Straddle injury b. Pelvic fracture 6. Drugs: spinal anesthesia, anticholinergics, smooth muscle depressants

onset of obstruction, pressures in the renal pelvis and tubules increase, resulting in dilatation of these structures and flattening of the renal papilla. Renal damage is probably initiated by high intraureteral and high intratubular pressures. Decreases in renal blood flow cause ischemia, cellular atrophy, and necrosis. In addition, parenchymal infiltration by macrophages and T lymphocytes may cause scarring of the kidney. Superimposed infection may accelerate the destruction of the kidney in this setting.

Normal urine flow from the renal pelvis to the bladder depends on ureteral peristalsis and a progressive decrease in hydrostatic pressure from Bowman's space to the renal pelvis. Ureteral peristalsis generates high intraluminal pressures, which propel the bolus of urine along the ureter. Contraction of circular muscle fibers in the ureter prevents transmission of this pressure to the kidney. Impaired urine flow in the urinary tract leads to a rise in the pressure and volume of urine proximal to the obstruction. In this setting, contraction of the circular muscle fibers may be lost, and high intraureteral pressures are transmitted to the kidney. This situation results in increased intratubular pressure. The rise in intratubular pressure without a similar rise in intraglomerular pressure decreases the net hydrostatic filtration pressure across glomerular capillaries, resulting in a fall in the glomerular filtration rate (GFR) (Fig. 81–1).

After the onset of complete obstruction, there is an initial period of renal vasodilatation lasting 1 to 3 hours, which is followed by progressive vasoconstriction of the renal circulation. This renal vasoconstriction leads to a decrease in renal blood flow, a decrease in intraglomerular pressure, and a decrease in the GFR (Fig. 81–1). The vasoconstriction is mediated by angiotensin II and thromboxane A_2. These two compounds, through their effects on mesangial cell contraction, may also decrease the glomerular surface area available for filtration. The decrement in glomerular surface area may explain the greater decrease in the GFR than in renal plasma flow observed in obstruction.

As a consequence of increased intrarenal levels of angiotensin II, there is an increase in the synthesis of prostaglandin E_2 (PGE_2) and prostacyclin. These eicosanoids are vasodilatory substances that also antagonize the effects of angiotensin II on mesangial cell contraction. Hence, in the setting of obstruction, the increased synthesis of both PGE_2 and prostacyclin tends to prevent the GFR and renal blood flow from decreasing further. After the release of obstruction in experimental animals, the administration of inhibitors of prostaglandin synthesis, such as nonsteroidal anti-inflammatory agents, decreases the GFR and renal blood flow.

Partial obstruction of the urinary tract may also decrease renal blood flow and the GFR. In addition, functional tubular defects are prominent. There is an inability to concentrate the urine and a decreased excretion of hydrogen ion and potassium. The concentrating defect is due in part to decreased osmolality of the renal medulla, probably related to decreased sodium reabsorption in the thick ascending limb of Henle's loop, and to the removal of medullary solutes (sodium, urea) as a consequence of the initial increase in medullary blood flow seen in obstruction. A decrease in the hydro-osmotic response of the cortical collecting duct to vasopressin also contributes to the concentrating defect. The decreased hydrogen ion and potassium excretion is due to impaired secretion of these ions in distal segments of the nephron, presumably as a consequence of a diminished response to the action of aldosterone. Secondary to increased tubular pressure and dilatation, there is also disruption of intercellular tight junctions, resulting in increased tubular permeability to solutes and in inhibition of sodium reabsorption.

CLINICAL MANIFESTATIONS

The clinical manifestations of urinary tract obstruction depend on the location (upper or lower urinary tract), degree (complete or partial), and duration (acute or chronic) of the obstruction (Table 81–2).

The symptoms of upper and lower urinary tract obstruction differ. Patients with acute complete obstruction may present with acute renal failure. Patients with chronic partial obstruction (chronic hydronephrosis) may be asymptomatic, may have intermittent pain, or may present with symptoms and laboratory findings of impaired renal function, including inability to concentrate the urine, manifested as nocturia and/or polyuria, with or without elevated levels of blood urea nitrogen (BUN) and serum creatinine.

Pain and Renal Colic

Pain, due to distention of the bladder or to stretching of the collecting system or the renal capsule, is a common presenting symptom in obstructive uropathy, particularly in patients with ureteral calculi. Classic "renal colic" is a steady crescendo, severe pain located in the flank (in the case of stones lodged in the upper third of the ureter) or radiating to the labia, testicles, or groin (stones in the lower two thirds of the ureter) and may be associated with sweating and vomiting. The acute attack may last less than 30 minutes or as long as a day. Pain radiating into the flank during micturition is said to be pathognomonic of vesicoureteral reflux. Chronic partial obstruction may cause intermittent flank pain. Pain may be elicited in some of these patients by administration of diuretics and/or excessive fluid intake. Physical examination may be normal or may reveal flank tenderness in patients with acute upper urinary tract obstruction. In patients with lower urinary tract obstruction, a distended, palpable, and occasionally painful bladder may be found. Careful rectal examination in men or pelvic examination in women should be performed, since it may reveal prostatic enlargement or pelvic masses.

Changes in Urinary Output

Anuria and acute renal failure occur in patients with complete bilateral ureteral obstruction, with complete lower urinary tract obstruction, or with unilateral ureteral obstruction when there is a solitary kidney. In patients with partial or incomplete obstruction of the urinary tract, the urinary output may be normal or increased (polyuria). Occasionally, such patients may develop marked polyuria and increased thirst (a diabetes insipidus–like syndrome). This condition may cause hypernatremia. A pattern of oliguria or anuria alternating with polyuria or the acute onset of anuria strongly suggests the presence of obstructive uropathy.

Hematuria

Gross hematuria may be seen in obstruction, particularly when it is due to stones. In the presence of gross hematuria, clots may cause ureteral obstruction.

Palpable Masses

Longstanding obstructive uropathy may increase kidney size. Such patients may have increased abdominal girth or a palpable flank mass. Hydronephrosis is a common cause of a palpable

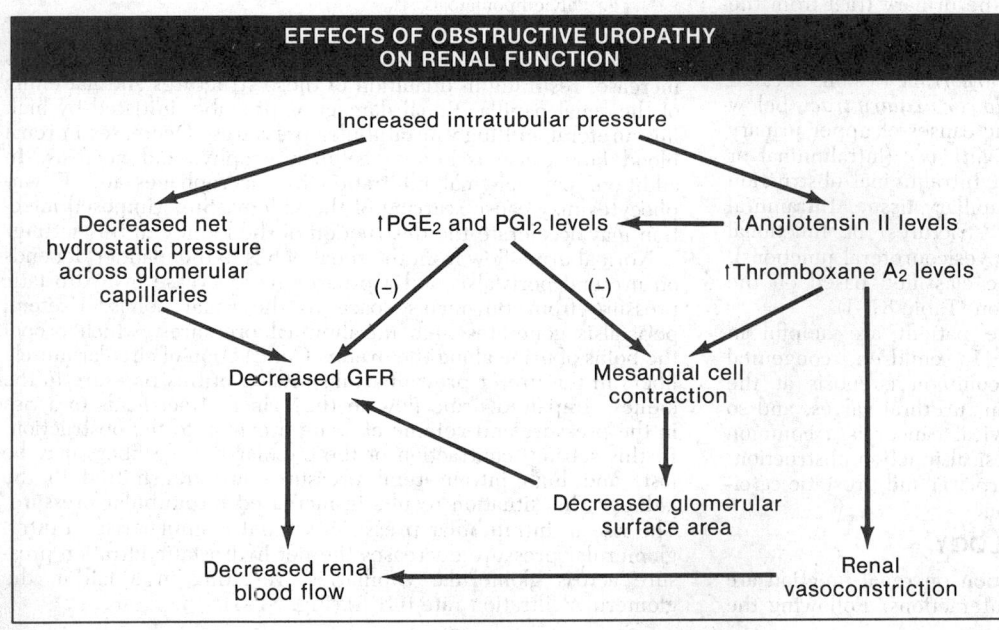

EFFECTS OF OBSTRUCTIVE UROPATHY ON RENAL FUNCTION

FIGURE 81–1. Increased levels of prostaglandin E_2 (PGE_2) and prostacyclin (PGI_2) tend to antagonize (−) the effects of angiotensin II and thromboxane A_2 on mesangial cell contraction and renal vasoconstriction. Hence, they tend to prevent GFR from decreasing further.

TABLE 81–2. CLINICAL MANIFESTATIONS AND LABORATORY FINDINGS IN URINARY TRACT OBSTRUCTION

1. No symptoms (chronic hydronephrosis)
2. Intermittent pain (chronic hydronephrosis)
3. Elevated levels of BUN and serum creatinine with no other symptoms (chronic hydronephrosis)
4. Renal colic (usually due to ureteral stones or papillary necrosis)
5. Changes in urinary output
   a. Anuria or oliguria (acute renal failure)
   b. Polyuria (incomplete or partial obstruction)
   c. Fluctuating urinary output
6. Hematuria
7. Palpable masses
   a. Flank (hydronephrotic kidney; usually in infants)
   b. Suprapubic (distended bladder)
8. Hypertension
   a. Volume dependent (usually due to chronic bilateral obstruction)
   b. Renin dependent (usually due to acute unilateral obstruction)
9. Repeated urinary tract infections or infection that is refractory to treatment
10. Hyperkalemic, hyperchloremic acidosis (usually due to defective tubular secretion of hydrogen and potassium)
11. Hypernatremia (seen in infants with partial obstruction and polyuria)
12. Polycythemia (increased renal production of erythropoietin)
13. Lower urinary tract symptoms: hesitancy, urgency, incontinence, postvoid dribbling, decreased force and caliber of urinary stream, nocturia

abdominal mass in children. In patients with lower urinary tract obstruction, particularly that due to benign prostatic hyperplasia, a suprapubic mass may be caused by a distended bladder. This part of the physical examination should not be neglected in patients with anuria and suspected obstructive uropathy. This type of obstruction is readily reversed by the placement of a catheter in the bladder.

Hypertension

Hypertension is commonly associated with renal disease regardless of its etiology. Patients with urinary tract obstruction may have hypertension due to (1) fluid retention and expansion of the extracellular fluid volume, (2) increased renin secretion, and (3) possibly decreased synthesis of medullary vasodepressor substances. In some patients with obstructive uropathy, the hypertension may be coincidental. Hypertension may occur in about one third of patients with acute unilateral obstruction and is usually, but not always, renin dependent. Release of acute obstruction should ameliorate the hypertension when the two are causally related.

In patients with chronic bilateral obstruction, the hypertension is usually due to impaired sodium excretion and expansion of the extracellular fluid volume (volume-dependent hypertension). In such patients, the circulating levels of renin are usually suppressed.

Urinary Tract Infections or Infection That Is Refractory to Treatment

Repeated urinary tract infections without apparent cause are suggestive of obstruction. Infection is more common in patients with lower urinary tract obstruction. This may be due to decreased bacterial "washout" and increased bacterial adherence to the mucosa of the bladder. Moreover, in the presence of obstruction, eradication of the infection is difficult. In noninstrumented patients, the finding of unusual organisms (Proteus, Pseudomonas) in urine cultures should suggest the presence of underlying obstruction. Thus, in patients with repeated urinary tract infections or persistent infection refractory to treatment, the possibility of underlying urinary tract obstruction should be considered.

Increased Levels of Blood Urea Nitrogen and Serum Creatinine

Obstructive uropathy is a potential cause of impaired renal function and end-stage renal disease and should be considered in the differential diagnosis, particularly in patients with a normal urinary sediment and no previous history of renal disease. Ob-

struction of the urinary tract may occur in patients with established renal parenchymal disease and cause an acceleration in the rate of progression.

Hyperkalemic Hyperchloremic Metabolic Acidosis

A hyperkalemic, hyperchloremic (non–anion gap) metabolic acidosis may be present in patients with urinary tract obstruction. It is seen more frequently in elderly individuals. The abnormality is due to decreased hydrogen ion and potassium secretion by distal segments of the nephron and may be caused by a decrease in aldosterone production and/or refractoriness of the distal tubule to the actions of this mineralocorticoid. Hyperchloremic metabolic acidosis may occur in the absence of hyperkalemia and results from a selective defect in hydrogen ion secretion.

Polycythemia

Polycythemia that subsides after relief of obstruction is a rare manifestation of urinary tract obstruction. Increased renal production of erythropoietin, presumably due to ischemia, may account for the development of polycythemia.

Lower Urinary Tract Symptoms

Patients with obstruction of the lower urinary tract may develop symptoms such as decreased force and caliber of the urine stream, intermittency, incontinence, postvoid dribbling, hesitancy, and urgency. Alterations in the process of micturition due to neurogenic bladder disease may also result in urgency, frequent urination, and urinary incontinence (overflow incontinence).

DIAGNOSTIC APPROACH

The presence of obstructive uropathy may not be obvious. Definitive tests are needed to exclude this diagnosis in suspected cases. Early diagnosis and prompt treatment are essential, since the degree of renal impairment resulting from obstructive uropathy is related to its severity and duration. The diagnostic approach to obstructive uropathy depends on the symptoms and the clinical findings of patients presenting with asymptomatic renal insufficiency, renal colic, or acute renal failure and anuria (Fig. 81–2).

When obstruction is suspected, the history may be of value: previous urinary tract infections, drugs ingested, and the presence of lower urinary tract symptoms (see above). In the hospital setting, the pattern of urinary output can be ascertained from input and output records. The physical examination may yield some clues: tenderness in the costovertebral angle, a mass in the flank area, and muscle rigidity over the kidney area. Abdominal distention and diminished peristalsis accompany acute renal colic. A suprapubic mass may be due to bladder outlet obstruction. The urinalysis may yield important clues: Is there hematuria, bacteriuria, or a urinary pH greater than 7.5 to indicate stones and/or infection with urea-splitting organisms? The urinary sediment should be carefully examined for the presence of crystals (uric acid, cystine, and so forth). Laboratory studies should include an assessment of renal function (BUN, serum creatinine).

The tests utilized to diagnose obstructive uropathy are summarized in Table 81–3. Ultrasound is a noninvasive diagnostic test used as the initial procedure in suspected obstruction. The main finding detected by ultrasound is dilatation of the urinary tract. In a few instances, the ultrasound may give false-negative results because dilatation does not occur as a consequence of dehydration or too recent an onset of obstruction (Fig. 81–2). Plain films of the abdomen (kidneys, ureter, bladder [KUB]) are particularly useful in patients with renal colic because ureteral calculi may be visualized (Fig. 81–2). They also provide information on renal and bladder morphology, such as size differences between the two kidneys or an enlarged bladder suggestive of outlet obstruction. The intravenous pyelogram (IVP) is used to investigate acute renal colic (Fig. 81–2). The excretion of contrast media may be delayed in patients with a low GFR because of a decrease in the filtered load of the dye. In such patients, the procedure should be extended until the collecting system and the site of obstruction are identified. This identification may require obtaining delayed films. The IVP is not useful in patients with compromised renal function, particularly those with serum

TABLE 81–3. DIAGNOSTIC TESTS UTILIZED IN OBSTRUCTIVE UROPATHY

Upper Urinary Tract Obstruction
Sonography (ultrasound)
Plain films of the abdomen (KUB)
Excretory or intravenous pyelography (IVP)
Retrograde pyelography
Isotopic renography
Computed tomography
Magnetic resonance imaging
Pressure flow studies (the Whitaker test)
Lower Urinary Tract Obstruction
Some of the tests listed above
Cystoscopy
Voiding cystourethrogram
Retrograde urethrogram
Urodynamic tests
  Debimetry
  Cystometrography
  Electromyography
  Urethral pressure profile

Reproduced by permission from Klahr S: Obstructive uropathy. *In* Jacobson HR, Striker GE, Klahr S (eds.): The Principles and Practice of Nephrology. Philadelphia, B.C. Decker, 1991, pp 432–441.

creatinine levels greater than 3 to 4 mg per deciliter. It also has the risk of potential nephrotoxicity. *Retrograde pyelography* requires the retrograde injection of radiocontrast and is used to visualize the ureter and collecting system when the IVP cannot be done or is not justified because of a history of allergic reaction to contrast material or other contraindications. This procedure can identify both the site and the cause of the obstruction. *Isotopic renography* can be used to diagnose upper urinary tract obstruction. It requires the intravenous injection of a radionuclide and subsequent imaging with a gamma scintillation camera. This imaging can be combined with intravenous furosemide administered 20 to 30 minutes after injection of the isotope. Other diagnostic procedures for obstructive uropathy include *computed tomography* and *magnetic resonance imaging.* Computed tomography is particularly useful in the diagnosis of causes of obstruction. Occasionally, obstruction of the upper urinary tract is difficult to diagnose using the techniques described above, and *pressure flow studies* (the Whitaker test) may be required. This test consists of measuring pressure differences between the renal pelvis and the bladder during the infusion, at a known rate, of fluid into the renal pelvis.

A number of diagnostic tests are useful in the diagnosis of lower urinary tract obstruction. These include a *voiding cystourethrogram,* which is utilized to investigate the presence of vesicoureteral reflux as a cause of dilatation of the urinary tract. *Cystoscopy* allows visual inspection of the entire urethra and bladder during the same procedure. However, this procedure requires the use of anesthesia in children and young adults. The anterior urethra can be assessed by *retrograde urethrogram,* which is performed by occluding the urethral meatus using a syringe or a catheter and injecting contrast medium. However, a retrograde urethrogram is not adequate to evaluate the posterior urethra. This anatomic area is best examined by an *excretory or retrograde cystogram.* The two tests combined usually provide a complete study of the urethra. *Urodynamic* tests with measurements of urine flow rate per unit time are useful to evaluate bladder outlet obstruction. Measurement of *urine flow rate (debimetry)* is a noninvasive test that examines the interplay between the expulsive force of the detrusor muscle and urethral resistance. *Cystometrography* can be used to assess the force of the detrusor muscle in the bladder, and it quantifies the pressure-volume relationships of this organ. Dyssynergy of the bladder sphincter refers to the inability of the sphincter to relax during contraction of the detrusor muscle and is seen in patients with neurologic disorders. This type of resistance is better analyzed by *electromyography* and *urethral pressure profiles.* About 25 per cent of children with spina bifida have detrusor sphincter dyssynergia at birth.

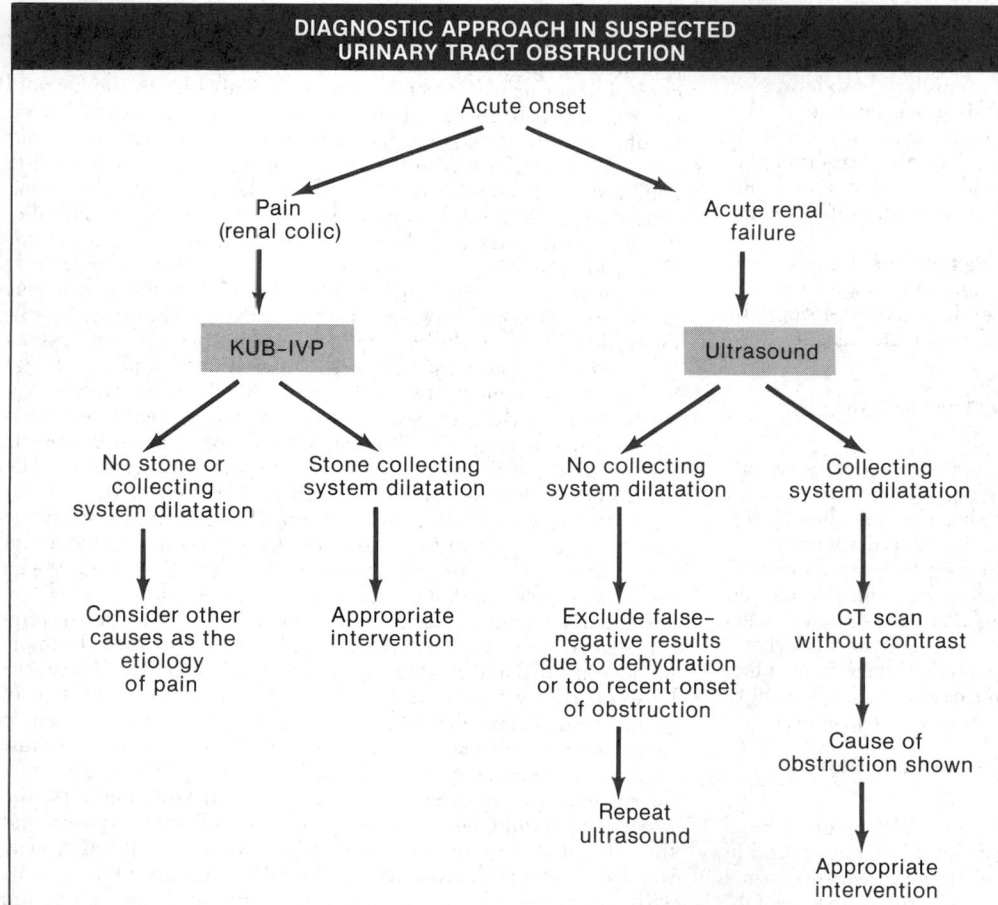

DIAGNOSTIC APPROACH IN SUSPECTED URINARY TRACT OBSTRUCTION

FIGURE 81–2. Scheme of diagnostic approach to urinary tract obstruction. KUB (kidney, ureter, bladder) = a flat film of the abdomen without contrast material; IVP = intravenous pyelography; CT = computed tomography.

TREATMENT

After the diagnosis of obstructive uropathy is established, it is necessary to decide whether or not surgery or instrumentation is required. The goals of therapy are (1) restoration and/or preservation of renal function, (2) relief of pain and/or other symptoms of obstruction, and (3) prevention or eradication of infection.

Acute Obstruction (Complete)

Complete bilateral ureteral obstruction presenting as acute renal failure requires prompt intervention. The site of obstruction determines the approach in these patients. If the obstruction is distal to the bladder, the placement of a urethral catheter may suffice. In some cases a suprapubic cystostomy is required. If the obstruction is located in the upper urinary tract, placement of percutaneous nephrostomy tubes or passage of a retrograde ureteral catheter may be necessary. Nephrostomy tubes not only provide drainage of the urine but also can be used for the local infusion of pharmacologic agents to treat infection, calculi, and so on. In patients with urinary tract infection and generalized sepsis, prompt relief of the obstruction is necessary, and appropriate antibiotic therapy is indicated. Sometimes dialysis may be required prior to instrumentation or surgery in patients with obstruction and acute renal failure.

Acute Obstruction (Partial)

Calculi are the most common cause of ureteral obstruction. Their treatment includes relief of pain, elimination of obstruction, and treatment of infection. Pain can be relieved by intramuscular injection of a narcotic analgesic. Stones less than 5 mm in diameter do not usually require surgical intervention or instrumentation. About 90 per cent of these stones are passed spontaneously. If the stones are 5 to 7 mm, however, only about half will pass, and stones larger than 7 mm usually are not passed spontaneously. High fluid intake to increase the urinary volume to at least 2 liters per day may help to mobilize the stone. The urine must be strained through a gauze sponge to recover the calculi for analysis. If the stone completely occludes the ureter and does not move, surgical treatment is necessary. Endourology refers to the closed controlled manipulation of the entire urinary tract. Endourologic methods can be used in the successful treatment of stones obstructing the ureter in about 98 per cent of patients. In addition, this approach shortens the hospital stay to 3 to 4 days and the convalescence period to only 4 to 7 days. Extracorporeal shock wave or ultrasound lithotripsy involves the focusing of electrohydraulic or ultrasonically generated shock waves to disintegrate the stone. The method is effective for ureteral calculi of 7 to 15 mm that lie above the pelvic brim. The stone is disintegrated in 90 per cent of patients, and all particulate matter passes within a 3-month period. Morbidity is low. However, all patients should be followed up for stone recurrence and should be given preventive therapy. In addition, there is a question of posttreatment hypertension, which requires follow-up. In selected individuals, the procedure can be done on an outpatient basis. Most patients are back at work 2 to 3 days after shock wave therapy. Calculi located distal to the pelvic brim can be approached from below. Antibiotics are useful when infections complicate renal calculi. The choice of antibiotic depends on appropriate urine cultures and sensitivity studies.

Chronic Partial Obstruction

Surgical intervention can be delayed sometimes for weeks or even months in patients with low-grade obstruction or partial chronic obstruction. However, prompt relief of partial obstruction is indicated when (1) there are repeated episodes of urinary tract infection, (2) the patient has significant symptoms (dysuria, voiding dysfunction, flank pain), (3) there is urinary retention, or (4) there is evidence of recurrent or progressive renal damage.

Lower Urinary Tract Obstruction

Urethral and bladder neck obstruction requires surgery in patients with recurrent infections who are ambulatory, particularly when reflux, renal parenchymal damage, marked urinary retention, repeated bleeding, or other symptoms are present. Obstruction secondary to benign prostatic hyperplasia is not always progressive. Therefore, a patient with minimal symptoms, no infection, and a normal upper urinary tract may be followed safely until he or she and the physician agree that surgery is desirable. Urethral strictures in men can be treated by dilatation or direct visual internal urethrotomy. The incidence of bladder neck and urethral obstruction in women is low. Hence, urethral dilatation, internal urethrotomy, meatotomy, and revision of the bladder neck in women are seldom indicated.

When obstruction is the result of neuropathic bladder function, dynamic studies are essential to determine therapy. The main goals of therapy should be (1) to establish the bladder as a urine storage organ without causing renal injury and (2) to provide a mechanism for bladder emptying that is acceptable to the patient. Patients fall into two categories, those with atonic bladders secondary to lower motor neuron injury and those with unstable bladder function due to upper motor neuron disease. The neurogenic bladder seen in diabetes mellitus is usually the result of lower motor neuron disease. Requesting these patients to void at regular intervals achieves satisfactory emptying of the bladder. Occasionally, these individuals respond to cholinergic agents, such as bethanechol chloride (Urecholine). Alpha-adrenergic blockers relax urethral sphincter tone but have only limited success because of side effects. The best treatment for patients with significant residual urine and recurrent urosepsis is the establishment of clean, intermittent self-catheterization at regular intervals. The goal is to catheterize four or five times per day so that the amount of urine drained from the bladder does not exceed 400 ml. This technique may be successful but requires the patient's acceptance and adequate training. In patients with a hypertonic bladder, the major goal is to improve its storage function. The use of anticholinergic agents may be indicated. Occasionally, chronic, clean, intermittent self-catheterization is necessary. In all patients with neurogenic bladders, chronic indwelling catheters should be avoided if possible, owing to risk of infection and other complications.

POSTOBSTRUCTIVE DIURESIS

Postobstructive diuresis refers to the marked natriuresis and diuresis that occasionally follow the relief of obstruction. This diuresis is characterized by excretion of large amounts of sodium, potassium, magnesium, and other solutes. Although usually self-limited, the losses of solutes and water may result in hypokalemia, hyponatremia or hypernatremia, hypomagnesemia, and marked volume depletion. In many patients, a brisk diuresis after relief of obstruction may represent a physiologic response to expansion of the extracellular fluid volume occurring during the period of obstruction. This postobstructive diuresis is appropriate and does not compromise the volume status of the patient. Postobstructive diuresis in this setting can be prolonged by overzealous replacement of salt and water after relief of obstruction.

Fluid replacement is justified only when excessive losses of sodium and water occur that are inappropriate for the volume status of the patient and are presumably due to an intrinsic tubular defect in sodium and water reabsorption. Fluid replacement in these patients is guided in large part by what is excreted. Intravenous fluid administration may be necessary, but urinary losses should be replaced only to the extent necessary to prevent extracellular fluid volume contraction or electrolyte imbalance.

PROGNOSIS

The return of renal function after relief of obstruction is variable and is influenced by the severity and duration of obstruction. Other events that condition the degree of recovery of renal function include the presence of infection, stones, pre-existing renal disease, and/or the underlying cause of the obstruction. Renal cortical thickness is a prognostic indicator of residual renal function in patients with chronic hydronephrosis. Patients with a very thin cortex have lost considerable renal function.

In experimental animals, the GFR reached 70 per cent of normal 2 years after relief of ureteral obstruction of 1 week's duration, 50 per cent of normal after 2 weeks of obstruction, and 20 per cent of normal after 4 weeks of obstruction. In rats with unilateral ureteral obstruction of 24 hours' duration, 15 per cent of nephrons were nonfunctional 2 months after relief of obstruction. The normalization of the GFR in these animals was due to hyperfiltration in the remaining functional nephrons. If similar changes occur in humans, short-term obstruction may result in loss of functional nephrons, which may go undetected because the GFR returns to normal owing to hyperfiltration in the remaining nephrons.

Klahr S, Bander SJ: Obstructive nephropathy. In Massry SG, Glassock RJ (eds.): Textbook of Nephrology. Vol I. 2nd ed. Orlando, Fla., The Williams and Wilkins Company, 1989, pp 889–909. *A recent and detailed discussion of clinical, pathologic, and diagnostic issues in obstructive nephropathy.*

Klahr S, Clayman RV, Bahnson RR: Obstructive uropathy. In Glassock RJ (ed.) Current Therapy in Nephrology and Hypertension. Vol 2. Toronto, B.C. Decker Publishers, 1987, pp 67–72. *Discusses the therapeutic approach to the patient with urinary tract obstruction or postobstructive diuresis.*

Klahr S, Harris K, Purkerson ML: Effects of obstructive uropathy on renal functions. Pediatr Nephrol 2:34, 1988. *A recent review on the pathophysiology of obstructive nephropathy with numerous references.*

82 Specific Renal Tubular Disorders

Martin G. Cogan

The diverse reabsorptive functions of the kidney are generally segregated so that specific nephron segments are responsible for specific transport functions. As described in Ch. 73, the proximal nephron is responsible for the reabsorption of most of the filtered bicarbonate, glucose, amino acids, uric acid, phosphate, and low molecular weight proteins. The loop of Henle reabsorbs over half the filtered sodium chloride as well as divalent cations. The distal nephron (including the cortical and medullary collecting ducts), under the influence of aldosterone, reabsorbs the final quantity of sodium and secretes hydrogen and potassium ions. The terminal collecting ducts can be induced by antidiuretic hormone to permit water reabsorption and thereby cause urinary concentration.

Genetic and acquired conditions can affect one or more of the reabsorptive or secretory transport processes within each of these nephron segments, as illustrated in Table 82–1. Depending on the transport sites affected, these diseases lead to abnormal wastage or retention of specific solutes. For instance, within a given nephron segment, there may be a selective transport defect for a single solute (e.g., bicarbonate in proximal renal tubular acidosis or glucose in renal glycosuria) or for a class of solutes (e.g., dibasic amino acids in cystinuria). Alternatively, those solutes whose transport is modulated by a specific hormone may be affected by a hormone-deficient or -resistant state (e.g., in hypoaldosteronism or diabetes insipidus). Finally, there are diseases that affect all solutes normally transported by a given nephron segment (e.g., all proximal transported solutes in Fanconi's syndrome). Luminal, cellular, or peritubular components of the overall transport process can be responsible for each of these situations. The following sections, and other chapters as identified in Table 82–1, describe some of the more common transport defects of the individual nephron segments.

DISORDERS OF PROXIMAL NEPHRON FUNCTION

The proximal nephron is responsible for reabsorbing 80 to 99 per cent of several filtered solutes, including glucose, amino acids, and bicarbonate. Detection of one or more of these solutes in the urine at normal filtered loads implies a disorder of proximal transport.

Renal Glycosurias

The renal glycosurias are caused by inherited or acquired defects in proximal tubule glucose reabsorption such that glycosuria occurs in the absence of hyperglycemia.

PATHOPHYSIOLOGY. Glucose is reabsorbed across the luminal membrane of the proximal tubule by a stereospecific carrier that requires sodium. The amount of glucose reabsorbed changes in proportion to filtered glucose load until a maximal reabsorptive capacity, or "Tm," is reached, as shown in Figure 82–1. Some-

what before saturation is attained, glucose reabsorption is incomplete, representing the "splay" in the response. The initial point of the splay represents that filtered glucose concentration or load, called the "threshold," at which reabsorption no longer equals filtration and glucose appears in the urine. The normal threshold concentration is 200 to 240 mg per deciliter, well above the normal plasma glucose concentration, so little glucose (< 125 mg per day) appears in the urine of a normal individual. The kinetics of glucose reabsorption have been compared with the behavior of an enzyme system: The Tm is equivalent to the $\dot{V}$max, whereas the Km is related to the degree of splay. In the two major types of renal glycosurias, either the capacity (type A, $\dot{V}$max or Tm mutation) or the affinity (type B, Km, or degree of splay mutation) of glucose reabsorption is altered (Fig. 82–1). In either case, the threshold is reduced, so that glucose is spilled into the urine at a normal plasma glucose concentration. The glycosuria is markedly exaggerated when filtered glucose concentration is elevated by intravenous hypertonic glucose infusion.

SYMPTOMS AND ETIOLOGIES. Renal glycosurias (Table 82–1) are relatively unusual, with a prevalence (depending on the stringency of diagnostic criteria) of about 0.2 to 0.6 per cent. They are usually inherited in an autosomal recessive manner. Homozygotes have more severe glycosuria than heterozygotes. Usually, but not invariably, $\dot{V}$max and Km variants of the syndrome are inherited separately. On renal biopsy, there are no consistent distinguishing pathologic features. In contrast to the aminoacidurias, there is no coexisting intestinal transport defect for glucose. Renal glycosuria is completely asymptomatic (i.e., affected individuals do not have polydipsia or polyuria).

Intermittent glycosuria is not unusual during pregnancy (second and third trimesters) and during the terminal phases of chronic renal insufficiency. In both cases, an increase in tubular flow rate, due to an increase in total or in single-nephron glomerular filtration rate (GFR), is probably the primary cause of the functional alteration in glucose transport kinetics. In a rare syndrome in children, malabsorption of two sugars, glucose and galactose, in both the jejunum and the kidney, causes diarrhea and mellituria.

DIAGNOSIS AND TREATMENT. Diagnosis should be based on finding a urinary glucose excretion of greater than 500 mg per 24 hours (on a diet containing 30 kcal per kilogram, of which 50 per cent is carbohydrate) in the absence of hyperglycemia (plasma glucose < 140 mg per deciliter). The glucose oxidase method should be used to confirm that the excreted sugar is glucose in order to exclude other mellituric conditions (pentosuria, fructosuria, sucrosuria, maltosuria, galactosuria, and lactosuria). Appropriate tests should be performed to rule out coexistent tubular transport defects (of amino acids, bicarbonate, phosphate, and uric acid) typical of the Fanconi syndrome, and diabetes mellitus must be excluded, using standard clinical and laboratory evidence. If desired, differentiation of the $\dot{V}$max or Km variants can be accomplished by glucose loading.

The condition is completely benign with respect to symptoms and to renal functional deterioration. Treatment is unnecessary. Prolonged fasting should be avoided to prevent the unusual complication of hypoglycemia and ketosis.

Renal Aminoacidurias

The renal aminoacidurias are inherited disorders in which one or a group of amino acids are excreted by the kidney (in the absence of hyperaminoacidemia) and are usually also malabsorbed by the intestine (Table 82–1).

GENERAL CONSIDERATIONS. Amino acids are avidly reabsorbed in the proximal nephron, so that only about 2 per cent of the filtered amino acid load is excreted in the urine (except for glycine, 5 per cent, and histidine, 8 per cent). In general, most amino acids are transported by a stereospecific carrier across the luminal membrane of the proximal nephron, accompanied by sodium and driven by the lumen-to-cell sodium concentration gradient. Under some circumstances, amino acids can also be secreted. Reabsorptive kinetics are similar to those of glucose (Fig. 82–1). Five major luminal membrane carriers for reabsorption exist, each of which transports a specific group of amino acids: basic amino acids (cystine, lysine, arginine, and ornithine); acidic amino acids (glutamic and aspartic acids); neutral amino acids (alanine, serine, threonine, valine, leucine, isoleucine, phenylalanine, tyrosine, tryptophan, and histidine); iminoglycine amino acids (proline, hydroxyproline, and glycine); and

TABLE 82–1. CLINICAL SYNDROMES ASSOCIATED WITH NEPHRON TRANSPORT DEFECTS

Proximal Nephron

I. *Selective transport defects*
   A. Renal glycosurias
      1. Primary
      2. Combined:
         a. Glucose/galactose malabsorption
         b. Glucoglycinuria
   B. Renal aminoacidurias
      1. Basic aminoacidurias
         a. General: cystinuria (cystine, lysine, arginine, ornithine)
         b. Specific: hypercystinuria, dibasic aminoaciduria (lysine, arginine, ornithine), lysinuria
      2. Neutral aminoacidurias
         a. General: Hartnup disease
         b. Specific: methioninuria, tryptophanuria, histidinuria
      3. Iminoglycinuria
         a. General (proline, hydroxyproline, glycine)
         b. Specific: glycinuria
      4. Dicarboxylic aminoaciduria
         a. General (glutamic, aspartic acids)
   C. Proximal renal tubular acidosis
      1. Primary: idiopathic or genetic
      2. Transient (infants)
      3. Carbonic anhydrase deficiency, inhibition, alteration
         a. Drugs: acetazolamide, sulfanilamide, mafenide acetate
         b. Idiopathic?
   D. Renal uric acid disorders (see Ch. 183, 184)
   E. Phosphate and calcium disorders (see Ch. 234, 235)
II. *Nonselective transport defects: Fanconi's syndrome*
   A. Primary: idiopathic or genetic
   B. Genetically transmitted systemic diseases
      1. Cystinosis
      2. Lowe's syndrome
      3. Wilson's disease
      4. Tyrosinemia
      5. Hereditary fructose intolerance
      6. Pyruvate carboxylase deficiency
   C. Dysproteinemic states
      1. Multiple myeloma
      2. Monoclonal gammopathy
   D. Secondary hyperparathyroidism with chronic hypocalcemia
      1. Vitamin D deficiency or resistance
      2. Vitamin D dependency
   E. Drugs and toxins
      1. Outdated tetracycline
      2. Methyl-3-chromone
      3. Streptozotocin
      4. Glue
      5. Gentamicin
   F. Heavy metals
      1. Lead
      2. Cadmium
      3. Mercury
   G. Tubulointerstitial diseases
      1. Sjögren's syndrome
      2. Medullary cystic disease
      3. Renal transplantation
   H. Other diseases
      1. Nephrotic syndrome
      2. Amyloidosis
      3. Osteopetrosis
      4. Paroxysmal nocturnal hemoglobinuria

Loop of Henle

I. *Bartter's syndrome*
II. *Drugs*
   A. Furosemide
   B. Bumetanide
   C. Ethacrynic acid

Distal Nephron

I. *Selective transport defects*
   A. Classic distal RTA
      1. Primary: genetic or idiopathic
      2. Genetically transmitted systemic diseases
         a. Ehlers-Danlos syndrome
         b. Hematologic disorders: hereditary elliptocytosis, sickle cell anemia, carbonic anhydrase I deficiency or alteration
         c. Medullary cystic disease
         d. With nerve deafness
         e. Glycogenosis type III
      3. Autoimmune diseases
         a. Hypergammaglobulinemia: hyperglobulinemic purpura, cryoglobulinemia, familial
         b. Sjögren's syndrome
         c. Thyroiditis
         d. Pulmonary fibrosis
         e. Chronic active hepatitis
         f. Primary biliary cirrhosis
         g. Systemic lupus erythematosus
      4. Diseases associated with nephrocalcinosis
         a. Primary hyperparathyroidism
         b. Vitamin D intoxication
         c. Hyperthyroidism
         d. Hypercalciuria: idiopathic or genetic
         e. Hereditary fructose intolerance
         f. Medullary sponge kidney
         g. Fabry's disease
         h. Wilson's disease
      5. Drug or toxic nephropathies
         a. Amphotericin B
         b. Toluene
         c. Glue
         d. Analgesics
         e. Cyclamate
      6. Tubulointerstitial diseases
         a. Chronic pyelonephritis secondary to urolithiasis
         b. Obstructive uropathy
         c. Renal transplantation
         d. Leprosy
         e. Hyperoxaluria
      7. Miscellaneous
   B. RTA of glomerular insufficiency
   C. Hypermineralocorticoid and other potassium secretory disorders (see Ch. 217)
II. *Nonselective transport defects: generalized distal RTA, hyperkalemia, and renal salt wasting*
   A. Primary mineralocorticoid deficiency (see Ch. 217)
   B. Hypoangiotensinemia
      1. Converting enzyme inhibitors: captopril, enalapril
      2. Angiotensin receptor blockers
   C. Hyporeninemic hypoaldosteronism
      1. Diabetic nephropathy
      2. Tubulointerstitial nephropathies
      3. Nephrosclerosis
      4. Nonsteroidal anti-inflammatory agents
      5. Acquired immunodeficiency syndrome (AIDS)
   D. Mineralocorticoid-resistant hyperkalemia
      1. Without salt wasting: genetic
      2. With salt wasting
         a. Childhood forms
         b. Tubulointerstitial nephropathies: methicillin, obstructive nephropathy, transplantation, sickle cell disease, cyclosporine
         c. Drugs: spironolactone, amiloride, triamterene

Loop and Medullary Collecting Ducts

I. *Diabetes insipidus* (see Ch. 214)
II. *SIADH* (see Ch. 214)
III. *Other concentrating and diluting disorders*

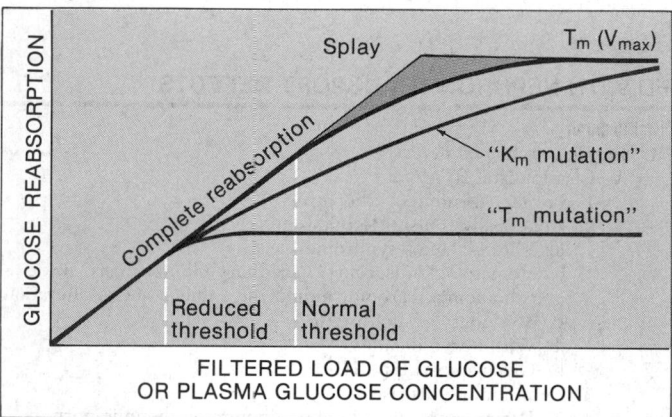

FIGURE 82–1. Kinetics of renal glucose reabsorption and the two variants of renal glycosuria. (Modified from Cogan MG: Disorders of proximal nephron function. Am J Med 72:278, 1982; with permission.)

beta-amino acids (beta-aminoisobutyric acid, beta-alanine, and taurine). Inherited dysfunction of a carrier results in urinary loss of the entire amino acid group: cystinuria (basic aminoaciduria); dicarboxylic aminoaciduria; Hartnup disease (neutral aminoaciduria); and iminoglycinuria. There is no clinical disorder yet described of beta-amino acid transport. There are also other carriers (>25 are estimated to exist) that selectively transport only one or several members of a given amino acid group. Disorders of these carriers cause even more selective aminoaciduria: hypercystinuria, histidinuria, and lysinuria.

Many of the amino acid carriers in the proximal nephron are also expressed on the luminal membrane of gastrointestinal epithelial cells. Defective gastrointestinal absorption therefore occurs conjointly with increased renal excretion of the amino acid or acids in question. Amino acid dimers can be normally absorbed by the gut, however, so that nutritional problems arising from amino acid malabsorption are unusual. Furthermore, gut absorption is not so constrained by time as that in the renal tubule, i.e., does not require such rapid response.

For diagnosis of a renal aminoaciduria, a high plasma level of the amino acid must first be excluded. Excessive filtration of an amino acid can overwhelm the tubular transport carrier for it and other members of its amino acid family and result in one or more aminoacidurias. These "overflow" aminoacidurias are discussed in Ch. 176 to 181. By contrast, the renal aminoacidurias are associated with low or normal levels of plasma amino acid concentrations because the aminoaciduria is due to defective proximal tubular transport.

CYSTINURIA. One of the most common aminoacidurias is *cystinuria* (basic aminoaciduria), an autosomal recessive disease estimated to affect about 1:7000 individuals (between 1:1000 and 1:20,000, depending on the population studied). Urinary spillage of lysine, arginine, and ornithine is asymptomatic. Cystine, however, is the least soluble of naturally occurring amino acids, and it therefore tends to precipitate to form cystine urolithiasis. Cystinuria accounts for about 1 to 2 per cent of all urinary calculi. Stone formation usually becomes manifest during the second and third decades of life, though presentation may occur from infancy to the ninth decade, and males are more severely affected. Cystine stones are yellow-brown and have a granular appearance. Such stones are radiopaque, can create staghorn calculi, and frequently form a nidus for calcium oxalate stone formation. Symptoms include renal colic, which may be associated with obstruction or infection or both. Evidence associating cystinuria with central nervous system disorders has been tenuous. A more general discussion of nephrolithiasis is found in Ch. 88.

The diagnosis of cystinuria should be considered in any patient with a renal calculus, even if the stone is composed primarily of calcium oxalate (since cystine might have been the formation nidus). The typical hexagonal crystals may be recognized on urinalysis, especially in a concentrated, acidic, early morning specimen. A useful screening test is the cyanide-nitroprusside test, which detects a cystine concentration of about 75 to 125 mg

per liter. Because of false-positive results, a definitive diagnosis requires thin-layer or ion-exchange chromatography or high-voltage electrophoresis. Excretion ratios in an adult of greater than 18 mg of cystine per gram of creatinine confirm the diagnosis. The dibasic amino acids will also be increased in excretion per gram of creatinine: lysine >130 mg; arginine >16 mg; and ornithine >22 mg. Persons with homozygous cystinuria routinely excrete more than 250 mg of cystine per gram of creatinine, usually about 0.5 to 1.0 gram per day. Cystinuria has three allelic variants, classified according to whether coexisting intestinal and renal basic amino acid transport is completely absent (types I and II) or variably reduced (type III) and whether heterozygotes have normal (type I) or supernormal (types II and III) urinary cystine and basic aminoaciduria.

Medical therapy of cystinuria is aimed at decreasing the urinary concentration below the solubility limit of 300 mg of cystine per liter. The most practical approach is to increase fluid intake to about 3 to 4 liters per day. The polyuria must be maintained at all times, including nighttime, when the urine otherwise tends to become concentrated and acidic. Cystine solubility can also be increased by alkalinizing urinary pH, but a urinary pH of greater than 7.5 is necessary to achieve a salutary effect. Avoidance of excessive intake of methionine, the metabolic precursor of cystine, is a reasonable adjunctive therapy but is ineffective as a sole therapy. When conservative measures fail, D-penicillamine is recommended, usually in a dose of 1 to 2 grams per day. This drug forms a mixed disulfide of penicillamine-cysteine, which is much more soluble than cystine alone. Free cystine excretion then falls to an acceptable level. Unfortunately, penicillamine causes fever and a rash in as many as 50 per cent of patients, and sometimes arthralgias and severe hypersensitivity reactions. In some cases the drug can be readministered at a lower dose following an adverse reaction. Pyridoxine should be given as a supplement, since penicillamine can deplete this cofactor. Other investigational agents, such as N-acetyl-D-penicillamine, mercaptopropionylglycine, glutamine, and chlordiazepoxide, have also been found to reduce cystine excretion.

HARTNUP DISEASE. Hartnup disease, a neutral aminoaciduria, is a rare autosomal recessive disorder (1:16,000 births) in which the clinical presentation is dominated by nicotinamide deficiency. Since up to 50 per cent of nicotinamide is normally supplied by metabolism of tryptophan, malabsorption and renal loss of tryptophan contribute to nicotinamide deficiency, especially when dietary nicotinamide is insufficient. Thus, this disorder exemplifies the importance of both the intestinal and the renal transport defects. Clinical signs of nicotinamide deficiency are intermittent and usually worse in children and include pellagra in sun-exposed areas, cerebellar ataxia, and sometimes psychiatric disturbance.

Hartnup disease should be suspected in a patient with pellagra or cerebellar symptoms who does not have a history of niacin deficiency. The diagnosis can be confirmed by chromatography of the urine. Sibs of an affected individual should be examined for heterozygosity. Supplemental nicotinamide (40 to 250 mg per day) suffices to prevent pellagra and neurologic problems.

OTHER AMINOACIDURIAS. Less common aminoacidurias lacking clinical manifestations include iminoglycinuria, isolated hypercystinuria (without hyperexcretion of other basic amino acids), isolated glycinuria, and dicarboxylic aminoaciduria. Mental retardation predominates in the rare disorders of hyperdibasic aminoaciduria, isolated lysinuria, histidinuria, and methioninuria.

Proximal Renal Tubular Acidosis (RTA)

Proximal RTA is a hyperchloremic, hypokalemic metabolic acidosis caused by a selective defect in proximal acidification, which is characterized by a normally acidic urine during acidosis but marked bicarbonate wasting when plasma bicarbonate concentration is normalized.

PATHOPHYSIOLOGY. The proximal nephron reabsorbs 85 to 90 per cent of the filtered bicarbonate, predominantly by Na^+/H^+ exchange and the enzymatic degradation of H_2CO_3 to CO_2 and H_2O by carbonic anhydrase (Fig. 82–2). Interference with the normal operation of Na^+/H^+ exchange or of carbonic anhydrase activity therefore results in excess delivery of bicarbonate to the distal nephron and, because of the limited distal bicarbonate reabsorption capacity, into the urine. Thus, the

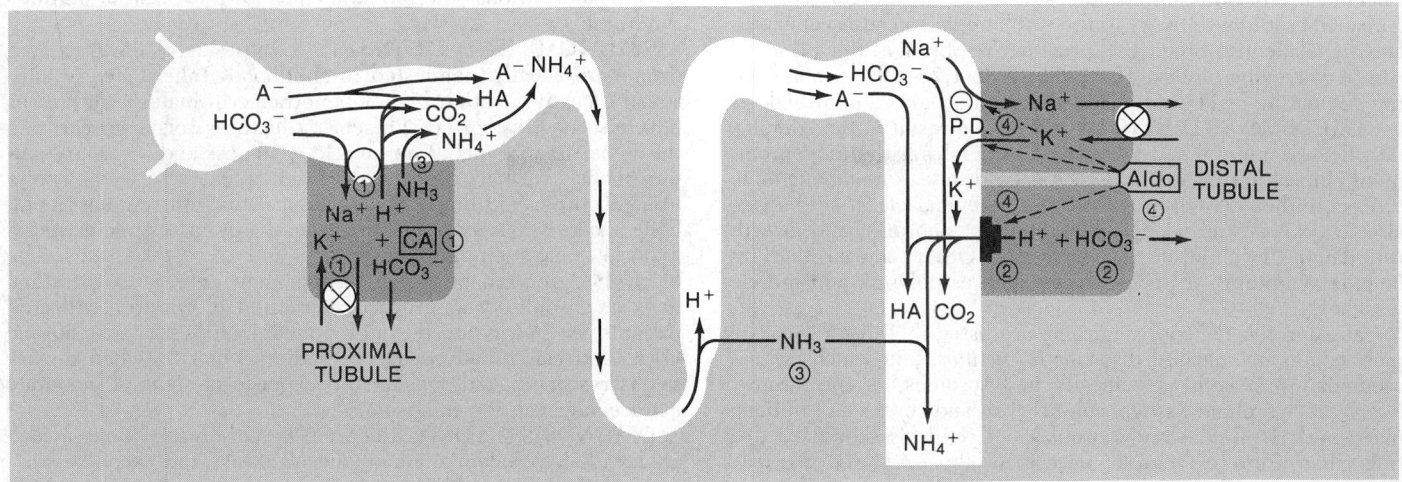

FIGURE 82–2. Sites of impaired renal acidification (RTA). The proximal tubule reabsorbs most of the filtered bicarbonate by hydrogen ion secretion. Proximal acidification is dependent on sodium and carbonic anhydrase and is energetically driven by the lumen-to-cell sodium gradient. Disorders of proximal acidification, proximal RTA, may result from defects (labeled 1) in the Na^+/H^+ exchanger, carbonic anhydrase activity, or the activity of the basolateral Na^+-K^+ ATPase. The distal nephron is regulated by aldosterone to reabsorb sodium and secrete hydrogen ions. Distal acidification is responsible for titrating both remaining filtered buffer (labeled A^-) to form titratable acids (HA) and proximally produced ammonia (NH_3) to form ammonium (NH_4^+). Disorders of distal acidification include defects of the proton pump or basolateral bicarbonate exit step (labeled 2) in classic distal RTA, in ammonia production or delivery (labeled 3) in the RTA of glomerular insufficiency, or in aldosterone levels or target sites (labeled 4) in generalized distal RTA.

urinary wastage of 15 per cent or more of the filtered bicarbonate load at a normal blood bicarbonate concentration is pathognomonic of proximal renal tubular acidosis (RTA). The excess delivery of the relatively impermeant bicarbonate to the distal nephron also results in accelerated potassium secretion and hypokalemia. As the plasma bicarbonate concentration and filtered load fall owing to defective proximal bicarbonate reabsorption and subsequent urinary bicarbonate wastage, absolute bicarbonate delivery to the distal nephron progressively decreases. At a certain point, usually when the plasma bicarbonate concentration is 15 to 18 mM, the distal nephron can cope with the delivery from the proximal tubule. At this stage, bicarbonaturia disappears, urinary pH can be lowered normally, and net acid excretion is equivalent to endogenous acid production. Acid-base homeostasis is re-established at the expense of metabolic acidosis.

SYMPTOMS AND ETIOLOGIES. Manifestations of proximal RTA are attributable to acidemia (growth retardation, anorexia and malnutrition, volume depletion), potassium depletion (muscular weakness, polyuria, nocturia, polydipsia), and disordered calcium/phosphate/parathormone/vitamin D metabolism (osteomalacia and other bone diseases). Proximal RTA is a rare disorder, usually found when carbonic anhydrase is defective or is inhibited, or in conjunction with the full Fanconi syndrome (Table 82–1).

DIAGNOSIS AND TREATMENT. Laboratory findings of proximal RTA are those of a hyperchloremic, hypokalemic metabolic acidosis. When the patient is acidemic, the urine is acidic and net acid excretion equals endogenous acid load (Table 82–2). When bicarbonate is infused to normalize the plasma bicarbonate concentration, massive bicarbonaturia results (≥ 15 per cent of the filtered load). Proximal RTA is usually not isolated but rather associated with the full Fanconi syndrome.

Therapy of the underlying disease should be undertaken if possible (e.g., multiple myeloma) or offending drugs or toxins discontinued (e.g., heavy metals). When this is not possible, proximal RTA is treated with large amounts of sodium and potassium bicarbonate. As the plasma bicarbonate concentration rises with treatment, distal bicarbonate delivery increases, causing more potassium wasting and the need for further potassium supplementation. Because of the inability to correct the disorder fully with bicarbonate alone, volume contraction utilizing diuretics, especially thiazides, is also used to stimulate fractional proximal bicarbonate reabsorption. Therapy with vitamin D is indicated when signs of vitamin D deficiency exist.

Nonselective Proximal Nephron Dysfunction: The Fanconi Syndrome

In the Fanconi syndrome, the entire array of proximal transport functions is impaired, resulting in glycosuria, generalized aminoaciduria, proximal RTA, phosphaturia, and uricaciduria.

PATHOPHYSIOLOGY. The lumen-to-cell sodium gradient provides the driving force in the proximal tubule for the absorption of glucose, amino acids, phosphate, and organic acids and for secretion of hydrogen ions needed to reabsorb bicarbonate. Disruption of this common driving force serves as an attractive hypothesis to explain the global functional impairment of reabsorption of solutes in the proximal tubule observed in the Fanconi syndrome. Collapse of the sodium gradient could arise by several mechanisms: a primary disturbance of the Na^+-K^+ adenosinetriphosphatase (ATPase), increased permeability of the cell to sodium, or reduced metabolic energy due to an abnormality in the redox potential or in intracellular phosphate supply.

In addition to the solutes described above, there is disordered reabsorption, and sometimes depressed serum concentrations, of

TABLE 82–2. RENAL TUBULAR ACIDOSES

Type	Renal Defect	GFR	Plasma [K⁺]	Proximal Acidification HCO₃⁻ Reabsorption (During HCO₃⁻ Loading)	Distal Acidification Minimal Urinary pH (During Acidosis)	UAG ≈ − Urine [NH₄⁺] (During Acidosis)
Proximal	↓ Proximal acidification	N	↓	↓	< 5.5	0 or +
Classic distal	↓ Distal pH gradient	N	↓	N	> 5.5	0 or +
Glomerular insufficiency	↓ NH₃ production	↓	N	N	< 5.5	0 or +
Generalized distal	↓ Aldosterone action	↓	↑	N	< 5.5	0 or +

N = normal; UAG = urinary anion gap = [Na] + [K] − [Cl] ≈ − [NH₄]; GFR = glomerular filtration rate.

calcium, magnesium, citrate, and low molecular weight proteins. Enhanced sodium delivery to the distal nephron causes kaliuresis and hypokalemia. Since the proximal nephron is the principal site of conversion of 25-OH vitamin D to 1,25-$(OH)_2$ vitamin D, the circulating level of this latter hormone is also diminished.

SYMPTOMS AND ETIOLOGIES. As a result of the complex disorders of mineral and vitamin D metabolism, the most prominent clinical finding of the Fanconi syndrome is metabolic bone disease, either rickets in children or osteomalacia in adults (see also Ch. 234). Nausea, episodic vomiting, anorexia, and growth retardation in children are frequent. Other clinical findings include symptoms of hypokalemia, such as polyuria and muscle weakness.

Causes of the Fanconi syndrome are listed in Table 82–1. The most common inherited disorder is *cystinosis,* in which cystine accumulates in cells, specifically in lysosomes, of the kidney, liver, gut, lymphoid tissues, conjunctiva, and cornea and in bone marrow–derived cells and fibroblasts. Cystinosis should be distinguished from cystinuria, described above. Cystinosis may present as the Fanconi syndrome, followed by renal failure, in the first 2 years of life (infantile nephropathic form) or in the adolescent years. It is usually relatively benign if it first appears in adulthood, causing only asymptomatic cystine deposits in the conjunctiva, cornea, and bone marrow. An interesting inducible form of the Fanconi syndrome is *hereditary fructose intolerance* (HFI), caused by a deficiency of aldolase B activity. Ingestion of fructose in affected individuals causes acute symptoms, including nausea, vomiting, abdominal pain, and neurologic dysfunction (Ch. 170).

In adults, acquired Fanconi's syndrome is most often caused by dysproteinemias, heavy metal (especially chronic cadmium or acute lead) exposure, or immunologic diseases (Table 82–1). An older adult presenting with the Fanconi syndrome should be assumed to have multiple myeloma until proved otherwise.

DIAGNOSIS AND TREATMENT. Diagnosis of the Fanconi syndrome is established by finding consequences of the full array of proximal nephron dysfunction: glycosuria, generalized aminoaciduria, proximal RTA, phosphaturia, hypouricemia, hypovitaminosis D, and secondary hypokalemia. Underlying causes of the Fanconi syndrome (Table 82–1) should be sought. Serum and urine electrophoresis should be obtained in adults to rule out multiple myeloma.

Treatment of the Fanconi syndrome requires supplements of bicarbonate (up to 15 to 20 mEq per kilogram of body weight per day), potassium, phosphate, magnesium, and vitamin D. Treatment of the underlying disease, of course, varies widely. Effective results have been reported in the treatment of cystinosis with cysteamine, of Wilson's disease with penicillamine, of hereditary fructose intolerance with fructose restriction, and of heavy metal intoxication with removal from metal exposure or chelation (for lead).

DISORDERS OF FUNCTION OF THE ASCENDING LIMB OF THE LOOP OF HENLE

The thick ascending limb of the loop of Henle reabsorbs sodium chloride by means of a luminal Na-K-2Cl system. A lumen-positive potential difference and parallel transport systems effect potassium, calcium, and magnesium reabsorption. Defective reabsorption by the thick ascending limb of Henle occurs during diuretic treatment or in Bartter's syndrome.

Bartter's Syndrome

Bartter's syndrome consists of a constellation of findings, including hypokalemia and metabolic alkalosis with hyperreninemic hyperaldosteronism. Hypertension and edema are absent.

PATHOPHYSIOLOGY. Evidence that dysfunction of the thick ascending limb of Henle is the proximate cause of Bartter's syndrome comes primarily from free-water clearance studies. Mild extracellular volume depletion causes hyperreninemic hyperaldosteronism and the juxtaglomerular hyperplasia found on renal biopsy. Enhanced sodium chloride delivery to the collecting duct stimulates potassium secretion (exacerbated by concurrent hyperaldosteronism) leading to hypokalemia, as well as hydrogen ion secretion resulting in metabolic alkalosis. Accelerated kinin

and prostaglandin (especially PGE_2 and prostacyclin) production occurs and may account for the vascular unresponsiveness to pressors and various other phenomena known to occur in Bartter's syndrome.

SYMPTOMS AND ETIOLOGY. Symptoms of Bartter's syndrome are usually manifested in childhood. Inheritance is autosomal recessive, with a higher penetrance in males. Adult cases have also been reported. Presenting features relate primarily to the hypokalemia, including muscle weakness and a vasopressin-unresponsive urinary concentrating defect, characterized by polyuria, nocturia, and enuresis. Divalent cation wasting and metabolic alkalosis may conspire to cause symptoms characteristic of hypocalcemia, including Trousseau's and Chvostek's signs. The electrolyte abnormalities can also present acutely as intestinal ileus or chronically as growth retardation in children. Affected patients are normotensive and nonedematous, have a normal GFR, and can usually conserve sodium chloride when dietary salt is restricted, although at the expense of signs of moderate extracellular volume compromise.

DIAGNOSIS AND TREATMENT. Other conditions associated with hypokalemia, metabolic alkalosis, and secondary hyperreninemic hyperaldosteronism must be excluded before making a diagnosis of Bartter's syndrome. Surreptitious vomiting, chronic diarrheal states, or surreptitious diuretic or laxative administration can cause symptoms indistinguishable from those of Bartter's syndrome. These disorders are associated with extracellular volume depletion, and therefore the urinary chloride level is less than 20 mEq per liter, unless diuretics are being actively consumed. Thus, the diagnosis of Bartter's syndrome must be preceded by confirmation that urinary chloride concentration is more than 20 mEq per liter and by negative screening test results for diuretics in the urine and for laxatives in the stool (phenolphthalein test). States of primary hyperreninism or hypermineralocorticoidism can be readily excluded, since they are usually associated with hypertension.

Therapy of Bartter's syndrome is primarily aimed at ameliorating the hypokalemia by disrupting the renin-angiotensin-aldosterone and kinin-prostaglandin axes. Potassium supplementation, magnesium repletion, propranolol, spironolactone, prostaglandin inhibition, and captopril have all been used, but each has usually been met with incomplete success.

DISORDERS OF DISTAL NEPHRON FUNCTION

The distal nephron, including the distal convoluted tubule and the collecting ducts, is responsible for reabsorbing the final quantity of sodium in the tubular fluid and for secreting potassium and hydrogen ions. Inherited and acquired defects exist for selective or combined disorders of sodium, potassium, and acid-base regulation.

Classic Distal Renal Tubular Acidosis (RTA)

Classic distal RTA is a hypokalemic, hyperchloremic metabolic acidosis owing to a selective defect in distal acidification. It is characterized by an inability to lower the urinary pH normally and therefore by subnormal urinary net acid excretion.

PATHOPHYSIOLOGY. The distal nephron (especially the cortical and medullary collecting ducts) is normally capable of lowering the urinary pH fully 2 to 3 pH units below that of blood to titrate filtered buffers (principally phosphate) to form titratable acids and endogenously produced ammonia to form ammonium (Fig. 82–2). If the distal nephron is incapable of lowering the luminal pH below 5.5 when challenged by metabolic acidosis, a classic distal RTA is present. Because of the inappropriately high urinary pH, net acid excretion (titratable acid plus ammonium minus bicarbonate) is subnormal, less than acid production by the body. Accelerated potassium secretion occurs, presumably because there is reduced competition by proton secretion for the electrochemical driving forces in the distal nephron. The acidification defect may result from an insufficient number of proton-secreting pumps in the distal nephron. Alternatively, there may be backleak of acid across the luminal membrane, so that establishment of a pH gradient is prevented even when proton secretion is normal.

SYMPTOMS AND ETIOLOGIES. Distal RTA is found in infants, children, and adults. Symptoms may be those of acidosis or hypokalemia, as described above. Nephrocalcinosis and nephrolithiasis are common, either as a cause or as a result of classic distal RTA. However, bone disease is not as frequent as in proximal RTA. Classic distal RTA may also be genetic (most frequently autosomal dominant) or due to autoimmune diseases, drugs and toxins, and various tubulointerstitial diseases (Table 82–1).

DIAGNOSIS AND TREATMENT. The findings of hyperchloremic, hypokalemic metabolic acidosis with an inappropriately high urinary pH (>5.5) and diminished net acid excretion confirm the diagnosis (Table 82–2). Laboratory features of classic distal RTA sometimes resemble those of diarrhea, since both are associated with hyperchloremic, hypokalemic metabolic acidosis with a urinary pH greater than 5.5. If differentiation cannot be made on clinical grounds, it can be facilitated by measuring the urinary anion gap, defined as urinary [Na] + [K] − [Cl], which is proportionate to the negative value of urinary [NH$_4$]. Diarrhea has a large, negative urinary anion gap, and thus a high urinary ammonium concentration (accounting for the high urinary pH), while classic distal RTA has a zero or positive urinary anion gap and a low urinary ammonium concentration (because of impaired acidification). In individuals with a normal plasma bicarbonate concentration, the failure to lower urinary pH below 5.5 following an acute acid challenge with NH$_4$Cl defines the syndrome of incomplete classic distal RTA (see Ch. 75 for details of the NH$_4$Cl test). Treatment with alkali is generally very effective. The daily dose of alkali in adults is 1 to 3 mEq per kilogram, to compensate for the normal acid production by the body plus a small amount of urinary bicarbonate wastage. In contrast to proximal RTA, urinary potassium wasting is ameliorated with alkali therapy. Children require more alkali than adults, about 5 to 14 mEq per kilogram per day. Prognosis with respect to stabilization of GFR in adults or growth in children is excellent with provision of adequate alkali therapy.

RTA of Glomerular Insufficiency

This disorder is a normokalemic, hyperchloremic metabolic acidosis associated with moderate renal insufficiency (GFR of 20 to 30 ml per minute). It results from deficient ammonia delivery and is characterized by an appropriately low urinary pH but subnormal urinary net acid (ammonium) excretion.

PATHOPHYSIOLOGY. When the GFR falls to about 20 to 30 ml per minute owing to any intrinsic glomerular or tubulointerstitial disease, a normokalemic metabolic acidosis is frequently found. The cause of this acidosis is thought to be either deficient ammonia production or impairment in the urinary trapping of ammonia as ammonium (Fig. 82–2). In either case, proximal bicarbonate reclamation and the ability to lower the urinary pH to less than 5.5 are intact, but the failure to generate sufficient acid excretion to equal intake results in systemic acidosis.

SYMPTOMS AND ETIOLOGY. The degree of metabolic acidosis is generally mild, and plasma bicarbonate concentration is usually greater than 15 mEq per liter. Acidemia exacerbates the osteodystrophy of progressive renal disease. Although tubulointerstitial diseases are thought to produce this form of RTA more commonly than glomerular diseases, this distinction has been difficult to verify. This hyperchloremic metabolic acidosis should be distinguished from the high anion gap (normochloremic) uremic metabolic acidosis secondary to retained organic acids that usually occurs when glomerular insufficiency is more severe (GFR <20 ml per minute). The two acidoses may coexist.

DIAGNOSIS AND TREATMENT. A hyperchloremic, normokalemic metabolic acidosis that occurs when the GFR falls to about 20 to 30 ml per minute is typical of the RTA of glomerular insufficiency. Although net acid, specifically ammonium, excretion is subnormal (reflected by a zero or positive urinary anion gap) the urinary pH is appropriately acidic (Table 82–2). Mineralocorticoid levels are not diminished. Treatment consists of 1 to 3 mEq per kilogram per day of alkali therapy to compensate for daily acid ingestion and production.

Nonselective Distal Nephron Dysfunction: Generalized Distal RTA, Hyperkalemia, and Renal Salt Wasting

These disorders arise from global dysfunction of the distal nephron due to aldosterone deficiency or antagonism and are characterized by hyperkalemic, hyperchloremic metabolic acidosis caused by subnormal net acid excretion and frequently by renal salt wasting.

PATHOPHYSIOLOGY. When sodium is reabsorbed in the distal nephron under the influence of aldosterone, luminal sodium concentration can be reduced to very low levels, less than 10 mEq per liter (sometimes ≤1 mEq per liter). Sodium reabsorption creates a lumen-negative potential difference, favoring secretion of potassium and hydrogen ions (Fig. 82–2). Disruption of sodium reabsorption and of potassium and hydrogen secretion may therefore be ascribable to a defect in the integrity of the distal nephron cell, deficient aldosterone production or action, diminished sodium reabsorption, or blunting of the lumen-negative potential by enhanced chloride reabsorption. Any of these processes lead to diminished total hydrogen ion and potassium excretion and therefore metabolic acidosis with hyperkalemia. The hyperkalemia also serves to depress renal ammoniagenesis independently, which exacerbates the defect in renal acidification. The ability to lower the urinary pH normally (a qualitative distal nephron function at low buffer strength) remains intact (Table 82–2).

SYMPTOMS AND ETIOLOGIES. The symptoms of generalized distal RTA in children or adults usually relate to the acidosis itself or occasionally to the neuromuscular consequences of hyperkalemia. Renal salt wasting can cause extracellular volume depletion and hypotension when sodium chloride intake is reduced. The most common forms of generalized distal RTA result from a reduction in aldosterone level or prevention of its action (Table 82–1). The adrenal synthesis of aldosterone may be directly impaired, as in Addison's disease or in inherited enzymatic defects, such as 18- or 21-hydroxylase deficiencies. More commonly, primary hyporeninemia caused by diabetic nephropathy, hypertensive nephrosclerosis, or tubulointerstitial diseases can also reduce aldosterone levels. Finally, end-organ unresponsiveness to mineralocorticoid with high circulating levels of aldosterone occurs in various tubulointerstitial diseases, especially those that have a predilection for the medulla and papilla of the kidney (e.g., analgesic abuse, sickle cell disease, and obstructive nephropathies).

DIAGNOSIS AND TREATMENT: HYPERKALEMIC, GENERALIZED DISTAL RTA. Generalized distal RTA is unique among the hyperchloremic metabolic acidoses in being a hyperkalemic disorder (Table 82–2). Glomerular filtration rate is invariably reduced in the forms associated with hyporeninemia or tubulointerstitial nephropathy but may be at levels (≥30 ml per minute) above those typically found in the RTA of glomerular insufficiency.

Treatment of the hyperkalemia and generalized distal RTA is effected with 9-α-fludrocortisone, 0.1 mg per day, when mineralocorticoid is deficient. When hyporeninemia is the cause, high doses of the synthetic mineralocorticoid are required (up to 0.5 mg per day) because of associated mineralocorticoid resistance. Hypertension can be precipitated with this treatment. A loop diuretic (furosemide or ethacrynic acid) is also useful, especially when hypertension precludes administration of mineralocorticoid, because it enhances urinary potassium excretion even when endogenous aldosterone is low. Useful adjuncts to diuretic therapy include dietary potassium restriction (≤50 mEq per day), alkali therapy to compensate for daily acid generation (sodium bicarbonate, 1 to 3 mEq per kilogram per day), and sometimes short-term use of cation exchange resin.

DIAGNOSIS AND TREATMENT: RENAL SALT WASTING. Renal salt wasting becomes apparent when dietary sodium chloride intake becomes less than the minimal threshold for sodium chloride excretion. Renal salt wasting is diagnosed when, in response to acute reduction of sodium intake (10 mEq per day), urinary sodium excretion remains inappropriately elevated, typically greater than 50 mEq per day, and weight loss is significant (>3 kg). Progressively severe extracellular volume depletion occurs with development of hypotension and renal insufficiency. This diagnostic maneuver is not without hazard, since symptomatic hypovolemia or hyperkalemia can be precipitated and should be performed only under close supervision.

Therapy for renal salt wasting secondary to aldosterone deficiency or partial resistance requires physiologic or supraphysiologic mineralocorticoid replacement, as described above. In all other cases, sodium chloride supplementation is indicated to prevent volume depletion in the event sodium intake is curtailed. The dose of sodium chloride prescribed, in the diet and salt tablets, should exceed that amount of sodium chloride spilled into the urine by the patient when dietary salt was restricted.

General

Cogan MG: Disorders of proximal nephron function. Am J Med 72:275, 1982. *This paper presents an overview of the physiology, pathophysiologic mechanisms, and clinical disorders of proximal nephron function.*

Sebastian A, Hulter HN, Kurtz I, et al.: Disorders of distal nephron function. Am J Med 72:289, 1982. *This article is a thoughtful, pathophysiologically oriented overview of the various clinical dysfunctions of potassium and hydrogen ion secretion.*

Renal Glycosurias

Wen S-F: Glycosurias. *In* Gonick HC, Buckalew VM Jr (eds.): Renal Tubular Disorders. New York, Marcel Dekker, 1985, pp 159–199. *This chapter presents an excellent discussion of the physiology of glucose transport and the pathophysiology and clinical spectrum of the renal glycosurias.*

Renal Aminoacidurias

Foreman JW, Segal S: Aminoacidurias. *In* Gonick HC, Buckalew VM Jr (eds.): Renal Tubular Disorders. New York, Marcel Dekker, 1985, pp 131–157. *This chapter presents an excellent overview of the physiology of amino acid transport and the clinical spectra of the aminoacidurias.*

Segal S, Thier SO: Cystinurias. *In* Scriver CR, Beaudet AL, Sly WS, et al. (eds.): The Metabolic Basis of Inherited Disease. 6th ed. New York, McGraw-Hill Book Company, 1989, pp 2479–2496. *This is an authoritative review of the most common of the aminoacidurias.*

Fanconi's Syndrome

Brewer ED: The Fanconi syndrome: Clinical disorders. *In* Gonick HC, Buckalew VM Jr (eds.): Renal Tubular Disorders. New York, Marcel Dekker, 1985, pp 475–544. *This is a superb, exhaustive review of the pathophysiology, clinical presentations, and principles of treatment of the multiple causes of the Fanconi syndrome.*

Roth KS, Foreman JW, Segal S: The Fanconi syndrome and mechanisms of tubular transport dysfunction. Kidney Int 20:705, 1981. *An excellent review of the pathogenetic mechanisms of this syndrome.*

Bartter's Syndrome

Gill JR, Bartter FC: Evidence for a prostaglandin-independent defect in chloride reabsorption in the loop of Henle as a proximal cause of Bartter's syndrome. Am J Med 65:766, 1978. *This paper describes in vivo studies pinpointing the tubular site of the reabsorptive defect in Bartter's syndrome.*

Stein JH: The pathogenetic spectrum of Bartter's syndrome. Kidney Int 28:85, 1985. *This article reviews the variety of clinical presentations and current concepts of pathogenesis of this heterogeneous syndrome.*

Renal Tubular Acidosis

Batlle DC, Hizon M, Cohen E, et al.: The use of the urinary anion gap in the diagnosis of hyperchloremic metabolic acidosis. N Engl J Med 318:594, 1988. *The use of the urinary anion gap to distinguish hyperchloremic acidosis of diarrhea from classic distal RTA is clearly explained.*

Cogan MG, Arieff AI: Sodium wasting, acidosis and hyperkalemia induced by methicillin interstitial nephritis. Evidence for selective distal tubular dysfunction. Am J Med 64:500, 1978. *This article describes the standard evaluation and treatment of a patient with marked renal salt wasting.*

Cogan MG, Rector FC Jr: Acid-base disorders. *In* Brenner BM, Rector FC Jr (eds.): The Kidney. 4th ed. Philadelphia, W. B. Saunders Company, 1991. *This chapter is a comprehensive review of acid-base homeostasis, including the RTA's.*

Harrington JT, Cohen JJ: Metabolic acidosis. *In* Cohen JJ, Kassirer JP (eds.): Acid-Base. Boston, Little, Brown and Company, 1982, pp 121–126. *This chapter describes the pathophysiology and clinical manifestations of metabolic acidoses.*

Schambelan M, Sebastian A, Biglieri EG: Prevalence, pathogenesis and functional significance of aldosterone deficiency in hyperkalemic patients with chronic renal insufficiency. Kidney Int 17:89, 1980. *This paper provides one of the most comprehensive reviews of the heterogeneous causes of generalized distal (type IV) RTA.*

83 Diabetes and the Kidney

Bryan D. Myers

INCIDENCE AND PREVALENCE

Among the 15,000 patients entering chronic dialysis and kidney transplantation programs in the United States each year, the development of end-stage renal failure can be attributed to diabetes mellitus in approximately 25 per cent. Diabetic glomerulopathy, a complex disorder associated with a diffuse expansion of collagenous components of the glomerulus, is the predominant cause of the renal failure. The diabetic patient is also prone to other renal diseases, such as pyelonephritis, papillary necrosis, and obstructive nephropathy, that occasionally cause or exacerbate renal failure (Ch. 81 and 84). Diabetic patients with glomerulopathy are more susceptible to these associated renal disorders than are those who do not have glomerulopathy. Most victims of end-stage diabetic renal disease have longstanding type I diabetes, defined here as juvenile-onset and insulin-dependent diabetes (see Ch. 218). Patients with type II diabetes, characterized by a more advanced age of onset and not requiring insulin for control of hyperglycemia, are not spared from diabetic glomerulopathy but constitute a substantial minority among diabetic patients in end-stage renal failure programs.

CLINICAL AND LABORATORY FEATURES OF DIABETIC GLOMERULOPATHY

The natural history of diabetic glomerulopathy has been best documented in type I patients. Early abnormalities of glomerular function and structure appear to be invariable in all type I diabetics, but only 30 to 50 per cent will develop a progressive, proteinuric form of diabetic glomerulopathy. The evolution of the glomerulopathy in this subset of type I diabetics may be thought of as a continuum of glomerular injury divisible into three stages (Fig. 83–1). The first stage of occult glomerulopathy cannot be diagnosed by conventional laboratory techniques and lasts for approximately 10 years. It is followed by two clinically evident stages of increasingly severe glomerular injury. Both are identified by the presence of proteinuria, while the milder, intermediate second stage merges with the advanced third stage with the development of azotemia. The clinical and laboratory features of this prolonged and progressive glomerular disease are reviewed by each stage separately.

Stage 1—Occult Diabetic Glomerulopathy

During this stage, the type I diabetic patient is devoid of clinical symptoms and signs of glomerulopathy. The most striking laboratory finding is a 20 to 40 per cent *elevation of the glomerular filtration rate* (GFR) above that found in age-matched normal control subjects. Such hyperfiltration could be partly attributable to a generalized hypertrophy of glomeruli, with an ensuing increase in the glomerular capillary filtration surface area. However, striking elevations of GFR in poorly controlled diabetic patients can be lowered within a matter of hours following restoration of normoglycemia, though not fully corrected. A parallel *increase in renal plasma flow*, measured by the clearance of p-aminohippurate, and also reversible by lowering blood glucose levels, points to a contribution by hemodynamic factors to the hyperfiltration. Notwithstanding the responsiveness of vasomotor regulation in the kidney to alterations in the metabolic milieu, GFR tends to remain elevated even with good metabolic control of the diabetic state. Not until proteinuria ushers in the intermediate second stage of the glomerulopathy does the GFR fall into the normal range.

The stage 1 glomerular hyperfiltration is sometimes accompanied by transient increases in the urinary albumin excretion rate that are measurable only by sensitive, immunochemical techniques. Healthy adolescents and young adults excrete albumin in their urine at rates of up to 15 µg per minute. Some patients with type I diabetes of short duration excrete albumin at rates in excess of 15 µg per minute but less than 100 µg per minute, which is roughly the threshold detectable by conventional techniques. This *microalbuminuria* is inferred to represent an increase in the transglomerular filtration of albumin rather than a decrease in tubular reabsorption of a normal, filtered albumin load. Microalbuminuria tends to be associated with the most striking degrees of hyperfiltration observed among type I diabetics, suggesting that it may also have a hemodynamic basis. It is exaggerated by exercise, which causes an increase in the intraluminal hydraulic pressure of the glomerular capillaries, and is blunted, although not abolished, by restoration of normoglycemia.

Early in the course of type I diabetes, hypertrophy of nephrons results in a consistent increase in kidney size. Hyperfiltration, renal hyperemia and enlargement, and intermittent microalbuminuria are all characteristic of this early occult stage, but hypertension, an important complication of diabetic glomerulopathy, is not prevalent. The incidence of hypertension in large diabetic populations without proteinuria is no different from that in nondiabetic populations.

Stage 2—Intermediate Diabetic Glomerulopathy

Stage 2, intermediate diabetic glomerulopathy, is characterized by *increasing proteinuria, declining GFR*, and the development of *hypertension* and *edema*. This stage is heralded by the development of sustained microalbuminuria, which increases over 2 or more years into a range (>250 µg per minute) that is easily measurable by dipstick. Once overt proteinuria has become manifest, its magnitude tends to reflect the rate of deterioration of glomerular capillary wall function that typifies the second stage of diabetic glomerulopathy. As indicated in Figure 83–1, proteinuria tends to increase exponentially with time and to be related inversely to GFR.

The onset of proteinuria is also accompanied by an increasing prevalence of hypertension and by the development of edema. Edema becomes clearly evident long before urinary protein losses reach nephrotic proportions (>3.5 grams per 24 hours). It worsens and often becomes refractory to diuretic therapy once proteinuria is sufficient to cause hypoproteinemia, however.

The proteinuria of stage 2 diabetic glomerulopathy has no pathognomonic characteristics, but several features distinguish it from other glomerular diseases: (1) From the onset of the second stage, immunoglobulins and other large plasma proteins are excreted in the urine in large quantities along with albumin, signifying an early loss of barrier size-selectivity in this disorder. (2) Persistent and even heavy urinary losses of plasma proteins in stage 2 diabetic glomerulopathy are often not accompanied by hypoproteinemia. Inasmuch as the conventional definition of the nephrotic syndrome requires hypoproteinemia in addition to heavy proteinuria and edema, stage 2 diabetic glomerulopathy does not always exemplify the nephrotic syndrome. An important role in edema formation is ascribed to reduction of plasma oncotic pressure in patients with the nephrotic syndrome as classically defined; the absence of hypoproteinemia, and hence the maintenance of normal plasma oncotic pressure, in much of stage 2 diabetic glomerulopathy implicates alternate mechanisms of edema formation. (3) Neither edema formation nor, for that matter, hypertension can be related unambiguously to a stimulated renin-angiotensin-aldosterone system. Rather, diabetic glomerulopathy is usually associated with normal or low circulating levels of active renin. In contrast, the circulating level of prorenin is frequently enhanced. Since prorenin is an inactive prohormone, the biologic significance of this finding is uncertain. The plasma concentration and urinary excretion rate of aldosterone tend, like active renin, also to be normal or depressed, despite the presence of edema. In fact, proteinuric diabetic glomerulopathy probably constitutes the most common example of hyporeninemic hypoaldosteronism, and such patients not infrequently exhibit the syndrome of generalized distal type IV renal tubular acidosis (see Ch. 82). Thus, both the mechanism by which edema is formed and the basis for the widespread prevalence of hypertension in stage 2 diabetic glomerulopathy remain obscure.

Stage 3—Advanced Diabetic Glomerulopathy

The third, advanced stage represents the terminal 2 or 3 years of what is typically a 20- to 25-year process. Its onset is delineated by the development of *azotemia*. Retention of urea, creatinine, and other nitrogenous compounds generally becomes apparent once the GFR has declined to less than one third of normal levels. As with the intermediate stage that precedes it, GFR in the third and terminal stage of diabetic glomerulopathy has been observed to decline at rates that are rather predictable for a given patient. Whereas the actual rate of GFR decline varies widely among individuals, it averages 1 ml per minute per month when hypertension is poorly controlled and can be halved by efficacious lowering of blood pressure. The prototypical case in Figure 83–1 is illustrative of a patient with poorly controlled hypertension, in whom GFR is predicted to decline from a normal value approximating 120 ml per minute at the onset of stage 2 to zero at the end of stage 3 over a period of 10 years. Not only does GFR decline irrevocably, resulting in progressive azotemia, but also *edema* and *hypertension* tend to worsen in the third and final stage of the disease. Similarly, *proteinuria* continues to be massive and *hypoproteinemia* finally results. Although reduced plasma protein concentration and the lowered GFR serve to lower the filtered protein load, urinary protein excretion rate is maintained at massive levels, reflecting increasing leakiness of the glomerular capillary wall to large plasma proteins.

By the time the third, advanced stage of diabetic glomerulopathy is reached, *widespread microangiopathy* involving the retinae and peripheral nerves is invariable. Although its extent varies among patients, retinopathy is frequently associated with

FIGURE 83–1. The glomerular filtration rate (*black line*) and albumin excretion rate (*red line*) have been plotted against time to chart a hypothetical course typical of diabetic glomerulopathy. The course of the disease has been divided into three stages, which are described in the text.

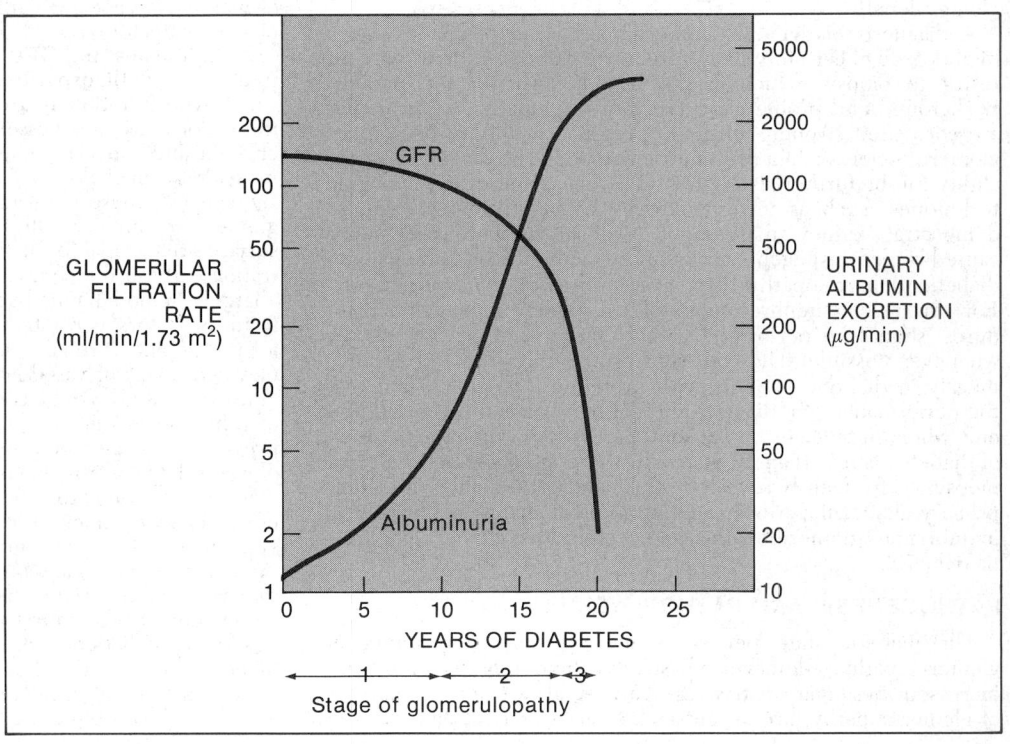

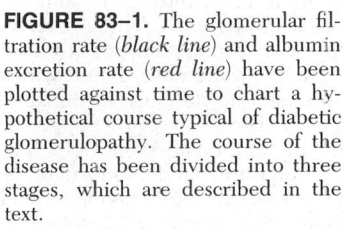

visual impairment sufficient to result in functional blindness. The effects of peripheral and more particularly of autonomic neuropathy may be equally devastating. This is particularly true when autonomic neuropathy results in partial paresis of the bladder. Progressive urinary retention may exacerbate renal insufficiency in stage 3 glomerulopathy by resulting in a superimposed obstructive nephropathy. Obstructive nephropathy in turn may predispose the already vulnerable patient to ascending pyelonephritis and/or ischemic papillary necrosis, thereby compromising renal function even further. (For more detailed discussion of obstructive nephropathy, see Ch. 81.)

Given the prolonged duration of diabetes mellitus, by the time stage 3 glomerulopathy is reached, many patients will be 40 years of age or more, an age group in which exuberant atherosclerosis is accelerated in part by the presence of longstanding hypertension and in part by lipid abnormalities that attend the diabetic state. Coronary artery disease, cerebrovascular disease and stroke, and peripheral vascular disease are all common in the third stage of diabetic glomerulopathy and account collectively for the majority of fatalities. The eventual need for substitution therapy in end-stage renal failure programs occurs in a setting, therefore, in which serious extrarenal complications are prevalent and impair the effectiveness of rehabilitation generally achieved by such therapy.

DIAGNOSIS

Proteinuria due to diabetic glomerulopathy is accompanied by typical changes of glomerular histopathology. These include a striking accumulation of extracellular matrix, which results in an expansion of the mesangium and a widening of the glomerular capillary wall caused by a thickened glomerular basement membrane. The acellular expansion of the mesangium tends to affect all glomeruli in a global fashion; thus, the histopathologic term used for this variety of diabetic glomerular disease is diffuse intercapillary glomerulosclerosis. Not infrequently, mesangial matrix accumulation occurs in a segmental fashion, however, resulting in the formation of acellular spherical nodules at the center of single or multiple peripheral glomerular lobules (Fig. 83–2) and termed nodular glomerulosclerosis. A nodular accumulation of mesangial matrix material, indistinguishable from that observed in diabetic subjects, has been associated with dysproteinemia, notably that associated with a monoclonal proliferation of B lymphocytes or plasma cells. Provided that the latter entity is excluded, however, the finding of diffuse or nodular glomerulosclerosis in a proteinuric diabetic subject is diagnostic of diabetic glomerulopathy.

A diagnosis of diabetic glomerulopathy can be made with a high degree of certainty in a proteinuric diabetic patient, without resort to biopsy, which carries a finite risk for the patient. Background and proliferative types of retinopathy, for example, are correlated strongly with the presence of diffuse or nodular glomerulosclerosis in a proteinuric diabetic. The diagnostic probability can be further strengthened by using noninvasive imaging techniques, such as ultrasonography or nephrotomography, to demonstrate kidney enlargement. Nephrotoxic acute renal failure caused by contrast agents occurs more commonly in patients with diabetic glomerulopathy than in any other category of patients. For this reason nephrotomography (or other radiologic procedures) should be performed without the use of contrast agents whenever possible. The coexistence of retinopathy and nephromegaly in diabetic patients with proteinuria is so constant that the performance of a diagnostic renal biopsy need be considered only when these factors are absent, particularly when the duration of diabetes is less than 10 years. In these circumstances, a renal biopsy has frequently revealed other, and presumably unrelated, primary glomerulopathies, such as minimal change nephropathy, membranous glomerulopathy, and proliferative glomerulonephritis (Ch. 79).

PATHOGENESIS AND PATHOPHYSIOLOGY

The diabetic state per se is the presumed forerunner of glomerulopathy. Glomerular basement membrane widening and increased mesangial matrix, the earliest ultrastructural markers of glomerulopathy, are absent at the onset and can be detected

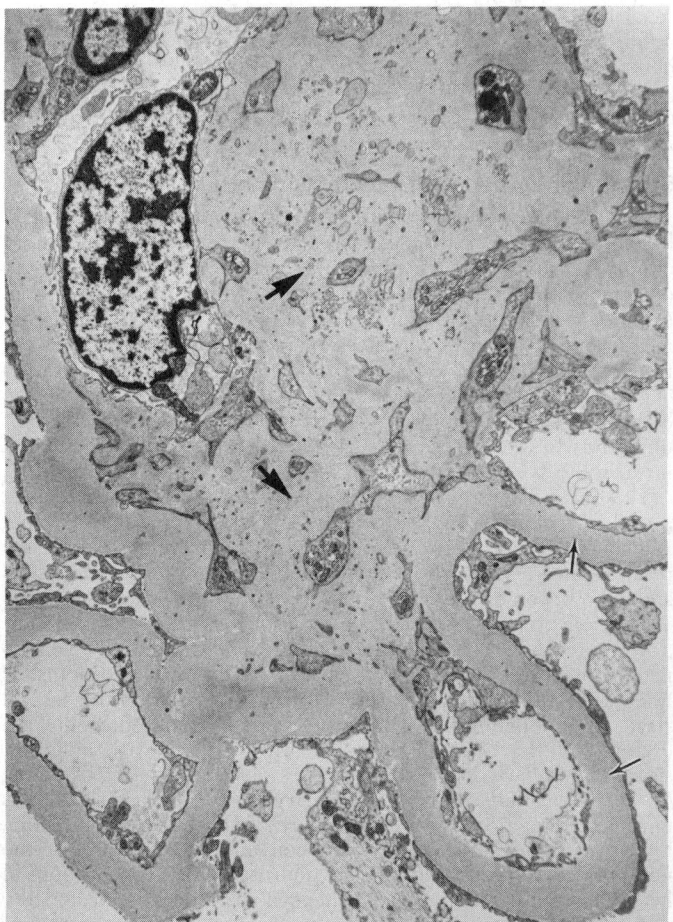

FIGURE 83–2. Electron photomicrograph of a portion of a glomerulus from a patient with proteinuric, diabetic glomerulopathy (magnification ×5000). A striking increase in collagenous components has resulted in (1) widening of the basement membrane of peripheral capillary loops (*small arrows*), and (2) expansion of the matrix of the glomerular mesangium (*large arrows*). The latter alteration is responsible for compressing and ultimately obliterating the glomerular capillary network.

only after some years of type I diabetes. An identical sequence has been observed in experimental diabetes induced in a variety of mammalian species with the use of pancreatic beta cell toxins or pancreatectomy.

As in humans, the GFR is substantially elevated in the insulin-treated rat with experimental diabetes of short duration. The early hyperfiltration is a consequence of altered vasomotion in the major resistance vessels of the renal cortex. Dilatation of the efferent and especially the afferent glomerular arterioles results in an elevation of glomerular capillary perfusion rate and pressure. By contrast, those determinants of GFR that are intrinsic to the glomerular capillary wall, namely, hydraulic conductivity and the surface area available for filtration, are unaltered. Thus hyperfiltration early in the course of diabetes in rodents appears to have a largely hemodynamic basis. It remains to be determined which factor or factors associated with the diabetic state are responsible for the deranged renal vasoregulation. Hyperglycemia per se, or elevated levels of vasodilator glucoregulatory hormones, such as glucagon and growth hormone, may be implicated. Abnormalities of other hormonal regulators of glomerular perfusion rate and pressure have also been identified. Thus, increased production of vasodilator prostaglandins by glomerular cells isolated from diabetic rats points to an imbalance in favor of local vasodilatation of renal cortical microvessels. Experimental maneuvers that prevent glomerular hyperemia and hypertension—such as the administration of an angiotensin-converting enzyme inhibitor or dietary protein restriction—largely prevent the subsequent development of proteinuria as well as the histopathologic damage observed in diabetic rats not so protected. These findings are taken to indicate that hemodynamic factors serve as a stimulus for an ensuing accumulation of extracellular matrix components and, hence, subsequent glomerulosclerosis.

Whether or not glomerular capillary hypertension and hyperperfusion are unique causes of an accumulation of extracellular matrix components, there seems little doubt that this lesion is responsible for the progressive reduction of GFR that typifies the second and third stages of clinical diabetic glomerulopathy. As shown in Figure 83–2, expansion of the mesangial matrix occurs at the expense of the surrounding glomerular capillary loops, with progressive reduction of the surface area available for filtration. By the time the end of the third stage of diabetic glomerulopathy has been reached, the mesangium will have encroached upon most glomerular capillary loops to the point that they have become almost totally obliterated.

The process by which the glomerular basement membrane becomes widened has been presumed to be responsible for the alteration in the glomerular capillary wall, causing it to become permeable to large plasma proteins. Surprisingly, however, no correlation whatsoever exists between glomerular basement membrane width and proteinuria. While the structural basis of proteinuria remains obscure, the functional nature of the disturbance in glomerular permselectivity has been elucidated by the use of physiologic techniques in vivo in which the clearance of probe filtration markers of graded size has been used to define the size-selective properties of the glomerular filter. One such study has revealed that proteinuria in diabetic glomerulopathy can be accounted for by the development within the glomerular capillary wall of a subpopulation of enlarged, protein-permeable pores. In contradistinction to the diffuse widening of the basement membrane seen by electron microscopy (Fig. 83–2), the enlarged pores can be estimated to be few in number and to behave as isolated defects in the glomerular capillary wall.

PROGNOSIS AND TREATMENT

The profound loss of filtering surface area and the disruption of glomerular membrane pore structure that underlie stage 2 and 3 glomerulopathy in diabetics are unlikely to be reversible. Attempts to maintain blood glucose in such patients in a normal range have failed to prevent or attenuate the progression of renal insufficiency. Meticulous control of hypertension, however, may slow the rate of decline of the GFR. Together with antihypertensive therapy, attention to and correction of coexistent cardiac failure, obstructive nephropathy, pyelonephritis, and other events that may lower the GFR independently of the glomerulopathy represent the mainstay of therapy of proteinuric glomerulopathy.

On the basis of our current understanding of the pathophysiology and pathogenesis of diabetic glomerulopathy, a strong case can be made for identifying early stage 2 disease by the detection of sustained microalbuminuria, particularly when it is associated with ophthalmoscopic evidence of diabetic retinopathy. The institution of measures that are likely to lower glomerular perfusion rate and pressure are regarded also to be likely to attenuate the rate of progressive glomerular injury. Such protective measures include dietary protein restriction and lowering of blood pressure, even within the so-called normal range established by the World Health Organization (<169/95 mm Hg). A growing body of evidence suggests that converting enzyme inhibitors have a more marked antiproteinuric effect than other antihypertensive agents, and studies are currently under way to determine whether they are also uniquely or disproportionately GFR sparing. Notwithstanding the absence of evidence for increased activity of the circulating (endocrine) renin-angiotensin system, it could be that a local (paracrine) system is implicated in the genesis of progressive glomerular injury in diabetic subjects. Inhibition of this local system provides a possible basis for a specific renoprotective effect of converting enzyme inhibitors. It should be emphasized, however, that the rationale for protective therapy with converting enzyme inhibitors is at the moment based on purely theoretical considerations. Prolonged and carefully controlled trials with this class of agents have yet to be conducted to confirm that it indeed has a GFR-sparing effect.

Once end-stage renal failure has supervened, the diabetic patient should be referred for treatment to a dialysis and/or transplantation center (Ch. 77 and 78). Many diabetic patients respond favorably to and enjoy a good quality of life with these modalities of treatment. With special attention to the unique problems of the diabetic patient with renal failure, the survival rates achieved with dialysis, particularly chronic ambulatory peritoneal dialysis, or following renal transplantation, are today approaching those achieved for nondiabetic patients.

Hostetter TH, Rennke HG, Brenner BM: The case for intrarenal hypertension in the initiation and progression of diabetic and other glomerulopathies. Am J Med 72:375, 1982. *A lucid review of the pathophysiology of diabetic glomerulopathy, citing virtually every important reference to this subject.*

Hostetter TH, Troy JL, Brenner BM: Glomerular hemodynamics in experimental diabetes mellitus. Kidney Int 19:410, 1981. *An elegant micropuncture study demonstrating the hemodynamic basis for glomerular hyperfiltration in early experimental rat diabetes.*

Luetscher JA, Kraemer FB, Wilson DM: Increased plasma inactive renin in diabetes mellitus. N Engl J Med 312:1412, 1985. *The abnormalities in the renin-angiotensin system in diabetic glomerulopathy are clearly delineated.*

Mauer SM, Steffes MW, Ellis EN, et al.: Structural-functional relationships in diabetic nephropathy. J Clin Invest 74:1143, 1984. *A review of the authors' use of electron microscopy and elegant morphometric techniques to chart the evolution and progression of diabetic glomerulopathy.*

Morelli E, Loon N, Meyer TW, et al.: Effects of converting enzyme inhibition on barrier function in diabetic glomerulopathy. Diabetes 39:76, 1990. *The sieving behavior of glomeruli was analyzed in 16 glomerulopathic patients in whom a 12-week course of enalapril lowered the urinary protein excretion rate. A theoretical analysis of dextran sieving profiles revealed that enalapril shifted the glomerular pore size distribution to pores of smaller radius. The improved barrier size-selectivity was unaccompanied by changes in glomerular hemodynamics, suggesting that inhibition of converting enzyme may modulate the intrinsic membrane properties of the glomerular barrier.*

Myers BD, Winetz JA, Chui F, et al.: Mechanisms of proteinuria in diabetic nephropathy: A study of glomerular barrier function. Kidney Int 21:96, 1982. *Modern physiologic techniques and mathematical modeling are used to describe the glomerular capillary wall as an ultrafiltration membrane; the defect in the glomerular filter of proteinuric diabetics is elucidated.*

Omachi R: The pathogenesis and prevention of diabetic nephropathy. West J Med 145:222, 1986. *This summary of a recent medical grand rounds offers a review of the topic with 57 references.*

Parving HH, Hommel E, Smidt UM: Protection of kidney function and decrease in albuminuria by captopril in insulin-dependent diabetics with nephropathy. Br Med J 297:1086, 1988. *A demonstration that chronic inhibition of converting enzyme with captopril lowers albuminuria and halves the rate at which GFR declines over a 24-month interval.*

Viberti GC, Bilous RW, Mackintosh D, et al.: Monitoring glomerular function in diabetic nephropathy. Am J Med 74:256, 1983. *A careful prospective study of the effects of metabolic control on proteinuric glomerulopathy. Its message is pessimistic.*

Zatz R, Meyer TW, Rennke HG, et al.: Predominance of hemodynamic rather than metabolic factors in the pathogenesis of diabetic glomerulopathy. Proc Natl Acad Sci USA 82:5963, 1985. *The protective effect of lowering glomerular pressures and flows on sclerosing diabetic glomerulopathy is well documented.*

84 Urinary Tract Infections and Pyelonephritis

Vincent T. Andriole

DEFINITION

Urinary tract infection refers to both microbial colonization of the urine and tissue invasion of any structure of the urinary tract. Bacteria are most commonly responsible, although yeast, fungi, and viruses may produce urinary infection. Urinary tract infections may be relatively mild, such as the "honeymoon cystitis" syndrome, or catastrophic, such as a perinephric abscess in a diabetic. Urinary tract infections are often categorized by the site of infection, which is convenient for the purpose of discussion. However, it is often not possible to diagnose the various types of infections on clinical grounds alone.

Significant bacteriuria refers to sufficient numbers of bacteria in the urine to denote active infection rather than contamination. A bacteria count over 100,000 organisms per milliliter in a fresh "clean-catch" midstream specimen is a reliable indicator of active urinary tract infection but does not indicate whether the infection is cystitis or pyelonephritis. In addition, women with acute cystitis may have more than 10^3 but less than 10^5 bacteria per milliliter in midstream urine cultures.

Asymptomatic bacteriuria refers to large numbers of bacteria in the urine without producing symptoms. Dysuria and frequency in the absence of significant bacteriuria are common problems among young women. This entity has been called the *acute urethral syndrome* and in 25 per cent of patients is caused by *Chlamydia trachomatis*.

Cystitis and *acute pyelonephritis* are symptomatic infections of the bladder and kidney, respectively. *Perinephric and renal abscesses*, uncommon complications of urinary infections, usually occur in (1) urinary tract obstruction; (2) bacteremia, particularly staphylococcal or candidal bacteremia; and (3) immunocompromised individuals, particularly diabetics.

Complicated infections refer to bacteriuria in association with structural or neurologic defects in the voiding mechanism (vesicoureteral reflux, neurogenic bladder), foreign bodies (stones or indwelling catheter), or intrinsic renal disease (diabetic nephropathy or polycystic kidney disease).

Chronic pyelonephritis refers to the pathologic and radiologic findings of chronic cortical scarring, tubulointerstitial damage, and deformity of the underlying calix. Chronic bacterial pyelonephritis can be *active*, which occurs in patients with persistent *complicated* infection, or *inactive*, which consists of focal sterile scars of a past infection. Recurrent infection can result in multiple scars combined with active foci of infection. In the absence of obstruction, reflux, foreign bodies, or an immunocompromised host (notably the diabetic patient), urinary tract infections rarely cause the shrunken, scarred kidneys of end-stage chronic pyelonephritis.

Other disease states can produce renal lesions that mimic "chronic pyelonephritis." Identical characteristics can be observed, in the absence of infection, in patients who suffered from severe vesicoureteral reflux in childhood. This entity, *reflux nephropathy*, refers to the radiographic triad of intrarenal reflux and vesicoureteral reflux, scarring, and loss of parenchymal mass in the absence of other obstructive lesions and can ultimately lead to end-stage renal failure with scarred, shrunken kidneys. "Reflux nephropathy" may result from "autoimmune" renal damage rather than bacterial infection of the kidney. Nevertheless, the combination of recurrent infection and reflux nephropathy can also result in chronic pyelonephritis. *Analgesic nephropathy* may produce papillary necrosis and may also mimic bacterial pyelonephritis on radiography.

PATHOGENESIS

The normal urinary tract is free of bacteria except for some organisms normally present near the external meatus and some staphylococci and diphtheroids normally found in the distal urethra. Urine, as a culture medium, generally supports bacterial multiplication. However, high concentrations of urea and hyperosmolality (which are present in the renal medulla), an acid pH, and urinary organic acid are generally unfavorable to bacterial growth. In addition, the dynamics of the urinary flow (washout) and antibacterial properties of the lining membrane of the urinary tract and of the vaginal and periurethral epithelial cells appear to be important defense mechanisms.

Urinary tract infections result most commonly from ascending transurethral invasion of the bladder by pathogenic gram-negative aerobic bacilli normally present in the large bowel and perineum, particularly of women. Sequentially, bacteria migrate from the anus to the periurethral area and along the urethra into the bladder, where infections occur if the organisms become established. This pathogenic mechanism helps explain the higher rate of urinary tract infection in women, whose urethras are shorter than those of men, and the marked frequency of the urinary tract infection associated with instrumentation of the urethra and the bladder. In addition, the increased vaginal fluid pH and altered vaginal microflora present in bacterial vaginosis are associated with *Escherichia coli* introital colonization and acute symptomatic urinary tract infection in young women who use diaphragms.

Other pathways from the large bowel to the urinary passages and kidneys include the hematogenous and lymphatic routes. The hematogenous route, a less common mechanism for renal infection, generally, but not always, requires antecedent structural damage to the kidney. Staphylococcal bacteremia can produce multiple microabscesses in the kidney (*renal carbuncle*). Disseminated *Candida albicans* infections in the immunocom-

promised host can involve the kidney. Finally, septic emboli, particularly in the setting of bacterial endocarditis, represent a classic mode for hematogenously disseminated infection of the kidney.

The renal medulla, because of its unique hypertonicity, is much more susceptible to infection than is the cortex. In experimental pyelonephritis, as few as 10 to 100 *E. coli* organisms may produce infection in the medulla, whereas 100,000 are required to infect the cortex. The increased susceptibility of the medulla is thought to be due to impaired leukocyte mobilization and phagocytosis in the hypertonic environment.

Microbial virulence factors are also important in the pathogenesis of symptomatic urinary infections. *E. coli* strains isolated from patients with pyelonephritis are more likely to (1) possess large amounts of K (capsular) antigen, (2) adhere in larger numbers to human urinary epithelial cells, and (3) possess surface pili, than are strains found in asymptomatic bacteriuria. The virulence of *Proteus* species may be related to their urease content and ammonia production.

CLINICAL MANIFESTATIONS

The symptoms of acute urinary tract infections are varied and include frequency, dysuria, burning pain on urination, suprapubic discomfort, passage of cloudy and occasionally blood-tinged urine, fever, costovertebral angle tenderness or flank pain, and rigors. Urinary tract symptoms, particularly dysuria, occur in 20 per cent of women each year, although only half seek medical attention. Approximately equal numbers of these women have the acute urethral syndrome (urethritis), bladder bacteriuria (cystitis), or renal infection.

In general, clinical grounds form an uncertain basis for separating patients with the acute urethral syndrome from those with either bladder or renal bacteriuria because frequency, burning, and suprapubic pain are found approximately equally in all three groups of patients. Costovertebral angle tenderness and fever may be present as frequently in patients with the acute urethral syndrome as in those with renal bacteriuria. Rigors occur almost equally (15 per cent) in patients with the acute urethral syndrome and those with cystitis. Similarly, tenderness in the region of one or both kidneys occurs not infrequently in lower urinary tract infections. However, sudden fever to 38.9° to 40.6°C, shaking chills, aching costovertebral or flank pain, and symptoms of sepsis are more characteristic of acute pyelonephritis than of cystitis or urethritis.

Laboratory tests show a polymorphonuclear leukocytosis in both cystitis and pyelonephritis. Pyuria is seen in urethritis, cystitis, and pyelonephritis, but white blood cell casts are more typical of pyelonephritis. Stain of the sediment and urine cultures reveal numerous bacteria, usually gram-negative bacilli. Cultures of blood may also be positive in some cases of pyelonephritis. A simple but convenient way of identifying infection of the urinary tract is by examining the urine (see below): The microscopic presence of bacteria in the urine generally indicates more than 100,000 colonies per milliliter of urine. However, the microscopic absence of bacteria does not exclude the diagnosis of urinary infection.

Impaired renal function or acute hypertension is rarely seen in acute pyelonephritis, but renal concentrating ability may be impaired. Also, subclinical forms of acute pyelonephritis may occur because tests that differentiate "upper" (kidney) from "lower" (bladder) infection may indicate the presence of renal infection in the absence of flank pain or fever. However, the only reliable tests, ureteral catheterization and bladder washout, are considered to be research maneuvers. A search for antibody-coated bacteria in the urine as a marker of renal bacteriuria may be performed, but the sensitivity and specificity of this test are not optimal. Pyelonephritis at times presents with symptoms that do not point to the urinary tract. Some patients may have only backache without demonstrable renal tenderness. Others have upper or lower abdominal pain, together with symptoms of disturbed gastrointestinal function. Some complain only of general fatigue.

In the absence of obstructive lesions of the urinary tract or host immunocompromise, as in diabetics, upper or lower urinary tract infections are generally self-limited, lasting 10 to 14 days. When obstruction or host immunocompromise is present, pyelonephritis may be complicated by papillary necrosis, perinephric abscess, or renal carbuncle. These complications should be suspected when persistent flank pain, fever, and leukocytosis are unresponsive to otherwise adequate chemotherapy (see below).

Acute urinary tract infection complicated by pyelonephritis may occur in patients subjected to urethral instrumentation, particularly long-term indwelling catheters. Sepsis from pyelonephritis is a major cause of death in individuals having neurologic disorders requiring long-term indwelling catheters.

DIAGNOSIS

Microscopic Methods

Rapid diagnostic methods are available either (1) by preparation of a Gram's stain of either centrifuged or uncentrifuged urine and examination with an oil immersion lens or (2) by study of either centrifuged or uncentrifuged urine, employing the high-dry objective under reduced light, with or without methylene blue stain. The presence of any bacteria on Gram's stain of centrifuged urine correlates best (97 per cent) with quantitative culture (100,000 bacteria per milliliter of urine). Examination of the unstained sediment for the presence of any bacteria is also very helpful and can be done during routine examination for formed elements. Pyuria, arbitrarily defined as 10 or more leukocytes per high-power field in the centrifuged specimen, can also be detected by the leukocyte esterase dipstick test. The presence of pyuria in a midstream urine sample suggests the likelihood of a urinary tract infection. Some erythrocytes may be seen in the urine, and gross hematuria may occur when inflammation in the bladder is intense. Proteinuria is not common in urinary tract infections, but in fulminant pyelonephritis, as in other severe acute interstitial nephritides, significant degrees of proteinuria may occur transiently.

Significant Bacteriuria

The concept of "significant bacteriuria" was introduced to distinguish between those bacteria that actually multiply in the urine and bacteria that are contaminants. This distinction can be made by knowledge of the site and manner in which the urine is collected from the patient and by enumeration of the number of organisms present in the sample. The criterion of 100,000 or more organisms per milliliter of urine for the diagnosis of significant bacteriuria is an excellent operational definition when the clear-voided method is used, in both males and females, to collect specimens that are processed promptly. However, bacterial counts lower than 100,000 colonies per milliliter may occur in patients with true bacteriuria. Specifically, some women with acute bacterial cystitis, who present with dysuria and frequency (the acute urethral syndrome), may have as few as 100 bacteria per milliliter of urine. Isolation of multiple species from the urine usually indicates contamination, especially in the asymptomatic person.

Urine collected by suprapubic aspiration or bladder catheterization is less likely to be contaminated. In this instance, bacterial counts of fewer than 100,000 organisms per milliliter are likely to be significant.

Bacteriologic Findings

The species of bacteria most likely to be recovered from individuals with bacteriuria depends upon prior history of infection, prior antimicrobial therapy, hospitalization, and instrumentation of the urinary tract. Enterobacteriaceae are the most common organisms identified. *E. coli* accounts for more than 80 per cent of all species recovered in uncomplicated cases, whereas *Proteus, Klebsiella, Enterobacter, Pseudomonas*, enterococci, and staphylococci are more often found in patients who have had previous infection or instrumentation. Occasionally, *Serratia marcescens, Acinetobacter, Candida albicans*, and *Cryptococcus neoformans* may produce infection of the urinary tract in diabetics and in immunosuppressed or corticosteroid-treated patients. Coliforms are also the most common organisms responsible for the acute urethral syndrome in women who have fewer than 10^5 bacteria per milliliter of urine, although *Staphylococcus saprophyticus* and *Chlamydia trachomatis* are responsible for some cases. Patients with the acute urethral syndrome caused by *Chlamydia trachomatis* have pyuria but sterile bladder urine when cultured with standard bacteriologic media.

Anaerobes are commonly present in the distal urethra and the vagina and are abundant in the gut, but they rarely produce urinary tract infection. Suprapubic aspiration of urine or examination of tissues is needed to prove anaerobic infections. When responsible, anaerobes are usually associated with complicated, longstanding infections.

Radiology

Radiographic evaluation of the urinary tract is undertaken to detect correctable lesions that may contribute to the severity or recurrence of urinary tract infections. Evaluation is indicated in men with any type of urinary tract infection or in instances of documented bacteremia. In women, urography is not indicated unless a complication, such as papillary necrosis, perinephric abscess, renal carbuncle, or tumor, is suspected because the patient is unresponsive to otherwise adequate chemotherapy.

EPIDEMIOLOGY AND NATURAL HISTORY

Bacteriuria in the newborn population has been difficult to study because of problems inherent in urine collection. Cultures of urine obtained by bladder puncture suggest an incidence of 1 to 2 per cent. Infection of the urinary tract in this age group may be part of a generalized, life-threatening gram-negative sepsis and is more common in boys than girls. Symptomatic urinary tract infections are more prevalent among girls in preschool years and are often associated with obstructive or neurogenic lesions. Urologic investigation is valuable in this age group. *Urologic evaluation is mandatory in males of any age because of the high frequency of structural abnormalities found* (valves, malformation, and obstructive and neurogenic lesions).

The incidence of bacteriuria among school girls is 1 to 2 per cent; it is only 0.03 per cent in boys of the same age. The incidence of bacteriuria in females rises about 1 per cent per decade.

Urinary tract infection is common after marriage. The pathogenesis of the "honeymoon cystitis" syndrome remains unclear. Physical factors associated with sexual activity in previously sexually nonactive women may play a prominent role. Many patients with "honeymoon cystitis" (up to 50 per cent) have dysuria due to local irritation rather than infection, and this should be clearly differentiated by culture.

Bacteriuria of pregnancy varies from 2 to 6 per cent, depending upon age, parity, and socioeconomic group. Acute symptomatic pyelonephritis develops later in pregnancy in approximately 20 per cent of these women. However, there is no evidence that isolated episodes of pyelonephritis in pregnant women lead to chronic urinary tract infections after these women cease childbearing activities. Early detection and treatment of bacteriuria in pregnancy prevent the emergence of symptomatic infection.

Elderly women may have frequencies of bacteriuria as high as 10 per cent; this rate may increase in hospitalized patients, particularly diabetics. Bacteriuria in men begins to appear in "prostate years" and is often initiated by instrumentation.

Role of Instrumentation

Bacteriuria persists in 1 to 2 per cent of relatively healthy individuals following a single catheterization; the risk is higher in the debilitated patient and in men with prostatic obstruction. With open indwelling catheter drainage, bacterial colonization exceeds 90 per cent within 3 to 4 days. This may lead to life-threatening pyelonephritis and gram-negative sepsis. Fortunately, it is largely preventable by (1) careful criteria for catheterization and (2) use of aseptic closed drainage. The catheter should be removed as soon as it is no longer needed.

Intermittent self-catheterization coupled with abdominal pressure may be of benefit in patients with neurogenic bladders and may result in minimal urinary tract infections.

TREATMENT

The goal of treatment is to eradicate bacteria from the urinary tract in order to relieve symptoms, prevent renal damage, and diminish the likelihood of spread of infections to other sites. Prophylaxis is used to prevent recurrent symptomatic infection. Suppression, although rarely effective, is used to diminish the number of bacteria in the urine or tissue. Indications for therapy depend on the potential of infection to give rise to symptoms or damage to the urinary tract and the likelihood that treatment will be effective (Fig. 84–1).

Asymptomatic Bacteriuria

Asymptomatic bacteriuria should probably not be treated except in those patients who are at high risk of developing symptomatic infections. Thus, treatment of asymptomatic bacteriuria is indicated in pregnant patients to prevent symptomatic illness in the third trimester; in patients who may have major predisposing factors to renal disease, such as diabetic or polycystic kidneys, or who have anatomic or neurologic abnormalities; and in patients who are immunocompromised or who will undergo urologic manipulation. If the treatment fails to eradicate asymptomatic infections in such individuals, further treatment should be reserved for acute symptomatic episodes. In contrast, asymptomatic bacteriuria in females should not be treated in the absence of underlying structural or neurologic lesions, since the likelihood that renal damage will occur is slight. Furthermore, short courses of therapy, when effective, are commonly followed by reinfection. In addition, asymptomatic bacteriuria in patients with indwelling catheter and in the very elderly or nonambulatory patients should not be treated, because the toxicity and expense of therapy may outweigh the risk of disease.

Symptomatic Urinary Tract Infection

Acute uncomplicated episodes of symptomatic bacteriuria localized to the lower urinary tract (bladder or urethra) can be treated effectively with oral single-dose therapy: amoxicillin–clavulanic acid (Augmentin), 3 grams (given as one 500-mg Augmentin tablet plus 2.5 grams of amoxicillin); co-trimoxazole (trimethoprim, 0.32 gram, plus sulfamethoxazole, 1.6 grams), two double-strength tablets; or the newer quinolones—ciprofloxacin (100 mg or 250 mg) or norfloxacin (800 mg). Single-dose therapy usually fails to eradicate either renal bacteriuria or complicated infections. In addition, single-dose therapy is more effective in suburban then in inner-city women with cystitis and in women less than 25 years of age than in women more than 40 years of age. Higher cure rates may be achieved in inner-city or older women with trimethoprim, 0.16 gram, plus sulfamethoxazole, 0.8 gram, or ciprofloxacin, 250 mg, or norfloxacin, 400 mg, twice daily for 3 days. Symptomatic urethritis caused by *Chlamydia trachomatis* should respond to oral doxycycline (100 mg twice daily) or tetracycline (500 mg four times per day) for 7 days.

Pyelonephritis requires a 7- to 14-day or longer course of therapy. Acute uncomplicated pyelonephritis can be treated orally with co-trimoxazole for 14 days on an outpatient basis. Complicated infections in which obstruction or a foreign body is not removed may not respond to such a course. Hematogenous pyelonephritis requires specific therapy directed at the invading organism.

The choice of an oral or parenteral agent depends upon the severity of the infection and the patient's ability to take the oral agent. Drugs are selected on the basis of cost, side effects, and antibacterial spectrum. Antimicrobial susceptibility tests should be used to guide therapy of recurrent episodes. Effective oral agents include sulfonamides, tetracyclines, ampicillin, amoxicillin, cinoxacin, ciprofloxacin, norfloxacin, cephalosporins, co-trimoxazole, trimethoprim, and nitrofurantoin. The last three drugs are useful in recurrent infections, because emergence of resistant strains occurs infrequently.

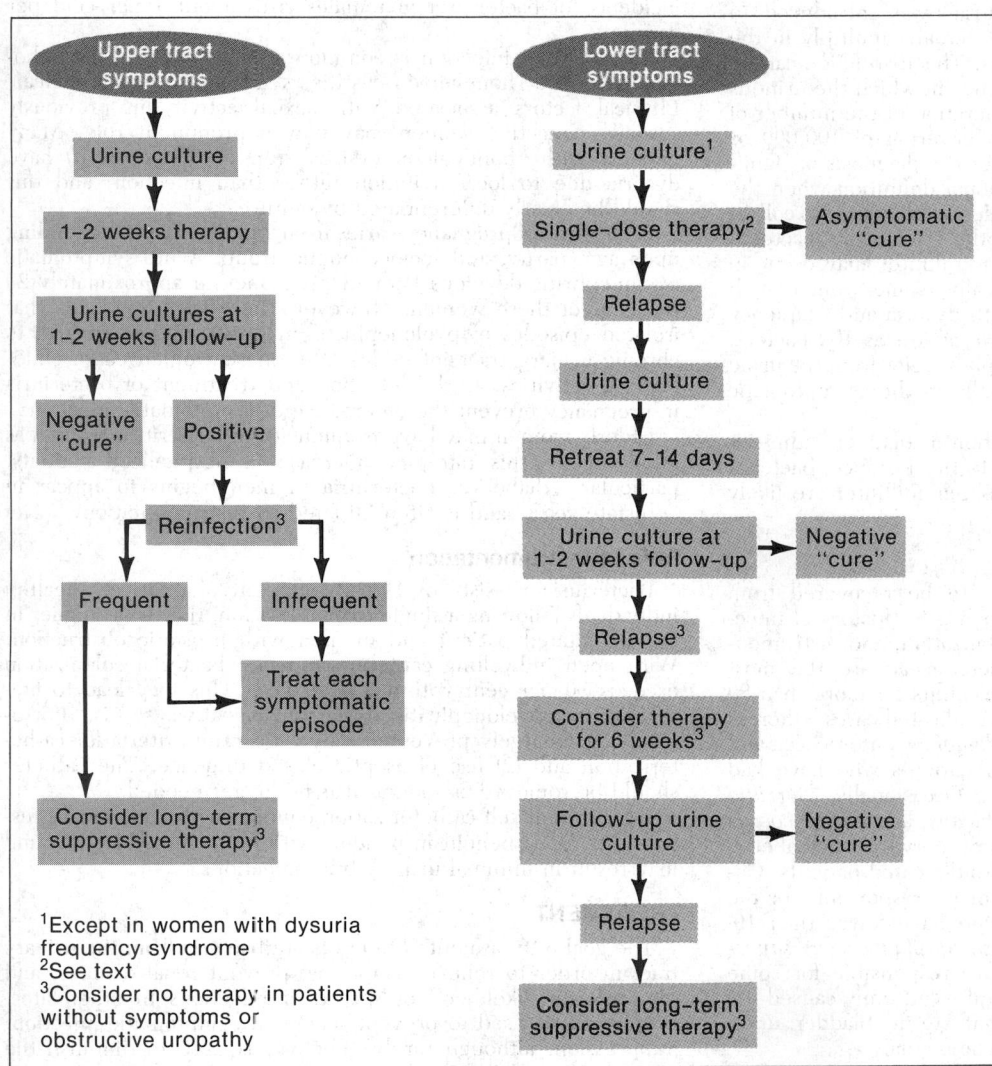

FIGURE 84–1. Management of urinary tract infections.

The initial attack of urinary tract infection is usually due to *E. coli*, which is sensitive to most antimicrobial agents and therefore may be treated "blindly" with the agents described above, with equal success. However, the widespread use of these agents for other infections has decreased their previous reliability. For example, approximately 40 per cent of *E. coli*, including those that are community acquired, are now resistant to ampicillin and amoxicillin.

Microscopic examination of urine and urine cultures have been the mainstay for accurate diagnosis of urinary tract infections. Pretreatment urine cultures are probably not essential, however, and are not cost effective in selected young women with acute dysuria and pyuria, in whom the probability of uncomplicated bacterial cystitis is high. These patients respond to short-course empiric therapy. Urine cultures can be reserved for those in whom therapy has failed. In contrast, pretreatment urine cultures should be obtained in symptomatic infants, children, men, and the elderly; patients with suspected pyelonephritis or complicated infection; patients with relapsing infections; those with *symptomatic* catheter- or instrument-associated nosocomial infection; and pregnant women to detect covert bacteriuria of pregnancy.

When therapy is successful, bacteriuria should disappear within 24 hours even if pyuria and symptoms continue. A repeat urine culture should be obtained after 72 hours of treatment in those patients who have had a pretreatment culture. A positive culture at this time denotes treatment failure. It is important to recognize bacteriologic failure early and to change to another drug. Parenteral agents, such as ampicillin, a cephalosporin, or an aminoglycoside, may be required in some instances or when the patient is too ill to receive an oral agent. A follow-up culture 1 week after the completion of antimicrobial therapy is recommended to document a cure.

Some authors recommend routine follow-up cultures several times over the ensuing year to detect recurrent bacteriuria, but this practice is prohibitively expensive and difficult to justify on medical grounds in asymptomatic patients.

Recurrent Infections

Recurrence of infection in the few weeks after treatment is usually due to persistence of the same focus, whereas later recurrence, particularly in women, is more often a result of reinfection. Frequent recurrent infections may be managed either by close follow-up and treatment of each episode or by prophylaxis with nitrofurantoin, trimethoprim, or co-trimoxazole as a single bedtime dose.

Urinary antiseptics, such as methenamine mandelate or hippurate, require an acidic urine, preferably at pH 5.5, and are of little value unless their use is accompanied by agents that consistently lower urinary pH, such as high-dose ascorbic acid (1000 mg daily). Methenamine, however, is an effective "suppressant" agent and is best used after infection is eradicated by a more effective drug.

Prophylaxis, when given for 3 to 6 months, is effective for recurrent infections of the reinfection type in women. Cessation of prophylaxis, however, results in a significant incidence of recurrence in individuals having structural abnormalities of the urinary tract or intrinsic renal structural defects. In those circumstances, prophylaxis should be reinstituted. Generally, the therapeutic agent should be changed if bacteriuria persists during treatment. This latter circumstance usually means an organism resistant to the agent is now colonizing the urine. Prophylaxis is ineffective in patients with indwelling catheters and will only lead to emergence of resistant bacteria.

The patient should be instructed to drink fluids generously and void frequently. Double voiding in patients with vesicoureteral reflux is recommended. Voiding after sexual intercourse is felt by some to decrease the chance of recurrent infection, but postcoital use of prophylactic agents is probably more effective.

Complicated Infections

Complex urinary infections, i.e., those in the presence of obstructive uropathy, neurogenic bladders, or catheters, are exceedingly difficult to eradicate. They are often best left untreated except for management of acute episodes. Suppressive therapy should be considered ineffective if bacterial populations in the urine are not reduced to less than 1000 per milliliter. The key to management is relief of obstruction or the removal of foreign bodies. Intermittent catheterization has benefited some patients with neurogenic bladders.

COMPLICATIONS

While most urinary tract infections, including pyelonephritis, are self-limited and easily treated, there are three severe complications of pyelonephritis with which the clinician must be familiar: *renal papillary necrosis, renal abscess* (renal carbuncle), and *perinephric abscess*. These complications are uncommon and occur most often in patients with underlying structural renal abnormalities or host immunocompromise (particularly diabetes).

Renal Papillary Necrosis

Renal papillary necrosis, an ischemic necrosis of the renal papilla and adjacent portions of the renal medulla, may be seen in association with severe pyelonephritis, diabetes mellitus, sickle cell anemia, obstructive uropathy, and analgesic abuse. Although infection appears to be the most important factor in the pathogenesis of this lesion, the peculiarities of blood supply of the medulla must also be a factor. This helps explain the frequent occurrence of the lesion in patients with diabetes and generalized vascular disease, as well as the role of obstruction, which must impair blood supply to this area. The zone of necrosis may occur from the extreme tip of the pyramid as far proximal as the corticomedullary junction. Eventually this may slough, with migration of chunks of necrotic tissue down the urinary passages.

The clinical manifestations of renal papillary necrosis are intensification of symptoms of pre-existing pyelonephritis. There may be pain in the lumbar region, colicky pain along the ureteral radiation, hematuria, and high fever. Manifestations of gram-negative bacteremia may supervene. This lesion should be considered in elderly patients with diabetes who show rapid deterioration in clinical status with signs of active pyelonephritis and increasing renal decompensation.

The diagnosis can sometimes be made by finding pieces of renal medullary tissue in the urinary sediment. Pyelography may demonstrate cavities and sinuses in the region of the papillae. The classic ring-shadow pattern results from detachment of a papilla and its outline within the contrast-filled cavity.

Therapy should be directed toward control of infection and measures employed to improve the status of patients who have diabetes mellitus or who are habitual abusers of analgesic agents.

Renal Abscess

Renal abscesses usually occur as a result of extension of a pyelonephritis process. Up to one half of the cases, however, arise from hematogenous spread, by virulent organisms such as *Staphylococcus aureus*, from a distant focus.

A renal abscess may be identified by intravenous pyelography, ultrasonography, computed tomography, or magnetic resonance imaging. It should be suspected whenever a urinary tract infection fails to respond to an adequate course of appropriate antibiotics. Blood and urine cultures may be negative, so empiric antibiotic regimens may be needed to cover gram-negative rods and staphylococci. Surgical drainage is usually required in addition to parenteral antibiotics, although early diagnosis may eliminate the need for surgery in some patients.

Perinephric Abscess

Perinephric abscesses are notoriously difficult to diagnose. They have an insidious onset, with symptoms usually present for over 2 weeks at the time of presentation. Fever and unilateral flank pain are common presenting symptoms. The diagnosis should be considered in the evaluation of any patient with a fever of unknown origin. A recent history of urinary tract infection should alert one to the possibility of a perinephric abscess, although this piece of history is often absent. More than two thirds of patients with perinephric abscesses have either diabetes or kidney stone disease.

Perinephric abscesses occur almost exclusively from the rupture of an intrarenal abscess. Diagnosis can be established by ultrasonography, computed tomography, or magnetic resonance imaging. Surgical drainage is mandatory.

Andriole VT: Current concepts of urinary tract infections. *In* Weinstein L, Fields BN (eds.): Seminars in Infectious Disease. Vol III. New York, Thieme-Stratton, 1980, pp 89–130. *The author's review of practical diagnostic methods, microbiologic concepts, host defenses, clinical syndromes, and treatment of urinary tract infections.*

Andriole VT: Renal and perirenal abscesses. *In* Schrier RW, Gottschalk CW (eds.): Diseases of the Kidney. 4th ed. Boston, Little, Brown and Company, 1987, pp 1049–1064. *A detailed review of the pathogenesis, diagnosis (including the value of diagnostic radiology), and treatment of infections in and around the kidney.*

Andriole VT: Urinary tract infections. Infect Dis Clin North Am 1:713, 1987. *A multiauthored text on all aspects of urinary tract infections in adults and children.*

Andriole VT: Urinary tract infections: Recent developments. J Infect Dis 156:865, 1987. *An update on current theories on the pathogenesis of urinary tract infections.*

Jenkins RD, Fenn JP, Matsen JM: Review of urine microscopy for bacteriuria. JAMA 255:3397, 1986. *An update on the value of urine microscopy.*

Johnson JR, Stamm WE: Urinary tract infections in women: Diagnosis and treatment. Ann Intern Med 111:906, 1989. *A current guide for antimicrobial therapy in urinary tract infections.*

Kunin CM: Detection, Prevention and Treatment of Urinary Tract Infections. 4th ed. Philadelphia, Lea & Febiger, 1986. *An excellent text that describes the pathogenesis, management, and prevention of urinary tract infections.*

Mayrer AR, Miniter P, Andriole VT: Immunopathogenesis of chronic pyelonephritis. Am J Med 75 (Suppl 1B):59, 1983. *Recent studies describing immunologic mechanisms of renal injury and scarring, which produce a histopathologic picture of chronic pyelonephritis.*

Stamm WE, Hooten TM, Johnson JR, et al.: Urinary tract infections: From pathogenesis to treatment. J Infect Dis 159:400, 1989. *A review of our understanding of the pathogenesis of urinary tract infections.*

85 Vascular Disorders of the Kidney

Jordan J. Cohen

RENAL ARTERY OCCLUSION

Partial occlusion (stenosis) of the main renal artery, or one or more of its branches, is common and typically results in hypertension. The clinical features of renovascular hypertension are discussed in Ch. 44. This section considers total or nearly total occlusion of the arterial supply to all or a portion of the kidney.

CAUSES (Table 85–1). Thrombosis in situ rarely occurs in the absence of a severely diseased or damaged vessel. Macroemboli of the renal circulation are far more common as a cause of complete occlusion than are in situ thrombi. (Atheroemboli are

TABLE 85–1. CAUSES OF RENAL ARTERY OCCLUSION

Thrombosis, in situ
    Progressive atherosclerosis
    Blunt trauma
    Inflammation (e.g., polyarteritis, thromboangiitis obliterans)
    Aortic or renal artery aneurysm
    Aortic or renal artery dissection
    Angiographic catheter
    No obvious cause ("spontaneous")

Macroemboli
    Atrial fibrillation
    Mitral stenosis
    Mural thrombus
    Atrial myxoma
    Infective endocarditis
    Prosthetic valve
    Paradoxical emboli (patent foramen ovale)

Atheroemboli
    Abdominal aorta surgery
    Blunt trauma
    Angiographic catheters
    Anticoagulation (?)
    No obvious cause ("spontaneous")

considered in the following section.) Approximately 90 per cent of renal artery emboli originate in the heart. Of these, most arise from the left atrium and are a consequence of atrial fibrillation due to arteriosclerotic heart disease. Although 20 per cent of the cardiac output normally goes to the kidney, only 2 to 3 per cent of the systemic emboli derived from the heart lodge in the renal circulation. The number, the size, and the consistency of individual embolic particles vary with the nature of the underlying process and determine the extent of renal involvement. Large emboli can occlude the main renal artery, but, more frequently, embolic material reaches primary or secondary branches of the vessel. Thus, total infarction of the kidney is much less common than is ischemia or segmental infarction. The presence of one or more accessory renal arteries in 20 to 30 per cent of people and of a generally rich capsular circulation also reduces the likelihood of extensive infarction. In most instances, the embolic event involves only one kidney; bilateral emboli and emboli to a solitary kidney do occur and are associated with greater morbidity.

CLINICAL MANIFESTATIONS. Sudden occlusion of a renal artery, whether from embolus or thrombosis, results in a wide spectrum of clinical manifestations in accordance with the caliber of the vessel or vessels involved and with the pre-existing status of the renal circulation. Occlusion of a primary or secondary branch of the renal artery in a patient with well-established collateral circulation due to chronic, high-grade stenosis may produce little or no infarction and, hence, few or no signs or symptoms; conversely, occlusion of the main renal artery in an otherwise normal kidney may result in immediate infarction of most of the organ and in a dramatic clinical presentation. Renal infarction typically results in the acute onset of vague, nonspecific flank pain that is described as dull and aching in character. The pain may, however, resemble that due to renal colic, cholecystitis, or pancreatitis. Nausea and vomiting are frequent; gross hematuria is *not* common. The symptoms usually subside within 3 to 4 days.

Fever is an infrequent finding at onset but often appears within 1 to 2 days. Hypertension is often present. The white blood cell count is usually elevated, and a leftward shift in the differential count is characteristic. Microscopic hematuria is common but may be absent. Striking elevations of serum lactate dehydrogenase (LDH) levels and lesser elevations of serum glutamic-oxaloacetic transaminase (SGOT) are characteristic. The blood urea nitrogen (BUN) and serum creatinine levels typically rise transiently in unilateral infarction; more severe and protracted degrees of renal functional impairment, including acute oliguric renal failure, may follow bilateral renal infarction or infarction of a solitary kidney.

DIAGNOSIS. The diagnosis of renal artery occlusion and infarction is often difficult because the clinical findings are frequently meager and nonspecific. As a result, fewer than 1 per cent of autopsy-proven cases may be diagnosed ante mortem. The intravenous pyelogram typically reveals reduced or absent function in the involved kidney or kidneys; retrograde pyelography usually reveals no abnormality. Indeed, a normal retrograde study in a kidney that makes no urine and fails to visualize on intravenous pyelography is virtually diagnostic of arterial occlusion. Radionuclide scanning of the kidney may show segmental perfusion defects or complete absence of perfusion. Definitive diagnosis of renal artery occlusion, however, requires renal angiography. In addition, angiography can often distinguish between embolic and thrombotic occlusion. Angiography should be reserved for those patients in whom the diagnostic information is crucial for making management decisions because the risk of the procedure in this setting is appreciable.

TREATMENT. The choice of therapy for acute renal artery occlusion varies widely with individual circumstances (Table 85–2). As a rule, unilateral renal artery occlusion should be treated conservatively, especially if a branch vessel or vessels are in-

TABLE 85–2. TREATMENT OPTIONS FOR RENAL ARTERY OCCLUSION

Observation
Anticoagulation
Thrombolytic therapy followed by anticoagulation
Percutaneous transluminal angioplasty
Surgical embolectomy or endarterectomy
Partial or total nephrectomy

volved; observation alone or coupled with anticoagulation often results in recanalization and avoids the high risk of surgery. Patients with bilateral occlusion or occlusion in a solitary kidney generally fare better with operative intervention. Mortality rates as high as 35 per cent have been reported in patients undergoing acute revascularization procedures. Fibrinolytic therapy followed by anticoagulation can be considered an alternative to surgery in selected cases. Recovery of renal function is a complex function of the duration and magnitude of the occlusion, the extent of collaterals, the degree of associated cardiovascular disease, and the skill and experience of the operative team. Hemodialysis can be used as a temporizing maneuver if the degree of renal functional impairment warrants. Recovery of renal function has been reported to occur after as long as 1 month of oliguric renal failure due to renal artery occlusion. Given that irreversible renal damage occurs within 60 minutes of total renal ischemia induced experimentally, such occurrences of recovery after lengthy delay underscore the important role of renal collaterals.

Percutaneous transluminal angioplasty has proved successful as an alternative to surgery for stenotic lesions of the renal artery and for occlusive lesions as well. Nephrectomy should not be considered unless unequivocal evidence of total infarction is present or hypertension is uncontrollable.

RENAL ARTERY ATHEROEMBOLI

CAUSES. Renal artery atheroembolization is a complication of severe erosive (ulcerative) atheromatosis of the abdominal aorta. Atheroemboli may occur with great frequency in patients with this condition, but, fortunately, in only a small fraction does the process culminate in significant clinical abnormalities. Events that can trigger the release of cholesterol-laden embolic material from ulcerative plaques are listed in Table 85–1.

CLINICAL MANIFESTATIONS. Atheroemboli characteristically lodge in vessels smaller than the interlobular arteries. As a consequence, macroscopic renal infarction does not usually occur, and the clinical picture is usually bland. The insidious development of renal insufficiency is the mode of presentation in most instances of severe atheroemboli. Hypertension is frequently present and may be severe. Distal embolization in the lower extremities, occasionally associated with livedo reticularis, is frequent. Acute pancreatitis and gastrointestinal bleeding can occur and indicate more widespread embolization. Laboratory findings are nonspecific and give evidence of steady or episodic decline in renal function over a period of days, weeks, or even months. Eosinophilia is common, but its cause is unknown. Urinalysis reveals nothing characteristic and is frequently normal. Kidney size is usually normal or only slightly reduced.

DIAGNOSIS. The diagnosis frequently goes undetected, and a high index of suspicion is warranted in the appropriate clinical setting. Diagnosis is made by renal biopsy. Cholesterol crystals contained in the embolic material are dissolved during routine preparation of the histologic sections, leaving pathognomonic biconvex, cleftlike structures in the occluded vessels. Skin and muscle biopsies of the lower extremities, especially from clinically affected sites, may contain similar lesions.

TREATMENT. No effective therapy is available for this condition. Anticoagulants are *not* helpful and may in fact foster atheroemboli by delaying healing of the atheromatous ulcers in the aorta. Unfortunately, once renal manifestations are evident, the process often progresses unrelentingly to renal failure.

RENAL VEIN THROMBOSIS

CAUSES (Table 85–3). Renal vein thrombosis in infants is typically an acute catastrophic event triggered by a volume-depleting illness, such as profuse diarrhea. The consequences are sudden cessation of renal function, engorgement and enlargement of the kidneys, and ultimate renal infarction and atrophy if venous obstruction is not relieved. Fortunately, acute renal vein thrombosis of such magnitude is rare in older children and adults.

TABLE 85–3. CAUSES OF RENAL VEIN THROMBOSIS

Reduced renal blood flow (especially in infants)
Nephrotic syndrome (especially in membranous glomerulopathy)
Renal cell carcinoma
Inferior vena caval thrombosis
External compression (e.g., retroperitoneal fibrosis, tumor)

Renal vein thrombosis in adults is typically of insidious onset and is almost always superimposed on an established disease. It occurs most frequently in association with idiopathic nephrotic syndrome, especially that due to membranous glomerulopathy. Predisposing factors may include reduced antithrombin III levels, reduced intravascular blood volume (often aggravated by diuretic therapy), thrombocytosis, and elevated liver-derived clotting factors. Patients with renal cell carcinoma often develop renal vein thrombosis consequent to tumor invasion of the renal vein.

CLINICAL MANIFESTATIONS. In the typical circumstance in which gradual occlusion of the renal vein occurs, the process may progress without any outward sign. Mild abdominal or back pain may be present, but severe pain is uncommon. Pulmonary emboli occur during the course of approximately half of all patients with chronic renal vein thrombosis and are frequently the initial manifestation of the condition. Renal vein thrombosis can also cause unexplained deterioration in renal function in patients with the nephrotic syndrome. Chronic renal vein thrombosis itself results in no characteristic findings on physical examination or laboratory testing. Heavy proteinuria occurs frequently in patients with this condition but reflects the presence of pre-existing nephrotic syndrome; it is not the result of renal vein thrombosis itself.

DIAGNOSIS. The index of suspicion may be heightened greatly by the clinical setting (e.g., recurrent pulmonary emboli in a patient with nephrotic syndrome) or by findings on intravenous pyelography (e.g., large kidneys with splayed calices due to interstitial edema, notching of the upper ureters due to collaterals). Definitive diagnosis, however, requires visualization of the renal vein. Selective renal venography is generally relied upon for unequivocal visualization of the vessel and its branches, but adequate visualization of the main vein can often be obtained with ultrasound, computed tomography, or magnetic resonance imaging.

TREATMENT. Long-term anticoagulation remains the treatment of choice in chronic, subtotal renal vein thrombosis. Fibrinolytic therapy for a few days prior to instituting anticoagulation should be considered in patients with more serious manifestations of renal vein thrombosis (e.g., acute flank pain coupled with a rising serum creatinine level, rapidly recurring pulmonary emboli).

Harrington JT, Kassirer JP: Renal vein thrombosis. Ann Rev Med 33:255, 1982. *An excellent, clinically relevant review.*

Keating MA, Althausen AF: The clinical spectrum of renal vein thrombosis. J Urol 133:938, 1985. *A well-referenced review of historical and modern concepts of the etiology and management of renal vein thrombosis.*

Lessman RK, Johnson SF, Coburn JW, et al.: Renal artery embolism: Clinical features and long-term follow-up of 17 cases. Ann Intern Med 89:477, 1978. *An excellent detailed review and follow-up of one of the larger series of patients with renal artery embolism; emphasizes the nonoperative management.*

Llach F: Hypercoagulability, renal vein thrombosis, and other thrombotic complications of nephrotic syndrome. Kidney Int 28:429, 1985. *An editorial review of the coagulation abnormalities and clinical features of renal vein thrombosis in patients with the nephrotic syndrome.*

Ouriel K, Andrus CH, Ricotta JJ, et al.: Acute renal artery occlusion: When is revascularization justified? J Vasc Surg 5:348, 1987. *Retrospective analysis of a single medical center's 20-year experience with the management of acute renal artery occlusion.*

Stanley JC, Whithouse WMJ: Occlusive and aneurysmal disease of the renal arterial circulation. DM 30:7, 1984. *A readable review emphasizing the diagnosis and therapy of common afflictions of the renal arteries.*

86 Renal Disease in Pregnancy

John P. Hayslett

The detection and clinical management of renal disease in the gravid woman are complicated by concern for fetal development and survival, as well as for the health of the patient. In addition, clinical evaluation requires knowledge of the physiologic changes in volume status and renal function that accompany pregnancy.

RENAL FUNCTION IN PREGNANCY. Pregnancy is characterized by a gradual, cumulative retention of 500 to 900 mEq of sodium and 6 to 8 liters of water, which are distributed between maternal extracellular fluid and the fetus. Despite an expansion in plasma volume of 30 to 45 per cent, mean blood pressure falls approximately 15 per cent owing to a reduction in peripheral vascular resistance. The glomerular filtration rate (GFR) and plasma flow increase by 30 to 50 per cent by the twelfth week of gestation, an elevation that is sustained until term (Fig. 86–1). Evaluation of GFR, therefore, should take into account expected levels during gestation and should not compare measured values with normal levels in the nonpregnant population. Since renal hemodynamics may be affected by position, a convenient way of measuring GFR in later pregnancy is with a timed (e.g., 4 hours) water-loaded creatinine clearance with the woman lying on her side, a position associated with the highest values.

Because of the increase in GFR, the levels of creatinine and blood urea nitrogen (BUN) fall to approximately 0.5 mg per deciliter and 9 mg per deciliter, respectively. Plasma concentrations above 0.8 mg per deciliter of creatinine and 13 mg per deciliter of urea nitrogen should alert the physician to the possibility of renal insufficiency. Plasma osmolality falls from approximately 280 mOsm • kg H_2O to 270, owing to a resetting of the osmostat; the plasma uric acid level falls to 3 to 4 mg per deciliter and plasma bicarbonate to approximately 20 mEq per liter (because of mild respiratory alkalosis). Glucosuria and aminoaciduria may occur during pregnancy owing, in part, both to increases in filtered load and to a transient reduction in the renal threshold of absorption. The ureters dilate during pregnancy and may remain dilated for as long as 12 weeks post partum with no implication of outflow obstruction.

PREECLAMPSIA (PREGNANCY-INDUCED HYPERTENSION)

DEFINITION. Preeclampsia, unique to human pregnancy, is characterized by hypertension in late pregnancy, usually accompanied by edema, and by proteinuria. It may rapidly progress to a convulsive phase, called eclampsia. Onset is usually insidious after the thirty-second week of pregnancy, but it may occur as early as the twenty-fourth week. In women with a hydatidiform mole, preeclampsia has been reported to occur in the first two trimesters. The usual sequence is edema and hypertension, followed by proteinuria, although proteinuria may occasionally precede hypertension. The disease usually subsides rapidly after delivery. Clinical criteria for diagnosis vary, depending on changes in blood pressure considered to be abnormal in preg-

nancy. In general, hypertension in the third trimester is defined by a blood pressure measurement of 140/85 mm Hg or greater if sustained for 4 to 6 hours, or an increase of 30 mm Hg or more in systolic blood pressure and 15 mm Hg or more in diastolic pressure above values measured during the early stages of pregnancy. The major differential diagnosis involves a distinction among preeclampsia, essential hypertension, and primary renal disease, although preeclampsia can be superimposed on the other two clinical entities.

INCIDENCE. Preeclampsia occurs worldwide with an incidence that varies between 2 per cent and 25 per cent in different populations. In the United States, the quoted incidence is 6 to 7 per cent. Individuals with a poor socioeconomic status may be at higher risk for developing the syndrome; the incidence is reduced by adequate prenatal care, with special attention to weight gain and monitoring of blood pressure. The syndrome occurs predominantly in primigravidas and especially at the extremes of reproductive age.

CLINICAL MANIFESTATIONS. Clinical symptoms of severe disease may include headache, epigastric pain, apprehension, and visual disturbances. While diastolic hypertension may be prominent, systolic blood pressure seldom exceeds 160 mm Hg, except when associated with underlying essential hypertension. Funduscopic examination may reveal segmental arteriolar narrowing and a generalized glistening fundus indicative of retinal edema. The ocular changes reflect vasoconstriction. Signs of central nervous system hyperexcitability are regarded as ominous, since they often precede convulsions, which account for most of the fetal and maternal morbidity and mortality associated with the disease. Laboratory findings include a rate of protein excretion exceeding 300 mg per day but most often below 2 grams per day, although occasionally reaching nephrotic levels of greater than 3 grams per day. There is a reduction in GFR and renal plasma flow to about 30 to 35 per cent of that in pregnancy control subjects. Owing to elevated levels of the GFR in normal pregnancy, however, BUN and serum creatinine levels may not appear to be elevated in toxemic patients, especially if compared with nonpregnant control values. Plasma uric acid levels rise in preeclampsia to about 5.0 mg per deciliter in mild toxemia and to over 7.0 mg per deciliter in severe states, because of a fall in its renal clearance. Some women with preeclampsia manifest coagulation abnormalities, thrombocytopenia, and/or liver function abnormalities.

PATHOGENESIS AND PATHOLOGY. The cause of preeclampsia is not understood. Plasma levels of aldosterone and renin are lower than in normal pregnant individuals but still may be inappropriately high in relation to salt intake and volume status. Many primigravidas who eventually develop toxemia exhibit increased sensitivity to the pressure effects of infused

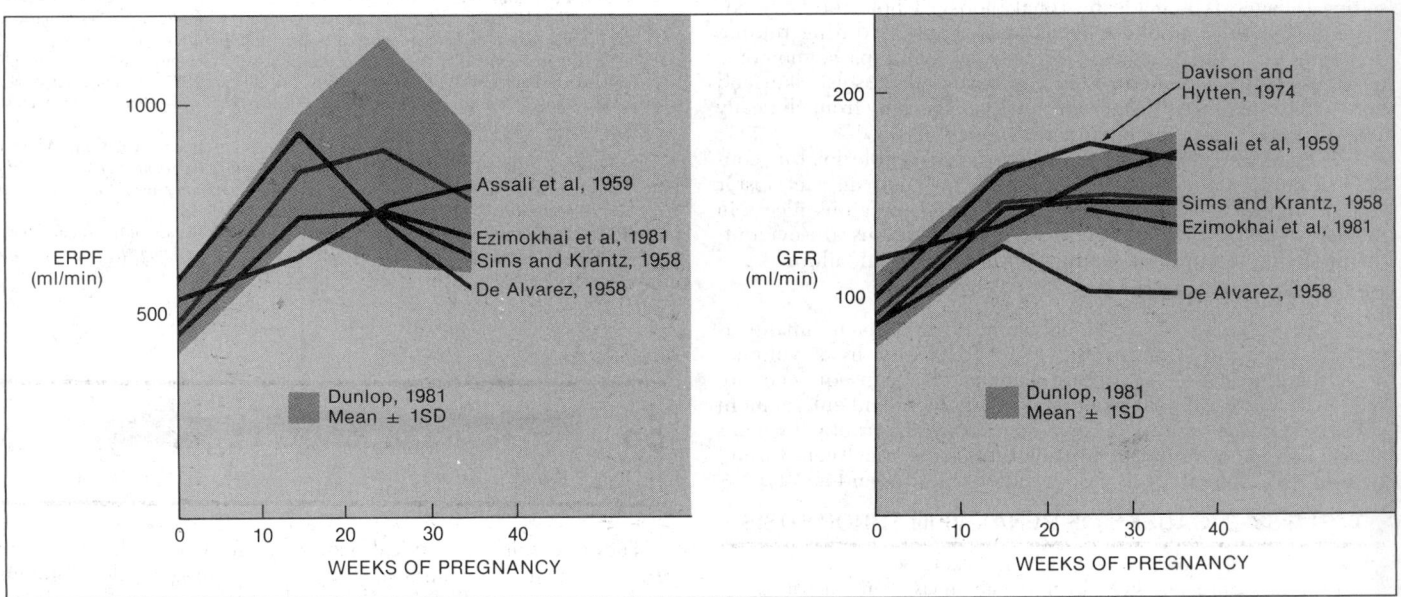

FIGURE 86–1. Changes in effective renal plasma flow (ERPF) and glomerular filtration rate (GFR) during the course of normal pregnancy. (From Davison JM, Dunlop W: Changes in renal hemodynamics and tubular functions enclosed by normal human pregnancy. Semin Nephrol 4:198, 1989; with permission.)

angiotensin many weeks before they become hypertensive. Most recently, evidence has suggested that abnormalities in eicosanoid metabolism may play a role in the pathogenesis of preeclampsia, reflecting an imbalance between production of vasodilating prostacyclin and the vasoconstrictor effects of thromboxane.

The histopathologic renal changes in toxemia, primarily confined to the glomerulus, are termed *glomerular capillary endotheliosis*. The glomeruli are large and swollen, with encroachment on capillary lumina by swollen and vacuolated endothelial and mesangial cells. Occasionally, small subendothelial deposits and fibrin deposits may be seen, but immunofluorescence studies are often negative for deposition of immunoglobulins. The characteristic lesion of endotheliosis seems to be invariably present, even when preeclampsia is mild, resolving a few weeks or months after delivery.

TREATMENT AND PROGNOSIS. All patients suspected of having preeclampsia should be hospitalized. The majority of patients with mild preeclampsia respond to bed rest and sedation. If the fetus is mature, delivery is induced. When gestational age is less than 34 weeks and disease is mild, one may temporize. In patients with diastolic blood pressure levels higher than 95 to 100 mm Hg, antihypertensive agents are administered, usually in the form of alpha-methyldopa, which can be combined with vasodilators or beta-blocking agents. In general, diuretic agents are avoided in the treatment of hypertension in pregnancy because of the risks of reducing placental blood flow. The definitive treatment for toxemia is delivery, which is indicated as soon as fetal maturity is achieved. Hyperreflexia or convulsions require immediate efforts to reduce the level of hypertension and depress central nervous system hyperexcitability. Most obstetric units employ parenteral magnesium sulfate to achieve these aims, along with monitoring of plasma magnesium levels to ensure that therapeutic levels of approximately 6 to 8 mEq per liter are maintained.

RENAL PARENCHYMAL DISEASES

Pregnancy occurs in women with pre-existing renal disease, and pregnant women are susceptible to the same kinds of disease that exist in the nongravid state. Three important clinical questions concerning these patients warrant further discussion: (1) What are the criteria that help to distinguish preeclampsia from other causes of renal dysfunction? (2) Does pregnancy adversely influence the course of the underlying renal or systemic disease? (3) Does the presence of renal insufficiency or nephrotic syndrome significantly reduce the likelihood for a successful fetal outcome?

DIFFERENTIAL DIAGNOSIS OF RENAL DISEASE IN PREGNANCY. Since the clinical hallmarks of preeclampsia— e.g., hypertension, proteinuria, and edema—are also manifested by most other types of renal parenchymal disease, a diagnostic evaluation cannot be based on these clinical features alone. Preeclampsia does not occur before the twentieth week of gestation, except in hydatidiform mole or multiple-gestation pregnancies. The differential diagnosis is therefore simplified if clinical signs of renal disease are known to exist prior to conception or in the early stages of pregnancy. In patients who are not observed until the last trimester of pregnancy, however, identification of the cause of renal dysfunction is often difficult. Multisystem involvement resulting in abnormal liver function tests and coagulation studies suggests preeclampsia. Renal biopsy, which could demonstrate the pathognomonic changes of preeclampsia, provides the only absolute method of confirming the diagnosis of preeclampsia, but few investigators advocate this procedure during gestation. When there is urgency about establishing the nature of the renal injury lesion because of treatment strategies, renal biopsy should be performed during the week immediately following delivery. During pregnancy, therefore, management in most cases must rely on a presumed clinical diagnosis. Since the clinical manifestations of preeclampsia usually resolve spontaneously within 4 to 6 weeks post partum, persistence of hypertension, proteinuria, or renal insufficiency strongly suggests a primary renal disease.

Information on the relative incidence of the various causes of hypertension and proteinuria during gestation has been reported in a large series of patients in whom the diagnosis was confirmed by renal biopsy performed within 6 days of delivery. These studies highlight the difficulty in establishing the correct diagnosis by clinical criteria. In most of these patients, a presumed diagnosis of preeclampsia was made during pregnancy. Among primigravidas, the incidence of preeclampsia, primary renal disease, and hypertensive glomerulosclerosis was 83 per cent, 12 per cent, and 5 per cent, respectively. In multiparous patients, in contrast, preeclampsia occurred in only 38 per cent of patients, while renal disease accounted for 26 per cent of cases and hypertensive renal disease for 24 per cent.

INFLUENCE OF PREGNANCY ON UNDERLYING RENAL DISEASE. Pregnancy does not significantly alter the course of pre-existing primary renal disease due to either glomerular or tubulointerstitial injury in patients with normal or nearly normal renal function. The effect of pregnancy on underlying disease, when renal insufficiency is more severe, (serum creatinine > 1.5 mg per deciliter) is less certain because of insufficient data. Although increased proteinuria, often to nephrotic levels, occurs in nearly one half of patients with a glomerulonephropathy, there is no constant relationship between pregnancy and long-term changes in the GFR. In general, the course of renal disease in these patients follows the expected course defined by the underlying pattern of injury.

There is less information on the effect of pregnancy on renal disease associated with systemic disorders. Pregnancy in diabetic patients does not appear to accelerate the onset of diabetic glomerulosclerosis or alter the natural course of renal disease in subjects with signs of renal disease before conception. In contrast, pregnancy may adversely influence systemic lupus erythematosus (SLE), as reflected in relapses and exacerbations of this disease in patients with an established diagnosis and a relatively high incidence of de novo onset of SLE during pregnancy and in the immediate postpartum period. In patients with established SLE but no clinical signs of active SLE for 6 to 12 months before conception, the clinical course during pregnancy is relatively mild and the live birth rate is approximately 90 per cent. In contrast, about half of all patients with clinical evidence of active SLE at the time of conception have subsequent exacerbations, which are often severe and associated with increased fetal loss.

An increase in urinary protein excretion in subjects with glomerulonephropathies is common during pregnancy and frequently results in the clinical manifestations of nephrotic syndrome. Sodium retention usually tends to become more severe in the last trimester. In most cases, proteinuria spontaneously returns to pregestational levels after delivery. An increase in the rate of edema formation should be anticipated during the later stages of pregnancy in patients with moderate or severe proteinuria and can be blunted by the introduction of a diet with low sodium content. The use of diuretics in pregnancy is controversial because of the possible induction of reduced placental blood flow. Conservative measures to control edema formation, including dietary measures and bed rest, are preferred. The judicious use of natriuretic agents, however, may be useful in patients with severe edema who fail to respond to conservative measures.

INFLUENCE OF RENAL DISEASE ON FETAL OUTCOME. Numerous studies have shown a live birth rate of 90 to 95 per cent in pregnancies associated with primary renal disease with normal or nearly normal renal function (serum creatinine < 1.4 mg per deciliter) and an absence of severe hypertension. These pregnancies, however, are characterized by high rates of preterm deliveries and fetal growth retardation. Analysis has shown an inverse correlation between the severity of blood pressure elevation and rates of fetal survival and birth weight. In patients with moderate or severe renal insufficiency (serum creatinine ≥ 1.5 mg per deciliter), live birth rates are reduced by 20 to 40 per cent, with proportional changes in morbidity. Fetal outcome in pregnancies associated with diabetic nephropathy is affected by the same factors found in primary renal disease and by complications present in all diabetic pregnancies, which include increased rates of macrosomia, major congenital defects, and neonatal complications.

ACUTE RENAL FAILURE IN PREGNANCY

Acute renal failure during pregnancy results from severe injury to tubular epithelial cells because of renal ischemia or the action of nephrotoxic agents. The cell injury may be reversible, with an eventual complete restoration of renal function; or it may be irreversible and lead to renal cortical necrosis. Renal cortical necrosis is characterized by the development of fibrosis within the cortex in a diffuse or patchy pattern, with relative sparing of the medullary portions of the kidney. Cortical necrosis is uncommon in nonpregnant individuals but occurs more often in pregnancy, especially in patients more than 30 years of age with third trimester abruptio placentae. It has been suggested that increased reactivity of the renal vasculature to vasoactive amines in pregnancy and local activation of coagulation may play an important role in the induction of tissue injury leading to cell death.

In addition to the usual causes of acute renal failure, some types of renal insults are unique to pregnancy. Septic abortion and hyperemesis gravidarum may cause renal failure in early pregnancy, while severe preeclampsia, placenta previa, and abruptio placentae are causative factors in the later stages of pregnancy. Clinical management of acute renal failure in pregnancy is comparable to that in nonpregnant patients. There is a high incidence of fetal loss associated with acute renal failure, but outlook has improved because of advances in dialytic therapy during pregnancy.

Barron WM, Murphy MB, Lindheimer MD: Management of hypertension during pregnancy. *In* Laragh JH, Brenner BM (eds.): Hypertension: Pathophysiology, Diagnosis and Management. New York, Raven Press, 1990, pp 1809–1827. *This chapter reviews blood pressure in normal pregnancy, the classification of hypertension in pregnancy, the pathogenesis and management of preeclampsia, and treatment of hypertension in pregnancy.*

Katz AI, Davison JM, Hayslett JP, et al.: Pregnancy in women with kidney disease. Kidney Int 18:192, 1980. *An analysis of a large series of pregnancies associated with primary renal disease. An excellent source for references.*

Reece EA, Coustan DR, Hayslett JP, et al.: Diabetic nephropathy: Pregnancy performance and feto-maternal outcome. Am J Obstet Gynecol 159:56, 1988. *An analysis of a large series of patients with diabetic nephropathy that compares risk factors associated with primary and diabetic renal disease.*

87 Hereditary Chronic Nephropathies

Wadi N. Suki

Several genetically transmitted renal disorders of unknown pathogenesis may fall under this heading. This chapter will discuss two of these disorders, Alport's syndrome and the nail-patella syndrome. Some hereditary disorders of renal tubular function are described in Ch. 82. Other genetic disorders that may be associated with renal disease are listed in Table 87–1 and discussed in the section on Metabolic Diseases (Part XIV).

ALPORT'S SYNDROME

DEFINITION. Also known as "chronic hereditary nephritis," this syndrome is characterized by the familial occurrence in successive generations of a progressive nephritis, more severe in males, manifested invariably by hematuria and frequently associated with a sensorineural hearing deficit.

GENETICS. The mode of transmission in most kindreds is consistent with X-linked dominant inheritance, and the gene has been localized to the middle of the long arm of the X-chromosome. Autosomal recessive and autosomal dominant inheritances have also been described in certain kindreds, suggesting that this disorder may be genetically heterogeneous.

INCIDENCE AND PREVALENCE. Several hundred kindreds of all races and geographic origins have been described. Alport's syndrome accounts for nearly 5 per cent of patients with end-stage renal disease.

PATHOLOGY AND PATHOGENESIS. Early in the disease, the kidneys may be normal or large in size, but they shrink with progression of the disease. Under light microscopy, the glomeruli may be normal or show some hypertrophy of epithelial cells and increase in mesangial matrix. Later changes consist of mesangial cell proliferation, thickening and splitting of glomerular and tubular basement membranes, thickening of Bowman's capsule, tubular cell atrophy, interstitial fibrosis, and the presence of foam

TABLE 87–1. INHERITED RENAL DISEASES*

Disorders of Tubular Function
Proximal tubule
  Cerebro-oculorenal syndrome of Lowe
  Cystinosis (Fanconi's syndrome)
  Cystinuria
  Galactosemia
  Glycogen storage (von Gierke's) disease
  Glycinuria
  Hartnup disease
  Hepatolenticular degeneration (Wilson's disease)
  Hereditary fructose intolerance
  Hypophosphatemic vitamin D–resistant rickets
  Iminoaciduria
  Proximal renal tubular acidosis
  Pseudohypoparathyroidism
  Renal glucosuria
Distal/collecting tubule
  Distal renal tubular acidosis
  Nephrogenic diabetes insipidus

Disorders of Renal Structure
Agenesis
Cystic disorders
  Hepatocerebrorenal syndrome of Zellweger
  Medullary sponge kidney
  Medullary cystic disease
  Polycystic kidney disease, adult type
  Polycystic kidney disease, infantile type
  Renal retinal dysplasia
Duplication
Renal malformations with extrarenal anomalies

Biochemical Disorders
Alkaptonuria
Cystinosis
Diabetes mellitus
Glycosphingolipidosis (Fabry's disease)
Hepatolenticular degeneration (Wilson's disease)
Hyperuricemia
Primary hyperoxaluria (oxalosis)
Xanthine oxidase deficiency

Systemic Disorders
Amyloidosis
Asphyxiating thoracic dystrophy (Jeune's disease)
Charcot-Marie-Tooth disease
Laurence-Moon-Biedl syndrome
Osteo-onychodysplasia (nail-patella syndrome)

Hereditary Chronic Nephropathies
Benign recurrent hematuria
Hereditary chronic nephritis
Hereditary chronic nephritis with hyperprolinemia
Hereditary chronic nephritis with thrombocytopathy
Hereditary immune nephritis
Infantile nephrosis

*Includes diseases that affect the kidney secondarily.

cells. Electron microscopy characteristically reveals both thinning and irregular thickening of the glomerular and tubular basement membranes, with splitting of the lamina densa into several lamellae separated by lucent zones containing electron-dense round granulations.

The etiology of Alport's syndrome appears to be the absence of a 28-kilodalton peptide component of the noncollagenous domain of the alpha$_1$ chain of type IV collagen in basement membrane. This peptide has been labeled the Goodpasture antigen (see below).

CLINICAL MANIFESTATIONS. The disease is discovered in 70 per cent of patients by the age of 6 years, the rest of the cases being discovered at any age thereafter up to and well into adulthood. Persistent or intermittent microscopic hematuria is universally present. Gross hematuria, especially after exercise or respiratory infections, may occur in 60 per cent of affected children but rarely in adults. Proteinuria is present in 70 per cent of patients. It is usually mild but reaches the nephrotic range in 30 to 40 per cent of patients. Sensorineural hearing loss in the high-frequency (4000 to 8000 Hz) range is observed in 40 to 60 per cent of patients, predominantly in males. Its detection may require audiometric testing, but it may progress to clinical deafness. Ocular disorders, especially anterior and posterior lenticonus and spherophakia, are seen in 15 per cent of patients. The renal disease may be mild and nonprogressive, especially in women, or may progress with the development of azotemia and hypertension, culminating in chronic renal failure and uremia. Progression occurs predominantly in males, with a predilection to those with massive proteinuria, deafness, and lenticonus. Renal failure may occur in childhood or in adulthood, and in affected males usually before age 40 years. Affected females may experience decline of renal function during pregnancy.

In several kindreds, patients with classic Alport's syndrome have been reported to have thrombocytopenia with giant platelets manifested clinically by bruising, epistaxis, and gastrointestinal bleeding and in the laboratory by prolonged bleeding time. A few cases have also been associated with hyperprolinemia (Ch. 172), leiomyomatosis, and a variety of other disorders.

DIAGNOSIS. The presence of progressive renal disease in one family member younger than age 50, other than the proband, and the presence of neural hearing loss in the patient or a relative form the basis for the diagnosis of Alport's syndrome in a patient with hematuria with or without proteinuria, azotemia, or hypertension. Differential diagnosis includes benign familial hematuria, a nonprogressive disorder characterized by a uniformly thin glomerular capillary basement membrane, and IgA nephropathy (Berger's disease), a glomerulonephritis with distinctive findings on light, electron, and especially immunofluorescent microscopic examination of the renal glomerulus. The audiometric findings, ocular manifestations, and family history, coupled with the changes in the glomerular and tubular basement membranes, usually should distinguish Alport's syndrome from other renal disorders.

TREATMENT. There is no specific treatment for Alport's syndrome, and no therapy is known to alter its course. Only conventional management of progressive renal disease is available. Peritoneal dialysis or hemodialysis and related or cadaveric donor kidney transplantation have been utilized with degrees of success at least matching those in other renal disorders. In fact, improvement of hearing deficit has been reported after renal transplantation. Recurrence of the renal lesion has not been observed following transplantation, but several patients have developed Goodpasture's syndrome in the renal graft caused by an antibody directed against the basement membrane antigen, which is absent in Alport's syndrome.

NAIL-PATELLA SYNDROME

An autosomal dominant trait also known as osteo-onychodysplasia, this disorder of mesenchymal tissue is characterized by atrophic or absent fingernails, hypoplasia or aplasia of the patella, accessory conical iliac horns, thickening of the scapula, and subluxation of the radial heads at the elbow. In 40 per cent of patients, the kidneys may be involved, as manifested by mild proteinuria and, rarely, hematuria. Occasionally, the nephrotic syndrome and progression to renal failure (27 per cent) may be observed. Light microscopy shows glomerular cellular proliferation, mesangial sclerosis, and basement membrane thickening. Electron microscopy reveals areas of rarefaction in the lamina densa of the glomerular basement membrane filled with bundles of curvilinear fibrils having the typical periodicity of collagen. No specific therapy exists for this disorder. Renal transplantation has been carried out without evidence of recurrence of the disease in the transplanted organ.

Bennett WM, Musgrave ME, Campbell RA, et al.: The nephropathy of the nail-patella syndrome. Am J Med 54:304, 1973. *A good description of the renal disorder in the nail-patella syndrome.*

Kashtan CE, Michael AF: Hereditary nephritis. Semin Nephrol 9:135, 1989. *An excellent review of the biochemical defect in, and the genetic transmission of, Alport's syndrome.*

88 Renal Calculi

Charles Y.C. Pak

DEFINITION

Renal calculi (kidney stones, nephrolithiasis) are abnormal concretions occurring in the kidneys, consisting of crystalline components and an organic matrix. They are typically located within the calices or pelvis and may become lodged in the ureter or bladder as they are passed. Nephrolithiasis should be differentiated from nephrocalcinosis, which is calcification of renal parenchyma. Stones originating in the bladder (bladder stones) are rare in industrialized countries, although they were common in antiquity and are still frequent in certain countries in Southeast Asia.

Nephrolithiasis affects 1 to 5 per cent of the population, with a recurrence rate in afflicted individuals of 50 to 80 per cent and an annual incidence rate of 0.1 to 0.3 per cent. Calcareous (calcium-containing) renal stones account for 80 to 95 per cent of stones and are principally composed of calcium oxalate and calcium phosphate, usually occurring as mixtures. The remaining stones are composed of uric acid, cystine, magnesium ammonium phosphate (struvite), and, rarely, xanthine, 2,8-dihydroxyadenine, triamterene, or silicate (Table 88–1).

ETIOLOGY AND PATHOGENESIS

Renal stones form by an initial crystallization of a nidus (termed nucleation) from a supersaturated urine with subsequent crystal growth and aggregation of the nidus into a macroscopic stone. Kidney stones are not simply masses of crystals. They usually have an organic matrix that gives form, cohesiveness, and sometimes a remarkably regular structure to the stone. At the present time, abnormalities in the amount or composition of stone matrix have not been demonstrated to be important in stone pathogenesis. It is impossible to dissolve the amounts of calcium, oxalate, and phosphate present in normal urine in 1 or 2 liters of distilled water. Obviously, therefore, there are substances present in normal urine that impede crystallization and sustain supersaturation. These normal inhibitors are not fully characterized but seem to include pyrophosphate, citrate, magnesium, and certain organic macromolecules (such as glycosaminoglycans and glycoproteins).

All patients with stones are presumed to have some physiologic derangements that make them susceptible to stone formation, although no cause can be demonstrated by current techniques in 3 per cent of patients. These derangements alter urinary concentration of stone-forming constituents and of inhibitors to cause supersaturation and facilitate crystallization (Table 88–2).

Crystallization involves three steps: *nucleation* (formation of nidus), *crystal growth* (enlargement of crystal size), and *crystal agglomeration* (clumping of crystals that are formed to attain a large size). It requires supersaturation of urine and reduced urinary content of inhibitors.

Supersaturation can result from (1) too little urine output (a concentrated urine), (2) an absolute increase in the amount of a stone constituent excreted over a period of time, such as calcium, oxalate, or uric acid, or (3) an alteration in urine pH. Low urinary pH (< 5.5) increases urinary saturation of uric acid, whereas high urinary pH raises that of calcium phosphate and magnesium ammonium phosphate.

Reduction in the concentration of inhibitors of crystallization in the urine may be of great importance in stone pathogenesis, by facilitating crystallization. Some inhibitors (such as citrate) may be directly measured in urine, providing diagnostic utility. Other inhibitors (such as glycoproteins) that are difficult to analyze

TABLE 88–1. COMPOSITION OF RENAL STONES*

Type	Percentage
Calcium oxalate	70
Calcium phosphate	10
Hydroxyapatite	
Brushite	
Tricalcium phosphate	
Carbonate apatite	
Magnesium ammonium phosphate	5–10
Uric acid	< 5
Cystine	1
Xanthine and other	< 1

*Some stones occur as mixtures. Percentages are calculated for the predominant stone types.

can sometimes be assessed indirectly from the overall inhibitor activity against crystallization of stone-forming salts.

Other factors may be important in stone formation. (1) *Stasis*: Most embryonic stones are probably harmlessly washed out in the urine. Stasis allows time for nascent stone to grow. (2) *Heterogeneous nucleation*: Crystallization may begin in a supersaturated solution that is seeded with a crystal of a different (heterogeneous) composition but one that has an analogous surface topography. This process of one crystal growing on the surface of another is known as epitaxy. Many stones are mixed in composition and perhaps represent epitaxial growth.

HYPERCALCIURIA. As noted, calcium is a constituent of 80 to 95 per cent of kidney stones. Hypercalciuria is the single most frequent abnormality found in patients with stone diathesis. Hypercalciuria is often statistically defined and varies with body size and diet. In general, the normal upper limit for urinary calcium is 300 mg per day on a diet containing 1000 mg of calcium per day (some authorities use a figure of 4 mg per kilogram per day) and 200 mg per day on a diet with a daily composition of 400 mg of calcium and 100 mEq of sodium (urinary calcium tends to parallel urinary sodium so that dietary sodium should ideally be controlled). Hypercalciuria can result from (1) enhanced absorption from dietary sources, (2) primary renal wastage with secondary enhanced absorption, (3) excessive resorption from storage in bone, or (4) a combination of the above (Fig. 88–1). These different forms will be discussed briefly.

Absorptive hypercalciuria, the most common abnormality, is encountered in 30 to 40 per cent of patients with kidney stones. Increased absorption of dietary calcium may rarely occur from excessive ingestion of milk and other dairy products, from vitamin D excess (Ch. 233), or from the altered vitamin D metabolism associated with sarcoidosis (Ch. 67). Absorptive hypercalciuria usually refers, however, to a primary idiopathic increase in intestinal absorption of calcium. The consequent rise in serum calcium concentration tends to suppress parathyroid function (PTH ↓). Hypercalciuria ensues from the increased renal filtered load of calcium and the reduced renal tubular reabsorption of calcium associated with suppression of the secretion of parathyroid hormone (PTH). Serum calcium is typically maintained within the normal range because of compensatory hypercalciuria. In its usual presentation, the disorder tends to be familial and is believed to occur independently of hypophosphatemia or altered vitamin D metabolism. There is some evidence that it represents a jejunal disease characterized by a selective intestinal hyperabsorption of calcium in this intestinal segment.

Renal hypercalciuria, as a form of "idiopathic hypercalciuria," occurs less commonly than absorptive hypercalciuria and originates from an impaired renal tubular reabsorption (renal leak) of calcium. The ensuing decline in serum calcium causes secondary hyperparathyroidism, which in turn stimulates the renal synthesis of 1,25-dihydroxyvitamin D (Fig. 88–1). Thus, the skeletal mobilization and intestinal absorption of calcium may be secondarily increased, effects that restore serum calcium concentration to normal and further contribute to the hypercalciuria. The possibility that there may be a more generalized disturbance in proximal tubular function is shown by an exaggerated natriuretic response to thiazide and calciuric response to a carbohydrate load.

Resorptive hypercalciuria results from excessive bone resorption, most commonly from the hypersecretion of PTH. Three to 5 per cent of all kidney stones are caused by primary hyperparathyroidism (Table 88–2); conversely, 10 to 30 per cent of patients with primary hyperparathyroidism present with renal stones. The hypercalcemia of hyperparathyroidism causes hypercalciuria by augmenting the renal filtered load of calcium. The intestinal calcium absorption may also be increased secondarily, consequent to parathyroid hormone-dependent stimulation of the synthesis of 1,25-dihydroxyvitamin D; this increased calcium absorption further contributes to the hypercalciuria. Hypercalciuria secondary to net bone resorption is also seen in thyrotoxicosis, multiple myeloma, pseudohyperparathyroidism of malignancy, metastatic disease of bone, and immobilization (acute osteoporosis) and with spontaneous or iatrogenic Cushing's syndrome.

Fasting hypercalciuria with normal levels of serum PTH is neither absorptive hypercalciuria (because of the presence of apparent renal calcium leak) nor renal hypercalciuria (since parathyroid stimulation is lacking). This picture may result from several disturbances. (1) *Enhanced 1,25-dihydroxyvitamin D synthesis*: It may cause parathyroid suppression and an acquired renal calcium leak. (2) *Renal phosphate leak*: It may produce hypophosphatemia and increased synthesis of 1,25-dihydroxyvitamin D. (3) *Combined renal proximal tubular defect*: Renal calcium leak may coexist with high 1,25-dihydroxyvitamin D production occurring primarily or secondarily from renal phosphate leak.

HYPEROXALURIA. Oxalate is the second most common constituent of kidney stones, after calcium (Table 88–1), but the great majority of patients with calcium oxalate stones have no abnormality of oxalate metabolism. Sustained hyperoxaluria, which may be defined as the excretion of greater than 60 mg of oxalate per 1.73 square meters per 24 hours, occurs only (1) in primary hyperoxaluria, a rare genetic disorder described in Ch. 171, (2) in pyridoxine deficiency, (3) rarely with excessive ingestion of ascorbic acid, and (4) from enhanced absorption of dietary oxalate, termed enteric hyperoxaluria.

TABLE 88–2. PATHOGENESIS OF NEPHROLITHIASIS

Cause	Percentage of Patients with Stones	Sex Predominance	Stone Composition
Hypercalciuria			
Absorptive hypercalciuria	20–40	Male	Ca oxalate, Ca phosphate
Renal hypercalciuria	5–8	Equivalent	Ca oxalate, Ca phosphate
Fasting hypercalciuria with normal PTH*	15–25	Male	Ca oxalate, Ca phosphate
Primary hyperparathyroidism	3–5	Female	Ca phosphate, Ca oxalate
Hyperoxaluria			
Primary	Rare	Equivalent	Ca oxalate
Enteric	<2	Equivalent	Ca oxalate
Dietary	2–15	Male	Ca oxalate
Hyperuricosuric calcium nephrolithiasis	10–40	Male	Ca oxalate, Ca phosphate
Hypocitraturic calcium nephrolithiasis			
Renal tubular acidosis	1–10	Equivalent	Ca phosphate, Ca oxalate
Other	9–40	Male	Ca oxalate, Ca phosphate
Uric acid stone diathesis	15–30	Male	Uric acid, Ca oxalate, Ca phosphate
Hypomagnesiuric calcium nephrolithiasis	5–10	Equivalent	Ca oxalate
Cystinuria	<1	Equivalent	Cystine
Infection lithiasis	1–5	Female	Struvite, carbonate apatite
Low urine volume	10–50	Female	Ca oxalate
No physiologic disturbance	< 5	Female	Ca oxalate

*PTH = parathyroid hormone.

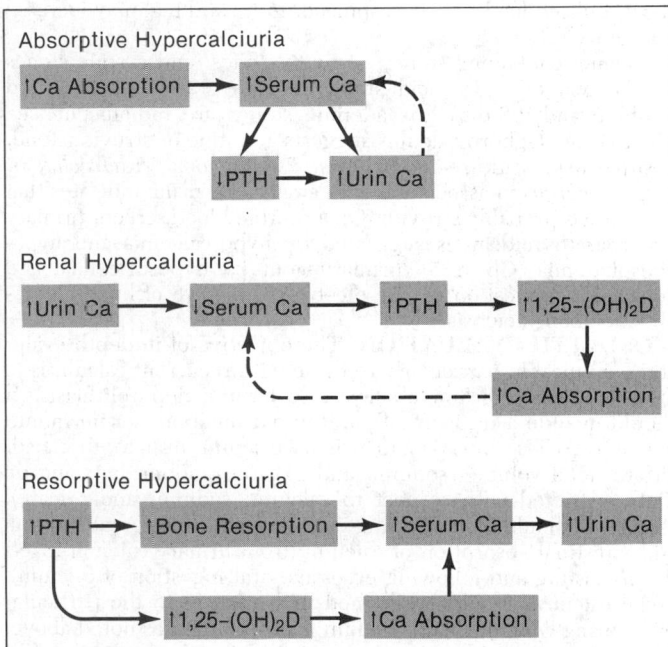

Absorptive Hypercalciuria

Renal Hypercalciuria

Resorptive Hypercalciuria

FIGURE 88–1. Pathophysiologic schemes for hypercalciuria. (After Pak CYC: Kidney stones. *In* Foster DW, Wilson JE [eds.]: Williams Textbook of Endocrinology. Philadelphia, W. B. Saunders Company, 1985, pp 1256–1273.)

Enteric hyperoxaluria, which is encountered in approximately 2 per cent of patients with stones, occurs typically in patients with ileal disease (ileal resection, jejunoileal bypass surgery, inflammatory disease of the small bowel). In ileal disease in which there is malabsorption of fat, the intraluminal content of divalent cations, particularly calcium, may be reduced by being bound to unabsorbed fatty acids. Thus, calcium is not normally available to bind and limit oxalate absorption. The resulting enlarged free intestinal oxalate pool increases absorption and renal excretion of oxalate. Oxalate absorption may be stimulated primarily as well, especially in the colon, since patients with ileostomies do not have hyperoxaluria. Low urine volume (from an excessive intestinal loss of fluid) and defective urinary inhibitor activity (from an impaired renal excretion of citrate and magnesium) probably contribute to calcium stone formation in ileal disease. Low urinary pH (from intestinal alkali loss) may cause formation of uric acid stones.

In hypercalciuria associated with increased calcium absorption (e.g., absorptive hypercalciuria), a mild increase in oxalate excretion may be found (up to 50 mg per day). The total amount of oxalate absorbed from the gut may be high because more calcium is absorbed and less calcium is available intraluminally to bind oxalate.

HYPERURICOSURIC CALCIUM OXALATE STONE DIATHESIS. Hyperuricosuria may be the only discernible biochemical abnormality associated with calcium oxalate stones (10 per cent), although it often coexists with hypercalciuria or hypocitraturia (40 per cent). Most patients with hyperuricosuric calcium oxalate nephrolithiasis do not suffer from clinical gout. The hyperuricosuria is usually dietary in origin, since a history of high purine intake may often be disclosed and normal urinary uric acid excretion values may be restored by purine restriction. Less commonly, hyperuricosuria results from a primary overproduction of uric acid. The urinary pH typically exceeds 5.5, so that dissociated urate rather than uric acid predominates. It is believed that urates facilitate crystallization of calcium oxalate, either directly by inducing heterogeneous nucleation or indirectly by removing macromolecular inhibitors through adsorption.

HYPOCITRATURIA. Citrate reduces urinary saturation of calcium salts by complexing calcium, as well as inhibits the crystallization of these salts. Crystal agglomeration of calcium oxalate is particularly retarded by citrate. Thus, hypocitraturia would be expected to increase the tendency toward the formation of calcium-containing kidney stones. Hypocitraturia is encountered in any acidotic condition, such as renal tubular acidosis,

chronic diarrheal states, thiazide-induced hypokalemia (which causes intracellular acidosis), ingestion of excessive animal protein (which has a high acid-ash content), and strenuous physical exercise (which produces lactic acidosis). Distal (type I) renal tubular acidosis, often in an incomplete form, may first manifest with nephrolithiasis. The cause for stone formation is multifactorial and probably includes hypercalciuria (from induced renal leak of calcium by acidosis), enhanced dissociation of phosphate, an increased saturation of calcium phosphate (from high urinary pH), as well as an impaired inhibitor activity (from defective excretion of citrates). Renal tubular acidosis is described in greater detail in Ch. 82. Hypocitraturia of excessive intestinal alkali loss has been found not only in ileal disease (enteric hyperoxaluria) but also in postgastrectomy states and ulcerative colitis. Hypocitraturia should be suspected in patients with hypercalciuric nephrolithiasis who continue to form stones while on thiazide therapy. Another cause of hypocitraturia is urinary tract infection (probably from bacterial degradation of citrate). The cause for hypocitraturia often remains unknown. Hypocitraturia may occur as a sole abnormality (10 per cent) but is usually associated with other causes of nephrolithiasis (50 per cent).

URIC ACID STONES. Approximately two thirds to three fourths of the uric acid synthesized in the body is excreted in the urine. The rest is excreted in the intestine and largely destroyed by bacterial degradation. Uric acid excretion varies widely with diet. Urinary values greater than 600 mg per 1.73 square meters per 24 hours after 3 days of a diet moderately restricted in purine probably represent endogenous overproduction. In the study of patients with kidney stones, it is more important to measure uric acid excretion on the patient's usual diet. In this case, an excretion of more than 750 mg for women and more than 800 mg for men would be considered abnormally high.

Uric acid stones usually form in urines with a pH of less than the dissociation constant for uric acid (5.5), especially when there are absolute increases in uric acid (hyperuricosuria). Thus, the amount of urinary free uric acid is increased. Uric acid stones often occur in primary gout, which may be accompanied by low urinary pH and hyperuricosuria (Ch. 183), or in secondary causes of purine overproduction, such as myeloproliferative states, glycogen storage disease, and malignancy. Chronic diarrheal syndromes (ulcerative colitis, regional enteritis, jejunoileal bypass surgery) may cause uric acid stones by inducing net alkali deficit (thereby reducing urinary pH) and lowering urine volume (thereby augmenting urinary concentration of uric acid).

Most patients with uric acid stones do not have clinical gout, secondary purine overproduction, or diarrheal syndromes. Urinary pH is invariably low without dietary excess of animal proteins. Some of them may have asymptomatic hyperuricemia or family history of gouty arthritis and may also form calcium-containing stones. The term *gouty diathesis* has been used to describe this condition.

CYSTINURIA. A cystine kidney stone forms only in a patient with the genetic disorder cystinuria (Ch. 82). Other forms of aminoaciduria are not associated with the excretion of enough cystine to form stones. Cystinuria is characterized by a disturbance in renal and intestinal handling of lysine, arginine, ornithine, and cystine. Stone formation, occurring in a minority of patients with cystinuria, is the result of an excessive renal excretion of cystine and its low solubility in urine. Cystine solubility is pH dependent; at pH 5, 170 to 300 mg of cystine may be dissolved in each liter of urine, whereas at pH 7.5, 220 to 500 mg of cystine may go into the solution. Many patients with homozygous cystinuria who are prone to cystine stone formation excrete more than 250 mg of cystine per day.

INFECTION. Urinary tract infections with urea-splitting organisms may be associated with renal stones of struvite (magnesium ammonium phosphate) and varying amounts of calcium phosphate. Ammonia formed by enzymatic degradation of urea by bacterial urease undergoes hydration to form ammonium and hydroxyl ions. The resulting alkalinity of urine augments dissociation of phosphate to form more triphosphate ions and reduces the solubility of struvite. Thus, the urinary environment becomes supersaturated with respect to struvite. Although struvite stones may form de novo from infection alone, they may sometimes occur as a complication of other causes of renal calculi, such as hypercalciuria. The presence of a struvite stone is presumptive evidence for concurrent or previous urinary tract infection.

MISCELLANEOUS. A minority of patients (10 per cent) present with low urine volume (< 1 liter per day) without any of the previously mentioned causes. Habitual decreased drinking of fluids may have contributed to stone formation. It has been reported that oxalate exchange in peripheral red blood cells is significantly increased in patients with "idiopathic" calcium oxalate nephrolithiasis and that this disturbance may be corrected by treatment with thiazide or amiloride. The significance of this finding is uncertain, since intestinal absorption and renal excretion of oxalate (given without calcium) are normal, and urinary oxalate is not affected by thiazide in patients with absorptive or renal hypercalciuria.

RENAL STRUCTURAL ABNORMALITIES. Nephrolithiasis may also be found in association with *renal structural abnormalities,* such as ectopic kidney, polycystic kidney, and horseshoe kidney. In this situation, it is generally believed that stones, usually composed of struvite or calcium phosphate, form secondarily to urinary tract infection. Medullary sponge disease is often associated with calcareous renal calculi. There is no convincing evidence that the structural abnormality causes stone formation, since metabolic abnormalities (such as the three forms of hypercalciuria) are usually found in medullary sponge disease, in similar distribution to that of patients without this disease.

IDIOPATHIC STONE DIATHESIS. In less than 5 per cent of patients, no physiologic abnormality can be discerned. The cause for stone formation remains unknown.

CLINICAL MANIFESTATIONS

Patients with renal stones may be asymptomatic; may pass small, sandlike concretions with relatively little pain; or may experience severe symptoms from ureteral obstruction, localized trauma, or infection. Renal colic is the manifestation of ureteral spasm produced by the irritation of a stone and accompanying obstruction. Microscopic hematuria is almost invariably present; gross hematuria, even clots, may sometimes accompany renal colic. Pain may begin in the costovertebral angle or the flank and may migrate toward the groin; sometimes pain moves into, and may be most severe in, the testis or penis in the male. Pain may subside after the stone or clot has passed, but the process may take several hours, even days, if the stone is impacted or if ureteral swelling impedes migration. Women frequently report that the pain of renal colic is more severe than that of labor. Infection arising from stones may lead to fever, flank tenderness, dysuria, and frequency of urination.

DIAGNOSIS

INITIAL SCREEN. The first step in the diagnosis of the cause of a kidney stone is to secure the stone for analysis, if at all possible. The analysis should preferably be carried out by a crystallographic technique, which can sometimes reveal the sequence of stone formation from the central nidus to the periphery.

All patients with renal stones should have a carefully taken history, abdominal roentgenographic examination, urinalysis and culture, and a routine blood screen.

A positive family history of renal calculi suggests absorptive hypercalciuria or, more rarely, cystinuria, primary hyperoxaluria, or type I renal tubular acidosis. Absorptive hypercalciuria should be suspected in middle-aged white men who have a history of recurrent calcium-containing stones and a family history of renal stones. Renal hypercalciuria may be present in patients with a history of recurrent urinary tract infection, especially if the infection preceded the onset of the stone disease. A high-calcium diet may aggravate the stone disease in those with an intestinal hyperabsorption of calcium. Patients with gout may form stones of either uric acid or calcium oxalate. A history of chronic diarrhea, ileal disease, or intestinal surgery should arouse the suspicion of uric acid or calcium oxalate stones (enteric hyperoxaluria or hypocitraturic calcium nephrolithiasis). A high purine intake may cause hyperuricosuria and contribute to stone formation in hyperuricosuric calcium oxalate nephrolithiasis. Acetazolamide may impair renal acidification and cause formation of calcium phosphate stones. Excessive ingestion of vitamin D and of oxalate-rich foods (such as spinach, nuts, and tea) may increase oxalate excretion.

Calcium-containing stones, struvite stones, and cystine stones are radiopaque. Uric acid stones and the rarely encountered xanthine and 2,8-dihydroxyadenine stones are radiolucent (see Ch. 184). A staghorn calculus suggests a cystine or struvite stone. Positive urine culture for *Proteus, Pseudomonas, Klebsiella,* or *Staphylococcus* in association with an alkaline urine indicates that the stone is probably struvite. On a routine blood screen, primary hyperparathyroidism is suggested by hypercalcemia and hypophosphatemia (Ch. 235); primary gout by hyperuricemia; and defective acidification by the electrolyte picture of hyperchloremic metabolic acidosis.

IN-DEPTH EVALUATION. The objective of in-depth evaluation, applicable particularly to those with recurrent calculi, is to discern the specific metabolic cause for the nephrolithiasis. It should include a measure of parathyroid function (serum immunoreactive PTH) and 24-hour urinary calcium, oxalate, uric acid, citrate, total volume, sodium, and pH (on random diets and on diets restricted with respect to calcium, sodium, and oxalate). Ideally, it should include a measure of renal tubular reabsorption and intestinal absorption of calcium (from urinary calcium levels during fasting and following excessive oral ingestion of calcium). Hypercalciuria should be defined with respect to the particular diet during which urinary calcium is determined as noted above. If the stone is not known to contain calcium, a qualitative test for urine cystine is indicated.

The nature of parathyroid function distinguishes the three forms of *hypercalciuria.* Primary hyperparathyroidism is suggested by parathyroid stimulation in the setting of hypercalcemia, absorptive hypercalciuria by normal or suppressed parathyroid function with normocalcemia and hypercalciuria, and renal hypercalciuria by parathyroid stimulation with normocalcemia and hypercalciuria. The fasting urinary calcium level is invariably increased in renal hypercalciuria and is frequently elevated in primary hyperparathyroidism, whereas it is typically normal in absorptive hypercalciuria. Intestinal calcium absorption is always increased in absorptive hypercalciuria and is often high in renal and resorptive hypercalciurias. Fasting hypercalciuria with normal parathyroid function is suggested by high fasting urinary calcium levels in the setting of normal levels of serum calcium and PTH.

In *enteric hyperoxaluria,* the urinary calcium level is typically low (< 100 mg per day) and the urinary oxalate level is high (often > 80 mg per day). Serum calcium and magnesium levels may be low, parathyroid function may be stimulated, metabolic acidosis may be present, and the urinary citrate level is low (< 320 mg per day). Hypocitraturia is also found in hypocitraturic calcium nephrolithiasis.

Urinary uric acid consistently exceeds 600 mg per day (and often > 750 to 800 mg per day), and pH is greater than 5.5 in *hyperuricosuric calcium oxalate nephrolithiasis.* Urinary pH is usually low (< 5.5) *in uric acid lithiasis* and high (> 7.5) in *struvite lithiasis.* Urine pH is high (> 6.9) in complete type I *renal tubular acidosis* and high normal or high (> 6) in the incomplete form.

TREATMENT

Kidney stones are heterogeneous in pathogenesis and not infrequently are manifestations of a generalized multisystem disorder. By and large, kidney stones cannot be treated medically in the sense of causing their dissolution. The goal of medical treatment is to stop growth or new formation of stones by correcting the specific underlying physicochemical and physiologic derangements. Stone prophylaxis often entails a prolonged program. It is particularly important, therefore, to ensure patient compliance, few complications, and reasonable costs.

GENERAL TREATMENT. The initial treatment program, applicable to all patients with renal calculi, consists of a high fluid intake to ensure a minimum urine volume of 2 liters per day. At least 3 liters of fluids should be drunk each day, distributed throughout the day. In general, any fluid (with the exception of milk and oxalate-rich tea in certain disorders to be enumerated) may be consumed. In patients with intestinal hyperabsorption of calcium, intake of dairy products and certain calcium-rich foods should be limited. Oxalate intake should be restricted in patients with calcium oxalate stones. An excessive dietary intake of sodium should be discouraged, since this may enhance calcium excretion. Urinary tract infection should be vigorously treated.

Activity of Stone Diathesis. As noted, as many as 5 per cent of the population may have a kidney stone at some time. Some patients, usually men, have a single calcium oxalate stone in middle life and are not subsequently affected. Clearly, it would not be wise to begin a lifetime program of pharmacologic intervention without some knowledge of the prognosis of the stone diathesis in the individual patient. In the absence of remediable disorders, such as primary hyperparathyroidism, it is often wise following a first stone episode to institute the general measures noted above and then to follow patients carefully to document whether new stones are forming or old stones are enlarging before more vigorous measures are instituted.

SPECIFIC MEDICAL TREATMENT. Specific programs may be required when the aforementioned conservative measures are ineffective in controlling stone formation and there is continued activity of stone diathesis.

Treatment of Hypercalciuria. The surgical removal of abnormal parathyroid tissue is clearly the treatment of choice for kidney stones secondary to the hypercalciuria of primary hyperparathyroidism. Following parathyroidectomy, serum 1,25-dihydroxyvitamin D levels, intestinal calcium absorption, and urinary calcium levels decline toward normal. Parathyroidectomy may also ameliorate the extrarenal manifestations of primary hyperparathyroidism, such as bone disease and peptic ulcer disease (Ch. 235). Similarly, the hypercalciuria of vitamin D excess, sarcoidosis, thyrotoxicosis, multiple myeloma, and malignancies may respond to specific therapies directed toward those systemic entities. The main problem is in the management of remaining forms of hypercalciuria. Several agents that have proved to be useful will be individually discussed.

Thiazides (and related compounds such as chlorthalidone) are unique among diuretics in their ability to augment the renal tubular reabsorption of calcium and therefore to reduce urinary calcium. At a dosage of hydrochlorothiazide of 50 mg once or twice a day, or an equivalent amount of related drugs, thiazides represent the treatment of choice for renal hypercalciuria. Thiazides correct the renal leak of calcium and thereby reverse the sequence of parathyroid hyperactivity, increased synthesis of 1,25-dihydroxyvitamin D, and enhanced absorption of intestinal calcium. The urinary saturations of calcium oxalate and calcium phosphate are reduced. Thiazides may be equally effective in the control of absorptive hypercalciuria, at least during the first 2 years of therapy. However, some patients may show an attenuation of the hypocalciuric response with chronic treatment. Moreover, thiazide therapy may cause hypokalemia and hypocitraturia. To overcome these problems, urinary calcium levels should be monitored, and potassium supplement (preferably as potassium citrate) should be provided.

Sodium cellulose phosphate (Calcibind) should be used only in patients with normophosphatemic absorptive hypercalciuria without bone disease in whom hypercalciuria cannot be controlled by dietary calcium restriction or by thiazide. When given orally, it forms a nonabsorbable complex with calcium that is then excreted in the feces. About 2.5 to 5 grams of this resin with each meal is sufficient to limit the amount of luminal calcium available for absorption and to restore normal urinary calcium levels. This reduces urinary saturation of calcium salts, particularly that of calcium phosphate, without overly stimulating parathyroid function or causing bone disease. Urinary oxalate may increase, because less calcium may be available intraluminally to complex oxalate, so that a moderate dietary restriction of oxalate is recommended. Oral magnesium supplementation should be provided, since this drug also binds magnesium. Sodium cellulose phosphate is contraindicated in primary hyperparathyroidism, in other states of excessive skeletal calcium mobilization, in renal hypercalciuria, in growing children or postmenopausal women, and in states of normal intestinal calcium absorption because it tends to stimulate parathyroid function and thereby produces or aggravates bone disease.

Orthophosphates, as neutral or alkaline soluble salts of sodium or potassium or both, are potentially absorbable from the intestinal tract, unlike sodium cellulose phosphate. When given orally (at a dosage of 1.5 to 2.0 grams of phosphorus per day in divided doses), they decrease urinary calcium and increase urinary phosphate levels. They reduce urinary saturation of calcium oxalate, although they may increase that of calcium phosphate. Moreover, urinary inhibitor activity may be increased, probably consequent to the increased renal excretion of inhibitors, such as pyrophosphate and citrate. Orthophosphates are optimally indicated in the management of renal phosphate leak because of the possibility that they may restore normal levels of serum 1,25-dihydroxyvitamin D and calcium absorption. Orthophosphates are contraindicated in moderate or severe hypercalcemia and in renal failure because of the danger of metastatic calcification and in urinary tract infection because of the danger of struvite or calcium phosphate stone formation.

Treatment of Enteric Hyperoxaluria. A limitation of dietary oxalate intake and potassium citrate therapy (to be discussed) may be helpful in lowering oxalate and increasing pH and citrate levels in urine, respectively. A high fluid intake is essential to overcome intestinal fluid loss. Oral administration of large amounts of calcium or magnesium has been recommended for the control of nephrolithiasis of enteric hyperoxaluria. Although urinary oxalate levels may decrease, the concurrent rise in urinary calcium may obviate the beneficial effect of this therapy in some patients. Cholestyramine does not generally cause a sustained reduction in oxalate excretion.

Treatment of Hyperuricosuric Calcium Nephrolithiasis. This form of hyperuricosuria usually results from a diet high in purine precursors of uric acid. It should therefore be subject to effective dietary therapy. Unfortunately, many patients cannot or do not choose to maintain this dietary restraint. Allopurinol, 300 mg per day orally, will produce normal or subnormal levels of urinary uric acid and thereby may inhibit urate-induced crystallization of calcium oxalate.

Treatment of Hypocitraturic Calcium Nephrolithiasis. In renal tubular acidosis (distal), sodium citrate or potassium citrate (60 to 120 mEq per day in divided doses) may augment citrate excretion (see Ch. 82 for details). In the absence of renal insufficiency, potassium citrate is preferable because it could reduce urinary calcium and correct potassium deficiency. In *chronic diarrheal states,* potassium citrate in a liquid form is recommended to allow for rapid absorption (60 to 120 mEq per day). Hypocitraturia is sometimes very severe and recalcitrant to alkali therapy. In *thiazide-induced hypocitraturia,* potassium citrate (30 to 40 mEq per day in two divided doses in a slow-release tablet form) is generally sufficient to correct both hypokalemia and hypocitraturia. In other causes of hypocitraturia, a sufficient dose of potassium citrate may be provided to restore normal urinary citrate levels. The efficacy of potassium citrate is shown in Figure 88–2.

Treatment of Uric Acid Stones. In uric acid diathesis, administration of potassium citrate may increase urinary pH and create an environment in which uric acid is more soluble. Moderate amounts of alkali (30 to 60 mEq of potassium citrate per day in divided doses), sufficient to raise urinary pH to a range of 6 to 6.5, may be effective in preventing formation of both uric acid and calcium stones. Sodium alkali, especially in high dosages, may cause formation of calcium stones. If hydration and alkali therapy are ineffective, allopurinol should be used to decrease uric acid stone formation. See the discussion in Ch. 183 on gout for more details.

Treatment of Cystinuria (see Ch. 82). If a high fluid intake and alkali therapy are ineffective in reducing cystine concentration below saturation of cystine, D-*penicillamine* (1 to 2 grams per day in divided doses) may be required. This compound reduces urinary cystine content by forming a more soluble mixed disulfide with cysteine. Unfortunately, penicillamine treatment may be complicated by serious side effects, including nephrotic syndrome, dermatitis, and pancytopenia. Alpha-mercaptopropionylglycine, which lowers urinary cystine by a similar mechanism, may be advantageous because of its apparent reduced toxicity.

Treatment of Struvite (Magnesium Ammonium Phosphate) Stones. If a longstanding effective control of infection with urea-splitting organisms can be achieved, there is some evidence that new struvite stone formation can be averted or some dissolution of existing stones may be achieved. Unfortunately, such a control is difficult to obtain with antibiotic therapy alone. It is difficult

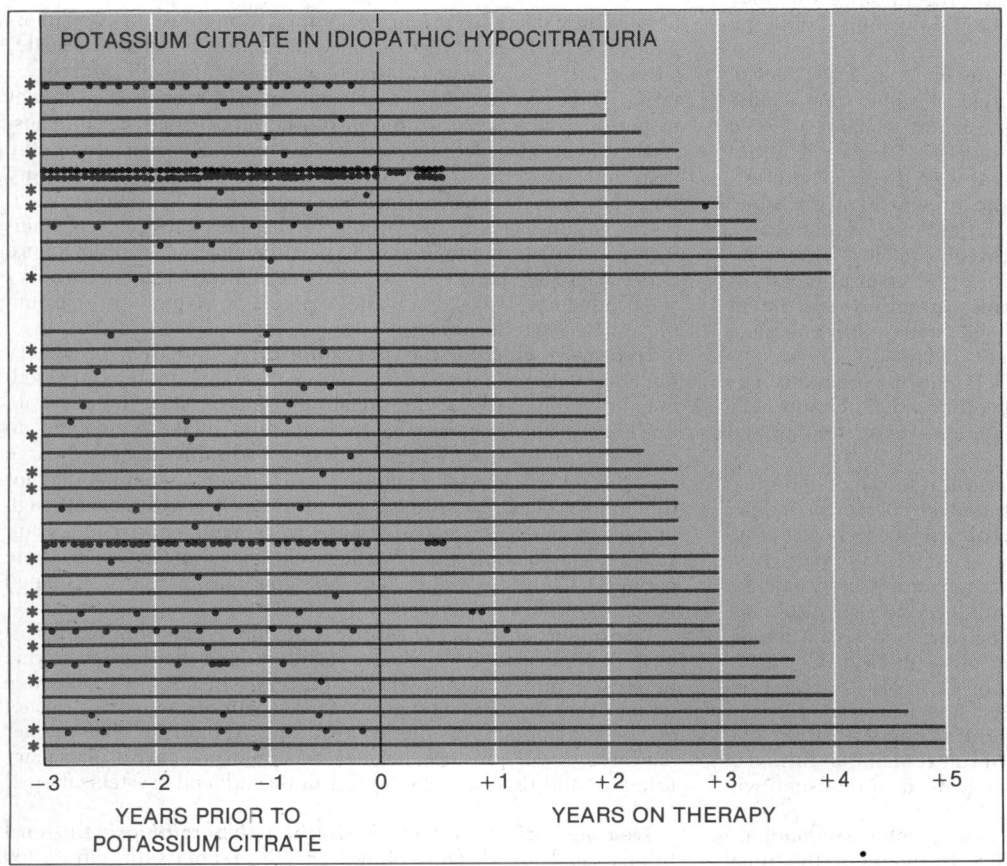

FIGURE 88–2. Effect of potassium citrate therapy on new stone formation. Each line represents one patient. An asterisk before the line indicates the presence of pre-existing stone(s). Each point shows new stone formation.

to eliminate the infection completely from an existing struvite stone because the stone often harbors the organisms within its interstices. Even if sterilization of urine is achieved by antibiotic therapy, reinfection often occurs from harbored organisms. Addition of acetohydroxamic acid, a urease inhibitor, at a dosage of 250 mg three times per day, may be more effective in controlling struvite stone formation. If not, surgical removal of stones should be considered.

Surgical Treatment

The goal of surgical treatment is removal of existing stones, whereas that of medical treatment is prevention of recurrent stone formation.

Removal of stones may become mandatory when nephrolithiasis is complicated by obstruction, infection, gross hematuria, or intractable pain. Dramatic progress has been made in techniques for stone removal. Certain stones may now be removed less invasively via percutaneous nephroscopy and by extracorporeal shock wave lithotripsy. The latter procedure, now widely introduced in the United States, utilizes focused, electrically generated shock waves to fragment stones within a human kidney without incision. Single stones of moderate size ($\leq$ 1 cm in diameter) located in the renal pelvis are particularly amenable to this treatment. The risk of obstruction, pain, and retained fragments is higher for multiple stones and larger stones. Not all stones are amenable to shock wave lithotripsy alone (e.g., staghorn calculi and stones in lower ureter). The criteria for the choice of different methods are undergoing rapid refinement as further experience is gained with new approaches.

Coe FL: Nephrolithiasis: Pathogenesis and Treatment. Chicago, Year Book Medical Publishers, 1979. *A detailed review of current concepts of cause and treatment of calcareous as well as noncalcareous stones.*

Drach GW, Dretler S, Fair W, et al.: Report of the United States cooperative study of extracorporeal shock wave lithotripsy. J Urol 135:1127, 1986. *A review of results of extracorporeal shock wave lithotripsy among 2501 patients undergoing this procedure in the United States.*

Millman S, Strauss AL, Parks JH, et al.: Pathogenesis and clinical course of mixed calcium oxalate and uric acid nephrolithiasis. Kidney Int 22:366, 1982. *A useful review of the intriguing and important interactions of uric acid and oxalate in stone pathogenesis.*

Pak CYC: Ch. 1, 3–7, 9–12. *In* Resnick MI, Pak CYC (eds.): Nephrolithiasis. Philadelphia, W. B. Saunders Company, 1990. *A comprehensive discussion of the pathogenesis and treatment of renal calculi.*

Pak CYC: Citrate and renal calculi. Miner Electrolyte Metab 13:257, 1986. *A review of the utility of the use of potassium citrate in the management of renal calculi.*

Pak CYC, Britton F, Peterson R, et al.: Ambulatory evaluation of nephrolithiasis: Classification, clinical presentation and diagnostic criteria. Am J Med 69:19, 1980. *A detailed description of the outpatient protocol that provides diagnostic criteria for different causes of nephrolithiasis.*

89 Cystic Disease of the Kidney

Patricia A. Gabow

Renal cystic diseases are characterized by epithelium-lined cavities filled with fluid or semisolid debris within the kidneys. The cysts may be single or multiple, inherited or acquired, occurring in infancy or old age, clinically silent or symptomatic, producing renal insufficiency. This discussion focuses on simple cysts, polycystic kidney disease, acquired cystic disease, and medullary cystic disorders.

Certain clinical settings suggest specific cystic disorders (Fig. 89–1 and Table 89–1). An abdominal mass in a neonate or infant should raise the consideration of either autosomal dominant (ADPKD) or recessive polycystic kidney disease (ARPKD). Renal failure in adolescence suggests ARPKD or medullary cystic disease. The finding of a solitary cyst in a 50-year-old person is most compatible with a simple cyst. A history of renal disease in a family raises the possibility of ADPKD, ARPKD, or medullary cystic disease. Recurrent renal stones can occur in ADPKD or medullary sponge kidneys. The onset of gross hematuria in a patient undergoing chronic hemodialysis raises the possibility of acquired cystic disease.

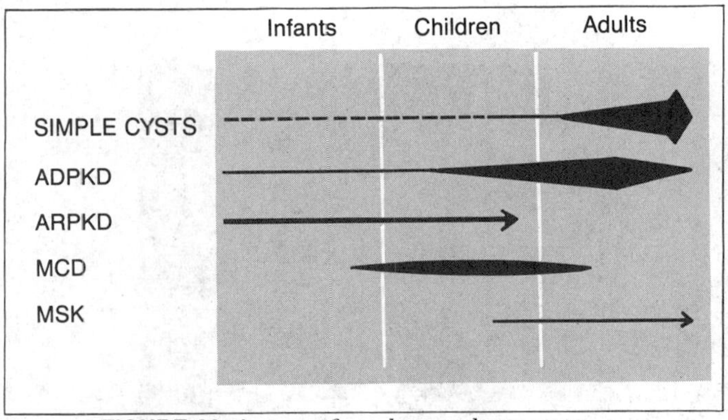

FIGURE 89–1. Ages of renal cystic disease patients.

SIMPLE CYSTS

Simple renal cysts, the most common and clinically least significant of all the cystic disorders, increase in frequency with age from 0.1 to 4 per cent in children to 50 per cent of the population over 50 years of age. Often simple cysts are asymptomatic and an incidental finding during abdominal imaging studies. Occasionally, patients with simple cysts present with hematuria or flank pain, thereby raising the question of malignancy within the cyst. With renal ultrasonography, a simple cyst demonstrates smooth walls, good sound transmission, and no intracystic debris. If the ultrasonographic pattern differs from this, computed tomography (CT) should be performed. Information from the two modalities should permit accurate differentiation of benign from malignant lesions in almost all cases. The CT scan has obviated cyst puncture for diagnosis. Occasionally, simple cysts with benign characteristics cause pain or are associated with renin-dependent hypertension. Such cysts can be punctured with ultrasonographic guidance, drained, and sclerosed with instillation of alcohol into the cyst. For another discussion of renal masses, see also Ch. 91.

Bosniak M: The current radiological approach to renal cysts. Radiology 158:1, 1986. *A comprehensive review of the subject.*

Ozgur S, Cetin S, Ilker Y: Percutanecus renal cyst aspiration and treatment with alcohol. Int Urol Nephrol 20:481, 1988. *A discussion of the role of sclerotherapy of simple cysts.*

POLYCYSTIC KIDNEY DISEASE

Polycystic kidney disease includes ADPKD and ARPKD, which were previously labeled adult polycystic kidney disease and infantile or childhood polycystic kidney disease, respectively.

Since ADPKD can be detected in childhood or even in infancy or in utero, the pattern of inheritance rather than age of onset distinguishes these disorders.

Autosomal Dominant Polycystic Kidney Disease (ADPKD)

ADPKD has a worldwide prevalence of 1 in 200 to 1 in 1000. It is the most common hereditary disease in the United States, affecting 500,000 people. The clinical disorder can be caused by at least two different genes. The most common type, ADPKD1, is carried on chromosome 16. The location of the other gene has not been determined. Complete penetrance of the gene is estimated to occur by 90 years of age. The gene defect produces a systemic disease with cysts in the kidneys and other organs, most commonly in the liver, and occasionally in the pancreas and ovaries and with frequent structural abnormalities in the gastrointestinal tract, the vascular tree, and the cardiac valves.

PATHOGENESIS AND PATHOLOGY. The pathogenesis of ADPKD has not been established. However, altered epithelial cell growth, secretion, and extracellular matrix have all been shown to occur in ADPKD. These abnormalities could, in fact, contribute to cyst development and extrarenal manifestations. Cells are not simply stretched to permit a tubular outpouching to become a cyst; cell numbers must increase. With electron microscopy, polypoid lesions have been noted throughout the cyst walls in both experimental cystic disease and human ADPKD.

The hyperplasia, exemplified by the polyps, illustrates the altered growth that is present in ADPKD. Fluid secretion must also be altered to form a cyst; altered growth without secretion would result in adenomas rather than cysts. The basement membrane also appears abnormal in cell culture systems of human ADPKD renal cyst epithelium. In fact, a primary or secondary disorder of extracellular matrix formation—e.g., basement membrane and other collagen types—offers the best current pathogenetic explanation for the extrarenal manifestations. Thus, studies of cyst epithelium suggest that the genetic defect either directly or indirectly alters cell growth, secretion, and/or matrix formation.

CLINICAL MANIFESTATIONS. Patients usually present either for screening because of a family history of the disease or for evaluation of symptoms. Pain and hematuria are the most common clinical manifestations. Flank pain and back pain are common and can be constant or intermittent, mild or severe and disabling. Both microscopic hematuria and gross hematuria occur. One third of patients have microscopic hematuria on a random

TABLE 89–1. CHARACTERISTICS OF RENAL CYSTIC DISORDERS

Feature	Simple Cysts	ADPKD	ARPKD	ACKD	MCD	MSK
Inheritance pattern	None	Autosomal dominant	Autosomal recessive	None	Often present, variable pattern	None
Incidence or prevalence	Common, increasing with age	1/200 to 1/1000	Rare	40% in dialysis patients	Rare	Common
Age of onset	Adult	Usually adults	Neonates, children	Older adults	Adolescents, young adults	Adults
Presenting symptom	Incidental finding, hematuria	Pain, hematuria, infection, family screening	Abdominal mass, renal failure, failure to thrive	Hematuria	Polyuria, polydipsia, enuresis, renal failure, failure to thrive	Incidental, urinary tract infections, hematuria, renal calculi
Hematuria	Occurs	Common	Occurs	Occurs	Rare	Common
Recurrent infections	Rare	Common	Occurs	No	Rare	Common
Renal calculi	No	Common	No	No	No	Common
Hypertension	Rare	Common	Common	Present from underlying disease	Rare	No
Method of diagnosis	Ultrasound	Ultrasound, gene linkage analysis	Ultrasound	CT scan	None reliable	Excretory urogram
Renal size	Normal	Normal to very large	Large initially	Small to normal, occasionally large	Small	Normal

ADPKD = autosomal dominant polycystic kidney disease; ARPKD = autosomal recessive polycystic kidney disease; ACKD = acquired cystic kidney disease; MCD = medullary cystic disease; MSK = medullary sponge kidney.

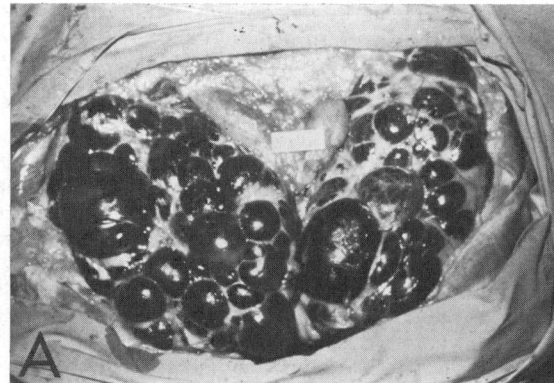
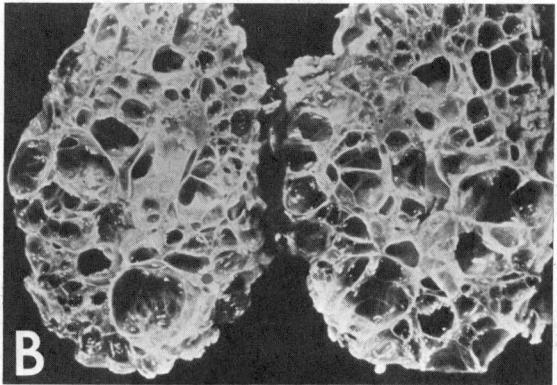

FIGURE 89–2. Autosomal dominant polycystic kidney disease (ADPKD) in situ *(A)* and on cut section *(B)*. Note diffuse, bilateral distribution of cysts. (Courtesy of F. E. Cuppage, Kansas City, Kan.; from Brenner BM, Rector FC Jr [eds.]: The Kidney. 3rd ed. Philadelphia, W. B. Saunders Company, 1986, p 1346.)

urinalysis, and a similar percentage have at least one episode of gross hematuria. Some patients present with complications, such as urinary tract infections, renal calculi, or retroperitoneal bleeding. Early in the course of ADPKD, the kidneys can be normal in size with only a few cysts. Ultimately, the kidneys enlarge and may attain the size of a football, weighing as much as 8 kg. The end-stage kidney appears to be virtually replaced by cysts throughout the renal parenchyma (Figs. 89–2 and 89–3).

The extrarenal manifestations of ADPKD are detailed in Table 89–2. The most common is hepatic cysts, which occur in 40 to 60 per cent of patients. Like renal cysts, hepatic cysts increase in number and/or size over time; however, unlike renal cysts,

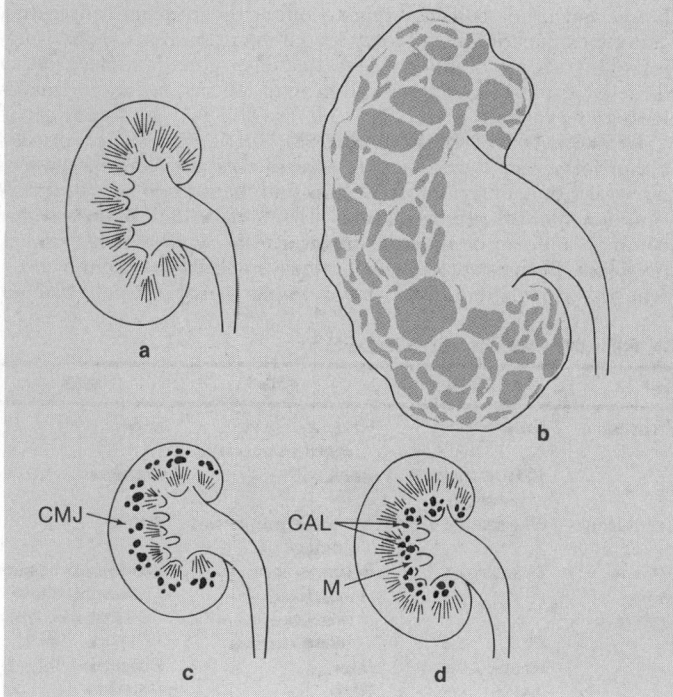

FIGURE 89–3. Schematic drawing of a cut section of *(a)* a normal kidney, measuring 12 cm with normal papilla, cortex, medulla, and corticomedullary junction, and *(b)* a kidney from a patient with ADPKD. The kidney is large, measuring 29 cm, and contains cysts throughout the cortex and medulla, which vary in size from 1 mm to 5 cm. *c,* A kidney from a patient with medullary cystic disease. The kidney is small, measuring 8 cm with a scarred surface. The cysts are at the corticomedullary junction (CMJ) and are small, measuring 1 to 5 mm across. *d,* A kidney from a patient with medullary sponge kidney; these are multiple ductal dilations measuring 1 to 5 mm in diameter, giving the medulla (M) a porous appearance. Some dilations contain calculi (CAL). (*c* and *d* from Spence HM, Singleton R: What is sponge kidney disease and where does it fit in the spectrum of cystic disorders? J Urol 107:176, © by Williams & Wilkins, 1972.)

hepatic cysts rarely occur before puberty, appear to increase in size and number from pregnancy, and very rarely produce functional impairment. Hepatic cysts can also become infected. Colonic diverticulosis appears to be another clinically important gastrointestinal manifestation and may be complicated by perforation and intra-abdominal abscess.

Hypertension, the most common cardiovascular manifestation of ADPKD, occurs in 60 per cent of patients before the onset of renal insufficiency. The hypertension appears to be related to the renin-angiotensin system. Intracranial aneurysms occur in 10 to 40 per cent of patients with ADPKD. Rarely, a subarachnoid hemorrhage is the presenting manifestation of ADPKD. Cardiac valve abnormalities are common; 26 per cent of all patients with ADPKD have mitral valve prolapse, often accompanied by palpitations and atypical chest pain. Myxomatous degeneration occurs in some patients and may require valve replacement.

As might be expected in a disorder with altered cell growth, renal adenomas are common, but it is not certain whether renal cell carcinoma is more common in ADPKD than in the general population. However, malignancy may present with asymmetric renal enlargement, increasing frequency or amount of hematuria, and weight loss; the frequency of these symptoms, as well as the underlying structural abnormalities in the kidney, often make the diagnosis of renal malignancy difficult in patients with ADPKD.

The natural history of renal functional impairment with ADPKD is variable. Renal failure may occur as early as the first decade of life, or renal function may be well maintained into the eighth decade. End-stage renal disease rarely occurs before 40 years of age. Approximately 50 per cent of patients have well-preserved renal function at 70 years of age. Renal function is less well maintained in ADPKD patients with hypertension. Other factors that influence long-term prognosis are less well defined.

DIAGNOSIS. The method of diagnosing ADPKD depends upon the level of certainty needed, the patient's symptoms, and the need for anatomic information (Table 89–3). A screening algorithm utilizing blood pressure, serum creatinine concentra-

TABLE 89–2. SYSTEMIC INVOLVEMENT IN AUTOSOMAL DOMINANT POLYCYSTIC KIDNEY DISEASE (ADPKD)

I. Genitourinary
  Polycystic kidney
  Renal adenoma/hypernephroma
  Renal calculi
  Ovarian cysts

II. Gastrointestinal
  Hepatic cysts
  Pancreatic cysts
  Diverticula

III. Cardiovascular
  Hypertension
  Cardiac valvular abnormalities
  Intracranial aneurysms

IV. Musculoskeletal
  Hernia formation

TABLE 89–3. METHODS OF DIAGNOSIS IN ADPKD

Method	Limitation
Renal concentrating ability in algorithm	Untested in children No anatomic information
Ultrasonography	May miss 2–6% of patients with cysts Highly operator and reader dependent Will not identify precystic gene carriers May miss rare patient with small cysts
CT scan	Radiation and contrast exposure Difficult to perform in children Expense Will not identify precystic gene carriers
Gene linkage analysis	Requires other family members to participate Requires that physician understand interpretation of results Expense Provides no anatomic information on organs involved

From Gabow PA: Autosomal dominant polycystic kidney disease—more than a renal disease. Am J Kidney Dis 16:403–413, 1990.

tion, and renal concentrating ability is inexpensive and easy but is the least reliable method. Imaging studies depend upon detectable cysts. The demonstration of the characteristic bilateral renal cystic involvement is best accomplished by renal ultrasonography. Occasionally, in children or young adults screening studies demonstrate only a few cysts in one or both kidneys. In adults, CT scan with contrast medium occasionally reveals more cystic involvement than is apparent by ultrasonography. Nonetheless, imaging studies that reveal only a few cysts require differentiation of early ADPKD from multiple simple cysts (Table 89–4). The patient's age and the presence of extrarenal involvement are helpful in this instance (Fig. 89–1). Since simple cysts are uncommon in children, the finding of any cysts in a child in an ADPKD family strongly suggests the disorder. However, in an individual over age 50 with similar ultrasonographic findings, the diagnosis is much less certain. The presence of extrarenal involvement, particularly hepatic cysts, lends support to the diagnosis of ADPKD. The information on gene location now permits identification of presymptomatic carriers of ADPKD1 through gene linkage analysis. If there is a need for definitive diagnosis, this technique can be utilized in many families and can predict gene status with 99:1 likelihood. As gene linkage is expensive, requires the cooperation of other family members, and supplies no anatomic information, it is probably best reserved for patients with nondiagnostic imaging studies.

It is not necessary to establish the presence of extrarenal involvement in all patients with ADPKD. Currently, total abdominal ultrasonography for detection of extrarenal cysts, echocardiography for diagnosis of cardiac valve lesions, carotid angiography, and CT scan of the head in search of intracranial aneurysm are not recommended in ADPKD patients without specific clinical indications.

TREATMENT. The treatment for patients with ADPKD is aimed at preventing complications of the disease and preserving renal function. Patients and family members should be educated about the inheritance and manifestations of the disease. Episodes of gross hematuria should be managed conservatively with bed rest, analgesics, and hydration. Urinary tract instrumentation, including Foley catheter placement, should be avoided because of the increased risk of serious urinary tract and renal cyst infections. Patients suspected of having a urinary tract infection should have urine and blood cultures. Selection of antibiotic therapy depends upon the presumed site of infection. Bladder and renal parenchymal infections can be treated as they are in other patients. Failure to respond to appropriate antibiotic treatment suggests cyst infections. In this instance, the antibiotic must be one that enters cyst fluid. These agents include chloramphenicol, trimethoprim-sulfamethoxazole, and ciprofloxacin.

Hypertension should be aggressively treated. The role of phosphorus and/or protein restriction or of cyst decompression in the preservation of renal function has not yet been established in ADPKD. Repeat imaging studies need not be performed unless new clinical symptoms occur. CT scan is the method of choice for establishing the diagnosis of complications, such as intracystic or retroperitoneal hemorrhage, renal calculi, or renal malignancy. A serum creatinine analysis should be performed yearly prior to the development of renal insufficiency and at least every 6 months thereafter. Patients with ADPKD and renal failure respond as well as patients with other renal disease to renal replacement therapy. A more general discussion of the treatment of renal failure is found in Ch. 78.

Chapman AB, Johnson A, Gabow PA, et al.: The renin-angiotensin-aldosterone system and autosomal dominant polycystic kidney disease. N Engl J Med 323:1091, 1990. *A study of mechanisms of hypertension in ADPKD.*

Gabow PA: ADPKD—more than a renal disease, Am J Kidney Dis 16:403, 1990. *A review of both renal and extrarenal manifestations of ADPKD.*

Gabow PA, Johnson AM, Kaehny WD, et al.: Risk factors for the development of hepatic cysts in autosomal dominant polycystic kidney disease. Hepatology 11:1033, 1990. *A comprehensive study of the correlates of hepatic cysts in ADPKD.*

Gardner KD, Bernstein J (eds.): The Cystic Kidney. Dordrecht, Kluaer Academic Publishers, 1990. *This comprehensive book addresses the genetic, clinical, and pathogenetic aspects of all types of cystic disease.*

Reeders ST, Germino GG, Gillespie GAJ: Recent advances in the genetics of renal cystic disease. Mol Biol Med 6:81, 1989. *A review of human genetic data in ADPKD and experimental genetic data as they relate to pathophysiology of disease.*

Autosomal Recessive Polycystic Kidney Disease (ARPKD)

ARPKD is a rare disorder that has been classified as perinatal, neonatal, infantile, and juvenile types based on age of onset. The presenting manifestations include abdominal masses, failure to thrive, or urinary tract infections. The pathogenetic mechanism is not understood. The kidneys are large early in life and may diminish in size with time. The cut surface of the kidney reveals radially oriented fusiform cysts. As in ADPKD, ultrasonography is the diagnostic method of choice. Examination of the parents and in some instances liver biopsy of the affected child are necessary to distinguish ARPKD from the childhood presentation of ADPKD. Normal renal ultrasonography in the parents strongly suggests ARPKD. In addition, children with ARPKD, particularly the juvenile form, often have hepatic fibrosis, frequently resulting in portal hypertension. As with other forms of renal disease, aggressive early treatment of hypertension may be important in the preservation of renal function. Children with ARPKD usually progress to end-stage renal disease before adolescence; in the perinatal form, this occurs within the first few weeks of life. Treatment of the chronic renal failure of ADPKD is similar to that for other childhood renal diseases.

Kaariainen H: Polycystic kidney disease in children: A genetic and epidemiological study of 82 Finnish patients. J Med Genet 24:474, 1987. *A review of presentation of both ADPKD and ARPKD in a population.*

TABLE 89–4. COMPARISON OF MULTIPLE SIMPLE CYSTS AND EARLY ADPKD

Feature	Multiple Simple Cysts	ADPKD
Family history	No	60%
Ultrasonographically demonstrable cysts in other family member(s)	No	90%
Sex distribution	M > F	M = F
Renal size	Normal	Normal to mildly enlarged
Kidneys involved	Usually unilateral, may be bilateral	Usually bilateral, may be unilateral early
Cyst distribution	Cortical	Cortical and medullary
Cyst size	Usually <2 cm, occasionally larger	<2 cm early
Blood in cysts	Rare	Common
Hepatic cysts	No	40–60%; likelihood increases with age
Intracranial aneurysm	No	10–40%
Mitral valve prolapse	No	26%
Hypertension	Rare	60%
Gene linkage analysis for chromosome 16	No	Likely

ACQUIRED CYSTIC KIDNEY DISEASE (ACKD)

Acquired cystic disease refers to the development of cysts in previously noncystic kidneys in patients with end-stage renal disease, almost exclusively in those undergoing dialysis. Reported frequencies range from 40 to almost 100 per cent, increasing with the years of dialysis. Although most patients have no symptoms from the cysts, others develop bleeding, which can be retroperitoneal, intrarenal, or into the pelvocaliceal system with resulting hematuria. Renal tumors, most commonly adenomas, but occasionally carcinomas, complicate this disorder. Although the diagnosis can be established with ultrasonography, CT scan is the diagnostic method of choice in ACKD because the kidneys and cysts are often small. Episodes of hematuria can be treated as in ADPKD. Severe, recurrent hematuria can be treated with renal arterial embolization, as it is not critical to preserve renal parenchyma in patients on dialysis. Renal tumors less than 3 cm in diameter can be followed with a yearly CT scan; larger tumors require surgery because of their greater propensity for malignancy.

Matson MA, Cohen EP: Acquired cystic kidney disease: Occurrence, prevalence, and renal carriers. Medicine 69:217, 1990. *A comprehensive review of the subject.*

MEDULLARY CYSTIC DISORDERS

Medullary cystic disease and medullary sponge kidney are the most common of the medullary cystic disorders. Medullary cystic disease has also been labeled nephronophthisis, cystic medullary complex, and renal-retinal dysplasia (because of the coincidence of retinitis pigmentosa in some families). Medullary cystic disease is uncommon; only about 300 cases have been reported. A familial pattern appears to be present in a majority of cases. Both the autosomal recessive and dominant forms of inheritance occur. Recessive transmission appears more common in the childhood presentation, and dominant inheritance is more frequent with the adult presentation.

PATHOGENESIS AND PATHOLOGY. No pathogenetic theory has been defined. The kidneys are small and generally display some cysts at the corticomedullary junction and in the medulla (Fig. 89–3). An acystic form of the disorder appears to occur. The glomeruli are hyalinized, and the tubules vary in appearance, from atrophic to tortuous. The tubular basement membrane is often irregular, with some areas thickened and others thinned and split; in addition, the composition of the tubular basement membrane appears abnormal. The interstitium reveals fibrosis and mononuclear cell infiltrate. This interstitial involvement suggests some as yet undefined relationship with other immune and nonimmune tubulointerstitial disease. It has been postulated that medullary cystic disease may be the end stage of other tubulointerstitial disease.

CLINICAL MANIFESTATIONS AND DIAGNOSIS. A majority of patients present in childhood or early adolescence with polydipsia, polyuria, and enuresis; this constellation presumably reflects a defect in urinary concentrating ability and secondary polydipsia. Often the children demonstrate growth retardation and anemia.

It has been suggested that renal salt wasting occurs in the disorder in excess of the impaired sodium conservation that accompanies any end-stage renal disease. The possibility of salt wasting should be considered prior to sodium restriction.

Diagnosis of the disorder is often difficult. The urinalysis is frequently unremarkable, and proteinuria is generally minimal. Imaging studies reveal only small end-stage kidneys. The disease in some patients is simply labeled "chronic renal failure" or "chronic pyelonephritis." The disorder should be considered in children or young adults who present with renal insufficiency, small kidneys, and a family history of renal disease. No specific treatment exists. Management is that appropriate for any child with renal insufficiency, with attention to growth, to bone disease, and in particular to sodium balance. The possibility of retinal abnormality must also be considered in the initial evaluation.

Cohen AH, Hoyer JR: Nephronophthisis: A primary tubular basement membrane defect. Lab Invest 55:564, 1986. *Data supporting abnormal basement membrane composition are presented.*

Helczyski L, Landing BH: Tubulointerstitial renal diseases of children: Pathologic

features and pathogenetic mechanisms of Fanconi's familial nephronophthisis, antitubular basement membrane antibody disease, and medullary cyst disease. Pediatr Pathol 2:1, 1984.

Chapman AB, Johnson A, Gabow PA, et al.: The renin-angiotensin-aldosterone system and autosomal dominant polycystic kidney disease. N Engl J Med 323:1091, 1990. *A review of both renal and extrarenal manifestations of ADPKD.*

MEDULLARY SPONGE KIDNEY

Medullary sponge kidney is a relatively common disorder, affecting between 1 in 5000 and 1 in 20,000 individuals. There is no known pathogenetic mechanism. Tubular dilatations occur within the medullary collecting ducts (Fig. 89–3). Patients present with recurrent hematuria, urinary tract infections, or renal calculi. The diagnosis is established with excretory urography, which reveals normal-sized kidneys with medullary ductal ectasia. The appearance on excretory urogram has been described as a "bouquet of flowers" or a "paintbrush." Often a plain film of the abdomen reveals renal calculi or calcification in the cystic areas. For this reason, other causes of nephrolithiasis and nephrocalcinosis need to be considered. Coincident hyperparathyroidism is common in medullary sponge kidney, and therefore both serum calcium and 24-hour urinary calcium determinations should be obtained and, if indicated, a serum parathyroid hormone level (Ch. 235). Conversely, as many as 20 per cent of patients presenting with nephrolithiasis may have medullary sponge kidney. Other clinical manifestations of medullary sponge kidney reflect the structural alterations in the renal papillae, with a consequent decreased renal concentrating ability, impaired acidification with an incomplete renal tubular acidosis, and an impairment in renal potassium excretion in response to acute potassium loading. Despite these defects, serum electrolyte concentrations are almost always normal. Treatment includes appropriate management of renal infections and renal calculus disease (Ch. 88). Urinary tract obstruction must be considered during acute episodes of renal colic. In the absence of obstruction, renal function remains normal.

Green J, Szylman P, Sznajder II, et al.: Renal tubular handling of potassium in patients with medullary sponge kidney. Arch Intern Med 144:2201, 1984. *Presentation of renal tubular defects in medullary sponge kidney.*

Morris RC, Yamaughi H, Palubinskas AJ, et al.: Medullary sponge kidney. Am J Med 38:883, 1965. *Twenty patients with medullary sponge kidney and some related abnormalities are discussed.*

Parks JH, Coe FL, Strauss AL: Calcium nephrolithiasis and medullary sponge kidney in women. N Engl J Med 306:1088, 1982.

Zawada ET Jr, Sica DA: Differential diagnosis of medullary sponge kidney. South Med J 77:686, 1984. *Differential diagnosis—a case report with excretory urography.*

90 Anomalies of the Urinary Tract

Richard D. Williams

Congenital aberrations of the urinary tract occur in more than 10 per cent of the population. They vary in severity from lesions incompatible with life to those that are insignificant and detected only incidentally during studies prompted by unrelated causes. Often the anomalies, although not intrinsically detrimental, predispose to infection, lithiasis, and chronic renal failure, which lead to their recognition.

KIDNEY

ANOMALIES OF NUMBER. *Bilateral renal agenesis* is rare (1 in 4800 births), more frequent in males (3:1 ratio), and typically accompanied by oligohydramnios, Potter's facies, and pulmonary hypoplasia; this complex results in death within a few days of birth. *Unilateral renal agenesis* is more common (1 in 1100 births), generally involves the left kidney, and is seen more often in males (ratio 1.8:1). Renal absence is considered secondary to lack of a ureteral bud. Occasionally, a presumptive diagnosis of unilateral renal absence may be made in males when an ipsilateral vas deferens is absent on palpation. In only 10 per cent of renal agenesis cases is the adrenal absent. Extrarenal tissue or *supernumerary kidneys* are extremely rare (no more than 66 cases have been described); they are distinct from ureteral and caliceal duplication, to be described further on.

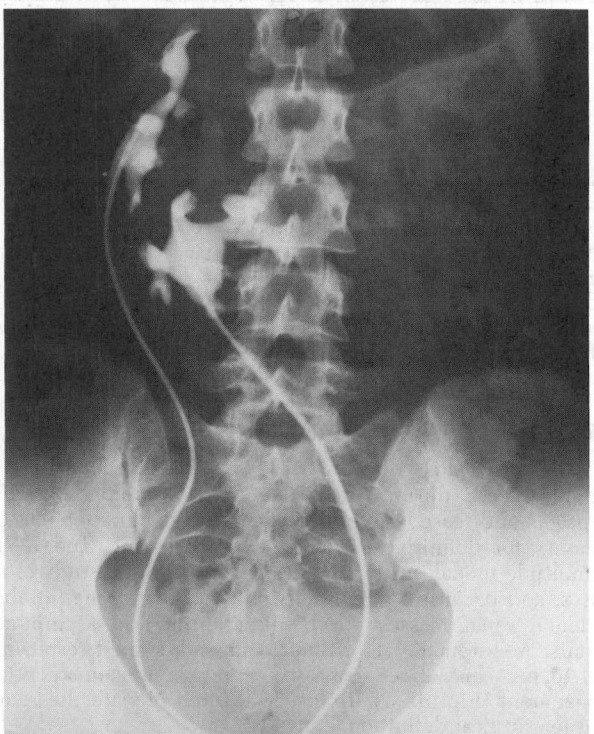

FIGURE 90–1. Bilateral retrograde ureteropyelogram of crossed renal ectopia.

ANOMALIES OF POSITION (ECTOPIA). These are due to abnormal renal ascent: They include lumbar and pelvic and the less common thoracic or crossed ectopic varieties (Fig. 90–1). As a group they occur in 1 in 900 cases and reach clinical significance only when they are mistaken for tumor during exploratory surgery or because of associated genital anomalies. Anomalies of fusion fall into this same category, since the abnormality leads to lack of ascent; *fused pelvic kidneys* or *horseshoe kidneys* (typically fused at their lower poles) are prevented from normal ascent by the inferior mesenteric artery (Fig. 90–2). These latter two anomalies are associated with recurrent infection and calculi in 10 to 20 per cent of patients and with a 30 per cent incidence of ureteropelvic junction obstruction. *Nephroptosis* is the descent toward the pelvis of a normally ascended kidney when the upright posture is assumed; it is seen in adults and is perhaps due to poor renal fixation in the retroperitoneum. This condition, which is not an anomaly per se, is usually asymptomatic and does not require surgical correction. Anomalies of rotation, commonly termed *malrotation,* are due to incomplete ventromedial rotation during ascent and are rarely related to any functional abnormality.

ANOMALIES OF THE RENAL PARENCHYMA. There is a heterogeneous group of cystic and dysplastic lesions of the kidney. The most important group of disorders comprises those that produce cystic abnormalities, described in detail in Ch. 89. *Renal dysplasia* occurs in several forms: (1) *Multicystic kidneys* are malformed, nonfunctioning, generally unilateral, and invariably associated with ipsilateral ureteral atresia. When both kidneys are involved, the manifestations and prognosis are similar to those in patients with bilateral renal agenesis. (2) *Segmental dysplasia* or *hypoplasia* is rare; it is not usually associated with significant renal complications, except in the bilateral and generalized form. (3) *Total renal dysplasia* is associated with lower urinary tract obstruction, such as *posterior urethral valves* or functional bladder outlet obstruction, as in the "*prune-belly*" syndrome.

RENAL VASCULATURE

Multiple renal arteries occur in 15 to 20 per cent of the population. They are of little significance, except when they are inadvertently injured during an operation or (rarely) when they cause caliceal infundibular obstruction or (more often) *uretero-pelvic junction obstruction. Congenital renal artery aneurysms* are infrequent; they are differentiated from acquired lesions by their location at the bifurcation of the main renal artery or at a distal branch point. The lesions require surgical treatment only if resulting hypertension is uncontrolled or if they are calcified and/or have a diameter of more than 2.5 cm. *Congenital arteriovenous fistulas* are rare but may result in hematuria, hypertension, and/or cardiac failure (if large), necessitating surgical intervention.

COLLECTING STRUCTURES AND URETER

Caliceal anomalies include *diverticuli, hydrocalycosis, megacalycosis,* and *infundibular stenosis.* They are clinically important only when urinary stasis results in recurrent infection and/or stone formation. *Ureteropelvic junction obstruction* is one of the more frequent causes of hydronephrosis in childhood. Bilaterality is not unusual, and the condition is often asymptomatic; however, flank pain (particularly following diuresis), urinary infection, and gross hematuria (following minor trauma) are frequent findings on presentation. Relief of symptoms as a rule follows surgical repair (pyeloplasty), although normalization of the radiologic abnormality is infrequent.

Ureteral duplication is the most common ureteral anomaly; it may be incomplete, with the duplicated ureters combining to form only one entrance per side into the bladder, or complete, with two or more ureters coursing toward the bladder on one or both sides (Fig. 90–3). Most often, completely duplicated ureters enter the bladder. The ureter from the upper pole is always placed inferior in the bladder to that of the lower pole ureter and often drains in an ectopic site, such as the bladder neck, prostate, or seminal vesicle in the male or mid-urethra in the female, resulting in obstruction and hydroureteronephrosis. The ureter from the lower pole often obtains poor implantation within the bladder, which may result in vesicoureteral reflux and possibly recurrent infection and hydroureteronephrosis. Ureteral ectopia can also occur in the absence of duplication but results in similar sequelae.

Ureteral reflux can be unrelated to duplication but may instead be due to an abnormal implantation of the ureter into the bladder, with a resulting poorly developed trigone and deficient lower ureteral muscle. This condition can cause recurrent urinary infection in children; however, surgical reimplantation is necessary only in severe cases, while newer transurethral injection methods may be sufficient in milder forms. Other ureteral anomalies include *ureterocele,* a congenital distal ureteral meatal stenosis; *megaloureter,* an abnormality of the ureteral musculature allowing massive ureteral dilatation, often without caliceal distortion; *ureteral valves; ureteral diverticuli;* and *retrocaval ureter,* an anomaly of the formation of the vena cava causing the ureter to course behind the cava.

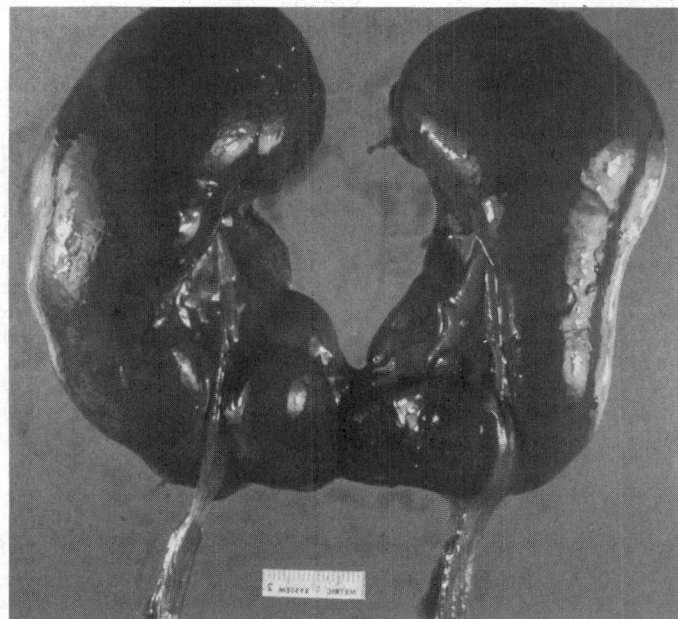

FIGURE 90–2. Gross pathologic specimen of horseshoe kidneys.

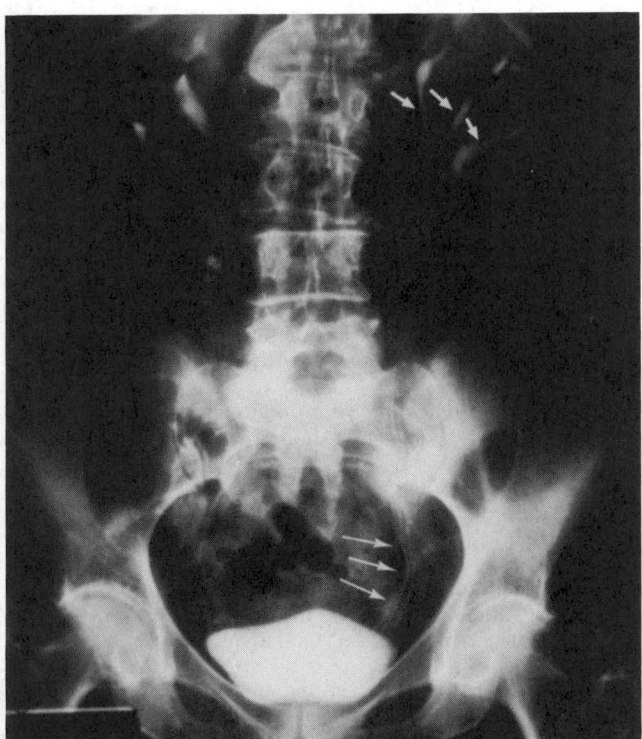

FIGURE 90–3. Intravenous urogram showing right ureteral triplication (*arrows*). (Courtesy of John Dyhrberg, M.D., Portland, Maine.)

BLADDER

Anomalies of the bladder are very infrequent and include (1) *complete absence* (agenesis), which results in a persistent cloaca; (2) *duplication*, which may be complete with separate ureteral openings drained by separate urethras, or incomplete with a septum or hour-glass deformity; (3) *urachal* anomalies, which may appear as a patent connection to the umbilicus, a *diverticulum* at the dome of the bladder, or a *urachal cyst* along the course of the partially obliterated urachus; and (4) *exstrophy*, which is the most common severe anomaly of the bladder. Exstrophy represents a midline defect in closure of the bladder wall, lower abdominal muscles, pubic bones, and anterior urethra (*epispadias*). The *"prune-belly" syndrome* is a complex anomaly in which absence of the abdominal muscles is associated with bilateral cryptorchidism, ureteral dilatation and reflux, and an irregular, capacious bladder with a dilated proximal urethra.

URETHRA

Hypospadias is the most common urethral anomaly in males (1 in 300 live births). The lesion results from failure of ventral fusion of the urogenital folds. It may present as a ventrally displaced meatus on the distal penile shaft or, in more severe forms, with the meatus opening more proximal on the shaft or in the perineum. These latter forms are often associated with a ventral penile chordee. Isolated *epispadias* (failure of dorsal closure of the urethra) occurs in males or females and is usually associated with incontinence. Congenital *urethral strictures* are infrequent. Although *meatal stenosis* is common, it is thought to be acquired, inasmuch as it generally is seen only in circumcised boys. Congenital *urethral diverticuli* are not rare, yet they generally are small and of no consequence. Finally, *megalourethra,* a markedly dilated anterior urethra, often associated with poor development of the erectile corpora, is rarely seen.

Arey LB: Developmental Anatomy. 7th ed. Philadelphia, W. B. Saunders Company, 1974. *The most complete text describing the derivation of congenital anomalies.*

Caldamone AA: Anomalies of the bladder and cloaca. *In* Gillenwater JY, et al. (eds.): Adult and Pediatric Urology. Chicago, Year Book Medical Publishers, 1987, p 1809. *An excellent discussion of the subject in a comprehensive textbook.*

Perlmutter AD, Retik AA, Bauer SB: Anomalies of the upper urinary tract. *In* Walsh PC, et al. (eds): Campbell's Urology. 5th ed. Philadelphia, W. B. Saunders Company, 1986, p 1665. *A complete and well-referenced treatise on the subject.*

91 Tumors of the Kidney, Ureter, and Bladder

Richard D. Williams

Benign and malignant renal tumors are either primary in the kidney and its surrounding connective tissue or collecting structures, or secondary (involving the kidney from adjacent organs or distant sites of origin). By definition, any mass within the kidney is a "renal tumor," but only solid masses are considered in this chapter. Cystic lesions of the kidney are discussed in Ch. 89. A classification of renal tumors is presented in Table 91–1.

APPROACH TO THE PATIENT WITH A RENAL MASS

In the past, most renal masses were detected on excretory urograms (IVP) during an evaluation prompted by signs or symptoms of disease (Table 91–2). Surgical exploration was often necessary for definitive diagnosis and treatment. Today, there are multiple modalities for the accurate diagnostic study of renal masses, and because of their sensitivity an increasing number of incidental renal masses are being identified in asymptomatic patients. A systematic algorithmic approach should result in less than 10 per cent of renal masses being indeterminate prior to management (Fig. 91–1). Its use will often obviate the requirement for surgical definition.

The IVP with nephrotomography is still the study of first choice and can accurately define 75 per cent of renal masses. A demonstrated renal mass will require renal ultrasonography (US) to determine more accurately whether the mass is cystic or solid (Fig. 91–2). If the mass fulfills all US criteria for a simple cyst (65 per cent of renal masses) there is no need for further workup, inasmuch as US is over 95 per cent accurate (Ch. 89). In the symptomatic patient, however, initial workup by computed tomographic (CT) scan, bypassing US, is appropriate. When a mass is suspected on IVP but not confirmed on US (15 per cent of cases), either an isotopic scan of the renal cortex with ^{99m}Tc dimercaptosuccinic acid (DMSA) or renal CT is required, particularly in symptomatic patients.

If the mass on US is solid or complex (20 per cent of cases), a renal CT scan (both with and without intravenous injection of iodine contrast) has replaced renal arteriography as the next diagnostic step. CT is as accurate as, and obviates the potential morbidity of, angiography in defining renal masses. Contrast enhancement of the usually highly vascular renal cancer on a CT study leaves little doubt as to the nature of a solid mass. In addition, CT can usually give sufficient local staging information to allow definitive surgical management. When contrast enhancement on CT is coupled with areas of a negative CT number (relative tissue density in Hounsfield units) typical of fat, a diagnosis of angiomyolipoma is appropriate and no further workup is required. In indeterminate cases, arteriography or needle aspiration cytology or both may be needed to define the diagnosis

TABLE 91–1. CLASSIFICATION OF RENAL TUMORS

Benign Tumors
  Adenoma
  Oncocytoma
  Mesoblastic nephroma
  Hamartoma-angiomyolipoma
  Leiomyoma
  Hemangioma
Primary Malignant Tumors
  Renal cell carcinoma (adenocarcinoma)
  Nephroblastoma (Wilms' tumor)
  Urothelial carcinoma (renal collecting system and pelvis)
  Sarcoma
Secondary Malignant Tumors (Direct Extension or Metastatic)
  Adrenal carcinoma
  Retroperitoneal sarcoma, pancreas, colon
  Lung, stomach, breast
  Reticuloendothelial—lymphoma and Hodgkin's disease, and
    hematologic—leukemia and multiple myeloma

TABLE 91–2. PRESENTING SYMPTOMS, LABORATORY FEATURES, OR PHYSICAL FINDINGS IN PATIENTS WITH RENAL CELL CARCINOMA

Finding	Occurrence (%)
Hematuria	50–60
Elevated erythrocyte sedimentation rate (ESR)	50–60
Abdominal mass	24–45
Anemia	21–41
Flank pain	35–40
Hypertension	22–38
Weight loss	28–36
Pyrexia	7–17
Hepatic dysfunction	10–15
Classic triad (gross hematuria, flank pain, and palpable abdominal mass)	7–10
Hypercalcemia	3–6
Erythrocytosis	3–4
Acute varicocele	2–3

Data from Skinner DG, et al.: Diagnosis and management of renal cell cancer. Cancer 28:1165, 1971; Chisholm GD: Nephrogenic ridge tumors and their syndromes. Ann NY Acad Sci 230:402, 1974; Fallon B: Renal parenchymal tumors. *In* Culp DA, Loening SA (eds.): Genitourinary Oncology. Philadelphia, Lea & Febiger, p 202, 1985.

further; however, in these unusual cases, final definition will likely require surgery.

In general, the nature of primary renal parenchymal masses in adults is readily defined via this algorithm. While MRI is equal to CT in diagnosing renal masses and is better in local tumor staging, other than defining the presence and cephalad extent of intravascular tumor thrombi, this information does not obviate or change the surgical approach. Thus, the less expensive CT is favored.

Cronan JJ, Zeman RK: Renal mass imaging: The internist's role. Am J Med 81:1026, 1986. *A succinct discussion of the imaging modalities available for renal mass evaluation, including cost and efficacy considerations.*

Cronan JJ, Zeman RK, Rosenfeld AT: Comparison of computerized tomography, ultrasound and angiography in staging renal cell cancer. J Urol 127:712, 1982. *A definitive study showing CT to be the most accurate modality for staging renal cell carcinoma (RCC).*
Hricak H, Thaeii RF, Carroll PR, et al.: Detection and staging of renal neoplasms: A reassessment of MRI. Radiology 166:643, 1988. *A definitive discussion of the role of MRI in defining solid renal masses.*
Richie JP, Garnick MD, Seltzer D, et al.: CT scan for diagnosis and staging of renal cell cancer. J Urol 129:1114, 1983. *A substantial series of patients studied by CT with surgical correlation of results.*

BENIGN RENAL TUMORS

Renal adenoma is the most common benign solid parenchymal lesion. Those under 3 cm in size have been designated as "benign," yet they tend to occur in circumstances similar to lesions larger than 3 cm (which are considered cancerous), i.e., in patients above 40 years of age, with a male to female ratio of 2 or 3 to 1. Small "renal adenomas" (<3 cm) are virtually indistinguishable histologically from renal adenocarcinomas and a few have in fact metastasized. Since the biology of these small tumors cannot be predicted preoperatively, most urologic oncologists consider them to be malignant and recommend radical nephrectomy. In highly selected lesions (solitary kidney, bilateral tumors, renal insufficiency, von Hippel–Lindau syndrome) subtotal nephrectomy is appropriate, however.

Renal oncocytoma, a subtype of adenoma accounting for 3 to 5 per cent of renal tumors, has a characteristic pale brown gross appearance and contains cells with an acidophilic cytoplasm that are thought to arise from the intercalated cells of the collecting ducts. These tumors, although sometimes several centimeters in size, are generally asymptomatic. The typical spoke-wheel pattern on angiography is not sufficiently specific to exclude a malignant lesion preoperatively, and therefore treatment continues to be radical nephrectomy.

Acquired renal cystic disease has been described in up to 45 per cent of patients with end-stage renal disease with an increas-

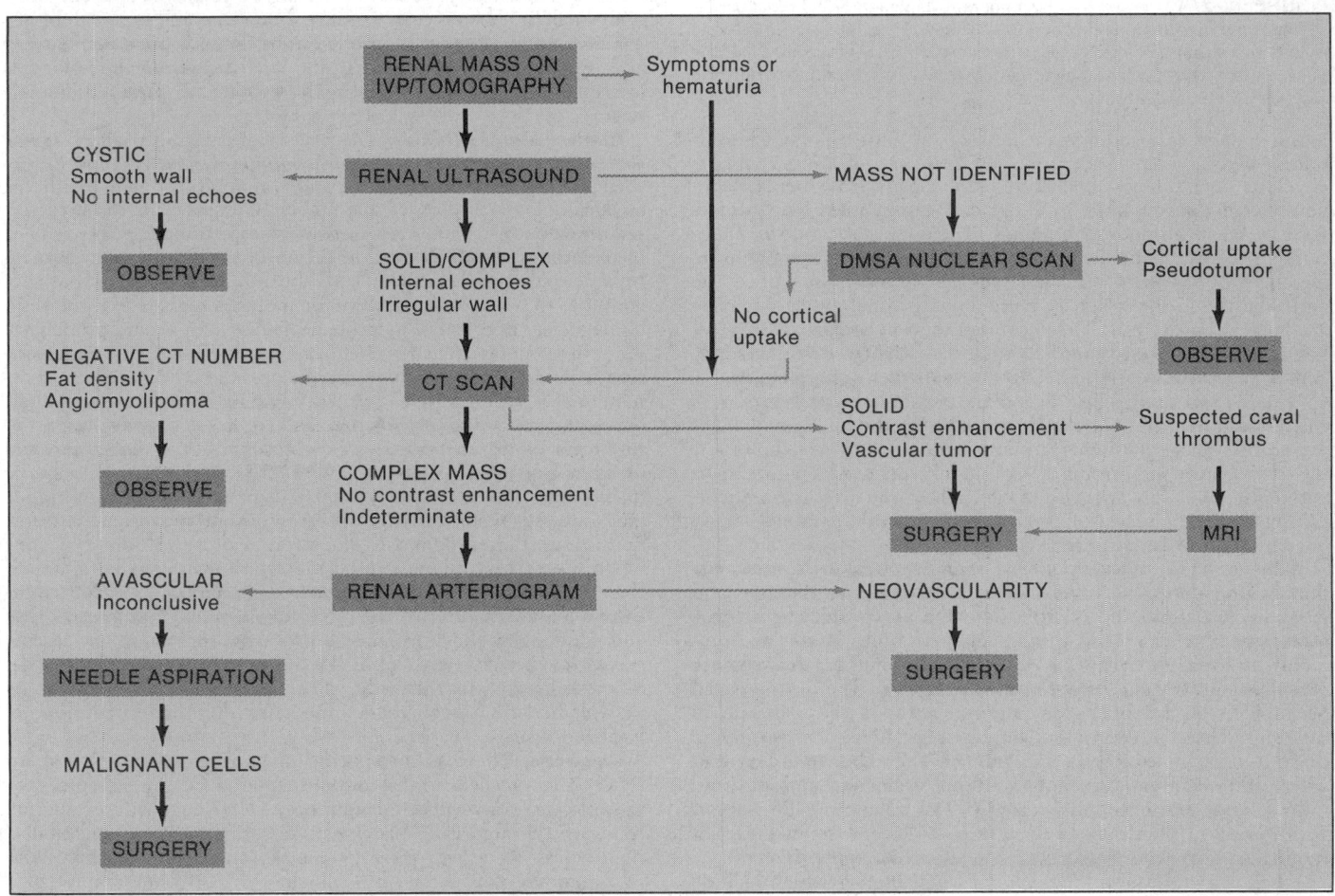

FIGURE 91–1. Algorithm for the workup of a renal mass.

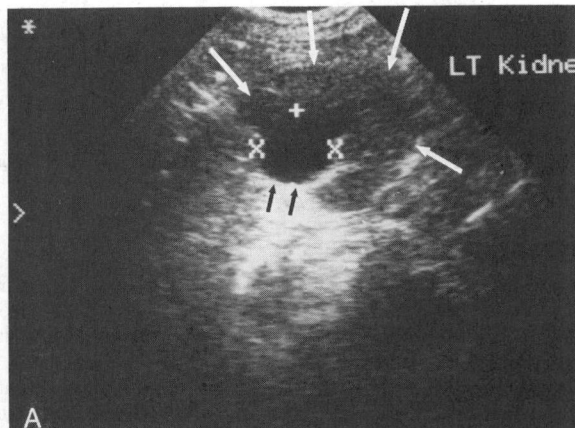

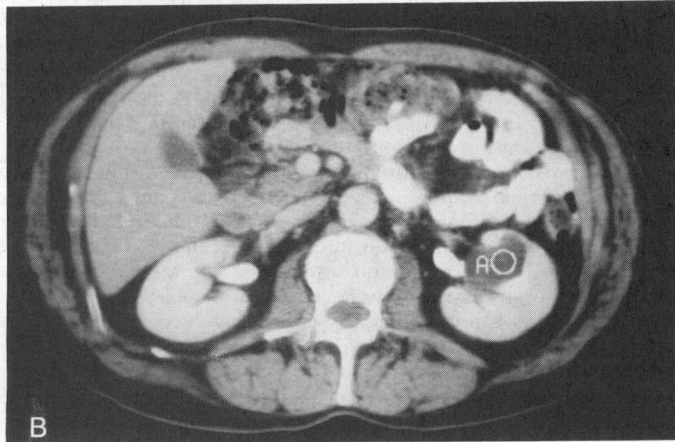

FIGURE 91–2. *A,* Left renal ultrasonogram showing normal renal parenchyma *(long arrows),* parapelvic cyst (× and +) exhibiting no internal echoes and strong posterior wall *(short arrows). B,* Transaxial CT of the same patient showing parapelvic cyst (A). The CT number within the cyst was 10 Hounsfield units.

ing incidence correlated with duration of either hemo- or peritoneal dialysis. Approximately 10 per cent of these patients develop renal tumors that vary histologically from benign adenomas and oncocytomas to renal cell carcinomas. The tumors tend to be multiple and bilateral. The metastatic rate of these tumors is only about 6 per cent. The etiology is thought to be due to a poorly excreted, nondialyzable metabolite, since the entity has been described in patients with renal failure but who are not yet on dialysis. These tumors tend to present with gross hematuria. It is recommended that all patients be screened by annual renal ultrasonography after 3 years of chronic dialysis.

Mesoblastic nephroma, a benign congenital renal tumor of early childhood, must be distinguished from the highly malignant nephroblastoma, or Wilms' tumor. Unlike the latter, however, the mesoblastic nephroma is commonly diagnosed at birth or within the first few months of life. The prognosis is excellent; complete surgical resection is curative, and neither chemotherapy nor radiotherapy is required.

Hamartoma-angiomyolipoma is seen most often in adult patients with tuberous sclerosis (adenoma sebaceum, epilepsy, and mental retardation) and is often detected as a result of retroperitoneal hemorrhage. The tumors may be quite large and commonly multiple and bilateral. As their name implies, they contain vascular, adipose, and smooth muscle elments. The diagnosis can be difficult to establish for patients without the stigmata of tuberous sclerosis. Computed tomography, however, can define these tumors by exhibiting a negative CT number in areas of fat within the mass and can in addition delineate multiple and bilateral tumors with more clarity. The asymptomatic patient with typical CT findings of fat within a < 5 cm tumor does not require surgery; the prognosis is excellent without treatment.

There is a variety of *other benign renal tumors* which include *fibroma,* a renal medullary fibrous mass most commonly found

in females; *lipoma,* adipose deposition within or around the kidney, often perihilar or within the renal sinus; *leiomyoma,* a not uncommon retroperitoneal tumor that may arise from the renal capsule or renal vessels; and *hemangioma,* occasionally accounting for hematuria with an elusive cause. Because these and other less common benign tumors are not frequently seen, it is often quite difficult to establish a diagnosis. When these tumors are accompanied by symptoms or produce a renal mass with caliceal distortion, the final diagnosis is generally made by the pathologist after the kidney is removed.

Fallon B, Williams RD: Renal cancer associated with acquired cystic disease of the kidney and chronic renal failure. Semin Urol 4:228, 1989. *A complete review of the literature and discussion of the probable causes of ARCD.*

Oesterling JE, Fishman EK, Goldman SM, et al.: The management of renal angiomyolipoma. J Urol 135:1121, 1986. *An excellent discussion of presenting findings and conditions for conservative management.*

Storkel S, et al.: The human chromophobe cell renal carcinoma: Its probable relationship to intercalated cells of the collecting duct. Virchows Arch 56:237, 1989. *Early data suggesting that oncocytomas may originate from collecting tubules.*

PRIMARY MALIGNANT TUMORS

RENAL CELL CARCINOMA. Renal cell carcinoma is the most common renal malignancy in adults, accounting for 3 per cent of all malignancies and approximately 9000 deaths per year in the United States. The tumor is also called renal adenocarcinoma, Grawitz' tumor, hypernephroma, and nephrocarcinoma, although renal cell carcinoma (RCC) has become a universally accepted designation. RCC appears to arise from cells of the proximal convoluted tubule. Risk factors include cigarette smoking and maleness (ratio of 2 or 3 to 1). Persons with HLA antigen types BW44 and DR8 may be more prone to develop renal cancer, and evidence suggests that oncogenes localized to the short arm of chromosome 3 may have etiologic implications. RCC is occasionally familial and is more common in patients with von Hippel–Lindau disease, horseshoe kidneys, adult polycystic kidney disease, and acquired renal cystic disease from renal failure. Histologically, RCC is of three varieties: the classic "clear cell" type characterized by uniformly large, cholesterol-laden cells with small nuclei and rare mitoses; a granular cell type exhibiting a darker staining cytoplasm containing numerous mitochondria, and more numerous mitoses; and an uncommon spindle cell (sarcomatoid) variety that has fusiform cells and variability in cell size.

Clinical Manifestations. The classic presenting triad of *hematuria, flank pain,* and a *palpable abdominal mass* is found in less than 10 per cent of patients and among those only with far advanced local tumors (Table 91–2). Gross or microscopic hematuria alone, however, is present in approximately 60 per cent of patients with RCC. The detection of renal tumors in asymptomatic patients has increased, but 30 per cent of patients continue to have local extension or metastatic disease at the time of diagnosis. Because of its protean manifestations and propensity for curious metastatic sites, RCC has been dubbed the "internist's tumor" (Table 91–3). Indeed, paraneoplastic syndromes are common in patients with RCC: *pyrexia* (fever as a presenting symptom occurs in approximately 15 per cent of cases), *hypertension* (20 to 40 per cent), *erythrocytosis* (3 to 4 per cent), *hypercalcemia* (3 to 6 per cent), *anemia* (20 to 40 per cent), and *hepatic dysfunction* (10 to 15 per cent). The paraneoplastic syndromes may raise suspicion of RCC but they do not suggest metastases; neither are they prognostic, since removal of the primary tumor when there is no demonstrated metastasis will usually eliminate the associated syndrome. Hepatic dysfunction (Stauffer's syndrome), characterized by elevated levels of alkaline phosphatase and alpha$_2$-globulin, prolonged prothrombin time, and a low serum level of albumin, all in the absence of hepatic metastases, is an exception to this rule, since in such cases there is an unexplained high recurrence rate after definitive treatment of localized disease.

Diagnosis. There is no specific diagnostic laboratory test for RCC. The physician must often suspect RCC in patients with unexplained constitutional symptoms. The diagnostic evaluation relies on the algorithm previously described for investigation of renal mass (see Fig. 91–1). A mass suspected on IVP with nephrotomograms should be confirmed by ultrasonography. If it is solid on US, an abdominal CT scan (Fig. 91–3) will, in

TABLE 91–3. SOME UNUSUAL OR SYSTEMIC MANIFESTATIONS OF RENAL CELL CARCINOMA

Fever
Weight loss, inanition
Anemia
Erythrocytosis
Leukemoid reaction, eosinophilia
Thrombocytosis
Hypercalcemia
Hypertension (with or without renin ↑)
Cushing's syndrome (ACTH)
Stauffer's syndrome (hepatopathy)
Galactorrhea (prolactin)
Amyloidosis
Congestive heart failure (AV fistula)
Thrombophlebitis
Inferior vena cava obstruction
Left varicocele
Budd-Chiari syndrome
von Hippel–Lindau disease

Adapted from Cronin RE, et al.: Renal cell carcinoma: Unusual systemic manifestations. Medicine 55:191, 1976. © 1976, The Williams & Wilkins Company, Baltimore. ACTH = adrenocorticotropic hormone; AV = arteriovenous.

approximately 95 per cent of cases, be sufficient to establish the diagnosis. MRI can also establish the diagnosis and be useful for staging. A renal vein or caval thrombus is common and may change the surgical approach to treatment, so the presence of a thrombus should be determined by US or MRI. In equivocal cases a venacavogram may be necessary for definition and/or determination of the cephalad extent of the thrombus before operation. The CT scan is sufficient for determining local extension and/or local lymph node involvement, although if nodal findings would obviate surgical management, needle biopsy confirmation is recommended.

Staging and Treatment. It is important to determine the presence of metastases before determining therapy. No benefit has been ascribed to removal of the primary tumor in patients with known metastases unless the patient is symptomatic, the metastasis is solitary and amenable to resection, or a promising medical therapeutic protocol is planned (see below). Spontaneous regression of metastases following surgical removal of the primary tumor is calculated at 0.5 per cent, whereas the surgical mortality is nearly 2 per cent in these patients. The common primary metastatic sites beyond the ipsilateral adrenal and local lymph nodes are lung and long bones. A chest roentgenogram and CT and a radionuclide bone scan are routine staging modalities.

Therapy of RCC depends entirely on the staging system summarized in Table 91–4. In patients with Stages I (T_1–T_2), II (T_{3a}), and IIIa (T_{3b}, T_{3c}, T_{4b}), treatment consists of a radical nephrectomy, which includes removal of the kidney and ipsilateral adrenal intact within its surrounding fascia, as well as removal of a possible intracaval thrombus. The local hilar lymph nodes are included, but a formal para-aortic node dissection is not warranted. The prognosis for patients so treated approximates a 50 to 70 per cent 5-year survival (Table 91–4). Patients with lymph node involvement (Stage IIIb, c [T_{1-3} N_{1-4}]) have a 15 to 35 per cent 5-year survival despite surgical treatment, and those with distant metastases (Stage IV [T_{1-4} N_{1-4} M_-]) generally have less than a 5 per cent 5-year survival no matter what treatment is employed.

Treatment of metastatic disease has included radiotherapy, chemotherapy, and immunotherapy, with none of these modalities emerging as clearly beneficial in effecting long-term survival. Hormonal therapy with medroxyprogesterone has less than a 5 per cent response rate. A variety of other hormonal agents, including testosterone, tamoxifen, nafoxidine, and estramustine, have similarly shown few responses. Approximately 20 per cent of patients with metastatic RCC were reported to respond to vinblastine. Immunotherapy with bacille Calmette-Guérin (BCG), *Corynebacterium parvum*, and xenogeneic immune ribonucleic acid (RNA) has been tried with limited success. Recent trials of recombinant alpha-interferon show up to a 20 per cent response rate with an occasional complete remission. Adoptive immunotherapy entails production of augmented autologous lymphocytes (LAK cells) by incubation with interleukin-2 in vitro. LAK cells are then reinfused into the patient. Early results showed a 33 per cent response rate in patients with pulmonary metastases, but confirmatory studies showed only a 16 per cent response rate and the toxicity of the treatment was great, and the duration of remissions was brief. Isolation of lymphocytes from the tumor incubated in IL-2 (TIL cells) was hoped to be more efficacious, although, to date, specificity of the cells produced toward autologous tumor cells is low; attempts to enhance specificity are in progress. Recent data suggest that alpha-interferon and IL-2 combined have an objective response rate of 30 per cent, but long-term data are not yet available. Although radiation therapy is not important in primary treatment, it can provide short-term control of symptomatic bone metastases.

Crusinberry R, Williams RD: Immunotherapy of renal cell carcinoma. Semin Surg Oncol (in press). *A review of the current treatment modalities and results.*
DeKernion JB: Treatment of advanced renal cell cancer—traditional methods and innovative approaches. J Urol 130:2, 1983. *A superb and inclusive review of the treatment of disseminated RCC.*
Fisher RI, Coltman CA, Doroshow JH, et al.: Metastatic renal cancer treated with interleukin-2 and lymphokine-activated killer cells A phase II clinical trial. Ann Intern Med 108:518, 1988. *Adoptive immunotherapy data in perspective.*
Garnick MB, Richie JP: Renal neoplasia. *In* Brenner BM, Rector FC Jr. (eds.): The Kidney. 3rd ed Philadelphia, W. B. Saunders Company, 1986, pp 1533–1550. *An excellent general review of renal cell carcinoma, sarcomas of renal origin, and Wilms' tumor, with 141 references.*
Holland JM: Cancer of the kidney—natural history and staging. Cancer 32:1030, 1973. *The classic article on RCC containing a complete description of the staging system.*
Krown SE: Interferon treatment of renal cell carcinoma. Cancer 59:64, 1986. *An exhaustive and authoritative review of interferon therapy for renal cancer.*
Williams RD: Renal, perirenal, and ureteral neoplasms. *In* Gillenwater JY, et al. (eds.): Adult and Pediatric Urology. Chicago, Year Book Medical Publishers, 1987, p 513. *A treatise on all aspects of upper urinary tract tumors.*

NEPHROBLASTOMA. Nephroblastoma (Wilms' tumor) is the most common malignant neoplasm of the urinary tract in childhood. It is diagnosed in one third of cases when the child is under the age of 2 and in two thirds of cases when the child is under the age of 4.

Clinical Manifestations and Diagnosis. The tumor is palpable in as many as 80 per cent of cases, often noted by a parent. Pain is initially present in 50 per cent of cases, hematuria (usually microscopic) in 10 to 20 per cent, and hypertension due to high renin levels in up to 60 per cent. The diagnosis is established first by IVP, which commonly shows caliceal distortion. Calcification within the mass occurs in 10 to 15 per cent of cases. Abdominal US or CT scans are useful to determine tumor extension and the possibility of bilaterality (this occurs in approximately 10 per cent of patients). Arteriography is necessary only in bilateral cases.

If there still is doubt about the differential diagnosis (after the studies just described are done), measurement of urine vanillylmandelic acid should help rule out neuroblastoma. The metastatic workup should be directed to the lungs, liver, and opposite kidney. A chest roentgenogram and CT and an abdominal CT are sufficient. Nephroblastoma, as is the case with RCC, often

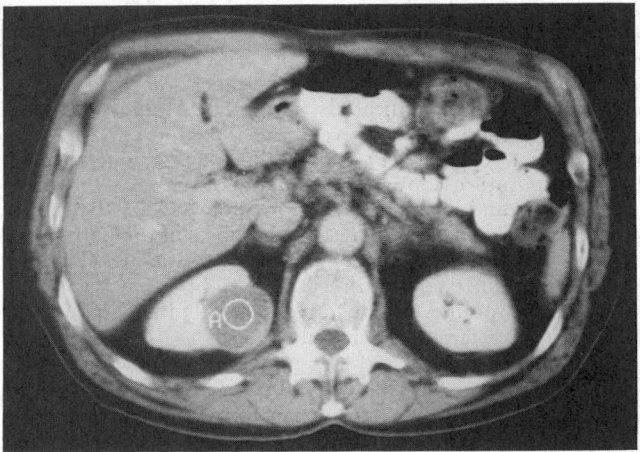

FIGURE 91–3. Transaxial CT showing enhanced solid renal cancer in left kidney (A). The CT number within the mass was 59 Hounsfield units.

TABLE 91–4. STAGING SYSTEMS AND PROGNOSIS FOR RENAL CARCINOMA

Conventional Stage		TNM Stage			5-Year Survival (%)
I. Tumor confined to renal parenchyma	T_1 (small tumor with minimal calyceal distortion) T_2 (large tumor with calyceal deformity)				60–70
II. Tumor extension to perirenal fat or ipsilateral adrenal, but confined within Gerota's fascia	T_{3a}				50–65
IIIa. Tumor thrombus in renal vein or vena cava	T_{3b} (renal vein involvement) T_{3c} (renal vein and caval involvement below the diaphragm) T_{4b} (caval involvement above the diaphragm)	N_0 (nodes negative)		M_0 (lack of distant metastases)	50–60 (renal vein) 25–35 (vena cava)
IIIb. Regional nodal involvement	T_{1-3}	N_1 (single homolateral regional node involved) N_2 (multiple regional, contralateral, or bilateral nodes involved) N_3 (fixed regional nodes involved) N_4 (juxtaregional nodes involved)			15–35
IIIc. Combination of IIIa and IIIb	T_{3-4}	N_{1-4}			15–35
IVa. Spread to contiguous organs except ipsilateral adrenal	T_{4a}	N_{0-4}			0–5
IVb. Distant metastases	T_{1-4}	N_{0-4}		M_1	0–5

Data from Robson CJ, Churchill BM, Anderson W: The results of radical nephrectomy for renal cell carcinoma. J Urol 101:297, 1969; Skinner DG, Colvin RB, Vermillion CD, et al.: Diagnosis and management of renal cell carcinoma. Cancer 28:1165, 1971; Johnson DE, Swanson DA, Von Eschenbach AC: Tumors of the genitourinary tract. In Smith DR (ed.): General Urology. Los Altos, Calif., Lange Medical Publications, 1984.

produces a tumor thrombus in the inferior vena cava, which may have to be delineated by venacavography. Abdominal US or MRI is also a reasonable alternative to establish this possibility.

Treatment. The development of successful treatment of nephroblastoma is rightfully heralded as one of the most significant advances in cancer therapy of the past few years. The prognosis has improved from a 25 per cent survival in the 1960's to a current rate of over 85 per cent disease-free survival, if there is no distant dissemination or unfavorable histology.

The initial treatment of nephroblastoma is complete surgical removal of the primary tumor and kidney, even when there are metastases. A transabdominal approach will allow the safest access and the necessary visibility of the liver, para-aortic nodes, and contralateral kidney for complete staging. Occasionally radiotherapy or chemotherapy may be required preoperatively to decrease the bulk of massive tumors. Needle biopsy is necessary to establish the diagnosis first, however. Combined therapy is indicated postoperatively in all patients but is dependent upon accurate staging, completeness of surgical extirpation, and tumor histology. A tumor confined to the kidney or Gerota's fascia requires only postoperative administration of actinomycin D and vincristine, whereas for all others the best results are obtained with radiation therapy to the tumor bed plus administration of actinomycin D, vincristine, and doxorubicin. Additional areas of current investigation include radiation therapy with triple drug versus quadruple drug (addition of cyclophosphamide) for cases with unfavorable histology (anaplasia or sarcomatous elements). Wilms' tumor may occasionally be seen in adults; similarly, RCC occurs but rarely in children.

D'Angio GJ, et al.: Treatment of Wilms' tumor: Results of the third National Wilms' Tumor Study. Cancer 64:349, 1989. *The most current study results and description of ongoing protocols.*

Pizzo PA, et al.: Solid tumors of childhood. *In* DeVita VT Jr, Hellman S, Rosenberg SA (eds.): Cancer Principles and the Practice of Oncology. Philadelphia, J. B. Lippincott, 1989. *An excellent discussion of pediatric solid tumors in the definitive cancer textbook.*

UROTHELIAL TUMORS. Malignant tumors of the urothelial lining of the urinary tract include those involving the collecting structures of the kidney (renal pelvis and calices), ureter, and bladder. These tumors are transitional cell cancers (TCC) in over 90 per cent of cases, with an occasional squamous cell carcinoma (often in association with chronic inflammation due to stone formation in the upper tracts and with *Schistosoma haematobium* infestation in the bladder) and rarely adenocarcinoma (commonly associated with embryologic hindgut remnants such as a persistent urachus in the dome of the bladder). TCC tends to be multifocal, occurring bilaterally in the upper tracts in a few cases but with an increasing frequency of simultaneous occurrence or recurrences in the ureter and particularly in the bladder. In each location there is a strong association of TCC with cigarette smoking, exposure to certain industrial chemicals (particularly aromatic amines), and chronic abuse of phenacetin-containing analgesics.

TCC of the Renal Pelvis and Calices. Clinical Manifestations and Diagnosis. The presenting finding is gross or microscopic hematuria in more than 60 per cent of cases. In contrast to RCC, constitutional symptoms and paraneoplastic syndromes are few. Generally the diagnosis is made by the finding of a filling defect in a calix, infundibulum, or renal pelvis on IVP. US can be utilized to eliminate the possibility of a nonopaque calculus. Examination of the urine by an experienced cytologist can be diagnostic of TCC, although the site will be undetermined. Cystoscopy with retrograde pyelography, including ureteral wash or brush cytology, may be required to establish the diagnosis. Ureteroscopy may be useful in equivocal cases. CT scanning may be useful in determining local extent of tumor. Arteriography is not diagnostically useful. The tumors tend to metastasize to lung and bone, and therefore a chest roentgenogram and CT and a bone scan are often indicated. Since these tumors tend to be multifocal, careful preoperative scrutiny of the opposite side of the urinary tract (on IVP) and of the bladder and urethra by direct cystourethroscopy is recommended.

Treatment and Prognosis. Treatment of renal urothelial cancer is radical nephroureterectomy, with removal of the entire ureter. Because 40 to 50 per cent of patients have or develop similar tumors within the bladder, direct cystourethroscopy is a necessary postoperative routine, usually done quarterly the first year, twice the second year, and then annually.

Most of these tumors are low grade and noninvasive, and the 5-year tumor-free survival rate after complete removal of the ipsilateral upper tract is more than 90 per cent. Patients with high-grade and/or invasive lesions, however, have a poor prognosis (<15 per cent 5-year survival). Chemotherapeutic combinations, which have begun to show activity in TCC of the bladder,

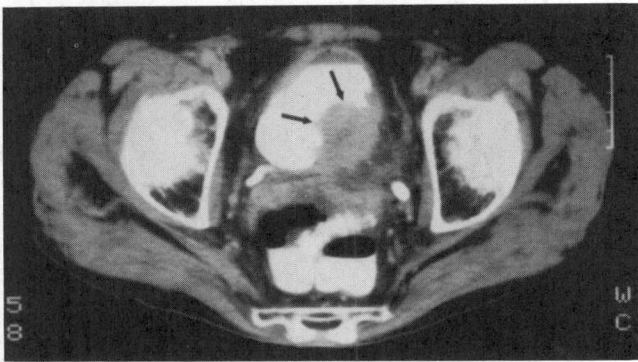

FIGURE 91–4. Transaxial CT of large bladder cancer invasive into perivesical fat (*arrows*).

are also efficacious in metastatic TCC from the upper tracts (see below).

TCC of the Ureter. Clinical Manifestations and Diagnosis. These tumors are most often detected secondary to gross or microscopic hematuria, but occasionally present with renal colic due to obstructing blood clots. Diagnosis is commonly made by the finding of a ureteral filling defect on IVP. If the ureter is totally obstructed with a resultant lack of contrast excretion, cystoscopy with retrograde ureterography or ureteroscopy is required to demonstrate the lesion. As in renal pelvis TCC, ureteral urine or brush cytology can be diagnostic. Abdominal CT scans can aid in local staging, as can chest roentgenograms, and CT and bone scanning assist in detecting distant metastases.

Treatment and Prognosis. Prognosis is determined by the histologic grade of the lesion and the depth of invasion. Selected low-grade lesions may be successfully treated by segmental resection, particularly in patients with renal insufficiency or a solitary kidney, but the definitive approach remains nephroureterectomy, as in renal pelvis TCC. Prognosis of low-grade noninvasive lesions is greater than 70 to 80 per cent 5-year survival, but for the higher grade, usually invasive lesions the prognosis is dismal. Treatment of metastatic disease is rarely successful; however, as with TCC of the renal pelvis, the newer combinations of chemotherapy are promising (see below).

TCC of the Bladder. Bladder cancer affects over 20,000 people and accounts for nearly 10,000 deaths annually in the United States. Men are affected at least twice as often as women.

Clinical Manifestations and Diagnosis. Hematuria occurs at presentation in 68 per cent of patients and classically is total (throughout the stream) whether microscopic (as tested by a three-glass test) or gross. The degree of hematuria does not parallel the size of the lesion. Bladder irritability (frequency and dysuria) in the absence of infection is also a common (25 per cent) presenting complaint, particularly in males.

Intravenous pyelography is not sufficiently sensitive to detect small bladder tumors, but it is helpful in detecting upper tract TCC in the 10 per cent of patients with simultaneous lesions and in predicting bladder wall invasion in patients with concomitant unilateral ureteral obstruction. Urine cytology may establish the diagnosis of TCC but not the site. Definitive diagnosis requires cystoscopy and transurethral bladder biopsy under anesthesia, at which time a bimanual examination can predict whether the tumor has extended beyond the bladder wall. Metastases are local into adjacent pelvic structures and lymph nodes and distant to lungs and bones, and therefore staging of deeply invasive tumors is by chest roentgenograms, CT of the chest and abdomen (Fig. 91–4), and bone scanning.

Treatment and Prognosis. Nearly 80 per cent of bladder TCC's are low grade and noninvasive (stage 0, T_a) or invade only into the lamina propria (stage A, T_1). Patients with such lesions have an 85 per cent 5-year survival rate when treated by complete transurethral resection of the tumor(s). The lesions tend toward multiple recurrences in more than 50 per cent of patients, and

therefore cystoscopic surveillance is a mandatory postoperative routine. Intravesical chemotherapy with thiotepa, doxorubicin, mitomycin-C, BCG, or more recently alpha interferon has been used successfully for prophylaxis in patients with multiple or recurrent superficial low-grade tumors, resulting in 50 to 70 per cent reduction in recurrences. Importantly, only about 20 per cent of patients presenting with superficial bladder TCC subsequently develop high-grade and/or invasive disease.

Unfortunately, 80 per cent of patients with invasive bladder TCC are found so at initial presentation. In patients with deeply invasive disease, stage B_1 (T_2) refers to superficial muscle invasion, stage B_2 (T_{3a}) to deep muscle invasion, and stage C (T_{3b}) to full-thickness bladder wall invasion. In the absence of metastases current best efforts at cure of invasive disease require pelvic lymphadenectomy and radical cystectomy (complete removal of the bladder and prostate in males and the bladder, urethra, and uterus in females). This approach affords a 50 to 60 per cent 5-year survival rate in patients with stage B_1, B_2 or C disease. Patients with pelvic lymph node (stage D_1, T_{2-4} N_+) or distant metastases (stage D_2, T_{2-4} N_+ M_+) have less than a 15 per cent 5-year survival rate. Recent advances in therapy include potency-sparing bladder removal and continent urinary diversion to the abdominal skin (external) or to the urethra (internal), obviating the necessity of wearing a stomal appliance.

Metastatic disease is difficult to treat, but combination chemotherapy with vinblastine, methotrexate, and cisplatin with or without doxorubicin is showing a durable 30 to 50 per cent complete remission rate. This significant advance, if consistent, may alter the surgical approach to bladder TCC in the future. Indeed, research protocols, including precystectomy chemotherapy or combined radiation and chemotherapy in the hope of bladder salvage, are in progress. As yet, evidence is not available to suggest that either is better than cystectomy alone.

SARCOMAS. Renal sarcomas are rare; they include rhabdomyosarcoma, liposarcoma, fibrosarcoma, osteogenic sarcoma, and, most commonly, leiomyosarcoma (60 per cent). In general, sarcomas are quite malignant and usually detected at a late stage, and thus have a poor prognosis. The diagnostic approach is similar to that for RCC. Treatment is surgical with wide local excision; however, local recurrence and subsequent distant metastases are the rule.

Catalona WJ: Bladder cancer. *In* Gillenwater JY, et al. (eds.): Adult and Pediatric Urology. Chicago, Year Book Medical Publishers, 1987, p 1000. *A superb discussion of all aspects of bladder cancer in the definitive urology textbook.*

Droller MJ: Transitional cell cancer: Upper tracts and bladder. *In* Walsh PC, Gittes RF, Perlmutter AD (eds.): Campbell's Urology. Philadelphia, W. B. Saunders Company, 1986, pp 1343–1440. *A detailed and complete discussion of uroepithelial cancer diagnosis and treatment.*

Wahle S, et al.: CMV chemotherapy for extensive urothelial carcinoma. World J Urol 6:158, 1988. *A comprehensive review of the newer and more effective chemotherapeutic regimens for urothelial cancer.*

SECONDARY MALIGNANT TUMORS

Tumors of the lung, stomach, and breast most commonly metastasize to the kidney, but the metastases are usually clinically silent except for microscopic hematuria. More than 50 per cent of patients with primary lung cancer have renal metastases at autopsy. Routine use of staging abdominal CT in a variety of primary malignancies is expected to increase the premorbid diagnosis of secondary renal tumors. Adjacent tumors of the adrenal, colon, and pancreas, and sarcomas may spread contiguously into the kidney. Reticuloendothelial tumors, such as lymphoma and Hodgkin's disease, and hematologic malignancies, such as leukemia and multiple myeloma, may infiltrate the kidney, but this type of renal involvement is almost never primary or symptomatic. Other forms of renal involvement in multiple myeloma are described in Ch. 151.

Mayer RJ: Infiltrative and metastatic disease of the kidney. *In* Riesselback RE, Garnick MB (eds.): Cancer and the Kidney. Philadelphia, Lea and Febiger, 1982, p 707. *A complete review of secondary cancers in the kidney.*

PART X
GASTROINTESTINAL DISEASES

92 Introduction to Gastrointestinal Diseases

Robert K. Ockner

In gastroenterology, as in most fields of medicine, the decade of the 1980's witnessed remarkable advances in understanding of the etiology, pathogenesis, diagnosis, and treatment of disease. For example, three distinct hepatitis viruses were newly characterized, liver transplantation became an established form of treatment for advanced liver disease, neuropeptides and the enteric nervous system became more fully defined as key elements in the control of gastrointestinal function, and potent new inhibitors of gastric acid secretion became firmly established in the management of acid-peptic disease.

Despite these and other notable examples of progress, however, new challenges have appeared, and previously recognized ones have continued to resist the advance of science and technology. Thus, the newly recognized and characterized agents of hepatitis C and D and the acquired immunodeficiency syndrome remain unresolved scientific and clinical issues, while more familiar diseases pose new challenges as their respective natural histories and epidemiologies are more fully appreciated. For example, genetic hemochromatosis is far more common than had been recognized (Ch. 193), and the major problem in the management of peptic ulcer disease appears to be prevention of recurrence rather than induction of initial healing (Ch. 98).

These fundamentally scientific issues, albeit of profound impact, have arisen in the context of equally profound changes in the socioeconomic, cultural, and political milieu. Increasing awareness of the limitation of fiscal and other resources, coupled with a massive increase in new information, has forced major changes in medical research, training, practice, and financing, and these seem likely to continue unabated into the next century. Clearly the solution to many of today's most important health problems will depend upon international efforts and cooperation that, in some respects, are only beginning.

The cornerstone of medicine will remain, however, the thoughtful, compassionate, and efficient care of the patient. This, in turn, continues to depend on a careful and thorough history and physical examination in order that an appropriate differential diagnosis be formulated and that the proper diagnostic and therapeutic options be selected.

HISTORY

A carefully obtained history usually provides information important to an understanding of the basis for the patient's symptoms and for the planning of indicated diagnostic studies. Systemic symptoms, such as anorexia, weight loss, fatigue, fever, and emotional changes, are nonspecific but may be prominent. When caused by digestive disorders, these symptoms are usually associated with other evidence, such as abdominal pain, diarrhea, or jaundice, that more directly links them to digestive disease. Occasionally, however, systemic symptoms may be the only clinical manifestations of such diseases as inflammatory bowel disease, abdominal lymphoma, or pancreatic cancer. Similarly, systemic diseases that secondarily involve the digestive organs, such as sarcoidosis and vasculitis, may be manifested only by general and constitutional symptoms. In these settings, special diagnostic studies, such as liver "function" tests, liver biopsy, or abdominal angiography, may be needed to document digestive system involvement. When symptoms more directly suggest digestive disease, their clinical and diagnostic significance requires a careful and systematic approach.

Abdominal pain, one of the most important and frequent presenting symptoms, must be carefully explored for location, quality, and temporal characteristics. Thus, epigastric pain typically arises from the stomach, proximal duodenum, or pancreas, whereas that in the right upper quadrant may reflect liver or biliary tract disease. Periumbilical pain is suggestive of small intestinal origin, the right lower quadrant of the cecum or appendix, and the lower mid-abdomen of the colon and rectum. The quality of the pain is also significant and reflects the dual nature of pain fibers and pathways that serve the intra-abdominal structures, as noted later. Intermittency of abdominal pain is often characteristic and warrants an exploration of factors that precipitate or alleviate it, such as its relationship to eating, bowel pattern, sleep, or emotional state. For example, duodenal ulcer pain is not usually present in the morning on arising but typically begins 30 minutes to 1 hour after meals or during the night, when it may awaken the patient and elicit the desire for food or antacid. Atypical manifestations of digestive disorders are not uncommon, especially among older patients and those taking certain medications such as corticosteroids. In both of these settings, for example, acute cholecystitis may be painless.

Mood and emotional stress may aggravate or even seem to produce many digestive symptoms. Because of the substantial role that emotions may play, digestive complaints are often more difficult to interpret than are symptoms referable to other organ systems. While emotional factors within the range of "normal" may influence many gastrointestinal functions and symptoms, certain eating disorders, such as anorexia nervosa and bulimia (Ch. 202) and some cases of morbid obesity (Ch. 203), are usually associated with clinically significant psychopathology. A patient's psychological profile may sometimes provide significant positive evidence pointing toward the diagnosis of irritable bowel syndrome, for example, which otherwise depends entirely on the exclusion of demonstrable "organic" pathology. Notably, disorders of swallowing, unlike other complaints such as abdominal discomfort or change in bowel habit, are almost always attributable to demonstrable organic disease. Although emotional factors may profoundly influence digestive function and the management of digestive diseases, there is no evidence that they alone account for the etiology or pathogenesis of diseases that in the past have been so represented, such as peptic ulcer disease or ulcerative colitis. Nor is there convincing evidence that certain personality types are predisposed to these disorders.

Other symptoms that must be specifically addressed include dysphagia (difficulty in swallowing), odynophagia (painful swallowing), heartburn, nausea, vomiting, hematemesis, melena, diarrhea, and constipation. For all symptoms, it is necessary to be as quantitative as possible (e.g., with respect to frequency, duration, or severity of a symptom, volume of stool or vomitus, or interval between aggravating or mitigating factors and the onset of their effects).

The background upon which a symptom occurs is also quite important. Thus, abdominal pain or melena in a patient with a documented history of peptic ulcer suggests ulcer recurrence.

Pain, bilious vomiting, or diarrhea in a patient with previous ulcer surgery, on the other hand, may be evidence of a complication of the surgery itself. And jaundice in a patient with chronic ulcerative colitis could be consistent with any of several possible explanations, including medication-induced hemolysis or liver injury, viral hepatitis transmitted by blood transfusion, or primary sclerosing cholangitis. Finally, a history of alcohol ingestion or abuse may provide the critical information to account for any of several manifestations of digestive disease, including jaundice, gastrointestinal hemorrhage, or severe abdominal pain caused by acute pancreatitis.

In the initial evaluation of the patient who presents with manifestations of digestive disease, the medical history must not be limited to matters directly related to gastroenterology. Thus, epigastric pain or gastrointestinal hemorrhage in a patient taking nonsteroidal anti-inflammatory agents suggests the presence of gastric erosions induced by the medication. And sudden onset of severe abdominal pain in a patient with known systemic vasculitis or advanced atherosclerosis immediately raises the possibility of intestinal ischemia.

In many instances, the patient and those close to him or her are unable to provide sufficient detail or documentation. In such cases, diagnosis and management may depend critically on access to medical records, including previous clinical and laboratory findings, biopsy and imaging studies, diagnoses, and treatments.

PHYSICAL EXAMINATION

A thorough physical examination is also an essential part of the initial evaluation of the patient with apparent digestive disease. It may provide crucial information about the patient's general health, for example, to determine if a patient is a suitable candidate for urgent surgery. It may also provide clues to a systemic explanation for abdominal complaints; for example, intestinal pseudo-obstruction may develop in a patient with progressive systemic sclerosis. Significant weight loss may reflect anorexia, dysphagia, malabsorption, or the catabolic effects of inflammatory or neoplastic disease. Finally, it may provide clues to the extent or severity of newly recognized digestive disease, such as cutaneous spider angiomata or asterixis in a patient with liver disease or uveitis or erythema nodosum in a patient with inflammatory bowel disease.

Examination of the abdomen may disclose distention caused by ileus, intestinal obstruction, ascites, or mass or may demonstrate the abdominal venous collaterals associated with portal hypertension or inferior vena cava obstruction. On palpation, the patient may intentionally tense the muscles of the abdominal wall in order to mitigate the actual or feared discomfort resulting from pressure of the examiner's hand on a tender organ or mass ("voluntary guarding"), or the musculature may be reflexly in spasm or rigid because of peritonitis-induced irritation of nerve endings in the parietal peritoneum. Midline tenderness in the epigastrium is typical of peptic ulcer disease or pancreatitis, whereas right upper quadrant tenderness suggests disease of the liver or biliary tract. If the tenderness is well localized to the region of the mid-clavicular line below the right costal margin, inflammation of the gallbladder is suggested, whereas tenderness just below and along much of the costal margin, especially if associated with the liver edge, suggests hepatic inflammation or a distended liver capsule. Tenderness of the right lower quadrant, possibly associated with guarding or spasm, is consistent with acute appendicitis, whereas a tender mass in this area suggests Crohn's disease or other chronic inflammatory or neoplastic process involving the ileocecal area, such as tuberculosis or lymphoma. Similar findings in the left lower quadrant, on the other hand (i.e., suggestive of a "left-sided appendicitis") are consistent with sigmoid diverticulitis. Examination of the liver should include not only an attempt to identify its lower edge, but also to characterize it with regard to form (i.e., sharp and nontender as in normal individuals, or rounded and possibly irregular as in cirrhosis) and consistency (firm as in cirrhosis or hard as in cancer), to determine whether it is tender, and to measure its cephalad-caudad span by defining its upper and lower borders. The clinical detection of ascites is often possible by demonstrating flank dullness, shifting dullness, or fluid wave, but if the volume of ascites is small, the relative nonspecificity of these signs makes their interpretation uncertain, in which case

sonography may be necessary. Auscultation may detect an hepatic friction rub, suggesting malignancy. Abdominal bruits indicate turbulent vascular flow, usually in the mesenteric vessels or the splenic or renal arteries, but their correlation with intestinal ischemia is poor. Abdominal aortic aneurysms can be detected by deep palpation in the epigastrium. Their size and the presence or absence of symptoms are important determinants of their prognosis with respect to the probability of rupture and the possible need for elective resection. An abdominal mass may be found in association with pancreatic pseudocyst, Crohn's disease, abdominal aortic aneurysm, abscess, or malignancy.

LABORATORY EVALUATION AND SPECIAL TESTS

Certain tests, such as the complete blood count and tests for fecal occult blood, are sufficiently informative and inexpensive that they may be considered routine in the evaluation of virtually all patients with digestive disease. Other studies, including those to assess intestinal absorption or the status of the liver, are employed as indicated (laboratory tests for the liver are discussed in Ch. 116). Endoscopy and the various methods for imaging play an essential role in the diagnosis of certain disorders, and therapeutic endoscopy and interventional radiology are increasingly contributing to treatment of some conditions, replacing more conventional surgical approaches (Ch. 93 and 94). Rapid scientific and technologic progress in these areas will require continuing evolution of clinical decision-making with respect to their use. Various biopsy and fine-needle aspiration techniques are available for the histopathologic characterization of known or suspected disease, and esophageal manometry may be useful in the diagnosis of certain esophageal diseases (Ch. 96). The decision to employ these options may be straightforward or complex. Without exception, such decisions need to take into consideration available alternatives, accuracy, safety, cost, and their possible impact on management.

MAJOR SYMPTOMS OF DIGESTIVE DISEASE

The symptoms discussed in the following section may occur in many digestive diseases. For a discussion of malabsorption syndromes and the causes of jaundice, the reader is referred to Ch. 102 and 115, respectively.

Disorders of Appetite and Feeding Behavior

The control of feeding behavior is complex and is often disturbed as an early manifestation of digestive disease. Subjectively, several sensations are involved. **Appetite** is the desire to ingest food, whether or not there is a physiologic need for nutrient. **Hunger,** in contrast, is the perceived need for nutrient replacement and is usually associated with a particular epigastric sensation of food craving ("hunger pangs"). **Satiety** is the diminished sensation of appetite and of hunger produced by feeding, whereas **anorexia** is the absence of appetite and hunger, usually because of illness, physiologic or pharmacologic factors, or emotion. "Feeding" and "satiety" centers in the hypothalamus play an important role in the regulation of feeding behavior. These centers appear to respond to changes in plasma levels of glucose and free fatty acids, as well as, directly or indirectly, to concentrations of humoral or paracrine mediators, including insulin, glucagon, α_2 agonist sympathomimetic amines, opioids, growth hormone–releasing factor, pancreatic polypeptide, and other neuropeptides. Cholecystokinin, released from enterocytes in the proximal intestine by the action of luminal fatty acids and amino acids, is thought to influence the sensation of satiety via its effect in the hypothalamus.

The pathophysiologic basis for the appetite-suppressant effects of many illnesses, and of digestive diseases in particular, is not well understood, although presumably the regulatory factors noted above and possible other factors as well are involved. Anorexia nervosa, bulimia, and hyperphagia seem to represent instances of a predominantly emotional basis for abnormal feeding behavior, but the pathophysiology of these illnesses is not known. Rarely, hyperphagia may reflect hypothalamic disease.

Nausea and Vomiting

The unpleasant triad of nausea, retching, and vomiting serves teleologically as a method to eliminate potentially injurious substances from the upper gastrointestinal tract. The process can also occur as the result of various chemical, humoral, or physical influences or disease states. **Nausea,** an undefinable and unmistakable sensation mediated via unknown neural pathways, is associated with hypersalivation, diminished gastric tone and peristalsis, increased duodenal tone, and duodenal-gastric reflux. **Retching** is characterized by spasmodic respiratory movements against a closed glottis with contractions of the abdominal musculature, during which the pyloric sphincter is closed and the lower esophageal sphincter relaxed (Fig. 92–1). Repeated herniations of the abdominal esophagus and gastric cardia during this phase may account for the occasional occurrence of Mallory-Weiss tears or the Boerhaave syndrome (Ch. 96). During **vomiting** itself, a sustained contraction of the abdominal musculature associated with the status of the gastric sphincters noted above results in a forceful expulsion of gastric contents. Other physiologic phenomena may accompany the process, including changes in cardiac rhythm and in intestinal and colonic motility.

The initiation and coordination of these events depend on two specialized areas of the brain, i.e., the vomiting center in the lateral reticular formation and the chemoreceptor trigger zone (CTZ) in the area postrema in the floor of the fourth ventricle. The vomiting center, which is directly excited by visceral afferent fibers from the gastrointestinal tract, serves to coordinate other medullary centers in producing the patterned response to the wide variety of noxious stimuli and disease processes that affect the digestive tract, mesentery, peritoneum, and ureters and that are associated with vomiting. An intact vomiting center is also required for the CTZ to cause vomiting. Because the CTZ is in a region in which the blood-brain barrier is poorly developed, it is influenced by a wide variety of endogenous and exogenous substances in plasma, including various chemical agents and transmitters. It also mediates radiation sickness and, in some species, motion sickness.

The timing of vomiting and the characteristics of the vomitus should be noted. For example, psychogenic vomiting typically occurs during or soon after a meal and rarely if ever is delayed as long as 12 hours. Conversely, vomiting due to gastric outlet obstruction or impaired motility tends to be somewhat delayed and usually occurs more than an hour after a meal. Vomiting that occurs in the morning before breakfast is typical of pregnancy and may also be associated with alcohol ingestion, uremia, or increased intracranial pressure. The presence of old food suggests impaired gastric emptying, whereas undigested food may possibly have come from an esophageal or Zenker's diverticulum. The presence of bile in vomitus excludes obstruction at the gastric pylorus or in the proximal duodenum. A feculent odor suggests prominent bacterial overgrowth, as may occur in intestinal obstruction, gastrocolic fistula, or longstanding intestinal stasis syndrome.

The causes of vomiting are many and not limited to the digestive system or the abdomen (Table 92–1). Psychogenic vomiting is often associated with anorexia nervosa or bulimia. Intracranial diseases, especially those associated with increased pressure, are typically associated with projectile vomiting, but more ordinary emesis also occurs. Many drugs and toxins cause vomiting, either through a direct effect on the CTZ or indirectly through their effects on the digestive tract, for example the gastric mucosa. Vomiting is frequently a problem confined to the first trimester of pregnancy but in severe cases (hyperemesis gravidarum) may persist through the third trimester. The mechanism for cyclic vomiting of childhood is unknown. Certain metabolic diseases, including disorders of fatty acid and amino acid metabolism, may be associated with episodic vomiting and possibly stupor or coma. The intra-abdominal causes of vomiting include inflammation, obstruction, ischemia, and perforation involving virtually any portion of the digestive tract, as well as peritonitis.

TABLE 92–1. MAJOR CAUSES OF VOMITING

Psychogenic (including anorexia nervosa and bulimia)
Pain
Intracranial disease
Drugs and toxins
Pregnancy
Metabolic disorders
Cyclic vomiting of childhood
Gastric retention (including gastric dysmotility and pyloric obstruction)
High small intestinal obstruction
Visceral inflammation, ischemia, or perforation
Peritonitis

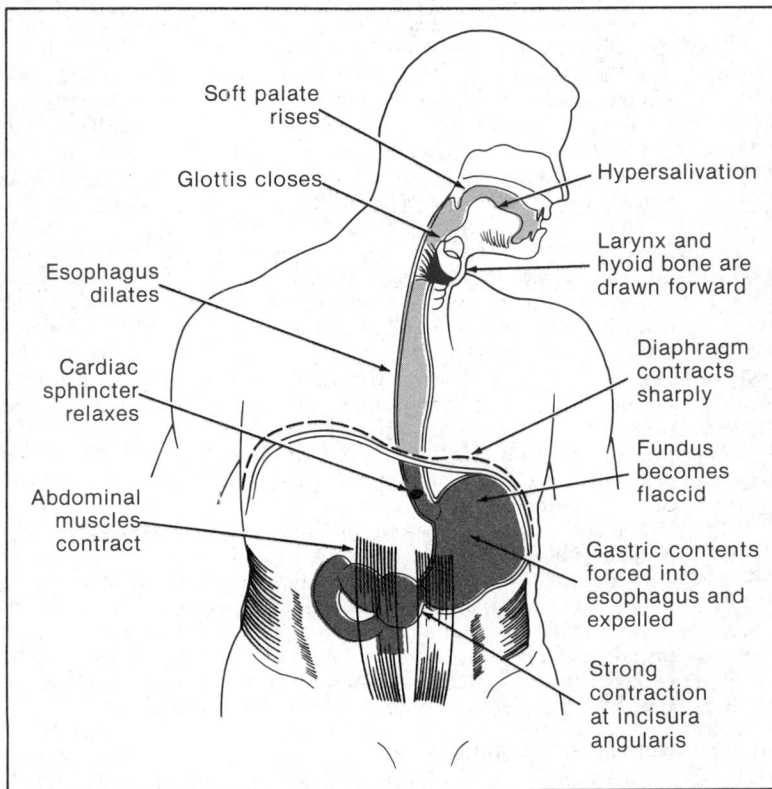

FIGURE 92–1. A diagrammatic summary of the act of vomiting in man. (From Feldman M: Nausea and vomiting. *In* Sleisenger M, Fordtran J [eds.]: Gastrointestinal Disease: Pathophysiology, Diagnosis, Management. 4th ed. Philadelphia, W. B. Saunders Company, 1989.)

Complications of Vomiting

Although it occasionally serves to eject noxious material from the stomach, vomiting usually accomplishes little of evident value. Moreover, it may be associated with both mechanical and metabolic complications. During vomiting, the gastroesophageal junction and the esophagus itself are subjected to substantial pressures and shearing forces. Occasionally, these mechanical forces produce the Mallory-Weiss or, rarely, the Boerhaave syndrome, which are associated with upper gastrointestinal bleeding and esophageal perforation, respectively (Ch. 96).

The metabolic complications of vomiting result from sustained losses of water and electrolytes in the vomitus, leading to hypokalemic metabolic alkalosis (Fig. 92–2). Hypokalemia reflects the combined effects of K^+ losses in vomitus, lack of K^+ intake, and K^+ loss in urine as the result of exchange of K^+ for Na^+ in the renal tubule (Ch. 75). The latter process is in turn a result of depletion of volume and Na^+, leading to extracellular fluid volume contraction and activation of the renin-angiotensin-aldosterone system. Alkalosis reflects loss of H^+ in vomitus, together with a K^+ depletion–induced shift of H^+ into cells in exchange for K^+ and into the urine in response to the aldosterone effect in the presence of K^+ depletion. The clinical manifestations of these changes are described in Ch. 75.

Heartburn and Dysphagia

Heartburn is a retrosternal burning sensation that may be accompanied by excessive salivation ("waterbrash"). It results usually from acid-peptic irritation of the esophageal mucosa, which may or may not be associated with histopathologic evidence of esophagitis. Thus, it is most commonly a manifestation of hiatal hernia or disorders that result in diminished lower esophageal sphincter pressure, so that it fails to prevent flow (reflux) of gastric contents down the hydrostatic pressure gradient from stomach to intrathoracic esophagus. It may be aggravated by bending over or by recumbency, especially after a meal.

Dysphagia (difficult or impaired swallowing) and **odynophagia** (painful swallowing) virtually always reflect organic disease involving the esophagus, proximal stomach, gastroesophageal junction, or pharynx. Disease processes that can produce these symptoms include mucosal inflammation (e.g., esophagitis), mechanical obstruction (e.g., stricture or tumor), or motility disorder (e.g., achalasia or systemic sclerosis). In dysphagia, the patient complains of the sensation of food "sticking," "stopping," or "hanging up," usually felt above or at the level of the abnormality.

Chest pain may also be an important and confusing symptom of esophageal disease, usually reflecting spasm or severe inflammation. Because of its retrosternal location, radiation, and often squeezing or constricting quality, it may be very difficult to distinguish clinically from pain of cardiac origin and may even be associated with electrocardiographic abnormalities. Many individuals with so-called noncardiac chest pain are found to have motility disorders of the esophagus, including "nutcracker esophagus," or diffuse esophageal spasm (Ch. 96). Patients with long-standing esophageal disease may develop respiratory complications, such as bronchospasm, resulting from chronic, recurrent, and often subclinical aspiration.

Abdominal Pain

Abdominal pain, or a variant of it, such as indigestion, is one of the most important symptoms of digestive disease, often providing to the patient the first hint that something is amiss and providing to the physician information that is often helpful in diagnosis. Many aspects of abdominal pain have been discussed previously under the topic of the medical history. Abdominal pain varies widely in severity, quality, and location. Because it is, by definition, "subjective," the significance of pain in relation to other symptoms and to underlying disease processes can be evaluated only by thoughtful and systematic discussions with the patient.

Abdominal pain is diverse in type, reflecting the dual sensory innervation of the abdominal structures and the characteristics of each of the fiber types and pathways involved: (1) *Visceral fibers,*

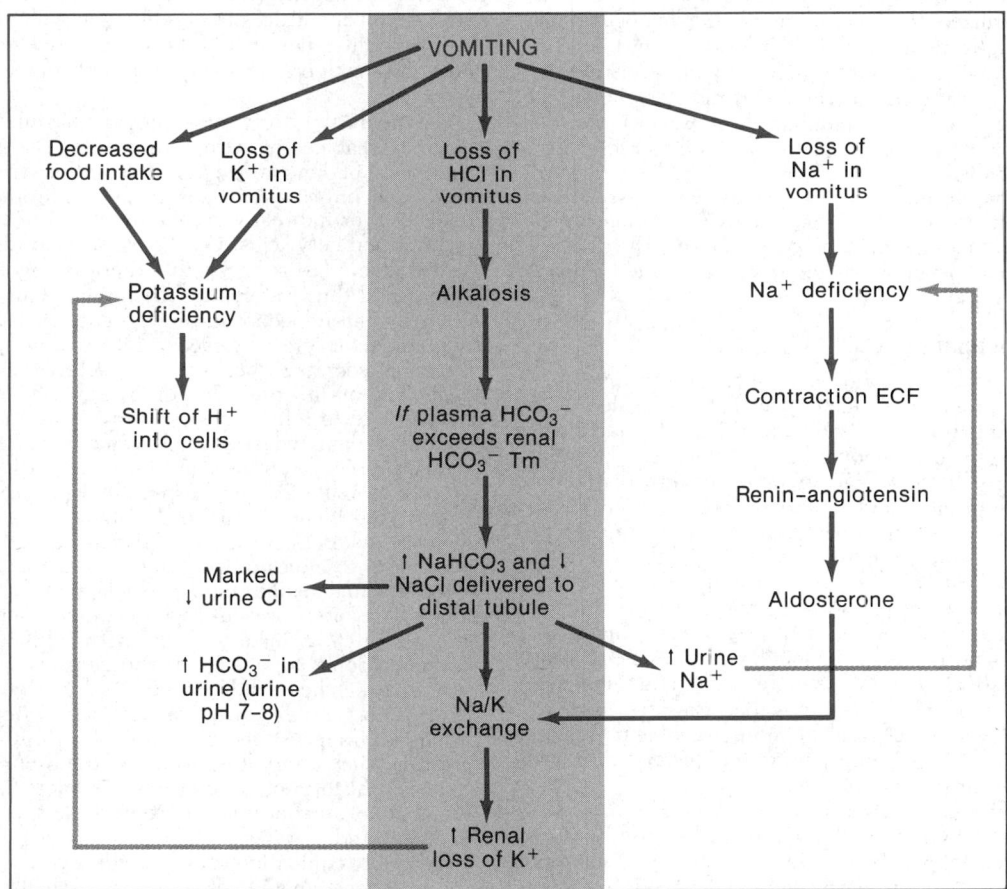

FIGURE 92–2. Metabolic consequences of vomiting. (From Feldman M: Nausea and vomiting. *In* Sleisenger M, Fordtran J [eds.]: Gastrointestinal Disease: Pathophysiology, Diagnosis, Management. 4th ed. Philadelphia, W. B. Saunders Company, 1989.)

largely type C, are present in the muscular walls of the hollow viscera and in the capsule of the solid organs and conduct afferent impulses from these sources via the vagus nerve. Innervation is usually bilateral. Pain conducted by these fibers is often perceived as midline in location, poorly localized but generally dull, cramping, or burning in quality, gradual in onset, prolonged in duration, and associated with autonomic manifestations such as nausea, vomiting, and diaphoresis. (2) *Somatic fibers*, largely type A-delta present in skin and muscle, innervate principally the parietal peritoneum and enter the spinal cord via the intercostal nerves. Pain conducted by these fibers tends to be sharper, more intense, more sudden in onset, and far more precisely localized than visceral pain. For example, the pain associated with intestinal obstruction, early acute cholecystitis, or uncomplicated peptic ulcer is typically visceral, whereas that associated with an acute peritonitis resulting from ulcer perforation is usually somatic.

Abdominal pain can be caused by (1) tension, stretching, or forceful contraction of the musculature of a hollow viscus, such as the intestine or gallbladder, (2) ischemia, presumably mediated by the local accumulation of metabolites and chemical mediators of inflammation, (3) local or generalized inflammation of the parietal peritoneum, (4) neoplastic or fibrotic involvement of nerve fibers, or (5) extra-abdominal causes, such as certain metabolic disorders (e.g., acute intermittent porphyria) or extra-abdominal pain referred to an intra-abdominal location.

Beyond the explanations that can be derived from these basic principles, certain empiric observations have related specific pain patterns to a particular organ or other site of origin. Esophageal pain, such as occurs in spasm or esophagitis, is located retrosternally, usually at or above the level of disease. If the pain is severe, it may be felt in the back. Pain arising from the stomach or duodenum is also midline and usually perceived in the epigastrium; if severe, it too may be felt in the back, a phenomenon that does not necessarily imply perforation of an ulcer. Small intestinal pain, as occurs with obstruction or ischemia, is usually periumbilical and, if severe, may also be felt in the back. Colonic pain is localized to the midline in the hypogastrium, whereas pain arising from the gallbladder or common bile duct is felt in the right upper quadrant. Pancreatic pain is localized to the mid- to left side of the epigastrium, but may also be felt in the back or the left shoulder, depending on its severity and on whether there is involvement of diaphragmatic nerves, e.g., during acute pancreatitis.

Significant information may be derived from an assessment of the temporal characteristics of the pain and its relationship to certain events such as eating or sleeping (see above). The physical examination of the patient in whom abdominal pain is a dominant symptom is described in Ch. 112.

Diarrhea and Constipation (Ch. 101 and 109)

Changes in bowel habit may be among the most difficult of gastrointestinal symptoms to evaluate. This is because the range of what is considered to be normal is very broad among individuals and because in any given individual bowel habits may be influenced by a similarly broad range of determinants that differ greatly in their significance and in the immediacy with which they must be addressed. Thus, changes in bowel habit may be caused not only by acute or chronic diseases of the digestive system and by medications, for example, but also by extra-abdominal diseases and by phenomena not considered to be "organic," such as mood and emotional stress. In many instances, the approach to diagnosis and management of the recent onset of diarrhea or constipation may be deliberate, and involve a gradual, stepwise investigation of possible causative factors; whereas in others the approach must be more urgent and possibly requires invasive studies in addition to the history, physical examination, and routine laboratory tests.

Definitions of normality or abnormality for bowel habits are of necessity somewhat arbitrary and imprecise, because what is normal for one individual may be decidedly abnormal for another. Stool frequency has an extraordinarily wide range of normal, from perhaps two or three per day to only one per week or longer, averaging one to two per day. Stool weight, accounted for mostly by water, is normally 50 to 200 grams per day but is not well correlated with stool frequency, because the extent to which the fecal mass is dehydrated during its passage through the colon varies considerably. Diarrhea can be defined as a stool weight of more than 200 grams or as more than three bowel movements per day (Ch. 101). Constipation is more difficult to define, as it involves not only stool frequency but also stool dehydration in the colon, i.e., its hardness. This and other characteristics, such as the ease or discomfort of stool passage or the sensation of a need to pass stool, are more difficult to quantify and therefore not very helpful. Perhaps the most reliable indicator of possibly disturbed physiology is the perception by the patient that an established pattern has changed, either to a degree or for a duration that seems beyond the range of variation which he or she considers normal. Such a change can reflect a change in either the amount of water excreted in the stool or the motility of the colon, or both.

Approximately 9 liters of water enter the gastrointestinal tract from exogenous and endogenous sources each day. Stool frequency and weight are therefore directly influenced by the extent to which water is absorbed from or secreted into the lumen of the small and large intestines. Essentially all water movement into and out of the intestinal lumen is passive. It is driven by osmotically active solutes that have been secreted, absorbed, or generated within the lumen through the breakdown of larger molecules by digestive enzymes or intestinal flora. Thus, abnormalities of fecal water excretion (i.e., diarrhea, or, to a lesser extent, constipation) reflect corresponding abnormalities in the digestion, absorption, or secretion of solutes. On this basis, diarrhea can be classified according to the source of these solutes. For example, the maldigestion or malabsorption of ingested nutrient solutes may occur in the malabsorption syndrome or in disaccharidase deficiency (so-called osmotic diarrhea). Or diarrhea may result from excessive secretion of inorganic ions such as Cl^- (so-called secretory diarrhea), as may occur in tumors that produce hormonal secretagogues, (e.g., "pancreatic cholera") or through the effects of bacterial enterotoxins, and the effects of nonabsorbed fatty acids and bile acids on the colonic mucosa. Changes in motility alone tend to influence stool frequency but have relatively little direct effect on volume. Suppression of bowel motility, however, retards the movement of luminal contents and may permit increased absorption of solutes and thus of water.

The medical history may provide useful clues to diagnosis. Diarrhea that ceases with fasting suggests that a nonabsorbed component of diet may be causative, either directly via an osmotic effect (e.g., intestinal malabsorption syndrome or disaccharidase deficiency) or indirectly via the induction of colonic secretion by nonabsorbed fatty acids. On the other hand, diarrhea that continues through a fast suggests that there is ongoing active secretion of ions, and thus water, into the lumen. This could be mediated either by an endogenous secretagogue, such as a tumor-derived humoral factor (e.g., vasoactive intestinal polypeptide), or by an exogenous secretagogue, such as a bacterial enterotoxin produced in cholera or in "traveler's diarrhea." Stools that are large in volume tend to reflect processes involving the small intestine or proximal colon, whereas small volume diarrhea suggests a left colonic or rectal source. The duration of diarrhea is often very important. Acute diarrhea, especially when associated with fever, cramps, and blood or pus in the stool, suggests invasive enteric infection, whereas chronic diarrhea associated with weight loss is more likely to indicate neoplastic or inflammatory bowel disease. Extraintestinal manifestations, such as arthritis or skin or eye lesions, are often present in idiopathic inflammatory bowel disease (Ch. 103). A history of recent travel is especially important and may point to one of the organisms associated with the traveler's diarrhea syndrome (Ch. 101). Homosexual contact or other factors predisposing to acquired immunodeficiency syndrome may suggest the presence of an opportunistic intestinal infection, such as cryptosporidiosis. In obscure cases of diarrhea, a careful history of laxative use is most important, and the possibility of surreptitious abuse of these substances must always be considered.

Physical examination may provide evidence of extraintestinal manifestations, an abdominal mass, perianal pathology associated with inflammatory bowel disease, or a neuropathy or other evidence of vitamin deficiency, reflecting a malabsorption syndrome. Laboratory evaluation of clinically significant diarrhea should routinely include examination of the stool for occult blood, leukocytes, enteric pathogens, and ova and parasites. Sigmoidoscopy with biopsy or swab and culture of rectal lesions may be indicated in selected cases, such as those in which symptoms are especially severe or protracted.

Sleisenger M, Fordtran J (eds.): Gastrointestinal Disease: Pathophysiology, Diagnosis, Management. 4th ed. Philadelphia, W. B. Saunders Company, 1989.

Zakim D, Boyer T (eds.): Diseases of the Liver. 2nd ed. Philadelphia, W. B. Saunders Company, 1990. *Two recent, authoritative, and extensively referenced texts.*

93 Diagnostic Imaging Procedures in Gastroenterology

Susan D. Wall

With the development of increasingly complex diagnostic imaging procedures in gastroenterology, the importance of direct communication with the consulting radiologist has increased. Clinical information regarding each diagnostic question is essential to tailoring the studies; none is "routine." In addition to conventional plain films of the abdomen and barium examination of the gastrointestinal tract, radiographic procedures of interest to the gastroenterologist include computed tomography, ultrasonography, endoscopic retrograde cholangiopancreatography, percutaneous transhepatic cholangiography, enteroclysis, radionuclide scanning, and magnetic resonance imaging.

COMPUTED TOMOGRAPHY

The faster scan time (2 to 3 seconds) and higher spatial resolution available with current computed tomography (CT) have improved greatly the images of the alimentary tract as well as of the pancreas (Fig. 93–1), liver, and gallbladder. Computed tomography continues to be an important modality for the investigation of possible hepatic tumor, pancreatic carcinoma, and retroperitoneal adenopathy. Less recognized is its contribution to the evaluation of the acute abdomen. When the diagnosis is unclear, CT is helpful in diagnosing possible pancreatitis (Fig. 93–2), perforated viscus, and subdiaphragmatic abscess, and in assessing the extent of Crohn's disease or bowel ischemia. It can detect extraluminal abscess associated with appendicitis and

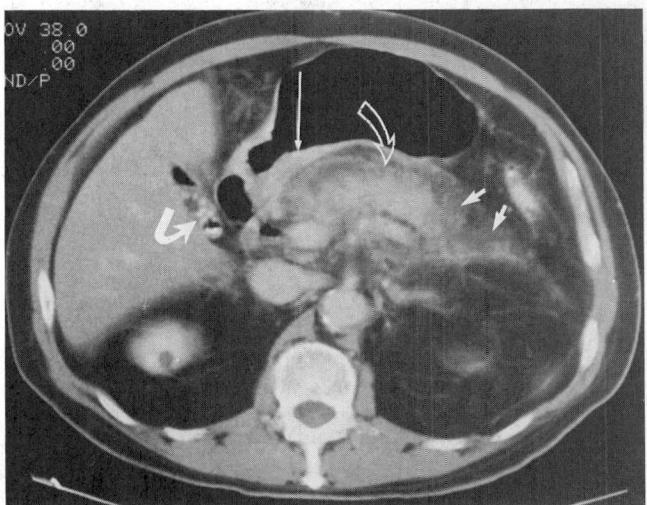

FIGURE 93–2. Computed tomography of acute pancreatitis. Abnormally dense fat surrounds the swollen pancreas *(open curved arrow)*. Free pancreatic fluid *(short arrows)* is present in the left anterior pararenal space, and the air-distended stomach has a thickened antral wall *(straight arrow)*. Note cholelithiasis *(closed curved arrow)*.

diverticulitis (Fig. 93–4) and can sometimes help in the decision regarding surgical versus nonsurgical management. Computed tomography also can detect free intra- or retroperitoneal air and small amounts of contrast material that have extravasated from the gastrointestinal tract (Fig. 93–3); it provides excellent visualization of the mesentery. It is the modality of choice for evaluation of suspected complications of pancreatitis, such as necrosis, abscess, pseudocyst, and colonic or mesenteric inflammation (Ch. 106).

Percutaneous fine needle aspiration (PFNA) with CT guidance can diagnose pancreatic carcinoma, primary and metastatic tumor of the liver, and sometimes tumor involvement of enlarged lymph nodes. False-negative results occur, but this procedure often obviates the need for diagnostic laparotomy. Furthermore, PFNA can diagnose a suspected abscess (Fig. 93–3), which can be variable and nonspecific in its radiographic appearance. Percutaneous drainage of an intra-abdominal or pelvic abscess with CT guidance is a nonsurgical treatment option for selected patients; it can palliate others until surgery is performed.

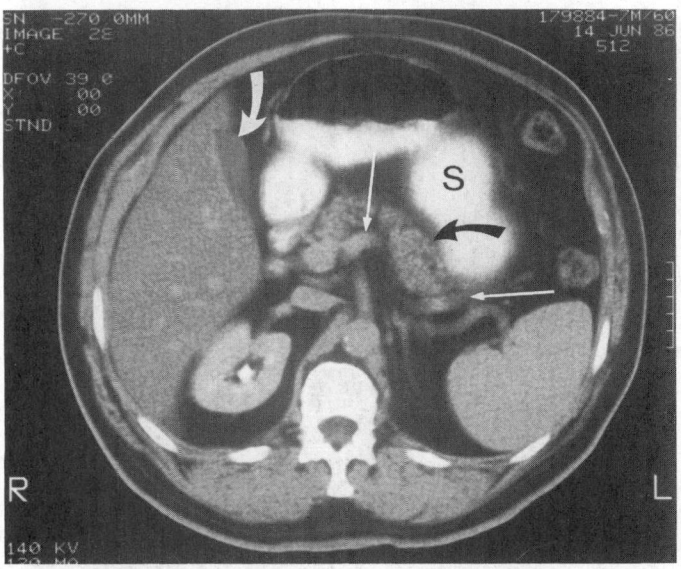

FIGURE 93–1. Normal computed tomogram. One cm thick transverse image (supine, patient's right to reader's left) is at the level of the pancreas *(black arrow)*, which is behind the contrast-filled stomach (S). The splenic artery is posterior to the splenic vein *(straight white arrows)*, which abuts the posterior margin of the tail and neck of the pancreas. The density of the right kidney is enhanced because of intravenous contrast material. *Curved white arrow* points to gallbladder.

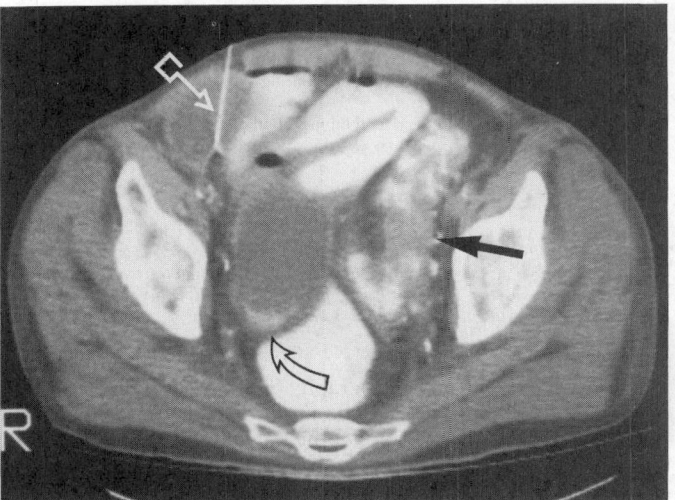

FIGURE 93–3. Computed tomography of diverticular abscess. Percutaneous fine-needle aspiration *(boxed white arrow)* of pelvic fluid collection diagnosed abscess in this patient with thickening of the wall of the sigmoid colon *(straight black arrow)* and diverticulitis. Note second fluid collection with small amount of contrast material *(curved black arrow)* extravasated from the diseased colon. Abscesses were drained percutaneously until the patient was well enough for surgery.

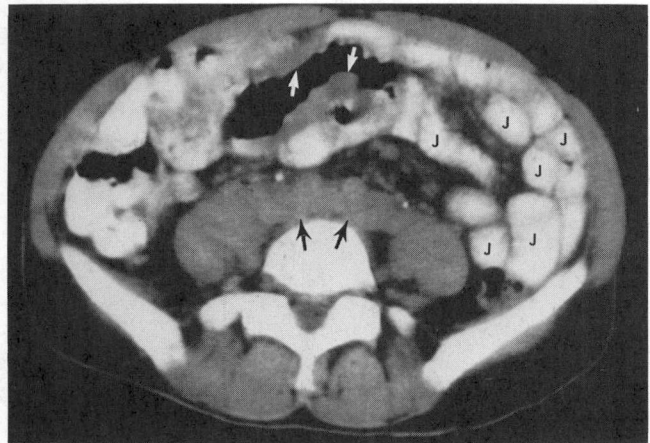

FIGURE 93–4. Small bowel Kaposi's sarcoma. Focal thickening *(arrows)* of a single segment of small bowel is due to Kaposi's sarcoma in this patient with acquired immunodeficiency syndrome. Note the normal jejunum (J) proximal to the tumor and the retroperitoneal lymphadenopathy *(black arrows)* anterior to the spine.

Computed tomography sometimes replaces barium contrast examination as the initial study of the gastrointestinal tract. Barium examination, which provides mucosal detail and delineation of the intraluminal contour, cannot demonstrate thickening of the wall, and the barium causes severe artifacts on CT images, precluding the possibility of a diagnostic study. Moreover, even unsuspected disease in the gastrointestinal tract, both primary and secondary, often is detected initially with CT. Assessment of thickening of the esophageal, gastric, and bowel wall is possible with current CT (Fig. 93–4), and surrounding organs may also be evaluated, especially regarding inflammatory processes, such as diverticulitis, appendicitis, Crohn's disease, pancreatitis, and possible perforated ulcer. Computed tomography has limited value in the regional staging of gastrointestinal malignancies because of its limited accuracy in determining tumor invasion into adjacent tissues. Indications for preoperative evaluation of patients with rectosigmoid colon carcinoma, for example, include suspected extensive disease or complications such as perforation. Computed tomography is more helpful in determining recurrence postoperatively. A baseline study is performed 2 to 4 months after resection, with follow-up comparison studies every 6 months for 2 years. New or enlarging masses in the pelvis suggest recurrent tumor; CT-guided biopsy can be performed for tissue diagnosis.

Balthazar EJ, Robinson DL, Megibow AJ, et al: Acute pancreatitis: Value of CT in establishing prognosis. Radiology 174:331, 1990. *A prospective study of 88 patients demonstrating radiographic findings predictive of serious complications.*

Moss AA: Imaging of colorectal carcinoma. Radiology 170:308, 1989. *Editorial overview of both preoperative staging and detection of postoperative recurrence.*

Sugarbaker PH: Surgical decision making for large bowel cancer metastatic to the liver. Radiology 174:621, 1990. *A superb summary of the current radiologic, laboratory, and medical considerations regarding this issue.*

Welch TJ, Sheedy PF II, Johnson CD, et al: CT-guided biopsy: Prospective analysis of 1,000 procedures. Radiology 171:493, 1989. *A valuable report documenting the high sensitivity, specificity, and predictive value of this safe alternative to more invasive diagnostic procedures such as laparotomy.*

ULTRASONOGRAPHY

Abdominal pelvic ultrasonography (US) is noninvasive, requires no ionizing radiation, and can be performed with a portable unit. Ultrasonography is superior to other modalities in differentiating cystic from solid lesions and is highly sensitive in detecting ascites. Because of the superb ability to demonstrate gallstones (Fig. 93–5), US has replaced oral cholecystography for the diagnosis of cholelithiasis. Interest in oral cholecystography has been renewed, however, with the development of extracorporeal shock wave lithotripsy and the attending need to determine the number and size of gallstones. Ultrasound is an effective and efficient first examination of suspected liver tumors (Ch. 124). It is the primary screening examination for hepatobiliary disease

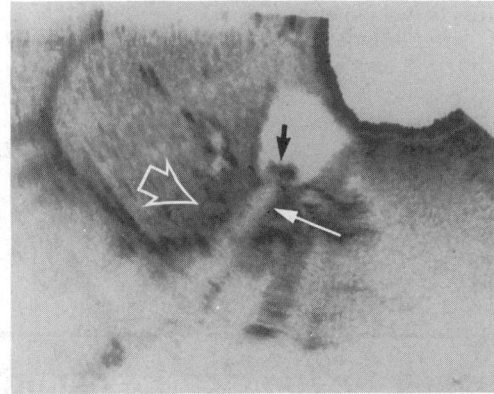

FIGURE 93–5. Ultrasound of cholelithiasis. Sagittal image (patient's head to reader's left) demonstrates a single gallstone *(black arrow)*. The sound waves easily pass through the fluid (bile) in the gallbladder—hence the "posterior acoustical enhancement" *(open arrow)* characteristic of a cystic structure. The echogenic stone impedes the sound waves—hence the "posterior shadowing" *(straight white arrow)* characteristic of a gallstone. This "static" ultrasound image produces black echoes on white background.

and often is the only study needed. Dilatation of the intra- and extrahepatic biliary system can be detected (Fig. 93–6), but the distal common bile duct often is not seen adequately with US. Similarly, the tail or body of the pancreas or both are well visualized less often than the head, principally because of interference by the overlying gas-filled bowel. Ultrasonography, which plays a complementary role with CT in many diseases, often is the preferred modality when follow-up examination is needed, as in pancreatic pseudocyst, abdominal aortic aneurysm, and drained fluid collections. Percutaneous fine needle aspiration and drainage procedures can be performed with ultrasonographic guidance with greater ease and less cost than with CT.

Recent advances in ultrasound involve the application of a transducer to an exposed organ at surgery or through an endoscope. Ultrasonography has facilitated the intraoperative search for pancreatic islet cell tumor and occasionally demonstrates unsuspected multiple tumors. Endosonography requires an endviewing fiberoptic gastroscope, which is modified to incorporate a transducer. This new imaging procedure can demonstrate the wall thickness of the esophagus, stomach, and duodenum and identify both diffuse and focal intramural lesions. It may also be valuable for the diagnosis of early pancreatic lesions. Preoperative assessment of rectal carcinoma with a high-frequency, 7.5 to 10 MHz endorectal transducer is reported to be at least as accurate as CT and magnetic resonance imaging in local staging of tumor.

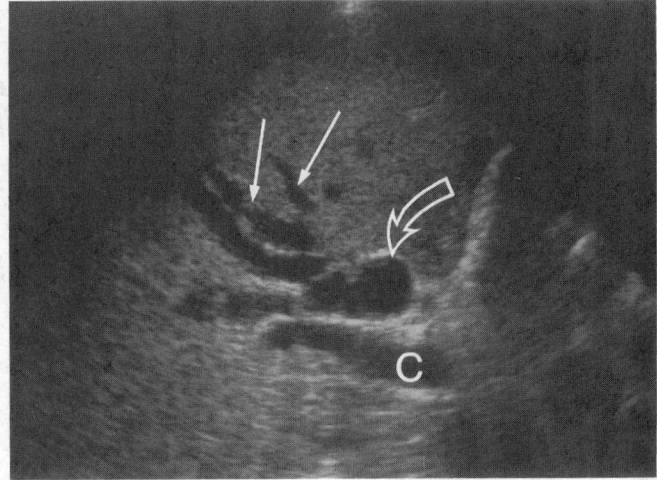

FIGURE 93–6. Ultrasound of dilated bile ducts. Dilatation of the intrahepatic *(straight arrows)* and extrahepatic *(curved arrow)* bile ducts is well demonstrated on the sagittal ultrasound image of a patient with distal biliary obstruction. (C indicates the inferior vena cava.) This realtime ultrasound image produces white echoes on black background.

Carroll BA: US of the gastrointestinal tract. Radiology 172:605, 1989. *An excellent review of the state of the art.*

Rifkin MD, Erlich MS, Marks G: Staging of rectal carcinoma: Prospective comparison of endorectal US and CT. Radiology 170:319, 1989. *Comparison of 102 consecutive patients demonstrated US to be as accurate as CT, or more so, in the preoperative staging of rectal cancer.*

ENDOSCOPIC RETROGRADE CHOLANGIOPANCREATOGRAPHY

Endoscopic retrograde cholangiopancreatography (ERCP) is performed with the fluoroscopic guidance of the radiologist. The papilla of Vater is visualized through a fiberoptic endoscope, and the common bile duct or the pancreatic duct or both are cannulated. Water-soluble iodinated contrast material is injected, and images are taken of the opacified biliary tree or pancreatic duct (Fig. 93–7). ERCP is performed specifically to evaluate the pancreatic duct or follows US or CT in demonstrating distal biliary obstruction. When a constricting or obstructing lesion is seen in the distal common bile duct, biopsy or papillotomy can be performed. A further discussion of ERCP is contained in Ch. 106.

TRANSHEPATIC CHOLANGIOGRAPHY

Percutaneous transhepatic cholangiography is used to visualize the intra- and extrahepatic biliary tree following CT, US, or ERCP that has demonstrated proximal obstruction of the common hepatic or common bile duct. It is performed by injecting water-soluble iodinated contrast material through a flexible 23-gauge

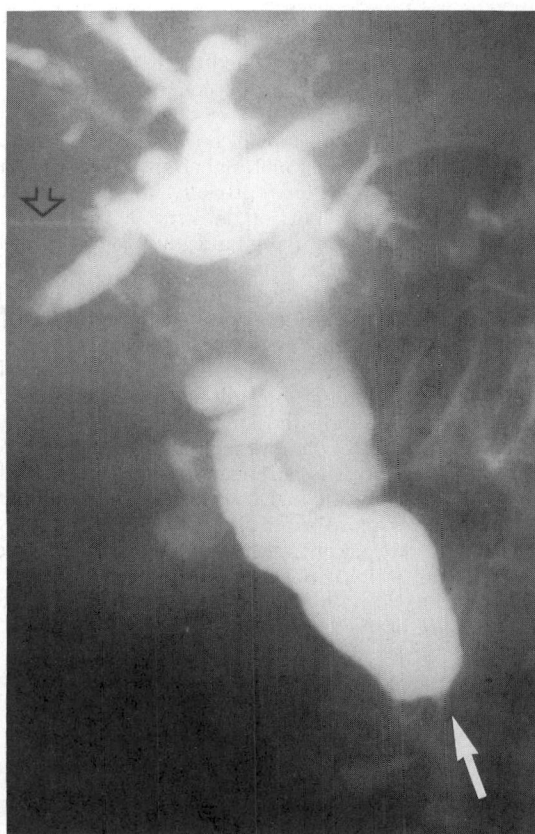

FIGURE 93–8. Percutaneous transhepatic cholangiogram. Dilatation of the biliary tree is demonstrated after percutaneous puncture and opacification of a dilated intrahepatic duct with a long 23-gauge needle *(open black arrow)*. The distal common bile duct is abruptly narrowed and obstructed *(white arrow)* owing to cholangiocarcinoma.

needle introduced percutaneously into the intrahepatic biliary tree under fluoroscopic guidance. After the biliary tree is opacified, multiple radiographs are taken in order to characterize the suspected site of blockage or narrowing (Fig. 93–8). This study provides the surgeon with the best demonstration of possible anastomotic sites of the biliary tree in the porta hepatis. Serious complications such as bile peritonitis or intraperitoneal hemorrhage occur in less than 2 per cent of cases. Biliary obstruction can be treated in patients who are poor surgical risks by several interventional procedures, including percutaneous stricture dilatation, percutaneous drainage, or insertion of a biliary endoprosthesis. The last procedure can be performed percutaneously or via an ERCP in conjunction with a percutaneous transhepatic technique.

McLean GK, Burke DR: Role of endoprostheses in the management of malignant biliary obstruction. Radiology 170:961, 1989. *State-of-the-art review of endoscopic versus percutaneous approaches to biliary drainage.*

Steinberg HV, Torres WE, Nelson RC: Gallbladder lithotripsy. Radiology 172:7, 1989. *Approach to extracorporeal shock wave lithotripsy (ESWL) described by experts in the field.*

ENTEROCLYSIS

Procedures used to study the small bowel include the "dedicated" small bowel follow-through, single- and double-contrast enteroclysis, and the peroral pneumocolon. Examination of the small bowel should not accompany most studies of the esophagus, stomach, and/or duodenum because the high-density barium used for the latter interferes with visualization of detail of the small bowel, especially the jejunum. Consequently, lesions that are present may be seen poorly or may be missed, and often it is nearly impossible to exclude abnormality. Hence, the traditional "upper gastrointestinal series with small bowel follow-through" is no longer the examination for small intestinal disease. An exception to this is the patient in whom the terminal ileum is the only suspected site of involvement. In this case, the peroral

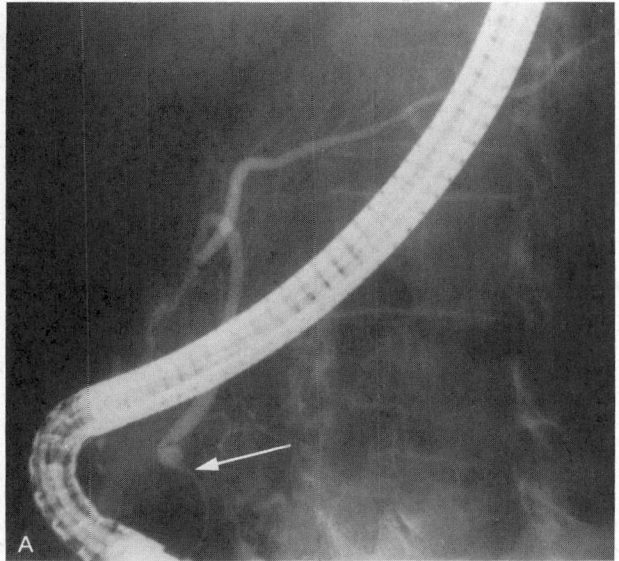

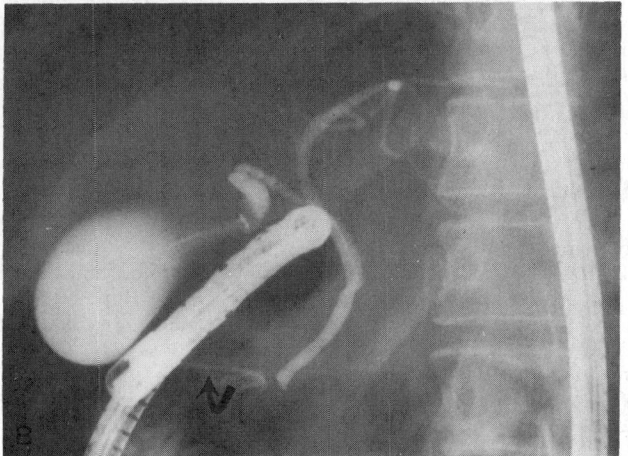

FIGURE 93–7. Normal endoscopic retrograde cholangiopancreatogram. *A,* Normal pancreatogram. The cannula *(arrow)* at the tip of the fiberoptic endoscope has been inserted into the papilla of Vater under direct visualization and the pancreatic duct opacified. *B,* Normal cholangiogram. The gallbladder, cystic duct, common hepatic duct, and common bile duct are visible. *Arrow* indicates cannula in the papilla of Vater.

pneumocolon may be the most precise approach. It is performed with introduction of insufflated air per rectum when orally administered thin barium has reached the cecum. With reflux of air across the ileocecal valve, double-contrast images of the terminal ileum are obtained.

Enteroclysis, also known as small bowel enema, refers to the direct introduction of contrast material after peroral intubation of the first loop of jejunum or, less optimally, the distal duodenum. It allows for a controlled rate of delivery of contrast material independent of gastric emptying and thus optimizes luminal distention. The double-contrast method uses air or methylcellulose to provide fine detail to the folds of the small bowel. Enteroclysis has been advocated as the most accurate method for the detection of focal lesions in the small bowel. However, it is comparable to a dedicated (tubeless) small bowel study for the detection of lesions due to Crohn's disease and tumor and is only slightly more sensitive for adhesions. A dedicated small bowel study does not immediately follow examination of the esophagus, stomach, or duodenum; it is performed with frequent, intermittent spot films by the radiologist. Enteroclysis, which is more lengthy and requires more expertise by the radiologist, is tolerated less well by the patient and, most importantly, involves a much greater radiation exposure. Preparation requires colon cleansing as well as 24 hours of clear liquid diet in order to clear the small bowel of particulate matter.

Dehn TCB, Nolan DJ: Enteroclysis: The diagnosis of intestinal obstruction in the early postoperative period. Gastrointest Radiol 14:15, 1989. *Demonstrates the efficacy of enteroclysis regarding this clinical problem.*

RADIONUCLIDE IMAGING

Acute cholecystitis is usually due to obstruction of the cystic duct by a calculus. Scanning with technetium-labeled iminodiacetic acid (^{99m}Tc HIDA), which is excreted by the hepatobiliary system, is valuable when such a diagnosis is in question. Visualization of the liver, bile ducts, gallbladder, and bowel occurs within 60 minutes of injection in normal, fasting patients (Fig. 93–9). Visualization of the gallbladder excludes the diagnosis of obstruction of the cystic duct. Nonvisualization of the gallbladder with normal visualization of the common bile duct and bowel indicates cystic duct obstruction (Fig. 93–10). Nonvisualization of both the gallbladder and the bowel can occur in conditions involving cholestasis without cystic duct obstruction, such as hepatocellular disease, total parenteral nutrition, and obstruction of the distal common bile duct. Ultrasonography is more sensitive regarding the detection of cholelithiasis but is less accurate in the diagnosis of acute cholecystitis.

Gastric mucosa secretes ^{99m}Tc pertechnetate. It can be used to detect ectopic gastric mucosa, especially in Meckel's diverticulum and sometimes in Barrett's esophagus. Ectopic gastric mucosa is present in most symptomatic Meckel's diverticula and in nearly all that bleed, but only half of the bleeding Meckel's diverticula in adults are detected by this study. False-positive results are common. This method of detecting Meckel's diverticulum is far more useful in children.

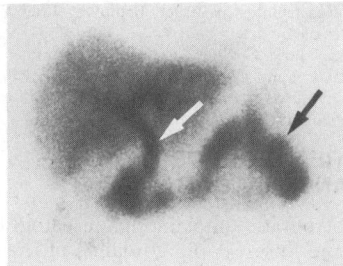

FIGURE 93–10. Tc HIDA of acute cholecystitis. Visualization of the common bile duct (*white arrow*) and small bowel (*black arrow*) without visualization of the gallbladder indicated obstruction of the cystic duct in this fasting patient with acute cholecystitis.

There are two nuclear medicine procedures available for the detection of acute and chronic gastrointestinal bleeding sites, both of which rely upon the extravasation of the radionuclide into the intestinal lumen. Injected ^{99m}Tc sulfur colloid remains in the circulation only briefly, and therefore its use requires active bleeding (approximately 2 ml per minute) at the time of the study. This disadvantage, which is shared with angiography, does not apply to ^{99m}Tc-labeled autologous erythrocytes because they remain in circulation. With the latter procedure, intermittent bleeding of 10 to 20 ml per hour may be detected on delayed views. The reliability of both procedures is greater for the colon and small bowel than for the esophagus, stomach, and duodenum because of overlapping structures in the upper abdomen. *Angiography* for gastrointestinal hemorrhage is used when the site of bleeding cannot be identified by endoscopy or radionuclide imaging or when transcatheter infusion or embolization therapy is indicated. Visceral angiography of most abdominal pathologic conditions has been replaced by other diagnostic procedures, but it is indicated still in the evaluation of vascular occlusive disease, in polysystemic vasculitis, and preoperatively for hepatic tumors.

Disorders of gastric motility are not well evaluated by barium radiographic techniques because these techniques are not quantitative, are relatively insensitive, and are not physiologic. Procedures using radiolabeled food with continuous gastric monitoring may yield quantitative data, such as gastric half-emptying time. Furthermore, with radionuclide imaging gastric emptying of solids versus liquids can be assessed simultaneously.

Liver scanning with ^{99m}Tc sulfur colloid is used for the assessment of size, shape, and position; identification of space-occupying lesions such as tumor, abscess, or hematoma; and evaluation of hepatocellular disease. Sensitivity for the detection of primary and metastatic tumor is comparable to that of CT (which is slightly more accurate) and that of US (which is slightly less sensitive). The newer technique of liver scanning with SPECT (single photon emission computed tomography) imaging produces three-dimensional cross-sectional tomographic images and eliminates the overlapping influences of the surrounding radioactivity. Thus, the sensitivity for small (2 cm) space-occupying lesions is increased.

McAtee JG, Kopecky RT, Frymoyer PA: Nuclear medicine comes of age: Its present and future roles in diagnosis. Radiology 174:609, 1990. *An overview of current uses of radionuclide imaging with an up-to-date list of references.*

MAGNETIC RESONANCE IMAGING

A very brief and simplified summary of the physics of magnetic resonance (MR) imaging is presented here as a background. Hydrogen nuclei (protons) have a dipole moment and therefore behave as would a magnetic compass. In MR scanning, the protons align with the strong magnetic field but are easily disturbed by a brief radiofrequency (rf) pulse of very low energy and then are altered in their alignment. As the protons return to their orientation with the magnetic field, they release energy of a rf that is strongly influenced by the biochemical environment. T_1 and T_2 relaxation times are a description of the released energy, which is detected, mathematically analyzed, and displayed as a two-dimensional proton-density map according to the "signal intensity" of each tissue. Because the water molecule contains two hydrogen nuclei, changes in distribution of water in tissue, as well as its overall concentration, strongly influence the "intensity" of the MR signal. Hence, MR can provide superior

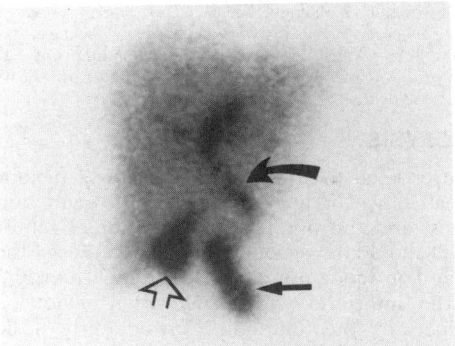

FIGURE 93–9. Normal Tc HIDA scan. Technetium-99m labeled iminodiacetic acid (HIDA) has been excreted by the liver in this normal, fasting patient. Within 60 minutes of intravenous injection, there is visualization of the common bile duct (*curved arrow*), gallbladder (*open arrow*), and duodenum (*straight arrow*).

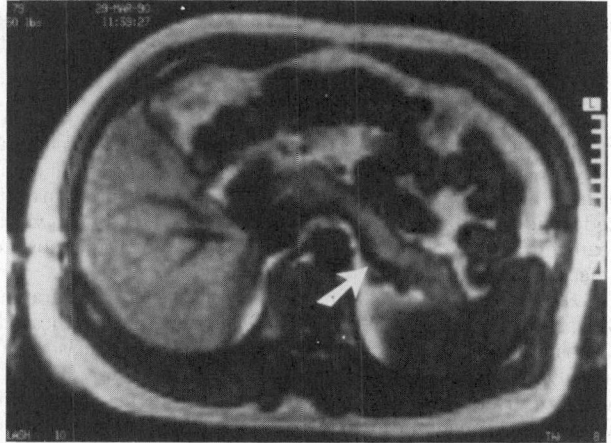

FIGURE 93–11. Normal abdominal magnetic resonance. TurboFlash (Seimens, Magnetom Imager, 1.5 Tesla) (TR = 507 msec, TE = 4 msec) transaxial image of the upper abdomen was acquired in less than 1 second. The tail of the pancreas abuts the splenic hilum and the body is seen anterior to the splenic vein *(arrow)*. Multiple segments of small bowel are seen posterior to the transverse colon.

contrast differentiation of tissues with varying amounts of water compared with conventional radiographic modalities, which depend only upon the attenuation of the roentgenographic beam. In addition, fat emits a strong signal because of the abundance of lipid protons. Other advantages of MR include its noninvasiveness, lack of ionizing radiation, and ability to image directly in transaxial, sagittal, coronal, and nonorthogonal planes. Its disadvantages include cost, limited availability, slow scanning time, and problems associated with the powerful magnetic field. The

last-named precludes imaging patients with a cardiac pacemaker or metallic clips on intracranial blood vessels. Moreover, critically ill patients cannot easily be monitored because of limited access to the patient during the study and because the strong magnetic field prohibits the presence of resuscitative equipment made of metal.

Physiologic motion limits the diagnostic capability of MR in the abdomen. With current imaging times of minutes for most scanners (as opposed to a few seconds for CT), respiration and peristalsis cause blurring and artifact, especially of pancreatic and bowel images. Several recently developed techniques have decreased the scan time to seconds and sometimes milliseconds. This makes it possible to image the pancreas (Fig. 93–11) and the mesenteric alimentary tract with MR in addition to the fixed segments as in the rectum (Fig. 93–12) and distal esophagus. Magnetic resonance imaging may have a greater sensitivity to primary and metastatic liver tumors compared with CT, US, and nuclear medicine; but whether it has greater specificity has not been established. The very long T_2 value of most cavernous hemangiomas makes it possible to noninvasively differentiate this common, incidentally noted, benign liver tumor from hepatic malignancy, either primary or metastatic. Magnetic resonance can also image blood vessels noninvasively, and as such may be useful to evaluate the patency of surgical shunts for portal hypertension. The effect of the presence of a paramagnetic substance, such as ferric iron, on the T_1 and T_2 relaxation times alters the MR signal intensity of involved tissue. Hence, MR can detect hemosiderosis and hemochromatosis (Ch. 193) and intravenously introduced ferric iron can enhance the detection of hepatic and splenic metastases. Similarly, paramagnetic substances such as gadolinium-DTPA can be used as contrast-enhancing agents. Magnetic resonance can image the gallbladder,

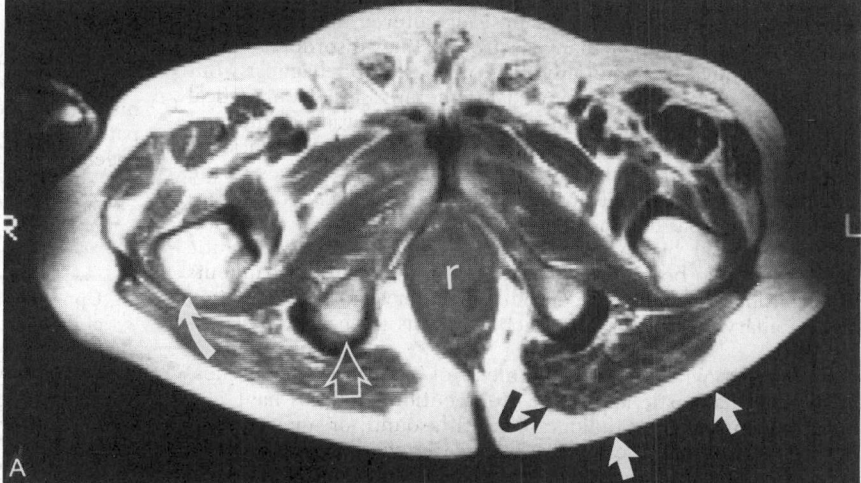

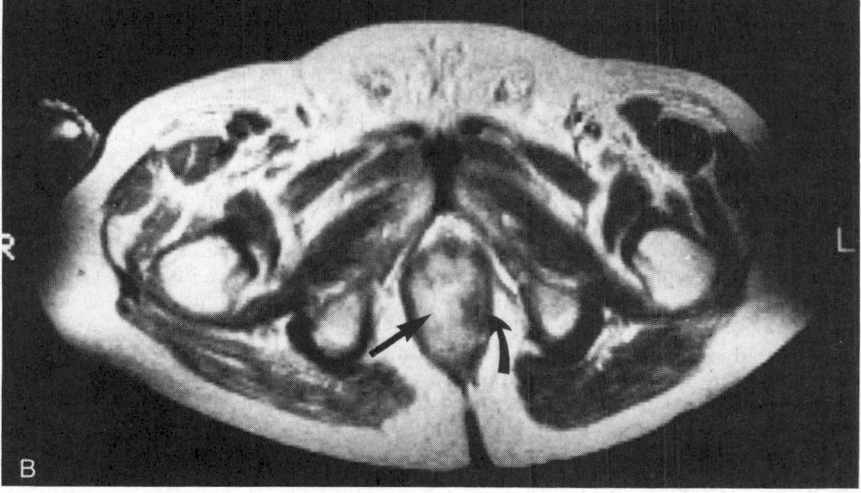

FIGURE 93–12. Magnetic resonance of rectal tumor. *A*, Transverse T_1 weighted image (TR = 0.5 sec, TE = 30 msec) demonstrates thickening of the rectum (r) due to cloacogenic carcinoma, which is isointense with the surrounding uninvolved muscle. Normal structures demonstrated include the gluteus muscle *(curved black arrow)*, which is emitting a low-intensity signal, subcutaneous fat *(white arrows)*, which is emitting a high-intensity signal, the right ischium *(open arrow)* and the right femoral head *(curved white arrow)*. *B*, T_2 weighted image of the same area demonstrates a relative increase in the signal intensity of the tumor *(straight arrow)* because of prolongation of its T_2 relaxation time. It now can be differentiated from the adjacent, noninvolved muscle *(curved arrow)*, which has retained a normal low-intensity signal.

detect cholelithiasis, and differentiate concentrated from nonconcentrated bile. With further development, it may become the procedure of choice for assessing not only morphology but also function of the gallbladder and for diagnosing acute cholecystitis.

Magnetic resonance spectroscopy (MRS) of tissue specifically localized by imaging techniques is a new procedure that is still in the research stage of development. It has not yet achieved clinical applicability in the abdomen, but early work indicates some promise of diagnostic value in the study of high-energy phosphate metabolism (^{31}P) and in imaging sodium (^{23}Na), fluorine (^{19}F), and carbon (^{13}C) Such a procedure, which would facilitate the in vivo study of the biochemistry of normal and diseased organs, is technically more demanding than proton imaging. Because of great potential clinical impact, research is progressing rapidly.

deLange EE, Fechner RE, Wanebo HJ: Suspected recurrent rectosigmoid carcinoma after abdominoperineal resection: MR imaging and histopathologic findings. Radiology 170:323, 1989. *Early work demonstrates limitations, especially regarding specificity.*

Hahn PF, Stark DD, Weissleder R, et al: Clinical application of superparamagnetic iron oxide to MR imaging of tissue perfusion in vascular liver tumors. Radiology 174:361, 1990. *Demonstrates improved diagnostic accuracy in the detection and characterization of focal liver lesions.*

Pykett IL: NMR imaging in medicine. Sci Am 246:78, 1982. *An excellent, understandable review of the physical principles of MRI.*

94 Gastrointestinal Endoscopy

Jack A. Vennes

Remarkable progress in optical engineering and in fiberoptics during the past two decades has basically altered the understanding and management of many gastrointestinal disorders. Fiberoptic techniques were initially used primarily for diagnosis, but increasingly they have been used for therapy. Excellent optical resolution and tip control permit direct visualization of mucosal abnormalities, with photographic record as desired. End-viewing instruments are adapted to visualize all mucosal surfaces of the esophagus, stomach, and duodenum or, alternatively, the entire colon. An internal channel permits routine aspiration, air insufflation, mucosal biopsy, or cytologic examination. Therapeutic devices can also be precisely directed. Side-viewing instruments are used for visualizing the ampulla of Vater and for cannulation of the biliary and pancreatic ductal systems for contrast visualization.

Coincident with the development of fiberoptic techniques, other new diagnostic and often therapeutic modalities have also been developed using radiographic, ultrasound, or nuclear scanning. The problem is often to decide, therefore, which of these diagnostic and therapeutic alternatives is best and most cost effective for patients. Proper sequencing of radiologic, ultrasonic, nuclear, and endoscopic techniques requires an understanding of relative procedural strengths by both the referring physician and the consultant. Procedural choices may also be influenced by factors of cost and available skill.

The diagnostic accuracy and therapeutic success of most procedures are dependent on operator skill and experience. Inexperience not infrequently results in increased complications—including the complication of an erroneous diagnosis. Endoscopic training programs are generally available, integrated with the disciplines of gastroenterology or colorectal or general surgery.

Endoscopy is contraindicated if a perforated viscus is suspected or if the diagnostic results are unlikely to affect management. Endoscopic procedures should be carefully discussed with patients in advance for reassurance. Procedures done by trained personnel are generally well tolerated after light parenteral sedation and analgesia. Topical pharyngeal anesthesia usually improves acceptance of upper tract endoscopy and indeed is often the only medication required for safe, minimally uncomfortable examinations with modern small-caliber endoscopes.

Discussions in this chapter focus on the clinical attributes and capacities of endoscopic procedures and only secondarily on the diseases being investigated. Disease and discovery are intertwined as usual.

ESOPHAGOGASTRODUODENOSCOPY

Endoscopic examination of the entire esophagus, stomach, and duodenum (EGD) is accomplished with routine examination to the deep descending duodenum. All mucosal surfaces are visualized, and photographic records are often made of visually recognized abnormalities. Histologic and cytologic diagnosis can be made as indicated.

INDICATIONS. Indications for diagnostic and therapeutic EGD are listed in Table 94–1. EGD is most often indicated in the evaluation or discovery of possible acid-peptic disease, malignancy, or gastrointestinal bleeding (see Color Plate 1). Endoscopy used "just in case" disease is found leads to overutilization, but management of a presumed disease without diagnostic confirmation often turns out to be underutilization. Both extremes are frequently cost *in*effective. Therapeutic use of endoscopic techniques is briefly discussed with each procedure in this chapter.

Patients frequently seek medical help for upper abdominal discomfort and associated dyspeptic symptoms of relatively recent onset. If other findings indicative of serious disease are absent, a trial of therapy may be indicated as a first diagnostic test. Most respond to a trial of therapy directed toward their presumed acid-peptic problem. EGD is therefore indicated for the perhaps 30 per cent of all patients with dyspeptic symptoms because symptoms continue despite 14 days of therapy.

Irritable bowel syndrome does not usually require endoscopy, but there are occasional exceptions. Other problems that usually do not require endoscopy include intermittent dyspepsia, heartburn responding to medical therapy, and asymptomatic or uncomplicated hiatal hernia. Uncomplicated duodenal bulb ulcer seen on radiograph that responds to therapy does not usually require endoscopy unless symptoms recur quickly.

Acid-Peptic Disease

Acid-peptic disease, i.e., reflux esophagitis, gastric ulcer, or duodenal ulcer, can be strongly suspected on the basis of the history, but one cannot confidently predict the specific site or pathologic condition. Symptoms of reflux esophagitis are quite specific, but other gastroduodenal lesions frequently coexist (Ch. 96). The presence of esophageal reflux symptoms correlates

TABLE 94–1. INDICATIONS FOR ESOPHAGOGASTRODUODENOSCOPY (EGD)

A. Upper abdominal distress that persists despite an appropriate trial of therapy
B. Upper abdominal distress associated with signs suggesting serious organic disease (e.g., anorexia and weight loss)
C. Dysphagia or odynophagia
D. Esophageal reflux symptoms that are persistent or progressive despite appropriate therapy
E. Persistent vomiting of unknown cause
F. Other system disease in which the presence of upper gastrointestinal pathologic conditions might modify other planned management; examples include patients with a history of gastrointestinal bleeding who are scheduled for renal transplantation, long-term anticoagulation, and chronic nonsteroidal therapy for arthritis
G. Radiographic findings of:
  1. A neoplastic lesion, for confirmation and specific histologic diagnosis
  2. Gastric or esophageal ulcer
  3. Evidence of upper tract stricture or obstruction
  4. Mass
H. Gastrointestinal bleeding:
  1. As the first procedure in most actively bleeding patients
  2. When surgical therapy is contemplated
  3. When rebleeding occurs after acute, self-limited blood loss
  4. When portal hypertension or aortoenteric fistula is suspected
  5. For endoscopic therapy of upper gastrointestinal bleeding
  6. For presumed chronic blood loss and iron deficiency anemia when colonoscopy findings are negative

Modified from Appropriate Use of Gastrointestinal Endoscopy. American Society for Gastrointestinal Endoscopy, 1989.

well with the presence of endoscopic findings and less well with histologic findings. Local symptoms in the mid or lower esophagus are usually predictive of disease location, whereas high substernal symptoms may be due to disease anywhere in the esophagus. Gastric or duodenal ulcers are usually symptomatic, but in patients with previous gastric or duodenal ulcer, asymptomatic recurrences are discovered in 5 per cent or more of patients who have had endoscopy in long-term studies.

EGD is more sensitive and specific than radiographic studies in evaluating disease of the upper gastrointestinal tract, although neither is infallible. Radiographic studies are least sensitive in evaluating lesions without apparent depth, such as flat stomal postgastrectomy ulcers, giant duodenal ulcers involving an entire wall of the duodenal bulb, or erosive esophagitis.

Cancer

Malignant lesions of the upper gastrointestinal tract are generally evident as exophytic masses protruding into the lumen (Ch. 99). Flat, infiltrative lesions do occur occasionally, however. In the esophagus, such lesions may resemble a benign stricture, and in the stomach (linitis plastica), the primary features are stiffness and poor distensibility. Malignancy may occasionally present as ulceration; accurate evaluation of all esophageal and gastric ulcers is therefore mandatory and challenging. At least 75 per cent of malignant ulcers are correctly identified by endoscopic visual criteria, as asymmetric folds or nodules that randomly form the crater rim and extend irregularly into surrounding mucosa. Malignant tissue is often seen as multihued. Benign ulcers are typically smoother with more crater depth and with more symmetry and less randomness, and a zone of erythema is present at the junction of the crater and rim.

Histologic and cytologic data should be added to the endoscopic evaluation of all suspicious lesions and most gastric ulcers. This results in a sensitivity (positive when disease is present) and specificity (negative when disease is absent) of 95 per cent. Brush or lavage cytology is a particularly important adjunct in evaluating the smooth, infiltrative esophageal stricture or the linitis plastica gastric lesion or the occasional superficial, spreading, flat gastric cancer. Primary gastric lymphoma may present as an ulcer, ulcerated mass, or large, asymmetric folds. Specific histologic features are frequently present only in submucosal tissue.

Mucosal polyps are rare in the stomach and rarer still in the duodenum and esophagus. Submucosal or intramucosal polypoid defects overlain with normal mucosa are usually pancreatic rests or leiomyomas and can be left in place. Adenomatous polyps have premalignant potential, which increases with size. All polypoid lesions should be endoscopically visualized, with biopsy or removal with snare cautery. Multiple small, hyperplastic polyps are not premalignant and need not all be removed, and no surveillance is indicated. Adenomas should be excised endoscopically when feasible. Very large lesions may require surgical removal. Surveillance is indicated after removal of gastric adenomatous polyps.

Other upper gastrointestinal malignancies originating in the pancreas or biliary tree do not usually extend into gastric or duodenal mucosa, and they require other diagnostic studies (see below). Ampullary carcinoma is usually visible *if* the papilla of Vater is adequately seen via a conventional end-viewing endoscope or a side-viewing instrument (see below).

Upper Gastrointestinal Bleeding (see Ch. 111)

EGD is the most informative procedure when further information is indicated for management of the acutely bleeding patient, particularly if done within 12 hours of admission. Information obtained includes (1) location and identity of the bleeding source; (2) whether bleeding is continuing; (3) whether bleeding is arterial; (4) which of multiple lesions is bleeding; and (5) whether a visible vessel is present in an ulcer base. These endoscopic observations are available in 85 per cent of patients with acute bleeding and influence prognosis and management decisions. There is no evidence that endoscopy initiates further bleeding. A precise diagnosis of the status and source of gastrointestinal bleeding is requisite for successful management. Endoscopic methods for controlling active bleeding are often effective. When indications for these techniques become clearer, more

early endoscopy of acute bleeding will likely be indicated (see below).

The source of chronic gastrointestinal blood loss or iron deficiency anemia in men is usually discovered in the colon. EGD may be indicated by history suggesting upper tract sources or after negative findings on colonoscopy in patients with chronic blood loss.

Therapeutic Applications of Esophagogastroduodenoscopy

Therapeutic endoscopic procedures commonly carried out in the upper gastrointestinal tract include removal of foreign bodies, dilation of benign or malignant esophageal strictures, sclerotherapy of bleeding esophageal varices, placement of percutaneous gastrostomies, and electrocoagulation of focal bleeding lesions. Foreign bodies in the esophagus or stomach can usually be removed by techniques that employ snares or forceps as grasping devices. Protective overtubes may be used to prevent soft tissue injury or aspiration. Impaction of food may occur because of an underlying esophageal abnormality, and careful esophagoscopy after removal of food may reveal a benign or malignant stricture or may suggest a motility disorder.

Esophageal strictures found to be benign on careful evaluation can be successfully dilated. If the course of the esophagus is tortuous, if the stricture is tight and does not admit the endoscope, or if epiphrenic diverticula are present, dilation is safely done over a guide wire passed under fluoroscopic control. Tapered bougies, metal olives, or inflatable balloons of progressively increasing diameter may be passed over the wire. Following this, endoscopy and biopsy are done to assess whether there is a malignant lesion. Less complex strictures that only partially occlude the lumen may, after endoscopy, be safely dilated with tapered bougies without wire guidance and without further endoscopy. A maintenance dilation schedule with individualized intervals is important. Dilation intervals can often be lengthened as stricture inflammation subsides.

Management of malignant esophageal strictures is directed to the goal of reducing tumor mass and allowing the unobstructed passage of food, liquids, and oral secretions. The options available include surgery, radiation therapy, or such endoscopic procedures as repeated esophageal dilation, dilation and endoscopic placement of a stent across the malignant narrowing (or across a tracheoesophageal fistula), or use of laser energy to restore the lumen by tumor destruction. All of these latter procedures have good reported results; all require skill for success and safety, and all can be done without prolonged hospitalization. Local skills are often valid determinants. Quality survival time is usually brief, but 85 to 90 per cent of patients can be helped, with a complication rate of about 5 per cent.

Several endoscopic measures have proved effective in controlling upper gastrointestinal bleeding. Endoscopic variceal sclerosis by intravariceal and perivariceal injection of various sclerosants controls the acute variceal hemorrhage of portal hypertension in 90 per cent of patients. Prophylactic sclerosis may also prevent future hemorrhage. Endoscopic variceal sclerosis reduces the risk of rebleeding, with fewer hospital days and transfusions, but survival is not significantly prolonged.

Focal nonvariceal bleeding can often be controlled using electrocoagulation with monopolar or bipolar current delivery or combined electrocoagulation and thermal heater probe techniques or laser photocoagulation. Neodymium yttrium aluminum garnet (YAG) laser energy is carried through the endoscope via a flexible wave guide and converted to thermal energy when precisely directed to an absorptive (bleeding) area. Bleeding is controlled in up to 90 per cent of lesions, including those with brisk arterial bleeding, but rebleeding rates are significant with all methods. Laser equipment is expensive and not portable. Perforation, although of low risk, is a definite hazard with all techniques.

Diagnostic endoscopy is urgently indicated if one or more of several clinical risk factors are present: a large volume bleed as evidenced by orthostasis, copious hematemesis, and need for transfusions. Urgent endoscopy is also indicated if portal hypertension and variceal bleeding are suspected with an active rebleed in the hospital or if there is a history of previous aortic aneurysm repair. Endoscopic observations include the site of bleeding and whether bleeding persists.

Eighty-five per cent or more of upper gastrointestinal bleeding episodes stop spontaneously; how then do we select those patients who need endoscopic control of bleeding? A pigmented, elevated visible vessel in the ulcer base, a fresh adherent clot, or continuing active bleeding are all observable risk factors for further bleeding and are indications for endoscopic therapy, most frequently with electrocoagulation or heater probe techniques. Surgery or angiographic occlusion of bleeding vessels is required for some whose bleeding is unusually brisk.

Percutaneous endoscopic gastrostomy (PEG) is a useful method for providing selected patients with long-term enteral feeding. Candidates are those with a functioning gut and chronically inadequate oral intake. Some may have recurrent aspiration secondary to upper esophageal dysfunction. Specific indications include neurologic disorders that affect the swallowing mechanism or that result in diminished food intake secondary to a decreased sensorium, or cancer of the pharynx or upper esophagus that does not totally obstruct (so that an endoscope can be passed). Percutaneous endoscopic gastrostomy is not indicated in postgastrectomy patients or in those with midline abdominal scar, severe, uncorrectable coagulopathy, or respirator dependency. The decision to initiate chronic enteral feeding can be a difficult one, involving the wishes of patient and family and the gravity of the underlying disease. Once the decision is made, however, PEG is a simple and safe method.

COMPLICATIONS. Complications from EGD are rare with modern small-caliber, flexible instruments but do occur. A morbidity of 0.13 per cent and a mortality of 0.0004 per cent have been reported. During or following endoscopic examination, perforation has occurred in the upper esophagus near the cricopharyngeus, through Zenker's diverticula, and through areas of tumor. Use of sedative or analgesic drugs may transiently suppress respiration, especially in elderly patients or those with severe obstructive pulmonary disease. Aspiration during endoscopy is very unlikely unless there is vomiting due to massive bleeding or gastric outlet obstruction. Cardiovascular complications, sepsis, prolonged bleeding, or thrombophlebitis from intravenous medications occur rarely.

COLONOSCOPY AND FLEXIBLE SIGMOIDOSCOPY

The entire colon is now routinely accessible to high-resolution viewing with biopsy, brush cytology, polypectomy, and photography of observed lesions. Much has been learned of the polyp-cancer progression, and significant control of colon cancer is within cost-effective reach of the trained endoscopist.

INDICATIONS. The indications for colonoscopy are listed in Table 94–2. As with EGD, colonoscopic examination is primarily used to evaluate possible cancer, inflammation, and bleeding. The procedure is contraindicated in the presence of fulminant colitis; acute, severe diverticulitis; or probable perforated viscus. Colonoscopy is generally not indicated for stable irritable bowel syndrome, acute diarrhea, upper gastrointestinal bleeding, or rectal bleeding with an anorectal source on anoscopy or sigmoidoscopy. Other nonindications include routine follow-up of inflammatory bowel disease (except as noted in Table 94–2) and routine preoperative examination of patients undergoing elective abdominal surgery for noncolonic disease.

Flexible fiberoptic sigmoidoscopy (FFS) is usually carried out with 60-cm instrumentation, although a 35-cm endoscope is available. Training requirements are less rigorous than those for colonoscopy. Indications for FFS are listed in Table 94–3. At least 60 per cent of colon cancers and potential colon cancers (neoplastic polyps) are located in the rectosigmoid and lower descending colon and thus are in reach of the "screening" FFS. FFS has the same contraindications as colonoscopy and is generally not indicated when colonoscopy is indicated (see Table 94–3). FFS is specifically not indicated for polypectomy because colonoscopy is needed, and full colonic preparation is necessary to prevent possible explosions during electrocautery. Preparation for FFS is simple, using two enemas, whereas preparation for colonoscopy requires a two-day liquid diet preparation or total

TABLE 94–2. INDICATIONS FOR COLONOSCOPY

A. Evaluation of an abnormality on barium enema that is likely to be clinically significant, such as a filling defect or stricture
B. For discovery and excision of colonic polyps:
  1. When polyps are seen on barium enema radiograph
  2. When neoplastic polyps are detected by proctosigmoidoscopy
C. Evaluation of unexplained gastrointestinal bleeding:
  1. Clinically significant hematochezia
  2. Melena with a negative upper gastrointestinal workup
  3. Presence of unexplained fecal occult blood
D. Unexplained iron deficiency anemia
E. Surveillance for colonic neoplasia
  1. Examination to "clear" entire colon of synchronous cancer or neoplastic polyps in a patient with a treatable cancer or neoplastic polyp
  2. Follow-up examination at two- to three-year intervals after resection of a colorectal cancer or neoplastic polyp and an adequate initial "clearing" colonoscopy
  3. Patients with a strongly positive family history of colonic cancer
  4. In patients with chronic ulcerative colitis: colonoscopy every one to two years with multiple biopsies for detection of cancer and dysplasia in patients with:
    a. Pancolitis of greater than seven years' duration
    b. Left-sided colitis of over 15 years' duration (no surveillance needed for disease limited to rectosigmoid)
F. Chronic inflammatory bowel disease of the colon if more precise diagnosis or determination of the extent of activity of disease will influence immediate management
G. Therapeutic colonoscopy, as control of bleeding or colonic decompression

Modified from Appropriate Use of Gastrointestinal Endoscopy. American Society for Gastrointestinal Endoscopy, 1989.

gut lavage with large volumes of an isotonic solution. The place for FFS is assured as a more comfortable, more informative replacement for rigid proctosigmoidoscopy at nearly equivalent cost.

Polyps and Cancer of the Colon (see Ch. 105)

Colonoscopy to evaluate the possibility of colon cancer or its precursor polyps is usually indicated after an abnormality is detected by barium enema or proctosigmoidoscopy or if there is unexplained lower gastrointestinal bleeding. If occult blood is detected in the interior of a passed stool, colonoscopy will identify an age-related 20 to 30 per cent incidence of adenomatous polyps and 8 to 15 per cent incidence of cancers. During active bleeding, colonoscopy may present technical difficulties in accurately locating the bleeding source. Repeat colonoscopy may be necessary after cessation of bleeding for accurate colonic assessment.

After endoscopic removal of neoplastic polyps or after resection of colon cancer, continued surveillance is indicated, since the patient is now identified as being at risk for later colon cancer. A "clearing" examination may be optionally done once within 12 months to be certain no polyps or cancers were missed at the first examination. Thereafter, follow-up examination every 3 years will detect new lesions before they become infiltrating carcinomas, since the process from polyp inception to infiltrating cancer appears to take up to 7 years. The only way to rule out cancer within a polyp is to remove it completely for histologic examination. Other conditions associated with increased risk for cancer also require surveillance (Table 94–2).

Most colonic polyps are hyperplastic and are not premalignant. In neoplastic polyps, cancer risk increases with increasing dysplasia and villoglandular transformation and also with size. Pedunculated polyps with an uninvolved stalk and with cancer confined to the mucosa can be cured by snare cautery removal.

TABLE 94–3. INDICATIONS FOR FLEXIBLE FIBEROPTIC SIGMOIDOSCOPY (FFS)

A. Screening of asymptomatic patients at risk for colonic neoplasia
B. Evaluation of suspected distal colonic disease when there is no indication for colonoscopy
C. Evaluation of the entire colon in conjunction with barium enema radiographs

Modified from Appropriate Use of Gastrointestinal Endoscopy. American Society for Gastrointestinal Endoscopy, 1989.

Most colonoscopists remove all polyps greater than 5 mm in diameter. Polyps less than 5 mm may be neoplastic; coagulation or a coagulation biopsy technique during colonoscopy is used to remove them.

Inflammatory Bowel Disease (see Ch. 103)

Most patients with inflammatory bowel disease do not require colonoscopy for diagnosis. At times, however, colonoscopy may provide unique and important information. Differentiation between granulomatous colitis (Crohn's disease) and ulcerative colitis is usually possible with colonoscopy and multiple biopsies. The anatomic extent of disease can be determined. The presence or absence of inflammatory bowel disease can be determined more accurately when clinically suspected despite absence of radiographic or sigmoidoscopic findings.

Diagnostic colonoscopy in ulcerative colitis is at times necessary to evaluate a stricture or a mass seen on barium enema. Occasionally, strictures are malignant with submucosal tumor spread. Pseudopolyps are not premalignant and need not be histologically examined. Polyps may be neoplastic or malignant, however, and those that are larger than 1 cm in diameter and are friable and irregular in color or configuration should be biopsied. In surveillance examinations of patients with ulcerative colitis, multiple biopsies are obtained throughout the involved colon. When moderate to severe dysplasia is consistently found, colectomy is usually recommended.

Polypectomy is the main therapeutic use of colonoscopy. Endoscopic control of bleeding is not usually feasible. Electrocautery of angiodysplastic lesions in the cecum and ascending colon has been successful, but new lesions may appear within months. Dilation of anastomotic strictures by balloons passed over a guide wire or through the endoscope is occasionally useful.

COMPLICATIONS. Diagnostic colonoscopy has a complication rate of 0.5 per cent, which rises to 1 per cent when polypectomy is added, with hemorrhage and perforation being the principal complications.

ENDOSCOPIC RETROGRADE CHOLANGIOPANCREATOGRAPHY (ERCP)

The side-viewing endoscope and the technique for identifying and cannulating the ampulla of Vater result in diagnostic quality radiographic study of both the common bile duct and the pancreatic duct in 90 per cent of attempts (Fig. 93–7). Failure may result from anatomic distortions due to prior surgery, tumor infiltration, or the duodenal edema of acute pancreatitis.

INDICATIONS. Indications for ERCP are listed in Table 94–4. Endoscopic retrograde cholangiopancreatography is generally not helpful in evaluating abdominal pain of obscure origin in the absence of objective findings suggesting pancreatic or biliary disease. Known or suspected gallbladder disease is not an indication for ERCP in the absence of evidence for bile duct involvement. Study of patients with acute pancreatitis is usually deferred until a second episode has established its recurrent nature, unless there is evidence to suggest gallstone disease.

TABLE 94–4. INDICATIONS FOR ENDOSCOPIC RETROGRADE CHOLANGIOPANCREATOGRAPHY (ERCP)

A. Evaluation of the jaundiced patient suspected of having treatable biliary obstruction

B. Evaluation of the patient without jaundice (with or without prior cholecystectomy) whose clinical presentation suggests bile duct disease

C. Therapeutic pancreatic or biliary endoscopy, e.g., endoscopic sphincterotomy, balloon dilatation of strictures, stent placement across strictures; these procedures frequently require follow-up endoscopy

D. Evaluation of signs or symptoms suggesting pancreatic malignancy when results of ultrasound (US) and/or computed tomography (CT) are equivocal or normal

E. Evaluation of recurrent or persistent pancreatitis of unknown etiology

F. Preoperative evaluation of the patient with chronic pancreatitis

G. Evaluation of possible pancreatic pseudocyst undetected by CT or US and for known pseudocyst prior to planned surgical therapy

Modified from Appropriate Use of Gastrointestinal Endoscopy. American Society for Gastrointestinal Endoscopy, 1989.

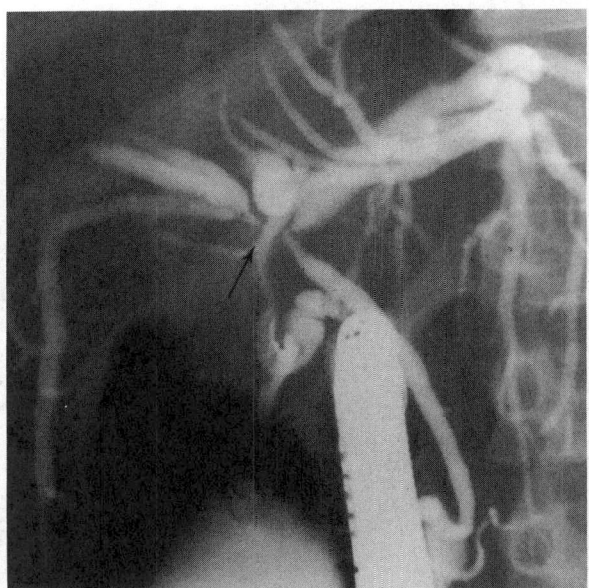

FIGURE 94–1. Retrograde cholangiogram: bile duct cancer. Multiple strictures at the bifurcation of the common hepatic duct (*arrow*) are due to a primary bile duct cancer (Klatskin tumor). Intrahepatic ducts are dilated and partially obstructed. The extrahepatic ductal system distal to the tumor is of normal caliber, here seen coursing medial to the endoscope.

Pancreatic malignancy clearly demonstrated on CT or ultrasonography need not be further evaluated with ERCP except for stent placement.

Other tests besides ERCP provide diagnostic evidence of pancreatic and biliary disease: percutaneous transhepatic cholangiography (PTC), computed tomography (CT), and ultrasonography (US). Transabdominal fine-needle aspiration cytology with CT, US, or ERCP guidance is also helpful, as malignant cells are found by this means in 85 per cent of patients with pancreatic cancer.

In evaluating suspected biliary obstruction, a cholangiogram is usually obtained prior to therapy (Fig. 94–1). When the patient has fever, pain, and icterus, choledocholithiasis is suspected with high clinical accuracy. One may then proceed directly to cholangiography by PTC or preferably by ERCP if endoscopic sphincterotomy is planned. Ultrasonography is usually performed to assess ductal dilatation, but this is of limited value, as calculi often reside in undilated ducts.

When the presence of extrahepatic obstruction and its etiology are less certain, US as the initial study provides useful information at reasonable cost. For example, a normal gallbladder without calculi makes choledocholithiasis unlikely. Masses in the pancreas, bile duct, or porta hepatis, diffuse pancreatic enlargement, or grossly dilated bile ducts direct an appropriate specific disease evaluation.

Ultrasonography and CT have improved greatly in their ability to detect pancreatic malignancy (Ch. 107). Equivocal results at times require confirmation by ERCP. Cut-off or stenosis of pancreatic duct and often of bile duct (double duct sign) is a reliable ERCP finding of carcinoma (Fig. 94–2). Patients with chronic pain and suspected chronic pancreatitis who are surgical candidates should have preoperative pancreatography and cholangiography to assess patency of the main pancreatic duct and to assess possible stricture of the intrapancreatic bile duct. Differentiating chronic pancreatitis from pancreatic cancer may be impossible, as the pancreatic duct is often dilated and tortuous with dilated, stubby lateral branches in both diseases (Fig. 94–3). Downstream ductal stricturing in the pancreatic head is the hallmark of malignancy, however.

Therapeutic Applications of Endoscopic Retrograde Cholangiopancreatography

In endoscopic retrograde sphincterotomy (ERS), soft tissues and sphincter fibers of the papilla and intraduodenal portion of

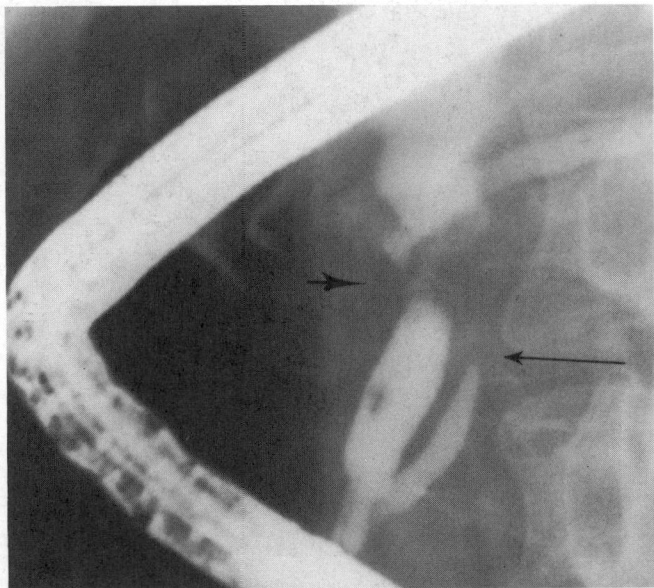

FIGURE 94–2. Pancreatogram and cholangiogram: pancreatic cancer. Both ducts are outlined by retrograde instillation of contrast at the bottom of the picture. Both the common bile duct (*large arrow*) and the pancreatic duct (*small arrow*) are strictured in the classic "double duct sign" of pancreatic cancer.

the common bile duct are divided with electrocautery to relieve ductal obstruction due to common duct stones or papillary stenosis. Endoscopic retrograde sphincterotomy has assumed a major role in the management of choledocholithiasis and offers a relatively safe and simple alternative to surgical management.

Biliary calculus obstruction is relieved by ERS in 85 to 90 per cent of attempts. Complications of hemorrhage, pancreatitis, perforation, and cholangitis occur in 3 to 8 per cent of cases with a mortality rate of 0.4 per cent. Late complications of re-stenosis or re-formed stones occur in 1 to 8 per cent of patients.

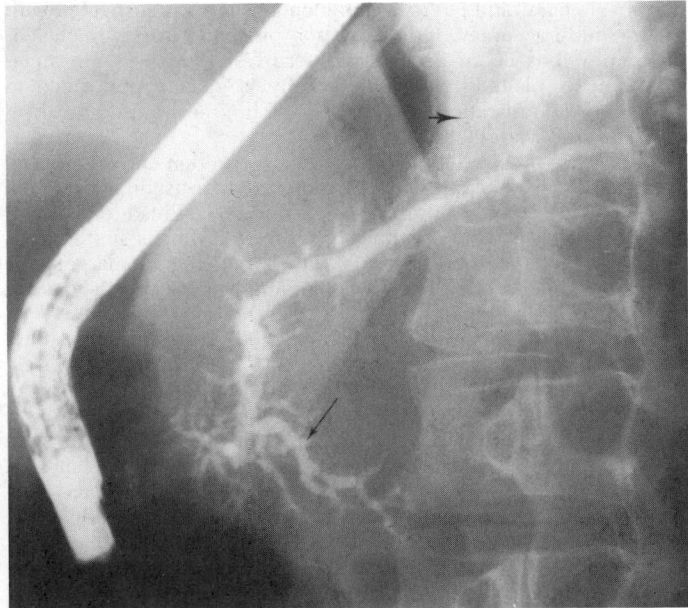

FIGURE 94–3. Pancreatogram: chronic pancreatitis. The main pancreatic duct is moderately dilated and unobstructed. The lateral branches are dilated, tortuous, and stubby. The duct from the uncinate process is prominent (*small arrow*). A small pseudocyst (*large arrow*) is barely visible overlying the spine in this oblique view. Filling defects in the main pancreatic duct may be calculi or air bubble artifact. With progression of the disease the main pancreatic duct may become more tortuous and dilated.

Endoscopic retrograde sphincterotomy is now widely considered the therapy of choice for patients with symptomatic stones in the common bile duct. The procedure is often carried out immediately following ERCP as soon as the presence of stones in the duct is confirmed. It is clearly safer and cheaper than surgery in these generally elderly patients and more successful than percutaneous transhepatic extraction. Cholangitis and gallstone pancreatitis usually respond dramatically to decompression. About 40 per cent of patients with symptomatic choledocholithiasis have never had cholecystitis, and therefore their gallbladders are intact. Almost all contain calculi. After removing duct calculi with ERS, should the gallbladder be electively removed to preclude further cholecystitis or migration of stones into the now open biliary tree? Or may the gallbladder be left in place and removed only as future symptoms dictate? Experience with patients at high surgical risk suggests the safety and success of waiting, as the probability of cholecystitis does not exceed 5 per cent per year in these generally elderly patients.

Papillary stenosis is a poorly defined disorder or group of disorders in which recurrent biliary colic or occasionally pancreatitis is thought to result from papillary fibrosis or sphincter dysfunction. Diagnostic criteria include a dilated bile duct, slow ductal drainage, cholestasis following painful episodes, and elevated basal sphincter of Oddi pressure during manometry. The problem arises most commonly in women who have had a cholecystectomy either for cholelithiasis or for biliary colic-like pain without stones. Endoscopic retrograde sphincterotomy is often curative for carefully selected patients with papillary stenosis.

Placement of plastic stents across biliary strictures is the second major therapeutic extension of ERCP. Most strictures are caused by inoperable pancreatic or bile duct carcinoma, and other treatment options are surgical or transhepatic decompression. A catheter containing a guide wire is introduced via the endoscope through the stricture, and a stent is passed over the catheter. The distal end is left in the duodenum, bile drainage is restored, and barbed flaps prevent dislodgment of the stent. The procedure is successful in 90 per cent of attempts. Present-day stents remain patent for 5 months or more and can be rather easily replaced.

COMPLICATIONS. In 1 per cent of patients, acute pancreatitis follows ERCP, usually beginning within 2 hours of the procedure as a clinically mild complication. Biliary sepsis occurs less commonly but is more serious and even life threatening. Introduction of even a few bacteria into a semiclosed space—bile duct, gallbladder, pancreatic pseudocyst—may occasionally have serious septic consequences. Organisms may be introduced from the unsterile gastrointestinal tract or from instruments. Stringent cleaning and disinfection techniques are mandatory, including periodic cultures of equipment. Sepsis is prevented by prompt surgical, endoscopic, or transhepatic decompression of discovered obstruction within 24 hours of ERCP, plus judicious use of appropriate parenteral antibiotics.

LAPAROSCOPY

Laparoscopy permits direct inspection of much of the anterior abdominal space. A pneumoperitoneum is created and a rigid or flexible laparoscope is introduced through a puncture in the abdominal wall, with the patient under local anesthesia and mild sedation. The procedure is well tolerated; complications of bleeding or bowel perforation occur in only 0.1 to 0.2 per cent. When it is clinically important to assess focal or diffuse liver disease, laparoscopy, by combining assessment of gross appearance and guided biopsy, is 90 per cent accurate, substantially better than percutaneous blind liver biopsy. This is true whether the disease is diffuse (cirrhosis) or focal (metastatic nodules). More than two thirds of the liver and variable parts of the gallbladder, spleen, peritoneum, and diaphragm can usually be visualized. The colon and small bowel are variably open to inspection.

The major indications for laparoscopy are (1) inspection and guided biopsy of the liver in suspected diffuse or focal disease, when the information will affect therapy and (2) evaluation of exudative ascites (malignancy versus inflammation). Determination of the presence or absence of abdominal metastases may be important in assessing operability. The procedure is contraindicated in the presence of acute peritonitis, intestinal obstruction, severe coagulopathy, infection of the abdominal wall, or severe

PLATE 1   GASTROINTESTINAL DISEASES

Endoscopy and colonoscopy in gastrointestinal hemorrhage.

A, Esophageal varices. Large serpiginous dilated submucosal veins *(arrows)* are noted coursing longitudinally down the distal esophagus.

B, Gastric varices. The endoscope has been turned around on itself to examine the gastric cardia, where large submucosal masses are seen projecting into the lumen *(arrows)*.

C, Duodenal bulbar ulcer. A white excavated base is noted just inside the pylorus *(large arrows)* containing a dark red central artery oozing blood *(small arrow)*.

D, Esophagitis. The normal pink esophageal mucosa is replaced by white exudate overlying extensive superficial erosions in a patient with reflux esophagitis.

E, Colonic cancer. Nearly all the lumen is obstructed by a fungating, bleeding colonic malignancy.

F, Vascular ectasia of the cecum. The normal delicate branching mucosal vessels are altered by a "coral reef" *(arrow)* telangiectatic lesion in an elderly patient with recurrent bouts of hematochezia.

G, Diverticulum of colon. Clotted blood can be seen within an outpouching of the colonic wall *(arrow)* in a patient with massive hematochezia.

H, Colonic polyp. An irregular fleshy mass on a pedicle *(arrow)* is noted projecting into the bowel lumen. Polypectomy subsequently removed and retrieved an adenomatous polyp.

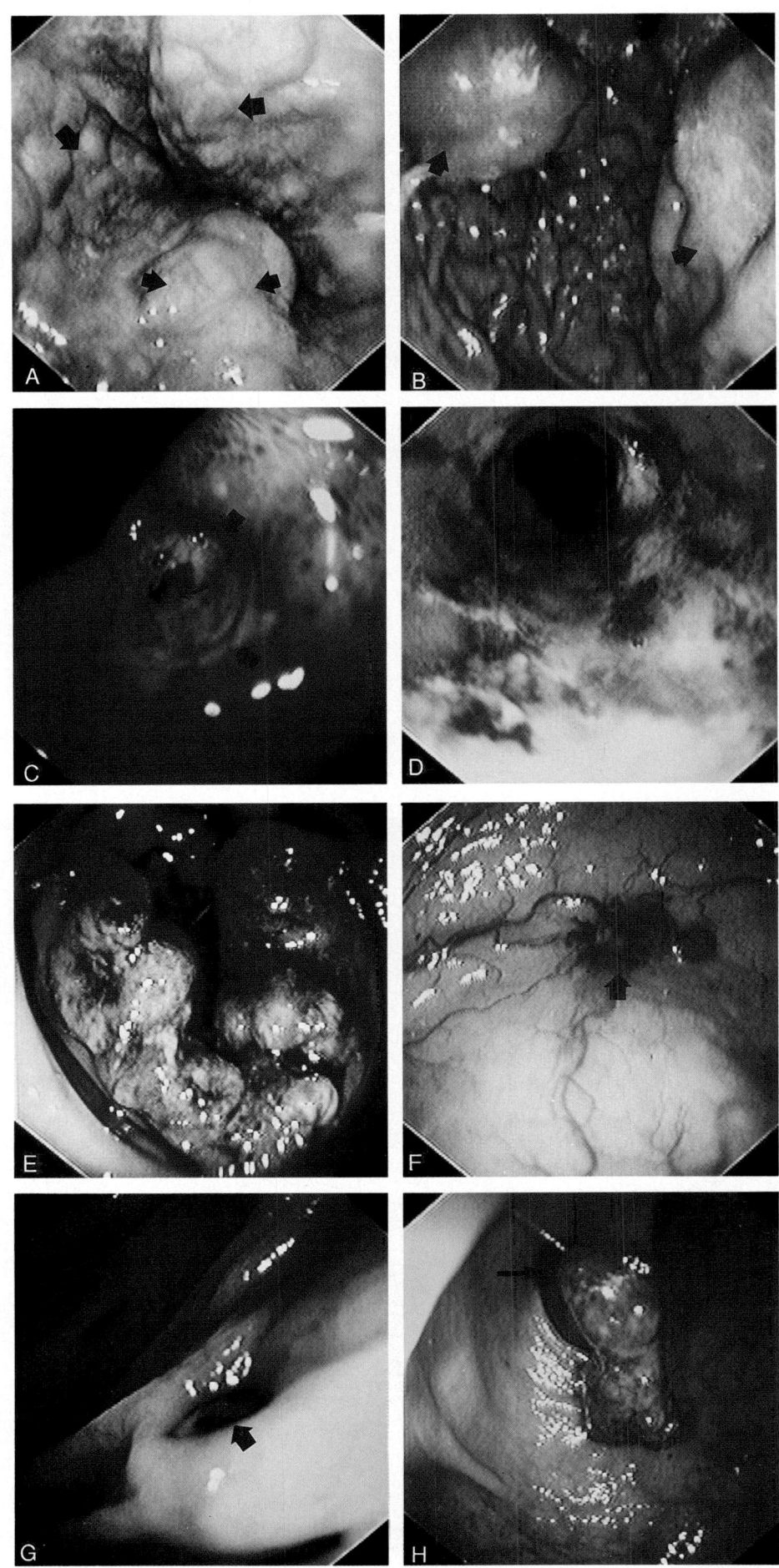

PLATE 2   GASTROINTESTINAL DISEASES

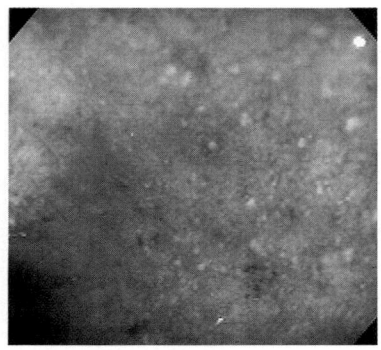

A, Mild ulcerative colitis seen on endoscopy. Granular-appearing mucosa with friability and pinpoint ulceration.

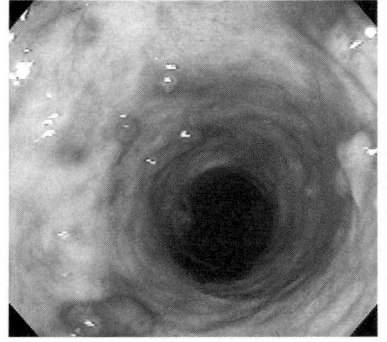

B, Quiescent ulcerative colitis seen on endoscopy. Distorted vascular pattern with residual "pseudopolyps."

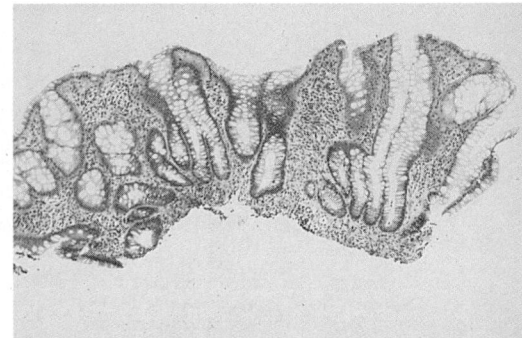

C, Mucosal biopsy of quiescent ulcerative colitis. Distorted, branching glands with reduced goblet cell mucus and minimal chronic inflammation.

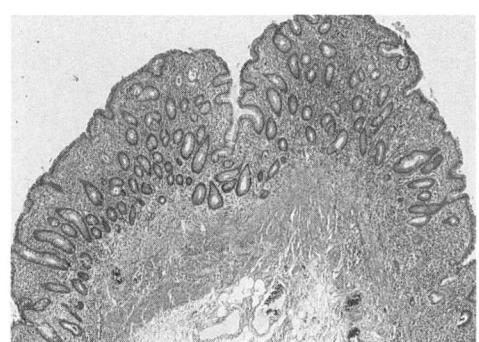

D, Mucosal biopsy of active ulcerative colitis. *Left,* Low power. Acute and chronic inflammation. *Right,* High power. Crypt abscess.

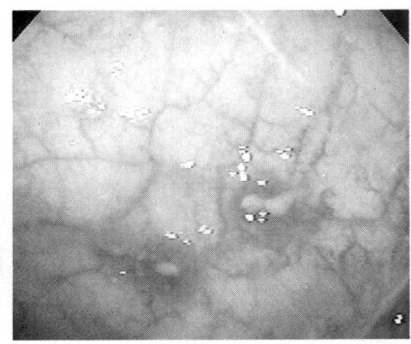

E, Aphthoid ulcer of Crohn's disease. Note normal surrounding mucosa.

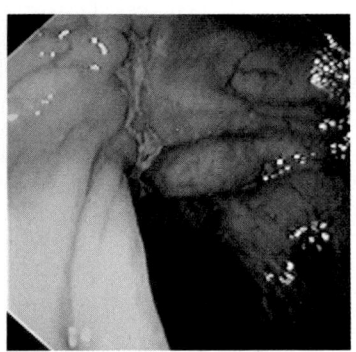

F, Crohn's disease. Linear ulceration.

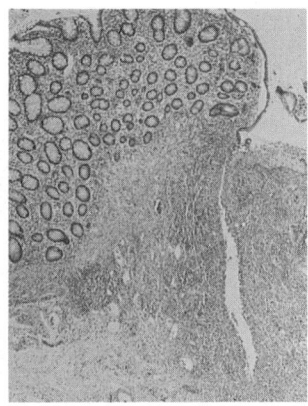

G, Mucosal biopsy of Crohn's disease. Focal inflammation with fissuring ulceration.

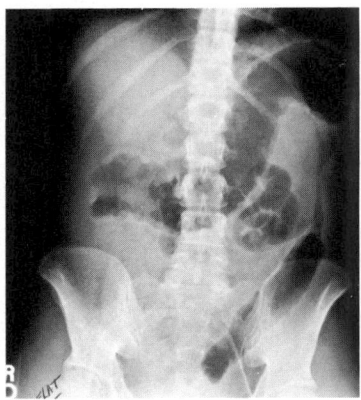

H, Abdominal flat-plate demonstrating toxic megacolon with dilated, ahaustral colon.

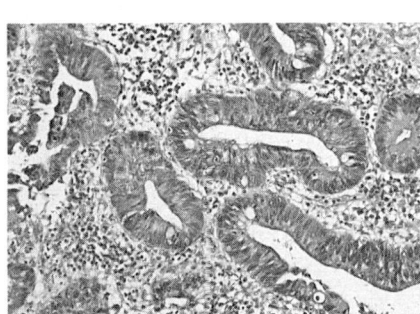
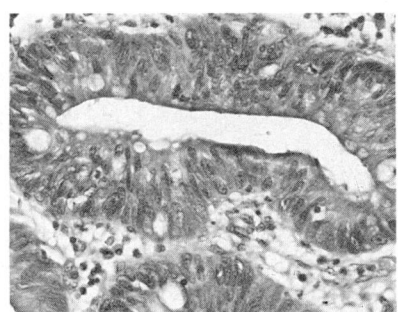

I, Low-power *(left)* and high-power *(right)* views of mucosal dysplasia with hyperchromatic epithelial cells and mucus depletion with stratification and loss of polarity.

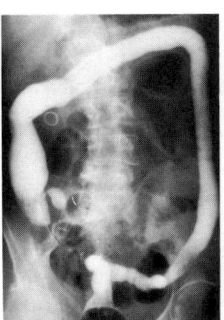
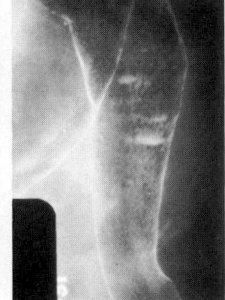

J, Left and *right,* Air-contrast barium enema of ulcerative colitis with contiguous loss of haustration and sandpaper-like granularity.

PLATE 3 GASTROINTESTINAL DISEASES

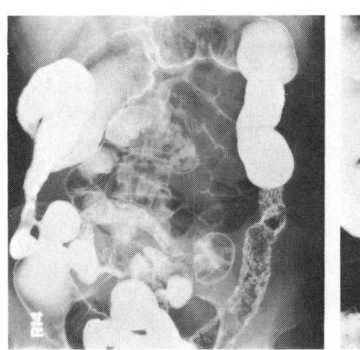 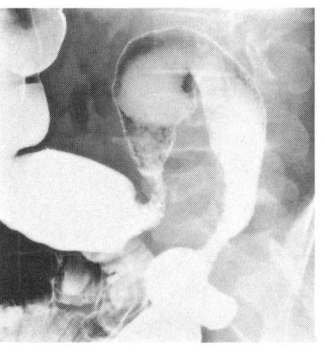

A, Left and *right,* Air-contrast barium enema of Crohn's disease of the colon with asymmetric linear ulceration, cobblestone mucosa, and rectal sparing.

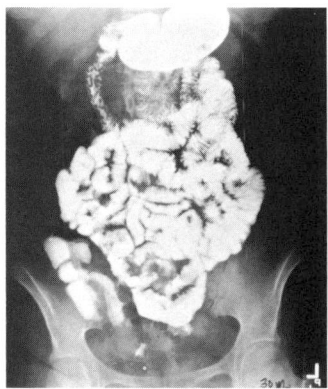 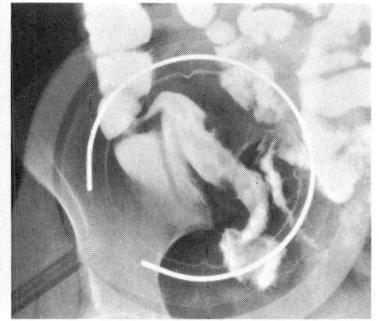

B, Left and *right,* Small bowel follow-through of ileal Crohn's disease, showing separation of loops of distal ileum and cobblestone appearance.

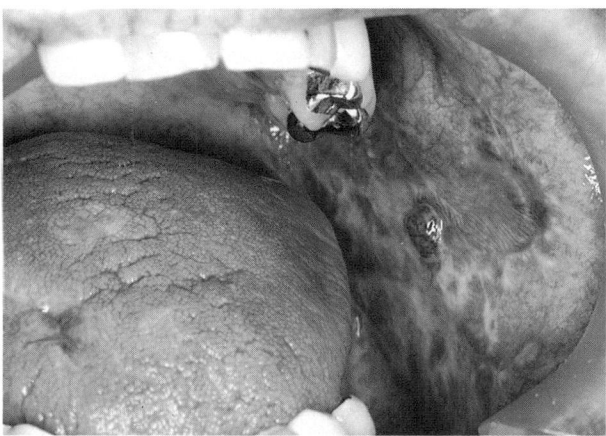

C, Erosive lichen planus in a 62-year-old woman. Note the white striae and central ulceration. Similar lesions were present on the opposite buccal mucosa.

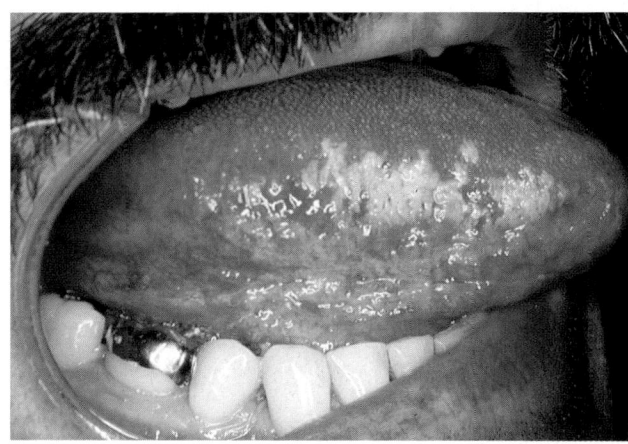

D, Hairy leukoplakia in a 38-year-old man. This was the first sign of HIV infection. One year later he developed *Pneumocystis carinii* pneumonia. (Courtesy of Dr. D. Greenspan.)

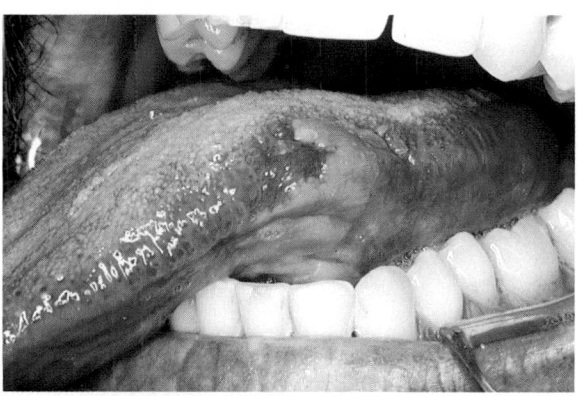

E, Erythroplakia anterior to leukoplakia in a 40-year-old man with a history of frequent cigarette smoking for many years. Histologically, the white area showed epithelial thickening and hyperkeratosis, whereas the red area showed moderately severe dysplasia.

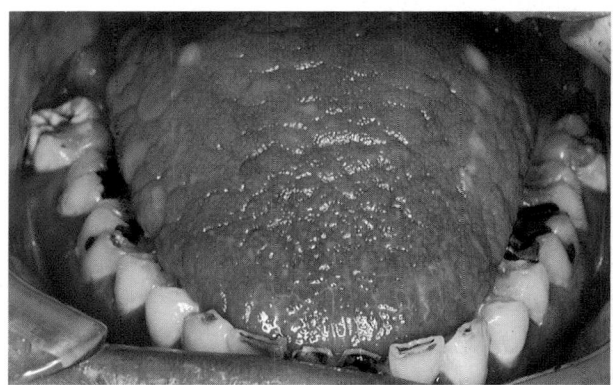

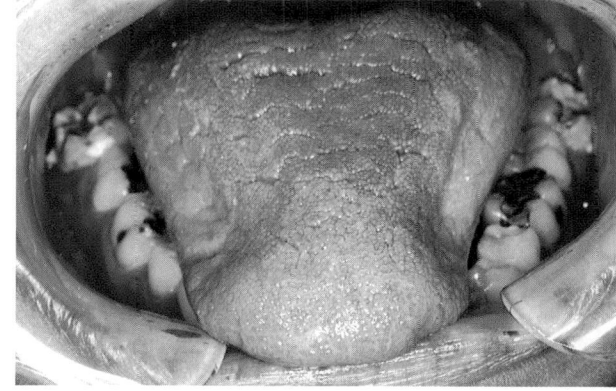

F, Chronic erythematous candidiasis in a 28-year-old woman with severe xerostomia from primary Sjögren's syndrome. *Top,* Dorsal tongue before treatment, showing erythema, atrophy of filiform papillae, and fissuring. Note caries in incisors. *Bottom,* Resolution of most of these changes after 4 months of intermittent topical antifungal therapy.

PLATE 4 CARDIOLOGY AND RHEUMATOLOGY

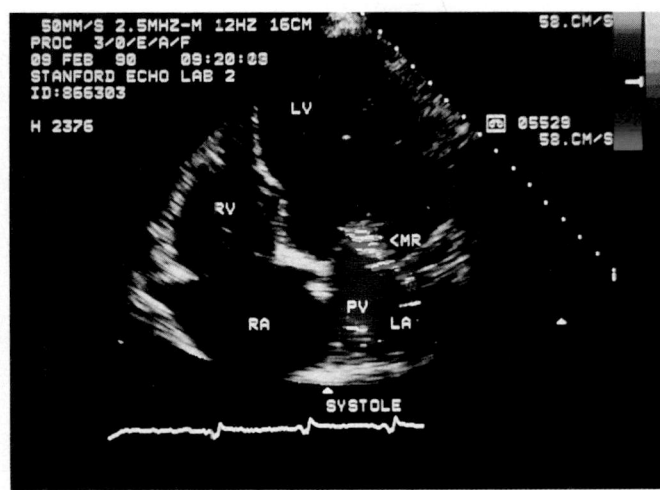

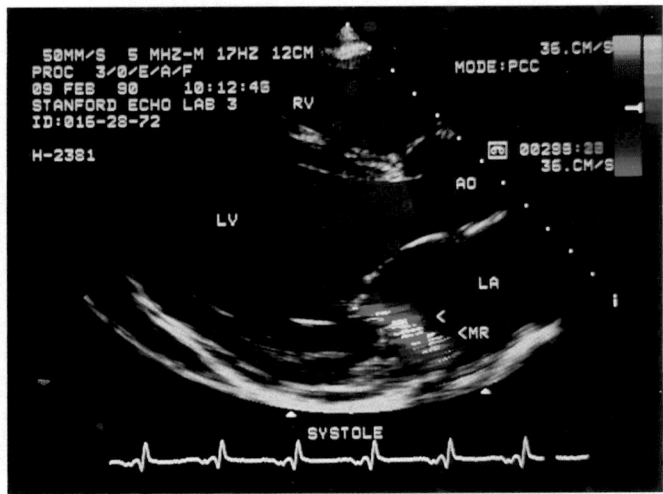

A, A two-dimensional echocardiographic image with Doppler color flow mapping superimposed to indicate blood flow. A portion of the image contains color-coded information regarding the direction and velocity of flow. Shades of orange represent flow toward the transducer, and shades of blue represent flow away from the transducer. Pulmonary venous (PV) flow into the left atrium is noted in orange during systole, while mitral regurgitation (MR) is indicated by the eccentric color at the lateral left atrial wall, extending from the area of the mitral valve. The mitral regurgitation signal contains blue, orange, and white, giving a mosaic pattern that is typical of high-velocity turbulent flow. LA = Left atrium; LV = left ventricle; RA = right atrium; RV = right ventricle.

B, A two-dimensional echocardiogram with Doppler flow mapping superimposed on a portion of the image. The color information is represented in the sector of the imaging plane extending from the apex of the triangular plane to the two small arrows at the bottom of the image plane. Mitral regurgitation (MR) is indicated *(open arrows)*, extending from the mitral valve leaflets toward the posterior aspect of the left atrium (LA) during systole. The mosaic of colors representing the mitral regurgitant signal is typical of high-velocity turbulent flow. The low-intensity orange-brown signal represents flow directed away from the transducer on the chest wall, and the blue shades represent blood in the left ventricular outflow tract moving toward the transducer. AO = Aorta; LV = left ventricle; RV = right ventricle.

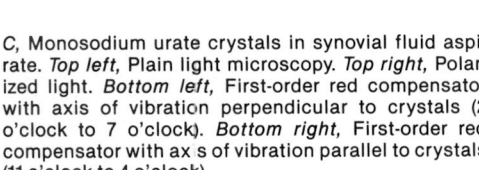

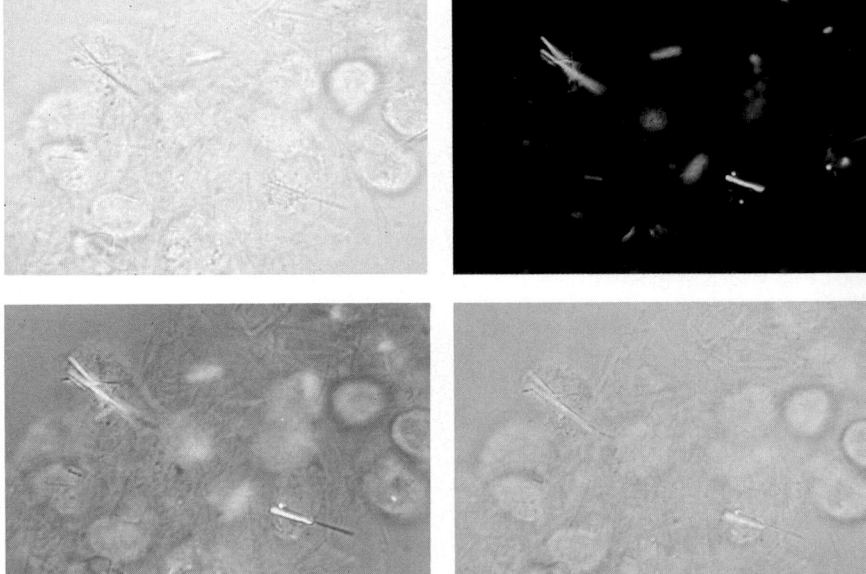

C, Monosodium urate crystals in synovial fluid aspirate. *Top left,* Plain light microscopy. *Top right,* Polarized light. *Bottom left,* First-order red compensator with axis of vibration perpendicular to crystals (2 o'clock to 7 o'clock). *Bottom right,* First-order red compensator with axis of vibration parallel to crystals (11 o'clock to 4 o'clock).

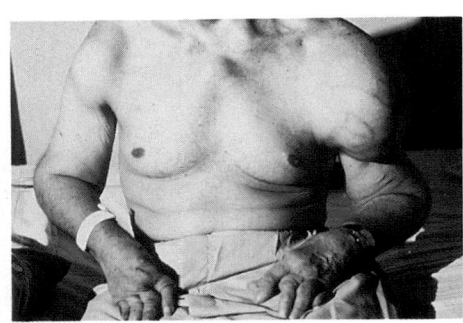

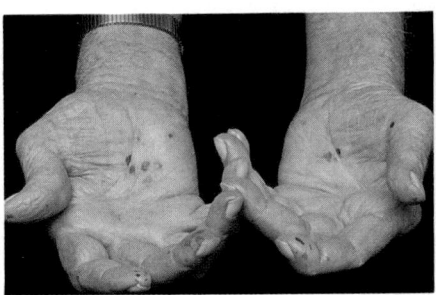

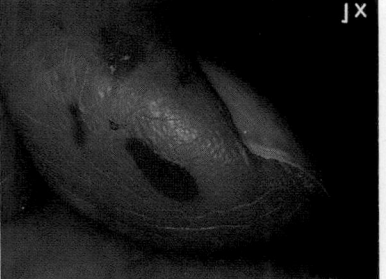

D, Large synovial cysts of the shoulders, especially on the left, in a patient with chronic deforming rheumatoid arthritis.

E, Left and *right,* Rheumatoid vasculitis with small brown infarcts of palms and fingers in chronic rheumatoid arthritis. (Courtesy of Dr. Martin Lidsky, Houston, Texas.)

ascites in patients with portal hypertension. Peritoneal adhesions as a result of peritonitis are absolute contraindications. The relative risks of postoperative adhesions and surgical scar must be weighed against the diagnostic importance.

FUTURE OF ENDOSCOPY

Endoscopic instrumentation is approaching optimal size and optical resolution, in both fiberoptic and emerging electronic video endoscopy equipment. The number of skilled endoscopists has increased so that precise diagnostic studies are generally available to most patients.

Endoscopy is contributing enormously to management of gastrointestinal disease and will continue to do so. A clearer understanding of the colonic polyp-cancer progression will likely be available in the next few years. Colonoscopic polypectomy will play a key role in altering the course of this major malignancy. It is likely that nearly all cases of common duct stones will be treated endoscopically in the near future. Removal of the gallbladder via a laparoscopic approach is attracting wide interest. Measures for successful control of gastrointestinal bleeding are greatly improving. Their influence on mortality should soon become clear.

Optimal management of patients with benign or malignant biliary obstruction is not clearly dependent on a single technique. Endoscopists, radiologists, and surgeons working together will likely evolve an integrated approach with indications for each of several options.

Fleischer DE, Goldberg SB, Brunning TH, et al.: Detection and surveillance of colorectal cancer. JAMA 261:580, 1989. *A current discussion of a topic slowly coming into focus.*

Infante-Riward C, Esnaola S, Villeneuve J-P: Role of endoscopic variceal sclerotherapy in the long-term management of variceal bleeding: A meta-analysis. Gastroenterology 96:1087, 1989. *The final role of endoscopic variceal sclerosis is not yet clear.*

Proceeding of the consensus conference on therapeutic endoscopy in bleeding ulcers. Gastrointest Endosc Suppl 36, 1990. *An important position statement on the current role of endoscopy.*

Ranshohoff DF, Lang CA, Kuo HS: Colonoscopic surveillance after polypectomy: Considerations of cost effectiveness. Ann Intern Med 114:177, 1991. *Useful analysis of the effectiveness of routine follow-up colonoscopy.*

Soll AH: Pathogenesis of peptic ulcer and implication for therapy. N Engl J Med 322:909, 1990. *Our understanding of acid-peptic disease is finally providing a rational basis for effective therapy.*

Vaira D, Ainley C, Williams S, et al.: Endoscopic sphincterotomy in 1000 consecutive patients. Lancet 2:431, 1990. *A broad review of experience with endoscopic sphincterotomy for choledocholithiasis.*

Van Stielmann G, Pearman NW, Goff JS, et al.: Endoscopic cholangiography and stone removal prior to cholecystectomy. Arch Surg 124:787, 1989. *Endoscopic retrograde sphincterotomy for bile duct stone removal poses a question—what to do with the often silent remaining gallbladder.*

95 Diseases of the Mouth and Salivary Glands

Troy E. Daniels

At least 200 primary lesions or diseases occur in the oral mucosa, gingiva, teeth, jaws, and minor or major salivary glands. In addition, many systemic diseases or drugs can cause secondary abnormalities of the oral mucosa or salivary glands. This chapter briefly discusses only the most common and important of the mucosal and salivary gland diseases, to provide a basis for developing a differential diagnosis and guiding treatment and referral. More complete coverage of these topics can be found in specialized texts cited at the end of the chapter.

ORAL MUCOSAL DISEASES

Acute Ulcerations

Painful short-term ulcerations, the most common oral mucosal lesions, are usually caused by mechanical trauma, immunologic mechanisms, and bacterial or viral infections (Table 95–1). Soon after formation, ulcers in the mouth become covered by a white to gray pseudomembrane, analogous to the scab that forms on

TABLE 95–1. COMMON AND SIGNIFICANT ORAL MUCOSAL LESIONS

Ulcers
  Acute (many are self-limiting)
    Mechanical trauma
    Recurrent aphthous ulcers/Behçet's syndrome
    Viral (herpes simplex,* varicella-zoster,* hand-foot-and-mouth disease,* herpangina,* rubeola*)
    Erythema multiforme/Stevens-Johnson syndrome
    Drug reaction
    Primary syphilis (chancre)
    Gonorrhea
  Chronic
    Squamous cell carcinoma
    Mucocutaneous diseases (pemphigus,* pemphigoid,* erythema multiforme, lichen planus,† lupus erythematosus†)
    Microbial infections (tuberculosis, leprosy, actinomycosis, noma, various fungi)
White lesions
  Squamous cell carcinoma (early)
  Leukoplakia
  Frictional keratosis
  Smokeless tobacco–associated lesions
  Nicotine stomatitis (palate)
  Lichen planus (reticular and plaque types)
  Pseudomembranous candidiasis (thrush)
  Hyperplastic candidiasis (candidal leukoplakia)
  Hairy leukoplakia (HIV-associated) (usually on lateral tongue)
  Geographic tongue
  Pseudomembrane-covered ulcers (see above)
  Mucous patch or condyloma latum of secondary syphilis
Red lesions
  Squamous cell carcinoma (early)
  Erythroplakia (epithelial dysplasia)
  Erythematous (atrophic) candidiasis
  Median rhomboid glossitis
  Mucocutaneous diseases (see above)
  Angular cheilitis
  Telangiectasias and purpuras
  Kaposi's sarcoma (blue to purple color)

*Vesicles present in early lesion formation
†Ulcers usually associated with white-red lesions

dry epidermis. Pseudomembrane-covered ulcers are usually distinguished from the white hyperkeratotic lesions described below by their clinical features of pain, a flat surface, and an erythematous periphery. Traumatic ulcers are characterized by their location on the tongue or inside of the cheeks or lips, their proximity to the chewing surfaces of the teeth, and the irregularity of their borders.

APHTHOUS ULCERS. These idiopathic recurrent ulcers, which afflict at least 20 per cent of the population, occur on all areas of the oral mucosa except the hard palate, gingiva, and vermilion. They are well-defined circles and may be single or multiple. There are three clinical forms: (1) minor, which are flat, less than 1 cm in diameter, and last only 5 to 10 days; (2) major, which have raised borders, are larger than 1 cm, and often last for weeks or months; and (3) herpetiform, which are usually clusters of very small ulcers that resemble recurrent herpetic lesions but are not preceded by vesicles and do not contain detectable viruses. Lesions clinically identical to minor aphthous ulcers occur in Behçet's syndrome (Ch. 269). Aphthous ulcers are occasionally associated with macrocytic anemias or gluten-sensitive enteropathy and may become more frequent and severe in association with human immunodeficiency virus (HIV) infection (Table 95–2).

Minor or herpetiform aphthous ulcers may not require treatment. Topical steroids, such as fluocinonide ointment in Orabase, can reduce the severity and duration of the lesions only if used with prodromal symptoms or early signs. Major aphthae usually require treatment by topical or systemic corticosteroids and occasionally are biopsied to rule out neoplasia.

VIRAL ULCERS. Several types of virus (most commonly herpes simplex) may cause oral mucosal vesicles that, after lasting a few days at most, quickly become shallow ulcers. In the initial infection by herpes simplex virus, usually in children, numerous

TABLE 95–2. ORAL LESIONS ASSOCIATED WITH HIV INFECTION

Kaposi's sarcoma
Candidiasis
  Pseudomembranous
  Hyperplastic
  Erythematous
Other opportunistic fungal infections (e.g., histoplasmosis or coccidioidomycosis)
Epithelial lesions
  Aphthous ulcers (increased frequency, duration, or size)
  Virus-associated epithelial hyperplasias
    Hairy leukoplakia
    Oral wart
    Focal epithelial hyperplasia (Heck's disease)
    Condyloma acuminatum
  Herpes zoster
Exaggerated forms of gingivitis and inflammatory periodontal disease
Decreased salivary gland function
Parotid gland enlargement (benign lymphoepithelial lesion)
Non-Hodgkin's lymphoma

vesicles may appear on any oral mucosal site (primary herpetic gingivostomatitis), accompanied by malaise, headache, fever, and cervical lymphadenopathy. Many patients previously exposed to this virus develop recurrent lesions, most commonly as clusters of small vesicles on the lips (herpes labialis); only a few develop intraoral recurrent herpes, as clusters of vesicles on the keratinized mucosa of the gingiva or hard palate. Such lesions tend to recur at the same site, but the frequency decreases with age.

Oral mucosal vesicles/ulcers may also accompany the initial infection by the varicella-zoster virus in children with chickenpox (Ch. 374), and unilateral lesions may occur with herpes zoster (Ch. 476), affecting branches of the trigeminal nerve. Uncommonly, oral mucosal lesions may be caused by different types of coxsackievirus (Ch. 377), appearing on any oral site in hand-foot-and-mouth disease (Ch. 380) or on the soft palate or pharynx in herpangina. After infection by the measles (rubeola) virus, small ulcers (Koplik's spots) form on the inside of the cheeks 1 to 2 days before development of the skin rash (Ch. 367).

ERYTHEMA MULTIFORME. In this mucocutaneous disease, painful oral mucosal ulcerations develop rapidly in as many as half of the patients. The lesions may be confined to the mouth, with no skin involvement. The affected patients, usually young adults with minimal or no systemic symptoms, present with irregularly shaped ulcers that can be small and few in number or involve large areas of the mucosa, most commonly the lower labial mucosa. These lesions may be distinguished from those of primary herpes by the absence of oral vesicles and systemic symptoms or the presence of characteristic skin lesions (Ch. 293). A major variant of this disease is the Stevens-Johnson syndrome.

VENEREAL INFECTIONS. Primary syphilis may present as a solitary, indurated, painless ulcer on the oral mucosa which resolves spontaneously in 4 to 6 weeks (Ch. 340). Uncommonly, *Neisseria gonorrhoeae* may cause oral ulcers, usually in the pharynx, that may be confused with oral ulcers of other causes.

Oral Squamous Cell Carcinoma

Approximately 4 per cent of all cancers occur in the mouth, largely squamous cell carcinomas of the mucosal epithelium. Oral carcinoma occurs usually in the fifth decade or beyond, in men twice as frequently as in women, and with long-term use of tobacco (more than 80 per cent of cases). The tongue is the most common site, followed by the lip, oropharynx, and mouth floor.

Oral carcinoma usually presents as a chronic, indurated, cratered ulcer, but early lesions of squamous cell carcinoma may appear as white or red macules (see Table 95–1). Most oral carcinomas develop on normal-appearing mucosa, but about 15 per cent arise within a pre-existing oral mucosal leukoplakia or erythroplakia (described below). The overall 5-year survival is approximately 50 per cent, but early treatment of small, localized lesions can lead to survival rates as high as 90 per cent.

Other Chronic Ulcerations

Chronic multifocal oral mucosal lesions composed of ill-defined areas of erythema and ulceration may be caused by several of the mucocutaneous diseases. They are among the most difficult oral mucosal lesions to diagnose and are discussed below with the red lesions (see Table 95–1). Several microbial infections can lead to indurated, chronic oral mucosal ulcerations with moderate symptoms—e.g., ulcers overlying granulomas associated with tuberculosis, leprosy, actinomycosis, histoplasmosis, or coccidioidomycosis.

White Lesions

White plaques are commonly found in the mouth but, like ulcerations, have a wide variety of causes and outcomes. The term "leukoplakia" applies to a white plaque that does not rub off and whose appearance is not indicative of another disease. Leukoplakia can occur in any area of the mouth and usually exhibits benign hyperkeratosis on biopsy. On long-term follow-up, between 2 and 6 per cent of these lesions will have undergone malignant transformation into squamous cell carcinoma. Areas of leukoplakia with a corrugated surface or mixed with areas of erythema are often found in the lower labial or buccal vestibule of those who use smokeless tobacco.

Frictional keratoses are often found posterior to the lower third molar teeth as irregular white plaques and on the buccal mucosa as white lines adjacent to the dental occlusion. Unlike leukoplakia, these lesions rarely become malignant.

LICHEN PLANUS. Oral lesions of lichen planus occur in about 1 per cent of the population, usually as a bilateral reticular network of linear white plaques, with or without adjacent areas of erythema (atrophy or erosion) or ulcers (see Color Plate 3C). The presence of mucosal atrophy, erosion, or ulceration usually causes pain or sensitivity to certain foods. Most lesions can be adequately controlled by topical application of fluocinonide ointment mixed with an equal weight of Orabase for periods of several weeks to several months, although recurrence is common.

ORAL CANDIDIASIS. This fungal disease has three clinical forms: pseudomembranous (thrush), erythematous (atrophic), and hyperplastic (candidal leukoplakia). Pseudomembranous candidiasis, usually of relatively short duration, occurs on any site and consists of white plaques that can be rubbed off, leaving a red or bleeding base. The lesion of hyperplastic candidiasis has fungal hyphae within the surface layers of hyperkeratotic epithelium; it does not rub off and is most frequently located on the anterior buccal mucosa or on the tongue. All forms of oral candidiasis represent overgrowth of *Candida* species from the oral flora, induced by a variety of causes. These include suppression of bacterial flora by systemic antibiotics, chronic xerostomia, uncontrolled diabetes mellitus or anemia, and immunosuppression (especially in HIV-infected patients) (Table 95–2). Treatment of erythematous candidiasis is discussed below with the red lesions.

HAIRY LEUKOPLAKIA. This recently identified lesion is a white plaque occurring most frequently on the lateral surfaces of the tongue, mainly in HIV-infected persons (see Color Plate 3D). *Candida* may be present in the surface layers, but the lesion is not eliminated by effective antifungal therapy and contains large quantities of Epstein-Barr virus. Its diagnosis should be followed by determination of whether HIV antibody is present in the patient's serum.

GEOGRAPHIC TONGUE. Also called "benign migratory glossitis," this is a benign idiopathic condition affecting the dorsal tongue of about 2 per cent of the population. It is characterized by well-defined circular areas of relatively atrophied filiform papillae bordered by arcs of normal or hyperplastic filiform papillae; the lesions change in location, or "migrate," over time. Treatment is usually not necessary.

SECONDARY SYPHILIS. Secondary syphilis may present well-defined white plaques on the labial or palatal mucosa, called "condyloma latum" (or "split papule," because of their lobulated periphery).

Red Lesions

Solitary red macules or plaques ("erythroplakia") are less common in the mouth than white lesions but should be viewed with concern because many exhibit microscopic dysplasia or carcinoma in situ (see Table 95–1). They are often associated with areas of leukoplakia (see Color Plate 3E). However, a red macule occurring in the midline of the posterior dorsal tongue, classified as median rhomboid glossitis, is an idiopathic but uniformly benign condition that is often associated with localized overgrowth of *Candida* species.

ERYTHEMATOUS (ATROPHIC) ORAL CANDIDIASIS. This chronic condition is characterized by diffuse mucosal erythema and atrophy of the filiform papillae on the dorsal tongue (see Color Plate 3*F*) or by ill-defined red macules on the palate, tongue, or buccal mucosa. Symptoms of oral mucosal burning and sensitivity to certain foods accompany the condition, which is frequently associated with xerostomia. In patients wearing removable dentures, there may be mucosal erythema confined to the denture-bearing area.

These lesions can be resolved with topical nystatin or clotrimazole-containing preparations or with systemic ketoconazole; these are usually administered for several months. In patients with xerostomia who have remaining natural teeth, topical antifungal preparations containing sucrose or glucose must be avoided to prevent caries. Oral use of vaginal tablets is safe and effective. Systemic ketoconazole may not be effective in patients with severe xerostomia. Effective treatment leads to significant improvement in oral symptoms, regardless of the cause of the candidiasis. Treatment of denture-associated candidiasis also requires appropriate treatment of the denture to remove the organisms; failure to do so leads to recurrence.

ANGULAR CHEILITIS. Erythema or crusting of the labial angles is usually caused by *Candida*. It is usually associated with intraoral candidiasis and in such cases topical treatment of the angular cheilitis should be accompanied by intraoral or systemic antifungal treatment.

MUCOCUTANEOUS DISEASES. Some mucocutaneous diseases involving immunologic abnormalities affect the oral mucosa—e.g., pemphigus vulgaris, mucous membrane pemphigoid, atrophic or erosive lichen planus, and lupus erythematosus. The appearance of oral lesions caused by these diseases is frequently similar. The diagnosis requires examination of a biopsy specimen by routine histopathology and usually also by direct immunofluorescence examination to identify characteristic depositions of immunoglobulins and complement components in the basement membrane zone with pemphigoid, lupus, or lichen planus or in the inter–epithelial cell spaces with pemphigus.

Pemphigus vulgaris usually presents as oral mucosal vesicles that rapidly rupture, leaving painful erosions or ulcerations. These are followed by development of skin lesions (Ch. 525). Rarely, the lesions remain confined to the mouth.

Lesions of mucous membrane pemphigoid are usually confined to the oral mucosa or conjunctivae and occur in patients over 50 years of age. They begin as vesicles that quickly rupture, leaving ulcers and areas of atrophic epithelium that are chronic but only moderately symptomatic. Use of topical fluocinonide for several months, as described above for lichen planus, is sometimes sufficient treatment of the oral lesions, but some patients need systemic treatment (Ch. 525).

Some cases of atrophic or erosive lichen planus do not show the characteristic reticular keratotic lesions described above and may be clinically indistinguishable from mucous membrane pemphigoid. In those cases, direct immunofluorescence examination of a biopsy specimen of intact mucosa is required for diagnosis.

Oral mucosal lesions of lupus may occur in patients who have systemic lupus erythematosus (SLE), in patients who do not have SLE but later develop that disease, or in patients who do not develop SLE. In this latter group, the lesions of mucosal lupus may be analogous to the skin lesions of chronic discoid lupus. Lesions of oral lupus are characterized by reticular hyperkeratotic figures associated with erythema and may resemble atrophic lichen planus. The lesions may be controlled by topical fluocinonide or intralesional triamcinolone.

Lesions of Kaposi's sarcoma associated with HIV infection frequently appear first on the oral mucosa, especially the palate. They begin as macules with a blue or purple color, at which time they need to be distinguished from purpura. Later, they spread radially and expand vertically (Table 95–2).

Pigmentations

Brown or gray-black macules on the oral mucosa are relatively common and may be caused by localized increase in melanin production, proliferation of melanin-producing cells, or deposition of local or systemically distributed pigmented substances

TABLE 95–3. PIGMENTATIONS OF THE ORAL MUCOSA (BROWN OR GRAY-BLACK IN COLOR)

Increased melanin production (flat lesions)
  Oral melanotic macule
  Ephelis (lip)
  Systemic diseases: Addison's disease, von Recklinghausen's disease of skin, Albright's syndrome, Peutz-Jeghers syndrome
Proliferation of melanin-producing cells (flat or raised lesions)
  Pigmented cellular nevi (benign and premalignant types)
  Atypical melanocytic hyperplasia
  Malignant melanoma
Nonmelanin pigmentation
  Amalgam tattoo
  Focal deposition of systemically distributed heavy metal (lead, bismuth, mercury, others) at sites of chronic inflammation
  Systemically administered drugs (chloroquine, minocycline, cyclophosphamide)

(Table 95–3). Mucosal pigmentation may occur after long-term administration of chloroquine, minocycline, or cyclophosphamide. Malignant melanoma can occur at any oral mucosal site but develops most frequently on the mucosa or gingiva covering the maxilla. Diagnosis of any of these is usually established by biopsy and knowledge of relevant underlying conditions.

ORAL SOFT TISSUE TUMORS

Connective Tissue Hyperplasias

The most common oral soft tissue tumors are small, pedunculated masses of hyperplastic fibrous connective tissue covered by normal-appearing mucosa (Table 95–4). These lesions are usually found on the inside of the cheeks or lips, in areas where they are subject to frequent irritation by the teeth. Similar lesions may be present at the border of an ill-fitting denture or may occur in clusters on the hard palate under an ill-fitting denture ("palatal papillomatosis").

Generalized enlargement of the gingiva may be caused by chronic administration of phenytoin, cyclosporine, or nifedipine. It can also be associated with a hereditary defect or be caused by an infiltration of white blood cells in some types of leukemia, especially acute monocytic. The drug-associated cases apparently represent an exaggerated response in susceptible patients to commonly occurring local irritants, such as dental plaque and calculus. The cause of this susceptibility is unknown.

TABLE 95–4. ORAL SOFT TISSUE TUMORS

Connective tissue hyperplasia (normal-appearing overlying mucosa)
  Irritation fibroma
  Denture-associated hyperplasia
  Palatal papillomatosis
  Generalized gingival hyperplasia
    Drug-induced (phenytoin, nifedipine, cyclosporine)
    Hereditary
Reactive hyperplasia (erythematous overlying mucosa)
  Pyogenic granuloma/pregnancy tumor
  Peripheral giant cell granuloma
  Inflammatory gingival hyperplasia
  Hyperplastic lingual tonsil
Epithelial masses (usually irregular white surface)
  Papilloma/oral wart
  Squamous cell carcinoma
  Verrucous carcinoma
  Focal epithelial hyperplasia (Heck's disease)
  Condyloma acuminatum (venereal wart)
  Keratoacanthoma (on lips)
Salivary duct obstruction (minor salivary glands)
  Mucocele/ranula (usually fluctuant)
  Salivary stone (sialolith)
Underlying connective tissue or salivary gland neoplasms
Other malignant diseases
  Metastatic lesions
  Local or generalized leukemic infiltrates in the gingiva (esp. with acute monocytic leukemia)

Reactive Hyperplasias

Small masses with surfaces that are ulcerated or only partially covered by normal-appearing mucosa usually represent reactive lesions in the form of pyogenic granulomas (whose frequency increases during pregnancy), peripheral giant cell granulomas, or lymphoid hyperplasia of the lingual or other tonsillar tissue. The granulomas are most often located on the gingiva. Rarely, such lesions may represent a metastatic neoplasm.

Epithelial Tumors

Small, white, wartlike epithelial masses are common and can occur in any area of the oral mucosa. They are occasionally classified as epithelial neoplasms, but most do not continue to grow. Human papillomavirus types 2, 6, 11, and 13 have been identified in some but not all of these wartlike lesions. Usually, these lesions are classified generically as papillomas but require identification of virus or further clinical evidence to confirm the diagnosis of a viral disease. A large wartlike lesion on the oral mucosa should raise the suspicion of verrucous carcinoma.

Salivary Duct Obstruction

Mucoceles are small, fluctuant, frequently recurring nodules that occur commonly on the inside of the cheeks and lips, the posterior palate, and the mouth floor. They are caused by injury and blockage of the excretory duct of one of the numerous minor salivary glands. Sialoliths may be apparent as hard nodules covered by normal-appearing mucosa in the submandibular or sublingual ducts of the mouth floor or, uncommonly, in areas of minor salivary glands. Both types of lesions require conservative surgical excision.

SALIVARY GLAND DISEASES

Primary Diseases of Salivary Glands

Patients with enlargement of a major or minor salivary gland usually bring the clinician a diagnostic challenge (Table 95–5). More than 20 types of benign or malignant salivary gland neoplasms may present as unilateral enlargement of a major gland that is firm and nontender to palpation. Most of these tumors can also arise in minor glands as a firm submucosal nodule on the palate or the labial or buccal mucosa. Uncommonly, unilateral major gland enlargement may be caused by an inflammatory lesion, such as benign lymphoepithelial lesion or other chronic sialadenitis. Observation of any of these lesions should be followed by appropriate imaging and biopsy.

Major salivary gland enlargement that is markedly painful and tender to palpation suggests bacterial sialadenitis and usually requires administration of systemic antibiotics, initially oral penicillin.

Bilateral Salivary Gland Enlargement and Decreased Salivary Secretion Associated with Systemic Diseases

The best-known cause of bilateral salivary gland enlargement is infection by the mumps virus in children (Table 95–5). The incidence of mumps has decreased in the United States by more than 90 per cent since the introduction of an effective vaccine in 1967, but the number of cases began to rise again in the late 1980's, apparently as a result of reduced use of the vaccine (Ch. 16). Uncommonly, a less acute, mumpslike illness may occur in adults in association with cytomegalovirus, influenza, or coxsackie A virus infection.

Sjögren's syndrome is characterized in about one third of patients by the development of firm, nontender or only slightly tender enlargement of major salivary glands (Ch. 263). The enlargement is bilateral but often asymmetric and may slowly wax and wane. Salivary secretion usually decreases gradually, and the resulting xerostomia can impair speech and swallowing and be associated with rapidly progressive dental caries, symptomatic oral candidiasis, and difficulty in wearing dentures. In severe cases, the oral mucosa may appear dry and sticky and saliva will not be expressible from the major ducts. Signs of erythematous candidiasis (see above) are seen in about one third of patients with Sjögren's syndrome.

The salivary component of Sjögren's syndrome is most reliably diagnosed in a labial salivary gland biopsy specimen of at least

TABLE 95–5. CAUSES OF SALIVARY GLAND ENLARGEMENT

Usually unilateral
  Benign or malignant salivary gland neoplasms (more than 20 different histopathologic types)
  Bacterial infection
  Chronic sialadenitis (single gland)
Usually bilateral, often asymmetric (associated with decreased salivary secretion)
  Viral infection (mumps, cytomegalovirus, influenza, coxsackie A)
  Sjögren's syndrome (benign lymphoepithelial lesion)
  Chronic granulomatous diseases (sarcoidosis, tuberculosis, leprosy, syphilis)
  Recurrent parotitis of childhood
  Human immunodeficiency virus infection
Bilaterally symmetric, soft, nontender, parotid only
  Sialadenosis (asymptomatic parotid enlargement), idiopathic or associated with:
    Diabetes mellitus
    Hyperlipoproteinemia
    Hepatic cirrhosis
    Anorexia/bulimia
    Chronic pancreatitis
    Acromegaly
    Gonadal hypofunction
    Phenylbutazone use

five glands. Examination must show focal lymphocytic sialadenitis in most or all of the specimen and exclude nonspecific chronic sialadenitis or pathology indicative of another disease, such as noncaseating granuloma. A patient's symptoms of oral dryness are important, but, being subjective and nonspecific (Table 95–6), they are not diagnostic. Results from functional studies or imaging of salivary glands are not specific to Sjögren's syndrome.

Several chronic granulomatous diseases, such as sarcoidosis, tuberculosis, leprosy, and syphilis, can cause bilateral enlargement and decreased function of salivary glands. The clinical and serologic features of sarcoidosis may closely mimic those of Sjögren's syndrome, and the distinction must be made by salivary gland biopsy.

Some patients with HIV infection develop major salivary gland enlargement and reduced salivary secretion associated with lymphocytic infiltration of a different type than in Sjögren's syndrome. Solitary benign lymphoepithelial lesions may occur in parotid glands of intravenous drug–abusing patients (see Table 95–2).

Recurrent parotitis of childhood includes episodes of unilateral or bilateral parotid enlargement. Salivary secretion may be reduced during flares of this illness, but usually without prominent secondary symptoms or signs. This condition, of unknown cause, usually subsides after puberty. Some serologic evidence suggests an association with Epstein-Barr virus infection.

TABLE 95–6. CAUSES OF DECREASED SALIVARY SECRETION (XEROSTOMIA)

Temporary
  Effects of short-term drug use (e.g., antihistamines)
  Virus infections (esp. mumps)
  Dehydration
  Fear
Chronic
  Effects of chronically administered drugs (especially antidepressants, MAO inhibitors, neuroleptics, parasympatholytics, some combinations of drugs for treating hypertension)
  Chronic diseases (with gland enlargement in some patients)
    Sjögren's syndrome
    Granulomatous diseases (sarcoidosis, tuberculosis, leprosy, syphilis)
    Amyloidosis
    Human immunodeficiency virus infection
  Graft-versus-host disease
  Therapeutic radiation to the head and neck
  Depression
  Absent or malformed glands (rare)

Asymptomatic Parotid Enlargement (Sialadenosis)

Parotid glands can develop bilateral, symmetric enlargement that is soft and nontender to palpation and not associated with xerostomia (see Table 95–5). Usually, results of sialography and salivary scintigraphy are within normal limits. Histopathologic examination reveals only serous acinar cell hypertrophy with vacuolation and loss of granulation in the secretory cell cytoplasm, but biopsy of the affected glands is not indicated for diagnosis. Diagnosis is established by the clinical presentation and (if necessary to rule out Sjögren's syndrome or sarcoidosis) a normal labial salivary gland biopsy.

This chronic, noninflammatory, and non-neoplastic condition may occur alone or may be associated with a variety of systemic diseases, including diabetes mellitus, hyperlipoproteinemia, hepatic cirrhosis, anorexia/bulimia, chronic pancreatitis, acromegaly, and gonadal hypofunction. It can also result from use of phenylbutazone or be a reaction to iodine-containing contrast media.

Impaired Salivary Secretion (Xerostomia) Without Gland Enlargement

The very common symptom of dry mouth is most often a side effect of chronically administered drugs. Many classes of drugs reduce unstimulated salivary secretion through anticholinergic or other mechanisms (Table 95–6). At least initially, most of these drugs do not interfere with stimulated salivary production in response to gustatory, olfactory, or masticatory stimuli. This means that patients experience the symptoms soon after beginning to use the drug, but produce sufficient amounts of saliva during a meal for normal chewing and swallowing. The effects are dose-dependent and are frequently seen in those patients using several of the tricyclic antidepressants, most neuroleptics, monoamine oxidase inhibitors, and all parasympatholytics. A combination of drugs for treatment of hypertension may cause symptoms of dry mouth, but usually not to the extent of the drugs listed above.

Several systemic diseases affect salivary secretion. As noted above, most patients with Sjögren's syndrome, some with sarcoidosis, and a few patients with HIV infection experience symptoms of dry mouth of various degrees of severity, with or without salivary gland enlargement (see Table 95–2). In addition, patients who have primary or secondary amyloidosis with salivary gland deposition may develop impaired secretion. Depressed patients not receiving drug treatment for their depression are thought by some to have decreased resting salivary secretion and to complain more frequently of symptoms of dry mouth.

Radiation to the head and neck region for treatment of a malignant tumor usually produces profound xerostomia before therapy is completed, with only a slight recovery of secretory capacity in the months following treatment. Graft-versus-host disease following bone marrow transplantation can also produce xerostomia, but it is usually less severe than that following radiation therapy to the head and neck. Secretory capacity usually recovers when the reaction resolves.

Clinical Management of Patients with Chronic Xerostomia

Severe chronic xerostomia from any cause produces a risk for dental caries in approximate proportion to the impairment of salivary secretion. This secondary caries can largely be prevented if appropriate measures are taken as soon as the xerostomia begins. Remaining teeth should be protected by an adequate dental caries prevention program, monitored by a dentist, that includes daily application of an appropriate topical fluoride and removal of dental plaque, counseling on control of dietary carbohydrates that can cause caries, and placement of dental restorations as necessary.

Chronic erythematous oral candidiasis is a frequent sequela of chronic xerostomia, and its treatment and retreatment, as noted above, improve the patient's oral symptoms.

Symptomatic treatment of mild to moderately severe chronic xerostomia can include sialogogues such as sugarless hard candies or chewing gum, frequent sips of water, and use of saliva substitutes at night. Severe xerostomia, especially that following radiation, can be improved by systemic pilocarpine, 10 to 15 mg three times a day, if not contraindicated.

Ellis GL, Auclair PL, Gnepp DR (eds.): Pathology of the Salivary Glands. Philadelphia, W. B. Saunders Company, 1991. *This current text includes comprehensive discussion of neoplastic, infectious, reactive, and autoimmune salivary gland diseases.*

Genco RJ, Goldman HM, Cohen DW (eds.): Contemporary Periodontics. St Louis, C. V. Mosby Company, 1990. *This text provides thorough and current coverage of the etiology and treatment of localized periodontal diseases and devotes a large section to the effect of systemic conditions on the periodontium.*

Jones JH, Mason DK (eds.): Oral Manifestations of Systemic Diseases 2nd ed. London, Bailliere Tindall, 1990. *This international reference text provides comprehensive coverage of essentially all oral manifestations of systemic diseases.*

Newbrun E: Cariology. 3rd ed. Chicago, Quintessence Books, 1989. *A concise and readable monograph on the causes, prevention, and management of dental caries.*

Regezi JA, Sciubba JJ: Oral Pathology: Clinical-pathologic Correlations. Philadelphia, W. B. Saunders Company, 1989. *This useful and comprehensive text discusses and illustrates the clinical features, differential diagnosis, pathogenesis, and pathology of most diseases affecting the mouth and salivary glands.*

96 Diseases of the Esophagus

Sidney Cohen

The esophagus, a relatively simple organ, is responsible for the transport of materials from the mouth to the stomach and for the prevention of retrograde flow of gastric contents. Antegrade flow is achieved by the act of swallowing with the initiation of primary peristalsis. Gastroesophageal reflux is prevented by the physiologic lower esophageal sphincter.

Disorders of the esophagus occur when one or both of the major esophageal functions become impaired. Abnormalities in esophageal transport may be due to disruption of peristalsis by a neuromuscular disorder or by an organic obstructing lesion. The physiologic lower esophageal sphincter may contribute to transport disorders when relaxation of its tonically elevated pressure is impaired. Disorders of peristaltic function such as achalasia occur together with abnormalities in sphincter relaxation. When the lower esophageal sphincter fails to function as an effective barrier to reflux, the patient develops gastroesophageal reflux with the associated complications of mucosal inflammation (peptic esophagitis).

The symptoms of esophageal disease relate closely to the abnormality in function. Disorders in transport lead to difficulty in swallowing or dysphagia. Abnormal esophageal contraction may cause chest pain. Gastroesophageal reflux leads to heartburn and postural regurgitation of food into the mouth.

The esophagus and its sphincters function through complex neural, humoral, and myogenic mechanisms. The upper esophageal sphincter, pharynx, and upper one third of the esophagus are composed of skeletal muscle. The lower two thirds of the esophagus and the lower esophageal sphincter are smooth muscle. Disorders of skeletal muscle such as polymyositis affect the upper portions of the swallowing mechanism. Disorders of smooth muscles such as scleroderma affect the distal esophagus and the lower esophageal sphincter.

The neurohumoral control of the esophagus is incompletely understood. The initiation of peristalsis by swallowing involves both cholinergic and noncholinergic pathways as well as myogenic mechanisms. The relaxation of the lower esophageal sphincter during swallowing is initiated by nonadrenergic inhibitory nerves in the vagus. These nerves may release vasoactive intestinal peptide (VIP). The sphincter responds to many peptides including gastrin, secretin, substance P, and glucagon. The role of these peptides in the physiologic control of the sphincter is not clear, but they may cause the wide fluctuations in sphincter pressure that follow a meal.

DYSPHAGIA. Consciousness of bolus arrest during swallowing, even if transient, indicates esophageal dysfunction. The patient usually uses the term "sticks," "hesitates," "pauses," or "hangs up" and often indicates the site of arrest with a finger.

Bolus arrest closely associated with the act of swallowing is dysphagia. The sensation of a substernal lump (globus hystericus) present one-half hour after eating is not dysphagia. Most patients consider mild dysphagia a normal phenomenon. "I just swallowed something that was too big." Thus, often they do not spontaneously mention the presence of dysphagia unless questioned closely.

A specialized type of dysphagia occurs when the bolus cannot be propelled from the mouth or hypopharynx into the esophagus, so-called "transfer dysphagia." This type of dysphagia is most commonly related to neurologic disease or to pharyngeal muscle weakness.

The sensation of dysphagia is localized to the suprasternal notch or substernal region. The exact location of the sensation is of little use in pinpointing the site of bolus arrest. Dysphagia for a liquid bolus usually indicates an esophageal motor disorder. Dysphagia for solids can be seen either with an organic obstruction (stricture or cancer) or secondary to esophageal motor disorders.

The patient's response to dysphagia can also provide useful information about the cause of dysphagia. If the bolus must be regurgitated, and if an attempt to force the bolus down with water is met by a sudden return of the fluid, then an organic obstruction should be suspected. If the patient is able to force the bolus down by posturing, by performing a Valsalva's maneuver, by repeated swallowing, or by ingesting fluid, then a motor disorder is more likely. Inexorable progression of dysphagia over months usually signals the presence of organic narrowing, either a lumen-obliterating carcinoma or a stricture caused by active peptic esophagitis.

Dysphagia is never an expression of a purely psychiatric disorder; it is not a manifestation of hysteria. Some patients with well-established esophageal disease such as achalasia report that their dysphagia is often worse at a time of severe emotional tension. Such observations have led many patients (and unfortunately some physicians) to believe that dysphagia is a matter for the psychiatrist rather than the gastroenterologist. Such an opinion can lead to subsequent embarrassment or tragedy, especially if an esophageal carcinoma is overlooked.

ODYNOPHAGIA. Pain upon swallowing, odynophagia, is another cardinal symptom of esophageal disease. Bolus arrest producing dysphagia can sometimes progress to a sensation of pain as esophageal obstruction continues. However, odynophagia usually occurs during the transit of the bolus and disappears once the swallowed material has left the esophagus. It may be mild in intensity so that the patient is merely aware of the location of the swallowed bolus. This is most commonly seen in patients with reflux disease. It can be of such intensity that the patient refuses to swallow any solids or liquids and expectorates saliva. Odynophagia can be seen after involvement of the mucosa by *reflux*, by *radiation*, or by *viral* or *fungal infections*. Odynophagia can be an uncommon manifestation of carcinoma or of a localized ulcer caused by a lodged tablet. Odynophagia thus localizes a process to the esophagus but gives no clue to pathogenesis.

HEARTBURN (PYROSIS). Heartburn or pyrosis is the most common manifestation of esophageal disease, so much so that it is difficult to recruit "normal" subjects, if strict histories are taken to eliminate any who have ever had heartburn. The term "burning" rather than "pain" is usually used, although heartburn can increase in intensity until it is perceived as pain. Patients commonly illustrate heartburn with a movement of the open hand up and down the sternum. This is in contrast to the stationary tightly clenched fist of angina pectoris. Heartburn is usually relieved, even if only temporarily, by taking antacids. A constant burning, unrelieved by antacids, may well be of esophageal origin, but it does not represent heartburn. Heartburn is often worse after recumbency or lifting and may follow overeating or alcoholic indiscretion.

REGURGITATION. Regurgitation of fluid contents into the mouth often accompanies heartburn. Sometimes such regurgitation is associated with eructation; often it accompanies bending over, lifting, or lying down at night. The bitter regurgitated fluid is often described as yellow-brown or green. Regurgitation at night may lead to stridor or to wheezing, a hoarse voice, and other respiratory symptoms from unrecognized reflux. Less commonly, regurgitated fluid is not from the stomach or duodenum, but from fluid retained in an *achalasic esophagus* or in a large

pharyngeal diverticulum. An uncommon but fascinating process that can be confused with regurgitation is *rumination*. In this condition, recently eaten food is propelled back into the mouth from the stomach by a strong contraction of the abdominal wall musculature. The food commonly is rechewed, reswallowed, and again returned to the mouth (Ch. 202).

ESOPHAGEAL COLIC (SPONTANEOUS ESOPHAGEAL PAIN). In addition to the discomfort from severe reflux, which can advance from heartburn into pain, abnormal motor activity of the esophageal muscle can cause severe pain clinically indistinguishable from angina pectoris in terms of intensity, radiation, relationship to exercise, and even response to nitroglycerin. Chest pain of esophageal origin can radiate directly through to the back and is often found in patients who also notice dysphagia. Esophageal colic can last from 5 to 10 seconds to hours.

HEMATEMESIS. Although vomiting blood is less specific for esophageal disease than are many of the symptoms listed above, hematemesis can signal the presence of esophageal varices, of mucosal ulceration resulting from esophageal reflux, of a rent of the mucosa of the lower esophagus, or, uncommonly, of an ulcerating carcinoma or leiomyoma of the esophagus. Although bleeding from the esophagus may be life threatening, more often it is a slow ooze, usually caused by esophageal reflux disease, which presents clinically as an iron deficiency anemia.

Berk JE (ed.): Bockus' Gastroenterology. 4th ed. Philadelphia, W. B. Saunders Company, 1985, pp 666–850. *Reference textbook chapters on esophagus. Good source for recent references.*

Pope CE II: Chapters on the esophagus. *In* Sleisenger MH, Fordtran JS (eds.): Gastrointestinal Disease. 4th ed. Philadelphia, W. B. Saunders Company, 1989. *Reference textbook on esophageal disease.*

GASTROESOPHAGEAL REFLUX DISEASE

DEFINITION. Gastroesophageal reflux disease (GERD) refers to the varied clinical manifestations of reflux of stomach and duodenal contents into the esophagus. It is preferable to the term "reflux esophagitis" because the latter expression tends to mean different things to the clinician, the endoscopist, and the pathologist. Although it may be associated with a sliding hiatus hernia, "symptomatic hiatus hernia" is a term that tends to put the emphasis on the wrong anatomic entity and pathophysiology. Gastroesophageal reflux disease can be characterized by any combination of symptoms and radiologic, endoscopic, or pathologic changes. In its milder manifestations, it is a common disease; its most florid state is uncommon but may be life threatening.

PATHOGENESIS. Several factors must work in concert to produce clinical effects of esophageal reflux. All persons will demonstrate short bursts of reflux if monitored with an intraesophageal pH probe over 24 hours. This reflux is seen postprandially and usually in the upright position. Those in whom reflux has produced symptoms or pathologic changes will demonstrate more prolonged episodes of reflux, which tend to occur at night. The factor or factors that cause this difference are not known. However, important differences between persons with and without reflux might help explain these findings.

The *lower esophageal sphincter* (LES) is a specialized bundle of circular muscle at the lower end of the esophagus with different physical and pharmacologic characteristics when compared with the circular muscle above and below it. There is a tendency for mean LES pressure to be significantly lower in subjects with GERD compared with normal persons, but LES pressures are not very useful in predicting whether reflux is present in an individual patient unless the pressure is very low. The most common event associated with reflux appears to be an *inappropriate relaxation of the lower esophageal sphincter*, i.e., LES relaxation unassociated with either swallowing or the distention of the esophageal body by refluxed fluid. Thus, two abnormalities of LES may be associated with reflux: a sphincter with very low tone, as measured by lower esophageal sphincter pressure, or inappropriate relaxation of a normally competent sphincter.

Several factors are important in removing refluxed material. The upright position facilitates esophageal emptying by gravity. Peristaltic waves initiated by swallowing or by esophageal distention help remove the refluxed material. Acid placed within the esophagus is cleared less well by patients with GERD than by normal subjects, even though the manometric tracings seen in both groups seem identical. Clearing occurs in two phases. The bulk of the fluid is returned to the stomach by a peristaltic contraction; the remainder of the acid film clinging to the esophageal wall is neutralized by swallowed saliva.

The composition and perhaps the quantity of the refluxed material also play a role in the production of GERD. Gastric acid and pepsin seem clearly important in the pathogenesis of GERD. Bile salts and possibly pancreatic enzymes may be responsible in those patients in whom acid is absent. The combination of bile salts plus acid is more injurious to the esophagus than either agent alone. Other less well-studied factors such as altered or abnormal esophageal mucus, swallowed saliva of high bicarbonate content, and diminished resistance of the esophageal mucosa to digestion may be important in determining the amount of mucosal damage in GERD.

Esophageal squamous epithelium reacts to reflux by an increase in the basal cell or germinative layer. The dermal pegs are increased in height and may become more vascular. If the process becomes more severe, the epithelial layer is destroyed, with the appearance of microulcers and classic signs of inflammation in the lamina propria, such as infiltration with polymorphonuclear leukocytes and edema. Even deeper lesions cause first submucosal, then muscular inflammation and fibrosis, resulting in an esophageal stricture. Why reflux is so common, yet inflammation and stricture formation so relatively uncommon, is not known.

Other conditions can be associated with the pathogenesis of reflux. Reflux during pregnancy, once thought to be due to the increased abdominal pressure from the fetus, may be due mainly to diminished LES strength caused by extra estrogen and progesterone. Weight gain also tends to aggravate reflux through an unknown mechanism. As expected, resection of the lower esophageal area for cancer or myotomy for achalasia can lead to severe postoperative reflux (see below). Gastroesophageal reflux with stricture formation is especially severe in patients with progressive systemic sclerosis.

ROLE OF HIATUS HERNIA. The presence of a hiatus hernia is now considered to be much less of a factor in GERD than previously thought. Some radiologists find hiatus hernias in a large percentage of patients, no matter what the reason for the examination. Others rarely demonstrate a hiatus hernia. It is not appropriate to spend a great deal of time trying to define whether a hiatus hernia is present or absent in dealing with most patients with GERD. The important entity to investigate is reflux, not hiatus hernia.

SYMPTOMS OF GASTROESOPHAGEAL REFLUX DISEASE. *Heartburn* is the most common manifestation of GERD. It can vary from an occasional mild burning after overeating to an ever-present, severe discomfort that severely limits a patient's lifestyle. It may be accompanied by *regurgitation* of gastric contents either into the mouth or into the respiratory tree. This latter group of patients may complain of nocturnal wheezing, hoarseness, a need to clear the throat repeatedly, and a sensation of deep pressure at the base of the neck. This group of symptoms may be the primary clinical presentation and more prominent than the classic symptoms of GERD.

Dysphagia is often present in those with significant GERD. Although dysphagia may be severe and even mark the onset of stricture formation, it usually is mild and must be carefully sought. Dysphagia of GERD is for solids, and the dysphagia is usually overcome by swallowing repeatedly or by washing down the bolus with some water. Dysphagia without anatomic strictures has been noted in about three fourths of patients scheduled for antireflux surgery. Many patients with GERD do not complain of bolus arrest, but rather of being aware of the location of each solid morsel as it travels down the esophagus.

Blood loss may result from esophageal erosion and shallow ulcers. Rarely producing life-threatening hemorrhage, the erosions are much more likely to weep quietly over a prolonged period of time, producing iron deficiency anemia. Some of these patients have very few other clinical manifestations of GERD, and the condition is discovered by endoscopy during an evaluation of occult gastrointestinal bleeding. Patients who vigorously and repeatedly abuse alcohol seem prone to develop severe erosive esophagitis with bleeding; this lesion heals with abstinence from alcohol without other major antireflux therapy.

DIAGNOSIS. The history and clinical manifestations of GERD are the most important aids in the establishment of the diagnosis; objective testing is used to quantify the extent and severity of the process. In the evaluation of an individual, questions to be answered dictate the appropriate test.

Does reflux exist and, if so, to what degree? This question might arise either if another condition such as pulmonary disease is present and a causal relationship is being sought, or if some idea of the frequency and extent of reflux is important. Reflux during a barium swallow in adults is uncommon unless vigorous provocative maneuvers are employed. When spontaneous reflux of barium is seen, it usually denotes free reflux. Children reflux barium more easily than do adults. The pH probe can be used either for short-term studies of 15 to 30 minutes or for more prolonged periods (24 hours). If repeated bursts of reflux are demonstrated during a 15-minute period, then severe reflux is present. At the same time, the ability of the esophagus to clear itself of refluxed acid can be evaluated. Usually a manometric catheter is attached to the pH probe in order to locate it in the esophagus; this catheter can also estimate the LES pressure. Very low values of LES pressure such as 1 to 2 mm Hg (normal, about 20 mm Hg) are of prognostic value.

Twenty-four-hour pH monitoring can be performed with a portable unit, which allows the patient to follow an almost normal lifestyle. During the prolonged monitoring period, the relationship between symptoms (heartburn, pain, wheezing) and episodes of reflux can be ascertained, and calculations can be made of the number of episodes of reflux and the amount of time the esophagus is acidified.

Reflux can be measured noninvasively by scanning of the esophageal area with a gamma camera after placing a solution of ^{99m}Tc sulfur colloid in the stomach. An abdominal binder is used to stress the gastroesophageal junction if free reflux is not seen. This technique seems to be of most value in infants and children, who tolerate esophageal tubes very poorly.

Could reflux be responsible for the patient's symptoms? This question might be asked if pain is the predominant symptom rather than more classic heartburn. This question can be answered with the same catheter assembly used to measure LES pressure and acid reflux. After a 5-minute period of dripping normal saline through one of the pressure catheters whose opening has been localized to the upper esophagus, this infusion is changed to 0.1 N hydrochloric acid without the patient's knowledge. Reproduction of the symptoms within 30 minutes of acid infusion (usually 4 to 5 minutes into the infusion) and rapid disappearance of the symptom with a switch back to saline infusion suggests an esophageal cause of the discomfort.

As another approach, the patient is asked to signal the time of discomfort during prolonged pH monitoring of the esophagus. If the patient signals discomfort at the same time that reflux is demonstrated by the pH probe, then a causal relationship is made more likely. Prolonged pH monitoring has shown good correlation between periods of reflux and heartburn as well as other unexplained chest pain syndromes.

What has reflux done to the esophageal mucosa? A barium swallow detects gross changes such as stricture formation or a deep esophageal ulcer but misses the much more common shallow ulcerations and erosions. These are detected by direct inspection with the endoscope. Only discrete lesions such as erosions and ulcerations should be taken as proof of esophageal damage; such endoscopic findings as erythema, edema, or friability are subject to wide interobserver variation. If the mucosa appears absolutely normal, as it is in approximately one third of patients with moderate to severe symptoms of GERD, a biopsy can demonstrate the changes of reflux.

A logic tree of how these tests might be used is shown in Table 96–1. A patient whose symptoms are severe enough to seek medical attention might be screened with a barium swallow. Uncommonly, reflux is demonstrated, a stricture found, or a deep ulcer seen. This might lead to immediate endoscopy for more complete evaluation. If a patient presents with hematemesis and reflux symptoms, endoscopy might appropriately be used as the first step. After first evaluation, it is appropriate to begin therapy (see Treatment, below). Only if there is a poor response to therapy should an acid perfusion test be used to confirm the diagnosis. At the same time, the presence of reflux can be checked, an estimate of LES pressure and acid clearance obtained, and the presence or absence of peristaltic waves determined.

More intensive therapy should be instituted at this point. If it

TABLE 96–1. DIAGNOSIS OF REFLUX

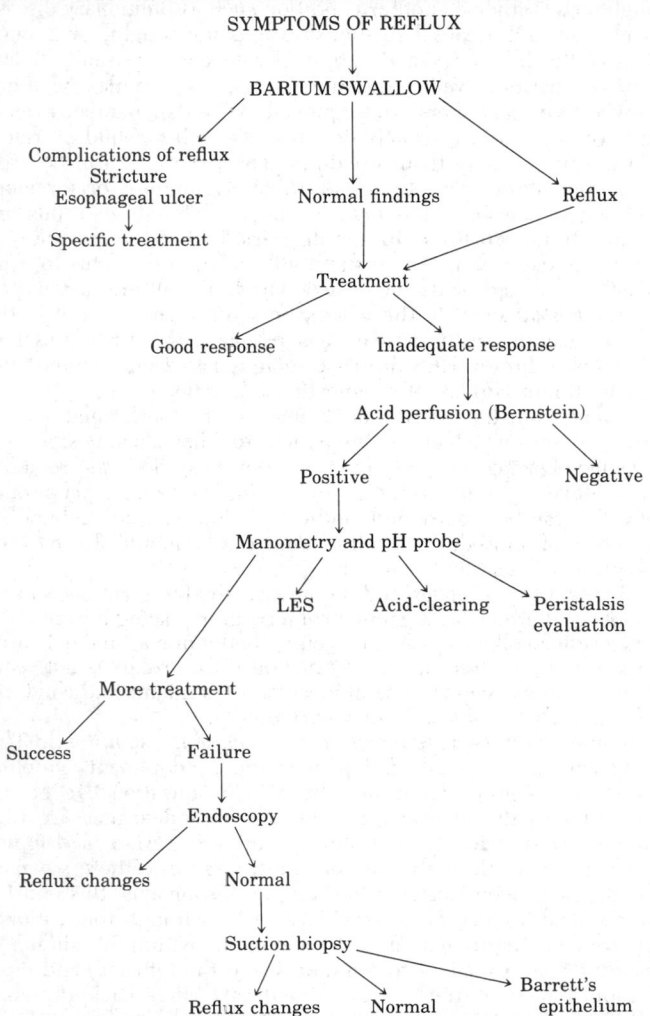

SYMPTOMS OF REFLUX

BARIUM SWALLOW

Complications of reflux
Stricture
Esophageal ulcer

Specific treatment

Normal findings

Reflux

Treatment

Good response

Inadequate response

Acid perfusion (Bernstein)

Positive

Negative

Manometry and pH probe

LES

Acid-clearing

Peristalsis evaluation

More treatment

Success

Failure

Endoscopy

Reflux changes

Normal

Suction biopsy

Reflux changes

Normal

Barrett's epithelium

---

fails and the patient is still symptomatic, endoscopy can be employed to see if gross disease is still present in the face of maximal therapy. If the appearance of the mucosa is normal grossly in the presence of overwhelming symptoms, biopsies can be obtained to search for objective evidence of reflux damage. This scheme will restrict extensive testing to those who have failed medical therapy and who are presumably candidates for surgical treatment. This algorithm can be modified if the patient has blood loss or severe dysphagia. Endoscopy is now being more widely used as the initial diagnostic study because of its overall sensitivity and specificity.

COMPLICATIONS OF GASTROESOPHAGEAL REFLUX DISEASE. Esophageal Stricture. Of the many who complain of symptoms of GERD, only a few develop esophageal strictures. Usually beginning at the lower end of the esophagus, strictures may migrate over years to the midesophagus or higher. Columnar epithelium is found below the stricture. Presumably those who develop strictures have had deep circumferential ulceration of the esophageal mucosa due to reflux damage. Instead of healing with only minimal submucosal and muscular fibrosis, these patients develop esophageal obstruction with a narrowed esophageal lumen. If reflux can be controlled, these strictures disappear.

Dysphagia is the clinical hallmark of esophageal stricture formation. Unlike the relatively mild dysphagia seen in uncomplicated GERD, the dysphagia in patients with strictures tends to be constant and slowly progressive, causing the patient to alter the type of food taken. If a bolus becomes arrested in the stricture, it is usually necessary for the bolus to be regurgitated back into the mouth before further intake of food or fluids is possible.

Strictures are most easily evaluated by barium swallow. Sometimes the extent of the strictured area is overestimated unless the esophagus below the stricture can be fully distended by barium. For mild strictures, the ingestion of a bread or marshmallow bolus can draw attention to slight luminal narrowing when the bolus impacts there. Once demonstrated, endoscopy with biopsy and/or brush cytology is in order to make certain that the stricture is benign.

Esophageal Ulcer. In addition to the more common shallow ulcerations, deep esophageal ulcers may complicate severe GERD. These ulcers, which retain barium and usually project outside the wall of the esophagus, characteristically produce severe and unrelenting pain, often with radiation of the pain through to the back. Brisk hemorrhage is another manifestation, from erosion either through to an esophageal artery or, more catastrophically, into the nearby aorta. The presence of an ulcer can be suspected on a barium swallow and confirmed endoscopically. The ulcer is usually found to reside in columnar (Barrett's) epithelium.

Columnar Epithelium. In some patients who have suffered severe esophageal ulceration as a result of GERD, the healing epithelium is replaced not with squamous epithelium but with a specialized columnar epithelium. The junctional zone between squamous and columnar epithelium can progress orad over years. Columnar epithelium is found at and below midesophageal strictures and around deep esophageal ulcers, although it can be found on routine biopsy of patients with severe GERD. Its major clinical importance is not only as a marker of severe reflux but also as a precursor for adenocarcinoma of the esophagus (see under Esophageal Tumors).

Pulmonary Aspiration. If refluxed material breaches the upper esophageal sphincter, it may easily spill into the larynx and tracheobronchial tree. Some patients react to such a spill with intense respiratory stridor. Others seem to tolerate the presence of refluxed contents in the larynx and tracheobronchial tree with milder laryngeal or respiratory symptoms. It is even possible that the gastric contents do not have to reach the larynx; instillation of acid in the esophagus of susceptible individuals while they are in the upright posture can be shown to cause closing of small bronchial airways by a vagal reflex.

None of the clinical features of pulmonary aspiration (Table 96–2) is pathognomonic. Taken together they point toward reflux and aspiration as a possible etiology. Diagnostic proof of the relationship is difficult with current techniques. Radioisotopes placed in the stomach have been demonstrated the next morning to be in the lungs by gamma camera scanning, but this cannot be demonstrated in the majority of patients. Only correction of reflux with subsequent disappearance of pulmonary symptoms can prove the relationship.

TREATMENT OF GASTROESOPHAGEAL REFLUX DISEASE AND ITS COMPLICATIONS. Medical Management. Most mildly symptomatic patients with reflux and some moderately afflicted individuals can be helped by manipulations designed to alter the frequency or type of esophageal reflux. Many patients respond to the simple measures outlined in Table 96–3. Elevation of the head of the bed by 6 to 8 inches is the simplest and most effective form of therapy. Twenty-four-hour pH monitoring has shown that this simple measure decreases the frequency and length of reflux episodes. The use of pillows to elevate the thorax does not work well, as patients tend to roll off the pillows during the night. A foam rubber wedge can be used if the bed frame cannot be moved. Avoiding food and fluid for at least 3 hours before retiring decreases the amount of material available for reflux at night. Avoidance of food that the patient finds distressing, such as fatty foods, chocolate, and onions, makes sense but has never been subjected to clinical trial.

TABLE 96–2. CLINICAL FEATURES OF PULMONARY ASPIRATION

1. Onset of "asthma" in patients over 30 years of age without a family history of asthma or industrial exposure
2. Nocturnal or early morning cough
3. Nocturnal wheezing
4. Hoarseness, especially on arising
5. The need to clear the throat repeatedly
6. A feeling of constant pressure deep in the neck

TABLE 96-3. TREATMENT OF GASTROESOPHAGEAL REFLUX DISEASE

Simple measures
1. Elevation of head of the bed
2. Avoidance of food and fluid intake before bedtime
3. Reduction of fat in diet
4. Liquid antacid (aluminum hydroxide, magnesium hydroxide) 1 and 3 hours after meals and at bedtime
5. Avoidance of cigarettes and alcohol
6. Weight loss

Measures for resistant cases
1. Alginic acid–antacid (Gaviscon), 15 ml four times a day
2. Bethanechol (Urecholine),* 10 or 25 mg four times a day
3. Metoclopramide (Reglan),* 10 mg three times a day
4. Cimetidine,* 300 mg four times a day
5. Ranitidine,* 150 mg twice a day
6. Famotidine,* 20 mg twice a day
7. Omeprazole,* 20 mg every day
8. Fundoplication

*Higher doses of an H_2 antagonist or omeprazole may be required in some cases.

Neutralization of acid is approached by taking 30 ml of aluminum hydroxide-magnesium hydroxide antacid 1 and 3 hours after meals and at bedtime. In recalcitrant cases, hourly antacids may be tried, with substitution of pure aluminum hydroxide gel to control diarrhea produced by the magnesium ion. Most patients do not tolerate such a regimen for long.

An attempt should be made to have the patient stop smoking, drinking alcohol, and overeating. Most patients, however, apparently prefer to suffer with reflux symptoms rather than to give up these mainstays of life.

If these simple measures are not effective, more vigorous treatment is indicated. Alginic acid-antacid, 15 ml after each meal and at bedtime, is more effective than placebo and as effective as antacids. It is worth trying but often does not control symptoms of severe reflux. Bethanechol, a parasympathomimetic agent, can be used in doses of 10 or 25 mg four times a day. Metoclopramide, 10 mg three times a day, can be helpful, but central nervous system side effects limit its usefulness.

The H_2 antagonists in the usual dosage range for duodenal ulcer improve symptoms of heartburn better than a placebo. Higher dosage regimens, cimetidine 800 mg, ranitidine 300 mg, or famotidine 40 mg, each twice per day, have been more effective for control of symptoms and healing of peptic esophagitis. Healing of esophageal erosions with H_2 antagonists usually takes 12 to 16 weeks.

The potassium-hydrogen ATPase inhibitor, omeprazole, 20 mg once per day, can sometimes give dramatic symptom relief and healing of esophagitis in 4 to 8 weeks.

Once healing has been achieved with either an H_2 antagonist or omeprazole, recurrence rates exceed 80 per cent if no maintenance therapy is utilized. Maintenance therapy for esophagitis generally requires full dosage, in contrast to the reduced maintenance dose used for duodenal ulcer.

Surgical Management. In a patient in whom adequate trial of medical management as outlined above has not brought good results in a 6-month period, and in whom there is good objective evidence of reflux, surgical correction of reflux should be considered. Current surgical therapy, regardless of exact techniques, attempts to restore sphincter competence by surrounding the lower end of the esophagus with a cuff of gastric fundal muscle. This is done either completely, as in the Nissen fundoplication, or partially (Hill repair, Belsey repair).

A well-done fundoplication can restore a competent lower esophageal sphincter, reduce gastroesophageal reflux, heal peptic esophagitis, and even lead to reversal of peptic stricture. Barrett's epithelium may regress in a limited number of cases, but usually the columnar epithelium does not disappear. The Nissen fundoplication seems to provide the most satisfactory long-term improvement.

A surgeon experienced in the techniques of antireflux surgery is necessary for good postoperative results. Technique is all important. Although some individual surgeons have enviable postoperative results, antireflux surgery has a relatively poor reputation in many medical communities. Currently, a conservative approach toward antireflux surgery seems indicated.

Treatment of Complications. Esophageal strictures, if only mildly symptomatic, can be handled by careful attention to dietary intake, improvement of dentition, and institution of medical therapy. Techniques of dilation have proliferated in recent years, but they still require an experienced operator. Short, simple strictures can be dilated with weighted rubber or Teflon dilators (Hurst, Maloney). Tortuous or angulated strictures are more easily approached over a previously placed guide wire. This, in turn, can be passed through an endoscope or under radiographic control. Graded steel olives (Eder-Peustow), a dilator with graded increases of size (Celestin), or a balloon with a fixed maximal diameter (Cooke) can be passed over the previously placed wire. Alternatively, a balloon of fixed maximal diameter can be passed through the large channel of an endoscope during diagnostic endoscopy, and dilation can be done under direct vision. Once the lumen is restored to a diameter of 13 to 15 mm, most patients swallow without difficulty. If the stricture is stable and requires dilation only every 4 to 6 months, nothing else is necessary.

Some patients do not tolerate dilation or require vigorous dilation every 3 to 4 weeks. This is an indication for definitive antireflux operation, following which the stricture may regress. Unfortunately, many strictures persist after attempts at antireflux surgery. Esophageal replacement by colon, jejunum, or stomach is a surgical maneuver of last resort; such procedures have relatively high morbidity and mortality. Those afflicted by strictures may have significant lung and cardiovascular disease that makes them unsuitable operative candidates. The use of high-dose H_2 antagonists or preferably omeprazole along with dilation of the stricture has led to healing of the mucosa and lower requirements for repeated stricture dilation.

Esophageal ulcers also represent a major therapeutic problem. Although cimetidine therapy may heal an ulcer, antireflux surgery, if tolerated, is a more reliable mode of treatment. If not, gastric radiation can be employed as in esophageal stricture.

Columnar epithelium may be premalignant. There is no way short of esophageal resection to make certain that the epithelium can be removed. Adequate antireflux therapy causes regression of columnar epithelium in a rare patient, but further study is necessary before antireflux surgery can be recommended as a treatment for columnar epithelium. The effect of omeprazole therapy on the columnar epithelium is not known. Currently, columnar epithelium is followed closely with periodic endoscopic biopsies to look for dysplasia and early changes of adenocarcinoma. Dysplasia can be graded using specific criteria. The persistence of confirmed high-grade dysplasia is an indication for esophagectomy.

Treatment of the pulmonary complications of reflux depends on the age of the patient. Infants who present with recurrent bronchitis can be treated by postural methods and by thickening the formula. In adults, attention to posture at night is most important (see above). Since diagnostic methods that establish a direct causal relationship between reflux and lung disease are lacking, caution is advised in offering surgery to those who present with primary pulmonary problems and in whom reflux is demonstrated.

Castell DO, Wu WC, Ott DS: Gastroesophageal Reflux Disease. Mt. Kisco, NY, Futura Publishing Company, 1985, pp 1–324. *Monograph with good literature review.*

Spechler SJ, Goyal RK: Barrett's esophagus. N Engl J Med 315:362, 1986. *Up-to-date review of columnar epithelium.*

MOTOR DISORDERS OF THE ESOPHAGUS

DEFINITION AND PATHOGENESIS. The muscular tube of the esophagus is guarded at both ends by specialized bundles of muscle, the upper and lower esophageal sphincters (UES, LES). Material from the oropharynx is injected at a high velocity (in the case of liquids), and precise coordination is required to link the muscles of the oropharynx, UES, body of the esophagus, and LES into a functional unit. Failure of any or all of these components results in an esophageal motor disorder.

Failure of the oropharyngeal and UES units can be caused either by primary muscle disease such as *myotonia dystrophica* or *dermatomyositis* or by neurologic lesions involving the innervation of these muscle groups. *Brain stem infarcts, multiple sclerosis,* and *amyotrophic lateral sclerosis* serve as examples for the latter process.

The pathogenesis of motor abnormality of the esophageal body is less well understood. The striated muscle that constitutes the upper one quarter to one third of the body can be affected by primary muscle disease, such as *myotonia dystrophica,* or by metabolic disease affecting muscle function, such as *hypothyroidism.* The smooth muscle seems more resistant to muscular disease, but the intrinsic nervous network can be involved in *Chagas' disease* and *achalasia.* In the latter disease, there is infiltration of Auerbach's plexus with lymphocytes or actual disappearance of the neuron cell bodies in the plexus.

The motor disorders of the body of the esophagus have historically been classified as *achalasia* or *diffuse spasm.* In achalasia, dysphagia and esophageal retention predominate; the radiograph shows a dilated esophagus with a distal beak, and manometry reveals a high pressure in the LES with no or incomplete relaxation as well as only simultaneous low-amplitude contractions in response to a swallow. Diffuse spasm has been characterized as a clinical syndrome of esophageal colic or dysphagia or both; segmental contractions seen by radiograph; and a manometric picture of some peristaltic waves interspersed with periods of slight simultaneous elevation of the baseline pressure in several leads surmounted by simultaneous contractions. Another common manometric abnormality is high-amplitude, long-duration waves that are peristaltic and can be associated with either esophageal colic or dysphagia or both (nutcracker esophagus). There are many variations of these "classic" diseases, and progression from diffuse spasm to achalasia has been documented in the same individual. Many nonspecific motor disorders of the esophagus do not fit these syndromes. The pathophysiology of these nonspecific disorders has not been described. It seems best at the present state of knowledge to be descriptive of the features of a motor disorder without being too precise about an actual name of the disorder.

SYMPTOMS. The type of symptom produced is a function of the level and extent of the problem. *Weakness of the oropharyngeal musculature* may cause *transfer dysphagia*—the inability to propel a solid or liquid bolus from the pharynx to the esophagus. Patients are aware usually that they cannot begin the act of deglutition. Solids are usually more troublesome than liquids. Palatal weakness may lead to *nasal regurgitation* of fluids or to *laryngeal aspiration* because of muscular failure to seal off the larynx. Such weakness may be signaled by a nasal quality of the voice.

Incoordination of UES relaxation has been suggested as a cause of transfer dysphagia and for the production of Zenker's diverticulum, but current high-fidelity methods fail to show such incoordination. Transfer dysphagia accompanied by a prominent cricopharyngeal impression on a barium swallow ("cricopharyngeal achalasia") similarly shows no defect in relaxing or in timing when studied by modern manometric methods.

Motor disorders in the body of the esophagus produce either *dysphagia* or *pain,* or both. The dysphagia may be intermittent or continuous. It may be manifest both for solids and for liquids. It is rare for the arrested material to be regurgitated; often posturing (throwing the shoulders back and extending the neck) or a Valsalva maneuver helps the material pass into the stomach.

Pain or esophageal colic is the other major clinical presentation of motor disorders. The pain is usually substernal, described as a feeling of pressure or aching, radiating to the back as well as to the neck, jaw, and arms. It can range in intensity from a transient discomfort to an overwhelming, agonizing pain similar to that of a major myocardial infarction or dissecting aortic aneurysm. The pain may last for only 5 to 10 seconds or may be present for hours. The differentiation between angina pectoris and esophageal colic may be impossible on clinical grounds; both may be related to exercise, have the same intensity and distribution, and respond to sublingual nitroglycerin.

Failure of the lower esophageal sphincter may present with two separate symptom complexes. If the sphincter fails to relax on deglutition (as occurs in achalasia), dysphagia and retention of contents in the body of the esophagus occur. This failure, coupled with loss of peristalsis (achalasia), leads to marked esophageal

retention, regurgitation, and overflow of esophageal contents into the tracheobronchial tree. If there is primary muscle failure of the sphincter, as occurs in *scleroderma,* massive reflux and the consequences of GERD follow.

DIAGNOSIS. A careful history is essential in choosing the correct diagnostic tools for evaluating esophageal motor disorders. If the difficulty is thought to be in the oropharynx and upper esophageal sphincter, a cineradiograph would offer the most information. The cine film allows for frame-by-frame analysis of this rapidly moving portion of the gastrointestinal tract. Incoordination of tongue and palate, unilateral pharyngeal weakness, and aspiration of small amounts of barium into the trachea on swallowing can be shown. Air double-contrast examinations of the pharynx can elucidate an unsuspected hypopharyngeal carcinoma. A diverticulum or prominence of the cricopharyngeal muscle can also be seen. Manometric examination of the hypopharynx and upper esophageal sphincter has not been helpful.

Radiology offers the best chance of diagnosis when the motor disorders have relatively static changes. In achalasia the body of the esophagus commonly dilates with retention of food, secretions, and barium (Fig. 96–1). Special attention can be paid to the terminal end of the esophagus. In achalasia, there is a smooth, tapering beak. Any irregularity of this beak should lead to a vigorous search for an infiltrating neoplasm of the cardia, which can exactly mimic achalasia clinically and radiologically.

If the esophageal muscle is atonic, as is seen in far-advanced scleroderma, barium and even air are retained for long periods of time in the supine position. Assumption of the upright position rapidly clears the barium from the esophagus and leaves a double-contrast view of a dilated esophagus.

The radiologist has more difficulty when the motor abnormality is more intermittent (Fig. 96–2). Such a radiologic appearance is not always evidence for a clinically important motor disorder; elderly patients often show similar radiologic findings and yet are totally asymptomatic.

Manometric examination allows more prolonged evaluation of esophageal motor function and is the only method that allows lower esophageal sphincter function to be directly determined. Normally, a swallow causes a peristaltic wave to be detected sequentially by pressure detectors spaced along the esophagus.

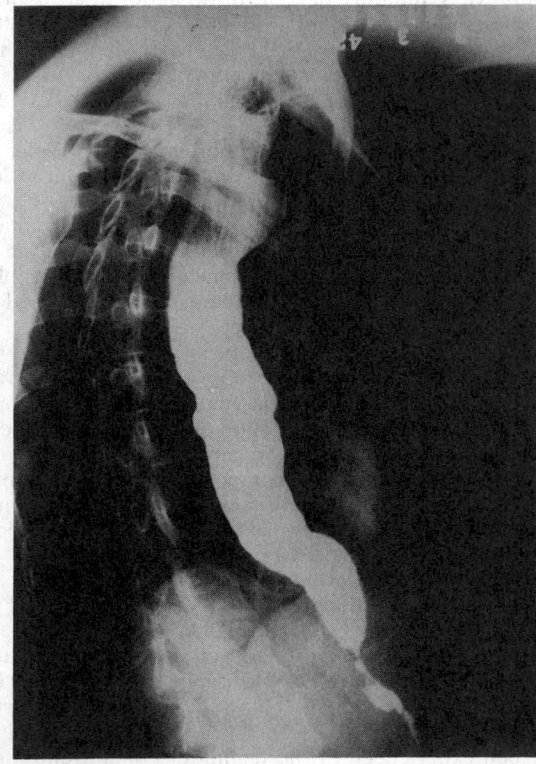

FIGURE 96–1. Radiologic appearance of achalasia. The esophageal body is dilated and terminates in a narrowed segment. (Courtesy of Dr. FE Templeton. From Pope CE II: *In* Sleisenger MH, Fordtran JS [eds.]: Gastrointestinal Disease. 3rd ed. Philadelphia, W. B. Saunders Company, 1983.)

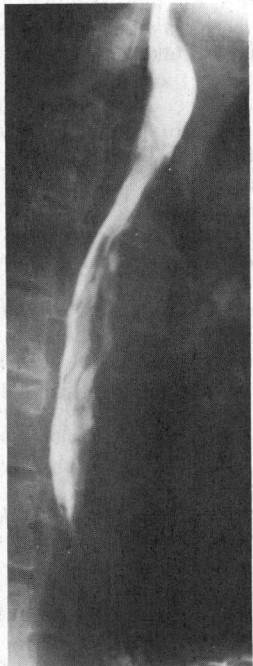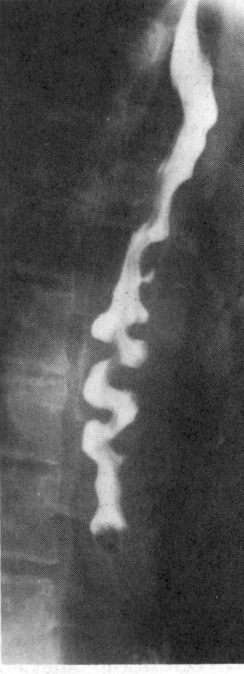

FIGURE 96–2. Radiologic appearance of diffuse spasm. Two spot films were taken within 10 seconds of each other. A fairly normal appearance on the left changes rapidly to an appearance of numerous contractions. (Courtesy of Dr. CA Rohrmann. From Pope CE II: *In* Sleisenger MH, Fordtran JS [eds.]: Gastrointestinal Disease. 3rd ed. Philadelphia, W. B. Saunders Company, 1983.)

Aperistalsis (no response to a swallow), simultaneous single or multiple contractions, prolonged contractions of high amplitude and low velocity, and spontaneous activity not related to swallowing can be recorded. Some of the "classic" patterns associated with diseases are shown in Figure 96–3. Many subjects present with dysphagia and/or chest pain in different patterns. It is best to describe the radiologic and manometric findings in the individual patient and then try to relate them to the classic syndrome most closely resembled. Also, one syndrome (diffuse spasm) may progress over time to another (achalasia).

Manometric examination can be of special benefit in the evaluation of chest pain if the patient happens to have an attack of chest pain during the examination. If the chest pain is accompanied by motor activity that allows the manometrist to predict onset, intensity, and disappearance of the chest pain by watching the manometric tracing, the diagnosis of an esophageal origin of chest pain is firmly established. Similarly, if pH is being simultaneously monitored and the episodes of chest pain correlate closely with drops in intraesophageal pH, an esophageal origin of pain is likely. Conversely, if typical chest pain occurs but there is no change in motor activity or pH over control values, an esophageal cause of pain is unlikely. Unfortunately, such definitive statements can be made only in about 20 per cent of the patients examined.

Pharmacologic stimulation of the esophagus has been employed for diagnostic purposes using such agents as mecholyl, pentagastrin, bethanechol, and edrophonium. Edrophonium (Tensilon) is the most widely used provocative agent for inducing chest pain along with simultaneous esophageal spasm. The cholinesterase inhibitor is short acting and extremely safe in clinical usage. Provocative testing has been helpful in delineating the cause of chest pain in patients with normal baseline esophageal manometry.

Endoscopy is useful in the evaluation of motor disorders, for inspection of the cardia with a retroflexed view from the stomach to rule out an infiltrating carcinoma, and for excluding inflammatory disorders.

TREATMENT. Of the various motor disorders of the esophagus, *achalasia* seems most amenable to relief. Since the problem in achalasia is one of obstruction of the lower end of the esophagus by a sphincter that does not relax, all forms of therapy are directed at relief of this obstruction. Short-term improvement in clinical symptoms and in scintigraphic esophageal emptying may occur with isosorbide dinitrate, a long-acting nitrate, or with nifedipine, a calcium channel blocker. The place of long-term pharmacologic management of achalasia has not been established. Dilation with a large Hurst bougie may give temporary relief; a few patients have been maintained for long periods of time with weekly self-dilations, but this treatment is no longer recommended. Much more effective is dilation with a pneumatic bag under radiographic control. This should be performed by an expert, since perforation even in good hands may occur in about 5 per cent of patients. Pneumatic dilation is preferable initially for all patients.

Surgery is reserved for those in whom bag dilation fails or those who do not wish to be exposed to the risk of perforation. Direct section of the lower esophageal sphincter muscle (my-

FIGURE 96–3. Idealized manometric patterns. *A,* The normal swallow consists of a progressive wave with a wave of short duration and rapid rise time in the striated upper esophagus. The lower esophageal sphincter shows a fall in pressure coincident with swallowing. *B,* In achalasia the striated muscle sometimes, but not always, produces a typical wave. The smooth muscle portion of the esophagus has a simultaneous low-amplitude contraction that follows the striated muscle contraction. The elevated pressure in the LES shows either incomplete or no relaxation. *C,* Diffuse spasm shows an elevation of the baseline after swallowing, on top of which are superimposed repetitive simultaneous contractions. LES pressure may be high and relaxation may terminate prematurely. *D,* High-amplitude, long-duration waves (nutcracker esophagus). The wave is peristaltic but of high amplitude. Duration is increased and velocity of propagation may be decreased. *E,* Scleroderma. Striated muscle contraction is normal, but the amplitude of contraction in the smooth muscle is reduced or may be absent. Sphincter pressure is low.

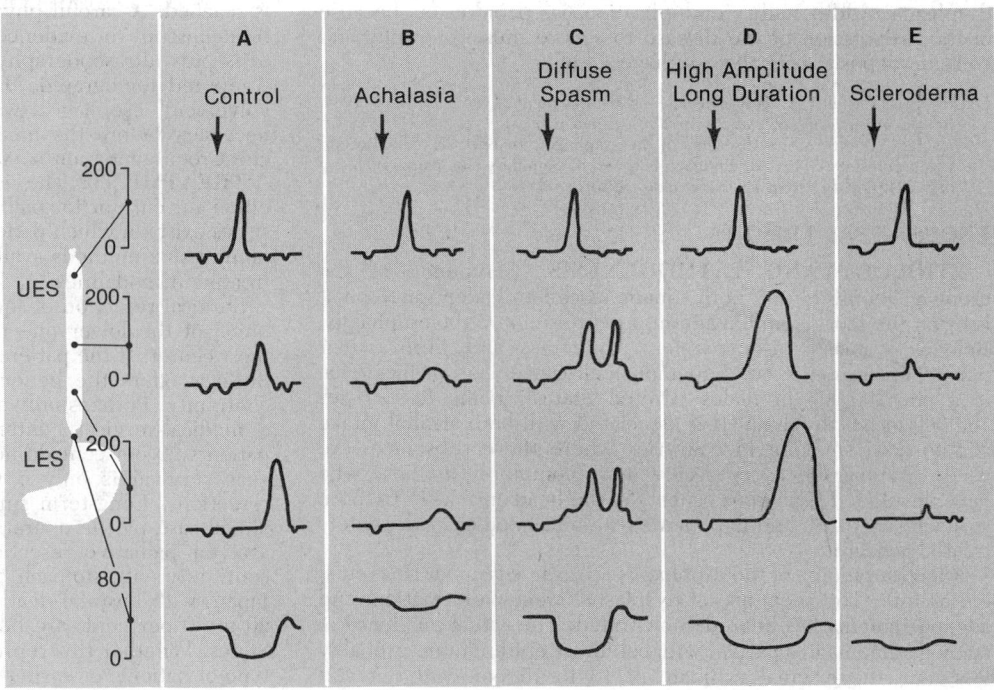

otomy) is carried out, sparing some gastric muscle fibers to prevent postoperative reflux (Heller procedure). Amazingly, after both bag dilation and myotomy, manometry reveals return of normal peristalsis in 10 per cent of those with achalasia. Many surgeons currently combine a "loose" fundoplication along with the Heller myotomy. Postoperative gastroesophageal reflux with esophagitis and peptic stricture of the esophagus may occur in patients if the myotomy abolishes all lower esophageal sphincter pressure and if no fundoplication is performed. This observation is difficult to explain in view of the degeneration of Auerbach's plexus in the intramural nervous network, thought to explain the pathogenesis of this disease.

Treatment of most other motor disorders is much more difficult. Patients with diffuse spasm can be given nitroglycerin, anticholinergics, or calcium channel antagonists. Balloon dilation has also been suggested to be of benefit in diffuse spasm and has been helpful in those patients with abnormal lower esophageal function, high basal tone with impaired relaxation. Division of all the circular muscle with a long myotomy has been tried, but the long-term results of this procedure are not always favorable.

Treatment of other nonspecific motor disorders associated with chest pain can be equally frustrating. Prescribing sublingual nitroglycerin is justifiable. If it is ineffective, long-acting nitrate therapy will probably not work. Anticholinergic drugs benefit only a few. Calcium channel antagonists reduce the force of the esophageal contractions and relieve pain. Meperidine (Demerol) has been uniformly useful. Obviously this medication is not a good long-term solution to the problem. Long myotomies have been tried in selected patients; occasional good long-term results have been obtained. It would seem wise not to subject any patient to myotomy until that patient has been observed manometrically during an attack and an esophageal origin of pain has been firmly established. Recently, a form of microvascular coronary artery disease has been suggested as a cause of chest pain in patients with "nutcracker" esophagus. The description of this new cardiac disease has further confused this field and has emphasized the reluctance to perform long esophageal myotomies in patients with esophageal chest pain.

The treatment of *scleroderma* and other conditions marked by aperistalsis revolves mostly around the associated reflux. If there is no obstruction at the lower end of the esophagus, either by a malfunctioning sphincter or by an organic narrowing, aperistalsis is amazingly well tolerated, usually with only mild dysphagia for solids. Caution should be employed in offering antireflux surgery to patients with scleroderma, as a tight fundoplication without any peristalsis in the body of the esophagus leads to severe dysphagia. Additionally, fundoplication has poor results because of the progression of the disease to severe muscle atrophy and collagen deposition in the esophageal wall.

Blackwell JN, Castell DO: Oesophageal chest pain: A point of view. Gut 25:1, 1984. *Review of the esophagus as a source of anginal pain.*
Ouyang A, Cohen S: Motor disorders of the esophagus. *In* Berk JE (ed.): Bockus' Gastroenterology. 4th ed. Philadelphia, W. B. Saunders Company, 1985, pp 690–704. *Good current review of motor disorders.*

ESOPHAGEAL TUMORS

ETIOLOGY AND PATHOGENESIS. Carcinoma of the esophageal epithelium, both squamous cell and adenocarcinoma, is by far the most common and important tumor of the esophagus. Benign neoplasms (leiomyoma, papilloma, and fibrovascular polyps) are rarer by far. Squamous cell cancer has an incidence of 4 per 100,000 in males (United States), rising to 130 per 100,000 in North China. It is associated with both alcohol intake and tobacco smoking in countries where these substances are used. Esophageal cancer occurs more commonly in those who have developed squamous cancers of the head and neck, in those with lye strictures, and in patients with untreated or inadequately treated achalasia.

Adenocarcinoma of the esophagus arises in columnar (Barrett's) epithelium. The sequence of dysplasia, adenoma formation, and adenocarcinoma has been demonstrated. The actual incidence of adenocarcinoma in a patient with columnar epithelium is probably less than the original estimate of 10 to 15 per cent but still represents a significant problem.

SYMPTOMS. In Western countries, the most common clinical symptom of carcinoma is *progressive dysphagia* over a 6- to 8-month period until only liquids can be taken. The obstruction reflects circumferential involvement of the esophageal wall by tumor and does not occur until the cancer is biologically rather far advanced. The dysphagia may be accompanied by a *steady, boring pain*, which signals mediastinal involvement and inoperability. In the Orient but not in the United States, pain is often a relatively early sign of a localized and thus resectable tumor. Unexplained persistent chest pain should always be investigated by a careful double-contrast radiographic view of the esophagus or by endoscopy.

More advanced lesions manifest themselves with *halitosis, weight loss,* and *coughing after drinking fluid*. The last-named symptom is caused either by nearly complete esophageal lumen obstruction with overspill into the larynx or by the development of a tracheoesophageal fistula. Hoarseness from involvement of the recurrent laryngeal nerve by tumor and hematemesis are unusual symptoms. Nail bed clubbing can be seen with both benign and malignant tumors.

Since dysphagia is the most common presenting symptom of neoplasm of the esophagus, the physician is responsible for making absolutely certain that cancer is not the cause of dysphagia. Early diagnosis affords the only chance for cure. Early diagnosis allows the patient, family, and physician to plan better all aspects of the patient's future.

DIAGNOSIS. The clinical suspicion of a cancer of the esophagus should lead immediately to an esophagogram, possibly with double-contrast techniques. Any irregularity, especially if it narrows the lumen, mandates further evaluation. If dysphagia is present, the radiologist should give a bolus of barium-soaked bread or a large marshmallow to discover any possible sites of arrest.

In the presence of symptoms but a normal barium swallow, endoscopy with biopsy and brushing of any suspicious lesion for examination of tissue and of exfoliated cells is indicated. The endoscopist should always obtain a good retroflexed view of the cardia from below to make certain that an adenocarcinoma of the gastroesophageal junction has not been overlooked.

If narrowing has been seen by barium swallow, endoscopy with biopsy and cytologic brushings of the involved area must be done. With the fiberoptic endoscope, numerous blind biopsies from as deep in the lesion as possible will be most helpful. Biopsy of visible tissue will often reveal only inflammatory tissue. Sometimes as many as eight or nine biopsies must be obtained before tumor is recovered.

Once a tumor is identified, certain procedures in addition to chest films are essential for staging before a therapeutic decision is reached. A careful physical examination for nodal metastases, bronchoscopy for evidence of tracheal involvement, liver function tests plus ultrasonography for evidence of liver metastases, and computed tomographic (CT) scanning for mediastinal nodal involvement, esophageal wall thickness, and liver metastases are necessary before the final therapeutic plan is decided upon. A chest roentgenogram is mandatory.

TREATMENT. The ideal treatment of esophageal cancer, either for cure or for palliation, has not yet been developed. No series exists in which patients were carefully staged with the best noninvasive methods available and then randomized to different treatment modalities.

Surgical resection of squamous cell carcinoma and adenocarcinoma of the lower one third of the esophagus is preferred in most centers if the patient does not have widespread metastases. Surgery offers the benefit of rapidly restoring esophagogastric continuity. Perhaps only one quarter of all patients presenting to a medical-surgical center have a resectable tumor; of these patients 20 per cent do not survive the operative period, and 5-year survival is only 5 to 10 per cent, even with extensive resections. Long-term survival cannot be predicted in the individual case by the operative findings. There is growing enthusiasm for palliative resection with restoration of gastrointestinal continuity with stomach or colon. Surgical results in China and Japan, with hospital deaths of 5 per cent and 5-year survivals of 20 to 30 per cent, are better than those quoted for the United States. Whether this represents better technical skill, a different type of patient, or earlier diagnosis is not certain.

Radiotherapy is employed in lesions of the upper one third of the esophagus and often in middle third tumors as well. This form of therapy has little hospital mortality, although it carries some short-term and long-term morbidity. With ideal home situations, radiotherapy can be carried out on an outpatient basis. Approximately 40 per cent of tumors cannot be destroyed with conventional 6000-rad therapy. Combination of pre- and postoperative radiation with resective therapy has been employed, but there is no good evidence that such combined therapy is better. Adenocarcinomas occasionally respond to radiotherapy but are not as radiosensitive as squamous cell carcinomas.

When obvious extraesophageal spread is present, palliation with bougienage to restore and maintain an adequate esophageal lumen may be done. If performed with a guide wire under fluoroscopic guidance, such therapy is not hazardous in skilled hands. If dilation does not offer lasting relief, then a Silastic tube can be placed perorally for relief of esophageal obstruction. Such tubes are also of great benefit in the treatment of a malignant tracheoesophageal fistula. Another useful approach is the destruction of intraluminal tumor and restoration of an adequate lumen by laser therapy or an intraluminal heatcoagulating probe.

Choice of therapy will depend on the location and size of the lesion, presence or absence of spread, cell type, and the skills of the medical community. Until an adequate randomized trial after adequate staging is carried out, choice of treatment modality will continue to be a matter of preference.

Earlam R, Cunha-Melo JR: Oesophageal squamous cell carcinoma. Br J Surg 67:381, 457, 1980. *Two articles present exhaustive literature reviews of surgical and radiotherapy of esophageal carcinoma.*

Livstone EM: General considerations of tumors of the esophagus. *In* Berk JE (ed.): Bockus' Gastroenterology. 4th ed. Philadelphia, W. B. Saunders Company, 1985, pp 818–840. *Review of diagnostic and therapeutic considerations in esophageal carcinoma.*

OTHER CONDITIONS

RINGS AND WEBS. During early development, the lumen of the esophagus becomes completely obliterated and then is recanalized to form the adult hollow viscus. A failure of this process leads to atresia or a residual web. Such webs usually occur in the upper esophagus, often with eccentric openings; occasionally they are multiple. A much more common web or ring is located in the terminal esophagus, has a symmetric opening, and is usually at the junction between squamous and the normal transitional or columnar epithelium of the stomach (Fig. 96–4). This latter ring (Schatzki's ring) can be demonstrated in many individuals if cine studies of the lower esophageal zone are used. It produces symptoms infrequently but in a character-

istic manner. An acquired web located in the postcricoid area is sometimes associated with iron deficiency anemia (Plummer-Vinson syndrome).

All these types of webs or rings cause dysphagia for solids, and the impacted bolus usually has to be regurgitated. The lower esophageal ring (Schatzki's ring) has a characteristic clinical presentation that allows the diagnosis to be made by history. Every 3 to 4 months, after a bolus of meat or bread, the patient complains of dysphagia and total inability to swallow solids or liquids. The bolus is regurgitated, and then the patient can continue to eat normally. If the patient comes to the emergency room with an impacted bolus of meat, nothing is seen after the impacted bolus is removed with the operating endoscope, and the disorder is labeled "hysterical dysphagia." The lower esophageal ring is not well seen with the rigid endoscope. Lower esophageal rings may be dilated using a through-the-endoscope balloon or a bougie. Rings of less than 12.0 mm across their narrowest diameter cause symptoms and require rupture.

Treatment of all webs involves mechanical disruption either with a dilator or with the endoscope. Treatment of iron deficiency anemia causes the postcricoid webs to disappear. Only very rarely is a surgical approach to a web or ring necessary.

DIVERTICULA OF THE ESOPHAGUS. Zenker's diverticulum of the pharynx is not anatomically an esophageal diverticulum, as its neck is above the upper esophageal sphincter muscle, but custom has dictated its inclusion in description of esophageal diverticula. An epiphrenic diverticulum usually occurs on the right side of the esophagus just above the lower esophageal sphincter. Other diverticula are at the level of the carina and are known as traction diverticula, although traction by scar tissue is rarely demonstrated. Scleroderma is occasionally associated with numerous wide-mouthed diverticula scattered along the length of the esophagus. Large-amplitude motor waves have been associated with midbody diverticula and either achalasia or motor incoordination with epiphrenic diverticula.

Symptoms vary widely; many diverticula are found by accident during barium examination of the esophagus. If a patient with dysphagia is found to have a diverticulum, it is difficult to tell whether the diverticulum or the associated motor disorder is the cause. Zenker's diverticulum often has a classic symptom complex, particularly when it becomes large. It retains saliva and food particles, which may either be aspirated or cause repeated postprandial throat clearing with production of liquid and food particles. Patients with this type of diverticulum can often press on the neck and empty the diverticulum. The pouch can become so large that it can compress the esophagus anteriorly and obstruct it. In the presence of diverticula great caution must be exercised in passing tubes into the esophagus or stomach. Zenker's diverticulum is a special problem, since tubes naturally enter it rather than the esophageal opening, and the risk of perforation into the mediastinum is great. Traction and epiphrenic diverticula do not require treatment. Zenker's diverticulum, if large, may require diverticulectomy or diverticulopexy with coincident section of the cricopharyngeus muscle. Most techniques for diverticulectomy automatically accomplish cricopharyngeal section at the same time. If the diverticulum is small, it may regress after section of the cricopharyngeus.

INFECTIONS OF THE ESOPHAGUS. Two major infections involve the esophagus: *Candida* and *herpesvirus* infections. Although both are most common in immunocompromised hosts, such as those on steroids undergoing cancer chemotherapy or those afflicted with AIDS, either or both can invade apparently healthy hosts. Both can be found incidentally at autopsy or during endoscopy for other indications. Most commonly, infection of the mucosa leads to odynophagia of rather marked degree. Dysphagia for both solids and liquids usually accompanies the odynophagia and can be of such intensity that weight loss is rapid. Herpes esophagitis may present with hematemesis.

Although the radiograph occasionally reveals a shaggy mucosa in the case of monilial involvement, and occasionally even a stricture, endoscopy is the best method of detecting and confirming infectious involvement. *Candida* can present as isolated white plaques, which can be confused with glycogenic acanthosis, or progress to form confluent ulcerations with an overlying membrane. Herpesvirus tends to produce isolated ulcers, but exten-

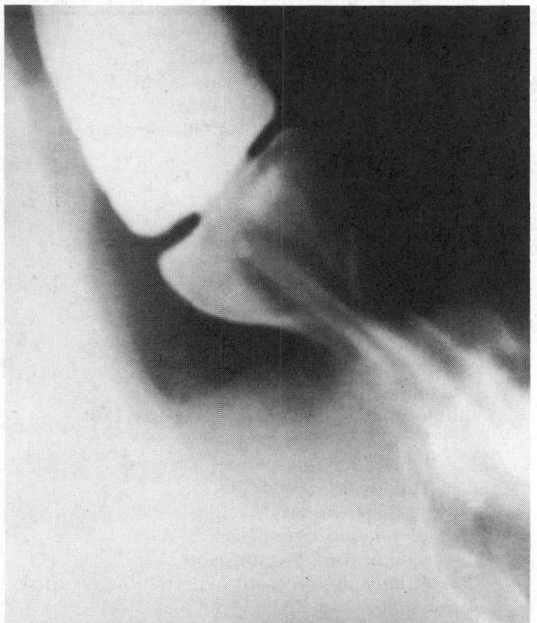

FIGURE 96–4. Lower esophageal ring (Schatzki's ring). This ring consists of a symmetric thin web located in the terminal esophagus. (From Pope CE II: *In* Sleisenger MH, Fordtran JS [eds.]: Gastrointestinal Disease. 3rd ed. Philadelphia, W. B. Saunders Company, 1983.)

sive involvement can produce confluent ulcerations. Biopsy of the ulcerated area usually shows either invasive hyphae of *Candida* or characteristic nuclear changes of the squamous cells when herpesvirus is present. Cytologic washings occasionally demonstrate the same change.

Treatment depends on correct identification of the etiologic agent. For *Candida* infection, an assessment of the degree of severity is needed. For mild noninvasive disease, topical therapy with 250,000 units of nystatin (Mycostatin) every 2 hours suffices. For more serious infections, low-dose intravenous amphotericin therapy has been successful, the dose being individualized on the basis of weight and renal status. Treatment with miconazole and ketoconazole appears promising. For severe esophageal infections, ketoconazole should be given in doses of 200 mg to 400 mg per day for 8 to 10 days. Herpesvirus infection is treated with acyclovir.

ESOPHAGEAL INJURIES. *Caustic Ingestion.* Caustic burns of the esophagus occur in children by accident; adults usually suffer such burns because of suicide attempts. Lye crystals, and especially liquid lye preparations for drain cleaning, are the most common cause. The speed of lye injury is so great that attempts to neutralize the caustic are futile. Detergents and Clorox also find their way into the esophageal lumens of both children and adults. The history is all important, but the degree of esophageal injury still must be assessed endoscopically as an emergency. Significant esophageal damage has been seen even without oral burns; conversely, oral burns do not necessarily mean that the material has reached the esophagus. If there is no esophageal reaction after apparent caustic ingestion, further care directed toward the esophagus will not be necessary.

The accepted therapy of a definite lye or caustic burn remains unsupported by clinical trials. For burns with solid lye or other solid agents, steroids have been recommended, at an initial dose of 80 mg per day, tapering to 20 mg per day until esophageal healing. Most clinicians also use broad-spectrum antibiotics. If liquid lye has been the damaging agent, serious consideration of emergency esophagogastrectomy is in order, as lesser measures have met with unacceptably high mortality.

Damage by Medication. A new form of iatrogenic illness of the esophagus has recently become evident. Ingested pills tend to lodge in the esophagus and damage the mucosa in a localized area. Tetracycline, doxycycline, ascorbic acid, and quinidine have all been indicted, and the list will undoubtedly grow. Normal individuals can retain small capsules in the esophagus, even when swallowing in the upright position. The clinical syndrome consists of steady burning or chest pain, accompanied by local odynophagia, all occurring 4 to 6 hours after ingestion of one of the offending capsules or tablets. Endoscopy usually shows a localized mucosal ulcer, which heals without a scar or may lead to a stricture requiring dilation. Symptomatic therapy is adequate, but prophylaxis seems to be a more practical idea. Pills of the offending class should be taken in the upright position with several swallows of water.

Esophageal Trauma. The esophagus is well protected by the thoracic cage but can be involved either by blunt trauma (automobile accidents) or by penetrating missiles (gunshots, knives). Often the surgeon's attention is directed toward more life-threatening damage to heart, lungs, or major blood vessels, and it is understandable that a rent in the esophagus may thus be overlooked. This unfortunate oversight, however, is followed by mediastinitis, which may worsen an already grave situation. Iatrogenic perforation with endoscope, dilator, or, very rarely, nasogastric tube leads to a similar complication.

Vomiting itself can cause esophageal injury, either mucosal (*Mallory-Weiss*) or through-and-through rupture (*Boerhaave's syndrome*). The mucosal lesion first described by Mallory and Weiss has been recognized much more frequently since the advent of rapid emergency endoscopy with fiberoptic endoscopes. Classically, the patient has repeated attacks of retching, productive at first of gastric contents and later of bright red blood. One quarter of patients shown to have a Mallory-Weiss tear have no prior history of vomiting. The tear is usually in the gastric mucosa just below the gastroesophageal junction, although it can extend through the junction and up into the esophageal mucosa. Diagnosis of this condition is almost always made at endoscopy; the

rent is usually seen as the endoscope is being withdrawn from the stomach into the esophagus. The majority of such lesions heal with conservative therapy. Angiographic or surgical therapy is necessary in less than 5 per cent. Bleeding has been stopped by direct application of electrocoagulation through the endoscope.

Vomiting can also cause a complete tear in the esophageal wall. Unlike the Mallory-Weiss lesion, the tear in Boerhaave's syndrome is located above the gastroesophageal junction on the left side. It usually follows vomiting, but other marked increases in intra-abdominal pressure such as lifting a heavy weight or straining at stool have been associated with a tear. The clinical diagnosis can be extremely difficult; often patients with esophageal rupture are thought to have a myocardial infarct, pneumothorax, a perforated viscus, or pancreatitis. Air in the mediastinum or the rapid appearance of a hydrothorax on the left usually leads to the correct diagnosis.

The diagnosis of esophageal perforation can usually be established by a cautious radiographic examination with water-soluble material. Barium may be used only if a rent is not demonstrated by the water-soluble agent. Immediate surgical repair is the accepted method of treatment of esophageal perforation. In those too ill for surgery, treatment consists of nasogastric suction, antibiotics, and subsequent mediastinal drainage if necessary.

Pope CE II, McDonald GB: Rings and webs; Diverticula; Involvement of the esophagus by infections, systemic illnesses, and physical agents. *In* Sleisenger MH, Fordtran JS (eds.): Gastrointestinal Disease. 4th ed. Philadelphia, W. B. Saunders Company, 1989. *Textbook review of these various conditions.*

97 Gastritis
Andrew H. Soll

Gastritis can be defined by gross appearance, histopathology or clinical presentation, thus defying simple categorization (Table 97–1). The term "gastritis," which implies inflammation, is a misnomer, for some of the entities considered lack appreciable inflammatory change—e.g., erosions due to aspirin or other nonsteroidal anti-inflammatory drugs (NSAID's). The terms "acute" and "chronic" have not been used here to segregate gastritis because these distinctions are rarely useful. The normal gastric mucosa has a remarkable ability to resist acid-peptic injury;

TABLE 97–1. CLASSIFICATION OF "GASTRITIS"

Erosive/hemorrhagic gastric disease
  NSAID-induced gastric damage
  Stress-related mucosal disease (SRMD)
  Alcohol-induced mucosal damage
  Chronic erosive (diffuse varioliform) gastritis
Nonerosive gastritis
  Fundal gland gastritis
    Atrophic gastritis
    Pernicious anemia
  Antral gland gastritis
  Gastritis and *Helicobacter pylori*
  Postoperative alkaline gastritis
Unusual or specific forms of gastritis
  Infectious gastritis
    Phlegmonous gastritis
    Syphilis, tuberculosis, anisakiasis
    Infections in immunocompromised host
      Viral (CMV, herpes)
      Fungal (*Candida*, histoplasmosis)
      Tuberculosis, syphilis
  Gastric ischemia
  Radiation-induced gastritis
  Ingestion of corrosive substances
  Ménétrier's disease (giant hypertrophic gastritis)
  Eosinophilic gastritis
  Granulomatous gastritis
  Vascular ectasia
    Watermelon stomach (antral vascular ectasia)
    Other vascular anomalies

TABLE 97–2. MECHANISMS IN MUCOSAL DEFENSE

Pre-epithelial mechanisms
   Mucus secretion/layer
   Bicarbonate output
Cellular mechanisms
   Apical membrane barrier to acid backdiffusion
   Cellular disposal of acid load
   Cellular defense against injury
   Restitution (resealing of injury areas of epithelium)
   Cellular replication
Post-epithelial mechanisms
   Blood flow
   Mesenchymal and inflammatory cells

The mucous layer creates a physical barrier to pepsin diffusion and stabilizes a pH gradient generated by bicarbonate output. The apical surface of mucosal cells resists acid backdiffusion, and cells are capable of disposing of an acid load. Intrinsic cellular mechanisms resist some forms of injury, but are poorly understood. Epithelial cells rapidly move across intact basement membrane to seal defects in the epithelium. Epithelial cells rapidly regenerate to replenish sloughed daughter cells. Blood flow is critical to maintaining mucosal integrity, proving nutrients and removing backdiffused acid. Lastly, mesenchymal cells and macrophages contribute to the critical wound-healing process.

several components mediate its defense (Table 97–2 and see Fig. 98–4). Efforts to establish the key element have not been successful, probably because the mechanisms are multiple, thus providing important redundant lines of defense.

CLINICAL PERSPECTIVES. Gastritis is often blamed for chronic abdominal pain, but the link between symptoms and gastritis is poorly established. For example, NSAID's produce both gastric damage and symptoms, yet neither is predictive of the other. In patients who have dyspeptic symptoms not linked to macroscopic ulcers, i.e., "nonulcer dyspepsia," it is helpful to distinguish those patients with postprandial indigestion, fullness, belching, bloating, nausea, early satiety, epigastric pain, and fatty food intolerance. This symptom complex is often indicative of *gastroparesis*, a diagnosis that can be confirmed with a nuclide gastric emptying study. This entity is frequently idiopathic but may be associated with diabetes, drug ingestion, or connective tissue diseases. An association between nonerosive gastritis and gastroparesis has been hypothesized, although not firmly established. Chronic abdominal pain is occasionally associated with back, chest, and abdominal wall musculoskeletal symptoms and can be reproduced by pressure on a paraspinous trigger point. This suggests the presence of a "back-gut" syndrome; an exhaustive workup can often be avoided, particularly if symptoms are relieved with a trial of local therapy (trigger point injection with lidocaine or physical therapy). Caution is necessary, since visceral pathology may trigger secondary musculoskeletal symptoms.

DIAGNOSIS. The diagnosis of gastritis may be suspected by a careful history, e.g., the prior ingestion of NSAID's or alcohol. Although barium radiographs may be suggestive, endoscopy coupled with the history is much more likely to establish a diagnosis by providing characteristic macroscopic or biopsy findings.

EROSIVE/HEMORRHAGIC GASTRIC DISEASE

NSAID-INDUCED GASTRIC DAMAGE. NSAID use is associated with petechiae, erosions, and ulcers in the gastric mucosa. In contrast to non-NSAID ulcers, however, only about half of NSAID-associated gastric ulcers occur in a surrounding area of diffuse gastritis. In these latter individuals, *Helicobacter pylori*, a putative factor in nonerosive gastritis, is also found, leaving no reason to implicate NSAID's as a causative factor for the gastritis. Thus, neither acute nor chronic inflammation is a major part of the spectrum of NSAID-induced gastroduodenal damage. Petechiae due to bleeding into the mucosa are frequent but of little clinical significance. Erosions, unlike ulcers, are superficial breaks that do not extend deeper than the mucosa itself and therefore do not cause perforation or severe bleeding. Superficial gastric lesions from NSAID ingestion may occasionally lead to iron deficiency anemia from chronic blood loss or to an acute upper gastrointestinal hemorrhage from a severe erosive process. Gastric erosions are often blamed for occult blood in the stool of patients taking NSAID's, but a thorough workup is appropriate. The incidence of other lesions (e.g., colonic polyps)

is the same in such patients as in those with occult blood in their stool who are not taking NSAID's.

STRESS-RELATED MUCOSAL DISEASE (SRMD). SRMD occurs during severe illness, most frequently in the intensive care unit setting, as a function of the severity of the underlying acute medical or surgical illness (e.g., respiratory or renal failure, sepsis, hypotension, trauma, or the postsurgical state). Mucosal lesions also occur in patients with severe burns (Curling's ulcers) and with central nervous system disease, trauma, or surgery (Cushing's ulcers). The etiology is multifactorial, resulting from a compromise in mucosal blood flow or in other elements of mucosal defense in the presence of acid/peptic activity in gastric juice (Table 97–2). The lesions are diffuse, superficial breaks in the acid-secreting mucosa. Bleeding, generally a slow ooze, may become severe because of the widespread mucosal involvement. Cushing's ulcers tend to be deeper and occasionally perforate, possibly reflecting the acid hypersecretion that can occur with central nervous system lesions. Lesions begin rapidly; for example, erosive changes can be found in the majority of patients examined endoscopically immediately after completion of open heart surgery. About 10 to 20 per cent of ICU patients develop gastric bleeding; the risk increases with severity of the underlying illness. Once bleeding has started, the mortality rate of the underlying condition doubles or triples.

Diagnosis. Gastrointestinal bleeding in the ICU setting requires accurate diagnosis; the initial step entails determining if bleeding is from an upper gastrointestinal source (Ch. 111). Melena may occur with right-sided colonic bleeding and hematochezia may occur with brisk upper gastrointestinal bleeding. Blood may be absent from the nasogastric aspirate if bleeding is intermittent or from a duodenal source. The consistent finding of bile without blood in the nasogastric aspirate argues for a bleeding site distal to the ligament of Treitz. If the nasogastric aspirate is bloody, it is worth determining how rapidly this blood clears with lavage and gravity drainage (suction aspiration may induce artifacts endoscopically indistinguishable from acute erosions). The only practical method for diagnosis is endoscopy. In the decision to do endoscopy the potential benefits of making a specific diagnosis must be weighed against the risks of endoscopy (premedication, respiratory and circulatory compromise, and possible bleeding or perforation). Any patient who has begun to bleed deserves aggressive medical management (see below), with endoscopy reserved for those patients in whom bleeding is brisk enough to warrant consideration of additional measures. Endoscopy can reveal a discrete ulcer or a focal lesion other than SRMD, which may respond to specific therapy.

Treatment and Prevention. Medical, endoscopic, and surgical treatment of bleeding due to SRMD all yield discouraging results, so prevention is of particular importance. Patients sick enough to be at risk deserve prophylaxis. Since gastric ischemia is a likely causative factor in SRMD, efforts to improve volume status, cardiac output, and respiratory function are critical to both treatment and prevention. The incidence of bleeding is generally decreased if the gastric pH is maintained above 3.5, a pH level above which pepsin activity is markedly reduced. An antacid drip or hourly antacids (15 to 30 ml) via a nasogastric tube can neutralize the gastric lumen. H_2 blockers are approved for intravenous use; slow bolus infusion is effective in increasing gastric pH (cimetidine 300 mg every 8 hours; ranitidine 50 mg every 12 hours; famotidine 20 mg every 12 hours). Continuous infusion may provide smoother control of pH; for example, an infusion of cimetidine (300 mg priming dose, 37.5 mg per hour) produces effective gastric neutralization. Omeprazole, the H^+-K^+-ATPase inhibitor, is likely to be effective for preventing SRMD, but it is not yet approved by the Food and Drug Administration for parenteral use, nor has efficacy for this indication been established. Sucralfate is also effective in reducing bleeding due to SRMD; nasogastric administration is required (1 gram every 6 hours).

ALCOHOL AND MUCOSAL DAMAGE. Characteristic subepithelial hemorrhages, with the endoscopic appearance of "blood under a plastic wrap," are commonly found in individuals abusing alcohol. Although termed "hemorrhagic gastritis," these lesions are composed of hemorrhage and edema in the interstitial space under the surface epithelium, without inflammation. Usually the bleeding is mild. If more severe bleeding is found, associated lesions, such as portal hypertension, peptic ulcer, or a Mallory-Weiss tear, should be sought (Ch. 98).

CHRONIC EROSIVE (DIFFUSE VARIOLIFORM) GASTRITIS. This entity, of unknown pathogenesis, which consists of erosive changes usually involving the antrum, can be diagnosed only in the absence of the use or abuse of NSAID and/or alcohol. Symptoms are nonspecific and include abdominal pain, nausea, vomiting, anorexia, weight loss, and sometimes bleeding. Occasionally isolated antral erosions are found without symptoms or progression to other entities.

NONEROSIVE GASTRITIS

CLASSIFICATION. Nonerosive gastritis refers to inflammatory change in a mucosa that is often grossly normal, and lacks, as the name implies, erosive changes. Nonerosive gastritis can be classified by whether the fundus (type A) or antrum (type B) is primarily involved and by whether the inflammation is superficial (involving the foveolar or gastric pit region and upper portion of the lamina propria), deep (involving the gastric glands that contain parietal and chief cells), or atrophic (with decreased or absent glandular elements and mucosal thinning). The term "active" reflects infiltration by polymorphonuclear leukocytes. Once glandular atrophy develops, the inflammatory infiltrate may be minimal. Other important features are intestinal and pseudopyloric metaplasia and dysplastic epithelial changes. With intestinal metaplasia, gastric mucosal cells may be replaced by typical goblet cells and absorptive cells; rudimentary intestinal villi may form. With pseudopyloric metaplasia the parietal and chief cells of fundic glands are replaced by mucous glands indistinguishable from normal antral glands. Fundal and antral gland gastritis constitute two distinct forms of nonerosive gastritis.

With *fundal or type A gastritis,* the inflammatory changes are usually maximal along the greater curvature in the fundus and body. Characteristic parietal cell antibodies occur in most patients, and pernicious anemia may develop (Ch. 132). Inflammatory change is usually much less marked in the antrum than in the fundus. Hyposecretion of acid occurs as a function of fundal glandular atrophy; the relative absence of glandular atrophy in the antrum accounts for the ability of many of these patients to develop marked hypergastrinemia as the feedback inhibition of acid on gastrin release is lost. Fundal gastritis and a decrease in maximal acid secretion may be a normal concomitant of aging, but only a small proportion of affected individuals go on to develop pernicious anemia.

Antral or type B gastritis has several features distinguishing it from fundal gastritis, including the predominance of antral inflammatory change, a lack of progression to atrophic gastritis, and an association with both peptic ulcer and *H. pylori.*

ETIOLOGY AND ASSOCIATIONS. The cause(s) of chronic gastritis remains unknown. Factors hypothesized to cause or exacerbate gastritis include chronic trauma, gastric bacteria, toxins, and thermal insult. A role for reflux of duodenal juice, containing bile and pancreatic enzymes, has been postulated but without supporting data. Lysolecithin, formed by the action of the pancreatic enzyme phospholipase A on biliary lecithin, can be refluxed from the duodenum. The detergent action of lysolecithin may disrupt the surface epithelial barrier to acid backdiffusion, thus creating a chronic insult that could provoke an inflammatory response. Chronic infection with *H. pylori,* as discussed below, is a leading candidate for causing nonerosive antral gastritis; the association with fundal gastritis is less well founded. Multiple factors probably interact in the pathogenesis of nonerosive gastritis; for example, the inflammatory infiltrate induced by *H. pylori* may disrupt normal mucosal architecture, thus interfering with mucosal resistance to acid/peptic injury and to refluxed bile. End-stage gastric atrophy may be accompanied by an intact surface epithelium and little inflammatory infiltrate, possibly because with achlorhydria the acid-peptic exacerbation of the inflammatory response is removed.

Pernicious anemia (Ch. 132) is on the end of the spectrum of fundal gastritis, although fundal gastritis may not reflect only a single disease mechanism. Despite histamine-fast achlorhydria, some patchy nests of parietal and chief cells may still be found.

Hypergastrinemia is present in about three fourths of patients with pernicious anemia. The absence of hypergastrinemia in achlorhydric patients suggests extensive antral gastritis.

Immunologic mechanisms appear to be operative in fundal, but not antral, gastritis. About 90 per cent of patients with pernicious anemia (fundal gastritis) have antibodies against parietal cells, which appear to react with the parietal cell H^+-K^+-ATPase. Antibodies reacting with intrinsic factor also occur, and such antibodies may block the vitamin B_{12} binding site. Whether these antibodies mediate immunologic damage or simply reflect a secondary reaction is unclear. Sera from patients with pernicious anemia contain an antibody reported to be cytotoxic to canine gastric mucosal cells. Pernicious anemia is also associated with other diseases in which immunologic mechanisms appear operative, such as Hashimoto's thyroiditis, hypothyroidism, hyperthyroidism, insulin-dependent diabetes mellitus, and vitiligo.

Genetic factors are important in pernicious anemia; family members of patients have an increased incidence of atrophic gastritis, achlorhydria, vitamin B_{12} malabsorption, and antibodies to parietal cells and intrinsic factor. There are no data regarding genetic factors in gastritis without pernicious anemia.

CLINICAL PRESENTATION. Nonerosive gastritis is frequently found in asymptomatic individuals; blaming this entity for dyspeptic symptoms is not justified. Despite this disclaimer, it has been hypothesized that altered motility resulting in symptomatic gastroparesis may be associated with nonerosive gastritis. An association between reflux esophagitis and altered esophageal motility (esophageal spasm) is well recognized. If symptoms suggestive of gastroparesis are elicited, a gastric emptying study should be performed. If gastric emptying is delayed, endoscopy is necessary to exclude a mechanical gastric outlet obstruction. Patients with pernicious anemia may develop symptoms secondary to vitamin B_{12} deficiency (Ch. 132). Macroscopic endoscopic findings (erythema, petechiae, nodularity, pallor, and atrophy) are generally nonspecific. Diagnosis requires biopsy, and multiple biopsies may be required, since the histopathology may be patchy. The ratio of pepsinogen I (present in fundic chief cells) to pepsinogen II (present in both chief cells and surface epithelial cells) falls with the degree of glandular atrophy.

NATURAL HISTORY OF GASTRITIS. About half of "normal" subjects over 50 years of age are thought to have superficial gastritis, which can progress to an atrophic pattern over the subsequent 10 to 20 years.

Enterochromaffin-like cells may undergo hyperplasia in atrophic gastritis, as in the Zollinger-Ellison syndrome (Ch. 98). It is probable that the severe and sustained hypergastrinemia found in these conditions has a trophic effect on enterochromaffin-like (ECL) cells, a population of endocrine cells identified by characteristic granules and silver staining properties. Carcinoid tumors composed of ECL cells have been described in atrophic gastritis and in the Zollinger-Ellison syndrome, the latter primarily in association with multiple endocrine neoplasia (MEN) type I. ECL cells do not contain serotonin, and thus these tumors do not produce the carcinoid syndrome found with tumors composed of serotonin-containing enterochromaffin (EC) cells (Ch. 230). Gastric carcinoids occurring without hypergastrinemia are solitary, aggressive tumors, whereas carcinoids associated with hypergastrinemia and ECL cell hyperplasia are generally indolent and multifocal. Antrectomy coupled with local excision deserves consideration as an alternative to total gastrectomy in atrophic gastritis with carcinoid tumor formation, since achlorhydria-induced hypergastrinemia exerts a trophic effect on these ECL tumors. This situation provides a logical indication for a gastrin receptor antagonist, when one becomes available for clinical use.

Gastric adenocarcinomas have been reported to occur with increased frequency with atrophic gastritis, but the assessment of increased risk is variable, ranging from nil to threefold in different series (Ch. 99).

TREATMENT. No specific therapy exists for fundal gastritis. Replacement of vitamin B_{12} is, of course, indicated in pernicious anemia. Delayed gastric emptying can be treated with the prokinetic agent metoclopramide (5 to 20 mg, 1 hour before meals and at bedtime). The liquid preparation (5 mg per milliliter) is generally more effective, since gastric emptying of tablets is also delayed. Parenteral administration may also be of benefit, particularly during the first few days of therapy. Metoclopramide has a high incidence of central nervous system side effects. Its use should be restricted to instances in which therapy is clearly warranted and effective and patients should be monitored closely for these side effects.

It is reasonable to evaluate family members of patients with pernicious anemia for gastritis and vitamin B$_{12}$ deficiency. Some advocate performing endoscopy at the time of an initial diagnosis of pernicious anemia, obtaining sufficient antral and fundal biopsies to assess the severity of intestinal metaplasia and epithelial dysplasia. Although imperfect, these findings are the best indicators of the cancer risk. Using this approach, only those patients with severe dysplasia would warrant close follow-up and/or surgical intervention.

GASTRITIS AND *Helicobacter pylori*. *H. pylori*, a gram-negative microaerophilic organism, may be the most common worldwide human infective agent. No reservoir other than the human stomach has been identified and the epidemiology is unknown. The organism is fastidious but can be cultured with careful technique. *H. pylori* can be identified as a bent or spiral rod on specific silver stains (Warthin-Starry or Giemsa) or by careful examination of routine hematoxylin and eosin–stained sections. Serology sensitively detects antibodies to *H. pylori*. The organism has a very high urease activity, which allows identification in biopsies by a rapid test or in vivo by using a breath test for $^{13}CO_2$ following an oral ^{13}C-urea load. *H. pylori* is found embedded in the mucous layer and tends to cluster over intracellular junctions. *H. pylori* is found in nearly all biopsies showing active antral gastritis with polymorphonuclear infiltration, whereas the organism is unusual in the histologically normal stomach (Table 97–3). Since it is unethical to experimentally administer an organism that may cause disease and may be difficult to eradicate, studies of causality must be indirect. Two investigators have self-administered *H. pylori*, however, with subsequent development of acute superficial gastritis associated with epigastric pain, nausea, and vomiting. Thus, it appears that *H. pylori* can induce a form of acute, superficial gastritis. Additional evidence that *H. pylori* causes active gastritis is that eradication of the organism reduces active inflammation, which remains unchanged following similar treatment without its eradication. It is possible, of course, that the gastritis comes first, creating an environment suited for colonization with *H. pylori*. Although *H. pylori* and antral gastritis are clearly associated, no such association has been shown between *H. pylori* and fundal gastritis, gastric atrophy, or gastric cancer.

Although *H. pylori* is clearly associated with antral gastritis, no clinical benefit has been established to result from eradication of this organism. The organism is difficult to treat; delayed recurrences with the same strain are frequent, and thus multiple antibiotic regimens, usually including colloidal bismuth and metronidazole, have been evaluated. Since there are other effective modalities for ulcer healing, therapy directed at the eradication of *H. pylori* should await demonstration of beneficial effects on the natural history of gastritis or peptic ulcer disease.

Two "epidemics" of acute, superficial gastritis, have been reported. Despite the absence of glandular gastritis and the presence of histologically robust parietal cells, acid secretion was markedly reduced, suggesting release of a factor inhibiting acid secretion. These epidemics occurred before recognition of *H. pylori*, but retrospective analysis revealed histology and serology consistent with *H. pylori* infection.

GASTRITIS ASSOCIATED WITH PEPTIC ULCER. Antral

TABLE 97–3. ANTRAL GASTRITIS AND *H. PYLORI*

		Antral Gastritis	
		+	−
H. pylori Status	+	233	5
	−	2	87

Normal subjects and individuals with duodenal and gastric ulcer or with ulcer-negative dyspepsia underwent endoscopic biopsy, which was then graded for active antral gastritis. *H. pylori* status was also ascertained using culture. Note the very tight association between the presence of *H. pylori* and antral gastritis. (Data from Rauws EAJ, Lagenberg W, Houthoff HJ, et al.: Campylobacter pyloridis–associated chronic active gastritis. A prospective study of its prevalence and the effects of antibacterial and antiulcer treatment. Gastroenterology 94:33, 1988.)

gastritis has been associated with both gastric and duodenal ulcer. Some of the differences between gastric and duodenal ulcer may be explained by the patterns of the associated gastritis. In patients with ulcers, antral gastritis is not age-related, in contrast to normal subjects. The fundic mucosa in patients with duodenal ulcer is usually robust and "juvenile" (they generally secrete more acid than normals) and lacks the development of the fundal gastritis that is often seen with aging. Patients with gastric ulcer, in contrast to duodenal ulcer, tend to have more severe antral gastritis. Mild to moderate superficial fundal gland gastritis is also more common with gastric than with duodenal ulcer. There is a close association between antral gastritis, peptic ulcer, and *H. pylori*; the causal nature of these interactions will remain controversial until properly designed, controlled trials firmly establish that the presence or absence of the bacterium alters that natural history of the gastritis and ulcer disease.

POSTOPERATIVE ALKALINE GASTRITIS. Macroscopic gastritis with a dramatic red color may rapidly develop after gastric resection or pyloroplasty, but this endoscopic appearance does not correlate with symptoms, bile reflux, or histologic inflammation. The occurrence of this difficult-to-treat complication of surgery for peptic ulcer is another indication to do the least physiologically disruptive operation (i.e., highly selective vagotomy), when possible.

UNUSUAL OR SPECIFIC FORMS OF GASTRITIS

PHLEGMONOUS GASTRITIS. This is a rarely encountered, purulent process involving the gastric submucosa and wall. Streptococci, but also staphylococci, *E. coli*, and *Proteus*, have been implicated. The course is fulminant and medical management is ineffective, leaving surgery as a drastic, but unavoidable, last resort.

OTHER INFECTIONS. As with infections in all other sites, the spectrum of gastric infections is expanded and altered in the immunocompromised host. Gastric tuberculosis, diagnosed by finding caseating granulomas and positive cultures, occurs in AIDS. Secondary syphilis may involve the stomach with thickened folds and erosions. Despite the frequency of esophageal candidiasis, gastric ulcers appear to be only colonized by these organisms. Mycelia may occur at the ulcer margin, but antifungal therapy does not alter ulcer healing, suggesting a lack of clinical importance. Cytomegalovirus can involve the stomach in the immunocompromized host. The ascaris-like larva, *Anisakis*, present in raw fish, may infect the normal gastric mucosa, producing pain and dyspepsia. *Strongyloides stercoralis* involves the small intestine much more frequently than the stomach and can cause dyspepsia. The diagnosis is made by examining duodenal aspirates or stool specimens.

GASTRIC ISCHEMIA. Ischemic gastric injury is rarely recognized, although erosive changes have been reported with vasculitis and atheromatous embolization. Whether chronic gastric ulcers have an ischemic component remains speculative.

MÉNÉTRIER'S DISEASE. Ménétrier's disease (giant hypertrophic gastritis) is a specific entity of unknown etiology characterized by the triad of giant folds, in the fundus and body of the stomach, hypoalbuminemia secondary to a protein-losing gastropathy, and the histologic features of foveolar (gastric pit region) hyperplasia with gland atrophy, cystic dilation, and increased mucosal thickness. Tortuous gastric folds may resemble the cerebral cortex. Hypochlorhydria is generally present, but a hypersecretory variant has been described. Symptoms are variable and may include abdominal pain, nausea, vomiting, weight loss, and edema. The disease is more common in men than in women, generally presenting after age 50, although a childhood form exists. Large folds, especially involving the greater curvature of the gastric body, are found on radiography. Typical biopsies can confirm the diagnosis, but variant patterns warrant the less specific diagnosis of idiopathic hypertrophic gastropathy. The differential diagnosis includes gastrinoma syndrome, infiltrating carcinoma, lymphoma, and amyloidosis. Large gastric folds are found without any associated pathology and also have been reported associated with *H. pylori* infection; the relevance of this organism to hypertrophic gastritis remains unclear. Usually no therapy is indicated, but anticholinergics and H$_2$ blockers may reduce gastric protein loss. Accompanying ulcers and erosions usually respond to standard antiulcer therapy (Ch. 98). No increased risk of cancer has been established.

EOSINOPHILIC GASTRITIS. Eosinophils may infiltrate the gastrointestinal mucosa and muscular layers, especially with antral involvement, in association with peripheral eosinophilia as an idiopathic syndrome. Thickening of gastric mucosal folds and wall rigidity are common. Antral motility may be altered, leading to gastric retention. Patients may present with eosinophilia, nausea, vomiting, or pain. Rarely, serosal involvement results in ascites. Milk-sensitive enteropathy of infancy, connective tissue disorders, and parasitic infections should be ruled out. Glucocorticoid therapy may be useful, and surgery may be needed if mechanical outlet obstruction occurs.

GRANULOMATOUS GASTRITIS. Granulomas in the gastric mucosa may occur in association with generalized diseases such as sarcoidosis, Crohn's disease, or infections. Crohn's disease may involve the duodenum, pylorus, antrum, and gastric body (in that order) in association with disease in the small intestine or colon. Mucosal granulomas may also be incidental findings or occur in eosinophilic granulomas or in isolated, idiopathic granulomatous gastritis. Involved portions of the stomach may be rigid or narrow or have thickened folds on radiographic examination, findings that must be distinguished from malignancy. The antrum is most often involved, and granulomas may occur in all layers of the stomach. Ulcerated lesions may perforate. Patients are often operated upon because of the difficulties in differentiating this entity from malignancy. Once the diagnosis is made, it is important to exclude potentially curable diseases (e.g., tuberculosis, histoplasmosis, syphilis) or treatable processes (e.g., sarcoidosis, Crohn's disease). With malignancy and associated diseases excluded, the patient can be followed, since spontaneous resolution has been reported.

WATERMELON STOMACH. This entity, also known as gastric antral vascular ectasia, represents another nongastric condition. At endoscopy, the antrum has erythematous folds or linear angioid streaks; the convergence of the latter at the pylorus in a pattern reminiscent of a watermelon prompted the naming of this entity. Biopsy can be diagnostic, demonstrating dilated antral vasculature with intravascular fibrin thrombi and fibromuscular hyperplasia. This uncommon lesion can present with either acute gastrointestinal bleeding or with chronic iron deficiency anemia. Corticosteroid therapy has been tried with uncertain success. Antrectomy is effective in eliminating bleeding; however, success has also been reported with repeated coagulation using endoscopic laser or heater probes.

Dooley CP, Cohen H: The clinical significance of *Campylobacter pylori.* Ann Intern Med 108:70, 1988. *Basic review of Helicobacter pylori in relationship to gastrointestinal disease. This field is rapidly changing, so conclusions will be different when new studies are available.*

Laine L, Weinstein WM: Histology of alcoholic hemorrhagic "gastritis": A prospective evaluation. Gastroenterology 94:1254, 1988. *Critical assessment of histopathology of alcohol-related gastric damage.*

Petrini JL Jr., Johnston JH: Heat probe treatment for antral vascular ectasia. Gastrointest Endosc 35:324, 1989. *Description of heat probe therapy for this entity. Provides references for description of the lesion.*

Robert A, Kauffman GL Jr.: Stress ulcers, erosions, and gastric mucosal injury. *In* Sleisenger MH, Fordtran JS (eds.): Gastrointestinal Disease. 4th ed. Philadelphia, W. B. Saunders Company, 1989, pp 772–791. *Good overview of the pathophysiology and therapy of gastric mucosal injury and stress related mucosal damage.*

Soll AH, Kurata JH, Walsh JH: Ulcer epidemiology conference. Gastroenterology 96:561, 1989. *Compendium of articles summarizing the consequences of NSAID-associated ulcers.*

Weinstein WM: Gastritis. *In* Sleisenger MH, Fordtran JS (eds.): Gastrointestinal Disease. 4th ed. Philadelphia, W. B. Saunders Company, 1989, pp 792–813. *Comprehensive summary of the various forms of gastritis.*

98 Peptic Ulcer

98.1 PATHOGENESIS

Charles T. Richardson

DEFINITION

Ulcers are defects in the gastrointestinal mucosa that penetrate the muscularis mucosa. This distinguishes them from superficial erosions, which do not extend through the muscularis mucosa. Peptic ulcers usually occur in the stomach, pylorus, or duodenal bulb but also can develop in the esophagus and the postbulbar duodenum. In patients with markedly increased acid secretion (as in Zollinger-Ellison syndrome) ulcers sometimes develop in the distal duodenum and jejunum. Peptic ulcers occasionally occur in the ileum in or near Meckel's diverticula.

Originally, all ulcers in the upper gastrointestinal tract were believed to be caused by the aggressive action of hydrochloric acid and pepsin on the mucosa. Thus they became known as "peptic ulcers." Although acid and pepsin are secreted by most patients with benign ulcers, they are not the only causes of ulcers. Thus, the term "peptic ulcer" may be a misnomer. Ulcers probably result from several different pathogenetic mechanisms. In general, ulcers occur when luminal aggressive factors overcome opposing mucosal defenses. Mechanisms believed important in the pathogenesis of ulcer disease are discussed in greater detail below.

NORMAL PHYSIOLOGY

STRUCTURE. The stomach is divided into four anatomic regions: the cardia, fundus, body, and antrum (Fig. 98–1). *Parietal cells,* which secrete hydrochloric acid, and *chief cells,* which secrete pepsinogen, are located primarily in the fundus and body, although a few are found in the antrum. *Gastrin (G) cells* are located in the antrum.

Gastric mucosa is made up of a series of pits and glands (Fig. 98–2). The pits contain surface epithelial cells, whereas the glands contain mucous, parietal, endocrine, and chief cells. Normal gastric juice is a mixture of parietal secretion (acid and intrinsic factor) and nonparietal secretions (mucus, bicarbonate, sodium, potassium, and pepsinogen). Pepsinogen is converted to pepsin in the presence of hydrochloric acid.

CONTROL OF GASTRIC SECRETION. Three endogenous chemicals (acetylcholine, gastrin, and histamine) stimulate acid secretion (Fig. 98–3): (1) *Acetylcholine,* believed to be a neural transmitter, is released by vagal efferent neurons. Vagal stimulation of acid secretion occurs when humans see, smell, taste, chew, or think about appetizing food. (2) *Gastrin* is a hormone responsible for acid secretion. Protein in food is the most potent stimulant of gastrin release, but vagal stimulation, calcium, other cations such as magnesium and aluminum, and alkalinization of the antrum also release gastrin. Gastrin release is inhibited by acid within the lumen of the antrum. (3) *Histamine* stimulates acid secretion via a paracrine mechanism. Mastlike cells that contain histamine are located in the lamina propria of the stomach in close proximity to parietal cells. When histamine is liberated from mast cells, it diffuses through intercellular spaces to reach parietal cells. Acetylcholine, gastrin, and histamine are believed to act on receptors on parietal cell membranes to cause acid secretion (see Ch. 98.3, on medical therapy of peptic ulcer disease).

Mechanisms within parietal cells that lead to acid secretion are not well defined. It is believed that cyclic adenosine monophosphate (AMP) is important in the mediation of histamine-stimulated acid secretion, while calcium entry into parietal cells is believed to play a role in gastrin- and acetylcholine-stimulated secretion. A hydrogen/potassium adenosine triphosphatase (ATPase) enzyme is located on the luminal surface of parietal cells (Ch. 98.3). This enzyme serves as a proton pump, which is the final step in secretion of hydrogen ions.

PRODUCTS OF GASTRIC SECRETION. In the pathogenesis of peptic ulcer the two most important products of gastric secretion are hydrochloric acid and pepsin.

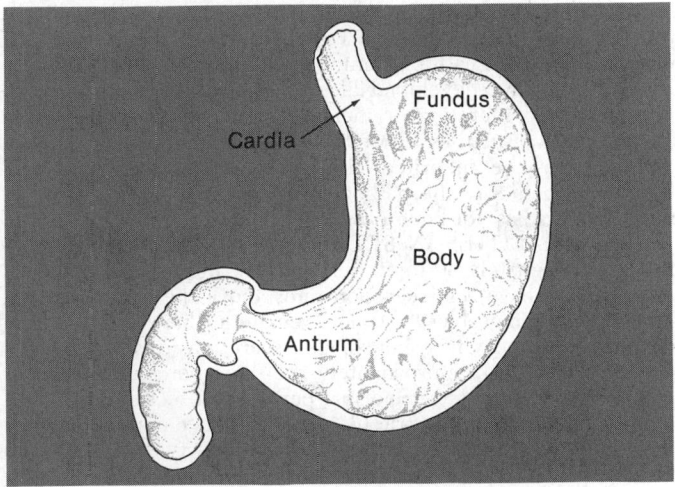

FIGURE 98–1. Anatomic divisions of the stomach.

Secretion of Acid. Basal acid output (BAO) is the amount of acid secreted under fasting or unstimulated conditions. Peak acid output (PAO) or maximum acid output (MAO) is acid secreted in response to an injection of either pentagastrin or histamine, the maximal amount of acid that a normal subject or patient with ulcer disease can secrete. MAO reflects the number of parietal cells in an individual, and the ratio of BAO to MAO represents the fraction of parietal cell mass functioning under basal conditions. Thus, if a patient has an increased amount of gastrin, acetylcholine, or histamine near parietal cells or if there is increased sensitivity of parietal cells to normal amounts of these stimulants, BAO will be increased, as will the BAO/MAO ratio. Such a patient is said to have a basal acid hypersecretory state, such as the Zollinger-Ellison syndrome (see below).

Upper and lower limits of normal acid secretion are shown in Table 98–1. Men usually secrete more acid than do women. This can be explained, in part, by differences in body size, but men secrete more acid than do women even when corrections are made for weight and lean body mass.

Secretion of Pepsin. Pepsin is secreted into the lumen as an inactive precursor, pepsinogen. Pepsinogen secretion usually accompanies acid secretion. Although mechanisms controlling pepsinogen secretion are less well understood, cholinergic stimulation is believed to be a major mediator. Once pepsinogen is secreted into the gastric lumen, it is converted by acid to pepsin,

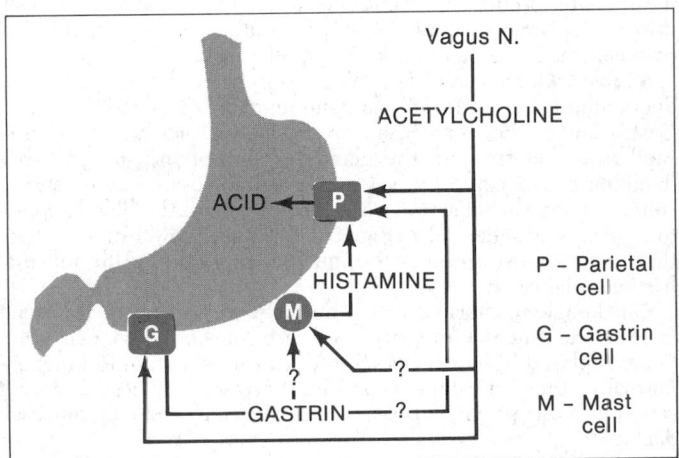

FIGURE 98–3. Model illustrating the chemical stimulants of acid secretion. Acetylcholine originates in the vagus nerves; gastrin is released from gastrin cells in the antrum; and histamine is liberated from mast cells in the lamina propria of the gastric mucosa.

the active enzyme. The optimal pH for conversion of pepsinogen to pepsin ranges between 1.8 and 3.5.

MAINTENANCE OF NORMAL MUCOSAL INTEGRITY.

Several mechanisms are believed important in protecting gastric and duodenal mucosa from damage by acid, pepsin, bile, pancreatic enzymes, and other possible aggressive factors. These defensive mechanisms include mucus, bicarbonate, mucosal blood flow, and cell renewal after injury. Endogenous prostaglandins currently are the most likely candidates as mediators to control these defensive mechanisms.

Mucus. This secretory product is a gel that forms a thin, protective coat over superficial mucosal cells (Fig. 98–4). Mucus has several functions: (1) to protect underlying cells from mechanical forces of digestion; (2) to lubricate the mucosa, assisting movement of food over mucosal surfaces; (3) to retain water within the mucous gel and thereby provide an aqueous environment for underlying cells; and (4) to form an unstirred layer impeding, but not blocking, diffusion of hydrogen ions from the lumen to the apical membrane of epithelial cells. Under normal conditions, mucus is constantly being produced but also is being removed continuously by mechanical forces during mixing and grinding of food and by pepsin, which degrades mucus into soluble glycoprotein subunits. However, secretion and degradation of mucus remain in equilibrium under normal conditions.

Bicarbonate. This is secreted by surface epithelial cells in the stomach and duodenum and also by Brunner's glands in the duodenum. Although some bicarbonate reaches the lumen, much of the secreted bicarbonate remains below or within the mucous layer (Fig. 98–4). Thus, the mucosal surface is in contact with fluid that contains a high pH relative to the lumen of the stomach. Under normal conditions, hydrogen ions are neutralized by

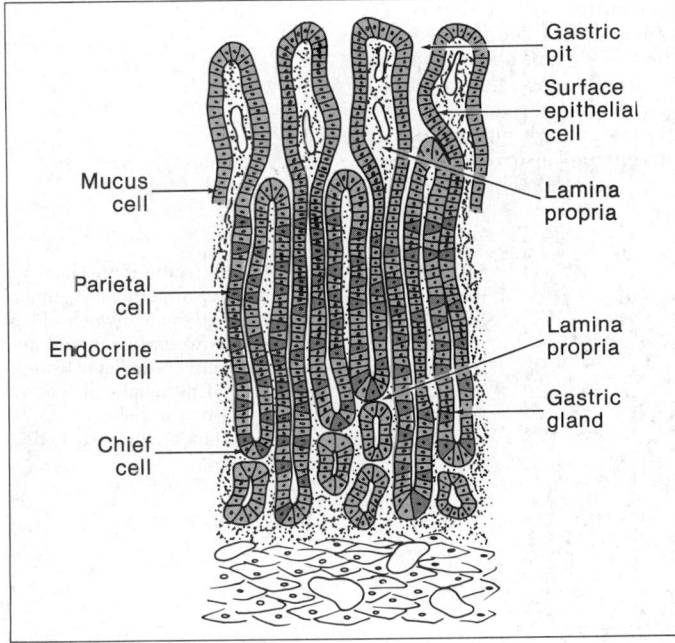

FIGURE 98–2. Diagram demonstrating the cell types lining the pits and glands of the gastric mucosa.

TABLE 98–1. UPPER (ULN) AND LOWER (LLN) LIMITS OF NORMAL ACID SECRETION IN HEALTHY MEN AND WOMEN

	Acid Output (mmol/hr)*			Basal/Maximum
	Basal	*Peak*	*Maximum*	
Men (N = 172)				
ULN	10.5	60.6	47.7	0.31
LLN	0	11.6	9.3	0
Women (N = 76)				
ULN	5.6	40.1	31.2	0.29
LLN	0	8.0	5.6	0

*Acid output (volume of gastric juice times concentration of acid) is measured in 15-minute intervals and is expressed in mmol/hr. Basal acid output is the sum of acid secreted during four 15-minute periods. Peak acid output is the sum of the highest two 15-minute periods after pentagastrin or histamine stimulation multiplied by two. Maximum acid output is the sum of four 15-minute intervals after pentagastrin or histamine stimulation.

bicarbonate (producing carbon dioxide and water) as they diffuse through the mucous gel layer. A pH gradient is thus established between the lumen and surface epithelial cells.

Mucosal Blood Flow. The blood supply of the stomach and duodenum is important in maintaining normal mucosal integrity. Gastric and duodenal mucosae are supplied by arborizing mucosal capillaries that traverse the glandular area of the stomach and duodenum. An extensive system of submucosal arteries and a submucous plexus of arteries and veins regulate the blood supply to surface epithelial cells (Fig. 98–4). Blood flow removes acid that might diffuse through the mucosa, especially if the mucosa has been damaged.

Cell Renewal. Normal cell renewal is an important factor in maintaining mucosal integrity. Cells are constantly dying and are being replaced by new cells. In order for this system to function normally, there must be a balance between cell loss and cell renewal. Disruption of this steady state may lead to mucosal damage.

Endogenous Prostaglandins. Prostaglandins of the E, F, and I types are found in the gastric and duodenal mucosa. When administered exogenously, prostaglandins stimulate secretion of mucus and bicarbonate, increase mucosal blood flow, and enhance mucosal regeneration after injury. Prostaglandins also may have a trophic effect on the mucosa. Duodenal mucosal prostaglandins appear to stimulate basal duodenal bicarbonate secretion. Exogenously administered prostaglandins protect the mucosa of animals against a variety of noxious agents, including boiling water, ethanol, bile acids, and aspirin, a property termed "cytoprotection." On the basis of such studies of exogenously administered prostaglandins, it is presumed that endogenous prostaglandins also possess cytoprotective properties and that they may help regulate the defensive mechanisms described above.

ABNORMALITIES IN PATIENTS WITH DUODENAL OR GASTRIC ULCERS

GENETIC PREDISPOSITION. Heredity has been postulated to play a role in the pathogenesis of ulcer disease in some patients. Several rare genetic syndromes are associated with peptic ulcer disease. Multiple endocrine neoplasia I syndrome is the most common example (Ch. 228). Additionally, several pathophysiologic abnormalities believed to be associated with increased acid and pepsin secretion or increased gastric emptying have been discovered, and several of these have been found in "ulcer families." For example, in several families an increased level of

serum pepsinogen I was inherited as an autosomal dominant trait. Since serum pepsinogen I concentrations reflect chief cell mass and correlate with maximum acid output, members of these families may have developed ulcers because of either increased pepsin or acid secretion or increased secretion of both. Other abnormalities, such as those leading to diminished mucosal defense, may be inherited also. The importance, if any, of hereditary factors in the pathogenesis of peptic ulcer disease in most patients has not been established.

ABNORMALITIES IN SECRETION OF ACID AND PEPSIN. Approximately 30 to 40 per cent of patients with duodenal ulcer disease have acid secretion rates above the upper limits of normal shown in Table 98–1. The remainder have values within the normal range. Since pepsinogen secretion usually accompanies acid secretion, approximately the same percentage of ulcer patients have increased or normal pepsinogen secretion.

Most patients with gastric ulcers have either normal or lower than normal acid secretion rates. Only a minority of patients with gastric ulcer disease (for example, a few patients with Zollinger-Ellison syndrome) have secretion rates above the normal range. The fact that most gastric ulcer patients have normal or lower than normal acid secretory rates does not exclude acid and pepsin as the cause of gastric ulcer disease in an individual patient but suggests that other factors may be involved (see below). This same concept applies to patients with duodenal ulcers who have normal rates of acid secretion. In fact, the role that acid or pepsin or both play in the pathogenesis of either gastric or duodenal ulcers is not known. It is assumed that acid is involved in the pathogenesis of ulcer disease in patients with higher than normal rates of acid secretion (see below). It is also assumed that pepsin is an essential factor in acid-mediated ulcer disease.

Three mechanisms for increased basal acid secretion are known: (1) increased stimulation by *gastrin* (Zollinger-Ellison syndrome, retained antrum syndrome, and antral gastrin [G] cell hyperplasia or hyperfunction); (2) increased stimulation by *acetylcholine* (vagal hyperfunction); and (3) increased *histamine* stimulation (systemic mastocytosis or basophilic leukemia). Other causes of basal hypersecretion may exist, but so far they have not been described. Ulcers presumably occur in patients with these disorders because of increased levels of acid and pepsin. All of the currently recognized syndromes causing increased basal acid secretion are rare. Of the group Zollinger-Ellison syndrome is the most common and will be discussed separately (see Ch. 98.6).

REFLUX OF BILE AND PANCREATIC JUICE. Bile acids, lysolecithin, and pancreatic enzymes are believed to be aggressive factors that lead to ulceration in some patients, especially some

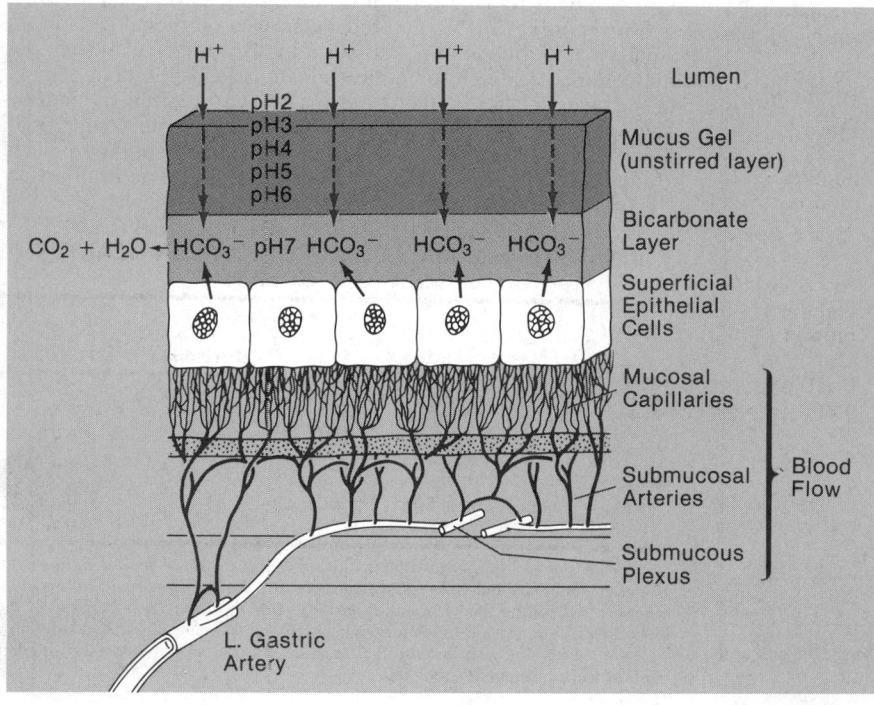

FIGURE 98–4. Model illustrating mechanisms maintaining mucosal integrity. Superficial epithelial cells secrete mucus and bicarbonate, which aid in maintaining a pH gradient between lumen and mucosa and protect the underlying epithelial cells from damage by acid and pepsin. Epithelial cell renewal and mucosal blood flow also are believed to be important mechanisms in maintaining mucosal integrity.

of those with gastric ulcers. It has been postulated that duodenal contents reflux into the stomach causing gastritis that, in turn, predisposes to gastric ulceration. Some patients with gastric ulcers may have an incompetent pyloric sphincter that allows reflux of bile or pancreatic enzymes or both into the stomach.

Two mechanisms have been proposed whereby bile and pancreatic juice may damage gastric mucosa: first, alteration of mucus overlying surface epithelial cells, reducing its protective effect; and second, damage to the so-called gastric mucosal barrier (the ability of the stomach to maintain electrical and hydrogen ion concentration gradients between lumen and blood). When these protective mechanisms are disrupted, the mucosa becomes more permeable to the damaging effects of acid and pepsin. Although bile and pancreatic juice have been postulated as the cause of gastric ulcers in some patients, a cause-and-effect relationship has not been clearly established.

ABNORMALITIES OF MUCOSAL DEFENSE. Little is known at the present time about how disruptions in mucosal integrity may lead to ulceration, although there are several theoretic ways in which this might occur. For example, some patients may secrete *reduced amounts of mucus* or *structurally abnormal mucus*. Both could lead to a weaker mucous gel layer.

Diminished blood flow may lead to cell injury and ulceration in some patients. Gastric mucosal ischemia is believed to be a factor in the pathogenesis of acute mucosal injury, as occurs in patients with severe medical or surgical illnesses (stress ulceration). Whether similar reductions in blood flow contribute to the development of chronic gastric or duodenal ulcers is not known. There are fewer collateral blood vessels on the lesser curvature of the stomach compared with the greater curvature. Whether this anatomic difference in blood supply leads to reduced blood flow to the lesser curvature with subsequent ulceration in some patients is not known, but most gastric ulcers do occur on the lesser curvature.

Decreased bicarbonate secretion is a possible cause for diminished mucosal defense. Gastric bicarbonate secretion has been measured in patients with duodenal ulcer disease and found not to be significantly different from that in normal subjects. However, bicarbonate secretion from the duodenum is decreased in some duodenal ulcer patients. Reduced pancreatic bicarbonate secretion into the lumen of the duodenum could theoretically lead to increased acidity in the duodenal bulb with subsequent duodenal ulceration, but patients with pancreatic insufficiency seem not to have a higher incidence of duodenal ulcers. The role of possible *abnormalities in cell renewal* in the pathogenesis of peptic ulcer is entirely speculative at the present time.

Prostaglandin content in gastric or duodenal mucosa might be diminished, leading to abnormalities of mucosal defense (see above) and ulceration. Studies have led to conflicting reports, however, so that it is impossible at this time to evaluate adequately the possible role of endogenous prostaglandins in the pathogenesis of gastric or duodenal ulcers.

EMOTIONAL STRESS. The mechanism or mechanisms by which emotional stress might contribute to ulcer disease in some patients are unclear. Certain emotions such as hostility, resentment, guilt, and frustration are associated with increased gastric acidity. Furthermore, basal acid secretion has been reported to increase during stressful interviews and prior to surgery in ulcer patients or before difficult school examinations in healthy subjects. Patients have been described who developed acid hypersecretion and gastric ulcer disease during periods of severe emotional stress. With alleviation of stress, acid secretion diminished and symptoms and ulcerations disappeared. Thus, certain emotions can cause increased acid secretion that in turn may lead to ulceration in certain patients. Emotional stress may alter factors that maintain mucosal integrity and thereby result in ulcers because of decreased mucosal defense. Although controlled studies suggest a relationship between emotional stress and ulcer disease in some patients, its exact role is uncertain.

DELAYED GASTRIC EMPTYING. Delayed gastric emptying has been postulated to have a role in the pathogenesis of gastric ulcer disease, possibly through retention of food in the stomach, which, in turn, might increase gastrin release and acid secretion. Prolonged gastric emptying, perhaps due to antral hypomotility, has also been thought to cause stasis and delayed clearing of duodenal contents (bile and pancreatic enzymes) that had refluxed into the stomach. This in turn could damage gastric mucosa,

cause gastritis, and lead to ulceration. Currently, delayed emptying is believed to be related to ulceration in only a minority of patients.

EXOGENOUS FACTORS. The most important exogenous factors that have been associated with peptic ulcer disease are cigarette smoking and the use of nonsteroidal anti-inflammatory drugs. Interest has increased during the past several years in the possible relationship between *Helicobacter pylori* and peptic ulcer disease. The possible association with adrenocorticosteroid therapy, alcohol, or caffeine is more tenuous.

Cigarette Smoking. Whether cigarette smoking is related to the pathogenesis of ulcer disease is unclear, although epidemiologic data suggest an association between the two: (1) Smoking is more common among patients with ulcers than among control subjects. (2) There is a positive correlation between the quantity of cigarettes smoked and the prevalence of ulcer disease. (3) Death due to peptic ulcer disease is more likely among patients who smoke than among those who do not. (4) Duodenal ulcers are less likely to heal in cigarette smokers than in nonsmokers. (5) Duodenal ulcers recur more frequently in smokers than in nonsmokers. Whether this applies also to patients with gastric ulcers is not known.

Nonsteroidal Anti-inflammatory Drugs (NSAID's). These medications inhibit prostaglandin synthesis and cause decreased mucus and bicarbonate secretion, diminished mucosal blood flow, and perhaps reduced cell renewal. Aspirin and other NSAID's cause superficial mucosal erosions in the stomach, presumably by reducing the factors believed important in maintaining mucosal integrity and likely cause chronic gastric or duodenal ulcers. NSAID's are an important cause of upper gastrointestinal bleeding from gastric and duodenal erosions and ulcers. Bleeding secondary to these drugs appears to be more common in elderly patients.

Adrenocorticosteroid Therapy. An association between treatment with glucocorticoids (especially prednisone) and peptic ulcer disease has been both supported and denied in conflicting studies. There appears to be a higher incidence of ulcer disease in patients taking large doses of glucocorticoids for long periods of time.

Infectious Agents. Cytomegalovirus (CMV) has been isolated from gastric ulcers in a few patients receiving immunosuppressive drugs and in patients with post-transfusion CMV mononucleosis. *Candida albicans* also has been found in gastric ulcers in several patients. Whether these organisms caused the ulcers or whether the organisms were there secondarily is not known. Herpesviruses have never been isolated from gastric or duodenal ulcers, but one study indicated that antibodies to Herpesvirus type I occurred more frequently and in higher titers in patients with duodenal ulcers than in control subjects.

Helicobacter pylori has been associated with gastric antral gastritis. There is circumstantial evidence that this organism may be related to the pathogenesis of peptic ulcer disease. How the organism might cause ulcers is unclear. It could disturb the normal defense mechanisms described above and this, in turn, lead to ulceration. The organism might produce a toxin that disrupts normal mucosal integrity which, in turn, would predispose to ulceration. More studies are needed before *H. pylori* can be established as an important cause of gastric or duodenal ulcers.

Alcohol or Caffeine-Containing Beverages. Even though both of these substances stimulate acid secretion, there is no evidence that either causes gastric or duodenal ulcers.

Peterson WL: Current concepts: *Helicobacter pylori* and peptic ulcer disease. N Engl J Med 324:1043, 1991. *This is a succinct summary of this topic of great current interest concerning the possible role of infection in gastritis and peptic ulcer.*

Richardson CT: Gastric ulcer. *In* Sleisenger MH, Fordtran JS (eds.): Gastrointestinal Disease. 4th ed. Philadelphia, W. B. Saunders Company, 1989. *The factors involved in the pathogenesis and therapy of gastric ulcer are discussed.*

Soll AH: Duodenal ulcer diseases. *In* Sleisenger MH, Fordtran JS (eds.): Gastrointestinal Disease. 4th ed. Philadelphia, W. B. Saunders Company, 1989. *The pathophysiologic abnormalities found in various groups of duodenal ulcer patients are discussed as well as the therapy of duodenal ulcer.*

Soll AH: Pathogenesis of peptic ulcer and implications for therapy. N Engl J Med 322:909, 1990. *This is an excellent, current review of factors believed important in the pathogenesis of peptic ulcer diseases.*

98.2 EPIDEMIOLOGY, CLINICAL MANIFESTATIONS, AND DIAGNOSIS

Lawrence R. Schiller

EPIDEMIOLOGY

Peptic ulcer disease is a common disorder; 5 to 10 per cent of all individuals develop peptic ulcer in their lifetime. Although ulcer disease is a common cause of morbidity, it is a relatively rare cause of death. The annual prevalence of symptomatic peptic ulcer disease in the United States is approximately 18 per 1000 adults, but the current mortality rate is only 2.5 per 100,000. Approximately 350,000 new cases of ulcer present each year in the United States.

Ulcer incidence varies by site, sex, and age. Symptomatic duodenal ulcer is more common than symptomatic gastric ulcer in both men (5.5 to 1) and women (2.8 to 1). Men are twice as likely as women to develop a duodenal ulcer but equally likely to develop a gastric ulcer; sex differences may be narrowing, however. Duodenal ulcer usually first produces symptoms between the ages of 25 and 55 years (peak occurrence at age 40) and gastric ulcer most commonly between 40 and 70 years of age (peak occurrence at age 50).

Hospitalization and mortality rates for duodenal ulcer disease seem to be declining in the United States, suggesting that the prevalence of duodenal ulcer may be declining. It is unclear whether this reflects an actual change in the prevalence of duodenal ulcer, a change in the criteria for hospitalization, or a change in the way mortality data are recorded. Hospitalization and mortality rates for gastric ulcer seem to be stable or increasing slightly, especially among the elderly. This has been attributed to increasingly widespread use of nonsteroidal anti-inflammatory drugs by these patients. Substantial differences in ulcer prevalence from country to country remain unexplained at present.

Epidemiologic studies have suggested strong associations between the occurrence of peptic ulcer and (1) cigarette smoking, (2) genetic factors, such as blood group O, (3) personality profiles, and (4) infection with *Helicobacter pylori*. Both gastric and duodenal ulcer are associated with active infection by *Helicobacter* in the gastric antrum, but the issue of cause and effect is not yet settled. There is no convincing evidence that alcohol ingestion or diet is associated with the development of peptic ulcer. Peptic ulcer is more prevalent than normal in patients with chronic obstructive pulmonary disease, cirrhosis, renal failure or transplantation, and renal stone (even when hyperparathyroidism is not present). Less firm associations have been suggested with coronary heart disease and polycythemia vera.

SYMPTOMS

DYSPEPSIA. Peptic ulcer usually presents as a painful upper abdominal disorder with the constellation of symptoms known as *dyspepsia*. Dyspepsia is poorly defined by both patients and physicians and often includes such symptoms as nausea, vomiting, anorexia, and fullness and bloating in addition to pain or discomfort. Most patients thought to have ulcers because of "typical dyspepsia" are not found to have peptic ulcer by radiography or endoscopy but instead have other diseases or are classified as having "non-ulcer" (functional) dyspepsia. The opposite can also be true; patients with symptoms such as heartburn, which might suggest gastroesophageal reflux, may actually have peptic ulcer. Thus it is impossible to differentiate ulcer reliably from any other condition causing dyspepsia on the basis of history alone.

PAIN. The clinical diagnosis of ulcer disease has usually been based on the location of pain, its character, and the factors aggravating or alleviating it. For example, ulcer pain is classically described as being located in the epigastrium and as burning or gnawing in character. Pain in this location also occurs in a majority of patients with "non-ulcer" dyspepsia, however, and pain of this character actually occurs in a minority of patients with either gastric or duodenal ulcer. Some patients describe ulcer pain as a cramping sensation not unlike hunger pangs, but descriptions of the character of pain are often hard to obtain in an unbiased way

and are difficult to assess. Typical ulcer pain is said to be relieved by ingestion of food or antacids, but this is also quite variable. A better predictor of the presence of peptic ulcer (especially duodenal ulcer) is an episodic pattern of pain. Individual episodes of pain usually are short lived, lasting for minutes rather than hours. Episodes of pain usually occur in clusters lasting from days to weeks, interspersed with long symptom-free periods. Recurrence is typical for peptic ulcer; some patients with ulcer report annual recurrences of pain during particular seasons such as spring or fall. Changes in the character of ulcer pain may herald ulcer complications, such as penetration or perforation (see Ch. 98.5).

The cause of ulcer pain remains unknown. Ulcer pain is usually attributed to increased acidity at the ulcer site and the relief of pain to a decrease in luminal acidity. This theory is consistent with the classic onset of pain several hours after a meal, when gastric emptying has reduced the buffering capacity of gastric contents and intraluminal acidity rises. Attempts to induce pain by perfusing the ulcer site with acid have not uniformly produced pain, however. In several studies ingestion of placebo with no buffering capacity was as effective as ingestion of active antacid in relieving ulcer pain. In addition, ingestion of food sometimes worsens pain. Alternative mechanisms for the production of ulcer pain have been proposed, such as abnormal gastric or duodenal motor function, but are similarly unproved.

COMPLICATIONS. Peptic ulcers frequently fail to produce dyspepsia or pain (perhaps as often as one third of the time) and therefore may present de novo as a complication, such as bleeding, obstruction, or perforation. These are discussed in Ch. 98.5.

PHYSICAL EXAMINATION

The physical examination is usually not helpful in uncomplicated peptic ulcer disease. Epigastric tenderness is an insensitive and nonspecific finding and correlates poorly with the presence of an active ulcer crater. When ulcer disease is complicated by obstruction, perforation, penetration, or bleeding, important physical findings may be present (see Ch. 98.5).

Rarely, peptic ulcer is associated with multisystem syndromes that may produce physical findings. For instance, systemic mastocytosis, stiff skin syndrome, pachydermoperiostosis, and multiple lentigines-ulcer syndrome may have cutaneous findings. Ulcer-tremor-nystagmus syndrome and amyloidosis may produce both peptic ulcer and neurologic findings.

DIAGNOSTIC VISUALIZATION

The definitive diagnosis of ulcer depends on visualizing the ulcer crater by radiography or endoscopy. Radiography is well tolerated (even in patients in fragile condition), readily available, and comparatively inexpensive, making it an excellent screening test. However, radiography may miss as many as 20 per cent of peptic ulcers. Endoscopy is more accurate and allows directed biopsy and cytologic study of suspicious lesions but cannot always be done safely in uncooperative patients or those whose condition is unstable. In the United States, where endoscopy currently costs from three to five times as much as radiography, upper gastrointestinal radiographs, preferably with both single-contrast and double-contrast techniques, are often the initial diagnostic test. In symptomatic patients with no radiographic abnormalities or with equivocal evidence of ulcer, endoscopy can establish or exclude the diagnosis of active ulcer disease. In situations in which there is little difference in cost between endoscopy and radiography, endoscopy is preferable in the investigation of patients with dyspepsia because of its greater sensitivity in diagnosis. Endoscopy is also preferable in patients with acute gastrointestinal bleeding because the risk of rebleeding can be assessed better and therapy can be delivered, if necessary.

DUODENAL ULCER. If a duodenal ulcer is demonstrated radiographically (Fig. 98–5), no further diagnostic evaluation is necessary and treatment can be started. Since duodenal ulcers are rarely malignant, endoscopic biopsy is not necessary. Follow-up examinations to assess healing of a duodenal ulcer need not be done routinely. However, if symptoms fail to subside with therapy, endoscopy should be done to prove the diagnosis of ulcer before considering surgery (see Ch. 98.4).

GASTRIC ULCER. If a gastric ulcer is found on the radiograph (Fig. 98–6), malignancy should be rigorously excluded, particularly if there is any suspicion by the radiologist that the ulcer

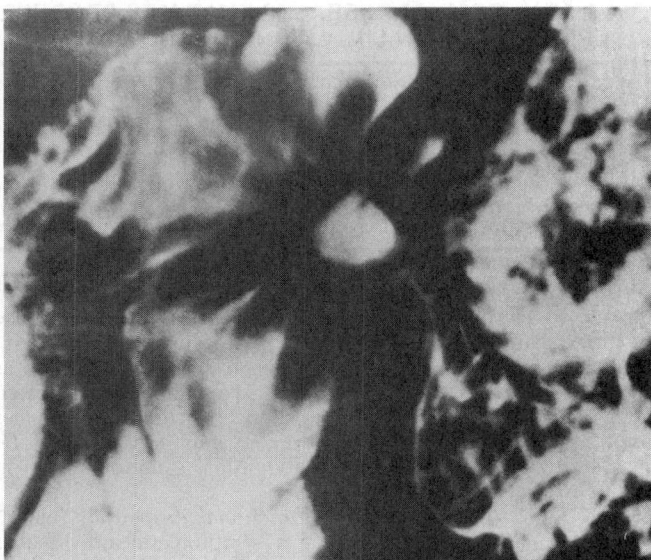

FIGURE 98–5. Duodenal ulcers are recognized when barium is retained within an ulcer niche. In this example barium has collected in an ulcer at the base of the duodenal bulb along the posterior wall. Folds radiate to the margin of this ulcer. (From Goldberg HI: *In* Sleisenger MH, Fordtran JS [eds.]: Gastrointestinal Disease. 2nd ed. Philadelphia, W. B. Saunders Company, 1978.)

may be malignant. Malignancy should be suspected if (1) the ulcer is located completely within the gastric wall or in an intraluminal mass, (2) there is nodularity of the ulcer base or of adjacent gastric mucosa, (3) there are no folds radiating to the ulcer margin, or (4) the ulcer is large. Malignancy can best be excluded by direct endoscopic visualization of the gastric ulcer to obtain brush cytologic specimens and to obtain a minimum of six

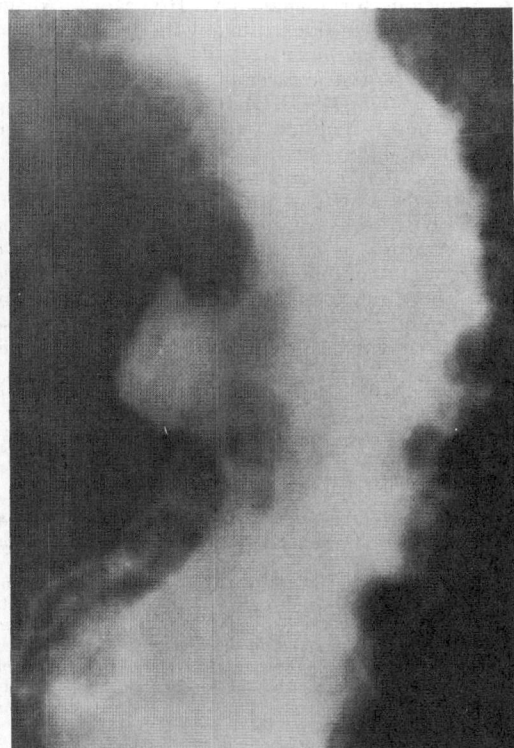

FIGURE 98–6. This ulcer of the lesser curve of the stomach demonstrates several features typical of benign gastric ulcers: The ulcer crater projects beyond the contour of the gastric wall, the margin of the ulcer crater is sharply defined and smooth, the ulcer is surrounded by a broad lucent band—an ulcer collar—resulting from edema at the ulcer orifice, and mucosal folds radiate from the ulcer collar. (From Goldberg HI: *In* Sleisenger MH, Fordtran JS [eds.]: Gastrointestinal Disease. 2nd ed. Philadelphia, W. B. Saunders Company, 1978.)

to eight pinch biopsy specimens for careful pathologic examination. This approach will lead to an accurate diagnosis in more than 95 per cent of cases. Some investigators recommend that patients with radiographically benign-appearing gastric ulcers not have endoscopy initially but that malignancy be excluded by repeating a radiographic study or by endoscopy after a period of therapy to prove that the ulcer has healed completely. Whether initially endoscoped and found benign or not, all gastric ulcers should be followed to healing to exclude malignancy. This can be done best by endoscopy after treatment for 8 to 12 weeks to allow healing to occur. Surgery may be needed to exclude malignancy in nonhealing gastric ulcer even if multiple endoscopic biopsies yield negative results (Ch. 98.4).

LABORATORY STUDIES

SERUM GASTRIN LEVELS. Radioimmunoassay of gastrin is useful in screening patients with known ulcer disease for Zollinger-Ellison syndrome (Ch. 98.6) and other rare hypersecretory states. The reasons for identifying these patients are (1) they may have a more severe course marked by excessive complications such as bleeding, obstruction, or perforation; (2) therapy is different, particularly surgical therapy (see Ch. 98.4); (3) associated but undiagnosed diseases of other organs, such as multiple endocrine neoplasia type I, may cause morbidity; and (4) gastrinomas associated with Zollinger-Ellison syndrome may be malignant and cause death from metastasis. Early recognition of Zollinger-Ellison syndrome makes possible effective control of symptoms and sometimes allows resection of tumor and cure of the disease (Ch. 98.6).

Measurement of serum gastrin concentrations in all patients with peptic ulcer disease is not cost effective because the incidence of Zollinger-Ellison syndrome is low (less than 1 per cent of patients with peptic ulcer disease). Table 98–2 lists the selective clinical situations in which obtaining a fasting serum gastrin level may be useful, although even with this selectivity the likelihood of identifying a patient as having Zollinger-Ellison syndrome is low.

If fasting serum gastrin concentrations are elevated (> 200 pg per milliliter) in patients not taking medications that alter intragastric pH such as high-dose antacids, H_2-receptor antagonists, or omeprazole, gastric acid secretion should be measured in order to prove that gastrin levels are not elevated in response to hypochlorhydria or achlorhydria, such as that due to pernicious anemia, atrophic gastritis, gastric cancer, or vagotomy. A finding of high serum gastrin levels and increased basal acid output limits the differential diagnosis to only a few entities (Table 98–3). If both fasting gastrin levels and basal acid secretion are very high (> 1000 pg per milliliter and > 15 mmol per hour, respectively), a diagnosis of Zollinger-Ellison syndrome is likely.

When fasting gastrin levels or basal acid outputs or both are less markedly elevated and the diagnosis of Zollinger-Ellison syndrome is unclear, the response of serum gastrin concentration to an intravenous injection of secretin may be helpful. In individuals with Zollinger-Ellison syndrome, intravenous injection of pure Secretin-Kabi, 2 U per kilogram of body weight, results in a prompt and pathognomonic rise of gastrin of greater than 200 pg per milliliter within 2 to 10 minutes. Patients with other hypergastrinemic conditions (Table 98–3) and normal individuals do not

TABLE 98–2. CLINICAL SITUATIONS IN WHICH MEASUREMENT OF SERUM GASTRIN LEVELS IS INDICATED

Family history of peptic ulcer
Ulcer associated with hypercalcemia or other manifestations of multiple endocrine neoplasia type I
Multifocal peptic ulcer
Peptic ulceration of postbulbar duodenum or jejunum
Peptic ulceration associated with diarrhea*
Chronic unexplained diarrhea*
Enlarged gastric folds on upper GI radiograph
Before surgery for "intractable" ulcer
Recurrent ulcer after ulcer surgery

*Not due to antacid ingestion.
GI = Gastrointestinal.

show this elevation. Gastrin secretion rises with calcium infusion also, but this rise is less reliable diagnostically than that following injection of secretin.

Differentiation of other rare hypergastrinemic syndromes (Table 98–3) can be made on the basis of (1) history of ulcer surgery (retained antrum syndrome, discussed in Ch. 98.4) or small bowel resection, (2) demonstration of gastric outlet obstruction by radiography or endoscopy, (3) laboratory evidence of renal failure, or (4) response of serum gastrin levels to a meal. Patients with antral G cell hyperplasia or hyperfunction more than double their already elevated fasting gastrin levels after ingestion of a protein meal. Patients with Zollinger-Ellison syndrome do not usually have this exuberant response to a meal.

ACID SECRETORY TESTING. Gastric acid secretion is measured by placing a vented nasogastric tube in the gastric antrum under fluoroscopic guidance and aspirating gastric juice with a suction pump. By measuring the volume and acid concentration (determined either by titration to pH 7.0 or indirectly from pH measurements), the quantity of acid secreted by the stomach can be calculated. Basal acid output (BAO) is defined as the amount of acid produced during four consecutive 15-minute periods. Vmax for acid secretion is estimated by injecting a maximally effective dose of gastric secretagogue. Pentagastrin (6 μg per kilogram), the biologically active carboxyl-terminal fragment of gastrin, is preferred for this purpose. Histamine or betazole (Histalog) can also be used. Stimulated secretion is expressed as peak acid output (PAO, the sum of the two highest consecutive 15-minute periods after injection multiplied by 2) or as maximal acid output (MAO, the sum of four consecutive 15-minute periods after injection). Values for acid secretion in healthy subjects and ulcer patients are shown in Table 98–1. In the absence of hypergastrinemia, measurement of gastric acid secretion is usually unnecessary in patients with peptic ulcer. Basal and peak acid output are increased in duodenal ulcer patients as a group (see Ch. 98.1), but knowledge of the level of acid secretion has no therapeutic implications for the individual patient at present. Measurement of acid secretion rates is sometimes useful preoperatively so that postoperative values can be compared and the effect of the operation on acid secretion can be assessed (see Ch. 98.4). When ulcer disease occurs in the presence of achlorhydria, malignancy should be suspected.

OTHER LABORATORY TESTS. The interest in *H. pylori* as a possible etiologic factor in peptic ulcer has spawned a number of tests for the presence of this organism. These include biopsy of antral mucosa with special stains, bacterial culture, immunologic tests, and tests based on bacterial metabolism, such as the ^{13}C-urea breath test. The clinical indications for any of these tests are unclear at present, since the implications of a positive test for subsequent management have not yet been defined.

In patients with recurrent gastric ulcer, blood salicylate levels may be helpful in detecting surreptitious aspirin ingestion.

Measurement of serum pepsinogen concentrations has been proposed as a surrogate test for direct measurement of gastric acid secretion. While the correlation of the two tests is good in large groups, individual values show too much variation to be useful for most clinical purposes.

DIFFERENTIAL DIAGNOSIS

Peptic ulcer can usually be distinguished from painful intestinal disorders that customarily produce discomfort in the periumbilical or lower quadrants of the abdomen (e.g., appendicitis or diverticulitis). Disorders affecting the viscera of the upper abdomen or chest are more difficult to differentiate from peptic ulcer

TABLE 98–3. CAUSES OF INCREASED FASTING SERUM GASTRIN CONCENTRATIONS AND INCREASED BASAL ACID OUTPUT

Zollinger-Ellison syndrome
Retained antrum syndrome
Massive small bowel resection (?)
Chronic gastric outlet obstruction (?)
Renal failure
Antral G cell hyperplasia or hyperfunction

TABLE 98–4. COMMON DISEASES THAT MAY PRODUCE EPIGASTRIC PAIN SIMULATING PEPTIC ULCER

Myocardial infarction
Pleurisy
Pericarditis
Esophagitis
Cholecystitis
Pancreatitis
Irritable bowel syndrome

disease (Table 98–4). Differentiation of these disorders can often be made by considering the acuteness of pain, lack of response to eating or antacids, changes of pain with changes in position, radiation of pain, and the presence of physical findings such as rebound tenderness, all of which are atypical in uncomplicated peptic ulcer disease. Because ulcer disease is common and ulcer symptoms are often variable, however, peptic ulcer must be considered as a possible cause of abdominal symptoms even in patients with atypical symptoms.

FUNCTIONAL DYSPEPSIA. *Functional dyspepsia* ("nonulcer" dyspepsia) is diagnosed when a symptomatic individual is not found to have an ulcer or other structural disease, such as cholelithiasis. The causes of this syndrome are unknown. It is likely that several different problems can lead to dyspepsia. It has been estimated that 20 to 30 per cent of patients with this diagnosis eventually develop peptic ulcer; therefore, some of these patients may really have evanescent ulcers that evade diagnosis. Some of these patients have a disruption of normal gastric motor function. Gastrokinetic agents such as metoclopramide or domperidone reverse both symptoms and motor dysfunction in some of these patients. Longer clinical trials are needed before such therapy can be generally recommended for patients with functional dyspepsia.

GASTRIC CANCER. Many patients with gastric cancer present with dyspepsia (Ch. 99). This diagnosis should be considered in particular when dyspepsia is associated with weight loss or evidence of occult gastrointestinal blood loss in an elderly individual or when radiographic or endoscopic appearances of gastric ulcer are suspicious for malignancy. However, a diagnosis of cancer should also be considered in any individual with a benign-appearing gastric ulcer, since roughly 2 to 5 per cent of such ulcers contain foci of gastric carcinoma.

MISCELLANEOUS DISORDERS. A variety of other diseases can produce dyspepsia that may mimic that of peptic ulcer. These conditions include *infiltrative diseases* of the stomach such as hypertrophic gastritis, tuberculosis, syphilis, Crohn's disease, and other granulomatous gastritides (see Ch. 97); *duodenal obstruction* by polyps, webs, or an annular pancreas; and *intestinal parasitosis* by *Giardia* or *Strongyloides*. More common diseases causing dyspeptic symptoms include *biliary tract disease* and *pancreatitis*. These can often be suspected by history, but tests such as sonography, cholecystography, and serum amylase determinations are usually necessary to confirm their diagnosis.

Graham DY: *Campylobacter pylori* and peptic ulcer disease. Gastroenterology 96:615, 1989. *Detailed review of possible relationships of infection by* Helicobacter pylori *and peptic ulcer disease.*

Kurata JH: Ulcer epidemiology: An overview and proposed research framework. Gastroenterology 96:569, 1989. *Introductory review and critique of epidemiologic techniques in ulcer disease.*

Richardson CT: Gastric ulcer. *In* Sleisenger MH, Fordtran JS (eds.): Gastrointestinal Disease: Pathophysiology, Diagnosis, Management. 4th Ed. Philadelphia, W. B. Saunders Company, 1989, pp 879–909. *Excellent review of clinical aspects of gastric ulcer disease.*

Soll AH: Duodenal ulcer and drug therapy. *In* Sleisenger MH, Fordtran JS (eds.): Gastrointestinal Disease: Pathophysiology, Diagnosis, Management. 4th Ed. Philadelphia, W. B. Saunders Company, 1989, pp 814–879. *Encyclopedic review of current knowledge about duodenal ulcer.*

Talley NJ, McNeil D, Piper DW: Discriminant value of dyspeptic symptoms: A study of the clinical presentation of 221 patients with dyspepsia of unknown cause, peptic ulceration, and cholelithiasis. Gut 28:40, 1987. *Analysis of symptoms in dyspepsia.*

98.3 MEDICAL THERAPY

Walter L. Peterson

In the healthy human stomach and duodenum, the potential for acid and pepsin to damage epithelium is effectively balanced by mucosal defense factors that act to prevent such damage.

Peptic ulcers occur when mucosal defense is disrupted in the presence of acid and pepsin. Potential mechanisms for this disruption include, but are not limited to, depletion of endogenous prostaglandins and *Helicobacter pylori* gastritis. Once formed, an ulcer remains as long as acid and pepsin overwhelm attempts at cellular regeneration. The goal of therapy is to shift the balance in favor of cell regeneration to effect healing of the ulcer, the clinical benefits of which are (a) relief of ulcer pain and (b) prevention of complications. Once an ulcer has healed, these early objectives may be extended by therapy designed to prevent recurrence.

Therapeutic agents used to accomplish these goals include antisecretory agents, antacids, sucralfate, and bismuth.

ANTISECRETORY AGENTS

Acid secretion may be reduced either by blocking the interaction of histamine or acetylcholine with their receptors on parietal cells (histamine H_2-*receptor antagonists* or *antimuscarinic drugs*) or by interfering with the intracellular machinery of the parietal cell (*prostaglandins* or *substituted benzimidazoles*) (Fig. 98–7).

H_2-RECEPTOR ANTAGONISTS. The effects of histamine are mediated through H_1 and H_2 receptors. H_1 receptors are located in the smooth muscle of the bronchus and small bowel, and H_2 receptors are located on parietal cells and the uterus. H_1 receptors are blocked by classic antihistamines such as diphenhydramine (Benadryl); H_2 receptors are blocked by specific H_2-receptor antagonists, which effectively lower both fasting and food-stimulated gastric acid secretion. There are four commercially available H_2-receptor antagonists for the acute treatment of duodenal or gastric ulcers. *Cimetidine* (Tagamet) is highly effective in the treatment of peptic ulcers in doses of 300 mg four times a day, 400 mg twice a day, or 800 mg at bedtime. *Ranitidine* (Zantac), used as 150 mg twice a day or 300 mg at bedtime, *famotidine* (Pepcid), used as 20 mg twice a day or 40 mg at bedtime, and *nizatidine* (Axid), used as 150 mg twice a day or 300 mg at bedtime, have subsequently become available. These agents are equal to cimetidine in effectiveness, with no clinical advantage of any one over the other three. Ulcers heal in over 80 per cent of patients after 6 to 8 weeks of therapy. Maintenance therapy with half-doses at bedtime also reduces the incidence of recurrent ulceration. These agents are remarkably safe, although side effects have been reported. Most reports deal with cimetidine and ranitidine, since the other two agents have not been in use long enough for a confident assessment of side effects. Central nervous system side effects (e.g., headache, mental confusion) are rare, reversible, and seen more often in patients with liver and renal failure. Gynecomastia and impotence have been reported, but in general the incidence is not significantly different from that of control groups. A number of drug interactions have been reported, predominantly with cimetidine, whereby concomitant administration with the H_2-receptor antagonist leads to increased levels of the agent in question. While there is potential for problems with drugs that have low therapeutic-to-toxic ratios (e.g., theophylline, warfarin, and phenytoin), the impact on patient management is minimal.

ANTIMUSCARINIC DRUGS. The classic antimuscarinic drugs reduce fasting and food-stimulated acid secretion by about 50 per cent and 30 per cent, respectively. However, these drugs also block other muscarinic receptors and produce unwanted side effects such as drowsiness, blurred vision, and urinary hesitancy. Therefore, these drugs (as well as the centrally active tricyclic antidepressant drugs trimipramine and doxepin, which possess antimuscarinic properties) have no role as first-line therapy for peptic ulcers.

PROSTAGLANDINS. Several methylated analogues of prostaglandin E_1 and E_2 have been developed which, when given in high doses, reduce gastric acid secretion by interfering with the generation of cyclic adenosine monophosphate (cAMP) in the parietal cell (Figure 98–7). Results of ulcer healing with these agents have been unimpressive, however, when compared to H_2-receptor antagonists. In addition, there has been a substantial incidence of diarrhea as well as the potential for abortion. Unfortunately, when lower doses (i.e., "cytoprotective" doses) of prostaglandin analogues are used, there is no effect on ulcer healing. Thus, most companies have abandoned their agents.

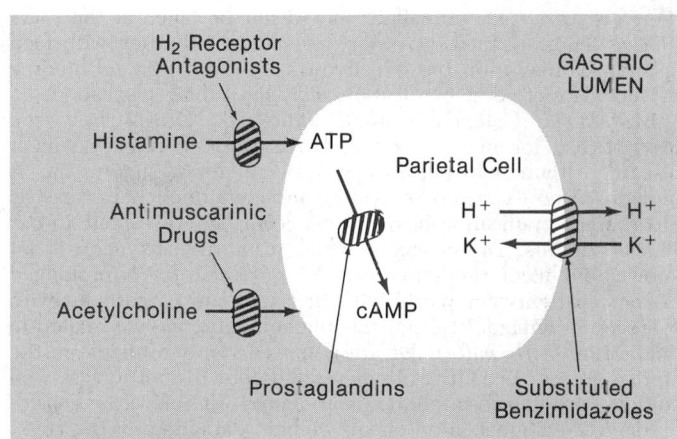

FIGURE 98–7. Sites of action of four drugs employed to inhibit acid secretion.

Only misoprostol (Cytotec) is commercially available and it is approved in doses of 200 µg four times a day only for the prevention of NSAID-induced gastric ulcers in patients at high risk of ulcer complications. The prostaglandin story is one of unfulfilled promises.

SUBSTITUTED BENZIMIDAZOLES. Drugs of this class, the prototype of which is omeprazole, are extremely potent inhibitors of gastric acid secretion. These drugs inhibit H^+-K^+– adenosine triphosphatase (ATPase), an enzyme found at the acid secretory surface of parietal cells that mediates final transport of hydrogen ions (via exchange with potassium ions) into the gastric lumen (Fig. 98–7). There is a prolonged duration of action, even when blood levels of drug are undetectable.

Omeprazole (Losec) in doses of 20 mg once daily produces ulcer healing modestly better than do H_2-receptor antagonists when the latter are given in standard doses. Because the cost of omeprazole is $0.50 to $1.00 higher per day than standard regimens of H_2-receptor antagonists, its major role should be in patients who might require larger than usual doses of H_2-receptor antagonists (e.g., patients with refractory ulcer, Zollinger-Ellison syndrome, severe esophagitis). The sustained hypochlorhydria produced by omeprazole results in hypergastrinemia, which, in rats, has led to the development of enterochromaffin-like cell hyperplasia and carcinoid tumors. The hypergastrinemia is reversible, however, and no such drug-related tumors have been documented in humans. Nevertheless, this drug should be used judiciously until more experience has been gained.

ANTACIDS. Antacids react with hydrochloric acid to form a salt and water, thereby reducing gastric acidity. Large doses (1000 mmol per day neutralizing capacity) of aluminum and magnesium hydroxide antacids are highly effective in healing gastric and duodenal ulcer, as effective as H_2-receptor antagonists. Such large doses often result in diarrhea, however. This property of antacids, as well as the advent of more convenient H_2-receptor antagonists, has relegated antacids to a position as supplemental rather than primary therapy for peptic ulcer. Interestingly, more recent studies from outside the United States suggest that low-dose antacids (e.g., one tablet, 25 mmol neutralizing capacity, four times daily) are as effective as large dose regimens. No such studies have been performed in this country.

SUCRALFATE

Sucralfate (Carafate) is the aluminum hydroxide salt of a sulfated disaccharide, sucrose octasulfate. Its mechanisms of action are uncertain. It has been suggested that sucralfate (1) forms a viscous shield over an ulcer crater, preventing acid from reaching regenerating ulcer tissue, (2) adsorbs bile acids or pepsin or both in the lumen, (3) stimulates the generation of local prostaglandins, (4) binds epidermal growth factor to the ulcer, or (5) acts as a scavenger of toxic free radicals. However it acts, sucralfate is effective for the acute therapy of duodenal ulcer in doses of 1 gram four times a day or 2 grams twice a day and as maintenance therapy in a dose of 1 gram twice a day. Results with gastric ulcer are less well studied. The drug is not absorbed and is therefore very safe. Sucralfate should not be taken at the same time as food, antacids, or other medications. Binding with food or antacids may limit the effectiveness of the drug, and binding by sucralfate of other medications may limit their absorption.

BISMUTH. Colloidal bismuth subcitrate (DeNol) has been used abroad for many years in the treatment of peptic ulcer disease. Although bismuth is bactericidal to *H. pylori*, this is unlikely to be its means of healing an active duodenal or gastric ulcer, since eradication of *H. pylori* occurs in only about 25 per cent of patients. The means by which bismuth heals ulcers is not known, but ulcer remission after bismuth therapy is prolonged in some patients compared with that seen after treatment with H_2-receptor antagonists, and this phenomenon may be related to eradication of *H. pylori*. DeNol is not currently available in the United States. Bismuth subsalicylate (Pepto-Bismol) is less well studied, and its use in peptic ulcer should, therefore, be considered investigational. Side effects include darkening of the stool, and, because of the potential for bismuth encephalopathy, long-term administration of bismuth is to be avoided.

If *H. pylori* is proven to have a role in the pathogenesis of peptic ulcers, its eradication may become a goal of treatment. Accomplishment of this goal, however, will likely require therapy with both a bismuth compound and at least one antibiotic.

TREATMENT OF PATIENTS WITH PEPTIC ULCER

At this writing, drugs available in the United States as therapy for patients with peptic ulcers include the H_2-receptor antagonists and sucralfate. Antimuscarinic agents, omeprazole, misoprostol, and antacids are also marketed but, for the reasons detailed above, are not recommended for first-line therapy. A physician should also be aware of several factors that at one time or another have been considered important in ulcer therapy.

COMPLEMENTARY FACTORS IN PEPTIC ULCER THERAPY. Factors to consider in this category include diet, smoking, alcohol or analgesic use, sedatives, and the need for hospitalization.

Diet. Diet therapy was once the standard treatment of peptic ulcer disease. Now, it is clear that no specific diet is of proven benefit in ulcer therapy. Patients should avoid whatever foods cause them discomfort but otherwise eat whatever they like. Because food, especially milk, stimulates acid secretion, between meal or bedtime snacks should be taken in moderation.

Smoking. There are many important reasons (other than the presence of a peptic ulcer) to encourage patients to stop smoking. Patients who do not smoke heal ulcers more often and more rapidly than those who smoke. The mechanism of this adverse effect on peptic ulcers is not known, although components of cigarettes may reduce endogenous generation of prostaglandins.

Alcohol. There is no evidence that alcohol ingestion retards ulcer healing. Nevertheless, because alcohol damages gastric mucosa, patients with ulcers who choose to drink should be advised to drink in moderation.

Analgesics. Drugs that inhibit prostaglandin synthesis (aspirin, nonsteroidal anti-inflammatory drugs [NSAID's]) are not only ulcerogenic but may predispose an ulcer to bleed. Therefore, patients with documented ulcer disease should be advised to discontinue the agent if at all possible. Patients with nonhealing ulcers should be queried regarding NSAID or aspirin use, and patients with documented ulcer who must continue taking NSAID's should be given prophylactic therapy with misoprostol (gastric ulcer) or an H_2-receptor antagonist (duodenal ulcer).

Sedatives. Although emotional stress may play a role in the pathogenesis of peptic ulcers in some patients, routine use of sedative drugs is of no proven benefit in ulcer therapy.

Hospitalization. Hospitalization should be reserved for patients with complications of ulcer disease (bleeding, perforation, penetration, obstruction) (see Ch. 98.5) or patients with ulcer pain refractory to routine medical management. In other situations, hospitalization is not warranted and has not been shown to lead to more rapid healing.

INITIAL MANAGEMENT OF PEPTIC ULCER. Patients should be treated initially with a single-drug, full-dose regimen of an H_2-receptor antagonist or sucralfate for duodenal ulcer and

an H_2-receptor antagonist for gastric ulcer. Duodenal ulcers are usually treated for 4 to 6 weeks; if at that time the patient is symptom-free, therapy is stopped with no further evaluation by radiography or endoscopy. Gastric ulcers are treated for 8 weeks, at which time assessment of healing is made, preferably with endoscopy or barium radiography. Follow-up evaluation to document ulcer healing is done to ensure that the ulcer is benign. Biopsies are taken any time an unhealed gastric ulcer is noted.

MANAGEMENT OF PATIENTS WITH UNHEALED ULCER. If a symptomatic duodenal ulcer or any gastric ulcer remains unhealed after initial therapy, the first steps are to ensure that the diagnosis of benign peptic ulcer is correct, to redouble efforts to have the smoking patient cease, and to inquire regarding aspirin or NSAID use. For duodenal ulcer, one will wish to increase the dose of H_2-receptor antagonist (if that was initial therapy) or change to omeprazole. Since medical therapy today can reduce gastric acidity as well as or better than can surgery, surgical therapy is almost never indicated for nonhealing duodenal ulcer. Of course, development of complications (e.g., bleeding) on medical therapy or noncompliance may mandate surgery. For patients with unhealed gastric ulcer, the first step is to treat longer with the same regimen, since gastric ulcers are usually larger than duodenal ulcers and, of necessity, take longer to heal. If healing still does not occur, the dose of H_2-receptor antagonist may be increased or therapy changed to omeprazole. If at any time the fear of cancer is overriding or if intensive therapy still fails to heal the ulcer, surgery should be considered. For patients who are not operative candidates, misoprostol has been reported to produce healing where H_2-receptor antagonists had not.

LONG-TERM MAINTENANCE THERAPY. Once an ulcer has healed with full-course therapy, long-term treatment with any of the H_2-receptor antagonists or sucralfate significantly reduces the high incidence of recurrent ulcer (as high as 70 to 80 per cent in 1 year). Not every patient requires such therapy, however. Patients who have bled from an ulcer should receive maintenance therapy with H_2-receptor antagonists in the hope that rebleeding will not occur and that surgery will not be necessary. Maintenance therapy is also given to those patients with frequent or especially severe recurrences for whom surgery might otherwise be considered. Unless a patient is a poor operative candidate, surgery is recommended if the ulcer recurs during maintenance therapy.

TREATMENT OF PATIENTS WITH ZOLLINGER-ELLISON SYNDROME. Patients with Zollinger-Ellison syndrome (ZES) pose a special problem. Because of constant gastrin-induced hypersecretion of acid, they are always at risk of ulceration and ulcer complications. The treatment is discussed in Ch. 98.6.

Feldman M, Burton ME: Drug therapy: Histamine$_2$-receptor antagonists—standard therapy for acid-peptic disease. N Engl J Med 323:1672, 1749, 1990. *Excellent recent review.*

Graham DY: Prevention of gastroduodenal injury induced by chronic nonsteroidal anti-inflammatory drug therapy. Gastroenterology 96:675, 1989. *Concise review of a controversial area.*

Lipsy RJ, Fennerty B, Fagan TC: Clinical review of histamine$_2$ receptor antagonists. Arch Intern Med 150:745, 1990. *Concise review of available H_2-receptor antagonists with long list of references.*

Maton PN: Omeprazole. N Engl J Med 324:965, 1991. *This is an excellent recent article in the* Drug Therapy *review series; with 181 references. It is the best starting point for reading about this new class of inhibitors of gastric acid secretion.*

Richardson CT: Gastric ulcer. *In* Sleisenger MH, Fordtran JS (eds.): Gastrointestinal Disease. 4th ed. Philadelphia, W. B. Saunders Company, 1989, pp 879–909. *Includes a detailed discussion of clinical results with therapeutic agents for gastric ulcer.*

Soll AH: Duodenal ulcer. *In* Sleisenger MH, Fordtran JS (eds): Gastrointestinal Disease. 4th ed. Philadelphia, W. B. Saunders Company, 1989, pp 814–879. *Excellent, detailed discussion of all aspects of duodenal ulcer disease.*

Wagstaff AJ, Benfield P, Monk JP: Colloidal bismuth subcitrate. A review of its pharmacodynamic and pharmacokinetic properties, and its therapeutic use in peptic ulcer disease. Drugs 36:132, 1988. *Encyclopedic review of bismuth subcitrate, a drug that may gain increased prominence in ulcer therapy if the* H. pylori *story holds up.*

Walan A, Bader J-P, Classen M, et al.: Effect of omeprazole and ranitidine on ulcer healing and relapse rates in patients with benign gastric ulcer. N Engl J Med 320:69, 1989. *Documents the results with omeprazole, 40 mg daily, in benign gastric ulcer. Also suggests a role for omeprazole in healing gastric ulcer in patients receiving concurrent NSAID therapy.*

98.4 SURGICAL THERAPY

Richard C. Thirlby

INDICATIONS

Peptic ulcers can be managed medically in most patients. Surgery may be required, however, to treat patients with complications of ulcers (hemorrhage, perforation, or obstruction) or patients with intractable ulcer disease. The decision to operate for intractability is difficult and is made primarily on subjective criteria. The physician and the patient must decide when pain and multiple ulcer recurrences become intolerable or intractable. Failure of medical therapy occurs when an ulcer does not heal on medication, when ulcers recur during maintenance medical treatment, or after multiple ulcer recurrences. Pain, interruption of livelihood or lifestyle, and history of major complications all influence the decision to refer patients for surgery. Pain per se is not an indication. Endoscopy should be performed before elective surgery to document the presence of an active ulcer in a patient with intractable pain, because the pain may arise from another cause. Although the frequency of elective operations for peptic ulcers continues to decline, the frequency of emergency operations for complications of peptic ulcers (e.g., bleeding, perforation) remains nearly constant.

SURGICAL PROCEDURES

SUBTOTAL GASTRECTOMY. Subtotal gastrectomy (65 to 75 per cent gastrectomy) was the standard operation for duodenal ulcer disease for many years. This procedure was effective in preventing ulcer recurrence in 90 to 95 per cent of cases, but the incidence of long-term postoperative complications was excessive (Table 98–5). This procedure is no longer recommended for treating patients with duodenal ulcers but is occasionally necessary in treating patients with gastric ulcers (see below).

TRUNCAL VAGOTOMY AND PYLOROPLASTY. Vagotomy eliminates cephalic (vagal) stimulation of acid secretion and reduces basal acid output by 80 to 90 per cent and maximal (peak) acid output by 50 to 60 per cent. Truncal vagotomy also denervates the antral pump mechanism, leading to delayed gastric emptying. This can be overcome by adding a drainage (gastric emptying) procedure to vagotomy either as a pyloroplasty (Fig. 98–8) or a gastrojejunostomy.

Operative mortality with vagotomy and pyloroplasty is less than 1 per cent (Table 98–5). Even when this procedure is performed as an emergency, operative mortality is relatively low in contrast to an operative mortality of 9 to 15 per cent after emergency vagotomy and antrectomy (see below). Vagotomy and pyloroplasty is the surgical treatment of choice for most patients with bleeding ulcers and is also used by some surgeons to treat patients with intractable ulcer disease.

TRUNCAL VAGOTOMY AND ANTRECTOMY. Resection of the gastric antrum, or antrectomy, removes gastrin-containing mucosa and diminishes the gastric phase of food-stimulated acid secretion. Antrectomy alone reduces acid secretion, and the combination of an antrectomy with a vagotomy leads to an even greater reduction of acid output (reducing basal acid output by 90 per cent and peak acid output by 70 to 80 per cent).

The combination of truncal vagotomy and antrectomy (Fig. 98–8) is frequently considered the standard elective operation for duodenal ulcer disease because ulcers recur rarely after this procedure. However, operative mortality is approximately 1 per cent, and long-term postoperative complications occur frequently

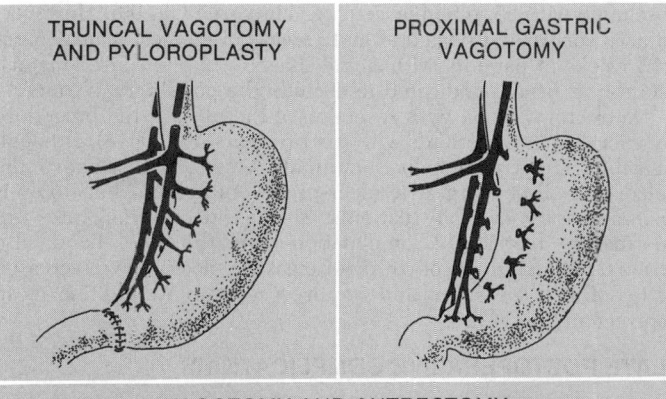

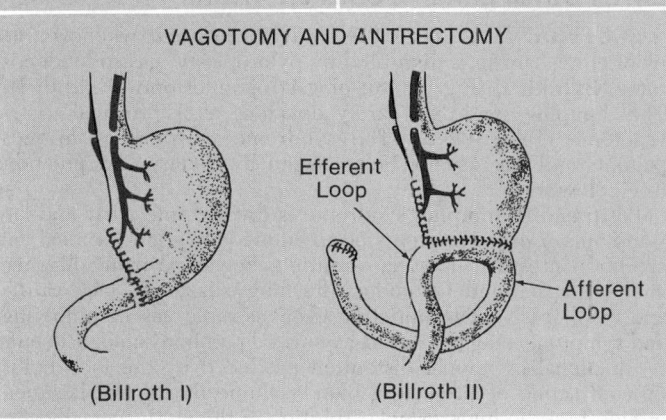

FIGURE 98–8. Model illustrating surgical procedures for peptic ulcer disease.

(Table 98–5). Therefore, proximal gastric vagotomy is gaining favor in some centers.

PROXIMAL GASTRIC VAGOTOMY. The parietal cell mass can be selectively denervated (proximal gastric vagotomy) (Fig. 98–8) while antral innervation and motor function remain intact. This operation reduces acid secretion while maintaining normal gastric emptying. Since many of the late sequelae of other acid-reducing procedures (e.g., dumping, diarrhea) are secondary to abnormal gastric emptying, the theoretic advantage of proximal gastric vagotomy is to reduce acid secretion with minimal mortality and long-term postoperative morbidity (Table 98–5).

Proximal gastric vagotomy is not indicated in patients with gastric outlet obstruction, active pyloric channel ulcers, prepyloric ulcers, or most patients with actively bleeding ulcers. Complicated peptic ulcer disease (history of bleeding or perforation) or high acid outputs do not contraindicate this procedure. Proximal gastric vagotomy is the operation of choice in many hospitals for patients undergoing elective operations for duodenal ulcers.

SPECIAL CONSIDERATIONS IN PATIENTS WITH GASTRIC ULCERS

The indications for operation and the surgical management of gastric ulcers are the same as for duodenal ulcers except that gastric cancer is a concern in patients with nonhealing gastric ulcers. If endoscopy with multiple biopsies and brush cytology specimens indicates that a gastric ulcer is benign, cancer is

TABLE 98–5. SURGICAL PROCEDURES FOR TREATMENT OF PEPTIC ULCER DISEASE

| | Operative Mortality | | Late Postoperative Complications | | | | | |
| | | | Dumping | | Diarrhea | | | |
	Elective	Emergency	MILD*	SEVERE	MILD*	SEVERE	Weight Loss	Incidence of Recurrent Ulcers
Subtotal gastrectomy	1%	10%	60%	5%	15%	0%	50%	5–10%
Truncal vagotomy and pyloroplasty	<1%	<7%	20%	2%	20%	2%	5–39%	7–10%
Truncal vagotomy and antrectomy	1%	9–15%	30%	2–5%	20–30%	2%	10–42%	1%
Proximal gastric vagotomy	0.1%	1%	0.5%	0%	1–2%	0%	0–5%	10%

*Nearly all patients have some change in bowel habits. Numbers are averages of many series and reflect clinically important symptoms.

excluded with 95 to 98 per cent certainty (see Ch. 99). However, if an ulcer has not healed after 12 weeks of medical management (15 weeks in patients with initial ulcers > 2.5 cm in diameter), surgery is usually indicated to exclude the possibility of cancer.

Antrectomy alone with resection of the ulcer is the procedure of choice in most patients with gastric ulcers (Fig. 98–8), although a subtotal gastrectomy is sometimes necessary to remove the ulcer and all of the gastric ulcer-prone epithelium. Vagotomy is not necessary in many patients, since acid secretion rates are normal or decreased. Some patients, on the other hand, also have duodenal ulcers or prepyloric gastric ulcers, have increased rates of acid secretion, and require vagotomy in addition to an antrectomy.

LATE POSTOPERATIVE COMPLICATIONS

POSTPRANDIAL DUMPING. This can occur whenever the pyloric mechanism is disrupted by pyloroplasty, gastroduodenostomy (Billroth I) (Fig. 98–8), or gastrojejunostomy (Billroth II). The dumping syndrome rarely develops after proximal gastric vagotomy (Table 98–5). The syndrome is transient in most patients and can usually be managed by dietary manipulations (see below).

Postprandial dumping syndrome is divided into early and late symptoms. *Early* symptoms occur immediately after a meal and are both intestinal (nausea, vomiting, epigastric pain, diarrhea, and dyspepsia) and vasomotor (flushing, dizziness, tachycardia, and diaphoresis). The initiating event is rapid gastric emptying, and symptoms may be caused by several pathophysiologic events: (1) duodenal or jejunal distention produced by the food bolus, (2) contraction of circulating blood volume due to displacement of fluid into the hyperosmolar solution in the gut (especially after consumption of refined carbohydrates), and (3) release of vasoactive hormones (serotonin, bradykinin, vasoactive intestinal peptide).

Late postprandial dumping symptoms occur 1 to 3 hours after a meal and are believed to result from hypoglycemia. The mechanism is presumed to be a rapid rise in blood glucose after ingestion of a large carbohydrate meal. This leads to an exaggerated insulin response followed by reactive hypoglycemia.

Treatment of the dumping syndrome is largely dietary (Table 98–6). Medications such as serotonin antagonists or antimuscarinic drugs are ineffective in most patients, although somatostatin analogues may prove efficacious. Reconstructive surgery aimed at slowing the transit of food through the small intestine using reversed intestinal segments or Roux-en-Y jejunal interpositions is indicated in the 2 to 5 per cent of patients who are severely disabled (Fig. 98–9).

POSTVAGOTOMY DIARRHEA. Diarrhea is common following gastric surgery, especially when vagotomy is included. In 20 to 30 per cent of patients, diarrhea is clinically important and in 2 per cent it is incapacitating (see Table 98–5). The pathogenesis is unclear, and diagnosis of postvagotomy diarrhea should not be made without excluding *inflammatory bowel disease*, *lactose deficiency*, *celiac sprue*, or other causes of diarrhea, because gastric surgery may unmask previously silent diseases.

Treatment of postvagotomy diarrhea is largely dietary (Table 98–6). Medications (antidiarrheal agents, opiates, cholestyramine, and aluminum hydroxide–containing antacids) may be helpful in some patients. Approximately 2 per cent of patients require reoperation (using reversed intestinal segments) to control disabling diarrhea.

WEIGHT LOSS. Weight loss occurs frequently after antrectomy (see Table 98–5). In general, it develops in proportion to the extent of gastric resection and occurs most commonly after a Billroth II gastrojejunostomy (see Fig. 98–8). Weight loss after gastric surgery most commonly results from inadequate caloric intake. Early satiety resulting from a small gastric remnant may cause patients to limit meal size. Fear of eating because of postprandial symptoms or diarrhea may also prevent patients from consuming adequate calories. Other causes of weight loss include bacterial overgrowth that can occur in the afferent limb (blind loop) of a Billroth II anastomosis (see Fig. 98–8), delayed and reduced mixing of pancreatic secretions with meals, and in rare cases celiac sprue. Bacterial overgrowth leads to hydrolysis

TABLE 98–6. DIETARY TREATMENT OF DUMPING SYNDROMES AND POSTVAGOTOMY DIARRHEA

1. Follow low-carbohydrate, high-protein, high-fat diet.
2. Avoid refined carbohydrates and concentrated carbohydrates such as sugar, jelly, cake, pie, pudding, candy; substitute complex carbohydrates such as starch.
3. Eat six small meals a day.
4. Drink fluids between meals rather than immediately before or during meals.
5. Eat slowly.

of conjugated bile salts and also damage to small intestinal absorptive cells. In turn, this causes malabsorption of fat, fat-soluble vitamins, and other nutrients. Malabsorption of calcium and vitamin D may combine to produce osteomalacia and osteoporosis. Bacteria also utilize vitamin B_{12}; this may lead to B_{12} deficiency.

Antibiotics (metronidazole, 250 mg three times a day) or surgical conversion of a Billroth II to a Billroth I anastomosis reduces bacterial overgrowth and may restore vitamin B_{12}, fat, and fat-soluble vitamin absorption toward normal. Weight loss and malabsorption may be helped also by dietary manipulations (Table 98–6), calcium and vitamin supplementation, antidiarrheal drugs, pancreatic enzymes, or a gluten-free diet in patients with celiac sprue.

ANEMIA. Anemia after surgery for ulcer disease can be caused by deficiency of iron, vitamin B_{12}, or folate. Iron deficiency is frequent after gastric resection. Malabsorption of iron and bleeding from recurrent ulcers or peristomal gastritis contribute to iron deficiency. Vitamin B_{12} deficiency may occur either because of atrophic gastritis (loss of parietal cells that secrete intrinsic factor) or because of bacterial overgrowth in the afferent loop of a Billroth II anastomosis (see Fig. 98–8). Folate deficiency is uncommon and presumably is caused by malabsorption of folate from food and by decreased ingestion of dietary folate.

Evaluation of anemic patients after surgery for peptic ulcer requires measurements of serum iron, vitamin B_{12}, and folate and assessment of stool for occult blood. Parenteral administration of vitamin B_{12} (1000 μg per month intramuscularly) and oral or intravenous iron (Imferon) may be required if deficiencies are documented. If bacterial overgrowth is suspected in patients with a Billroth II anastomosis, antibiotics (e.g., metronidazole, 250 mg three times a day) may be helpful.

ALKALINE REFLUX GASTRITIS AND ESOPHAGITIS. Reflux of duodenal contents, particularly bile, into the gastric remnant is believed to cause gastritis and esophagitis (see Ch. 97). Symptoms include continuous, burning abdominal pain,

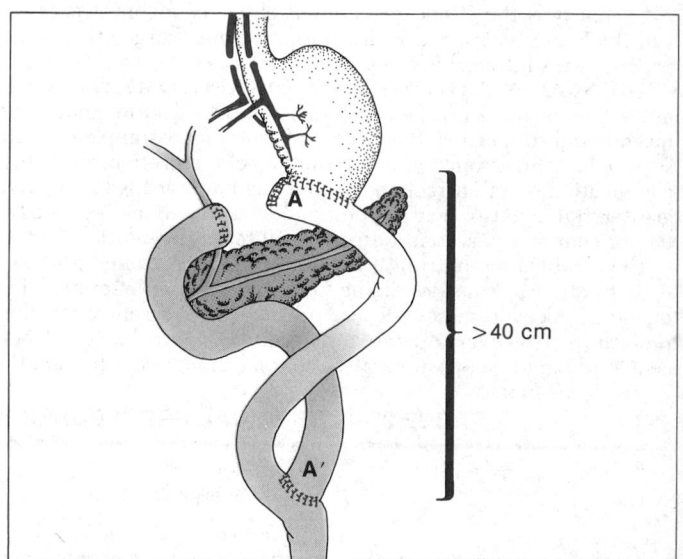

FIGURE 98–9. Model illustrating truncal vagotomy, antrectomy, and Roux-en-Y gastrojejunostomy (see text). Jejunum is divided at A-A' with distal end (A) anastomosed to stomach. Pancreaticobiliary secretions are thus diverted from the stomach by at least 40 cm of interposed intestine (pancreaticobiliary secretions shown in red).

nausea, and vomiting of bile-containing material. Establishing reflux and inflammation as the cause of pain is difficult, since many asymptomatic postgastrectomy patients have similar endoscopic or histologic findings. No test definitively confirms that pain is caused by reflux.

Results of medical treatment with drugs that bind bile salts (cholestyramine or aluminum hydroxide–containing antacids) are poor. Roux-en-Y jejunal interposition prevents reflux of duodenal contents into the gastric remnant and esophagus and relieves symptoms in most patients (Fig. 98–9). However, many patients with alkaline reflux gastritis have slow gastric emptying and do poorly after Roux-en-Y diversion, developing a syndrome of nausea, vomiting, and abdominal pain.

AFFERENT LOOP SYNDROME. This can occur in patients who have a Billroth II–type gastroenterostomy (Fig. 98–8). Symptoms occur when pancreatic and biliary secretions collect in a partially obstructed afferent loop, causing distention and pain. Eventually, the fluid bypasses the partial obstruction, rushes into the stomach, and provokes vomiting. Thus, the symptom complex is characterized by postprandial cramping epigastric pain followed by projectile vomiting. Pain is relieved after vomiting. The vomitus is voluminous, contains bile, and does not contain food because food has left the stomach and passed through the efferent loop. Management of severe symptoms requires operative revision of the gastrojejunal anastomosis.

POSTOPERATIVE RECURRENT PEPTIC ULCER

Postoperative ulcers can develop in the stomach, the duodenum, or the jejunum in patients with a Billroth II gastrojejunostomy (marginal ulcer) (Fig. 98–8). The incidence varies for the different operations (Table 98–5). The clinical presentation is characterized by pain in only one half of patients, and complications, especially bleeding, are frequent. Diagnosis of postoperative recurrent ulcer is best made by endoscopy because upper gastrointestinal barium studies are poor at identifying postoperative ulcers.

Incomplete vagotomy is responsible for postoperative recurrent ulcers in the majority of patients. Other uncommon causes include *Zollinger-Ellison syndrome, retained antrum syndrome, ulcerogenic drugs* (aspirin or other nonsteroidal anti-inflammatory drugs), *silk surgical sutures* at the anastomosis, or *antral G cell hyperplasia.* Serum gastrin concentrations should be measured in all patients with recurrent ulcers to rule out Zollinger-Ellison syndrome (see Ch. 98.6) or retained antrum syndrome.

Sham feeding is the best test for diagnosis of incomplete vagotomy (see Ch. 98.1). An appetizing meal is presented to a patient, and the meal is chewed but not swallowed. Acid output is measured during the test by aspirating gastric secretions through a nasogastric tube. Acid output induced by sham feeding greater than 10 per cent of pentagastrin-stimulated peak acid output implies intact vagal innervation of the stomach.

The use of histamine H$_2$-receptor antagonists is the first choice for the treatment of postoperative recurrent ulcers caused by incomplete vagotomy. Postoperative recurrent ulcers heal with standard doses of histamine H$_2$-receptor antagonists in 60 to 90 per cent of patients, and reoperation may not be necessary. Lifetime maintenance therapy (e.g., ranitidine, 150 mg, at bedtime) is required in all patients to prevent further recurrence and complications. The indications for reoperation in patients with recurrent ulcer secondary to incomplete vagotomy are (1) failure to heal with H$_2$-receptor antagonists, (2) recurrence on maintenance therapy with H$_2$-receptor antagonists, (3) a complication (bleeding, obstruction, or perforation) associated with recurrent ulcer, or (4) noncompliance with long-term medical therapy. The choice of reoperation should be individualized. If sham feeding confirms incomplete vagotomy, and if the patient has had an emptying procedure such as a pyloroplasty or a gastroenterostomy at the initial operation, transthoracic revagotomy usually should be performed. Antrectomy (or re-resection) is indicated in patients who have a complete vagotomy as judged by sham feeding.

Jordan PH Jr.: Indications for parietal cell vagotomy without drainage in gastrointestinal surgery. Ann Surg 210:29, 1989. *Review of a single institution's experience with 658 parietal cell (proximal gastric) vagotomies. Overall results were excellent in patients with intractable, perforated, and even bleeding duodenal ulcers.*
Jordan PH Jr.: Operations for peptic ulcer disease and their early postoperative complications. In Sleisenger MH, Fordtran JS (eds.): Gastrointestinal Disease. 4th ed. Philadelphia, W. B. Saunders Company, 1989. *A general review of the surgical treatment of peptic ulcer disease, including indications for surgery and a description of the operations.*
McConnell DB, Baba GC, Deveney CW: Changes in surgical treatment of peptic ulcer disease within a Veterans Hospital in the 1970s and the 1980s. Arch Surg 124:1164, 1989. *Current status of trends in rates of elective and emergency operations for peptic ulcers.*
Meyer JA: Chronic morbidity after ulcer surgery. In Sleisenger MH, Fordtran JS (eds.): Gastrointestinal Disease. 4th ed. Philadelphia, W. B. Saunders Company, 1989. *Detailed review of pathophysiology and treatment of postgastrectomy syndromes.*
Schirmer BD: Current status of proximal gastric vagotomy. Ann Surg 209:131, 1989. *Excellent review of historical, physiological, clinical, and technical aspects of proximal gastric vagotomy.*

98.5 COMPLICATIONS
Mark Feldman

Approximately one of three patients with peptic ulcer disease experiences *bleeding, perforation,* or *obstruction* at some point in the course of his or her disease. Patients with a peptic ulcer in the pyloric channel or postbulbar duodenum, with combined duodenal and gastric ulcer, and with Zollinger-Ellison syndrome are especially likely to experience complications. The incidence of complications has not changed since introduction of histamine (H$_2$) blockers. Complications may cause death before the patient can be brought to a hospital or before definitive treatment can be carried out.

BLEEDING

Bleeding is the most common complication of peptic ulcer disease, occurring in 15 to 20 per cent of patients with duodenal ulcer and 10 to 15 per cent of patients with gastric ulcer. Risk of bleeding is unrelated to duration of ulcer disease; one of three to one of four patients have no history of ulcer disease when he or she presents with bleeding. The mortality rate for a single bleeding episode (5 to 10 per cent) has not changed in the past several decades.

Hemorrhage results from erosion of the ulcer into a blood vessel. The most common sign of acute bleeding is melena, with or without hematemesis. Although these symptoms usually indicate major blood loss (> 1000 ml), melena may occur with loss of as little as 50 to 75 ml of blood. In some patients with major hemorrhage, gastrointestinal transit of blood may be so rapid that the stool is bright red or maroon. Moreover, a nasogastric aspirate may not contain blood if active bleeding from a duodenal ulcer does not reflux into the stomach. Thus, the combination of hematochezia and a bloodless nasogastric aspirate can occur in patients with bleeding peptic ulcer. The hemoglobin and hematocrit on admission may not reflect the severity of bleeding if sufficient time has not elapsed to allow for compensatory hemodilution. Therefore, the severity of acute bleeding is better assessed by the blood pressure and pulse rate. A systolic blood pressure of less than 100 mm Hg and a pulse rate of more than 100 beats per minute, both taken with the patient supine, suggest major blood loss, as do a fall in blood pressure of greater than 10 mm Hg and an increase in pulse of more than 20 beats per minute after the patient assumes an upright position.

Peptic ulcer is the most common source of acute upper gastrointestinal bleeding (accounting for 40 to 50 per cent of cases). The differential diagnosis, however, includes esophagogastric varices, erosive and hemorrhagic gastritis, and Mallory-Weiss laceration. Less common causes include benign and malignant gastric neoplasm, esophagitis, duodenitis, vascular anomaly (e.g., angiodysplasia and arteriovenous malformation), and aortoenteric fistula, usually in patients with a prosthetic aortic graft. Peptic ulcers may also cause chronic or intermittent bleeding, resulting in iron deficiency anemia. In such instances, it is mandatory to exclude other causes of chronic blood loss, such as colonic cancer, before attributing the bleeding to a peptic ulcer (Ch. 105).

Certain factors may, if present, adversely affect clinical outcome in patients with bleeding peptic ulcers: (1) severe, continuing hemorrhage; (2) early rebleeding, usually occurring within 3 to 5 days of initial stabilization; (3) age greater than 60 years; (4) associated diseases, especially involving the cardiovascular system, lungs, and liver; (5) history of ingestion of nonsteroidal anti-inflammatory drugs; and (6) endoscopic visualization of a blood vessel in the base of the ulcer.

Various therapeutic measures have been employed in patients with bleeding ulcers, including nasogastric suction, antacid therapy, and inhibition of gastric acid-pepsin secretion with histamine H_2-receptor antagonist drugs or with somatostatin. None of these measures, alone or in combination, has been proved to stop active bleeding, to prevent rebleeding, to decrease need for surgery, or to reduce mortality.

Ulcers that are actively bleeding or that have a visible vessel are sometimes treated endoscopically using electrodes (monopolar, multipolar, heater probes), laser (argon, neodymium: yttrium aluminum garnet), or by injecting alcohol, epinephrine, or other agents into the ulcer base. While all of these modalities can usually stop active bleeding, it is not yet clear which is most effective in preventing rebleeding, reducing transfusion requirements, and reducing the need for emergency surgery. It is also uncertain whether any of these newer modalities will reduce mortality rates.

Continuous bleeding from an ulcer or major bleeding that recurs in the hospital commonly is an indication for surgery. Urgent surgery in patients with bleeding peptic ulcers carries a mortality rate two- to threefold higher than elective surgery. Emergency surgical therapy for bleeding duodenal ulcer consists of suture ligation of the bleeding vessel, along with truncal vagotomy and pyloroplasty, parietal cell vagotomy, or truncal vagotomy and antrectomy. Vagotomy without gastric resection has a higher in-hospital rebleeding rate than truncal vagotomy and antrectomy but a lower operative mortality rate. For bleeding gastric ulcer, the distal stomach, including the ulcer, is usually resected. If the ulcer is quite proximal in the stomach, the ulcer is usually biopsied and oversewn, followed by distal gastrectomy. Emergency surgery stops bleeding in 90 to 95 per cent of cases. In poor surgical candidates, angiography with arterial embolization using Gelfoam or autologous clot may stop bleeding.

Following discharge from the hospital, patients should receive an H_2 blocker by mouth for 4–8 weeks to facilitate ulcer healing. Once medical therapy is stopped, a patient has a 30 to 50 per cent chance of bleeding again from an ulcer. The severity of the initial bleeding event is not correlated with the severity of subsequent bleeding. Late rebleeding may be partly preventable by prolonged, nocturnal therapy with an H_2 blocker (e.g., 150 mg ranitidine), but more studies are needed.

Armstrong CP, Blower AL: Non-steroidal anti-inflammatory drugs and life threatening complications of peptic ulceration. Gut 28:527, 1987. *One of several case-controlled studies from the United Kingdom linking NSAID use and life-threatening ulcer complications (bleeding, perforation).*

Christensen A, Bousfield R, Christiansen J: Incidence of perforated and bleeding peptic ulcers before and after the introduction of H_2-receptor antagonists. Ann Surg 207:4, 1988. *Study shows nearly constant annual incidences of ulcer bleeding (5 to 10 per 100,000) and perforation (4 to 10 per 100,000) from 1974 to 1984 in Denmark, despite introduction of H_2 blockers in 1977.*

Christensen J, Ottenjann R, Arx FV: Placebo-controlled trial with the somatostatin analogue SMS 201-995 in peptic ulcer bleeding. Gastroenterology 97:568, 1989. *Demonstrates no benefit of a 5-day intravenous course followed by subcutaneous somatostatin analogue (octreotide) in stopping ulcer bleeding or preventing rebleeding.*

Laine L: Multipolar electrocoagulation in the treatment of active upper gastrointestinal tract hemorrhage. A prospective controlled trial. N Engl J Med 316:1613, 1987. Multipolar electrocoagulation in the treatment of peptic ulcers with nonbleeding visible vessels. A prospective, controlled trial. Ann Intern Med 110:510, 1989. *Two controlled trials showing benefit of multipolar electrocoagulation of actively bleeding ulcers or ulcers with a visible vessel.*

Murray WR, Laferla G, Cooper G, et al.: Duodenal ulcer healing after presentation with haemorrhage. Gut 27:1387, 1986. *Controlled study showing 4-week healing rate of 80 per cent with ranitidine (150 mg twice a day) compared to 25 per cent with placebo after a duodenal ulcer hemorrhage.*

Therapeutic endoscopy and bleeding ulcers. JAMA 262:1369, 1989. *NIH consensus development conference which reviews different endoscopic techniques available for control of bleeding ulcers.*

PERFORATION

An ulcer may penetrate the wall of the duodenum or stomach, resulting in (1) *free perforation*—rupture into the peritoneal cavity with spillage of duodenal or gastric contents; (2) *penetration*—erosion into and confinement by a solid organ, such as pancreas, liver, or spleen; or (3) *fistula formation*—extension into a hollow viscus, such as the common bile duct, pancreatic duct, gallbladder, or intestine.

Free perforation occurs in 6 to 11 per cent of patients with duodenal ulcer and in 2 to 5 per cent of patients with gastric ulcer, during the course of known peptic ulcer disease or as the initial manifestation. Free perforation occurs more commonly in men, in elderly patients, and in patients who ingest nonsteroidal anti-inflammatory agents. Ulcers on the anterior duodenal wall are more likely to perforate, while ulcers on the posterior wall are more likely to bleed. A posterior duodenal ulcer may occasionally perforate into the lesser sac and cause back pain rather than signs of generalized peritonitis. Most perforated gastric ulcers arise from the lesser curvature. In approximately 10 per cent of cases, peptic ulcer perforation is complicated by significant bleeding.

Free perforation characteristically causes sudden, severe, constant abdominal pain that reaches maximal intensity rapidly. The pain is initially present in the upper abdomen but quickly becomes generalized. Movement exacerbates the pain so that the patient prefers to lie on his or her back without moving. Marked abdominal tenderness to palpation and diffuse, boardlike rigidity of the abdominal wall musculature are present. Hypotension and tachycardia usually occur owing to intraperitoneal fluid losses. Hemoconcentration and leukocytosis are usually present, whereas fever often is absent. The serum amylase level is mildly elevated in one of six patients. Upright abdominal or chest radiographs show free air (pneumoperitoneum) in approximately 75 per cent of cases. If pneumoperitoneum is not evident and there is clinical suspicion of perforation, it may be helpful to insufflate 400 to 500 ml of air into the stomach through a nasogastric tube and then to obtain upright radiographs of the chest and abdomen (pneumogastrography) or to administer a contrast agent such as meglumine diatrizoate (Gastrografin) through the tube or by mouth. Free air can also be diagnosed by sonography. However, definite diagnosis of perforated peptic ulcer often is not established until surgery is performed, and radiologic studies should be done expeditiously to avoid delays in therapy. The differential diagnosis of perforated ulcer is discussed in Ch. 98.2.

The presentation of free perforation may be atypical: (1) A perforation may close rapidly with only minimal contamination of the peritoneal cavity and with rapid, spontaneous clinical improvement. (2) Abdominal pain and physical findings may be less impressive in elderly patients and in patients with neurologic or psychiatric problems or both. Such patients may present with unexplained shock. (3) Fluid may leak into the peritoneal cavity slowly and collect in the right paracolic gutter, resulting in a clinical presentation simulating that of acute appendicitis.

Treatment of free perforation is usually surgical. In most cases, surgery is carried out to establish the diagnosis and to patch the perforation with a piece of omentum (Graham's closure). Whether definitive ulcer surgery should be carried out also at the time of patching a perforation is controversial. Many physicians will perform parietal cell vagotomy, truncal vagotomy and pyloroplasty, or truncal vagotomy and antrectomy for perforated duodenal ulcer (or distal gastrectomy for perforated gastric ulcer) if there has been a long history of ulcer disease or previous ulcer complications. If perforation occurred more than 8 to 12 hours earlier, definitive surgery is usually not performed because of extensive peritoneal soiling. If a perforated gastric ulcer is not resected, the ulcer should be biopsied because 10 per cent of perforated gastric ulcers are malignant. Medical therapy of free perforation, usually reserved for high-risk patients, consists of nasogastric suction and intravenous fluids and broad-spectrum antibiotics. In a recent study, about two thirds of patients could be treated medically, while one third required surgery. Whether perforation is treated surgically or medically, H_2 blockers should be prescribed orally for 4 to 8 weeks to facilitate ulcer healing.

Mortality from free perforation is approximately 5 to 15 per cent for duodenal ulcer and somewhat higher for gastric ulcer, especially if the gastric ulcer is near the cardia. Factors associated with a poor outcome in perforated duodenal ulcer are longstanding (> 48 hours) perforation prior to surgery; preoperative shock; serious concurrent illnesses; and old age.

Penetration into solid organs such as the pancreas occurs with unknown frequency, since penetration can be diagnosed with certainty only at surgery or autopsy. These patients almost always have a long history of ulcer disease and usually present with intractable ulcer pain. Serum amylase and lipase levels may be elevated with posterior penetrating ulcers.

A *fistula*, an uncommon form of perforation, from a duodenal ulcer usually extends into the common bile duct; one from a gastric ulcer usually extends into the colon or duodenum. Patients with duodenocholedochal fistula may be asymptomatic but have air in the biliary tree, or they may present with cholangitis and abnormal liver function tests. The fistula is usually demonstrated by an upper gastrointestinal series, in which case barium refluxes from the duodenal bulb into the biliary tree. The fistula may close during medical treatment, although surgery may be required in some cases. Gastrocolic or gastrojejunocolic fistula caused by perforated gastric ulcer is often associated with ingestion of nonsteroidal anti-inflammatory drugs. These patients may present with diarrhea and malabsorption. The usual treatment is surgical. A gastric ulcer in the antrum may also perforate into the duodenal bulb, resulting in two or even three channels from the stomach to the duodenum.

Chang-Chien C, Lin H, Yen C, et al.: Sonographic demonstration of free air in perforated peptic ulcers: Comparison of sonography with radiography. J Clin Ultrasound 17:95, 1989. *Since many patients with abdominal pain now receive abdominal sonography, the ability to detect free air with this method is important to recognize.*

Crofts TJ, Park KGM, Steele RJC, et al.: A randomized trial of nonoperative treatment for perforated peptic ulcer. N Engl J Med 320:970, 1989. *Controlled study which suggests that an initial period of careful observation and medical therapy is often safe, except in patients above age 70.*

Simpson CJ, Lamont G, Macdonald I, et al.: Effect of cimetidine on prognosis after simple closure of perforated duodenal ulcer. Br J Surg 74:104, 1987. *Controlled trial showing that cimetidine is superior to placebo in relieving symptoms and preventing morbidity after simple closure of perforated duodenal ulcer.*

Svanes C, Salvesen H, Larssen TB, et al.: Trends in and value and consequences of radiologic imaging of perforated gastroduodenal ulcer. A 50-year experience. Scand J Gastroenterol 25:257, 1990. *Compares plain film and use of water-soluble contrast agents in diagnosis of ulcer perforation and emphasizes that these procedures delay treatment by at least 2 hours.*

OBSTRUCTION

Gastric outlet obstruction occurs in approximately 5 per cent of patients with duodenal or gastric ulcer and is especially common if the ulcer is located in the pyloric channel. Obstruction is caused by edema, smooth muscle spasm, fibrosis, or a combination of these processes. Obstruction usually occurs after ulcer disease of many years duration but may occasionally occur as the initial manifestation. Mortality rates from obstruction in peptic ulcer disease are 7 to 26 per cent, depending on the age of the patient and the presence or absence of associated diseases.

Obstruction delays gastric emptying and commonly causes nausea, vomiting, epigastric fullness or bloating, anorexia, early satiety, and a fear of eating (sitophobia). Significant weight loss may result. Epigastric pain is frequent and may be relieved temporarily by vomiting. Symptoms have usually been present for weeks or months. Vomiting, which may be delayed an hour or more after eating, is often copious and may contain undigested food but usually no bile. Physical examination may reveal volume depletion (hypotension, tachycardia, and dry skin and mucous membranes), visible peristalsis in the epigastrium, or a succussion splash over the stomach.

Any of the following objective measurements support the diagnosis of gastric retention: (1) aspiration of more than 300 ml of gastric fluid 4 or more hours after a meal (a large-bore tube may be necessary for measuring this); (2) aspiration of more than 200 ml of gastric fluid the morning after an overnight fast; or (3) removal of more than 400 ml of gastric fluid 30 minutes after instilling 750 ml of isotonic saline into the empty stomach (*saline load test*). Gastric retention may be appreciated on a plain abdominal radiograph (large, dilated stomach containing solid debris) and documented by an upper gastrointestinal series or radionuclide scintigraphy. Gastric retention is not always caused by gastric outlet obstruction. It may result from gastric atony, as in diabetic gastroparesis, from vagotomy, or as a side effect of medications. Gastric outlet obstruction, which is caused by peptic ulcer disease in 80 to 90 per cent of cases, can usually best be established by endoscopy. The other common cause is carcinoma of the antrum. Less common causes include gastric lymphoma,

pancreatic carcinoma, pancreatitis, hypertrophic pyloric stenosis, eosinophilic gastritis, Crohn's disease, antral caustic stricture, antral polyp, and annular pancreas.

Laboratory studies usually reflect intravascular volume depletion (hemoconcentration, prerenal azotemia) and a hypokalemic, hypochloremic metabolic alkalosis due to vomiting. If extensive weight loss has occurred, hypoalbuminemia, cutaneous anergy, and a low serum transferrin concentration may be present. The urine is usually concentrated and contains less than 10 mEq of chloride per liter, but the urinary sodium concentration and pH are variable, depending on the renal tubular threshold for bicarbonate reabsorption.

Therapy of gastric outlet obstruction has three goals: gastric decompression and resolution of obstruction; replacement of fluids and electrolytes; and nutritional support. Gastric decompression is accomplished by continuous nasogastric suction for at least 72 hours. With prolonged obstruction, gradual gastric dilation occurs, and this interferes with the contractile function of gastric smooth muscle. Electrolyte disturbances such as hypokalemia can also contribute to gastric motor dysfunction. Saline load tests, performed serially, may have prognostic value. For example, a return of more than 300 ml after 24 hours of nasogastric suction suggests that obstruction will not resolve and that surgery may be required. After 72 hours, a return of less than 200 ml is a favorable sign and usually indicates that the tube can be removed and the patient can be fed liquids. Intravenous fluids and electrolytes are given to replace pre-existing and current losses. Isotonic saline containing 10 to 20 mEq of potassium chloride per liter is satisfactory in most cases. Losses of gastric acid from continuous gastric aspiration can be curtailed by administering H_2-receptor antagonists (cimetidine, ranitidine, or famotidine) intravenously. If suction is carried out for only a few days, 5 per cent dextrose solution administered intravenously, along with soluble vitamins, may suffice. If prolonged suction proves necessary, parenteral intravenous hyperalimentation should be instituted. This is especially valuable if the patient has lost significant lean body mass.

Approximately 50 per cent of patients with obstruction improve with medical management. If obstruction does not resolve in 3 to 7 days, surgery may be necessary. There is controversy over which operation is best: truncal vagotomy and antrectomy, truncal vagotomy and drainage (pyloroplasty or gastrojejunostomy), or subtotal gastrectomy. Some surgeons are reluctant to perform truncal vagotomy for fear of postoperative gastric atony, although this complication is uncommon. Gastrojejunostomy (without gastric resection or truncal vagotomy) is associated with a high rate (30 to 40 per cent) of recurrences of ulcer. Nonsurgical dilation of the obstructed pylorus using balloons passed through an endoscope is a newly introduced therapy that has not yet been compared with surgery in a controlled study. Nevertheless, approximately 80 per cent of patients can be successfully treated by dilation followed by oral H_2 blockers. Follow-up of patients receiving dilation is short, however (<2 years), and thus the long-term effectiveness remains to be established.

Graham D: Complications of peptic ulcer disease and indications for surgery. *In* Sleisenger MH, Fordtran JS (eds.): Gastrointestinal Disease. 4th ed. Philadelphia, W. B. Saunders Company, 1989, p 925. *Comprehensive review with extensive references.*

Griffin SM, Chung SCS, Leung JWC, et al.: Peptic pyloric stenosis treated by endoscopic balloon dilatation. Br J Surg 76:1147, 1989. *Uncontrolled study of 25 patients with gastric outlet obstruction dilated endoscopically with 9 months of median follow-up. Excellent results in 20 patients.*

98.6 ZOLLINGER-ELLISON SYNDROME

Charles T. Richardson

DEFINITION

The Zollinger-Ellison syndrome is defined by both chemical and clinical criteria: (1) an increased serum gastrin concentration, (2) an increased basal acid output, (3) an increased ratio of basal to peak (pentagastrin-stimulated) acid output, (4) the presence of peptic ulcer disease or diarrhea or both, and (5) a gastrin-producing tumor. Not all patients with an elevated serum gastrin concentration and hypersecretion of acid have tumors that can be identified at surgery or by noninvasive tests such as sonography or computed tomography. Presumably, such patients have tumors that are too small to be identified, or they have hyperplasia of the islets of Langerhans, a condition known as microadenomatosis.

CLINICAL MANIFESTATIONS

Zollinger-Ellison syndrome occurs most frequently between ages 35 and 65 years and more commonly in men than in women. *Abdominal pain* resulting from an ulcer is the most common clinical finding. Ulcers usually occur in the duodenal bulb but also may develop in the postbulbar duodenum, jejunum, stomach, or esophagus. Complications of ulcer disease, such as bleeding or perforation, occur in 40 to 50 per cent of patients at some time during their course and may be the presenting manifestation. Forty-five per cent of patients have esophageal symptoms consisting of heartburn, dysphagia, or both. *Diarrhea* is a frequent complaint and may precede ulceration in some patients or occur without ulcers in others (5 to 10 per cent). *Fat malabsorption* (steatorrhea) is occasionally noted.

About 20 to 30 per cent of patients with Zollinger-Ellison syndrome have multiple endocrine neoplasia (MEN I) syndrome and thus have a hereditary form of peptic ulcer disease (Ch. 228). These patients may have parathyroid or pituitary tumors and clinical findings such as hypercalcemia, renal stones, or increased prolactin levels. It is unlikely that peptic ulcer disease occurs with increased frequency in association with parathyroid adenomas except in patients who also have MEN I syndrome.

In some patients, Cushing's syndrome can develop as a result of either pituitary disease or ectopic adrenocorticotropic hormone (ACTH) production by gastrinomas. Patients with ectopic ACTH production frequently have metastatic gastrinoma, for example, in the liver.

PATHOPHYSIOLOGY

Peptic ulcers in patients with Zollinger-Ellison syndrome presumably result from increased secretion of acid and pepsin driven by excessive amounts of circulating gastrin. Gastrin also has a trophic effect on parietal (acid-secreting) cells that leads to an increased parietal cell mass.

Diarrhea results almost exclusively from the large volumes of fluid secreted by the stomach and is relieved in most patients by aspirating gastric juice via a nasogastric tube or more conveniently by treating patients with H_2-receptor antagonists or omeprazole (see below).

Steatorrhea may occur for several reasons: (1) excess acid damages small bowel epithelial cells, causing a mucosal defect that limits transport of fat and perhaps other nutrients across the mucosa; (2) pancreatic lipase is inactivated by acid, which impairs hydrolysis of triglycerides and contributes to fat malabsorption; (3) acid may decrease the amount of conjugated bile acids in the duodenum and upper jejunum, resulting in inadequate formation of micelles for fat absorption (Ch. 102).

DIAGNOSIS

Zollinger-Ellison syndrome should be suspected in patients who have (1) ulcers in unusual locations, such as the postbulbar duodenum or jejunum, (2) ulcers that persist despite medical treatment, (3) ulcers and diarrhea, (4) abnormally large gastric folds or thickened duodenal and/or jejunal folds, (5) ulcers and manifestations of other endocrine tumors such as renal stones, (6) a family history of ulcer disease, and (7) recurrent ulcers after ulcer surgery.

These criteria call for measurement of the serum gastrin concentration (see Table 98–2). If the level is abnormally high, a gastric analysis should be performed. Zollinger-Ellison syndrome is a likely diagnosis if the serum gastrin level is elevated, basal acid output is increased (>10.6 mmol per hour in men and 5.6 mmol per hour in women), and the ratio of basal to peak acid output (pentagastrin stimulated) is greater than 0.40:1.0. The diagnosis can be confirmed by performing a secretin stimulation test (see Ch. 98.2). This test is especially helpful in patients with serum gastrin concentrations or basal acid outputs that are only slightly increased. A positive secretin test, along with an increased serum gastrin concentration and basal acid output, establishes the diagnosis of Zollinger-Ellison syndrome in over 95 per cent of patients.

Tumors are found at surgery in 40 to 70 per cent of patients with Zollinger-Ellison syndrome and are usually located in the pancreas. Tumors have also been found in the duodenum, stomach, greater omentum, transverse mesocolon, and other areas of the peritoneal cavity. Computed tomography (CT) is useful in detecting gastrinomas and therefore should be performed in patients suspected of having the Zollinger-Ellison syndrome. A positive CT scan is almost always correct, whereas a negative CT scan is less reliable. Angiography and sonography are helpful adjuncts to CT. Since some gastrinomas have been found in the stomach or duodenum, upper endoscopy also should be performed to look for tumors. Techniques such as intraoperative sonography or transhepatic venous sampling to measure gastrin from tributaries draining the pancreas or duodenum have been helpful in localizing tumors.

THERAPY

For many years total gastrectomy was the treatment of choice for patients with Zollinger-Ellison syndrome. All of the acid-secreting mucosa as well as the antrum is removed, with subsequent cure of peptic ulcers and diarrhea. However, many of the late postoperative complications that occur in patients with ordinary peptic ulcer disease develop after total gastrectomy (see Ch. 98.4). Furthermore, in some centers mortality is higher with total gastrectomy than with other surgical procedures for ulcer disease.

With the advent of H_2-receptor antagonists and omeprazole, it has become possible to treat patients medically. Reducing acid secretion with an H_2-receptor antagonist or omeprazole effectively treats symptoms related to the disease in most patients. However, larger than normally prescribed doses, as well as more frequent administration, are often required. For example, 600 mg of cimetidine every 4 hours or 300 mg of ranitidine every 8 hours may be necessary to reduce acid secretion adequately.* A few patients have required even larger and more frequent doses of H_2-receptor antagonist. For example, a few patients have required as much as 5 to 10 grams of cimetidine daily. The dose of H_2-receptor antagonist may be reduced by treating patients concomitantly with an antimuscarinic drug such as glycopyrrolate or isopropamide (see Fig. 98–7), since antimuscarinic drugs have been shown to enhance the inhibitory effect on acid secretion of H_2-receptor antagonists. Many patients can be treated with once-daily doses of omeprazole (see Ch. 98.3). Even when using this more potent inhibitor of acid secretion, higher than normal doses must be prescribed in many patients. For example, doses as high as 60 to 120 mg have been required in some patients and doses of 60 mg twice daily have been needed in a few patients to reduce acid secretion effectively.

Medical treatment alone with H_2-receptor antagonists or omeprazole is not ideal for two reasons: First, complications of ulcer disease have occurred in some patients, and second, medical therapy does not provide an opportunity to search for resectable tumors, more than half of which are believed to be malignant. Because of this, a reasonable approach to treating patients with Zollinger-Ellison syndrome is laparotomy to search for resectable tumors present in about 20 to 30 per cent of patients, followed by medical therapy with H_2-receptor antagonists or omeprazole. At laparotomy a careful search for resectable tumors should be carried out. This includes intraoperative endoscopy with transillumination of the stomach and duodenum and intraoperative sonography.

Vagotomy may be combined with medical therapy in some patients to reduce acid secretion and to add to the inhibitory effect of medication. Treatment with a drug is still necessary, although the dose of H_2-receptor antagonist or omeprazole can sometimes be reduced. Regardless of the therapy used (tumor search followed by medical therapy alone or medical therapy combined with vagotomy), close follow-up to ensure compliance with the regimen is mandatory.

---

*May exceed maximum recommended daily dose.

Jensen RT, Doppman JL, Gardner JD: Gastrinoma. *In* Brooks F, Dimagno E, Gardner JD, et al.: The Exocrine Pancreas: Biology, Pathology and Disease. New York, Raven Press, 1986, pp 727–745. *An excellent review of the clinical manifestations, diagnosis, and treatment of patients with Zollinger-Ellison syndrome.*

McGuigan JE: The Zollinger-Ellison Syndrome. *In* Sleisenger MH, Fordtran JS (eds.): Gastrointestinal Disease. 4th ed. Philadelphia, W. B. Saunders Company, 1989.

Wolfe MM, Jensen RT: Zollinger-Ellison syndrome: Current concepts in diagnosis and management. N Engl J Med. 317:1200, 1987. *Both of the last two references review the pathophysiology, diagnosis, and treatment of Zollinger-Ellison syndrome and give extensive references to the recent literature for this disorder.*

99 Neoplasms of the Stomach

Sidney J. Winawer

The majority of gastric neoplasms are malignant, in contrast to the colon, where the reverse is true. Although gastric carcinoma is steadily decreasing in the United States, it still represents a major public health problem throughout the world. In some countries it is the most frequent cancer and the leading cause of death from cancer. In the United States gastric carcinoma is responsible for 90 to 95 per cent of malignant disease of the stomach. Approximately 5 per cent of all primary gastric malignancy is Hodgkin's disease (HD) and non-Hodgkin's lymphoma, particularly the latter, since HD rarely involves the stomach as a primary site. The sarcomas, including leiomyosarcoma, liposarcoma, neurogenic sarcoma, and fibrosarcoma, are all relatively rare malignant tumors that may involve the stomach. Leiomyosarcoma of the stomach represents about 1 per cent of gastric cancers.

CARCINOMA OF THE STOMACH

EPIDEMIOLOGY. The incidence of gastric cancer varies markedly in different areas of the world. It is extremely common in Japan, Latin America west of the Andes, some parts of the Caribbean, and Eastern Europe; moderately common in Finland, Austria, and Czechoslovakia; and uncommon in the United States, Australia, New Zealand, and other Anglo-Saxon countries. Colorectal cancer tends to be rare where gastric cancer is common and vice versa. The low incidence in the United States is a recent development (Fig. 99–1), since gastric cancer was the most common known cancer in the United States 40 to 50 years ago. Other countries that previously had a high incidence have also begun to show a decrease. The reasons for this are unknown. Environmental factors are considered important in the etiology of gastric cancer, as evidenced by populations migrating to areas of either low or high risk and taking on the risk of the area of migration. Japanese moving to Hawaii have a decreased incidence of gastric cancer in subsequent generations, and there is a further reduction with migration to the mainland. The incidence of colonic cancer increases with this migration.

ETIOLOGY. *Dietary influences* are thought to be important, but without direct proof. Consumption of barbecued meals, smoked or pickled fish and sauces, and alcohol and deficiencies of magnesium and vitamin A have all been postulated but unproved as causes of gastric cancer (Table 99–1).

Nitrosamines are powerful carcinogens for animals. They can be formed easily from common, secondary, tertiary, and quaternary amines by combining these with nitrite (the nitrosation reaction). This reaction can take place under varying conditions of pH and temperature, so that nitrosamines may be formed in the soil, under conditions of food storage, during food preparation such as frying bacon, or in the body. Bacteria may play a role by catalyzing the amine nitrite union or by reducing nitrate to nitrite. Thus the achlorhydric stomach is considered a favorable site for nitrosamine synthesis. The necessary amines can be found in many foods and medications, whereas nitrate and nitrites are found naturally in food and water and are present in food preservatives. Ascorbic acid (vitamin C) blocks the nitrosation reaction in the test tube. The increased intake of vitamin C and refrigeration have been postulated to be responsible for the

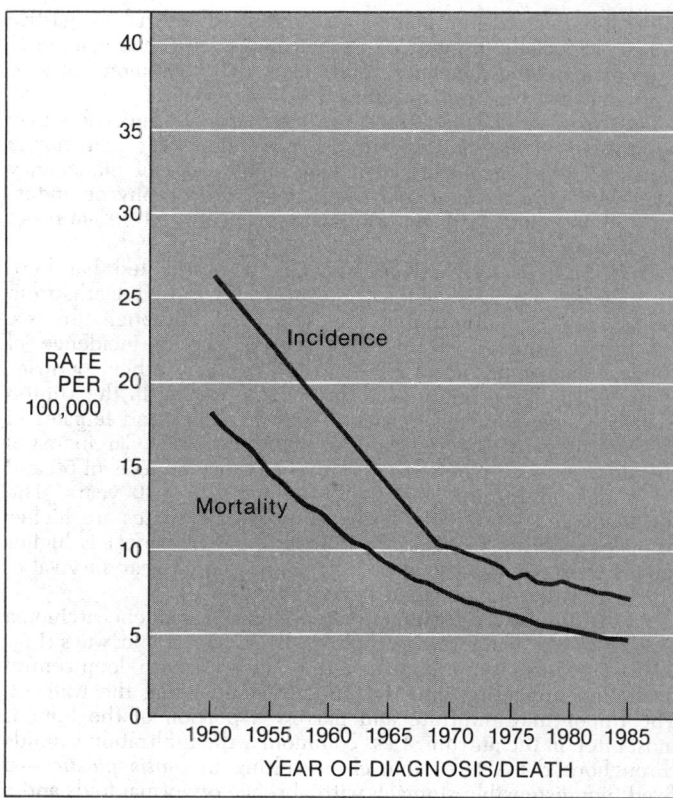

FIGURE 99–1. Incidence and mortality of gastric adenocarcinoma in the United States. (Data obtained and modified from the NCI Annual Cancer Statistics Review including Cancer Trends: 1950–1985 and is representative of the United States population.)

decrease in gastric cancer in the United States over the last few decades, but the nitrite hypothesis itself remains to be validated.

Blood group A is associated with a higher incidence of gastric cancer even in areas of the world where gastric cancer is rare. This fact and the threefold increase in gastric cancer among first-degree relatives, (parents, siblings, children) of gastric cancer patients has raised the possibility of an inherited or familial component.

Pernicious anemia had been considered a premalignant condition, but the prior high incidence of gastric cancer seen in this disease is no longer seen. This may be a reflection of the progressively decreasing incidence of gastric cancer being observed worldwide. Although atrophic gastritis is usually seen in association with gastric cancer, this disorder is extremely common, and the vast majority of such patients never develop cancer.

Adenomatous polyps of the stomach, especially those larger than 2 cm, may occasionally give rise to carcinoma. Most stomach polyps, however, are hyperplastic and do not become malignant.

Subtotal resection for benign disease results in chronic atrophic gastritis from either bile reflux or removal of the gastrin trophic factor. This has been shown to produce gastric cancer in animals. It has also been shown to result in gastric cancer after a 10-year

TABLE 99–1. DIETARY FINDINGS FROM CASE CONTROL STUDIES OF GASTRIC CANCER*

Positive Association	Negative Association
Salted fish	Vegetables
Pickled vegetables	Fruit
Salty foods	Milk
Smoked fish	Meat
Starchy foods	Squash
Cabbage, potatoes	Eggplant
Cooked cereals	Lettuce
Bacon	Celery
	Animal fat

*United States (including Hawaii), Japan, Norway, England, and Israel.

interval in persons living in countries at increased risk for gastric cancer, especially in men, who are at higher risk than women.

Immunologic deficiencies, particularly the common variable type, may cause a predisposition to gastric cancer.

Gastric ulcer does not transform into cancer. Cancer foci may be present in association with an ulcer, however. All gastric ulcers must be suspected of having small areas of malignancy even when the ulcer appears benign by radiography or endoscopy. Biopsy and cytologic examination reveal the true nature of the lesion.

INCIDENCE AND PREVALENCE. It is estimated that there were 20,000 new cases of gastric cancer and 14,000 deaths from gastric cancer in the United States in 1990. Although this is a substantial number, a dramatic decline in the incidence of stomach cancer has occurred here and in many other countries (Fig. 99–1). The magnitude of the decline varies. In the United States the age-adjusted mortality rate for males and females of all races decreased 25 per cent from 1973 to 1985. Carcinoma of the stomach occurs most frequently between the ages of 50 and 70 years and is rare in patients younger than 30 years. The incidence and mortality rise steeply with age. Rates are higher in males than females by 2 to 1. Risk of gastric cancer is higher among those of low socioeconomic status. The 5-year survival of 16 per cent has not changed in recent years.

PATHOLOGY. Carcinoma of the stomach is adenocarcinoma that usually is manifested pathologically in one of four ways (Fig. 99–2): (1) Most often it appears as a bulky mass with deep central ulceration projecting into the lumen and invading the wall. (2) The tumor may infiltrate and narrow a portion of the lumen, most often in the antrum. Less commonly, the infiltration extends throughout the entire stomach, resulting in *linitis plastica*—a fixed, nondistensible stomach with absence of normal folds and a narrowed lumen. (3) Polypoid or exophytic carcinoma with or without a stalk may occur and be difficult to distinguish from a benign polyp on radiograph. (4) More rarely, carcinoma of the stomach may occur as a superficially spreading tumor involving only the mucosal surface and producing a granular appearance. This is unlike linitis plastica, which extends through the entire thickness of the wall. *Early gastric cancer* is a term used to characterize very superficial cancer that is detected by screening radiography or endoscopy primarily in asymptomatic people. This has the same anatomic and male-female distribution as the more advanced stage. Prognosis is excellent even with lymph node involvement. It is commonly seen in Japan and rarely in the United States.

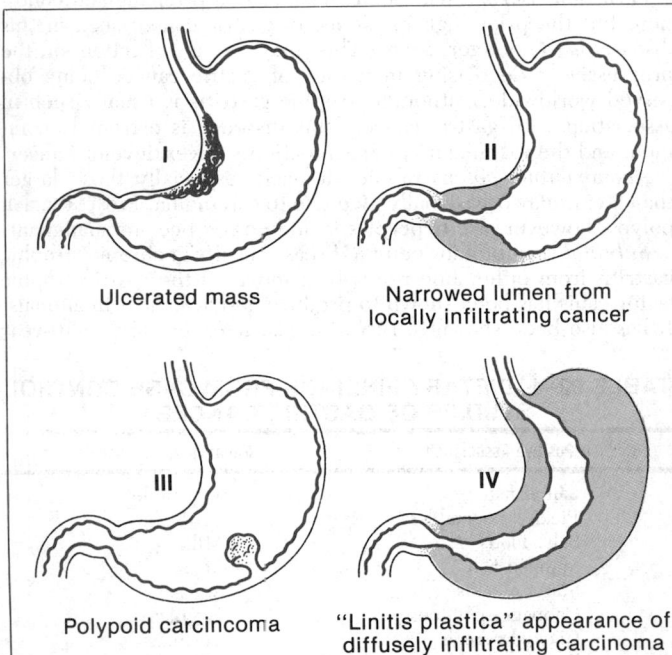

FIGURE 99–2. Diagrammatic representation of various presentations of gastric carcinoma.

TABLE 99–2. STAGING OF GASTRIC CANCER*

Stage		Tumor, Nodes, Metastasis
0	(T_{is}, N_0, M_0)	T_{is}—Limited to mucosa
I	(T_1, N_0, M_0)	T_1—Limited to mucosa and submucosa
II	$(T_{2,3}; N_0, M_0)$	T_2—To but not through serosa
		T_3—Through serosa but not adjacent structures
III	$(T_{4a}, N_0, M_0; T_{1-4}, N_{1-2}, M_0)$	T_{4a}—Through serosa and involves adjacent structures
		N_1—Perigastric nodes within 3 cm of tumor
		N_2—Perigastric nodes more than 3 cm from tumor (within celiac group)
IV	$(T_{4b}, N_{0-3}, M_0; T_{1-3}, N_3, M_0;$ Any T, Any N, $M_1)$	T_{4b}—Involves liver, diaphragm, pancreas, abdominal wall, retroperitoneum, small bowel, or duodenum via serosa
		N_3—Other intra-abdominal nodes (retroperitoneal, mesenteric, etc.)
		M_1—Distant metastasis

*From American Joint Committee on Cancer: Manual for Staging of Cancer. Philadelphia, J.B. Lippincott Company, 1983

Gastric carcinomas may be well-differentiated adenocarcinomas or may be so anaplastic as to resemble diffuse histiocytic lymphoma or sarcoma. A true carcinoma in situ is rarely found and is confined entirely to the glands (Table 99–2). This is more commonly seen at the surface of large adenomatous polyps of the stomach.

In about 75 per cent of patients with carcinoma of the stomach the tumors are found in the distal third. The lymphatic flow from such tumors is in the direction of the subpyloric nodes and porta hepatis and along both curvatures. The tumor very rarely spreads to the pancreaticolineal nodes, in contrast to proximal and mid-stomach lesions. Celiac and pancreatic nodal involvement occurs from lesions in all areas. In addition to invasion of lymph nodes, gastric carcinoma invades local structures: the lower end of the esophagus by submucosal spread, the pancreas, the transverse colon, the peritoneum, and, rarely, the duodenum. Hematogenous spread results in pulmonary, pleural, liver, brain, and bone metastases.

CLINICAL MANIFESTATIONS (Table 99–3). Early carcinoma of the stomach is frequently asymptomatic. *Anorexia* and *weight loss* are nonspecific symptoms and not well correlated with the size of the tumor. *Early satiety*, particularly with linitis plastica; *bloating; dysphagia; epigastric distress*; or more severe epigastric boring pain may be later symptoms. *Vomiting* is commonly a later symptom that may be caused by pyloric obstruction but may occur with other levels of obstruction. Vomiting also occurs without obstruction and may be secondary to the motility disturbance that a fixed mass in the wall produces. The pain is similar to that of peptic ulcer in about one fourth of patients, particularly when the tumor has ulcerated. In most patients, however, the pain usually occurs after eating and is not relieved by foods or antacids. Boring pain radiating to the back may indicate penetration of the tumor into the pancreas.

Dysphagia may occur with more proximal lesions, particularly

TABLE 99–3. ADENOCARCINOMA OF THE STOMACH

Associated With	Clinical Manifestations
Environment—geographical differences	Anorexia, early satiety, weight loss
Diet—? nitrosamines	Dysphagia, vomiting, weakness
Blood group A—genetic	Epigastric distress to severe, boring pain
Atrophic gastritis	Anemia, occult blood in stools
Adenomatous polyps (>2 cm)	Epigastric mass, signs of metastases
Subtotal resection for benign ulcer disease in high-risk countries	Rare—Virchow's node, Blumer's shelf, Trousseau's syndrome, acanthosis nigricans

when they have invaded the area around the cardioesophageal junction or spread submucosally to the esophagus, which is common in fundal lesions. Weakness and fatigue from *anemia* caused by chronic occult blood loss are common, although acute massive bleeding and hematemesis are unusual. Angina pectoris, congestive heart failure, and rarely cerebral ischemia may occur because of the anemia. Perforation occurs in a very small percentage of patients and can simulate peptic ulcer. When the tumor metastasizes, additional symptoms may include jaundice or right upper quadrant pain from liver metastases, cough from lung metastases, hiccups, and vague abdominal discomfort and bloating from peritoneal seeding and ascites.

Physical examination during the early stages of gastric carcinoma may be completely unremarkable. Later there may be signs of weight loss and anemia. When the tumor has disseminated, hepatomegaly from metastases, jaundice, or ascites may be present. Splenomegaly may occur if the portal or splenic vein is invaded. A palpable *epigastric mass* is present in less than one half of patients and usually, but not always, indicates extensive involvement. Rarely, left supraclavicular adenopathy (Virchow's node), a nodular perirectal wall (Blumer's shelf), or umbilical nodules give evidence of metastatic spread.

Several extragastric signs may precede the detection of an underlying malignancy. These include recurrent thrombophlebitis (Trousseau's syndrome); acanthosis nigricans, a verrucous, hyperpigmented, elevated skin lesion involving primarily the flexor spaces of the body; neuromyopathy characterized by localized sensory and/or motor disturbances; and profound central nervous system involvement with abrupt onset of confusion, memory defects, hostility, or ataxia. More detailed descriptions of the paraneoplastic syndromes are contained in specific chapters in Part XIII.

Laboratory studies usually disclose iron deficiency, or megaloblastic anemia if the tumor is associated with untreated pernicious anemia. *Occult blood in the stool* is present in less than half of the patients. Most patients have gastric acid present but in reduced amounts. A few have achlorhydria after maximal stimulation with pentagastrin. A few have hypersecretion, especially with antral tumors. Therefore the presence of acid does not ensure that carcinoma is not present. Abnormalities in liver function, particularly a markedly elevated alkaline phosphatase and 5'nucleotidase level, suggest liver metastases. Microangiopathic hemolytic anemia has been reported in several patients with gastric cancer. Rarely, protein-losing enteropathy occurs with ulcerated carcinomas of the stomach. Elevation of carcinoembryonic antigen is a late finding, usually in the presence of metastatic disease.

DIAGNOSIS. Roentgenologic Diagnosis. Most gastric cancers will be suspected on roentgenologic examination. The standard upper gastrointestinal series has been refined to include barium contrast studies capable of detecting very small lesions. With the gastric mucosa covered by a thin layer of barium and distended with air or gas, multiple projections are taken, which outline almost the entire stomach surface. Refinement of technique can be accomplished by using high-density barium, CO_2, simethicone for gas dispersion, and glucagon to induce gastroparesis. With such methods films showing fine detail may be produced and small mucosal lesions visualized.

The radiologist is usually able to define the characteristics of a benign versus malignant lesion and suggest a histologic diagnosis. For example, lymphoma of the stomach may be suspected by the extensive involvement, multiple shallow ulcerations, and giant rugal hypertrophy caused by infiltrative disease, and by the fact that the duodenum may be involved in the neoplastic process. A gastric ulcer often gives difficulty, but radiologic accuracy is in the range of 80 per cent. Characteristic radiographic signs that suggest a malignant lesion are the presence of an ulcer in a mass, irregular folds stopping short of the ulcer crater, and an irregular ulcer base. It is essential, however, to determine the nature of the ulcer by endoscopy with biopsy and cytology. Generally the location of an ulcer is not important in determining malignancy. Ulcers on the greater and lesser curvatures have about equal frequency of malignancy. Rigidity, loss of distensibility, unchanging contour, and irregular peristalsis are characteristic of a malignant lesion; when extensive infiltration from linitis plastica is present, a "leather bottle" appearance may result.

Endoscopy with Biopsy and Cytology. Fiberoptic endoscopy has increased the diagnostic yield over radiology alone. When combined with biopsy and brush cytology, the diagnostic accuracy is in the range of 95 to 99 per cent in various series. About one half of early gastric cancers present as small ulcerations; some have slight elevation or depression of the adjacent mucosa. The next most common type is a small polyp. Appearance at endoscopy may be misleading. Directed tissue sampling techniques, such as biopsy or brush cytology, should be used on any suspicious area, whether it is raised, depressed, or ulcerated. With more advanced carcinoma a specific tissue diagnosis can also be achieved with high accuracy by directed biopsy and cytology. Endoscopy is now being used also to stage and treat gastric cancer. Endoscopic ultrasonographic probes are highly accurate in evaluating depth of penetration of the cancer through the wall and extension to lymph nodes. This information can complement CT scans or standard ultrasonography in defining the extent of the tumor. The use of endoscopy to diagnose malignancies of the stomach is described in greater detail in Ch. 94.

TREATMENT. At present *surgery* provides the only satisfactory curative treatment for gastric cancer. The high frequency of regional node metastases plays a major role in the choice of the surgical procedure and the results of various therapeutic efforts. When the tumor is localized in the distal portion of the stomach, the omentum as well as nodes in the region of the porta hepatis and the pancreatic head are dissected, and a generous subtotal gastrectomy is performed. For tumors in the pars media and the proximal stomach, total gastrectomy may be indicated to obtain an adequate margin and for dissection of the predictable lymphatic spread in all directions. Distal pancreatectomy and splenectomy are usually necessary. There is little doubt that operative mortality is greater after total gastrectomy than after subtotal resection, and the procedure should be avoided whenever possible.

With extensive bleeding or obstruction, a palliative limited subtotal gastric resection can be done even in the presence of residual cancer. Palliative total gastrectomy should almost never be done. Resection of recurrent cancer in the gastric remnant may be of palliative value even when a cure is not obtained.

Chemotherapy is often suggested for unresectable gastric adenocarcinoma in an effort to decrease symptoms and prolong survival. The most widely used drug has been 5-fluorouracil (5FU), with an overall partial response rate of 15 to 20 per cent. Other agents such as mitomycin-C, doxorubicin (Adriamycin), and the various nitrosoureas have also been used as single agents with varying response. Combined use of several agents such as 5FU, doxorubicin, and mitomycin-C has resulted in some studies in a better response rate but has not improved survival.

Adjuvant chemotherapy following apparently curative surgery is an attractive concept for gastric carcinoma because of its high recurrence rate. Micrometastases are undoubtedly frequently present after surgery, and it has been postulated that chemotherapy might be most effective against such minimal disease. However, multiple trials with single agents have not shown success. Several trials using adjuvant chemotherapy with combinations of agents are in progress and may provide an answer to this very important question, although to date no effective adjuvant program has been demonstrated.

Radiation therapy is generally unsatisfactory, since gastric carcinomas are not very radiosensitive. Occasionally palliation may be obtained for persistent bleeding, obstruction, or pain. An occasional patient with inoperable gastric carcinoma has had prolonged survival with radiation therapy. Combining 5FU with radiation can provide a synergistic response.

Patients with gastrointestinal cancer frequently have complications associated with their disease or its treatment that require vigorous supportive treatment. Many aspects of the patients' general condition require consideration and treatment, including the management of infection; anemia; gastrointestinal bleeding; fluid and electrolyte loss secondary to vomiting, diarrhea, or fistula formation; disabling ascites; pain; and poor nutrition. Endoscopic laser treatment is also being evaluated as a palliative approach to keeping the lumen open in unoperated upon or recurrent cancer in order to maintain nutrition. Total parenteral nutrition is being utilized more frequently to supply the daily caloric requirement of patients with gastric cancer. Preoperative and postoperative use of this modality enables patients to withstand the rigors of surgery and to tolerate more effectively the postoperative period, including the use of chemotherapy.

PROGNOSIS. The 5-year survival rate depends upon whether or not adjacent lymph nodes contain cancer. The presence of perigastric lymph node metastases indicates a less than 15 per cent chance for survival. Early diagnosis plays a role in prognosis because a long period of time between the onset of cancer and its diagnosis favors lymphatic spread. In the Japanese studies, resection of gastric cancer limited to the mucosa and submucosa had a more than 80 per cent cure rate; when disease was limited to the mucosa, cure rate was 90 to 95 per cent. Linitis plastica and infiltrating lesions have a very poor prognosis compared with polypoid or exophytic disease.

PREVENTION. Until we learn more of the etiologic factors in gastric carcinoma we cannot practice primary prevention. We can only practice a limited degree of secondary prevention, i.e., detect the disease at an earlier stage in minimally symptomatic people in order to prevent its devastating consequences. The mass survey approach utilized in Japan is not practical in the United States because of the relatively low incidence of gastric cancer.

LYMPHOMA OF THE STOMACH (Ch. 147 and 148)

Primary lymphoma represents about 5 per cent of all primary malignant tumors of the stomach, and non-Hodgkin's lymphoma accounts for most of these. It is extremely rare for Hodgkin's disease (HD) to involve the stomach as a primary lesion. Patients with lymphoma are generally about a decade younger than those with carcinoma of the stomach, and males are affected more frequently. Pain is the most frequent symptom, and mild anemia is common, owing to gastrointestinal bleeding (which on occasion can be massive). A palpable mass is the most common presenting physical finding. Studies of maximal stimulation of gastric acid secretion have not been done in a large group of patients, but achlorhydria seems to be unusual. Secondary lymphoma involving the stomach is common in the course of disseminated lymphoma but is difficult to diagnose.

Lymphoma of the stomach frequently presents radiographically as a bulky mass and less frequently as a diffusely infiltrating tumor—the most common form of secondary lymphoma—giving the appearance of large folds on upper gastrointestinal series, frequently associated with multiple nodular defects and ulcerations. Lymphoma of the stomach often resembles superficially spreading carcinoma, linitis plastica, or solitary adenocarcinoma. Gastroscopy with directed biopsy and brush cytology gives a higher yield than was previously appreciated. Exophytic lesions provide a diagnosis in about 88 per cent of cases; the infiltrative type does not yield as high an accuracy.

Pseudolymphoma is a gastric lesion that may be confusing. This diffuse or discrete lesion is an atypical inflammatory response in the region of benign gastric ulcers. It is frequently difficult for the pathologist to differentiate pseudolymphoma from a true lymphoma.

In patients with lymphoma of the stomach there is a significant incidence of nontumorous lesions such as stress ulcer, hemorrhagic gastritis, and monilial gastritis. Therefore in such patients with upper gastrointestinal bleeding or other symptoms referable to the stomach, it is important that a careful diagnostic approach be undertaken to determine the possible nontumor cause of the sign or symptom.

Treatment of primary lymphoma of the stomach is usually surgical resection followed by 3600 to 4000 rads of radiotherapy, particularly if lymph nodes are involved. Some have advocated radiotherapy alone because of the marked sensitivity of lymphoma to radiation. If lymphoma involves the stomach secondarily, radiotherapy or chemotherapy or both are indicated. The 5-year survival following surgery for primary lymphoma of the stomach is in the range of 50 per cent for non-Hodgkin's lymphoma and less for HD, suggesting that HD is already disseminated when initially found in the stomach. The best prognosis for primary tumors occurs with small lesions confined to the stomach, differentiated into tumor follicles without lymph node involvement and with only superficial infiltration of the wall.

OTHER MALIGNANT TUMORS OF THE STOMACH

Leiomyosarcoma of the stomach represents about 1 per cent of gastric cancers and may present with a large intramural mass with central ulceration. Systemic symptoms are minimal, but massive bleeding or a palpable mass of which the patient is aware may be the presenting complaints. The tumor may be slow growing; 5-year survival following resection is in the range of 50 per cent. Metastases to the liver and nodes are common, but these patients have a better prognosis than those with other metastatic tumors. Liposarcoma, fibrosarcoma, myxosarcoma, and neurogenic sarcoma are extremely rare and present with symptoms similar to those of leiomyosarcoma. Neurogenic sarcoma can be associated with von Recklinghausen's disease.

Metastatic disease to the stomach from other sites is not common but may simulate primary gastric cancer. Malignant melanoma and breast and lung carcinomas are the most frequent offenders. In breast cancer the metastatic lesions may be ulcerative, of linitis plastica type, or polypoid.

LEIOMYOMAS AND BENIGN TUMORS

Leiomyomas are commonly found at postmortem examination but are rarely of clinical significance. They occur equally in men and women, and are usually found in the midportion and antrum of the stomach. They may grow toward the mucosa, encroach on the lumen, and cause mucosal effacement and secondary ulceration. They may grow in the direction of the serosa, producing a mass that is predominantly extrinsic. Simultaneous inward and outward growth results in a dumbbell shape. These features are also characteristic of leiomyosarcomas, and differentiation on radiography or gastroscopy is difficult. Bleeding is common and epigastric pain may simulate peptic ulcer disease. On roentgen examination the findings are usually an intramural filling defect with or without secondary ulceration. Gastroscopic examination reveals effaced but normal mucosa overlying the mass. Central ulceration may be seen.

Asymptomatic leiomyomas need not be removed while symptomatic lesions are excised locally.

Neurofibroma occasionally associated with von Recklinghausen's disease, neuroma, lymphangioma, ganglioneuroma, lipoma, carcinoid, and hamartoma associated with Peutz-Jeghers syndrome all may involve the stomach. About 10 per cent of hamartomas of the stomach and duodenum in Peutz-Jeghers syndrome become malignant.

ADENOMAS

Adenomas of the stomach are relatively rare lesions. Most polyps of the stomach are hyperplastic, not neoplastic, and do not become malignant. Adenomatous polyps are the usual neoplastic type of polyp. These are more frequent in men than in women and are generally seen in patients over 50. Patients with familial adenomatous polyposis or Gardner's syndrome (Ch. 105) have a 30 per cent probability of having polyps in the upper gastrointestinal tract. These are usually hyperplastic in the stomach and adenomatous in the duodenum. Patients with Peutz-Jeghers syndrome occasionally have similar findings. Bleeding, dyspepsia, and nausea are the most common symptoms, but most patients are asymptomatic. The diagnosis may be strongly suspected when a rounded smooth defect in the stomach on upper gastrointestinal series or a mass covered by mucosa with or without a stalk is detected by radiograph or endoscopy.

The size of polyps strongly influences management. It is rare for a polyp under 2 cm to show malignant change. In view of their potential for malignancy (present and future), polyps larger than 2 cm or polyps of any size causing significant symptoms should be removed. Pedunculated polyps can now be safely removed by cautery-snare technique through the fiberoptic endoscope. For sessile polyps more than 2 cm in diameter, a segmental gastric resection may be necessary. If carcinoma is diagnosed histologically at the time of surgery, subtotal gastric resection should be done. Multiple gastric polyps are usually hyperplastic and of no significance.

TUMORS OF THE DUODENUM

Adenocarcinoma of the duodenum is rare but is more common than lymphoma, which, in turn, arises more commonly in the jejunum and ileum. The second and third portions of the duodenum are the usual sites of adenocarcinoma except when associated with Crohn's disease, in which it is in the ileum. Cancer in the duodenal bulb is exceedingly rare. Adenocarcinoma of the duodenum more frequently affects men and develops at a younger age than carcinoma of the stomach or colon. The tumor tends to grow into the lumen or to invade the wall of the duodenum. Cramping abdominal pain, anorexia, weight loss, vomiting, and melena are common. Jaundice or fever may result from obstruction of the ampulla of Vater or the common bile duct when the carcinoma involves the second portion of the duodenum. The tumor may simulate benign postbulbar ulceration. The diagnosis is usually made by radiologic examination and confirmed by endoscopy. Pancreaticoduodenectomy is necessary. Five-year survival ranges between 4 and 15 per cent.

Lymphoma, leiomyosarcoma, carcinoid, metastatic cancer, and benign tumors may involve the duodenum, and these are discussed in more detail in Ch. 105. In general, these lesions are manifested as an intramural and submucosal mass with the exception of lymphoma and metastatic cancer, which frequently are exophytic and ulcerate. Any tumor, benign or malignant, may occur in a diverticulum at the descending portion of the duodenum. Aberrant pancreatic tissue may produce a submucosal filling defect in the duodenum, which may resemble a neoplastic lesion. Also, hyperplasia or adenoma of Brunner's glands may produce multiple polypoid defects in the duodenal bulb and is frequently associated with hypersecretion, duodenal ulcer and, rarely, Zollinger-Ellison syndrome. A prominent ampulla of Vater may resemble a neoplastic lesion radiographically. Endoscopy may be necessary to clarify the situation.

Brooks JJ, Enterline HT: Primary gastric lymphomas. A clinicopathologic study of 58 cases with long-term follow-up and literature review. Cancer 51:701, 1983. *A large series of primary gastric lymphomas with long-term follow-up (average 12.8 years). Five- and 10-year survival rates were 57 and 46 per cent, respectively. Statistically significant prognostic variables were smaller tumor size, superficial mural invasion (submucosal only), and pathologic stage 1 disease.*

Fleischer D, Sivak MV: Endoscopic Nd:YAG laser therapy as palliative treatment for advanced adenocarcinoma of the gastric cardia. Gastroenterology 87:815, 1984. *Endoscopy has taken on therapeutic potential for palliative treatment of gastric cancer with lasers, especially in the relief of obstruction at the gastroesophageal junction.*

Kurtz RC, Lightdale CJ, Winawer SJ, et al.: Endoscopy and gastrointestinal neoplasm: Diagnosis and management. Curr Probl Cancer 5:4, 1980. *This monograph describes the techniques and applications of endoscopy in patients with cancer of the gastrointestinal tract, including the stomach.*

Lawrence W Jr.: Gastric cancer. CA 36:5, 1986. *This monograph reviews the status of epidemiology, etiology, staging, pathology, and prognosis from a clinician's point of view.*

Le Chevalier T, Smith FP, Harter WK, et al.: Chemotherapy and combined modality therapy for locally advanced and metastatic gastric carcinoma. Semin Oncol 12:46, 1985. *An overview of therapeutic results. Response rates are still disappointing, and combination protocols have not as yet been dramatically better.*

Lightdale CJ, Botet JF, Kelsen DP, et al.: Diagnosis of recurrent upper gastrointestinal cancer at the surgical anastomosis by endoscopic ultrasound. Gastrointest Endosc 35:407, 1989. *The fiberoptic endoscope has advanced from solely a diagnostic instrument to one that has the capability of staging. Incorporation of an ultrasonographic probe into the scope now permits the endoscopist to see beyond the mucosal surface.*

Nomura A: Stomach. *In* Schottenfeld D, Fraumeni Jr. (eds.): Cancer Epidemiology and Prevention. Philadelphia, W. B. Saunders Company, 1982, pp 624–637. *A comprehensive dissertation on all aspects of gastric cancer from a worldwide epidemiologic point of view.*

O'Brien MJ, Burakoff R, Robbins EA, et al.: Early gastric cancer, clinicopathologic study. Am J Med 78:195, 1985. *Early gastric cancer as seen in United States patients is discussed. The disease is not seen often in the United States because of late diagnosis but is the same disease as early gastric cancer seen in Japan.*

Schafer LW, Larson DE, Melton LJ, et al.: Risk of development of gastric carcinoma in patients with pernicious anemia: A population-based study in Rochester, Minnesota. Mayo Clin Proc 60:444, 1985. *This study demonstrates the present lack of significant risk of gastric cancer in patients with pernicious anemia. The prior association was probably related to the higher incidence of gastric cancer worldwide. The risk for gastric cancer is no longer being expressed in this population.*

Shiu MH, Karas M, Nisce LZ, et al.: Management of primary gastric lymphoma. Ann Surg 195:196, 1982. *The surgical management of primary gastric lymphoma is presented in this paper and put into clinical perspective.*

Shiu MH, Moore E, Sanders M, et al.: Influence of the extent of resection on survival after curative treatment of gastric carcinoma. Arch Surg 122:1347, 1987. *Surgery varies with the size and location of the gastric cancer. This paper presents data and concepts underlying a rational operative approach to patients.*

Sonenberg A: Endoscopic screening for gastric stump cancer—would it be beneficial? Gastroenterology 87:489, 1984. *This paper provides a good perspective as well as a useful review of literature. Gastric stump cancer is a real entity but*

is expressed primarily in individuals living in countries at high risk for gastric cancer.

Winawer SJ, Posner G, Lightdale CJ, et al.: Endoscopic diagnosis of advanced gastric cancer. Factors influencing yield. Gastroenterology 69:1183, 1975. *Diagnostic yield was higher for exophytic lesions than for infiltrative tumor, and directed brush cytology alone was more productive than directed biopsy alone. Combination of infiltrative character and location in antrum or cardia often resulted in nondiagnostic biopsy and cytology specimens.*

100 Disorders of Gastrointestinal Motility

William J. Snape, Jr.

NORMAL MOTILITY IN STOMACH, SMALL INTESTINE, AND COLON

Motility of the gastrointestinal tract regulates the orderly movement of ingested material through the gut to ensure adequate absorption of nutrients, electrolytes, and fluid. Transit of intraluminal contents through the stomach, small intestine, and colon depends on the coordination of regional control of intraluminal pressure. Sphincters, interposed at several discrete areas along the length of the bowel, not only regulate the forward movement of intraluminal contents but impede the retrograde flow of intestinal contents. Unlike in the esophagus, external physical forces such as gravity have little impact on the movement of gastrointestinal intraluminal contents. Coordinated gastrointestinal motility depends on neural and hormonal control of sphincter, longitudinal, and circular smooth muscle contraction and relaxation.

SMOOTH MUSCLE. Changes in tension of the smooth muscle wall control regional intraluminal pressures, which in return regulate movement of intraluminal contents through the bowel. Movement of luminal contents from the stomach to the distal colon requires coordination between phasic and tonic contractions and relaxation of the intrinsic smooth muscle tone (peristaltic reflex), since luminal contents move from a high-pressure zone to a lower one. Differences in the physiologic control of contraction or relaxation of the muscle in each region determine the local pressure gradients. Myoelectric activity, including slow waves and spike potentials, coordinates regional intestinal smooth muscle contractions by controlling their frequency and by electrically linking neighboring smooth muscle cells (Fig. 100–1). The slow wave is a cyclic change in membrane potential that

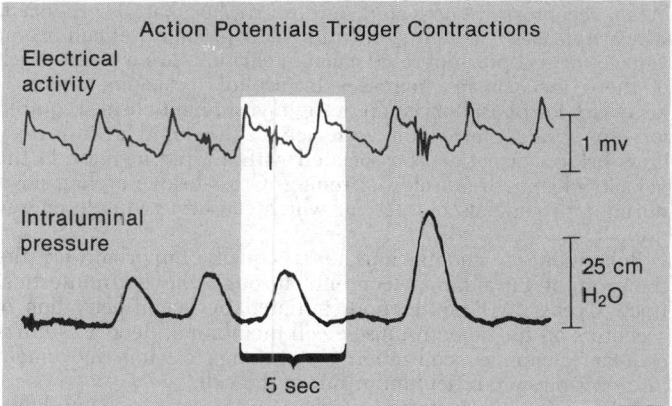

FIGURE 100–1. Simultaneous electrical and mechanical activity in the canine jejunum. The electrical signal was recorded from an extracellular electrode in the tunica muscularis; it shows a regular cycle of depolarization-repolarization at 12 to 14 cycles per minute. Superimposed on some of these cycles (basic electrical rhythm, slow wave, or pace-setter potential) are more rapid oscillations (fast waves, spikes). When spiking occurs, the smooth muscle contracts, causing intraluminal pressure to rise (lower tracing).

occurs in smooth muscle from the stomach, small bowel, and colon. The slow wave frequency of a smooth muscle cell is intrinsic to the cell, but it can be modified by the activity in neighboring cells. A pacemaker region sets the dominant frequency of each region of the gastrointestinal tract. Calcium influx during spike potentials, superimposed upon the slow waves, results in smooth muscle cell contraction.

Tight electrical coupling of gastric smooth muscle cells is responsible for progressive propagation of the slow waves, oral to caudal, along the proximal to distal slow wave gradient. Therefore, without a change in the slow wave frequency, contractions also propagate in an oral to caudal direction. In the small intestine and colon, in addition to tight intercellular coupling, regional differences in slow wave and contraction frequency maintain the forward movement of intraluminal contents. A higher contraction frequency elevates mean pressure, stimulating movement of intraluminal contents distally into the lower pressure area. Higher intraluminal pressure in the descending colon creates a pressure gradient that regulates the movement of intraluminal contents back to the transverse colon and forward to the sigmoid colon. Therefore, a pressure amplitude gradient, rather than a frequency gradient, determines colonic transit. In the colon the dominance of contractions in the proximal descending colon and splenic flexure mixes the intraluminal contents and is responsible for a storage area in the transverse colon. Another motility pattern, the propagating contraction, is under neural control and propagates the fecal content distally from the transverse colon for further storage in the sigmoid colon.

Circular and longitudinal muscles have different functions. Throughout the gut, circular contractions segment the lumen, mixing the contents to expose the mucosa to continually different contents. The longitudinal muscle shortens the bowel, moving intraluminal contents forward.

Sphincters are high-pressure zones interposed through the gastrointestinal tract. The upper esophageal and external anal sphincters are localized bands of skeletal muscle. The lower esophageal sphincter is not an anatomically distinct structure; in contrast, the pylorus is a localized collection of smooth muscle. The ileocecal valve, a valvelike structure separating the colon and the ileum, responds like a sphincter. The internal anal sphincter is a localized collection of circular smooth muscle surrounded by the external anal sphincter. Contraction or relaxation of the sphincters is controlled by enteric neurotransmitters or by circulating peptide hormones, in response to changes in pressure in the surrounding bowel or physiologic stimuli, such as eating or emotional stress. In general, proximal distention relaxes all sphincters; distal distention contracts sphincters.

Contraction of gastrointestinal smooth muscle requires an increase in the intracellular calcium concentration. Regulation of intracellular calcium begins at the smooth muscle cell membrane. When receptors are activated, inositol triphosphate is produced, which releases calcium from the sarcoplasmic reticulum, or voltage- or receptor-operated calcium channels are opened. Each of these mechanisms increases intracellular calcium, which is necessary for phosphorylation of the myosin light chain, required for cross-bridge formation with actin. The rapid actin-myosin cross-bridge formation is associated with a rapid increase in the velocity of smooth muscle shortening. Cross-bridge cycling slows during a prolonged contraction, which conserves muscle energy use.

Relaxation of smooth muscle is equally important for the transport of intraluminal contents through the gastrointestinal tract. Cyclic AMP production, initiated by ligand activation of receptors on the smooth muscle cell membrane, decreases intracellular calcium concentration by initiating calcium movement into sarcoplasmic reticulum or out of the cell.

Enteric Nervous System. Enteric neurons contain many different excitatory and inhibitory neurotransmitters (Table 100–1). Many nerve cells release more than one neurotransmitter upon stimulation. The complex interaction among inhibitory and excitatory neurotransmitters coordinates bowel activity. Although some neurotransmitters are generally stimulating (e.g., acetylcholine) and others inhibitory (e.g., vasoactive inhibitory polypeptide [VIP]), some neurotransmitters may control the motility pattern through different effects on nerve and muscle (opiates

TABLE 100–1. ENTERIC NEUROTRANSMITTERS AFFECTING GASTROINTESTINAL MOTILITY

Excitatory	Inhibitory
Acetylcholine	Vasoactive intestinal polypeptide (VIP)
Neurokinins	Calcitonin gene-related peptide
Gastrin-releasing peptide	Adenosine triphosphate
Neurotensin	Neurotensin
Enkephalin	Enkephalin
Cholecystokinin	Somatostatin
5-Hydroxytryptamine	Neuropeptide Y

stimulate muscle and inhibit acetylcholine release) or by different regional effects (neurotensin relaxes gastric muscle and stimulates small intestinal and colonic muscles). In addition to the efferent neurons, afferent neurons provide important signals for control of the motility through relaying sensations from one region of the gut to other regions or to the central nervous system (CNS).

The intrinsic enteric neurons of the gastrointestinal tract have numerous interconnections (Fig. 100–2). Input comes from the CNS, internuncial neurons, and interaction with afferent neurons via the prevertebral ganglia. Sympathetic and cholinergic fibers, which originate in the CNS and travel in the vagus, splanchnic, lumbar colonic, or sacral nerves, regulate the output of neurotransmitters from the myenteric plexus. Control of the myenteric plexus is mediated by intestinal afferent neurons and CNS neurons, interacting in the celiac, superior mesenteric, and inferior mesenteric ganglia. The interaction of interneurons within the myenteric plexus controls neural output to the gut. Each site of neural interconnection may be a potential target for future therapeutic intervention.

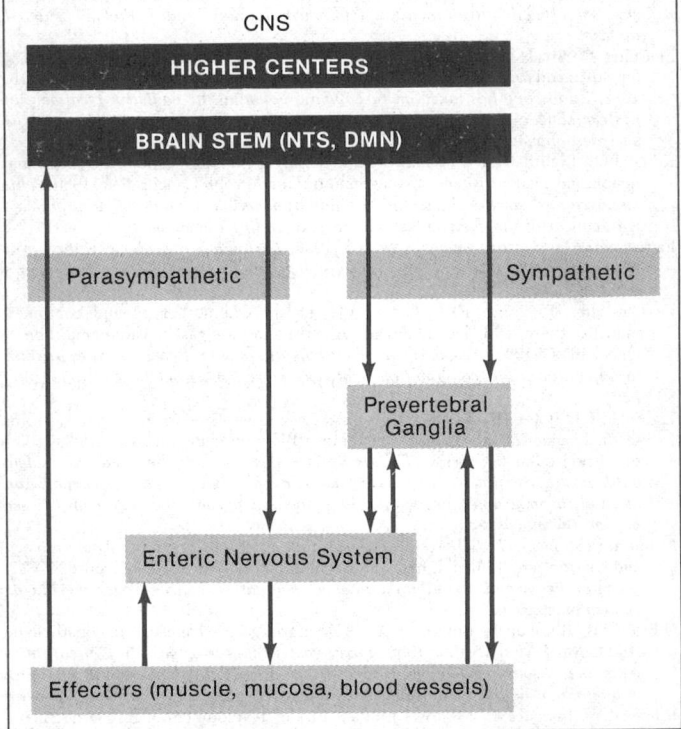

FIGURE 100–2. Schematic diagram showing control levels for neural regulation of gastrointestinal effector function. The enteric nervous system integrates information from the periphery and the central nervous system and modulates effector function. In prevertebral ganglia, afferent inputs from the gut and descending inputs through the sympathetic branch of the autonomic nervous system are integrated into output that has primarily inhibitory effects on gut motility. Autonomic nuclei of sympathetic and parasympathetic nerves located in the brain stem integrate inputs from the periphery and the cortex. Output reaches the gut via the parasympathetic and sympathetic nerves. NTS = Nucleus tractus solitarius; DMN = dorsal motor nucleus. (Adapted from Mayer EA, Raybould H: Role of neural control in gastrointestinal motility and visceral pain. *In* Snape WJ Jr. [ed.]: Pathogenesis of Functional Bowel Disease. New York, Plenum Medical Book Company, 1989, pp 13–35.)

Enteric Peptide Hormones. Peptides, released from the gastrointestinal mucosa into the blood after eating, act as hormones and affect gastric, small intestinal, and colonic smooth muscle contractions. As in the enteric nervous system, a counterbalance between stimulating peptides (gastrin, cholecystokinin, and motilin) and inhibitory peptides (enteroglucagon and peptide yy) controls motility. Further flexibility is gained in the peptide hormone modulation of motility by regional variation in response to a peptide (e.g., cholecystokinin stimulates gallbladder emptying and inhibits gastric emptying). Blood levels of the enteric hormonal peptides reach their maximum approximately 30 to 60 minutes after eating. In contrast to the enteric neurotransmitters, which affect motility soon after the stimulus does, the hormones may mediate a delayed gastrointestinal response to eating.

In summary, the neurohumoral control of gastrointestinal smooth muscle involves interactions among the CNS, local neural reflexes, and circulating hormones. This control mechanism modulates smooth muscle contraction and regulates the coordinated movement of intraluminal contents through the entire gastrointestinal tract.

Gastrointestinal Transit. Regulated smooth muscle contractions result in coordinated changes in gut intraluminal pressure, which controls the transit of chyme through the gastrointestinal tract. Each of the major sections of the gastrointestinal tract has a specific function that requires a different transit pattern. Different transit patterns exist during fasting and after eating. Eating ends the fasting motility pattern and initiates a postprandial transit pattern in each segment of the alimentary tract. Emotional stress and physical exercise modulate these patterns but are not the primary controls.

Stomach. As an initial response to eating, the proximal stomach relaxes to accommodate the volume of a meal. The distal stomach grinds the masticated chunks of food to less than 1-mm diameter and regulates the delivery of the processed gastric contents to the intestine synchronous with the release of digestive enzymes. Gastric emptying adjusts to the different physical and chemical characteristics of the food. Emptying of liquids is faster ($T_{1/2}$ = 6 to 12 min) than that of solids ($T_{1/2}$ = 45 to 70 min). Specific chemoreceptors regulate gastric emptying of different substances. Gastric emptying of glucose solutions is regulated so that approximately 2 kcal of glucose is emptied per minute; an equiosmolar solution of saline empties more rapidly. The gastric fundal tone regulates liquid emptying, whereas antral contractions control the rate of solid food emptying. Therefore, the stomach prepares as well as transports the gastric contents.

Small Intestine. The small intestine slowly moves the chyme distally, which allows mixing of the contents with digestive enzymes and absorption of the nutrients, electrolytes, and water. The transit time for material to move through the small intestine and appear in the cecum is approximately 40 to 180 minutes. In addition to controlling the distal transit of nutrients, the small intestine must clear the extruded dead cells and bacteria. The migrating motor complex (MMC) (Fig. 100–3), which occurs during fasting, removes these indigestible luminal contents. The MMC consists of three different phases: Phase 1 is a period of inactivity; phase 2 is a period of intermittent phasic contractions similar to the postprandial pattern; and phase 3 is a continuous period of contractions, which are at the slow wave frequency indigenous for that region of the bowel. The entire complex migrates from the stomach to the ileum. Phase 3 propels the intestinal contents that remain during fasting.

Colon. Regulation of colonic transit allows the colon to absorb additional water and electrolytes and to store the fecal waste for elimination. Eating stimulates aborad and orad movement of luminal contents. This back and forth shuttling mixes the luminal contents and allows greater time for absorption by the colonic mucosa. The transverse and rectosigmoid colons are separate sites of storage. Propagating contractions transport the luminal contents distally and appear necessary for normal bowel movements. The transit time is approximately 40 to 80 hours for excretion of one-half of the colonic content.

CLINICAL ASSESSMENT OF GASTROINTESTINAL MOTILITY

HISTORY AND CLINICAL EXAMINATION. Although symptoms can originate from disturbances of any part of the gastrointestinal tract, particular symptoms may suggest dysfunction of a specific site. In motility disturbances of each of the distinct organs (stomach, small intestine, colon), cramping abdominal pain occurs frequently, often after eating. The location of the pain can indicate the most likely source—epigastric for stomach, periumbilical or generalized for small intestine, or lower quadrants for the colon. In fact, pain referred from the anatomic location of the colon may occur in any of the abdominal quadrants. Colonic pain resolves after a bowel movement or passing flatus.

Early satiety or postprandial vomiting occurs in patients with delayed transit through the stomach and upper small bowel. Both symptoms can also result from organic nonmotility disorders (e.g., gastritis), which are not discussed in this chapter. Because receptive relaxation of the stomach is usually intact, postprandial vomiting secondary to obstruction of the gastric outlet is characteristically voluminous and may not occur until after eating several meals. When disturbed motility causes either symptom, the pathophysiologic defect may be secondary to reduced receptive relaxation, a low threshold for sensory nerve recognition of gastric distention, or uncoordinated antroduodenal contractions. Rapid gastric emptying causes symptoms of the "dumping syndrome," which include sweating, weakness, occasional orthostasis, tachycardia, and diarrhea (Ch. 98.5).

If massive gastric retention (>750 ml) is present, findings include a soft mass in the left upper quadrant. In a fasting patient, recovery of more than 150 ml of gastric contents via nasogastric tube, especially if old food is present, suggests gastric retention. An abdominal radiograph shows a large fluid-filled viscus in the left upper quadrant. If the patient is vomiting acutely, nasogastric suction should be initiated for therapy, and the hypovolemia and metabolic alkalosis should be treated.

Intestinal pseudo-obstruction may present with symptoms that are difficult to differentiate from those of true obstruction. Abdominal distention and pain occur in both anatomic and functional disorders of the gastrointestinal tract. Distention is an objective physical sign in patients with pseudo-obstruction, but in patients with the irritable bowel syndrome, the sensation of bloating may be secondary to a defect in sensory recognition. Tightly fitting clothes are uncomfortable to these patients. There is no increase in bowel gas in patients with the irritable bowel syndrome complaining of abdominal bloating.

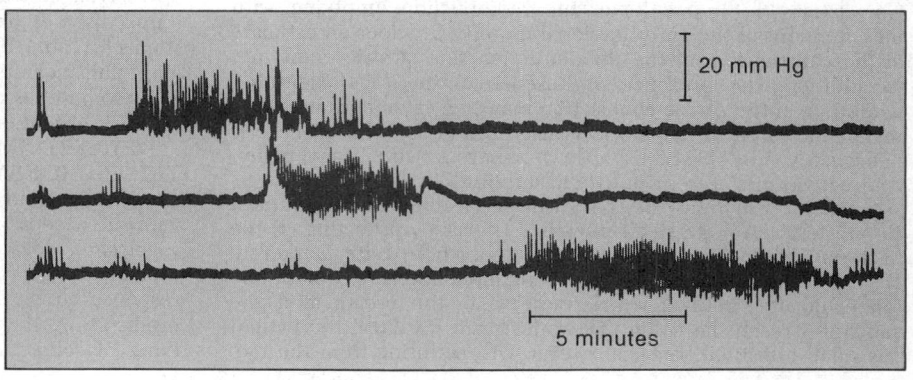

FIGURE 100–3. The activity front of the interdigestive motor complex is characterized on manometric tracings by a burst of rhythmic contraction waves that progress down the intestine. The top tracing is in the distal duodenum. The pressure ports are 25 cm apart. (From Van-Trappen G, Janssen SJ, Hellmans J, et al.: The interdigestive motor complex of normal subjects and patients with bacterial overgrowth of the small intestine. J Clin Invest 59:1158, 1977, by copyright permission of the American Society for Clinical Investigation.)

20 mm Hg

5 minutes

Bowel sounds are loud with high-pitched rushes in patients with obstruction. If the obstruction has been present a long time, the bowel sounds are quieter or absent. In acute ileus or pseudo-obstruction the bowel sounds are quiet but usually present. If the ileus is associated with a severe abdominal insult, such as peritonitis or surgery, the bowel sounds are absent.

Vomiting is a common symptom of intestinal pseudo-obstruction, acute ileus, and a high anatomic obstruction. If the obstruction is in the distal small intestine, distention is a more prominent complaint than vomiting. In distal obstructions the vomitus, when present, has a feculent odor. An abdominal radiograph usually shows a cut-off between dilated and nondilated bowel in a true obstruction. In acute ileus or pseudo-obstruction the bowel is dilated throughout, with air visible in the rectum.

Alterations in bowel habit (diarrhea or constipation) are the cardinal symptoms of motor disorders of the gastrointestinal tract, but they do not specifically identify the pattern of motility. In the absence of a defect in mucosal absorption, diarrhea results from more rapid transit of intestinal contents through either the small intestine or the colon (Ch. 101). The mechanism of rapid transit through the small intestine is unclear, but diarrhea due to altered colonic motility is associated with an increased frequency of propagating contractions. Constipation generally results from slow colonic transit due to either colonic inertia or increased segmenting contractions, which impede the forward movement of the intraluminal contents. Propagating contractions are markedly decreased or absent in patients with constipation.

The frequency, character, and volume of bowel movements should be carefully defined in each patient. More than three bowel movements a day defines excessive frequency. Stool volume is increased in small bowel–mediated diarrhea, whereas low-volume stools result from disordered colonic motility. Stools may vary in consistency from liquid to merely soft. Constipation is defined as fewer than three bowel movements each week. The constipated stool generally has a lower volume (weight) and is firmer than normal stools, since more water has been absorbed. These strict definitions may exclude the patient complaining of constipation who has stools of normal size and consistency but who strains to defecate. The patient who has only increased straining may have a functional anal outlet obstruction.

MOTILITY TESTS. Regional differences in anatomy and physiologic controls in the gastrointestinal tract require distinct procedures to measure motility and transit. In addition to identifying the motility disturbance responsible for the patient's symptoms, standardized motility tests allow objective assessment of response to treatment.

Gastric emptying of liquids and solids must be measured independently to provide a full description of the organ's function. Gastric emptying is best assessed using standardized measurements of the respective emptying rates of liquids and solids. These measurements can be performed simultaneously using different radionuclides to tag the liquid and the solid phases. The bedside assessment of the gastric transit of a bolus of isotonic saline may be a useful and inexpensive screening test. After a period of 30 minutes, the residual should be less than 40 per cent of an oral volume of 750 ml administered. Estimation of gastric emptying from an upper gastrointestinal barium study often does not provide useful information. Changes in gastric fundic pressure can be measured by placing a large balloon in the fundus and measuring the tone before and after a meal. Correlation of the results of the radionuclide emptying with measurement of the antroduodenal motility provides an estimate of the contribution of the duodenum to slow gastric emptying. In addition, the presence or absence of the MMC and the amplitude of the phasic contraction may suggest a neuropathic or myopathic cause of the motility disorder. Thus, with an enteric neuropathy, the MMC is absent, whereas with a myopathy, contractions are present but their amplitude is decreased.

Small intestinal transit is measured by different techniques. Breath tests estimate small intestinal transit by reflecting (1) the bacterial metabolism of nonabsorbable carbohydrate marker to H_2, or (2) the bacterial release of a radionuclide label from a bile salt conjugate, both of which increase in the breath after the substrates reach the colon. These tests are invalid if the patient has small intestinal bacterial overgrowth resulting from the mo-

tility dysfunction or a blind loop of intestine, since the bacteria release the marker proximal to the ileocecal valve. The appearance in the right lower quadrant (cecum) of a radionuclide-labeled nonabsorbable marker ingested with a meal also provides an estimate of small intestinal transit. Measurement of intraluminal pressures in the small intestine may document abnormalities in the fasting MMC and the postprandial motility response. As in the stomach, concomitant use of transit and manometric studies allows the contribution of the enteric nerves and smooth muscle to the motility disorder to be estimated objectively.

Global colonic transit can be easily measured by orally administering radiopaque markers and measuring the distribution of the markers throughout the colon 5 days later. If no markers are then present within the colon, the patient probably is not constipated. In the constipated patient the localization of the markers to the rectosigmoid region suggests that the patient has a rectoanal outlet dysfunction. If the markers are distributed throughout the colon, there is a colonic motility disturbance. Regional emptying times can be calculated from this test. Once the motility defect has been localized to the colon, more specific transit and motility tests, measuring increases in intraluminal pressure and segment transit times with radionuclide markers, are available in specialized centers. The absence of a postprandial increase in segmenting contractions suggests a neural lesion, whereas low amplitude postprandial contraction suggests a disturbed smooth muscle function. Anorectal manometry shows whether the anal sphincter contributes to outlet dysfunction. The internal anal sphincter relaxes and the external anal sphincter contracts after the rectum is distended. If this spinal reflex is absent, an abnormality of the enteric neurons controlling the internal anal sphincter is suggested.

Cohen S, Snape WJ Jr.: Movement of the small and large intestine. *In* Sleisenger MH, Fordtran JS (eds.): Gastrointestinal Disease: Pathophysiology, Diagnosis, Management. 4th ed. Philadelphia, W. B. Saunders Company, 1989, pp 1088–1105. *Complete review of associations between alteration in physiology and presentation of small intestinal and colonic disease.*

Meyer JH: Motility of the stomach and gastroduodenal junction. *In* Johnson LR (ed.): Physiology of the Gastrointestinal Tract. 2nd ed. New York, Raven Press, 1987, pp 613–630. *Comprehensive review of physiology of the region; contains all major references and basic mechanism.*

Sarna SK, Otterson MF: Small intestinal physiology and pathophysiology. Gastroenterol Clin North Am 18:375, 1989. *Excellent review of pathophysiology of intestinal motility disorders.*

Szurszewski JH: Electrophysiological basis of gastrointestinal motility. *In* Johnson LR (ed.): Physiology of the Gastrointestinal Tract. 2nd ed. New York, Raven Press, 1987, pp 383–422. *Comprehensive review of physiology of the region; contains all major references and basic mechanism.*

DISORDERS OF GASTRODUODENAL MOTILITY

Delayed Gastric Emptying

Delayed gastric emptying is a more frequent source of symptoms than is excessively rapid emptying. The only significant cause of excessively rapid emptying, resulting in the "dumping syndrome," is partial gastric resection, the incidence of which is decreasing as the indications for gastric surgery diminish (Ch. 98.5). Chronic delayed gastric emptying (gastroparesis) is caused most often by an intrinsic disturbance in gastric or upper gastrointestinal motility and requires specific therapy of the underlying neuromuscular disorder. Acute gastroparesis, which is most frequently associated with an electrolyte disturbance, ketoacidosis, systemic infection, or an acute abdominal insult, is managed by treating the underlying disease, not the gastric motility disorder.

Delayed gastric emptying may be associated with other systemic diseases or may be due to a primary dysfunction of the stomach (Table 100–2). The typical symptoms of delayed gastric emptying include early satiety, nausea, and vomiting. Phytobezoars sometimes occur in these patients as well, especially if the MMC is absent.

DELAYED GASTRIC EMPTYING COMPLICATING GASTRIC SURGERY. Delayed gastric emptying not infrequently complicates gastric surgery for peptic ulcer disease. Vagotomy, with the exception of the highly selective vagotomy (parietal cell vagotomy), decreases fundic relaxation, antral contractions, and coordinated relaxation of the pylorus. The expected physiologic response to vagotomy is rapid emptying of liquids, possibly predisposing the patient to dumping syndrome, and slow emptying of solids. Although most often patients have no gastric

Delayed gastric emptying
Postvagotomy
Diabetes mellitus
Viral infections
Reflux esophagitis
Brain stem lesions
Anorexia nervosa
Tachygastria

Rapid gastric emptying
Dumping syndrome
Pancreatic insufficiency
Celiac sprue
Zollinger-Ellison syndrome
Duodenal ulcer

symptoms following abdominal vagotomy, approximately 5 to 10 per cent have delayed gastric emptying. This complication is more likely to occur if the patient had gastric outlet obstruction due to his or her primary disease. Antral contractions are poorly coordinated owing to irregular antral slow wave activity. Gastric MMC activity is often absent, although intestinal MMC remains normal.

Metoclopramide, a putative dopamine receptor antagonist, improves symptoms in many patients with delayed gastric emptying after a vagotomy. The usual dose of metoclopramide (10 mg orally, four times a day) causes anxiety, fatigue, or sedation in about 15 per cent of patients. Domperidone, also a dopamine antagonist, does not cross the blood-brain barrier and has fewer CNS side effects. Cisapride, which releases acetylcholine from the enteric neurons, may be useful, but this agent is currently approved only for investigational use in the United States.

Roux-en-Y anastomoses after gastric resection occasionally cause poor gastric emptying, especially of solids (Ch. 98.4). The MMC and the postprandial motor response are abnormal in the roux limb. Delayed gastric emptying of solids is the major functional disturbance; liquid gastric emptying may be normal. Patients with severe vomiting can be treated with subcutaneous bethanechol, further gastric resection, or elimination of the roux loop. The patient's symptoms may be recalcitrant to other prokinetic agents, such as metoclopramide or cisapride. Leuprolide may reduce symptoms in some patients.

DIABETIC GASTROPARESIS. Delayed gastric emptying complicating diabetic ketoacidosis resolves as the patient improves, but the stomach is sometimes massively distended, exhibits mucosal bleeding, and may require decompression by nasogastric tube. Chronic delayed gastric emptying, associated with longstanding insulin-dependent diabetes mellitus, is a greater clinical problem. Such patients have frequent episodes of nausea and vomiting, which affect food intake and complicate insulin requirements. Retinopathy, nephropathy, peripheral neuropathy, and other complications are commonly present. Absence of the gastric MMC, necessary for the emptying of nondigestible material larger than 1 mm, predisposes the diabetic patient to the development of bezoars, causing abdominal discomfort, early satiety, and vomiting. Vagal neuropathy is thought to be the pathogenesis of gastric stasis in diabetes mellitus, although a demonstrable autonomic neuropathy is not always present. Early in the patient's course gastric emptying of liquids may be rapid, although in many patients emptying of liquids is slow from the initiation of symptoms. Gastric emptying of solids is slow throughout the course of the disease.

Metoclopramide improves the symptoms of gastric stasis in patients with diabetes mellitus both by increasing gastric emptying and by decreasing the CNS recognition of nausea and distention. Gastric emptying is rarely normalized after treatment with metoclopramide, even though symptoms may be completely alleviated. Bethanechol also stimulates an increase in gastric motility and improves symptoms in patients with diabetic gastric stasis. Cisapride, which has no demonstrated CNS effect, improves both symptoms and gastric emptying. Cisapride also improves the emptying of nondigestible solids and may prevent the occurrence of bezoars. Erythromycin improves gastric emptying by increasing MMC activity in recent studies.

ANOREXIA NERVOSA. This psychiatric disorder, which oc-

curs predominantly in young women, is characterized by excessive weight loss (Ch. 202). The gastric emptying of solids, but not of liquids, is slowed in patients with anorexia nervosa, but not in patients with bulimia nervosa. The delayed gastric emptying is associated with antral dysrhythmia, fundal hypotonia, decreased postprandial plasma concentrations of norepinephrine and neurotensin, and impaired autonomic function (decreased resting diastolic blood pressure and skin conductance). The mechanism causing delayed gastric emptying is unclear. Patients with equal weight loss but without the psychiatric disorder do not have delayed gastric emptying. Interestingly, gastric emptying in obese patients is more rapid than in healthy subjects.

Repletion of the patient's calories improves gastric emptying in the absence of prokinetic medicine. Bethanechol, metoclopramide, and cisapride increase the emptying of solids by stimulating antral motility. The ultimate success of prokinetic drugs for anorexia nervosa is unclear, since they treat only the peripheral symptom of gastric emptying. Reversal of the underlying psychiatric disturbance appears necessary for complete resolution of symptoms.

MISCELLANEOUS CAUSES. *Tachygastria* is a condition of unknown etiology which presents as intractable vomiting that causes failure to thrive in infants and as vomiting in young adults. Tachygastria is caused by rapid slow wave activity in the antral smooth muscle segment, which becomes the dominant pacemaker initiating orad propagating contractions. Parvovirus-like agents (Norwalk or Hawaii viruses) can slow gastric emptying. The decreased gastric emptying associated with an acute viral infection usually resolves quickly. Up to 25 per cent of patients with reflux esophagitis, associated with an incompetent lower esophageal sphincter, have delayed gastric emptying, which must be corrected in order to treat the reflux esophagitis adequately. Lesions such as tumors, infarction, or viral encephalitis that affect the vagal complex in the medulla can delay gastric emptying.

Rapid Gastric Emptying

Rapid gastric emptying occurs in some patients with duodenal ulcer disease and Zollinger-Ellison syndrome as a result of duodenal insensitivity to an acid load. Rapid liquid emptying occurs in patients with pancreatic insufficiency and possibly with celiac sprue because of poor feedback inhibition of gastric motility by fat due to a maldigestion or malabsorption. The dumping syndrome is discussed in Ch. 98.5.

McCallum RW: Motor function of the stomach in health and disease. *In* Sleisenger MH, Fordtran JJ (eds.): Gastrointestinal Disease. 4th ed. Philadelphia, W. B. Saunders Company, 1989, pp 675–712. *Comprehensive review of pathophysiology of gastroduodenal motility disorder; complete bibliography.*

DISORDERS OF SMALL INTESTINAL MOTILITY

Motility disorders of the small intestine can most usefully be categorized by their respective motility patterns, although some symptom complexes (e.g., postprandial bloating) foil simple categorization. Small intestinal motility may be hypoactive, hyperactive, or uncoordinated. Decreased intestinal motility reflects either absent or fewer MMC's during fasting or a minimal increase in postprandial motility in the different regions of the small bowel. Conversely, increased motility is reflected in increased numbers of fasting MMC's or an augmented intraluminal pressure response to eating. Uncoordinated intestinal motility can be caused by retrograde MMC's and clustered contractions. For rational therapy it is important to determine if the decreased intestinal motility is due to a neuropathy or a myopathy. In general, increased or uncoordinated motility is secondary to neural dysfunction. A disease may affect both the enteric nerves and smooth muscle and may present with different abnormalities in motility during its course (e.g., progressive systemic sclerosis). Table 100–3 lists the conditions associated with chronic disordered small intestinal motility.

In patients with motility disorders, qualitatively similar transit patterns may result in different symptoms. For example, patients with the irritable bowel syndrome may have delayed small intestinal transit that results in constipation. In contrast, a patient with pseudo-obstruction may have a greater delay in intestinal transit that results in diarrhea due to bacterial overgrowth.

TABLE 100–3. SMALL INTESTINAL MOTILITY DISORDERS

Decreased motility
Hollow visceral myopathy (primary intestinal
  pseudo-obstruction)
Progressive systemic sclerosis (late)
Amyloidosis
Muscular dystrophy
  Duchenne s
  Myotonic
Hypothyroidism
Jejeunal diverticulosis
Jejeunoileal bypass

Increased or uncoordinated motility
Primary visceral neuropathy
Carcinoma-associated visceral neuropathy
Progressive systemic sclerosis (early)
Irritable bowel syndrome
Diabetes mellitus
Infectious diarrhea
Mass lesion of brain stem
Amyloidosis
Hyperthyroidism
Carcinoid syndrome
Shy-Drager syndrome

Therefore, symptoms may not be helpful in determining the etiology of a disease process.

Patients with slow intestinal transit tend to complain of nausea, vomiting, abdominal distention, and periumbilical abdominal cramps. Although constipation can occur with delayed intestinal transit, diarrhea is more common. The MMC, which propels bacteria and sloughed, dead epithelial cells from the small intestine into the colon, is often absent or severely deranged by an enteric neuropathy. Bacterial overgrowth due to a diminished number of MMC's deconjugates bile salts, causing steatorrhea and diarrhea. The absence of postprandial motility impedes the normal transit through the small intestine.

Diarrhea is generally the result of rapid intestinal transit because of decreased time of contact of the luminal contents with the mucosa. The patients also may have maldigestion and malabsorption due to poor mixing of the dietary material with the digestive enzymes and bile salts. Borborygmi may also disturb the patient.

Decreased Intestinal Motility

HOLLOW VISCERAL MYOPATHY (INTESTINAL PSEUDO-OBSTRUCTION). This disorder is the prototype for myopathic diseases of the small intestine. The disease generally displays vacuolization or degeneration of the smooth muscle in the circular or longitudinal layers, separately or together, without affecting the enteric nerves. In some cases the muscle is not histologically altered. Defective slow wave generation or actin-myosin cross-bridge formation may cause the myopathy. The contractions are decreased in amplitude and number, but usually the MMC is present because the nerves are unaffected (Fig. 100–4). The MMC may function poorly, however, because of the low-amplitude contractions. The motility pattern differs from that associated with a partial small bowel obstruction in which 3 to 10 clustered contractions occur regularly, separated by 1-minute intervals of quiescence.

Patients usually present with symptoms and signs of small intestinal stasis without evidence of an anatomic obstruction or of a secondary cause for pseudo-obstruction (Table 100–3). Hollow visceral myopathy is familial, but random, nonfamilial cases are probably more common. With familial primary intestinal pseudo-obstruction, parts of the urinary system (bladder, renal pelvis) may also be dilated as a result of abnormal smooth muscle contraction. Familial visceral myopathy is also associated with a high incidence of intestinal malrotation.

Anatomic bowel obstruction or acute ileus must be excluded before making the diagnosis of pseudo-obstruction. Acute adynamic ileus occurs most frequently after abdominal surgery, peritonitis, intra-abdominal vascular accidents, or a severe electrolyte imbalance. Ileus or obstruction can cause hypovolemia or

third-space accumulation of fluid. The signs and symptoms of acute ileus are similar to those of chronic disorders of decreased intestinal motility, but in contrast treatment of the initiating cause results in resolution of the symptoms. Acute ileus or obstruction is treated by decompression via a nasogastric tube, replacement of fluid volume, and correction of electrolyte and acid-base imbalances.

The therapy of hollow visceral myopathy is generally highly unsatisfactory. Metoclopramide has little efficacy in treating patients with pseudo-obstruction, but the newer prokinetic agent cisapride shows promise in the therapy of severe small intestinal motility disorders, especially in those patients with postprandial hypomotility with a normal fasting pattern. Intestinal bypass surgery should be avoided in patients with pseudo-obstruction. Occasionally antibiotics may be of help if a blind loop syndrome with bacterial overgrowth is present.

PROGRESSIVE SYSTEMIC SCLEROSIS (Ch. 262). This is the most common "collagen vascular disease" to cause disordered intestinal motility, although polymyositis and systemic lupus erythematosus may rarely do so. Approximately 40 per cent of patients with progressive systemic sclerosis have intestinal in-

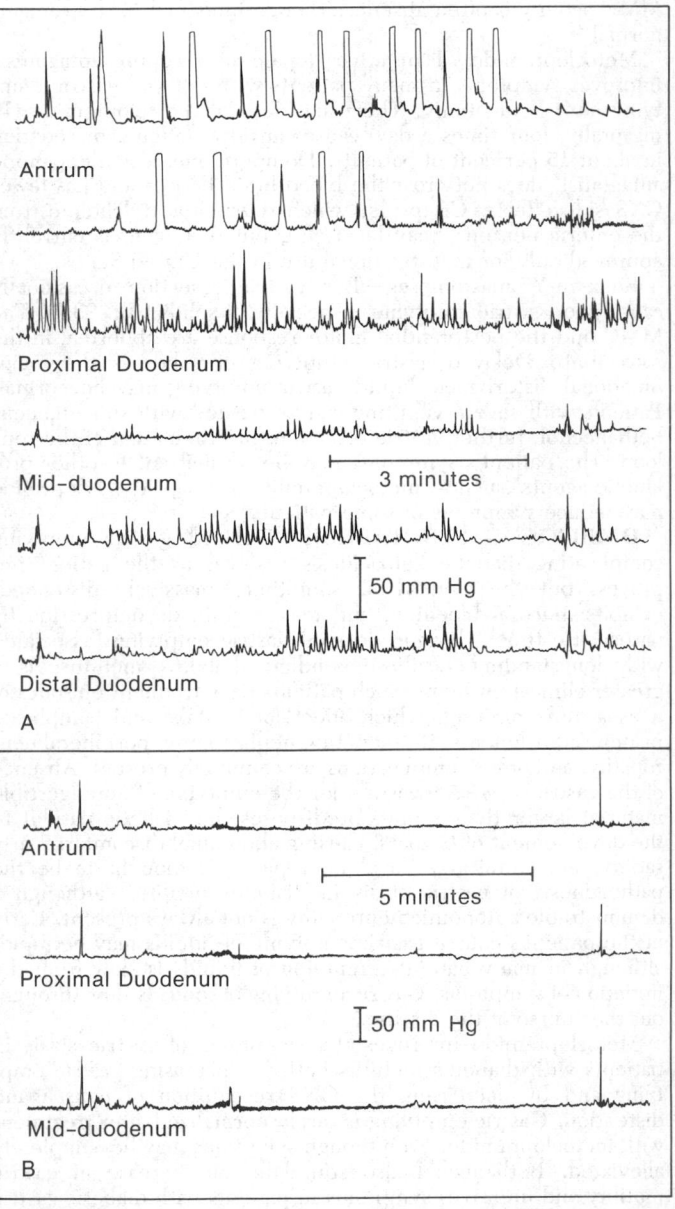

FIGURE 100–4. Postprandial gastroduodenal manometry recordings from a healthy subject (*A*) and a patient with myopathic pseudo-obstruction (*B*). The postprandial response is decreased in the patient with pseudo-obstruction. (From Hyman PE: Absent postprandial duodenal motility in a child with cystic fibrosis: Correction of the symptoms and manometric abnormality with cisapride. Gastroenterology 90:1274, 1986.)

volvement consisting of defects in both neural and smooth muscle. Early in the course of the disease, signs of a neuropathy predominate, whereas collagen later replaces smooth muscle and a myopathy becomes the major component of the disease. In symptomatic patients, characteristically postprandial motility is markedly reduced. Since a neuropathy is often present, the MMC's are absent. In general, patients become symptomatic only after extensive replacement of the smooth muscle with collagen. In contrast to hollow visceral myopathy, muscle cells in progressive systemic sclerosis are decreased in number but morphologically normal. Since the number of functional smooth muscle cells is decreased, pharmacologic stimulation with prokinetic drugs is generally unsuccessful.

OTHER CONDITIONS. *Amyloidosis* of the small intestine may cause either a myopathy or a neuropathy, depending on its distribution. Several of the *muscular dystrophy* syndromes may affect the intestinal smooth muscle in addition to skeletal and cardiac muscle. *Hypothyroidism* decreases the slow wave frequency and amplitude of contraction of the intestine, which may result in atony. *Jejunal diverticulosis* is secondary to pseudo-obstruction, which predominantly involves the small intestine. The histologic pattern is similar to that of progressive systemic sclerosis in most patients, although some patients have a neuropathy.

Increased or Uncoordinated Motility

VISCERAL NEUROPATHY. Intestinal motility can be increased, as well as uncoordinated, in patients with visceral neuropathy because of a decrease in neural inhibition. The hallmark of visceral neuropathy is a patchy loss of nerve tracts, a decreased number of neurons, or fragmentation and dropout of axons. Specialized silver stains are needed for the accurate histologic diagnosis of an enteric neuropathy.

Primary visceral neuropathy can be familial or random. Familial cases may be associated with other neural lesions, including mild autonomic insufficiency, mental retardation, altered sensory recognition of position, and absent deep tendon reflexes. Random cases may be secondary to injury from a viral infection or an environmental toxin or to carcinomatous neuropathy (Ch. 162). The motility patterns associated with visceral neuropathy are variable, probably because different disease complexes have not been separated at this time. In general, during fasting a neuropathy disrupts either the propagation or configuration of the MMC. In some patients the MMC may be absent. Eating may initiate no contractions or uncoordinated contractions or may fail to inhibit MMC's in patients with neuropathy.

IRRITABLE BOWEL SYNDROME. In this common disorder, to be discussed more fully under colonic disorders, symptoms of abdominal pain and an altered bowel habit consistent with the irritable bowel syndrome may be associated with abnormal motility in the small intestine as well as in the colon. Balloon distention of the small intestine provokes characteristic abdominal pain in some patients. Two patterns of contractions, "discrete clustered contractions" and "prolonged propagated contractions," are associated with abdominal pain more frequently in patients with the irritable bowel syndrome than in healthy control subjects.

DIABETES MELLITUS. The diarrhea associated with diabetes mellitus is most likely due to small intestinal motility disturbances. Abnormal manometric patterns in diabetics, who also have gastroparesis, include decreased motility or uncoordinated bursts of small intestinal contractions. The MMC's can be present, deranged, or absent in diabetic patients. Patients with a central autonomic nervous system disturbance, Shy-Drager syndrome, have similar findings to patients with diabetes (Ch. 452). Diabetic diarrhea may respond to treatment with the α_2-adrenergic agent clonidine.

OTHER DISORDERS. *Infectious diarrhea* (e.g., due to enterotoxigenic *E. coli* or *Shigella*) initiates a significant motility disorder, characterized experimentally by powerful aborad migrating contractions. *Brain stem mass lesions* can either slow the small intestinal MMC or initiate an activity front simultaneously at different levels of the small intestine, through an effect on the vagal motor complex and the autonomic nuclei in the medullary reticular formation. *Amyloid* can affect the enteric nerves of the small intestine as well as replace smooth muscle. *Hyperthyroid-ism* increases the slow wave frequency of the bowel, which is a possible cause of the frequently associated diarrhea. *Carcinoid syndrome* with increased 5-hydroxytryptamine production increases the migration velocity of the MMC and increases the cycling frequency.

Malagelada J-R, Camilleri M, Stanghellini V: Manometric Diagnosis of Gastrointestinal Motility Disorders. New York, Thieme-Stratton, 1986. *A monograph on the diagnosis of motility disorders but dealing also with normal physiology and the pathophysiology of the common and uncommon disorders of motility. The bibliography is extensive and will guide the reader into any area.*
Kellow JE, Phillips SF: Functional disorders of the small intestine. In Snape WJ Jr. (ed.): Pathogenesis of Functional Bowel Disease. New York, Plenum Medical Book Company, 1989, pp 171–198. *Extensive discussion of pathophysiology of small intestinal motility disturbance; extensive bibliography.*

DISORDERS OF COLON MOTILITY

Orderly transit of contents through the colon "fine tunes" the absorption of salt and water. If the transit is too slow, the mucosa can extract too much water and the stool becomes hard, resulting in constipation. Rapid transit causes frequent, soft stools. Diarrhea caused by colonic motility disorders is low in volume (less than 400 ml per day), since most intestinal fluid is absorbed in the small intestine (Ch. 101). Table 100–4 lists the diseases or syndromes that cause disordered colonic motility. Many of the systemic diseases that affect gastric and small intestinal motility also alter colonic motility.

Either increased or decreased segmenting contractions can slow transit through the colon. A functional partial obstruction results from increased segmenting contractions, since the movement of the colonic contents is impeded by the segmentation. The colonic contents also move slowly if colonic segmenting activity is decreased (colonic inertia). Propagating contractions are invariably absent in patients with slow colonic transit and constipation, suggesting that these contractions are necessary for net forward movement of feces into the distal rectosigmoid.

Patients with diarrhea and rapid colonic transit have decreased colonic segmenting contractions and increased numbers of contractions propagating into the rectum. As a result, intraluminal contents are rapidly transported distally. When these powerful contractions carry the colonic contents into the rectum, the patient experiences urgency.

Cramping abdominal pain referable to the colon occurs predominantly in the lower abdominal quadrants, but it can be felt anywhere over the anatomic distribution of the colon. This pain is characteristically relieved by flatus or a bowel movement. Although the patients feel bloated, ascribed to increased gastrointestinal gas, they actually have normal amounts of bowel gas. Tenesmus, a feeling of incomplete evacuation, is associated with rectosigmoid spasm.

Slow Transit with Increased Segmenting Contractions

PRIMARY CONSTIPATION. Most people experience brief periods of constipation during their lives; treatment is usually not

TABLE 100–4. PATHOGENESIS OF COLONIC MOTILITY DISORDERS

Slow transit
Increased segmenting contraction
Primary constipation
Irritable bowel syndrome (spastic)
Diverticular disease
Anal outlet obstruction
Congenital—Hirschsprung's disease
Acquired
Decreased segmenting contractions
Irritable bowel syndrome (inertia)
Primary colonic pseudo-obstruction
Ogilvie's syndrome
Diabetes mellitus
Progressive systemic sclerosis
Spinal cord injury
Rapid transit
Functional diarrhea
Bile salt diarrhea
Surreptitious abuse of laxatives

necessary unless the symptoms last for several months. Infrequent bowel movements (less than every other day) result in hard fecal pellets, which require straining to eliminate, because of slow colonic transit and the ensuing desiccation of the stool. Patients do not complain of abdominal pain but rather have nonspecific symptoms of bloating, increased flatus, and mild malaise. Fecal impactions, which rarely occur except in elderly or sedentary patients, may cause overflow diarrhea or bleeding from stercoral rectal ulcers.

Although the pathophysiology of primary constipation is poorly understood, most patients respond quickly to increasing fiber in their diet. The chronic use of osmotic laxatives, dioctyl sodium sulfosuccinate, or stimulant laxatives has the potential to damage the myenteric plexus, causing an unresponsive "cathartic colon."

IRRITABLE BOWEL SYNDROME (SPASTIC). Symptoms of the irritable bowel syndrome occur in up to 25 per cent of otherwise healthy individuals. Although most common in women in early adulthood, the irritable bowel syndrome can begin after the age of 45 years. In such older patients, however, it is extremely important to exclude other disease, including carcinoma of the colon or colonic diverticular disease.

Cramping abdominal pain of colonic origin and an altered bowel habit are the hallmarks of the irritable bowel syndrome. The symptoms are intermittent with variable periods of remission. Eating, especially a large meal with a high fat content, or episodes of emotional stress increase the pain. Constipation alternating with an increased frequency of low-volume stools is the "classic" bowel pattern, although patients may have more frequent looser stools at the onset of an attack of the irritable bowel or may complain only of constipation. A perception of uncomfortable abdominal distention and increased fecal mucus are common adjunctive symptoms.

Patients with constipation-predominant irritable bowel syndrome have an increased prevalence of colonic slow waves at a frequency of 3 cycles per minute compared with normal individuals. In approximately 60 per cent of patients with constipation-predominant irritable bowel syndrome, segmenting contractions are increased after eating a meal, whereas in the remainder no increase in motility and little mixing movement of the fecal contents in the colon occur. The increased segmenting contractions shuttle the colonic contents back and forth in the transverse and descending colon. When present, the normal increase in postprandial motility is delayed. There are subtle differences in symptoms in the two groups of patients; nausea and vomiting are more prominent symptoms in patients with little postprandial motility (colonic inertia). Propagating contractions are absent in both groups of patients.

Balloon distention of the rectum or other regions of the colon causes abdominal pain at a lower threshold in patients with the irritable bowel syndrome than in healthy people. This is not a generalized increase in pain perception because the patients generally feel less somatic pain. The abnormal pathophysiology in visceral sensory nerves and in colonic motility combines to cause the classic symptoms of the irritable bowel syndrome.

The diagnosis of the irritable bowel syndrome requires exclusion of other diseases. Functional diarrhea, variably lumped into the irritable bowel syndrome, is discussed in detail later in reference to rapid transit. The rigor used to exclude the diagnosis of other diseases depends on the age and clinical presentation of the patient. The major differential diagnoses include carcinoma of the colon, diverticulitis, and inflammatory bowel disease. After a careful history and physical examination, the stool should be examined for occult blood. Patients over the age of 40 years definitely should have colonoscopy or barium enema to exclude anatomic colonic disease. If the symptoms persist, especially that of diarrhea, the terminal ileum should be visualized to exclude inflammatory bowel disease (Ch. 103).

Once organic disease is excluded, the irritable bowel syndrome is best treated by reassuring the patient, explaining the cause of symptoms, and instituting some alterations of the diet. Decreasing dietary fat reduces colonic intraluminal pressure. An increase in soluble and insoluble dietary fiber decreases water net absorption and intraluminal pressure, respectively. Pharmacologic agents should be used only if counseling and dietary changes have no effect on symptoms. Anticholinergics, the next line of

therapy, decrease the colonic contractions and may relieve symptoms. Combined therapy with dietary fiber supplements and anticholinergics has enhanced efficacy. Diarrhea and fecal continence may improve following a dietary fiber supplement owing to increased bulk. Anxiolytics or antidepressants should be used only after documenting a psychoneurosis.

ACQUIRED DIVERTICULAR DISEASE OF THE COLON. Diverticular disease, mucosal outpouchings through the colonic wall that occur as the patient ages, results in a spectrum of abnormalities extending from no symptoms to diverticulitis. Diverticular disease may occur more often in patients who had the irritable bowel syndrome in their youth.

Acquired diverticula, which occur most frequently in the left colon, result from increased intraluminal pressure pushing sleeves of mucosa through perivascular weaknesses in the wall of the colon juxtaposed to the taeniae coli. The predilection for the left colon results from the decreased colonic diameter there leading to increased pressures, as predicted by Laplace's law: Intraluminal pressure is directly correlated with wall tension and inversely correlated with bowel diameter. Decreased dietary fiber and distal colonic smooth muscle hypertrophy contribute to elevation in distal colonic intraluminal pressure.

The symptoms of *painful colonic diverticular disease* are similar to those of irritable bowel syndrome but are more likely to be localized in the left lower quadrant. When *diverticulitis* occurs as a complication, the patient may have similar symptoms with the addition of fever, left lower quadrant mass, leukocytosis, and occult blood in the stool (Ch. 112). Gross hematochezia is more frequent in asymptomatic patients with diverticula (Ch. 112). Diverticula can be diagnosed by barium enema or colonoscopy. Muscular hypertrophy gives a saw-tooth pattern visible on barium enema. Narrowing due to diverticular inflammation can be difficult to differentiate from carcinoma of the colon.

Painful diverticular disease of the colon is best treated by decreasing the intraluminal pressure, similar to the therapy in the irritable bowel syndrome. Narcotics, especially morphine, should be avoided because of an exaggerated increase in smooth muscle contraction.

ANAL OUTLET OBSTRUCTION. Constipation may result from a disturbance in the elimination of stool through the anal sphincter. Elimination normally begins by the involuntary relaxation of the internal anal sphincter after distention of the rectum. The patient uses voluntary control to open the rectoanal angle and relax the external anal sphincter. A disturbance of any component of this mechanism leads to constipation.

Hirschsprung's disease is the congenital absence of enteric neurons in the submucosal and myenteric plexuses, due to an arrest of the embryonic caudad migration of the enteric neurons along the gut. The aganglionic segment remains contracted, causing dilatation of the proximal normal bowel. The severity of symptoms and the age at diagnosis are related to the length of the aganglionic segment. Involvement of the rectum or additional parts of the colon results in constipation or obstipation in infancy, requiring emergent resection of the aganglionic bowel and a pull-through anastomosis to the anus.

Abnormalities in anal physiology are a significant cause of constipation; impaired anal sphincter relaxation occurs relatively frequently in adults. The absent rectoanal reflex may be secondary to a short aganglionic segment (short-segment Hirschsprung's disease), to chronic distention with a fecal impaction, or to an insufficient distention stimulus due to an enlarged rectal vault. In acquired megacolon, relaxation of the internal anal sphincter may be impaired if a large volume is not used to distend the rectum. Some patients have subtle histologic abnormalities in the myenteric plexus, suggesting that an acquired neuropathy may also account for the abnormal sphincter response. In the spastic pelvic floor syndrome (animus) the external anal sphincter and the puborectalis relax poorly or the levator ani contracts poorly, leading to impaired opening of the rectoanal angle. This acquired condition, which occurs more often in multiparous women, can prevent the patient from normal stool evacuation. Anal outlet dysfunction can be diagnosed as a cause of constipation by observing the accumulation of the fecal markers in the rectum and by abnormal anal manometry.

Impaired internal anal sphincter relaxation in an adult patient may respond to a posterior anal sphincter myomectomy. Patients who have difficulty in opening the rectoanal angle or who have animus may sometimes respond to biofeedback training.

Patients with decreased segmenting contractions have symptoms similar to those in patients with increased contractions. The colonic inertia form of the irritable bowel syndrome and primary colonic pseudo-obstruction may be the same pathophysiologic disturbance. Postprandial increases in colonic motility are absent in both, but the colon is dilated in primary intestinal pseudo-obstruction, explaining the increased incidence of abdominal distention. Constipation is a major symptom in both conditions. Ogilvie's syndrome is the primary colonic pseudo-obstruction, usually paraneoplastic.

Constipation is present in many patients with longstanding, insulin-requiring diabetes mellitus, progressive systemic sclerosis, or thoracic spinal cord lesions. Colonic motility is not increased postprandially in these patients. In the patients with diabetes or spinal cord lesions, colonic smooth muscle can be stimulated with exogenous drugs, suggesting a neural lesion, not a myopathy. In progressive systemic sclerosis the colon cannot increase intraluminal pressure after drug stimulation, as expected in a neuropathy.

It is difficult to treat patients with decreased colonic motility. In patients with neuropathy and normal smooth muscle function, prokinetic drugs have had some success. In patients with a myopathy it is unlikely that pharmacologic stimulation will have much effect.

Rapid Transit

FUNCTIONAL DIARRHEA. Some patients have functional, painless diarrhea with fecal urgency but with no associated anatomic or histologic abnormality of the gastrointestinal tract. These patients present with small frequent stools, consistent with a large bowel abnormality, and fecal incontinence is relatively frequent because their anal sphincters cannot retard evacuation of a liquid stool. Lactose intolerance must be excluded either by history or by a lactose tolerance test. The diarrhea is greater than that in the spastic irritable colon syndrome, and abdominal pain may be absent.

Segmenting postprandial contractile activity is decreased in functional diarrhea. Propagating contractions are increased and propagate into the rectum, possibly accounting for the increased urgency and fecal incontinence that occur in these patients. The lack of segmenting contractions to impede forward movement or transit may exacerbate the urgency. Specific foods may stimulate an increase in prostaglandin E_2 production by the colon, which could initiate the diarrhea. Increased concentrations of fecal bile salts, which occur in some patients, may contribute to the functional diarrhea also. Bile salts irritate colonic sensory nerves and thereby stimulate frequent propagating contractions in the colon through irritation of sensory nerves.

Microscopic or collagenous colitis presents as functional diarrhea without obvious anatomic abnormalities. The diagnoses can be made by histologic examination of the rectal biopsy.

In the treatment of functional diarrhea, antidiarrheal agents such as the opioid analogues, loperamide, or diphenoxylate are used to decrease symptoms. Fecal continence improves as the stool consistency becomes firmer. Some patients may require biofeedback training to maintain continence. If excess bile salts contribute to the diarrhea, low doses of cholestyramine may decrease the diarrhea. Microscopic and collagenous colitis may respond to 5-aminosalicylic compounds.

Surreptitious Laxative Abuse. Surreptitious laxative abuse is a common cause of functional diarrhea (Ch. 101). Oxyphenisatin and bisacodyl stimulate increased numbers of propagating contractions and diarrhea. Patients may take these or other laxatives as a manifestation of a psychiatric disorder. It is a challenge to the physician to make the correct diagnosis.

Ulcerative Colitis. There is rapid transit of colonic contents through the colon, in addition to increased mucosal secretion, in patients with active ulcerative colitis. As in the other colonic causes of diarrhea, propagating contractions are increased in number and propagate into the rectum, accounting for the significant incidence of fecal incontinence. The rapid transit improves as the mucosal inflammation decreases after therapy for the underlying inflammation (Ch. 103).

Devroede GJ: Constipation: Mechanism and management. *In* Sleisenger MH, Fordtran JS (eds.): Gastrointestinal Disease. 4th ed. Philadelphia, W. B. Saunders Company, 1989, pp 331–368. *This is a complete examination of the pathophysiology and treatment of constipation.*
Snape WJ Jr.: Irritable bowel syndrome. *In* Snape WJ Jr. (ed.): Pathogenesis of Functional Bowel Disease. New York, Plenum Medical Book Company, 1989. *This summarizes the field, providing 150 references for further study.*

DRUGS THAT AFFECT GASTROINTESTINAL MOTILITY

As understanding of the pathophysiology of gastrointestinal motility disorders grows, the number and the diversity of the drugs that are available for therapy increase (Table 100–5). Drugs that stimulate motility may indiscriminately increase smooth muscle contractions or increase a specific motility function, such as MMC initiation. Many of the drugs on the list, used for treatment of other systemic diseases, may precipitate gastrointestinal symptoms as a side effect.

Excitatory Agents

Drugs that excite the gastrointestinal tract should be used to treat decreased motility when the smooth muscle can functionally contract. In general, patients who benefit from these agents have an enteric neuropathy with decreased release of endogenous stimulatory neurotransmitters or an increased release of inhibitory neurotransmitters. When the smooth muscle is absent or severely damaged, the prokinetic drugs are rarely helpful. Acetylcholine analogues, such as bethanechol, stimulate both longitudinal and circular gastrointestinal smooth muscle by directly binding to the M_2 muscarinic receptor to release inositol triphosphate or to open

TABLE 100–5. EFFECTS OF DRUGS ON SMALL AND LARGE INTESTINAL CONTRACTILITY

Drug	Effect on Stomach	Effect on Small Intestine	Effect on Colon	Mechanism of Action
Acetylcholine analogues	Excitatory	Excitatory	Excitatory	Agonist of muscarinic receptors on muscle cells
Neostigmine	Excitatory	Excitatory	Excitatory	Acetylcholine esterase inhibitor
Metoclopramide	Excitatory	Excitatory	Excitatory	Dopamine antagonist (central, peripheral)
Domperidone	Excitatory	Excitatory	No effect	Dopamine antagonist (peripheral)
Cisapride	Excitatory	Excitatory	Excitatory	Unknown
Macrolide antibiotic	Excitatory	Excitatory	?	Binds to motilin receptor
Leuprolide acetate	?	Excitatory	?	Reduces progesterone and relaxin
Atropine	Inhibitory	Inhibitory	Inhibitory	Antagonist of muscarinic receptor
Secoverine	?	Inhibitory	Inhibitory	Antagonist of M_2 muscarinic receptors on muscle cells
Papaverine	?	?	Inhibitory	Unknown
Calcium channel blockers	Inhibitory	Inhibitory	Inhibitory	Blocks voltage-operated calcium channels
Nitrate compounds	?	Inhibitory	Inhibitory	Blockade of receptor-operated calcium channels; Increase of intracellular cGMP
Peppermint oil	?	Inhibitory	Inhibitory	Unknown
Cholecystokinin antagonists	?	?	?	Blocks CCK receptors

receptor-operated or voltage-dependent calcium channels. Drugs that block acetylcholinesterase increase endogenous acetylcholine concentration at the myoneural junction. These drugs have a theoretical advantage in regulating as well as in increasing motility, since the distribution of acetylcholine release is predetermined by the autonomic nervous system.

Dopamine antagonists can variably increase motility throughout the gastrointestinal tract. Metoclopramide, a centrally and peripherally acting dopamine antagonist, increases gastric emptying and transit through the small intestine and the colon. Metoclopramide is useful in diabetic gastroparesis, in the placement of small intestinal tubes in patients with ileus, and in diabetic constipation. It has little therapeutic value in symptomatic patients with progressive systemic sclerosis or in many patients with pseudo-obstruction. Domperidone, a peripherally acting dopamine antagonist, mainly increases gastric emptying and has little therapeutic effect in small intestinal or colonic motility disorders.

Cisapride may stimulate motility through antagonism of a serotonin (5-hydroxytryptamine) receptor in the bowel. Cisapride stimulates gastric emptying, increases small intestinal transit, and stimulates colonic contractility. Cisapride may improve symptoms in patients with decreased gastric emptying, small intestinal pseudo-obstruction, or colonic inertia. This drug is not currently available in the United States.

Erythromycin, one of the macrolide antibiotics, stimulates MMC activity by binding at the motilin receptor on the small intestinal smooth muscle cell. Normal MMC activity is absent in many patients with neuropathic pseudo-obstruction. The clinical usefulness of this agent remains to be established.

Leuprolide acetate may improve symptoms secondary to functional disturbances of small intestinal motility. This drug is believed to work by decreasing the concentrations of the smooth muscle inhibitory hormones progesterone and relaxin.

Inhibitory Agents

Inhibitory drugs should be most useful for treating patients whose symptoms result from increased motility, which causes uncoordinated movement of the intestinal contents. The inhibitory drugs may block the receptors for excitatory neurotransmitters or block the increase in intracellular calcium necessary for normal smooth muscle contraction.

Anticholinergic drugs, which inhibit muscarinic receptor stimulation, are sometimes effective in the treatment of the small intestinal or colonic variants of the irritable bowel syndrome. The anticholinergics must be used with care in patients who may develop urinary retention (e.g., prostatism) or glaucoma.

Calcium channel blockers inhibit the increase in intracellular calcium that is necessary for smooth muscle contraction. Several classes of calcium channel blockers, including verapamil and the dihydropyridines, are available. The dihydropyridine, nifedipine, decreases smooth muscle contraction and may be used in some patients with increased small intestinal or colonic motility.

Nitrate compounds inhibit smooth muscle contraction, probably through an increase in the intracellular concentration of cyclic guanosine monophosphate and a decrease in calcium influx into the smooth muscle cell.

Peppermint oil is a relaxant of smooth muscle, which improves symptoms in some patients with the irritable bowel syndrome. In the future, a new class of agents, cholecystokinin antagonists, may prove useful in the treatment of multiple gastrointestinal motility disorders.

Burks TF: Actions of drugs on gastrointestinal motility. *In* Johnson LR (ed.): Physiology of the Gastrointestinal Tract. 2nd ed. New York, Raven Press, 1987, pp 723–744. *Extensive references are provided for the background of drug action.*

Camilleri M, Malageladn JR, Abell TL, et al.: Effect of six weeks of treatment with Cisapride in gastroparesis and intestinal pseudo-obstruction. Gastroenterology 96:704, 1989. *Report of efficacy for the new class of prokinetic drugs.*

Corazziari E, Ricci R, Biliodtti D, et al.: Oral administration of loxiglumids (CCK antagonist) inhibits postprandial gallbladder contraction without affecting gastric emptying. Dig Dis Sci 35:50, 1990. *Interesting study showing the potential of the new medication.*

101 Diarrhea

Guenter J. Krejs

Diarrhea is defined as the presence of stool liquidity (instead of formed or soft stool) and an increase in daily stool weight, the upper normal limit of which is 200 grams in industrialized societies. Diarrhea is usually associated with increased stool frequency (more than three bowel movements per day) and is often accompanied by urgency, perianal discomfort, and incontinence. Some patients may have increased frequency and liquidity of stools, however, when their daily stool weights are less than 200 grams. Since diarrhea results from a disturbance in the normal flow and transport of gut fluids, the normal physiology of absorption in the digestive tract is first considered.

NORMAL PHYSIOLOGY

DELIVERY, FLOW, AND ABSORPTION RATES. During fasting, the intestine contains very little fluid, but when three normal meals per day are eaten, about 9 liters of fluid are delivered to the proximal duodenum. Approximately 2 liters of this fluid are from ingested food and liquids, the rest being digestive secretions.

The volume of chyme that passes through different segments of the small bowel depends on the type of food that has been eaten. For example, meals containing high concentrations of sugar are hypertonic, and when such meals are ingested, the volume of material passing through the jejunum is even greater than the volume that enters the proximal duodenum. On the other hand, after isotonic or hypotonic meals (such as a meal of steak, potatoes, and tea), the volume of fluid traversing the jejunum is much less than that which was delivered to the duodenum. (These considerations are especially important in patients who have had gastric surgery or intestinal resection.) In either case, the osmolality of chyme is adjusted toward that of plasma as fluid travels through the duodenum and upper jejunum, and by the time chyme reaches the ileum, most of the dietary sugars, amino acids, and fats have been absorbed. Fluid arriving at the ileum is mainly an isotonic salt solution and therefore similar in its ionic composition to plasma. The ileum absorbs much, but not all, of this salt solution. About 1 liter per day of this isotonic unabsorbed ileal fluid enters the colon. Although ileal fluid resembles plasma with regard to its sodium and potassium concentrations, the concentrations of chloride and bicarbonate are quite different, being approximately 70 and 60 mEq per liter, respectively.

The colon can absorb 2 to 4 liters of isotonic salt solution per day (even more in patients with secondary hyperaldosteronism associated with salt depletion). The presence of nonabsorbable and osmotically active solutes from the diet and from bacterial action, a relatively slow rate of absorption from the rectosigmoid, and timely bowel movements prevent complete fluid absorption and desiccation of the fecal mass. About 100 ml of fluid is excreted in the feces; its sodium and chloride concentrations are about 50 mEq per liter, while the potassium concentration is about 90 mEq per liter. This fluid also contains a high concentration of volatile fatty acids (from bacterial action on nondigestible carbohydrates), which dissipate most of the unabsorbed or secreted bicarbonate ions and which often cause stool fluid to be hypertonic to plasma. Since the gastrointestinal tract does not have a diluting mechanism, the osmolality of fecal fluid is never less than the osmolality of plasma.

To summarize, daily volumes of fluid traversing the duodenum are 9 liters, traversing the ileocecal valve area are 1 liter, and traversing the anal sphincter are 0.1 liter. Stated in another way, the small bowel absorbs 8 liters of fluid per day and empties 1 liter into the colon, and the colon absorbs 0.9 liter. Theoretically 2 to 4 liters of fluid would have to be delivered to the colon per day before diarrhea would ensue, provided that delivery rates were steady, the fluid contained no abnormal solutes, and colon function was normal. Unfortunately, the latter qualifications do not apply in many gastrointestinal diseases.

TRANSPORT PHYSIOLOGY. The mechanisms responsible for fluid absorption differ in different regions of the gut and in different species. According to the model for the ileum shown in Figure 101–1, the brush border membrane contains a carrier that facilitates the simultaneous entry of Na^+ and glucose into the cells; Na^+ cannot enter without glucose. A separate pair of exchange carriers works together to facilitate the simultaneous and electrically neutral entry of Na^+ and Cl^-. Na^+ enters in exchange for H^+, and Cl^- enters in exchange for HCO_3^-. If these two exchange carriers operate at the same rate, Na^+ and Cl^- are absorbed in equal amounts, and H^+ and HCO_3^- are secreted in equal amounts and react in the lumen to form CO_2 and water. However, the anion carrier usually operates more rapidly than the cation carrier, and there is a net secretion of HCO_3^-. (This accounts for the high concentration of HCO_3^- and the low concentration of Cl^- in fluid that the ileum delivers to the colon.) Once inside the cell (via either the Na^+-H^+ exchange or the Na^+-glucose carrier), Na^+ is pumped out of the cell across the basolateral membrane by a pump that is probably an Na^+-K^+ adenosine triphosphatase (ATPase). Chloride and glucose exit the basolateral membrane by facilitated or passive diffusion.

Sodium pumping at the basolateral membrane causes a potential difference (PD) across the mucosa (serosal side positive). However, the tight junctions between small bowel mucosal cells (the "shunt pathway") are "leaky," and passive diffusion of anions (in the absorptive direction from lumen to plasma) or cations (in the secretory direction) readily dissipates the PD. Therefore, the residual PD across small bowel mucosa is only 2 to 4 mV.

Colonic cells and colonic transport are somewhat different. The brush border membrane apparently has a carrier for Na^+ that is not influenced by glucose or other actively absorbed nonelectro-

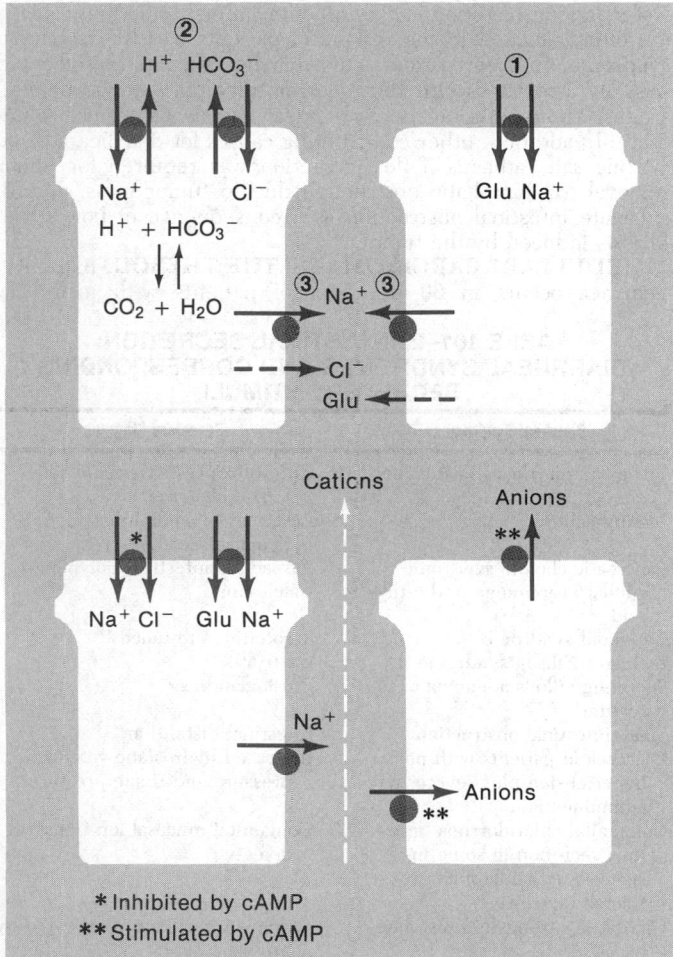

FIGURE 101–1. *Top,* Active transport mechanisms in the human ileum. *1,* Brush border glucose-sodium carrier. *2,* Double exchange carriers for neutral NaCl entry. *3,* Basolateral membrane sodium pump. *Bottom,* Model of cyclic AMP–mediated change in intestinal transport. Active anion secretion is stimulated (**), and there is inhibition of neutral NaCl entry across the brush border membrane (*). The glucose-sodium entry carrier and the basolateral membrane sodium pump are intact. Cations are secreted passively via the tight junction pathway.

lytes (glucose is not absorbed in the colon). There is no convincing evidence for Na^+-H^+ exchange, but the brush border membrane appears to have an anion exchange carrier that facilitates chloride absorption and bicarbonate secretion. The tight junctions are "tight," so the electrical gradient generated by the basolateral membrane pump is sustained. The PD is, therefore, about 30 mV (serosal side positive).

Potassium movement in all regions of the gut is passive, in response to electrochemical gradients. Thus, passive potassium absorption in the colon is retarded (owing to the high lumen-negative PD), and the potassium concentration in fecal fluid is much higher than in plasma (up to 100 mEq per liter). Water movement throughout the gut is passive, secondary to osmotic pressure gradients generated by active solute transport.

NORMAL SMALL BOWEL SECRETION. Small intestinal cells normally secrete as well as absorb electrolytes and water, with the secretory rate normally being of less magnitude than the absorptive rate, so that the net effect of small bowel transport processes is absorption of fluid. (Although it is possible that the same cell might both absorb and secrete, the putative small bowel secretion probably originates in crypt cells, whereas absorption takes place from villous cells.) This is an extremely important concept, because it means that a hormone or toxin might reduce net absorption rate in either of two ways: (1) by stimulating secretion, or (2) by inhibiting absorption. In either case, the observed effect is reduced absorption. Similarly, a hormone or a toxin might cause small bowel secretion by stimulating active secretion, so that it overwhelms the normal absorptive process; or a hormone or a toxin could cause secretion by inhibiting absorption, so that the normal small bowel secretion is unmasked. In fact, many toxins and hormones appear capable of both stimulating secretion and inhibiting normal absorption (see below). In patients with diarrhea caused by toxins or hormones, it is difficult to ascertain which of these factors is predominant.

In the colon, absorption takes place from the surface epithelial cells. There is no evidence for or against a normal colonic secretion.

PATHOPHYSIOLOGY OF DIARRHEA

Diarrhea may result from one or more of the following four mechanisms. There is, in addition, a miscellaneous group for which a single mechanism cannot currently be identified:

1. Poorly absorbable, osmotically active solutes in the intestinal lumen.
2. Active ion secretion.
3. Deranged intestinal motility.
4. Altered mucosal morphology or loss of absorptive surface.
5. Miscellaneous (several mechanisms or pathophysiology not clearly understood).

Osmotic Diarrhea

Osmotic diarrhea is caused by the accumulation of nonabsorbed solutes in the gut lumen. There are three main subtypes: (1) ingestion of poorly absorbable solutes, such as saline purgatives; (2) maldigestion of ingested food, such as in lactase deficiency; and (3) failure of a mucosal transport mechanism, such as in glucose-galactose malabsorption (Table 101–1). Being osmotically active, these solutes cause water and salts to be retained within the intestinal lumen, resulting in diarrhea.

Osmotic diarrhea stops when the patient fasts (or stops ingesting the poorly absorbable solute). Furthermore, the fecal fluid has a large solute gap; i.e., normal electrolytes do not account for much of the fecal fluid osmolality (fecal solute gap = [osmolality] $-$ 2[(Na^+) + (K^+)]; the factor of 2 is to account for anions in stool water). An exception is congenital chloridorrhea, in which unabsorbed chloride prevents water absorption. In chloridorrhea the chloride concentration in fecal fluids exceeds the sum of the concentration of sodium and potassium. Such fecal fluid analysis is performed on supernatant stool water following centrifugation of a stool sample in a test tube (30 minutes at 2000 g). In most instances, electrolytes and osmolality will provide meaningful information only if the stools are liquid enough that at the end of centrifugation the supernatant stool water constitutes at least one third of the total sample. In osmotic diarrhea resulting from

TABLE 101–1. CAUSES OF OSMOTIC DIARRHEA

Ingestion of poorly absorbable solutes
  Magnesium sulfate, sodium sulfate, citrate-containing laxatives
  Some antacids—Mg(OH)$_2$
  Mannitol, sorbitol (chewing gum, diet candy)
Maldigestion
  Disaccharidase deficiencies (lactose, sucrose-isomaltose, trehalose intolerance)
  Gastrocolic fistula, jejunoileal bypass, short bowel syndrome
  Postgastrectomy, postvagotomy state
  Chronic intestinal ischemia
  Lactulose therapy
Mucosal transport defects
  Glucose-galactose malabsorption
  Chloridorrhea
  Congenital sodium diarrhea
  General malabsorption in diffuse disease of small bowel mucosa

carbohydrate malabsorption, the concentration in stool of short-chain fatty acids is high, and thus the pH is low (pH 4.0 to 6.0). In some instances it is necessary to measure magnesium (normal less than 12 mM), sulfate (normal less than 5 mM), and phosphate (normal less than 12 mM) in stool water to identify the cause of osmotic diarrhea, especially in surreptitious laxative abuse.

Normal fecal fluid, which can be isolated from stool by dialysis methods, often has a modest solute gap (mainly because of unabsorbed carbohydrates and their bacterial products). Therefore, the presence of a solute gap is suggestive of osmotic diarrhea only if stool volume losses are substantially higher than normal. For example, a modest osmotic gap with a stool weight of only 200 grams per 24 hours would not by itself be suggestive of osmotic diarrhea.

Secretory Diarrhea

The net effect of a secretory stimulus on intestinal mucosa can be either inhibition of absorption or a net luminal gain (secretion) of water and electrolytes. This sequence of net movement changes may follow a dose-response curve, with a low secretagogue dose (e.g., circulating vasoactive intestinal polypeptide [VIP] concentration) inhibiting intestinal water and ion absorption and a high dose causing net secretion. On a cellular level, both processes can occur at the same time, with inhibition of villus absorption and enhancement of crypt secretion in the small bowel.

Secretory diarrhea is recognized clinically by certain features: Stools are large in volume and watery (more than 1 liter per day), and diarrhea persists with fasting. The stool osmolality can be totally accounted for by normal ionic constituents: ([Na$^+$] + [K$^+$]) × 2 equals stool osmolality, which is close to the osmolality of plasma. Table 101–2 gives the major causes of secretory diarrhea. A few examples are discussed in detail.

ENTEROTOXIN-INDUCED SECRETION. The classic disease in this category is Asiatic cholera (Ch. 317). Intestinal secretion is caused by cholera toxin; the morphologic appearance of intestinal mucosa, however, remains normal. An increase in intracellular cyclic adenosine monophosphate (cAMP) in cholera mediates active ion secretion by the enterocytes (Fig. 101–1B). Patients may lose 10 to 20 liters of watery stool per day. Mortality was high prior to the introduction of oral rehydration solutions. This therapy is successful because glucose-stimulated sodium absorption remains normal despite ongoing secretion.

Enterotoxigenic *Escherichia coli* strains can produce one or more of at least three types of toxins (one heat-labile and two heat-stable toxins). Intestinal secretion caused by these toxins is responsible for many episodes of acute diarrhea, including traveler's diarrhea (Ch. 319). Enterotoxin is produced by a large number of other bacteria, some of which are also capable of tissue invasion (*Campylobacter jejuni, Yersinia enterocolitica, Salmonella, Shigella, Clostridium difficile, Staphylococcus aureus, Klebsiella pneumoniae, Aeromonas, Plesiomonas*).

PANCREATIC CHOLERA SYNDROME (Ch. 220). High circulating levels of VIP cause intestinal water and electrolyte secretion that results in large-volume diarrhea. In adults, VIP production usually comes from tumors originating in pancreatic islet cells, whereas in children these tumors are often gangli-

oneuromas or ganglioneuroblastomas. The disease can be mimicked by prolonged intravenous VIP infusion in healthy subjects. This syndrome is also known as Verner-Morrison syndrome, VIP-oma syndrome, or watery diarrhea-hypokalemia-hypochlorhydria (WDHH) syndrome. Diarrhea disappears when plasma VIP levels return to normal following tumor resection. Fifty per cent of patients have metastatic disease at diagnosis, however, so that resection is not possible.

In one study of patients with pancreatic cholera, mean daily stool weights averaged 4224 grams during a regular diet and 1817 grams during fasting. Hypokalemia and metabolic acidosis due to large fecal potassium and bicarbonate losses are prominent features, whereas hypochlorhydria is variable. Cosecretion of calcitonin, pancreatic polypeptide, PHM (peptide histidine methionine), or helodermin by these tumors has been found in a number of patients.

IDIOPATHIC SECRETORY DIARRHEA. Patients with this syndrome present with the large-volume secretory diarrhea and other clinical features of pancreatic cholera, but no evidence of tumor or of an abnormally elevated concentration of a circulating secretagogue can be found. These patients undergo extensive negative investigations that often include exploratory laparotomy. Autopsy examination may also be unrevealing, and the etiology remains unknown. Both the severity of this syndrome and the prognosis vary widely. Spontaneous resolution of the diarrhea may occur after several months. A few patients respond to opiates.

CARCINOID SYNDROME (Ch. 230). Diarrhea is a common manifestation of the carcinoid syndrome, occurring in about 70 to 80 per cent of patients. In most patients, intestinal secretion can be demonstrated. Serotonin and substance P elicit intestinal water and ion secretion in experimental animals, and these agents are often elevated in the plasma of patients with the carcinoid syndrome. In other patients, the diarrhea appears episodic and possibly associated with the hypermotility that can be demonstrated when serotonin is given intravenously to normal volunteers. In addition, other contributing causes for diarrhea may be (1) bile salt catharsis if ileal resection was required for tumor removal, (2) lymphatic obstruction due to tumor mass, and (3) subacute intestinal obstruction as a consequence of bowel wall fibrosis induced by the tumor.

MEDULLARY CARCINOMA OF THE THYROID (Ch. 216). Diarrhea occurs in 30 per cent of patients with medullary

TABLE 101–2. INTESTINAL SECRETION: DIARRHEAL SYNDROMES AND CORRESPONDING SECRETORY STIMULI

Diarrheal Syndromes	Secretory Stimulus
Traveler's diarrhea, Asiatic cholera	Enterotoxins (*Escherichia coli, Vibrio cholerae*)
Laxative abuse	Laxatives (phenolphthalein, senna, bisacodyl)
Pancreatic cholera syndrome	Vasoactive intestinal polypeptide
Medullary carcinoma of the thyroid	Calcitonin
Carcinoid syndrome	Serotonin, substance P
Zollinger-Ellison syndrome	Gastrin
Secreting villous adenoma of the rectum	Prostaglandins
Small intestinal obstruction	Intestinal distention
Diarrhea in patients with portal hypertension plus severe hypoalbuminemia	Increased hydrostatic vascular pressure and tissue pressure
Congenital chloridorrhea (intestinal secretion in some instances); lethal familial protracted diarrhea	Congenital mucosal ion transport defects
Giardiasis, strongyloidosis, amebiasis	Unknown mechanism activated by protozoa
Idiopathic chronic secretory diarrhea (pseudopancreatic cholera syndrome)	Unknown
Collagen vascular diseases (scleroderma, systemic lupus erythematosus, mixed connective tissue disease)	Unknown
Intestinal lymphoma	Unknown

carcinoma of the thyroid and may precede the presence of a palpable thyroid mass. Circulating calcitonin is the major mediator of intestinal secretion in this syndrome. Since this tumor may be part of multiple endocrine neoplasia syndromes (Ch. 228), first-degree relatives need to be investigated by measuring basal and postprovocation (intravenous pentagastrin) plasma calcitonin concentrations. Other than in medullary carcinoma of the thyroid, calcitonin is also found in high concentrations in the plasma and tumor tissue of a number of patients with endocrine pancreatic tumors (VIPoma, somatostatinoma), but usually it is not the predominant peptide.

ZOLLINGER-ELLISON SYNDROME (Ch. 98.6). The secretory diarrhea that occurs in gastrinoma (Zollinger-Ellison syndrome) has a unique pathophysiology. Owing to the gastric hypersecretion caused by high concentrations of circulating gastrin, an excessive load of acidic fluid enters the small bowel and overwhelms the intestinal absorptive capacity. In such patients, daily delivery of up to 24 liters of acidic fluid to the jejunum can occur in the fasting state. Although the percentage of decrease in luminal flow rates in the intestine is similar to that in healthy subjects, the remaining fecal volume is often still in excess of 1 liter per day. Other factors that may play a role in causing diarrhea in gastrinoma are the functional or morphologic impairment of the mucosal brush border by the abnormal acid milieu, the direct effect of excessive gastrin on the small bowel mucosa (reducing absorption), and inactivation of pancreatic lipase by the acidic fluid, causing a mild degree of steatorrhea. Low intraluminal pH may also cause some of the primary bile acids to become insoluble, leading to a reduction of micelle formation and a mild degree of steatorrhea.

BILE ACID DIARRHEA. Watery diarrhea in cholerrheic enteropathy results from the secretory effect of malabsorbed bile acids on colonic mucosa. Interruption of the normal enterohepatic circulation of bile acids can be caused by three types of bile acid malabsorption. Type I is due to ileal disease or resection. Type II, which is less common, consists of a selective ileal transport defect for bile acids. Type III is bile acid malabsorption in the postcholecystectomy and postvagotomy state. Cholestyramine is the treatment of choice for type I and type II bile acid diarrhea. Patients with type III are rarely found to have secretory concentrations of fecal bile acids and rarely respond to cholestyramine.

Deranged Intestinal Motility

On a priori grounds, three major derangements might cause diarrhea: (1) Abnormally reduced peristalsis may allow bacterial overgrowth in the small bowel. (2) "Intestinal hurry" may reduce contact time between the small bowel mucosa and its contents and thus result in delivery of abnormally large and qualitatively abnormal fluid loads to the colon. This occurs in spite of the fact that absorption in the small bowel is normal per unit of time. (3) Premature emptying of the colon caused by an abnormality of its contents, or by intrinsic colonic "irritability" or inflammation, results in a reduced contact between luminal contents and colonic mucosa and therefore increased volume and liquidity of the stools.

Some diarrheal diseases due, at least in part, to deranged motility are irritable bowel syndrome, malignant carcinoid syndrome, postvagotomy diarrhea, diarrhea resulting from diabetic neuropathy, diarrhea resulting from thyrotoxicosis, and the diarrhea associated with postgastrectomy dumping syndrome. Abnormal motility may also contribute to acute diarrhea caused by infections. Stool analysis in diarrhea due to a motility disturbance may be consistent with that in osmotic diarrhea if nutrient absorption is impaired in the small bowel or may resemble that in secretory diarrhea, if, following nutrient absorption, the ileocecal transit volume remains largely unabsorbed. Alternatively, a mixed pattern can exist, with electrolytes accounting for an osmolality equal to that of plasma and an additional component making stool water hyperosmolar, owing mainly to bacterial metabolism of malabsorbed carbohydrates in the collection unit following passage of the stool. Irritable bowel syndrome and fecal incontinence are discussed in more detail.

IRRITABLE BOWEL SYNDROME. In the United States, up to 50 per cent of all patients seen by primary care physicians for digestive tract problems have irritable bowel syndrome. Diarrhea is usually referred to as functional diarrhea, since no obvious cause can be found on extensive routine clinical testing. On special investigations, altered myoelectric activity in the large bowel and a significant acceleration in small bowel transit have been demonstrated in patients with irritable bowel syndrome and diarrhea. At the present time, however, it is unclear what clinical relevance these findings may have in the diagnostic and therapeutic management of such patients.

Although functional diarrhea as part of the irritable bowel syndrome is generally considered a diagnosis by exclusion, this does not mean that extensive testing is necessary when one is initially confronted with such a patient. Rather, a positive diagnosis can often be made at the first interview. This is based mainly on a typical history: abdominal pain of long duration (often for several years), discomfort and pain in different areas of the abdomen, bloating associated with various so-called food intolerances, and alternating diarrhea and constipation. Functional diarrhea may show a temporal relation to meal intake, and nocturnal diarrhea is typically absent. Furthermore, signs of systemic disease, such as weight loss, are usually absent. Classically, patients are female and in their 20's and 30's, and a history of emotional conflict, stress, or anxiety is common.

In functional diarrhea, stool weight rarely exceeds 500 grams per day (normal less than 200 grams). In a patient who complains of an increased frequency of defecation, a normal or nearly normal 24-hour stool weight may be the first clue to fecal incontinence, a diagnosis often confused with functional diarrhea.

INCONTINENCE. Most patients whose major disability is due to fecal incontinence present to their physician with "diarrhea." Either they are embarrassed to mention the incontinence, or they interpret it as a manifestation of severe diarrhea. If patients do mention incontinence, the physician also usually attributes it to voluminous diarrhea. In most instances, however, these patients are suffering primarily from a defect in the continence mechanisms rather than from severe diarrhea. As a matter of fact, quantitative stool collections usually reveal rather small fecal volumes, even though stools are soft to liquid in consistency. In any case, the major problem in most such patients is in the anal continence mechanisms. The most frequent causes for sphincter dysfunction are previous anal surgery for fissures, fistulas, or hemorrhoids; episiotomy or tear during childbirth; anal Crohn's disease; and diabetic neuropathy.

Anal sphincter training may improve sphincter function and reduce the frequency of incontinent episodes. It is also important to establish the cause of diarrhea if possible, since effective therapy of the diarrhea usually prevents further incontinence. Symptomatic therapy with opiate drugs is helpful in some patients. There is recent interest in surgical treatment for incontinence, but no good prospective studies have been done. No therapy for incontinence in patients with diarrhea, whether involving drugs, biofeedback, or surgery, has included objective data that convincingly establish its benefit.

Morphologic Alterations

Efficient intestinal absorption requires that the intestinal mucosa be intact with a well-functioning blood supply and intact neural connections. A large number of diseases can cause diarrhea by disrupting the normal anatomy of the intestine (Table 101-3).

VIRAL GASTROENTERITIS. It is estimated that every year 5 million children less than 2 years of age die in developing countries as a consequence of acute diarrhea. Rotavirus is responsible for at least 50 per cent of these infections. The pathogenesis of viral diarrhea is thought to be as follows. The virus enters the absorptive epithelial cells on the tip of the villus, and these cells are sloughed off. Crypt cells then move quickly to replace the lost enterocytes. These cells, however, are immature and cannot absorb effectively. Their sucrase and lactase activities are low, whereas adenylate cyclase activity and cAMP content are normal (in contrast to cholera, in which sucrase and lactase activities are normal and adenylate cyclase activity and cAMP content are increased). There is no enhanced water and electrolyte secretion in viral gastroenteritis; however, sodium-stimulated glucose absorption is markedly diminished. Malabsorption of water, electrolytes, and nutrients results until the infection subsides and mature enterocytes again coat the surface of the villus.

TABLE 101–3. DIARRHEA DUE TO DISRUPTION OF STRUCTURAL INTEGRITY OF THE INTESTINE

Viral gastroenteritis
Bacterial infection with tissue invasion
Sprue (tropical, nontropical, collagenous)
Whipple's disease
Radiation enteritis
Drugs (e.g., chemotherapeutic agents)
Amyloidosis
Collagen vascular diseases (systemic lupus erythematosus, scleroderma, mixed connective tissue disease)
Inflammatory bowel disease (Crohn's disease, ulcerative colitis, microscopic and collagenous colitis)
Eosinophilic gastroenteritis
Intestinal lymphoma
Ileocecal tuberculosis
Intestinal ischemia, mesenteric vasculitis
Diverticulitis
Pelvic inflammatory disease
Acquired immunodeficiency syndrome (AIDS)

SPRUE (Ch. 102). The changes associated with sprue involve villous atrophy and a marked diminution in the effective absorptive surface of the bowel. When studied with intestinal perfusion techniques, such patients demonstrate jejunal secretion. This can be expected from the observation that the mucosa in total villous atrophy consists only of crypts, and crypts normally secrete fluid and electrolytes. Diarrhea is a result of fat and carbohydrate malabsorption. Typically, there is no diarrhea when these patients fast, suggesting that the colon reabsorbs the small bowel secretions. In rare cases patients with sprue have severe secretory diarrhea; a stool output as high as 5 liters a day has been observed.

RADIATION ENTERITIS. Acute radiation enteritis usually occurs within the initial weeks of radiation exposure and is characterized by abdominal cramping, diarrhea, nausea, and vomiting. With the passage of time, symptoms abate, and a quiescent period ensues. The average onset of further symptoms is 1 year, but symptoms may occur at any time. Malabsorption of varying degree for bile acids, fat, carbohydrate, and vitamin B_{12} is observed. Interference with absorption occurs owing to infiltration of the mucosa by inflammatory cells and luminal narrowing of the submucosal arterioles with fibrin plugs. Disturbances in motility due to the effects of radiation on the muscularis propria can also contribute to the diarrhea. Late-appearing structural changes with intermittent obstruction, mucosal ulceration, and fistula formation may also lead to diarrhea. Medical therapy with antidiarrheal agents, broad-spectrum antibiotics for bacterial overgrowth, and prednisone rarely provides total control of symptoms. Ultimately, 15 per cent of patients require surgical intervention, such as segmental resection or fistula closure.

LOSS OF ABSORPTIVE SURFACE. The diarrhea that results from intestinal resection may be on the basis of the region removed (e.g., ileum, with its special transport sites for active bile acid absorption) or of the length of bowel resected. At least 50 per cent of the small bowel is required in order to avoid diarrhea and malnutrition associated with the short bowel syndrome.

AIDS (ACQUIRED IMMUNODEFICIENCY SYNDROME) (Part XXI). Small intestinal morphologic alterations and consequent malabsorption and diarrhea are common among patients with AIDS. Infectious agents (*Giardia*, *Salmonella*, *Cryptosporidium*, and *Stronglyoides*) and Kaposi's sarcoma can cause gastrointestinal disturbances in AIDS. There remains a group of patients, however, who do not have identifiable infectious or parasitic agents or Kaposi's sarcoma but who still manifest diarrhea, malabsorption, and weight loss. Such patients have abnormal D-xylose and fat absorption. Duodenal biopsies reveal blunting of the villi and an inflammatory infiltrate in the lamina propria. This condition is referred to as AIDS enteropathy. Other patients with AIDS may demonstrate a histiocytic infiltrate (pseudo-Whipple's disease) containing numerous acid-fast organisms. *Mycobacterium avium-intracellulare* has been isolated in these patients.

MICROSCOPIC COLITIS. Some patients with chronic diarrhea demonstrate inflammation of colonic mucosa despite a normal appearance of the colon on barium enema and colonoscopy. The histologic changes consist of excess neutrophils and round cells in the lamina propria, cryptitis, and reactive changes of surface epithelial cells. When colonic absorption is measured in these patients by perfusion techniques, water and electrolyte absorption is either abolished or abnormally low. Thus, the normal ileocecal transit volume (1 liter per day) remains largely unabsorbed, and stool weights are typically in the range of 400 to 800 grams per day.

Miscellaneous Causes of Diarrhea

Table 101–4 gives a list of diseases in which several of the discussed mechanisms may cause diarrhea or in which the pathophysiology is not clearly understood.

DIAGNOSIS

Although the cause of diarrhea is obvious in many clinical situations, in many others it is not. Here we are concerned with a diagnostic approach to the patient with diarrhea in whom the cause is unknown.

History and Physical Examination

When the stools are consistently large in volume, the underlying cause of diarrhea is likely to be located in the small bowel or in the proximal colon. By contrast, in small-volume diarrhea, in which the patient has frequent urges to defecate but passes only small amounts of feces or mucus, the disorder is usually in the left portion of the colon and rectum. Passage of blood mixed in with the diarrheal stool usually indicates inflammation of the mucosa, less often a neoplasm. Passage of nonbloody mucus suggests irritable bowel syndrome, as does a history of small-volume diarrhea alternating with constipation. Frothy stools and excessive flatus suggest fermentation of unabsorbed carbohydrates. Excessively foul stools suggest putrefaction of unabsorbed amino acids. Visible oil or fat indicates severe steatorrhea. Fecal soiling (incontinence) suggests an anal sphincter defect. Diarrhea in a patient with features of anorexia nervosa suggests laxative abuse.

There are, of course, many other pertinent facts obtainable from the history, including previous surgery, drug intake (Table 101–4), symptoms of systemic illness, travel, and related illnesses in family members. In chronic and recurrent diarrhea, an association of exacerbation of diarrhea with emotional stress should be sought, an association that may suggest irritable bowel syndrome. The patient's sexual history should be discussed, as male homosexuals have a high incidence of shigellosis, giardiasis, other intestinal infections, and the usually recognized venereal diseases. Diarrhea may be the presenting manifestation of AIDS.

The physical examination may provide clues to the cause of diarrhea. Some physical findings, as well as other clinical associations that may assist in the diagnosis of diarrhea, are listed in Table 101–5.

Diagnostic Tests

ROUTINE EXAMINATION OF STOOL. Unless the diagnosis is readily apparent from the history and physical examination, certain relatively simple studies on the stool should routinely be

TABLE 101–4. MISCELLANEOUS CAUSES OF DIARRHEA

Drugs
    Diuretics, cardiac glycosides, propranolol, quinidine, colchicine, antibiotics, methotrexate, 6-mercaptopurine, 5-fluorouracil, guanethidine, ethanol
Endocrine disorders
    Addison's disease, hypoparathyroidism
Neurologic diseases
    Tabes dorsalis, multiple sclerosis, myelitis, encephalitis, heat stroke, Charcot-Marie-Tooth disease, myotonia dystrophica, orthostatic hypotension
Toxicologic disorders
    Lead poisoning
Immunoglobulin deficiency
Allergy
Systemic mastocytosis

TABLE 101–5. CLUES TO DIAGNOSIS OF DIARRHEA FROM OTHER SYMPTOMS, SIGNS, AND LABORATORY TESTS

Symptom or Sign Associated with Diarrhea	Diagnoses To Be Considered
Arthritis	Ulcerative colitis, Crohn's disease, Whipple's disease
Liver disease	Ulcerative colitis, Crohn's disease, bowel malignancy with metastasis to liver
Fever	Ulcerative colitis, Crohn's disease, amebiasis, lymphoma, tuberculosis
Marked weight loss	Malabsorption, inflammatory bowel disease, cancer, thyrotoxicosis
Eosinophilia	Eosinophilic gastroenteritis, parasitic disease
Lymphadenopathy	Lymphoma, Whipple's disease, AIDS
Neuropathy	Diabetic diarrhea, amyloidosis
Postural hypotension	Diabetic diarrhea, Addison's disease, idiopathic orthostatic hypotension
Flushing, large liver	Malignant carcinoid syndrome
Proteinuria	Amyloidosis
Perianal disease or right lower quadrant abdominal mass	Crohn's disease
Purpura	Celiac disease
Peptic ulcer	Zollinger-Ellison syndrome, antacid therapy, gastrocolic fistula
Following cholecystectomy	Bile acid malabsorption
Frequent infections	Immunoglobulin deficiency, AIDS
Immunodeficiency	Giardiasis, nodular lymphoid hyperplasia, celiac sprue
Hyperpigmentation	Whipple's disease, celiac disease, Addison's disease
Good response to corticosteroids	Ulcerative colitis, Crohn's disease, Whipple's disease, Addison's disease, pancreatic cholera, eosinophilic enteritis
Good response to antibiotics	Bacterial overgrowth in small intestine, tropical sprue, Whipple's disease, celiac disease

performed. Regardless of the clinical classification, the information obtained usually narrows the diagnostic possibilities.

Stain for Pus. The presence or absence of intestinal inflammation can often be ascertained by examination of a stained stool specimen. Wright's or methylene blue stains are satisfactory. The presence of large numbers of white blood cells is diagnostic of inflammation. The presence of rare, scattered white cells is within normal limits.

In patients with acute or traveler's diarrhea, pus in the stool suggests invasion of the mucosa by *Shigella, E. coli, Entamoeba histolytica, Salmonella, Campylobacter,* gonococci, or other invasive organisms. In general, shigellosis and invasive *E. coli* infections cause more pus than do *Salmonella* and *E. histolytica* infections. Antibiotic-related colitis may or may not be associated with pus. Diarrhea caused by noninvasive organisms that produce enterotoxins (toxigenic *E. coli,* for example), viruses, and *Giardia* is not associated with pus in the stool.

In patients with chronic and recurrent diarrhea or diarrhea of unknown etiology, pus suggests colitis of some type—idiopathic ulcerative colitis, Crohn's colitis, antibiotic-associated colitis, amebic colitis, ischemic colitis, or tuberculous colitis. Pus is especially abundant in idiopathic ulcerative colitis and tends to be less so in amebic colitis. It is usually absent in microscopic colitis. Absence of pus on a single examination does not, of course, absolutely rule out any of these entities. Radiation-induced disease of the large or small bowel and Crohn's disease limited to the small intestine may or may not be associated with pus in the stool. Pus is not present in the stools of patients with irritable bowel syndrome, most causes of malabsorption syndrome, laxative abuse, viral gastroenteritis, and giardiasis.

Occult Blood. Occult (or gross) blood in association with diarrhea usually indicates inflammation and therefore usually has the same significance as pus in the stools (see above). When blood is present in diarrheal stools that do not contain pus, one should consider neoplasms of the colon, heavy metal poisoning, and acute ischemic damage to the gut.

Sudan Stain for Fat. If excess fat is evident on Sudan stain, steatorrhea is probably present, and the various causes of malabsorption syndromes should be considered (see Ch. 102). Most such patients have chronic and recurrent diarrhea; steatorrhea in a patient with acute or traveler's diarrhea suggests giardiasis.

Alkalinization. A pink color following alkalinization of a stool or urine sample indicates phenolphthalein ingestion as the cause of diarrhea. The test is so easily and quickly done, and the significance of a positive result is so great, that it should be carried out routinely in female patients with chronic diarrhea. Surreptitious laxative ingestion is rarely seen in males.

OTHER TESTS. Evidence of systemic illness has obvious implications in the etiology of diarrhea (Table 101–5). For instance, a history of flushing and diarrhea leads to determination of urinary 5-hydroxyindoleacetic acid (Ch. 230). The order in which tests are carried out, assuming that further tests are necessary, varies according to the physician's intuition regarding a particular patient. Certain of the diagnostic tests deserve brief discussion here.

Search for Infectious and Parasitic Organisms. It is important to complete the examination for parasites and to have adequate bacterial cultures in progress prior to examination of the patient with radiologic contrast media because barium interferes with successful demonstration of pathogens. Failure to find *Giardia* in stool samples is not strong evidence against giardiasis; sometimes it is necessary to examine duodenal fluid in order to demonstrate this organism. *Cryptosporidium* can be revealed by acid-fast stain of feces subjected to a flotation technique for concentration. Special culture methods are required if the presence of infection by *Gonococcus, Campylobacter,* or *Yersinia* is to be established. A microimmunofluorescent test with monoclonal antibodies can be used on a rectal mucosal smear to assess for chlamydial proctitis. Serologic tests for amebae and lymphogranuloma venereum may assist in the diagnosis in some patients. Finally, tests for clostridial toxin in fecal fluid help in the diagnosis of pseudomembranous colitis.

Proctosigmoidoscopy. Proctosigmoidoscopy is helpful in establishing the presence or absence of mucosal inflammation. In antibiotic-associated diarrhea, it may reveal pseudomembranes. Proctosigmoidoscopy is often essential in patients with chronic and recurrent diarrhea and in patients with diarrhea of unknown etiology. The findings are especially apt to be abnormal in those whose stools contain pus or blood or both; they are usually normal in patients with diarrhea caused by the various malabsorption syndromes.

Proctosigmoidoscopy to investigate diarrhea should be done without enemas, laxatives, or suppositories. Such preparation may wash away exudate, distort the mucosa, induce trauma, and possibly obscure evidence of disease or create the false impression of disease. In almost all instances, fecal matter can easily be aspirated or pushed aside, and since most abnormalities are diffuse, fecal matter does not interfere greatly with a satisfactory examination. The presence of solid stool in the rectum of a patient who supposedly has diarrhea is also revealing, suggesting that an acute diarrhea is subsiding, that the patient may have irritable bowel syndrome, that the diarrhea is an illusion, or that the diarrhea is secondary to fecal impaction.

Since proctitis may not be evident grossly, even to the experienced eye, mucosal smears should always be obtained and stained for pus. The mucosa should be carefully examined for melanosis coli, although melanosis may be present microscopically even if it is not present grossly.

Rectal Biopsy. Biopsy can often be helpful in the evaluation of patients with diarrhea. The main disorders that might be detected by biopsy, but not by smears and stool examination, are amyloidosis, Whipple's disease, microscopic colitis, granulomatous inflammation, melanosis coli, intestinal spirochetosis (other than that caused by *Treponema pallidum*), and schistosomiasis. Biopsy is indicated in patients with diarrhea of unknown origin, especially in a search for melanosis coli and unsuspected colitis that may not have been evident grossly. It is the opinion of this author that irritable bowel syndrome should not be diagnosed until after a rectal mucosal smear has shown that pus is not present and a rectal biopsy is found to reveal no abnormality. The biopsy should be taken from the posterior wall of the rectum on a valve.

Although the risk is uncertain, some clinicians believe that a rectal biopsy with large forceps predisposes to a colonic perforation if a barium enema is done within 10 days of the biopsy.

Quantitative Fecal Fat. Collected stools (usually for 72 hours) should be quantitatively analyzed for fat content (1) when malabsorption is suggested by the history and physical examination, (2) when the qualitative test for fecal fat is positive, or (3) routinely in patients with diarrhea of unknown origin. If steatorrhea is present, the differential diagnosis of malabsorption syndrome can be pursued (see Ch. 102). Of course, the results of this test must be interpreted with knowledge of the approximate intake of dietary fat. Stool weight in grams (which is equivalent to stool volume in milliliters) should also be noted and recorded (see below).

Twenty-four-hour Stool Volume. For reasons indicated under History and Physical Examination above, knowledge of stool volume helps localize the region of the intestine that is most likely responsible for diarrhea, and in several instances specific information on stool volume is of great diagnostic help. For example, stool volumes greater than 500 ml per day are rarely seen in patients with irritable bowel syndrome, and stool volumes of less than 1000 ml per day provide evidence against pancreatic cholera syndrome. In addition, very large measured stool volumes will alert the physician to the need for vigorous fluid replacement therapy.

Collection of 24-hour stool specimens is easy to do in the initial phases of a diarrhea workup, prior to barium radiographs, enemas, or other preparations. With a little effort, it can be accurately done on an outpatient basis. If a record of stool frequency is kept, the average volume of each stool can be calculated, and the results may give useful insight.

In special instances, e.g., in diarrhea of unknown origin, it is useful to measure stool electrolytes and osmolality and to determine whether or not the diarrhea persists during a 48-hour fast (while the patient is given glucose and salt solutions intravenously). These results help establish whether the diarrhea is secretory or osmotic in type (see Pathophysiology, above). If the osmolality of stool water is less than 250 mOsm per kilogram, water has been added to the stool to simulate diarrhea. A sodium concentration in fecal water that is higher than that of plasma indicates contamination by urine.

Vasoactive Intestinal Polypeptide (VIP) and Other Circulating Agents. The pancreatic cholera syndrome should be considered if diarrhea of unknown origin has lasted longer than 4 weeks, is secretory in type, and is severe (more than 1 liter per day and/or associated with hypokalemia and salt and water depletion), and if surreptitious laxative abuse and organic disease of the gastrointestinal tract have been excluded. The incidence of this syndrome is 1 in 10 million population per year. Only in this rare subgroup of patients is serum assay for VIP, PHM, and calcitonin likely to be helpful. Other gastrointestinal hormones such as pancreatic polypeptide (PP) may be elevated in plasma and serve as markers of endocrine pancreatic malignancy. In the United States, Dr. O'Dorisio's laboratory (Columbus, Ohio) and, in England, Dr. Bloom's laboratory (London) offer a gastrointestinal hormone profile that can be obtained from a single plasma sample. Blood needs to be drawn in iced tubes containing ethylenediamine tetra-acetic acid (EDTA) with aprotinin added to inhibit serum peptidases (aprotinin [Trasylol], 0.5 ml [5000 Kallikrein Inactivator Units] per 10 ml of blood). After immediate centrifugation in a refrigerated centrifuge, plasma is stored at $-25°C$ or lower until sent in a frozen state on Dry Ice to the appropriate laboratory.

Therapeutic Trials. In some instances therapeutic trials are indicated as diagnostic tests. (Obviously, in most instances, the results must be considered suggestive rather than conclusive.) These trials may include pancreatic enzymes, antibiotics (also as part of the Schilling test), metronidazole or quinacrine (for giardiasis), cholestyramine (for bile acid malabsorption), indomethacin (for prostaglandin synthetase inhibition), and various diets (lactose free, carbohydrate free, low fat, and avoidance of any specific food to evaluate the unlikely possibility of food allergy).

THERAPY

The most satisfactory therapy is to cure the underlying disease. When this is not possible, certain drugs may ameliorate the disease and thus reduce the severity of diarrhea (prednisone for inflammatory bowel disease is an example). In a few instances, the disease cannot be ameliorated, but there is fairly specific therapy for the diarrhea, such as cholestyramine for bile acid malabsorption.

At present, unfortunately, in many patients the disease process responsible for diarrhea cannot be satisfactorily suppressed, and specific therapy is lacking. Supportive and symptomatic therapy is required in such instances.

Fluid Replacement

The most important aspect of therapy in acute and traveler's diarrhea, and in some patients with chronic diarrhea, is prevention or correction of salt and water depletion. This can be done by oral ingestion of liquids and salty foods, oral glucose-saline solutions, or intravenous fluid therapy, as dictated by the clinical situation. Two points deserve emphasis. First, soft drinks, tea, and citrus juices contain little, if any, sodium chloride (even Gatorade contains only 23 mEq per liter of sodium chloride). Second, oral glucose-saline solutions or liquids plus salty foods will actually worsen the diarrhea (in terms of stool volume) as they help correct fluid depletion. The oral rehydration solution recommended by the World Health Organization contains the following in millimoles (grams) per liter: glucose, 111 (20); NaCl, 60 (4); KCl, 20 (2); NaHCO$_3$, 30 (2); and osmolality is 331 mOsm per kilogram. In some patients, particularly those with short bowel syndrome, a high sodium concentration is needed in the oral rehydration solution to achieve a positive sodium and fluid balance. To prevent hypertonicity of such a solution, glucose is best given as a polymer. Glucose polymer consists of linear chains of mostly five to nine glucose units and is obtained from hydrolysis of starch. Glucose polymer is available as Polycose (Ross Laboratories, Columbus, Ohio) or Moducal (Mead Johnson, Evansville, Indiana) and in England as Caloreen (Roussel Ltd., Wembly Park, England). Glucose polymer is readily hydrolyzed in the gut lumen, providing glucose to the sodium-glucose carrier in the brush border. The solution contains the following in millimoles (grams) per liter: glucose polymer, 20 (20); NaCl, 120 (7); KCl, 10 (1); and osmolality is 280 mOsm per kilogram. Various flavoring substances can be added to this solution (e.g., Kool Aid).

Avoidance or Treatment of Perianal Discomfort

Helpful therapy consists of the following: (1) avoidance of soap, toilet paper, washcloths, and towels; (2) gentle washing with warm water on absorbent cotton after each bowel movement, followed by gentle, thorough drying with absorbent cotton; (3) if seepage is present, absorbent cotton retained next to the anal orifice and held in place by snug underwear; (4) sitz baths for 10 minutes two or three times a day; and (5) hydrocortisone creams (1 per cent). In addition to these measures, patients may obtain relief by additional gentle cleaning with soft pads containing witch hazel (Tucks). Locally applied anesthetic ointments may be transiently helpful, but ointments restrict perspiration and anesthetics may irritate the perianal skin, so these agents should be used only for short periods of time. It is important to recognize specific treatable conditions, such as perianal moniliasis.

Opiates

Codeine, diphenoxylate with atropine (Lomotil), and loperamide reduce urgency, bowel movement frequency, and stool volume in a wide variety of acute or chronic diarrheal illnesses. This is not to say that they have a beneficial effect in every patient; but they do in most, so that when groups of patients are studied, both stool frequency and stool volume are reduced to a statistically significant extent. Of the three drugs, loperamide and codeine are usually somewhat superior to diphenoxylate; loperamide may have less tendency than codeine to cause addiction. Codeine, however, is much less expensive. In chronic diarrhea, the drugs may be given once a day in a maximally tolerated dose or several times daily in smaller doses.

Opiate drugs are generally thought to reduce diarrhea through reducing the propulsive activity of the gut and thereby reducing stool frequency. This mechanism might also enhance contact time between intestinal mucosa and luminal contents. Assuming that at least part of the gut mucosa is in an absorbing and not a secretory state, this would allow greater absorption of fluid and thereby reduce stool volume. In vitro opiates have also been reported to stimulate sodium chloride absorption and to have antisecretory action against several secretagogues. These effects cannot be demonstrated in clinical situations using therapeutic doses of opiate drugs.

Opiates should not be used in patients with severe ulcerative colitis with impending toxic megacolon, and there is evidence suggesting that they may prolong the diarrhea in shigellosis and perhaps in diarrheal diseases caused by other invasive bacteria and in antibiotic-associated diarrhea. These reservations notwithstanding, opiates are often of benefit in the symptomatic relief of diarrhea in patients with less severe ulcerative colitis and with many acute infectious diarrheal illnesses. Obviously, they should be prescribed only when diarrhea is causing significant disability.

There are rare case reports suggesting that opiate drugs can be a cause of paradoxical diarrhea.

Bismuth Subsalicylate

Bismuth subsalicylate may prevent infection with enterotoxin-producing E. coli organisms. In addition, this agent brings mild symptomatic relief in patients with acute infectious diarrhea, whether bacterial or viral in origin. The mechanism of the effect is unknown. The dose is 30 to 60 ml every 30 minutes for eight doses. Patients should be warned that this medication may turn their stools black. If the patient is on other medications, possible drug interaction should be considered.

Antibiotics in Acute and Traveler's Disease (Ch. 319)

For at least two reasons, antibiotics should not usually be used. First, in most patients they do not shorten the duration of illness. Second, their use risks the development of antibiotic-associated diarrhea or colitis, superimposed on whatever was causing the diarrhea initially. This greatly confuses the problem if the diarrhea becomes chronic.

In mild disease (small-volume diarrhea, no chills or fever, no blood or pus in the stool), antibiotics should not be prescribed unless a specific indication emerges from the bacteriology and parasitology laboratory. In patients who are severely ill, especially if they have blood or pus in the stool, antibiotic therapy aimed at shigellosis is reasonable, pending the result of stool culture.

Antisecretory Drugs

A specific and potent inhibitor of intestinal secretion is not available. On the basis of in vitro observations and individual case reports, a number of agents can be tried on an empiric basis. Phenothiazines inhibit secretion caused by cholera toxin and E. coli enterotoxins; aspirin, indomethacin, and other non-steroidal anti-inflammatory agents reduce secretion mediated by prostaglandins (inhibition of prostaglandin synthesis); glucocorticoids decrease mucosal inflammation and enhance NaCl absorption (increase in Na-K-ATPase activity); nicotinic acid, clonidine, lidamidine,* and lithium carbonate may increase intestinal NaCl absorption (inhibition of adenylate cyclase); and cromoglycate may inhibit release of mediators of allergic reaction in the intestine. When diarrhea is due to circulating agents (VIPoma, carcinoid), a somatostatin analogue given subcutaneously may abolish diarrhea by decreasing secretagogue release from tumor tissue.

Bo-Linn GW, Vendrell DD, Lee E, et al.: An evaluation of the significance of microscopic colitis in patients with chronic diarrhea. J Clin Invest 75:1559, 1986. First description of microscopic colitis as a separate disease entity. Patients reveal abolished water and electrolyte absorption during colonic perfusion studies.

Field M, Fordtran JS, Schultz SG (eds.): Secretory Diarrhea. Bethesda, Md., American Physiological Society, 1980. Sixteen chapters by different experts on various aspects of the pathophysiology of secretory diarrhea. The emphasis is on basic research, although there is a highly original chapter on the pharmacology of antidiarrheal drugs.

Fine KD, Krejs GJ, Fordtran JS: Diarrhea. In Sleisenger MH, Fordtran JS (eds.): Gastrointestinal Disease. 4th ed. Philadelphia, W. B. Saunders Company, 1989, pp 290–315. A detailed description of the physiology of the human intestinal tract with regard to water and electrolyte movement and the pathophysiology of chronic diarrhea.

Krejs GJ (ed.): Diarrhoea. Clin Gastroenterol 15, No 3, 1986. Thirteen chapters on the pathophysiology and clinical investigation of diarrhea. Contains re-evaluation of criteria for defining secretory diarrhea and extensive description of diarrhée motrice (diarrhea due to motility derangement).

Krejs GJ: VIPoma syndrome. Am J Med (in print). An extensive description of pancreatic cholera syndrome, the most prominent example of secretory diarrhea caused by a circulating agent.

Lambert HP (ed.): Infections of the GI tract. Clin Gastroenterol 8, No 3, 1979. Twelve excellent chapters by different experts dealing with the pathophysiology of diarrhea, viral infections, pathogenic mechanisms in bacterial diarrhea, E. coli, Shigella, food poisoning, typhoid and paratyphoid fever, Campylobacter enteritis, traveler's diarrhea, antibiotic-associated colitis, antibiotic resistance, and antimicrobial agents. The book contains much practical and clinically useful information.

Read NW, Krejs GJ, Read MG, et al.: Chronic diarrhea of unknown origin. Gastroenterology 78:264, 1980. A detailed account of the clinical problems encountered in patients with intractable and difficult-to-diagnose chronic diarrhea.

Santangelo WC, Krejs GJ: Gastrointestinal manifestations of the acquired immunodeficiency syndrome. Am J Med Sci 292:328, 1986. Complete review of enteric infections, parasitic infestations, enteropathy, gastrointestinal bleeding, and neoplasms in patients with AIDS.

102 Malabsorption
Phillip P. Toskes

The malabsorption syndrome refers to a clinical condition in which a number of nutrients and minerals are not normally absorbed; almost always, however, lipids fail to be normally absorbed. At times the absorption of a single nutrient may be selectively impaired. A sound knowledge of normal absorptive processes allows the physician to pursue a logical approach to the diagnosis and treatment of the patient with malabsorption.

NORMAL ABSORPTION OF NUTRIENTS

Absorption is the integration of those processes whereby the products of digestion pass from the lumen of the intestine through the small intestinal enterocyte to appear in the general circulation via the lymphatics or the portal vein. Although the digestive process is initiated by acid and pepsin within the stomach, the exocrine pancreas has the major role in digesting fat, carbohydrate, and protein by its secretion of lipase, amylase, and proteases. Fat is eventually broken down to monoglycerides and fatty acids; carbohydrate, to disaccharides and monosaccharides; and proteins, to peptides and amino acids. These forms of nutrients are absorbed through the intestinal enterocyte. The villi and microvilli of the small intestine provide an enormous area for absorption. The motility of the intestine and the contraction of the microvilli allow molecules to pass through an "unstirred layer" adjacent to the microvilli.

Nutrients pass through the enterocyte by several processes: active transport, passive diffusion, facilitated diffusion, and endocytosis. Active transport and passive diffusion are the main mechanisms whereby nutrients pass through membranes. *Active transport* moves nutrients against a chemical or electrical gradient, requires energy, is carrier mediated, and is subject to competitive inhibition. *Passive diffusion* does not require energy and allows nutrients to pass through a membrane according to chemical concentration and electrical gradients. Passive diffusion, best typified by water absorption, is not carrier mediated and does not demonstrate competitive inhibition. *Facilitated diffusion* is similar to passive diffusion but may be carrier mediated and may be subject to competitive inhibition. *Endocytosis* is a process whereby nutrients are engulfed by parts of the cell membrane. Although endocytosis may be most important in the neonatal period, this absorptive mechanism may also occur to some extent in the adult and may be involved in the absorption of antigens.

Absorption of nutrients may be regionalized (Table 102–1). Although many nutrients can be absorbed throughout the small intestine, each nutrient has a major site of absorption. When areas of the intestine are damaged or resected, the remaining intestine usually adapts effectively to absorb the nutrients that

*Investigational agent.

TABLE 102–1. REGIONALIZATION OF NUTRIENT ABSORPTION

Nutrient	Major Site of Absorption
Fat	Proximal small intestine
Protein	Mid small intestine
Carbohydrate	Proximal and mid small intestine
Iron	Proximal small intestine
Calcium	Proximal small intestine
Folic acid	Proximal and mid small intestine
Cobalamin (vitamin B_{12})	Distal small intestine (ileum)
Other water-soluble vitamins	Proximal and mid small intestine
Bile salts	Distal small intestine (ileum)
Water and electrolytes	Small intestine and colon (especially cecum)

would normally have been absorbed by those areas. Two noteworthy exceptions to this adaptation process are cobalamin (vitamin B_{12}) and bile salts. If the distal ileum has been resected, the subject can *never* actively absorb these two nutrients again. This has important clinical implications, especially for cobalamin. Patients who have had their distal ileum resected must receive monthly parenteral cobalamin or they will develop macrocytic anemia and neuropathy secondary to cobalamin deficiency (Ch. 132).

Fat Absorption

Dietary fat is ingested largely as long-chain triglycerides, the absorption of which is a complex process involving the pancreas, liver, small intestine, and lymphatics (Fig. 102–1). Nevertheless, the process is very efficient; the coefficient of fat absorption is greater than 93 per cent, i.e., less than 7 per cent of ingested fat escapes absorption and appears in the stool per day. A breakdown in any one of these steps (Fig. 102–1) leads to malabsorption of fat (steatorrhea). A thorough knowledge of this physiologic process allows a logical approach to be pursued in the evaluation of the patient with steatorrhea.

Some triglyceride digestion begins in the stomach by lingual and gastric lipases. Triglyceride is emulsified in the stomach, and fat is slowly emptied into the duodenum, where its entry, and that of acid, release cholecystokinin-pancreozymin and secretin. As a result, the pancreas secretes enzymes and bicarbonate, and the gallbladder contracts to release bile salts. Bicarbonate maintains the pH of the intestinal lumen above 4, allowing pancreatic lipase to be effective in hydrolysis of triglycerides to yield free fatty acids and monoglycerides. Another pancreatic protein, colipase, facilitates the interaction between lipase and triglyceride for effective lipolysis. Fatty acids and monoglyceride interact with conjugated bile salts to form molecular aggregates or micelles (Fig. 102–1). A critical concentration of bile salts for micelle formation (5 to 15 μmol per milliliter) is maintained by a very efficient enterohepatic circulation of bile salts. Although the total

bile salt pool is only 2 to 4 grams, 95 per cent of bile salts is actively absorbed in the ileum and returned to the liver by the portal venous system. Each day 20 to 30 grams of bile salts recirculate in this enterohepatic circulation. Only about 200 to 600 mg of bile salts is excreted in the feces per day and must be replaced by hepatic biosynthesis from cholesterol.

Micellar fat passes through the "unstirred" water layer covering the surface of the enterocyte. Because of their solubility in the lipid-rich surface membrane, the fatty acids and monoglycerides are released and diffuse into the enterocyte. Fatty acid–binding protein (low molecular weight cytosolic protein) avidly binds long-chain fatty acids in the enterocyte and transports them to the smooth endoplasmic reticulum, where they are re-esterified with monoglyceride to form triglyceride. Absorbed cholesterol is also largely esterified with fatty acids for optimal transport. The intestine must also synthesize phospholipids and specific proteins (apoproteins) in order to incorporate these nonpolar lipids into lipoproteins, the major transport vehicles for fat transport in lymph and plasma (Ch. 172). These polar components are added to the surface of the lipid droplet, producing lipoproteins called chylomicrons. Chylomicrons are concentrated in the Golgi apparatus and then discharged through the lateral basal portion of the cell to the interstitium and mesenteric lymph to be delivered via the thoracic duct to the vena cava.

Medium-chain triglycerides (C-6 to C-12 fatty acids) are absorbed quite differently and more effectively than are long-chain triglycerides (C-16 to C-18 fatty acids) described above. Medium-chain triglycerides (MCT) (1) are more completely hydrolyzed by pancreatic lipase, (2) do not require bile salts for absorption, (3) can be directly taken up into the enterocyte and hydrolyzed by a mucosal lipase to fatty acids, (4) do not need to be re-esterified, (5) are not incorporated into lipoproteins, and (6) can pass directly into the portal venous system, transported as fatty acids bound to albumin. These characteristics of MCT allow its therapeutic use to improve fat absorption in a number of diseases in which dietary triglyceride absorption is impaired.

Fat-soluble vitamins (A, D, E, K) are absorbed after micellar solubilization and are transported into lymph with chylomicrons. In the case of vitamin A, the free vitamin is esterified within the enterocyte with palmitic acid, transported via chylomicrons in the lymph and stored as retinol palmitate in the liver. Vitamin metabolism is described more fully in Ch. 204.

Carbohydrate Absorption

Carbohydrate is ingested in the form of starch, sucrose, and lactose. Salivary and pancreatic amylases hydrolyze starch to oligosaccharides and disaccharides. All carbohydrate must be digested to a final monosaccharide product before it can be absorbed. Disaccharides are split by membrane-bound disaccharidases located on the microvilli of the enterocyte. Lactose is digested by lactase to glucose and galactose; sucrose, by sucrase to glucose and fructose; and maltose by maltase to two molecules of glucose. These monosaccharides are then transported through the enterocyte to the portal blood. Glucose and galactose are

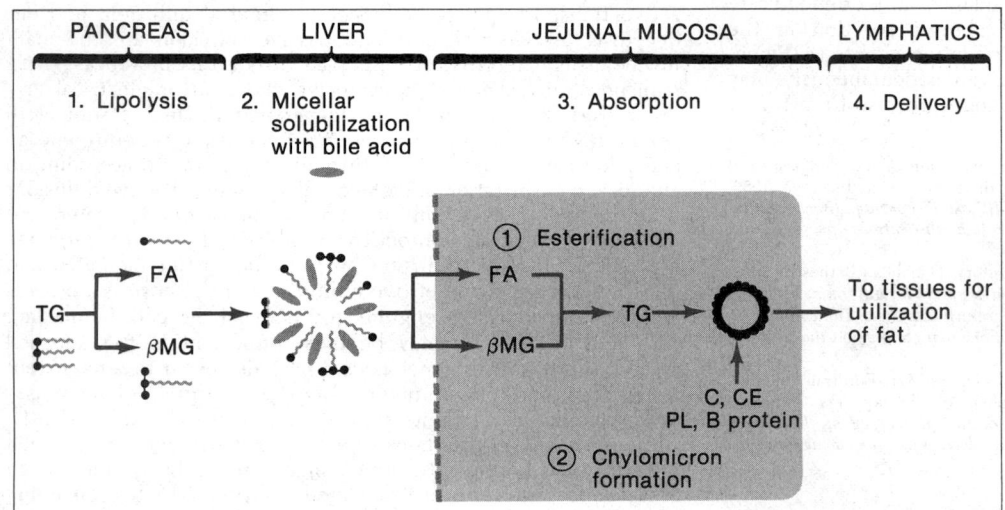

FIGURE 102–1. Schematic of intestinal absorption, showing the participation of the pancreas, liver, and intestinal mucosal cell in fat absorption. (From Wilson FA, Dietschy JM: Gastroenterology 61:911, 1971. Copyright 1971, The Williams & Wilkins Company, Baltimore.)

absorbed by active transport requiring sodium. Fructose is transported by facilitated diffusion. Glucose is transported into the enterocyte, probably bound along with sodium to a protein carrier. These monosaccharides are transported out of the cell by active sodium extrusion across the basolateral aspect of the enterocyte via a sodium pump.

Protein and Amino Acid Absorption

The digestion of dietary protein is initiated in the stomach by acid and pepsin but is largely completed by pancreatic proteases, both endopeptidases (trypsin, chymotrypsin, elastase) and exopeptidases (carboxypeptidase). Pancreatic proteases secreted in inactive forms (zymogens) must be activated. Enterokinase from the small intestinal mucosa activates trypsin from trypsinogen, and trypsin then activates all of the other protease precursors. The digestive products of pancreatic proteases are peptides containing two to six amino acids as well as single amino acids. Peptidases on the microvillus membrane or in the cytosol of the enterocyte further hydrolyze oligopeptides to free amino acids, which are directly absorbed in the portal vein.

The L forms of amino acids are actively transported in the enterocyte by specific energy-requiring, sodium-dependent processes. There are several specific transport systems for amino acids: (1) the dibasic amino acid system, which is often abnormal in cystinuria; (2) the neutral amino acid system, which is abnormal in Hartnup disease; (3) the iminoglycine system; and (4) the dicarboxylic acid system. Intact di- and tripeptides are also actively transported across the enterocyte membrane without hydrolysis by peptidases on the microvillus membrane. These peptides are hydrolyzed in the cytosol of the enterocyte to amino acids, which are then released into the circulation.

Water and Electrolyte Absorption

Over 7 liters of water (both ingested and reabsorbed from intestinal secretion) is absorbed by the small intestine per day through the process of passive diffusion. Absorption of water often follows that of glucose and electrolytes in order to maintain isotonicity of intraluminal contents

Sodium is actively transported linked to an exchange with H^+ in the jejunum and ileum and with Cl^- and HCO_3^- in the ileum. Na^+ transport is enhanced by glucose absorption in the jejunum (via the glucose-Na^+ carrier on the microvillus membrane) and by solvent (water) drag. Some Na^+ also moves down a gradient across the mucosa, i.e., by passive diffusion. Changes in the concentration of sodium in the lumen depend on relative rates of exchange of both sodium and water between blood and lumen. Potassium passively diffuses from the lumen of the proximal small intestine and into the lumen of the distal small intestine.

Calcium Absorption

Calcium is actively absorbed in the duodenum largely regulated by the active form of vitamin D_3–1,25-dihydroxycholecalciferol (calcitriol). Vitamin D_3 from the diet is metabolized first by the liver (25-hydroxylation) and then by the kidney (1-hydroxylation) to form 1,25-dihydroxycholecalciferol ($1,25[OH]_2D_3$) (Ch. 233). This process is influenced by parathyroid hormone levels, which are regulated by plasma levels of ionized calcium. Calcitriol stimulates the synthesis of calcium-binding protein, alkaline phosphatase, and a calcium-activated ATPase—all involved in active calcium transport. Absorption of vitamin D, a fat-soluble vitamin, is often impaired in the malabsorptive syndromes such that calcium absorption is diminished. Fatty acids within the lumen of the intestine may also directly impair absorption by binding calcium. In turn, the unavailability of ionized calcium in the lumen leads to excessive absorption of oxalate and a resulting propensity to form calcium oxalate kidney stones.

Iron Absorption (Ch. 131)

The average intake of iron from dietary sources is 15 to 25 mg per day, of which 0.5 to 2.0 mg is normally absorbed. Iron is absorbed as inorganic iron (cereals, vegetables) or as heme iron (meat). For optimal absorption, inorganic iron must be released from dietary components to soluble iron complexes in the intestinal lumen. Gastric acid enhances the absorption of inorganic iron (both Fe^{3+} and Fe^{2+}) by facilitating its chelation with sugars, amino acids, bile, and ascorbic acid. Such iron complexes remain in solution at the alkaline pH of the duodenum—the major site of iron absorption. Inorganic iron is absorbed from the intestinal lumen by the mucosa and then transported to the blood by mechanisms that are still not clear. A mucosal regulatory system keeps much of the iron trapped within the enterocyte, to be excreted into the feces depending on the need for iron, as determined by body stores of iron or by the rate of erythropoiesis. Organic iron (heme iron) is absorbed more efficiently than is inorganic iron. Heme is split from globin and absorbed as an intact metalloporphyrin at an alkaline pH. Iron is released from heme by heme oxygenase intracellularly. In plasma, iron is transported bound to transferrin, a specific globulin, to various tissues for use or storage.

Iron absorption is increased in iron deficiency, pregnancy, idiopathic hemochromatosis, and any conditions in which there is active erythropoiesis. Absorption is decreased in chronic infection and after the ingestion of large amounts of iron. Diffuse disease of the duodenum such as nontropical sprue may impair iron absorption and lead to iron deficiency.

Folic Acid Absorption

Dietary folic acid is conjugated with glutamyl peptides; prior to its absorption, these polyglutamates must be deconjugated to monoglutamates by folic deconjugase, an enzyme found on the microvillus membrane. Folate monoglutamates are absorbed by active transport at low concentrations of folate and by passive diffusion at high concentrations of folate. Folic acid undergoes an enterohepatic circulation. Since its body stores are limited, the major cause of folate deficiency is poor dietary intake of fresh fruits and vegetables. Folic acid deficiency may also occur if there is extensive damage to the proximal small intestine (e.g., nontropical sprue) or secondary to the use of a number of medications (sulfasalazine, phenytoin, trimethoprim) that inhibit its absorption. Other causes of folate deficiency are listed in Table 132–1.

Cobalamin (Vitamin B₁₂) Absorption (Ch. 132)

The current concept of cobalamin absorption and transport is depicted in Figure 102–2. Cobalamin, found in animal protein, is released from protein in the stomach by the synergistic action of both acid and pepsin. Cobalamin initially binds to a cobalamin-binding protein (R binder or cobalophilin), also secreted by the stomach. The cobalophilin-cobalamin complex is degraded by pancreatic proteases within the duodenal lumen, with release of cobalamin to bind with gastric intrinsic factor (a glycoprotein secreted by the parietal cells). After intrinsic factor binds cobalamin, the intrinsic factor–cobalamin complex passes down the small intestine until it reaches the distal 60 cm of the ileum, where it binds to a specific receptor of the brush border. In the absence of the terminal ileum, intrinsic factor–mediated cobalamin absorption ceases, although large doses of cobalamin (milligram in contrast to microgram amounts) may lead to adequate absorption by passive diffusion throughout the gastrointestinal tract.

Intrinsic factor does not enter the ileal cell and is not absorbed. Transcobalamin II (TCII), the most important transport protein for cobalamin, picks up cobalamin in the ileal mucosa and promotes its uptake by tissues throughout the body. The TCII-cobalamin complex enters tissues via endocytosis, with cobalamin being released by lysosomal proteolysis.

At equilibrium, the majority of circulating cobalamin is attached to cobalophilin, which is also found in saliva, gastric secretions, intestinal secretions, semen, and tears. It also moves continuously in an enterohepatic circulation. The function of the ubiquitous cobalophilins is unclear, but they may prevent or retard the absorption and dissemination of a variety of cobalamin analogues, either produced by bacteria or even found within multivitamin supplements.

CLASSIFICATION AND CLINICAL MANIFESTATIONS OF MALABSORPTION

Causes of Malabsorption

Table 102–2 divides the causes of the malabsorption syndrome into nine categories, based upon its pathophysiology (see Fig. 102–1). Some conditions have multiple reasons for malabsorption

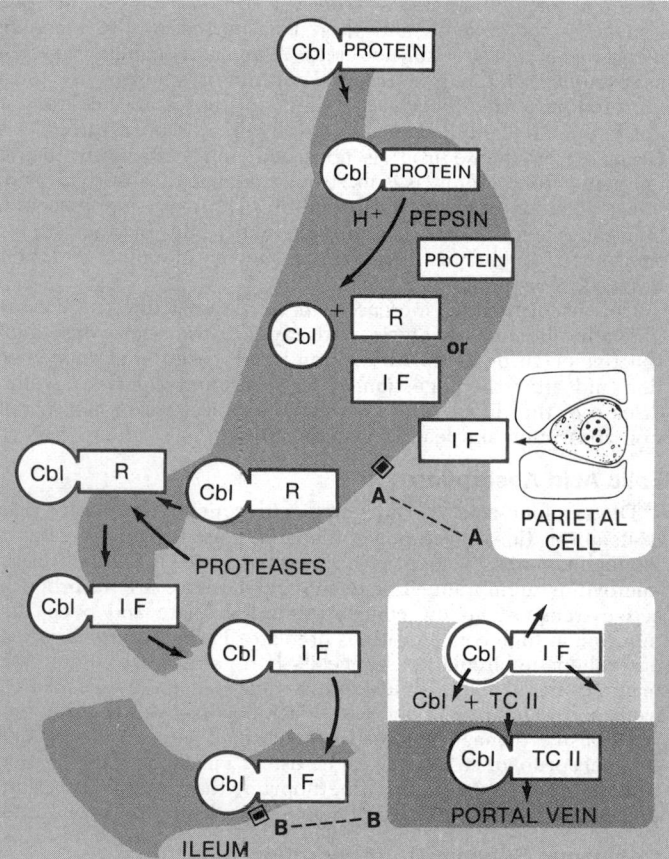

FIGURE 102–2. Cobalamin absorption and transport. Cbl = Cobalamin, R = R-protein or cobalophilin, IF = intrinsic factor, TC II = transcobalamin II. (From Toskes PP: J Clin Gastroenterol 2:287, 1980.)

but are arbitrarily classified under one major category. The differential features and management of important types of this syndrome are detailed later in the chapter.

Clinical Manifestations

Patients with the malabsorption syndrome usually present with diarrhea, weight loss, and malnutrition. These patients often complain that their stools are bulky, greasy, and excessively malodorous and that they float and are difficult to flush down the toilet. Steatorrheal stools float not because of their fat content but because of their high gas content. Patients with severe malabsorption, as exemplified by that secondary to pancreatic insufficiency, may complain of oil seeping out of the rectum. The symptoms and signs of malabsorption are varied and involve a number of organ systems. Patients may demonstrate one or more of these manifestations depending on the severity of their malabsorption. The different symptoms and signs that such patients may show and the causes of these symptoms and signs are detailed in Table 102–3. These aspects of the history and physical examination are crucial in evaluating a patient with malabsorption.

DIAGNOSIS OF MALABSORPTION

Although there may be selective malabsorption of nutrients, most patients with clinically relevant malabsorption have steatorrhea. Consequently, documentation of steatorrhea is important and is the cornerstone of the diagnostic evaluation of patients with malabsorption. The only truly reliable means to document the presence of steatorrhea is the quantitative chemical analysis of fat in a 72-hour stool collection while the patient is ingesting a high-fat diet (at least 100 grams per day). On such a diet normal subjects excrete less than 7 grams of fat per day (coefficient of absorption of >93 per cent). Unfortunately, the quantitative fecal fat determination is cumbersome to perform and difficult to

obtain in most hospitals. Furthermore, the documentation of steatorrhea only indicates that the patient has the malabsorption syndrome—it does not indicate the pathophysiology or confer a specific diagnosis.

Table 102–4 details some alternative tests (other than the quantitative fecal fat determination) that can be employed to detect the presence and the cause of malabsorption in a given patient. The tests are categorized into screening tests and those that are more specific in localizing the site of the malabsorption. It is usually necessary to utilize a number of malabsorptive tests to establish the cause of the malabsorption.

Qualitative Stool Fat

The microscopic examination of stool for the presence of fat is a helpful test if performed properly and if the patient is ingesting a high-fat diet. Two specimens of stool are placed on two slides. To the first slide, two drops of water and two drops of 95 per cent ethyl alcohol are added, followed by two drops of a fat stain (e.g., Sudan III). The specimen is microscopically examined for orange neutral fat (triglyceride) globules. The globules should be larger than a red cell and should be numerous per high-power field. To the second slide, several drops of 36 per cent acetic

TABLE 102–2. CLASSIFICATION OF THE MALABSORPTION SYNDROME

1. Impaired digestion
   a. Primary pancreatic exocrine insufficiency
   b. Gastric surgery (Billroth I and II, vagotomy, and pyloroplasty)*
   c. Gastrinoma*
2. Reduced bile salt concentration
   a. Liver disease
   b. Small intestine bacterial overgrowth (scleroderma, diabetes mellitus, primary motility disturbances, postgastrectomy, achlorhydria)*
   c. Ileal disease or resection*
3. Abnormalities of intestinal mucosa
   a. Disaccharidase deficiency
   b. Impaired monosaccharide transport
   c. Folate or cobalamin deficiency
   d. Nontropical sprue
   e. Nongranulomatous ileojejunitis
   f. Amyloidosis
   g. Crohn's disease*
   h. Eosinophilic enteritis
   i. Radiation enteritis*
   j. Abetalipoproteinemia
   k. Cystinuria
   l. Hartnup disease
4. Inadequate absorptive surface
   a. Short bowel syndrome
   b. Jejunoileal bypass*
5. Infection
   a. Tropical sprue
   b. Whipple's disease*
   c. Acute infectious enteritis
   d. Parasitic infections
6. Lymphatic obstruction
   a. Lymphoma*
   b. Tuberculosis
   c. Lymphangiectasia
7. Cardiovascular disorders
   a. Congestive heart failure
   b. Constrictive pericarditis
   c. Mesenteric vascular insufficiency
8. Drug-induced
   a. Cholestyramine
   b. Neomycin
   c. Colchicine
   d. Phenindione
   e. Irritant laxatives
9. Unexplained
   a. Carcinoid syndrome
   b. Diabetes mellitus*
   c. Adrenal insufficiency
   d. Hyper- and hypothyroidism
   e. Mastocytosis
   f. Hypogammaglobulinemia

* Multiple reasons for malabsorption.

TABLE 102–3. SYMPTOMS AND SIGNS OF MALABSORPTION

History	Pathophysiology	Physical Examination	Pathophysiology
Diarrhea	Increased secretion and impaired absorption of water and electrolytes, unabsorbed dihydroxy bile acids, unabsorbed fatty acids	Pallor	Anemia secondary to iron, folate, or cobalamin deficiency
Greasy, bulky, malodorous stools that are difficult to flush	Increased fat in stool	Glossitis, stomatitis, cheilosis	Iron, folate, cobalamin, and other vitamin deficiencies
Oil seeping from rectum	Unabsorbed triglyceride (pancreatic insufficiency)	Ecchymosis, purpura	Vitamin K malabsorption
Weight loss despite good appetite	Loss of calories from malabsorption	Acrodermatitis	Zinc and fatty acid deficiency
		Dehydration, hypotension	Water and electrolyte malabsorption
Excessive flatus	Fermentation of unabsorbed carbohydrates by colonic bacteria	Edema	Protein malabsorption (decreased serum albumin)
Diffuse abdominal pain	Inflammation or infiltration of tissue (pancreatic insufficiency, Crohn's disease, lymphoma)	Peripheral neuropathy	Cobalamin deficiency
Postprandial (30 minutes after eating) midabdominal pain	Intestinal ischemia		
Abnormal bruisability	Vitamin K malabsorption		
Weakness and fatigue	Protein, electrolyte, fat, iron, folate, cobalamin malabsorption		
Milk intolerance	Lactase deficiency		
Bone pain	Calcium and protein malabsorption		
Tetany, paresthesias	Calcium and magnesium malabsorption, cobalamin deficiency (paresthesias only)		
Night blindness	Vitamin A malabsorption		
Nocturia	Delayed absorption of water, hypokalemia		
Amenorrhea	Protein malabsorption		

TABLE 102–4. TESTS FOR MALABSORPTION

Test	Normal Values	Comments Relevant to Patients with Malabsorption
Screening Tests		
1. Serum carotene	>0.06 mg/dl	Decreased; very good test if poor oral intake has been excluded
2. Serum calcium	9.0 to 10.5 mg/dl	Decreased, not very sensitive
3. Serum cholesterol	150 to 250 mg/dl	Decreased, not very sensitive
4. Serum albumin	4.0 to 5.2 mg/dl	Decreased, not very sensitive
5. Serum magnesium	1.7 to 2.0 mEq/L	Decreased, not very sensitive
6. Prothrombin time	Control value	Increased, not very sensitive
7. Qualitative stool fat	No fat globules per hpf*	Numerous fat globules per hpf; part 1 for neutral fats, part 2 for split fats (see text)
Specific Tests		
1. Serum iron	80–150 μg/dl	Malabsorbed in proximal small bowel disease
2. Serum folate	5–21 ng/ml	Decreased in proximal small bowel disease, may be increased in bacterial overgrowth
3. Serum cobalamin (vitamin B_{12})	200–900 pg/ml	Malabsorbed in distal small bowel disease, pernicious anemia, bacterial overgrowth, chronic pancreatitis
4. Urinary D-xylose	>5 grams/5 hr	Decreased in small bowel disease and bacterial overgrowth, normal in pancreatic disease
5. Bentiromide test	Arylamine excretion >57% in 6 hr	A value of <50 per cent is diagnostic of pancreatic insufficiency
6. Serum trypsin–like immunoreactivity (TLI)	29–80 ng/ml	A value of <20 ng/ml is specific for pancreatic insufficiency
7. Secretin test	HCO_3^- conc >80 mEq/L Vol >1.8 ml/kg/hr	Most sensitive test of pancreatic function
8. [57]Cyanocobalamin urinary excretion test	>8%/24 hr	Decreased in pernicious anemia, chronic pancreatitis, bacterial overgrowth, ileal disease
9. Urine 5-HIAA*	1.7–8.0 mg/24 hr	Markedly elevated in carcinoid syndrome, minimally elevated in any kind of malabsorption
10. Breath tests		
a. ^{14}C-xylose	<0.0013% of administered dose as breath $^{14}CO_2$ at 30 min	Elevated in bacterial overgrowth
b. cholyl-1-^{14}C-glycine	<1% of administered dose as breath $^{14}CO_2$ at any interval over 4 hr	Elevated in bacterial overgrowth or bile acid malabsorption
c. Lactulose H_2	<10 ppm rise in breath H_2 over baseline at any interval for 120 min	Elevated in bacterial overgrowth; increase in fasting breath H_2 suggests bacterial overgrowth; up to 27% of subjects may not have flora that produces H_2
d. Lactose-H_2	<20 ppm rise in breath H_2 over baseline at any interval for 180 min	Elevated in lactase deficiency
11. Small intestinal culture	≤10^5 organisms per ml jejunal secretions	>10^5 organisms per ml jejunal secretions indicates bacterial overgrowth
12. Small intestinal biopsy	See Figure 102–4	See Table 102–7

*hpf = High-power field; 5-HIAA = 5-hydroxyindoleacetic acid.

acid are added, then several drops of Sudan III. The slide is heated until it begins to boil. Microscopically, the presence of large orange globules or spicules represents free fatty acids. Part 1 is positive in patients with pancreatic insufficiency, detecting undigested triglyceride; part 2, in patients with small bowel disease, detecting free fatty acids. Figure 102–3 demonstrates a positive part 1 test in a patient with pancreatic insufficiency. There is a 25 per cent false-negative rate when steatorrhea is mild, i.e., <10 grams per 24 hours. The false-positive rate is about 15 per cent. This test is simple to perform and inexpensive.

Urinary D-Xylose Test

The urinary xylose excretion test distinguishes between malabsorption due to small intestinal disease and that due to pancreatic exocrine insufficiency. A 5-hour urinary excretion of 5 grams or greater is normal following the oral administration of 25 grams of D-xylose to a well-hydrated subject. Decreased xylose absorption and excretion are found in patients with damage to the proximal small intestine and in bacterial overgrowth in the small intestine (the bacteria catabolize the xylose). Patients with pancreatic steatorrhea usually have normal xylose absorption. As with any urinary excretion test, decreased renal function or incomplete collection of the urine may invalidate the test. Impaired renal function is most important when evaluating an elderly patient who may not have obvious renal disease, but whose creatinine clearance may be low. Decreased urinary xylose values may also be seen in patients with ascites. Although a blood level of 30 mg per deciliter or greater 1 hour after ingestion of xylose may indicate normal absorption, there appears to be a great deal of overlap between control subjects and those with malabsorption.

Bentiromide Urinary Excretion Test

Bentiromide is a synthetic peptide attached to para-aminobenzoic acid (PABA). The bond between the peptide and PABA is easily split by chymotrypsin. Following the oral administration of 500 mg of bentiromide, PABA is absorbed in the proximal small intestine, partially conjugated in the liver, and excreted in the urine as arylamines. A cumulative 6-hour arylamine excretion of less than 50 per cent of that ingested as bentiromide is virtually diagnostic of pancreatic insufficiency. In a patient with symptomatic diarrhea or steatorrhea or both, a normal bentiromide test result virtually excludes pancreatic disease as the cause of the symptoms. The use of bentiromide offers a simple, reliable confirmatory test (high specificity, few false-positive results) for the diagnosis of pancreatic insufficiency. The test is not accurate when the serum creatinine level exceeds 2.0 mg per deciliter.

Serum Trypsin-like Immunoreactivity (TLI)

TLI, a radioimmunoassay, measures serum levels of this pancreas-derived protein. Although not as sensitive as the bentiro-mide or secretin test, a decreased value appears to be completely specific for pancreatic insufficiency.

Secretin Test

The most sensitive tests of impaired pancreatic function are direct measurements of its exocrine function; unfortunately, these are the most complex to perform. The patient swallows a tube that is fluoroscopically placed, with the aspiration site within the second part of the duodenum near where the pancreatic duct enters the duodenum. A hormone is given intravenously, and a component of pancreatic secretion (bicarbonate after secretin; trypsin, amylase, or lipase after cholecystokinin) is measured. False-positive tests are virtually nonexistent if the tube has been properly positioned, and false-negative tests are not relevant because the secretin test will invariably be abnormal if the steatorrhea is secondary to pancreatic insufficiency.

Tests for Cobalamin (Vitamin B$_{12}$) Absorption (Ch. 132)

In the Schilling test, 1.0 μg of ^{57}Co-cyanocobalamin is administered orally, followed by 1000 μg of nonlabeled cobalamin given intramuscularly to help "wash out" that fraction of the isotope that has been absorbed. If the subsequent 24-hour urinary excretion of the radioactivity is less than 8 per cent of that administered, cobalamin malabsorption is present. There are four common clinical causes of cobalamin malabsorption, which can be sorted out by a differential Schilling test (Table 102–5). If an abnormal test result improves with the concomitant administration of hog intrinsic factor or pancreatic extract (six to eight conventional tablets or three enteric-coated microsphere capsules), the cobalamin malabsorption is secondary to pernicious anemia or exocrine pancreatic insufficiency, respectively. If cobalamin malabsorption still persists, the tests should be repeated after 4 days of antimicrobial therapy (metronidazole, 250 mg three times daily). If the malabsorption of labeled cobalamin is corrected by this therapy, bacterial overgrowth was the etiology. Metronidazole is the antimicrobial agent of choice because anaerobes such as *Bacteroides* are usually responsible for the cobalamin malabsorption. If the malabsorption still persists, damage to the ileal receptor (Crohn's disease, ileal resection, lymphoma, Imerslund's syndrome) is probably present and the patient must always receive a monthly injection of cobalamin (100 μg). In the face of renal impairment, 4 ml of plasma may be obtained 8 hours after the administration of labeled cobalamin. A value greater than 0.6 per cent of the orally administered dose is considered normal.

There are two caveats concerning the Schilling test: (1) Severe cobalamin deficiency itself may damage the ileum such that the ileal receptors may not bind the intrinsic factor–cobalamin complex. This may confuse interpretation of the Schilling test. Thus, it is advisable to wait until 1 week of cobalamin therapy (100 μg per day intramuscularly) has been completed before performing the differential Schilling test. (2) Two other clinical conditions

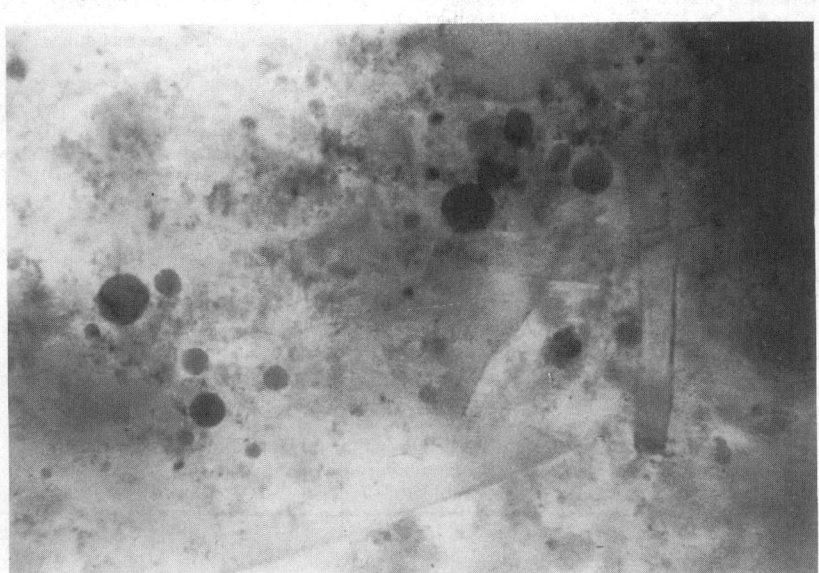

FIGURE 102–3. Positive fecal fat stain. Note the many globules of undigested triglycerides.

TABLE 102–5. THE DIFFERENTIAL SCHILLING (^{57}CO-CYANOCOBALAMIN) TEST

	Stage 1: Free Cobalamin	Stage 2: Free Cobalamin and Intrinsic Factor	Stage 3: Free Cobalamin and Pancreatic Extract	Stage 4: Free Cobalamin and Antibiotics	Comment
Pernicious anemia	Abnormal	Normal	Abnormal	Abnormal	In face of severe cobalamin deficiency, test should be performed only after a week of cobalamin therapy
Chronic pancreatitis	Abnormal	Abnormal	Normal	Abnormal	Although cobalamin malabsorption is common, cobalamin deficiency is rare
Bacterial overgrowth	Abnormal	Abnormal	Abnormal	Normal	Anaerobicidal antibiotic is needed
Ileal disease	Abnormal	Abnormal	Abnormal	Abnormal	Once receptor is permanently damaged, cobalamin malabsorption is permanent
Complete vegetarian* (vegan)	Normal	Normal	Normal	Normal	Cobalamin deficiency secondary to poor intake, absorption normal
Hypo- or achlorhydria*	Normal	Normal	Normal	Normal	Absorption of cyanocobalamin (free B_{12}) does not depend on acid; food B_{12} (protein-bound) does; must employ protein-bound cobalamin absorption test

*Cobalamin deficiency with normal Schilling test.

are associated with cobalamin deficiency—cobalamin deficiency secondary to lack of intake (as in complete vegetarians) and the failure to absorb food-bound cobalamin because of decreased acid secretion—that are not associated with an abnormal Schilling test (Table 102–5). The patient's history is the key to the former, and a test of protein-bound cobalamin absorption detects the latter.

Breath Tests

Two breath tests are reliable enough to receive routine clinical use—the lactose-H_2 breath test for detecting lactase deficiency and the ^{14}C-xylose breath test for the diagnosis of small intestine bacterial overgrowth.

The *lactose-H_2 breath test* has replaced the lactose intolerance test because of superior sensitivity and specificity. Lactose (1 gram per kilogram) is administered orally, and an increase in breath H_2 of more than 20 ppm over basal breath H_2 indicates lactose malabsorption. This test depends upon the release of H_2 from unabsorbed lactose by bacterial metabolism.

The *^{14}C-xylose breath test* is a sensitive and specific test for bacterial overgrowth. Following the oral administration of xylose (1 gram, 5 to 10 μCi), breath $^{14}CO_2$ concentration is monitored at 30 and 60 minutes, with an increase of $^{14}CO_2$ at 30 minutes being the most reliable assessment. Neither false-negative nor false-positive results appear to be a clinically significant problem. Xylose is catabolized by gram-negative aerobes, which are always part of the overgrowth flora, whereas other breath tests often utilize substrates that are catabolized by gram-negative anaerobes, which may or may not be present in the overgrowth of bacteria. The small dose of xylose (1 gram) is either catabolized by the overgrowth flora or absorbed in the proximal bowel, leaving very little xylose to "dump" into the colon, causing a possible false-positive result. An abnormal xylose breath test indicates, similar to a culture, the presence of increased numbers of bacteria within the lumen of the proximal small intestine. Whether or not the abnormal test indicates that therapy is necessary is a decision the clinician must make. Table 102–6 lists two other breath tests used to diagnose bacterial overgrowth, both of which suffer from inadequate sensitivity and specificity.

A ^{14}C-triolein breath test has received some use as a test of fat absorption, but it does not appear to separate control subjects from those with malabsorption very reliably, especially if the steatorrhea is not severe.

Culture of the Small Intestine

The proximal small intestine of normal subjects has fewer than 10^5 organisms per milliliter of jejunal fluid—usually fewer than 10^3, largely streptococci and staphylococci, and only an occasional coliform or *Bacteroides*. The ileocecal area is a transition zone with both a qualitative and a quantitative change toward the pattern that is found in the colon. In the colon, there is a marked increase in both aerobes (>10^7 organisms per milligram of stool) and anaerobes (>10^{10} organisms per milligram of stool). The qualitative change is also remarkable, with a preponderance of anaerobes (*Bacteroides*, *Clostridium*, enterococci) and coliforms (*Escherichia coli*, *Klebsiella*). In small intestine bacterial overgrowth, the small intestine becomes populated with a colon-like flora. Cultures should be considered suspicious if more than 10^3 organisms per milliliter are present (especially when anaerobes are identified) and clearly abnormal when more than 10^5 organisms per milliliter are present.

Biopsy of the Small Intestine

Biopsy of the small intestine is an important test in the evaluation of malabsorption presumed to be secondary to disease of the small intestine itself. Most instruments (Rubin's tube, Crosby's capsule, Carey's capsule) utilize a blind suction biopsy technique, but biopsies can be obtained endoscopically as well. Figure 102–4 illustrates the findings of a normal biopsy. Note the long, frondlike villi. The lining columnar epithelium is regular with basal orientation of the nuclei. There is not much cellular infiltration of lamina propria. The villus/crypt ratio favors the villus, with villus height normally being three to four times the height of the crypts.

For contrast, note Figure 102–5, which represents a biopsy from a patient with nontropical sprue (adult celiac disease). There is total villus atrophy, elongated crypts, and a dense infiltration

TABLE 102–6. BREATH TESTS FOR BACTERIAL OVERGROWTH

Procedure	Simplicity	Sensitivity	Specificity	Safety
^{14}C-xylose	Excellent	Excellent	Excellent	Good
Cholyl-1-^{14}C-glycine	Excellent	Fair	Poor	Good
Lactulose-H_2	Excellent	Fair–good	Fair	Excellent

Modified from King CE, Toskes PP: The use of breath tests in the study of malabsorption. Clin Gastroenterol 12:591, 1983.

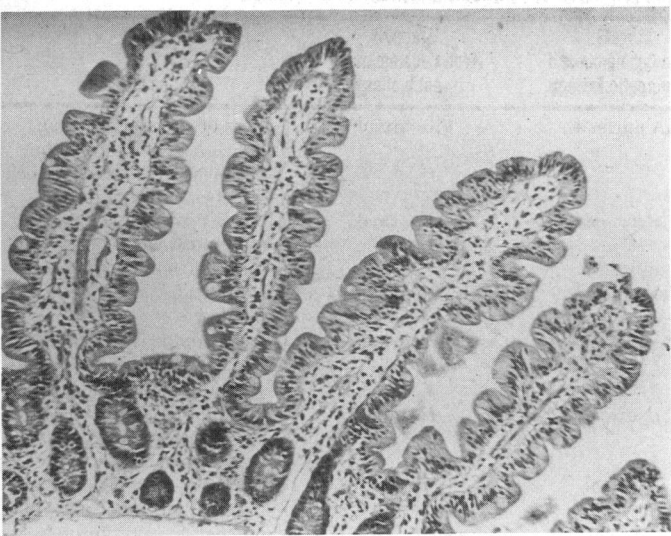

FIGURE 102–4. Appearance of normal small intestine on biopsy.

of chronic inflammatory cells in the lamina propria, and at higher magnification the surface epithelial cells are cuboidal, not columnar. Total villus atrophy, as shown in Figure 102–5, is almost always nontropical sprue (adult celiac disease), but it is not a specific lesion, since it may occasionally be observed in other diseases such as lymphoma, Whipple's disease, tropical sprue, ileojejunitis, or bacterial overgrowth. Table 102–7 lists disorders associated with abnormalities in the biopsy of the small intestine and points out that there are very few disorders in which multiple biopsies are consistently abnormal and diagnostic, i.e., a diagnostic diffuse lesion.

Gastrointestinal Radiology

With the possible exception of pancreatic calcification on plain film of the abdomen, radiographs of the intestinal tract do not play a primary role in the diagnostic evaluation of malabsorption. Function tests as described previously are more sensitive and more specific and afford the patient little, if any, radiation exposure. The radiation exposure received from a small bowel series may be considerable. The traditional signs of malabsorption on small bowel radiographs—segmentation or clumping of the barium (moulage sign)—were noted when thick barium was used in contrast to the thin barium commonly employed now. Small bowel radiographs are most frequently used now to determine why bacterial overgrowth has occurred (e.g., the presence of

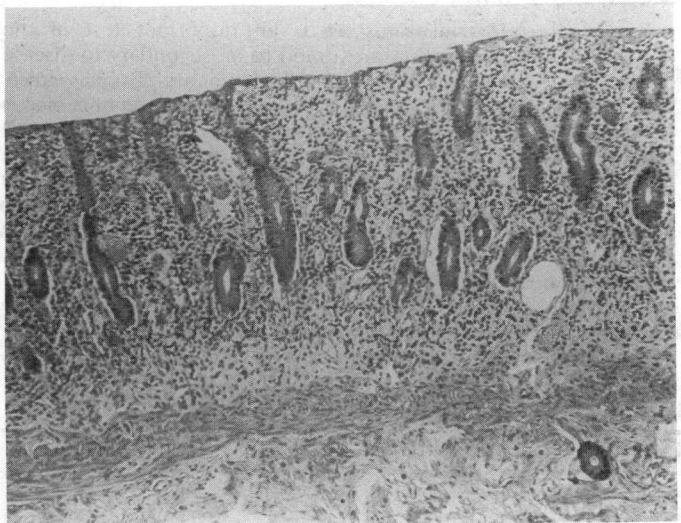

FIGURE 102–5. Small intestinal biopsy from a patient with nontropical sprue showing total villus atrophy.

TABLE 102–7. VALUE OF SMALL INTESTINAL BIOPSY

I. **Conditions in which the biopsy is consistently abnormal and diagnostic:**
   Abetalipoproteinemia
   Immunodeficiency syndrome
   Whipple's disease

II. **Conditions in which the biopsy is diagnostic but the lesion is often patchy:**
   Amyloidosis
   Capillariasis
   Coccidiosis
   Crohn's disease
   Cryptosporidiosis
   Eosinophilic enteritis
   Giardiasis
   Lymphangiectasia
   Lymphoma
   Mastocytosis
   Strongyloidiasis

III. **Conditions in which the biopsy is often abnormal but not diagnostic:**
   Bacterial overgrowth
   Cobalamin (vitamin B_{12}) deficiency
   Celiac sprue (nontropical)
   Drug enteritis
   Folate deficiency
   Infectious gastroenteritis
   Protein-calorie malnutrition
   Radiation enteritis
   Tropical sprue
   Unclassified sprue
   Zollinger-Ellison syndrome

IV. **Conditions in which the biopsy is invariably normal:**
   Functional bowel disease
   Liver disease
   Pancreatic disease
   Primary disaccharidase deficiency
   Ulcerative colitis

diverticula or dilation of the small intestine in scleroderma) or to confirm a clinical diagnosis of Crohn's disease.

Algorithm for Evaluation of Malabsorption

An algorithm for evaluating patients with malabsorption is presented in Table 102–8. The algorithm complements a thorough history and physical examination. A serum carotene determination and a microscopic fat stain of the stool are the best screening tests and together detect the presence of steatorrhea about 85 per cent of the time, especially if the patient is excreting more than 15 grams of fat per day. Once steatorrhea has been confirmed, the clinician should ask whether the steatorrhea is secondary to pancreatic disease or to small bowel disease. The urinary xylose test helps differentiate between these two categories. If xylose absorption is normal, tests of pancreatic function should be pursued. If diffuse calcification of the pancreas is present on a plain film of the abdomen, there is likely to be approximately 80 per cent damage to the exocrine pancreas. The bentiromide test has about the same sensitivity as plain film calcification and is abnormal 80 to 90 per cent of the time if the steatorrhea has a pancreatic cause. A serum trypsin level complements the bentiromide test, adding specificity to the evaluation. If these simple tubeless tests of pancreatic function are not diagnostic, a direct tube test like the secretin test should be performed.

If the xylose test is abnormal, small bowel tests should be performed. A breath test (^{14}C-xylose, lactulose H_2) detects bacterial overgrowth. If normal, a small bowel radiograph, culture, and biopsy should be done, with the radiograph suggesting the site to be biopsied. If steatorrhea is not present, tests designed to detect selective malabsorption of single nutrients can be pursued (lactose H_2 breath test, the Schilling test, and so on).

The algorithm is logical and cost effective, emphasizing inexpensive, noninvasive, outpatient evaluation. A specific diagnosis can often be made for less than $300 with minimal or no discomfort to the patient. If more complicated tests are needed, such as the secretin test or small bowel biopsy, the expense and discomfort to the patient increase. The algorithm also emphasizes initial testing for the more common causes of malabsorption (pancreatic insufficiency, bacterial overgrowth) and delayed testing for less common disorders (nontropical sprue, Whipple's disease, and so on).

DIFFERENTIAL FEATURES AND TREATMENT OF INDIVIDUAL FORMS OF THE MALABSORPTION SYNDROME

Numerous disorders can be associated with malabsorption (see Table 102–2). Although there may be specific therapy for individual disorders (gluten-free diet for nontropical sprue, pancreatic enzymes for pancreatic insufficiency), there are many nonspecific therapies for malabsorption (Table 102–9).

Impaired Digestion

PANCREATIC EXOCRINE INSUFFICIENCY (Ch. 106). Pancreatic exocrine insufficiency is a relatively common cause of severe malabsorption. It is not rare to note steatorrhea in excess of 50 grams of fat per day.

Steatorrhea in pancreatic disease is relatively well treated with administration of pancreatic extract. Large doses of pancreatic extract are required: six to eight conventional tablets (Viokase, Cotazym) or three enteric-coated, microsphere preparations (Creon, Pancrease MT, Entolase, Zymase) with each meal. Adjuvant therapy (sodium bicarbonate, H_2-receptor antagonists) along with conventional tablet therapy may lead to the best results by raising duodenal pH. The adjuvant of choice is sodium bicarbonate (650-mg tablet before and after each meal) because of its effectiveness, low cost, and lack of side effects at this dose. Antacids containing calcium or magnesium are not to be used as adjuvant therapy because they may increase steatorrhea. Adjuvant therapy is not recommended with enteric-coated preparations, for it may cause the enteric coat to open up within the stomach and the released enzymes may then be destroyed by gastric acid before they can enter the duodenum.

POSTGASTRECTOMY STATES (Ch. 98.4). The pathogenesis of the malabsorption noted in patients with gastric surgery (Billroth I, Billroth II, vagotomy and antrectomy, vagotomy and pyloroplasty) is multifactorial: (1) loss of reservoir function with rapid emptying and dispersion of food through the small intestine, thereby diluting the normal output of pancreatic enzymes; (2) postcibal asynchrony, i.e., in a patient who has undergone a Billroth II procedure, food may get to the jejunum before bile salts and pancreatic enzymes do; and (3) occurrence of stasis, leading to bacterial overgrowth of the small intestine. Postgastrectomy steatorrhea is usually mild (<10 grams of fat per day) but occasionally may be marked. Severe steatorrhea in this setting is usually the result of bacterial overgrowth or rarely is secondary to pancreatic insufficiency. Because the duodenum (the major site for calcium and iron absorption) is bypassed when a Billroth II procedure is performed, clinically significant problems related to calcium and iron malabsorption may result.

GASTRINOMA (Ch. 98.6). Multiple mechanisms contribute to the malabsorption observed in patients with a gastrinoma (Zollinger-Ellison syndrome). The extreme hypersecretion of acid irreversibly inactivates lipase, causing a secondary pancreatic insufficiency. In addition, this acid environment precipitates bile salts and may cause abnormal small bowel histologic findings. All of these abnormalities have been shown to revert to normal after effective therapy with large doses of H_2-receptor antagonists (cimetidine or ranitidine).

Reduced Concentration of Bile Salts

LIVER DISEASE. Steatorrhea (usually mild) may occur in acute or chronic liver disease, presumably owing to impaired synthesis and excretion of conjugated bile salts. Patients with liver disease who manifest clinically significant steatorrhea should have their pancreatic function evaluated, since these patients often have pancreatic exocrine insufficiency responsive to pancreatic extract therapy. Metabolic bone disease (bone pain, spontaneous pathologic fractures) resulting from malabsorption of calcium and vitamin D may occur, particularly in those with biliary cirrhosis (Ch. 234).

BACTERIAL OVERGROWTH. Overgrowth of bacteria within the small intestine accompanied by nutrient malabsorption is called the stasis, stagnant loop, or blind loop syndrome. The normal subject usually has sparse bacterial growth in the proximal small intestine (see section on Diagnosis—Culture of the Small Intestine). In the stasis syndrome, the proximal small intestinal flora resembles that of the colon and the overgrowth flora competes with the human host for ingested nutrients. The resultant malabsorption is due to a disturbed intraluminal environment (catabolism of carbohydrate by gram-negative aerobes, deconjugation of bile salts by anaerobes, binding of cobalamin by anaerobes) and patchy damage to the small intestinal enterocyte, perhaps secondary to toxins secreted by the overgrowth flora.

In healthy persons, bacteria within the small intestine are controlled by the cleansing motion of the small intestine, gastric acid secretion, and luminal immunoglobulins. Any alteration of these protective factors may lead to bacterial overgrowth (Table 102–10). In the past, bacterial overgrowth was thought to be related largely to blind loops and other structural abnormalities. Now the emphasis is on motor disturbances, often with no structural abnormality, and on states of decreased acid secretion. Indeed, bacterial overgrowth is one of the major, if not the major, cause of clinically significant malabsorption in the elderly, who often have both decreased acid secretion and a motility disturbance of the small intestine.

The diagnosis has become much more practical with the development of noninvasive breath tests (see section on Diagnosis—Breath Tests, Tables 102–4 and 102–6). This has greatly increased the awareness of this syndrome. Intestinal cultures have been expensive, awkward to perform, and usually not utilized extensively in clinical practice.

In the past, treatment was often empiric, not based on a firm diagnosis but dictated by a clinical impression. Broad-spectrum antibiotics (tetracycline) were prescribed for 7 to 10 days and the clinical response monitored. Up to 60 per cent of the anaerobes (Bacteroides) now may be resistant to tetracycline. It behooves the physician to establish the diagnosis firmly, for the antibiotics needed may have serious side effects.

The mainstays of therapy are antimicrobial therapy and nutritional support. If there is a surgically correctable cause of the overgrowth, surgery should be performed if possible. Most patients with overgrowth do not have a surgically correctable

TABLE 102–8. ALGORITHM FOR EVALUATION OF MALABSORPTION

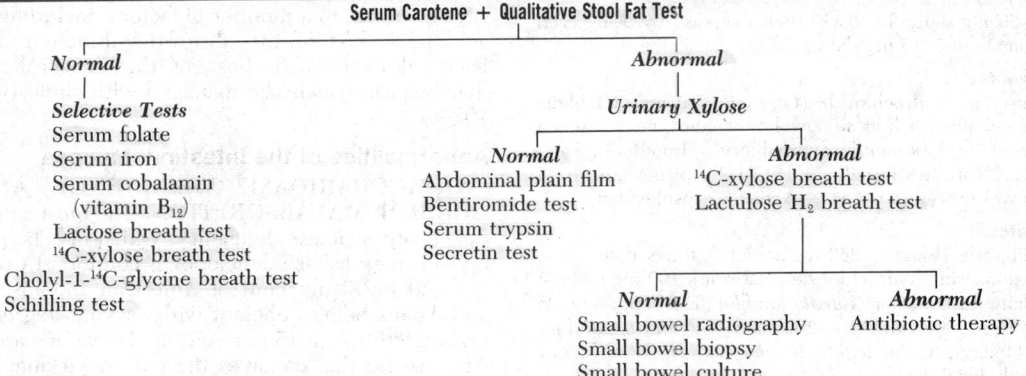

TABLE 102–9. AGENTS USED IN THE TREATMENT OF MALABSORPTION

1. Calcium
Oral: Requires 1200 mg elemental calcium daily. Preparations:
a. Calcium gluconate (91 mg Ca^{2+}/gm), 5–10 gm 3 times per day
b. Calcium carbonate (500 mg Ca^{2+}/tablet),1–2 gm per day in divided doses
c. Calcium carbonate, 2 tablets supplied as Caltrate or 2½ tablets as Os-Cal 500
Intravenous: Calcium gluconate injection (10% solution, 9.1 mg Ca^{2+}/ml), 10–30 ml administered slowly

2. Magnesium
Oral: Magnesium gluconate, 500-mg tablets (20 mg Mg^{2+}/tablet), 1–4 gm daily in divided doses
Intramuscular: (20% sol.) 10 ml 2–3 times daily
Intravenous: Magnesium sulfate, 0.5 per cent sol., up to 1000 ml at a rate not faster than 1.0 mEq/min

3. Iron
Oral: Ferrous sulfate, 325 mg (65 mg elemental iron) 3 times daily
Intramuscular: Imferon must be calculated according to severity of anemia

4. Cyanocobalamin (vitamin B_{12})
Intramuscular: 100 µg daily for 2 weeks, then 100 µg monthly

5. Folic acid
Oral: 5 mg daily for 1 month; maintenance 1 mg daily

6. Vitamin B complex
Any multivitamin preparation that contains US RDA amounts; use 2 tablets daily; intramuscular preparations are available

7. Fat-soluble vitamins
a. Vitamin A
Capsules (25,000 units of Vitamin A per capsule), 100,000–200,000 units daily in severe deficiencies; maintenance, 25,000–50,000 units daily. *Caution:* Vitamin A toxicity can occur with recommended doses if hypertriglyceridemia is present
b. Vitamin D
Vitamin D_2 or D_3, 30,000 units daily; dosage varies considerably depending on response as determined by level of serum calcium and urinary calcium
c. Vitamin K
Oral: Menadione, 4–12 mg daily; vitamin K tablets (Mephyton), 5–10 mg daily
Intravenous: Acute bleeding episodes: vitamin K (Mephyton), 50-mg ampule administered slowly over 10-min period; repeat in 8–12 hr if prothrombin time has not returned to normal

8. Cholestyramine
4-gm pk, 1–2 pk before breakfast and lunch

9. Medium-chain triglyceride (MCT oil)
Administer 60% of fat intake as MCT oil

10. Human albumin, salt poor (0.25 gm/ml)
Intravenous administration of 50–100 gm daily for 3–7 days to elevate a severely depressed serum albumin level

11. Immune serum globulin (0.165 gm/ml)
Intramuscular injection of 0.05 ml/kg each 3–4 wk in patients with hypogammaglobulinemia and recurrent infection

12. Adrenocorticosteroids
Prednisone, 40–60 mg daily for 2 wk, then decrease by 5 mg each week to maintenance of 5–15 mg daily

13. Antidiarrheal agents
Oral: Diphenoxylate hydrochloride (Lomotil), 5.0 mg (2 tablets) initially and after each loose bowel movement, not to exceed 8 tablets daily; loperamide hydrochloride (Imodium), 2-mg capsules, 2 capsules initially and then 2 capsules after each loose bowel movement, not to exceed 8 capsules daily

14. Drugs for parasites
Oral: Metronidazole (Flagyl), 250-mg tablet 3 times daily for 1 wk, or quinacrine hydrochloride (Atabrine), 100-mg tablet 3 times daily for 1 wk for *Giardia lamblia.* Thiabendazole (25 mg/kg/day): strongyloidiasis, 2–3 days; *Capillaria philippinensis*, 30 days; *A. duodenale, N. americanus*, 25 mg/kg/day twice daily for 2 days

TABLE 102–10. CLINICAL CONDITIONS ASSOCIATED WITH BACTERIAL OVERGROWTH

I. Gastric proliferation of bacteria
Hypo- or achlorhydria, especially when combined with motor or anatomic disturbances
II. Small intestinal stagnation
Anatomic
Afferent loop of Billroth II partial gastrectomy
Duodenal or jejunal diverticulosis
Surgical blind loop (end-to-side anastomosis)
Surgical recirculating loop (side-to-side anastomosis)
Obstruction (stricture, adhesion, inflammation, cancer)
Motor
Scleroderma
Idiopathic intestinal pseudo-obstruction
Derangements of interdigestive motor complex
Diabetic autonomic neuropathy
III. Abnormal communication between proximal and distal gastrointestinal tract
Gastrocolic or jejunocolic fistula
Resection of ileocecal valve
IV. Miscellaneous
Hypogammaglobulinemia
Chronic pancreatitis

Modified from King CE, Toskes PP: Small intestine bacterial overgrowth. Gastroenterology 76:1035, 1979.

cause (e.g., they have scleroderma, diverticulosis, or diabetes) and must receive lifelong antimicrobial and nutritional therapy.

A 10-day course of a cephalosporin (Keflex), 250 mg four times a day, and metronidazole (Flagyl), 250 mg three times a day, is very effective in suppressing the flora and correcting malabsorption, as is the clavulonic acid derivative Augmentin, 250 mg three times a day. Tetracycline is an alternative, but the resistance problem must be appreciated. If these fail, chloramphenicol (50 mg per kilogram per day in four divided doses) is also very effective. Anaerobicidal agents by themselves (metronidazole, clindamycin) do not seem to be as effective as the combination of an aerobicidal and an anaerobicidal agent.

Three therapeutic patterns occur. Usually a 10-day course of an effective antimicrobial program corrects the malabsorption for months; some patients may need cyclic therapy (1 week out of every 6); rarely a patient may need continuous therapy for several months. Antibiotic sensitivity assays of the overgrowth flora are not recommended because of the multitude of organisms present.

Nutritional therapy (especially with medium-chain triglyceride oil) is very important but often ignored. Medium-chain triglyceride administration is ideal therapy for this condition, since this form of fat does not need bile salts for absorption. Other agents such as cobalamin, vitamin D, and calcium are given in doses detailed in Table 102–9.

ILEAL DISEASE OR RESECTION. Disease of the distal ileum leads to an interruption of the enterohepatic circulation of conjugated bile acids, resulting in a diminished bile acid pool and steatorrhea. The degree of steatorrhea is proportional to the amount of diseased or resected intestine. When less than 100 cm of intestine is damaged or resected, proximal to the ileocecal valve, the steatorrhea is mild and choleretic diarrhea tends to be the most frequent problem. The malabsorbed bile acids dump into the colon and impair water and electrolyte absorption. When more than 100 cm of small intestine is resected, the steatorrhea is large owing to a number of factors, including a diminished bile acid pool, loss of the absorptive function of the ileum, and bacterial overgrowth (loss of the ileocecal valve). Choleretic diarrhea can usually be managed with cholestyramine (see Table 102–9).

Abnormalities of the Intestinal Mucosa

DISACCHARIDASE DEFICIENCY AND MONOSACCHARIDE MALABSORPTION. The most common disaccharide deficiency is lactase deficiency, which may be primary or secondary. Primary lactase deficiency is common throughout the world, with 60 to 90 per cent of American Indians, black Americans, and Asians being deficient with varying degrees of lactose intolerance. Only 5 to 15 per cent of Caucasians are lactase deficient. Any disease that damages the enterocyte may lead to secondary lactase deficiency.

Lactase-deficient subjects are intolerant to milk, experiencing bloating, abdominal cramps, and diarrhea. The lactose within milk cannot be hydrolyzed to glucose and galactose. It remains in the intestinal lumen, where it is fermented by bacteria, producing organic acids, which increase the osmotic load, inducing shifts of water into the intestinal tract. The end result is distention of the intestine and diarrhea.

Primary lactase deficiency may not manifest itself until adulthood, yet the reason for this delayed appearance is not clear. Subtotal gastrectomy or pyloroplasty and vagotomy may unmask the condition by increasing the load of ingested lactose on the jejunal mucosa. Although the diagnosis is often made by taking a history, the lactose-H_2 breath test is the best way to document lactose intolerance (see Diagnosis section and Table 102–4). Treatment of primary lactase deficiency is avoidance of milk products or the ingestion of one to two capsules of Lactrase when dairy products are ingested. Lactrase, derived from *Aspergillus oryzae*, is commercially available.

Sucrase deficiency is quite rare. In afflicted patients, diarrhea occurs after ingesting sucrose. Elimination of sucrose, dextrins, and starches from the diet is effective.

Monosaccharide (glucose-galactose) malabsorption is a rare disorder present from birth. All sugars metabolized to glucose or galactose cannot be tolerated. Therapy consists of utilizing fructose as a source of sugar.

NONTROPICAL SPRUE (ADULT CELIAC DISEASE, CELIAC SPRUE, GLUTEN-SENSITIVE ENTEROPATHY). Nontropical sprue is a disease of unknown etiology characterized by malabsorption resulting from gluten-induced damage to the differentiated villus epithelial cells of the small intestine. Gluten is a high molecular weight protein found in wheat, rye, oats, and barley. The mechanism for this toxic effect is not known, but the most accepted theory at present is that metabolites of gluten initiate an immunologic reaction in the enterocyte. The enterocyte is often strikingly damaged, and biopsy of the small intestine demonstrates characteristic changes (see Fig. 102–5 and discussion of small bowel biopsy in Diagnosis section). Malabsorption is secondary to the impaired transport of nutrients through the damaged enterocyte. In addition, a net secretory state for water and electrolytes has been noted in the jejunum, and pancreatic exocrine function may be secondarily diminished owing to a decreased release of secretin and cholecystokinin from the damaged small bowel mucosa.

Genetic factors appear important in this disease. Nontropical sprue is closely linked to two histocompatibility antigens, HLA-B8 and HLA-DRw3. These antigens are present in 60 to 90 per cent of patients with this disease and in only 20 to 30 per cent of the general population. An additional antigen has been found on the surface of B lymphocytes in 70 to 80 per cent of patients with nontropical sprue and in 15 per cent of normal controls. The same antigen is present in 100 per cent of the patients' parents. Perhaps these antigens evoke antibodies to gluten, which result in the binding of gluten to the enterocyte with subsequent mucosal damage.

Patients with nontropical sprue usually have severe malabsorption—steatorrhea, diarrhea, weight loss, and many of the other symptoms and signs detailed in Table 102–3. Symptoms typically begin in infancy, disappear in late childhood, and reappear in the third to sixth decade of life. The proximal small intestine is usually the most severely damaged organ, and the symptoms, signs, and laboratory evaluation reflect this (Tables 102–3 and 102–4). At times, the clinical presentation may be quite subtle, e.g., anemia secondary to iron deficiency or bone pain from osteomalacia without obvious diarrhea or steatorrhea. Small bowel biopsy is essential in this disease, for a diagnosis of nontropical sprue commits the patient to a very restricted diet indefinitely. Evidence is accumulating that increased levels of serum antibodies to gliadin may be of considerable diagnostic benefit. Elevated serum IgA antigliadin may spare patients unnecessary small bowel biopsies.

The cornerstone of therapy is the withdrawal of all gluten from the diet, i.e., all grains must be eliminated except rice and corn. Most patients respond to dietary restriction with a remarkable decrease in symptoms and signs within a few days to a week. In some patients, however, it may take months before a significant improvement is noted. Function tests such as urinary xylose excretion return to normal within a few weeks of gluten withdrawal. Post-treatment biopsies demonstrate marked improvement in most patients and completely normal histologic findings in many. The patient with the characteristic syndrome and biopsy findings who does not respond to gluten withdrawal is usually not adhering to the diet. Some patients may have the characteristic clinical picture and flat biopsy and in reality are not responding because they have another disease such as Whipple's disease, nongranulomatous ileojejunitis, giardiasis, lymphoma, or collagenous sprue. Collagenous sprue, a variant of nontropical sprue, demonstrates not only the characteristic changes in the small intestinal biopsy but also masses of eosinophilic hyaline material in the lamina propria. Such patients have a poor prognosis. Corticosteroid therapy (see Table 102–9) or parenteral hyperalimentation may be needed in some patients.

Small bowel lymphoma and carcinoma in general seem to be increased in patients with nontropical sprue. The appearance of abdominal pain in a patient with sprue should suggest lymphoma. Whether or not these complications are fewer in those who adhere strictly to a gluten-free diet is controversial.

Two other associated abnormalities in patients with sprue are (1) ulcers of the jejunum and ileum with abdominal pain, bleeding, and perforation, which are unresponsive to therapy, and (2) dermatitis herpetiformis. Some patients with this skin lesion may have latent sprue. The dermatitis is pruritic, vesicular, and papular and responds to sulfone treatment. Sulfone does not improve the intestinal lesion, but some of these lesions may respond to gluten withdrawal.

NONGRANULOMATOUS ILEOJEJUNITIS. This disease has features of both Crohn's disease and nontropical sprue, even a flat small intestinal biopsy. There is an abrupt onset with fever, abdominal pain, at times splenomegaly, and elevated white count—all suggesting lymphoma. Malabsorption may be profound, resulting in a therapeutic trial of steroids and a gluten-free diet—often to no avail.

CROHN'S DISEASE (Ch. 103). Malabsorption in Crohn's disease results from several problems: (1) decreased absorptive surface from active disease or surgical resection, (2) bile salt depletion from ileal disease, and (3) bacterial overgrowth secondary to dilatation of the bowel and resection of the ileocecal valve.

EOSINOPHILIC ENTERITIS. Peripheral blood eosinophilia and infiltration of the gastrointestinal tract by eosinophils characterize this disease. Three patterns of involvement are seen: (1) involvement of the muscle layers of the stomach and small intestine causing obstruction, (2) involvement of the mucosa of the small intestine causing malabsorption, and (3) involvement of the subserosa causing ascites. Most patients have no evidence of allergy or food sensitivity. Corticosteroids and occasionally surgery are employed successfully.

RADIATION ENTERITIS (Ch. 112 and 530). Radiation injury to the intestine may lead to malabsorption from (1) extensive mucosal damage, (2) lymphangiectasia from lymphatic obstruction, and (3) bacterial overgrowth. Malabsorption may occur shortly after exposure to radiation or years later. Most patients with clinically significant malabsorption appear to respond to therapy for bacterial overgrowth.

ABETALIPOPROTEINEMIA (Ch. 172). This rare disease represents a defect in chylomicron formation. The intestinal cells are lacking apoprotein B, and therefore fat absorption cannot occur normally. Biopsy of the small intestine shows the epithelial cells to be engorged with fat even after an overnight fast. The clinical manifestations are steatorrhea, neurologic disease (ataxia, retinitis pigmentosa), very low serum cholesterol and triglyceride levels, and "spiny red cells" (acanthocytes). Therapy consists of substitution of dietary fat with medium-chain triglyceride and administration of fat-soluble vitamins, especially vitamin E.

Inadequate Absorptive Surface

SHORT BOWEL SYNDROME. Extensive resection of the small intestine is usually performed for Crohn's disease, intestinal infarction, or trauma. Acute hyperalimentation in these patients has been life-saving, and the ability of the remaining gut to adapt for increased nutrient absorption by hypertrophy of residual small intestinal villi is remarkable. Patients do rather well despite extensive resection if approximately 90 to 100 cm of duodenum and jejunum and the terminal ileum (intact ileocecal valve) remain.

Treatment consists of parenteral hyperalimentation for weeks to months until evidence exists that the remaining gut is functional. Gradual introduction of oral feedings, high in protein content, vitamins, and minerals, as well as medium-chain triglyceride (MCT), forms the basis for maintenance therapy. Antidiarrheal agents and cholestyramine may help (see Table 102–9). Occasionally, pancreatic extract therapy and H_2-receptor antagonists are necessary to treat the transient acid hypersecretion and secondary pancreatic insufficiency that may occur. Steroids may increase water absorption. Some patients must receive hyperalimentation at home indefinitely. Diarrhea resistant to all other therapy may respond to somatostatin analogues (Sandostatin).

JEJUNOILEAL BYPASS. Some patients with morbid obesity have had a surgical procedure performed (14 inches of proximal jejunum is anastomosed to 4 inches of terminal ileum) that induces malabsorption. In addition to many of the problems detailed above in the short bowel syndrome, other serious complications occur, such as oxalate kidney stones, intestinal pseudo-obstruction, cirrhosis, and arthritis. Because of these complications, the operation has been abandoned.

Infection

TROPICAL SPRUE. The pathogenesis of this malabsorptive disorder occurring in tropical regions (Far East, India, Caribbean) is poorly understood. An overgrowth of coliforms within the jejunum has been demonstrated in these patients. Such organisms have been shown to elaborate an enterotoxin that induces fluid secretion. Tropical sprue is not a true bacterial overgrowth, since anaerobes (particularly *Bacteroides*) are conspicuously absent. Malabsorption of many nutrients occurs, especially folic acid, cobalamin, and fat. The intestinal biopsy does not demonstrate total villus atrophy, but rather nonspecific changes in the villi (shortening, thickening) and cellular infiltration of the lamina propria. Successful therapy has been achieved with cobalamin, folic acid, or antibiotics. A two-month course of a broad-spectrum antibiotic (e.g., tetracycline, 250 mg orally four times daily) and folic acid, 5.0 mg daily, is most effective. In those patients with cobalamin deficiency, 1000 µg of cobalamin should be given intramuscularly for 2 consecutive days. Improvement of malabsorption following therapy with folic acid or cobalamin alone casts doubt upon infection as the sole etiology.

WHIPPLE'S DISEASE. Patients (usually male) who present with Whipple's disease manifest steatorrhea, weight loss, abdominal pain, nondeforming arthritis, fever, peripheral lymphadenopathy, and neurologic abnormalities (nystagmus, ophthalmoplegia, cranial nerve defects). Protein-losing enteropathy may be present because of lymphatic obstruction.

Small bowel biopsy is diagnostic, demonstrating heavy infiltration of the mucosa and lymph nodes by macrophages that stain positive with periodic acid–Schiff reagent (PAS). Biopsy of the small intestine also shows blunting of villi and dilated lymphatics. The macrophages are filled with rod-shaped bacilli, which disappear after antibiotic therapy and reappear prior to an exacerbation of the disease. Although these rodlike structures resemble bacilli, no bacteria have been consistently cultured from patients with this disease—hence the bacterial etiology of Whipple's disease has not been proved.

Untreated, this is a fatal disease. These patients should be treated for at least a year and probably indefinitely. The antibiotic of choice appears to be trimethoprim-sulfamethoxazole, 500 mg given orally four times daily.

Lymphatic Obstruction

LYMPHOMA (INTESTINAL). Malabsorption occurs in patients with intestinal lymphoma from (1) mucosal invasion, (2) lymphatic obstruction, and (3) bacterial overgrowth secondary to dilatation of the bowel with stasis. Antibiotic therapy often completely corrects the clinical manifestations of malabsorption (diarrhea, steatorrhea), suggesting that bacterial overgrowth is an important cause of malabsorption in these patients. Abdominal pain, fever, and steatorrhea are principal complaints; lymphadenopathy and hepatosplenomegaly are uncommon. The small

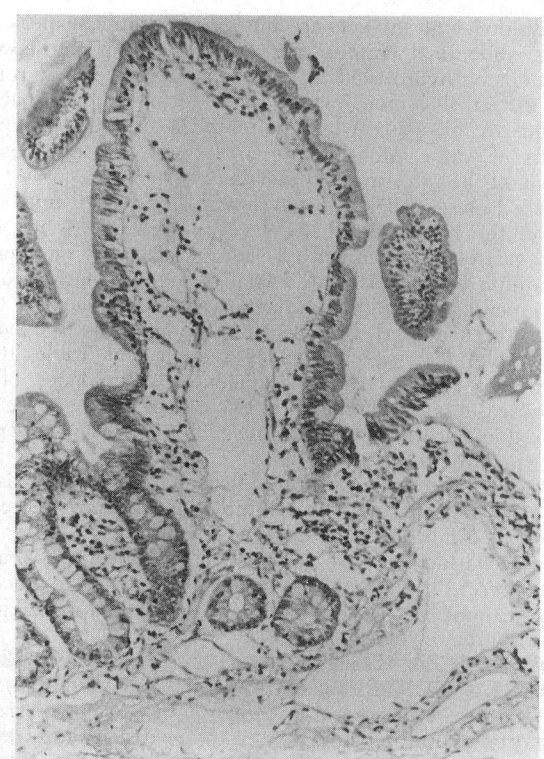

FIGURE 102–6. Small intestinal biopsy from a patient with intestinal lymphangiectasia. Note the dilated lymph channels (clear spaces).

bowel biopsy may mimic nontropical sprue but not respond to a gluten-free diet. The diagnosis is usually made by the finding of malignant lymphoid cells in the mucosa or submucosa via small bowel biopsy or by full-thickness biopsy at surgery. As many as 10 per cent of patients with nontropical sprue may develop lymphoma.

LYMPHANGIECTASIA. Primary or congenital lymphangiectasia is characterized by diarrhea, mild steatorrhea, edema, enteric loss of protein (protein-losing enteropathy), and abnormal dilated lymphatic channels on small intestinal biopsy (Fig. 102–6). The main clinical feature of this disorder, which affects primarily children and young adults, is asymmetric edema secondary to the hypoplastic peripheral lymphatics and chylous effusions. Lymphocytopenia and depressed serum protein levels are a result of the protein-losing enteropathy. The hypoplastic lymphatics lead to an obstruction in lymph flow, increased pressure within lymphatics, dilated lymphatic channels in the intestine, and finally rupture of the lymphatic channels, discharging lymph into the bowel lumen. Therapy is directed to decreasing lymph flow via a low-fat diet and substitution of dietary fat with medium-chain triglycerides (MCT), which are transported by the portal venous system rather than the lymphatic system.

Although protein-losing enteropathy is a hallmark of intestinal lymphangiectasia, many other disorders can also cause enteric protein loss. The mechanisms are multifactorial: (1) exudation of protein through inflamed or engorged mucosa (gastric cancer, hypertrophy of gastric mucosa, ulcerative colitis), (2) loss of protein because of abnormal enterocytes (nontropical sprue, scleroderma), and (3) passage of proteins into the intestine secondary to increased pressure within lymphatics (lymphangiectasia, constrictive pericarditis, lymphoma).

Enteric protein loss can be detected by intravenously administering various labeled macromolecules and measuring the radioactivity in the feces. These tests are cumbersome to perform and not readily available. Recently, α_1-antitrypsin has been used as a marker for this disorder. Alpha$_1$-antitrypsin (similar size as albumin) can be measured in the feces by immunodiffusion.

Cardiovascular Disorders

Any disorder causing poor perfusion of the intestine may lead to steatorrhea. Atherosclerosis and vasculitis may both affect the mesenteric blood supply.

Drug-Induced Malabsorption

This entity is not very common and usually produces clinically insignificant malabsorption. Steatorrhea secondary to therapy with cholestyramine and neomycin is thought to be a result of precipitation of bile salts. The mechanism or mechanisms of most drug-induced malabsorption are not well understood.

Unexplained Malabsorption

Other than that in diabetes and perhaps in the carcinoid syndrome, the malabsorption occasionally observed in endocrine disorders (adrenal insufficiency, thyroid disease) is not at all understood. In diabetes, malabsorption may result from neuropathic changes (diarrhea) or bacterial overgrowth (steatorrhea). In systemic mast cell disease, there may be massive infiltration of the small intestine with mast cells, blunting of intestinal villi, and marked acid hypersecretion (Ch. 252). Malabsorption, however, does not appear to correlate well with any of these abnormalities. Hypogammaglobulinemia is at times associated with severe malabsorption. Although the pathogenesis is not well defined, such patients may have giardiasis, bacterial overgrowth, and histologic abnormalities of the small intestine (patchy villus atrophy, nodular lymphoid hyperplasia). Plasma cells are absent within the intestine.

Malabsorption in the Elderly

Elderly patients may develop malabsorption from any of the disorders listed in Table 102–2, but bacterial overgrowth appears to be the most common cause of clinically significant steatorrhea in this population. The elderly often have decreased gastric acid secretion and abnormalities in intestinal motility that predispose them to malabsorption from bacterial overgrowth. The hypo- or achlorhydria may lead to cobalamin (vitamin B_{12}) deficiency from malabsorption of food-bound cobalamin (see Table 102–5). Such patients may be treated effectively just with tablets of cyanocobalamin (unbound B_{12}), since they have intrinsic factor in adequate amounts. Recognition of this problem may avoid parenteral administration of cobalamin.

Malabsorption in the Acquired Immunodeficiency Syndrome (AIDS) (Ch. 416)

Patients with AIDS often have diarrhea, malabsorption, and weight loss. A number of infectious agents, including *Giardia lamblia, Mycobacterium avium-intracellulare, Cryptosporidium, Microsporidium, Strongyloides stercoralis,* and *Isospora belli,* may cause malabsorption in patients with AIDS. Although these patients often have enteric infections and intestinal involvement with Kaposi's sarcoma, there are significant numbers of patients with AIDS who have malabsorption without these two abnormalities. In some patients with AIDS, biopsy of the small intestine demonstrates large numbers of histiocytes within the lamina propria. Although such findings on biopsy may be confused with Whipple's disease, in patients with AIDS these histiocytes contain acid-fast bacilli, representing *Mycobacterium avium-intracellulare*. Still other patients with AIDS have malabsorption with the only abnormality found being that of a nonspecific mild to moderate chronic inflammatory response in the small bowel biopsy. The malabsorption in this last group of patients may be due to bacterial overgrowth or other unidentified enteric infections.

Brasitus TA, Sitrin MD: Intestinal malabsorption syndromes. Ann Rev Med 41:339, 1990. *New developments in malabsorption associated with AIDS, celiac sprue, bacterial overgrowth, and old age.*

Donaldson RM, Toskes PP: The relation of enteric bacterial populations to gastrointestinal function and disease. *In* Sleisenger MH, Fordtran JS (eds.): Gastrointestinal Disease. 4th ed. Philadelphia, W. B. Saunders Company, 1989, p 107. *Thorough review of human intestinal flora.*

Keinath RD, Merrell DE, Vlitstra R, et al.: Antibiotic treatment and relapse in Whipple's disease. Long-term follow-up of 88 patients. Gastroenterology 88:1867, 1985. *Current discussion of therapy in this disease.*

Kelly CP, Feighery CF, Gallagher RB, et al.: Diagnosis and treatment of gluten-sensitive enteropathy. Adv Intern Med 35:341, 1990. *Current thorough review of clinical features of celiac disease.*

King CE, Toskes PP: Comparison of the 1-gram ^{14}C-xylose, 10-gram lactulose-H_2, and the 80-gram glucose-H_2 breath tests in patients with small intestine bacterial overgrowth. Gastroenterology 91:1447, 1986. *Direct comparison of ^{14}C breath tests and H_2 breath tests for diagnosing bacterial overgrowth.*

King CE, Toskes PP: The use of breath tests in the study of malabsorption. Clin Gastroenterol 12:591, 1983. *Thorough overall review of clinical usefulness of these tests.*

Ladefoged K, Christensen KC, Hegnhoj J, et al.: Effect of a long-acting somatostatin analogue SMS 201-995 on jejunostomy effluents in patients with severe short bowel syndrome. Gut 30:943, 1989. *Somatostatin analogues offer new therapy for intractable diarrhea of short bowel syndrome.*

Montgomery RD, Haboubi NY, Mike NH, et al.: Cause of malabsorption in the elderly. Age Ageing 15:235, 1986. *Points out importance of bacterial overgrowth in the elderly.*

Rich EJ, Christie DL: Anti-gliadin antibody panel and xylose absorption test in screening celiac disease. J Pediatr Gastroenterol Nutr 10:174, 1990. *Role of serum antibodies to gliadin in the diagnosis of celiac disease.*

Sleisenger MH, Fordtran JS (eds.): Gastrointestinal Disease. 4th ed. Philadelphia, W. B. Saunders Company, 1989, Ch. 18, 19, 57, 61, 66–68. *Normal absorption and malabsorption in well-referenced text of gastroenterology.*

Toskes PP: The bentiromide test for pancreatic endocrine insufficiency. Pharmacotherapy 4:74, 1984. *Review of worldwide experience with this noninvasive test of pancreatic function.*

Toskes PP, Donaldson RM: The blind loop syndrome. *In* Sleisenger MH, Fordtran JS (eds.): Gastrointestinal Disease. 4th ed. Philadelphia, W. B. Saunders Company, 1989, p 1289. *Complete review of pathophysiology, diagnosis, and treatment of small intestine bacterial overgrowth.*

103 Inflammatory Bowel Disease

Stephen B. Hanauer

DEFINITION

The term "inflammatory bowel disease" applies to the idiopathic, chronic inflammatory bowel diseases (IBD): Crohn's disease (CD) and ulcerative colitis (UC). These are distinguished from IBD of established origin such as viral, bacterial, and parasitic infections; diverticulitis; radiation enteritis or colitis; drug or toxin-induced enterocolitis; or vasculitis of the intestinal tract. CD and UC are disorders of unknown etiology involving genetic and immunologic influences on the gastrointestinal tract's ability to distinguish foreign from self-antigens and/or to downregulate the mucosal immune response. They share many overlapping epidemiologic, clinical, and therapeutic features. Both are chronic, medically incurable conditions. Whereas a proctocolectomy cures UC, surgery for CD is limited to treatment of complications.

Ulcerative colitis encompasses a spectrum of diffuse, continuous, superficial inflammation of the colon, which begins within the rectum and extends to a variable proximal level. The inflammatory features are constant within the involved segment of the colon and, once established, the upward margin of inflammation usually remains constant in the same individual. Occasionally, the disease progresses to more proximal areas, usually within the first several years after diagnosis. The condition never involves the small intestine except when the distal terminal ileum is inflamed in a similar, superficial fashion (backwash ileitis) in patients with inflammation throughout the colon (pancolitis). The inflammation extends beneath the lamina propria only in severe cases, when submucosal involvement produces a thinning of the circular and longitudinal muscles leading to colonic distention (toxic megacolon). UC is primarily a mucosal process, and removal of the entire mucosa is curative.

Crohn's disease is characterized by focal, asymmetric, transmural inflammation affecting any portion of the gastrointestinal tract from the mouth to the anus. The ileum and right colon are most often involved, but any segment of the gastrointestinal tract can be inflamed. The focal, transmural inflammation and the potential for proximal gastrointestinal tract involvement distinguish CD from UC. The presence of noncaseating granuloma also distinguishes CD from UC but is not necessary for the diagnosis. Microscopic changes are present throughout the gastrointestinal tract, distant from grossly involved segments of intestine.

ETIOLOGY

The cause(s) of UC and CD is not known. Although genetic, biochemical, and immunologic patterns are recognized in patients, a definitive etiopathogenesis remains elusive. The absence of an appropriate animal model for chronic IBD has hampered progress in determining pathogenesis. Spontaneously occurring chronic colitis in the cotton-top tamarin, *Sanguinus oedipus*, shares many biochemical, pathologic, and chronic features with UC, including the increased frequency of colonic adenocarcinoma. Unfortunately, these animals are an endangered species, and their rarity and the difficulty of breeding them in captivity complicate investigations. An alternative animal model is needed.

No infectious agent has been linked to UC or to CD, although it is speculated that exposure to a common bacterial antigen stimulates an autoimmune reaction against a shared host antigen via molecular mimicry.

EPIDEMIOLOGY (Table 103–1)

UC and CD occur among all age groups but have a peak incidence in the second and third decades. The incidence of CD has risen over the past 20 years and now shares incidence and prevalence rates with UC of 5 per 100,000 and 50 per 100,000, respectively. The combined prevalence of the two diseases is approximately 100 per 100,000 population. These disorders are seen most commonly in Northern Europe and North America and in relatives of European immigrants in the cities of South Africa, Australia, and New Zealand. IBD is rare in Central America, South America, Africa, the Middle East, and Asia. Although IBD can be seen in all ethnic groups, there is an increased prevalence in Jews who have emigrated from Northern Europe. This Jewish predisposition is not seen in Sephardic (Mediterranean or Middle-Eastern) Jews. Although less common in the nonwhite population, more cases are being recognized in the black population in American cities and in Asian immigrants to Great Britain.

A presumed genetic influence is derived from family studies, in which approximately 20 per cent of individuals with IBD have a relative with UC or CD. The pattern of inheritance is more complicated than that of a simple mendelian trait, and the risk is spread across families. In children with IBD the likelihood of another family member having the diagnosis is greater than 40 per cent. Although the risk to a child of a parent with IBD is less than 5 per cent, when both parents have IBD the risk to offspring is greater than 50 per cent. There is a stronger concordance within families and in twin studies for CD than for UC. The only epidemiologic difference between UC and CD pertains to cigarette smoking. Cigarette smoking appears to protect against the development of UC and is associated with CD. More than 80 per cent of patients with UC are nonsmokers, whereas 80 per cent of patients with CD smoke cigarettes. Often, UC begins after a "predisposed" individual stops smoking.

Attempts have been made to implicate a number of environmental factors in the development of IBD, including atypical mycobacterium, diets high in refined sugar (including corn flakes), increased consumption of polysaturated fats (margarine), and oral contraceptive pills, but none has been proven.

PATHOGENESIS

The absence of an etiologic factor leaves a gap in our understanding of the pathogenesis of IBD. Although a number of potential factors may influence the *initiation* of the inflammatory response, a popular view is that there is a defect in the "downregulation" of immune events, allowing persistent *amplification* of the tissue-damaging process. The inflammatory reaction in IBD closely mimics infectious enterocolitis with the exception of the failure to halt progressive tissue destruction. Subtle differences exist between the immunologic findings of UC and CD,

TABLE 103–1. EPIDEMIOLOGY OF INFLAMMATORY BOWEL DISEASE

More common in whites than nonwhites
Increased frequency among European stock
More common among Jews (especially Ashkenazic)
  than non-Jews (three to six times)
Most frequent age of onset: 15 to 30 years
Aggregation in families (25–40%)
Concordance for Crohn's disease in twins
Cigarette smokers—Crohn's disease
Nonsmokers—ulcerative colitis

such as the production of immunoglobulin heavy-chain allotypes or neutrophil-cytoplasmic antibodies; however, pathognomonic findings to classify these disorders remain elusive. Nosology is currently based on descriptive clinical, endoscopic, and histologic criteria, and misclassification often is recognized as the clinicopathologic process evolves over time. When the diagnosis changes, it is almost always from UC to CD and virtually never the converse.

Potential initiating events in IBD include increased intestinal permeability, aberrant epithelial processing of antigen, improper epithelial utilization of short-chain fatty acids, and molecular mimicry between a luminal antigen and components of intestinal mucosa. There is evidence of increased intestinal permeability to small or medium-sized molecular particles in patients and relatives of patients with IBD, which may be affected by qualitative differences in intestinal mucus glycoprotein. Similar alterations in colonic mucin fraction IV from patients with UC are present in cotton-top tamarins with spontaneous colitis. Cigarette smoking can also influence mucin production and intestinal permeability, and nonsteroidal anti-inflammatory drugs damage proximal and distal intestinal epithelium, increase intestinal permeability, and tend to exacerbate IBD.

Intestinal epithelial cells stimulated by interferon express class II major histocompatibility complexes and become antigen-presenting cells. The processing and presentation of antigens to T8 (suppressor T cells) are altered in patients with IBD such that the presentation of antigen is preferentially directed toward the T4 (helper T cell) system. This could be a primary, genetically mediated event that stimulates the gut immune system rather than induces tolerance.

A defect in the ability of the gut epithelium to metabolize short-chain fatty acids derived from the intestinal lumen or injury to the epithelium by an infectious or toxic injury may alter or expose cell proteins that are perceived as foreign by the mucosal immune system. A conclusive target antigen has not been identified for either UC or CD. A variety of antibodies to epithelial cell components, some of which cross-react with enterobacterial antigens, are present but are not specific for IBD. In addition, serum antibodies against enteric bacteria or food-related antigens (e.g., milk protein) are increased in a nonspecific manner. There is also evidence of autoimmune lymphocyte-mediated cytotoxicity against epithelial cells, but a consistent abnormality in mucosal or systemic immune regulation has not been identified. Most of the local (mucosal) or systemic immunologic parameters represent secondary rather than primary changes.

Once initiated, many of the pathophysiologic events in IBD are related to amplification of the inflammatory process. When antigens are presented to mucosal macrophages, cytokines and other inflammatory mediators are activated and released. IL1 is released and induces T-cell activation and proliferation. Activated T cells become cytotoxic and/or release IL2, which induces clonal expansion of helper T cells, B-cell proliferation, and antibody synthesis. IgG production by B cells invokes complement activation and subsequent activation of the kinin system. The arachidonic acid cascade of inflammatory mediators is shifted toward the proinflammatory, lipoxygenase pathway with enhanced production of leukotriene B_4, a potent chemotactic agent for neutrophils, and platelet-activating factor (PAF) is produced. When neutrophils accumulate and are stimulated, they further damage tissue by releasing reactive oxygen species, amplifying the inflammatory process via recruitment of additional acute inflammatory cells, whether or not the primary initiating sequences have been halted.

The release of inflammatory mediators, including prostaglandins and leukotrienes, histamine from mast cells, and neuropeptides such as substance P or vasoactive intestinal peptide, alters epithelial function and contributes to the intestinal secretory process inducing diarrhea. The enteric nervous system participates in the regulation of the local and systemic immune system, linking the association of "stress" and psychological factors with flare-ups of disease activity.

PATHOLOGY

UC and CD encompass a spectrum of clinicopathologic findings. Many of the macroscopic and microscopic changes are not specific and overlap with those of acute and chronic infectious enteritides, toxin- or radiation-induced damage to the intestine, ischemic changes, and, on rare occasion, malignancy.

ULCERATIVE COLITIS. Ulcerative colitis, primarily a mucosal disease, begins in the anorectum and involves a variable contiguous proximal segment of colonic mucosa. In approximately one quarter of patients the disease is limited to the rectum (proctitis); in another 25 to 50 per cent the rectum and sigmoid (proctosigmoiditis) or the descending colon (left-sided colitis) is involved. In approximately one third of patients the inflammation extends proximal to the splenic flexure (extensive colitis) or involves the entire colon (pancolitis). The small intestine occasionally is involved by superficial inflammation (backwash ileitis) in a small group of patients with pancolitis. Once the upper demarcation of disease has been identified, it usually remains constant. Approximately 10 to 15 per cent of patients develop proximal extension of colonic involvement, usually within the first few years after diagnosis. With treatment, healing typically begins proximally, with the rectum being the last segment to improve. Occasionally, UC may heal in a patchy distribution, although interval segments demonstrate chronic histologic changes. Some patients with proctitis have patches of endoscopic or histologic changes in the cecum or right colon. The prognostic implications of these findings are uncertain.

The gross or endoscopic appearance of the colonic mucosa in UC ranges from normal-appearing mucosa to complete denudation. Mild inflammatory changes include absence of the mucosal vascular pattern, fine granularity of the mucosa, pinpoint hemorrhage to mucosal swabbing, and exudation of mucopus (see Color Plate 2A). Moderate changes include coarse granularity and pinpoint ulceration, confluent hemorrhage, confluent mucopus that progresses to gross ulcerations, spontaneous hemorrhage, and exudation of pus (see Color Plate 2A). With healing the mucosal vascular pattern remains distorted. Islands of postinflammatory "pseudopolyps" may appear as filamentous projections or mucosal bridges that may be quite friable or indistinguishable from adenomatous polyps (see Color Plate 2B).

Early histologic changes include vascular congestion, increased inflammatory cells in the lamina propria, and distortion of the crypts of Lieberkühn. The degree of the inflammatory reaction determines the "activity" of disease. In inactive colitis the mucosal architecture is distorted with branching or regenerating crypts, and epithelial cells are depleted of goblet cell mucus (see Color Plate 2C). In the active phase of inflammation, acute inflammatory cells, primarily polymorphonuclear leukocytes, accumulate near the epithelium, invade the crypts, and are concentrated within the crypt lumen (crypt abscess) (see Color Plate 2D). Progressive changes include degeneration or necrosis of the crypt epithelium with coalescence of crypt abscesses to produce shallow ulcerations extending to the lamina propria. Only rarely, in severe UC or toxic megacolon, do inflammation and necrosis extend below the lamina propria to involve the submucosa and circular or longitudinal muscles. Then the bowel wall may become "tissue paper" thin with a significant risk of spontaneous perforation.

Typically with acute disease, reversible changes in the colonic musculature lead to loss of haustrations, thickening of the smooth muscle of the colon, and the "lead pipe" appearance of the colon or, occasionally, the appearance of a stricture on radiographic examination.

Epithelial dysplasia may occur in longstanding UC and is highly associated with the presence of colonic malignancy as a long-term complication (see below).

CROHN'S DISEASE. CD involves any segment or combination of segments of the alimentary tract from the mouth to the anus. Unlike UC, microscopic changes often are identified distant from sites of macroscopic disease. These focal changes and the tendency of CD to recur after segmental resection suggest that subtle changes of CD exist throughout the alimentary tract. Most commonly the distal ileum and right colon are macroscopically inflamed (ileocolitis). The colon is involved, exclusively, in about 20 per cent of patients (Crohn's colitis or granulomatous colitis); approximately 15 to 20 per cent of individuals have gross disease limited to the small bowel (ileitis or regional enteritis). The stomach or duodenum is involved in fewer than 10 per cent of patients and usually in association with more distal disease. Diseases of the anal canal, including deep fissures, fistulas, and prominent "hemorrhoidal" skin tags, are common and distinguish CD confined to the colon from UC. Unlike UC, the mucosa in

CD is involved in a focal, discontinuous fashion, both microscopically and macroscopically. Rarely, lesions indistinguishable from those of CD occur in the skin or urogenital mucosal surfaces (miliary CD).

The earliest lesion of CD is the aphthoid ulcer (see Color Plate 2E), a minute ulceration that invariably occurs over a lymphoid aggregate. These ulcerations extend in a linear fashion (see Color Plate 2F), often isolating normal islands of mucosa to produce a "cobblestone appearance," or extend deep throughout the layers of the bowel wall, producing a fissure that can become a fistula into the mesentery or a contiguous organ. Inflammatory changes in CD are typically transmural, accounting for the thickening of the bowel wall and narrowing of the lumen. As CD heals, fibrotic changes replace acute inflammation, creating permanent, focal strictures. In gross specimens, changes include the thickened, "sausage-shaped" appearance of the bowel with serosal hyperemia, "creeping fat" along the antimesenteric border, and thickening and lymphoid hyperplasia of the adjacent mesentery. The inflammatory process is focal in all layers of the bowel (see Color Plate 2G). Acute and chronic inflammatory cells invade isolated or contiguous single crypts (including the production of crypt abscesses) with normal adjacent glands. Lymphoid aggregates are common throughout all layers of the mucosa, submucosa, and serosa, with characteristic aggregations of histiocytes forming noncaseating granulomas in up to 50 per cent of resected specimens. Mucosal biopsies, however, reveal granuloma formation in fewer than 20 per cent of patients. The presence of granulomas differentiates CD from UC, but they are not necessary to distinguish the two diseases. Rather, the focal, transmural involvement of CD associated with aphthoid or linear ulcers, fissures, fistulas, perianal disease, or small intestinal involvement morphologically distinguishes CD from UC. In approximately 20 per cent of patients with colitis, "indeterminant" features do not allow classification between UC and CD. In this setting, the response to therapy and repeated observations over the course usually allow eventual classification.

CLINICAL MANIFESTATIONS

ULCERATIVE COLITIS. The symptoms of UC depend upon the extent and severity of inflammation within the colon. UC always involves the rectum; patients with proctitis present with rectal bleeding, tenesmus, and the passage of mucopus. The consistency of stools is variable, and many patients with ulcerative proctitis are constipated. Abdominal cramping is common, but abdominal pain or tenderness is not a typical finding of UC. The inflammatory process is limited to the mucosa, while pain receptors are located on the serosa or peritoneum. The greater the extent of colon involved, the more likely the patient is to suffer from diarrhea. Rectal urgency reflects reduced compliance of the inflamed rectum.

As the severity of inflammation increases, the patient is more likely to suffer from systemic symptoms. Low-grade fever, malaise, occasional nausea and vomiting associated with defecation, night sweats, and arthralgias are frequent complaints. With severe UC, patients present with fever, dehydration, tachycardia, and symptoms of abdominal tenderness, reflecting progressive inflammation into deeper layers of the colon. A distended abdomen and tympanic bowel sounds accompanied by fever, tachycardia, and vomiting are ominous signs of fulminant colitis or toxic megacolon.

Patients with UC in remission have normal bowel habits, although many patients suffer from an accompanying irritable bowel syndrome with occasional cramping, irregular bowel habits, and the passage of mucus without blood or pus.

Laboratory studies reflect the severity of colitis. Iron deficiency anemia secondary to chronic blood loss is the most common abnormality. A low serum ferritin confirms the presence of iron deficiency anemia and better documents iron stores than do serum iron and iron-binding capacity, which are reduced by chronic disease. Elevation of the erythrocyte sedimentation rate and other acute phase reactants are inconstant features in UC and are of no value in the evaluation of individual patients. A low serum albumin occurs with extensive colitis as a manifestation of protein exudation from the inflamed colon. Serum alkaline phosphatase and GGTP may be modestly elevated (less than twice normal) in patients with pericholangitis; greater changes in bilirubin or hepatocellular enzymes suggest sclerosing cholangitis or chronic hepatitis.

CROHN'S DISEASE. The symptoms and signs of CD also are determined by the site and extent of inflammation. Gastroduodenal CD mimics peptic ulcer disease, with nausea, vomiting, and epigastric pain. Patients with small intestinal involvement present with abdominal cramping, diarrhea, and abdominal tenderness. The pain and tenderness of CD are due to transmural inflammation. Transmural inflammation leads to fibrosis and narrowing of the intestinal lumen, which produce symptoms of obstruction: nausea, vomiting, waves of abdominal pain, and a reduced output of stool. This is appreciated as a thickened, tender loop of bowel or an abdominal mass, if the mesentery is involved. Patients with colonic CD present with abdominal pain, cramping or localized pain, rectal bleeding, and diarrhea.

Weight loss is more common in CD than in ulcerative colitis due to small bowel–related malabsorption or a reduced intake of food to minimize postprandial symptoms. Systemic symptoms, including fever, night sweats, malaise, and arthralgias, are common.

Laboratory features in CD reflect blood loss, malabsorption, protein-losing enteropathy, and elevation of acute phase reactants. Anemia may be due to iron deficiency (blood loss or malabsorption), folic acid deficiency, or vitamin B_{12} deficiency. Serum albumin and total protein are reduced with either malnutrition or protein-losing enteropathy. Electrolyte abnormalities reflect the severity of diarrhea, and lowered serum calcium may reflect reduced serum albumin, calcium malabsorption, or vitamin D deficiency. Patients with ileal disease often malabsorb fat-soluble vitamins (A, D, E, and K), deficiency of which can produce clinically significant symptoms or signs.

COMPLICATIONS

INTESTINAL COMPLICATIONS. *Rectal bleeding* is a common manifestation of both UC and CD. In UC the superficial inflammation induces capillary hemorrhage, manifested as bright red coating of stool or blood-tinged mucopus. In severe UC the bleeding can be more prominent and on rare occasions is profuse. Iron deficiency anemia is a common secondary association due to the chronic blood loss. In CD, hemorrhage may be profuse as a result of deeper inflammation and ulceration into larger vessels. Recurrent bleeding occurs in a small subset of patients with CD and is sometimes the single indication for surgery.

Toxic megacolon, once thought only to occur with UC, also occurs in CD and infectious colitis. Toxic megacolon develops in seriously ill individuals when transmural inflammation extends into the muscular layer, thinning the intestinal wall. The entire colon, or segments of the colon, can dilate as a result of disruption of the neural and muscular elements that maintain normal tone. Dilatation of the diameter of the colon on a plain abdominal radiograph to greater than 6 cm (see Color Plate 2*H*), associated with clinical symptoms of increasing abdominal pain, distention, rebound tenderness, and signs of fever, tachycardia, dehydration, and a reduction in bowel sounds, is diagnostic of toxic megacolon. Even in the absence of prominent dilatation, similar symptoms and signs are sufficient to diagnose severe colitis with an identical risk of perforation and the hazard of peritonitis. Precipitating circumstances include severe colitis, instrumentation with barium studies or endoscopic procedures in severe inflammation, potassium depletion, anticholinergic medications, or narcotics, which are thought to reduce neuromuscular activity of the gut. Associated laboratory findings include leukocytosis, hypokalemia, anemia, and hypoalbuminemia.

Toxic megacolon should be anticipated in any patient with severe colitis, including segmental colitis, and these individuals require careful monitoring of vital signs, abdominal examinations for rebound tenderness, flat-plate abdominal radiographs for dilatation or free air, and laboratory studies to maintain an adequate hematocrit and electrolyte status. Toxic megacolon should be treated with intensive medical therapy, and failure to improve within 12 to 24 hours is an indication for colectomy.

Early colectomy can prevent the morbidity and mortality of a perforation, which may exceed 20 per cent.

Crohn's disease, being transmural, is associated with additional intestinal complications. Thickened segments of inflamed bowel become fibrotic, and stricturing is common. Whereas bowel narrowing in UC is due to reversible muscular hypertrophy, the scarring in CD is largely irreversible. Transmural fissures extend into adjacent structures, producing an inflammatory mass, abscess, or fistula. Entero-enteric, -vesicular, -mesenteric, or -cutaneous fistulas are common, as are rectovaginal fistulas, perianal fistulas, and abscesses.

CANCER (Table 103–2, also Ch. 105). Cancer of the colon not infrequently complicates longstanding UC, depending upon two factors: the extent of mucosal involvement (pancolitis greater than left-sided colitis) and the duration of disease. Severity of the initial attack, subsequent course, and specific medical therapies are not related to the cancer risk. Colonic adenocarcinomas may occur in patients who have had quiescent UC for decades. Indeed, these may be the patients at highest risk. In European countries where colectomy is performed earlier, the risk of cancer is reduced.

Mucosal dysplasia is a precursor of cancer. Dysplasia can be identified with colonoscopic biopsies by experienced pathologists (see Color Plate 2*I*) and must be distinguished from inflammatory or regenerative epithelial changes. Repeat biopsies and aggressive medical therapy should be considered when there is doubt about pathologic interpretation. Confirmed epithelial dysplasia is an indication for colectomy, as malignancies are often identified separate from the dysplastic foci. Routine screening for dysplasia and neoplasia is now recommended in longstanding UC. Surveillance colonoscopies and biopsies throughout the length of the colon should be initiated after 8 to 10 years of extensive colitis and repeated at 1- to 2-year intervals. The finding of dysplasia warrants confirmation by an experienced pathologist or repeat examination. Dysplasia in a nodular or polypoid lesion has an extremely high (greater than 50 per cent) association with concurrent malignancy. Dysplasia and cancers in UC can occur in normal flat mucosa, with ulceration or stricture formation, or within a polyp or mass.

CD also increases the incidence of adenocarcinomas of the intestine. The same risk factors (extent and duration) probably apply but have not been as clearly established for CD. Patients with inactive CD should be monitored for a change in symptoms, bleeding, or obstruction; endoscopic or radiographic evaluation should be pursued for a change in an otherwise inactive phase. There is also a small increased risk of leukemia, lymphoma, and bile duct carcinomas in patients with IBD.

EXTRAINTESTINAL COMPLICATIONS (Table 103–3). The extraintestinal manifestations of IBD can be divided into complications of gastrointestinal inflammation or diseases associated with IBD. The latter occur most often with "colitis" but can occur in either UC or CD when the colon is inflamed.

Nutritional and metabolic abnormalities occur with chronic disease, inadequate intake of calories, maldigestion, and malabsorption. Blood and protein loss contribute to iron deficiency anemia and hypoalbuminemia. Deficiencies of calcium, magnesium, or zinc are most often noted with small intestinal CD in the presence of active inflammation or extensive surgical resections. Calcium deficiency may be aggravated by milk-free diets or vitamin D deficiency. Deficiency of folic acid can be secondary to inadequate intake, proximal small bowel disease, or competitive inhibition of folate absorption by sulfasalazine. Treatments for these nutritional deficiencies require appropriate diagnosis,

TABLE 103–2. CANCER IN ULCERATIVE COLITIS

Risk factors
 Extent of colon involved
 Duration of disease after 10 years

Surveillance
 Begin after 10 days
 Increase frequency of surveillance with increased duration of disease

Warning
 Dysplasia; low grade, low grade with mass, high grade; requires confirmation and follow-up in 3 to 6 months

Surgical indication
 Confirmed high-grade dysplasia, or dysplasia-associated lesion or mass (DALM)

TABLE 103–3. EXTRAINTESTINAL MANIFESTATIONS OF THE INFLAMMATORY BOWEL DISEASES

Nutritional and metabolic abnormalities
Weight loss, growth retardation in children
Hypoalbuminemia—nutritional, protein-losing enteropathy
Vitamin deficiencies*
Deficiencies of calcium, magnesium, or zinc*

Hematologic abnormalities
Anemia—Fe, folate, B_{12}* deficiency
Leukocytosis, thrombocytosis

Skin and mucous membranes
Pyoderma gangrenosum
Erythema nodosum
Stomatitis with multiple aphthous ulcers

Musculoskeletal
Ankylosing spondylitis, sacroiliitis (HLA-B27 associated)
Peripheral arthritis of large joints
Osteoporosis
Osteomalacia*

Hepatic and biliary manifestations
Fatty liver
Pericholangitis
Sclerosing cholangitis
Gallstones*
Carcinoma of the bile ducts

Renal complications
Kidney stones
  Uric acid
  Calcium oxalate*
Obstructive uropathy*
Fistulas to urinary tract*
Amyloidosis (rare)

Eye complications
Conjunctivitis, episcleritis, iritis
Uveitis (HLA-B27)

*Crohn's disease.

treatment of the underlying inflammation, and enteral or parenteral repletion. Deficiencies in fat-soluble vitamins (vitamins A, D, E, and K) are most often produced by ileal disease or resection. Low vitamin D levels can aggravate metabolic bone disease and calcium malabsorption. Vitamin B_{12} deficiency can be avoided by regular injections of intramuscular vitamin B_{12} (Ch. 132).

Diarrhea is aggravated by malabsorption of fat or bile salts due to ileal disease or resection. Diarrhea with fat malabsorption is diagnosed by increased fecal fat (greater than 5 grams per day) and treated with a low-fat diet (Ch. 101). Additional calories can be supplied by medium-chain triglycerides, which are absorbed more proximally and do not require bile salts. Ileal resection also can deplete the bile salt pool owing to inadequate reabsorption and recirculation. Bile salt malabsorption induces diarrhea after bile salts are converted into bile acids in the colon, which stimulate secretion. Bile acid–induced diarrhea can be treated with small amounts of cholestyramine, which binds to bile salts and prevents its conversion to bile acids. Malabsorption of fat and bile salts in Crohn's disease increases the incidence of gallstones and kidney stones. Gallstones form because cholesterol levels are more saturated in the gallbladder secondary to a reduced bile salt pool. Calcium oxalate kidney stones are increased by fat malabsorption (Ch. 102). Normally dietary oxalate binds to calcium within the lumen of the small intestine and is excreted as insoluble calcium oxalate in the feces. With fat malabsorption, calcium alternatively binds to long-chain fatty acids rather than to oxalate. Free oxalate is then abnormally absorbed from the colon and excreted in the urine as "enteric hyperoxaluria." In CD kidney stones are due more often to hyperabsorption of oxalate than to increased urinary excretion of calcium. In addition, patients with IBD have low levels of urinary citrate, a nonspecific solubilizer that reduces mineral saturation in the urine. The treatment of calcium oxalate kidney stones includes reduction of fat intake to reduce fat malabsorption; maintenance of fluid intake and hydration; a low-oxalate diet; supplementation of citrate; supplementation with oral calcium as

an intestinal oxalate binder; and the addition of cholestyramine as an alternative binder for intestinal oxalate. Enteric hyperoxaluria is discussed further in Ch. 88.

Skin and mucous membrane changes are common in IBD. Oral aphthae occur in CD, and fissuring of the lips or mouth may be due to zinc deficiency or *Candida* infection. Inflammatory skin disorders associated with IBD, pyoderma gangrenosum and erythema nodosum, tend to correlate with the disease activity in the colon, although, on occasion, skin changes may precede symptomatic colitis. Erythema nodosum presents usually as a painful, tender, erythematous, or violaceous nodule, most commonly on the leg. The lesions may be multiple, may develop on any extremity, and may be induced by minor trauma. Erythema nodosum usually responds to treatment of the underlying inflammation in the bowel but may respond more rapidly to topical or systemic steroids. Pyoderma gangrenosum, a more serious, necrotizing ulceration, occasionally runs an independent course from the intestinal inflammation. It also typically occurs on the lower extremities but can be noted anywhere on the skin and occasionally on surgical incisions or adjacent to a stoma. These lesions should not be biopsied, since this may lead to cutaneous breakdown and ulceration. Effective treatment of the underlying IBD, as well as topical antibiotics and potent topical steroids, should be implemented immediately. Systemic steroids may be necessary; pyoderma gangrenosum also responds to oral sulfone therapy. On rare occasions resection of the active IBD is necessary to prevent progressive skin breakdown from extending into muscle or, rarely, into bone.

Ocular complications of IBD share many inflammatory components with the intestinal inflammation. Conjunctivitis, episcleritis, and iritis often occur in conjunction with active intestinal inflammation and respond to topical steroids. Uveitis, an HLA-B27–associated complication, may run an independent course from the IBD.

Hepatic and biliary complications of IBD are frequent. Gallstones are related to bile salt malabsorption in Crohn's disease, and steatosis may be secondary to malnutrition, corticosteroid therapy, or excessive parenteral carbohydrates from total parenteral nutrition solution. There is a spectrum of bile duct inflammation ranging from pericholangitis to sclerosing cholangitis and associated biliary cirrhosis. Pericholangitis (portal triaditis) is a nonprogressive inflammation of intrahepatic bile ductules manifested as a minor elevation of the alkaline phosphatase and GGTP with minimal elevation of the serum transaminases. Bilirubin remains normal, and inflammation is confined to the portal triads. Sclerosing cholangitis is a progressive form of bile duct inflammation involving the intrahepatic and/or extrahepatic biliary tree. Elevations of serum alkaline phosphatase and GGTP are greater than two times normal, and transaminase elevation can occur. Intermittent cholangitic episodes or asymptomatic jaundice may be the first manifestation. Visualization of the biliary tree via ERCP or transhepatic cholangiography confirms the extent of bile duct abnormalities. There are no proven therapies to limit the biliary inflammation, although preliminary studies using ursodeoxycholic acid or methotrexate are encouraging. Occasionally, endoscopic dilatation of a prominent stricture can relieve obstruction, although the disease is typically multifocal. Rarely, carcinoma of the bile duct mimics sclerosing cholangitis limited to the extrahepatic biliary system.

Kidney stones are a common complication of IBD. Hyperoxaluria and calcium oxalate stones are related to steatorrhea, whereas uric acid stones are more commonly associated with dehydration in patients with diarrhea or ileostomies. Obstructive uropathies can occur as a complication of an inflammatory mass. Fistula to the bladder occurs frequently with ileal CD in association with ileo-sigmoid-bladder communication, manifested as urinary frequency, dysuria, sterile pyuria, or recurrent cystitis. Amyloidosis is a rare, occasionally reversible complication of longstanding intestinal inflammation.

The metabolic bone diseases, osteoporosis and osteomalacia, occur commonly in chronic IBD. Osteoporosis is a frequent complication of long-term steroid therapy. Reduced bone mineralization also is a complication of malabsorption of vitamin D and calcium. Clubbing of the fingers and two distinct syndromes of enteric arthropathy may occur: (1) Peripheral arthritis frequently involves larger joints (knees, elbows, ankles) in an asymmetric fashion with swelling, erythema, and an inflammatory synovial analysis. It precedes or coincides with bowel symptoms and usually responds to treatment of the intestinal inflammation. Joint destruction does not occur, and serologic studies for rheumatoid factors are negative. (2) Central arthritis of the spine, ankylosing spondylitis, and sacroiliitis are HLA-B27–associated arthropathies that run an independent course from the bowel disorders. Progressive calcification and joint fusion proceed despite treatment of the IBD and require independent therapy (physical therapy and anti-inflammatory drugs). Nonsteroidal anti-inflammatory drugs must be used with caution in patients with IBD because of the potential for aggravating intestinal inflammation while attempting to treat arthritic symptoms.

Children are susceptible to several unique complications of IBD. Often the initial manifestations of IBD in children occur without intestinal symptoms. Growth retardation, delayed sexual maturation, peripheral arthritis, fevers of undetermined origin, or anemia can precede abdominal symptoms. Impairments of growth and development usually are associated with inadequate nutritional status. Improved caloric intake can reverse growth failure in conjunction with treatment of intestinal inflammation. Surgical resection is sometimes necessary to reverse growth failure. Children also are susceptible to delayed psychological development because of chronic illness and may require additional supportive therapy from the physician and other health care providers. Family counseling can also provide an important service for the patient and family.

Fertility, pregnancy, and lactation are important aspects for young adults with IBD. In general, IBD does not reduce fertility. Women with active IBD or high-dose steroid therapy, however, often have anovulatory menstrual cycles or secondary amenorrhea, which temporarily impairs fertility. Women with active IBD are more likely to miscarry, but usually fetal development is normal in those carried to term. Medicinal and nutritional support for the pregnant woman should be continued throughout pregnancy. Corticosteroids and sulfasalazine should not be discontinued if they are successful in managing the mother's intestinal symptoms. Occasionally, total parenteral nutrition may be necessary to supply adequate calories. Metronidazole and immunosuppressive agents are not recommended during pregnancy. Immunosuppressive therapies have been used with success in patients following transplantation and in several patients with IBD. Approximately one third of women with quiescent IBD experience flare-ups during the postpartum period. Corticosteroids and sulfasalazine are secreted in small quantities in breast milk, but nursing is generally safe during their use.

DIAGNOSIS

There are no pathognomonic clinical, endoscopic, or histologic features of the idiopathic IBD's. The physician must therefore consider the entire clinical picture and the evolution of the illness. It is particularly important to exclude other disorders that may mimic the broad range of symptoms and findings that may be present in IBD. It is important first of all to establish the presence of intestinal inflammation. A cardinal feature is the exudation of inflammatory cells into the lumen, reflected in the presence of fecal leukocytes or red blood cells on examination of the stool. Symptoms of rectal bleeding, tenesmus associated with the passage of pus, nocturnal pain and diarrhea, fever, night sweats, weight loss, or extraintestinal symptoms or signs generally exclude an uncomplicated "irritable bowel syndrome." The presence of anemia, electrolyte disorders, hypoalbuminemia, or an elevated erythrocyte sedimentation rate or C-reactive protein is sufficient, but not necessary, to suggest IBD. On physical examination, evidence of significant weight loss or extraintestinal signs, a palpable abdominal mass or tenderness, or significant perianal disease suggests IBD. When suspicion of the diagnosis warrants, endoscopic and radiographic studies, in conjunction with histologic interpretation of biopsy specimens, confirm the diagnosis. The degree of illness at the time of presentation should determine the aggressiveness of the diagnostic workup. Acutely ill patients should be stabilized before invasive studies are pursued.

ENDOSCOPY. Patients presenting with colitic symptoms of rectal bleeding, cramping, tenesmus, mucopus, or watery diarrhea in conjunction with fecal leukocytes warrant a colonic examination. A proctoscopic examination or flexible sigmoidoscopy reveals the presence and pattern of distal colonic inflammation. In the absence of perianal disease, diffuse, continuous mucosal changes with a distinct upper boundary to adjacent normal-appearing mucosa are typical of ulcerative proctitis or proctosigmoiditis. Focal inflammation with aphthoid ulcers, linear or stellate ulcers with normal intervening mucosa, or inflammatory changes beginning above the rectum (rectal sparing) in previously untreated patients suggest Crohn's disease. If the patient is not acutely ill, colonoscopy demonstrates more proximal colonic changes and allows examination and intubation of the ileocecal valve to evaluate terminal ileal findings. Patients with upper abdominal symptoms can be diagnosed with upper gastrointestinal endoscopy when typical mucosal changes of Crohn's disease involve this area. Findings can be correlated with mucosal biopsy studies and radiographic evaluation of the small and large intestine.

RADIOGRAPHY. Radiographic examination should begin with a supine and upright view of the abdomen. Associated findings of nephrolithiasis, cholelithiasis, or arthritis of the spine or sacroiliac joints may be identified. Intestinal dilatation or air-fluid levels suggesting obstruction preclude aggressive barium studies until the patient's clinical condition is stabilized. In colitis, a plain view of the abdomen often demonstrates a tubular, ahaustral segment of colon in the presence of distal UC with fecal matter proximal to diseased mucosa. Intestinal edema, ulceration, or thumb-printing may give a gross estimate of disease activity. Air-contrast barium studies of the colon reveal diffuse, contiguous granularity, superficial ulceration, and absent haustration in active UC (see Color Plate 2J). Pseudopolyps or a tubular-appearing "lead pipe" colon may be found in chronic UC. Focal, asymmetric ulceration with linear or fissuring ulcers, the presence of fistulas, rectal sparing, or a diseased terminal ileum with reflux of the barium defines the radiographic extent and severity of colonic CD (see Color Plate 3A). A small bowel follow-through or enteroclysis (small bowel enema) demonstrates the extent of small intestinal involvement in CD (see Color Plate 3B) and is normal in the absence of backwash ileitis in UC.

Specialized diagnostic imaging studies are occasionally useful to diagnosis the extent or complications of IBD. Ultrasonography or a computed tomography (CT) examination can clarify the presence of thickened bowel wall and mesentery versus an abscess cavity in an abdominal mass. Perineal CT scan or rectal ultrasonography demonstrates the degree of perianal involvement and the complexity of anorectal fistulas. Occasionally, ultrasound- or CT-guided aspiration of a cavity can reduce the morbidity of abdominal or retroperitoneal suppuration. Injected indium- or technetium-labeled leukocytes localize in sites of intestinal inflammation, and fecal excretion of radiolabeled leukocytes can be a measure of inflammatory activity.

DIFFERENTIAL DIAGNOSIS. Patients with irritable bowel syndrome rarely present with "inflammatory" features. Persistent symptoms despite therapy for presumed irritable bowel syndrome, especially in the presence of weight loss, bleeding attributed to "hemorrhoids," or a family history of IBD, deserve a more comprehensive evaluation to exclude IBD. Most enteric infections are self-limited. Viral gastroenteritis typically lasts 1 to 4 days without the presence of rectal bleeding or fecal leukocytes. Most bacterial pathogens produce self-limited disease lasting less than 7 to 14 days, despite the presence of intermittent rectal bleeding, fevers, fecal leukocytes, and a mucosal appearance that may be indistinguishable from that of UC or CD. Occasionally, *Campylobacter jejuni* produces protracted symptoms (Ch. 316), and *Clostridium difficile* toxin–induced colitis can mimic the symptoms, signs, and endoscopic appearance of UC or CD (Ch. 308). When a patient with IBD presents with new or exacerbated symptoms, stool cultures for enteric pathogens and studies for *Clostridium difficile* toxin should be obtained, especially if the patient has been recently treated with antibiotics. In Northern Europe and Canada, *Yersinia enterocolitica* infection can mimic terminal ileitis (Ch. 321). If the clinical suspicion warrants, cultures and serologic studies for *Yersinia* should be obtained. Similarly, tuberculosis of the gastrointestinal tract may mimic CD in areas where intestinal tuberculosis is endemic, and, rarely, *actinomycosis* simulates fistulizing CD.

TABLE 103–4. COMPARISON OF CLINICAL AND PATHOLOGIC FEATURES OF CROHN'S COLITIS AND ULCERATIVE COLITIS

Feature	Crohn's Colitis	Ulcerative Colitis
Clinical		
Smoker	+ +	+/−
Malaise, fever	+ +	+
Rectal bleeding	+ +	+ + +
Abdominal tenderness	+ +	−
Abdominal mass	+ +	−
Abdominal pain	− + +	+
Perianal disease	+ + +	−
Endoscopic		
Rectal disease	+	+ + +
Diffuse, continuous, symmetric involvement	+	+ + +
Aphthous or linear ulcers	+ +	−
Cobblestoning	+ +	−
Friability	+ +	+ + +
Radiologic		
Continuous disease	+	+ + +
Ileal involvement	+ +	−
Asymmetry	+ + +	−
Strictures	+ +	+
Fistulas	+ +	−
Pathologic		
Discontinuity	+ +	−
Transmural involvement	+ + +	+/−
Lymphoid aggregates	+ + +	−
Crypt abscesses	+ + +	+ + +
Granulomas	+ +	−
Sinus tract/fistula	+ + +	−

+ + + = Always
+ + = Common
+ = Occasional
− = Never

Chronic intestinal infections usually are parasitic. Amebiasis may present with diarrhea, rectal bleeding, and a sigmoidoscopic appearance similar to that of idiopathic IBD (Ch. 431). Deep "collar button" ulcerations are similar to focal ulcerations of CD. Fresh stool specimens should be examined repeatedly for amebic cysts or trophozoites; and biopsies may be indicated in patients who have been exposed to endemic environments (including nursing homes and the homosexual population). Syphilis, gonorrhea, and lymphogranuloma venereum also induce proctitis in the gay population. HIV diarrhea should be excluded by serologic studies in patients with suspected exposure.

Occasionally, with an acute onset, Crohn's ileitis is diagnosed at laparotomy performed for presumed appendicitis. Likewise, in young individuals with acute right lower quadrant pain, mesenteric adenitis may mimic the symptoms of CD. In the older population, ischemic bowel disease, especially chronic mesenteric ischemia, or recurrent diverticulitis can mimic Crohn's colitis.

Persistent rectal bleeding should not be attributed to hemorrhoids unless a flexible sigmoidoscopy has excluded IBD (Ch. 94). In the older population, colonic carcinomas also can present with chronic symptoms and intermittent rectal bleeding (Ch. 111). Intestinal lymphoma may be very difficult to distinguish from CD and often requires a surgical diagnosis when suspected. Radiation enteritis is limited to patients with a history of that therapy. Some patients receiving chemotherapy or gold develop diarrhea and mucosal ulceration. Nonsteroidal anti-inflammatory drug–induced ulceration of the ileum and colon mimics the aphthous ulcers of CD. Eosinophilic gastroenteritis presents with diarrhea, malabsorption, and protein-losing enteropathy, but the associated peripheral blood eosinophilia and biopsies are distinguishing. The diffuse, proximal malabsorptive pattern of celiac sprue, associated with diffuse villous atrophy, is distinct from the focal, distal small bowel changes of CD. Table 103–4 outlines the distinguishing features between UC and CD confined to the colon.

TREATMENT

The therapy of either UC or CD depends upon the extent and severity of intestinal involvement (Table 103–5). The patient/physician team must embark upon treatment with due consideration of the entire clinical picture and the chronic nature of the illness. Both the patient and the family should participate in the decision making, and this requires education and support. Although the therapies for UC and CD overlap in many ways, they are considered separately to clarify the differences. A primary difference is that UC can be cured by removing the colon and all colonic mucosa. CD is not cured by surgery and has a predictable tendency to recur after removal of an involved segment of intestine. Medical alternatives are discussed first, followed by specific IBD syndromes.

Medical Alternatives

SULFASALAZINE AND MESALAMINE. Sulfasalazine was developed 50 years ago to combine a known antibiotic (sulfapyridine) with a salicylate (5-aminosalicylic acid, mesalamine) for delivery into the connective tissue of the colon. It is now recognized that the azo bond between sulfapyridine and 5-aminosalicylic acid is split by colonic bacteria, releasing both separate components in the colon. The majority of the sulfapyridine is absorbed from the colon, acetylated by the liver in a genetically determined fashion, and excreted in the urine. The majority of the mesalamine remains within the colon and is excreted within the feces. Mesalamine delivered into the colon has therapeutic efficacy similar to that of sulfasalazine, but without the potential adverse consequences of the sulfa moiety.

Sulfasalazine is effective in a dose-dependent manner for the treatment of acute UC and for maintaining remission of quiescent UC. Sulfasalazine also has been effective for mild to moderate CD when the colon is involved. It has not been clearly shown that sulfasalazine maintains a remission in CD, although patients with CD who respond symptomatically to sulfasalazine may have flare-ups when the drug is discontinued.

Many patients develop side effects from sulfasalazine before achieving therapeutic doses. Nausea, malaise, headache, and myalgias are common side effects that reduce patient compliance. Sulfa-induced hemolysis, allergic reactions, and toxic pancreatitis, pneumonitis, hepatitis, or colitis are rare, but reversible abnormalities of sperm motility and morphology are seen in up to 80 per cent of males taking sulfasalazine. Sulfasalazine also competitively inhibits intestinal absorption of folate, occasionally producing folate deficiency (Ch. 132). Folic acid supplementation (1 mg daily) is therefore recommended for patients on long-term therapy. Sulfasalazine seems to be safe for both the mother and the infant during pregnancy and with breast feeding.

Because 5-ASA (mesalamine) is an active moiety of sulfasala-

TABLE 103–5. INFLAMMATORY BOWEL DISEASE: SEVERITY CRITERIA

	Mild	Severe	Fulminant / Toxic
Bowel frequency	<4/day	>6/day	>10/day
Blood in stool	+/−	+ +	Continuous
Fever	Normal	>37.5° C	>37.5° C
Pulse	Normal	>90/min	>90/min
Hemoglobin	Normal	<75%	Transfusion required
Erythrocyte sedimentation rate	<30 mm/hr	>30 mm/hr	>30 mm/hr
Abdominal radiograph	Normal	Colonic edema, thumb-printing, air-fluid levels	Dilated colon or small bowel
Clinical sign		Abdominal tenderness	Rebound tenderness, distention, diminished bowel sounds

TABLE 103–6. ULCERATIVE COLITIS: MEDICAL THERAPY

Therapy	Mild/Moderate	Severe*	Fulminant*	Maintenance
Diet	Symptomatic	PO + PN	NPO/TPN	Symptomatic
Oral anti-inflammatory				
Sulfasalazine	2–6 g/day	2–6 g/day	—	2–4 g/day
Olsalazine	1.5–3.0 g/day	1.5–3.0 g/day	—	0.75–1.5 g/day
Mesalamine	1.5–4.8 g/day	1.5–4.8 g/day	—	1.5–3.0 g/day
Topical anti-inflammatory				
Mesalamine enema or suppository	1–4 g/day	—	—	—
Corticosteroid enema or foam	80–200 mg/day	100–200 mg/day	—	—
Systemic anti-inflammatory†				
Prednisone	20–60 mg/day	40–60 mg/day IV	40–60 mg/day	—
ACTH	—	80–120 U/day IV	80–120 U/day	—
Antibiotics	—	—	+	—
Surgical consultation	—	+	+ +	

*Avoid anticholinergics, antidiarrheals, narcotics, and invasive procedures.
†Not warranted for proctitis.

zine, topical mesalamine has been used as a substitute for sulfasalazine in the treatment of distal colitis. Mesalamine enemas are effective for active UC confined to the left colon when administered nightly, and they prolong remissions of left-sided UC if therapy is maintained. Mesalamine suppositories (500 mg administered two to three times daily) are also effective for ulcerative proctitis, and nightly therapy with 500-mg suppositories maintains remissions.

Free mesalamine is rapidly absorbed from the proximal gastrointestinal tract. Several delayed or sustained-release preparations are currently under development in the United States. Asacol, which contains 400 mg of mesalamine coated with a resin that breaks down at pH 7, supplies the same amount of mesalamine present in 1 gram of sulfasalazine. Pentasa, which contains mesalamine encapsulated into microgranules of ethylcellulose, releases mesalamine throughout the small and large intestine. Dipentum (olsalazine), an azo-bonded dimer of two 5-ASA molecules, releases two molecules of mesalamine in the colon in a manner similar to that of sulfasalazine.

Mesalamine has fewer side effects than sulfasalazine. Except for topical therapy with mesalamine enemas in distal UC, mesalamine has no therapeutic advantage over sulfasalazine. Mesalamine preparations are tolerated in 80 per cent of patients who cannot tolerate sulfasalazine. The sperm abnormalities associated with sulfasalazine are reversed when the patient is transferred to mesalamine treatment. Olsalazine may increase intestinal secretion to produce diarrhea that is sufficiently severe to stop therapy in approximately 6 per cent of patients. Diarrhea can be minimized or avoided by gradual titration of the therapeutic doses.

CORTICOSTEROIDS. Corticosteroids are indicated for the induction of remission in either UC or CD, but they should not be used for maintenance therapy because of their inability to prevent relapse and their associated side effects (Ch. 27). In UC, hydrocortisone enemas are useful for the treatment of distal colonic symptoms, and cortisone acetate foam can be applied for the relief of rectal inflammation. Oral prednisone is indicated for moderate to severe UC at doses of 40 mg daily initially, followed by gradual tapering according to the clinical course. Severe UC should be treated with parenteral corticosteroids in intravenous daily doses comparable to 40 mg of prednisone. Alternatively, intravenous ACTH may be administered for patients who have not previously received steroid therapy. In CD, corticosteroids are useful in similar doses for acute disease and, again, are not recommended for maintenance therapy.

Corticosteroid therapy is also limited by its well-recognized adverse effects. Cushingoid features, acne, facial hair, and elevations of blood pressure are common early side effects. Cataract formation, osteoporosis (aggravated by vitamin D deficiency and calcium malabsorption in CD), and aseptic necrosis limit high-dose or long-term therapy. In children, corticosteroid therapy may further aggravate growth retardation.

ANTIBIOTICS. Antibiotic therapy for UC is limited to the presurgical treatment of severe or toxic colitis. Antibiotics have not been useful for less severe UC or to prevent relapse. In CD, metronidazole is as effective as sulfasalazine for colonic CD and

may be more beneficial for small intestinal disease and perianal complications of CD. Metronidazole (10 to 20 mg per kilogram administered orally in divided doses) can relieve symptoms of CD, reduce acute phase reactants, and heal perianal disease. Metronidazole therapy is limited by coating of the tongue, nausea, alcohol intolerance, and peripheral neuropathy. The latter may be most troublesome, with documented abnormalities on neurologic examination and nerve conduction studies before clinical symptoms arise. Alternative antibiotics have not been adequately studied in CD, although many clinicians continue to use broad-spectrum antibiotics, such as tetracycline, sulfa-trimethoprim, or cephalexin, for symptomatic therapy of mild to moderate CD.

IMMUNOSUPPRESSIVES. 6-Mercaptopurine and azathioprine are effective in the long-term therapy of UC and CD. In both settings, these agents are useful in doses (50 to 150 mg per day) that are not immunosuppressive but probably have anti-inflammatory activity. There has been a reluctance to use these agents in UC because immunosuppressives have been found to be carcinogenic in patients who have received organ transplants. These medications, which require 3 to 6 months to have a maximal therapeutic effect, are largely useful for patients who are steroid-dependent, for disease refractory to standard medical therapies, for the healing of some intestinal and perianal fistulas, and possibly for maintenance therapy for patients who fail treatment or who cannot tolerate mesalamine. Allergic pancreatitis occurs in up to 15 per cent of patients receiving these drugs (Ch. 106). Blood counts should be monitored for the risk of neutropenia, although this is rarely found in patients receiving low-dose therapy for IBD. Immunosuppressives are not recommended during pregnancy, and the long-term potential carcinogenic effects should limit therapy to the above-stated indications.

Specific Syndromes

ULCERATIVE COLITIS

The medical therapy of UC depends upon the extent and severity of mucosal ulceration. It is advisable early in the course to define the colonic extent of disease with either colonoscopy or a combination of proctosigmoidoscopy and air-contrast barium enema. The treatment of UC can be divided into that for acute disease and that for maintaining remission (Table 103–6). Maintenance therapy is indicated because 80 per cent of patients who are seen to improve by endoscopic or histologic examination experience an exacerbation of their disease within a year after cessation of active therapy.

ULCERATIVE PROCTITIS. Mild ulcerative proctitis can be treated with topical corticosteroids or topical mesalamine. Hydrocortisone enemas (Cortenema) or cortisone acetate foam (Cortifoam), administered intrarectally at night, generally provides prompt relief. Patients should be treated until the symptoms resolve and the mucosa has healed (absence of granularity, friability, and mucopus at proctoscopy). After healing, the topical corticosteroids should be discontinued and used intermittently for mild relapses, or oral mesalamine* should be substituted for

---

*For purposes of discussion, sulfasalazine, olsalazine, and mesalamine preparations are all included as "mesalamine."

maintenance therapy. Some patients prefer oral mesalamine therapy as initial treatment for mild disease. Patients with more severe symptoms of proctitis with profound urgency, tenesmus, and frequent stooling may require a combination of topical corticosteroids and oral mesalamine or a combination of oral and topical mesalamine. Rarely, systemically active steroids are required for distal proctitis.

PROCTOSIGMOIDITIS. Proctosigmoiditis also responds to hydrocortisone or mesalamine enemas but more often requires combination therapy with oral mesalamine. Patients with severe symptoms require oral corticosteroids at a dose equivalent to 40 mg of prednisone daily. As the inflammation resolves and the mucosa heals, the steroids should be tapered with maintenance by either oral or topical mesalamine. Steroids generally can be withdrawn according to the acuteness of symptoms. A reduction by 5 to 10 mg per week from 40 down to 20 mg, followed by a reduction of 2.5 mg per week, is a reasonable approach that should be modified according to the individual's response. Again, mesalamine maintenance therapy is beneficial.

EXTENSIVE COLITIS. Patients with extensive colitis but mild symptoms should be treated with oral mesalamine. More severe symptoms (e.g., greater than 5 to 10 bowel movements per day, weight loss, abdominal tenderness, night sweats) require the addition of corticosteroids, with mesalamine as a maintenance therapy.

SEVERE COLITIS OR TOXIC MEGACOLON. Either of these conditions is a medical emergency. Patients presenting with more than 10 bowel movements per day accompanied by fever, leukocytosis, anemia, and tachycardia should be hospitalized. Appropriate fluid and electrolyte resuscitation should be instituted, and patients with significant anemia should receive transfusions to keep up with continued blood loss until the inflammation is stabilized. Patients who have not received prior corticosteroid therapy may be treated with parenteral ACTH or corticosteroids. Rectal application of steroid enemas or foam provides relief from severe tenesmus in conjunction with systemic steroids. Patients with a dilated colon should not be fed until their condition improves. Less severely ill patients may continue an oral intake of elemental feedings or a light diet, as tolerated, if there is no nausea or vomiting. Parenteral nutrition should be added for malnourished patients. Severely ill patients require constant monitoring because of the potential of toxic megacolon. Abdominal flat-plate examination should be performed at 12- to 24-hour intervals if there is evidence of colonic dilatation or any worsening. Patients with evidence of transmural disease, such as abdominal tenderness, fever, or leukocytosis, should receive broad-spectrum antibiotic treatment (e.g., metronidazole and an aminoglycoside) as if they had a bowel perforation. Failure to improve, evidence of rebound tenderness, or free air under the diaphragm requires surgical intervention.

MAINTENANCE THERAPY. Corticosteroids are not useful for the maintenance therapy of UC because they do not prevent relapse and they have many undesirable, long-term side effects. Sulfasalazine, olsalazine, and mesalamine are effective as maintenance therapies and should be continued "indefinitely" at the lowest dose that prevents relapse, with any withdrawal being carried out at a very gradual pace. Any recurrent symptoms require resumption of therapeutic doses.

SUPPORTIVE THERAPY. Dietary therapy has a limited role in the treatment of inflammation in UC, but diet should not be ignored as a symptomatic therapy. Patients who present with constipation improve with an increase in the fiber content of their diet. Patients with abdominal cramping or diarrhea have symptomatic improvement with a low-fiber diet with the exclusion of nonabsorbed carbohydrates (sorbitol, fructose, and lactose in lactose-intolerant patients). Iron replacement is necessary for patients with continued blood loss, and folic acid should be supplemented in patients taking sulfasalazine. In patients with mild disease, antispasmodics or antidiarrheal agents improve associated symptoms of bowel "irritability," but these should be used cautiously in severe disease because of the potential of inducing toxic megacolon.

SURGERY. UC can be cured by colectomy, which alleviates the symptoms, medication requirements, and potential long-term complications of colitis (cancer). Indications for surgery include toxic megacolon, perforation, intractable hemorrhage, complications of medical therapy, failure to improve with medical therapy, or evidence of confirmed dysplasia or cancer.

Surgical alternatives include proctocolectomy and ileostomy, which is the standard operation, or sphincter-saving operations, which remove the abdominal colon and rectal mucosa (saving the distal rectal musculature) and which create an ileal pouch and ileoanal anastomosis. This novel surgical approach is performed satisfactorily in two or three stages with an expected outcome of four to eight liquid bowel movements per day and full continence in 80 per cent of patients. The operation is limited to patients with confirmed UC and may be complicated by inflammation of the ileal pouch ("pouchitis"), which often requires therapy with metronidazole, sulfasalazine, or corticosteroids. The cause of pouchitis is not yet known, although it occurs only in patients with ileoanal anastomoses performed for IBD.

CROHN'S DISEASE

Medical therapy for CD must be individualized according to the disease location, severity, and complications. Unlike UC, nutritional therapies have a more prominent role in the treatment of CD and the prevention of complications. Furthermore, it has been difficult to prove any maintenance therapy effective in CD clinical trials. Corticosteroids should not be continued once clinical benefit has been obtained, because of their severe long-term sequelae and their lack of benefit in preventing relapse. Many patients who respond to sulfasalazine or mesalamine worsen upon withdrawal, and chronic therapy has a much larger benefit/risk ratio. Metronidazole has unique long-term toxicity (neuropathy), and other antibiotics can induce vitamin K deficiency or growth of *C. difficile*. Immunosuppressives have the best record in maintaining remission, but their long-term risks have not been established.

Symptomatic *gastroduodenal* CD is uncommon and usually responds to short-term corticosteroid therapy in conjunction with acid reduction with an H_2-receptor antagonist or omeprazole (Ch. 98.3). Gastric outlet obstruction unresponsive to corticosteroids requires surgical diversion with a gastrojejunostomy. *Jejunoileitis* often presents with diarrhea and protein-losing enteropathy. Mild symptoms respond to oral mesalamine or alternating antibiotics, which control associated small bowel bacterial overgrowth. Corticosteroids and an elemental diet have equal beneficial effects on persistent symptoms and laboratory studies, including albumin and acute phase reactants. Immunosuppressives are sometimes necessary for control of this diffuse form of small intestinal CD when steroids cannot be withdrawn. *Ileitis* and *ileocolitis* are more common variants of CD. Mild symptoms respond to adjustments in the diet to control diarrhea and abdominal cramping. If a low-residue diet is not sufficient, elemental feedings can be useful to reduce symptoms. Sulfasalazine, mesalamine, or antibiotics control mild symptoms, but patients presenting with fever, abdominal tenderness, or the presence of an inflammatory mass usually require short-term corticosteroids. Immunosuppressives or total parenteral nutrition can be useful for patients who cannot be tapered off steroids or who remain refractory with active disease. *Colonic* CD also responds to sulfasalazine, mesalamine, antibiotics, or, if necessary, corticosteroids. Immunosuppressives should be reserved for steroid-dependent or refractory patients.

NUTRITION IN CROHN'S DISEASE. The panenteric nature of CD can lead to a variety of nutritional deficiencies. Besides the enhanced requirements for iron due to blood loss and protein due to inflammatory exudation from the digestive tract, patients with small bowel CD who malabsorb calcium and magnesium, folic acid, and water-soluble vitamins require supplementation. Ileal CD requires monitoring and therapy for malabsorption of fat-soluble vitamins and vitamin B_{12}.

Some symptoms can be treated with dietary alterations, e.g., avoidance of fiber in patients with intestinal narrowing or diarrhea, the addition of fiber to patients who are constipated, avoidance of fat in patients with fat malabsorption, and avoidance of lactose for lactose-intolerance. Dietary modifications can also sometimes reduce the inflammatory features of CD. Elemental diets and corticosteroid therapy have equal therapeutic benefit. Elemental feedings can be administered by nasoenteric tube at night and are most beneficial for children with impaired growth. Total parenteral nutrition also benefits patients who cannot tolerate elemental feedings, who have a short bowel syndrome, or who have refractory symptoms despite medical therapy. Bowel rest does not affect the natural history of CD after therapy is discontinued.

SURGERY IN CROHN'S DISEASE. Active CD recurs at a predictable rate at the margins of a surgical resection. Virtually all patients develop some endoscopic and microscopic inflammation at an anastomotic site by 1 year after an operation. Usually, the course of a recurrence is similar to the initial manifestations; e.g., inflammatory or suppurative CD tends to recur as an inflammatory mass or fistula, whereas chronic, fibrosing CD recurs at a slower rate, evolving to intestinal obstruction. The recurrence rate is lower after exteriorization of the bowel with an ileostomy or colostomy than after reanastomosis.

Since surgery does not cure CD, the indications for surgery are for treatment of complications rather than as a "cure." Surgery is indicated for recurrent intestinal obstruction, complicated fistulas, intractable hemorrhage, disease refractory to medical therapy or complicated by inability to withdraw corticosteroids, growth retardation that does not respond to medical or nutritional intervention in children, or cancer. Unfortunately, the recurrence of CD cannot be prevented after resection, although mesalamine or immunosuppressives may possibly delay the time to recurrence.

PROGNOSIS

ULCERATIVE COLITIS. The course of UC depends upon the severity of the initial attack and the response to medical treatment. Fewer than 5 per cent of patients succumb to fulminant UC or require immediate colectomy, and a small percentage of patients have a single attack without recurrence. The majority of patients have periods of remission maintained by medical therapy interrupted by spontaneous, acute exacerbations induced by stress, intercurrent illness, pregnancy, infectious diarrhea, or the injudicious use of nonsteroidal anti-inflammatory drugs. Noncompliance or cessation of maintenance therapy may lead to recurrence. Approximately 15 per cent of patients have refractory UC with continuous symptoms, despite all attempts at medical therapy, and 20 per cent of patients in the United States require a colectomy at some time in their course.

Advances in medical and surgical therapies have greatly improved the prognosis for patients with UC. Patients who are properly managed rarely succumb to acute disease, and supportive long-term treatment can reduce chronic morbidity and mortality. Death, when it occurs, is usually due to complications of colonic perforation when surgery is deferred, to postoperative complications after colectomy, or to colonic carcinoma. The life expectancy after recovery from an initial attack of UC is no different from that of the general population. Long-term morbidity from UC is usually due to complications of medical therapy, especially when chronic corticosteroid therapy is required or abused. Changes in lifestyle may be required after colectomy and ileostomy, although, in general, there is an improvement in well-being after surgery undertaken for protracted or complicated illness. The long-term outcome of ileoanal anastomoses needs to be evaluated. By and large, patients who have undergone the sphincter-saving operations prefer to accommodate to frequent stooling and the occasional need for medical treatment of pouchitis rather than to life with a stoma.

CROHN'S DISEASE. The prognosis for CD depends upon the site and extent of intestinal involvement, as well as upon complications of the disease. Approximately 50 per cent of patients require surgical intervention, the risk being higher for patients with small intestinal disease than large bowel CD. Fifty per cent of patients undergoing an operation require a second operation, and 50 per cent of these, a third procedure. Periodic remissions and exacerbations are common, although disease-free intervals may extend for years or decades after surgery for chronic, fibrotic strictures. Relapses after acute inflammatory CD are more common and occur earlier. The tendency for recurrence is a frustrating psychosocial feature. Additionally, physical changes associated with surgical or medical therapy can greatly affect self-image, especially in adolescents or socially active patients. Perianal disease can be an especially troublesome feature.

Fortunately, recent advances in medical and supportive therapy have limited mortality in CD to that of the general population. Death usually occurs as a complication of surgical therapy, related to pulmonary emboli or sepsis. Morbidity, however, may be significant in patients requiring dietary modifications, frequent medical therapy, or recurrent surgeries or in individuals troubled by refractory diarrhea or perianal disease. The quality of life with CD is lower than with UC, often because of uncertainties related to recurrence after operations. Corticosteroid therapy adds significant morbidity to the long-term treatment of CD, and the increasing recognition of intestinal cancer as a long-term complication may have increasing significance as patients survive over longer intervals.

SUMMARY

Inflammatory bowel disease extracts a substantial cost in altered patient lifestyle and in regular, often intensive medical and surgical care. The outlook for patients with ulcerative colitis and Crohn's disease has improved steadily with advances in medical and surgical treatment, and further progress is anticipated as scientific advances in the understanding of the genetic influence on the gut immune response evolve. In the meantime, the treatment of patients with inflammatory bowel disease requires an optimistic physician working in conjunction with the patient and the family and with nursing, dietary, and psychosocial ancillary staff. Patient support groups and educational material from the Crohn's Disease and Colitis Foundation of America have offered substantial benefit to patients and their families.

Bayless TM: Current Therapy in Gastroenterology and Liver Disease. Philadelphia, B. C. Decker, Inc., Publishers, 1990. *Individual aspects of medical and surgical management are discussed by experts.*

Camilleri M, Proano M: Advances in the assessment of disease activity in inflammatory bowel disease. Mayo Clin Proc 64:800, 1989. *A review of methods of disease assessment.*

Ginsberg AL: Management of Inflammatory Bowel Disease. Gastroenterol Clin North Am 18(1):March, 1989. *Recent reference on inflammatory bowel disease.*

Hanauer SB, Kirsner JB: Inflammatory Bowel Disease: A Guide for Patients and Their Families. New York, Raven Press Publishers, 1985. *A helpful text for patient and family information.*

Hawthorne AB, Hawkey CJ: Immunosuppressive drugs in inflammatory bowel disease: A review of their mechanisms of efficacy and place in therapy. Drugs 38:267–288, 1989. *Discussion of immunosuppressives, possible mechanisms of action and efficacy.*

Peppercorn M: Therapy of Inflammatory Bowel Disease: New Medical and Surgical Approaches. New York, Marcel Dekker Publishers, 1990. *A thorough review of medical therapies for IBD.*

Riddell RH, Goldman H, Ransahoff DF, et al.: Dysplasia in inflammatory bowel disease: Standardized classification with provisional clinical implications. Human Pathol 14:931, 1983. *The outcome of a multispecialty work-group on classification and management of dysplasia and cancer in IBD.*

Shorter RG, Kirsner JB: Inflammatory Bowel Disease. 3rd ed. Philadelphia, Lea & Febiger, 1988. *A comprehensive, inclusive text covering all aspects of IBD.*

104 Vascular Diseases of the Intestine

James H. Grendell

ANATOMY, PHYSIOLOGY, AND PATHOPHYSIOLOGY OF THE MESENTERIC CIRCULATION

The intra-abdominal portions of the digestive tract receive their blood supply almost entirely from three relatively large arteries arising from the aorta. The anatomy of these vessels, including their anastomotic interrelationships and potential for collateral formation, determines the consequences of acute or chronic vascular occlusion.

The *celiac axis*, the most cephalad of the three major arteries, usually originates at a level between the twelfth thoracic and the first lumbar vertebrae, passing next to the median arcuate ligament of the diaphragm (Fig. 104–1). Its branches supply the liver and biliary structures (hepatic artery), the spleen (splenic artery), and the stomach (left gastric and gastroepiploic, short gastrics, and branches of the gastroduodenal, including the right gastroepiploic). The gastroduodenal artery gives rise to the superior

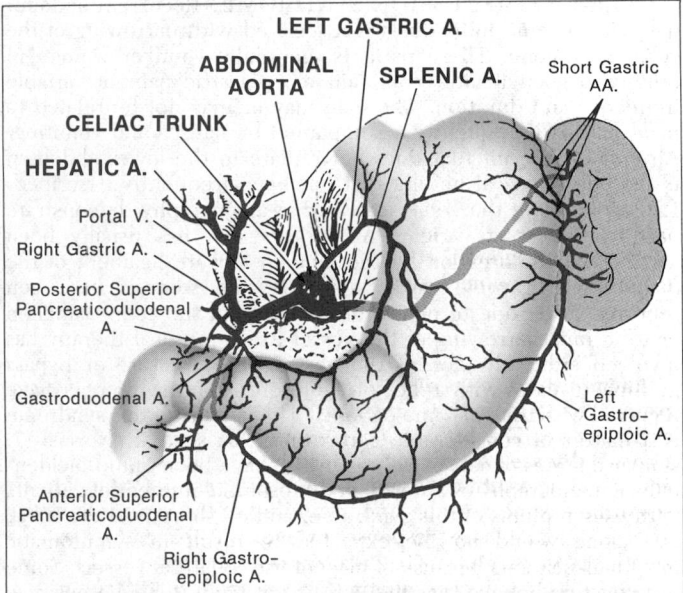

FIGURE 104–1. Arterial supply to the stomach and duodenum, showing major branches of the celiac axis and the superior portion of the pancreaticoduodenal arcades. (From Grendell JH, Ockner RK: *In* Sleisenger MH, Fordtran JS [eds.]: Gastrointestinal Disease. 3rd ed. Philadelphia, W. B. Saunders Company, 1983.)

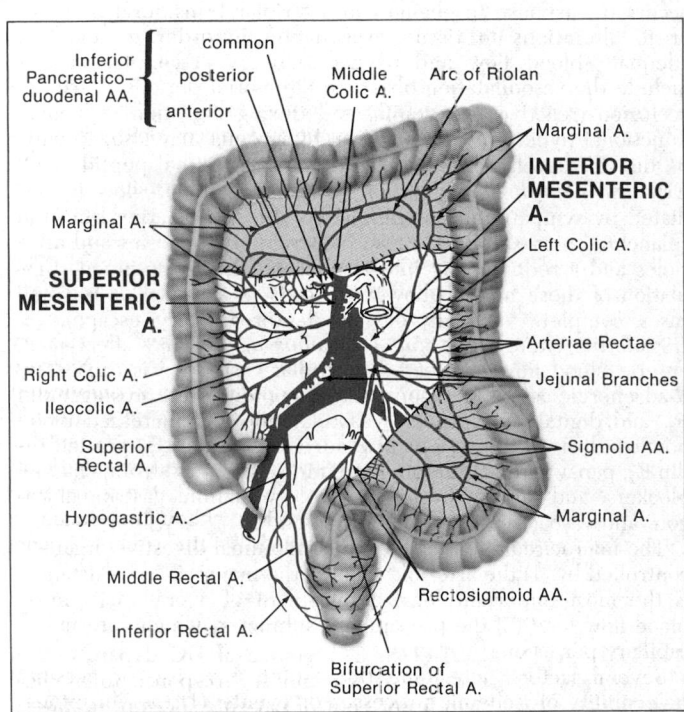

FIGURE 104–2. Arterial supply to the small and large intestines, showing the inferior portion of the pancreaticoduodenal arcades and the anastomoses between superior and inferior mesenteric arteries (arc of Riolan or "meandering mesenteric," and the marginal artery). (From Grendell JH, Ockner RK. *In* Sleisenger MH, Fordtran JS [eds.]: Gastrointestinal Disease. 3rd ed. Philadelphia, W. B. Saunders Company, 1983.)

pancreaticoduodenal arteries, which not only provide part of the blood supply to the pancreas and duodenum but also form anastomoses with the inferior pancreaticoduodenal arteries, which are derived from the superior mesenteric artery. These interconnections, the pancreaticoduodenal arcades, are an important potential route for collateral blood flow between the celiac and the superior mesenteric arteries.

The *superior mesenteric artery* originates behind the pancreas at the level of the first lumbar vertebra, just caudal to the celiac axis (Fig. 104–2). In addition to the inferior pancreaticoduodenal arteries, the superior mesenteric artery gives rise to branches supplying the small and large intestines from the distal duodenum to the distal transverse colon. These intestinal branches form a series of three or four arcades before entering the wall of the intestine as arteriae rectae. Although there is considerable potential for collateral flow within the primary and secondary arcades, the arteriae rectae appear to represent end-arteries, and few, if any, important anastomotic connections are present within the bowel wall itself. Accordingly, selective occlusion of these more distal vessels, as may occur in vasculitis, may lead to segmental infarction.

The *inferior mesenteric artery*, the smallest of the three major arteries, supplies the distal transverse colon, the descending and sigmoid colon, and the proximal portions of the rectum. Its branches form a series of arcades ending in arteriae rectae similar to what is found in the superior mesenteric artery's distribution. Branches of the inferior mesenteric artery connect with those of the superior mesenteric artery via the arc of Riolan ("meandering mesenteric artery") and the marginal artery (Fig. 104–2), and with the inferior and middle rectal branches of the hypogastric (internal iliac) arteries.

In general, veins parallel arteries in the smaller branches and for portions of the main mesenteric trunks (Fig. 104–3). However, rather than entering the vena cava directly, the superior mesenteric and splenic veins join to form the portal vein, which enters the liver after receiving additional blood from the gastric circulation via the coronary vein. The inferior mesenteric vein usually drains into the splenic vein.

The blood supply to the intra-abdominal portion of the gastrointestinal tract is richly endowed with anastomotic interconnections that help protect against the consequences of occlusive vascular disease. If the occlusive process is chronically progressive, these interconnections usually permit sufficient collateral flow to maintain intestinal viability. In fact, it is possible for *all* of the intra-abdominal digestive tract to be adequately supplied by only one of its three primary arterial sources. Conversely, the

collateral supply may be only marginally adequate or nonexistent in certain areas, such as the arteriae rectae and intramural arteries. Also potentially vulnerable are the "watershed" areas in the distal transverse colon and splenic flexure and at the junction of the superior and middle portions of the rectum, where branches of the inferior mesenteric artery anastomose with branches of the superior mesenteric and hypogastric arteries, respectively. This may, in part, explain why segmental infarction of the colon occurs most commonly in the region of the splenic flexure and rectosigmoid.

The *mesenteric circulation* is regulated by three different means: (1) *Intrinsic regulation* or local modulation of blood flow

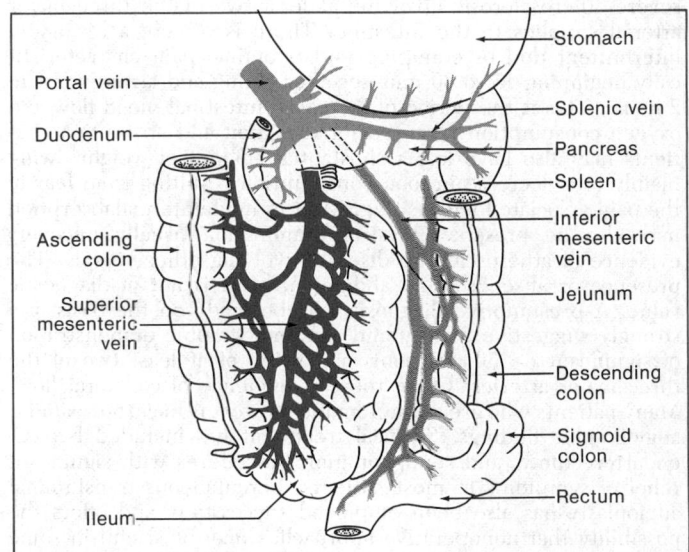

FIGURE 104–3. Venous drainage of the small intestine and colon showing the superior and inferior mesenteric veins, which, along with the splenic vein, constitute the major tributaries of the portal vein.

occurs in response to changes in arteriolar transmural pressure or to alterations in tissue oxygenation in order to maintain adequate blood flow and oxygen delivery. Examples of this include the vasodilatation observed after brief periods of arterial occlusion (reactive hyperemia) and during digestion of a meal (functional hyperemia). Functional hyperemia may also, in part, be due to the effects of regulatory gastrointestinal peptides. (2) *Extrinsic neurologic regulation* of intestinal blood flow is mediated by sympathetic postganglionic fibers originating from the splanchnic nerves, which cause constriction of arteries and arterioles and a reduction in intestinal blood flow. Continued stimulation of these nerves, however, leads to a partial or in some cases complete recovery of flow (autoregulatory escape). (3) *Circulating endogenous and exogenous agents* may affect mesenteric blood flow. Increased arteriolar resistance is caused by α-adrenergic agonists, vasopressin, angiotensin II, prostaglandin F_2, and digitalis glycosides. Vasodilatation and increased blood flow result from the actions of β-adrenergic agonists, prostaglandin E_2, papaverine, aminophylline, nitroglycerin, calcium channel blockers, and the gut hormones cholecystokinin, gastrin, glucagon, and vasoactive intestinal polypeptide.

The microcirculation of the intra-abdominal digestive organs is controlled by (1) the arteriole that, as the major site of resistance, is the most important local determinant of overall mesenteric blood flow, and (2) the precapillary sphincter, which determines capillary perfusion.

Several factors determine the extent, severity, or possible reversibility of ischemic processes or events: (1) the abruptness of a vascular occlusion; more gradually occlusive processes may permit development of collaterals; (2) size and configuration of a vessel; emboli most commonly enter the large, obliquely situated superior mesenteric artery; (3) the level of involvement of a localized occlusive process; vasculitis involving arteriae rectae or intramural arteries does not allow for development of collateral blood flow and may result in ischemia of a limited segment of intestine.

Intestinal ischemia may occur in hypoxic or low cardiac output states in the absence of an anatomic obstruction to blood flow (nonocclusive intestinal infarction). It is postulated that this may result from (1) the formation of toxic superoxide anions, (2) loss of the protective function of small intestinal brush border glycoproteins against the deleterious effects of luminal pancreatic proteases and bacterial toxins, or (3) shunting of oxygen from the villus tip caused by a countercurrent exhange resulting from the arrangement of blood vessels in the villus.

CHRONIC INTESTINAL ISCHEMIC SYNDROMES

ABDOMINAL ANGINA. This uncommon syndrome is due to severe atherosclerosis involving at least two of the three major arterial supplies to the intestine. There is usually a history of intermittent dull or cramping midabdominal pain characteristically beginning 15 to 30 minutes after eating and lasting for 1 to 2 hours. This is the period of increased intestinal blood flow and oxygen consumption required for digestion and absorption. Patients may also have lost a substantial amount of weight owing mainly to a decrease in food consumption resulting from fear of the pain associated with eating. Mild to moderate malabsorption may also be present. Physical examination usually uncovers evidence of atherosclerotic disease involving other vessels. The presence or absence of an abdominal bruit is not of diagnostic value. A presumptive diagnosis may be made on the basis of a strongly suggestive history and the angiographic demonstration of significant (> 50 per cent) narrowing of at least two of the three major arteries. Often there is evidence of collateral flow. Many patients who are asymptomatic, however, may show similar angiographic findings. Surgical treatment has included bypass, endarterectomy, and reimplantation procedures with significant relief of symptoms in most patients. Percutaneous transluminal angioplasty has also been employed successfully and offers the possibility that nonoperative approaches may be useful in some patients. As many as 50 per cent of patients with acute mesenteric arterial occlusion (see below) give a history suggestive of previous abdominal angina. Successful treatment of chronic intestinal ischemia may prevent such a catastrophic outcome.

CELIAC COMPRESSION SYNDROME. Recurrent abdominal pain in some individuals is associated with narrowing of the celiac axis alone. These patients, generally younger women in otherwise good health, complain of epigastric pain of variable frequency and duration. The pain may or may not be related to meals and is infrequently accompanied by nausea and vomiting. An epigastric bruit that does not radiate to the lower abdomen is the only physical finding that has been frequently described. Lateral views of the celiac axis during angiography demonstrate narrowing near its origin. At surgery this has usually been ascribed to compression by the median arcuate ligament of the diaphragm. In some cases, however, the stenosis has been reported to be due to neurofibrous tissue of the celiac ganglion or to intimal narrowing of the vessel itself. Surgical therapy has involved either division of the obstructing structure or bypass grafting, usually with relief of symptoms. The symptoms have recurred with time in some patients. The validity of this syndrome is a matter of considerable controversy for several reasons: (1) similar degrees of celiac axis narrowing have been found incidentally at angiography or autopsy in a substantial number of patients without symptoms of this syndrome, and (2) stenosis of the celiac axis alone would not be expected to result in symptomatic intestinal ischemia because of mesenteric collateral vessels. Some investigators believe that the pain is not truly ischemic but may arise in the celiac ganglion, which is removed or disrupted by most surgical treatments for this syndrome. In view of this controversy, surgery should be reserved for those patients with preoperative angiographic evidence of celiac stenosis who would otherwise undergo exploratory laparotomy for disabling and unexplained abdominal pain. At operation a thorough search for other disorders should precede treatment for presumed celiac compression syndrome.

CHRONIC RECTAL ISCHEMIA. A syndrome of rectal or sacral pain, at times associated with fecal incontinence, has been reported in some patients with occlusive disease involving both the inferior mesenteric artery *and* the internal iliac arteries.

ACUTE INTESTINAL ISCHEMIC SYNDROMES

ACUTE BOWEL INFARCTION: MESENTERIC ARTERIAL OCCLUSION. Gradual occlusion of one or sometimes even two of the three major mesenteric arteries may be asymptomatic because of the development of adequate collateral circulation. However, when intestinal blood flow falls below a critical level, ischemic necrosis of the supplied areas results. Most commonly this is due to advanced *atherosclerotic disease* affecting at least two of the major visceral branches of the aorta. Generally the most proximal segments of these arteries are most severely involved. In addition to *embolism*, which is discussed below, other causes of mesenteric arterial occlusion include dissecting *aortic aneurysm, fibromuscular hyperplasia*, and *systemic vasculitides*, which may involve the mesenteric arteries at any level from the major arterial trunks to the intramural arteries. An association has also been reported with the use of *oral contraceptives*.

Diagnosis. The early diagnosis of acute intestinal infarction is often difficult. The history usually is not very helpful, but evidence of "abdominal angina" (see above) or other conditions predisposing to thrombosis may aid in the evaluation. Patients frequently have *severe abdominal pain* that initially may be colicky in nature and periumbilical in location. Bowel sounds not only may be present but may even be hyperactive. At this stage the patient's complaint of pain often appears out of proportion to physical findings or laboratory studies. As ischemia progresses, pain becomes constant and poorly localized. Systemic manifestations become prominent and severe, including *tachycardia, hypotension, fever, leukocytosis, acidosis*, and the presence of *blood* in nasogastric aspirate, vomitus, or stool. It has been suggested that an elevation in serum and peritoneal fluid phosphate concentration may be a sensitive indicator of intestinal infarction. Because an elevation in serum phosphate concentration in this setting is often associated with extensive bowel injury, acute renal insufficiency, and acidosis, it implies a poor prognosis. Abdominal radiographs usually show evidence of an *ileus* with distended, thick-walled loops of bowel and air-fluid levels (Fig. 104–4). Gas in the intestinal wall or portal vein is a late finding. Ultimately, when ischemic necrosis becomes transmural, signs of

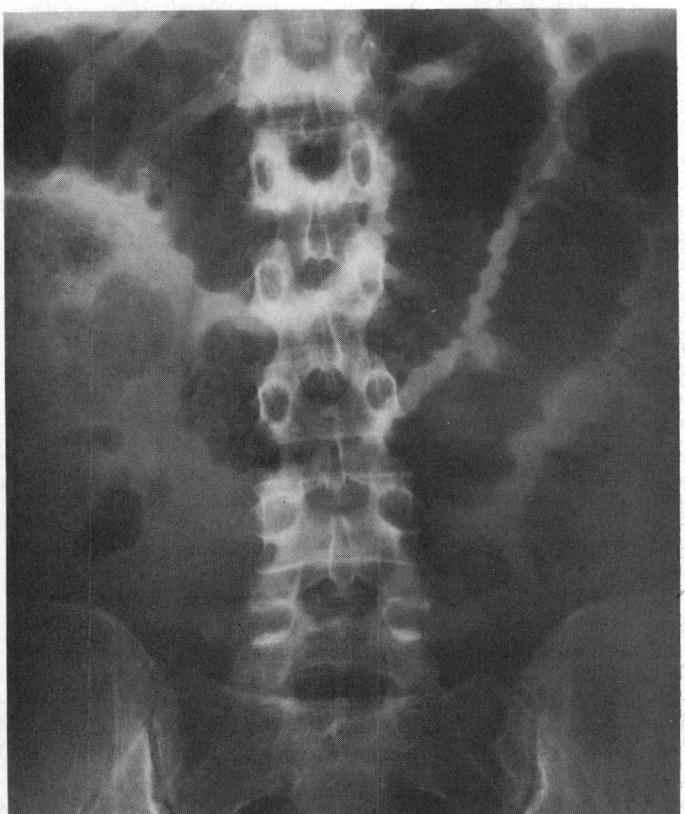

FIGURE 104–4. A supine abdominal radiograph in a patient with acute infarction of the small intestine showing dilated loops of small bowel with irregular thickening of the bowel wall.

peritonitis, including bloody peritoneal fluid, appear. At this point, the prognosis (with or without surgery) is extremely poor.

The early diagnosis of bowel infarction depends upon a high index of suspicion and exclusion of other intra-abdominal conditions that can manifest virtually identically (e.g., acute pancreatitis, perforated viscus, bowel obstruction). A decision regarding extensive radiographic studies, especially angiography, in patients with suspected bowel infarction must be individualized. For the patient in whom hypotension, acidosis, or signs of peritonitis are present, suggesting that perforation may have already occurred, the information to be obtained from further studies may not justify the necessary delay in surgical management. However, earlier in the course, angiography may help define the nature and extent of the occlusive process or, in the absence of major vessel occlusion, suggest the diagnosis of nonocclusive infarction. Interpretation, however, is often difficult, and clinical judgment is based only in part on angiographic findings. Abdominal sonography and, in particular, computed tomography show promise as rapid, noninvasive means of confirming the diagnosis of acute bowel infarction by identifying characteristic changes in the appearance of the bowel wall and mesentery. The sensitivity and specificity of these imaging techniques remain to be defined, however.

Treatment. Initial supportive therapy, aimed at stabilization of the patient's condition prior to surgery, includes nasogastric suction, replacement of fluid and electrolyte deficits, administration of broad-spectrum antibiotics after blood cultures have been obtained, and cardiopulmonary support, if needed. In the treatment of patients judged to be sufficiently stable to tolerate angiography, the use of vasodilators infused through a catheter placed at angiography has been advocated to treat the severe vasospasm frequently observed in the setting of intestinal ischemia. Papaverine is most commonly employed, although tolazoline has also been used in this setting. Although appealing on a theoretical basis, the efficacy of this use of vasodilators has not been conclusively established. As soon as the patient's condition is adequately stabilized and the diagnosis strongly suspected, prompt surgical exploration should be performed. At surgery, resection of necrotic bowel is the primary objective. An attempt

may be made to revascularize the remaining viable intestine by bypass graft or endarterectomy if the patient's condition is sufficiently stable to permit the additional surgery.

At the time of operation the limits of viable bowel must be defined in order to resect completely irreversibly diseased intestine while at the same time avoiding unnecessary development of the short bowel syndrome. It is often necessary to perform a "second-look" operation 12 to 36 hours after the initial exploration to identify and resect any additional bowel that in the interim proves to be nonviable. Infarction of large segments of intestine carries essentially a 100 per cent mortality rate without surgery. Even with surgery the mortality rate is greater than 50 per cent in most series because of delay in diagnosis or because of other complicating factors such as advanced age or atherosclerotic disease involving other vital organs.

Mesenteric vasculitis (e.g., as may occur in lupus erythematosus, polyarteritis nodosa, dermatomyositis, rheumatoid vasculitis, and Henoch-Schönlein purpura) may cause segmental intestinal infarction not conforming to the distribution of the major arteries. Vascular occlusion may not be demonstrable angiographically if only intramural arteries and arterioles are involved. Although some patients may require emergency surgery for intestinal necrosis and perforation, these complications are less common than with occlusions of the major arteries or their principal branches. In some cases the acute episode may resolve spontaneously, which may leave the patient with a segmental stricture demonstrable by barium contrast studies.

MESENTERIC ARTERY EMBOLISM. Emboli to the mesenteric circulation most commonly involve the superior mesenteric artery because of its size and the oblique angle of its origin from the aorta. These emboli usually arise from mural thrombi in the heart in patients with atherosclerotic or valvular heart disease but may also arise from vegetations of bacterial endocarditis, atrial myxomas, valvular prostheses, or atherosclerotic plaques in the thoracic or upper abdominal aorta, either spontaneously or during angiography. Patients may have a history of previous embolic episodes or exhibit evidence of simultaneous peripheral embolization (e.g., to the brain or extremities). Typically patients describe the *abrupt onset of severe midabdominal cramping pain*, accompanied by vomiting or diarrhea. Although patients may feel and appear severely ill, early in the course objective physical findings are sparse. If the diagnosis is not made promptly and appropriate treatment undertaken, a mesenteric embolus leads to bowel infarction. Angiography may demonstrate mesenteric artery occlusion in the absence of collateral circulation, indicating the acute nature of the process. The use of intra-arterial infusion of vasodilators has been advocated, although its value has not been clearly proven. Computed tomography may also strongly suggest the diagnosis early in the course of the disease in a patient with acute onset of abdominal pain of unknown source. Following supportive measures as needed to stabilize the patient's condition, immediate exploration with embolectomy and resection of any infarcted bowel is indicated. A "second-look" procedure is sometimes necessary. The characteristic setting in which mesenteric embolism occurs, as well as its abrupt onset, offers a greater opportunity for early diagnosis and treatment. For this reason, and because the patients generally are younger, the prognosis is more favorable than for most nonembolic causes of bowel infarction. Some patients who are successfully treated by embolectomy without need for bowel resection may develop a transient malabsorption syndrome persisting for several months.

NONOCCLUSIVE INTESTINAL INFARCTION. In some patients clinical findings suggestive of mesenteric arterial occlusive disease or embolism occur without a demonstrable obstruction to arterial flow. This syndrome, now recognized with increasing frequency, usually occurs in the setting of severe congestive heart failure, shock, hypoxia, or a recent myocardial infarction. In addition, it has been reported following cocaine use, possibly related to α-adrenergic stimulation due to the drug. The clinical course often evolves more slowly than is seen with occlusive processes. Occasionally a precipitating event is not identifiable. The use of α-adrenergic vasoconstrictors (and possibly digitalis glycosides) may also contribute to the development of this process. Because of its high degree of metabolic activity, the mucosa has the greatest requirement for intestinal blood flow of the various layers of the bowel wall. Thus it shows the earliest evidence of ischemic injury. At times, it may be the only portion to undergo hemorrhagic infarction. However, infarction may ultimately become transmural and occur in a patchy and irregular distribution, not conforming to the area supplied by a major vessel. Early angiography is useful to exclude a major vessel occlusion, which would usually require vascular surgery. In at least 50 per cent of such patients angiography reveals irregular narrowing of the major arterial branches and arcades (due to spasm) and impaired filling of the intramural vessels. Therapy consists of supportive measures and surgical exploration to resect infarcted bowel if the patient's situation suggests the need for this. Selective infusion of vasodilators into the mesenteric circulation has been suggested, but its therapeutic efficacy remains to be established. This syndrome generally carries a very poor prognosis, primarily because it is usually associated with shock or severe cardiopulmonary disease.

ISCHEMIC COLITIS. Ischemic injury to the colon may be caused by advanced atherosclerosis or interruption of the colonic blood supply during surgery (e.g., abdominal aortic aneurysmectomy, aortoiliac reconstruction, abdominoperineal resection) or may occur in association with "hypercoagulable" states, amyloidosis, vasculitis, ruptured aortic aneurysm, colorectal cancer, or the use of oral contraceptive agents. In addition, nonocclusive colonic ischemia may occur in states of low cardiac output or hypoxia. Nonocclusive colonic ischemia may be mediated primarily by the renin-angiotensin system, to which the colonic vasculature appears to be remarkably sensitive. The syndrome of ischemic colitis may be quite variable in its extent, severity, and prognosis. However, extensive infarction and perforation appear to be infrequent. Localized or segmental ischemia is more common, particularly affecting those areas of the colon that lie on the "watershed" between two adjacent arterial supplies, i.e., the splenic flexure (superior and inferior mesenteric arteries) and the rectosigmoid (inferior mesenteric and internal iliac arteries). Characteristically, patients over the age of 50 are most often affected with *abrupt onset of lower abdominal cramping pain, rectal bleeding,* and, to variable degrees, *vomiting* and *fever.* Some patients give a history of similar symptoms occurring intermittently for weeks to months before presentation. Left-sided abdominal tenderness and peritoneal signs may be present, as well as evidence of generalized atherosclerotic disease. Sigmoidoscopy may be normal; may show evidence of mild, nonspecific proctitis; or may reveal a spectrum of findings, including multiple discrete ulcers, blue-black hemorrhagic submucosal blebs, or an adherent pseudomembrane. Angiography generally has not proved useful in the diagnosis of patients in this setting. The differentiation of ischemic colitis from infections of the colon,

diverticulitis, and idiopathic inflammatory bowel disease (ulcerative colitis, Crohn's disease of the colon) may be very difficult. Initial management consists of general supportive measures, including antibiotics. In those patients in whom perforation or infarction of the colon appears likely, early surgical exploration is indicated; however, many patients improve without surgery. Subsequent barium enema often shows a characteristic picture of intramural hemorrhage and edema, including "thumb-printing," tubular narrowing, and "sawtooth" irregularity (Fig. 104–5). Some patients proceed to complete resolution of the clinical process and radiographic abnormalities. Others develop a residual stricture that eventually may require surgical resection.

MESENTERIC VENOUS THROMBOSIS. This condition, which accounts for about 5 to 15 per cent of patients with intestinal ischemia, almost always involves the superior mesenteric vein. It is associated with a variety of conditions: stasis in the mesenteric venous bed (portal hypertension, congestive heart failure), abdominal neoplasms, intra-abdominal inflammation (peritonitis, abscess, inflammatory bowel disease), abdominal surgery and trauma, a variety of presumed hypercoagulable states (antithrombin III deficiency, polycythemia vera), and use of oral contraceptives. Occasionally a predisposing condition is absent. Patients may have abrupt onset of a clinical picture indicative of acute bowel infarction; however, many others have a more gradual course with development of progressive abdominal discomfort over a period of weeks. Physical findings are nonspecific. The presence of a small amount of bloody peritoneal fluid is typical and may be an important clue to the diagnosis in patients with a subacute clinical course. Selective superior mesenteric angiography shows intense spasm of the arteries to the involved segment of bowel and absence of venous drainage.

Following initial supportive care to stabilize the patient's condition, an operation should be performed to resect infarcted or severely ischemic bowel. Reconstructive venous surgery is not generally possible. Because there is about a 25 per cent rate of recurrent thrombosis within the first several weeks postoperatively, anticoagulation is recommended except in patients who have underlying disease processes that would make this too hazardous. A "second-look" operation to search for recurrent thrombosis may also be required if there is unexplained clinical deterioration following initial surgery. In general, the prognosis is more favorable than for patients with mesenteric arterial disease, with reported mortality as low as 20 per cent.

MISCELLANEOUS DISORDERS

INTRAMURAL INTESTINAL HEMORRHAGE. This may follow abdominal trauma or may occur in the setting of ischemic bowel injury, vasculitis, or bleeding diatheses. Some patients have a picture suggesting a perforated viscus (severe abdominal pain, tenderness, leukocytosis), but most have cramping abdom-

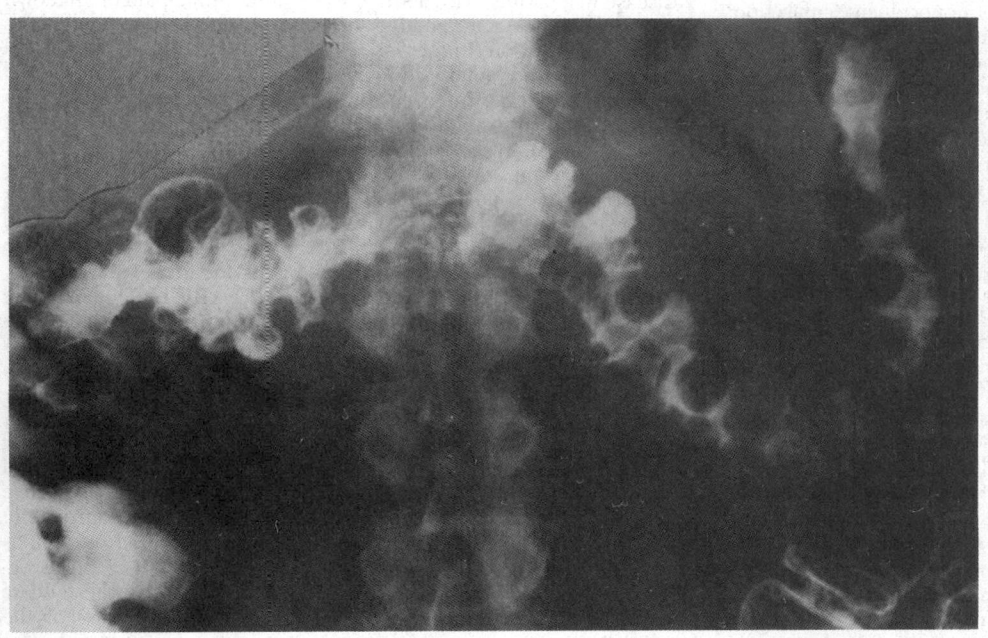

FIGURE 104–5. A barium enema in a patient with ischemic colitis showing narrowing and "thumb-printing" (nodular indentations of the bowel wall) in the distal transverse colon. This is one of the "watershed" areas of the colon between two adjacent arterial supplies (superior and inferior mesenteric arteries) where ischemia is more likely to develop.

inal pain and vomiting suggestive of partial or complete bowel obstruction. Hematemesis or melena and fever may be present. Occasionally a palpable abdominal mass caused by the presence of a hematoma may be noted. Barium studies of the small intestine typically show a "stacked coins" or "thumb-print" appearance. Usually intramural intestinal hemorrhage can be managed conservatively with nasogastric suction, intravenous hydration and electrolytes, and correction of any underlying coagulopathy, when possible. In those patients with high-grade or unremitting intestinal obstruction, or in whom signs of peritonitis develop (suggesting perforation), surgery is necessary.

PARAPROSTHETIC-ENTERIC AND AORTOENTERIC FISTULAS. Following aortic aneurysmectomy and other procedures in which vascular prostheses are placed in the abdomen or retroperitoneum, fistulas may form between the graft and adjacent bowel. This may occur as early as several weeks postoperatively but in most cases is delayed by at least 2 years. This complication usually results from local infection or damage to the intestine or its blood supply at surgery, with subsequent erosion of the bowel wall by the graft. Patients may present with massive upper or lower gastrointestinal bleeding or both that may be rapidly fatal without emergency surgery. In a number of patients, however, bleeding may be initially intermittent, resembling that from a number of more common lesions. In these patients, early consideration of this diagnosis with urgent evaluation by upper endoscopy to exclude other lesions and computed tomography, if the patient's condition permits, may be required to establish the diagnosis and need for surgical intervention.

Unoperated abdominal aortic aneurysms and aneurysmal dilatations of other major abdominal arteries may erode into the gastrointestinal tract, causing upper or lower gastrointestinal bleeding or both of various degrees of severity.

SUPERIOR MESENTERIC ARTERY SYNDROME. This uncommon syndrome of postprandial epigastric pain, distention, and vomiting has been attributed to compression of the third portion of the duodenum between the superior mesenteric artery anteriorly and the fixed retroperitoneal structures posteriorly. This has been described as occurring most commonly in individuals who have lost a substantial amount of weight or are of "asthenic habitus," and in children with rapid growth in the absence of corresponding weight gain or who have been fixed in a position of hyperextension by a cast following spinal injury or surgery. Barium contrast studies show distention of the proximal duodenum, and lateral aortograms or abdominal sonograms have shown a narrowing of the angle between the aorta and the superior mesenteric artery. The differential diagnosis includes generalized disorders of gastrointestinal motility, such as scleroderma, and anorexia nervosa. Recommended treatment has included the use of small feedings and elemental diets with the patient lying prone or on the left side in the knee-chest position after eating. In refractory cases duodenal mobilization or duodenal-jejunal bypass has reportedly been effective in relieving symptoms. Since apparent compression of the duodenum by the superior mesenteric artery does not prove to be a clinically significant obstruction, the diagnosis of this syndrome must be made only after other possible causes of duodenal stasis have been excluded. This entity is frequently overdiagnosed unless strict diagnostic criteria are employed.

VASCULAR MALFORMATIONS INCLUDING VASCULAR ECTASIA. Hemangiomas of the small intestine are very uncommon vascular tumors found throughout the bowel, particularly the jejunum. They represent one of the causes of gastrointestinal bleeding that may be very difficult to locate. These lesions are most reliably diagnosed by abdominal angiography. Surgical removal of the involved segment of bowel is the usual treatment.

Vascular malformations can occur in the gastrointestinal tract in association with diseases involving the skin, such as the *hereditary hemorrhagic telangiectasia (Osler-Weber-Rendu) syndrome, blue rubber bleb nevus syndrome,* and the *CREST syndrome* (calcinosis, Raynaud's phenomenon, esophageal hypomotility, sclerodactyly, and telangiectasia). In addition, vascular malformations may occur as a primary process (*vascular ectasia, angiodysplasia*) chiefly involving the colon but also occurring in the stomach or small intestine. This is a frequent cause of lower intestinal bleeding, especially in patients over the age of 60. An association of angiodysplasia with aortic stenosis has also been reported but not fully established. Vascular ectasias of the stom-

ach and small intestine may be the most common source of upper gastrointestinal bleeding in patients with chronic renal failure.

Vascular ectasias consist of ectatic, tortuous submucosal veins and groups of ectatic mucosal vessels lying just under the gastric, intestinal, or colonic epithelium or at times on the luminal surface unprotected by any intestinal epithelium. The etiology of these lesions remains uncertain. One theory suggests that they develop as a result of chronic low-grade obstruction of the submucosal veins as they penetrate the muscularis propria; another theory proposes that these lesions develop because of chronic mucosal ischemia.

Larger vascular malformations, including some vascular ectasias, may be visualized by selective mesenteric arteriography. However, most of these lesions are small and are best demonstrated by endoscopy. Such lesions are present in a large number of older individuals without apparent gastrointestinal blood loss. For those patients who have severe anemia due to chronic or recurrent gastrointestinal blood loss without other apparent cause, surgery has been recommended if vascular malformations could be identified and localized (e.g., right colectomy for lesions in the cecum). This approach is often unsatisfactory, and bleeding may recur either because some lesions in other parts of the gastrointestinal tract may not have been appreciated at the initial evaluation or because new lesions may subsequently develop. For these reasons, nonoperative endoscopic approaches have been developed to obliterate vascular malformations by such techniques as laser photocoagulation, electrocoagulation, or thermal coagulation (heater probe).

Baur CM, Millay DJ, Taylor CM, et al.: Treatment of chronic visceral ischemia. Am J Surg 148:138, 1984. *Illustrates the efficacy of surgical treatment for abdominal angina in properly selected patients.*

Cello JP, Grendell JH: Endoscopic laser treatment for gastrointestinal vascular ectasias. Ann Intern Med 104:352, 1986. *Demonstrates the effective use of nonoperative therapy for this disorder.*

Croft RJ, Menon GP, Marston A: Does "intestinal angina" exist? A critical study of obstructed visceral arteries. Br J Surg 68:316, 1981. *A provocative report demonstrating the difficulty in relating gastrointestinal symptoms to angiographic findings.*

Federle MP, Chun G, Jeffrey RB, et al.: Computed tomographic findings in bowel infarction. AJR 142:91, 1984. *This report demonstrates the potential value of computed tomography in the diagnosis of vascular diseases of the intestine.*

Fiddian-Green RG: Splanchnic ischaemia and multiple organ failure in the critically ill. Ann R Coll Surg Engl 70:128, 1988. *Interesting discussion of the pathophysiology, diagnosis, and treatment of nonocclusive intestinal ischemia.*

Grendell JH, Ockner RK: Vascular diseases of the bowel. *In* Sleisenger MH, Fordtran JS (eds.): Gastrointestinal Disease. 4th ed. Philadelphia, W.B. Saunders Company, 1989, p 1903. *A comprehensive survey including pathophysiology, diagnosis, and management.*

Hines JR, Gore RM, Ballantyne GH: Superior mesenteric artery syndrome: Diagnostic criteria and therapeutic approaches. Am J Surg 148:630, 1984. *Emphasizes the importance of strict diagnostic criteria to avoid overdiagnosis of this entity.*

Hunter GC, Guernsey JM: Mesenteric ischemia. Med Clin North Am 72:1091, 1988. *This review emphasizes diagnostic and therapeutic considerations in managing the different types of mesenteric ischemic processes.*

Kiernan PD, Pairolero PC, Hubert JP Jr, et al.: Aortic graft–enteric fistula. Mayo Clin Proc 55:731, 1980. *A detailed review of clinical features, management, and prognosis.*

Reinus JF, Brandt LJ, Boley SJ: Ischemic diseases of the bowel. Gastroenterol Clin North Am 19:319, 1990. *A thorough and up-to-date review emphasizing the approach to diagnosis and management.*

Zuckerman GR, Cornette GL, Clouse RE, et al.: Upper gastrointestinal bleeding in patients with chronic renal failure. Ann Intern Med 102:588, 1985. *Demonstrates the importance of angiodysplastic lesions as a source of upper gastrointestinal bleeding in patients with chronic renal failure.*

105 Neoplasms of the Large and Small Intestine

Bernard Levin

NEOPLASMS OF THE LARGE INTESTINE

Cancer of the large bowel (colon and rectum) is the most common malignancy of the gastrointestinal tract and together with breast and lung cancer is one of the three most frequent malignancies in the United States. It is also a worldwide health problem of great importance, particularly in other Western countries. Approximately 155,000 cases of cancer of the colon and rectum were diagnosed in the United States in 1990, only one half of whom will survive 5 years or longer. The mortality from colorectal cancer has slowly declined over the past 10 years while the incidence has been stable. New understanding about the genetics and molecular biology of this neoplasm has been recently gained, and advances have also been made in methods of prevention, diagnosis, and treatment.

The large bowel also may be involved by other malignant tumors. These include anal carcinoma (squamous or transitional types), lymphoma, leiomyosarcoma, malignant carcinoid tumor, and Kaposi's sarcoma. The large bowel may also be involved through direct invasion by malignancies from adjacent sites such as prostate, ovary, uterus, and stomach. The most frequent tumors that occur in the large intestine are benign adenomas (adenomatous polyps). Except for lipomas of the ileocecal valve, other benign tumors are very unusual.

POLYPS OF THE COLON

A polyp is any lesion that arises from the surface of the gastrointestinal tract and protrudes into the lumen. In the large intestine, polyps noted at sigmoidoscopy or colonoscopy or during barium enema may be single or multiple, pedunculated or sessile, and sporadic or part of an inherited syndrome. They become significant because of bleeding or because of their potential for malignant transformation.

PATHOLOGY. In addition to adenocarcinoma, which may present as a polypoid mass, three distinct types of benign polyps arise from colonic epithelium: hyperplastic (metaplastic), inflammatory, and neoplastic (adenomatous). Hyperplastic polyps, which tend to be small and asymptomatic, account for about one fifth of all polyps in the colon and for most of the polyps in the rectum and distal sigmoid. They are not considered neoplastic. Inflammatory polyps occur in chronic ulcerative colitis and also are not neoplastic (Ch. 103). Juvenile polyps are hamartomas of the lamina propria and may be single or multiple and occur most commonly in the rectum. They are susceptible to hemorrhage and autoamputation.

Adenomatous Polyps

PREVALENCE AND DISTRIBUTION. The incidence of colonic adenomas increases with age in countries with a high or intermediate risk for colorectal cancer, occurring in 40 to 50 per cent of individuals over the age of 60 in the United States. Adenomas are uncommon in areas where the incidence of cancer is low; for example, the prevalence of adenomas varies from almost zero among black South Africans to 10 per cent in Japan and in Cali, Colombia. The presence of adenomas does not necessarily convey a high risk because the propensity for neoplastic transformation is related to size. The low incidence of cancer in some countries, such as Japan, is probably related to the small number of large adenomas as well as to the total number of adenomas.

MACROSCOPIC AND MICROSCOPIC APPEARANCES. Adenomas may be separated into tubular, villous, and intermediate tubulovillous types. The typical tubular adenoma is small and spherical and has a stalk. Its surface is roughly separated into lobules by intercommunicating clefts. In contrast, the villous adenoma may be large and sessile with a velvety surface. Histologically the tubular adenoma consists of closely packed tubular glands that divide and branch. In the villous adenoma, finger-like projections of neoplastic epithelium project toward the bowel lumen. The tubulovillous lesions consist of a mixture of tubular and villous patterns. About 60 per cent of adenomas are tubular, 20 to 30 per cent are tubulovillous, and about 10 per cent are villous. All adenomas are dysplastic, and dysplasia in adenomas may be graded into mild, moderate, and severe. This classification is based on the presence of cytologic (mainly nuclear) abnormalities and glandular architectural changes.

DEVELOPMENT OF ADENOMAS. In the normal adult, the epithelial tissue of the colon actively renews itself with a turnover of about 3 to 8 days. DNA synthesis occurs primarily in cells in the lower one third of crypts. Normally cells replicate and migrate up the crypt to be subsequently exfoliated from the mucosal surface. In adenomas immature cells are found higher up the colonic crypt than normal, associated with unrepressed DNA synthesis, representing abnormal cell renewal along the surface of the crypt and the entire length of the crypt. DNA-synthesizing cells can accumulate on the luminal surface, thus forming new adenomatous tissue.

RELATIONSHIP OF COLONIC ADENOMAS TO CANCER. Colonic adenomas appear to have malignant potential: (1) The epidemiology of adenomas and carcinoma is similar; (2) adenocarcinomas and adenomas occur in the same anatomic distribution in the colon; (3) residual adenomatous tissue is observed quite commonly in small cancers; (4) the incidence of cancer increases as the size of the adenoma increases; (5) the adenoma-to-cancer transition has been observed in familial polyposis and in experimental animals treated with a carcinogen; (6) the risk for colorectal cancer is higher in patients with a history of adenomas and may be lessened if the adenoma is removed; (7) a period of approximately 5 years elapses between the diagnosis of adenoma and the development of carcinoma.

Less than 5 per cent of adenomas develop into carcinomas. Several important factors in this transformation can be identified, especially size, histologic type, and epithelial dysplasia. The frequency of cancer in adenomas under 1 cm is 1 to 3 per cent, those between 1 to 2 cm have a rate of 10 per cent, whereas those over 2 cm have a rate of malignancy over 40 per cent. The highest malignancy rate is associated with a villous growth pattern. Invasive neoplasm has been found in 40 per cent of the villous tumors, in less than 5 per cent of the tubular ones, and in 23 per cent of the tubulovillous variety. The malignant potential of adenomas increases with increasing degrees of dysplasia. Most adenomas smaller than 1 cm show only mild dysplasia and have a low malignant potential. With severe dysplasia, the rate of malignant transformation rises to 27 per cent.

Cancer in adenomas is usually well differentiated and occurs most commonly in the tip of a pedunculated adenoma without invasion of the muscularis mucosae. These lesions are usually satisfactorily treated by polypectomy. Occasionally cancers in adenomas invade the muscularis mucosae, grow down the stalk, invade lymphatics and adjacent lymph nodes, and metastasize. The roles of autocrine factors, tumor suppressor genes, and oncogenes in the development of adenomas and their malignant transformation are currently under study.

CLINICAL MANIFESTATIONS. Most adenomatous polyps are asymptomatic. Some adenomatous polyps are diagnosed by detection of occult blood loss in asymptomatic individuals being screened for colon cancer. Adenomas may also be detected by double contrast barium enema examination or by fiberoptic sigmoidoscopy or colonoscopy. Adenomas may also cause hematochezia and rarely iron deficiency anemia (Ch. 131). Large villous adenomas may very rarely cause watery diarrhea (with severe potassium depletion).

MANAGEMENT AND FOLLOW-UP. Because of the association of adenomas with the development of adenocarcinomas, colonic polyps should usually be removed or destroyed. In individual clinical circumstances (e.g., age of patient, location of lesion) this rule may rarely have to be modified. Pedunculated polyps, even if large, can be removed by electrocautery snare while small sessile polyps (1 to 8 mm in size) should be biopsied and destroyed with the "hot biopsy" forceps. For sessile polyps with a wide-based attachment to the colonic wall, several electrocautery sessions may be required for complete excision. Endoscopic removal may not be safe or possible if a sessile lesion is larger than 3 cm or if it is in a relatively inaccessible location. In general, benign-appearing polyps are removed by electrosurgery and not biopsied and the entire lesion is submitted for histopathologic examination.

The endoscopic appearance of a polyp that suggests carcinomatous invasion includes ulceration, an irregular surface contour, firm consistency, and friability. If a diagnosis of malignancy is made after polypectomy, a decision has to be made about the adequacy of the polypectomy. In the presence of a poorly differentiated histology, penetration of the muscularis mucosa, vascular or lymphatic invasion, and a resection margin containing cancer, the risk of regional lymph node involvement is approximately 5 per cent. The mortality from surgical resection is less than 2 per cent in patients aged 50 to 69 years and 4.4 per cent for those over 70 years, so any decision to recommend surgical resection must take into account individual operative risk.

FOLLOW-UP AFTER COLONOSCOPIC POLYPECTOMY. Ideally, the colon should be cleared of all synchronous adenomas at the time of the initial examination. A follow-up colonoscopy is appropriate at 1 year to evaluate for the presence of any lesions missed at the time of the previous procedure as well as new lesions that may have arisen. If this examination is normal, an interval of 2 to 3 years is appropriate for the next colonoscopy. Nutritional and chemotherapeutic strategies aimed at prevention of adenoma recurrence are being studied.

Inherited Polyposis Syndromes

Recent advances in genetics and molecular biology have accentuated our interest in the inherited risk of colorectal cancer. The polyposis syndromes account for approximately 1 per cent of colorectal cancer, whereas the nonpolyposis inherited conditions may be responsible for up to 6 per cent.

ADENOMATOUS POLYPOSIS SYNDROMES. The adenomatous polyposis syndromes include familial adenomatous polyposis and Gardner syndrome, in both of which hereditary disorders hundreds to thousands of colonic adenomas are present (Fig. 105–1). The adenomas begin to appear early in the second decade of life. Gastrointestinal symptoms occur in the third or fourth decade. Almost all patients with familial polyposis develop carcinoma of the colon by age 40 if the colon has not been removed.

Some cases occur without a family history and may represent spontaneous mutations.

Gardner syndrome differs from familial adenomatous polyposis in that affected individuals exhibit benign extraintestinal growths, including osteomas (especially mandibular) and soft tissue tumors (lipomas, sebaceous cysts, fibrosarcomas). Other associated features include supernumerary teeth, desmoid tumors, and mesenteric fibromatosis (Fig. 105–2). The colonic adenomas are similar to those of familial adenomatous polyposis and have the same potential for malignancy.

In both familial adenomatous polyposis and Gardner syndrome, upper gastrointestinal polyps are commonly found. Gastric polyps are hyperplastic and rarely cause symptoms. Adenomatous duodenal polyps are present in up to 80 per cent of individuals with familial adenomatous polyposis or Gardner syndrome, and approximately 10 per cent develop periampullary cancer. Adenomas occur in the small bowel distal to the duodenum but rarely undergo malignant transformation.

Familial adenomatous polyposis and Gardner syndrome are inherited as autosomal dominant disorders with incomplete penetrance. The mutant adenomatous polyposis coli (APC) gene on the long arm of chromosome 5 has recently been identified in both conditions. DNA markers can be used to ascertain whether a specific individual in a polyposis family is likely to express the phenotype.

For screening purposes, flexible proctosigmoidoscopy should

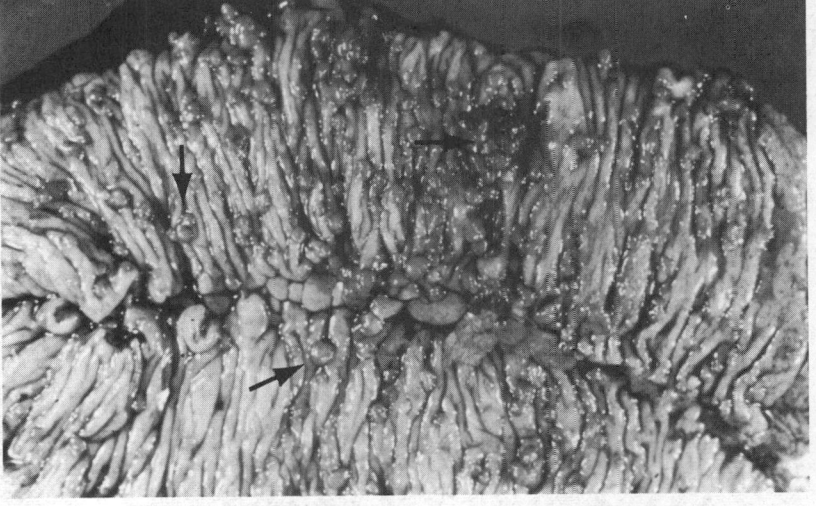

FIGURE 105–1. *A*, Patients with familial polyposis have multiple adenomatous polyps carpeting the colon, as demonstrated in this gross specimen. Note that the colon is diffusely studded with sessile and occasional pedunculated adenomatous polyps (*arrows*). Many of the larger polyps contain villous elements, and occasionally villous adenomas are found. Although no carcinoma was seen in this patient, nearly all patients eventually develop colorectal carcinoma if surgery is not performed. *B*, This barium enema examination of a patient with familial polyposis represents diffuse studding of the large bowel with adenomatous polyps. Note the marked variation in size of these polyps. Although this patient did not have osteomas or soft tissue tumors, the barium enema is similar to that seen in Gardner syndrome. (From Boland CR, Kim YS: *In* Sleisenger MH, Fordtran JS [eds.]: Gastrointestinal Disease. 3rd ed. Philadelphia, W. B. Saunders Company, 1983.)

A

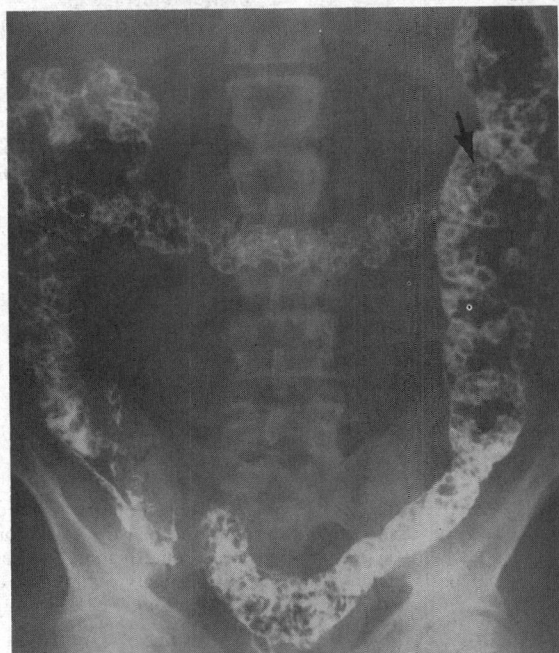

B

be performed annually in all first-degree relatives, beginning at 12 years of age until age 40, and every 3 years thereafter. This screening is appropriate for those with the mutant gene. Until gene markers are 100 per cent specific and sensitive, screening is also indicated for those without the mutant gene, although less often. Surveillance with a side-viewing endoscope for gastric and duodenal polyps should begin when the diagnosis of colonic polyposis is made and should continue every 2 to 3 years thereafter.

HEREDITARY NONPOLYPOSIS COLORECTAL CANCER (LYNCH SYNDROMES I AND II).

In both of the Lynch syndromes, colon cancer is inherited in a highly penetrant, autosomal dominant manner. Several adenomas, which are occasionally flat, may be present (in spite of the name), but myriads of adenomas are not found. The average age of diagnosis of cancer is in the mid 40's, and it is characteristic to find a majority of lesions proximal to the splenic flexure as well as multiple synchronous cancers. In Lynch syndrome I (site-specific colon cancer) only inherited colonic neoplasms occur, whereas Lynch syndrome II (cancer family syndrome) includes female genital (uterine, ovarian) and breast cancer. Individuals in families with hereditary nonpolyposis colorectal cancer should have colonoscopy every 2 years beginning at an age 5 years younger than the age of the earliest colon cancer diagnosed in the family. Mammography (at an earlier age than the general population) and ovarian ultrasonography are also appropriate in Lynch syndrome II families in whom there is a preponderance of breast or ovarian malignancies.

PEUTZ-JEGHERS SYNDROME.

This syndrome is characterized by melanotic spots on the lips, buccal mucosa, and skin and by multiple hamartomatous polyps throughout the gastrointestinal tract from the stomach to the rectum (Fig. 105–3). It is generally believed to be inherited in an autosomal dominant fashion but with variable expressivity. Usually polyps are fewer in number than in familial adenomatous polyposis. Microscopically, these polyps consist of elongated branching glands lined by benign epithelium native to the location of the polyps. The most distinctive feature is the presence of an arborizing proliferation of smooth muscle in the lamina propria. Rarely, malignancies have been described in the intestine with a preponderance in

the small intestine. Other manifestations include ovarian sex cord stromal tumors and polyps of the gallbladder, ureter, and nose. Intestinal symptoms of recurrent, colicky abdominal pain may appear in adolescence, and intussusception may require surgical removal of a polyp. Gastrointestinal bleeding may occur, causing iron deficiency anemia.

OTHER POLYPOSIS SYNDROMES.

Turcot's syndrome, inherited as an autosomal recessive condition, is rare and is characterized by hereditary adenomatous polyposis with a low number of polyps (20 to 300) and tumors of the central nervous system. These neoplasms include medulloblastoma, glioblastoma, and ependymoma.

Juvenile polyposis is inherited as an autosomal dominant trait, with an occasional case occurring spontaneously. The number of polyps is less than in familial adenomatous polyposis, averaging 25 to 40. Polyps may be found throughout the gastrointestinal tract or may be restricted to the colon. Symptoms may begin in childhood or adolescence with rectal bleeding, anemia, abdominal pain, or intussusception. A variety of extraintestinal symptoms including congenital abnormalities and pulmonary arteriovenous malformations have been described in association with juvenile polyposis. Foci of adenomatous epithelium may be present in these polyps, or adenomas may coexist. The true risk of malignancy in these patients is unknown, but 10 per cent of the reported patients with juvenile polyposis have developed carcinoma of the gastrointestinal tract. Subtotal colectomy may occasionally be warranted in those with severely dysplastic adenomas.

Cronkite-Canada syndrome is a nonfamilial disorder of adults characterized by diffuse gastrointestinal polyposis, alopecia, dystrophy of the fingernails, and cutaneous hyperpigmentation. The polyps resemble juvenile polyps and are in greatest density in the stomach and colon. Watery diarrhea, anorexia, abdominal pain, cachexia, protein-losing enteropathy, and carcinoma of the gastrointestinal tract (in up to 14 per cent of cases) have been reported.

Cowden's syndrome (multiple hamartoma syndrome) is transmitted in an autosomal dominant manner and is characterized by multiple facial tricholemmomas, oral papillomas, keratoses of the hands and feet, and a high rate of associated systemic malignancies, particularly of thyroid and breast. The polyps are not dysplastic, and the risk of gastrointestinal malignancy is not increased.

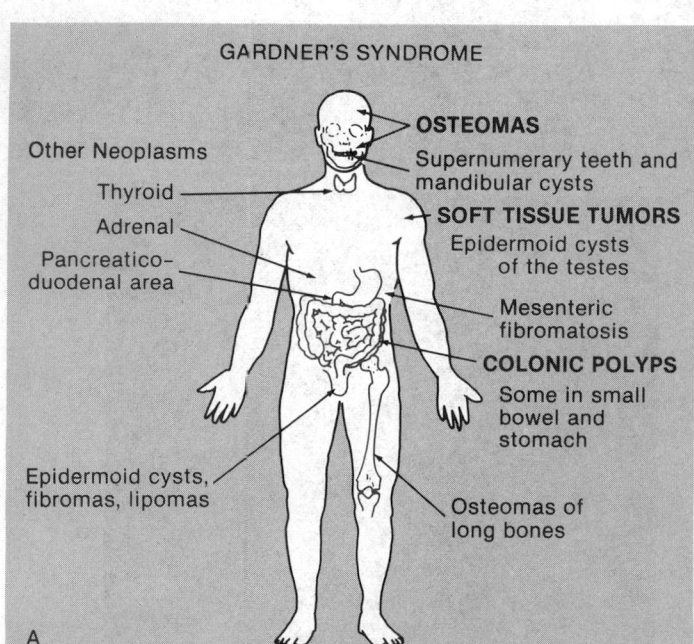

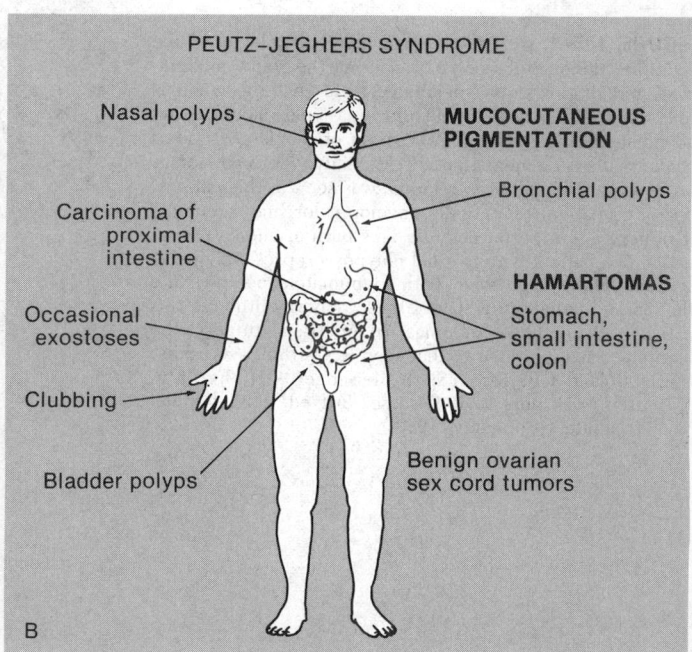

FIGURE 105–2. *A,* Schematic representation of Gardner syndrome. The triad of colonic polyposis, bone tumors, and soft tissue tumors (heavy print) constitutes the primary features; other features are indicated in lighter print. *B,* Schematic presentation of the Peutz-Jeghers syndrome. Mucocutaneous pigmentation and benign gastrointestinal polyposis (heavy print) are the primary features of this syndrome. Lighter print shows the secondary features. (From Boland CR, Kim YS: *In* Sleisenger MH, Fordtran JS [eds.]: Gastrointestinal Disease. 3rd ed. Philadelphia, W. B. Saunders Company, 1983.)

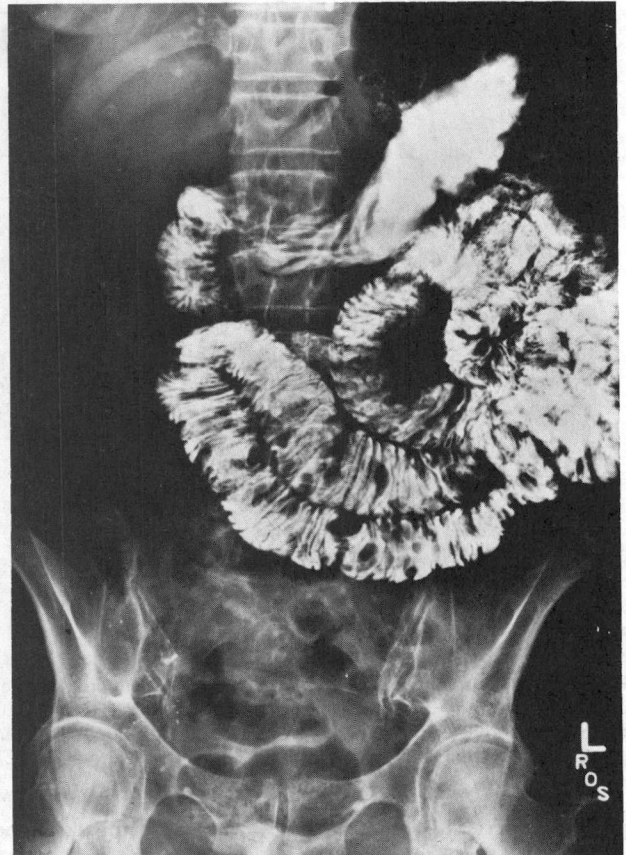

FIGURE 105–3. Barium study of the upper gastrointestinal tract showing multiple polyps of the small bowel in a patient with Peutz-Jeghers syndrome.

ADENOCARCINOMA OF THE LARGE BOWEL

Carcinoma of the colon and rectum varies widely in frequency in different parts of the world. Large bowel cancers occur commonly in North America, northwestern Europe, and New Zealand, whereas in South America, southwest Asia, equatorial Africa, and India the risk is much less. The incidence varies from 3.5 per 100,000 in India to 32.3 per 100,000 in Connecticut. Colorectal cancers display regional differences within the United States, with the highest incidence in the Northeast. Rectal cancer is more common in men in most, but not all, areas of the world. In the United States rectal cancer incidence has declined over the past 50 years.

Migrants from parts of the world with a low incidence to regions with a higher risk, such as the United States or Canada, show a rapid increase in incidence. This is exemplified by the higher incidence in Puerto Ricans who have migrated to the mainland compared with those in Puerto Rico and in first- and second-generation Chinese and Japanese immigrants to Hawaii and the mainland United States compared with Japanese in Japan and Chinese in the Peoples' Republic of China.

ETIOLOGY. Both inherited predisposition and environmental factors seem to be implicated in carcinogenesis in the colon and rectum, but in ways yet to be clearly delineated. Of the environmental factors, diet has been the most extensively studied. Fat intake, not only the amount, but also the type of fat, has been correlated with the risk for colorectal cancer in many but not all studies. Consumption of saturated fat (with a high content of animal fat) has been reported to be positively correlated with colon cancer incidence. Other studies suggest that monounsaturated fatty acids may exert a protective effect against the development of colon cancer. In countries with a high incidence of colon cancer, the average fat content in the diet is about 40 per cent of total calories, in contrast to the dietary fat content of 15 to 20 per cent or less of total calories in countries with a low cancer incidence. If fat in the colon does in fact promote cancer, the effect might be related to increased biliary sterol excretion,

leading to increased colonic epithelial proliferation, to modification of cell membranes, or to stimulation of the synthesis of prostaglandins that induce cellular proliferation. The possible role of *dietary fiber* in reducing colonic carcinogenesis has been suggested but not firmly established. Fiber is not a single chemical substance. Certain components of fiber found in cereals, fruits, and vegetables may be helpful in reducing the risk of cancer by diluting and binding carcinogens in the lumen, by modifying colonic bacterial flora, and by acidifying the colonic lumen by short-chain fatty acids. Naturally occurring anticarcinogens found in fruits and vegetables (indoles, thioethers, dithiothiones, retinoids) are being investigated. Other factors that have been postulated to play a role in colonic carcinogenesis are excess caloric intake and obesity and inadequate intake of calcium and vitamin D.

AGE. Risk factors for colorectal cancer are listed in Table 105–1. The relationship of age to adenomas has been previously discussed. The risk of colorectal cancer begins to increase from the age of 40 and rises sharply at age 50 to 55; with each succeeding decade the risk doubles, reaching a peak by age 75.

INFLAMMATORY BOWEL DISEASE (Ulcerative Colitis and Crohn's disease—Ch. 103). Among all patients diagnosed as having a large bowel adenocarcinoma, only about 1 per cent give an antecedent history of inflammatory bowel disease. In chronic ulcerative colitis, carcinoma of the colon occurs more commonly (approximately 10 to 20 times) than in the general population. The duration of disease and the extent of colonic involvement correlate with the subsequent development of colon cancer. Approximately 2 to 4 per cent of all patients with chronic ulcerative colitis develop colorectal carcinoma, with a cumulative incidence of about 12 per cent after 25 years. Patients with ulcerative proctitis have no increase in risk, and the risk for patients with left-sided colitis may be delayed until approximately 10 years later. In ulcerative colitis, mucosal dysplasia, defined as an unequivocal neoplastic alteration of the colonic epithelium, is the recognized precursor for the development of carcinoma. Dysplastic epithelium may itself overlie an area of malignancy associated with direct invasion into the submucosa. The dysplastic area may be flat or proliferative, and the likelihood of carcinoma increases significantly in the presence of a dysplasia-associated lesion or mass. Whether routine colonoscopic surveillance is useful in patients with inflammatory bowel disease is not settled. Nevertheless, many authorities favor periodic colonoscopy with multiple biopsies for dysplasia in individuals with over 8 years of symptoms and extensive colonic involvement. The availability of newer surgical procedures, such as ileoanal pouches, favors a trend toward earlier colectomy in high-risk individuals. The demonstration of high-grade dysplasia or a dysplasia-associated lesion or mass, even in the presence of low-grade dysplasia, warrants prophylactic colectomy because the risk of an associated carcinoma may be as high as 50 or 60 per cent. Newer epithelial markers, such as flow cytometry, lectins, oncogene mutations, and mucins, are being studied in an attempt to define the biology of neoplastic transformation and to identify individuals at high risk before cancer develops.

Patients with Crohn's colitis are also at higher risk (approximately 4 to 7 times that of the general population) for the development of colorectal cancer, but this is probably lower than

TABLE 105–1. RISK FACTORS FOR COLORECTAL CANCER

Standard Risk: Age over 40 years in men and women
Higher Risk
   Associated disease
      Ulcerative colitis
      Crohn's colitis
   Personal history
      Colorectal cancer
      Colorectal adenomas
      Female genital or breast cancer
   Family history
      Familial polyposis syndromes
      Hereditary nonpolyposis colorectal cancer
        (Lynch syndromes I and II)

in ulcerative colitis. Colonic surveillance has not been widely used.

HEREDITY AND COLONIC CANCER. Inherited risk has become very important in colonic cancer screening. The adenomatous polyposis syndromes and hereditary nonpolyposis colorectal cancer, previously discussed, together account for approximately 7 per cent of colon cancers. The remainder of colon cancers are referred to as "sporadic," but this term may be a misnomer. Population studies have demonstrated a two- or threefold increased risk for colon cancer in first-degree relatives of individuals with colon cancer. A similar risk is present in first-degree relatives of individuals with adenomatous polyps. In fact, as many as 50 per cent or more of "sporadic" adenomas and cancers may exhibit a partially penetrant autosomal dominant inheritance.

MOLECULAR GENETICS OF COLORECTAL CANCER. The genetic events surrounding the development of colorectal cancer are now being studied with increasing sophistication. The gene for familial adenomatous polyposis has been identified on chromosome 5. Deletions of DNA sequences at the same locus are also frequently observed in adenocarcinomas from "sporadic" cases. This may be the earliest change in the neoplastic process. K-*ras* mutations follow the chromosome 5 changes and are observed more commonly on larger adenomas and cancers (Ch. 157). Chromosome 17 (p53 gene) and chromosome 18 (DCC gene) deletions are often present and may be important in malignant transformation. Overexpression of the c-*myc* gene has also been reported in colonic cancers. The total accumulation of genetic changes (allelic deletions, oncogene mutations) may be more important than a particular sequence of events in the development of invasive cancer.

PATHOLOGY. The vast majority of colorectal cancers are adenocarcinomas. The tumors exhibit varying degrees of glandular differentiation and produce variable amounts of mucin. Cross morphologic features may be divided into two major groups, polypoid and annular constricting lesions. The polypoid lesion is most commonly found on the right side, and the annular constricting lesion is more common on the left side of the colon. Adenocarcinomas of the rectum may be sessile or polypoid. Approximately 75 per cent of colorectal cancers occur in the descending colon, rectosigmoid, and rectum. Approximately 50 per cent are within the reach of the 60-cm fiberoptic sigmoidoscope. The cecum and ascending colon are involved in 15 per cent and the transverse colon in 10 per cent (Fig. 105–4). Carcinoma of the colon spreads by direct extension through the wall of the bowel into the pericolonic fat and mesentery, by invasion of surrounding organs, by way of the lymphatics to the regional lymph nodes, and via the portal vein to the liver. Additionally, the tumor may spread throughout the peritoneal cavity and to the lungs and bones. Rectal cancers may directly invade the perirectal fat, vagina, prostate, bladder, ureters, and bony pelvis and may metastasize to the lungs and liver.

CLINICAL MANIFESTATIONS. The major symptoms of colorectal cancer are *rectal bleeding, pain,* and *change in bowel habit.* The clinical presentation in an individual patient is related to the size and location of the tumor. Those on the right side are often asymptomatic, and bleeding may be occult. Tumors of the cecum and ascending colon rarely obstruct early. Changes in bowel habit, with reduction in stool caliber or progressive constipation, and hematochezia are more common with left-sided lesions. Adenocarcinomas of the colon may present with a localized perforation and with signs of peritonitis. An abdominal mass or symptoms and signs of liver metastasis may be the earliest clinical manifestations of an underlying colorectal cancer.

Rectal or anal cancers may present with rectal bleeding, perineal pain, or change in bowel habit. Presenting symptoms may also include those referable to invasion of adjacent organs, including hematuria, renal insufficiency (obstructive uropathy), and vaginal fistulas.

Colorectal cancer must be suspected when patients present with rectal bleeding, a change in bowel habit, decrease in stool caliber, iron deficiency anemia, or unexplained abdominal pain. Rectal bleeding may be caused by other conditions, including hemorrhoids, angiodysplasia, diverticulosis, and other benign and malignant tumors (Ch. 111). Over the age of 40, the frequency

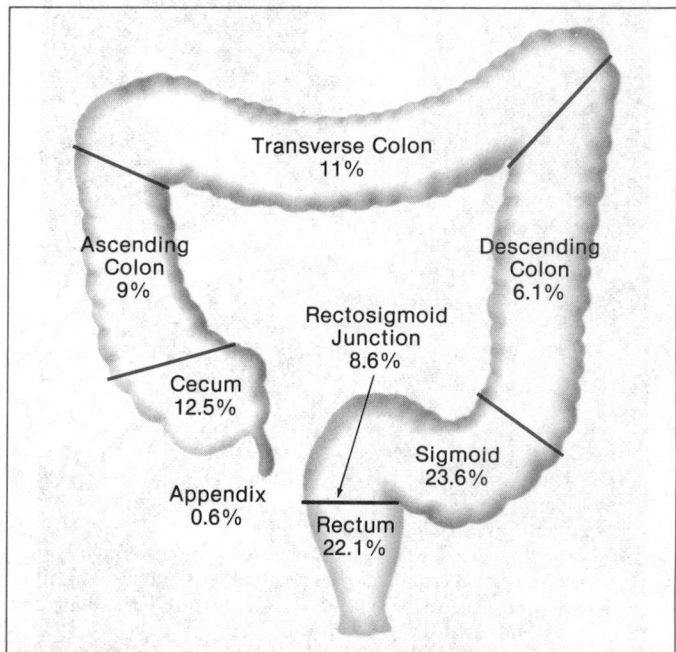

FIGURE 105–4. Distribution of large bowel cancer by anatomic segment according to the third national cancer survery (segment unspecified). (From Shottenfeld D, Fraumeni J Jr [eds.]: Cancer Epidemiology and Prevention. Philadelphia, W. B. Saunders Company, 1982, pp 703–727.)

of neoplasia increases significantly. Unexplained iron deficiency in both older men and women always requires a thorough evaluation to exclude gastrointestinal cancer (Ch. 131).

METASTATIC COLON CANCER. Metastases may be clinically apparent before or after resection of the primary colorectal cancer. Massive hepatomegaly may occur with pain due to distention of the liver capsule. Spread within the abdomen may cause small and large bowel obstruction and ascites. Pelvic spread may cause bladder dysfunction, sacral or sciatic nerve pain, and vaginal discharge or bleeding. Distant spread to lungs and bone may be silent until very advanced. Intestinal recurrences are uncommon and usually result from tumor implants related to the original resection growing from the serosa into the lumen.

DIAGNOSIS. A careful history, physical examination, and selected use of laboratory and radiologic tests facilitate the diagnosis of colorectal cancer. The history includes the patient's symptoms, prior removal of an adenoma or cancer, previous or present inflammatory bowel disease, or a family history of one of the inherited colorectal cancer syndromes. Special emphasis should be paid to first-degree relatives with a history of colorectal neoplasia. Physical examination may reveal evidence for Peutz-Jeghers or Gardner syndrome and may provide substantiation of spread to lymph nodes, liver, or peritoneal cavity. A digital rectal examination is essential in determining the presence of a distal rectal cancer or of perineal or pelvic spread. A complete pelvic examination should not be omitted. Laboratory tests may reveal iron deficiency anemia or an abnormality of liver enzymes. Radiologic studies may include a chest roentgenogram or computed tomographic scan of the abdomen and pelvis.

In the evaluation of patients with symptoms or signs of colorectal cancer, the digital rectal examination is followed by colonoscopy or double-contrast barium enema following sigmoidoscopy. Endoscopic ultrasonography is being used with increasing frequency to help in the staging of rectal cancers. Depth of invasion can often be accurately determined. Flexible sigmoidoscopy has replaced rigid proctoscopy and is particularly useful in evaluating a patient with a rectosigmoid neoplasm or an individual who presents with rectal bleeding and in whom active inflammatory bowel disease is suspected. In the latter case a barium enema or even colonoscopy may be undesirable.

Colonoscopy is more sensitive than double-contrast barium enema in detecting small adenomas and cancers and is also of value in evaluating patients who have had an abnormality detected by barium enema. In addition, the presence or absence of synchronous cancers and adenomas can be determined. Colonoscopy can be used to remove adenomas, to biopsy suspected cancers, and to obtain brush biopsy for cytology of suspected malignancies and colonic strictures.

MANAGEMENT. The modern approach to management is a multidisciplinary one and includes consideration not only of the immediate clinical problem but also a long-term approach to the patient. This may include postoperative adjuvant treatment, future plans for assessment of local recurrence or distant metastasis, and attention to family members at increased risk.

Surgery. The most important goal of treatment for primary malignancies of the colon and rectum is complete removal. Surgical resection of the affected segment, including omentum and lymph nodes, is performed. Cancers of the right and left colon are treated by hemicolectomies; cancer of the sigmoid and upper rectum above 6 cm from the anal verge are resected anteriorly with removal of a margin of normal colon above and below the tumor. Stapling techniques have facilitated anastomoses within the pelvis. While 3-cm proximal and distal margins have been previously emphasized, an adequate radial margin is equally important.

Lesions within 5 cm of the anal verge are usually treated by a combined abdominoperineal resection and permanent colostomy. Newer approaches for small, early rectal cancers include sphincter-saving procedures utilizing local excision followed in some instances by radiation therapy to the pelvis.

For anal cancers the standard approach is to utilize a combination of radiation and chemotherapy, which will usually shrink or obliterate the cancer. Surgical resection is now usually reserved for lesions that do not respond to chemoradiation or that recur.

Surgery may be required for palliation as well as for cure. Colonic obstruction may necessitate a palliative colostomy, although a primary resection and colostomy can often be accomplished at the same operation. A perforated carcinoma is usually managed by primary resection and colostomy with later closure of the colostomy. For selected medically fit patients with one to three hepatic metastases, surgical resection of part of the tumor-bearing liver is often possible. Careful preoperative radiologic staging as well as intraoperative ultrasonography facilitates these technically demanding procedures. Laser photoablation is being increasingly used to relieve colonic or rectal obstruction or bleeding in patients with unresectable tumors or those with extensive metastatic disease.

Radiation Therapy. Radiation therapy plays an important role in the postoperative management of rectal cancer. The combination of radiation (50 Gy) and chemotherapy, 5-fluorouracil (5-FU), is now standard therapy and has been shown to decrease local recurrence and distant metastasis. Preoperative radiation therapy decreases postoperative local recurrence but does not prolong overall survival. It may also be used to reduce tumor size and enable otherwise unresectable lesions to be resected. Radiation therapy is useful in palliating recurrent rectal cancer (pain or bleeding) or bone or brain metastases. Intraoperative radiation therapy is being evaluated in several centers.

Chemotherapy. Patients with resected colonic cancer with lymph node spread may have improved survival if treated with the combination of 5-FU and levamisole for a period of 1 year. For patients with metastatic spread, the combination of 5-FU and leucovorin increases tumor shrinkage compared to 5-FU alone. Combinations of chemotherapeutic agents and cytokines are under study.

In patients with liver metastases, hepatic arterial therapy with implantable pumps or via injection ports using floxuridine (FUDR) alone or in combination with other drugs such as leucovorin produces an enhanced tumor shrinkage in the liver, but increased survival has not been demonstrated.

PROGNOSIS AND FOLLOW-UP. The 10-year survival for patients with colorectal cancer after surgical resection is approximately 50 per cent. The survival correlates well with the stage of the disease: cancer confined to the mucosa, 80 to 90 per cent 10-year survival; cancer extending through all areas of the bowel wall, 70 to 80 per cent; and cancer involving the regional lymph nodes, 30 to 55 per cent. Cancers of the distal rectum with lymph node involvement have a poorer prognosis. Several histopathologic staging systems (e.g., Dukes' or TNM) are in use to describe the extent of the malignancy (Table 105–2).

Prior to surgical resection, the entire colon should be examined, preferably by colonoscopy, for the presence of synchronous

TABLE 105–2. AMERICAN JOINT COMMITTEE ON CANCER: CLASSIFICATION OF COLON/RECTAL CANCER

Stage 0	Carcinoma in situ; the cancer does not extend beyond the smooth muscle that separates the mucosa from the submucosa. (T_{is}, N_0, M_0)
Stage I	Cancer confined to the mucosa, submucosa, or external muscle; the cancer does not extend through the bowel wall. (T_1 or T_2, N_0, M_0)
Stage II	Cancer that penetrates all layers of the bowel wall, with or without invasion of adjacent tissues. (T_3, N_0, M_0)
Stage III	Cancer involving regional lymph nodes or extending into nearby tissues or organs without spread to lymph nodes. (Any T, N_1–N_3, M_0; or T_4, N_0, M_0)
Stage IV	Cancer that has spread to distant sites, usually the liver or lungs. (Any T, any N, M_1)

T = Tumor size; N = lymph node involvement; M = degree of metastasis.

adenomas. If not possible preoperatively, colonoscopy should be performed postoperatively, usually within 2 to 3 months of the surgical procedure. Colonoscopy should be repeated a year later and every 2 to 3 years thereafter because new adenomas require 3 years or more to develop into large adenomas with malignant potential.

After surgical resection, patients without known systemic metastases are evaluated for adjuvant therapy. Patients with colonic cancer and lymph node involvement should receive 5-FU and levamisole, and those with rectal cancer and spread through the wall or with lymph node involvement should receive radiation plus chemotherapy. While receiving chemotherapy or radiation therapy, patients are followed very carefully according to protocol guidelines. For those not receiving any specific therapy, periodic follow-up including interim history, physical examination, and laboratory tests (liver enzymes, hematocrit) are performed every 3 to 6 months for the first 3 years, then every 6 months until the fifth year. Controversy exists concerning the cost-effectiveness of obtaining periodic chest radiographs or computed tomography (CT) scans of the abdomen and pelvis as part of routine follow-up care in the absence of symptoms or laboratory test abnormalities.

Carcinoembryonic Antigen (CEA). CEA levels in the blood may rise before symptoms or other laboratory test abnormalities are evident in patients with recurrent or metastatic colonic cancer. Some authorities favor periodic CEA determinations (e.g., every 3 months) after colorectal cancer resection, but this is very expensive and helpful only in a minority of patients. Occasionally, a rising CEA may detect a localized, surgically resectable metastasis. In conjunction with conventional radiologic techniques (CT scan or MRI), radiolabeled monoclonal antibodies to CEA may be helpful in localizing such metastases. In the absence of defined lesions, a "second look" laparotomy based on a rising CEA has not been shown to prolong survival.

In screening large patient groups for colon cancer, CEA elevation was found to have a false-positive rate of 15 per cent and a false-negative rate of about 50 per cent in nonmetastatic disease. The test is thus unsuitable for screening, lacking both appropriate specificity and sensitivity.

PREVENTION OF COLORECTAL CANCER

Many colorectal cancers are first brought to medical attention by the patient's recognition of symptoms. For improved survival, the diagnosis should ideally be made earlier, in an asymptomatic phase. A greater emphasis is now being placed on preventive measures. Primary prevention is the identification of factors, either genetic or environmental, responsible for colorectal cancers. Secondary prevention refers to the identification and eradication of premalignant lesions and the detection and resection of cancer while still curable.

Although definitive evidence of effectiveness is still lacking, the National Cancer Institute has issued certain dietary guidelines to try to reduce the risk of colorectal cancer: (1) a reduction of fat intake to less than 30 per cent of calories; (2) an increase of dietary fiber to 20 to 30 grams per day; (3) inclusion in the diet of a variety of vegetables and fruits; (4) avoidance of obesity; and

(5) moderate consumption of alcohol, if at all. In addition, regular exercise may also reduce risk.

Implicit in the concept of secondary prevention is the need for improved techniques for screening for early cancer or premalignant adenomas. Effective screening requires the availability and application of simple and economic measures to a large number of asymptomatic individuals to identify those with these lesions. Screening for colorectal cancer can be classified as follows: general screening of patients at average risk and screening of patients in high-risk groups. (For discussion of high-risk groups see *Polyposis Syndromes* and *Ulcerative Colitis.*)

AVERAGE-RISK PATIENTS. Currently, testing for fecal occult blood and flexible sigmoidoscopy in asymptomatic individuals are used for detecting early colorectal cancer. Testing for occult blood using guaiac-based methods seems to detect earlier lesions in those screened compared to controls, but whether cancer mortality is reduced has not yet been demonstrated. Newer immunochemical tests for human hemoglobin in the stool, currently under clinical trial, are likely to be more specific. Randomized controlled trials of flexible sigmoidoscopy have not been performed on a large scale. Flexible sigmoidoscopy can not only identify and eradicate premalignant and malignant lesions in the area examined but also can identify individuals who may have more proximal synchronous adenomas and carcinomas.

In the absence of definitive data concerning the value of mass screening, many physicians have accepted interim guidelines for their own patients: (1) annual digital rectal examination after age 40; (2) testing for fecal occult blood annually after age 50; and (3) flexible sigmoidoscopy every 3 to 5 years after age 50. Patients with abnormal findings require careful diagnostic evaluation, including colonoscopy. A critical evaluation of a screening program for colorectal cancer requires that important issues be addressed: (1) What are the expected benefits in terms of survival of patients whose disease is discovered by screening tests and treated? (2) Is there a mortality reduction from colorectal cancer in the entire screened population? (3) What are the psychological, economic, and other factors influencing patient compliance? (4) Are there adequate health resources available for the diagnostic workup and treatment of patients with a positive screening test? (5) What are the costs and risks of such screening?

Adenomas

Haggitt RC, et al.: Prognostic factors in colorectal carcinomas arising in adenomas: Implications for lesions removed by endoscopic polypectomy. Gastroenterology 89:328, 1985. *A practical discussion of cancers arising in adenomas.*

Risk

Burt RW, et al.: Dominant inheritance of adenomatous colonic polyps and colorectal cancer. N Engl J Med 312:1540, 1985. Cannon-Albright LA, et al.: Common inheritance of susceptibility to colonic adenomatous polyps and associated colorectal cancers. N Engl J Med 319:533, 1988. *These two papers present data concerning the inheritance of sporadic adenomas and cancer.*

Levin B, et al.: Surveillance of patients with chronic ulcerative colitis. WHO Bulletin (in press). *A review of the current approach to surveillance for dysplasia in high-risk individuals and an evaluation of the relationship between inflammatory bowel disease and cancer.*

Lynch HT, et al.: Differential diagnosis of hereditary nonpolyposis colorectal cancer (Lynch syndrome I and Lynch syndrome II). Dis Colon Rectum 31:372, 1988. *A review of hereditary nonpolyposis colorectal cancer.*

Molecular Biology

Nishisha I, Nakamura Y, Miyoshi Y, et al.: Mutations of chromosome 5 q 21 genes in FAP and colorectal cancer patients. Science 253:665, 1991. *One of several exciting recent papers on the molecular biology of polyps and colon cancer.*

Therapy

Moertel CG, et al.: Levamisole and fluorouracil for adjuvant therapy of resected colon carcinoma. N Engl J Med 322:352, 1990. *An encouraging report of a trial of adjuvant therapy in 1300 patients, demonstrating a benefit for adjuvant therapy.*

Poon MA, et al.: Biochemical modulation of fluorouracil: Evidence of significant improvement of survival and quality of life in patients with advanced colorectal carcinoma. J Clin Oncol 7:1407, 1989. *A description of biochemical modulation with apparent clinical benefit.*

Rosenberg SA, et al.: Principles and applications of biologic therapy in cancer. *In* DeVita VT, Hellman S, Rosenberg SA (eds.): Principles and Practice of Oncology. Philadelphia, J. B. Lippincott Company, 1989, pp 301–347.

Dietary Factors

Garland C, Shekelle RB, Barrett-Connor E, et al.: Dietary vitamin D and calcium and risk of colorectal cancer: A 19 year prospective study in men. Lancet 1:307, 1985. *An intriguing epidemiologic study suggestive of an important role for calcium in the prevention of colorectal cancer.*

Physiological Effect and Health Consequences of Dietary Fiber. Federation of American Societies for Experimental Biology, Life Science Research Office, 1987. *A critical evaluation of the interactions of fiber and intestinal physiology.*

Wargovich MJ, et al.: Dietary factors and colorectal cancer. Gastroenterol Clin 17:727, 1988. *A review of naturally occurring anticarcinogens and other factors that may influence the development of colorectal cancer.*

Screening

Hardcastle JD, Pye G: Screening for colorectal cancer: A critical review. World J Surg 13:38, 1989.

Winawer SJ, St. John J, Bond J, et al.: Risks and screening of average risk individuals for colorectal cancer. WHO Bull 68:505, 1990. *These two papers evaluate current approaches to screening for large bowel cancers.*

NEOPLASMS OF THE SMALL BOWEL

Benign and malignant tumors of the lining epithelium and mesenchymal tissues may arise in the small intestine, or these areas may be secondarily involved by direct invasion from surrounding structures or by metastases. The small bowel represents almost 90 per cent of the mucosal surface of the gut, but small intestinal cancers account for only 1 to 2 per cent of all gastrointestinal neoplasms. Only about 2000 cases occur in the United States each year.

RISK FACTORS. Patients with regional enteritis, especially those who have had segments of intestine surgically bypassed, have an increased incidence of small bowel carcinoma. Individuals with Gardner syndrome have an increased risk of periampullary adenocarcinoma. In patients with Peutz-Jeghers syndrome, the relative risk of small intestinal adenocarcinoma is 16 times that expected, with a lifetime incidence of 2 per cent. Patients with celiac disease of long duration have an increased incidence of intestinal lymphoma, as do patients with the acquired immunodeficiency syndrome and other immunodeficiency states. Mediterranean abdominal lymphoma (immunoproliferative small intestinal disease) has been widely reported among Arabs and Jews of Middle Eastern origin and also occurs sporadically throughout the world, including blacks in southern Africa.

Why small bowel neoplasms, especially adenocarcinomas, are so uncommon compared with large bowel cancers is uncertain. It is possible that the rapid transit time with a resultant decreased exposure time to carcinogens, lower numbers of bacteria, and dilution of potential carcinogens by the large volume of enteric liquids may contribute.

PATHOLOGY. Benign. These lesions include adenomas, leiomyomas, lipomas, and angiomas. Brunner's gland adenomas are not neoplastic but represent a hyperplasia or hypertrophy of submucosal duodenal glands. These appear as small nodules in the duodenal mucosa detected at endoscopy or on barium radiographs.

Malignant. Adenocarcinomas, carcinoids, lymphomas, and leiomyosarcomas account for over 90 per cent of malignant small bowel tumors. Adenocarcinomas are most common in the proximal small intestine, whereas lymphomas and carcinoids are most common in the distal small intestine.

CLINICAL MANIFESTATIONS. Over one half of all benign bowel tumors remain asymptomatic and may only be discovered incidentally at laparotomy or autopsy. Lack of symptoms is attributable to the liquid contents of the small intestine and distensibility of the small intestine. Large tumors may lead to partial or complete mechanical obstruction from intussusception or volvulus. Adenocarcinomas account for about half of the malignant tumors of the small intestine, with a peak incidence in the sixth and seventh decades. The duodenum is the most frequently affected site. When postbulbar in location, adenocarcinoma may simulate peptic ulcer disease; when in the periampullary region, it may cause obstructive jaundice. More distally, adenocarcinomas may remain silent until symptoms of intestinal obstruction or gastrointestinal hemorrhage occur.

Carcinoids are the most frequent small intestinal neoplasm, with over half found incidentally either at autopsy or at operation for other diseases. Small carcinoid tumors may be asymptomatic, but larger carcinoid tumors can obstruct the lumen or bleed. Once metastasis occurs to the liver, features of the carcinoid syndrome become apparent (Ch. 230). Weight loss, intestinal obstruction, fever, bleeding, and evidence of malabsorption syndrome are features of lymphoma. Massive hemorrhage and intestinal perforation may be the presenting symptoms of large sarcomas.

SIGNS. Physical examination may be unremarkable in patients with benign tumors, unless the neoplasms are large enough to present with a mass. Loud borborygmi, visible peristalsis, and abdominal distention may be present in intestinal obstruction. In patients with malignant small bowel neoplasms, more obvious physical findings may be evident. Cachexia, hepatomegaly, ascites, and jaundice may be found. Peripheral lymphadenopathy or splenomegaly may be found in those with extensive lymphoma.

DIFFERENTIAL DIAGNOSIS. The initial symptoms may be vague and poorly defined. Once bleeding occurs, causes such as peptic ulceration, Meckel's diverticulum, and vascular anomalies need to be considered (Ch. 111). Obstructive jaundice may occur with periampullary neoplasms, bile duct cancer, impacted common duct stones, pancreatitis, and pancreatic cancer (Ch. 107). Intestinal obstruction may be due to adhesions, particularly in patients who have had prior abdominal operations, internal hernias, volvulus, or intussusception.

LABORATORY AND RADIOLOGIC STUDIES. A hypochromic, microcytic anemia is quite common. Elevation of alkaline phosphatase and bilirubin may recur if the ampulla of Vater is obstructed or if liver metastases are present. Elevated levels of plasma serotonin or urinary 5-hydroxyindoleacetic acid occur in the carcinoid syndrome (Ch. 230). Dysproteinemia is a typical feature of Mediterranean lymphoma and is characterized by the presence of abnormal fragments of IgA in the serum and urine that is devoid of light chains (Ch. 151).

Upper gastrointestinal barium radiographs and selective nasoenteric intubation (enteroclysis), which permits the introduction of barium and air into a relatively localized segment, may be useful in localizing tumors. Abdominal ultrasonography and computed tomography may determine the extent of hepatic involvement, aid in the workup of jaundice, and assess intraabdominal and retroperitoneal spread. Intestinal lymphoma may occasionally be diagnosed by peroral intestinal biopsy, but the disease mainly involves the lamina propria and usually requires a full-thickness surgical biopsy. A thorough staging of lymphoma involves bone marrow biopsy, laparotomy with splenectomy, and biopsies of regional lymph nodes and liver.

ENDOSCOPIC EVALUATION. Front-viewing and side-viewing fiberoptic endoscopes are used to examine the duodenum; suspicious lesions can be biopsied and brushed. Periampullary lesions can be well visualized; the pancreatic and biliary trees can be studied by contrast radiography after endoscopic cannulation. The terminal ileum can also be viewed at colonoscopy. Small bowel enteroscopy, a relatively new technique, is sometimes helpful in localizing a small bleeding lesion.

THERAPY. Treatment is primarily surgical for symptomatic benign tumors, adenocarcinomas, leiomyosarcomas, malignant carcinoids, and those with secondary involvement of the small intestine. Duodenal carcinomas or large villous adenomas are treated by pancreaticoduodenal resection (Whipple procedure). In patients with localized lymphoma (stage I) surgical excision is recommended. Combination chemotherapy is used for more extensive lymphoma (Ch. 147). Radiation therapy may be helpful for bulky tumors or localized recurrences.

PROGNOSIS AND PREVENTION. The prognosis for benign tumors of the intestine is good if surgical resection can alleviate bleeding and obstruction. The prognosis of small intestinal adenocarcinomas is generally poor. The prognosis for leiomyosarcoma and primary lymphomas is good if surgical resection is complete, but this is rarely possible. Patients with malignant carcinoid tumors may survive for long periods even in the presence of extensive hepatic involvement (Ch. 230).

Primary small intestinal lymphomas occurring in the Middle East could possibly be decreased by public health measures that decrease parasitic infestation. Earlier diagnosis and adequate treatment of celiac disease (gluten free diet) may reduce the frequency of malignancy. Surgical bypass should not be performed in patients with Crohn's disease. In patients with familial polyposis syndromes, duodenal and periampullary adenomas should be monitored periodically. Prophylactic endoscopic or surgical removal may be appropriate.

Ashley SW, Wells SA: Tumors of the small intestine. Semin Oncol 15:116, 1988. *An updated review of pathology, natural history, and epidemiology.*

Lightdale CJ, Koepsell TC, Sherlock P: Small intestinal cancer. *In* Schottenfeld D, Fraumeni J (eds.): Cancer Epidemiology and Prevention. Philadelphia, W. B. Saunders Company, 1982. *A comprehensive discussion of the topic, including epidemiologic and etiologic aspects.*

Moertel CG: An odyssey in the land of small tumors. J Clin Oncol 5:1503, 1987. *New insights into the biology, natural history, and management of carcinoid tumors.*

106 Pancreatitis

William M. Steinberg

Normal Anatomy and Physiology of the Pancreas

The dorsal pancreas forms in the fetus as an outpouching from the duodenum at approximately 4 weeks of gestation. Several days later, the ventral pancreas forms from the hepatic diverticulum. At 7 to 8 weeks of gestation, the rotation of the duodenum leads the two pancreatic buds and their main ducts to fuse. If the two buds fuse incompletely, the duct of Wirsung drains only the ventral pancreas and the duct of Santorini the dorsal pancreas. This common anomaly, termed pancreas divisum, is present in 5 to 10 per cent of the general population.

The exocrine pancreas consists of acinar, centroacinar, and ductular cells. The acinar cells, the majority of cells, synthesize approximately 20 digestive enzymes, which are secreted from zymogen granules in the apical portions of the cell into the central ductule of the acinus by exocytosis. The ductules coalesce to form larger ducts, which empty into the duodenum at the ampulla of Vater. The ductular cells exchange bicarbonate for chloride, especially at increased rates of secretion. This ensures an alkaline milieu in the duodenum, which is necessary for optimal activity of pancreatic enzymes. Pancreatic secretion is stimulated by the vagus nerve (cerebral, gastric, and intestinal phases) and by the action of two hormones secreted by the duodenum: (1) secretin, which is released in response to acid in the duodenum and stimulates a pancreatic juice high in bicarbonate concentration, and (2) cholecystokinin (CCK), which is released in response to fatty acids and amino acids in the duodenum and results in a secretion rich in enzymes.

The enzymes from the pancreas digest starch (amylase), fats (lipase), and protein (trypsin and many other proteolytic enzymes). Although amylase and lipase are secreted in active forms, the proteolytic enzymes are secreted as inactive zymogens that must be activated in the duodenum. Trypsinogen is activated by the small bowel mucosal enzyme enterokinase to form trypsin. Trypsin then activates the other proteolytic enzymes. The pancreas is protected from autodigestion by three mechanisms: (1) secretion of proteolytic enzymes in an inactive form; (2) packaging of pancreatic proenzymes and lysozomes in separate compartments, preventing premature activation, and (3) concomitant secretion of protease inhibitors to neutralize any prematurely activated enzyme.

ACUTE PANCREATITIS

Pathogenesis

The precise mechanisms that trigger the autodigestive processes causing acute pancreatitis are not known. Some of the factors that may play a role include transient obstruction of the pancreatic duct, reflux of duodenal contents into the pancreatic duct, ischemia, altered pancreatic duct permeability, and intracellular coalescence of zymogen granules with lysozomal enzymes, such as cathepsin B, causing premature acinar cell activation of trypsin. The autodigestive process starts with the intraacinar activation of trypsin, which in turn activates other enzymes, such as phospholipase A_2 and elastase. These active enzymes disrupt cellular membranes and cause intrapancreatic edema, peripancreatic fat necrosis, parenchymal hemorrhage, and necrosis of acinar cells. Furthermore, activated enzymes, liberated into the peritoneal space and systemic circulation, may overwhelm host defenses (α-antitrypsin and α_2-macroglobulin) and cause distant end-organ dysfunction by as yet unknown mechanisms.

Etiologic Associations (Table 106–1)

In the United States, acute pancreatitis is most commonly associated with *alcoholism* and *gallstones;* a large number of cases are also *idiopathic.* The pathogenesis of alcoholic pancreatitis is discussed in the section on chronic pancreatitis. Most alcoholics who present with a first attack of alcoholic pancreatitis probably already have superimposed chronic pancreatitis, as evidenced by reduced bicarbonate or enzyme secretion when tested with sensitive methods. In these patients the trigger for the acute attacks of pain is unknown.

Gallstone-associated pancreatitis, especially common in elderly women, is thought to occur when gallstones transiently obstruct the common bile duct in or near the orifice of the pancreatic duct. In fact, a gallstone can usually be found if stools are carefully collected and examined immediately after attacks of gallstone pancreatitis. The mechanism by which choledocholithiasis causes pancreatitis is unclear. Theories include (1) obstruction of the ampulla of Vater by a stone, allowing bile to reflux into the pancreatic duct, injuring the parenchyma, and (2) transient obstruction of the pancreatic duct without bile reflux.

TABLE 106–1. ETIOLOGIC ASSOCIATIONS WITH ACUTE PANCREATITIS

I. Obstructive causes
  A. Choledocholithiasis
  B. Ampullary or pancreatic tumors
  C. Worms or foreign bodies obstructing the papilla
  D. Pancreas divisum with accessory duct obstruction
  E. Choledochocele
  F. Periampullary duodenal diverticula
  G. Hypertensive sphincter of Oddi
  H. Duodenal loop obstruction
II. Toxin/drug causes
  A. Toxins
    1. Ethyl alcohol
    2. Methyl alcohol
    3. Scorpion venom
    4. Organophosphorus insecticides
  B. Drugs
    1. Definite association (documented with rechallenges): azathioprine/6-mercaptourine, valproic acid, estrogens, tetracycline, metronidazole, nitrofurantoin, pentamidine, furosemide, sulfonamides, methyldopa, cytarabine, cimetidine, sulindac
    2. Not definite (no rechallenges reported): thiazide diuretics, ethacrynic acid, phenformin, procainamide, chlorthalidone, L-asparaginase, acetaminophen
III. Metabolic causes
  A. Hypertriglyceridemia
  B. Hypercalcemia
IV. Trauma
  A. Accidental—blunt trauma to the abdomen
  B. Iatrogenic—postoperative, ERCP, endoscopic sphincterotomy, sphincter of Oddi manometry
V. Inherited
VI. Infection
  A. Parasitic—ascariasis, clonorchis
  B. Viral—mumps, hepatitis A, hepatitis B, coxsackie B, Epstein-Barr
  C. Bacterial—*Mycoplasma, Campylobacter jejuni*
VII. Vascular
  A. Ischemia—hypoperfusion (e.g., post–cardiac surgery).
  B. Atherosclerotic emboli
  C. Vasculitis—systemic lupus erythematosus, polyarteritis nodosa, malignant hypertension
VIII. Miscellaneous
  A. Penetrating peptic ulcer
  B. Crohn's disease of the duodenum
  C. Pregnancy associated
  D. Pediatric association—Reye's syndrome, cystic fibrosis
IX. Idiopathic

Whether pancreas divisum predisposes to acute pancreatitis is controversial. Some believe that both the congenital abnormality and stenosis of the accessory papilla (which obstructs the flow of juices draining the duct of Santorini) must be present to cause pancreatitis. Other conditions that obstruct the pancreatic duct (either Wirsung or Santorini) have been reported to cause acute pancreatitis (e.g., foreign bodies, parasites, tumors) (Table 106–1). Hypertensive sphincter of Oddi as determined by pressure measurements has been reported to be a cause of recurrent acute pancreatitis and based on this presumption has been treated by endoscopic sphincterotomy. In elderly patients, gallstones are usually the cause of a first attack of acute pancreatitis, but a small tumor of the ductular or periampullary region must also be considered.

Toxins other than ethanol that may cause acute pancreatitis include methyl alcohol (Ch. 28), scorpion stings, and organophosphorus insecticides.

Drug-induced pancreatitis usually reflects hypersensitivity rather than excessive dosage. Characteristically, it occurs within the first month of exposure and is usually mild and self-limited. The most commonly implicated drugs in adults are azathioprine and its congener 6-mercaptopurine. Three to 5 per cent of individuals taking these drugs develop pancreatitis. In children, valproic acid is most commonly implicated.

Hypertriglyceridemia with levels exceeding 1000 mg per deciliter may be associated with moderate to severe acute pancreatitis (Ch. 172). If triglyceride levels are reduced to below 500 mg per deciliter, recurrent attacks are greatly reduced in frequency. *Hypercalcemia* from any cause is another rare metabolic cause of acute pancreatitis (Ch. 235).

Trauma to the pancreas, either accidental (e.g., blunt abdominal trauma in an automobile accident) or iatrogenic (surgical abdominal trauma), can lead to pancreatitis. Postoperative acute pancreatitis can also follow extra-abdominal surgery and may occasionally be severe. The trauma of endoscopic retrograde cholangiopancreatography (ERCP) produces acute pancreatitis in about 1 to 5 per cent of patients.

A propensity for pancreatitis may be inherited as a rare autosomal dominant trait. Characteristically, attacks of acute pancreatitis begin in childhood or young adulthood and progress to chronic pancreatitis and pancreatic insufficiency. Pancreatolithiasis may be prominent, and an associated aminoaciduria has been described in some families.

Infections as precipitating events in initiating acute pancreatitis have been reported secondary to mumps, hepatitis A and B, and Epstein-Barr and coxsackie B viruses, as well as from *Mycoplasma* and *Campylobacter jejuni.* Further documentation to confirm many of these associations is needed.

Vascular insufficiency (hypoperfusion, atherosclerotic plaques) and vasculitis have also been implicated as causes of acute pancreatitis, consistent with experimental evidence that reducing blood flow to the pancreas can cause or exacerbate pancreatitis.

Clinical Presentation

Severe knifelike epigastric *pain* with radiation to the back associated with nausea and vomiting is the classic presentation of acute pancreatitis. The pain tends to come on rapidly over seconds to minutes, is constant, and can last from days to more than a week. The latter distinguishes acute pancreatitis from peptic ulcer and biliary colic, in which painful episodes are shorter. The pain of pancreatitis can sometimes be partially relieved by flexing the trunk. Rarely, acute pancreatitis may be painless.

Physical findings include mild fever, tachypnea, tachycardia, and hypo- or hypertension. The abdomen may be distended because of the presence of ileus or a pseudocyst or phlegmon (an inflammatory mass), which may be palpable. If ileus is present, the bowel sounds are hypoactive or absent. Epigastric tenderness is usually marked and occasionally is associated with rigidity and guarding suggestive of an acute surgical abdomen. Rarely, with hemorrhagic pancreatitis, blood dissects from the retroperitoneal location of the pancreas around fascial planes and appears as a large ecchymosis in the flanks (Grey Turner sign) or umbilical area (Cullen sign). With hemorrhagic or other forms of severe pancreatitis, patients may present in shock with marked hypotension due to loss of blood into the pancreas, or exudation of large amounts of plasma into the retroperitoneal space, or changes in vascular tone mediated in part by vasoactive peptides.

The differential diagnosis is that of the acute abdomen and includes peptic ulcer with or without perforation, biliary colic, renal colic, small bowel obstruction and infarction, and suppurative cholangitis.

Diagnosis

LABORATORY TESTS

AMYLASE. The diagnosis of acute pancreatitis relies heavily on the demonstration of an increased serum amylase activity. Serum amylase, however, can be mildly elevated in many diseases not affecting the pancreas (e.g., those involving the salivary glands, small intestine, biliary tract, and Fallopian tubes), as well as in macroamylasemia (aggregated circulating amylase with or without immunoglobulin A). Amylase elevations of more than two- or threefold above the upper limit of normal in the setting of acute abdominal pain most often indicate acute pancreatitis. The amylase returns to normal more rapidly than do other pancreatic enzymes (e.g., lipase) so that a normal amylase by no means excludes the diagnosis of pancreatitis. This is especially true in a patient with acute pancreatitis superimposed on chronic pancreatitis (e.g., a chronic alcoholic) in whom a normal amylase level presumably reflects a "burnt out" pancreas with extensive destruction of acinar cells. The height of the rise of the serum amylase does not correlate with the severity of the pancreatitis. Patients with alcoholic pancreatitis tend to have lower serum levels of amylase (usually < 1000 IU per liter) than patients with other forms of pancreatitis. Amylase can be fractionated into pancreatic and salivary isoamylase components by different techniques. Several simple-to-use chemical kits have been developed to semiquantitatively measure pancreatic isoamylase, but technical difficulties with these kits have limited their usefulness. In general, amylase fractionation gives no more useful clinical information than that which can be obtained from other enzyme markers such as the serum lipase.

In the typical attack of pancreatitis, the serum amylase tends to normalize 4 to 7 days after the onset of pain. If the amylase is elevated beyond 7 days, complications such as a pseudocyst may be present. Renal failure, in the absence of pancreatitis, may raise the serum amylase (as well as lipase and other enzyme markers) to as high as four to six times the upper limit of normal. Elevations above this level in a patient with renal failure suggest concurrent pancreatic inflammation. Hypertriglyceridemia associated with turbid serum can mask an elevated serum amylase, thus obscuring the diagnosis of acute pancreatitis. In these circumstances, diluting the serum leads to a paradoxical rise in the measured serum amylase value.

LIPASE. Serum lipase tests, especially those that employ colipase as a cofactor, have the advantage of greater sensitivity and specificity than the amylase levels. Lipase is elevated as early as amylase but stays elevated for much longer periods of time. This allows a diagnosis to be made after the amylase level may have returned to normal. An initial lipase determination is often helpful in confirming pancreatitis in patients who are hyperamylasemic or who have symptoms of pancreatitis but a normal serum amylase level.

OTHER BLOOD TESTS. Immunologic blood tests (radioimmunoassays and ELISA assays) of other enzymes or proenzymes such as trypsinogen or elastase are more sensitive and specific than amylase in detecting pancreatic injury. They offer few, if any, advantages over the lipase assay, however. Immunoassays are more helpful in detecting pancreatic exocrine insufficiency (see below) than are the enzymatic lipase or amylase assays.

The white blood cell count is frequently elevated moderately (< 20,000 per microliter). Acute pancreatitis characteristically lowers the serum calcium concentration (see below under complications). A patient presenting with a high normal level of serum calcium during acute pancreatitis may actually have an underlying hypercalcemia. Serum triglyceride levels should be obtained in all patients with acute pancreatitis because of potential etiologic importance and also to aid in interpreting amylase levels. Gallstone pancreatitis is suspected if patients with acute pancreatitis present with bilirubin levels greater than 2.5 mg per deciliter and alkaline phosphatase and aminotransferase levels greater than three times normal. Other blood tests are discussed under risk factors.

URINARY TESTS. Plasma amylase is filtered by the renal glomerulus; normally most is resorbed or metabolized by the renal tubules, and the remainder is excreted in the urine. During acute pancreatitis, increased amounts of amylase are excreted into the urine owing to inhibition of renal tubular resorption. Timed 2-hour or 24-hour measurements of urinary amylase content or of the amylase-to-creatinine clearance ratio have been used as diagnostic markers of acute pancreatitis. These urinary measurements, however, are not as sensitive or specific as the easier-to-obtain serum lipase or immunologic blood tests and add little clinical information.

OTHER DIAGNOSTIC TESTS. A diagnostic peritoneal tap with lavage can occasionally be helpful in diagnosing acute pancreatitis and in differentiating this condition from other intra-abdominal processes. Acute pancreatitis frequently is accompanied by sterile, straw- to prunish-colored peritoneal fluid with a high amylase content. Dark prune-colored fluid suggests severe necrotizing or hemorrhagic pancreatitis. Fluid that is foul smelling and has bacteria or vegetable matter on Gram's stain suggests a perforated viscus.

IMAGING TESTS

Plain and upright films of the abdomen are important in ruling out a perforated viscus, e.g., as suggested by the finding of free air under the diaphragm. Pancreatitis may sometimes be difficult to differentiate from small bowel obstruction because it may lead to diffuse or localized ileus (sentinel loop). In rare circumstances, an acutely inflamed pancreas may cause localized obstruction of the transverse or descending colon (colon "cutoff" sign). Calcification of the pancreas suggests that the bout of acute disease is superimposed on chronic pancreatitis. Later in the course of severe pancreatitis, a plain film may rarely detect air bubbles ("soap bubble sign") in the retroperitoneum, suggestive of a pancreatic abscess with gas-producing organisms.

Chest roentgenograms may show some of the pulmonary findings seen in association with pancreatitis, including pleural effusions (left side more often than right), atelectasis, and acute pulmonary edema patterns. Barium contrast studies of the upper gastrointestinal tract may show anterior displacement of the stomach due to a pancreatic phlegmon or edema and spiculation of the duodenal C loop due to the adjacent pancreatic inflammatory process.

The two most important imaging modalities in the field of pancreatitis are *ultrasonography* and *computed tomography* (CT scan) of the abdomen. These two techniques have important complementary roles in the diagnosis and management of acute pancreatitis (Figs. 106–1, 106–2, and 93–2). Ultrasonography is especially helpful in detecting the presence of cholelithiasis and in determining if there is dilatation of the biliary tree to suggest choledocholithiasis and gallstone pancreatitis (see Figs. 93–5 amd 93–6). Ultrasonography is less sensitive in detecting stones in the common bile duct and tends not to visualize the pancreas well because of overlying bowel gas. The CT scan does not visualize the gallbladder as completely as does ultrasonography, but it visualizes the pancreas and peripancreatic spaces with greater accuracy. A CT scan of the pancreas is frequently normal in mild cases of acute pancreatitis but is especially helpful in determining if phlegmonous pancreatitis is present or if extra- or intrapancreatic fluid collections are forming. Serial scans may delineate the formation of abscesses, which may require drainage. CT scanning with high-bolus intravenous contrast (dynamic CT scanning) may demonstrate areas of low or no perfusion, suggestive of necrosis. This may be helpful in prognosis, as greater than 50 per cent necrosis of the pancreas is associated with high mortality.

ASSESSMENT OF RISK FACTORS IN PROGNOSIS. Several blood tests alone or in combination (multiple criteria tests) are used to delineate severe forms of acute pancreatitis (Table 106–2). Ranson's criteria have been modified over time to separate those patients with gallstone from nongallstone pancreatitis. If three or more risk factors are present from the Ranson or Glasgow list (Table 106–2), the patient's course tends to have much greater morbidity and mortality. For instance, patients who have up to two Ranson risk factors have a mortality of less than 5 per cent; those with three to four risk factors, a mortality of 15 to 20 per cent; five to six risk factors, a mortality of 40 per

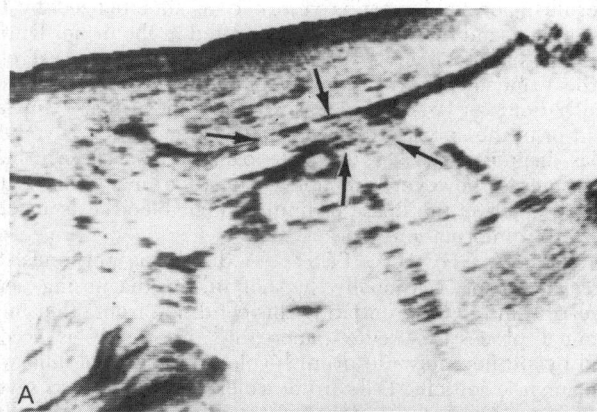

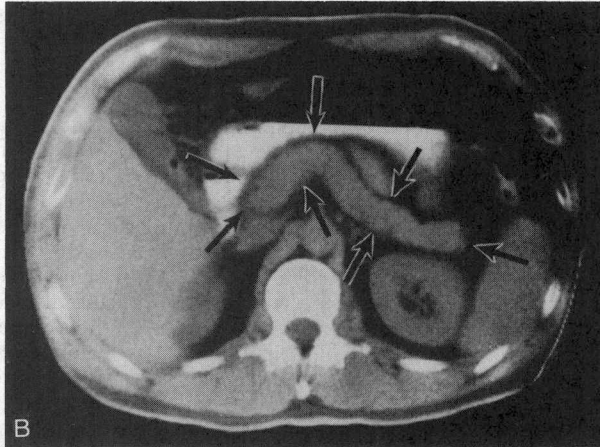

FIGURE 106–1. Normal pancreas demonstrated by ultrasound (A) and computed tomography (B). (Courtesy of Dr. Eugene P. DiMagno, Mayo Medical School, Rochester, Minnesota.)

cent; seven to eight risk factors, a mortality approaching 100 per cent.

Other blood tests, such as phospholipase A_2, methemalbumin, α_1-antitrypsin, α_2-macroglobulin, and, most recently, the C-reactive protein and trypsinogen-activated peptide, have been reported to be helpful in predicting severity of disease.

Course and Complications

In most patients acute pancreatitis is mild, requiring less than 1 week of hospitalization, but 5 to 25 per cent of patients have a more complicated course. The complications of pancreatitis (Table 106–3) can be divided into those that occur early (within the first week or two after admission) and those that occur late (more than 2 weeks after admission). The most serious of the early complications, usually found with necrotizing pancreatitis, are shock and pulmonary failure.

The pathogenesis of shock in acute pancreatitis can be hemorrhage into the substance of the pancreas or extravasation of massive amounts of plasma into the retroperitoneum. Release of vasoactive substances that cause vasodilation or myocardial depression may play an ancillary role. *The adult respiratory distress syndrome* (Ch. 70), the most serious of the pulmonary complications, is thought to be caused by injury of pulmonary capillaries and surfactant by circulating pancreatic enzymes, such as phospholipase A_2. The autodigested, necrotic pancreas may be sterile or secondarily infected with enteric organisms (infected necrosis). Severe hypocalcemia (serum calcium < 7 mg per deciliter) is associated with a more serious prognosis. The etiology of hypocalcemia is thought to be multifactorial, including concomitant hypoalbuminemia (the most prevalent cause), complexing of calcium to fatty acids released in the vicinity of the pancreas, and inadequate secretion or increased inactivation of parathyroid hormone or refractoriness to its action. Fluid collections and inflammatory debris may form between the pancreas and adjacent organs (Fig. 106–3). Most of these pseudocysts resolve sponta-

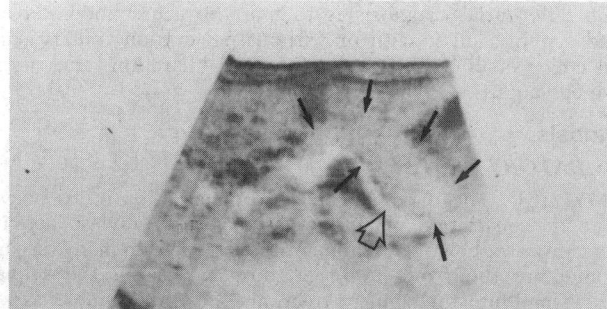

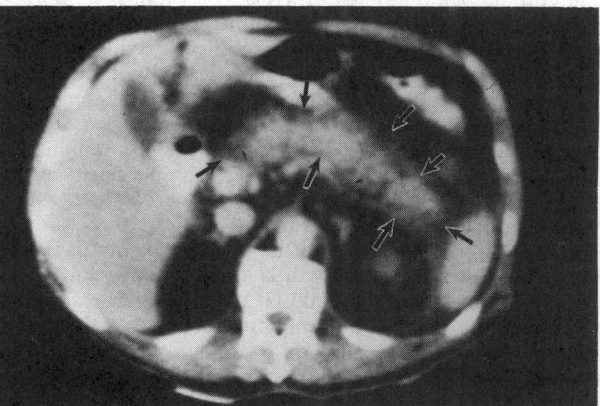

FIGURE 106–2. Diffusely enlarged pancreas of acute pancreatitis demonstrated by ultrasonography (*above*) and computed tomography (*below*). The large arrow on the sonogram points to the splenic vein. (Courtesy of Dr. Henry I. Goldberg, Department of Radiology, University of California at San Francisco.)

neously, but some may persist and become infected. Infected pseudocysts or abscesses, the most common causes of late morbidity and mortality in acute pancreatitis, should be suspected in patients who have recurrent or persistent fever into the second or third week of illness. Serial CT scans can detect most, but not all, fluid collections but cannot conclusively confirm or exclude infection. Fever spikes within the first week are common in severe pancreatitis and may be seen with either sterile or infected necrosis.

TABLE 106–2. ADVERSE PROGNOSTIC FACTORS IN SEVERE ACUTE PANCREATITIS

Ranson's Criteria[1, 2]		Modified Glasgow Criteria[3]
Nongallstone	*Gallstone*	
On admission	**On admission**	**Within 48 hours**
Age >55	Age >70	Age >55
WBC >16,000/μl	WBC >18,000/μl	WBC >15,000/μl
Glu >200 mg/dl	Glu >220 mg/dl	Glu >180 mg/dl
LDH >350 IU/L	LDH >400 IU/L	BUN >96 mg/dl
AST >250 IU/L	AST >250 IU/L	LDH >600 IU/L
		Albumin <3.3 gm/dl
Within 48 hours	**Within 48 hours**	Calcium <8 mg/dl
HCT decrease >10 pts	HCT decrease >10 pts	Po₂ <60 mm Hg
BUN increase >5 mg/dl	BUN increase >2 mg/dl	
Calcium <8 mg/dl	Calcium <8 mg/dl	
Po₂ <60 mm Hg		
Base deficit >4 mEq/L	Base deficit >5 mEq/L	
Fluid deficit >6 L	Fluid deficit >4 L	

[1]Ranson JH, Rifkind KM, Roses DF, et al.: Prognostic signs and the role of operative management in acute pancreatitis. Surg Gynecol Obstet 139:69, 1974.
[2]Ranson JHC: Etiological and prognostic factors in human acute pancreatitis: A review. Am J Gastroenterol 77:633, 1982.
[3]Blamey SL, Imrie CW, O'Neill J, et al.: Prognostic factors in acute pancreatitis. Gut 25:1340, 1984.
Glu = Glucose; LDH = lactic dehydrogenase; AST = aspartate aminotransferase; HCT = hematocrit; BUN = blood urea nitrogen.

TABLE 106–3. COMPLICATIONS OF ACUTE PANCREATITIS

Early
  Vascular instability, shock
  Pulmonary insufficiency—atelectasis, effusions, adult respiratory
    distress syndrome
  Renal insufficiency—acute tubular necrosis
  Metabolic disturbances—hypergylcemia, acidosis, hypocalcemia,
    hypomagnesemia
  Acute fluid collections—pseudocysts
  Infected necrosis
  Colonic obstruction and necrosis
  Pancreatic hemorrhage
  Disseminated intravascular coagulation
  Miscellaneous—metastatic fat necrosis (skin, bone, brain), psychosis,
    sudden blindness due to retinal artery occlusion
Late
  Fluid collections—pseudocysts, abscess

Management

Patients with mild pancreatitis, who have few poor prognostic factors (see Table 106–2), are easily managed by avoidance of oral intake, intravenous hydration, and analgesia with meperidine. Pain usually subsides in 2 to 4 days and oral feedings can be resumed.

Patients with severe pancreatitis and more than three risk factors (see Table 106–2) frequently require close monitoring in an intensive care unit with specific attention to the complications that develop. Hypotension and vascular instability require intensive and frequently massive fluid resuscitation monitored by a central venous line. Metabolic complications such as hyperglycemia, hypocalcemia, and hypomagnesemia may require insulin and appropriate calcium or magnesium supplementation. Pulmonary failure may require mechanical ventilation with positive end-expiratory pressure therapy. When performed within the first few days of hospitalization, peritoneal dialysis has been reported to ameliorate and stabilize the severe vascular and pulmonary complications of early acute pancreatitis. Unfortunately, overall survival is not improved, as patients succumb from pancreatic abscess later in the course of their disease. The use of agents known to suppress pancreatic secretion, either directly or indirectly (e.g., glucagon, somatostatin, cimetidine, or nasogastric suction), or of enzyme inhibitors (e.g., aprotinin or gabexate mesilate) has also failed to improve the morbidity or mortality of acute pancreatitis in controlled studies. Whether antibiotics are useful in the treatment of acute pancreatitis has not been well defined. Many authorities use broad-spectrum antibiotics in patients having a complicated course, but without documentation of their effectiveness.

If gallstone pancreatitis is suspected (gallstones on sonogram, dilated common bile duct, elevated serum bilirubin and alkaline phosphatase), and the patient has severe disease (three or more Ranson criteria) without improvement within 48 hours, emergency endoscopic retrograde pancreatography should be considered. Emergent sphincterotomy with extraction of the common duct stone can improve the prognosis in this setting.

Patients with acute pancreatic fluid collections should be followed with serial CT scans. Most cysts subside spontaneously. Cysts that are greater than 5 to 6 cm in diameter after 6 weeks of observation usually do not resolve spontaneously. They should be drained percutaneously, endoscopically, or surgically to prevent complications such as perforation, infection, or hemorrhage. Early fluid collections accompanied by signs of sepsis in a toxic-appearing patient should be aspirated percutaneously under CT scan guidance. If bacteria are found on Gram's stain, prompt percutaneous or surgical drainage is indicated.

Surgery in acute pancreatitis is usually reserved for the following indications: (1) patients with an acute abdomen in whom a surgical emergency, such as a perforated viscus, cannot be excluded; (2) patients who require elective biliary surgery after gallstone pancreatitis has resolved (usually within 7 to 10 days after presentation); and (3) patients who require drainage of an infected fluid collection. In the absence of these indications, the role of surgery is more controversial. Patients with early pulmonary or vascular complications, who do not respond to intensive medical management, are sometimes operated upon with necrosectomy, total or partial pancreatectomy, wide debridement with sump drainage, multiple decompressions of adjacent organs, or a feeding jejunostomy. Dynamic CT scanning for evidence of extensive necrosis and percutaneous needle aspiration of pancreatic phlegmons for evidence of bacterial invasion may indicate which patients might benefit most from surgery.

CHRONIC PANCREATITIS

Pathogenesis

The pathogenesis of chronic pancreatitis is usually obscure, except for that of alcohol-induced disease. In an animal chronically fed large amounts of ethanol, the pancreas hypersecretes protein, which may precipitate as proteinaceous plugs in the small ductules. These plugs combine with the supersaturated solutions of calcium carbonate in pancreatic fluid to form small calcium carbonate stones, further obstructing the small ductules. There is some debate as to whether the pancreas normally secretes a

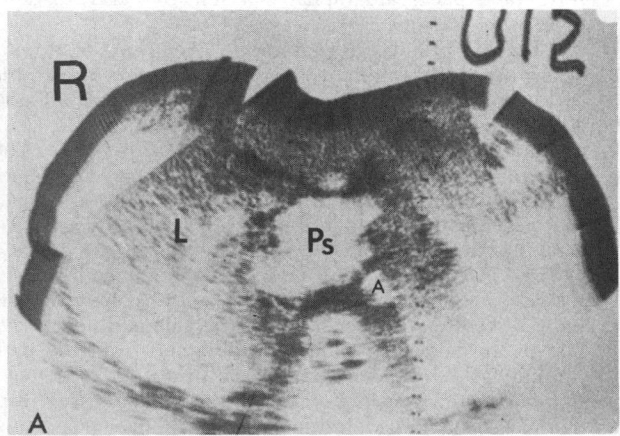 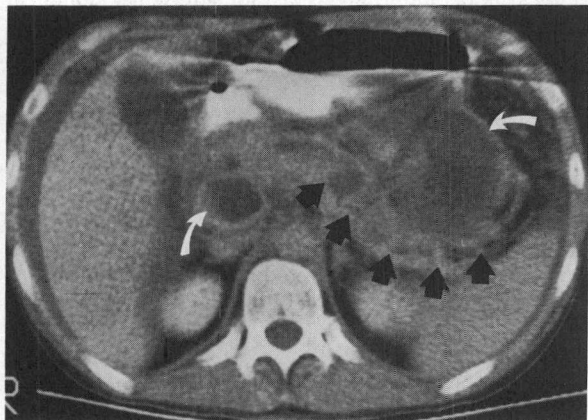

FIGURE 106–3. *A*, A pseudocyst demonstrated by ultrasonography. Ps = pseudocyst; A = aorta; L = liver; R = right of patient. (Courtesy of Dr. Dennis A. Sarti, Dept. of Radiological Sciences, University of California at Los Angeles, and Radiology 125:789, 1977.) *B*, A CT scan through the region of the tail, body, and head of the pancreas demonstrates the presence of two pancreatic pseudocysts (*curved white arrows*). The larger of the two extends from the tail of the pancreas anteriorly to compress a portion of the greater curvature of the stomach, here denoted by contrast material in the dependent portion and an air-fluid level. The smaller of the two is well circumscribed and located in the head of the pancreas. Both pseudocysts are of low CT density and well-described margins. In addition, the pancreatic duct (*black arrows*) is dilated and irregular in contour, a finding typical of a chronic pancreatitis. (Courtesy of Dr. Henry Goldberg, University of California at San Francisco.)

TABLE 106–4. ETIOLOGIC ASSOCIATIONS WITH CHRONIC PANCREATITIS

Nonobstructive
Chronic alcoholism
Tropical/nutritional
Inherited
Traumatic
Metabolic—hypertriglyceridemia, hypercalcemia
Idiopathic
Obstructive
A. Benign obstruction—localized fibrosis of the duct, pancreas divisum with obstruction of accessory ampulla
B. Neoplastic obstruction—tumors of the ampulla or ductal system

specific protein inhibitor of stone formation, insufficient secretion of which leads to a stone-forming diathesis. Blockage of the ductules, and later of the large ducts including the main pancreatic duct, leads to periductular and intralobular fibrosis, to loss of acinar parenchyma, and eventually to destruction of the islets of Langerhans. Chronic pancreatitis secondary to alcohol sometimes progresses even if alcohol ingestion is discontinued.

When the pancreatic ductal system is obstructed by other processes, such as by benign or malignant tumors, the duct distal to the obstruction becomes dilated and the acinar parenchyma becomes atrophic and fibrotic. This form of pancreatitis, termed obstructive pancreatitis, can be partially reversed if the obstruction is relieved.

Etiologic Associations (Table 106–4)

The most common cause of chronic pancreatitis is chronic alcoholism, usually present for more than 10 years by the time of presentation. Most alcoholics do not develop pancreatitis, so that unknown genetic, dietary, or environmental factors may play protective roles. Diets either high or low in fat content are thought by some to be additional risk factors in the development of alcoholic pancreatitis. Some alcoholics with pancreatitis develop hypertriglyceridemia after ingesting alcohol; possibly this metabolic aberration initiates pancreatitis in this subset of patients.

If alcoholism is excluded, most patients with chronic pancreatitis in the United States have no demonstrable cause, and therefore the disorder is classified as idiopathic. Idiopathic pancreatitis can present at any age and be associated with a spectrum of findings from mild functional disturbances of the pancreas with a normal ductal system to advanced calcific disease with markedly abnormal ducts. Notably, acute pancreatitis associated with gallstones rarely if ever leads to chronic pancreatitis.

Pancreatitis can be inherited as a rare autosomal dominant trait, presenting as acute or chronic pancreatitis with prominent pancreatolithiasis. Rarely, chronic pancreatitis may result from trauma or from metabolic disturbances, such as hypertriglyceridemia and hyperparathyroidism.

A form of calcific chronic pancreatitis, termed nutritional or tropical pancreatitis, occurs in children and young adults in southern India and some other parts of the developing world. It is speculated that this puzzling form of pancreatitis may be caused by a combination of factors, including genetic factors, protein and calorie deficiency, and/or ingestion of potentially injurious dietary factors, such as cassava. Affected individuals present most frequently with signs and symptoms of diabetes mellitus.

Clinical Presentation

Chronic pancreatitis presents most often with *abdominal pain*. Pain can occur either in discrete episodes lasting hours to days or can persist for months or even years at a time. On occasion, chronic pancreatitis is painless and patients present with the sequela of exocrine or endocrine insufficiency: steatorrhea, weight loss, or diabetes mellitus. Weight loss may also be due to avoidance of food, as pain is frequently exacerbated after eating. Pain may be due to (1) perineural irritation of the nerves supplying the pancreas, (2) dilatation of the pancreatic duct, (3) the presence of a pancreatic pseudocyst, or (4) a combination of these factors. Chronic pancreatitis and cancer of the pancreas

may present in a similar manner, making it difficult to differentiate between them.

Diagnosis

BLOOD TESTS. Serum amylase and lipase are often mildly elevated during acute exacerbations of abdominal pain in chronic pancreatitis, but not to the degree seen in acute pancreatitis. These enzyme markers are frequently normal, however, as a result of loss of pancreatic parenchyma. The immunoassays, such as the radioimmunoassay for trypsinogen, are better markers of pancreatic insufficiency. With severe pancreatic insufficiency leading to steatorrhea, the serum trypsinogen level falls below normal in 80 to 85 per cent of patients. With milder forms of the illness, trypsinogen levels are low in only 15 to 20 per cent of patients. A low trypsinogen level is highly specific for chronic pancreatic exocrine deficiency.

URINE TESTS. The bentiromide (Chymex) absorption test measures the chymotrypsin component of pancreatic exocrine function. This test, described in Ch. 102, can detect about 90 per cent of patients with steatorrhea, but its specificity is only about 80 per cent. The pancreo-lauryl test, similar in principle to the bentiromide test, is commonly employed in Europe, but not in the United States.

TUBED PANCREATIC FUNCTION TESTS. In the most sensitive test to detect chronic pancreatitis, a double-lumen tube is placed fluoroscopically into the C loop of the duodenum. Careful collection of pancreatic and intestinal juices is made after a stimulus (secretin or cholecystokinin) is given. Analysis of duodenal contents for bicarbonate or enzyme concentrations can determine mild, moderate, or severe exocrine insufficiency of the pancreas. In the simpler Lundh test, a defined liquid meal with various nutrients is used to stimulate pancreatic secretion, and trypsin concentrations are measured in duodenal secretions.

STOOL TESTS. The qualitative and quantitative tests for stool fat and the use of these and other tests for detecting pancreatic exocrine deficiency are described in Ch. 102.

IMAGING TESTS. The plain film of the abdomen can visualize calcifications within the pancreas. Calcifications, which may be localized or diffuse, represent calcium carbonate stones in the small or large ducts, not calcium in the parenchyma of the pancreas. Oblique views, as well as anteroposterior views, allow the calcifications to be seen best. Pancreatic calcification is usually diagnostic of chronic pancreatitis. Small amounts of calcium may be missed on plain films of the abdomen but detected on the more sensitive CT scans of the pancreas. Other findings on CT scan include masses within the organ and dilatations of the main pancreatic duct (see Fig. 94–3). The latter two findings can occur also with cancer of the pancreas (Ch. 107). Early in chronic pancreatitis the small secondary ductules become blunted and dilated, changes that later extend to the major ducts. Endoscopic retrograde pancreatography is a sensitive way to detect these diagnostic changes.

OTHER TESTS. An abnormal Schilling test (vitamin B_{12} absorption), corrected by pancreatic enzyme preparations, is a highly specific but not a sensitive test (sensitivity of about 30 to 40 per cent) for diagnosing chronic pancreatitis (Ch. 132). Clinical vitamin B_{12} deficiency in chronic pancreatitis is rare. The CA 19-9 radioimmunoassay blood test, a tumor-associated marker, may be helpful in differentiating chronic pancreatitis from cancer of the pancreas. Very high blood levels of this antigen suggest cancer of the pancreas.

SEQUENCE OF TESTS. A logical sequence in ordering these tests is to advance from the simple and less invasive ones to the more difficult and expensive tests, as deemed necessary. A plain film of the abdomen should be obtained from the patient presenting with chronic abdominal pain in order to detect calcification. A serum trypsinogen level and a urinary bentiromide test might also be considered simple, inexpensive, and noninvasive tests. Symptoms of steatorrhea suggest pancreatic exocrine insufficiency and may be evaluated as described in Ch. 102. If the simple tests are not diagnostic, CT scanning, endoscopic pancreatography, and/or tubed function tests may be employed as indicated.

Course and Complications

Usually in chronic pancreatitis, attacks of abdominal pain precede calcification of the gland. With time, calcification may become evident and with further progression, steatorrhea and/or diabetes may develop. Secretion of pancreatic lipase must be diminished by more than 90 per cent before steatorrhea develops. Despite fat malabsorption, deficiency of fat-soluble vitamins is uncommon. The painful attacks tend to diminish over time (5 to 10 years), as endocrine and exocrine insufficiencies worsen. Abstinence from alcohol also lessens the frequency of painful attacks, but exocrine and endocrine insufficiencies may progress notwithstanding. Diabetes secondary to pancreatitis may exhibit with time some of the microvascular complications seen with other causes of diabetes (Ch. 218).

Chronic pancreatitis may be complicated by pseudocysts, pancreatic ascites, or biliary obstruction. Pseudocysts usually occur anterior to the pancreas. If a pseudocyst develops posteriorly, however, it may dissect down or up fascial planes and appear in atypical locations, such as the mediastinum, neck, or pelvis. Moderate to large pseudocysts (>5 to 6 cm in diameter) that do not resolve by 6 weeks will probably not resolve spontaneously and drainage procedures are advised (Fig. 106–3). In practice, if a CT scan obtained within several days of a painful attack of pancreatitis demonstrates a large pseudocyst with a thick wall, it probably is chronic rather than acute. Percutaneous drainage usually results in recurrence unless drainage catheters are left in place for some time. Endoscopic techniques using electrocautery or laser can create drainage fistulas between the cyst and adjacent stomach or duodenum, but surgical drainage with anastomosis to an adjacent organ is usually the procedure of choice. If large pseudocysts are not drained, they may become infected or perforated or bleed internally or into adjacent structures, such as the stomach, intestine, or retroperitoneum.

Pancreatic ascites occurs when a tear in the pancreatic duct or pseudocyst communicates with the peritoneal cavity. This most frequently occurs gradually in the absence of significant abdominal pain. Analysis of peritoneal fluid shows an elevation in protein content and in amylase concentration (higher than its serum concentration).

Biliary obstruction, an insidious complication of chronic pancreatitis, is caused by compression of the distal common bile duct as it passes through the fibrotic head of the pancreas. It is suspected in patients with chronic pancreatitis who have persistent elevations of serum alkaline phosphatase activity. Some of these patients develop dilatation of the common bile duct, jaundice, pruritus, biliary sepsis, and, rarely, secondary biliary cirrhosis.

Management

The most difficult task in the treatment of chronic pancreatitis is the control of abdominal pain. Exacerbations of pain frequently require hospitalization. The acute attacks usually respond to abstinence from oral intake and the use of intravenous fluids and parenteral analgesics. Oral narcotic analgesics are usually required for chronic unremitting pain, and addiction is common. Abstinence from alcohol may lessen the frequency and severity of pain. In a few patients with mild forms of chronic pancreatitis, pain may be improved by the oral administration of large doses of oral pancreatic proteolytic enzyme preparations, which tend to reduce endogenous pancreatic secretion by a negative feedback mechanism, thus "putting the pancreas at rest." Non–enteric-coated pancreatic enzyme preparations, such as Viokase, Cotazyme, or Ilozyme, five to eight pills with meals, may be helpful. Failure of response may be due to destruction of the enzymes by gastric acid. Concomitant use of preparations to neutralize acid, such as sodium bicarbonate or aluminum antacids, or of histamine receptor blockers (e.g., cimetidine or ranitidine) to inhibit acid secretion, may improve results. Magnesium- and calcium-containing antacids should not be used, as these complex with fatty acids and interfere with their absorption. Alternatively, enteric-coated enzyme preparations, such as Pancrease, Entolase, or Creon, two to three pills with meals, may be tried. Unfortunately, pancreatic enzyme therapy is usually unsuccessful in managing the painful attacks of chronic pancreatitis. Percutaneous CT-guided celiac nerve blocks with phenol or alcohol have been tried to control pain with some degree of success, as have biofeedback and endoscopically placed pancreatic stents. Improvement of pain has been reported to result from endoscopic sphincterotomy followed by basket removal of pancreatic stones,

and from extracorporeal shock wave lithotripsy of large stones with subsequent endoscopic removal. For intractable pain, different surgical approaches are sometimes attempted after endoscopic retrograde pancreatography delineates the pancreatic ductal anatomy: celiac ganglionectomies, splanchnicectomies, various resections of the pancreas (distal pancreatectomy to 95 per cent or total pancreatectomy), drainage of pseudocysts, and lateral pancreaticojejunostomy (Puestow procedure). Surgical series report a 70 to 90 per cent success rate in alleviating abdominal pain.

Pancreatic steatorrhea is treated with adequate doses of oral pancreatic enzyme therapy as described above. If symptomatic steatorrhea persists, a low-fat diet (<40 grams per day) can improve symptoms. Supplementation of the diet with medium-chain triglycerides can improve caloric intake. The diabetes mellitus that accompanies chronic pancreatitis usually requires treatment with insulin.

Medical management of pancreatic ascites consists of large-volume paracentesis and total parenteral nutrition. If medical management is unsuccessful, an endoscopic retrograde pancreatogram should be performed to define the site of leakage for surgical repair. Internal drainage of pseudocysts, anastomosis between bowel and pancreas, or pancreatic resection is performed in this setting.

The need and timing of any intervention with regard to biliary obstruction depend on the level of symptoms (jaundice, pruritus, fever) and the fear of the possible development of the complications (sepsis, biliary cirrhosis). Endoscopic placement of biliary stents or surgical bypass of the obstructed ducts (e.g., choledochoduodenostomy, choledochojejunostomy) can successfully decompress the duct.

Bradley EL, Clements JL, Gonzalez AC: The natural history of pancreatic pseudocysts: A unified concept of management. Am J Surg 137:135, 1979. *The classic paper on the natural history of pseudocysts.*
DiMagno EP, Go VLW, Summerskill WHJ: Relations between pancreatic enzyme outputs and malabsorption in severe pancreatic insufficiency. N Engl J Med 288:813, 1973. *The classic paper on the pathophysiology of fat malabsorption in chronic pancreatitis.*
Neoptolemos JP, Carr-Locke DL, London NJ, et al.: Controlled trial of urgent endoscopic retrograde cholangiopancreatography and endoscopic sphincterotomy versus conservative treatment for acute pancreatitis due to gallstones. Lancet 2:979, 1988. *An important study delineating the usefulness of urgent endoscopic sphincterotomy in gallstone pancreatitis.*
Ranson JHC: Etiological and prognostic factors in human acute pancreatitis: A review. Am J Gastroenterol 77:633, 1982. *Ranson describes his classification of risk factors that guide the early prognosis of acute pancreatitis in a given patient.*
Rattner DW, Warshaw AL: Surgical intervention in acute pancreatitis. Crit Care Rev 16:89, 1988. *A good review of the surgical management of acute pancreatitis, its indications and limitations.*
Sarner M, Cotton PB: Classification of pancreatitis. Gut 25:756, 1984.
Singer MV, Gyr K: Revised classification of pancreatitis; report of the second international symposium on the classification of pancreatitis in Marseille, France, March 28–30, 1984. Gastroenterology 89:683, 1985. *Two important international meetings defined and classified the different forms of pancreatitis.*
Slaff J, Jacoson D, Tillman CR, et al.: Protease specific suppression of pancreatic exocrine secretion. Gastroenterology 87:44, 1984. *This paper explains the rationale for the use of oral enzymes to relieve the pain of chronic pancreatitis.*
Steer ML: Classification and pathogenesis of pancreatitis. Surg Clin North Am 69:467, 1989. *A good review of the different theories of the pathogenesis of acute pancreatitis.*
Steinberg WM, Schlesselman S: Treatment of acute pancreatitis: Comparison of animal vs. human studies. Gastroenterology 93:1420, 1987. *An analysis of the controlled medical trials in acute pancreatitis, giving the reasons for the negative results.*

107 Carcinoma of the Pancreas

Eugene P. DiMagno

DEFINITION

Ductal adenocarcinoma, comprising 90 per cent of pancreatic cancers, is a relentlessly progressive and fatal disease. Most tumors are moderately well differentiated mucinous carcinomas arising from the cuboid epithelium of pancreatic ducts. The remaining 10 per cent of pancreatic cancers are endocrine tumors (Ch. 220); acinar cell, giant cell, and epidermoid cancers; adenocanthomas; sarcomas; or cystadenocarcinomas.

INCIDENCE AND EPIDEMIOLOGY

Pancreatic cancer kills more Americans than any other neoplasm except breast, colorectal, lung, and prostate cancers. Each year approximately 27,000 Americans develop pancreatic cancer and 25,000 die. Median survival after diagnosis is only 4 to 8 months. Overall 5-year survival remains less than 1 per cent. Resection of the tumor improves median survival to 17 to 20 months, but 5-year survival remains less than 10 per cent. For reasons that are unclear, the incidence of pancreatic cancer has more than doubled during the past generation (from less than 5 to between 11 and 12 per 100,000 population).

Pancreatic cancer is associated with certain demographic characteristics and risk factors (Table 107–1). Pancreatic cancer occurs more frequently in men (1.5:1). Eighty per cent occur between ages 60 and 80; the disease is unusual under age 40. Patients with hereditary pancreatitis, members of families with the nonpolyposis colon cancer syndrome, and patients with diabetes mellitus of greater than 2 to 3 years' duration are at increased risk. The major environmental factors associated with an increased risk of pancreatic cancer are ingestion of a high-fat and cholesterol diet rich in linoleic acid and exposure to coal tar derivatives, coke, benzidine, and β-naphthylamine. It is unlikely that consumption of coffee, alcohol abuse, or a previous cholecystectomy or gastrectomy increases the risk of pancreatic cancer. The risk for pancreatic cancer may be reduced by eliminating cigarette smoking and eating a diet low in cholesterol and containing olive oil and fish as the main sources of fat.

PATHOPHYSIOLOGY AND CLINICAL MANIFESTATIONS (Table 107–2)

In pancreatic ductal adenocarcinoma, well-differentiated to poorly differentiated duct glands are embedded in a dense network of fibrous tissue. As it extends in the pancreas and surrounding tissue, the tumor envelops and fixes vessels and invades fat, lymph channels, and perineural areas. Symptoms and signs of pancreatic cancer are related to the location of the tumor within the gland and to the extension of the tumor to stomach, duodenum, bile duct, retroperitoneum, and porta hepatis. The presenting symptoms are nonspecific and most commonly consist of pain, jaundice, weight loss, and, rarely, diabetes mellitus.

Pain occurs in 90 per cent of patients. It may be vague and rather nonspecific and may occur up to 3 months before the onset of jaundice. Early in the course the pain may be ignored both by the patient and by the physician to whose attention it is brought. The tumor most commonly extends to the retroperitoneal space, producing visceral pain variously described as persistent, disagreeable, aching, increased by lying supine or by eating, and causing the patient to awaken at night. Relief is sometimes obtained by bending forward, lying on the side, and

TABLE 107–1. RISK FACTORS FOR PANCREATIC CANCER

Definite
Age >60
Male sex
Cigarette smoking
Hereditary pancreatitis
Nonpolyposis colon cancer syndrome
Diabetes mellitus

Probable
High-fat diet
Chemical exposure

Unlikely
Coffee
Alcohol
Prior cholecystectomy or
gastrectomy

TABLE 107–2. CLINICAL MANIFESTATIONS OF PANCREATIC CANCER

Clinical Manifestations	Pancreatic Cancer of Head (%)	Pancreatic Cancer of Body and Tail (%)
Symptoms		
Weight loss	92	100
Jaundice	82	7
Pain	72	87
Anorexia	64	33
Dark urine	63	—
Light stools	62	—
Nausea	45	37
Vomiting	37	37
Weakness	35	43
Pruritus	24	—
Signs		
Jaundice	87	13
Palpable liver	83	33
Palpable gallbladder	29	—
Ascites	14	20
Abdominal mass	13	23

Data from Howard JM, Jordan GL: Cancer of the pancreas. Curr Probl Cancer 2(3):1, 1977; and DaVita VT Jr., Hellman S, Rosenberg SA (eds.): Cancer: Principles and Practice of Oncology. Philadelphia, J. B. Lippincott Company, 1985, p 100.

drawing the knees to the chest or chin and sometimes by crouching forward on four extremities.

Jaundice secondary to obstruction of the bile duct occurs early in the course of the disease in the 60 to 70 per cent of patients with carcinoma of the head of the pancreas. When carcinomas of the head of the pancreas arise in its central part or in the uncinate process, jaundice is usually not an early presentation. In cancer of the body and tail of the pancreas jaundice occurs late and is secondary to hepatic metastases or obstruction of the bile duct at the porta hepatis by lymphadenopathy. Painless jaundice is not a manifestation of pancreatic cancer.

Weight loss of more than 10 per cent of ideal body weight, almost universal, is usually due to both malabsorption and decreased food intake. Seventy-five per cent of patients malabsorb fat and 50 per cent malabsorb protein. Malabsorption occurs in patients who have a carcinoma of the head of the pancreas that obstructs the pancreatic duct and thereby produces pancreatic exocrine insufficiency. The particular features of pancreatic malabsorption are described in Ch. 102.

Glucose intolerance may be present in up to 80 per cent of patients with pancreatic cancer, but in most such patients diabetes is mild. Less than 5 per cent of patients have hyperphagia, polydipsia, and polyuria.

Other symptoms and signs include *depression*, *light-colored stools* (60 per cent of patients with carcinoma of the pancreatic head), *constipation*, and *emotional lability* (27 per cent of patient with carcinoma of the tail). *Vomiting* and *weakness* occur in one third of patients. More rarely patients exhibit superficial thrombophlebitis (Trousseau's syndrome) or gastrointestinal bleeding due either to direct extension of the tumor into the stomach or duodenum or to varices secondary to splenic vein obstruction.

Metastases from pancreatic cancer of the body and tail may cause testicular enlargement and pain, whereas metastases to the temporal bone may produce sudden profound hearing loss, and metastases to the esophagus may lead to dysphagia.

Hepatomegaly and *jaundice* are present in 80 and 30 per cent of patients with pancreatic carcinoma of the head and body and tail, respectively. A palpable gallbladder (Courvoisier's sign) is present in 30 per cent of patients with carcinoma of the head of the pancreas. An abdominal mass or ascites is present in less than 20 per cent of patients. Ascites, splenomegaly, and peripheral edema may occur secondary to occlusion of the portal vein by tumors, whereas compression of the aorta or splenic artery may produce an abdominal bruit.

DIAGNOSIS

In patients suspected of having pancreatic cancer, an initial screening series of blood tests should be obtained, as well as a chest radiograph and an abdominal film to look for calcification

TABLE 107–3. DIAGNOSTIC ACCURACY OF IMAGING TESTS IN THE DIAGNOSIS OF PANCREATIC CANCER

	Sensitivity (%)	Specificity (%)	Predictive Value	
			Positive (%)	*Negative (%)*
Ultrasonography	74	84	78	79
Computed tomography	79	64	76	78
Endoscopic retrograde cholangiopancreatography	95	90	87	97

of the pancreas. As a group, patients with pancreatic cancer have higher values for serum lipase, amylase, and glucose than do other patients, but these tests do not distinguish between pancreatic cancer and pancreatitis. Similarly, serum alkaline phosphatase, aspartate aminotransferase, and bilirubin are commonly elevated, but these tests lack specificity in excluding hepatic disorders. Nonspecific findings on the chest radiograph and abdominal films may be present in patients with pancreatitis or pancreatic cancer. Pancreatic calcifications have a sensitivity of 95 per cent for the diagnosis of chronic pancreatitis, but primary ductal carcinomas, mucosal pancreatic cancers such as a mucinous cystadenocarcinoma (curvilinear calcification), and solid and papillary epithelial neoplasms can calcify. If obvious pulmonary or bony metastases are found, one may opt to perform no further diagnostic tests.

No sensitive serologic marker with tumor and organ specificity has been established as a routine diagnostic or screening test for pancreatic cancer. Currently available serologic tests include carcinoembryonic antigen (CEA), galactosyltransferase, monoclonal antibodies CA 19-9, CA-50, and DU-PAN-2, pancreatic oncofetal antigen, and pancreatic cancer–associated antigen. These tests have ranged in sensitivity from 50 to 85 per cent, but positive tests occur in up to 46 per cent of patients with benign diseases and in up to 65 per cent of those with other malignancies.

Pancreatic cancer is most readily diagnosed by imaging the pancreas with ultrasonography, computed tomography (CT), or endoscopic pancreatography. The diagnosis is usually confirmed by ultrasonographic or CT-guided percutaneous aspiration cytology of the pancreatic mass or biopsy of liver metastases. This technique is 90 per cent sensitive for the diagnosis of pancreatic cancer.

The sensitivity and specificity of ultrasonography and CT are approximately 80 per cent for the detection of a pancreatic mass or cancer (Table 107–3). Endoscopic retrograde cholangiopancreatography is 90 to 95 per cent sensitive and specific (Table 107–3). In practice, ultrasonography is commonly the first test used to diagnose pancreatic cancer (Fig. 107–1) because it is least expensive. When ultrasonography fails for technical reasons (10 per cent), or if the diagnosis is uncertain (20 per cent), CT is then performed. If doubt still exists, endoscopic retrograde pancreatography should be performed (see Fig. 94–2). Rarely is it necessary to perform an invasive pancreatic function test, in which either secretin or cholecystokinin is administered intravenously and pancreatic secretion is obtained through a tube placed into the duodenum. Patients with pancreatic cancer have a low volume of pancreatic secretion, but a normal bicarbonate concentration after secretin stimulation or reduced enzyme outputs after cholecystokinin stimulation. The algorithm in Figure 107–1 has a sensitivity and specificity of greater than 90 per cent.

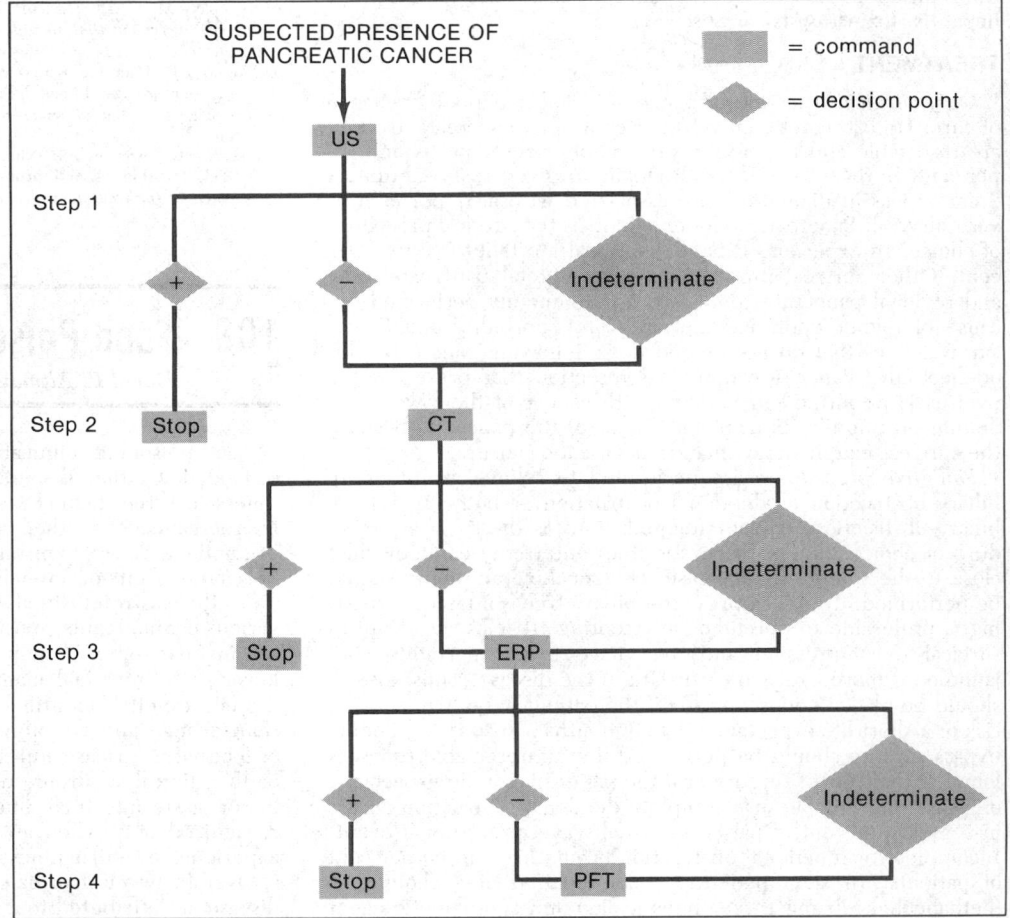

FIGURE 107–1. Algorithm for the diagnosis of pancreatic cancer. US = Ultrasonography; CT = computed tomography; ERP = endoscopic retrograde pancreatography; PFT = pancreatic function tests. (From DiMagno EP: Overview: Biology and diagnosis of pancreatic cancer. *In* Levin B [ed.]: Annual Clinical Conference on Cancer, Vol. 30, Gastrointestinal Cancer: Current Approaches to Diagnosis and Treatment. Houston, University of Texas Press, 1988, pp 299–308.)

TABLE 107–4. DIFFERENTIAL DIAGNOSIS OF PANCREATIC CANCER

Nonmalignant conditions
Chronic pancreatitis
Extrahepatic jaundice
  Common bile duct stones
  Bile duct stricture (secondary to previous biliary tract surgery or
    sclerosing cholangitis)
  Cholecystitis
Intrahepatic cholestatic jaundice
  Alcoholic hepatitis
  Toxins
  Cysts
  Abscess
Posterior penetrating duodenal or gastric ulcers
Depression
Functional bowel disorders

Malignant conditions
Retroperitoneal lymphomas
Bile duct cancer
Ampullary cancer
Gynecologic malignancies
Carcinoma of the duodenum or small intestine

DIFFERENTIAL DIAGNOSIS (Table 107–4)

The presenting symptoms and signs of pancreatic cancer are nonspecific. Indeed, most patients presenting with weight loss and abdominal pain, with or without jaundice, do not have pancreatic cancer. In patients without jaundice, the abdominal pain and weight loss of pancreatic cancer may be difficult to distinguish from an extensive list of disorders (Table 107–4). In jaundiced patients, it is extremely important to differentiate pancreatic cancer from potentially treatable conditions, such as common bile duct stones, chronic pancreatitis obstructing the common bile duct, bile duct stricture secondary to previous biliary tract surgery or sclerosing cholangitis, cholecystitis, and from intrahepatic cholestatic jaundice secondary to alcoholic hepatitis, toxins, cysts, or abscesses.

TREATMENT

Only *surgical resection* of pancreatic cancer offers any chance of cure. Unfortunately, only 10 per cent of all pancreatic cancers are resectable and the 5-year survival after resection is only 10 per cent. In recent studies from Japan, however, resected tumors 2 cm or less in diameter were associated with a 37 per cent 5-year survival. Pancreaticoduodenectomy is the surgical procedure of choice. In experienced hands, surgical mortality is 2 to 5 per cent. Other surgical procedures, such as total pancreatectomy and regional pancreatectomy, are not commonly performed because of higher operative mortality and morbidity and 5-year survival rates that do not exceed those following pancreaticoduodenectomy. Pancreaticoduodenal resection that preserves the pylorus is performed in patients with cancer of the lower duodenum or ampulla, but not for cancer of the pancreas, because the surgical margins may include pancreatic cancer.

Palliative procedures are performed to relieve symptoms of biliary obstruction or duodenal obstruction or both. To relieve biliary obstruction, cholecystojejunostomy is the surgical procedure of choice, unless the cystic duct enters the common duct close to the tumor. In this case, choledochojejunostomy should be performed. To decompress the biliary tree, endoscopic stenting is preferable to percutaneous stenting. It is as successful as surgical decompression and may have lower morbidity, but jaundice is more likely to recur late in the disease. Thus, a stent should be placed endoscopically if the patient has a high surgical risk or a short life expectancy (1 to 3 months). In contrast, double bypass surgery should be performed if an unresectable tumor is found at the time of surgery or if the patient has a life expectancy of 6 to 7 months, because complete duodenal obstruction occurs in 5 to 15 per cent of patients—usually as a preterminal event. Incomplete or functional obstruction occurs in 40 to 60 per cent of patients. In such patients, a combination of a cholinergic (bethanechol, 25 mg three times a day) and a prokinetic agent

(metoclopramide, 10 mg four times a day) may alleviate symptoms of gastric stasis by enhancing gastric emptying.

No single agent or combination of *chemotherapeutic drugs* significantly prolongs or enhances the quality of life of patients with pancreatic cancer. 5-Fluorouracil (5-FU) produces a partial response rate in 10 to 15 per cent of patients, but its use is associated with a median survival of less than 20 weeks. Other agents have a similar limited effect (mitomycin C), even less effect (streptozotocin, doxorubicin, Epirubicin, ifosfamide, methyl-CCNU and high-dose methotrexate), or no effect (actinomycin D, carmustine, standard-dose methotrexate, cisplatin, melphalan, and L-asparaginase).

The combination of 5-FU or SMF (streptozotocin, mitomycin C, and 5-FU) and external beam radiation improves survival compared to radiation or chemotherapy alone. Intraoperative electron-beam radiation and ^{125}I implants do not improve survival in comparison to external-beam radiation. Even though these modalities may limit local tumor extension, they do not control liver and peritoneal metastases.

Pain can usually be successfully managed if analgesics are prescribed on a regular basis, adequate doses are used, and adjuvant drugs are used when necessary. Mild to moderate pain can be controlled with aspirin, acetaminophen, and nonsteroidal anti-inflammatory agents. If these drugs fail to relieve pain, opioid analgesics should be used (codeine or morphine). Addition of an antihistamine or an amphetamine to an opiate increases analgesia. Intraoperative or percutaneous neurolytic celiac plexus block is remarkably effective in controlling pain. If patients have intolerable pain, subcutaneous patient-controlled analgesia or epidural administration of narcotics affords pain relief.

Malabsorption can be reasonably well controlled by the ingestion of eight tablets of pancreatin with meals (total dose of lipase should be 30,000 IU). Two tablets should be taken immediately after eating a few bites, two tablets at the end of the meal, and four tablets interspersed during the meal (Ch. 102).

Cello JP: Carcinoma of the pancreas. *In* Sleisenger MH, Fordtran JS (eds.): Gastrointestinal Disease. Pathophysiology, Diagnosis, and Management. Philadelphia, W. B. Saunders Company, 1989, pp. 1872–1884. *A complete review of pancreatic cancer, with 67 references.*
DiMagno EP: Early diagnosis of chronic pancreatitis and pancreatic cancer. *In* Geokas MC (ed.): Difficult Diagnoses. Med. Clin. North Am. 72:979–992, 1988. *A review that includes the epidemiology and diagnosis of pancreatic cancer.*
DiMagno EP: Exocrine pancreatic neoplasia. *In* Yamada T (ed.): Textbook of Gastroenterology. Philadelphia, J. B. Lippincott Company, 1990. *This recent review is a general overview of pancreatic cancer and includes over 170 references.*
Warshaw AL, Swanson PS: What's new in general surgery. Pancreatic cancer in 1988. Possibilities and probabilities. Ann Surg 208:541, 1988. *A thorough review of the treatment of pancreatic cancer, with 164 references.*

108   Food Poisoning

David F. Altman

Food poisoning, clinical syndromes arising from the ingestion of food that either is contaminated or is itself toxic, may cause illness in three distinct ways: (1) by contamination of food with microorganisms or their products (most common); (2) by its contamination with poisonous chemicals; or (3) by ingestion of poisonous plants or animals.

As the gastrointestinal tract is the mode of entry for these various contaminants, most illnesses associated with food poisoning involve some form of gastroenteritis, with either upper or lower gastrointestinal manifestations predominating. Other syndromes are often identifiable by extraintestinal (particularly neurologic) signs and symptoms. It is difficult to identify single cases of foodborne disease unless the incubation period is very short or the clinical syndrome distinctive because of the frequency of minor gastrointestinal illnesses. Foodborne disease is usually recognized only when an outbreak occurs and several persons experience a similar illness after ingesting a common food.

Overall, fewer than half of the known outbreaks of foodborne disease are attributed to a specific etiologic agent. Nevertheless, it is important to attempt to define the etiology of such an outbreak. Prophylaxis against secondary spread of an infection may be important (e.g., in shigellosis). A more accurate prognosis for the victim may become available, as some illnesses are self-limited and short-lived, whereas others may have a chronic residual effect. Perhaps most important, faulty food handling or storage techniques may be identified and further outbreaks prevented.

To facilitate identification of possible agents in foodborne illness, such syndromes can be classified by their incubation period and the type of clinical symptoms (see Table 108–1). With the possibilities thus limited, specific sampling of food or bacteriologic cultures of blood or stool may quickly lead to the correct diagnosis.

BACTERIAL FOOD POISONING

As an aid to diagnosis and therapy, bacterial food poisoning can be conveniently classified as (1) that due to the ingestion of living microorganisms, (2) that due to the ingestion of a toxin produced by microorganisms in food prior to its ingestion, or (3) that due to enterotoxins produced in the gut by pathogens only after their ingestion.

The most important "infectious" types of food poisoning, requiring ingestion of living organisms, are *Salmonella* gastroenteritis and *Shigella* dysentery, which are dealt with in Ch. 314 and 315, respectively. Other organisms responsible in this way include *Campylobacter jejuni, Escherichia coli, Vibrio cholerae, Vibrio parahaemolyticus, Bacillus cereus,* and *Clostridium perfringens.* In addition, epidemics of listeriosis transmitted by food and a foodborne outbreak of streptococcal pharyngitis have both been reported.

The "toxin" type of food poisoning most often identified is due to *Staphylococcus aureus.* The syndrome of botulism caused by ingestion of the toxin produced by *Clostridium botulinum* is discussed in Ch. 309.

Staphylococcal Food Poisoning

ETIOLOGY. This form of food poisoning is caused by an enterotoxin produced by multiplying staphylococci before the contaminated food is ingested. Most but not all strains known to elaborate enterotoxins are coagulase-positive *Staphylococcus aureus.* The two major sources of contamination are human carriers (90 per cent, usually nasal or skin) and cows with mastitis. Staphylococcal food poisoning requires not only contamination of food with the microorganisms but also a period of some hours during which they may multiply, as may occur during slow cooling after cooking or if food is held at ambient temperature. Subsequent reheating may destroy the organism but not the remarkably heat-resistant toxin, the proximate cause of the clinical illness.

PATHOGENESIS, CLINICAL MANIFESTATIONS, AND TREATMENT. In experimental animals enterotoxins destroy gastrointestinal mucosal cells, evoke an inflammatory response, and may affect other organ systems, including the emetic centers in the brain. Symptoms usually begin 2 to 4 hours after ingestion of the toxin, heralded by salivation and followed rapidly by nausea, vomiting, abdominal cramping, and diarrhea. The illness usually is short, rarely lasting 24 hours, and often is subsiding by the time medical attention is sought. It may occasionally be life-threatening, especially in the elderly or in persons with other serious illness. Therapy is supportive and symptomatic, the primary goal being to restore extracellular fluid volume with parenteral fluids as necessary. Antibiotic therapy may worsen the course of the illness.

PREVENTION. Proper food handling prevents staphylococcal food poisoning. Sanitary measures and personal hygiene can prevent contamination of the food to some degree. More importantly, enterotoxin is not produced at ordinary domestic refrigerator temperatures. Foods should not be left to cool slowly, especially in large containers, and should be taken from the refrigerator (and reheated, if required) immediately before serving.

Clostridial Food Poisoning

ETIOLOGY. *Clostridium perfringens* type A is the third most common bacterial cause of food poisoning in the United States. Clostridial poisoning typically occurs in fairly large outbreaks. The organism is ubiquitous, being found in most samples of raw meat, human and animal feces, flies, soil, and dirt from kitchens. Both heat-sensitive and heat-resistant strains can cause outbreaks. Usually outbreaks follow the cooking of meat, poultry, or beans at a temperature (usually less than 100°C) high enough to kill vegetative forms but insufficient to destroy heat-resistant spores. Oxygen is driven out of the food, thereby lowering the oxidation-reduction potential of the medium. During slow cooling the spores germinate, encouraged by the relatively anaerobic environment and the rich supply of amino acids and other growth factors. If the food is not reheated to a temperature high enough to inactivate the recently multiplied organism, ingestion may result in illness.

PATHOGENESIS AND CLINICAL MANIFESTATIONS. Clostridial food poisoning follows ingestion of living organisms, as the production of the enterotoxin responsible for the clinical manifestations occurs with sporulation in the alkaline environment of the small intestine. The incubation period is usually 7 to 15 hours after ingestion but may be as long as 24 hours. The usual symptoms are abdominal cramps and diarrhea; nausea, vomiting, and fever are much less common. The illness is self-limited, rarely lasting more than 24 hours. Treatment rarely is necessary and should always be confined to efforts at symptomatic relief. The few deaths recorded have been in elderly or debilitated patients.

PREVENTION. Food is best served immediately after cooking. If it is to be kept, it should be cooled rapidly. Cooked meat should always be kept either cold, below 5°C, or hot, over 60°C. This is especially true of food prepared in large batches.

Vibrio parahaemolyticus Food Poisoning

V. parahaemolyticus, a gram-negative facultative anaerobe found in marine water and fauna throughout the world, lives in sediment of coastal and estuarian waters during cold winter months. As the temperature rises in spring and summer, the organism leaves the sediment and colonizes animal life, especially shellfish and crustaceans. Not all strains are pathogenic.

TABLE 108–1. CLINICAL INDICATORS OF THE ETIOLOGY OF FOODBORNE ILLNESS

Predominant Symptomatology	Mean Incubation Period			
	< 2 Hours	2–7 Hours	8–14 Hours	> 14 hours
Upper intestinal	Heavy metals	S. aureus B. cereus		
Lower intestinal			C. perfringens B. cereus	V. cholerae Enterotoxic or invasive E. coli Shigella spp. V. parahaemolyticus Salmonella
Both upper and lower gastrointestinal				V. parahaemolyticus
Extragastrointestinal, i.e., some gastrointestinal plus others, usually paresthesias or other abnormal sensory complaint	Scombrotoxin Shellfish toxin Mushroom toxin (early)	Ciguatoxin	Mushroom toxin (delayed)	C. botulinum

The pathogenesis of the illness is not clearly defined, and different serotypes may produce disease by different mechanisms. The presence of fecal leukocytes and occasionally bloody diarrhea implies bacterial invasion and damage of the gut mucosa.

Virtually all outbreaks of V. parahaemolyticus food poisoning occur during warm months of the year and are associated with the ingestion of raw or improperly refrigerated seafood. Although originally described in Japan, cases have occurred in other parts of Asia and on the Atlantic, Gulf, and Pacific coasts of the United States. The incubation period is usually between 12 and 24 hours but has been as long as 96 hours. Explosive watery diarrhea is present in more than 90 per cent of cases, with nausea, vomiting, and abdominal cramps as common accompaniments. Fever, headache, and chills occur less often. The diagnosis is suspected when a typical illness occurs after eating seafood and is confirmed by recovery of the organism from stool. Treatment is rarely necessary, as the illness infrequently lasts more than 3 days. However, in protracted cases, antibiotic treatment with tetracycline or ampicillin may shorten the illness.

Prevention depends on the recognition both of the potential for contamination of seafood with V. parahaemolyticus during warm months and of the predisposition of organisms to multiply under conditions of inadequate refrigeration. Cooked seafood may also become cross-contaminated when stored under proper conditions with a raw source.

Bacillus cereus Food Poisoning

Bacillus cereus, an anaerobic, motile, spore-forming, gram-positive rod, causes two separate clinical forms of the foodborne disease. An emetic form, clinically identical to staphylococcal food poisoning, is associated with contaminated fried rice. A diarrheal form has a longer incubation period and predominantly lower gastrointestinal symptoms, reminiscent of Clostridium perfringens food poisoning. Cell-free filtrates derived from B. cereus strains responsible for this latter form of illness stimulate the adenylate cyclase–cyclic adenosine monophosphate (cAMP) system in intestinal epithelial cells. This activity is destroyed by heat, thus resembling cholera enterotoxin. The illnesses are usually mild and self-limited, and antibiotics are not indicated. No fatalities have been reported. As the organism commonly occurs in soil and in many dried or processed foods, careful food handling is most important in prevention of the disease. B. cereus may be found in uncooked rice, for example, and heat-resistant spores may survive boiling. If the rice is left unrefrigerated, the spores may then germinate and produce toxin. Flash frying or rewarming before serving is often not sufficient to destroy the preformed, heat-stable toxin. The disease thus can be prevented by prompt refrigeration of boiled rice.

Benenson AS (ed.): Foodborne intoxication. In Control of Communicable Diseases in Man. 14th ed. Washington, D.C., American Public Health Association, 1985, pp 142–152. A brief compendium of information on foodborne illness, with emphasis on identification and prevention.
Centers for Disease Control: Foodborne disease outbreaks, annual summary, 1982. In CDC Surveillance Summaries, 35:7ss, 1986. An annual compendium of reports of foodborne diseases in the United States, with analysis of vehicles of transmission and contributing factors to contamination for each type of infection identified.
Linnan MJ, Mascola L, Lou XD, et al.: Epidemic listeriosis associated with Mexican-style cheese. N Engl J Med 319:823, 1988. A classic description of an epidemiologic investigation of a recently recognized cause of foodborne illness.
Morris JG Jr., Black RE: Cholera and other vibrioses in the United States. N Engl J Med 312:343, 1985. This article reviews both common and more obscure illnesses caused by these organisms.
Shandera WX, Tacket CO, Blake PA: Food poisoning due to Clostridium perfringens in the United States. J Infect Dis 147:167, 1983. This article provides a thorough review of the pathogenesis of this cause of food poisoning, as well as information on epidemiology and diagnosis.
Terranova W, Blake PA: Bacillus cereus food poisoning. N Engl J Med 298:143, 1978. A brief but comprehensive review of the various forms of this illness.

CHEMICAL FOOD POISONING

Chemicals may cause food poisoning following accidental contamination of food prior to its preparation or during storage or as food additives or preservatives. Thus various forms of metallic poisoning, discussed in Ch. 533, can occur when food, particularly acid liquids, comes in contact with certain metals, especially cadmium, copper, tin, or zinc.

The so-called Chinese restaurant syndrome, in which individuals develop sensations of burning skin, facial pressure, chest pressure, and headaches 10 to 20 minutes after eating certain Chinese foods (especially won ton soup), has been attributed to the use of monosodium L-glutamate (MSG). The symptoms appear to be a pharmacologic effect of MSG, obeying a dose-effect relationship, but with a widely variable threshold for an oral dose.

Sodium nitrite, widely used as a preservative in smoked meats, has been blamed for the "hot dog headache" seen in some persons. In addition, because of its metabolism to nitrosamines it is suspected to be a potential carcinogen, although evidence for this is inconclusive.

L-Tryptophan, an essential amino acid, is available as an over-the-counter nutritional supplement and has been recommended for the treatment of depression, insomnia, and the premenstrual syndrome. It has now been associated with a potentially fatal disorder called the eosinophilia-myalgia syndrome. This illness is characterized by diffuse, severe myalgias and skin changes ranging from a morbilliform rash to scleroderma-like changes, all associated with peripheral blood eosinophilia. Some patients also develop a hypersensitivity pneumonitis, myocarditis, cerebral vasculitis, and a progressive polyneuropathy. Onset may be months to years after beginning use of L-tryptophan–containing products, and at least in some patients discontinuation leads to resolution of the symptoms. Some deaths have been reported, however. The syndrome is now believed to have been caused by the ingestion of a chemical constituent that arose from the manufacturing conditions of L-tryptophan at one company. This compound apparently decomposes to a carboxylic acid derivative in the presence of gastric acid. The syndrome is strikingly similar to the toxic oil syndrome that was epidemic in Spain in 1981 and that was linked to the consumption of denatured rapeseed oil sold as cooking oil.

Food additives such as aspartame and pesticides have been incriminated as a cause of foodborne disease. Although the former have not been conclusively identified as the source of illness, outbreaks of the latter have been documented. Contamination of watermelons by aldicarb caused gastrointestinal and neurologic symptoms in over 1000 individuals.

Martin RW, Duffy J, Engel AG, et al.: The clinical spectrum of the eosinophilia-myalgia syndrome associated with L-tryptophan ingestion. Ann Intern Med 113:124, 1990. A description of a new syndrome, including clinical features and speculation on pathogenesis.
Schaumburg HH, Byck R, Gerstil R, et al.: Monosodium L-glutamate: Its pharmacology and role in the Chinese restaurant syndrome. Science 163:826, 1969. A careful analysis of MSG pharmacology and its dose-effect relationships.

POISONOUS ANIMALS AND PLANTS

Fish and Shellfish Poisoning

Various toxins from vertebrate fish are capable of causing human illness. Most commonly this is due to toxin contained in musculature (ichthyosarcotoxins), of which nine types have been described. The most common fish poisonings worldwide—ciguatera, scombroid, and puffer fish poisoning—are attributable to ichthyosarcotoxins.

Two forms of shellfish poisoning, paralytic and neurotoxic, have been described. These are caused by toxins derived from dinoflagellates contaminating the shellfish.

CIGUATERA FISH POISONING. Ciguatera poisoning, the most common illness brought on by the ingestion of fish and seafood, follows the ingestion of ciguatoxin produced by the dinoflagellate Gambierdiscus toxicus. This marine organism is passed up the food chain, and more than 400 fish species, generally bottom-dwelling shore fish in temperate and tropical zones, have been implicated.

Ciguatoxin is a lipid-soluble, heat-stable substance that is resistant to gastric acid. It is believed to inhibit the calcium regulation of passive cell membrane sodium channels.

The onset of the illness usually occurs 1 to 6 hours after ingestion of toxic fish, but this time interval may vary from as soon as a few minutes to as long as 30 hours. Gastrointestinal symptoms, including abdominal cramps, nausea, vomiting, and diarrhea, predominate at the outset, along with numbness, pruritus, and paresthesias of the lips, tongue, and throat. Paresthesias may later involve the extremities, and in severe cases there may be abnormal temperature sensations, cranial nerve palsies, hypotension, bradycardia, and even respiratory paralysis. Acute symptoms usually subside within a few days and require only symptomatic, supportive therapy. Intravenous mannitol has been reported to provide rapid symptomatic relief, as has oral tocainide. Neither therapy has been subjected to careful clinical trials. The return of pruritus with alcohol ingestion is thought to be almost pathognomonic of this syndrome. Weakness and sensory disturbances may persist for months or years.

SCOMBROID FISH POISONING. Scombroid fish poisoning is the only form of ichthyosarcotoxism in which toxins are formed by the action of bacteria, in this case particularly *Proteus morgani*, on fish flesh. Scombrotoxin is thought to consist of histamine and related substances. Most fish that have caused outbreaks are members of the suborder Scombroidae, most commonly mahimahi, tuna, mackerel, and bonito. Symptoms begin within a few minutes of ingestion and resemble those of a histamine reaction: flushing, headache, dizziness, abdominal cramps, nausea, vomiting and diarrhea, and occasionally urticaria and generalized pruritus. The illness has a median duration of 4 hours in the reported outbreaks. Both intravenous cimetidine and antihistamines have provided symptomatic relief. Production of the toxin is inhibited by proper refrigeration, perhaps reflecting the temperature optimum of 20 to 30°C for the enzymatic conversion of histidine to histamine. Improper refrigeration of fresh-caught fish has been observed in most outbreaks of this illness.

PUFFER FISH POISONING (TETRODOTOXIN POISONING). Many puffer fish found in the Pacific, Atlantic, and Indian Oceans are inherently toxic. The tetrodotoxin found in their viscera is a neurotoxin, and its effects are nearly identical to the saxitoxin that produces paralytic shellfish poisoning (see below).

PARALYTIC SHELLFISH POISONING. Paralytic shellfish poisoning is caused by the ingestion of bivalve mollusks contaminated with the neurotoxin of the dinoflagellates *Gonyaulax catanella* or *Go. tamarensis*. Although a "red tide," related to "blooming" of the dinoflagellates, has been associated with paralytic shellfish poisoning, not all red tides are toxic, and some outbreaks have occurred in the absence of a red tide. The toxin of *Go. catanella*, saxitoxin, appears to act by inhibiting sodium channels on excitable membranes, thus blocking the propagation of nerve and muscle action potentials.

The illness begins within 30 minutes of ingestion of a toxic mollusk and is characterized by paresthesias of the mouth, lips, face, and extremities and by nausea, vomiting, and diarrhea. In more severe cases, muscle weakness or paralysis and respiratory embarrassment may occur. The fatality rate is 8 to 9 per cent, with deaths occurring within the first 12 hours. Treatment consists of a cathartic or enema in severe cases to remove unabsorbed toxin. Gastric lavage may be used if vomiting has not occurred. Mechanical ventilatory assistance may be required.

NEUROTOXIC SHELLFISH POISONING. *Ptychodiseus breve*, a toxic dinoflagellate, causes a red tide off both the Gulf and Atlantic coasts of Florida. Within 3 hours of the consumption of shellfish contaminated with this toxin, patients experience paresthesias, abnormal temperature sensations, ataxia, nausea, vomiting, and diarrhea. The disease is self-limited and milder than paralytic shellfish poisoning. No deaths have been reported.

MUSHROOM POISONING

Of the more than 2000 identified species of mushrooms, fewer than 50 are poisonous. However, even expert mycologists may have difficulty identifying poisonous species. Moreover, with the increased interest in "organic" foods and in the hallucinogenic substances found in certain species, poisoning from the ingestion of wild mushrooms has been increasing in frequency.

The principal toxin is α-amanitin, which contains cyclic octapeptides. It selectively inhibits nuclear ribonucleic acid (RNA) polymerase II. Phalloidin, another putative toxin, appears to have some hepatocellular toxicity, but probably is primarily responsible for the gastroenteritis seen early in the course. Mushrooms containing these toxins belong to the genera *Amanita* and *Galerina*. *Amanita verna* (the "destroying angel"), *A. virosa*, and *A. phalloides* (the "death cap") are the species most often associated with mushroom poisoning in the United States, and *A. phalloides* accounts for more than 90 per cent of such deaths in Europe.

Symptoms of *A. phalloides*–type mushroom poisoning characteristically occur in three stages. The first is characterized by the abrupt onset of abdominal pain, nausea, vomiting, and diarrhea 6 to 24 hours after ingestion. This may be accompanied by severe fluid and electrolyte disturbances and fever. The second stage, occurring during the next 24 to 48 hours, involves worsening of hepatic and renal function despite resolution of the initial symptoms. Finally, during the third and fourth days after ingestion, hepatic and renal functions rapidly deteriorate, accompanied occasionally by cardiomyopathy and coagulopathy, convulsions, coma, and death. The mortality rate is between 40 and 90 per cent.

The diagnosis of mushroom poisoning may be difficult. The delayed onset of symptoms may cause patients not to associate the illness with the ingestion of wild mushrooms. The mushroom toxins can be detected in blood, gastric aspirate, vomitus, or stool by thin-layer chromatography or by radioimmunoassay in some laboratories. Treatment remains supportive, including dialysis for the renal insufficiency. A number of medical therapies, including cytochrome C, sulfamethoxazole, penicillin G, thioctic acid, and silibinin, have been recommended, but none has been subjected to controlled trials. Careful attention to the complications of hepatic failure and consideration of orthotopic liver transplantation are particularly critical. Early identification of those patients at highest risk of fulminant hepatic failure—a rapidly rising prothrombin time or the development of stage II encephalopathy, for example—is critical, since early hepatic transplantation can be life-saving.

Plant Alkaloids, Mycotoxins, and Other Poisonings

These various forms of food poisoning remind us of historic knowledge of the pharmacologic effect of plant alkaloids and other toxicants found naturally in foods. Although formerly used with therapeutic intent, plant alkaloids are now more often ingested accidentally and often in large doses: e.g., digitalis intoxication from home-brewed teas made with foxglove or oleander; diarrhea from senna tea, which contains the stimulant cathartic anthraquinone; and liver failure from *Senecio longilobus*, which contains highly hepatotoxic pyrrolizidine alkaloids. Other highly toxic plants include *Atropa belladonna* (deadly nightshade) and *Datura stramonium* (thorn apple, jimson weed), whose berries and seeds can cause an atropine effect; *Conium maculatum* (hemlock), which contains several alkaloids with severe central nervous system depressant effects; and *Phytolacca americana* (pokeweed), whose leaves and berries have strong emetic properties. Finally, the ingestion of fava beans can trigger hemolysis in those with G6PD deficiency (Ch. 134).

Lathyrism, a slowly progressive spastic paraplegia, is associated with the ingestion of sweet peas of the species *Lathyrus sativus*. Large amounts of this may be ingested during famines in Africa and Asia. The toxic principle appears to be β-aminoproprionitrile. Interestingly, this substance, when given to poultry and other experimental animals, causes degeneration of the aortic media, with resulting dissecting aortic aneurysms or aortic rupture. This effect is not seen in humans.

Mycotoxins may contaminate some moldy foods. Ergotism, characterized by intense vasospasm, is the most familiar syndrome caused by this ingestion. Aflatoxin, a product of *Aspergillus flavus*, contaminates grains stored in warm, damp areas and has been associated with the development of hepatocellular carcinoma. Small amounts of aflatoxin have been found in commercial peanut butter in the United States.

Eastaugh J, Shepherd S: Infectious and toxic syndromes from fish and shellfish consumption. Arch Intern Med 149:1735, 1989. *An up-to-date review with thorough discussion of pathogenesis and treatment of these diseases.*

Klein A, Hart J, Brems JJ, et al.: *Amanita* poisoning: Treatment and the role of liver transplantation. Am J Med 86:187, 1989. *Case presentations and analysis of therapeutic options. Recommended treatment protocol explained in detail.*

Poisoning associated with herbal teas. MMWR 26:257, 1977. *Case reports and discussions of several types of herbal poisonings.*

Wogan GN: Mycotoxins. Ann Rev Pharmacol 15:437, 1975. *A review of the current understanding of the pharmacology and health impact of mycotoxins.*

109 Diseases of the Rectum and Anus

Theodore R. Schrock

ANATOMY

The rectum and anus fuse over a zone several centimeters long, and together these structures are termed the "anorectum" (Fig. 109–1). The distal anal canal is lined by modified skin (anoderm), the epithelium of the upper anal canal is columnar, and the transitional zone (cuboidal epithelium) lies between the two. The anoderm is exquisitely sensitive, but the upper anal canal is relatively insensitive.

At the dentate line, an important site of pathologic problems, anal papillae project into the lumen. Flaps of skin connecting anal papillae are termed anal valves; behind these valves lie anal crypts, each containing in its depths an anal gland.

The internal anal sphincter is the thickened lower portion of the circular smooth muscle layer of the gut. This involuntary muscle is encircled by skeletal muscle bundles comprising the external sphincters. The levators ani form the muscular floor of the pelvis. One of the levators, the puborectalis, passes around the rectum as a sling and is easily palpable posteriorly on digital rectal examination.

EXAMINATION OF THE ANORECTUM

The anorectum is examined with the patient in the left lateral decubitus position or in the prone jackknife position, if a special table is available for that purpose. Good lighting is essential. The buttocks are retracted to expose the anal orifice. Digital rectal examination is performed. Anoscopy is required for thorough evaluation of the anal canal. Rigid or flexible sigmoidoscopy completes the examination in some patients, but others (e.g., those with bleeding) need colonoscopy or a barium enema.

HEMORRHOIDS

Hemorrhoids are masses of areolar tissue containing numerous small arteries and veins. These congenital vascular cushions are located above the dentate line and are termed "internal hemorrhoids." External hemorrhoids are dilated vessels below the dentate line; they rarely cause symptoms by themselves, but they are enlarged in association with prolapsing internal hemorrhoids.

Intrarectal pressure pushes hemorrhoids downward, the anchoring fibromuscular structures attenuate, and the tissues congest, bleed, and eventually prolapse. Small hemorrhoids that protrude a short distance into the anal canal are first-degree hemorrhoids. Second-degree hemorrhoids prolapse but reduce spontaneously. Third-degree hemorrhoids must be manually reduced, and fourth-degree hemorrhoids are irreducible. Internal hemorrhoids occur in three primary locations: right posterior, right anterior, and left lateral.

Bleeding and *prolapse* are the most common symptoms of internal hemorrhoids. Blood is typically bright red, and it may spurt or drip from the anus. Nonspecific discomfort is noted, but pain is usually caused by some other associated condition such as fissure or abscess.

Anoscopy reveals a mass of tissue above the dentate line; large hemorrhoids prolapse to the outside as the anoscope is withdrawn. Differential diagnosis includes skin tags, hypertrophied anal papillae, and rectal prolapse.

Acute prolapse and thrombosis of internal hemorrhoids are severely painful. The entire circumference of the anus appears to protrude, and there is extreme pain from the edema and inflammation.

Initial treatment of internal hemorrhoids involves a high-bulk diet and avoidance of prolonged sitting at stool. Proprietary remedies have little benefit. Small bleeding hemorrhoids can be treated by a "fixation procedure" that promotes adherence of the vascular cushions to the underlying sphincter. These outpatient procedures require no anesthetic. One popular method is the injection of a sclerosing agent (e.g., 5 per cent phenol in oil) into the submucosa of the hemorrhoid above the dentate line. This painless injection evokes fibrosis and eventual adherence of the sliding mucosa. Another method is rubber band ligation, in which tiny bands are slipped over each internal hemorrhoid using a special instrument. The banded tissue sloughs and fixation results. Photocoagulation using an infrared device is also effective. Lasers can be used for the same purpose, but they are more expensive and more hazardous. Electrocoagulation with a bipolar electrode or a direct current device and thermocoagulation with a "heater probe" are new alternatives. All of these procedures have the same objective, and they are similarly effective.

Fourth-degree hemorrhoids with large external components are not responsive to fixation procedures, and if the symptoms warrant, hemorrhoidectomy is advised. Surgical excision can be performed in an outpatient setting. Results are good, although the operation is painful, and there is loss of time from work. Complications are uncommon and recurrences are unusual.

Thrombosed external hemorrhoid is a blood clot within a complex of subcutaneous external veins. This problem develops in young adults, often related to heavy exercise. A painful bluish mass is present at the anal verge. If pain does not subside after 48 hours, the thrombosed hemorrhoid can be excised under local anesthesia.

ANAL FISSURE

Anal fissure (fissure in ano, anal ulcer) is a tear in the anoderm just inside the anal verge. Acute fissures are common, but in some patients the tiny laceration does not heal and it becomes chronic. Severe pain with defecation and spots of blood on the toilet tissue are the symptoms.

The diagnosis is made by inspection. Pain is so severe that the patient may not tolerate digital rectal examination. Lateral trac-

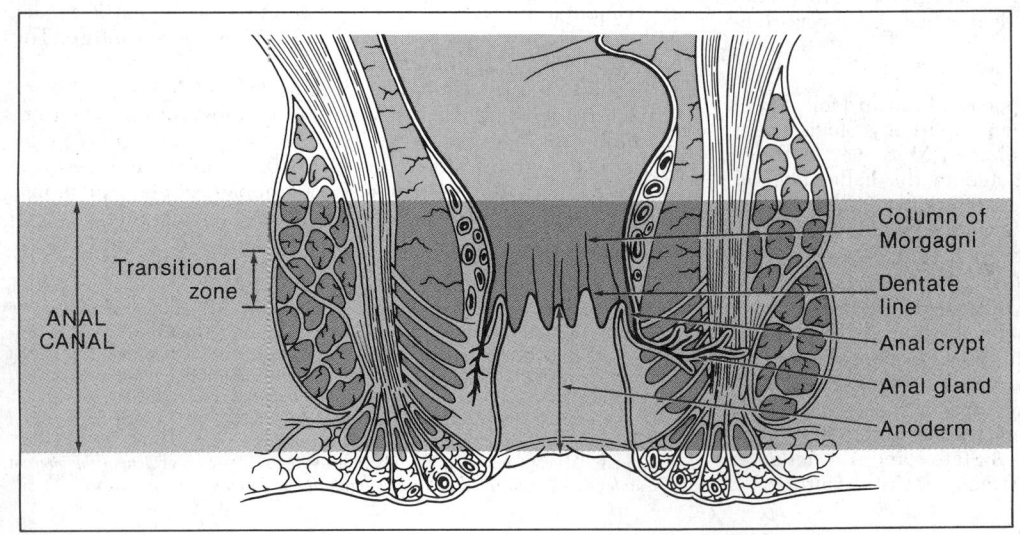

ANAL CANAL
Transitional zone

Column of Morgagni
Dentate line
Anal crypt
Anal gland
Anoderm

FIGURE 109–1. The lining of the anal canal. (Redrawn from Goldberg SM, Gordon PH, Nivatvongs S: Essentials of Anorectal Surgery. Philadelphia, J. B. Lippincott Company, 1980. Used by permission.)

tion on the buttocks exposes the fissure in nearly every instance. Acute fissures are red, but chronic fissures may have eroded completely through the anoderm to expose the white fibers of the internal sphincter in the base. The fissure triad seen in chronic lesions includes the fissure, an edematous sentinel tag at the anal verge, and a hypertrophied anal papilla at the dentate line.

Fissures are located in the posterior midline in 98 per cent of men and 90 per cent of women. The remaining fissures are in the anterior midline. A fissure off the midline should raise a suspicion of cancer, Crohn's disease, or a sexually transmitted infection.

Measures to improve bulk and softness of stools are important, and sitz baths are soothing. Acute fissures usually heal. Chronic fissures may require lateral subcutaneous internal anal sphincterotomy. This simple procedure reduces pressure in the anal canal and allows the fissure to heal. The long-term cure rate exceeds 95 per cent.

ANORECTAL ABSCESS

Infections arising in anal glands at the dentate line may develop into abscesses in the adjacent tissue spaces (Fig. 109–2). Abscesses near the skin surface cause throbbing pain that is worse with walking. Deeper abscesses may produce insidious symptoms including abdominal pain. Patients with large abscesses are febrile. An indurated tender mass is apparent on examination in a patient with a perianal or ischiorectal abscess, and the anus is pushed to one side. Intersphincteric abscesses are invisible on the outside, but they are palpable as a firm, tender area on digital rectal examination. Supralevator abscesses are also palpable.

Prompt surgical incision and drainage are required. A neglected abscess may extend, and necrotizing infections can be lethal. Abscesses in immunocompromised patients pose special problems, and standard treatment may not be appropriate.

ANORECTAL FISTULAS

A hollow fibrous tract lined by granulation tissue develops after spontaneous or surgical drainage of an anorectal abscess. The primary orifice is usually at the dentate line where the infection originated. The secondary orifice is most often external at the site of drainage. The patient has pus, blood, mucus, and discomfort. One or more reddish papules on the perianal skin mark the sites of secondary openings. Gentle pressure may produce a drop of pus from the orifice. A firm tract may be palpated with a well-lubricated finger as it travels from the secondary orifice toward the anal verge.

Anoscopy reveals the primary opening; a hooked probe confirms its patency. At times it is difficult to identify the primary orifice. Goodsall's rule describes the usual relationship of primary

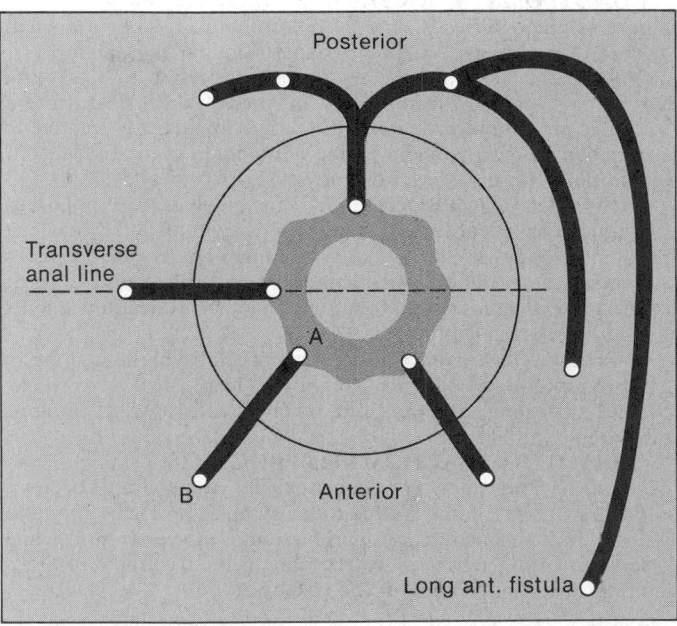

FIGURE 109–3. Goodsall's rule indicates the usual relationship of primary (A) and secondary (B) fistula orifices. The long anterior fistula is an exception to the rule. (Redrawn from Schrock TR: *In* Fromm D [ed.]: Gastrointestinal Surgery. New York, Churchill Livingstone, 1985. Used by permission.)

and secondary fistula orifices (Fig. 109–3). Crohn's disease, carcinoma, tuberculosis, and chlamydial infections should be considered in the differential diagnosis. Proctosigmoidoscopy is done routinely, and barium studies or even colonoscopy may be indicated in some cases.

Fistulas do not heal spontaneously, and operation is required (fistulotomy). The tissue overlying the tract is incised and the base is curetted. The defect heals secondarily. High fistulas encompass important sphincters and require special techniques.

Rectovaginal fistulas most commonly result from childbirth injuries. Fecal incontinence may be associated. The patient complains of passage of flatus and occasionally feces through the vagina. Surgical repair is usually successful.

PRURITUS ANI

Pruritus ani is perianal itching. It is a symptom, not a diagnosis, and the causes are many and varied. Responsible conditions include anorectal diseases, dermatologic diseases, contact dermatitis, infections by bacteria or fungi, parasites, oral antibiotics, systemic diseases (e.g., diabetes), poor or excessively zealous hygiene, warmth and moisture, dietary intolerance (coffee, cola, tomatoes, chocolate), and psychological problems. Leakage of mucus or tiny amounts of stool onto the perianal skin is perhaps the most frequent cause of pruritus, and usually there is no significant sphincter defect.

A thorough history should be obtained. Examination may disclose no abnormality, or at the other extreme there may be moist, macerated, excoriated perianal skin. Dermatologic diseases should be looked for elsewhere on the trunk and extremities. Parasites are rare.

If a specific cause of pruritus is identified, appropriate therapy is given. Antibiotics should be stopped, topical agents discontinued, and diet modified. Cleansing after defecation should be accomplished with moist cotton followed by gentle drying. Nonmedicated talcum powder is applied to combat moisture. A small bit of cotton applied to the anal verge may absorb excess moisture. More severe cases may require application of corticosteroid creams.

SEXUALLY TRANSMITTED DISEASES

Homosexually active men have a high incidence of anorectal infections, and women who practice anal intercourse also are at risk for development of these conditions.

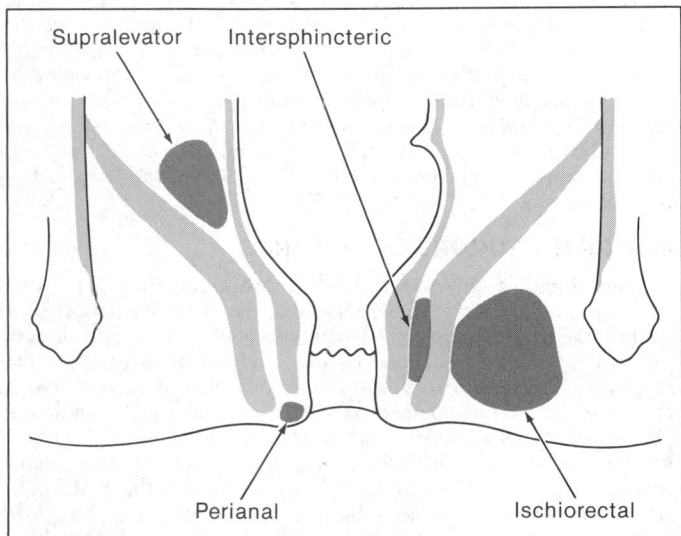

FIGURE 109–2. Classification of anorectal abscesses. (Redrawn from Gordon PH: Management of anorectal abscesses and fistulous disease. *In* Kodner IJ, Fry RD, Roe JP [eds.]: Colon, Rectal and Anal Surgery. St. Louis, The C. V. Mosby Company, 1986.)

CONDYLOMATA ACUMINATA. These are warts caused by human papillomaviruses. usually types 6 and 11. They are small, discrete excrescences on the perianal skin, on the anoderm, or just above the dentate line. In the latter location they are pink and velvety, but on the skin they are pearly white. Pruritus and bleeding are common symptoms. Condylomata are treated by application of 25 per cent podophyllin in tincture of benzoin, fulguration with electrocautery devices, or surgical excision.

GONOCOCCAL PROCTITIS. This involves the mucosa of the upper anal canal and rectum. Pain, frequent defecation, and purulent bloody discharge are symptoms. The rectal mucosa is edematous and friable with ulcerations and thick pus. Cultures confirm the diagnosis but treatment may be warranted even if the cultures are negative (Ch. 336).

SYPHILIS. The primary lesion of anorectal syphilis is an ulcer. Mild symptoms resolve as the lesion heals in a few weeks. Secondary lesions are multiple plaques with a white odorous discharge (Ch. 340).

CHLAMYDIA TRACHOMATIS PROCTITIS. *Chlamydia trachomatis* is the most common sexually transmitted bacterial pathogen in the United States today (Ch. 345). Three immunotypes of this organism cause lymphogranuloma venereum, which resembles Crohn's disease. Tetracycline is the treatment of choice after culture confirmation of the organism.

FOREIGN BODIES AND RECTAL TRAUMA

Foreign bodies are introduced into the anus for erotic purposes, for concealment, for self-treatment, accidentally, or by assault. Complications include perforation of the rectum or colon and injuries of the sphincters. Removal of a rectal foreign body can be difficult because the sphincters tighten and trap the slippery object in the rectal ampulla. Most objects can be removed through the rectum with the aid of local or occasionally general anesthesia.

DISORDERS OF THE PELVIC FLOOR

Disorders of the pelvic floor are a group of conditions arising from abnormal structure or function of the levators ani and anal sphincters.

ANAL INCONTINENCE. Anal incontinence has many causes (Table 109–1). Partial incontinence is occasional loss of flatus or loose stool, and major incontinence is abnormal control of stool of normal consistency. Thorough history should be obtained. The anus may be deformed and gaping, and an obvious anatomic defect may be visible and palpable. In other instances the

TABLE 109–1. CAUSES OF ANAL INCONTINENCE

Normal sphincters and pelvic floor
  Diarrhea
  Fistula
Abnormal function of sphincters and/or pelvic floor
  Partial incontinence
    Deficient internal sphincter
      Trauma
      Rectal prolapse
      Third-degree hemorrhoids
    Fecal impaction
      Elderly
      Neurologic disorders
    Minor external sphincter and pelvic floor denervation
  Major incontinence
    Congenital anomalies
    Trauma
    Complete rectal prolapse
    Rectal carcinoma
    Anorectal infection
    Idiopathic
    Drug intoxication
    Neurologic
    Upper motor neuron
      Cerebral
      Spinal
    Lower motor neuron

Modified from Henry MM, Swash M (eds.): Coloproctology and the Pelvic Floor. Pathophysiology and Management. Boston, Butterworths, 1985.

structures seem intact but function is inadequate. Special investigations include anorectal manometry and electromyography.

The underlying systemic intestinal disorder, if any, should be treated. Loose stools are managed with bulk agents and constipating drugs. Elderly patients who soil because of fecal impaction may need regular laxatives and/or enemas. Biofeedback may improve patients with organic neuromuscular impairment. Surgical repair is successful for traumatically disrupted sphincters.

SOLITARY RECTAL ULCER SYNDROME. Solitary rectal ulcer syndrome is a chronic, benign condition characterized by anal pain, bleeding, mucous discharge, and obsessive straining to defecate. It affects mainly young women. Excessive straining forces the anterior rectal mucosa downward where it becomes traumatized.

On examination the anterior rectal mucosa 6 to 10 cm above the anal verge is indurated and may be grossly ulcerated. Biopsies confirm the diagnosis. Treatment should be directed toward avoidance of straining by education of the patient and the use of bulk agents. Unfortunately, current methods of therapy are often disappointing, and patients must live with the chronic condition. Surgical repairs are unsatisfactory unless the patient has a true rectal prolapse.

DESCENDING PERINEUM SYNDROME. Some patients, mostly parous women, complain of a sense of incomplete evacuation and a constant desire to defecate. They are, in effect, attempting to evacuate their own rectal mucosa. The diagnosis is made if the patient strains and the plane of the perineum balloons downward below a line connecting the ischial tuberosities. Education, bulk agents, and occasionally local surgical procedures are helpful.

RECTAL PROLAPSE. Partial prolapse is protrusion of the mucosa alone, and complete rectal prolapse (procidentia) is protrusion of the entire thickness of the rectum. Prolapse is much more common in women than in men, and it appears with increasing frequency after age 40. Surgical or other traumatic injuries are causative in a few patients, but laxity of the pelvic musculature as a result of aging or neurologic disease is more commonly responsible.

With the patient sitting on the edge of the examining table or, even better, on a toilet seat, straining produces the prolapse. Mucosal prolapse is a small symmetric projection 2 to 4 cm long with radial folds. True procidentia may protrude as much as 12 cm from the anus, and the mucosal folds are concentric. Palpation reveals a large mass of tissue anteriorly. Proctosigmoidoscopy and barium enema are required.

Procidentia must be repaired surgically to avoid further weakening of the anal sphincters. Repairs can be accomplished abdominally or through the perineum, depending on the circumstances. Mucosal prolapse is managed by fixation procedures or excision, as described for hemorrhoids.

CHRONIC ANAL PAIN SYNDROMES. *Proctalgia fugax* (levator syndrome) is episodic rectal pain of varying severity. Examination discloses spasm and tenderness of the levator ani muscles. Warm baths and periodic massage of levators may be helpful. *Coccygodynia* is throbbing or aching pain in the coccygeal region. Some patients have abnormal mobility of the coccyx and respond to local anesthetic injections. A number of patients with chronic idiopathic anal pain seem to defy diagnosis and satisfactory treatment.

MALIGNANT TUMORS OF THE ANUS

Epidermoid carcinomas of the anus are uncommon (2 per cent of cancers of the large bowel). Human papillomavirus is etiologically linked to anal cancer. Anal carcinoma may extend directly into the sphincters, perianal tissues, vagina, or prostate, and it tends to metastasize to lymph nodes behind the rectum and in the groins. Bleeding, pain, and a mass are the usual complaints. Often symptoms are mistakenly attributed to hemorrhoids until examination reveals the lesion. Biopsy provides proof. A combination of radiation therapy and chemotherapy is the first line of treatment, and it is followed by local or radical surgical excision if the tumor is not controlled. Overall 5-year survival rates of 60 per cent are expected.

Malignant melanoma in the anorectum is rare but highly lethal. *Mucinous adenocarcinoma* in the glands is also rare. *Bowen's disease* is chronic squamous cell carcinoma in situ. Local excision is required to prevent progression to invasive cancer. Extramammary *Paget's disease* is an intraepithelial mucinous adenocarcinoma. It is treated by wide local excision. It tends to recur locally and can metastasize.

Adams YG, Efron G: Current concepts and controversies concerning the etiology, pathogenesis, diagnosis, and treatment of malignant tumors of the anus. Surgery 101:253, 1987. *A review of most of the current issues regarding anal malignancies.*

Gordon PH: Management of anorectal abscesses and fistulous disease. *In* Kodner IJ, Fry RD, Roe JP (eds.): Colon, Rectal and Anal Surgery. Current Techniques and Controversies. St. Louis, The C. V. Mosby Company, 1985, pp 91–107. *An authoritative discussion of a complex topic.*

Henry MM, Swash M (eds.): Coloproctology and the Pelvic Floor. Pathophysiology and Management. Boston, Butterworths, 1985, pp 193–392. *This monograph helped establish the importance of the pelvic floor in pathogenesis of anorectal diseases.*

Motson RW, Clifton MA: Pathogenesis and treatment of anal fissure. *In* Henry MM, Swash M (eds.): Coloproctology and the Pelvic Floor. Pathophysiology and Management. Boston, Butterworths, 1985, pp 340–349. *An excellent review of the pathophysiology and treatment of anal fissure.*

Rompao AM, Stamm WE: Anorectal and enteric infections in homosexual men. West J Med 142:647, 1985. *An excellent review of the myriad of sexually transmitted anorectal and enteric infections.*

Schrock TR: Hemorrhoids: Nonoperative and interventional management. *In* Barkin JS, O'Phelan CA (eds.): Advanced Therapeutic Endoscopy. New York, Raven Press, 1990. *A thorough review of the subject with details of therapeutic procedures.*

Smith LE, Henrichs D, McCullah RD: Prospective studies on the etiology and treatment of pruritus ani. Dis Colon Rectum 25:358, 1982. *Analysis of the causes and management of this symptom.*

110 Diseases of the Peritoneum, Mesentery, and Omentum

Michael D. Bender

ANATOMY AND PHYSIOLOGY. The peritoneum, a continuous mesothelial membrane, lines the abdominal cavity and its contained viscera. The peritoneal cavity is subdivided by peritoneal reflections and mesenteric attachments into several compartments or recesses, which are clinically important because they determine the location and spread of pathologic processes such as abscesses and metastases. The omentum, a double layer of fused peritoneum, plays an important role in peritoneal defense mechanisms by closing perforations, containing infection, and providing blood supply. The microvascular anatomy of the peritoneum consists of long, straight vessels arranged in two layers at right angles to each other, which helps account for the efficiency of the peritoneal membrane as an exchange interface.

The visceral peritoneum does not contain pain receptors; afferent stimuli are transmitted via the visceral autonomics. In contrast, the parietal peritoneum is supplied by spinal nerves that also innervate the abdominal wall. As a result, irritation of the parietal peritoneum produces well-localized somatic pain, whereas irritation of the visceral peritoneum produces a less well-defined discomfort that is poorly localized. The diaphragmatic portion of the peritoneum is supplied by the phrenic nerve centrally and by intercostal nerves peripherally. As a result, pain caused by diaphragmatic irritation may be referred either to the shoulder or to the thoracic and abdominal wall.

The peritoneal surface, a semipermeable membrane, allows for the passive diffusion of water and solutes between the abdominal cavity and the subperitoneal vascular (blood and lymphatic) channels. In general, water and solutes of molecular weight less than 2000 are absorbed from the peritoneal cavity via the blood vascular system; larger molecules and particulate substances enter the lymphatics. Movement of particles from the peritoneal cavity into the subdiaphragmatic lymphatics is facilitated by discontinuities that exist between the peritoneal mesothelial cells and the lymphatic endothelial cells. Basement membranes are scanty or absent so that particles of substantial size may move freely from the abdominal cavity into the subdiaphragmatic lymphatics, a process that may be facilitated by respiratory motion of the diaphragm itself. Water and electrolytes equilibrate rapidly (within 2 hours) between the blood vascular compartment and the free peritoneal cavity. *Net* fluid movement from the abdominal cavity into the plasma occurs at a maximal rate of approximately 30 to 35 ml per hour both in normal persons and in patients with portal hypertension and ascites. This rate cannot be exceeded despite vigorous diuresis; rather, such diuresis serves only to remove fluid from other body compartments and may cause hypovolemia. The importance of transperitoneal fluid exchange is also illustrated in peritonitis, in which fluid movement into the peritoneal cavity caused by increased vascular permeability can be rapid and massive and may lead to hypotension and shock.

The peritoneum heals readily after damage. Peritoneal injuries normally heal without the formation of adhesions, but in the presence of infection, ischemia, or foreign bodies, adhesions may result. In these situations, fibrinogen released into the peritoneal cavity is converted to fibrin, and then to fibrous adhesions.

DIAGNOSIS. The cardinal symptoms of peritoneal disease are *abdominal pain* and *ascites*. More variable in their occurrence are fever, distention, nausea and vomiting, and altered bowel habits. Direct tenderness, rebound tenderness, and involuntary spasm of the abdominal musculature are the major signs of peritoneal irritation. These signs and symptoms may be minimal or absent in the elderly or debilitated patient and vary, with the location, cause, and acuteness of the underlying process. Because of this, peritoneal disease should be considered in any patient whose abdominal pain is difficult to diagnose.

Radiographically, ascites may be manifested by abdominal haziness, separation of bowel loops, or widening of the flank stripe on plain abdominal films. Otherwise, peritoneal disease reflects itself indirectly on barium contrast studies. Angulation, separation, or rigidity of bowel loops may indicate visceral peritoneal involvement. *Ultrasonography* and *computed tomography* demonstrate inflammatory or neoplastic masses more directly, and may be useful in demonstrating relatively small amounts of peritoneal fluid, and especially in distinguishing free fluid from cystic masses. Computed tomography also has occasionally been successful in the demonstration of peritoneal implants and in the examination of the retroperitoneum. At present, magnetic resonance imaging is rarely indicated in evaluating ascites or peritoneal disease.

If ascites is present, *abdominal paracentesis* is essential to establish its cause (see below). *Peritoneal biopsy*, particularly with the Cope needle, is a relatively simple and safe bedside technique that may yield a positive diagnosis of neoplastic or infectious causes in 50 to 60 per cent of cases. *Peritoneoscopy*, performed under the proper circumstances by a physician experienced in this technique, can be accomplished with little morbidity or mortality. A successful examination may obviate the need for exploratory surgery and may permit biopsy under direct vision of involved portions of the peritoneum or liver. If a diagnosis cannot be made in a patient with obvious peritoneal disease by means of the aforementioned procedures, *exploratory laparotomy* may be necessary.

Patients with mesenteric disease usually have nonspecific symptoms such as abdominal pain, distention, or intestinal obstruction. The most frequent physical finding is a mass, which may be mobile. There are no specific laboratory findings, but mesenteric disease may be suspected if calcifications, displacement of bowel loops, or pressure deformities are observed radiographically. Ultrasonography and computed tomography are useful in identifying mesenteric and omental masses. However, definitive diagnosis usually depends on direct inspection and biopsy, either surgically or by peritoneoscopy.

ASCITES

CLINICAL FEATURES. The accumulation of fluid within the peritoneal cavity is a common clinical finding with a wide range of causes. Its pathophysiology varies with the cause; possible factors are outlined in Table 110–1. The pathophysiology of ascites associated with portal hypertension is considered in Ch. 122.

Small amounts of ascites may be asymptomatic, but as it increases the patient becomes aware of abdominal distention and a sense of fullness and discomfort. Larger amounts of ascites,

TABLE 110–1. FACTORS IN ASCITES FORMATION

Cirrhotic Ascites
Increased portal venous hydrostatic pressure
Decreased portal venous colloid osmotic pressure
Increased hepatic lymph formation
Decreased renal sodium excretion
Decreased renal free water excretion

Noncirrhotic Ascites
Increased subperitoneal capillary permeability
Decreased peritoneal lymphatic drainage
Leakage from disrupted abdominal viscera

especially if the abdomen is tensely distended, may cause respiratory distress, anorexia, nausea, early satiety, pyrosis, or frank pain. Body weight may vary, depending on the state of nutrition and the underlying disease process. On physical examination the flanks bulge, and a fluid wave may be demonstrable. Shifting dullness is somewhat more sensitive but may be nonspecific. Although it is difficult to detect less than 1.5 to 2 liters of fluid, placing the patient on his or her hands and knees and percussing flatness over the dependent abdomen (puddle sign) may demonstrate smaller amounts. Indirect evidence such as penile or scrotal edema, umbilical herniation, or pleural effusion may suggest the presence of ascites.

The diagnosis of ascites may be facilitated by plain abdominal films, ultrasonography, or computed tomography.

EVALUATION OF ASCITIC FLUID. Once the diagnosis of ascites is made by examination, imaging techniques, or paracentesis, laboratory analysis of the fluid removed is essential to determine its cause. Evaluation of ascitic fluid consists of routine studies to characterize the fluid and other studies that may be chosen depending on the clinical situation, as noted in Table 110–2.

Fluids with protein concentrations *exceeding 3 grams per 100 ml* are designated exudates, and below these values, transudates. Other characteristics that may help separate transudates from exudates include ascites–lactate dehydrogenase (LDH), and ascites–serum protein and LDH ratios. The *serum–ascites albumin gradient* (serum albumin − ascites albumin), which reflects the oncotic pressure gradient between the vascular bed and the ascitic fluid, is elevated in association with increased portal pressure, whereas a low gradient occurs in conditions in which portal hypertension is not a factor in the genesis of ascites. Conditions associated with a wide gradient usually are transudative, and conditions with a low gradient usually are exudative. Tests that help distinguish transudates from exudates, and their common causes, are listed in Table 110–3. Although this classification is useful, exceptions in both directions occur not infrequently. For this reason, ascitic fluid chemistries must be interpreted only in the context of all other clinical and laboratory findings.

A large number of red cells suggests the diagnosis of neoplasm, especially hepatocellular or ovarian carcinoma. Other causes of bloody ascites include tuberculosis, trauma, perforated viscus, and spontaneous bleeding associated with cirrhosis. An ascitic fluid leukocyte count of more than 500 per cubic millimeter is strongly suggestive of a peritoneal inflammatory process, such as infection or tumor infiltration. A predominance of polymorphonuclear leukocytes suggests acute bacterial infection, whereas lymphocytes and monocytes characterize chronic inflammatory disease, especially tuberculosis, but there are exceptions. Cytologic examination is essential if malignancy is suspected and may be expected to yield accurate results in more than half of cases. Samples of fluid should be cultured for bacteria, acid-fast bacilli, or fungi in the appropriate clinical setting, such as fever, undiagnosed pain, or deterioration in a patient with cirrhosis. Other chemical determinations that may be helpful in diagnosis are listed in Table 110–2.

TREATMENT: GENERAL CONSIDERATIONS. Although small or moderate amounts of ascites are often only esthetically displeasing, ascites frequently has a detrimental effect on the overall sense of well-being of the patient. Massive ascites may require urgent removal for severe abdominal discomfort, respiratory distress, cardiac dysfunction, or ulceration or impending

TABLE 110–2. LABORATORY ANALYSIS OF ASCITIC FLUID

Test	Abnormal Values	Clinical Situations
Red cell count	> 10,000/mm³	Routine
White cell count and differential	> 500/mm³	Routine
Total protein*	> 3 gm/dl	Routine
LDH*	> 200 IU/liter	Routine
Albumin†	< 1.1 gm/dl	Routine
Bacterial culture	+	Routine
Acid-fast, fungal culture	+	History or findings of Tbc; cirrhosis; immunosuppressed patient
Cytology	+	Neoplasm
Amylase‡	Ascites > serum	Pancreatitis, alcoholism, cirrhosis
Glucose‡	Ascites < serum	Tuberculosis, neoplasm, secondary bacterial peritonitis
Triglycerides‡	Ascites > serum	Chylous (milky) ascites
Starch granules (polarizing microscopy)	+	Postoperative abdominal pain
pH§	< 7.35	Spontaneous bacterial peritonitis
Lactate§	> 25 mg/dl	Spontaneous bacterial peritonitis
CEA	> 10 ng/ml	Adenocarcinoma
Hyaluronic acid¶	> 0.25 mg/ml	Mesothelioma

*Simultaneous blood value for ratio.
†Serum albumin − ascites albumin = gradient. See text.
‡Simultaneous blood value for comparison.
§Also abnormal in neoplastic, tuberculous, and pancreatic ascites.
¶Liquid chromatographic method.
LDH = lactate dehydrogenase; CEA = carcinoembryonic antigen; Tbc = tuberculosis.

rupture of an umbilical hernia. Paracentesis is the method of choice for rapid removal of fluid, as it rapidly reduces intra-abdominal pressure and improves cardiac performance. The risk to the patient of a single, large paracentesis of 2 to 5 liters is minimal and is not associated with a change in plasma volume in cirrhotic patients with edema. One should not hesitate to remove ascites in sufficient volume to treat the complications of tense ascites noted above, but repeated paracentesis to control ascites is rarely warranted.

In patients with intractable, disabling, massive ascites that does not respond to repeated paracentesis or diuretic therapy, peritoneovenous shunting has been successful. Because of numerous complications, careful consideration must be given before recommending peritoneovenous shunting (see Ch. 122). Details of nutritional and diuretic management of ascites are discussed in Ch. 122.

DIFFERENTIAL DIAGNOSIS OF ASCITES. More than 90 per cent of patients with ascites have *cirrhosis, neoplasm, congestive heart failure,* or *tuberculosis.* Causes of ascites may be

TABLE 110–3. DIAGNOSIS OF TRANSUDATIVE VERSUS EXUDATIVE ASCITES

	Transudate	Exudate
Protein	< 3 gm/dl	> 3 gm/dl
LDH	< 200 IU/liter	> 200 IU/liter
Protein ascites/serum ratio	< 0.5	> 0.5
LDH ascites/serum ratio	< 0.6	> 0.6
Albumin gradient*	> 1.1	< 1.1
Common causes	Congestive heart failure	Neoplasm
	Constrictive pericarditis	Tuberculosis
	Inferior vena cava obstruction	Pancreatitis
		Myxedema
	Budd-Chiari syndrome	Vasculitis
	Cirrhosis	
	Nephrotic syndrome	
	Hypoalbuminemia	

*Serum albumin − ascites albumin.
LDH = lactate dehydrogenase.

TABLE 110–4. CAUSES OF ASCITES NOT ASSOCIATED WITH PERITONEAL DISEASE*

I. **Portal hypertension**
  A. Cirrhosis
  B. Hepatic congestion
    1. Congestive heart failure
    2. Constrictive pericarditis
    3. Inferior vena cava obstruction
    4. Hepatic vein obstruction (Budd-Chiari syndrome)
  C. Portal vein occlusion
II. **Hypoalbuminemia**
  A. Nephrotic syndrome
  B. Protein-losing enteropathy
  C. Malnutrition
III. **Endocrine**
  A. Myxedema
  B. Ovarian disease
    1. Meigs' syndrome
    2. Struma ovarii
    3. Ovarian overstimulation syndrome
IV. **Visceral leakage**
  A. Pancreatic ascites
  B. Bile ascites
  C. Chylous ascites
  D. Urine ascites and nephrogenic ascites

*Modified from Bender MD, Ockner RK: *In* Sleisenger MH, Fordtran JS (eds.): Gastrointestinal Disease. 4th ed. Philadelphia, W. B. Saunders Company, 1988.

divided into diseases not involving the peritoneum (Table 110–4) and diseases of the peritoneum (Table 110–5). Of those cases not associated with peritoneal disease, cirrhosis is by far the most common (Ch. 122). Portal hypertension caused by diseases of the heart and great veins accounts for a substantial number of patients with ascites of obscure origin. Included in this group are patients with congestive heart failure, constrictive pericarditis, and inferior vena cava and hepatic vein obstruction (Budd-Chiari syndrome). Clinically, patients with these conditions may not be readily distinguishable from those with hepatic cirrhosis; a high index of suspicion is necessary, and special procedures may be required in order to establish or exclude the diagnosis.

Hypoalbuminemia of any cause, including nephrotic syndrome and protein-losing enteropathy, may be associated with a classically transudative ascites. Ascites occurs only when the serum albumin is very low, usually less than 2 mg per deciliter.

Various endocrine conditions may be associated with ascites. These include *myxedema,* in which the fluid is typically protein rich, and diseases of the ovary, among them *Meigs' syndrome,* in which transudative ascites is associated with ovarian fibroma or cystadenoma, struma ovarii, ovarian edema, and "ovarian overstimulation syndrome."

Pancreatic ascites usually occurs in the presence of chronic pancreatitis or pseudocyst. The most common etiologic factors are alcohol and trauma. The ascitic fluid amylase concentration is elevated, often to extremely high levels. Diagnosis of ductal disruption and pseudocyst leakage is usually possible with endoscopic retrograde pancreatography. Drainage of the pseudocyst and repair of duct injury often have been effective in managing this complication, particularly in traumatic cases. In the chronic alcoholic with pancreatic ascites, a trial of conservative management is indicated before surgery is undertaken. Leakage of bile may be associated with the development of *bile ascites,* a condition for which surgical repair of the biliary tract is usually necessary. This situation is not necessarily associated with the fulminant clinical picture of fever, leukocytosis, and peritonitis, i.e., *bile peritonitis*, which appears to result from superimposed infection.

Chylous ascites is due to the presence of lipoproteins and chylomicrons in the peritoneal cavity and is the result of lymphatic obstruction or leakage. These lipid-rich particles impart a turbidity to the fluid that facilitates its diagnosis. However, not all turbid abdominal fluids are "chylous." Establishment of the diagnosis requires direct evidence that the turbidity is indeed the result of neutral lipid, a determination best made by analysis of the fluid for triglyceride concentration. Other turbid abdominal fluids may be due to cellular debris and are designated *pseudochylous ascites,* a condition occasionally associated with abdominal neoplasm or infection. The differential diagnosis of true chylous

ascites depends upon its chronicity and the age of the patient. *Chronic chylous ascites* in adults is caused in over 80 per cent of cases by abdominal neoplasm, usually lymphoma, with associated obstruction and disruption of the abdominal lymphatics resulting from extensive lymph node involvement. Inflammatory causes include tuberculosis, pancreatitis, cirrhosis, and adhesions. *Acute chylous ascites* ("chylous peritonitis") is associated with abrupt onset of abdominal pain. In some cases, this syndrome is due to trauma, intestinal obstruction, or rupture of a chylous cyst, but identifying a specific cause may not be possible even at laparotomy. In children, congenital malformations of the lymphatics, including intestinal lymphangiectasia, account for a higher proportion of the cases of chylous ascites. Treatment of chylous ascites depends on the underlying cause. General measures include (1) the use of low-fat diets with medium-chain triglyceride supplementation (these are transported by the portal vein rather than the lymphatics); (2) total parenteral nutrition, to achieve bowel rest and allow healing of damaged lymphatics; and occasionally (3) peritoneovenous shunting, if other measures are unsuccessful.

Urine ascites may result from trauma to the urinary tract, high-grade obstruction caused by posterior urethral valves in the neonate, or renal transplantation. Ascites also may occur in a few patients maintained on chronic hemodialysis. The cause appears to reflect a number of factors including prior peritoneal dialysis or infection, fluid overload, hypertension, poor nutrition, or hypoalbuminemia. Management may be difficult, but if aggressive dialysis does not help, renal transplantation seems to offer the best chance of relieving this form of chronic ascites.

TABLE 110–5. DISEASES OF THE PERITONEUM

I. **Infections**
  A. Bacterial peritonitis
  B. Tuberculous peritonitis
  C. Fungal diseases
    1. Candidiasis
    2. Histoplasmosis
    3. Coccidioidomycosis
    4. Cryptococcosis
  D. Parasitic diseases
    1. Schistosomiasis
    2. Enterobiasis
    3. Ascariasis
    4. Strongyloidiasis
    5. Amebiasis
II. **Neoplasms**
  A. Secondary malignancy
  B. Mesothelial hyperplasia and benign mesothelioma
  C. Primary malignant mesothelioma
  D. Pseudomyxoma peritonei
III. **Granulomatous peritonitis**
  A. Exogenous
  B. Endogenous
  C. Iatrogenic
IV. **Sclerosing peritonitis**
  A. Toxic
  B. Indwelling foreign bodies
  C. Idiopathic
V. **Miscellaneous**
  A. Vasculitis
  B. Familial paroxysmal peritonitis (familial Mediterranean fever)
  C. Eosinophilic gastroenteritis
  D. Whipple's disease
  E. Gynecologic disease
    1. Endometriosis
    2. Deciduosis
    3. Gliomatosis
    4. Leiomyomatosis
    5. Dermoid cyst
    6. Melanosis
  F. Splenosis
  G. Peritoneal lymphangiectasia
  H. Peritoneal cysts
  I. Peritoneal encapsulation

*Modified from Bender MD, Ockner RK: *In* Sleisenger MH, Fordtran JS (eds.): Gastrointestinal Disease. 4th ed. Philadelphia, W. B. Saunders Company, 1988.

INFECTIONS OF THE PERITONEUM

ACUTE BACTERIAL PERITONITIS. Bacterial peritonitis most commonly results from perforation of an abdominal viscus caused by trauma, obstruction, infarction, neoplasm, foreign bodies, or primary inflammatory disease (Ch. 51). Peritonitis may also be associated with chronic indwelling catheters used for chronic ambulatory peritoneal dialysis, peritoneovenous shunting, and intraperitoneal chemotherapy. The peritoneum has several defense mechanisms in response to bacterial contamination: (1) Bacteria may be cleared from the peritoneum via the diaphragmatic lymphatics. (2) Opsonins, polymorphonuclear leukocytes, and macrophages enter the peritoneal cavity, where phagocytosis of bacteria can occur. (3) The peritoneum and omentum can contain localized infections and enclose small visceral perforations, in part by exudation of fibrin-containing fluid.

Regardless of etiology, abdominal pain, nausea, vomiting, tachycardia, and fever are usually present. The severity of these symptoms is related to the extent of contamination; in generalized peritonitis, shock is often present and may be profound, whereas signs and symptoms may be minimal if infection is localized. In severe cases, there may be exquisite, diffuse, direct, and rebound tenderness and rigidity of the abdomen; bowel sounds are usually diminished or absent, and distention may be present. Despite its dramatic presentation, recognition of acute peritonitis may be difficult in those patients in whom the clinical manifestations are masked or suppressed, such as the elderly patient or those receiving corticosteroids. In these patients, a high index of suspicion is necessary, since minor or isolated signs such as tachycardia or unexplained hypotension may herald peritonitis.

Laboratory findings are nonspecific and may include leukocytosis, hemoconcentration (from fluid loss into the peritoneum), and subdiaphragmatic air or distended intestinal loops on plain abdominal films. In debilitated or obtunded elderly patients, *peritoneal lavage* may help establish or rule out the presence of peritonitis. One liter of fluid is instilled through a peritoneal dialysis catheter; a positive lavage fluid contains more than 500 white blood cells per cubic milliliter of fluid or more than 50,000 red blood cells per milliliter or, on Gram's stain, reveals bacteria.

The principal systemic complications of peritonitis are septicemia, shock, ileus, and widespread organ failure, including respiratory, renal, hepatic, and cardiac failure. Local complications include wound infection, abscess, anastomotic breakdown, and fistula formation.

The initial management of peritonitis includes restoration of fluid and electrolyte balance, institution of nasogastric suction to reduce distention and improve pulmonary function, oxygen, analgesics to control pain, and early antibiotic therapy. In advanced peritonitis, polymicrobial aerobic and anaerobic organisms are usually found, requiring broad-spectrum coverage. A frequently used regimen combines an aminoglycoside for aerobes with clindamycin or metronidazole for anaerobes. Cephalosporins are popular for their low toxicity and broad-spectrum coverage, especially the third-generation compounds such as cefoxitin and ceftazidime, which provide broad aerobic and anaerobic coverage. Total parenteral nutrition may be necessary in severe peritonitis with major catabolic losses.

In patients who are seen early after a recognized perforation of a viscus and who are good operative candidates, early surgery is usually indicated. In a few patients who are very poor operative risks, it may be desirable to attempt to control the process nonoperatively and to encourage its localization by antibiotic drugs and other conservative measures. Localized abscesses so formed may be drained later when circumstances are more favorable.

Despite the use of antibiotics, modern anesthesia, and intensive support systems, the mortality of generalized peritonitis remains at 50 per cent. Factors adversely affecting prognosis include older age, malnutrition, shock, and organ failure.

ABDOMINAL ABSCESSES. Intra-abdominal abscesses form from a collection of necrotic tissue, bacteria, and white blood cells contained in one of the spaces of the peritoneal cavity and walled off from the rest of the peritoneal cavity by inflammatory adhesions. The contamination is almost invariably derived from endogenous gut flora that escapes as a result of inflammatory perforation, ischemia, traumatic injury, or a surgical procedure. Abscesses within the abdomen localize in three distinct areas: the subphrenic spaces, the intermesenteric area (including the paracolic gutters and interloop areas), and the pelvis. The subphrenic and pelvic localizations reflect the dependent position of these spaces in the recumbent patient and the effect of diaphragmatic movement in drawing fluid up into the subphrenic spaces.

The diagnosis of intra-abdominal abscesses is often a difficult challenge, particularly in immunologically depressed patients with malignancy or malnutrition or patients receiving perioperative antibiotics; all of these may mask clinical signs of sepsis. Fever is the most reliable finding. Other signs and symptoms include malaise, pain, nausea, vomiting, anorexia, tachycardia, abdominal tenderness, and abdominal distention. A subphrenic localization is suggested by thoracic symptoms and signs, including dyspnea, chest pain, decreased breath sounds, dullness, and radiologic evidence of impaired diaphragmatic motion, pleural effusion, or atelectasis. Pelvic localization is suggested by urinary or rectal symptoms and careful vaginal or rectal examination. Leukocytosis with a left shift in the differential count, the usual finding, may be absent. Elevated bilirubin or hepatic enzymes may be a clue to the presence of intra-abdominal sepsis. In summary, a high degree of suspicion is important, and the possibility of an abdominal abscess should be suggested by otherwise unexplained fever, sepsis, leukocytosis, ileus, poor postoperative recovery, or organ dysfunction.

Diagnosis is facilitated by imaging procedures. Plain films may reveal nonmovable gas bubbles, often with air-fluid levels, and barium contrast studies may suggest a mass by displacement of normal structures. Ultrasonography, computed tomography, and gallium citrate-76 or indium-111 leukocyte labeling are newer modalities to diagnose and visualize abscesses. Of these, computed tomography is the most sensitive and specific. Occasionally the diagnosis is made only at the time of abdominal exploration.

Antimicrobial therapy usually suppresses the process and helps to contain it but may also obscure its recognition. Prior computed tomography–guided percutaneous aspiration, with Gram's stain and culture of the obtained fluid, may quickly confirm the presence or absence of an abscess and expedite selection of the proper antibiotic.

Appropriate drainage is indispensable for treatment of an intra-abdominal abscess. Computed tomography–guided percutaneous drainage has increasingly been utilized but may be less successful in complex abscesses associated with multiple cavities, viscous debris, or a source of continued contamination, such as a perforated viscus or fistula. If percutaneous drainage is inappropriate, surgical drainage should be undertaken.

PRIMARY (SPONTANEOUS) BACTERIAL PERITONITIS. Bacterial peritonitis may occur in the absence of an acute intra-abdominal precipitating factor. In this circumstance, the offending organism may not be enteric, and the syndrome is more likely to occur in patients who have pre-existing ascites, impaired immunologic defenses, or a cause for bacteremia such as localized infection elsewhere in the body or indwelling catheters. A widely recognized example of this circumstance is the child with nephrotic syndrome and ascites who develops primary peritonitis. The pathogenesis is probably hematogenous seeding of the peritoneum, particularly suggested by the frequent identification of extra-abdominal pathogens such as *Streptococcus pneumoniae*. The mortality rate associated with this entity has diminished considerably during recent decades because of the availability of antimicrobial drugs.

More common is spontaneous bacterial peritonitis in patients with advanced, decompensated cirrhosis and ascites. This syndrome is discussed in Ch. 122.

OTHER INFECTIONS. *Tuberculous peritonitis* is discussed in detail in Ch. 332. This disorder may present in a variety of ways, ranging from an acute abdomen to an insidiously developing, otherwise unexplained ascites resembling cirrhosis. Accordingly, its presence should be suspected in all patients with ascites, particularly in patients from endemic areas, in cirrhotic patients, and in immunosuppressed patients. Fewer than half of the patients have active disease elsewhere in the body, and tuberculosis skin testing and appropriate cultures of ascitic fluid for tubercle bacilli should be regarded as routine in the evaluation of ascites. The diagnosis is strongly suggested by a high percentage of lymphocytes in the abdominal fluid and may be confirmed by means of a positive culture, peritoneal biopsy, laparoscopy, or, if necessary, exploratory laparotomy. The very satisfactory response of this condition to appropriate chemotherapy adds to the importance of early diagnosis.

N. gonorrhoeae and *C. trachomatis* may enter the peritoneal cavity through the female genital tract and cause peritonitis, or rarely, ascites. This usually presents with right upper quadrant pain, tenderness, and fever (perihepatitis, Fitz-Hugh-Curtis syndrome) (see Ch. 336). *Fungal and parasitic diseases* may be associated with peritoneal involvement and occasionally with ascites. The most common fungal peritonitis is due to *candidiasis*, which may occur after contamination of the peritoneal cavity caused by perforated ulcer, trauma, surgery, or peritoneal dialysis. Other disorders, including histoplasmosis, coccidioidomycosis, cryptococcosis, ascariasis, amebiasis, and schistosomiasis, are quite uncommon, but deserve consideration in otherwise unexplained cases of peritoneal disease with or without ascites.

TUMORS OF THE PERITONEUM

SECONDARY CARCINOMATOSIS. Secondary malignancy is the most common form of neoplastic involvement of the peritoneum. More than 75 per cent of such tumors are classified as adenocarcinoma, mainly from ovary, pancreas, and colon, but peritoneal involvement by sarcoma, lymphoma, leukemia, carcinoid, and multiple myeloma has been described. Ascites formation in these patients appears to result from the combination of increased capillary permeability and obstruction of channels that drain the peritoneal cavity by way of the subdiaphragmatic lymphatics. The clinical picture is usually that associated with advancing malignancy, including weakness and weight loss, and variable complaints referable to the abdomen such as pain, distention, nausea, or vomiting. Radiographic findings may include angulation, fixation, or displacement of intestinal loops, or submucosal edema reflecting lymphatic obstruction. Ultrasonography or computed tomography may help confirm the presence of ascites and associated mass lesions. On abdominal paracentesis, the fluid obtained usually has a high LDH and protein content (more than 3.0 grams per deciliter) and low albumin gradient; cellular composition is variable, and occasionally the fluid is grossly bloody (see Tables 110–2 and 110–3). The diagnosis is made by cytology in approximately 50 per cent of patients, and, if that is negative, by computed tomography–guided percutaneous biopsy or peritoneoscopy. The diagnostic yield of fluid and tissue studies may be increased by new techniques such as flow cytometry and immunologic determination of a variety of tumor or tissue markers. Occasionally surgical exploration may be necessary.

Malignant ascites formation is a grave prognostic sign, with few patients surviving beyond 6 months after onset. Treatment of this condition involves the intraperitoneal administration of antitumor agents, including alkylators, antimetabolites, or radioactive isotopes. The standard intracavitary treatments use a small drug volume, but recent trials have used a large volume (2 liters) administered through a semipermanent indwelling catheter to allow for uniform drug distribution, high local drug levels, and repetitive treatments. Intra-abdominal quinicrine or other sclerosing agents have occasionally been successful in producing a fibrous serositis, thereby obliterating the free peritoneal space and reducing further fluid exudation, but the usefulness of this approach is limited by the frequent occurrence of fever, nausea, vomiting, and abdominal pain.

Salt restriction and diuretics may be tried but are often unsuccessful. Paracentesis is useful, and removal of large volumes may be well tolerated; although it may reduce body protein stores, it is often indispensable for patient comfort. In selected patients, peritoneovenous shunting affords palliation in 75 per cent of cases.

PRIMARY MESOTHELIOMA. The mesothelium may undergo hyperplasia or metaplasia, and rare benign cystic and papillary mesotheliomas have been described, but most mesothelial neoplasms are malignant. Primary mesotheliomas are tumors arising from the epithelial and mesenchymal elements of the mesothelium. Approximately 25 per cent involve the peritoneum, often in association with the more frequent pleural localization. Exposure to asbestos is the most established etiologic factor (see

Ch. 527), although it is unclear if asbestos fibers produce peritoneal disease by passage from the intestinal lumen, penetration of the diaphragm, or via retrograde lymphatic transport.

Mesothelioma is most common in males over the age of 50 and is associated with the gradual onset of abdominal pain and distention, anorexia, nausea, vomiting, weight loss, and ascites. Blood counts and chemistries are rarely helpful, and barium contrast films reveal nonspecific findings. Ultrasonography and computed tomography demonstrate ascites and sheetlike masses that may suggest the diagnosis. Paracentesis yields an exudate that may be hemorrhagic, and high fluid hyaluronic acid concentrations suggest the diagnosis. Peritoneoscopy reveals extensive studding of peritoneal surfaces with nodules and plaques. However, laparotomy is often necessary to provide adequate biopsies and rule out a primary neoplasm. Even with biopsy or cytologic specimens, the variable histologic characteristics of epithelial and mesenchymal elements may make it difficult to differentiate from other malignancies.

The prognosis of peritoneal mesothelioma is exceedingly poor, with a median survival of about 1 year after diagnosis. Death usually results from cachexia or obstruction rather than metastatic disease. Tumor response and increased survival have been reported after chemotherapy (especially doxorubicin) and/or radiotherapy. Intensive combination therapy with surgical debulking, whole abdominal radiotherapy, and intraperitoneal doxorubicin and cisplatin may provide substantial palliation in selected, early cases.

PSEUDOMYXOMA PERITONEI. Pseudomyxoma peritonei is a rare condition in which the peritoneal cavity becomes distended with a mucinous, semisolid, translucent material. The two major causes of this "mucinous ascites" are mucinous cystadenomas and cystadenocarcinomas of the ovary and appendix, although other tumors of the genitourinary and gastrointestinal tract have been associated with the process. Extensive pseudomyxoma is invariably associated with cystadenocarcinomas, although they may be low grade.

The condition usually presents as an increase in abdominal girth with little in the way of other clinical signs of disease. At surgery, the abdominal cavity is found to contain gelatinous material existing in a variety of states, including cystic masses, lying freely without apparent attachment or anchored to the peritoneal surface. If the tumor is indeed malignant, it appears to be low grade and rarely metastasizes. As a result, the course of the disease is prolonged and is characterized by recurrent episodes of intestinal obstruction and fistula formation. Surgical removal of the ovary, appendix, and as much mucin as possible and intraperitoneal instillation of an alkylating agent are usually indicated. More aggressive combination therapy with surgical debulking and intra-peritoneal chemotherapy is also being investigated.

GRANULOMATOUS PERITONITIS. The peritoneum responds to a wide variety of stimuli with a granulomatous inflammatory reaction. *Exogenous* causes include mycobacteria, parasites, fungi, or organic material; *endogenous* causes are rare and include keratin in squamous tumors, meconium, sarcoidosis, and Crohn's disease. The most common etiology is *iatrogenic*, due to contamination at the time of surgery from starch, talc, cotton, or wood fibers used in surgical gloves, gowns, or drapes. *Starch granulomatous peritonitis* presents 2 to 9 weeks postoperatively with pain, tenderness, fever, distention, nausea, and vomiting and may suggest adhesions or abscesses. If it is considered, the diagnosis can be made by demonstrating starch granules in peritoneal fluid. Short-term indomethacin or corticosteroids often speed recovery.

SCLEROSING PERITONITIS. This unusual form of peritonitis manifests with symptoms of intestinal obstruction caused by the encasement of the entire small bowel in a fibrotic membrane or "cocoon." Several causes have been reported: (1) *Toxins*, such as practolol, a β-blocker; (2) *foreign bodies*, such as indwelling peritoneal catheters for shunts, chemotherapy, or dialysis, and (3) *idiopathic*, occurring in young females. The etiology is unclear but may involve toxins or subacute infections that stimulate fibroblast proliferation.

MISCELLANEOUS DISEASES OF THE PERITONEUM. The peritoneal membrane may be affected by a wide variety of systemic diseases, including systemic lupus erythematosus (see Ch. 261) and other collagen vascular diseases, Whipple's disease (see Ch. 102), familial Mediterranean fever (see Ch. 196), and eosinophilic gastroenteritis. Rarely, unusual tissues deposit on the peritoneum, which may cause low-grade peritoneal symptoms or be mistaken for metastatic carcinoma. Examples include endometrial, decidual, glial, and splenic tissue. Several other unusual conditions affecting the peritoneum have been described (Table 110–5).

MESENTERIC INFLAMMATORY DISEASE. This syndrome includes a spectrum of conditions ranging from acute inflammation to a chronic fibrosing process associated with intestinal obstruction, ascites, and steatorrhea. Included are such conditions as "mesenteric panniculitis" and "retractile mesenteritis." The cause of this syndrome is not known, but it is believed to represent the sequel to some inciting event such as trauma, infection, or ischemia in the mesentery. Fat necrosis occurs, evoking an inflammatory reaction with subsequent scarring and granuloma formation.

The condition is most commonly seen in males and in late adulthood. The acute syndrome ("mesenteric panniculitis"), which constitutes the presentation of 60 per cent of cases, is characterized by recurring abdominal pain, weight loss, nausea, vomiting, and fever. In most patients, a tender abdominal mass is palpable; leukocytosis may or may not be present. The remaining 40 per cent of cases are identified by the discovery of a mass on examination or at surgery. Radiographic examination is nonspecific, showing the effects of an abdominal mass and variable scarring that includes displacement and separation of intestinal loops with angulation, stenosis, and extrinsic compression. In some patients the condition evolves into a more chronic process ("retractile mesenteritis"), characterized by continuing pain, fever, weight loss, and various signs of intestinal obstruction, ascites, and steatorrhea. At surgery, the small bowel mesentery is found to be the principal site of involvement; it is thickened and fibrotic, particularly at the root. Resection of the mass is often not possible and generally should not be attempted. Microscopically in mesenteric panniculitis there is infiltration of adipose tissue by foamy macrophages and lymphocytes, with fat necrosis, fibrosis, and calcification. In retractile mesenteritis, the thickening and fibrosis are more pronounced, and there is less evidence of acute necrosis and inflammation. Infrequently, the mesocolon or parietal peritoneum may be involved, or the process may occur in association with retroperitoneal fibrosis.

Most patients seem to have prolonged survival and become asymptomatic after a period of months to years. A minority exhibits the more chronic symptoms noted earlier. The role of corticosteroids is uncertain; although they may be effective in the management of those patients in whom acute symptoms predominate, there is no evidence that they affect the long-term prognosis or progression of the disease. In 15 per cent of patients, malignant lymphomas develop; the basis for this apparent association is not known.

MESENTERIC AND OMENTAL CYSTS AND TUMORS. Mesenteric cysts usually develop as the result of anomalies in the mesenteric lymphatic system but may also be of mesothelial origin. They may spontaneously wax and wane in size; usually they do not cause symptoms in patients less than 10 years of age. Symptoms are related to the size and position of the cyst, which on physical examination is nontender, round, and mobile. Spontaneous rupture, hemorrhage, or infection may occur, but these complications are unusual. Treatment consists of surgical enucleation or excision.

Mesenteric tumors are rare and usually arise from the cellular elements normally present in the mesentery. They include fibromas, myxomas, lipomas, and other less common neoplasms of mesenchymal or neural origin. Most are well differentiated, low-grade fibrosarcomas that produce symptoms such as pain, weight loss, abdominal mass, and compression of adjacent organs. They may be treated successfully by surgical excision. Others are more highly malignant and may metastasize distantly. *Mesenteric lymphoid tumors* also occur, and certain of these have been associated with unexplained abnormalities in iron metabolism with hypochromic microcytic anemia. *Metastatic tumors* of the mesentery are more common than primary tumors and are usually due to enlarged lymphomatous or carcinomatous lymph nodes.

Tumors of the omentum, unlike those of the mesentery, are chiefly muscular in origin (leiomyomas, leiomyosarcomas). About 40 per cent of these are malignant and cause symptoms by virtue of local invasion and development of an abdominal mass; distant metastasis is unusual.

MISCELLANEOUS DISEASES OF OMENTUM AND MESENTERY. *Torsion of the omentum* is an acute surgical condition that mimics acute appendicitis or cholecystitis. It usually occurs in patients over age 30 and causes right-sided abdominal pain with nausea, vomiting, fever, leukocytosis, and occasionally a mass. Omentectomy is indicated. *Idiopathic primary omental infarction* presents a similar clinical picture and is invariably diagnosed only at laparotomy. *Mesenteric fibromatosis* (desmoid tumor) is a benign, noninflammatory fibrous proliferation of the mesentery, which occurs mainly in patients with familial polyposis of the colon or Gardner's syndrome.

Bender MD, Ockner RK: Ascites. *In* Sleisenger MH, Fordtran JS (eds.): Gastrointestinal Disease. 4th ed. Philadelphia, W. B. Saunders Company, 1989.

Bender MD, Ockner RK: Diseases of the peritoneum, mesentery and diaphragm. *In* Sleisenger MH, Fordtran JS (eds.): Gastrointestinal Disease. 4th ed. Philadelphia, W. B. Saunders Company, 1989. *A broad review, extensively referenced.*

Hoefs JC: Diagnostic paracentesis: A potent clinical tool. Gastroenterology 98:230, 1990. *A complete review of the role of paracentesis in the diagnosis of peritonitis and the differential diagnosis of ascites. The utility of the albumin gradient is thoroughly explained and stressed.*

Malangoni MA, Shumate CR, Thomas MA, et al.: Factors influencing the treatment of intra-abdominal abscesses. Am J Surg 159:167, 1990. *A comparison of radiologic and surgical drainage, and the best time to use each.*

Piceigallo E, Jeffer LJ, Reddy KJ, et al.: Malignant peritoneal mesothelioma. Dig Dis Sci 33:633, 1988. *An analysis of 10 cases collected over 20 years from two institutions. Laparoscopic findings are well described.*

Press OW, Press NO, Kaufman SD: Evaluation and management of chylous ascites. Ann Intern Med 96:358, 1982. *An analysis of 28 cases from one institution, seen over 20 years.*

Reddy KJ, DiPrima RE, Raskin JB, et al.: Tuberculous peritonitis: Laparoscopic diagnosis of an uncommon disease in the United States. Gastrointest Endosc 34:422, 1988. *Review of 15 cases found over 15 years from one institution.*

Rodgers PN, Wright IH, Ledingham IM: Critical abdominal sepsis. J R Coll Surg Edinb 34:1, 1989. *A thorough review of the pathophysiology and treatment of severe peritonitis.*

Vanek VW, Phillips AK: Retroperitoneal, mesenteric and omental cysts. Arch Surg 119:838, 1984. *Surveys the literature and gives a complete overview of cystic lesions.*

Weaver DW, Walt AJ, Sugawa C, et al.: A continuing appraisal of pancreatic ascites. Surg Gynecol Obstet 154:845, 1982. *Reviews a series of 42 alcoholic patients with chronic pancreatitis. Preoperative endoscopic retrograde cholangiopancreatography (ERCP) is emphasized to plan the surgical approach.*

111 Gastrointestinal Hemorrhage

John P. Cello

Bleeding from the gastrointestinal tract is one of the most common causes of admission to urban medical centers in the Western world. While in some countries the number of patients admitted for peptic ulcer disease has gradually decreased, the overall mortality for gastrointestinal tract hemorrhage has remained largely unchanged over the past several decades. A multiplicity of lesions can cause bleeding from the gastrointestinal tract (Tables 111–1 and 111–2). Although the specific bleeding lesion and pathophysiology of hemorrhage may vary considerably, the initial therapeutic and diagnostic approach to the bleeding patient remains largely the same (Fig. 111–1).

SIGNS AND SYMPTOMS

Gastrointestinal tract hemorrhage usually produces dramatic clinical signs and symptoms that bring patients to the attention of physicians. *Hematemesis* is the term applied to vomiting of gross blood. Usually, vomiting of bloody material is indicative of bleeding from the upper gastrointestinal tract, but blood passing into the gastrointestinal tract from anywhere proximal to the ligament of Treitz (duodenojejunal junction) can be vomited by the patient (Table 111–1). Hematemesis most frequently follows bleeding *from* the esophagus, stomach, or duodenum, but occasionally nasopharyngeal, pulmonary, and even pancreaticobiliary

TABLE 111–1. ETIOLOGY AND SEVERITY OF UPPER GASTROINTESTINAL TRACT HEMORRHAGE*

Source of Hemorrhage	Severity of Hemorrhage	
	Mild-Moderate (246 cases)	Severe (140 cases)
Esophagus		
Esophagitis	12%	7%
Ulcer	2%	2%
Mallory-Weiss tear	5%	19%
Esophageal varices	5%	31%
Total Esophagus	24%	59%
Stomach		
Gastric ulcer	15%	14%
Prepyloric ulcer	2%	4%
Pyloric channel ulcer	4%	2%
Gastric erosions	2%	0
Gastritis	7%	0
Varices	1%	2%
Portal-hypertensive gastropathy	2%	
Gastric cancer	2%	2%
Polyp	0	
Dieulafoy lesion	0	
Total Stomach	35%	24%
Duodenum		
Ulcer	31%	15%
Duodenitis	8%	
Diverticulum		
Aortoenteric fistula	2%	2%
Pancreatic pseudocyst		
Post-sphincterotomy		
Total Duodenum	41%	17%
	100%	100%

*All patients underwent diagnostic endoscopy at the San Francisco General Hospital over 3 years.

tract bleeding can be manifested initially by hematemesis. *Melenemesis*, or "coffee grounds" vomiting, occurs when blood has had an appreciable period of time in contact with gastric acid. Patients vomiting "coffee grounds" material are usually bleeding at a slower rate than those who have bloody emesis. As with hematemesis, "coffee grounds" emesis follows bleeding into the gastrointestinal tract from a site proximal to the duodenojejunal junction. As with hematemesis, however, it too can follow bleeding from the nasopharynx, tracheobronchial tree, liver, or pancreas. *Melena*, usually noted by patients with bleeding from the proximal gastrointestinal tract, is characterized by dark black, liquid, tarry, metallic-smelling stools. Melenic stools usually indicate upper gastrointestinal tract bleeding, but not infrequently mid- to distal small bowel and even proximal colonic bleeding can be manifested by dark, black, liquid stools. *Hematochezia*, bright red stools, is usually a sign of distal small bowel or colonic hemorrhage (Table 111–2). Brisk hemorrhage from the proximal gastrointestinal tract with accelerated transit may, however, present with dark red blood in the stools. Up to 10 per cent of patients with hemodynamically significant hematochezia are actually bleeding from an upper, not lower, gastrointestinal tract lesion. The remaining 90 per cent of patients with hemato-

TABLE 111–2. ETIOLOGY OF HEMATOCHEZIA IN 72 HOSPITALIZED PATIENTS*

Source of Hemorrhage	Per Cent
Colonic cancer	7
Colonic polyps	11
Diverticula	23
Colitis	11
Vascular ectasia	1
Large hemorrhoids only	12
Ulcer/tear (rectum)	10
Upper gastrointestinal or small bowel source	10
No site identified	15
	100

*Patients underwent colonoscopy (and endoscopy if colonoscopy was negative) at the San Francisco General Hospital

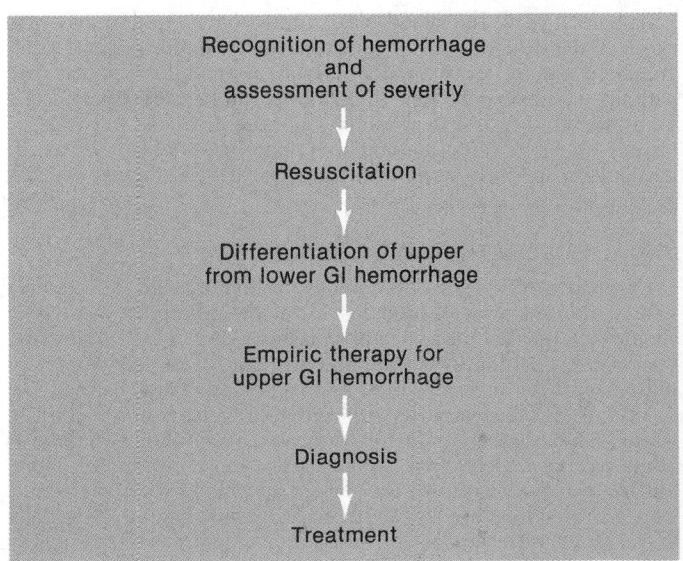

FIGURE 111–1. Approach to the patient with gastrointestinal hemorrhage.

chezia are bleeding from some site distal to the ileocecal valve, with the majority, particularly in those without orthostatic signs or symptoms, bleeding from superficial mucosal lesions in the sigmoid, rectum, or anorectal junction. In addition to signs of gross blood loss, patients with hemodynamically significant gastrointestinal tract bleeding often present with lightheadedness, dizziness, diaphoresis, or frank syncope if hypovolemia has occurred. Patients with slow but persistent gastrointestinal tract bleeding may present with signs and symptoms of profound iron deficiency anemia, including pallor, dyspnea, angina, and exertional weakness (Ch. 131).

DETERMINATION OF THE SEVERITY OF THE HEMORRHAGE

Patients with gastrointestinal tract bleeding often present very dramatically with the above-indicated signs and symptoms. First, the severity of bleeding must be rapidly assessed and resuscitation instituted. In all patients with brisk gastrointestinal tract hemorrhage, these measures take priority over any diagnostic or specific therapeutic approaches. The most accurate noninvasive indicator of the severity of blood loss is the presence of *shock* or changes in *postural vital signs*. Shock is indicative of an acute blood volume loss of at least 15 to 20 per cent. Postural vital sign changes, i.e., upright tachycardia, widening of the pulse pressure, and/or upright systolic hypotension, are indicative of acute intravascular volume loss of at least 10 to 15 per cent. It is therefore essential to determine the blood pressure and pulse in the sitting and standing positions in patients who report signs and symptoms of gastrointestinal tract blood loss but who have normal *supine* vital signs.

Other bedside diagnostic findings may indicate the severity of hemorrhage in patients with upper gastrointestinal tract bleeding. Brisk hemorrhage with hematemesis and/or "coffee grounds" emesis is usually associated with *increasing stool frequency, hyperactive bowel sounds*, and a *change in the color of the stools* from dark black to dark red color. With bleeding from a postpyloric duodenal ulcer, relatively small amounts of blood may be vomited or lavaged by nasogastric tube, most passing distally into the gastrointestinal tract. *Nasogastric lavage* is helpful but highly inaccurate in estimating the severity of upper gastrointestinal tract bleeding. Young patients with duodenal ulcers in particular may exhibit a small amount of bloody emesis and/or "coffee grounds" on nasogastric tube lavage. However, the absence of significant blood by nasogastric lavage (particularly when the lavage does not contain bile) does not rule out upper gastrointestinal tract bleeding. With profuse hematemesis, the return of large amounts of clots or bright red blood is obviously indicative of vigorous active upper gastrointestinal tract hemorrhage. In the face of fresh bleeding, the *hematocrit and hemoglobin levels* are not reliable indicators of the severity of bleeding. For the hematocrit to fall, the blood plasma must have equilibrated with extracellular fluid or with administered intravenous fluids. Exsanguination can occur with a relatively normal hematocrit, and patients with extremely low hematocrits can be hemodynamically quite stable. For these reasons, one should avoid relying too heavily upon the initial hemoglobin concentration or hematocrit, particularly in those patients with other manifestations of brisk gastrointestinal tract hemorrhage.

INITIAL EVALUATION AND TREATMENT

Regardless of the site or etiology of hemorrhage, all patients with significant active blood loss from the gastrointestinal tract should be approached in a similar fashion (Fig. 111–1). Initially, vital signs, including supine and upright blood pressure and pulse, must be measured to assess hemodynamic severity of blood loss. If blood loss is significant, intravenous fluids must be started immediately to restore intravascular volume. Saline or other balanced electrolyte solutions are most rapidly available, but there is no substitute for packed red blood cells in patients who are bleeding briskly. With brisk hemorrhaging, especially in patients with known cardiopulmonary disease, pulmonary artery and peripheral arterial catheters may be helpful in monitoring the severity of bleeding and the adequacy of resuscitation. Nasal oxygen should be administered to these patients to improve blood oxygen transport.

The history of the bleeding episode and of any previous gastrointestinal tract hemorrhage should be rapidly obtained after the initial evaluative and resuscitative measures noted above. A personal or family history of gastrointestinal tract illness, particularly from peptic ulcers, cancer, or vascular ectasias (e.g., Osler-Weber-Rendu syndrome) is helpful, as is a history of previously documented gastrointestinal tract disease as determined by radiography, endoscopy, or surgical procedures. Patients with a longstanding history of alcohol abuse or known or suspected chronic active liver disease may present with painless hematemesis from esophageal varices. Substernal burning pain, regurgitation, or reflux symptoms may indicate longstanding reflux esophagitis. Patients with forceful, dry retching or multiple episodes of vomiting of food prior to the onset of hematemesis may be bleeding from Mallory-Weiss tears of the gastroesophageal junction. A history of epigastric burning pain promptly relieved by food or antacids or nocturnal pain suggests peptic ulcer disease, particularly duodenal ulcer (Ch. 98). Dyspepsia may not always occur in patients with bleeding from peptic ulcer disease, however.

A history of known diverticular disease supports the possibility of colonic diverticular hemorrhage in patients with brisk hematochezia (Ch. 112). Colorectal malignancy is often suggested by a history of gradual weight loss, intermittent blood in the stools, or altered bowel habits (Ch. 105). Patients with idiopathic inflammatory bowel disease often have longstanding mucous and bloody diarrhea (Ch. 103). Hemorrhoidal bleeding is often suggested by the presence of bright red blood surrounding well-formed normal-appearing stools.

The physical examination is sometimes helpful in suggesting the etiology of hemorrhage. Patients with stigmata of chronic liver disease (e.g., spider angiomata, ascites, gynecomastia) and upper gastrointestinal tract bleeding often bleed from esophageal varices, but almost half are found to be bleeding from lesions other than varices. Localized epigastric tenderness to palpation may indicate peptic ulcer disease or gastritis. Occasionally patients with lower gastrointestinal tract bleeding from a malignancy have a palpable lower abdominal mass, signs of obvious weight loss, or adenopathy. A rectal examination is essential to document stool color as well as to palpate for gross anorectal mass lesions such as polyps, cancers, or large hemorrhoids.

Following rapid resuscitation and an expedited history and physical examination, nasogastric tube lavage should be carried out, not only for obvious signs and symptoms of upper gastrointestinal tract hemorrhage but also for hemodynamically significant hematochezia. Blood or "coffee grounds" material in a nasogastric lavage may indicate that bright red blood per rectum is coming from an upper gastrointestinal tract site. Nasogastric tube lavage using room temperature water may also decrease the bleeding rate by vasoconstricting smaller gastric vessels.

Following the initial evaluation, the hematocrit or hemoglobin, the prothrombin time, and the partial thromboplastin time should be measured and a specimen of blood obtained for typing and cross-matching for transfusions. For patients with shock or postural vital sign changes, four to six units of packed red cells should be cross-matched urgently. A serum electrolyte and chemistry panel should likewise be requested. A disproportionate elevation of the BUN:creatinine ratio may indicate bleeding from a proximal gastrointestinal site. In addition, gross abnormalities of liver function tests may suggest the presence of varices as the cause of hemorrhage.

UPPER GASTROINTESTINAL TRACT

Peptic ulcer disease, including both duodenal and gastric ulcers, is the most common cause of upper gastrointestinal tract bleeding (see Color Plate 1C). It is responsible for 50 per cent of moderately severe and 35 per cent of severe bleeding episodes (Table 111–1). Bleeding from peptic ulcers may not always be associated with heartburn or epigastric burning pain, especially in older patients. *Hemorrhage from esophageal or gastric varices* (responsible for nearly one third of the episodes of massive upper gastrointestinal hemorrhage) is usually, but not always, associated with known or suspected chronic liver disease (see Color Plate 1A and B). Most patients with variceal hemorrhage due to alcohol abuse have physical stigmata of liver disease such as a large, firm liver, gross ascites, scleral icterus, palmar erythema, and evidence of peripheral muscle wasting. However, patients with postnecrotic cirrhosis due to viral hepatitis often lack overt peripheral stigmata of chronic liver disease. Variceal hemorrhage usually presents with brisk bleeding, occasionally with regurgitation of large amounts of dark, clotted blood without emesis. However, variceal hemorrhage may present occasionally with only "coffee grounds" emesis and melena. *Mallory-Weiss tears* of the gastroesophageal junction (causing 5 per cent of minor and 20 per cent of severe upper gastrointestinal hemorrhage) are usually associated with antecedent, forceful retching. Nearly half of patients with Mallory-Weiss tears abuse alcohol and report "dry heaves" followed by small and then progressively larger amounts of bloody emesis. *Gastritis* due to alcohol or nonsteroidal anti-inflammatory agents is usually manifested by epigastric discomfort not relieved by food or antacids (Ch. 97). The signs and symptoms of gastritis-associated bleeding may be identical to those of gastric ulcer disease. *Esophagitis* (see Color Plate 1D), particularly in the patient with longstanding reflux or regurgitation, is suggested by substernal burning pain occasionally relieved by the ingestion of food or antacids (Ch. 96). Alcohol abusers or patients with prolonged recumbency may sometimes have brisk bleeding from esophagitis without any antecedent substernal burning. *Gastrointestinal tract malignancies,* such as esophageal, gastric, or duodenal cancer or carcinoma of the ampulla of Vater, rarely cause hemodynamically significant upper gastrointestinal tract bleeding (Table 111–1). Rare causes of upper gastrointestinal tract bleeding include (1) *aortoduodenal fistulae* in patients with atherosclerotic aneurysms of the abdominal aorta, usually following prosthetic grafting; (2) chronic renal disease and *acquired vascular ectasias,* or (3) ectasias associated with other systemic conditions, such as hereditary hemorrhagic telangiectasias (Osler-Weber-Rendu syndrome). Patients with trauma to the liver or with pancreatic pseudocysts may present with signs and symptoms suggestive of upper gastrointestinal tract bleeding but are actually bleeding from adjacent organs. Even rare causes include ectatic superficial arteries (Dieulafoy lesions), duodenal diverticula, and endoscopic sphincterotomy.

Diagnostic and Therapeutic Approach

ENDOSCOPY

Multiple diagnostic procedures are available to localize the site of hemorrhage in patients with upper gastrointestinal bleeding. For patients with hemodynamically significant upper gastrointestinal tract bleeding (bleeding associated with shock, postural vital sign changes, multiple units of transfusion), endoscopy is the diagnostic procedure of choice because of its high accuracy and immediate therapeutic potential. Endoscopy, however, must be performed only following adequate resuscitation and clinical assessment of the patient (Fig. 111–1). If bleeding is severe, the patient should be transferred to an intensive care unit or an operating room where adequate monitoring and resuscitation can be maintained. Endoscopy can document the site of brisk hemorrhage in at least 95 per cent of patients. In patients with significant cardiopulmonary disease, however, endoscopy is not without risk, since it does require sedation and analgesia. Furthermore, endoscopy is considerably more expensive than other means of evaluation, such as an upper gastrointestinal barium series. An endoscopic evaluation of a vigorously bleeding, unstable patient should be performed by an expert because it requires careful sedation, lavage, selection of instruments, and the use of accessory therapeutic endoscopic procedures. Although endoscopy is used in virtually all patients with manifestations of acute gastrointestinal tract hemorrhage, its urgent use is indicated primarily for patients with any of the following: postural vital sign changes or shock, multiple transfusions, hematocrits diluting below 30 per cent, a high index of suspicion of variceal hemorrhage, recurrent hemorrhage from unknown sources, and high risk for surgery (prior to undertaking a surgical procedure). Contraindications to endoscopy include acute myocardial infarction, severe chronic lung disease, hemodynamic instability, and patient agitation. Furthermore, endoscopy is strongly contraindicated in any patient whose underlying disease is so severe as to preclude effective treatment. This latter contraindication to endoscopy is the only absolute one, since patients with other contraindications can often undergo endoscopy safely with expert attention.

In addition to documenting the site and probable cause of hemorrhage, endoscopy may provide definitive short-term or long-term therapy. Acute variceal bleeding, for example, can be controlled with endoscopic sclerotherapy in nearly 90 per cent of patients and the likelihood of recurrent bleeding diminished. The long-term effect of this treatment on survival is less well established. Endoscopic multipolar (or bipolar or "bicap") electrocoagulation and heater probe coagulation are inexpensive, widely available, and highly reliable techniques for controlling upper gastrointestinal tract hemorrhage, particularly for patients with actively bleeding ulcers. These techniques, essentially comparable to one another in effectiveness, not only control acute hemorrhage but also decrease transfusion requirements, the necessity for surgery, and the duration and cost of hospitalization. Endoscopic injections of sclerosants or dilute solutions of epinephrine directly into the bleeding site of an ulcer also show early promise. Endoscopic laser photocoagulation has been advocated, but its expense, logistic constraints, lack of general availability, and absence of advantages over the use of contact coagulation probes have greatly reduced its employment. Endoscopic sclerotherapy for varices and coagulation and injection hemostasis for peptic ulcers are now widely accepted therapies, particularly for patients with hemodynamically significant bleeding.

BARIUM RADIOGRAPHY

An "upper G.I. series," when performed with a double-contrast technique, identifies at least 70 to 80 per cent of lesions confirmed to be associated with upper gastrointestinal tract bleeding. Barium radiography is noninvasive, lower in cost than endoscopy, and readily available but has significant disadvantages, particularly in patients who are bleeding briskly. Large amounts of retained blood in the upper gastrointestinal tract impede the mucosal coating by barium and therefore the localization of superficial mucosal lesions. In patients who are briskly bleeding and hemodynamically unstable, contrast radiography is also impractical. Moreover, on occasion, multiple lesions may be detected by barium radiography and the actual site of bleeding may be difficult to assess. Barium contrast radiography is an acceptable means of diagnosing upper gastrointestinal lesions, however, in patients who have not bled excessively, who have no stigmata of chronic liver disease, and who are not in need of endoscopic hemostasis.

ANGIOGRAPHY

The site of upper gastrointestinal tract bleeding may occasionally be missed on endoscopy. In these patients, angiography may localize the site of bleeding. In addition, selective infusion with vasopressin or coil embolization of actively bleeding arteries may control bleeding. In most instances, angiography localizes the bleeding site but does not establish its etiology. Bleeding must

also be active because angiography detects only extravasation of contrast into the gastrointestinal tract. Angiography is expensive, time consuming, and invasive and requires transportation of the patient to a specialized unit, but it is particularly helpful if bleeding is brisk in the face of a negative evaluation of the upper or lower gastrointestinal tract.

NUCLEAR SCINTIGRAPHY

For patients with less active blood loss, technetium red cell nuclear scintigraphy ("red cell scan") can be helpful in localizing the site of bleeding, with a reported sensitivity of as little as 3 ml of blood loss per hour. Scintigraphy is noninvasive and can be performed with portable gamma cameras. As with angiography, the sensitivity of technetium scintigraphy is limited, since active hemorrhage is needed; therefore, frequent repeat scanning is necessary. Technetium red cell scanning is often performed prior to any angiographic evaluation to assist in the localization of the bleeding focus.

LOWER GASTROINTESTINAL TRACT (Table 111–2)

Colonic diverticula (see Color Plate 1G) are responsible for nearly one quarter of all episodes of hemodynamically significant bleeding from the lower gastrointestinal tract (Table 111–2). Diverticular hemorrhage is characteristically painless and associated with large-volume hematochezia. Patients with clinical diverticulitis rarely bleed significantly (Ch. 112). *Colonic cancers and polyps* (see Color Plate 1E and H) often present with gross blood loss, particularly with lesions in the distal sigmoid colon and rectum. Colonic neoplasms cause nearly 20 per cent of lower gastrointestinal bleeding episodes. Proximal colonic polyps and cancers, however, often present with iron deficiency anemia and less frequently with dark black or bloody stools. *Idiopathic ulcerative colitis and Crohn's colitis* commonly present with bloody diarrhea and tenesmus, and usually with a longstanding history of inflammatory bowel disease (Ch. 103). Significant lower gastrointestinal tract bleeding also occurs from abnormal, superficial vessels called *vascular ectasias*, previously called angiodysplasia (see Color Plate 1F). As noted above, up to 10 per cent of hemodynamically significant hematochezia is secondary to bleeding from upper gastrointestinal sites, particularly from duodenal bulbar ulcers (Table 111–2). Other uncommon causes of "lower" gastrointestinal blood loss include aortoenteric fistulae, Meckel's diverticula of the ileum, and mesenteric varices.

Diagnostic and Therapeutic Approach

Proctoscopy (whether by rigid or flexible instruments) with a careful evaluation of the anorectal junction is the initial diagnostic step for all patients with hematochezia. The anus and anorectal junction must be carefully examined for hemorrhoids or lacerations, since documented brisk bleeding from one of these sources can obviate the need for further invasive or noninvasive imaging. Blood from a very distal site in the rectum may retrogress into the colon and appear as blood coming from above the maximal depth of insertion of the proctoscope or sigmoidoscope. In addition to hemorrhoids, diverticula, and rectal lacerations, colitis and many polyps and cancers are found within reach of a sigmoidoscope.

Following anorectal and sigmoidoscopic examination, the evaluation of patients with lower gastrointestinal tract hemorrhage depends upon the clinical presentation. If blood loss is modest (as evidenced by a normal hematocrit and vital signs), sigmoidoscopy may be followed by *double-contrast barium radiography*, which is highly accurate for detecting even smaller polyps and superficial mucosal abnormalities such as colitis. Single-contrast barium enemas have a high false-negative rate, particularly for modest-sized polyps. If signs and symptoms indicate lower gastrointestinal tract hemorrhage together with anemia, *colonoscopy* should be performed as the next step in evaluation. The colon can be rapidly cleaned within a few hours, using oral, nonabsorbable electrolyte solutions, in order to make colonoscopy technically feasible. Colonoscopic evaluation not only allows the site of hemorrhage to be accurately determined but also allows for biopsy of suspicious mass lesions, polypectomy for modest-sized polyps, and the use of coagulation techniques for the control of bleeding from vascular ectasias. If brisk bleeding continues, as evidenced by profuse hematochezia, rapid *upper endoscopic evaluation* should be considered. Certainly this should be performed in all patients with "coffee grounds" nasogastric lavage and in patients with known or suspected peptic ulcer disease.

If bleeding is brisk, colonoscopy is usually not possible and other means of determining the site of hemorrhage are required. *Technetium red blood cell scintigraphy* can be employed in patients in whom there is substantial active bleeding (at least 3 to 10 ml per hour for a positive scan). Frequent repeat scanning may be needed over the first several hours. Technetium red cell scintigraphy usually localizes the site but not the etiology of active hemorrhage. If bleeding continues at a rate exceeding 30 to 50 ml per hour, *angiography* can be extremely helpful in localizing the site of hemorrhage. In addition, angiographic therapy is possible with vasopressin or embolization techniques. An obvious advantage for technetium scintigraphy or angiographic localization is that surgical resection of the site of hemorrhage, regardless of etiology, is usually very effective.

UNKNOWN ORIGIN

Rarely patients continue to bleed from the gastrointestinal tract without any lesion being detected by upper gastrointestinal endoscopy or pancolonoscopy. In these cases bleeding is usually from a lesion distal to the inferior duodenal angle and proximal to the ileocecal valve. In such patients, technetium scintigraphy, often repeated frequently, can be extremely helpful in localizing the site of hemorrhage. In addition, angiography may determine the site of active blood loss. Other techniques that are sometimes useful in patients with persistent gastrointestinal tract blood loss are *small bowel enteroclysis* and operative *panenteroscopy*. Small bowel enteroclysis, or small bowel enema, is performed by passing a nasoduodenal tube to facilitate the direct instillation of barium and methylcellulose. Radiographic evaluation of the entire small bowel can be completed by enteroclysis in less than 1 hour. Mass lesions such as polyps or cancers and diverticula such as Meckel's diverticula can thus be detected with a high degree of reliability. In patients who have bled repeatedly and profusely from the gastrointestinal tract and have negative evaluations by upper and lower endoscopy, operative panenteroscopy should be considered. At laparotomy, a sterilized endoscope is passed, usually through an enterotomy, and the entire small bowel is passed over the endoscope while the operator and assistant visualize the entire luminal surface. This is most commonly employed in detecting and treating patients with multiple vascular ectasias of the small bowel.

Cello JP, Grendell JH: Endoscopic laser treatment of gastrointestinal vascular ectasias. Ann Intern Med 104:352, 1986. *Review of clinical presentation, therapy, and outcome of patients with bleeding vascular ectasias.*

Cello JP, Grendell JH, Crass RA, et al.: Endoscopic sclerotherapy versus portacaval shunt in patients with severe cirrhosis and acute variceal hemorrhage. Long-term follow-up. N Engl J Med 316:11, 1987. *Randomized trial of endoscopic therapy and surgical shunting in cirrhotic patients with acute hemorrhage from esophageal varices.*

Cello JP, Thoeni RF: Gastrointestinal hemorrhage—comparative values of double-contrast upper gastrointestinal radiology and endoscopy. JAMA 243:685, 1980. *Study of endoscopy and radiography in diagnosing sites of acute upper gastrointestinal hemorrhage.*

Jensen DM, Machicado GA: Diagnosis and treatment of severe hematochezia. The role of urgent colonoscopy after purge. Gastroenterology 95:1569, 1988. *Prospective study of 80 patients admitted with severe rectal bleeding.*

Laine L: Multipolar electrocoagulation in the treatment of active upper gastrointestinal tract hemorrhage. A prospective controlled trial. N Engl J Med 316:1613, 1987. *Endoscopic coagulation reduces rebleeding, transfusions, duration of hospitalization, and hospital costs.*

Laine L: Multipolar electrocoagulation in the treatment of peptic ulcers with nonbleeding visible vessels. A prospective controlled trial. Ann Intern Med 110:510, 1989. *Endoscopic treatment of nonbleeding vessels in ulcer bases decreases morbidity, hospital stay, and hospital costs.*

Lewis BS, Waye JD: Chronic gastrointestinal bleeding of obscure origin: Role of small bowel enteroscopy. Gastroenterology 94:1117, 1988. *Endoscopic examination of the small bowel discloses additional lesions missed by standard endoscopy and colonoscopy.*

Rex DK, Lappas JC, Maglinte DD, et al.: Enteroclysis in the evaluation of suspected small intestinal bleeding. Gastroenterology 97:58, 1989. *Small bowel enemas may diagnose specific lesions in up to 20 per cent of patients with occult hemorrhage.*

112 Miscellaneous Inflammatory Diseases of the Intestine

Marvin H. Sleisenger

ACUTE APPENDICITIS (INCLUDING THE ACUTE ABDOMEN)

DEFINITION. Appendicitis is acute inflammation of the vermiform appendix. It is rare before the age of 2 and reaches a peak incidence in the second and third decades. The vast majority of patients are between the ages of 5 and 30. Although incidence of the disease declines after the age of 40, the annual incidence is about 1.5 per thousand for males and 1.9 per thousand for females between the ages of 17 and 64. The disease is important because it is common and curable; it therefore constitutes the most important entity in the differential diagnosis of the acute abdomen.

PATHOLOGY. Usually, the appendix is swollen, hyperemic, warm, and covered with exudate. However, in the early stages it may appear only slightly discolored and, in the late stages, gangrenous with perforation. Microscopically, the picture ranges from some acute inflammatory cells in the lumen and mucosa to acute inflammatory changes transmurally with superficial mucosal ulcerations; in advanced stages, one or more perforations may be noted, particularly in patients over the age of 60.

ETIOLOGY AND PATHOGENESIS. Although the vast majority of cases have no obvious cause for obstruction, identifiable etiologies include *calculi, Enterobius vermicularis, Kaposi's sarcoma, Burkitt's lymphoma, adenocarcinoma, schistosomiasis,* and *carcinoid tumors.* The initiating event in acute appendicitis appears to be obstruction, followed by increased intraluminal pressure, reduced venous drainage, thrombosis, hemorrhage, edema, and bacterial invasion of the wall. The appendiceal artery (an end-artery) becomes occluded and perforation results.

Calculi are thought to be the most common cause of the initial obstruction. A small percentage of inflamed appendices contain a radiologically demonstrable calculus, compared with 2.7 per cent of normal ones. Gangrene and perforation are more common in appendices with calculi. The calculi are composed of inspissated fecal material, calcium phosphate–rich mucus, and inorganic salts. Although fecaliths are more common in populations eating a low-fiber diet, the incidence of appendicitis is decreasing in the West, and 70 per cent of patients with acute appendicitis do not have calculi. Etiology when the lumen is not obstructed is unclear. Whether the increasing use of high-fiber diets underlies this reduction of incidence is not yet proved.

CLINICAL PICTURE AND DIAGNOSIS. The duration of appendicitis is usually 12 to 48 hours from onset to hospitalization. Over 95 per cent of patients complain of *pain* at onset, classically referred to the epigastric or periumbilical areas and later localizing in the right lower quadrant. This sequence, however, is not found in all patients and is notably absent in *retrocecal appendicitis.* Further, in a significant number of patients, particularly women in the late second or third trimester of pregnancy, the pain does not localize clearly to the right lower quadrant, being either diffuse or in the lower abdomen. In *pelvic appendicitis* the pain may be in the left lower quadrant. When retrocecal, the pain may be referred to the thigh or right testicle. Dysuria is present frequently in both types of appendicitis.

Pain referred to the mid-epigastrium is due to stretching of the organ during early inflammation. Initially it is vague and mild, but it gradually increases over about 4 hours and may be colicky. It tends to subside, and when the process has reached the serosa and the peritoneum, it localizes over the site of disease. In some patients distress appears to be alleviated at the time of perforation; after perforation, localization of pain depends on whether or not the process is quickly walled off locally. Thus if the spreading infection is not contained, generalized abdominal discomfort of variable severity results. *Anorexia* and *nausea* (with or without vomiting) are the second and third most frequent symptoms. In almost all instances, pain precedes the appearance of these other complaints, and its principal feature is *persistence*. About 10 per cent of patients have constipation; diarrhea is uncommon. Temperature usually ranges between 38 and 38.6°C; higher levels usually indicate perforation.

PHYSICAL EXAMINATION. The findings on physical examination depend not only upon the stage of the inflammation but also upon the age of the patient. Tenderness to palpation is the most common (99 per cent), important, and reliable sign; indeed, without it, diagnosis is unlikely. It is usually confined to McBurney's point (one finger) in the right lower quadrant, corresponding to the usual location of the organ. However, although rectal tenderness is present in about one third of patients, it may be so severe as to indicate pelvic peritonitis and thus probable *pelvic appendicitis*. On initial examination in a minority of patients, a mass may be felt in the right lower quadrant or in the pelvis or transrectally. Localized rebound pain is found in 75 per cent. Generalized rebound tenderness indicates diffuse peritonitis. Bowel sounds may be present or absent; absence associated with distention and generalized rebound tenderness is consistent with perforation and diffuse peritonitis. The patient with acute appendicitis often does not seem ill. The physician must not be deceived; the diagnosis rests upon persisting pain and localized tenderness.

On occasion, tenderness may be elicited in the case of retrocecal appendicitis by stretching the psoas by hip extension. Very rarely, because of the odd location of the appendix, tenderness may be in the right upper quadrant or even the left lower quadrant.

LABORATORY FINDINGS. Laboratory studies consistently show a leukocytosis, with an increase in polymorphonuclear cells—over 10,000 per cubic millimeter and greater than 75 per cent, respectively. Urinalysis is usually normal; however, about 15 per cent of patients have either a slight amount of protein or mild pyuria or hematuria. Presence of a calcified fecalith in the right lower quadrant on flat film of the abdomen is helpful, but it is present in only a small percentage of patients. Other findings on flat film include possible obliteration of the right psoas shadow, right lower quadrant sentinel loop ileus, and a right lower quadrant soft tissue mass with or without gas bubbles. With perforation and generalized peritonitis, fluid in the peritoneal cavity and obliteration of the peritoneal lines may be noted.

DIFFERENTIAL DIAGNOSIS OF APPENDICITIS AND OF THE ACUTE ABDOMEN. Appendicitis is first on the list of conditions causing acute abdominal pain that require surgery or immediate consultation with a surgeon. Computed tomography (CT) is now increasingly used in diagnosis, demonstrating swelling, perforation, and fecaliths in a high proportion of cases, and appears to be more helpful than a plain film early in the disease. About 15 per cent of patients operated upon for acute appendicitis have a normal appendix; in view of the gravity of unoperated upon disease, this figure is entirely acceptable. Here a few principles regarding the acute surgical abdomen in the setting of the differential diagnosis of acute appendicitis are reviewed.

Pain Characteristics. Conditions associated with pain of sudden onset include *perforated viscus*, more commonly a *peptic ulcer* or a *colonic diverticulum*, or, rarely, a *carcinoma of the colon* or *acute ischemia* (although acute ischemia does not always cause acute or severe pain in the elderly). The onset of pain in *acute small bowel obstruction, choledocholithiasis, ureteral obstruction, rupture of an abdominal aortic aneurysm*, and *dissection of the abdominal aorta* may also be abrupt. The more gradual onset of pain usually indicates an inflammatory lesion—*cholecystitis, acute pancreatitis, diverticulitis*, and *appendicitis*. However, the pain of diffuse *inflammatory bowel disease* is not localized as it is in appendicitis, except as a consequence of perforation or fistulization in Crohn's disease. The pain of pelvic inflammatory disease is usually associated with menstruation and has been present for 24 or more hours, whereas appendicitis pain is more often intermenstrual and rarely persists so long except with perforation.

The type and radiation of the pain also help in differential diagnosis. For example, evidence of irritation of the diaphragm may be found on the right in *acute cholecystitis* and on the left in *acute pancreatitis*. Sudden, severe pain referred to the tips of the shoulders, associated with diffuse intra-abdominal pain and, later, distention, is more typical of perforated viscus, particularly *peptic ulcer*. *Ureteral obstruction* causes pain that is frequently referred to the genitalia or groin. Steady, continuous pain is more characteristic of inflammation, as in appendicitis; on the other hand, intermittent or crampy pain is more characteristic of *obstruction of a hollow viscus* such as the gallbladder or small bowel.

Pain precedes nausea and vomiting in *appendicitis*; on the other hand, vomiting may be an early symptom of *acute cholecystitis* or *acute pancreatitis*. Bile-stained vomitus associated with acute cramping upper abdominal pain suggests *small bowel obstruction*; blood in the vomitus points toward a mucosal lesion proximal to the third portion of the duodenum. Relief of pain by vomiting suggests *gastric outlet obstruction*. Vomiting, of course, may accompany any intra-abdominal conditions, particularly if the patient is in great pain and has ileus or generalized peritonitis.

Physical Findings. Physical examination of the patient with an acute abdomen is of great importance, and the range of findings expected in acute appendicitis has been discussed. Unlike many causes of acute and severe abdominal pain, *mesenteric ischemia* is not associated with notable abdominal tenderness for 6 or more hours after onset. Localized tenderness and temperature elevation associated with continuing pain over a period of hours reflect either *localized peritonitis*, with or without perforation, or *vascular necrosis* of an ischemic organ. In such instances, the temperature is approximately 38.5 to 39.5°C. Higher temperatures are more often associated with urinary tract infections or bacterial pneumonias. Marked epigastric tenderness in a patient with a steadily increasing boring type of epigastric pain for several hours, particularly if accompanied by falling blood pressure, suggests *acute pancreatitis*. A rapidly rising pulse rate strengthens this possibility but is present with *perforation of a viscus*, a *gangrenous bowel*, or *rupture of an aneurysm*, as well.

Diffuse peritonitis is reflected by resistance of movement and change in position because of accentuation of pain; on the other hand, colic caused by *obstruction* of bile ducts, ureter, or small bowel early in its course is associated with restless movement. Later, in biliary tract and small bowel obstruction, infection and compromise of the blood supply may ensue and cause the appearance of signs of localized tissue necrosis and peritonitis. The abdomen should be carefully examined for scars of previous surgery that may now underlie an *intestinal obstruction* caused by adhesions; hernias must be sought. A succussion splash indicates marked *gastric outlet obstruction*. A large, pulsatile mid-abdominal mass points to *dissection of the abdominal aorta*. *Rupture of an aortic aneurysm* is usually very sudden; pain is brief, since shock quickly supervenes. Abdominal examination reveals distention.

In examining the patient with an acute abdomen, the physician should palpate in the quadrant farthest removed from the site of distress. The important findings that indicate a surgical condition include persistent, localized tenderness with unequivocal rebound, indicating localized peritonitis, and guarding. Guarding must be interpreted circumspectly, because it may be voluntary or involuntary. If it is the latter, underlying peritoneal irritation is likely. Generalized involuntary guarding is a classic finding for a perforated intra-abdominal viscus. The presence of an abdominal mass not previously noted, particularly when associated with other findings of inflammation, gangrene, or perforation, is very strong evidence for a surgical condition. Likewise, free air in the abdominal cavity, as evidenced by distention, absence of bowel sounds, and absence of liver dullness in the setting of acute abdominal pain, reflects a perforated viscus. Bowel sounds may be more active and high pitched in early obstruction or continuously active in diffuse acute inflammation (nonsurgical) of the small bowel. With increasing distention of small bowel loops, the sounds become less frequent and more high pitched. Bruits are an important finding, because they may reflect the presence of *arterial aneurysms*, the dissections of which may be the cause for the abdominal pain.

Rectal examination is crucial in differential diagnosis. Unequivocal tenderness indicates pelvic inflammation, and a mass usually reflects the presence of an abscess. As noted above, this examination often reveals positive findings in *acute appendicitis*. A glove specimen of stool must always be examined for occult blood. In females with acute abdominal pain, pelvic examination is essential to complement a careful gynecologic history.

Laboratory Aids in Diagnosis. The laboratory examination, consisting of urinalysis, complete blood count, serum electrolytes, blood urea nitrogen (BUN) and creatinine, serum amylase, radiographic examination of the abdomen and chest, and sonography of the abdomen, is essential in the differential diagnosis of the acute abdomen.

A *polymorphonuclear leukocytosis* strongly substantiates an acute intra-abdominal process with inflammation or necrosis; a low hematocrit reflects a disorder that is also capable of producing bleeding—*mucosal ulcerations, intestinal carcinoma, ischemia, dissecting aneurysms,* or, uncommonly, *acute hemolysis* associated with acute abdominal pain. An elevated hematocrit and BUN suggest dehydration, usually caused by vomiting and deficient fluid intake.

Urinalysis is vital in differential diagnosis, because the presence of pyuria, particularly white cell casts and bacteria on the smear of urinary sediment, is strong evidence for urinary tract infection and interdicts surgical exploration. Microscopic hematuria (numerous red cells) suggests stone or tumor of the genitourinary tract; red cell casts, on the other hand, suggest glomerulitis. A few scattered white and red cells may be seen in the sediment of about 20 per cent of patients with acute appendicitis. Examination of a *stool specimen* for blood and white blood cells is indicated in patients with right lower quadrant pain, fever, and *diarrhea. Salmonella* enterocolitis (and other bacterial infections) may be confused with acute appendicitis.

Important blood chemistries are *serum amylase,* elevation of which usually reflects acute pancreatitis; however, it may not be elevated in chronic relapsing pancreatitis, and it is elevated in other conditions such as *perforated peptic ulcer, strangulated obstruction* of the small bowel with perforation, *acute cholecystitis, cholangitis, acute renal failure,* and *ruptured tubal pregnancy.*

Visual Aids in Diagnosis. Roentgenologic examinations of importance include chest and flat films of the abdomen and CT scans, including contrast films with water-soluble, iodine (1 to 2 per cent)-containing substances. Radionuclide studies and ultrasonography are often useful as well. The flat and upright films of the abdomen may show free air in the peritoneal cavity, reflecting a perforation of a hollow viscus (80 per cent of cases are due to perforated ulcer, followed by perforated diverticulum and appendicitis). They also support the diagnosis of acute small bowel obstruction, indicate the likelihood of calculus disease of either gallbladder or urogenital tract, outline a large obstructed stomach, and reveal a variety of soft tissue masses that may reflect cysts or abscesses. Collections of extraintestinal gas often point to abscesses; occasionally, the biliary tree may be outlined by air, thus revealing a fistula to bowel. Diffuse calcification of the region of the pancreas indicates chronic pancreatitis. As noted, calculi in the right lower quadrant may rarely help in the diagnosis of acute appendicitis. Flat film of the abdomen also may yield findings characteristic of acute pancreatitis, including "sentinel" loops and a "cut-off" of the colon. A cross-table lateral view will outline an abdominal aortic aneurysm. A routine chest radiograph is essential in order to reveal free intraperitoneal air under the diaphragm, to demonstrate pneumonia, or to show an elevated diaphragm on the left with or without pleural effusion and partial atelectasis, as noted in acute pancreatitis, or on the right, reflecting subphrenic abscess.

Sonography is particularly helpful in demonstrating gallstones, obstruction of the extrahepatic biliary tract (dilated intrahepatic ducts), collections of fluid including abscesses, defects in the liver, and obstruction of the urinary tract. Compression sonography demonstrating a noncompressible appendix larger than 6 mm in diameter is very sensitive in the diagnosis of *acute appendicitis.* A diameter less than 6 mm accurately rules out *acute appendicitis.* Overall accuracy is about 90 per cent, limited, of course, by inability to visualize retrocecal appendices that are inflamed. Ultrasonography may also indicate *colonic diverticulitis, Crohn's disease, intramural hemorrhage,* or *intussusception* by revealing a thickened bowel wall. It may also help in diagnosing "closed loop" obstruction.

CT scans are increasingly used in difficult cases, especially when flat films and sonograms are not helpful. CT may detect choledocholithiasis, the swollen pancreas of acute pancreatitis; inflammatory pseudocyst of the pancreas; intra-abdominal and pancreatic abscess; enlarged lymph nodes; subcapsular hematomas of liver, spleen, or kidney; dissection of the aorta; colonic diverticulitis; and with contrast, perforated or thickened bowel of Crohn's disease or cancer.

Radionuclides given intravenously may help by visualizing the gallbladder (technetium-99m–labeled iminodiacetic acid or derivative compounds) or by localizing an intra-abdominal abscess (gallium citrate-67). Visualization of the gallbladder by technetium-99m scan renders the diagnosis of acute cholecystitis highly unlikely. Radiolabeled agents may also detect localized inflammation and abscess. Gallium-67 collects in granulocytes and mononuclear cells; indium-111-labeled white cells of the patient are given intravenously. These agents are most useful when CT scanning and ultrasonography yield negative findings in the search for an inflamed organ or mass.

Nonsurgical conditions that cause acute abdominal pain are important in the differential diagnosis of acute appendicitis. Chief among these are *pyelonephritis, pneumonia, pulmonary infarction, acute myocardial infarction,* and *pericarditis,* all of which may cause acute upper abdominal pain. Acute distention of the liver and its capsule resulting from *acute right heart failure* may stimulate *acute cholecystitis. Acute hepatitis,* viral or toxic (including alcohol), may closely stimulate acute biliary tract disease. In these instances, however, an enlarged, tender liver will be felt. Further, serum glutamic-oxaloacetic transaminase (SGOT) determinations will be markedly elevated when the liver has been acutely damaged by virus, carbon tetrachloride, or acetaminophen. Alcoholic hepatitis usually demonstrates only modest elevations of SGOT. (However, acute obstruction of the common duct with cholangitis may transiently raise SGOT to levels of 1000 units or more for 24 to 48 hours.)

Systemic diseases, such as *sickle cell disease, acute intermittent porphyria, tabes dorsalis, heavy metal poisoning,* and *diabetic neuropathy,* all may present pictures simulating an acute surgical abdomen.

Acute pancreatitis usually is characterized by pain of many hours' to days' duration, associated with a history suggestive of biliary tract disease or indicative of acute and chronic alcoholism, and in its early stages abdominal tenderness is usually localized to the epigastrium. Markedly elevated plasma amylase (within 48 hours of onset) will help establish the diagnosis. Elevation of serum bilirubin above 3.0 mg per deciliter and of alkaline phosphatase indicates obstruction of the common bile duct, and occasionally ultrasonography or CT scan, in addition to indicating obstruction, may help in establishing choledocholithiasis as the cause of the pancreatitis.

SPECIAL CONSIDERATIONS IN DIFFERENTIAL DIAGNOSIS OF ACUTE APPENDICITIS. Great care must be extended to establish the diagnosis of this condition in the very young and very old. Children with diffuse abdominal pain that is preceded by anorexia, nausea, and vomiting and is often associated with diarrhea are more likely to have *acute infectious gastroenteritis,* in some cases due to *Yersinia enterocolitica, Campylobacter,* or *Salmonella.* Acute enteric infection with *Salmonella* must always be suspected, particularly in young adults with right lower quadrant pain, fever, and diarrhea. *Acute mesenteric adenitis,* presumably caused by viral illnesses and often associated with diffuse abdominal pain, is frequently confused with acute appendicitis in children. The difficulty is in those patients in whom there is some right lower quadrant tenderness and slight elevation of the white count. In such instances a diagnosis must be established at operation, because it is far safer to undertake a negative exploration than to neglect removal of an acutely inflamed appendix. Clinical differentiation of acute appendicitis from *Meckel's diverticulitis* is impossible. The acute onset of *Crohn's disease* involving terminal ileum may be very difficult to distinguish from acute appendicitis, although such patients usually have cramping abdominal pain and diarrhea.

In young women diagnosis is confused by problems in the reproductive system, such as *ruptured graafian follicles, twisted ovarian cysts, ectopic pregnancy, dysmenorrhea, ruptured endometrioma,* and *acute pelvic inflammatory disease. Ruptured ectopic pregnancy* is usually of dramatic suddenness and is often associated with shock and massive blood loss; these findings in a pregnant woman make the diagnosis virtually certain. The *ruptured graafian follicle* is noted in mid-cycle; fever and leukocytosis are uncommon. Tenderness on moving of the cervix on vaginal examination points toward a *twisted ovarian cyst*, the pain of which is out of proportion to the general well-being of the patient. The pain of *gonococcal salpingitis* is more diffuse, and tenderness is not so well localized as in appendicitis. Localized pain and tenderness in a pregnant woman whose pregnancy remains normal and who is not bleeding indicate probable appendicitis.

The differential diagnosis of appendicitis in the elderly may also be difficult. The classic picture is seldom noted, the history may be inadequate or misleading because of infirmity or the effects of medication, and the appendix perforates early. Findings on physical examination are usually not as dramatic, and, despite complications, fever may be only slightly elevated. Accuracy in diagnosis of patients over 60 years of age is below 70 per cent, and the incidence of perforation without a localized or generalized peritonitis at surgery is nearly 70 per cent—more than twice as high as all other age groups combined.

In elderly patients the principal problems in differential diagnosis are *cholecystitis, diverticulitis, mesenteric thrombosis, intestinal obstruction, incarcerated hernia,* and *perforated ulcer.*

Right-sided acute diverticulitis, particularly *cecal diverticulitis,* may simulate acute appendicitis in every respect. In a few instances, *left-sided diverticulitis* may localize tenderness to the right lower quadrant, because the sigmoid is often more redundant in the elderly. Rarely perforation of a *cecal carcinoma* presents a picture indistinguishable from that of acute appendicitis. The patient also may have an episode of diarrhea associated with cramping or steady lower abdominal pain, slight temperature elevation, and, later, evidence of moderate-to-complete large bowel obstruction. When differential diagnosis is difficult, a cautiously administered barium enema or a CT scan with contrast may help greatly in excluding acute diverticulitis as the cause of the problem.

In all instances, elderly patients must not be subjected to the risk of exploration falsely. Accordingly, all efforts should be extended to make certain that *acute myocardial* or *pulmonary infarction, pneumonia,* or other systemic disease or toxin, in addition to intra-abdominal conditions that do not require immediate surgery, are not responsible for acute abdominal pain simulating appendicitis.

TREATMENT. Unless strongly contraindicated, the principal therapy for acute appendicitis is surgical removal of the appendix. Recently appendectomies via laparoscopy have been successfully performed. Since mortality correlates with perforation and, except in elderly patients, perforation correlates with duration of symptoms, early diagnosis and appendectomy are essential for the lowest acceptable morbidity and mortality for the disease. To avoid the catastrophe of unoperated-upon acute appendicitis, normal appendices may have to be removed in 10 to 15 per cent of patients.

In patients in whom complications (*perforation, peritonitis,* and *abscess*) have already occurred or are suspected, dehydration must be corrected; continuous nasogastric suction should be started; and gentamicin, 1.0 to 1.5 mg per kilogram, clindamycin, 1.6 to 2.5 grams, and metronidazole, 2.0 grams, given parenterally per day in divided doses, should be administered prior to surgery.

Patients with obvious acute appendicitis for whom no surgeon is available may be treated with head-up position of the bed; intravenous fluids; gentamicin, 1.0 to 1.5 mg per kilogram, clindamycin, 1.6 to 2.4 grams, and ampicillin, 2.0 grams, intravenously in divided doses daily; and nasogastric suction. The chance for recovery in otherwise healthy individuals with this program is surprisingly good. However, these patients must be scheduled for appendectomy 6 weeks later, or appendicitis is likely to recur.

MORBIDITY AND MORTALITY OF SURGERY. Overall, about 15 per cent of patients with acute appendicitis develop complications postoperatively; this figure is about 35 per cent in those with perforation and localized peritonitis at the time of surgery and is 70 per cent in those with perforation and generalized peritonitis. The complications include *wound infection, intra-abdominal abscess,* mechanical *small bowel obstruction, fecal fistula,* and, much more rarely, *intraperitoneal hemorrhage. Pylephlebitis* is extremely rare (1 in 1000).

The overall mortality of acute appendicitis ranges from 0.18 to 1.6 per cent and is due principally to the interrelated factors of age and perforation. Indeed, mortality over the age of 60 ranges from 6.4 to 14 per cent. The cause of death in this group may be attributed equally to septic and nonseptic complications.

Alvarado A: A practical score for the early diagnosis of acute appendicitis. Ann Emerg Med 15:557, 1986. *Predictive factors for diagnosis in order of importance are localized tenderness in the right lower quadrant, leukocytosis, migration of pain, shift to the left in the neutrophils, temperature elevation, nausea, vomiting, anorexia, and direct rebound pain.*

Jeffrey RB Jr., Laing FC, Townsend RR: Acute appendicitis; sonographic criteria based on 250 cases. Radiology 167:327, 1988. *A new compression technique shows an accuracy of about 90 per cent in ruling the diagnosis in or out.*

Lau WY, Fan ST, Yiu TF, et al.: Acute appendicitis in the elderly. Surg Gynecol Obstet 161:157, 1985. *A prospective study of 104 patients more than 60 years old with appendicitis showed clinical features similar to those of the younger patient; however, the elderly patient may have little or no pain, and the incidence of appendiceal perforation is increased.*

Schrock TR: Acute appendicitis. *In* Sleisenger MH, Fordtran JS (eds.): Gastrointestinal Disease. 4th ed. Philadelphia, W. B. Saunders Company, 1989. *A concise yet comprehensive article on every aspect of the subject. A handy reference.*

Way LW: Abdominal pain and the acute abdomen. *In* Sleisenger MH, Fordtran JS (eds.): Gastrointestinal Disease. 4th ed. Philadelphia, W. B. Saunders Company, 1989. *An excellent chapter containing all important information on diagnosis of the acute abdomen, identifying the cause and the accepted approaches to management.*

DIVERTICULITIS OF THE COLON

DEFINITION. *Diverticulitis* of the colon is a focal inflammation in the wall of the apex of a diverticulum, most commonly of the sigmoid, caused by inspissated feces. It is more common in those with multiple diverticula that have appeared at an early age. Peridiverticulitis results from necrosis with micro- or macro-perforation. An abscess then forms, its size depending on the size of the rupture; small ones may subside with scarring, whereas larger abscesses involve pericolonic tissue and may even dissect along, or within, the bowel wall. Occasionally they rupture into contiguous organs (bladder, ureter, vagina, and small bowel).

CLINICAL PICTURE. The predominant clinical symptoms of diverticulitis are *pain* and *fever*. The pain is usually prominent and is frequently constant. Most commonly, it is localized in the left lower quadrant, because the sigmoid and descending colon are the sites of the largest number of diverticula; however, it may be suprapubic or in the right lower quadrant if the sigmoid is redundant or a right-sided diverticulum is involved. The patient may have a few loose stools or become constipated, and only rarely is rectal bleeding noted. Bleeding from diverticula is not associated with inflammation and perforation. It is usually bright red and may be copious. Bleeding colonic diverticula must be differentiated from ischemic colitis, acute amebic and *Shigella* dysenteries, *ulcerative colitis,* and *tumors of the colon* (see Ch. 111). When the perforation and sepsis are of sufficient magnitude, the patient may also have chills with fever as high as 39 to 39.5°C. Usually, however, the fever is low grade, between 38 and 39°C.

Although the pain may be somewhat intermittent and even colicky at onset, it usually becomes steady and is of the same quality as noted in acute appendicitis. Indeed, acute diverticulitis has often been referred to as "left-sided appendicitis." The patient may seek medical help after only a few hours or, when the situation is not so severe, after a few days of lingering but nagging lower quadrant pain and low-grade fever. Rarely, a *diverticulum of the right colon* perforates, causing right lower quadrant pain with fever, closely simulating appendicitis. Diagnosis is usually made at laparotomy.

Physical examination is extremely important in establishing the diagnosis. Since the process usually quickly involves the serosal surface and peritoneal cover, marked, localized tenderness is found, both direct and rebound. Frequently, a tender mass may be discerned. When present for more than a few days, this mass may be astonishingly firm, even hard, and the distinction grossly from carcinoma is almost impossible. The abdomen is often slightly distended. Rectal examination is also painful, because inflamed bowel is often within reach of the finger; also, a mass may be palpable if a sizable abscess has formed.

In some instances the patient presents with complications of diverticulitis; *dysuria, pyuria, pneumaturia,* or *passing gas or feces through the vagina.* These symptoms are due to perforation of bladder or vagina by the diverticulitis (colovesical and colovaginal fistulas). The vast majority of these patients, usually elderly, do not relate these symptoms to a prior attack of severe pain. The presenting symptom may be septic fever, caused by pericolic, pelvic, or subdiaphragmatic abscess. The inflammatory process may penetrate other pelvic organs, but such fistulization is often clinically undramatic. Rarely, the diverticulum perforates freely. In this instance the signs of free perforation are evident—that is, distention of the abdomen, generalized rebound tenderness, and absent bowel sounds. It is unusual also for diverticulitis to cause persistent colonic obstruction (see below). Very rarely arthritis and pyoderma gangrenosum accompany acute diverticulitis—symptoms more commonly associated with Crohn's disease (see below). The disease may also underlie *polymicrobial septicemia.*

DIAGNOSIS. Diverticulitis should be suspected particularly in patients with known diverticula who develop fever, leukocytosis, and signs of pericolic and peritoneal inflammation in the left lower quadrant. The diagnosis is even more likely if a mass is palpable. Fever between 38.5 and 39°C is also compatible with the diagnosis. When the process is more extensive and with formation of a *pericolic abscess* and its complications, the temperature is usually over 39°C, and the white count is proportionately higher. Urinalysis reflects varying degrees of involvement of the urinary tract by this septic process; that is, with mild ureteral irritation a few red and white cells may be seen in the urinary sediment, but with direct involvement of the ureter or invasion of the ureter or the bladder, the urine may be frankly septic and contain large numbers of red cells.

Some patients suffer much left flank pain owing to *hydronephrosis* resulting from obstruction of the ureter by a *pericolic abscess.* An intravenous pyelogram shows no function or an obstructed kidney on the left, and a sonogram or CT scan demonstrates unilateral hydronephrosis.

The use of radiographs is of crucial importance in the diagnosis, especially a flat film of the abdomen. Pericolic perforation and abscess formation may be suspected from collections of air and fluid in the left lower quadrant. Free air may be seen under the diaphragm in instances of free perforation. Sonography may reveal a localized thickening of the wall or pericolic abscess, particularly in the sigmoid abutting the wing of the ilium. CT scans are particularly helpful by showing inflamed pericolic fat, fistulas, and pericolic abscess in nearly all cases, the involved diverticula in 85 per cent, and thickening of the bowel wall in 75 per cent. A small volume of Hypaque (200 ml) may be instilled to enhance tomographic definition. A fistula to the bladder or ureteral obstruction may be seen with ultrasonography or by CT scan.

Flexible sigmoidoscopy, carefully performed without preparation and air insufflation, helps to exclude other conditions (see below). Usually with diverticulitis the instrument cannot be passed beyond the rectosigmoid junction, which is occluded by fixation, angulation, and spasm.

Clinicians debate the advisability of using a barium or Hypaque enema in the diagnosis of diverticulitis. The concern is that the increased intraluminal pressure may cause perforation. The history, physical examination, laboratory information, cautious Hypaque enema, and, in appropriate instances, ultrasonography or CT scan are sufficient to make the clinical diagnosis. Hypaque enema is safer than barium enema (in the event of extravasation) and, if cautiously performed, is a sensitive method for diagnosis of uncomplicated diverticulitis. It also helps to rule out *acute ischemic colitis* of the left colon and perforation of a left colonic carcinoma.

The roentgenographic features characteristic of diverticulitis are the presence of contrast agent outside a diverticulum, the delineation of a pericolic mass, or the demonstration of a fistula originating in the colon. In some instances the distinction between diverticulitis and carcinoma or Crohn's disease may be difficult (see below). The presence of irregularity, thickening, or even a sawtooth appearance of the bowel is not sufficient to make the diagnosis of diverticulitis, because these are typical for diverticula without perforation.

CT scan with contrast is a sensitive method for diagnosis of complications of diverticulitis, particularly *fistulas* and *pericolic abscess* (Fig. 112–1). It and sonography are also important in ascertaining *ureteral obstruction* or contiguous inflammation, particularly left sided.

DIFFERENTIAL DIAGNOSIS. For many years symptoms of *diverticulosis* have been attributed incorrectly to *diverticulitis. Diverticulosis* may periodically be associated with marked local tenderness, a palpable sigmoid loop, and some degree of large bowel obstruction, and thus the picture suggests diverticulitis. However, such patients do not have fever, the localized tenderness gradually recedes, the white count is not elevated, and there is no evidence of involvement of contiguous organs. Barium enema reveals an irregular luminal contour with a narrowed sigmoid, possibly even a so-called sawtooth appearance of the mucosa. Barium or Hypaque must be noted outside the diverticulum, a fistula seen, or evidences of a pericolic or intramural mass detected before the diagnosis of *diverticulitis* is definitely made.

Carcinoma of the colon must be distinguished from diverticulitis because of similarity of age during which both diverticulitis and cancer of the colon appear. The differential diagnosis is especially difficult, because in about 25 per cent of patients with diverticulitis the lumen is narrowed, suggesting carcinoma. Differentiation from cancer is more difficult if diverticulitis has appeared insidiously. Chronic obstruction, more persistent rectal bleeding, and weight loss are more characteristic of *cancer.* However, the tumor may be obscured on barium enema in 50 per cent of patients with diverticula. Localized tenderness with rebound, leukocytosis, and fever support the diagnosis of diverticulitis. In some cases, however, it may be impossible to

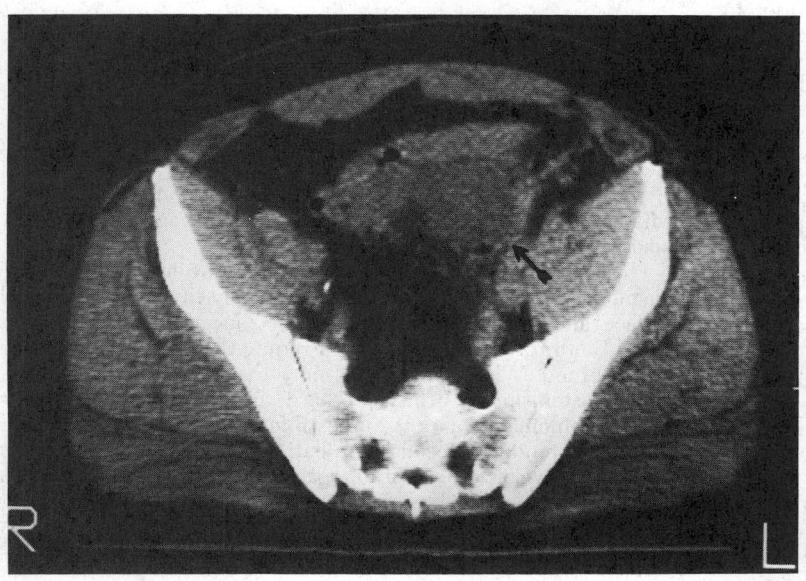

FIGURE 112–1. CT scan showing air-filled diverticula in a contracted segment of sigmoid colon lying just anterior to a paracolic abscess, indicated by a circumscribed area of uniform low density *(arrow).* (From Sleisenger MH, Fordtran JS (eds.): Gastrointestinal Disease. 4th ed. Philadelphia, W. B. Saunders Company, 1989.)

distinguish the two conditions, especially when the contrast enema has features common to both—i.e., a mass, luminal irregularities, and partial obstruction. In such patients CT scan with contrast and colonoscopy may be very helpful in excluding cancer. Rapid disappearance of the obstruction strongly suggests diverticulitis. In some patients correct diagnosis can be made only at surgery, and, in a few, only from surgical biopsy or by the disappearance of the occlusion following colostomy.

Crohn's disease of the colon may be difficult to exclude in the face of marked luminal narrowing or multiloculated channels parallel to the bowel wall on radiograph. Clinically, although both may produce pain, partial obstruction and lower abdominal mass, some rectal bleeding, fever, and leukocytosis, the past history differs. The patient with Crohn's colitis usually has had previous episodes of lower abdominal pain, fever, and diarrhea. Sigmoidoscopy may reveal the rectum to be involved with granulomatous disease. Also, evidence elsewhere in the bowel of granulomatous disease, such as cobblestoning, long intramucosal sinus tracts, and skip areas, help in the differential diagnosis (see Ch. 103).

Ischemic colitis of the left colon in elderly patients may produce signs and symptoms of bowel necrosis and localized peritonitis that are difficult to distinguish from diverticulitis. In these instances, gross rectal bleeding is prominent, and a barium enema is of crucial importance, because so-called thumb-printing is found in ischemic colitis, especially in the area of the splenic flexure and descending colon (see Ch. 104).

TREATMENT OF DIVERTICULITIS. Patients with low-grade fever and no evidence of mass, fistula, or obstruction may be treated with clear liquids by mouth and ampicillin (2.0 grams) or a cephalosporin (4.0 to 6.0 grams) per day in divided dosage intravenously. If the patient has fever of 39°C or more or has a tender mass or other evidence of greater extent of infection, gentamicin, 1.0 to 1.5 mg per kilogram, clindamycin, 1.6 to 2.4 grams, and metronidazole, 2.0 grams, are given parenterally in divided doses daily. In such patients nasogastric suction and intravenous fluids are given to maintain intravascular volume, urinary output, and electrolyte balance. About 50 per cent of complicated cases require surgery. Surgical consultation must be obtained early in all cases in which a mass is palpable or when there is suspicion of peritonitis or involvement of a contiguous organ.

Most patients respond well to this type of therapy with abatement of the fever, tenderness, and evidence of partial obstruction. Long-term therapy becomes identical with that for diverticulosis (see Ch. 100).

COMPLICATIONS AND INDICATIONS FOR SURGERY. Intervention is necessary for the complications of diverticulitis, such as an *enlarging mass* despite therapy, *generalized peritonitis*, *persisting intestinal obstruction*, or the development of a *fistula*. Fistulas extend most commonly to the urinary bladder, occasionally to the vagina, and rarely to other contiguous structures, such as the left hip, infecting joint or bone. Unresolving pericolic abscesses are best drained transabdominally by an interventional radiologist under sonographic or CT guidance. For more complicated or multiple abscesses, fistulas, or obstruction, surgery is recommended. If possible, a one-stage procedure is carried out; if not, a temporary colostomy is established after resection of a fistula or drainage of a septic area. More definitive resection and reanastomoses are carried out later. Elective surgery is indicated for recurrent attacks of diverticulitis and for the inability to exclude a carcinoma as the cause for persisting deformity after recovery from the acute phase.

Almy TP, Naitove A: Diverticula of the colon. *In* Sleisenger MH, Fordtran JS (eds.): Gastrointestinal Disease. 4th ed. Philadelphia, W. B. Saunders Company, 1989. *A complete description of etiology, pathogenesis, and clinical pictures and complications of colonic diverticula, including diverticulitis.*
Chappins CW, Cohn I Jr.: Acute colonic diverticulitis. Surg Clin North Am 68:301, 1988. *A comprehensive review of the disease with a good summary of the modern tools for diagnosis and of the evolving relationship of CT scanning, percutaneous drainage, and surgical management of complications.*
Johnson CD, Baker ME, Rice RP, et al.: Diagnosis of acute colonic diverticulitis: Comparison of barium enema and CT. AJR 148:541, 1987. *A careful analysis of the sensitivities of barium enema and CT in diagnosis of this disease and its complications.*

RADIATION ENTEROCOLITIS

Damage to the small intestine and colon may result from radiation therapy for abdominal and pelvic malignancy.

INCIDENCE. Incidence of severe radiation injury varies

between 2.5 and 25 per cent of patients treated with radiotherapy for pelvic and intra-abdominal malignancy. Minor degrees of damage are common, as evidenced by impaired ileal absorption of conjugated bile acids in many women who are irradiated for pelvic cancer. It is noted most commonly after the total dosage exceeds 5000 rads. Transient histologic inflammatory change may, however, be found in the rectal mucosa of nearly 75 per cent of individuals receiving such therapeutic irradiation. The small intestine is more frequently affected than the rectum.

PATHOGENESIS AND PATHOLOGY. Damage results from interference with replication of radiosensitive epithelial cells, particularly of the crypt, leading to varying degrees of damage to the mucosal surface. Often it is reversible if dosage is not too great or treatment is not prolonged. Such damage may follow dosage of less than 5000 rads. Damage to the mesothelial cells of the small submucosal arterioles results in varying degrees of occlusion and mucosal transmural necrosis. Accordingly, hyperemia and ulceration of the mucosa are frequent. With extreme damage, diffuse edema is followed by extensive fibrosis with multiple strictures and irreversible damage. Such serious damage is more common in diabetics, in those with previous abdominal surgery, previous fixation of intestines, and serious vascular disease.

The pathologic changes range from diminution of crypt cell mitosis and shortening of villi of the small intestine to varying degrees of hyperemia, edema, and inflammatory cell infiltration of the mucosa. Mucosal thickness decreases. Progress of damage is marked by crypt abscesses, sloughing of epithelial cells, and, later, mucosal ulcerations, diffuse or localized, are found. Two to 12 months after radiotherapy, the damage to the blood vessels becomes prominent. In these instances, repair of acute damage does not ensue. The mucosa and submucosa become progressively ischemic and fibrotic. *Abscesses* and *fistulas* may form with sinus tracts between loops of intestine and between intestine and neighboring organs. A more general discussion of radiation injury is found in Ch. 530.

CLINICAL PICTURE. Symptoms may appear early, that is, during the first or second week of therapy, or late, that is, 6 months or more after completion of therapy. Early, diarrhea and mild rectal bleeding may appear, resembling ulcerative colitis. Sigmoidoscopy reveals acute proctitis with an edematous mucosa that may be friable; in more extreme instances, the acute changes also reveal a patchy or diffusely necrotic mucosa.

Later, symptoms of radiation include gross rectal bleeding, decrease in stool caliber, and progressive difficulty in defecation with marked constipation, all indicating severe rectal involvement. Small intestinal symptoms result from either fibrosis and obstruction or fistulization and abscess formation. These serious complications are clinically apparent, on the average, 20 to 24 months after the insult; however, serious symptoms due to obstruction, fistula, or abscess may appear 10 to 15 years after therapy. Those with fistulas are more likely to have synchronous lesions; areas most severely affected are the mid and distal small intestine and the rectosigmoid. If the damage is especially diffuse, malabsorption may be noted. Malabsorption also follows resections of small intestine, as described in Ch. 102. Impaired motility, in addition to mucosal damage, contributes to impaired absorption.

DIAGNOSIS. Diagnosis of *radiation enteritis* is suspected with any of the aforementioned symptoms in patients who have received significant radiation. Sigmoidoscopy shows a picture that ranges from variable degrees of edema to a markedly inflamed and necrotic mucosa. Multiple telangiectases are common, as is rectal stricture. Since most cases are fairly clear cut, biopsy is usually not indicated.

Barium studies of the intestine are not specific and range from changes of diffuse edema and spasm to diffuse fibrosis with strictures, fistulas, and ulceration in more severe cases. Thus the picture may resemble localized malignancy in the colon or diffuse granulomatous disease in the small intestine. Long strictured areas may also be noted, however, in the colon. CT scans are useful if complications such as fistulas or abscesses are suspected.

Differential diagnostic usefulness of small vessel angiography of the intestine in radiation enteritis remains to be confirmed.

TREATMENT. Improving methods for monitoring radiotherapy and delivering rads in small increments will probably reduce the incidence of this complication; however, the increasing incidence of malignancy and of the efficacy of radiotherapy will probably increase the total number of such patients.

Symptoms caused by early reaction consist of mild diarrhea and perhaps some minimal bleeding that can be managed by reduction of dose by 10 per cent, with the judicious use of tranquilizers, anticholinergic drugs, local analgesics, agents that increase stool bulk, and warm sitz baths for those with rectal involvement. An elemental diet free of gluten, milk protein, and lactose may benefit patients with early radiation reaction. If watery diarrhea is a problem, treatment with cholestyramine (4 to 6 grams per day) to bind bile salts may help greatly. If rectal bleeding is prominent, treatment with steroid retention enemas should be initiated as in ulcerative colitis (see Ch. 103). If the bleeding is more significant, transfusions may be required and even, possibly, surgery. Rectal strictures may be dilated, provided that it is early in their course and they are not extensive. Lubricants and stool softeners are often helpful; however, the progress to symptomatic occlusion of the lumen may necessitate proximal colostomy. Fistulas should be resected and abscesses drained. Resection of bowel and anastomoses are hazardous in view of the impaired blood supply, and anastomoses should always be made to uninvolved intestine.

In patients with malabsorption, treatment is as outlined in Ch. 102.

PROGNOSIS. Prognosis depends on the extent and degree of damage, the age of the patient, the course of the underlying malignancy, and whether or not the patient has systemic vascular disease. Unfortunately extensive disease of the colon usually means significant disease in the small intestine. The prognosis is guarded in those with ulceration, fibrosis, or fistulas in whom repeated resections or other major surgical procedures must be carried out. In such cases, age and cardiovascular status are also crucial determining factors. Life expectancy is shorter in those with perforation or fistulas than in those with stricture or bleeding.

Earnest DH, Trier JS: Radiation enterocolitis. *In* Sleisenger MH, Fordtran JS (eds.): Gastrointestinal Disease. 4th ed. Philadelphia, W. B. Saunders Company, 1989. *A comprehensive discussion of the radiation damage to small and large gut.*

Galland RB, Spencer J: Radiation-induced gastrointestinal fistulae. Ann R Coll Surg Engl 68:5, 1986. *Of 70 patients with radiation enteritis, 10 (14 per cent) had 14 radiation-induced fistulas. The median latent period between radiotherapy and presentation of the fistula was 20 months. The fistulas were often multiple and/or associated with other radiation-induced lesions, patients presenting with fistulas being significantly more likely to have synchronous lesions compared with those who presented with strictures.*

Harling H, Balslev I: Long-term prognosis of patients with severe radiation enteritis. Am J Surg 155:517, 1988. *An important follow-up of 136 patients with radiation enteritis over nearly 5 years. Twelve died within 3 months of operation; 68 became asymptomatic. The remaining 56 continued to have problems.*

Miholic J, Vogelsang H, Schlappack D: Small bowel function after surgery for chronic radiation enteritis. Digestion 42:30, 1989. *A study of 22 patients with diarrhea, 16 of whom had resection of small intestine or terminal ileum for complications of radiation injury. Studies of absorption and motility indicate that impaired motility of intestine due to radiation injury contributes to malabsorption caused by resection.*

SMALL INTESTINAL ULCERATION: ISOLATED AND DIFFUSE

ISOLATED NONSPECIFIC ULCERS

In most patients with this rare inflammatory disease, the etiology is unknown. About 75 per cent are ileal and 25 per cent jejunal. Often they are multiple. These ulcers may be caused by ingestion of enteric-coated potassium chloride. Such ulceration may also be associated with *vascular disease* (systemic lupus erythematosus, polyarteritis nodosa, rheumatoid arthritis), *hematologic disorders, granulomatous diseases, trauma, infections, Behçet's syndrome, neoplasia* (including acute leukemia), and *tuberculosis.* Rarely, they result from blunt abdominal trauma and are associated with strictures.

The clinical picture consists of periumbilical colicky pain and perhaps nausea and vomiting. Frequently, however, the patient presents with small bowel obstruction, bleeding, or perforation. Duration of illness is usually weeks to months but may be years. Accordingly, examination may show signs of obstruction, or peritonitis may be present.

Laboratory investigation is normal unless the patient has been bleeding or has had protracted vomiting; plain films of the abdomen are of great value if small bowel is obstructed or has perforated. Barium contrast studies in the uncomplicated cases are most often unrevealing, although in rare instances ulceration and narrowing may be noted. Upper endoscopy may reveal the ulcer or ulcers if located in the high jejunum.

Treatment for the disease is conservative if no complications have occurred. If the involved segment is bleeding, perforated, or stenotic, it should be resected.

Bayless T: Small intestinal ulcers and strictures. *In* Sleisenger MH, Fordtran JS (eds.): Gastrointestinal Disease. 4th ed. Philadelphia, W. B. Saunders Company, 1989. *An up-to-date summary of all the types of cases.*

Thomas WE, Williamson RC: Nonspecific small bowel ulceration. Postgrad Med J 61:587, 1985. *Good report of clinical and radiologic features of this entity.*

DIFFUSE ULCERATION OF JEJUNUM AND ILEUM

Diffuse ulceration of the small bowel may be found in *gluten-sensitive enteropathy (celiac sprue), lymphoma,* and *idiopathic chronic ulcerative enteritis* (also known as *chronic ulcerative nongranulomatous jejunoileitis*). It may also be found after oral administration of flucytosine. Patients with *gluten-sensitive enteropathy* may develop diffuse ulceration of jejunum and ileum, usually signaling a rapid decline in their clinical course despite elimination of gluten from the diet, with increased diarrhea, malabsorption, and, in some patients, perforation or hemorrhage. In instances of mild degrees of ulceration, steroids may induce remission; however, the majority are refractory to medical therapy. Mortality in this group is high. The condition in patients with *lymphoma* and diffuse ulceration also is often refractory to localized resection and radiotherapy.

Chronic ulcerative enteritis and *eosinophilic gastroenteritis* affect the small intestine, usually in patients under 50. They are characterized by diarrhea, weight loss, variable degrees of malabsorption, and protein-losing enteropathy. *Chronic ulcerative enteritis* is a much graver illness, often with fever, ascites and edema, a rapidly progressive course unresponsive to steroids, and a high mortality. It has been reported in association with skin rash, pancytopenia, and hepatitis. The etiology is unknown. Biopsy, peroral or at laparotomy, reveals nonspecific diffuse inflammation and mucosal ulcers. Prednisolone, 60 to 100 mg intravenously daily over 2 to 3 weeks, may be associated with remission in about one half of these patients. Infection, intraperitoneal or systemic, is the common cause of death.

Eosinophilic gastroenteritis may be localized to stomach, small intestine, or colon—so-called *eosinophilic granuloma.* It appears in the fourth to sixth decades and consists of infiltration by sheets of eosinophils into the submucosal and muscle layers. Epigastric pain, anorexia, and nausea are common complaints; it may obstruct the gastric outlet or even the duodenum and terminus of the common bile duct. It may be associated with other diseases, including malignancy. Steroids are often effective, but surgery may be indicated. *Universal eosinophilic gastroenteritis,* on the other hand, is a disease of younger persons, is often associated with allergies, always has a peripheral eosinophilia (greater than 20 per cent), affects stomach and small intestine diffusely, and is associated with diarrhea, crampy pain, weight loss, hypoalbuminemia, and often occult bleeding. Rarely, it responds to elimination of certain foods, particularly fish or meat. Most patients, however, require treatment with steroids, usually short-term (10 days to 2 weeks), but some may require long-term administration of 10 mg of prednisolone daily.

Bayless TR: Small intestinal ulceration: Isolated and diffuse. *In* Sleisenger MH, Fordtran JS (eds.): Gastrointestinal Disease. 4th ed. Philadelphia, W. B. Saunders Company, 1989. *Excellent clarification and description of isolated and diffuse ulceration of the small gut.*

Heyman IN: Allergic disorders of the intestine and eosinophilic gastroenteritis. *In* Sleisenger MH, Fordtran JS (eds.): Gastrointestinal Disease. 4th ed. Philadelphia, W. B. Saunders Company, 1989. *A concise review of eosinophilic disease of the gut.*

PART XI

DISEASES OF THE LIVER, GALLBLADDER, AND BILE DUCTS

113 Clinical Approach to Liver Disease

Robert K. Ockner

The liver plays a central and varied role in many essential physiologic processes. It is the sole source of albumin and many other plasma proteins, and of blood glucose in the postabsorptive state; it is the major site of lipid synthesis and source of plasma lipoproteins; and it is the principal organ in which a wide variety of endogenous and exogenous substances such as ammonia, steroid hormones, drugs, and toxins undergo biotransformation. To the extent that biotransformation "detoxifies" or inactivates a substance, the liver may be viewed as serving a regulatory or protective function for the whole organism. To the extent that such biotransformation results in the formation of toxic products, as in the case of certain drugs, the liver may bear the brunt of their adverse effects.

The clinical manifestations of liver diseases are also varied. Moreover, the clues by which the clinician may be first alerted to the existence of liver disease, even when advanced, may be subtle, consisting of seemingly trivial information gleaned during a careful history (e.g., increased fatigue, or the reversal of sleep pattern or personality change of early hepatic encephalopathy), physical examination (e.g., prominence of breast tissue and small testes in a man with cirrhosis, or excoriation reflecting pruritus), or routine laboratory screening tests (e.g., mild decreases in one or more of the formed elements of the blood because of portal hypertension-associated hypersplenism). Careful assessment is equally important in the patient with obvious liver disease, to address more complex questions. For example, does what seems to be acute hepatitis in fact represent relapse of previously subclinical chronic hepatitis, or delta-agent (hepatitis D) infection in a hepatitis B carrier? (See Ch. 117.) Or does the deteriorating course of a patient with known cirrhosis represent the natural progression of the disease, or a superimposed common bile duct stone, adverse drug reaction, or hepatocellular carcinoma?

HISTORY. Some very *nonspecific symptoms* may be important evidence of liver disease, including fatigue, malaise, fever, change in sleep pattern or behavior, diminished libido, anorexia, weight loss, nausea, and vomiting. *Pruritus* is an important symptom of *cholestasis* (impaired bile secretion), and may be present in the absence of jaundice. *Jaundice* is often first noted by family members or friends, and, especially in dark-skinned individuals, may appear first as a yellow discoloration of the conjunctivae, ("*scleral icterus*"). Since jaundice in most forms of liver and biliary disease reflects cholestasis (see below), such patients will often observe that stool color lightens; while urine gets darker as the excretion of "bile pigments" is diverted from bile to urine. Right upper quadrant *abdominal discomfort* or *pain* may reflect a rapidly enlarging liver with distention of Glisson's capsule because of acute hepatic inflammation or congestion, an acutely inflamed gallbladder, common bile duct obstruction by an impacted gallstone, or abscess or tumor in the liver or adjacent areas.

The history may provide important clues to the presence of *complications of liver disease*, especially those reflecting *portal hypertension* and *portal-systemic shunting*. Early hepatic *encephalopathy* may cause subtle changes in affect or sleep pattern. More overt symptoms include episodic somnolence, confusion, combativeness, ataxia, incoordination, or obtundation. A history of *abdominal swelling* suggests ascites and may be most easily recalled by the patient as a change in the fit of clothing, possibly associated with *edema*. Ascites may also occur in many other conditions, including hepatic vein or inferior vena cava occlusion, congestive cardiac failure, and constrictive pericarditis, and a wide variety of neoplastic and inflammatory processes (see Ch. 110). A history of *gastrointestinal bleeding* in a patient with liver disease may suggest esophageal varices but can also reflect other lesions such as *gastritis, Mallory-Weiss syndrome,* and *peptic ulcer*.

The history is of major importance in the identification of potentially significant *etiologic* or *predisposing factors*. Viral hepatitis is suggested by a history of contact with jaundiced persons, exposure to persons known to have hepatitis or to a common source of hepatitis, ingestion of uncooked or partially cooked shellfish, prior blood transfusion, work with subhuman primates, employment in certain health professions (especially in dialysis or transplantation units), accidental inoculation, sexual promiscuity (especially in the homosexual community), sharing of needles, travel to geographic areas with inadequate public health programs, and consumption of water or uncooked vegetables in such areas. Foreign travel may also suggest parasitic disease such as amebic liver abscess. Q fever hepatitis may occur in individuals in proximity to livestock. Exposure to drugs, ethanol, and other potential dietary, occupational, or environmental toxins must be reviewed in detail. The information obtained may require supplementation or corroboration by family members or other close associates, especially in regard to ethanol consumption. It is often possible to document previous liver function through recourse to *medical records*, and this is particularly useful in evaluating the chronicity of liver disease. A *family history* of jaundice, liver disease, or neonatal jaundice may suggest an inherited disorder such as Wilson's disease, α_1-antitrypsin deficiency, or hemochromatosis.

PHYSICAL EXAMINATION. Scleral *icterus* may be detected at a serum bilirubin concentration as low as 2.0 to 2.5 mg per deciliter. Although *spider telangiectasias*, most prominent around the shoulders and upper trunk, and *palmar erythema* are nonspecific and may be present to a limited extent in normal subjects (especially women in pregnancy), they are potentially important signs of liver disease and usually imply chronicity. Excoriations reflect pruritus and suggest significant cholestasis, not necessarily accompanied by jaundice. *Xanthomas* and *xanthelasmas* are not specific for hepatobiliary disease, but may be a sign of prolonged cholestatic hypercholesterolemia. Changes in hair pattern, gynecomastia, and small or soft testes may reflect the *hormonal changes* that accompany cirrhosis in men. Prominence of cutaneous veins in the epigastrium or around the umbilicus may indicate a *portal-systemic collateral circulation* and, therefore, portal hypertension.

Examination of the heart and lungs may provide evidence of congestive cardiac failure, constrictive pericarditis, or diseases of the lungs or pleura that may be associated with liver dysfunction, cause pain referred to the abdomen, or reflect processes involving the subdiaphragmatic regions such as tumor or abscess.

Examination of the *liver* should include documentation of its *size* and is best recorded both as the distance to which the lower edge extends below the costal margin and its overall vertical span as determined by percussion. These dimensions should be related to a reproducible landmark such as the mid-clavicular line. The *form* and *consistency* of the liver should be noted: e.g., smooth, with a sharp edge; nodular and rock-hard; firm with a rounded and irregular edge. A rapidly decreasing liver size during the course of severe acute hepatitis may be a sign of massive hepatic necrosis. An abdominal mass, tenderness, or muscular spasm may suggest secondary involvement of the liver or biliary passages by a neoplastic or inflammatory process. *Ascites*, most readily detected as dullness or bulging in the flanks, fluid wave, or shifting dullness, may be caused by advanced liver disease, or superimposed infectious or neoplastic processes. Unfortunately, physical findings of ascites may be unreliable, and in equivocal cases abdominal ultrasound may be helpful.

A diffusely tender and enlarged liver suggests hepatitis or congestion, whereas tenderness in a relatively limited area at or below the lower margin in the region of the interlobar fissure may reflect acute cholecystitis. A visible or palpable gallbladder is abnormal and may be an important sign of primary gallbladder pathology or of cystic or common bile duct obstruction, the latter usually neoplastic in jaundiced patients (Courvoisier's sign). Splenomegaly may be the first evidence of portal hypertension of any cause, or may reflect primary splenic pathology such as neoplasm or infection.

Neurologic evaluation is of particular importance with respect to signs of hepatic encephalopathy. These are discussed in detail in Ch. 123, but, as noted, these may be very subtle, consisting initially of a personality change, a mild confusional state, or lethargy. A *flapping tremor* (asterixis), characteristic of metabolic encephalopathy of any cause, is usually present in more obvious cases. In advanced hepatic encephalopathy almost any form of neurologic abnormality may be present, including seizures, lateralizing signs, and abnormal posturing. Despite this, it is essential in patients with liver disease to consider other causes of central nervous system pathology such as the effects of ethanol, sedatives or other toxins, hypoglycemia, trauma, hemorrhage, infection, and primary or secondary neoplasms.

LABORATORY AND IMAGING STUDIES. These special studies, which may play an essential role in the evaluation and management of diseases of the liver and biliary tract, are discussed in Ch. 116 and 126.

Schiff L, Schiff E (eds.): Diseases of the Liver. 6th ed. Philadelphia, J. B. Lippincott Company, 1987.
Sherlock S: Diseases of the Liver and Biliary System. 7th ed. Oxford, Blackwell Scientific Publications, Ltd., 1985.
Wright R, Millward Sadler GH, Alberti KGMM, et al. (eds.): Liver and Biliary Disease. 2nd ed. London, W. B. Saunders Company, 1985.
Zakim D, Boyer T (eds.): Hepatology: A Textbook of Liver Disease. 2nd ed. Philadelphia, W. B. Saunders Company, 1990. *Four current and comprehensive textbooks that serve to introduce the topic and provide literature references dealing with the broad field of hepatobiliary structure, function, and disease.*

114 Hepatic Metabolism in Liver Disease

Richard A. Weisiger

Intermediary metabolism may be profoundly disturbed in liver disease. In some instances, the resulting changes may overshadow the underlying disease process.

CARBOHYDRATE METABOLISM. Except during the absorption of dietary carbohydrate, maintenance of normal blood glucose levels depends entirely on the liver. Two distinct mechanisms are involved: *glycogenolysis* and *gluconeogenesis*. In glycogenolysis, glucose is released from hepatic glycogen by activated glycogen phosphorylase. The process is triggered by the action of glucagon or epinephrine on specific liver cell surface receptors, which activate glycogen phosphorylase kinase via the calcium messenger system. Conversely, insulin stimulates the incorporation of glucose into hepatic glycogen. Normal hepatic glycogen stores are sufficient to sustain blood glucose levels for only about 24 hours. Beyond that, maintenance of blood glucose in the fasting state depends entirely on hepatic gluconeogenesis: the de novo synthesis of glucose from precursors including lactate, pyruvate, and amino acids. This process is stimulated by glucagon and epinephrine and inhibited by insulin.

The normally functioning liver continually responds to changes in its nutritional and hormonal milieu. In the fed state (relative excess of insulin and glucose), glucose production by gluconeogenesis and glycogenolysis is minimal. Instead, dietary glucose is either stored as glycogen or converted to fatty acids (*lipogenesis*), largely to be secreted from the liver in the form of triglyceride-rich lipoproteins and destined for storage in adipose tissue. In the fasting state the process is reversed, resulting in mobilization rather than storage of energy substrates. High glucagon levels relative to insulin trigger glycogenolysis and gluconeogenesis. The resulting glucose is no longer diverted to lipogenesis but is released into the plasma. The decrease in fatty acid synthesis is associated with increased fatty acid oxidation, which becomes the principal energy source for the liver.

Failure of these homeostatic mechanisms in liver disease may produce *hypoglycemia* or *glucose intolerance*. Mild hypoglycemia (blood glucose concentrations between 45 and 60 mg per deciliter) occurs in about 50 per cent of patients with uncomplicated acute viral hepatitis. As a rule, these patients are not hyperinsulinemic. Instead, hypoglycemia may reflect several metabolic abnormalities, including diminished glycogen stores, diminished glycogenolytic response to glucagon, diminished gluconeogenesis, and impaired repletion of hepatic glycogen during the fed state. In most cases, the hypoglycemia is not clinically significant, but in severe acute liver injury of any cause, such as virus- or toxin-induced necrosis and Reye's syndrome, hypoglycemia may be profound and life threatening. Hepatic hypoglycemia may also occur in the absence of overt liver damage. For example, *alcoholic hypoglycemia* classically occurs in persons whose only important source of calories over a period of days is ethanol, which cannot be metabolically converted to glucose and may inhibit gluconeogenesis. Hypoglycemia should be considered in the differential diagnosis of altered mental status in any patient with significant acute liver disease or exposure to ethanol or other toxins.

Glucose intolerance, on the other hand, is more typically associated with chronic liver disease and cirrhosis. Plasma insulin concentrations tend to be high, suggesting a state of *insulin resistance*. Both the number of insulin receptors and their binding affinity may be diminished in peripheral blood monocytes in liver disease, suggesting a more generalized receptor defect. In addition, insulin resistance may in part reflect increased plasma glucagon concentrations and in part a diminished insulin effect on the liver owing to diversion of insulin from the liver by portal-systemic shunts. Regardless of the mechanism, the glucose intolerance associated with chronic liver disease is rarely of clinical significance. Occasionally, patients with chronic liver disease may also have other disorders such as *hemochromatosis* (Ch. 193) and *chronic pancreatitis* (Ch. 106), in which *diabetes mellitus* may contribute to glucose intolerance.

LIPID METABOLISM. The liver plays a central role in the metabolism of fatty acids and other lipids and lipoproteins. Of the total daily turnover of plasma nonesterified (free) fatty acids derived from adipose tissue, about one third enter the liver, where they are esterified to triglycerides or other esters or undergo oxidation. The balance between esterification and oxidation is closely regulated, as is the rate of de novo fatty acid synthesis. In the fasting state, fatty acid synthesis is inhibited, whereas fatty acid oxidation is increased at the expense of the esterification pathways. In the fed state, de novo fatty acid synthesis and esterification are favored, whereas oxidation is diminished. Exclusive of dietary sources and de novo synthesis, a total of approximately 60 to 70 grams of plasma nonesterified fatty acid (>200 mmol) is taken up by the liver each day in the average adult. This provides the major energy source for the liver in the fasting state. Interference with hepatic fatty acid metabolism may either cause or be caused by clinically significant abnormalities of hepatic structure and function.

Fatty liver usually reflects excess accumulation of triglyceride, which may be deposited as large vacuoles displacing the nucleus, or as small droplets surrounding a central nucleus. It usually reflects an imbalance between the rate of triglyceride biosynthesis and secretion into the plasma, primarily as very low density lipoproteins. This imbalance may result from many factors that can affect synthesis, secretion, or both. Conditions associated with large fat droplets in liver cells include obesity, protein-calorie malnutrition (e.g., kwashiorkor, jejunoileal bypass), diabetes mellitus, corticosteroid therapy, and ethanol ingestion (Ch. 118). Small-droplet fat accumulation (see below) is characteristic of acute fatty liver of pregnancy, Reye's syndrome, Jamaican vomiting sickness, and tetracycline and valproic acid hepatotoxicity but is occasionally ethanol related. Accumulation of triglyceride in the liver cell is usually associated with hepatomegaly and reflects abnormal liver function but does not *by itself* appear to cause severe, progressive, or lasting liver damage.

Conversely, interference with fatty acid oxidation at any of several stages may have profound consequences. For example, *alcoholic ketosis* is attributed to an ethanol- or acetaldehyde-mediated impairment of the tricarboxylic acid cycle, resulting in incomplete oxidation of the products derived from β-oxidation of fatty acids. Metabolites of hypoglycin, a low molecular weight compound present in the unripened fruit of the ackee tree and the cause of *Jamaican vomiting sickness*, are converted to coenzyme A thioesters and to carnitine derivatives. Since these cannot be metabolized further, they effectively sequester the cellular carnitine pool. Fatty acid oxidation is inhibited, and there is a corresponding decrease in ATP production and gluconeogenesis. Continuing fatty acid esterification under these conditions leads to a form of fatty liver characterized by *small-droplet fat* deposition, associated in severe cases with liver failure and hypoglycemia. This entity is clinically similar to *Reye's syndrome, obstetric fatty liver,* and *tetracycline* and *valproic acid hepatotoxicity,* but in none of these latter conditions has the pathogenesis been fully elucidated.

The liver is the major source of endogenously synthesized cholesterol (approximately 0.5 gram per day). Together with cholesterol of dietary origin, this newly synthesized cholesterol enters a "metabolically active" hepatic cholesterol pool, from which is derived the cholesterol destined for secretion into bile or into plasma (in lipoproteins), for synthesis of liver cell membranes, and for conversion to bile acids. Bile acid synthesis accounts for the disposition of approximately half of the total daily turnover of cholesterol and, as such, is an important determinant of body cholesterol stores. Relative rates of secretion of bile acids, cholesterol, and phosphatidyl choline (lecithin) into bile are important factors in the pathogenesis of cholesterol gallstones (Ch. 126), but the mechanism(s) by which the secretion of these substances is effected and controlled is incompletely understood.

AMINO ACID AND PROTEIN METABOLISM. Except for the immunoglobulins, most plasma proteins, including albumin, clotting factors, transferrin, α_1-antitrypsin, and the nonalimentary lipoproteins, are synthesized in the liver. The synthesis of each is controlled by specific regulatory mechanisms. In all cases, however, synthesis and secretion are dependent on the integrity of many aspects of cell function, including the transcriptional mechanisms in the nucleus, the translational mechanisms in the rough endoplasmic reticulum, and the secretory mechanisms in the Golgi apparatus. Despite these common features, individual proteins are affected differently in liver disease. This nonuniformity may result from several factors such as the availability of an essential *nutritional* component (e.g., the vitamin K–dependent clotting factors), *hormonal* influences (e.g., very low density lipoproteins), *genetic* determinants (e.g., ceruloplasmin or α_1-antitrypsin), the effects of drugs or toxins (e.g., the warfarin-like anticoagulants or ethanol), or the response of selected proteins such as fibrinogen (and other "acute phase reactants," including C-reactive proteins, ceruloplasmin, haptoglobin, and transferrin) to inflammatory processes. In addition, the *kinetics* of synthesis and turnover of a particular protein are major determinants of

response of its plasma concentration to acute liver injury. In general, plasma concentrations of proteins of which the turnover is rapid (e.g., clotting factors, plasma half-time of hours to days) are more likely to be depressed by severe acute liver injury than are those proteins that turn over more slowly (e.g., albumin, plasma half-time about 3 weeks). Finally, *catabolism* of certain plasma proteins may be accelerated (e.g., clotting factors in *disseminated intravascular coagulation,* or albumin in *protein-losing enteropathy*). For these reasons, although liver disease generally tends to depress the plasma concentration of proteins of hepatic origin, plasma concentrations of such proteins may not accurately reflect the severity of the liver disease in a given patient. Interpretation of the prothrombin time, partial thromboplastin time, and serum albumin concentrations in the evaluation of liver disease is discussed in Ch. 116.

Amino acids, in addition to their obvious importance in protein synthesis, also participate in other reactions in the liver. Of special significance is the role of certain amino acids as precursors for gluconeogenesis, as discussed above. Amino acids may undergo *transamination,* in which the α-amino group is transferred to an α-keto group, as in the alanine transaminase (ALT)–mediated deamination of alanine to pyruvate; the resulting transfer of the amino group to α-ketoglutarate converts this acceptor to glutamate. Alternatively, amino acids may undergo *oxidative deamination.* In this case, an α-keto acid is formed as the amino group is converted to ammonium ion and, ultimately, to urea (see below).

BIOTRANSFORMATION AND DETOXIFICATION. The liver is the major site of chemical modification of a wide variety of exogenous drugs and toxins, as well as endogenous substances such as hormones. The reactions potentially involved are numerous and, in many instances, involve the cytochrome P-450–dependent microsomal mixed function oxidase system. The basic principles of drug disposition are discussed in Ch. 118, but several aspects warrant special emphasis in the context of liver function disease. First, while biotransformation of an endogenous or exogenous substance may *inactivate* it or render it more suitable for urinary or biliary excretion, there are many examples of compounds that are rendered toxic by this process. A number of clinically significant hepatotoxins are *activated* in this way, and some "idiosyncratic" drug reactions may reflect individual differences in drug metabolism rather than an immunologic response (see Ch. 118). Second, diseases of the liver may seriously impair the biotransformation of exogenous substances, thereby resulting in an *increased sensitivity* to certain drugs (e.g., sedatives and opiates) or may enhance the biologic effect of endogenous hormones (e.g., contributing to the feminizing effects of chronic liver disease) or toxins (e.g., diminished hepatic conversion of ammonia to urea in hepatic encephalopathy). Finally, one substance may significantly influence the hepatic biotransformation of another. Examples of this particular form of *drug-drug interaction* include the well-recognized induction of the microsomal drug-metabolizing system by prior administration of phenobarbital and its inhibition by various toxins.

A particularly important hepatic detoxification pathway converts *ammonium ion* to urea via the Krebs-Henseleit *urea cycle,* in which ornithine, citrulline, argininosuccinate, and arginine are intermediates and which involves both mitochondrial and cytosolic components (see Fig. 180–1). Glutamate, formed from NH_4^+ and α-ketoglutarate, is the principal NH_3 donor. Ammonium ion is produced in abundance in the intestinal tract, especially the colon, by the bacterial degradation of luminal proteins and amino acids and of endogenous urea, 25 per cent of the daily production of which diffuses into the intestinal lumen. The NH_4^+ diffuses into the portal circulation and is transported to the liver, where it is converted to urea by the mechanism described above. *Hepatic encephalopathy* in part reflects the failure of this important detoxification process (or of analogous pathways for other *enterogenous toxins*) because of extensive acute liver cell necrosis or direct entry of portal blood into the peripheral circulation via spontaneous or surgically created portal-systemic shunts (Ch. 123).

Arias IM, Jakoby WB, Popper H, et al. (eds.): The Liver Biology and Pathobiology. New York, Raven Press, 1988. *An in-depth and well-referenced presentation of many basic aspects of normal and abnormal hepatic structure and function.*

Arky RA: Hypoglycemia associated with liver disease and ethanol. Endocrinol Metab Clin North Am 18:75, 1989. *Comprehensive review of this important clinical complication.*

Howden CW, Birnie GG, Brodie MJ: Drug metabolism in liver disease. Pharmacol Ther 40:439, 1989. *Includes practical information on adjusting drug dosages in liver disease.*

Zakim D, Boyer T (eds.): Hepatology: A Textbook of Liver Disease. 2nd ed. Philadelphia, W. B. Saunders Company, 1990. *A comprehensive and well-written clinical text with a good foundation in basic metabolism.*

115 Bilirubin Metabolism and Hyperbilirubinemia

Bruce F. Scharschmidt

BILIRUBIN METABOLISM (See Fig. 115–1)

BILIRUBIN CHEMISTRY. Bilirubin consists of four pyrrole rings linked by three carbon bridges. Unconjugated bilirubin is virtually water-insoluble at physiologic pH because its —COOH and —NH groups are involved in strong intramolecular hydrogen bonds and are therefore unable to interact with water. These intramolecular hydrogen bonds are disrupted by conjugation of the —COOH groups with glucuronic acid as occurs in the liver cell, thus greatly enhancing the aqueous solubility of the molecule and altering its biologic properties. In contrast to the more polar water-soluble conjugates, relatively nonpolar unconjugated bilirubin diffuses across most biologic membranes such as the blood-brain barrier, placenta, and intestinal and gallbladder epithelium. It is excreted in bile in only trace amounts. Thus, hepatic conjugation confers upon bilirubin the properties that permit its elimination from the body and thereby prevents damage to the central nervous system. Exposure of unconjugated bilirubin to light causes the formation of polar photoisomers and "lumirubin," which results from intramolecular cyclization. These compounds are excreted by the liver without conjugation; their formation is the mechanism by which phototherapy lowers serum bilirubin concentration in neonatal hyperbilirubinemia.

BILIRUBIN FORMATION. Bilirubin is formed from the breakdown of heme. Daily bilirubin production in adults averages about 4 mg per kilogram. About 70 per cent is derived from the heme moiety of hemoglobin in senescent erythrocytes, which are sequestered and degraded in the mononuclear phagocytic cells of the spleen, liver, or bone marrow. Most of the remainder results from the breakdown of nonhemoglobin hemoproteins in the liver, principally the cytochromes P-450. A minor fraction of bilirubin production results from ineffective erythropoiesis; i.e., premature destruction of newly formed erythrocytes in the bone marrow or circulation.

Microsomal heme oxygenase, the heme-cleaving enzyme, is most abundant in the liver, spleen, and bone marrow and exhibits substrate-mediated induction by heme or hemoglobin. The conversion of heme to biliverdin, which is rate limiting for bilirubin formation, is followed by reduction of biliverdin to bilirubin by cytosolic biliverdin reductase. Tin-protoporphyrin, a synthetic metalloporphyrin, is a potent competitive inhibitor of heme oxygenase. This compound may prove useful in reducing bilirubin production and preventing kernicterus in selected infants with hyperbilirubinemia. Mammals, unlike birds, reptiles, and amphibia, convert nontoxic, water-soluble biliverdin to water-insoluble bilirubin. This may reflect the fact that bilirubin, unlike biliverdin, is able to cross the placenta. Moreover, bilirubin may be more than a waste product and serve as a potent physiologic antioxidant.

BILIRUBIN BINDING TO PLASMA PROTEINS. Unconjugated bilirubin is bound reversibly to albumin at a primary high-affinity site (10^8 M^{-1}). At plasma concentrations exceeding its molar equivalence with albumin (about 35 mg per deciliter), bilirubin also binds to at least two low-affinity sites. A variety of compounds, including certain sulfonamides, penicillin derivatives, furosemide, and radiographic contrast media, may displace bilirubin from its albumin-binding sites and increase the risk of kernicterus in neonates. Presumably because of its tight albumin binding and low water solubility, unconjugated bilirubin is not excreted in urine. Conjugated bilirubin is somewhat less tightly bound to albumin than is bilirubin. It is filtered to a greater extent at the glomerulus, is incompletely reabsorbed by the renal tubules, and therefore does appear in the urine in small amounts in patients with conjugated hyperbilirubinemia.

In addition to the reversible binding to albumin just described, another bilirubin fraction binds very tightly, perhaps covalently, to albumin. This pigment fraction has a serum half-life of about 17 days, similar to that of albumin. It has been detected only in patients with conjugated hyperbilirubinemia, in whom it accounts for a varying (8 to 90 per cent) fraction of total bilirubin (see below). The identification of this protein-bound fraction helps explain the occasionally slow resolution of hyperbilirubinemia in patients convalescing from hepatitis or in whom biliary obstruction has been relieved, as well as the disappearance of bilirubinuria in these patients prior to the resolution of jaundice.

HEPATIC BILIRUBIN TRANSPORT. Uptake of bilirubin and other substances tightly bound to protein is facilitated by large fenestrations in the cells of the sinusoidal lining that permit plasma proteins to enter the space of Disse and directly contact the hepatocyte plasma membrane. Uptake of bilirubin and other organic anions such as sulfobromophthalein across the sinusoidal membrane of the hepatocyte displays several features characteristic of carrier-mediated transport, including saturability and competition. Once inside the liver cell, bilirubin and other organic anions appear to bind to cytoplasmic proteins such as ligandin. Ligandin, which constitutes 2 per cent of cytoplasmic protein in human liver, may alter net uptake by reducing bilirubin efflux back into plasma. In addition to transport through the

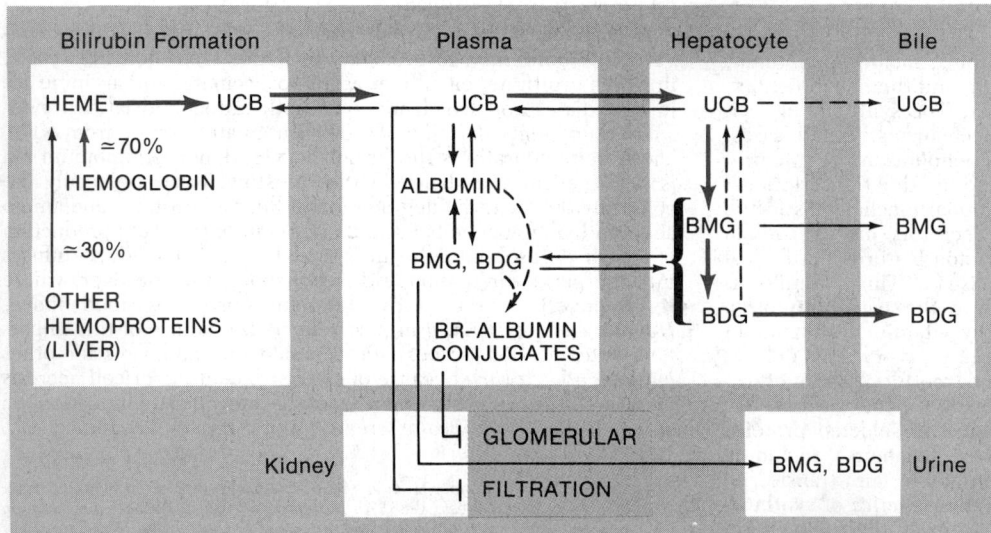

FIGURE 115–1. Overview of bilirubin metabolism. Unconjugated bilirubin (UCB) formed from the breakdown of hemoglobin heme and other hemoproteins is transported in plasma reversibly bound to albumin and is converted in the liver to bilirubin monoglucuronide (BMG) and diglucuronide (BDG), the latter being the predominant form secreted in bile. BMG and BDG together normally account for less than 5 per cent of serum bilirubin. In the presence of hepatobiliary disease, BMG and BDG accumulate in plasma and appear in urine. Bilirubin glucuronides in plasma also react nonenzymatically with albumin and possibly other serum proteins to form protein conjugates, which do not appear in urine and have a plasma half-life similar to that of albumin.

cytoplasm, bilirubin may be directly transferred from the plasma membrane to the membranes of the endoplasmic reticulum, where conjugation occurs.

In the process of conjugation, the carboxyl groups of one or both propionic acid side chains of bilirubin are esterified, usually with glucuronic acid. Glucose and xylose conjugates are formed in trace amounts only. Formation of bilirubin monoglucuronide and diglucuronide is catalyzed by microsomal UDP-glucuronyl-transferase. Transport of conjugated bilirubin from the hepatocyte into bile, like the uptake step, exhibits saturability and competition and is presumably carrier mediated. The carrier responsible for excretion of conjugated bilirubin may also transport conjugated sulfobromophthalein as well as certain sulfate and glucuronide bile acid conjugates. Excretion and/or conjugation, but not uptake, appears to be rate limiting for overall bilirubin transport from blood to bile. Bilirubin diglucuronide predominates in human bile (70 to 80 per cent), with the isomeric monoglucuronides present in small amounts.

ENTEROHEPATIC CIRCULATION. Absorption of conjugated bilirubin from the gallbladder and small intestine is negligible. In the terminal ileum and colon, conjugated bilirubin is hydrolyzed by bacterial enzymes to form unconjugated bilirubin, which is converted into colorless urobilinogens and related products, including urobilins. Most urobilinogen that is absorbed from the intestine is re-excreted in bile and ultimately in feces; a small fraction appears in urine. Urobilinogen is absent from the bile and urine of patients with complete biliary obstruction; however, fecal and urinary urobilinogen levels correlate poorly with bilirubin production rate and are of little clinical utility. In addition to urobilins, the normal brown color of stool may reflect the presence of nonbilirubin pigments, perhaps of plant origin, which are also excreted in bile and undergo enterohepatic circulation.

CONCENTRATION IN PLASMA. Plasma bilirubin concentration, which ranges normally between 0.3 and 1.0 mg per deciliter, varies directly with bilirubin production and inversely with hepatic bilirubin clearance. About 95 per cent of circulating bilirubin in healthy adults is unconjugated. In contrast, circulating bilirubin in patients with hepatocellular or biliary tract disease consists predominantly of monoconjugates and diconjugates. The conventional diazoassay, which is employed in most clinical laboratories, tends to overestimate the conjugated fraction, particularly at low concentrations of total bilirubin. The tightly, perhaps covalently bound conjugated bilirubin fraction reacts directly with the diazoreagent but is often removed by the deproteinizing step used in many laboratories. Nonetheless, for practical clinical application, conventional laboratory techniques are generally adequate. While more accurate methods for measurement of conjugated and unconjugated serum bilirubin have been developed, they are not readily automated and therefore not widely available.

APPROACH TO THE PATIENT WITH HYPERBILIRUBINEMIA

Differential Diagnosis (Table 115–1)

The differential diagnosis of hyperbilirubinemia can be divided into two major pathophysiologic categories: bilirubin overproduction and decreased bilirubin clearance.

BILIRUBIN OVERPRODUCTION. Bilirubin overproduction

TABLE 115–1. DIFFERENTIAL DIAGNOSIS OF HYPERBILIRUBINEMIA

I. **Increased bilirubin production**
   Examples: hemolysis, ineffective erythropoiesis, resorption of hematomas
II. **Decreased bilirubin clearance**
   A. Inherited disorders of bilirubin metabolism
      Examples: Gilbert's syndrome, Crigler-Najjar syndrome, Dubin-Johnson syndrome, Rotor's syndrome
   B. Fasting hyperbilirubinemia
   C. Cholestasis
      1. Hepatocellular disease
         Examples: viral, drug-induced, or alcoholic hepatitis
      2. Biliary tract obstruction
         Examples: choledocholithiasis, tumor, sclerosing cholangitis, chronic pancreatitis

is most commonly caused by hemolysis (see also Ch. 133). Chronic steady-state hemolysis does not, by itself, usually account for a sustained bilirubin concentration greater than 4 to 5 mg per deciliter. Concentrations consistently above this level typically indicate the additional presence of hepatic dysfunction. In contrast to chronic hemolysis, acute hemolysis can result in a rate of bilirubin production that transiently exceeds the excretory capacity of even a normal liver and may cause striking bilirubin elevation and occasionally conjugated hyperbilirubinemia. Ineffective erythropoiesis may also be increased in certain disease states and can cause hyperbilirubinemia. Examples include megaloblastic anemia from either vitamin B_{12} or folic acid deficiency, iron deficiency anemia, sideroblastic anemia, thalassemia minor, polycythemia vera, aplasia, and lead poisoning. Markedly increased ineffective erythropoiesis is the basis of the rare disorder known as *shunt hyperbilirubinemia* or *idiopathic dyserythropoietic jaundice*. Bilirubin overproduction may also result from the resorption of large hematomas.

INHERITED DISORDERS OF BILIRUBIN METABOLISM. The hereditary disorders of hepatic bilirubin metabolism are characterized by impaired ability of the liver to transport or conjugate bilirubin (Table 115–2). The common, benign entity of *Gilbert's syndrome* and the rare, almost uniformly lethal type I *Crigler-Najjar syndrome* represent opposite ends of this spectrum. Routine tests of liver function are generally normal in all these disorders, but a variety of abnormalities in the hepatic handling of bilirubin and other compounds such as sulfobromophthalein have been described. Many of these disorders, including Gilbert's syndrome, the *Dubin-Johnson syndrome*, and *Rotor's syndrome*, may be mistaken for acquired hepatobiliary disease.

Gilbert's Syndrome. Because of its frequency (up to 7 per cent of the population), Gilbert's syndrome is the disorder most likely to be encountered by the clinician. Mild unconjugated hyperbilirubinemia is recognized most commonly during the second and third decades of life because of the presence of scleral icterus, often first noted with fasting or as an incidental laboratory finding. Although a variety of nonspecific symptoms have been described, it is unlikely that any significant symptoms are attributable to Gilbert's syndrome itself. Gilbert's syndrome results from a decrease in the hepatic clearance of unconjugated bilirubin, probably due to impaired conjugation. Up to one half of patients with Gilbert's syndrome have a very slight decrease in red cell survival detectable by ^{51}Cr labeling. The principal clinical importance of this disorder is that it may be confused with more serious acquired hepatobiliary disease. From a practical standpoint, the diagnosis of Gilbert's syndrome is made by demonstrating low-grade unconjugated hyperbilirubinemia in a patient with a normal physical examination and otherwise repeatedly normal laboratory tests of liver function. Liver biopsy to demonstrate normal histology is usually not necessary. An exaggerated hyperbilirubinemic response to fasting, lipid withdrawal, or nicotinic acid administration has been found to be helpful by some investigators, but these tests are neither sensitive nor specific enough to warrant routine use. In patients with overt hemolysis, direct measurement of hepatic bilirubin clearance may be necessary to establish the diagnosis. Gilbert's syndrome and the other inherited disorders of hepatic bilirubin metabolism are outlined in Table 115–2.

FASTING HYPERBILIRUBINEMIA. Fasting causes an increase in the plasma concentration of unconjugated, indirect-reacting bilirubin owing primarily to a decrease in hepatic bilirubin clearance. This effect may be particularly marked in patients with Gilbert's syndrome and the type II Crigler-Najjar syndrome. Both dietary composition and total caloric intake are important, since a normocaloric but lipid-free diet produces a response similar to that observed with complete fasting, and the effect of complete fasting is reversed by feeding small amounts of lipid. The mechanism of the decrease in hepatic bilirubin clearance with fasting is unclear. A slight increase in bilirubin production contributes to fasting hyperbilirubinemia.

CHOLESTASIS. In most patients, hyperbilirubinemia and jaundice reflect the presence of cholestasis, that is, impaired bile formation and/or bile flow resulting from extrahepatic biliary tract obstruction or hepatic parenchymal disease. Even in cholestasis, however, increased bilirubin production may be an important

TABLE 115–2. THE HEREDITARY DISORDERS OF HEPATIC BILIRUBIN METABOLISM

	Gilbert's Syndrome	Type I Crigler-Najjar Syndrome	Type II Crigler-Najjar Syndrome	Dubin-Johnson Syndrome	Rotor's Syndrome
Incidence	Up to 7% of population	Very rare	Uncommon	Uncommon	Rare
Inheritance	? Autosomal dominant	Autosomal recessive	? Autosomal dominant	Autosomal recessive	Autosomal recessive
Defect(s) in bilirubin metabolism	Decreased hepatic UDP-glucuronyltransferase activity, (?) slow hepatic bilirubin uptake, associated mild hemolysis in up to 50% of patients	Absence of hepatic UDP-glucuronyltransferase activity	Markedly decreased or undetectable UDP-glucuronyltransferase activity	Impaired biliary excretion of conjugated bilirubin	Impaired biliary excretion of conjugated bilirubin
Plasma bilirubin concentration (mg/dl)	≤3 in absence of fasting or hemolysis, predominantly unconjugated	17–50, usually >20, all unconjugated	6–45, usually <20, all unconjugated	1–25, usually <7, about 60% conjugated	1–20, usually <7, about 60% conjugated
Clinical sequelae	None	Death in infancy from kernicterus in almost all cases	Usually none, rarely kernicterus	Probably none	Probably none
Plasma sulfobromophthalein disappearance rate	Mildly abnormal in some patients (45-min retention <15%)	Usually normal	Usually normal	Slow initial disappearance with frequent secondary rise (45-min retention <20%)	Markedly slowed, no secondary rise (45-min retention 30–50%)
Oral cholecystography	Normal	Normal	Normal	Faint or nonvisualization	Usually normal
Hepatic histology (light microscopy)	Normal, occasionally increased lipofuscin	Normal	Normal	Coarse pigment in centrolobular cells	Normal
Reduction of plasma bilirubin concentration by phenobarbital	Yes	No	Yes	Minimal	Unknown
Diagnosis	Clinical and laboratory findings, response to fasting occasionally helpful, liver biopsy not usually necessary	Clinical and laboratory findings, lack of response to phenobarbital	Clinical and laboratory findings, response to phenobarbital	Clinical and laboratory findings, sulfobromophthalein disappearance, urinary coproporphyrin excretion	Clinical and laboratory findings, sulfobromophthalein disappearance, urinary coproporphyrin excretion
Treatment	None necessary	Liver transplantation; other measures not uniformly effective	Phenobarbital if bilirubin concentration markedly elevated	None available, avoid estrogens (may worsen jaundice)	None available

contributing factor (e.g., hemolysis complicating viral hepatitis or ineffective erythropoiesis caused by folate deficiency complicating alcoholic hepatitis).

Cholestasis can be subdivided into intrahepatic and extrahepatic causes. Intrahepatic causes include conditions in which the hepatocyte is unable to excrete bile even though the major ducts are patent. Included are acute and chronic viral hepatitis, drugs or toxins (in particular. alcohol, phenothiazines, and estrogens), primary biliary cirrhosis, congestive heart failure, sepsis, pregnancy, infiltrative diseases of the liver, and liver disease in infancy. The other major cause of cholestasis is extrahepatic biliary obstruction, most commonly due to gallstones or a neoplasm.

Evaluation of the Patient

CLINICAL EVALUATION. Most conditions causing hyperbilirubinemia can be diagnosed by means of the clinical history, physical examination, and routine laboratory tests. Certain aspects of the *patient history* may be particularly helpful in the differential diagnosis. Itching should alert one to the presence of cholestasis. Although the identity of the "pruritogen(s)" is controversial, bile salts in the skin are the most likely candidates. A history of dark urine implies an increased level of bilirubin conjugates in the serum and represents a clue to the presence of cholestasis, Rotor's syndrome, or Dubin-Johnson syndrome. The presence of clay-colored (acholic) stool implies severe cholestasis. Abdominal pain suggestive of biliary or pancreatic disease, previous biliary surgery, intermittent cholestasis, and abdominal pain all represent clues to the presence of biliary disease.

Physical examination is also important. A serum bilirubin concentration of 3 mg per deciliter or greater is usually required for the detection of scleral icterus; mucous membrane or cutaneous icterus generally requires higher concentrations. Chronic cholestasis also may produce markedly elevated cholesterol levels, which may result in cutaneous xanthomas. The presence of occult blood in the stool may represent a clue to a periampullary neoplasm or hemobilia. Additional clues to biliary obstruction include a palpable gallbladder or abdominal mass, fever suggestive of cholangitis, or abdominal tenderness.

Biochemical tests are of particular value and should include a complete blood count, reticulocyte count in selected cases, and hepatic function tests. If hepatic function tests apart from bilirubin

are normal, one should think of either hemolysis, ineffective erythropoiesis, or a selective defect in hepatic bilirubin transport, such as Gilbert's syndrome. If hepatic function tests are abnormal, the jaundice is very likely a manifestation of cholestasis. Cholestasis is characteristically accompanied by increased serum activities of γ-glutamyl transpeptidase, 5'-nucleotidase, leucine aminopeptidase, and alkaline phosphatase, and variable increases in alanine and aspartate aminotransferase. Unlike bilirubin or bile acids, an elevated alkaline phosphatase activity in serum does not reflect diminished biliary excretion, but rather increased synthesis and possibly increased release of this enzyme into the circulation. Alkaline phosphatase activity may also be increased in certain bone disorders and in pregnancy. γ-Glutamyl transpeptidase activity may be increased by certain enzyme-inducing drugs or alcohol, even in the absence of a hepatic disorder. It is not found in bone, and a normal value therefore suggests that an elevated alkaline phosphatase activity is of bony origin. Leucine aminopeptidase is also present in virtually all tissues, but elevated serum levels are seen only in hepatobiliary disease, particularly biliary obstruction, and pregnancy. Again, the primary use of this enzyme is in evaluating the significance of an elevated alkaline phosphatase activity. Elevated serum bile acids are a sensitive indicator of cholestasis, but this test is not widely available. Biochemical *clues to the presence of biliary obstruction* include a disproportionate elevation of bilirubin concentration and alkaline phosphatase activity with mildly abnormal transaminase activities, an elevated amylase suggestive of pancreatic disease, and normalization of a prolonged prothrombin time following vitamin K administration. The latter is indicative of vitamin K malabsorption due to intestinal bile acid deficiency, with normal hepatic synthetic function.

IMAGING STUDIES. If extrahepatic obstruction is suspected, further evaluation to determine the site and nature of the obstruction is warranted (Fig. 115–2). A reasonable next step is the use of a noninvasive study such as *ultrasonography* or *computed tomography* (CT) to determine whether the intra-and/or extrahepatic biliary system is dilated, implying mechanical obstruction. Because of its lesser expense and the lack of radiation exposure, ultrasonography is often preferred to CT as a first procedure. Ultrasonography and CT both demonstrate ductal dilatation in 85 per cent or more of patients with jaundice due to biliary obstruction. Both techniques may also yield additional

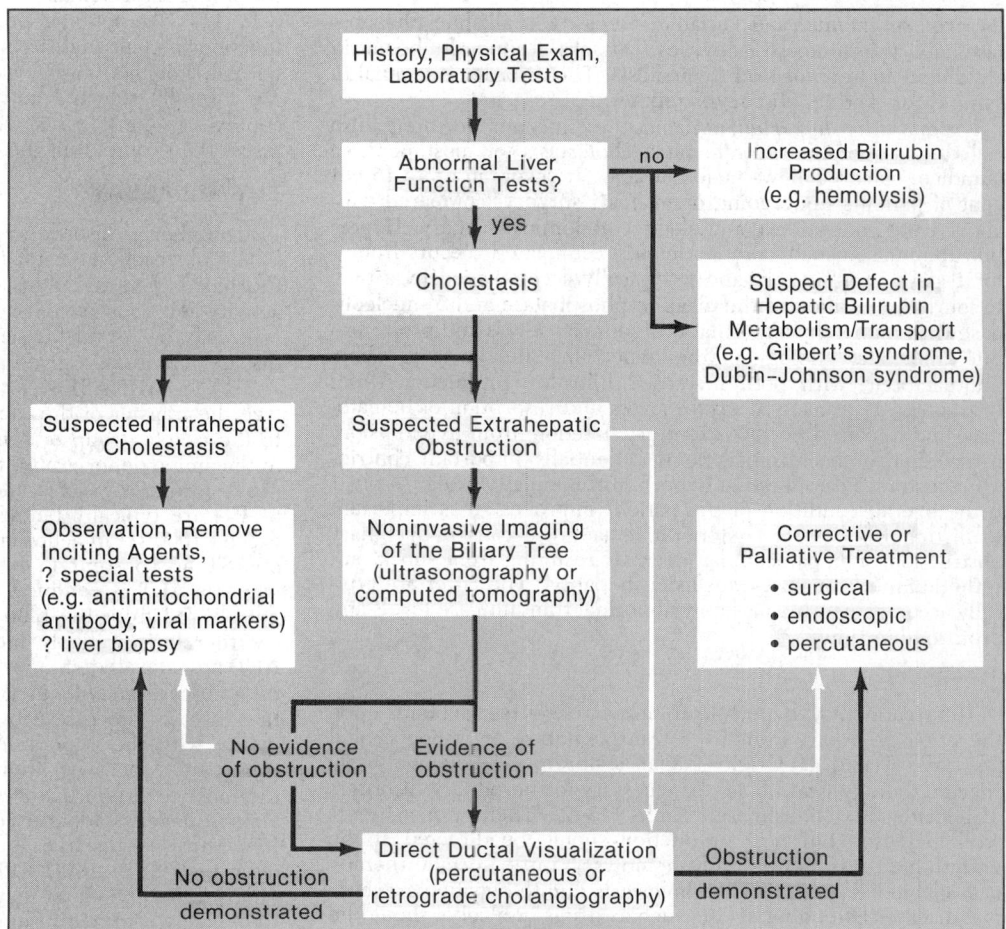

FIGURE 115–2. Approach to the patient with cholestasis. (From Scharschmidt BF, Way LW: The jaundiced patient: Differential diagnosis and clinical approach. *In* Way LW, Pellegrini CA (eds.): Surgery of the Gallbladder and Bile Ducts. Philadelphia, W.B. Saunders Company, 1987.)

information such as the presence of stones in the gallbladder or the presence of a pancreatic mass. CT may be preferable in instances in which precise definition of anatomic structures and level of obstruction is desired. False-negative examinations may occur in patients with sclerosing cholangitis or cirrhosis, presumably because of poor distensibility of the biliary tree, and in patients with gallstones, which commonly produce only partial or intermittent biliary obstruction.

If dilated bile ducts are detected, it is generally appropriate to further define the location and nature of the obstruction with direct cholangiography. Direct cholangiography is also appropriate even when noninvasive imaging studies are negative, if the clinical suspicion of biliary obstruction is high. Indeed, in selected situations such as the evaluation of a patient who has previously undergone biliary surgery, direct ductal visualization may be appropriate as a first procedure. Because of its lower morbidity, *endoscopic retrograde cholangiography* is often preferred to *percutaneous transhepatic cholangiography* as the initial procedure for direct visualization. In an individual patient, the choice between these procedures reflects a variety of factors, including the suspected location of the lesion (proximal versus distal); the presence of a coagulation disorder or prior gastroduodenal surgery which might, respectively, preclude a percutaneous or retrograde approach; anticipation of a therapeutic maneuver such as stent placement or sphincterotomy; and the availability of skilled personnel.

Other tests are occasionally employed in the evaluation of suspected biliary obstruction but are of lesser value. *Hepatobiliary scintigraphy* using derivatives of iminodiacetic acid, which are taken up by hepatocytes and excreted into bile, are of value primarily in the evaluation of cystic duct obstruction and acute cholecystitis (Ch. 126). However, radionuclide scans are unable to provide the resolution available with direct cholangiography and are of limited value in the evaluation of cholestasis. *Intravenous cholangiography* is also unreliable and usually fails to produce ductal visualization if the bilirubin concentration exceeds

3 mg per deciliter. *Oral cholecystography*, while useful in identifying gallbladder stones, is of little value in the evaluation of cholestasis. *Liver biopsy* is not indicated in the routine workup of suspected obstruction, because diagnostic histologic findings are often absent even in the presence of proven obstruction, and the biopsy generally provides no information regarding the location or nature of the obstruction. The principal role of a liver biopsy is in the differential diagnosis of difficult or confusing cases of intrahepatic cholestasis (Fig. 115–2).

HEPATIC DISORDERS THAT MAY MIMIC OBSTRUCTION. It is important for the clinician to be aware of certain hepatic disorders that may present with severe cholestasis suggestive of extrahepatic obstruction (Table 115–3). In some instances (e.g., alcoholic hepatitis, amyloidosis), liver biopsy usually permits a specific diagnosis. In other instances (e.g., cholestatic hepatitis, drug- or estrogen-induced cholestasis, benign recurrent cholestasis, cholestasis related to sepsis), liver biopsy typically demonstrates only cholestasis with variable hepatocellular necrosis, findings that by themselves do not permit a specific diagnosis.

Benign recurrent cholestasis is a particularly confusing disorder. Patients with this rare entity have recurrent episodes of cholestasis which last from weeks to months and recur at highly irregular intervals. These are manifested by pruritus, conjugated

TABLE 115–3. CHOLESTATIC DISORDERS THAT CAN MIMIC EXTRAHEPATIC OBSTRUCTION

Viral hepatitis	Primary biliary cirrhosis
Alcoholic hepatitis	Postoperative cholestasis
Benign recurrent cholestasis	Parenteral nutrition
Pregnancy	Hodgkin's disease
Sepsis	Drugs (e.g., estrogens,
Infiltrative liver disease (e.g.,	phenothiazines, rifampin)
amyloidosis, sarcoidosis)	Inherited disorders (e.g., arterio-
Hepatic neoplasia	hepatic dysplasia)
Hepatic abscess	Sickle cell disease

hyperbilirubinemia, and variable increases in alkaline phosphatase and transaminase activities. Attacks frequently begin in childhood and do not lead to cirrhosis. The disorder is familial in some cases, and its etiology is unknown.

Postoperative hyperbilirubinemia (>2 mg per deciliter), also called postoperative intrahepatic cholestasis or postoperative jaundice, usually follows major surgery. It occurs in up to 15 per cent of patients undergoing open heart surgery, compared with about 1 per cent undergoing elective abdominal surgery. Hyperbilirubinemia, usually predominantly conjugated, occurs from 1 to 10 days after surgery and is typically accompanied by a two- to fourfold elevation of the alkaline phosphatase and 5'-nucleotidase with minimally abnormal transaminase levels and prothrombin time. The etiology of the hyperbilirubinemia is probably multifactorial, with both increased bilirubin production (from breakdown of transfused erythrocytes and resorption of hematomas) and impaired hepatic excretory function (from hypotension, hypoxemia, or bacteremia) being potentially important contributing factors. Postoperative hyperbilirubinemia typically resolves if the overall condition of the patient improves. It is important to distinguish it from postoperative jaundice caused by biliary obstruction or hepatocellular necrosis resulting from shock, anesthetic injury, or post-transfusion hepatitis. The latter are typically accompanied by markedly abnormal transaminase levels and prothrombin time.

Treatment

The treatment of hyperbilirubinemia, of course, depends upon the etiology. Apart from liver transplantation or phenobarbital for types I and II Crigler-Najjar syndrome, respectively, no specific therapy is available or necessary for hereditary disorders of bilirubin metabolism (see Table 115–2). Therapy in patients with increased bilirubin production should be directed at the underlying disorder, typically hemolysis. Little specific therapy is available for patients with cholestasis due to hepatic parenchymal disease. Offending agents such as drugs or alcohol should be withdrawn when possible, and transplantation is appropriate for patients with progressive cholestasis and hepatic dysfunction due to primary biliary cirrhosis or other disorders. Biliary tract disease typically requires direct intervention via surgery or a percutaneous or endoscopic approach.

In patients with prolonged cholestasis and fat malabsorption, oral or parenteral administration of fat-soluble vitamins may be necessary, as well as alteration in the type or amount of dietary fat (Ch. 102). Mild pruritus may be relieved by less frequent bathing and the use of skin softeners. Cholestyramine should be tried in patients with more severe pruritus. Other agents (oral charcoal administration, rifampin, plasma exchange) have also been advocated for refractory pruritus but are not proven modalities.

Gollan JL (ed.): Pathobiology of bilirubin and jaundice. Semin Liver Dis 8:105, 1988. *An entire volume containing nine thoroughly referenced articles focusing on all aspects of bilirubin metabolism.*

La Russo NF (ed.): Medical and surgical aspects of biliary tract disease. Semin Liver Dis 7:311, 1987. *Six review articles outlining the evaluation and treatment of the patient with suspected biliary disease.*

Scharschmidt BF, Way LW: The jaundiced patient: Differential diagnosis and clinical approach. *In* Way LW, Pellegrini CA (eds.): Surgery of the Gallbladder and Bile Ducts. Philadelphia, W. B. Saunders Company, 1987. *A thoroughly referenced review of the diagnosis and treatment of the jaundiced patient.*

116 Laboratory Tests in Liver Disease

Richard A. Weisiger

Many "liver function" tests provide only indirect evidence of hepatic integrity, unlike most tests used for evaluating other organ systems. Specific functions of the liver include clearance of toxic substances from the blood (including drugs, metabolites,

and bacterial toxins), synthesis of plasma proteins and lipoproteins, and intermediary metabolism (e.g., glucose and ammonia) (Ch. 114). Depending on the disease process, some of these functions may be highly compromised while others remain nearly normal. For this reason, liver tests are most valuable when they are carefully selected and interpreted within the total clinical context. In most cases, serial determinations are required to assess the evolution of the disease.

ENZYME ASSAYS

A number of disorders, including inflammation, necrosis, and biliary obstruction, result in the release of hepatic enzymes into the blood. Enzyme release is an indirect indication of disease activity and does not measure liver function. Nevertheless, these tests may be useful for screening and for following the level of disease activity in a given patient.

TRANSAMINASES. *Transaminases (aminotransferases)* catalyze the transfer of the α-amino group from aspartate or alanine to the α-keto group of ketoglutarate; they are named according to the amino donor group. Serum levels of aspartate transaminase (AST, formerly SGOT) and alanine transferase (ALT, formerly SGPT) are typically below 40 IU per liter in normals but may exceed 1000 IU in acute viral or toxic injury. Different isozymes of AST are present in liver cell mitochondria and cytoplasm, whereas ALT is confined to the cytoplasm. Transaminases are not cleared from the blood by excretion into urine or bile and are therefore probably metabolized. Serum levels of AST and ALT are elevated in most hepatic diseases; the height of the transaminase activity in general reflects the current activity of the disease process. However, transaminase levels correlate poorly with the overall severity of the liver disease and with prognosis. Moreover, there are important exceptions. Even in the most severe forms of *alcoholic hepatitis*, for example, transaminase levels seldom exceed 200 to 300 IU per liter (Ch. 118). In contrast, serum transaminase activities of 1000 IU or more are often present in mild acute *viral hepatitis* or shortly after acute *biliary obstruction*, as may occur during passage of a gallstone. Conversely, serum transaminase levels may fall during the clinical course of massive hepatic necrosis, suggesting that the liver is so severely damaged that little enzyme activity remains (Ch. 123). Spuriously low transaminase levels may also occur in renal failure due to chemical interference with the assay.

Despite these caveats, serum transaminase activities may be helpful in certain circumstances. First, they are useful as *screening tests* for liver disease. Elevation of the ALT is relatively specific for hepatobiliary disease. Although AST levels may be increased in diseases of other organs (e.g., myocardium and skeletal muscle), values more than 10 times the upper limit of the normal range usually reflect hepatic or biliary pathology. In the context of other clinical and laboratory findings, identification of the source of increased serum transaminase activity is not usually difficult. Second, transaminase values are useful in monitoring the course of acute or chronic parenchymal liver disease, although they may be misleading in certain cases, as noted earlier. Finally, they may be useful diagnostically: It is distinctly uncommon for the AST to exceed 15 times the upper limit of normal in bile duct obstruction, except when it occurs suddenly or is associated with cholangitis. Because hepatic ALT is a cytoplasmic enzyme while most AST is sequestered in mitochondria, a high ratio of AST to ALT usually indicates severe hepatocellular necrosis (such as *alcoholic hepatitis*). Milder insults that cause leakage of cytoplasmic enzymes commonly produce a ratio of 1 or less.

ALKALINE PHOSPHATASE. *Alkaline phosphatases*, present in many tissues (e.g., liver, bile ducts, intestine, bone, kidney, placenta, and leukocytes), catalyze the release of orthophosphate from ester substrates at alkaline pH. The normal serum level of activity in adults is 25 to 85 IU per liter, although higher levels are normal in children and in pregnancy. The biologic function of alkaline phosphatase is unknown, except for an apparent role in the deposition of hydroxyapatite in osteoid to form bone. Normally, serum alkaline phosphatase activity reflects mainly the hepatic and bone isozymes, although occasionally the intestinal form may account for 20 to 60 per cent of the total. In the later stages of pregnancy, the placental contribution may be substantial. A less common variant, called the *Regan isozyme*, is associated with tumors (especially hepatoma and lung cancer) and appears identical to the placental form (Ch. 125).

Serum alkaline phosphatase activity may be increased in many conditions not associated with hepatobiliary disease, including bone disorders (e.g., Paget's disease, osteomalacia, metastases to bone), pregnancy, normal growth, and occasionally the presence of malignancy not involving bones or liver. In some cases, the source is obvious because of other clinical and laboratory findings. When the source is less apparent, several methods, such as heat stability and electrophoretic separation, are available to differentiate hepatobiliary from other isozymes. However, it is usually more practical to measure serum levels of *5'-nucleotidase, leucine aminopeptidase,* or *γ-glutamyl transpeptidase,* which tend to parallel alkaline phosphatase in hepatobiliary disease but do not usually increase in bone disease (see below). The increased serum activity in liver disease reflects increased enzyme synthesis rather than decreased biliary excretion or leakage from damaged cells and may be triggered by high tissue bile salt concentrations.

Slight to moderate increases in serum alkaline phosphatase activity (one to two times normal) occur in many parenchymal disorders of the liver such as *hepatitis* and *cirrhosis.* In the absence of bone disease, larger increases (3 to 10 times normal) usually indicate obstruction of bile flow. Although the highest levels usually occur with extrahepatic bile duct obstruction, very high values may also be seen with *intrahepatic cholestasis* and with infiltrative or mass lesions (primary or metastatic *cancer, lymphoma, leukemia,* or *sarcoidosis*). The serum alkaline phosphatase level rarely remains normal in the presence of significant bile duct obstruction. Increased alkaline phosphatase may be the only clinically apparent abnormality in bile duct stricture or in lesions that produce obstruction of a single hepatic lobe or segment. Its measurement, therefore, offers a relatively sensitive screening test for tumors involving the liver. As many as one third of patients with isolated elevations of serum hepatobiliary alkaline phosphatase activity may have no demonstrable underlying liver or biliary disease.

OTHER HEPATIC ENZYMES. *Leucine aminopeptidase* (LAP) is an ubiquitous cellular peptidase, while *5'-nucleotidase* (5'-NT) is a plasma membrane enzyme that cleaves orthophosphate from the 5' position on the pentose sugar of adenosine or inosine phosphate. The serum activity of both enzymes usually increases in cholestasis, and their major clinical value is to help determine if an elevated serum alkaline phosphatase activity originates from the liver. A parallel elevation of the serum activity of either of these enzymes suggests an hepatobiliary origin of the alkaline phosphatase, but the converse is not true. Serum levels of liver alkaline phosphatase may occasionally be increased while LAP and 5'-NT levels remain normal. Because both of these enzymes may be increased in late pregnancy, they are most useful in the nonpregnant patient.

γ-Glutamyl transpeptidase (GGTP), present in many tissues, increases in serum not only in hepatobiliary disease, but also after myocardial infarction, in neuromuscular diseases, in pancreatic disease (even in the absence of biliary obstruction), in pulmonary disease, in diabetes, and during the ingestion of ethanol and other inducers of microsomal enzymes. Measurement of GGTP has been proposed as a sensitive screening test for hepatobiliary disease and for the monitoring of abstinence from ethanol, but its high sensitivity ensures that many who test positive have no identifiable liver disease on further study. It offers no clear advantage over LAP or 5'-NT for identifying the source of increased serum alkaline phosphatase activity except in pregnancy.

Lactate dehydrogenase (LDH) is often elevated in liver disease but is usually not helpful in diagnosis because it is also found in most other body tissues.

CLEARANCE OF METABOLITES AND DRUGS

As a major function, the liver removes various metabolites and absorbed toxins from the blood (Ch. 118). In liver disease, clearance of these compounds may be impaired as a result of loss of parenchymal cells, obstruction of bile flow, reduced cellular transport, or reduced hepatic blood flow. When a metabolite is produced at a relatively constant rate (as is usually true for bilirubin), its serum level can be a sensitive indicator of liver function. The rate of clearance of certain drugs and dye com-

pounds from the plasma following a single dose can be used similarly.

BILIRUBIN. The metabolism of bilirubin and its measurement are discussed in detail in Ch. 115.

BILE ACIDS. Bile acids, absorbed from the ileum in an active recycling process, are nearly completely removed by the liver before they reach the systemic circulation. Impaired hepatic uptake or reflux from blocked bile ducts can lead to high plasma levels of bile acids and result in severe pruritus. Quantitation of serum bile acids has little proven clinical utility at present, however.

AMMONIA. The liver clears ammonia from blood by converting it to urea via the Krebs-Henseleit cycle for excretion by the kidney (Fig. 180–1). In the setting of severe hepatic dysfunction (e.g., fulminant hepatic failure) or portosystemic shunting, serum ammonia levels rise. The level of serum ammonia is widely used to confirm the diagnosis of hepatic encephalopathy and to monitor the success of therapy, but the correlation of the ammonia level with the degree of encephalopathy is only approximate (Ch. 123). Elevated ammonia levels may also be seen when ammonia production is increased by intestinal flora (e.g., following a high-protein meal or gastrointestinal bleeding), by the kidney (in response to metabolic alkalosis or hypokalemia), or in certain rare genetic diseases affecting the pathway of urea synthesis (Ch. 180). Arterial or cerebrospinal fluid levels of ammonia are not more useful than venous levels for clinical purposes.

DRUG CLEARANCE. The liver is primarily responsible for clearing many drugs from blood, particularly those that are poorly filtered by the kidney because of binding to albumin or to other blood components. Clearance of certain drugs has therefore been used to quantitate this function. Indocyanine green clearance provides a useful estimate of hepatic blood flow. The retention of sulfobromophthalein in blood 45 minutes following bolus injection is normally 5 per cent or less but is increased by even mild hepatic dysfunction. Unfortunately, this drug has produced occasional anaphylactic reactions and is no longer routinely available in the United States. Other drugs that have been used to quantitate hepatic function include antipyrene, caffeine, and rose bengal.

SYNTHETIC FUNCTIONS

PROTHROMBIN TIME. The prothrombin time, usually performed by the one-stage (Quick) method, measures the rate at which prothrombin in citrated plasma is converted to thrombin in the presence of added calcium, tissue thromboplastin, and activated clotting factors (Ch. 155). This test depends on the plasma concentration not only of prothrombin, but also of other clotting factors synthesized in the liver, including Factors V, VII, and IX, and fibrinogen. Results may be expressed in seconds, percentage of a standardized control sample, or prothrombin content. The test is abnormal in the setting of reduced synthesis (e.g., liver failure, vitamin K deficiency), increased consumption (e.g., disseminated intravascular coagulation), or both.

Synthesis of fibrinogen, prothrombin, and Factors II. V, IX, X, XI, XII, and XIII occurs in the liver. Synthesis of prothrombin and Factors VII, IX, and X depends on an adequate supply of *vitamin K,* which activates certain hepatic polypeptides by stimulating the synthesis of the calcium-binding residue, γ-carboxyglutamic acid. An abnormal prothrombin time is commonly caused by *vitamin K deficiency, liver disease,* or both and may rarely be seen with *inherited abnormalities.* Vitamin K, a fat-soluble vitamin that is found in many foods, is also produced by intestinal bacteria (Ch. 204). Deficiency is most commonly seen in *malabsorption syndromes,* including failure to absorb dietary fat due to biliary obstruction or other causes of cholestasis (Ch. 102). It may also be seen with antimicrobial suppression of intestinal bacteria, especially when the patient is receiving inadequate oral or parenteral vitamin K replacement.

Any acute or chronic liver disease may cause an abnormal prothrombin time if the synthesis of essential clotting factors is impaired. The plasma half-life of these factors is typically less than 1 day; the prothrombin time therefore responds rapidly to changes in hepatic synthetic function. This property makes the prothrombin time particularly useful for following the course of acute liver diseases; significant elevation often indicates an unfavorable prognosis.

An abnormal prothrombin time may be of diagnostic value in the evaluation of the jaundiced patient. In general, when it is prolonged on the basis of vitamin K deficiency alone (as in fat malabsorption due to cholestasis), it returns to normal within hours of parenteral administration of vitamin K. In contrast, when the synthesis of clotting factors is diminished because of parenchymal liver disease, response to vitamin K may be slight or absent. Both factors may coexist, however. In severe liver failure, elevation of the prothrombin time may also reflect disseminated intravascular coagulation (Ch. 155). Because of these shortcomings, the prothrombin time must be interpreted in the context of all available information.

The *partial thromboplastin time* is used to assess the "intrinsic" clotting mechanism and reflects the activity of all clotting factors except for platelet factor 3, Factor VII, and Factor XII. For this reason, the test is complementary to the prothrombin time and may indicate deficiencies of other clotting factors or the presence of a circulating anticoagulant (Ch. 155).

ALBUMIN. *Albumin,* synthesized exclusively in the liver at a rate of 100 to 200 mg per kilogram of body weight per day, has a long half-life in plasma (about 3 weeks in healthy adults). The synthesis rate is influenced by many factors, including nutritional state, the presence of systemic and/or liver disease, thyroid and glucocorticoid hormones, plasma colloid osmotic pressure, and toxins such as alcohol and carbon tetrachloride. The normal mechanism of albumin turnover is not well understood, although losses are increased in nephrotic syndrome, protein-losing enteropathy, severe burns, exfoliative dermatitis, and gastrointestinal bleeding.

The serum albumin concentration reflects a balance between synthesis and loss and is therefore not specific for the functional state of the liver. Because the serum half-life is long, abnormalities are slow to develop and may persist for weeks after correction of the underlying problem. On the other hand, when other factors can be excluded, hypoalbuminemia may be an important indicator of chronic liver disease. In patients with cirrhosis and ascites, hypoalbuminemia commonly reflects diminished synthesis, but in some synthesis is normal and hypoalbuminemia is caused by a redistribution among the extracellular fluid compartments, including the peritoneal cavity.

SERUM LIPIDS AND LIPOPROTEINS. Parenchymal liver disease and bile duct obstruction may produce significant abnormalities in serum lipids and lipoproteins. In acute parenchymal liver disease, the serum electrophoretic band of α_1-lipoprotein may be lost, reflecting an abnormal composition and altered physical properties of the high density lipoproteins. A transient hypertriglyceridemia may also occur because of the presence in serum of abnormal low density lipoproteins rich in triglycerides. These changes appear attributable in part to deficient activity of plasma lecithin–cholesterol acyltransferase (LCAT), an enzyme of hepatic origin that esterifies plasma cholesterol. The changes are transient, and with resolution of the acute liver injury plasma lipids and lipoproteins return to their previous state.

The liver is primarily responsible for removing cholesterol from the body by its direct secretion into bile or its conversion to bile acids. In cholestasis, the serum concentrations of unesterified cholesterol and phospholipids increase, and *xanthomas* and *xanthelasma* may develop if these abnormalities are severe and sustained. A major fraction of the increased plasma unesterified cholesterol is accounted for by an abnormal low density lipoprotein, designated LPX. LPX consists mainly of unesterified cholesterol and phosphatidyl choline (lecithin) with a small amount of protein, largely albumin and C apolipoproteins. LPX is not of value in the differential diagnosis of jaundice, but it may contribute to an elevated plasma cholesterol concentration in patients with liver disease.

IMMUNOLOGIC TESTS

GLOBULINS. *Serum globulins* are of limited diagnostic utility in hepatobiliary diseases. As a group, they are heterogeneous with respect to site and regulation of production, physical properties, and physiologic function. Their concentration, as measured by serum protein electrophoresis or salt fractionation, may be influenced by a wide variety of hepatic and extrahepatic factors and disease states. The mechanism of their increased serum concentration in liver disease is not fully understood but may include stimuli to increased antibody production resulting from decreased removal of bacterial antigens from the portal blood or release of antigenic material from damaged liver cells. An important exception is the finding of a diminished concentration of the α_1-globulin fraction as demonstrated by serum protein electrophoresis. Since approximately 85 per cent of this fraction is accounted for by α_1-antitrypsin, a decrease in its concentration may be an important sign of α_1-antitrypsin deficiency, an inherited disorder associated with neonatal hepatitis, cirrhosis, and pulmonary emphysema (Ch. 121). Elevated IgM concentrations are common in primary biliary cirrhosis, but other clinical, laboratory, and imaging procedures are of greater diagnostic value. Diffuse increases in globulin concentrations are commonly seen in cirrhosis and may be especially pronounced in chronic active hepatitis in the absence of serum markers for active infection by hepatitis B or C viruses.

MITOCHONDRIAL ANTIBODY. In approximately 90 per cent of patients with primary biliary cirrhosis, the serum contains antibodies directed against a lipoprotein component of the inner mitochondrial membrane (Ch. 122). The antibodies are neither organ nor species specific and are demonstrated by immunofluorescent techniques employing rat kidney, liver, and stomach and human thyroid, stomach, and kidney. These antibodies include the three main immunoglobulin classes, are complement fixing, and bind to at least seven different components of the inner and outer mitochondrial membranes. In patients with primary biliary cirrhosis, the titer is not related to the increased level of serum IgM or to the stage or severity of the disease.

Mitochondrial antibodies are also present in up to 25 per cent of patients with chronic active hepatitis and postnecrotic cirrhosis and in 7 to 8 per cent of asymptomatic relatives of patients with primary biliary cirrhosis. They are rarely present in extrahepatic biliary obstruction. A small percentage of patients with nonhepatic diseases may also exhibit positive tests; these include the collagen-vascular disorders, thyroiditis, myasthenia gravis, Addison's disease, autoimmune hemolytic anemia, and chronic biologic false-positive reactions for syphilis. Of the several types of mitochondrial antibodies thus far identified, M_2 is the type usually found in primary biliary cirrhosis. Mitochondrial antibodies are demonstrable in only 0.4 to 0.7 per cent of the general population.

The mitochondrial antibody is useful in the differential diagnosis of jaundice for two reasons. First, a negative result renders the diagnosis of primary biliary cirrhosis unlikely, although it does not exclude it. Second, because of its rarity in extrahepatic biliary obstruction, a positive result helps confirm parenchymal disease. Since the incidence of gallstones in patients with primary biliary cirrhosis is approximately 40 per cent and is also increased in other forms of cirrhosis, the mitochondrial antibody test does not reliably exclude extrahepatic obstruction.

ANTINUCLEAR AND SMOOTH MUSCLE ANTIBODIES. Either or both of these tests are positive in a variable percentage of patients with chronic active hepatitis, usually in cases not associated with hepatitis B or C infection. These antibodies also occur in a minority of patients with primary biliary cirrhosis. As is true of the mitochondrial antibody, these factors are neither organ nor species specific. They probably do not play a role in pathogenesis. The presence of these antibodies in serum does not exclude bile duct obstruction.

TESTS FOR HEPATITIS VIRUS INFECTION. These tests and their clinical significance are discussed in Ch. 117.

EXAMINATIONS OF URINE AND STOOL

The presence of bilirubin in urine indicates that a significant fraction of plasma bilirubin is conjugated and is strong evidence of hepatobiliary disease. Jaundice in the absence of bilirubinuria indicates an exclusively unconjugated hyperbilirubinemia, i.e., reflecting hemolysis, ineffective erythropoiesis, or an inherited disorder of bilirubin conjugation. For several reasons, urine and fecal urobilinogen determinations usually do not provide useful information in the evaluation of hepatobiliary disease (Ch. 115). Testing of stool for occult blood is essential and may provide the first evidence of an alimentary tract lesion related or unrelated to hepatobiliary disease, a bleeding diathesis, or an explanation for the appearance of hepatic encephalopathy. In selected cases, depending on the clinical circumstances, stool culture or examination for ova and parasites may provide information of importance in the diagnosis of liver disease.

HEMATOLOGIC TESTS IN LIVER DISEASE

Diseases of the liver may be associated with a wide variety of hematologic abnormalities, including qualitative and quantitative changes in the formed elements and in clotting function. The abnormalities depend not only on the etiology of the liver disorder but also on whether it is acute or chronic or associated with complications such as liver failure or portal hypertension.

In acute liver disease not associated with liver failure, major changes in the formed elements are uncommon and consist primarily of mild anemia, reflecting either low-grade hemolysis or marrow depression. Slight leukopenia is not uncommon and is often associated with atypical lymphocytes.

Severe aplastic anemia may sometimes complicate acute viral hepatitis, especially following liver transplantation for fulminant hepatitis C infection. In other forms of acute liver disease, hematologic abnormalities such as marrow suppression may be caused by toxins such as ethanol or drugs. In the alcoholic, Zieve's syndrome, consisting of hemolytic anemia and hypertriglyceridemia, may rarely be found. Coagulopathy may complicate massive hepatic necrosis, reflecting depressed hepatic synthesis of clotting factors and, frequently, disseminated intravascular coagulation.

In chronic liver disease, erythrocytic target cells, often associated with cholestasis, result from an expansion of the cell membrane, with relative preservation of the cholesterol-phospholipid ratio. Spur cells (acanthocytes), most often found in advanced alcoholic cirrhosis, reflect a more profound relative and absolute increase in membrane cholesterol.

Red cells, white cells, and platelets may be decreased in patients with portal hypertension, primarily because of hypersplenism (Ch. 152). A number of other abnormalities may be present, but to a large extent these are caused by associated nutritional, pathologic, or pharmacologic influences. Examples include iron deficiency, megaloblastic, and sideroblastic anemias.

LIVER BIOPSY

Liver biopsy is of value in the diagnosis of diffuse or localized parenchymal diseases, including cirrhosis, chronic hepatitis, and mass lesions. It is commonly performed by the blind percutaneous technique but may be done under direct visualization during laparoscopy or with sonographic or radiologic guidance when specific areas must be sampled. Because the histologic changes are usually nonspecific in acute hepatitis or acute cholestatic jaundice, the value of liver biopsy in this setting is primarily prognostic. Liver biopsy requires the cooperation of the patient, except in infants, and normal clotting function. Relative or absolute contraindications include the presence of biliary sepsis or high-grade biliary obstruction, ascites, severe coagulopathy, and right pleural disease.

IMAGING TECHNIQUES AND CHOLANGIOGRAPHY

These techniques are discussed in detail in Ch. 126.

McKenna JP, Moskovitz M, Cox JL: Abnormal liver function tests in asymptomatic patients. Am Fam Physician 39:117, 1959. *Many enzyme abnormalities are detected during routine screening, such as for blood donation. Here is a cost-effective method for evaluating these patients.*

Reichling JJ, Kaplan MM: Clinical use of serum enzymes in liver disease. Dig Dis Sci 33:1601, 1988. *Comprehensive review of the use of serum enzymes for diagnosis and monitoring liver disease. Over 150 references.*

Zakim D, T Boyer (eds.): Hepatology: A Textbook of Liver Disease. 2nd ed. Philadelphia, W. B. Saunders Company, 1990. *A comprehensive and well-written text covering all aspects of liver function and dysfunction.*

Zaloga GP, Prough DS: Monitoring hepatic function. Crit Care Clin 4:591–603, 1988. *Well-written review with an emphasis on clearance tests.*

117 Acute Viral Hepatitis

Robert K. Ockner

DEFINITION. Acute viral hepatitis is caused by any of several agents and presents as a spectrum of syndromes ranging from entirely subclinical and inapparent to rapidly progressive and fatal. In most cases, it is self-limited and uncomplicated, but, depending on the viral agent involved, there is a variable incidence of clinically significant extrahepatic manifestations or of progression to chronic liver disease. These diseases represent infections by viral agents with relative or absolute predilection for the hepatocyte. After a variable incubation period, viral replication in the liver cell approaches a maximum, leading to the appearance of viral components in body fluids and/or excreta, liver cell necrosis with an associated inflammatory response, changes in laboratory tests of liver function, and symptoms and signs of liver damage. The immunologic response of the host appears to play an important but not fully defined role in pathogenesis.

ETIOLOGY. Viral hepatitis is caused by five major agents which differ in structure and in the epidemiology and natural history of the diseases they cause, and several minor agents. The vast majority of cases in the United States are accounted for by hepatitis viruses A, B, C, and D. In addition hepatitis E has been identified as a cause of severe disease in Asia, Africa, and Mexico. Selected characteristics are summarized in Table 117–1, and each is considered in greater detail below. Other viral agents that cause an acute hepatitis syndrome include the Epstein-Barr virus (infectious mononucleosis), cytomegalovirus, herpes simplex, yellow fever, and rubella; the clinical disorders caused by these agents are considered in greater detail elsewhere in the text.

PATHOLOGY. The lesion of acute hepatitis consists of focal necrosis of individual hepatocytes associated with a mononuclear inflammatory response and expanded portal areas that are infiltrated predominantly by lymphocytes and in which bile ducts may be especially prominent (bile duct "proliferation"). There is often a variable, but usually minor, degree of necrosis of hepatocytes bordering the portal areas (so-called periportal hepatitis or piecemeal necrosis). Necrosis of an individual liver cell, whether periportal or within the lobule, is usually reflected in its replacement by a cluster of mononuclear cells, or it may be represented by balloon degeneration or by a shrunken cell with homogeneously eosinophilic cytoplasm and a condensed pyknotic nucleus ("acidophil body"). The regular pattern of the cords of hepatocytes is disrupted, mitotic figures and cholestasis are common, and Kupffer cells are prominent. Although these features are characteristic of typical acute viral hepatitis, they are not specific, individually or collectively. Thus, the same overall pattern of injury is seen in certain forms of drug-induced liver disease, and its individual components are seen in many processes of diverse etiology and duration. Mononuclear cell portal infiltrates, periportal hepatitis, and bridging or confluent necrosis may be especially prominent in chronic forms of hepatitis.

More severe variants of the acute necrotic process include "bridging" necrosis, "confluent" or "submassive" necrosis, and massive necrosis. In these, the necrotic process simultaneously involves contiguous groups of cells rather than single cells in isolation. As a result, there may be variable collapse or condensation of stroma. Bridging necrosis, so named because the continuous zones of necrosis may extend between (i.e., "bridge") adjacent portal and/or central areas, may be a necessary, if not sufficient, antecedent to evolution to a subacute form of hepatitis with progressive deterioration of liver function leading over several months to death in liver failure or to chronic hepatitis or to cirrhosis. Such a predisposition is not conclusively established, however. Thus, bridging necrosis is compatible with complete clinical and histologic recovery and therefore does not per se constitute evidence of chronic or progressive liver disease.

Submassive and massive forms of hepatic necrosis are reflected in a more severe clinical course and a less favorable prognosis. Massive necrosis, in which broad areas of hepatocytes are destroyed, with condensation of stromal elements and portal structures (bile ducts and vessels), is usually manifested clinically as fulminant hepatic failure (see Ch. 123). This syndrome is characterized by severely deranged liver function, hepatic encephalopathy, and a high case fatality rate. In survivors, however, despite the severity of the acute process, a chronic course is unusual, and liver histology typically returns nearly to normal.

In the recovery phase there is regeneration of hepatocytes and a largely complete restoration of normal lobular architecture. It

TABLE 117–1. CHARACTERISTICS OF COMMON CAUSATIVE AGENTS OF ACUTE VIRAL HEPATITIS

	Hepatitis A	Hepatitis B	Hepatitis D	Hepatitis C	Hepatitis E
Causative agent	27 nm RNA virus	42 nm DNA virus; core and surface components	36 nm hybrid particle with HBsAg coat	Flavivirus-like RNA agent	27–34 nm non-enveloped RNA virus
Transmission	Fecal-oral; H_2O-, food-borne	Parenteral inoculation, or equivalent; direct contact	Similar to HBV	Similar to HBV	Similar to HAV
Incubation period	2–6 weeks	4 weeks–6 months	Similar to HBV	5–10 weeks	2–9 weeks
Period of infectivity	2–3 weeks in late incubation and early clinical phases	During HBsAg positivity (occasionally only with anti-HBc positivity)	During HDV RNA or anti-HDV positivity	During anti-HCV positivity	Similar to HAV
Massive hepatic necrosis	Rare	Uncommon	Yes	Uncommon	Yes
Carrier state	No	Yes	Yes	Yes	No
Chronic hepatitis	No	Yes	Yes	Yes	No
Prophylaxis (see text)	Hygiene; immune serum globulin	Hygiene; hepatitis B immune globulin; vaccine	Hygiene; HBV vaccine	Hygiene; ? immune serum globulin	Hygiene, sanitation

is distinctly uncommon for the healing that follows a circumscribed acute hepatitis to be accompanied by fibrous scar formation or by nodular regeneration. In the latter, hepatocytes cluster in an abnormal configuration lacking a central vein and other components of the normal lobular architecture. These two manifestations of an *abnormal* healing process (fibrosis and nodular regeneration) are the essential components of cirrhosis, a form of chronic liver disease that almost always reflects ongoing injury and repair rather than a single acute event.

CLINICAL AND LABORATORY MANIFESTATIONS. The earliest symptoms of acute viral hepatitis typically are nonspecific, predominantly constitutional and gastrointestinal. They may include malaise, fatigue, anorexia, nausea, vomiting, and arthralgias and may suggest a "flu" or upper respiratory syndrome to both patient and physician. Classically, the patient may describe a loss of taste for coffee or cigarettes. Fever, if present, is usually mild. Abdominal discomfort may reflect an enlarged tender liver. Arthritis occurs in 10 to 15 per cent of cases; in hepatitis B it appears to represent immune complex deposition. Skin rash and arthritis occur with similar frequency in hepatitis A, in which circulatory immune complexes also have been demonstrated. Urticaria may occur occasionally.

After a period of several days to a week or more, the prodromal phase may lead to an icteric phase. The earliest clinical manifestation of a rising serum concentration of direct-reacting bilirubin is bilirubinuria, followed by a lightening of stool color, scleral icterus, and, in light-skinned individuals, frank jaundice. Constitutional symptoms often abate during the icteric phase, especially in children, in whom the disease is characteristically less severe. In adults, the gastrointestinal components of the prodrome may persist or even increase for a time. If cholestasis worsens, pruritus may cause increasing discomfort.

Physical findings are variable and depend on the stage of the illness. The only objective finding during the prodrome, apart from mild fever, may be an enlarged and tender liver, associated in perhaps 20 per cent with splenomegaly. Jaundice may or may not appear; indeed, it is likely that the majority of cases remain anicteric, especially among children with hepatitis A. Excoriations reflect the intensity of pruritus. Spider nevi occasionally develop during an acute hepatitis, but since this is unusual, it should suggest the possibility of a more chronic process.

Laboratory studies are highly variable, but almost by definition the clinical onset is accompanied by rising activities of serum aminotransferases; usually the ALT (SGPT) exceeds the AST (SGOT). An elevated serum bilirubin is predominantly direct reacting; very high concentrations, e.g., greater than 15 to 20 mg per deciliter, indicate a severe lesion or may reflect associated hemolysis. The alkaline phosphatase is usually moderately increased, whereas serum albumin concentration may decrease slightly. A diffuse hyperglobulinemia is common. Prothrombin time is prolonged in more severe cases, and a persisting or increasing prolongation is an unfavorable prognostic sign. Mild

and clinically insignificant hypoglycemia occurs in perhaps 50 per cent of cases; more profound hypoglycemia may complicate fulminant hepatic failure. Hematologic tests are also quite variable. Usually the total leukocyte count is normal or slightly decreased and atypical lymphocytes may be present. In more severe cases, total leukocytes may be increased, with relative or absolute neutrophilia. Hemoglobin and hematocrit are usually relatively normal, but occasionally there may be a coincidental hemolytic process, and rarely the course is complicated by aplastic anemia, especially following hepatitis C (non-A, non-B). Urinalysis is usually nonspecific except for the presence of bilirubin.

An important aspect of the laboratory approach to acute viral hepatitis is the etiologic serodiagnosis. Although establishing a specific etiologic diagnosis does not usually influence management, it may have a bearing on prognosis and is particularly useful epidemiologically and for preventing transmission. These tests are considered below, in the discussions of hepatitis A, B, C, and D, and of prevention.

After an icteric phase lasting usually from several days to several weeks, the patient enters a convalescent phase in which there is gradual improvement in symptoms and laboratory tests. The healing process may require several weeks, during which time residual weakness and malaise are common. Normalization of laboratory tests is usually complete within 4 months. Persistence of abnormalities beyond 6 to 12 months suggests that for hepatitis B, C, or D, the process may have become chronic; in this circumstance, liver biopsy may be indicated if there is no evidence of continuing improvement.

COMPLICATIONS AND EXTRAHEPATIC MANIFESTATIONS. The two most important complications of acute viral hepatitis are massive hepatic necrosis (fulminant hepatitis) and progression to chronic hepatitis. Fortunately, these are uncommon, especially in hepatitis A, in which chronicity does not occur and massive necrosis is less common and has a somewhat more favorable prognosis than in hepatitis B, C, and D.

Massive hepatic necrosis with fulminant hepatic failure occurs in fewer than 1 per cent of cases of acute viral hepatitis and is usually signaled by deepening jaundice, increasing prothrombin time, and hepatic encephalopathy, which, in its earliest stages, may appear only as a subtle personality change. Serum transaminase levels may remain high, but in many cases will fall, often in association with a decrease in liver size. These changes are assumed to reflect extensive loss of parenchymal mass and, in the presence of other evidence of a deteriorating course, are unfavorable prognostic signs suggesting fulminant hepatic failure, and the possible need to consider urgent orthotopic liver transplantation. The diagnosis and management of acute hepatic failure and encephalopathy are considered in greater detail in Ch. 123.

Evolution to chronic hepatitis is a more common complication of acute hepatitis B, C, and D. It is suggested by persistence of abnormal serum transaminases, with or without other laboratory abnormalities and clinical symptoms, beyond an arbitrarily selected endpoint. Authorities differ as to where that endpoint belongs; guidelines range from 4 to 12 months, but most would accept 6 months as reasonable. Clearly, however, judgments must be individualized as to when an acute process becomes chronic (or, more pragmatically, when investigations such as liver biopsy should be performed). For example, as long as the patient continues to show evidence of clinical and laboratory improvement, there is little to be gained from a more vigorous diagnostic or therapeutic approach. Conversely, evidence suggestive of chronic liver disease (e.g., signs of portal hypertension or progressive deterioration of laboratory tests) appearing before 6 months may justify earlier diagnostic intervention. Since many of the histopathologic features associated with chronic hepatitis also may be components of an acute process, however, liver biopsies obtained too early in the course may be difficult to interpret and potentially misleading. Chronic hepatitis is also considered in the discussions of hepatitis B, C, and D below, and in greater detail in Ch. 119.

The *cholestatic hepatitis syndrome* occurs occasionally as a complication of acute viral hepatitis, especially hepatitis A. Patients may exhibit a relatively prolonged course of several months dominated by cholestatic features, including pruritus, dark urine, light stools, direct-reacting hyperbilirubinemia, and elevation of alkaline phosphatase. Almost without exception, the prognosis is favorable. The major problem in management posed by this variant is the occasional need to exclude disorders such as biliary stones, stricture, and tumors by means of appropriate imaging and cholangiographic techniques. Brief corticosteroid therapy may be useful symptomatically.

Aplastic anemia may very rarely complicate the icteric or convalescent phase of acute viral hepatitis, especially non-A, non-B (presumably some of which are C). Its pathogenesis is unknown, and its prognosis is poor. Among the relatively few survivors, there is no clear evidence of a beneficial effect of glucocorticoids or anabolic steroid treatment. Other formed elements may also be depressed, and pancytopenia, agranulocytosis, and thrombocytopenia have been reported.

Extrahepatic manifestations of acute viral hepatitis also include *arthralgias* and *arthritis,* and *urticaria.* These are usually most prominent during the prodromal phase and, in hepatitis A and B, appear to reflect deposition of immune complexes. They also may occur in hepatitis C. Other manifestations of hepatitis B infection, such as *glomerulonephritis* and *vasculitis,* are also associated with immune complex deposition and are discussed in Ch. 79 and 60, respectively. A tentative association of *essential mixed cryoglobulinemia* with hepatitis B infection also has been reported. *Pancreatitis* is found in 12 to 40 per cent of cases of fatal acute viral hepatitis, and serum amylase activity may be elevated in up to 30 per cent of nonfatal cases; the true overall incidence and mechanism of pancreatitis in viral hepatitis are not known. Myocarditis, pneumonitis, and other extrahepatic manifestations are rare, and in their presence other systemic disorders should be considered.

SPECIFIC ETIOLOGIC CATEGORIES OF VIRAL HEPATITIS

HEPATITIS A. This form of hepatitis also has been referred to as infectious hepatitis, short-incubation hepatitis, or MS-I hepatitis. The causative agent (hepatitis A virus) is a 27-nm diameter RNA virus that is readily and almost exclusively transmitted via the fecal-oral route. In this important respect it differs significantly from other forms of hepatitis except E (see below). Accordingly, when the etiology of water-borne, point-source, food-handler-related, and institutional hepatitis outbreaks in North America and Europe has been defined, hepatitis A almost invariably has been implicated. In addition, hepatitis A occurs sporadically and is spread by direct person-to-person contact; there appears to be an increased incidence among promiscuous homosexuals. Spread of hepatitis A in day care centers may involve not only children but also the staff and the families of affected children. Although parenteral transmission is theoretically possible, it is rare. The incidence of the disease appears to correlate in a general way with personal hygiene and the efficacy of public health measures, as suggested by the apparent influence of socioeconomic status on the prevalence of hepatitis A antibodies (anti-HAV), which averaged 45 per cent in one study of an urban population in the United States and approximated 90 per cent in residents of Costa Rica. There is no evidence for the existence of a chronic form of hepatitis A or a carrier state. The "reservoir" for the virus appears to consist of clinically inapparent acute cases, in which the disease is not recognized at the time of viral shedding.

Hepatitis A infection typically has an incubation period of 2 to 6 weeks. Fecal shedding of virus occurs over a 2- to 3-week period beginning during the final week of the incubation period and the prodromal phase, and declines as serum transaminases reach maximal levels (Fig. 117–1 and Table 117–1). Although there is a transient viremia during this interval, parenteral transmission of the disease is very rare. Viral shedding in stool declines as antibody (anti-HAV) appears in serum. Initially, antibody is predominantly of the IgM class, but an IgG antibody soon appears. The IgG antibody persists in serum for many years; its exclusive presence indicates prior experience with, and immunity to, the hepatitis A virus. The presence of the IgM antibody, on the other hand, almost always indicates recent infection (within a few months) (Table 117–2), although occasionally this antibody may persist for up to 1 year or more. An IgA antibody to HAV appears in the feces of patients at about the time fecal shedding of virus ceases and persists for several weeks.

The acute illness itself is quite diverse in its clinical manifestations and course. The majority of cases probably are clinically inapparent, especially in children, or are perceived as a nonspecific "flu" syndrome. Jaundice, when it occurs, is usually mild. Symptoms usually subside, and serum transaminases return to normal within 3 to 4 months. Hepatitis A virus infection has been

FIGURE 117–1. Sequence of clinical and laboratory findings in a patient with hepatitis A. Fecal shedding of virus is brief in duration and ends with the appearance of anti-HAV in serum. IgM anti-HAV, usually present for a few months, may persist in serum for a year or more after the acute illness. (From Krugman S, Gocke DJ: Viral Hepatitis. Philadelphia, W. B. Saunders Company, 1978.)

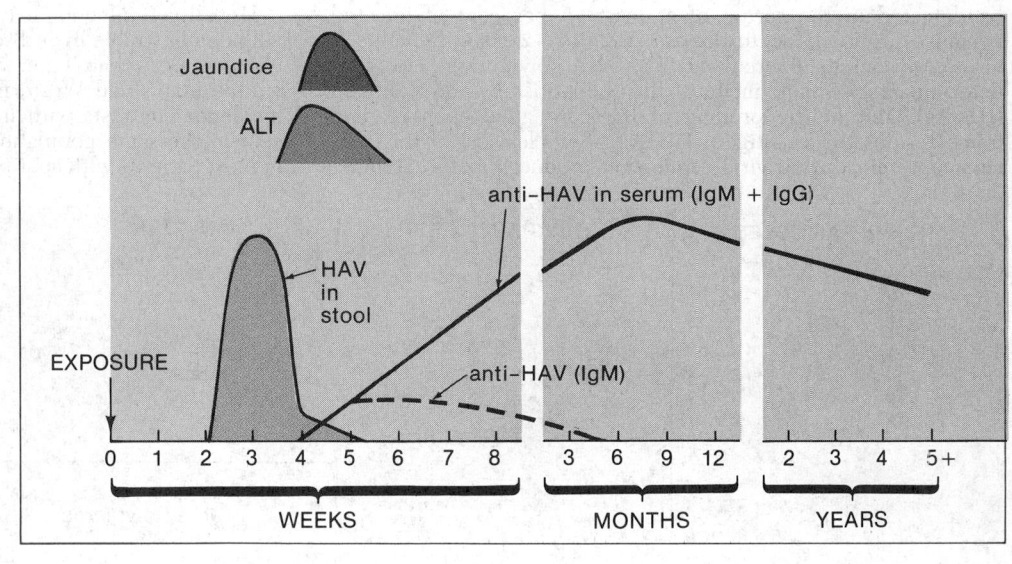

TABLE 117–2. SEROLOGIC TESTS IN VIRAL HEPATITIS

Agent	Terminology	Definition	Significance
Hepatitis A (HAV)	Anti-HAV IgM type	Antibody to HAV	Current or recent infection or convalescence
	IgG type		Current or previous infection; indicates immunity
Hepatitis B (HBV)	HBsAg	HBV surface antigen	Positive in most cases of acute or chronic infection
	HBeAg	e antigen; HBV core component	Transiently positive during active virus replication, acute hepatitis, and in some chronic cases; reflects Dane particle concentration and infectivity
	Anti-Hbc (IgM or IgG)	Antibody to HBV core antigen	Positive in all acute and chronic cases and in carriers; thus, marker of HBV infection; not protective; IgM anti-HBc may reflect active virus replication
	Anti-HBe	Antibody to e antigen	Transiently positive during convalescence and in some chronic cases and carriers; not protective; reflects low infectivity
	Anti-HBs	Antibody to surface antigen	Becomes positive late in convalescence in most acute cases; protective
Hepatitis C (HCV)	Anti-HCV	Antibody to cloned C100-3 polypeptide	Becomes positive on average 15 weeks after clinical onset; not protective; may be infectious
Hepatitis D (HDV)	Anti-HDV (IgM or IgG)	Antibody to HDV antigen	Similar to anti-HBc in indicating infection; not protective

implicated in some cases of acute cholestatic hepatitis and may exhibit a relapsing or protracted course. Rarely, hepatitis A causes massive hepatic necrosis and fulminant hepatic failure, but this complication is less common and more favorable in prognosis than that in hepatitis B and C.

The ease with which hepatitis A is transmitted among contacts and via water and food, as well as the demonstrated efficacy of immune serum globulin in prevention or amelioration of the disease, underscores the value of individual and public health measures to control the spread of infection. The application of these to the management of the individual patient and his or her contacts is discussed below.

HEPATITIS B. In contrast to hepatitis A, hepatitis B virus infection may cause a wide variety of acute or chronic hepatic and extrahepatic diseases, as well as a chronic carrier state. Its presentation as an acute hepatitis is typical of those cases that previously were designated serum hepatitis, homologous serum jaundice, long-incubation hepatitis, or MS-II hepatitis, although it is now apparent that some of these cases represented hepatitis C (see below). The hepatitis B virus (HBV) differs in almost every respect from hepatitis A (Tables 117–1 and 117–2; Fig. 117–2). The complete infective virion, or *Dane (HBV) particle*, is a DNA virus of 42 nm diameter, consisting of antigenically distinct surface and core components. The *surface coat* is largely lipid and protein and may exist in serum or other body fluids either as a component of the Dane particle or as separate 20-nm diameter spheres or cylinders. Its major antigenic determinant (hepatitis B surface antigen, HBsAg) includes several subtypes (d, y; w, r), and it can be detected in the serum of at least 75 per cent of infected persons during the acute disease (Fig. 117–2). The hepatitis B virus *core* consists of circular DNA, DNA polymerase, and other determinants, which include the hepatitis B core antigen (HBcAg). Within the product of the core gene open reading frame resides the e antigen (HBeAg). Self-cleavage of this precursor protein during viral replication produces mature HBcAg

and HBeAg. HBcAg remains an intrinsic part of the complete virion, while HBeAg is secreted from the hepatocyte and exists separately in plasma. Each elicits a humoral antibody response (anti-HBc and anti-HBe, respectively) during the course of the hepatitis B infection. HBV-DNA can be detected in serum by molecular hybridization techniques, including polymerase chain reaction, and is the most sensitive indicator of the presence of infective virus.

Also unlike hepatitis A, *transmission* of hepatitis B by the fecal-oral route is relatively unimportant; infection may follow oral ingestion, but large doses appear necessary. Instead, the virus is present in virtually all body fluids and excreta, and transmission of this disease occurs primarily via parenteral routes. Therefore, it usually requires either overt inoculation (e.g., transfusion, or injection via a contaminated needle) or intimate personal contact (e.g., between sexual partners, patients and health professionals, and mother and newborn infant). The disease occurs with an increased frequency among sexual partners of acutely infected individuals, as well as among chronically exposed persons, including health professionals and patients exposed to blood and blood products (e.g., workers and patients in clinical laboratories, dialysis and oncology units), the sexually promiscuous (especially male homosexuals), drug users who share needles, and handlers of primates (which are susceptible to infection). In urban centers, hepatitis B may account for up to 50 per cent of sporadic cases of acute hepatitis, even in the absence of documented parenteral inoculation. This attests to the importance of person-to-person contact in the spread of this disease.

Hepatitis B infection may become chronic, either in association with demonstrable liver disease or in otherwise seemingly healthy carriers. Less than 1 per cent of the general population of the United States and Western Europe is HBsAg-positive. This low incidence contrasts with incidence of anti-HBs of about 10 per cent in the same population, providing additional evidence that in most patients with acute hepatitis B the infection is self-limited

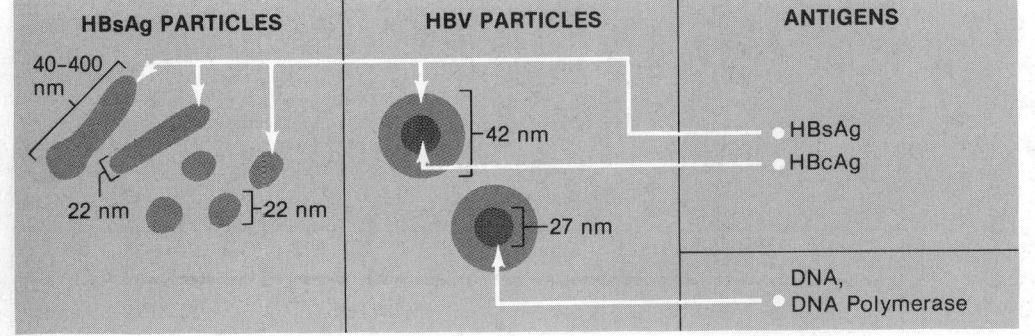

FIGURE 117–2. Forms of HBV in plasma, showing location of the various components and antigenic determinants. HBeAg, probably not a component of the complete virus particle, is not shown. (Adapted from Koff RS: *In* Sanford JP, Luby JP [eds.]: The Science and Clinical Practice of Medicine. Infectious Diseases. Vol. 8. New York, Grune & Stratton, 1981; by permission.)

and followed by immunity and only infrequently leads to chronic liver disease or a carrier state. The incidence of HBsAg positivity is much higher in less-developed areas (up to 15 per cent) and among certain subpopulations with increased exposure and/or impaired immunity, such as patients with Down's syndrome, leprosy, or lymphoproliferative disorders; addicts; and patients undergoing dialysis. In addition to acute cases, therefore, these chronically infected individuals constitute the "reservoir" that serves to perpetuate the virus. Historically, it is likely that transmission of the disease has occurred not so often via overt parenteral inoculation but rather via close personal and sexual contact or from mother to newborn. In the latter instance (*vertical transmission*), i.e., in infants born to mothers with acute or chronic infection, there is a high probability that the neonate will acquire the disease. This is especially likely when the mother develops acute hepatitis B in late pregnancy or in the early postpartum period or has chronic hepatitis. Transmission appears to correlate with the presence of HBeAg in maternal serum, reflecting the concentration of infective virions. Characteristically, these infants remain chronically infected for many years, either as "carriers" or with a persisting low-grade and chronic hepatitis. They are at increased risk of developing hepatocellular carcinoma (see Ch. 125). Vertical transmission may be an important mechanism by which the reservoir of the virus is sustained from generation to generation.

The *incubation period* of acute hepatitis B, as defined by the appearance of clinical symptoms, varies between 4 weeks and 6 months, with an average of about 50 days. If the incubation period is defined instead in terms of the interval between exposure and the first *serologic* evidence of viremia, it may be as brief as 2 weeks, especially after exposure to large parenteral doses. Two weeks to 2 months prior to the clinical onset, HBsAg becomes detectable in serum (see Fig. 117–3 and Table 117–2). At about the time of the clinical onset and the rise in serum transaminase activities, anti-HBc becomes detectable. Initially, an IgM anti-HBc is present in high titer and persists for several months to 1 year; thereafter IgG anti-HBc predominates. In chronic HBV infections, IgM anti-HBc may be detectable during periods in which the virus is actively replicating. IgG anti-HBc persists for up to several years after acute hepatitis and is present in all chronic carriers. It appears to play no role in host defenses; rather, it serves as a reliable marker of hepatitis B infection currently or within the preceding few years. The Dane particle markers (HBeAg and DNA polymerase) usually become detectable in serum prior to the increase in transaminase. The duration of HBsAg positivity is highly variable. It may persist for a few days to 2 to 3 months; persistence beyond this time may indicate a chronic course. Characteristically, HBsAg becomes undetectable prior to the appearance of anti-HBs. This antibody can be demonstrated in 80 to 90 per cent of patients, usually late in convalescence, and indicates relative or absolute immunity. Its appearance suggests a successful response to the infection, but there are exceptions to this in certain patients with chronic hepatitis (see Ch. 119).

Several important qualifications should be noted in interpreting the results of hepatitis B serologic tests. First, in a significant number of patients with acute hepatitis B the serum is negative for HBsAg, presumably because the antigen is very low in titer or evanescent. For this reason, a single negative HBsAg test does not exclude the diagnosis. Anti-HBc is more sensitive in this regard and may be the only serologic indication of hepatitis B infection. A negative test for anti-HBc effectively excludes the diagnosis. On the other hand, a positive test for anti-HBc in an HBsAg-negative serum could merely reflect a prior episode of hepatitis B. These HBsAg-negative, anti-HBc–positive patients may be classifiable on the basis of the anti-HBs: a positive test early in the course of an acute hepatitis is evidence against the diagnosis of acute hepatitis B. Detection of IgM anti-HBc suggests recent acute or chronic HBV infection during a phase of active virus replication, as noted above. In those IgM-anti-HBc–negative subjects in whom HBV infection appears to have antedated the acute illness, the possibility of superimposed infection by hepatitis D (delta-agent), a non-A, non-B virus, or other causes of an acute hepatitis syndrome must be considered. With the advent of more sensitive methods for detecting HBV-DNA, perceptions of the relationship of serology to host-virus interactions are evolving.

The *clinical course* of acute hepatitis B is more variable and usually more prolonged than that of hepatitis A. It is also associated with extrahepatic manifestations, including urticaria and other rashes, arthritis, and, much less commonly, glomerulonephritis and vasculitis. The immune complexes that appear to cause these extrahepatic manifestations consist of HBsAg, anti-HBs, and complement components. Glomerulonephritis and vasculitis are also associated with chronic hepatitis B infection and are not necessarily accompanied by apparent liver disease. Indeed, up to one third of all cases of polyarteritis nodosa may be associated with hepatitis B virus infection.

Approximately 90 per cent or more of otherwise healthy adult patients with acute hepatitis B recover completely and become HBsAg negative. Fewer than 1 per cent develop massive hepatic necrosis, but this complication is more common than in hepatitis A. The 5 to 10 per cent of patients who remain HBsAg positive beyond 4 to 6 months are at risk of developing chronic hepatitis (see Ch. 119).

HEPATITIS C ("NON-A, NON-B"). The ability to document hepatitis A and B virus infection made it clear that many cases of acute hepatitis were caused by one or more other agents,

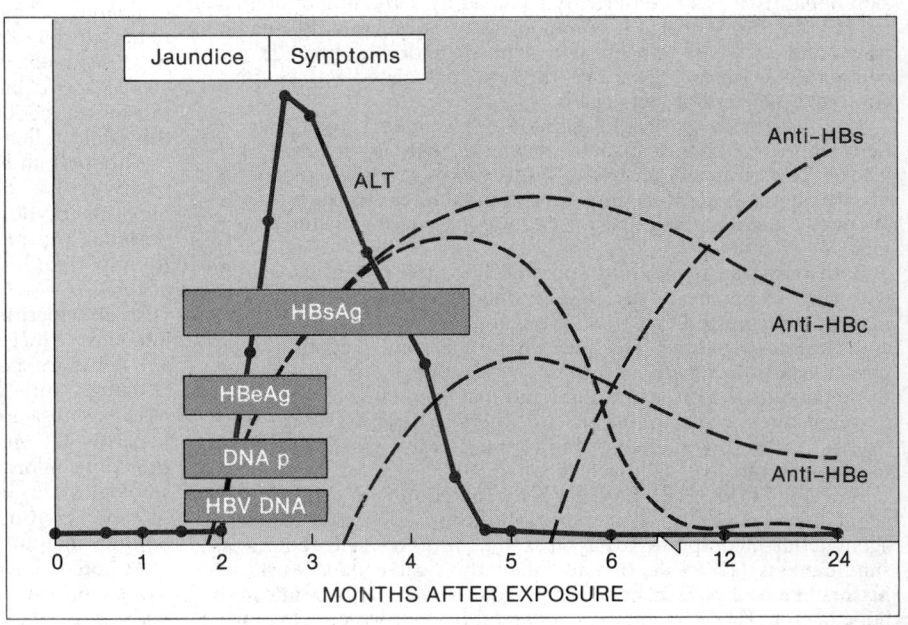

FIGURE 117–3. Sequence of clinical and laboratory findings in a patient with acute hepatitis B, followed by recovery. HBsAg-emia is the initial manifestation. "Dane particle markers" (HBeAg, DNA polymerase, and HBV DNA) precede the ALT rise and are transient. Anti-HBc (IgM, then IgG) appears during the acute illness; after the disappearance of HBsAg and before the appearance of anti-HBs, anti-HBc may be the only marker of hepatitis B infection. Specific timing of the detection of a given variable will depend to some extent on the method used. (Adapted from Hoofnagle J, Schafer DF: Serologic markers of hepatitis B virus infection. Semin Liver Dis 6:4, 1986.)

Jaundice | Symptoms

ALT
Anti-HBs
HBsAg
HBeAg
DNA p
HBV DNA
Anti-HBc
Anti-HBe

MONTHS AFTER EXPOSURE
0   1   2   3   4   5   6   12   24

designated "non-A, non-B." One of these, hepatitis C virus, has been characterized and appears to account for the great majority of such cases. Accordingly, the designation hepatitis C, as used here, includes cases previously referred to as non-A, non-B (except for the water-borne epidemic disease now referred to as hepatitis E, noted below). It remains likely that a few cases of non-A, non-B hepatitis may ultimately be attributed to one or more as yet unidentified agents.

Hepatitis C virus (HCV) was identified by a novel and painstaking application of the techniques and concepts of molecular biology, initially utilizing the sera of chimpanzees known to carry post-transfusion non-A, non-B hepatitis infection in high titer. Nucleic acid sequences from chimpanzees' sera were cloned and screened for in vitro expression of a polypeptide antigen recognized by antibodies present in the sera of patients with well-characterized post-transfusion non-A, non-B hepatitis. These efforts led to the development of an assay for an antibody to one viral epitope (C100-3) and to the characterization of the virus itself. HCV is an RNA agent related to the flaviviruses, a family that includes dengue fever and yellow fever. The agent appears to be readily transmitted parenterally; vertical transmission probably occurs, and transmission to sexual and household contacts appears to occur less frequently than in hepatitis B. In adults, it causes an illness with an average incubation period of 7 weeks (range 5 to 10). The antibody test does not become positive until 15 weeks after the clinical onset; among acute resolving cases only 15 per cent were positive. Thus, the antibody test is not useful in the early diagnosis of acute resolving hepatitis, and additional assays are under development. These confirmatory tests are important for identifying false-positive standard tests for the anti–C100-3 antibody, which is commonly found during screening of normal populations, e.g., in blood donors, and in patients with hyperglobulinemia. They include a recombinant immunoblot assay (RIBA) for the C100-3 epitope and polymerase chain reaction assays for HCV-RNA. The latter may detect viral sequences in acute hepatitis and in many cases that are positive for anti–C100-3, indicating that this antibody may be present in the infectious serum of patients with ongoing disease. In chronic cases worldwide, the antibody test is positive in 70 to 100 per cent of post-transfusion and in 22 to 90 per cent of community-acquired non-A, non-B hepatitis. It is positive in 65 per cent or more of patients with hepatocellular carcinoma.

Hepatitis C is the major cause of *post-transfusion hepatitis*. It occurs in approximately five to ten cases per 1000 transfusions and can be transmitted in whole blood, packed cells, platelets, plasma, and especially clotting factor concentrates. The recent availability of tests to screen donor units for HCV antibodies, and eventually components of the virus itself, should decrease the incidence substantially, just as the incidence of post-transfusion hepatitis B has been greatly reduced by screening of donors for HBsAg. HCV also is a common cause of hepatitis in needle users and accounts for 50 per cent or more of sporadic or community-acquired cases, i.e., those not associated with obvious contact or parenteral inoculation.

The incubation period of hepatitis C is longer than that of hepatitis A, ranging from 5 to 10 weeks, with an average of 7 weeks. The acute illness is also quite variable. The incidence of massive hepatic necrosis appears comparable to that of hepatitis B, and together these two categories account for the great majority of cases.

Both post-transfusion and sporadic hepatitis C are associated with both an apparent carrier state (inferred from the fact that it may be transmitted by blood from apparently healthy donors) and chronic hepatitis. The incidence of chronic hepatitis after post-transfusion hepatitis C approaches 50 per cent. In some of these patients the disease is mild and may spontaneously subside or remit after a year or more. In others, a "carrier" state may evolve, or the process may exhibit a progressive course and lead to cirrhosis and liver failure (see Ch. 119).

HEPATITIS D (DELTA-AGENT). Infection with this unusual agent may be regarded as a complication of hepatitis B. The agent is an incomplete RNA virus that requires antecedent or simultaneous HBV infection to infect the host cell. It exists in plasma in a coat of HBsAg and is present in the nuclei of infected hepatocytes. HDV infection is reflected by the presence of anti-

HDV antibody (IgM acutely; IgG chronically) or HDV-RNA in serum. Almost invariably the serum is positive for HBsAg and anti-HBc and, in most, anti-HBe. It is most commonly found among intravenous drug addicts and recipients of multiple transfusions. In subjects who are acutely and simultaneously infected with HBV and HDV there is no apparent increase in the probability that chronic hepatitis will ensue, but the likelihood of fulminant hepatic failure is greater than for acute hepatitis B alone. In individuals chronically infected with HBV, however, superimposed acute HDV infection usually also becomes chronic and is associated with the histopathologic findings of chronic active hepatitis.

HEPATITIS E. In recent years, an *epidemic form of non-A, non-B hepatitis* has been described, associated with outbreaks in India, Southeast Asia, Burma, North Africa, and the Soviet Union. The responsible agent is an RNA virus distinct from HAV and the enteroviruses. Serologic tests for it are not yet generally available. The illness affects young adults primarily and is associated with a mortality approaching 20 per cent in pregnant women. There is no evidence that this illness becomes chronic.

GENERAL APPROACHES TO DIAGNOSIS AND MANAGEMENT

DIAGNOSIS. In its classic presentation, the presumptive diagnosis of acute viral hepatitis is readily suggested by a compatible history and physical examination, in association with laboratory evidence of hepatocellular injury, i.e., significantly increased serum aminotransferase activities. Because all of these features are nonspecific, however, it is essential that other possible etiologic factors be considered, such as use of medications or illicit drugs, alcohol, exposure to environmental or industrial toxins, and the possible acquisition of unusual infections as suggested by travel or residence in rural or less well-developed areas. Exposure to viral hepatitis itself is suggested by contact with jaundiced persons or persons known to have developed hepatitis, sexual promiscuity (especially among male homosexuals), transfusion of blood or blood products, or the sharing of needles by drug users. Among health professionals, workers in dialysis and oncology units, surgeons, dentists, and clinical laboratory technicians are at increased risk, as is anyone in direct contact with blood, blood products, or other body fluids. Despite the importance of a careful inquiry into these possible risk factors, many patients with acute viral hepatitis report no significant exposures.

A careful and complete physical examination helps establish the diagnosis (tender hepatomegaly is the most common finding) and helps exclude other processes that occasionally mimic acute viral hepatitis, such as acute hepatic congestion, disseminated sepsis or liver abscess, or biliary tract disease with or without cholangitis.

Serodiagnosis of viral hepatitis is an important part of the initial evaluation. A positive test for the IgM class of anti-HAV or a rising titer of total anti-HAV is strong evidence for acute hepatitis A. Conversely, if the test for anti-HAV is negative well into the convalescent phase, the diagnosis is excluded. A single positive test for unfractionated anti-HAV is of little diagnostic value, since this could reflect a previous infection.

Although an acute hepatitis syndrome associated with HBsAg positivity has been taken as presumptive evidence for acute hepatitis B, none of the tests generally available at this time permits early and unequivocal diagnosis or exclusion of this entity. An important but not routinely available exception is the presence of HBV-DNA. Also, the presence of anti-HBs early in the course of acute hepatitis tends to suggest chronic rather than acute HBV infection. Since the classic pattern in which both HBsAg and anti-HBc are positive acutely may not be present in all cases (although anti-HBc itself is virtually always positive), a single negative test for HBsAg does not definitively exclude acute hepatitis B. Medical records, if available, may be of help by providing information about prior liver function tests, hepatitis serologies, or blood donation. Since donated blood has been screened routinely for HBsAg since 1972, such information may be quite helpful in the evaluation of hepatitis B serologies.

As noted above, early acute hepatitis C is not usually associated with a positive test for the C100-3 antibody, which does not become reactive until an average of 15 weeks after the clinical onset. Moreover, a positive result indicates only that the patient has been or is infected with HCV, possibly chronically, and does not necessarily reflect the etiology of an acute hepatitis syndrome. Serologic characterization of hepatitis C infection will be facilitated by the development of direct assays for viral components. Hepatitis D may be documented by a positive test for serum IgM anti-HDV or for HDV-RNA.

If a *liver biopsy* is performed, it may demonstrate the pathologic features of acute viral hepatitis. However, these are non-specific, and in the vast majority of cases biopsy is not indicated. Its use should be reserved for patients in whom the diagnosis is uncertain or in whom there is concern regarding chronicity or a deteriorating course, or any circumstance in which documentation of the histopathology may influence management. In the most severely ill patients biopsy may not be possible because of abnormalities of clotting function.

DIFFERENTIAL DIAGNOSIS. Acute viral hepatitis may be mimicked by a large number of other acute infections and noninfectious processes. Infections include other viruses such as cytomegalovirus, Epstein-Barr virus (infectious mononucleosis), and yellow fever virus; and nonviral processes such as Q fever, secondary syphilis, leptospirosis, salmonellosis, pyogenic and amebic liver abscess, malaria, and toxoplasmosis. A wide variety of drugs and toxins may injure the liver and cause a clinical syndrome that can resemble viral hepatitis (see Ch. 118). Inborn errors of metabolism such as Wilson's disease may also lead to acute hepatic necrosis. Acute hepatic congestion secondary to cardiac failure or venous occlusion, cholecystitis, and acute biliary obstruction should also be excluded. Finally, the possibility that what appears to be acute hepatitis may in fact represent the exacerbation of chronic hepatitis should be considered.

MANAGEMENT. There is no specific treatment for acute viral hepatitis. Major emphasis is placed on symptomatic and supportive care and on the prevention of transmission. Prevention is considered in detail below.

Most patients with acute viral hepatitis do not require hospitalization and are appropriately managed at home. Rest is advisable, but strict confinement to bed is not necessary beyond what is dictated by the patient's own sense of fatigue and malaise. No specific dietary measures are indicated, but most patients find a low-fat, high-carbohydrate diet more palatable. During the most severe phases of the illness, anorexia and nausea may be so extreme that oral intake of any kind is minimal. In such instances, attention to fluid balance is important, and it may be necessary to advise the intake of small amounts of clear fluids at frequent intervals. Although there is an appropriate reluctance to administer medication to the patient with liver disease, judicious use of small doses of antinausea agents such as hydroxyzine, trimethobenzamide, and even prochlorperazine is occasionally necessary and usually well tolerated. As the patient's symptoms decrease and appetite improves, intake can be liberalized, usually according to taste. Alcoholic beverages should be avoided throughout the course of the acute illness. Ambulation and activity may be increased as symptoms and laboratory tests improve; the most useful advice is that such activity should be limited so as to avoid causing fatigue. The decision to return to employment or school must take into consideration the patient's symptoms, the strenuousness of the work, and the potential for transmission of the disease; this, in turn, is a function of the viral etiology and the closeness of contact with others. In general, transmission is quite unlikely after 2 to 3 weeks in hepatitis A, whereas spread of hepatitis B or C ordinarily requires direct person-to-person contact.

Hospitalization is indicated for those patients in whom severe nausea and vomiting prevent maintenance of adequate fluid balance, in whom there is evidence of progressive deterioration, especially with encephalopathy or prolongation of prothrombin time, or in whom invasive diagnostic studies are indicated.

There is no convincing evidence to justify the use of corticosteroids in acute hepatitis, regardless of its severity. The management of fulminant hepatitis poses special problems in patient monitoring and support and should take place in a center with liver transplantation capability. It is discussed in detail in Ch. 124.

PREVENTION. The entire area of hepatitis prophylaxis has been dramatically changed by the availability of an effective vaccine for hepatitis B. In this vaccine, the immunizing antigen is HBsAg, prepared from donor sera or, more recently, by recombinant DNA technology employing yeast. An appropriate immune response is reflected by the appearance of anti-HBs. Immunization for hepatitis B also prevents hepatitis C. Hepatitis A virus has been propagated in tissue culture, and a vaccine is undergoing clinical trials. Finally, continuing progress in the identification, isolation, and characterization of hepatitis C, D, and other non-A, non-B agents suggests the possibility of active immunization, although not for some time. Pending the advent of generally available and effective vaccines for all of the viral causes of acute hepatitis, prevention must depend mainly on personal hygiene and public health measures directed at minimizing the exposure of potentially susceptible individuals, and on the appropriate use of passive immunization.

The use of public health and hygienic measures rests on the premise that body fluids and excreta of infected individuals are potentially infective. Clearly there are certain exceptions, depending on the specific virus involved, the clinical stage of the infection, the amount of potentially infective material involved, and the nature of the exposure. For example, because of the ease with which hepatitis A and E are spread via the fecal-oral route, contact of such patients with others should be minimized, and their excreta and essentially all materials handled by them during their brief period of infectivity should be carefully disposed of. In contrast, hepatitis B, C, and D are not commonly spread via the fecal-oral route. Although excreta are to be regarded as infective in these patients, the more important concern is transmission via puncture by contaminated needles (or equivalent exposure to infective material) or intimate personal (sexual) contact, especially during the period of HBsAg positivity. Because of these differences among the agents and differences in the approach to passive immunization, serologic diagnosis of the acute viral hepatitis case is useful, even though most patients with these disorders may be expected to do well regardless of etiology. In practice, rapid serodiagnosis is not always possible, and for this reason certain generalizations regarding the early management of the patient and his or her contacts are appropriate and are discussed below, along with measures for specific agents.

Hepatitis A. Since the infection is spread primarily via the fecal-oral route, including transmission by handling food, in drinking water, and potentially by fomites, strict attention to hygiene on the part of the patient and his or her attendants, whether in home or hospital, is of utmost importance during the period of viral shedding (Fig. 117–1). Direct body contact should be limited to that necessary for care; attendants should wear gloves, and careful handwashing is appropriate. Food, utensils, clothing, linen, needles, and excreta should be handled separately and carefully, also by gloved attendants. The virus is readily inactivated by boiling or by exposure to formalin, chlorine, or ultraviolet irradiation. In the hospital setting, strict isolation is not usually required for cooperative and informed patients with hepatitis A. In the home, similar measures should be implemented to the extent possible.

Close contacts of patients with hepatitis A should receive passive immunization with immune serum globulin as soon as possible, preferably within the first few days. The official recommended dose is 0.02 ml per kilogram up to a maximum of 2 ml, although up to 5 ml has been advocated. This would apply to immediate family members, sexual contacts, or others with whom the patient has been in close contact during the presumed period of infectivity. Casual contacts in the workplace or school probably do not require passive immunization unless there is reason to suspect mutual handling of food, beverages, or contaminated items. On the other hand, it is important to inquire about other possible cases among work or classroom associates. If there is reason to suspect a possible point-source outbreak, then all similarly exposed persons should receive immune serum globulin and appropriate epidemiologic information should be obtained.

The mode of transmission of hepatitis A also renders its prevention a matter of concern for those who intend to travel in areas where public health and sanitation measures may be suboptimal. In such circumstances, drinking water, fresh fruits and vegetables, and shellfish may be contaminated and should be avoided if possible. For these persons, administration of a standard dose (0.02 ml per kilogram) of immune serum globulin may be expected to afford protection for up to 3 months; for longer periods, a dose of 0.06 ml per kilogram is recommended and should be repeated at 4 to 6 month intervals.

Hepatitis B. Although this agent is less readily transmitted via the fecal-oral route, due consideration should be given to the general hygienic measures outlined for hepatitis A, in both home and hospital. Transmission ordinarily requires direct contact with the patient or the equivalent of a parenteral inoculation of infective material. Thus, in the home, children are far less likely than the spouse to acquire hepatitis B from an acutely infected adult. In the hospital, strict isolation may not be necessary if excreta, needles and other medical supplies, and personal utensils are identified, carefully handled, and discarded.

Passive immunization with immune serum globulin enriched in anti-HBs (hepatitis B immune globulin, or HBIG) is protective against hepatitis B infection in certain circumstances and when used in accordance with established guidelines. Because this material is expensive, it should not be used indiscriminately. At present, its use is officially recommended in the following specific situations:

1. Inoculation of material known to be contaminated with the hepatitis B virus, e.g., inadvertent puncture of a health professional by a needle from an HBsAg-positive patient, or accidental transfusion of HBsAg-positive blood or blood products.

2. Splash of HBsAg-positive material into the eye or on an open skin wound or eruption, as may occur in a laboratory accident or during a surgical or diagnostic procedure.

3. Ingestion of HBsAg-positive material, as may occur during a laboratory pipetting accident.

4. Sexual partners of patients with *acute* hepatitis B (partners of patients with chronic hepatitis B presumably have been previously exposed) within 14 days of contact.

5. Infants born to HBsAg-positive mothers, especially those who have had acute hepatitis B during the final trimester of pregnancy or first 2 months post partum or who are positive for both HbsAg and HBeAg at the time of delivery.

The rational use of HBIG depends on two essential components. First, it must be documented that the material to which the person has been exposed contains HBsAg, and this requires identification of the source and appropriate serologic confirmation. For example, accidental puncture of the skin by one of several used needles in a disposal container effectively precludes meeting this requirement and, therefore, the use of HBIG. Second, the exposed person must actually be at risk. If, at the time of exposure, he or she is already positive for HBsAg (i.e., infected) or anti-HBs (i.e., immune if the s/n value by radioimmunoassay exceeds 10), nothing will be gained from the administration of anti-HBs (HBIG). Ideally, therefore, the serologic status of both "donor" and "recipient" should be documented before the decision to administer HBIG is made. In practice, however, this is not usually possible within the few days' interval after exposure in which HBIG appears to be most effective. As a practical alternative to this dilemma, one possible approach is to immediately obtain serum from both the "donor" and the person at risk. Pending results of the HBsAg assays, the latter may be given 5 ml of ordinary immune serum globulin. HBIG may be administered later, if indicated by the test results. This approach represents a compromise between the need to institute early passive immunization on the one hand and to avoid indiscriminate use of HBIG on the other, and at a cost that is small relative to that of the HBIG itself. Other approaches are possible. In the family situation, the value of administering HBIG to the spouse remains controversial, but it is generally accepted that its use is not required for children, since they are at low risk.

Hepatitis B Vaccine. Safe and effective vaccines have been developed for the prevention of hepatitis B, consisting either of highly purified and triple-inactivated HbsAg obtained from the serum of chronic carriers or a recombinant preparation utilizing HBsAg synthesized in yeast. The vaccine is administered in three doses: initially and 1 month and 6 months later, and usually elicits production of anti-HBs in the recipient. Intramuscular injection is important and is more likely effective with deltoid than with gluteal administration. (Smaller doses are used for children, and larger doses for dialysis and immunocompromised patients.) The recombinant vaccine is safe for use in pregnant

women. Although most subjects who have completed the three-dose immunization are protected against hepatitis B infection, there are important exceptions, especially among immunosuppressed subjects. The duration of this protection varies, but probably is of the order of 5 years. No firm recommendations exist regarding booster doses.

The vaccine is recommended for use in high-risk groups and individuals. These include, but are not limited to, health professionals (especially those with high exposure risk such as surgeons, dentists, and dialysis workers), susceptible dialysis patients, and those subject to multiple transfusions (e.g., hemophiliacs), certain residents and staff of custodial care institutions, parenteral illicit drug users, heterosexual and household contacts of HBsAg carriers, Alaskan Eskimos, and sexually active and promiscuous male homosexuals. Available evidence suggests that it is also effective, when the first vaccine dose is combined with HBIG, in the passive-active immunization of health professionals after accidental needle stick and of infants born to HBsAg-positive mothers. The cost-effectiveness of screening of potential vaccine recipients (e.g., anti-HBs determination) varies with the circumstance. In general, in those groups in which prevalence of hepatitis B is relatively low, screening is not cost effective, whereas it is useful in groups with a high prevalence (e.g., the homosexual community). For most health professionals, screening is marginally cost effective and depends on the prevalence of hepatitis B infection in the particular subgroup. In any case, it is established that administration of the vaccine to individuals already infected or immune is not harmful.

Hepatitis D. There is no established method for active or passive immunization. Since HDV infection requires simultaneous or antecedent HBV infection, prevention of HBV, e.g., by the vaccine, protects against HDV. Since previously infected HBV subjects are at risk for HDV infection, care should be taken to minimize exposure to HDV-containing materials, e.g., HBV-positive serum or secretions.

Hepatitis C. It appears to be transmitted in a manner that more closely resembles that of hepatitis B than hepatitis A. Thus close personal contact and parenteral inoculation appear necessary, suggesting that prophylactic measures suitable for hepatitis B are appropriate, although available evidence suggests that it is not as readily transmitted to sexual and household contacts.

A problem largely confined to hepatitis C at present is that of post-transfusion hepatitis. The single most effective means of reducing the incidence of this disorder has been the exclusion of blood obtained from commercial (paid donor) sources. There is a correlation between both elevated aminotransferase activity and anti-HBc positivity in donor unit plasma and the probability of post-transfusion hepatitis in a recipient, and exclusion of such units is desirable. The advent of wide-scale screening of donor units for anti-HCV is expected to diminish the incidence of post-transfusion hepatitis further. The possible role of pre-exposure (i.e., pretransfusion) immune serum globulin in the prevention of the disorder remains unclear, and at present immune serum globulin is not officially recommended for its prevention.

Advisory Committee on Immunization Practices: Recommendations for protection against viral hepatitis. MMWR 34:313, 1985. Ibid: Update on hepatitis B prevention. Ann Intern Med 107:353, 1987. Ibid: Prevention of perinatal transmission of hepatitis B virus: Prenatal screening of all pregnant women for hepatitis B surface antigen. MMWR 37:341, 1988. *Three papers that summarize current policy regarding hepatitis B immunization, including the most recent revisions concerning vertical transmission.*

Alter MJ, Hadler SC, Judson FN, et al.: Risk factors for acute non-A, non-B hepatitis in the United States and association with hepatitis C virus infection. JAMA 264:2231, 1990. *Useful trends derived from sentinel counties survey.*

Alter HJ, Purcell RH, Shih JW: Detection of antibody to hepatitis C virus in prospectively followed transfusion recipients with acute and chronic non-A, non-B hepatitis. N Engl J Med 321:1494, 1989. *Important information regarding the natural history of hepatitis C infection and the utility of screening blood for hepatitis C antibody.*

Dienstag JL (ed.): Viral hepatitis. Semin Liver Dis, Vol. 11, May 1991. *A minisymposium in which clinically relevant aspects of acute and chronic hepatitis are critically reviewed by recognized experts.*

Everhart JE, DiBisceglie MD, Murray LM, et al.: Risk for non-A, non-B (type C) hepatitis through sexual or household contact with chronic carriers. Ann Intern Med 112:544, 1990. *Evidence suggesting that hepatitis C is less readily transmitted via these kinds of personal contact than is hepatitis B.*

Favero MS, Maynard JE, Leger RT, et al.: Guidelines for the care of patients hospitalized with viral hepatitis. Ann Intern Med 91:872, 1979. *Specific recommendations that provide a useful guide.*

Gocke D: Hepatitis A revisited. Ann Intern Med 105:960, 1986; Lemon SM: Type

A viral hepatitis. New developments in an old disease. N Engl J Med 313:1059, 1985. *Two useful reviews and summaries of some more recently recognized clinical features of the disease.*

Miller RH, Kaneko S, Chung CT, et al.: Compact organization of the hepatitis B virus genome. Hepatology 9:322, 1989. *Authoritative and comprehensive summary.*

Ramalingaswami V, Purcell RH: Waterborne non-A, non-B hepatitis. Lancet 1:571, 1988. *An authoritative review of epidemiologic and clinical aspects of hepatitis E.*

Reyes GR, Purdy MA, Kim JP, et al.: Isolation of a cDNA from the virus responsible for enterically transmitted non-A, non-B hepatitis. Science 247:1335, 1990. *Further progress in the characterization of hepatitis E and a useful summary of the status of the field.*

Zuckerman A (ed.): Viral Hepatitis and Liver Disease. New York, Alan R. Liss, 1988. *Proceedings of a recent symposium in which clinical and basic aspects of all forms of viral hepatitis are addressed.*

118 Toxic and Drug-Induced Liver Disease

Nathan M. Bass

In clearing and biotransforming xenobiotics, the liver is exposed to a large variety of potentially toxic chemical agents and metabolites: naturally occurring plant alkaloids and mycotoxins, industrial chemicals, and, most commonly, pharmacologic agents used in the treatment of disease. The manifestations of toxic and drug-induced liver disease also constitute a spectrum of clinical, laboratory, and histopathologic changes and prognoses virtually as broad as the entire range of acute and chronic hepatobiliary disorders. The severity may range, at one extreme, from asymptomatic abnormalities in liver function tests to fatal massive liver necrosis at the other. Viral hepatitis and biliary obstruction may be closely mimicked by several types of hepatotoxic drug reactions, and exposure to certain agents may also lead to chronic hepatitis, cirrhosis, and liver tumors.

PATHOGENESIS

It is rare for a parent chemical to be directly responsible for drug- and toxin-induced liver disease; more commonly a toxic metabolite(s) formed by the drug-metabolizing enzymes within the liver is the immediate causative agent. Drug biotransformation appears to be a common requirement in the pathogenesis of many different types of drug-induced liver injury. Individual susceptibility to the injury produced by some drugs varies considerably. Potentially hepatotoxic agents are therefore conventionally divided into two categories based on the predictability with which they produce liver disease: *intrinsic hepatotoxins* and *idiosyncratic hepatotoxins*.

Intrinsic hepatotoxins typically produce acute liver damage after a relatively brief latent period (usually a few days) in a predictable, dose-dependent fashion that is largely independent of host susceptibility factors and that is readily reproducible in experimental animals. Examples of this group include the industrial solvents *carbon tetrachloride, 2-nitropropane, trichloroethane,* the octapeptide toxins of the *Amanita* mushroom species, and the antipyretic *acetaminophen.* In most instances, toxic metabolites formed from the parent compound by the cytochrome P-450 drug-metabolizing enzymes produce liver damage by covalent modification of liver macromolecules, or through the generation of reactive oxygen species and subsequent peroxidation of cell membrane lipids.

Idiosyncratic hepatotoxins, in contrast, produce liver disease in an infrequent, unpredictable fashion after a variable latent period, often only after several months of administration of the drug. A large number of therapeutic agents are capable of producing idiosyncratic hepatotoxic reactions in a small proportion of patients who receive them (e.g., halothane, isoniazid, phenytoin, and chlorpromazine). Although severe liver disease occurs infrequently with these drugs, milder hepatic dysfunction may occur frequently (e.g., with isoniazid and chlorpromazine), or toxic liver disease may be reproduced in animal models (e.g., halothane) Many of these agents may therefore be "intrinsic hepatotoxins" which lead to severe "idiosyncratic" liver disease in a few susceptible individuals, possibly because of variations in

the pathways of drug biotransformation, immune-mediated hypersensitivity ("drug allergy"), or both. In a given individual, genetic polymorphism in drug-metabolizing enzymes may increase activity of subsidiary pathways that form toxic metabolites and thereby increase the risk of severe toxicity from drugs that are processed in part via these pathways. In idiosyncratic drug-induced liver disease, fever, arthralgias, rash, and eosinophilia are often prominent, indicative of a hypersensitivity-based mechanism. Furthermore, in some cases of drug-induced hepatitis (e.g., halothane), antibodies that recognize liver cell macromolecules covalently modified by metabolites of the implicated drug antibodies have been detected. Adducts formed on the liver cell surface between drug metabolites and liver cell membrane proteins may therefore constitute neoantigens that are capable of provoking immune-mediated liver damage.

MORPHOLOGIC PATTERNS OF DRUG-INDUCED LIVER DISEASE

Drugs and toxins produce a wide variety of pathologic lesions in the liver (Table 118–1). Some agents may injure the liver in more than one way. For example, isoniazid may produce a nonspecific focal hepatitis, an acute viral hepatitis–like lesion, or chronic active hepatitis, whereas oral contraceptives may cause cholestasis or liver cell adenoma and have been implicated in hepatic vein thrombosis.

ZONAL NECROSIS. Intrinsic hepatotoxins typically cause liver cell necrosis, largely confined within a particular zone of the liver lobule. Centrilobular necrosis, the most common pattern of zonal injury, is produced by *carbon tetrachloride, acetaminophen,* and *Amanita* toxins (see Ch. 108). This pattern of injury is explained in part by the greater abundance of cytochrome P-450 drug-metabolizing enzymes in the central region of the liver lobule and possibly also by the relative hypoxemia of the centrilobular region. *Halothane*, despite its classification as an idiosyncratic hepatotoxic agent, also frequently produces centrilobular necrosis. Periportal zonal necrosis, a much rarer lesion, is produced by *allyl alcohol* and *yellow phosphorus*. Extremely high elevations of serum transaminases usually accompany this type of liver injury, and in severe cases, acute liver failure may result. Acute zonal necrosis is either fatal or is followed by complete recovery. Chronic exposure to some toxins may produce a similar lesion, but it is not certain that this ultimately progresses to cirrhosis.

NONSPECIFIC FOCAL HEPATITIS. Nonspecific focal hepatitis consists of scattered foci of liver cell necrosis with mononuclear cell infiltrates, without the characteristic features of viral hepatitis. Nonspecific hepatitis may result from many forms of drug injury including the dose-dependent, intrinsic hepatotoxicity of *aspirin* and *oxacillin*. This lesion has an excellent prognosis and resolves completely upon discontinuation of the responsible drug.

VIRAL HEPATITIS–LIKE REACTIONS. Diffuse hepatocellular degeneration and necrosis with variable inflammatory infiltration and acidophil bodies, resembling the acute pathologic lesion of viral hepatitis and producing similar clinical manifestations, is another common pattern of idiosyncratic injury. In severe

TABLE 118–1. CLASSIFICATION OF DRUG-INDUCED LIVER DISEASE

Category	Examples
Zonal necrosis	Acetaminophen, carbon tetrachloride
Nonspecific hepatitis	Aspirin, oxacillin
Viral hepatitis-like reactions	Halothane, isoniazid, phenytoin
Cholestasis	
Noninflammatory	Estrogens, 17α-substituted steroids
Inflammatory	Chlorpromazine, antithyroid agents
Fatty liver	
Large droplet	Ethanol, corticosteroids
Small droplet	Tetracycline, valproic acid
Granulomas	Phenylbutazone, allopurinol
Chronic hepatitis	Methyldopa, nitrofurantoin
Fibrosis	Methotrexate, hypervitaminosis A
Tumors	Estrogens, vinyl chloride
Vascular lesions	6-Thioguanine, anabolic steroids

cases this lesion may progress to bridging, submassive or massive liver necrosis, and fulminant liver failure. Drugs producing viral hepatitis–like reactions include *halothane, isoniazid, ketoconazole, methyldopa, sulfonamides,* and *phenytoin.* In some instances, the presence of fever, rash, and serum and tissue eosinophilia, as well as other evidence of immunologic dysfunction, are important clues to the drug etiology of the disease and also implicate a hypersensitivity-based mechanism. In other examples, such as halothane and isoniazid, features of hypersensitivity are highly variable or distinctly rare.

CHOLESTASIS. Cholestasis is characterized by clinical symptoms of pruritus and jaundice and biochemically by elevated serum alkaline phosphatase and minimal or modest increases in serum transaminases. Two distinct forms of this very common manifestation of drug-induced liver injury are recognized. In the first, caused principally by *natural and synthetic estrogens* and by *17α-substituted androgenic and anabolic steroids,* there is usually little or no evidence of hepatocellular necrosis or inflammation. The injury is most simply viewed as the impaired secretion of bile by the liver cell, probably reflecting a direct steroid effect on the physical properties of cellular membranes or the activities of enzymes involved in this process. The lesion is completely and rapidly reversible.

In the second form of cholestatic injury, there is significant hepatocellular necrosis and portal and lobular inflammation; acidophil bodies and eosinophils are variably present. Systemic features, including fever, rash, and arthralgias, are not uncommon. This form of injury is produced by a broad group of agents, including the *phenothiazines, oral hypoglycemic* and *antithyroid* agents, and the *macrolide antibiotics* (e.g., erythromycin estolate). Its prognosis is generally favorable and complete recovery may be expected, except in very few individuals in whom chlorpromazine leads to a prolonged but ultimately resolving cholestatic course; rarely, the reaction may prove fatal. Marked differences in individual susceptibility associated with systemic features have suggested drug allergy as the basis for this form of injury. Chlorpromazine, however, is converted to a number of variably toxic metabolic products; this may account not only for the frequently abnormal liver function observed in patients receiving large doses for prolonged periods but also for the smaller number who develop the overt inflammatory and necrosing cholestatic injury.

FATTY LIVER. Triglycerides may accumulate within hepatocytes in two forms. Most commonly, fat accumulates as large droplets that displace the liver cell nucleus and confer an adipocyte-like appearance. Hepatomegaly and mildly elevated transaminases are typically found, but liver function is usually well preserved. This form of fatty liver typically occurs with direct hepatotoxins including *ethanol, halogenated hydrocarbons, acetaminophen,* and also with *corticosteroids* and is similar in appearance to the fatty liver seen in other systemic conditions such as *protein-calorie malnutrition, obesity,* and uncontrolled *diabetes mellitus.*

A much less common pattern is seen in association with *tetracycline* or *valproic acid* hepatotoxicity, and occasionally with *alcoholic liver disease,* and superficially resembles that seen in *Reye's syndrome, obstetric fatty liver,* and *Jamaican vomiting sickness.* It consists of fat deposited in smaller droplets throughout the liver cell, the nucleus remaining central. This pattern is usually associated with significant, occasionally fatal, disturbances in liver function. A distinctive type of hepatic lipid accumulation in the form of lysosomal phospholipid storage occurs as a direct effect of the drugs *amiodarone* and *perhexilene maleate.*

GRANULOMAS. Therapeutic agents are probably responsible for up to one third of cases of granulomatous hepatitis. Drug-induced granulomas are typically noncaseating and are often associated with extrahepatic granulomas and prominent systemic features of hypersensitivity. Responsible agents include *phenylbutazone, quinidine, allopurinol, phenytoin, hydralazine, sulfonamides,* and *sulfonylurea derivatives.*

CHRONIC HEPATITIS. Chronic hepatitis has been associated with an increasing number of drugs, including *amiodarone, dantrolene, isoniazid, methyldopa, nitrofurantoin, oxyphenisatin, perhexilene maleate, phenytoin, propylthiouracil, sulfonamides, acetaminophen,* and *aspirin.* Although these agents more often

cause acute liver injury, prolonged use may occasionally result in a chronic progressive process leading in some instances to cirrhosis. The histologic abnormalities usually resemble those seen in idiopathic autoimmune or viral chronic active hepatitis. In the case of amiodarone, a lesion strikingly similar to that of alcoholic hepatitis with prominent Mallory bodies may be produced. In many cases, the lesion is largely or completely reversible, but in severe cases this may require many months after the drug is discontinued. Rarely, progressive liver failure and death may ensue despite cessation of the drug.

FIBROSIS. Chronic liver injury from some agents increases collagen deposition, often with minimal or absent evidence of hepatocellular necrosis or inflammatory response. Fibrosis may progress to cirrhosis and portal hypertension, although the latter may occur as a result of hepatic portal fibrosis even in the absence of cirrhosis. This type of injury may occur following the chronic administration of *methotrexate* in the treatment of psoriasis or exposure to *inorganic arsenicals* and in *hypervitaminosis A.*

TUMORS. Tumors caused by drugs and other chemical agents may be of several types, including *hepatic adenoma (and possibly hepatocellular carcinoma)* associated with *oral contraceptive* use, and *angiosarcoma* caused by prolonged exposure to *vinyl chloride* monomer or Thorotrast. The mechanisms by which these tumors are produced are not known, but their clinical and laboratory features generally resemble those of similar tumors occurring "spontaneously." A possible exception is the apparently greater size, vascularity, and tendency to sudden hemorrhage of hepatic adenomas associated with oral contraceptive use (see Ch. 125).

VASCULAR LESIONS. Vascular lesions of several kinds occasionally are caused by drugs. Oral contraceptives have been implicated as a cause of hepatic vein thrombosis. Hepatic *veno-occlusive disease,* a process that affects the smaller tributaries of the hepatic veins, has been associated with the use of *antitumor agents,* including *6-thioguanine, cytarabine,* and *azathioprine,* as well as with ingestion of *pyrrolidizine alkaloids,* e.g., from plants of *Senecio* and *Crotalaria* species ("bush tea poisoning"). *Oral contraceptives* and *anabolic steroids* have been identified as causes of *peliosis hepatis,* a condition in which the liver lobule contains extrasinusoidal blood-filled spaces; this lesion is also seen in certain chronic wasting neoplastic and inflammatory diseases.

PRINCIPLES OF DIAGNOSIS AND MANAGEMENT

A causal relationship between the use of a drug and liver injury may be difficult to establish. Drugs may produce abnormalities very similar to those of other common disorders such as viral hepatitis or biliary disease, and some drugs may produce more than one kind of lesion. A detailed drug history is essential, and information about past exposure and the response to a suspect agent may be of considerable value in diagnosis. Because a number of industrial chemicals are potential hepatotoxins, details of the patient's occupation and work environment should be routinely obtained. The diagnosis of drug-induced liver disease ultimately depends on (1) a history of exposure, (2) consistent clinical, laboratory, and occasionally liver biopsy findings, and (3) resolution of the problem after the presumed toxin is discontinued. In some instances, when only a single agent is involved and a characteristic histologic type of injury is found, the diagnosis based on laboratory and biopsy findings is relatively straightforward. Examples include the small-droplet fatty liver caused by *tetracycline* or the centrilobular necrosis produced by *acetaminophen* (usually associated with significant blood levels of the drug). Conditions are more complex when several drugs are being used, any one of which or even the underlying disorder for which the drugs were prescribed may be responsible for a nonspecific or viral hepatitis–like type of liver injury. The causal role of a particular drug in idiosyncratic liver disease can usually be established through rechallenge with the drug. Rechallenge is rarely justified, however, because of the risk of a severe or even fatal outcome. Furthermore, it is not necessary to incriminate the drug unambiguously if alternative drugs are available.

Drug-induced liver disease is managed by discontinuing the implicated drug(s) and giving supportive care for acute hepatitis and hepatic failure as needed. In the case of severe, acute drug- or toxin-induced liver failure, urgent liver transplantation may be life-saving (Ch. 124). Specific pharmacologic intervention is generally limited to the administration of *N*-acetylcysteine in acetaminophen overdosage (see below). Corticosteroids have no established value in the treatment of drug-induced liver disease, although they may suppress the serum sickness–like syndrome associated with certain idiosyncratic reactions.

SELECTED EXAMPLES OF DRUG-INDUCED LIVER DISEASE

ACETAMINOPHEN. This readily available analgesic and antipyretic is a classic example of an intrinsic, dose-dependent hepatotoxin causing zonal necrosis and acute liver failure, often associated with renal failure. Significant liver injury usually occurs with doses in excess of 10 to 15 grams, most frequently taken in a suicide attempt. Within a few hours, patients develop nausea, vomiting, and diarrhea. These initial symptoms soon subside and are followed by a relatively asymptomatic phase. Clinical and laboratory signs of liver damage become evident 24 to 48 hours following ingestion. Serum transaminase levels in excess of 5000 U per liter are common, whereas severe liver injury may lead to progressive liver failure with encephalopathy, prolongation of the prothrombin time, hypoglycemia, and lactic acidosis.

The liver injury is caused by a toxic metabolite of acetaminophen formed by the cytochrome P-450–dependent drug-metabolizing system. Below threshold doses, this metabolite is efficiently detoxified by conjugation with glutathione. In the toxic dose range, glutathione stores are rapidly exhausted and the metabolite reacts with essential cellular constituents, leading to cell dysfunction and death. The rate at which reactive acetaminophen metabolites are formed is influenced not only by the dose ingested but also by the activity of the cytochrome P-450 enzymes (which may be stimulated by inducers such as phenobarbital and ethanol) and by the availability of glutathione, which may be reduced by fasting and ethanol. A combination of both enzyme induction and glutathione depletion may underlie the particular susceptibility of patients with chronic alcoholism to acetaminophen hepatotoxicity. In such individuals, doses of acetaminophen within the therapeutic range occasionally produce significant liver damage.

The initial treatment of acetaminophen overdose consists of supportive measures and gastric lavage. N-Acetylcysteine should be administered to high-risk patients, in whom it may significantly reduce the severity of liver necrosis and its attendant mortality. The plasma level of acetaminophen is the most reliable means for assessing prognosis. Levels in excess of 200 mg per liter at 4 hours, 100 mg per liter at 8 hours, or 50 mg per liter at 12 hours after ingestion are predictive of severe liver damage and are indications for treatment with N-acetylcysteine. This agent appears to act mainly by providing cysteine for glutathione synthesis and is most effective when given within 10 hours of acetaminophen ingestion. N-Acetylcysteine may afford some benefit after 10 hours, but not after 24 hours have elapsed. Intravenous preparations have been used in Britain, but only the oral form of N-acetylcysteine is currently available in the United States. The recommended oral dose is 140 mg per kilogram initially, followed by maintenance doses of 70 mg per kilogram every 4 hours for 72 hours.

Survivors of acute acetaminophen toxicity usually recover completely without progressive or residual liver damage. Chronic ingestion of acetaminophen at doses in the range of 3 to 8 grams per day may produce a largely subclinical liver injury with centrilobular necrosis or chronic hepatitis found on liver biopsy. This injury reverses fully after the drug is discontinued.

AMIODARONE. This iodinated benzofuran, used in the treatment of refractory arrythmias, is capable of producing an unusual form of liver injury, in addition to its recognized pulmonary, thyroid, ocular, and cutaneous toxicity. A number of patients who receive amiodarone develop mild increases in serum transaminases levels, which may normalize despite continuation of therapy, accompanied by engorgement of lysosomes with phospholipid. Between 1 and 3 per cent of patients receiving amiodarone develop a more severe liver injury that histologically resembles acute alcoholic hepatitis, with fat infiltration of hepatocytes, focal necrosis, fibrosis, polymorphonuclear leukocyte infiltrates, and Mallory bodies. This lesion may progress to micronodular cirrhosis, with portal hypertension and liver failure. The pseudoalcoholic lesion and its progression to cirrhosis often occur in a clinically insidious manner, with minimal elevation of

serum transaminases. Hepatomegaly may be found, but jaundice is rare. Evidence of hepatotoxicity may persist for several months after the drug is discontinued.

Amiodarone concentrates in lysosomes and inhibits lysosomal phospholipases, causing the characteristic phospholipidosis. How amiodarone causes pseudoalcoholic hepatitis and how this relates to phospholipid accumulation are unknown; the processes appear to be independent. Liver biopsy is helpful in diagnosis and should be considered in patients receiving amiodarone who develop persistent or significant (greater than twofold) elevation of serum transaminases or hepatomegaly. The decision to discontinue amiodarone in the presence of histologic evidence of hepatotoxicity is often difficult in view of the more ominous risk of sudden death from cardiac arrhythmias which may be increased by abrupt withdrawal of the drug.

CHLORPROMAZINE. This agent, and less frequently other phenothiazines, produces a cholestatic reaction in approximately 1 per cent of patients after 3 to 5 weeks of treatment. Symptoms of fever, anorexia, nausea, upper abdominal pain, rash, and arthralgias may occur at the onset, preceding the development of pruritus and jaundice. Eosinophilia is commonly present. Liver biopsy reveals cholestasis with canalicular bile plugs, a prominent portal inflammatory cell infiltrate of mononuclear, polymorphonuclear, and eosinophilic leukocytes with variable focal liver cell necrosis. The systemic accompaniments of this idiosyncratic type of hepatotoxicity suggest a drug hypersensitivity mechanism, but chlorpromazine is also an intrinsic hepatotoxin. Thus, subclinical abnormalities of liver function tests occur frequently among patients treated with high doses or for prolonged periods with this drug. In addition, chlorpromazine impairs bile secretion in experimental animals at doses approximating those used clinically, and certain metabolites of this drug adversely affect several factors necessary for bile formation.

The symptoms of chlorpromazine cholestasis usually subside over a period of weeks following discontinuation of the drug. Rarely, a syndrome of prolonged cholestasis resembling primary biliary cirrhosis may occur, but eventual recovery, even after a period of years, is also the rule. Fatalities are rare. Apart from discontinuing the drug, treatment is supportive, with cholestyramine for severe pruritus and fat-soluble vitamin supplementation in cases of prolonged cholestasis.

ERYTHROMYCIN. A cholestatic reaction with components of inflammatory cell infiltration and liver cell necrosis may complicate the use of erythromycin. In most instances, this has occurred with erythromycin estolate; other erythromycins including the ethylsuccinate and lactobionate have been less frequently implicated. Hepatotoxicity typically presents as an acute syndrome of right upper quadrant pain, fever, and variable cholestatic symptoms. The clinical picture may closely mimic acute cholecystitis or cholangitis and has prompted surgical exploration in some instances. The prognosis is uniformly excellent, but the reaction may recur within days of readministration of the drug. The mechanism of the injury is unknown.

HALOTHANE. This halogenated alkane anesthetic rarely causes a viral hepatitis–like reaction which, in severe cases, may progress to fatal massive hepatic necrosis. Susceptibility to halothane hepatitis appears to be increased in older persons, women, and obese individuals, and severe reactions usually occur after previous or multiple exposures to this anesthetic. Symptoms usually indistinguishable from viral hepatitis occur between 7 and 10 days after anesthesia, but this interval may shorten considerably after repeated exposure. Fever, which may be hectic, with chills and sweats, commonly precedes the onset of jaundice; rash and eosinophilia are less consistent features. The course may terminate fatally within days, or recovery occurs, which is usually rapid and complete. Some patients run a more protracted course before either recovery or the development of liver failure. Metabolites of halothane formed by the cytochrome P-450 system are clearly important in the mechanism of the hepatic injury. Some of these metabolites may be directly toxic; others may form haptens with cell membrane proteins, provoking an immune-mediated attack on the liver. Cross-sensitization may occur between halothane, methoxyflurane, and enflurane, although hepatic injury appears to be less common with the latter two anesthetic agents.

ISONIAZID (INH). Among persons taking isoniazid (INH) for single-drug chemoprophylaxis against tuberculosis, there is approximately a 10 to 20 per cent incidence of subclinical liver injury. This manifests during the first few weeks of therapy as a mild to moderate increase in serum transaminase levels. These laboratory abnormalities, which reflect a focal nonspecific hepatitis, subside in the majority of patients despite continued administration of the drug. About 1 per cent of patients receiving isoniazid develop significant liver injury, which clinically and histologically resembles the wide spectrum of viral hepatitis. The liver disease may present as a relatively mild, acute process, a subacute or chronic hepatitis, or fatal massive liver necrosis. The onset usually occurs within 2 to 3 months after commencing the drug, and initial symptoms are often nonspecific, with malaise and anorexia preceding signs of liver disease. Clinical features of "drug allergy" are distinctly unusual. Age influences the incidence of severe isoniazid liver injury, which increases significantly after the age of 35, and probably exceeds 2 per cent among persons over the age of 50.

Isoniazid appears to injure the liver through the formation of a toxic metabolite. Liver injury is more frequent in persons who are slow acetylators (as opposed to rapid acetylators) of the drug. The conversion of the isoniazid metabolite acetylhydrazine to the nontoxic diacetylhydrazine may be impaired in slow acetylators, thus favoring the formation of a toxic derivative of acetylhydrazine via the cytochrome P-450–dependent drug-metabolizing system. Induction of P-450 enzymes by rifampin may account for occurrences of a precipitous and severe form of isoniazid hepatitis when the two drugs have been administered together.

Patients receiving isoniazid should be followed at regular intervals and advised to report intercurrent symptoms. If these are associated with evidence of disturbed liver function, the drug should be discontinued, pending further evaluation. Since liver enzyme abnormalities are common early in the course of isoniazid treatment and reflect, in the vast majority (especially in younger patients), a transient and self-limiting event, routine monitoring of liver function tests in patients taking isoniazid is not generally recommended. The risk:benefit ratio of isoniazid chemoprophylaxis rises rapidly after the age of 35, however, warranting a conservative approach to the institution of chemoprophylaxis in this group. A several-fold elevation in transaminases in a patient over 35 years of age, even in the absence of symptoms, should be regarded as potentially serious and may justify discontinuation of the drug.

METHYLDOPA. This antihypertensive drug is similar to isoniazid in that minor and apparently inconsequential abnormalities in liver function occur in up to 6 per cent of treated patients. Clinically overt hepatotoxicity is much less common and usually resembles acute viral hepatitis or chronic active hepatitis, as a rule developing within 20 weeks after methyldopa is started. The Coombs' test is not infrequently positive in users of this drug but does not correlate with the occurrence of hepatic injury. Furthermore, clinical manifestations of drug hypersensitivity are unusual in methyldopa-induced liver disease, which may be mediated by a toxic drug metabolite. Hepatitis usually abates when the drug is discontinued, but full recovery may be delayed by months while progression to a fatal outcome has occurred in some cases despite stopping the drug.

PHENYTOIN. This anticonvulsant has been rarely associated with a severe, viral hepatitis–like liver injury with pronounced accompanying hypersensitivity features. The onset, usually within 6 weeks of starting the drug, is characterized by malaise, marked fever, lymphadenopathy, and a striking rash. Leukocytosis may be marked, with atypical lymphocytosis and eosinophilia. Liver histology resembles that of acute viral hepatitis except with a greater abundance of eosinophils. In the most severe cases, progressive liver failure and death may ensue. In spite of the marked serum sickness–like syndrome that characterizes phenytoin hepatotoxicity, a toxic metabolite may participate in its pathogenesis. Phenytoin is partly converted in the liver to highly reactive arene oxides. A genetically determined impairment in the ability to detoxify arene oxides may underlie individual susceptibility to toxicity from these metabolites via their covalent and hence immunologic modification of hepatic macromolecules.

SODIUM VALPROATE. This branched, medium-chain fatty acid used principally in the treatment of petit mal epilepsy may produce severe hepatotoxicity, most commonly in children under the age of 10 years. Similar to isoniazid, sodium valproate treatment is accompanied by a high incidence of transient, slight, and asymptomatic increases in serum transaminase activity, usually after several weeks of therapy. In rarer cases of severe liver injury, nonspecific systemic and digestive symptoms are followed by jaundice and evidence of liver failure, including encephalopathy and coagulopathy. Rash and eosinophilia are absent. The liver injury is characterized histologically by centrilobular necrosis and small-droplet fat infiltration, and bile duct injury may also be evident. The clinical and histologic features of sodium valproate hepatotoxicity are, to a degree, reminiscent of Reye's syndrome, although the former is distinguished by a greater frequency of jaundice, bile duct injury, and liver necrosis. The mechanism of sodium valproate–induced liver disease is uncertain, but available evidence has implicated the impairment of mitochondrial oxidation of long-chain fatty acids by a metabolite of the drug. Spontaneous recovery after stopping sodium valproate is the rule; fatalities are rare.

ORAL CONTRACEPTIVES. These hormonal agents produce several adverse effects on the hepatobiliary system: (1) hepatocellular cholestasis, (2) liver cell neoplasms, (3) increased predisposition to cholesterol gallstone formation, and (4) hepatic vein thrombosis (Budd-Chiari syndrome). In many cases of hepatic vein thrombosis associated with oral contraceptives, a latent myeloproliferative disorder appears to be present and undoubtedly predisposes to the thrombogenic disorder.

The cholestatic effects of oral contraceptives are largely attributable to the estrogenic component. Estrogens appear to affect directly several aspects of the formation of bile. Indeed, most users of oral contraceptives exhibit subtle disturbances in hepatic excretory function as evidenced, for example, by impaired plasma clearance of sulfobromophthalein. A small number of patients develop clinical cholestasis with pruritus and jaundice in a matter of weeks to months after commencing the pill. Manifestations of drug hypersensitivity are absent, and histologically, cholestasis without inflammation or liver cell necrosis is found. This condition is highly analogous to the clinical syndrome of *intrahepatic cholestasis of pregnancy*, which manifests as subclinical to overt cholestasis in the later stages of gestation, resolving rapidly in the postpartum period. Women with either a personal or family history of cholestasis occurring during pregnancy are particularly susceptible to cholestasis induced by estrogenic preparations. A genetic predisposition to estrogen-induced cholestasis is also suggested by the high incidence of this disorder in certain populations (e.g., Scandinavian and Chilean women).

Treatment of oral contraceptive–induced cholestasis consists of discontinuation of the drug and symptomatic support (e.g., cholestyramine for pruritus) as needed. Complete resolution within 2 to 3 months is the rule. Abnormalities persisting or worsening beyond this period suggest the unmasking of a pre-existing subclinical condition such as primary biliary cirrhosis and indicate the need for additional diagnostic evaluation.

Bass NM, Ockner RK: Drug-induced liver disease. *In* Zakim D, Boyer TD (eds.): Hepatology: A Textbook of Liver Disease. 2nd ed. Philadelphia, W. B. Saunders Company, 1990, pp 754–791. *A detailed current classification and summary of pharmacologic agents that may cause liver injury, including consideration of mechanisms and clinical aspects.*

Gitlin N: Clinical aspects of liver diseases caused by industrial and environmental toxins. *In* Zakim D, Boyer TD (eds.): Hepatology. 2nd ed. Philadelphia, W. B. Saunders Company, 1990, pp 791–821. *A well-referenced summary of industrial and environmental agents that may cause liver disease, including clinical and pathophysiologic aspects.*

Kaplowitz N, Aw TY, Simon FR, et al.: Drug-induced hepatotoxicity. Ann Intern Med 104:826, 1986. *A useful review of mechanisms and clinical aspects of drug hepatotoxicity.*

Lewis JH, Ranard RC, Caruso A, et al.: Amiodarone hepatotoxicity: Prevalence and clinicopathologic correlations among 104 patients. Hepatology 9:679, 1989. *A careful prospective study of the prevalence, as well as clinical and histopathologic aspects, of amiodarone hepatotoxicity, with a detailed, well-referenced discussion.*

Lewis JH, Zimmerman HJ: Drug-induced liver disease. Med Clin North Am 73:775, 1989. *A concise summary of current perspectives on prevalence, mechanisms, and clinical aspects of drug hepatotoxicity.*

McMaster KR, Hennigas GR: Drug-induced granulomatous hepatitis. Lab Invest 44:61, 1981. *A summary of implicated agents, with histopathologic documentation.*

Seeff LB, Cuccherini BA, Zimmerman HJ, et al.: Acetaminophen hepatotoxicity in alcoholics. A therapeutic misadventure. Ann Intern Med 104:399, 1986. *This paper and an accompanying editorial by M. Black and J. Raucy provide and review evidence regarding the mechanism by which alcohol use increases susceptibility to acetaminophen hepatotoxicity.*

Zimmerman HJ: Hepatotoxicity. The Adverse Effects of Drugs and Other Chemicals on the Liver. New York, Appleton-Century-Crofts, 1978. *Although this classic monograph is now outdated, it remains a comprehensive and authoritative source. Well organized, readable, and thoroughly referenced.*

119 Chronic Hepatitis

Robert K. Ockner

GENERAL CONSIDERATIONS

DEFINITION. Chronic hepatitis, a syndrome characterized by liver cell necrosis and inflammation lasting more than 6 months to 1 year, encompasses a spectrum of disorders differing in etiology, pathogenesis, histopathology, and clinical manifestations. Patients with chronic hepatitis may be entirely asymptomatic and exhibit only minimal abnormalities on routine laboratory tests or may be incapacitated by progressive liver failure and the complications of portal hypertension. At any given time, the clinical and laboratory features may not correlate well with histopathology or long-term prognosis. On biopsy, there is variable hepatocellular necrosis and an inflammatory response that may be predominantly portal, periportal, or lobular in its distribution. When severe, this lesion may include collapse of stromal elements, distortion of the lobular architecture, and a reparative process consisting of fibrosis and nodular regeneration (i.e., cirrhosis). These disorders may be classified on the basis of either etiology or histopathology.

ETIOLOGIC CLASSIFICATION (Table 119–1). Chronic hepatitis can be caused by hepatitis B (with or without superimposed hepatitis D) and hepatitis C virus infection, drugs and toxins (see below and Ch. 118), and inborn errors of metabolism, such as Wilson's disease and α_1-antitrypsin deficiency. In addition, some types are of unknown etiology (idiopathic) in which clinical and laboratory features may suggest but do not prove an immunologically mediated process ("autoimmune"). The prevalence of these categories of chronic hepatitis varies and depends in part on the prevalence of hepatitis virus infection in the general population. Genetic hemochromatosis, while not typically associated with biopsy findings of chronic hepatitis, is a more common cause of chronic liver disease than had been appreciated and deserves consideration in the differential diagnosis.

HISTOPATHOLOGY AND HISTOPATHOLOGIC CLASSIFICATION. Because the clinical and laboratory features are nonspecific, the diagnosis of chronic hepatitis cannot be established without liver biopsy. In most forms of chronic hepatitis, hepatic portal areas are prominently inflamed and are infiltrated mainly by mononuclear cells, especially small lymphocytes and plasma cells. Necrosis and inflammation may also involve hepatocytes immediately adjacent to the portal area. In this *periportal hepatitis* (or *"piecemeal necrosis"*), the inflammatory process involves the peripheral portions of the hepatic lobule, so that individual liver cells or nests of cells become isolated. Periportal hepatitis is not specific for chronic hepatitis and often is present in uncomplicated acute hepatitis and several other processes. For this reason it does not necessarily reflect a chronic or progressive process, and its significance can be judged only in the context of associated histopathologic, laboratory, and clinical findings.

The lobular architecture may be substantially disrupted. The portal inflammatory and necrotic process may extend into the lobule to a depth sufficient to span adjacent portal and/or central areas, i.e., *"bridging necrosis."* Although bridging necrosis can occur as part of an otherwise uncomplicated and self-limited acute hepatitis, it reflects a more severe injury that may have a greater propensity to lead to progressive deterioration over a period of weeks to months (*"subacute hepatic necrosis"*) or to chronic active hepatitis and cirrhosis. Thus, its presence, or the presence of submassive necrosis or significant fibrosis, in a patient with liver disease lasting more than 6 to 12 months, suggests a chronic and progressive process. Paradoxically, among survivors of the most severe form of acute liver injury (i.e., massive hepatic necrosis) chronic progressive liver disease is uncommon. The histopathologic classification of chronic hepatitis that follows is useful for descriptive purposes, but overlap is common, and differentiation of one from the other may be difficult. Most importantly, any of the histopathologic types may be associated with any of the causes of chronic hepatitis, and its significance may vary among them.

Chronic Persistent Hepatitis. Chronic persistent hepatitis, the most common form of chronic hepatitis, is an inflammatory process largely confined to the portal areas. There is little or no periportal or lobular hepatitis; significant fibrosis and cirrhosis are absent. Of the small number of patients with acute hepatitis B whose illness becomes chronic, most are found to have this lesion. By definition, the diagnosis of persistent hepatitis is not appropriate if there is significant stromal collapse, fibrosis, or nodular regeneration.

Chronic persistent hepatitis of most etiologies is usually associated with mild clinical manifestations. Patients have nonspecific symptoms, including fatigue, anorexia, abdominal discomfort, or right upper quadrant pain. Extrahepatic manifestations such as arthritis, glomerulonephritis, and vasculitis are unusual. Jaundice, if present, is usually mild. Physical findings are usually limited to palmar erythema, a few spider telangiectasias, and mildly tender hepatomegaly; the spleen occasionally is slightly enlarged. By definition, complications of advanced liver disease and portal hypertension, such as evidence of a collateral circulation, ascites, and encephalopathy, are absent.

Laboratory abnormalities are also mild and include moderate increases in serum aminotransferase activities, bilirubin, and globulins. Albumin concentration and prothrombin time are usually normal.

The outlook for persistent hepatitis usually is favorable, in that progression to chronic active hepatitis, cirrhosis, or liver failure is uncommon. However, the syndrome may last for 10 years or more and may cause continuing or intermittent discomfort or disability. Because of the difficulties inherent in the biopsy diagnosis of this group of disorders, continuing observation is important. Evidence of significant clinical deterioration may indicate the presence of a more serious process such as chronic active hepatitis, cirrhosis, or hepatocellular carcinoma and would be reason to consider repeat liver biopsy. In chronic hepatitis B infection, for example, increased activity of virus replication may be associated with clinical and histopathologic deterioration (see below).

The possible role of antiviral therapy in chronic hepatitis B, C, and D has been examined in recent clinical trials (see below). Symptomatic and nutritional support is appropriate, and exposure to potential hepatotoxins should be avoided. For patients in whom alcohol has been excluded etiologically, small amounts of alcoholic beverages are permissible if these do not cause worsening of symptoms or laboratory tests. A form of chronic persistent hepatitis may be found in those patients in whom corticoste-

TABLE 119–1. CAUSES OF CHRONIC HEPATITIS

Chronic viral infections
  Hepatitis B
  Hepatitis B with superimposed hepatitis D
  Hepatitis C (non-A, non-B)
Drugs and toxins, including
  Acetaminophen
  Amiodarone
  Aspirin
  Dantrolene
  Ethanol
  Isoniazid
  Methyldopa
  Nitrofurantoin
  Oxyphenisatin
  Perhexilene maleate
  Phenytoin
  Propylthiouracil
  Sulfonamides
Wilson's disease
α_1-Antitrypsin deficiency
Idiopathic ("autoimmune")

roid treatment of idiopathic or "autoimmune" chronic active hepatitis has induced a remission (see below).

Chronic Lobular Hepatitis. This is a less well-defined category of chronic hepatitis in which the predominant lesion is a scattered single-cell necrosis in the lobule, with a relatively minor portal inflammatory component. It is, in effect, a variant of chronic persistent hepatitis, appearing not to progress to cirrhosis or liver failure except in those subjects in whom the underlying disease becomes more active.

Chronic Active Hepatitis. This most serious form of chronic hepatitis has the potential for progression to cirrhosis and liver failure. Approximately 20 per cent of cases are associated with, and presumably caused by, *chronic hepatitis B infection*, with or without superimposed *hepatitis D* infection (see Ch. 117). Chronic active hepatitis may also follow post-transfusion or community-acquired *hepatitis C* or *non-A, non-B*. Drugs that can cause the syndrome include *amiodarone, dantrolene, isoniazid, methyldopa, nitrofurantoin, oxyphenisatin, perhexilene maleate, phenytoin, propylthiouracil,* and *sulfonamides* (Table 119–1). Long-term use of acetaminophen, aspirin, and ethanol occasionally may cause similar changes, as may *Wilson's disease* and α_1-*antitrypsin deficiency*. In a large number of cases, the etiology is unknown, although many patients in this group exhibit clinical features and serologic abnormalities suggestive of autoimmunity. Despite such suggestive evidence, however, a truly "autoimmune" basis for chronic hepatitis has not been established conclusively, and in many instances phenomena that might be considered to reflect such a mechanism are also found in those forms of the disease associated with chronic hepatitis virus infections. The syndrome is characterized by expansion of portal areas, which are infiltrated by lymphocytes and plasma cells, by periportal hepatitis, and by a variable degree of bridging necrosis, collapse, and fibrosis. In one third or more of patients, macronodular cirrhosis is present at the time of diagnosis. Except for the characteristic features of α_1-antitrypsin deficiency, which can be demonstrated histochemically, the various causes of chronic active hepatitis cannot be differentiated on the basis of histopathology.

The course of chronic active hepatitis may be highly variable. The onset is usually insidious but in perhaps one third of cases may resemble an acute hepatitis. It may affect all age groups and both sexes. However, HBsAg-negative cases, sometimes associated with a more severe course and "autoimmune" features, occur mainly in young adult females, whereas HBsAg-positive cases are more common in males and are often minimally symptomatic.

Patients with chronic active hepatitis may be asymptomatic or may exhibit a wide range of local or constitutional symptoms typical of liver disease, such as fatigue, malaise, fever, anorexia, jaundice, or ascites. *Extrahepatic manifestations* are often quite prominent, especially in young females with the idiopathic ("autoimmune") type. These include amenorrhea, various skin rashes, glomerulonephritis, polyserositis, thyroiditis, vasculitis, Sjögren's syndrome, pneumonitis, depression of the formed elements of the blood, and an apparently increased incidence of ulcerative colitis.

Physical findings may also be quite variable. Patients may exhibit only a few spider telangiectasias, possibly with mild enlargement of liver and/or spleen, and may or may not be jaundiced. In advanced cases with cirrhosis, patients may have ascites, evidence of collateral circulation, or encephalopathy. In young women, acne and hirsutism may reflect the hormonal effects of chronic liver disease. Evidence of other extrahepatic manifestations may also be prominent, as noted above.

Serum aminotransferase activities are usually increased over a range from minimally abnormal to over 1000 IU per liter. Globulins usually are diffusely increased, and the albumin value often is low. The alkaline phosphatase is usually only slightly to moderately increased; major increases should suggest the possibility of biliary tract disease or infiltrative or mass lesions. Prothrombin time generally reflects the severity of the disease but may also be influenced by vitamin K deficiency. Because of their variability, the laboratory tests often poorly reflect the pathologic process; for this reason they do not always provide a reliable basis for the assessment of natural history or response to treatment. Serologic tests, including autoantibodies and viral antigen/antibody markers, are discussed below.

The diagnosis of chronic active hepatitis requires liver biopsy. In addition to the histopathology, it is essential to establish a specific etiology, if possible (e.g., chronic hepatitis B/D or C infection, drugs, ethanol, Wilson's disease, or α_1-antitrypsin deficiency). Exposure to drugs and toxins usually can be identified by means of a careful history, including, when appropriate, questioning of family members or friends. Tests for chronic viral hepatitis are discussed below. Wilson's disease should be excluded in any patient with chronic hepatitis who is under the age of 40. Appropriate tests for this purpose include slit-lamp examination for Kayser-Fleischer rings and measurement of serum ceruloplasmin and urinary copper excretion. If all tests are negative, additional studies are not necessary; when the suspicion persists, measurement of liver copper concentration or incorporation of radioactive copper into serum ceruloplasmin may be necessary (see Ch. 192). α_1-Antitrypsin deficiency can be demonstrated by protease-inhibitor phenotyping of serum and, in liver biopsy specimens, by the presence of PAS-positive material in hepatocytes after diastase treatment of the tissue section.

The differential diagnosis includes chronic persistent hepatitis, postnecrotic cirrhosis, and some cases of primary biliary cirrhosis in which clinical and pathologic features may resemble those of chronic active hepatitis. Treatment options for the various forms of chronic active hepatitis, which now include orthotopic liver transplantation, are discussed below.

IDIOPATHIC ("AUTOIMMUNE") CHRONIC ACTIVE HEPATITIS. The general characteristics of this syndrome, including its propensity to affect young women and to be associated with extrahepatic manifestations, have been noted above. The syndrome has been characterized in addition by the presence in serum of several autoantibodies, of uncertain role in etiology and pathogenesis. These include smooth-muscle antibodies (antiactin), positive in approximately two thirds of patients; antinuclear antibodies (SMA; anti–DNA–histone complex) in about one half; anti–double-stranded DNA; and anti–mitochondrial (AMA) antibodies in about one third each. These autoantibodies also occur with increased frequency in family members, although there is no evidence of a simple genetic basis for this observation. A high incidence of HLA-B8 and -DR3 has also been noted. Additional variants of the syndrome have been described, based on recognition of novel autoantibodies and, to a variable extent, distinctive clinical features. These autoantibodies include an anti–nuclear lamin antibody and an anti–liver/kidney microsomal (anti-LKM1) antibody in idiopathic chronic hepatitis, an anti-LKM2 associated with tricrynafen hepatitis, and an anti-LKM3 associated with chronic hepatitis D. Anti-LKM1 and anti-LKM2 are directed against the hepatic microsomal drug-metabolizing enzymes cytochrome P-450IID6 and P-450IIC, respectively; the significance of this is unknown. Also identified in autoimmune chronic hepatitis have been antibodies to liver-specific proteins (LSP), liver membrane antigen (LMAg), and soluble liver antigen (anti-SLA) or liver cytosol antigen (anti-LC1). Although there are some clinical differences among the syndromes associated with these autoantibodies, there is no clear evidence that they either reflect the etiology of the disease or are involved in its pathogenesis.

In fact, the syndrome of chronic hepatitis with autoimmune features can be caused by chemical agents such as nitrofurantoin. Moreover, an unexpectedly high incidence of antimeasles antibodies and of persistent measles virus genome in peripheral blood mononuclear cells has been reported in patients with autoimmune chronic active hepatitis, raising the possibility that some of these cases represent a persistent viral infection. Finally, chronic hepatitis C infection is present in some patients with autoimmune chronic hepatitis, although the C100-3 antibody test may be falsely positive when serum globulins are highest, and a confirmatory test, such as the recombinant immunoblot assay (RIBA), may be required. Whether any cases of this syndrome are truly the result of a primary immune attack on a previously normal liver has not been established.

In the treatment of idiopathic chronic active hepatitis, *corticosteroids*, with or without low-dose azathioprine, usually reduce symptoms, improve laboratory test results, suppress the inflammatory process seen on biopsy, and decrease short-term and long-term morbidity and mortality. For example, in a Mayo Clinic study, a favorable clinical, biochemical, and histologic response was seen initially in 56 per cent of patients, whereas spontaneous improvement occurred in only 20 per cent of placebo controls; early mortality and progression to cirrhosis were also decreased.

Despite this seemingly beneficial overall response, several factors that importantly influence the natural history and response to treatment must be considered in making the decision to institute a chronic treatment plan with potentially significant adverse effects. First, chronic hepatitis does not usually progress to cirrhosis or liver failure in the absence of bridging necrosis on liver biopsy; the absence of such changes would weigh significantly against the use of corticosteroids. Second, there is no evidence that corticosteroids are of benefit in asymptomatic chronic active hepatitis. Third, since the reported series include an unknown number of patients with chronic hepatitis C, and since the natural history of this disorder is variable, it is difficult to assess the impact of corticosteroids in this subset. Fourth, the presence or absence of autoimmune features seemed to be of little consequence in the Mayo Clinic series, in regard to prognosis or response to treatment. Finally, since many patients with chronic active hepatitis would fail to meet the criteria for inclusion in some of the published series, any decision regarding their treatment is necessarily an extrapolation from a selected study population.

In view of this substantial uncertainty concerning the value of corticosteroids in certain subsets of chronic active hepatitis, it is very difficult to make broadly applicable recommendations concerning their use. In general, however, an initially favorable response would most likely be expected in a young symptomatic female with progressive disease and no recent transfusion or other exposure to or evidence for hepatitis B or C.

In the Mayo Clinic study, the following regimen was found to be most effective: an initial daily dose of 60 mg of prednisone or of 30 mg of prednisone combined with 50 mg of azathioprine, tapered gradually over several weeks to months to a daily maintenance dose of 20 mg of prednisone or 10 mg of prednisone plus 50 mg of azathioprine. Azathioprine was of no value when given alone but permitted use of the lower prednisone dose, thereby reducing the incidence of significant steroid-related complications, which otherwise approximated 60 per cent. Alternate-day treatment was less effective. If a favorable response is not observed within 2 to 3 months, treatment should be discontinued.

Patients being treated for chronic active hepatitis should be examined and have liver tests periodically. The possible side effects of drug treatment should be monitored, and liver biopsies may need to be repeated at intervals of 6 months to 1 year, depending on the circumstances. Repeated biopsies serve little purpose in a stable patient. Return of liver enzymes to a level less than twice the upper limit of normal, together with a liver biopsy showing subsidence of the inflammatory and necrotic process to a picture similar to that of persistent hepatitis, is considered a successful response and warrants an attempt gradually to discontinue treatment. In about 50 per cent of patients, this attempt succeeds and additional corticosteroid treatment is not needed. In the remainder, evidence of relapse may suggest the need for reinstitution of therapy.

Unfortunately, the disease may eventually progress to cirrhosis or liver failure despite an apparently favorable initial clinical response, especially in those patients in whom repeated recurrences of activity require treatment over a period of 3 years or longer. Over these longer intervals the advisability of continued corticosteroid therapy must be judged not only on the basis of symptoms and laboratory and biopsy findings but also in recognition of the successful treatment of many of these patients with orthotopic liver transplantation (Ch. 124).

CHRONIC HEPATITIS B. Up to 10 per cent of otherwise healthy individuals remain chronically infected with hepatitis B virus after acute hepatitis caused by this agent (Ch. 117). Approximately two thirds develop the lesion of chronic persistent hepatitis and the remainder chronic active hepatitis. Chronicity is more common in men than women, is predisposed to by immune suppression, and is, in general, a clinically more subdued disease process than its autoimmune counterpart. Nevertheless, chronic hepatitis B clearly may evolve to cirrhosis, liver failure, and hepatocellular carcinoma. The severity of the course is largely dependent on the activity of virus replication in the hepatocyte

and the response of the host immune system. In somewhat simplified terms, the process can be described as follows: Active replication of episomal (i.e., nonintegrated viral DNA) results in the presence in serum of markers of the complete virion, or Dane particle (i.e., HBeAg, DNA polymerase, and HBV DNA). Viral antigens are also expressed on the surface of the hepatocyte in association with Class I HLA determinants, thereby eliciting lymphocyte cytotoxicity and a resulting hepatitis. When replication subsides, fewer complete virions are produced; HBeAg gives way to anti-HBe (seroconversion); and a brief flare in the hepatitis ushers in a period of relative clinical and histopathologic quiescence. This may occur in 10 to 30 per cent of patients each year. The reverse may also occur, if an increase in viral replication leads to increases in the production of virions and markers and in the severity of the hepatitis (reactivation).

This dynamic host-virus interaction has important diagnostic implications. Thus, an HBsAg-positive patient with a syndrome of apparent acute hepatitis may in fact have chronic hepatitis B undergoing either seroconversion or reactivation. Other factors, such as superimposed viral or drug-induced hepatitis, may lead to similar confusion. Active HBV replication and chronic hepatitis B are suggested by HBsAg, HBeAg, and anti-HBc positivity and anti-HBs negativity. (In a small number of patients, usually with active disease, an heterotypic anti-HBs may be present simultaneously with HBsAg.) Definitive evidence of active replication would be provided by demonstration of DNA polymerase in serum or HBV DNA in serum, but these tests are not available routinely.

The treatment of chronic hepatitis B remains frustrating. Corticosteroids are not beneficial and may be harmful, possibly in part reflecting their demonstrated enhancement of HBV replication. In trials of antiviral therapy, patients selected have usually exhibited active viral replication (i.e., HBeAg, DNA polymerase, and HBV DNA positivity). In these trials adenine arabinoside (ara-A) and ara-AMP have proven to be unacceptably toxic. α-Interferon, however, has proven more promising in that about one third of patients respond to a variable extent by decreasing replicative activity (e.g., loss of HBeAg), although only approximately 10 per cent seem to eradicate the virus. Factors predisposing to a favorable response included female sex, a clinically mild course, relatively brief duration, high serum aminotransferase and HBV DNA levels, and immune competence (e.g., HIV negativity), whereas less favorable results have been obtained in male homosexuals, HIV-positive and Asian subjects, and individuals with neonatally acquired infections. Unfortunately, it is unclear in those patients in whom treatment appears successful whether the longer-term course of the disease is substantially altered; thus, α-interferon use at present should remain limited to controlled trials. Other antiviral and immunomodulatory agents are also undergoing clinical trials. Orthotopic liver transplantation has been successfully employed in the management of liver failure secondary to chronic hepatitis B (Ch. 123). Results thus far suggest that there is a somewhat increased early postoperative mortality, possibly related to sepsis, and virtually universal reinfection of the transplanted liver. In most centers, liver failure in chronic hepatitis B is considered an appropriate indication for liver transplantation despite the fact that the overall outlook for this group is less favorable.

CHRONIC HEPATITIS C. Acute post-transfusion or community-acquired hepatitis C becomes chronic in about 50 per cent of cases (Ch. 117). Typically, chronic hepatitis C exhibits an intermittent course, in which episodes of increased symptoms and laboratory abnormalities are separated by periods of relative quiescence, but 10 to 20 per cent of patients evolve to cirrhosis or progressive liver failure. Furthermore, 65 per cent or more of patients with primary hepatocellular carcinoma test positive for the antibody to HCV.

Treatment of chronic hepatitis C remains undefined. It seems likely but undocumented that a significant number of these patients were included in the various treatment trials of autoimmune hepatitis and responded to corticosteroids; α-interferon has been used with limited success and with an unknown overall effect on the natural history of the disease. Thus, normalization or near normalization of the serum aminotransferase activity was achieved in 46 per cent of patients with chronic post-transfusion hepatitis C treated with 3 million units three times weekly for 24 weeks, as compared with untreated controls, and was associated with histologic improvement. Unfortunately, 51 per cent of the responders relapsed within 6 months after the end of the treatment.

Patients with liver failure resulting from HCV-induced chronic active hepatitis or cirrhosis have successfully undergone orthotopic liver transplantation and are regarded as appropriate candidates for the procedure in virtually all centers. Unlike chronic hepatitis B, disease recurrence in the transplanted organ appears to be mild and evidently of limited clinical impact. The actual recurrence rate is not yet known and will require more sensitive assays such as polymerase chain reaction or immunologic tests for viral antigens.

CHRONIC HEPATITIS D. Hepatitis D infection depends on antecedent or simultaneous infection with the hepatitis B virus. When HDV infection is superimposed on pre-existing chronic hepatitis B, it also becomes chronic in most cases. Simultaneous infection with both HBV and HDV does not increase the probability of chronic disease but is associated with an increased incidence of fulminant hepatic failure. Trials involving α-interferon treatment of chronic HBV with HDV have met with limited temporary success and a high probability of relapse after cessation of treatment. There is also a high probability of recurrent disease after orthotopic liver transplantation.

SPECIAL CLINICAL PROBLEMS

Two circumstances are encountered in clinical practice with sufficient frequency that they deserve particular comment with reference to diagnostic approach and management.

UNEXPECTED INCREASE OF SERUM AMINOTRANSFERASE. The advent and common use of multiphasic laboratory screening techniques have led to the identification of individuals in whom aminotransferase activities are abnormal but who lack clinical evidence of liver disease. If the abnormal finding is confirmed, and if it does not reflect muscle or other extrahepatic disease, it may have either of two possible implications: (1) It may reflect a subclinical acute process (e.g., acute viral hepatitis) or (2) it may reflect a chronic process (e.g., chronic toxic or viral hepatitis or nonalcoholic steatohepatitis). If the patient is asymptomatic or nearly so, a period of observation is appropriate, and follow-up studies and hepatitis serologies should be obtained. Alcohol and potentially hepatotoxic drugs and toxins should be avoided. Improvement would presumably reflect resolution of a self-limited process or the response to removal of a toxin (e.g., ethanol). Worsening of the test results during observation may herald the onset of overt disease, the proper evaluation of which would depend on the circumstances. Persistence of the abnormality beyond 6 to 12 months may reflect a chronic hepatitis and may justify liver biopsy.

HEPATITIS B SURFACE ANTIGEN POSITIVITY. Approximately 0.1 to 0.2 per cent of the population of the United States is positive for HBsAg. At any given time, most of these persons exhibit no overt evidence of liver disease and are designated carriers. The meaning of the term *carrier* varies, however, and has been used to include all chronically positive individuals, or only those who have no apparent liver disease.

The practical question of significance concerns the management of the otherwise apparently healthy patient with a positive test. If the result is confirmed, it could indicate (1) a subclinical acute hepatitis B, (2) chronic hepatitis (persistent or active) or cirrhosis, or (3) a "healthy" carrier state. Although differentiation of these conditions may require liver biopsy, HBsAg-positive persons who have no other clinical or laboratory evidence of liver disease usually have normal or nonspecific biopsy findings. There is no conclusive evidence that treatment is indicated for the few among this group of asymptomatic persons with normal liver function tests who may have chronic active hepatitis on biopsy. Therefore, these individuals can be followed at intervals without first obtaining a liver biopsy. Those HBsAg-positive persons who do have clinical and/or laboratory signs of liver disease should be managed in accordance with the severity and duration of the process; persistence of the abnormalities beyond 6 months may suggest a chronic hepatitis and the need to consider liver biopsy.

Carman WF, Jacyma MR, Hadziyannis S, et al.: Mutation preventing formation of hepatitis B e antigen in patients with chronic hepatitis B infection. Lancet 2:588, 1989. *An important description of the molecular basis for a clinically severe variant of chronic hepatitis B.*

Czaja AJ, Hay, JE, Rakela J: Clinical features and prognostic implications of severe corticosteroid-treated cryptogenic chronic active hepatitis. Mayo Clin 65:23, 1990. *Recent demonstration, in a large series of cases, of the apparent lack of effect of autoimmune features on disease severity, histopathology, response to treatment, and survival.*

Czaja AJ, Taswell HF, Rakela J, et al.: Frequency and significance of antibody to hepatitis C virus in severe corticosteroid-treated cryptogenic chronic active hepatitis. Mayo Clin Proc 65:1303, 1990. *Evidence that hepatitis C virus infection is uncommon in this population.*

Davis GL, Balart LA, Schiff ER, et al.: Treatment of chronic hepatitis C with recombinant interferon alpha. N Engl J Med 321:1501, 1989; DiBisceglie AM, Martin P, Kassianides C, et al.: Recombinant interferon alpha therapy for chronic hepatitis C. N Engl J Med 321:1506, 1989. *Two controlled trials demonstrating a potential role for antiviral therapy.*

Dienstag JL (ed.): Viral hepatitis. Semin Liver Dis, Vol. 11, May 1991. *A minisymposium in which clinically relevant aspects of acute and chronic hepatitis are critically reviewed by recognized experts.*

Hoofnagle JH: Type D (delta) hepatitis. JAMA 261:1321, 1989. *A brief but well-referenced and informative review.*

Liaw Y-F, Chu C-M, Chen T-J, et al.: Chronic lobular hepatitis: A clinicopathological and prognostic study. Hepatology 2:258, 1982. *A histopathologic category with generally benign prognostic implications, but for which continuing observation is indicated.*

Maddrey WC: Chronic hepatitis. In Zakim D, Boyer T (eds.): Hepatology: A Textbook of Liver Disease. Philadelphia, W. B. Saunders Company, 1989, pp 1025–1061. *A comprehensive and well-referenced review, emphasizing clinical aspects.*

Meyer zum Buschenfelde K-H (ed.): Autoimmune hepatitis. Semin Liver Dis, Vol. 11, August 1991. *A collection of authoritative, critical reviews of autoimmunity and liver disease.*

Perillo RP, Schiff, Davis GL, et al.: A randomized, controlled trial of interferon alpha-2b alone and after prednisone withdrawal for the treatment of chronic hepatitis B. N Engl J Med 323:295, 1990. *Results of a multicenter trial demonstrating the efficacy of interferon in certain patients.*

Scott J, Gollan JL, Samourian S, et al.: Wilson's disease presenting as chronic active hepatitis. Gastroenterology 74:645, 1978. *A thorough clinical and pathologic description of 17 patients presenting with features of chronic active hepatitis. Emphasis is placed on the often difficult problem of differential diagnosis.*

Vitirski-Trepo L, Kay A, Pichoud C, et al.: Early and frequent detection of HBxAg and/or anti-HBx in hepatitis B infection. Hepatology 12:1278, 1990. *Useful information concerning detection of hepatitis B x-gene markers.*

Zuckerman A (ed.): Viral Hepatitis and Liver Disease. New York, Alan R. Liss, 1988. *Proceedings of a recent symposium in which clinical and basic aspects of all forms of viral hepatitis are addressed.*

120 Parasitic, Bacterial, Fungal, and Granulomatous Liver Disease

Teresa L. Wright

Fungal and parasitic diseases of the hepatobiliary system are more commonly associated with underdeveloped countries, but their frequency is increasing in the United States. Contributing factors include the growing number of patients with AIDS, as well as patients receiving cancer chemotherapy or immunosuppressive therapy following organ transplantation.

PARASITIC DISEASES OF THE LIVER AND BILIARY TRACT

Clinical features of parasitic infections that involve the liver and biliary tract are summarized in Table 120–1. A history of travel to areas where these infections are endemic should be obtained and the appropriate diagnostic tests ordered. Geographic distributions of these diseases, as well as specific therapies, are discussed elsewhere in this book.

Helminthic Infections

PATHOGENESIS. Humans are important intermediate hosts in the life cycles of many helminths, and the liver and biliary tract are commonly involved in both the larval stage (toxocariasis, ascariasis, strongyloidiasis, schistosomiasis, echinococcosis, and fascioliasis) and the adult stage (ascariasis, clonorchiasis, fascioli-asis). In addition, adult worms residing in mesenteric vessels or the biliary tract lay eggs, which form a nidus for granuloma formation (schistosomiasis, ascariasis, clonorchiasis). The liver responds to the larvae in a variable manner. Ascariasis usually causes little tissue injury, whereas larval migration in toxocariasis results in a marked inflammatory response with tissue eosinophilia (visceral larva migrans). Damage from the adult worms is also variable. In ascariasis, migration of adult worms into the bile ducts may be accompanied by acute pain. Biliary tract obstruc-tion, cholangitis, and biliary calculi may occur; treatment involves surgical or endoscopic removal of worms. In clonorchiasis, the adult worm migrates up the bile duct from the duodenum and lays its eggs in the intrahepatic ducts. Little inflammation occurs within the liver itself, and eosinophilia is rare. Infection may remain silent for years until patients present with cholangitis (recurrent Oriental cholangiohepatitis) or cholangiocarcinoma. Despite surgical drainage of the bile ducts, recurrent stone

formation is common. In schistosomiasis, adult worms migrate from the portal vein into the mesenteric vessels where they lay eggs (Ch. 434). Subsequently blood carries the eggs into portal venules, where they lodge and elicit an immune response from the host. Granuloma formation, fibrosis, and portal hypertension result. Treatment of chronic infection may include sclerosis of bleeding esophageal varices or portacaval shunt.

CLINICAL MANIFESTATIONS. The clinical features of hel-minthic infections are variable. Tender hepatomegaly and eosin-ophilia are common findings during larval migration. Fever, jaundice, and abdominal pain accompany the biliary tract obstruc-tion caused by adult worms of ascariasis and clonorchiasis. Bleed-ing from esophageal varices is a common manifestation of the portal hypertension that results from infection with schistosomi-asis.

DIAGNOSIS. Diagnosis of helminthic disorders relies on iden-

TABLE 120–1. COMMON PARASITIC DISEASES OF THE LIVER AND BILIARY TRACT

Disorder (Organism)	Predisposition to Infection*	Nature of Hepatic Involvement		
		Pathophysiology	*Manifestations*	*Diagnosis*
Helminthic disorders				
Ascariasis (*Ascaris lumbricoides*) (roundworm)	Ingestion of raw vegetables	Larval migration through portal vein to liver; later adult invasion of biliary tract with egg production	Abdominal pain, fever, jaun-dice during larval migra-tion; bile duct obstruction, cholangitis, perforation later; granuloma formation around eggs	Ova or adult worm in stool; worms in duodenum on contrast studies or endo-scopic examination
Toxocariasis (*Toxocara carris, cati*) (roundworm)	Contact with dogs and cats	Larval migration in hepatic parenchyma (visceral larva migrans)	Granuloma formation with eosinophilia	Demonstration of larvae in tissue; serology: ELISA
Strongyloidiasis (*Strongyloides stercoralis*)	Immunodeficiency (AIDS, organ transplant, cancer chemotherapy)	Larval penetration through intestine into liver	Occasional jaundice, hepato-megaly, larvae in portal tract and liver lobule	Larvae in stool or duodenal aspirate; serology not use-ful
Echinococcosis (*Echinococcus granu-losa, multilocularis*) (tapeworm)	Sheep and cattle raising	Larval migration to liver where encystment occurs (hydatid cyst)	Asymptomatic; symptoms of hepatic mass lesions, bili-ary tract obstruction, cyst rupture	Serologic tests (indirect hemagglutination, ELISA); CT scans: hepatic cysts
Schistosomiasis (*Schistosoma mansoni, Japonicum*) (flatworm)		Host immune response to ova in portal vein, result-ing in fibrosis	*Acute:* eosinophilic infiltrate *Chronic:* hepatosplenomeg-aly, complications of por-tal hypertension, granu-loma formation	Identification of ova in stool or on liver biopsy
Clonorchiasis (*Clonorchis sinensis*) (flatworm)	Ingestion of raw fish	Migration of worms through ampulla of Vater; eggs produced in bile ducts	Bile duct obstruction, cho-langitis, choledocholithia-sis, cholangiocarcinoma	Ova in stool; multiple bile duct stones at ERCP
Fascioliasis (*Fasciola hepatica*) (flatworm)	Ingestion of fresh-water plants	Larval migration through liver, penetration of bile ducts	*Acute:* fever, abdominal pain, jaundice, hemobilia *Chronic:* asymptomatic hep-atomegaly, choledocholi-thiasis	Eosinophilia, elevated liver tests; ova in stool; adult flukes in bile ducts at ERCP
Protozoan disorders				
Amebiasis (*Entamoeba histolytica*)	Poor sanitation, sexual con-tact	Hematogenous spread with tissue invasion; abscess formation	Fever, RUQ pain, peritoni-tis, elevated right hemidi-aphragm	Cysts in stool; serologic tests (counterimmuno-electrophoresis, indirect hemagglutination); techne-tium-99 liver scan
Malaria (*Plasmodium vivax, fal-ciparum, ovale, ma-lariae*)	Blood transfusion, parenteral drug use	Sporozoites cleared from cir-culation by hepatocytes; exoerythrocytic replication in liver	Tender hepatomegaly; rarely hepatic failure (*P. falcipa-rum*)	Identification of organism on blood smear
Cryptosporidiosis (*Cryptosporidium*)	Immunodeficiency (AIDS)	Unknown; biliary tract in-volvement only in immu-nodeficient patients	Fever, RUQ pain, cholecys-titis	Elevated alkaline phospha-tase; bile duct dilatation at ERCP
Toxoplasmosis (*Toxoplasma gondii*)	Intrauterine infection; im-munodeficiency (AIDS, organ transplant)	Multiplication in liver caus-ing necrosis and inflamma-tion	Fever, hepatosplenomegaly	Transaminase elevation; iso-lation of organism from tissue; Sabin-Feldman dye test
Visceral leishmaniasis (*Leishmania donovani*)	Immunodeficiency (AIDS, organ transplant)	Infection of reticuloendothe-lial cells of liver	Fever, leukopenia, hepato-splenomegaly	Organism in bone marrow; immunoserologic tests
Trypanosomiasis (*Trypanosoma cruzi, rhodesiense, gam-biense*)		*Acute:* parasites in reticulo-endothelial cells of liver *Chronic:* passive congestion secondary to heart failure	*Acute:* fever, hepatospleno-megaly *Chronic:* hepatomegaly	Organisms in blood, tissue; immunofluorescent tests

*Travel in endemic areas predisposes to infection with all protozoa and helminths. Additional predisposing factors are listed.

tification of ova in stool. Serologic tests are usually unhelpful (except in the diagnosis of echinococcosis or toxocariasis). Occasionally liver biopsy demonstrates organisms. Adult worms may be found at laparotomy, performed for biliary tract obstruction (e.g., for clonorchiasis or ascariasis).

Protozoan Infections

Protozoa commonly infect the liver, with organisms in both reticuloendothelial cells (leishmaniasis and trypanosomiasis) and hepatocytes (toxoplasmosis and malaria).

CLINICAL MANIFESTATIONS. These are usually nonspecific and may resemble viral hepatitis (toxoplasmosis and malaria). In certain infections, extrahepatic manifestations predominate (e.g., cardiomyopathy with chronic trypanosomiasis, diarrhea with cryptosporidiosis). Extrahepatic features may be prominent early in the course (e.g., amebic colitis), and hepatic symptoms predominate later (e.g., with hepatic abscess formation).

DIAGNOSIS. In contrast to helminthic infections, serologic tests are useful in making a specific diagnosis (Table 120–1). Amebic liver abscess is discussed below.

FUNGAL INFECTIONS OF THE LIVER

The liver is frequently involved in disseminated fungal infection. Prevalence of these infections varies geographically. *Coccidioides immitis* is endemic in the southwest region of the United States, whereas *Histoplasma capsulatum* is endemic in the eastern and central regions.

CLINICAL MANIFESTATIONS. Patients present with fever, hepatomegaly, and an elevated serum level of alkaline phosphatase. Hepatic involvement in histoplasmosis, coccidioidomycosis, North American blastomycosis, and cryptococcosis occurs in immunocompetent patients, most commonly with granuloma formation (Table 120–2). In contrast, hepatic involvement in candidiasis, aspergillosis, and mucormycosis occurs in immunocompromised patients, often with abscess and granuloma formation.

DIAGNOSIS. The diagnosis of all fungal infections relies on identification of the organism on liver biopsy. Serologic tests are not helpful. Because of diagnostic difficulty with systemic fungal infections, antifungal therapy is frequently started empirically in an immunocompromised patient with persistent fever. The diagnosis may only be made at postmortem examination.

THERAPY. Despite therapy, mortality in disseminated fungal infection remains high (25 to 100 per cent). Amphotericin B (0.6

mg per kilogram per day intravenously for at least 42 days) may be effective in the treatment of candidiasis, histoplasmosis, coccidioidomycosis, and cryptococcosis. Newer antifungal agents (e.g., ketoconazole or fluconazole, 200 mg per day) may be as effective as amphotericin, with fewer side effects (Ch. 398). *Aspergillus* is poorly responsive to amphotericin and should be treated with miconazole or fluconazole.

HEPATIC MANIFESTATIONS OF SYSTEMIC BACTERIAL INFECTION

Liver abnormalities are associated with a wide variety of bacterial infections (Table 120–2). The mechanism by which jaundice occurs is unclear but has been postulated to be due to effects of bacterial endotoxin on hepatocyte function (e.g., *Escherichia coli*), direct mechanical effects (e.g., right lower lobe pneumonia), nonspecific inflammation and necrosis (e.g., typhoid fever), or associated hemolysis (e.g., pneumococcal pneumonia). Organisms may directly infect the liver (e.g., actinomycosis, tuberculosis, and syphilis) with granulomas or abscess formation. With successful antibiotic therapy, liver function abnormalities usually resolve.

LIVER ABSCESS

DEFINITION. Liver abscesses are focal collections of organisms and pus within the hepatic parenchyma. Although frequently multiple, abscesses may coalesce to form a single abscess. There is geographic variation in causative organisms, with amebae more prevalent in developing countries and pyogenic organisms more common in developed nations, including the United States.

Pyogenic Liver Abscess

ETIOLOGY. Multiple hepatic abscesses are most frequently due to underlying biliary tract infection (cholecystitis, cholangitis). Infection in organs drained by the portal vein (e.g., appendicitis, diverticulitis) may cause pylephlebitis and secondary abscess formation. Abscesses also result from seeding of the liver with bacteremia from a nonabdominal source as well as from abdominal trauma with hematoma formation. Causative organisms include enteric bacteria (*Escherichia coli, Klebsiella pneumoniae, Streptococcus faecalis*) and pyogenic gram-positive cocci (*Staphylococcus aureus*). Careful culture techniques have demonstrated anaerobic bacteria (*Bacteroides, Clostridium*) in approximately 50 per cent of abscesses.

CLINICAL MANIFESTATIONS. Hepatic abscesses present with fever, anorexia, and abdominal pain. No feature of the fever pattern distinguishes hepatic abscesses from any other intra-

TABLE 120–2. HEPATOBILIARY MANIFESTATIONS OF BACTERIAL INFECTIONS

Disease	Organism	Clinical Features	Liver Histology
Lobar pneumonia	*Pneumococcus*	Jaundice, hepatomegaly	Focal necrosis, inflammation
Toxic shock syndrome; osteomyelitis	*Staphylococcus*	Jaundice	Abscess formation; granulomas
Fitz-Hugh-Curtis syndrome	*Gonococcus*	RUQ pain, tender hepatomegaly, peritoneal adhesions	Perihepatitis; organism seen on liver biopsy
Neonatal infection	*Esherichia coli*	Jaundice	Focal necrosis, inflammation
Typhoid fever	*Salmonella typhi*	Hepatomegaly, jaundice; asymptomatic (carrier state)	Focal necrosis; chronic cholecystitis
Brucellosis	*Brucella abortis, melitensis, suls*	Tender hepatomegaly, splenomegaly	Granulomas
Gas gangrene; pylephlebitis	*Clostridium welchii*	Jaundice, high mortality	Abscess formation; portal vein gas
Melloidosis	*Pseudomonas pseudomallei*	Hepatomegaly only with septicemia	Focal necrosis, abscess formation
Legionnaire's disease	*Legionella pneumophilia*	Hepatosplenomegaly	Focal necrosis
Actinomycosis	*Actinomyces israelii, bovis*	Fever, abdominal pain	Multiloculated abscess with pus, organisms
Mycobacteria			
Miliary tuberculosis	*Mycobacterium tuberculosis*	Fever, weight loss, hepatomegaly	Caseating granulomas, tuberculomas, tuberculous cholangitis
Atypical mycobacterial infection	*Mycobacterium avium-intracellulare*	Fever, hepatomegaly, alkaline phosphatase elevation	Caseating granulomas, frequent organisms
Leprosy	*Mycobacterium leprae*	Asymptomatic	Granulomas, "foamy histiocytes," frequent organisms
Spirochetes			
Syphilis (congenital, secondary, tertiary)	*Treponema pallidum*	Hepatomegaly	Organisms, granulomas; gummatous necrosis
Leptospirosis (Weil's disease)	*Leptospira icterohaemorrhagiae*	Fever, jaundice, renal failure, hemolysis	Hemorrhagic necrosis, cholestasis

abdominal infection. Presentation may be insidious, with fever for weeks, or more acute. Jaundice occurs in 20 per cent of cases and is often associated with underlying biliary tract disease. Patients typically have hepatomegaly with point tenderness on palpation of the liver. Rales and percussion dullness may be found at the base of the right lung.

DIAGNOSIS. Leukocytosis, anemia, hypoalbuminemia, and elevation of serum alkaline phosphatase are invariably present. Other liver tests are usually only mildly abnormal. Blood cultures are positive in 60 per cent of patients with hepatic abscesses. Liver ultrasonography is highly sensitive in detecting hypoechoic mass lesions. Abcesses can usually be distinguished from cysts by their irregular borders and increased echogenicity within the lesion. Computed tomography (CT) scan with intravenous contrast can detect lesions of 1 cm or greater, which typically appear as low-density lesions with a surrounding "rim" of tissue. CT scan is also useful in identifying other intra-abdominal processes (e.g., diverticular abscess). However, neither ultrasonography nor CT scan can reliably distinguish abscesses from necrotic tumors in the liver. Diagnosis should be confirmed by ultrasound-guided fine-needle aspiration with Gram's stain, culture, and histology (Fig. 120–1).

TREATMENT. When the diagnosis of hepatic abscess is suspected, blood cultures should be drawn and ultrasound-guided fine-needle aspiration performed prior to institution of antibiotics. Aspiration should be both diagnostic and therapeutic. Initial therapy should include anaerobic coverage (e.g., with ampicillin, an aminoglycoside, and metronidazole). Treatment can be modified when results of cultures are obtained and should be continued for 10 to 14 days. Percutaneous catheter drainage of large abscesses plays an adjunctive role to antibiotics and may obviate surgical intervention. Although surgical drainage has been advocated in the past, this is necessary only if there is an associated intra-abdominal process (e.g., diverticular abscess, appendiceal abscess, or biliary tract disease). Patients with multiple small abscesses who fail to respond to an initial course of antibiotics may require treatment for months. With early diagnosis and aggressive treatment, mortality has improved from 80 per cent to less than 10 per cent.

Amebic Liver Abscess

ETIOLOGY. Although several types of amebae are found in the colon in man, only *Entamoeba histolytica* is known to be pathogenic (Ch. 431). Amebae may remain dormant in the colon for years before tissue invasion with hematogenous spread that results in hepatic abscess formation. The reason for the male predominance of this disease is unknown.

CLINICAL MANIFESTATIONS. Amebic liver abscess should be suspected in a patient with fever, malaise, right upper quadrant pain, and a history of travel to an endemic area. Signs

of infection include tender hepatomegaly and percussion dullness at the base of the right lung. Jaundice is rare. A minority of patients have symptoms of amebic colitis (bloody diarrhea). Complications of amebic abscess include rupture into the chest (empyema), peritoneum, or pericardium and obstruction of the common bile duct or inferior vena cava. The development of complications carries a poor prognosis and may require surgical intervention.

DIAGNOSIS. Serologic tests are positive in the majority of patients with amebic liver abscess (Table 120–1). Because titers may remain elevated for years, they provide supportive rather than definitive evidence of acute infection. Liver function abnormalities are nonspecific. Imaging studies (ultrasonography, CT scan, and technetium-99 liver scan) demonstrate the abscess. In contrast to pyogenic abscesses, amebic abscesses are usually single. An elevated right hemidiaphragm and a pleural effusion are often present on chest radiography. Aspiration of the abscess is usually not required for diagnosis and carries the risk of causing bacterial superinfection.

TREATMENT AND PROGNOSIS (also see Ch. 431). Medical therapy with metronidazole (750 mg three times per day for 10 days) is usually adequate both for treatment of the abscess and for eradication of amebae from the colon. Concomitant treatment with the intestinal amebicide diiodoquine (650 mg three times daily for 20 days) has also been advocated. In the past, surgical drainage of amebic abscesses was routine but is now rarely required. Aspiration may be necessary for abscesses extending into the pleura, peritoneum, or pericardium but is not required routinely. Aspiration, if performed, reveals straw-colored fluid (described as "anchovy paste") and amebae on microscopic examination.

GRANULOMATOUS LIVER DISEASE

ETIOLOGY. Reticuloendothelial cells in the liver remove circulating antigens, microorganisms, and immune complexes from the systemic circulation. These in turn form the nidus of the inflammatory reaction that results in granulomas. The large number of Kupffer cells (tissue macrophages), as well as the strategic location of the liver, probably account for the frequent finding of granulomas in liver biopsy specimens (2 to 10 per cent). Some of the numerous causes of hepatic granulomas are listed in Table 120–3. The relative frequency of causes varies geographically. Sarcoidosis and tuberculosis account for approximately two thirds of all causes of hepatic granulomas in the United States. In endemic areas, the predominant granulomas are those surrounding the eggs of *Schistosoma mansoni* in portal vein tributaries (Ch. 434). Hepatic granulomas associated with lepromatous leprosy are also frequent in underdeveloped countries. Commonly, no specific cause of the granuloma can be identified.

PATHOLOGY AND PATHOGENESIS. As in other organs, granulomas in the liver are focal collections of inflammatory cells that are distinct from the adjacent tissue. As granulomas develop, macrophages, the predominant cell type in the granuloma, fuse to form multinucleate giant cells. Histologic features of the granuloma may point toward a specific etiology. For example, a fibrinoid ring in a fat granuloma is highly suggestive of *Coxiella burnetii* infection, Q fever; acid-fast organisms may be found in tuberculosis or *Mycobacterium avium-intracellulare* infection; ova may be present in schistosomiasis; and birefringent granules indicate starch granulomas associated with intravenous drug use. The presence of central necrosis or "caseation" within the granuloma, although suggestive of tuberculosis, is not pathognomonic. The location within the hepatic lobule may be suggestive of certain etiologies. For example, granulomas associated with primary biliary cirrhosis or sarcoidosis tend to be well circumscribed and are found in the periportal region, whereas those associated with lymphomas tend to be poorly formed and are scattered throughout the lobule.

CLINICAL MANIFESTATIONS. Most frequently hepatic granulomas are found in a patient with fever of unknown etiology and an elevated serum alkaline phosphatase. Patients have hepatomegaly but rarely have evidence of portal hypertension (splenomegaly, ascites, or esophageal varices).

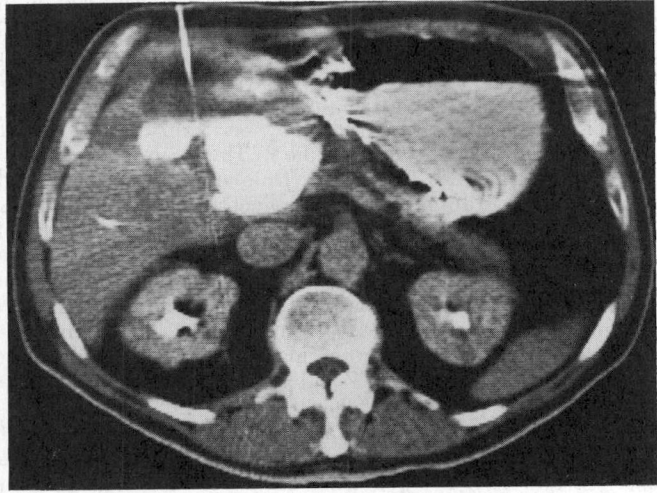

FIGURE 120–1. Computed tomogram showing CT-directed needle aspiration of a liver abscess. The needle is seen as the thin dense linear object entering the liver from the anterior abdominal wall. Contrast material has been introduced into the abscess cavity through the needle in order to outline the extent of the abscess.

TABLE 120–3. CAUSES OF HEPATIC GRANULOMAS

I. Infection
  A. Bacterial
    *Tuberculosis   Salmonellosis
    *Brucellosis   Listeriosis
    *Leprosy   Nocardiosis
    **Mycobacterium avium-*   Melioidosis
      intracellulare
  B. Fungal
    *Histoplasmosis   Candidiasis
    *Coccidioidomycosis   Blastomycosis
    Aspergillosis   Cryptococcosis
  C. Viral
    Mononucleosis   Lymphogranuloma venereum
    Cytomegalovirus   Influenza B
    Chickenpox   Psittacosis
  D. Parasitic
    *Schistosomiasis   Visceral larval migrans
    Ascariasis   Toxoplasmosis
    Stronglyloides   Giardiasis
    Clonorchiasis   Cryptosporidiosis
  E. Rickettsial
    *Q fever
  F. Spirochetal
    Secondary syphilis
II. Systemic diseases
  *Sarcoidosis   Lymphoma
  *Hodgkin's disease   Polymyalgia rheumatica
  Crohn's disease   Systemic lupus erythematosus
  Wegener's granulomatosis
III. Drugs
  Sulfonamides   Halothane
  Penicillin   Allopurinol
  Cephalosporines   Carbamazepine
  Methyldopa   Phenytoin
  Hydralazine   Chlorpropamide
  Procainamide   Phenylbutazone
  Quinidine   Contraceptive pill
  Tocainide
IV. Miscellaneous conditions
  Berylliosis
  Jejunoileal bypass   Parenteral drug abuse
                     Primary biliary cirrhosis

*Denotes more common causes.

DIAGNOSIS. Diagnosis ultimately depends on pathologic or culture confirmation. Serial sections of the biopsy should be examined and tissue cultured for mycobacteria and fungi. Determining a specific cause of hepatic granulomas often relies on demonstration of extrahepatic disease (e.g., granulomas of the uvea in sarcoidosis or acid-fast bacilli in sputum with tuberculosis). Thus, liver biopsy plays an adjunctive rather than a primary role in identifying a specific etiology in patients with fever of unknown origin. Serum angiotensin-converting enzyme is elevated in granulomatous liver disease of any etiology and is not specific for sarcoidosis.

TREATMENT. This is dependent on the etiology of the granulomas. Histologic or culture evidence of infection with a specific infectious agent (e.g., schistosomiasis, Q fever) should prompt specific therapy with praziquantel and tetracycline, respectively. The presence of hepatic granulomas in patients with tuberculosis is evidence of miliary disease, and if the suspicion of tuberculosis is high, therapy should be initiated prior to culture confirmation. Response to treatment of *Mycobacterium avium-intracellulare* in patients with AIDS has been disappointing. Demonstration of hepatic involvement in sarcoidosis, particularly in association with systemic symptoms, should prompt treatment with corticosteroids (Ch. 67). Although patients with hepatic sarcoidosis may develop symptoms of portal hypertension (e.g., bleeding esophageal varices), hepatic failure is rare. Treatment of systemic mycoses is discussed above.

PROGNOSIS. Prognosis is dependent on the underlying condition. With treatment and resolution of associated bacterial, viral, and rickettsial infections, prognosis is excellent. Disseminated fungal infections carry a poor prognosis despite therapy. Patients with hepatic sarcoidosis usually respond symptomatically

to steroid therapy, although progressive fibrosis and cirrhosis may occur. In patients with primary biliary cirrhosis, the presence of granulomas is indicative of improved prognosis.

Barnes PF, De Cock KM, Reynolds TN, et al.: A comparison of amebic and pyogenic abscess of the liver. Medicine 66:472, 1987. *Clinical and radiologic features, diagnosis, and outcome of 146 patients with hepatic abscesses admitted to a county hospital.*

Elliot DL, Tolle SW, Goldberg L, et al.: Pet-associated illness. N Engl J Med 313:985, 1985. *Review of parasitic, bacterial, and rickettsial illnesses acquired from cats and dogs.*

El-Rooby A: Management of hepatic schistosomiasis. Semin Liver Dis 5:263, 1985. *Summary of pathology, clinical manifestations, diagnosis, and treatment of acute and chronic schistosomiasis.*

Greenstein AJ, Sachar DB: Pyogenic and amebic abscesses of the liver. Semin Liver Dis 8:210, 1988. *Concise summary of clinical features, diagnosis, and current recommendations for treatment of pyogenic and amebic liver abscesses.*

Harrington PL, Gutierrez JJ, Ramirez-Rhondra CH, et al.: Granulomatous hepatitis. Rev Infect Dis 4:638, 1982. *Complete review of disorders associated with hepatic granulomas.*

Schneiderman DJ: Hepatobiliary abnormalities of AIDS. Gastroenterol Clin North Am 17:615, 1988. *Complete review of infectious agents causing liver and biliary tract disease in patients with AIDS, with a summary of the recent literature.*

Thaler M, Pastakia B, Shawker TH, et al.: Hepatic candidiasis in cancer patients: The evolving picture of the syndrome. Ann Intern Med 108:88, 1988. *Presentation, diagnosis, and treatment of eight patients with hepatic candidiasis, and review of 60 patients in the literature.*

121 Inherited, Infiltrative, and Metabolic Disorders Involving the Liver

Bruce F. Scharschmidt

The liver is involved in a variety of inherited, infiltrative, and metabolic disorders. Most of the disorders included in this chapter, e.g., Wilson's disease, hemochromatosis, the glycogen and lipid storage diseases, and amyloidosis, are discussed here only with respect to their hepatic involvement. A more comprehensive treatment of these entities can be found elsewhere in this textbook.

ALPHA₁-ANTITRYPSIN DEFICIENCY

Alpha$_1$-antitrypsin (A_1AT) deficiency is an inherited disorder associated with a decreased concentration of A_1AT in serum (see Ch. 58). This glycoprotein, which is found in other body fluids as well as in serum, inhibits a variety of proteolytic enzymes, including pancreatic trypsin, chymotrypsin, and elastase, as well as certain proteases produced by macrophages and leukocytes, in particular neutrophil elastase. It is produced primarily by the liver and released into the bloodstream, where it is normally present in a concentration of about 200 mg per deciliter and accounts for 90 per cent of total antitrypsin activity and a major portion of the α_1-globulin fraction.

A_1AT production is controlled by codominant alleles, with about 75 different alleles identified. There are four common (normal) "M" alleles. They differ from each other by a single amino acid substitution, have a collective allele frequency of about 0.95 in the United States, and are associated with normal plasma A_1AT levels. The deficiency state results from mutations that cause the A_1AT gene to encode for defective proteins. Homozygous and heterozygous combinations of at least 17 different mutations are associated with abnormally low serum levels and an increased risk of emphysema (Ch. 58), but only a subset of these mutant alleles (the "Z" allele, in particular) is associated with liver disease.

The pathogeneses of lung and liver disease in patients with A_1AT deficiency appear to differ from each other. Lung disease likely results from the deficiency state per se, possibly due to the lack of inhibition of neutrophil elastase. Liver disease, associated only with alleles encoding for proteins that cannot be effectively secreted, likely results from accumulation of defective α_1-antitrypsin within the endoplasmic reticulum of hepatocytes. This is supported by the observations that transgenic mice that express the abnormal human Z gene develop liver disease despite the presence of normal endogenous A₁AT levels and that patients with the "null" phenotype who have no α_1-antitrypsin in serum or in hepatocytes do not develop liver disease.

The presence of the mutant genes is not, by itself, sufficient to produce disease. Only up to 10 per cent of individuals with P₁ZZ phenotype develop overt liver disease in childhood and have signs and symptoms of cholestasis in the first few days to weeks of life. In a minority of infants, cholestasis persists or worsens and is associated with liver failure and death in a few years. Cholestasis typically remits by 6 months in the remaining patients, about half of whom nevertheless develop cirrhosis. The long-term prognosis for these children is uncertain. An as yet undefined proportion of infants with P₁ZZ phenotype who do not develop neonatal cholestasis have also been shown to have elevated transaminase levels in serum and fibrosis or cirrhosis on liver biopsy. Severe deficiency, P₁ZZ phenotype, is associated with a several-fold increase in the risk of developing both cirrhosis and hepatocellular carcinoma, particularly in males. Heterozygous A₁AT deficiency (phenotypes MZ and SZ) may also be associated with an increased incidence of liver disease and cancer, although the link is less clear than for severe deficiency.

The diagnosis of A₁AT deficiency is made by measurement of A₁AT in serum either as trypsin inhibitory activity or by immunoassay. Individuals with heterozygous A₁AT deficiency may have serum levels of A₁AT in the low normal range. More definitive diagnosis requires determination of protease inhibitor phenotype by isoelectric focusing, and genotype can be determined using molecular biologic techniques including polymerase chain reaction to identify specific alleles. On liver biopsy, patients with the Z allele, with or without liver disease, also exhibit characteristic rounded eosinophilic cytoplasmic inclusions in periportal hepatocytes. These inclusion bodies are immunologically related to A₁AT but differ in certain amino acids as well as in their content of sialic acid and other sugars. Importantly, such eosinophilic inclusions occur as an apparently acquired defect in patients with alcoholic liver disease and are thus not diagnostic of inherited A₁AT deficiency.

There is currently no specific therapy for patients with A₁AT deficiency and liver disease. While direct administration of A₁AT or gene therapy to increase serum levels may help prevent or retard lung disease, it is unlikely to prevent liver disease. Liver transplantation (Ch. 124) should be considered in patients with progressive deterioration in hepatic function. Following transplantation, serum A₁AT levels increase and assume the genotype of the donor.

WILSON'S DISEASE

Wilson's disease is an autosomal recessive disorder with a prevalence worldwide of about 1 in 30,000 (Ch. 192). Its clinical and pathologic manifestations result from excessive accumulation of copper in many tissues, including the brain, liver, cornea, and kidneys. The abnormal gene responsible for Wilson's disease is on chromosome 13 and is manifested as impaired hepatic excretion of copper into bile, which is the cause of the copper accumulation. Unfortunately the diagnosis of this treatable disorder is often missed or delayed because of its rarity and diverse presentations. Hepatic disease is a common initial clinical manifestation in childhood and adolescence and may take the form of a self-limited illness resembling viral hepatitis, fulminant hepatic failure, or chronic active hepatitis; thus, biochemical screening for Wilson's disease is imperative in all patients under the age of 35 years who have liver disease of uncertain etiology. Biochemical clues to the presence of Wilson's disease include an alkaline phosphatase to bilirubin ratio of <2 and AST to ALT ratio of >4. Hemolysis represents an important clinical clue to the presence of Wilson's disease and predisposes to the development of cholelithiasis. Neurologic manifestations typically appear between the ages of 12 and 30 years and are almost invariably accompanied by the presence of Kayser-Fleischer rings.

The diagnosis and treatment of Wilson's disease are discussed in detail in Ch. 192; however, certain points merit special emphasis here. First, while the combination of an abnormally low ceruloplasmin level in serum and Kayser-Fleischer rings establishes the diagnosis, about 15 per cent of patients having Wilson's disease presenting with hepatic manifestations have serum ceruloplasmin concentrations in the low normal range, and low concentrations are seen in some heterozygotes as well as in occasional patients with severe hepatic dysfunction but without Wilson's disease. Moreover, about one half of patients who seek medical help with chronic active hepatitis or fulminant hepatic failure have not yet developed Kayser-Fleischer rings. If the diagnosis of Wilson's disease is uncertain, a liver biopsy should be performed for quantitative copper determination. If coagulation abnormalities preclude a biopsy, measurement of incorporation of orally administered radiolabeled copper into ceruloplasmin or measurement of serum copper or urinary copper excretion may be useful. Finally, patients with hepatic failure due to Wilson's disease frequently do not respond to chelation therapy, and liver transplantation should be considered. Because the genetic defect is expressed in the liver, successfully transplanted patients are effectively "cured" of their disease.

HEMOCHROMATOSIS

Hemochromatosis is among the more common genetic disorders, with a calculated homozygous frequency of about 1 in 300 to 1 in 400 in certain high-prevalence areas. The molecular basis of the underlying defect responsible for enhanced intestinal iron absorption remains undetermined. Males homozygous for the hemochromatosis allele, which is in close linkage with HLA-A3 on chromosome 6, show progressive accumulation of hepatic iron, and clinical evidence of disease usually develops in the fourth, fifth, or sixth decades of life. Most homozygous females do not develop clinical evidence of disease, presumably because of iron loss through menses and pregnancy. Heterozygotes may also show abnormal accumulation of hepatic iron, but the absolute amounts present are much less than in homozygotes, and clinical evidence of iron overload rarely develops.

Hepatic iron overload is most commonly manifested as moderate to marked hepatomegaly with initially well-preserved liver function. Esophageal varices, ascites, and impaired hepatic synthetic function are present in more advanced cases. Other important clinical features include abnormal skin pigmentation, glucose intolerance, cardiac involvement, hypogonadism, and arthropathy. Hepatocellular carcinoma develops in up to one third of patients. These classic manifestations are present in only a minority of homozygotes. Indeed, there is considerable variability in the expression of the disorder, and some homozygotes never develop overt disease. With appropriate phlebotomy therapy hepatic function frequently improves, and there are case reports that suggest regression of apparent cirrhosis.

Screening for hemochromatosis is probably best accomplished by measurement of transferrin saturation and serum ferritin. A saturation exceeding 50 per cent is present in nearly all homozygotes over 20 years of age, and a value less than 50 per cent largely precludes the diagnosis. However, the positive predictive value of a transferrin saturation exceeding 50 per cent is relatively low. In contrast, a transferrin saturation exceeding 80 per cent is a more reliable indicator of hemochromatosis, and a large study in Utah suggests that a transferrin saturation greater than 62 per cent most reliably separates homozygotes from heterozygotes and normal persons. Serum levels of ferritin are a generally accurate reflection of tissue iron stores and exceed 1000 ng per ml in most patients. However, occasional families with hemochromatosis and normal serum ferritin levels have been described and, conversely, serum ferritin is typically increased out of proportion to tissue iron stores in patients with hepatocellular necrosis. If either of these tests suggests iron overload, liver biopsy with quantitative iron determination and histochemical stains for iron should be performed.

Patients with alcohol-induced liver injury frequently have an abnormally elevated transferrin saturation and serum ferritin level and therefore represent a problem in differential diagnosis. Liver biopsies in such patients typically demonstrate hepatic iron levels well below those seen in patients with genetic hemochromatosis, and these patients are not benefited by phlebotomy. Conversely, an abnormally elevated hepatic iron level is indicative of genetic hemochromatosis, irrespective of a history of alcohol abuse.

A variety of noninvasive methods for measurement of hepatic iron have been proposed for use in patients who cannot undergo a liver biopsy. Dual-energy computed tomography appears particularly promising, and nuclear magnetic resonance and magnetic susceptibility measurement are also undergoing evaluation. Hemochromatosis is discussed in detail in Ch. 193.

STORAGE DISEASES

The *glycogen storage diseases* may present as disorders of the liver as well as of the heart and musculoskeletal system. Hepatomegaly is a prominent feature of most of these disorders, whereas splenomegaly is found primarily in type IV and less commonly in type III. Most of these disorders are not distinguishable on clinical grounds, and tissue analysis for glycogen content and enzyme activity are required for definitive diagnosis. Patients with type I or III glycogen storage disease frequently survive childhood and may be encountered by the physician treating adults. Patients with type I glycogen storage disease have an increased incidence of hepatic adenoma as well as hepatocellular carcinoma. Portacaval anastomosis may improve growth and reverse certain metabolic abnormalities in selected type I patients, although the mechanism for these beneficial effects is uncertain. Cirrhosis invariably develops in patients with type IV disease, as well as some patients with type III. The glycogen storage diseases are discussed in detail in Ch. 169. In addition to glycogen, the liver abnormally stores fatty acids, cholesterol, or complex lipids in the lipid storage disorders as well as various mucopolysaccharides and mucolipids. Although hepatomegaly is common to most of these disorders, the clinical consequences are attributable to involvement of the nervous and musculoskeletal systems.

PROTOPORPHYRIA

Protoporphyria is a disorder characterized by increased protoporphyrin content in erythrocytes, plasma, feces, and liver. It is usually classified as an autosomal dominant trait and results from a deficiency of heme synthase (ferrochelatase), the enzyme that catalyzes the formation of heme from protoporphyrin and iron. It is most conveniently diagnosed by demonstrating an elevated level of erythrocyte protoporphyrin. Protoporphyria is usually manifested by mild photosensitivity and, rarely, hemolysis. Hepatobiliary complications include pigment gallstones and, in less than 30 reported cases, hepatic failure. The hepatic failure, typically heralded by cholestasis, is associated with and presumably results from massive hepatic accumulation of birefringent crystals of protoporphyrin. Interruption of the enterohepatic circulation of protoporphyrin with cholestyramine or activated charcoal has been reported to deplete hepatic protoporphyrin deposits and restore liver function to normal in some patients with mild disease. Oral iron therapy has also been reported to decrease protoporphyrin production. The value of such treatments in patients with severe cholestasis and established hepatic failure is unknown, however, and hepatic transplantation should be considered in such instances. At present there is no way of identifying the small proportion of patients with protoporphyria who will develop significant hepatic disease.

CYSTIC FIBROSIS

In infants with cystic fibrosis, amorphous eosinophilic material in bile ducts and ductules, presumably representing inspissated secretions, may produce cholestasis (Ch. 64). Later manifestations include cholangitis, fibrosis, and obstructive biliary cirrhosis. Up to 20 per cent of patients who survive to adolescence have cirrhosis with portal hypertension, and bleeding from esophageal varices represents a significant cause of morbidity in this older age group. Patients who have bled from varices and have good pulmonary function are candidates for shunt surgery. Since liver disease with portal hypertension has even been reported as a first manifestation of cystic fibrosis, the diagnosis should be considered in a young patient with otherwise unexplained liver disease.

AMYLOIDOSIS

Amyloid deposition in the liver is common in amyloidosis of all types (Ch. 156). Hepatomegaly is present in approximately one half of patients with systemic amyloidosis; splenomegaly is present in about 10 per cent of patients; and mild elevation of the serum alkaline phosphatase is the most common biochemical abnormality. Cutaneous stigmata of chronic liver disease (e.g., spider angiomas, palmar erythema) and portal hypertension are unusual. Intrahepatic cholestasis with marked elevation of the serum bilirubin and alkaline phosphatase concentrations occurs in about 5 per cent of patients. The diagnosis of amyloidosis can usually be established without resorting to liver biopsy.

SARCOIDOSIS

Hepatic involvement in sarcoidosis represents a continuum from the presence of asymptomatic granulomas to cases in which hepatic involvement represents a prominent part of the overall clinical picture (Ch. 67). Approximately two thirds to three quarters of patients with sarcoidosis have hepatic granulomas, making the liver one of the most commonly involved organs in this disease, and liver biopsy is often of value in establishing the diagnosis of sarcoidosis.

About 20 per cent of patients with sarcoidosis have hepatomegaly. A higher proportion have abnormal liver function tests, most commonly elevation of alkaline phosphatase. Overt hepatic involvement is present in fewer than 20 per cent of patients. This may take several forms, including (1) hepatomegaly, generally with splenomegaly, and multiple abnormal liver function tests; (2) portal hypertension and its manifestations; and (3) chronic cholestasis, which may closely mimic primary biliary cirrhosis. Primary biliary cirrhosis can usually be distinguished from sarcoidosis based on the absence of systemic disease and presence of antimitochondrial antibody. The characteristic histologic feature of hepatic sarcoidosis is the presence of granulomas, frequently located in portal tracts. Chronic portal tract inflammation, hepatocyte poikilocytosis and anisocytosis, fibrosis, and even cirrhosis may be accompanying findings. Fever and systemic symptoms typically respond to corticosteroid treatment. It is less certain whether corticosteroids retard hepatic fibrosis and progression to portal hypertension, but a therapeutic trial is justified if significant symptoms are present and tuberculosis and other disorders producing hepatic granuloma have been excluded.

ENTERIC BYPASS

Hepatic disease related to enteric bypass surgery has typically been reported in patients who have had extensive bypass procedures for treatment of marked obesity. Jejunocolic bypass, an early operation, has now largely been abandoned because of a high incidence of complications, including cirrhosis and hepatic failure. Hepatic abnormalities are also common following jejunoileal bypass and may take several forms. Fatty change is present in up to two thirds of markedly obese patients prior to bypass surgery, and hepatic lipid content increases during the period of weight loss. Cirrhosis ensues in up to 5 per cent of patients, and death from liver failure accounts for a substantial proportion of the early postoperative mortality of 2 to 4 per cent. Histologic features may mimic those of alcoholic liver disease, including the presence of alcoholic hyalin. Longer-term follow-up studies suggest that hepatic abnormalities may not appear until several years after surgery in some patients.

The pathogenesis of these hepatic changes is unclear. Weight loss itself does not account for the progressive postoperative fat accumulation, since this does not occur in nonoperated obese patients who lose weight through dietary measures. However, hepatic disease resembling alcoholic hepatitis and even cirrhosis have been described in abstinent patients with obesity who have not undergone bypass surgery. Protein depletion, leading to a kwashiorkor-like state, may contribute to the fatty change. Increased production in the gut of potentially toxic substances may also play a role. For example, increased delivery of chenodeoxycholate to the colon results in increased production of the potentially hepatotoxic bile salt, lithocholate. The bypassed segment may also serve as a site for bacterial overgrowth and production of potentially toxic bacterial products.

Laboratory studies of hepatic function are frequently abnormal in the first few postoperative months following bypass surgery even in the absence of serious liver disease. Conversely, the absence of abnormal hepatic function tests or clinical evidence of liver disease during the first postoperative year does not preclude the possible later development of significant liver disease. Deterioration of synthetic or excretory function as evidenced by an abnormal prothrombin time that does not respond to vitamin K administration, hypoalbuminemia, or hyperbilirubinemia is an ominous sign. Biopsy is the only reliable way of assessing the severity of hepatic disease, and some advocate follow-up biopsies in all patients. Serious and persistent hepatic disease is an indication for re-establishing normal bowel continuity, which may be required in up to 25 per cent of patients. Currently, alternative procedures such as gastroplasty, which are associated with fewer hepatic and metabolic complications, are preferred in the morbidly obese patients.

INFLAMMATORY BOWEL DISEASE

Liver function tests may be transiently abnormal in up to one half of patients with chronic ulcerative colitis and less commonly in Crohn's disease, but significant and persistent biochemical abnormalities are present in fewer than 10 per cent of patients (Ch. 103).

A variety of hepatic abnormalities occur in patients with inflammatory bowel disease, the most important of which is *primary sclerosing cholangitis* (PSC). With increasing use of direct cholangiography, bile duct abnormalities characteristic of PSC have been identified in up to 5 per cent of patients with ulcerative colitis (much less commonly in Crohn's disease), and many hepatic histopathologic abnormalities in these patients appear to be manifestations of PSC. *Pericholangitis*, a histologic diagnosis, denotes a spectrum of acute and chronic portal tract changes including edema, inflammatory infiltration, bile duct damage, periductal and periportal fibrosis, and cirrhosis. Most patients with these findings have radiologic evidence of PSC. In those patients without abnormalities in radiologically demonstrable ducts, pericholangitis may represent *small duct sclerosing cholangitis*. Although PSC has been postulated to be secondary to inflammatory bowel disease or to the accompanying presence of bacteria or other toxins in portal blood, the high frequency of HLA-B8 and -DR3 in PSC and occasional association with thyroiditis implicate an immune pathogenesis in genetically predisposed individuals. There is evidence that more than 90 per cent of patients with PSC have, or will develop, ulcerative colitis. Apart from the tendency of PSC to accompany inflammatory bowel disease with extensive colonic involvement, there is no clear relationship between the severity of PSC and the accompanying inflammatory bowel disease. Similarly, treatment of the inflammatory bowel or colectomy does not predictably alter the course of PSC.

Patients with radiologically documented PSC have highly variable biochemical and clinical manifestations ranging from asymptomatic, in which case the disorder may be accompanied only by elevation of alkaline phosphatase activity, to deeply jaundiced with clinical and biochemical features of cirrhosis and hepatic decompensation. Although a variety of medical and surgical treatments have been tried, none has been proven to be effective for this disorder, and liver transplantation should be considered for patients with advanced disease.

Chronic active hepatitis also occurs in patients with inflammatory bowel disease, but the histologic changes of PSC can mimic those of chronic active hepatitis, and the latter diagnosis should not be made unless a cholangiogram is normal. Even then, the distinction between small duct PSC and chronic active hepatitis is difficult. Other hepatic abnormalities in patients with inflammatory bowel disease include fatty liver (which often parallels disease severity), amyloidosis (present in a small percentage of patients with Crohn's disease), and cholangiocarcinoma (closely linked to PSC).

TOTAL PARENTERAL NUTRITION

Total parenteral nutrition has been associated with a spectrum of hepatic abnormalities, including mild elevations in alkaline phosphatase and transaminase levels, cholestasis with jaundice, and, rarely, progressive hepatic disease resulting in death. Liver biopsy in these patients has frequently revealed fatty change, cholestasis, and mild periportal inflammation, with fibrosis or cirrhosis found in a minority. Some of these abnormalities have been due to the underlying disease or complicating infection, but total parenteral nutrition, by itself, can produce elevated serum bile salt levels and occasionally hyperbilirubinemia in both infants

and adults. The degree of abnormality appears related to the duration, type, and amount of parenteral alimentation. In infants, cholestasis associated with parenteral nutrition also increases in frequency with decreasing gestational age and birth weight, and adults with the short-bowel syndrome appear particularly at risk for severe liver disease. Hepatic function generally returns gradually to normal after total parenteral nutrition is discontinued. Modifying the infusate by lowering the calorie:nitrogen ratio or decreasing the total caloric intake has reportedly produced improvement in some patients, but this has not been systematically studied, and no one component of the parenteral formula has been clearly implicated as causative. Total parenteral nutrition also appears to predispose patients to the development of gallstones and both calculous and acalculous cholecystitis, and these possibilities should be kept in mind when one is evaluating a patient receiving parenteral nutrition for hepatobiliary disease.

In patients with mild biochemical abnormalities, adjustments in the infusion regimen may be helpful, including increasing the proportion of nonprotein calories supplied as lipid (versus glucose) or cyclic parenteral nutrition, in which the infusion is stopped for 8 to 12 hours per day. Copper and manganese, which are secreted in bile, should be decreased or eliminated in patients with cholestasis. Progressive liver disease in patients requiring chronic parenteral nutrition is a serious problem. While alteration of the infusion regimen or antibiotics such as metronidazole to alter gut flora may be tried, their usefulness is unproven. Finally, daily stimulation of gallbladder contraction by infusion of cholecystokinin or (if possible) oral administration of lipid and protein meals may be useful in preventing complications with biliary stasis.

PREGNANCY

Liver size and liver histology remain normal during uncomplicated pregnancy. Serum levels of alkaline phosphatase and leucine aminopeptidase typically rise in the second and third trimesters and are of placental origin; aminotransferase and bilirubin levels are normal.

EFFECT OF PREGNANCY ON COEXISTING LIVER DISEASE. In the United States and Western Europe, pregnancy does not appear to alter the course of acute viral hepatitis. In underdeveloped countries, however, an epidemic form of non-A, non-B viral hepatitis appears to run a more severe course in pregnancy, particularly during the third trimester, and is associated with an unusually high incidence of fulminant hepatic failure with high fetal and maternal mortality. Pregnancy has not been shown to alter the course of chronic persistent or chronic active hepatitis, although maternal and fetal morbidity and mortality may be increased because of variceal bleeding and postpartum hemorrhage. Vertical transmission of hepatitis B virus infection occurs commonly when the mother contracts acute hepatitis B during the third trimester or is a chronic carrier (particularly if she also is HBeAg positive), and it is important that the infant receive appropriate passive and active prophylaxis at delivery (Ch. 117).

LIVER DISEASES ASSOCIATED WITH PREGNANCY. *Hyperemesis gravidarum* of sufficient severity to require hospitalization may be accompanied by minor abnormalities in standard liver function tests. *Acute fatty liver of pregnancy* can be defined as a syndrome of acute hepatic dysfunction that develops in late pregnancy, is associated with microvesicular fat accumulation in hepatocytes, and resolves with delivery. It is more common in twin gestations and is associated with pre-eclampsia in up to one half of cases. It typically becomes apparent after the 30th week of gestation and is manifested initially by constitutional symptoms, often with abdominal pain, followed in many instances by overt evidence of hepatic failure, including encephalopathy and jaundice. In the past, intravenous tetracycline therapy was incriminated in some cases, but this is rarely true at present. The only known treatment is termination of the pregnancy. Early reports suggested that the disorder was associated with a very high mortality rate, but more recent reports suggest that there is a spectrum of disease severity and that milder cases without frank hepatic failure occur and have a favorable prognosis. At least 15 women who survived this disorder have had normal subsequent pregnancies. It also appears that acute fatty liver may, at least in some instances, fall within the spectrum of hepatic dysfunction associated with *pre-eclampsia* or *eclampsia*, as these two disorders occasionally share certain features, including onset in late pregnancy, increased incidence in young primiparas, the presence of coagulopathy, hypertension, and proteinuria, and resolution upon delivery. Focal necrosis and, rarely, hepatic rupture may occur in women with *eclampsia. Cholestasis of pregnancy* generally occurs in the last 4 months of gestation (range 27 to 39 weeks). It is characterized by pruritus, sometimes followed by jaundice. It typically resolves within 2 weeks of delivery and frequently recurs in subsequent pregnancies or with administration of oral contraceptives. Serum alkaline phosphatase and bile salts are increased, and hyperbilirubinemia may be present. Serum transaminase is also frequently mildly increased. Although generally considered a benign condition, cholestasis of pregnancy has been associated with an increased incidence of premature labor and postpartum hemorrhage.

CIRCULATORY DISTURBANCE

Hepatic function and histology are commonly altered in patients with cardiovascular disease. Disorders associated with an elevation of systemic venous pressure typically produce hepatic venous congestion manifested by hepatomegaly, minor abnormalities of liver function tests, and centrolobular congestion without necrosis. Longstanding hepatic congestion may lead to cardiac cirrhosis with fibrous bands joining centrilobular areas (Ch. 122). When hypotension is superimposed, even transiently, on hepatic congestion, severe centrilobular to midzonal necrosis, transaminase levels exceeding 1000 units, marked hyperbilirubinemia, and hypoprothrombinemia may result. Differentiating this disorder from viral hepatitis may be difficult, since the clinical features are similar and hepatic dysfunction often is not recognized until several days after the resolution of the circulatory failure. Unlike viral hepatitis, however, serum transaminase levels frequently fall very rapidly and may approach normal within days. If the circulatory insult is brief, patients usually recover from their hepatic injury uneventfully. Fatal fulminant hepatic failure has been reported, however. A similar form of acute hepatic injury is occasionally seen in persons without pre-existing cardiovascular disease who suffer severe or prolonged hypotension or in patients with severe isolated left-sided heart failure.

Adams PC, Halliday JW, Powell LW: Early diagnosis and treatment of hemochromatosis. Adv Intern Med 34 111, 1989. *A comprehensive review with a practical orientation.*

Crystal RG: Alpha-1-antitrypsin deficiency, emphysema and liver disease: Genetic basis and strategies for therapy. J Clin Invest (In press, 1990). *A thoroughly referenced and current review which focuses on the pathogenesis and prospects for treatment.*

Faloon WW: Hepatobiliary effects of obesity and weight-reducing surgery. Semin Liver Dis 8:229, 1988. *A concise review with 77 references.*

Klein S, Nealon WH: Hepatobiliary abnormalities associated with total parenteral nutrition. Semin Liver Dis 8:237, 1986. *A well-written review dealing with practical aspects of diagnosis and management.*

Shrumpf E, Fausa O, Elgjo K, et al.: Hepatobiliary complications of inflammatory bowel disease. Semin Liver Dis 8:201, 1988. *A well-referenced review focusing in particular on primary sclerosing cholangitis and its pathologic and clinical manifestations.*

Smith LH Jr: Overview of hemochromatosis. West J Med 153:296, 1990.

van Theil DH: Effects of pregnancy and sex hormones on the liver. Semin Liver Dis 7:1, 1987. *An entire volume with eight chapters covering various liver problems associated with pregnancy and steroid hormones.*

122 Cirrhosis of the Liver and Its Major Sequelae

Thomas D. Boyer

GENERAL CONSIDERATIONS. Cirrhosis is an irreversible alteration of the liver architecture, consisting of hepatic fibrosis and areas of nodular regeneration. When the nodules are small (less than 3 mm), uniform, and encompass one lobule, the term micronodular or unilobular cirrhosis is applied. In macronodular or multilobular cirrhosis the nodules exceed 3 mm, vary in size, and encompass more than one lobule. Frequently, features of both micronodular and macronodular cirrhosis are present in the same liver. Etiologic diagnosis may be impossible from the gross and microscopic appearance of the cirrhotic liver and must therefore be based on history, physical examination, biochemical and serologic tests, and histochemical stains. The causes of cirrhosis are listed in Table 122–1.

Patients with cirrhosis may have one of two general types of manifestations: (1) signs or symptoms related to hepatocellular necrosis, which are similar to those of acute hepatitis and include jaundice, nausea and vomiting, and tender hepatomegaly; or (2) signs or symptoms of the complications of cirrhosis, which are largely due to the rise in intrahepatic vascular resistance that leads to portal hypertension and its complications (ascites, formation of portal-systemic collaterals, encephalopathy, splenomegaly, and bleeding esophageal and gastric varices). Other, less specific manifestations of cirrhosis include gynecomastia, spider angiomas, parotid hypertrophy, and testicular atrophy. Patients frequently present a mixed picture with features of both hepatocellular necrosis and portal hypertension.

Agents that cause cirrhosis may have systemic effects as well. Extrahepatic features may dominate the clinical picture with little or no evidence of liver disease. For example, patients with alcoholic liver disease frequently have complaints referable to the central nervous system, peripheral nerves, heart, muscles, and gastrointestinal tract. Patients with disease such as primary biliary cirrhosis may have prominent eye and skin disorders. Patients with hemochromatosis may present with diabetes mellitus or arthritis, and patients with Wilson's disease, with central nervous system dysfunction, before liver disease becomes apparent. Thus, cirrhosis is frequently a subclinical illness, and a high index of suspicion may be necessary to establish a correct diagnosis.

ALCOHOLIC LIVER DISEASE

DEFINITION AND INCIDENCE. Alcoholic liver disease, a frequent and serious sequela of the chronic abuse of ethanol, occurs singly or intermingled in three forms: *fatty liver, alcoholic hepatitis*, and *cirrhosis*. Alcohol is the most common cause of liver disease in the Western world. Alcoholic cirrhosis is discovered in 1.6 to 9.9 per cent of all necropsies in the United States. The peak incidence is in patients 40 to 55 years of age; however, patients in their 20's may be seen with advanced alcoholic liver disease. The male to female ratio is 2:1.

ETIOLOGY AND PATHOGENESIS. *The relationship between alcohol abuse and cirrhosis* is well established. The incidence of cirrhosis and the per capita consumption of alcohol are directly related; countries with the greatest alcohol consumption also have the highest incidence of cirrhosis. Neither the pattern

TABLE 122–1. CAUSES OF CIRRHOSIS

Drugs and Toxins	Metabolic
Alcohol	Wilson's disease
Methyldopa	Hemochromatosis
Methotrexate	Erythropoietic protoporphyria
Isoniazid	Pediatric—α_1-antitrypsin
Perhexiline maleate	deficiency, galactosemia,
Amiodarone	hereditary fructose
Oxyphenisatin	intolerance, glycogen storage
Vitamin A	disease type IV, tyrosinosis
Carbon tetrachloride	**Cardiovascular**
Infections	Chronic right heart failure
Hepatitis B and C	Budd-Chiari syndrome
Syphilis (tertiary)	Veno-occlusive disease
Schistosoma japonicum	**Miscellaneous**
Biliary Obstruction	Chronic active hepatitis
Carcinoma (pancreatic or bile duct)	Primary biliary cirrhosis
Chronic pancreatitis	Sarcoidosis
Common duct stones	Jejunoileal bypass
Strictures	Neonatal hepatitis
Cystic fibrosis	Indian childhood cirrhosis
Biliary atresia	Hereditary hemorrhagic telangiectasia
Sclerosing cholangitis	**Cryptogenic**

of drinking (spree versus daily) nor the type of alcoholic beverage consumed appears to be important in the genesis of liver disease. The single most important factor is the average daily consumption of ethanol. Levels of daily ethanol consumption exceeding 40 to 80 grams (36 to 72 oz of beer, 4.5 to 9 oz liquor, 15 to 30 oz of wine) for 10 to 15 years are associated with an increase in the incidence of cirrhosis. Women may be more susceptible to the toxic effects of ethanol than men, and a lower (20 grams) daily consumption of ethanol by women may lead to cirrhosis. As the daily level of alcohol consumed rises, the time required for the development of cirrhosis is reduced.

Ethanol is a hepatotoxin. Administration of alcohol to humans or animals leads to the development of fatty liver (hepatic steatosis). The mitochondria and endoplasmic reticulum of hepatocytes are altered morphologically and functionally. Many of the effects of ethanol reflect its metabolism, which is catalyzed primarily by the cytosolic enzyme alcohol dehydrogenase as shown:

$$CH_3CH_2OH \xrightarrow[\text{NAD} \longrightarrow \text{NADH + H}^+]{\text{Alcohol dehydrogenase}} CH_3CHO$$
Ethanol   Acetaldehyde

(Other metabolic pathways via a microsomal ethanol oxidizing system or a catalase system appear to be of minor importance, except perhaps at high ethanol concentrations.) The acetaldehyde formed from ethanol is then oxidized to acetate by acetaldehyde dehydrogenase with NAD^+ as a cofactor. The lack of the active high-affinity form of acetaldehyde dehydrogenase (50 per cent of Japanese) leads to high blood levels of acetaldehyde following ethanol ingestion. The high levels of acetaldehyde in these individuals are associated with flushing, vasodilatation, tachycardia, and aversion to ethanol. A similar but more severe reaction is seen in patients who ingest ethanol while taking the acetaldehyde dehydrogenase inhibitor disulfiram. The limiting step in the rate of metabolism of ethanol is the availability of the cofactor NAD^+, which is converted to NADH during the aforementioned two reactions. This increased reducing potential in the cell favors the conversion of pyruvate to lactate. When blood levels of ethanol are high (more than 200 mg per deciliter), the resulting lactic acidemia decreases the clearance of urate by the kidneys and hyperuricemia develops. Inhibition of gluconeogenesis and fasting hypoglycemia may also follow ethanol abuse (Ch. 114). Fatty acid oxidation is impaired, and the esterification of fatty acids to triglycerides is increased. The latter effects, acting in concert with less well defined events, lead to the development of a fatty liver. Chronic use of ethanol also leads to an increase in the activity of some P-450 isozymes, and alcoholics may manifest altered metabolism of drugs that are normally degraded by these P-450 isozymes (Ch. 24).

The metabolic effects of ethanol are relatively well understood, but the mechanism by which it causes chronic liver disease is not. There is evidence for impaired protein synthesis and secretion, mitochondrial injury, lipid peroxidation, interaction of acetaldehyde with cellular proteins and membrane lipids, cellular hypoxia, and cell-mediated and antibody-mediated cytotoxicity, but the relative importance of each of these in producing sustained cell injury is unknown.

Ethanol fed to animals receiving an otherwise balanced diet has not been shown to cause alcoholic hepatitis. In addition, only 10 to 20 per cent of alcoholics and about 30 per cent of ethanol-fed baboons develop cirrhosis despite similar levels of ethanol ingestion. Thus, *genetic, nutritional,* or *environmental* factors may act in concert with ethanol to cause liver disease.

Malnutrition is a common finding in alcoholics who have both poor diet and reduced intestinal absorption of dietary nutrients. Lesions identical to those of alcoholic hepatitis may develop following jejunoileal bypass for obesity, a condition in which protein malnutrition is common. Thus, malnutrition appears to potentiate the adverse effects of alcohol. Other factors, such as simultaneous exposure to other hepatotoxins, may also be important in the genesis of liver injury. For example, because of the effects of alcohol on drug metabolism, alcoholics are more susceptible to injury by direct hepatotoxins such as acetaminophen. Alcoholism and alcoholic liver disease are more common in certain populations, in twins, and within families, but there is no evidence of a genetically determined abnormality in the metabolism of ethanol that renders them more susceptible to liver injury.

DIAGNOSIS. The diagnosis of alcoholic liver disease should be considered in any patient who consumes more than 40 grams of ethanol daily. Tender hepatomegaly, fever, and jaundice are suggestive of alcoholic hepatitis, whereas ascites and venous collaterals suggest cirrhosis. Many patients, however, lack any distinctive clinical features such that a firm diagnosis cannot be established without liver biopsy. In addition, up to 20 per cent of patients with clinical features of alcoholic liver disease are found on liver biopsy to have another type of hepatic disorder.

PATHOLOGY, CLINICAL PRESENTATION, AND THERAPY. Alcohol causes three major pathologic lesions and clinical illnesses: *fatty liver, alcoholic hepatitis, and cirrhosis.* Each of these may occur as an isolated event, or they may be present in any combination in a single patient. Therefore, although the three lesions are described as single entities, many patients have all three and have a mixed clinical picture. The histologic pattern is not specific for alcohol alone but may also be found in the livers of patients who have undergone jejunoileal bypass for obesity or as an unusual accompaniment of obesity or diabetes mellitus. Patients treated with the vasodilator perhexiline maleate or the antiarrhythmic drug amiodarone also may develop a lesion identical to alcoholic liver disease (Ch. 118).

Fatty Liver. Fatty liver is the most common biopsy finding in alcoholics. The fat, either centrilobular or diffuse in location, is present in large droplets, which occupy most of the volume of the hepatocyte. Occasionally the fat is present in small droplets, resembling the lesion of Reye's syndrome or fatty liver of pregnancy. Patients with fatty liver are usually asymptomatic, but on occasion they may have abdominal pain, icterus, or vague gastrointestinal complaints. The liver is enlarged and may be tender but is of normal consistency. Ascites, venous collaterals, and the stigmata of chronic liver disease, if present, are not attributable to the fatty liver per se but reflect more serious lesions. The laboratory tests are only mildly abnormal in fatty liver. Jaundice, when present, is usually mild (bilirubin below 5 mg per deciliter), although intense cholestasis occasionally develops in patients with fatty liver. The AST, if elevated, is only modestly so (less than five times normal). The serum albumin and globulin levels are abnormal in about 25 per cent of patients. Patients with alcoholic fatty liver alone have an excellent prognosis unless there is fibrosis around the central veins. Withdrawal of the alcohol leads to a rapid resolution of the clinical illness and histologic lesion (fat disappears within 3 to 6 weeks). On rare occasions, these patients die suddenly from multiple fat emboli to the lungs (Ch. 66).

Alcoholic Hepatitis. Alcoholic hepatitis (acute sclerosing hyaline necrosis) is a serious sequela of alcoholism because it may lead to hepatic failure or to cirrhosis. The pathologic lesion is most severe in central areas and consists of hepatocellular necrosis and the triad of (1) *alcoholic hyalin,* (2) *infiltration by polymorphonuclear leukocytes,* and (3) *increased intralobular connective tissue* in the space of Disse and sclerosis of terminal hepatic (central) veins. Alcoholic hyalin (Mallory body), an eosinophilic intracellular aggregate of proteinaceous material characteristically perinuclear in location, is present in only 30 per cent of liver biopsies in which the diagnosis of alcoholic hepatitis can be made on clinical and other histologic criteria. Alcoholic hyalin is not specific for alcoholic liver disease, since it has also been found in the livers of patients with Wilson's disease, primary biliary cirrhosis, hepatocellular carcinoma, and diabetes mellitus, as well as following jejunoileal bypass. Central vein sclerosis may be severe enough to cause a severe outflow block and portal hypertension in the absence of cirrhosis.

The clinical features of alcoholic hepatitis range from absence of symptoms to hepatic failure. Patients commonly complain of anorexia, nausea, vomiting, abdominal pain, and weight loss. Tender hepatomegaly is present in at least 80 per cent of hospitalized patients. Ascites, jaundice, fever (temperature 37.2 to 39.4°C), splenomegaly, and encephalopathy are common but not invariable. Although fever is common, bacterial infection should be excluded, since such patients are at an increased risk for developing pneumonia, urinary tract infections, sepsis, and bacterial peritonitis. The AST is elevated frequently; however, the degree of elevation is modest (less than 10 times normal) although on occasion it can exceed 15 times normal. The ALT may be normal and is almost always less than the AST. The AST/ALT ratio frequently exceeds two. This is in contrast to viral hepatitis, in which the AST frequently exceeds 15 to 25 times normal and the ALT is equal to or greater than the AST. Hyperbilirubinemia is common (60 to 90 per cent) in alcoholic hepatitis, and it may be marked (20 to 30 mg per deciliter). The alkaline phosphatase is usually elevated to less than three times normal, but an occasional patient has a cholestatic picture in which the alkaline phosphatase is unusually high. Prolongation of the prothrombin time, hypoalbuminemia, and hyperglobulinemia may be present. The white blood cell count frequently is elevated (>10,000) and may exceed 30,000 to 40,000 per cubic millimeter. Patients with alcoholic hepatitis may develop the hepatorenal syndrome, and a rising BUN and creatinine are poor prognostic signs.

Treatment for alcoholic hepatitis is nonspecific. Patients should receive a well-balanced diet, high in calories (2500 to 3000 kcal). Protein should be included in the diets unless encephalopathy is present. Anorexia is frequent, and tube or intravenous alimentation may be necessary. Improvement in the patient's nutritional state may be associated with more rapid resolution of the liver test abnormalities; however, the effect of nutritional support on survival is unclear. Prednisone has not been shown to decrease the morbidity or mortality in patients with mild to moderate disease. Use of steroids to treat patients with severe alcoholic hepatitis is controversial and cannot be recommended on the basis of available evidence. Propylthiouracil, penicillamine, anabolic steroids, and colchicine also have been used in the treatment of alcoholic hepatitis, but without clear success.

The *prognosis* for patients with alcoholic hepatitis is much worse than for those with fatty liver. Some patients who stop drinking may have complete resolution of the lesion. In most patients, however, alcoholic hepatitis persists (with clinical improvement), progresses to diffuse fibrosis or cirrhosis, or leads to hepatic failure and death. The hospital mortality for patients with severe disease (who cannot have a biopsy or who have encephalopathy) exceeds 40 per cent, whereas for those with milder disease the expected death rate is 10 per cent or less.

Alcoholic Cirrhosis. *Alcoholic cirrhosis* usually consists of micronodules of regular size, but it can be macronodular or of a mixed type. Micronodular cirrhosis is not specific for alcoholic liver disease. Histologically, dense bands of connective tissue join portal and central areas. Scarring is most severe in the central regions, and collagen may deposit in the space of Disse. In addition, alcoholic hepatitis frequently coexists, as well as varying amounts of cholestasis, iron, and fat.

Clinically, cirrhosis is an asymptomatic disease in 10 to 20 per cent of patients. It is also commonly present in association with alcoholic hepatitis, and signs of acute liver injury may dominate the clinical picture. Patients may also have ascites, gastrointestinal bleeding, or encephalopathy, to be discussed later. The liver may be large or small and usually has a firm consistency. Spider angiomas, palmar erythema, parotid enlargement, testicular atrophy and gynnecomastia (men), menstrual irregularities (women), and muscle wasting are found frequently; however, these findings are not specific for alcoholic cirrhosis. Upper abdominal pain associated with bloody ascitic fluid, right upper quadrant bruit, or a friction rub over the liver suggests hepatocellular carcinoma.

The *laboratory abnormalities* present in patients with cirrhosis may be similar to those of alcoholic hepatitis. The AST is normal to mildly elevated, and bilirubin is only slightly increased unless the picture is complicated by alcoholic hepatitis, hemolysis, sepsis, hepatic failure, or carcinoma. Anemia is a common finding. The cause of the anemia is multifactorial, including blood loss, folate and pyridoxine deficiency, hemolysis, and the toxic effect of ethanol on the bone marrow. Hypersplenism or bone marrow suppression by ethanol may lead to thrombocytopenia or leukopenia. The serum sodium and potassium may be low in patients with ascites. Hypomagnesemia and hypophosphatemia are common, as is a mild respiratory alkalosis. The BUN and creatinine are increased in patients who have been treated with excessive diuretics or who are developing hepatorenal failure.

The *treatment* of alcoholic cirrhosis is also nonspecific. Colchicine, when used for several years, may improve survival, but further study is warranted before its use can be recommended. Deficiencies of vitamins (folate, thiamine, pyridoxine, vitamin K) and minerals (magnesium, phosphate) should be corrected. The sodium content of the diet need not be reduced unless there is sodium retention by the kidneys. Protein restriction is necessary only when there is clinical evidence of hepatic encephalopathy.

The *prognosis* for patients with alcoholic cirrhosis depends upon two features: presence of complications and continued abuse of alcohol. Patients without ascites, jaundice, or gastrointestinal bleeding have a better prognosis than those with these complications. Continued alcohol abuse reduces the expected 5-year survival to only 40 per cent, whereas it is 60 per cent or greater in those who abstain.

D'Amico G, Morabito A, Pagliaro L, et al.: Survival and prognostic indicators in compensated and decompensated cirrhosis. Dig Dis Sci 31:468, 1986. *Analysis of variables associated with a poor prognosis in alcoholic and nonalcoholic cirrhosis.*

Kershenobich D, Vargas F, Garcia-Tsao G, et al.: Colchicine in the treatment of cirrhosis of the liver. N Engl J Med 318:1709, 1988. *This paper describes the treatment of alcoholic liver disease with colchicine. The results of this study were encouraging, but the accompanying editorial should be read, as it discusses some of the difficulties with the study.*

Rothschild MA, Oratz M (eds.): Alcohol, alcoholism and alcoholic liver disease. Semin Liver Dis 8:1, 1988. *Contains a series of articles that discuss the metabolism of ethanol, the genetics of alcoholism, and the diagnosis and management of alcoholic liver disease.*

Zakim D, Boyer TD, Montgomery C: Alcoholic liver disease. *In* Zakim D, Boyer TD (eds.): Hepatology: A Textbook of Liver Disease. 2nd ed. Philadelphia, W. B. Saunders Company, 1990, pp 821–869. *A complete review of the pathogenesis, diagnosis, and treatment of alcoholic liver disease.*

PRIMARY BILIARY CIRRHOSIS

DEFINITION AND ETIOLOGY. Primary biliary cirrhosis, a cholestatic disorder, develops because of progressive destruction of small and intermediate-sized intrahepatic bile ducts. The extrahepatic biliary tree and larger intrahepatic bile ducts are patent. The cause of primary biliary cirrhosis is unknown. The injury to the bile ducts is thought to be on an immunologic basis, as there is a high frequency of serum autoantibodies, elevated levels of immunoglobulins (especially IgM), circulating immune complexes, and a reduced cell-mediated immune response in patients with this disease. In addition, the injured bile ducts are surrounded by lymphocytes and, on occasion, by granulomas. These findings, however, are nonspecific and do not establish the etiologic agent or agents responsible for the disease. Genetic factors may also be important, as the disease has been described in a mother and daughter, in siblings, and in twins. In addition, the incidence of positive tests for antimitochondrial antibodies in relatives of patients with primary biliary cirrhosis is increased. The high female preponderance suggests that estrogens or progesterone may be important in the pathogenesis of this disease.

PATHOLOGY. Primary biliary cirrhosis is characterized by progressive, nonsuppurative, destructive cholangitis, which occurs in four histopathologic stages: *ductal, ductular, scarring,* and *cirrhotic.* The lesions in the first two stages are distributed unevenly and may therefore be absent in needle biopsies of the liver. The characteristic lesion (ductal or Stage 1) consists of damaged interlobular and septal bile ducts surrounded by a dense infiltrate of lymphocytes and plasma cells. Well-formed granulomas are seen frequently near the injured bile ducts. In Stage 2 (ductular) of the disease, bile ductules proliferate and bile ducts are reduced in number. Portal fibrosis may be present or absent, and granulomata are found less often than in Stage 1. Later, as the inflammation subsides, scarring increases, most marked in portal areas with fibrous septa extending into the lobule (Stage 3). When cirrhotic (Stage 4), the liver may lose all of the characteristic lesions. Bile ducts are few in both Stages 3 and 4, and this paucity of bile ducts may be the only clue to the diagnosis of primary biliary cirrhosis. In one quarter of the cases, alcoholic hyalin is identifiable in the biopsy. Histologic features of chronic active hepatitis may also be present, leading to difficulties in diagnosis.

CLINICAL MANIFESTATIONS (Table 122–2). Ninety per cent of patients with primary biliary cirrhosis are female. The disease has been found in patients as young as 23 and as old as 72; however, the majority of patients are of ages 40 to 60. The

TABLE 122–2. CLINICAL FEATURES OF PRIMARY BILIARY CIRRHOSIS

Signs and Symptoms	Laboratory
Female preponderance (> 90%)	Antimitochondrial antibodies (> 90%)
Pruritus	Elevated alkaline phosphatase, cholesterol, IgM, serum bile acids, and bilirubin
Jaundice (late)	
Skin hyperpigmentation	
Hepatosplenomegaly	
Xanthelasma/xanthoma	**Associated Diseases**
Bleeding diathesis (vitamin K deficiency)	Sjögren's syndrome
	Scleroderma/CREST syndrome
Bone pain (osteoporosis/ osteomalacia)	Arthritis
	Autoimmune thyroiditis
Ascites/variceal hemorrhage (late)	Renal tubular acidosis

onset is usually marked by *pruritus* or by discovery of asymptomatic hepatomegaly. Sometimes the first abnormality is an elevated alkaline phosphatase noted on an automated screening panel. The itching may start during pregnancy or with the use of birth control pills. Following delivery or withdrawal of the medication, the itching usually continues; this is in contrast to *cholestasis of pregnancy*, in which pruritus resolves following parturition. Itching leads to excoriative dermatitis and thickening and darkening of the skin. Hepatomegaly and less frequently splenomegaly may be found at the time of diagnosis. *Jaundice* rarely precedes the onset of pruritus and may follow it by several years. *Portal hypertension* and *hepatic failure* are usually late events, and ascites or bleeding esophageal varices are uncommon presenting features. *Hypercholesterolemia*, secondary to the decreased biliary excretion of cholesterol, may be severe enough to produce xanthomas. *Osteomalacia* or more commonly *osteoporosis* may develop in these patients. The cause of the bone disease is incompletely understood; however, malabsorption of vitamin D and calcium are important pathogenic factors. Copper accumulates in the livers of patients with primary biliary cirrhosis because it cannot be efficiently secreted into the bile. The levels of hepatic copper may reach levels equal to those found in Wilson's disease, and rarely *Kayser-Fleischer rings* have been described.

ASSOCIATED DISEASES. Primarily biliary cirrhosis is associated with a variety of disorders. *Sjögren's syndrome* with dryness of the eyes and mouth is present in at least 70 per cent of patients when specific tests (Schirmer test, buccal biopsy, and others) are used (Ch. 263). These same patients may have hyposecretion by the pancreas. *Scleroderma* and the *CREST syndrome* (calcinosis, Reynaud's phenomenon, esophageal hypomotility, sclerodactyly, telangiectasia) are both increased in frequency in patients with primary biliary cirrhosis. The prevalence of *arthritis*, both seropositive and seronegative, is increased in these patients. *Thyroid autoantibodies* are found in about 25 per cent of patients, and in the antibody-positive patients thyroid dysfunction (primarily hypothyroidism) is common. *Renal tubular acidosis* also is present in patients with primary biliary cirrhosis. The pathogenesis of the renal tubular acidosis is unknown, but it may be secondary to deposition of copper in renal tubules. There also appears to be an increase in the frequency of breast cancer and celiac disease in these patients.

LABORATORY FINDINGS. The *alkaline phosphatase* is elevated in almost all patients with primary biliary cirrhosis, although it may be normal in asymptomatic patients. The elevation is usually two to six times normal, but can be more than 10 times normal. The serum bilirubin is usually normal or mildly elevated until the later stages of the disease are reached. Serum bile acids and cholesterol are increased frequently. Serum *immunoglobulin M* levels are increased in 75 per cent of patients with primary biliary cirrhosis. The finding, however, is not specific. Hypoprothrombinemia and hypocalcemia may be present and reflect deficiencies of vitamins K and D. The serum transaminases are normal to mildly elevated. Eighty-four to 98 per cent of patients with primary biliary cirrhosis have *circulating antimitochondrial antibodies*. There are a number of different antimitochondrial antibodies, but the one most specific for primary biliary cirrhosis is termed M2 and is directed toward an antigen in the inner mitochondrial membrane. The antibody is neither species nor organ specific. Antimitochondrial antibodies

may be present in patients with HBsAg-negative chronic active hepatitis, cryptogenic cirrhosis, and collagen vascular diseases; however, test results are normal in patients with extrahepatic obstruction unless they also have primary biliary cirrhosis or chronic active hepatitis. A small percentage of patients (5 to 30 per cent) with primary biliary cirrhosis have antinuclear antibodies in their serum.

DIAGNOSIS. The diagnosis of primary biliary cirrhosis is established by finding a positive antimitochondrial antibody test and the characteristic pathology (Stage 1 or 2) on liver biopsy. It may be necessary to exclude extrahepatic obstruction in some patients in whom the diagnosis of primary biliary cirrhosis cannot be made with certainty, as *extrahepatic biliary obstruction* can clinically mimic primary biliary cirrhosis. Also, patients with primary biliary cirrhosis have an increased incidence of gallstones, which may cause biliary obstruction. Biliary tract disease may be excluded by either transhepatic or endoscopic retrograde cholangiography.

THERAPY AND PROGNOSIS. No specific therapy for primary biliary cirrhosis is available. Corticosteroids are not known to be effective in this disease and will aggravate the bone disease. D-Penicillamine, azathioprine, ursodeoxycholic acid and colchicine have been used in the treatment of primary biliary cirrhosis. D-Penicillamine cannot be recommended because its use is associated with numerous complications without improvement in survival. Treatment with colchicine has been shown to improve liver tests but not hepatic histology as compared to placebo-treated controls. Similarly, treatment with ursodeoxycholic acid improves liver tests but not symptoms, and its effects on survival are unclear. Further experience is required in the use of colchicine and ursodeoxycholic acid before they can be recommended. Patients with advanced clinical disease (e.g., jaundice, ascites) are excellent candidates for liver transplantation (Ch. 124). Successful transplantation is associated with resolution of all hepatic symptoms.

The treatment of primary biliary cirrhosis is directed toward its complications and includes correction of specific deficiency states and reduction in the pruritus. Dietary fat may be reduced to 40 grams daily to decrease steatorrhea and improve calcium absorption. Medium-chain triglycerides, which are absorbed directly into the portal vein without the requirement for intraluminal bile salts, may be given as a dietary supplement. If the prothrombin time is prolonged, vitamin K (10 mg) is given intramuscularly every 4 weeks. Osteomalacia can be prevented by exposure to sunlight (10 to 20 minutes daily) and dietary supplementation with vitamin D and calcium. The serum 25(OH)D level should be measured, and, if low, it should be increased to the normal range with oral vitamin D (Ch. 233). Hepatic osteomalacia, but not the more common osteoporosis, responds to treatment with metabolites of vitamin D. Patients with thyroid antibodies should be tested for hypothyroidism.

The cause of the pruritus is unknown, but it may be secondary to increased tissue levels of bile salts. Cholestyramine and colestipol are anion exchange resins that bind bile salts in the intestines, preventing their reabsorption in the terminal ileum. Eight to 12 grams of cholestyramine is given daily in divided doses with breakfast and dinner. Fat-soluble vitamins should not be given at the same time as the resin. The hypercholesterolemia may also respond to cholestyramine therapy. Clofibrate should not be used in these patients, as there may be a paradoxical increase in the serum cholesterol.

Asymptomatic patients with primary biliary cirrhosis have a good prognosis, with a 10-year survival similar to age-matched controls. Patients who present with symptoms have, in contrast, an average life expectancy of 5.5 to 11 years. The development of jaundice, ascites, or cirrhosis is associated with a poor prognosis.

Dickson ER, Grambsch PM, Fleming TR, et al.: Prognosis in primary biliary cirrhosis: Model for decision making. Hepatology 9:1, 1989. *The prognosis of individual patients with primary biliary cirrhosis can be determined with reasonable accuracy by using symptoms and laboratory test results. This study has developed a model for this type of analysis.*

Gershwin ME, Mackay IR (eds.): Primary biliary cirrhosis. Semin Liver Dis 9:1, 1989. *A series of articles about primary biliary cirrhosis including discussions of antimitochondrial antibody tests, medical therapy, and liver transplantation.*

Kaplan M: Primary biliary cirrhosis. N Engl J Med 316:521, 1987. *A succinct Medical Progress article with an excellent bibliography of 124 references. A good place to start.*

Leuschner U, Fischer H, Kurtz W, et al.: Ursodeoxycholic acid in primary biliary cirrhosis: Results of a controlled double-blind trial. Gastroenterology 97:1268, 1989. *One of the first controlled trials on the use of ursodeoxycholic acid in the treatment of primary biliary cirrhosis. There was a significant improvement in some liver tests during treatment with ursodeoxycholic acid, and following withdrawal of therapy liver tests worsened.*

Vierling J: Primary biliary cirrhosis. In Zakim D, Boyer TD (eds.): Hepatology: A Textbook of Liver Disease. 2nd ed. Philadelphia, W. B. Saunders Company, 1990, pp 1158–1205. *An up-to-date review of the pathogenesis, diagnosis, and treatment of primary biliary cirrhosis.*

SECONDARY BILIARY CIRRHOSIS

DEFINITION, ETIOLOGY, AND PATHOLOGY. Secondary biliary cirrhosis is an uncommon sequela of longstanding obstruction of the biliary tree. Obstruction is usually present for more than 1 year (mean of about 6 years) before cirrhosis develops; however, intervals as short as 4 months from the onset of obstruction (jaundice) to the diagnosis of cirrhosis have been reported. Cirrhosis or fibrosis may also develop in the absence of jaundice in patients with prolonged partial biliary tract obstruction, as may be seen in chronic pancreatitis. In adults, obstruction is due most commonly to gallstones, strictures, carcinoma, chronic pancreatitis, or sclerosing cholangitis. In children, biliary atresia and cystic fibrosis are common causes of secondary biliary cirrhosis.

The liver is usually enlarged and dark green. The surface is granular or occasionally nodular. The lobular pattern is usually preserved until the cirrhosis is advanced. The portal tracts are widened owing to fibrosis and proliferation of bile ducts. The hepatic parenchyma may contain bile plugs, infarcts, or lakes. There is focal hepatocellular necrosis. As the cirrhosis progresses, the fibrous septa extend into the hepatic parenchyma, forming pseudolobules. In advanced cirrhosis, there is nodular regeneration.

CLINICAL MANIFESTATIONS. *Jaundice* is common but not invariable, and the level of jaundice may fluctuate. Patients with strictures or stones may have suffered recurrent bouts of cholangitis or biliary colic. *Pruritus* is also a common complaint and may precede the onset of icterus. If the pruritus is severe, itching may lead to thickening and darkening of the skin. Xanthelasma and xanthomas may appear. *Steatorrhea* with diarrhea may be a major complaint, and *bone disease* may develop owing to malabsorption of vitamin D and calcium. Splenomegaly is common. Ascites and gastrointestinal bleeding develop later in the course of the disease and are uncommon presenting complaints.

LABORATORY TESTS. The serum bilirubin is usually moderately increased (3 to 15 mg per deciliter). The alkaline phosphatase is also almost always increased; however, in 25 to 30 per cent, the elevation is less than twice normal. The AST is usually elevated, but the elevations are moderate. The prothrombin time may be prolonged and may improve with vitamin K administration. Hypoalbuminemia and hyperglobulinemia may also be present. Serum cholesterol and bile acids are frequently increased. *Lipoprotein X*, an abnormal lipoprotein, is found commonly in patients with extrahepatic obstruction (see Ch. 116). Lipoprotein X is also present in other forms of liver disease, and its absence does not exclude extrahepatic obstruction. Elevations of the white blood cell count in patients with extrahepatic obstruction suggest the presence of cholangitis or a hepatic abscess.

THERAPY AND PROGNOSIS. Relief of the biliary obstruction is the only specific form of treatment. In patients in whom the obstruction cannot be relieved, the correction of vitamin deficiencies and the use of cholestyramine to relieve itching, as outlined for the treatment of primary biliary cirrhosis, is warranted. In addition, there may be recurrent episodes of cholangitis requiring antibiotic treatment. Liver transplantation is an excellent option for patients with benign diseases such as sclerosing cholangitis and biliary atresia.

The prognosis for patients with carcinoma is poor, with most dying because of the malignancy and not because of the liver disease. The mortality for patients with benign obstructions (stone or stricture) depends on whether or not the obstruction can be relieved. When the obstruction cannot be relieved, mortality is high; however, survival may be prolonged (years) before the patient dies from hepatic failure or bleeding esophageal varices. Surgical relief of the biliary obstruction improves survival, although ascites and esophageal varices may develop later. The development of these complications, usually many years after apparently successful surgery, may be due to subclinical recurrence of partial biliary obstruction.

Littenberg G, Afroudakis A, Kaplowitz N: Common bile duct stenosis from chronic pancreatitis: Clinical and pathologic spectrum. Medicine 58:385, 1979. *Reviews the effects on the liver of biliary obstruction secondary to chronic pancreatitis.*

CRYPTOGENIC CIRRHOSIS

DEFINITION AND ETIOLOGY. Cryptogenic (macronodular or postnecrotic) cirrhosis is any cirrhosis for which the etiology is unknown. The liver contains little or no necrosis or inflammation and has no diagnostic pathologic lesions (for example, alcoholic hepatitis). It lacks any specific lesions demonstrable by histochemical stains, e.g., α_1-antitrypsin or iron; and specific serologic tests, e.g., HBsAg, anti-HBc, AMA, and ceruloplasmin, are normal. It is assumed that most cases represent the end stage of a previously active, chronic, or recurrent hepatitis, but alcoholic and other chronic liver diseases give rise to a very similar form of coarsely nodular cirrhosis. At least half of patients with cryptogenic cirrhosis have antibodies against the recently identified hepatitis C virus, and it may be that the development of cirrhosis in these patients is due to chronic infection with this virus. Cryptogenic cirrhosis should become a less frequent diagnosis as our understanding of the causes of liver disease increases and we develop tests for agents such as the hepatitis C virus.

PATHOLOGY. The size of the liver is variable and its surface distorted by large regenerative nodules (macronodular), which may be several centimeters in diameter. The liver between the nodules appears to be collapsed and fibrotic. The microscopic appearance of the liver is one of regenerative nodules separated by connective tissue. The portal areas may be infiltrated by mononuclear cells, but the liver cells are well preserved, and active hepatocellular necrosis or hepatic steatosis is minimal or absent.

CLINICAL MANIFESTATIONS. Cryptogenic cirrhosis may remain clinically silent for many years and frequently is discovered unexpectedly, often during the evaluation of an unrelated condition. When the disease becomes "clinically manifest," its signs and symptoms are usually nonspecific (malaise, lethargy) or related to portal hypertension and include ascites, splenomegaly, hypersplenism, or bleeding esophageal varices. The liver frequently is of normal size or small. Splenomegaly is common; spider angiomas, ascites, and abdominal wall venous collaterals may also be present. Serum transaminases and bilirubin are usually normal to slightly increased. Hyperglobulinemia is common and may be the only laboratory abnormality.

DIAGNOSIS. Cryptogenic cirrhosis is a diagnosis of exclusion and is based on histologic and clinical evidence of cirrhosis in the absence of a definable etiology (see Table 122–1). Wilson's disease and hemochromatosis are specifically treatable and should therefore be carefully excluded (see Ch. 192 and 193). Hepatitis B and C should be excluded by appropriate serologic tests. A small number of patients with cryptogenic cirrhosis may have chronic hepatitis B infection despite the absence in the serum of detectable levels of HB_sAg. Measurement of anti-HB_c may be helpful in identifying these patients. Testing for antimitochondrial antibodies, ANA, and an LE preparation helps exclude primary biliary cirrhosis and chronic active hepatitis. Alpha$_1$-antitrypsin deficiency may be excluded by appropriate histochemical stains and serologic tests (see Ch. 121). Findings of hepatic congestion on biopsy may be indicative of occult cardiac disease or hepatic vein occlusion. A previous history of alcoholism may be the only evidence for alcohol as the cause of the cirrhosis.

TREATMENT AND PROGNOSIS. Specific therapy for this type of cirrhosis is lacking. Complications such as ascites, encephalopathy, and gastrointestinal bleeding should be managed as discussed in Ch. 110, 111, and 123. Patients who have asymptomatic cirrhosis may do quite well with a good 5-year prognosis; however, the onset of ascites or bleeding esophageal varices is a poor prognostic sign.

Bruix J, Barrera J, Calvet X, et al.: Prevalence of antibodies to hepatitis C virus in Spanish patients with hepatocellular carcinoma and hepatic cirrhosis. Lancet

CARDIAC CIRRHOSIS

ETIOLOGY. Cardiac cirrhosis is an uncommon complication of severe, prolonged, recurrent right heart failure of any cause, although it is usually due to rheumatic heart disease (mitral or aortic stenosis with tricuspid regurgitation), cardiomyopathy, or constrictive pericarditis.

PATHOLOGY. The gross appearance of the liver in acute hepatic failure is one of alternating red and pale areas (nutmeg liver). The red areas are congested central areas of the hepatic lobule, whereas the pale areas are the preserved hepatocytes. With recurrent bouts of heart failure, the centrilobular hepatocytes atrophy and fibrosis develops. The fibrosis is most marked in the central areas, and with time fibrous septa extend out into the rest of the lobule. Regenerative nodules develop later, and they arise from the periphery of the hepatic lobule.

CLINICAL MANIFESTATIONS, DIAGNOSIS, AND THERAPY. The clinical picture is usually dominated by the cardiac disease. Differentiation of patients with acute hepatic congestion from those with cardiac cirrhosis is difficult, as the clinical features are similar (see Ch. 121). The liver may be small or enlarged and firm. When tricuspid regurgitation is present, the absence of hepatic pulsation suggests cirrhosis. Ascites and splenomegaly are common. The bilirubin is usually only mildly increased, and either the unconjugated or conjugated pigment may predominate. The AST is often moderately elevated but may be normal if the heart failure is controlled. The prothrombin time may be prolonged, and in the presence of significant liver disease coumarin anticoagulants should be used with caution. The diagnosis of cardiac cirrhosis is established by performing a liver biopsy. However, in most situations, this is not warranted.

Reduction in the incidence of rheumatic fever and tuberculosis as well as advances in cardiovascular surgery in the Western world have made cardiac cirrhosis an uncommon disease. Its prognosis depends largely upon the course of the cardiac disease. If the latter can be successfully treated, hepatic function improves and liver disease stabilizes.

Cello JP, Grendell J: The liver in systemic conditions. *In* Zakim D, Boyer TD (eds.): Hepatology: A Textbook of Liver Disease. 2nd ed. Philadelphia, W. B. Saunders Company, 1990, pp 1415–1422. *A portion of this chapter reviews the effects of acute and chronic heart failure on the liver.*

MAJOR SEQUELAE OF CIRRHOSIS

The major sequelae of cirrhosis are summarized in Table 122–3. Portal hypertension, bleeding esophageal and gastric varices, ascites, and the hepatorenal syndrome are discussed here. Liver failure, portosystemic encephalopathy, hepatocellular carcinoma, and hypersplenism are discussed elsewhere (Ch. 123 and 125).

Portal Hypertension

ANATOMY AND PHYSIOLOGY OF PORTAL VENOUS SYSTEM. The portal venous system begins in the capillaries of the intestines and terminates in the hepatic sinusoids. The portal vein is formed by the confluence of the superior and inferior mesenteric veins and splenic vein.

The liver receives about 1500 ml of blood each minute, two thirds of which is provided by the portal vein. The hepatic artery provides 40 to 60 per cent of the oxygen supply to the liver. The liver offers little resistance to the flow of blood, and the pressure within the sinusoids is low (less than 5 mm Hg above the pressure in the inferior vena cava). Since the veins in the portal system

TABLE 122–3. MAJOR SEQUELAE OF CIRRHOSIS

1. Portal hypertension
   a. Bleeding esophageal and gastric varices
   b. Splenomegaly and hypersplenism (Ch. 152)
   c. Ascites
   d. Spontaneous bacterial peritonitis
2. Hepatorenal syndrome
3. Liver failure (Ch. 123)
4. Portosystemic (hepatic) encephalopathy (Ch. 123)
5. Hepatocellular carcinoma (Ch. 125)

lack valves, increased resistance to flow at any point between the splanchnic venules and the heart increases pressure in all vessels on the intestinal side of the obstruction.

DEFINITION AND PATHOGENESIS. Portal hypertension represents an increase in the hydrostatic pressure within the portal vein or its tributaries. This is manifested clinically by the development of *portal-systemic collaterals, splenomegaly,* and/or *ascites.* Since portal hypertension may be present in the absence of clinical findings, it may be detectable only by measurement of pressures in the portal system. Pressures within the hepatic sinusoids may be measured by catheterizing the hepatic veins (wedged hepatic vein pressure), or the portal vein pressure may be measured directly by transhepatic or umbilical vein catheterization or at surgery. Portal hypertension is present when the wedged hepatic vein pressure is more than 5 mm Hg higher than the inferior vena cava pressure. Although generally considered to be a progressive disorder, portal hypertension may in fact decrease as the liver disease improves, i.e., alcoholic hepatitis. Portal hypertension also can be an acute and transient phenomenon, as may occur with acute right heart failure. Since the pressure in any vascular system is directly proportional not only to resistance but also to flow, portal hypertension may result from either increased blood flow in the portal vein or increased resistance to flow within the portal venous system.

Increased portal venous blood flow is an unusual cause of portal hypertension for two reasons: (1) Increases in portal vein flow cause a reflex decrease in hepatic artery blood flow, thereby tending to maintain relatively normal sinusoidal pressure. (2) The outflow resistance from the liver is so low that increases in portal vein flow must be very large to cause a significant increase in portal venous pressure.

Increased resistance to venous flow is the most common mechanism for the development of portal hypertension. Liver disease accounts for the majority of cases; however, occlusion of the portal or hepatic veins and cardiac disease also cause increased resistance to flow and increases in portal pressure. The diseases causing portal hypertension are listed in Table 122–4 and are discussed below.

CLINICAL MANIFESTATIONS. The clinical presentation of portal hypertension depends to a certain extent upon its cause. Essentially all forms may present with either *bleeding esophageal varices* or *splenomegaly* with or without *hypersplenism.* In portal vein thrombosis, as the liver is normal, ascites and jaundice are unusual. *Ascites* and other signs of hepatic disease (jaundice, spiders, encephalopathy) are common clinical features of cirrhosis. Occlusion of the hepatic veins almost always leads to development of ascites and varying degrees of hepatic dysfunction. Thus, the clinical findings may be important clues to the cause of the portal hypertension.

The development of portal-systemic collaterals is the major complication of portal hypertension. Several vessels may form collaterals. The veins that lie in the mucosa of the gastric fundus and esophagus are of greatest clinical interest because, when

TABLE 122–4. CAUSES OF PORTAL HYPERTENSION

I. **Increased resistance to flow**
   Liver diseases
     Cirrhosis—all causes
     Congenital hepatic fibrosis
     Schistosomiasis
     Idiopathic portal hypertension
     Sarcoidosis
     Alcoholic hepatitis
     Partial nodular transformation
   Diseases of cardiovascular system
     Portal vein occlusion
     Splenic vein occlusion
     Hepatic vein occlusion
     Veno-occlusive disease
     Web lesion or thrombosis of inferior vena cava
     Congestive heart failure—constrictive pericarditis
II. **Increased portal blood flow**
     Splenomegaly not due to liver disease
     Arteriovenous fistula

dilated, they form gastric and esophageal varices (Fig. 122–1 and Color Plate 1A and B). The remnant of the umbilical vein may also dilate. If flow through this vessel becomes great enough, a loud venous hum may be audible over the path of the umbilical vein (Cruveilhier-Baumgarten syndrome). The umbilical vein enters the left portal vein, and therefore, if a venous hum is present, the cause of the portal hypertension must be intrahepatic or in the hepatic veins or inferior vena cava. Large collaterals also may form between the splenic and renal (chiefly left) veins. Dilated abdominal wall veins are common in patients with portal hypertension and are especially prominent when the patient stands. The hemorrhoidal veins may also act as collaterals. Varices may also form in unusual locations within the intestines (e.g., ileostomies, upper small bowel, and ascending, descending, and sigmoid colons), and these may bleed.

DISEASES CAUSING PORTAL HYPERTENSION (see Table 122–4).

Arteriovenous fistulas may form between an artery and the portal vein or one of its tributaries as a consequence of abdominal trauma, liver biopsy, carcinoma (either intrahepatic or extrahepatic), or rupture of an arterial aneurysm (e.g., splenic). An upper abdominal bruit or a palpable thrill at surgery suggests this diagnosis in any patient with portal hypertension. The fistula can be localized by celiac angiography and is usually surgically correctable.

Splenomegaly resulting from hematologic diseases such as polycythemia rubra vera and myelofibrosis or an infiltrative process such as Gaucher's disease may, in rare instances, lead to portal hypertension. The enlarged spleen receives high blood flow from the splenic artery, leading to high flow within the splenic vein which is thought to cause the rise in portal pressure. These diseases also frequently involve the liver, and the infiltrative process may increase intrahepatic resistance. However, the principal event in the genesis of the portal hypertension appears to be the high portal vein blood flow, since splenectomy usually cures the portal hypertension.

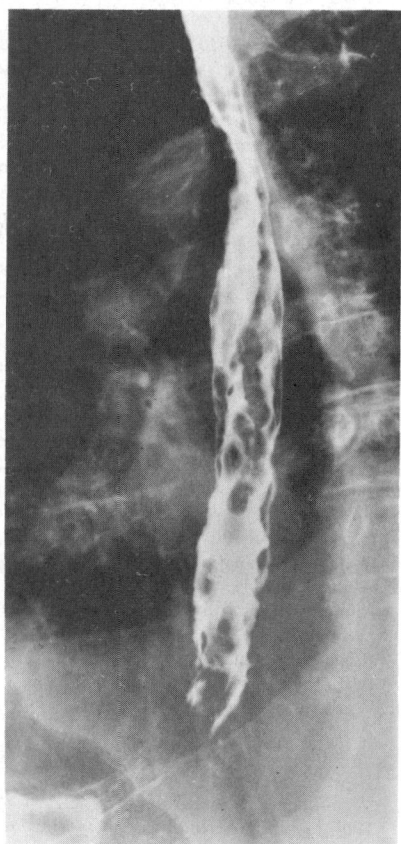

FIGURE 122–1. Barium esophagogram, demonstrating large varices involving the lower two thirds of the esophagus. (Courtesy of T. Munyer. *From* Zakim D, Boyer TD [eds.]: Hepatology: A Textbook of Liver Diseases, 2nd ed. Philadelphia, W. B. Saunders Company, 1990.)

Splenic vein thrombosis may be caused by pancreatitis, abdominal trauma, or a locally invasive tumor. Pressure is increased only in areas drained by the splenic vein, whereas pressure in the portal vein is normal. The diagnosis should be suspected in a patient with gastric or esophageal varices but a normal liver biopsy and is established by celiac angiography. Splenectomy is curative.

Portal vein thrombosis may develop following abdominal trauma or intra-abdominal sepsis, or in association with cirrhosis or hepatocellular carcinoma. In the majority of cases, however, the cause is unknown. This is primarily a disease of children, although adults may also develop portal vein thrombosis. The diagnosis again is suggested by the presence of portal hypertension in a patient with a normal liver biopsy. The diagnosis is established by angiography. Thrombi also may be identified by ultrasonography or CT scan. The surgical management of these patients may be difficult because of the absence of a patent vein to use for making a portal-systemic shunt.

Thrombosis of the hepatic veins (Budd-Chiari syndrome) may follow abdominal trauma or the use of birth control pills or may occur in patients with diseases such as polycythemia rubra vera, myeloproliferative disorders, and paroxysmal nocturnal hemoglobinuria, which have an associated hypercoagulable state. Patients with hepatic vein thrombosis may develop an acute, subacute, or chronic illness in which abdominal pain and ascites are the major features. The liver is usually enlarged and tender. Elevations of the serum transaminases and bilirubin are usually mild, although they can be increased significantly in patients who have an acute illness. The initial clinical diagnosis is usually cirrhosis, and the correct diagnosis is not suspected until centrilobular congestion is seen on liver biopsy. Catheterization of the inferior vena cava and hepatic veins is a useful test in the evaluation of this condition. The presence of thrombi in the inferior vena cava can be established. The diagnosis of hepatic vein thrombosis is made by finding the characteristic pathology on liver biopsy, excluding cardiac disease that causes a similar histologic lesion, and inability to catheterize the hepatic veins. The outlook for patients with hepatic vein thrombosis is poor, with mortality of 50 to 90 per cent. The use of side-to-side portacaval shunts in these patients has been thought to prolong survival. Further experience is required before the proper role of this procedure can be evaluated. The use of anticoagulants has not been shown to affect survival. Liver transplantation is an effective therapy, but anticoagulation is required to prevent recurrent hepatic vein thrombosis.

Veno-occlusive disease (nonthrombotic occlusion of hepatic venules) also causes a Budd-Chiari–like syndrome. Veno-occlusive disease develops in patients who have ingested plants containing pyrrolidizine alkaloids, who have been treated for malignant disease with certain chemotherapeutic agents, or following bone marrow transplantation. It also is a common pathologic finding in patients with alcoholic hepatitis and cirrhosis. The disease is thought to be due to a toxic injury to the endothelium of the affected vessels. The occluded venules may be present in a liver biopsy, and an abnormal vascular pattern is found when contrast material is injected into the hepatic veins.

Thrombi, tumor, or a membrane in the inferior vena cava may obstruct the hepatic veins and give a clinical picture similar to that of hepatic vein thrombosis, with the additional features of peripheral edema and stasis dermatitis. Membranous obstruction near the terminus of the inferior vena cava has been described in all areas of the world but is most frequently observed in South Africa and Asia. These patients also have a high incidence of hepatocellular carcinoma. The reasons for this latter association are unclear. Catheterization of the inferior vena cava identifies the obstructing lesion. Removal of the membrane surgically is sometimes possible and leads to resolution of the portal hypertension. Thrombectomy is usually not helpful.

Cirrhosis causes portal hypertension by increasing the intrahepatic vascular resistance. The increased resistance is thought to occur because of compression of vessels by regenerative nodules, distortion and reduction of the sinusoidal bed, and narrowing of portal vessels by the fibrous tissue. In alcoholic liver disease, serious portal hypertension may develop without cirrhosis. In some patients with acute alcoholic hepatitis, there is progressive obliteration of the central veins with resultant centrilobular fibrosis. These patients develop a severe outflow block, which leads to the formation of ascites or esophageal varices.

Portal hypertension due to noncirrhotic portal fibrosis may occur in four conditions. In *schistosomiasis*, the adult worm resides in the intestinal venules. The eggs are shed into these vessels and are swept into the portal vein and into the liver, where they lodge in and obstruct the portal venules. The host's immune response to the eggs leads to periportal fibrosis and the development of portal hypertension. (Schistosomiasis is discussed more fully in Ch. 434). *Idiopathic portal hypertension* (Banti's syndrome) is a disease in which there is portal hypertension, no cirrhosis, and a patent portal vein. The liver biopsy may be normal, or there may be fibrosis in the periportal areas and in the space of Disse. The disease process is progressive, with the liver eventually becoming small and fibrotic. A similar clinical picture may be seen in patients exposed to arsenic, vinyl chloride, and copper salts. *Congenital hepatic fibrosis* also causes portal hypertension without cirrhosis. In the portal areas, there is marked hyperplasia of the bile ducts and stellate fibrosis. This condition may be present in association with cystic liver disease and Caroli's disease (intrahepatic ductal ectasia), with an associated polycystic renal lesion in many patients. The development of portal hypertension is the major consequence of this form of liver disease, as hepatic function is well maintained. Hepatic *sarcoidosis* may rarely lead to hepatic fibrosis and portal hypertension.

DIAGNOSTIC APPROACH TO PORTAL HYPERTENSION. Portal hypertension should be suspected in any patient with ascites or splenomegaly, and its presence is established when portal-systemic collaterals are found. One may find collaterals on physical examination (dilated abdominal wall or umbilical veins), or they may be identified in the esophagus or stomach by a gastrointestinal series or by endoscopy. It is important that the etiology of portal hypertension be identified, since some causes (splenic vein thrombosis) may be curable. A liver biopsy will provide useful information as to the presence of liver disease; central venous congestion suggests hepatic vein thrombosis or cardiac disease. If the biopsy is not diagnostic, then catheterization of the hepatic veins may be performed. Elevated pressure establishes the presence of liver disease. Also, inferior vena cava or hepatic vein thrombosis may be found during catheterization of the hepatic veins. If the wedge pressure and right atrial pressure are normal, then the cause of the portal hypertension is (1) occlusion of the portal vein or its tributaries, (2) liver disease that involves the periportal areas and portal venules (schistosomiasis or idiopathic portal hypertension) and therefore does not increase the wedge pressure, or (3) increased flow in the portal vein. Celiac angiography usually differentiates among this group of patients. Ultrasonography or CT also may be used to identify thrombi in the portal vein.

Bleeding Esophageal and Gastric Varices

PATHOGENESIS. Hemorrhage from esophageal varices is a major complication of portal hypertension. The mortality in adult patients with cirrhosis varies from 30 to 60 per cent for each bleeding episode. The varices form because of increased pressure in the portal vein. Bleeding from varices may occur when the portal pressure exceeds 11 to 12 mm Hg above inferior vena cava pressure. However, not all patients with pressures above these levels have bleeding varices. The tension on the vessel wall is greater in large than in small varices for a given level of pressure. Therefore, large varices are more likely to rupture and bleed than are smaller ones; reflux esophagitis and ascites do not appear to be important in the genesis of bleeding.

CLINICAL MANIFESTATIONS. The most common presentation is hematemesis. The bleeding may be massive with the rapid development of shock, or the bleeding may stop spontaneously only to recur later. On occasion, the patient may only complain of hematochezia or melena without an antecedent history of hematemesis. Features suggesting underlying liver disease such as hepatomegaly, ascites, or jaundice may be present or absent, depending on the etiology of the portal hypertension and the activity of the underlying hepatic disease.

DIAGNOSIS AND TREATMENT. The care of the patient with gastrointestinal bleeding is discussed in detail in Ch. 111. The restoration of the patient's blood volume takes precedence over all other therapy and diagnostic tests. The blood volume should be corrected rapidly but not excessively, since overexpansion may lead to the development of ascites or renewed bleeding. Proof that esophageal or gastric varices are the source of hemorrhage depends on endoscopy, since, even in those with known varices, 30 to 50 per cent are bleeding from other lesions (especially gastritis).

The bleeding from varices in many patients stops without any specific therapy. The *medical management* of patients who continue to bleed includes *vasopressin, endoscopic sclerosis of varices,* and *balloon tamponade.* Long-term therapy with *propranolol* for the prevention of variceal hemorrhage is controversial and cannot be recommended.

Vasopressin, a potent vasoconstrictor, is believed to act by constricting the splanchnic arterioles, which results in a fall in portal flow and thus a drop in portal pressure. This drug should be given only to patients who can be carefully monitored, preferably in an intensive care unit. Vasopressin is infused into a peripheral vein at a rate of 0.2 to 0.4 unit per minute. This therapy provides temporary control in about 60 per cent of patients. Unfortunately, about half of those initially controlled have rebleeding, and the use of vasopressin has little effect on morbidity or mortality. The intravenous use of somatostatin or combined use of vasopressin and nitroglycerin may be as effective as vasopressin alone in controlling variceal hemorrhage, with fewer side effects. The gastric and esophageal varices lie in the mucosa of the gastric fundus and esophagus and are therefore susceptible to *balloon tamponade.* Tamponade is best accomplished by inserting a tube that has a gastric balloon with or without an esophageal balloon (Sengstaken-Blakemore tube). Once placed in the stomach, the gastric balloon is inflated and pulled into the cardia of the stomach, tamponading the varices. If bleeding does not stop, then the esophageal balloon is inflated. This therapy is effective in controlling hemorrhage in 70 to 90 per cent of patients. There is a significant risk of aspiration during balloon tamponade, and 50 to 60 per cent of the patients hemorrhage again. During endoscopy, the *direct injection of esophageal varices* with sclerosing agents has been described as a method for the control of acute bleeding and for the long-term management of these patients. Repeated injections over several weeks are required to obliterate the varices, and rebleeding during this period is common. Once they are obliterated the rate of rebleeding from the varices is reduced, and survival may be improved. Endoscopic sclerotherapy is associated with serious side effects (esophageal ulcers and strictures, pleural effusions), but it is an important form of therapy for the management of recurrent bleeding esophageal varices.

In *surgical therapy* for portal hypertension the high-pressure portal system is anastomosed to the low-pressure systemic venous system to create a *portal-systemic shunt.* There are two basic types of shunts. One is *nonselective,* in that the entire portalvenous system is decompressed. The end-to-side and side-to-side portacaval and mesocaval shunts are nonselective. *Selective* shunts decompress only the varices. The pressure remains high in the portal vein, and portal flow into the liver is preserved. Thus the varices are decompressed with minimal disruption of the normal hepatic circulation. The distal splenorenal shunt is of this type. The selective shunt may cause less encephalopathy than the nonselective types of shunts without improving survival.

Portal-systemic shunts have been used in four clinical situations: (1) *Hypersplenism* is not an indication for a portal-systemic shunt, because the reduction in formed elements in the blood is usually not of clinical significance. (2) The *prophylactic shunt* is made in patients with cirrhosis and varices who have never bled. Prophylactic shunts shorten survival compared to unoperated controls, with death from hepatic encephalopathy and liver failure. Thus prophylactic shunts should not be performed. (3) *Emergency shunts* may be used to control hemorrhage in actively bleeding patients. However, the operative mortality may exceed 50 per cent, so that emergency shunts should be used rarely and in a select group of patients. The indications for this operation are still controversial. (4) *Therapeutic portal-systemic shunts* are used in patients who have bled at least once from varices. Operations in these patients have been shown to effectively stop further bleeding from varices. Unfortunately, the patient's survival is not improved significantly because of an increased incidence of hepatic encephalopathy and liver failure when compared to unoperated controls. Possibly these results could be improved by better selection of patients for the operations. As might be expected, the majority of patients with poor hepatocellular function, i.e., those who are jaundiced with hypoalbuminemia, ascites, encephalopathy, and poor nutrition, tolerate a portal-systemic shunt less well than do patients without these complications of liver disease. Patients with more severe liver disease may well be better managed by sclerosis of their varices or liver transplantation than by shunt operations. The choice of therapy (sclerosis or shunt) for bleeding varices in patients with well-compensated cirrhosis is controversial. The morbidity and mortality from bleeding esophageal varices will remain high until current therapies are refined and new ones developed.

Bass NM: Preventing variceal hemorrhage. N Engl J Med 317:893, 1987. *An editorial that reviews the controversy of the effectiveness of β-blockers in preventing variceal hemorrhage.*

Boyer TD: Portal hypertension and bleeding esophageal varices. *In* Zakim D, Boyer TD (eds.): Hepatology: A Textbook of Liver Disease. 2nd ed. Philadelphia, W. B. Saunders Company, 1990, pp 572–615. *A current review of portal hypertension and treatment of bleeding varices.*

de Franchis R, et al.: Prediction of the first variceal hemorrhage in patients with cirrhosis of liver and esophageal varices. N Engl J Med 319:983, 1988. *Patients at greatest risk of hemorrhage had poor hepatic function and large varices.*

Groszman RJ (ed): Portal hypertension: Circulatory and renal abnormalities. Semin Liver Dis 6:277, 1986. *Contains a number of excellent articles on the portal circulation and the changes in portal hemodynamics that occur with liver disease.*

Smith JL, Graham D: Variceal hemorrhage: A critical evaluation of survival analysis. Gastroenterology 82:968, 1983. *A careful evaluation of survival following an episode of hemorrhage from varices.*

Ascites

DEFINITION. Ascites is the presence of excess fluid in the peritoneal cavity. It is most frequently due to cirrhosis, but there are numerous other causes (see Ch. 110), and it cannot be assumed that the appearance of ascites is indicative of cirrhosis. For this reason, patients with a recent onset of ascites must be thoroughly evaluated to establish its cause.

PATHOGENESIS (Table 122–5). Ascites forms in patients with portal hypertension because of changes in the formation and reabsorption of hepatic and splanchnic lymph and because of alterations in the metabolism of salt and water by the kidneys.

Splanchnic Lymph Formation. Increases in portal venous pressure cause a rise in the pressure within the splanchnic capillaries, resulting in loss of fluid into the interstitial space. The capillaries of the intestine restrict the loss of protein to the interstitial space, and an oncotic gradient develops between the capillary and the extravascular space. This oncotic gradient returns the majority of the fluid to capillary, and any fluid loss is usually removed by the intestinal lymphatics. For this reason, diseases that elevate the pressure only in the splanchnic bed, e.g., portal vein thrombosis, cause ascites uncommonly.

Hepatic Lymph Formation. In the noncirrhotic liver the endothelial lining of the hepatic sinusoids is discontinuous and does not effectively restrict plasma protein loss with even slight increases in sinusoidal pressure. Thus, in contrast to the intestines, the oncotic gradient between the sinusoids and extravascular space is small, and much of the fluid entering the interstitial space is not returned to the vascular space. These large amounts of fluid lost into the interstitial space must be returned to the

TABLE 122–5. FACTORS IN THE PATHOGENESIS OF CIRRHOTIC ASCITES

1. Increased hydrostatic pressure in hepatic sinusoids and splanchnic capillaries.
2. Overproduction of hepatic and splanchnic lymph secondary to (1), leading to a transudation of lymph into peritoneal space.
3. Limited or reduced reabsorption of water and protein by peritoneal lymphatics.
4. Sodium retention by the kidney secondary to hyperaldosteronism, increased sympathetic activity, alterations in metabolism of prostaglandins and kinins, and altered renal hemodynamics.
5. Impaired renal water excretion, in part caused by increased levels of ADH.

vascular space via hepatic lymphatics. When the rate of formation of lymph exceeds the rate of removal, then fluid "weeps" out of the lymphatics and into the peritoneal cavity. Diseases that cause marked elevations of the sinusoidal pressure in an otherwise normal liver, e.g., congestive heart failure and hepatic vein thrombosis, therefore commonly cause ascites. With cirrhosis the situation is more complex in that there is "capillarization" of the sinusoids such that an oncotic gradient forms between plasma and lymph. Large amounts of lymph are formed by the cirrhotic liver with overflow into the peritoneal space; however, the protein content of this fluid is low.

Peritoneal Reabsorption. The peritoneum plays an active role in the reabsorption of the ascitic fluid. Water and protein are reabsorbed by the lymphatics in the peritoneal membrane. The intra-abdominal pressure and character of the peritoneum are important factors in determining the rate of ascitic fluid removal. The amount of fluid removed by the peritoneal lymphatics is variable but usually does not exceed 800 to 1000 ml every 24 hours.

Renal Function. An important factor in the genesis of ascites is the *retention of sodium* by the kidney. During the formation of ascites there is a positive sodium balance despite a total body sodium that is greater than normal. The pathogenesis of the sodium retention by the kidney is understood poorly; however, there is increased reabsorption of sodium by both proximal and distal tubules. The increased reabsorption of sodium may be mediated, in part, by increased plasma levels of aldosterone, increased sympathetic activity, and alterations in the renal production of prostaglandins and kinins. Reduced renal blood flow resulting from vasoconstriction also leads to enhanced sodium reabsorption.

CLINICAL MANIFESTATIONS AND DIAGNOSIS. Patients with ascites complain of increasing abdominal girth. The presence of ascites on physical examination is suggested by the findings of shifting dullness, a ballotable liver, or a fluid wave. Small amounts of ascites may be identified by abdominal ultrasonography. Once the presence of ascites is suspected, diagnostic paracentesis should be performed. The character of the ascitic fluid in cirrhosis is variable; however, 80 to 90 per cent of patients have an ascitic fluid protein concentration of less than 2.5 grams per deciliter. The ascitic fluid lactic dehydrogenase is low, and the difference between the serum and ascitic albumin exceeds 1.1 grams per deciliter. The ascitic fluid white blood cell count is less than 500 per cubic millimeter in 90 per cent of patients with cirrhosis, and mononuclear cells predominate (>75 per cent). Patients with cirrhosis who have high protein ascites and a low serum/ascites albumin difference or a high ascitic fluid white blood cell count require further evaluation.

MANAGEMENT. Resolution of the acute hepatic injury, following withdrawal of ethanol or a specific course of therapy, may reduce portal pressure, and ascites may resolve spontaneously. In many patients, however, ascites is chronic and specific therapy is warranted. Accumulation of ascitic fluid occurs only in patients who are in positive sodium balance; therefore, *restricting sodium intake* diminishes or stops the accumulation of ascitic fluid. Diets containing 250 to 500 mg of sodium (10 to 20 mEq) are adequate to achieve sodium balance in most patients. The kidney is also unable to excrete a water load normally in some patients with ascites, in part because of high blood levels of antidiuretic hormone. *Fluid restriction* (1000 to 1500 ml daily) is sometimes necessary, therefore, to prevent hyponatremia. Many patients do not lose their ascites or edema with sodium restriction, and the use of *diuretics* becomes necessary. Spironolactone, amiloride, and triamterene act on the distal tubule and cause natriuresis with sparing of potassium. Spironolactone, 150 to 400 mg daily, causes diuresis in patients with mild to moderate sodium retention and is used as initial therapy. Furosemide, thiazides, and ethacrynic acid are more potent diuretics and cause both natriuresis and potassium wasting. If the patient fails to respond to treatment with spironolactone, furosemide, 40 to 80 mg daily, is added to the diuretic regimen. All diuretics cause a loss of fluid from the plasma. This fluid is then replaced by the reabsorption of ascitic or edema fluid. The rate of fluid lost should therefore not exceed the rate at which the ascites and edema fluids may be reabsorbed. The maximal rate of reabsorption of ascitic fluid varies widely; however, fluid losses of 1 kg daily in patients with edema and ascites and 0.3 to 0.5 kg daily in those with only ascites are well tolerated. The BUN and electrolytes must be monitored for the development of azotemia and hypokalemia. The use of diets very low in sodium (250 to 500 mg) is possible in the hospital; however, this is rarely possible in an outpatient setting. Therefore, preceding discharge from the hospital, the patient's sodium intake should be increased (1 to 2 grams daily) and diuretics adjusted so that he or she is still in negative sodium balance.

A few patients with cirrhosis do not respond to diuretic therapy. It is important to establish that failure is not due to an inappropriately high sodium intake. This can be determined by measuring the urine sodium. If this value is high (greater than prescribed sodium intake), the patient's diet requires adjustment. Alternately, if the urine sodium is low and treatment in the hospital with increasing doses of diuretics leads to azotemia or hepatic encephalopathy, the patient is resistant to diuretic therapy. Repeated large-volume (4 to 5 liters) paracentesis in combination with an infusion of albumin (40 grams) to maintain plasma volume has been used to manage patients with cirrhotic ascites. Although relief of ascites is more rapid and complications fewer than are observed with diuretic therapy, survival and frequency of readmission to the hospital for recurrent ascites are unaffected. The use of repeated large-volume abdominal paracentesis should be limited to patients who are refractory to diuretic therapy or who require relief of tense ascites because of difficulty in breathing. If these refractory patients are incapacitated by the ascites, they may be candidates for other therapies. The *peritoneovenous (LeVeen) shunt* consists of a tube placed subcutaneously between the peritoneal cavity and the superior vena cava. There is a pressure-activated one-way valve that allows peritoneal fluid to enter the vascular space but prevents the backflow of blood into the tube. This shunt may be effective in controlling ascites; however, its use is associated with episodes of disseminated intravascular coagulation, sepsis, and frequent shunt thrombosis, thus limiting its application only to patients who have severe and incapacitating ascites. The shunt should not be used in patients whose condition can be managed by other therapies including repeated paracentesis. Attempts to increase the venous oncotic pressure by infusions of albumin or plasma are not likely to cause sustained diuresis and are an expensive form of therapy.

SPONTANEOUS BACTERIAL PERITONITIS. Patients with cirrhosis and ascites may develop spontaneous bacterial peritonitis without obvious cause, i.e., perforation of the bowel. Possibly peritonitis occurs because of bacterial seeding of the ascitic fluid via the lymph or blood or by bacteria traversing the bowel wall. The frequency of this complication in patients with ascites may be increasing, and its early recognition is essential (mortality exceeds 60 to 90 per cent even if treated). Patients with very low ascitic fluid protein levels (less than 1 gram per deciliter) appear to be at greater risk for developing peritonitis because of a low level of opsonic activity in the fluid. The clues to the diagnosis are the presence of fever, abdominal pain or tenderness, or decreased bowel sounds in a patient with ascites. The diagnosis should also be suspected in patients with the sudden onset of hepatic encephalopathy or hypotension. Patients may be asymptomatic and the diagnosis suggested only by finding an elevated ascitic fluid white blood cell count, or by a positive ascitic fluid culture. The diagnosis is established by abdominal paracentesis, which should be performed in patients with onset of new ascites or in those with a change in their clinical course. The ascitic fluid white blood cell count in peritonitis is usually above 500 per cubic millimeter (93 per cent of cases), and more than 50 per cent of the cells are polymorphonuclear leukocytes. The ascitic fluid pH also is lower than the blood pH. Bacteria may be identified on Gram's stain. The ascitic fluid and blood should be cultured and treatment instituted before the results of culture are known, as delays in therapy may increase mortality. The organisms most frequently cultured are Enterobacteriaceae (mainly *E. coli*) and Group D streptococci, *Streptococcus pneumoniae*, and *Streptococcus viridans*. Other bacteria are cultured less frequently, and anaerobic bacteria are uncommon isolates. Initial antibiotic therapy should therefore include both an aminoglycoside and ampicillin or a newer cephalosporin antibiotic such as cefotaxime. When using an aminoglycoside, blood levels of the drug must be obtained to minimize the risk of renal injury. The response to therapy is monitored by the fever pattern and by changes in the ascitic fluid leukocyte count. If therapy is effective, the ascitic fluid leukocyte count falls and the predominant cell again becomes mononuclear. Antibiotic therapy is continued for 7 to 10 days.

Hepatorenal Syndrome

DEFINITION AND PATHOGENESIS. The hepatorenal syndrome (functional renal failure) is a decrease in renal function that develops in a patient with serious liver disease in whom all other causes of renal dysfunction are excluded. The kidneys lack serious pathologic lesions. If the liver disease improves, normal renal function returns. The pathogenesis of the hepatorenal syndrome is unknown. There is intense intrarenal vasoconstriction and redistribution of blood flow. In addition, the plasma levels of renin, aldosterone, and prostaglandins are increased, and there is increased sympathetic activity. These changes may be due to reduced "effective" plasma volume in some patients.

CLINICAL MANIFESTATIONS. Patients developing the hepatorenal syndrome frequently have severe hepatic disease and therefore are jaundiced and have other signs and symptoms of liver disease. Almost all of the patients with this syndrome have ascites. The illness is marked by oliguria. The urine is usually free of protein, and the urine sediment is normal. The urine sodium level is low (<10 mEq per liter), the urine:plasma creatinine ratio is high (>30:1), and the urine:plasma osmolality ratio is greater than 1.0. These urine findings are different from those of acute tubular necrosis, in which the urine sodium content is high (>30 mEq per liter), the urine:plasma creatinine ratio is low (<20:1), and the urine is isosmotic to plasma. The progression of the renal failure is variable, with some patients having a complete loss of renal function over several days, whereas in others the serum creatinine slowly increases over several weeks as the liver function gradually worsens.

DIFFERENTIAL DIAGNOSIS (Ch. 76). Patients with liver disease may develop renal failure for a variety of reasons. These patients commonly receive diuretics and may develop prerenal azotemia. Renal function will improve with withdrawal of the medication. Acute tubular necrosis may occur following an episode of hypotension (bleeding or sepsis) or during fulminant hepatitis and can be distinguished from hepatorenal failure by the urine findings. Drugs (antibiotics, especially aminoglycosides, and nonsteroidal anti-inflammatory medications) may cause worsening of renal function in patients with cirrhosis. Acute pyelonephritis, with or without papillary necrosis, may also cause renal failure in patients with liver disease.

THERAPY AND PROGNOSIS. Specific causes of renal failure should be looked for and excluded. Any medications that are potential nephrotoxins should be withdrawn. A brief trial of plasma expansion with monitoring of urine output and serum creatinine may be attempted, to exclude hypovolemia as a cause of the renal failure. The volume of fluid infused should be limited (1000 ml), as overexpansion of the plasma volume may precipitate variceal hemorrhage. Infusions of vasodilators may transiently improve renal function; however, this does not improve survival. Uremia may be treated by dialysis; again, overall survival is not improved. The use of peritoneovenous shunts in these patients is being investigated, but their efficacy is as yet unproven. The prognosis for patients with the hepatorenal syndrome is poor, with over 90 per cent dying during hospitalization, usually from liver failure or complications of portal hypertension. Definitive therapies must await a better understanding of the pathogenesis of this syndrome.

Akriviadis EA, Runyon BA: Utility of an algorithm in differentiating spontaneous from secondary bacterial peritonitis. Gastroenterology 98:127, 1990. *Reviews the criteria used to diagnose spontaneous bacterial peritonitis and how to tell it from secondary bacterial peritonitis.*

Epstein M: Functional renal abnormalities in cirrhosis: Pathophysiology and management. *In* Zakim D, Boyer TD (eds.): Hepatology: A Textbook of Liver Disease. 2nd ed. Philadelphia, W. B. Saunders Company, 1990, pp 493–513. *A review of the renal abnormalities present in patients with cirrhotic ascites.*

Schrier RW: Pathogenesis of sodium and water retention in high-output and low-output cardiac failure, nephrotic syndrome, cirrhosis, and pregnancy. N Engl J Med 319:1127, 1988. *A brief discussion of some of the factors thought to be important in the formation of cirrhotic ascites.*

Tito L, Gines P, Arroyo V, et al.: Total paracentesis associated with intravenous albumin in management of patients with cirrhosis and ascites. Gastroenterology 98:146, 1990. *Describes the use of a single large-volume paracentesis to remove all of a patient's ascitic fluid. This therapy was associated with few side-effects and rapid relief of the ascites.*

Wright TL, Boyer TD: Diagnosis and management of cirrhotic ascites. *In* Zakim D, Boyer TD (eds.): Hepatology: A Textbook of Liver Disease. 2nd ed. Philadelphia, W. B. Saunders Company, 1990, pp 616–636. *Discusses the pathogenesis and treatment of cirrhotic ascites and spontaneous bacterial peritonitis.*

123 Acute and Chronic Hepatic Failure

Bruce F. Scharschmidt

This chapter begins with a discussion of hepatic encephalopathy, one of the most characteristic features of liver failure. This is followed by discussions of the approach to the patient with acute or chronic hepatic failure.

THE SYNDROME OF HEPATIC ENCEPHALOPATHY

DEFINITION AND SIGNIFICANCE. Hepatic encephalopathy (also called hepatic coma or portal-systemic encephalopathy) is a reversible neuropsychiatric syndrome which can accompany advanced, decompensated liver disease of all types and/or extensive portal-systemic shunting. Recognition of the signs and symptoms of encephalopathy represents an important clue to the presence of deteriorating liver function or superimposed complications. In addition, repeated neurologic evaluation of the encephalopathic patient provides valuable information regarding the patient's course and prognosis.

PATHOGENESIS. The pathogenesis of hepatic encephalopathy remains unclear, and possible mechanisms are outlined in Table 123–1. The encephalopathy is at least partially attributable to toxic materials that are derived from the metabolism of nitrogenous substrate in the gut and that bypass the liver through anatomic or functional shunts. This is the origin of the term *portal-systemic encephalopathy,* often used interchangeably with hepatic encephalopathy. *Ammonia* and *mercaptans* result from the degradation of urea or protein and sulfur-containing compounds, respectively, and both can produce coma when administered in large doses to animals. The presence of mercaptans in the breath of some encephalopathic patients probably accounts for the characteristic sweetish musty odor termed *fetor hepaticus.* While often present in increased amounts in the blood or cerebrospinal fluid or both, the absolute concentration of ammonia, ammonia metabolites including glutamine, and mercaptans correlates only roughly with the presence or severity of encephalopathy. *Gamma-aminobutyric acid* (GABA), the principal inhibitory neurotransmitter in the mammalian brain, is also produced in the gut and is present in increased amounts in the blood of patients and animals with hepatic failure. A role for GABA in hepatic encephalopathy is supported by the observation that visual evoked potentials in animals with hepatic failure mimic those produced by benzodiazepines or barbiturates, both of which act on the GABA receptor, but differ from those of comatose states caused by administration of ether, ammonia, or mercaptans. Moreover, recent studies suggest a beneficial effect of GABA receptor antagonists. Their use should still be regarded as experimental, however. A separate hypothesis holds that accelerated entry of *aromatic amino acids* into the central nervous system results in decreased synthesis of normal neurotransmitters such as norepinephrine and enhanced synthesis of *false neurotransmitters* such as octopamine. Other compounds such as short-chain *fatty acids* are also present in blood in increased amounts and have been proposed as potentially toxic. Finally, there is impaired integrity of the *blood-brain barrier* in animals with acute hepatic failure. It is possible that hepatic encephalopathy may represent the synergistic effects of a number of toxins acting on an unusually susceptible nervous system.

NEUROLOGIC MANIFESTATIONS. Patients with hepatic encephalopathy display a characteristic spectrum of mental and motor changes which are frequently divided into stages (Table 123–2). Although useful, individual variations occur, and many patients do not show an orderly progression of symptoms. Moreover, the clinical grading scale is relatively insensitive. Standardized testing has revealed psychomotor abnormalities in a high proportion of patients with cirrhosis in whom conventional neurologic examination is normal. Such *subclinical encephalopathy* is potentially important inasmuch as it may be associated with impaired functional capacity, including job performance and ability to drive an automobile.

In addition to the acute, reversible signs and symptoms already mentioned, rare patients with longstanding liver disease and portal-systemic shunting develop *irreversible neurologic dysfunction.* Acquired *hepatocerebral degeneration* is characterized by tremor, rigidity, dysarthria, oral-facial dyskinesia, choreoathetosis, and ataxic gait. *Myelopathy* is another rare manifestation of advanced chronic liver disease and portal-systemic shunting and may be manifested by spastic paraparesis, hyperreflexia, and incontinence.

As with other types of metabolic encephalopathy, asymmetric neurologic findings are unusual, and brain stem reflexes such as the pupillary light response, oculovestibular response, and oculocephalic response are typically preserved. Thus, asymmetric

TABLE 123–1. HEPATIC ENCEPHALOPATHY: PROPOSED PATHOGENIC MECHANISMS

Mechanism	Hypothesis	Evidence For	Evidence Against	Therapeutic Implications
Toxins (ammonia and mercaptans)	Produced by action of intestinal bacteria on urea, protein; decreased clearance from portal blood by diseased liver	Increased levels of these substances or their metabolites in blood, CSF; administration can produce coma	Poor correlation of plasma levels with encephalopathy; EEG changes produced by administration of these agents differ from those in hepatic encephalopathy	Oral administration of poorly absorbable antibiotics, lactulose
False neurotransmitters (increased brain octopamine and phenylephrine; decreased dopamine and norepinephrine)	Increased brain influx of aromatic amino acid precursors for false neurotransmitters	Increased ratio of plasma aromatic amino acids to branched-chain amino acids	Inconsistent findings regarding brain levels of neurotransmitters; lack of effect of false neurotransmitter administration on neurologic function	Administration of branched-chain amino acids (no consistent benefit in clinical trials)
Enhanced GABA (-ergic) neurotransmission	Decreased hepatic clearance of gut bacteria-derived GABA, which enters brain and inhibits neurotransmission	Increased plasma levels of GABA; increased brain entry of GABA-like substances; visual evoked responses in encephalopathy mimic those produced by GABA; increased brain GABA receptors	Inconsistent evidence regarding serum GABA levels and GABA receptor density in brain	Administration of poorly absorbable antibiotics; improved mental status with experimental use of GABA receptor antagonists

neurologic signs or abnormal brain stem reflexes may suggest a structural lesion of the central nervous system such as a subdural hematoma. Seizures are also uncommon in the absence of alcohol withdrawal and should alert the clinician to the possibility of a structural lesion or hypoglycemia. The disappearance of pupillary reactivity, of the oculocephalic or oculovestibular response, or of deep tendon reflexes is associated with a very poor prognosis in all types of metabolic encephalopathy, including hepatic encephalopathy (but excluding drug overdose). Electroencephalographic changes are sensitive indicators of hepatic encephalopathy, being present in most patients with subclinical disease (Table 123–2), but are not specific for this disorder. They include symmetric slowing observed initially over the frontal areas with later spreading laterally and posteriorly.

DIAGNOSIS. The diagnosis of hepatic encephalopathy is based upon the presence of compatible neurologic signs and symptoms in a patient with advanced liver disease and exclusion of other possible causes of the neurologic abnormalities. The diagnosis is most difficult when liver disease is not obvious. Routine laboratory studies, including electrolytes, calcium, blood urea nitrogen, creatinine, glucose, and standard liver function tests, are of help primarily in excluding other causes of metabolic encephalopathy and evaluating the presence and severity of hepatic disease. Toxicologic screening is also appropriate when ingestion of sedatives or toxins capable of altering neurologic function is suspected. Blood ammonia and cerebrospinal fluid levels of glutamine correlate only roughly with mental status and are therefore of limited value in most circumstances. Structural lesions such as a subdural hematoma are often a consideration and may require special radiologic studies. Other causes of encephalopathy such as the Wernicke-Korsakoff syndrome, sepsis, or meningitis must also be excluded, depending on the clinical circumstances.

TREATMENT. The management of patients with hepatic encephalopathy is largely supportive and has as its goals (1) improvement, when possible, of hepatic function, (2) prevention or correction of factors that may precipitate or aggravate encephalopathy (Table 123–3), and (3) decreasing the production of putative toxins that result from enteric bacterial metabolism of nitrogenous substrates. All nonessential drugs should be stopped—particularly sedatives and potentially hepatotoxic agents. For the occasional patient who demonstrates manic disorientation as an early manifestation of encephalopathy, soft restraints are preferable to sedative hypnotic agents.

Decreasing Production and Absorption of Enteric Toxins. Gut cleansing should be accomplished by enema, and oral administration of cathartics such as magnesium citrate is appropriate unless lactulose (see below) is administered. It is also generally appropriate to restrict dietary protein to about 40 grams per day in mildly encephalopathic patients and eliminate it in patients

TABLE 123–3. HEPATIC ENCEPHALOPATHY—COMMON PRECIPITATING FACTORS

Deterioration in hepatic function
Drugs (sedative or potentially hepatotoxic agents)
Gastrointestinal hemorrhage
Increased dietary protein
Azotemia
Hypokalemia
Infection
Constipation
Anesthesia and surgery
Hypoxia
Diuretics (hypokalemia, alkalosis, and hypovolemia)

with more advanced or progressive encephalopathy. *Vegetable protein* appears somewhat less likely to induce encephalopathy than animal protein and may be useful in the long-term management of patients with chronic or recurrent encephalopathy. While oral or parenteral administration of *branched-chain amino acids* has been reported to be beneficial in the treatment of hepatic encephalopathy, controlled trials have not provided clear evidence of efficacy, and their use is not generally recommended (see Table 123–1).

In addition to these measures aimed at decreasing nitrogenous substrate, production of enteric toxins should be further inhibited by oral administration of a poorly absorbable antibiotic, such as neomycin in a dose of 1 to 2 grams every 6 hours, or by administration of lactulose. Lactulose is neither metabolized nor absorbed in the upper small bowel and is metabolized by ileal and colonic bacteria to organic acids. It is as effective as neomycin in lowering blood ammonia and reversing encephalopathy in patients with chronic liver disease. Because prolonged neomycin administration may produce ototoxicity or malabsorption, lactulose is preferable as chronic therapy. The mechanisms of action of lactulose may include increased bacterial assimilation of ammonia, decreased ammonia production, and possibly trapping of ammonia as NH_4^+ in the bowel lumen. Therapy is commonly initiated by administering 30 to 45 ml of the syrup orally every 2 hours until diarrhea ensues. Thereafter, the dose is decreased to that amount necessary to produce two to four soft stools per day. Lactulose can also be given by retention enema. Concomitant administration of neomycin and lactulose may be useful in selected patients.

FULMINANT HEPATIC FAILURE

DEFINITION. *Fulminant hepatic failure* is defined as hepatic failure with encephalopathy developing in less than 8 weeks in a patient without pre-existing liver disease. *Subacute* or *late-onset hepatic failure* refers to a slightly slower-paced illness, also occurring in patients without pre-existing disease, in whom the time from jaundice to onset of encephalopathy ranges from 8 weeks to 6 months.

ETIOLOGY. Among the various causes of hepatic failure (Table 123–4), acute viral hepatitis, particularly hepatitis B with or

TABLE 123–2. STAGES OF HEPATIC ENCEPHALOPATHY

Stage	Mental Status	Motor Changes
Subclinical	No changes on routine examination; may be associated with impaired work performance or driving ability	Impaired performance on standardized psychomotor tests or bedside tests such as figure drawing or number connection
I	Mild confusion, apathy, agitation, anxiety, euphoria, restlessness, sleep disorder	Fine tremor, slowed coordination, asterixis
II	Drowsiness, lethargy, disorientation, inappropriate behavior	Asterixis, dysarthria, primitive reflexes (suck and snout), ataxic paratonia
III	Somnolent but rousable, marked confusion, incomprehensible speech	Hyperreflexia, Babinski's sign, incontinence, myoclonus, hyperventilation
IV	Coma	Decerebrate posturing; brisk oculocephalic reflexes; response to painful stimuli present early; may progress to flaccidity and absence of response to stimuli

TABLE 123–4. CAUSES OF FULMINANT HEPATIC FAILURE

Common	Uncommon
Viral hepatitis	Ischemia
A	Hepatic vein obstruction
B	Veno-occlusive disease
D (coinfection with B or superinfection)	Malignant infiltration
Non-A, non-B (presumed)	Wilson's disease
Drugs	Fatty liver of pregnancy
Necrosis: acetaminophen, halothane, isoniazid, methyldopa;	Reye's syndrome
Steatosis: tetracycline, valproate	Hyperthermia
Toxins	
Amanita phalloides, chlorinated hydrocarbons, phosphorus, aflatoxins	

without coexistent D hepatitis, is the most common both in the United States and elsewhere. Many cases are attributed to non-A, non-B hepatitis based on an absence of known causes and negative serologic tests for hepatitis A and B. Recently developed serologic tests for hepatitis C are just beginning to be used in these patients. The course of the illness differs depending on the cause. Acetaminophen overdose, exposure to toxins, *Amanita phalloides* ingestion, and ischemia typically produce a fulminant illness with encephalopathy in less than a week. Most patients with late-onset hepatic failure, by contrast, have presumed non-A, non-B hepatitis. Finally, combined hepatic and renal failure should alert one to the possibility of toxic exposure.

DIAGNOSIS. The diagnosis of fulminant hepatic failure requires the presence of encephalopathy in a patient with severe, acute liver disease. Synthetic function of the liver as reflected by the prothrombin time is nearly always markedly abnormal. Serum bilirubin concentration is less helpful, since some patients may become very ill rapidly and progress to coma before the serum bilirubin is markedly elevated. Serum transaminase levels are usually elevated early in the illness but do not reliably distinguish between fulminant hepatic failure and acute hepatitis without encephalopathy.

TREATMENT. *Supportive Measures.* A thorough search should be made to detect and correct factors that may precipitate (Table 123–3) or complicate hepatic failure (Table 123–5); several points merit emphasis. Encephalopathy in fulminant hepatic failure primarily reflects the severe nature of the underlying liver injury, and correcting potential precipitating factors is less likely to produce objective benefit than it is in patients with encephalopathy complicating chronic liver disease. *Cerebral edema* is present in over half of patients dying of fulminant hepatic failure. It is often detectable on CT scan and may result in intracranial herniation. Moreover, in conjunction with systemic hypotension, it reduces cerebral perfusion and may cause brain death. Treatment of clinically evident intracranial hypertension, manifested by unequal or abnormally reactive pupils, myoclonus, and/or decerebrate posturing, is certainly appropriate. Unfortunately, clinical signs may be an insensitive way of detecting intracranial hypertension, and invasive monitoring of intracranial pressure is advocated by some. The decision regarding invasive intracranial pressure monitoring must thus be carefully individualized. Coagulation abnormalities should be corrected before monitor insertion.

Experimental Measures. Because the mortality of fulminant hepatic failure is high even with optimal supportive care, a variety of other forms of therapy have been tried. These include *corticosteroid administration, exchange transfusion,* administration of L-*dopa* or *hepatitis B hyperimmune globulin* (for hepatitis B), *charcoal hemoperfusion, amino acid infusion, plasmapheresis, hemodialysis, total body washout, cross circulation* with a human volunteer or baboon, or *extracorporeal perfusion* through a human cadaver liver, pig liver, or baboon liver. However, these experimental forms of therapy offer *no advantage* over conventional supportive care. Thiopental, as well as osmotic agents such as mannitol, are effective at least temporarily in reducing intracranial pressure. The utility of these agents and intracranial pressure monitoring are still under evaluation.

Liver Transplantation. Liver transplantation may yield favorable results (60 to 70 per cent survival) in patients with fulminant hepatic failure. While the follow-up in such patients is limited, most deaths following liver transplantation occur in the first 3 postoperative months. Physicians caring for patients with fulminant and late-onset hepatic failure who are likely to have a poor prognosis with supportive care alone should therefore contact a liver transplant center as soon as possible for consideration of transfer (Ch. 124).

PROGNOSIS. The short-term prognosis for patients with fulminant hepatic failure that progresses to coma is poor, the average reported survival being 10 to 40 per cent. Factors associated with an especially poor prognosis include age of less than 10 or greater than 40 years, illness due to presumed non-A, non-B hepatitis or idiosyncratic drug reaction, a slow course with encephalopathy following jaundice by more than 7 days, Stage IV encephalopathy, marked biochemical abnormalities (bilirubin exceeding 20 mg per deciliter, prothrombin time exceeding 30 seconds), or the presence of complications (Table 123–5). In contrast, the outlook for those patients who do survive an episode of fulminant hepatic failure with coma is quite good. Virtually all patients have returned to their previous state of health within 2 to 3 months, and follow-up liver biopsies have usually demonstrated no or minimal abnormalities. Patients with persistent biochemical or histologic abnormalities have frequently been found to have had pre-existing liver disease or to have continuing exposure to toxic or infectious agents.

CHRONIC LIVER DISEASE WITH ENCEPHALOPATHY

ETIOLOGY. Hepatic encephalopathy may also occur in patients with chronic liver disease, usually cirrhosis with portal-systemic shunting. Some patients with cirrhosis may be chronically encephalopathic. In most, however, encephalopathy tends to occur acutely and intermittently. In this latter group, the occurrence of encephalopathy reflects a worsening of hepatic function and/or the presence of one or more precipitating factors (Table 123–3).

DIAGNOSIS. As with fulminant hepatic failure, diagnosis requires the presence of signs and symptoms compatible with

TABLE 123–5. HEPATIC FAILURE: COMPLICATIONS AND MANAGEMENT

Complications	Pathophysiology	Management
Aspiration	Decreased mental status, emesis	Endotracheal intubation with onset of coma
Azotemia	Volume depletion, acute tubular necrosis, hepatorenal syndrome	Assess volume (may require invasive monitoring or fluid challenge), fluid administration if appropriate
Cerebral edema	?Altered vascular permeability, circulating toxins	Clinical assessment insensitive; intracranial pressure monitoring advocated by some, but entails risk and not of proven value; elevation of head of bed; hyperventilation; mannitol; barbiturates
Encephalopathy	See Table 123–1	See Table 123–1
Gastrointestinal bleeding	Stress gastritis aggravated by coagulopathy and portal hypertension	Prophylaxis (e.g., with H_2-receptor antagonists, antacids or sucralfate; fresh frozen plasma if overt bleeding occurs
Hypoxemia	Right to left shunting, noncardiogenic pulmonary edema	Increased inspired O_2; intubation with positive end-expiratory pressure
Hypotension	Decreased vascular resistance, sepsis, gastrointestinal bleeding	Identify and treat underlying cause, pressors if necessary
Infection	Via intravenous lines, enteric origin	Blood cultures, empiric treatment if infection suspected
Metabolic		
Acidosis	Decreased perfusion, decreased hepatic clearance of organic acids	Identify and treat underlying cause; administration of HCO_3^-
Alkalosis	Hyperventilation, presumably central	No treatment necessary
Hypoglycemia	Decreased glycogenolysis and gluconeogenesis	Frequent glucose monitoring, 1–2 liters of 5% or 10% glucose daily
Hypokalemia	Renal or gastrointestinal K^+ loss	KCl administration
Hyponatremia	Decreased renal free water clearance, fluid administration	Minimize administration of free water

hepatic encephalopathy in a patient with underlying chronic liver disease. Routine tests of liver function are typically abnormal but are of little value in differential diagnosis. Unlike fulminant hepatic failure, encephalopathy in patients with chronic liver disease may be accompanied by only minimally abnormal liver function tests. A markedly elevated or rising prothrombin time in an encephalopathic patient with known chronic liver disease suggests superimposed acute hepatocellular necrosis. It is extremely important in patients with chronic alcoholic liver disease to exclude other causes of metabolic encephalopathy (e.g., hypoglycemia, alcohol intoxication, Wernicke-Korsakoff syndrome), meningitis, or structural lesions such as subdural hematoma.

TREATMENT. *Supportive Measures.* Unlike fulminant hepatic failure, encephalopathy in the patient with chronic liver disease frequently results from one or more potentially reversible precipitating factors. These should be sought and, when possible, corrected (Table 123–3). Additional general measures as outlined earlier for the treatment of hepatic encephalopathy should be undertaken.

The complications and additional supportive care required for these patients are similar to those described for fulminant hepatic failure. Overall, however, the severity and frequency of complications (e.g., hypoglycemia) are less than with fulminant hepatic failure. The various forms of experimental therapy that have been tried in fulminant hepatic failure also have no established role in the management of patients with chronic liver disease with encephalopathy.

Liver Transplantation. Patients with chronic, progressive liver disease of all types may be candidates for transplantation. The presence of encephalopathy or other complications should prompt the physician to consider this option and contact a transplant center (Ch. 124).

PROGNOSIS. Because encephalopathy in patients with chronic liver disease is frequently precipitated by potentially reversible factors, the short-term prognosis is better than in fulminant hepatic failure, particularly if the encephalopathy is not attributable to a sudden deterioration of hepatic function. However, because the underlying chronic liver disease is commonly irreversible and slowly progressive, the long-term prognosis is guarded.

Gammal SH, Jones EA: Hepatic encephalopathy. Med Clin North Am 73:793, 1989. *A comprehensive review with a particular focus on manifestations and pathogenesis.*

Katelaris PH, Jones DB: Fulminant hepatic failure. Med Clin North Am 73:955, 1989. *A complete treatment of this topic, including the role of transplantation.*

Munoz SJ, Maddrey WC: Major complications of acute and chronic liver disease. Gastroenterol Clin North Am 17:265, 1989. *An exhaustive review with over 150 references focusing on prevention, diagnosis, and management of complications.*

O'Grady J, Alexander GJM, Hayllar KM, et al.: Early indicators of prognosis in fulminant hepatic failure. Gastroenterology 97:439, 1989. *A very important article summarizing information on nearly 600 patients, the largest series reported.*

Rothstein JD, Herlong HF: Neurologic manifestations of hepatic disease. Neurol Clin 7:563, 1989. *A thoroughly referenced review that deals with neurologic manifestations of specific hepatic disorders as well as hepatic encephalopathy.*

124 Liver Transplantation

John Paul Roberts

In the last 25 years liver transplantation has moved from an experimental procedure to an accepted medical therapy for patients with both acute and chronic liver failure. Survival following liver transplantation has improved from approximately 30 per cent in the 1970's to 80 per cent or better in the closing years of the 1980's. The procedure is currently underwritten by many states and most private insurance companies, and recently Medicare has decided to pay for liver transplantation for specific indications. Although liver transplantation is still an expensive procedure, the cost has decreased such that it now offers a better outcome and lower cost than many therapies for acute and chronic liver failure.

More than 1800 liver transplantations were carried out in the United States during 1989. The improvement in patient and graft survival following liver transplantation has resulted from changes in (1) patient selection, (2) operative techniques, and (3) immunosuppressive drugs and their use. As newer immunosuppressive medications become available, it appears likely that the morbidity, mortality, and costs of liver transplantation will continue to decrease. With improvement in survival and with more patients undergoing liver transplantation, availability of donor organs has become rate-limiting in its use.

PATIENT SELECTION

The indications for liver transplantation have broadened with improved postoperative survival. When 1-year survival was 50 per cent, liver transplantation was indicated only in those patients who were expected to have less than a 50 per cent 1-year survival from their primary disease. Predictability for survival based on natural history data has been reasonably well established for primary biliary cirrhosis and for fulminant liver failure, but the natural histories of other liver diseases (e.g., chronic active hepatitis with cirrhosis or sclerosing cholangitis) vary widely, making it difficult to select patients with a less than 50 per cent 1-year survival. Fortunately, the current marked improvement in survival after liver transplantation has made it possible to broaden the criteria and to include quality-of-life issues in making the decision for liver transplantation. These issues include extreme fatigue or pruritus in patients with chronic liver disease, recurrent cholangitis in patients with sclerosing cholangitis, portal-systemic encephalopathy, ascites refractory to medical management, and correction of certain metabolic diseases.

Liver transplantation has also changed the indications for or replaced many of the operations previously done for complications of chronic liver disease, such as portal-systemic shunting for recurrent variceal hemorrhage, LeVeen shunting for intractable ascites, and radical biliary tract surgery for patients with sclerosing cholangitis. These operations, which were once the only option for the patient with liver disease, are now assuming a secondary role. As an example, portacaval shunting has a poor outcome in patients with severe liver dysfunction, whereas these patients can do very well following liver transplantation. It is therefore important that patients who would otherwise be suitable candidates for transplantation and in whom another surgical procedure is contemplated be discussed with a liver transplantation center regarding the appropriateness of the planned procedure.

Early referral is extremely important in patients with *fulminant liver failure* (Ch. 123). This diagnosis can only be made in patients with evidence of hepatic failure, including Stage III or IV encephalopathy developing less than 8 weeks after onset in the absence of pre-existing liver disease (Table 124–1). Viral hepatitis is the most common cause of fulminant liver failure, but other etiologies include toxins (e.g., *Amanita phalloides*), medications (e.g., acetaminophen), or metabolic disorders (e.g., fulminant Wilson's disease). If a patient has reached Stage IV coma or has a prothrombin time greater than 20 seconds, limited survival without hepatic replacement can be expected. These patients are at high risk for developing cerebral edema followed by brain herniation if not properly managed. Pretransplantation management includes elevation of the head, monitoring intracranial pressure, and aggressive therapy using mannitol, hyperventilation, and barbiturate coma for increased intracranial pressure.

The most common indication for liver transplantation is chronic active hepatitis (Table 124–1). The role of the hepatitis C virus in this group of disorders is becoming increasingly clear as the ability to identify this infection has improved. Other common diseases for which transplantation is performed include primary biliary cirrhosis, autoimmune hepatitis, sclerosing cholangitis, Wilson's disease, extrahepatic biliary atresia, α_1-antitrypsin deficiency, alcoholic liver disease, cholangiocarcinoma, and primary hepatic malignancy. Contraindications to liver transplantation include systemic sepsis, active substance abuse, extrahepatic malignancy, and advanced cardiopulmonary disease. Transplantation for cholangiocarcinoma is controversial because survival of these patients following transplantation is poor, although disease limited to the extrahepatic ducts without lymph node involvement

TABLE 124–1. INDICATIONS FOR LIVER TRANSPLANTATION AND POSTOPERATIVE SURVIVAL*

Disease	Per Cent of Patients	(n)	6-month Actuarial Survival	12-month Actuarial Survival
Chronic active hepatitis/cryptogenic cirrhosis	22	(37)	97%	88%
Alcoholic liver disease	16	(26)	100%	100%
Fulminant liver failure	13	(21)	95%	95%
Subacute fulminant liver failure	2	(3)	100%	100%
Primary biliary cirrhosis	10	(17)	94%	85%
Sclerosing cholangitis	8.5	(14)	100%	92%
Chronic active hepatitis B	9	(15)	80%	69%
α_1-Antitrypsin disease	3	(5)	100%	100%
Extrahepatic biliary atresia	3	(5)	60%	60%
Cancer	3	(5)	80%	60%
Hemochromatosis	2	(4)	100%	100%
Autoimmune hepatitis	2	(4)	100%	100%
Miscellaneous†	5	(8)	50%	50%

*Based on 164 patients who underwent liver transplantation at the University of California, San Francisco.
†Includes Budd-Chiari, Crigler-Najjar, fatty liver, Wilson's disease, unknown etiology.

has a more favorable prognosis. Although theoretically liver transplantation is a logical therapy for hepatocellular carcinoma, (Ch. 125), an effective adjuvant chemotherapy is lacking, and hepatic and systemic relapse of the disease is common. Thus, only 20 per cent of patients with hepatocellular carcinoma survive 3 years following liver transplantation. As an exception, the fibrolamellar variant of hepatocellular carcinoma carries a much better prognosis. End-stage liver disease caused by chronic ethanol abuse has been increasingly recognized as an appropriate indication for transplantation; results in these patients are the same as those for patients with chronic liver failure of other causes. The 6- and 12-month actuarial survival is given for different disease entities in Table 124–1. The overall patient survival is given in Figure 124–1.

Liver transplantation has also been performed for a variety of metabolic conditions, including those that directly lead to chronic liver disease (e.g., Wilson's disease) and those that do not produce liver disease but for which transplantation removes all or much of the metabolic defect leading to disease expression systemically (e.g., primary hyperoxaluria). At this time liver transplantation has been carried out for the following genetic diseases: α_1-antitrypsin deficiency, Wilson's disease, hemochromatosis, homozygous familial hypercholesterolemia, Crigler-Najjar syndrome, erythropoietic protoporphyria, glycogen storage disease types I and IV, tyrosinemia, primary hyperoxaluria, and genetic diseases of the urea cycle.

DONOR SELECTION

Selection of the appropriate organ donor for liver transplantation is primarily based on ABO blood type and body size compatibility between donor and recipient. In general, donors for large non-O recipients tend to be more available than for small O recipients. This discrepancy reflects a higher accident rate for young adult males, and the ability to utilize type O livers in recipients of other blood types. In October, 1987, a nationwide organ-sharing system was instituted in the United States. In this system potential organs are first offered to local transplantation programs; if no local recipient is available, the organ is offered to centers within a defined geographic region. If no regional recipient is available, the organs are then offered nationally. Selection of a recipient is based upon criteria that include the level of care that potential recipients currently require. Those in intensive care or with fulminant hepatic failure are assigned the highest priority; those still able to work, the lowest.

IMPROVEMENTS IN OPERATIVE TECHNIQUE

A number of operative advances have contributed to the improved results seen with liver transplantation. The use of choledochocholedochostomy or choledochojejunostomy has decreased the incidence of biliary leak and sepsis. The liver from a large donor can be pared down to fit a smaller recipient; this procedure has increased the donor pool for small recipients. Further, this technique has led to the recent use of liver segments from living related donors. Finally, the use of multiple organ transplants in patients with multiorgan disease involvement has increased the access of patients who otherwise would not be candidates for transplantation.

POST-TRANSPLANTATION COMPLICATIONS

Complications of liver transplantation are primarily vascular (e.g., thrombosis of the anastomosed hepatic artery or portal vein), biliary (relating to reconstruction of the biliary tract), infectious, or those relating to organ rejection. Early postoperative hepatic artery thrombosis requires retransplantation, since it usually results in necrosis of the liver and/or biliary tree. Portal vein thrombosis can be asymptomatic or present with complications of portal hypertension. Biliary tract complications usually appear as strictures within the biliary tree or as leakage of bile from the biliary reconstruction. Renal failure may complicate the post-transplantation period, resulting from pre-existing renal dysfunction, intraoperative renal ischemia, postoperative cyclosporine toxicity, or a combination of these factors.

Postoperative infections commonly occur. The average patient develops at least one episode of bacterial infection and has a 40 to 50 per cent chance of developing a fungal or viral infection following liver transplantation. Bacterial infections may involve the biliary tree, intra-abdominal abscesses, pneumonia, or may be related to central venous catheters. Fungal infections include systemic candidiasis, usually occurring during the early transplant period and related to intravascular catheters or intra-abdominal candidal abscesses. Other opportunistic fungal infections, such as aspergillosis, predominate later, and all can represent a serious threat to the patient's life. Viral infections following liver transplantation are most often caused by members of the Herpesvirus family. Mucocutaneous herpes simplex and varicella zoster can

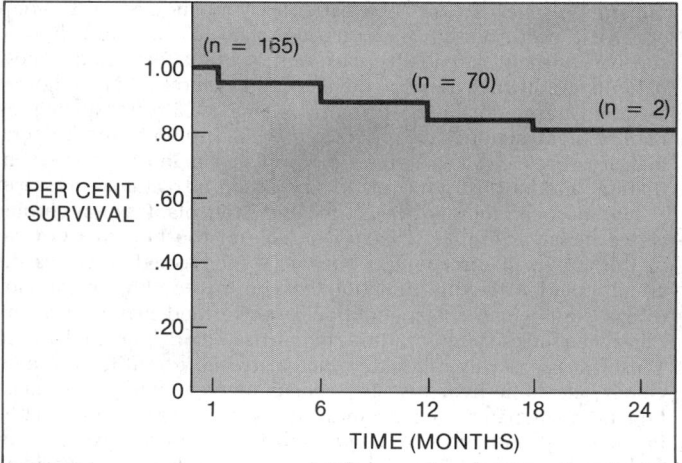

FIGURE 124–1. Survival following hepatic transplantation (adult and pediatric) at the University of California, San Francisco, from January 31, 1988 to June 27, 1990.

occur following transplantation, and either prophylactic or therapeutic acyclovir is effective in preventing and treating these infections. Post-transplantation cytomegalovirus (CMV) infections represent either a reactivation of disease in a previously infected, immunosuppressed recipient or a primary infection arising from transmission of the agent via the donor liver or a blood transfusion. In general, primary disease appears to be more serious than reactivation. In renal transplantation recipients, high doses (3200 mg per day) of acyclovir are effective prophylaxis for CMV infections, and it is hoped that this approach will also prove effective in liver transplantation recipients. Gancyclovir, a congener of acyclovir, appears to be effective in treatment of systemic CMV disease in liver recipients. As one of the major complications of immunosuppression is infection, the use of prophylactic anti-infectives is a method of improving the therapeutic index of the immunosuppressive agents. *Pneumocystis carinii* infection was previously a problem in all forms of solid organ transplantation, but with the use of prophylactic trimethoprim-sulfamethoxazole, it is expected that morbidity and mortality related to this protozoal agent will be eliminated in transplantation recipients.

IMMUNOSUPPRESSION

Immunosuppression in the liver transplantation recipient is largely based on the use of cyclosporine, a cyclic polypeptide that binds to and inhibits the action of an intracellular prolyl peptidyl isomerase. As a result the production of interleukin-2 (IL-2) by T helper cells is sharply diminished; this in turn prevents cell proliferation and the generation of cytotoxic T cells. Cyclosporine is usually started in the early post-transplantation period and is continued indefinitely. Because the intestinal absorption of oral cyclosporine depends on the presence of bile, external biliary diversion or postoperative liver dysfunction can interfere with this process. Cyclosporine is metabolized by the cytochrome P-450–dependent mono-oxygenases and, therefore, systemic levels can be decreased by drugs that induce this pathway, such as rifampin, barbiturates, or phenytoin. Major side effects of cyclosporine include neurotoxicity, manifested by headache and tremor; nephrotoxicity, manifested by increase in BUN and creatinine; sensitivity to volume depletion; hypertension; and hyperkalemia. Chronic cyclosporine administration can result in renal interstitial fibrosis and an increased risk of post-transplantation lymphoproliferative disorders.

Prednisone is generally used in combination with cyclosporine to prevent rejection. Prednisone reduces the release of interleukin-1 (IL-1) by macrophages and in this fashion inhibits IL-1's amplification of IL-2 production. The complications of the use of glucocorticoids are described elsewhere (Ch. 27).

Azathioprine, a third agent used for post-transplantation immunosuppression, blocks proliferation of white blood cells and thereby decreases the proliferative or amplification response of the rejection process. The major adverse effect of azathioprine is marrow depression.

Several new drugs are being evaluated for use in liver transplantation. The most promising of these, FK-506, appears to act similarly to cyclosporine, but through binding to a different intracellular peptidyl prolyl isomerase in the cell. This results in a marked increase in potency. Its primary benefits appear to be less nephrotoxicity and its ability to achieve adequate immunosuppression without concomitant azathioprine and with relatively small doses of prednisone.

Rejection occurs commonly after liver transplantation, but with prompt diagnosis and therapy it is rarely a cause of graft loss. Its histologic features include periportal infiltrate, bile duct epithelial damage, and endothelialitis. Treatment for rejection includes additional steroids or the use of antilymphocyte preparations.

Kusne S, Dummer JS, Singh N, et al.: Infections after liver transplantation. An analysis of 101 consecutive cases. Medicine 67:132, 1988. *Compilation of infectious complications at the University of Pittsburgh.*

Roberts JP, Forsmark C, Lake JR, et al.: Liver transplantation today. Ann Rev Med 40:287, 1989. *Report from a single institution performing liver transplantation.*

Starzl TE, Demetris AJ, Van Thiel DH: Liver transplantation. N Engl J Med 321:1014, 1092, 1989. *A comprehensive review of the history of clinical liver transplantation and a summary of advances in the field.*

125 Hepatic Tumors
Bruce F. Scharschmidt

Characteristic aspects of hepatic neoplasms encountered commonly in adults are summarized in Table 125–1 and selectively described in more detail below. The approach to the patient with a neoplasm and the role of imaging studies are outlined at the end of this section.

BENIGN HEPATIC TUMORS
Hepatocellular Adenoma

Hepatocellular adenomas occur almost exclusively in women. These tumors are most frequently detected during the third and fourth decades of life but are occasionally found in postmenopausal women as well. Adenomas most commonly occur in the right lobe of the liver, are frequently solitary, and are often quite large, with up to one half being 10 cm or more in diameter. Hepatocellular adenomas are usually well circumscribed, may be surrounded by a pseudocapsule, and often show areas of bile stasis, hemorrhage, and necrosis. Microscopically, these tumors consist of a monotonous sheet of normal to slightly atypical hepatocytes without portal tracts or bile ducts. Kupffer cells are markedly reduced in number or absent, and a few arteries and thin-walled veins are present.

The preponderance of this tumor in women suggests a hormonal role in its pathogenesis, and there is strong evidence implicating oral contraceptives. Nearly 90 per cent of cases are associated with oral contraceptive use, and some adenomas have regressed in a period of months to years after use of oral contraceptives was discontinued. The annual incidence is estimated to be 3 to 4 per 100,000 in women who have taken oral contraceptives continuously for several years. Although not generally regarded as a premalignant lesion, there are instances in which hepatocellular carcinoma appears to have arisen in an hepatocellular adenoma.

Symptomatic patients with hepatocellular adenomas present with signs and symptoms of an abdominal mass, tumor infarction, intratumor hemorrhage (pain, fever, leukocytosis), or, in about one third of cases, tumor rupture (pain, hemoperitoneum, circulatory collapse). The mortality in this last group is approximately 20 per cent. Because the true incidence of these tumors is unknown, the actual proportion that ruptures cannot be determined.

The management of hepatocellular adenomas is a matter of some debate. In patients taking oral contraceptives that can be discontinued, a several-month period of observation with repeated imaging studies is justifiable, particularly if the location, size, or number of tumors would make resection hazardous. Surgery is appropriate for most persistent resectable lesions.

Focal Nodular Hyperplasia

Focal nodular hyperplasia, which shows a female to male predominance of 2:1 to 7:1, has also been referred to as pseudotumor, focal cirrhosis, and hepatic hamartoma. Unlike hepatocellular adenoma, a firm link between focal nodular hyperplasia and oral contraceptives has not been established. Focal nodular hyperplasia generally is a solitary tumor in the right lobe measuring 5 cm or less in diameter. On cut section it has a characteristic grossly lobulated appearance, which is produced by a central fibrous core with septa radiating in a stellate pattern. Hemorrhage and necrosis are rare. Microscopically, these fibrous septa contain bile ductules and inflammatory cells and are surrounded by normal or slightly atypical hepatocytes as well as Kupffer cells.

Unlike hepatocellular adenomas, focal nodular hyperplasia does not usually produce symptoms and is generally found incidentally at surgery or necropsy. In up to 20 per cent of the cases, it presents as an upper abdominal mass. Portal hypertension has been reported in association with multiple lesions, and rupture is rare. Since focal nodular hyperplasia has no known malignant potential, asymptomatic lesions can be followed nonoperatively. If the lesion is encountered unexpectedly at surgery, simple wedge biopsy is appropriate if complete excision would be difficult.

Hemangioma

Cavernous hemangioma is probably the most common benign hepatic tumor, occurring in up to 7.3 per cent of necropsies with a predominance in females. The great majority are asymptomatic and are found incidentally at surgery or necroscopy. These lesions can, however, present with signs and symptoms of an abdominal mass, infarction, rupture, or thrombocytopenia and hypofibrinogenemia. Because of the accuracy of current imaging techniques in distinguishing hemangioma from other tumors (Table 125–1),

resection is not usually necessary to establish a diagnosis and is appropriate only for large symptomatic lesions. There are also case reports of regression following radiotherapy or hepatic artery ligation.

Other Benign Tumors

A variety of less common benign liver tumors may also occur in adults. They usually produce no symptoms unless very large. Included in this group are *bile duct adenomas, bile duct cystadenomas, fibromas, lipomas, leiomyomas, mesotheliomas, teratomas,* and *myxomas. Nodular regenerative hyperplasia* (also called *nodular transformation* or *multiple adenomatosis*) is a condition characterized by multiple nodules of varying size typically occurring throughout a noncirrhotic liver. The nodules are composed

TABLE 125–1. CHARACTERISTICS OF HEPATIC NEOPLASMS

	Predisposing Factors	M/F Ratio	Manifestations and Complications	Imaging/Diagnostic Studies	Treatment
Benign tumors					
Hepatocellular adenoma	Oral contraceptives; glycogen storage disease type I	<1:10	Abdominal mass; intratumor or intraperitoneal hemorrhage; rare transition to malignancy	Detectable by US, CT, or MRI and may show areas of hemorrhage or necrosis; cold spot on colloid scan; typically hypervascular on AG; may be difficult to diagnose on biopsy	Must be individualized: discontinue oral contraceptives and observe if no symptoms; resection if symptomatic or diagnosis uncertain
Focal nodular hyperplasia	None established	1:2–7	Typically none; occasionally mass effect and rarely portal hypertension	Detectable by US, CT, or MRI and may show central scar; has Kupffer cells and may not be visible on colloid scan; typically hypervascular on AG; may be difficult to diagnose on biopsy	Usually none; resection if symptomatic
Hemangioma	None established	<1:1	Typically none; occasionally mass effect, rarely infarction, rupture, or thrombocytopenia	Characteristic appearance on MRI, CT with bolus contrast, or radionuclide blood pool scan; typically hyperechoic on US; biopsy not necessary if imaging studies show typical findings and probably associated with increased risk of hemorrhage	None if asymptomatic; resection if symptomatic; radiotherapy or hepatic artery ligation in unusual circumstances
Malignant tumors					
Hepatocellular carcinoma	Cirrhosis; hepatitis B or C virus infection; hemochromatosis; mycotoxin exposure; α_1-antitrypsin deficiency; androgenic steroids; Thorotrast; possibly oral contraceptives; tyrosinemia; glycogen storage disease type II	3:1	Abdominal mass; tumor infarction, intratumor or intraperitoneal hemorrhage; portal or hepatic vein occlusion; rarely hypercalcemia, hypercholesterolemia, carcinoid syndrome, hypoglycemia, acquired porphyria	Detectable by US, CT, MRI, or colloid scan (cold spot); often multicentric with vascular invasion; takes up gallium; biopsy or aspiration cytology often diagnostic; elevated or rising α-fetoprotein suggestive	Resection if technically feasible and permitted by hepatic function; transplantation curative in less than one third of even selected cases; palliative chemotherapy
Fibrolamellar carcinoma (variant of hepatocellular carcinoma)	None established	About equal	Mass effect	Detectable by US, CT, MRI (may show calcifications on CT and central scar); cold spot on colloid scan; α-fetoprotein typically not elevated	As for hepatocellular carcinoma; resection or transplantation more likely to result in cure
Cholangiocarcinoma	Primary sclerosing cholangitis; clonorchiasis or opisthorciasis	—	Mass effect; obstructive jaundice	Direct cholangiography often helpful in jaundiced patients; also detectable by US or CT, which may show dilated biliary radicles; aspiration cytology may be diagnostic	As for hepatocellular carcinoma; resection or transplantation rarely curative
Angiosarcoma	Exposure to vinyl chloride, arsenic, or Thorotrast	>1:1	Mass effect; intraperitoneal hemorrhage; thrombocytopenia	Detectable by US, CT; MRI or AG particularly helpful; biopsy	As for heptocellular carcinoma; resection or transplantation rarely curative

Abbreviations: US = ultrasonography; CT = computed tomography; MRI = magnetic resonance imaging; AG = angiography.

of liver plates that are two cells thick. An association with rheumatoid arthritis, Felty's syndrome, CREST syndrome, oral contraceptives, and a variety of drugs is reported. The most common manifestation of nodular regenerative hyperplasia is portal hypertension.

MALIGNANT HEPATIC TUMORS

Hepatocellular Carcinoma

EPIDEMIOLOGY. Hepatocellular carcinoma (hepatoma) is relatively uncommon (less than 2.5 per cent of all malignancies) in the United States and Western Europe. In certain other areas of the world, including parts of sub-Saharan Africa, Southeast Asia, Japan, Oceania, and Greece, hepatocellular carcinoma is among the most frequent malignancies. Hepatocellular carcinoma is predominantly a disease of males and usually arises in a cirrhotic liver. The risk appears to be greatest in cirrhosis associated with hemochromatosis and hepatitis B and C virus infection, low in primary biliary cirrhosis and Wilson's disease, and intermediate in alcoholic and cryptogenic cirrhosis. There is a particularly strong association between chronic hepatitis B virus infection and hepatocellular carcinoma, and prospective epidemiologic studies suggest that the incidence of hepatocellular carcinoma is about 100-fold higher in individuals with hepatitis B virus infection than in noninfected controls. Moreover, tumor tissue in patients with serologic evidence of hepatitis B virus infection frequently has hepatitis B virus integrated into the genome, and woodchucks and ducks infected with viruses that are related to the human hepatitis B virus also develop hepatocellular carcinoma. Infection with the recently identified hepatitis C virus is also associated with an increased prevalence of hepatocellular carcinoma.

Epidemiologic evidence has also suggested a link between hepatocellular carcinoma and ingestion of aflatoxins, mycotoxins produced by *Aspergillus flavus*, a mold that can grow in warm moist areas and contaminate peanuts and stored grains. Case reports also suggest a link between hepatocellular carcinoma and α_1-antitrypsin deficiency and administration of androgenic steroids, Thorotrast, and possibly estrogenic steroids in the form of oral contraceptives (Table 125–1).

CLINICAL FEATURES. The most common presenting features of hepatocellular carcinoma are *abdominal pain,* the presence of an *abdominal mass,* and *weight loss.* Hepatocellular carcinoma may also present with rupture and hemoperitoneum, obstructive jaundice, unexplained deterioration in a patient with cirrhosis, or a variety of paraneoplastic syndromes, including erythrocytosis, persistent fever, hypercalcemia, and hypoglycemia. Hepatomegaly is present in about two thirds of patients. Other suggestive physical findings include the presence of a bruit, hepatic friction rub, or bloody ascites. Hepatocellular carcinoma may invade and obstruct the portal and hepatic veins and metastasizes most often to regional lymph nodes and the lungs. Alpha-fetoprotein levels in serum greater than 1000 ng per milliliter or progressively rising levels are highly suggestive of hepatocellular carcinoma. Unfortunately, only a minority of patients with asymptomatic hepatocellular carcinoma in most parts of the world, including the United States, have elevations of this magnitude. Elevations up to about 200 ng per milliliter are a more sensitive indicator of early tumors but are also less specific. For this reason, α-fetoprotein has proved disappointing in the screening of high-risk populations. Ultrasonography is also used for screening in certain centers throughout the world. While these screening modalities do identify some tumors at an early stage, they have not yet been proven to improve survival in high-risk populations.

TREATMENT AND PROGNOSIS. The results of current treatment for hepatocellular carcinoma are discouraging. In the United States, median survival from the time of diagnosis is about 6 months. Because of the advanced stage of the disease at the time of diagnosis and the frequent coexistence of severe liver disease, less than 20 per cent of patients are candidates for hepatic resection. The presence of coexisting cirrhosis in a patient with well-preserved hepatic function does not altogether preclude surgery; however, such patients may not tolerate more than limited resection of a localized tumor. Adriamycin alone or in combination with other agents has produced objective tumor response in up to 50 per cent of patients but has minimally affected survival. Radiation therapy has also yielded disappointing results. Other approaches (e.g., hormonal therapy, hepatic artery ligation or embolization, radiolabeled antibodies to tumor-specific antigens) have been tried but have not yet been shown to improve survival. As discussed in Ch. 123, liver transplantation for unresectable hepatocellular carcinoma is curative in only a minority of patients.

A variant of typical hepatocellular carcinoma termed *fibrolamellar carcinoma* differs from the typical form of the disease in that it usually occurs in young adults without underlying cirrhosis, lacks the usual male predominance, is associated with a longer survival (32 to 68 months) when untreated, and has been cured surgically in between 10 and 30 per cent of cases.

Other Primary Hepatic Malignancies

Cholangiocarcinoma occurs much less frequently than hepatocellular carcinoma and shows an association with sclerosing cholangitis and with clonorchiasis and opisthorchiasis in the Far East. It may present with obstructive jaundice when it involves major ducts in the area of the hepatic hilum. Truly mixed hepatocellular cholangiocarcinomas are rare. Angiosarcoma, an unusual tumor associated with vinyl chloride exposure as well as arsenic and Thorotrast administration, frequently causes thrombocytopenia and has a propensity to rupture, causing hemoperitoneum and circulatory collapse. Other unusual primary hepatic malignant tumors of adults include cystadenocarcinoma, squamous carcinoma, and hepatoblastoma.

As with hepatocellular carcinoma, treatment of these malignant hepatic tumors has been unsatisfactory. Resection is seldom possible. Of patients with cholangiocarcinoma who have undergone liver transplantation, the 3-year survival is less than among patients with hepatocellular carcinoma.

Tumors Metastatic to Liver

The liver and lung are the most frequent sites of metastatic cancer, and metastases constitute the largest group of hepatic tumors in adults. Necropsy studies have demonstrated hepatic metastases in more than half of patients with primary malignant tumors having portal venous drainage (e.g., stomach, colon, and pancreas). Other solid tumors that frequently metastasize to the liver include melanoma and tumors of the lung, oropharynx, and bladder. Next to the spleen, the liver is also the most common extranodal site of involvement by Hodgkin's disease, the non-Hodgkin's lymphomas, and malignant histiocytosis (histiocytic medullary reticulosis).

Pseudotumors

A variety of nonneoplastic lesions may mimic hepatic tumors. These include regenerative nodules, anomalous hepatic lobulation, cysts, and focal fatty deposits. In many cases, imaging studies can distinguish these from true neoplasms.

DIAGNOSTIC APPROACH TO THE PATIENT WITH A SUSPECTED HEPATIC NEOPLASM

CLINICAL EVALUATION. Most hepatic neoplasms present as a right upper quadrant or epigastric mass. Additional clinical features that may provide clues regarding the specific type of tumor are summarized above and in Table 125–1. Cholangiocarcinoma and hepatocellular carcinoma can cause biliary obstruction, but this may potentially result from strategically located tumors of all types. Physical examination most commonly reveals hepatomegaly or a discrete mass. The presence of a bruit or friction rub may suggest hepatocellular carcinoma but is not specific. Elevations of alkaline phosphatase and transaminase levels are the most common biochemical abnormalities; however, liver function tests are not particularly helpful in diagnosis and may be entirely normal in some patients. A markedly elevated and/or rising α-fetoprotein level is strongly suggestive of hepatocellular carcinoma.

IMAGING TECHNIQUES. The detection of hepatic neoplasms has been improved by modern imaging modalities. Ultrasonography (US), computed tomography (CT), and magnetic resonance imaging (MRI) have gradually replaced hepatic scintigraphy. Unlike scintigraphy, these other modalities visualize structures outside the liver, and US and CT can be used for directed biopsy. Because of its lesser expense and lack of radiation exposure, US is often a useful initial study. As compared with US, CT provides sharper definition of other abdominal structures, is not hindered by bowel gas, and probably detects smaller hepatic lesions. MRI appears comparable to CT, but its role in hepatic imaging is still being defined. Angiography, which entails more risk and discomfort for the patient, may be particularly helpful in planning surgical resection. Because of the rapidly evolving capabilities of current imaging modalities, radiologic consultation is often appropriate.

METASTATIC TUMORS. In a patient with a known extra-hepatic malignant tumor and clinical or biochemical evidence of hepatic metastases, US is a reasonable screening study. The finding of single or multiple defects is consistent with metastatic disease, and a percutaneous biopsy can be expected to recover tumor in 50 to 75 per cent of such cases. Two biopsies performed through the same skin site and cytologic examination of the tissue core and aspirated fluid appear to enhance the yield without increasing the risk of bleeding. In patients with lymphoreticular malignant disease, percutaneous biopsy is less sensitive in demonstrating hepatic involvement than wedge biopsy obtained at laparotomy, and histologic evidence of hepatic involvement may be found even in the absence of clinical, biochemical, or radio-nuclide scan abnormalities.

PRIMARY TUMORS. The workup in suspected primary hepatic tumor must be individualized on the basis of the relative risks and benefits of establishing a diagnosis. Asymptomatic patients in whom imaging studies yield findings characteristic of hemangioma (Table 125–1) may not require additional evaluation. In most other instances, however, examination of tissue is appropriate. In a patient who is a candidate for operation and who has an apparently resectable lesion of uncertain or suspicious nature based on imaging studies, preoperative biopsy may not be necessary. In the patient who is not a candidate for surgery or in whom information regarding tumor type will importantly influence decisions regarding further evaluation and therapy, biopsy is usually appropriate. Several factors should be considered in this regard. First, needle biopsy of lesions such as hemangioma, angiosarcoma, and possibly hepatocellular adenoma is probably associated with increased risk of hemorrhage, and biopsy of a possible echinococcal cyst is contraindicated. Second, definitive diagnosis of hepatocellular adenoma and focal nodular hyperplasia, which consist predominantly of normal or minimally abnormal hepatocytes, may be difficult from examination of a needle biopsy alone. Third, compared with percutaneous biopsy, laparoscopic approach permits directed biopsy of visible tumor deposits and may facilitate control of bleeding. Finally, a CT- or US-directed fine needle percutaneous aspiration biopsy has yielded excellent results in many centers and appears to be associated with a lower risk of hemorrhage than standard biopsy. It is particularly helpful for lesions not accessible to blind percutaneous biopsy.

Colombo M, Choo QL, Del Ninno E, et al.: Prevalence of antibodies to hepatitis C virus in Italian patients with hepatocellular carcinoma. Lancet 2:1006, 1989. *This is one of two companion articles in the same issue that implicates hepatitis C in the pathogenesis of hepatocellular carcinoma.*

DiBiscegli AM, Rustgi VK, Hoofnagle JH, et al.: Hepatocellular carcinoma. Ann Intern Med 108:390, 1988. *Proceedings of a National Institutes of Health Conference dealing with all aspects of this topic.*

Ishak KG: Benign tumors and pseudotumors of the liver. J Appl Pathol 6:82, 1988. *A review oriented toward histopathology drawn from the uniquely rich experience of the Armed Forces Institute of Pathology.*

Reading NG, Forbes A, Nunnerly HB, et al.: Hepatic hemangioma: A critical review of diagnosis and management. Q J Med 67:431, 1988. *An excellent recent review of this most common hepatic neoplasm.*

Regan LS: Screening for hepatocellular carcinoma in high-risk individuals: A clinical review. Arch Intern Med 149:1741, 1989. *A brief review of an important topic.*

Rothschild MA, Oratz M: Hepatic imaging. Semin Liver Dis 9:1, 1989. *An entire issue with nine thoroughly referenced chapters dealing with all aspects of hepatic imaging.*

126 Diseases of the Gallbladder and Bile Ducts

Peter F. Malet and Roger D. Soloway

Biliary tract disorders result from a variety of congenital, inflammatory, metabolic, infectious, and neoplastic conditions. These conditions often present in subtle ways and can pose challenging diagnostic problems. Ongoing improvements in diagnostic and therapeutic techniques have allowed the clinician to diagnose biliary tract disease more quickly and to treat patients more effectively.

NORMAL PHYSIOLOGY OF BILE FORMATION

Bile is an isotonic aqueous mixture consisting primarily of electrolytes, proteins, bile salts, cholesterol, phospholipids, and bilirubin. Secretion across the canalicular membrane of the hepatocyte accounts for about two thirds of total bile flow. Bile salt-dependent secretion comprises about one half of canalicular bile formation, while the other half is termed bile salt independent and consists mainly of electrolytes. The remaining one third of bile flow is an alkaline fraction generated by the epithelial cells lining the bile ducts; ductular secretion is stimulated by secretin, cholecystokinin, and gastrin. An as yet unquantitated contribution to canalicular bile flow consisting mainly of water and electrolytes occurs by way of the interhepatocytic space (paracellular pathway). The total volume of bile produced ranges from 500 to 800 ml per day.

Under basal (fasting) conditions, tonic contraction of the sphincter of Oddi diverts about half of the flow of hepatic bile into the gallbladder; the other half flows into the duodenum assisted by phasic peristaltic action of the sphincter. The gallbladder actively reabsorbs Na^+, Cl^-, and HCO_3^+ and passively resorbs H_2O. It is capable of concentrating bile 10-fold within about 4 hours. The gallbladder mucosa secretes H^+ and mucin.

Cholecystokinin, released from the intestinal mucosa after meals by fat, amino acids, and H^+, simultaneously stimulates the gallbladder to contract and the sphincter of Oddi to relax, emptying bile into the duodenum.

Bile salts are synthesized by hepatocytes (Fig. 126–1) from cholesterol by a multistep process, the rate-limiting step of which is catalyzed by 7α-hydroxylase, which is under inhibitory feedback control. Cholate and chenodeoxycholate, the two *primary* bile salts (that is, they are synthesized in the liver), are conjugated with either glycine or taurine before secretion to improve solubility. Bile salts are secreted by active transport across the biliary canalicular membrane. After entering the proximal small intestine, bile salts aid in fat absorption by forming *micelles* (Ch. 102) and then are largely reabsorbed in the mid and distal small intestine. Bile salts that reach the colon are partially deconjugated, which makes them more lipid soluble and facilitates their reabsorption. Cholate and chenodeoxycholate are also partially converted by bacterial 7α-dehydroxylation to the *secondary* bile salts, deoxycholate and lithocholate, respectively. Deoxycholate is absorbed from the colon, reconjugated in the liver, and excreted in bile. Lithocholate is poorly reabsorbed; it is sulfated as well as reconjugated during hepatic transfer. Sulfation increases aqueous solubility and further reduces intestinal reabsorption. The average bile salt composition of bile is 35 per cent chenodeoxycholate, 35 per cent cholate, 25 per cent deoxycholate, 2 per cent ursodeoxycholate, and 2 per cent lithocholate. Each is conjugated with either glycine or taurine in a ratio of 2 to 3:1. Bile salts are secreted in the form of micelles containing phospholipids (mainly lecithin), and cholesterol. These lipids account for 90 per cent of biliary solids.

Intestinal reabsorption of bile salts, which is about 95 per cent for a single passage, occurs by passive diffusion throughout the intestine and by active transport within the terminal ileum. The reabsorbed bile salts are largely bound to albumin in portal blood and are then almost completely removed by the hepatocytes in a single passage through the liver sinusoids. The bile salt pool, normally 1.8 to 3.0 grams, passes through the liver and intestine two or three times during each meal, producing six to nine cycles

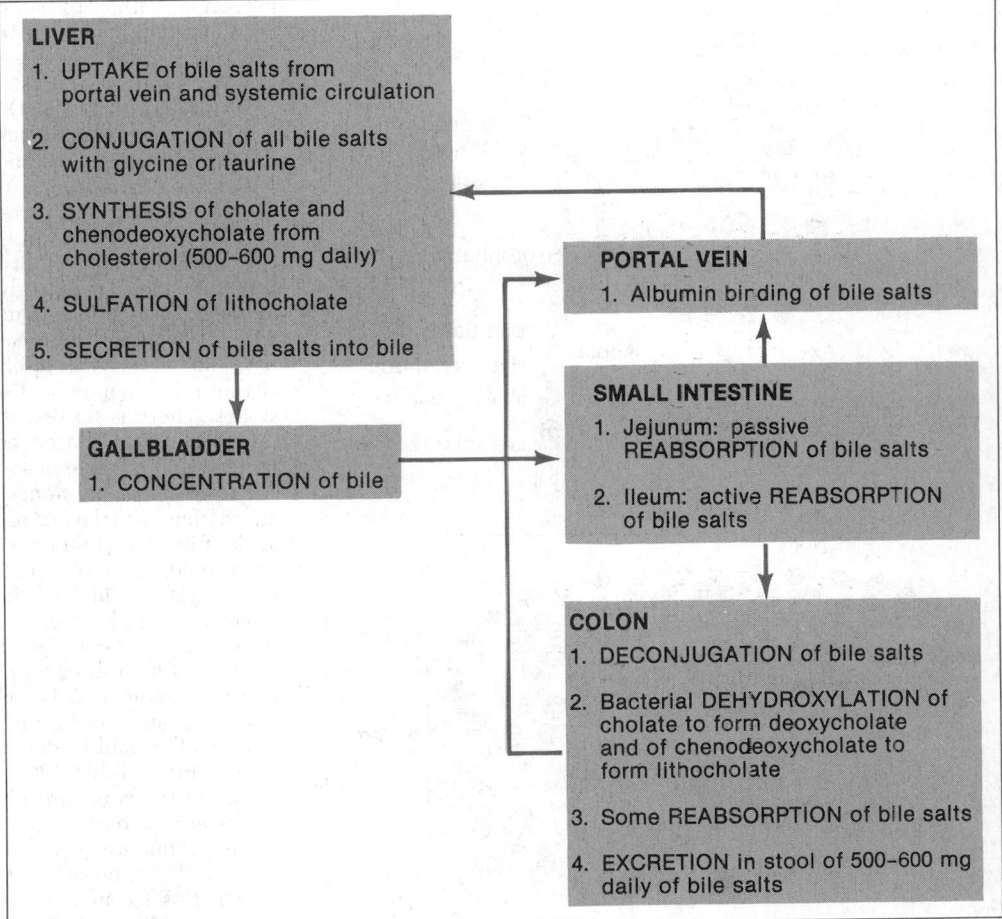

FIGURE 126–1. The major steps in the enterohepatic circulation of bile salts. This cycle provides for conservation of bile salts by an effective reabsorption mechanism in the intestine.

daily (i.e., each day about 20 to 25 grams of bile salts enter the duodenum); this cycling is termed the *enterohepatic circulation*. During an average day involving three meals, bile salts are in continuous motion with peaks of secretion during and following meals. At night, when the majority of the secreted hepatic bile eventually enters the gallbladder, and there is no stimulus for gallbladder contraction, the intestinal concentration of bile salts is much lower. Conservation of bile salts in this enterohepatic circulation is so efficient that only 15 to 25 per cent (500 to 600 mg) of the bile salt pool must be replaced by hepatic synthesis of new bile salts daily. If the efficiency of enterohepatic conservation is impaired by conditions such as biliary fistula, ileal Crohn's disease, or ileal resection, hepatic synthesis of bile salts increases. The maximal synthetic rate (5 grams per day) is insufficient to restore intraluminal concentrations to normal if external losses exceed this amount.

Bile salts are *amphophiles*, possessing water-soluble and fat-soluble sides. In an aqueous medium they are distributed randomly until a critical concentration (about 2 mM) is reached, at which point spontaneous aggregation forms multimolecular structures called micelles. In micelles the bile salt molecules line up with their hydrophilic portions facing the solvent (water) and their hydrophobic portions facing each other (Fig. 126–2). The hydrocarbon center of the micelle can incorporate biliary lecithin and cholesterol, and the entire aggregate remains water soluble. The addition of lecithin expands micellar size and enhances the ability of bile salt micelles to incorporate other lipids. In addition, a variable amount of cholesterol is carried in lecithin-cholesterol vesicles. The ultimate cholesterol-carrying capacity of bile depends on the relative amounts of bile salts and lecithin as well as the total lipid concentration.

Besides electrolytes, other solutes in bile are bilirubin that has been conjugated in the liver with glucuronic acid (Ch. 115), proteins, and cations such as calcium, iron, copper, and zinc, and low concentrations of the end-products of drug and hormone metabolism.

PATHOPHYSIOLOGY OF GALLSTONE DISEASE

In Western nations about 75 per cent of gallstones are composed principally of cholesterol (*cholesterol gallstones*) and 25 per cent of calcium bilirubinate and other calcium salts (*pigment gallstones*). Overall, about 15 per cent of gallstones are radiopaque, about two thirds of which are pigment and one third are cholesterol stones. The symptoms caused by gallstones are the same regardless of the chemical composition and to a large extent are independent of size. Stones can cause pain and jaundice by passage into the common bile duct or can cause pain by intermittently becoming impacted in the neck of the gallbladder.

CHOLESTEROL GALLSTONES. Cholesterol stones are usually yellow-green to tan or brown and are round or faceted. They may be single or multiple; most range in size from 1 mm to 3 to 4 cm. Cholesterol accounts for 50 to 100 per cent of stone weight, the remainder consisting of mucin glycoproteins and less than 10 per cent calcium bilirubinate and/or other calcium salts. These stones occur two to three times as frequently in women as men, the difference beginning at puberty and declining after menopause. In the United States, 20 per cent of 75-year-old men and 35 per cent of 75-year-old women have stones at autopsy. The incidence is higher with multiparity and with the use of birth control pills. About 75 per cent of American Indian women over the age of 25 years and 90 per cent of those over age 60 are affected. Obesity and hereditary influences are also important in stone formation.

Cholesterol, which is insoluble in water, is normally carried in bile within bile salt–lecithin micelles and lecithin-cholesterol vesicles. A completely clear micellar solution of bile is one in which cholesterol is completely solubilized. A prerequisite for cholesterol gallstone formation is an excess of cholesterol in relation to carrying capacity, a condition that may result from decreased bile salt or increased cholesterol concentration in bile. When the cholesterol-solubilization capacity of bile is exceeded, bile is termed *supersaturated* or *lithogenic*.

Bile of patients with gallstones has relatively more cholesterol

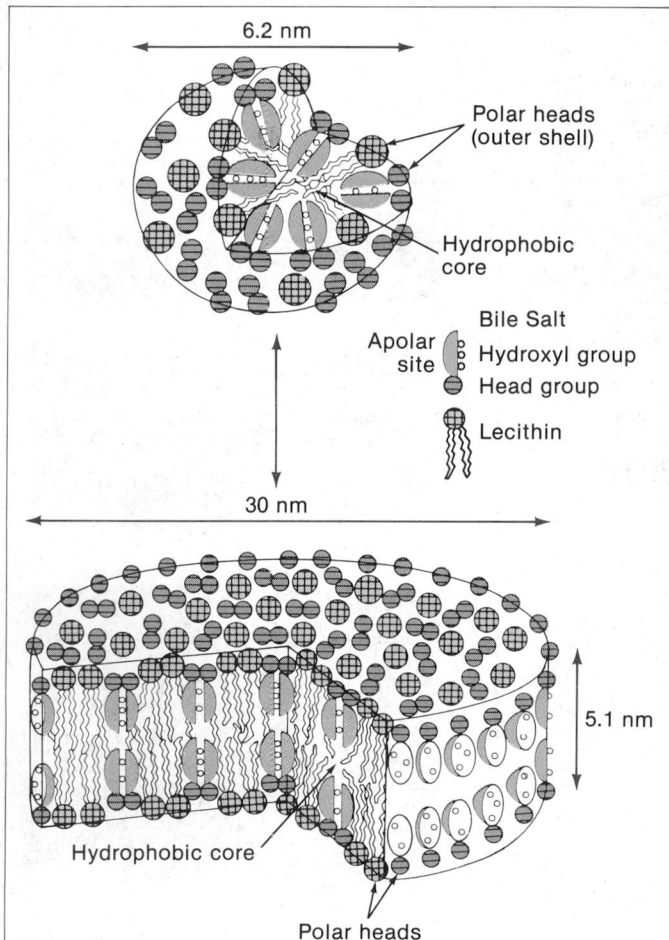

FIGURE 126–2. Dimorphic structure of a biliary mixed lipid micelle, which has been shown to exhibit a sphere → disc transition, depending upon whether the solution is bile salt-rich (*sphere*) or lecithin-rich (*disc*). The lecithin-rich micelle is larger and capable of dissolving and transporting a much larger amount of cholesterol. The transition depends upon the bile salt–lecithin molar ratio present in the micelle but may also be influenced by other constituents present in native bile. Bile salt molecules in both micellar forms are thought to form pairs (dimers) to avoid contact of the hydroxyl groups (*small clear circles*) with the nonpolar environment of the micellar core. (Adapted with permission from Muller K: Biochemistry 20:404, 1981. Copyright 1981 American Chemical Society.)

than that of normal persons, although the overlap is great. In patients with gallstones, bile is supersaturated with cholesterol as it emerges from the liver, implicating the hepatocytes as the cause of the abnormality. In some patients with gallstones the total bile salt pool is decreased in size, and the hepatocytes have decreased amounts of the enzyme 7α-hydroxylase. Another factor, particularly associated with obesity, is increased cholesterol secretion into hepatic bile.

The relationship between cholesterol and bile salt output is hyperbolic, so that when bile salt secretion declines, the cholesterol–bile salt ratio climbs and the bile becomes more supersaturated. During fasting, bile salts are sequestered in the gallbladder, hepatic secretion of bile salts declines, the rate of cholesterol secretion persists, and the bile becomes more lithogenic. Supersaturation of bile with cholesterol is therefore common even in normal persons after overnight or prolonged fasting.

Cholesterol saturation of bile appears to be a necessary but not a sufficient condition for cholesterol gallstone formation. Supersaturated bile from patients without gallstones forms cholesterol crystals slowly on prolonged incubation (long nucleation time), while bile of identical lipid composition from patients with stones usually forms such crystals quickly (short nucleation time). Normal human bile contains *solubilizing* or *antinucleating factors*,

for example, apolipoprotein A-1, that inhibit cholesterol crystallization. The gallbladder is considered to be important in gallstone formation, either by supplying a nidus (*nucleating factor*) for crystallization, such as mucin glycoproteins or other smaller proteins secreted by the epithelium, or by providing an area of stasis to facilitate precipitation.

PIGMENT GALLSTONES. Pigment stones are subdivided into two categories, black and brown stones, on the basis of differing compositional and microstructural characteristics.

Black pigment stones, much more common in the West, are usually under 1 cm, irregular in shape, and homogeneous on cross-section. They form in the gallbladder and are composed of calcium bilirubinate, bilirubin polymers, calcium phosphate and carbonate, and mucin glycoproteins. There is no relationship between black stones and obesity, parity, or saturation of bile with cholesterol. The great majority of patients with black stones have no underlying disease, but the elderly or patients with cirrhosis and hemolytic diseases are predisposed to develop these stones. There is no sexual predisposition. American Indians are rarely affected. The concentration of unconjugated bilirubin is increased in the bile of some patients with these stones.

Brown pigment stones have layers of calcium bilirubinate alternating with layers of cholesterol and calcium salts of fatty acids. Bilirubin is thought to precipitate with calcium because β-glucuronidase of bacterial, biliary epithelial, or hepatic origin deconjugates bilirubin diglucuronide to less soluble bilirubin monoglucuronide or unconjugated bilirubin. The fatty acids of biliary lecithin may be similarly precipitated as calcium salts because of hydrolysis by phospholipases. These stones are much more common in Asia, where bacterial infection of the biliary tract is thought to be involved in their pathogenesis. They can form in the gallbladder and/or in intrahepatic or extrahepatic biliary ducts (Table 126–1). In Western nations they form primarily in the common bile duct years after cholecystectomy for cholesterol or black pigment stones. Unlike in the West, in Asia stones frequently recur after removal and are associated with massive dilatation of the biliary tract and accompanying cholangiohepatitis (recurrent pyogenic cholangitis), often resulting in secondary biliary cirrhosis and hepatic failure.

DISSOLUTION OF GALLSTONES. Cholesterol gallstones can be dissolved by reversing some of the above pathogenetic mechanisms. Ursodeoxycholate (urso), 10 to 12 mg per kilogram per day orally, dissolves a proportion of radiolucent cholesterol gallbladder stones within 2 years. Urso causes the bile to become unsaturated, thereby allowing absorption of cholesterol from the surface of the stone. Minor problems with urso therapy include diarrhea and elevation of serum ALT in about 1 per cent of patients. Urso is ineffective for dissolution of stones greater than 20 mm diameter, of pigment stones, radiopaque stones, and stones in gallbladders nonopacified by oral cholecystography. Candidates for dissolution treatment are mildly to moderately symptomatic patients who wish to avoid surgery or are bad risks for surgery because of other illnesses. Stones usually dissolve in 1 or 2 years in 30 to 40 per cent of patients. Higher success rates

TABLE 126–1. CONDITIONS ASSOCIATED WITH A PROPENSITY FOR GALLSTONE FORMATION

1. **Cholesterol**
   Obesity
   Ileal disease or resection
   Multiparity
   Drugs: clofibrate, estrogens
   Race: American Indian
   Cystic fibrosis
   Rapid weight loss
2. **Black pigment**
   Old age
   Cirrhosis
   Hemolysis
   Intravenous hyperalimentation
3. **Brown pigment**
   Oriental cholangiohepatitis
   Sclerosing cholangitis
   Caroli's disease
   Choledochal cysts
   Duodenal diverticula (perivaterian)

are seen in patients with small (less than 5 mm diameter) floating gallstones. Women who may become pregnant should not be treated because of the potential (though not proven) for harmful effects of urso on the fetus. When treatment is discontinued after initial dissolution, gallstones re-form in about two thirds of patients within 12 years. Prophylactic therapy with urso (300 mg per day orally) can halve this recurrence rate.

Current research into new methods of gallstone dissolution includes direct instillation of methyl-tert-butyl ether into the gallbladder lumen by percutaneous transhepatic catheter placement. This technique usually dissolves cholesterol gallstones within 1 to 2 days. Another technique undergoing study is extracorporeal shock-wave lithotripsy in which gallstones are fragmented into fine particles. These particles are easier to dissolve with urso than are the intact stones.

PATHOPHYSIOLOGY OF BILIARY OBSTRUCTION

Obstruction caused by a stone is the primary cause of all manifestations of gallstone disease. Obstruction of the cystic duct by gallbladder stones distends the gallbladder, producing biliary pain. If the obstruction persists, acute cholecystitis or hydrops may ensue. Whether complications such as empyema or perforation develop depends on whether secondary infection occurs. Cholecystectomy cures cholecystitis, but cholecystostomy, which only relieves the obstruction, eliminates all the clinical manifestations of the disease.

Obstruction of the common duct may produce pain, jaundice, pruritus, infection, and biliary cirrhosis. Surgical procedures that decompress the duct upstream from the stone eliminate these manifestations. The situation in the ductal system differs from that in the gallbladder, however, because when ductal pressure exceeds about 25 cm/H$_2$O, bile is refluxed into blood. Pressures in this range and even higher commonly accompany mechanical obstruction. Regurgitation of ductal bacteria into the systemic circulation may explain why cholangitis is often accompanied by systemic bacteremia, chills, and high fever. Fortunately obstruction of the common duct by stones is rarely complete. With unrelieved ductal obstruction, biliary cirrhosis gradually develops. Three months is the shortest time in which cirrhosis occurs, and the earliest cases follow neoplastic (high-grade) obstruction.

OBSTRUCTIVE JAUNDICE. Patients with biliary obstruction often present with jaundice. The approach to the clinical evaluation of jaundice is described in detail in Ch. 115.

ROENTGENOLOGIC AND OTHER IMAGING TESTS

Since biliary disease usually results from obstructive lesions, radiologic techniques, if successful in outlining the system, are often diagnostic. The choice and timing of these direct and indirect procedures depend upon the diagnostic strategy of the clinician. They are discussed in greater detail in Ch. 93 and 113.

Plain roentgenograms can demonstrate the 10 to 15 per cent of gallstones that contain enough calcium to be radiopaque, but the relationship of the stones to the gallbladder or bile ducts is not always obvious. Emphysematous cholecystitis, air in the bile ducts, and calcium in the wall of the gallbladder also have diagnostic appearances on plain films.

Oral cholecystography requires that the night prior to the examination the patient swallow tablets of iopanoic or tyropanoic acid, which are then absorbed from the gut, excreted in bile, and concentrated in the gallbladder. If the gallbladder is opacified, stones in the lumen are shown as radiolucent defects (Fig. 126–3). Oral cholecystography is 90 to 95 per cent accurate in detecting gallstones. Nonopacification of the gallbladder occurs if the cystic duct is blocked or if the diseased gallbladder mucosa cannot concentrate the contrast material. The gallbladder may not be opacified for several reasons not related to gallbladder disease: if the patient has been vomiting, if the patient has been fasting for several days immediately before taking the tablets, or if absorption by the gut or excretion by the liver is faulty. If extrabiliary causes of a nonopacified gallbladder are excluded, nonopacification is 95 per cent reliable in indicating gallbladder disease.

Ultrasonography of the biliary tree may demonstrate gallstones or dilatation of the intrahepatic or extrahepatic ductal system (Fig. 126–4). It also has the advantage of being able to examine the liver and pancreas at the same time. Real-time ultrasonog-

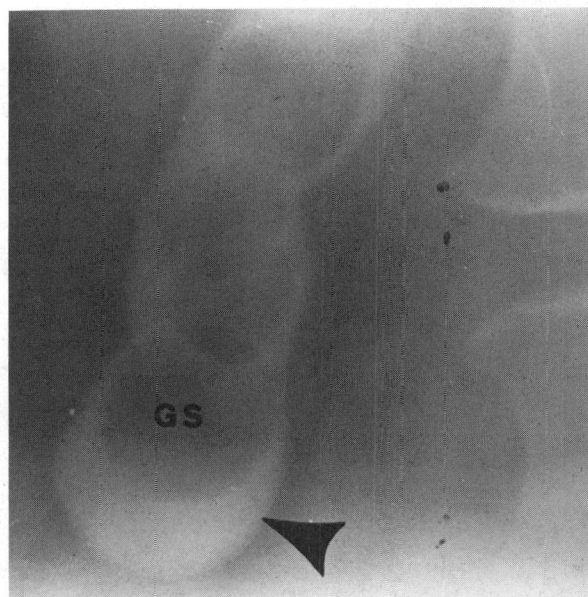

FIGURE 126–3. Oral cholecytogram showing a gallbladder (*arrowhead*) opacified by an orally administered contrast agent. The gallbladder is filled with four large round gallstones (GS).

raphy is very reliable in detecting gallbladder stones (false positives are uncommon); it should be used as the first test for screening for gallstones. Ductal dilatation is detected in about 90 per cent of cases of proven obstruction. Unfortunately, less than one third of common duct stones are actually identified. Ductal dilatation usually indicates distal obstruction by neoplasm, stricture, or stone. The correlation between dilatation and obstruction is inexact because (1) the ducts may be dilated from previous disease or surgery although currently unobstructed, (2) cirrhosis or scarring from previous cholangitis may stiffen the ducts enough to prevent dilatation, and (3) lesions characterized by intermittent obstruction (e.g., common duct stones, stricture) may result in dilatation followed by spontaneous decompression; ducts may appear undilated if the patient is examined after such decompression.

Percutaneous transhepatic cholangiography (PTC) involves direct percutaneous puncture of an intrahepatic duct by a needle inserted through the eighth or ninth right intercostal space into the center of the liver. An abnormal clotting mechanism, significant ascites, and severe cholangitis are contraindications. PTC has proved particularly valuable in diagnosing gallstones within the intrahepatic biliary tract, biliary strictures, and neoplastic obstruction of the bile ducts (Fig. 126–5). A technically successful study can be obtained in nearly all patients with dilated ducts and in 70 per cent of patients with normal-sized ducts.

Endoscopic retrograde cholangiopancreatography (ERCP) involves cannulation of the common bile duct and pancreatic duct through the ampulla of Vater via the endoscope (see Fig. 93–7). With experience, a successful study of one or both ducts is possible in 90 per cent of attempts. ERCP is particularly useful in patients with normal-sized bile ducts or in whom pancreatic disease as a cause of bile duct obstruction is strongly suspected.

Both PTC and ERCP are usually contraindicated in active cholangitis unless a therapeutic maneuver is planned because as ductal pressure increases during injection of the contrast material, severe uncontrollable sepsis may be produced. Patients undergoing either of these procedures should usually receive premedication with antimicrobial agents if biliary obstruction is known or suspected.

Radionuclide imaging of the biliary tree may be accomplished by intravenous injection of a ^{99m}Tc-labeled derivative of iminodiacetic acid (e.g., HIDA or DISIDA). Normally, a high-quality image of the biliary tree appears within 30 minutes after administration of the radionuclide agent (see Fig. 93–9). This test is the procedure of choice in verifying the diagnosis of acute cholecystitis. Filling of the ducts but not of the gallbladder

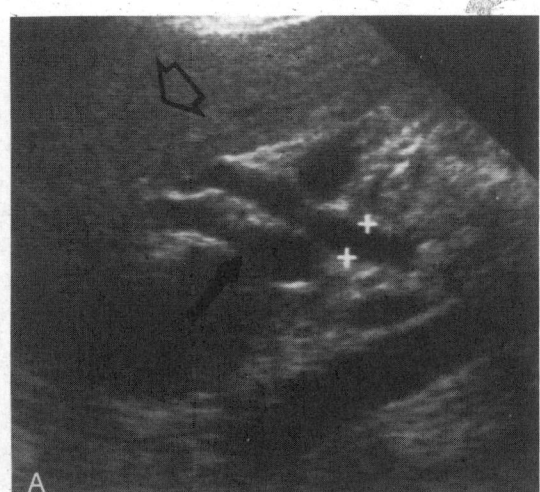

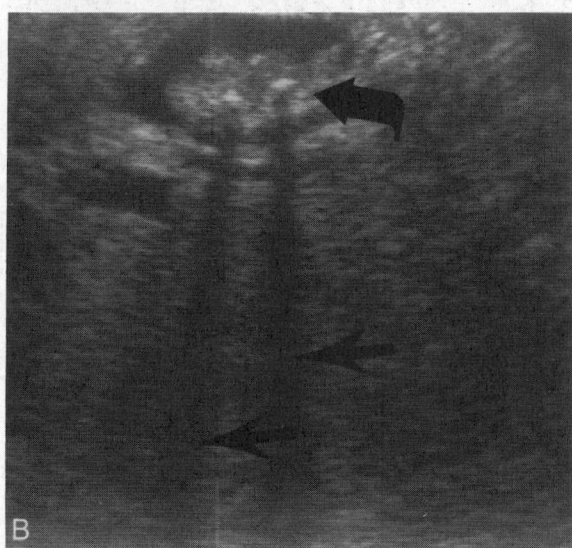

FIGURE 126–4. A, Real-time ultrasonography of the extrahepatic biliary tract showing a dilated common bile duct (the width of the duct measured between the two white crosses is 9 mm); the portal vein is seen as the anechoic area (solid arrow) directly beneath the common bile duct. The liver parenchyma is indicated by the arrowhead. B, Ultrasonography of a gallbladder containing gallstones and sludge (curved arrow) that appear as echogenic foci within the gallbladder lumen. The gallstones exhibit acoustic shadowing (lower two arrows), that is, paucity of echoes distal to the stones due to blockage of the echo waves by the solid stones. (Courtesy of Dr. Peter Arger.)

supports the diagnosis of cholecystitis due to obstruction of the cystic duct by a stone or edema. A false-negative study is rare; however, false-positive (nonfilling) studies are seen in patients with severe illnesses such as pancreatitis and in those receiving intravenous hyperalimentation. Ultrasonography is more useful in detecting common bile duct obstruction than is radionuclide imaging.

Computed tomography is usually performed after evidence of biliary ductal disease has been ascertained by ultrasonography or cholangiography. It is useful in defining pancreatic causes of biliary tract obstruction, in detecting paraductal lymph node enlargement, and in examining the liver for abscesses, intrahepatic ductal dilatation, and neoplasms.

CLINICAL CATEGORIES OF GALLBLADDER AND BILIARY TRACT DISEASES

Asymptomatic Gallstones

Approximately 60 to 80 per cent of patients with gallstones are asymptomatic, based on surveys using ultrasonography. In the past, patients with asymptomatic gallstones were advised to have a cholecystectomy. The trend now is to observe such patients

and not to recommend surgery unless they develop biliary pain. Prophylactic cholecystectomy is reserved for patients with *calcified gallbladders*, often associated with carcinoma of the gallbladder. Asymptomatic patients with gallstones have approximately a 20 per cent chance of developing biliary pain in 20 years. Even with symptomatic patients, the decision to perform surgery is not always clear-cut. Patients with infrequent mild pain may prefer not to undergo cholecystectomy, or the physician may be hesitant to recommend surgery because of serious coexisting illnesses. Such patients are suitable candidates to consider for medical dissolution with ursodeoxycholate.

Symptomatic Gallstones

PATHOLOGY. The pathologic findings in the gallbladder wall and the clinical manifestations of gallstone disease often correlate poorly. In some patients the gallbladder is severely affected as the result of previous attacks of acute cholecystitis, with shrinking, scarring, and thickening of the wall, adhesions to adjacent viscera, and patchy replacement of the mucosa by granulation tissue or collagen. Nonopacification following oral cholecystography is frequent in such patients. At the other extreme the gallbladder may be grossly normal with only slight thinning of the mucosa, mild patchy scarring and inflammation, and a normally visualized oral cholecystogram. The term *chronic cholecystitis* is a descriptive pathologic term for such changes, although it has been used to describe the clinical manifestations of chronically symptomatic gallstones.

CLINICAL MANIFESTATIONS. Symptomatic gallstones commonly produce a steady pain most often located in the epigastrium or right upper quadrant, thought to be caused by gallbladder distention arising from transient obstruction of the cystic duct by a stone. The onset of pain takes only a few minutes; it quickly reaches a plateau in intensity that may range from mild to moderate to excruciating. After 30 minutes to several hours the pain subsides gradually. The pain does not wax and wane like intestinal colic; hence the preferred term is *biliary pain*, not biliary colic. Nausea and vomiting may accompany the attack, and a vague residual ache or soreness may remain after the acute pain has dissipated. Tenderness, muscular guarding, a palpable mass, fever, and leukocytosis are absent, distinguishing this condition from acute cholecystitis. Many patients have simultaneous pain referred to the back near the scapula or to the right shoulder area. Attacks may occur daily or as seldom as once every few years. Not uncommonly, patients with symptomatic gallstones have pain that does not exactly fit this "textbook description." Dyspepsia, intolerance to fatty food, flatulence, heartburn, and belching may occur but are not helpful diagnostically because they often occur in persons with normal gallbladders.

Hydrops (mucocele) of the gallbladder refers to its distention with mucus (white bile) and gallstones; it may develop from cystic duct obstruction. Hydrops produces constant discomfort in the right upper quadrant and a palpable mass without the clinical findings of acute cholecystitis.

DIAGNOSIS. Real-time *ultrasonography* is the preferred test because it is 95 to 99 per cent sensitive in detecting gallbladder stones. It also has the advantage of allowing examination of the common bile duct, pancreas, and liver at the same time without radiation exposure. An oral cholecystogram after a double dose of contrast material (that is, taken on the two nights prior to the examination) identifies 90 to 95 per cent of gallstones. In about 5 to 10 per cent of patients with gallstones, opacification of the gallbladder is adequate during oral cholecystography, but calculi are not demonstrated, usually because the stones are too small to be seen.

In patients with typical biliary pain in the absence of demonstrable gallstones by cholecystography or ultrasonography, examination of bile for crystals may prove helpful. A sample of bile is obtained from an orally placed duodenal tube or via endoscopy and is examined microscopically for the presence of cholesterol crystals. The significance of calcium bilirubinate crystals is uncertain. In the presence of what seems to be biliary pain, a positive duodenal drainage test is highly suggestive that tiny stones are present or, in rare cases, that cholesterolosis is present.

The *differential diagnosis* includes other common causes of chronic abdominal symptoms such as peptic ulcer, gastroesophageal reflux, esophageal spasm, and pancreatitis, which may have manifestations similar to those of gallstones. Radicular pain from spinal lesions or rib pain from bone lesions may mimic biliary pain. Angina pectoris may cause pain thought to be abdominal, just as biliary pain may be felt in the precordial region. Postprandial pain or discomfort may result from the irritable bowel syndrome or intestinal tumors.

COMPLICATIONS. *Choledocholithiasis* is the most common complication, affecting about 15 per cent of patients with cholecystolithiasis. The incidence of common duct stones increases with advancing age. Patients with symptomatic gallstones may eventually develop an attack of *acute cholecystitis*. About two thirds of patients with acute cholecystitis have previously had symptomatic gallstones. *Acute pancreatitis* may develop when stones migrate through the distal common bile duct. *Mirizzi's syndrome* results from extrinsic compression of the common hepatic or common bile duct by a large stone in the cystic duct. Obstructive jaundice may develop. Calcification of the gallbladder *(porcelain gallbladder)* is an uncommon condition, but of special significance because of its frequent association with carcinoma of the gallbladder. The diagnosis is made from the radiographic demonstration of an eggshell-like rim of calcium in the gallbladder wall. *Adenocarcinoma* of the gallbladder is found mainly in elderly patients with cholelithiasis, most of whom have had biliary symptoms for many years.

TREATMENT. Dietary changes, anticholinergics, and antispasmodics have no effect on the course of the disease, but they sometimes provide temporary symptomatic relief. Analgesics should be used for relief of pain. *Cholecystectomy* is the treatment of choice. An attempt to dissolve the stones with urso is an appropriate alternative in selected cases. At operation the common bile duct is inspected, a cholangiogram is obtained, and the duct is explored if there is evidence of choledocholithiasis.

Cholecystectomy relieves symptoms from gallstones; the postcholecystectomy syndrome is discussed later in this chapter. Removal of the gallbladder does not impair gastrointestinal function. The mortality in elective cholecystectomy is less than 0.5 per cent. In patients over 70 years of age, however, mortality rises to 2 to 3 per cent; most of the postoperative deaths are a result of pre-existing cardiopulmonary diseases.

Acute Cholecystitis

PATHOGENESIS. Acute cholecystitis is the result of cystic duct obstruction and chemical inflammation rather than of bacterial infection. Filling the gallbladder of a dog with concentrated bile and obstructing the cystic duct produce acute inflammation. If the gallbladder is empty or distended with physiologic saline solution instead of bile, cystic duct obstruction is tolerated without inflammation. Obstruction is associated with the release of phospholipase from the gallbladder epithelium that can hydrolyze lecithin, resulting in lysolecithin, an epithelial toxin. Simultaneously the epithelial barrier coating of mucin glycoproteins may be acutely disrupted, making the epithelium susceptible to injury by the detergent action of the concentrated bile salts.

Bacterial infection is secondary to biliary obstruction rather than being primary. Bacteria are not present in the gallbladders of asymptomatic or chronically symptomatic patients with cholesterol or black pigment gallstones. Early in acute cholecystitis, the gallbladder bile is sterile, but within a week after onset, bacteria may be present in bile in over 50 per cent of cases. Although infection is secondary, it may be ultimately responsible for the most serious sequelae of acute cholecystitis—empyema, gangrene, and perforation.

Acalculous cholecystitis accounts for less than 5 per cent of cases. Most cases have been associated with prolonged fasting after major trauma, e.g., war or automobile accident injuries, surgical operations, multisystem organ failure, sepsis, or severe burns. Rare cases are caused by *Salmonella typhosa*, polyarteritis nodosa, or ischemia of other causes. At operation the bile is viscous and full of sludge. Gangrene and perforation are more frequent, and the outcome is worse than in acute calculous cholecystitis.

PATHOLOGY. Early inflammation with subserosal edema, mucosal ulcerations, and submucosal hemorrhages progresses slowly to cellular infiltration of the wall after 3 to 4 days, which reaches its greatest intensity at the end of the first week. During the second week, patchy mural gangrene, small intramural ab-

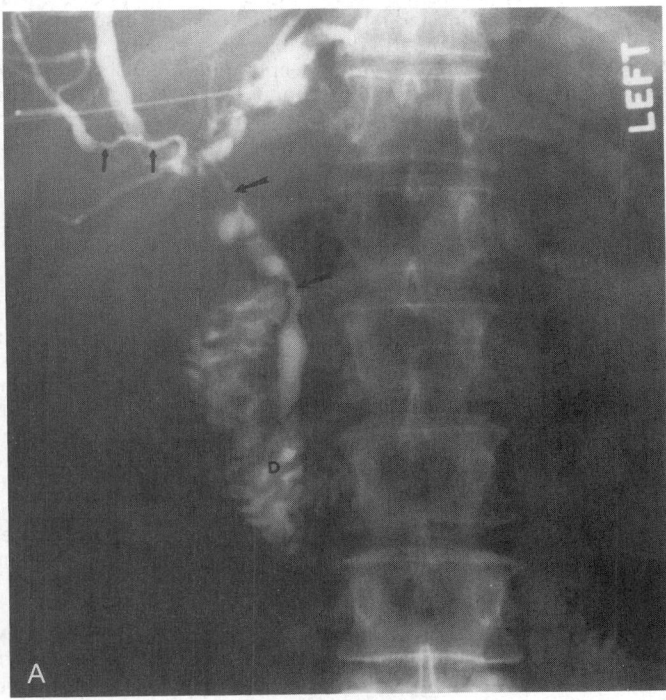
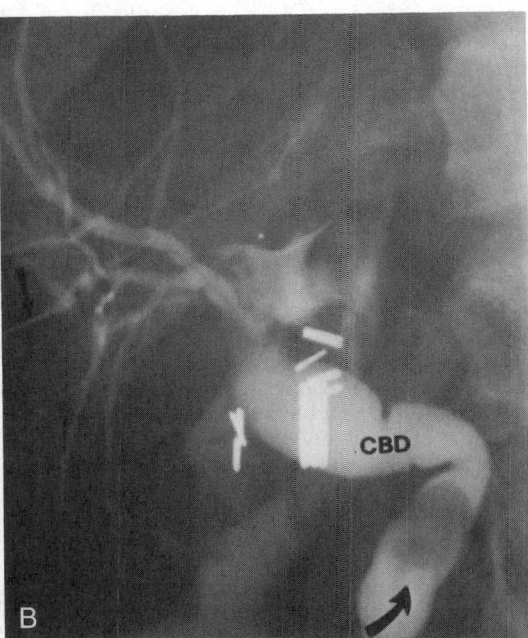

FIGURE 126–5. *A,* Percutaneous transhepatic cholangiogram demonstrating primary sclerosing cholangitis in a 54-year-old woman with a long history of Crohn's disease and biochemical evidence of cholestasis. There are strictures *(arrows)* scattered throughout her intra- and extrahepatic biliary tract; dye is seen to flow into the duodenum (D). *B,* Percutaneous transhepatic cholangiogram (skinny needle used for dye injection is indicated by arrow on left) showing a 1.5 × 2.0 cm gallstone *(curved arrow)* in the distal common bile duct (CBD) causing dilatation of the extrahepatic biliary tract. The metallic clips are from a prior cholecystectomy. The patient presented with a 3-day history of RUQ pain and jaundice with a total bilirubin of 5.6 mg per deciliter. (Courtesy of Dr. Gordon McLean.)

scesses, and collagen deposition appear. Resolution of the acute changes takes another week or more.

The term *empyema* describes the rare entity of a pus-filled gallbladder characterized clinically by a septic form of acute cholecystitis. Gangrene and perforation are most common in the fundus where the blood supply is meager or in the neck where stones become impacted. With perforation, gallbladder contents may spill into the free abdominal cavity (bile peritonitis) or, more often, are confined by adhesions (pericholecystic abscess). Sometimes an adherent viscus is penetrated, forming a cholecystenteric fistula through which the gallstones and pus may be discharged. Fistulization is most frequent with the duodenum, but jejunal and colonic fistulas have been described.

CLINICAL MANIFESTATIONS. An attack of acute cholecystitis begins with *abdominal pain* that increases gradually in severity. The pain is usually located in the right subcostal region from the start, but it sometimes begins in the epigastrium or left upper quadrant and then shifts to the region of the gallbladder as inflammation progresses. Two thirds or more of patients have had previous episodes of typical biliary pain. Early in the attack the patient may expect the symptoms to subside spontaneously as had happened before with similar pain, and medical aid is often not sought until 24 to 48 hours or more. Referred pain may be experienced in the back at the scapular level. Patients in their 70's and 80's may have few or no localizing symptoms.

Anorexia, nausea, and vomiting are often present, but vomiting is rarely severe enough to be confused with bowel obstruction and is generally less than in acute pancreatitis. In the absence of complications, chills are rare, and the temperature is about 38°C. Chills and high temperature suggest suppurative cholecystitis or associated cholangitis.

The right subcostal region is tender to palpation, and involuntary muscle spasm generally limits the examination. If the patient takes a deep breath while the subhepatic area is being palpated, heightened tenderness arrests inspiration (*Murphy's sign*).

In somewhat less than a quarter of the patients, a distended, tender gallbladder can be distinctly felt, an important finding that confirms the suspected diagnosis. The gallbladder cannot be felt in the rest of the patients because of obesity, rigidity of the abdominal wall, or deep subhepatic location or because it is small and shrunken from previous inflammation. Other related conditions characterized by a tender mass in the same area are pericholecystic abscess, acute cholecystitis complicating carcinoma of the gallbladder, or gallbladder distention in obstructive cholangitis.

About 10 per cent of patients with acute cholecystitis have *mild jaundice* caused by edema of the nearby common duct or by common duct stones.

With treatment, improvement is usually noticeable within the first 12 to 24 hours, and the signs and symptoms gradually subside over 3 to 7 days. Persistent severe pain, a rise in temperature or leukocyte count (>10,000 per cubic millimeter), and appearance of shaking chills or of more severe local or generalized abdominal tenderness all indicate progression of the disease and the need for immediate surgery.

Empyema (suppurative cholecystitis) can produce systemic toxicity and mild increases in bilirubin, alkaline phosphatase, and the transaminases and may herald perforation.

DIAGNOSIS. The diagnosis is strongly suggested by the clinical manifestations just described. Roentgenograms of the abdomen may show calcified gallstones. Ultrasonography is the simplest and most reliable method of detecting gallbladder stones in these patients.

Radionuclide scanning following intravenous administration of ^{99m}Tc DISIDA or related compounds is the procedure of choice to verify a clinical impression of acute cholecystitis. If the gallbladder fills, the diagnosis of acute cholecystitis is quite unlikely. If the bile duct fills but the gallbladder does not, the diagnosis is strongly supported.

In the differential diagnosis, acute pancreatitis, acute appendicitis, and penetrated or perforated peptic ulcer are the conditions that most often cause major problems. Furthermore, acute cholecystitis and acute pancreatitis may coexist.

In women, *gonococcal perihepatitis* (Fitz-Hugh-Curtis syndrome), caused by intra-abdominal spread of the infection from the reproductive tract to the right upper quadrant, may be mistaken for acute cholecystitis, but adnexal tenderness is usually present on pelvic examination. A cervical smear usually reveals gonococci, and the patients are younger, often have higher temperature, and are in less distress than would be expected with cholecystitis.

Acute hepatitis, either viral or alcoholic, sometimes produces marked right upper quadrant pain and tenderness. A history of recent binge drinking, high transaminase levels, and liver biopsy aid differentiation. Pneumonitis, pyelonephritis, and acute cardiac disease (particularly right-sided failure) all on occasion may cause acute pain suggestive of cholecystitis. The use of ^{99m}Tc DISIDA distinguishes between the unusual location of pain in these disorders and acute cholecystitis.

TREATMENT. Most patients with acute cholecystitis improve with either expectant treatment or cholecystectomy performed during the acute attack. In general, the decision regarding the kind of treatment should include the following considerations (Fig. 126–6): (1) whether the diagnosis is secure, (2) whether biliary complications have occurred or appear imminent, and (3) the overall condition of the patient (operative risk).

Upon the patient's admission to the hospital, nasogastric suction should be started if the patient has significant vomiting, and fluids should be given intravenously to correct dehydration. In many elderly patients the acute biliary condition may aggravate pre-existing cardiac, pulmonary, or renal disease and produce a more ominous prognosis if surgery is delayed or if adequate treatment is not given.

Antimicrobials are of principal value to prevent bacteremia and to treat suppurative complications. If the patient is seen shortly after symptoms begin, and if local signs and symptoms are mild, antimicrobial therapy need not be given. Otherwise, an antimicrobial regimen with coverage for gram-negative aerobes as well as enterococci is preferred. One that is often used is ampicillin plus gentamicin given parenterally. In seriously ill patients, such as those with empyema or perforation, it is wise to also add an antimicrobial with anaerobic coverage, such as clindamycin.

Cholecystectomy is the optimal therapy for acute cholecystitis, but only after the diagnosis is secure and the patient adequately prepared for operation. Some physicians still prefer to reserve surgery during the acute attack for those patients who develop complications and for those who become worse or fail to improve. Although this is still done, about 25 per cent of patients managed in this way require urgent operation for worsening disease. For patients who respond to nonoperative management, cholecystectomy is recommended. The timing of cholecystectomy in such patients has been debated, but the trend is to perform surgery early on during the same hospitalization.

In about 30 per cent of patients, the diagnosis is obvious within 12 to 24 hours, they are good operative risks, and cholecystectomy can be scheduled promptly. Another 30 per cent are good surgical candidates, but the diagnosis is not quite firm. In this situation, a ^{99m}Tc DISIDA scan should be obtained to verify the clinical impression. Another 30 per cent of patients have serious coexistent cardiac, respiratory, or other disease for which treatment takes precedence. The cholecystitis should be treated expectantly while the other problems are being corrected. Progression of local abdominal findings requires continued re-evaluation, balancing the risks of operation with the risks of continued delay.

About 10 per cent of patients require emergency intervention for complications present on admission or that appear later during observation and medical management. When emergency operation becomes necessary, cholecystostomy may sometimes be preferable to cholecystectomy in the seriously ill patient. In this procedure the fundus is incised, stones and pus are removed from the lumen, and the organ is decompressed by catheter drainage, allowing the acute infection to resolve. Cholecystostomy can also be performed using radiologic techniques. Patients who recover should undergo cholecystectomy 6 to 8 weeks later. Those who continue to be poor surgical risks may be followed expectantly if postoperative cholecystography shows that the gallbladder and common duct contain no residual stones. If stones are present, interventional radiologic techniques can be used to remove gallbladder stones through the cholecystomy tract after 4 to 6 weeks of tract maturation, and endoscopic sphincterotomy can be utilized to remove ductal stones. In seriously debilitated patients the cholecystostomy tube can be left in place indefinitely.

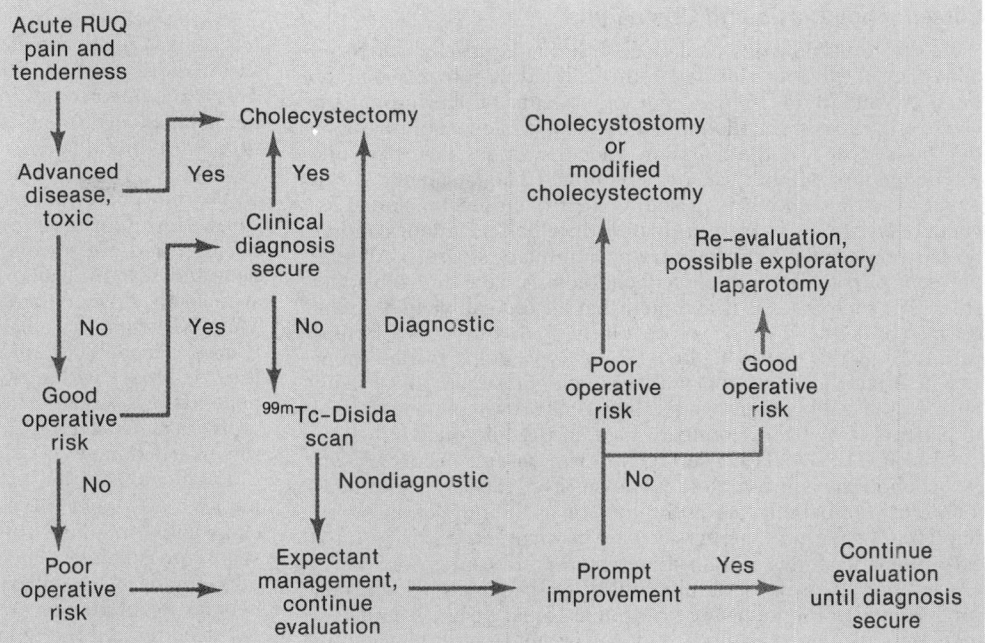

FIGURE 126–6. Schema for managing patients with right upper quadrant pain and tenderness who are thought possibly to have acute cholecystitis. This approach is based on a policy of early operation for appropriate patients and distinguishes between patients who are good versus poor operative risks.

After the cholecystostomy tube is removed from a patient whose biliary system contains no calculi, within several years about 50 per cent of patients develop new stones.

COMPLICATIONS. *Emphysematous Cholecystitis.* In emphysematous cholecystitis, a rare variant of acute cholecystitis, gas of bacterial origin can be seen in the gallbladder lumen and adjacent tissues. Clinically, emphysematous cholecystitis causes the same signs and symptoms as acute cholecystitis. About 30 per cent of patients have diabetes mellitus, and the gallbladder is acalculous in about half the cases. Gas does not develop until 24 to 48 hours after the attack begins, at which time a radiolucent halo outlines the lumen, and an air-fluid level may be seen on upright films. Subserosal and then pericholecystic emphysema appear with time. Differential diagnosis of the radiographic findings includes cholecystenteric fistula and appendiceal, perinephric, or subhepatic abscess. In about half the cases the gas-forming organisms are clostridia, and the rest are *Escherichia coli*, streptococci, and other bacteria of intestinal origin. Treatment is the same as for acute cholecystitis, but the more aggressive nature of emphysematous cholecystitis mandates prompt surgery.

Perforation. Perforation is usually manifested by greater sepsis and more marked abdominal signs. Perforation may take any of three forms: (1) free perforation into the abdominal cavity, (2) localized (contained) perforation with pericholecystic abscess, and (3) perforation into another viscus with fistula formation.

Free perforation, which has a 25 per cent mortality, is the least common type. It usually occurs early in the attack, often within the first 3 days, suggesting that when gangrene develops this quickly it cannot be walled off by adjacent viscera or the omentum. Clinically, free perforation classically causes toxicity with high temperatures (greater than 39°C), leukocytosis (over 15,000 per cubic millimeter), and diffuse abdominal tenderness and rigidity. In more than half the cases the correct diagnosis is unsuspected until laparotomy or autopsy, because a clear-cut history of preliminary right upper quadrant pain is often lacking. Treatment consists of intravenous antimicrobial therapy and emergency cholecystectomy.

Localized perforation most often appears in the second week of the attack at the peak of the inflammatory reaction. The diagnosis should be suspected with increasing local signs, especially when a mass suddenly appears. In most cases cholecystectomy can be performed, but in a severely ill patient cholecystostomy and drainage of the abscess may be wiser.

Fistula formation usually involves the nearby second portion of the duodenum or, less commonly, the colon, jejunum, stomach, or common bile duct. Rare fistulas have entered the renal pelvis or bronchus or extended through the abdominal wall (empyema necessitatis). After intestinal fistulization the contents of the gallbladder are discharged into the gut, often aborting the acute attack. Clinically, the fistula itself may not be suspected because it produces no unique findings; many are discovered incidentally later. In the absence of biliary obstruction a cholecystenteric fistula is not necessarily of pathophysiologic significance. Cholecystocolonic fistulas may cause malabsorption from diversion of bile or from bacterial overgrowth in the upper gut.

Gallstone Ileus. If a particularly large gallstone enters through the fistula, it may obstruct the intestine, a condition called gallstone ileus. The stone, passing through a cholecystenteric fistula, most often enters the gut in the duodenum, less commonly in the jejunum, ileum, colon, or stomach. It is often assumed that the initial event responsible for fistula formation is an attack of acute cholecystitis, but only 30 per cent of patients with gallstone ileus give a history of recent right upper quadrant pain. After entering the gut, the gallstone moves downstream until it encounters an area of intestinal lumen too narrow to accommodate it. Gallstones, usually more than 2.5 cm in diameter, most frequently obstruct the terminal ileum; they block the colon only if its lumen has been narrowed by intrinsic disease.

On physical examination the findings are those of small-bowel obstruction. Rarely can the stone be felt as a mass on abdominal, vaginal, or rectal examination. Roentgenograms usually show air in the biliary tree if the films are carefully examined, and in some cases a radiopaque gallstone can be identified at the leading edge of the obstruction. Treatment consists of removing the obstructing gallstone through a small enterotomy. It is generally wise to leave the biliary disease undisturbed initially, because these often elderly patients tolerate long procedures poorly, and nothing much is gained by repairing the fistula primarily. Postoperatively, many patients remain asymptomatic, and the fistula may even close spontaneously; for them, expectant management is best. Some patients may require cholecystectomy later because of symptoms related to gallstones.

The mortality is 15 to 20 per cent because of delay in diagnosis and because of cardiopulmonary complications.

PROGNOSIS. The mortality in acute cholecystitis of 5 to 10 per cent is almost totally confined to patients over 60 years of age with serious associated disease. Suppurative complications are more common in the elderly, who can tolerate them least. In most instances, localized perforation can be managed satisfactorily at operation. Free perforation is considerably more ominous (25 per cent mortality) but is rare.

Choledocholithiasis and Cholangitis

In Western countries choledocholithiasis is usually the result of passage of gallstones formed in the gallbladder into the common duct. About 10 to 15 per cent of patients with symptomatic cholecystolithiasis are thought to develop choledocholithiasis on this basis. Once in the common duct the stones may pass into the duodenum without causing symptoms. The frequency of this event is not known but is probably greatly underestimated. Less commonly, stones form in a dilated duct behind a longstanding obstruction caused by a stricture or ampullary stenosis. About 5 per cent of patients with choledocholithiasis have no gallbladder stones; in such cases it is assumed that all the gallbladder stones escaped into the duct or, more rarely, that the stones formed primarily in the common duct. Stone type helps to determine site of origin: Cholesterol or black pigment stones more likely form in the gallbladder, while almost all brown pigment stones in patients in Western countries form in the bile ducts.

CLINICAL MANIFESTATIONS. The natural history of choledocholithiasis is incompletely known (Fig. 126–7). About 30 to 40 per cent of patients are asymptomatic at the time of diagnosis, implying a relatively benign course in many cases. How often asymptomatic stones remain undetected is, of course, unknown. Obstruction by stones of the biliary or pancreatic ducts may produce any of the following syndromes: biliary pain, jaundice or increased alkaline phosphatase alone (without pain), cholangitis, pancreatitis, or a combination of these. Secondary hepatic effects of persistent obstruction include biliary cirrhosis or hepatic abscesses.

Intermittent *cholangitis*, consisting of biliary pain, jaundice, and fever and chills (*Charcot's triad*), is a common presenting symptom complex. In the absence of previous biliary surgery it is almost diagnostic of choledocholithiasis. Intermittency of symptoms is quite characteristic, a manifestation of intermittent partial obstruction. Whenever pain, chills with fever, and jaundice fluctuate together over a span of a few days or a week, cholangitis from biliary obstruction is almost certainly the cause. In a typical attack, chills may precede the other symptoms, and bilirubinuria may follow. Epigastric or right upper quadrant pain, indistinguishable from biliary pain caused by gallbladder stones, is steady and severe. Pain may be referred to the right infrascapular area, the upper back, the right shoulder, or even the precordium, suggesting coronary artery or esophageal disease.

The severity of cholangitis varies widely from the usual mild transient illness to overwhelming sepsis with shock (see Suppurative Cholangitis, below). In the average case, the temperature rises to 38.5 to 40°C, preceded by chills and positive blood cultures. Localized tenderness in the subcostal region may be associated with extreme guarding and rigidity, but more often

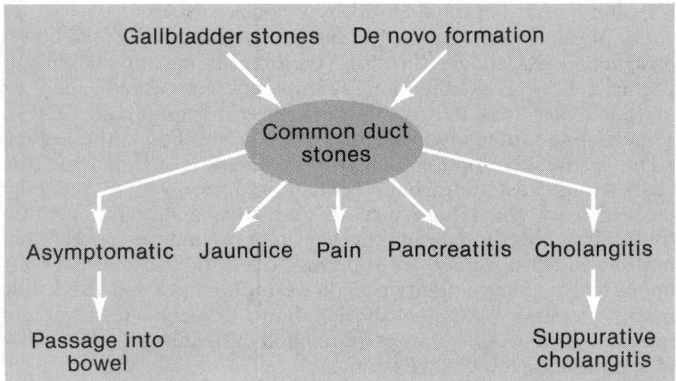

FIGURE 126–7. Natural history of choledocholithiasis. In most cases, common duct gallstones originate in the gallbladder. In some cases, particularly after the gallbladder has been surgically removed, stones may form in the common duct. The majority of stones in the common duct remain asymptomatic and may either remain in the duct without causing symptoms, pass into the bowel through the ampulla of Vater and be excreted in stool, or eventually result in symptoms, the most common of which are indicated. The exact frequency of each of these occurrences is not known.

the local findings are minimal or intermittent and are usually less severe than in acute cholecystitis.

In most cases of common duct obstruction caused by stones the gallbladder does not become distended, because it is scarred and inelastic, and the obstruction is recent, partial, or transient. This is the obverse of Courvoisier's law; i.e., a distended nontender gallbladder in a jaundiced patient signifies neoplastic obstruction of the bile duct.

DIAGNOSIS. In cholangitis the leukocyte count averages 15,000 per cubic millimeter but may go much higher in severe cases. Bilirubin values are usually in the range of 2 to 4 mg per deciliter and are uncommonly higher than 10 mg per deciliter. Elevated serum alkaline phosphatase and 5'-nucleotidase levels are usually greater than three times the upper limit of normal. The ALT generally remains below 200 units; however, transiently it may exceed 1000 units. In these instances the prompt drop of the ALT level within 48 hours allows differentiation from viral hepatitis and suggests the diagnosis of obstruction. Ultrasonography usually demonstrates a dilated ductal system proximal to the obstruction.

The demonstration of gallbladder stones does not necessarily imply that stones in the bile ducts are responsible for the cholangitis, although this is usually true. When the presenting syndrome is painless cholestatic jaundice, other causes, especially periampullary and biliary neoplasms, must be considered. With neoplastic obstruction, the bilirubin averages about 15 to 20 mg per deciliter and rarely fluctuates. Although jaundice from stones may be as intense, the level of bilirubin is characteristically less than 10 mg per deciliter, and it may rise and fall episodically. The diagnosis of intrahepatic cholestasis from causes such as drugs, viral hepatitis, or pregnancy should follow the schema outlined in Ch. 115. In such cases, opacification of normal bile ducts by PTC or ERCP may ultimately be required. Gallstone disease is common in cirrhosis, so choledocholithiasis and liver disease may coexist. In patients who have had cholecystectomy, differentiation between choledocholithiasis and biliary stricture as the cause of cholangitis depends on direct radiologic demonstration of the ducts.

Common duct stones may cause acute pancreatitis indistinguishable clinically from that resulting from alcohol or other causes and unaccompanied by specific signs of biliary disease (Ch. 106). Pancreatitis caused by biliary calculi, despite numerous attacks, rarely progresses to pancreatic calcification, chronic pain, and pancreatic insufficiency, as often occurs in the alcoholic variety. Gallstone disease should be ruled out in every patient with acute pancreatitis, because further damage during such an episode and future attacks can be avoided if the gallstones are removed.

TREATMENT. The potential seriousness of cholangitis necessitates hospitalization for diagnosis and treatment. After blood cultures are obtained, antimicrobial drugs effective against enteric organisms are given by the parenteral route. A regimen consisting of an aminoglycoside plus ampicillin for mild attacks with the addition of clindamycin in severe infection is usually successful. A shift from the initial regimen on the basis of the result of cultures and drug susceptibility tests may be necessary. The margin between mild and severe illness is small; antimicrobial therapy should be expected to control the acute attack within 24 to 48 hours, and if there is no improvement or worsening after this period, emergency surgery or endoscopic sphincterotomy must be considered seriously.

More than 90 per cent of patients respond satisfactorily to treatment, allowing an orderly attempt at diagnosis. Ultrasonography should be performed first to detect ductal dilatation. Direct opacification of the ducts can be attempted by PTC or ERCP. Both kinds of direct cholangiography are potentially hazardous in active cholangitis and should be postponed if possible until infection is well controlled; then one proceeds only under the protection of antimicrobial therapy. However, rapid decompression of the bile duct using a percutaneous transhepatic catheter or by endoscopic sphincterotomy may provide the control needed in advanced cases.

Deciding between endoscopic and surgical approaches to the management of choledocholithiasis should be on a case-by-case basis. If the gallbladder is present, cholecystectomy is performed and the common duct is opened and emptied of stones. A T tube is left in the duct to decompress biliary pressure in the postoperative period and to provide a route for subsequent cholangiography. Recurrent ductal stone formation occurs infrequently.

Selected patients with choledocholithiasis such as the elderly, poor operative risks, or those who have already had a cholecystectomy may be satisfactorily treated by endoscopic sphincterotomy. By means of the side-viewing duodenoscope, a wire (papillotome) is passed into the bile duct and the sphincter divided by electrocautery. Common duct stones 1.5 cm or smaller usually pass into the duodenum. This technique may be unsuccessful with very large stones. Bleeding and pancreatitis are the principal complications but are infrequent. Mortality in the procedure is less than 1 per cent in experienced hands. When endoscopic sphincterotomy is successfully used for cholangitis in patients with gallbladder stones, there is debate about whether to perform cholecystectomy at a later date. In our opinion this decision should be based on whether the patient subsequently develops symptoms referable to the gallbladder stones.

RETAINED COMMON DUCT STONES. The methods for detecting duct stones at operation are about 95 per cent reliable, which means, unfortunately, that a few are overlooked only to be discovered on postoperative T-tube cholangiograms. There are several approaches to remove residual stones without another laparotomy. Instrumental extraction is the treatment of choice. Under image-intensification fluoroscopy the T tube is pulled out, a basket is passed into the duct, and the stone is grasped and withdrawn. This method should not be tried until 4 to 6 weeks postoperatively to allow for maturation of the T-tube tract. If mechanical extraction is not successful, endoscopic sphincterotomy may allow the stone to pass into the duodenum. Another uncommonly used technique depends on the ability of mono-octanoin (glyceryl-1-mono-octanoate) to dissolve cholesterol gallstones. Mono-octanoin is infused into the duct at 2 to 5 ml per hour. The retained stones disappear in about one half of patients within a 4- to 8-day treatment period. If all these are unsuccessful, reoperation is necessary.

SUPPURATIVE CHOLANGITIS. The most severe form of cholangitis, suppurative cholangitis, involves the same causative factors as the "nonsuppurative" form but differs in that obstruction is complete, ductal contents become purulent, and clinically the manifestations of sepsis overshadow those of cholestasis. Hypotension and mental changes such as lethargy or confusion appear in addition to right upper quadrant pain, chills, fever, and jaundice. Some elderly patients may be hypothermic and have minimal clinical signs. Because infection in the face of the high-grade obstruction progresses so rapidly, the serum bilirubin does not reach very high levels before the patient becomes moribund from sepsis. Costly delays in diagnosis are frequent, a consequence of failure to recognize the significance of mild icterus and abdominal pain in a patient with sepsis. All but a few cases involve complications of choledocholithiasis, the others occurring with biliary stricture or neoplastic obstruction, usually from bile duct carcinoma.

Laboratory tests reveal evidence of cholestasis with bilirubin values between 2 and 5 mg per deciliter and elevated serum levels of alkaline phosphatase, 5'-nucleotidase, and transaminases. The leukocyte count varies from subnormal to 40,000 per cubic millimeter. Hypoglycemia may sometimes be present.

Tenderness to palpation is present in the right upper quadrant, but rigidity is uncommon. In some cases secondary cholecystitis develops, and an enlarged tender gallbladder may be found on abdominal examination. Ultrasonography shows dilated bile ducts. Diagnosis rests on recognizing the evidence of biliary obstruction and its relationship to the sepsis and on verifying the initial impression by ultrasonography. After initial resuscitation—consisting of intravenous infusions, antimicrobial drugs (gentamicin plus ampicillin and clindamycin parenterally), and measures to restore cardiac, pulmonary, or renal function—decompression of the duct by emergency laparotomy, percutaneous transhepatic catheter placement, or endoscopic sphincterotomy offers the only hope of saving the patient. Biliary stents have also been placed endoscopically to reduce obstruction and systemic sepsis.

At surgery when choledochotomy is performed, pus often squirts from the duct as a result of the high pressure. If the patient's condition permits, thorough exploration can be carried out to correct the obstruction by removing stones, repairing a stricture, or bypassing a tumor. Insertion of a T tube proximal to the obstruction is sufficient in patients who are unable to tolerate a longer operation, but sometime later it will be necessary to perform a second, more definitive procedure before the T tube can be removed. The mortality is about 50 per cent, resulting from septic shock, renal or respiratory failure, acute hepatic insufficiency, or a combination of these complications.

Other Causes of Bile Duct Obstruction

Duodenal and pancreatic tumors are common causes of obstruction in the middle-aged or elderly (Ch. 105 and 107). Common bile duct obstruction may also be caused by a variety of uncommon disorders such as sclerosing cholangitis or by Oriental cholangiohepatitis. Rare causes are compression by neoplastic paraductal lymph nodes or by duodenal Crohn's disease.

SCLEROSING CHOLANGITIS. Sclerosing cholangitis, a condition of unknown cause, consists of benign nonbacterial chronic inflammatory narrowing of the bile ducts. The entire ductal system is involved in most cases; less commonly the process may be confined to the extrahepatic or intrahepatic portion. The ratio of males to females is 3:2, and the peak incidence occurs in the third and fourth decades. More than half of the cases are associated with *ulcerative colitis* (Ch. 103) or *regional enteritis*. The severity of sclerosing cholangitis does not parallel the activity of the colitis, and colectomy does not improve the cholangitis. Other rarely associated diseases are retroperitoneal fibrosis and Riedel's thyroiditis.

The initial complaint may be jaundice or pruritus, although more cases are being discovered at an asymptomatic stage. There may be mild upper abdominal pain and sometimes fever, but a clinical picture resembling bacterial cholangitis is uncommon in the absence of previous surgical exploration or instrumentation of the ducts. Hepatomegaly may be present in some cases; when secondary cirrhosis develops, ascites or splenomegaly may be found.

Jaundice may be constant or fluctuating, and bilirubin values are usually in the range of 2 to 10 mg per deciliter. The alkaline phosphatase is always increased, usually greater than three times the upper limit of normal, and remains increased despite variations in clinical manifestations. Transaminases are usually mildly increased. Antimitochondrial antibodies are normal.

Percutaneous transhepatic cholangiography or preferably endoscopic retrograde cholangiopancreatography is required to establish the diagnosis. The radiographs show diffuse or focal irregular ductal narrowing with intervening areas of normal caliber or dilatation; this "beaded" appearance is characteristic. Some patients develop gallstones behind the strictured areas as a result of stasis; these are usually brown pigment gallstones. Localized strictures may be difficult to distinguish from ductal carcinoma. A radiographic appearance similar to that of sclerosing cholangitis may be seen in some patients with AIDS and CMV infection of the biliary tract and in some patients after intra-arterial infusion of FUDR for liver metastases.

In asymptomatic patients, no therapy is warranted. Treatment with corticosteroids or immunosuppressants has not been proved to be generally effective. Cholestyramine is useful for pruritus. Antimicrobials are necessary if bacterial cholangitis develops.

In symptomatic patients the aim of therapy is to relieve biliary obstruction if technically possible and if the benefit is thought to outweigh the risk. If a segmental stricture is present, balloon dilatation can be attempted either percutaneously or, if the lesion is in the common bile duct, endoscopically. This involves the insertion into the bile duct of a balloon-tipped catheter; inflation of the balloon stretches the narrowed area and allows greater bile flow. Balloon dilatation may have to be repeated intermittently to provide sustained relief of obstruction; there is the risk of inducing bacterial cholangitis, particularly with the endoscopic approach. Percutaneous catheter drainage is another option but often does not provide adequate drainage of all obstructed areas in diffuse disease. Surgical therapy is warranted in some cases to provide stenting in diffuse disease or to bypass severe distal common bile duct disease. Significant palliation follows surgery in most cases, but is not usually permanent. Most patients have episodic remissions and exacerbations, during which secondary biliary cirrhosis develops. Death may follow uncontrollable biliary sepsis with hepatic abscesses, liver failure, or bleeding from esophageal varices. Liver transplantation is now an option for those with advanced disease.

STRUCTURAL ABNORMALITIES. *Choledochal cysts* occasionally produce their initial clinical manifestations in young adults, presenting with jaundice, pain, or cholangitis. Diagnosis requires direct ductal visualization with PTC or ERCP; computed tomography or ultrasonography can provide information about surrounding structures. The most definitive surgical procedure is excision of the cyst, followed by Roux-en-Y choledochojejunostomy.

Caroli's disease, consisting of saccular intrahepatic bile duct dilations, most often becomes symptomatic in patients between the ages of 20 and 50 years, because of intrahepatic stone formation and cholangitis. Two forms are recognized: (1) disease of the ducts only and (2) ductal disease associated with hepatic fibrosis and medullary sponge kidney (more common). The latter patients often have complications of portal hypertension before cholangitis or obstructive jaundice appears. Antimicrobial therapy may control attacks of cholangitis, and surgical procedures to facilitate ductal emptying or to extract stones may help in some cases, but the intrahepatic anomaly cannot be definitively corrected unless lobectomy is possible for single lobe involvement.

PANCREATITIS. Acute pancreatitis can produce transient jaundice by obstruction of the distal common duct where it is surrounded by pancreatic tissue. Prolonged obstruction can result from pressure by an adjacent *pseudocyst* or entrapment of the distal common bile duct in severe pancreatic scarring from *chronic pancreatitis.* Diagnosis may be delayed in alcoholic patients in whom elevated alkaline phosphatase or bilirubin values are usually attributed to hepatocellular disease. Persistent elevation of the alkaline phosphatase value in an alcoholic should raise suspicion of the possibility of biliary obstruction, particularly if pancreatic calcification is present on plain abdominal radiographs. Jaundice resulting from chronic pancreatitis requires choledochoduodenostomy or Roux-en-Y anastomosis of the jejunum to the common bile duct.

HEMOBILIA. Hemobilia classically presents with biliary pain, obstructive jaundice, and occult or gross intestinal bleeding. Most cases are caused by hepatic injury from external or operative trauma, with secondary bleeding into the ductal system. Other causes include biliary or hepatic neoplasms, ductal rupture of a hepatic artery aneurysm, hepatic abscess, and gallstones, or it may follow percutaneous needle biopsy of the liver or cholangiography. Hemobilia following trauma is best treated by hepatic artery ligation, which is well tolerated except when there is advanced parenchymal disease; otherwise, direct management of the causative lesion is necessary.

PARASITIC DISEASE. An *echinococcal hepatic cyst* can rupture into the ducts and can give rise to biliary colic, jaundice, and cholangitis (Ch. 433). *Ascariasis* may produce biliary colic, jaundice, and cholangitis by worm invasion into the bile ducts from the duodenum (Ch. 433).

ORIENTAL CHOLANGIOHEPATITIS. Oriental cholangiohepatitis or *recurrent pyogenic cholangitis* is a common form of recurrent cholangitis in Asia associated with brown pigment gallstone formation throughout the biliary tract. The cause is unclear, but the parasite *Clonorchis sinensis* is found in very few cases so does not seem to be a major causative factor. Most patients present with acute cholangitis; those with recurrent cholangitis may develop liver abscesses, biliary-enteric fistulas, or sepsis. In advanced cases, one (usually the left) or both lobar ducts may become honeycombed with scars or abscesses, producing atrophy of the hepatic parenchyma.

Direct cholangiography is necessary for a definitive diagnosis. Sphincteroplasty or choledochojejunostomy is usually performed to remove stones and sludge and provide adequate biliary drainage. Cholecystectomy or partial hepatic resection is required when the gallbladder or localized hepatic segments are involved.

BILIARY STRICTURE. Biliary stricture almost always results from *surgical injury* to the duct and usually follows cholecystectomy rather than procedures on the duct itself such as common duct exploration. Biliary stricture may also result from external trauma or scarring produced by choledocholithiasis.

The symptoms resemble those of cholangitis with choledocholithiasis. Differential diagnosis includes all the various causes of

obstructive jaundice and cholangitis. Laboratory evidence consists of leukocytosis and elevated serum levels of bilirubin, alkaline phosphatase, and transaminases. The jaundice and cholangitis are generally mild and transient, and infection generally responds promptly to antimicrobial therapy. Diagnosis can be made with visualization of the biliary tract by either PTC or ERCP. With persistent obstruction over several years, secondary biliary cirrhosis or multiple intrahepatic abscesses may develop.

In almost all cases an attempt should be made to repair the stricture surgically by creating a new unobstructed conduit between normal duct on the hepatic side of the lesion and the proximal intestine rather than attempting direct end-to-end anastomosis of the duct after excision of the lesion. The overall success rate of these operations is about 75 per cent with an operative mortality of 10 per cent.

Balloon catheter dilatation of a short stricture at the time of either PTC or ERCP may be useful in some patients, particularly those who are poor operative risks.

Carcinoma of the Gallbladder

In the United States there are approximately 2500 deaths annually from carcinoma of the gallbladder, a number equal to the mortality from benign disease of the biliary tract. Women are affected more frequently than men by a ratio of 3:1, and the average age is 70 years. Because 70 to 80 per cent of cases occur in patients with gallstones, cholelithiasis or lithogenic bile is thought to be etiologically important, but the mechanism involved is unclear. Gallbladder cancer develops in fewer than 1 per cent of patients with cholelithiasis. The disease is 5 to 10 times more frequent in American Indian populations.

Almost all gallbladder carcinomas are *adenocarcinomas;* the earliest spread is usually by metastasis to the hilar lymph nodes and adjacent hepatic parenchyma followed by direct extension to the liver and hilar structures. Distant metastases appear relatively late.

Patients have one of the following clinical pictures: (1) unremitting deep jaundice from common duct and hepatic involvement; (2) acute cholecystitis, often with a palpable mass; (3) chronic intermittent right upper quadrant pain; and (4) advanced disseminated carcinoma. The diagnosis is not often considered preoperatively, but in some instances clinical clues are present. In about two thirds of patients a mass can be felt, and in one third there is local tenderness. In all but a few cases the gallbladder is not opacified during oral cholecystography, and even when it is, the tumor can rarely be demonstrated. The diagnosis can be suspected on ultrasound study if an intraluminal gallbladder mass is identified that does not change with position. The differential diagnosis is that of a cholesterol polyp or of a stone adherent to the gallbladder wall. Pathologic studies indicate that all apparent tumor would be removed in 25 per cent of cases by cholecystectomy, resection of a rim of adjacent liver, and dissection of the common duct lymph node chain. Even in this favorable group the 5-year survival rate is 5 per cent. Most patients live for only a few months after the diagnosis.

Benign Tumors and Pseudotumors of the Gallbladder

Adenomyomatous hyperplasia, also called *adenomyomatosis*, is the most common of the benign conditions of the gallbladder; there is hyperplasia of the mucosa with formation of intramural diverticula. The cause is unknown. Typically, neoplastic or inflammatory changes are absent. Adenomyomatosis is usually diagnosed by oral cholecystography as a diffuse, segmental, or focal sessile filling defect with a central umbilication and small peripheral opaque areas representing diverticula. Most often adenomyomatosis is asymptomatic. Rare cases are associated with biliary pain that can be cured by cholecystectomy.

Cholesterolosis (strawberry gallbladder) is a condition of unknown cause characterized by an accumulation of cholesterol and other lipids in macrophages in the gallbladder mucosa. Unlike cholesterol gallstones, it does not appear to be necessarily related to biliary supersaturation with cholesterol. *Cholesterol polyps* are a focal form of cholesterolosis consisting of a core of macrophages filled with cholesterol covered by epithelium located at a villous tip. Generally, multiple polyps are present. The polyp is attached to the mucosa by a fragile stalk that can easily be broken. Cholesterol polyps appear on oral cholecystography or ultrasonography as a fixed filling defect on the gallbladder wall that does not change with position; in contrast to gallstones, no acoustic shadowing is seen on ultrasonography. Unless cholesterol polyps are present, cholesterolosis is difficult to detect by oral cholecystography. Most patients with cholesterolosis are asymptomatic. Some patients have concomitant gallstones and, if symptoms are present, they are attributed to the stones. Those few patients with cholesterolosis without gallstones who have typical biliary pain are often relieved by cholecystectomy.

Papillary and nonpapillary adenomas are benign neoplasms of the gallbladder. They are much less common than cholesterol polyps. Most adenomas are pedunculated; about two thirds are multiple. They appear as filling defects on oral cholecystography. Carcinoma in situ is found in about 5 per cent of adenomas, but the relationship between gallbladder adenomas and carcinoma is not clear.

Tumors of the Bile Duct

The main cause of early morbidity from tumors of the bile duct is biliary obstruction with gradual hepatocellular damage or secondary hepatobiliary infection. Tumors of the bile ducts are rarely benign. Papilloma, the most frequent benign tumor, is often multifocal and therefore difficult to cure. Adenomas and granular cell tumors are localized, but are often difficult to treat surgically without radical excision. This section is directed primarily to discussion of malignant tumors, but many of the same principles of pathophysiology and diagnosis apply to the rare benign tumors.

Except for a rare squamous cell tumor, malignant bile duct tumors are adenocarcinomas with either a scirrhous or a papillary pattern. Grossly, three types of pathologic presentations occur: *focal stricture, diffuse thickening,* and *nodular mass.* The first two varieties can easily be mistaken for a benign process such as post-traumatic stricture or sclerosing cholangitis. In many cases, spread is confined to local lymph node metastases or hepatic invasion for months or years before there is more widespread abdominal or systemic involvement. The common hepatic duct or common bile duct is the site of origin in about two thirds of the cases. The eponym *Klatskin tumor* is often used to refer to adenocarcinoma at the bifurcation of the common hepatic duct. In contrast with carcinoma of the gallbladder, cholelithiasis is found in only one third of patients, and men slightly outnumber women. The average age at diagnosis is 70 years. A number of cases have been reported in younger patients with ulcerative colitis. Since some of these patients have previously undergone colectomy, it is thought that elimination of the diseased colon is not protective. Sclerosing cholangitis is a complication in these same patients and may have identical clinical features, especially when it primarily affects the extrahepatic bile ducts. Caroli's disease and choledochal cysts are also associated with the development of carcinoma in a small percentage of cases. In Asia, infestation with *Clonorchis sinensis* probably contributes to the higher incidence of bile duct carcinoma.

CLINICAL MANIFESTATIONS. The typical patient presents with unremitting severe jaundice, mild deep-seated upper abdominal pain, and weight loss. Pruritus is reported by many, usually but not always after the onset of jaundice. Pain, present in more than half the patients, is not colicky and tends to be steady; fever and chills are absent. Hepatomegaly without splenomegaly is found on abdominal examination. Tumors of the common duct sparing the cystic duct often produce in addition to jaundice a distended nontender palpable gallbladder (*Courvoisier's law*).

The serum bilirubin value exceeds 10 mg per deciliter in most cases, with a mean between 15 and 20 mg per deciliter. Complete obstruction of the ductal system results in a bilirubin value of 30 mg per deciliter or higher. The alkaline phosphatase is almost always increased, often more than 10-fold, and ALT may be slightly elevated, although rarely higher than 200 units per liter. Obstruction of the right or left hepatic system alone causes a 10- to 30-fold increase in alkaline phosphatase with normal levels of bilirubin. The prothrombin time may be prolonged, but responds to parenteral vitamin K.

DIAGNOSIS. Ultrasonography or computed tomography shows dilatation of the bile ducts. Transhepatic or retrograde cholangiography can demonstrate the site of the block.

The differential diagnosis includes primary biliary cirrhosis and drug-induced cholestatic jaundice. Antimitochondrial antibodies can be demonstrated in the serum of 95 per cent of patients with primary biliary cirrhosis. Sclerosing cholangitis shows a characteristic pattern on cholangiography, although it may be difficult to distinguish focal disease from carcinoma. Choledocholithiasis and postoperative biliary stricture are less likely to present with deepening jaundice and weight loss. The jaundice fluctuates, is milder, and is usually associated with fever. PTC or ERCP helps to differentiate these diseases from carcinoma.

Cytologic examination of tissue obtained by brushing the suspected tumor at the time of PTC or ERCP or by radiologically guided skinny needle aspiration may reveal malignant cells. Not uncommonly, however, a preoperative tissue diagnosis may not be made because of the scirrhous nature of many of these carcinomas.

TREATMENT. Unfortunately, complete excision of the tumor is often impossible, because nonexpendable anatomic structures are involved early. Nevertheless, a few cures can be expected when radical surgery is judiciously employed, and palliation is often lengthy and of excellent quality.

Distal lesions require pancreaticoduodenectomy (Whipple's procedure) for complete removal. Because this operation has a 10 to 15 per cent mortality, it should be performed only if no gross tumor would be left behind. Tumors of the midportion of the common bile duct are sometimes amenable to complete resection. Localized tumors of the bifurcation of the hepatic duct can sometimes be treated by excision, even though microscopic deposits of tumor usually remain in the bed of the dissection. Reconstruction involves use of a Roux-en-Y hepaticojejunostomy. Radiotherapy with either external beam or intraluminal rods may provide some benefit.

For tumors with local or distant spread the goal is palliation. The treatment of choice is percutaneous or endoscopic stenting of the biliary tract with catheters having multiple portholes above and below the point of bile duct obstruction. Either type of tube can be changed periodically to prevent clogging. Distal tumors can be bypassed by cholecystojejunostomy or other types of biliary-enteric anastomoses.

PROGNOSIS. Cure is achieved in 5 to 10 per cent, and many patients survive in good condition for several years or more following palliative surgery. If biliary drainage can be maintained with a catheter, patients with unresectable lesions occasionally do well for a year or two. Death eventually results from hepatic replacement with tumor or intrahepatic sepsis from ductal obstruction.

Postcholecystectomy Syndrome

After cholecystectomy, 10 per cent of patients continue to have significant abdominal symptoms. In most patients the explanation for continued postoperative symptoms is that the gallstone disease was not the cause of their preoperative complaints. Patients with typical biliary pain are more often relieved by cholecystectomy than are those with atypical pain or vague symptoms such as fatty food intolerance, dyspepsia, or flatulence. Postcholecystectomy complaints can often be attributed to overlooked disease such as choledocholithiasis, pancreatitis, peptic ulcer, esophageal or small-bowel disease, or irritable bowel syndrome. These possibilities must be investigated by appropriate studies.

Neuroma of the cystic duct stump and other cystic duct remnant lesions are uncommon conditions that may be responsible for postcholecystectomy symptoms. A few patients with episodic typical biliary pain in the absence of stones or other bile duct abnormalities have hypertension, dysmotility, and/or stenosis of the sphincter of Oddi. The appearance of a narrowed sphincter alone is insufficient to document either stenosis or dyskinesia. Dyskinesia of the sphincter without stenosis is very difficult to establish as a cause of the syndrome. Clinicians should remain skeptical about a diagnosis of ampullary stenosis or dyskinesia when the principal finding is abdominal pain. The diagnosis is more secure in patients with recurrent pancreatitis, increase of transaminases, cholangitis, and/or a dilated bile duct whose sphincter appears tight radiographically and will accept only a small probe.

The usual evaluation of such patients, after other more common conditions have been ruled out, starts with ultrasonography of the right upper quadrant. Typically, ERCP is performed next. Manometric recordings of sphincter of Oddi pressures obtained transendoscopically show hypertension or dysmotility in some but not all cases.

In the management of such patients with chronic abdominal pain thought to be due to dyskinesia, treatment can be tried with nitrates, antispasmodics, anticholinergics, or calcium channel blockers. If this is unsuccessful, consideration can be given to endoscopic sphincterotomy, although its efficacy remains uncertain. Exploratory laparotomy has a very low rate of success for diagnosis, and surgical correction of minor variations in the gut anatomy usually fails to cure.

Barkun ANG, Ponchon T: Extracorporeal biliary lithotripsy. Review of experimental studies and a clinical update. Ann Intern Med 112:126, 1990. *Excellent review of this topic, with 72 references.*

Carey MC, Cahalane MJ: Whither biliary sludge? Gastroenterology 95:508, 1988. *An in-depth treatise on the biochemical and physicochemical events leading to cholesterol stone formation.*

Duane WC: Pathogenesis of gallstones: Implications for management. Hosp Pract 25:65, 1990. *Succinct review of cholesterol and pigment gallstone formation.*

Neoptolemos JP, Carr-Locke DL, Fossard DP: Prospective randomised study of preoperative endoscopic sphincterotomy versus surgery alone for common bile duct stones. Br Med J 294:470, 1987. *Routine precholecystectomy endoscopic sphincterotomy for removal of concomitant common bile duct stones was not shown to be better (or worse) than conventional surgery.*

Neoptolemos JP, Carr-Locke DL, London NJ, et al.: Controlled trial of urgent endoscopic retrograde cholangiopancreatography and endoscopic sphincterot-omy versus conservative treatment for acute pancreatitis due to gallstones. Lancet 2:979, 1988. *This prospective study of 121 patients demonstrated that urgent ERCP with endoscopic sphincterotomy was safe and effective for acute gallstone pancreatitis; the decision to perform ERCP in this setting remains an individualized one, however.*

Pessa ME, Hawkins IF, Vogel SB: The treatment of acute cholangitis. Percutaneous transhepatic biliary drainage before definitive therapy. Ann Surg 205:389, 1987. *Percutaneous cholangiography performed early can provide an accurate diagnosis and allow stabilization of the patient before definitive therapy.*

Podda M, Battezzati PM, Ghezzi C, et al.: Efficacy and safety of a combination of chenodeoxycholic acid and ursodeoxycholic acid for gallstone dissolution: A comparison with ursodeoxycholic acid alone. Gastroenterology 96:222, 1989. *Comprehensive study of bile salt dissolution of gallstones in 120 patients; 53 references.*

Ransohoff DF, Gracie WA: Management of patients with symptomatic gallstones: A quantitative analysis. Am J Med 88:154, 1990. *An erudite analysis of strategies for treating symptomatic patients.*

Savoca PE, Longo WE, Zucker KA, et al.: The increasing prevalence of acalculous cholecystitis in outpatients. Results of a 7-year study. Ann Surg 211:433, 1990. *Although most often thought of as a problem associated with sepsis, burns, severe trauma, and the postoperative period, acalculous cholecystitis can also be seen in outpatients. Thirty-six of 47 patients seen over a 7-year period developed it at home without evidence of these predisposing conditions; most were elderly with vascular disease.*

Sievert W, Vakil NB: Emergencies of the biliary tract. Gastroenterol Clin North Am 17:245, 1988. *Good review of acute cholecystitis, cholangitis, and gallstone pancreatitis, with 83 references.*

Sivak MV: Endoscopic management of bile duct stones. Am J Surg 158:228, 1989. *An extensive, authoritative review of the use of endoscopic sphincterotomy, with 105 references.*

van Erpecum KJ, van Gerge Henegouwen GP, Stoelwinder B, et al.: Bile concentration is a key factor for nucleation of cholesterol crystals and cholesterol saturation index in gallbladder bile of gallstone patients. Hepatology 11:1, 1990. *An important contribution to our understanding of cholesterol crystal nucleation from supersaturated bile.*

HEMATOLOGIC DISEASES

127 Introduction to Hematologic Diseases

David G. Nathan

This introduction is primarily intended to provide a general background to diagnostic hematology and marrow function. The remaining chapters in Part XII emphasize fundamental physiologic principles and provide descriptions of relatively common hematologic disorders. It is hoped that the entire part will influence the reader to consider such diseases broadly and systematically.

The nonmalignant disorders of erythrocytes, phagocytes, and platelets, including their precursors and progenitors, are initially discussed. Then follows a description of the acute and chronic proliferative disorders that involve the cells of the marrow and lymphoid systems, a series of chapters that ends with a discussion of bone marrow transplantation. The final chapters of Part XII are devoted to a review of the disorders of the fluid phase of blood coagulation and the vascular purpuras.

DIAGNOSTIC HEMATOLOGY. The circulating blood cells are the products of the terminal differentiation of recognizable precursors. In fetal life, hematopoiesis occurs throughout the reticuloendothelial system. In the normal adult, terminal differentiation of the recognizable precursors of erythrocytes, granulocytes, and platelets occurs exclusively in the marrow cavities of the axial skeleton, with some extension into the proximal femora and humeri. The space is highly expandable, however, when the demand for blood cell production is accelerated (Fig. 127–1).

Observations of differentiated blood cells by enumeration and relatively simple morphologic studies of properly prepared blood films provide the essential cornerstone of diagnostic hematology.

Automated blood counts and cell sizing now provide both reproducibility and enhanced diagnostic capacity. For example, early failure of red cell production may be heralded by unexpected macrocytosis. Peripheral blood cell counts and morphology offer insight into the rate of effective hematopoiesis; the state of marrow nutrition with respect to vitamin B_{12}, folic acid, and iron; the presence of acquired and congenital disorders of the erythrocyte membrane; the energy metabolism or the hemoglobin of erythrocytes, which influences the rate of their destruction; the differential diagnosis of infections; the presence of allergic reactions; the acquired or congenital abnormalities of intracellular organelles; and the invasion of the marrow by malignant cells or infectious agents. The contributions of morphologic techniques to hematologic diagnosis depend entirely upon the adequacy of specimen preparation and the skill of the observer. Egregious errors are made when diagnostic pronouncements are based on inadequate material. The slavish enumeration of individual cells is rarely of aid without careful overall inspection and positive searches for diagnostic clues that are relevant to the case at hand. Morphology can be particularly misleading if the observer does not understand that many kinds of disorders induce similar changes in shape, particularly in the red cells.

Although circulating lymphocytes appear to be terminally differentiated cells, they are instead capable of rapid proliferative responses to appropriate stimuli, during which they resume the appearance of relatively undifferentiated precursors. At this stage, they are often called atypical. The functional subsets of lymphoid cells are not readily demonstrable by inspection, although "killer" lymphocyte function may be associated with larger cells that contain granules. Obtaining useful information about lymphocyte subsets requires studies of lymphocyte function and measurements with specially prepared antibodies reactive with lymphocytes.

Well-prepared marrow films and biopsy specimens also contribute important information, such as total marrow cellularity, the presence of invading malignant cells or infectious granulomas,

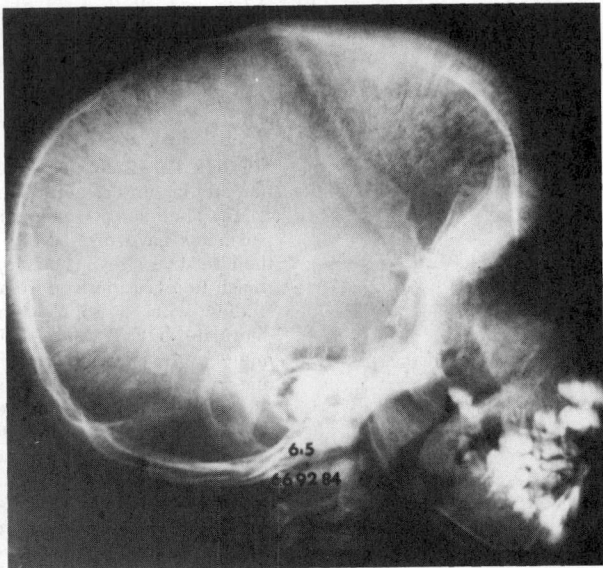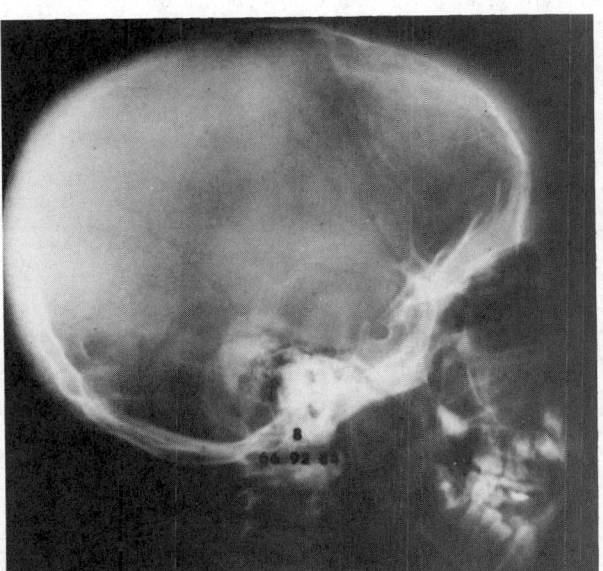

FIGURE 127–1. Roentgenograms of the skull of a patient with homozygous beta-thalassemia at the age of 6½ years *(left)*, before splenectomy and transfusion therapy, and at the age of 8 years *(right)*, after splenectomy and transfusion therapy to control anemia. Note the marked "hair-on-end" appearance in the left-hand radiograph, signifying expansion of the marrow space. (From Nathan DG: N Engl J Med 286:586, 1972. Reprinted by permission of the New England Journal of Medicine.)

the adequacy of the numbers of megakaryocytes, the ratio of myeloid to erythroid precursors, the state of marrow cell nutrition, the presence of abnormal storage cells, and even the deposition of abnormal crystals in metabolic diseases. In brief, the blood and marrow lend themselves to biopsy and to structural, chemical, and functional studies far more readily than do any other human organs. Their mature cellular elements are diverse, bearing in common only a joint ancestral cell, origin in the marrow, and the property of being transported through vessels suspended in plasma.

PRECURSORS OF CIRCULATING BLOOD CELLS. *Erythrocytes.*

Much of the progress of differentiation of erythroid precursors can be appreciated morphologically, particularly the onset of hemoglobin synthesis and the maturation and extrusion of the nucleus. During this process, each proerythroblast may give rise to approximately eight erythrocytes. The transit time from proerythroblast to emergence of reticulocytes is approximately 5 days. The transit time may decrease during anemic stress to as few as 2 days by means of skipped divisions. The red cells that emerge under conditions of stress are macrocytic and may contain as much as 25 per cent fetal hemoglobin (F cells). They may also bear additional fetal characteristics, particularly the presence of i antigen on their surfaces. More quantitative analyses of the transit of erythroid precursors during the process of maturation may be appreciated from the use of radioactive iron that, when injected intravenously, accumulates preferentially in the newly synthesized ferritin of proerythroblasts and ultimately emerges in peripheral blood incorporated into reticulocyte hemoglobin. The use of surface scanning following infusion of ^{59}Fe-labeled transferrin reveals the site as well as the rate of intramedullary erythropoiesis, and the rate of erythropoiesis may be estimated from the level of transferrin receptors in plasma. The use of ^{59}Fe transferrin is largely an investigative and not a clinical tool, except for cases in which the anatomic site of erythropoiesis needs to be determined, such as in myeloid metaplasia. A qualitative clinical assessment of erythroid precursor activity throughout the body may be gained from injection of indium chloride and marrow scintigraphy. Indium–111 binds to transferrin and is incorporated into immature marrow erythroid precursors. Body scanning then reveals the distribution of marrow.

Granulocytes. The process of intramedullary granulocyte maturation involves changes in nuclear configuration and the accumulation of specific intracytoplasmic granules. A model that describes the production and kinetics of neutrophils is shown in Figure 127–2 (see also Ch. 138). It is highly compartmentalized. The relatively small peripheral blood pool is divided into two compartments in equilibrium, the circulating and the marginated pools. These pools provide entrance into the tissues. The level

of peripheral cells is buffered by an immense marrow reserve of identifiable precursors, some of which are in the mitotic compartment and some in the maturing and storage compartment. The kinetics of proliferation of these recognizable precursors have been studied using labeled precursors of DNA. These so-called labeling indices, from which estimates of cell cycle times can be derived, have served as important approaches to the study of pharmacology and toxicity of chemotherapeutic agents.

Platelets. The differentiation of committed megakaryocytes, the precursors of platelets, involves a nuclear endoreduplication phenomenon that produces 16N and 32N megakaryoblasts. The endoreduplication ceases at the stage of the mature megakaryocyte. Platelet shedding from megakaryocytes is accomplished by the formation of multiple demarcation membranes within the cytoplasm of the cell, usually visible only by electron microscopy. Although the platelet appears to be a simple tissue fragment, its functions are diverse and hemostatically versatile. It must selectively adhere to abnormal surfaces and then sequentially secrete, aggregate, fuse, and retract to ensure a firm platelet-fibrin plug. In the process, it assists in the coagulation cascade, synthesizes prostaglandins, and releases adenosine diphosphate (ADP) and a variety of other substances of known and unknown function (Ch. 154).

Lymphocytes. The geography of lymphocyte precursor maturation and differentiation is considerably more complex than that of the other hematopoietic cells. Primitive lymphoid precursors of B cell origin arise in the marrow, spleen, and lymph nodes, where they continue their maturation and differentiation. Primitive T cell precursors arise in the marrow; travel to the thymus, where they undergo further differentiation; and are finally exported to the spleen, lymph nodes, and marrow, where they establish their final residence and perform many of their functions. Both T and B cells enter the peripheral blood circulation, which delivers them to tissue sites at which their functions may be required or their unbridled activity may cause disease. T cells previously "educated" in the thymus give rise to progeny that may survive for the life of the individual. Circulating lymphocytes represent only a tiny fraction of the total lymphocyte pool. Therefore, analysis of these circulating cells may not reflect the nature of the total pool.

THE HEMATOPOIETIC MICROENVIRONMENT.

For clarity, we have separately described each class of blood precursor cells, but in reality they are closely packed together. The bone marrow is a vast mesh that is best described as millions of fronds of fibroblasts and endothelial cells (to be described below), which provide a lacy framework in which are embedded differentiating progenitor cells, developing precursors bound by fibronectin to the mesh, tissue macrophages, and T cells.

The fronds of developing marrow cells float in a bog of sluggishly moving venous blood, the so-called sinusoids. Figure 127–3 demonstrates one of the least understood, but most dra-

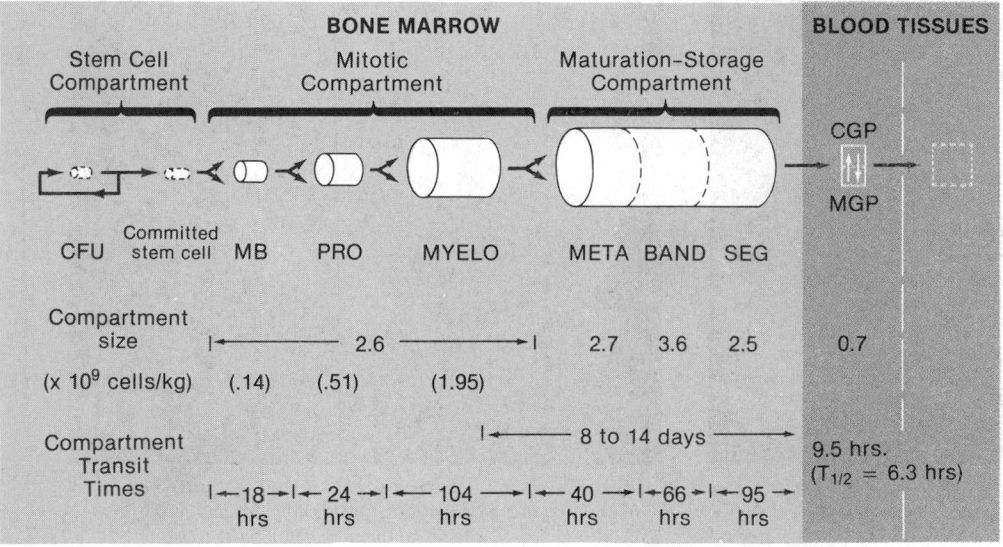

FIGURE 127–2. Model of the production and kinetics of neutrophils in humans. The marrow and blood compartments have been drawn to show their relative sizes. The compartment transit times, as derived from labeling studies with di-isopropyl phosphofluoridate (DF^{32}P) and tritiated thymidine, are shown on the next to last line and the last line. The less obvious symbols in the figure include CGP, the circulating granulocyte pool; MGP, the marginating granulocyte pool; CFU (colony-forming unit), the tripotential stem cell; MB, myeloblast; and PRO, promyelocyte. (From Wintrobe MM, Lee RG, et al.: Clinical Hematology. 7th ed. Philadelphia, Lea & Febiger, 1974, p 244.)

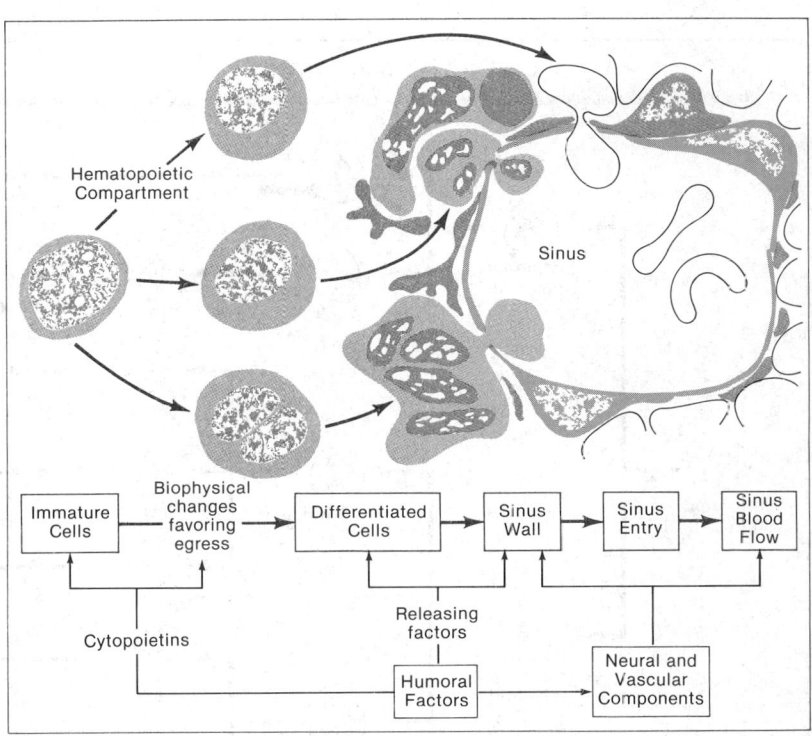

FIGURE 127–3. A schematic diagram of the factors that may be involved in controlling the release of marrow cells. The central relationship between the hematopoietic compartment and the marrow sinus is depicted. The drawing highlights the similarity of the egress process for the three major hematopoietic cells: reticulocytes in the top pathway, granulocytes and monocytes in the center pathway, and platelets in the lower pathway. Immature cells undergo biophysical changes under the influence of cytopoietins that favor egress. In the case of reticulocytes, enucleation precedes egress. This is shown by the solid black inclusion in the perisinal macrophage, representing nucleophagocytosis antecedent to digestion of the erythroblast nucleus. The cytoplasmic protrusion of the megakaryocyte presumably detaches itself from the cell and will further fragment into platelets in the circulation. (From Lichtman MA, Chamberlain JK, Santillo PA: *In* Silber R, LoBue J, Gordon AS [eds.]: The Year in Hematology, 1978. New York, Plenum Medical Book Company, 1978, p 274.)

matic, aspects of hematopoiesis, the migration of completed blood cells in the fronds through gaps that exist between endothelial cells and fibroblasts to gain access to the sinusoids and on to the general circulation. Bone marrow aspiration disrupts the fronds and eliminates a view of this microanatomy, while marrow biopsy provides only a two-dimensional aspect that sacrifices cytology for a better, albeit imperfect, representation of architecture. The fronds of hematopoietic tissue are lined by reticular cells that form the adventitial surfaces of the vascular sinuses and extend cytoplasmic processes to create a lattice for the mesh of endothelial cells and fibroblasts on which blood cells reside. The lattice is revealed by reticulin stains of marrow sections and scanning electron photomicrographs. To escape the fronds, the developing blood cells must lose their adhesiveness and do so, at least with respect to the erythroid system, by shedding fibronectin receptors to escape the sticky embrace of the microenvironment and pass into the circulation. Clumps of megakaryocytes are found adjacent to marrow sinuses. They shed platelets, the products of their cytoplasm, directly into the lumen. This situation avoids the requirement for movement of bulky megakaryocytes, a mobility characteristic of the granuloid and erythroid differentiated precursors as they approach the point at which they egress from the marrow.

KINETICS OF HEMATOPOIESIS. The marrow microenvironment supporting the progenitors and precursors must provide for the normal steady-state rates of renewal of the cellular elements of blood. Under homeostatic conditions, the production rates precisely equal destruction rates. The average lifespan of a human red cell is approximately 120 days. This means that approximately 5×10^4 red cells must be produced per day per microliter of blood in an adult. The average lifespan of platelets is 7 to 10 days, for a daily production rate of 2×10^4 platelets per microliter of blood. The white blood cell compartment exhibits more complex kinetics. Granulocytes are rapidly turned over, with an approximate intravascular lifespan of 6 to 12 hours in humans. To maintain a level of circulating granulocytes of 5 $\times 10^3$ per microliter requires a daily production that is roughly comparable to that of red cells and platelets, approximately 2 $\times 10^4$ cells per microliter of blood. At the opposite extreme in terms of lifespan are lymphocytes, some of which can exhibit lifetimes measured in months, or even years. This long lifespan of lymphocytes suggests that the daily renewal of certain lymphocyte progenitors occurs at a rate substantially lower than that of the

progenitors of the other formed elements of blood. The various symptoms of complete marrow failure are closely related to the lifespan and the turnover of the peripheral cells of the blood. Thus, patients with complete marrow failure initially lose granulocytes and therefore usually present with enhanced susceptibility to infection. Bleeding caused by platelet deficiency rapidly follows, and finally pallor and symptoms of anemia occur. Loss of circulating lymphocytes and cellular immune function is an unusual event in such circumstances and represents severe and longstanding marrow failure.

The turnover of red cells and platelets can be measured for diagnostic purposes, using $Na_2^{51}CrO_4$ as a labeling agent. Both the red cell and the platelet lifespans can be estimated and the site of the red cell destruction determined. This can be a useful maneuver in decisions regarding splenectomy.

HEMATOPOIETIC PROGENITORS. The recognizable marrow precursors of the differentiated peripheral blood cells tend to occupy the attention of hematologists, but they are rarely primary causes of the hematopoietic cytopenias. It is true that various toxins, cytotoxic antibodies, or nutritional deficiencies can so seriously damage the orderly progression of precursor differentiation that effective production of fully differentiated cells is embarrassed. In general, however, deficient or excessive production of blood cells is due to abnormalities of *undifferentiated progenitor cells*. They must themselves undergo vital processes of maturation and amplification to give rise to the recognizable precursors of circulating differentiated blood cells.

Progenitor Maturation. The hematopoietic progenitor system can be envisaged as a continuum of functional compartments (Fig. 127–4). The most primitive compartment is made up of very rare cells with high self-renewal capacity. These are so-called pluripotent stem cells (PSC's). These PSC's randomly (or stochastically) give rise to more mature stem cells that are committed to either lymphoid or myeloid development. But the fidelity of these commitments is not absolute. Hence, lymphoid surface markers may be expressed on myeloid leukemic cells. Lymphoid stem cells give rise to T and B cell precursors and their mature progeny (see Ch. 242). Trilineage myeloid stem cells are called CFU-S, for the spleen colony-forming unit first described in mice. Hematopoietic colonies were observed in the spleens of lethally irradiated mice rescued with bone marrow cells of histoidentical donors. The spleen colonies contained megakaryocyte, granulocyte, and erythroid precursors. Following

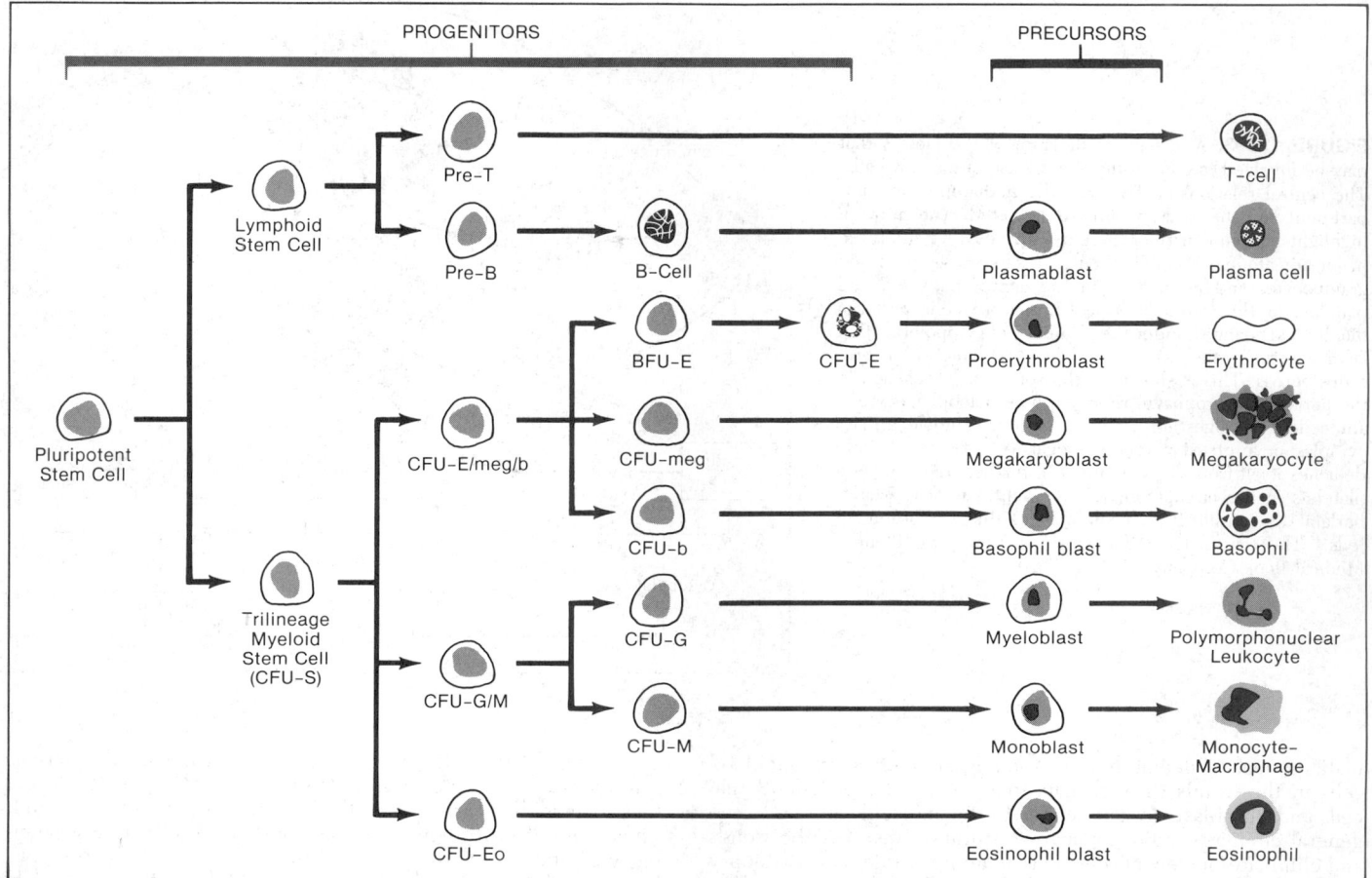

FIGURE 127–4. A schematic outline of the progenitor basis of hematopoiesis. Note the progressive restriction in the potential for terminal differentiation of the progenitors as they mature from left to right in the drawing. They finally form the recognizable marrow precursors from which the circulating blood cells, shown on the far right, are derived. Not shown in this outline is the process of self-renewal of fractions of the progenitor cell populations, particularly the immature progenitors. Also not shown is the progressive amplification of progenitors and precursors as they mature and differentiate. The bipotential erythroid-megakaryocyte progenitor shown in this drawing and referred to in the text has been demonstrated in the mouse, but not definitely in humans.

bone marrow transplantation in mice with a limited number of PSC's, a process of so-called clonal equilibration takes place, in which the progeny of some PSC's are extinguished while other PSC's begin to populate the marrow. A subset of the grafted pluripotent stem cells then dominates hematopoiesis.

Trilineage myeloid stem cells (CFU-S) eventually give rise to the committed single-lineage progenitors of the recognizable precursors through a random process of lineage restriction, shown in Figure 127–4 as a stepwise process. Actually, this represents a random set of choices that eventuate in progenitors that are restricted to single-lineage development. The restriction is probably due to the cell-surface expression of lineage-specific growth factor receptors. These single-lineage progenitors, including erythroid burst-forming units (BFU-E), erythroid colony-forming units (CFU-E), megakaryocyte colony-forming units (CFU-Meg), and basophil, granulocyte, monocyte, and eosinophil colony-forming units (CFU-Baso, CFU-G, CFU-M, and CFU-Eo, respectively), proliferate and differentiate to their respective precursors in response to the growth factors that bind to their unique receptors. The capacity of lineage-specific committed progenitors

TABLE 127–1. CHARACTERISTICS OF HUMAN HEMATOPOIETIC GROWTH FACTORS

Growth Factor	Cellular Source	Progenitor Cell Target*	Mature Cell Target
Interleukin 3 (IL3)	T lymphocytes	CFU-Blast, CFR-GEMM, CFU-GM, CFU-G, CFU-M, CFU-Eo, CFU-Meg, CFU-Baso, BFU-E	Eosinophils, monocytes
GM-CSF	T lymphocytes, monocytes, fibroblasts, endothelial cells	CFU-Blast, CFU-GEMM, CFU-GM, CFU-G, CFU-M, CFU-Eo, CFU-Meg, BFU-E	Granulocytes, eosinophils, monocytes
G-CSF	Monocytes, fibroblasts, endothelial cells	CFU-G	Granulocytes
M-CSF	Monocytes, fibroblasts, endothelial cells, uterus	CFU-M	Monocytes
Erythropoietin	Peritubular cells of the kidney, Kupffer cells	CFU-E, late BFU-E?, CFU-Meg	None
IL5	T lymphocytes	CFU-Eo	Eosinophils

*CFU-Blast = colony-forming unit—blast; CFU-GEMM = colony-forming unit—granulocyte, erythrocyte, monocyte, and megakaryocyte; CFU-GM = colony-forming unit—granulocyte and macrophage; CFU-Eo = colony-forming unit—eosinophil; CFU-Meg = colony-forming unit—megakaryocyte; BFU-E = burst-forming unit—erythroid; CFU-G = colony-forming unit—granulocyte; CFU-M = colony-forming unit—macrophage; CFU-E = colony-forming unit—erythroid; and CFU-Baso = colony-forming unit —basophil.

to proliferate and differentiate in response to demand constitutes the most important buffer of the hematopoietic system against increased requirement for mature blood cell production. Little is known about the cell biology of progenitors because their rarity makes their purification extremely difficult. Such purification has been recently accomplished to a considerable extent in mice, and the antibody to the cell-surface antigen CD–34 has been useful in achieving partial purification of progenitors in humans.

Hematopoietic Growth Factors. The proliferation, differentiation, and survival of immature hematopoietic progenitor cells are sustained by a family of glycoproteins, the hematopoietic growth factors (HGF's) (see Table 127–1). In addition to their effect on the proliferation and differentiation of progenitors, these factors also influence the survival and function of mature blood cells. The HGF's are also known collectively as the colony-stimulating factors (CSF's), a term derived from the in vitro observation that they stimulate progenitor cells to form colonies of recognizable maturing cells. It is important to recognize that the lineage-specific HGF's, erythropoietin, G-CSF, M-CSF, and interleukin 5 (IL5), are not active alone except in their interactions with the most mature committed progenitor cells. The majority of lineage-specific progenitors demand the presence of either IL3 or GM-CSF in addition to a lineage-specific HGF to produce the colonies for which they are programmed. Hence, immature committed progenitors bear receptors for both IL3 and GM-CSF. They differ from one another with respect to their lineage-specific receptors.

The genes for several human HGF's have been cloned, and this, in turn, has led to the production and purification of the respective recombinant proteins. This advance in molecular biology has allowed intensive investigations of the actions of purified HGF's, their cellular origins, and their regulatory mechanisms (Fig. 127–5), while the availability of large quantities of highly purified HGF's has led to preclinical and clinical evaluation of their effectiveness in vivo. In general, IL3 and GM-CSF stimulate the survival, proliferation, and differentiation of a broad range of progenitors, if lineage-specific HGF's are also present. Stem cells may also be stimulated by three other interleukins, IL1, IL4, and IL6, but the actions of these factors may be indirect or may require the presence of other cytokines. Interleukin 6 is particularly interesting because in combination with IL3 it reduces the time during which blast cells in culture begin to divide to form colonies, suggesting that the combination influences stem cell cycling. It may also synergize with IL3 or GM-CSF to induce megakaryocyte differentiation. Figure 127–5 emphasizes the interaction of the most important HGF's with progenitor cells. Note the requirement for combinations of IL3 and/or GM-CSF

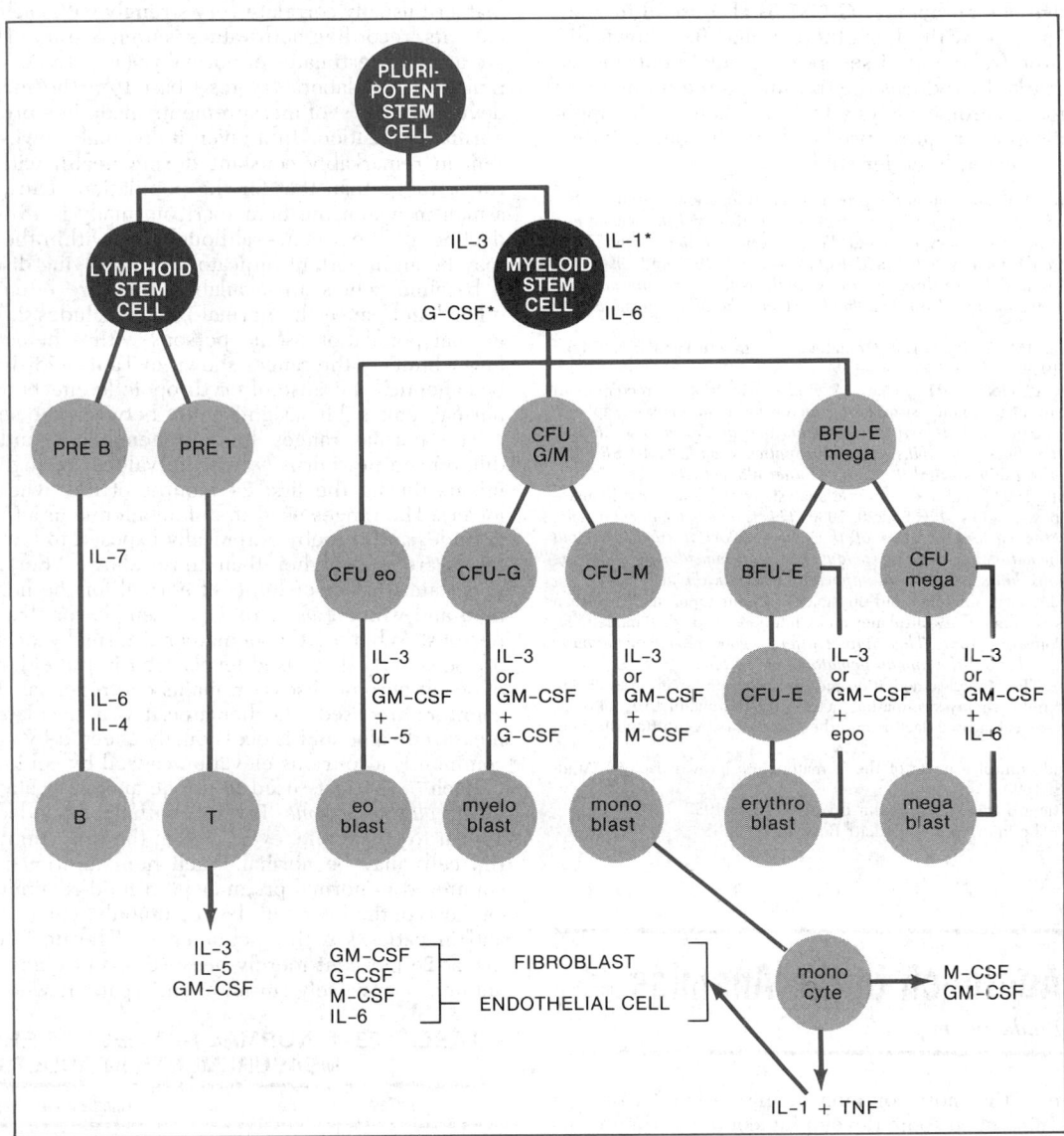

FIGURE 127–5. The hematopoietic progenitors and growth factors. The differentiation of hematopoietic progenitors is shown, beginning with the pluripotent stem cell. The myeloid stem cell differentiates randomly into the CFU-G/M, BFU-E/mega, and CFU-Eo lineages. The rate of differentiation is influenced by IL3 (interleukin 3) and IL6 and perhaps by G-CSF (colony-stimulating factor) and IL1. The synergistic effects of IL5, G-CSF, M-CSF, and IL6 with either IL3 or GM-CSF are shown. The production of growth factors is demonstrated at the bottom of the figure. See footnote to Table 127–1 for definition of the growth factors.

with lineage-specific growth factors for the induction of specific precursors.

The bottom of Figure 127–5 summarizes the cells of origin of the HGF's and demonstrates that the monocyte and T cell play an important role in progenitor differentiation. Monocytes produce IL1 and tumor necrosis factor (TNF) in response to bacterial products. These in turn stimulate fibroblasts and endothelial cells to produce all of the HGF's except IL3 and IL5. Antigens of various kinds stimulate T cells to produce IL3 and IL5, as well as GM-CSF. All of these growth factors in turn interact with their specific progenitors to produce the developing blood cells. As mentioned above, fibroblasts and endothelial cells are not merely factories of growth factors. They also provide a critically important adherent layer on which progenitor differentiation must take place. Fibronectin is a key component of the microenvironment because it binds progenitors to fibroblasts and endothelial cells through fibronectin receptors.

THERAPEUTIC APPLICATIONS. Thus far, three HGF's have shown promise in clinical trials. GM-CSF regularly elevates the granulocyte count in a dose-dependent fashion in patients with acquired immunodeficiency syndrome (AIDS) and shows promise as well in the management of aplastic anemia in children. It may also be useful in protocols involving autotransplantation following intensive chemotherapy. G-CSF is also useful in granulocytopenia associated with chemotherapy and has shown distinct promise in the treatment of severe congenital neutropenia. Erythropoietin markedly reduces the transfusion requirements of patients undergoing chronic dialysis for renal failure. Its application in other disorders requiring red cell transfusion, including autotransfusion, is currently under study.

Cannistra SA, Griffin JD: Regulation of the production and function of granulocytes and monocytes. Semin Hematol 25:173, 1988. *This article and the second and sixth through tenth references offer excellent reviews of the status of the hematopoietic growth factors as the field evolved between 1987 and 1990. The article by Strober and James discusses the growth factors that interact with progenitors and precursors of the lymphoid system. The others focus on the myeloid system.*

Groopman JE, Molina JM, Scadden DT: Hematopoietic growth factors. N Engl J Med 321:1449, 1989.

Guinan EC, Sieff CA, Oette DH, et al.: A Phase I/II trial of recombinant granulocyte-macrophage colony stimulating factor for children with aplastic anemia. Blood, in press. *This article represents one of the more optimistic results of the treatment of aplastic anemia patients with GM-CSF. The bibliography is also useful in that it describes other clinical trials.*

Jordan CT, Lemischka IR: Clonal and systemic analysis of the long-term hematopoiesis in the mouse. Genes Devel 4:220, 1990. *This is a very technical article, but it explores the various theories of the contribution of stem cells and progenitors to hematopoiesis in the steady state and immediately following bone marrow transplantation. It is an important article in the field.*

Lipton JM, Nathan, DG: The anatomy and physiology of hematopoiesis. *In* Nathan DG, Oski F (eds.): Hematology of Infancy and Childhood. 3rd ed. Philadelphia, WB Saunders Company, 1987. *This chapter offers a good review of the basic anatomy and physiology of the human hematopoietic system.*

Nathan DG, Sieff CA: The biological activities and uses of recombinant granulocyte macrophage and multi-colony stimulating factors. Prog Hematol 15:1, 1987.

Nicola NA: Hemopoietic cell growth factors and their receptors. Annu Rev Biochem 58:45, 1989.

Sieff CA: Biology and clinical aspects of the hematopoietic growth factors. Annu Rev Med 41:483, 1990.

Sieff C: Hematopoietic growth factors. J Clin Invest 79:1549, 1987.

Strober W, James S: The interleukins. Pediatr Res 24:549, 1988.

128 An Approach to the Anemias

John Lindenbaum

Anemia is one of the most common manifestations of disease the world over. Indeed, in some developing countries the majority of apparently normal people in certain population groups are anemic. Even in technologically advanced nations, a third or more of patients admitted to the medical service of a hospital are anemic. Yet a low hematocrit is often ignored or is put aside to be dealt with at a later time while other, more pressing medical problems are managed on an urgent basis. This practice is frequently a mistake, since anemia is usually a clue that should not be ignored. In fact, the clinician should almost always think of anemia in a manner similar to the way in which he or she regards symptoms like chest pain or diarrhea—as an indicator or a manifestation of an underlying disease, rather than an entity in itself.

Physicians often use laboratory tests inappropriately in the evaluation of anemic patients. In some instances, the small number of crucial tests needed to diagnose the cause of any anemia is not obtained. In others, blood is withdrawn for a long list of unnecessary tests, often worsening the anemia without elucidating it. In this chapter a logical and orderly approach to anemia is advocated. Commonly encountered diagnostic challenges receive greater emphasis than the rarer entities. The strategy outlined allows the clinician to diagnose the cause of anemia in the great majority of patients, using a small number of laboratory tests (since most anemias are caused by only a handful of conditions). The strategy also furnishes clues to the less common or more esoteric causes of anemia.

DEFINITION OF ANEMIA

In Table 128–1, normal ranges are listed for the hematocrit, hemoglobin concentration, and red blood cell count in adults. Any of these three tests can be used as an estimate of the presence or absence of anemia. Since the hemoglobin and hematocrit usually correlate very strongly with each other in anemic patients, recording both values is unnecessary. The ranges shown are arbitrary estimates of normality (as is the case for the normal range for any laboratory test) based on the mean ±2 standard deviations (SD's) of measurements made in a presumably healthy normal population. In a given individual, however, these values remain remarkably constant during health within a much narrower range than that for the population. Thus, for example, in a man in whom the hematocrit normally is 48 to 50 per cent, a decline to 40 per cent—although still within the normal range—may be an important indicator of underlying disease. Therefore, if baseline values are available, they are often useful. On the other hand, since the normal range excludes 2.5 per cent of the normal population, some persons with a hematocrit below the lower limits of the ranges shown in Table 128–1 may not actually be "anemic." Because of erythropoietic effects of androgens, the normal ranges differ significantly between the sexes.

The normal ranges for the hematocrit and the MCV are different in newborns (when the values are higher) as well as in infants during the first 24 months of life (when the values are lower). The ranges used to define anemia in adults living at high altitudes and thereby chronically exposed to low ambient oxygen levels are also higher than those shown. For reasons that are uncertain, the lower limits of normal for the hematocrit in black men and women are 1 to 2 per cent lower than those for white persons. Whether the hematocrit normally declines with aging or the slightly decreased levels seen in the elderly are indicators of occult chronic disease remains controversial. When electronic counters are used, the hematocrit is a calculated rather than a measured value and is occasionally affected by artifacts; the most common is a spurious elevation caused by cold agglutinins.

Each of the tests used to define anemia is affected by changes in the *plasma volume*. Patients with an expanded plasma volume appear to be anemic, even though the total number of circulating red cells may be normal. Such hemodilution is frequently encountered in normal pregnancy; in fluid-retaining states, such as cirrhosis of the liver and, less commonly, congestive heart failure; and in patients with splenomegaly. The hematocrit may fall as low as 28 per cent merely because of an expansion of the plasma volume. Conversely, in an anemic patient who has a decreased

TABLE 128–1. NORMAL RANGES* OF ERYTHROCYTE MEASUREMENTS IN ADULTS

Test	Females	Males
Hematocrit (%)	36–48	40–52
Hemoglobin (grams/dl)	12.0–16.0	13.5–17.7
Red blood cells ($\times 10^6/\mu l$)	4.0–5.4	4.5–6.0
Mean cell volume (fl)	80–100	80–100

*Ranges of values measured by Coulter electronic counting, representing 2 SD's above and below the mean for healthy white adults living at sea level.

plasma volume (e.g., due to dehydration), the hematocrit may lie within the normal range. If necessary, the total number of circulating red cells can be measured by a radioisotope dilution method, yielding a value known as the "red cell mass." This test is usually not necessary clinically and is more often employed in the evaluation of polycythemia.

CARDIOVASCULAR ADJUSTMENTS TO ANEMIA

The circulating erythrocyte is a nonreplicating, differentiated cell with a normal average lifespan of 120 days. Its function is to deliver oxygen to the tissues. Therefore, the main consequence of anemia is tissue hypoxia. When anemia develops slowly, several adjustments tend to maintain tissue oxygenation. The plasma volume increases, tending to maintain the total blood volume at a normal or only slightly reduced level. Early in the development of anemia, there is increased generation of the glycolytic intermediate, 2,3-diphosphoglycerate (2,3-DPG), in erythrocytes. The 2,3-DPG binds to hemoglobin, causing a rightward shift in the oxyhemoglobin dissociation curve, which allows more oxygen to be unloaded from the erythrocyte at any given blood oxygen tension.

As anemia becomes more severe, compensatory peripheral vascular dilatation increases blood flow to the tissues, through a fall in the systemic vascular resistance and an increase in the cardiac output. The latter mainly results from an increased cardiac stroke volume, since the heart rate increases only slightly, if at all, in most anemic patients. An increase in cardiac output is usually seen only in severe anemia, when the hematocrit falls to levels of about 20 per cent or less. As a result of the decrease in peripheral resistance, the blood pressure falls modestly, especially the diastolic component, leading to an increased pulse pressure. The systolic pressure, although often reduced from the normal baseline of the patient, typically remains normal. Not infrequently, a patient with previous hypertension who develops severe anemia (due, for example, to deficiency of iron or vitamin B_{12}) becomes unexpectedly normotensive; hypertension then recurs after the anemia is corrected. Similarly, correction of anemia due to renal failure by treatment with erythropoietin may cause or exacerbate hypertension. In a minority of anemic patients (usually but not invariably those with underlying cardiovascular disease), the demands of the high output state coupled with impaired coronary oxygenation lead to circulatory congestion, in some cases without an associated fall in output ("high output failure").

The cardiovascular adjustments described above are those seen when anemia develops slowly. In patients with acute blood loss, however (e.g., massive gastrointestinal bleeding), there is no time for them to occur. Instead, there is a sudden marked contraction of the intravascular volume, which may result in severe postural hypotension, a fall in cardiac output, the shunting of blood from the skin to central organs, sweating, restlessness, thirst, and air hunger (Ch. 111). This life-threatening emergency must be managed by immediate restoration of the intravascular volume, usually by transfusion of red cells. In contrast, in the chronically anemic patient, who often has a relatively well maintained central intravascular volume, blood transfusions (particularly if given rapidly to an elderly patient with underlying heart disease) may expand the central blood volume and precipitate or worsen congestive heart failure.

SYMPTOMS AND SIGNS OF ANEMIA

The complaints caused by anemia are related to tissue hypoxia. In patients with chronically developing anemia, the hematocrit level at which symptoms appear varies widely, influenced by the rate of development of anemia, the age of the patient, and the presence of underlying vascular disease. Frequent symptoms include dyspnea with exertion, dizziness, light-headedness, throbbing headaches, tinnitus, palpitations, syncope, easy fatigability, disruption of sleep patterns, decrease in libido, disturbances of mood, and impaired ability to concentrate. In elderly patients with vascular disease, angina pectoris may be a prominent complaint, even with only modest reductions in hematocrit. Anemia also frequently worsens or precipitates dementia or intermittent claudication. Anorexia is common and may be accompanied by significant weight loss. *Common physical findings* in severely anemic patients include pallor of the skin and mucous membranes (a sign of limited sensitivity and specificity), modest tachycardia and increased pulse pressure, systolic ejection murmurs, venous hums, and mild peripheral edema. Retinal hemorrhages, often flamelike, may occur in severe anemia, most commonly in association with thrombocytopenia.

THE HISTORY

As in almost all other clinical disorders, *a careful history usually provides information crucial to diagnosing the underlying cause of anemia.* The duration and time of onset of anemia or its symptoms should be determined. Onset during childhood is seen with congenital hemolytic disorders, although when anemia is not severe, these conditions may first manifest in adult life. A history of scleral icterus or gallstones, or the presence of jaundice, gallstones, or anemia in a sibling or a parent, suggests hemolysis. A history of blood loss or blood donation should be sought. Onset of the anemia during or soon after pregnancy is consistent with iron or folate deficiency. Recurrences and remissions of anemia are frequent in iron, cobalamin (vitamin B_{12}), and folate deficiencies. Pica, or excessive craving for certain (sometimes bizarre) food items, occurs with lack of iron. A history of alcohol intoxication raises a number of diagnostic considerations (see below). Paresthesia or ataxia suggests cobalamin deficiency; a sore tongue may indicate lack of cobalamin, folate, or iron. If these deficiencies are caused by celiac or tropical sprue, diarrhea or other gastrointestinal symptoms are commonly present. The patient

TABLE 128–2. DRUGS AND OTHER AGENTS THAT MAY CAUSE ANEMIA

Anemia	Type of Agent	Example
Marrow aplasias	Anticancer	Antimetabolites, alkylating agents
	Anti-inflammatory	Phenylbutazone, gold
	Antibiotic	Chloramphenicol
	Anticonvulsant	Phenytoin
	Other	Benzene, insectides
Macrocytic or megaloblastic states	Dihydrofolate reductase inhibitors	Methotrexate, pyrimethamine, trimethoprim, triamterene, pentamidine
	Antiviral	Zidovudine
	Anticancer	Hydroxyurea, cytosine arabinoside, alkylating agents
	Immunosuppressive	Azathioprine
	Other	Alcohol, sulfasalazine
Hemolytic	Antibiotic	Penicillin,* cephalosporins,* sulfonamides*†
	Antiarrhythmic	Procainamide,* quinidine*
	Antihypertensive	Alpha-methyldopa*
	Antimalarials	Primaquine*
	Other	Fava beans,† naphthalene,† dapsone†
Blood loss	Anti-inflammatory	Aspirin, nonsteroidal drugs
	Anticoagulants	Warfarin, heparin

*Causes antibody-induced hemolysis.
†Causes hemolysis in glucose-6-phosphate dehydrogenase (G6PD)–deficient persons. Sulfonamides also cause hemolysis in patients with unstable hemoglobins.

TABLE 128–3. THE INITIAL LABORATORY DATA BASE IN THE EVALUATION OF ANEMIA

Hematocrit
Reticulocyte count (absolute)
MCV
Blood smear
Serum ferritin level
White blood cell count and differential
Platelet count (or estimate)

MCV = mean cell volume.

must be questioned, sometimes repeatedly, about the possible intake of various medications (Table 128–2). The most important aspect of the history in an anemic patient, however, is often the search for underlying disease: for evidence of renal, liver, or endocrine disturbances; the acquired immunodeficiency syndrome (AIDS), tuberculosis, or other infections; chronic inflammatory disorders, such as rheumatoid arthritis or lupus erythematosus; or malignancies.

THE PHYSICAL EXAMINATION

Findings on physical examination that point to specific underlying etiologic mechanisms include atrophy of the tongue (in cobalamin, folate, or iron deficiencies); abnormal gait or impaired vibration sense or other sensory modalities (in cobalamin lack); scleral icterus, splenomegaly, or leg ulcers (in certain hemolytic anemias); petechiae (with thrombocytopenia of any cause, e.g., acute leukemia); and the myriad signs of primary diseases (e.g., infections, malignancies, liver disorders, hypothyroidism) that may cause a secondary anemia.

THE INITIAL LABORATORY DATA BASE

A small number of tests should be obtained on every anemic patient: the complete blood count (CBC), including the white blood cell count and differential, a platelet count, or an estimate on the smear of the numbers of platelets; a careful evaluation of red blood cell morphology on the Wright-stained blood smear; the reticulocyte count; the mean cell volume (MCV); and some measure of iron stores—the serum ferritin (preferably) or the combined determination of the serum iron and total iron-binding capacity (Table 128–3). In at least three quarters of patients, the cause of the anemia will be apparent when the results of these tests are combined with the history, physical examination, and other diagnostic studies that are guided by complaints not caused by the anemia.

THE BLOOD SMEAR. In the current era of automation and high technology, the value of careful, expert assessment of the red cell morphology on the peripheral blood smear tends to be forgotten. The blood smear, however, is essential to the diagnosis of many anemias and virtually always provides useful information, even when unremarkable or normal. Proper identification of the full range of clinically useful abnormalities requires a certain expertise. Blood smears are subject to both *overinterpretation* (usually because of frequent artifacts in poorly prepared smears

or in inappropriate areas of well-prepared ones) and *underinterpretation* (most frequently the result of hurried interpretation by an overwhelmed routine laboratory). Therefore, the clinician must take the time to develop expertise in this area or, in most instances, demand that the hospital laboratory provide an expert assessment of the blood smear.

Some characteristic red cell abnormalities useful in the diagnosis of various anemias are listed in Table 128–4. The *context* in which a particular morphologic finding is noted must be emphasized. If red cell fragmentation is the most striking abnormality on the blood smear of a patient with a high reticulocyte count, hemoglobinuria, and a poorly functioning aortic valve prosthesis, the morphologic changes strongly support the diagnosis of a traumatic hemolytic anemia. In contrast, an occasional fragmented cell in the blood smear of a patient with marked hypochromia, microcytosis, a low reticulocyte count, and a history of recent blood loss is much more likely to be caused by iron deficiency. The widely used term *poikilocytosis*, to indicate variation in cell shape, is of limited usefulness. The clinician really desires to know precisely which abnormalities in shape have been noted, e.g., sickle cells, oval macrocytes, elliptocytes, or fragments. Although *polychromasia* (see Color Plate 5F, left) is indicative of the presence of young reticulocytes (see below), the abundance of polychromatic cells is important. An occasional polychromatic cell is often seen in severe anemias due to bone marrow failure (e.g., megaloblastic anemia, marrow infiltration by tumor). The presence of blasts in the differential white count suggests acute leukemia as the cause of a patient's anemia; decreased numbers of platelets or white cells point toward conditions in which anemia is associated with other cytopenias (e.g., megaloblastic anemia, hypersplenism, acute leukemia, aplastic anemia).

ERYTHROPOIETIC RESPONSE TO ANEMIA. As tissue hypoxia develops with increasing anemia, a major homeostatic system attempts to return the number of circulating red cells to normal. Although a number of other hormones and growth factors may influence erythrocyte production, erythropoietin, a glycoprotein, is probably the most important. Erythropoietin appears to be predominantly produced by peritubular cells of the kidney (most likely capillary endothelial cells). Other cells, possibly including hepatocytes and macrophages, may be less important sources of the hormone. A heme protein present in cells sensitive to hypoxia may undergo a conformational change that in some way activates the gene for erythropoietin production. Erythropoietin released into the circulation acts mainly to stimulate the differentiation of erythroid stem cells in the bone marrow, cells that are already committed to form red cells (so-called CFU-E, or colony-forming units–erythroid). The hormone also acts on later erythroid precursors. The result is the enhanced production and release of young red cells, or *reticulocytes* (see Color Plate 5F, right).

THE RETICULOCYTE COUNT. A key test that should be included as part of the initial workup of every anemic patient is the reticulocyte count. The reticulocyte, a 1- to 2-day-old cell that is continuing to synthesize protein (unlike more elderly erythrocytes), contains aggregates of ribosomes, demonstrated by a supravital stain (new methylene blue). The reticulocyte count is the percentage of such cells per 500 or 1000 cells counted,

TABLE 128–4. ABNORMALITIES ON BLOOD SMEARS IN ANEMIC PATIENTS

Abnormality	Characteristic Disorder	Found Also in Other Conditions
Hypochromia, microcytosis	Iron deficiency, thalassemias	Anemia of chronic disease, sideroblastic anemias
Macro-ovalocytes	Cobalamin and folate deficiencies	Myelodysplasias, myelofibrosis, autoimmune hemolysis
Hypersegmented neutrophils	Cobalamin and folate deficiencies	Renal failure, iron deficiency, chronic myelocytic leukemia, congenital hypersegmentation
Teardrop cells, nucleated red blood cells	Myelofibrosis	Marrow replacement by tumor, autoimmune hemolysis, megaloblastic anemias, thalassemia major
Microspherocytes	Autoimmune hemolysis, hereditary spherocytosis	Microangiopathic hemolysis, hypophosphatemia
Sickle cells	Hemoglobin SS, SC, S-thalassemia	Hemoglobin C$_{Harlem}$
Red cell fragments (schistocytes)	Microangiopathic or traumatic hemolysis	Iron deficiency, megaloblastic anemias, cancer chemotherapy
Target cells	Hemoglobin C, SC, thalassemias, liver disease	Artifact, SS disease, iron deficiency, splenectomy
Elliptocytes	Hereditary elliptocytosis	Iron deficiency, myelofibrosis, megaloblastic anemias
Burr cells (echinocytes)	Renal failure	Artifact, pyruvate kinase deficiency
Spur cells (acanthocytes)	Liver disease, abetalipoproteinemia	

TABLE 128–5. CAUSES OF ANEMIA

Cause	Absolute Reticulocyte Count
Bone marrow failure	Low or normal
Acute blood loss	High
Hemolysis	High

rather than an absolute number. It therefore needs to be "corrected" to make it a better index of total production of young cells. This can be done by multiplying the reticulocyte percentage times the red blood cell count. Thus, for example, in a normal person with a reticulocyte count of 1 per cent and a red cell count of 5 million per microliter, the absolute numbers of circulating reticulocytes would be $0.01 \times 5,000,000 = 50,000$ reticulocytes per microliter. The upper limit of normal is approximately 100,000 per microliter. In contrast, in an anemic patient with a red cell count of 2 million per microliter and a reticulocyte count of 1 per cent, the number of circulating reticulocytes would be $0.01 \times 2,000,000$, or 20,000 per microliter. Although the reticulocyte percentage is the same (1 per cent) in this instance, the absolute number is markedly below normal, indicating that the bone marrow has failed to respond to the severe anemia by increasing its production of young cells.

INITIAL EVALUATION OF ANEMIA

Calculation of the absolute numbers of reticulocytes allows the clinician to make an important early decision that will shape further diagnostic thinking (Table 128–5). Anemias can be divided into those in which the marrow response to the anemia is appropriate, that is, red cell production is increased, and those in which there is an inappropriate failure of the marrow to augment cell output. An anemia in which the absolute number of reticulocytes is not increased is defined as one in which *bone marrow failure* is present (Table 128–5). *In most anemic patients encountered in clinical medicine, the underlying cause of the anemia is marrow failure.* The subsequent diagnostic workup of the patient with marrow failure differs markedly from that of one in whom the reticulocyte count is elevated.

The classification shown in Table 128–5, although extremely useful clinically, is an oversimplification. It emphasizes the *predominant* cause of the anemia. In many anemias, more than one mechanism is operative. Thus, for example, in the anemia of chronic disease, the red cell lifespan is modestly shortened, although the primary cause of the anemia is the failure of the bone marrow to increase the number of circulating reticulocytes. Similarly, in severe anemias due to deficiencies of iron, vitamin B_{12}, or folate, or in beta-thalassemia major, the red cell lifespan may be shortened, although the primary problem is one of cell production. In addition, in many chronic hemolytic anemias, even though the bone marrow has increased its output of new cells, the marrow response is less than maximal and an element of inadequate marrow compensation may contribute to the anemia. Furthermore, when acute hemolysis or blood loss develops, the maximal reticulocyte response may be delayed for several days or as long as a week. Thus, approximately 20 per cent of patients with an acute episode of autoimmune hemolytic anemia do not have an elevated absolute reticulocyte count at the time of admission to the hospital, although reticulocytosis develops subsequently. In patients hospitalized for several weeks, the equivalent of a unit of whole blood is often obtained as part of an intensive diagnostic workup for various disorders. In this situation, acute blood loss caused by multiple venesections may be superimposed upon a marrow failure anemia, frequently without an adequate reticulocyte response.

ANEMIA DUE TO BONE MARROW FAILURE

RED CELL SIZE IN PATIENTS WITH MARROW FAILURE. The first question that should be asked about a patient with a marrow failure anemia is, *what is the average size of the red cells?* The MCV is measured directly by electronic counters and is usually available as part of the initial hemogram. Although the mean cell hemoglobin (MCH) and mean cell hemoglobin concentration (MCHC) are also routinely provided, they add little information of diagnostic value. The MCH varies in the same direction as the MCV in microcytic or macrocytic anemias. The MCHC is of very limited value and is often normal in

TABLE 128–6. CLASSIFICATION OF ANEMIAS DUE TO MARROW FAILURE

Type	MCV (fl)
Normocytic	80–100
Microcytic	<80
Macrocytic	>100

patients with frank microcytic anemias. The normal range for the MCV in adults is 80 to 100 fl (femtoliters), a better working range in the classification of anemias than the more narrow ones often reported by hospital laboratories. The MCV determination may be falsely elevated by laboratory artifacts, which may be caused by cold agglutinins, marked hyperglycemia, and extreme leukocytosis.

On the basis of the MCV, anemias due to marrow failure should be classified as normocytic, microcytic, or macrocytic (Table 128–6). In normocytic or microcytic anemias, the subsequent diagnostic evaluation differs markedly from that in macrocytic anemias.

Normocytic Anemias Due to Marrow Failure

Normocytic anemias due to marrow failure account for the largest group of patients with anemia seen in clinical practice. The most common causes of normocytic anemia due to decreased cell production (Table 128–7) are iron deficiency, the anemia of chronic disease, and anemias secondary to renal, hepatic, and endocrine disorders. Less frequently, a normocytic marrow failure anemia may result from one of a variety of "primary" marrow disturbances.

IRON DEFICIENCY ANEMIA (Ch. 131). Iron deficiency anemia is usually considered microcytic and hypochromic. As iron deficiency develops, however, the hematocrit often falls before the MCV becomes subnormal. Therefore, iron lack (especially when the hematocrit is above 30 per cent) must always be considered in patients with normocytic marrow failure anemia. In outpatient practice, iron deficiency is a frequent cause of such an anemia. Blood smears may be entirely normal except for mild anisocytosis; or there may be a minority population of microcytic cells, even though the MCV is still normal. Since most of the iron in the body is found in red cells, loss of blood (commonly from gastrointestinal or uterine sources) is usually the underlying cause of iron deficiency. Imbalances between demand and dietary supply frequently cause iron deficiency anemia in normal pregnancy, infancy, and adolescence. Rare causes include loss of hemoglobin and hemosiderin in the urine in certain hemolytic anemias (e.g., with malfunctioning valve prostheses or in paroxysmal nocturnal hemoglobinuria), intrapulmonary hemorrhage (in idiopathic pulmonary hemosiderosis), and malabsorption of iron (usually secondary to gastrectomy or to celiac or tropical sprue). Iron deficiency anemia due to primary inadequacy of iron intake in the diet is an unusual cause of anemia in adults in industrialized countries. In many developing nations, however, in addition to blood loss, anemia may be caused by a diet that is adequate in total iron content but that contains iron in poorly bioavailable form.

ANEMIA OF CHRONIC DISEASE (Ch. 131). In patients who have chronic infections (e.g., tuberculosis, lung abscess), chronic inflammation (e.g., rheumatoid arthritis, systemic lupus

TABLE 128–7. CAUSES OF NORMOCYTIC MARROW FAILURE ANEMIAS

Iron deficiency
Anemia of chronic disease
Renal failure
Liver disease
Endocrine disorders
"Primary" marrow disorders*
  Aplasias
  Myelodysplasias
  Myelofibrosis
  Hematologic or solid tumors
  Granulomas
  HIV infection

*Marrow aspiration and biopsy are useful.

erythematosus, inflammatory bowel disease), or underlying malignancies that are not necessarily metastatic to the bone marrow, or who have recently had major trauma or surgery, a characteristic anemia that is gradual in onset and is usually normocytic often develops. Typically, the anemia is mild, although in 10 per cent of patients (usually with very severe chronic illnesses) the hematocrit may be below 20 per cent. Red cell morphology is little changed from normal, although there may be modest anisocytosis with a few microcytes. Marked anisocytosis, poikilocytosis, or nucleated red blood cells are not seen. The primary problem is failure of cell production. Relative lack of erythropoietin, sequestration of iron in macrophages, and inhibitory effects of cytokines are among the postulated causes of the marrow failure. The anemia remits when the underlying disorder clears. The presence of one of the associated chronic disorders is usually obvious. Occasionally, however, the anemia of chronic disease is the only apparent illness, and a careful search for an occult disorder, such as a malignancy or polymyalgia rheumatica, is indicated. The anemia of chronic disease does not occur in all chronic conditions, however. Uncomplicated diabetes mellitus, hypertension, asthma, ischemic heart disease, or congestive heart failure should not be considered a satisfactory explanation for an anemia of this type.

DIFFERENTIATION OF IRON DEFICIENCY ANEMIA FROM THE ANEMIA OF CHRONIC DISEASE.

Since iron deficiency is usually accompanied by greater variation in red cell size than is seen in the anemia of chronic disease, it has been proposed that a quantitative assessment of the degree of anisocytosis, as measured by electronic cell sizing (the "red cell distribution width," or RDW), can be helpful in distinguishing these two common causes of marrow failure anemia. This assessment has not proved to be reliable. The differentiation is often aided, however, by serum tests that are influenced by the amount of iron in body stores. The most useful screening measure for this purpose is the *serum ferritin* level (Ch. 131), which is low in the majority of patients with iron deficiency and normal or elevated in the anemia of chronic disease. A low serum ferritin value virtually always indicates iron deficiency. Unfortunately, there is an overlap zone (approximately 20 to 150 ng per milliliter) in the lower end of the normal range that is compatible with *either* condition. Other tests frequently used for estimating iron stores are the *serum iron* and the *serum total iron-binding capacity* (TIBC). The serum iron level is typically low in both disorders, however. In chronic disease, the TIBC (an indicator of circulating levels of the iron-binding protein transferrin) is usually depressed, and in iron deficiency it is often elevated. Unfortunately, many patients with iron deficiency anemia, especially if complicated by a chronic disease, may have normal or even low levels of the TIBC. In both conditions, *the per cent saturation of serum transferrin* (i.e., the serum iron divided by the TIBC × 100) is low. The test is not helpful unless the value is higher than 25 per cent, which argues against iron deficiency. The interpretation of these laboratory measures is summarized in Table 128–8. If these tests are equivocal, direct examination of the bone marrow with histochemical staining of iron stores in macrophages is needed to exclude iron deficiency definitely. Alternatively, a therapeutic trial of iron can be given, repeating the hematocrit after 3 to 4 weeks. This practice may be reasonable

TABLE 128–8. RELIABILITY OF SERUM TESTS IN PREDICTING IRON STORES

Test	Interpretation
Definitive	
Low ferritin	Deficient
High TIBC	Deficient
High normal or high ferritin	Not deficient*
Equivocal	
Low normal ferritin	Uncertain
Low serum iron	Uncertain
Low or normal TIBC	Uncertain
Low per cent of transferrin saturation	Uncertain

*Even if inflammation, malignancy, liver disease, or renal failure is present.
TIBC = total iron-binding capacity.

in a patient with uncomplicated iron deficiency anemia (for example, a menstruating woman who is otherwise well but with a serum ferritin level of 35 ng per milliliter). In a patient with an underlying chronic disorder, however, if iron is given at the same time as the chronic disease is treated or spontaneously improves, the "response" of the hematocrit to iron will be difficult to interpret. It is preferable to assess marrow iron stores directly before treatment, since once lack of iron is proved, a search for an underlying cause of blood loss is mandated.

The serum ferritin is an acute phase reactant; it is elevated out of proportion to the amount of iron in stores in acute and chronic inflammatory disorders or malignancies (as well as liver and kidney disease). Nonetheless, the presence of some iron in stores appears to be necessary for a marked increase in the serum ferritin level to occur in association with these conditions. Therefore, *an elevated or high normal serum ferritin is not seen in patients who are iron deficient*, even though they have associated inflammation, malignancy, liver disease, or renal failure. Such a value rules out the presence of coexistent iron deficiency.

ANEMIAS SECONDARY TO OTHER SYSTEMIC CONDITIONS. In addition to iron deficiency and the anemia of chronic disease, normocytic marrow failure anemias are frequently encountered in association with renal failure, hepatic disease, and a variety of endocrine disturbances. The anemia in such patients often resembles the anemia of chronic disease but is commonly of multifactorial etiology.

Renal Failure. A normocytic marrow failure anemia occurs in chronic renal insufficiency. Its severity is roughly (but not invariably) proportional to the degree of the renal failure. Erythrocyte survival is modestly decreased, although the absolute reticulocyte count is not elevated. Serum iron levels and TIBC are either low or normal, and the serum ferritin level is typically increased. Red cells with scalloped outlines ("burr" cells) (see Color Plate 6F, right) may be seen on blood smears. Failure of the kidney to elaborate erythropoietin in amounts appropriate to the degree of anemia appears to be a major (if not the principal) cause of the anemia. In most cases, the anemia responds completely to the regular parenteral administration of recombinant human erythropoietin, thereby obviating blood transfusions. Resistance to erythropoietin is also likely to contribute to the marrow failure state, although circulating inhibitors of erythropoiesis have not been clearly identified. In individual patients with renal failure, however, other mechanisms may contribute to anemia, such as iron deficiency. A serum ferritin level below 60 ng per milliliter in the presence of renal insufficiency strongly suggests lack of iron. Anemia in renal disease may also be caused by folate deficiency (much less frequently); aluminum toxicity, in which case the anemia is typically *microcytic;* partial fibrous replacement of the bone marrow in patients with severe hyperparathyroidism and osteitis fibrosa, which may be associated with leukopenia and thrombocytopenia; hypersplenism, which occasionally develops with chronic hemodialysis; and "microangiopathic hemolytic anemia" accompanied by fragmentation on blood smears and an elevated absolute reticulocyte count (with malignant hypertension, vasomotor nephropathy, acute glomerulonephritis, thrombotic thrombocytopenic purpura, and the hemolytic-uremic syndrome).

Liver Disease. Any chronic liver disease may cause an associated anemia of the type seen in other chronic diseases, but additional mechanisms are also often important. For example, anemia caused by acute blood loss may occur, and iron deficiency may eventually supervene owing to continuing hemorrhage. A variety of hemolytic states are also seen, including "spur cell" anemia, in which irregularly contracted red cells, or *acanthocytes*, are seen on blood smears in tandem with brisk hemolysis in advanced liver disease; autoimmune hemolytic anemia accompanying acute viral or chronic active hepatitis; acute hemolysis caused by profound hypophosphatemia in alcoholics; and, rarely, acute hemolytic states associated with alcoholic hepatitis. Chronic alcoholics (independent of the presence of liver disease) are highly prone to develop megaloblastic anemia due to folate deficiency, as well as sideroblastic anemia. Chronic infections, such as tuberculosis and lung abscesses, may cause an anemia of chronic disease. Therefore, in anemic patients with liver disease, careful evaluation of the patient, with particular attention to the MCV, reticulocyte count, and blood smear, is essential to determine the likely contributory factors. In alcoholics the anemia is *usually* multifactorial. The clinician should avoid the casual attribution of

PLATE 5   HEMATOLOGY

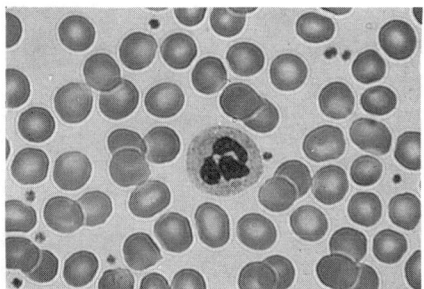

A, A normal peripheral blood smear. The red cells are normocytic with a good hemoglobin content. A normal segmented neutrophil is in the center of the field. A normal platelet is immediately adjacent. (L.O.)

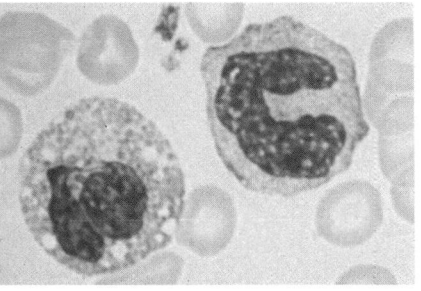

B, A normal eosinophil *(left)* and band *(right).* The eosinophil shows orange granules, vacuoles, and a segmented nucleus. The band has gray-pink cytoplasm and a reticular, horseshoe-shaped nucleus. (V.H.O.)

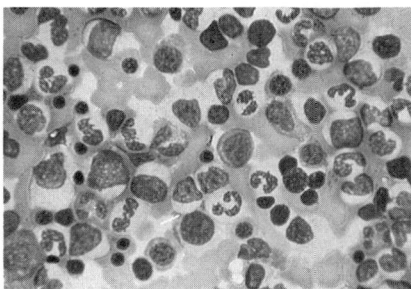

C, Normal bone marrow aspirate seen at low power. There is a 2:1 ratio between myeloid and erythroid precursors. The latter are identified by their shrunken, pyknotic ("coal black") nuclei. (L.P.)

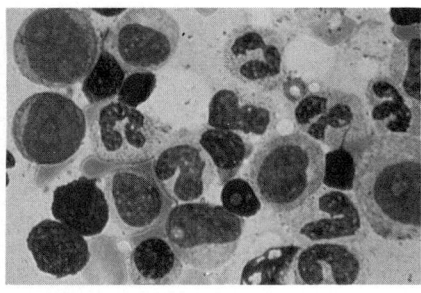

D, A bone marrow aspirate. Five erythroid precursors (with pyknotic nuclei) are present. The remaining cells are myeloid precursors in various stages of maturation, ranging from myeloblast to segmented neutrophil. (L.O.)

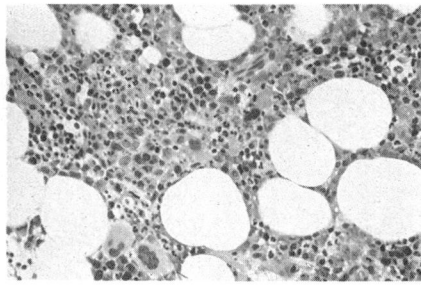

E, A hematoxylin and eosin (H & E)-stained normal bone marrow biopsy. Normal distribution and cellularity are seen. Several distinct megakaryocytes can be recognized because of their large size and multiple nuclear lobes. (L.P.)

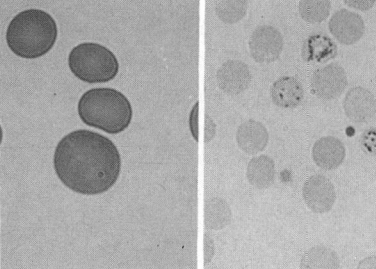

F, Left, The larger, gray-pink erythrocyte in the center of this field is called a polychromatophilic or "shift" cell. (H.O.) *Right,* Reticulocytes. The dark purple reticulin in red blood cells newly entering the blood is demonstrated by this new methylene blue stain. (L.O.)

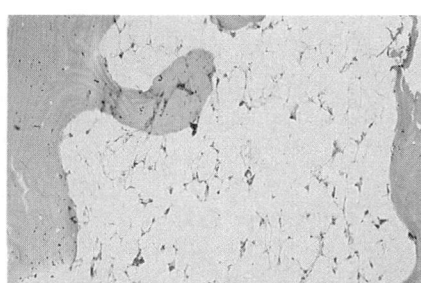

G, This low-power view of an H & E-stained bone marrow biopsy is from a patient with severe aplastic anemia. The virtually empty marrow can be appreciated by comparing with frame *E.* Even the marrow stroma is scanty. (L.P.)

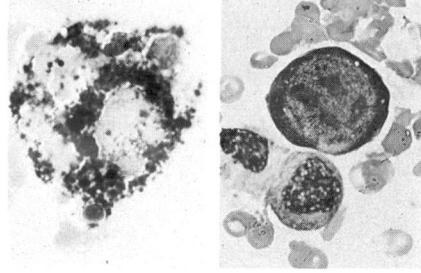

H, Left, Anemia of chronic disease; iron-stained bone marrow aspirate. Heavy dark blue globules of iron are seen in the storage cells. *Right,* Giant pronormoblast is from the bone marrow aspirate of a patient with red cell aplasia due to parvovirus infection. (H.O.)

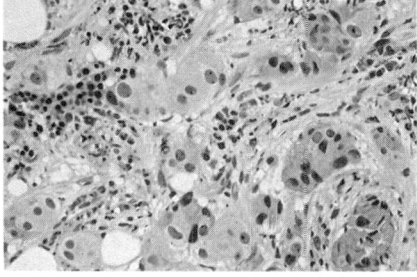

I, Metastatic breast carcinoma is seen in this view of an H & E-stained bone marrow biopsy. The malignancy has virtually replaced normal marrow elements. (L.P.)

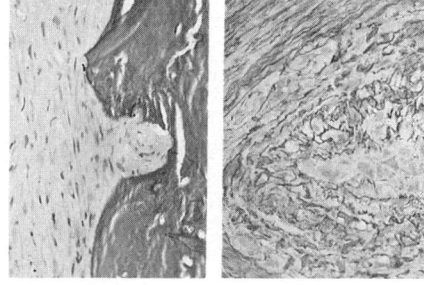

J, Agnogenic myeloid metaplasia with myelofibrosis. *Left,* This H & E-stained preparation shows virtual replacement of the marrow cavity with light pink-staining fibrous tissue. *Right,* A reticulin stain demonstrates the fibrosis as well. (L.P.)

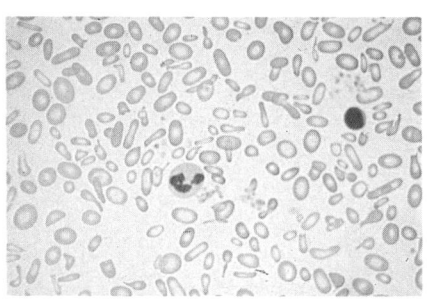

K, The peripheral blood in a patient with severe iron deficiency anemia. A normal lymphocyte is present (for comparison purposes) to the right of center. Marked anisocytosis and poikilocytosis can be appreciated, as can microcytosis and hypochromia. (L.P.)

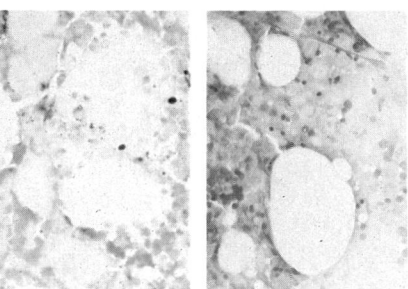

L, These are views of iron-stained bone marrow. *Left,* Normal iron stores are seen as dark blue-staining material. *Right,* The absence of iron is a characteristic finding in iron deficiency anemia. (L.P.)

PLATE 6   HEMATOLOGY

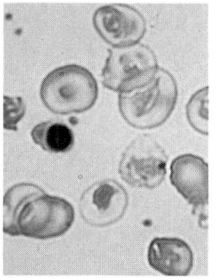 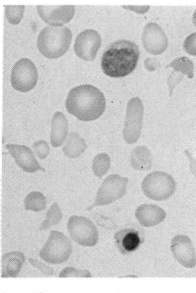

A, Left, Beta-thalassemia. Smear shows an orthochromic normoblast to the left. Also seen are targeting, hypochromia, and a Howell-Jolly body. (H.O.) *Right,* Alpha-thalassemia, E hemoglobinopathy. A normoblast and lymphocyte and anisocytosis are present. (L.O.)

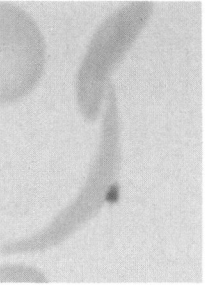 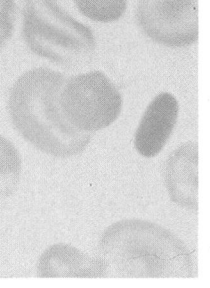

B, Left, Sickle cell disease. A classic sickle cell is seen in this field. *Right,* The cell to the right of center is a classic finding in hemoglobin C disease. It represents crystallized hemoglobin C. Also present are targeting and anisocytosis. (V.H.O.)

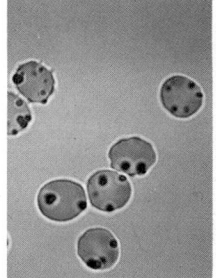 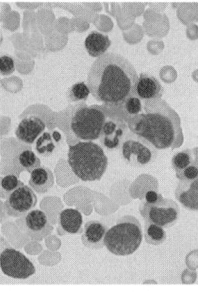

C, Hemolytic anemia. *Left,* Heinz body preparation showing dark-staining denatured globin intraerythrocytic particles. (H.O.) *Right,* The ratio of erythroid to myeloid cells in the bone marrow aspirate is less than 1, indicating increased erythroid activity. (L.O.)

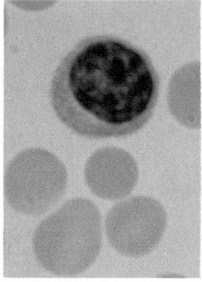 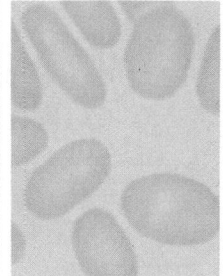

D, Left, This view of the peripheral blood in a patient with hereditary spherocytosis (HS) shows microspherocytes and a normal lymphocyte. *Right,* Hereditary elliptocytosis. Significant numbers of elliptocytes (oval erythrocytes) are seen in this field. (V.H.O.)

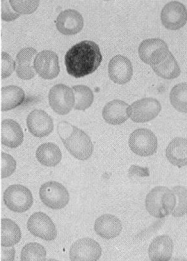 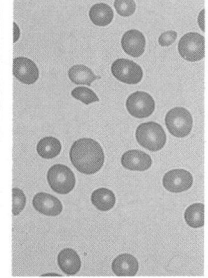

E, Left, G6PD deficiency. Central to the normal lymphocyte is a red cell with a blistered appearance secondary to portions of denatured hemoglobin being "bitten" off. *Right,* Microangiopathy. A shift cell and fragments are seen centrally. (L.O.)

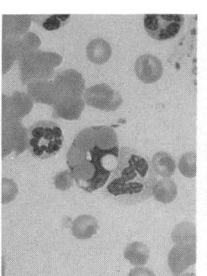 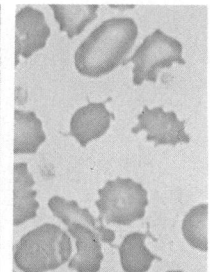

F, Hemolytic anemia. *Left,* Erythrophagocytosis. Four red blood cells (center) have been engulfed by a cell of the monocyte-macrophage line. *Right,* Marked red cell membrane abnormalities in severe hepatorenal failure, with burr cells and spur cells. (L.O., H.O.)

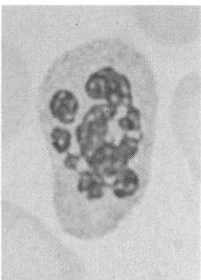 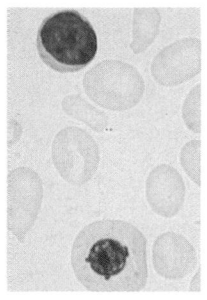

G, Pernicious anemia. *Left,* Marked neutrophil hypersegmentation. *Right,* Peripheral blood with large lymphocyte (top), macrocytosis, and orthochromic megaloblast (bottom). The latter has nuclear-cytoplasmic disproportion and beaded nuclear chromatin. (V.H.O.)

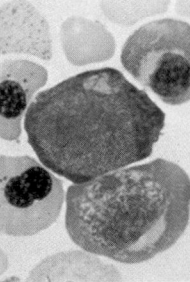

H, Pernicious anemia megaloblasts. Typical nuclear chromatin changes are seen in both frames. *Left,* Large central cell is a promegaloblast. *Right,* Large cell below is a basophilic megaloblast. Two cells above are polychromatophilic megaloblasts. (V.H.O.)

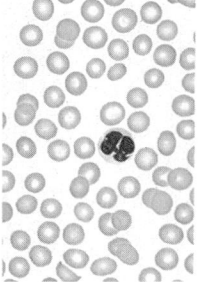 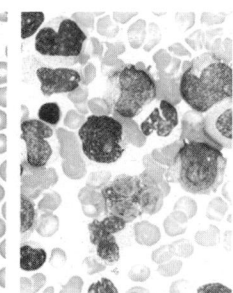

I, Myelodysplasia. *Left,* Therapy-related myelodysplasia. Dysmorphic red cells and a markedly abnormal granulocyte are seen. *Right,* Refractory anemia with excess blasts in transition (RAEBT). Several blasts and other dyspoietic changes are seen. (H.P.)

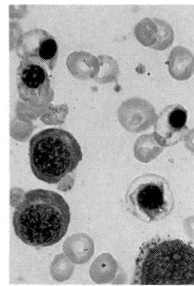 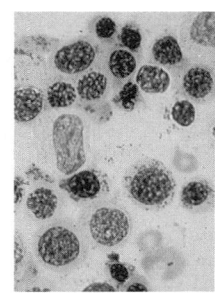

J, Myelodysplasia. *Left,* Marked erythroid dyspoiesis. Diagnosis was refractory anemia with ring sideroblasts (RARB). *Right,* An iron stain in the same patient showing perinuclear rings of iron-laden mitochondria. (L.O.)

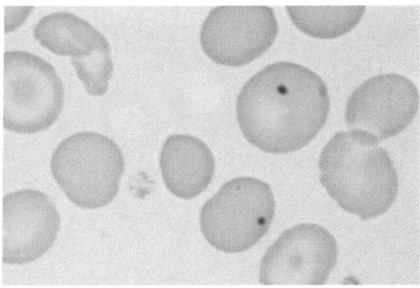

K, Postsplenectomy changes. This view of the peripheral blood shows three deeply basophilic granules peripherally in three different red cells—Howell-Jolly bodies. Targeting is also seen. (V.H.O.)

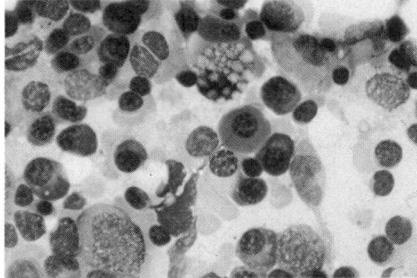

L, A bone marrow aspirate in a patient with Felty's syndrome. Maturation arrest is at the metamyelocyte stage. There is significant reactive plasmacytosis (30 per cent). A "Mott cell" with grapelike inclusions is seen top center. (L.O.)

PLATE 7 HEMATOLOGY

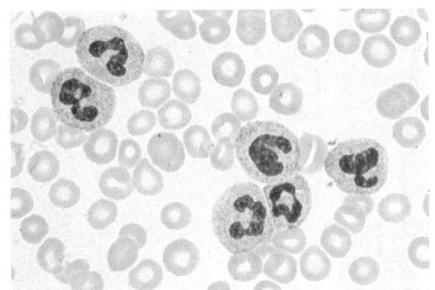

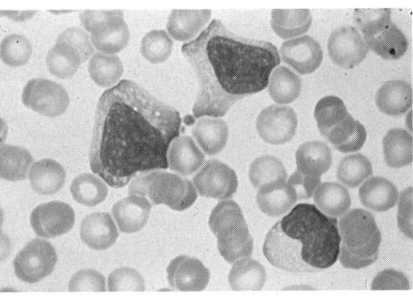

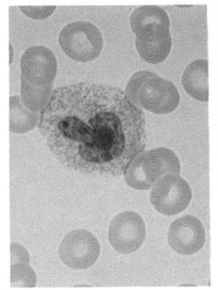 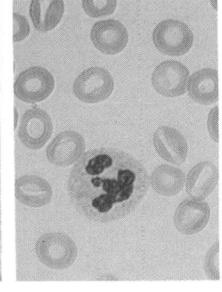

A, Neutrophilia. Four segmented and two band neutrophils are seen in this view of the peripheral blood. Some red blood cells are slightly hypochromic. (L.O.)

B, Infectious mononucleosis. Reactive (or atypical) lymphocytosis is seen in this peripheral blood smear. Pleomorphic reticular nuclei, peripheral basophilia of cytoplasm, and scalloped cell borders are characteristic. Slight rouleaux are also present. (H.O.)

C, Left, This band neutrophil shows basophilic or toxic granulation. *Right*, This segmented neutrophil shows some toxic granulation and a grayish Döhle body at 7 o'clock. Both are blood changes seen in bacterial infection. (H.O.)

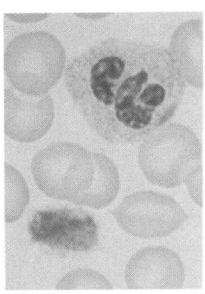 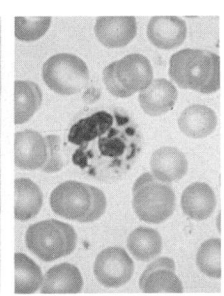

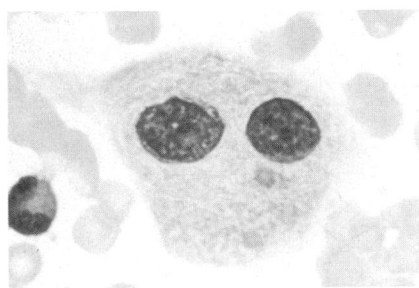

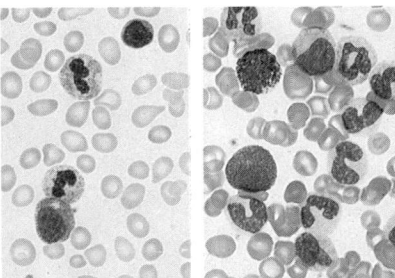

D, Left, May-Hegglin anomaly. The segmented neutrophil at the top of this field has a gray, spindle-shaped Döhle body at 4 o'clock. A giant platelet is seen at the bottom. (V.H.O.) *Right*, Chédiak-Higashi syndrome. Characteristic giant neutrophilic lysozymes are seen. (H.O.)

E, Gaucher's disease. This bone marrow aspirate shows a giant binucleate storage cell filled with glucocerebrosides. The fibrillar pattern is characteristic. (H.O.)

F, Left, Agnogenic myeloid metaplasia. This blood smear shows some teardrop-shaped red cells and a characteristic leukoerythroblastic reaction. *Right*, Chronic myelogenous leukemia (CML). Marked neutrophilia with left shift and two abnormal eosinophils are seen. (H.P.)

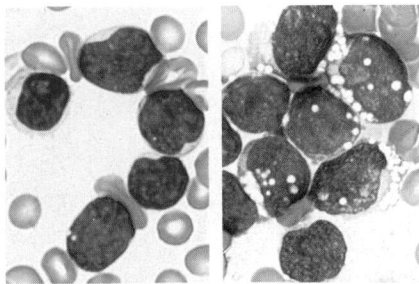

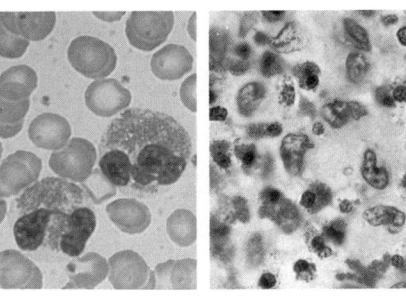

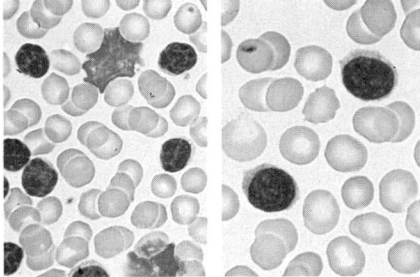

G, Left, Chronic myelogenous leukemia, blast crisis. The blasts have very immature nuclear chromatin. The patient was Ph-1 chromosome positive. *Right*, Ph-1 chromosome–positive acute lymphoblastic leukemia. These blasts are shown for comparison. (H.O.)

H, Left, Two eosinophils are shown from the peripheral blood of a patient with the hypereosinophilic syndrome. (H.O.) *Right*, Eosinophilic granuloma. In this lymph node, eosinophils and histiocytes are seen. (H.P.)

I, Left, Chronic B cell lymphocytic leukemia. The neoplastic lymphocytes are B cells. Two destroyed lymphocytes are in the center. (L.O.) *Right*, Chronic T cell lymphocytic leukemia. The neoplastic lymphocytes have been identified as T cells. (H.O.)

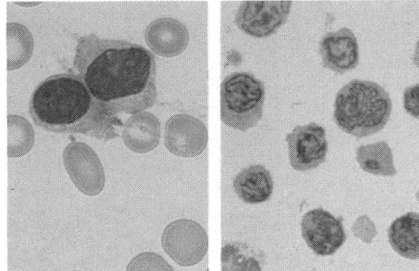

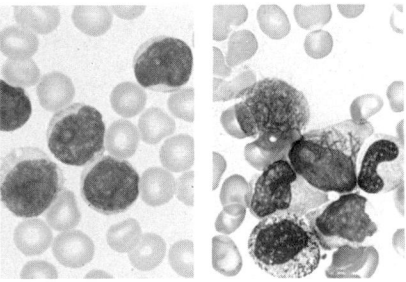

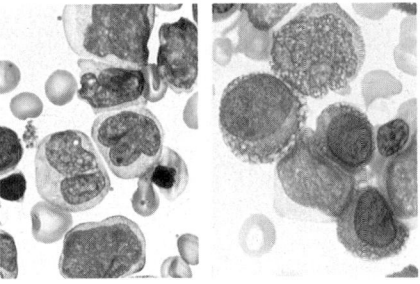

J, Left, Hairy cell leukemia (HCL). This frame shows two "hairy cells" with thin cytoplasmic projections and reticular nuclear chromatin. (H.O.) *Right*, Sézary's syndrome. This buffy coat preparation shows nuclear pleomorphism and convolutions.

K, Acute nonlymphoblastic leukemia (ANLL). *Left*, M-1 type. The blasts have round or slightly indented nuclei, fine nuclear chromatin, and very little cytoplasmic granulation. *Right*, M-3 type. Three leukemic promyelocytes with multiple Auer rods and cytoplasmic inclusions are seen. (H.O.)

L, ANLL (continued). *Left*, M-4 type. Blasts in the center of this field have both monocytic and myeloid features. *Right*, M-6 type. This field shows abnormalities seen in erythroleukemia. Most blasts have marked nuclear dyspoiesis. The central blast could be myeloid. (H.O.)

PLATE 8   HEMATOLOGY

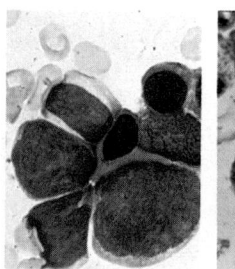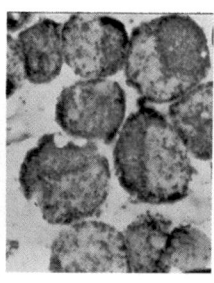

A, ANLL (continued). *Left,* M-7 type. This bone marrow aspirate shows characteristic large blasts. *Right,* The myeloperoxidase stain is often useful in identifying myeloid blasts. Dark granules are characteristic of a positive reaction. (H.O.)

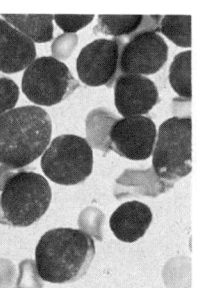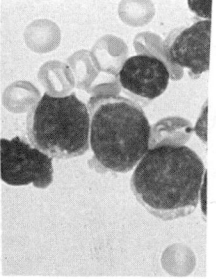

B, Acute lymphoblastic leukemia (ALL). *Left,* L-1 type. This bone marrow aspirate shows L-1 lymphoblasts that are moderately uniform in size. *Right,* L-2 type. In this bone marrow aspirate, the pleomorphism of the blasts is apparent. (H.O.)

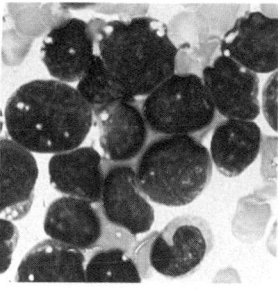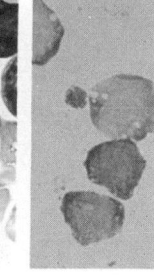

C, ALL (continued). *Left,* L-3 type. This bone marrow aspirate shows characteristic blasts. Cytoplasmic and nuclear vacuoles are seen. *Right,* Coarse, red-pink cytoplasmic granules characterize periodic acid–Schiff (PAS)–positive lymphoblasts.

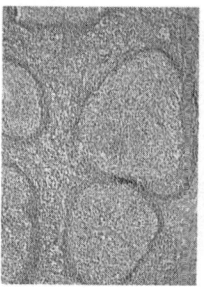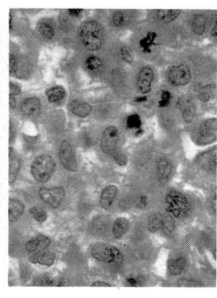

D, Left, Non-Hodgkin's lymphoma (follicular, small cleaved cell type). Lymph node. The follicular pattern is seen. (L.P.) *Right,* Non-Hodgkin's lymphoma (diffuse, T immunoblastic type). Lymph node, H & E stain. A diffuse pattern of large neoplastic cells is seen. (H.P.)

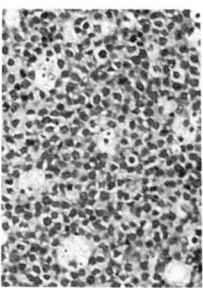

E, Left, Non-Hodgkin's lymphoma (B cell type) in a patient with AIDS. Lymph node biopsy, H & E stain. *Right,* Non-Hodgkin's lymphoma in a patient with AIDS. Brain involvement is present. (L.P.)

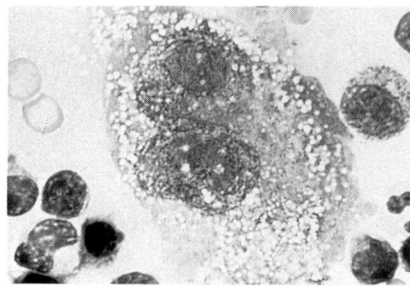

F, Hodgkin's disease. This bone marrow aspirate shows a classic Reed-Sternberg cell. The "mirror-image" nuclei are characteristic, as are the large nucleoli. It is unusual to find these cells in the bone marrow aspirate. (H.O.)

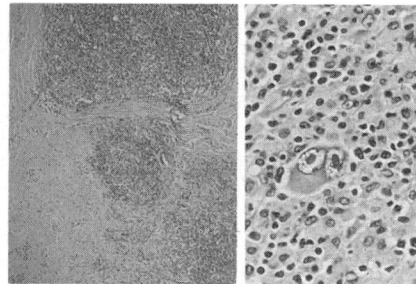

G, Left, Hodgkin's disease (nodular sclerosis type). Large fibrotic nodules enclose the cellular areas of Hodgkin's disease. (L.P.) *Right,* Hodgkin's disease (lymphocyte-depleted type). Lymph node biopsy. A Reed-Sternberg cell is near the center of the field. (H.P.)

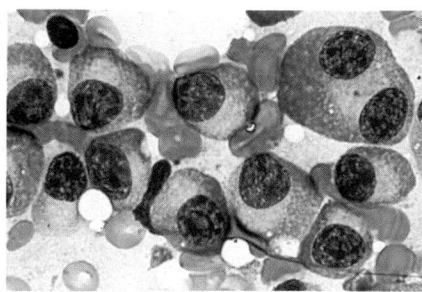

H, This bone marrow aspirate is from a patient with multiple myeloma. All plasma cells in this field are neoplastic myeloma cells. The nuclei are pleomorphic and eccentric, and the cytoplasm is gray-blue. One cell is binucleate. (H.O.)

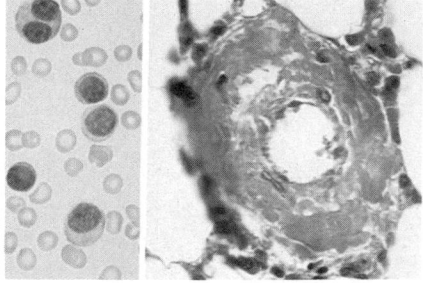

I, Left, Plasma cell leukemia. Five neoplastic plasma cells (one of which is binucleate) are seen in this field. (L.O.) *Right,* Amyloid. Bone marrow biopsy. A small blood vessel is heavily infiltrated with the pink-staining, waxy amyloid material. (H.P.)

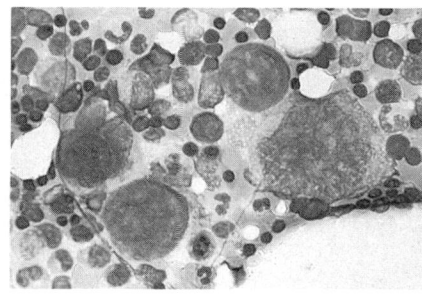

J, Immune thrombocytopenic purpura (ITP). Bone marrow aspirate. Megakaryocytosis is reflected in this field, where four are seen. These range from a megakaryoblast (top) to a mature megakaryocyte (middle right).

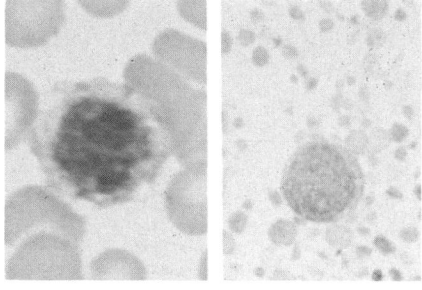

K, Left, Bernard-Soulier syndrome. A typical giant platelet is seen in the center of the field. *Right,* Essential thrombocythemia. Massive thrombocytosis is noted, as is variation in platelet size and a giant platelet. (H.O.)

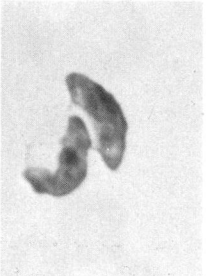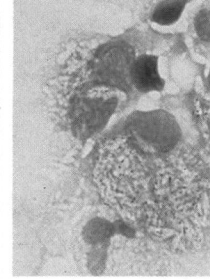

L, Left, Falciparum malaria. Peripheral blood showing two crescent-shaped gametocytes. *Right,* AIDS, *Mycobacterium avium-intracellulare* infection. Massive numbers of red, acid-fast organisms are seen in the macrophages of this marrow aspirate. (H.O.)

anemia in a patient with hepatic dysfunction to "the anemia of liver disease." The term should be abandoned in favor of more precise diagnostic thinking. In addition, in many patients with portal hypertension and an expanded plasma volume, the hematocrit may be moderately decreased, even though the number of circulating red cells is normal ("hemodilution").

Endocrine Disorders. A mild normocytic anemia occurs in some patients with endocrine disturbances. One quarter of patients with *hypothyroidism* are anemic. The red cell lifespan is normal, and there is no reticulocytosis. In many patients the anemia responds to hormone replacement therapy. Such anemias are usually normocytic, although in a minority the MCV may be mildly elevated and may return to normal after treatment with thyroid preparations. Another cause of macrocytic marrow failure anemia in hypothyroidism is pernicious anemia due to associated autoimmune gastritis. When microcytic anemia is seen, iron deficiency is the rule. Ferritin synthesis may be depressed as a result of insufficient thyroid hormone action, and the serum ferritin level may not be a reliable indicator of iron stores in hypothyroid patients.

A mild normocytic marrow failure anemia is a characteristic feature of *hypopituitarism* and may also occur in *primary adrenal insufficiency*, although it is often masked by a contracted plasma volume due to dehydration. A normocytic marrow failure anemia is also encountered in a few patients with *thyrotoxicosis*, although in some the MCV may be low. In either event, the anemia remits after suppression of thyroid hyperactivity. An occasional patient with *hyperparathyroidism* has a mild normocytic anemia due to marrow failure.

"PRIMARY MARROW DISORDERS." When iron deficiency and anemia related to systemic diseases have been excluded, there remains a minority of normocytic marrow failure anemias that are caused by primary disturbances of the bone marrow (see Table 128–7). These include rare disorders in which developing red cells are absent or markedly diminished in the bone marrow (aplastic anemia, pure red cell aplasia) or in which there are increased marrow erythroid precursors that fail to mature normally, so-called "ineffective erythropoiesis" (sideroblastic anemias, other myelodysplasias); replacement of the bone marrow by fibrosis or a variety of hematologic and solid tumors or granulomas; and a poorly understood marrow failure state that may be associated with AIDS. In many patients with AIDS, the anemia is typical of that seen with other chronic infections; in others, ineffective erythropoiesis (often associated with neutropenia) is present, possibly related to human immunodeficiency virus (HIV) infection of marrow stem cells. In most patients with these marrow disturbances, certain features of the initial laboratory data base strongly suggest that the patient has something other than iron deficiency, the anemia of chronic disease, or anemia secondary to renal, hepatic, or endocrine dysfunction. These clues include depression of the platelet count, white blood cell count, or both; abnormalities in the white cell differential; significant numbers of nucleated erythrocytes on the blood smear; marked abnormalities in red cell morphology, especially significant poikilocytosis; and a normal or increased serum iron level with a per cent saturation of transferrin that is above normal. In the normocytic anemias due to primary disturbances of marrow function, *bone marrow aspiration and biopsy* (see Color Plates 5 to 8) often provide highly useful diagnostic information, whereas in the previously discussed causes of normocytic anemia, marrow examination is rarely useful (except for the estimation of iron stores when the serum indicators of iron status give equivocal results). These primary marrow disorders may, on occasion, also present as a *macrocytic* marrow failure anemia.

Microcytic Anemias Due to Marrow Failure

In contrast to the potentially complex considerations in normocytic anemias, the differential diagnosis of marrow failure associated with a low MCV is relatively straightforward (Table 128–9). Two major conditions commonly cause marrow failure with microcytic anemia—iron deficiency and the anemia of chronic disease. Although most patients with the anemia of chronic disease have a normal MCV, in approximately 30 per cent, mean red cell size is slightly decreased, with the MCV in the range of 70 to 80 fl. An MCV lower than 70 fl is almost always due to iron deficiency or thalassemia. With severe iron

TABLE 128–9. CAUSES OF MICROCYTIC MARROW FAILURE ANEMIAS

Common	Rare
Iron deficiency	Aluminum toxicity
Anemia of chronic disease	Thyrotoxicosis
Thalassemias	Hereditary sideroblastic anemias

deficiency, the MCV may fall as low as 50 fl, and marked anisocytosis and poikilocytosis may be seen. The results of the serum tests of iron status are similar to those seen when iron deficiency and the anemia of chronic disease manifest with a normal MCV (Table 128–8).

THALASSEMIAS (Ch. 136). In these disorders, decreased synthesis of either the alpha or the beta chain of hemoglobin occurs, with the resultant imbalance in globin chain formation leading to a decreased rate of hemoglobin production as well as microcytosis. In *homozygous beta-thalassemia*, which manifests in childhood, a severe microcytic anemia results owing to a combination of ineffective erythropoiesis and a shortened red cell lifespan. Reticulocytosis is modest, although grossly inadequate. In *heterozygous beta-thalassemia*, anemia is frequently absent, or only mild in degree, although the MCV is low. In some patients the blood smear may show target cells, basophilic stippling, anisocytosis, and poikilocytosis; in others the smear is unremarkable because there is a uniform population of small red cells with little anisocytosis. The reticulocyte count is normal or minimally elevated, and the serum ferritin, iron, and TIBC values are normal. The disorder is usually detected when a CBC, including an MCV, is obtained during the evaluation of some other medical problem. *Alpha-thalassemia* is more varied because there are four genes for alpha globin chain synthesis. When three alpha chain genes are deleted or abnormal, a moderate hemolytic anemia develops, with microcytosis and the formation of "β_4" tetramers (hemoglobin H disease). This anemia sometimes occurs as an acquired disorder in association with acute leukemia or myelodysplastic states. Much more commonly, *heterozygous alpha-thalassemia* with two-chain deletion is encountered, particularly in American blacks, 3 per cent of whom are affected. Typically, these patients have a low MCV, have a normal blood smear and iron studies, and are not anemic, although in some the hematocrit may be slightly decreased. A common error in attempting to diagnose heterozygous thalassemic states is to obtain a routine hemoglobin electrophoresis, which is normal. Instead, the conditions can be differentiated by specific measurement of the hemoglobin A_2 concentration, which is usually elevated in patients with beta-thalassemia but is normal or reduced in those with alpha-thalassemia. There is no readily available test for alpha-thalassemia. It should be suspected in blacks and patients from Southeast Asia with microcytosis. Family members also often have microcytosis without anemia. Even though, as a rule, anisocytosis is more striking in iron deficiency than in the heterozygous thalassemias, there are so many exceptions that measurement of the RDW is not a useful screening test.

RARE CAUSES OF MARROW FAILURE WITH MICRO-CYTIC ANEMIAS. *Aluminum toxicity* in patients with renal failure who receive aluminum-containing phosphate binders can result in a microcytic marrow failure anemia by an unknown mechanism. Aluminum overload may cause resistance to erythropoietin therapy in chronically hemodialyzed patients (even those with a normal MCV). *Thyrotoxicosis* may occasionally result in a mild microcytic anemia. Although in most sideroblastic anemias (which are almost always acquired in nature) the MCV is normal or elevated, mean red cell size is decreased in the much rarer *hereditary sideroblastic anemias*, which may present in childhood or adult life.

Macrocytic Anemias Due to Marrow Failure

Macrocytic anemias due to bone marrow failure (Table 128–10) are common. The history, physical examination, and blood smear are the cornerstones of the initial approach to a patient with an elevated MCV and in most cases indicate its cause. Major clues include the recent use of alcohol, exposure to chemother-

TABLE 128–10. CAUSES OF MACROCYTIC MARROW FAILURE ANEMIAS

Megaloblastic anemias
    Cobalamin and folate deficiencies
    Congenital disorders
Alcoholism
Drugs (see Table 128–2)
Liver disease
"Primary" marrow disorders (see Table 128–7)
Hypothyroidism
Splenectomy
Artifactual MCV elevations

apeutic or immunosuppressive drugs, and evidence of liver disease, glossitis, or neurologic signs and symptoms. In most macrocytic anemias, the blood smear contains round macrocytes without multilobed granulocytes. On the other hand, *the combination of macro-ovalocytes and hypersegmented neutrophils strongly suggests the presence of cobalamin or folate deficiency* (although rarely this dual abnormality may be seen after chemotherapy with methotrexate or cytosine arabinoside, in myelodysplasias, or in acute myelocytic leukemia) (see Color Plate 6G and H). The reticulocyte count is also a useful early test in patients with macrocytosis. Because of the slightly increased size of young erythrocytes, brisk *reticulocytosis* (an uncorrected count of ≥10 per cent) caused by hemolysis or blood loss often causes a modest elevation of the MCV.

MEGALOBLASTIC ANEMIAS (Ch. 132). Megaloblastic anemias due to a disturbance in DNA synthesis caused by cobalamin or folate deficiency account for only 5 to 10 per cent of macrocytic anemias with marrow failure. Early recognition is extremely important, however, because of their responsiveness to therapy and the need to prevent irreversible neurologic damage caused by lack of cobalamin. As with most other causes of macrocytic anemia, the MCV becomes elevated early in the development of cobalamin or folate deficiency, before a lowered hematocrit is evident. A distinction should be made between the hematologic and biochemical profiles of patients with *early* cobalamin or folate deficiency (with little or no anemia) and the classic textbook manifestations of severe megaloblastic anemia. With severe anemia, marked anisocytosis and poikilocytosis (often including teardrop erythrocytes, microcytes, and red cell fragments) are found on blood smears. The consequences of ineffective erythropoiesis (destruction of red cell precursors in the bone marrow) may simulate a hemolytic anemia, with decreased or absent plasma haptoglobin values, elevated serum unconjugated bilirubin levels, sometimes exceptionally high serum lactate dehydrogenase (LDH) levels, and an elevated serum iron level with an increased transferrin saturation. In such severely deficient patients, marrow failure often causes thrombocytopenia and (sometimes) neutropenia. In any moderately or severely anemic patient with pancytopenia, cobalamin and folate deficiency should always be considered. In contrast, patients with deficiency of cobalamin or folate who have little or no anemia often have minimal changes on the blood smear, with few macro-ovalocytes and only rare hypersegmented neutrophils that may not be identified by routine hospital laboratories. In addition, there may be normal values for serum LDH, bilirubin, haptoglobin, white cell count, and platelet count. In cobalamin deficiency, severe involvement of the tongue or nervous system may occur early or late relative to the hematologic manifestations, so that a patient with advanced neurologic impairment may not have developed anemia or even a clear-cut elevation of the MCV.

Radioisotopic assays of serum cobalamin and folate levels are valuable in the diagnosis (Ch. 132). A serum cobalamin level should be measured in any patient with neutrophil hypersegmentation, macro-ovalocytes, atrophic glossitis, or a neurologic disorder compatible with cobalamin deficiency, as well as in virtually all patients with an elevated MCV in the absence of reticulocytosis. Possible exceptions to this rule are those treated with drugs that interfere with DNA synthesis (e.g., zidovudine, azathioprine, methotrexate) in whom the MCV has been clearly documented to be normal immediately prior to beginning drug therapy. There are problems with both the specificity and the sensitivity of the vitamin assays. The serum cobalamin level is often low in patients who are not deficient in the vitamin, and it may also be depressed as a result of folate deficiency. At least 5 per cent of patients with unequivocal clinical evidence of cobalamin deficiency have normal serum cobalamin concentrations (usually in the range of 200 to 350 pg per milliliter). The measurement of *methylmalonic acid* and *total homocysteine* in serum is very useful in the interpretation of low or low-normal serum cobalamin values when the presence of deficiency of the vitamin is not clinically obvious (Ch. 132). There are similar problems with the *serum folate* level. The *red cell folate* concentration is a better indicator of tissue folate stores; however, it is diminished in 50 per cent of patients with primary cobalamin deficiency and may be normal in some patients deficient in folate. Serum total homocysteine levels are almost always elevated in clinically significant folate depletion (as well as in cobalamin deficiency); however, the serum methylmalonic acid value remains normal in deficiency of folate. With the combined use of a careful history and physical examination, as well as examination of the blood smear, serum vitamin levels, and (if needed) serum metabolites, it is rarely necessary to perform a bone marrow examination to show the presence of a megaloblastic anemia. The determination of *antibodies to intrinsic factor* in serum is a useful early test in patients with cobalamin deficiency, since it is positive in approximately half of those with pernicious anemia (the most common cause of lack of cobalamin) and is specific for that diagnosis, eliminating the need for a Schilling test when such antibodies are present.

Iron deficiency frequently coexists with lack of cobalamin (e.g., in patients with pernicious anemia) or folate (e.g., in pregnant patients or alcoholics). In such combined deficiency states, the MCV may be low, normal, or high, and macro-ovalocytes and hypersegmented neutrophils on blood smear may be the most important clues to the presence of a "masked" megaloblastic anemia when the MCV is low or normal.

MACROCYTOSIS OF ALCOHOLISM. The most common cause of an elevated MCV in chronic alcoholic patients is not folate deficiency, but the *macrocytosis of alcoholism*. This condition appears to be an effect of chronic alcohol intoxication that is not related to the presence of liver disease, reticulocytosis, or vitamin deficiency (which are all part of the differential diagnosis of an elevated MCV in an alcoholic). The macrocytosis of alcoholism does not respond to vitamin B_{12} or folic acid and will disappear only after months of abstinence. The degree of MCV elevation is modest (usually ≤110 fl), and anemia is often absent. Round macrocytes are seen on blood smears. In many anemic patients with the macrocytosis of alcoholism, the anemia is due to some other cause (e.g., lung abscess, hepatic inflammation, or even iron deficiency), and the patient only apparently has a macrocytic anemia.

DRUG-INDUCED MACROCYTOSIS. In current clinical practice, this is the most common cause of an elevated MCV in nonalcoholic patients. Frequent offending agents are listed in Table 128–2. Most of the drugs that cause macrocytosis interfere with DNA synthesis by erythroid precursors. These agents most commonly cause macrocytosis without anemia; a low hematocrit is typically seen only after prolonged high dosage. The reticulocyte count is characteristically not increased, although slight elevations are not uncommon with sulfasalazine and azathioprine.

LIVER DISEASE. In patients with hepatic dysfunction, because of a poorly understood abnormality in serum lipoproteins, increased amounts of cholesterol and phospholipids are deposited on the membranes of circulating erythrocytes, causing an increase in surface area, which results in macrocytosis. Blood smears typically show round macrocytes and target cells. This is a benign abnormality that does not affect the red cell lifespan and is unrelated to any of the causes of anemia seen in liver disease.

PRIMARY MARROW DISTURBANCES. All of the derangements involving the bone marrow that are occasional causes of normocytic anemias resulting from decreased cell production (see Table 128–7) may also cause a macrocytic marrow failure anemia. The mechanisms underlying the macrocytosis in such diverse disorders as marrow aplasia, sideroblastic anemia, myelodysplasias, acute myeloblastic leukemia, and infiltration of the marrow by myeloma, lymphoma, or solid tumors have not been established. Macro-ovalocytes may be present in these conditions, but neutrophil hypersegmentation is extremely unusual. Aspiration and biopsy of the marrow are often crucial to establishing the cause of macrocytosis in this group of patients. Cytogenetic studies on material obtained by marrow aspiration may also be useful.

ANEMIAS ASSOCIATED WITH INCREASED RED CELL PRODUCTION

Assuming that recovery from marrow failure (e.g., pernicious anemia recently treated with an injection of vitamin B_{12}) has been excluded, the patient with an absolute reticulocytosis usually has underlying blood loss or hemolysis. In these conditions, the MCV is normal or increased, although very rarely in hemolytic anemias it may be low. Owing to the presence of reticulocytes, modest increments in red cell volume (usually MCV's in the range of 100 to 110 fl) are common in patients with increased cell production. Rarely, an even higher MCV is caused by artifactual clumping of red cells by a cold agglutinin. Elevations in the MCV are more common in hemolytic anemias than in acute blood loss. The diagnostic approach to the patient with an elevated reticulocyte count differs from that in patients with marrow failure. The very first consideration is to rule out obvious or occult blood loss. In the absence of bleeding, evidence of an underlying hemolytic disorder must be sought utilizing a different set of diagnostic tests than are used in the patient with marrow failure. Even in the absence of reticulocytosis, a rapidly developing anemia cannot be due primarily to marrow failure, because of the long lifespan of the red cell. When the marrow fails, anemia develops gradually over many weeks. Thus, if a marked fall in hematocrit (e.g., 10 per cent over a period of a few days) is noted, a search for blood loss or hemolysis should be initiated, regardless of the reticulocyte count.

HEMOLYTIC ANEMIAS (Ch. 133)

Anemias primarily due to red cell destruction are much less common than those caused by marrow failure or blood loss. Nonetheless, after blood loss has been excluded, the possibility of a hemolytic anemia takes center stage in the patient with an absolute reticulocytosis. At this point, a very long list of laboratory tests might be ordered. Therefore, the clinician needs to make a fundamental distinction. One group of tests (Table 128–11) attempts to answer the question, *is hemolysis present?* An entirely separate set of laboratory determinations, to be obtained only subsequently, addresses the question, *what is the cause of hemolysis?* Examples of the latter type would include the Coombs test or a hemoglobin electrophoresis. Such studies are often inappropriately ordered in the assessment of marrow failure or blood loss anemias. It is much more rational to obtain evidence first that the patient is actually hemolyzing before undertaking a search for various disorders that are known to cause hemolysis.

IS HEMOLYSIS PRESENT? Unfortunately, no one measure has been shown to be 100 per cent sensitive in detecting clinically significant hemolysis. Therefore, to answer the first question, a number of tests should be obtained (Table 128–11). Hemoglobin liberated into the circulation after red cells are damaged forms a complex with circulating haptoglobin, which is rapidly removed by hepatocytes. If the capacity of the liver to compensate by synthesizing new haptoglobin is exceeded, the plasma concentration will fall. Once the plasma haptoglobin reaches zero, free hemoglobin circulates and is filtered by the kidney. Modest amounts of filtered hemoglobin are taken up by renal tubular cells, which convert the iron in hemoglobin to a storage form, hemosiderin. This can be detected days later by histochemical staining of renal tubular cells that have been shed in the urine. If the amount of hemoglobin filtered exceeds the renal tubular uptake capacity, hemoglobin itself will appear in the urine. This hemoglobin may be detected by specific laboratory assays or may

TABLE 128–11. COMMONLY USED TESTS INDICATING THE PRESENCE OF HEMOLYSIS

Test	Result
Plasma haptoglobin	Decreased
Urine hemosiderin	Present
Urine hemoglobin	Present
Serum unconjugated bilirubin	Increased
Serum lactate dehydrogenase	Increased

be suspected when a routine urinalysis is positive for occult blood in the absence of hematuria. If the amount of hemoglobin excreted is great, the patient will pass urine that is red, reddish-purple, or even black. In contrast, when red cells are engulfed by macrophages and digested intracellularly, the heme moiety of hemoglobin is processed to unconjugated bilirubin, which is transferred to the circulation (Ch. 115). Lactate dehydrogenase is also released from hemolyzed cells. A distinction is sometimes made between *intravascular* and *extravascular* hemolytic states, but this is only occasionally useful. Acute intravascular hemolysis certainly occurs with a severe hemolytic transfusion reaction after ABO-incompatible blood is given. The plasma haptoglobin, however, is often decreased in states such as hereditary spherocytosis, in which red cell destruction is believed to occur primarily in splenic macrophages. Probably most hemolytic anemias reflect a combination of intravascular and extravascular events. The presence of hemoglobin or hemosiderin in the urine may reflect the *rate* of hemolysis as much as its location.

Any of the tests listed in Table 128–11 may be normal in patients with a clear-cut hemolytic anemia. The ability of the liver to clear a load of unconjugated bilirubin is greater in some individuals than in others. The plasma haptoglobin level is often normal in acutely hemolyzing patients who have an associated illness, since it is an acute phase reactant and hepatic synthesis may be markedly stimulated. Many of the tests are also not specific for hemolysis. The LDH may be released from many different injured organs; unconjugated bilirubin elevations are commonly due to Gilbert's disease; the plasma haptoglobin may be reduced on a genetic basis or due to liver dysfunction; myoglobin may cause a positive urine test for occult blood. It is possible to demonstrate that the red cell lifespan is shortened by performing a cumbersome and time-consuming study with radioisotopically labeled erythrocytes, but this is rarely necessary. In almost all patients with a hemolytic anemia, one or more of the tests listed in Table 128–11 are positive.

WHAT IS THE CAUSE OF HEMOLYSIS? Once there is a positive answer to one or more of the tests that determine whether hemolysis is present, the clinician must then ask, what is the cause of hemolysis? The list of possible causes of hemolytic states is formidably long. Many of these disorders are discussed in Ch. 134 to 136. For example, deficiencies of 14 different red cell enzymes may lead to a congenital hemolytic anemia. Table 128–12 lists some hemolytic conditions that are likely to be encountered over the course of a year in an adult medical service. It is representative but not necessarily exhaustive. With so many possible causes of hemolytic anemia, the clinician must be judicious in the choice of laboratory tests to answer this second question. Diagnostic strategy must be based on clues provided by the history, physical examination, and blood smear. For example, a young black man with a history of episodes of bone

TABLE 128–12. SOME RELATIVELY COMMON CAUSES OF HEMOLYTIC ANEMIA

Mechanism	Examples
Congenital	
Enzyme deficiency	Glucose-6-phosphate dehydrogenase, pyruvate kinase
Membrane skeletal protein abnormalities (e.g., spectrin)	Hereditary spherocytosis, hereditary elliptocytosis
Hemoglobinopathies	Hemoglobin SS, SC, CC, S-thalassemia
Acquired	
Antibody-induced	Autoimmune hemolysis (warm antibodies), cold agglutinin disease, hemolytic transfusion reaction
Mechanical fragmentation	Intravascular coagulation, malignant hypertension, cancer chemotherapy, malfunctioning valve prosthesis, thrombotic thrombocytopenic purpura
Membrane protein anchoring abnormality	Paroxysmal nocturnal hemoglobinuria

pain and sickle cells on the smear needs a hemoglobin electrophoresis, not a Coombs test or sucrose hemolysis determination. A previously healthy middle-aged woman who suddenly develops a severe anemia with many microspherocytes on the smear should have a Coombs test, not a hemoglobin electrophoresis, as part of the initial evaluation. In a man with malignant hypertension, evidence of hemolysis, and many red cell fragments on the blood smear, no further diagnostic studies may be required to conclude that a microangiopathic hemolytic anemia has developed secondary to damage to small blood vessels. Therefore, rather than following a rigid algorithm, the physician is guided by the clinical context and the blood smear in ordering laboratory tests for the individual patient. Morphologic abnormalities (see Table 128–4) often provide highly useful clues, although in some hemolytic anemias (e.g., glucose-6-phosphate dehydrogenase [G6PD] deficiency, paroxysmal nocturnal hemoglobinuria), the blood smear may be unremarkable or nondiagnostic. In some cases, clinical judgment may supersede the laboratory results. About 10 per cent of patients with autoimmune hemolytic anemias have a negative Coombs test but this diagnosis may still be considered on the basis of clinical and morphologic findings.

Hemolytic anemias may appear in deceptive disguises. Hereditary spherocytosis, a common congenital disorder that can be caused by a variety of abnormalities of the major red cell skeletal protein, spectrin, is frequently so mild that there is little or no anemia (Ch. 134). Only an elevated reticulocyte count, microspherocytes on smear, and minimal splenomegaly may bear witness to a state of *compensated hemolysis*. Such a patient may present as an adult with bilirubin gallstones or may develop anemia for the first time when a parvovirus B19 infection of committed red cell marrow precursors (CFU-E) causes an *aplastic crisis* with a sudden loss of the compensatory reticulocytosis. This virus is the most common cause of aplastic crisis, which may occur in a number of hemolytic anemias, including sickle cell disease. Continuing hemolysis that is no longer accompanied by reticulocytosis may rapidly lead to a life-threatening worsening of the anemia and require immediate transfusion. In the most common type of G6PD deficiency, the A-variant seen in 11 per cent of American blacks, there is no chronic hemolytic state. Anemia and hemolysis occur only acutely, after exposure to an oxidant stress, such as infection, acidosis, or certain drugs, e.g., antimalarials or sulfonamides.

ANEMIA DUE TO ACUTE BLOOD LOSS

The causes and management of blood loss are discussed in other chapters. A few points are worth noting here. In the bleeding patient, a reticulocytosis will be sustained until iron stores are depleted by continued chronic blood loss. In acute blood loss, however, a high reticulocyte count may not occur until a few days after the onset of bleeding. In most patients, the source of hemorrhage is clinically obvious, e.g., the gastrointestinal or genitourinary tract. The clinician must be alert to more occult sites of potentially massive blood loss, e.g., into a fractured hip or the retroperitoneal area, especially in patients with coagulation disorders or those receiving anticoagulants. Even though hemorrhage may be documented, it is worthwhile to obtain the entire initial laboratory base. The blood smear may reveal unexpected findings. It is not unusual in a bleeding alcoholic to find evidence of other coexistent causes of anemia (e.g., macroovalocytes and hypersegmented neutrophils). In the hemorrhaging patient with AIDS, absence of reticulocytosis may point to a coexistent marrow failure anemia.

Since red cells are lost from the body in most bleeding patients, the tests used to determine whether hemolysis is present are usually negative. With hemorrhage into an internal space, however, (as with a hemothorax, hemoperitoneum, or hip fracture), the decomposed blood in the body cavity is handled in similar ways to red cells that are hemolyzed. The plasma haptoglobin may be absent and the LDH and unconjugated bilirubin elevated in patients bleeding internally. Combined with the increased reticulocyte count, these findings may lead the unwary clinician to misdiagnose a hemolytic anemia.

EXAMINATION OF THE BONE MARROW IN ANEMIC PATIENTS

In more than 90 per cent of patients with anemia, it is unnecessary to obtain a bone marrow aspiration or biopsy if the approach advocated here is followed. In certain situations, however, the test is quite useful, such as in marrow failure anemias for definitive estimation of marrow iron stores when serum tests of iron status are equivocal. In all of the primary marrow disorders that cause normocytic and macrocytic marrow failure states (see Table 128–7), marrow aspiration and biopsy are often diagnostic. In a pancytopenia of unknown cause, it is wise to obtain an early marrow examination. If aplasia, marrow infiltration by tumor, myelofibrosis, or granulomatous infection is suspected, a greater diagnostic yield is obtained by biopsy than by aspiration (see Color Plate 5). A marrow aspirate may resolve diagnostic conundrums in patients suspected of having combined or dimorphic anemias (e.g., simultaneous iron and cobalamin deficiency, megaloblastic anemia accompanying the anemia of chronic disease). Marrow aspiration and biopsy are also indicated in monoclonal gammopathies and in any patient with a severe or unexplained anemia.

BLOOD TRANSFUSION

In contrast to patients with acute hemorrhage, those with chronic anemia often have few symptoms, particularly while at rest in the hospital, and the physician should always think twice before exposing them to the many risks of blood transfusion, some of them potentially fatal, which are discussed in Ch. 137. There is no threshold level of hematocrit that mandates transfusion, and the decision to administer red blood cells must be based on the functional status and symptomatology of the patient. Transfusion should never be used as a substitute for careful diagnostic evaluation that may lead to more definitive and less dangerous therapy. However, it may be necessary to transfuse elderly anemic patients before they undergo rigorous procedures, such as colonoscopy or barium enema.

ABNORMAL MEAN CELL VOLUMES IN THE ABSENCE OF ANEMIA

With the widespread availability of electronic cell counting, patients are frequently seen with increased or decreased MCV's in the absence of anemia. Not uncommonly, the MCV elevation is ignored because the hematocrit is normal—a potentially dangerous practice, especially in patients with macrocytosis. In some instances, a minimal increase or decrease in the MCV may be compatible with no underlying disorder, since the normal range excludes 2.5 per cent of healthy individuals at either extreme. However, an *elevated MCV* in the absence of anemia is most commonly a sign of chronic alcoholism (often in patients who deny it). Cobalamin or folate deficiency is another frequent cause of such an MCV increment; correct diagnosis may prevent subsequent hospitalization for anemia, or may avert serious nervous system damage (in the case of lack of cobalamin). Therefore, it is worth obtaining a serum cobalamin level in any patient with an unexplained increase in the MCV. Another common cause of nonanemic macrocytosis is the administration of drugs (Table 128–2). An MCV elevation may precede the development of anemia in a patient with a myelodysplasia (e.g., a sideroblastic anemia or refractory anemia following antimetabolite therapy) or marrow aplasia (e.g., a congenital Fanconi anemia manifesting in a young adult) (see Color Plate 6I and J). Occasionally, a modest rise in the MCV without anemia is caused by reticulocytosis in a compensated hemolytic state.

A *decreased MCV* associated with a normal hematocrit is almost always caused by heterozygous alpha- or beta-thalassemia. In some patients with polycythemia vera or polycythemia secondary to chronic hypoxia, iron stores may be outstripped by the expanding erythroid marrow. The previously elevated hematocrit then falls to the normal range as the MCV decreases. Studies of iron status are typically diagnostic of iron deficiency in these patients, and iron administration causes a return of the hematocrit to polycythemic levels. Blood loss should be ruled out, however, before the iron depletion is merely attributed to increased internal demands. Occasionally, a patient with microcytosis and a normal hematocrit is recovering from a self-limited or treated episode of iron deficiency anemia.

Cook JK: Clinical evaluation of iron deficiency. Semin Hematol 19:6, 1982. *A clinically sophisticated review of the use of laboratory tests in the diagnosis of iron deficiency and related conditions.*

Erslev AJ, Schuster SJ, Caro J: Erythropoietin and its clinical promise. Eur J Hematol 43:367, 1989. *An excellent review of the physiology of erythropoietin and the therapeutic use of the recombinant hormone.*

Liesveld JL, Rowe JM, Lichtman MA: Variability of the erythropoietic response in autoimmune hemolytic anemia: Analysis of 109 cases. Blood 3:820, 1987. *An interesting series of antibody-induced anemias with a focus on the lag in the response of the erythroid marrow to hemolytic stress.*

Lindenbaum J: Hematologic complications of alcohol abuse. Semin Liver Dis 7:169, 1987. *A comprehensive review of the pathophysiology and clinical features of the effects of ethanol on blood cells and the hematologic syndromes seen in liver disease.*

Petz LD, Swisher SW (eds.): Clinical Practice of Transfusion Medicine. 2nd ed. New York, Churchill Livingstone, 1989. *An up-to-date and well-written text centered on the transfusion of blood components. Contains many nuggets of clinical wisdom and a number of interesting chapters on the pathophysiology and immunologic aspects of various anemias.*

Stabler SP, Allen RH, Savage DG, et al.: Clinical spectrum and diagnosis of cobalamin deficiency. Blood 76:871, 1990. *A large series of patients with clinically significant cobalamin deficiency as seen in current practice, including many with "atypical" presentations. Data are presented that support the use of serum metabolite values as ancillary tests in the diagnosis of deficiency of this vitamin.*

129 Aplastic Anemia and Related Bone Marrow Failure Syndromes

Neal S. Young

Blood counts may be low because cells are prematurely removed from the peripheral circulation or are inadequately produced in the bone marrow. Bone marrow failure occurs commonly but is often classified by other dominant clinical or morphologic features (like the leukemias) or by specific etiology (like pernicious anemia). The term "bone marrow failure" is vague and inclusive, and it awaits redefinition with more precise understanding of pathophysiologic processes. By default, therefore, the disorders discussed in this chapter are currently defined by their marrow pathology: the fatty bone marrow of aplastic anemia, the disordered hematopoiesis of the myelodysplasias, and the fibrosis of myelofibrosis. Making inferences about disease processes from the appearance of the bone marrow is as misleading as it is inevitable, and an effort is made here to distinguish what is understood from what is conjecture.

APLASTIC ANEMIA

Definition (Table 129–1)

APLASTIC ANEMIA. Aplastic anemia is a disease of the young, with a median incidence at about 25 years of age (excluding aplasia secondary to cancer chemotherapy). It must be a leading diagnosis in the pancytopenic adolescent or young adult. The bone marrow is usually readily aspirated but appears dilute on smear. The biopsy specimen (see Color Plate 5G), often grossly pale, shows mainly fat under the microscope, with hematopoietic cells occupying by definition less than 25 per cent of the marrow space and, in the most serious cases, 0 to 5 per cent (Fig. 129–1). Prognosis is determined by the degree of blood count depression. The commonly accepted standard for severe disease requires two of the following three values: (1) absolute neutrophil count (percentage of polymorphonuclear and band forms multiplied by the total white blood cell count) of less than 500 per cubic millimeter; (2) platelets less than 20,000 per cubic millimeter; and (3) reticulocyte count (corrected for hematocrit) in the presence of anemia of less than 1 per cent (or an absolute reticulocyte count less than 40,000 per cubic millimeter).

BICYTOPENIA AND SINGLE-LINEAGE FAILURE STATES. Some patients present with bone marrow hypocellularity and depression of only two of the three major blood lines; many progress to typical aplastic anemia. Failure of a single lineage also occurs, as in pure red blood cell aplasia (rare), amegakaryocytic thrombocytopenia (extremely rare), and agranulocytosis (not rare but usually an idiosyncratic drug reaction). Single-lineage failures show a characteristic absence of a single set of recognizable precursor cells in an otherwise cellular bone marrow, and in this way they are differentiated from the much more common causes of anemia (such as vitamin or iron deficiency

TABLE 129–1. CLASSIFICATION OF APLASTIC ANEMIA AND SINGLE CYTOPENIAS

I. Acquired aplastic anemia
    Radiation
    Drugs and chemicals
        Regular effects
        Idiosyncratic reactions
    Viruses
        Epstein-Barr virus (infectious mononucleosis)
        Hepatitis C virus (non-A non-B hepatitis)
        Parvovirus (transient aplastic crisis, pure red cell aplasia [PRCA])
        Human immunodeficiency virus (AIDS)
    Immune diseases
        Eosinophilic fasciitis
        Hypoimmunoglobulinemia
        Thymoma and thymic carcinoma
        Graft-versus-host disease in immunodeficiency
    Paroxysmal nocturnal hemoglobinuria
    Pregnancy
    Idiopathic—the most frequent diagnosis
II. Inherited aplastic anemia
    Fanconi's anemia
    Dyskeratosis congenita
    Schwachman-Diamond syndrome
    Reticular dysgenesis
    Amegakaryocytic thrombocytopenia
    Familial aplastic anemias
        Preleukemia (e.g., monosomy 7)
    Nonhematologic syndromes (Down's, Dubovitz's, Seckel's)
	I. Acquired cytopenias
	    Anemias
	        Pure red cell aplasia (see Table 129–3)
	        Transient erythroblastopenia of childhood
	    Neutropenias
	        Idiopathic
	        Drugs, toxins
	    Thrombocytopenias
	        Drugs, toxins
	II. Inherited cytopenias
	    Anemias
	        Congenital pure red cell aplasia
	    Neutropenias
	        Kostmann's syndrome
	        Schwachman-Diamond syndrome
	        Reticular dysgenesis
	    Thrombocytopenias
	        Thrombocytopenia with absent radii
	        Idiopathic amegakaryocytic

and hemolysis) or thrombocytopenia (from peripheral destruction of platelets). The pathophysiology of the more restricted marrow failure states is probably similar to that of general bone marrow failure, but with a more mature target cell.

CONSTITUTIONAL (FANCONI'S) ANEMIA. Fanconi described children with inherited pancytopenia and marrow hypocellularity with associated anomalies of the skeletal and urogenital systems. Fanconi's anemia now is defined by specific chromosomal aberrations in cultured cells after clastogenic stress. Indeed, cytogenetic analysis of families of children with Fanconi's anemia has shown that the majority of patients lack associated anomalies and that the disease can manifest in adults, in the third and fourth decades or even later. Congenital pure red cell aplasia (Diamond-Blackfan syndrome) lacks a cytogenetic marker or associated physical abnormalities, and distinction from acquired aplastic anemia after infancy is possible only by family history. Isolated neutropenia or thrombocytopenia occurs in a number of pediatric syndromes.

Etiology

In the majority of patients, aplastic anemia is diagnosed as "idiopathic." There is little to distinguish these cases clinically from those with a presumed etiology, like exposure to a drug or chemical. Even when clinical associations are established, they should not automatically be equated with etiology and pathophysiology: Association is not equivalent to cause, nor does it define a mechanism.

RADIATION. Marrow aplasia is a major acute sequela of radiation exposure. Radiant energy damages DNA. The bone marrow, as a tissue dependent on active mitosis, is particularly susceptible to its effects. Nuclear accidents and radiation injury

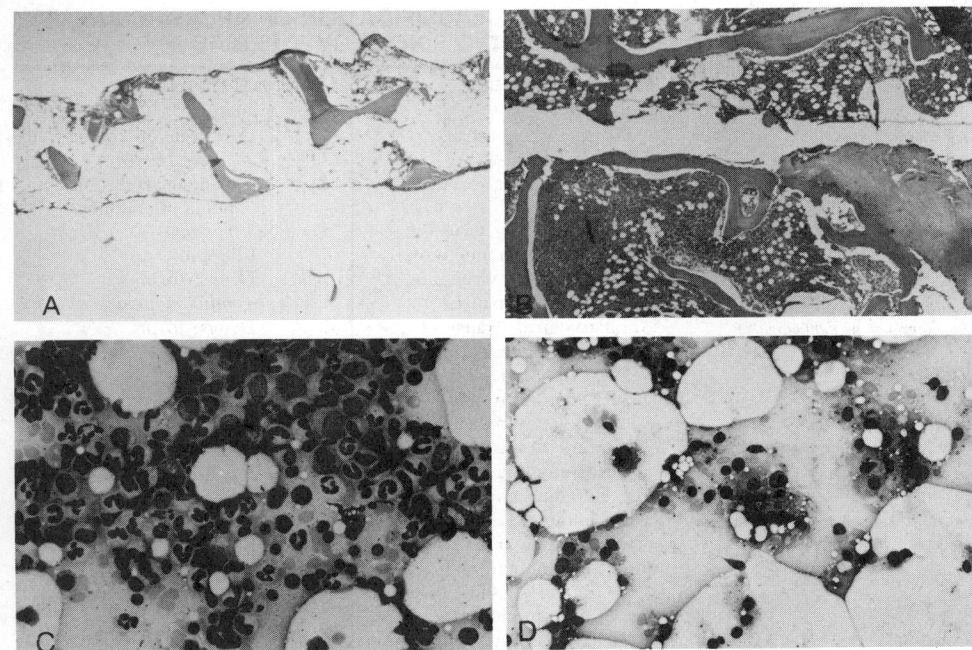

FIGURE 129–1. The bone marrow is normally 30 to 70 per cent cellular, and there is a heterogeneous mix of myeloid, erythroid, and lymphoid cells. Marrow biopsies show (A) severe hypocellularity of aplastic anemia and (B) hypercellularity of myelodysplasia. Normal aspirate smear (C) shows variety of hematopoietic precursor cell types, replaced in aplastic anemia (D) by fat and only residual stromal and lymphoid cells.

can involve not only power plant workers but also employees of hospitals, laboratories, and industry (e.g., food sterilization, metal radiography, and so forth), as well as those innocent persons exposed to stolen, misplaced, or misused radiation sources. The radiation dose can be approximated from the rate and degree of decline in blood counts; dosimetry by reconstruction of the exposure can help to estimate the patient's prognosis and also to protect medical personnel from contact with radioactive tissue and excreta. Myelodysplasia and leukemia, but not aplastic anemia, are late effects of irradiation.

CHEMICALS (Table 129–2). Benzene has been clearly linked to bone marrow failure, including aplastic anemia, acute leukemias, and probably multiple myeloma. The occurrence of hematologic abnormalities is roughly correlated with cumulative exposure, but there must also be an important element of susceptibility, as only a minority of even heavily exposed workers develop evidence of benzene myelotoxicity. A history of past employment is important, especially in "open" industries in which benzene is used for a secondary purpose (usually as a solvent) rather than in "closed" industries for chemical production. Benzene-related blood diseases have declined with regulation of industrial exposure, and benzene is not generally available as a household solvent. However, the benzene content of gasoline has been increased with its unleading. The association of marrow failure with other chemicals that contain a benzene ring is much less well substantiated; some, like the insecticide lindane, were probably contaminated with benzene during manufacture.

DRUGS (Table 129–2). Many of the common cancer chemotherapeutic drugs suppress the bone marrow. The mechanisms by which these drugs act offer useful clues to the pathophysiology of "idiopathic" aplastic anemia (see below). A very large and diverse group of drugs is related to aplastic anemia by rare but serious idiosyncratic reactions. These associations, which rest mainly on case reports, are tenuous at best. For example, some incriminated drugs may have been used to treat the first symptoms of bone marrow failure (antibiotics for fever or the preceding viral illness) or may have provoked the first symptom of a pre-existing disease (petechiae produced by nonsteroidal anti-inflammatory agents administered to a thrombocytopenic individual). In the context of total drug employment, idiosyncratic reactions, while individually devastating, are very rare events.

Chloramphenicol, the most infamous culprit, reportedly produced aplasia in only about 1 of 60,000 therapeutic courses, and even this number is almost certainly an overestimate. Chloramphenicol also consistently causes a dose-related, rather modest marrow depression, mainly reticulocytopenia and altered marrow morphology and iron kinetics. This effect of chloramphenicol use is mechanistically unrelated to and clinically not predictive of the rare, severe reaction, which occurs 1 to 2 months or longer after its routine use. The introduction of chloramphenicol was thought to have produced a notable increase in the number of cases of aplastic anemia, but its diminished use has not been followed by a reduced frequency of aplastic anemia. Chloramphenicol remains a popular antibiotic in less developed countries.

Suspected drug reactions account for only about 20 per cent of cases of aplastic anemia, while virtually all instances of agranulocytosis in the adult are drug related. The drugs associated with agranulocytosis are similar but not identical to those related to generalized bone marrow failure. Myeloid cells may be uniquely susceptible because of their ability to metabolize drugs, often to toxic intermediate compounds. In contrast to drug-associated aplastic anemia, agranulocytosis should spontaneously resolve with removal of the drug, and the severely neutropenic patient should survive if infection is adequately treated.

INFECTIONS. Hepatitis is the most common infection preceding aplastic anemia, accounting for about 5 per cent of Western cases and perhaps twice that proportion in Asian series. Typically,

TABLE 129–2. SOME DRUGS AND CHEMICALS ASSOCIATED WITH APLASTIC ANEMIA

I. Agents that regularly produce marrow depression as the major toxicity in commonly employed dose or normal exposures:
    Cytotoxic drugs used in cancer chemotherapy: alkylating agents, antimetabolites, antimitotics
    Some antibiotics

II. Agents that frequently but not inevitably produce marrow aplasia:
    Benzene (and benzene-containing chemicals like kerosene, carbon tetrachloride, Stoddard's solvent, chlorophenols)

III. Agents probably associated with aplastic anemia but with a relatively low probability:
    Chloramphenicol
    Insecticides
    Antiprotozoals: quinacrine and chloroquine, mepacrine
    Nonsteroidal anti-inflammatory drugs (including phenylbutazone, indomethacin, ibuprofen, sulindac, aspirin)
    Anticonvulsants (hydantoins, carbamazepine, phenacemide)
    Heavy metals (gold, arsenic, bismuth, mercury)
    Sulfonamides: some antibiotics, antithyroid drugs (methimazole, methylthiouracil, propylthiouracil), antidiabetes drugs (tolbutamide, chlorpropamide), carbonic anhydrase inhibitors (acetazolamide and methazolamide)
    Antihistamines (cimetidine, chlorpheniramine)
    D-Penicillamine
    Estrogens (in pregnancy and in high doses in animals)

severe aplasia occurs in a young man who has recovered from a mild bout of hepatitis 1 to 2 months earlier. The hepatitis is most often the non-A, non-B type, and some cases may represent aberrant responses to hepatitis C virus infection. Aplastic anemia can rarely follow infectious mononucleosis, and Epstein-Barr virus has been found in the marrow of some patients with aplastic anemia, with or without a suggestive preceding history. Parvovirus B19 has not been associated with generalized bone marrow failure. Moderate marrow depression occurs commonly in the course of many viral and bacterial infections, but the primary disease is usually overt.

IMMUNOLOGIC DISEASE. Aplasia occurs in immunodeficient children who develop graft-versus-host disease after infusion of unirradiated blood products. Pure red blood cell aplasia is associated with thymoma, and patients with red cell aplasia or pancytopenia may be hypoimmunoglobulinemic. Immunologic aspects of aplastic anemia are discussed in greater detail below.

OTHER ASSOCIATIONS. Aplastic anemia may occur during pregnancy and has sometimes resolved with delivery or with spontaneous or induced abortion. Pancytopenia occurs in about one third of patients with paroxysmal nocturnal hemoglobinuria (Ch. 135), and perhaps 5 per cent of patients with aplastic anemia have a positive Ham's test, often with hematopoietic recovery.

Pathophysiology

TYPES OF INJURY. Most bone marrow failure almost certainly results from damage to the hematopoietic stem cell compartment; little evidence exists that aplastic anemia results from defective stroma or from inadequate production of growth factors. Two different routes to stem cell damage are derived from animal experiments and models of the stem cell compartment. The paradigm for type I damage is the effect of drugs that directly damage DNA. The administration of busulfan in the mouse is followed by a long latent period and then severe aplasia. DNA damage is random and will affect late precursor cells and primitive stem cells alike; the consequences for the earlier cell may be graver, owing to its necessity to transit more mitotic cycles to mature. In humans, examples of type I aplasia are Fanconi's anemia, the result of defective DNA repair (the same chromosomal phenotype and recessive inheritance might result from genetic defects in different DNA repair enzymes), and aplasia caused by irradiation, benzene, and perhaps also chloramphenicol. Type I aplasia is associated with both early aplasia (immediate, direct cytotoxicity) and later myelodysplasia and leukemia (the sequelae of mutational events).

Type II aplasia is illustrated by the effect of a cycle-active agent like 5-fluorouracil, which mainly depletes later progenitor cells and leaves relatively intact the most quiescent and also most proliferatively capable stem cells. Most environmental damage would be expected to affect preferentially the mitotically and metabolically active cells, although massive disruption of hematopoiesis may severely dysregulate the spared stem cells. The drug- and virus-associated marrow failure syndromes are probably type II, mediated either by chemical injury to the hematopoietic cell's metabolic machinery or by immunologic injury to the cell membrane.

Cases of aplastic anemia can be apportioned roughly equally between types I and II, based on indirect evidence (the failure to cure about half of identical twins with simple bone marrow infusion, the 50 per cent response rate to nonreplacement therapies like antithymocyte globulin [ATG]). The severity of injury in both types is probably related to the duration, repetition, or specific type of the damaging agent.

METABOLIC DRUG INJURY. Many drugs and chemicals, especially if they are polar and have limited water solubility, are metabolized to highly reactive electrophilic intermediates that bind to cellular macromolecules. Excessive generation of such toxic intermediates or failure to detoxify them may be genetically determined and apparent only on drug challenge. The complexity and specificity of the pathways imply multiple susceptible loci. In one case of phenytoin-associated aplastic anemia, a defect in detoxification of that drug's metabolites was detected in the patient after recovery, and cells from the patient's mother were intermediately susceptible; cells from both normally detoxified metabolites generated from closely related drugs.

IMMUNE-MEDIATED INJURY. The recovery of their own marrow function by some patients being prepared for bone marrow transplantation with immunosuppressive horse antilymphocyte globulin first suggested that aplastic anemia might be immune mediated. Blood and bone marrow of patients often suppress normal bone marrow growth in progenitor assays, and removal of T cells from the bone marrow of those with aplastic anemia can improve colony formation in vitro. Patients with aplastic anemia may have increased numbers of activated cytotoxic lymphocytes (CD8+ cells bearing HLA-DR and interleukin 2 [IL2] receptors) that overproduce lymphokines (particularly gamma-interferon), and these abnormalities usually improve with successful immunosuppressive therapy. The clinical effectiveness of cyclosporine is further evidence that T cells play a pathogenic role in many cases of bone marrow failure.

In some cases, the inciting cause of the immune response may be an antecedent viral infection. Hepatitis C is a member of the flavivirus family, and other similar viruses, like that causing dengue, can both infect hematopoietic cells and stimulate a lymphocyte-lymphokine reaction similar to that observed in aplastic anemia. A similar final immune pathway may occur following infections with herpesviruses and retroviruses. Presumably, disease is the result of genetically determined features of the immune response that convert a normal physiologic response to a sustained and abnormal pathologic process.

PURE RED BLOOD CELL APLASIA (Table 129–3). Like aplastic anemia, pure red blood cell aplasia results from diverse mechanisms. Immune mechanisms have been implicated when pure red cell aplasia is associated with thymoma, systemic lupus erythematosus, and chronic lymphocytic leukemia, but not in failed erythropoiesis secondary to myelodysplasia, myeloproliferative diseases, and distinct cytogenetic abnormalities. Antibodies to red blood cell precursors can be detected in the blood of some patients, but T cell inhibition is probably the more common mechanism. Cytotoxic lymphocyte activity restricted by histocompatibility locus or specific for cells infected by human T cell lymphotropic virus (HTLV1) has been demonstrated in particularly well studied individual cases.

Parvovirus B19 (see Color Plate 5H, right) represents the best example of the interaction of virus, host hematologic target cell, and immune response. This common virus causes "fifth disease," a benign exanthema of childhood and a polyarthralgia syndrome in adults. In persons with underlying hemolysis, parvovirus infection causes abrupt but temporary worsening of anemia resulting from failed erythropoiesis, a syndrome called transient aplastic crisis. Parvovirus B19 has extraordinary tropism for human erythroid progenitor cells. Direct cytotoxicity of the virus causes anemia if demands on erythrocyte production are high. In normal individuals, the temporary cessation of red cell production is not clinically apparent, and disease is mediated entirely by immune complex deposition. In persons unable to mount an

TABLE 129–3. CLASSIFICATION OF PURE RED BLOOD CELL APLASIA

Self-limited
  Transient erythroblastopenia of childhood
  Transient aplastic crisis of hemolysis (B19 parvovirus infection)

Fetal red blood cell aplasia
  Nonimmune hydrops fetalis (in utero parvovirus infection)

Hereditary pure red cell aplasia
  Congenital pure red cell aplasia (Diamond-Blackfan syndrome)

Acquired pure red cell aplasia
  I. Thymoma and malignancy: thymoma, lymphoid malignancies (and more rarely other hematologic diseases), paraneoplastic to solid tumors
  II. Connective tissue disorders with immunologic abnormalities: systemic lupus erythematosus, juvenile rheumatoid arthritis, rheumatoid arthritis, multiple endocrine gland insufficiency
  III. Virus: B19 parvovirus, hepatitis, adult T cell leukemia virus, Epstein-Barr virus
  IV. Pregnancy
  V. Drugs: especially phenytoin, azathioprine, chloramphenicol, procainamide, isoniazid
  VI. Idiopathic

adequate antibody response, parvovirus B19 persists in the bone marrow and causes a chronic anemia that resembles pure red blood cell aplasia. The presence of giant pronormoblasts (Fig. 129–2), the cytopathic sign of the virus, should suggest the diagnosis. Persistent parvovirus infection should be sought in anemic patients with congenital and acquired immunodeficiency syndromes and in patients iatrogenically immunosuppressed because it can be effectively treated with immunoglobulin infusions.

Incidence and Epidemiology

The incidence of aplastic anemia is approximately 1.5 to 2 per million, but the disease may be more frequent in Asia. Mortality statistics indicate an equal sex ratio and a preponderance of older persons, but at referral centers the median age is about 24 years.

Agranulocytosis has an incidence of 3.4 per million. Pure red blood cell aplasia is a very rare disease, with only a few hundred reported cases, and amegakaryocytic thrombocytopenia is rarer still, with fewer than 20 cases in the literature.

Clinical Description

HISTORY. Bleeding is the most common early symptom of aplastic anemia: A complaint of days to weeks of easy bruising, including oozing from the gums, nose bleeds, or heavy menstrual flow is made, and sometimes petechiae will have been noticed. With thrombocytopenia, massive hemorrhage is unusual, but small amounts of bleeding in the central nervous system can result in serious intracranial or retinal hemorrhage. In cases of more gradual onset, symptoms of anemia are also described, usually lassitude, weakness, shortness of breath, and a pounding sensation in the ears. Infection is unusual as a first symptom in aplastic anemia, in contrast to agranulocytosis, in which pharyngitis, anorectal infection, or frank sepsis may be presenting syndromes. A striking feature of aplastic anemia is the restriction of symptoms to the hematologic system. Patients often feel and look remarkably well despite drastically reduced blood counts; systemic complaints and weight loss should point to other etiologies of pancytopenia. Drug use, chemical exposure, and preceding viral illnesses must often be elicited with repeated questioning; prompt cessation of drug or chemical exposure is especially important in agranulocytosis, which is usually self-limited.

PHYSICAL EXAMINATION. Petechiae and ecchymoses are frequently present, and there may be retinal hemorrhages. Pelvic and rectal examinations should be performed infrequently and gently to avoid trauma; these examinations often show bleeding from the cervical os and blood in the stool. Pallor of the skin and mucous membranes is also common except in the most acute cases or in those patients already transfused. Although infection on presentation is uncommon, by the time the patient reaches a referral center, fever and signs of systemic or local infection may well be present. Lymphadenopathy and splenomegaly are very unusual in aplastic anemia. Café au lait spots and short stature point to Fanconi's anemia; peculiar nails suggest dyskeratosis congenita.

Diagnosis and Differential Diagnosis (Table 129–4)

The diagnosis of aplastic anemia is usually straightforward, based on the combination of pancytopenia with a fatty, empty bone marrow. Prompt arrival at the appropriate diagnosis is part of the effective management of the patient with aplastic anemia.

BLOOD. The smear typically shows large erythrocytes and a paucity of platelets and granulocytes. Macrocytosis determined by automated cell counting is very common. Lymphocyte numbers may be normal or also reduced. The presence of immature myeloid forms should suggest leukemia or myelodysplasia; nucleated red blood cells suggest marrow fibrosis or invasion; and abnormal platelets suggest either peripheral destruction or dysplasia.

BONE MARROW (Fig. 129–2). "Watery" marrow can almost always be obtained, and a "dry tap" occurs in fibrotic or myelophthisic disease. In severe aplasia, the smear of the aspirated specimen shows only residual lymphocytes and stromal cells; in milder cases, the remaining hematopoietic cells can show "megaloblastoid" erythropoiesis. Megakaryocytes are invariably greatly reduced, usually absent. The areas adjacent to the spicule should be searched for myeloblasts. Total cellularity is assessed by biopsy (see Color Plate 5G) of a core more than 1 cm in length, which in the most severe cases is virtually 100 per cent fat and in more moderate disease less than 20 per cent cellular. Nonetheless, the correlation between marrow cellularity and severity is imperfect: Some patients with moderate disease according to blood counts have empty iliac crest biopsies, and there may be "hot spots" of hematopoiesis in severe cases. In unilineage failure states, the bone marrow reflects the absence of a specific morphologic subtype, but in both pure red blood cell aplasia and agranulocytosis, early and midmature precursor cells may be present. Granulomas (in cellular specimens) may indicate an infectious cause of the marrow failure.

ANCILLARY STUDIES. Cytogenetic studies of peripheral blood should be performed on patients younger than 35 years (at least) to exclude Fanconi's anemia. Testing for abnormal sensitivity of erythrocytes to complement (Ham's test) establishes paroxysmal nocturnal hemoglobinuria (Ch. 135). Serologic studies may show evidence of viral infection, especially antibodies to human immunodeficiency virus, Epstein-Barr virus, and hepatitis viruses. Parvovirus should be sought by DNA hybridization in chronic pure red cell aplasia. Hypoimmunoglobulinemia and thymoma are also associated with pure red blood cell aplasia; a thymoma should be sought by computed tomography, less because the hematologic disease remits with thymectomy (it often does not) than because a potentially malignant tumor should be removed. The size of the spleen should be determined by scanning if the physical examination of the abdomen is unsatisfactory.

DIFFERENTIAL DIAGNOSIS. Pancytopenia occurs in many

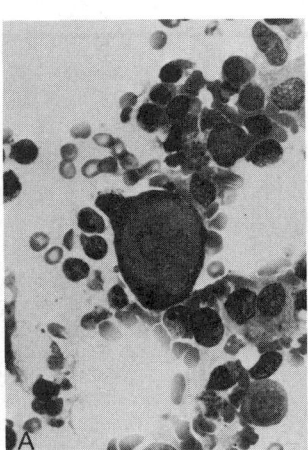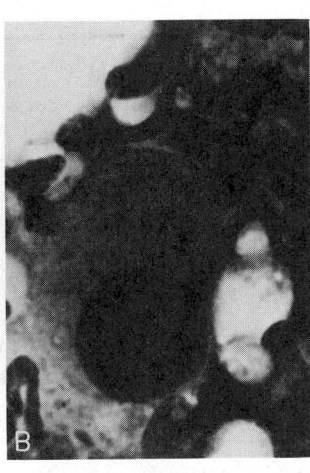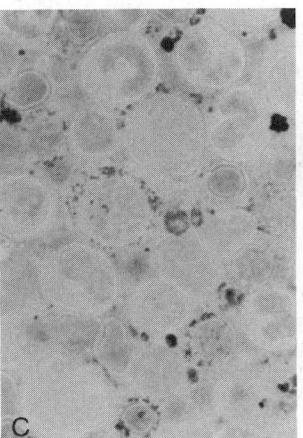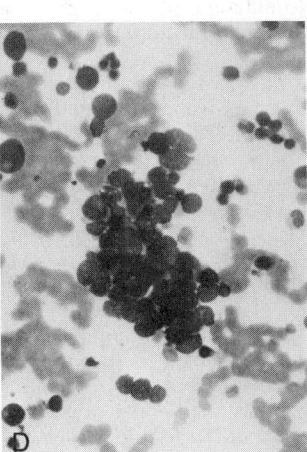

FIGURE 129–2. Four pathognomonic cells in the bone marrow. A, Giant pronormoblast, the cytopathic effect of B19 parvovirus infection of the erythroid progenitor cell. B, Uninuclear megakaryocyte and microblastic erythroid precursors typical of the 5q-myelodysplasia syndrome. C, Ringed sideroblast showing perinuclear iron granules. D, Clump of nonhematopoietic cells forming syncytium of metastatic tumor cells.

TABLE 129–4. DIFFERENTIAL DIAGNOSIS OF PANCYTOPENIA

Pancytopenia with hypocellular bone marrow
- Acquired aplastic anemia
- Inherited aplastic anemia (Fanconi's anemia)
- Some myelodysplasia syndromes
- Rare aleukemic leukemia (acute myelogenous leukemia [AML])
- Some acute lymphoblastic leukemias
- Some lymphomas of bone marrow

Pancytopenia with cellular bone marrow
- Myelodysplasia syndromes
- Paroxysmal nocturnal hemoglobinuria
- Myelofibrosis
- Some aleukemic leukemias   } Primary bone marrow diseases
- Myelophthisis
- Bone marrow lymphoma
- Hairy cell leukemia

- Systemic lupus erythematosus
- Hypersplenism
- Vitamin B_{12}, folate deficiency
- Overwhelming infection   } Secondary to systemic diseases
- Alcohol
- Brucellosis
- Sarcoidosis
- Tuberculosis

Hypocellular bone marrow ± cytopenia
- Q fever
- Legionnaires' disease
- Anorexia nervosa, starvation
- Mycobacterial infection

diseases, but when secondary blood count depression rivals that of severe aplastic anemia, the primary diagnosis is usually obvious from either the history or the physical examination (e.g., the massive spleen of alcoholic cirrhosis, the history of metastatic cancer or systemic lupus erythematosus, or obvious miliary tuberculosis on the chest radiograph).

Treatment

BONE MARROW TRANSPLANTATION (Ch. 153). This offers the best therapy for a young patient with a fully histocompatible sibling donor. Survival of patients younger than 20 years old following bone marrow transplantation is about 80 per cent. Early consideration of the transplantation option in a child or adolescent can avoid unnecessary transfusions. Transfusions increase the risk of graft rejection, already peculiarly high in patients with aplastic anemia, and graft rejection is the major determinant of a successful clinical outcome. Survival of minimally transfused patients approximates that of patients who have had an identical twin as donor. Graft-versus-host disease increases progressively with age and occurs in about 90 per cent of adults over 30 years old. In older persons, marrow transplantation also carries significant risks from interstitial pneumonitis and opportunistic infections secondary to the conditioning regimen. As a result, it is usually not recommended for patients with aplastic anemia who are more than 40 years old. Management of patients in the intermediate range, 20 to 40 years old, depends on their transfusion history, on their general clinical condition, and, unfortunately, often on their medical insurance. Use of alternative donors, unrelated histocompatible volunteers or closely but not perfectly matched family members, remains experimental but has been occasionally successful.

IMMUNOSUPPRESSION. Most patients with aplastic anemia lack a suitable marrow donor. Antithymocyte globulin therapy leads to recovery of autologous bone marrow function in about 50 per cent of patients, usually with independence from transfusion and a leukocyte count adequate to prevent infection. Improvement in granulocyte number is generally apparent within 2 months of treatment. In most patients who recover with this treatment, the blood counts remain somewhat depressed, the mean corpuscular volume continues to be high, and the bone marrow cellularity returns only very slowly toward normal, if at all. Relapse is infrequent, although 5 to 10 per cent of patients may suffer recurrent severe pancytopenia or myelodysplasia, paroxysmal nocturnal hemoglobinuria, or acute leukemia. Bone

marrow examinations should therefore be performed annually or when there is an unfavorable change in blood counts, and a Ham test should be obtained periodically. About 50 per cent of patients in whom therapy with ATG fails will respond to a 3- to 6-month course of cyclosporine. The combination of ATG and cyclosporine may be superior to ATG alone as initial therapy for severe aplastic anemia.

Antithymocyte globulin can be given intravenously in a regimen of 40 mg per kilogram per day for 4 days. Anaphylaxis is a rare but occasionally fatal complication of ATG treatment; allergy should be tested for by a prick test with an undiluted solution and immediate observation. Antithymocyte globulin binds to peripheral blood cells, and therefore platelet and granulocyte numbers may fall further during active treatment. Serum sickness often develops about 10 days after initiating treatment (Ch. 249). Most patients receive methylprednisolone (1 mg per kilogram per day for 2 weeks) to ameliorate the immune consequences of heterologous protein infusion. Cyclosporine is administered orally at an initial dose of 12 mg per kilogram per day in adults and 15 mg per kilogram per day in children, with subsequent adjustment according to blood levels obtained every 2 weeks. Nephrotoxicity, hypertension, seizures, and opportunistic infections, especially *Pneumocystis carinii* pneumonia, are the most serious complications of cyclosporine treatment.

Immunosuppression is also effective in pure red blood cell aplasia and probably in amegakaryocytic thrombocytopenia as well. Treatments include corticosteroids, azathioprine, or cyclophosphamide, followed by ATG or cyclosporine.

OTHER THERAPIES. Androgen therapy has not been verified as effective in controlled trials, but occasional patients respond or even demonstrate blood count dependence on continued therapy. For patients with moderate disease or for those with severe pancytopenia in whom immunosupression has failed, a 3- to 4-month trial of an androgen is appropriate: nandrolone decanoate at 5 mg per kilogram per week given intramuscularly (with firm pressure at the injection site to prevent hemorrhage) or oxymetholone at 150 mg per day by mouth.

Hematopoietic growth factors, GM-CSF and G-CSF, have not been shown to induce remissions in aplastic anemia, although they may increase the white blood cell count during the period of administration in some patients.

PRINCIPLES OF SUPPORT. Meticulous medical care is required so that the patient can survive to benefit from definitive therapy or, having experienced a treatment failure, can maintain a reasonable existence in the face of pancytopenia. First and most important, infection in the patient with severe neutropenia must be aggressively treated (see also Ch. 140). Parenteral, broad-spectrum antibiotics should be started promptly, usually a combination of an aminoglycoside, cephalosporin, and semisynthetic penicillin (monotherapy with ceftazidime is a reasonable alternative). Therapy is empiric and must not await results of culture, although specific foci of infection, like oropharyngeal or anorectal abscesses, pneumonia, sinusitis, and typhlitis, should be sought on physical examination and with suitable radiographic studies. When indwelling plastic catheters become contaminated, vancomycin should be added. Persistent or recrudescent fever implies fungal disease; candidiasis and aspergillosis are common, especially after several courses of antibacterial antibiotics, and a progressive course may be averted by the timely initiation of amphotericin. Granulocyte transfusions are seldom indicated (Ch. 140). Handwashing, the single most effective method of preventing the spread of infection in the hospital, remains a neglected practice. Nonabsorbed antibiotics for gut decontamination may be effective but are rarely tolerated because of their gastrointestinal side effects. Total reverse isolation is difficult, expensive, psychologically debilitating, inhibitory of nursing and medical attention, and not clearly beneficial in reducing mortality from infections.

Platelets and erythrocytes can be maintained by transfusion. Candidates for bone marrow transplantation should be transfused sparingly and, of course, never with blood products from a family member. Alloimmunization limits the usefulness of prophylactic platelet transfusions, and single-donor platelets from which leukocytes have been removed by filtration are the best product (Ch. 140). There are no direct studies of the value of prophylaxis versus demand platelet transfusions in chronic bone marrow failure. Any rational regimen of prophylaxis requires transfusions once or twice weekly to maintain the platelet count above 10,000 per microliter (oozing from the gut, and presumably also from other vascular beds, increases precipitously at values lower than 5000 per microliter). About one third of patients become refractory to platelet transfusions, sometimes to HLA-matched as well as to random-donor platelets. Inhibitors of fibrinolysis, like aminocaproic acid, may help reduce mucosal oozing. Menstruation should be suppressed by either oral estrogens or nasal follicle-stimulating hormone (FSH)/luteinizing hormone (LH) antagonists. Aspirin and other nonsteroidal anti-inflammatory agents that inhibit platelet function must be avoided.

Red blood cells should be transfused to allow a normal level of activity, usually to a hemoglobin value of 70 grams per liter (90 grams per liter if there is underlying cardiac disease). A regimen of 2 units every 2 weeks replaces the normal loss of erythrocytes in a patient without a functioning bone marrow. In chronic anemia, the iron chelator deferoxamine should be added at about the time the patient receives the fiftieth transfusion to avoid secondary hemochromatosis.

Prognosis

The natural course of untreated severe aplastic anemia is rapid deterioration and death resulting from infection or hemorrhage. Survival in patients with severe disease treated with transfusions only is poor, probably about 20 per cent at 1 year. In most large unselected series, bone marrow transplantation leads to a 60 to 80 per cent survival rate at 1 year. In Europe, immunosuppression has given overall results equivalent to marrow transplantation in adults, although survival was better with transplantation if severe neutropenia (<200 per microliter) was present. The physician has the responsibility of informing the patient of the relative values of bone marrow transplantation, which cures the hematologic disease but at great cost and often with significant morbidity, and immunosuppressive therapy, which is easier but often not completely effective.

Red cell aplasia is compatible with long life. Patients with congenital anemias have survived for decades with a combination of transfusions and iron chelation. Probably more than half of patients with acquired red cell aplasia can be cured by immunosuppression.

MYELODYSPLASIA

Definition

Myelodysplasia describes a heterogeneous group of hematologic disorders that are defined only broadly by cytopenias associated with a dysmorphic or abnormal-appearing bone marrow (Table 129–5) (see Color Plate 6I and J). The classification scheme marks the convergence of two areas of investigation: preleukemia, the cytopenic phase sometimes observed to precede frank malignancy, and refractory anemia, states that resemble megaloblastic anemia but without evidence of vitamin deficiency. The French-American-British nomenclature, while based on morphologic features, has real predictive value. (Sideroblastic anemia is also discussed in Ch. 131 as an example of hypochromic anemias.)

Etiology and Pathophysiology

The myelodysplastic syndromes are clonal disorders and have been convincingly linked to exposure to radiation, benzene, and many drugs employed in the treatment of cancer, particularly the radiomimetic alkylating agents. Cytogenetic abnormalities are common in patients with myelodysplasia. Some of the same specific chromosomal lesions also occur in frank leukemia and can be a transient stage in the development of a fully malignant phenotype. The presence and number of gross cytogenetic abnormalities in myelodysplasia are strongly correlated with the probability of leukemic transformation and therefore inversely with survival. One stereotypical karyotypic finding is deletion of a portion of the short arm of the fifth chromosome, or 5q-syndrome (Fig. 129–2), particularly provocative because the genes for multiple hematopoietic growth factors and their receptors are found in the affected region (including granulocyte-macrophage and macrophage colony-stimulating factors; interleukins 3, 4, 5, and 9; and the cell-surface receptors for macrophage colony-stimulating factor [the c-fms gene] and platelet-derived growth factor). Mutations that activate the ras oncogene and the c-fms gene have also been implicated in other cases of myelodysplasia. A mutation in a cell-surface receptor might result in a continuous proliferative stimulus and the uncoupling of signal transduction required for normal differentiation. The dysfunction measured in erythrocyte enzyme pathways for heme synthesis or in platelet aggregation in myelodysplasia is likely a secondary effect of mutations that dysregulate progenitor cell growth.

Incidence and Epidemiology

Idiopathic myelodysplasia is a disease of the elderly; the average mean age at onset is approximately 68 years, with a slight male preponderance. The exact incidence of myelodysplasia is unknown, but this is not a rare syndrome in our aging population. Therapy-related myelodysplasia, which is not age-related, may occur in 10 to 15 per cent of patients within a decade following intensive treatment, especially following a combination of irradiation and drugs like busulfan, nitrosourea, or procarbazine.

Clinical Description

Anemia dominates the early course. Most symptomatic patients complain of the gradual onset of fatigue and weakness, dyspnea, and pallor, but half are asymptomatic, with the myelodysplasia being discovered only incidentally. Previous chemotherapy or radiation exposure is an important historical fact. Fever and weight loss are more indicative of a myeloproliferative than of a myelodysplastic process. A family history may indicate a hereditary form of sideroblastic anemia. The physical examination is remarkable for signs of anemia and, in about 20 per cent of cases, splenomegaly. In addition, some unusual skin lesions, like those of Sweet's syndrome (febrile neutrophilic dermatosis), have been associated with myelodysplasia.

Diagnosis and Differential Diagnosis

BLOOD. Anemia is present in the majority of cases, either alone or as part of bicytopenia or pancytopenia, but isolated neutropenia or thrombocytopenia is unusual. Macrocytosis is common, and the smear may be dimorphic with a distinctive population of large cells. Platelets are large and lack granules. Neutrophils may be hypogranulated, show Pelger-Huët, ringed, or abnormally segmented nuclei, and contain Döhle's bodies. Circulating myeloblasts usually correlate with the number of marrow blasts, and their quantitation is important for classification and prognosis. The total white blood cell count is usually normal or low, with the exception of the monocytosis observed in chronic myelomonocytic leukemia.

TABLE 129–5. CLASSIFICATION OF MYELODYSPLASIA

Subtype	Blood	Marrow	Per Cent of Cases	Median Survival (mo)	Leukemic Evolution (%)
Refractory anemia	Blasts <1%	Blasts <5%	27	50	16
Refractory anemia with ringed sideroblasts	Blasts <1%	Blasts <5%	20	65	15
Refractory anemia with excess blasts	Blasts ≤5%	Blasts 5–20%	26	15	48
Refractory anemia with excess blasts in transformation	Blasts >5%	Blasts 20–30% or Auer rods	13	9	62
Chronic myelomonocytic leukemia	≥1 × 10⁹/L monocytes	Any number	14	23	29

By definition, the bone marrow of acute myelogenous leukemia contains more than 30 per cent blasts. Leukemic evolution refers to the percentage of cases that transform into acute myelogenous leukemia. Data derived from published series after Dunbar and Nienhuis.

TABLE 129–6. CAUSES OF MYELOPHTHISIS

A. Neoplastic infiltration of the marrow
1. Hematologic malignancies
   Leukemias—acute and chronic
   Lymphomas—Hodgkin's and non-Hodgkin's
   Plasma cell myeloma
   Hairy cell leukemia
2. Nonhematologic malignancies
   Carcinomas—especially breast, prostate, lung, stomach
   Neuroblastoma

B. Myelofibrosis
1. Primary (idiopathic)
2. Secondary—chronic myeloid leukemia, cancers, vasculitis (lupus, rheumatoid arthritis)

C. Granulomatous infections
1. Tuberculosis
2. Fungi

D. Metabolic abnormalities
1. Lipid storage diseases, e.g., Gaucher's disease
2. Osteopetrosis

BONE MARROW. The bone marrow is usually normocellular or hypercellular, but in 20 per cent of patients with myelodysplasia, it is sufficiently hypocellular to be confused with aplasia. No single characteristic feature of marrow morphology distinguishes myelodysplasia. Megaloblastoid and dyserythropoietic changes in the red blood cell precursors, a left shift with an increase in myeloblasts, and abnormal megakaryocytes with reduced numbers of disorganized nuclei are common features. The specific diagnosis is based on the presence of ringed sideroblasts (Fig. 129–2), the percentage of blasts, and increased immature myelomonocytic forms. A hematologist helps delineate myelodysplasia from acute myelogenous leukemia on the one hand and aplastic anemia on the other. Analysis of chromosomes from cultured bone marrow cells should always be performed, as cytogenetic abnormalities are unusual in aplasia and common in myelodysplasia. Complex chromosomal abnormalities imply poor survival.

Treatment

Therapy for myelodysplasia has generally been unsatisfactory. Occasional patients with sideroblastic anemia, usually hereditary, respond to pyridoxine. Androgens and corticosteroids may improve blood counts but have not been shown to influence survival. Older patients suffer a high mortality during induction with high-dose chemotherapy for leukemia and have a lower remission rate than do patients with acute myelogenous leukemia. Reported good responses using low-dose chemotherapy (in particular, cytosine arabinoside) or retinoids to induce marrow differentiation have not been widely confirmed.

A substantial proportion of patients with myelodysplasia have been found to respond with significant blood count improvement to granulocyte or granulocyte-macrophage colony-stimulating growth factors. Leukocytes almost always increase during factor therapy, and in some cases blast numbers have been significantly reduced and cytogenetic abnormalities have resolved. Unfortunately, sometimes progression to acute leukemia has also occurred. Platelet and reticulocyte numbers respond less consistently. Current long-term trials of these factors, as well as interleukin 3 and factors in combination, should provide an indication of optimal regimens and long-term benefits.

The same principles of supportive care described for aplastic anemia apply to myelodysplasia. Because many patients will be anemic for years, erythrocyte transfusion support should be accompanied by iron chelation to prevent hemochromatotic damage to the heart, liver, and pancreas.

Prognosis

The median survival for a patient with myelodysplasia is about 2 years, but survival varies greatly with the specific subtype. Most patients die as a result of complications of pancytopenia and not because of leukemic transformation. Approximately one third succumb to other diseases unrelated to myelodysplasia. Precipitous worsening of pancytopenia, acquisition of new chromosomal abnormalities detected on serial cytogenetic determination, and increase in the number of blasts are all obviously poor prognostic indicators. The outlook in therapy-related myelodysplasia is particularly poor, with many patients rapidly progressing to refractory acute myelogenous leukemia.

MYELOPHTHISIC ANEMIAS AND MYELOFIBROSIS

Marrow fibrosis, usually accompanied by a characteristic blood smear presentation called leukoerythroblastosis (see Color Plate 7F, left), can occur as a primary hematologic disease, called myelofibrosis or myeloid metaplasia (see Color Plate 5J), and as a secondary process, called myelophthisis, which represents reaction to invading tumor cells (see Color Plate 5I), infectious agents like mycobacteria or fungi, intracellular lipid deposition in Gaucher's disease (see Color Plate 7E), and the granulomas of sarcoidosis (Table 129–6). In secondary fibrosis, the infectious or malignant underlying processes are usually obvious. The pancytopenia of human immunodeficiency virus may be associated with moderate marrow fibrosis. Modest degrees of fibrosis can also be a feature of a variety of other hematologic syndromes, especially chronic myelogenous leukemia, poorly differentiated lymphomas, myeloma, and hairy cell leukemia. Marrow fibrosis also occurs in the bony proliferative disease of childhood called osteopetrosis.

The pathophysiology of myelofibrosis has three distinct features: proliferation of fibroblasts in the marrow space; extension of hematopoiesis into the long bones and most peculiarly into extramedullary sites, usually the spleen, liver, and lymph nodes (myeloid metaplasia); and ineffective erythropoiesis. The etiology of fibrosis is unknown but most likely involves dysregulated production of growth factors. Many cell types in the marrow produce growth factors for fibroblasts: Platelet-derived growth factor is one example, and profuse megakaryocytopoiesis and thrombocytosis are often seen early in the course of idiopathic myelofibrosis. Abnormal regulation of other hematopoietins would lead to the localization of blood-producing cells in nonhematopoietic tissues and uncoupling of the usually balanced processes of stem cell proliferation and differentiation. Myelofibrosis is remarkable for pancytopenia despite extraordinarily large numbers of circulating hematopoietic progenitor cells.

Idiopathic (or agnogenic) myelofibrosis is one of the myeloproliferative syndromes, a category that also includes polycythemia vera, essential thrombocythemia, and chronic myelogenous leukemia. It is discussed in Ch. 143 in the context of the myeloproliferative disorders.

Deeg HJ, Klingemann H-G, Phillips GL: A Guide to Bone Marrow Transplantation. Berlin, Springer-Verlag, 1988. *Multifaceted and balanced approach.*

Dunbar C, Nienhuis A: The myelodysplastic syndromes. *In* Handin R, Lux S, Stossel T (eds.): Blood, Principles and Practice of Hematology. Philadelphia, J.B. Lippincott, in press. *Good clinical descriptions and in-depth considerations of mechanisms.*

Young NS: Drugs and chemicals as agents of bone marrow failure. *In* Testa NG, Gale RP (eds.): Hematopoiesis: Long-term Effects of Chemotherapy and Radiation. New York, Marcel Dekker, 1988, 131 pp. *Detailed review of epidemiologic and mechanistic aspects.*

Young NS: Hematologic and hematopoietic consequences of B19 parvovirus infection. Semin Hematol 25:159, 1988. *The story of this virus, from its discovery to the genetic engineering of a vaccine, should make good reading.*

Young NS, Alter BA: Bone marrow failure. *In* Handin R, Lux S, Stossel T (eds.): Blood, Principles and Practice of Hematology. Philadelphia, J.B. Lippincott, in press. *Exhaustive review of aplastic anemia, both acquired and constitutional, and single-lineage failures.*

130 Normochromic, Normocytic Anemias

James P. Kushner

The normocytic, normochromic anemias are those in which the average cell size (mean corpuscular volume [MCV]) and the average cell hemoglobin concentration (mean corpuscular hemoglobin concentration [MCHC]) are normal. These anemias occur in association with a large number of diseases, and the mechanisms responsible for the anemia are quite diverse. Frequently, the anemia is only a minor manifestation of a systemic disease.

The anemia, however, may be the first detected evidence of disease, and the finding of anemia may lead to studies resulting in correct diagnosis of an underlying disorder.

In spite of their highly variable causes, it is possible to approach normocytic, normochromic anemias with a classification scheme that can direct the diagnostic investigation (Table 130–1). Central to this classification is the determination of whether the bone marrow is responding appropriately to a given degree of anemia. Normally functioning bone marrow can accelerate the rate of erythropoiesis up to eightfold. Accelerated erythropoiesis is reflected by an increase in the reticulocyte count. Reticulocytosis can be detected on routinely stained smears by the finding of a population of large polychromatophilic red cells. When reticulocytosis is pronounced, the MCV may be moderately elevated because of the contribution of the large young erythrocytes to the measurement of the average cell size. Reticulocytosis (see Color Plate 5F, right) is a manifestation of an appropriate marrow response to hemolytic anemia (see Ch. 133) and to acute posthemorrhagic anemia. These two conditions can generally be differentiated on clinical grounds.

When evidence of accelerated erythropoiesis in response to anemia is *not* found, it is likely that the underlying disorder is directly or indirectly affecting the bone marrow. Intrinsic marrow disease should be strongly suspected when leukopenia and thrombocytopenia are also found, or when morphologic abnormalities are found on the blood smear. These morphologic abnormalities include nucleated red cells, teardrop-shaped poikilocytes, immature granulocytes, and large platelets or megakaryocyte fragments (dwarf megakaryocytes). Marrow aspiration and biopsy are nearly always indicated when these findings are present.

When anemia is found in association with an impaired marrow response and no signs of intrinsic marrow disease are detected, it is likely that an underlying disease is producing an indirect effect on red cell production. Renal disease, liver disease, and a variety of endocrine disorders indirectly affect erythropoiesis in association with a reduction of erythropoietin production. The pathogenesis of the anemia of chronic disease may also involve this mechanism, in addition to the defect in the mobilization of reticuloendothelial iron stores (Ch. 131).

ACUTE POSTHEMORRHAGIC ANEMIA

DEFINITION. The anemia caused by loss of a large volume of blood may occur as a result of trauma or because of an underlying disease that affects blood vessels or the coagulation mechanism. Bleeding may be obvious when profuse hemorrhage occurs from a body orifice or from an external wound. If bleeding occurs within a body cavity, tissue space, or the gastrointestinal tract, the nature of the problem may not be immediately appreciated (Ch. 111). The manifestation of hemorrhage depends on the rate and magnitude of the bleeding and the time elapsed between the acute hemorrhage and the first clinical observations.

CLINICAL MANIFESTATIONS AND DIAGNOSIS. The events following a single acute hemorrhage can be divided into two phases. The first, lasting up to 3 days, reflects the volume of blood loss and is dominated by the manifestations of hypovolemia. Anemia may not be detected by measurement of the hematocrit or hemoglobin. The second phase occurs after the body has restored the blood volume to normal or nearly normal and is characterized by the findings of anemia and reticulocytosis.

As outlined in Table 130–2, a normal individual can rapidly lose up to 20 per cent of the blood volume without any signs or symptoms. Limited signs of cardiovascular distress appear with losses up to 30 per cent of the blood volume, but shock gradually appears only when the blood loss exceeds 30 to 40 per cent of the blood volume. As the plasma volume and red cell mass are reduced in proportional amounts, the hematocrit and hemoglobin fail to reflect the magnitude of blood lost. Clinical signs and symptoms must be used initially to estimate the degree of blood volume depletion and to plan emergency treatment. When blood loss is more gradual, the plasma volume may be restored by endogenous mechanisms, and very large volumes of blood can be lost without clinical manifestations of shock.

Anemia is first detected following expansion of the plasma volume. In recumbent patients most of the plasma volume expansion has occurred by 24 hours; this expansion mainly is caused by movement of water and electrolytes into the intravascular space. In ambulatory patients plasma volume expansion occurs more slowly, mainly through the mobilization of albumin from extravascular sites. The hematocrit may not reach the minimum value until 3 or 4 days after the hemorrhagic episode. Erythropoietin secretion is stimulated shortly after the appearance of the anemia, and hyperplasia of marrow erythroid elements then begins.

Reticulocytosis is usually detected 3 to 5 days after the hemorrhagic episode, and maximal reticulocyte counts are reached at 6 to 11 days. The degree of reticulocytosis is related to the magnitude of hemorrhage but rarely exceeds 14 per cent. During the period of maximal reticulocytosis, polychromatophilia and macrocytosis can be detected on the peripheral blood smear, and the MCV may become transiently increased. If the initial evaluation is done during this state, the findings may be mistaken for those of hemolytic anemia. Differentiation from hemolytic anemia may be difficult if bleeding has occurred into a body cavity or tissue space, because resorption of blood from these areas often results in an increased production of unconjugated bilirubin and even mild jaundice. In contrast to the reticulocyte response, both the platelet count and the leukocyte count may rise dramatically within hours of hemorrhage. Platelet counts as great as 1000×10^9 per liter may be detected within 1 to 2 hours, and leukocyte counts of 20 to 35×10^9 per liter may be reached by 2 to 5 hours. Elevated platelet and leukocyte counts generally return to normal within 3 to 5 days.

TREATMENT. During the hypovolemic phase, therapy should be directed at stopping the hemorrhage, combating shock,

TABLE 130–1. CLASSIFICATION OF THE NORMOCYTIC, NORMOCHROMIC ANEMIAS

I. **Anemia with appropriate marrow response**
   A. Acute posthemorrhagic anemia
   B. Hemolytic anemia (may be macrocytic when there is pronounced reticulocytosis) (Ch. 133–135)
II. **Anemia with impaired marrow response**
   A. Marrow hypoplasia
      1. Aplastic anemia (Ch. 129)
      2. Pure red cell aplasia (Ch. 129)
   B. Marrow infiltration
      1. Infiltration by malignant cells
      2. Myelofibrosis (Ch. 143)
      3. Inherited storage diseases
   C. Decreased erythropoietin production
      1. Kidney disease
      2. Liver disease
      3. Endocrine deficiencies
      4. Malnutrition
      5. Anemia of chronic disease (Ch. 131)

TABLE 130–2. CLINICAL MANIFESTATIONS OF ACUTE BLOOD LOSS IN OTHERWISE HEALTHY INDIVIDUALS

Percentage of Blood Volume Lost	Amount Lost (ml)	Clinical Manifestations
10–20	500–1000	Usually none; vasovagal syncope may occur in 5%; tachycardia in response to exercise; mild postural hypotension may be noted
20–30	1000–1500	Few changes in the supine position; light-headedness and hypotension commonly occur when the patient is upright; marked tachycardia in response to exertion
30–40	1500–2000	Blood pressure, cardiac output, central venous pressure, urine volume reduced even when supine; thirst, shortness of breath, clammy skin, sweating, clouding of consciousness and rapid, thready pulse may be noted
40–50	2000–2500	Severe shock, often resulting in death

and restoring the blood volume. Restoration of the blood volume may be achieved by intravenous infusion of crystalloid (electrolyte) solutions; colloid solutions of plasma protein, albumin, or dextran; or fresh whole blood. Complete reliance on fresh whole blood in the emergency situation is unwise for several reasons. First, large amounts of type O Rh-negative whole blood are required. If typing and crossmatching are done prior to transfusion, there may be a dangerous delay in therapy. Second, allergic transfusion reactions may restrict volume expansion or even produce plasma volume contraction. For the emergency situation, crystalloid solutions are preferred.

A nonprotein crystalloid solution with a sodium concentration approximating that of plasma is the most widely used fluid therapy for hemorrhagic shock. Ringer's lactate, Ringer's acetate, or normal saline supplemented with 90 mmol of sodium bicarbonate (2 ampules) per liter may be used. Crystalloid solutions containing large amounts of glucose should be avoided, as they may induce osmotic diuresis, further depleting the vascular volume. An initial infusion of two to three times the volume of the estimated blood loss is administered. When larger volumes of crystalloid solutions are administered, peripheral edema often develops, as these solutions are rapidly distributed throughout the intravascular and extravascular compartments.

The use of protein-containing solutions (albumin or fresh frozen plasma) has been supported by some who claim that increasing the oncotic pressure within the vascular space is beneficial. There is little evidence to support this contention, as protein is extravasated into interstitial spaces throughout the body in patients in shock. Dextran solutions have been widely used in the treatment of hemorrhagic shock, but there is no convincing evidence to suggest they are superior to crystalloid solutions in acute emergencies. Acute renal failure has occurred in a few patients receiving dextran solutions. Dextran may cause difficulty in crossmatching and may interfere with platelet adhesiveness and the normal coagulation cascade.

The administration of 3 liters of a crystalloid solution over 15 to 20 minutes generally resuscitates any patient in hemorrhagic shock if the hemorrhage has been arrested. Continued signs and symptoms of hypovolemia indicate continued bleeding and usually indicate the need for surgical intervention to control the hemorrhage.

Once the emergency has been dealt with, the bleeding lesion identified, and the bleeding stopped, attention can be directed to the anemia. The anemia itself rarely requires specific therapy, and provision of a high-protein diet and oral iron supplementation suffices in most cases. Blood transfusions may be reserved for those situations in which rapid correction of the anemia is required, as in preparation of the patient for surgery.

Billhardt RA, Rosenbush SW: Cardiogenic and hypovolemic shock. Med Clin North Am 70:853, 1986. *A useful review of the crystalloid versus colloid controversy in the acute management of hypovolemic shock.*
Mollison PL: Blood Transfusion in Clinical Medicine. 8th ed. St. Louis, C.V. Mosby, 1988. *The "bible" for detailed analysis of the measurement of blood volume and its restoration by transfusions.*

OTHER NORMOCYTIC, NORMOCHROMIC ANEMIAS
ANEMIA OF CHRONIC RENAL INSUFFICIENCY.
In contrast to the anemia found in association with most chronic diseases, the anemia associated with renal failure may be quite severe. Many factors may contribute to the anemia. Folate may be lost into the dialysate in patients receiving long-term dialysis therapy. Iron deficiency may develop because of blood loss from the genitourinary or gastrointestinal tracts or into the hemodialysis coil. Microangiopathic hemolytic anemia (see Color Plate 6E, right) may occur in patients with renal failure because of malignant hypertension, or in the hemolytic-uremic syndrome. In the absence of any of these mechanisms, the degree of anemia correlates roughly with the increase in the blood urea nitrogen and creatinine levels. Although red cell survival may be moderately shortened, the mechanism underlying the anemia is mainly reduced red cell production. Failure of the erythropoietin-secreting function of the kidney appears to be responsible for the impaired marrow response to the anemia.

Blood transfusions are infrequently required. The hematocrit rarely drops below 15 per cent, and most patients tolerate this degree of anemia remarkably well. Long-term dialysis therapy may result in a modest reduction in the degree of anemia,

provided that folate or iron deficiency does not develop as a complicating factor. Human erythropoietin derived from recombinant DNA is extremely effective in treating the anemia of chronic renal disease in patients maintained by hemodialysis. An initial intravenous dose of 150 units per kilogram of body weight three times per week usually raises the hematocrit to 35 per cent or greater in 6 to 8 weeks. Most patients require a maintenance dose between 50 and 125 units per kilogram of body weight three times per week. Intravenous injections of erythropoietin are generally administered after each dialysis treatment. Following a successful renal homograft, normal and even supranormal hematocrit values may be achieved.

ANEMIA IN CIRRHOSIS AND OTHER LIVER DISEASE. Anemia is a frequent manifestation of liver disease; the pathogenetic mechanisms responsible may be more varied than those underlying the anemia of chronic disease. The anemia is generally normocytic and normochromic, but occasionally it may be mildly macrocytic. It is unusual for the MCV to exceed 115 fl in the absence of advanced folate deficiency with frank megaloblastic changes in the marrow. Etiologic factors implicated in the pathogenesis of the anemia associated with liver disease include chronic alcoholism and its effect on erythropoiesis; iron deficiency due to blood loss from gastritis, peptic ulcer, varices, and deficient coagulation factors; sequestration of erythrocytes and other formed elements of the blood by the enlarged spleen resulting from portal hypertension; exaggeration of the degree of anemia because of the increased plasma volume associated with cirrhosis; and alterations in the lipid composition of erythrocyte membranes.

ANEMIAS ASSOCIATED WITH ENDOCRINE DISORDERS. Anemia frequently accompanies disorders of the pituitary gland, the thyroid gland, the adrenal glands, and the gonads. In general, the anemia is mild and by itself produces few symptoms. Reduced tissue oxygen requirements as a result of the endocrine disturbance may result in diminished renal production of erythropoietin. Loss of the stimulating effect of androgens on erythrocyte production may be a factor in some cases. Endocrine disorders tend to begin insidiously; the early symptoms are generally no more specific than fatigue and lassitude. When initial laboratory testing reveals anemia, the diagnostic studies may be directed to the hematopoietic system. Unless endocrine disease is included in the differential diagnosis of a normocytic, normochromic anemia, the primary diagnosis may be overlooked.

Anagnostou A, Kurtzman NA: Hematological consequences of renal failure. *In* Brenner BM, Rector FC (eds.): The Kidney. 3rd ed. Philadelphia, W. B. Saunders Company, 1986. *A comprehensive treatise on the subject, with over 500 references.*
Eschbach JW: The anemia of chronic renal failure: Pathophysiology and the effects of recombinant erythropoietin. Kidney Int 35:134, 1989. *Clinical features and the application of erythropoietin in the treatment of the anemia of chronic renal failure presented in the format of a clinical conference.*
Savage D, Lindenbaum J: Anemia in alcoholics. Medicine 65:322, 1986. *A review of factors causing anemia in alcoholics, the group of patients most likely to manifest advanced liver disease.*
Williams WJ, Beutler E, Erslev AJ, et al. (eds.): Hematology. 4th ed. New York, McGraw-Hill Book Company, 1990. *Extensive references to the anemias associated with renal and endocrine disorders.*

131 Hypochromic Anemias
James P. Kushner

Anemias associated with a subnormal average cell hemoglobin concentration (mean corpuscular hemoglobin concentration [MCHC]) are classified as hypochromic. When the average cell size (mean corpuscular volume [MCV]) is also reduced, the anemia is classified as hypochromic, microcytic. Hypochromia and microcytosis can be detected either by examination of the stained blood smear (see Color Plate 5K) or by calculation of the erythrocyte indices (Table 131–1). The widespread use of electronic cell counting equipment makes available the erythrocyte

TABLE 131–1. RED CELL INDICES*
IN HYPOCHROMIC AND MICROCYTIC ANEMIAS

	MCV (fl)	MCHC (gm/dl)	MCH (pg)
Normal	83–96	32–36	28–34
Hypochromic	83–100	28–31	23–31
Microcytic	70–82	32–36	22–27
Hypochromic-microcytic	50–79	24–31	11–29

*Variations in the methods for measuring the red blood cell count, the volume of packed red cells, and the hemoglobin concentration could change the values slightly.

indices at the same time that anemia is usually detected by the finding of subnormal values for the hemoglobin concentration and the hematocrit.

The developing erythrocyte requires iron, protoporphyrin, and globin for the biosynthesis of hemoglobin. Hypochromic anemias, characterized by deficient hemoglobin synthesis, can be divided into three groups, depending on which of the three components required for hemoglobin biosynthesis is deficient (Table 131–2).

IRON DEFICIENCY ANEMIA

DEFINITIONS. Iron deficiency anemia occurs when body iron stores become inadequate for the needs of normal erythropoiesis. Body iron stores must be exhausted before red cell production is restricted; therefore, anemia occurs at a late stage of iron deficiency. In its fully developed form, iron-deficient erythropoiesis is characterized by hypochromia and microcytosis of the circulating erythrocytes, low plasma iron and ferritin concentrations, and a transferrin saturation of about 15 per cent or less. Iron deficiency anemia is a sign of disease and is not in itself a complete diagnosis.

PREVALENCE. Iron deficiency is the most common cause of anemia throughout the world, although it is difficult to define its prevalence precisely. In parts of Africa and India, where marginal dietary intake and excessive iron loss due to intestinal parasites are present together, over half the population may suffer from iron deficiency anemia.

In most developed countries, about 3 per cent of men, 20 per cent of women, and over 50 per cent of pregnant women are deficient in iron, as judged by plasma iron levels. As judged by serum ferritin levels, iron stores are greatly reduced in about 25 per cent of children, 30 per cent of adolescents, 30 per cent of menstruating women, 60 per cent of pregnant women, and 3 per cent of men.

IRON METABOLISM. The total iron content of a healthy human subject remains within relatively narrow limits. Loss of iron from the body is precisely matched by absorption of iron from food. Iron loss is not due to "excretion" in the usual sense but rather to loss of intact cells containing iron. Epithelial cells

TABLE 131–2. CLASSIFICATION OF ANEMIAS CHARACTERIZED BY DEFICIENT HEMOGLOBIN SYNTHESIS AND THE PRESENCE OF HYPOCHROMIC ERYTHROCYTES

I. Disorders of iron metabolism
  A. Iron deficiency anemia
  B. Anemia of chronic disease
  C. Hereditary atransferrinemia
  D. Congenital hypochromic-microcytic anemia with iron overload (Shahidi-Nathan-Diamond syndrome)
II. Disorders of porphyrin and heme synthesis: sideroblastic anemias
  A. Acquired sideroblastic anemias
    1. Idiopathic refractory sideroblastic anemia
    2. Complicating other diseases
    3. Associated with drugs or toxins—ethanol, INH, lead
  B. Hereditary sideroblastic anemias
    1. X chromosome–linked
    2. Autosomal recessive
III. Disorders of globin synthesis
  A. The thalassemias (Ch. 136)
  B. Hemoglobinopathies characterized by unstable hemoglobins (Ch. 136)

from the gastrointestinal and urinary tracts, and from the skin, account for the normal daily iron loss in men of about 1 mg. In women, menstrual flow, childbearing, and lactation are additional routes of iron loss.

The body iron content in normal adult men is about 50 to 55 mg per kilogram of body weight and in women is about 35 to 40 mg per kilogram. This difference reflects the high incidence of iron deficiency in women and does not indicate any fundamental differences in iron metabolism between the sexes. Most of the body iron is found in hemoglobin, with smaller amounts in myoglobin and iron storage compounds (Table 131–3). Only a minute portion is found in plasma, where it is bound to transferrin.

The metabolism of iron is dominated by its role in hemoglobin synthesis. Iron incorporated into hemoglobin is utilized over and over again through an internal cycle, the *iron cycle* (Fig. 131–1). The plasma iron compartment, in which iron is bound to the transport protein transferrin, is central to this cycle. Iron moves from the plasma to erythroid precursor cells in the marrow. These cells synthesize hemoglobin and, with maturation, are released into the circulation. At the end of their 120-day lifespan, the red cells are ingested by macrophages, principally in the splenic sinusoids, and the iron is extracted from hemoglobin by the enzyme heme oxygenase. A small portion of this iron is stored in macrophages as ferritin, but most is returned to the plasma, where it becomes bound to transferrin, completing the cycle. In the normal adult male about 30 mg of iron completes the iron cycle daily. One to 2 mg of iron leaves the plasma daily and enters the liver and other tissues, where it is utilized for the synthesis of other hemoproteins such as cytochromes and myoglobin.

ABSORPTION. The average intake of iron in the meat-containing diet in the United States is about 10 to 30 mg per day, but much greater variations occur in different parts of the world. Only 5 to 10 per cent of dietary iron (about 1 mg) is absorbed daily to balance precisely the amount lost. The amount of iron absorbed can increase up to fivefold if body iron stores are depleted or if erythropoiesis is accelerated. The amount absorbed decreases in states of iron overload or if there is erythroid hypoplasia. Total body iron balance is thus regulated at the absorptive step; the precise mechanism by which this control is accomplished has not been defined. Iron is absorbed chiefly in portions of the intestine proximal to the mid-jejunum, and very little is absorbed in more caudal intestinal segments.

Iron is absorbed by two distinct pathways in humans, one for iron in heme and the other for iron in ferrous and ferric iron salts. Heme iron is derived from the hemoglobin, myoglobin, and other heme proteins in foods of animal origin. Exposure to the acid and proteases of gastric juice liberates the heme from its apoprotein. Heme is rapidly taken up by gastrointestinal epithelial cells, and the iron is made available by enzymatic degradation of the porphyrin macrocycle. The absorption of heme iron is influenced very little by other dietary components.

The "bioavailability" of nonheme dietary iron, however, varies greatly. Availability is dependent on the oxidation state and solubility of the iron and the presence of chelating substances in the diet. Factors modifying the form in which iron is presented to the intestinal mucosal cell play an important role in the amount of iron that can be absorbed. At the acidic pH normally found in the stomach, both ferrous and ferric iron are soluble. Patients who have undergone gastrectomy, or who are achlorhydric for other reasons, demonstrate impaired absorption of iron. In the duodenum, as the pH rises, ferric iron is readily converted to

TABLE 131–3. DISTRIBUTION OF IRON IN THE BODY

Compound	Iron Content (mg)		Per Cent of Total Body Iron	
	Men (70 kg)	Women (50 kg)	Men	Women
Hemoglobin	2670	1500	69.6	73.1
Myoglobin	350	220	9.1	10.7
Heme enzymes	8	7	0.2	0.3
Transferrin	6	5	0.2	0.2
Ferritin-hemosiderin	800	320	20.9	15.7
Total	3834	2052	100.0	100.0

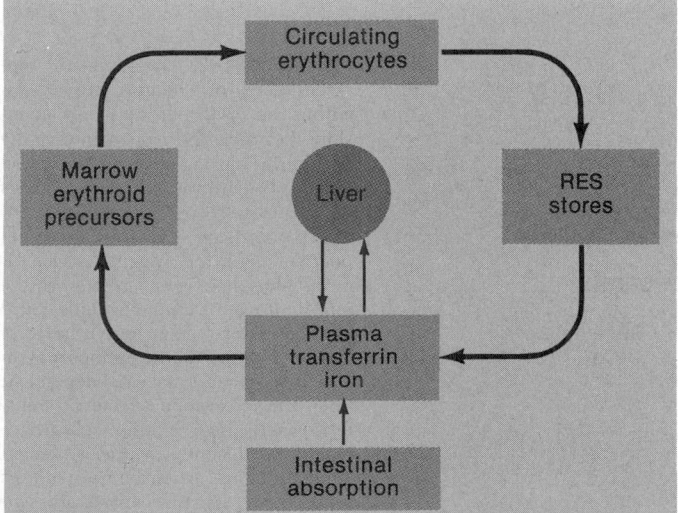

FIGURE 131–1. The internal iron cycle. In the plasma, iron bound to transferrin is transported to the marrow where it is transferred to developing red blood cells and incorporated into hemoglobin. The mature red blood cells are released into the circulation and after 120 days are ingested by macrophages in the reticuloendothelial system (RES). Here the iron is extracted from hemoglobin and returned to plasma, completing the cycle.

insoluble ferric hydroxides. Agents such as ascorbic acid may promote iron absorption by reducing some ferric iron to ferrous iron, which remains soluble at neutral pH. Dietary constituents such as citrate may enhance the solubility of inorganic iron and hence enhance absorption. Phytates, neutral detergent fibers, and other substances present in cereals, grain, and corn impair iron absorption by binding iron as relatively insoluble complexes.

The clinical significance of the various luminal factors that influence iron absorption may be minimal in U.S. society, where the diet provides relatively large amounts of heme iron. In developing countries, however, diets are generally characterized by low meat content and high content of grains and vegetables. Such diets, with low heme iron content and high content of substances that impair nonheme iron absorption, may not meet the iron demands of many individuals. The manipulation of dietary iron content by large-scale iron supplementation programs has been instituted in both developed and underdeveloped countries. The incidence of iron deficiency in the population is decreased by such programs, but the risks to individuals predisposed to iron loading remain to be determined (Ch. 193).

The uptake of iron from the intestinal lumen is both energy dependent and regulated. The uptake of ^{59}Fe by duodenal mucosal cells in iron-deficient individuals exceeds that in normal subjects by twofold or threefold. Although correction of the anemia in iron-deficient subjects by red cell transfusion does not decrease iron uptake, repletion of body iron stores restores the kinetics of iron uptake to normal. Once iron enters the mucosal cell, it must be transported to the serosal surface of the intestine, where iron enters the plasma. Iron within the mucosal cell can have two fates. One is to be incorporated into ferritin within the cytosol of the mucosal cell. Most ferritin iron does not ultimately reach the plasma but is lost from the body when the intestinal mucosal cell is sloughed after its 3- to 4-day lifespan. Iron not incorporated into mucosal cell ferritin is transported across the cell and ultimately appears in plasma as ferric iron bound to transferrin. The process of intracellular transport is unclear. Although transferrin plays a central role in transporting iron from sites of entry into plasma to tissue sites of utilization, it may not play an important role in iron absorption. Rare patients with congenital atransferrinemia show no evidence of deficient iron absorption.

TRANSPORT. Transferrin, the iron transport protein in plasma, is a glycoprotein with an approximate molecular weight of 80,000. The liver is the major source of transferrin synthesis, and the protein is equally distributed in the intravascular and extravascular spaces. Transferrin is capable of binding two iron atoms in the ferric state. In normal subjects the plasma

concentration of transferrin is about 2.5 to 3.0 grams per liter. Plasma transferrin is usually quantified in terms of the amount of iron it will bind, a measure called the *total iron-binding capacity* (TIBC). In normal subjects only about one third of the available transferrin binding sites are occupied (transferrin saturation = 33 per cent). Plasma iron concentration varies diurnally, with the highest values in the morning and the lowest in the evening, but no diurnal variation occurs in the TIBC. Transferrin has no known function other than as a transport protein and is reused for many cycles of iron transport. With the exception of very small amounts of iron in ferritin, all the iron in plasma is carried by transferrin. The affinity of transferrin for iron is sufficiently high that, theoretically, less than one free iron atom might be present in a liter of blood.

CELLULAR UPTAKE. The initial event in the transfer of iron to cells is binding of diferric transferrin to specific, high-affinity receptors on the cell surface. When receptors are lost because of cell maturation (as occurs in developing erythrocytes in vivo) or artificial manipulations in vitro, the ability of the cell to take up iron from transferrin is lost. Cellular iron uptake is directly proportional to the number of transferrin cell-surface receptors. The biosynthesis of hemoglobin by erythroid cells has a high iron requirement, and the human reticulocyte may have as many as 300,000 receptors per cell. Developing erythroid cells in the bone marrow may have even more.

In the process of iron uptake by cells, the transferrin receptor–diferric transferrin complex is internalized into an acidic, nonlysosomal vesicle (Fig. 131–2). At the acidic pH of the vesicle, iron is readily dissociated from diferric transferrin, but the resulting apotransferrin remains bound to the receptor. The transferrin receptor–apotransferrin complex is transported back to the cell surface, where, at neutral pH, the apotransferrin is liberated and becomes available for another cycle of iron binding and release.

Once iron enters the cell, two events occur. One is the delivery of iron to the mitochondria, where it is enzymatically incorporated into protoporphyrin to form heme. The other is the incorporation of iron into ferritin. Ferritin iron is a storage form of iron and is probably not utilized by the cell for heme synthesis. Ferritin iron may, however, be recycled for use by other cells.

STORAGE. Iron-free apoferritin is a spherical protein made up of 24 subunits that surround a central cavity. The central cavity of each apoferritin molecule can potentially store more than 4000 molecules of iron. When iron is present in the central cavity, the protein is termed ferritin. The importance of ferritin as an iron storage compound is emphasized by the wide distribution of structurally similar ferritins in both plant and animal tissues. Two different ferritin subunits exist, termed H (the major subunit of heart ferritin) and L (the major subunit of liver ferritin). These may be present in differing quantities within a given ferritin molecule, leading to heterogeneity. The H and L subunits are derived from different genetic loci.

Ferritin meets the requirement of cells for an efficient form of iron storage. It has a large capacity to store iron, maintains a reserve storage capacity (few ferritin molecules are iron replete), and can quickly both take up and release iron. Ferritin aggregates are visible by light microscopy in developing erythroid cells when bone marrow smears are stained with Prussian blue. These "siderotic granules" are found in the cytosol of normal developing erythroblasts and are absent in erythroblasts obtained from subjects with iron deficiency anemia (see Color Plate 5L).

Small amounts of iron-poor ferritin (mostly apoferritin) circulate in plasma and can be accurately measured by a widely available radioimmunoassay. Under most conditions, the concentration of ferritin in the plasma correlates directly with body iron stores. Normal values range from 12 to 325 ng per milliliter, with a mean of about 125 ng for men and 55 ng for women. The concentration of ferritin in iron-deficient individuals is less than 10 ng per milliliter, whereas in individuals with iron overload, the concentration is proportional to the increase in tissue storage iron.

Hemosiderin is an insoluble iron aggregate with a ratio of iron to protein that is high. It is derived from ferritin; however, the reactions leading from ferritin to hemosiderin have not been resolved. Iron in hemosiderin disappears from tissues after repeated venesections, but the mechanism by which iron is mobilized is unknown.

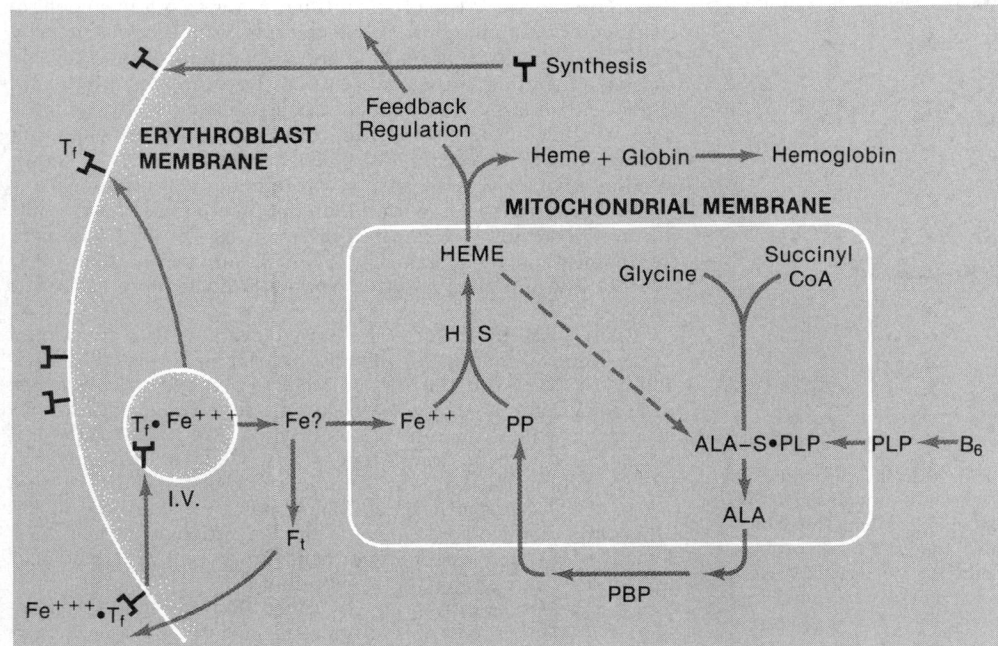

FIGURE 131–2. Diagrammatic representation of heme biosynthesis within the erythroblast. The relationships between the iron pathway, the porphyrin biosynthetic pathway, the vitamin B_6 pathway, and the synthesis of transferrin receptors are illustrated. The biosynthesis of porphyrins is dependent upon the availability of pyridoxal phosphate as a cofactor at the rate-limiting Δ-aminolevulinic acid synthase step. The biosynthesis of heme requires both protoporphyrin and iron. Iron uptake is dependent upon the interaction of diferric transferrin with high affinity cell-surface receptors. Receptor synthesis is regulated by heme; when heme synthesis is impaired, more receptors are synthesized and the cell takes up more iron. T_f = transferrin ⊤ receptors for diferric T_f; I.V. = the acidic, non-lysosomal intermediate vesicle; Fe^{+++} = ferric iron; PP = protoporphyrin; PBP = porphyrin biosynthetic pathway; ALA = Δ-aminolevulinic acid; ALA-s = Δ-aminolevulinic acid synthase; PLP = pyridoxal-5'-phosphate; and B_6 = vitamin B_6.

THE MACROPHAGE. While net iron uptake occurs through the intestinal mucosa, most transferrin-bound iron (over 95 per cent) reflects iron recycled from damaged or aged red blood cells by macrophages in the spleen and other organs. Within the macrophage, the membrane of ingested erythrocytes is disrupted and the iron in hemoglobin is oxidized to the trivalent state, forming methemoglobin. The heme and globin are dissociated, and the iron is liberated from hemin (ferric-protoporphyrin) by the microsomal enzyme heme oxygenase, yielding iron and biliverdin. To meet a variable demand for iron, macrophages maintain a storage pool in ferritin and hemosiderin. Under normal conditions, the amount of iron entering the macrophage approximates that leaving, and there is little interchange between iron newly liberated from hemin and iron in the storage pool. Iron from recently destroyed erythrocytes passes quickly through the macrophage and appears in the plasma bound to transferrin.

When the red cell mass is expanding and erythrocytes are being produced more rapidly than they are being destroyed (e.g., following an acute hemorrhage), iron is mobilized from macrophages. The amount of iron leaving the macrophage under these conditions exceeds that entering. When red cell destruction exceeds production (e.g., in aplastic anemia), the amount of iron entering the macrophage exceeds that leaving and iron is deposited in stores. The control mechanism coupling the rate at which iron leaves the macrophage to the rate of erythrocyte production is unknown. Mobilization of iron from the storage pool is interfered with by infection, inflammation, and malignancy; such interference may be responsible for the anemia associated with chronic disease (see Color Plate 5*H*, left).

FERROKINETICS. Ferrokinetic studies, based on tracking ^{59}Fe as it moves from the plasma transferrin to the bone marrow and into circulating erythrocytes, make it possible to assess rates of both effective erythropoiesis and ineffective erythropoiesis. The term *ineffective erythropoiesis* refers to the production of defective erythrocytes that are destroyed before they leave the marrow (or very shortly thereafter). A small proportion of erythropoiesis is ineffective even in normal subjects, but in conditions such as megaloblastic anemia, thalassemia, and sideroblastic anemias, ineffective erythropoiesis becomes greatly exaggerated. The plasma ^{59}Fe disappearance, expressed as the half-life (t½), is normally between 60 and 120 minutes. More rapid disappearance (a shorter t½) is found in iron deficiency and conditions with accelerated erythropoiesis (such as polycythemia and hemolytic anemias). A long t½ indicates erythroid hypoplasia. The *plasma iron transport* (PIT) rate is a measure of the rate at which iron

leaves the plasma. The PIT is a good index of total erythropoiesis, whether effective or ineffective. The PIT correlates well with the total nucleated red cell mass and the rate of red cell production. However, when erythropoiesis is reduced, or when the degree of transferrin saturation is high, the interpretation of the PIT is complicated by transfer of iron to tissues other than marrow.

The *erythrocyte iron turnover* (EIT) rate measures the rate at which iron moves from marrow to circulating red cells and correlates well with the reticulocyte index.

The *marrow transit time* (MTT) evaluates the responsiveness of the marrow to erythropoietin. In general, there is an inverse correlation between the MTT and the degree of erythropoietic stimulation. In situations characterized by an appropriate marrow response to anemia, the MTT may be less than 24 hours.

Ferrokinetic measurements are useful for clinical and investigational purposes but are only approximations. Sophisticated computer analysis of plasma iron disappearance curves, coupled with body surface counting over the liver, spleen, and sacrum, may yield a more accurate assessment of the rates at which iron moves through the iron cycle, but such analyses are not routinely employed for clinical purposes.

PATHOGENESIS. Iron deficiency comes about as a late manifestation of prolonged negative iron balance caused by one or a combination of the following factors: inadequate dietary intake, malabsorption, blood loss, repeated pregnancies, and rapid growth during childhood. As daily iron loss under normal conditions is very small (about 1 mg), assigning the cause of iron deficiency in adults to inadequate intake or malabsorption implies chronicity measured in years. Iron losses that occur from the gastrointestinal tract or through excessive menstrual bleeding are far more important factors. Factors leading to negative iron balance can be divided into two broad categories: decreased iron uptake and increased iron loss (Table 131–4).

Decreased Iron Uptake. The daily dietary iron requirement for healthy adult men is about 5 to 10 mg. For premenopausal women the daily dietary requirement is higher, roughly 7 to 20 mg per day. In the United States the average diet contains about 6 mg per 1000 calories. The average man therefore consumes more iron than needed, but many women subsist on a marginal iron uptake. Because of the adequacy of their diets and their larger iron stores, men in the United States rarely develop iron deficiency solely on the basis of an inadequate dietary intake of iron. Even in women, some factor in addition to poor diet is usually necessary before overt anemia develops.

Gastric acid facilitates the absorption of ferric iron in the diet

TABLE 131–4. FACTORS PRODUCING NEGATIVE IRON BALANCE AND IRON DEFICIENCY

I. **Decreased iron uptake**
  A. Inadequate diet
  B. Impaired absorption
    1. Achlorhydria
    2. Gastric surgery
    3. Celiac disease
    4. Pica
II. **Increased iron loss**
  A. Gastrointestinal bleeding (Ch. 111)
    1. Neoplasm
    2. Duodenal and gastric ulcers
    3. Hiatal hernia
    4. Gastritis from salicylates, other drugs, or toxins
    5. Diverticulosis
    6. Ulcerative colitis and regional enteritis
    7. Hookworm
    8. Meckel's diverticulum
    9. Hemorrhoids
    10. Arteriovenous malformations
  B. Menometrorrhagia
  C. Repeated blood donations
  D. Repeated pregnancies
  E. Hemoglobinuria due to chronic intravascular hemolysis
  F. Hereditary hemorrhagic telangiectasia
  G. Idiopathic pulmonary hemosiderosis
  H. Disorders of hemostasis

(although it has little effect on heme iron or ferrous iron), and iron deficiency is a frequent complication following gastric operations. Additional factors that impair iron absorption after gastrectomy include rapid intestinal transit and bypass of the most active sites of iron absorption in the duodenum (as occurs in the Billroth II or Polya procedures). Malabsorption of iron may also occur in patients with adult celiac disease, and rarely iron deficiency anemia may be the dominant manifestation of celiac disease.

Impaired absorption of iron because of interactions with food substances such as phytates and vegetable fibers has been discussed. The ingestion of unusual substances, a practice known as *pica*, may also impair iron absorption. Although pica may be a manifestation of iron deficiency, in certain cultural groups the compulsive ingestion of substances such as clay (geophagia) or starch (amylophagia) may lead to iron deficiency. Clay interferes with iron absorption by acting in the gut as an ion exchange resin. Laundry starch is a carbohydrate with a very low iron content. When it is consumed in large quantities to the exclusion of other foods, a dietary deficiency of iron results.

Increased Iron Loss. Gastrointestinal bleeding is by far the most common cause of iron deficiency in men and is second only to menstrual loss as a cause in women. Repeated pregnancies without iron supplementation are a less common cause of iron deficiency in women.

Although any hemorrhagic lesion of the gastrointestinal tract may cause iron deficiency (Table 131–4), those most likely to do so are associated with chronic occult bleeding and the steady loss of small amounts of blood. To estimate the effect of blood loss on iron balance, it is convenient to consider that 1.0 ml of blood contains about 0.4 mg of iron. A steady blood loss of as little as 4 to 5 ml per day (1.6 to 2.0 mg of iron) can result in negative iron balance and depletion of iron stores over several years. Failure to detect occult blood in the stool, even after repetitive testing, does not exclude gastrointestinal blood loss as the cause of iron deficiency. *Iron deficiency in men and in postmenopausal women must be considered to result from blood loss unless some other cause can be proved.* This is a critical dictum because iron deficiency anemia may be the first sign of a cancer of the gastrointestinal tract, and the anemia may lead to the diagnosis when the tumor is in an operable stage. Carcinoma of the cecum, for example, is often clinically silent until the symptoms of anemia appear.

Blood loss from erosive gastritis due to aspirin ingestion is a frequent cause of iron deficiency. Chronic ingestion of as few as two aspirin tablets daily may lead to blood loss of up to 4.5 ml per day.

CLINICAL MANIFESTATIONS. Iron deficiency anemia is not a disease; it is a sign of disease. In some patients, iron deficiency anemia is discovered incidentally when the presenting signs and symptoms are those of the disease that led to the deficiency. In some patients, signs and symptoms of both the underlying disease and the iron deficiency are found together. In others, only the symptoms of iron deficiency are present, and the disease leading to the deficiency is occult.

The onset of iron deficiency anemia is insidious, and the progression of symptoms is gradual. Patients are often able to accommodate quite well to the anemia and may continue to perform strenuous work with few symptoms. Fatigue, irritability, palpitations, dizziness, breathlessness, and headache are all common complaints of symptomatic individuals with anemia of any type and do not in themselves suggest iron deficiency as the cause of the anemia. However, some clinical findings do specifically suggest the presence of iron deficiency.

Chlorosis, a peculiar greenish pallor of iron-deficient adolescent girls, was frequently described in the decades between 1890 and 1910, although now is rarely noted. Oral lesions associated with iron deficiency include angular stomatitis (ulcerations or fissures at the corners of the mouth), atrophy of the lingual papillae, and varying degrees of glossitis. *Ozena* (chronic atrophy of the nasal mucosa associated with a foul-smelling discharge) occurs in some patients with iron deficiency anemia, particularly in southeastern Europe. Thinning and flattening of nails and finally the development of spoon-shaped nails (koilonychia) have been described in patients with advanced iron deficiency.

The association of dysphagia, angular stomatitis, and lingual abnormalities with iron deficiency anemia (Plummer-Vinson or Paterson-Kelly syndrome) is rarely noted in the United States but is quite common in Great Britain and Scandinavia. The dysphagia is due to the development of a mucosal web at the juncture of the hypopharynx and esophagus. Multiple webs may develop, usually extending from the anterior wall of the esophagus into the lumen. Occasionally, they may encircle the lumen, forming a cufflike structure. In other patients a stricture with or without a web may be found, drastically constricting the opening into the esophagus at the level of the cricoid cartilage. Relief of the dysphagia requires rupturing of the webs or dilatation of the stenosis, because repletion of the iron stores alone is not effective. Other gastrointestinal complaints, such as anorexia, pyrosis, flatulence, nausea, belching, and constipation, are common in association with advanced iron deficiency anemia.

Pica, as already mentioned, can be a cause of iron deficiency but it also may be a striking manifestation of iron deficiency. The ingestion of ice (pagophagia) is particularly common. Many patients compulsively eat one or other food items; oddly, the object of the unnatural dietary craving usually contains very little iron.

The spleen is slightly enlarged in about 10 per cent of patients with iron deficiency anemia. There are no specific pathologic changes in the organ, and the splenomegaly recedes with correction of the iron deficiency. Neuralgic pains, numbness, and tingling without objective neurologic abnormalities are reported by 15 to 30 per cent of patients, and rarely iron deficiency anemia may lead to increased intracranial pressure, papilledema, and the clinical picture of pseudotumor cerebri.

LABORATORY FINDINGS. The degree of anemia is variable and depends upon the duration of iron-limited erythropoiesis. Because of the hypochromia, the hemoglobin concentration is usually reduced to a greater degree than the hematocrit. The mean corpuscular volume (MCV), mean corpuscular hemoglobin (MCH), and mean corpuscular hemoglobin concentration (MCHC) are all usually reduced. The degree of change in the red cell indices is related to both the duration and the severity of the anemia. Average values for patients with hemoglobin concentrations of 8 to 9 grams per deciliter are MCV of 74 fl, MCHC of 28 grams per deciliter, and MCH of 20 pg.

A well-stained blood smear reveals an increase in the area of central pallor in the individual red corpuscles (hypochromia), microcytes, and marked variations in cell size (anisocytosis) and shape (poikilocytosis) (Fig. 131–3 and Color Plate 5*K*). The plasma iron concentration is generally less than 50 μg per deciliter, and the plasma TIBC (the transferrin concentration) is greater than 350 μg per deciliter. As a result, the transferrin saturation is less

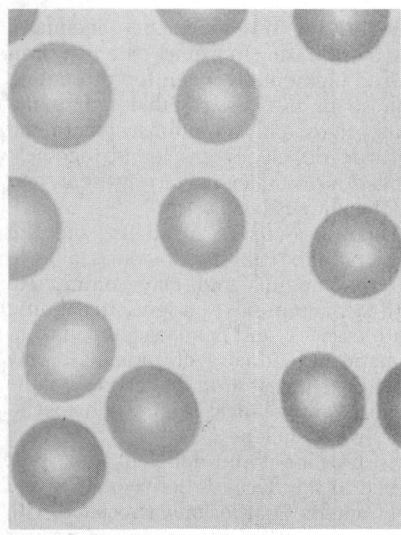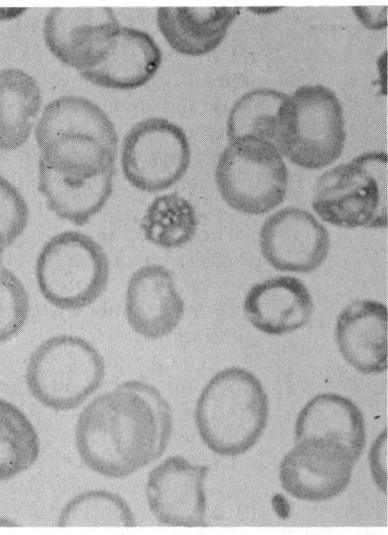

FIGURE 131–3. Blood smear from a patient with advanced iron deficiency anemia (*right*) and from a normal subject (*left*). The red cells from the iron-deficient subject are poorly hemoglobinized (hypochromic), are smaller than normal (microcytic), and vary in size and shape (anisocytosis and poikilocytosis). (Wright's stain, × 1000.)

than 15 per cent. The plasma ferritin concentration is generally less than 10 ng per milliliter. The last enzymatic reaction leading to the biosynthesis of heme (the ferrochelatase or heme synthase reaction) requires both iron and protoporphyrin as substrates. In iron deficiency excess protoporphyrin accumulates in the developing erythrocyte and is retained by the circulating erythrocytes. As a result, the free erythrocyte protoporphyrin (FEP) is increased, generally about five times normal (normal range, 30 to 80 µg per deciliter of red cells).

Both the percentage and the absolute number of reticulocytes are usually normal. The osmotic fragility of the erythrocytes may be normal, but more often there is increased resistance to hemolysis in hypotonic salt solutions. Although the leukocyte count is usually normal, in very chronic iron deficiency a slight decrease in the absolute number of granulocytes may be seen. The platelet count is usually elevated to levels of about two to three times normal and returns to normal after therapy. Rarely, in severe, longstanding iron deficiency anemia, mild thrombocytopenia may be noted.

Examination of the bone marrow is generally not required to establish a diagnosis of iron deficiency anemia. An exception is the clinical situation when suspected iron deficiency coexists with a chronic disease. Although anemias associated with chronic disease may mimic iron deficiency (see below), they can be distinguished by examination of the marrow. In iron deficiency the marrow is usually normocellular and there is mild erythroid hyperplasia. Macrophage iron is absent or severely reduced. Fewer than 10 per cent of the marrow normoblasts contain siderotic granules visible with Prussian blue staining. In the anemia of chronic disease, macrophage iron stores are normal or increased; however, as in iron deficiency, very few normoblasts contain siderotic granules.

The sequence of laboratory changes in slowly developing iron deficiency is fairly predictable. Initially, as iron stores are depleted, the serum ferritin concentration falls. At the earliest stage of iron deficiency, the transferrin concentration rises, the plasma iron concentration falls, and the FEP increases. When anemia first appears, the morphology of the circulating erythrocytes and the erythrocyte indices are generally normal. As the anemia progresses, the morphology becomes clearly hypochromic and microcytic, and the indices reflect this.

TREATMENT. *Every effort must be made to recognize and, if possible, correct the underlying cause.* This should be possible in most patients. A simpler goal is correcting the anemia and replenishing body iron stores.

Iron is highly effective in treating iron deficiency but has no other legitimate therapeutic use. Iron exerts no beneficial effect on any of the anemias not caused by iron deficiency. A large number of preparations containing iron have been promoted for the oral treatment of iron deficiency, but none has any advantage over simple ferrous salts (ferrous sulfate, ferrous gluconate, and ferrous fumarate). Ferrous sulfate is the standard preparation for oral use. A daily dose of about 200 mg of elemental iron produces an optimal response. This dose is achieved with three ferrous sulfate tablets (each tablet contains 60 mg of elemental iron) given in divided doses with or just after a meal. Iron is best absorbed when the stomach is empty, but gastric irritation is extremely common when iron is taken this way. In spite of some reduction in absorption when iron is taken with meals, the gain in patient compliance is worth this slight disadvantage. Enteric-coated preparations, designed to reduce gastric irritation by retarding dissolution of the iron, cannot be recommended because with them the most actively absorbing regions of the intestine are bypassed and absorption is markedly reduced. Although large doses of ascorbic or succinic acid increase iron absorption as much as 20 to 30 per cent, they add greatly to the expense of therapy.

Some patients given oral iron therapy complain of gastrointestinal symptoms (nausea, epigastric pain, cramps, diarrhea); however, it is rare that these symptoms are severe enough to require discontinuation of therapy. Gastric symptoms appear to be dose related, and patients intolerant of full therapeutic doses may be able to take a dose of 120 mg per day. Gastric symptoms may be minimized by gradually increasing the dose during the first week of therapy. Regardless of the form of oral therapy used, it is important to continue treatment for 6 to 12 months after the anemia has been corrected. The prolonged therapy allows for repletion of iron stores.

When adequate doses of iron are given, there is often a rapid subjective improvement with a reduction of fatigue, lassitude, and other nonspecific symptoms. This response may occur within 2 or 3 days, before any evidence of a hematologic response can be detected. An increase in the number of reticulocytes is the first sign of hematologic response, and a maximal value of 5 to 10 per cent is usually achieved after about 10 days of therapy. The height of the reticulocyte peak and the rate of hemoglobin regeneration are proportional to the severity of the anemia. With only slight to moderate degrees of anemia, a pronounced reticulocyte response cannot be expected. Although the hemoglobin concentration increases more rapidly at low levels than at high, it takes about 2 months to reach normal values regardless of the starting level.

It is not rare to encounter patients said to have iron deficiency anemia unresponsive to oral iron therapy. The following possible explanations for failure to respond to iron should be considered: (1) The diagnosis is incorrect and the anemia is not due to iron deficiency; (2) a complicating illness is present that dampens the expected response to iron therapy; (3) the patient failed to take the iron preparation as prescribed; (4) an ineffective iron preparation was prescribed; (5) the patient is continuing to lose iron in excess of intake; and rarely (6) there is malabsorption of iron.

Parenteral iron therapy should be reserved for patients who

(1) are unable to tolerate iron compounds given orally, (2) repeatedly fail to heed instructions or are incapable of following them, (3) are losing blood at a rate too rapid to be compensated for by oral iron intake, (4) have a disorder such as ulcerative colitis or regional enteritis in which symptoms may be aggravated by oral iron therapy, or (5) are unable to absorb iron from the gastrointestinal tract.

Iron-dextran complex (Imferon) containing 50 mg of iron per milliliter is the preparation of choice for parenteral administration. The total dose required to correct the anemia and to replenish stores can be calculated by the following formula:

$$\text{Iron to be injected (mg)} = [15 - \text{patient's Hb (gm/dl)}] \times \text{body weight (kg)} \times 3$$

Iron-dextran can be given intramuscularly or intravenously. Intravenous administration does not appear to have a higher incidence of adverse effects than the intramuscular route. Anaphylactic reactions are rare (0.1 to 0.6 per cent), but fever, arthralgia, myalgia, and regional adenopathy occur in about 5 per cent of patients. Intramuscular injections should be made into the upper outer quadrant of the buttock, and the skin displaced laterally prior to injection to prevent staining of the skin by reflux of the dark-brown iron solution along the injection path. A test dose of 0.5 ml should be given initially to test for hypersensitivity. Generally, 2.5 ml is injected into each buttock (total of 5 ml or 250 mg of iron) daily. Intravenous administration permits larger doses to be given in a single injection; thus, the discomfort and inconvenience of repeated intramuscular injections can be avoided. After testing for hypersensitivity, 10 ml (500 mg of iron) of undiluted iron-dextran may be administered over about a 5-minute period. In Great Britain and Europe, it is usual to administer the entire dose calculated by the formula in a single intravenous infusion. A 1:20 dilution of iron-dextran in saline is prepared and administered at an initial flow rate of 20 drops per minute. After 5 minutes, if no side effects are observed, the rate is increased to 40 to 60 drops per minute. Dextrose solutions should not be used as a diluent because the incidence of superficial phlebitis may be as high as 25 per cent with this vehicle.

PROGNOSIS. The prognosis in iron deficiency relates only to the underlying disorder causing the anemia. Patients rarely, if ever, die of iron deficiency anemia itself, but they may die of the underlying cause. Recurrence of iron deficiency anemia after treatment is common, emphasizing the importance of identifying and effectively treating the cause of the iron deficiency.

HYPOCHROMIC ANEMIAS NOT CAUSED BY IRON DEFICIENCY

Once iron deficiency has been excluded as the cause of a hypochromic anemia, a limited number of diagnostic possibilities remain. A presumptive diagnosis is generally possible after analysis of the history and physical examination and the basic hematologic parameters. If the diagnosis remains obscure, a useful approach is to segregate the diagnostic possibilities on the basis of an accurate determination of the serum iron level. When the serum iron is reduced to levels at which the transferrin saturation is less than about 15 per cent, only iron deficiency and the anemia of chronic disease need be considered.

Hypochromic anemias due to defects in globin biosynthesis (the thalassemias and hemoglobinopathies characterized by unstable hemoglobins) are discussed in Ch. 136.

THE ANEMIA OF CHRONIC DISEASE

The anemia of chronic disease is not always hypochromic; however, because of its association with hypoferremia, it is best discussed under the heading of hypochromic anemias. Although the anemia of chronic disease is usually normocytic and normochromic, hypochromia and even microcytosis may be the dominant morphologic abnormalities. When microcytosis is present, it is usually not as marked as in iron deficiency. The MCV rarely falls below 72 fl.

DEFINITION. A mild to moderate anemia frequently accompanies chronic infections, inflammatory diseases such as rheumatoid arthritis, and cancers. Since these are so common, the anemia of chronic disease is frequently encountered and may be second only to iron deficiency anemia in overall incidence. The anemia of chronic disease is defined by the presence of a chronic disease, anemia, and hypoferremia despite abundant quantities of iron in macrophage stores.

ETIOLOGY AND PATHOGENESIS. Three factors seem to interact in the pathogenesis of the anemia: (1) impaired flow of iron from macrophages to plasma, (2) decreased erythrocyte lifespan, and (3) inadequate marrow response to the mild hemolysis.

Characteristically, the serum iron level is decreased, TIBC is reduced (a point often useful in differentiating the anemia from iron deficiency anemia), and transferrin saturation is subnormal. Injection of ^{59}Fe-labeled red cells (or labeled hemoglobin) reveals rapid clearance by reticuloendothelial cells but defective reutilization of the iron for new hemoglobin synthesis. In bone marrow aspirates stained for iron, there is an increase in hemosiderin and ferritin in the macrophages; however, the number of red cell precursors containing siderotic granules is reduced. A decrease in the amount of iron available for heme biosynthesis results in the production of hypochromic erythrocytes and, as in iron deficiency, an increase in FEP to levels of three to five times normal. In contrast to iron deficiency anemia, in the anemia of chronic disease, the FEP increases slowly and does not become clearly abnormal until significant anemia has developed. Humoral factors are probably involved in the pathogenesis of the abnormal iron metabolism. These factors include the cytokines interleukin 1, interleukin 6, and tumor necrosis factor–alpha (TNF-α). TNF-α, when injected into humans, produces the abnormalities of iron metabolism that characterize the anemia of chronic disease. It is not known if this is a direct effect or an indirect effect mediated through other factors produced in response to TNF-α.

The erythrocyte lifespan is about 80 days rather than the normal 120 days. When red cells from a patient with the anemia of chronic disease are transfused into normal subjects, they survive normally. Conversely, normal red cells have a shortened survival when transfused into patients with anemia. This finding suggests that an extracorpuscular factor is involved in the pathogenesis of the hemolysis. However, no such factor has yet been identified. Normally, the bone marrow should be able to compensate for such a modest reduction in erythrocyte survival. Failure of the marrow to do so implies that impaired production capacity is important in the pathogenesis of the anemia. The marrow response to anemia is under the control of erythropoietin. In patients with the anemia of chronic disorders, erythropoietin levels are usually lower than expected for the degree of anemia. The marrow, however, is capable of responding appropriately to erythropoietin when the hormone is injected or when erythropoietin production is stimulated by hypoxia or cobalt administration. The precise mechanism causing failure of erythropoietin release in response to the slowly developing anemia is unknown.

The three basic abnormalities are interrelated in the pathogenesis of the anemia. For example, the response to erythropoietin suggests that the hormone directly or indirectly affects the block in iron metabolism. It appears that balance is eventually reached among the three factors, and thus the anemia is only mild to moderate and does not generally progress to the point at which transfusion therapy is required.

CLINICAL MANIFESTATIONS. Because this type of anemia occurs in association with so many diseases, the clinical manifestations vary widely. Although the signs and symptoms of the underlying disorder usually overshadow those of the anemia, in occasional patients the anemia is the first sign of the underlying disease.

DIAGNOSIS. The anemia develops during the first few months of the underlying illness and rarely progresses thereafter. The hematocrit generally remains constant in a range between 25 and 40 per cent. The red cell morphology is usually normal, as is the reticulocyte count. The characteristic iron determinations are a transferrin saturation less than 15 per cent and a normal serum ferritin level. In the marrow the number of erythroid precursors containing cytoplasmic iron granules (sideroblasts) is decreased, but reticuloendothelial cells contain normal or increased iron stores (see Color Plate 5H, left). Despite the hemolysis, the usual manifestations of increased blood destruction are absent. The serum bilirubin and the excretion of urobilinogen are generally normal.

TREATMENT. Correction of the anemia depends upon successful treatment of the underlying disease. Blood transfusions are not usually necessary because the anemia is generally mild to moderate and is not progressive. Therapy with cobalt, androgenic steroids, and corticosteroids offers more potential for harm than good. The block to iron flow cannot be bypassed, and the administration of oral or parenteral iron is of no benefit. When bleeding causes superimposed iron deficiency, the administration of iron will restore hemoglobin levels to those of the underlying chronic disorder but not back to normal.

SIDEROBLASTIC ANEMIA

DEFINITION. When hypochromic anemia is associated with hyperferremia and increased transferrin saturation, a diagnosis of sideroblastic anemia is suggested. The sideroblastic anemias are a heterogeneous group of disorders associated with various defects in the porphyrin biosynthetic pathway. Porphyrin biosynthetic defects lead to diminished synthesis of heme, which in turn may be associated with an increase in cellular iron uptake (Fig. 131–2). The sideroblastic anemias are characterized by the association of anemia with the presence of an abnormal erythroid precursor in the marrow. The abnormal precursor, the ringed sideroblast, is a normoblast containing excessive deposits of iron within mitochondria. These iron-laden mitochondria, because of their perinuclear distribution, account for the Prussian blue–positive granules forming a full or partial ring around the nucleus of the ringed sideroblast (see Color Plate 6J, right). Normal sideroblasts contain one to four Prussian blue–positive ferritin aggregates in the cytoplasm and no visible iron in mitochondria.

PATHOGENESIS AND CLASSIFICATION. Mitochondrial iron excess appears to be a consequence of defective heme synthesis. A population of hypochromic erythrocytes, common to all the sideroblastic anemias, is morphologic evidence of the synthetic defect. Other common characteristics include abnormalities in porphyrin biosynthesis; an increase in total body iron stores; an increase in the serum iron concentration, often to the point of complete saturation of transferrin; and kinetic evidence of ineffective erythropoiesis. It is customary to divide the sideroblastic anemias into two groups, depending on whether the disorder appears to be acquired or inherited (see Table 131–2).

Acquired Sideroblastic Anemias

IDIOPATHIC REFRACTORY SIDEROBLASTIC ANEMIA. This acquired disease of older adults has an unknown pathogenesis. The anemia develops insidiously and is often discovered during a routine examination. The anemia is usually slightly macrocytic. Examination of the peripheral blood smear reveals two populations of erythrocytes. One is entirely normal, and the other is macrocytic and quite hypochromic with prominent basophilic stippling. Leukocyte and platelet counts are usually normal, but leukopenia is occasionally noted, and either moderate thrombocytopenia or thrombocytosis has been reported. The FEP is increased, but the precise enzymatic defect (or defects) in porphyrin biosynthesis has (or have) not been defined. About 30 to 40 per cent of patients have a palpable spleen. Therapy with pyridoxine or folic acid is not successful, and only rare patients respond to androgens. The median survival for patients with idiopathic refractory sideroblastic anemia is about 10 years; most patients require no therapy. Transfusion therapy should be kept to a minimum because the chronic administration of erythrocytes has led to transfusional hemochromatosis. Therapy with daily subcutaneous infusions of deferoxamine may be of value to selected patients who require repeated transfusion. The condition in about 10 per cent of patients eventually shows evidence of transformation to acute leukemia. No reliable indicators predict the likelihood of leukemic transformation. The closest association between the development of leukemia and the presence of ringed sideroblasts is noted when sideroblastic anemia occurs following chemotherapy for a variety of malignant disorders. Alkylating drugs such as cyclophosphamide, nitrogen mustard, and melphalan are the most common offenders.

SIDEROBLASTIC ANEMIA COMPLICATING OTHER DISEASES. Acquired sideroblastic anemia associated with other diseases and with drugs or toxins is quite common; however, the anemia is usually only mild. Inflammatory diseases such as rheumatoid arthritis, neoplasms, and a variety of primary hematologic disorders have all been associated with a secondary sideroblastic anemia. The treatment, course, and prognosis are all related to the nature of the associated disease.

SIDEROBLASTIC ANEMIA ASSOCIATED WITH DRUGS OR TOXINS. Sideroblastic anemia is a common complication in hospitalized alcoholics. Withdrawal of alcohol results in a reticulocytosis and disappearance of the ringed sideroblasts within 5 to 10 days. *Alcohol* may cause sideroblastic anemia by interfering with pyridoxine metabolism and thus indirectly affecting the activity of Δ-aminolevulinic acid synthetase, the rate-limiting enzyme in the porphyrin biosynthetic pathway. This mechanism likely also underlies the sideroblastic anemia occasionally seen in association with the administration of the antituberculous agent *isonicotinic acid hydrazide* (INH). The sideroblastic anemia that occurs in *lead poisoning* is caused by the inhibition by lead of the enzyme that converts Δ-aminolevulinic acid to porphobilinogen (Δ-aminolevulinic dehydratase) and the enzyme heme synthetase (ferrochelatase). As a result of these two enzymatic defects, it is possible to screen for lead poisoning by detecting either increased urinary excretion of Δ-aminolevulinic acid or a markedly increased FEP.

Hereditary Sideroblastic Anemias

Hereditary sideroblastic anemia is almost always a disease of males and is most likely inherited as an X-linked recessive trait. Although the anemia is usually detected in the late teenage years, in rare cases the anemia is found first in either infancy or adult life. The anemia is severe (average blood hemoglobin, 6.5 grams per deciliter), and the red cell indices indicate marked microcytosis and hypochromia. The inherited defect in some way involves the interaction between Δ-aminolevulinic acid synthetase and its cofactor pyridoxal phosphate. Individuals with hereditary sideroblastic anemia are not pyridoxine deficient; however, large amounts of vitamin B_6 produce partial correction of the anemia. There is an erythroid-specific form of Δ-aminolevulinic acid synthetase that is coded for by a gene on the X chromosome. It seems likely that mutations at this locus will prove to be the cause of many cases of hereditary sideroblastic anemia.

Beutler E, Fairbanks VF: The effects of iron deficiency. *In* Jacobs A, Worwood M (eds.): Iron in Biochemistry and Medicine II. New York, Academic Press, 1980, pp 394–428. *An extensive review of both the hematologic and the nonhematologic manifestations of iron deficiency.*

Miescher PA, Jaffe ER, Finch CA (eds.): Semin Hematol, vol. 19, no. 1, 1984. *An issue of a respected review journal devoted to the clinical aspects of iron deficiency and excess.*

Ward JH, Kushner JP, Kaplan J: Iron: Metabolism and clinical disorders. *In* Fairbanks VF (ed.): Current Hematology and Oncology. Vol. 3. New York, John Wiley & Sons, 1984, pp 1–50. *A review of basic iron metabolism with an extensive list of references.*

Williams WJ, Beutler E, Erslev AJ, et al. (eds.): Hematology. 4th ed. New York, McGraw-Hill Book Company, 1990. *A comprehensive textbook of hematology with an excellent presentation of basic iron metabolism and its application to clinical medicine.*

Wintrobe MM, Lee GR, Boggs DR, et al. (eds.): Clinical Hematology. 8th ed. Philadelphia, Lea & Febiger, 1981. *The oldest standard textbook of hematology with an exhaustive description of the clinical manifestations of iron deficiency anemia.*

132 Megaloblastic Anemias

Robert H. Allen

DEFINITION

The megaloblastic anemias are caused by various defects in DNA synthesis that lead to a common set of hematologic abnormalities of the bone marrow and peripheral blood. The term "megaloblastic" refers to a morphologic abnormality of cell nuclei that is readily recognizable but difficult to describe (see Color Plate 6G and H). The erythrocytic, granulocytic, and megakaryocytic cell lines are all involved, and a pancytopenia may develop. Recognition of megaloblastic anemia is important because two of its most common causes, cobalamin (vitamin B_{12}) deficiency and folate deficiency, are completely corrected with appropriate therapy. The recognition of cobalamin deficiency is of particular importance because it also causes a wide variety of neurologic and psychiatric abnormalities that are preventable or reversible if the diagnosis is made at an early stage.

ETIOLOGY

The four major etiologic categories of megaloblastic anemia are (1) cobalamin deficiency, (2) folate deficiency, (3) drugs, and (4) miscellaneous, which includes rare enzyme deficiencies and unexplained disorders (Table 132–1). The etiology of cobalamin deficiency can be subdivided into causes of decreased ingestion, impaired absorption, or impaired utilization of the vitamin. Folate deficiency can also be caused by decreased intake, by impaired absorption, by impaired utilization, and, in addition, by a number of conditions in which there is an increased requirement for folic acid or an increased loss of folic acid. Drugs that cause megaloblastosis can be categorized as those that are purine or pyrimidine antagonists and those that inhibit some other aspect of DNA synthesis. The miscellaneous category includes enzyme defects and some cases of myelodysplastic syndrome and acute leukemia.

It is important to determine the correct etiology of megalo-

blastic anemia. For example, if a cobalamin-deficient patient is misdiagnosed as having a myelodysplastic syndrome, the use of chemotherapy for the latter condition might result in the early death of a patient who could have been completely cured with cobalamin therapy. Similarly, some causes of cobalamin and folate deficiency require therapy for the underlying disease in addition to replacement therapy with the appropriate vitamin.

INCIDENCE AND PREVALENCE
Cobalamin Deficiency

The term "pernicious anemia," often used as a synonym for cobalamin deficiency, should be reserved for conditions in which a gastric mucosal defect results in insufficient intrinsic factor to facilitate the absorption of physiologic amounts of cobalamin. It is by far the most common cause of cobalamin deficiency in the Western Hemisphere. Pernicious anemia was originally believed to be primarily a disease of elderly individuals of northern European ancestry. It is now clear that it also occurs in individuals in their 20's and in all ethnic groups, including blacks and Hispanics. Before the discovery of liver therapy in 1926, perni-

TABLE 132–1. ETIOLOGIC CLASSIFICATION OF THE MEGALOBLASTIC ANEMIAS

Category	Etiologic Mechanisms
I. Cobalamin deficiency	
A. Decreased ingestion	Poor diet, lack of animal products, strict vegetarianism

B. Impaired absorption	1. Failure to release cobalamin from food protein
	  Old age
	  Gastrectomy (partial)
	2. Intrinsic factor (IF) deficiency
	  Pernicious anemia
	  Gastrectomy (total)
	  Destruction of gastric mucosa by caustics
	  Congenital abnormal or absent IF molecule
	3. Chronic pancreatic disease
	4. Competitive parasites
	  Bacteria in diverticula of bowel, blind loops
	  Fish tapeworm infestations (*Diphyllobothrium latum*)
	5. Intrinsic intestinal disease
	  Ileal resection, Crohn's disease, radiation ileitis
	  Tropical sprue, celiac disease
	  Infiltrative intestinal disease (e.g., lymphoma, scleroderma)
	  Drug-induced malabsorption
	  Congenital selective malabsorption (Imerslund-Gräsbeck syndrome)

C. Impaired utilization	Congenital enzyme deficiencies Lack of transcobalamin II Nitrous oxide administration
II. Folate deficiency	
A. Decreased ingestion	Poor diet, lack of vegetables Alcoholism Infancy
B. Impaired absorption	Intestinal short circuits Tropical sprue, celiac disease Anticonvulsants, sulfasalazine, other drugs Congenital malabsorption
C. Impaired utilization	Folic acid antagonists: methotrexate, triamterene, trimethoprim, pyrimethamine, ethanol Congenital enzyme deficiencies
D. Increased requirement	Pregnancy, infancy Hyperthyroidism Chronic hemolytic disease Neoplastic disease, exfoliative skin disease
E. Increased loss	Hemodialysis
III. Drugs—metabolic inhibitors	Purine synthesis: methotrexate, 6-mercaptopurine, 6-thioguanine, azathioprine Pyrimidine synthesis: methotrexate, 6-azauridine Thymidylate synthesis: methotrexate, 5-fluorouracil Deoxyribonucleotide synthesis: hydroxyurea, cytosine arabinoside
IV. Miscellaneous	
A. Inborn errors	Lesch-Nyhan syndrome Hereditary orotic aciduria Others
B. Unexplained disorders	Pyridoxine-responsive megaloblastic anemia Thiamine-responsive megaloblastic anemia Some cases of myelodysplastic syndrome Some cases of acute myelogenous leukemia

cious anemia was invariably fatal. About 1.0 per cent of individuals in the United States will develop pernicious anemia at some time during their life. With a population of 250 million, an average lifetime of 75 years, and the assumption that cobalamin deficiency exists for an average of 5 years before it is treated or the patient dies, there should be about 150,000 patients at various stages of cobalamin deficiency in the United States at any point in time. Approximately 10 per cent of the U.S. population over age 70 have low or low-normal serum cobalamin levels *and* metabolic evidence of cobalamin deficiency (elevated levels of serum methylmalonic acid and homocysteine that fall to normal with cobalamin therapy). The etiology and the hematologic and neuropsychiatric significance of these findings are unknown at the present time. These estimates of the actual and potential incidence of cobalamin deficiency further emphasize the importance of recognizing this eminently treatable disease.

Folate Deficiency, Drugs, and Other Causes

The incidence of folate deficiency and of drug-related megaloblastic anemia is less well established. Through its association with alcoholism, folate deficiency is far from a rare condition. The marked increase in the use of chemotherapeutic agents to treat malignancies and immune disorders suggests that these drugs may now be the most common cause of megaloblastic anemia in the Western Hemisphere.

PATHOGENESIS AND PATHOLOGY
Mechanism of Megaloblastosis

FOLATE DEFICIENCY. Folate functions to transfer one-carbon units, such as methyl, methylene, and formyl groups, to various substrates in a variety of enzymatic reactions that are intimately related to the synthesis of DNA, RNA, and proteins. In folate deficiency, all forms of folate are reduced within cells, which impairs the growth and maturation of rapidly growing cells, such as those in the bone marrow. For example, thymidylate synthase catalyzes the synthesis of thymidine (dTMP) from deoxyuridine (dUMP) and 5,10-methylenetetrahydrofolate. Inhibition of thymidylate synthase leads to increased intracellular concentrations of deoxyuridine triphosphate (dUTP), which is incorporated into DNA in positions that normally arise from deoxythymidine triphosphate (dTTP). Attempts to repair this abnormal DNA increase DNA fragmentation, which may play a major role in causing the abnormalities of cell growth and maturation that are present in folate deficiency.

COBALAMIN DEFICIENCY. Cobalamin functions as an essential cofactor for only two enzymes in human cells, methionine synthase and L-methylmalonyl-CoA (coenzyme A) mutase (Figs. 132–1 and 132–2). Methionine synthase catalyzes the recycling of homocysteine to methionine, using 5-methyltetrahydrofolate as a required coenzyme (Fig. 132–1). Methionine, an essential amino acid for protein synthesis, also serves in the form of S-adenosylmethionine as the major methyl donor in numerous

important enzymatic reactions. In cobalamin deficiency, increasing amounts of intracellular folate are converted to 5-methyltetrahydrofolate in an attempt to prevent intracellular methionine deficiency. The "trapping" of intracellular folate as 5-methyltetrahydrofolate is augmented by the fact that this is the major component of plasma folate and is the form that enters cells and must be converted to tetrahydrofolate by methionine synthase before it can enter the folate pool. Thus, cobalamin deficiency results in a secondary intracellular deficiency of all forms of folate except for 5-methyltetrahydrofolate. As a result, the activities of all of the enzymes that utilize folate to transfer one-carbon moieties, including thymidylate synthase, are impaired. This concept of "methylfolate trapping" explains why cobalamin deficiency and folate deficiency produce indistinguishable hematologic abnormalities and why the hematologic abnormalities seen in cobalamin deficiency can be completely reversed by pharmacologic amounts of folic acid. The latter oxidized, nonphysiologic form of folate can be reduced directly to tetrahydrofolate without first being converted to 5-methyltetrahydrofolate. This concept also explains why the hematologic abnormalities caused by folate deficiency respond only slightly, if at all, to large amounts of cobalamin.

DRUGS AND OTHER CAUSES. Drugs that cause megaloblastic anemia inhibit a variety of enzymes involved in DNA synthesis. 5-Fluorouracil (5-FU) inhibits thymidylate synthase directly. The addition of 5-formyltetrahydrofolate (Leucovorin) to 5-FU regimens actually increases the inhibition of thymidylate synthase, since 5-formyltetrahydrofolate is readily converted to 5,10-methylenetetrahydrofolate, which is involved in the formation of inhibitory ternary complexes between 5,10-methylenetetrahydrofolate, 5-FU, and thymidylate synthase. Why megaloblastic changes occur in some cases of the myelodysplastic syndrome and acute leukemias is unknown, but this is probably due to a variety of mutations that alter DNA synthesis.

Mechanism of Neuropsychiatric Abnormalities in Cobalamin Deficiency

A wide variety of neuropsychiatric abnormalities are seen in cobalamin deficiency and appear to be due to an undefined defect involving myelin synthesis. These abnormalities are not seen in folate deficiency. It has therefore been tempting to ascribe them to deficient activity of the second cobalamin-dependent enzyme, L-methylmalonyl-CoA mutase, which is unrelated to any folate-dependent enzyme or pathway. This enzyme catalyzes the conversion of L-methylmalonyl-CoA to succinyl-CoA, utilizing adenosylcobalamin as a required coenzyme (Fig. 132–2). Abnormal odd-carbon and branched-chain fatty acids are formed when the mutase is impaired. The neuropsychiatric abnormalities of cobalamin deficiency are not seen, however, in individuals with genetic defects of the mutase reaction, caused either by primary defects in the enzyme itself or by defects in the formation of adenosylcobalamin. Impairment of methionine synthase has also been postulated as the cause of the neuropsychiatric abnormalities because of the importance of methionine and s-adenosylmethionine for the many methylation reactions that take place in the nervous system. As noted, however, the neuropsychiatric abnormalities caused by cobalamin deficiency are not seen in folate deficiency, even though methionine synthase appears to be equally impaired in both vitamin deficiencies (based on similar marked elevations in serum homocysteine concentrations). Genetic defects in which the synthesis of adenosylcobalamin and methylcobalamin are both impaired do lead to neuropsychiatric abnormalities of the kind seen in cobalamin deficiency. These observations suggest that both cobalamin-dependent enzymes must be impaired for the neuropsychiatric abnormalities to develop and that the two cobalamin-dependent enzymes or pathways are connected or interrelated in some way that has not yet been discovered.

Mechanisms of Cobalamin Deficiency

Cobalamin is not present in plants; until recently, humans obtained their cobalamin exclusively from animal products. Cobalamin is synthesized only by certain microorganisms. During the past 40 years, humans have received increasing amounts of their dietary cobalamin from multivitamin supplements taken in the form of pills and as additives to many food preparations. Most

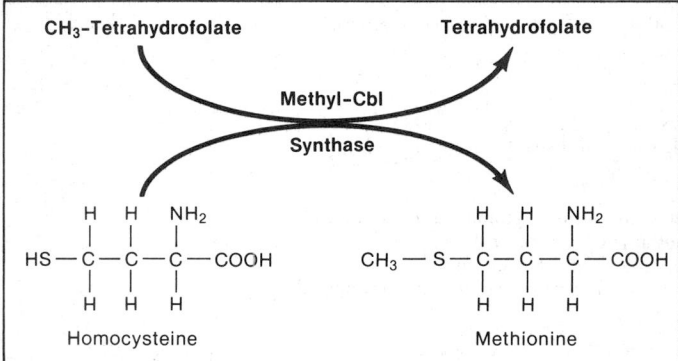

FIGURE 132–1. Reaction catalyzed by methionine synthase that requires methylcobalamin (methyl-Cbl) and transfers the methyl group of 5-methyltetrahydrofolate (CH_3-tetrahydrofolate) to homocysteine to form methionine and tetrahydrofolate. Homocysteine accumulates in cobalamin deficiency owing to a lack of methylcobalamin and in folate deficiency owing to a lack of 5-methyltetrahydrofolate.

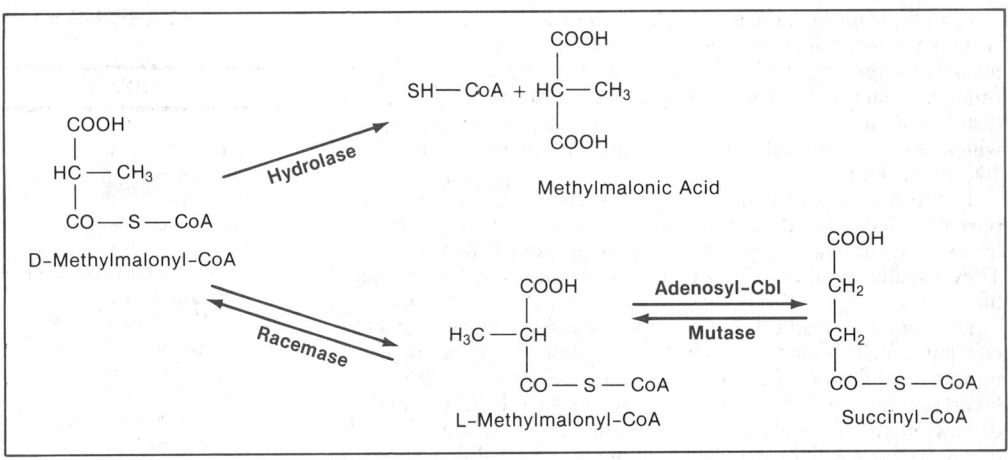

FIGURE 132–2. Reactions involved in the metabolism of D- and L-methylmalonyl-CoA (CoA = coenzyme A). Methylmalonic acid accumulates in cobalamin deficiency owing to a lack of adenosylcobalamin (adenosyl-Cbl), which leads to an increase of L-methylmalonyl-CoA, which is converted to D-methylmalonyl-CoA and hydrolyzed to methylmalonic acid.

cobalamin in animal products is tightly bound to proteins, i.e., the two cobalamin-dependent enzymes, and is released from them in the stomach by the concerted action of HCl and pepsin. The stomach is also the site of synthesis of intrinsic factor (IF), which binds free cobalamin with high affinity and plays an essential role in cobalamin absorption (Fig. 102–2). Gastric juice contains another cobalamin-binding protein that originates in saliva and has a more rapid or "R"-type electrophoretic mobility than does IF. R protein binds cobalamin with a higher affinity than does IF, particularly at an acid pH. Thus, under normal conditions of gastric acidity, dietary cobalamin enters the duodenum bound to R protein. Additional cobalamin bound to R protein enters the duodenum after it is secreted into bile by the liver (this is the only significant route by which cobalamin is lost from the body). Pancreatic proteases partially degrade salivary and biliary R protein–cobalamin complexes in the jejunum, and only after this occurs is cobalamin bound to IF. The IF-cobalamin complex remains intact until it reaches the distal ileum, where it binds with high affinity to specific receptors located on ileal mucosal cells. Cobalamin then enters these cells and reaches the portal plasma, which contains three cobalamin-binding proteins known as transcobalamin I (TC I), transcobalamin II (TC II), and transcobalamin III (TC III). Their roles are summarized in Table 132–2. Although it contains only about 10 per cent of the plasma cobalamin, TC II is the important transport protein because of its rapid clearance and its ability to deliver cobalamin to all cells within the body. TC II–cobalamin is taken up by cells by endocytosis during a process in which the TC II moiety is degraded and the cobalamin is reduced and eventually converted to its two coenzyme forms, i.e., methylcobalamin and adenosyl-cobalamin. Cobalamin is not stored intracellularly; all of the intracellular vitamin is bound to the two enzymes, which are present in greater amounts than is cobalamin. Additional information concerning the gastrointestinal phase of cobalamin absorption is found in Ch. 102.

A large number of acquired and genetic diseases affect the pathway of cobalamin absorption and transport and result in cobalamin deficiency (see Table 132–1). Strict vegans, i.e., those who ingest neither meat nor other animal products, such as milk, cheese, and eggs, and who do not ingest multivitamin supplements, become cobalamin deficient on a dietary basis. Approximately 10 to 15 years are required for clinical signs to develop, since the absorption of biliary cobalamin remains intact. The secretion of biliary cobalamin ranges from 5 to 10 μg per day, and approximately 90 per cent is reabsorbed by strict vegans and other normal individuals. Thus, only 0.5 to 1.0 μg of the 5 to 10 μg of cobalamin present in a normal diet must be absorbed each day to maintain the total body content of cobalamin in the normal range of 2000 to 5000 μg.

Achlorhydria and the loss of pepsin secretion are very common in elderly subjects (>50 per cent of individuals > age 70) and in those with partial gastrectomies. These individuals develop cobalamin deficiency because of an inability to liberate cobalamin from its protein-bound form in foods of animal origin. Secretion of IF is reduced, but because it is normally formed in vast excess, sufficient IF usually remains for the reabsorption of biliary R protein–cobalamin, which is not dependent upon HCl and pepsin. The same time span of 10 to 15 years is required for these subjects to develop clinical signs of cobalamin deficiency as for those with dietary lack. Many of them never develop cobalamin deficiency, apparently because of the availability of free, non–protein-bound cobalamin in multivitamin pills and supplements and because some natural animal products contain small amounts of free cobalamin.

A complete lack of IF occurs in individuals who have undergone total gastrectomy or who have pernicious anemia, in which there is an idiopathic and essentially complete atrophy of the gastric mucosa in association with autoantibodies to parietal cells and IF. Only about 3 to 5 years are required for clinical signs of cobalamin deficiency to develop because these individuals malabsorb biliary as well as all forms of dietary cobalamin.

Cobalamin malabsorption occurs commonly in severe pancreatic exocrine insufficiency because of an inability to degrade R protein–cobalamin complexes in the jejunum. Clinically evident cobalamin deficiency rarely occurs, however, probably because oral therapy with pancreatic extract is usually instituted in these patients during the 3 to 5 years that are necessary for the signs of cobalamin deficiency to develop.

TABLE 132–2. DISTRIBUTION OF ENDOGENOUS COBALAMIN AMONG THE VARIOUS TRANSCOBALAMINS AND THEIR RELATIVE IMPORTANCE TO COBALAMIN TRANSPORT*

Cobalamin Transport Protein	Endogenous Cobalamin (pg/ml)	T½ for Cobalamin Clearance (hr)	Cobalamin Clearance (pg/ml/24 hr)	Site of Specific Uptake
R proteins†:				
Transcobalamin I	425–450	240.0	30	None
Transcobalamin III	0–25	0.1	0–4000	Hepatocytes
Transcobalamin II‡	50	0.1	8000	All cells

*In a typical normal subject with a serum cobalamin level of 500 pg per milliliter.

†In congenital R protein deficiency, the total serum cobalamin level is very low, but no hematologic abnormalities are present because R proteins do not transport cobalamin to rapidly dividing cells, such as those in the bone marrow.

‡In congenital transcobalamin II deficiency, the total serum cobalamin level is well within the normal range, but severe megaloblastic anemia develops because only transcobalamin II transports cobalamin to rapidly dividing cells, such as those in the bone marrow.

The abnormal presence of high concentrations of bacteria and certain parasites in the small intestine can result in cobalamin malabsorption, since these organisms can avidly take up and retain cobalamin. Diseases that interfere with the integrity of the distal ileal mucosa can also result in cobalamin malabsorption, which occurs invariably after the surgical removal of the distal 100 cm of ileum.

A large number of genetic disorders involve the plasma transport of cobalamin, its intracellular conversion to its coenzyme forms, or its utilization by the two cobalamin-dependent enzymes. They usually manifest themselves within the first few weeks of life.

The general anesthetic nitrous oxide causes multiple defects in cobalamin utilization that include the following: (1) rapid (within minutes) inhibition of methionine synthase activity, with a slow (over several days) recovery when nitrous oxide is stopped; (2) displacement of cobalamin from methionine synthase; (3) a decrease in the level of methylcobalamin; (4) irreversible conversion of cobalamin to inactive and inhibitory cobalamin analogues; (5) the gradual (over many weeks) development of cobalamin deficiency; (6) an eventual decrease in L-methylmalonyl-CoA mutase activity; and (7) a further decrease in methionine synthase activity.

Mechanisms of Folate Deficiency

Folate is widely distributed in plants and products of animal origin. Green vegetables are particularly rich sources of folate. Excessive cooking can destroy or remove a high percentage of folate in foods. Folate either is missing or is present in relatively small amounts (≤ 400 µg) in nonprescription multivitamin pills and supplements because of the justified concern that its presence in larger amounts could mask the diagnosis of cobalamin deficiency by correcting its hematologic abnormalities without having any beneficial effect on the neuropsychiatric abnormalities. Folates in natural foods are conjugated to chains of polyglutamic acid. Enzymes in the lumen of the small intestine convert the polyglutamate forms of folate to the monoglutamate and diglutamate forms, which are much more readily absorbed in the proximal jejunum. Absorption involves active and passive transport. Most of the folate in plasma is present as 5-methyltetrahydrofolate in the monoglutamate form. The majority is loosely bound to albumin, from which it is readily taken up by high-affinity folate receptors that are present on cells throughout the body. Once it enters the cell, the 5-methyltetrahydrofolate must be converted to tetrahydrofolate by the cobalamin-dependent enzyme methionine synthase before it can be converted to the polyglutamate form and take part in the other folate-dependent enzymatic reactions (Fig. 132–1). In addition to being secreted in the bile and reabsorbed in the small intestine, folates are also degraded and excreted in the urine.

Decreased intake is by far the most common cause of folate deficiency. Normal individuals have about 5000 to 20,000 µg of folate in body stores. Because folate is degraded within the body and is excreted in both the bile and the urine, approximately 50 to 100 µg must be absorbed each day from the average Western diet, which contains about 200 to 500 µg of folate. Clinical signs of folate deficiency develop in about 4 months of decreased intake, as can occur readily in chronic alcoholics.

Absorption of folate is impaired in a variety of diseases that affect the mucosa of the jejunum, including tropical sprue and celiac disease. Certain drugs, such as anticonvulsants and sulfasalazine, may impair folate absorption in some individuals. Ethanol and drugs such as triamterene impair the utilization of folate. Certain conditions associated with hypermetabolism or rapid cell growth lead to an increased requirement for folate that often cannot be met by a normal diet. These conditions include hyperthyroidism, pregnancy, chronic hemolytic disease, and various exfoliative skin diseases. An increased loss of folate from the body is caused by hemodialysis.

CLINICAL MANIFESTATIONS OF MEGALOBLASTIC ANEMIA

Hematologic Manifestations

All of the causes of megaloblastic anemia produce a common set of hematologic, laboratory, and other abnormalities that are

TABLE 132–3. HEMATOLOGIC AND OTHER ABNORMALITIES THAT MAY BE CAUSED BY ANY OF THE VARIOUS ETIOLOGIES OF MEGALOBLASTIC ANEMIA*

Hematologic	Other
Anemia	Glossitis
Reticulocytopenia	Stomatitis
Macrocytosis ($\uparrow$ MCV)	Gastrointestinal symptoms
Neutropenia	Hyperpigmentation
Thrombocytopenia	Infertility
Peripheral blood smear:	Orthostatic hypotension
Neutrophil hypersegmentation	Weight loss
Erythrocytes:	
Variation in size	
Variation in shape	
Macro-ovalocytes	
Serum:	
Elevated lactate dehydrogenase	
Elevated bilirubin	
Elevated iron	
Decreased haptoglobin	
Bone marrow:	
Hypercellular	
Megaloblastic morphology	
Giant bands and metamyelocytes	

*These abnormalities may be present in any number or combination in a given patient. The absence of any one or more of them occurs commonly in individual patients with all causes of megaloblastic anemia, including cobalamin deficiency and folate deficiency.

summarized in Table 132–3. None of the abnormalities are specific for the various diseases that cause megaloblastic anemia. The abnormalities may also be present in any combination, which can vary greatly from patient to patient. In addition, none of the abnormalities are always seen in conditions that cause megaloblastic anemia, and the absence of any one or more of them cannot be used to exclude any of the diseases that cause megaloblastic anemia, including cobalamin or folate deficiency, in a given patient.

The anemia typically develops slowly over many months and may not cause symptoms until the hematocrit is less than 20 per cent. The reticulocyte count is not elevated, in either absolute or relative (percentage) terms, even when the anemia is severe. The mean cell volume (MCV) is often increased (normal, 80 to 100 fl), and values as high as 140 fl may be seen. A review of previous blood counts often reveals a steady increase in the MCV over several months or years, often within the normal range. Neutropenia and thrombocytopenia occur less commonly than anemia and are usually not severe. On occasion, however, neutrophil counts less than 1000 per microliter and platelet counts less than 50,000 per microliter are seen. The peripheral blood smear frequently shows neutrophil hypersegmentation (Fig. 132–3 and Color Plate 6G, left), which can be documented by

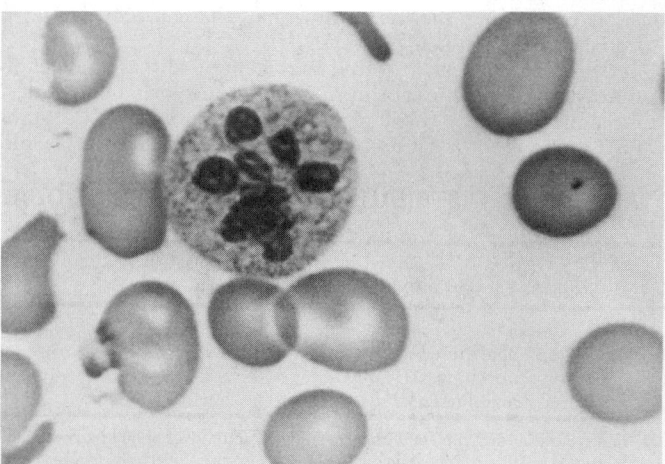

FIGURE 132–3. A hypersegmented neutrophil on a peripheral blood smear from a patient with megaloblastic anemia.

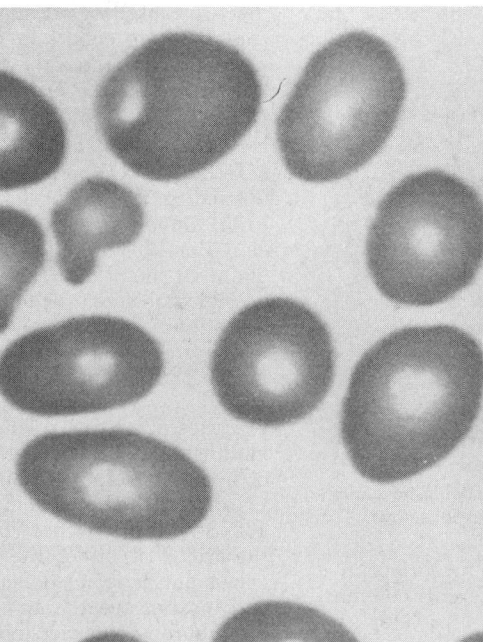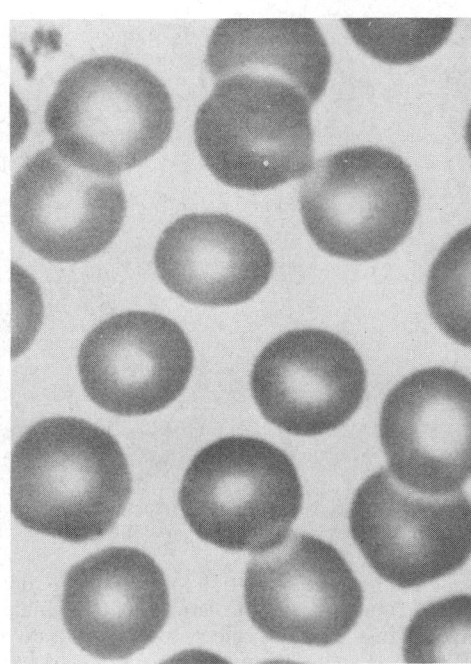

FIGURE 132–4. Peripheral blood smears from a patient with megaloblastic anemia (*left*) and from a normal subject (*right*), both at the same magnification. The smear from the patient shows variation in the size and shape of erythrocytes and the presence of macro-ovalocytes.

observing one or more of the following: (1) the presence of at least one neutrophil containing 6 or more lobes; (2) the presence of 5 per cent or more of 5-lobe neutrophils; or (3) an increased neutrophil lobe average, which is normally fewer than 3.4 lobes per neutrophil. Erythrocytes often vary markedly in size and shape, and macroovalocytes, large, oval erythrocytes, are frequently present (Fig. 132–4 and Color Plate 6G, right). When the hematocrit is low, nucleated red cells may be seen on the peripheral smear, and then the megaloblastic morphology of the nuclei can be observed without performing a bone marrow aspiration or biopsy.

Although the reticulocyte count is normal or low, a number of serum abnormalities are often present that are usually seen and associated with hemolytic anemia. These include elevated serum levels of lactate dehydrogenase, indirect bilirubin, and iron and decreased levels of haptoglobin. Red cell production and destruction can be markedly increased in megaloblastic anemia, but both are confined to the bone marrow, described as "intramedullary hemolysis" or "ineffective erythropoiesis."

The bone marrow is usually hypercellular with an increase in all cellular elements. Megaloblastic morphologic changes are often seen in all cells within the bone marrow but are usually more prominent in the erythroid series. All cells in the erythroid series are larger than their normal counterparts, their cytoplasm appears more mature than their nuclei (nuclear-cytoplasmic asynchrony), and the nuclear chromatin has a distinctive open and fine-grained texture (Fig. 132–5 and Color Plate 6H). Similar abnormalities are seen in neutrophil precursors and are usually most striking at the metamyelocyte and band stage, in which "giant metamyelocytes" and "giant bands" are seen. All of these features are much more prominent in the Wright stain smear of bone marrow aspirates than in fixed sections of the bone marrow biopsy. The use of the latter alone can lead to disastrous clinical consequences because even the most experienced hematopathologist can, on the basis of fixed bone marrow sections only, have difficulty in distinguishing the hypercellularity and abnormal morphology of megaloblastosis from the changes seen in the myelodysplastic syndromes and some cases of acute leukemia. Coexisting iron deficiency may also cause diagnostic problems, since all of the erythroid megaloblastic changes may be absent even in the Wright stain smears of aspirated bone marrow. Thus, the diagnosis of megaloblastic anemia should never be excluded after a bone marrow examination has been performed unless bone marrow aspirates have been examined and the presence of bone marrow iron has been established.

Megaloblastic abnormalities may occur in other proliferating body cells, all of which share the underlying defect in DNA synthesis. These changes have been documented in the epithelial cells of the buccal mucosa, stomach, intestine, and vagina and account for such phenomena as glossitis, stomatitis, and secondary malabsorption. Similar changes may account for the infertility that is sometimes seen.

Few, if any, patients with cobalamin or folate deficiency or other causes of megaloblastic anemia have all or even most of the hematologic and other abnormalities listed in Table 132–3. Even the classic abnormalities, such as anemia and an elevated MCV, are frequently absent, even in patients with otherwise severe deficiencies of cobalamin or folate. This point is often overlooked despite being well documented by several studies, including a recent prospective study of 86 consecutive patients with low serum cobalamin levels (<200 pg per milliliter) *and* one or more objective hematologic and/or neuropsychiatric responses to cobalamin therapy. These patients failed to display the abnormalities listed in Table 132–3 with the following frequencies: (1) lack of anemia (44 per cent); (2) MCV of 100 fl or less (36 per cent); (3) normal white blood cell count (86 per cent); (4) normal platelet count (79 per cent); (5) normal peripheral smear on routine laboratory study (33 per cent); (6) normal serum lactate dehydrogenase (43 per cent); and (7) normal serum bilirubin level (83 per cent).

Neuropsychiatric Abnormalities Caused by Cobalamin Deficiency

Cobalamin deficiency, unlike folate deficiency and other causes of megaloblastic anemia, produces a wide variety of neuropsychiatric abnormalities (Table 132–4). None of these abnormalities are specific for cobalamin deficiency, and they may be present alone or in any combination, which can vary greatly from patient to patient. In addition, none of the abnormalities are always seen in cobalamin deficiency, and the absence of any one or combination of them does not rule out cobalamin deficiency. The neuropsychiatric abnormalities may occur early or late in the course of cobalamin deficiency and with or without any of the hematologic or other abnormalities listed in Table 132–3. How the deficiency of a single substance, such as cobalamin, can produce a clinical picture with such wide differences in the severity and dissociation of various hematologic and neuropsychiatric abnormalities is unknown.

Pathologic studies show loss of myelin with axonal degeneration, most frequently in the dorsal and lateral columns of the spinal cord but also in peripheral and cranial nerves and the cerebral cortex. *Combined systems disease* designates a spinal cord disorder marked by an insidiously beginning and a gradually

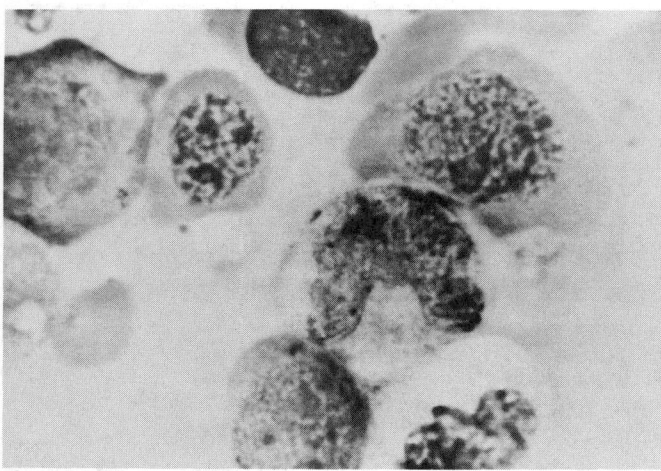

FIGURE 132–5. Erythroid precursors with marked megaloblastic features on a bone marrow smear from a patient with megaloblastic anemia.

progressing demyelination of, first, the dorsal (proprioceptive afferent) and, later, the lateral (corticospinal efferent) columns. Axonal degeneration affects the same pathways as a late, irreversible change. Demyelinative neuropathy of large peripheral fibers may precede or develop concurrently with the cord changes. Signs and symptoms are usually symmetric and often include paresthesias in the extremities, together with impaired vibration and position sense, which may progress to an abnormal gait, spastic ataxia, and quadriparesis. Urinary and fecal incontinence may be seen, as well as impotence. Cerebral and cranial nerve abnormalities include irritability, memory loss, disorientation, obtundation, and changes of taste, smell, and vision, with the last-named sometimes progressing to severe optic atrophy and near-blindness. Psychiatric abnormalities may be prominent and isolated. They include depression, hallucinations, agitation, marked personality change, abnormal behavior, and suicide.

The neuropsychiatric abnormalities caused by cobalamin deficiency frequently bear no relationship to the presence or degree of hematologic abnormalities. The severity of neuropsychiatric abnormalities actually bears a striking *inverse correlation* to the degree of anemia. The frequency with which hematologic and neuropsychiatric abnormalities are dissociated is often unappreciated. For example, several clinical studies document that a

normal hematocrit, MCV, or both occur in at least 25 per cent to 50 per cent of patients with neuropsychiatric abnormalities that are caused by cobalamin deficiency *and* respond partially or completely to cobalamin therapy. Other hematologic and laboratory abnormalities of the kind outlined in Table 132–3 are lacking in a similar or even higher percentage of these patients.

DIAGNOSIS

INDICATIONS. If drugs are excluded as a cause, the differential diagnosis of megaloblastic anemia in adults is usually limited to the important task of distinguishing between cobalamin deficiency and folate deficiency and firmly establishing the presence of one or the other. The diagnostic approach to the patient with possible cobalamin or folate deficiency is outlined in Table 132–5. Patients should always be evaluated for these two conditions in the presence of any unexplained hematologic or other abnormality of the kind listed in Table 132–3. In addition, patients should always be evaluated for cobalamin deficiency in the presence of any unexplained neuropsychiatric abnormality of the kind listed in Table 132–4, regardless of the presence or absence of hematologic abnormalities. The yield may be relatively low because of the nonspecific nature of the abnormalities in Tables 132–3 and 132–4, but such evaluations are clearly justified by the fact that all of the hematologic abnormalities caused by cobalamin or folate deficiency are completely corrected by safe and inexpensive therapy with the proper vitamin. In addition, the neuropsychiatric abnormalities caused by cobalamin deficiency are usually partially or completely corrected by cobalamin therapy, and in the small minority of patients who do not improve, cobalamin therapy always prevents them from getting worse. It is particularly important that the diagnosis of cobalamin deficiency be established with a high degree of certainty because parenteral cobalamin therapy must almost always be given for the lifetime of the patient. The distinction between cobalamin deficiency and folate deficiency is also very important because the treatment of cobalamin deficiency with folate does not improve the neuropsychiatric abnormalities, even though hematologic responses often occur.

SERUM COBALAMIN AND FOLATE. Radiodilution assays for serum cobalamin and serum folate are used as the initial screening tests because they are widely available and relatively inexpensive. Essentially all serum cobalamin assays today utilize cobalt-57–cobalamin and purified IF, which does not bind and measure the serum cobalamin analogues that caused problems with earlier assays. Radiodilution assays for serum folate utilize iodine-125–folate and a milk folate-binding protein. Because of the composition of commercial assay kits, and because cobalt-57 and iodine-125 are readily distinguished from each other, assays for serum cobalamin and serum folate are almost always performed in the same test tube. Values for serum levels of both vitamins are thereby recorded by laboratories, even though they

TABLE 132–4. NEUROPSYCHIATRIC ABNORMALITIES* THAT MAY BE CAUSED BY COBALAMIN DEFICIENCY

Neurologic Abnormalities:	Psychiatric Abnormalities:
Paresthesia	Depression
Impaired vibration sense	Paranoia
Impaired position sense	Listlessness
Impaired touch or pain perception	Acute confusional state
Ataxia	Hallucinations
Abnormal gait	Delusions
Fatigue	Insomnia
Memory loss	Apprehensiveness
Disorientation	Psychosis
Obtundation	Slow mentation
Decreased reflexes	Paraphrenia
Weakness	Mania
Decreased muscle strength	Panic attacks
Romberg's sign	Suicide
Increased reflexes	
Spasticity	
Babinski's sign	
Lhermitte's phenomenon	
Urinary or fecal incontinence	
Urinary urgency or nocturia	
Impotence	
Abnormal smell or taste	
Decreased vision or optic atrophy	

*These abnormalities may be present in any number or combination in a given patient. They are seen frequently with *or without* any of the hematologic or other abnormalities listed in Table 132–3.

TABLE 132–5. DIAGNOSTIC APPROACH TO THE PATIENT WITH COBALAMIN OR FOLATE DEFICIENCY

I. **Initial approach**
   A. Indications
      1. Any unexplained hematologic or other abnormality of the kind listed in Table 132–3 (cobalamin and folate deficiency)
      2. Any unexplained neuropsychiatric abnormality of the kind listed in Table 132–4 (cobalamin deficiency)
   B. Initial tests
      1. Serum cobalamin (normal, 200–900 pg/ml)
      2. Serum folate (normal, 2.5–20 ng/ml)

II. **Follow-up**
   A. Indications
      1. Serum cobalamin <300 pg/ml, *or*
      2. Serum folate <5 ng/ml, *or*
      3. Clinical condition:
         a. Serious unexplained hematologic or neuropsychiatric abnormalities, *or*
         b. Very suggestive of cobalamin or folate deficiency
   B. Follow-up tests
      1. Serum methylmalonic acid (normal, 70–270 nM)—elevated in cobalamin deficiency
      2. Serum homocysteine (normal, 5–16 μM)—elevated in cobalamin and folate deficiency

will report only the cobalamin or the folate level if only one was ordered by the physician. This point can be of practical importance because the physician can usually obtain the value for the other vitamin many weeks or months later if questions arise about the possible deficiency of the other vitamin and the original serum is no longer available.

Normal ranges are defined as the mean ± 2 standard deviations for normal subjects and thus include only 95 per cent of normal individuals. Such normal ranges for serum cobalamin are approximately 200 to 900 pg per milliliter and for serum folate, approximately 2.5 to 20 ng per milliliter. By definition, 2.5 per cent of normal subjects who have no evidence of cobalamin deficiency and who will not benefit in any way from cobalamin therapy have low values for serum cobalamin of less than 200 pg per milliter (false-positive readings). One can calculate that approximately 6,250,000 normal subjects in the United States have serum cobalamin levels lower than 200 pg per milliliter (2.5 per cent $\times$ 250,000,000 = 6,250,000). This number is much greater than the estimate of approximately 150,000 cobalamin-deficient patients who are present in the United States at any point in time (see above). The number of false-positive readings will remain large even if cobalamin testing is restricted, as it should be, to individuals with one or more unexplained abnormalities of the kind contained in Tables 132–3 and 132–4. Similar calculations can be made with respect to serum folate values. Serum cobalamin and folate levels cannot, therefore, be used alone to establish unequivocally the diagnosis of cobalamin or folate deficiency. The problem is compounded by the fact that not all patients with clinically confirmed cobalamin or folate deficiency (defined as those who have objective clinical responses to appropriate therapy) have low values for serum cobalamin or folate (false-negative readings). The following distribution of serum cobalamin levels has been noted in clinically confirmed cobalamin-deficient patients: less than 100 pg per milliliter, approximately 50 per cent; 100 to 200 pg per milliliter, approximately 40 per cent; 200 to 300 pg per milliliter, approximately 10 per cent; and higher than 300 pg per milliliter, approximately 0.1 to 1 per cent. The distribution of serum folate levels in patients with clinically confirmed folate deficiency has been less well studied, but currently available data indicate that only about 75 per cent of such patients have serum folate levels lower than 2.5 ng per milliliter, with almost all of the remaining 25 per cent being in the 2.5 to 5.0 ng per milliliter range.

Perhaps it is not surprising that many patients with clinically confirmed cobalamin or folate deficiency have serum vitamin levels within the normal range. Both vitamins, after all, function within cells and not in plasma. In the case of cobalamin, furthermore, serum levels of the vitamin are greatly influenced by levels of plasma binding proteins, which bear no relationship to cellular cobalamin levels. In fact, TC I has no apparent function (Table 132–2). Thus, the assays for serum cobalamin and serum folate are useful as initial screening tests that allow the physician to exclude from consideration almost all patients with serum cobalamin levels of 300 pg per milliter or higher and serum folate levels of 5.0 ng per milliliter or higher. Additional follow-up tests are required for serum cobalamin levels lower than 300 pg per milliliter, serum folate levels less than 5.0 ng per milliliter, or clinical conditions that are serious or very suggestive of cobalamin or folate deficiency. Examples of such conditions include (1) a patient with marked myelodysplasia who is about to be started on chemotherapy; (2) a young patient with incapacitating urinary and fecal incontinence of unknown cause; (3) a patient with pancytopenia and an elevated MCV and serum lactate dehydrogenase level; and (4) a patient with symmetric paresthesias in the hands and feet who also has spastic ataxia and a recent change in personality.

SERUM METHYLMALONIC ACID AND HOMOCYSTE-INE. The most useful follow-up tests for diagnosing and distinguishing between cobalamin and folate deficiency are serum levels of methylmalonic acid (normal, 70 to 270 nM) and homocysteine* (normal, 5 to 16 μM). These tests, which can be

performed on serum that remains after cobalamin and folate levels have been determined, are now widely available in the United States through a number of laboratories, including all of the large national reference laboratories. The combined cost of the two tests, which are usually performed together, is similar to the cost of a Schilling test or a bone marrow examination. The serum methylmalonic acid level is elevated in more than 95 per cent of patients with clinically confirmed cobalamin deficiency (Fig. 132–2). Values as high as 2,000,000 nM have been observed, with a median value in the range of 3500 nM. Serum methylmalonic acid levels are not elevated in folate deficiency. In contrast, serum homocysteine concentrations are elevated in both cobalamin and folate deficiency (Fig. 132–1). Values as high as 500 μM have been observed in cobalamin deficiency, with a median value of 70 μM. Values as high as 250 μM have been observed in folate deficiency, with a median value of 50 μM. Except for rare inborn errors of metabolism involving cobalamin- and folate-dependent enzymes or pathways, the only other conditions that also give rise to elevations of serum methylmalonic acid or serum homocysteine are renal failure and intravascular volume depletion. Broad-spectrum antibiotics can lower an elevated serum methylmalonic acid level to normal in patients with cobalamin deficiency by inhibiting the gut microflora, an important source of precursors of methylmalonic acid. Antibiotics do not affect elevated homocysteine levels in these patients, nor do they change any clinical parameters.

Elevated levels of methylmalonic acid and homocysteine due to cobalamin deficiency return to normal within 5 to 10 days of starting cobalamin therapy. Elevated levels of homocysteine due to folate deficiency fall to normal during the same period following folate therapy. Elevations of serum methylmalonic acid and homocysteine due to cobalamin deficiency do not respond to pharmacologic doses of folate therapy even in cobalamin-deficient patients in whom folate causes a marked hematologic improvement (together with no response or a worsening of neuropsychiatric abnormalities). Elevations of homocysteine due to folate deficiency do not respond to pharmacologic doses of cobalamin therapy. Elevations of methylmalonic acid and homocysteine due to renal insufficiency or intravascular volume depletion are not corrected with therapy with either vitamin unless vitamin deficiency coexists. Thus, repeat determinations of serum methylmalonic acid and homocysteine levels after a short course of therapy with a single vitamin may provide additional information of diagnostic usefulness.

With few exceptions, patients with serum cobalamin levels lower than 300 pg per milliliter or serum folate levels less than 5.0 ng per milliliter do not show objective hematologic or neuropsychiatric responses to cobalamin or folate therapy if their serum levels of methylmalonic acid and homocysteine are normal. Thus, the use of serum levels of cobalamin and folate as initial screening tests, together with the use of serum methylmalonic acid and homocysteine determinations as follow-up tests, makes it possible to diagnose cobalamin or folate deficiency and to distinguish between them in the vast majority of patients (Table 132–5). If in doubt, one can always start empiric therapy, but such therapeutic trials can be difficult to perform (see below) and should be monitored carefully in an attempt to establish a definitive diagnosis. As an alternative, patients can be followed carefully with repeat determinations of methylmalonic acid and homocysteine after 6 months or a year. The usual patterns of serum cobalamin, folate, methylmalonic acid, and homocysteine concentrations in cobalamin and folate deficiency are summarized in Table 132–6.

OTHER TESTS. A number of other tests have been used as diagnostic or follow-up tests in cobalamin deficiency. Serum antibodies to IF are present in about 50 per cent of patients with pernicious anemia and are highly specific for that condition. They fail to diagnose about 50 per cent of such patients, however, as well as all patients with other causes of cobalamin deficiency. The standard Schilling test (see Ch. 102) for a complete description of this test) requires a reliable 24-hour urine collection, and since it uses free, i.e., non–protein-bound, cobalamin, it fails to diagnose cobalamin deficiency not only in patients who are strict vegans but also the much more common patients who malabsorb cobalamin from food sources. Both the IF antibody test and the

---

* What is actually measured is "total homocysteine," which consists of the sum of homocysteine and the homocysteine that is linked via disulfide bond formation in a variety of compounds that include homocystine (homocysteine–homocysteine disulfide), homocysteine-cysteine mixed disulfide, proteins via their cysteine moieties, and peptides such as glutathione via their cysteine moieties.

TABLE 132–6. TYPICAL SERUM FINDINGS IN MEGALOBLASTIC ANEMIA

	Normal Levels	Deficiency of	
		Cobalamin	Folate
Cobalamin	200–900 pg/ml	↓ *	N
Folate	2.5–20 ng/ml	N	↓ *
Methylmalonic acid	70–270 nM	↑ ↑	N
Homocysteine	5–16 μM	↑ ↑	↑ ↑

*A significant number of patients with cobalamin deficiency will have serum cobalamin levels in the lower portion of the normal range (see text). The same is true with respect to folate deficiency and serum folate levels.

Schilling test actually provide information about the etiology of cobalamin deficiency rather than information about the presence or absence of cobalamin deficiency per se. The etiology of cobalamin deficiency (and of folate deficiency) should be pursued in unusual patients and those with gastrointestinal symptoms that do not respond to cobalamin therapy because such studies may disclose the presence of a disease that requires additional therapy. It is acceptable practice to institute lifetime cobalamin therapy in individuals with anti-IF antibodies or abnormal Schilling tests who lack evidence of current cobalamin deficiency, since they will likely become deficient in the future. A normal result with either test should never be used, however, to exclude the diagnosis of cobalamin deficiency or to withhold lifetime therapy.

RESPONSE TO THERAPY. Therapeutic trials with cobalamin or folate must be performed with physiologic levels of either vitamin (1 μg per day for cobalamin and 100 μg per day for folate), since larger amounts can give hematologic responses even if the incorrect vitamin is employed. Such trials may require months before responses can be completely evaluated. They can be particularly difficult to interpret in patients with neuropsychiatric abnormalities, since these do not always respond to even large doses of cobalamin, even if cobalamin deficiency is the cause of the abnormalities. Therapeutic trials with pharmacologic doses of folate are potentially dangerous, since partial or even complete hematologic responses may be seen in cobalamin-deficient patients. The continuation of folate therapy in such patients is extremely dangerous, since folate does nothing for the neuropsychiatric abnormalities, which may progress or develop during folate therapy.

THERAPY

COBALAMIN DEFICIENCY. Therapy consists of the intramuscular or subcutaneous administration of either cyanocobalamin or hydroxocobalamin. Because cobalamin is inexpensive and free of any side effects, it is better to give too much than too little. The regimen used in our clinic consists of injections of 1000 μg of cyanocobalamin given once a week for 8 weeks and then once a month for life. More frequent injections are often used in hospitalized patients or those with marked neuropsychiatric abnormalities, but there is no evidence that this is beneficial. Once the weekly injections are completed, one can often teach the patient or a family member or friend to give the injections. The absolute requirement of lifetime therapy must be well understood by the patient. Oral therapy with cobalamin in a dose of 10 μg per day can be used with strict vegans. In theory, such therapy could also be used in individuals who malabsorb food cobalamin, but this is not recommended, since their IF production is often precarious and may decrease further over the years. Oral therapy with cobalamin in doses of 500 to 1000 μg per day should be reserved for the occasional patient who, for some reason, cannot receive cobalamin injections. Future measurements of serum levels of methylmalonic acid and homocysteine under various treatment and maintenance regimens may lead to changes in these recommendations.

FOLATE DEFICIENCY. Therapy is usually administered orally in the form of 1-mg tablets of folic acid. Oral therapy is almost always satisfactory, even in the presence of intestinal malabsorption. The usual dose is 1 to 2 mg daily. Therapy limited to several weeks is usually adequate in an alcoholic who begins to eat a normal diet. In patients with chronic conditions, such as malabsorption, hemolysis, exfoliative skin diseases, or renal fail-ure requiring hemodialysis, oral folate is continued indefinitely and usually given prophylactically.

COBALAMIN OR FOLATE DEFICIENCY. Red cell transfusions are rarely required because of the well-compensated state of moderately, and even severely, anemic patients. Such transfusions should be avoided if at all possible because of the cost and risk associated with them. If transfusions are required, they should be given very slowly, since fluid overload occurs commonly and can precipitate lethal congestive heart failure. The only additional therapy is that required for certain underlying causes of cobalamin or folate deficiency, such as antibiotics in bacterial overgrowth or dietary changes in celiac disease.

DRUGS OR OTHER CAUSES. When drugs are responsible, either they can be stopped or the dosages can be reduced if necessary. In other cases, pyridoxine or thiamine can be tried in pharmacologic doses, since an occasional patient will respond.

PROGNOSIS

The hematologic abnormalities due to cobalamin or folate deficiency respond rapidly to therapy with the appropriate vitamin. Reticulocytosis begins by day 5, followed shortly by an increase in the hematocrit, which returns to normal within several months. Neutrophil and platelet counts and other laboratory abnormalities usually return to normal within a week to 10 days. If a complete correction of all hematologic abnormalities does not occur, a search should be made for other conditions, such as iron deficiency or hypothyroidism.

The response of the neuropsychiatric abnormalities caused by cobalamin deficiency is less predictable. Cobalamin therapy always prevents such patients from getting worse and most often results in a partial or complete correction. Responses may be seen within several days but may take as long as 12 or 18 months before improvement can be ruled out or is maximal. Patients with pernicious anemia have an approximately twofold elevated risk of developing gastric carcinoma, an increased association with hyperthyroidism and hypothyroidism, and other manifestations of the polyglandular failure syndrome (Ch. 228).

Allen RH, Stabler SP, Savage DG, et al.: Diagnosis of cobalamin deficiency I: Usefulness of serum methylmalonic acid and total homocysteine concentrations; II: Sensitivity of serum cobalamin, methylmalonic acid and total homocysteine concentrations. Am J Hematol 34:90, 1990. *A review of the development of serum cobalamin, methylmalonic acid, and homocysteine assays and their use in diagnosing cobalamin deficiency and distinguishing it from folate deficiency.*

Babior BM: Metabolic aspects of folic acid and cobalamin. Erythrocyte disorders—anemias related to disturbance of DNA synthesis (megaloblastic anemias). In Williams WJ, Beutler E, Erslev AJ, et al. (eds.): Hematology. 4th ed. New York, McGraw-Hill Book Company, 1990, pp 339–355, 453–481. *Sections of a leading hematology text that cover the megaloblastic anemias in detail. Extensive bibliographies through part of 1988.*

Carmel R: Pernicious anemia—the expected findings of very low serum cobalamin levels, anemia, and macrocytosis are often lacking. Arch Intern Med 148:1712, 1988. *The important message of this article is stated in its title.*

Carmel R, Sinow RM, Siegel ME, et al.: Food cobalamin malabsorption occurs frequently in patients with unexplained low serum cobalamin levels. Arch Intern Med 148:1715, 1988. *This article provides a convincing explanation for the normal results that are frequently obtained with standard Schilling tests in patients with proven cobalamin deficiency and underscores the important point that a normal Schilling test should never be used to exclude the diagnosis of cobalamin deficiency.*

Castle WB: The conquest of pernicious anemia. In Wintrobe MM (ed.): Blood, Pure and Eloquent: A Story of Discovery, of People, and of Ideas. New York, McGraw-Hill Book Company, 1980, pp 283–318. *An engrossing historical essay by the one who, in 1929, discovered intrinsic factor.*

Healton EB, Savage DG, Brust JCM, et al.: Neurologic aspects of cobalamin deficiency. Medicine 70:229, 1991. *Detailed description of 143 patients seen from 1968 to 1985, together with an excellent review of the literature; 57 references.*

Hector M, Burton J: What are the psychiatric manifestations of vitamin B_{12} deficiency? J Am Geriatr Soc 36:1105, 1988. *An excellent review of the psychiatric abnormalities that are caused by cobalamin deficiency and respond to cobalamin therapy, although I disagree with the definition and conclusions about dementia; 85 references.*

Lindenbaum J, Healton EB, Savage DG, et al.: Neuropsychiatric disorders caused by cobalamin deficiency in the absence of anemia or macrocytosis. N Engl J Med 318:1720, 1988. *Detailed description of 42 patients with serious neuropsychiatric abnormalities that responded to cobalamin therapy despite the lack of one or more of the classic hematologic abnormalities that are also caused by cobalamin deficiency.*

Stabler SP, Allen RH, Savage DG, et al.: Clinical spectrum and diagnosis of cobalamin deficiency. Blood 76:871, 1990. *A total of 145 patients with serum cobalamin levels lower than 200 pg per milliliter were studied before and after cobalamin therapy; 86 had objective clinical responses and 59 did not. The two groups are compared in detail.*

133 Hemolytic Disorders: Introduction

Manuel E. Kaplan

PATHOPHYSIOLOGY OF HEMOLYSIS. Human red blood cells normally survive for approximately 120 days after they are released from the bone marrow as reticulocytes, being destroyed only after they have become senescent. With advancing cell age the activities of various red cell enzymes decline, and the cells become denser and less deformable. Phagocytic cells of the spleen and liver are believed to recognize and destroy effete red cells, although splenectomy does not extend the red cell lifespan beyond 120 days.

A hemolytic disorder is defined by premature destruction of red cells, which may occur either because inherently defective red cells are produced or because noxious factors are present in the intravascular environment. Intrinsic abnormalities that predispose to hemolysis may occur in the red cell membrane or in its contained hemoglobin or enzymes. These are, for the most part, genetically determined. In contrast, the environmental abnormalities that curtail red cell survival are almost all acquired. A classification of the causes of hemolytic anemia is given in Table 133–1.

To measure red cell survival, anticoagulated venous blood is incubated with radioactive chromium (^{51}Cr), which combines primarily with intracellular hemoglobin, and is then reinfused. Normally, 50 per cent of the injected ^{51}Cr activity disappears from the blood (t½) in 29 ± 3 days rather than at 60 days, because ^{51}Cr is an imperfect label and slowly elutes from the red cells. Nevertheless, the results of such studies are clinically informative because rates of hemolysis are reliably quantified and the sites of red cell destruction can be identified by external scanning utilizing a collimated gamma scintillation counter.

CONSEQUENCES OF HEMOLYSIS. Accelerated destruction of red cells may occur intravascularly or, much more commonly, after the cells have been culled from the circulation (sequestered).

Intravascular Hemolysis. Following intravascular hemolysis, hemoglobin is released into the plasma and is bound by haptoglobin, an alpha globulin synthesized by the liver. The haptoglobin concentration of blood, normally about 100 mg per 100 ml, reflects the rate of haptoglobin synthesis and catabolism. Haptoglobin synthesis is usually diminished in patients with parenchymal liver disease and may be increased in various inflammatory disorders, since it acts as an acute-phase protein. Free (uncomplexed) haptoglobin has a half-life of approximately 4 days. In contrast, hemoglobin-haptoglobin complexes are removed from the plasma within minutes, primarily by hepatic reticuloendothelial cells that catabolize both components of the complex. Haptoglobin catabolism usually exceeds haptoglobin synthesis in

TABLE 133–1. CLASSIFICATION OF THE CAUSES OF HEMOLYTIC ANEMIA

   I. **Congenital hemolytic disorders (see Ch. 134)**
     A. Membrane defects
     B. Enzyme defects
       1. Embden-Meyerhof pathway defects
       2. Hexose monophosphate shunt defects
     C. Hemoglobin defects
       1. Structural (hemoglobinopathies) (see Ch. 136)
       2. Synthetic (thalassemias) (see Ch. 136)
     D. Other
  II. **Acquired hemolytic disorders (see Ch. 135)**
     A. Sequestrational hemolysis (hypersplenism)
     B. Immune hemolytic disorders
       1. Alloimmune
       2. Autoimmune
       3. Drug-induced
     C. Paroxysmal nocturnal hemoglobinuria
     D. Due to toxins and metabolic abnormalities
     E. Due to red cell parasites
     F. Due to red cell trauma

patients with intravascular hemolysis, and plasma haptoglobin levels fall, frequently to undetectable levels. If the quantity of hemoglobin entering the plasma exceeds the binding capacity of haptoglobin, hemoglobin appears in the glomerular filtrate, primarily as a 32,000-dalton alpha-beta dimer. The dimers are readily absorbed by cells of the proximal tubules, which convert heme iron into ferritin and hemosiderin. After the tubular cells are sloughed, hemosiderin can be detected in the urinary sediment with a Prussian blue stain. Hemoglobinuria, which occurs only when the filtered load of alpha-beta dimer exceeds the absorptive capacity of the tubular cells, connotes very rapid intravascular hemolysis. Persistent urinary loss of hemosiderin or hemoglobin may result in iron deficiency.

Hemoglobin in the plasma is unstable. Its ferrous (Fe^{2+}) heme prosthetic groups tend to dissociate, oxidize to metheme (Fe^{3+}), and bind either to hemopexin, a beta globulin, or to albumin, forming methemalbumin. Neither of these heme-protein complexes appears in the urine unless significant proteinuria is present. Because heme-hemopexin complexes are cleared rapidly from the blood, serum levels of hemopexin, like haptoglobin, are typically reduced or absent in the presence of significant intravascular hemolysis.

Since erythrocytes are rich in the enzyme lactate dehydrogenase (LDH), very high serum LDH levels are found in patients with intravascular hemolysis.

Extravascular Destruction. In most hemolytic disorders red cell destruction occurs extravascularly rather than intravascularly. Red cells are sequestered primarily within the spleen and/or liver and are phagocytized in situ. Although only a small fraction of the hemoglobin they contain escapes into the plasma, plasma haptoglobin levels characteristically fall, particularly when hemolysis is longstanding. Because plasma hemoglobin levels do not rise significantly, no hemoglobinuria or hemosiderinuria occurs. Serum LDH levels may be elevated, but not to the degree seen in intravascular hemolysis.

Hemoglobin derived from destroyed red cells is normally catabolized by reticuloendothelial cells to unconjugated, indirect-reacting bilirubin. As each heme tetrapyrrole ring is opened, one molecule of carbon monoxide is elaborated. Thus, the rate of formation of endogenously produced carbon monoxide can be used to quantify red cell destruction in vivo. However, this may not accurately reflect the rapidity of hemolysis, since ineffective erythropoiesis (destruction of immature red cells in the bone marrow) also contributes to carbon monoxide formation. The unconjugated bilirubin produced by phagocytic cells is bound by albumin, and its concentration in the patient's serum reflects the quantity of heme catabolized and the rate at which the liver is able to convert it into the direct-reacting, water-soluble product (Ch. 115). Serum levels of conjugated bilirubin are typically normal in patients with uncomplicated hemolysis, and bilirubinuria does not occur unless there is concomitant hepatocellular or biliary disease.

Bone Marrow Response. The loss of circulating red cells results in an erythropoietic stimulus to the bone marrow proportional to the decline in the oxygen-carrying capacity of the blood. The normal bone marrow responds by increasing commensurately its erythropoietic activity. When examined morphologically, the bone marrow of patients with hemolysis characteristically exhibits erythroid hyperplasia (see Color Plate 6C, right). Consequently, unless an underlying neoplastic disorder such as leukemia or lymphoma is suspected, bone marrow studies are usually not informative. The marrow's effective erythropoietic response to hemolysis, which may reach a maximum of approximately eight times normal, is reflected by the number of reticulocytes in the peripheral blood. The reticulocyte percentage alone does not adequately mirror the degree of marrow compensation (see Color Plate 5F, right). This may be more reliably gauged by calculating the reticulocyte index (patient's hematocrit times the percentage of reticulocytes/normal hematocrit). In some patients, a sustained reticulocytosis may compensate fully for the increased red cell destruction, and there is no anemia. More commonly, bone marrow compensation is incomplete, so that anemia, of greater or lesser severity, supervenes. If, in the presence of hemolysis, bone marrow function is compromised by such factors as infection or folate deficiency, the resultant reticulocytopenia will herald a rapidly worsening anemia.

DIFFERENTIAL DIAGNOSIS OF HEMOLYTIC DISORDERS.

Recognition and Diagnosis of Hemolysis. The recognition of clinically significant hemolysis is generally not difficult. Commonly, a nonbleeding patient presents with a sustained reticulocytosis but exhibits no evidence of a rising hemoglobin or hematocrit. Some or all of the following findings may be seen:

1. *Evidence of enhanced marrow response:* reticulocytosis, polychromasia, erythroid hyperplasia of the bone marrow
2. *Evidence for excessive release and catabolism of red cell constituents:*
   a. in plasma—unconjugated bilirubin ↑, LDH ↑, haptoglobin ↓, hemopexin ↓, methemalbumin +, free hemoglobin ↑;
   b. in urine—hemosiderin +, methemalbumin +, hemoglobin +
3. *Decreased* ^{51}Cr *red cell survival*

The problem remains to determine the etiology of the hemolytic process (see Table 133–1). Hemolysis is caused either by an intrinsic abnormality of the red cell or an abnormality in its environment, the circulatory system in which the red cell resides. Red cell abnormalities that predispose to hemolysis may be congenital (genetically determined) or acquired. The congenital red cell defects may involve the membrane, the cellular enzymes, or the contained hemoglobin. Acquired red cell defects that predispose to hemolysis occur less commonly (1) under conditions of grossly abnormal (dysplastic) red cell maturation within the marrow (such as occurs in marked deficiencies of iron, vitamin B$_{12}$, or folate) with resultant release into the circulation of severely misshapen erythrocytes and (2) in paroxysmal nocturnal hemoglobinuria (Ch. 135). More commonly, acquired hemolytic disorders are due to the presence in the circulation of such noxious factors as red cell antibodies, immune complexes that provoke complement activation, microthrombi, chemical or metabolic "toxins," or parasites.

Clinical Findings. A patient with hemolysis may present with diverse complaints and physical findings that reflect the rapidity, underlying etiology, and pathophysiologic mechanism of red cell destruction. Patients with congenital hemolytic disorders are commonly anemic and intermittently jaundiced early in life. A suggestive family history of anemia, jaundice, cholelithiasis, splenomegaly, and/or therapeutic splenectomy can usually be elicited. A significant proportion of patients with acquired hemolysis have an identifiable underlying disease such as systemic lupus erythematosus (SLE) or chronic lymphocytic leukemia (CLL). A patient with rapidly falling hemoglobin due to hemolysis, whatever its cause, frequently presents with fatigue, palpitations, breathlessness, postural dizziness, and worsening of pre-existing angina. Physical examination commonly discloses pallor, mild jaundice, and splenomegaly. When hemolysis occurs secondary to an underlying disease, signs and symptoms of the latter may also be present: joint discomfort, rash, and pleuritis in SLE and lymphadenopathy in CLL.

Laboratory Findings. As previously noted, patients with significant hemolysis typically exhibit reticulocytosis with polychromasia on peripheral smear, unconjugated hyperbilirubinemia, serum haptoglobin levels ranging from decreased to absent, erythroid hyperplasia of the bone marrow, and elevated serum LDH levels. Indeed, these findings form the basis of recognizing a hemolytic anemia. Hemoglobinemia, hemoglobinuria, and hemosiderinuria occur only as a result of rapid intravascular hemolysis, which occurs in relatively rare situations, e.g., glucose-6-phosphate dehydrogenase (G6PD) deficiency exacerbated by oxidant drugs, certain infections (*Clostridium welchii,* falciparum malaria), paroxysmal nocturnal hemoglobinuria, paroxysmal cold hemoglobinuria, incompatible transfusions, and as a result of

TABLE 133–2. MORPHOLOGIC ABNORMALITIES OF RED CELLS IN VARIOUS HEMOLYTIC DISORDERS

Abnormality	Hemolytic Disorder	
	Congenital	*Acquired*
Permanently sickled cells	Sickle cell anemia	
Fragmented cells (schistocytes)	Unstable hemoglobins (Heinz body anemias)	Microangiopathic processes
		Prosthetic heart valves
Spur cells (acanthocytes)	Abetalipoproteinemia	Severe liver disease
Spherocytes	Hereditary spherocytosis	Immune, warm antibody (immunoglobulin G, IgG) type
Target cells	Thalassemia Hemoglobinopathies (Hb C)	Liver disease
Agglutinated cells	—	Immune (immunoglobulin M, IgM), cold agglutinin disease

traumatic disruption of red cell membranes by excessive heat or mechanical stress.

Frequently, the morphologic appearance of red cells is abnormal in patients with hemolysis. Occasionally, the abnormalities are so typical that they indicate the correct diagnosis (Table 133–2).

Further Studies. The overall clinical picture in an individual hemolyzing patient is usually sufficiently informative to suggest a rational diagnostic approach. Laboratory studies that are frequently useful in elucidating the cause of a putative congenital hemolytic process include measurement of osmotic fragility, G6PD and pyruvate kinase screening, and hemoglobin electrophoresis. Where the hemolytic disorder is presumably acquired, a direct antiglobulin (Coombs') test should always be performed.

TREATMENT OF HEMOLYTIC ANEMIA. Only general supportive measures are discussed here, since optimal therapy requires precise definition of the etiology and pathophysiologic mechanism underlying the hemolytic process in the individual patient, as described in the subsequent two chapters.

Poorly compensated anemic patients should limit their activities to reduce cardiac output. Bed rest and nasal oxygen may afford symptomatic relief. Transfusions with packed red cells should be utilized to correct hemodynamic abnormalities rather than to treat low hemoglobin or hematocrit values. Transfusions, when necessary, should be administered slowly to avoid iatrogenically induced hypervolemia. The physician must consider the potential dangers of transfusion, particularly in patients with autoimmune hemolytic disorders (see Ch. 135).

To maintain maximal erythropoietic activity in patients with chronic hemolysis, supranormal quantities of folic acid are required. Therefore, daily oral supplementation with folic acid, 1 to 2 mg per day, is recommended. Serum cobalamin concentrations should also be measured if concomitant vitamin B$_{12}$ deficiency is suspected; when low, parenteral vitamin B$_{12}$ should also be administered.

SPECIFIC HEMOLYTIC DISORDERS. The purpose of this brief introduction is only to provide a pathophysiologic background to the hemolytic anemias and their general classification (Table 133–1). The anemias are discussed more extensively in Ch. 131 and 132. Specific hemolytic diseases resulting from intracorpuscular abnormalities caused by genetic abnormalities of the red cell membrane, of red cell enzymes, or of hemoglobin are presented in the following chapter. Ch. 135 summarizes the acquired hemolytic disorders.

134 Hereditary Defects in the Membrane or Metabolism of the Red Cell

Samuel E. Lux

MEMBRANE DISORDERS

Normal Red Cell Membrane

STRUCTURE

Membrane Lipids. The red cell membrane, or *ghost*, is a mixture of phospholipids, unesterified cholesterol, and glycolipids, arranged in a bilayer, and traversed randomly by transmembrane protein channels and receptors. The phospholipids are asymmetrically arranged. Choline phospholipids (phosphatidyl choline and sphingomyelin) are found primarily in the outer half of the bilayer; amino phospholipids (phosphatidyl serine and phosphatidyl ethanolamine) and phosphatidyl inositols are confined to the inner half. The mechanism that maintains this arrangement is poorly understood, but there is evidence that an adenosine triphosphate (ATP)–dependent aminophospholipid translocase ("flippase") is involved. It is probably important to sequester amino phospholipids, since their exposure triggers coagulation and causes red cells to adhere to phagocytes. The lipids are mobile in the plane of the membrane. This gives the membrane properties of a viscous two-dimensional fluid.

Membrane Proteins. The red cell membrane contains 10 to 15 major proteins and innumerable minor ones (Fig. 134–1). The proteins fall into two classes. (1) *Integral membrane proteins* traverse the bilayer, interact with the hydrophobic lipid core, and are tightly bound. They include functionally important transport proteins (e.g., the anion exchange protein) and glycoprotein surface antigens (e.g., glycophorin). (2) *Peripheral membrane proteins* are confined to the cytoplasmic membrane surface and include structural proteins, such as spectrin and actin, and some red cell enzymes (e.g., glyceraldehyde-3-phosphate dehydrogenase). These proteins bind to each other and to anchoring sites on integral proteins.

The major peripheral membrane proteins form a two-dimensional protein network that laminates the cytoplasmic membrane surface (Fig. 134–1). The principal components of this *membrane skeleton* are spectrin, actin, protein 4.1, and ankyrin. *Spectrin*, the major skeletal protein, is composed of two long, flexible chains, the alpha and beta subunits. The chains are mostly a series of successive 106 amino acid repeats, the result of ancient gene duplications. The two subunits are aligned antiparallel and are twisted about each other. These heterodimers interact at their "head" end to form heterotetramers or higher order oligo-

mers (spectrin self-association) (Fig. 134–1). At the opposite ("tail") end, spectrin binds to *short filaments of actin*. This interaction is greatly strengthened by *protein 4.1*, which attaches to beta spectrin near the actin-binding site. Because multiple spectrins can bind to each actin filament, the spectrin-actin-4.1 complex is a molecular junction that allows spectrin filaments to branch and form a two-dimensional membrane skeleton.

The skeleton is anchored to the overlying lipid bilayer by *ankyrin*, which binds to spectrin near the self-association site and links it to the cytoplasmic portion of protein 3, the anion exchange protein. Protein 4.2, which binds to both ankyrin and protein 3, may strengthen this interaction (Fig. 134–1). Interactions between protein 4.1 and some of the glycophorins and between various skeletal proteins and membrane lipids also occur but are less well characterized.

MAJOR FUNCTIONS

Membrane Strength and Durability. In humans the red cell must be flexible enough to negotiate splenic and capillary channels less than half its diameter and still be strong and durable enough to survive the turbulent journey through the heart approximately 500,000 times during its 120-day lifespan. These properties are *determined by the membrane skeleton*. The membrane spontaneously vesiculates when spectrin and actin are selectively extracted or when spectrin is denatured (at 49°C). Mice with hereditary deficiencies of alpha or beta spectrin or ankyrin have extremely fragile red cells that rapidly fragment in the circulation, leading to marked spherocytosis and severe hemolysis.

Maintenance of Cell Volume. The red cell controls its volume and water content by regulating its intracellular concentration of Na^+ and K^+. This is possible because the membrane is relatively impermeable to cations. Normally, small passive cation leaks are balanced by the active transport of Na^+ outward and K^+ inward. These ion movements are powered by a pump that is fueled by the membrane enzyme Na^+-K^+-ATPase. Normally, this system maintains intracellular Na^+ and K^+ at about 10 mEq per liter and 100 mEq per liter, respectively. The pump is regulated by the intracellular Na^+ concentration and has considerable ability to compensate for an increased leak of Na^+ into the cell. If this capacity is surpassed and the inward leak of Na^+ exceeds the K^+ leak out, red cells gain cations and water and swell. Unfortunately, the pump does not compensate nearly as well to a decrease in intracellular K^+. Any increase in the outward leak of K^+ relative to Na^+ leads to loss of total monovalent cations and water and results in cellular dehydration.

Calcium Homeostasis. Excessive intracellular Ca^{2+} is very deleterious, and the red cell actively extrudes it with an efficient, calmodulin-regulated calcium pump that is driven by a Ca^{2+}-ATPase. Intracellular Ca^{2+} is normally almost undetectable (about 0.1 μM). If ATP levels fall below about 20 per cent of normal or if Ca^{2+} leakage exceeds the capacity of the pump, Ca^{2+} accumulates and changes the red cell from a biconcave disc to an echinocyte—a spiculated sphere with numerous short, regular projections. Elevated intracellular Ca^{2+} also causes a selective loss of K^+ and water. The result is a crenated, dehydrated, almost indeformable cell that is highly susceptible to splenic sequestration and destruction.

Anion Exchange. Physiologically, the red cell is a critical component of CO_2 transport. Red cells normally convert tissue CO_2 to HCO_3^- and carry the HCO_3^- to the lungs, where they exchange it for Cl^-. The process is massive and requires a large number of transport channels (~1 million per red cell). These are formed by *protein 3* (Fig. 134–1).

Interactions Between Red Cells and the Spleen

Red cells that enter the spleen must squeeze their 7-μ wide bodies through narrow elliptical fenestrations that separate the splenic cords and sinuses to return to the circulation (Ch. 152). Normal red cells make this journey about 120 times per day and complete it in about 30 seconds, but abnormal cells may be detained for minutes to hours in the hypoxic, acidic, hypoglycemic environment of the splenic cords. This taxing metabolic stress is often fatal for old or defective erythrocytes.

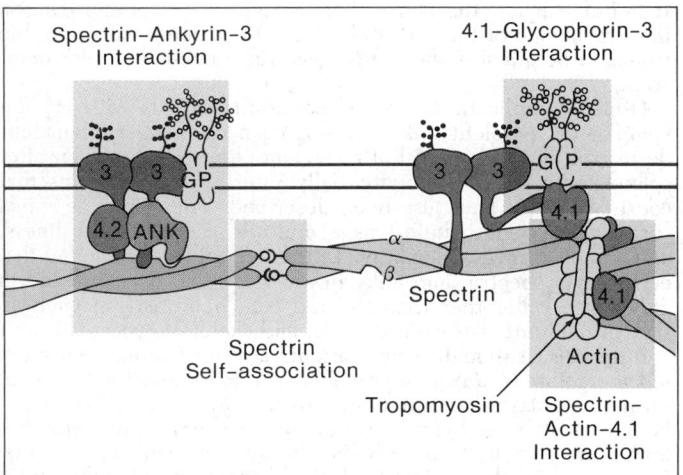

FIGURE 134–1. Schematic illustration of the organization of the major proteins of the red cell membrane and membrane skeleton. ANK = ankyrin; GP = glycophorin.

Red cells are detained in the spleen if they are rigid or if they are coated with proteins such as immunoglobulin G1 (IgG1), immunoglobulin G3 (IgG3), or C3b that bind to receptors on splenic macrophages. Probably other, less well defined, changes in the red cell surface also attract phagocytes and lead to red cell death. Increased rigidity may result from (1) increased cytoplasmic viscosity (e.g., sickled cells and other dehydrated red cells); (2) intracellular rubbish (e.g., Heinz bodies); (3) membrane rigidity (e.g., secondary to oxidative crosslinking of the membrane skeleton); or (4) a decrease in the red cell surface-volume ratio.

SURFACE-VOLUME RATIO: OSMOTIC FRAGILITY TEST

Spherocytes are caused by a decrease in the surface-volume ratio of the red cell. Target cells form when this ratio is increased. Because the area of the red cell membrane is fixed (i.e., the membrane is not stretchable), the cell becomes progressively more rigid as its spheroidicity increases. Surface-volume ratio is assessed clinically by the *unincubated osmotic fragility test*. This test measures the ability of red cells to swell in a graded series of hypotonic solutions. Spherocytes are osmotically fragile; that is, they can tolerate less osmotic swelling than normal cells before they hemolyze. Target cells are osmotically resistant.

Hereditary Spherocytosis (HS)

Hereditary spherocytosis is an inherited hemolytic anemia characterized by osmotically fragile, partially spherical, spectrin-deficient red cells that are selectively trapped by the spleen (see Color Plate 6D, left). The disease occurs in all races but is particularly common in northern Europeans, in whom the prevalence is about 1 in 5000. There are at least two patterns of inheritance: 75 per cent of the families show a classic autosomal dominant pattern. Most of the remainder have a nondominant (probably autosomal recessive) form.

Pathogenesis. Hereditary spherocytes transfused into normal subjects show impairment of survival, demonstrating clearly that they are intrinsically defective. The primary physiologic defect appears to be membrane instability. Red cell membranes from most HS patients fragment more easily than normal when stressed. This weakness suggests defects of the membrane skeleton.

Most HS red cells are spectrin deficient, and many are also ankyrin deficient. The degree of spectrin deficiency correlates closely with the degree of spherocytosis, as measured by osmotic fragility, and with the severity of hemolysis and response to splenectomy. In general, patients with dominant HS have only mild deficiency (spectrin content is 75 to 90 per cent of normal) and mild to moderate hemolysis. Patients with recessive HS often have a more severe deficit—rarely so severe (30 to 50 per cent of normal) that it produces life-threatening, transfusion-dependent hemolysis.

The causes of spectrin and ankyrin deficiency are an active topic of investigation. Preliminary evidence suggests that alpha spectrin defects are common in recessive HS, while ankyrin and beta spectrin defects predominate in the dominant form of the disease. Recessive HS associated with *absence of protein 4.2* and dominant HS with partial *deficiency of protein 3* also occur. However, in these variants, red cell spectrin content is normal.

It is speculated that HS red cells gradually lose portions of the lipid bilayer and become progressively more spherocytic as they age in the circulation (Fig. 134–2). Eventually, they are detained in the splenic cords, where, for unknown reasons, their membrane loss is accentuated by the toxic cordal environment. This *"splenic conditioning"* can be mimicked in vitro by incubating red cells in the absence of glucose for 24 hours. Under these conditions, hereditary spherocytes lose membrane fragments more rapidly than do normal red cells. This is the basis of the *incubated osmotic fragility test*. In vivo, conditioned spherocytes are prevalent in the splenic pulp, and some escape into the peripheral circulation as the characteristic HS hyperchromic microspherocytes. These impaired cells form the hyperspherical tail on osmotic fragility curves. Undoubtedly, many HS red cells never escape the conditioning process. Those that do are especially susceptible to recapture and destruction by the spleen.

Clinical Features (Table 134–1). The hallmarks of HS are *anemia, jaundice,* and *splenomegaly.* The disease may present at any age. In neonates, excessive jaundice is frequent (~50 per cent) and sometimes requires an exchange transfusion. In addition, some HS infants respond sluggishly to their anemia during the first few months of life and require intermittent booster transfusions. After the neonatal period most patients develop partially compensated hemolysis with only mild to moderate anemia (hemoglobin [Hb] = 9 to 11.5 grams per deciliter), intermittent mild jaundice (especially during viral infections), and splenomegaly. *Clinical severity can vary widely,* sometimes even within the same family. A small proportion of patients have life-threatening hemolysis and are transfusion dependent. A much larger proportion, roughly 25 per cent, have unusually mild disease. In these patients marrow erythropoiesis is sufficient to balance the modest rate of spherocyte destruction, and there is no anemia, little or no jaundice, and minimal splenomegaly. However, severe hemolysis and anemia may develop with illnesses that cause the spleen to hypertrophy, such as infectious mononucleosis. Hemolysis may also be exacerbated by long-term intensive physical activity, possibly because of increased splenic blood flow. Finally, in old age, when bone marrow function becomes sluggish, previously well compensated nonsplenectomized patients may become dangerously anemic.

Complications. Crises. The clinical course is interrupted in most patients by occasional crises, characterized by worsening anemia. *Hemolytic crises* are the most frequent but usually are mild and clinically insignificant. They are presumably secondary to the reticuloendothelial hyperplasia that accompanies many infections. *Aplastic crises* are less prevalent but are often severe enough to threaten heart failure and require transfusion. They are frequently caused by a human parvovirus (see Color Plate 5H, right) (Ch. 129) that invades erythropoietic stem cells and inhibits their growth. The infection typically presents in young children as a febrile illness or as fifth disease, a viral exantham; however, some older children and adults are also susceptible to the virus and aplastic crises. Parvovirus is contagious and is especially dangerous to the fetus. All patients with aplastic crises should be isolated from contact with women who are or might be pregnant. *Megaloblastic crises* (see Color Plate 6H) occur when dietary intake of folic acid is inadequate for the increased needs of the erythroid HS bone marrow. This need is particularly acute during pregnancy. To prevent megaloblastic crises, all HS patients should receive daily supplements of folic acid (1 mg per day).

Gallstones. Untreated older children and adults with HS often develop bilirubinate gallstones secondary to increased bilirubin production. Only 5 per cent of children less than 10 years old are affected, but the prevalence rises to 40 to 50 per cent in the second to fifth decades and 55 to 75 per cent thereafter. The frequency after age 30 parallels the frequency in the general population, which suggests that gallstones in HS patients form primarily in the second and third decades. Ultrasonography is the most reliable method for detecting bilirubin stones. Only 50 per cent are radiopaque. Concern about cholecystitis and biliary obstruction is the major impetus for splenectomy in most patients. It is unfortunate, therefore, that there are no accurate data on the prevalence of these complications in patients with bilirubin stones to help assess the indications (risk-benefit ratio) for operation.

Other Complications. Occasional adult patients with HS develop gout, indolent ankle ulcers, or a chronic erythematous dermatitis on the legs. All of these complications disappear after splenectomy. Rarer but potentially interesting syndromes that coexist with HS have also been described. These include spinal cord dysfunction, manifest as a multiple sclerosis–like illness, and a familial myocardiopathy. In this regard it is intriguing that erythrocyte spectrin and ankyrin are known to be expressed in only three cells other than the red cell: neurons (especially in the cerebellum), cardiac myocytes, and skeletal myocytes.

Diagnosis. Although many patients are not anemic, the *reticulocyte count is always increased* prior to splenectomy (except during an aplastic crisis). It is a much more dependable sign of hemolysis than is hyperbilirubinemia, since indirect bilirubin levels are elevated in only 50 to 60 per cent of patients. *Spherocytosis,* the hallmark of the disease, is the other most reliable finding (see Color Plate 6D, left). However, spherocytes are a frequent artifact in normal blood smears, so the physician must take care to examine only areas of the smear in which the

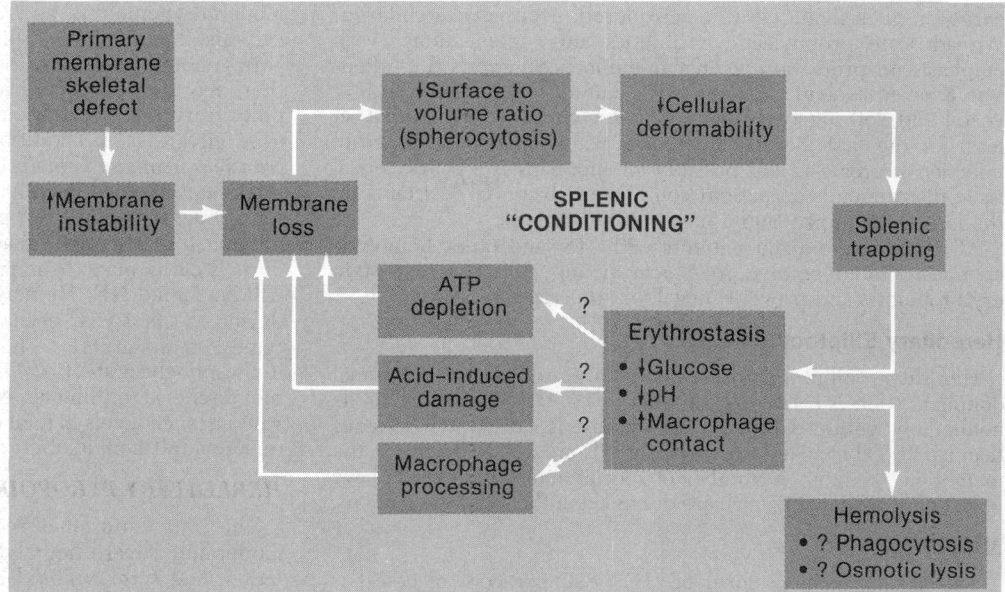

FIGURE 134–2. Currently favored model of the pathophysiology of hereditary spherocytosis. ATP = adenosine triphosphate.

red cells are well separated and some cells with central pallor are evident. Spherocytosis is also observed in a variety of other conditions (Table 134–2); however, with the exception of certain *immunohemolytic anemias* (which can be excluded with a Coombs test), most of these do not present any diagnostic difficulty.

In 20 to 25 per cent of patients, classic microspherocytes are sparse, and it may be difficult to recognize spherocytosis from the blood smear alone. In these patients, the *unincubated* osmotic fragility (OF) test is sometimes normal or only slightly increased, since it simply quantifies what is visible on the smear. The *incubated* OF, however, is almost always abnormal and is the most reliable available diagnostic test. HS red cells are quite dehydrated and therefore have an *increased mean corpuscular hemoglobin concentration (MCHC)*. An MCHC level of 36 or greater is present in 50 per cent of HS patients and is useful confirmatory evidence of the disease. Since deficiencies of spectrin, ankyrin, protein 3, or protein 4.2 appear to be the primary defects in HS, quantitation of these proteins should provide the most accurate diagnostic test; however, at present these measurements are available in only a few research laboratories.

Once HS is diagnosed, *a careful search for the disease should always be made in all close relatives*. It is tragic to see HS become symptomatic in elderly patients with a poor operative risk, in whom this condition could have been discovered earlier.

Treatment. *Splenectomy* dependably blunts both red cell conditioning and hemolysis in HS and is the recommended therapy. Following surgery, spherocytosis persists because the basic red cell defect is unchanged, but conditioned microspherocytes disappear and changes typical of the postsplenectomy state (Howell-Jolly bodies, target cells, siderocytes, and acanthocytes) become evident on the blood smear (see Color Plate 6K). During the

operation the surgeon must be careful to search for accessory spleens, which occur in 20 to 30 per cent of patients. Recurrence of hemolysis due to regrowth of an accessory spleen is occasionally observed after years or even decades and should be suspected if reticulocytosis recurs or Howell-Jolly bodies disappear from the blood smear.

Splenectomy increases susceptibility to sepsis from pneumococci and certain other encapsulated bacteria. The major issues today are who should undergo splenectomy and how should they be treated postoperatively. It is impossible to answer either question absolutely. In general, *we recommend splenectomy for all HS patients with either anemia or significant hemolysis* (reticulocyte counts repeatedly greater than 5 per cent). We defer splenectomy in patients with mild compensated hemolysis, but if these patients subsequently develop bilirubin gallstones and require cholecystectomy, we advocate splenectomy to prevent the recurrence of common duct stones. The risk of sepsis after splenectomy is very high in infancy and early childhood; splenectomy should therefore be delayed until the age of 6 or 7 years if possible and to at least 2 to 3 years in all cases, even if chronic transfusion is required in the interim. There is no evidence that delay beyond 7 years is useful, and it may be harmful, since the risk of gallstones increases dramatically after the age of 10 years.

It is difficult to estimate accurately the risk of postsplenectomy sepsis in older children and adults. The incidence of fulminant infection in splenectomized adults appears to be about 0.2 cases per 100 person-years, and the incidence of all serious infections is about 7 cases per 100 person-years.

All splenectomized patients should receive *polyvalent pneumococcal vaccine* (Pnu-Immune 23 or equivalent, 0.5 ml given subcutaneously or intramuscularly), preferably given preoperatively. Immunization with meningococcal and *Haemophilus influ-*

TABLE 134–1. HEREDITARY SPHEROCYTOSIS

Clinical Manifestations	Laboratory Features
Anemia	Reticulocytosis
Splenomegaly	Spherocytosis
Intermittent jaundice	Elevated MCHC
From hemolysis	Increased osmotic fragility
From biliary obstruction	(especially incubated osmotic
	fragility test)
Aplastic crises	Normal Coombs' test
Often dominant inheritance	Decreased red cell spectrin or
	spectrin and ankyrin or protein
	3 or protein 4.2
Rare manifestations	
Leg ulcers	
Spinal cord dysfunction	
Myocardiopathy	
Good response to splenectomy	

TABLE 134–2. DISEASES WITH SPHEROCYTOSIS AS THE PREDOMINANT MORPHOLOGIC ABNORMALITY ON THE BLOOD SMEAR

Common
  Hereditary spherocytosis
  Immunohemolytic anemias (warm antibody type)
  ABO incompatibility in neonates
Uncommon to rare
  Hemolytic transfusion reactions
  Clostridial sepsis
  Severe burns and other red cell thermal injuries
  Spider, bee, and snake venoms
  Acute red cell oxidant injury*
  Severe hypophosphatemia
  Hawkinsinuria

*Acute red cell oxidant injury is common, but spherocytosis is rarely the predominant morphology.

enzae vaccines should also be considered, especially in children. We advocate prophylactic antibiotics after splenectomy, with emphasis on protection against pneumococcal sepsis (i.e., Pen-Vee K or equivalent, 125 mg twice daily in young children [<7 years] and 250 mg twice daily in older children and adults), at least for the first 2 years after surgery, when the incidence of infection is greatest, and possibly for life. This is a controversial issue that depends on patient compliance, bacterial resistance in the local community, and a host of other factors.

All unsplenectomized patients with HS (and other hemolytic anemias) should receive *folic acid* (1 mg per day) to sustain erythropoiesis and prevent megaloblastic crises.

Hereditary Elliptocytosis (HE)

Hereditary elliptocytosis, usually inherited as an autosomal dominant trait, is relatively common (~1:2500), particularly in its nonhemolytic form. Clinically, the disease is more heterogeneous than is HS (Table 134–3). All types of HE are due to defects in the membrane skeleton. A number of specific molecular defects have been defined, some of which are discussed in the following sections.

MILD HE

This most prevalent form of HE (~90 per cent of cases) is usually caused either by defects in the head end of spectrin that interfere with spectrin self-association or by the partial absence or dysfunction of protein 4.1. Practically, it is little more than a morphologic curiosity. Most patients have no anemia or splenomegaly and only mild hemolysis (reticulocyte counts of 1 to 3 per cent). The blood smear shows prominent elliptocytosis (usually

TABLE 134–3. HEREDITARY ELLIPTOCYTOSIS

Clinical Manifestations	Laboratory Features
Mild HE	
Asymptomatic	Blood smear: elliptocytes, few or no poikilocytes
Dominant inheritance: one parent with HE	No anemia, little or no hemolysis (reticulocytes = 1 to 3%)
Variants:	Normal osmotic fragility
Some neonates with moderately severe hemolytic anemia and HPP-like smear. Converts to typical common HE by 1 to 2 years	Often defect in spectrin self-association or partial deficiency or dysfunction of protein 4.1
Some patients with mild chronic hemolysis	
Hereditary Pyropoikilocytosis (HPP)	
Anemia	Blood smear: bizarre poikilocytes, fragments, spherocytes, ± elliptocytes
Splenomegaly	
Intermittent jaundice	Reticulocytosis
Aplastic crises	Decreased MCV due to red cell fragmentation
Recessive inheritance: both parents normal or one or both parents with HE	Increased osmotic fragility
Good response to splenectomy	Decreased red cell heat stability
	Marked defect in spectrin self-association
Spherocytic HE	
Anemia	Blood smear: rounded elliptocytes, ± spherocytes
Splenomegaly	Reticulocytosis
Intermittent jaundice	Increased osmotic fragility
Dominant inheritance pattern	Primary defect unknown
Good response to splenectomy	
Southeast Asian Ovalocytosis	
Asymptomatic	Blood smear: rounded elliptocytes, some with a transverse bar that divides the central clear space
Dominant inheritance	
Lowland aboriginal tribes in Melanesia and Malaysia	No anemia or hemolysis
	Very rigid red cells that resist invasion by malarial parasites
	Increased ankyrin binding to a mutant protein 3 molecule

>40 per cent; normal <15 per cent) (see Color Plate 6*D*, right). Osmotic fragility is normal. A few cases (10 to 20 per cent) have moderate hemolysis and are classified as sporadic hemolytic variants. The reason for this variation is unknown.

In general, patients with common HE require no therapy; but they may develop significant hemolysis if the spleen hypertrophies in response to various stimuli (e.g., infectious mononucleosis, cirrhosis). In addition, the physician must be alert for *transient neonatal hemolysis*. Neonates in some HE families have moderately severe hemolytic anemia with marked red cell budding, fragmentation, and poikilocytosis. The relative paucity of elliptocytes may create diagnostic confusion; however, the diagnosis is easily made from family studies, since one of the parents will have mild HE. Hemolysis gradually declines in these infants during the first year or so of life, and the disorder evolves into typical common HE. This susceptibility may be due to 2,3-diphosphoglycerate (2,3-DPG), which destabilizes the red cell membrane at millimolar concentrations. Free 2,3-DPG is elevated to such levels in fetal erythrocytes because fetal hemoglobin (unlike adult hemoglobin) does not bind 2,3-DPG.

HEREDITARY PYROPOIKILOCYTOSIS (HPP)

This rare autosomal recessive disorder is characterized by moderately severe hemolytic anemia, marked red cell fragmentation, and *bizarre poikilocytosis*. It is most common in blacks. When heated for short periods, HPP red cells fragment (and their isolated spectrin denatures) at 45 to 46°C instead of the normal 49°C. This *exceptional heat sensitivity* is one of the primary tests for the disease. Hemolysis decreases after splenectomy, the treatment of choice, but the bizarre red cell morphology and heat sensitivity are unchanged. HPP is related to common HE in that all HPP patients have a *defect in spectrin self-association* that is qualitatively identical to the defect in common HE, but more severe. In addition, patients with HPP often have first-degree relatives with HE. A current hypothesis is that HPP patients are homozygous or compound heterozygous for mild HE, homozygous for a related "silent" mutation, or doubly heterozygous for mild HE and the putative silent gene defect.

SPHEROCYTIC HE

This variant (~10 per cent of cases) is clinically and pathophysiologically similar to hereditary spherocytosis. It is inherited in an autosomal dominant pattern. The primary molecular defect is unknown. Patients typically have moderate hemolysis, mild anemia, and splenomegaly. Elliptocytes are less prominent and are more rounded than in typical common HE. Spherocytes are often evident and occasionally may predominate; however, at least one family member will usually have clear-cut elliptocytosis. Patients with this form of HE, like those with HS, have osmotically fragile red cells and respond dramatically to splenectomy. The indications for splenectomy are the same as for HS.

SOUTHEAST ASIAN OVALOCYTOSIS

This curious autosomal dominant disorder is very prevalent in Melanesian and Malaysian aborigines but is rarely seen in other populations. It is characterized by *extraordinarily rigid* red cells that resist invasion by a variety of malarial parasites. The rigidity appears to be caused by increased binding of ankyrin to a mutant protein 3. Surprisingly, the red cells circulate freely, despite their rheology, and there is no associated hemolysis or anemia. Blood smears show rounded elliptocytes, some of which have a characteristic transverse bar that crosses the long axis of the cells and divides the area of central pallor.

Hereditary Defects in Membrane Permeability
HEREDITARY XEROCYTOSIS

In this rare autosomal dominant disorder of red cell membrane permeability, the ratio of K^+ loss to Na^+ gain exceeds the normal ratio of 2:3; as a result, total cation content and cell water decrease. This occurs as a secondary event in a variety of conditions (e.g., sickle cell disease, hereditary spherocytosis, hemoglobin C disease, and glycolytic enzyme deficiencies). Morphologically, dehydrated red cells are typically either targeted or contracted and spiculated. Because dehydration increases intracellular viscosity, these cells are relatively rigid and risk splenic sequestration and hemolysis.

HEREDITARY HYDROCYTOSIS (HEREDITARY STOMATOCYTOSIS)

In this rare autosomal dominant disease, an inherited defect in Na^+ permeability causes massive Na^+ influx, which overwhelms the Na-K pump and leads to an increase in intracellular cations and water. In some families this results in severe hemolysis. In others, for unknown reasons, hemolysis is much milder. Patients with the severe variant respond well to splenectomy. The partially swollen red cells appear on blood smears as stomatocytes (i.e., red cells with a mouthlike band of pallor across the center of the stained cell). Stomatocytes are much more frequently seen as an acquired defect, without hydrocytosis, cation changes, or hemolysis, in patients with acute alcoholism or with various types of liver disease.

ENZYME DEFICIENCIES

Normal Red Cell Metabolism

Reticulocytes have no nuclei and lose their mitochondria and microsomes as they mature; consequently, mature red cells consume little oxygen and do not synthesize protein. Glucose, the main metabolic substrate of the cells, is metabolized via two major pathways: the *Embden-Meyerhof pathway* and the *hexose monophosphate shunt* (Fig. 134–3).

THE EMBDEN-MEYERHOF (EM) PATHWAY

Approximately 90 to 95 per cent of metabolized glucose is converted to lactate via the EM pathway. This is the *major pathway of ATP synthesis in mature red cells.* Only two moles of ATP are generated from glycolysis per mole of glucose consumed, very inefficient compared with cells that possess mitochondria and an active Krebs cycle (that generates 38 moles of ATP per mole of glucose). Nevertheless, the meager amount of ATP produced permits renewal of 150 to 200 per cent of the total red cell ATP every hour. Red cell ATP is used to transport monovalent cations and calcium, to phosphorylate various proteins, to synthesize glutathione, to salvage nucleotides, and to produce the hexose phosphates needed to fuel glycolysis.

The EM pathway is also the major source of red cell nicotinamide-adenine dinucleotide, reduced form (NADH). This cofactor is essential for the maintenance of heme iron in the reduced state, an enzymatic process that is mediated by *NADH methemoglobin reductase.* Oxidation of heme iron to Fe^{3+} produces methemoglobin, which does not transport oxygen (Ch. 136).

Red cells have a uniquely high concentration of *2,3-DPG;* only traces of this metabolic intermediate are present in other cells. This intermediate, formed by the Rapaport-Luebering shunt (Fig. 134–3), decreases the oxygen affinity of hemoglobin and increases oxygen delivery to peripheral tissues (Ch. 136).

HEXOSE MONOPHOSPHATE (HMP) SHUNT

Approximately 5 to 10 per cent of utilized glucose is normally directed through the HMP shunt. This pathway is the *major source of nicotinamide-adenine dinucleotide phosphate, reduced form (NADPH)* in human red cells: Two moles of NADPH are produced for each mole of glucose metabolized. Under conditions in which the oxidation of NADPH is accelerated, diversion of glucose through the shunt can increase up to 10- or 20-fold.

The most important reactions associated with NADPH oxidation are those related to glutathione. Red cells contain relatively high concentrations (2 mM) of *reduced glutathione (GSH),* a tripeptide (gamma-glutamylcysteinylglycine) that is synthesized by mature red cells (Fig. 134–3). GSH protects red cells from injury by oxidants such as superoxide anion (O_2^-), hydrogen peroxide (H_2O_2), and hydroxyl radical ($OH^\bullet$), which are produced continuously in normal red cells as by-products of the oxidation of heme by its dangerous oxygen cargo. Large amounts of oxidants are generated by activated phagocytes (e.g., during infections) and by red cells in the presence of certain drugs. Injury to cell lipids and proteins occurs if these agents accumulate. Normally, this is prevented by GSH. Detoxification of H_2O_2 can occur spontaneously, but it is enhanced by *glutathione peroxidase.* Catalase also degrades H_2O_2, but under physiologic conditions it is less important. In these reactions GSH is converted to *oxidized glutathione (GSSG)* and to mixed disulfides with protein thiols (Fig. 134–3). GSH levels are restored by *glutathione reductase.* In the process, NADPH is oxidized to NADP, which stimulates the HMP shunt, regenerating NADPH. This tight coupling of

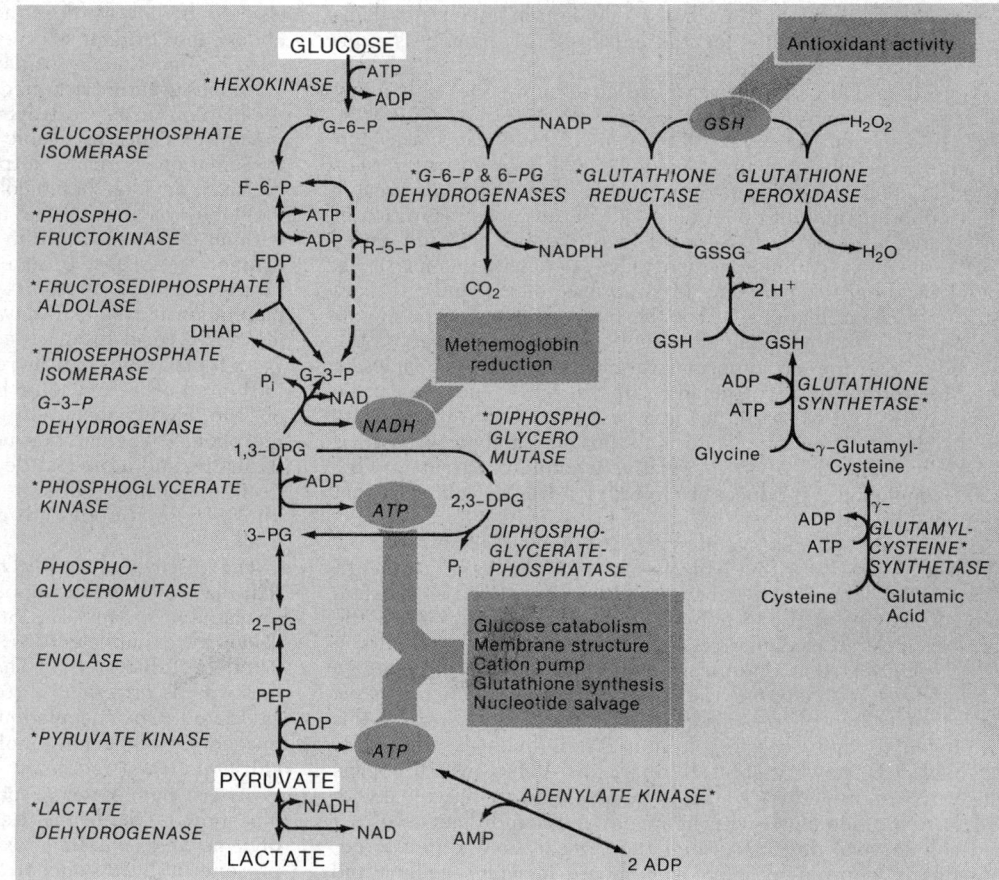

FIGURE 134–3. Glycolytic pathways and glutathione metabolism in the human erythrocyte. Asterisks indicate enzymes for which severe deficiency has been established. G-3-P = glucose-3-phosphate; G-6-P = glucose-6-phosphate; ATP = adenosine triphosphate; ADP = adenosine diphosphate; AMP = adenosine monophosphate; 1,3-DPG = 1,3-diphosphoglycerate; 2,3 DPG = 2,3-diphosphoglycerate; PG = phosphogluconate; PEP = phosphoenolpyruvate; NAD = nicotinamide-adenine dinucleotide; NADH = nicotinamide-adenine dinucleotide (reduced form); NADP = nicotinamide-adenine dinucleotide phosphate; NADPH = nicotinamide-adenine dinucleotide phosphate (reduced form); R-5-P = ribose-5-phosphate; GSH = reduced glutathione; GSSG = oxidized glutathione. (From Valentine WN: Hemolytic anemia and inborn errors of metabolism. Blood 54:549, 1979. Reprinted by permission.)

the HMP shunt with glutathione metabolism normally protects red cells from oxidant injury.

Defects in the HMP Shunt or Glutathione Metabolism

Almost all HMP shunt defects are due to *glucose-6-phosphate dehydrogenase (G6PD)* deficiency, the most common enzyme abnormality associated with hemolytic anemia. It affects millions of people throughout the world. In contrast, pyruvate kinase deficiency, the most common glycolytic defect, affects only hundreds to thousands of patients.

GLUCOSE-6-PHOSPHATE DEHYDROGENASE (G6PD) DEFICIENCY

Pathophysiology. Defects in the HMP shunt or glutathione metabolic pathways impair the ability of red cells to defend themselves against oxidative assault. Oxidants produced by infections or oxidant drugs are normally detoxified by GSH, but GSH levels are not maintained in G6PD deficiency because of the diminished ability to generate NADPH. As a consequence, the oxidants are free to damage vital cell constituents. Oxidation of hemoglobin produces the functionless *methemoglobin* and intracellular precipitates of denatured hemoglobin that are known as *Heinz bodies* (see Color Plate 6C, left). Heinz bodies are not visible in ordinary Wright's-stained blood smears but are revealed with supravital stains such as *methyl violet*. They attach to the membrane and damage it in various ways. Among other things, they cause protein 3 molecules and immunoglobulin to cluster on the cell surface, opsonizing the cells for phagocytes. In vitro, they also increase membrane leakiness to cations and decrease osmotic fragility and cellular deformability. In vivo, Heinz bodies are "pitted" from circulating red cells by the spleen and thus are more plentiful in splenectomized patients. *"Bite cells"*—that is, red cells with a localized invagination, possibly at the site of Heinz body damage or removal—appear in the circulation during acute hemolytic episodes. Red cells with a submembranous hemoglobin-free area, *"blister cells,"* may also be seen (see Color Plate 6E, left). In addition to damage from Heinz bodies, G6PD-deficient red cells suffer oxidative crosslinking of spectrin and peroxidation of membrane lipids. Spectrin crosslinking decreases membrane flexibility and promotes splenic trapping. Lipid damage may be responsible for the intravascular hemolysis seen during acute hemolytic episodes.

More than 300 G6PD variants are now known, but only a few of these are common. The normal enzyme is termed G6PD^B or *Gd^B*. It is present in about 70 per cent of American blacks and in more than 99 per cent of whites. *Gd^{A+}* is a normal variant found in about 20 per cent of American blacks. It has a greater electrophoretic mobility than does Gd^B because of substitution of an asparagine for an aspartic acid in the amino acid sequence. *Gd^{A-}*, the most common variant associated with hemolysis, is found in about 10 per cent of American blacks and in many African black populations. It has the same electrophoretic mobility as Gd^{A+}, but its catalytic activity is decreased. *Gd^{Med}*, the second most common abnormal variant, is found in peoples of the Mediterranean area (Italians, Greeks, Sardinians, Sephardic Jews, Arabs, and so forth), in India, and in southeastern Asia. Its electrophoretic mobility is normal, but its catalytic activity is markedly reduced. *Gd^{Canton}*, a relatively common variant in Oriental populations, produces a clinical syndrome similar to that produced by Gd^{A-}.

As normal red cells age in vivo, the activity of intracellular Gd^B decays slowly, with a half-life of about 60 days (Fig. 134–4). Despite this loss of active enzyme, older normal red cells retain enough activity to produce NADPH and maintain GSH in the face of almost all oxidant stresses. The defect in Gd^{A-} results in a *labile enzyme* that disappears and has a half-life of about 13 days. *Young red cells thus have normal enzyme activity, while older red cells are grossly deficient.* As a consequence of this heterogeneity, hemolysis is self-limited in individuals with Gd^{A-}.

This fact is shown graphically in Figure 134–5, which depicts the course of primaquine-induced hemolysis in an individual with Gd^{A-}. Acute hemolysis with hemoglobinuria and decreased ^{51}Cr red cell survival develops when the drug is first administered, but this is followed by a recovery phase in which anemia and

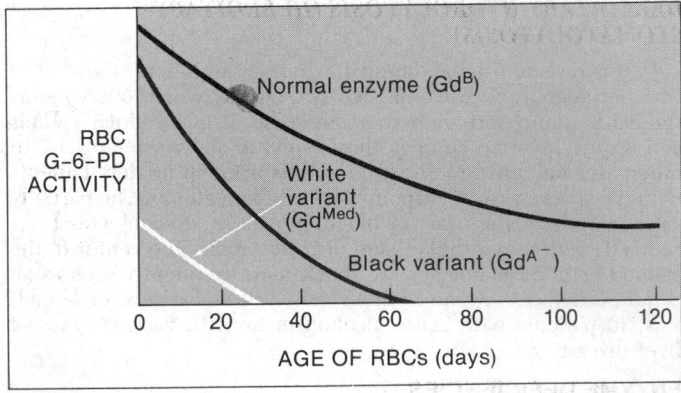

FIGURE 134–4. Intracellular decay of red cell G6PD as a function of cell age. The top curve shows the decay rate for Gd^B, the normal enzyme. The middle and lower curves show the greater than normal decay rates for the unstable Gd^{A-} and Gd^{Med} variants. Note that only the oldest Gd^{A-} red cells are markedly G6PD deficient and susceptible to hemolysis, whereas nearly all Gd^{Med} erythrocytes are vulnerable. Note also that after the most deficient Gd^{A-} red cells have been destroyed, the average G6PD level in the remaining cells will be near normal. This explains why G6PD assays after a hemolytic episode often fail to disclose the defect in Gd^{A-} males. (Modified from Lux SE: Hemolytic anemias. Metabolic disorders. In Beck WS [ed.]: Hematology. 4th ed. Cambridge, MA, The MIT Press, 1985, p 223. Reprinted with permission.)

reticulocytosis abate and red cell survival improves despite continued administration of the drug. The reason is that once the oxidant-sensitive older red cells are destroyed, the remaining young cells are oxidant resistant. Since only about 50 per cent of the cells are oxidant sensitive to begin with in Gd^{A-}, the bone marrow can compensate by simply doubling its output. This apparent drug resistance persists as long as the offending drug is continuously administered. Note, however, that if the drug is stopped for 2 to 3 months, older red cells will survive and accumulate, and the patient will again become drug sensitive.

Gd^{Med} is considerably more unstable than Gd^{A-} (Fig. 134–4). Very little activity is present in mature red cells. Despite this, chronic hemolysis does not occur, which must indicate that endogenous oxidant stresses are normally very low. When threatened by infections or oxidant drugs, however, these patients are at much greater risk because virtually their entire red cell population can be destroyed.

Clinical Features (Table 134–4). The most dramatic clinical presentation is acute intravascular hemolysis. These patients typically develop hemoglobinemia (pink to brown plasma), hemoglobinuria (red-brown to black urine), and jaundice acutely with an infection or within 1 to 3 days of exposure to an oxidant drug or fava beans. In severe cases, abdominal or back pain may be prominent. Symptoms of acute anemia (dizziness, headache, palpitations, dyspnea) may also develop, and if hemoglobinuria is severe, renal tubular necrosis and renal failure are risks (Ch. 76). Heinz bodies and increased levels of methemoglobin appear in the red cells, and some bite cells and blister cells may be seen on the blood smear. In many cases, however, the red cell morphology is relatively normal. More often, hemolysis is less dramatic, and a modest decline of hemoglobin (3 to 4 grams per deciliter) occurs, without hemoglobinuria or prominent symptoms. These episodes are easily overlooked unless the physician is alert.

The discovery of G6PD deficiency followed the observation that black soldiers developed explosive hemolysis after receiving primaquine for malaria. Subsequently, numerous other oxidant drugs were implicated as causative agents, some of which are listed in Table 134–5. The most common cause of hemolysis, however, is *infection*. Virtually every type of infection has been associated. One speculation is that oxidants generated by warring phagocytes trigger hemolysis by impinging on neighboring G6PD-deficient red cells.

Severe hemolytic episodes occur in some patients following ingestion of *fava beans* (Italian broad beans), probably caused by divicine and isouramil, oxidant pyrimidine derivatives that are present in high concentrations in the beans. This dangerous

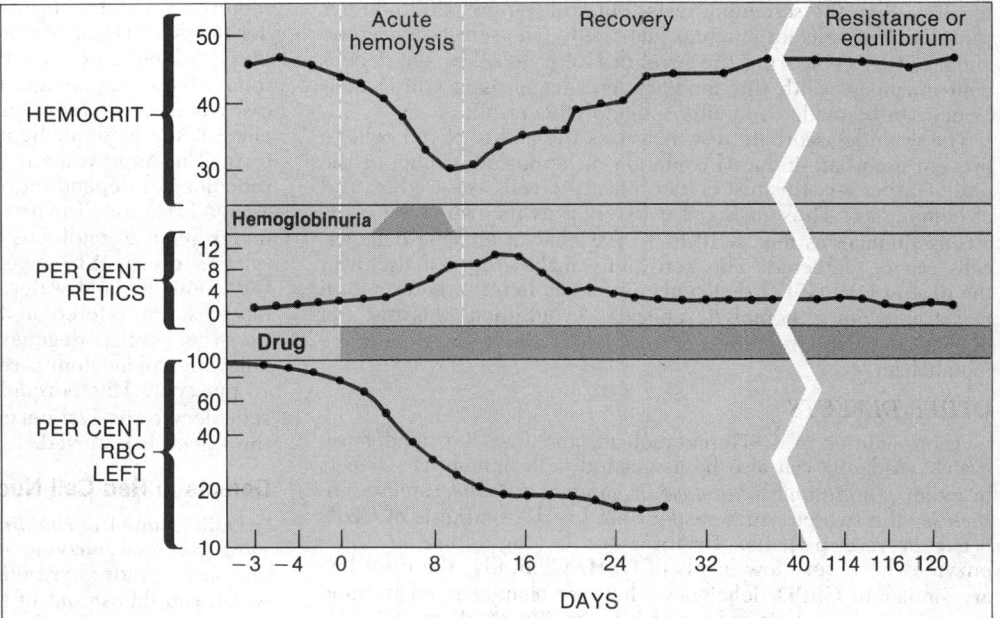

FIGURE 134–5. Course of drug-induced hemolysis in an individual with Gd^{A-}. Note that hemolysis abates and apparent resistance to the drug develops after the initial hemolytic episode owing to repopulation with young red cells. (Adapted from Alving AS: Bull World Health Organ 22:621, 1960. Reprinted with permission.)

phenomenon occurs mainly in individuals with Gd^{Med}; it is not seen in Gd^{A-}. This, and the fact that not all patients with Gd^{Med} are susceptible, indicates that other unknown factors must be involved.

Neonatal jaundice is a common complication of G6PD deficiency. It typically develops at 1 to 4 days of age and may require an exchange transfusion. In most cases, however, the jaundice is adequately controlled with phototherapy.

In some patients with rare variants of G6PD, *chronic hemolysis* occurs in the absence of obvious oxidants. These cases are characterized by enzymes that are unable to maintain basal NADPH production. Variants generally have a low substrate affinity for G6P or nicotinamide-adenine dinucleotide phosphate (NADP) and decreased affinity for the inhibitor, NADPH.

Genetics. The gene for G6PD is located on the X chromosome, so its inheritance is sex linked. Males have one type of G6PD; females can have two types. For example, 70 per cent of black males have Gd^B, 20 per cent have Gd^{A+}, and 10 per cent have Gd^{A-}. Black females, however, can be heterozygous for any two of these enzymes. According to the *Lyon hypothesis*, only one X chromosome is active in any somatic cell; thus any given red cell in heterozygous females is either normal or deficient. Mean enzyme activity in females who are heterozygous for G6PD deficiency may be normal, moderately reduced (usual), or grossly deficient, depending on the degree of lyonization. Deficient cells in heterozygous females are just as susceptible to oxidant injury as enzyme-deficient cells in males; however, the overall magnitude of hemolysis is less because of the smaller population of vulnerable cells.

TABLE 134–4. CLINICAL COMPARISON OF THE TWO COMMON FORMS OF G6PD DEFICIENCY

	Gd^{A-}	Gd^{Med}
Frequency	Common in black populations	Common in Mediterranean populations
Chronic hemolysis	None	None
Degree of acute hemolysis	Moderate	Severe
G6PD defect	Old red cells	All red cells
Hemolysis with:		
Drugs	Unusual	Common
Infection	Common	Common
Need for transfusions	Rare	Sometimes

Despite the disadvantages of a gene for G6PD deficiency, it remains common in many geographic areas. Its prevalence has been attributed to a selective advantage heterozygotes are believed to enjoy against malaria caused by *Plasmodium falciparum*. This proposal is supported by a large body of data, including epidemiologic studies, observations in heterozygous females demonstrating the resistance of cells containing the abnormal enzyme to malarial infection, and poor growth of *P. falciparum* parasites in G6PD-deficient red cells in vitro.

Diagnosis. Several tests for the diagnosis of G6PD deficiency are currently available. Their sensitivity varies, and their usefulness is determined by the clinical situation (sex of patient, type of G6PD deficiency, and proximity to the hemolytic episode).

Commonly used screening tests are based on NADPH-mediated dye decolorization or on the reduction of methemoglobin in the presence of methylene blue. These tests are of limited sensitivity, since 30 to 40 per cent of the cells must be abnormal for the deficient state to be detected. This criterion may not be met in patients with Gd^{A-} or Gd^{Canton} after a severe hemolytic episode, since most of their enzyme-deficient, older red cells will have been destroyed.

Definitive assay of the enzyme depends on direct spectrophotometric measurement of NADPH production. This test is more

TABLE 134–5. DRUGS COMMONLY LEADING TO HEMOLYSIS IN G6PD DEFICIENCY*

Antimalarials	*Analgesics*
Primaquine	Acetanilid
Quinacrine (Atabrine)	Acetylsalicylic acid†
	Acetophenetidin (Phenacetin)†
Sulfonamides	
Sulfanilamide	*Sulfones*
Salicylazosulfapyridine (Azulfidine)	Diaminodiphenylsulfone (Dapsone)
Sulfisoxazole (Gantrisin)†	
	Miscellaneous
Other Antibacterials	Dimercaprol (BAL)
Nitrofurantoin (Furadantin)	Naphthalene (moth balls)
Nitrofurazone (Furacin)	Methylene blue†
Chloramphenicol†	Vitamin K (water-soluble analogues)†
Para-aminosalicylic acid	
Nalidixic acid	Ascorbic acid†

*A more comprehensive list of drugs implicated in oxidant hemolysis appears in Beutler E: Pharmacol Rev 21:73, 1969.

†Hemolysis is infrequent and generally requires a high concentration of the drug. Probably a risk in Gd^{Med} but not in Gd^{A-} or Gd^{Canton}.

sensitive than the screening tests, but still requires 20 to 30 per cent deficient cells for an abnormal result. The sensitivity can be enhanced by comparing the level of G6PD to other age-dependent enzymes. With this modification, diagnosis of G6PD deficiency can be made even after a hemolytic episode.

The cyanide-ascorbate test measures the ability of red cells to prevent ascorbate-induced oxidation of hemoglobin. One of the unique aspects of this test is that intact red cells are used instead of hemolysate. Thus each red cell serves as its own cuvette. As a consequence, as few as 10 to 15 per cent of enzyme-deficient cells can be detected. This sensitivity makes the test useful in the diagnosis of G6PD deficiency in female heterozygotes and in males following a hemolytic episode. In addition, this test can detect other abnormalities of the HMP shunt or glutathione metabolism.

OTHER DEFECTS

Abnormalities of GSH metabolism, the first line of defense against oxidants, can also be associated with hemolysis. Defects in either *glutathione synthetase* or *gamma-glutamylcysteine synthetase*, the two enzymes responsible for the synthesis of GSH, occur in rare patients. Erythrocytes lacking either of these enzymes have very low levels of GSH. Clinically, the disorders are similar to G6PD deficiency; they are characterized by mild to moderate hemolytic anemia that is sensitive to drugs. Chronic neurologic disease also occurs in some patients with glutathione synthetase deficiency, but it is not certain that the enzyme disorder and neurologic defect are causally related.

Inherited deficiencies of *GSSG reductase* are thought to exist, but they are rare, and no case of hemolysis due to this disorder has been proved. Many individuals (including all newborn infants) are relatively deficient in *GSH peroxidase*, but they do not have excessive hemolysis. This probably reflects the fact that nonenzymatic reduction of peroxide by GSH occurs at a significant rate.

Defects in Glycolysis

General Features. Abnormalities in most glycolytic enzymes have been described, but pyruvate kinase (PK) deficiency accounts for about 90 per cent of the cases associated with hemolysis.

Almost all of the glycolytic defects are inherited in an autosomal recessive pattern. Hemolysis is observed in homozygotes. Heterozygotes are normal, although their red cells contain less than normal amounts of enzyme. Phosphoglycerate kinase (PGK) deficiency is an exception, since this enzyme is located on the X chromosome.

Hemolysis caused by glycolytic defects is thought to be due to lack of ATP. However, red cell ATP concentrations are often not decreased because (1) the mean cell age is very young and reticulocytes have high ATP levels; (2) defective cells with low ATP content are probably removed promptly from the circulation; and (3) ATP may be compartmentalized within reticulocytes, in which case a decline in ATP at one critical locus may be sufficient to cause cell injury.

Clinical Features. Hemolysis is chronic and is not affected by drugs. *Splenomegaly* is usually present because of stagnation of red cells in this organ. The acidic, hypoxic, and nutrient-poor environment of the spleen is an added insult to the metabolically abnormal cells. Thus the hemolytic rate often decreases after splenectomy. In most cases red cell morphology is relatively unremarkable prior to splenectomy. After splenectomy the blood smear typically contains a small number of *dense, spiculated red cells*, but this is not invariable or unique to these disorders.

Diagnosis. Definitive diagnosis requires spectrophotometric enzyme assays performed under a variety of conditions (i.e., with varying substrate and cofactor concentrations) to detect enzymes with abnormal kinetics. Measurements of glycolytic intermediates may reveal subtle enzyme abnormalities, since the concentration of an intermediate usually increases proximal to a defect and decreases distal to it.

PYRUVATE KINASE (PK) DEFICIENCY

PK catalyzes one of the major reactions responsible for ATP production in glycolysis; it is not surprising, therefore, that deficiency of this enzyme causes hemolytic anemia. Hemolysis can be mild and completely compensated or severe enough to require frequent transfusions. The distal glycolytic block in PK deficiency causes a twofold to threefold increase in red cell 2,3-DPG, which enhances tissue oxygenation and may minimize some of the physiologic consequences of the anemia. In most cases hemolysis improves following splenectomy, although the effect is not as dramatic as in diseases like hereditary spherocytosis. The improvement is related to the fact that PK-deficient reticulocytes depend on mitochondrial oxidative phosphorylation as an ATP source. In vitro incubation of PK-deficient reticulocytes under hypoxic conditions or with inhibitors of oxidative phosphorylation causes ATP levels to fall. The cells subsequently gain Ca^{2+}, lose K^+ and water, and become rigid. PK-deficient reticulocytes sequestered in the hypoxic splenic cords presumably undergo similar degeneration. Even when anemia improves following splenectomy, reticulocytes may rise to levels of 50 to 70 per cent. This *paradoxical reticulocytosis* is due to increased reticulocyte survival once the adverse metabolic environment of the spleen is removed.

Defects in Red Cell Nucleotide Metabolism

Deficiency of *pyrimidine-5'-nucleotidase* is the third or fourth most common enzyme deficiency leading to hemolysis. This enzyme degrades pyrimidine nucleotides to cytidine and uridine, which can diffuse out of the cell. Lacking this activity, red cells accumulate partially degraded messenger and ribosomal RNA, and up to 5 per cent of the cells develop *prominent basophilic stippling*. Apparently, the basophilic stippling in lead poisoning is produced by a similar mechanism, since pyrimidine-5'-nucleotidase is markedly inhibited by lead. Patients with an inherited (autosomal recessive) deficiency of this enzyme have chronic, moderately severe hemolytic anemia. The mechanism of hemolysis is unknown. Splenomegaly is common, but splenectomy produces little discernible benefit.

Finally, a rare disorder characterized by *overproduction of adenosine deaminase* illustrates the importance of ATP in red cell integrity. In affected patients, excessive deamination of adenosine apparently reduces the amount of this purine sufficiently to impair ATP synthesis. A chronic hemolytic anemia results. The disorder seems to be caused by hyperefficient translation of an adenosine deaminase mRNA that is present in normal amounts and produces a qualitatively normal enzyme. This extraordinary result suggests that a defect will be found in the 5' untranslated region of the mRNA that enhances binding of the message to ribosomes or initiation factors.

Agre P, Asimos A, Casella JF, et al.: Inheritance pattern and clinical response to splenectomy as a reflection of erythrocyte spectrin deficiency in hereditary spherocytosis. N Engl J Med 315:1579, 1986. *By comparing red cell spectrin content with clinical manifestations in 33 HS patients, the authors find that the dominant form of the disease is milder than the nondominant form and that spectrin content correlates closely with spheroidicity, hemolytic rate, and response to splenectomy.*

Arese P, DeFlora A: Pathophysiology of hemolysis in glucose-6-phosphate dehydrogenase deficiency. Semin Hematol 27:1, 1990. *Review of the mechanisms of red cell damage in G6PD deficiency, with an emphasis on favism.*

Bennett V: The spectrin-actin junction of erythrocyte membrane skeletons. Biochim Biophys Acta 988:107, 1989. *Recent review of the structure of the normal red cell membrane skeleton by one of the most accomplished investigators in the field.*

Beutler E: Current concepts: Glucose-6-phosphate dehydrogenase deficiency. N Engl J Med 324:169, 1991. *Review of the molecular defects responsible for G6PD deficiency and the insight they provide about the structure and function of the normal enzyme.*

Delaunay J, Alloisio N, Morle L, et al.: The red cell skeleton and its genetic disorders. Mol Aspects Med 11:161, 1990. *Comprehensive review of the structure of the normal red cell membrane skeleton and its derangement in HS and HE.*

Lux SE, Becker PS: Disorders of the red cell membrane skeleton: Hereditary spherocytosis and hereditary elliptocytosis. In Scriver CR, Beaudet AI, Sly WS, et al. (eds.): The Metabolic Basis of Inherited Disease. 6th ed. New York, McGraw-Hill, 1989, pp 2367–2408. *Comprehensive review of the etiology and clinical features of HS and HE.*

Lux SE, Tse WT, Menninger JC, et al.: Hereditary spherocytosis associated with deletion of human erythrocyte ankyrin gene on chromosome 8. Nature 345:736, 1990. *First direct evidence that ankyrin deficiency causes HS.*

Palek J: Hereditary elliptocytosis, spherocytosis and related disorders: Consequences of a deficiency or a mutation of membrane skeleton proteins. Blood Rev 1:147, 1987. *Review of membrane skeleton disorders with an emphasis on molecular defects responsible for HE.*

Schwartz PE, Sterioff S, Mucha P, et al.: Postsplenectomy sepsis and mortality in adults. JAMA 248:2279, 1982. *The only good epidemiologic study of postsplenectomy sepsis. Indicates that the risk of serious infection is much lower than previously thought.*

Valentine WN, Tanaka KR, Paglia DE: Hemolytic anemias and erythrocyte enzymopathies. Ann Intern Med 103:245, 1985. *One of the best recent reviews of the biochemical and clinical abnormalities in glycolytic enzyme deficiency.*

135 Acquired Hemolytic Disorders

Manuel E. Kaplan

Hemolysis resulting from congenital, intrinsic defects of the red cell has been discussed in Ch. 134. Hemolysis can also result from a variety of acquired abnormalities of the erythrocyte or of its extracellular environment (see Table 133–1). In these disorders, red cells are destroyed prematurely as a result of immunologic, physical, or chemical injury. The general manifestations of the acquired hemolytic anemias do not differ from those resulting from inherited intracorpuscular defects.

SEQUESTRATIONAL HEMOLYSIS (HYPERSPLENISM)

By virtue of its unique vascular architecture, the normal spleen carefully sieves circulating red cells (Ch. 152). Arterial blood enters the spleen via arterioles in the white pulp. In the red pulp these arterioles communicate with either endothelium-lined sinuses which communicate directly with the splenic venous system or with closed, nonendothelialized cords that end blindly and contain numerous fixed macrophages. To enter the splenic venous circulation, red cells in the cords must squeeze through narrow (3 μ) fenestrations between the endothelial cells that line the splenic sinuses. Poorly deformable red cells are unable to meet this challenge and are destroyed by splenic cord macrophages. The splenic filtration barrier does not significantly jeopardize the survival of normal nonsenescent red cells. However, when the spleen becomes enlarged, it may randomly entrap and destroy normal red cells. This pathologic process is called *hypersplenism*. The differential diagnosis of splenomegaly is discussed in Ch. 152. In patients with hypersplenism the rapidity of hemolysis is poorly correlated with overall spleen size. Indeed, patients with marked splenomegaly may exhibit little evidence of hemolysis.

Hypersplenism is best treated by effectively managing the underlying disease process. Splenectomy is rarely indicated; the procedure should be limited to transfusion-dependent patients who are reasonable operative risks and whose condition is refractory to medical therapy. Splenectomized individuals, particularly the young (under age 10), are statistically more likely to develop fulminant bacterial or protozoal infections and are less able to mount an effective primary IgM immune response to certain antigens. Consequently, the indications for splenectomy and its inherent risks should be carefully weighed before it is recommended.

IMMUNOHEMOLYTIC DISORDERS: PATHOPHYSIOLOGY

In patients with immune hemolysis, red cell destruction results from the binding of antibodies and/or complement components to the erythrocyte membrane. This may occur as a result of autoimmunization, alloimmunization, or exposure to certain drugs.

TYPES OF ANTIBODIES. Antibodies induce red cell destruction in vivo by mechanisms that are largely determined by their structure, concentration, and immunologic properties (complement-fixing activity, the optimal temperature at which they are active) as well as by the density and topographic distribution of the membrane antigens with which they combine. IgM red cell antibodies are generally agglutinating ("complete"), complement fixing, and active at colder temperatures. In contrast, most IgG red cell antibodies are fully active at 37°C ("warm"), have little or no agglutinating activity ("incomplete"), and vary in their ability to fix complement. IgA red cell antibodies usually occur in conjunction with IgG and/or IgM, have little complement-fixing activity, and rarely cause red cell destruction.

ROLE OF COMPLEMENT. Most IgM and some IgG red cell antibodies, after combining with membrane antigens, activate the classic complement pathway. After C1 binds to the Fc region of immunoglobulin heavy chains, it develops proteolytic C1 esterase (1S) activity, splits C4 into two fragments, C4a and C4b (Ch. 243). Nascent C4b may covalently attach to the red cell membrane and bind C2, which is then cleaved by C1s into C2a and C2b. The C4b, 2a membrane complex acts as the classic pathway C3 convertase, binding and cleaving C3 into C3a and C3b. Nascent C3b may also be covalently bound to the red cell membrane, where it completes assembly of the classic pathway C5 convertase (C4b,2a,3b). C5, after binding to C3b, is cleaved by C2a, thereby activating the terminal "membrane attack complex" (C5–9) of the complement cascade. Insertion of activated C9 into the red cell membrane produces its osmotic destabilization, resulting in egress of hemoglobin. If unopposed complement activation were to occur, life-threatening intravascular hemolysis could ensue. However, the process is restrained by inhibitors and inactivators of complement normally present in the plasma (Factor I, Factor H, C4-binding protein) and within the red cell membrane itself, i.e., CR1 (the receptor for C3b), DAF (decay-accelerating factor), HFR (homologous restriction factor or C8-binding protein), and MIRL (membrane inhibitor of reactive lysis). Red cells bearing covalently bound fragments of activated complement, i.e., C4b, C3b, and C3bi (C3b cleaved by Factor I), are prematurely removed from the circulation and destroyed, primarily by hepatic macrophages bearing complement receptors (CR1 and CR3). A more detailed description of complement is given in Ch. 243.

HEMOLYSIS WITHOUT COMPLEMENT ACTIVATION. Red cells sensitized with IgG antibodies without complement are sequestered and destroyed primarily within the splenic cords. Here they come into prolonged and intimate contact with macrophages bearing membrane receptors (FcγR) for the Fc portion of the IgG molecule. The sensitized cells may be damaged by a cytotoxic process (antibody-dependent cell-mediated cytotoxicity, or ADCC), be totally engulfed, or undergo partial phagocytosis. Incompletely phagocytized red cells may reseal their membranes and, having lost proportionately more membrane than cytoplasm, become microspherocytic. If these cells re-enter the systemic circulation, their spherocytic shape testifies to their previous encounter with splenic macrophages. They are particularly vulnerable to resequestration, since their deformability has been impaired and they retain significant membrane antibody.

DETECTION OF ANTIBODIES. The presence of red cell antibodies may be suspected from the appearance of the patient's anticoagulated venous blood and perusal of the peripheral blood film. IgM antibodies may induce such marked red cell agglutination at room temperature that anticoagulated blood samples may appear "clotted." Red cell clumping is readily apparent in the blood smear. Although IgG antibodies are usually nonagglutinating, they may so markedly reduce the negative charge (zeta potential) of the red cell that the cells are aggregated by fibrinogen and other plasma macromolecules. This condition appears as rouleaux in the blood film.

The *direct antiglobulin (Coombs') test* is most frequently used to detect immunoproteins present on the red cell membrane. A polyspecific antiserum containing antibodies against human immunoglobulins and complement components is added to a washed, dilute suspension of the patient's red cells. If agglutination is observed, the test is positive. More precise identification of the membrane-bound immunoprotein may help to delineate the etiology and pathophysiologic mechanisms underlying the hemolytic disorder. This is accomplished by exposing the patient's red cells to monospecific antisera reactive with individual immunoglobulin classes or complement components. Almost all patients with immunohemolytic disorders exhibit positive direct antiglobulin tests. In the small number of patients (< 5 per cent) in whom this test is negative, more sensitive immunologic techniques may disclose increased concentrations of red cell–associated immunoproteins.

The *indirect antiglobulin test*, important when considering red cell transfusions, detects serum antibodies capable of attaching to normal red cells. The patient's serum is incubated with a panel of serologically defined normal red cells; the cells are then washed, and membrane-associated immunoprotein is sought by the antiglobulin reaction. Although in clinical situations, both direct and indirect Coombs' tests are frequently ordered simultaneously, only the former provides unequivocal evidence of an immune hemolytic process.

HEMOLYSIS DUE TO ALLOANTIBODIES. Alloantibodies capable of destroying transfused, but not autologous, red cells are products of immunologic responses to (1) bacteria that normally colonize the large intestine (giving rise to so-called natural antibodies that cross-react with allogeneic erythrocyte antigens), (2) transfused, imperfectly matched red cells, or (3) antigens of fetal red cells that entered the maternal circulation during pregnancy or at delivery.

Alloimmune red cell antibodies present in a patient's serum may be detected by agglutination of normal cells or by the indirect antiglobulin reaction. Since these antibodies have specificity for nonself antigens, they are harmless unless the patient receives red cells that contain the immunizing antigen, or is pregnant. In the latter situation, the IgG red cell alloantibodies that gain access to the fetal circulation may induce erythroblastosis fetalis.

AUTOIMMUNE HEMOLYTIC ANEMIAS. Autoimmune hemolytic disorders are characterized by antibodies directed against autologous red cell antigens. The pathophysiologic mechanisms that result in autoantibody production are not fully understood. B lymphocyte clones capable of producing red cell autoantibodies probably are present normally. However, in health, they fail to synthesize detectable quantities of autoantibody because their activities are suppressed by immunoregulatory T lymphocytes. If this mechanism is deranged, such autoantibodies may be produced in quantities sufficient to trigger red cell destruction. Certain diseases—infections, neoplasms, or collagen vascular disorders—appear to predispose to increased synthesis of red cell autoantibodies. The hemolytic disorders that result are therefore categorized as secondary. In primary or idiopathic autoimmune hemolytic anemia, no underlying disease can be detected.

AUTOIMMUNE HEMOLYTIC DISEASE DUE TO IgG WARM-REACTING ANTIBODIES

CLINICAL MANIFESTATIONS. *Disease Associations.* In approximately 40 per cent of patients with IgG-mediated autoimmune hemolytic anemia, the process is secondary to an underlying disease, usually neoplastic or collagen vascular in origin. Chronic lymphocytic leukemia (see Color Plate 7*I*, left) and, less frequently, other lymphoproliferative disorders are the most commonly associated malignancies. There is a well-documented relationship between warm autoimmune hemolytic anemia and ovarian teratoma as well as adenocarcinoma of the stomach. Systemic lupus erythematosus is the most frequently associated collagen vascular disorder; less common are systemic sclerosis and rheumatoid arthritis. Occasional patients with ulcerative colitis present with warm autoimmune hemolysis. Certain drugs, the most commonly used being methyldopa, may give rise to this problem as well.

Symptoms and Signs. Since the rate of red cell destruction, degree of anemia, and presence of underlying disease differ from patient to patient, a highly variable clinical picture can result. If hemolysis is sudden in onset and rapid, the patient usually presents with symptoms and signs related to severe anemia, i.e., pallor, fatigue, exertional dyspnea, dizziness, and palpitations. When hemolysis starts more gradually, the anemia is usually less severe, and the patient may be relatively asymptomatic. On physical examination mild jaundice and splenomegaly are commonly present.

Laboratory Findings. The degree of anemia is variable, and there are usually normal numbers of white cells and platelets. In occasional patients significant thrombocytopenia or neutropenia, or both, occurs in conjunction with immune hemolysis (*Evans' syndrome*). The mean corpuscular volume (MCV) may be increased, sometimes strikingly so (> 115 fl). When spherocytosis is prominent, the mean corpuscular hemoglobin concentration (MCHC) is usually elevated. In addition to rouleaux formation, the peripheral blood film typically discloses significant anisocy-

tosis with numerous microspherocytes and increased numbers of large polychromatophilic reticulocytes. Normoblasts may be present, particularly when hemolysis is rapid. The reticulocyte count is almost always elevated. Reticulocytopenia may be encountered in occasional patients and requires additional diagnostic evaluation, including bone marrow aspiration and biopsy as well as search for an infectious etiology, including parvovirus (B19) (see Color Plate 5*H*, right). Other typical laboratory findings include hyperbilirubinemia of the unconjugated type, diminished to absent serum haptoglobin, normal or slightly elevated plasma hemoglobin levels, and no urine hemosiderin. The direct antiglobulin test discloses only IgG or IgG and complement (C3dg). The indirect antiglobulin test may be positive or negative, a positive result generally indicating that excess red cell autoantibody has been produced. Antibody eluted from the patient's red cells may occasionally exhibit specificity for a well-defined antigen, particularly Rh. More commonly, the eluted antibody is found to be a "panagglutinin," reacting with all normal red cells tested.

DIFFERENTIAL DIAGNOSIS. Since identifiable underlying disorders are present in about half the patients with warm autoimmune hemolytic anemia, appropriate diagnostic studies should be undertaken. If hemolysis appears to be acquired but the direct antiglobulin test is negative, a previously undiagnosed congenital hemolytic process, paroxysmal nocturnal hemoglobinuria, and various nonimmunologic causes (hypersplenism, microangiopathy, and so on) must be considered (Table 135–1). If there is no evidence for these, the patient may have an immunohemolytic process that can be demonstrated only by immunologic studies more sensitive than the antiglobulin test. Alternatively, this process may be inferred from a patient's objective clinical response to an empiric therapeutic trial of steroids.

TREATMENT. If an underlying disease process is identified and treated, marked improvement of the accompanying hemolysis frequently results. Slow, well-compensated hemolysis may require no therapy.

Glucocorticoids. Patients with more rapid hemolysis should be treated with oral steroids equivalent to 1 to 1.5 mg prednisone per kilogram per day, in daily single or divided doses. If the patient is very symptomatic because of severe anemia, initial treatment with intravenous hydrocortisone, 400 to 800 mg per day, may be preferred, followed by daily oral prednisone in divided doses. Improvement usually occurs within 5 to 10 days, evidenced by increasing hemoglobin and hematocrit levels and decreasing reticulocytosis. At this time steroid therapy can be consolidated into a single daily dose. Over the succeeding 3 to 4 weeks, as hemoglobin levels approach normal, the daily steroid dosage can usually be tapered, at 5- to 7-day intervals, to a daily prednisone dose of approximately 20 mg. Blood counts and reticulocyte counts should be checked periodically. Thereafter, the dose of steroids should be decreased more slowly, every 2 to 3 weeks, by 5 mg per day as long as the reticulocyte count does not rise significantly and the hemoglobin level remains stable. In occasional patients it may be possible to discontinue steroids

TABLE 135–1. DIAGNOSTIC APPROACH TO ACQUIRED COOMBS-NEGATIVE HEMOLYTIC ANEMIA

Reassess patient's history
Re-evaluate red cell morphology
Deduce most likely site(s) of hemolysis,
    i.e., extravascular (E), intravascular (I)

Morphology	*Site(s)*	*Possible diagnosis*
Fragments	I	Microangiopathy (TTP/HUS)
		Cardiac/valvular abnormality
		DIC
Spherocytes*	E	Hypersplenism
		Immunohemolytic anemia†
	I(E)	Paroxysmal cold hemoglobinuria†
		Toxins (clostridial, drugs, etc.)
Inclusions		
Parasites	E(I)	Malaria, etc.
Heinz bodies‡	I(E)	Oxidant drugs/toxins (consider G6PD deficiency)
Normal	I	Paroxysmal nocturnal hemoglobinuria

*Hereditary spherocytosis must always be considered.
†Characteristically Coombs-positive.
‡Requires special stain.

entirely without exacerbating the hemolysis. More commonly, significant hemolysis persists and patients require daily maintenance steroid therapy, 5 to 15 mg of prednisone, or 10 to 30 mg on alternate days, which results in fewer undesirable side effects.

The mechanism of the corticosteroid effect in warm autoimmune hemolytic disorders is not fully understood. Steroids appear to diminish the number, and possibly the binding strength, of monocyte and macrophage Fcγ receptors, thereby decreasing the ability of these cells to bind and destroy IgG-sensitized red cells. Prolonged therapy with steroids suppresses antibody synthesis; however, this effect certainly does not explain the prompt, frequently dramatic clinical improvement seen in most patients.

If the response to corticosteroid therapy is unsatisfactory, i.e., if (1) hemolysis and anemia are not significantly improved within 2 weeks after initiating high-dose steroid therapy or (2) unacceptably large daily doses of steroids (> 15 to 20 mg of prednisone) are required to maintain hematologic improvement, other therapeutic approaches must be considered.

Splenectomy. ^{51}Cr red cell survival and sequestration studies should be performed, if possible, before splenectomy is undertaken. Typically, they disclose significantly reduced red blood cell survival (t ½ = 5 to 15 days), and the spleen will be the major, if not exclusive, site of red cell destruction. In such a patient splenectomy is advisable and should result in marked hematologic improvement. Occasionally, significant hemolysis persists after splenectomy. This results from intense red cell sensitization with IgG autoantibody and usually responds to small maintenance doses of steroids. If ^{51}Cr sequestration studies reveal the liver to be a major site of red cell destruction, the direct antiglobulin test usually discloses complement (C3dg) as well as IgG. Splenectomy results in less effective control of hemolysis in such patients, favorable responses being achieved in only 30 per cent. Consequently, a trial of an immunosuppressive drug and/or high-dose intravenous gamma globulin may be preferred prior to splenectomy.

Immunosuppressive Drugs. Oral azathioprine* (Imuran), 50 to 200 mg per day, and cyclophosphamide* (Cytoxan), 50 to 150 mg per day, are frequently employed in patients with refractory, warm immunohemolytic anemia. Responses are variable and usually not very dramatic. However, their use in patients whose hemolysis is resistant to steroids may permit reduction in the excessive steroid dosages required for maintenance. Significant toxicities include marrow suppression evidenced by leukopenia, thrombocytopenia, or reticulocytopenia with worsening anemia. Chronic treatment with immunosuppressive agents predisposes to development of malignancies.

Large amounts of intravenously administered gamma globulin (0.5 to 1.0 gram per kilogram), when infused daily for 5 consecutive days, has been shown to mitigate hemolysis in a small number of well-studied patients with IgG-mediated immunohemolytic anemia. The observed therapeutic responses have not been striking, appear slowly (7 to 10 days), and have been transient. Indeed, the majority of patients so treated have failed to respond. High-dose gamma globulin therapy induces hemolysis in some patients with immune thrombocytopenia or immunodeficiency disorders, probably because of its anti-Rh antibody content.

Transfusion. Before hemolysis is adequately controlled by steroid therapy, severely anemic patients may require red cell transfusions. Transfusion carries an increased risk when the patient has a positive indirect antiglobulin test because donor-patient compatibility cannot be ensured by crossmatching techniques. The serum of such a patient frequently contains a panagglutinating autoantibody reactive with red cells from all prospective donors. More important, the serum autoantibody may mask the presence of a red cell alloantibody that may be capable of provoking intravascular hemolysis of transfused red cells. To distinguish these possibilities, the patient's red cells from which autoantibody has been eluted are used to absorb all autoantibody from the patient's serum. The absorbed serum is then tested for alloantibody activity with potential donor cells. In addition, blood banks usually attempt to identify possible blood group specificity of antibody eluted from a patient's red cells and of the serum antibody. Following these studies, donor

---

*This use is not listed in the manufacturer's directive.

red cells "most compatible" with the patient are selected for transfusion. Usually, patients with warm autoimmune hemolysis can be safely transfused when these precautions are taken. Donor cells should be administered slowly, with the patient being closely observed for symptoms and signs suggestive of a possible hemolytic transfusion reaction, the diagnosis and treatment of which are described in Ch. 137.

COURSE AND PROGNOSIS. In patients with secondary IgG-mediated autoimmune hemolytic disorders, the clinical course and ultimate prognosis are generally determined by how effectively the underlying disease process can be controlled. In 75 per cent of patients with primary (idiopathic) immune hemolysis due to IgG autoantibodies, anemia can be abrogated with corticosteroid therapy or splenectomy or both. Uncontrollable hemolysis resulting in death rarely occurs. All evidence of hemolysis may disappear in rare patients. More commonly, a positive direct antiglobulin test persists, and the patient may experience recurrent episodes of mild hemolysis requiring intermittent steroid therapy. Splenectomized patients are generally more stable hematologically than are patients managed by medical therapy alone. Major causes of death include thromboembolic complications and sequelae of chronically impaired host defense mechanisms caused by corticosteroids, splenectomy, or immunosuppressive drugs.

AUTOIMMUNE HEMOLYTIC DISEASE DUE TO COLD-REACTING ANTIBODIES

Cold-reacting red cell antibodies combine most avidly with erythrocyte membrane antigens at grossly subphysiologic temperatures (0 to 4°C). They exhibit characteristic "thermal amplitudes," i.e., maximum temperatures beyond which they are unable to combine effectively with their antigens. Pathologically significant cold antibodies produce clinical hemolysis because they retain significant immunologic reactivity at temperatures that are achievable in vivo (30 to 32°C). Thus, if the thermal amplitude of a red cell antibody does not extend to 30°C, the antibody will have no pathophysiologic relevance. IgM cold-reacting antibodies occur most commonly. Because they strongly agglutinate red cells in the cold, they are designated *cold agglutinins.* Rare IgA cold agglutinins have been described; however, these antibodies do not produce hemolysis in vivo because they lack complement-fixing activity. Cold-reacting IgG red cell autoantibodies are occasionally encountered. They are intensely complement fixing and produce the disease picture of paroxysmal cold hemoglobinuria.

COLD AGGLUTININ DISEASE. *Pathophysiology.* IgM cold agglutinins are normally present in low concentrations in human serum. They have no known function and may represent byproducts of polyclonal immunologic responses to viruses and other microorganisms. They are quantified by the cold agglutinin titer, i.e., the maximal serum dilution, at 4°C, that induces red cell agglutination. Normal cold agglutinins are harmless because they are present in low titer (≤ 1:32) and exhibit low thermal amplitude. Usually, but not always, the higher the patient's titer, the higher the thermal amplitude of the cold agglutinin, and the greater the probability that the patient will experience hemolysis.

The synthesis of polyclonal cold agglutinins may increase in response to certain infections, especially with mycoplasma, various viruses (Epstein-Barr [EB] cytomegalovirus), and protozoans (trypanosomiasis, malaria). Cold agglutinin titers usually peak within 2 to 3 weeks of onset, but rarely do they rise sufficiently to provoke clinically apparent hemolysis.

Secondary cold agglutinin disease occasionally appears in patients with lymphoproliferative disorders (see Color Plates 6 to 8), particularly large cell lymphomas. Indeed, hemolytic anemia may be the initial manifestation of the lymphoma. In these patients the cold agglutinins are predictably monoclonal, containing either kappa or lambda light chains. Occasionally, the antibody may be present in such high concentrations that it is detectable as a monoclonal spike on serum protein electrophoresis.

Idiopathic cold agglutinin disease occurs most frequently in elderly patients in whom, by definition, no underlying infectious or neoplastic process can be identified. The cold agglutinin is almost always monoclonal kappa IgM.

Cold agglutinins react with polysaccharide constituents of red cell membranes, glycolipids and glycoproteins immunochemically related to human ABO blood group antigens. One of these polysaccharide antigens (I) is better expressed on adult erythrocytes and another (i) on fetal red cells. Cold agglutinins that react more strongly with adult red cells are said to exhibit anti-I specificity, whereas those that preferentially combine with fetal (cord) erythrocytes are designated anti-i. I and i are not alleles, and both antigens are usually expressed on adult, as well as on fetal, red cells. However, infrequently, the red cells of otherwise normal individuals express only I or i. Rare patients with cold agglutinin disease have antibodies that exhibit exclusive anti-I or anti-i reactivity. Some cold antibodies that react equally well with adult and cord cells fail to agglutinate red cells pretreated with proteolytic enzymes; they are said to show anti-PR specificity. Identification of the major reactivity of a cold agglutinin (anti-I, -i, or -PR) and its clonal diversity may be clinically informative, since cold agglutinins produced in various diseases show different characteristic patterns of reactivity (Table 135–2).

Mechanisms of Hemolysis. When high thermal amplitude cold agglutinins bind to red cells in the cooler portions of the circulation, they initiate agglutination and complement activation via the classic pathway so that intra-vascular hemolysis may ensue. However, in most patients, this occurs minimally, or not at all, because propagation of the complement cascade is effectively aborted before membrane damage occurs. Activation of the earlier components of the classic pathway (C1, 4, 2, and 3), as previously described, results in the binding of nascent C3b to the red cell membrane (EC3b). EC3b is usually so rapidly cleaved by the plasma C3 inactivator (Factor I) that it is unable to support effective activation of the membrane attack components of complement (C5–9). Factor I activity is greatly enhanced by cofactors in the plasma (Factor H) and in the red cell membrane itself (CR1). EC3b is sequentially cleaved into EC3bi and ECdg, which are incapable of supporting further complement activation. Indeed, EC3dg appears to inhibit binding of additional cold agglutinin to the red cell membrane. Although significant intravascular hemolysis is prevented, red cells bearing C3b or C3bi are sequestered primarily within the liver and destroyed by hepatic macrophages.

Clinical Manifestations. In patients with cold agglutinin disease secondary to infections, hemolysis is usually self-limited and mild. In contrast, idiopathic and lymphoma-associated cold agglutinin syndromes are characterized by persistent hemolysis that is usually worse in winter. After exposure to cold, the patient may experience painful acrocyanosis, resembling Raynaud's phenomenon, induced by intense red cell agglutination. Unlike Raynaud's, there is usually no antecedent blanching or reactive hyperemia, and local gangrene does not occur. Severe chilling may accelerate hemolysis to such a degree that hemoglobinuria results.

Diagnosis. On physical examination the patient may be mildly jaundiced. When the patient's blood is drawn, the red cells may clump so rapidly that it appears to clot despite the presence of an anticoagulant. Warming the anticoagulated blood to 37°C rapidly restores its normal appearance. Electronically measured

TABLE 135–2. RELATIONSHIP BETWEEN COLD AGGLUTININ STRUCTURE AND SPECIFICITY IN VARIOUS DISEASES

Structure	Specificity		
	Anti-I	Anti-i	Anti-PR
Polyclonal/ oligoclonal (α + λ)	Mycoplasma pneumoniae	Infectious mononucleosis	—
Monoclonal κ	Idiopathic cold agglutinin disease	Lymphoma	Idiopathic cold agglutinin disease
λ	—	Lymphoma	—

blood counts are frequently inaccurate because of the intense autoagglutination at room temperature. The red count and MCV are particularly affected, leading to distortion of the calculated hematocrit. This situation should be recognized by alert laboratory personnel. Not uncommonly, the reticulocyte count is only mildly increased, indicating suboptimal bone marrow compensation. The cold agglutinin titer is invariably elevated, and the direct antiglobulin test discloses only EC3dg. Typically, serum haptoglobin levels are decreased, and lactate dehydrogenase (LDH) concentrations are increased.

Treatment. An underlying disease process should be sought and, when identified, should be treated appropriately. Patients must avoid exposure to the cold and dress warmly. Treatment with daily chlorambucil,* 2 to 4 mg orally, decreases the rate of hemolysis in some patients, probably by reducing the synthesis of cold agglutinin. Glucocorticoids and splenectomy are generally of no benefit. If rapid hemolysis persists, the daily chlorambucil dosage may be increased to as much as 10 mg, with careful monitoring for toxicity. It may be advisable for the patient to move to a warmer climate. Although transfusions are not absolutely contraindicated, they should be avoided unless the patient is critically ill, i.e., exhibiting evidence of cardiovascular decompensation (tachyarrhythmias, angina, congestive failure) or cerebral hypoxia (e.g., confusion and visual disturbances) that responds poorly to bed rest and oxygen therapy. In addition to the transfusion-associated risks previously described in patients with warm autoimmune hemolysis, the following must be considered: (1) Transfused compatible red cells will be hemolyzed as rapidly, or even more rapidly, than the patient's own cells; the latter, having membrane-associated C3dg, appear to be more resistant to additional IgM cold agglutinin binding. By increasing the circulating red cells at risk of complement-mediated destruction, transfusion may exacerbate intravascular hemolysis, resulting in hemoglobinemia and hemoglobinuria. This situation may further jeopardize the patient's renal function and predispose to thromboembolic complications, red cell stroma being thrombogenic. (2) Although theoretically hazardous, the actual danger of administering refrigerated donor blood to a patient with cold agglutinin disease has been debated. Some experts strongly advise that a properly functioning, in-line blood warmer be utilized. Uncontrolled warming of donor erythrocytes must be avoided, since this is more hazardous than the slow administration of refrigerated blood. (3) The usual risks of transfusion therapy (Ch. 137) must be considered. By expanding the patient's blood volume, transfusion may exacerbate congestive heart failure. Transmission of hepatitis, cytomegalovirus, or human immunodeficiency virus (HIV) infections may occur. When transfusions are administered, the patient must be kept warm, a limited volume of red cells (designed to alleviate life-threatening symptoms, not simply to improve the hemoglobin concentration) should be infused slowly, and the patient's response monitored carefully. In life-threatening situations, plasmapheresis with plasma exchange should be considered. When this procedure is performed, the blood tubing and centrifugation apparatus should be maintained at 37°C.

PAROXYSMAL COLD HEMOGLOBINURIA (DONATH-LANDSTEINER HEMOLYTIC ANEMIA). Paroxysmal cold hemoglobinuria (PCH) is an exceedingly rare autoimmune hemolytic disorder caused by IgG cold-reacting antibodies directed against the ubiquitous P blood group antigen. It was first described in patients with tertiary syphilis who, following exposure to cold, developed paroxysms of chills, fever, headache, and diffuse pain in the abdomen, back, and legs accompanied by hemoglobinuria. PCH now more commonly occurs as a complication of certain viral infections, particularly infectious mononucleosis, measles, or mumps. In this context, hemolysis is rarely paroxysmal, and a history of cold exposure is seldom obtained. Consequently, it has been proposed that the syndrome be renamed Donath-Landsteiner (DL) hemolytic anemia to honor the investigators who first described the offending antibody. The diagnosis of PCH is made by demonstrating in the patient's serum the biphasic DL cold hemolysin. This IgG, nonagglutinating autoantibody activates complement so efficiently that intravascular hemolysis results. Normal red cells are mixed with the patient's serum and a source of complement, briefly chilled (0 to 4°C) and then warmed to

---

*This use is not listed in the manufacturer's directive.

37°C. If hemolysis is observed, this is presumptive evidence of the DL antibody. The patient's direct Coombs' test may be negative or may disclose only small amounts of complement, with or without traces of IgG. When PCH occurs secondary to a viral infection, hemolysis is usually transient, requiring only supportive therapy. If hemolysis recurs or becomes chronic, it may respond to treatment with glucocorticoids or to immunosuppressive drugs, such as cyclophosphamide.*

IMMUNOHEMOLYTIC ANEMIA DUE TO DRUGS. A number of drugs, or their in vivo metabolic derivatives, may induce immune hemolysis. Three distinct mechanisms have been described (Fig. 135–1):

1. *Drug binding to red cells.* When administered intravenously, certain immunogenic drugs, exemplified by penicillin, bind tightly to erythrocyte membranes. If drug-specific antibodies are produced, they attach to the cells at membrane sites containing the drug, triggering red cell destruction. In the case of penicillin-induced immune hemolysis, a non–complement-fixing, IgG antipenicillin antibody is characteristically involved. In vivo, it binds to penicillin-modified red cells and causes their destruction by a mechanism essentially identical to that seen in warm autoimmune hemolytic anemia, i.e., IgG-sensitized red cells are sequestered primarily within the spleen and destroyed by Fcγ receptor–bearing macrophages. The direct antiglobulin test discloses only IgG, whereas the indirect Coombs test is characteristically negative. The antipenicillin specificity of the red cell antibody can be demonstrated by eluting it and showing that it fails to combine with normal erythrocytes unless they have been pretreated with penicillin. Since hemolysis promptly ceases soon after penicillin is discontinued, corticosteroid therapy is usually unnecessary.

2. *Innocent bystander hemolysis.* Other drugs that induce immune hemolytic anemia in humans (e.g., sulfonamides, phenothiazines, quinine and quinidine) are bound primarily by plasma proteins rather than red cells. Although they are weakly immunogenic, they stimulate the synthesis of drug-specific, complement-fixing antibodies in some patients. As a result, the patient's erythrocytes are bathed in plasma containing drug-antibody immune complexes that may bind to the cells and activate complement. Nascent C3b may covalently bind to the red cell membrane and facilitate activation of the alternative complement pathway by binding factor B, which is then cleaved into Bb by factor D, a proteolytic enzyme normally present in plasma. C3b,Bb, the alternative pathway C3 convertase, cleaves additional C3, generating more nascent C3b that is available to bind to the red cell membrane. C3b,Bb,C3b complexes, acting as the alternative pathway C5 convertase, cleave C5, thereby triggering activation of the terminal (C5–9) membrane attack complex of complement. If inadequately restrained by the complement inactivators and inhibitors previously described, this process will result in life-threatening intravascular hemolysis. Even if activation of the membrane attack complex is effectively prevented, red cells bearing C4b, C3b, and C3bi are at risk of sequestration and destruction by hepatic macrophages. The direct antiglobulin test reveals only membrane-associated complement cleavage products, primarily C3dg. Efforts to elute immunoprotein from the patient's red cells are usually unsuccessful. The indirect antiglobulin test is characteristically negative. However, when the offending drug, or an appropriate metabolic derivative thereof, is added to normal erythrocytes that have been suspended in the patient's serum with a source of complement, hemolysis may be provoked. Coombs' testing of the nonhemolyzed cells may disclose membrane-associated complement fragments. After the patient discontinues the drug, hemolysis usually subsides promptly, and no additional therapy is required.

3. *Drug-induced autoimmune hemolytic anemia.* A pure IgG direct antiglobulin test appears in approximately 15 per cent of patients undergoing long-term treatment with methyldopa (Aldomet). However, only 10 per cent of these Coombs-positive patients develop clinically apparent hemolysis. The IgG eluted from patient's red cells combines readily with normal erythrocytes in the absence of methyldopa, thereby displaying true autoimmune reactivity. Patients treated with levodopa or mefenamic

---

*This use is not listed in the manufacturer's directive.

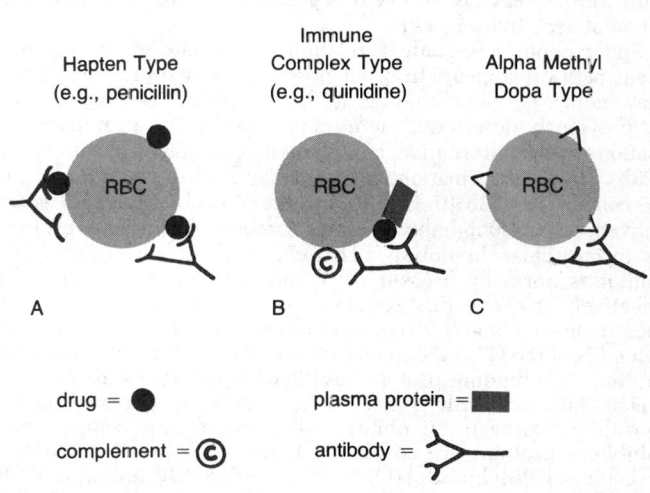

FIGURE 135–1. Mechanisms of drug-induced, immune hemolysis. *A,* The drug, or its metabolite, binds to the red cell membrane and acts as a hapten. Antibodies to the drug-membrane complex can induce red cell destruction either via FcγR-mediated sequestration by macrophages or by activating complement. *B,* A drug capable of acting as a hapten binds to plasma protein(s). After antibodies are formed, the Ab-drug-protein complex binds to the red cell membrane and activates complement, resulting in lysis. *C,* Long-term treatment with drug appears to induce a change in the red cell membrane, often altering its Rh specificity. Antibodies that develop bind to the altered membrane, producing a positive direct Coombs test and, rarely, hemolysis. (Adapted from Andreoli TE, Carpenter CCJ, Plum F, et al. [eds.]: Cecil Essentials of Medicine. 2nd ed. Philadelphia, W. B. Saunders Company, 1990, p 357.)

acid (Ponstel), a nonsteroidal anti-inflammatory drug, may develop similar erythrocyte autoantibodies. By unknown mechanisms these agents may interfere with immunoregulatory processes that suppress synthesis of red cell autoantibodies. Moreover, it is not clear why hemolysis occurs in only a small percentage of Coombs-positive, methyldopa-treated patients. The mechanism of cell destruction appears identical to that seen in warm autoimmune hemolytic anemia, i.e., splenic sequestration and red cell destruction by Fcγ receptor–positive macrophages. Hemolysis usually subsides within 1 to 3 weeks after methyldopa is discontinued, but a positive direct antiglobulin test may persist for many months. Although the hemolysis responds to steroid therapy, it is rarely required. If methyldopa is readministered to a patient who has fully recovered from methyldopa-induced hemolysis, no anamnestic autoimmune response usually occurs. Hemolysis may recur, but only after a prolonged treatment period.

PAROXYSMAL NOCTURNAL HEMOGLOBINURIA

Paroxysmal nocturnal hemoglobinuria (PNH) is an acquired hemolytic disorder resulting from the proliferation of an abnormal clone of stem cells whose progeny are uniquely susceptible to complement-mediated membrane damage. Its etiology is not known. Since patients with PNH are unusually prone to develop aplastic anemia or acute leukemia, the disease may represent a "preneoplastic" transformation of hematopoietic stem cells. PNH is quite rare; however, it is probably underdiagnosed because of its frequently protean manifestations. It occurs with greatest frequency in early adulthood but has been described in young children and in the very elderly.

PATHOPHYSIOLOGY. PNH red cells are inordinately sensitive to the lytic effects of complement. A patient's peripheral blood usually contains two or three subpopulations of red cells differing in their complement sensitivity (I = normally sensitive cells, II = cells of intermediate sensitivity, and III = very sensitive cells). In vitro, when PNH red cells are exposed to complement activated by either the classic or the alternative pathway, PNH II and III cells bind more C3b than do normal red cells. The in vivo rate of red cell destruction correlates well with the percentages of erythrocytes that exhibit extreme complement-sensitivity in vitro.

Spontaneous low-grade activation of the alternative complement pathway appears to occur normally in vivo. This activation may induce covalent binding of C3b to the red cell membrane. As previously described, membrane-bound C3b can initiate formation of the alternative complement pathway C3 convertase (C3b, Bb). This formation, in turn, may lead to assembly of the C5 convertase (C3b,Bb,C3b). Cleavage of C5 by the latter would activate the C5–9 membrane attack complex, potentially resulting in intravascular hemolysis. The complement inactivators and inhibitors normally present in plasma and red cell membranes effectively prevent this sequence of events. Normal red cell membranes contain a glycoprotein, DAF or CD55, that inhibits assembly of the C3 and C5 convertases. Two additional membrane proteins, C8 binding protein (also known as HRF) and MIRL or CD59, interfere with hemolysis by preventing insertion of C9 into the erythrocyte membrane. All three of these complement-inhibitory proteins are covalently linked to red cell membrane glycophosphatidylinositol (GPI): each is essentially absent in PNH III and present in markedly reduced concentrations in PNH II red cells. This situation accounts for the marked susceptibility of these cells to complement-mediated hemolysis.

Platelets and granulocytes in paroxysmal nocturnal hemoglobinuria are also deficient in these GPI-anchored, complement-regulatory proteins. These cells also exhibit increased vulnerability to complement activation in vitro. Although the in vivo survival of PNH platelets has been reported to be normal, their enhanced susceptibility to complement activation may underlie the thrombotic diathesis commonly seen in these patients. Functional abnormalities of the PNH granulocyte, which has been found to be deficient in the GPI-linked Fcγ receptor (type III), have also been described.

CLINICAL MANIFESTATIONS. The diagnosis of PNH must be considered in all patients with chronic hemolysis, particularly when associated with hemoglobinuria, pancytopenia, or unusual veno-occlusive events. During episodes of rapid hemolysis, patients commonly experience diffuse abdominal and back pain that has been attributed to ischemia resulting from microcirculatory thrombi. Not infrequently, major thromboses occur, involving the hepatic, splenic, portal, or cerebral veins. On physical examination, pallor and scleral icterus are common. The degree of anemia is highly variable, ranging from mild to severe. The reticulocyte count may be inappropriately low, given the severity of the anemia. The MCV may be normal, slightly increased, or diminished, depending upon the degree of reticulocytosis and the presence of accompanying iron deficiency due to prolonged urinary loss. Mild thrombocytopenia and granulocytopenia occur commonly. The peripheral blood smear reveals no autoagglutination, spherocytosis, or red cell fragmentation. The direct antiglobulin test is usually negative. Bone marrow cellularity varies from markedly hypoplastic to profoundly hyperplastic, and iron stores are usually reduced or absent. Erythroid elements predominate, and cell maturation is typically normoblastic.

Because red cell destruction occurs intravascularly, the serum LDH is elevated, serum haptoglobin levels are reduced or absent, and hemosiderinuria is present. Frank hemoglobinuria usually occurs only intermittently and is most apparent after periods of sleep.

DIAGNOSIS. The diagnosis of PNH requires that the patient's red cells show excessive susceptibility to complement-mediated hemolysis in vitro, usually demonstrated by mixing the patient's red cells with freshly collected normal human serum that has been mildly acidified (*Ham's test*). The hemolysis observed results from activation of the alternative pathway. The Ham test is highly specific but is too insensitive to detect all patients with PNH. The simpler sucrose hemolysis test, which induces complement activation via the classic pathway, is much more sensitive than Ham's test. However, it is less specific, false-positive results occurring in some patients with myeloproliferative disorders. Neutrophil alkaline phosphatase and erythrocyte acetylcholinesterase are characteristically reduced in PNH. Although these findings are not specific for PNH, both enzymes are GPI linked, strengthening the concept that PNH results from defective anchoring of various membrane constituents to GPI.

Other causes of intravascular hemolysis and hemoglobinuria that should be considered in the differential diagnosis include (1) drug-induced immunohemolytic anemia; (2) paroxysmal cold hemoglobinuria; (3) red cell hemolysins such as those present in snake venoms and *Clostridium welchii* exotoxin; (4) traumatic intravascular hemolysis as occurs in thrombotic thrombocytopenic purpura, hemolytic-uremic syndrome, or march hemoglobinuria; and (5) glucose-6-phosphate dehydrogenase (G6PD) deficiency exacerbated by oxidant drugs (Ch. 134).

TREATMENT. Erythropoiesis may be enhanced with folic acid, iron, and androgen therapy. In some patients iron administration may provoke increased hemolysis and hemoglobinuria. This situation may be prevented by prior transfusion and probably results from the destruction of increased numbers of newly produced, complement-sensitive reticulocytes. Androgen administration may significantly improve the anemia. A 6- to 8-week trial of oral fluoxymesterone or oxymesterone (5 to 50 mg per day), or of intramuscular nandrolone decanoate (25 to 200 mg once weekly), is usually sufficient to identify androgen-responsive patients.

Glucocorticoids (equivalent to 0.25 to 1 mg of prednisone per kilogram per day) slow the acute hemolytic episodes in some patients. Continuous treatment with low-dose steroids may reduce chronic hemolysis. However, daily steroids should not be administered except in life-threatening situations because of their unacceptable side effects and the increased danger of overwhelming bacterial or fungal sepsis. Alternate-day prednisone, in doses ranging from 15 to 40 mg, has been reported to improve the majority of patients so treated.

Most patients with PNH eventually require blood transfusions. Initially, donor red cells survive normally and suppress the production of the patient's abnormal red cells, resulting in marked clinical improvement. Following repetitive transfusions, however, patients are prone to develop hemosiderosis and to produce alloantibodies to red cell, neutrophil, platelet, and even plasma protein antigens. Once alloimmunization has occurred, further transfusion therapy is difficult, since in vivo complement activation triggered by alloantigen administration may result in rapid destruction of the patient's red cells. Even compatible transfusions may accelerate hemolysis of the patient's red cells and induce hemoglobinuria, probably because the donor material contains small quantities of activated complement. If evidence of increased hemolysis follows transfusion of packed donor red cells, administration of washed or frozen and reconstituted red cells may circumvent this problem.

Patients with PNH are predisposed to major venous thromboses and therefore require anticoagulation not infrequently. Since heparin therapy has been reported to exacerbate hemolysis in some patients, it must be used with caution. Vitamin K antagonists can usually be employed without difficulty, but it is not clear whether continuous prophylactic anticoagulation with warfarin (Coumadin) derivatives is clinically beneficial.

Bone marrow transplantation has successfully eradicated the PNH clone in a small number of patients.

PROGNOSIS. The course of PNH is exceedingly variable. Most patients die within 10 years of diagnosis. In a small percentage of patients, all disease manifestations spontaneously subside, possibly reflecting disappearance of the aberrant clone. More commonly, patients experience waxing and waning hemolysis, which may be exacerbated by immunologic stress, such as infection, transfusion, and immunization. Thrombotic events, primarily venous, account for much of the morbidity and mortality. With time, marrow function progressively deteriorates, not infrequently evolving into a clinical picture of aplastic anemia. In approximately 5 per cent of patients, acute myeloblastic leukemia develops.

HEMOLYSIS CAUSED BY CHEMICALS

A number of chemical toxins may directly injure and destroy red cells. These range in complexity from inorganic cations (arsenic and copper) and simple organic compounds such as chloramine to complex biologic substances produced by microorganisms, plants, and lower animals. Arsenic and copper damage red cells probably by binding to membrane sulfhydryl groups. Copper-induced hemolysis has been observed in hemodialyzed patients and may be responsible for the transient hemolytic episodes observed in patients with Wilson's disease.

Purification of urban water supplies with alum and chlorine results in the generation of chloramine, a potent oxidant. If chloramine is not effectively removed from tap water used for hemodialysis, it may swiftly oxidize hemoglobin to methemoglobin, resulting in Heinz body formation and rapid hemolysis.

Amphotericin B is a lipophilic fungal product that binds avidly to red cell membrane lipids rendering them more permeable to sodium. In occasional patients it may provoke hemolysis.

Clostridium welchii, spiders, and snakes produce potent lipolytic toxins capable of damaging red cell membrane integrity. They provoke rapid intravascular hemolysis characterized by marked spherocytosis. Hemolysis of uncertain etiology may accompany severe infections with other bacteria (*Streptococcus pneumoniae*, *Escherichia coli*, *Staphylococcus aureus*). Castor beans and certain species of mushrooms contain hemolysis-inducing toxins.

HEMOLYSIS CAUSED BY METABOLIC ABNORMALITIES

SPUR CELL HEMOLYTIC ANEMIA. Patients with a significant hepatocellular disease are frequently anemic. Blood loss, folate deficiency, alcohol-induced marrow dysfunction, and hypersplenism may contribute to the etiology of the anemia. However, in a small percentage of patients with end-stage cirrhosis, a clinical picture of rapid hemolysis develops with the appearance of numerous acanthocytes (spiculated, spur-shaped red cells).

Pathophysiology. Red cell membrane cholesterol and phospholipids exist in dynamic equilibrium with plasma lipids. In many patients with severe parenchymal liver disease, plasma lipoproteins appear to unload excessive cholesterol and phospholipid onto the erythrocyte membrane. As a result, the membranes spread and the cells thin, becoming target cells. However, the molar ratio of cholesterol to phospholipids in target cells remains normal, and the cells usually survive normally in vivo. In patients with spur cell hemolytic anemia, excess cholesterol relative to phospholipid accumulates in the red cell membrane. This condition may be caused by an abnormal high-density plasma lipoprotein. Red cell deformability becomes markedly reduced and hemolysis results.

Clinical Manifestations. Patients with spur-cell hemolytic anemia characteristically exhibit marked splenomegaly and signs of advanced cirrhosis, including jaundice, ascites, varices, and neurologic manifestations of hepatic encephalopathy. The anemia is usually severe, and the peripheral smear contains numerous acanthocytes and polychromatophilic reticulocytes. The direct antiglobulin test is negative. Red cell survival is short, the cells being sequestered by the spleen.

Diagnosis. The presence of a significantly elevated reticulocyte count and numerous spur cells on peripheral smear in a patient with end-stage cirrhosis is diagnostic of this syndrome. When normal compatible red cells are incubated with the patient's plasma in vitro, they become echinocytic in shape.

Prognosis and Treatment. Spur cell hemolytic anemia carries an exceedingly poor prognosis, almost all patients dying within months as a result of underlying liver disease. The benefits of transfusion are limited, since normal erythrocytes survive no better than patient's cells. Splenectomy may slow the rate of hemolysis but is exceedingly hazardous because of the severe liver disease.

HYPOPHOSPHATEMIA. Hemolysis may occur in patients with profoundly depressed serum phosphorus levels (< 1 mg per 100 ml) (Ch. 194). Hypophosphatemia of this degree occurs primarily in severely malnourished patients, particularly when they ingest excessive quantities of phosphate-binding antacids. Erythrocyte adenosine triphosphate (ATP) levels fall, the cells become poorly deformable, and hemolysis occurs primarily within the spleen.

HEMOLYSIS CAUSED BY RED CELL PARASITES

MALARIA. *Malarial infections*, particularly with *Plasmodium falciparum*, are probably the most common cause of hemolytic anemia worldwide (see Color Plate 8L, left) (Ch. 424). Merozoites invade red cells and utilize for their own purposes the contained hemoglobin, enzymes, and substrates. The metabolically deprived erythrocytes are unable to maintain normal cation fluxes and become osmotically fragile. Moreover, infected red cells may display new membrane antigens that incite host immune responses, resulting in positive direct antiglobulin tests. IgG antibodies eluted from the Coombs-positive red cells exhibit specificity for malarial antigens. Red cell destruction appears to occur primarily in the spleen, and splenomegaly is almost universally present in patients with chronic malarial infection. Rarely, rapid intravascular hemolysis with hemoglobinuria (blackwater fever) occurs soon after antimalarial therapy is initiated. It is not clear whether the infection or the drug plays the more important role in this phenomenon.

BABESIOSIS. *Babesia* are protozoans that parasitize red cells of many animal species (Ch. 432). Several cases of babesia-induced hemolytic anemia have been reported in humans, the disease being particularly fulminant in previously splenectomized individuals. Such patients may present with thrombocytopenia, disseminated intravascular coagulation, and renal insufficiency. Although deer ticks are the usual vector, the disease may be transmitted by transfusion of infected red cells. The disease has been reported most frequently in the northeastern United States (Martha's Vineyard and Nantucket). Intraerythrocytic parasites can usually be seen in Giemsa-stained peripheral blood films.

BARTONELLOSIS. *Bartonella bacilliformis*, a gram-negative pleomorphic bacterium, is endemic to Peru, Ecuador, and Columbia. It grows on the surface of red cells rather than within them (Ch. 331). The disease is transmitted by the bite of the sand fly and usually appears 3 weeks thereafter. The patient develops hectic fever and chills, headache, and musculoskeletal pain before hemolysis begins. The hemolytic episode is acute in onset and rapid. The red cells are Coombs-negative and are sequestered by both liver and spleen. The peripheral blood smear typically discloses rod-shaped organisms on the erythrocyte surface and large numbers of spherocytes, normoblasts, and reticulocytes. The infection responds well to various antibiotics.

HEMOLYSIS RESULTING FROM TRAUMA TO RED CELLS

When subjected to excessive mechanical stress, circulating red cells may undergo fragmentation and hemolyze. The forces responsible may be generated extracorporeally or intravascularly. For example, fragmentational hemolysis may result from excessive intravascular shear stress originating around critically narrowed heart valves, pathologic shunts (arterial or arteriovenous), cardiac valve prostheses, poorly endothelialized vascular surfaces, or microvascular thrombi. In these situations hemolysis is accompanied by characteristic morphologic evidence of red cell fragmentation. Similarly, red cells may be injured by excessive heat, resulting in hemolysis. Temperatures exceeding 49°C destabilize the human red cell membrane. In vitro, they are observed to undergo budding and fragmentation. Patients who have suffered extensive third-degree burns may show prominent spherocytosis on the peripheral smear, and in some cases hemoglobinemia and hemoglobinuria may occur acutely. The major syndromes associated with traumatic hemolysis are summarized briefly.

MARCH HEMOGLOBINURIA. As red cells circulate through narrow vessels overlying the bones of the hands and feet, they may be traumatized by repetitive, relatively uncushioned forces generated, for example, by prolonged marching, running, and karate blows. Intravascular hemolysis accompanied by hemoglobinemia and hemoglobinuria may result. Interestingly, no red cell morphologic abnormalities are apparent in the peripheral blood film during, or immediately following, the physical activity that precipitated the hemolytic episode.

FRAGMENTATIONAL HEMOLYSIS DUE TO CARDIAC PATHOLOGY OR ABNORMALITIES OF LARGE VESSELS. Cardiac abnormalities primarily involving the left side of the heart, where pressures are high, may predispose to hemolysis. These include severe aortic stenosis or regurgitation and ruptured sinus of Valsalva. Significant red cell fragmentation may also result from traumatic arteriovenous fistulas or therapeutic aortofemoral bypass procedures. In such patients the hemolysis is usually low grade.

More rapid hemolysis may occur in patients with prosthetic heart valves. It occurs more frequently with aortic than mitral prostheses, with artificial valves rather than those of biologic (porcine) origin, with metallic rather than Silastic valves, and with defective or poorly functioning valves that exhibit ball variance or paravalvular leaks.

Clinical Manifestations. Patients rarely present with rapid intravascular hemolysis. A common clinical picture is one of increasing anemia, low-grade reticulocytosis, and numerous fragmented red cells (schistocytes) on peripheral blood film (see Color Plate 6E, right). Some findings typical of significant intravascular hemolysis are usually present, i.e., low to absent haptoglobin levels, increased serum LDH concentrations, and hemosiderinuria. Chronic urinary iron loss may result in iron deficiency. Although the direct Coombs test is usually negative, a poorly understood positive result has been observed in a few patients.

Treatment. Patients should be advised to limit their physical activity in an effort to reduce cardiac output and, thereby, to slow the rate of hemolysis. Oral iron, 300 mg of ferrous sulfate three times a day, should be given to correct iron deficiency. Rarely, parenteral iron (iron-dextran) or transfusions may be required. If the rate of hemolysis necessitates repeated transfusion, replacement of the prosthesis should be considered.

FRAGMENTATIONAL HEMOLYSIS DUE TO ABNORMALITIES WITHIN THE MICROCIRCULATION (MICROANGIOPATHIC HEMOLYTIC DISORDERS). **Pathophysiology.** Red cells may be fragmented by being forced to flow through small vessels partially occluded by microthrombi. Excessive shear forces are generated as the cells encounter and become tethered to fibrin strands that bisect and fragment the erythrocytes. The microthrombi may result from (1) an underlying coagulopathy, i.e., disseminated intravascular coagulation (DIC), (2) injury to the vascular endothelium, or (3) unknown mechanisms. Pathophysiologic processes that trigger DIC commonly induce endothelial injury as well; however, the reverse is frequently not true. Diseases accompanied by diffuse microvascular pathology may present with none of the laboratory findings characteristic of DIC. Consequently, in many patients with microangiopathic hemolytic anemia, the predominant etiologic factor (i.e., coagulation or vascular injury) can be discerned.

Disseminated intravascular coagulation results when procoagulant is introduced into the systemic circulation (Ch. 155). Coagulation factors are consumed, thrombus formation occurs, and fibrinolytic mechanisms are secondarily activated. Patients with significant DIC typically present with thrombocytopenia and abnormal plasma coagulation studies, i.e., prolonged prothrombin, activated partial thromboplastin, and thrombin times, reflecting decreased concentrations of certain clotting factors (particularly V, VIII, and fibrinogen) and increased plasma concentrations of fibrin degradation products. These abnormalities are generally poorly corrected by addition of normal plasma to that of the patient. DIC may be triggered by infections, particularly with gram-negative endotoxin-containing bacteria, amniotic fluid embolism, and disseminated neoplasms (Trousseau's syndrome) that elaborate potent procoagulants such as mucin, tissue factor, or cysteine proteases that activate clotting Factors VII or X. Although patients with severe DIC may be critically ill, rapid hemolysis is unusual.

Diffuse or localized vascular lesions associated with a variety of diseases may induce red cell fragmentation, e.g., cavernous hemangiomas (Kasabach-Merritt syndrome), renal allografts undergoing rejection, malignant hypertension, eclampsia, diseases associated with vasculitis (rickettsial infections, periarteritis nodosa, Wegener's granulomatosis), and certain disseminated neoplasms. The severity of hemolysis ranges from mild to severe. Coagulation abnormalities mimicking those of DIC are frequently absent.

Thrombotic thrombocytopenic purpura (TTP) (Ch 154), the hemolytic uremic syndrome (HUS) (Ch. 79), and mitomycin C–induced HUS of cancer patients are life-threatening disorders of unknown etiology. They closely resemble one another clinically, and are characterized by fragmentational hemolysis, thrombocytopenia, and renal failure. The patients are frequently febrile, manifest mild to moderate jaundice reflecting unconjugated hyperbilirubinemia, have petechiae and ecchymoses, and exhibit a variety of CNS abnormalities, including seizures. Gastrointestinal bleeding is commonly present. In patients presenting with bloody diarrhea, infections with verotoxin-producing *Escherichia coli* may be responsible for the clinical picture of HUS/TTP. Biopsies disclose characteristic microscopic findings of hyaline thrombi within small arterioles and capillaries.

Diagnosis. The diagnosis of a microangiopathic hemolytic disorder is based on the demonstration of schistocytes, grossly misshapen, sharply angulated erythrocytes that occasionally appear helmet shaped (see Color Plate 6E, right), usually in association with reticulocytosis, unconjugated hyperbilirubinemia, serum haptoglobin levels that are diminished to absent, increased serum LDH concentrations, and hemosiderinuria. Hemoglobinemia and hemoglobinuria occur much less frequently. The direct Coombs test is characteristically negative. If significant thrombocytopenia is present, laboratory evidence of DIC should be sought but is frequently absent.

Treatment. Treatment of the patient with microangiopathic hemolysis must be highly individualized. Efforts should be made to reverse the underlying triggering mechanism (i.e., withdrawal of potentially offending drugs or treatment with antibiotics or chemotherapeutic agents) and the patient supported with red cell transfusions, platelet packs, and cryoprecipitate as required. Occasional patients may benefit from anticoagulation with heparin. Although antiplatelet drugs and high-dose adrenocorticoid therapy are frequently employed, their efficacy is less certain. Vigorous plasma exchange (plasmapheresis combined with infusion of normal plasma) may induce dramatic remissions in TTP. TTP, HUS, and mitomycin-associated microangiopathy have also been reported to respond to intravenous administration of high-dose gamma globulin.

Jandl JH: Blood: Textbook of Hematology. Boston, Little Brown and Company, 1987. *Contains crystal clear, succinct expositions of the various topics covered in this chapter—especially recommended for its discussions of the hemolytic anemias associated with red cell trauma, liver disease (spur cell hemolysis), and infections (malaria, Babesia, Bartonella).*

Moake JL: Hypercoagulable states. Adv Intern Med 35:235, 1990. *A brief, incisive review of the pathophysiology of this complex and confusing topic—includes discussion of DIC.*

Rosse WF: Clinical Immunohematology: Basic Concepts and Clinical Applications. Boston, Blackwell Scientific Publications, 1990. *This authoritative treatise, encyclopedic in scope and lucidly written, includes masterful discussions of all the immunohemolytic anemias as well as paroxysmal nocturnal hemoglobinuria. Enthusiastically recommended as a primary reference.*

Ruggenenti P, Remuzzi G: Thrombotic thrombocytopenic purpura and related disorders. Hematol/Oncol Clin North Am 4:219, 1990. *A thorough, beautifully organized discourse on the pathophysiology, diagnosis, and treatment of these disorders.*

136 Hemoglobin and Hemoglobinopathies

136.1 STRUCTURE, FUNCTION, AND SYNTHESIS OF THE HUMAN HEMOGLOBINS

Edward J. Benz, Jr.

The structure, genetics, physiology, and pathology of human hemoglobins are topics important to the internist for several reasons. First, hemoglobins and the erythrocytes in which they circulate are well characterized at the cellular, biochemical, and genetic levels. Second, hemoglobinopathies are extremely common disorders in many areas of the world. Third, elucidation of the molecular basis of hemoglobinopathies has been the result of the most thorough and successful application to date of recombinant DNA technology to the understanding of human disease. The derived principles have enhanced the understanding of many other clinical conditions. Finally, the mechanisms by which abnormal amounts or functions of hemoglobin derange other organ systems demonstrate uniquely well the pathophysiologic principles by which disordered function of a single gene can lead to multisystem disease.

THE STRUCTURE OF HEMOGLOBIN

Each human hemoglobin consists of a tetramer of globin polypeptide chains: a pair of "α-like" and a pair of "non-α" chains (Table 136–1). The major adult hemoglobin (Hb), Hb A, for example, has the following structure: $\alpha_2\beta_2$. Each chain enfolds a single heme moiety, consisting of a protoporphyrin IX ring complexed with a single ferrous ion atom (Fe^{2+}). The heme moiety resides within each polypeptide chain in a configuration optimal for reversible binding of oxygen. One heme moiety can bind a single oxygen molecule, so that every molecule of hemoglobin can transport up to four oxygen molecules. The α-like globin chains (α and ζ) are 141 amino acids long, whereas the non-α chains (ε, γ, δ, β) are 146 amino acids long.

The *primary structures* (amino acid sequences) of globins are highly homologous to one another, suggesting that all of the proteins arose from a common ancestral gene.

Each globin has a largely helical *secondary structure*. About 80 per cent of each polypeptide exists in the form of α helix. The non-α chains contain eight helical segments, designated A to H, separated from one another by short nonhelical stretches. The α-like chains contain seven helices; D helix is absent. The helices fold into three-dimensional globular *tertiary structures* (Fig. 136–1).

Each globin chain folds in a manner that causes the exterior surface to be rich in polar (hydrophilic) amino acids that enhance solubility; the hydrophobic interior forms a cleft between the E and F helices into which the heme ring is deeply buried. This "heme pocket" excludes water from the vicinity of the heme, allowing numerous noncovalent hydrophobic "weak" bonds to form. These in turn stabilize the interaction between heme and globin chains. In particular, a histidine in the F helix forms a strong covalent bond with the iron atom; in the presence of oxygen, the iron also bonds with a histidine in the E helix. These histidine iron-oxygen bonds are critical for reversible oxygenation.

The *quaternary structure* of normal adult Hb A is also complex and clinically important. The tetramer consists of two αβ dimers. The two α chains in the complete tetramer interact indirectly by means of numerous tight interactions ($\alpha_1\beta_1$ contacts) between the α and β chain within each dimer. The tetramer is held together by noncovalent bonds ($\alpha_1\beta_2$ contacts) between the α-like chain of one dimer and the non-α chain of the other dimer. These contact points undergo major conformational shifts during binding and release of oxygen.

In its oxygen transport function, hemoglobin undergoes complex conformational and solubility changes secondary to the changes that occur within the heme groups, the globin chains, and the contact points between dimers during binding and release of oxygen. The hydrophilic surface amino acids, the hydrophobic amino acids lining the heme pocket, the F8 and E7 histidines, the $\alpha_1\beta_1$ and $\alpha_1\beta_2$ contact points, and the contacts between αβ dimers represent particularly critical regions within the globin polypeptide chains. Mutations in residues that influence these strategic sites tend to be the ones associated with significant changes in clinical phenotype.

OXYGEN-CARRYING FUNCTION OF HEMOGLOBIN

Hemoglobins are physiologically useful oxygen transport proteins because of their reversible interaction with oxygen. They bind avidly to oxygen at the P_{O_2} of the alveolar capillary bed, retain the bound oxygen as the red cells traverse the circulation, and unload the ligand to the tissues at the lower oxygen tensions of tissue capillary beds. Hemoglobins provide for the necessary

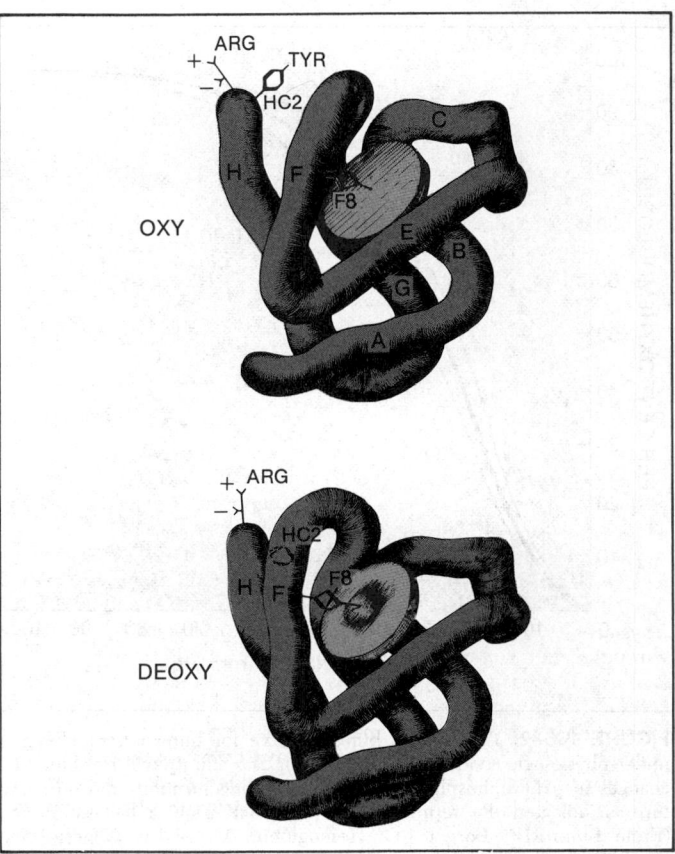

FIGURE 136–1. Structure of the oxy and deoxy states of a globin chain. Note that the amino acid sequence of globin dictates folding of eight helical segments (A–H) around the "heme" pocket in which the heme residue resides. In the deoxy state, the "F8" histidine is bound to the heme group, but this bond is broken in the oxy state. Also shown is an allosteric effect of this change on the topology of the arginine and tyrosine residues in the H helix (not discussed in the text).

amounts of oxygen acquisition and delivery over a relatively narrow range of oxygen tensions because of a property called "cooperativity" or "heme-heme interaction." This property is inherent in the tetrameric arrangement of the heme and globin subunits.

Monomeric globin-like peptides, e.g., individual globin subunits or myoglobin, acquire oxygen readily but cannot release it except at very low oxygen pressures incompatible with life. In contrast, complete hemoglobin tetramers exhibit an **S**-shaped oxygen dissociation curve (Fig. 136–2). At low oxygen tensions, the hemoglobin is deoxygenated. As the oxygen tension rises, oxygen binds to the tetramer; each heme group in the tetramer can bind one oxygen moiety. The binding of the first oxygen to deoxyhemoglobin requires a considerable amount of free energy (see below). Fully deoxygenated hemoglobin is thus said to be in the T (tense) state. As soon as one oxygen has been bound by the hemoglobin molecule, however, affinity for the binding of the remaining oxygen moieties increases, causing an increased slope in the binding curve. In other words, oxygen binding begets more oxygen binding. Oxyhemoglobin is said to be in the "R," or relaxed, state.

The cooperative mechanism of oxygen binding has been clarified by x-ray crystallography. The completely deoxy form is stabilized in its T state by the formation of several strong salt bonds (electrostatic bonds), especially within each α chain. To bind the first oxygen, these bonds must be broken. The first oxygen to bind must overcome significant resistance. As the bonds are broken, the oxygen affinity approaches that of the individual subunits, resulting in a marked increase in the affinity for the remaining oxygen molecules. This situation results in the physiologically more useful **S**-shaped oxygen equilibrium curve. Substantial amounts of oxygen are thus loaded and unloaded over a narrow range of oxygen tensions.

TABLE 136–1. COMPOSITION OF NORMAL HUMAN HEMOGLOBINS

Name of Hemoglobin	Subunit Structure	Time of Expression
Hemoglobin Portland	$\zeta_2\gamma_2$	Embryonic life
Hemoglobin Gower I	$\zeta_2\epsilon_2$	Embryonic life
Hemoglobin Gower II	$\alpha_2\epsilon_2$	Embryonic life
Hemoglobin F	$\alpha_2 G\gamma_2$	Fetal life*
	$\alpha_2 A\gamma_2$	
Hemoglobin A_2	$\alpha_2\delta_2$	Minor adult hemoglobin
Hemoglobin A	$\alpha_2\beta_2$	Major adult hemoglobin

*Produced in small amounts in a limited subpopulation of cells (F cells) in adults.

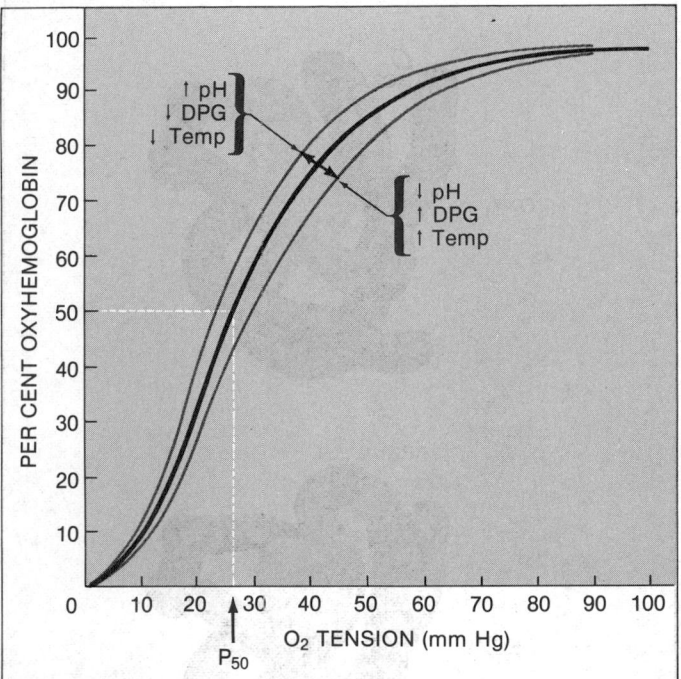

FIGURE 136–2. The oxygen binding curve for human hemoglobin A under physiologic conditions (*dark curve*). The affinity will be shifted by changes in pH, diphosphoglycerate (DPG) concentration, and temperature as indicated. P_{50} represents the oxygen tension at half saturation. (From Bunn HF, Forget BG: Hemoglobin: Molecular, Genetic, and Clinical Aspects. Philadelphia, W. B. Saunders Company, 1986.)

The oxygen affinity of normal hemoglobin is affected by many factors. Maintenance of the iron in the ferrous (Fe^{2+}) rather than the ferric (Fe^{3+}) form is critical. Hemoglobin carrying ferric iron is called methemoglobin. The classic effect of pH on oxygen affinity, known as the Bohr effect, arises from the stabilizing action of protons on the deoxy confirmation. Deoxyhemoglobin binds protons more readily than oxyhemoglobin because it is a weaker acid. Protons tend to stabilize the salt bonds that make deoxyhemoglobin more resistant to oxygen binding. Hemoglobin thus has a lower oxygen affinity at lower pH.

Allosteric effectors are small molecules that bind hemoglobin and alter oxygen affinity. The best characterized of these is 2,3-diphosphoglycerate (2,3-DPG), generated and destroyed enzymatically as an intermediate of glycolysis in red cells. In its interaction with deoxyhemoglobin, 2,3-DPG stabilizes the deoxy state. High levels of 2,3-DPG or other conditions that increase the affinity of hemoglobin for 2,3-DPG tend to result in *lower* oxygen affinity.

The major adult hemoglobin, Hb A, has a reasonably high affinity for 2,3-DPG. The oxygen affinity of Hb A is thus sensitive to the presence of 2,3-DPG. In contrast, Hb F, the major fetal hemoglobin, has very little ability to bind 2,3-DPG. Thus, Hb F and Hb A exhibit identical oxygen binding curves when analyzed as "stripped" hemoglobins in solution, but Hb F tends to have a higher oxygen affinity than does Hb A in vivo because Hb F does not interact with 2,3-DPG very well.

In brief, the structure-function features just outlined provide an exquisitely adaptive form of oxygen binding. Proper oxygen transport depends on the tetrameric structure of the proteins, the proper arrangement of charged and hydrophobic amino acids, and interaction with low molecular weight substances, such as protons or 2,3-DPG.

ONTOGENY OF HUMAN HEMOGLOBINS

Hemoglobin synthesis begins during the second month of gestation. Red cells first appear in yolk sac erythroblastic islands; these erythrocytes, called the primitive cell line, are large and nucleated. The predominant hemoglobins produced are Hb Portland ($\zeta_2\gamma_2$), Hb Gower I ($\zeta_2\epsilon_2$), and Hb Gower II ($\alpha_2\epsilon_2$), but small amounts of Hb F and Hb A can be detected even at these early stages. At about 10 to 11 weeks of gestation, erythropoiesis moves to the liver and spleen. Coincidentally, the embryonic hemoglobins decline (Fig. 136–3), to be replaced by fetal hemoglobin (Hb F: $\alpha_2\gamma_2$), a mixture of two hemoglobins differing in the composition of the γ chain component. $^A\gamma$ chains have alanine and $^G\gamma$ chains have glycine at position 136. Red cell production shifts to bone marrow during the sixth to seventh month of gestation, but Hb F continues to predominate until late in the third trimester (about 38 weeks of gestation). At that time, a switch (Hb F → Hb A switch) to the predominant synthesis of Hb A (Hb A: $\alpha_2\beta_2$) occurs. The switch causes an abrupt increase in Hb A production accompanied by a reciprocal rapid decline in Hb F production (Fig. 136–3). Synthesis of a minor Hb (Hb A_2: $\alpha_2\delta_2$) also commences at this time. Hb A (95 to 98 per cent) predominates throughout the rest of life under normal conditions. Hb F is usually present in minute amounts of 0.5 to 1.5 per cent, while Hb A_2 comprises 1.5 to 3.5 per cent of total hemoglobin in normal subjects.

Fetal and adult erythrocytes differ from each other in several ways, in addition to hemoglobin content. Fetal red cells tend to be larger (macrocytes) and have shorter circulating lifespans. Fetal red cells express the i, rather than the I (adult), surface antigen; lack the β isozyme of carbonic anhydrase present in adult cells; and produce the $^G\gamma$ and $^A\gamma$ forms of Hb F at a $^G\gamma{:}^A\gamma$ ratio of 7:3, whereas the adult $^G\gamma{:}^A\gamma$ ratio is 2:3.

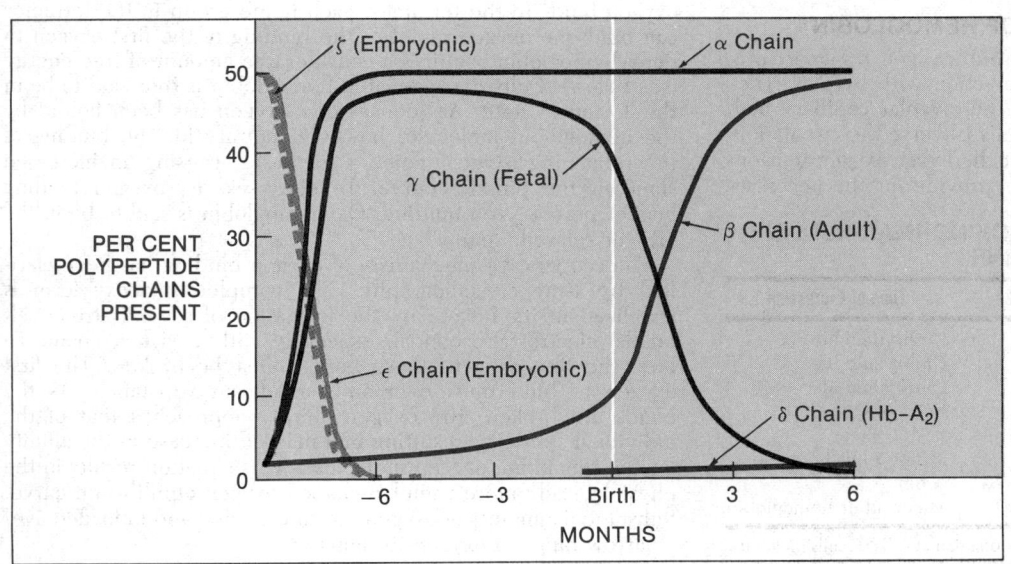

FIGURE 136–3. A diagram of the relative abundance of various human globin chains during development. (From Bunn HF, Forget BG: Hemoglobin: Molecular, Genetic, and Clinical Aspects. Philadelphia, W. B. Saunders Company, 1986.)

How hemoglobin switching is regulated is unclear. The potential of a given primitive erythroid stem cell (burst-forming unit–erythrocyte, or BFU-E) to express a particular globin gene is determined early in differentiation. By the time the stem cell has differentiated to the proerythroblast stage, when globin gene expression begins, the genetic program has been fixed and is not particularly susceptible to further modulation. The regulation of hemoglobin switching appears to result from a complex series of events. Changes in stem cell pools with varying potential for Hb F expression have profound effects, as does the chromatin configuration of the γ and β genes. The latter genes modulate transcriptional potential during the erythroblast phase of erythropoiesis. Gene expression of Hb F and Hb A is regulated largely at the stage of the primitive stem cell rather than the maturing erythroblast. Elevated Hb F levels in adults are thus often encountered in states of disordered erythropoiesis.

Small amounts of Hb F are produced during postnatal life but are confined to a small subpopulation of red cells called "F" cells. Both the numbers of F cells produced and the Hb F content of each F cell appear to be genetic polymorphisms. F cells are not truly fetal cells; they express other features of fetal cells incompletely. Changes in Hb F after birth result from altered stem cell dynamics. The most immature committed erythroid stem cell precursors (BFU-E) proceed through a series of proliferative and differentiating cell divisions before they actually form a pool of more fully differentiated progenitors (colony-forming units–erythrocyte, or CFU-E) ready to become proerythroblasts (Fig. 136–4). To a first approximation, the most immature or undifferentiated BFU-E's retain the highest potential to express Hb F in adult subjects. Under normal conditions of erythropoiesis, these cells continue to proliferate slowly and to differentiate into more mature BFU-E's before being "recruited" into the pool of maturing progenitors (CFU-E's and proerythroblasts). By this time, they have largely lost their ability to produce Hb F. Only a small number of "early" BFU-E's are actually recruited into the maturing pool, thus accounting for the small number of F cells produced under normal conditions.

Under conditions of marked erythroid stress or deranged erythropoiesis (e.g., as in chronic congenital hemolytic anemias, recovery from bone marrow transplantation or chemotherapy, or certain myelodysplastic syndromes), many BFU-E's are recruited into the pool of maturing progenitors before they have undergone their normal series of differentiating cell divisions. These cells still retain considerable potential to produce Hb F, resulting in higher than normal levels of F cells and Hb F. The molecular mechanisms mediating these complex events remain poorly understood.

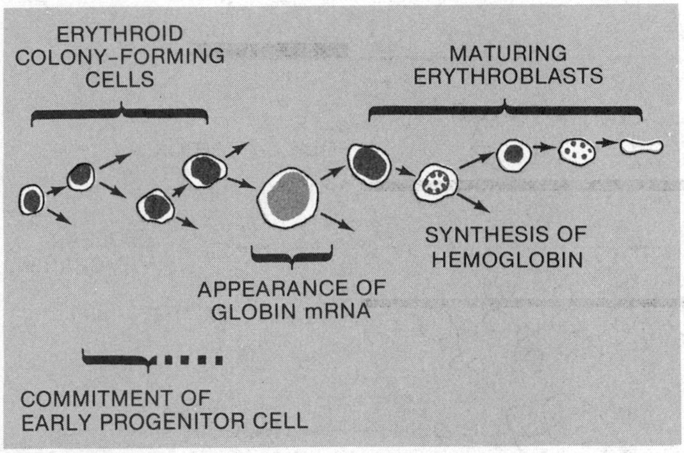

FIGURE 136–4. Regulation of hemoglobin synthesis during erythropoiesis. Two general classes of cells are the precursors of circulating red cells. Erythroblasts at various stages of maturation may be recognized within the bone marrow; these cells and circulating reticulocytes are engaged in hemoglobin synthesis. Erythroid stem cells, the progenitors of erythroblasts, are present within the bone marrow in very small numbers but may be detected by virtue of their ability to form colonies of erythroblasts in semisolid media in vitro. Current evidence suggests that commitment to expression of either the γ or the β globin genes occurs in erythroid stem cells prior to the initial appearance of globin messenger RNA (mRNA).

GENETICS AND BIOSYNTHESIS OF HUMAN HEMOGLOBIN

The production of the various human hemoglobins is controlled by two tightly linked gene clusters (Fig. 136–5). The α-like globin genes are clustered on the short arm of chromosome 16, between band 13.2 and the telomere, and the non-α genes are found on chromosome 11 at band P15, near the terminus of the short arm. The α-like cluster consists of two α globin genes and a single copy of the ζ gene. The non-α gene cluster consists of a single ε gene, the $^G\gamma$ and $^A\gamma$ fetal globin genes, and the adult δ and β genes. The functional anatomy of globin genes is typical of most eukaryotic genes. Each globin gene contains three blocks of nucleotide sequences (exons) that ultimately code for mature messenger RNA (mRNA); these are arrayed in tandem with two intervening sequences (introns). The non-α globin genes contain a small (130 bases) and large (900 to 1100 bases) intervening sequence, whereas both of the intervening sequences in the α and ζ globin genes are small (100 to 200 bases).

Flanking sequences at each end of the globin genes are important for regulating their activity. Immediately upstream (30 to 70 base pairs [bp]) are typical eukaryotic promoter elements facilitating entry of mRNA polymerase (Fig. 136–6). Regions 100 to 500 bases upstream are important for proper developmental expression. Sequences in the 5′ flanking region of the γ genes and the β genes influence, but do not exclusively control, the developmental regulation of these genes.

Important regulatory elements are also found in the 3′ flanking regions. The regions in which these regulatory sequences exist exhibit the structural features of highly active genes in bulk chromatin, such as DNase hypersensitivity. The methylation state of the γ globin genes also changes during development. In fetal erythroblasts, the promoter regions are relatively devoid of methyl group modification of cytosines (hypomethylation). In general, this characteristic correlates with higher levels of gene activity. In adult erythroblasts, the genes are heavily methylated, a feature associated with inactivity. Whether this correlation is causally related to the level of γ gene expression in fetuses and adults is unclear.

In proerythroblasts, globin synthesis comprises at most 0.5 to 1 per cent of total protein synthesis. During the subsequent maturation steps, globin gene expression increases enormously. For example, in reticulocytes generated during this 3- to 5-day period, globin mRNA and globin synthesis comprise 90 to 95 per cent of total mRNA content and protein synthesis, respectively. To achieve this remarkable degree of activation, globin genes are highly adapted for expression in erythroid cells.

Tissue and developmental activation of individual globin genes depends in part upon short DNA sequences called enhancers. These are located in the 5′ and 3′ flanking sequences and possibly in the introns of the genes. An important enhancer activating the entire non-α gene complex (called the "locus activating region" [LAR] or "dominant control region" [DCR]) has been tentatively identified several thousand bases upstream of the ε gene. These regulatory DNA sequences are called "cis" acting elements. They achieve their biologic effects via their interaction with "trans" acting factors, i.e., nuclear DNA binding proteins that specifically bind to these sequences, thereby promoting or inhibiting transcription.

Several "transcription factors" have been found to bind the globin gene promoters and enhancers. Many of these protein factors appear to be nonspecific in that they can activate a number of genes in many tissues if they gain access to their binding sites. At least one factor, however, called NFe-1 or GF-1, is largely erythroid specific (it is also found in megakaryocytes). It recognizes a consensus DNA sequence called "AGATAAG" found near many genes that are expressed specifically in erythroid cells, including the globin genes and the erythropoietin receptor gene. Although *important* for activation of the erythroid program of gene expression, GF-1 alone is probably not sufficient to trigger the process. The activity of GF-1 may depend on interaction with other transcription factors.

Each globin gene possesses structural features that are essential for the normal function of most genes (Fig. 136–6). These include the presence of a "CAP" site necessary to mark the beginning of

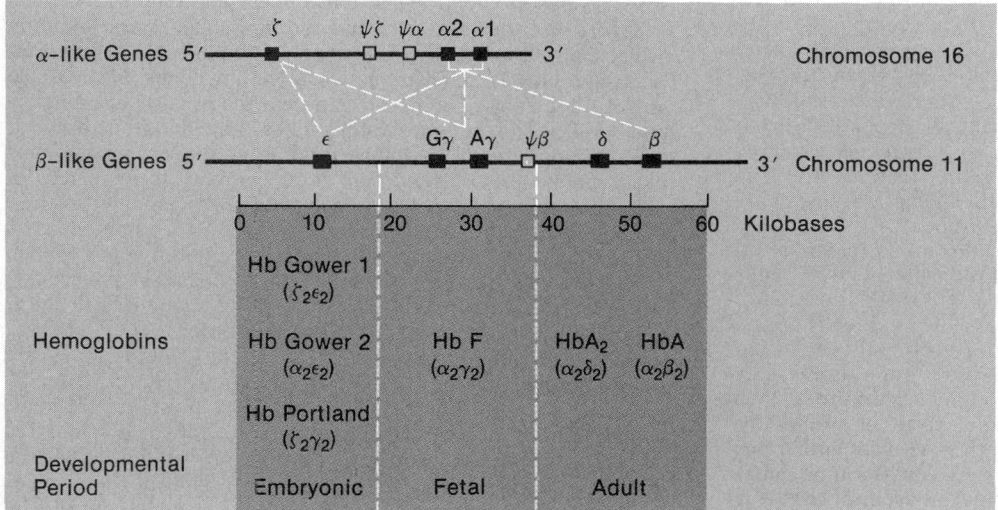

FIGURE 136–5. A diagram of the arrangement of the clusters of human α-like and β-like globin genes on chromosomes 16 and 11 and the embryonic, fetal, and adult hemoglobins that result from the combinations of the various globin chains encoded by these genes. The ψ genes are similar to globin genes but do not code for protein. Distances along the chromosome are expressed in terms of 1000 nucleotide pairs (a kilobase).

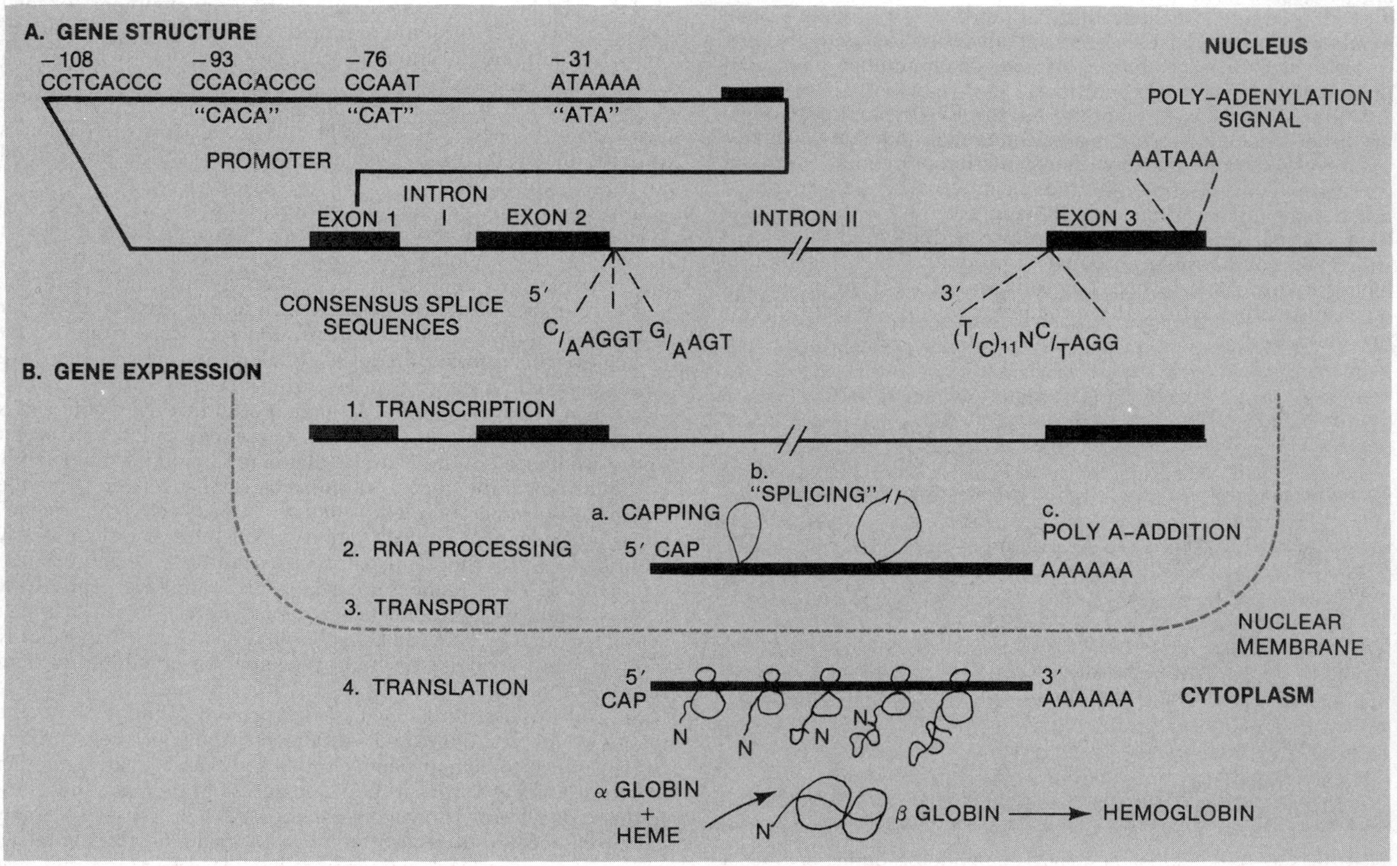

A. GENE STRUCTURE

NUCLEUS

−108 CCTCACCC   −93 CCACACCC   −76 CCAAT   −31 ATAAAA

"CACA"   "CAT"   "ATA"

PROMOTER

POLY-ADENYLATION SIGNAL

AATAAA

EXON 1   INTRON I   EXON 2   INTRON II   EXON 3

CONSENSUS SPLICE SEQUENCES

$5'$ $C_{/A}AGGT$ $G_{/A}AGT$

$3'$ $(T_{/C})_{11}NC_{/T}AGG$

B. GENE EXPRESSION

1. TRANSCRIPTION

2. RNA PROCESSING
   a. CAPPING
   b. "SPLICING"
   c. POLY A-ADDITION
   5' CAP   AAAAAA

3. TRANSPORT

NUCLEAR MEMBRANE

4. TRANSLATION
   5' CAP   3' AAAAAA   CYTOPLASM
   N   N   N   N   N

α GLOBIN + HEME   β GLOBIN ⟶ HEMOGLOBIN

FIGURE 136–6. Structure and expression of the normal human β globin gene. The three exons encode for β globin; these coding sequences are interrupted by two introns or intervening sequences. Certain segments of the promoter region ("boxes") are conserved in many globin genes. The actual sequence of these "boxes" in the β globin gene promoter is shown. The splice sequences shown represent the consensus of those found at many exon-intron boundaries. Those actually found in the β globin gene resemble the consensus sequence but are not identical. The processes involved in gene expression include transcription of the gene, processing of the primary RNA transcript, transport of the mRNA from nucleus to cytoplasm, and translation of the mRNA into β globin. C = cytosine; T = thymine; A = adenine; G = guanine.

transcription of the mRNA precursor; properly located initiation and termination codons to signal the beginning and end of translation of the mature mRNA; the presence in the appropriate locations, but nowhere else, of the donor (GT) and acceptor (AG) splicing sites that mark the points in the mRNA precursor at which the introns should be removed while the exons are ligated together; "consensus" sequences surrounding the donor and acceptor dinucleotides that form the functional splicing signal; and the presence of 5' and 3' untranslated sequences whose significance remains unclear. Like many other eukaryotic mRNA's, globin RNA's are polyadenylated. Their 3' untranslated sequences contain appropriate polyadenylation signals. As discussed in Ch. 136.4, these regions are mutated in various forms of thalassemia.

The pathway of globin gene expression is typical of most eukaryotic genes (Fig. 136–6). Each gene is initially transcribed into an mRNA precursor. Through a series of splicing reactions, the introns are removed and the exons are spliced together. At an early step in this process, the mRNA is modified at the 5' end by the "5' CAP" structure and the addition of a poly A tail. Mature mRNA is then transported from nucleus to cytoplasm. It associates with ribosomes, transfer RNA's (tRNA's), and proteinaceous initiation and elongation factors needed for translation on polyribosomes. The newly synthesized globin polypeptide chains combine rapidly with heme and then with one another to form hemoglobin tetramers. These posttranslational steps proceed rapidly and spontaneously (i.e., nonenzymatically). As hemoglobin "ages" in circulating erythrocytes, it is susceptible to further modification, such as acetylation (especially Hb F) and nonenzymatic glycosylation (Hb A_{1-C}). The latter has been used to follow control of diabetes mellitus, since A_{1-C} levels increase when the blood glucose level is high.

The hemoglobin tetramer, the final product of this complex process, is a highly soluble molecule. In contrast, the individual globin chains are rather insoluble. To prevent the globin chains from precipitating, it is essential that α and non-α globins be synthesized in approximately equal, or balanced, amounts. Each newly synthesized α or non-α globin chain will then have a "mate" with which to pair. The pathophysiology of severe thalassemia syndromes involves imbalance of globin chain synthesis and precipitation of the unpaired chains.

RELATIONSHIP OF IRON ACCUMULATION AND HEME SYNTHESIS TO HEMOGLOBIN PRODUCTION

The successful synthesis of hemoglobin requires coordination and regulation of the expression not only of the globin genes but also of the many genes responsible for heme and iron metabolism. The considerable amount of iron required for hemoglobin synthesis is provided to the erythroblast via membrane receptors specific for the iron transport protein transferrin. Iron is ultimately inserted into protoporphyrin to form heme. Synthesis of protoporphyrin IX occurs by a series of reactions catalyzed by enzymes found in relatively high concentrations in erythroblasts (Ch. 191). Excess iron is stored as ferritin and may later become available for heme synthesis or may be transferred from erythroid to phagocytic cells in bone marrow.

Heme has important roles in the process of hemoglobin synthesis in addition to being an essential component of the hemoglobin molecule. Heme deficiency leads to inactivation of a critically required initiation factor, thereby markedly reducing the rate of protein synthesis. Furthermore, heme may stimulate the synthesis and accumulation of globin mRNA directly and thus may have a regulatory role in modulating globin gene expression.

Globin biosynthesis and heme biosynthesis are coupled and cross-regulated in a poorly understood fashion. Disorders in which either iron or the protoporphyrin component of heme accumulates in inadequate amounts generally result in a secondary reduction in the amount of hemoglobin being synthesized. For complex reasons, a mild imbalance in globin chain synthesis also occurs: α Chain synthesis is more impaired by heme or iron deficiency than is β chain synthesis. Anemias characterized by inadequate iron or heme accumulation thus tend to be *mildly* α-thalassemic. With the exception of this phenomenon, interactions among heme and globin biosynthetic pathways remain poorly understood. The mechanisms whereby heme, α, and non-α globin are constrained to be expressed in equal amounts remain totally obscure. Since imbalances in this regulatory scheme occur reg-

ularly in the thalassemic syndromes, iron deficiency anemia, and disorders of heme biosynthesis, it can be inferred that the normal regulatory mechanisms are rather easily overcome.

Rodgers GP, Schechter AN: Molecular pathology of the hemoglobin molecule. *In* Hoffman R, Benz EJ Jr, Cohen H (eds.): Hematology: Basic Principles and Practice. New York, Churchill Livingstone, 1991, pp 441–449.
Steinberg MH, Benz EJ Jr: Hemoglobin synthesis, structure, and function. *In* Hoffman R, Benz EJ Jr, Cohen H (eds.): Hematology: Basic Principles and Practice. New York, Churchill Livingstone, 1991, pp 291–302.

136.2 CLASSIFICATION AND BASIC PATHOPHYSIOLOGY OF THE HEMOGLOBINOPATHIES

Edward J. Benz, Jr.

In patients with hemoglobinopathies, clinical abnormalities are attributable to altered structure, function, or production of hemoglobin. These disorders are usually inherited disorders that arise from mutations within the globin gene clusters described above (Ch. 136.1), but "acquired hemoglobinopathies" can occur as the result of toxic exposures (e.g., methemoglobinemia) or hematologic neoplasms. Hemoglobinopathies range in clinical severity from asymptomatic laboratory abnormalities to profound multisystem syndromes that result in death in utero or in early childhood. Hemoglobinopathies are the most common inherited disorders in humans. In many geographic areas, they constitute significant public health problems because of their prevalence and chronicity. The hemoglobinopathies demonstrate extremely well the complex pathophysiologic consequences that can arise from deranged function of single genes. Hemoglobinopathies frequently manifest as clinical syndromes in childhood, but with improved supportive care, many of these patients now survive well into adult life. The molecular basis, pathophysiology, epidemiology, and clinical features of the major hemoglobin disorders are therefore issues of increasing importance to internists.

CLASSIFICATION OF HEMOGLOBINOPATHIES

Hemoglobinopathies can be classified into five major groups:

1. *Structural hemoglobinopathies* (Table 136–2) are due to mutations altering the amino acid sequence and, thereby, the physiochemical properties of a particular globin polypeptide chain. The altered properties of the resulting abnormal hemoglobin produce the characteristic clinical syndrome. Some hemoglobins polymerize abnormally, e.g., those in sickle cell anemia (see Color Plate 6B, left); others exhibit abnormal solubility, while others have altered oxygen affinity.

2. The *thalassemia syndromes* are characterized by defective *biosynthesis* of globin chains, caused by mutations that impair production and/or translation of globin messenger RNA (mRNA). Symptoms result from the inadequate supply of hemoglobin and from imbalances in the production of individual globin chains.

3. *Thalassemic hemoglobin variants* exhibit features of both thalassemia, i.e., defective globin biosynthesis, and structural hemoglobinopathies, i.e., an abnormal amino acid sequence (see Color Plate 6A, left).

4. *Hereditary persistence of fetal hemoglobin*, as the name implies, represents continued synthesis of Hb F at high rates after the perinatal period.

5. *Acquired hemoglobinopathies* are secondary to other disease processes, rather than resulting from genetic derangements of hemoglobin structure or synthesis. Common examples include modifications of the hemoglobin molecule by toxins (acquired methemoglobinemia). Abnormal hemoglobin synthesis, e.g., high levels of Hb F production in preleukemia, also occurs sporadically in blood cell dyscrasias.

More than 400 structural variants and 100 thalassemia mutations have been identified. Only a few cause significant morbidity. Most of these involve the α and β globin chains that constitute the major adult hemoglobin, Hb A ($\alpha_2\beta_2$). Disorders of fetal and embryonic hemoglobins that are not lethal in utero are asymp-

TABLE 136–2. CLASSIFICATION OF HEMOGLOBINOPATHIES

I. Structural hemoglobinopathies—hemoglobins with altered amino acid sequences that result in deranged function or altered physical or chemical properties

Abnormal hemoglobin polymerization—Hb S

Altered O₂ affinity

High affinity—polycythemia

Low affinity—cyanosis, pseudoanemia

Hemoglobins that oxidize readily

Unstable hemoglobins, hemolytic anemia, jaundice

M hemoglobins—methemoglobinemia, cyanosis

II. Thalassemias—defective production of globin chains

α-Thalassemias

β-Thalassemias

δβ-, γδβ-, αβ-Thalassemias

III. Structural hemoglobinopathies—structurally abnormal Hb associated with co-inherited thalassemia phenotype

Hb E

Hb Constant Spring

Hb Lepore

IV. Hereditary persistence of fetal hemoglobin—persistence of high levels of Hb F into adult life

Pancellular—all red cells contain elevated Hb F levels

Nondeletion forms

Deletion forms

Hb Kenya

Heterocellular—only specific subpopulations of red cells contain elevated levels of Hb F

Acquired—see below

V. Acquired hemoglobinopathies

Methemoglobin due to toxic exposures

Sulfhemoglobin due to toxic exposures

Carbonoxyhemoglobin

Hb H in erythroleukemia

Elevated Hb F in states of erythroid stress and bone marrow dysplasia, usually heterocellular

---

tomatic after birth because these hemoglobins are not normally expressed then.

DISTRIBUTION AND EPIDEMIOLOGY OF HEMOGLOBINOPATHIES

Hemoglobinopathies are especially common in areas where malaria is endemic. The clustering of hemoglobinopathies in the "malaria belt" suggests that heterozygotes enjoy a selective advantage if infected with the malaria parasite. Presumably, their erythrocytes provide a less hospitable environment during the obligate intraerythrocytic stages of the parasitic life cycle (Ch. 424). For example, malarial parasites grow poorly in sickle cell trait erythrocytes. This selective advantage fixes the mutant genes in the population. One should thus be especially alert to the presence of hemoglobinopathies in Asians, blacks, and ethnic groups derived from the Mediterranean basin. Hemoglobinopathies do occur in every ethnic group, however.

INHERITANCE OF HEMOGLOBINOPATHIES

Hemoglobinopathies are "autosomal co-dominant" traits; thus, compound heterozygotes, who inherit a different abnormal globin allele from each parent, exhibit composite features of each abnormal allele. For example, patients inheriting a β-thalassemia gene from one parent and a β⁵ (sickle cell) allele from the other have sickle cell/β-thalassemia, which exhibits features of both β-thalassemia and sickle cell anemia. Each hemoglobinopathy is transmitted in families as a tightly linked allele of a globin gene. A thorough family history is thus an important part of the general approach to hemoglobinopathies, regardless of type.

Globin gene mutations behave like "co-dominant" traits in that some evidence of the abnormality, even if it be only laboratory evidence, can be detected in the heterozygote. The dominance of individual mutations with respect to clinical symptoms varies in different types of hemoglobinopathies. For example, patients with thalassemia trait and sickle cell anemia are, for the most part, asymptomatic. In each case, the amount of normal Hb A generated by the normal β globin allele, coupled with the lessened impact of abnormal globin production from the affected allele, protects patients from the complications of these diseases under normal conditions. Certain provocative stresses, such as very high altitude (low partial pressure of oxygen) for the patient with sickle cell trait, or pregnancy (for the patient with thalassemia trait), can occasionally produce symptoms characteristic of these disorders, i.e., sickling or anemia.

Some hemoglobinopathies behave like dominant traits, especially the structural mutations causing reduced solubility or profoundly altered oxygen affinity of the hemoglobin. In these cases, the absolute amount of the abnormal hemoglobin arising from the single affected allele is often sufficient to alter the behavior of the red cell.

In some hemoglobinopathies, the homozygous state is clinically benign, but compound heterozygous states are associated with severe disease. For example, homozygous hemoglobin C disease is only minimally symptomatic, but inheritance of β⁵ on one chromosome and β⁶ on the other (hemoglobin sickle cell [SC] disease) behaves like a moderately severe form of sickle cell anemia, exhibiting certain unique and distinctive features, to be described subsequently. Similarly, homozygous Hb E disease is very mild, but co-inheritance of Hb E and β-thalassemia produces a moderately severe β-thalassemia–like syndrome. These considerations illustrate the complexity of hemoglobin genetics. The ultimate clinical phenotype is determined not only by the type of change resulting from the globin gene mutation but also by a composite effect of the altered properties of the abnormal chain, the amount produced (or the severity of the production deficit), and the interaction between the product of one abnormal allele and that of the normal allele or of a different type of abnormal allele present on the complementary chromosome. These principles, important for understanding individual syndromes, also offer the best existing examples of gene interactions in determining the ultimate clinical phenotype.

Spontaneous mutations occur at a measurable frequency within the globin gene cluster, producing symptomatic or asymptomatic hemoglobinopathies in patients with negative family histories. The unstable (insoluble) hemoglobin disorders seem especially prone to arise by de novo spontaneous mutation. Thus, while family history is an extremely important part of the evaluation of patients with potential hemoglobinopathies, a negative family history does not necessarily rule out the diagnosis.

BASIC PRINCIPLES OF PATHOPHYSIOLOGY

The α globin genes are duplicated; the β gene is a single-copy locus. In the diploid erythroblast, there are thus four copies of the α and only two copies of the β gene. Mutation of a single α globin gene thus affects only about 25 per cent of the hemoglobin produced, while β mutations affect about 50 per cent. Consequently, β chain mutations tend to be encountered more frequently than α variants as causes of symptomatic hemoglobinopathies.

Globin genes are expressed exclusively in developing erythroid cells. During the terminal stages of erythroid maturation, one might expect symptoms to be confined to the red cell compartment, e.g., anemia. The clinical manifestations of hemoglobinopathies are protean, however. In most cases, it has been possible to trace these changes to the impact of specific mutations on particular properties of the hemoglobin molecule. Homeostasis of hemoglobin and the homeostasis of the red cells in which it circulates are closely linked. Deranged production or function of globin frequently deranges erythropoiesis, and the converse is also often true. Hemoglobin accumulates to extremely high concentrations within red cells, where it must remain soluble and chemically reduced. Individual globin chains are insoluble and have extraordinarily high oxygen affinities. If globin or hemoglobin molecules precipitate within red cells, the resulting inclusions cause premature destruction of the red cells (hemolytic anemia) with all of its attendant stigmata. Lesions affecting oxygen affinity perturb the erythropoietin circuit by which red cell production is regulated. The signal for release of erythropoietin is based upon *oxygen delivery* to cells within the kidney rather than to the *red cell mass*. Inappropriate secretion of erythropoietin as well as premature destruction of red cells can thus be caused by hemoglobinopathies. These consequences of deranged hemoglobin structures, amount, or structure-function relationships, rather than mere reduction in the amount or normal function of hemoglobin, tend to dominate the pathophysiology of the disorders.

The behavior of particular hemoglobinopathies is also influenced by the ontogeny of hemoglobin synthesis. α Chain hemoglobinopathies cause abnormalities of Hb A, Hb A$_2$, and Hb F, because the α chain is present in all of these hemoglobins. The α globin hemoglobinopathies are symptomatic both in utero and after birth because normal function of the α globin gene is required throughout gestation as well as adult life. In contrast, β globin gene expression is not abundant until after birth. Infants with β globin hemoglobinopathies thus tend to be asymptomatic until 3 to 9 months of age, the time at which Hb F is largely replaced by Hb A.

Schecter AN: Molecular pathology of the hemoglobin molecule. In Hoffman R, Benz EJ Jr, Cohen H (eds.): Hematology: Basic Principles and Practice. New York, Churchill Livingstone, 1990, in press.
Steinberg MH, Benz EJ Jr: Hemoglobin: Structure and synthesis. In Hoffman R, Benz EJ Jr, Cohen H (eds.): Hematology: Basic Principles and Practice. New York, Churchill Livingstone, 1990, in press.

136.3 HEMOGLOBINOPATHIES WITH ALTERED SOLUBILITY OR OXYGEN AFFINITY

Edward J. Benz, Jr.

Structural hemoglobinopathies are due to mutations that alter the amino acid sequence and, thereby, the functional properties of the hemoglobin molecule: (1) mutations causing abnormal polymerization, of which hemoglobin (Hb) S (sickle cell hemoglobin) is the most important example; (2) mutations causing altered solubility of hemoglobin within circulating erythrocytes; (3) mutations causing altered affinity of the hemoglobin molecule for oxygen; and (4) methemoglobinemia, which represents a subclass of hemoglobins with altered oxygen affinity. Sickle cell syndromes are so common, serious, and protean in their manifestations that they merit extended separate coverage (Ch. 136.5). In this chapter, we shall consider hemoglobins exhibiting abnormal solubility and altered oxygen affinity. Methemoglobins are considered a separate category within this chapter, even though they could be considered a subclass of hemoglobins with altered oxygen affinity. The altered interaction with oxygen is far more severe in methemoglobin than in most other types of oxygen affinity mutations; moreover, methemoglobin is important as one of the few acquired hemoglobinopathies (carbon monoxyhemoglobin being another) that can develop by exposure to selected toxins. Finally, methemoglobins can arise by inherited mechanisms in other genes as well as globin genes. Therefore, these syndromes receive special consideration.

HEMOGLOBINS EXHIBITING REDUCED SOLUBILITY— UNSTABLE HEMOGLOBINS

Pathogenesis and Clinical Manifestations

"Unstable" hemoglobins arise from amino acid substitutions that render the hemoglobin less soluble or more susceptible to oxidation of its amino acid residues (Fig. 136–7). Both α and β globin variants can cause this condition; about 100 such variants have been described. The mutations that produce insoluble hemoglobins tend to disrupt hydrogen bonding and hydrophobic interactions holding the tetramer together. Some alter the helical segments [Hb Geneva, (β$^{28leu→pro}$)]; others disrupt contact points between the α- and β-subunits [Hb Philadelphia, (β$^{35Tyr→Phe}$)], while others disrupt interactions of the hydrophobic pockets of the globin subunits for heme [e.g., Hb Köln, (β$^{98Val→Met}$)]. The most common biochemical basis for reduced solubility is reduced strength of the binding of heme to globin. An actual loss of heme groups can occur, e.g., in Hb Gun Hill, in which five amino acids, including the F8 histidine, are deleted.

Precipitation of hemoglobin in circulating red cells produces intracellular inclusions called "Heinz bodies" (see Color Plate 6C, left). The spleen attempts to remove these inclusions, leading to formation of pitted, rigid cells that eventually become seques-

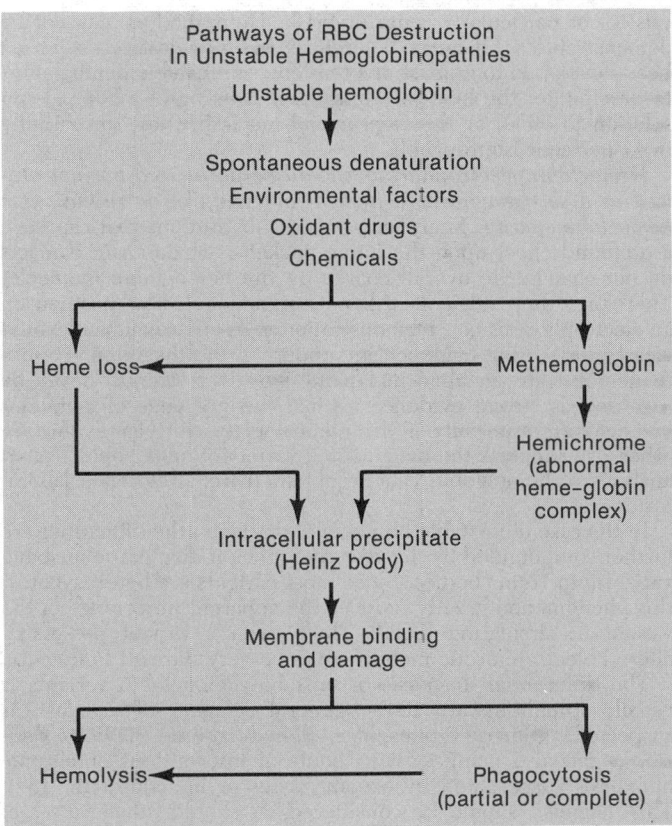

FIGURE 136–7. The presumed mechanisms by which denaturation of hemoglobin leads to erythrocyte destruction are outlined. The rate of travel through the various pathways probably differs for different hemoglobin variants and for a variety of stresses to which the protein is subjected.

tered, thus producing a hemolytic anemia. In severely affected patients, the anemia may require chronic transfusion therapy. Splenectomy is often effective for relief of anemia. Leg ulcers and premature gallbladder disease occur with high frequency.

Unstable hemoglobins are quite rare in comparison to sickle cell anemia and the thalassemias. They occur sporadically in many ethnic groups, often by spontaneous mutation. The heterozygous state is usually symptomatic ("dominant") because significant numbers of Heinz bodies form even when the unstable variant accounts for only half of the total hemoglobin. Most of the symptomatic unstable hemoglobins are β globin variants, since sporadic mutations affecting the α globin loci would usually involve only one of the four alleles, thus generating only 20 to 30 per cent abnormal hemoglobin. The propensity of unstable hemoglobins to precipitate is exaggerated by "oxidative" stress, such as infection or exposure to oxidizing drugs (e.g., quinine). Indeed, some of these variants are symptomatic only when oxidant stress occurs.

Diagnosis

The presence of an unstable hemoglobin should be suspected in individuals with chronic hemolytic anemia, unexplained jaundice, premature biliary tract disease (caused by bilirubin gallstones generated by excess red cell turnover), unexplained reticulocytosis, or bouts of intermittent hemolysis that can be related to exposure to oxidant drugs or infections. Other suggestive symptoms include dark urine, transient jaundice, or leg ulcers. These findings are stigmata of chronic or intermittent hemolysis.

Laboratory diagnosis is based upon identification of a mutant hemoglobin that precipitates more easily than normal hemoglobin. The in vivo evidence for precipitated hemoglobin is the Heinz body, which is an intraerythrocytic inclusion body detectable by staining of a peripheral blood film with a supravital dye, usually brilliant cresyl blue or new methylene blue. Since the spleen can remove Heinz bodies efficiently, especially if hemolysis is not particularly acute or brisk, Heinz bodies may not be demonstrable at all times. Therefore, two provocative tests have been developed to unmask the tendency of unstable hemoglobins to precipitate: the heat instability test (heating of a hemoglobin solution to 50°C) or the isopropanol instability test (insolubility in 17 per cent isopropanol).

Hemoglobin electrophoresis should be performed but not utilized as a sole diagnostic criterion for ruling in or ruling out a hemoglobinopathy. Many amino acid substitutions that can have a profound effect upon the heme pocket or chain-chain contacts do not change the overall charge on the hemoglobin molecule. Therefore, these variants will not migrate to a new position on an electrophoresis gel. Demonstration of an abnormal band would clearly add strong evidence in support of the diagnosis. Failure to demonstrate an abnormal band, however, should never be regarded as strong evidence against the presence of a mutant hemoglobin, especially if the clinical picture or family history otherwise supports the diagnosis. A variety of more sophisticated analyses of hemoglobin can be obtained from reference laboratories.

In the case of unstable hemoglobin variants, the difficulties are further compounded by the selective precipitation of the unstable variant into Heinz bodies. Since most patients are heterozygotes, this phenomenon greatly reduces the apparent percentage of the variant in circulating blood. Thus, even a variant possessing altered electrophoretic mobility may be very difficult to detect.

The differential diagnosis of unstable hemoglobin variants is usually straightforward if the general category of diagnosis is suspected. Glucose-6-phosphate dehydrogenase (G6PD) deficiency can also manifest with bouts of intermittent or chronic hemolysis exacerbated by oxidant drugs or infection (Ch. 134). This diagnosis should be considered, as should other causes of chronic or intermittent hemolytic anemia, such as red cell membrane disorders (e.g., hereditary spherocytosis) or immune hemolytic anemias. Spherocytes are relatively rare in unstable hemoglobin disorders; this is sometimes a useful discriminant.

Management

The severity of the clinical complications of unstable hemoglobins varies enormously. Many patients can be managed adequately by expectant monitoring and avoidance of drugs provoking hemolysis. Occasional patients may require transfusions during bouts of severe acute hemolytic anemia. Individuals who suffer significant morbidity because of chronic anemia or repeated episodes of severe hemolysis should be considered candidates for splenectomy, especially if hypersplenism has developed. Finally, the tendency of infection to exacerbate hemolysis should prompt one to monitor these patients closely during those episodes.

HEMOGLOBINS WITH INCREASED OXYGEN AFFINITY

Hemoglobin functions as a biologically useful oxygen transport pigment because of the sigmoidal shape of its oxygen affinity curve. In the transition from the fully deoxygenated (tense, or T) to the fully oxygenated (relaxed, or R) state, the initial oxygenation steps occur with difficulty. In fact, the act of binding the first oxygen molecule increases the affinity of the molecule for subsequent oxygen binding events, thus creating the sigmoidal shape of the curve. The necessary intramolecular reorganization occurs only when the proper arrangement of hydrogen bonds, hydrophobic interactions, and salt bridges is broken and formed in the proper sequence during R-T transitions.

Mutant hemoglobins exhibiting altered oxygen affinity usually arise when amino acid substitutions occur at the interface between α and β chains or in regions affecting the hydrogen bonds, hydrophobic interactions, or salt bridges. A second major class of mutations comprises those affecting interaction with 2,3-diphosphoglycerate (2,3-DPG) (Ch. 136.1), which alters oxygen affinity when bound to hemoglobin.

Pathogenesis and Clinical Manifestations

"High-affinity" hemoglobins exhibit higher avidity for oxygen, causing the oxygen dissociation curve to "shift to the left"; an example is Hb Zurich ($\beta^{63his \rightarrow arg}$) (Fig. 136–8). These hemoglobins bind oxygen more readily but are less able to deliver the oxygen

to tissues at normal capillary oxygen pressures. Since the Po_2 in the lung ($Po_2 = 90$ to 100 mm Hg) is normally well above that needed to saturate hemoglobin fully with oxygen (60 mm Hg), these variant hemoglobins cannot acquire any additional oxygen in the lung despite their higher affinity. At capillary Po_2 (35 to 45 mm Hg), however, high-affinity hemoglobins deliver less oxygen. The resultant mild tissue hypoxia stimulates erythropoietin release and leads to inappropriately high red cell production and polycythemia (Ch. 142). In extreme cases, hematocrits of 60 to 65 per cent can be encountered.

High-affinity variants arise from several forms of mutations. Some alter interactions within the heme pocket, others disrupt the Bohr effect or the salt-bond site, and others impair the interaction of Hb A with 2,3-DPG. The 2,3-DPG binding lowers the oxygen affinity of Hb A. Reduced 2,3-DPG binding results in an effective increase in oxygen affinity. As a good example of a high-affinity hemoglobin, a single amino acid substitution in Hb Kempsey blocks the hydrogen bond formation with the tyrosine at α^{42} needed to stabilize the T (deoxy) state. This and numerous other examples that have been analyzed at the molecular level have greatly aided our understanding of the molecular basis for reversible oxygen binding.

Diagnosis

"High-affinity" hemoglobins should be considered in patients with unexplained erythrocytosis, especially if there is a positive family history (Ch. 142). Oxygen affinity is usually measured as the P-50, the partial pressure of oxygen at which a hemoglobin preparation (either in the form of a red cell suspension or in the form of a hemoglobin solution) is 50 per cent saturated with oxygen (Fig. 136–2). The hemoglobin preparation is exposed to increasing oxygen pressures in the laboratory, and the relative percentages of oxyhemoglobin and deoxyhemoglobin are determined optically, forming a curve from which the 50 per cent saturation point is determined. A "shift to the left" means that the hemoglobin reaches 50 per cent saturation at a *lower* partial pressure of oxygen. *High-affinity variants are thus associated with a lower than normal P-50 value.* Hemoglobin electrophoresis should be performed but may not be revealing.

The most common cause of a low P-50 value is carbon monoxide poisoning. Hemoglobin–carbon monoxide has an extremely "left-shifted" oxygen affinity curve, which reflects stabilization of hemoglobin in the R state without benefit of oxygen binding. The clinical impact is the same as that of a very high oxygen affinity hemoglobin. The most common cause of hemoglobin–carbon monoxide is cigarette smoking, although chronic carbon monoxide exposure in individuals such as caisson workers or tunnel toll booth collectors is encountered sporadically.

P-50 curves should be performed with both whole-blood suspensions and isolated hemoglobin solutions. In the latter circumstance, the contribution of 2,3-DPG is eliminated. This can eliminate the potential confounding artifact and reveal those variants arising from abnormal interaction with this ligand.

Management

Most patients with high-affinity hemoglobins have mild erythrocytosis not requiring treatment. Very rarely, the hematocrit and, therefore, the blood viscosity are sufficiently elevated to warrant treatment by phlebotomy.

HEMOGLOBINS WITH DECREASED OXYGEN AFFINITY

Pathogenesis and Clinical Manifestations

Low-affinity hemoglobin variants, such as Hb Kansas ($\beta^{102Asn \rightarrow Thr}$), represent the pathophysiologic "mirror image" of the high-affinity hemoglobins (Fig. 136–8). In Hb Kansas, the threonine position β^{102} cannot form a hydrogen bond with aspartic acid at position α^{94}, which normally stabilizes the R (oxy) state. Thus, Hb Kansas has less tendency to bind oxygen and exhibits a "right-shifted" P-50 value.

In all but the most severe examples of low-affinity variants, oxygen affinity remains high enough that the hemoglobin becomes fully saturated in the highly oxygen-abundant environment of the pulmonary capillary. At the Po_2 of the capillary bed in most tissues, however, these hemoglobins "dump" excessive amounts of oxygen and become more desaturated than normal hemoglobin. There are two pathophysiologic consequences of this higher than normal level of oxygen delivery. First, since tissue oxygen delivery is so efficient, the erythropoietin "thermostat" can be set lower, resulting in normal oxygen transport at lower than normal hematocrits. This situation produces a state of "pseudoanemia." In other words, the hematocrit appears to be abnormally low, even though homeostasis of oxygen transport and the patient are completely normal. Second, the amount of desaturated hemoglobin circulating in capillaries can be greater than 5 grams per deciliter, producing clinically apparent cyanosis. In contrast to most other causes of cyanosis, this usually ominous finding is entirely benign in these individuals.

Diagnosis

A low-affinity variant should be suspected in patients with unexplained anemia or cyanosis who, by all other criteria, appear to be entirely well, especially if there is a positive family history. Testing for the abnormal variant follows the same reasoning as that just described for high-affinity variants, except that the P-50 value will be shifted to the right.

Management

Patients with low-affinity hemoglobins are usually asymptomatic. No treatment is required. It is important to document that a low-affinity hemoglobin is the cause of an apparent anemia and that this finding is only a physiologic response to the altered oxygen affinity. Cyanosis in some individuals can pose a cosmetic problem, but correction with transfusions is rarely, if ever, justified.

METHEMOGLOBINEMIAS

Methemoglobin is generated by oxidation of the iron moieties in hemoglobin from the ferrous (Fe^{2+}) to the ferric (Fe^{3+}) state. Oxygen transport by hemoglobin requires that iron be present in the ferrous state in deoxyhemoglobin. Yet oxygenation of hemoglobin causes a partial transfer of an electron from the iron to the bound oxygen; iron in this state thus resembles ferric iron. The oxygen resembles superoxide (O_2^-). Deoxygenation returns the electron to the iron, with release of oxygen. When this electron return fails to occur, methemoglobin forms. Normally methemoglobin constitutes 3 per cent or less of the total hemoglobin content. Indeed, reduction of methemoglobin levels to less than 1 per cent is routinely accomplished in vivo by the activity of an enzyme called methemoglobin reductase (nicotinamide-adenine dinucleotide [NADH]–dehydratase, NADH-diaphorase, erythrocyte cytochrome b_5). This enzyme reduces hemoglobin iron by transfer of an electron from NADH to oxidize cytochrome b_5; cytochrome b_5 then converts ferric to ferrous iron by direct interaction with hemoglobin. The generation of NADH depends on the glycolytic pathway.

A second reducing enzyme, nicotinamide-adenine dinucleotide phosphate (NADPH)–dependent methemoglobin reductase, does not normally function in erythrocytes because there is no electron carrier available to interact with NADPH as the "go-between" with hemoglobin iron. Artificial electron carriers, such as methylene blue, can provide this missing link. As discussed later, methylene blue is therefore an important agent for the treatment of methemoglobinemia. Reduced glutathione and ascorbic acid can also reduce methemoglobin directly; however, these nonenzymatic reactions are considerably slower than the reductase pathways.

Pathogenesis and Clinical Manifestations

Methemoglobinemias of clinical import arise by one of three distinct mechanisms: (1) globin chain mutations that result in increased formation of methemoglobin, (2) deficiencies in the reductase pathways described above; and (3) "toxic" methemoglobinemia in which even normal red cells endowed with normal hemoglobin and normal methemoglobin reductase can be "overwhelmed" by exposure to substances that oxidize hemoglobin iron (Table 136–3).

Abnormal hemoglobins causing methemoglobinemia ("M hemoglobins") tend to arise from mutations that alter the heme

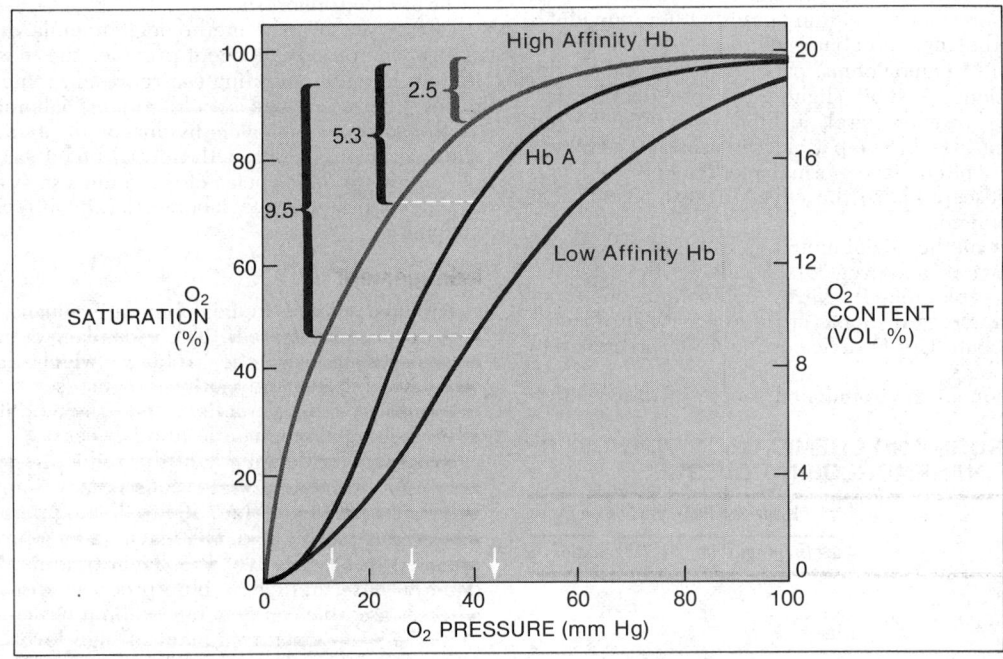

FIGURE 136–8. Hemoglobin-oxygen dissociation curves are illustrated for normal hemoglobin (Hb A) and for model abnormal hemoglobins with high and low oxygen affinities. On the abscissa the partial pressure of oxygen is indicated in millimeters of mercury. On the left ordinate the saturation of hemoglobin with oxygen is indicated as a percentage; on the right ordinate the oxygen content of the hemoglobin is expressed as volumes per cent. The three inverted arrows show the P_{50} for the three hemoglobins (the partial pressure of oxygen at which the hemoglobin is 50 per cent saturated). This value is lowest for the high-affinity hemoglobin. As the partial pressure of oxygen drops from 100 (arterial) to 40 (tissues), hemoglobin desaturates, giving up a portion of its bound oxygen; the numbers on the brackets indicate the amount of oxygen unloaded by the three hemoglobin types expressed in volumes per cent. Note that the high-affinity hemoglobin delivers less than half the oxygen that Hb A gives to the tissues, resulting in tissue anoxia, increased erythropoietin secretion, and erythrocytosis. Conversely, the low-affinity hemoglobin is even more efficient than Hb A in supplying the tissues with oxygen, resulting in diminished erythropoietin production and anemia.

TABLE 136–3. TYPES OF METHEMOGLOBINEMIA

A. Congenital
  1. Defective enzymatic reduction of Fe^{+3}-hemoglobin to Fe^{+2}-hemoglobin
     a. NADH–methemoglobin reductase (cytochrome b_5 reductase) deficiency
     b. Cytochrome b_3 deficiency
  2. Abnormal hemoglobins resistant to enzymatic reduction (M hemoglobins)
B. Acquired
  1. Excessive (toxic) oxidation of Fe^{+2}-hemoglobin
     a. Environmental chemicals
     b. Drugs

pocket in a fashion that favors stabilization of the iron in the ferric state. In the majority of these, a histidine is replaced by a tyrosine; the hydroxyl group of the tyrosine forms a complex that stabilizes the iron in the ferric state in a fashion resistant to reduction by the methemoglobin reductase system. A few of the variants tend to lose heme and thus also exhibit features of a mildly unstable hemoglobin disorder.

Methemoglobin has a brownish to blue color, which does not become red upon exposure to oxygen. These individuals thus appear to be cyanotic. In contrast to truly cyanotic individuals, however, arterial Po_2 values are normal. These individuals are otherwise asymptomatic, because methemoglobin is rarely above 30 to 50 per cent, the levels at which symptomatology becomes apparent, as described below.

Hereditary methemoglobinemia resulting from methemoglobin reductase deficiency is rare; 100 to 200 cases have been described. Numerous recessive mutations cause a variety of defects in the resulting variant enzymes, including catalytic activity, electrophoretic mobility, and structural stability. Hispanics, Eskimos, and Native Americans in particular are frequently affected. In some individuals, neurologic defects are also present, suggesting that the mutation affects isoforms of the enzyme common to both erythrocytes and other tissues, including brain. Other individuals exhibit only the methemoglobin abnormality.

Like patients with M hemoglobins, patients with methemoglobin reductase deficiency exhibit slight gray "pseudocyanosis." Even homozygotes, however, rarely exhibit more than 25 per cent methemoglobin, a level compatible with absence of symptoms. Heterozygotes often have normal methemoglobin levels but are especially susceptible to the effects of toxic agents that cause methemoglobinemia.

The third form of methemoglobinemia is caused by exposure to certain chemical agents and drugs that accelerate the oxidation of methemoglobin (Table 136–4). Nitrite compounds are especially notorious in this regard. Some of these agents also have a propensity to exacerbate G6PD deficiency and the precipitation of unstable hemoglobins.

Nitrates are a frequent environmental source of toxic methe-

TABLE 136–4. DRUGS AND CHEMICALS HAVING TOXIC EFFECT ON HEMOGLOBIN MOLECULE

	Hemoglobin Derivative Observed	
Agent	Methemoglobin	Sulfhemoglobin
Acetanilid, phenacetin	+	+
Nitrites (amyl, sodium, potassium, nitroglycerin)	+	+
Trinitrotoluene, nitrobenzene	+	+
Aniline, hydroxylamine, dimethylamine	+	+
Sulfanilamide	+	+
Para-aminosalicylic acid	+	
Dapsone	+	
Primaquine, chloroquine	+	
Prilocaine, benzocaine, lidocaine	+	
Menadione, naphthoquinone	+	
Naphthalene	+	
Resorcinol	+	
Phenylhydrazine	+	+

moglobinemia, even though nitrates do not directly interact with either hemoglobin or the reductase system. Rather, nitrates are converted to nitrites in the gut. Well water is the most frequently encountered source of excessive nitrates. In general, substantial intake of these agents is required before significant amounts of methemoglobin are generated. Very young infants are more susceptible to these agents than are adults, but all age groups are at risk if exposure is sufficient.

Toxic or acquired methemoglobinemia is virtually the only situation in which life-threatening amounts of methemoglobin accumulate. In general, the only symptom produced when methemoglobin comprises less than 30 per cent of total hemoglobin is the cosmetic effect of cyanosis. As levels of methemoglobin rise above 30 per cent, however, patients begin to exhibit symptoms of oxygen deprivation, such as malaise, giddiness, and other alterations of mental status. The symptoms reflect a true lack of oxygen availability at the tissue level, since a substantial number of hemoglobin molecules are no longer delivering oxygen to the tissues. At levels of methemoglobin greater than 50 per cent, loss of consciousness, coma, and death can ensue rapidly. At this level of methemoglobin, "cyanosis" is severe, and the blood is chocolate brown.

Diagnosis

Methemoglobinemia should be suspected in patients with unexplained cyanosis. One should be especially alert to the potential medical emergency inherent in a patient with cyanosis and altered mental status, despite a normal arterial Po_2. The ingestion of nitrites as a suicide gesture, especially in individuals knowledgeable with respect to chemistry, medicine, or pharmacology, is not uncommon. The diagnosis of methemoglobinemia can be suspected from the brownish color of blood when it is drawn. In the laboratory, methemoglobin exhibits characteristic peaks of absorption at 630 and 502 nm, rendering it easily distinguishable from normal hemoglobin. In addition, the inherited M hemoglobins are frequently detectable by altered electrophoretic mobility, especially if ferricyanide treatment in vitro is used to convert all of the hemoglobin solution to methemoglobin prior to electrophoresis.

In the case of toxic methemoglobinemia, recognition of exposure to an appropriate agent provides the most important historical clue. Acute poisoning can represent a life-threatening emergency; therefore, one should request laboratory evaluation for methemoglobin in any individual with atypical cyanosis or cyanosis occurring along with normal blood gas values. Methemoglobin due to deficiencies of the reductase system can be further evaluated in reference laboratories by direct analysis of these enzymes.

Management

Patients with M hemoglobins are usually asymptomatic and require no management. The secondary cyanosis can represent an unfortunate cosmetic problem, which cannot be reversed, since ascorbic acid and methylene blue (see below) are ineffective with most of these variants despite their utility in the treatment of methemoglobinemia due to other causes.

Patients with deficiency of the reductase system generally do not require treatment, but cyanosis can be improved by treatment with oral methylene blue, 100 to 300 mg per day, or 500 mg per day of oral ascorbic acid. Riboflavin (20 mg per day) has also been reported to be effective. Riboflavin treatment has been championed because methylene blue produces discolored (blue) urine, whereas ascorbic can generate sodium oxalate stones.

In the emergency treatment of high levels of toxic methemoglobinemia, 1 to 2 mg per kilogram of methylene blue is given as a 1 per cent solution in saline, usually administered rapidly (10 to 15 minutes) intravenously. The dose may be repeated if necessary. This treatment is usually effective. As noted above, methylene blue acts via the NADPH reductase system, which in turn requires G6PD activity. The method is thus not effective in patients who also have G6PD deficiency. These patients, or patients who are severely affected, may require exchange transfusion. Oral ascorbic acid, at doses noted earlier, is not useful in emergency situations because it acts too slowly. Follow-up maintenance management, however, can be accomplished with either ascorbic acid or oral methylene blue.

Mild cases of methemoglobin intoxication do not require treatment. The patient can be monitored for 1 to 3 days, during which time methemoglobin levels will gradually return to normal if the offending agent is eliminated. The most important follow-up therapy of patients with toxic methemoglobinemia involves a thorough search for the offending agent and its removal from the environment.

Bunn HF, Forget BG: Hemoglobin: Molecular, Genetic and Clinical Aspects. Philadelphia, W.B. Saunders Company. 1986. *Chapter 13 discusses unstable hemoglobins; Chapter 14, hemoglobins with altered oxygen affinity; and Chapters 15 and 16, various forms of methemoglobinemia.*

Mansouri A: Methemoglobinemia. Am J Med Sci 289:200, 1985.

Weatherall DJ, Clegg JB, Higgs DR, et al.: The hemoglobinopathies. *In* Scriver CR, Beaudet AL, Sly WS, et al. (eds.): The Metabolic Basis of Inherited Disease. 6th ed. New York, McGraw-Hill Book Company, 1989, pp 2281–2339.

136.4 THE THALASSEMIAS

Arthur W. Nienhuis

The thalassemias are hereditary anemias that occur because of mutations that affect the synthesis of hemoglobin. In β-thalassemia there is deficient synthesis of β globin, whereas in α-thalassemia there is deficient synthesis of α globin (see Color Plate 6A). Reduced synthesis of one of the two globin polypeptides leads to deficient hemoglobin accumulation, resulting in hypochromic and microcytic red cells. These red cell abnormalities are the most constant and characteristic features of this group of disorders. Table 136–5 contains a clinical classification of the thalassemias presented in the order in which they are discussed in this chapter.

The incidence and prevalence of these conditions are highly variable. Most common is thalassemia trait, a mild, clinically insignificant anemia that apparently protects individuals from malaria (see below), and therefore through natural selection it has become extremely common in certain parts of the world. Thalassemia trait generally represents the heterozygous form of either α- or β-thalassemia. Hence where thalassemia trait is common, homozygous, more severely affected patients will be found frequently. In the United States, the incidence of β-thalassemia is highest among ethnic groups originating from the Mediterranean area, parts of Africa, and Asia, whereas the incidence of α-thalassemia is highest among those from Asia. Generally, the incidence of thalassemia trait in these ethnic groups is 3 to 5 per cent. Approximately 1000 patients with more severe forms of thalassemia are known in the United States.

SEVERE β-THALASSEMIA (Cooley's Anemia)

Severe β-thalassemia occurs in patients who are homozygous for mutations that lead to a decrease in β globin synthesis. Because both β globin genes are affected, there is marked deficiency in β globin synthesis, but α globin synthesis continues at an approximately normal rate. Accumulation of a large excess of α chains for which there are no β chains with which to combine has several serious deleterious effects. α Globin is highly insoluble and forms large intracellular inclusions. These interfere with the cell cycle in the bone marrow, retard the passage of red cells

TABLE 136–5. CLINICAL CLASSIFICATION OF THE THALASSEMIAS

I. Severe β-thalassemia (Cooley's anemia)	Severe anemia, growth retardation, hepatosplenomegaly, bone marrow expansion, and bone deformities
A. Thalassemia major	Transfusion dependent
B. Thalassemia intermedia	No regular transfusion requirement
II. Thalassemia trait (α or β)	Mild anemia with microcytosis and hypochromia
III. Hb H disease (α-thal)	Moderately severe hemolytic anemia, icterus, and splenomegaly
IV. Hydrops fetalis (α-thal)	Death in utero caused by severe anemia
V. Silent carrier (α or β)	Hematologically normal

from the bone marrow, and reduce the survival of red cells in the circulation by virtue of membrane damage and splenic trapping. Marked ineffective erythropoiesis is the hallmark of this disorder because α inclusions interfere with erythroblast maturation, leading to intramedullary death of many red cell precursors. Severe anemia stimulates erythropoietin production, leading to erythroid stem cell and erythroblast proliferation. The vastly expanded erythroid cell mass results in osteoporosis with a potential for pathologic fractures. Extramedullary hematopoiesis is also often seen, and compression of vital structures, particularly the spinal cord, may occur as a consequence. Because of marrow expansion and deformities of the skull and facial bones, patients with severe β-thalassemia often have an abnormal appearance with prominent epicanthal folds, referred to as a chipmunk facies.

Patients with severe β-thalassemia may be divided into two groups on the basis of their requirement for blood transfusion. Those with thalassemia major have an absolute requirement for blood without which severe anemia leads to death in infancy or early childhood. In contrast, patients with thalassemia intermedia are able to maintain their hemoglobin at 6 to 7 grams per deciliter without transfusion. This level is compatible with fairly normal growth and development, and many of these patients survive into adulthood.

Thalassemia Major

CLINICAL FEATURES. At birth patients with thalassemia major are nearly normal hematologically, since γ globin synthesis is normal and hemoglobin (Hb) F production is therefore adequate. However, as the switch from Hb F to Hb A is completed during the first year of life, the deficiency in β globin production becomes evident. By 6 to 9 months of age, severe anemia reflected by pallor, poor growth, or inadequate food intake leads the anxious parents to bring the infant to the physician, at which time examination reveals the presence of marked hepatosplenomegaly. The hemoglobin may be 3 to 6 grams per deciliter, and the red cells exhibit the characteristic severe microcytosis, hypochromia, and fragmentation (see Color Plate 6A, left). Demonstration of thalassemia trait (see below) in both parents is usually sufficient to establish the diagnosis. Study of the infant's blood shows absence of or low Hb A, a large amount of Hb F, and an increase in the amount of Hb A_2 to 4 to 10 per cent of the total (normal <2.5 per cent). Biosynthetic studies, a tool of the research laboratory, may be employed to show the deficiency of β globin production.

CLINICAL COURSE. Prior to the use of regular blood transfusions, these children were grossly deformed because of expansion of the marrow spaces of the skull (see Fig. 127–1). Severe osteoporosis led to pathologic fractures, and anemia caused weakness and inanition. Death by 2 to 3 years of age was common. Blood transfusions were initially given infrequently for palliation, but gradually physicians interested in this condition came to recognize that regular transfusion to nearly normal hemoglobin levels could be used to suppress all disease manifestations. Growth and bone development are normal in children who have undergone hypertransfusion, and in fact they are virtually indistinguishable from other children if the hypertransfusion regimen is started at a very early age. If transfusions are given less frequently, the patient may exhibit some stigmata of the untreated disorder—bone deformities, growth retardation, and hepatosplenomegaly.

THE PROBLEM OF IRON OVERLOAD. Because humans have a very limited ability to excrete iron, regular blood transfusions inevitably lead to a vast accumulation. Each unit of packed red cells contains approximately 200 mg of iron, so that by the age of 12 the average thalassemic, having received 125 to 150 units of packed cells, will have accumulated 25 to 30 grams of excess iron. This amount compares with the normal 3 to 4 grams found in adults, 75 per cent of which is present in red cells as hemoglobin. Even in the patient with thalassemia intermedia who has not had transfusions, excess iron absorption leads inevitably to the manifestations of hemochromatosis, although at a later age than in the patient with transfusion-dependent thalassemia. Excess iron deposition occurs in virtually all organs. Most cells have a considerable ability to cope with this extra iron by making ferritin and its partial degradation product hemosiderin. Nonetheless, cell damage occurs by virtue of iron-catalyzed peroxidation of membrane lipids and release of the enzymes from lysosomes rendered labile by their content of hemosiderin granules. Thus tissue hemosiderosis (excess iron) leads ultimately to the clinical condition of secondary hemochromatosis. The liver, endocrine glands, and particularly the heart are the primary target organs (see Ch. 193).

Liver dysfunction is mild in the thalassemic patient with secondary hemochromatosis. Typically the liver is enlarged several centimeters below the right costal margin, and the transaminases are two to four times above the normal limits. Despite a 20- to 30-fold increase in iron concentration over normal, liver biosynthetic function as reflected by the concentration of serum albumin and various clotting factors is preserved. Fibrosis, invariably present on liver biopsy, may progress to frank cirrhosis anatomically, but clinical evidence of cirrhosis is rare.

As noted above, the course of adequately tranfused thalassemic patients is essentially normal until the age of 10 to 12. Then growth failure is a frequent and distressing complication for both the child and parents. The mechanism for this growth failure is not known; growth hormone levels are generally normal, but the serum somatomedin concentration may be low. Failure of growth is accompanied by lack of pubescence. Primary hypogonadism is exceedingly common. The mechanism is usually a failure of the pituitary to produce adequate amounts of follicle-stimulating hormone (FSH) and luteinizing hormone (LH). Diabetes mellitus, hypothyroidism, and, rarely, hypoparathyroidism with tetany are additional complications that may occur, particularly in patients who are in their late teenage years or early 20's.

Cardiac disease in the patients with severe β-thalassemia may take three forms: pericarditis, congestive heart failure, and cardiac arrhythmias. Recurrent attacks of acute pericarditis are manifested by chest pain, often pleuritic and affected by a change of position, accompanied by fever and occasionally a pericardial friction rub. These attacks are usually self-limited, lasting 4 to 7 days. Treatment consists of bed rest, aspirin, and other anti-inflammatory agents, such as indomethacin in appropriate doses. Rarely, constrictive pericarditis may require a pericardiectomy.

Congestive heart failure is to be expected ultimately in patients with secondary hemochromatosis unless death occurs early by virtue of cardiac arrhythmias. Careful echocardiographic studies have suggested that iron deposition begins by the age of 5 to 6 years. By 10 or 12 years, when the patient has received more than 100 units of blood, left ventricular dysfunction may be demonstrated by radionuclide cineangiography during the physiologic stress of exercise. Clinical congestive heart failure is usually a late complication; most patients die within 12 months of the onset of definite evidence of heart failure. Treatment with digoxin in doses adequate to achieve therapeutic blood levels may be quite helpful. Appropriate use of diuretics and vasodilator therapy may be extremely useful in providing palliation and extending the lifespan of these patients.

Atrial and ventricular ectopy is present in 24-hour electrocardiographic recordings in virtually all patients who have received more than 150 units of packed red cells. High-grade ventricular ectopy with couplets, short runs of ventricular tachycardia, and multiple ventricular foci are of ominous prognostic significance. Ectopy may be extremely distressful to the patient, particularly at night, when it is often most severe. Tachyrhythmias such as ventricular tachycardia and/or ventricular fibrillation occur despite therapy and are frequent causes of death in patients with severe thalassemia who are undergoing regular transfusions. The pharmacologic treatment of cardiac arrhythmias is described in Ch. 42.

The prognosis of patients with thalassemia major is determined by the cardiac disease. The average age of death is 17 years, although a few patients may survive to their mid-20's. Because of this grim prognosis, a considerable effort has been focused on attempts to reduce the iron burden in these patients.

THE ROLE OF SPLENECTOMY. Splenic enlargement is frequent and often causes functional hypersplenism as manifested by an increasing transfusion requirement. Careful documentation of the patient's needs often alerts the physician to the development of hypersplenism as the need for blood rises. An average patient on a hypertransfusion regimen designed to maintain the hemoglobin at a level greater than 10 grams per deciliter requires 250 ml of packed cells per kilogram per year. If substantially more blood is required, the spleen should be removed. Leukopenia and thrombocytopenia, if present, are indicators of the presence of hypersplenism and should lead to prompt splenectomy.

The complication of splenectomy in this patient population is a risk of sudden overwhelming sepsis by encapsulated organisms. For this reason, delay of splenectomy until after the age of 4 is highly desirable. Splenectomized patients should receive Pneumovax and may be placed on a regimen of daily penicillin prophylaxis. More important, each patient should be given a small supply of a broad-spectrum antibiotic, such as ampicillin, to be taken orally in appropriate doses if a high temperature develops and immediate medical attention cannot be obtained.

CHELATION THERAPY. The only drug available for use in removal of iron is deferoxamine (Desferal). This drug has an extremely high affinity for trivalent iron, and despite extensive clinical use it appears to be relatively free of serious toxicity when given subcutaneously. It must be given parenterally and it has a very short serum half-life. Thus, most of the drug, given as a single intramuscular injection, is rapidly excreted without binding any iron. To maximize the efficacy of the drug, a technique has been devised to administer it subcutaneously by using a small mechanical infusion pump. A needle is inserted into the subcutaneous tissue of the abdomen, and the drug is infused very slowly over a period of 8 to 12 hours. With 1.5 to 2.0 grams of Desferal, two to three times more iron may be removed than by a single daily intramuscular injection. Often daily excretion of 30 to 40 mg of iron may be achieved in older patients and may lead to overall negative iron balance despite continued transfusion therapy, provided that the drug is used at least five times per week. This regimen retards the rate of iron accumulation in the liver and reduces liver fibrosis.

Clinical evidence indicates that cardiac disease may be delayed. Indeed, reversal of established congestive heart failure with documented left ventricular dysfunction has been observed in patients treated intensively with intravenous deferoxamine. This may be accomplished by placement of a Hickman catheter. Well-motivated patients may be taught to administer the drug daily by the intravenous route in doses of 3 to 4 grams per day given over 18 to 20 hours. Gastrointestinal disturbances and reversible renal dysfunction have been observed. Reduction of dose eliminates these complications. Significant neurosensory toxicity affecting sight and auditory function has been observed at high intravenous doses. The greatest probability of successfully preventing iron damage is in patients in whom treatment is begun early, preferably by the age of 5 years. Vitamin C in small doses (150 to 250 mg per day) given orally may increase the amount of iron excretion in response to deferoxamine infusions, although some evidence suggests that this agent may enhance tissue iron toxicity, particularly to the heart, and therefore it should be used with caution in older patients.

Various oral chelations have been developed, and two have reached the stage of clinical trials in limited numbers of patients. The efficacy of Desferal is well established, however, and therefore substitution of untested therapy is problematic, since the outcome cannot be known for several years.

Thalassemia Intermedia

Those patients with severe β-thalassemia who maintain their hemoglobin levels above 6.0 to 7.0 grams per deciliter have a generally better prognosis. Individual patients with thalassemia intermedia generally have large amounts of Hb F, significant amounts of Hb A_2, and variable amounts of Hb A in their red cells. Iron accumulation may occur because of increased gastrointestinal absorption and ultimately may lead to secondary hemochromatosis with endocrine and cardiac dysfunction, but most patients with thalassemia intermedia survive into adulthood and many have children. Splenectomy may become necessary if evidence of hypersplenism is present. Osteoporosis may be severe, as these patients' erythroid mass is not suppressed. A disabling form of arthritis has been described. Large masses of erythroid tissue in extramedullary sites may cause organ dysfunction. Particularly distressing is spinal cord compression with paraplegia, although usually local radiation reverses this condition. Any or all of these complications may ultimately lead to the use of a regular transfusion regimen in patients with thalassemia intermedia despite their marginally adequate hemoglobin levels. Such treatment has the added benefit of preventing the disfiguring facial abnormalities.

Genetically this condition is heterogeneous. Often the red cells of both parents exhibit stigmata of thalassemia trait, although frequently one parent may be a silent carrier of the thalassemia gene (see below). In such persons the impairment of β globin synthesis is so mild that the red cells are normal, but when the abnormal β gene is paired with another affected by a more severe β-thalassemia mutation, thalassemia intermedia results. Elucidation of any thalassemia mutations at the molecular level has revealed marked quantitative variability ranging from 50 to 100 per cent reduction of β globin messenger RNA (mRNA) production (see below). Many patients are doubly heterozygous for two different mutations. The clinical heterogeneity of the β-thalassemias reflects the many combinations of mutations that may be present in individual patients. Other genetic modifiers of the β-thalassemia phenotype include α-thalassemia mutations and genetic variants characterized by increased Hb F production. Co-inheritance of an α-thalassemia gene decreases α globin production, leading to partial correction of the highly deleterious imbalance in α and β biosynthesis. Increased γ globin synthesis, resulting in increased Hb F production, compensates directly for deficient β globin production.

THALASSEMIA TRAIT

CLINICAL CHARACTERISTICS. Common to both α- and β-thalassemia is a condition referred to as thalassemia minor or trait. This condition generally occurs in individuals who are heterozygous for a mutation affecting α or β globin synthesis (see below). Characteristically the red blood cells are small and contain less hemoglobin than normal; the mean corpuscular volume averages 65 μm^3 (range, 56 to 74), whereas the mean corpuscular hemoglobin averages 21 pg (range, 20 to 23). Normal values for these parameters are 88 ± 5 and 30 ± 2, respectively. The total red cell count is often increased to 10 to 20 per cent above the normal range, so that anemia, if present, is mild. Rarely the packed cell volume may be as low as 30 per cent; values of 32 to 38 per cent are more typical. Splenomegaly is said to occur but is distinctly unusual, and other causes should be sought if this physical finding is present. No clinical symptoms may be attributed to the presence of thalassemia trait.

DIFFERENTIAL DIAGNOSIS. A characteristic feature of β-thalassemia trait is an elevation of the level of Hb A_2. This minor hemoglobin accounts for only 2 or 3 per cent of the total in normal red cells, but in thalassemia trait it may be elevated in the range of 4 to 8 per cent in more than 90 per cent of persons with this condition. Similarly, the level of Hb F is often elevated to 1.5 to 2.5 per cent, although in rare types of thalassemia trait it may be as high as 10 to 15 per cent. In normal red cells, Hb F accounts for less than 1 per cent of the total. The minor hemoglobins, Hb A_2 and Hb F, are either normal or slightly decreased in patients with α-thalassemia.

The differential diagnosis of thalassemia trait includes a consideration of iron deficiency. This diagnosis can be excluded only by measurement of the serum iron, total iron-binding capacity, and serum ferritin. If these values are normal in patients whose red cells are severely microcytic, but in whom anemia, if present, is mild, the diagnosis of thalassemia trait can be considered established. The distinction between α- and β-thalassemia depends on the measurement of the minor hemoglobins. If these are normal, the diagnosis of α-thalassemia is most likely, although rare subjects with β-thalassemia also have normal levels of Hb A_2 and Hb F.

GENE FREQUENCY. Thalassemia trait is thought to protect persons from malaria, particularly during the early years of life when immunity is not yet established and fatal cerebral malaria caused by *Plasmodium falciparum* may occur. This selective advantage accounts for the high frequency of thalassemia genes in regions where malaria has been endemic for the past two millennia. These include the Mediterranean basin particularly, but also large parts of Asia and Africa. The gene frequency may be as high as 20 per cent in certain populations.

HEMOGLOBIN H DISEASE

PATHOPHYSIOLOGY. An anemia of moderate severity characterized by hypochromia, microcytosis, striking red cell frag-

mentation, and the presence of a fast migrating hemoglobin on electrophoresis occurs in patients who have a moderately severe deficiency in α globin production. The genetics of this condition are considered later in this chapter. The fast migrating "hemoglobin" has the globin subunit composition β_4. It may account for up to 30 per cent of the total hemoglobin in these patients. Because the β_4 tetramer exhibits no cooperativeness and has an extremely high oxygen affinity, it is functionally useless in oxygen transport. Thus patients with a significant amount of Hb H functionally have a more severe anemia than measurement of the hemoglobin concentration might suggest.

Hb H is an unstable tetramer. Thus as the red cell ages and loses its ability to withstand oxidative stress, Hb H may precipitate, forming inclusions that cause hemolysis (see Color Plate 6C, left). Oxidant drugs such as the sulfonamides may exacerbate hemolysis. Because the β_4 tetramer is soluble during the early phases of the red cell's lifespan, erythropoiesis in the bone marrow is effective and the anemia is generally not as severe as that seen in patients with β-thalassemia who have an equivalent impairment in β globin production.

CLINICAL FEATURES. The average patient with Hb H disease maintains gainful employment, marries, and reproduces. Usually the anemia is moderate, with a hemoglobin concentration of 7 to 10 grams per deciliter, although occasional patients may have more severe anemia. Moderate splenomegaly is often present. Splenectomy may be considered, but the occurrence of severe postoperative thrombocytosis with a propensity for recurrent pulmonary emboli makes this procedure inadvisable except in patients with unequivocal clinical evidence of hypersplenism, as manifested by leukopenia, thrombocytopenia, and a worsening anemia or a transfusion requirement in a previously stable patient. Other therapeutic measures include prescription of folic acid, avoidance of oxidant drugs and iron salts, prompt treatment of infection, and judicious use of transfusions. Acquired Hb H disease has been described as a complication in patients with various forms of myeloproliferative and myelodysplastic disorders. In such patients, treatment and prognosis are related to the primary disorder.

HYDROPS FETALIS

The birth of stillborn infants from parents who both have α-thalassemia trait reflects the severest form of α-thalassemia. These infants are grossly edematous or hydropic because of the congestive heart failure that occurs as a result of severe anemia. Their failure to produce any α globin results in the production of only Hb Barts (γ_4) and Hb H (β_4) during the later parts of gestation. Both these hemoglobins are nonfunctional in oxygen transport, so that once the embryonic hemoglobins disappear from the circulation early in fetal development, life is no longer possible. A high incidence of toxemia of pregnancy has been noted in mothers of hydropic infants. Prenatal diagnosis of this condition is possible (see below) and should be followed by prompt termination of the pregnancy.

SILENT CARRIER

The silent carrier state was first recognized among the α-thalassemia syndromes. One parent of a patient with Hb H disease usually has all the features of α-thalassemia trait, whereas the other has normal-appearing red cells with no anemia. Similarly, progeny of persons with Hb H disease fall into two groups: those having α-thalassemia trait and those with apparently normal hemoglobin production. In the silent carrier, the defect in α globin synthesis is so mild that no impairment in hemoglobin synthesis is evident, although when the mutation is paired genetically with a more severe impairment of globin synthesis, e.g., α-thalassemia trait, Hb H disease occurs. A similar silent carrier state has also been described among the β-thalassemia syndromes. Thalassemia intermedia occurs in those who inherit one thalassemia gene from a silent carrier and a second from a person with thalassemia trait.

THE GENETICS OF THE α THALASSEMIA SYNDROMES

As described in Ch. 136.1, the α globin genes in humans are duplicated. Thus two genes are found on each chromosome 16, making a total of four in each diploid cell. Four clinical states are seen in α-thalassemia: silent carrier, thalassemia trait, Hb H disease, and hydrops fetalis. These conditions occur in persons who have, respectively, one, two, three, or four α globin genes affected by mutations that reduce α globin synthesis.

The most frequent mutation that leads to α-thalassemia is gene deletion. In the silent carrier one of the two genes on one chromosome 16 is missing, whereas the other two genes on the other chromosome 16 are normal. α-Thalassemia trait can occur by two mechanisms. Persons who have two chromosomes with only one α gene exhibit α-thalassemia trait. This form is most common in the black population. Hb H disease is distinctly uncommon in this population, since offspring of two persons each of whom is homozygous for the one α gene chromosome can have only α-thalassemia trait and not Hb H disease. In the Asian population, α-thalassemia trait occurs most commonly in those who lack both α genes on one chromosome and have the normal two on the other. Mating of such a person with a silent carrier who has one chromosome having only one α gene can lead to children with Hb H disease. Hydrops fetalis occurs among offspring of parents both of whom are heterozygous for chromosomes lacking both normal α globin genes.

In addition to the deletion mutations, many nondeletional types of α-thalassemia have been described. Molecular characterization of several has revealed a diversity of defects involving RNA splicing, polyadenylation, mRNA translation, or α globin stability. These mutations are similar to those in β-thalassemia globin genes; their effects on RNA metabolism are discussed in more detail in the next section.

THE MOLECULAR GENETICS OF THALASSEMIA

The β-thalassemia mutations may be separated into two classes: β^+-thalassemia, in which there is synthesis of a small amount of normal β globin, and β^0-thalassemia, which in the homozygote is manifested by no β globin production at all. Similarly, nondeletional types of α-thalassemia may abolish (α^0) or decrease (α^+) α globin production. Many mutations having specific effects on gene expression have been characterized by molecular cloning, DNA sequencing, and functional characterization. Each of the several steps in RNA metabolism—transcription, processing, transport, and mRNA translation—has been found to be affected by one or more individual mutations. The variable quantitative effect of the individual mutations on globin production has been clarified by these molecular studies.

PROMOTER MUTATIONS. Five globin genes, each of which has a single nucleotide substitution in the promoter region, have been isolated from different individuals with β-thalassemia. Three of the mutant genes have substitutions in the "ATA" box (see Fig. 136–6). These mutations reduce promoter function to 20 to 25 per cent of normal, but some β globin mRNA is produced from these genes; hence they cause β^+-thalassemia. The other two promoter mutants characterized to date have substitutions at 86 or 87 nucleotides from the start site for transcription in the first of the conserved "CACA" boxes.

SPLICING MUTATIONS. These are among the most common of mutations that cause thalassemia. Figure 136–9 contains a few illustrative examples classified by the manner in which they affect splicing of the globin mRNA precursor. Mutations that occur within the splice junction sequence decrease or abolish normal splicing at that site and often are accompanied by splicing at other sites that are not normally used. A substitution in the invariant GT, as shown in the example (Fig. 136–9A), abolishes splicing, making this a β^0 gene, whereas substitutions in consensus nucleotides at the splice junction have a quantitative effect on splicing and hence are β^+ mutations.

An interesting class of mutations consists of those that create an alternate site for splicing. These may occur within introns or, as shown in the examples in Figure 136–9B, within coding sequence (exons). These substitutions occur within regions of the precursor RNA molecule that resemble the consensus splice junction sequence (see Fig. 136–6) but lack some critical element necessary for splicing. Nucleotide substitutions that add that element to the potential splice junction sequence lead to its activation, causing abnormal splicing and hence a thalassemic

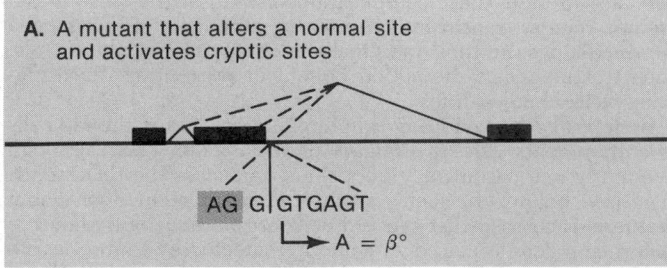

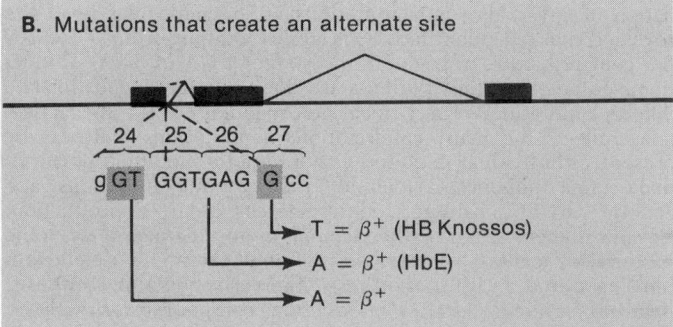

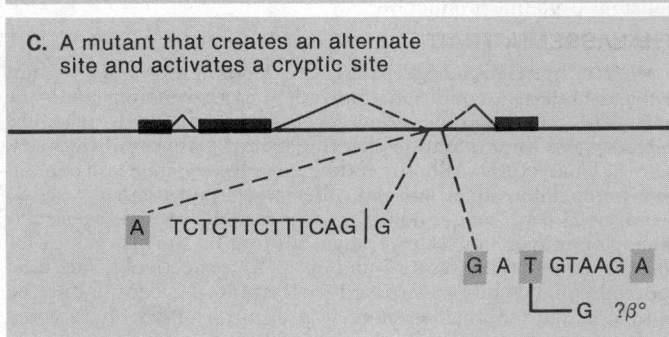

FIGURE 136–9. Thalassemia mutations that alter the splicing of the β globin gene transcript. *A*, The nucleotides guanine (G) and thymine (T) are obligatory for normal splicing. Replacement of the G with adenine (A) abolishes normal splicing and leads to abnormal splicing at otherwise cryptic sites. *B*, Several different mutations at this position in the transcript create an alternate site that leads to abnormal splicing. This segment of the normal transcript includes the obligatory dinucleotide, GT, and matches the consensus sequence in all but the nucleotides in the boxes. Single nucleotide substitutions activate this otherwise inactive site. *C*, A substitution toward the end of intron II creates an alternate splice site. A normally cryptic site farther upstream in the intron is also involved in a splicing reaction with exon 2–intron II splice junction, resulting in formation of a processed globin RNA that retains a portion of the sequence transcribed from intron II. Therefore, it cannot be translated into β globin.

effect. Substitution of A for T in codon 24 of the β globin gene does not alter the amino acid sequence (GGT and GGA both encode for glycine) but creates an alternate site for splicing. The other two mutations illustrated in Figure 136–9B (Hb E and Hb Knossos) alter both protein structure and the splicing pattern. Such structural mutants that are also characterized by decreased synthesis are referred to as *thalassemic hemoglobinopathies*.

A class of mutations that has interesting implications for control of splicing is made up of those that create an alternate site and also activate cryptic splice sites remote from the mutation. There is a potential for a cryptic splice site in the β globin gene transcript that matches the consensus splice junction sequence nearly perfectly, and yet this site is used rarely, if ever, during normal splicing. Use of an alternative site, created by a thalassemia mutation, apparently alters the secondary structure of the precursor RNA molecule, leading to splicing at the otherwise cryptic site (Fig. 136–9C).

A POLYADENYLATION MUTATION. The sequence "AATAAA" is one of the signals that leads to cleavage of the globin gene transcript and addition of the poly-A tail (see Fig. 136–9). An α-thalassemia gene isolated from an individual with Hb H disease has G substituted for A, altering the polyadenylation signal to "AATAGA." Most of the RNA transcript is not processed correctly and is prematurely degraded, although a small amount of normal α globin mRNA is produced by this mutant gene. Thus it is an α^+ thalassemia gene.

MUTATIONS THAT AFFECT mRNA TRANSLATION. Among the more common mutations in thalassemia genes are those that lead to premature termination of mRNA translation. Single nucleotide substitutions or small deletions that alter the mRNA reading frame introduce codons that signal the termination of protein synthesis on the abnormal mRNA. For example, substitution of thymine for cytosine in codon 39 introduces the stop codon UAG at that position. This abnormal β globin mRNA can be read only through codon 38, yielding a small, nonfunctional remnant of β globin. Premature termination mutations cause β^0- (or α^0-) thalassemia.

Common mutations that cause α-thalassemia are chain termination mutations. As described in Ch. 136.2, the completed globin molecule is released from the polyribosome when the protein synthetic apparatus encounters the normal terminator codon UAA. A single nucleotide change in this terminator codon converts it to a codon that is functional for the insertion of any one of several amino acids, depending on the exact nucleotide that is substituted. In this case protein synthesis continues into the part of the mRNA that is usually untranslated, leading to the synthesis of a protein that may be as many as 30 amino acids longer than normal. Such an elongated α globin is found in Hb Constant Spring. This protein accounts for only 1 to 2 per cent of the total α globin in the cells of patients with Hb Constant Spring, and their red cells exhibit the stigmata of thalassemia trait.

MUTATIONS THAT AFFECT GLOBIN STABILITY. Certain mutations may alter globin sequence and lead to instability and thus have a thalassemic effect despite a normal rate of synthesis of the mutant globin. Among the more dramatic of this class of mutations is one that leads to substitution of leucine for proline at position 125 of the α globin found in Hb Quong Sze. This mutation was discovered upon sequencing of the abnormal α gene and evidence of $\alpha^{Quong\ Sze}$ instability was subsequently obtained in vitro. Because of its marked instability, $\alpha^{Quong\ Sze}$ could not be detected in the red cells of the affected individual. Hb Quong Sze, like Hb E, is another of the thalassemic hemoglobinopathies characterized by both deficient net globin production and a structural abnormality.

DELETION MUTATIONS. Deletions causing α-thalassemia have been described earlier. Small deletions that leave one of the two α-globin genes intact on a chromosome are classified as α^+ mutations, while large deletions that remove both α genes are considered α^0 mutations. In contrast to α-thalassemia, in which gene deletion is the most common mutation, gene deletion is rarely the mechanism for β-thalassemia. A few patients of Indian ancestry have been found to have a deletion that has removed the 3′ half of the β globin gene and a small amount of flanking DNA. A special kind of deletion has resulted in the δβ fusion gene present in a few Italian patients who produce Hb Lepore. An unequal crossover during meiosis has led to the fusion gene that encodes for a globin that has the N-terminal sequence of δ globin and the C-terminal sequence of β globin. This globin is produced in very small amounts; hence this gene leads to thalassemia trait or thalassemia major in heterozygotes or homozygotes, respectively.

Several large deletions that have removed two or more genes from the β cluster have been characterized. The β-thalassemia mutations have resulted in loss of the δ and β genes; the $^A\gamma\delta\beta$- thalassemia deletions include the $^A\gamma$ gene in addition. Two interesting forms of γδβ-thalassemia have resulted in loss of all but the β gene, and yet this β gene does not function. These observations suggest that the DNA sequences remote from a gene can nonetheless influence its expression. Two deletions have resulted in loss of the entire β-like gene cluster.

MUTATIONS THAT INCREASE Hb F PRODUCTION

About 1 per cent of the hemoglobin in adult blood is Hb F. This fetal hemoglobin is found in 2 to 10 per cent of red cells; these cells—called F cells—contain roughly 4 to 8 pg of Hb F and 24 to 28 pg of adult hemoglobin. As discussed in Ch. 136.2, these F cells originate during the differentiation of erythroid progenitor cells. F cell number and therefore Hb F levels are genetically determined in humans.

Increased Hb F in individuals who are homozygous for β-thalassemia mainly reflects amplification of the F cell population. In the bone marrow, those erythroblasts producing small amounts of γ globin have less of an excess in α globin synthesis and therefore are more likely to survive and leave the bone marrow. By this mechanism, the 1 per cent of γ synthesis in the bone marrow cell population may be amplified 10- to 40-fold in the peripheral blood. Of more interest from the aspect of gene control are those mutations that alter Hb F production by genetic mechanisms.

There are two general classes of deletion mutations that increase Hb F production in adults. The δβ-thalassemia mutations are characterized by production of 5 to 12 per cent of Hb F in heterozygotes, while *hereditary persistence of fetal hemoglobin* (HPFH) deletion mutations are characterized by production of 25 to 30 per cent. Most of the red cells in heterozygous individuals with HPFH contain Hb F, whereas heterozygotes with δβ-thalassemia mutations have Hb F in only 30 to 70 per cent of their red cells. These mutations have been carefully characterized structurally in an attempt to define the basis at the DNA level for these differing phenotypes. Twenty-eight mutations have been studied, but no common patterns have emerged, with one exception. Deletions that remove the left side of the cluster (ε and γ genes) also inactivate the remaining intact β gene, whereas deletions that remove the right-hand portion of the cluster (δ and β genes) increase expression of the remaining γ globin genes. The removal of sequences within the cluster that normally modulate gene expression and the movement of "activating" sequences into the cluster by virtue of deletion are other possible mechanisms that may lead to increased Hb F production as a consequence of these deletions.

Another category of mutations that cause HPFH leave the β-like gene cluster intact and therefore are referred to as *nondeletion mutations*. Nondeletion HPFH mutations are often characterized by a heterogeneous distribution of Hb F in red cells (heterocellular) in contrast to the pancellular distribution of Hb F in heterozygotes with the deletion types of HPFH. There may be many different heterocellular HPFH mutations; genetic studies indicate that at least some are not linked to the β-like gene cluster. Ten different point mutations within the γ globin gene promoter region have been discovered in individuals with nondeletion HPFH.

PRENATAL DIAGNOSIS

Because of the serious consequences of severe β-thalassemia (Cooley's anemia), prenatal diagnosis of this condition with subsequent therapeutic abortion is thought by many to be highly desirable. Two general strategies have made this a feasible undertaking. The first approach is based on the fact that small amounts of β globin synthesis may be detected in the early mid-trimester fetus. In fetuses who have inherited two genes for β-thalassemia, no β globin or very small amounts are produced at a time when normal fetuses are producing approximately 10 per cent β globin. By using sophisticated obstetric techniques, blood may be obtained from the umbilical vein and used for biosynthetic measurements of the globin synthetic pattern. Absence of or low β globin synthesis occurs in homozygous fetuses, whereas intermediate levels are found in heterozygotes. This strategy has been widely applied in parts of Greece and Italy and has led to a significant reduction in the incidence of the severe form of β-thalassemia in certain populations.

A second and now more widely applied strategy relies on the use of fetal DNA for analysis. A chorionic villus biopsy late in the first trimester of pregnancy provides a simple noninvasive method to obtain DNA. Alternatively, amniotic fluid obtained at mid-pregnancy provides sufficient cells for extraction of fetal DNA. Major advances in our knowledge of mutations that cause thalassemia and in methods of detection of such mutations make DNA analysis the most useful approach for prenatal diagnosis.

More than 60 point mutations that cause β-thalassemia have been described. However, each ethnic group has two or three common mutations and three or four mutations that occur with lower frequency and that together account for the majority of disease in that ethnic group. Since the spectrum of mutations has been defined for each of the ethnic groups in which thalassemia is common, prenatal diagnosis can be directed to detection of a specific subset of known mutations.

The polymerase chain reaction has revolutionized DNA diagnosis. With the use of sequence-specific primers, a small segment of the entire genome can be amplified more than a million-fold within a few hours. Nanogram quantities of the amplified DNA are obtained. Usually the entire β globin gene is amplified in two segments. Detection of specific mutations is accomplished by annealing aliquots of the amplified DNA, immobilized on filter paper, to a series of mutation-specific oligonucleotides and the corresponding oligonucleotides having the normal sequence. Occasionally, it is necessary to sequence the amplified DNA if the patient carries a rare or new mutation. The parents can be prescreened with this methodology so that prenatal diagnosis can focus on the mutation or mutations for which the fetus is at risk.

Prenatal diagnosis of α-thalassemia often requires Southern blot analysis to detect deletion mutations. Again, the spectrum of mutations in individual ethnic groups has been defined so that probes and enzymes can be chosen that readily define the deletion breakpoint. Southern blot analysis is occasionally also required for β-thalassemia if the phenotype in the parents suggests the presence of a δβ-thalassemia mutation. Red cell microcytosis combined with Hb F of 5 per cent or greater is suggestive of this diagnosis.

The application of prenatal diagnosis requires appropriate screening and identification of persons at risk. Thalassemia trait can usually readily be identified by virtue of the morphologic changes in the red cells. Confirmation of the diagnosis depends on measurement of hemoglobin A_2 and Hb F.

EXPERIMENTAL THERAPY

Knowledge of globin gene structure and regulation has suggested a means to activate the structurally normal but inactive γ globin genes in individuals with severe β-thalassemia. Increased γ globin synthesis is desirable because it partially compensates for the deficiency of β globin production and decreases the relative excess of α globin. DNA is modified after synthesis by methylation of cytosine residues. Expressed genes are relatively undermethylated compared with unexpressed DNA sequences. For example, the γ globin genes are undermethylated in fetal erythroid cells, but after the switch to adult hemoglobin synthesis the γ globin genes are fully methylated in adult erythroid cells. 5-Azacytidine* inhibits DNA methylation and has been shown to activate genes in tissue culture cells and in experimental animals. Administration of 5-azacytidine to patients with severe β-thalassemia under defined experimental protocols has resulted in increased γ globin synthesis and improvement in red cell production and survival. The effect is transient, lasting only 2 to 3 weeks. Reluctance to administer a potentially carcinogenic and toxic drug for longer periods has limited the use of 5-azacytidine to experimental studies of a few severely affected patients. Nonetheless these encouraging results have prompted a search for other effective and less toxic drugs that may make pharmacologic stimulation of the γ globin genes a useful approach for treatment of severe β-thalassemia.

Cure of severe β-thalassemia can be achieved by bone marrow transplantation from an HLA-identical, unaffected sibling. Several patients have already been cured by this method. This procedure carries a 5 to 20 per cent risk of death or significant graft-versus-host disease (GVHD). Transplantation in infancy, preferably before transfusions are given, increases the probability of successful engraftment, although a high cure rate has also been achieved in older patients. However, adequate transfusion therapy and effective chelation may provide 20 or more years of good-quality life for newborns. Thus, the availability of bone marrow transplantation raises a significant ethical dilemma for parents and physicians. In the future, refinements in the treatment of GVHD and transplantation techniques may permit wider appli-

---

*Available from the National Cancer Institute.

cation of bone marrow transplantation as treatment for patients with severe β-thalassemia.

Insertion of intact globin genes into the bone marrow cells of patients with severe forms of thalassemia has become a feasible research objective. Gene transfer mediated by retroviral vectors is highly efficient and has resulted in the insertion and expression of genes in experimental animals. Many problems remain to be overcome before this strategy becomes clinically feasible, however.

Hershko C, Weatherall DJ: Iron-chelating therapy. Crit Rev Clin Lab Sci 26:303, 1988; Fosburg MT, Nathan DG: Treatment of Cooley's anemia. Blood 76:435, 1990; Nathan DG, Piomelli S: Oral iron chelators. Semin Hematol 27:83, 1990. *This series of articles provides a detailed account of current therapeutic recommendations for severe β-thalassemia, including the status of iron chelation therapy and new oral iron chelators.*

Kazazian HH Jr, Boehm CD: Molecular basis and prenatal diagnosis of beta-thalassemia. Blood 72:1107, 1988. *This is a definitive account of the mutations that could cause β-thalassemia and the modern strategies used for prenatal diagnosis.*

Lucarelli G, Galimberti M, Polchi P, et al.: Bone marrow transplantation in patients with thalassemia. N Engl J Med 322:417, 1990. *This article describes the most extensive experience with transplantation for severe β-thalassemia and provides a guide to patient selection and predicted outcomes.*

McDonagh KT, Nienhuis AW: The thalassemias: Disorders of hemoglobin synthesis. *In* Nathan DG, Oski F (eds.): Hematology of Infancy and Childhood. Philadelphia, W. B. Saunders Company, 1991. *This chapter contains a more detailed exposition of the thalassemia syndromes with a comprehensive account of the molecular basis of these disorders and the current status of prenatal diagnosis.*

Nienhuis AW, Ley TJ, Humphries RK, et al.: Pharmacological manipulation of fetal hemoglobin synthesis in patients with severe beta-thalassemia. Ann NY Acad Sci 445:198, 1985. Ley TJ, Nienhuis AW: Induction of hemoglobin F synthesis in patients with beta thalassemia. Ann Rev Med 36:485, 1985. *Reviews of the results achieved by using drugs in an effort to stimulate fetal hemoglobin synthesis for therapeutic benefit in patients with thalassemia.*

136.5 SICKLE CELL ANEMIA AND ASSOCIATED HEMOGLOBINOPATHIES

Bernard G. Forget

DEFINITION. The sickle cell syndromes are due to the inheritance of a gene for a structurally abnormal β globin chain subunit of adult hemoglobin (Hb), the β^S chain of Hb S ($\alpha_2\beta^S_2$). The structural abnormality of the β^S globin chain consists of a single amino acid substitution or replacement: valine instead of the normal glutamic acid at position number 6 of the β polypeptide chain. Hb S can be found in the heterozygous state (Hb AS or sickle cell trait), in the homozygous state (Hb SS, sickle cell anemia, or sickle cell disease) (see Color Plate 6B, left), in association with other structural hemoglobin variants (i.e., Hb SC and SD disease), in association with β-thalassemia (Hb S/β-thalassemia or sickle/β-thalassemia syndromes), or in association with the thalassemia-like disorder termed hereditary persistence of fetal hemoglobin (Hb SF or Hb S/HPFH). The structural abnormality of Hb C, a nonsickling hemoglobin, also consists of a single amino acid substitution at residue number 6 of the β globin chain: in the β^C chain lysine replaces glutamic acid. Clinical syndromes associated with the inheritance of Hb C include Hb SC disease and homozygous Hb C disease (see Color Plate 6B, right).

PREVALENCE AND GENETICS. The sickle cell syndromes are particularly prevalent in black persons of African or Afro-American ancestry. However, the gene is also found at a lower frequency in persons of Mediterranean ancestry (southern Italians, Sicilians, and Greeks), in Saudi Arabia, and in India. The highest gene frequencies occur in equatorial Africa, in the so-called malaria belt. The heterozygous state for Hb S (sickle cell trait) probably confers a biologic advantage against infection with *Plasmodium falciparum* malaria, and for this reason the gene frequency for Hb S has achieved high levels through natural selection in geographic areas of endemic malaria. In the United States the prevalence of the sickle cell trait in blacks is 8 to 10 per cent and the number of homozygous persons approaches 50,000, or 1 in 400 births. In certain areas of western Africa (Ghana and Nigeria), the prevalence of Hb AS can reach 25 to 30 per cent. The prevalence of Hb AC in black Americans is approximately 3 per cent. Gene mapping studies, using restriction endonuclease analysis of cellular DNA to identify polymorphisms of nucleotide sequence in the DNA around the β^s globin gene, have disclosed an unexpected heterogeneity of polymorphisms linked to the sickle β globin genes in different individuals, suggesting multiple independent origins of the sickle gene.

PATHOPHYSIOLOGY. Disease in the sickle syndromes results from aggregation or polymerization of Hb S molecules inside erythrocytes, which causes (1) chronic compensated hemolytic anemia, (2) chronic and progressive tissue and organ damage, and (3) acute painful vaso-occlusive crises. These clinical phenomena are directly related to the physicochemical behavior of the intracellular Hb S molecules and result from alterations of red cell rheology and, possibly, changes in the red cell membrane.

The polymerization process occurs only when the Hb S molecule is in the deoxy conformation (see Ch. 136.1). When Hb S is in the oxy conformation it has essentially normal physicochemical properties. In the deoxy conformation, Hb S molecules can aggregate with one another into long polymers and are aligned to form a gel of liquid crystals that are also called tactoids. The polymerization process goes through a number of stages, as illustrated diagrammatically in Figure 136–10. In the process of nucleation, Hb S molecules form small aggregates, which then grow by addition of successive Hb S molecules. The larger aggregates then align themselves to form linearly arranged fibers that constitute a paracrystalline gel. These fibers can be detected as helical electron-dense tube-like structures by electron microscopy (Fig. 136–10). The end result of the polymerization process is the transformation of the intracellular contents of the red cell from a fluid liquid to a viscous gel. The amount of Hb S polymer within red cells increases progressively as the percentage of oxygen saturation of the hemoglobin decreases. The viscous polymer decreases the flexibility of the erythrocyte and thus impairs its transit through the microcirculation. When the amount of polymer is sufficiently high, the red cells may assume the typical sickle or holly leaf shape associated with sickled erythro-

cytes (Fig. 136–11). The shape change of the erythrocyte is a passive phenomenon in which the red cell membrane conforms to the shape that is assumed by the intracellular gel of polymerized hemoglobin. The polymerization phenomenon is reversible: With reoxygenation of the Hb S molecules the aggregated molecules disassociate, the gel becomes liquid, and the erythrocyte, if it has sickled, can return to its normal shape, as long as the red cell membrane has not become altered to form an irreversibly sickled cell (see below).

A number of factors can influence the rate and degree of Hb S aggregation in red cells. One of the most important determinants is the concentration of Hb S and of total hemoglobin within the red cell. In general, the higher the percentage of Hb S, the more severe the sickle syndrome. Factors such as cellular dehydration that increase the mean corpuscular hemoglobin concentration (MCHC) greatly facilitate polymerization by increasing the opportunity and frequency of contact between Hb S molecules. The importance of hemoglobin concentration on polymerization is underscored by the clinical observation that the coinheritance of α-thalassemia together with sickle cell anemia is generally (but not universally) associated with less severe hemolysis. The milder clinical course of Hb S/β-thalassemia is also thought to be due in part to the associated hypochromia. The length of time during which Hb S remains deoxygenated is also very important; Hb S polymerization is enhanced with any increase in the transit time of the red cell through the microcirculation. The presence of other hemoglobins within the red cell can also influence sickling. In general, at a constant MCHC, any other non-S hemoglobin molecules in the red cell, by a simple dilution effect, decrease the opportunity of contact between Hb S molecules. In addition, the type of non-S hemoglobin present can differentially affect polymerization: Fetal hemoglobin (Hb F)

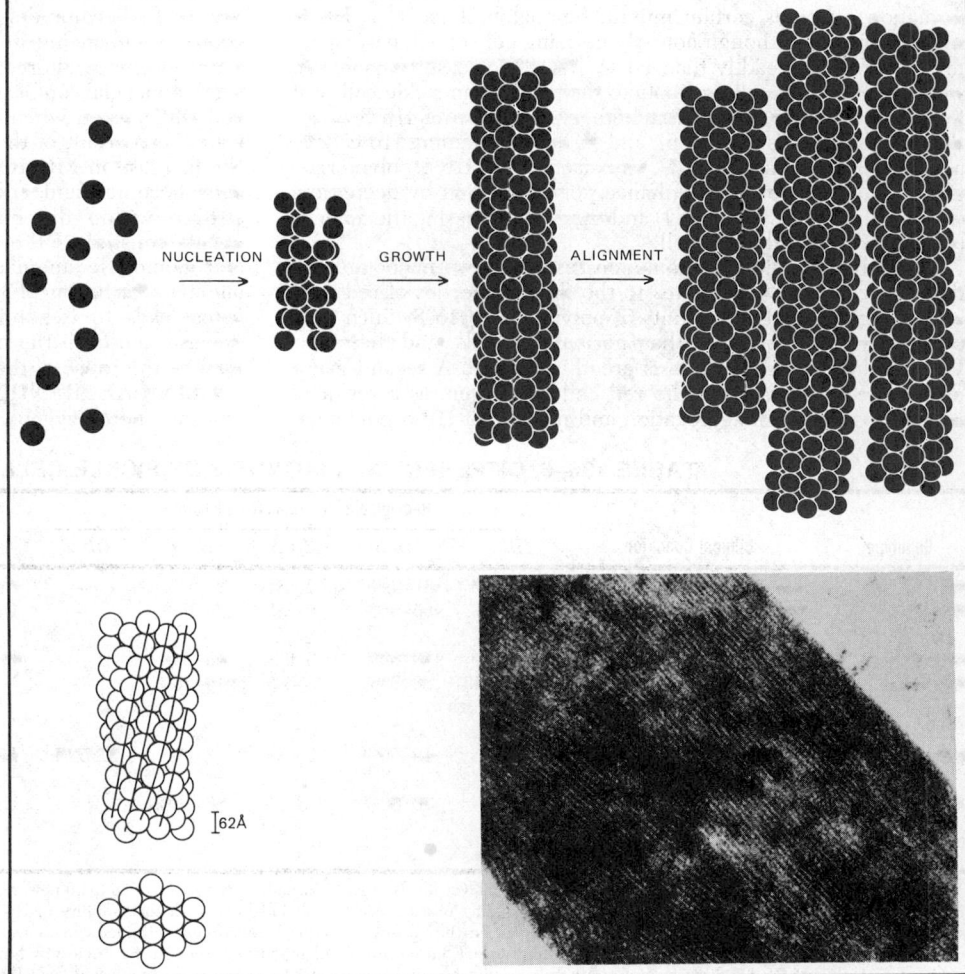

FIGURE 136–10. *Top,* Schematic representation of mechanism of deoxyhemoglobin S polymerization. Each circle represents a deoxyhemoglobin S tetramer: $\alpha_2\beta_2{}^s$. *Lower left,* Molecular model, based on electron microscopy, of the helical arrangement of deoxyhemoglobin S tetramers in a fiber of polymerized Hb S molecules; side view *(above)* and cross-section or end-on view *(below)*. *Lower right,* Electron micrograph (longitudinal section) of deoxyhemoglobin S gel in a sickled erythrocyte.

NUCLEATION → GROWTH → ALIGNMENT

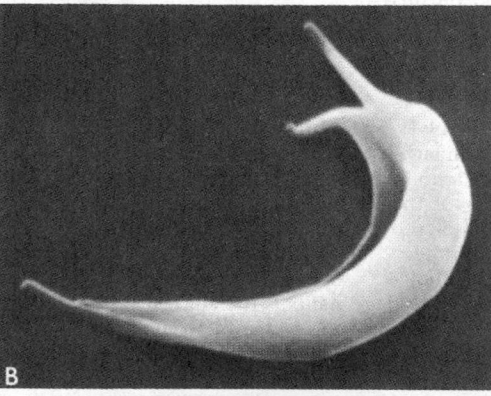

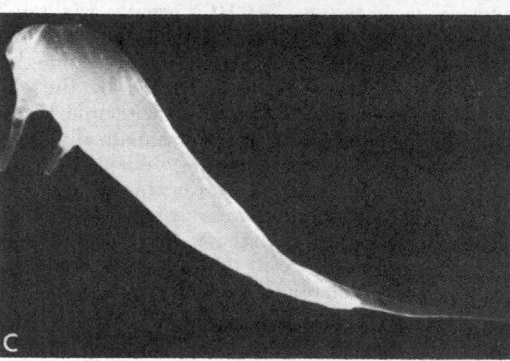

FIGURE 136–11. Scanning electron micrographs of oxygenated (*A*) and deoxygenated (*B* and *C*) SS erythrocytes. (Courtesy of Dr. James White. *In* Bunn HF, Forget BG: Hemoglobin: Molecular, Genetic, and Clinical Aspects. Philadelphia, W. B. Saunders Company, 1986.)

participates much less readily than normal Hb A in polymer formation, whereas certain mutant hemoglobins, such as Hb O Arab and Hb D, although nonpolymerizing per se, will participate in gelation more readily than Hb A. Hb SC disease is associated with a more severe clinical course than is seen in sickle cell trait for two reasons: (1) There is a higher proportion of Hb S in SC than in AS cells (Table 136–6); and (2) cells containing Hb C have a higher than normal MCHC, thus facilitating Hb S polymerization. Finally, acidosis can enhance polymerization by decreasing oxygen affinity (see Ch. 136.1) and thereby increasing the amount of deoxy Hb S in the red cell.

The polymerization phenomenon results in two major red cell disturbances. The first relates to the flow properties of red cells containing substantial amounts of polymerized Hb S. Such cells are much less deformable than normal red cells, and their flow through the microcirculation is greatly retarded. A second major disturbance is damage to the red cell membrane as a result of repeated episodes of aggregation and melting of Hb S polymers.

Sickle red cells are "leaky." They tend to lose K$^+$ and water and eventually become dehydrated, the resulting increase in MCHC probably enhancing further polymerization. The red cell membrane becomes altered in other ways, so that it may assume a rigid, abnormal conformation, thus forming an irreversibly sickled cell (ISC), even when the hemoglobin is not in the aggregated state. As a result of the intracellular polymerization of Hb S, of the increase in MCHC, and of the membrane changes, the red cells become rigid and are sequestered and prematurely destroyed within the reticuloendothelial system. This series of events constitutes the basis for the shortened red cell survival and hemolytic anemia that invariably accompany sickle cell anemia. Occlusion of the microvasculature by viscous erythrocytes leads to ischemia and eventual infarction of the tissue downstream from the obstruction, results in organ damage, and may be the cause of the characteristic painful "crises."

CLINICAL MANIFESTATIONS. *Sickle Cell Trait.* Persons who are heterozygous for Hb S are essentially asymptomatic.

TABLE 136–6. DIFFERENTIAL DIAGNOSIS OF SICKLE CELL SYNDROMES

| Genotype | Clinical Condition | Hemoglobin Electrophoresis Findings | | | | | Other Associated Findings |
		Hb A	Hb S	Hb A$_2$	Hb F	Hb C	
AS	Sickle cell trait	55–60%	40–45%*	2–3%	~1%	—	Asymptomatic; no anemia
SS†	Sickle cell anemia	0	85–95%	2–3%	5–15%	—	Usually clinically severe; Hb F distributed heterogeneously among red blood cells
S/β⁰-thal	Sickle cell/β-thalassemia	0	70–80%	3–5%	10–20%	—	Moderate severity; splenomegaly in over half of the cases; Hb F distributed heterogeneously among red blood cells; hypochromia and microcytosis
S/β⁺-thal	Sickle cell/β-thalassemia	10–20%	60–75%	3–5%	10–20%	—	
SC‡	Hb SC disease	0	45–50%	2–3%	~1%	45–50%	Moderate severity; splenomegaly; many target cells on blood smear
SF (S/HPFH)	Sickle/hereditary persistence of fetal hemoglobin	0	70–80%	1.5–2%	20–30%	—	Uniform distribution of Hb F among all red cells; asymptomatic; no anemia

*Persons with associated α-thalassemia trait (-α/-α) have lower levels of Hb S, usually in the range of 25 to 30 per cent; those with concomitant heterozygous α-thalassemia 2(-α/αα) have Hb S levels of 30 to 36 per cent. The finding of a (nonsickling) hemoglobin with the mobility of Hb S but in much lower amounts (5 to 15 per cent) is suggestive of the Hb Lepore trait (see Ch. 136.4). Except for the (-α/αα) genotype, hypochromia and microcytosis are usually associated with these conditions.

†Hb SD disease gives similar electrophoretic findings at pH 8.6 but can be distinguished from Hb SS disease by hemoglobin electrophoresis in citrate agar at pH 6.1.

‡Hb S/O-Arab and Hb SE diseases give similar electrophoretic findings at pH 8.6 but can be distinguished from Hb SC disease by hemoglobin electrophoresis in citrate agar at pH 6.1. Hb A$_2$ co-migrates with Hb C at pH 8.6 and can be quantitated only by column chromatography.

They should not have any anemia attributable to the hemoglobinopathy. Any anemia in such persons should be investigated for other secondary causes. Symptoms resulting from vaso-occlusion occur only in extreme circumstances of severe hypoxia such as flying in unpressurized aircraft. However, a universal finding in sickle cell trait is microinfarction of the renal medulla presumably owing to the ambient hyperosmolarity that is thought to lead to dehydration of the red cells, an increased MCHC, and sickling; as a result, in affected persons the urine is unconcentrated and isosthenuria is manifested. Painless hematuria can also occasionally be attributed to microinfarction of the renal medulla, although the other usual causes should be ruled out before painless hematuria in persons with sickle cell trait is attributed to the sickling phenomenon.

Sickle Cell Disease. The Anemia. Patients homozygous for Hb S invariably have a chronic compensated hemolytic anemia of variable severity. In general, the hematocrit ranges between 20 and 30 per cent and the hemoglobin between 6.5 and 10 grams per deciliter. The hemolysis is compensated for by increased erythropoiesis, manifested as an elevated reticulocyte count in the range of 10 to 25 per cent. Mild jaundice and indirect hyperbilirubinemia are also present as a reflection of the hemolysis. The degree of the anemia is usually stable in a given patient, although occasional hypoplastic or aplastic crises can occur owing to suppression of erythropoiesis at the time of infectious episodes and can result in a rapid decrease in the reticulocyte count and a precipitous drop in the hemoglobin and hematocrit levels. Infection with parvovirus B19 has been implicated in the pathogenesis of aplastic crises. Another cause of rapid worsening of the anemia is the acute splenic sequestration crisis (a sudden pooling of large volumes of blood in the spleen) that can occur in younger patients with sickle cell anemia before autoinfarction of the spleen or in older patients with Hb SC disease and Hb S/β-thalassemia in whom the spleen is not infarcted and may in fact be enlarged. There is some controversy whether or not a hyperhemolytic state can be associated with sickle cell anemia. From what is known of the basis for the hemolysis in this condition, there is no pathophysiologic mechanism for variable or accelerated hemolysis resulting from sickling alone. In general, the anemia and hemolysis in sickle cell disease do not increase or worsen during vaso-occlusive painful crises. If hemolysis suddenly worsens, one should look to other secondary causes that may be responsible, such as an associated glucose-6-phosphate dehydrogenase deficiency and exposure to an oxidant stress from drugs or an acute infection. Finally, in patients with marginal nutritional status and increased requirements, such as during pregnancy, folic acid deficiency can develop and aggravate the anemia—the so-called megaloblastic crisis of sickle cell disease.

Vaso-occlusive Crises. The major disabilities suffered by patients with sickle cell anemia are related to painful vaso-occlusive crises and to secondary end-organ damage as a direct consequence of the sickling phenomenon and occlusion of the microvasculature of one or another organ, most commonly the bones of the trunk and extremities. The episodes are characterized by sudden onset of excruciating pain in the back, chest, or extremities. There is frequently no identifiable precipitating event, although infections may be associated with the onset of the episode. Other predisposing factors include dehydration, acidosis, or increased hypoxia, as during a pulmonary infection. A low-grade fever may be associated with the painful attacks, although not necessarily. In general, the onset of fever occurs 1 or 2 days after the onset of pain and parallels the degree of tissue necrosis resulting from the ischemic infarction. The painful attacks last for variable periods, ranging from a few hours to a few days, depending on the extent of the vaso-occlusive phenomenon and the rapidity with which treatment is initiated and is successful in reversing the occlusive episode. In general there are no external signs, such as heat, swelling, or tenderness of the soft tissues over the affected bones. However, if the bone infarction occurs in proximity to a joint, an effusion can develop. Bone infarction may be difficult to differentiate from osteomyelitis, and definitive diagnosis of the latter must ultimately rely on positive bacterial cultures from aspirated material.

When the vaso-occlusive process occurs in the vasculature (including large vessels) of organs other than bones, the clinical manifestations are primarily related to damage of the affected organ. Common acute vaso-occlusive clinical syndromes include

cerebrovascular accidents (i.e., hemiplegia and seizures) caused by involvement of the cerebral vasculature; the acute chest syndrome associated with occlusion of the pulmonary vessels, which can be difficult to differentiate from acute pulmonary infarction caused by emboli or from acute pulmonary infections; hepatic crisis, with marked hyperbilirubinemia and other abnormal liver function tests, which can be difficult to differentiate from acute hepatitis or choledocholithiasis; priapism resulting from vaso-occlusion within the corpus cavernosum; and acute renal papillary infarction with hematuria and/or obstruction of the urinary collecting system.

More chronic complications include refractory skin ulcers of the leg, usually in the vicinity of the medial malleolus, an area that has poor collateral circulation, and variable degrees of renal insufficiency resulting from the combination of repeated infarctions and infectious episodes. All patients manifest the inability to concentrate the urine and have isosthenuria. Microinfarction in the peripheral retina is initially asymptomatic but may lead to the formation of new blood vessels that are fragile and can hemorrhage, causing retinal detachment and blindness. For this reason periodic eye examinations are important so that the early asymptomatic lesion may be recognized and treated before it progresses to the point of causing visual disturbances. Finally, repeated bone infarcts in the vicinity of joints can lead to secondary degenerative arthritis, and gradual infarction of the head of the femur results in aseptic necrosis of the hip.

Other Clinical Manifestations. Clinical manifestations of sickle cell anemia not directly related to the sickling phenomenon include increased susceptibility to infections, cholelithiasis, and abnormal growth and development. The increased susceptibility to infections is probably related at least in part to absence of splenic function and in some cases to an abnormality of the properdin opsonization pathway. In early childhood, septicemia and meningitis caused by encapsulated organisms such as *Streptococcus pneumoniae* and *Haemophilus influenzae* are common. In later life common infectious episodes include recurrent pneumonias, urinary tract infections, and osteomyelitis. The predisposition to osteomyelitis is probably related to the repeated bone infarcts that can form a nidus for infection. Although osteomyelitis caused by *Salmonella* occurs almost exclusively in patients with sickle cell anemia or one of the other sickle cell syndromes, *Staphylococcus aureus* is still the most common causative organism of osteomyelitis in these syndromes.

Cholelithiasis is very common and can be manifested at a young age; it is caused by the chronic hemolysis that results in increased bilirubin production. Episodes of cholecystitis and choledocholithiasis can easily be confused with abdominal and hepatic sickle cell crises. The causes of delayed growth and development are poorly understood. Delayed puberty can result in late closure of the epiphyses and an asthenic habitus.

Sickle/β-Thalassemia and Hb SC Disease. The anemia and the hemolysis are less severe in the other sickle syndromes, such as Hb SC disease and sickle/β-thalassemia, in which there is somewhat less propensity for sickling than in homozygous Hb SS disease. The degree of anemia is strongly related to the extent of intracellular Hb S polymerization. In these conditions the anemia frequently ranges between hemoglobin levels of 10 and 12 grams per deciliter, and the reticulocyte counts are usually less than 10 per cent, frequently in the range of 5 per cent.

In general the vaso-occlusive manifestations resulting from sickling are also less frequent and less severe in Hb SC disease and in sickle/β-thalassemia than in sickle cell anemia, although all of the complications previously described for sickle cell anemia can also occur in these conditions. However, in contrast to sickle cell anemia, splenomegaly in adults is usually present in these syndromes, and splenic infarcts and acute splenic sequestration crises can occur. The ocular complications of sickling also tend to occur more frequently in Hb SC disease than in sickle cell anemia and can in fact be the presenting symptoms. There is also increased frequency of aseptic necrosis of the femoral head in Hb SC disease. Sickle/β⁰-thalassemia, in which Hb A is totally absent, is generally more severe than sickle/β⁺-thalassemia and can be as clinically severe as sickle cell anemia.

DIAGNOSIS. The diagnosis of the various sickle syndromes relies on two types of tests: (1) screening tests to detect the presence of Hb S on the basis of its physicochemical properties, and (2) more definitive tests for the precise diagnosis of the particular genetic syndrome involved.

Two types of screening tests for the detection of Hb S are in current use. Both tests simply detect the presence of some Hb S in erythroid cells but do not differentiate sickle cell trait from the other sickle syndromes. The standard "sickle cell preparation" consists of mixing blood with a solution of sodium metabisulfate, which totally deoxygenates the blood and thus induces sickling that can be observed under the microscope. A second screening test is a solubility test that consists of mixing blood with a solution of high ionic strength and observing the mixtures for turbidity; normal hemoglobin gives a clear solution, whereas any Hb S in the solution precipitates to give a turbid solution through which one cannot see the lines of an indicator card. Both tests, if properly done, are highly specific and accurate. The solubility test has the advantages that a microscope is not needed and that the test solution is relatively stable.

Once Hb S is detected by screening tests, hemoglobin electrophoresis should be carried out for precise diagnosis of the sickle syndrome. Table 136–6 summarizes the results obtained by hemoglobin electrophoresis in the various sickle cell syndromes as well as other associated clinical and laboratory findings that are useful in the differential diagnosis. In general, routine hemoglobin electrophoresis at pH 8.6 will suffice to establish the diagnosis. However, a few exceptions to this rule require additional tests to confirm or establish the suspected diagnosis. Because other hemoglobin variants can have the same electrophoretic mobility as Hb S at pH 8.6, electrophoresis in citrate agar at pH 6.1 should be performed to confirm the diagnosis (see Table 136–6). The distinction between Hb SS disease and Hb S/β⁰-thalassemia can be very difficult to establish, since electrophoretic findings are similar in both cases. The Hb A_2 level should be elevated in Hb S/β-thalassemia, but precise quantitation of Hb A_2 in the presence of Hb S is sometimes unreliable. Findings that should establish the diagnosis of Hb S/β⁰-thalassemia rather than Hb SS disease include (1) the presence of hypochromia and microcytosis indicated by low mean corpuscular volume (MCV) and MCH; (2) family study showing that one parent or an offspring has β-thalassemia trait rather than sickle cell trait; (3) experimental studies of globin chain synthesis using labeled amino acid precursors (see Ch. 136.4), demonstrating decreased synthesis of βˢ chains relative to α chains (βˢ/α = 0.5 to 0.6); and (4) gene mapping studies to distinguish between βᴬ and βˢ globin genes in the patient's DNA (Fig. 136–12). The rare but interesting syndrome of Hb S/HPFH also gives hemoglobin electrophoretic findings similar to those of Hb SS disease, but with an unusually high level of Hb F in the range of 30 per cent. Such patients, however, are not anemic and should be asymptomatic. The diagnosis can be confirmed by family study showing the absence of sickle cell trait and the presence of heterozygosity for HPFH in a parent or offspring. Study of the distribution of Hb F within individual red cells, using the acid elution test of Betke and Kleihauer, shows uniform distribution of Hb F in Hb S/HPFH but heterogeneous distribution of Hb F in Hb SS disease. Inheritance of Hb D (another relatively common β chain hemoglobinopathy in blacks) along with Hb S can also mimic homozygosity for Hb S, since Hb D co-migrates with Hb S on electrophoresis at pH 8.6. Hb SD disease is not as clinically severe as sickle cell disease, and the diagnosis can be established by performing hemoglobin electrophoresis at neutral or acid pH, which separates the two hemoglobins. Similarly, Hb SC disease can be confused with the inheritance of Hb S along with a second hemoglobin variant that has an electrophoretic mobility similar to that of Hb C at pH 8.6, such as Hb O Arab or Hb E. These syndromes can be distinguished from Hb SC disease by electrophoresis in citrate agar at pH 6 to 7.

The peripheral blood smear in individuals with Hb SS disease shows variable numbers of ISC's, usually ranging between 5 and 10 per cent. In general, the number of ISC's is relatively stable for a given patient, and there is a rough correlation between the numbers of ISC's and the severity of the hemolytic anemia. There is no correlation between the number of ISC's and the frequency or presence of vaso-occlusive crises. The peripheral blood smear, in addition to ISC's, usually shows variable numbers of target cells and occasional Howell-Jolly bodies owing to absence of spleen function. Other hematologic findings related to functional asplenia include the presence of somewhat elevated leukocyte counts and platelet counts. Examination of the peripheral blood smear can also be helpful in the differential diagnosis of the sickle syndromes. In general, significant numbers of ISC's are found essentially only in homozygous SS disease and not in the other sickle syndromes. Large numbers of target cells are characteristic of the inheritance of Hb C in either the heterozygous or the homozygous state (see Color Plate 6B, right).

TREATMENT. Despite extensive knowledge of the molecular basis and physical chemistry of the polymerization and sickling phenomena, there is still no specific molecular therapy available for the treatment or prevention of sickling. A number of compounds have been tested, and new compounds continue to be sought, that might interfere with sickling in vivo and be useful clinically. Unfortunately no such compound is currently available. Another potential molecular approach to the prevention of sickling would be to reactivate or increase fetal hemoglobin synthesis in the majority of the erythroid cells of affected patients to render them similar to the red cells of patients with Hb S/HPFH, a clinically mild syndrome. Successful enhancement of Hb F levels in patients with sickle cell anemia and homozygous β-thalassemia (see Ch. 136.4) has been accomplished by the administration of the chemotherapeutic agents 5-azacytidine* and hydroxyurea to a number of patients. The rationale for 5-azacytidine therapy resided in the findings that the drug causes demethylation of DNA and that active genes are usually hypomethylated, whereas the inactive fetal γ globin genes of adults are hypermethylated. However, other mechanisms related to cell toxicity and depletion followed by regeneration, cell selection, and changes in gene expression resulting from disruption of the cell cycle probably also contribute to the increased levels of Hb F following administration of chemotherapeutic agents. These therapies should be considered investigational at this time and restricted in their general applicability until the long-term efficacy and toxicity of these drugs, including carcinogenicity, is established. Hydroxyurea is likely to be a less toxic agent for chronic administration. Clinical trials of the drug have revealed that it is effective in raising the Hb F levels of many, though not all, patients with sickle cell anemia. However, controlled clinical trials have not yet been carried out to determine the efficacy of the drug in decreasing the frequency of painful vaso-occlusive crises.

The cornerstones of therapy in sickle cell anemia have therefore not changed in recent years and continue to consist of the administration of the following supportive measures: large volumes of intravenous fluids (preferably hypotonic and alkaline); analgesics to control the pain; when indicated, antibiotics to treat any associated bacterial infection; and oxygen to treat hypoxemia.

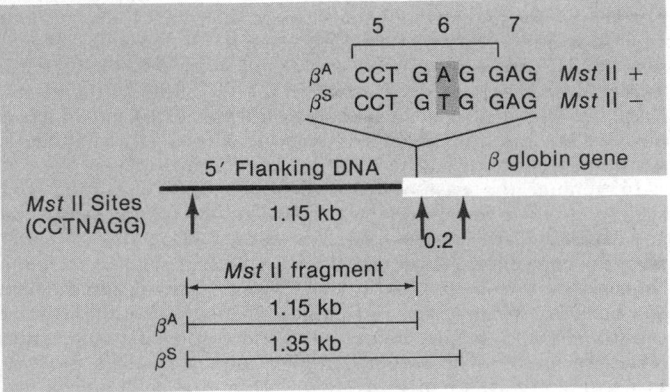

FIGURE 136–12. Direct identification of the sickle cell mutation in cellular DNA by restriction endonuclease digestion using the enzyme *Mst* II. The diagram shows the flanking region and 5' portion of the β globin structural gene. Arrows indicate the *Mst* II sites, including the one corresponding to amino acid portions 5, 6, and 7. The 1.15-kilobase (kb) fragment is seen in normal DNA, and the 1.35-kb fragment is seen in sickle DNA.

---

*Investigational agent available from the National Cancer Institute.

When administering fluids to patients with sickle cell anemia, one should remember that these patients have a fixed renal water loss owing to inability to concentrate urine and that they are frequently dehydrated on presentation because of associated infection and fever. The amounts of intravenous fluids administered should therefore be increased to two to three times what would be considered a normal maintenance volume. Patients with sickle cell disease are frequently hypoxic because of chronic pulmonary disease. Even though they do not appear to be cyanotic, monitoring of arterial PO_2 is important, especially if there is an associated chest syndrome, and oxygen should be administered if there is significant hypoxemia. In the absence of arterial hypoxemia, oxygen therapy is probably not beneficial in the treatment of vaso-occlusive crises and may result in suppression of erythropoiesis. The role of alkali is controversial, and certainly if the patient is mildly acidotic, this acidosis should be corrected, since it can potentiate the propensity of deoxy Hb S molecules to aggregate.

The role of blood transfusions and partial exchange transfusions is controversial in the treatment of acute vaso-occlusive crises of sickle cell disease. In general there is very little rationale for performing partial exchange transfusions simply for a painful vaso-occlusive crisis in a nonvital organ. Nevertheless such treatment may be occasionally indicated to interrupt an unusually prolonged painful crisis or when a patient is virtually continually disabled by frequent recurrent crises. In cases of life-threatening vaso-occlusive episodes or when there is a threat of severe organ damage, as in acute cerebrovascular accidents and priapism, partial exchange transfusions should be promptly carried out because no other effective form of therapy is available. It is also generally agreed that patients who have suffered one cerebrovascular accident are likely to have recurrent life-threatening or debilitating episodes, and a course of long-term maintenance blood transfusions to prevent recurrent sickling is indicated in such cases. Such a program should probably be associated with phlebotomies prior to transfusion and/or the institution of an iron chelation program to prevent or delay the complications of iron overload (see Ch. 136.4). Use of transfusions during pregnancy is controversial. It is common practice in many centers to give transfusions to pregnant women with sickle cell syndromes during the latter half of pregnancy to prevent fetal loss and postpartum complications. However, a controlled study has not documented that this practice is clearly beneficial. Finally, it is also general practice for patients with clinically significant sickle cell syndromes to receive a partial exchange transfusion to lower the Hb S value to less than 50 per cent prior to general anesthesia for surgical procedures because of the risk of a fatal or incapacitating sickling episode in the event of an anesthetic accident or transient hypoxia. With the exception of the hypoplastic crises and acute sequestration crises, blood transfusions are not usually required to maintain hemoglobin levels above 6.5 to 7 grams per deciliter, and transfusions are not required on a long-term basis simply to treat the anemia.

Because of the high risk of septicemia and other serious infections caused by *Streptococcus pneumoniae*, young children with sickle cell anemia should receive prophylactic oral penicillin. This approach has been shown to be highly effective in reducing morbidity and mortality in pediatric populations. Pneumococcal and *Haemophilus influenzae* vaccines may provide additional protection against such infections.

PROGNOSIS. The prognosis of patients with sickle cell syndromes is variable. A significant number of infants with sickle cell anemia and Hb SC disease may die in the first 2 to 3 years because of overwhelming sepsis and/or acute splenic sequestration crises. Cord blood screening programs and identification of affected individuals with subsequent close medical follow-up, including prophylactic penicillin and vaccinations, should prevent or decrease the incidence of these early fatalities. For the group of patients who survive the early years, improved general medical care has substantially prolonged survival in the past two decades. There are reports of patients surviving to the fifth and sixth decades, although the mean survival is probably to the fourth decade, with death resulting from cardiopulmonary complications and/or renal insufficiency. Other causes of death include sepsis and cerebrovascular accidents. In general, patients with Hb S/β-thalassemia and Hb SC disease have longer survival than do patients with sickle cell disease, although there are unexplained

cases of relatively mild disease with homozygous inheritance of Hb S.

PREVENTION. Sickle cell disease and other clinically significant sickle syndromes can be prevented in two general ways. First, genetic counseling of identified heterozygotes can alert couples at risk about the possibility of having affected offspring. However, no matter how good the program of genetic counseling and education, it rarely significantly affects the reproductive behavior of identified carriers and generally has little impact on the overall incidence of the disease.

An alternative approach is the availability of prenatal diagnostic services for pregnancies at risk for sickle cell anemia and other sickle hemoglobinopathies. Prenatal diagnosis for sickle cell anemia has gone through many stages in recent years, including fetal blood sampling by fetoscopy for assays of hemoglobin synthesis and analysis by gene mapping techniques of DNA from amniotic fluid cells, obtained after amniocentesis, for restriction fragment length polymorphisms shown to be linked to the sickle gene by prior study of DNA from family members. A restriction endonuclease enzyme (*Mst* II) can distinguish between a sickle and a nonsickle β globin gene because the recognition site for this enzyme is specifically abolished by the nucleotide base substitution that is associated with the sickle mutation (Fig. 136–10). Thus the most reliable and acceptable method for prenatal diagnosis of sickle cell anemia is analysis of fetal DNA by the enzyme *Mst* II. The source of DNA may be amniotic fluid cells obtained by amniocentesis between 14 and 20 weeks of gestation, or chorionic villi obtained by transcervical biopsy between 8 and 10 weeks of gestation. The latter has the advantage of allowing diagnosis, counseling, and decision making to occur much earlier in the pregnancy. Although DNA analysis may be accomplished by standard gene mapping techniques (Southern gel blotting), it is much more quickly and efficiently achieved by use of the polymerase chain reaction procedure, as in the case of prenatal diagnosis of β-thalassemia (see Ch. 136.4).

HOMOZYGOUS Hb C DISEASE. Individuals homozygous for Hb C usually have a mild to moderate hemolytic anemia characterized by splenomegaly and large numbers of target cells on peripheral blood smear. Occasionally, intraerythrocytic crystals of Hb C can be visualized in fixed blood smears. The clinical manifestations and general laboratory findings are those of any mild chronic hemolytic anemia. Diagnosis is established by hemoglobin electrophoresis (see Color Plate 6B, right).

Bunn HF, Forget BG: Sickle cell disease—clinical and epidemiological aspects; and molecular basis of sickle cell disease. *In* Hemoglobin: Molecular, Genetic and Clinical Aspects. Philadelphia, W. B. Saunders Company, 1986, pp 502–554. Platt OS, Nathan DG: Sickle cell disease. *In* Nathan DG, Oski FA (eds.): Hematology of Infancy and Childhood. 3rd ed. Philadelphia, W. B. Saunders Company, 1987, pp 655–698. *Comprehensive chapters in hematology textbooks covering the pathophysiology as well as the clinical manifestations and therapy of sickle cell disease.*

Fleming AF (ed.): Sickle Cell Disease: A Handbook for the General Clinician. New York, Churchill Livingstone, 1982. Serjeant GR: Sickle Cell Disease. New York, Oxford University Press, 1985. *Comprehensive and detailed clinical descriptions of the manifestations of sickle cell anemia.*

Francis RB Jr, Johnson CS: Vascular occlusion in sickle cell disease: Current concepts and unanswered questions. Blood 77:1405, 1991. *An up-to-date review of this major and serious complication of sickle cell disease.*

137 Blood Transfusion

Jay E. Menitove

Whole blood collected for transfusion contains approximately 450 ml of anticoagulated blood. From this, red blood cells (or packed cells) are separated from plasma to achieve a hematocrit of 65 to 80 per cent in 250 to 300 ml. Solutions containing adenine and saline, added to blood shortly after collection, extend the permissible storage time from 21 or 35 days to 42 days. Red blood cells, adenine-saline added, have a hematocrit of 55 to 65 per cent and a volume of approximately 325 ml.

TABLE 137–1. INDICATIONS FOR RED BLOOD CELL COMPONENTS

Whole blood
  Symptomatic deficit in oxygen-carrying capacity and significant hypovolemia
Red blood cells (packed cells)
  Symptomatic deficit of oxygen-carrying capacity in anemic patients
Leukocyte-depleted red blood cells
  Symptomatic anemia, prevention of recurrent febrile, nonhemolytic transfusion reactions
Washed red blood cells
  Symptomatic anemia, prevention of severe urticarial reactions and anaphylaxis in IgA-deficient patients
Frozen/thawed red blood cells
  Symptomatic anemia, inventory maintenance for rare blood types

Blood donors are questioned extensively, and their blood is tested to decrease the risk of transmitting retroviruses, hepatitis, syphilis, and, in some instances, cytomegalovirus. All hazards cannot be eliminated, however. Transfusion therapy must therefore be used appropriately to ensure that the benefit outweighs potential risk (Table 137–1).

INDICATIONS FOR WHOLE-BLOOD TRANSFUSION

Whole blood is indicated for patients with a symptomatic deficit in oxygen-carrying capacity and hypotension as a result of hypovolemia. Crystalloid or colloid solutions are used to restore intravascular volume in patients with moderate hemorrhage. It is appropriate to use whole blood when blood loss exceeds 25 to 30 per cent of blood volume.

Factors V and VIII are labile, but the activity of other coagulation factors is stable during the shelf-life of whole blood (Ch. 155). Since Factor V or VIII deficiency is unusual in patients resuscitated after massive blood loss, whole blood is appropriate replacement therapy for patients with coagulation factor deficiency who also require red cell augmentation. Currently, whole blood accounts for approximately 5 per cent of red cell component transfusions in the United States.

INDICATIONS FOR RED BLOOD CELLS

Red blood cells are indicated for anemic patients who require an increase in oxygen-carrying capacity. The hemoglobin/hematocrit level at which tissue oxygenation is compromised is the subject of debate. In the perioperative period, a hemoglobin concentration of 7 grams per deciliter (hematocrit of approximately 21 per cent) is usually tolerated in the absence of depleted intravascular volume. In patients with chronic anemia, decreased oxygen delivery is compensated for by an increase in cardiac output, redistribution of blood away from renal and splanchnic beds to muscle tissue, and enhanced oxygen extraction by tissues (Ch. 111). In addition, coronary artery blood flow increases, ventilatory volume and respiratory rates rise, and oxygen unloading is more rapid, since erythrocyte levels of 2,3-diphosphoglycerate (2,3-DPG) are elevated. Anemic patients are susceptible to fatigue, dyspnea on exertion, decreased exercise capacity, decreased mental acuity, and breathlessness. These symptoms usually become significant when the hemoglobin concentration is between 7 and 10 grams per deciliter but vary according to the patient's cardiac, respiratory, and cerebrovascular status. Increasing cardiac and respiratory rate, congestive heart failure, angina, or confusion may indicate that compensatory mechanisms are not able to meet tissue oxygen demands.

Symptomatic patients with chronic anemia should receive two to three units of red blood cells at 2- to 3-week intervals. One unit of red cells raises the hemoglobin by approximately 1 gram per deciliter (or a hematocrit increase of 3 per cent) in the average-size adult. In general, the "transfusion trigger" is a hemoglobin concentration of 8 or 9 grams per deciliter (hematocrit of 24 or 27 per cent). The efficacy of compensatory mechanisms is uncertain when the hemoglobin is lower than 7 grams per deciliter.

LEUKOCYTE-DEPLETED RED BLOOD CELLS. Leukocyte-depleted red blood cells are used to prevent the recurrence of nonhemolytic febrile transfusion reactions in patients who have a history of two or more such reactions.

Leukocytes are removed from red blood cells by filtration or centrifugation. Certain filters withhold more than 95 per cent of white cells while allowing 90 per cent of red cells to pass. In contrast, there is a 70 to 80 per cent decrease in leukocyte content and a 20 to 30 per cent red cell loss when leukocyte depletion is accomplished by centrifugation.

WASHED RED BLOOD CELLS. Washed red blood cells are indicated for patients with a history of severe allergic or anaphylactic reactions. Plasma is effectively removed from red cells by adding saline to blood, sedimenting the red cells by centrifugation, and decanting the supernatant. Washed blood cells are not currently recommended for patients with paroxysmal nocturnal hemoglobinuria.

RED BLOOD CELLS STORED IN THE FROZEN STATE. Frozen red blood cells are used to create repositories of "rare" red blood cell units for patients with alloantibodies directed against red cell antigens that occur at high frequency in the population. They may be used for patients who have febrile nonhemolytic transfusion reactions but leukocyte-depleted red blood cells by filtration are preferred.

Red blood cells are prepared for frozen storage for up to 10 years by adding glycerol as a cryoprotective agent. Prior to transfusion, red cells are thawed and washed to remove glycerol. Only minimal amounts of leukocytes and plasma remain.

AUTOLOGOUS TRANSFUSION

The procedure of collecting and reinfusing a patient's own blood is a recommended alternative to homologous transfusion for patients who have at least 2 weeks' notice prior to scheduled surgery, who are likely to need a transfusion during or after surgery, and who have a hemoglobin higher than 11 grams per deciliter. Patients providing autologous blood should receive oral iron supplementation. They may donate as frequently as every 3 days but no later than 72 hours before surgery.

Perioperative blood salvage is another approach for reducing homologous transfusion. Blood lost during and immediately after surgery is collected and reinfused. Intraoperative blood salvage is contraindicated if the operative field is contaminated with bacteria or tumor.

Acute normovolemic hemodilution is also an alternative to homologous transfusion. Blood is removed prior to anesthesia induction, concomitant with crystalloid/colloid infusion. Hence, patients must be able to tolerate rapid blood withdrawal. The removed blood is reinfused at the completion of surgery, or sooner if needed.

Used alone or in combination, these methods are effective in decreasing homologous blood use and should be considered for appropriate patients. Recombinant erythropoietin has been used to augment hemoglobin concentration in patients initiating autologous blood collections 3 weeks before surgery. It is effective in ameliorating transfusion requirements in patients with renal insufficiency and may increase erythropoiesis in the perioperative setting.

DIRECTED DONATIONS

A directed donation refers to blood provided by a donor (usually a family member or friend) selected by the patient. There is an impression that these donors are "safer" than those donating to the general blood supply. This hypothesis is not supported by data.

MINIMAL EXPOSURE TRANSFUSION CONCEPT

Reducing the number of donors to whom a patient is exposed has a theoretical advantage of decreasing transfusion-associated risk. For example, donor exposures are reduced by use of whole blood in lieu of red blood cells from one donor and fresh frozen plasma from another or by providing apheresis platelet transfusions collected from one donor instead of an equivalent dose of pooled platelet concentrates from six to eight donors. Minimal exposure transfusion is potentially more adaptable for pediatric patients, who use less blood than adults, or for supplying platelets to those with a self-limited condition (such as extensive coronary artery bypass surgery).

BLOOD GROUPS. Red blood cell antigenic determinants are under genetic control. Allelic relationships are assigned on the basis of family studies and population statistics that demonstrate different antigens or through gene mapping and biochemical analysis. The clinical importance of a particular blood group depends on its frequency in the population, the immunogenicity of the antigen, and whether alloantibodies directed against it are immunoglobulin G (IgG) or immunoglobulin M (IgM) or whether they activate complement.

Blood group nomenclature has been revised into systems, collections, and series. Each of the 19 distinct systems refers to red cell antigens controlled by a single gene or continuous homologous genes and include ABO, MNS, P, Rh, Lutheran (Lu), Kell (Kk), Lewis (Le), Duffy (Fy), Kidd (Jk), and so on. The nine collections comprise specificities that have serologic, biochemical, or genetic connections, e.g., Gerbich (Ge), Cromer (Cr), Auberger (Au), and Ii. Two series have determinants that cannot be assigned to systems or collections: One consists of 38 specificities of low incidence (<1 per cent in a random Caucasian population), and the other contains 13 specificities of high incidence (>90 per cent in a random Caucasian population). Examples of such low-incidence antigens are Wright (Wr^a), Batty (By^a), and Christiansen (Chr^a), and high-incidence markers include Vel, Langreis (Lan), JMH, Fritz (Wr^b), and Sid (Sd^a).

ABO is the most important blood group system, because anti-A and anti-B are found in all persons lacking the corresponding antigen (Table 137–2). Intravascular hemolysis is a significant hazard if these antibodies are present at high titer and incompatible blood is infused. Anti-A and anti-B are "naturally occurring" antibodies, i.e., are present in the absence of previous transfusion or pregnancy. They are probably formed in response to bacterial antigens.

The Rh system is next in importance. Approximately 70 per cent of Rh-negative persons exposed to Rh-positive blood form anti-Rh antibodies. Anti-Rh antibodies are implicated in hemolytic reactions and cross the placenta to cause hemolytic disease of the newborn. For practical purposes, the Rh system is divided into Rh-positive and Rh-negative types by testing red cells with the most frequent Rh antibody, anti-D. A commonly used classification further subdivides the Rh system into three pairs of closely linked allelic genes: Cc, Dd, Ee. For example, a person may inherit C, D, e from one parent and c, d, e from another. Although the symbol "d" is used, it is an amorph; i.e., there is no allele for D.

A, B, and D are the most immunogenic red cell antigens. Kell (K), c, and E are less potent immunogens, and Fy^a and Jk^a are even less immunogenic. As a result of differences in antigenic strength and the frequency that patients are exposed to non-self antigens, Rh antibodies other than anti-D account for approximately 50 per cent and anti-K, anti-Fy^a, and anti-Jk^a for approximately 45 per cent of alloantibodies detected by hospital transfusion services.

COMPATIBILITY TESTING. Compatibility testing involves confirming the donor's blood group, determining the recipient's ABO and Rh types, screening the patient's serum for unexpected antibodies (i.e., antibodies other than anti-A and anti-B), and performing a major crossmatch.

Recipients of whole blood must receive blood from a donor with the same ABO group, since anti-A and/or anti-B present in the plasma may cause destruction of recipient red cells. For example, group O whole blood must be given only to group O patients, and group AB patients must receive only group AB whole blood. Since the amount of plasma is reduced in red blood cells, the blood type of donor and recipient of packed cell transfusions may be compatible rather than identical; i.e., group O (universal donor) red cells may be given to group A, B, or AB patients, and group AB patients (universal recipients) may receive group O, A, or B red blood cells. Rh-negative patients should receive Rh-negative whole blood or red blood cells. Rh-positive recipients may receive either Rh-positive or Rh-negative blood.

The test for unexpected antibodies must include antiglobulin reagents to detect agglutinating and nonagglutinating antibodies.

The crossmatch detects incompatibility between donor red cells and antibodies in the recipient's serum or plasma. Donor cells and the patient's serum are incubated; subsequently, antiglobulin reagents are added. Incompatibility is recognized by red cell agglutination or hemolysis. An abbreviated or "type and screen" procedure is used in some laboratories to determine incompatibility. The patient's blood is typed for ABO and Rh, and the serum or plasma is screened for unexpected antibodies. In the absence of unexpected antibodies or a record of such antibodies, the patient's serum is made to react with donor red cells and centrifuged briefly. If agglutination or hemolysis does not occur, the blood is released for transfusion. The centrifugation step, or "immediate spin," is used to detect ABO incompatibility. If unexpected antibodies are present, blood that does not contain the corresponding antigen should be selected, and a crossmatch should be performed.

When there is an urgent requirement for blood, such as when a delay in transfusion may jeopardize the patient unduly, blood may be issued without performing compatibility testing. If the ABO type of the recipient is not known, group O red cells should be provided. If the ABO group was determined by the hospital transfusion service, ABO group–compatible red cells may be given. Whole blood must be ABO group identical. In these circumstances, the patient's record should contain a statement from the attending physician explaining the urgent nature of the clinical situation and the requirement to transfuse blood before completion of the compatibility testing.

ADVERSE EVENTS ASSOCIATED WITH BLOOD TRANSFUSION

Complications of blood transfusion are categorized into acute, delayed, or transfusion-transmitted disease-related events (Table 137–3).

ACUTE REACTIONS. Acute adverse events caused by transfusion occur within minutes or hours after infusing red blood cells or other components. The presenting signs and symptoms are not always sufficiently specific to indicate a definite diagnosis. Correlation of clinical findings and laboratory test results is needed to establish the pathogenic mechanisms and treatment plan.

Acute Hemolytic Transfusion Reactions. These serious complications of blood transfusion occur infrequently—1 per 6000 to 25,000 component infusions. Intravascular destruction of red cells is the result of complete complement activation. Osmotic red cell lysis occurs, and free hemoglobin and antibody-coated red cell stroma are released into the plasma. If this situation is caused by anti-A or anti-B, the associated mortality approaches 10 per cent.

TABLE 137–2. FREQUENCY (%) OF BLOOD GROUPS IN SELECTED POPULATIONS

	Whites‡	Blacks‡	Hispanics§	Asians§	Native Americans§	Antibody in Plasma
O*	40	51	57	34	60	Anti-A, anti-B
A	44	25	32	35	35	Anti-B
B	12	20	9	23	4	Anti-A
AB†	5	4	2	8	1	None
Rh-positive	84	95	97	99+	97	—
Rh-negative	16	5	3	<1	3	—

*Universal donor of red blood cells.
†Universal recipient of red blood cells.
‡Derived from unpublished observations, Blood Center of Southeastern Wisconsin, Milwaukee.
§Estimates based on selected populations.

Extravascular hemolysis is associated with antibodies that coat red cells without complement activation beyond C3b. Opsonized red cells are removed by tissue macrophages. Most antibodies directed against Rh, Kell, Kidd, and Duffy antigens behave in this manner.

Fever is observed in almost all patients suffering a hemolytic reaction. Nausea, vomiting, and chest pain occur less often. Also reported are wheezing and dyspnea, back pain, restlessness, and discomfort at the infusion site. Hypotension may be a prelude to disseminated intravascular coagulation (DIC).

Major adverse sequelae are a consequence of vasomotor instability, hypotension, bleeding diatheses, and renal impairment. Hypotension is caused by release of C3a, C4a, and C5a into plasma as a result of antibody-antigen interaction. The thromboplastic activity of red cell stroma activates the intrinsic clotting cascade and gives rise, in some patients, to DIC. Renal insufficiency and oliguria are caused by changes in renal blood flow brought about by hypotension and vasoconstriction.

Most hemolytic reactions are a consequence of clerical error or failure to observe proper procedures, such as misidentification of blood samples, donor units, or patients. The blood infusion must be stopped as soon as a hemolytic transfusion reaction is suspected. Therapy is directed at correction of hypotension, control of bleeding, and prevention of acute renal failure. Blood pressure maintenance is important, since hypotension is a prelude to DIC and acute renal failure. Intravenous fluids, mannitol, or other diuretics such as furosemide or ethacrynic acid are used to increase renal blood flow and maintain urine output at 100 ml per hour. If oliguria or anuria ensues, standard measures for renal failure management must be instituted (Ch. 76).

Febrile Nonhemolytic Transfusion Reactions. These chill-fever reactions occur at a frequency of approximately 1 per 200 component infusions. They are characterized by a posttransfusion temperature rise of 1°C or more in the absence of hemolysis. They are caused by cytotoxic or agglutinating antibodies stimulated by previous transfusions or pregnancies against antigens on donor lymphocytes, granulocytes, or platelets.

These reactions occur in three phases. Initially, there is a transient episode of flushing, palpitation, tachycardia, cough, chest discomfort, or neutropenia that often is unnoticed. A 15- to 60-minute latent period intervenes. The third part consists of a rise in diastolic blood pressure, headache, chilliness, or a frank rigor. The reactions cannot be distinguished from hemolytic reactions on the basis of clinical presentation. Hence, the infusion should be stopped immediately. Most febrile nonhemolytic reactions are self-limited, however, and subside with supportive measures and orally administered antipyretics. Fewer than 15

per cent of patients suffer a recurrence when transfused subsequently. After a second reaction, it is advisable to provide further transfusions with red blood cells that have been leukocyte depleted by filtration.

Transfusion-Related Acute Lung Injury. This occurs infrequently but has significant clinical consequences. It is probably caused by passive infusion of donor antibody directed against recipient leukocytes (anti–human leukocyte antigen [HLA] antibody). The symptom complex is marked by fever, substernal chest pain, severe dyspnea, cyanosis, cough, blood-tinged sputum, and hypoxemia that occur within 4 hours (usually 1 to 2 hours) after plasma-containing components are given. The presentation resembles pulmonary edema, but hemodynamic measurements indicate a noncardiogenic etiology. Rapid intervention with respiratory support and mechanical ventilation is required. If the pulmonary capillary wedge pressure is low and hypotension is present, fluid replacement may be indicated. Recovery usually ensues within 48 hours.

Allergic Reactions. Urticarial eruptions and pruritus occur in 1 to 3 per cent of transfused patients. They are caused by an interaction between donor plasma proteins and recipient immunoglobulin E (IgE) antibody. The reactions are usually mild and respond to antihistamines. The transfusion may be continued after hives subside.

Anaphylactic reactions occur with a frequency of 1 per 150,000 component transfusions, usually in immunoglobulin A (IgA)–deficient patients (approximately 1 per 1000 of the population) who have anti-IgA that is reacting against IgA in donor plasma. The dramatic clinical presentation includes apprehension, a feeling of doom, chest or lumbar pain, facial flushing, generalized urticaria, laryngeal or facial edema with bronchospasm, wheezing, dyspnea, hypotension, loss of consciousness, vomiting, or diarrhea. These reactions require urgent treatment with intravenous epinephrine. If subsequent transfusions are required, cellular components should be washed to remove plasma.

Hypervolemia. Patients with impaired myocardial reserve are at risk of congestive heart failure caused by overexpansion of intravascular volume. An average unit of whole blood contains 56 mEq of sodium; a unit of red cells, 8 to 20 mEq of sodium; and a unit of red cells with additive solutions, 24 to 30 mEq of sodium.

Bacterial Sepsis. Septicemia is a rare complication of blood transfusion. In these cases blood has been contaminated at the time of phlebotomy, and bacteria have proliferated during storage. Following infusion of as little as 50 to 70 ml of blood, patients develop chills or frank rigors, which may be associated with nausea, vomiting, and lethargy. Subsequently, fever, hypotension, shock, and DIC may occur. Profound symptoms are compatible with endotoxin produced by gram-negative organisms.

TABLE 137–3. SIGNS AND SYMPTOMS OF ACUTE AND DELAYED ADVERSE CONSEQUENCES OF TRANSFUSION

Fever	*Wheezing/dyspnea*
Acute and delayed hemolytic transfusion reactions	Acute hemolysis
Febrile, nonhemolytic reactions	Acute lung injury
Acute lung injury	Anaphylaxis
Anaphylaxis	Hypervolemia
Septic transfusions	Air embolus
Chills/rigors	*Back/lumbar pain*
Acute hemolysis	Acute hemolysis
Febrile, nonhemolytic reactions	Anaphylaxis
Anaphylaxis	Septic transfusions
Septic transfusions	*Discomfort at infusion site*
Nausea/vomiting	Acute hemolysis
Acute hemolysis	Septic transfusions
Anaphylaxis	*Hypotension*
Septic transfusions	Acute hemolysis
Chest discomfort/pain	Anaphylaxis
Acute hemolysis	Septic tranfusions
Febrile, nonhemolytic reactions	*Bleeding/DIC*
Acute lung injury	Acute hemolysis
Anaphylaxis	Complication of massive transfusion
Air embolus	*Hemoglobinuria*
Facial flushing	Acute hemolysis
Brisk, acute hemolysis	Nonimmune hemolysis
Febrile, nonhemolytic reactions	*Hives/pruritus*
Anaphylaxis	Allergic reactions

Less dramatic clinical presentations occur when gram-positive organisms are involved. The infusion must be stopped. Samples for microbacteriologic examination and a Gram stain of an aliquot of noninfused blood should be obtained, and broad-spectrum antibiotics must be started immediately.

DELAYED REACTIONS. Delayed or nonimmediate adverse consequences of blood transfusion occur days to years after the transfusion is given.

Delayed Hemolytic Transfusion Reactions. Destruction of red cells by an antibody not detected by compatibility testing occurs at a frequency between 1 in 300 and 1 in 1600 transfusions. Only 20 per cent of these patients experience clinical symptoms, however. The antibodies are a result of a secondary or amnestic response. Clinical symptoms appear 6 to 8 days (range, 3 to 21 days) after transfusion. The triad of anemia, fever, and a history of recent transfusion in a patient previously immunized by transfusion or pregnancy should alert the clinician to suspect a delayed hemolytic transfusion reaction. Jaundice is present in approximately two thirds of those who are symptomatic. The direct antiglobulin test is usually positive. Anti-E, anti-Jk^a, anti-K, anti-D, anti-C, anti-c, and anti-Fy^a are commonly associated with these reactions. Severe sequelae are uncommon, and specific therapy is rarely needed.

Graft-Versus-Host Disease. This reaction occurs when transfused lymphocytes recognize and react against the "host" (recipient). Graft-versus-host disease requires the transfer of viable immunocompetent T lymphocytes that are disparate in HLA type from those of the patient but are sufficiently similar to permit initial engraftment. Most patients developing graft-versus-host disease have severely impaired cellular immune function; however, this syndrome has occurred in patients undergoing therapy for Hodgkin's disease, non-Hodgkin's lymphoma, acute leukemia, and neuroblastoma. Immunocompetent patients recovering from cardiac surgery have also been affected. Transfusion-associated graft-versus-host disease occurs 4 to 30 days after transfusion. Patients develop fever that may be accompanied by erythema, diarrhea, liver function abnormalities, and bone marrow suppression marked by pancytopenia. Treatment is usually unsuccessful; the mortality rate is approximately 90 per cent. Hence, prevention, accomplished by gamma irradiation (1500 to 3000 cGy, 15 to 30 Gy) of blood and components, is the primary strategy.

Iron Overload. Endocrine, cardiac, and liver dysfunction occurs in adults who receive 60 to 210 (mean, 120) units of blood. Iron chelation therapy has been used successfully to reduce iron stores.

Posttransfusion Purpura. This syndrome is manifested by profound thrombocytopenia 5 to 9 days after transfusion. Most cases occur in multiparous women receiving their first blood transfusion, but nulliparous women as well as previously transfused women and men have had this complication. The etiology is not known precisely, but more than 90 per cent of patients are Pl^{Al} negative and make an anti-Pl^{Al} alloantibody. Pl^{Al} is a platelet-specific antigen present on the platelets of 98 per cent of the population. It is unclear why a Pl^{Al}-negative patient with Pl^{Al} alloantibody becomes thrombocytopenic. Potential mechanisms relate to production of autoantibodies in addition to alloantibodies, formation of immune complexes that bind to autologous platelets, or binding of soluble alloantigen to autologous platelets, which are destroyed subsequently by alloantibody. The syndrome also occurs in association with alloantibodies directed against Pl^{A2}, Bak^a, Bak^b, and other platelet-specific antigens. Posttransfusion purpura is a self-limited condition but may be fatal. Therapy involves corticosteroids, plasma exchange, whole blood exchange transfusions, or intravenous gamma globulin infusion.

TRANSFUSION-TRANSMITTED DISEASES. These complications are among the most feared consequences of transfusion. The recent introduction of screening tests for retroviruses and hepatitis has decreased the incidence of these infections.

Hepatitis (Ch. 117). Posttransfusion hepatitis A and hepatitis B are reported occasionally, and posttransfusion hepatitis C (previously non-A, non-B hepatitis) occurs most frequently. Recently introduced screening tests to detect potentially infectious donors should reduce the frequency of posttransfusion hepatitis C to 1 per 1000 to 1500 components transfused. Clinical illness, described in Ch. 117, occurs an average of 7 to 8 weeks after transfusion. Approximately 50 per cent of patients with hepatitis C develop chronic hepatitis, and, of these, 10 to 20 per cent are at risk for cirrhosis or hepatocellular carcinoma, which may occur several decades after transfusion.

Retroviral Infections. Approximately 3 per cent of acquired immunodeficiency syndrome (AIDS) cases are transfusion related, and 1 per cent have appeared in patients treated with coagulation factor concentrates. The median latent period between transfusion with an infected unit and clinical evidence of AIDS is at least 7 years. Screening tests to detect human immunodeficiency virus-1 (HIV-1) carriers, combined with donor screening measures, have reduced the risk of HIV infection to less than 1 per 150,000 components transfused.

HIV-2 is closely related to HIV-1 and causes a similar illness. The infection is endemic in West Africa; very few cases have been reported in the United States. Concern that transfusion could be a vector for further spread throughout the population led to development of screening tests combining anti–HIV-1 and anti–HIV-2 reagents.

The human T lymphotropic virus I (HTLV-I) is a transforming retrovirus associated with adult T cell leukemia/lymphoma and tropical spastic paraparesis. This cell-associated virus is transmitted to 60 to 70 per cent of recipients of infected units of whole blood, red cells, or platelet concentrates. Serologic tests for anti–HTLV-I are used routinely to identify donors at risk of transmitting the virus through transfusion. The HTLV-I screening test also detects donors infected with HTLV-II, an agent not currently linked to a specific disease entity. Confirmatory testing indicates the majority of volunteer blood donors found reactive by the screening test are infected with HTLV-II rather than HTLV-I.

Cytomegalovirus (CMV) (Ch. 372). This latent virus is found predominantly in polymorphonuclear (PMN) leukocytes and lymphocytes. Most immunocompetent patients exposed to CMV become infected but are rarely symptomatic. In contrast, bone marrow transplant recipients and low birth weight neonates are at risk for fever, arthralgias, enteritis, hepatitis, thrombocytopenia, leukopenia, encephalitis, and interstitial pneumonitis that may be fatal. Blood components from donors who are anti–CMV antibody negative do not transmit the virus and are indicated for seronegative bone marrow transplant patients who receive bone marrow from seronegative donors and neonates who weigh less than 1200 grams and who are born to seronegative women. Preliminary results indicate that CMV is not transmitted by blood passed through newly developed, highly effective blood filters.

Malaria (Ch. 424). This is an uncommon complication of transfusion. It occurs approximately 3 weeks (range, 7 to 50 days) following transfusion from an asymptomatic infected donor. Deferral of donors who are residents of geographic regions where malaria is endemic is an appropriate method for reducing the risk of this complication.

Chagas' Disease (Ch. 426). This infection, caused by *Trypanosoma cruzi*, may cause transfusion-associated illness in immunocompromised patients. The incubation period between transfusion and onset of symptoms is approximately 2 months. Epidemiologic studies to determine the prevalence of infection in U.S. blood donors are in progress.

Syphilis (Ch. 340). Syphilis is an extremely uncommon complication of blood transfusion because donors are screened by serologic tests for syphilis and spirochetes remain viable in blood stored at 4°C for only a few days. The period between infusion of spirochete-infected blood and symptoms is 1 to 4½ months.

Other Infectious Agents. Other infectious agents that are transmitted infrequently by blood transfusion include *Babesia, Bartonella*, Epstein-Barr virus, parvovirus, and *Toxoplasma*. It is possible, but unlikely, that *Borrelia* is transmitted by transfusion.

SUMMARY

Red blood cell transfusions are indicated when there is a clinical need to increase oxygen-carrying capacity in anemic patients. Transfusion of one unit of red cells increases the hemoglobin concentration by 1 gram per deciliter in the average adult patient. The "transfusion trigger" in the perioperative period may be as low as 7 grams per deciliter if physiologic compensatory mechanisms are adequate. In chronically anemic patients, transfusions should be given only if clinical symptoms are present or eminent. Since transfusion is associated with risks that are unavoidable, it must be used appropriately. Alternatives to homologous transfusion, such as autologous transfusion, should be considered and used whenever possible.

Huestis DW, Bove JR, Case S: Practical Blood Transfusion. 4th ed. Boston, MA, Little, Brown and Company, 1988. *Answers to day-to-day questions arising in hospital-based transfusion services are provided in this quick-reading text.*

Mollison PL, Engelfriet CP, Contreras M.: Blood Transfusion in Clinical Medicine. 8th ed. Oxford, Great Britain, Blackwell Scientific Publications, 1987. *This is an encyclopedic compendium about transfusion medicine and is considered the primary reference on this subject.*

Petz LD, Swisher SN: Clinical Practice of Blood Transfusion. 2nd ed. New York, Churchill Livingstone, 1988. *This text provides excellent in-depth discussions of clinical aspects of transfusion medicine.*

138 Function of Neutrophils and Mononuclear Phagocytes

Bernard M. Babior

Neutrophils and mononuclear phagocytes (see Color Plate 5*A* and *B*) are essential components of the host defense system. Both are made in the bone marrow, and both accomplish most of their purposes through the act of eating (Greek *phagein,* to eat). Mononuclear phagocytes are versatile cells whose functions include the destruction of invading pathogens, the elimination of debris from the bloodstream and from sites of tissue damage, the remodeling of normal tissues, and the assignment of targets to lymphocytes. Neutrophils, on the other hand, are singlemindedly dedicated to the destruction of invading pathogens.

THE NEUTROPHIL

ORIGIN. Like other cells in the circulation, neutrophils originate from pluripotential stem cells that reside in the bone marrow. Depending on environmental influences, a pluripotential stem cell may give rise to the committed progenitors of any of the blood cells. Under the influence of certain *colony-stimulating factors* (CSF's), this stem cell will give rise to a population of neutrophils.

Colony-stimulating factors are proteins that control the proliferation and differentiation of particular types of cells. Table 138–1 lists the four CSF's that promote the formation of neutrophils and monocytes. Multi-CSF (interleukin 3) and GM-CSF act on early as well as late progenitors and show broad specificity, stimulating the production of phagocytes, red cells, platelets, and eosinophils. The other two act only on late progenitors, M-CSF stimulating the production of monocytes and G-CSF of neutrophils. The four CSF's also function as partial activators of the mature cells.

The route from a committed progenitor to a neutrophil involves a series of precursors, some of which can be recognized under the microscope. The earliest identifiable neutrophil precursor is a myeloblast, a relatively large cell with a rim of pale blue cytoplasm surrounding a large nucleus containing dispersed chromatin and multiple nucleoli. As the cell progresses through later stages of differentiation, the chromatin condenses and the nucleoli are lost, while at the same time the cytoplasm acquires its characteristic granules. The various neutrophil precursors are listed in Figure 138–1 (see Color Plate 5*D*).

Through the myelocyte stage, neutrophil precursors divide as well as differentiate (Fig. 138–1). These proliferative forms constitute the *mitotic compartment* of the neutrophil precursor pool. Later precursors, which do not divide, constitute the *nonmitotic* or *storage compartment*. Cells in this compartment can be released into the bloodstream in response to infections or other stresses. As a rule, the only cells released from the storage compartment are neutrophils and bands, but if the stress is sufficiently severe, a few metamyelocytes may be liberated as well.

A newly committed stem cell requires 8 to 10 days to become a mature neutrophil. In the bloodstream, neutrophils are distributed evenly between two rapidly exchanging pools: the *circulating pool*, composed of neutrophils suspended in the circulation, and the *marginated pool*, consisting of cells that have settled onto the endothelium of the capillaries and postcapillary venules. Neutrophils in the circulation leave for the tissues randomly and rapidly; their half-time in the bloodstream is only 6 hours. In the tissues, however, the cells may sojourn for days.

STRUCTURE. The neutrophil is a terminally differentiated, nondividing cell that is well equipped for killing microorganisms. The cell is packed with granules whose contents are used to kill and degrade target microorganisms. The granules are of two types: *azurophil*, which contain proteases and other hydrolytic enzymes, defensins and other microbicidal peptides, and myeloperoxidase, a Cl⁻-oxidizing enzyme; and *specific*, which contain, among other things, a collagenase and an enzyme that releases C5a from the complement component C5. The nucleus is a vestigial structure that can no longer replicate its DNA. The plasma membrane contains some of the neutrophil's killing equipment as well as sensors that locate the microorganisms against which the neutrophil acts. The cytoskeleton of the neutrophil is a complex system of tubes and fibers that is responsible for the orderly movement of this highly motile cell.

FUNCTION. Neutrophils undergo radical changes in behavior in response to external stimuli. These changes include aggregation, degranulation (i.e., the discharge of granule contents through the plasma membrane), and the initiation of oxidant production. They are provoked by many stimuli, the most important of which are target microorganisms and chemotactic factors at high concentration (see below). These behavioral changes convert the neutrophil from a placid resident of the bloodstream to a powerful weapon. A cell that has undergone these changes is known as an *activated neutrophil*. The destruction of a microorganism by a neutrophil can be divided into three stages: finding the microorganism, ingesting it, and finally killing it and disposing of its remains.

Adhesion. Because neutrophils move by crawling, they must adhere to surfaces to migrate through the tissues to an inflammatory site. Adhesion is accomplished through a group of neutrophil surface glycoproteins known as the *CD11/CD18* family. Neutrophils bind to other cells through an interaction between CD11/CD18 and *ICAM-1* (intercellular adhesion molecule), a protein expressed on the surfaces of a variety of cells, including fibroblasts, epithelia, and vascular endothelium. Endothelium also expresses *ELAM-1* (endothelial leukocyte adhesion molecule), which binds neutrophils through an unknown mechanism not involving CD11/CD18. The activities of these adhesion molecules increase when cells bearing them are activated by inflammatory mediators, explaining the increase in neutrophil adhesiveness at sites of inflammation.

Chemotaxis. The neutrophil finds its target through a chemical sense that enables the cell to detect certain substances known as

TABLE 138–1. COLONY-STIMULATING FACTORS

CSF	Sources	Targets
Multi-CSF	T lymphocytes	Early and late progenitors (broad specificity)
GM-CSF	T lymphocytes	Early and late progenitors (broad specificity)
	Fibroblasts, monocytes, endothelium	
M-CSF	Fibroblasts, monocytes, endothelium	Late monocyte progenitors
G-CSF	Fibroblasts, monocytes, endothelium	Late neutrophil progenitors

Data from Groopman JE, Molina J-M, Scadden DT: Hematopoietic growth factors. N Engl J Med 321:1449, 1989. By permission of the New England Journal of Medicine.

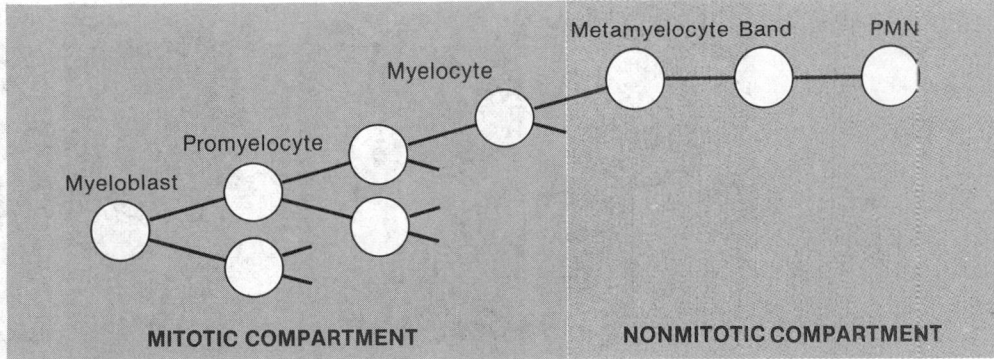

FIGURE 138–1. Neutrophil precursor pool.

chemotactic factors. These chemotactic factors are continuously released at sites where microorganisms have invaded tissues, diffusing away to set up a concentration gradient. Neutrophils in the circulation sense this gradient and travel toward its source. They begin their journey by marginating on the capillary and postcapillary endothelium. They then migrate outward through the vessel walls, penetrating the subendothelial basement membrane by local digestion, presumably with collagenase. Once outside the capillaries, they continue their directed migration, eventually reaching the site of origin of chemotactic factors—that is, the region of tissue that has been invaded by microorganisms. This process of migrating toward the source of a chemical attractant is known as *chemotaxis* (Fig. 138–2).

Neutrophils respond to a large number of chemotactic factors, but three are of primary importance: (1) *N-formylated oligopeptides*, (2) the complement fragment *C5a*, and (3), *leukotriene B₄* (LTB₄), a product of arachidonate oxidation. These chemotactic factors are produced both by the invading microorganisms (N-formylated oligopeptides and C5a) and by the neutrophils themselves (C5a and LTB₄). N-formylated oligopeptides are intermediates in bacterial protein synthesis and are released from damaged bacteria. C5a is produced by the complement system when it interacts with microorganisms and also by activated neutrophils through the release of the C5-splitting enzyme of the specific granules. LTB₄ is also produced by activated neutrophils, which manufacture it from arachidonic acid released from endogenous phospholipids. The production of C5a and LTB₄ by activated neutrophils lends a self-reinforcing character to the process of chemotaxis, since neutrophils at a site of inflammation generate chemotactic factors that attract more neutrophils to the inflamed region.

Bacteria in the circulation are thought to be handled primarily by the mononuclear phagocytes (see below). Neutrophils, however, may play a role in clearing the circulation of microorganisms that enter the bloodstream suddenly and in large numbers. During such episodes of bacteremia, the complement system is activated, releasing C5a into the circulation. Neutrophils react to this surge of C5a by marginating in the pulmonary capillaries, where they may act temporarily (15 to 30 minutes) as a filtration system, removing microorganisms from the blood as they pass through the pulmonary circulation. In this special situation, chemotaxis is not needed to help the neutrophils find their targets, because the targets are brought directly to the phagocytes by the flow of blood.

Ingestion. Once the neutrophil has come into contact with the microorganism, the stage is set for ingestion. For this to occur, the cell has to recognize the microorganisms as an edible target, not just a piece of random debris. Often it is not the microorganism itself that the cell recognizes, but certain plasma proteins that coat the microorganism once it has entered the bloodstream or tissue. These proteins are called *opsonins* (Greek, *opson*, seasoning), and their attachment to the surface of the microorganism is called *opsonization* (Fig. 138–3).

The proteins that are able to opsonize targets for ingestion by neutrophils include antibodies belonging to certain of the immunoglobulin G (IgG) subclasses (opsonizing antibodies) and the complement component C3b. These bind to the surface of the microorganism by mechanisms discussed elsewhere (see Ch. 243). The opsonized target then attaches to the neutrophil surface by means of these opsonins, which are recognized and bound by receptors in the neutrophil membrane: the Fc receptors, which recognize complexes between antigen and opsonizing antibody, and the C3 receptors, which recognize particle-associated C3b.

The attachment of the target to the neutrophil surface is the signal for ingestion (Fig. 138–4). The membrane in the region of the attached particle invaginates into the cell, carrying the particle in with it. When the particle is fully internalized, the invagination closes at its neck to form a vesicle that breaks away from the cell membrane. The end result is that a particle initially attached to the surface of the neutrophil is transferred to the cell's interior in a vesicle lined with what was originally neutrophil plasma membrane. This vesicle, known as the *phagocytic vesicle*, is the site of killing of the ingested organism.

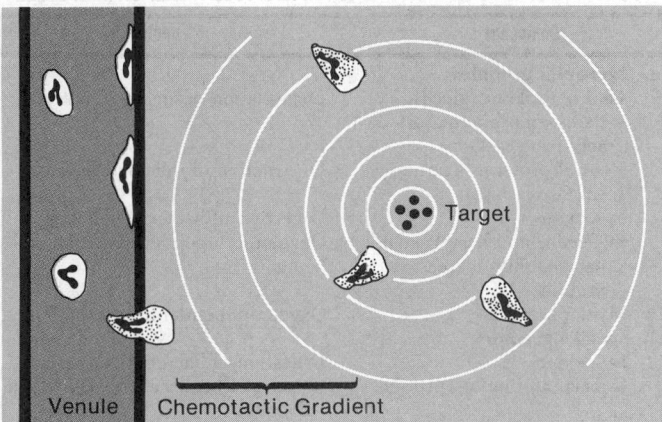

FIGURE 138–2. Chemotaxis. Neutrophils in the venule undergo margination in response to chemotactic factor, then leave the vessel by migrating between the endothelial cells (diapedesis) and travel up the chemotactic gradient toward the target.

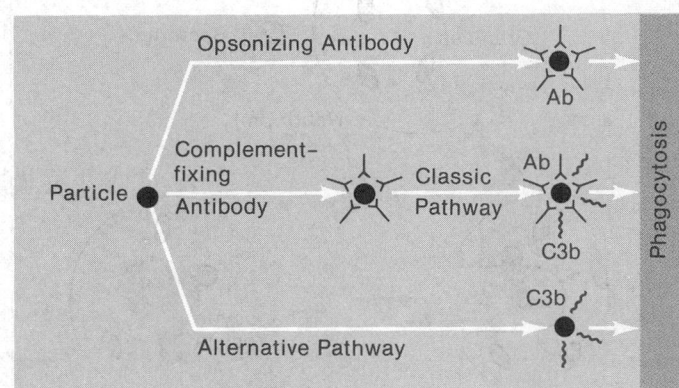

FIGURE 138–3. Opsonization. The coating of a particle by a plasma protein that is recognized by neutrophil receptors as a signal for ingestion is termed *opsonization*. Two classes of proteins are capable of opsonizing particles for ingestion by neutrophils: opsonizing antibodies and complement component C3b.

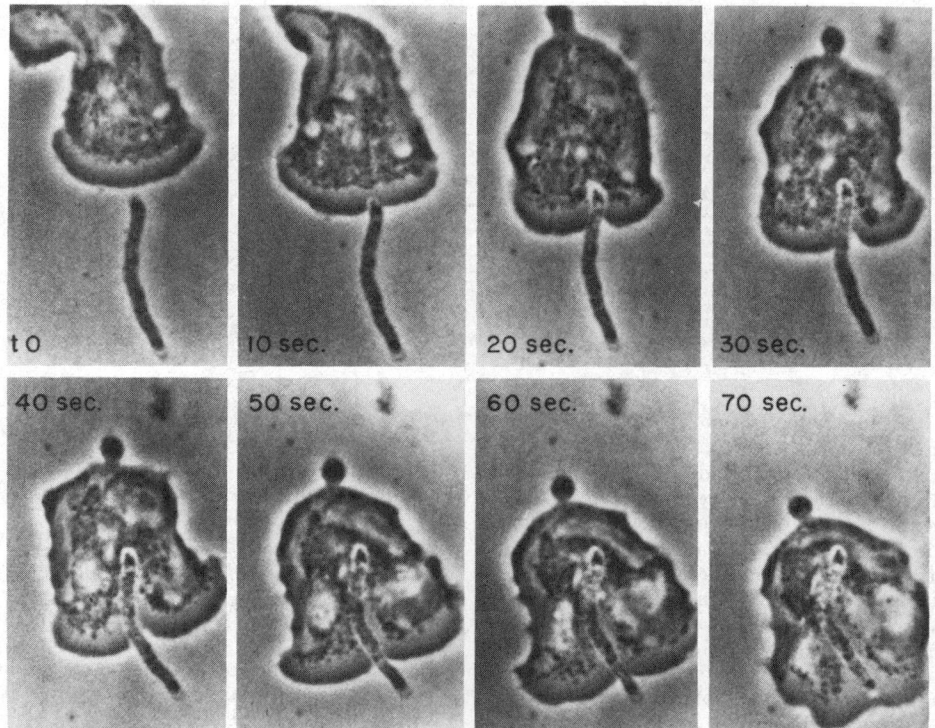

FIGURE 138–4. Ingestion of a target microorganism by a neutrophil. (Reproduced from Hirsch JG: Cinemicrophotographic observations of granule lysis in polymorphonuclear leucocytes during phagocytosis. J Exp Med 116:827, 1962, by copyright permission of the Rockefeller University Press.)

Killing. Killing involves two separate actions on the part of the neutrophils: *degranulation* and the *activation of the respiratory burst.* Degranulation refers to a process whereby the granule membrane fuses with the plasma membrane, releasing the granule contents into a transmembrane compartment—either a phagocytic vesicle (Fig. 138–5) or the external environment. Azurophil granules degranulate almost exclusively into the phagocytic vesicles, so their contents act principally against the ingested microorganism. Specific granules degranulate into both the phagocytic vesicles and the external environment, so their contents act exterior to the neutrophils as well as on the ingested microorganisms. Some of the constitutents of each of these granules are listed in Table 138–2, together with their actions.

The respiratory burst refers to a metabolic event whose purpose is the production of potent microbicidal oxidants through the partial reduction of oxygen. The burst is activated by the same stimuli that provoke degranulation of the specific granules—primarily contact with ingestible particles and exposure to chemotactic factors at high concentrations. These stimuli activate a plasma membrane–bound oxidase that catalyzes the reduction of oxygen to superoxide (O_2^-) at the expense of nicotinamide-adenine dinucleotide phosphate (NADPH) (Fig. 138–6). Most of the O_2^- reacts with itself to yield H_2O_2 while at the same time NADPH is regenerated by way of the hexosemonophosphate shunt.

The microbicidal oxidants are derived from the H_2O_2: (1) A portion of the H_2O_2 is used to oxidize Cl^- to the highly microbicidal hypochlorite ion (OCl^-), a reaction catalyzed by myeloperoxidase, an enzyme delivered into the phagocytic vesicle from the azurophil granules. (2) Another portion of the H_2O_2 is converted to the exceedingly reactive hydroxyl radical ($OH\cdot$) in a metal-catalyzed reaction with O_2^-. These and related oxidants

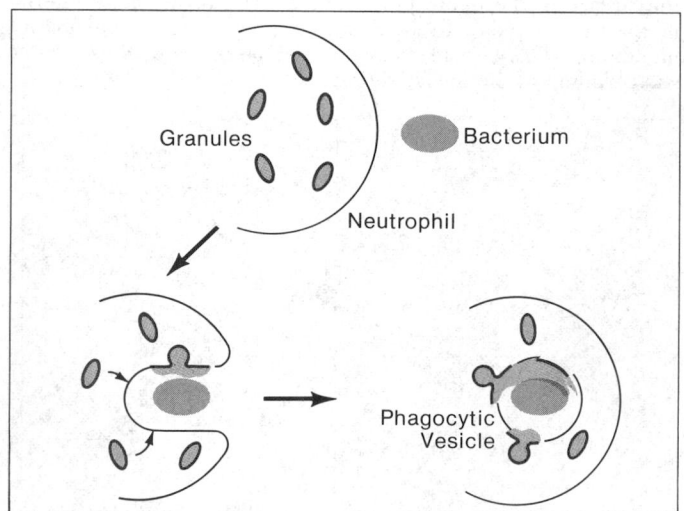

FIGURE 138–5. Degranulation into a phagocytic vesicle. Granules migrate toward a phagocytic vesicle, eventually fusing with it. Upon fusion, the contents of the granule are released into the vesicle, while the granule membrane becomes incorporated into the vesicle wall.

Table 138–2. CONTENTS OF NEUTROPHIL GRANULES

Compound	Function
I. Azurophil granules	
Acid hydrolases (glycosidases, phospholipases, acid proteases)	Degradation of ingested material
Neutral proteases (cathepsin G, elastase)	Destruction of inflamed tissue?
Lysozyme	Digestion of bacterial cell wall
Defensins and bactericidal/permeability-increasing protein	Oxygen-independent bacterial killing
Myeloperoxidase	Oxygen-dependent bacterial killing
II. Specific granules	
Lysozyme	Digestion of bacterial cell wall
Cobalamin-binding protein	Binding of bacterial cobalamin analogues
Apolactoferrin	Binding of free iron, control of granulopoiesis
Collagenase	Digestion of connective tissue
C5-splitting enzyme	Release of C5a

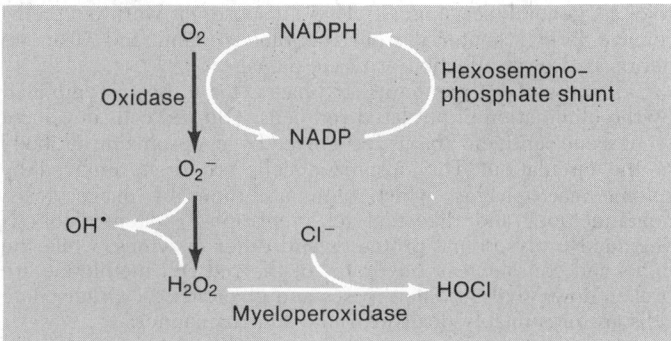

FIGURE 138–6. The respiratory burst.

TABLE 138–3. TISSUE MACROPHAGES

Fixed
    Kupffer cells
    Microglial cells (central nervous system)
    Macrophages of spleen, lymph nodes, and bone marrow sinusoids
    Mesangial cells (kidney)
    Osteoclasts
Wandering
    Macrophages of serosal cavities (pleural, peritoneal, pericardial)
    Alveolar macrophages

attack and kill ingested microorganisms by oxidizing their cellular constituents.

MONONUCLEAR PHAGOCYTES

Mononuclear phagocytes and neutrophils (see Color Plate 5A and B) are closely related. Both are descended from the same progenitor, and both share many functions, including the unusual ability to ingest particles as large as half or more their own diameter. There is, however, only one type of neutrophil, whereas there are many varieties of mononuclear phagocytes.

ORIGIN AND STRUCTURE. All mononuclear phagocytes are derived from a single circulating precursor: the monocyte. This cell and the neutrophil both arise from a single pluripotential stem cell. During differentiation, this stem cell first makes a general commitment to the phagocyte lineage. Later its descendants commit themselves further, some to the neutrophil and others to the monocyte line.

The first recognizable monocyte precursor is the *monoblast.* In normal marrow, this cell is indistinguishable from a myeloblast; it can be identified, however, in marrow from patients with monocytic leukemia. The next stage is the *promonocyte,* a somewhat larger cell with cytoplasmic granules and an indented nucleus containing finely divided chromatin. Finally, the fully developed *monocyte* appears. Larger than the neutrophil, and with a large horseshoe-shaped nucleus containing dispersed chromatin, the mature monocyte has cytoplasm that is filled with granules whose contents include hydrolytic enzymes and other proteins necessary for the cell's activities. It requires about 5 days to go from a monoblast to a mature circulating monocyte.

FURTHER DIFFERENTIATION. Unlike neutrophils, monocytes retain a limited capacity to divide and, in addition,

undergo considerable further differentiation. After circulating briefly in the bloodstream ($t_{1/2}$ ~12 hours), they enter the tissues, where they differentiate into mature macrophages that live for weeks to months. The properties of these macrophages depend on the tissues in which they reside. Those in the liver, for example, are the Kupffer cells, spidery phagocytes that bridge the sinusoids separating adjacent plates of hepatocytes (Fig. 138–7A). Those in the lungs are the large ellipsoidal alveolar macrophages (Fig. 138–7B). These and other tissue macrophages are listed in Table 138–3.

Macrophages are important components of the inflammatory reactions elicited by noxious agents (e.g., microorganisms or foreign bodies). Some of the macrophages that appear at a site of inflammation are recruited from surrounding tissues, while others are derived from monocytes that have migrated there from the bloodstream. Once at the inflamed site, macrophages are exposed to certain stimuli (e.g., *gamma-interferon,* a T lymphocyte product, and *lipopolysaccharide* from the bacterial cell walls) that induce them to undergo functional and morphologic changes that enable them to deal more effectively with the inciting agent. Initially, the cells enlarge, accumulate many new granules, and begin to secrete large quantities of certain specific proteases, including collagenase, elastase, and plasminogen activator, a component of the fibrinolytic system (see Ch. 146). CD11/CD18 increases on their surfaces. Their capacity for phagocytosis is increased, as is their ability to degrade ingested material. The cells become stickier and more motile and develop the ability to manufacture lethal oxidizing agents. Most important, their microbicidal power is greatly increased, so they can kill pathogens that they were unable to deal with in their former state. Cells that have attained this heightened degree of microbicidal potency are known as *activated macrophages.*

If the inciting agent has not been eliminated within the first few days, the activated macrophages begin to aggregate into a

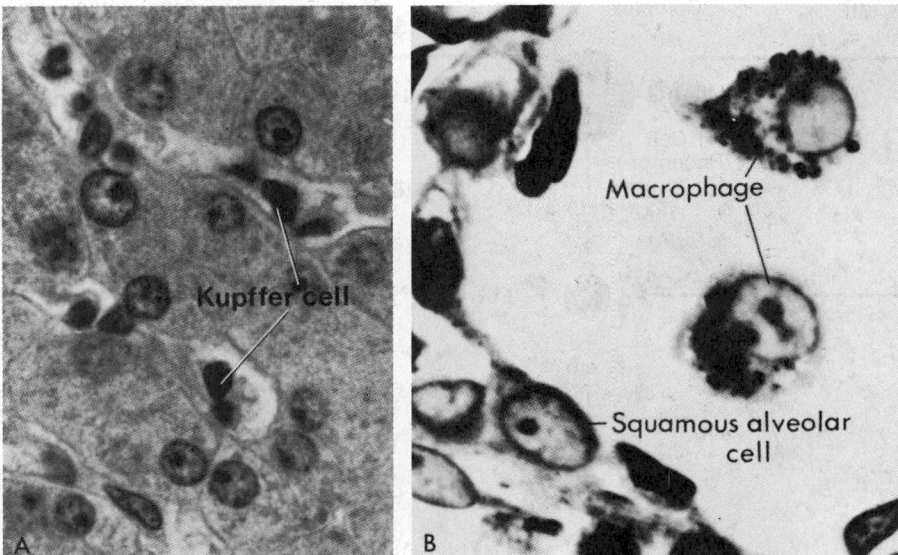

FIGURE 138–7. Some tissue macrophages. A, Kupffer cell. (Reprinted with permission from Popper H: Liver Structure and Function. New York, McGraw-Hill Book Company, 1957, p 97.) B, Alveolar macrophage. (From Sorokin SP: The respiratory system. *In* Weiss L, Greep RO: Histology. 4th ed., p 765. Copyright © 1977 by McGraw-Hill Inc. Used by permission of McGraw-Hill Book Company.)

TABLE 138–4. SUBSTANCES SECRETED BY MACROPHAGES

Substance	State of Macrophage	Additional Stimulus Needed
Lysozyme	Resident, activated	None
Neutral proteases Collagenase Elastase Plasminogen activator	Activated	None
Interleukin 1	Resident, activated	Lymphokine, endotoxin, others
Superoxide	Activated	Contact with particles or
Leukotrienes	Resident, activated	appropriate soluble stimulus
Complement components		

granuloma. Continued stimulation leads to additional growth of the aggregated cells and further augmentation in secretory capacity; the phagocytes have now turned into epithelioid cells, the characteristic constituents of mature granulomas. Eventually, giant cells appear, arising through the fusion of epithelioid cells with each other and with newly arrived macrophages. With the elimination of the inciting agent, the inflammatory process resolves and the macrophages disappear.

FUNCTIONS. Mononuclear phagocytes carry out three basic functions: secretion, ingestion, and interaction with lymphocytes.

Secretion. Mononuclear phagocytes secrete a large number of substances, some protein and others nonprotein in nature (Table 138–4). Lysozyme is secreted by mononuclear phagocytes regardless of their state of activation, but proteases active at neutral pH ("neutral proteases") are secreted only by activated cells. Activated cells also produce interleukin 8, a neutrophil chemotaxin. Other substances such as O_2^- and leukotrienes are secreted under even more specialized circumstances.

Ingestion. Mononuclear phagocytes (see Color Plate 6F, left) eat for two purposes: to eliminate waste and debris (scavenging) and to kill invading pathogens.

Scavenging. Mononuclear phagocytes play a highly important role as general scavengers. They dispose of worn-out cells, remove foreign material from the bloodstream, and clean up debris at sites of infection or tissue damage.

Cell disposal by mononuclear phagocytes is best exemplified by the elimination of outdated red cells. Old red cells develop a "senescence antigen" that is recognized by an opsonizing antibody in the circulation. The opsonized cells are then removed by splenic macrophages, which eliminate them by phagocytosis, degranulation, and digestion (cf. neutrophils). Hemoglobin is degraded by lysosomal proteases and other enzymes, while the lipids and complex carbohydrates of the red cell membrane are broken down by lysosomal lipases and glycosidases. Other effete cells are presumably dealt with in a similar manner.

Foreign material is removed from the bloodstream chiefly in the liver and spleen. In these two organs, the blood is forced to pass through a dense network of mononuclear phagocytes, which ingest foreign matter encountered in the flow. Bacteria and bacterial breakdown products (e.g., lipopolysaccharide) that enter the bloodstream from the large intestine are removed principally by the Kupffer cells of the liver, because these are the first mononuclear phagocytes encountered by the gastrointestinal venous drainage.

Dead cells and tissue fragments at sites of infection or injury are disposed of by macrophages recruited to the damaged area. Ingestion may be aided by circulating fibronectin, which opsonizes denatured collagen for phagocytosis by macrophages. The activated macrophages also secrete neutral proteases that break down damaged connective tissue (collagenase, elastase) and fibrin mesh (plasminogen activator), clearing the way for the reconstruction of injured tissues.

Mononuclear phagocytes also eliminate from the circulation denatured proteins, protein fragments, and certain native proteins (e.g., activated clotting factors). Some proteins are eliminated through *pinocytosis*, a process in which the material to be eliminated is taken into the cell along with a minuscule quantity of plasma via a tiny invagination of the cell membrane that buds off and enters the cytoplasm as a pinocytotic vesicle. (Mononuclear phagocytes are constantly engaged in pinocytosis; they take in and process several times their own volume of plasma every day.) Other proteins are eliminated by *receptor-mediated endocytosis*, a process similar to pinocytosis except that the ingested protein is bound to a surface receptor before internalization. The lipids of atherosclerotic lesions are derived in part from lipopro-

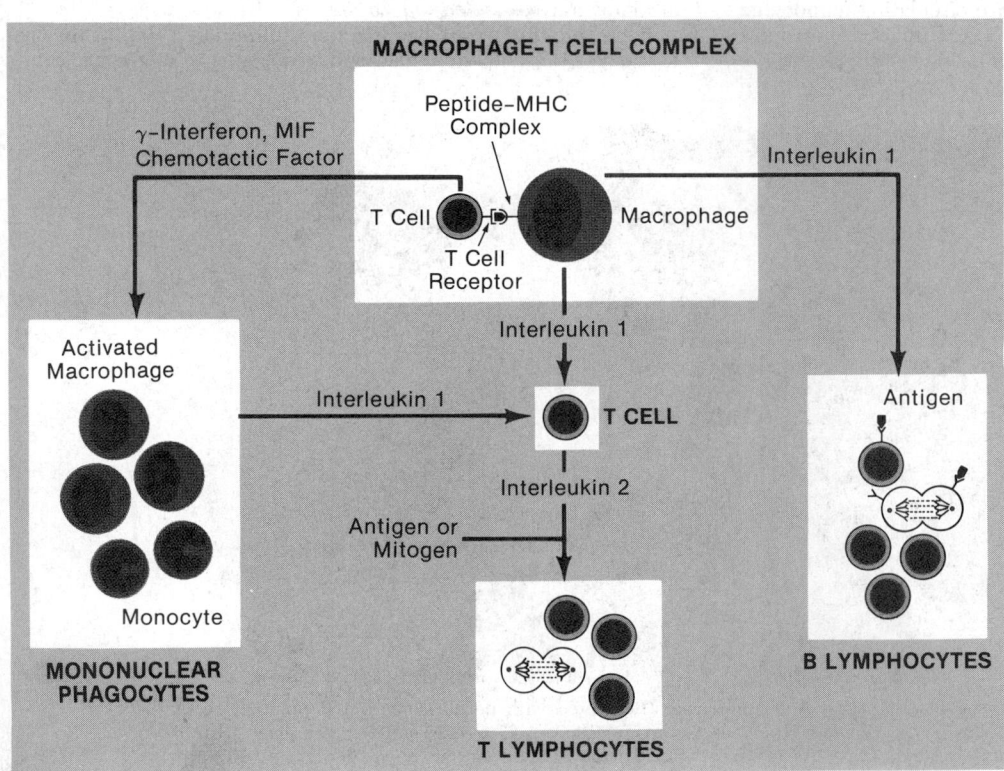

FIGURE 138–8. Macrophage-lymphocyte interactions. The macrophage, acting in its capacity as an "accessory cell," presents a peptide to a T cell equipped with specific receptors that recognize the complex between the peptide and a class II MHC molecule on the macrophage surface. The T cell to which the antigen has been presented undergoes activation and begins to secrete lymphokines. These lymphokines include γ-interferon, macrophage-immobilizing factor (MIF), and monocyte chemotactic factor; they cause macrophages to accumulate and undergo activation at the site of the initial macrophage–T cell interaction. Macrophages so activated secrete interleukin 1, a potent mediator capable, among other things, of inducing the proliferation of both B and T cells. B cells are directly stimulated by interleukin 1 to proliferate and to differentiate into antibody-secreting plasma cells. T cells, however, proliferate under the influence of a mediator known as interleukin 2 (T cell growth factor), itself a T cell product; interleukin 1 promotes the proliferation of T cells indirectly by inducing them to secrete interleukin 2.

TABLE 138–5. INTRACELLULAR PATHOGENS AGAINST WHICH MACROPHAGES PLAY A SPECIAL ROLE

Bacteria	*Chlamydia*
Brucella	*Rickettsia*
Listeria	Protozoan parasites
Legionella	*Leishmania*
Salmonella	*Trypanosoma*
Mycobacteria and systemic fungi	*Toxoplasma*
Coccidioides immitis	
Histoplasma capsulatum	
Mycobacterium tuberculosis	
Others	

teins that had been taken into macrophages by receptor-mediated endocytosis.

Killing. Like neutrophils, mononuclear phagocytes can kill invading microorganisms. Killing by both types of phagocytes involves the same general sequence of events—an initial encounter between the phagocyte and the target microorganism, ingestion, and finally the destruction of the target—but the events differ in detail between the two cell types. Monocytes, for example, attach to three endothelial adhesion molecules. ICAM-1, ELAM-1, and VCAM-1 (vascular cell adhesion molecule, which binds to VLA-4, a molecule found on monocytes but not neutrophils); neutrophils attach only to the first two. Neutrophils generally find their targets by migrating up a chemotactic gradient, while many mononuclear phagocytes (the fixed-tissue varieties, such as Kupffer cells and splenic macrophages) have their targets brought to them by the bloodstream. Those mononuclear phagocytes that find their targets by chemotaxis (e.g., monocytes) respond to a wider variety of attractants than neutrophils do. Monocytes, for instance, are attracted by lymphocyte-generated chemotactic factors that have no effect on neutrophils. With respect to ingestion, mononuclear phagocytes can take up particles opsonized by immunoglobulin E (IgE) as well as IgG; neutrophils will take up only the latter. Mononuclear phagocytes are also equipped with a mannose receptor that enables them to take up certain bacteria and other particles without the need for opsonization. With regard to microbial killing, mononuclear phagocytes lose their myeloperoxidase as they develop from monocytes into macrophages, so that oxygen-dependent killing by mature macrophages is accomplished by oxidants that can be generated in the absence of myeloperoxidase (e.g., hydroxyl radical).

Mononuclear phagocytes play a particularly important role in defending against nonviral pathogens that live and grow intracellularly (Table 138–5). For the destruction of these pathogens, macrophage activation is critical. The pathogens are readily killed by activated macrophages, but they are able to infect and multiply within unactivated macrophages, eventually killing them and spreading to infect fresh macrophages. Little is known about how the pathogens evade the microbicidal system of the unactivated macrophages.

Mononuclear phagocytes, particularly activated macrophages, are also able to kill malignant cells in vitro. The extent to which they perform this antitumor function in vivo is unknown.

Interactions Between Mononuclear Phagocytes and Lymphocytes. The activation of mononuclear phagocytes by gamma-interferon is one of a series of mutually potentiating interactions between mononuclear phagocytes and lymphocytes that take place at sites of inflammation (Fig. 138–8). Both T lymphocytes and B lymphocytes participate in these interactions.

The interaction with T lymphocytes begins with a special physical encounter between a T lymphocyte and a mononuclear

phagocyte. When an antigen-bearing particle is ingested by a mononuclear phagocyte, the antigen is degraded to small peptides, some of which are transferred to the phagocyte surface bound to class II proteins of the major histocompatibility complex (MHC; the MHC controls immune responses to such challenges as foreign proteins, virally infected cells, and tissue allografts [see Ch. 250]). If a T lymphocyte bearing a suitable receptor should encounter this peptide-bearing mononuclear phagocyte, it will recognize the peptide-MHC complex and bind to the phagocyte, and both cells will begin to secrete immunologic mediators. In this interaction, the mononuclear phagocyte is referred to as an *accessory cell* and is said to have "presented" the antigen to the lymphocyte.

Immunologic mediators secreted by T lymphocytes *(lymphokines)* include gamma-interferon, macrophage inhibitory factor, and monocyte chemotactic factor. Their net effect is to cause the accumulation and activation of mononuclear phagocytes in the vicinity of the initial interaction between the peptide-bearing phagocyte and its complementary T lymphocyte. Mediators secreted by mononuclear phagocytes are known as *monokines*. One of these is *interleukin 1;* among its other effects (for a list, see Table 138–6), it stimulates the proliferation of T lymphocytes indirectly by causing them to secrete *interleukin 2*, a substance that promotes their own growth. Another monokine, *tumor necrosis factor*, causes many of the manifestations of endotoxin shock, and may be responsible for the weight loss seen in patients with chronic wasting illnesses, such as tuberculosis and certain forms of cancer.

Macrophages also act upon B lymphocytes. They are not needed for the presentation of antigen to B lymphocytes, because B lymphocytes carry surface immunoglobulins that directly recognize the antigens against which the cells are programmed. Rather, the macrophages exert their effects after the antigen-recognition step. They operate through interleukin 1, which helps the antigen-primed B lymphocytes proliferate and differentiate into antibody-secreting plasma cells.

TABLE 138–6. SOME ACTIONS OF INTERLEUKIN 1

Site of Action	Effect
T lymphocytes	Secretion of interleukin 2 (T cell growth factor)
B lymphocytes	Proliferation, secretion of immunoglobulins
Hepatocytes	Production of acute phase reactants
Hypothalamus	Fever
Muscle	Catabolism of protein

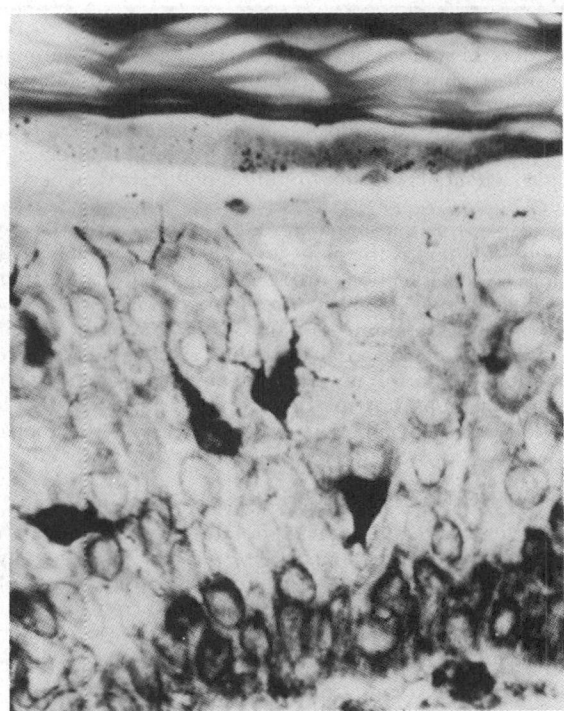

FIGURE 138–9. Langerhans cells in the skin. The darkly stained cells in the acanthocyte layer are the Langerhans cells. Their characteristic branching dendrites are easily seen. (Reproduced with permission from Breathnach AS, Wolff K: Structure and development of the skin. *In* Fitzpatrick TB, Eisen AZ, Wolff K, et al.: Dermatology in General Medicine. 2nd ed., p 56. Copyright © 1979 by McGraw-Hill, Inc. Used by permission of McGraw-Hill Book Company.)

Dendritic Cells. Antigens are also presented by *dendritic cells*. These cells are found in the follicles of the lymph nodes and spleen, in the thymus, and in the skin, where they are known as *Langerhans' cells* (Fig. 138–9). Like mononuclear phagocytes, they carry class II MHC molecules on their surfaces but are thought to be incapable of phagocytosis. Their major role seems to be to present new antigens to the T lymphocytes.

Adams DO, Hamilton TA: The cell biology of macrophage activation. Annu Rev Immunol 2:283, 1984. *A complete and clearly written review of this sometimes confusing topic.*

Gallin JI, Goldstein IM, Synderman R (eds.): Inflammation: Basic Principles and Clinical Correlates. New York, Raven Press, 1988. *A multiauthor text providing comprehensive coverage of all aspects of inflammation.*

Ganz T, Selsted ME, Szklarnek D, et al.: Defensins. Natural peptide antibiotics of human neutrophils. J Clin Invest 76:1427, 1985. *The structure and properties of these recently discovered antimicrobial agents.*

Groopman JE, Molina J-M, Scadden DT: Hematopoietic growth factors. Biology and clinical applications. N Engl J Med 321:1449, 1989. *An up-to-date survey of this rapidly moving field.*

Murray HW: Interferon-gamma, the activated macrophage, and host defense against microbial challenge. Ann Intern Med 108:595, 1988. *A recent review of macrophage activation, emphasizing the role of gamma-interferon.*

Patarroyo M, Makgoba MW: Leucocyte adhesion to cells in immune and inflammatory responses. Lancet: 2:1139, 1989. *A succinct discussion of the leucocyte adhesion molecules.*

Steinman RM: Dendritic cells. Transplantation 31:151, 1981. *A short review of dendritic cell structure and function.*

Unanue ER, Cerottini J-C: Antigen presentation. FASEB J 3:2496, 1989. *Recent developments in this area, including current views of antigen processing.*

Williams GT, Williams WJ: Granulomatous inflammation: A review. J Clin Pathol 36:723, 1983. *An excellent review of the development and function of granuloma.*

139 Disorders of Neutrophil Function

Bernard M. Babior

Disorders of neutrophil function are relatively common. For the most part, they are minor manifestations of systemic diseases, rarely diagnosed and of little clinical significance. In a few disorders, however, defective neutrophil function leads to serious clinical problems. Most of these are inherited disorders in which particular elements of neutrophil function are almost totally deficient.

The principal clinical manifestation of a serious disorder of neutrophil function is the repeated occurrence of major bacterial infections. Such infections are most commonly associated with severe neutropenia (<500 neutrophils per cubic millimeter) or an abnormality of immunoglobulins or complement. Occasionally, however, repeated bacterial infections cannot be accounted for by abnormalities in the neutrophil count, the immunoglobulins, or the complement system. In such a case, a qualitative abnormality in neutrophil function is likely to be at the root of the problem.

EVALUATING NEUTROPHIL FUNCTION

A complete evaluation of neutrophil function, including motility, granule content and function, respiratory burst activity, and bacterial killing, requires a specialized laboratory. Screening for functional abnormalities, however, can be carried out relatively simply (Table 139–1). Morphologic abnormalities (see Color Plate 7D), such as the large malformed granules of Chédiak-Higashi

TABLE 139–1. SCREENING FOR ABNORMALITIES OF NEUTROPHIL FUNCTION

Examination of blood film
Rebuck skin window test
NBT test
Special stains: myeloperoxidase, alkaline phosphatase

TABLE 139–2. ACQUIRED ALTERATIONS OF NEUTROPHIL ADHESIVENESS

1. Decreased ashesiveness
   A. With demargination
      Corticosteroids
      Epinephrine
   B. Without demargination
      Aspirin
      Alcohol
2. Increased adhesiveness
   A. Bacteremia
   B. Hemodialysis

disease, can be detected by *examination of a blood film* under the microscope. Chemotaxis and locomotion can be estimated by a *Rebuck skin window*, a test that measures the migration of phagocytes onto a glass coverslip applied to a superficial abrasion. The respiratory burst is evaluated by the *NBT test*, in which cells are activated in the presence of nitroblue tetrazolium (NBT), a dye that forms a dark precipitate on any cell engaged in the production of O_2^- (superoxide). Neutrophil enzymes can be detected by *special stains for myeloperoxidase and alkaline phosphatase*. One or more of these tests are abnormal in most symptomatic disorders of neutrophil function.

ACQUIRED DISORDERS

In acquired disorders of neutrophils, functional abnormalities are generally incomplete. Accordingly, signs and symptoms caused by neutrophil dysfunction are uncommon in these conditions.

ADHESION (Table 139–2). Neutrophils undergo frequent alterations in adhesiveness, with resulting changes in the size of the marginated pool (see Ch. 138). *Corticosteroids* and *epinephrine* reduce neutrophil adhesiveness, releasing the cells from the marginated pool into the circulation. Conversely, C5a and agents that release C5a (e.g., gram-negative bacteremia) increase neutrophil adhesiveness, causing cells to aggregate into clumps. These tend to be trapped in small vessels, particularly in the lungs.

Besides corticosteroids and epinephrine, *aspirin* and *alcohol* cause decreased adhesiveness of neutrophils. With these agents the decrease in adhesiveness occurs in vitro but is not associated with demargination. Evidently, neutrophil adhesiveness covers a broader range of functions than merely the ability to attach to an endothelial cell.

In patients undergoing *hemodialysis*, neutrophil counts fall sharply, rising a few minutes later to values that exceed the predialysis counts. Pulmonary symptoms may accompany these changes in neutrophil counts. The fall in the neutrophil count and the accompanying pulmonary symptoms occur because C5a is released when the complement system is activated by the passage of blood over the dialysis membrane, causing neutrophils to marginate and be trapped in the lungs. The subsequent neutrophilia reflects the release of cells from the marrow storage pool.

CHEMOTAXIS. Depressed neutrophil chemotaxis is seen in a large number of conditions (Table 139–3). In some of these conditions, chemotactic depression is caused by a circulating inhibitor, while in others the neutrophils themselves are defective. These chemotactic abnormalities contribute in only a minor way to the decreased resistance to bacterial infections characteristic of many of these disorders.

TABLE 139–3. CONDITIONS ASSOCIATED WITH DEPRESSED NEUTROPHIL CHEMOTAXIS

Diabetes mellitus	Anergy
Uremia	Hodgkin's disease
Cirrhosis of liver	Leprosy
Severe burns	Sarcoidosis
Bacterial infections	Hypophosphatemia
	Neonates

Various functional abnormalities are seen in neutrophils from patients with these conditions. Cells in *chronic myelogenous leukemia* are very sluggish, showing markedly reduced motility and chemotaxis. Granules are often abnormal in number and type (specific granules, for example, may be absent), the respiratory burst is frequently attenuated, and bacterial killing may be depressed. These cells, however, make up in numbers what they lack in function, so infections are unusual in patients with chronic myelogenous leukemia.

In patients with *acute myelogenous leukemia*, neutrophils may arise from residual normal stem cells or by differentiation of the leukemic clone; in the latter case, the neutrophils may show abnormalities similar to those seen in chronic myelogenous leukemia. *Myelodysplasia* (see Color Plate 6*I* and *J*) is a disease in which hematopoiesis is taken over by a nonmalignant but defective stem cell that gives rise to inadequate numbers of functionally abnormal blood cells. Bilobed nuclei (pseudo Pelger-Huët anomaly) and abnormal granulation are typical of myelodysplastic neutrophils. In both acute myelogenous leukemia and myelodysplasia, bacterial infections are frequent, but their frequency is due more to neutropenia than to functional abnormalities of the phagocytes.

CONGENITAL DISORDERS

CHRONIC GRANULOMATOUS DISEASE. Chronic granulomatous disease (CGD) refers to a group of inherited disorders in which phagocytes cannot express a respiratory burst (Ch. 138). The disease is caused by a major defect in the O_2^--forming nicotinamide-adenine dinucleotide phosphate (NADPH) oxidase of phagocytes. The oxidase consists of several components, and different types of CGD occur when different components are defective. The most common type of CGD, affecting two thirds of patients, is due to a mutation in an X chromosomal gene encoding a protein that forms part of a membrane-associated cytochrome found only in leukocytes. Patients with this type of CGD lack the leukocyte cytochrome, and transmission of the disease is X linked. Most of the remaining patients lack a cytosolic oxidase-activating protein; in these patients, the leukocyte cytochrome is present, and CGD is transmitted as an autosomal recessive trait.

Clinical Picture. The clinical picture of CGD is one of recurrent, severe bacterial infections that are slow to heal and difficult to

treat. The infections include sinusitis, pneumonia, and abscesses that usually involve the deep subcutaneous tissues, lymph nodes, or liver. Infections generally begin in infancy or early childhood, although the disease occasionally presents in adolescence or later. In its unmodified form, the course of CGD is characterized by frequent hospitalizations for repeated infections caused by bacteria that the defective phagocytes are unable to kill (mostly *Staphylococcus aureus* and enterobacteria), with death from infection in the first or second decade. With chronic antibiotic prophylaxis, however, the course of the disease has changed. Hospitalization is much less frequent, and survival seems to be prolonged, but patients develop serious complications owing to imperfectly suppressed infections—e.g., strictures of the bladder and gastrointestinal tract and chronic lung disease with fibrosis and bronchiectasis. Death often results from infections by fungi, particularly *Aspergillus*.

Diagnosis. The diagnosis is made by neutrophil function studies. Most of these are normal, but those that measure the respiratory burst are severely deranged: the NBT test is negative (Fig. 139–1), and O_2^- production and other manifestations of the respiratory burst are greatly reduced or absent. Many microorganisms are handled in a normal fashion by CGD neutrophils (including pneumococci and streptococci, accounting for the rarity of pneumococcal and streptococcal infections in patients with CGD), but those such as *S. aureus* or *Pseudomonas cepacia*, whose destruction is particularly dependent on oxidant production by phagocytes, are poorly killed by the defective cells. In CGD carriers the size of the respiratory burst is decreased by about half, so suspected carriers can often be identified by quantitation of the burst. Because carriers of X-linked CGD are mosaics, only a fraction of their neutrophils are able to make O_2^-; the NBT test stains only that fraction, leaving the rest of the cells unstained (Fig. 139–1).

A condition similar to CGD has been seen in a few patients with exceptionally severe *glucose-6-phosphate dehydrogenase* (G6PD) *deficiency*. G6PD is essential for the production of NADPH, the reducing agent used by the O_2^--forming oxidase. In neutrophils that are severely deficient in G6PD, the levels of NADPH may be so low that the O_2^--forming oxidase is starved for substrate, so the cells cannot express an adequate respiratory burst.

Treatment. Management of CGD consists of long-term antibiotic prophylaxis (trimethoprim-sulfamethoxazole at 5 to 10 mg

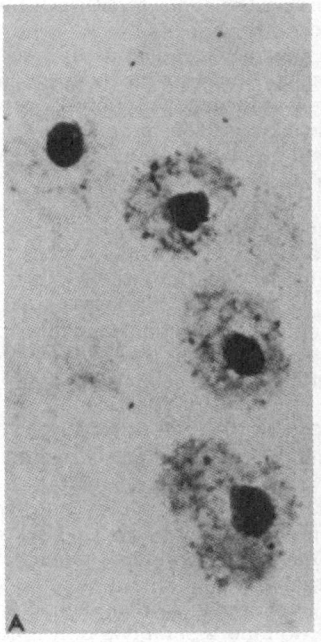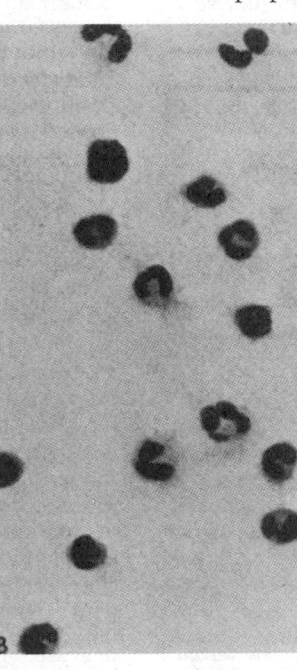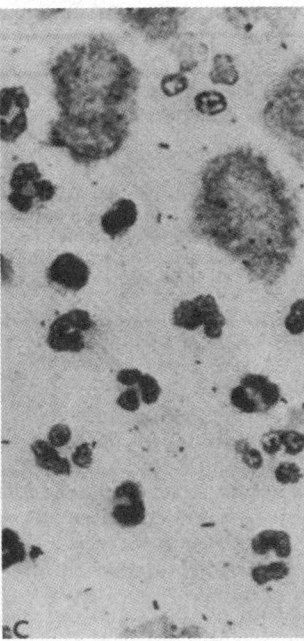

FIGURE 139–1. The NBT test in CGD. *A,* Normal. *B,* CGD. *C,* Carrier of X-linked CGD, showing an NBT-positive and an NBT-negative population of neutrophils. (From Babior BM, Crawley CA: Chronic granulomatous disease and other disorders of oxidative killing by phagocytes. *In* Stanbury JB, Wyngaarden JB, Fredrickson DS, et al. [eds.]: The Metabolic Basis of Inherited Disease. 5th ed., p 1972. Copyright © 1983 by McGraw-Hill Inc. Used by permission of McGraw-Hill Book Company.)

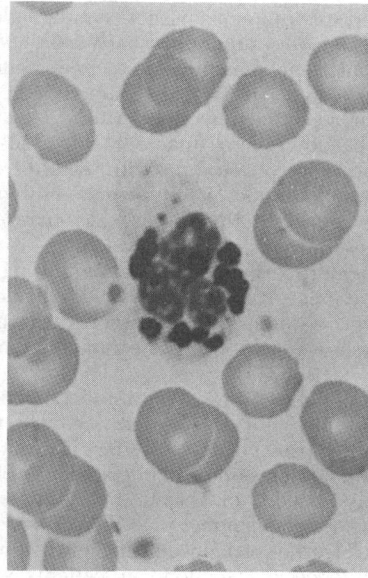
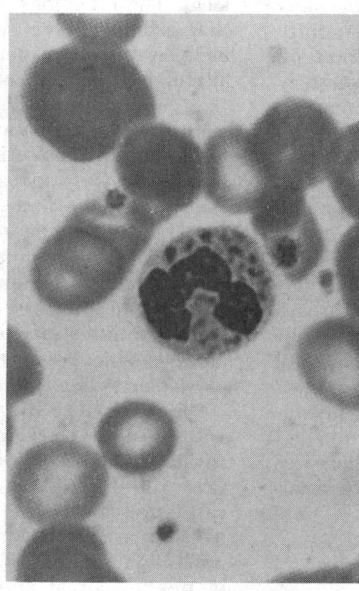

FIGURE 139–2. Neutrophils in Chédiak-Higashi disease, showing the giant granules that are the hallmark of the disease. *A*, A cell with unusually large and prominent granules. *B*, A more typical Chédiak-Higashi neutrophil. (Reprinted with permission from Miwa S, Watanabe Y [eds.]: Atlas of Blood Cells. 4th ed. Tokyo, Bunkodo Press, 1990.)

of trimethoprim per kilogram per day), long-term gamma-interferon (50 μg per square meter in adults or 1.5 μg per kilogram in children, given three times a week), and vigorous treatment of acute infections with antibiotics in adequate doses, plus surgery if indicated. Leukocyte transfusions may be helpful. Complications should be treated as conservatively as possible, although surgery may be required. Bone marrow transplantation has been performed in a few instances, but with its widely known hazards and the improvement in the outlook of CGD resulting from the use of long-term prophylaxis, marrow transplantation must be regarded as a last resort. Families of patients with CGD should be investigated to ascertain the mode of transmission of the disease, and genetic counseling should be offered to them. In pregnant carriers, CGD may be diagnosed prenatally through NBT tests of fetal blood or, in X-linked disease, through a restriction fragment length polymorphism in DNA obtained by amniocentesis or chorionic villus biopsy.

CHÉDIAK-HIGASHI DISEASE. Chédiak-Higashi disease is an autosomally inherited defect in lysosome production. Normally, these organelles are oval bodies of relatively uniform size, but in Chédiak-Higashi disease they are very irregular both in size and in shape, ranging from tiny spheres to huge, malformed bodies many times larger than normal. The molecular lesion responsible for Chédiak-Higashi disease is unknown, although there is some evidence that the condition may result from an abnormality in microtubule function.

Clinical Picture. The clinical features of Chédiak-Higashi disease result from the malfunction of three types of lysosome-containing cells: the melanocytes, the platelets, and the phagocytes. Melanocyte dysfunction leads to *partial albinism*, a uniform but incomplete loss of pigment from the irises, skin, and hair that can be detected even at birth. The platelet defect causes a mild *bleeding disorder* associated with a prolonged bleeding time. The most serious clinical problems, however, are caused by the abnormalities in the phagocytes. These lead to *marked lowering of resistance to bacterial infections,* so that patients with Chédiak-Higashi disease suffer from frequent deep tissue abscesses as well as recurrent attacks of severe bacterial sinusitis and pneumonia. These infections are difficult to treat and often lead to death in the first or second decade.

Patients with Chédiak-Higashi disease who survive into their teens or later are confronted with a further clinical problem, probably the most serious of all. In most of these patients, the disease ultimately evolves into a fatal form known as the accelerated phase. This is a peculiar lymphoma-like illness possibly caused by an out-of-control Epstein-Barr virus infection (see Ch. 373). The lymph nodes, liver, spleen, and bone marrow become infiltrated with small lymphocytes and histiocytes that look perfectly benign but behave in a malignant fashion, causing the

infiltrated organs to enlarge and producing through marrow infiltration and splenomegaly a rapid, relentless, and ultimately fatal progression of the mild granulocytopenia seen in the stable phase of the disease. Death from pancytopenia generally occurs within a few months after the onset of the accelerated phase.

In Chédiak-Higashi disease, the white blood cell count is typically low (2000 to 3000 per cubic millimeter), a result of ineffective granulopoiesis. The low white cell count is an important factor in the low resistance to infection that characterizes this condition. Neutrophil chemotaxis and degranulation are depressed, but phagocytosis and the respiratory burst are normal. Bacterial killing is defective, probably because the abnormality in degranulation hinders the delivery of microbicidal substances into the phagocytic vesicles.

Diagnosis. The diagnosis is made by demonstrating giant granules in neutrophils and eosinophils, a feature that is virtually pathognomonic of Chédiak-Higashi disease (Fig. 139–2) (see Color Plate 7D, right). The diagnosis of the accelerated phase depends on finding the characteristic infiltrate in a biopsy of the involved tissue.

Treatment. The management of the early stage of Chédiak-Higashi disease amounts to the management of the infectious complications. Prophylactic antibiotics (trimethoprim-sulfamethoxazole at the dose given previously) should be used, and infections should be treated vigorously with appropriate antibiotic therapy. Ascorbic acid (20 mg per kilogram per day) has corrected the microbicidal defect in some but not all patients with Chédiak-Higashi disease. Treatment of the accelerated phase is unsatisfactory; splenectomy has been tried, as has chemotherapy with a variety of agents, but nothing has proved to be of much benefit. Marrow transplantation has also been used in Chédiak-Higashi disease, though the indications for transplantation (e.g., the question of transplantation in early childhood as opposed to transplantation for the accelerated phase) are not yet clearly established.

DISORDERS OF NEUTROPHIL MOTILITY (Table 139–4). There are a number of conditions in which recurrent abscesses or other bacterial infections occur because of severe impairment in neutrophil mobility. Neutrophils from affected patients migrate poorly onto a glass coverslip in the Rebuck skin window test and show grossly impaired chemotaxis when tested in vitro. These disorders are thought to be inherited, although evidence for their heritability is often weak. For most of them (e.g., congenitally increased microtubule assembly), only one or two cases have been reported. A few, however, have been seen in several patients. These are discussed here.

Hyper-IgE Syndrome. In this condition, reduced neutrophil motility is associated with bacterial respiratory tract infections and cold staphylococcal abscesses (i.e., abscesses lacking much

TABLE 139–4. DISORDERS OF NEUTROPHIL MOTILITY

Disorder	Distinguishing Features
Job's syndrome	Cold abscesses, eosinophilia, greatly increased IgE
Juvenile periodontitis	Early severe gingival inflammation, systemic infections only in occasional patients
Leukocyte glycoprotein deficiency	Omphalitis or other infections in newborn, delayed separation of umbilical stump, leukemoid reactions
Congenital absence of specific granules	Abnormal segmentation of nucleus, alkaline phosphatase decreased or absent

of the swelling and redness associated with inflammation), eosinophilia, and greatly increased levels of IgE. Patients characteristically have very high blood levels of an antistaphylococcal IgE antibody. Neutrophils from these patients show greatly reduced chemotaxis if assayed immediately after isolation, but chemotaxis returns to normal if the cells are stored for a few hours in the absence of serum prior to assay. The abnormalities in leukocyte function and IgE production may be related to a defect in gamma-interferon production by T cells from affected patients.

Juvenile Periodontitis. In this familial disease, neutrophils show a chemotactic defect that is thought to be caused by a serum abnormality. Serious gingival inflammation develops in late childhood or adolescence, similar to but more severe than that seen in normal middle-aged adults with poor dental hygiene. Affected individuals will often have lost many of their teeth by the time they are 30 years old. Among the organisms infecting the gums of such patients is *Capnocytophaga*, an anaerobic bacillus that secretes a potent inhibitor of neutrophil chemotaxis. The antichemotactic agent enters the bloodstream, where, in a few patients with juvenile peridontitis, it reaches concentrations that impair systemic host defenses and result in repeated bacterial infections. Elimination of the *Capnocytophaga* organisms by long-term administration of antibiotics and vigorous local therapy corrects the impairment in host defenses and normalizes the patient's resistance to bacterial infections.

Leukocyte Adhesion Deficiency. In this inherited disease, a chemotactic defect is caused by a defect involving the CD11/CD18 adhesion glycoproteins. The first indication of this condition may be delayed separation of the umbilical stump. Patients are subject to recurrent infections, particularly with *Pseudomonas*. The first infection may occur in the newborn as an omphalitis. Infections are generally accompanied by a neutrophilic leukemoid reaction in which the white count may exceed 100,000. The diagnosis can be made with commercially available anti-CD11/CD18 antibodies, which bind to normal but not glycoprotein-deficient white cells. Vigorous and prolonged therapy is necessary for successful treatment of infections in leukocyte adhesion deficiency. Prophylactic antibodies are indicated in this condition; they maintain the patient's health and keep the white cell count at normal or near-normal levels.

Congenital Absence of Specific Granules. In this disorder a chemotactic defect results in recurrent, severe bacterial infections. The neutrophils show abnormalities in nuclear segmentation, most frequently a grotesque bilobed nucleus, and stain poorly for alkaline phosphatase. Certain granule-associated proteins (e.g., defensins, cobalamin-binding protein) are absent, and bacterial killing is impaired. Under the electron microscope, the neutrophils show normal azurophil granules, but specific granules are rare or absent.

MYELOPEROXIDASE DEFICIENCY. Deficiency of myeloperoxidase (MPO) is the most common inherited disorder of neutrophil function. Transmitted as an autosomal recessive trait, it affects 1 person in ~2000. Once thought rare, its true incidence was revealed through automated white cell differential counters that rely on the peroxidase stain to identify neutrophils.

Clinically, MPO deficiency is almost completely silent. The most frequent problem is an increase in *Candida* infections in occasional MPO-deficient patients with coincident diabetes mellitus. The original misconception about the incidence of MPO deficiency can probably be explained by the low incidence of clinical disease in patients with this condition.

MPO-deficient neutrophils show characteristic functional abnormalities. Chemotaxis, phagocytosis, and degranulation are normal, but the respiratory burst is prolonged because of an increase in the lifespan of the O_2^--forming oxidase, which is normally destroyed by myeloperoxidase during the course of the respiratory burst. Bacterial killing by MPO-deficient cells is delayed but eventually reaches completion, indicating that the myeloperoxidase-independent oxidants generated by the deficient cells kill more slowly but just as effectively as the myeloperoxidase-dependent oxidants of normal cells. The completeness of bacterial killing by MPO-deficient cells contrasts with the extensive failure of bacterial killing in CGD, and it explains why bacterial infections are such a serious problem in the latter but not the former condition.

The diagnosis is made from a peroxidase stain of the blood film. The stain normally shows activity in neutrophils, monocytes, and eosinophils. In MPO deficiency the activity is missing from neutrophils and monocytes. Eosinophils, however, stain normally, since their peroxidase, which is different from myeloperoxidase, is not affected in myeloperoxidase deficiency. Peroxidase levels can be quantitated spectrophotometrically if desired, but this is usually unnecessary. Treatment is generally not required for MPO deficiency.

Babior BM, Woodman RC: Chronic granulomatous disease. Semin Hematol 27:247, 1990. *The latest on CGD and the respiratory burst oxidase.*

Boogaerts MA, Nelissen V, Roelant C, et al.: Blood neutrophil function in primary myelodysplastic syndromes. Br J Haematol 55:217, 1983. *A thorough study of neutrophil dysfunction in myelodysplasia.*

Curnutte JT (ed.): Phagocytic defects. Hematol/Oncol Clin North Am, 1988, Vols. 1 and 2. *A series of reviews on the inherited disorders of phagocytes.*

Donabedian H, Gallin JI: The hyperimmunoglobulin E recurrent infection (Job's) syndrome. A review of the NIH experience and the literature. Medicine 62:195, 1983. *A detailed clinical study of Job's syndrome.*

Lehrer RI, Ganz T: Antimicrobial polypeptides of human neutrophils. Blood 76:2169, 1990. *A recent and excellent review of this important but rarely discussed topic.*

Lomax KJ, Malech HL, Gallin JI: The molecular biology of selected phagocyte defects. Blood Rev 3:94, 1989. *A clearly written and up-to-date review of the molecular defects in several inherited disorders of phagocytes.*

140 Leukopenia

Grover C. Bagby, Jr.

The peripheral blood white cell count ranges from 5.0 to 10.0 $\times$ 10^9 per liter in normal individuals. Circulating leukocytes consist of heterogeneous cell types (neutrophils, monocytes, basophils, eosinophils, and lymphocytes), each of which serves a unique purpose and each of which represents a different fractional component of the total peripheral leukocyte population. A rational discussion of leukopenia must therefore focus on specific leukocyte types. Nor can a normal white blood cell count ensure that substantial and serious deficiencies of leukocyte components do not exist. Patients may be severely neutropenic or lymphocytopenic despite total white blood counts that fall within the normal range. If there is a reason to order a white blood count, that reason is generally sufficient to justify performance of a differential count as well.

NEUTROPENIA

DEFINITION. Neutropenia exists when the peripheral neutrophil count is less than 2.0 $\times$ 10^9 per liter. Because the normal range in blacks and Yemenite Jews is somewhat lower, neutropenia in these populations is defined as counts less than 1.5 $\times$ 10^9 per liter. The role of the neutrophil in phagocytic defense of the host is generally met if the neutrophil count is above 1.0 $\times$ 10^9 per liter. If the neutrophil count drops below this number, particularly when the count falls below 0.5×10^9 per liter, the incidence of serious, recurrent, and difficult-to-treat infections rises markedly.

ETIOLOGY AND PATHOGENESIS. The multiple causes of neutropenia in pathophysiologic terms are best described in the context of the normal processes of neutrophil production and traffic. Such a description also simplifies the diagnostic and therapeutic approaches to patients with neutropenia. Neutrophils arise from a pool of marrow precursor cells through serial divisions and synchronous maturation steps (Fig. 140–1). The rate of neutrophil production is astonishingly high: more than 10^{11} cells per day. The bone marrow component of the neutrophil's life consists of a mitotic pool and a storage pool, the latter containing cells that no longer divide. Released after a few days in the bone marrow, neutrophils circulate freely for only a matter of hours before crawling into the extravascular space. For unknown reasons, half of the neutrophils in the peripheral blood are "marginated" along the endothelium and therefore are not measured in the white blood cell count. Accordingly, the true peripheral blood content of neutrophils, consisting of the circulating and the marginated pools, is ordinarily twice that measured by the neutrophil count (Fig. 140–1).

A simple etiologic classification of neutropenia can be derived from the three-compartment model, representing abnormalities in (1) the marrow compartment, (2) the peripheral blood compartment, (3) the extravascular compartment, or (4) combinations of the above (Fig. 140–2).

Abnormalities in the Marrow Compartment. Abnormalities in the marrow account for the majority of neutropenias in clinical practice. Failure of the marrow compartment can occur as a result of direct injury, in which case the marrow usually contains fewer than normal hematopoietic cells, or from maturation defects of hematopoietic cells, principally characterized by normal or increased numbers of morphologically abnormal hematopoietic cells. In either case, neutropenia most frequently occurs along with abnormalities in the number of platelets and red cells. Marrow injury can occur as a consequence of a variety of diseases (Fig. 140–2).

Drug-induced injury is most common (Table 140–1). Antineoplastic and immunosuppressive agents are generally *designed* to inflict injury on a proliferative population of cells; myelosuppressive toxicity is the rule but is generally predictable and dose related. Drugs that are well tolerated in the majority of patients, however, can induce either marrow injury or peripheral neutrophil destruction in certain patients. These drug-induced reactions can result from direct drug-mediated cytotoxicity or from an immune mechanism in which (1) neutrophils are destroyed in extramedullary sites (e.g., the penicillins) or (2) the marrow compartment is injured (e.g., procainamide, chloramphenicol, dapsone).

Radiation may result in acute self-limited and chronic marrow injury. Chronic radiation-induced injury can also result in the later development of myelodysplasia and nonlymphocytic leukemia, both of which often present with neutropenia. *Benzene* toxicity can also result in acute or chronic neutropenia and, like radiation-induced marrow failure, is associated with a high risk of acute nonlymphocytic leukemia.

Immune-mediated abnormalities may injure the marrow, either by autoantibody-mediated or by T lymphocyte–mediated mechanisms. Most patients with immune-mediated leukopenia have concurrent rheumatic or autoimmune diseases (see Color Plate 6L). *Infection* of the marrow per se is unusual and most often does not result in neutropenia; some exceptions include mycobacterial infection (especially those caused by *Mycobacterium tuberculosis* and *M. kansasii*) and certain viral infections.

Marrow invasion by abnormal cells can result in neutropenia. Carcinoma of the prostate, breast, stomach, and lung, as well as malignant hematopoietic disorders, can occupy enough of the medullary space to cause global marrow failure. Similarly, fibroblasts can proliferate in certain disease states to the extent that they dominate the marrow (Fig. 140–2).

Maturation arrest can result in bone marrow failure in the absence of granulopoietic hypocellularity. In *folate* and *vitamin B_{12} deficiency*, for example, the marrow is loaded with granulocyte precursors that, because of the effects of the deficiency states on nuclear replication, fail to mature normally and therefore suffer a high rate of intramedullary death (Ch. 132). The marrow is hypercellular, and hematopoiesis goes on actively, but this activity belies the inability of the marrow to deliver mature cells effectively—hence the term *ineffective hematopoiesis*. Certain congenital neutropenias also represent maturation abnormalities, as do the acute nonlymphocytic leukemias, myelodysplastic syndromes, and paroxysmal nocturnal hemoglobinuria.

Abnormalities in the Peripheral Blood Compartment. Perturbations of the peripheral blood compartment result from shifts in the circulating pool (Figs. 140–1 and 140–2). In *pseudoneutropenia*, neutrophil production and utilization are normal, but the size of the marginated pool is unusually large and substantially greater in size than the circulating pool. Patients with stable hereditary or constitutional pseudoneutropenia are not at increased risk of infection unless a neutrophil function abnormality coexists. Acquired pseudoneutropenia often occurs as an acute or subacute response to systemic infections. It is generally associated with acute changes in other compartments (Fig. 140–3) and

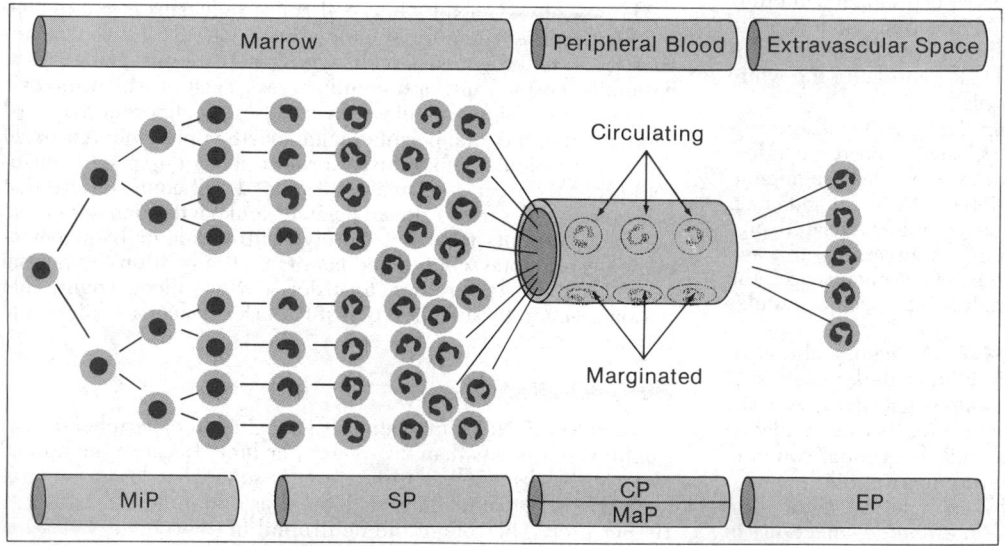

FIGURE 140–1. Production and distribution of neutrophils involve three compartments. Stem cells, committed progenitor cells, and morphologically recognizable precursor cells proliferate and mature (differentiate) under the influence of a variety of humoral regulatory factors, including GM-CSF (colony-stimulating factor) and G-CSF. These phenomena occur in the "mitotic pool" (MiP). Once the cells reach the intermediate maturation stage known as the metamyelocyte, they stop proliferating but continue differentiating to bands and segmented neutrophils. These cells, although capable of leaving the marrow if needed, generally spend about 5 days in the marrow, in the "storage pool" (SP). The neutrophils then enter the blood. Half of those cells in the blood circulate and can be measured in a blood sample by counting—the "circulating pool" (CP)—but the other half move about out of the main column of flowing blood, probably in close association with vascular endothelial cells. These latter cells are components of the "marginated pool" (MaP). After their brief sojourn in the peripheral blood, the neutrophils invade the extravascular compartments of most organs, where they either are utilized as defenders or garbage disposal systems or die within 1 or 2 days.

Figure labels: Marrow | Peripheral Blood | Extravascular Space | Circulating | Marginated | MiP | SP | CP/MaP | EP

THE CAUSES OF NEUTROPENIA

Marrow

ABNORMALITIES IN THE BONE MARROW COMPARTMENT

1. Bone Marrow Injury
   A. Drugs
      Cytotoxic and noncytotoxic agents
   B. Radiation
   C. Chemicals
      Benzene, DDT, dinitrophenol, arsenic, bismuth, nitrous oxide
   D. Certain congenital and hereditary neutropenias
   E. Immunologically mediated (largely seen in patients with rheumatic disorders)
      Cytotoxic T cell–mediated (T)
      Antibody–mediated (Ab)
      Mechanisms that require both T and Ab
   F. Infection
      Viral (hepatitis, parvovirus, AIDS)
      Bacterial (*M. tuberculosis, M. kansasii*)
   G. Bone marrow replacement (infiltrative diseases)
      Malignancies (lung, breast, prostate, stomach, lymphomas, and lymphoid leukemias)
      Fibrosis
      Agnogenic myeloid metaplasia
      Long-standing polycythemia vera
      Chronic myelogenous leukemia
      Radiation injury
      Injury from chronic cytotoxic drug therapy
      Acute megakaryocytic leukemia

2. Maturation Defects
   A. Acquired
      Folic acid deficiency
      Vitamin B_{12} deficiency
   B. Neoplastic and other clonal disorders
      Congenital neutropenias
      Acute nonlymphocytic leukemia
      Myelodysplastic syndromes
      Paroxysmal nocturnal hemoglobinuria

Peripheral Blood

ABNORMALITIES IN THE PERIPHERAL BLOOD COMPARTMENT

1. Shift of neutrophils from the circulating to the marginated pool (known as pseudoneutropenia)
   A. Hereditary or constitutional benign pseudoneutropenia
   B. Acquired
      Acute: Severe bacterial infection, frequently associated with endotoxemia
      Chronic: Protein-calorie malnutrition, malaria
2. Intravascular sequestration
   A. In lung (complement-mediated leukoagglutination)
   B. In spleen (hypersplenism)

Extravascular

ABNORMALITIES IN THE EXTRAVASCULAR COMPARTMENT

1. Increased utilization
   A. Severe bacterial, fungal, viral, or rickettsial infection
   B. Anaphylaxis

FIGURE 140–2. The causes of neutropenia have been arranged according to the compartment in which the abnormality usually resides. The approach to the neutropenic patient should begin by determining which of the three major compartments is likely at fault.

resolves when the infection is appropriately treated or spontaneously abates.

Demands of the Extravascular Compartment. Neutrophils and their precursors respond to infections in a highly coordinated and regulated fashion. The cellular responses are largely controlled by two granulopoietic factors, GM-CSF and G-CSF, and include (1) a rather prompt increase in the rate of production of neutrophils in the mitotic compartment, a response mediated by a complex network of cellular and humoral regulatory interactions, (2) the early release of neutrophils from the marrow storage pool to the peripheral blood pool, (3) an increase in the rate of neutrophil egress from the peripheral blood pool to the invaded tissue or tissues, and (4) increased phagocytic and bactericidal activity of the neutrophils. Rarely, increased demand for neutrophils in the extravascular compartment can lead to transient neutropenia, especially in patients with severe acute infections (Fig. 140–3). In such cases, the immediate demand for neutrophils completely utilizes the marrow storage pool before it can be restored by increased proliferative activity. The neutrophil count generally rises within a few days. The bone marrow is highly effective in responding to infectious events, so that the demand for neutrophils almost never exceeds the capacity of the mitotic pool to supply them. In contrast, neutrophil consumption in patients with autoimmune neutropenia and hypersplenism can

outstrip marrow production. Whether this reflects absence in such patients of the complete humoral stimulatory mechanisms that evolve in the infected host, or whether the rate of destruction in these patients actually exceeds the rate of utilization in patients with infections, is not known.

In summary, the causes of neutropenia are heterogeneous and best categorized in pathophysiologic terms (Fig. 140–3).

CLINICAL MANIFESTATIONS. Neutropenia can occur in a wide variety of systemic diseases (Fig. 140–2), the manifestations of which may dominate the clinical picture. Many neutropenic patients remain asymptomatic, most often those whose neutrophil count exceeds 1.0×10^9 per liter or those whose neutropenia is acute and self-limited in duration. When symptoms do occur, they generally result from recurrent, often severe, bacterial infections. This is not surprising in view of the pivotal importance of the neutrophil in the defense of the host against microorganisms (Ch. 138).

This risk of bacterial infection increases significantly as the peripheral neutrophil count falls below 1.0×10^9 per liter but is greatly increased at levels below 0.5×10^9 per liter. The degree to which monocytosis compensates for neutropenia may modify the risk. I have observed a patient with such severe congenital neutropenia that no neutrophil has ever been seen in her blood smears over an 18-year period. Her leukocyte count is, however,

TABLE 140–1. DRUGS THAT CAUSE NEUTROPENIA

Antiarrhythmics
  Procainamide, propranolol, quinidine
Antibiotics
  Chloramphenicol, penicillins, sulfonamides, trimethoprim-methoxazole, para-aminosalicylic acid (PAS), rifampin, vancomycin, isoniazid, nitrofurantoin
Antimalarials
  Dapsone, quinine, pyrimethamine
Anticonvulsants
  Phenytoin, mephenytoin, trimethadione, ethosuximide, carbamazepine
Hypoglycemic agents
  Tolbutamide, chlorpropamide
Antihistamines
  Cimetidine, brompheniramine, tripelennamine
Antihypertensives
  Methyldopa, captopril
Anti-inflammatory agents
  Aminopyrine, phenylbutazone, gold salts, ibuprofen, indomethacin
Antithyroid agents
  Propylthiouracil, methimazole, thiouracil
Diuretics
  Acetazolamide, hydrochlorothiazide, chlorthalidone
Phenothiazines
  Chlorpromazine, promazine, prochlorperazine
Immunosuppressive agents
  Antimetabolites
Cytotoxic agents
  Alkylating agents, antimetabolites, anthracyclines, vinca alkaloids, cis-platinum, hydroxyurea, actinomycin D
Other agents
  Recombinant alpha- and gamma-interferon, allopurinol, ethanol, levamisole, penicillamine

normal because of marked monocytosis; the frequency of infections in this patient has been low.

Lungs, genitourinary system, oropharynx, and skin are the most frequent sites of infection in neutropenic patients. The infecting organisms are the expected pathogens for the given anatomic site. In patients who have recurrent infections and require prolonged and recurrent antibacterial therapy, unusual organisms can colonize and subsequently cause infection. The antibiotic history of infected neutropenic patients is important to obtain. *The usual signs and symptoms of infection are often diminished or absent in patients with neutropenia because the cell that mediates much of the inflammatory response to infection is absent.* Thus, neutropenic patients with severe bilateral bacterial pneumonia can present with minimal infiltrates demonstrable by the chest radiograph and nonpurulent sputum; patients with pyelonephritis may not exhibit pyuria; patients with bacterial pharyngitis may not have purulence in the oropharynx; and patients with severe bacterial infection of the skin may present only with erythroderma rather than furunculosis. In the neutropenic patient, infections that in an otherwise normal individual might have been well localized become quickly disseminated. Therefore, not only is the infected neutropenic patient a diagnostic problem but, in addition, because any given infection is more apt to be widespread at the time of diagnosis, these patients are often dangerously ill.

DIAGNOSIS. The diagnostic evaluation of neutropenia is influenced by its severity and the clinical setting in which it occurs. The assessment of patients with neutrophil counts of less than 0.5 to 1.0 × 10⁹ per liter should obviously proceed briskly. The patient with fever, sepsis, or both, in whom neutropenia is discovered for the first time, presents a particularly difficult problem. In such patients it is impossible to determine immediately whether the neutropenia antedated sepsis, a situation with both prognostic and therapeutic implications, or whether the neutropenia is merely a short-lived response to the infection itself (Fig. 140–3). Examination of the peripheral blood smear and differential white blood count can be helpful in such cases. If the blood film has been prepared promptly after obtaining the sample, vacuolization of neutrophil cytoplasm suggests the presence of bacterial infection. An increase in the fraction of circulating band forms to levels above 20 per cent suggests that marrow granulopoietic activity is responding appropriately (Fig. 140–4). It is then presumed either that the marrow is recovering from injury or that the neutropenia is derived from a transient shift to the marginated pool or to the extravascular compartment.

The diagnostic evaluation of neutropenia must first address the question of the severity of the disorder and then whether the patient has fever, sepsis, or both. The patient with sepsis and severe neutropenia should be treated promptly with intravenous antibiotics following appropriate cultures, but *without waiting* for the results of those cultures. Once these important initial questions are answered, the remainder of the diagnostic evaluation

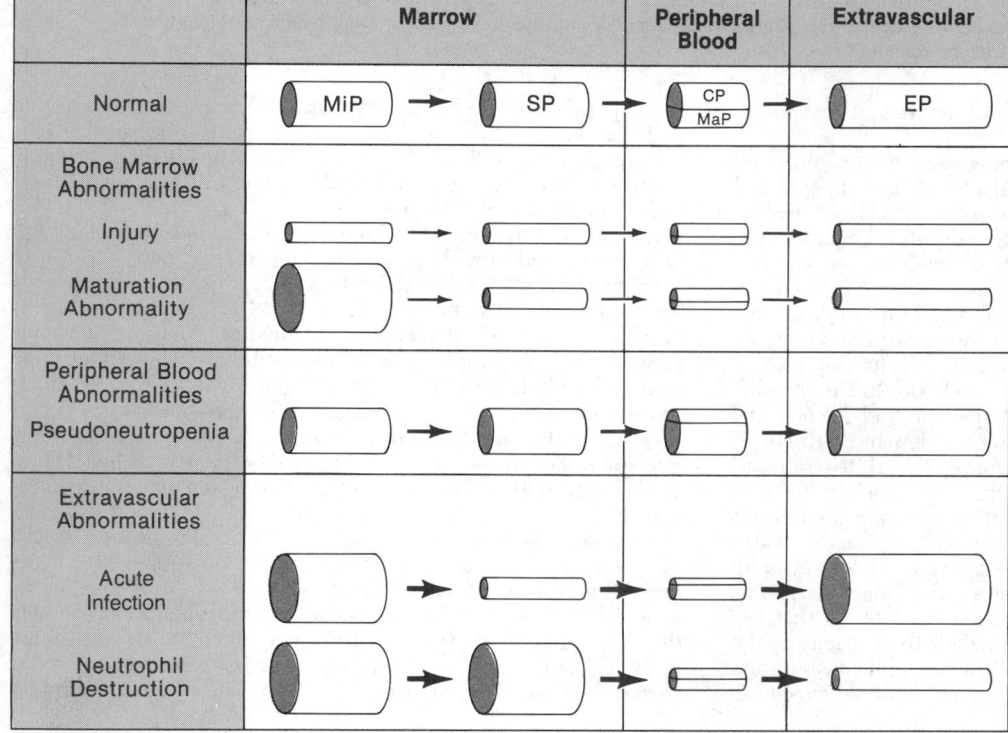

	Marrow		Peripheral Blood	Extravascular
Normal	MiP →	SP →	CP / MaP →	EP
Bone Marrow Abnormalities				
Injury				
Maturation Abnormality				
Peripheral Blood Abnormalities				
Pseudoneutropenia				
Extravascular Abnormalities				
Acute Infection				
Neutrophil Destruction				

FIGURE 140–3. Pathophysiologic mechanisms of neutropenia. The size of a given compartment is represented by the size of the corresponding cylinder. The number of cells leaving a compartment for the next compartment can vary substantially, but flow between compartments is unidirectional. Notice that in every case the circulating neutrophil pool is small, but the size of the other pools is variable. In marrow injury there is a global decline in the size of all pools. A maturation abnormality, however, is characterized by an increase in the number of precursor cells that do not mature. Pseudoneutropenia is characterized by a movement of circulating neutrophils to the marginated pool. In severe infections the acute demand for neutrophils in the infected extravascular site results in a transient loss of storage pool neutrophils before the hypercellular (but as yet immature) mitotic compartments can renew the storage pool. Finally, excessive destruction of neutrophils can result in neutropenia. MiP = mitotic pool; SP = storage pool; CP = circulating pool; MaP = marginated pool; EP = extravascular pool.

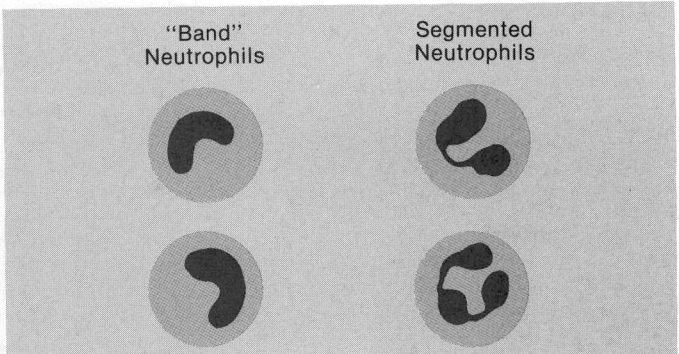

FIGURE 140–4. Band neutrophils are somewhat "younger" forms than segmented neutrophils. The nuclear lobes in a segmented form are separated by fine filaments absent in the band.

can proceed (Fig. 140–5): (1) identifying any potential drugs and toxins to which the patient might have been exposed; (2) determining, if possible, the chronicity of the neutropenia; (3) ascertaining whether there have been recurrent infections; (4) identifying any underlying systemic disease that might be causative; and (5) examining the blood counts and blood morphology and bone marrow (the latter is usually indicated) to determine the most likely pathophysiologic explanation. The latter is important even if a specific, likely causative, underlying disease is promptly identified. Felty's syndrome, for example, is a well-recognized cause of neutropenia, but there are at least two separate pathophysiologic mechanisms in groups of these patients, one mediated by antineutrophil antibodies, the other by T lymphocyte–mediated bone marrow failure. Each mechanism has different therapeutic implications.

One approach to the neutropenic patient is shown in algorithmic form in Figure 140–5. Once the severity of the neutropenia is determined, careful examination of the peripheral blood counts and blood smear is in order. Patients with selective neutropenia are approached differently from those with additional deficiencies of platelets and red cells, although drugs or toxins may be involved in either category. Patients with selective neutropenia but with no drug or toxin exposure, no history of recurrent sepsis, and no underlying chronic inflammatory or autoimmune disease may have stable and benign neutropenia. This category includes some cases of familial and congenital neutropenia and pseudoneutropenia. Any patient with selective neutropenia with a history of sepsis or toxin exposure should have a bone marrow examination to assess (1) the degree of cellularity of each compartment (storage and mitotic pools), (2) the distribution of differentiation stages found in each pool, and (3) whether any morphologic abnormality exists in the hematopoietic cells.

In patients with pancytopenia or bicytopenia, bone marrow examination, which must include not only aspiration but biopsy as well, is almost always indicated. The only regular exception to this rule would include patients with unambiguous evidence of vitamin B_{12} or folate deficiency (Ch. 132).

TREATMENT. Rational treatment of the neutropenic patient follows diagnosis and generally involves treatment of the underlying disease or discontinuation of suspected toxins or drugs. The nature of the specific therapy naturally depends on the pathophysiology of the neutropenia in a given patient.

Treatments Specifically Designed to Increase the Neutrophil Count. Trials of the few agents available for the purpose of increasing the neutrophil count must be considered only in patients with severe neutropenia and a history of infections and should be attempted only after the potential risks involved are explained to the patient.

Lithium carbonate, an agent that increases the neutrophil production rate in normal individuals, rarely has been effective in the management of chronic bone marrow failure. The dose used in adults is 300 mg by mouth three times daily. In view of the frequency of toxicity, trials of therapy should be considered only as a last resort. No test to predict individual responsiveness has yet been developed.

Immunosuppressive therapy, including glucocorticoids or azathioprine, almost always elicits a favorable response in patients with marrow failure mediated by cytotoxic T lymphocytes. In vitro clonogenic cultures of bone marrow cells in severely neutropenic patients can aid in the identification of patients apt to respond to such therapy. Some responses to immunosuppressive therapy have also occurred in patients whose neutropenia resulted from antineutrophil antibodies. Splenectomy is rarely helpful in the management of neutropenic patients, even those with Felty's syndrome. It is now reserved for patients with unambiguous hypersplenism in whom bone marrow function is normal.

Recombinant Human Granulopoietic Factors. The genes of many hematopoietic growth factors have been cloned, their sequences reported, and the biologic activities of the proteins encoded by them characterized in humans. Some of these recombinant proteins, including GM-CSF (colony-stimulating factor, granulocyte and macrophage) and G-CSF (colony-stimulating factor, granulocyte), are now in clinical trials for management of bone marrow failure. Both GM-CSF and G-CSF induce neutrophilic leukocytosis; GM-CSF also induces the appearance of eosinophils. GM-CSF and G-CSF have many similar therapeutic effects, but there are some differences. (1) Used in high doses, some GM-CSF preparations may induce fever and local thrombophlebitis (in the vein of administration) more frequently than does G-CSF. (2) G-CSF is effective in the treatment of children and adults with cyclic neutropenia and of children with severe congenital agranulocytosis. These growth factors have recently been approved by the Food and Drug Administration for use in selected clinical settings. However, they will probably be beneficial in the management of patients with neutropenia in specific clinical settings such as bone marrow transplantation. These clinical settings have yet to be defined completely. An important unresolved issue is the theoretical potential of these factors to worsen the underlying disease. Some in vitro models, for example, predict that therapy with certain recombinant granulopoietic factors might hasten the development of leukemia in selected types of myelodysplasia and may stimulate the growth of certain cancer cells. GM-CSF by itself might possibly induce the release of HIV-1 from latently infected cells, but in combination therapy GM-CSF enhances the net anti-HIV effect of azidothymidine. Recombinant granulopoietic factors can undoubtedly play an important therapeutic role in the near future, but the underlying cause of the neutropenia must be taken into account to ensure that short-term benefits are not ultimately complicated by acceleration of the primary disease process.

Bone Marrow Transplantation. In severe aplastic anemia the role of bone marrow transplantation is well established (Ch. 153). Other marrow failure states (e.g., myelodysplastic syndromes and congenital neutropenias) may also prove to respond to transplantation. Allogeneic transplantation is associated with high mortality; its use in patients with selective neutropenia is therefore uncertain. Before transplantation is seriously considered, the duration and severity of the neutropenia must be assessed; marrow failure must be established as the primary cause; and immunologically mediated marrow failure should be ruled out. If the patient has an identical twin, transplantation might be attempted with fewer constraints, but allogeneic transplantation should always be reserved for individuals with severe and symptomatic neutropenia caused by marrow failure.

Treatment of the Infected Neutropenic Patient. Each patient with neutropenia should understand the function of neutrophils, the consequences of neutrophil deficiency, and the importance of communicating with his or her physician the moment signs and symptoms of infection occur. If a neutropenic patient is afebrile and there is no sepsis, the diagnostic workup should generally take place in the outpatient clinic to avoid unnecessary exposure to nosocomial infections. Patients with severe neutropenia and fever, however, should be hospitalized. Cultures of urine, blood, and other relevant sites should be obtained, but broad-spectrum antibiotics should be given without waiting for the results of these cultures. One of three responses will be seen. (1) A causative organism will be identified, in which case the spectrum of antimicrobial agents can be appropriately narrowed.

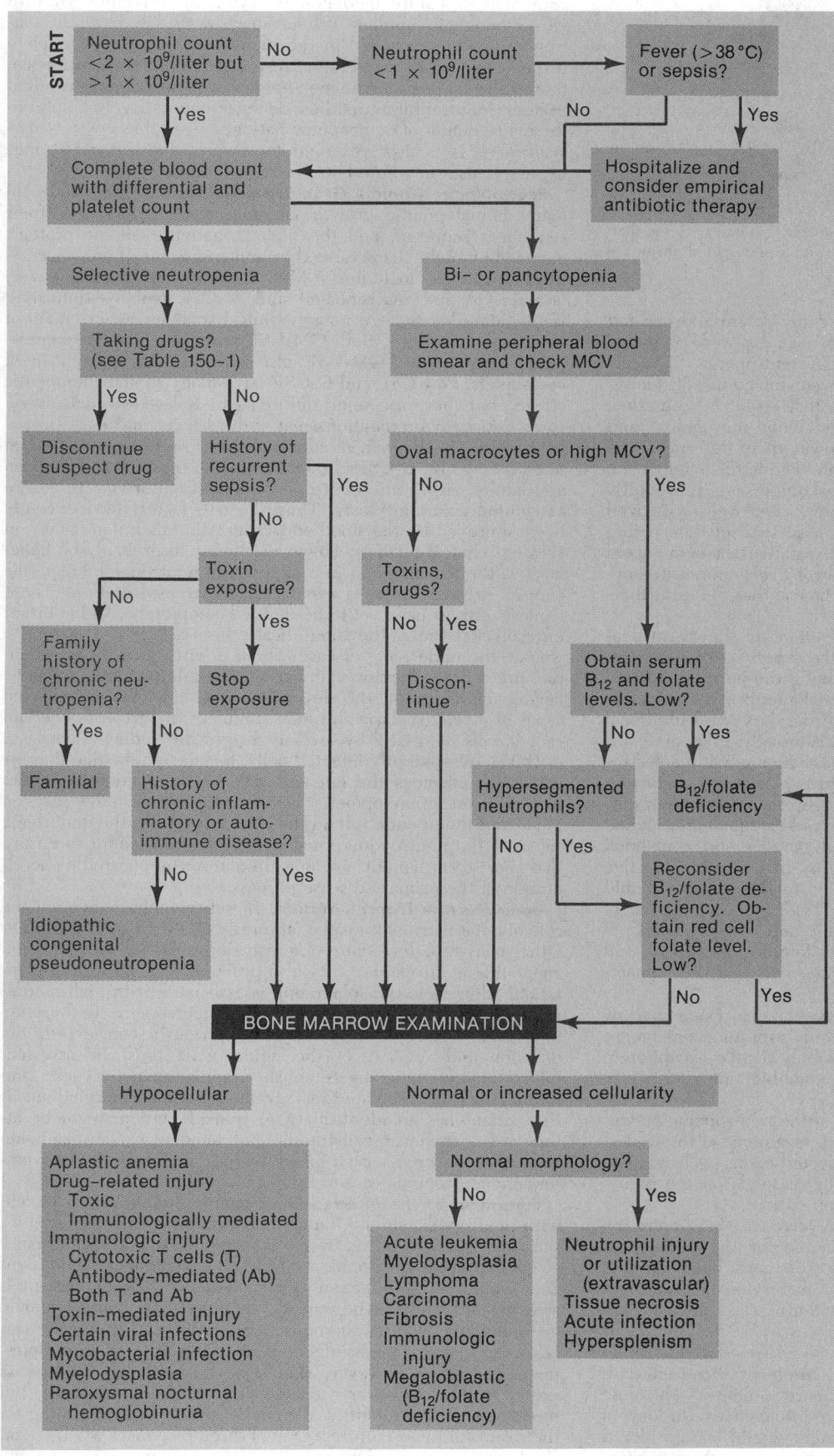

FIGURE 140–5. An algorithm for the evaluation of patients with neutropenia.

(2) A candidate organism will not be found, but the patient still improves with empiric therapy. In this type of setting a full course of broad-spectrum antibiotics should be given. Moreover, after a full course of parenteral antibiotics has been given, another 7 to 14 days of oral antibiotics should be considered, especially in patients with invasive infections associated with necrosis, in those whose initial response was slow, or in those with infections that have recurred in the same anatomic site. (3) No organism is found, and the clinical picture is not altered after 3 days of empiric treatment. This unsettling situation occurs with some regularity in practice. The approach to a patient at this point depends on the seriousness of the infection. For a patient with localized disease who is not critically ill, it is sometimes helpful for empiric therapy to be discontinued and for repeat cultures to be obtained. If the patient is critically ill, however, antibiotics should be discontinued *only* if other antibiotics are substituted. Among those antibiotics to consider in this situation is amphotericin B. Amphotericin B should be strongly considered for the therapeutic regimen in certain clinical settings, i.e., for patients with acute leukemia, diabetes, dysphagia and/or esophagitis, endophthalmitis, or defective cell-mediated immunity (including those receiving immunosuppressive therapy) and for those who have received prolonged treatment with broad-spectrum antibacterial agents in the recent past.

Neutrophil transfusions, when used specifically for the treatment of seriously infected neutropenic patients, are capable of providing enough phagocytes to make a difference in the course of some infections. They should not, however, be used prophylactically in uninfected neutropenic patients. Neutrophils survive briefly in the peripheral circulation and tissues, so that they must be given at least daily, probably for at least 3 days. The decision to use neutrophil transfusions is not a trivial one. White cells for transfusion are expensive, and if preformed antibodies exist in the recipient, a number of transfusion reactions can occur, including fever, chills, myalgia, and acute dyspnea with or without transient bilateral pulmonary infiltration. These same clinical manifestations can also result from invasion of the sites of infection by the transfused neutrophils and their subsequent release of mediators of inflammation that have hitherto been absent in the infected patient. In the absence of clear-cut signs of hypersensitivity (e.g., urticaria), therefore, one cannot be sure whether the infection is being better controlled or whether the transfused cells are being destroyed. For this reason, a decision to discontinue neutrophil transfusions cannot be made on the grounds that such reactions have occurred. Each patient's adverse response must be approached individually.

DEFICIENCIES OF OTHER CIRCULATING PHAGOCYTES

Monocytopenia, eosinopenia, and basophilopenia are seen in most of the bone marrow failure states associated with neutropenia. Selective *monocytopenia*, however, is very unusual. In view of the heterogeneous and critical roles played by the monocyte-macrophage in normal physiology (Ch. 138), complete failure of monocyte production for a period of more than 9 to 10 months (the estimated lifespan of tissue macrophages) may be incompatible with life.

Eosinopenia and *basophilopenia* are more common than monocytopenia in clinical practice and most often represent redistributional mechanisms resulting from stress, including acute infections, widespread neoplasms, and severe injury (e.g., burns). A variety of humoral factors, including glucocorticoids, prostaglandins, and epinephrine, are released in such settings and are known to induce eosinopenia. In view of the consistency of this stress response, if a patient with sepsis does not have eosinopenia, one should consider that adrenocortical insufficiency or a primary myeloproliferative syndrome may coexist.

LYMPHOCYTOPENIA. The life cycle of the neutrophil involves a well-defined and limited set of compartments and a unidirectional flow of cells from the marrow to the blood and from the blood to the tissues. Lymphocyte production and traffic are difficult to assess: (1) Both T and B lymphocytes replicate in heterogeneous anatomic sites, including the lymph nodes, spleen, tonsils, and bone marrow; (2) lymphocytes are capable of leaving and then later re-entering a given compartment. Given these variables, it is surprising that the lymphocyte counts in the peripheral blood are so tightly regulated; normal counts range from 2 to 4×10^9 per liter. Approximately 20 per cent of these are B lymphocytes, and 70 per cent are T lymphocytes. Lymphocytopenia is defined as a peripheral blood lymphocyte count below 1.5×10^9 per liter.

ETIOLOGY AND PATHOGENESIS. Lymphocytopenia can result from three types of abnormalities: (1) those of lymphocyte production, (2) those of lymphocyte traffic, and (3) those of lymphocyte loss and destruction (Table 140–2).

Reduced Production of Lymphocytes. The most common cause of reduced lymphocyte production in the world is *protein-calorie malnutrition* (Ch. 201). The immunologic paresis resulting from malnutrition contributes substantially to the high incidence of infection in malnourished populations. *Radiation* and *immunosuppressive agents*, including alkylating agents and antithymocyte globulin, can induce lymphocytopenia by injuring the progenitor pool and inhibiting replication of more well differentiated cells. A variety of *congenital lymphocytopenic immunodeficiency states* exist, some of which result in selective deficiencies of B lymphocytes, some of T cells, and, in other cases, combined deficiencies of both T cells and B cells (Ch. 244). The mechanisms by which production and maturation of B and T lymphocytes are impaired in these patients are heterogeneous; many are ill defined. Immunodeficiency states can clearly exist even in the absence of lymphocytopenia, because of abnormal lymphocyte function or selective deficiency of one component of the circulating lymphocyte population. Certain *viruses* are capable of inducing lymphocytopenia; some of these agents infect lymphoid cells and cause their destruction. Such viruses include measles, polio, varicella zoster, and HIV (human immunodeficiency virus, the acquired immunodeficiency syndrome [AIDS] virus) (Part XXI). HIV does not frequently cause lymphocytopenia but does infect the helper (T4$^+$) subset of T lymphocytes and destroys them, a process that results in a marked decline in the absolute numbers of helper (T4$^+$) T cells in the peripheral circulation. Patients with untreated Hodgkin's disease occasionally have lymphocytopenia, especially during the late stages of the disease and with the least favorable histologic subtypes (Ch. 148).

Alterations in Lymphocyte Traffic. Alterations are common and most frequently represent transient responses to a variety of stressful events, including bacterial infections and trauma. These responses are likely mediated by high levels of endogenous glucocorticoids that induce rapid declines in circulating levels of B and T lymphocytes. The lymphocytopenic response to this type of steroid results from a self-limited shift of lymphocytes away from the peripheral blood compartment. Lymphocyte values generally return to normal within 24 to 48 hours. For this reason, the transient declines induced by endogenous steroid production

TABLE 140–2. CAUSES OF LYMPHOCYTOPENIA

Abnormalities of lymphocyte production
  Protein-calorie malnutrition
  Radiation
  Immunosuppressive therapeutic agents
  Congenital immunodeficiency states
    Wiskott-Aldrich syndrome
    Nezelof's syndrome
    Adenosine deaminase deficiency
  Viral infections
  Hodgkin's lymphoma (?)
  Widespread granulomatous infection (mycobacterial, fungal)
Alterations in lymphocyte traffic
  Acute bacterial infection, trauma, stress, glucocorticoids
  Viral infection
  Widespread granulomatous infection
  Hodgkin's lymphoma (?)
Lymphocyte destruction or loss
  Viral infection
  Antibody-mediated lymphocyte destruction
  Protein-losing enteropathy
  Chronic right ventricular failure
  Thoracic duct drainage or rupture

are not associated with functional immunologic deficiency. Certain viruses can also bind to lymphocyte populations and cause their departure from the blood compartment into other sites.

More persistent lymphocytopenia has been described in patients with widespread granulomatous disease, a phenomenon that is likely multifactorial, deriving from both inhibition of production and alterations of traffic. Patients with these disorders are often difficult to treat. Establishing a cause-and-effect relationship between the infection and lymphocytopenia is difficult when one considers that the reverse might just as easily be true; consider, for example, the frequency of mycobacterial infection in patients with AIDS.

Increased Destruction of Lymphocytes. Lymphocytopenia can occur as a result of *viral infection*, as outlined above. In some patients lymphocytopenia results from *antilymphocyte antibodies.* As was the case in patients with immunologically mediated neutropenia, the majority of such individuals have underlying autoimmune or rheumatic diseases. Losses of viable lymphocytes can also occur because of *structural defects* in sites of high-density lymphocyte traffic, e.g., via thoracic duct fistulas. In such patients, both T cells and B cells decline in the peripheral blood. Loss of lymphocytes from intestinal lymphatics can occur in protein-losing enteropathies, severe congestive heart failure, or primary diseases of the gut or intestinal lymphatics (Table 140–2).

CLINICAL MANIFESTATIONS AND DIAGNOSIS. There are no specific clinical manifestations of lymphocytopenia per se. The signs and symptoms present in patients with lymphocytopenia are those characteristic of the disease with which the cytopenia is associated. Whether the patient exhibits signs of immunologic deficiency depends on the pathophysiology of the disorder, the duration of the disease, which subsets of lymphocytes are affected most significantly, and the degree to which cellular or humoral immunity is functionally perturbed. Accordingly, unless the clinical setting is clearly one in which transient lymphocytopenia is likely, the approach to diagnosis should involve comprehensive assessment of the integrity of the immune apparatus. Specifically, the subsets of lymphocytes remaining in the circulating blood should be identified and should at least include B cells, helper-inducer T cells, and cytotoxic-suppressor T cells. In addition, quantitative immunoglobulin levels should be measured in the serum, and a series of skin tests performed to detect deficiencies of cell-mediated immunity.

TREATMENT. Because lymphocytopenia ordinarily represents a response to an underlying disease, primary attention must be paid to establishing the nature of that disease and instituting therapy for it. Patients whose lymphocytopenia is accompanied by hypogammaglobulinemia may require immune globulin replacement therapy (Ch. 244). The treatment of severe deficiencies of cell-mediated immunity remains experimental. Responses have been described with transplantation of allogeneic marrow, fetal liver, or thymic epithelial cells.

Brandt SJ, Peters WP, Atwater SK, et al.: Effect of recombinant human granulocyte-macrophage colony-stimulating factor on hematopoietic reconstitution after high-dose chemotherapy and autologous bone marrow transplantation. N Engl J Med 318:869, 1988. Neta R, Oppenheim JJ: Cytokines in therapy of radiation injury. Blood 72:1093, 1988. Pluda JM, Yarchoan R, Smith PD, et al.: Subcutaneous recombinant granulocyte-macrophage colony-stimulating factor used as a single agent and in an alternating regimen with azidothymidine in leukopenic patients with severe human immunodeficiency virus infection. Blood 76:463, 1990. *The first paper provides good evidence that GM-CSF therapy can reduce the period of marrow failure in patients who have received high-dose chemotherapy followed by autologous bone marrow reinfusion. The second paper, one of many by this group, indicates that interleukin 1 (IL1) is radioprotective in mice and is capable of protecting mice from life-threatening marrow failure even when administered after radiation exposure. It is likely that clinical trials in humans will begin soon. The third paper supports, in a clinical study, the legitimacy of the concern that GM-CSF, used as a single agent, may activate proviral expression in latently infected cells and also demonstrates that GM-CSF enhances the antiviral activity of azidothymidine.*
Gabrilove JL, Jakubowski A, Scher H, et al.: Effect of granulocyte colony-stimulating factor on neutropenia and associated morbidity due to chemotherapy for transitional-cell carcinoma of the urothelium. N Engl J Med 318:1414, 1988. Bonilla MA, Gillio AP, Ruggeiro M, et al.: Effects of recombinant human granulocyte colony-stimulating factor on neutropenia in patients with congenital agranulocytosis. N Engl J Med 320:1574, 1989. Negrin RS, Haeuber DH, Nagler A, et al.: Maintenance treatment of patients with myelodysplastic

syndromes using recombinant human granulocyte colony-stimulating factor. Blood 76:36, 1990. *These three papers provide convincing evidence that G-CSF therapy will likely be part of future standard therapy for selected patients with the disorders discussed by the respective authors. GM-CSF and G-CSF not only stimulate granulocyte production but also activate neutrophils to become more potently phagocytic, another advantage for the neutropenic patient.*
Hoffman R, Benz EJ, Shattil FJ, et al.: Hematology: Basic Principles and Practice. New York, Churchill Livingstone, 1991. *This new textbook of hematology includes a number of informative and well-referenced chapters on phagocyte and lymphocyte production, granulopoietic factors, and phagocyte traffic and function.*
Jacob HS, Craddock PR, Hammerschmidt D, et al.: Complement-induced granulocyte aggregation. An unsuspected mechanism of disease. N Engl J Med 302:789, 1980. *This work documents very well the rapidity with which complement-induced aggregation can account not only for neutropenia but for significant respiratory dysfunction as well.*
Lelezari P, Jiang A-F, Yegen L, et al.: Chronic autoimmune neutropenia due to anti-NA2 antibody. N Engl J Med 293:744, 1975. *Despite the difficulties in documenting shortened survival of a cell whose survival is intrinsically short, this paper presents good evidence that chronic neutropenia can be mediated by antibodies directed at antigens expressed by neutrophils.*
Metcalf D: The molecular control of cell division, differentiation, commitment and maturation in haemopoietic cells. Nature 339:27, 1989. Clark SC, Kamen R: The human hematopoietic colony-stimulating factors. Science 236:1229, 1987. *These are two comprehensive reviews by investigators who have themselves contributed mightily to the development of new knowledge on the structure, function, and biologic activity of heterogeneous hematopoietic growth factors. Potential readers should not be daunted by the breadth of Metcalf's title; the article is short and focuses almost exclusively on humoral control.*
Vincent PC: Drug induced aplastic anaemia and agranulocytosis. Incidence and mechanisms. Drugs 31:52, 1986. *This comprehensive review is informative and is easy to read.*

141 Leukocytosis and Leukemoid Reactions

Grover C. Bagby, Jr.

Circulating leukocytes consist of neutrophils, monocytes, eosinophils, basophils, and lymphocytes. Any one or all of these cell types can rise to abnormal levels in peripheral blood in response to various stimuli. Each type of leukocyte is produced by the bone marrow in response to specific growth factors. The term *leukocytosis,* an increase in the total leukocyte count to a level above 11.0×10^9 per liter, is less meaningful clinically than are terms that identify the type of leukocyte that is predominantly increased. The terms *neutrophilia* (neutrophilic leukocytosis), *monocytosis, lymphocytosis, eosinophilia,* and *basophilia* suggest specific diagnostic considerations.

Leukocytosis is a common finding in acutely ill patients. When the leukocyte count exceeds 25 to 30×10^9 per liter, it is termed a *leukemoid reaction.* Leukemoid reactions generally reflect the response of healthy bone marrow to signals that evolve in the patient under the influence of trauma, inflammation, and similar stresses. Leukemoid reactions are *not* synonymous with *leukoerythroblastosis,* which indicates the presence of immature white cells and nucleated red cells in the peripheral blood irrespective of the total leukocyte count. Leukoerythroblastosis is less common than leukemoid reactions but often, especially in the adult patient, reflects serious marrow dysfunction (Table 141–1). Consequently, the finding of leukoerythroblastosis (see Color Plate 7F, left) represents a clear indication to perform bone marrow aspiration and biopsy, unless the clinical setting is acute severe hemolytic anemia, sepsis in a patient with hyposplenism, or massive trauma (with multiple fractures).

NEUTROPHILIA

PATHOPHYSIOLOGY. There are three major anatomic sites of neutrophil traffic: the bone marrow, the peripheral blood, and the extravascular space (Fig. 141–1). Traffic moves unidirectionally from marrow to blood to extravascular space. The number of neutrophils within each site can be independently regulated. The number of neutrophil precursors in the marrow mitotic pool (MiP) is largely influenced by the granulopoietic growth factors:

Normal marrow
  Severe acute hemolytic anemia
  Acute infection in hyposplenic patients
Abnormal marrow
  Multiple fractures
  Marrow infiltration
    Tuberculosis
    Fungal disease
    Fibrosis
    Malignant cells (carcinoma, sarcoma, lymphoma,
      myeloma, acute leukemia)
  Chronic myeloproliferative disorders
    Agnogenic myeloid metaplasia
    Chronic myelogenous leukemia
  Other disorders
    Osteopetrosis
    Gaucher's disease
    Amyloidosis
    Paget's disease of bone
    Severe tissue hypoxia

granulocyte-macrophage colony-stimulating factor (GM-CSF) and granulocyte colony-stimulating factor (G-CSF). These factors, the products of separate genes, not only function to stimulate the growth and differentiation of granulocyte and/or macrophage progenitor cells but also functionally activate neutrophils. The marrow storage pool is sufficient to provide the periphery with neutrophils for about 5 days in the steady state, even if it were unsupported by the MiP. Neutrophils are released from the storage pool into the circulating pool in response to a variety of physiologic stresses, including endogenous glucocorticoids (Fig. 141–1B). Peripheral neutrophils are normally equally divided between the circulating pool and the marginated pool. Neutrophilia can therefore result from a shift of neutrophils from the marginated to the circulating pool—"demargination" (Fig. 141–1C). This response is rapid and can be induced by injections of

epinephrine. In patients with acute inflammatory illnesses, storage pool release and demargination usually occur together (Fig. 141–1D).

A complex regulatory network of mononuclear phagocytes, stromal cells, lymphocytes, and granulocyte progenitors and their progeny responds to acute inflammatory events by augmenting production of the critically important CSF's (Fig. 141–2). The CSF's act on the granulopoietic progenitors to increase mitosis, which expands the storage pool and consequently increases the size of the blood and extravascular pools (Fig. 141–1E). This new state persists until the inflammatory process is resolved.

CAUSES. Neutrophilia (neutrophil counts greater than 7.5 × 10⁹ per liter), a common finding in clinical practice, usually reflects the inflammatory response to acute or subacute infection (Fig. 141–2, Table 141–2) (see Color Plate 7A). Indeed, while the presence of neutrophilia should initiate a search for the cause of this response, it should also be viewed as a sign that the patient is likely responding appropriately to the stimulus.

When neutrophilia occurs in the absence of evidence of acute inflammation or illness, three conditions should be considered: (1) Certain agents such as glucocorticoids, lithium chloride, or epinephrine commonly produce neutrophilia. (2) Malignant tumors may express certain of the CSF genes inappropriately and thereby increase CSF blood levels. When such cancers are effectively treated, the neutrophilia resolves. (3) The chronic myeloproliferative disorders—chronic myelogenous leukemia, agnogenic myeloid metaplasia, essential thrombocytosis, and polycythemia rubra vera—may result in substantial neutrophilia. Patients with these diseases can present with few symptoms. When there is an acute inflammatory illness, it is most prudent to await its resolution before seeking to rule out one of the myeloproliferative disorders.

DIAGNOSIS. The diagnostic approach to patients with neutrophilia is presented as an algorithm in Figure 141–3. Notice that the diagnostic path leads quickly to the performance of bone marrow aspiration and biopsy for patients with leukoerythroblastosis. In patients without leukoerythroblastosis, neutrophilic leu-

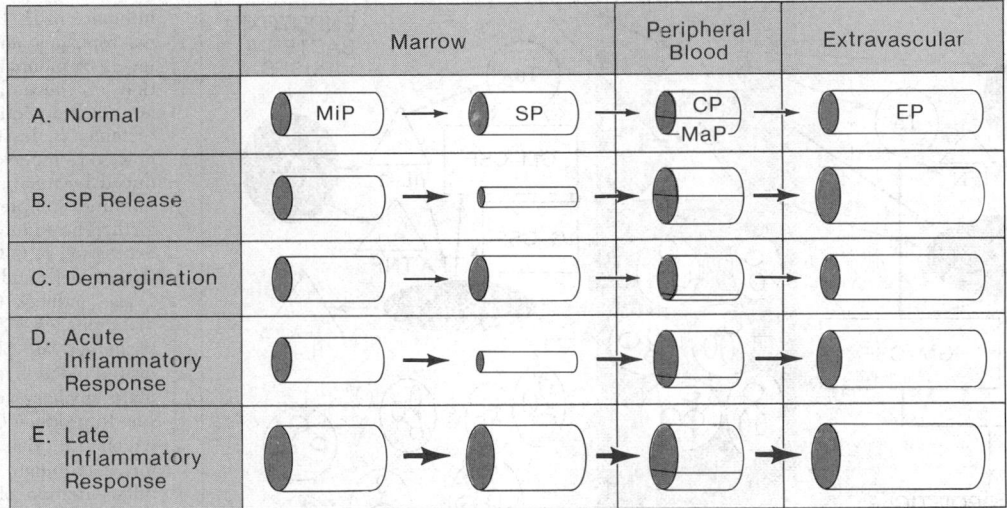

FIGURE 141–1. Pathophysiologic mechanisms of neutrophilia. In this figure the size of a given compartment is represented by the size of a given cylinder. The number of cells leaving a compartment for the next compartment is reflected by the size of the arrows between compartments. *A,* MiP = the mitotic pool of granulocyte precursor cells; SP = the granulocyte storage pool; CP = the circulating granulocyte pool; MaP = the marginated pool; EP = the extravascular pool. Notice that in every case the circulating neutrophil pool is large, but the size of the other pools is variable. *B,* A variety of stresses on the organism can result, perhaps through the action of glucocorticoid hormones, in the release of storage pool granulocytes. This occurs commonly as an acute response to acute infections. *C,* The circulating granulocyte pool can also increase in size by virtue of a shift of neutrophils from the marginated to the circulating pool. The demargination response can be regularly elicited by the administration of epinephrine and can also result from a variety of stresses, including acute infection. *D,* With most bacterial infections and other inflammatory processes, the acute demand for neutrophils in the infected extravascular sites results in the simultaneous release of storage pool neutrophils and demargination. *E,* Once the hematopoietic growth factor released in response to the inflammatory stimulus (see Fig. 141–2) has induced a few days of proliferation in the mitotic pool, the content of granulocytes in all pools increases, and delivery to the tissues becomes maximal.

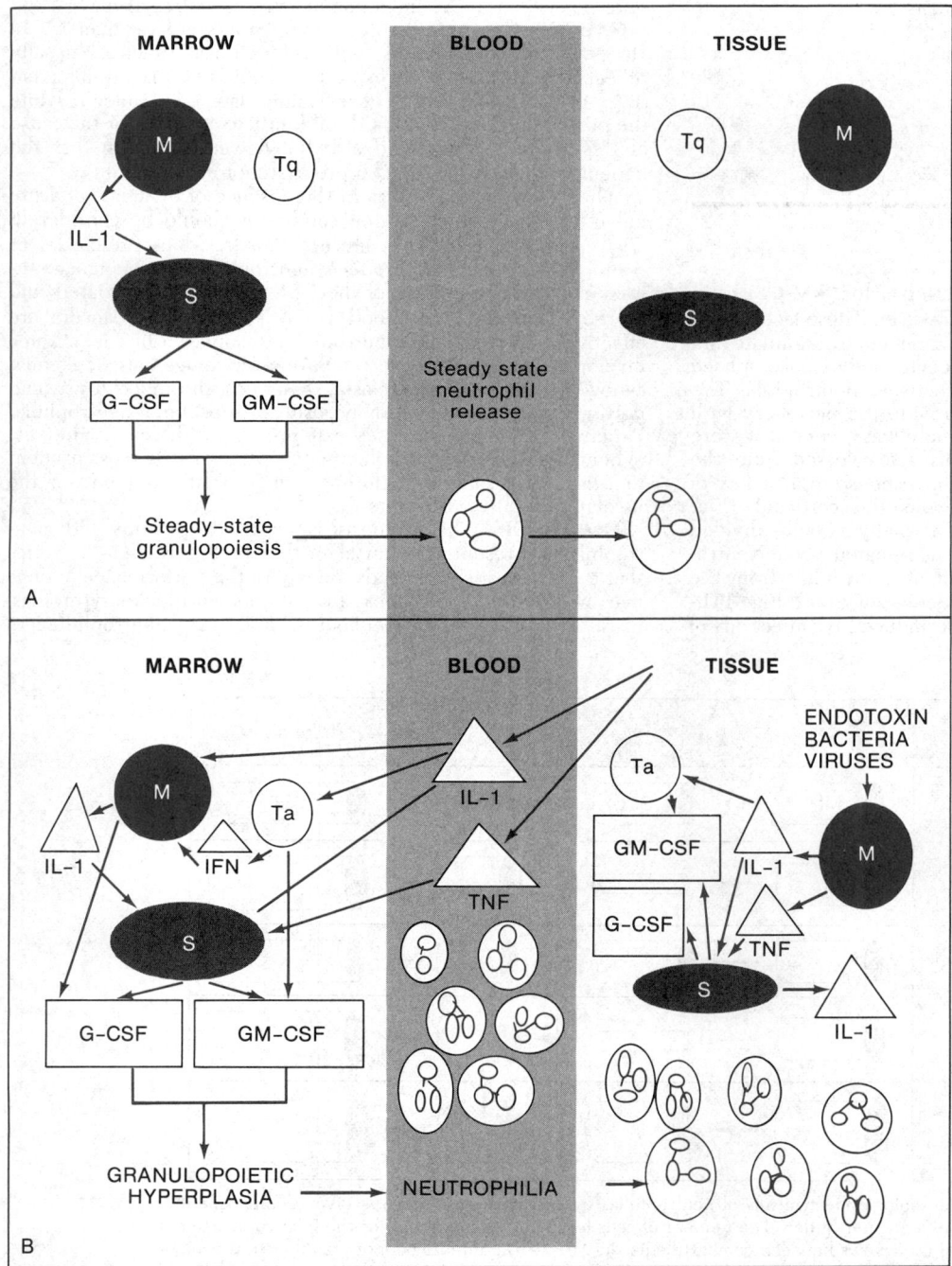

FIGURE 141–2. An intercellular regulatory network controls the production and function of phagocytes in inflammation. The figure represents the likely mechanisms by which neutrophil production and function are enhanced during the inflammatory response. The cells *(circles)* labeled M, S, and T represent monocytes/macrophages, stromal cells (e.g., fibroblasts and endothelial cells), and T lymphocytes, respectively. Tq are quiescent T cells (not activated), and Ta are activated T cells. Neutrophils have segmented trilobed nuclei. Two monokines, interleukin 1 (IL-1) and tumor necrosis factor–alpha (TNF), are depicted by triangles labeled IL-1 or TNF. The two granulopoietic factors—granulocyte colony-stimulating factor (G-CSF) and granulocyte-macrophage CSF (GM-CSF)—are symbolized by rectangles. Relative concentrations of monokines and CSF's are reflected by the size of the triangles or rectangles, respectively. *A,* In the steady state, stromal cells of the marrow produce both CSF's. The production of G-CSF and GM-CSF by stromal cells even in the steady state may be under the influence of IL-1 produced by marrow macrophages and monocytes. Blood levels of monokines are low. Production of these factors in uninflamed nonhematopoietic tissues is barely detectable. *B,* In states of inflammation, however, monokine production is induced by microorganisms, endotoxin, immune complexes, crystals, and so forth. The induced monokines induce expression of G-CSF and GM-CSF by stromal cells and activated T cells. IL-1 also induces G-CSF expression in macrophages. CSF's produced in the tissue activate phagocytes locally. Elevated blood levels of monokines stimulate auxiliary cells in the bone marrow to produce G-CSF and GM-CSF, which, in that microenvironmental niche, stimulate increased growth and differentiation of granulocyte precursors, with consequent granulocytic hyperplasia and neutrophilic leukocytosis.

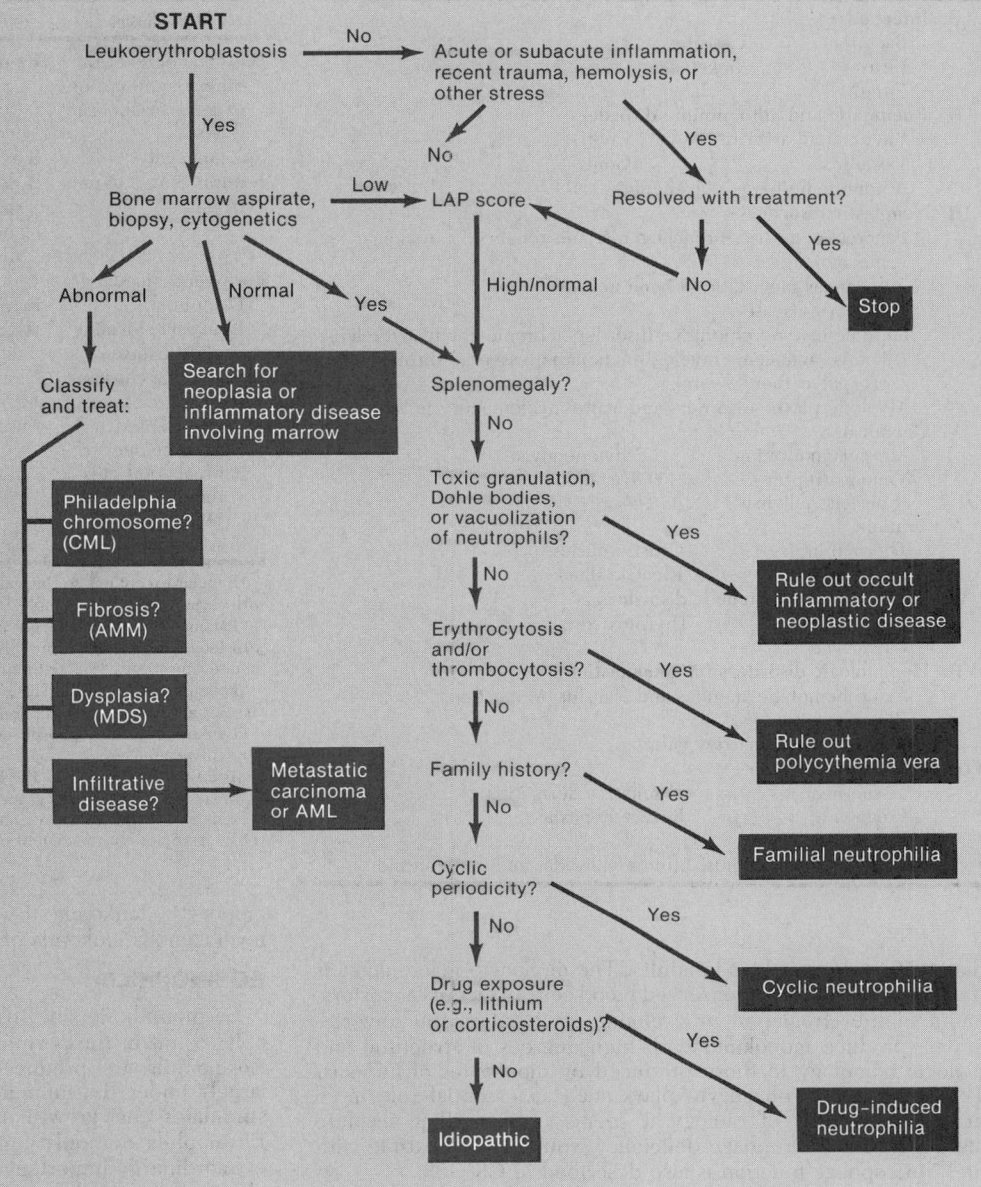

FIGURE 141–3. An algorithm for the evaluation of patients with neutrophilic leukocytosis (NL). LAP = leukocyte alkaline phosphatase; CML = chronic myelogenous leukemia; AMM = agnogenic myeloid metaplasia; MDS = myelodysplastic syndromes; AML = acute myelogenous leukemia. Branch termini are enclosed in boxes.

kocytosis generally results from acute toxic, inflammatory, or traumatic stresses, and it is usually best simply to observe the course of neutrophilia to determine its degree of linkage with the underlying disease. If the underlying disease resolves and the neutrophilia does not, other, less common, explanations must be pursued.

Neutrophil Morphology. Neutrophil morphology can lead to early diagnosis (Fig. 141–3). Toxic granulation of neutrophils, the presence of Döhle bodies (see Color Plate 7C), and the presence of vacuoles in the neutrophil cytoplasm suggest that overt or subclinical inflammation, exposure to a toxin, trauma, or neoplasia exists. Because glucocorticoids induce prompt eosinopenia and basophilopenia, these cells are almost universally absent in the blood of the acutely injured or infected patient. Thus their presence should indicate that (1) the acutely ill patient may have concomitant adrenocortical insufficiency, (2) the neutrophilia derives from the inappropriate production of GM-CSF (generally by malignant cells), or (3) the neutrophilia is one manifestation of a hematopoietic neoplasm (a chronic myeloproliferative disorder, myelodysplastic syndrome, or certain of the acute nonlymphocytic leukemias).

Leukocyte Alkaline Phosphatase. Leukocyte alkaline phosphatase (LAP) activity is restricted to the neutrophil. Simple histochemical techniques are used to measure LAP levels in neutrophils of the peripheral blood. When neutrophilia represents a

reaction to an acute illness, the LAP levels usually increase substantially. In chronic myelogenous leukemia (CML), however, the LAP score is markedly decreased. A low LAP level in a patient with neutrophilia should therefore lead to a diagnostic evaluation designed to rule out CML (Table 141–3 and Fig. 141–3).

Differential Diagnosis of Neutrophilic Leukemoid Reactions. Neutrophilic leukemoid reactions generally occur in patients who are obviously systemically ill. When the neutrophil count exceeds 80×10^9 per liter, or when the mildness of the systemic illness seems discordant with the extremely high level of neutrophils in the peripheral blood, the diagnosis most often considered is CML. A number of additional features distinguish leukemoid reactions from CML (Table 141–3). In the past, the most definitive test for CML has been a marrow chromosome analysis for the Philadelphia chromosome (see Ch. 144). In the near future, even more sensitive tests may be direct DNA analyses to detect structural changes in the bcr (breakpoint cluster region) locus on chromosome 22 or immunoassay for the abnormal c-abl gene product p210 (Table 141–3).

MONOCYTOSIS

Monocytosis is defined as absolute peripheral blood monocyte counts greater than 0.80×10^9 per liter in children and greater

TABLE 141–2. COMMON CAUSES OF NEUTROPHILIA

I. **Infections**
  Bacteria   Parasites
  Viruses   *Rickettsiae*
  Fungi
II. **Rheumatic and autoimmune disorders**
  Rheumatoid arthritis   Colitis
  Vasculitis   Gout
  Autoimmune hemolytic anemia
III. **Neoplastic disorders**
  Pancreatic, gastric, bronchogenic, and renal cell carcinoma; melanoma
  Any cancer metastatic to bone marrow
  Hodgkin's disease
  Chronic myeloproliferative disorders (chronic granulocytic leukemia, agnogenic myeloid metaplasia, essential thrombocytosis, polycythemia vera)
  Myelodysplastic disorders and acute myelomonocytic leukemia
IV. **Chemicals**
  Mercury poisoning   Ethylene glycol
  Venoms (reptiles,   Histamine
    insects, jellyfish)
V. **Trauma**
  Thermal injury   Crush injuries
  Hypothermia   Electric shock
VI. **Endocrine and metabolic disorders**
  Ketoacidosis   Thyrotoxicosis
  Lactic acidosis
VII. **Hematologic disorders (nonneoplastic)**
  Acute hemolytic anemias and transfusion reactions
  Postsplenectomy
  Recovery from marrow failure
VIII. **Other disorders**
  Tissue necrosis   Exfoliative dermatitis
  Pregnancy   Severe hypoxia
  Eclampsia
  Drugs: corticosteroids, lithium chloride, and epinephrine

TABLE 141–3. DISTINCTIONS BETWEEN NEUTROPHILIC LEUKEMOID REACTIONS AND CHRONIC MYELOGENOUS LEUKEMIA (CML)

Finding/Result	Leukemoid Reaction	CML
Presence of fever or other manifestations of acute or subacute illness	Usual*	Infrequent†
Splenomegaly	Rare	Frequent
Natural course of neutrophilia	Resolution linked temporally with abatement of underlying disease	Progressive slow increase over time
Peripheral blood:		
Basophilia	Rare‡	Common
Leukocyte alkaline phosphatase	High	Low§
Philadelphia chromosome	Never	Frequent (85%)
Abnormal DNA: Rearrangement of breakpoint cluster region in DNA (chromosome 22)	Absent‖	Frequent (>85%)

*Regular exceptions to this rule are patients with leukemoid reactions associated with certain carcinomas (Table 141–1).

†Patients with CML are not exempt from developing infections. Some patients with infectious processes may be found to have CML. The ideal time to evaluate them diagnostically is after the inflammatory process resolves.

‡Patients with acute allergic reactions and patients with widespread parasitic diseases are frequently exceptions to this rule.

§Leukocyte alkaline phosphatase scores are sometimes normal in CML patients after splenectomy.

‖As described in Ch. 144, the Philadelphia chromosome forms when chromosome 22 breaks in a region called the breakpoint cluster region (bcr). There are some patients with CML who have no Philadelphia chromosome on karyotypic analysis, yet do have bcr rearrangement on DNA analysis.

than 0.50×10^9 per liter in adults. The monocyte-macrophage is the most evolutionarily conserved blood cell. In fact, its ancestors, found in the circulation or coelomic cavity of marine invertebrates, produce monokines with high degrees of structural and biologic homology to those produced by monocytes of humans. The mononuclear phagocyte plays such an essential role in so many components of biology it seems unlikely that absolute monocyte and macrophage deficiency would be compatible with life. Macrophage function is also described in Ch. 138.

Monocytes present antigen to lymphocytes, mediate cellular cytotoxicity, release procoagulants, participate in bone remodeling and wound repair, dispose of damaged cells, and regulate immune and hematopoietic responses by producing interleukin 1 (IL1), tumor necrosis factor (TNF)–alpha, G-CSF, and certain alpha-interferons. Two factors stimulate the growth and differentiation of mononuclear phagocytes: M-CSF and GM-CSF (Fig. 141–3). Stromal cells, including endothelial cells and fibroblasts, constitutively produce M-CSF, a protein that acts only on cells of the monocyte lineage to stimulate their differentiation and survival. Steady-state monocyte production probably depends upon GM-CSF production. M-CSF production is not clearly inducible by factors released during the inflammatory response, but GM-CSF production is induced during inflammation (Fig. 141–2).

The mononuclear phagocyte is more sluggish than the neutrophil in moving toward and killing bacteria but is as effective, if not more so, in killing obligate intracellular parasites such as fungi, yeast, and viruses. In addition, it participates substantially in all types of granulomatous inflammation. Accordingly, monocytosis is often seen in patients with tuberculosis, syphilis, fungal infections, ulcerative and granulomatous colitis, and sarcoidosis (Table 141–4). Mild monocytosis is common in patients with Hodgkin's disease and a variety of cancers. High levels of monocytes in the blood are most often seen in patients with myeloid malignant diseases, including acute and chronic myelo-

monocytic leukemia, acute monocytic leukemia, and chronic myelogenous leukemia of the juvenile type.

EOSINOPHILIA

Eosinophilic leukocytosis (eosinophilia) exists when the eosinophil count in the peripheral blood exceeds 0.4×10^9 per liter. Eosinophils are produced by progenitor cells in the marrow largely under the influence of interleukin 5, a protein that also stimulates the growth and differentiation of B lymphocytes. Eosinophils not only function as phagocytes but also play an extraordinarily important role in modulating the potentially toxic effects of mast cell degranulation in hypersensitivity reactions.

The eosinophilic syndromes and the causes of eosinophilia are described in Ch. 150.

TABLE 141–4. CAUSES OF MONOCYTOSIS

I. **Infections**
  Tuberculosis   Syphilis
  Brucellosis   Fungal infections
  Bacterial endocarditis   Recovery from acute infections
  Typhoid and paratyphoid   Protozoal infections
    fevers
  Listeriosis
II. **Neoplastic disorders**
  Hodgkin's disease
  Carcinoma (many)
  Acute and chronic myelomonocytic leukemia, myelodysplastic syndromes, and chronic myelogenous leukemia of the juvenile type
III. **Gastrointestinal disorders**
  Ulcerative colitis   Cirrhosis
  Granulomatous colitis
IV. **Sarcoidosis**
V. **Drug reactions**
VI. **Recovery from marrow suppression**
VII. **Congenital neutropenia**

LYMPHOCYTOSIS

Lymphocytosis is defined as any lymphocyte count in excess of 5.0×10^9 per liter. Atypical lymphocytosis is present when atypical lymphocytes account for more than 20 per cent of the total peripheral blood lymphocyte population (see Color Plate 7*B*). The production and traffic of lymphocytes are clearly under tight control. A number of factors induce growth of T lymphocytes (IL2 and IL3), natural killer cells (IL2), and B lymphocytes (IL2, B cell stimulatory factor [BSF]–1, BSF–2, and B cell growth factor II).

DIAGNOSIS. Mild to moderate lymphocytosis (lymphocyte counts $< 12 \times 10^9$ per liter) is most commonly caused by viral infections, notably infectious mononucleosis and infectious hepatitis. Careful examination of the peripheral blood lymphocyte morphology can help distinguish between these two disorders. In infectious mononucleosis (see Ch. 373), many of the lymphocytes are large, with abundant cytoplasm and a ballerina skirt–like cytoplasmic border. These are the characteristic "atypical" lymphocytes that exceed 20 per cent of the total lymphocyte population during the course of this disease. Interestingly, while the B lymphocyte is the target of the causative Epstein-Barr (EB) virus, the majority of the cells in the peripheral blood of patients with this disease are T lymphocytes. This proliferative response of T cells probably plays a major role in coordinating the process of recovery from the viral infection.

Acute bacterial infections rarely cause lymphocytosis. One exception is pertussis (in children), in which profound lymphocytosis (up to 60×10^9 per liter) is sometimes seen. Interestingly, specific soluble factors derived from the causative organism, *Bordetella pertussis*, induce lymphocytosis in experimental ani-

mals. In Table 141–5 are listed a variety of additional disorders associated with mild to moderate lymphocytosis. Perhaps with the exception of those with early chronic lymphocytic leukemia, most patients have overt signs of an underlying illness involving anatomic sites other than the lymphohematopoietic system. This

TABLE 141–5. CAUSES OF LYMPHOCYTOSIS

I. High ($>15 \times 10^9$ per liter)
Infectious mononucleosis
Pertussis
Acute infectious lymphocytosis
Chronic lymphocytic leukemia
Acute lymphocytic leukemia

II. Moderate ($<15 \times 10^9$ per liter)
Many viral infections
  Infectious mononucleosis
  Measles
  Varicella
  Hepatitis
  Coxsackie
  Adenovirus
  Mumps
  Cytomegalovirus
Other infectious diseases
  Toxoplasmosis
  Brucellosis
  Tuberculosis
  Typhoid fever
  Syphilis (secondary)
Neoplastic disorders
  Carcinoma
  Hodgkin's disease
  Acute lymphocytic leukemia (early)
  Chronic lymphocytic leukemia (early)
Other disorders
  Graves' disease

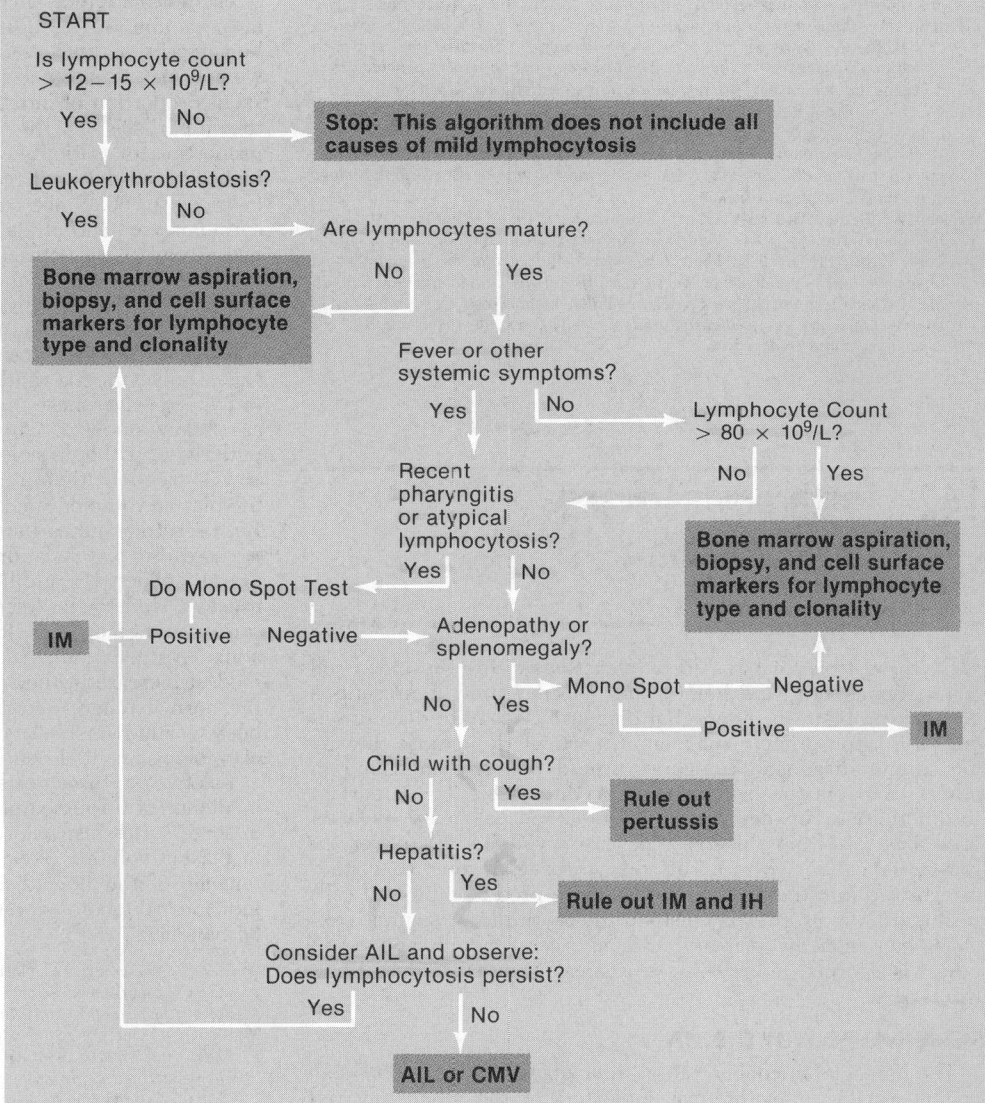

FIGURE 141–4. An algorithm for the evaluation of patients with lymphocytosis in excess of 12×10^9 per liter. IM = infectious mononucleosis; CMV = cytomegalovirus infection; AIL = acute infectious lymphocytosis; IH = infectious hepatitis. Branch termini are enclosed in boxes.

rule also holds true for patients with substantial lymphocytosis (>12 to 15×10^9 per liter), the differential diagnosis of which is limited (Table 141–5). The diagnostic approach presented as an algorithm in Figure 141–4 depends simply upon establishing a tissue diagnosis to rule out malignant disease in patients who do not have clear-cut evidence of one of the benign disorders.

An important adjunct to histologic diagnosis is immunophenotypic analysis of the lymphocyte surface. Not only will such studies provide evidence for or against dominance of one lymphocyte type, but they are also capable of determining whether B lymphocytes in the circulation are all members of a single (therefore, likely neoplastic) clone.

Bagby GC, Dinarello CA, Wallace P, et al.: Interleukin 1 stimulates granulocyte macrophage colony-stimulating activity release by vascular endothelial cells. J Clin Invest 78:1316, 1986. Broudy VC, Kaushansky K, Segal G, et al.: Tumor necrosis factor type alpha stimulates human endothelial cells to produce granulocyte/macrophage colony-stimulating factor. Proc Natl Acad Sci USA 83:7467, 1986. Zucali J, Dinarello C, Oblon D, et al.: Interleukin 1 stimulates fibroblasts to produce granulocyte-macrophage colony-stimulating activity and prostaglandin E$_2$. J Clin Invest 77:1857, 1986. *These three papers provide important evidence that the production of granulopoietic factors by stromal cells can be stimulated by the monokines IL1 and TNF-alpha. These in vitro observations provide insight into the importance of mononuclear phagocytes, the producers of monokines, as regulators of phagocyte production and function in inflammatory states. The reader is also referred to Figure 141–2.*

Clark SC: Biological activities of human granulocyte-macrophage colony-stimulating factor. Int J Cell Cloning 6:365, 1988. Metcalf D: The molecular control of cell division, differentiation, commitment and maturation in haemopoietic cells. Nature 339:27, 1989. Herrmann F, Schulz G, Lindemann A, et al.: Hematopoietic responses in patients with advanced malignancy treated with recombinant human granulocyte-macrophage colony-stimulating factor. J Clin Oncol 7:159, 1989. Sullivan R, Fredette JP, Socinski M, et al.: Enhancement of superoxide anion release by granulocytes harvested from patients receiving granulocyte-macrophage colony-stimulating factor. Br J Haematol 71:475, 1989. *For those readers interested in a short course on the biologic activities of G-CSF and GM-CSF, these papers will suffice. The first two are good reviews by two leaders in the field. The third and fourth papers provide direct experimental evidence of the two major in vivo activities of GM-CSF.*

Daley GQ, Van Etten RA, Baltimore D: Induction of chronic myelogenous leukemia in mice by the p210$^{bcr/abl}$ gene of the Philadelphia chromosome. Science 247:824, 1990. *This outstanding work provides the most up-to-date clarification of the exact role of the Philadelphia chromosome translocation in the pathophysiology of chronic myelogenous leukemia.*

Williams WJ, Beutler E, Erslev AJ, et al.: Hematology. 4th ed. New York, McGraw-Hill Book Company, 1990. Paul WE: Fundamental Immunology. 2nd ed. New York, Raven Press, 1989. *These textbooks include a number of chapters on phagocyte and lymphocyte production, traffic, distribution, and function. In the Williams text, the reviews of neutrophilia, monocytosis, eosinophilia, and lymphocytosis are comprehensive and clinically relevant. Reference lists are encyclopedic and informative.*

142 Erythrocytosis and Polycythemia

Paul D. Berk

Erythrocytosis, manifested by elevations of the red blood cell count, hematocrit, and hemoglobin concentration, represents a complex problem in differential diagnosis. Accurate diagnosis is crucial to appropriate management, particularly because therapy for certain diagnostic categories would be contraindicated in others. Early in the evaluation of erythrocytosis it is important to differentiate an increase in the total red cell mass (absolute erythrocytosis) from a decrease in plasma volume (relative erythrocytosis). Patients with absolute erythrocytosis must be further categorized into those in whom excessive production of red cells results from a disorder intrinsic to the erythroid progenitor cells of the bone marrow (primary) or from excessive stimulation of an otherwise normal marrow by substances such as erythropoietin (secondary).

RELATIVE POLYCYTHEMIA

The hemoglobin concentration, hematocrit, and red blood cell count, usually interpreted as indicators of the circulating red blood cell or hemoglobin masses, are in fact, merely measures of the extent to which the red cell mass is diluted in the plasma volume. The red cell mass and the plasma volume are regulated independently. Hence, a patient with an elevated hemoglobin concentration, hematocrit, or red cell count may have (1) an increase in the red cell mass, i.e., an absolute erythrocytosis; (2) a reduction in the plasma volume; or (3) a combination of a red cell mass at the upper end of the normal range and plasma volume at the lower end of the normal range. These last two situations have been termed relative or spurious polycythemia, since the elevated hemoglobin concentration, hematocrit, and red cell count do not reflect an absolute increase in the mass of circulating erythrocytes. Strictly speaking, the designation polycythemia should be reserved for conditions involving increased levels of other formed elements (granulocytes, platelets) in addition to erythrocytes; in fact, the term *polycythemia* is also widely applied to disorders characterized solely by abnormalities in erythroid parameters and is therefore employed in this chapter.

The most frequent cause of relative polycythemia is dehydration. Accordingly, fluid balance should be corrected before a hematologic evaluation of an elevated hematocrit is done. As an important first step, after dehydration is ruled out, patients with absolute polycythemia can be accurately distinguished from those with relative polycythemia by measurement of both the red cell mass and the plasma volume, using ^{51}Cr-labeled erythrocytes and ^{125}I-albumin, respectively. This is especially important because, in the absence of arterial hypoxemia (e.g., cyanotic congenital heart disease, chronic pulmonary disease), cases of relative polycythemia are at least as common as cases of absolute polycythemia but need not be subjected to the extensive and expensive investigations required to determine the cause of an absolute increase in the circulating red cell mass.

The normal red cell mass averages 30 ± 3 (SD) ml per kilogram in men and 27 ± 2 ml per kilogram in women. Although hematocrits as high as 54 per cent in men or 48 per cent in women may be normal, increased red cell masses are found in a small proportion of individuals of either sex with hematocrits in the upper 40's. As the hematocrit increases into the 50's, the proportion of patients with an increased red cell mass also increases but does not reach 100 per cent until the hematocrit is in excess of 60. Since approximately half of patients with polycythemia vera and other forms of true erythrocytosis and a large majority of those with spurious erythrocytosis present with hematocrits between 50 and 60, the need for direct measurement of the red cell mass to distinguish true polycythemia from spurious erythrocytosis is apparent.

Relative erythrocytosis, also called spurious polycythemia, stress polycythemia, and Gaisböck's syndrome, typically occurs in hypertensive obese middle-aged men, especially in those who are heavy smokers. The male-female ratio is at least 5:1. Its underlying pathophysiology remains obscure. Both hypertension and its frequent therapy with diuretics may lead to reduction in the plasma volume. Smoking may contribute by two mechanisms. Both nicotine and carboxyhemoglobin, which circulates in smokers because of inhalation of carbon monoxide, may have mild diuretic effects. In addition, the presence of carboxyhemoglobin causes a shift to the left in the oxygen dissociation curve of the remaining hemoglobin, leading to mildly impaired tissue oxygenation. Normal compensatory mechanisms, in turn, lead to a modest increase in the red cell mass that may not always exceed the normal range, particularly when expressed per kilogram of body weight in an obese patient. In some smokers discontinuation of smoking results in cure of the erythrocytosis.

Relative erythrocytosis is not always a benign condition, the incidence of thromboembolic events reaching almost 30 per cent in some series, especially in patients with an absolute reduction in plasma volume. Treatment remains controversial, but maintenance of the hematocrit at no more than 50 per cent by a judicious phlebotomy regimen is often recommended and may be beneficial.

Isbister JP: The contracted plasma volume syndromes (relative polycythemias) and their haemorheological significance. Clin Haematol 1:665, 1987. *A lucid review of a subject with a confusing and often contradictory literature.*

Watts EJ, Lewis SM: Spurious polycythemia—a study of 35 patients. Scand J Haematol 31:241, 1983. *An evaluation of factors, such as smoking and obesity, associated with spurious polycythemia. The authors argue in favor of treating the underlying condition rather than the hematocrit.*

ABSOLUTE POLYCYTHEMIA: PATHOPHYSIOLOGY AND CLINICAL EVALUATION

Regulation of the Red Cell Mass

The circulating red cell mass is determined by a balance between the rate at which new erythrocytes are produced and released from the bone marrow and the rate of peripheral red cell destruction. The latter, as measured by studies of the red cell lifespan, is ordinarily fixed, with a normal mean value of about 100 days. While red cell lifespan may be reduced in pathologic states, there are no mechanisms by which it may be increased. Hence, physiologic regulation of the red cell mass occurs entirely by changes in the rate of red cell production.

Alterations in the red cell mass are effected to provide for a critical level of tissue oxygenation (Fig. 142–1). The principal sensors of the state of tissue oxygenation in adults are probably located in the kidney, although the existence of extrarenal oxygen sensors has also been proposed. The kidney responds to the perceived adequacy of oxygen delivery by modulating the output of the hormone erythropoietin. The gene for this carbohydrate-rich glycoprotein has been successfully cloned, and its biologic activity has been found to reside in a polypeptide chain of 166 amino acids.

Normal hematopoiesis is regulated by a complex network of interactions between a hierarchy of bone marrow stem cells of differing proliferative capacity and potential to differentiate (see Ch. 127 and 143). The network includes a variety of soluble mediators (erythropoietin; granulocyte-macrophage colony-stimulating factor, granulocyte colony-stimulating factor, and macrophage colony-stimulating factor [GM-CSF, G-CSF, and M-CSF, respectively]; interleukins 1, 3, 5, and 6 [IL1,3,5, and 6]; insulin-like growth factor I; γ-interferon; and tumor necrosis factor [TNF]) as well as nonhematopoietic regulatory cells with both stimulatory and suppressor functions. The functions of each of these mediators in regulating hematopoiesis are still being elucidated.

Pluripotent bone marrow stem cells differentiate to the earliest erythroid-committed progenitors, the *erythroid burst-forming units* (BFU$_E$), under the influence of a T cell–derived growth regulator called *burst-promoting activity*. In vitro, such burst-promoting activity can be provided by IL3 and GM-CSF. By contrast, erythropoietin, the principal regulator of the subsequent stages of erythropoiesis, stimulates proliferation of the *erythroid colony-forming units* (CFU$_E$), the more differentiated but still morphologically unrecognizable progeny of the BFU$_E$. CFU$_E$ are primitive blastlike cells with large nuclei, a prominent nucleolus, a perinuclear clear zone, and an absence of granules. Since further differentiation of the CFU$_E$ to early, recognizable proerythroblasts is a stochastic process, expansion of the pool of CFU$_E$ results in an increase in the production of recognizable erythroid precursors in the marrow. Erythropoietin also shortens the overall maturation time of developing erythroid precursors and accelerates the release of reticulocytes into the circulation. Hence its net effect is to increase the output of red cells from the marrow and ultimately to expand the circulating red cell mass.

Mechanisms Producing Erythrocytosis

Erythrocytosis, or "polycythemia" reflects an increase in marrow red cell production caused by increased proliferation of erythroid progenitors. This proliferation could be either "autonomous," as a result of an intrinsic cellular defect permitting escape from normal regulatory mechanisms, or secondary to an external stimulus.

AUTONOMOUS PROLIFERATION. The increased erythroid activity in the primary polycythemias, including polycythemia rubra vera and the more recently described entity of primary erythrocytosis, is seemingly autonomous in that increased red cell production occurs despite low or undetectable levels of erythropoietin as measured by in vivo bioassay techniques. Moreover, "endogenous colonies" of erythroid progenitors from such patients may be successfully grown in various in vitro tissue culture systems without added erythropoietin, which is otherwise essential for erythroid progenitor growth in vitro. Finally, phlebotomy to low normal or anemic levels produces an increase in erythropoietin production, indicating that the "servomechanism" relating erythropoietin output to tissue oxygen delivery is intact. The apparent independence of erythropoiesis from erythropoietin in the primary polycythemias has been postulated to reflect a markedly increased sensitivity of erythroid progenitors to minute amounts of the hormone, rather than total independence from erythropoietin.

SECONDARY PROLIFERATION. Alternatively, the proliferation could result from abnormalities in the erythropoietic regulatory mechanism extrinsic to the erythroid progenitors themselves. The increased red cell production in these circumstances is driven by increased levels of erythropoietin or other erythroid stimulatory substances, and erythroid progenitors require exogenous erythropoietin to grow successfully in vitro. These features characterize the various secondary polycythemias.

The secondary polycythemias can be further subdivided into three categories. The *first* is disorders in which the signal resulting in erythrocytosis, most often an increase in erythropoietin production, represents a physiologically appropriate response to poor tissue oxygenation caused by arterial hypoxemia, genetically determined or "acquired" high-affinity hemoglobins that release oxygen to tissue inadequately, or reduced tissue perfusion. For these conditions, reduction of the red cell mass by phlebotomy, even to values still substantially greater than normal, may reduce tissue oxygen delivery and result in a further increase in erythropoietin output. The *second* category comprises disorders characterized by excessive autonomous production of erythropoietic stimulatory substances (erythropoietin, androgens, adrenal corticosteroids). Increased, autonomous erythropoietin production may occur in certain neoplasms, as a result of nonneoplastic lesions in the kidney (hydronephrosis, cysts, tumors, vascular lesions) that produce local ischemia involving the renal oxygen-sensing mechanism, or in certain rare familial syndromes, without a demonstrable anatomic lesion. For the disorders in this category, erythropoietin production is not influenced by phlebot-

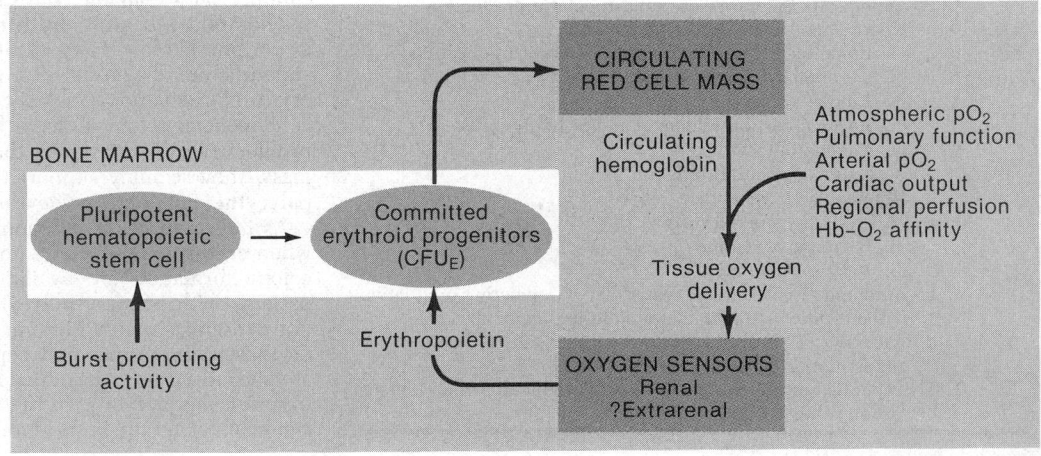

FIGURE 142–1. Relationship between tissue oxygen delivery, erythropoietin output, and the circulating red cell mass.

omy-induced changes in the red cell mass. The *third* category is the entity in which erythropoietin secretion remains under physiologic control in that it responds to phlebotomy, but at a level of production inappropriately high for the level of tissue oxygenation. A classification of the various absolute erythrocytoses, based on underlying mechanisms, is presented in Table 142–1.

Pathophysiology of Absolute Erythrocytosis

Irrespective of underlying etiology, all disorders characterized by an absolute erythrocytosis share certain common clinical manifestations resulting from the expanded blood volume and increased blood viscosity. The increased blood volume leads to generalized vascular expansion and venous engorgement, which are reflected by the characteristic ruddy cyanosis of the skin and mucous membranes. These factors are magnified by the marked decrease in cerebral blood flow that accompanies elevation of the hematocrit and in turn contributes to headaches, tinnitus, a frequently described feeling of fullness in the head and neck, and light-headedness. There appears to be an increase in thrombotic complications, particularly involving the cerebrovascular circulation, in patients with markedly elevated hematocrit and expanded blood volume. Epistaxis and upper gastrointestinal hemorrhage are also more frequent in the hypervolemic patient. The increase in viscosity accompanying hypervolemia and erythrocytosis may result in a decrease in cardiac output, in a reduction in regional blood flow, and ultimately in an impairment of tissue oxygenation, even in cases in which the underlying initial stimulus was poor oxygen delivery.

In contrast to the consequences of expanded blood volume and blood viscosity, the consequences of bone marrow hyperactivity and of increased red cell destruction are minimal. Because expansion of the red cell mass often occurs very slowly, increases in bone marrow volume, alterations in the myeloid-erythroid ratio, and changes in reticulocyte count or plasma iron turnover

TABLE 142–1. CAUSES OF ERYTHROCYTOSIS

I. Relative erythrocytosis (stress, spurious, or pseudopolycythemia; Gaisböck's syndrome)
II. Absolute erythrocytosis
  A. Primary (proliferative bone marrow disorder)
    1. Polycythemia vera
    2. Primary erythrocytosis
  B. Secondary (e.g., increased marrow stimulation by erythropoietin)
    1. Physiologically appropriate increased erythropoietin production
      a. Arterial hypoxemia
        i. High altitude
        ii. Chronic pulmonary disease
        iii. Cardiovascular shunt (right-to-left)
        iv. Massive obesity (pickwickian syndrome)
        v. Postural hypoxemia
      b. Abnormal release of oxygen from hemoglobin
        i. Hereditary hemoglobin with high oxygen affinity
        ii. Congenitally decreased red cell 2,3-DPG
        iii. Smoker's polycythemia (carboxyhemoglobinemia)
      c. Interference with tissue oxygen metabolism
        i. Cobalt
    2. Physiologically inappropriate erythropoietin production
      a. Neoplasms
        i. Renal, adrenal, hepatocellular, and ovarian carcinomas
        ii. Cerebellar hemangioblastomas (e.g., von Hippel–Lindau syndrome)
        iii. Adrenal cortical adenoma and/or hyperplasia
        iv. Pheochromocytoma
        v. Large uterine fibroids (rare)
      b. Nonneoplastic renal diseases
        i. Cysts, hydronephrosis
        ii. Bartter's syndrome
        iii. Posttransplantation
      c. Autonomous, fixed increased erythropoietin production without demonstrable anatomic lesion (familial)
      d. Excessive basal erythropoietin output with further augmentation following phlebotomy (familial)
    3. Therapeutic administration or excess production of androgens or certain other corticosteroids

may be difficult to appreciate. Similarly, although a doubling of the red cell mass results in a doubling of bilirubin production, this may be insufficient to drive the plasma unconjugated bilirubin concentration outside its relatively wide normal range.

Clinical Evaluation of the Patient with Erythrocytosis

ROLE OF CONVENTIONAL DIAGNOSTIC METHODS. A systematic approach to the evaluation of the patient with erythrocytosis is illustrated in Figure 142–2. This algorithm ensures the correct classification of patients with relative as opposed to absolute erythrocytosis. In the majority of instances, patients with absolute erythrocytosis can also be appropriately classified as having primary or secondary erythrocytosis, and in the latter case, the specific underlying cause can be identified on the basis of conventional, widely available diagnostic studies. The diagnosis of polycythemia vera is discussed later in this chapter.

SPECIAL STUDIES: ASSAY OF ERYTHROPOIETIN AND ENDOGENOUS COLONY FORMATION. Erythropoietin may be estimated by an in vivo bioassay in polycythemic mice. Injection of plasma or urine preparations from the patient into such animals stimulates the incorporation of ^{59}Fe into newly produced erythrocytes, to a degree proportional to the erythropoietin content of the injected material. When this assay is applied to urine samples, normal individuals have basal levels of erythropoietin excretion within a well-defined normal range. After phlebotomy, urinary erythropoietin excretion increases, and an inverse logarithmic relationship is observed between the hematocrit and the erythropoietin excretion rate. Patients with hypoxic secondary erythrocytosis have variable basal values ranging from normal to increased, but all have increased values following reduction of the hematocrit to normal by means of phlebotomy. In contrast, basal urinary erythropoietin excretion is very low in patients with polycythemia vera. Normal human plasma contains a mean of 25 mIU of erythropoietin per milliliter, as determined by current radioimmunoassay procedures. The lower limit of sensitivity of the polycythemic mouse assay is approximately 50 mIU per milliliter. Hence, when applied to plasma, this bioassay cannot distinguish normal subjects from those with polycythemia vera, since both groups fall below this sensitivity limit. The assay can detect the elevated levels seen in some cases of secondary polycythemia. After concentrating the plasma to increase the sensitivity of this technique, patients with polycythemia vera still had undetectable plasma levels of erythropoietin by bioassay, whereas most (but not all) normal subjects had detectable values, and the majority of patients with a clinical diagnosis of secondary polycythemia had elevated levels. Unfortunately, the concentration procedure is cumbersome and may introduce artifacts into the in vivo bioassay.

Several alternative procedures for measuring erythropoietin are now available. Radioimmunoassays (RIA's) give a well-defined normal range (typically, approximately 17 to 38 mIU per milliliter of plasma). Patients with polycythemia vera usually have significantly reduced values, and some patients with secondary erythrocytosis have appreciably elevated values, although there is overlap with the normal range in both groups. The problem of immunoreactive but biologically inert erythropoietin fractions or of other cross-reacting materials remains of concern with available RIA procedures. A hemagglutination inhibition assay is also commercially available, but its specificity has been questioned.

The ability to grow erythroid progenitors from bone marrow or peripheral blood in vitro without added erythropoietin strongly supports the diagnosis of a primary bone marrow disorder of erythroid regulation. Such seemingly erythropoietin-independent "endogenous colonies" have been reported in all of the myeloproliferative disorders. In the setting of an expanded red cell mass, they strongly support the diagnosis of one of the primary polycythemias, e.g., polycythemia vera.

As indicated in the foregoing discussion and in Figure 142–2, when erythropoietin assays and/or studies of in vitro endogenous colony formation are available, they may help to distinguish patients with primary polycythemias from those with secondary polycythemias. In addition, the influence of phlebotomy on erythropoietin output may separate the physiologically appropriate secondary polycythemias from those in which erythropoietin output is autonomous. In the majority of cases, these distinctions can be made on the basis of conventional diagnostic investigations.

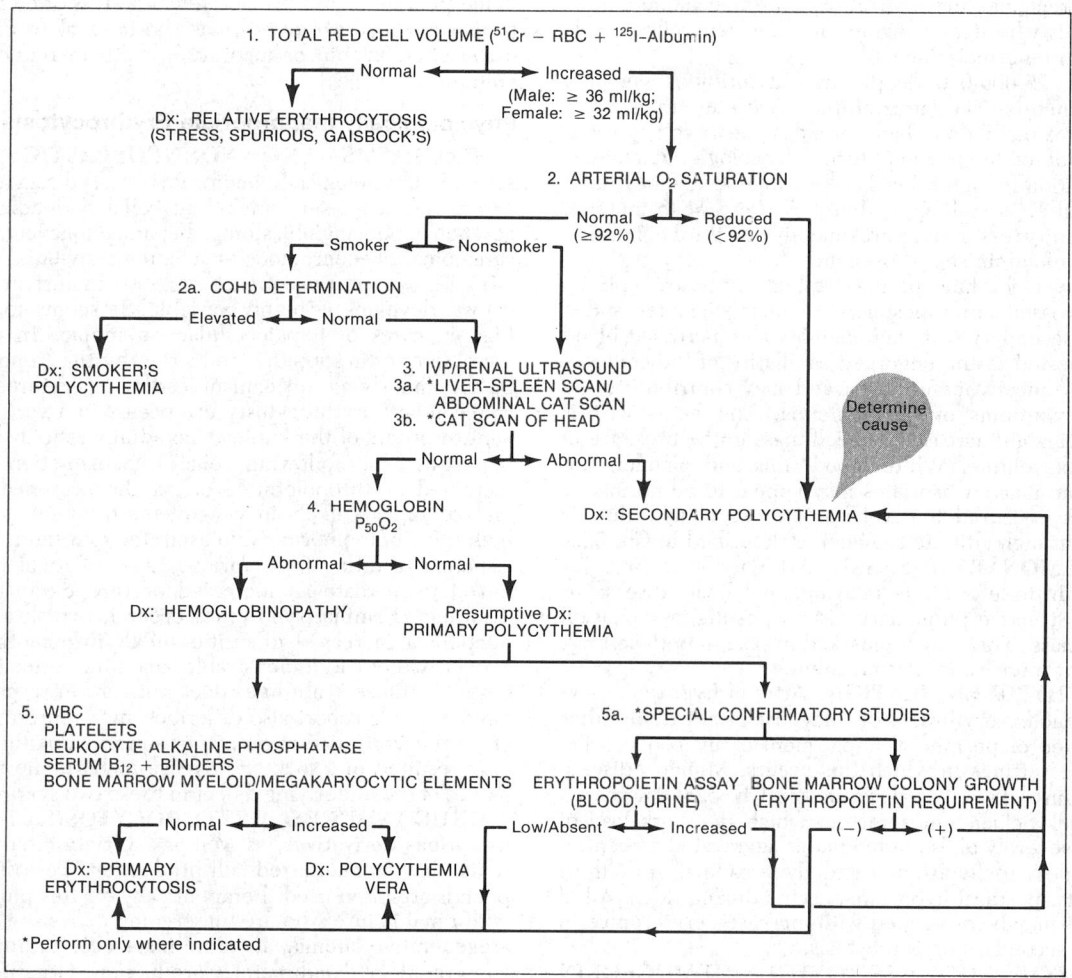

FIGURE 142–2. Algorithm for evaluation of an elevated hematocrit. Laboratory features suggestive of a myeloproliferative disease include elevated platelet and white blood cell counts and increased reticulin and clustered atypical megakaryocytes in a bone marrow biopsy. A careful history (e.g., ? family history of elevated hematocrit, ? heavy smoking) and physical examination (? splenomegaly, evidence of cardiac or pulmonary disease) provide indispensable information.

Cotes PM, Doré CJ, Liu Yin JA, et al.: Determination of serum immunoreactive erythropoietin in the investigation of erythrocytosis. N Engl J Med 315:283, 1986. *A careful examination of the value of measuring serum immunoreactive erythropoietin levels in patients with elevated hematocrits, with a useful bibliography.*

Erslev AJ, Caro J: Pure erythrocytosis classified according to erythropoietin titers. Am J Med 76:57, 1984. *Clear demonstration of both the uses and limitations of erythropoietin bioassays in diagnosis of polycythemic states.*

Groopman JE, Molina J-M, Scadden DT: Hematopoietic growth factors: Biology and clinical applications. N Engl J Med 321:1449, 1989. *An excellent review of the complex biology of hematopoietic regulation, indicating clinical applications of the five hematopoietic growth factors that have already been cloned and produced on a large scale through recombinant DNA technology: erythropoietin, GM-, G-, and M-CSF and IL3.*

Quesenberry PJ: Hemopoietic stem cells, progenitor cells and growth factors. *In* Williams WJ, Beutler E, Erslev AJ, et al. (eds.): Hematology. 4th ed. New York, McGraw-Hill, 1990, pp 129–147. *Another excellent review with the focus more on cell biology than clinical application. Outstanding bibliography.*

SECONDARY POLYCYTHEMIAS

In the secondary polycythemias, a normal bone marrow is stimulated to produce increased numbers of red blood cells, leading to an increase in the circulating red cell mass, as a result of increased production of erythropoietin or of other erythrostimulatory substances. These disorders all have in common the diverse symptomatic consequences of hypervolemia and increased blood viscosity described earlier. The secondary polycythemias may be classified into those in which the polycythemia is an appropriate physiologic response to inadequate tissue oxygenation and those in which the development of erythrocytosis is inappropriate to the oxygen balance of the patient (Table 142–1).

Physiologically Appropriate Polycythemias

HIGH ALTITUDE. In the presence of normal hemoglobin A and appropriate intraerythrocytic levels of 2,3-diphosphoglyceric acid (2,3-DPG), the partial pressure of oxygen in capillaries must be maintained close to 40 mm Hg to ensure adequate off-loading of oxygen to tissues. At sea level, where the atmospheric partial pressure of oxygen is approximately 160 mm Hg, oxygen is readily loaded onto the hemoglobin molecule, and the steep oxygen pressure gradient from the alveoli to the tissue capillaries ensures an adequate driving force for tissue oxygenation. In contrast, at elevated altitudes the atmospheric oxygen tension diminishes, and at approximately 5400 meters, the altitude of the highest permanent human settlement, atmospheric oxygen pressure is only 80 mm Hg, providing a much smaller alveolar-capillary oxygen pressure gradient. To provide adequate tissue oxygenation in the face of this reduced driving force, individuals constantly exposed to high altitude are acclimatized by two principal mechanisms, hyperventilation and the development of erythrocytosis. Hyperventilation causes a reduction in the pulmonary dead space and an increase in the surface area of adequately perfused alveoli. Erythrocytosis increases the oxygen-carrying capacity of circulating blood. Together, these two alterations permit acclimatization to occur without the need for a significant increase in cardiac output. In general, although a shift in the oxygen-hemoglobin dissociation curve to the right would also increase tissue oxygenation at a given capillary oxygen tension, such a change would also impair the on-loading of oxygen in the lungs at high altitudes. The latter appears to take precedence in that direct measurement of oxygen dissociation curves among individuals who live at higher altitudes generally reveals patterns within the normal range.

Approximately 25,000,000 people live at altitudes between 3000 and 5400 meters. The latter altitude, with an atmospheric pressure of approximately one-half normal, appears to represent the extreme limit of human long-term physiologic adaptation. Transient adaptation to higher levels is possible, as demonstrated by the successful 1978 scaling of Mount Everest (8848 meters), where atmospheric pressure is approximately one third of normal, without the use of administered oxygen.

Those who dwell for long periods at high altitudes typically develop an increased anteroposterior thoracic diameter and a ruddy cyanosis secondary to hypervolemia. The increased blood volume is manifested in the engorged capillaries of the conjunctivae, skin, and mucous membranes, and may contribute to all of the classic symptoms of hypervolemia. The hematocrit is elevated, reflecting an increased red cell mass in the presence of a normal plasma volume. White blood cells and platelets are normal, and bone marrow aspirates may appear to be normal or to show modest erythroid hyperplasia. The acute and chronic effects of living at high altitude are further described in Ch. 528.

CARDIOPULMONARY DISEASE. Arterial hypoxemia, resulting from right-to-left shunts in congenital heart disease or from chronic obstructive pulmonary disease results in expansion of the red cell mass. This may be masked in part in both settings by a concomitant increase in plasma volume.

ALVEOLAR HYPOVENTILATION. Arterial hypoxemia, cyanosis, and secondary erythrocytosis may also result from either centrally mediated or peripheral impairment of alveolar ventilation. One of the settings in which this occurs, Monge's disease (chronic mountain sickness), is described in Ch. 528. Another is the so-called pickwickian syndrome, in which the work load of ventilation in a severely obese individual is aggravated by central hyporesponsiveness to hypoxemia and hypercapnia. In a third group of patients, postural hypoxemia occurs during sleep. All of these conditions may be associated with increased erythropoietin production and secondary erythrocytosis.

ABNORMALITIES OF THE OXYGEN-HEMOGLOBIN DISSOCIATION CURVE. Abnormalities in the ability of hemoglobin to release oxygen to tissues, manifested by a shift in the oxyhemoglobin dissociation curve to the left, may occur on either a congenital or an acquired basis. At least 42 such hemoglobins have been described in association with erythrocytosis (Ch. 136.3). In most an amino acid substitution occurring in the contact area between the α and β chains interferes with the normal conformational changes that facilitate oxygen release from the molecule. The resulting hemoglobin with high oxygen affinity results in noncyanotic tissue hypo-oxygenation and ultimately in secondary erythrocytosis. High-affinity variants involving both α chain substitutions (hemoglobin Capetown, hemoglobin Chesapeake) and β chain substitutions (hemoglobin Ranier, hemoglobin Yakima) have been described. Most of these high-affinity mutations are electrophoretically silent because there is no charge difference between the normal and variant hemoglobin. Hence, determination of an oxygen-hemoglobin dissociation curve or determination of the P_{50} is essential in the evaluation of patients suspected of having a hemoglobin with high oxygen affinity. This suspicion particularly should be directed toward individuals in whom familial erythrocytosis is observed.

Secondary erythrocytosis may also occur in the presence of certain hereditary methemoglobinemias, disorders in which amino acid substitutions occur in the regions of the heme pockets. Most of these conditions are associated with hemolysis, but in the few in which the rate of red cell destruction is nearly normal, compensatory mechanisms may result in a secondary erythrocytosis. Several different congenital disorders involving a decreased ability to synthesize 2,3-DPG have been described. Since reductions in red cell 2,3-DPG content are associated with an increased oxygen affinity for hemoglobin, such patients may behave clinically as if they had a high-affinity hemoglobin disorder with resulting secondary erythrocytosis, even though they in fact have hemoglobin A. Finally, prolonged exposure to carbon monoxide, occasionally on an industrial basis but more frequently in chain smokers, results in erythrocytosis because carboxyhemoglobin has the effect of increasing the oxygen affinity of the remaining heme prosthetic groups. The hematocrit is often increased out of proportion to the red cell mass because of secondary effects of carboxyhemoglobin or nicotine or both in reducing the plasma volume.

Physiologically Inappropriate Erythrocytosis

NEOPLASMS AND NONNEOPLASTIC RENAL DISEASES. Physiologically inappropriate erythrocytosis is seen in a variety of neoplasms, including renal and adrenal carcinoma, cerebellar hemangioblastoma, hepatocellular carcinoma, ovarian carcinoma, pheochromocytoma, and massive uterine fibroids (Ch. 161). The proportion of each of these tumors in which erythrocytosis develops is highly variable. It seems to be particularly high in cases of hepatocellular carcinoma. In most instances, increased erythropoietin production by the tumor is believed to be the underlying mechanism leading to erythrocytosis.

Secondary erythrocytosis also occurs in a variety of nonmalignant disorders of the kidney, including cystic disease and hydronephrosis, and following renal transplantation. Production of increased erythropoietin levels in the presence of renal cystic disease appears likely in view of the frequent documentation of high titers of the hormone in aspirated cyst fluid. Local intrarenal ischemia resulting from various types of renal pathology is believed to mediate an increased erythropoietin output in these disorders. Familial syndromes occur in which autonomous production of increased quantities of erythropoietin has been observed without a demonstrable anatomic lesion. Erythropoietin output in these syndromes does not vary in response to phlebotomy. A single report also describes an inappropriately high level of basal erythropoietin output in an individual in whom phlebotomy resulted in a further increase in hormone production. The nature of the underlying defect in these two syndromes is unclear.

DRUG-INDUCED ERYTHROCYTOSIS. Testosterone and its various derivatives, as well as a variety of adrenal corticosteroids, may stimulate red cell production. Testosterone-like compounds are often used therapeutically for this purpose in patients with renal failure who are undergoing dialysis or in patients with aregenerative anemia. In some instances, androgens also stimulate granulocyte and platelet production. Occasionally, increased levels of steroid hormones, whether administered therapeutically or produced in the course of adrenal disorders, may result in secondary erythrocytosis.

Treatment of the Secondary Polycythemias

Hypervolemia and increased blood viscosity accompany the development of erythrocytosis. Accordingly, when a secondary erythrocytosis is not in response to an appropriate physiologic stimulus, reduction of hematocrit to less than 50 per cent by means of phlebotomy is an appropriate part of the treatment regimen, which should also address itself to the underlying disorder.

The issue is more complex in those secondary erythrocytoses that represent a physiologic response to poor tissue oxygenation. The beneficial effect of expansion of the red cell mass may ultimately be offset by the detrimental effect of increasing blood viscosity on cardiac output, systemic oxygen transport, and local tissue oxygen delivery. In a normovolemic state, oxygen transport is optimal at a hematocrit of 40 to 45 per cent. In the presence of hypervolemia, optimal oxygen delivery may occur at hematocrits close to 60 per cent. However, hematocrits higher than this inevitably impair oxygen delivery. Nevertheless, in a given patient, if an increase in the hematocrit to the region of 60 per cent does not achieve normal tissue oxygenation, a continued increase in erythropoietin output may result in overcompensation. This overcompensation may not only decrease net tissue oxygen delivery but may also impair regional blood flow in a number of organs, particularly within the cerebral circulation. In summary, in the physiologic secondary polycythemias, there is a balance between the beneficial effects of an increasing hematocrit and the negative consequences of an excessive increase in blood viscosity. In general, hematocrits in excess of 60 per cent are detrimental and should be reduced by phlebotomy. In patients with arterial hypoxemia resulting from pulmonary disease or right-to-left cardiac shunts, the optimal level of hemoglobin and hematocrit may be difficult to determine except by trial and error. In some cases, improvement in cerebral function and decrease in congestive heart failure may follow a reduction in blood volume to hematocrits in the mid 50's or even lower.

Bunn HF, Forget B: Hemoglobin: Molecular, Genetic and Clinical Aspects. Philadelphia, W. B. Saunders Company, 1986, pp 595–622. *This chapter presents an outstanding review of hemoglobin variants with abnormal oxygen binding and their clinical consequences, as well as a comprehensive bibliography.*

Chetty KG, Brown SE, Light RW: Improved exercise tolerance of the polycythemic lung patient following phlebotomy. Am J Med 74:415, 1983. *A detailed clinicophysiologic study documenting that patients with polycythemia due to chronic obstructive pulmonary disease benefit from reduction of hematocrit to the mid 50's by phlebotomy.*

Erslev AJ: Blood and mountains. *In* Wintrobe MM (ed.): Blood, Pure and Eloquent. New York, McGraw-Hill, 1980, pp 257–280. *A lucid and fascinating review of the evolution of current concepts of human adaptation to the hypoxemia of high altitudes. Excellent bibliography.*

Erslev AJ: Secondary polycythemia (erythrocytosis). *In* Williams WJ, Beutler E, Erslev AJ, et al. (eds.): Hematology. 4th ed. New York, McGraw-Hill, 1990, pp 705–715. *A detailed review of the causes, pathophysiology, and treatment of the different forms of secondary polycythemia. Good discussion of the rare familial syndromes associated with hypererythropoietinemia. Comprehensive bibliography.*

Wallis PJW: Effects of erythropheresis on pulmonary haemodynamics and oxygen transport in patients with secondary polycythemia and cor pulmonale. Clin Sci 70:91, 1986. *Outstanding clinical physiologic study of the benefits of phlebotomy in this setting.*

POLYCYTHEMIA VERA: A CLONAL STEM CELL DISORDER

Nature of the Defect in Polycythemia Vera

Polycythemia vera is a hematologic malignant disorder characterized by excessive proliferation of erythroid, myeloid, and megakaryocytic elements within the bone marrow, resulting in an increased red blood cell mass and, frequently, elevated peripheral granulocyte and platelet counts. Several lines of evidence, including cytogenetic observations and isoenzyme marker studies in glucose-6-phosphate dehydrogenase (G6PD) heterozygotes, indicate that the increased proliferation of all three hematopoietic cell lines can trace its origin to a single abnormal clone, which has presumably developed at the level of the pluripotent stem cell. B lymphocytes are also derived from the abnormal stem cell clone. Studies of the growth of both erythroid progenitors and granulocyte-macrophage progenitors (CFU-GM) in vitro have demonstrated the presence of residual normal stem cells in the marrow early in the disease, but a steady decline in the proportion of the normal elements as the duration of the illness lengthens.

Thrombotic episodes that are usually attributed to increased blood viscosity and/or thrombocytosis; hemorrhagic episodes associated with thrombopathy and/or the elevated platelet and erythrocyte counts; the development of a "spent" phase characterized by cytopenias, myelofibrosis, and myeloid metaplasia; and the transformation to acute leukemia are among the principal complications of this disorder. Polycythemia vera shares several clinical, pathophysiologic, and histologic features with agnogenic myeloid metaplasia, chronic myelogenous leukemia, and primary (essential) thrombocythemia, which are collectively classified as the myeloproliferative disorders (Ch. 143).

The excessive rate of erythropoiesis in polycythemia vera occurs despite bioassayable erythropoietin levels that are low or absent; endogenous erythroid colonies in this disorder can grow in vitro without added erythropoietin. These observations led to the concept that erythropoiesis in polycythemia vera was "autonomous." The growth of endogenous colonies from patients with polycythemia vera can be markedly reduced or eliminated by adding antierythropoietin antibody to the culture, however, and can be restored by the re-addition of minute quantities of the hormone. This suggests that erythroid progenitors in polycythemia vera, rather than being independent of the hormone, may be uniquely sensitive to trace levels of erythropoietin. However, studies of erythropoietin receptors on erythroid progenitors in polycythemia vera have not demonstrated an increase in either receptor number or hormone affinity, which could account for this observation. In blood and bone marrow of patients with polycythemia vera, increased numbers of pluripotent colony-forming stem cells give rise to mixed colonies of granulocytic, erythroid, macrophage, and megakaryocytic elements (CFU-GEMM). These CFU-GEMM undergo erythroid differentiation without added erythropoietin and, compared with normal CFU-GEMM, exhibit increased megakaryocyte formation. The "endogenous" erythroid differentiation is abolished with antibodies to erythropoietin. Hence, both the increased "erythropoietin-independent" erythropoiesis and the increased megakaryopoiesis characteristic of polycythemia vera reflect functional features of an identifiable abnormal pluripotent stem cell population. Long-term tissue cultures of bone marrow from patients with polycythemia vera demonstrate a population of abnormally replicating erythroid progenitors. These cells fail to respond to the normal inhibitory signals derived from nonhematopoietic elements within the marrow.

The mechanism of malignant transformation in polycythemia vera is unknown. The rare occurrence of documented polycythemia vera in monozygotic twins and the only marginally increased incidence in first-degree relatives of affected patients suggest a minimal genetic role in most cases, and neither toxic chemicals nor exposure to radiation is established as an etiologic factor. Although two documented cases occurred among exposed observers of a 1957 nuclear test explosion, the incidence of polycythemia vera has not been appreciably increased in survivors of the Hiroshima and Nagasaki atomic bomb explosions. Preliminary reports of reverse transcriptase activity and of retrovirus-like particles in platelets of patients with myeloproliferative disorders are intriguing, particularly in view of the murine polycythemia produced by one strain of Friend mouse erythroleukemia virus. These studies require extensive confirmation.

Clinical Manifestations

Polycythemia vera is typically a disease of later life, with the median age at presentation being close to 60 years. Nevertheless, patients in their second through fourth decades are not rare. The disorder is characterized by a slight preponderance in males and a propensity to occur with somewhat increased frequency in patients of Jewish ancestry.

Multiphasic screening is currently resulting in an increasing percentage of cases being detected prior to the development of symptoms. Alternatively, a routine blood count may demonstrate increased hematocrit and other abnormalities in patients who present with only mild headaches and plethoric facies. Further symptoms as they develop usually are referable to the combination of hypervolemia and hyperviscosity resulting from the increased red cell mass and blood volume, frequently aggravated by thrombocytosis and platelet dysfunction; to the local consequences of panhyperplasia of the bone marrow; or to the metabolic consequences of increased cell turnover.

SYMPTOMS. Headaches, tinnitus, light-headedness and vertigo, and blurred vision appear to result principally from increased blood viscosity and hypervolemia. Thrombotic complications, which may involve both arterial and venous occlusive events, are usually attributed to a combination of hyperviscosity, thrombocytosis, and platelet dysfunction. An increased incidence of epistaxis, spontaneous bruising, and upper gastrointestinal hemorrhage is also ascribed to the effects of hypervolemia and platelet dysfunction. Peptic ulcer disease seems to occur with increased frequency in patients with polycythemia vera, as does pruritus, sometimes aggravated after a hot bath or shower, and occasionally so severe as to be disabling. The increased frequency of both peptic ulcer and pruritus may be related to the increased histamine release caused by excessive turnover of granulocytes and, more specifically, basophils. Approximately one third of patients complain of sweating and weight loss, presumed to be on the basis of a hypermetabolic state. Patients with polycythemia vera often complain of severe pain in their feet, which is characteristically relieved by very low doses of aspirin or nonsteroidal anti-inflammatory agents.

PHYSICAL FINDINGS. In established cases, physical examination typically reveals plethora or dusky cyanosis of the face, hands, feet, and mucous membranes. Engorgement of the conjunctivae and retinal veins is frequently present, and in patients with markedly increased hematocrit, retinal hemorrhages are occasionally seen. Mild hypertension is noted in approximately one third of patients. Ecchymoses are not infrequently observed.

The most useful physical finding in terms of differential diagnosis is splenomegaly, which is present in approximately 75 per cent of patients with polycythemia vera and tends to exclude the diagnosis of most of the secondary polycythemias. Procedures such as abdominal computed tomography demonstrate splenomegaly in a percentage of those patients in whom the spleen is not palpably enlarged. Splenic enlargement appears to reflect principally the development of extramedullary hematopoiesis. Hepatomegaly is present in approximately 40 per cent of patients.

Symptomatic bone pain and tenderness on physical examination, particularly in the ribs and sternum, are occasionally severe and reflect intense panhyperplasia of the bone marrow. In addition to hyperhistaminemia, the cellular proliferation of polycythemia vera results in overproduction of uric acid, leading, not infrequently, to either uric acid stone diathesis or overt secondary gout.

Laboratory Data

The characteristic laboratory findings in polycythemia vera reflect the various consequences of increased bone marrow activity.

ERYTHROCYTES. Patients with this disorder typically present with an elevation of the hemoglobin concentration, hematocrit, and red blood cell count. Red blood cell morphology usually reveals hypochromic microcytic cells with a reduced mean corpuscular volume, suggestive of iron-deficient erythropoiesis (see Color Plate 5K). This suggestion is frequently confirmed by a low serum iron level and absence of bone marrow iron stores. These features may occur prior to the onset of therapeutic phlebotomy and without any history of gastrointestinal blood loss and result from the shift of iron from various body storage pools into the circulating erythron as the red cell mass is expanded. This phenomenon may of course be exaggerated in patients who have gastrointestinal bleeding or in whom therapeutic phlebotomies have been initiated. Of the three conventional parameters reflecting the red cell mass, the red blood cell count is often most strikingly elevated, and red cell counts of 10×10^6 per microliter may be seen in the newly diagnosed case. In contrast, the hematocrit probably provides the best, although imperfect, simple guide to the size of the circulating red cell mass and to blood viscosity. It is difficult to define the precise upper limit for the normal hematocrit. As noted earlier, increased red cell masses may be found in a small percentage of patients with hematocrits of 48 per cent or above, and an increase in the hematocrit to greater than 60 per cent is required before the hematocrit alone can be taken positively as evidence for an absolute erythrocytosis. The plasma volume in polycythemia vera has variously been reported to be normal, reduced, or increased and thus has no direct correlation with the red cell mass. The red cell lifespan is normal in the early phases of polycythemia vera, even in the presence of moderate splenomegaly. As the disease evolves, the development of increasingly ineffective erythropoiesis, as well as a larger element of extramedullary hematopoiesis with hepatomegaly and splenomegaly, results in progressive shortening of the red cell lifespan in some patients. This development is usually associated with the appearance of anisocytosis and poikilocytosis, nucleated red blood cells, and teardrop cells in the peripheral blood. When such studies are available, patients with untreated polycythemia vera will invariably demonstrate very low levels of plasma and urine erythropoietin and the ability to grow endogenous, erythropoietin-independent colonies of erythroid progenitors in vitro from either peripheral blood or bone marrow samples.

LEUKOCYTES. Sixty per cent of patients with polycythemia vera have an increased granulocyte count in the peripheral blood at the time of diagnosis. Early in the disease, elevations are usually modest and involve the presence of only normal granulocytes and bands. Subsequently, striking elevations in total white cell count may achieve leukemoid proportions, associated with the appearance of early myeloid forms, particularly myelocytes and metamyelocytes. When the appearance of these cells is accompanied by increasing splenomegaly and the appearance of abnormal erythroid elements in the periphery, a significant element of myeloid metaplasia is likely. The alkaline phosphatase

activity of circulating granulocytes is increased in polycythemia vera, in contrast to the reduction observed in chronic granulocytic leukemia. Increased granulocyte turnover is reflected by high serum and urine muramidase (lysozyme) levels and by an increase in serum B_{12} and unbound B_{12} binding capacity that results from high levels of transcobalamins 1 and 3. The basophil count and, to a lesser extent, the eosinophil count may also be increased in polycythemia vera. Increased excretion of histamine metabolites reflects increased turnover of the former cell line. Total lymphocyte counts in polycythemia vera are normal. However, a decreased number of suppressor T lymphocytes and an increase in the helper/suppressor T lymphocyte ratio have been reported.

PLATELETS. At diagnosis, the platelet count exceeds 500,000 per microliter in approximately half of patients with polycythemia vera, and striking elevations into the millions have been recorded. There is a tendency for the platelet count to increase with time, particularly in patients who are treated principally with phlebotomy. The platelets in polycythemia vera frequently appear morphologically abnormal, with megathrombocytes and megakaryocytic fragments being observed in the peripheral blood smear. As determined by electronic particle sizing, both the mean platelet volume and the platelet distribution width are increased in patients with polycythemia vera and other myeloproliferative disorders who have thrombocytosis. By contrast, the platelet distribution width is generally normal in reactive thrombocytosis. An appreciable fraction of patients with polycythemia vera also have abnormalities of conventional studies of platelet function, including aggregation; a prolonged bleeding time may be present. Studies of prostaglandin metabolism also demonstrate decreased lipoxygenase activity and increased thromboxane A_2 production by the platelets of patients with polycythemia vera and other myeloproliferative diseases. However, it has not been possible to correlate either the height of the platelet count or the presence of platelet functional abnormalities with the propensity to thrombosis in these patients. In contrast, there seems to be a crude association between the extent of the elevation of the platelet count and the propensity to hemorrhagic complications.

BONE MARROW. The bone marrow in polycythemia vera is typically hyperplastic and reveals a panmyelosis. Because of the parallel increase in all three cell lines, the myeloid/erythroid ratio may be normal. Megakaryocytes are not merely increased but typically are seen in sheets or clumps (Fig. 142–3), either in biopsy sections or in the spicules of bone marrow aspirates; this finding is strongly supportive of the diagnosis of a myeloproliferative disease. Bone marrow biopsy as well as aspirate is useful in the assessment of polycythemia vera, both because it gives a better indication of the extent of hypercellularity and because connective tissue staining illustrates the extent of myelofibrosis. Serum levels of the procollagen III amino terminal peptide, now

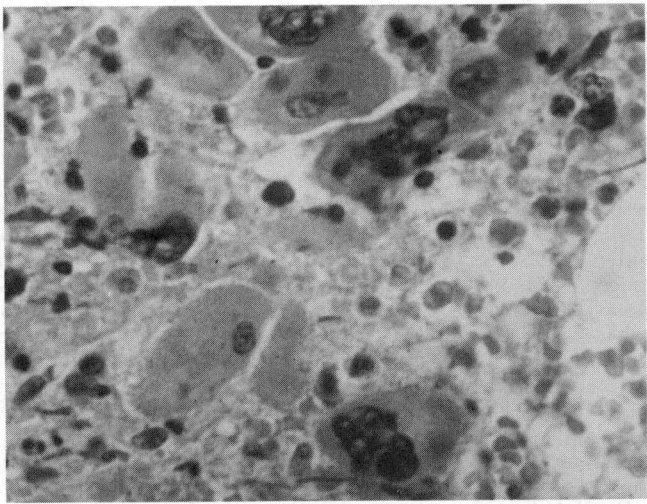

FIGURE 142–3. Bone marrow biopsy specimen from a patient with polycythemia vera. Increased numbers of atypical megakaryocytes present in clusters, as shown here, are indicative of a myeloproliferative disorder and, in the presence of an increased red cell mass, strongly support a diagnosis of polycythemia vera. Such megakaryocytic clusters may also be observed within the spicules obtained from a bone marrow aspirate.

measurable by commercially available RIA, also reflect the extent of myelofibrosis. Cytogenetic studies reveal various abnormalities in as many as 50 per cent of patients with polycythemia vera. Trisomy of chromosomes 8 and 9 and loss of chromosome 7 or its long arm (7q−) are the abnormalities most frequently observed in untreated patients; loss of chromosome 5 or of the long arms of chromosome 5 (5q−) or 20 (20q−) has been observed in some patients, especially those treated with myelosuppressives. However, no abnormality is either specific for or diagnostic of polycythemia vera. Interestingly, the presence of cytogenetic abnormalities at the time of diagnosis appears to be of no prognostic significance.

MISCELLANEOUS. Low serum cholesterol concentrations are frequently observed in patients with polycythemia vera; these reflect accelerated catabolism of low density lipoproteins, presumably by the spleen. Hyperuricemia, reflecting a general increase in cell turnover, and an increase in lactate dehydrogenase and the indirect serum bilirubin concentration, reflecting accelerated erythroid turnover, are other commonly found abnormalities.

Diagnosis and Differential Diagnosis

The diagnosis of polycythemia vera is based on the demonstration of an increased red cell mass that is not associated with excessive erythropoietin production, as well as evidence of a concomitant increase in bone marrow production of granulocytes and thrombocytes. Polycythemia is one of two disorders characterized by "autonomous" erythropoiesis. It differs from the entity designated *primary erythrocytosis* in its associated increase in granulocyte and megakaryocytic proliferation and the presence of related abnormalities such as elevated levels of leukocyte alkaline phosphatase and serum B_{12}–binding proteins. The abnormalities in primary erythrocytosis are limited to the erythroid series, but within this sphere the low bioassayable erythropoietin levels and the presence of endogenous colonies are similar to those seen in polycythemia vera. Some argue that primary erythrocytosis represents a disorder arising in the committed erythroid stem cell compartment, i.e., at a later stage than the pluripotent stem cell affected in polycythemia vera, but primary erythrocytosis has not yet been demonstrated to be a clonal disorder. Others believe that these patients represent a forme fruste of typical polycythemia vera and that granulocytic or thrombocytic abnormalities will be revealed if patients are observed for sufficient periods.

The diagnosis of a primary bone marrow disorder with autonomous erythropoiesis may be made in accordance with the algorithm illustrated in Figure 142–2 by systematically excluding the various secondary causes of an absolute erythrocytosis. Patients appearing to have increased erythroid proliferation due to a primary bone marrow defect would be classified as having polycythemia vera if they have concomitant granulocytic or platelet abnormalities in the peripheral blood, evidence of a panmyelosis in the bone marrow, or splenomegaly. In the absence of these features, when abnormalities are restricted solely to the erythroid series, the diagnosis of primary erythrocytosis would be made.

The Polycythemia Vera Study Group has developed a set of empiric criteria that permit the diagnosis of polycythemia vera to be established in many patients within one to two office visits (Table 142–2). In patients who meet these criteria, the diagnosis of polycythemia vera is highly likely, the false-positive rate having been found to be less than 0.5 per cent. False-positive results are most likely in patients who are excessive users of both alcohol and tobacco. In this setting, excessive erythroid proliferation associated with carboxyhemoglobinemia and splenomegaly, leukocytosis, and increased leukocyte alkaline phosphatase activity and serum B_{12} associated with alcoholic liver disease may confound the diagnosis. The false-negative rate for the Polycythemia Vera Study Group criteria is unknown. Patients with early disease who do not yet meet these criteria may ultimately prove to have polycythemia vera, or at least a form of primary erythrocytosis, when more extensive evaluation is carried out in accordance with the criteria of Figure 142–2.

Course

In the absence of treatment, polycythemia vera is a serious disease in which a high incidence of fatal thrombotic or hemor-

rhagic complications historically has led to a median survival of 6 to 18 months from diagnosis. Current treatment programs designed to maintain peripheral blood counts and the red cell mass at close to normal levels have achieved median survivals approximating 10 years, during the course of which aspects of the natural history of the disease have become more evident. In many patients, polycythemia vera is a readily managed disorder that remains asymptomatic for long periods. However, inadequate control of the red cell mass predisposes to both thrombotic and hemorrhagic complications, of which cerebrovascular, coronary, and abdominal vascular occlusions involving both arterial (e.g., mesenteric artery) and venous (Budd-Chiari syndrome) thromboses are most frequent. Expansion of the red cell mass is clearly not the only factor predisposing to thrombosis in polycythemia vera. The presence of endogenous erythroid progenitor colonies may be the only laboratory indicator of incipient myeloproliferative disease in young patients presenting initially with the Budd-Chiari syndrome. Thrombosis is the major cause of death overall in polycythemia vera, accounting for approximately one third of all fatalities. Some patients are particularly prone to thrombosis, suffering repeated events, one of which may ultimately prove fatal; others are spared. Unfortunately, there is no way at present to identify this thrombosis-prone subset prior to a thrombotic event. Transformation to acute leukemia, the development of other neoplasms, hemorrhage, and myelofibrosis are other major causes of fatality and collectively, along with thrombosis, account for 75 per cent of all deaths. Acute leukemia is clearly a part of the natural history of polycythemia vera, occurring with an incidence of up to 2 to 4 per cent even in patients who have not been exposed either to radiotherapy or to radiomimetic drugs.

Upper gastrointestinal hemorrhage, particularly from bleeding peptic ulcers, occurs with an increased incidence in patients with polycythemia vera. Underlying etiologic factors are believed to be increased acid secretion stimulated by hyperhistaminemia and vascular mucosal ischemia caused by increased blood viscosity and poor regional perfusion.

The complete natural history of polycythemia vera involves the ultimate transition from the proliferative phase, during which therapy is aimed at reducing peripheral blood counts, to a stable phase in which relatively normal blood counts may be maintained without therapy, to the so-called *burned out* or *spent phase*. Transition results predominantly from the gradual development of progressive myelofibrosis and, possibly, from a gradual reduction in the proliferative capacity of the abnormal hematopoietic clone. That myelofibrosis is a complication of polycythemia vera has long been recognized, but the nature of the association has been uncertain. The bulk of current evidence suggests that bone marrow fibroblasts in this setting are not part of the hematopoietic malignant clone. Similar conclusions have been reached in studies of the bone marrow fibroblast following transplantation. Hence, the increasing proliferation of fibroblasts and increased collagen deposition leading to myelofibrosis appear to be reactive phenomena rather than an intrinsic component of the neoplastic process. The clinical features and the management of postpolycythemic myelofibrosis do not differ appreciably from those of idiopathic myelofibrosis with myeloid metaplasia except that the incidence of acute leukemic transformation is markedly increased in the postpolycythemic setting, especially if the myelofibrosis follows

TABLE 142–2. PARAMETERS FOR THE DIAGNOSIS OF POLYCYTHEMIA VERA

A1 ↑ Red cell mass	B1 Thrombocytosis
Male: ≥36 ml/kg	Platelet count >400,000/μl
Female: ≥32 ml/kg	B2 Leukocytosis: >12,000/μl
A2 Normal arterial O_2	(no fever or infection)
saturation (≥92%)	B3 ↑ Leukocyte alkaline
A3 Splenomegaly	phosphatase (LAP) (>100)
	B4 ↑ Serum B_{12} (>900 pg/ml) or
	↑ $UB_{12}BC$ (>2200 pg/ml)*

Dx acceptable if following combinations are present:
    A1 + A2 + A3
    A1 + A2 + any two from category B
*$UB_{12}BC$ = unbound serum B_{12} binding capacity

treatment with radioactive phosphorus or chlorambucil (see Ch. 143).

Treatment

The initial treatment in any newly diagnosed case of polycythemia vera is phlebotomy. Efforts should be made to reduce the hematocrit to approximately 45 per cent, a level at which the complications of hypervolemia and hyperviscosity are minimized. In patients with appreciable splenomegaly, the hematocrit no longer reliably reflects the red cell mass, which may continue to be significantly increased despite hematocrits in the upper 40's. The initial phlebotomy regimen may involve removal of 500-ml aliquots of whole blood as often as every 2 to 3 days until a normal hematocrit is achieved. Subsequent phlebotomies should be carried out as frequently as necessary to maintain the hematocrit at or below 45 per cent. As iron deficiency supervenes, red cell production will be retarded, so that patients managed by phlebotomy alone may require as few as two or three phlebotomies per year.

Some investigators believe that phlebotomy alone, at rates sufficient to maintain a normal hematocrit and blood viscosity, is adequate to prevent the thrombotic complications of the disease and provides a minimal incidence of leukemic transformation. Others argue that some form of myelosuppression is preferable, in part because this offers an approach to the control of the thrombocytosis that is often a major clinical feature of the illness. Myelosuppression in this disorder has most often been carried out with radioactive phosphorus (^{32}P), with alkylating agents such as chlorambucil or busulfan and, more recently, with the nonalkylating myelosuppressive agent hydroxyurea.

In an ongoing randomized, controlled study in 431 patients, median survivals of 13.9 years with phlebotomy or 11.8 years with radioactive phosphorus therapy were significantly better than those achieved with chlorambucil (8.9 years), although the difference achieved statistical significance only after more than 10 years of treatment. Causes of death varied appreciably as a function of the treatment administered. Patients managed with phlebotomy alone had a significant excess incidence of severe and often fatal thrombotic complications, particularly in the first 2 to 4 years of treatment. Thrombotic complications were particularly frequent in more elderly patients (e.g., older than 70 years), in those with a high phlebotomy requirement (more than four to six per year), and in those who had had a prior history of a thrombotic event. Beyond 3 years, the incidence of thrombotic complications became the same in patients treated with phlebotomy alone as in those treated with myelosuppression, suggesting that a subset of patients particularly susceptible to thrombosis had been selected out by this time. By contrast, myelosuppression with either ^{32}P or alkylating agents effectively decreased the risk of thrombotic complications in thrombosis-prone patients early in the disease. However, both chlorambucil and ^{32}P were associated with a statistically significant increased risk of acute leukemia, which became particularly prominent after 5 to 7 years of treatment, and a somewhat later increased incidence of carcinomas of the skin and gastrointestinal tract. Thus, long-term myelosuppression with either of these agents is associated with an increased propensity for malignant transformation of the three rapidly proliferating tissues of the body: bone marrow, skin, and gastrointestinal mucosa. In addition, an increased incidence of intra-abdominal lymphocytic lymphoma has followed long-term treatment of polycythemia vera with chlorambucil.

Radioactive phosphorus, preferably given as an intravenous dose of 3 to 5 mCi, reliably produces a reduction in bone marrow proliferation with few immediate side effects. Chlorambucil or busulfan, administered either continuously or intermittently, also successfully controls peripheral counts in a high proportion of patients. In contrast to ^{32}P, myelosuppression with alkylating agents results in an appreciable incidence of cytopenias, which in the case of busulfan may be prolonged and troublesome. Because of these drug-related cytopenias and the fact that malignant complications occur both earlier and more frequently with chlorambucil than with ^{32}P, long-term treatment of polycythemia vera with alkylating agents can no longer be recommended. Although some argue that complications observed with chloram-

bucil should not preclude use of other alkylating agents, especially busulfan, there are sufficient anecdotal cases of leukemic transformation with all of the alkylating drugs that the burden of proof must be on those who argue for the safety of any such agent.

Hydroxyurea,* administered at a dose of 0.5 to 1.5 grams per day, has recently been shown to be an effective nonalkylating chemotherapeutic agent in the management of polycythemia vera. To date, this regimen has not been associated with an increased incidence of malignant transformation. However, the maximal follow-up with this agent, now approximately 10 years, is still too short for its full mutagenic potential to have been realized.

In patients with marked thrombocytosis refractory to conventional management, successful control of the platelet count has been achieved with experimental protocols employing either anagrelide or interferon.

Since no form of treatment for polycythemia vera is without some risks, the following recommendations would appear to provide the best control of the disease with the fewest treatment-related complications. Because of the increased risk of thrombosis associated with age, patients over 70 are most effectively treated with a combination of ^{32}P and supplemental phlebotomy. Patients below the age of 50, particularly those in the childbearing years, should be treated with phlebotomy alone whenever possible. Myelosuppression with hydroxyurea would seem advisable in such younger patients if they are particularly at risk for thrombotic complications because of a high phlebotomy requirement or a history of prior thrombotic events. The role of myelosuppression is most uncertain in the age group between 50 and 70. In the absence of thrombosis-associated risk factors, it is probably preferable to attempt to manage such patients by phlebotomy alone. If chemotherapy is deemed advisable, hydroxyurea would appear to be the agent of choice. Chlorambucil would now seem to be contraindicated for long-term therapy of polycythemia vera in view of its unacceptably high risk of leukemic and carcinogenic transformation, which may apply as well to other alkylating agents.

Although conclusive data are lacking, many physicians believe that a substantial increase in platelet count (i.e., in excess of 10^6 per microliter) is an indication for myelosuppressive therapy. Excessive splenic enlargement with local symptoms, bone tenderness, intractable pruritus, and poor veins may be other indications for the addition of myelosuppression to the treatment regimen. H_1 (cyproheptadine, 4 mg by mouth three times daily) and H_2 blockers (cimetidine, 300 mg by mouth three times daily), alone or in combination, provide relief from pruritus in some patients.

The results of attempts to reduce the incidence of thrombotic complications with the prophylactic use of platelet-antiaggregating agents have been controversial. Some investigators have reported a reduced incidence of such complications with the use of low-dose aspirin. A randomized, controlled trial of aspirin and dipyridamole, however, found not only no significant benefit from these agents in terms of thrombosis but also a statistically significant increase in the incidence of gastrointestinal hemorrhage, particularly with prolonged administration to patients with platelet counts greater than 1 million. Hence, long-term prophylactic use of this group of agents cannot be recommended at this time. Short-term use of platelet-antiaggregating agents may be helpful during transient attacks of digital or cerebral ischemia, but such episodes are an indication for, and often respond to, myelosuppression.

Patients with polycythemia vera are at increased risk for complications associated with surgery, including an appreciably increased surgical mortality rate. The incidence of complications appears to decrease with good control of the underlying disorder. Therefore, elective surgery in such patients should be undertaken only after careful consideration of the risk-benefit ratio and should always be delayed until optimal control of the peripheral blood counts has been achieved.

Treatment of the burned-out myelofibrotic stage of polycythemia vera can be extremely difficult but does not differ from that described for idiopathic myelofibrosis. The acute leukemias that develop in polycythemia vera, either spontaneously or following

---

*This use is not listed in the manufacturer's directive.

myelosuppressive therapy, may be myeloid, myelomonocytic, lymphoid, or biphenotypic in morphology. In those patients with lymphoid morphology and/or increased levels of terminal deoxyribonucleotidyl transferase (TdT), a trial of vincristine and prednisone is indicated. Nevertheless, response to any form of treatment in these patients is infrequent, and median survival in a relatively recent series of postpolycythemic acute leukemias was approximately 30 days.

Meticulous control of blood volume and viscosity with the use of phlebotomy, supplemented when specifically indicated by judicious use of myelosuppression, can ensure most patients with polycythemia vera a prolonged period of relatively symptom-free survival. Median survival in recent series has exceeded 10 years, and symptom-free survival of 15 to 20 years is no longer uncommon. The longest documented survival following a well-founded diagnosis is 34 years.

Berk PD, Goldberg JD, Donovan PB, et al.: Therapeutic recommendations in polycythemia vera based on Polycythemia Vera Study Group protocols. Semin Hematol 23:132, 1986. *A detailed report on a continuous 19-year randomized control study of a large cohort of patients with polycythemia vera and the therapeutic recommendations derived from it. Part of a useful eight-article symposium on polycythemia vera.*

Caldwell GG, Kelley DB, Heath CW Jr, et al.: Polycythemia vera among participants of a nuclear weapons test. JAMA 252:662, 1984. *A provocative report that illustrates some of the difficulties in conclusively linking relatively uncommon disorders to radiation exposure.*

Cashman JD, Eaves CJ, Eaves AC: Unregulated proliferation of primitive neoplastic progenitor cells in long-term polycythemia vera marrow cultures. J Clin Invest 81:87, 1988. *An interesting and important study emphasizing both the abnormal replicative potential of the primitive stem cells in polycythemia and the existence of inhibitory signals derived from nonhematopoietic marrow elements to which these stem cells fail to respond.*

Conley CL: Polycythemia vera, diagnosis and treatment. Hosp Practice 22:107, 1987. *An excellent overview by a senior hematologist with great experience.*

Ellis JT, Peterson P, Geller SA, et al.: Studies of the bone marrow in polycythemia vera and the evolution of myelofibrosis and second hematologic malignancies. Semin Hematol 23:144, 1986. *An important review of bone marrow findings in polycythemia vera, exploring such issues as the evolution of fibrosis and second malignant disorders.*

Malmaeus J, Akre T, Adami HO, et al.: Early postoperative course following elective splenectomy in haematological diseases: A high complication rate in patients with myeloproliferative disorders. Br J Surg 73:720, 1986. *A recent review that underscores the increased risks of surgery in patients with myeloproliferative disorders.*

Means RT Jr, Krantz SB, Sawyer ST, et al.: Erythropoietin receptors in polycythemia vera. J Clin Invest 84:1340, 1989. *One of the first studies employing purified erythropoietin to examine the state of receptors on erythroid progenitors in polycythemia vera. It provides no support for the hypothesis that abnormalities in receptor number or affinity explain the apparent increased sensitivity to erythropoietin observed in polycythemia vera.*

Murphy S: Polycythemia vera. *In* Williams WJ, Beutler E, Erslev AJ, et al. (eds.): Hematology. 4th ed. New York, McGraw-Hill, 1990, pp 193–202. *An excellent and comprehensive review of the pathophysiology, clinical features, and treatment, with an especially complete bibliography.*

Najean Y, Mugnier P, Dresch C, et al.: Polycythemia vera in young people: An analysis of 58 cases diagnosed before 40 years. Br J Haematol 67:285, 1987. *An important review that emphasizes the somewhat different biologic behavior of polycythemia in younger patients.*

Silverstein MM, Petitt RM, Solberg LA Jr, et al.: Anagrelide: A new drug for treating thrombocytosis. N Engl J Med 318:1292, 1988. *Preliminary report on a promising new agent with highly selective effects in controlling thrombocytosis in myeloproliferative disorders.*

143 Myeloproliferative Disorders

Paul D. Berk

The normal bone marrow contains self-replicating pools of morphologically undifferentiated stem cells, recognizable hematopoietic cells undergoing differentiation and maturation, as well as vascular and connective tissue stromal elements. There is a hierarchy of hematopoietic stem cell populations: (1) a pluripotent stem cell capable, under appropriate conditions, of producing erythroid, myeloid, megakaryocytic, macrophage, and B lymphocyte progeny; (2) intermediate stem cells capable of producing several but not all of these lineages; and (3) committed, unipotent stem cells giving rise exclusively to erythroid, myeloid, or megakaryocytic offspring. The rate of proliferation, pool size, and rate

of transition from less restricted to more restricted potential are carefully regulated so that the bone marrow can respond to the body's need for blood elements in a manner that is both selective in terms of the cell types produced and restricted or self-limited in duration (see Fig. 127–2). These selective responses are mediated by a complex and incompletely understood network of endocrine, paracrine, and possibly autocrine factors, including erythropoietin, various interleukins, interferons, and growth factors (Ch. 127 and 142), of which macrophages, as well as the endothelial cells lining the marrow vascular channels, may be the major sources. As a result, in hemolysis, pyogenic infection, and immune platelet destruction, specific needs for increased production of erythrocytes, granulocytes, and platelets, respectively, are met ordinarily by selective erythroid, myeloid, or megakaryocytic hyperplasia of the marrow. Stromal cells such as fibroblasts do not appear to play a significant role in these physiologic responses.

In the myeloproliferative disorders, in contrast, each of the three major marrow cell lines proliferates in an unregulated, essentially autonomous and self-perpetuating manner. Four disorders—polycythemia vera, agnogenic myeloid metaplasia, chronic myelogenous leukemia, and essential thrombocythemia—can usefully be classified under this heading. Although the proliferation of one particular cell line may dominate the clinical picture, each of these is a clonal hematopoietic malignant disorder arising at the level of the pluripotent stem cell. In each disorder, erythroid, myeloid, and megakaryocytic elements proliferate excessively, but to varying degrees, in the bone marrow and in sites of extramedullary hematopoiesis (often resulting in splenomegaly). In each disorder there is a variable tendency for reactive proliferation of the otherwise normal bone marrow fibroblast—which both cytogenetic and glucose-6-phosphate dehydrogenase (G6PD) isoenzyme studies confirm is not a part of the malignant clone—with the development of myelofibrosis, and for termination in an acute blastic leukemia. Despite differences in the predominant cell line released into the periphery, bone marrows at the time of presentation show many similarities and may be indistinguishable, with clumps or sheets of abnormal megakaryocytes being common to all. Hyperuricemia secondary to increased cell turnover and abnormal levels of serum B_{12} and its binding proteins and of leukocyte alkaline phosphatase activity are also common to this group. Some investigators include acute leukemias of various types (notably erythroleukemia) and paroxysmal nocturnal hemoglobinuria within the myeloproliferative syndromes; others consider these disorders sufficiently different from the basic four to warrant their exclusion.

The myeloproliferative syndromes have long been considered to exhibit transitions between the various entities. The evolution of polycythemia vera into a disorder characterized by myelofibrosis with myeloid metaplasia is well documented, as is the transition of all entities—albeit with varying frequency—to acute leukemia. Other transitions have been harder to document. Thus, Philadelphia chromosome (Ph¹)–positive chronic myelogenous leukemia may present transiently with elevated red cell and platelet counts but does not at this stage represent polycythemia vera. Similarly, a patient with polycythemia vera who has suffered a gastrointestinal hemorrhage may at initial examination have only an elevated platelet count, resembling essential thrombocythemia. Repletion of iron stores with resulting erythrocytosis does not represent a true transition from essential thrombocythemia to polycythemia vera.

Despite the failure to confirm true transitions among several of these disorders, the concept of a myeloproliferative syndrome involving the four basic entities just listed is now firmly supported by their clonal, morphologic, pathophysiologic, and clinical similarities. Various nonspecific cytogenetic abnormalities are also observed in each of these entities. The appearance of the Ph¹ chromosome, characteristic of chronic myelogenous leukemia, is a late event in the pathogenetic evolution of the disorder and follows the initial development of the malignant clone of pluripotent stem cells.

Gilbert HS: Myeloproliferative disorders. Clin Geriatr Med 1:773, 1985. *A reassessment of the myeloproliferative disease concept on its fortieth anniversary by an astute clinical observer.*

Lichtman MA: Classification and clinical manifestations of the hematopoietic stem cell disorders. *In* Williams WJ, Beutler E, Erslev AJ, et al. (eds.): Hematology. 4th ed. New York, McGraw-Hill, 1990, pp 148–157. *A useful classification of various types of hematopoietic stem cell disorders that places the chronic myeloproliferative disorders in proper perspective.*

Nathan CF: Secretory products of macrophages. J Clin Invest 79:319, 1987. *A concise yet lucid review of the diverse biologic properties of the numerous regulatory molecules now known to derive, at least in part, from macrophages, including modulation of cellular replication and differentiation.*

MYELOFIBROSIS WITH MYELOID METAPLASIA

Definition and Pathogenesis

Myelofibrosis with myeloid metaplasia is a syndrome in which morphologic evidence of excessive fibroblast proliferation and collagen deposition in the bone marrow is accompanied by myeloid metaplasia of organs such as the liver, spleen, and lymph nodes. These organs, involved normally in fetal but not adult erythropoiesis, become active sites of extramedullary hematopoiesis. Similar clinical syndromes may be seen in three distinct settings. The first of these is progressive hepatosplenomegaly and the evolution of a leukoerythroblastic peripheral blood picture indicative of myeloid metaplasia occurring in the absence of an apparent inciting cause. This disorder, termed *agnogenic myeloid metaplasia* (see Color Plates 5*J* and 7*F*, left), is a clonal stem cell hemopathy constituting one of the primary myeloproliferative syndromes. Second, a similar picture of myelofibrosis with myeloid metaplasia may evolve in the course of polycythemia vera or chronic granulocytic leukemia, either as a part of the natural history of the illness or as a consequence of the myelosuppressive therapies administered. The third setting is myeloid metaplasia with varying degrees of reactive myelofibrosis that may occur secondary to a wide spectrum of clinical disorders, including, among others, severe hemolytic anemia, Hodgkin's disease, various nonhematopoietic neoplasms metastatic to the bone marrow, infections such as tuberculosis, or following bone marrow injury caused by radiation, benzol, fluorine, phosphorus, or strontium.

In myelofibrosis with myeloid metaplasia, the extent of extramedullary hematopoiesis tends to parallel the extent of bone marrow fibrosis. Indeed, it was previously believed that the mesenchymal cells in the liver, spleen, and lymph nodes resumed their embryonic potential for hematopoiesis in an attempt to compensate for myelophthisis. However, in some cases there is a dissociation between the degree of marrow fibrosis and extramedullary hematopoiesis, resulting in (1) marrow fibrosis without evidence of significant myeloid metaplasia or (2) progressive hepatosplenomegaly with a leukoerythroblastic peripheral blood picture in the absence of significant fibrosis. Pluripotent hematopoietic stem cells, presumably of bone marrow origin, are constantly present in the circulation of normal individuals and appear in increased numbers in the peripheral blood of patients with myelofibrosis. It is more likely that these circulating stem cells take up residence in organs such as the liver and spleen to produce extramedullary hematopoiesis than that this represents the reactivation of hematopoietic capabilities in local mesenchymal cells.

Except in the secondary setting noted above, the primary pathogenetic event is believed to be a mutation leading to a malignant pluripotent hematopoietic stem cell clone. In black women with agnogenic myeloid metaplasia who are also heterozygous for two different G6PD isoenzymes, the presence of only one G6PD isoenzyme in all of their erythroid, myeloid megakaryocytic, macrophage, and B lymphoid cells and/or progenitor colonies confirms that all of these cells are derived from a single, mutated pluripotent stem cell. A similar cellular distribution of acquired cytogenetic abnormalities in the significant proportion of patients with abnormal karyotypes suggests the same conclusion. Endogenous colonies of erythroid progenitor cells can be grown from peripheral blood or bone marrow.

The development of myelofibrosis appears to be a reaction to the presence of this abnormal, proliferating hematopoietic clone. Marrow fibrosis in agnogenic myeloid metaplasia, as in the other myeloproliferative disorders, correlates with the presence in the marrow of increased numbers of often dysplastic megakaryocytes (Fig. 142–3). The release of increased quantities of megakaryocyte- and platelet-derived growth factor, and of transforming growth factor–β (TGF-β), from the markedly expanded bone marrow megakaryocyte pool appears to be primarily responsible for the increased fibroblast proliferation and collagen deposition that characterize these disorders. Possible roles for tumor necrosis factor–α and interleukin 1 (IL1), also potent stimulators of fibroplasia, remain to be established. Colonization of the liver, spleen, and lymph nodes may, in this setting, represent a form of metastasis of abnormal stem cells to organs that retain an intrinsic potential to support hematopoiesis.

Clinical Features

Myelofibrosis with myeloid metaplasia, whether agnogenic or secondary to another myeloproliferative syndrome, is primarily a disorder of the middle-aged or older adult. Although reported to occur as early as infancy, at least 60 per cent of cases occur in those between the ages of 50 and 70, with no predilection for either sex. The onset of symptoms is usually insidious over several years, and in most cases disease progression is slow. One quarter of cases are asymptomatic at diagnosis. Most commonly presenting symptoms are referable to anemia with its cardiovascular consequences or to increased abdominal girth or discomfort resulting from splenic and hepatic enlargement. Bone pain, often migratory, and gouty arthritis occasionally bring the patient to medical attention. Osteosclerosis is common; deafness resulting from otosclerosis occurs in a small minority of cases. Increasing numbers of asymptomatic patients are being detected today in the course of routine screening laboratory or physical examinations.

On physical examination, splenomegaly is an almost universal finding. In approximately 85 per cent of cases, the spleen extends 8 cm or more below the left costal margin and in one third of cases is enlarged more than 16 cm. Occasional patients without palpable splenomegaly are demonstrated to have splenic enlargement by means of an isotopic or computed tomographic (CT) imaging study. Rarely, significant myelofibrosis with cytopenia occurs, at least initially, without myeloid metaplasia and with no evidence of splenic enlargement. Hepatomegaly occurs in approximately 50 per cent of cases, frequently with mild abnormalities of liver function tests—especially elevation of alkaline phosphatase levels. Hepatomegaly in the absence of splenomegaly is extremely rare in agnogenic myeloid metaplasia or when the syndrome occurs secondary to another myeloproliferative disease and points to a diagnosis of secondary myeloid metaplasia. Extramedullary hematopoiesis is frequently demonstrable histologically in lymph nodes, but clinically significant lymph node enlargement occurs in only 10 per cent of cases. Extramedullary tumors of hematopoietic tissue, often with intense fibrosis, may occur virtually anywhere but are most commonly reported in the adrenal glands, kidneys, intestinal tract, lungs, mediastinum, breast, and skin. When they occur in the intracranial or intraspinal epidural spaces, they may lead to serious neurologic consequences. Ascites and pleural or pericardial effusions, often containing immature hematopoietic cells, may result from the implantation of hematopoietic foci on various serosal surfaces. A combination of increased splenic and portal blood flow, due to proliferation of extramedullary hematopoietic tissue within the spleen, and decreased intrahepatic vascular compliance, caused by both intrasinusoidal extramedullary hematopoiesis and perisinusoidal fibrosis, may lead to clinically significant portal hypertension, with consequent ascites, esophageal varices, and gastrointestinal hemorrhage. Jaundice, edema, and ascites occur in 10 to 20 per cent of cases. Petechiae, caused by both thrombocytopenia and platelet dysfunction, have been reported in up to 25 per cent of patients.

Laboratory Data

At diagnosis, a mild to moderate degree of anemia is typical, with the hemoglobin ranging between 9 and 13 grams per deciliter. Red cells are initially normocytic and normochromic with mild poikilocytosis. Polychromatophilia, a modest reticulocytosis of 2 to 5 per cent, and occasional teardrop erythrocytes are seen (see Color Plate 7*F*, left). The presence of at least a few normoblasts and occasionally even earlier erythroid precursors is extremely common. As the disease progresses and the spleen enlarges, more severe anisocytosis, poikilocytosis, polychromasia, basophilic stippling, and normoblastosis may be sufficiently characteristic to indicate the diagnosis. Red cell autoantibodies, with autoimmune hemolysis, may contribute to the anemia in some cases. The white blood cell count is initially normal in about one third of patients, elevated in approximately one half, and low in the remaining 15 per cent. Most typically, the count is in the range of 15,000 to 30,000 per cubic millimeter, but counts as high as 70,000 per cubic millimeter are observed. The white count tends to fluctuate with time and often does not show the downward trend observed for the hemoglobin concentration and platelet count. A degree of granulocyte immaturity in the peripheral blood is typical, including the presence of as many as 10 per cent blasts. This condition does not necessarily suggest the evolution of acute leukemia, particularly when there are proportionate numbers of promyelocytes, myelocytes, and metamyelocytes as well. Basophilia and an acquired Pelger-Huët anomaly are other typical features of the peripheral blood smear. The leukocyte alkaline phosphatase score is variable but is most often normal or increased. The platelet count initially is most often normal, although reduced or elevated counts are not uncommon. Exceedingly high counts in excess of 10^6 per microliter may cause this condition to be confused with the entity of primary thrombocytosis. Morphologically, megathrombocytes and megakaryocytic fragments are extremely common. Over time, the platelet count gradually tends to decrease, and thrombocytopenia is common late in the disorder. Overall, a peripheral blood smear demonstrating striking teardrop poikilocytosis, leukoerythroblastic nucleated cells, and megathrombocytes and megakaryocytic fragments is highly suggestive of the syndrome of myelofibrosis with myeloid metaplasia. Erythrocyte survival is almost invariably reduced, and splenic sequestration often is present. Erythrokinetic studies demonstrate markedly ineffective erythropoiesis. Platelet production is usually increased even in patients with thrombocytopenia, associated with a marked increase in splenic pooling.

Normal or slightly elevated serum levels of vitamin B_{12} and B_{12}-binding proteins occur both in agnogenic myeloid metaplasia and postpolycythemia myelofibrosis, but the values are not as striking in those seen in chronic granulocytic leukemia. Hyperuricemia, caused by increased uric acid production, is common. Miscellaneous laboratory abnormalities include high levels of lactate dehydrogenase (LDH), modest elevations of serum transaminase and bilirubin levels, increased serum alkaline phosphatase activity caused by both hepatic and bone isoenzyme fractions, and modest increases in muramidase (lysozyme). A variety of autoantibodies, circulating immune complexes, and complement activation have been reported, as have associations with systemic lupus erythematosus, periarteritis nodosa, scleroderma, and nonspecific vasculitis. These reports have suggested a possible autoimmune pathogenesis in some cases.

Cytogenetic abnormalities occur in up to 50 per cent of patients with agnogenic myeloid metaplasia, with trisomy of chromosomes 7, 8, and 9 being most commonly found. Abnormalities of chromosomes 1, 5, and 20 also occur with increased frequency. The Ph[1] chromosome is not present; cases in which this abnormality was reported most likely represent atypical examples of chronic myelogenous leukemia.

Osteosclerosis distributed primarily in the flat bones of the axial skeleton and in the metaphyseal ends of the femur and humerus may be recognized radiographically in up to 70 per cent of patients. The typical radiographic finding is the loss of definition of individual bony trabeculae, leading to a ground glass appearance.

Attempts to aspirate bone marrow almost invariably lead to a dry tap, even when the marrow is very cellular. Accordingly, bone marrow biopsy, either percutaneous or surgical, is usually required for diagnosis. Demonstration of bone marrow fibrosis (see Color Plate 5J), often with accompanying osteosclerosis, is the sine qua non, and the marrow content of types I, III, and IV collagen is increased. The bone marrow may sometimes be hypercellular, frequently demonstrating a panhyperplasia, in residual focal areas. Even in these areas, in which mature collagen may not be evident, an increase in reticulin fibers can usually be demonstrated by silver impregnation. Extramedullary hematopoiesis is demonstrable in both liver and spleen, but because of the risks involved in percutaneous biopsy of these organs, its diagnosis usually is based on the typical leukoerythroblastic blood picture and occasionally on isotopic erythrokinetic studies. The increase of bone marrow collagen content in myelofibrosis is principally the result of excessive collagen deposition and is reflected in an increase in the serum level of procollagen III amino-terminal peptide. Serum prolyl hydroxylase and plasma fibronectin are also increased.

Course of the Disease

The course of both agnogenic and postpolycythemic myelofibrosis is characterized by progressive splenic enlargement and, typically, by slightly less striking enlargement of the liver. The spleen often fills the entire left side of the abdomen, extending beyond the midline to the right and down into the pelvis. The resulting early satiety, associated with a hypermetabolic state from increased cell turnover, may result in appreciable weight loss. Painful splenic infarcts may also complicate the disease. The marked splenic enlargement and consequent increase in splenic blood flow, coupled with increased resistance to flow within the liver caused by extramedullary hematopoiesis, lead to portal hypertension and its various complications, including ascites, edema, and variceal hemorrhage in a small proportion of patients. Hepatic vein thrombosis with the Budd-Chiari syndrome is another recognized complication. The progressive splenomegaly is accompanied almost inevitably by progressive anemia and thrombocytopenia, the former occasionally complicated by iron deficiency of blood loss or, less frequently, by folic acid deficiency. Although granulocyte counts are usually better maintained than those of other blood cellular elements, eventually granulocytopenia may develop. In this setting, bacterial infections occur with increased frequency and may be a major factor leading to death. The association of myelofibrosis with tuberculosis is well documented, and this infection should be excluded by histologic and bacteriologic examination. Because of the almost inevitable hyperuricemia, attacks of gouty arthritis may develop in untreated patients.

Acute leukemic transformation is an occasional terminal event in agnogenic myeloid metaplasia. About 10 per cent of patients with polycythemia vera will develop a spent phase with advanced myelofibrosis. The likelihood of developing postpolycythemic myelofibrosis does not seem to be influenced by the type of therapy given for the underlying polycythemia, but evolution to the spent phase is a risk factor for subsequent development of acute leukemia. Once myelofibrosis has developed in this setting, the incidence of subsequent leukemic transformation (6 per cent in phlebotomy-treated patients, 45 per cent in those taking chlorambucil, and 25 per cent in those treated with ^{32}P) is 2½ to 4 times greater than in similarly treated polycythemic patients who have not developed myelofibrosis.

Treatment and Prognosis

No agreement has been reached concerning the optimal treatment of agnogenic myeloid metaplasia or of postpolycythemic myelofibrosis. There is thus far no effective treatment that inhibits the fibrotic process. Moreover, none of the conventional forms of treatment, including androgen therapy to stimulate erythropoiesis, chemotherapy, or splenectomy, has been shown to prolong life. Because of the relatively indolent progression of the disorder in most patients, a majority of hematologists undertake no specific treatment in the asymptomatic patient except for the administration of allopurinol at doses of 200 to 400 mg per day to avoid the complications of hyperuricemia.

In the presence of symptomatic anemia, androgens may be employed: testosterone enanthate, 200 to 600 mg weekly given intramuscularly, or oxymetholone, 50 to 150 mg daily by mouth. Treatment must be continued for at least 3 months to establish whether a particular preparation is effective, and some hematologists argue that patients who fail to respond to one androgen preparation may ultimately respond to another. Androgens seem most effective in women who have been splenectomized previously or who have never had massive splenomegaly. The doses employed inevitably lead to excessive fluid accumulation and, in female patients, to significant masculinization. Except in patients with a documented autoimmune component, the hemolytic anemia almost never responds to corticosteroids; these drugs may, however, increase the risk of infection in granulocytopenic patients. In patients with marked thrombocytosis, busulfan, in an initial dosage of 4 mg per day, followed by lower doses as the platelet count normalizes, or hydroxyurea, at a dosage of 500 to 1500 mg per day, is often effective in gaining control of the platelet count. Although busulfan is widely used in this setting, its potential mutagenic risks are a cause for concern. These agents may occasionally produce a beneficial reduction in spleen size and/or increase the hemoglobin concentration but equally frequently result in suppression of erythropoiesis and thrombopoiesis. Anagrelide and alpha- and gamma-interferons have also been used experimentally to reduce thrombocytosis (Ch. 142). Radiation therapy to the spleen has largely been abandoned because the doses required to produce a meaningful reduction in spleen size often cause severe leukopenia and thrombocytopenia. Radiotherapy remains useful for the treatment of areas of localized bone pain, serosal hematopoietic implants leading to serous effusions, or symptomatic extramedullary hematopoietic tumors, especially those compressing the brain or spinal cord.

The role of splenectomy in patients with agnogenic myeloid metaplasia or postpolycythemic myelofibrosis is highly controversial. As a high-risk procedure, it should probably be reserved for patients with severe hemolytic anemia, thrombocytopenia sufficient to produce bleeding, portal hypertension, or severe discomfort secondary to pressure symptoms or infarction. Striking thrombocytosis with thrombosis or hemorrhage or both may develop postoperatively and may require aggressive myelosuppression. In some patients splenectomy is followed by progressive and massive enlargement of the liver, with recurrent hemolysis and thrombocytopenia. The diagnosis of acute leukemia is often difficult to make in these patients, in whom the percentage of blasts in the peripheral blood may increase slowly and progressively for years.

Survival in agnogenic myeloid metaplasia and in postpolycythemic myelofibrosis is difficult to define with certainty. Several authors suggest that median survival in agnogenic myeloid metaplasia is approximately 10 years from the onset of the disease and 5 years from the time of diagnosis. However, there is considerable heterogeneity, with both shorter and longer survival frequently observed.

Bone marrow transplantation has been attempted both by conventional techniques and after surgical manipulation of bone marrow cavity spaces in attempts to provide an improved microenvironment for the transplanted marrow. Only occasional successes have been reported, and this procedure must be considered highly experimental.

Several additional suggested approaches to the treatment of myelofibrosis include the use of inhibitors of collagen synthesis (such as monoamine oxidase inhibitors and colchicine) and the vitamin D analogues 1,25-dihydroxyvitamin D and 1,25-dihydroxycholecalciferol. The latter are reported to decrease proliferation of megakaryocytes and, presumably, the consequent release of platelet- and megakaryocyte-derived fibroproliferative factors. The clinical value of these experimental approaches has not been established.

The syndrome of acute myelofibrosis, which is a rapidly progressive and fatal variant, has been shown by various cytologic marker studies to represent a form of acute megakaryocytic leukemia. It is believed that the release of platelet-megakaryocyte–derived growth factor from the malignant megakaryoblasts is responsible for the rapidly progressive marrow fibrosis. Induction chemotherapy may produce temporary hematologic remission, but only partial reversal of marrrow fibrosis. This is the one setting with myelofibrosis in which bone marrow transplantation deserves early consideration, particularly in patients under 40 years of age who have a suitable bone marrow donor.

Berk PD, Castro-Malaspina H, Wasserman LR (eds.): Myelofibrosis and the Biology of Connective Tissue. New York, Alan R. Liss, 1984. *This book contains 29 concise chapters by multiple authors who review the available information about the regulation of fibroblast proliferation, collagen biosynthesis, cell biology of marrow stromal cells, and other aspects of basic biologic science believed to be relevant to the pathogenesis of myelofibrosis.*

Carlo-Stella C, Cazzola M, Gasner A, et al.: Effects of recombinant α and γ interferons on the in vitro growth of circulating hematopoietic progenitor cells (CFU-GEMM, CFU-Mk, BFU-E and CFU-GM) from patients with myelofibrosis with myeloid metaplasia. Blood 70:1014, 1987. *An interesting study demonstrating an inhibitory effect of recombinant interferons on proliferation*

of abnormal hematopoietic progenitors in myelofibrosis with myeloid metaplasia. In concert with other studies showing that interferons decrease collagen synthesis, this study sets the stage for clinical trials of interferon therapy.

Lichtman MA: Agnogenic myeloid metaplasia. In Williams WJ, Beutler E, Erslev AJ, et al. (eds.): Hematology. 4th ed. New York, McGraw-Hill, 1990, pp 223–232. *A comprehensive review of the pathogenesis, clinical features, and management of the myelofibrosis syndromes, with a thorough and up-to-date bibliography.*

McCarthy DM: Fibrosis of the bone marrow: Content and causes. Br J Haematol 59:1, 1985. *An examination of the pathobiology of marrow fibrosis and of experimental approaches to its prevention and treatment.*

ESSENTIAL THROMBOCYTHEMIA

Essential (primary) thrombocythemia, also known as a hemorrhagic thrombocythemia or essential thrombocytosis, is a primary myeloproliferative disorder of the pluripotent hematopoietic stem cell in which the predominant laboratory feature is a persistent, striking elevation of the platelet count to values in excess of 1×10^6 per microliter (see Color Plate 8K, right). Megakaryocytic colony-forming units (CFU-M) in peripheral blood and bone marrow are both quantitatively increased and qualitatively altered, in that they can be grown in vitro in the absence of various normally required growth factors. The disorder shows many features of polycythemia vera, including an almost identical distribution of patient ages at the time of diagnosis, similar degrees of leukocytosis, morphologically similar bone marrow abnormalities, and the presence of endogenous erythroid progenitors in peripheral blood and bone marrow. Splenomegaly has been reported to occur in 30 to 75 per cent of cases. The criteria outlined in the following paragraph would restrict the diagnosis to patients who have either normal or reduced hemoglobin concentrations, those with concomitant erythrocytosis being classified as having polycythemia vera.

The Polycythemia Vera Study Group has proposed the following diagnostic criteria for essential thrombocythemia: (1) platelet count persistently greater than 1×10^6 per microliter in the absence of an identifiable cause, such as malignant disease, infection, chronic inflammatory disease, or previous splenectomy; (2) normal total red cell volume, the measurement of which may be omitted if the hemoglobin concentration is less than 13 grams per 100 ml; (3) presence of iron in the bone marrow; if iron is absent, failure of the hemoglobin concentration to increase by more than 1 gram per deciliter after a 1-month trial of oral iron therapy; (4) absence of collagen fibrosis in bone marrow biopsy; and (5) absence of the Ph[1] from unstimulated metaphases obtained from a bone marrow aspirate. Because of both morphologic and clinical similarities, criteria 2 and 3 are necessary to exclude a diagnosis of polycythemia vera, whereas criteria 4 and 5 distinguish the disorder from agnogenic myeloid metaplasia and chronic myelogenous leukemia, respectively.

Clinical Features

Essential thrombocythemia is generally a disease of later life, diagnosed most often in those between the ages of 50 and 70, and affecting both sexes equally, but a distinct second peak of incidence occurs in younger patients, particularly females, and childhood cases have been reported.

The predominant clinical manifestations of essential thrombocythemia result from hemorrhagic and/or thrombotic events. Some patients have easy bruising, epistaxis, unexplained gastrointestinal bleeding, and an excessive tendency to postoperative hemorrhage. Conversely, other patients present evidence for microvascular occlusion in sites such as the extremities, the central nervous system, and the coronary circulation. The most common manifestation of microvascular occlusion is burning pain in the feet, hands, and digits, which may progress to frank gangrene. Although these symptoms are striking when they occur, approximately two thirds of patients are asymptomatic at diagnosis, and large numbers of patients, particularly younger patients, may remain asymptomatic for long periods. Hence, the precise incidence of these complications is unknown. Similarly, transition to acute leukemia has been clearly documented, but there is no accurate estimate of its frequency, particularly in patients not previously exposed to mutagenic agents.

Course and Prognosis

The natural history of this disease is poorly appreciated, and most reports in the literature describe very small series of patients with a focus on a particular complication. Neurologic manifestations, ranging from headaches and paresthesias to visual disturbances, transient ischemic attacks, and strokes, are especially worrisome, but their overall frequency remains unclear. The most typical manifestation is erythromelalgia, a vaso-occlusive syndrome characterized by localized pain, burning, redness, and warmth of one or more distal extremities. It may progress to frank necrosis of a digit. When present, erythromelalgia typically responds dramatically to rapid reduction of the platelet count or to administration of nonsteroidal anti-inflammatory agents. These responses are consistent with a proposed pathogenesis involving the arteriolar vasospastic effects of metabolites of platelet arachidonic acid. Descriptions emphasizing hemorrhagic, thrombotic, and embolic episodes and a high fatality rate are directly contradicted by others emphasizing prolonged periods without complications. The largest series suggest a life expectancy perhaps analogous to that of polycythemia vera.

Therapy

Because of uncertainties about its natural history, there is a substantial lack of agreement about appropriate therapy for essential thrombocythemia. Despite strikingly high platelet counts, many hematologists recommend expectant management in asymptomatic patients under the age of 60, while others recommend the use of only platelet-antiaggregating agents (e.g., aspirin, 300 mg per day, with or without dipyridamole, 50 mg three times per day). However, the experience in polycythemia vera suggests that prolonged administration of platelet-antiaggregating agents may increase the risk of gastrointestinal hemorrhage. Chronic myelosuppression should be attempted in older patients and those who have a history of significant thrombotic episodes. In these cases, prevention of neurologic damage takes precedence over concern about long-term mutagenic effects of myelosuppression. Control of the thrombocytosis can usually be achieved with hydroxyurea* at an initial dose of 500 to 1500 mg per day, tapered to an individualized maintenance dose as the platelet count falls. Concerns about the long-term mutagenic effects of alkylating agents and of radioactive phosphorus have made hydroxyurea the initial drug of choice in this setting. Its short duration of action, however, requires strict adherence to the prescribed regimen to maintain control of the platelet count. In less compliant patients, adequate control can be obtained with a longer acting agent, such as melphalan,* 6 to 10 mg per day by mouth for 1 week, followed by 4 to 6 mg per day until the platelet count is in the normal range. Subsequent maintenance with 2 to 6 mg per week is continued indefinitely, the dose being adjusted according to the platelet count. Alternatively, particularly in the elderly patient, radioactive phosphorus, 2.9 mCi per square meter of body surface area given intravenously, repeated as necessary at intervals of not less than 3 months, is highly effective. Both anagrelide and interferons have been used experimentally to control the platelet count is essential thrombocythemia, as they have in polycythemia vera (Ch. 142), but their precise roles remain to be established. Patients presenting with serious thrombotic or hemorrhagic manifestations and uncontrolled thrombocytosis should be treated with platelet-antiaggregating agents, urgent plateletpheresis, and the initiation of a myelosuppressive regimen. Every effort should be made to avoid splenectomy in patients with essential thrombocythemia because of the extreme thrombocytosis and serious complications that often follow this procedure.

Barbui T, Buelli M, Cortelazzo S, et al.: Aspirin and risk of bleeding in patients with thrombocythemia. Am J Med 83:265, 1987. *A clinical study demonstrating that aspirin may excessively prolong the bleeding time in some patients with thrombocythemia associated with myeloproliferative disorders. The message is that chronic administration of aspirin as a platelet antiaggregating agent in this setting may be hazardous.*

Jabaily J, Iland HJ, Laszlo J, et al.: Neurologic manifestations of essential thrombocythemia. Ann Intern Med 99:513, 1983. *A contrary report suggesting that approximately two thirds have evidence of at least transient neurologic dysfunction.*

Kessler CM, Klein HG, Havlik RJ: Uncontrolled thrombocytosis in chronic myeloproliferative disorders. Br J Haematol 50:157, 1982. *A retrospective study suggesting that, at least in the younger patient, severe thrombocytosis in myeloproliferative disease may have fewer complications than previously believed.*

---

*This use is not listed in the manufacturer's directive.

Mazur EM, Cohen JL, Bogart L: Growth characteristics of circulating hematopoietic progenitor cells from patients with essential thrombocythemia. Blood 71:1554, 1988. *One of several recent studies demonstrating quantitative and qualitative abnormalities in both megakaryocytic and erythroid progenitor cells in essential thrombocythemia.*

Murphy S: Primary thrombocythemia. In Williams WJ, Beutler E, Erslev AJ, et al. (eds.): Hematology. 4th ed. New York, McGraw-Hill, 1990, pp 231–236. *A balanced critique of the often contradictory literature about this uncommon yet fascinating disease.*

144 The Chronic Leukemias

Michael J. Keating

CHRONIC MYELOGENOUS LEUKEMIA (Chronic Myeloid Leukemia, Chronic Myelocytic Leukemia, Chronic Granulocytic Leukemia)

Definition

Chronic myelogenous leukemia (CML) is a disease characterized by an overproduction of cells of the granulocytic, especially the neutrophilic, series and occasionally the monocytic series (see Color Plate 7F, right), leading to marked splenomegaly and very high white blood cell counts. Basophilia and thrombocytosis are common. A characteristic cytogenetic abnormality, the Philadelphia (Ph[1]) chromosome, is present in the bone marrow cells in more than 95 per cent of cases. The granulocytes usually appear relatively normal, although many patients exhibit dysplastic changes, including Pelger-Huët anomalies. Neutrophil functions, such as phagocytosis and bactericidal activity, are largely preserved. Before effective treatment was available, patients survived, on the average, approximately 2 years after diagnosis.

Etiology

Usually, no etiologic agent can be incriminated in CML. Exposure to ionizing radiation increases the risk of subsequent CML. Survivors of the atomic bomb explosions in Japan in 1945 have had an increased incidence of CML, with a peak occurring 5 to 12 years after exposure and seemingly dose related. The relative risk has been falling since that time but is still above the expected rate for Japan. Radiation treatment of ankylosing spondylitis and cervical cancer has increased the incidence of CML. No increase in the risk of CML has been demonstrated in individuals working in the nuclear industry. Radiologists working without adequate protection prior to 1940 were more likely to develop myeloid leukemia, but no such association has been found in recent studies. Benzene exposure increases the risk of acute myelogenous leukemia (AML) but not of CML. Patients with CML have an increased frequency of the Cw3 and Cw4 human leukocyte antigens (HLA's). Chronic myelogenous leukemia is not a frequent secondary leukemia following the treatment of other cancers with radiation and/or alkylating agents.

Incidence

Chronic myelogenous leukemia constitutes one fifth of all cases of leukemia in the United States. One or 2 persons per 100,000 are diagnosed as having CML per year, with a slight male preponderance. This incidence has not changed significantly in the past few decades. The incidence of CML increases with age; the median age at diagnosis is approximately 45 to 50 years. Ph[1]-positive CML is uncommon in children and adolescents. Patients who are older than 60 years have a poorer prognosis. No familial association of CML has been noted.

Molecular Pathogenesis

The striking feature in CML is the presence of Ph[1] chromosome in the bone marrow cells of more than 90 per cent of patients with typical CML. The Ph[1] chromosome results from a balanced translocation of material between the long arms of chromosomes 9 and 22. As more chromosomal material is lost from chromosome 22 than is gained from chromosome 9, the Ph[1] chromosome is a shortened chromosome 22 containing approximately 60 per cent of its normal complement of DNA. The break, which occurs at band q34 of the long arm of chromosome 9, allows translocation of the cellular oncogene *C-ABL* to a position on chromosome 22 called the breakage cluster region (bcr). The breakpoint in the bcr varies from patient to patient but is identical in all cells of any one patient. *C-ABL* is a homologue of *V-ABL*, the Abelson virus that causes leukemia in mice (Ch. 157). The apposition of these two genetic sequences produces a new hybrid gene (*abl/bcr*), which codes for a novel protein of molecular weight 210,000 kD (P210). The P210 protein, a tyrosine kinase, may play a role in triggering the uncontrolled proliferation of CML cells. The Ph[1] chromosome occurs in erythroid, myeloid, monocytic, and megakaryocytic cells, less commonly in B lymphocytes, rarely in T lymphocytes, but not in marrow fibroblasts. This extensive cellular distribution places the abnormality in CML close to the pluripotent stem cell. Studies of glucose-6-phosphate dehydrogenase (G6PD) isoenzymes support the finding of multilineage monoclonal proliferation, since a single isoenzyme is present in the above-mentioned cells in informative patients with CML. *C-sis*, the homologue of the simian sarcoma virus, is also translocated from chromosome 22 to chromosome 9 in CML but is distant from the breakpoint and not expressed in benign-phase CML. *C-sis* encodes for a protein identical to platelet-derived growth factor (PDGF). Insertion of a retrovirus encoding P210 (*abl/bcr*) into cells of mice has led to the development of a disease closely resembling CML in some of these animals, giving credence to the hypothesis that the (*abl/bcr*) hybrid gene is sufficient to cause CML.

The fusion *abl/bcr* gene and the P210 protein can be found in many cases of typical CML in which no cytogenetic abnormality occurs or in which changes other than typical t(9;22)(q34;q11) are identified. These patients have a survival rate and a response to therapy that are similar to those in Ph[1]-positive patients. Patients with atypical CML who are Ph[1] and *abl/bcr* negative have a different natural history than do patients who are either Ph[1] positive or Ph[1] negative with *abl/bcr* positivity. They resemble more closely patients with myelodysplastic syndrome (MDS) (Ch. 129). Thus, three groups of patients with CML can be identified: (a) positive for Ph[1] and *abl/bcr*, (b) Ph[1] negative and *abl/bcr* positive, and (c) negative for Ph[1] and *abl/bcr* (Table 144–1).

Although 100 per cent of the metaphases on cytogenetic analysis usually show the presence of the Ph[1] chromosome, some normal stem cells must remain. Normal diploid cells appear on long-term bone marrow culture and following treatment with interferon, high-dose chemotherapy, and autologous bone marrow transplantation.

Symptoms and Signs

Many asymptomatic patients are diagnosed as having CML because of the use of hematologic studies in routine annual physical examinations or in evaluations for other illnesses. In these patients, the white blood cell (WBC) count may be relatively low at the time of diagnosis. The WBC count correlates well with tumor mass as defined by spleen size. Patients with higher WBC counts and larger spleens have more symptoms. The symptomatology of CML, usually nonspecific, is secondary to anemia, spleen size, or an increased basal metabolic rate, but most patients are asymptomatic or only mildly symptomatic. Fatigue, weight loss, malaise, easy satiety, and a sense of left upper quadrant fullness are the major symptoms of CML. Rarely, bleeding (associated with a low platelet count and/or platelet dysfunction) or thrombosis (associated with thrombocytosis and/or marked leukocytosis) occurs. The serum uric acid level is commonly elevated at diagnosis, and acute gouty arthritis may follow treatment. An elevated blood histamine level (related to the basophil cell mass) can cause upper gastrointestinal ulceration and bleeding. Neutrophil function is usually normal or only modestly impaired, and neutrophil numbers are markedly increased; infections are therefore uncommon at the time of diagnosis. Headaches, bone pain, arthralgias, pain from splenic infarction, and fever are uncommon in the early stages of CML but become more common as the disease progresses. Priapism is occasionally noted, usually in patients with marked leukocytosis or thrombocytosis. Leukostatic symptoms, such as dyspnea, drowsiness, loss of coordination, or confusion, which are due to sludging in the pulmonary or cerebral vessels, are uncommon in the benign phase of CML despite WBC counts that may exceed 400,000 per microliter. These symptoms appear more frequently in later stages of the disease (i.e., in the accelerated or blast crisis phases, in which more premature cells predominate). All symptoms subside as the WBC count falls and the splenomegaly decreases as a result of effective treatment.

Splenomegaly, by far the most consistent physical sign in CML, occurs in more than 90 per cent of cases. The spleen may extend to the pelvic brim and across the midline of the abdomen in some cases. Hepatomegaly is less common and is usually minor (1 to 3 cm below the right costal margin). Lymphadenopathy is very uncommon, as is infiltration of skin and other tissues. If present, these findings suggest a Ph[1]-negative CML or an accelerated or blastic transformation of CML. Rarely, patients present initially with a blast crisis; these patients can have any of the clinical manifestations of acute leukemia.

Natural History

More than 90 per cent of patients present with CML in the benign phase, in which the disease behaves in a predictable fashion, with the symptoms, abnormal physical signs, and abnormal blood findings returning to normal following treatment. This satisfactory response is transient; all patients eventually develop a variety of changes in the behavior of the disease. Most frequently, there is a "blast crisis," a clinical picture resembling that of acute leukemia. This change can be abrupt, but more frequently it is preceded by a period of progressively greater difficulty in maintaining the WBC count at a level of less than 20,000 per microliter and of other manifestations, such as increasing splenomegaly, hepatomegaly, and infiltration of nodes, skin, bones, or other tissues; the appearance of blast cells or basophils in the peripheral blood; development of anemia and/or thrombocytopenia; or fever, malaise, and weight loss. This last group of features, termed the accelerated phase of CML, demands reevaluation of the bone marrow, which, in the accelerated phase, shows dysplastic changes in the myeloid and other cell lineages and may show an increase in the percentage of blast cells (5 to 29 per cent) and an increase in basophils. Aspiration of bone marrow may be difficult, especially in patients who have developed myelofibrosis subsequent to the CML. Chromosomal abnormalities, in addition to the Ph[1] chromosome, occur in both the accelerated and the blastic phases of CML. Blast crisis is diagnosed when 30 per cent or more blast cells are present in the bone marrow and/or peripheral blood.

When the accelerated phase or blast crisis is suspected (i.e., 10 to 40 per cent blasts in bone marrow), the patient should be further evaluated in 2 to 4 weeks, since the percentage of blasts in the blood and bone marrow can increase transiently after the treatment of CML is discontinued, especially with hydroxyurea or interferon. It is important to be cautious in classifying patients as having blast crisis or accelerated phase because of the adverse prognostic implications (Fig. 144–1). Criteria for the accelerated phase are the following: an increase in blast cells (>15 per cent or basophils (>20 per cent) in the blood or bone marrow, thrombocytopenia (<100,000 per microliter), serious anemia (hemoglobin [Hb] < 7 grams per deciliter); documented extramedullary leukemia, or development of clonal evolution (new chromosomal changes in addition to the Ph[1] chromosome).

The risk of developing accelerated phase or blast crisis in CML is relatively low in the first 2 years after diagnosis (~10 per cent per year) but then increases and remains constant (15 to 20 per cent per year) after that unless therapy such as bone marrow transplantation is used.

TABLE 144–1. CLASSIFICATION OF CHRONIC MYELOGENOUS LEUKEMIA (CML)

Disease	Ph[1] Present	abl/bcr Rearrangement	Prognosis
Classic CML	Yes	Yes	Median, 4 yr
bcr+, Ph[1]-	No	Most	Median, 4 yr
CMML/CMoL/bcr-CML	No	No	18–24 mo

bcr = Break cluster region; abl/bcr = a hybrid gene (see text); CMML = chronic myelomonocytic leukemia; CMoL = chronic monocytic leukemia.

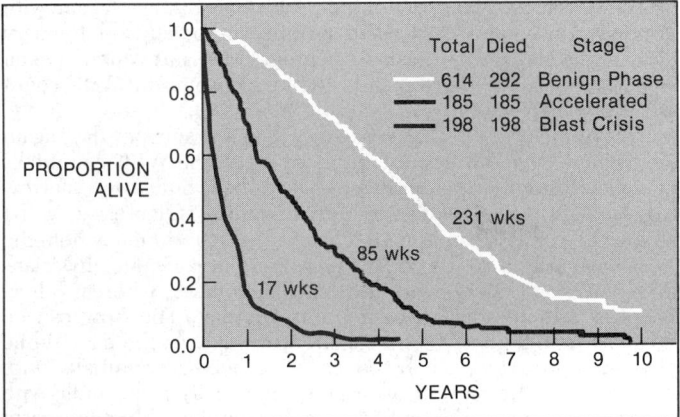

FIGURE 144–1. Survival of M. D. Anderson Cancer Center patients with chronic myelogenous leukemia (CML) by phase of disease.

Laboratory Findings

All patients with untreated CML have an elevated WBC count ranging from 10,000 per microliter to more than 1,000,000 per microliter. The predominant cells are of the neutrophil series, with a left shift extending to blast cells (see Color Plate 7F, right). In addition, eosinophils and basophils are commonly increased in number. Monocytes may be slightly increased in some cases that overlap with chronic myelomonocytic leukemia (CMML). The bone marrow is hypercellular with marked myeloid hyperplasia and sometimes shows evidence of increased reticulin or collagen fibrosis. The myeloid-erythroid ratio is 15:1 to 20:1. About 15 per cent of patients have 5 per cent or more blast cells in the peripheral blood or bone marrow at diagnosis. T cells (both T-helper and T-suppressor), but not B cells, are increased in number in CML. A hemoglobin of less than 11 grams per deciliter is present in one third of patients. The red cells are usually normochromic and normocytic, but nucleated red cells are present in the blood of one quarter of the patients at diagnosis. Autoimmune hemolytic anemia and thrombocytopenia (<100,000 per microliter) are rare in CML, but thrombocytosis (>450,000 per microliter) occurs in almost half of the patients.

Biochemical abnormalities in CML include a markedly decreased leukocyte alkaline phosphatase (LAP) score in the neutrophils of 90 per cent or more of patients, being completely absent in 5 to 10 per cent of cases. A low LAP score also occurs in some patients with agnogenic myeloid metaplasia, which is sometimes difficult to differentiate from CML (Ch. 143). The serum levels of transcobalamins I and III, cobalamin-binding glycoproteins produced by neutrophils, are elevated in accord with the increased neutrophils (Ch. 132). This elevation leads to extremely high serum cobalamin values (e.g., vitamin B_{12} levels >10 times normal). Serum levels of lactate dehydrogenase, uric acid, and lysozyme are often increased. The lysozyme levels are modestly increased in CML compared with CMML, in which the levels in blood and urine are often markedly increased. Kinetic studies show an increased neutrophil production rate related to a markedly expanded myeloid mass. The number of colony-forming cells in the blood in CML is increased, but the number in the bone marrow is in the normal range. Defective feedback control of WBC production is common in CML; some patients demonstrate a cyclic oscillation of the WBC count. The labeling index of myeloblasts in CML is lower than in normal bone marrow, and the generation time is prolonged, confirming the concept that CML is an accumulative rather than a proliferative disease. Neutrophils in CML survive intravascularly slightly longer than do normal granulocytes.

Diagnosis

The diagnosis of typical CML is not difficult. The presence of unexplained myeloid leukocytosis with splenomegaly should lead to a LAP test on the peripheral blood neutrophils and a bone marrow examination with a cytogenetic analysis. Marrow myeloid hyperplasia and hypercellularity further suggest the diagnosis. The ultimate test, however, remains the cytogenetic analysis; the presence of the Ph^1 chromosome in this clinical setting establishes the diagnosis. When the Ph^1 chromosome is not found in a patient with suspected CML, molecular evidence for the presence of the hybrid *abl/bcr* gene should be sought, as 40 to 50 per cent of Ph^1-negative patients with CML have *abl/bcr* rearrangement. The Ph^1 chromosome is usually present in 100 per cent of metaphases, ordinarily as the sole abnormality. Ten to 15 per cent of patients at initial presentation have an additional chromosomal change, such as loss of the Y chromosome, trisomy 8, an additional 22q−, or an atypical translocation. The patients who have atypical complex chromosomal changes, which may or may not involve chromosome 9 or 22 morphologically, demonstrate evidence of the hybrid *abl/bcr* gene when techniques of molecular biology are used.

Chronic myelogenous leukemia must be differentiated from leukemoid reactions, which usually produce WBC counts lower than 50,000 per microliter, toxic granulation vacuolation, Döhle bodies in the granulocytes, absent basophilia, a normal or increased LAP level, and a clinical history and physical examination suggesting the origin of the leukemoid reaction (Ch. 141). Corticosteroids can rarely cause extreme neutrophilia together with the left shift, but this response is self-limited and short in duration and thus seldom a cause of diagnostic difficulty.

Chronic myelogenous leukemia may be more difficult to differentiate from other myelodysplastic or myeloproliferative syndromes. Patients having agnogenic myeloid metaplasia with or without myelofibrosis present with splenomegaly and often with neutrophilia and thrombocytosis (Ch. 143). Polycythemia rubra vera with associated iron deficiency, which allows a normal hemoglobin level and hematocrit value, can manifest with an elevated neutrophil and platelet count (Ch. 142). Such patients usually have a normal or increased LAP score and a WBC count less than 25,000 per microliter, and the Ph^1 chromosome is not present.

The greatest diagnostic difficulty lies with patients who have splenomegaly and leukocytosis but who do not have the Ph^1 chromosome. Many of these patients have the usual blood and marrow findings of Ph^1-positive CML, and the *abl/bcr* hybrid gene can be demonstrated despite a normal or atypical cytogenetic pattern. Patients who are Ph^1 negative and *abl/bcr* negative are considered to have Ph^1-negative CML or CMML (Table 144–1). The cytogenetic findings in patients with CMML are normal or involve an additional chromosome 8 or findings other than the Ph^1 chromosome. Patients with CMML have *ras* mutations in 50 to 60 per cent of cases. Rarely, patients present with myeloid hyperplasia, which involves almost exclusively the neutrophil, eosinophil, or basophilic cell lineage. These patients are described as having chronic neutrophilic, eosinophilic, or basophilic leukemia and do not have evidence of the Ph^1 chromosome or *abl/bcr* gene. Isolated megakaryocytic hyperplasia can give rise to a syndrome called idiopathic thrombocythemia with marked thrombocytosis and splenomegaly (Ch. 143, 154). These conditions are considered to fall under the general category of myeloproliferative disorders and have a better prognosis than does CML.

Evolution of CML

Death occurs rarely during the chronic phase of CML, but over time the clinical behavior of the disease changes. One third of patients abruptly develop an acute transformation (blast crisis of CML); the other two thirds respond progressively less well in the control of the WBC count and spleen size with conventional agents such as busulfan and hydroxyurea. This loss of control (accelerated phase) is often associated with an increased proportion of blasts, promyelocytes, and basophils in the peripheral blood and bone marrow and is often accompanied by anemia and thrombocytopenia. Some patients develop bone marrow failure in which anemia and thrombocytopenia are accompanied by increasing evidence of dysplastic changes in the marrow and myelofibrosis. The median survival after developing a blast crisis of CML is only 3 months (Fig. 144–1). The survival after development of the accelerated phase of CML is 12 to 18 months if the blood and bone marrow contain more than 30 per cent blasts plus promyelocytes or more than 20 per cent basophils or if the platelet count falls to less than 100,000 per microliter. Most patients with blast crisis or accelerated phase have additional chromosomal abnormalities (clonal evolution), such as duplication of the Ph[1] chromosome, trisomy of chromosome number 8, or development of an isochromosome number 17. Clonal evolution usually presages the accelerated phase or blast crisis of CML. The blast cells in blast crisis are usually myeloblasts, but less commonly erythroid, monocytoid, or megakaryoblastic transformations occur. In one-quarter of cases, the blast cells are lymphoid in origin, as demonstrated by cytochemical stains (terminal deoxynucleotidyl transferase), immunophenotyping, and immunoglobulin heavy-chain rearrangement studies. In 10 per cent of cases, the blast cells are completely undifferentiated. Some patients who present with acute leukemia and the Ph[1] chromosome abnormality presumably have blast crisis that occurred before the diagnosis of CML was made. These cases have the P210 protein and 8.5-kb fusion messenger RNA. Patients with acute lymphoblastic leukemia (ALL) with a Ph[1] usually have a P190 protein or a 7.1-k fusion messenger RNA probably restricted to the lymphoid cells. Extramedullary blast crisis of CML can occur in the spleen, lymph nodes, skin, meninges, bone, and other sites. This initial extramedullary transformation is usually shortly followed by evidence of marrow involvement.

Chronic myelomonocytic leukemia and Ph[1]- and *abl/bcr*-negative CML appear to overlap clinically in some instances, and their clinical behavior, progress, and response to therapy resemble those of the MDS more than Ph[1]-positive CML. A male preponderance is noted, splenomegaly is common (60 to 70 per cent), and the WBC count, while elevated, is usually in the 25,000 to 100,000 per microliter range. Anemia and thrombocytopenia are more common than in Ph[1]-positive CML, and eosinophilia and basophilia are less common. The median survival is 18 to 24 months, with patients dying of infection, bleeding, or transformation to acute leukemia.

Treatment

Immediate treatment of CML is not necessary unless the WBC count exceeds 200,000 per microliter or there is evidence of leukostasis (priapism, venous thrombosis, confusion, or dyspnea) or unless painful splenomegaly suggests splenic infarction. Hyperuricemia is common at the diagnosis of CML and should be treated with allopurinol, 100 mg three times a day, and adequate hydration while the WBC count is higher than 25,000 per microliter to prevent renal dysfunction. Acute gouty arthritis is rare.

Palliative Treatment

Chronic myelogenous leukemia has been treated traditionally with oral busulfan, which, if used prudently, gives smooth, sustained control of the WBC count, platelet count, and spleen size. Since overdosage with busulfan can cause prolonged myelosuppression, another active oral agent, hydroxyurea, has been increasingly used. Both agents have a high level of acceptance by the patient, and both control the manifestations of the disease in 90 per cent of cases when first used, but over time they produce progressively shorter and less complete reductions in the WBC count and spleen size.

Busulfan is usually started at a dosage of 4 to 8 mg per day, depending on the WBC count and the patient's body size. Use of higher dosages of 12 to 16 mg per day should be restricted to patients with WBC counts greater than 200,000 per microliter. Leukapheresis can also be used on a short-term basis to decrease the leukocyte or platelet counts rapidly. When the initial WBC count halves, the starting dose should be decreased by 50 per cent. The leukocyte count decreases exponentially and is closely correlated with a reduction in spleen size. Since the WBC count continues to fall for 2 to 4 weeks after cessation of busulfan, the drug should be discontinued when the WBC count reaches 20,000 to 25,000 per microliter to prevent severe pancytopenia from marrow hypoplasia. The WBC count may not begin to rise again for several months or for more than a year, at which time a lower dose (2 to 4 mg per day) should be reinstituted. Few acute side effects are noted with busulfan, although premature menopause does occur in 20 to 40 per cent of young women and sterility is frequent in both men and women. Hyperpigmentation, weight loss, and fatigue, which can mimic Addison's disease, occur with prolonged use, and in a small number of patients pulmonary fibrosis develops. As the disease progresses, intervals between courses of busulfan shorten and the rate of rise in the WBC count at relapse increases.

Hydroxyurea is given at dosages of 1 to 4 grams per day, again according to the WBC count and body size. The WBC count falls in similar fashion to that induced by busulfan, but severe marrow hypoplasia is rare. The dosage of hydroxyurea is decreased as the leukocyte count decreases and can be discontinued when the WBC count is 5 to 10 × 10³ per microliter. Some physicians prefer to treat patients with intermittent courses, whereas others maintain patients on 0.5 to 2 grams per day. The drug can be given as a single dose or fractionated throughout the day. While close monitoring of the blood count is necessary initially with hydroxyurea, the pattern of response is usually predictable with repeated courses. Side effects are uncommon, although rash, mucositis, and diarrhea can occur. The survival of patients treated with busulfan or hydroxyurea is similar. Splenic irradiation is not recommended for the treatment of CML.

Cytogenetically Directed Therapy

Busulfan and conventional-dose hydroxyurea rarely eliminates the Ph[1] chromosome from marrow cells. With high-dose hydroxyurea, however, diploid metaphases have been observed in several patients. A return to a normal chromosomal pattern would seem to be a reasonable therapeutic goal, and it might be anticipated that patients who achieve a normal karyotype may survive better than those who do not. Three therapeutic initiatives have been developed based on this concept: the use of interferons, intensive chemotherapy, and bone marrow transplantation.

INTERFERON THERAPY. Both human leukocyte interferon and recombinant alpha-interferon (r-IFnα) have been demonstrated to produce hematologic and cytogenetic remissions in CML. Complete hematologic remissions are obtained in 75 to 80 per cent of patients treated with r-IFnα, and 30 to 40 per cent of the patients have a complete or partial suppression in the Ph[1] chromosome. Gamma-interferon alone or combined with alpha-interferon does not have a significant therapeutic effect. Return of normal metaphases following the use of r-IFnα is associated with a longer survival than is seen in patients without a cytogenetic response. The dosage of r-IFnα is 2 to 5 million units per square meter per day, administered subcutaneously or intramuscularly. The response rate is higher with the higher dose. The most common acute side effects—musculoskeletal discomfort, fever, and chills—subside in most patients but are often replaced by symptoms of fatigue, depression, lethargy, inattention, loss of weight, lack of libido, and mild alopecia. These toxicities are more common in patients over 60 years of age. Reactions at the injection site occur in approximately 5 per cent of patients. Thrombocytopenia, anemia, arthritis, nephrotic syndrome, and seizures occur rarely. Loss of disease control, together with lack of side effects, may signal the development of neutralizing antibodies to interferon.

AGGRESSIVE CHEMOTHERAPY. Regimens commonly employed for the treatment of acute myelogenous leukemia (AML) have been used in an attempt to suppress the Ph[1] chromosome. In more than 50 per cent of the treated patients, the percentage of Ph[1]-positive metaphases is greatly reduced, and about one third become transiently diploid for 2 to 12 months. Research protocols using chemotherapy induction therapy followed by r-IFnα maintenance are now under way.

ALLOGENEIC BONE MARROW TRANSPLANTATION. Marrow transplantation has been performed in patients with benign-phase CML (Ch. 153). The risk of early death due to complications of transplantation (20 to 30 per cent) is balanced against the observation that 50 to 60 per cent of patients will be in hematologic or cytogenetic remission 3 to 5 years after transplantation. Favorable factors for survival are age lower than 30 years, transplantation within 1 year of diagnosis, and absence of severe graft-versus-host disease (GVHD). Long-term survival rates after transplantation in accelerated and blast phases of CML are only approximately 10 to 15 per cent. After syngeneic (identical twin) bone marrow transplantations, 84 per cent of patients treated at the Fred Hutchinson Cancer Center (Seattle, Washington) are alive and 75 per cent continue in complete hematologic and cytogenetic remission. The possibility exists that many of these patients will be cured. Autologous marrow and peripheral blood stem cell support following ablative chemotherapy and radiation therapy is currently being evaluated.

Treatment of Accelerated and Blast Crisis of CML

Loss of control of CML with agents such as busulfan, hydroxyurea, or interferon is marked by development of increasing splenomegaly, leukocytosis, and thrombocytosis. Many of these patients developed additional cytogenetic abnormalities (clonal evolution). Some patients develop severe anemia and thrombocytopenia. Splenectomy occasionally corrects the thrombocytopenia. The bone marrow often develops increasing dysplasia of one or multiple cell lines, together with an increasing left shift (5 to 29 per cent blast cells), eosinophilia, and basophilia. Change of therapy from busulfan to hydroxyurea or vice versa is successful for a short time (3 to 6 months) in 10 to 25 per cent of patients. These patients are considered to have an accelerated phase of the disease. If the proportion of blast cells in bone marrow exceeds 30 per cent, the patient is considered to be in blast crisis (acute transformation of CML) (see Color Plate 7G). The blast crisis or refractory accelerated phase of CML is usually treated with regimens designed for the treatment of acute leukemia (Ch. 145). Treatment of myeloid, undifferentiated, or mixed-lineage blast crisis is usually unsatisfactory, with only 25 to 30 per cent of patients achieving a complete remission. Patients with a lymphoid blast crisis phenotype have a better chance (50 to 65 per cent) of achieving a complete remission on regimens utilizing vincristine, corticosteroids, asparaginase, and/or anthracyclines. The Ph[1] chromosome persists, and the duration of response is usually short (2 to 6 months), with no prospect of cure. Only 10 to 15 per cent of patients with blast crisis survive for more than 1 year (Fig. 144–1). Allogeneic marrow transplantation should be offered to patients with blast crisis (with active disease or after remission is obtained) if a suitable donor is available, since few of these patients have survived more than 5 years. The mortality rate and relapse rate after allogenic transplantation for CML blast crisis are much higher than for CML in the benign phase. Patients who have an HLA-compatible sibling should have an allogeneic transplantation performed before the accelerated or blast phases of CML develop.

Prognosis

The median survival of Ph[1]-positive CML was 3 to 4 years for patients treated in the 1970's, with a range of 1 to 20 years (Fig. 144–2). The median survival at the M. D. Anderson Cancer Center in Houston, Texas, for patients diagnosed after 1980 is greater than 5 years. The risk of death is 5 to 8 per cent per year for the first 24 months and increases to 15 to 20 per cent per year for the next 2 years and 25 per cent per year thereafter. No

TABLE 144–2. ADVERSE PROGNOSTIC FACTORS IN CHRONIC MYELOGENOUS LEUKEMIA

Older age
Large spleen size
Large liver size
Increase or decrease in platelets
High white count
Basophilia
Clonal evolution

From Kantarjian HM, Keating MJ, Smith TL, et al.: Proposal for a simple synthesis prognostic staging system in chronic myelogenous leukemia. Am J Med 88:1, 1990; with permission.

patients are projected to be cured with a palliative use of busulfan and/or hydroxyurea. The influence of treatment with interferon, aggressive chemotherapy, and allogeneic transplantation on the improved survival of patients diagnosed after 1980 is not certain at this time. Large spleen, increased liver size, elevated platelet counts, high marrow and blood blast and basophil percentages, advanced age, and clonal evolution are consistent adverse prognostic factors (Table 144–2) and have been combined into a simple staging system. This system identifies a high-risk group (30 to 40 per cent) of patients with a median survival of only 2 years. The quality of life of patients in the benign phase is usually excellent.

Bos JL: *Ras oncogenes in hematopoietic malignancies.* Hematol Pathol 2:55, 1988. *A review illustrating the frequency and pattern of mutations in the ras oncogene family in acute and chronic leukemias.*

Butturini A, Keating A, Goldman J, et al.: Autotransplants in chronic myelogenous leukemia: Strategies and results. Lancet 335:1255, 1990. *A recent review of the results and problems of autologous transplantation in CML.*

Daley GQ, Van Etten RA, Baltimore D: Induction of chronic myelogenous leukemia in mice by the P210abl/bcr gene of the Philadelphia chromosome. Science 247:824, 1990. *A seminal report of the role of the* abl/bcr *gene as a causative factor in CML.*

Fefer A, Thomas ED: Bone marrow transplantation for the treatment of chronic myelogenous leukemia. *In* DeVita VT, Hellman S (eds.): Important Advances in Oncology. Philadelphia, J.B. Lippincott, 1990, p 143. *A comprehensive overview of the results of allogeneic transplantation in CML.*

Kantarjian HM, Dixon D, Keating MJ, et al.: Characteristics of accelerated disease in chronic myelogenous leukemia. Cancer 61:1441, 1988. *A quantitative analysis of the impact on survival of various features of accelerated-phase CML.*

Kantarjian HM, Keating MJ, Walters RS, et al.: Clinical and prognostic features of Philadelphia chromosome–negative chronic myelogenous leukemia. Cancer 58:2023, 1986. *An analysis of the prognostic factors and clinical features of Ph[1] chromosome–negative CML, illustrating differences from Ph[1]-positive CML and similarities to the MDS.*

Kurzrock R, Gutterman JU, Talpaz M: The molecular genetics of Philadelphia chromosome–positive leukemias. N Engl J Med 319:990, 1988. *A detailed analysis of the current relevance of molecular genetic data in Ph[1] chromosome–positive acute and chronic leukemias.*

Strife A, Lambek C, Wisniewski D, et al.: Discordant maturation as the primary biological defect in chronic myelogenous leukemia. Cancer Res 48:1035, 1988. *An analysis of the morphologic changes associated with the various clinical stages of CML.*

Talpaz M, Kantarjian HM, McCredie K, et al.: Hematologic remission and cytogenetic improvement induced by recombinant human interferon alpha A in chronic myelogenous leukemia. N Engl J Med 314:1065, 1986. *Initial demonstration of the ability of interferon to induce cytogenetic remissions in CML.*

HAIRY CELL LEUKEMIA
Clinical Features

Hairy cell leukemia (HCL) is uncommon (1 to 2 per cent of all leukemias). The median age at diagnosis is 50 years, with a 4:1 male preponderance. Patients present with symptoms of fatigue due to anemia, fever, weight loss, and/or abdominal discomfort produced by splenomegaly. Sometimes the disease is diagnosed when patients present with infection secondary to granulocytopenia or monocytopenia. The only consistent physical findings are slight to marked splenomegaly (75 to 80 per cent of cases) caused by massive infiltration by hairy cells and slight to moderate hepatomegaly (33 per cent of cases). Clinical lymphadenopathy is very uncommon, although retroperitoneal lymphadenopathy is noted on computed tomography (CT) scans in 20 to 25 per cent of cases. More than two thirds of patients present with anemia (<10 grams per deciliter), neutropenia (<1500 per microliter),

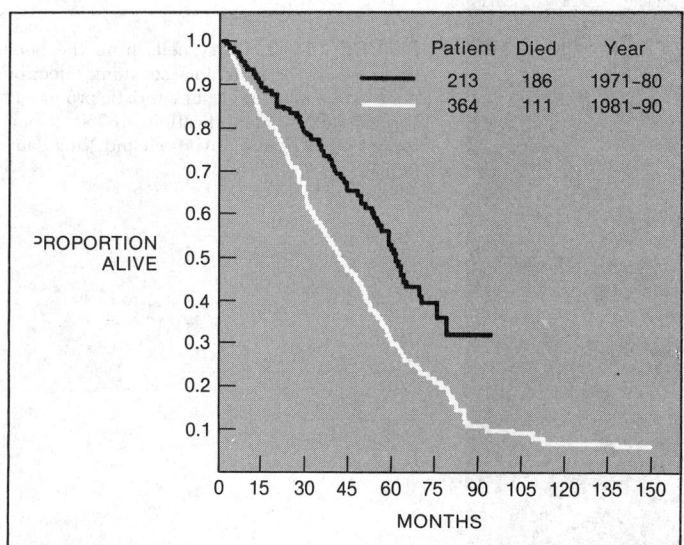

	Patient	Died	Year
	213	186	1971–80
	364	111	1981–90

FIGURE 144–2. Survival of M. D. Anderson Cancer Center patients with benign-phase CML by year of diagnosis.

thrombocytopenia (<100,000 per microliter), and monocytopenia (<100 per microliter). The WBC count is usually lower than 4000 per microliter at diagnosis, but marked thrombocytopenia is rare. The cytopenias are due to a combination of bone marrow production failure caused by leukemic infiltration and of hypersplenism. Marrow failure may be due in part to inhibitory factors (e.g., tumor necrosis factor) produced by the leukemic infiltrate, since the pancytopenia is often much more marked than would be anticipated from the degree of leukemic infiltration. During the course of the illness, patients often experience repeated infections and more rarely a systemic vasculitis resembling polyarteritis nodosa or osteolytic bone lesions, usually affecting the upper femora. Although gram-positive or gram-negative infections occur as expected with neutropenia, patients with HCL have a predilection to develop tuberculosis, atypical mycobacterial infections, or fungal infections, perhaps related to the severe monocytopenia that is characteristic of this disorder. Pneumonia and septicemia are common causes of death in HCL.

Diagnosis

In conjunction with the described clinical features, examination of the blood often suggests the diagnosis of HCL. In addition to the cytopenias described above, the peripheral blood film usually demonstrates a relative or absolute lymphocytosis, composed of cells with cytoplasmic projections, giving rise to the name "hairy cell" leukemia (Fig. 144–3) (see Color Plate 7J, left). The cytoplasmic projections are best seen using phase contrast or electron microscopy. The hairy cells are 10 to 15 μm in diameter with pale blue cytoplasm and a nucleus with a loose chromatin structure and one or two indistinct nucleoli. Bone marrow aspiration is usually inadequate owing to increased reticulin, collagen, and fibrin deposition, and a bone marrow biopsy is necessary. The biopsy demonstrates an increased cellularity with a diffuse or occasionally patchy infiltrate with hairy cells. The infiltrate is loose and spongy, with pale-staining cytoplasm surrounding bland, monotonous round or ovoid nuclei.

Hairy cells exhibit a strong acid phosphatase (isoenzyme 5) cytochemical reaction in 95 per cent of cases, a reaction that is resistant to the inhibitory effect of tartaric acid (TRAP). Other lymphoproliferative diseases are rarely TRAP positive. Electron microscopy exquisitely demonstrates the microvillar projections. Often, ribosomal-lamellar complexes can be identified; these are characteristic, but not diagnostic, of HCL. The peroxidase stain is negative, and lysozyme activity is absent in hairy cells, differentiating the cells from monocytes.

The cell of origin of HCL is the B lymphocyte, as documented by the demonstration of heavy- and light-chain immunoglobulin gene rearrangements. Hairy cells express CD19 and CD20, FMC7, and CD22, but not CD21 or CD5. Cell-surface immunoglobulins can be immunoglobulin G (IgG) or immunoglobulin A (IgA), which are rare in chronic lymphocytic leukemia (CLL). The cells demonstrate a kappa or lambda light-chain phenotype excess. The cells are CD25 (TAC or low-affinity interleukin 2 [IL+2] receptor) positive and anti-HC2 positive, and they are positive for an early plasma cell antigen PCA-1, but not a late plasma cell antigen PCl. These findings suggest that hairy cells are late B lymphocytes or early plasma cells. High levels of soluble IL-2 receptors (>5 times normal) are present in the sera of almost all patients with HCL, with extremely high levels being noted in many cases. Some cases of HCL have a 14q+ cytogenetic abnormality with a breakpoint at 14q32 (the locus of the Ig heavy-chain gene). Hairy cells have a low proliferative index, with fewer than 1 per cent being in the S phase of the cell cycle. Immune dysfunction is wide ranging in HCL. Monocytopenia is universal, B and T lymphocytes are decreased in number; the CD4/CD8 ratio is often inverted; and skin test reactivity to recall antigens is impaired, as is antibody-dependent cellular cytotoxicity. Humoral immunity is relatively preserved with normal immunoglobulin levels. A markedly impaired ability of patients with HCL to produce alpha-interferon has been reported.

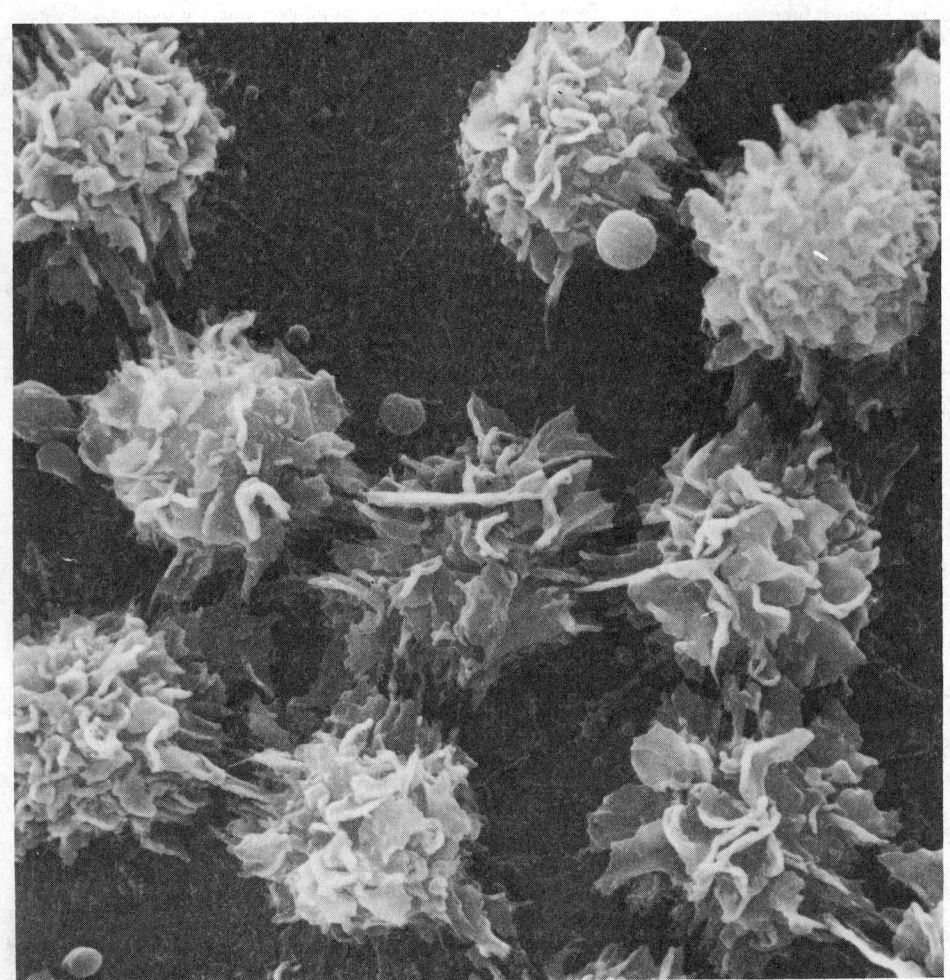

FIGURE 144–3. Hairy cells from the bone marrow as seen in the scanning electron microscope, showing characteristic prominent surface ruffles. Magnification ×8750. (Courtesy of Dr. Etienne deHarven and Nina Lampen.)

Differential Diagnosis

The differential diagnosis is most difficult between HCL and patients with lymphoma or CLL who have predominant splenomegaly and minimal lymphadenopathy. Some patients with a myelodysplastic or myeloproliferative syndrome have marked splenomegaly and pancytopenia with only a few atypical cells. Patients with other diseases, such as systemic lupus erythematosus and other autoimmune diseases, infiltrative splenomegaly, or tuberculosis, may present with splenomegaly and cytopenia, but these diagnoses can usually be made by history, physical examination, and appropriate blood and bone marrow tests. Splenomegaly, cytopenia, and an inaspirable marrow in a male should create a very high index of suspicion for HCL.

Other pathologic conditions to be differentiated from HCL requiring special tests are HCL variant, splenic lymphoma with villous lymphocytes, B cell and T cell prolymphocytic leukemia, and CLL with splenomegaly and no lymphadenopathy. Splenectomy and lymph node biopsy are sometimes necessary to establish the diagnosis in difficult cases. Cases of HCL variant manifest with higher WBC counts, are TRAP negative, have prominent nucleoli, and are only occasionally positive for antibodies against CD25. HCL variant responds poorly to interferon or deoxycoformycin, which are very effective agents in the management of typical HCL.

Prognosis and Treatment

A small proportion (<5 per cent) of patients with HCL do not require therapy. These patients have mild cytopenias, are not transfusion dependent, have no history of infections, and have a low level of marrow infiltration by hairy cells.

SPLENECTOMY. Because splenomegaly can itself cause pancytopenia, splenectomy was used in the past as the first treatment of most patients with HCL when complications such as splenic infarction or abdominal discomfort occurred, when infections became frequent, or when anemia, neutropenia, or thrombocytopenia worsened. Splenectomy was temporarily effective in improving blood counts in two thirds of patients, with improvement usually noted within 1 to 4 weeks. Splenectomy was usually ineffective if the spleen was not palpable. Removal of the spleen does not decrease the infiltration of hairy cells in the marrow or reduce the incidence of infections. Usually within 2 years, pancytopenia recurs owing to progressive marrow infiltration. The median survival of most patients in whom splenectomy alone was utilized was 4 to 5 years. Splenectomy is now recommended mainly for patients with splenic infarcts or massive splenomegaly.

INTERFERON. Chemotherapy for HCL with alkylating agents, corticosteroids, androgens, and anthracyclines is not effective and, when used in the past, was associated not infrequently with prolonged myelosuppression and severe infections. Low-dose chlorambucil was better tolerated but seldom resulted in significant clinical improvement. The use of human leukocyte interferon (HuIFn), however, has revolutionized the present approach to therapy. The use of HuIFn or r-IFnα rapidly improves (1 to 3 months) granulocyte, platelet, and hemoglobin levels; reduces spleen size; and consistently decreases marrow infiltration. Peripheral blood counts return to normal in 80 per cent of cases, and these patients achieve a complete remission (no hairy cells in the marrow) or a partial remission (>50 per cent reduction in marrow HCL infiltration). The most commonly used dosage of IFn is 3×10^6 units given subcutaneously three times a week, although daily schedules for 6 months reduce the marrow HCL infiltration more effectively. Higher doses (3 to 5 $\times 10^6$ units daily) increase the complete remission rate from 5 to 10 per cent to 25 per cent, with a partial remission rate of 55 to 65 per cent and a total failure rate of less than 5 per cent. Most patients achieve a partial remission by 6 months and a complete remission by 12 to 18 months. Response to therapy is most satisfactory in patients who are less anemic and monocytopenic and who have lower marrow cellularity. Lack of response or loss of an initial response may result from the development of neutralizing antibodies to r-IFnα, especially if the antibody titer is high. When treatment is discontinued, most patients relapse within 1 to 2 years, but most will again respond to treatment. Relapse occurs more quickly in patients who achieve only a partial remission than in those who respond completely. Treatment is usually reintroduced when patients become granulocy-

topenic. The presence of active, severe infection is not a contraindication to treatment with interferon. Indeed, the response to therapy provides patients with the best chance to recover from the infection.

INVESTIGATIONAL AGENTS. *Pentostatin* (2-deoxycoformycin), an adenosine deaminase inhibitor, has marked activity in HCL. At the low dosages used to treat HCL (4 mg per square meter every 2 weeks), pentostatin produces complete remissions in 50 to 60 per cent of patients and partial remissions in 40 per cent. Higher dosages of pentostatin are associated with a high rate of infections, usually with opportunistic infections, since the agent is very immunosuppressive, decreasing both T cell number and function. The response rate of the higher dose regimen is 80 to 90 per cent, with more than 60 per cent of patients achieving a complete response. The response to treatment is more rapid than for interferon, occurring within 2 to 4 months following the initiation of therapy. Pentostatin is active in patients previously treated with interferon. Responses appear to be more durable than those seen in interferon-treated patients. Toxicity includes nausea and vomiting, infection, renal and hepatic dysfunction, conjunctivitis, and photosensitivity.

2-Chlorodeoxyadenosine (2-CDA), an adenosine analogue, has been reported to produce complete remissions in more than 90 per cent of HCL patients with a single course of 0.1 mg per kilogram per day for 7 days by continuous intravenous infusion. Since the remissions appear to be very durable, 2-CDA promises to be the most effective agent developed to treat HCL. The drug is very well tolerated, with a low infection rate. *Granulocyte colony-stimulating factor (G-CSF)* has been reported to correct the granulocytopenia in HCL.

PROGNOSIS. The median survival of patients with HCL prior to interferon was 2 to 3 years. A return to normal leukocyte counts in HCL diminishes the risk of infection and is certain to improve the survival of patients with HCL. More than 90 per cent of interferon-treated patients are projected to be alive at 5 years.

Chilosi M, Semanzato G, Cetto G, et al.: Soluble interleukin-2 receptors in the sera of patients with hairy cell leukemia: Relationship with the effect of recombinant alpha-interferon therapy on clinical parameters and natural killer in vitro activity. Blood 70:1530, 1987. *Description of a clinically useful serum marker in the diagnosis and management of HCL.*

Piro LD, Carrera CJ, Carson DA, et al.: Lasting remissions in hairy-cell leukemia induced by a single infusion of 2-chlorodeoxyadenosine. N Engl J Med 322:1117, 1990. *Report of dramatic clinical activity of a purine analogue, 2-chlorodeoxyadenosine, in HCL, resulting in a high frequency of complete remissions.*

Quesada J: Hairy cell leukemia. In Freireich EJ, Kantarjian HM (eds.): *Therapy of Hematopoietic Neoplasia.* New York, Marcel Dekker, in press. *A balanced analysis of the biology, clinical features, treatment, and prognosis of HCL.*

Van Norman AS, Nagorney DM, Martin JK, et al.: Splenectomy for hairy cell leukemia. A clinical review of 63 patients. Cancer 57:644, 1986. *Describes the features associated with response to splenectomy in HCL.*

CHRONIC LYMPHOCYTIC LEUKEMIA

Chronic lymphocytic leukemia (CLL) is a neoplasm characterized by accumulation of monoclonal lymphocytes, usually of B cell immunophenotype (>95 per cent of cases), more rarely of T cell immunophenotype (see Color Plate 7I). The cells accumulate in the bone marrow, lymph nodes, liver, spleen, and occasionally other organs. Chronic lymphocyte leukemia is the most common leukemia (one third of all cases) in the Western world and is twice as common as CML. The disease occurs rarely in those below the age of 30; most patients with CLL are over 60 years of age. Chronic lymphocytic leukemia increases in incidence exponentially with age; by age 80 the incidence rate is 20 cases per 100,000 persons per year. The male-female ratio is approximately 2:1. Asian countries such as Japan and China have an incidence of CLL only 10 per cent of that in the United States and other Western countries. Intermediate incidence rates exist for persons of Hispanic origin.

Etiology

The cause of CLL is unknown. Ionizing radiation and viruses have not been associated with CLL. Familial clustering in CLL is more common than in other leukemias; first-degree relatives of patients have a twofold to fourfold higher risk than does the general population. Farmers have a higher incidence of CLL than do those in other occupations, raising the question of the possible etiologic role of herbicidal or pesticidal chemicals. No specific leukemogenic role of chemicals, including benzene, has been established for CLL.

Pathogenesis

Leukemia cells in CLL are usually remarkably homogeneous. The cells express monoclonal surface immunoglobulin (SmIg, usually immunoglobulin M [IgM] ± immunoglobulin D [IgD]) of a single kappa or lambda light-chain phenotype. A number of patients with CLL have SmIg molecules that cross-react with IgM rheumatoid factor paraprotein. CLL cells are early B cells and have lost terminal deoxynucleotidyl transferase activity. The CLL cells express the pan B antigens CD19, CD20, and CD24 in almost all cases and CD21 (which includes the receptor for the Epstein-Barr virus and the C3D component of complement) in more than 75 per cent of cases. In fewer than 20 per cent of cases is the C3B complement component receptor expressed. The vast majority of cells exhibit Ia antigen, have receptors for the Fc fragment of IgG, and spontaneously form rosettes with mouse erythrocytes. In 95 per cent of cases, the CLL cells coexpress pan B cell antigens and CD5 (Leu 1, T1, and T101), a pan T cell antigen. Other T cell antigens and common acute lymphocytic leukemia antigen (CALLA) (CD10) are absent. CD25 (TAC, IL2 receptor) antigen is positive in more than 20 per cent of cells in 20 per cent of cases.

Monoclonality of the B cells is demonstrated by a marked preponderance of kappa or lambda light chains, by evidence of immunoglobulin gene rearrangement, by the presence of monoclonal serum Ig peaks in some cases, and by glucose-6-phosphate dehydrogenase isoenzyme studies.

Chronic lymphocytic leukemia is an accumulative rather than a proliferative disease, since the CLL cells have a low proliferative index. Patients with higher WBC counts and more advanced stages have higher proliferative indices and shorter survivals. Most of the CLL cells in the blood and bone marrow are in the Go phase of the cell cycle, with only a small proportion of larger cells in the marrow and lymph nodes being in the other phases. The CLL cells have a longer lifespan in the blood than do normal B cells and have impaired egress from the blood. The CLL B cells have impaired responses to B cell mitogens and to B cell growth factors. The cells appear to be blocked in differentiation, with a high content of cytoplasmic IgM but a low surface IgM. Although most of the cells do not secrete immunoglobulins, in about 5 per cent of cases, a paraprotein of the same type as that on the surface of the CLL cells is present in the plasma or urine. The CLL cells have a low or absent stimulatory effect in allogeneic or autologous mixed lymphocyte cultures. The CLL cells can be stimulated to differentiate into cells resembling hairy cells or plasma cells under the influence of phorbol esters, B cell mitogens, or growth factors.

T cell function is invariably abnormal in CLL. T cells are increased in number in the blood, bone marrow, and lymph nodes of patients with CLL, but they are polyclonal, and T cell receptor gene rearrangement is rare. The CD4/CD8 (T-helper/T-suppressor) ratio is often close to unity or is inverted owing to a relatively greater increase in the CD8-positive cells. The T cells have a blunted response to T cell mitogens in unseparated blood and decreased delayed hypersensitivity reactions to recall antigens. The T cell defects worsen as the disease progresses to a more advanced stage. Purified T cells have a normal response to T cell mitogens.

Clinical Features

Many patients with CLL are asymptomatic, and the disease is diagnosed when an absolute lymphocytosis is noted in the peripheral blood during evaluation for other illnesses or when the patient undergoes a routine physical examination. Symptoms such as fatigue, lethargy, loss of appetite, weight loss, or reduced exercise tolerance are nonspecific. These features are occasionally greater than can be explained by the degree of anemia or extent of tumor burden. Many patients present with enlarged lymph nodes, usually cervical, noted by themselves or others. Fever

and night sweats, or documented infections, are uncommon initial symptoms (<5 per cent) but become more prominent as the disease progresses. Sinopulmonary infections are most common during the early phase of the disease, but as the disease progresses, the frequency of neutropenia, T cell deficiency, and hypogammaglobulinemia increases, resulting in gram-negative bacterial, fungal, and viral infections. Herpes zoster, herpes simplex, and cytomegalovirus infections usually occur later in the disease. An intriguing but unexplained common feature of CLL is an exuberant reaction to insect bites.

The major physical findings relate to infiltration of the reticuloendothelial system. Lymphadenopathy with discrete, rubbery, mobile lymph nodes is present in two thirds of patients at diagnosis. Later, as the lymph nodes enlarge, they become matted. Enlargement of the liver or spleen is less common at diagnosis (approximately 10 per cent and 40 per cent of cases, respectively). Less commonly, and usually late in the disease, clinically significant infiltration of skin, eyelids, heart, lungs, pleura, or gastrointestinal tract may occur. Organ failure due to infiltration with CLL is uncommon, with pulmonary symptoms being most likely to cause clinical problems. Infiltration of the central nervous system in CLL is rare, and central nervous system symptomatology is more likely to be due to opportunistic infections, such as cryptococcosis or listeriosis. The extent of involvement varies from only a single node or node group to enlargement of virtually all nodes. Later in the disease, massive adenopathy may develop and cause luminal obstruction, such as obstructive jaundice, obstructive uropathy, dysphagia, or partial bowel obstruction. Unilateral or bilateral leg edema can occur owing to obstruction of the lymphatic and/or venous systems. Pleural effusions and ascites can also develop and are associated with a poor prognosis.

Diagnostic Features

Chronic lymphocytic leukemia is characterized by an absolute lymphocytosis in the peripheral blood, a minimal level of more than 5000 per microliter, but more usually in the range of 40,000 to 150,000 per microliter. Extreme leukocytosis approaching 1 × 10⁶ per microliter occurs only late in the disease, and hyperviscosity symptoms can occur if the WBC count is higher than 500,000 per microliter. If the lymphocyte count is 5000 to 15,000 per microliter, supportive evidence for clonality (kappa or lambda light chain excess or immunoglobulin gene rearrangement) should be present before the diagnosis is made. Most physicians also document a lymphocytosis in the bone marrow (>30 per cent lymphocytes) and perform a bone marrow biopsy. Anemia (<11 grams per deciliter) is present in 15 to 20 per cent of patients at diagnosis and thrombocytopenia (<100,000 per microliter) in 10 per cent. Bone marrow replacement and hypersplenism contribute to the anemia and thrombocytopenia in most cases. The anemia is usually normochromic and normocytic, and the reticulocyte count is normal unless the patient has autoimmune hemolytic anemia, which usually results from the development of a warm-reacting IGg antibody (Ch. 135). The diagnosis of autoimmune hemolytic anemia, which occurs in the course of 8 to 10 per cent of cases, is confirmed by a positive direct Coombs test, reticulocytosis, a low serum haptoglobulin value, and an elevated unconjugated serum bilirubin level. In such patients, reactive erythroid hyperplasia as a response to the hemolysis may be masked in the bone marrow by the marked lymphocytic infiltration. Autoimmune thrombocytopenia can be diagnosed in some cases with a positive test for platelet antibodies. Cold agglutinin hemolysis occurs rarely in CLL. The antibodies causing the red cell and platelet destruction are not produced by the CLL cells, and the mechanism for the autoimmune diseases is not known. Pure red cell aplasia associated with T-suppressor cell activity is an additional reported cause of anemia in CLL.

The lymphocytes in CLL are indistinguishable on light or electron microscopy from normal small B lymphocytes. On bone marrow aspiration, the proportion of lymphocytes is greater than 30 per cent and may extend up to 100 per cent in newly diagnosed patients with CLL. The rest of the cells are normal myeloid and erythroid cells. Four patterns of lymphocyte infiltration on bone marrow biopsy occur and have prognostic value in CLL: (a) nodular (15 per cent), (b) infiltrative (30 per cent), (c) mixed nodular and infiltrative (30 per cent), and (d) diffuse (35 per cent).

Most early-stage patients have patterns a, b, or c; a diffuse histology is most common in advanced-stage disease and becomes more prominent as the disease evolves. A diffuse histologic pattern confers a poor prognosis regardless of the stage of disease. Hypogammaglobulinemia is common in CLL and predisposes to infections, especially with encapsulated microorganisms. Low levels of IgG, IgA, or IgM occur in 25 per cent of newly diagnosed patients, are more common in advanced stages, and increase in frequency to 50 to 70 per cent as the disease progresses.

Nonrandom cytogenetic abnormalities in CLL include trisomy 12 (40 per cent), 14q+ abnormalities (25 per cent), and abnormalities in the long arm of chromosomes 6 and 11. Single abnormalities are more common in early and recently diagnosed diseases, and additional changes develop with time (clonal evolution). The site of the breakpoint on chromosome 14 (q32) is close to the site of the Ig heavy-chain gene.

Staging Systems

Two major staging systems are used. The Rai staging system (1975) defines five stages and is most frequently used in the United States, whereas the Binet system (1981) defines three stages and is most frequently used in Europe (Table 144–3). Both systems have the advantage of simplicity, low cost, and reproducibility and have been prospectively validated (Figs. 144–4 and 144–5). Within the stages, outcome is variable and other prognostic factors, such as the bone marrow histologic pattern, provide additional prognostic information. Patients with anemia and thrombocytopenia (Rai stages III and IV, Binet C) have, on the average, a poor prognosis; patients with lymphocytosis alone (Rai 0, some Binet A patients) have an excellent prognosis. The prognosis of the other patients is heterogeneous and, as might be expected, is worse in patients with a greater tumor burden. Rai stage II patients who have splenomegaly without lymphadenopathy (pure splenic form) have a better prognosis than do other stage II patients. While useful in the design and analysis of clinical trials, the staging systems are not particularly useful for individual patients because of the heterogeneity of outcome. A group of patients with a lymphocyte count of less than 30,000 per microliter, a hemoglobin higher than 11 grams per deciliter, a platelet count lower than 100,000 per microliter, with fewer than three involved node areas, and a lymphocyte doubling time of greater than 12 months has been described as having "smoldering" CLL, with a survival equal to that of an age- and sex-matched population.

Patients tend to progress through stages, with many patients developing more sites of involvement with time and eventually experiencing marrow failure, but anemia and thrombocytopenia can develop abruptly even without antibody-mediated destruction or increasing tumor burden.

Differential Diagnosis

Many diseases can cause a lymphocytosis: pertussis, infectious lymphocytosis, cytomegalovirus and Epstein-Barr virus mononucleosis, tuberculosis, toxoplasmosis, chronic inflammatory disorders, and autoimmune syndromes. Although they may superficially resemble CLL, their clinical pictures seldom are confused with that of B cell CLL. Many of these patients are younger and

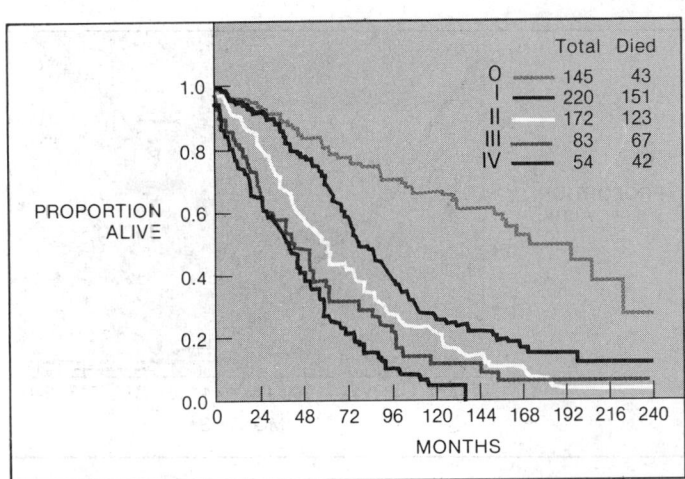

FIGURE 144–4. Survival of untreated patients with chronic lymphocytic leukemia (CLL) by Rai stage.

have fever or other acute symptoms, or exhibit other clinical features, such as rash and joint symptoms, that are uncommon in CLL. The lymphocytosis is usually less than 15,000 per microliter and not sustained. If doubt persists, monoclonal antibodies will distinguish the monoclonal lymphocytosis in CLL from the polyclonal B cell proliferation in the other disorders. The more difficult differential diagnosis is from other lymphoproliferative disorders, such as prolymphocytic leukemia, HCL, the leukemic phase of lymphoma, Waldenström's macroglobulinemia, and T cell CLL. While certain clinical features are more common in some of these disorders—for example, marked splenomegaly with minimal or no lymphadenopathy in prolymphocytic leukemia and HCL versus extensive lymphadenopathy with or without splenomegaly in CLL—none of these differential features is specific. The differential diagnosis therefore depends largely on histopathologic and more specifically immunophenotypic features (Table 144–4).

Small lymphocytic lymphoma (SLL) shares histopathologic and immunophenotypic features with CLL, differing only in lacking an absolute monoclonal lymphocytosis in the peripheral blood. The bone marrow in SLL may or may not have more than 30 per cent lymphocytes. LFA-1 adhesion protein is much more commonly expressed on SLL cells than CLL cells. Occasionally, other lymphomas, such as follicular small cleaved cell lymphoma (FSCCL), manifest in a leukemic phase. These cells are often cleaved on light microscopy, have bright staining for SmIg, and are commonly FMC7 and CD10 positive. Lymph node biopsy should be performed to identify these cases with greater precision. The presence of lymphoma cells in the blood in SLL and FSCCL is more common later in the disease. The WBC count in Waldenström's macroglobulinemia at diagnosis is usually much lower than in CLL (<10,000 per microliter), and many patients

TABLE 144–3. RAI AND BINET STAGING SYSTEMS IN CHRONIC LYMPHOCYTIC LEUKEMIA (CLL)

	Lymphocytosis	Lymphadenopathy	Hepatomegaly or Splenomegaly	Hemoglobin (grams/dl)	Platelets × 10³/μl
Rai stage					
0	+	—	—	≥11	≥100
I	+	+	—	≥11	≥100
II	+	±	—	≥11	≥100
III	+	±	±	<11	≥100
IV	+	±	±	Any	<100
Binet stage					
A	+	±	±	≥10	≥100
			(<3 Lymphatic groups* positive)		
B	+	±	±	≥10	≥100
			(≥3 Lymphatic groups* positive)		
C	+	±	±	<10 or	<100

*(1) Cervical, axillary, and inguinal nodes; (2) liver; and (3) spleen; each group is considered one group whether unilateral or bilateral.

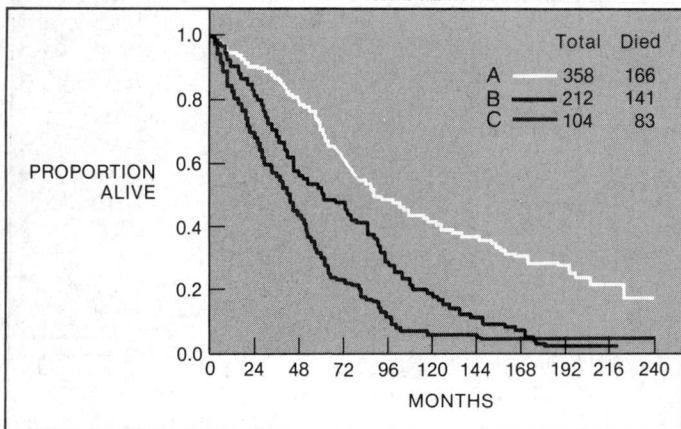

FIGURE 144–5. Survival of untreated patients with CLL by Binet stage.

are leukopenic (Ch. 151). The cells have a plasmacytoid appearance, CD38 and PCA-1 positivity, and more SmIg and cytoplasmic Ig. A monoclonal IgM plasma peak is present in almost all cases of Waldenström's macroglobulinemia but is rare in CLL. Prolymphocytic leukemia (PLL) is an uncommon disease (10 per cent of the incidence of CLL), and its characteristics of massive splenomegaly, minimal lymphadenopathy, WBC count commonly greater than 100,000 per microliter, with 10 to 90 per cent of the cells being prolymphocytes, distinguish this disease from typical B cell CLL. Prolymphocytes are larger cells than typical CLL lymphocytes; they have a distinct nucleolus and are often FMC7 positive. The male-female ratio is 4:1, and the median age at diagnosis is 70 years. Survival is shorter than in CLL (median, 3 years), and response is poor to therapies usually applied in CLL. A monoclonal spike, usually IgG or IgA, is present in one third of cases. The immunoglobulin on the surface of the cells is usually IgG or IgA, not IgM ± IgD, as in CLL. A specific karyotypic abnormality, t(6;12) (q15;q13), has been reported in PLL. One fifth of the cases are of T cell phenotype. The predominant clinical manifestation in Sézary's syndrome (a CD4+ T cell malignancy related to mycosis fungoides) is chronic exfoliative erythroderma with a low number of circulating monoclonal T cells. The clinical and laboratory differential diagnosis from CLL is not difficult. Other T cell malignancies with peripheral blood involvement are adult T cell leukemia-lymphoma and large granular lymphocytosis (LGL). Adult T cell leukemia-lymphoma is associated with a retrovirus (human T cell leukemia/lymphoma virus [HTLV-1]) and is common in Japan and the Caribbean. It is frequently manifested by lytic bone lesions and hypercalcemia. In LGL the absolute lymphocyte count is usually low (<5000 per microliter), with a CD2+, CD3+, and CD8+ (T-suppressor) phenotype (T-gamma cells). These patients often have spleno-

megaly, neutropenia, and rheumatoid arthritis–like symptomatology and serology. The lymphocytes have abundant cytoplasm with azurophilic granules. In most patients a benign course is noted, although repeated infections can occur.

Prognostic Factors

In addition to the impact of tumor burden and marrow function on prognosis, as reflected in the Rai and Binet staging systems, other adverse factors are as follows: (a) a diffuse pattern of lymphocytic infiltration observed on bone marrow biopsy; (b) an abnormal karyotype (e.g., trisomy 12 or multiple chromosomal abnormalities); (c) advanced age; (d) male sex; (e) elevated serum levels of thymidine kinase, uric acid, alkaline phosphatase, or lactate dehydrogenase; (f) rapid lymphocyte doubling time; and (g) an increased proportion of large or atypical lymphocytes in the peripheral blood. A poor response to therapy is an adverse factor in all phases of the disease. As the disease progresses, a worsening of stage and the development of a prolymphocytic leukemia (10 per cent of cases), large cell lymphoma, or myelomatous or acute lymphocytic leukemia (rare) are grave prognostic features. Multiple chromosomal abnormalities identify patients at risk of developing a large cell lymphomatous transformation (Richter's syndrome), which occurs in 5 to 10 per cent of CLL patients as a terminal event. Richter's syndrome should be suspected whenever a single lymph node area or the spleen begins to enlarge in CLL or when unexplained clinical deterioration occurs. The transformation does not always share immunophenotypic or cytogenetic features with the original CLL clone and may be a coincidental second tumor. Response to therapy in Richter's transformation is not usually as satisfactory as for de novo large cell lymphoma. A high incidence of second malignancies (10 to 20 per cent of patients) either precedes or follows the diagnosis of CLL, with the roles of therapy versus impaired immune surveillance as causative factors being unclear. Skin cancer, including melanoma, colorectal and lung cancers, and sarcomas are common in patients with CLL. Hypogammaglobulinemia may have an adverse impact on survival. Patients who develop repeated infections fare less well than other patients.

Treatment

The major therapeutic questions for CLL are when to treat and which therapeutic agent or agents to use.

WHEN TO TREAT. Patients with CLL are usually in later life, and the prognosis of the disease is variable (with some early-stage patients being stable for 5 to 20 years). It is traditional, therefore, to delay treatment of early-stage CLL (Rai 0, Binet A) until the disease progresses. Early treatment with alkylating agents does not prolong survival and may be associated with a heightened risk of developing second malignancies. Treatment of Rai stages III and IV (Binet stage C) patients is recommended at the time of diagnosis because of the poor survival of these patients (median, 2 years). Treatment of intermediate-stage disease (Rai stages I and II, Binet stage B) is recommended if symptomatic disease (fever, sweats, weight loss, severe fatigue), massive lymphadenopathy, or hepatosplenomegaly is present. Progressive

TABLE 144–4. DIFFERENTIAL DIAGNOSIS OF INDOLENT LYMPHOPROLIFERATIVE DISORDERS

Disease	Lymphadenopathy (%)	Splenomegaly (%)	Cell of Origin (B/T)	Positive Markers* SmIg	CD5	CD19, 20 (%)	Other Positive
CLL	75	50	B(20:1)	Weak	>90%	≥90	Mouse red blood cell (RBC) receptors
Prolymphocytic leukemia	33	95	B(4:1)	Bright	T cell PLL	75	FMC-7
Hairy cell leukemia	<10	80	B(T rare)	Bright	—	>90	CD25, CD11C
Lymphoma (leukemic phase)	90	80	B(T rare)	Bright	Some	>90	CD10
Waldenström's macroglobulinemia	33	33	All B	Weak	Some	Many	CD38, PCA-1
Large granular lymphocytosis	10	10	All T	Absent	—	—	CD2, CD3, CD8

*CD5 —pan T cell, B CLL CD8 —T cell (suppressor-cytotoxic)
CD19 —early pan B cell CD10 —early B cell
CD20 —pan B cell CD11C —hairy cells, activated T cell, NK cell
FMC7—PLL and hairy cells CD38 —activated B cell, thymocytes, plasma cells
CD2 —pan T cell PCA1 —plasma cell
CD3 —pan mature T cell CD25 —low-affinity interleukin 2 (IL2) receptor

organ and/or node enlargement and lymphocytosis (>100,000 per microliter) are other common indications for treatment. Development of anemia, thrombocytopenia, or neutropenia associated with infections is usually an indication for systemic antileukemic therapy unless an autoimmune cause of the cytopenia (positive direct Coombs' test, antiplatelet or antineutrophil antibodies) is found. In the latter group of cases, the use of corticosteroids, such as prednisone, should be tried prior to the initiation of cytotoxic therapy. A doubling of blood lymphocytes in less than 12 months is an adverse prognostic factor and suggests that treatment is indicated.

CHEMOTHERAPY. *Chlorambucil* (less commonly, cyclophosphamide) is usually the first chemotherapeutic agent used. Corticosteroids are often used concurrently, but with no clearly demonstrated advantage in therapeutic response or survival. Chlorambucil regimens vary widely. In the chronic low-dosage daily regimen, 0.1 to 0.2 mg per kilogram per day of chlorambucil is continued for 3 to 6 weeks until the desired effect is obtained or until thrombocytopenia or neutropenia develops. The dosage is then adjusted for maintenance and is continued for 6 to 12 months. For intermittent high-dosage (pulse) schedules, chlorambucil (0.5 to 2 mg per kilogram) is given over 1 to 4 days every 4 weeks or given at half dosage every 2 weeks. Neither dosage schedule for chlorambucil has been established as definitely superior. If prednisone is given concurrently with chlorambucil, the dosage is 60 to 100 mg per day in the pulse schedule. Continuous prednisone is not recommended in this elderly population but can be given at a dosage of 40 to 60 mg per day for 4 weeks initially, tapering to 10 to 20 mg per day when combined with chlorambucil in the continuous-therapy schedule. Following therapy, many patients remain stable for months to years before disease progression indicates the need for further treatment. The endpoints for response to therapy have not been well defined, since treatment is usually strictly palliative. Most physicians try to achieve the disappearance of lymphadenopathy and splenomegaly and the return to a normal WBC count, but rarely a normal bone marrow. Myelosuppression is the most common toxicity with chlorambucil, although occasionally rash, nausea, or pulmonary toxicity occurs.

The COP regimen (cyclophosphamide, 100 to 300 mg per square meter per day given orally on days 1 through 5; vincristine [Oncovin], 2 mg given intravenously on day 1; and prednisone, 100 mg administered orally on days 1 through 5) does not appear to have any advantage over chlorambucil. Indeed, vincristine has never been demonstrated to have activity in CLL. Sixty to 75 per cent of patients obtain at least a partial clinical response with these alkylating agents, but a complete remission, including fewer than 30 per cent lymphocytes in the bone marrow aspirate, is achieved in only 10 to 15 per cent of the cases. Repeated rechallenge with the same drug combinations is usually associated with less satisfactory and shorter responses. Damage to DNA gives rise to concern regarding the role of alkylating agents as contributory factors to the high incidence of second malignancies in CLL. Two recent sets of recommendations address response and eligibility criteria in CLL studies (Table 144–5).

Regimens utilizing cyclophosphamide, doxorubicin (Adriamycin), and prednisone with vincristine (CHOP) or without vincristine (CAP) have produced response rates of 50 to 70 per cent in previously untreated Binet stage C patients and are well tolerated in CLL despite the advanced age of most patients. The CAP regimen resulted in a complete remission rate of 45 per cent in CLL, with a median survival of 7 years in the Binet C patients.

CORTICOSTEROID THERAPY. Corticosteroids, usually prednisone (60 to 100 mg per day), are indicated as treatment for Coombs-positive autoimmune hemolytic anemia and for some cases of immune-mediated thrombocytopenia in CLL. If there is no response in 3 to 4 weeks, the treatment has failed and the dose should then be tapered over 1 to 2 weeks. If a response is obtained, the dose is usually reduced by 25 per cent each week over 4 weeks. Autoimmune hemolytic anemia and immune-mediated thrombocytopenia do not correlate closely with the activity of CLL.

RADIATION THERAPY. In CLL, radiation therapy is usually restricted to external irradiation of localized nodal masses or an enlarged spleen that has been refractory to chemotherapy. Repeated leukapheresis and extracorporeal irradiation of blood can decrease the tumor burden in CLL and occasionally increase hemoglobin and platelet levels but are not practical for long periods.

EXPERIMENTAL THERAPIES. Two adenosine analogues, fludarabine monophosphate and 2-CDA, and pentostatin (deoxycoformycin), an adenosine deaminase inhibitor, have exhibited therapeutic potential in CLL. Fludarabine monophosphate (25 to 30 mg per square meter per day for 5 days every 4 weeks) leads to complete remission in 70 per cent of untreated patients and 35 per cent of those previously treated with alkylating agents. The dose-limiting toxicity is myelosuppression. The course of therapy may be complicated by infections with organisms usually associated with immunodeficiency syndromes involving T lymphocytes (e.g., those caused by *Pneumocystis carinii*, herpesviruses). 2-CDA and deoxycoformycin have not been as widely studied in CLL.

Intravenous immunoglobulin (400 mg per kilogram every 3 to 4 weeks) significantly decreases the incidence of infections of minor to moderate severity in CLL patients with hypogammaglobulinemia, but the cost of this therapy is substantial. Although ineffective in patients with advanced-stage CLL, alpha-interferon may significantly decrease the lymphocyte count in 50 to 70 per

TABLE 144–5. DEFINITION OF REMISSION IN CLL: COMPARISON OF THE INTERNATIONAL WORKSHOP IN CLL (IWCLL) AND THE NATIONAL CANCER INSTITUTE WORKING GROUP (NCI-WG) CRITERIA

Criteria	Complete Remission (CR)		Partial Remission (PR)	
	IWCLL	*NCI-WG*	*IWCLL*	*NCI-WG*
Physical examination				
Nodes	None	None	Shift to a lower Binet stage, e.g., C → A or B, B → A	≥50% decrease
Liver/spleen	Not palpable	Not palpable		≥50% decrease
Symptoms	None	None		N/A
Peripheral blood				
Neutrophils	≥1500/μl	≥1500/μl		>1500/μl or ≥50% ↑ from baseline
Platelets	>100,000/μl	>100,000/μl		100,000/μl or >50% ↑ from baseline
Hemoglobin	Not specified	>11 grams/dl		>11 grams/dl or >50% ↑ from baseline
Lymphocytes	<4000/μl	<4000/μl		>50% decrease
Bone marrow				
Lymphocytes	Normal aspirate and biopsy*	<30%		N/A
		Normal*		N/A

*Nodules or focal aggregates of lymphocytes are comparable to CR.

cent of early-stage patients as well as increase the absolute granulocyte count, improve the serum immunoglobulin level, and improve T-helper/T-suppressor ratios. Interleukin 2 has been administered sparingly to patients with refractory CLL, with no consistent improvement in disease parameters. Similarly, monoclonal antibodies directed against CLL cells have not as yet resulted in consistent benefit to patients.

Prognosis in CLL (Figs. 144–4 and 144–5)

The median survival of patients with CLL is 4 to 5 years following the initiation of treatment. As expected, early-stage patients (Rai 0 to II) survive significantly longer, a median of 7 to 8 years. No current treatment strategy has demonstrated a survival advantage over conventional therapy with chlorambucil.

Chronic lymphocytic leukemia tends to develop in elderly patients; death often occurs, therefore, from other intercurrent illnesses of this age group. Younger patients (<60 years of age) almost all die as a result of CLL or one of its complications, especially infections. Gram-positive organisms usually cause nonfatal infections early in CLL, but most deaths due to infection are associated with gram-negative bacterial or fungal infections. Other opportunistic organisms such as *Mycobacterium tuberculosis*, herpesvirus, and *Pneumocystis carinii* may also contribute to death.

Bennett JM, Catovsky D, Daniel M-T, et al.: Proposals for the classification of chronic (mature) B and T lymphoid leukaemias. J Clin Pathol 42:567, 1989. *Classification of common and less common chronic leukemias using an integrated clinical, morphologic and immunophenotypic approach.*

Cheson BD, Bennett JM, Rai KR, et al.: Guidelines for clinical protocols for chronic lymphocytic leukemia: Recommendations of the National Cancer Institute–sponsored Working Group. Am J Hematol 29:152, 1988. *Standard guidelines for eligibility criteria, indications for treatment, and response criteria in B cell CLL.*

Foon KA, Rai KR, Gale RP: Chronic lymphocytic leukemia: New insights into biology and therapy. Ann Intern Med 113:525, 1990. *This is a useful general review of recent advances in our understanding of the pathogenesis of CLL and of new approaches to therapy; 227 references.*

Freedman AS, Boyd AW, Bieber FR, et al.: Normal cellular counterparts of B cell chronic lymphocytic leukemia. Blood 70:418, 1987. *Surface markers are used to indicate the differentiation arrest in CLL and to address the question of the cell of origin of the disease.*

French Cooperative Group on Chronic Lymphocytic Leukemia: Effects of chlorambucil and therapeutic decision in initial forms of chronic lymphocytic leukemia (Stage A): Results of a randomized clinical trial on 612 patients. Blood 75:1414, 1990. *Randomized trial comparing the outcome of early versus late treatment with chlorambucil in CLL. Disturbing data on second malignancies in the early treatment group.*

Juliusson G, Oscier DG, Fitchett M, et al.: Prognostic subgroups in B-cell chronic lymphocytic leukemia defined by specific chromosomal abnormalities. N Engl J Med 323(11):720, 1990. *A major report on the prognostic and biologic importance of cytogenetic abnormalities in CLL.*

Keating MJ, Kantarjian H, Talpaz M, et al.: Fludarabine: A new agent with major activity against chronic lymphocytic leukemia. Blood 74:19, 1989. *Report of the marked clinical activity of fludarabine, a new purine analogue, in refractory CLL.*

Montserrat E, Vinolas N, Reverte JC, et al.: Natural history of chronic lymphocytic leukemia: On the progression and prognosis of early clinical stages. Nouv Rev Fr Hematol 30:359, 1988. *Illustrates the features associated with risk of progression in early-stage CLL.*

Rozman C, Montserrat E, Rodriguez-Fernandex JM, et al.: Bone marrow histologic pattern—the best single prognostic parameter in chronic lymphocytic leukemia: A multivariate analysis of 329 cases. Blood 64: 642, 1984. *The bone marrow histologic pattern in CLL is shown to be a major prognostic factor for survival in all stages of disease.*

Ziegler-Heitbrock HWL, Schlag R, Flieger D, et al.: Favorable response of early stage B CLL patients to treatment with IFN-α₂. Blood 73:1426, 1989. *Despite modest antitumor activity in CLL, interferon enhances a variety of immune functions, including gamma globulin levels.*

145 The Acute Leukemias

Frederick R. Appelbaum

DEFINITION

Normal hematopoiesis requires the tightly regulated proliferation and differentiation of pluripotent hematopoietic stem cells to become mature peripheral blood cells. Acute leukemia is the result of a malignant event, or events, occurring in an early hematopoietic precursor. Instead of proliferating and differentiating normally, the affected cell gives rise to progeny that fail to differentiate and instead continue to proliferate in an uncontrolled fashion. As a result, immature myeloid cells (in acute myelogenous leukemia) or lymphoid cells (in acute lymphocytic leukemia), often called "blasts," rapidly accumulate and progressively replace the bone marrow, leading to diminished production of normal red cells, white cells, and platelets. This loss of normal marrow function in turn gives rise to the common clinical complications of leukemia: anemia, infection, and bleeding. With time the leukemic blasts pour out into the bloodstream and eventually occupy the lymph nodes, spleen, and other vital organs. If untreated, acute leukemia is rapidly fatal; most patients die within several months of diagnosis. With appropriate therapy, the natural history of acute leukemia can be markedly altered and many patients can be cured.

ETIOLOGY

In most cases acute leukemia develops for no known reason, but sometimes a possible cause can be identified.

Radiation

Ionizing radiation is leukemogenic. Acute lymphocytic leukemia (ALL), acute myelogenous leukemia (AML), and chronic myelogenous leukemia (CML) are all increased in incidence in patients given radiation therapy for ankylosing spondylitis and in survivors of the atomic bomb blasts of Hiroshima and Nagasaki. The magnitude of the risk depends on the dose of radiation, its distribution in time, and the age of the individual. Greater risk results from higher dose radiation delivered over shorter periods to younger patients. An increased incidence of leukemia is seen within several years of exposure and appears to peak between five and ten years after exposure. In areas of high natural background radiation (often due to radon), chromosomal aberrations have been reported to be more frequent, but an increase in acute leukemia has not been consistently found. Recently, concern has been raised about possible leukemogenic effects of extremely low-frequency nonionizing electromagnetic fields emitted by electrical installations. If such an effect exists at all, the magnitude of the effect is small.

Oncogenic Viruses

The search for a viral cause of leukemia has been intensely pursued, but not found, except for two rare leukemias associated with retroviruses. Human T cell lymphotropic virus type I (HTLV-I), an enveloped, single-stranded RNA virus, is considered the causative agent of adult T cell leukemia (ATL). This distinct form of leukemia is found within geographic clusters in southwestern Japan, the Caribbean basin, and Africa. The virus can be spread vertically from mother to fetus or horizontally by sexual contact or through blood products. In areas where ATL is found, infection with the virus is endemic, but only 1 to 2 per cent of those infected with HTLV-I develop ATL, and the latency period seems to be quite long (perhaps 10 to 30 years). Although previously rare in the United States, HTLV-I seropositivity has been found with increasing frequency among chronically transfused patients and intravenous drug users. Screening of blood products for antibodies to HTLV-I is now a routine practice in blood banks in the United States. A second human retrovirus, genetically distinct from HTLV-I, termed HTLV-II, has been isolated from several patients with a syndrome resembling hairy cell leukemia. The etiologic link between HTLV-II and malignancy is uncertain.

Genetics and Congenital Factors

A genetic predisposition to leukemia exists in some individuals. If leukemia develops before age 10 in a patient with an identical twin, the unaffected twin has a one in five chance of subsequently developing leukemia. In occasional families, multiple members have developed an identical form of leukemia. Several autosomal recessive disorders associated with chromosomal instability are prone to terminate in acute leukemia, including Bloom syndrome, Fanconi anemia, and ataxic telangiectasia. Other congenital disorders associated with an increased incidence of leukemia are Down syndrome and infantile X-linked agammaglobulinemia.

Chemicals

Heavy occupational exposure to benzene frequently results in marrow hypoplasia, which sometimes evolves into acute leukemia. Other associations between occupational exposure to chemicals and subsequent leukemia are not persuasive.

Prior exposure to alkylating agents, such as chlorambucil, melphalan, and nitrogen mustard, is associated with an increased risk of AML. The risk of secondary AML is greater with increasing exposure to the agent and with increased patient age. Patients often present with a myelodysplastic syndrome before developing secondary AML. Cytogenetic studies of secondary leukemias frequently reveal abnormalities of chromosomes 5, 7, and 8.

INCIDENCE

The annual new case incidence of all leukemias is 8 to 10 per 100,000. This rate has remained static over the past three decades. The relative incidences for the four categories of leukemia are as follows: ALL, 11 per cent; CLL, 29 per cent; AML, 46 per cent; and CML, 14 per cent. The leukemias account for about 3 per cent of all cancers in the United States. The impact of leukemia is heightened because of the young age of some patients. For example, ALL is the most common cancer and the second leading cause of death in children under 15 years of age. Acute lymphocytic leukemia has a maximal incidence between 2 and 10 years of age, with a second, more gradual rise in frequency in later life. The incidence of AML gradually increases with age, without an early peak. Approximately half of AML cases occur in patients under age 50.

PATHOPHYSIOLOGY

The precise molecular event or events that cause leukemic transformation are unknown; the end result, however, is the relentless proliferation of immature hematopoietic cells that have lost their capacity to differentiate normally. The development of leukemia may be a multistep process, as demonstrated by the fact that in many cases acute leukemia develops in patients with a pre-existing myelodysplastic disorder. The disease is monoclonal, i.e., the final leukemic event occurs in a single cell. The level of differentiation at which the malignancy becomes evident is variable. In some cases of AML, it appears that the malignancy occurs in a very undifferentiated cell similar to the normal hematopoietic stem cell, in that red cell, platelet, and myeloid precursors are all products of the malignant clone. In other cases of AML, the malignant event may occur in a more differentiated cell, and only granulocyte and monocyte precursors develop from the malignant cell, while red cell and platelet precursors do not. In almost all cases of ALL, the myeloid lineage is not malignant, suggesting that in ALL, the malignant event occurs in a cell that is at least partially differentiated. Although the majority of leukemic cells are relatively undifferentiated, some mature circulating cells may be products of the malignant clone.

As the malignant clone expands, it does so at the expense of normal hematopoiesis. The mechanism of normal marrow suppression in leukemia is complex; in many patients with hypercellular marrows, pancytopenia is probably the result, at least in part, of physical replacement of normal marrow precursors by leukemic cells. Some patients with acute leukemia develop pancytopenia with a hypocellular marrow, however, suggesting that marrow failure is not simply due to physical replacement of the marrow space but also may be due to substances released by the malignant cells.

CLASSIFICATION

The acute leukemias can be classified in a variety of ways, including morphology, cytochemistry, cell-surface markers, cytoplasmic markers, cytogenetics, and oncogene expression. The most important distinction is between AML and ALL, since these two diseases differ considerably in their clinical behavior, prognosis, and response to therapy. Within the various subgroups of AML or ALL, there are also some important differences. A summary of the major subtypes of acute leukemia is provided in Table 145–1.

Morphology

Leukemic cells in AML typically are 12 to 20 μm in diameter, with discrete nuclear chromatin, multiple nucleoli, and cytoplasm that usually contains azurophilic granules. Auer rods, which are slender, fusiform cytoplasmic inclusions that stain red with Wright-Giemsa Stain, are virtually pathognomonic of AML. The French-American-British (FAB) collaborative group has subdivided AML into eight subtypes based on morphology and histochemistry (Table 145–1). M0, M1, M2, and M3 reflect increasing degrees of differentiation of myeloid leukemic cells. M4 and M5 leukemias have features of the monocytic lineage, M6 has features of the erythroid cell lineage, and M7 is acute megakaryocytic leukemia (see Color Plates 7K and L and 8A).

The leukemic cells in ALL tend to be smaller than AML blasts and relatively devoid of granules. Acute lymphocytic leukemia can be divided, using FAB criteria, into L1, L2, and L3 subgroups. L1 blasts are uniform in size, with homogeneous nuclear chromatin, indistinct nucleoli, and scanty cytoplasm with few, if any, granules. L2 blasts are larger and more variable in size and may have nucleoli. L3 blasts are quite distinct, with prominent nucleoli and deeply basophilic cytoplasm with vacuoles (see Color Plate 8B and C).

Cell-Surface Markers

Monoclonal antibodies reactive with cell-surface antigens have been used to classify acute leukemias. Antibodies that react with antigens found on normal immature myeloid cells, including CD13, CD14, CD33, and CD34, also react with blast cells from most patients with AML. Exceptions are the M6 and M7 variants, which have antigens restricted to the red cell and platelet lineages, respectively. Myeloid leukemia blasts also express Ia antigens but usually lack T cell, B cell, and other lymphoid antigens. In 10 to 20 per cent of patients, however, the leukemic cells have characteristics of both myeloid and lymphoid cells. Such cases are termed "hybrid" leukemias. Although sometimes useful in discriminating myeloid from lymphoid leukemias and in defining M6 and M7 variants, cell-surface markers do not have other clearly defined, important clinical correlations in AML.

Acute lymphocytic leukemia can be divided into several forms based on cell-surface antigen expression. Approximately 60 per cent of cases of ALL express the common ALL antigen, or CALLA, on the cell surface. CALLA (CD10) is a glycoprotein also found on occasional normal early lymphocytes and other nonhematopoietic tissues. CALLA-positive ALL's are felt to represent a very early B cell differentiative state. About 20 per cent of CALLA-positive ALL's have intracytoplasmic immunoglobulin and are termed pre–B cell ALL. B cell ALL is signified by the presence of immunoglobulin on the cell surface and accounts for fewer than 5 per cent of cases of ALL. About 20 per cent of cases of ALL are of the T cell phenotype, expressing antigens found on normal early T cells, such as CD5, CD3, or CD2. Approximately 15 per cent of cases of ALL fail to express CALLA, B, or T cell markers and are termed null cell ALL. Leukemic cells in about 25 per cent of patients with ALL also express myeloid antigens.

Cytoplasmic Markers

Of the cytoplasmic markers identified, only one is commonly used clinically, deoxynucleotidyl transferase (TdT), a nuclear enzyme that is not found on normal mature myeloid or lymphoid cells. In more than 90 per cent of cases of ALL, however, the lymphoblasts contain large amounts of the enzyme. Only 4 per cent of cases of AML stain positively for TdT. Other cytoplasmic enzymes of occasional relevance include adenosine deaminase, which is elevated in T cell ALL; 5-nucleosidase, which is low in T cell ALL; and lysozyme, which is produced by monocytic leukemia cells.

Cytogenetics

In most cases of acute leukemia, there is a numerical or structural chromosomal abnormality within the leukemic cell population. The simplest chromosomal change is a gain or loss of a whole chromosome. Other common structural changes include translocations, which involve the exchange of material between two chromosomes; deletions, in which part of a chromosome is lost; or inversions, in which a single chromosome is broken in two places and the middle piece is inverted and rejoined. When

TABLE 145–1. CLASSIFICATION OF ACUTE LEUKEMIAS

| Subtype | Morphology | Histochemistry | | | Monoclonal Reactivity | Cytogenetic Abnormalities |
		Myeloperoxidase	Nonspecific Esterase	PAS		
M0, Acute undifferentiated leukemia	Uniform, very undifferentiated	–	–	–	For subtypes M0–M5b, approximately 90% of cases will react with at least one of the following antimyeloid antibodies: Anti-CD13 Anti-CD14 Anti-CD33 Anti-CD34	Various
M1, Acute myeloid leukemia with minimal differentiation	Very undifferentiated, few azurophilic granules	+/–	+/–	–		Various
M2, Acute myeloid leukemia with differentiation	Granulated blasts predominate; Auer rods may be seen	+++	+/–	+		Various
M3, Acute promyelocytic leukemia	Hypergranular promyelocytes predominate	+++	+	+		t(15;17)
M4, Acute myelomonocytic leukemia M4E	Both monoblasts and myeloblasts present; like M4 but with eosinophils	++	+++	++		Various inv/del(16)
M5, Acute monocytic leukemia M5a M5b	Monoblasts predominate type a >80% monoblasts type b >20% promonocytes	+/–	+++	++		t(9;11)
M6, Acute erythroleukemia	Erythroblasts and megaloblastic red cell precursors seen	–	–	++	Antiglycophorin, antispectrin	Various
M7, Acute megakaryocytic leukemia	Undifferentiated blasts	–	+/–	+	Antiplatelet GpIIb/IIIa	Various
L1, Acute lymphoid leukemia Childhood variant	Small, uniform blasts, nucleoli indistinct	–	–	+++	65% react with anti-CD10 (anti-CALLA)	Various
L2, Acute lymphoid leukemia Adult variant	Larger, more irregular nucleoli present	–	–	++	20% react with anti-CD5, 3, or 2 (anti–T cell)	Various
L3, Burkitt-like acute lymphoid leukemia	Large with strongly basophilic cytoplasm and vacuoles	–	–	–	Antisurface immunoglobulin, anti-CD19, anti-CD20	t(8;14)

PAS = periodic acid–Schiff.

patients with acute leukemia and a chromosomal abnormality are treated and enter a complete remission, the chromosomal abnormality disappears, but it reappears when patients relapse.

In more than 80 per cent of cases of AML, a clonal chromosomal abnormality is found. The most frequent changes are a gain of chromosome 8 or loss of part or all of chromosome 7 or 5. These abnormalities are each seen in approximately 7 to 12 per cent of cases of AML and are not associated either with a particular subtype of AML or with a particularly good or bad prognosis. Other chromosomal abnormalities are associated with specific syndromes of AML. Acute promyelocytic leukemia virtually always has a translocation involving chromosomes 15 and 17 [(t(15;17)]. Acute myelomonocytic (M4) leukemia with abnormal eosinophilia is associated with an inversion in chromosome 16. Patients with M2 AML who have t(8;21) have a particularly good outcome with chemotherapy.

Between 15 and 20 per cent of adults with ALL have a Philadelphia (Ph) chromosome [t(9;22)]; the precise breakpoint of the translocation in ALL differs from that in CML. The other two most common changes in ALL are t(4;11), an abnormality seen mostly in neonatal ALL, and t(8;14), an abnormality associated with the L3 variant of ALL. The leukemic cells in about 20 per cent of patients with ALL have a propensity to gain many chromosomes, often reaching an average of 50 to 60 chromosomes per cell. Patients with such hyperdiploid leukemias tend to respond well to chemotherapy.

Oncogenes (Ch. 157)

It is generally believed that the above-mentioned abnormalities in chromosomal structure are important in the development of leukemia, either by altering the expression of a normal gene (a proto-oncogene) necessary for cell growth and development or by causing the loss or inactivation of certain "tumor suppressor genes" (anti-oncogenes). To date, the specific changes caused by these chromosomal abnormalities have not been identified, but it is known that the *abl* proto-oncogene is affected in the t(9;22) translocation, while the *myc* proto-oncogene is altered with t(8;14). Approximately 25 per cent of AML samples and 10 per cent of ALL cases exhibit point mutations in the *N-ras* oncogene.

CLINICAL MANIFESTATIONS

The signs and symptoms of acute leukemia result from decreased normal marrow function and invasion of normal organs by leukemic blasts. *Anemia* is present at diagnosis in most patients, causing fatigue, pallor, and headache and, in predisposed patients, angina or heart failure. *Thrombocytopenia* is usually present, and approximately one third of patients have clinically evident bleeding at diagnosis, usually in the form of petechiae, ecchymoses, bleeding gums, epistaxis, or hemorrhage. Most patients with acute leukemia are significantly *granulocytopenic* at diagnosis. As a result, approximately one third of patients with AML, and slightly fewer patients with ALL, have significant or life-threatening infections at presentation, most of which are bacterial in origin.

In addition to suppressing normal marrow function, leukemic cells can infiltrate normal organs. The prevalence and degree of organ infiltration differ between ALL and AML. In general, ALL tends to infiltrate normal organs more often than AML. Enlargement of lymph nodes, liver, and spleen is common at diagnosis. Bone pain, thought to result from leukemic infiltration of the periosteum or expansion of the medullary cavity, is a common complaint, particularly in children with ALL, many of whom are originally diagnosed as having juvenile rheumatoid arthritis. Leukemic cells may infiltrate the leptomeninges, causing leukemic meningitis. Signs of leukemic meningitis are headache and nausea. As the disease progresses, central nervous system palsies and seizures may develop. Although fewer than 5 per cent of patients have central nervous system involvement at diagnosis, the central nervous system is a frequent site of relapse, particularly with ALL, and because of the so-called blood-brain barrier, the central nervous system requires special therapy, as will be discussed. Testicular involvement is also seen in ALL and is a frequent site of relapse. In AML, collections of leukemic blast cells, often referred to as chloromas or myeloblastomas, can occur in virtually any soft tissue, presenting as rubbery, fast-growing masses.

Certain clinical manifestations are unique to specific subtypes of leukemia. Patients with acute promyelocytic leukemia (M3) commonly present with subclinical or clinically evident disseminated intravascular coagulation, caused by tissue thromboplastins present in the leukemic cells, which are released as the leukemic cells die. Acute monocytic or myelomonocytic leukemias are the forms of AML most likely to have extramedullary involvement. M6 leukemia often has a long prodromal phase. Patients with T cell ALL often have mediastinal masses.

LABORATORY MANIFESTATIONS

Abnormalities of peripheral blood counts are usually the initial laboratory evidence of acute leukemia. Anemia is present in most patients. Most are also at least mildly thrombocytopenic, and up to one quarter have severe thrombocytopenia (<20,000 per microliter). Although most patients are granulocytopenic at diagnosis, the total peripheral white cell count is more variable, with approximately 25 per cent of patients presenting with very high white cell counts (>50,000 per microliter), approximately 50 per cent presenting with white cell counts between 5000 and 50,000, and 25 per cent presenting with a low white cell count (<5000 per microliter). In most cases, blasts are present in the peripheral blood, although in some patients the percentage of blasts may be quite low, or blasts may be absent.

The diagnosis of acute leukemia is generally established by marrow aspiration and biopsy, usually from the posterior iliac crest. Marrow aspirates and biopsy specimens are usually hypercellular and contain 30 to 100 per cent blast cells, which largely replace the normal marrow. Occasionally, in addition to the blast cell infiltrate, other findings are present, including marrow fibrosis (especially with M7 AML) or bone marrow necrosis.

Other laboratory abnormalities often seen are hyperuricemia, especially in ALL, and increased serum lactate dehydrogenase (LDH). Increased serum or urinary levels of muramidase, a hydrolytic enzyme present in the primary granules of primitive granulocytes and especially monocytes, are sometimes seen with M4 and M5 AML. Rarely, lactic acidosis may complicate acute leukemia, especially in patients with extreme hyperleukocytosis and L3 ALL.

DIFFERENTIAL DIAGNOSIS

The diagnosis of acute leukemia is usually straightforward but occasionally can be more difficult. Leukemia and aplastic anemia can both manifest with peripheral pancytopenia, but the finding of a hypoplastic marrow without blasts usually distinguishes aplastic anemia. Occasionally, a patient may present with a hypocellular marrow and a clonal cytogenetic abnormality, which establishes the diagnosis of myelodysplasia or hypocellular leukemia. A number of processes other than leukemia can lead to the appearance of immature cells in the peripheral blood. Although other small round cell neoplasms can infiltrate the marrow and sometimes mimic leukemia, immunologic markers are effective in differentiating between the two. Leukemoid reactions to infections such as tuberculosis can result in the outpouring of large numbers of young myeloid cells, but virtually never does the percentage of blasts in marrow or peripheral blood reach 30 per cent in a leukemoid reaction (Ch. 141). Infectious mononucleosis and other viral illnesses can sometimes resemble ALL, particularly when large numbers of atypical lymphocytes are present in the peripheral blood and when the disease is accompanied by immune thrombocytopenia or hemolytic anemia.

TREATMENT

With the development of effective programs of combination chemotherapy and advances in marrow transplantation, many patients with acute leukemia can be cured. These therapies are complex and therefore are best carried out at centers with appropriate support services and experience in treating leukemia. Because leukemia is a rapidly progressive disease, specific antileukemic therapy should be started as soon after diagnosis as possible, usually within 48 hours. Before starting therapy, hemorrhage and infection should be brought under control, if possible. To prevent uric acid nephropathy, patients should be hydrated and placed on allopurinol, 100 to 200 mg given orally, three times per day. The diagnosis of leukemia usually comes as a profound psychological shock to the patient and family. In addition to stabilizing the patient hematologically and metabolically, therefore, it is worthwhile having at least one formalized conference before treatment is initiated in which the patient and the family are advised about the meaning of the diagnosis of leukemia and the consequences of therapy.

Management of Emergencies

Patients sometimes present with treatable emergencies that require immediate attention before specific antileukemic therapy is begun. Severe bleeding usually results from thrombocytopenia, which can be reversed with platelet transfusions. Once thrombocytopenic bleeding is stopped, continued prophylactic transfusions of platelets to maintain the platelet count above 20,000 per microliter are warranted. Occasionally, patients also have evidence of disseminated intravascular coagulation (DIC), usually associated with the diagnosis of M3 AML. If active bleeding is due to DIC, the use of low doses of heparin (50 units per kilogram) given intravenously every 6 hours can often be of benefit. Whether heparin should be given prophylactically to patients with laboratory evidence of DIC but no active bleeding is an often debated, but unsettled, question. Patients who present with fever and granulocytopenia should have cultures, but infection should be assumed, and broad-spectrum antibiotics should be begun empirically. It is preferable to bring an infection under control before starting initial chemotherapy if the patient has an adequate granulocyte count. Patients often present with infection and essentially no granulocytes, and delaying chemotherapy in such patients is unlikely to be of benefit. Patients with very high blast counts (>150,000 per microliter) may develop symptoms attributable to the effect of masses of these immature cells on blood flow. The leukostasis may evolve into vascular injury and local hemorrhage. If this situation occurs in the central nervous system, the outcome may be fatal. Leukapheresis, immediate whole-brain irradiation (600 cGy in one dose), and administration of hydroxyurea, 3 grams per square meter given orally for 2 or 3 days, can usually prevent this complication. Patients with very high white cell counts may also present with uremia and anuria secondary to greatly increased serum uric acid levels, with subsequent intratubular crystallization. Rehydration, urine alkalinization with acetazolamide (500 mg per day), and prevention of uric acid production with allopurinol may lead to improved renal function. If patients do not respond and remain uremic, dialysis should be begun before instituting chemotherapy.

Treatment of ALL

After patients have been stabilized, antileukemic therapy should be started as soon as possible. Initial therapy for ALL can be divided into three phases: remission induction, postremission therapy, and central nervous system prophylaxis.

REMISSION INDUCTION. The initial goal of treatment is to induce a complete remission, which is usually defined as the reduction of leukemic blasts to undetectable levels and restoration of normal marrow function. A number of different chemotherapeutic combinations can be used to induce remission; all include vincristine and prednisone, and most add L-asparaginase and/or daunorubicin, administered over 3 to 4 weeks. With such regimens, 90 per cent of children and 75 per cent of adults achieve complete remission. Since vincristine, prednisone, and L-asparaginase are relatively nontoxic to normal marrow precursors, patients often enter complete remission after a relatively brief period of myelosuppression. Failure to achieve complete remission is usually due either to resistance of the leukemic cells to the drugs used or to progressive infection. These two complications occur with approximately equal frequency.

POSTREMISSION CHEMOTHERAPY. If no further therapy is given after induction of complete remission, virtually all patients relapse, most within several months. This fact demonstrates the need for further postremission therapy. Chemotherapy after complete remission can be given in a variety of combinations, dosages, and schedules. The term "consolidation chemotherapy" generally refers to short courses of further chemotherapy given at doses similar to those used for initial induction and thus requiring rehospitalization. Attempts are usually made to select drugs for consolidation that were not used in inducing the initial remission. In the case of ALL, such drugs include high-dose methotrexate, cyclophosphamide, and cytarabine, among others. "Maintenance" involves the administration of low-dose chemotherapy on a daily or weekly outpatient basis for long periods. The most commonly used maintenance regimens in ALL are daily 6-mercaptopurine and weekly or biweekly methotrexate. The optimal duration of maintenance chemotherapy is unknown, but maintenance is usually given for 2 to 3 years. Optimal chemotherapy for ALL requires both consolidation and maintenance chemotherapy.

CENTRAL NERVOUS SYSTEM PROPHYLAXIS. Most chemotherapeutic agents, when given intravenously or orally, do not penetrate the central nervous system well, making the central nervous system a common site of relapse unless specific measures are taken. Effective regimens for central nervous system prophylaxis include the use of intrathecal methotrexate alone, intrathecal methotrexate combined with 2400 cGy to the cranium, or 2400 cGy to the craniospinal axis.

PROGNOSIS AFTER INITIAL CHEMOTHERAPY. A number of factors are predictive of outcome in ALL, the two most consistent of which are age and white cell count at diagnosis. With currently available treatment regimens, 50 to 70 per cent of children and 25 to 45 per cent of adults who achieve a complete remission remain in complete remission for longer than 5 years and thus are probably cured of their disease. In both children and adults, a low white cell count at diagnosis predicts a favorable outcome, while a high white cell count at diagnosis does the reverse. Specific syndromes of ALL with a poor prognosis include the L3 variant of ALL or the presence of the Philadelphia chromosome or the t(4;11) chromosomal abnormality.

TREATMENT OF RELAPSED ALL. Most relapses occur within 2 years of diagnosis, and most occur in the marrow. Occasionally, a relapse may first be found in an extramedullary site, such as the central nervous system or testes. Extramedullary relapse is usually followed shortly by systemic (marrow) relapse and so should be considered part of a systemic recurrence. With the use of chemotherapeutic regimens similar to those used for initial induction, 50 to 70 per cent of patients achieve at least short-lived second remissions. A small percentage of patients whose first remission was longer than 2 years may be cured with salvage chemotherapy. If the central nervous system or testes were the initial site of the relapse, specific therapy to that site is also required along with systemic retreatment. Since the prognosis of relapsed leukemia treated with chemotherapy is so poor, marrow transplantation is now generally recommended in this setting.

MARROW TRANSPLANTATION (Ch. 153). The use of high-dose chemoradiotherapy followed by marrow transplantation from a human leukocyte antigen (HLA)–identical sibling can cure 20 to 40 per cent of patients with ALL who fail to achieve an initial remission or who relapse after an initial complete remission. The major limitations of transplantation are graft-versus-host disease, interstitial pneumonia, and disease recurrence. If an HLA-identical sibling is not available, alternative sources of marrow are from a partially matched family member; from an HLA-matched unrelated donor; or autologous marrow that has been removed during remission, treated in vitro to remove contaminating tumor cells, and then subsequently stored. The outcome of transplantation using either autologous marrow or alternative sources of marrow has not been as favorable as that using matched allogeneic family member donors.

Treatment of AML

REMISSION INDUCTION. Treatment with a combination of daunomycin and cytarabine leads to complete remission in 60 to 80 per cent of patients with AML. Profound myelosuppression always follows when these agents are used at doses capable of achieving complete remission. Failure to achieve complete remission is usually due either to drug resistance or to fatal complications of myelosuppression.

POSTREMISSION THERAPY. Intensive consolidation chemotherapy using repeated courses of daunomycin and cytarabine at conventional doses, high-dose cytarabine, or other agents prolongs the average remission duration and improves the chances for long-term disease-free survival. Unlike the situation in ALL, low-dose maintenance therapy is of no benefit after intensive consolidation treatment. In AML, leukemic recurrence occurs less often in the central nervous system, being seen in only approximately 10 per cent of cases, most commonly in patients with M4 or M5 variants. There is no evidence that central nervous system prophylaxis improves overall disease-free survival in AML.

PROGNOSIS AFTER INITIAL CHEMOTHERAPY. Among those patients who achieve complete remission, 15 to 30 per cent remain alive in continuous complete remission for more than 5 years, suggesting probable cure. As with ALL, younger patients and those with a low white cell count at diagnosis have a more favorable outcome. Patients whose disease is characterized by certain chromosomal abnormalities, particularly t(8;21), t(15;17), and inv 16, do somewhat better, whereas those with t(4;11) and t(9;22) do worse. Patients who have a long preleukemic phase before their condition evolves into acute leukemia and those whose leukemia is secondary to prior exposure to alkylating agents or radiation respond poorly to chemotherapy.

TREATMENT OF RECURRENT AML. Patients whose AML recurs after initial chemotherapy can achieve second remission in about 50 per cent of cases following retreatment with daunomycin-cytarabine or high-dose cytarabine. Unfortunately, these remissions tend to be short lived, and few patients who relapse after first-line chemotherapy are cured by salvage chemotherapy.

BONE MARROW TRANSPLANTATION (Ch. 153). For patients with AML who fail to achieve an initial remission or who relapse after chemotherapy, marrow transplantation from an HLA-identical sibling offers the best chance for cure. If carried out when patients have end-stage disease, approximately 15 per cent of patients can be saved. If the procedure is applied earlier, the outcome with marrow transplantation improves, with approximately 30 per cent of patients transplanted at first relapse or second remission being cured, and with cure rates of 50 to 60 per cent if transplantation is carried out in the first remission. Several studies have prospectively compared the outcome of marrow transplantation with that of chemotherapy in patients with AML in first remission. The trend in all of these studies has been in favor of transplantation, although in not all the studies was there a statistically significant difference. Currently, transplantation is the treatment of choice for patients with AML who have suffered an initial relapse, and it should be strongly considered for most patients while in first remission. The major limitations to transplantation are graft-versus-host disease, interstitial pneumonia, and disease recurrence. Since the incidence of graft-versus-host disease increases with age, most centers limit transplantation to patients age 50 or less. Alternative sources of marrow include the use of partially matched family members, matched unrelated donors, and autologous transplantation. As with ALL, these alternative sources of marrow, while sometimes successful, do not yield results as good as those obtained using a matched family member.

Supportive Care

Treatment of acute leukemia, especially AML, is accompanied by a number of complications, the two most serious and frequent being infection and bleeding. During the granulocytopenic period following induction and consolidation chemotherapy, most patients become febrile, and in approximately 50 per cent of cases, a bacterial infection can be documented. The most commonly isolated organisms vary somewhat from medical center to medical center, but usually gram-positive organisms, such as *Staphylococcus epidermidis*, and gram-negative enteric organisms, such as *Pseudomonas aeruginosa, Escherichia coli*, and *Klebsiella aerobacter*, are the most commonly isolated bacteria. Even if no cause for fever is found, bacterial infection should be assumed, and in general, all patients with fever and neutropenia should begin receiving broad-spectrum antibiotics. Commonly used antibiotic combinations include a cephalosporin and a semisynthetic penicillin or a semisynthetic penicillin and an aminoglycoside. Once begun, antibiotics should be continued until patients recover their granulocyte count, even if the patients become afebrile first. If documented bacterial infections persist despite appropriate antibiotics, removal of indwelling catheters and granulocyte transfusions should be considered. It may be possible to reduce the incidence of bacterial infection through the use of selective gastrointestinal decontamination, using, for example, ciprofloxacin or a combination of trimethoprim-sulfamethoxazole plus colistin. The use of protective environments can also reduce the incidence of infection, but it is costly and has not been shown to influence overall survival.

Frequently, patients on broad-spectrum antibiotics become afebrile for a time, only to develop a second fever. Such patients should be carefully reassessed with a high index of suspicion for fungal infection. Granulocytopenic patients who remain febrile for more than a week on broad-spectrum antibiotics should be treated empirically with amphotericin for presumed fungal infection.

In addition to being granulocytopenic, patients undergoing induction chemotherapy for leukemia have deficient cellular and humoral immunity, at least temporarily, and so are subject to those infections common in other immunodeficiency states, including *Pneumocystis carinii* infection and a variety of viral infections. *Pneumocystis carinii* infection can be prevented by prophylactic use of trimethoprim-sulfamethoxazole. Cytomegalovirus (CMV) infection can be prevented in the CMV-seronegative patient by the sole use of CMV-seronegative blood products. Herpes simplex can often complicate existing mucositis and can be treated successfully with acyclovir. Acyclovir is also useful for the treatment of disseminated varicella zoster.

Platelet transfusions from random donors often suffice to maintain platelet counts above 20,000 per microliter. In 30 to 50 per cent of cases, however, patients eventually become alloimmunized and require the use of HLA-matched platelets. Occasionally, cells (presumably T cells) within the blood product can engraft in the immunosuppressed leukemic patient and cause a graft-versus-host reaction. Transfusion-induced graft-versus-host disease manifests with a rash, low-grade fever, elevated values in liver function tests, and falling blood counts. This syndrome can be prevented by irradiating all blood products with at least 1500 cGy before transfusion.

Appelbaum FR, Fisher LD, Thomas ED, et al.: Chemotherapy and marrow transplantation for adults with acute nonlymphocytic leukemia: A five-year follow-up. Blood 72:179, 1988. *A comparison of the outcome of marrow transplantation with that of continued chemotherapy for adults with AML.*

Bennett JM, Catovsky D, Daniel MT, et al.: Proposed revised criteria for the classification of acute myeloid leukemia. Ann Intern Med 103:626, 1985. *An update of the French-American-British (FAB) classification of acute leukemia.*

Champlin R, Gale RP: Acute myelogenous leukemia: Recent advances in therapy. Blood 69:1551, 1987. *Very good review of therapy for AML with an excellent bibliography.*

Champlin R, Gale RP: Acute lymphoblastic leukemia: Recent advances in biology and therapy. Blood 73:2051, 1989. *Like above reference, but this time directed at ALL.*

Cheson BD, Cassileth PA, Head DR, et al.: Report of the National Cancer Institute–sponsored workshop on definitions of diagnosis and response in acute myeloid leukemia. J Clin Oncol 8:813, 1990. *A report of the recently adopted NCI definitions of diagnostic and response criteria for AML.*

Clarkson B, Ellis S, Little C, et al.: Acute lymphoblastic leukemia in adults. Semin Oncol 12:160, 1985. *A review of chemotherapy for adult ALL centering on the Sloan-Kettering experience.*

Mayer RJ: Current chemotherapeutic treatment approaches to the management of previously untreated adults with de novo acute myelogenous leukemia. Semin Oncol 14:384, 1987. *A comprehensive, balanced review of chemotherapy for adult AML.*

Rowley JD: Recurring chromosome abnormalities in leukemia and lymphoma. Semin Hematol 27:122, 1990. *Updated review of the chromosomal abnormalities seen in the hematologic malignancies.*

146 Introduction to Neoplasms of the Immune System

Carol S. Portlock

Neoplasms of the immune system are a heterogeneous group of tumors whose cells of origin may be the lymphocyte, the histiocyte, or other cell components of the immune system. Each neoplasm is thought to be a monoclonal expansion of malignant cells, although this has only been conclusively demonstrated for lymphocytic tumors. It is interesting that these neoplasms often retain many morphologic, functional, and migratory characteristics common to their normal cell counterparts.

With increasing understanding of the normal immune system, it has become possible to classify many malignant immune disorders according to their cell of origin. Monoclonal antibodies to cell-surface antigens permit the identification of B or T lymphocyte proliferations. By such immunophenotyping, malignant lymphocytic neoplasms can be related to stages of normal B or T lymphocyte development and maturation. Table 146–1 lists these diseases according to their normal cell lineage counterpart.

Establishing clonality of a B lymphocyte proliferation is usually accomplished by the demonstration of a single class of heavy-and/or light-chain cell-surface immunoglobulin. At the DNA level, clonality can be confirmed by the presence of a single immunoglobulin gene rearrangement. In precursor B lymphocyte neoplasms where surface immunoglobulin is not present, gene rearrangement studies are necessary to demonstrate clonality.

For T lymphocyte proliferations, clonality can be conclusively shown only by T lymphocyte receptor gene rearrangement studies. Studies of cell-surface antigens alone are not sufficient. Clonal lymphocyte proliferations are not always malignant, as exemplified by the chronic monoclonal T lymphocyte disorder of lymphomatoid papulosis.

Tumors of histiocytic lineage have not yet been shown to be monoclonal. These cells lack endogenous immunoglobulin but may acquire exogenous immunoglobulin on their cell surface. They may be rich in lysozyme or muramidase, and as phagocytic cells, they can be shown to ingest latex particles or sensitized erythrocytes. The cell lineage of the Reed-Sternberg cell in Hodgkin's disease is not known with certainty. It has in vitro characteristics in common with both histiocytes and lymphocytes. Recent molecular studies demonstrating immunoglobulin gene rearrangement and the presence of *bcl-2* oncogene suggest a B lymphocyte origin.

TABLE 146–1. LYMPHOMAS AS NEOPLASMS OF THE IMMUNE SYSTEM

Cell of Origin	Neoplasm
I. B cell	
Medullary B cell	Chronic lymphocytic leukemia, diffuse small lymphocytic lymphoma
Follicular B cell	Follicular lymphomas, diffuse mixed lymphoma, diffuse large cell lymphoma, Burkitt's lymphoma
Immunoblastic B cell	Diffuse immunoblastic lymphoma
II. T cell	
Thymic T cell	Lymphoblastic lymphoma
Mature T cell	Peripheral T cell lymphomas, chronic lymphocytic leukemia (rare), HTLV-I–associated lymphoma, mycosis fungoides, Sézary's syndrome
Immunoblastic T cell	Diffuse immunoblastic lymphoma
III. Histiocytic	
Histiocyte	Malignant histiocytosis, true histiocytic lymphoma (rare)
IV. Unknown	Hodgkin's disease

In addition to a specific immunotype and genotype, chromosomal abnormalities can be detected in the majority of immune system neoplasms. In many, the recurring karyotypic abnormality appears to be specific. Among B lymphocyte lymphomas, these abnormalities most often include translocations involving chromosome 14 q 32 (the heavy-chain immunoglobulin gene locus) and the cellular oncogenes *c-myc* (chromosome 8), *bcl-1* (chromosome 11), or *bcl-2* (chromosome 18). The 14;18 and 11;14 translocations are primarily associated with follicular lymphomas and t8;14 with Burkitt's lymphoma. Similarly, specific translocations of the T lymphocyte receptor gene loci appear to be involved in the recurring karyotypic changes identified among T-cell lymphocyte lymphomas. These include chromosome 14 q 11 (lymphocyte receptor alpha- and delta-chain genes) or chromosome 7 q 34–36 or chromosome 7 p 15 (T lymphocyte receptor beta- and gamma-chain genes). The presumed oncogene translocation partner is yet to be identified for the majority of T lymphocyte neoplasms. No specific chromosomal changes have been identified thus far in Hodgkin's disease. Reed-Sternberg cells are difficult to isolate, are few in number, and have complex hyperdiploid karyotypes. Another marker that appears to be specific is the presence of antibodies to the human retrovirus HTLV-1 (human T cell leukemia/lymphoma virus) found in patients with adult T cell leukemia/lymphoma. These and other in vitro methods may provide additional information for defining prognostically important patient subsets.

Each neoplasm of the immune system is a distinct clinicopathologic entity. However, these disorders tend to share some common clinical features. For example, systemic symptoms of fever, night sweats, and weight loss may be present and tend to correlate with advanced stage of disease. The neoplasm usually arises in one or more organs of the hematopoietic system (lymph nodes, spleen, liver, bone marrow), and if untreated or ineffectively treated, it tends to disseminate to all those organs, as well as to other sites. Bone marrow involvement with or without peripheral blood manifestation is common in certain disorders and may be the predominant feature. Meningeal infiltration is often present when aggressive neoplasms involve the bone marrow.

PATHOLOGY AND CLASSIFICATION

Neoplasms of B or T lymphocytic lineage are termed non-Hodgkin's lymphomas. They are a diverse group of diseases with varying clinical presentations, responses to therapy, and prognoses. The Rappaport histopathologic classification of non-Hodgkin's lymphomas (Table 146–2) has been used successfully in clinical trials and practice. It has permitted the identification of specific clinicopathologic entities and of favorable and unfavorable

prognostic groups since 1956. Nevertheless, the Rappaport classification, based exclusively upon morphologic concepts, does not take into account recent information regarding the immune system. For example, the term "histiocytic" lymphoma is generally incorrect because virtually all non-Hodgkin's lymphomas are of lymphocytic origin.

Table 146–2 juxtaposes a more recent National Cancer Institute Working Formulation with the Rappaport classification. Tumor architecture is an important feature in both: Rappaport's "nodular" is replaced by the more immunologically accurate term "follicular." Cell morphology is more descriptive in the Working Formulation, and "histiocytic" is replaced by "large cell." Prognostically favorable and unfavorable groups are termed low, intermediate, and high grade. The low-grade category includes small lymphocytic consistent with chronic lymphocytic leukemia; a miscellaneous category includes mycosis fungoides and true histiocytic lymphoma.

Many non-Hodgkin's lymphomas may exhibit two distinct histologic subtypes. Both the architecture and the cell type may change, usually evolving from a low-grade lymphoma to an intermediate- or high-grade lymphoma. Rarely, two histologic subtypes may be present at diagnosis in the same lymph node (composite lymphoma). More often, two histologic subtypes may be seen at diagnosis in two separate biopsy specimens; most frequently, one is seen at diagnosis and a second at relapse or autopsy. It is thought that such "transformation" represents clonal expansion of a more aggressive cell line. Its clinical importance is that both therapy and prognosis may be dramatically altered by its emergence.

In contrast to non-Hodgkin's lymphomas, the diagnostic malignant cells (Reed-Sternberg cells) of Hodgkin's disease appear similar in all four histologic subtypes of the neoplasm. Instead, distinguishing pathologic features include the number of Reed-Sternberg cells and the composition of normal background cells and stroma. The pathologic classification of Hodgkin's disease is fully discussed in Ch. 148.

DIAGNOSIS AND STAGING

The diagnosis of a neoplasm of the immune system is based upon pathologic classification of biopsy material. This classification requires adequate tissue (preferably lymph node, so that both architecture and cell type may be assessed), proper handling, and excellent hematopathologic interpretation. Special studies, such as imprints, immunotyping, gene rearrangement, karyotyping, deoxynucleotidyl transferase (TdT) determination, and electron microscopy, may provide additional information for classification. Since these latter studies require fresh tissue and special handling, it is important that the pathologist be involved *before* biopsy. Similarly, it is important that each case be evaluated jointly by a medical oncologist, radiation therapist, surgeon, and radiologist from the outset.

With the diagnosis established, the extent of disease should be completely defined. Since each neoplasm has distinct clinicopathologic features, the choice of staging studies will be based on that information. All patients should have a complete history, particularly assessing the presence or absence of systemic symptoms, and physical examination. All nodal areas should be examined, including Waldeyer's ring and preauricular, epitrochlear, and popliteal lymph nodes. In addition to liver and spleen, epigastric or other abdominal masses may be found. The lungs, skin, breasts, testicles, and central nervous system should be carefully examined for extranodal involvement. Blood counts and liver and renal function tests are necessary in all patients. In addition to chest radiography, computed tomography (CT) may be indicated in an abnormal chest. Abdominal CT and lymphography are often complementary and not mutually exclusive. Gallium-67 scanning may be useful but is not a diagnostic method. Liver and spleen scans are of minimal value. Studies of bone or gastrointestinal tract should be performed when symptoms are present. However, with Waldeyer's ring involvement, associated upper gastrointestinal disease may be asymptomatic, and therefore it should be screened for routinely. Bone marrow biopsy is often indicated, particularly if advanced clinical disease is present or the patient has a low-grade lymphoma. Cerebrospinal fluid cytology should be determined in all patients with intermediate- and high-grade lymphomas who have bone marrow involvement

TABLE 146–2. CLASSIFICATION OF NON-HODGKIN'S LYMPHOMAS

NCI Working Formulation (1982)	Rappaport Classification (1966)
Low-grade	
Small lymphocytic (SLL)	Diffuse lymphocytic, well differentiated (DLWD)
Follicular, small cleaved cell (FSCL)	Nodular lymphocytic, poorly differentiated (NLPD)
Follicular, mixed small cleaved and large cell (FML)	Nodular mixed lymphocytic-histiocytic (NML)
Intermediate-grade	
Follicular, large cell (FLCL)	Nodular histiocytic (NHL)
Diffuse, small cleaved cell (DSCL)	Diffuse lymphocytic, poorly differentiated (DLPD)
Diffuse, mixed small cleaved and large cell (DML)	Diffuse, mixed lymphocytic-histiocytic (DML)
Diffuse, large cell (cleaved and noncleaved) (DLCL)	Diffuse histiocytic (DHL)
High-grade	
Large cell immunoblastic (IBL)	Diffuse histiocytic (DHL)
Lymphoblastic (convoluted and nonconvoluted) (LL)	
Small noncleaved cell (Burkitt and non-Burkitt) (SNCL)	Diffuse undifferentiated (DUL)

and in all patients with Burkitt's lymphoma, lymphoblastic lymphoma, or malignant histiocytosis.

Several different staging systems are applied to neoplasms of the immune system. Their purpose is to define disease extent, to assist in treatment strategies, to evaluate therapeutic results, and to determine prognosis. In Hodgkin's disease the utility of staging has been elegantly demonstrated, and excellent clinical care demands careful clinical and often pathologic staging. Staging laparotomy with splenectomy and biopsy of liver, lymph nodes, and bone marrow was developed for adequate intra-abdominal assessment of Hodgkin's disease. It accurately identifies pathologic stage, and its results often dictate treatment strategy. The Ann Arbor staging system for Hodgkin's disease has also been applied to non-Hodgkin's lymphomas. In this setting it has less value in determining therapy but remains an important prognostic variable. Modified staging systems are used in pediatric lymphomas, chronic lymphocytic leukemia, Burkitt's and lymphoblastic lymphomas, and mycosis fungoides. Since pathologic intra-abdominal assessment is rarely needed to determine treatment in non-Hodgkin's lymphomas, staging laparotomy is usually unnecessary. Nonetheless, careful clinical staging is imperative in all cases.

DIFFERENTIAL DIAGNOSIS

The differential diagnosis of neoplasms of the immune system is usually that of lymphadenopathy. Reactive processes, infections, other malignant tumors, and collagen vascular disorders may all cause enlarged lymph nodes or hepatosplenomegaly or both. The location or locations of the lymph nodes, their size, shape, consistency, rapidity of onset, and other characteristics may aid in determining etiology.

Regional lymph node hyperplasia may be seen with acute or chronic infections of the extremities and with vaccinations or insect bites. Diffuse lymphadenopathy may occur following ingestion of phenytoin. Other diffuse reactive processes, such as acquired immunodeficiency syndrome (AIDS) angioimmunoblastic lymphadenopathy, and collagen vascular disorders, may be associated with an increased likelihood of developing lymphoma. Consequently, a single lymph node biopsy may not solve the diagnostic dilemma. That is why pathologic consultation before biopsy is recommended.

Among infectious etiologic factors, viral illnesses predominate and often produce bizarre pathologic material. Infectious mononucleosis may present with features common to Hodgkin's disease. Cytomegalovirus, cat-scratch disease, toxoplasmosis, tuberculosis, syphilis, and sarcoidosis are other considerations. Other malignant neoplasms usually involve lymph nodes by regional spread. For example, cervical lymphadenopathy may be the first symptom of a malignant tumor involving the oropharynx or nasopharynx. Similarly, breast cancer may manifest with axillary adenopathy and a microscopic primary tumor.

In virtually all instances, the only way to determine conclusively the cause of lymphadenopathy is by pathologic tissue examination. Low cervical and supraclavicular lymph nodes are more likely to yield diagnostic material than are axillary and inguinal nodes. When only intrathoracic or abdominal disease is present, bone marrow biopsy may provide diagnostic information and obviate surgery. Fine-needle aspiration is of lesser value in neoplasms of the immune system than in solid tumors, because cell morphology and architecture are both important diagnostic parameters.

Lippman ME, Yee D (eds.): The lymphomas: Current concepts in pathogenesis and management. J Natl Cancer Inst Monogr 10:1–82, 1990. *This monograph reviews basic science and clinical aspects of non-Hodgkin's lymphomas and Hodgkin's disease.*

Non-Hodgkin's lymphoma pathologic classification project. National Cancer Institute sponsored study of classifications of non-Hodgkin's lymphomas: Summary and description of a working formulation for clinical usage. Cancer 49:2112, 1982. *The Working Formulation is presented, and six pathologic classifications are compared.*

Simon R, Durrleman S, Hoppe RT, et al.: The non-Hodgkin's lymphoma pathologic classification project: Long-term follow up of 1153 patients with non-Hodgkin's lymphomas. Ann Intern Med 109:939, 1988. *A median follow-up of 11 years, again demonstrating the clinical relevance of the Working Formulation.*

147 Non-Hodgkin's Lymphomas

Carol S. Portlock

Non-Hodgkin's lymphomas are the single largest group of neoplasms of the immune system. Composed of more than 10 distinct disease entities, non-Hodgkin's lymphomas are best understood as a heterogeneous group of malignant diseases whose common link is a characteristic monoclonal expansion of malignant B or T cells.

EPIDEMIOLOGY

Non-Hodgkin's lymphomas may occur at any age, although they are rarely diagnosed during the first year of life. They occur with increasing frequency throughout adulthood. The incidence is estimated to be approximately 33,000 cases per year in the United States (1989), with males affected more often than females. Moreover, male predominance is most evident among young patients in association with the aggressive histologic subtypes of lymphoblastic and Burkitt's lymphomas.

Geographic clustering is characteristic of some non-Hodgkin's lymphomas: Burkitt's lymphoma in central Africa; adult T cell leukemia/lymphoma in southwestern Japan and the Caribbean; and small intestinal lymphoma with associated immunoglobulin disorders in the Middle East.

Preceding immune dysfunction has been associated with the development of aggressive non-Hodgkin's lymphomas. Congenital immunodeficiency states associated with lymphoma include severe combined immunodeficiency, ataxia-telangiectasia, Wiskott-Aldrich syndrome, X-linked lymphoproliferative syndrome, and common variable immunodeficiency (Ch. 244). Transplant recipients, patients with autoimmune states, and patients with AIDS (acquired immunodeficiency syndrome) also have increased risk of developing lymphoma.

ETIOLOGY AND PATHOGENESIS

The etiology of non-Hodgkin's lymphomas is unclear. Perhaps the best studied lymphoma is Burkitt's with which the Epstein-Barr virus (EBV) has been associated and for which specific chromosomal and oncogene translocations have been implicated in its pathogenesis.

Burkitt's lymphoma is the most common childhood malignant disorder in Uganda. The disease is found along a "lymphoma belt" lying approximately 10 degrees north and 10 degrees south of the African equator. Within the belt there are altitude, temperature, and rainfall restrictions; these climatic conditions are similar to those of Papua, New Guinea, where Burkitt's lymphoma is also commonly identified. Holoendemic or hyperendemic malaria follows the geographic distribution of the lymphoma belt and originally suggested to Burkitt a mosquito-borne vector and/or associated host immune dysfunction.

In addition to its geographic restrictions, endemic Burkitt's lymphoma is associated with time-space clustering. Nonendemic Burkitt's lymphoma, a similar disease occurring rarely and sporadically in other areas of the world (less than one case per million annually in the United States), has also been reported to occur in time-space clusters. Moreover, nonendemic Burkitt's lymphomas may be associated with preceding immune dysfunction (e.g., organ transplantation and AIDS).

The EBV is present in almost 90 per cent of African Burkitt's lymphoma but fewer than half of nonendemic cases. Whether the virus plays an etiologic role or is merely a passenger in Burkitt's lymphoma remains controversial. Typically, primary EBV infection precedes the development of Burkitt's lymphoma by at least 7 or more months. Ugandan children with high EBV capsid antigen titers have a 30-fold greater risk of developing Burkitt's lymphoma than do control subjects. Elevated EBV/VCA (viral capsid antigen) titers are also associated with a favorable prognosis in both African and nonendemic tumors.

Adult T cell leukemia/lymphoma (ATL), a rare and recently discovered disorder, is associated with a unique human retrovirus, HTLV-I (human T cell leukemia/lymphoma virus). This disease is endemic to southwestern Japan, where 12 to 15 per cent of normal persons have HTLV-I antibodies; it is also found in the Caribbean basin.

The specific chromosomal translocations seen in Burkitt's lymphoma have uniformly involved the *c-myc* oncogene on chromosome 8 and the immunoglobulin heavy- or light-chain genes on chromosomes 14, 2, or 22. These chromosomal translocations— t(8;14), t(8;2), and t(8;22)—deregulate the *myc* gene and result in the constitutive production of a DNA binding protein that appears to control aspects of gene expression or DNA replication. The biologic correlate of this molecular event is the finding of spontaneous B cell lymphomas in transgenic mice carrying DNA sequences from the 8;14 translocation breakpoint. Specific chromosomal translocations have also been reported in follicular lymphomas, involving chromosomes 11 and 14 or 18 and 14. The translocation site on chromosome 14 also involves the immunoglobulin heavy-chain locus and, by analogy, suggests that a transforming gene on chromosome 11 or 18 is activated when brought into proximity with this locus. These oncogenes, *bcl-1* (on chromosome 11) and *bcl-2* (on chromosome 18), have been identified and cloned.

In addition to the etiologic considerations of oncogenic viruses and oncogene transformation, other factors that have been associated with an increased incidence of lymphoma include ionizing radiation (whole-body dose greater than 100 cGy), hereditary predisposition, congenital or acquired immunodeficiency, and exposure to pesticides.

PATHOLOGY AND CLINICAL FEATURES

Many different pathologic classifications have been proposed for non-Hodgkin's lymphomas (Ch. 146). Rappaport's classification (see Table 147–2) has been the most successfully utilized and applied in clinical trials, while that of Lukes and Collins is more immunologically correct, classifying diseases based on their cell of origin. The National Cancer Institute Working Formulation (1982) is being increasingly accepted, since it is proving both clinically useful and immunologically correct.

Pathologic interpretation of non-Hodgkin's lymphomas can be supplemented with a variety of complementary studies. Immunophenotyping may identify the cell of origin by demonstrating B cell monoclonal surface immunoglobulin, T cell sheep erythrocyte rosettes (E rosettes), and B or T cell differentiation antigens. Clonality may also be ascertained by detection of the rearrangement of the B cell immunoglobulin genes or of the T cell receptor gene loci. Moreover, the karyotype may reveal a specific chromosomal translocation. The presence of antibody against HTLV-I suggests a T cell lymphoma, whereas human immunodeficiency virus (HIV) antibody suggests an aggressive B cell neoplasm (see Color Plate 8E).

Each disease entity of the Working Formulation has a distinct clinical presentation and prognosis, as noted below. The pathologic appearance and some of the clinical characteristics of each category, as outlined in the Working Formulation, are listed in Tables 147–1 and 147–2.

LOW GRADE (see Color Plate 8D, left). The low-grade lymphomas (small lymphocytic [SLL]; follicular, predominantly small cleaved cell [FSCL]; and follicular, mixed, small cleaved and large cell [FML]) have several clinical characteristics in common: (1) Each has a history of waxing and waning or of slowly progressive adenopathy. (2) These are rubbery, mobile lymph nodes that are rarely fixed and have no overlying skin infiltration; lymph nodes may be very bulky but are rarely painful. (3) Liver and spleen are frequently involved pathologically and may be enlarged; liver function tests are usually normal, although the alkaline phosphatase level may be mildly increased. (4) Bone marrow involvement is common; circulating lymphoma cells may be identified on smear or by cell-sorting techniques. (5) Blood counts are usually normal at diagnosis. Elevation of the white blood cell count with circulating cells, anemia with autoimmune hemolytic anemia, and cytopenias secondary to hypersplenism or bone marrow replacement are uncommon complications. (6) Other extranodal disease sites may include pleura, lung, skin, breast, and gastrointestinal tract. (7) Enlarged lymph nodes may cause lymphedema, ureteral obstruction, or epidural cord com-

TABLE 147–1. PATHOLOGIC CHARACTERISTICS OF NON-HODGKIN'S LYMPHOMAS

Subtype	Architectural Pattern	Malignant Lymphocyte Cytology	Immunophenotype/ Immunogenotype
SLL	Diffuse	Small round cells	B cell; rarely T cell
FSCL	Follicular	Small cleaved cells	B cell
FML	Follicular	Small cleaved cells admixed with large cells, cleaved or noncleaved	B cell
FLCL	Follicular	Large cells cleaved or noncleaved	B cell
DSCL	Diffuse	Small cleaved cells	B cell; occasionally T cell
DML	Diffuse	Admixture of small and large cells cleaved or noncleaved	B cell; T cell
DLCL	Diffuse	Large cells cleaved or noncleaved	B cell; T cell
IBL	Diffuse	Large cells; plasmacytoid, clear, or polymorphic cell variants	B cell; T cell
LBL	Diffuse "starry sky"	Lymphoblasts, convoluted or nonconvoluted nuclei	Thymic T cell
SNCL	Diffuse "starry sky"	Noncleaved cells, round nuclei with prominent nucleoli	B cell

pression. (8) Central nervous system (meningeal or parenchymal), renal, or testicular infiltration rarely occurs.

INTERMEDIATE GRADE AND HIGH GRADE (see Color Plate 8D, right). As a group, the intermediate (follicular, predominantly large cell [FLCL]; diffuse, small cleaved cell [DSCL]; diffuse, mixed small and large cell [DML]; and diffuse, large cell [DLCL]) and high-grade lymphomas (large cell immunoblastic [IBL]; lymphoblastic [LBL]; and small noncleaved cell, including Burkitt's lymphoma and diffuse and undifferentiated lymphoma, non-Burkitt's type [SNCL]) have several general clinical features in common: (1) There is a history of abrupt onset with rapidly enlarging lymph node masses. (2) Lymph nodes may be rubbery and mobile but may also be hard, fixed, and with overlying skin infiltration. Masses may be warm, erythematous, and painful. (3) Bulky lymph node masses (>10 cm) may be present in the mediastinum, retroperitoneum, and/or mesentery. (4) Waldeyer's ring may be involved and is often associated with extranodal disease of the stomach or small bowel or both. (5) Hepatosplenomegaly may be present, and liver function tests may be abnormal. Porta hepatis or even intrahepatic obstructive patterns may be seen. (6) Extranodal involvement is common: stomach, small bowel, lung, skin, bone, and central nervous system (particularly meningeal disease in association with bone marrow involvement). Rarely ovarian, testicular, or renal disease may be present. (7) Bone marrow involvement and circulating cells are less commonly seen at diagnosis than in low-grade lymphomas. A leukemic picture may emerge, however, when progressive disease develops. (8) Lymph node masses may cause lymphedema, ureteral obstruction, vascular obstruction (superior vena cava syndrome, thrombophlebitis), and epidural cord compression.

MISCELLANEOUS. A miscellaneous category of the Working Formulation includes mycosis fungoides (see Color Plate 7J, right)—a rare helper T cell lymphoma of the skin; composite lymphoma—multiple histologic subtypes (e.g., FSCL and IBL) occurring simultaneously; and true histiocytic lymphoma.

Since the Formulation's publication in 1982, additional mature T cell lymphomas have been recognized. The peripheral T cell lymphomas are a diverse group of "postthymic" neoplasms, whose cell of origin is the differentiated T cell. Their morphology includes diffuse small cell, mixed cell, large cell, or immunoblastic lymphoma, as well as subgroups with histologic features of angioimmunoblastic lymphadenopathy, lymphomatoid granulomatosis, Hodgkin's-like disease, or Lennert's lymphoma. Clinical features include a 2:1 male predominance, prominent extranodal disease (particularly lung involvement) in the majority, systemic symptoms, and skin rash. In general, response to treatment and

TABLE 147–2. CLINICAL CHARACTERISTICS OF NON-HODGKIN'S LYMPHOMAS*

Subtype	% All Lymphomas	Median Age (yr)	Sex Ratio M:F	% PS I, II	% PS III, IV	% Bone Marrow Involvement
SLL	3.6	61	1.2:1	11	89	71
FSCL	22.5	54	1.3:1	18	82	51
FML	7.7	56	0.8:1	27	73	30
FLCL	3.8	55	1.8:1	27	73	34
DSCL	6.9	58	2:1	28	72	32
DML	6.7	58	1.1:1	45	55	14
DLCL	19.7	57	1:1	46	54	10
IBL	7.9	51	1.5:1	52	49	12
LBL	4.2	17	1.9:1	27	74	50
SNCL	0.5	30	2.6:1	34	66	14

*PS = pathologic stage (according to the Working Formulation, 1982).

survival appear to parallel their counterparts in the Working Formulation.

HTLV-I–associated adult T cell leukemia/lymphoma is characterized by geographic clustering, the presence of antibody to HTLV-I, and a rapidly fatal clinical course. Clinical features include abrupt onset of generalized lymphadenopathy, hepatosplenomegaly, skin infiltration, lytic bone disease, bone marrow involvement with circulating cells, and hypercalcemia. In spite of intensive chemotherapy, median survival is less than 1 year. Although clinically distinct, this rare T cell lymphoma is not easily distinguishable pathologically from other T cell lymphomas. Diffuse small cell, mixed cell, large cell, and undifferentiated cell types have all been described. Therefore, clinical suspicion and the presence of HTLV-I antibody are necessary to confirm the diagnosis.

DIAGNOSIS AND STAGING

As discussed in Ch. 146, the diagnosis of non-Hodgkin's lymphoma requires skilled interpretation of adequate tumor tissue, preferably from an involved lymph node, so that tumor architecture as well as cell type may be assessed. B cell and T cell typing studies may complement the pathologic interpretation but do not supplant it. The clinical history and ancillary studies, e.g., HTLV-I or HIV antibody, may also contribute. Once a diagnosis has been established, then it is useful to determine the extent of disease through staging.

The Ann Arbor staging system utilized for Hodgkin's disease (see Ch. 148) is also used in the management of non-Hodgkin's lymphomas. Although of clinical value, this staging system has several shortcomings when applied to non-Hodgkin's lymphomas: Factors such as disease site, disease bulk, and extent of extranodal involvement are not considered. In addition, the presence of systemic symptoms plays a lesser role in influencing treatment planning and prognosis in non-Hodgkin's lymphoma. Nevertheless, thorough pretreatment staging is necessary in all patients.

Noninvasive studies, which should be obtained in all patients, are listed in Table 147–3.

On the basis of this information, the clinical stage of the lymphoma can be determined. Since bone marrow involvement is so common, particularly in low-grade lymphoma, bilateral percutaneous bone marrow biopsies are often the simplest way to establish pathologic stage IV disease.

Pathologic confirmation of other extranodal sites may be appropriate, as when gastroscopic biopsy, pleural cytology, or skin biopsy is obtained. Laparotomy or thoracotomy is indicated only in those patients with no other evident disease or when a gastrointestinal tumor is removed prior to treatment. Staging laparotomy as performed for Hodgkin's disease is rarely, if ever, indicated.

TREATMENT

In defining a treatment approach for the patient with non-Hodgkin's lymphoma, it is necessary to consider such factors as histologic subtype, stage, sites of disease, tumor bulk, thoroughness of initial staging, general medical condition, and age, as well as the goals and effectiveness of therapy. In practical terms, non-

Hodgkin's lymphomas can be considered in two broad categories: those diseases that progress slowly and have an indolent natural history (the low-grade lymphomas) and those diseases that present aggressively, progress rapidly, and, if unsuccessfully treated, are soon fatal (the intermediate- and high-grade lymphomas).

LOW-GRADE LYMPHOMAS. As outlined above, low-grade lymphomas infrequently present with truly localized disease (pathologic stage I or II). Only 11 to 27 per cent, depending upon histologic subtype, are therefore eligible for regional treatment with radiation therapy. Although uncommon, this disease presentation appears to be highly favorable, with more than 75 per cent of patients remaining free of disease for 10 years or longer after irradiation alone (3500 to 4400 cGy to the region).

Many more patients appear to have clinically localized disease after noninvasive staging and bone marrow biopsy but have not undergone complete laparotomy staging. Under these circumstances, radiation therapy may still accomplish good local control. Many patients, however, have undetected microscopic disease outside the treatment portal that will slowly progress and lead to disease recurrence several years after initial therapy. Nevertheless, irradiation may still be a reasonable choice, since relapse may occur years later, and salvage treatment at relapse may be effective. Patients eligible for this approach are those with peripheral lymph node presentations (stages I and II) involving cervical, supraclavicular, axillary, or inguinal regions. Abdominal masses usually require whole-abdominal irradiation in which this approach may not be justified. Thoracic presentations are rare.

The majority (74 to 89 per cent) of patients with low-grade lymphomas have advanced stage (III or IV) disease and are therefore ineligible for localized treatment approaches. Optimal management of such patients remains controversial. Complete disappearance of all known tumor (including bone marrow biopsy) may be induced in more than 80 per cent of patients with single-

TABLE 147–3. NONINVASIVE STUDIES IN NON-HODGKIN'S LYMPHOMA

History with assessment of systemic symptoms, predisposing epidemiologic factors
Physical examination
Complete blood count and platelet count; Coombs' test if anemic
Liver and renal function tests
Serum immunoglobulins in low-grade lymphomas
Antibody for HTLV-I or HIV, if indicated
Chest radiograph, posteroanterior and lateral
Chest computed tomography, if indicated
Abdominal and pelvic computed tomography
    If unavailable, abdominal ultrasound study
    If normal, lymphography possibly indicated
Bone scan and bone radiographs if clinical involvement suspected
Upper gastrointestinal series, if clinical involvement suspected or if Waldeyer's ring involved
Gallium scan, optional in aggressive histologies
Cerebrospinal fluid cytology (in all patients with intermediate- or high-grade lymphomas and known bone marrow disease)

agent or multiagent chemotherapy, with whole-body irradiation, or with combined chemotherapy-irradiation. Unfortunately, median remission durations are usually limited to 2½ to 5 years. Complete responders actually have persistent lymphoma cells in their peripheral blood and bone marrow that may be detected by sensitive methods. The presence of such cells correlates with subsequent relapse.

The most promising combination chemotherapy program is ProMACE-MOPP* followed by a total lymphoid irradiation of 2400 cGy in complete responders. Preliminary results reveal a high complete response rate, with more than 70 per cent remaining in remission at 4 years. It is premature to speculate on the ultimate remission durability of such combined-modality regimens. Sensitive molecular methods (utilizing the polymerase chain reaction) to detect residual cells may be helpful in assessing whether such programs can eliminate the malignant clone.

In summary, a standard treatment regimen in advanced low-grade lymphoma has not been established. Daily single-agent cyclophosphamide; daily or pulse chlorambucil; or combinations of cyclophosphamide, vincristine, prednisone with or without procarbazine or doxorubicin (Adriamycin) are reasonable choices, depending upon the clinical circumstances. Enrollment in a protocol regimen is encouraged whenever possible, since an optimal treatment regimen has not been identified.

Another management approach in patients with advanced low-grade non-Hodgkin's lymphomas is initial treatment deferral, with institution of therapy when there is disease progression. This approach is based on the premise that treatment at diagnosis does not appear curative. Many patients have indolent, slowly progressive disease, and treatment deferral does not appear to compromise therapeutic outcome. Approximately one half of all patients may be eligible for observation at diagnosis; the median treatment-free period correlates with histology: more than 8 years for SLL, 5 years for FSCL, and 10 months for FML.

Biologic therapies have also been investigated in low-grade lymphomas and appear to have transient efficacy. These include monoclonal antibody therapy directed specifically against the malignant B cell immunoglobulin idiotype, antibody against B cell differentiation antigens, and alpha-interferon.

In up to 50 per cent of patients, low-grade lymphomas may change with or without treatment from an indolent to an aggressive form by the eighth year following diagnosis. Most often the transformation manifests as rapidly growing disease in one or more sites, while the low-grade component remains stable or progresses slowly. Pathologic study reveals DLCL, IBL, or other aggressive subtypes, and studies of clonality are consistent with the low-grade histology (B cell primarily). Most transformations represent the emergence of an aggressive subclone from the original indolent disease, but some cases appear to represent the emergence of a completely new second neoplasm that is a clonally distinct, aggressive lymphoma in the setting of indolent lymphoma.

Histologic transformation is important to recognize, since it has prognostic and therapeutic implications. Median survival is less than 1 year following its emergence, and intensive treatment programs are necessary to gain disease control. Some patients appear to have the aggressive component eradicated by such measures, often with persistence or later relapse of the indolent histology.

INTERMEDIATE- AND HIGH-GRADE LYMPHOMAS. Intensive combination chemotherapy is the mainstay of curative treatment in aggressive non-Hodgkin's lymphomas. Of the half of all patients who may present with regional disease alone, only that small subset with pathologic stage I presentation may be eligible for radiation therapy alone. This is because the intent and realistic goal of treatment in the aggressive lymphomas is always cure, and relapse must be avoided whenever possible.

The expectation of cure in the majority of patients with aggressive lymphomas, regardless of stage, is based upon the

following observations in advanced disease: (1) Tumors are rapidly proliferating and initially very sensitive to combination chemotherapy. (2) Survival curves in advanced disease are biphasic, revealing a rapid death rate during the 2 first years (composed of partially responding and nonresponding patients) and then a plateau of cured cases (composed of complete responders). (3) With intensifying drug regimens, the proportion of complete responders may be increased and, similarly, the proportion cured. (4) Increasing tumor bulk correlates with decreased complete response, the emergence of drug resistance, and poor survival. (5) The highest complete response rates to combination chemotherapy are achieved in patients with regional or disseminated nonbulky disease.

Commonly used agents in combination regimens include cyclophosphamide, doxorubicin (Adriamycin), vincristine, prednisone, methotrexate, bleomycin, etoposide, and cytosine arabinoside. Representative regimens are listed in Table 147–4. Treatment should be initiated promptly after diagnosis and appropriate noninvasive staging; the regimen must be intensive (leading to at least moderate toxicity), administered in high and often escalating doses, on a rigorous schedule; attention must be paid to rapidity of response and any evidence of early drug resistance; and after a defined treatment course, complete restaging is undertaken. With these guidelines, at least 60 per cent of patients with advanced disease and more than 80 per cent with localized disease achieve complete response. The majority of complete responses (>70 per cent) are durable, and maintenance chemotherapy is unnecessary.

By increasing the relative dose intensity of combination chemotherapy regimens utilized in the treatment of aggressive lymphomas, the number of complete responders appears to have increased. To establish the validity of this concept, a national intergroup study is currently testing the relative efficacy of the four most commonly utilized regimens (each with a different dose intensity).

Another investigative approach has been the use of potentially lethal doses of chemotherapeutic agents with autologous bone marrow rescue in high-risk patients. Preliminary reports suggest that this approach is superior to standard combination chemotherapy.

SPECIAL CONSIDERATIONS. *Histopathologic Subtype.* Lymphoblastic lymphoma and SNCL are often treated with modified intensive drug programs, and all patients require central nervous system prophylaxis.

Mediastinal Disease. Superior vena cava syndrome may be present and is effectively managed with chemotherapy and/or irradiation. Biopsy of undetermined mediastinal masses must be accomplished with less than 750 to 1000 cGy (200 to 250 cGy fractions) of irradiation before biopsy.

Gastrointestinal Disease. Perforation and/or bleeding may be complications prior to or following treatment. To avoid this, surgical resection of the involved region is often recommended, prior to therapy.

Central Nervous System. All patients with lymphoblastic lymphoma and SNCL, as well as those with other aggressive histologic types and bone marrow involvement, are at risk for meningeal disease. Cerebrospinal fluid cytology is determined before therapy, and meningeal prophylaxis is given.

Primary brain lymphoma, as often identified in immunodeficient patients, requires high-dose whole-brain irradiation with or without chemotherapy.

Tumor Masses Larger than 10 cm. Supplementary irradiation is sometimes administered concurrently with or following chemotherapy. Residual fibrosis may occasionally persist after therapy. Surgical resection of tumor masses has been shown to be of value only with intra-abdominal Burkitt's lymphoma.

Tumor Lysis Syndrome. Rapid tumor shrinkage with excess urate production should be anticipated in all patients and allopurinol administered. With bulky or disseminated tumor or both, rapid cell lysis may lead to hyperkalemia, hypocalcemia, hyperphosphatemia, hyperuricemia, and acute renal failure. Patients with SNCL and lymphoblastic lymphoma are most often affected.

AIDS-Associated Lymphomas. The presence of significant immunodeficiency, multiple infections, and extranodal disease may make standard chemotherapy regimens excessively toxic and unsuccessful in this group of patients (see Color Plate 8E).

---

*ProMACE = prednisone, methotrexate, doxorubicin (Adriamycin), cyclophosphamide, etoposide; MOPP = Mechlorethamine (Mustargen), vincristine (Oncovin), procarbazine, prednisone.

TABLE 147–4. REPRESENTATIVE DRUG COMBINATIONS FOR INTERMEDIATE AND HIGH-GRADE NON-HODGKIN'S LYMPHOMAS

MACOP-B

Methotrexate	400 mg/m² IV	Weeks 2, 6, 10 with leucovorin
Adriamycin (doxorubicin)	50 mg/m² IV	Weeks 1, 3, 5, 7, 9, 11
Cyclophosphamide	350 mg/m² IV	Weeks 1, 3, 5, 7, 9, 11
Oncovin (vincristine)	1.4 mg/m² IV	Weeks 2, 4, 6, 8, 10, 12
Prednisone	75 mg PO	Daily, dose tapered over the last 15 days
Bleomycin	10 U/m² IV	Weeks 4, 8, 12
Co-trimoxazole	2 tab PO	Twice daily throughout

ProMACE-CytaBOM (21-day cycles)

Prednisone	60 mg/m² PO	Days 1–14
Adriamycin (doxorubicin)	25 mg/m² IV	Days 1 and 8
Cyclophosphamide	650 mg/m² IV	Day 1
Etoposide (VP-16)	120 mg/m² IV	Day 1
Cytarabine	300 mg/m² IV	Day 8
Bleomycin	5 mg/m² IV	Day 8
Oncovin (vincristine)	1.4 mg/m² IV	Day 8
Methotrexate	120 mg/m² IV	Day 8 with leucovorin
Co-trimoxazole	2 tab PO	Twice daily throughout

m-BACOD (28-day cycles)

Methotrexate	200 mg/m² IV	Days 8 and 15 with leucovorin
Bleomycin	4 mg/m² IV	Day 1
Adriamycin (doxorubicin)	45 mg/m² IV	Day 1
Cyclophosphamide	600 mg/m² IV	Day 1
Oncovin (vincristine)	1 mg/m² IV	Day 1
Dexamethasone	6 mg/m² PO	Days 1–5

CHOP (21- to 28-day cycles)

Cyclophosphamide	750 mg/m² IV	Day 1
Hydroxydaunomycin/ Adriamycin (doxorubicin)	50 mg/m² IV	Day 1
Oncovin	1.4 mg/m² IV	Day 1
Prednisone	100 mg PO	Days 1–5

IV = intravenous; PO = by mouth.

PROGNOSIS

The Working Formulation identifies more than 10 distinct disease entities and groups them according to prognosis. The survival curves upon which these prognostic groups were initially based are no longer entirely valid because of improved treatment methods. Nevertheless, it is still important to recognize a low-grade category in which the lymphoma progresses slowly and has an indolent natural history, as well as intermediate- and high-grade categories in which the disease presents aggressively, progresses rapidly, and, if unsuccessfully treated, is soon fatal.

In Figure 147–1A are the overall survival curves of the original Working Formulation (based on 1975 data) according to prognostic category. The median survivals are approximately 6½ years for the low-grade, 2½ years for the intermediate-grade, and 1½ years for the high-grade categories. Figure 147–1B illustrates representative overall survival curves based on 1985 data, according to prognostic category. The median survival in the low-grade category is 6½ years, unchanged from the original Working Formulation, whereas the median survival for the intermediate- and high-grade categories has not yet been reached, and at least 60 per cent of all patients remain alive and disease free at 5 years. Followed to 8 years, the curves overlap as patients in the low-grade category succumb to progressive lymphoma, while patients in the intermediate- and high-grade categories continue to be disease free.

This, then, is the prognostic paradox of non-Hodgkin's lymphomas: Initially favorable and indolent, the low-grade histologic types are, in fact, the unfavorable category with longer observation; and initially unfavorable and aggressive intermediate- and high-grade histologic types are, in fact, the favorable categories, since cure may be regularly achieved.

Armitage JO: Bone marrow transplantation in the treatment of patients with lymphoma. Blood 73:1749, 1989. *An excellent review of the topic of transplantation in lymphomas.*

DeVita VT Jr, Hubbard SM, Young RC, et al.: The role of chemotherapy in diffuse aggressive lymphomas. Semin Hematol 25 (Suppl 2):2, 1988. *A review of combination chemotherapy regimens, emphasizing the importance of prognostic factors and relative dose intensity in analyzing results.*

Haber DA, Mayer RJ: Primary gastrointestinal lymphoma. Semin Oncol 15:154, 1988. *A comprehensive review of pathology, clinical aspects, and therapeutic strategies.*

Knowles DM, Chamulak GA, Subar M, et al.: Lymphoid neoplasia associated with the acquired immunodeficiency syndrome (AIDS): The New York University

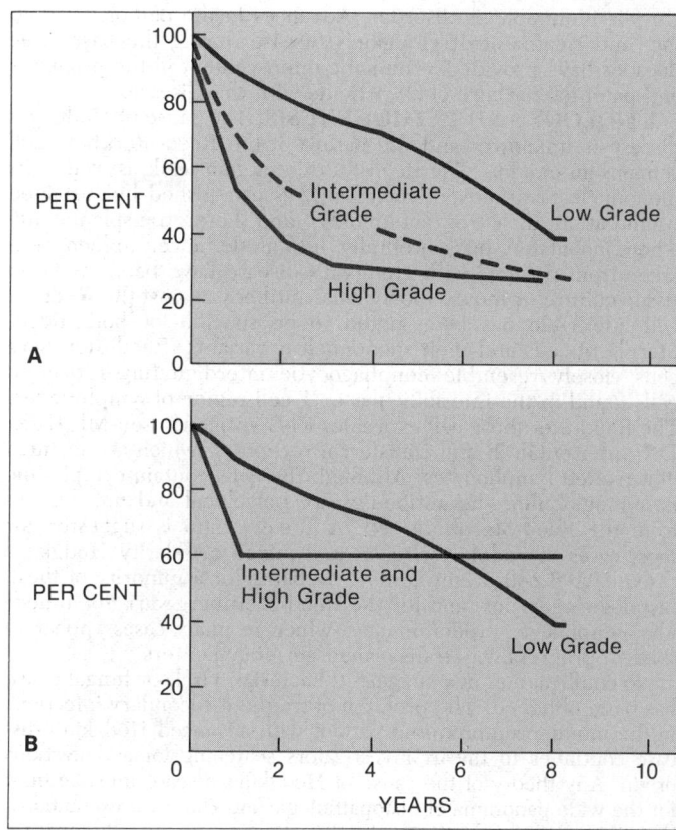

FIGURE 147–1. *A,* Actuarial survival according to histologic grade, based on 1975 data, as reported in the Working Formulation (1982). *B,* Hypothetical actuarial survival according to histologic grade, based on 1985 data (see text).

Medical Center experience with 105 patients (1981–1986). Ann Intern Med 108:744, 1988. *A comprehensive study of the epidemiology, clinical features, and treatment outcome of 105 patients with AIDS-associated lymphomas.*

The Non-Hodgkin's Lymphoma Pathologic Classification Project: National Cancer Institute sponsored study of classifications of non-Hodgkin's lymphomas: Summary and description of a working formulation for clinical usage. Cancer 49:2112, 1982. *The Working Formulation is presented in detail with pathologic and clinical analyses.*

Williams SF, Golomb HM (eds.): Non-Hodgkin's lymphoma. Semin Oncol 17:1–132, 1990. *A complete journal issue devoted to all aspects of non-Hodgkin's lymphomas: Pathology, basic science, clinical management, and complications of disease and therapy.*

Young RC, Longo DC, Glatstein E, et al.: The treatment of indolent lymphomas: Watchful waiting versus aggressive combined modality treatment. Semin Hematol 25 (Suppl 2):11, 1988. *The results of ProMACE-MOPP plus irradiation are presented in this preliminary report of a randomized trial.*

148 Hodgkin's Disease

John H. Glick

DEFINITION. Hodgkin's disease is a unique malignant disorder, usually arising in lymph nodes, with a characteristic histopathologic appearance. It is defined by the presence of the virtually pathognomonic Reed-Sternberg giant cell in an appropriate cellular background. The disease was first recognized as a distinct clinicopathologic entity in 1832 by Thomas Hodgkin, who described seven patients with a fatal illness involving "hypertrophy of the lymphatic system." Although the etiology is unknown, definitive evidence has emerged that Hodgkin's disease is indeed a malignant neoplasm and not a granulomatous infection or a chronic immunologic disorder. Advances in the pathology, staging, and treatment of Hodgkin's disease during the past three decades have provided a dramatic improvement in the prognosis and potential for cure of all patients with this disease.

ETIOLOGY AND PATHOGENESIS. The cause of Hodgkin's disease is unknown, and the nature of the Reed-Sternberg cell remains an enigma. The Reed-Sternberg giant cell, as well as its mononuclear variants, is malignant, as established by sustained proliferation in vitro, aneuploidy, and heterotransplantability when inoculated intracerebrally into nude mice. Spleen cells taken from patients with Hodgkin's disease have been grown in tissue culture. A mouse monoclonal antibody against the Hodgkin cell line L428 has been noted to be specific for both Reed-Sternberg cells and their mononuclear variants. Reed-Sternberg cells closely resemble nonphagocytic interdigitating reticulum cells found in the interfollicular or T cell region of lymph nodes. The Reed-Sternberg cell expresses Ki–1 antigens, Leu-Ml, HLA-DR, interleukin 2, and transferrin receptors, which are features of activated lymphocytes. Although the cells contain cytoplasmic immunoglobulin, the antibodies are polyclonal and not derived from the Reed-Sternberg cell. A T cell origin is suggested for most cases of nodular sclerosis and mixed cellularity Hodgkin's disease. A B cell origin is most probable for a minority of these histologic subtypes, and for the Reed-Sternberg variants in nodular lymphocyte predominance, which in many cases appear to arise in progressively transformed germinal centers.

No confirmation of a suggested bacterial, viral, or fungal cause has been obtained. The problem of frequent secondary infections in the immunocompromised patient with advanced Hodgkin's disease continues to thwart investigators searching for an infectious origin. Any theory of the cause of Hodgkin's disease must account for the wide panorama of histopathologic and clinical presentations, the variety of neoplastic giant cells, the signs of an inflammatory reaction and infection-like symptoms, the characteristic immunologic defects, and the specific epidemiologic patterns.

EPIDEMIOLOGY. Approximately 8000 new cases of Hodgkin's disease are diagnosed each year in the United States, with only 1600 deaths. These patients average 32 years of age and are more commonly male than female. The age-specific distribution curve is an unusual bimodal pattern for both sexes, with the first peak at ages 15 to 35 and the second after age 50. Hodgkin's disease is distributed throughout the world, but the age-specific rates differ markedly in different countries. The developed areas of the United States and Northern Europe have a prominent young adult peak, which is lower in less developed countries and absent in Japan.

There is an inverse risk with family size, with a rate 2.5 times greater among persons without siblings than those with four or more siblings. There is up to a sevenfold increased risk among siblings of young adults with Hodgkin's disease. Increased risk also occurs with early birth order position and improved living conditions. All these factors tend to decrease and delay exposure to infectious agents. It has been suggested that Hodgkin's disease may be an age-dependent host response to a common infection. Population-based studies have failed to document significant "clustering" of cases. No increased risk in medical personnel exposed to large numbers of patients with Hodgkin's disease has been observed. Thus, at the present time, there is no firm evidence for a contagious etiology.

PATHOLOGY. Histologic diagnosis of Hodgkin's disease requires the presence of characteristic Reed-Sternberg giant cells in association with an appropriate stromal background or cellular milieu. The classic Reed-Sternberg cell (Fig. 148–1A) is a large, bilobed cell with prominent eosinophilic nucleoli, perinucleolar clearing, thick nuclear membrane, and relatively abundant cytoplasm (see Color Plate 8F). Distinctive multinuclear giant cells in lacunar-like spaces (Fig. 148–1B) are associated with the nodular sclerosis subtype and are considered Reed-Sternberg variants. Mononuclear variants are also found on biopsy but cannot be considered as reliably diagnostic. Although the diagnosis of Hodgkin's disease is rarely made in the absence of Reed-Sternberg cells, the presence of such a cell is not pathognomonic of the disease. Cells indistinguishable from or closely resembling Reed-Sternberg cells may be found in reactive conditions such as infectious mononucleosis, in which immunoblasts, or trans-

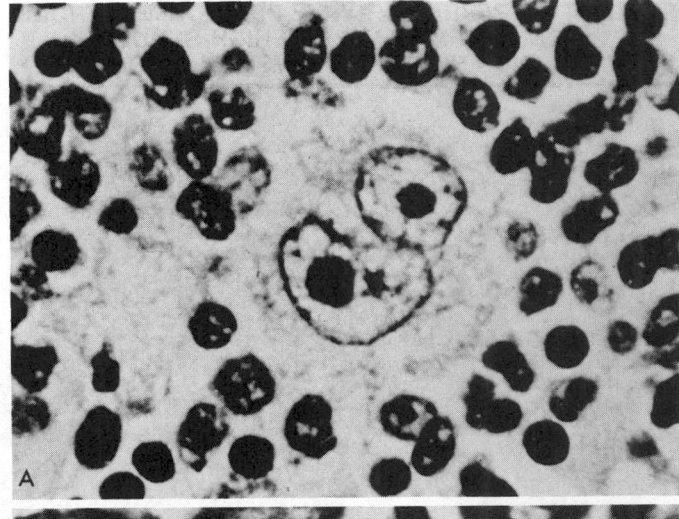

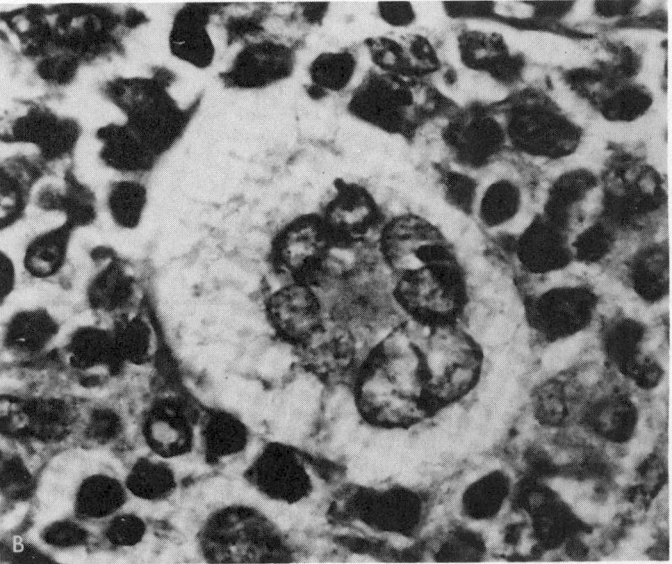

FIGURE 148–1. Pathologic diagnosis. *A*, Diagnostic Reed-Sternberg cell with large inclusion-like nucleoli, high power. *B*, Reed-Sternberg cell variant, lacunar cell type, high power. (Reprinted by permission from Tindle BH: Pathology of Lymphomas. *In* Bennett JM [ed.]: Lymphomas I. The Hague, Martinus Nijhoff, 1981, p. 70.)

formed lymphocytes, may mimic Reed-Sternberg cells. The character of the stromal background is as important for the diagnosis of Hodgkin's disease as is the Reed-Sternberg cell. This background consists of a mixed population of cytologically benign cells, including reactive lymphocytes, benign histiocytes, plasma cells, and eosinophils.

Frozen section material should not be used to make a definitive diagnosis when Hodgkin's disease is suspected because of the presence of artifacts. Formalin-fixed tissue is required for careful histologic review. If any uncertainty of diagnosis exists, consultation with an experienced hematopathologist is required. The monoclonal antibody Leu-M1, which reacts with granulocytes, stains Reed-Sternberg cells and their mononuclear variants. This immunodiagnostic marker may be particularly useful in distinguishing Hodgkin's disease from other lymphoproliferative disorders, such as peripheral T cell lymphomas. Needle aspiration of lymph nodes for diagnostic purposes is generally not reliable because insufficient tissue is obtained for accurate evaluation.

Hodgkin's disease is subclassified histopathologically into four subtypes according to the Rye classification (Table 148–1) (see Color Plate 8G). The relative frequency of the four groups is variable in different series, depending on epidemiologic and patient referral factors. The natural history of Hodgkin's disease correlates well with the histopathologic groups. The *lymphocyte predominance type* is the most favorable and is associated with early-stage disease in asymptomatic patients with nodal presentations. The *nodular sclerosis variety* has a relatively

TABLE 148–1. RYE HISTOPATHOLOGIC CLASSIFICATION OF HODGKIN'S DISEASE

Subgroup	Major Histologic Features	Relative Frequency
Lymphocyte predominance	Abundant normal-appearing lymphocyte infiltrate with or without benign histiocytes; occasionally nodular; rare Reed-Sternberg (R-S) cells	5–15%
Nodular sclerosis	Nodules of lymphoid infiltrate of varying size, separated by bands of collagen and containing numerous "lacunar" cell variants of R-S cells	40–75%
Mixed cellularity	Pleomorphic infiltrate of eosinophils, plasma cells, histiocytes, and lymphocytes with numerous R-S cells	20–40%
Lymphocyte depletion	Paucity of lymphocytes with numerous R-S cells, often bizarre in appearance; may have diffuse fiberosis or reticulum fibers	5%

favorable prognosis, usually occurs in young women with supradiaphragmatic nodes, and frequently involves the mediastinum. The *mixed cellularity pattern* tends to occur in middle-aged patients with systemic symptoms and more extensive disease than is first evident on initial presentation. The *lymphocyte depletion subtype* has the least favorable prognosis, as it generally occurs in patients with advanced-stage disease and systemic symptoms and frequently involves the bone marrow. Recent studies have indicated a lower incidence of lymphocyte depletion Hodgkin's disease than previously reported and have suggested that some cases formerly diagnosed as this histologic subtype may have represented large cell immunoblastic lymphomas. Advances in aggressive therapy, after precise staging, have obscured the prognostic value of histopathologic classification.

CLINICAL MANIFESTATIONS. The initial presentation and subsequent clinical course of patients with Hodgkin's disease can be extremely variable, depending on when in the natural history the patient first seeks medical attention.

Adenopathy. The majority of patients present with a painless and enlarging mass, most commonly in the neck, but occasionally in the axilla or inguinal-femoral region. This lymphadenopathy is usually discovered accidentally by the patient and is often the only manifestation of the disease at the time of diagnosis. Upon examination, this mass is found to be a discrete, rubbery, usually nontender lymph node or group of surrounding enlarged and matted lymph nodes. Asymptomatic lymphadenopathy may also be noted by the physician on a routine physical examination. In other instances, a chest roentgenogram, obtained either for a routine purpose or because of a persistent, dry, nonproductive cough, may demonstrate a mediastinal mass. Physical examination may then disclose lymphadenopathy of which the patient had been unaware. Although these typical presentations may occur at any age with any histopathologic type, they are more common in young patients, usually between 15 and 35 years of age with the nodular sclerosis histologic pattern.

The duration of lymphadenopathy prior to diagnosis is extremely variable. Typically, several weeks to several months elapse between the time of the patient's first observation of an asymptomatic mass and the diagnostic biopsy. However, some patients report that a particular mass has been present for many months to several years, with intermittent waxing and waning in size.

Fever and Systemic Symptoms. Although the asymptomatic presentation is most common, one quarter to one third of patients present with unexplained and persistent fever and/or night sweats as initial symptoms. Fatigue and weight loss may be associated complaints. Patients with these symptoms tend to be in the older age group, are more often men than women, and are generally discovered to have more widespread disease than the usual patient presenting without symptoms. Although superficial lymphadenopathy is present in most such patients, occasionally palpable lymphadenopathy is absent in the patient past the age

of 40 with severe systemic symptoms. These patients present with fever of undetermined origin. Extensive diagnostic efforts may be required to discover the presence of Hodgkin's disease, including lymphangiography, abdominal computed tomographic (CT) scanning, bone marrow biopsies, or even exploratory laparotomy.

The presence of fever, drenching night sweats requiring the changing of bed clothing, and weight loss exceeding 10 per cent of baseline body weight during the 6 months preceding diagnosis constitute systemic or B symptoms for staging purposes and confer an adverse prognosis.

Although fever secondary to Hodgkin's disease is usually low grade, occasional patients have intermittent evening fever lasting several days, alternating with afebrile periods lasting days or weeks. This cyclic fever has been labeled the *Pel-Ebstein type* but is rarely the presenting manifestation of the disease.

Pruritus. Pruritus is another characteristic systemic symptom of Hodgkin's disease. It may be mild and localized, but usually progresses and becomes generalized. Severe pruritus may result in extensive excoriations and inability to sleep. It is rarely relieved by topical medications or antihistamines. The prognostic significance of pruritus itself is unclear. It rarely occurs in the absence of fever and/or night sweats but is no longer considered a B symptom because its presence does not correlate with an adverse prognosis. Generalized, severe pruritus may occur in patients with non-Hodgkin's lymphomas and in other medical and dermatologic conditions, but its presence should always suggest Hodgkin's disease. Its cause is unknown.

SELECTED CLINICAL PROBLEMS. A wide variety of other symptoms may initially call the attention of patients and their physicians to the disease. These same problems occur more commonly as the course of Hodgkin's disease progresses. In addition, almost all patients receive treatment that profoundly affects the natural history of their illness, resulting in either apparent cure or persistent, relapsing Hodgkin's disease, or frequently in complications that become difficult to separate from the manifestations of the disease itself.

Pulmonary involvement occurs in only 10 to 20 per cent of patients at presentation. It appears to arise by spread along lymphatics from ipsilateral hilar lymph nodes. Hodgkin's disease frequently involves the lungs with a patchy pulmonary infiltrate without circumscribed borders. Its appearance is variable, and it must be distinguished from radiation effects, drug reactions, and the wide variety of pulmonary infections that occur in these immunocompromised patients. In a severely ill patient in whom the diagnosis is uncertain, the therapeutic significance of these lesions is so great that bronchoscopy with transbronchial biopsy or diagnostic thoracotomy may be justified. Pleural effusions—transudates, exudates, or chylous—are most frequently caused by central lymphatic and venous obstruction resulting from Hodgkin's disease in the mediastinum or obstruction of the thoracic duct. These effusions are rarely caused by direct pleural involvement, and cytologic examination of the fluid or pleural biopsy infrequently reveals diagnostic Reed-Sternberg cells.

Superior vena caval obstruction, upper airway compression, and recurrent laryngeal nerve involvement are rare despite bulky intrathoracic disease presentations. Myocardial involvement is extremely unusual, but pericardial effusions may occur from direct invasion by adjacent mediastinal Hodgkin's disease. Effusions rarely produce cardiac tamponade, and this complication is more often a consequence of radiation-induced pericarditis.

Spinal cord compression, usually caused by epidural spread of tumor from paravertebral lymph nodes through intervertebral foramina in the thoracic or lumbar regions, may be a devastating acute complication. This syndrome may be seen in patients with an otherwise favorable prognosis, although it usually occurs in patients with progressive tumor in whom primary treatment has failed. Back or neck pain, either directly over the vertebral body or occurring in a radicular pattern, should promptly raise the suspicion of cord compression. Symptoms suggestive of more advanced cord compression include numbness, tingling or weakness of an extremity, motor weakness, and bladder or bowel dysfunction. Prompt diagnostic evaluation, including magnetic resonance imaging (MRI) and/or CT scanning is mandatory, as is prompt therapeutic intervention with immediate radiotherapy to prevent permanent neurologic damage. Surgical decompression is rarely indicated.

Bone involvement may occur from hematogenous spread in advanced disease or by local nodal spread to adjacent bone. Bone involvement often produces pain but rarely fracture, since the bone lesion is generally osteoblastic or mixed osteoblastic and osteolytic.

Hepatic involvement is present in fewer than 5 per cent of patients at the time of diagnosis and is generally focal in nature. Liver involvement in Hodgkin's disease is almost always associated with splenic involvement. Massive hepatomegaly or jaundice is rarely seen at the time of initial presentation. However, as the liver becomes progressively involved, diffuse infiltration of the portal spaces may be associated with serious hepatic dysfunction and laboratory features of intrahepatic biliary obstruction. Rarely, enlarged lymph nodes in the porta hepatis may produce extrahepatic biliary obstruction. Direct *renal involvement* is rarely a clinically significant problem, and ureteral obstruction and hydronephrosis, secondary to massive retroperitoneal lymphadenopathy, suggest a non-Hodgkin's lymphoma. The nephrotic syndrome, presenting as lipoid nephrosis, is a rare manifestation of Hodgkin's disease and is occasionally accompanied by evidence of glomerular immune complex deposition.

Infectious complications are common in patients with Hodgkin's disease and may or may not be temporarily related to concurrent treatment. Virtually all patients with uncontrolled Hodgkin's disease who succumb to this disorder have episodes of serious infections at some point in the course of their disease. Localized or disseminated herpes zoster is the most frequently diagnosed serious viral infection, while cryptococcosis, especially of the lungs and meninges, is the most virulent of the fungal complications. *Pneumocystis carinii* pneumonia causes diffuse pulmonary infiltrates and may appear in patients whose disease is in remission between cycles of chemotherapy, as well as in patients in whom relapse occurs. Toxoplasmosis is being recognized with increasing frequency, while tuberculosis has become distinctly uncommon in this population. Children who have undergone splenectomy are particularly predisposed to overwhelming pneumococcal infections unless prophylactic antibiotics or pneumococcal vaccine is administered.

Immunologic abnormalities are common in patients with Hodgkin's disease even at the time of initial diagnosis and prior to initiation of any treatment. A significantly higher frequency of cutaneous anergy is observed than in a control population. The presence or absence of anergy, however, has been shown to have no influence on the prognosis within a specific stage, given the effectiveness of modern therapy. Thus, there is no role for the routine anergy panel. With refined immunologic techniques, a defect in delayed hypersensitivity and T cell transformation can be detected even in early stage I disease. These deficits are aggravated by therapy and persist for many years even after successful curative treatment. In addition, T cell number, T cell helper (CD4)/suppressor (CD8) ratio, and T cell in vitro response to antigen may also be reduced. Decreased production of interleukin 2 (IL2) by peripheral blood mononuclear cells and decreased natural killer cell activity have been reported. Although cell-mediated immunity may be abnormal, patients with Hodgkin's disease rarely develop opportunistic infections prior to treatment. Therapy for Hodgkin's disease undoubtedly accentuates the T cell abnormality. However, it is still unknown whether the observed immunologic abnormalities contribute to the pathogenesis of the disease or are merely secondary phenomena. B cell function and B cell numbers appear to be normal in Hodgkin's disease at the time of diagnosis. Pneumococcal vaccine, for example, results in normal antibody response as long as subsequent treatment is delayed 10 to 14 days. However, overwhelming bacterial sepsis with encapsulated organisms is still a potential risk following splenectomy, especially in children.

STAGING. The progress achieved in the treatment of Hodgkin's disease has paralleled the improvement in techniques for identifying the extent or stage of disease in the untreated patient. In view of the current choices of therapy, it is essential that all cases of Hodgkin's disease be completely evaluated before therapeutic decisions are made. The primary goals of staging are to assess the extent of disease, facilitate the selection of an appropriate treatment program, provide an accurate determination of prognosis, and establish a baseline for re-evaluation following completion of therapy.

The staging classification in current use is outlined in Table 148–2. Patients are assigned a *clinical stage* (CS) on the basis of their initial biopsy, systemic symptoms, physical examination, laboratory results, and radiologic procedures. However, treatment decisions are generally based on a *pathologic stage* (PS), after the extent of involvement has been documented with appropriate biopsies. The basic staging classification is modified by the adverse prognostic significance of systemic symptoms (B disease) and by the realization that localized contiguous extranodal extension (E disease) generally does not carry the same poor prognosis as hematogenous extranodal involvement (stage IV disease).

Within each stage of Hodgkin's disease there is a spectrum of patients who have a more or less favorable prognosis, depending on the site or sites of disease, size of the tumor masses, and degree of symptoms. The importance of these prognostic factors and substages within the Ann Arbor classification has become increasingly recognized, because treatment methods are now tailored to individual clinical situations. Controversy exists over the prognostic and therapeutic significance of the E lesion and the substaging of IIIA patients. Pathologic stage IIIA disease, for example, may be subdivided into a prognostically favorable III$_1$ group, in which abdominal disease is confined to the upper abdominal nodes and/or the spleen, and a less favorable III$_2$ group, with disease extending to the lower abdomen, including the para-aortic, iliac, or inguinal lymph nodes.

Further modifications in the Ann Arbor staging system have been recommended to reflect changes in clinical staging criteria, newly recognized prognostic factors, and their impact on therapeutic decisions. The value of CT scanning and other imaging modalities in defining the extent of lymph node, liver, and splenic involvement is now recognized. In regional disease, the number of involved sites is denoted by a subscript (e.g., II$_3$). Bulky disease is defined by maximal dimension (> 10 cm) or by mass to thorax ratio (≥ one third at T5–T6). In the setting of bulky intrathoracic disease, contiguous spread to adjacent extranodal tissues is clearly distinguished from disseminated extranodal involvement (such as multiple lung nodules). A complete knowledge of staging is vital to guide an efficient but thorough diagnostic evaluation. The tests performed as part of a staging evaluation must be individualized rather than obtained automatically.

DIAGNOSTIC EVALUATION. Recommended staging procedures are outlined in Table 148–3. This evaluation should

TABLE 148–2. MODIFIED ANN ARBOR STAGING CLASSIFICATION

Stage	
I	Involvement of a single lymph node region (I) or of a single extralymphatic organ or site (I$_E$)
II	Involvement of two or more lymph node regions on the same side of the diaphragm (II) or localized involvement of an extralymphatic organ or site and of one or more lymph node regions on the same side of the diaphragm (II$_E$)
III	Involvement of lymph node regions on both sides of the diaphragm (III), which may also be accompanied by involvement of the spleen (III$_S$) or by localized involvement of an extralymphatic organ or site (III$_E$) or both (III$_{SE}$)
III$_1$	Involvement limited to the lymphatic structures in the upper abdomen, that is, spleen, or splenic, celiac, or hepatic portal nodes, or any combination of these
III$_2$	Involvement of lower abdominal nodes, that is, para-aortic, iliac, inguinal, or mesenteric nodes, with or without involvement of the splenic, celiac, or hepatic portal nodes
IV	Diffuse or disseminated involvement of one or more extralymphatic organs or tissues, with or without associated lymph node involvement

E = extralymphatic site; S = splenic involvement

Note: The presence of fever, night sweats, and/or unexplained loss of 10 per cent or more of body weight in the 6 months preceding diagnosis is denoted by the suffix letter B. The letter A indicates the absence of these symptoms. Each patient is assigned a clinical stage (CS) on the basis of the initial biopsy, physical examination, and laboratory and radiologic results and a pathologic stage (PS) on the basis of subsequent biopsy results, whether normal or abnormal.

TABLE 148–3. DIAGNOSTIC EVALUATION

148 HODGKIN'S DISEASE / 959

A. Required procedures
1. Histologic confirmation by biopsy
2. Detailed history for unexplained fever, weight loss, night sweats, and pruritus
3. Physical examination to document all areas of lymphadenopathy, including Waldeyer's ring, size of liver and spleen, bone tenderness; neurologic evaluation
4. Laboratory studies
   a. CBC and platelet count, ESR
   b. Serum alkaline phosphatase, LDH
   c. Renal function, including uric acid
   d. Liver function
5. Radiologic studies
   a. Chest roentgenogram
   b. Bipedal lymphangiogram
   c. CT of the chest and whole abdomen, including the pelvis
B. Frequently performed procedures under specific clinical conditions
1. Bone marrow biopsy (needle or open surgical technique)
2. Bone roentgenography and scanning for areas of bone pain or tenderness
3. Gallium whole-body scanning
4. Staging laparotomy and splenectomy, if therapeutic decisions will depend on the identification of subdiaphragmatic disease

CBC = complete blood count; ESR = erythrocyte sedimentation rate; LDH = lactate dehydrogenase.

commence promptly after the initial biopsy establishes the diagnosis.

History and Physical Examination. A careful history and physical examination are essential to discover characteristic systemic symptoms and to describe all the lymph node areas of the body. Enlarged lymph nodes are not necessarily involved by disease; reactive lymphoid hyperplasia occasionally occurs in some patients with Hodgkin's disease. If confirmation of Hodgkin's disease in suspicious lymph nodes will change the therapeutic approach, then additional biopsies should be obtained. Although Waldeyer's ring involvement is uncommon in Hodgkin's disease, the lymphoid tissues in this region should be evaluated by physical examination. The size of the liver and spleen should be carefully determined, although mild enlargement of either organ may merely be a sign of nonspecific hypertrophy rather than involvement by Hodgkin's disease. A palpable abdominal mass caused by enlarged mesenteric or para-aortic lymph nodes is a rare initial finding. The bones should be examined for areas of tenderness, and a careful baseline neurologic examination performed.

Laboratory Studies. Routine laboratory tests include a complete blood count, erythrocyte sedimentation rate (ESR), urine analysis, renal and liver function tests, and serum alkaline phosphatase. Mild to moderate anemia may be found in patients with widespread disease and is often associated with normal indices, normal or low reticulocyte count, and a negative Coombs test. Anemia in a patient with Hodgkin's disease is usually caused by the typical chronic anemia of malignancy and rarely is secondary to hypersplenism, marrow involvement, or a Coombs-positive hemolytic anemia. A moderate to marked neutrophilic leukocytosis and thrombocytosis are characteristic of active, symptomatic Hodgkin's disease. Eosinophilia of a mild degree is common. In patients with severe and longstanding pruritus, moderate or marked eosinophilia frequently occurs. Absolute lymphopenia (<1000 per cubic millimeter) may be seen in a small percentage of patients with more advanced disease and is usually a poor prognostic sign.

The ESR is commonly elevated in patients with active disease but has limited sensitivity. An elevated serum alkaline phosphatase level may be a nonspecific finding or secondary to involvement of bone, bone marrow, or liver with Hodgkin's disease. Elevation of the serum uric acid level is rare at the time of initial presentation, except in advanced stages of disease with massive nodal or bone marrow involvement.

Radiologic Studies. Radiologic examinations should include routine chest roentgenograms, which demonstrate mediastinal involvement in 50 to 60 per cent of patients. In contrast, hilar disease is seen at presentation in fewer than 20 per cent of cases. In the absence of mediastinal involvement, hilar disease is unusual. Computed tomography of the chest provides better

definition of mediastinal, hilar, and paravertebral adenopathy, and pulmonary involvement, and is indicated for all patients. Its role is to define more precisely the extent of disease, including possible localized extension into the pulmonary parenchyma, as well as to assist in radiation treatment planning. The presence of a small pleural effusion in the patient with a mediastinal mass does not necessarily indicate malignant involvement of the pleura. Thoracentesis or pleural biopsy is rarely diagnostic of Hodgkin's disease in these situations.

Subdiaphragmatic sites are best evaluated by performing both bipedal lymphangiography and abdominal-pelvic CT. These examinations are complementary, and neither procedure should replace the other. Recently, with the advent of CT, the routine use of the lymphangiogram has been questioned. However, the specificity appears better for lymphangiography, in that abnormalities of intranodal architecture can be demonstrated in up to 25 per cent of cases at presentation (Fig. 148–2). The overall accuracy of this procedure is 80 to 90 per cent. Lymphangiography is also valuable in preparation for exploratory laparotomy, in that it directs the surgeon to potentially abnormal areas for lymph node biopsy.

Abdominal CT complements lymphangiography by demonstrating lymphadenopathy in the mesentery, porta hepatis, celiac nodes, and para-aortic nodes above the level of those opacified by the lymphangiogram. Computed tomography can assess nodal involvement only when there is an increase in lymph node size (Fig. 148–3). In contrast, lymphangiography provides information

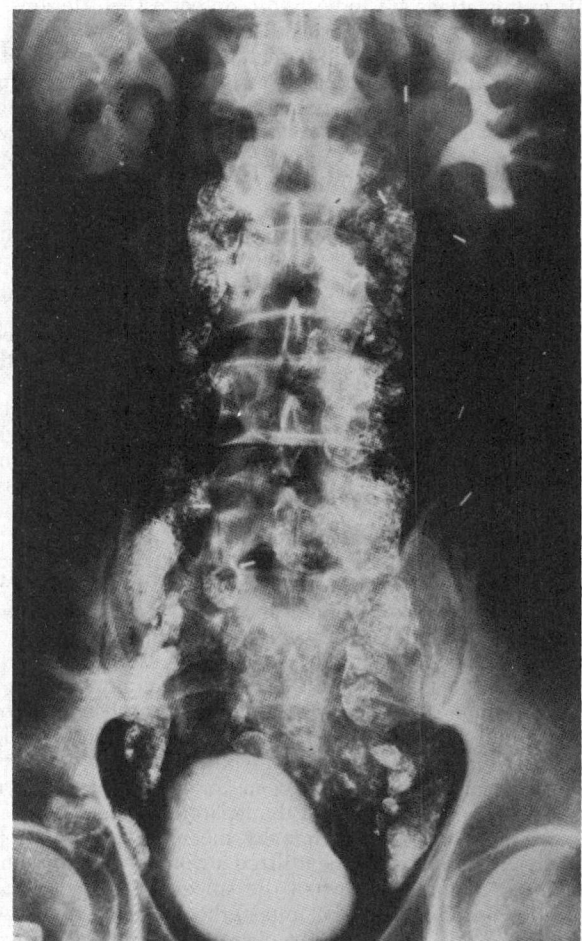

FIGURE 148–2. Abnormal lymphangiogram with enlargement and distortion of the internal architecture in the pelvic, iliac, and para-aortic lymph nodes. Despite the extensive lymphadenopathy, little displacement of the ureters and no obstruction of the upper urinary tracts were seen. (Reprinted, by permission of the publishers, from Hodgkin's Disease by Henry S. Kaplan, Cambridge, MA, Harvard University Press. Copyright © 1972, 1980, by the President and Fellows of Harvard College.)

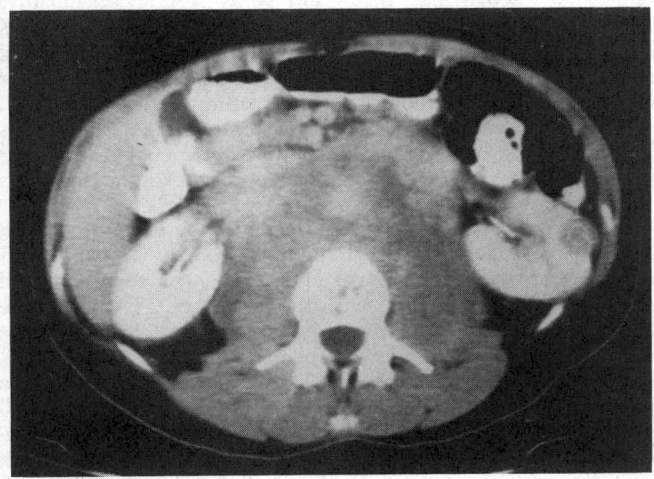

FIGURE 148–3. Abnormal abdominal CT scan with massive enlargement of retroperitoneal nodes.

on abnormal architecture even in unenlarged nodes. Thus, reliance on CT alone may lead to understaging.

Routine bone scans or skeletal radiographic examinations are not indicated in the asymptomatic patient with a normal alkaline phosphatase level. However, in those patients with areas of bone pain or tenderness, bone scans complemented by selective radiographic examinations are indicated to detect osseous lesions.

The liver is considered involved if multiple focal defects are detected by CT scan. A single percutaneous needle biopsy of the liver is rarely diagnostic, because of the focal nature of hepatic involvement. Gallium whole-body scans, particularly with higher dose (7 to 10 mCi) imaging on a triple-peak camera, may be occasionally helpful in determining sites of initial disease but is more useful in evaluating response to therapy (e.g., in the mediastinum) and in detecting areas of recurrence after therapy. Magnetic resonance imaging has not proved more useful than CT in determining sites of initial involvement, but MRI may be able to distinguish lymphomatous involvement from residual fibrosis of lymph nodes after treatment.

Bone Marrow Biopsy. This procedure should be performed in all patients with systemic symptoms or CS III disease or both. It is also useful in patients with significant peripheral blood count abnormalities, increased serum alkaline phosphatase level of bone origin, and abnormal bone roentgenograms or scans. Hodgkin's disease in the bone marrow is rarely demonstrable by simple marrow aspiration. Involvement is usually focal, is often associated with fibrosis, and is diagnosed more readily by either a unilateral or a bilateral bone marrow biopsy.

Staging Laparotomy. In the absence of medical contraindications, an exploratory laparotomy with splenectomy is frequently employed as part of the staging evaluation to identify and confirm the presence of Hodgkin's disease below the diaphragm. The purpose of the laparotomy is diagnostic, the results of which may alter treatment selection significantly. Laparotomy findings that frequently influence both the staging and the subsequent treatment include detection of Hodgkin's disease in the spleen, detection of the extent of splenic involvement, and detection of the presence of disease in the celiac or retroperitoneal lymph nodes. Secondary benefits from the laparotomy include attempting to preserve ovarian function by means of an oophoropexy when pelvic irradiation is to be utilized in young women, reducing required irradiation fields when the spleen is treated, and improving the peripheral blood counts in the occasional patient with hypersplenism. In one quarter of patients with normal-sized spleens on physical examination, Hodgkin's disease is found in the spleen removed at surgery. Conversely, approximately 50 per cent of patients with clinical or radiologic enlargement of the spleen do not have histologic involvement. The identification of Hodgkin's disease in the liver is especially difficult. Physical examination, routine liver function tests, and liver scans correlate poorly, if at all, with histologic verification. Liver involvement can be demonstrated at laparotomy on wedge or needle biopsy

and is more often found in patients with significant splenomegaly and/or abnormal lymphangiograms.

Staging laparotomy is not a routine diagnostic procedure and should be performed only in those patients in whom the results will potentially modify treatment selection. Discussion of potential treatment options with the radiotherapist or medical oncologist for each stage of Hodgkin's disease should be held prior to the decision to perform a laparotomy. Thus, staging laparotomy with splenectomy is generally recommended for patients with CS I to IIA/B or IIIA disease. Patients with stage IIIB or IV disease are not candidates for laparotomy because combination chemotherapy is used as their primary method of treatment.

Certain subgroups have a very low likelihood of change in stage with laparotomy. Female patients with CS IA at a single supradiaphragmatic site and patients with CS IA limited to a small mediastinal mass have less than a 10 per cent risk of intra-abdominal involvement. In other cases, such as patients with massive mediastinal disease, laporotomy is omitted because chemotherapy is employed as the primary treatment, eliminating the need for precise staging below the diaphragm.

As a result of staging laparotomy and splenectomy, approximately one third of patients with CS I and II are found to have either subdiaphragmatic lymph node disease or splenic involvement. The factors most likely to be associated with upstaging include male gender, B symptoms, and two or more sites of disease above the diaphragm. If extensive splenic involvement (> four nodules) is documented, either combination chemotherapy alone or a combined-modality program is required. Approximately one third of CS IIIA patients (i.e., those with suspicious lymphangiograms or abdominal CT scans) have a negative staging laparotomy that allows their pathologic stage to be downgraded to I or II. Although the results of the laparotomy allow change in the stage in as many as 35 per cent of patients, this change modifies the treatment plan in approximately 25 per cent, depending on the extent of disease found below the diaphragm. Even in the hands of experienced surgeons, staging laparotomy is associated with a small risk of perioperative morbidity, including infection, fever, and phlebitis. Rare fatalities have been reported. Because of occasional severe bacterial infections occurring after splenectomy, pneumococcal vaccine should be administered preoperatively.

MODE OF SPREAD. Careful mapping of initial sites of involvement of Hodgkin's disease and the use of lymphangiography, staging laparotomy, and splenectomy provide evidence that involvement of various lymph node groups is distinctly nonrandom. Two different theories have been proposed to account for the nonrandom patterns of spread: (1) The *contiguity theory* (Rosenberg and Kaplan) postulates that the disease is unifocal in origin, beginning in an initial focus within the lymphatic system and spreading via lymphatic channels to contiguous lymphatic structures. The contiguity theory has been challenged because of the frequency of cervical, supraclavicular, and retroperitoneal lymph node involvement without intervening mediastinal disease, as well as the common involvement of the spleen, which has no afferent lymphatics. (2) The *susceptibility theory* (Smithers) postulates that the disease is multifocal in origin. The giant cells of Hodgkin's disease are thought to migrate in and out of lymph nodes from the bloodstream but are thought to grow only in preferential sites, presenting an appearance of contiguous spread. Noncontiguous spread is more common in the mixed cellularity and lymphocyte depletion subtypes, when multiple sites are present and when vascular invasion is present. However, the role of vascular invasion in the spread of Hodgkin's disease is not fully understood. Vascular invasion in the spleen may lead to hematogenous dissemination, since the spleen is almost invariably involved when Hodgkin's disease is present in the liver or bone marrow.

TREATMENT. The prognosis for patients with Hodgkin's disease has improved dramatically during the past three decades because of (1) the advances in precise staging and an awareness of the important prognostic factors previously described, (2) the development of supervoltage radiotherapeutic techniques, and (3) the use of effective combination chemotherapy programs.

Radiotherapy. Important factors in determining the success of radiation therapy include the radiation dose per field, the extent of the fields employed, the beam energy, and precision of treatment planning. A tumoricidal dose of 3600 to 4400 cGy is required to eradicate the lesions of Hodgkin's disease. Lymphoid regions adjacent to areas of known disease or those that are contiguous via lymphatic channels are usually treated to full dose. Apparently uninvolved areas are treated prophylactically for subclinical disease with doses of 3600 cGy. Large fields, shaped to conform to the patient's anatomy, are designed to treat multiple contiguous lymph node regions. A *mantle* port covers the cervical, supraclavicular, infraclavicular, axillary, mediastinal, and hilar lymph nodes. The *para-aortic* field includes the para-aortic lymph nodes from the level of the diaphragm down to the aortic bifurcation but omits the pelvis and treats the splenic hilar lymph nodes in a patient with a prior splenectomy. An inverted-**Y** port in one field not only includes the para-aortic and splenic hilar lymph nodes but also extends into the pelvis to encompass the iliac and inguinal-femoral lymph nodes. The combination of a mantle and para-aortic field is also referred to as subtotal nodal or extended-field irradiation. *Total lymphoid irradiation* implies sequential treatment to both a mantle and an inverted-Y field.

The use of sequential large-field irradiation minimizes the risk of either overlap or underdosage, which could result in either undue normal tissue toxicity or inadequate therapy, respectively. Treatment of these large fields requires supervoltage radiation. This capability is available primarily with contemporary linear accelerators, which have the advantages over cobalt of skin sparing, increased depth dose, and sharp beam edges with reduced lateral scatter. The use of a treatment simulator to plan the radiotherapy fields and proper field verification (portal films) during the treatment process is essential.

Definitive radiation therapy alone is appropriate initial management for the majority of patients with PS I and II Hodgkin's disease. Mantle and para-aortic irradiation is the treatment of choice for most patients with PS IA and IIA disease, providing an 80 to 85 per cent chance of cure with irradiation alone. Selected patients with PS IA and IIA supradiaphragmatic disease of the nodular sclerosis or lymphocyte predominance histology who do not have mediastinal involvement can be treated with mantle radiotherapy alone. Many patients with stage IB and IIB disease can be treated effectively with mantle and para-aortic radiotherapy alone, with a 70 to 75 per cent chance of cure, provided they do not have both fever and weight loss and/or a large mediastinal mass. Controversy exists over the indications for using both radiotherapy and chemotherapy in stage I or II patients who present with large mediastinal masses, limited contiguous extranodal disease (the E lesion of the Ann Arbor system), or systemic symptoms. In each of these disease settings, the use of radiation alone results in a lower disease-free survival rate than when a combined-modality program is employed as the initial treatment, although the use of chemotherapy at relapse may provide an equivalent chance of cure. Patients with III_SA or III_1A Hodgkin's disease and minimal splenic involvement are usually treated with either mantle and para-aortic radiotherapy or total lymphoid irradiation alone. Controversy exists over whether prophylactic hepatic irradiation should be delivered to those patients with splenic involvement.

Subdiaphragmatic early-stage Hodgkin's disease is a relatively rare clinical presentation. These patients tend to be older and male and to have mixed cellularity pathology. Staging laparotomy is generally indicated with treatment based on pathologic findings. Patients with subdiaphragmatic stage IA are generally treated with inverted-Y radiotherapy. In patients with PS IIA, with or without limited splenic involvement, total lymphoid irradiation and combined-modality therapy appear to be of comparable efficacy, based on limited data.

Complications of radiation treatment are related to the technique employed, dosage administered, and irradiated volume. Acute side effects of radiotherapy include transient nausea and vomiting, dysphagia, and marrow suppression. These effects subside shortly after radiation therapy is completed. Late potential side effects of radiation include hypothyroidism, pneumonitis, transient myelitis (generally manifested as electric-like shocks in limbs on neck flexion known as *Lhermitte's sign*), and rarely pericarditis. Persistent myelosuppression is a rare late complication. Radiation-induced decreased bone growth has been noted in children.

Chemotherapy. The major advance in the treatment of stage IIIB and IV Hodgkin's disease was the development of curative combination chemotherapy. The initial studies from the National Cancer Institute demonstrated that a four-drug combination known as MOPP (nitrogen mustard [Mustargen], vincristine [Oncovin], procarbazine, and prednisone) was capable of producing documented complete remissions in 70 to 80 per cent of patients with advanced Hodgkin's disease. At least one half to two thirds of the patients who achieved complete remission with MOPP have not had recurrence after more than 10 to 20 years of observation. Thus, 50 per cent of all patients with stage IIIB and IV who underwent treatment were cured with MOPP chemotherapy alone.

The potential for clinical cure of Hodgkin's disease with chemotherapy exists for all histologic subtypes, stages, and extranodal sites of disease. Patients who have received prior radiotherapy and in whom relapse subsequently occurs have an equivalent chance of being cured with "salvage" chemotherapy. Older patients and those with bone marrow involvement, systemic symptoms, bulky disease, and poor performance status have a less favorable long-term response with chemotherapy. The best results have been reported for asymptomatic patients with disease limited to the lymph nodes and/or lung.

It is essential to administer the drugs in the MOPP regimen at full doses and in a timely fashion. Therapy is repeated every 4 weeks, for a minimum of six cycles. An additional two cycles are administered after a complete clinical remission is obtained. At that time, chemotherapy is discontinued only when repeat restaging studies document that a true complete remission has been obtained. The restaging diagnostic evaluation includes repeat radiologic procedures and biopsies as indicated to verify the complete response status. Maintenance chemotherapy beyond the documentation of a restaged complete remission is of no advantage in improving either disease-free or overall survival. Patients who have relapsed after definitive radiation treatment for early-stage disease are often salvaged and cured with the same chemotherapy regimens used for patients with previously untreated advanced disease.

No alternative four- or five-drug combinations have been demonstrated conclusively to be superior to MOPP, considering differences in patient selection, prognostic factors, restaging evaluation, and adequate follow-up. However, results comparable to those with MOPP have been achieved with a variety of alternative chemotherapy programs that offer significantly less toxicity than MOPP. Combinations that contain cyclophosphamide or chlorambucil instead of nitrogen mustard, vinblastine in place of vincristine, and/or the addition of a nitrosourea appear to be as efficacious as MOPP in producing durable complete responses but have substantially fewer side effects.

The identification of the active non–cross-resistant combination ABVD (doxorubicin [Adriamycin], bleomycin, vinblastine, and dacarbazine [DTIC]) in the patient who has had a relapse led to the investigation of sequential alternating chemotherapy regimens (i.e., MOPP alternating monthly with ABVD or a hybrid of seven drugs, MOPP/ABV, in one monthly cycle) as primary induction therapy. By exposing tumor cells to more drugs early in the course of disease, drug-resistant clones might be eradicated before growing too large to be cured. Recent randomized trials have demonstrated significantly improved relapse-free and overall survival with either alternating monthly MOPP/ABVD or the MOPP/ABV hybrid regimens compared with MOPP alone as first-line therapy. Thus, at the present time it now appears that MOPP can no longer be considered standard initial therapy for advanced-stage Hodgkin's disease. The use of ABVD alone is intriguing because of its apparently reduced long-term toxicity, but this regimen cannot be routinely recommended, as it is still being evaluated in controlled clinical trials.

The major complication of chemotherapy is bone marrow suppression with increased risk of infection and, rarely, hemorrhage. The peripheral blood counts are monitored carefully during chemotherapy, and drug doses are adjusted depending on the degree of myelosuppression. However, drug dose reductions made simply for the purpose of decreasing subjective toxicity are inappropriate because the opportunity for cure is also reduced. Sterility, more commonly seen in male patients, is a permanent side effect of chemotherapy. Significant nausea and vomiting are seen with the MOPP and ABVD regimens, requiring the use of antiemetic agents. These drug programs also often produce serious psychological problems that require effective counseling. Mild peripheral neuropathy is commonly seen with vincristine, but paresthesias are not an indication to reduce drug dosage. Acute leukemia as a late effect of chemotherapy alone is a recognized complication.

Combined-Modality Therapy. Combinations of irradiation and chemotherapy in the treatment of Hodgkin's disease have been utilized during the past 20 years with the goal of increasing the cure rate. It is logical to assume that combination chemotherapy, effective in curing a significant percentage of patients with advanced disease, should be even more effective for occult disease that might be present after radiation therapy. Patients who have recurrence after receiving MOPP chemotherapy frequently have relapse in sites of major pretreatment involvement, including bulky lymph node areas. An additional rationale for combined-modality therapy includes improved management of childhood Hodgkin's disease by reduction of radiation fields that may cause bone growth retardation, decreased requirement for staging laparotomy, and reduced complications from newer radiotherapy techniques involving larger treatment fields.

Adjuvant chemotherapy can substitute effectively for prophylactic irradiation of apparently uninvolved sites, but to date there is no clear justification for the routine use of a combined-modality approach for the overwhelming majority of patients with PS I or II disease. However, there are certain subsets of patients with early-stage Hodgkin's disease for whom combined-modality treatment is indicated because of an unacceptably high relapse rate, that is, patients with large mediastinal masses or contiguous extranodal involvement. In this subgroup of patients with early-stage disease who receive initial combined-modality therapy, staging laparotomy is not indicated, and treatment is initiated with one of the currently accepted regimens for advanced disease (e.g., MOPP/ABVD or the MOPP/ABV hybrid). Once maximal benefit from chemotherapy has been obtained, limited radiation therapy (generally to the mediastinum alone or a mantle field) is utilized. With this approach, approximately 80 to 85 per cent of patients remain relapse free beyond 5 years.

The treatment of PS IIIA Hodgkin's disease remains controversial. Retrospective studies have concentrated on identifying prognostic subgroups in which there is an unacceptably low disease-free survival with radiotherapy alone. At the present time, it would be premature for radiation therapists to abandon definitive irradiation in III₁A patients in whom the prognosis is favorable and who at laparotomy are found to have minimal involvement of the spleen or upper abdominal nodes. In this subgroup, mantle and para-aortic irradiation and total nodal irradiation appear equally effective as initial treatment, with chemotherapy reserved for those who relapse. However, for the majority of stage IIIA patients, chemotherapy alone or combined-modality therapy should be utilized. Patients to be treated in this manner should meet one or more of the following criteria: extensive splenic involvement (i.e., more than four splenic nodules), PS III₂A disease, unequivocal CS III₂A (grossly positive lymphangiogram and/or CT scan), and CS IIIA patients with large mediastinal masses. Although combination chemotherapy remains the mainstay for stage IIIB disease, both improved disease-free and overall survival may be obtained for those patients in whom initial chemotherapy followed by or sequenced with total nodal irradiation is utilized.

Significant improvement in survival rates as a result of combined-modality programs has not been clearly demonstrated for certain subsets of patients. In part, this is because of the long time (10 or more years) required to establish an overall survival benefit. Combined-modality programs generally demonstrate improved disease-free survival, but interpretation of current clinical trials must be tempered by the observation that patients who relapse after radiation alone are frequently salvaged or cured with chemotherapy administered only at the time of relapse. It may be more acceptable to treat patients conservatively at the onset of their disease with one method, reserving the more complicated combined-modality programs for those patients with poor prognostic factors and an unacceptably high relapse rate after primary irradiation alone.

The complications and morbidity of combined-modality programs are significant. The potential risk of acute complications, including profound and prolonged myelosuppression, sterility of both men and women, and demonstrated risk of second malignant tumors, has modified the enthusiasm for a combined-modality approach.

Second Neoplasms. Patients cured of their Hodgkin's disease are at an increased risk of developing second primary cancers. The most widely reported neoplasm is acute nonlymphocytic leukemia. The risk of leukemia is lowest in patients treated with radiotherapy alone, while the development of nonhematologic second neoplasms (e.g., lung cancer) increases significantly over time with this modality. The incidence of leukemia is approximately 3 to 9 per cent at 10 years in patients treated with chemotherapy alone using a MOPP-like regimen, with initial combined-modality therapy using adjuvant MOPP, and with salvage chemotherapy following relapse after radiotherapy. It is interesting that there does not appear to be an increased risk of leukemia after ABVD chemotherapy with or without radiotherapy.

Salvage Therapy for Advanced Disease. The choice of salvage therapy for patients relapsing after initial treatment must be individualized to the specific clinical circumstances of the relapse. Patients with early-stage disease relapsing after primary radiotherapy have a greater than 50 per cent chance of being cured with one of the accepted chemotherapy regimens used as initial treatment for stage III and IV disease (e.g., MOPP/ABVD or MOPP/ABV hybrid). For patients whose initial complete remission on chemotherapy lasted more than 1 year, retreatment with the same regimen results in a high rate of second complete response. Patients whose initial response to chemotherapy lasted less than 1 year and those who failed to achieve a complete response with initial chemotherapy represent a poor prognostic group. Recent experience with high-dose chemotherapy followed by autologous bone marrow transplantation now offers these patients a significant survival advantage and the possibility of cure.

Hodgkin's Disease in Acquired Immunodeficiency Syndrome (AIDS) Patients. There are increasing reports of Hodgkin's disease in AIDS patients. In these cases, Hodgkin's disease usually presents as stage IV, frequently with B symptoms and extranodal sites of involvement. Absence of mediastinal adenopathy is common, and marrow involvement in the absence of splenic disease has been reported. The presence of extranodal Hodgkin's disease alone should raise the suspicion of human immunodeficiency virus (HIV) infection. Although Hodgkin's disease in the AIDS patients responds to chemotherapy, these remissions are usually brief, and patients die of opportunistic infections or progressive Hodgkin's disease.

Recommended Therapy. The recommended therapy for a patient with Hodgkin's disease must be individualized. Important management considerations include stage and bulk of disease, age, prior therapy, medical complications, and availability of modern skills in radiotherapy and chemotherapy. The improved results of aggressive therapy after accurate clinical evaluation and pathologic staging are achievable only by experienced teams of physicians working closely together to achieve the excellent cure rates now possible while avoiding the risks of excesses in treatment. The recommended therapeutic approaches for the previously untreated adult patient with various stages of Hodgkin's disease are listed in Table 148–4. Estimated results are expressed as the percentage of patients likely to achieve a disease-free interval of 5 years. Careful evaluation of their condition and observation of a high proportion of patients, perhaps 90 or 95 per cent, who have survived free from relapse for 5 years demonstrate that they are cured of their disease.

A patient with early-stage disease who has relapsed after radiation therapy alone may be cured with salvage chemotherapy. Thus, freedom from a first or even second relapse must be considered in the evaluation of both disease-free and overall survival when the results of current clinical trials are analyzed. With dramatically improved treatment results, the challenge facing physicians and investigators caring for patients with all stages of Hodgkin's disease is to weigh carefully the toxicity-benefit ratio for each new recommended regimen.

PROGNOSIS. Hodgkin's disease is a curable malignant condition. Advances in histopathologic classification, precise diagnostic evaluation, and selection of appropriate aggressive therapy have led to continuous improvement in both disease-free and

TABLE 148–4. THE TREATMENT OF HODGKIN'S DISEASE IN ADULTS

Ann Arbor Pathologic Stage	Recommended Therapy	Estimated 5-Year Disease-Free Survival (%)
IA, I$_E$A, IIA, II$_E$A*†	Mantle and para-aortic radiotherapy	80–90
IB, I$_E$B, IIB, II$_E$B*	Mantle and para-aortic or total lymphoid radiotherapy	70–75
III$_1$A, III$_S$A*‡	Mantle and para-aortic radiotherapy ± chemotherapy or chemotherapy alone	60–85
III$_2$A	Combination chemotherapy (i.e., MOPP/ABVD or MOPP/ABV hybrid) ± total lymphoid radiotherapy	70–85
IIIB, III$_S$B, III$_E$B	Combination chemotherapy (i.e., MOPP/ABVD or MOPP/ABV hybrid) ± total lymphoid radiotherapy	60–80
IVA, IVB	Combination chemotherapy (i.e., MOPP/ABVD or MOPP/ABV hybrid)	55–70

*Patients with large mediastinal masses (>0.33 of the transverse diameter of the chest) are controlled by irradiation alone in approximately 40 to 50 per cent of cases and should receive combined-modality therapy (chemotherapy followed by irradiation) as primary management, with 5-year disease-free survival of 80 to 85 per cent.

†Patients with subdiaphragmatic state IA should receive inverted-Y radiotherapy, while patients with subdiaphragmatic stage IIA or II$_S$A with minimal splenic involvement are treated with either total lymphoid radiotherapy or chemotherapy plus inverted-Y radiotherapy.

‡Patients with extensive involvement of the spleen (> four nodules) are controlled by irradiation alone in approximately 40 per cent of cases and should receive combined-modality therapy (chemotherapy and irradiation) or chemotherapy alone as primary management.

overall survival. Survival figures and prognostic factors that were acceptable 10 or even 20 years ago are not acceptable today. The 5-year survival rate has increased from approximately 25 to 50 per cent 20 years ago to at least 75 per cent today.

The success of modern radiotherapy, chemotherapy, or combined-modality programs has obscured the significance of such important prognostic factors as histologic subtype, stage of disease, and the presence of systemic symptoms. In recent years, newer prognostic factors have been identified, including anatomic substage III$_2$A, extensive splenic disease, bulky mediastinal lymphadenopathy, and contiguous extranodal extension. Combined-modality treatment programs or chemotherapy alone is recommended for patients with these unfavorable prognostic factors. However, any potential disease-free survival advantage seen after combined-modality therapy must be balanced by the potential risk of late complications, particularly second malignant conditions, and must be translated into an overall survival benefit before general acceptance.

Table 148–4 presents a reasonable estimate of prognosis, recommended therapy, and current appropriate investigative approaches for the various stages of Hodgkin's disease. These treatment recommendations provide only the broadest of guidelines. Therapy must be individualized, depending on the specific clinical situation and the skill and experience of physicians treating the patient. Any treatment recommendations and estimates of cure must be viewed with the understanding that the management of Hodgkin's disease is dynamic, constantly undergoing change and refinement, and is designed to provide each patient with the best probability of cure and the least possibility of long-term toxicity.

Bonadonna G, Valagussa P, Santoro A: Alternating non–cross-resistant chemotherapy or MOPP in stage IV Hodgkin's disease: A report of 8-year results. Ann Intern Med 104:739, 1986. *The first report of the superiority of the MOPP/ABVD regimen over conventional chemotherapy. These results have now been confirmed.*

Crnkovich MJ, Leopold K, Hoppe RT, et al.: Stage I and IIB Hodgkin's disease: The combined experience at Stanford University and the Joint Center for Radiation Therapy. J Clin Oncol 5:1041, 1987. *The combined experience from two major institutions in the treatment of stage IB and IIB is reported, indicating that definitive radiotherapy is the preferred treatment for these patients.*

Glick JH, Portlock C: Hodgkin's disease: Clinical manifestations, staging, and treatment. In Benz EJ, Cohen HJ, Furie B, et al. (eds.): Hematology: Basic Principles and Practice. New York, Churchill Livingstone, 1991. *A thorough analysis and current review of staging and treatment for all stages of Hodgkin's disease are presented.*

Jagannath S, Armitage JO, Dicke KA, et al.: Prognostic factors for response and survival after high-dose cyclophosphamide, carmustine, and etoposide with autologous bone marrow transplantation for relapsed Hodgkin's disease. J Clin Oncol 7:179, 1989. *An important summary of the benefits of high-dose chemotherapy and autologous bone marrow transplantation for relapsed Hodgkin's disease, indicating that prolonged disease-free survival can be obtained in this subset of patients.*

Kadin ME: Pathology and origin of Hodgkin's disease. In Benz EJ, Cohen HJ, Furie B, et al. (eds.): Hematology: Basic Principles and Practice. New York, Churchill Livingstone, 1991. *A complete review of current concepts in the histopathology of Hodgkin's disease, as well as a thoughtful discussion of the controversies surrounding the origin of the Reed-Sternberg cell.*

Kaplan H: Hodgkin's Disease. 2nd ed. Cambridge, MA, Harvard University Press, 1980. *A detailed, extensively illustrated and referenced volume covering every aspect of the disease as seen by one of the acknowledged experts and pioneers in the field.*

Klimo P, Connors JM: An update on the Vancouver experience in the management of advanced Hodgkin's disease treated with the MOPP/ABV hybrid program. Semin Hematol 25:34, 1988. *A report on an important new chemotherapy regimen, MOPP/ABV hybrid, for advanced disease. The results from this single institution trial await long-term follow-up but are being confirmed in large multi-institutional trials.*

Lister TA, Crowther D, Sutcliffe SB, et al.: Report of a committee convened to discuss the evaluation and staging of patients with Hodgkin's disease: Cotswolds meeting. J Clin Oncol 7:1630, 1989. *Report of an international multidisciplinary committee recommending modifications in the Ann Arbor staging classification to reflect changes in clinical staging criteria, newly recognized prognostic factors, and their impact on therapeutic decisions.*

Longo D, Young R, Wesley M, et al.: Twenty years of MOPP therapy for Hodgkin's disease. J Clin Oncol 4:1295, 1986. *A classic and important long-term follow-up report of MOPP-treated patients by the National Cancer Institute group.*

Mauch P, Larson D, Osteen R, et al.: Prognostic factors for positive surgical staging in patients with Hodgkin's disease. J Clin Oncol 8:257, 1990. *An important retrospective analysis correlating clinical stage and histopathology with pathologic stage as documented by staging laparotomy. This analysis suggests that certain subgroups of patients can be treated with limited-field radiotherapy without staging laparotomy.*

Mauch P, Tarbell N, Weinstein H, et al.: Stage IA and IIA supradiaphragmatic Hodgkin's disease: Prognostic factors in surgically staged patients treated with mantle and para-aortic irradiation. J Clin Oncol 6:1576, 1988. *A retrospective analysis of a large series of PS IA and IIA patients treated with mantle and para-aortic irradiation. Correlation with prognostic factors, including large mediastinal masses, is reported with long follow-up.*

Rosenberg S, Kaplan H: The evolution and summary results of the Stanford randomized clinical trials of the management of Hodgkin's disease. Int J Radiat Oncol Biol Phys 11:5, 1985. *The long-term follow-up on the important Stanford controlled trials of the use of radiotherapy with or without adjuvant chemotherapy.*

Young RC, Bookman MA, Longo DL: Late complications of Hodgkin's disease management. Monogr J Natl Cancer Inst 10:55, 1990. *A concise but detailed review of the late complications of radiotherapy, chemotherapy, and combined-modality treatment for Hodgkin's disease.*

149 Langerhans Cell (Eosinophilic) Granulomatosis

Jerome E. Groopman

The numerous and sometimes confusing classifications of clinical disorders associated with Langerhans cell proliferation reflect our ignorance of both the cause and the pathophysiology of many of these diseases. The Langerhans cell belongs to the larger family of cells termed *histiocytes*. Histiocytes are tissue macrophages and include the hepatic Kupffer cell, the alveolar macrophage of the lung, the giant cell of granulomas, and the osteoclast, in addition to the dermal Langerhans cell. The microglial cell of the brain is probably of macrophage origin as well. All of these tissue macrophages derive from precursor cells that normally reside in bone marrow, mature into circulating blood monocytes, and then egress into tissues and differentiate into a particular type of histiocyte.

A number of benign disorders are associated with proliferation of histiocytes and their fusion into multinucleated giant cells that form granulomas. Langerhans cell (eosinophilic) granulomatosis is an idiopathic benign disease characterized by proliferation and infiltration of tissue by histiocytes and eosinophils. Although this disorder was previously termed eosinophilic granuloma, the proliferating cell that appears primarily responsible for the clinical manifestations of the disorder is the Langerhans cell. The eosinophils may take residence in the lesion because of potent eosinophilic chemotactic factors released secondarily by the histiocytes. Langerhans cell granulomatosis is a distinct disorder unrelated to the eosinophilic syndromes (Ch. 150).

The interaction of "activated macrophages" with surrounding normal tissues may form the pathophysiologic substructure of many of the clinical features of Langerhans cell granulomatosis.

Clinical conditions of unknown cause characterized pathologically by proliferation of tissue macrophages in sheetlike masses with interspersed eosinophils have been difficult to define as specific disease entities. There is great histologic variability within these disorders, and lesions taken from different sites in the same patient may differ pathologically. The clinical course and prognosis do not correlate with histopathologic findings. The concept of Langerhans cell granulomatosis, Hand-Schüller-Christian disease (the classic triad of exophthalmos, diabetes insipidus, and bone destruction) and Letterer-Siwe disease as elements of a continuum termed *histiocytosis X* fails to recognize important differences in clinical course, organ involvement, and therapeutic response. This chapter discusses unifocal Langerhans cell granulomatosis, multifocal Langerhans cell granulomatosis, and Letterer-Siwe disease. These are the best characterized idiopathic histiocytoses, yet in clinical practice many cases do not readily fit into these categories.

UNIFOCAL LANGERHANS CELL (EOSINOPHILIC) GRANULOMATOSIS

Unifocal Langerhans cell granulomatosis is a benign disorder generally occurring in males during childhood or early adult life. It may occur as late as the sixth or seventh decade of life.

CLINICAL MANIFESTATIONS. The most common presentation of the disorder is a single osteolytic lesion in a long or flat bone, most frequently in the calvarium or femur in children and in a rib in adults. The predilection for skull, femur, rib, pelvis, vertebra, and mandible is not understood. The small bones of the distal extremities are not generally involved. Although the lesions are usually purely lytic, mixed blastic and lytic lesions occur. Pain and swelling over the affected area are common presenting symptoms, although disruption of teeth with mandibular disease, fracture, and otitis media due to mastoid involvement are not infrequent. Many lesions are asymptomatic and diagnosed serendipitously during radiologic evaluation for unrelated problems. Unifocal Langerhans cell granulomatosis of lymph nodes, thymus, or salivary glands is very rare and has the same benign course as that of the more frequent bone lesions. Unifocal Langerhans cell granulomatosis is rarely associated with systemic symptoms, and there are no characteristic laboratory findings. Diagnosis is established by biopsy.

DIAGNOSIS. The bone scan is very useful in determining that the lesion is indeed unifocal and in following patients over time for development of new osteolytic lesions. An open biopsy should be performed for diagnosis. Pathologically, an infiltrate with foamy macrophage and admixed eosinophils favors the diagnosis of Langerhans cell granulomatosis. Langerhans histiocytes contain a cytoplasmic inclusion of unknown composition but with constant thickness and striation termed an *X body*. They also stain by immunoperoxidase for a cytoplasmic protein termed S–100; detection of S–100 assists the histopathologic diagnosis of Langerhans cell granulomatosis.

TREATMENT. At the time of biopsy, curettage, with or without bone chip packing, should be carried out. This simple surgical approach is almost uniformly successful as definitive therapy for an individual lesion. Lesions in anatomic sites that are difficult to approach surgically, such as weight-bearing bones or cervical vertebrae, are best treated by low-dose (300 to 600 cGy fractioned total dose) local supervoltage irradiation. This low-dose radiotherapy generally eradicates the proliferating histiocytes and allows for normal bone repair, while high-dose radiotherapy leads to tissue damage and resultant poor healing. Surgical decompression followed by low-dose irradiation is some-

times indicated for lesions requiring emergency intervention, such as those compressing the spinal cord. Patients should be carefully followed after therapy for the development of new lesions, which generally arise within the first year after diagnosis. Individuals with a lesion in the bones of the head, neck, or pelvis are more likely to have subsequent disease. Bone scans to detect new lesions and plain films to follow the known site of involvement should be obtained every 6 months for 1 to 2 years after therapy. Extraosseous Langerhans cell granulomatosis involving soft tissue is generally successfully managed by complete surgical excision, if possible, or by low-dose irradiation.

MULTIFOCAL LANGERHANS CELL (EOSINOPHILIC) GRANULOMATOSIS

CLINICAL MANIFESTATIONS. Similar to the unifocal form, multifocal Langerhans cell granulomatosis generally presents in children, predominantly in males, and often with *bone lesions*. In addition to the calvarium, the sphenoid bone, sella turcica, mandible, and long bones of the upper extremities may be involved. This tropism for the head is unexplained but may indicate local reaction to an inciting agent that enters via the nasopharynx or oropharynx. Complications of this disorder include chronic otitis media caused by destruction of temporal and mastoid bones, proptosis with orbital masses, loose teeth with infiltration of maxilla or mandible, and both anterior and posterior pituitary dysfunction with involvement of the sella turcica. This last complication may occur with focal disease of the hypothalamus or pituitary without bone involvement, and growth retardation of the patient may occur. Diabetes insipidus is caused by granulomatous involvement of the hypothalamus or pituitary and may be either transient or permanent. The classic triad of lytic skull lesions, exophthalmos, and diabetes insipidus, called *Hand-Schüller-Christian disease*, is best viewed as a subset of multifocal Langerhans cell (eosinophilic) granulomatosis. Dermal lesions may appear papulosquamous, seborrheic, eczematous, and rarely xanthomatous. Vulvar lesions with ulceration are not uncommon. Hepatosplenomegaly and lymphadenopathy are unusual in multifocal Langerhans cell granulomatosis.

In *Langerhans cell granulomatosis* the lung is an important extraosseous site of involvement. The disorder mainly affects young adult men and often manifests with a chronic cough, pneumothorax, and constitutional symptoms. The chest radiograph usually shows a diffuse micronodular and interstitial infiltrate involving the mid-zones and bases of the lungs with relative sparing of the costophrenic angles. Ultimately, a honeycomb appearance may occur; it is caused by coalescence of small parenchymal pulmonary cysts. Fibrosis is a late finding that may lead to chronic cor pulmonale. Pulmonary function tests may show restrictive impairment. Diagnosis is best made by biopsy that shows the mixed histiocytic-eosinophilic infiltrate with a variable degree of fibrosis. Pulmonary Langerhans cell granulomatosis has a highly variable natural history. Spontaneous remissions are not infrequent, but prognosis is poorer at the extremes of age and with involvement of extrapulmonary organs.

DIAGNOSIS. There are no distinctive laboratory abnormalities in multifocal Langerhans cell granulomatosis. The leukocyte count is generally normal, and eosinophilia is not present unless it is from another cause. Hypercalcemia generally does not result from bone lesions.

The diagnosis of multifocal Langerhans cell granulomatosis is definitively made by biopsy (see Color Plate 7*H*, right), usually of a bone lesion. Again, S–100 detected by the immunoperoxidase method may be useful in confirming the diagnosis. The extent of multifocal involvement is established by physical examination, chest radiography, bone scanning, and, if indicated, computed tomography of the brain. This last test is useful for hypothalamic or pituitary lesions associated with diabetes insipidus.

TREATMENT. The natural history of multifocal Langerhans cell granulomatosis is relatively favorable when cases best diagnosed as Letterer-Siwe disease (see below) are excluded. Destructive lesions of bone, when present early in the clinical course, may predict a better outcome. The therapy is guided by the particular organs involved. Diabetes insipidus and growth retardation should be treated by hormonal replacement with vasopressin (Ch. 213) and human growth hormone, respectively. Low-dose irradiation to the suprasellar area may restore endocrine function in certain individuals. The seborrheic dermal eruption is responsive to tar treatments. X-irradiation using doses generally below 600 cGy to symptomatic bone lesions is nearly always effective. Surgery may be necessary to relieve spinal cord compression and mastoid problems and to excise skull lesions eroding through skin. Oral granulomatosis can be treated with dexamethasone elixir used as a mouth rinse three times a day. Similarly, topical steroid creams may accelerate the healing of vulvar lesions.

Systemic therapy is indicated when either radiation fails or multiple sites demand treatment. Corticosteroids alone may achieve dramatic results. Prednisone at a single dose of 0.5 to 1.0 mg per kilogram can be used in the acute phase. Alternate-day corticosteroid therapy can be initiated after remission is achieved. Use of cytotoxic agents, such as vinblastine or methotrexate, is generally reserved for aggressive and refractory disease.

There is insufficient experience to recommend a single first-line chemotherapeutic regimen. Addition of vinblastine at a dose of 0.1 mg per kilogram intravenously every week for 4 to 8 weeks is generally successful in achieving remission. It is unclear whether maintenance chemotherapy with weekly vinblastine or prednisone is required to sustain remission. Should disease recur within several months after discontinuation of therapy for the acute phase, the patient should be re-treated with the initially successful regimen and receive maintenance therapy. The striking variability in clinical course makes it difficult to generalize with regard to therapeutic guidelines.

LETTERER-SIWE SYNDROME

In 1924 Letterer described a 6-month-old child with diffuse purpura, fever, otitis media, lymphadenopathy, and hepatosplenomegaly. Nine years later, Siwe included this case in a series of six similar cases. In all instances, there was diffuse tissue infiltration by histiocytes. The histiocytes of Letterer-Siwe disease have abundant acidophilic cytoplasm and are often vacuolated. There may be prominent hemophagocytosis. Generally, there is a relative paucity of eosinophils in the histiocytic infiltrates.

CLINICAL MANIFESTATIONS. Children are usually affected in the first years of life, although an adult form of the syndrome may exist. Liver, spleen, lymph nodes, lung, and bone are the most commonly affected areas. Laboratory evaluation often demonstrates leukocytosis, although pancytopenia caused by hypersplenism or bone marrow infiltration may be seen. The dermal lesion of Letterer-Siwe disease is generally a brown-red, scaly eczematoid or seborrheic eruption, and purpura secondary to thrombocytopenia may be present. Hepatosplenomegaly may occur with or without jaundice or elevated levels of hepatic parenchymal enzymes. There is no familial or hereditary predisposition, and that distinguishes Letterer-Siwe disease from another histiocytic disorder of infants, familial erythrophagocytic lymphohistiocytosis. A clinical pathologic syndrome nearly identical to Letterer-Siwe disease has been described in immunologically compromised children infected with a variety of viruses. In addition, certain cases termed Letterer-Siwe disease may actually be unusual forms of malignant lymphoma.

TREATMENT. The course of Letterer-Siwe disease is commonly fulminant and fatal. Spontaneous remissions are rare. It is important to distinguish Letterer-Siwe disease from disorders of infectious or clearly neoplastic origin before initiating therapy. Systemic symptoms of Letterer-Siwe disease often improve with corticosteroids, and focal lesions may be palliated with radiotherapy. Occasionally, clinical remission has been achieved with chemotherapy, particularly vinblastine and prednisone. If this regimen fails, methotrexate and 6-mercaptopurine may be used. Successful allogeneic bone marrow transplantation has been reported in a single case.

Chu T, D'Angio GJ, Favara, B, et al.: Histiocytosis syndromes in children. Lancet 1:208, 1987. *This brief article offers an up-to-date classification of this group of disorders "not only as a standard for diagnosis and patient management but also for research and for use in publications on the subject."*

Greenberger JS, Crocker AC, Vawter G, et al.: Results of treatment of 27 patients with systemic histiocytosis (Letterer-Siwe syndrome, Schuller-Christian syndrome and multifocal eosinophilic granuloma). Medicine 60:311, 1981. *A detailed analysis of therapy of histiocytic disorders at a single academic medical center.*

Groopman JE, Golde DW: The histiocytic disorder: A pathophysiologic analysis.

Ann Intern Med 94:95, 1981. *Comprehensive review of the histiocytic disorders, with emphasis on pathophysiologic mechanisms; extensive bibliography.*

Komp DM: Langerhans cell histiocytosis. N Engl J Med 316:747, 1987. *An informative editorial with an excellent bibliography.*

Novice FM, Collison DW, Kleinsmith DM, et al.: Letterer-Siwe disease in adults. Cancer 63:166, 1989. *An illustrative case report and comprehensive review of adult cases, with emphasis on treatment options; extensive bibliography.*

Sims DG: Histiocytosis X: Follow-up of 43 cases. Arch Dis Child 52:433, 1977. *A large series followed over a long period; illustrates the striking variability in clinical course.*

Zinkham WH: Multifocal eosinophilic granuloma: Natural history, etiology and management. Am J Med 60:457, 1976. *A comprehensive and well-written clinical paper; of great assistance in clinical management.*

150 Eosinophilic Syndromes

Peter F. Weller

Eosinophilia, often with heightened production of eosinophils as well as increased blood and tissue eosinophil accumulations, is associated with distinctive disease processes that include helminthic parasitic infections, allergic diseases, and a diversity of diseases of often ill-defined etiologies. Several eosinophil-related diseases are discussed in other chapters. This chapter provides an overview on eosinophils as a distinct class of leukocytes and considers the variety of diseases associated with eosinophilia.

STRUCTURE OF EOSINOPHILS. Eosinophils are distinguished from other leukocytes by their morphologies, constituents, products, and associations with specific diseases. Eosinophils are produced in the bone marrow. The cytokine interleukin 5, which specifically promotes the development and terminal differentiation of eosinophils, is principally responsible for increases in eosinophilopoiesis. Eosinophils normally dwell primarily in tissues, especially in tissues with an epithelial interface with the environment, including the respiratory, gastrointestinal, and lower genitourinary tracts. The lifespan of eosinophils, longer than that of neutrophils, may extend for weeks within tissues. Eosinophils, of a size similar to neutrophils but with usually bilobed nuclei, are morphologically characterized by their cytoplasmic granules. Specific granules, the most numerous of several types of cytoplasmic granules, have unique crystalloid cores and contain eosinophil-specific cationic proteins. These cationic granule proteins, which bind acidic dyes like eosin, are responsible both for the tinctorial properties and for many of the functional properties of eosinophils. The four eosinophil cationic proteins are major basic protein, eosinophil peroxidase, eosinophil cationic protein, and eosinophil-derived neurotoxin. Lysophospholipase, another predominant eosinophil protein, forms bipyramidal Charcot-Leyden crystals, often found in sputum, feces, and tissues as a hallmark of eosinophil-related diseases. In addition to their content of preformed granule proteins, eosinophils also elaborate newly synthesized lipid mediators, including the 5-lipoxygenase pathway–derived eicosanoid, leukotriene C_4, and platelet activating factor.

FUNCTION OF EOSINOPHILS. Eosinophils serve several immunologic functions. Eosinophils are capable of phagocytosing and killing bacteria and other small microbes. In vivo however, eosinophils do not have a major role in host defense against such microbial pathogens and cannot constitute an effective defense against bacterial infections when neutrophil function is deficient. Rather, eosinophils primarily defend against large, nonphagocytosable organisms, most notably the multicellular, helminthic parasites, utilizing several mechanisms, including their cytotoxic cationic granule proteins. In allergic diseases, including asthma, eosinophils elaborate specific lipid mediators, leukotriene C_4 and platelet activating factor, which can contract airway smooth muscle, promote mucus secretion, alter vascular permeability, and elicit eosinophil and neutrophil infiltration. Eosinophils can also elicit the release of allergic mediators from mast cells and from basophils. Some of the mechanisms beneficial in the eosinophil's role in host defense can prove detrimental to the host. Released eosinophil cationic proteins are toxic to host cells and may contribute to the pathogenesis of diseases in which heightened numbers of eosinophils are found within involved tissues. The effector functions of mature eosinophils, whether they be mediated by release of preformed granule proteins or by the synthesis of new lipid mediators, can be stimulated by cytokines, including interleukin 5 and granulocyte macrophage colony-stimulating factor. Additional immunologic functions, based on the eosinophil's capabilities to interact collaboratively with lymphocytes and other cells, are beginning to be defined, which may further contribute to our understanding of how eosinophils participate in normal mucosal immune responses and in eosinophil-related diseases.

Blood eosinophil numbers do not always reflect the extent of eosinophil involvement in affected tissues in various diseases. Eosinophils usually number less than 450 per microliter in the blood, with a mild diurnal variation, being higher in the early morning and falling as endogenous glucocorticosteroid levels rise. Eosinopenia occurs with corticosteroid administration and also is frequent with active bacterial and viral infections. Some patients with sustained blood eosinophilia develop organ damage, especially cardiac damage, as found in the idiopathic hypereosinophilic syndrome. Why this complication of sustained eosinophilia occurs in some patients but not others is unclear. It suggests that some other activating events, as yet ill-defined, promote eosinophil-mediated tissue damage in the face of eosinophilia. Patients with sustained eosinophilia should be monitored for evidence of cardiac disease (see below).

DISEASES ASSOCIATED WITH EOSINOPHILIA
(Table 150–1)

PARASITIC DISEASES. Eosinophilia is not elicited by infections with single-celled protozoan parasites (with the exception of the intestinal coccidian parasite *Isospora belli*), but rather by the multicellular helminthic parasites. The level of eosinophilia tends to parallel the magnitude and extent of tissue invasion, especially by larvae. Eosinophilia may be absent in established infections that are well contained within tissues or are solely intraluminal in the gastrointestinal tract (e.g., *Ascaris*, tapeworms). Even with helminthic diseases, superimposed bacterial infections (e.g., in disseminated strongyloidiasis) can suppress eosinophilia. In evaluating a patient with unexplained eosinophilia, geographic and dietary histories are germane in indicating potential exposures to helminthic parasites. The stool should be examined for diagnostic ova and larvae, although with some infections more than the usual three examinations may be needed. In addition, for a number of the helminthic parasites that cause eosinophilia, diagnostic parasite stages are never present in feces. Hence, normal stool examinations do not necessarily exclude a helminthic etiology for eosinophilia, and examination of appropriate blood or tissue biopsy specimens, as guided by the clinical findings and exposure histories, may be needed. Specific tissue or blood-dwelling infections capable of causing eosinophilia include trichinosis, filarial infections, and, in children, visceral larva migrans.

OTHER INFECTIOUS DISEASES. Acute bacterial and viral infections usually cause eosinopenia, although in the convalescent phase of these diseases eosinophil numbers return to normal and at times to above normal, as seen with scarlet fever. Two fungal

TABLE 150–1. DISEASES ASSOCIATED WITH EOSINOPHILIA

I. Infectious diseases
  A. Tissue-invasive helminths
    1. Principally outside North America
      a. Filariasis (especially in those from nonendemic regions)
      b. Schistosomiasis, acute and chronic
      c. Fascioliasis, acute
      d. Paragonimiasis
      e. Clonorchiasis
      f. Echinococcosis (often absent unless cyst fluid leakage)
    2. Indigenous to North America and other regions
      a. Trichinosis
      b. Toxocariasis (visceral larva migrans)
      c. Strongyloidiasis (may be suppressed with sepsis in hyperinfection syndrome)
      d. Ascariasis and hookworm disease (especially with early lung and tissue invasive stages)
  B. Other infections
    1. Coccidioidomycosis (acute and less commonly chronic)
    2. Bronchopulmonary aspergillosis
    3. Afebrile tuberculosis
    4. Convalescent phase of some infections, especially scarlet fever
    5. Chlamydial pneumonia of infancy
II. Allergic diseases
  A. Allergic rhinitis
  B. Asthma
  C. Atopic dermatitis
  D. Acute urticaria
  E. Hypersensitivity drug reactions
III. Myeloproliferative and neoplastic diseases
  A. Idiopathic hypereosinophilic syndrome
  B. Solid tumors, principally of mucin-secreting, epithelial cell origin, when metastatic to serosa or bone
  C. Lymphoid
    1. Lymphomas, especially T cell type and Hodgkin's disease
    2. Acute lymphoblastic leukemia, only uncommonly
    3. Occasionally with myeloma (heavy-chain disease)
  D. Myelogenous
    1. Eosinophilic leukemia—rare
    2. Chronic myelogenous leukemia
    3. Acute myelogenous leukemia, with some subtypes
  E. Other
    1. Angioimmunoblastic lymphadenopathy
    2. Histiocytosis with cutaneous involvement
    3. Angiolymphoid hyperplasia (Kimura's disease)

IV. Other cutaneous disease
  A. Bullous pemphigoid
  B. Herpes gestationis
  C. Scabies
  D. Eosinophilic cellulitis (Well's disease)
  E. Episodic angioedema with eosinophilia
  F. Pruritic urticarial papules and plaques of pregnancy
V. Other pulmonary diseases
  A. Transient pulmonary eosinophilic infiltrates (Löffler's syndrome)
  B. Hypersensitivity pneumonitis
  C. Allergic bronchopulmonary aspergillosis
  D. Tropical pulmonary eosinophilia
  E. Eosinophilic pneumonia—acute and chronic
VI. Connective tissue diseases
  A. Vasculitis
    1. Allergic granulomatosis with angiitis (Churg-Strauss syndrome)
    2. Hypersensitivity vasculitis
  B. Rheumatoid arthritis (severe)
  C. Eosinophilic fasciitis
VII. Immunodeficiency diseases
  A. Hyper-IgE syndrome
  B. Wiskott-Aldrich syndrome
  C. Nezelof's syndrome with thymic dysplasia and increased IgE
  D. Selective IgA deficiency, when associated with increased IgE
  E. Graft-versus-host reactions
VIII. Gastrointestinal diseases
  A. Eosinophilic gastroenteritis
  B. Inflammatory bowel disease
IX. Occasional causes of eosinophilia
  A. Cholesterol embolization
  B. Long-term peritoneal dialysis
  C. Postirradiation
  D. Hypoadrenocorticosteroidism: Addison's disease, hypopituitarism
  E. Other localized disorders with occasional blood eosinophilia
    1. Eosinophilic lymphadenitis
    2. Eosinophilic cystitis
    3. Eosinophilic cholecystitis
    4. Eosinophilic meningitis
  F. Toxic: L-tryptophan, toxic oil syndrome (Spain)

diseases may be associated with eosinophilia: aspergillosis, but only in the form of allergic bronchopulmonary aspergillosis and not as invasive disease (Ch. 406), and coccidioidomycosis, following primary infection, especially in conjunction with erythema nodosum and at times with progressive disseminated disease (Ch. 400). On occasion, eosinophilia may be present in chronic tuberculosis.

ALLERGIC DISEASES. These diseases, including allergic rhinitis and asthma, are discussed elsewhere (Ch. 246 and 57). Hypersensitivity drug reactions can elicit eosinophilia, not necessarily accompanied by other manifestations, such as drug fever or organ dysfunction. When organ dysfunction develops, the drug must be stopped. Drug-induced interstitial nephritis (Ch. 80) may be accompanied by blood eosinophilia, and eosinophils may be found in the urine.

MYELOPROLIFERATIVE DISEASES. The idiopathic hypereosinophilic syndrome (see Color Plate 7H, left) is a myeloproliferative disease characterized by sustained overproduction of eosinophils. The three diagnostic criteria for this disorder are (1) eosinophilia in excess of 1500 per microliter of blood persisting for longer than 6 months, (2) lack of an identifiable parasitic, allergic, or other etiologic cause for eosinophilia; and (3) signs and symptoms of organ involvement. Not all patients with prolonged eosinophilia develop organ involvement, and many have benign courses. Moreover, the above diagnostic criteria are sufficiently broad to include, potentially, eosinophilic disorders of other etiologies, currently unrecognized, that may have more favorable courses. The presence of angioedema was recognized as a good prognostic sign in hypereosinophilic patients, and this finding may be related to the more recent identification of a distinct clinical syndrome of recurrent episodic angioedema with eosinophilia, not complicated by the development of hypereosinophilic cardiac disease. The clinical signs and symptoms of the hypereosinophilic syndrome can be heterogeneous, since patients reflect the diversity of potential organ involvement. One of the most serious and more frequent complications in this disorder is cardiac disease due to endomyocardial thrombosis and fibrosis. Chordae tendineae may sustain progressive fibrotic damage, leading to mitral and tricuspid regurgitation and congestive heart failure from valvular incompetence and endomyocardial fibrosis. Echocardiography can facilitate detection and monitoring of these changes. Neurologic involvement can take three forms: embolic disease originating from the heart, diffuse encephalopathy, and peripheral neuropathy, especially mononeuritis multiplex. Other organ systems that can be involved include the skin, liver, spleen, gastrointestinal tract, and lungs. For patients with prominent organ involvement and no therapy, mortality is about 75 per cent after 3 years. Therapy is aimed at suppressing eosinophilia and is initiated with corticosteroids, to which about one third of patients respond. In those unresponsive to corticosteroids, hydroxyurea may be beneficial. For those unresponsive to or intolerant of hydroxyurea, vincristine or chlorambucil, alone or with lower doses of hydroxyurea, can control the disease. Similar cardiac involvement to that seen in the hypereosinophilic syndrome, which may require surgical valve replacement, may occur rarely with eosinophilias of other etiologies, including parasitic infections. A pathologically similar disease, Löffler's endocarditis and endomyocardial fibrosis, occurs in tropical regions, where it is possible that antecedent parasite-elicited eosinophilias are responsible for the development of this cardiac disease.

NEOPLASTIC DISEASES. Eosinophilic leukemia is distinctly uncommon. Eosinophilia may accompany chronic myelogenous leukemia (often with basophilia) and some subtypes of acute myelogenous leukemia but is uncommon with acute lymphoblastic leukemia. In a minority of patients with Hodgkin's disease, blood eosinophil levels are elevated, occasionally to high values. Increases in marrow and lymph node eosinophilia are more common. A small proportion of patients with carcinomas, especially those of mucin-producing epithelial cell origins, have associated blood eosinophilia. About a third of patients with angioimmunoblastic lymphadenopathy have eosinophilia. Eosinophilia may accompany mycosis fungoides, Sézary's syndrome, and lymphomatoid papulosis.

CUTANEOUS DISEASES. In addition to the neoplastic involvement of skin noted above, a number of cutaneous diseases can be associated with eosinophilia, including scabies, bullous pemphigoid, and two diseases associated with pregnancy, herpes gestationis and the syndrome of pruritic urticarial papules and plaques of pregnancy. In episodic angioedema with eosinophilia, recurrences are marked by blood eosinophilia; by prominent angioedema, at times with significant weight gain from fluid retention; and less frequently by fever. This entity is responsive to corticosteroids.

PULMONARY EOSINOPHILIAS (see Ch. 60). Blood eosinophilia can infrequently accompany pleural fluid eosinophilia, which is a nonspecific response seen with various disorders, including trauma and even repeated thoracenteses.

GASTROINTESTINAL DISEASES. Eosinophilic gastroenteritis (Ch. 112) and inflammatory bowel diseases (Ch. 103) are considered elsewhere. Although eosinophils are present in the lesions of ulcerative colitis, on occasion increased blood eosinophilia can accompany both ulcerative colitis and Crohn's disease.

IMMUNE DISEASES. Of the various forms of vasculitis (Ch. 264), only two are commonly associated with eosinophilia: hypersensitivity vasculitis and allergic granulomatous angiitis, the Churg-Strauss syndrome, in which asthma, eosinophilia, and pulmonary and neurologic involvement are frequent. Cholesterol embolization is at times associated with eosinophilia and hypocomplementemia, suggesting a secondarily elicited immunologic component. Some primary immunodeficiency syndromes are associated with eosinophilia, either commonly with the hyper–immunoglobulin E (IgE) syndrome, the Wiskott-Aldrich syndrome, and graft-versus-host disease or more selectively with Nezelof's syndrome and selective immunoglobulin A (IgA) deficiency when these are accompanied by increased levels of IgE. Eosinophilic fasciitis (Ch. 262) and rheumatoid arthritis (Ch. 258) are considered elsewhere. Eosinophilia may uncommonly accompany rheumatoid arthritis itself but is more commonly due to treatment medications.

OTHER DISEASES. Irritation of serosal surfaces can be associated with eosinophilia, e.g., Dressler's syndrome, eosinophilic pleural effusions, peritoneal and, at times, blood eosinophilia that develops during chronic peritoneal dialysis, and perhaps the eosinophilia that follows abdominal irradiation. Two notable apparently toxic diseases, the eosinophilia-myalgia syndrome due to contaminated L-tryptophan and the earlier toxic oil syndrome in Spain, were prominently associated with eosinophilia. Loss of normal adrenoglucocorticosteroid production in Addison's disease, adrenal hemorrhage, or hypopituitarism can cause modest eosinophilia (Ch. 217.6).

Fauci AS, Harley JB, Roberts WC, et al.: NIH Conference. The idiopathic hypereosinophilic syndrome. Clinical, pathophysiologic, and therapeutic considerations. Ann Intern Med 97:78, 1982. *Provides a review of the idiopathic hypereosinophilic syndrome with considerations of the prognosis and therapy for this disorder, based on experience at a referral center that has had the opportunity to evaluate many eosinophilic patients.*

Nutman TB, Ottesen EA, Cohen SG: The eosinophil, eosinophilia, and eosinophil-related disorders. III. Clinical assessments and eosinophil-related disorders. Allergy Proc 10:33, 1989.

Nutman TB, Ottesen EA, Cohen SG: The eosinophil, eosinophilia, and eosinophil-related disorders. IV. Eosinophil-related disorders (continued). Allergy Proc 10:47, 1989. *These articles discuss the approach to the patient with eosinophilia and provide a thorough consideration of the various diseases associated with eosinophilia.*

Weller PF: The immunobiology of eosinophils. N Engl J Med 324:1110, 1991. *A brief review of the structure and immunologic functions of eosinophilic leukocytes.*

151 Plasma Cell Disorders*

Robert A. Kyle

The plasma cell disorders are a group of neoplastic or potentially neoplastic diseases associated with proliferation of a single clone of immunoglobulin-secreting plasma cells derived from the B cell series of immunocytes. This group of disorders has been referred to as monoclonal gammopathies, immunoglobulinopathies, paraproteinemias, and dysproteinemias.

The plasma cell disorders are characterized by the secretion of electrophoretically and immunologically homogeneous (monoclonal) proteins. Each monoclonal protein (M-protein, myeloma protein, or paraprotein) consists of two heavy (H) polypeptide chains of the same class and subclass and two light (L) polypeptide chains of the same type (Fig. 242–1). The heavy polypeptide chains are designated by Greek letters: γ in immunoglobulin G (IgG), α in immunoglobulin A (IgA), μ in immunoglobulin M (IgM), δ in immunoglobulin D (IgD), and ε in immunoglobulin E (IgE). The subclasses of IgG are IgG1, IgG2, IgG3, and IgG4. There are two subclasses of IgA—IgA1 and IgA2. No subclasses of IgM, IgD, or IgE have been recognized. The light-chain types are kappa (κ) and lambda (λ). Both heavy chains and light chains have "constant" and "variable" regions with respect to amino acid sequence. Class specificity of each immunoglobulin is defined by a series of antigenic determinants on the constant regions of the heavy chains (γ, α, μ, δ, and ε) and the two major classes of light chains (κ and λ). The amino acid sequence in the variable regions of the immunoglobulin molecule corresponds to the active antigen-combining site of the antibody, whereas the constant regions convey other biologic properties (see Ch. 242).

RECOGNITION OF MONOCLONAL PROTEINS

Electrophoresis with cellulose acetate membrane is satisfactory for screening. High-resolution agarose gel electrophoresis is more sensitive for the detection of small monoclonal proteins. Immunoelectrophoresis or immunofixation with agarose gel or both should be used to confirm the presence of a monoclonal protein and to distinguish the immunoglobulin class and its light-chain type.

Analysis of Serum for Protein

Serum protein electrophoresis should be done when multiple myeloma, macroglobulinemia, or amyloidosis is suspected. Electrophoresis is also indicated in any patient with unexplained weakness or fatigue, anemia, back pain, osteoporosis, osteolytic lesions or spontaneous fracture, elevation of the erythrocyte sedimentation rate, hypercalcemia, Bence Jones proteinuria, renal insufficiency, immunoglobulin deficiency, or recurrent infections. It should also be performed in adults with sensorimotor peripheral neuropathy, carpal tunnel syndrome, refractory congestive heart failure, nephrotic syndrome, orthostatic hypotension, or malabsorption, because a spike or localized band is strongly suggestive of primary systemic amyloidosis (AL).

A monoclonal protein (M-protein) is usually seen as a narrow peak (like a church spire) in the densitometer tracing or as a dense, discrete band on the cellulose acetate membrane (Fig. 151–1A). Although the immunoglobulins (IgG, IgA, IgM, IgD, and IgE) compose the gamma component, they are also found in the β-γ or β region, and IgG may actually extend to the α₂-globulin area. Consequently, an IgG monoclonal protein may range from the slow gamma (cathode) to the α₂-globulin region. In contrast, an excess of polyclonal immunoglobulins (having one or more heavy-chain types and both κ and λ light chains) produces a broad-based peak or broad band. It is usually limited to the γ region (Fig. 151–1B). It is important to differentiate between a monoclonal protein and a polyclonal increase because the former is associated with a malignant process or a potentially neoplastic condition, whereas a polyclonal increase in immunoglobulins is associated with a reactive or inflammatory process. In 2 to 3 per cent of sera with a monoclonal peak, there is an additional monoclonal protein of a different immunoglobulin class. This condition is designated as a biclonal (double) gammopathy.

The presence of an M-protein is most suggestive of monoclonal gammopathy of undetermined significance (MGUS), multiple myeloma, primary amyloidosis, Waldenström's macroglobulinemia, or other lymphoproliferative disease. Rarely, other conditions may also simulate the presence of an M-protein in the serum, e.g., free hemoglobin-haptoglobin complexes resulting from hemolysis, large amounts of transferrin in patients with iron deficiency anemia, or the presence of fibrinogen. On the other hand, a monoclonal protein may appear as a rather broad band

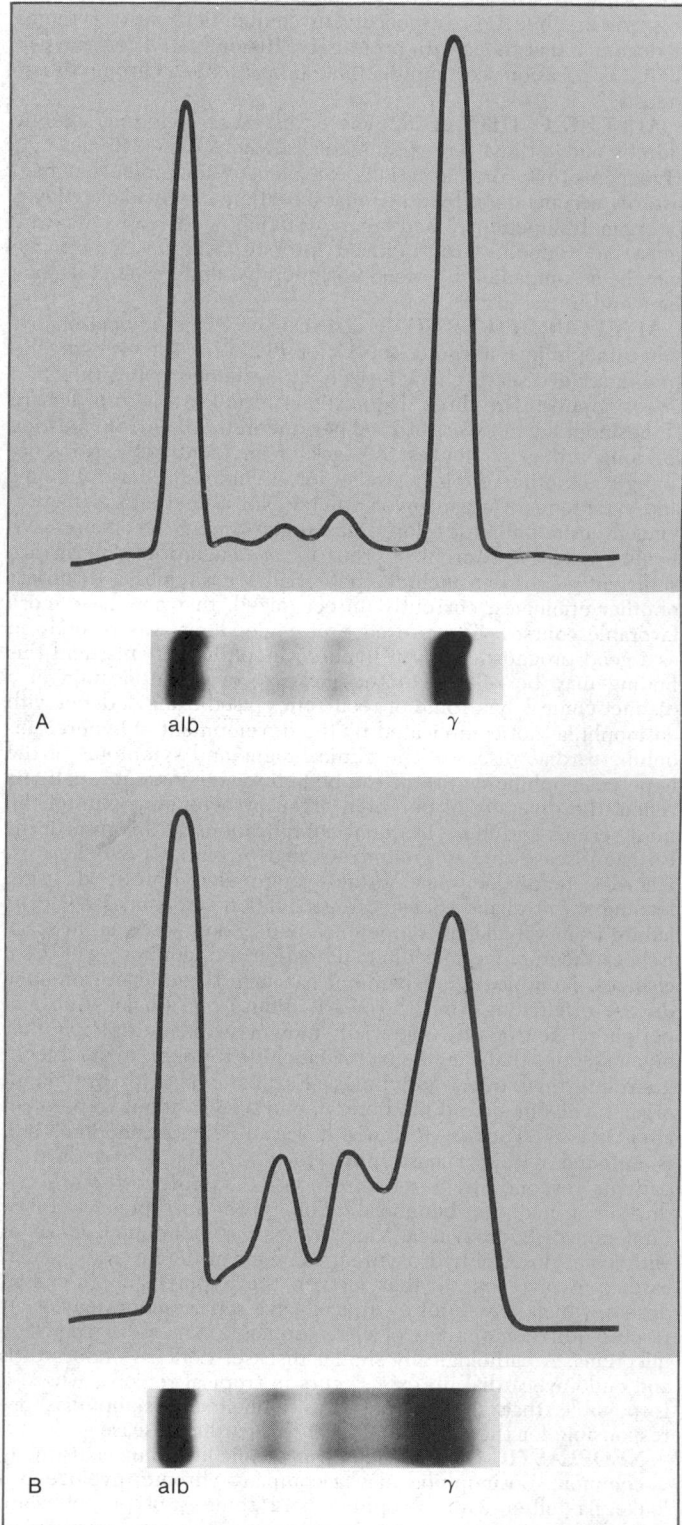

FIGURE 151–1. *A, top,* Monoclonal pattern of serum protein from densitometer tracing after electrophoresis on cellulose acetate (anode on left): tall, narrow-based peak of γ mobility. *Bottom,* Monoclonal pattern from electrophoresis of serum on cellulose acetate (anode on left): dense, localized band representing monoclonal protein in γ area. *B, top,* Polyclonal pattern of serum protein from densitometer tracing after electrophoresis on cellulose acetate (anode on left): broad-based peak of γ mobility. *Bottom,* Polyclonal pattern from electrophoresis of serum on cellulose acetate (anode on left): γ band is broad. (*A* and *B* from Kyle RA, Garton JP: Laboratory monitoring of myeloma proteins. Semin Oncol 13:310, 1986; with permission of W. B. Saunders Company.)

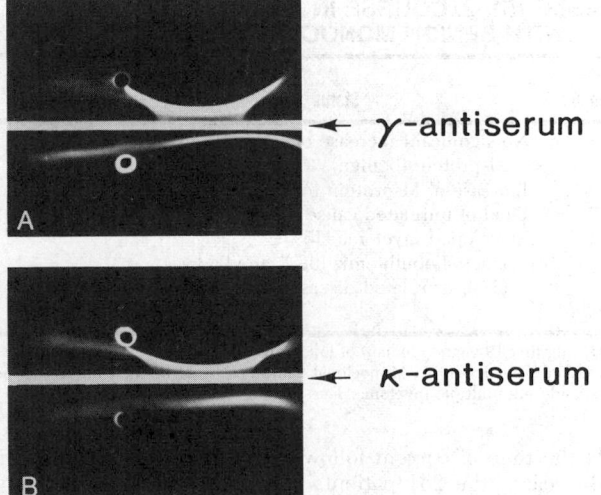

← γ-antiserum

← κ-antiserum

FIGURE 151–2. Immunoelectrophoretic pattern of serum. *A, top,* Antiserum to IgG (γ) shows a thickened arc. *B, top,* Antiserum to κ chains shows a thickened arc similar to the IgG arc. *A* and *B, bottom,* Antiserum to γ and to κ chains shows a faint normal arc. Patient's serum contains a monoclonal IgG κ protein. (From Kyle RA, Greipp PR: 3. The laboratory investigation of monoclonal gammopathies. Mayo Clin Proc 53:719, 1978; with permission of the Mayo Foundation, Rochester, MN.)

on the cellulose acetate membrane or as a broad peak in the densitometer tracing, owing to the complexing of a monoclonal protein with other plasma components or aggregates of IgG, polymers of IgA, or dimers of IgM.

An M-protein can be present when the total protein concentration, β and γ globulin levels, and quantitative immunoglobulin values are all within normal limits. A small M-protein may be concealed in the normal β or γ areas and may be overlooked. In addition, the presence of a monoclonal light chain (Bence Jones proteinemia) is rarely seen in the cellulose acetate tracing. In the heavy-chain diseases, the M-component is usually not apparent. Immunoelectrophoresis, a useful technique for identifying an M-protein, should be performed when a peak or band is seen in the cellulose acetate tracing or when multiple myeloma or related disorders are suspected (Fig. 151–2). Immunofixation, which is more sensitive, is useful when results of immunoelectrophoresis are equivocal or when one is searching for a small M-protein in primary amyloidosis, solitary plasmacytoma, or extramedullary plasmacytoma, or after successful treatment of multiple myeloma or macroglobulinemia.

Quantitation of Immunoglobulins

This procedure is more useful than immunoelectrophoresis or immunofixation for the detection of hypogammaglobulinemia. Quantitation can be performed by radial immunodiffusion, but this is tedious and subject to spurious abnormalities. Rate nephelometry is the preferred method for quantitation of immunoglobulins. The degree of turbidity produced by antigen-antibody interaction is measured by nephelometry in the near-ultraviolet region.

Serum Viscometry

Serum viscometry should be measured when the IgM monoclonal level is more than 3 grams per deciliter, when the IgA or IgG value is more than 4 grams per deciliter, or when the patient has oronasal bleeding, blurred vision, or other symptoms suggestive of a hyperviscosity syndrome.

Analysis of Urine

Dipstick tests are used in many laboratories to screen for protein, but unfortunately they are often insensitive to Bence Jones protein. Consequently, sulfosalicylic acid or Exton's reagent is best for the detection of protein.

Screening tests for Bence Jones proteins (monoclonal light chain in the urine) that utilize their unique thermal properties are not recommended because of their serious shortcomings. Characteristically, Bence Jones protein precipitates at 40°C to

60°C, dissolves at 100°C, and reprecipitates with cooling. Both false-positive and false-negative results occur. Immunoelectrophoresis or immunofixation of an adequately concentrated 24-hour urine specimen reliably detects Bence Jones protein, however. An M-protein appears as a dense, localized band on the cellulose acetate strip or a tall, narrow, homogeneous peak in the densitometer tracing, and its amount can be calculated on the basis of the size of the spike and the amount of total protein in the 24-hour specimen. It is not uncommon to have a negative reaction for protein and no obvious spike on electrophoresis and yet for immunoelectrophoresis or immunofixation of a concentrated urine specimen to show a monoclonal light chain. Immunoelectrophoresis or immunofixation should also be done on the urine of every adult older than 40 years who develops a nephrotic syndrome of unknown cause. The presence of a monoclonal light chain in a nephrotic urine is strongly suggestive of primary amyloidosis.

The differential diagnosis of a monoclonal protein in the serum or urine is given in Table 151–1.

Kyle RA, Garton JP: Laboratory monitoring of myeloma proteins. Semin Oncol 13:310, 1986. *This is a guide for the analysis of serum and urine for monoclonal proteins. Multiple illustrations of immunoelectrophoresis and immunofixation are provided.*

MONOCLONAL GAMMOPATHY OF UNDETERMINED SIGNIFICANCE (MGUS)

The term "monoclonal gammopathy of undetermined significance" (MGUS) (benign monoclonal gammopathy) denotes the presence of a monoclonal protein (M-protein) in persons without evidence of multiple myeloma, macroglobulinemia, amyloidosis, or other related diseases. The term "benign monoclonal gammopathy" is misleading because one does not know at the time of diagnosis whether a process producing a monoclonal protein will remain stable and benign or will develop into symptomatic multiple myeloma, macroglobulinemia, amyloidosis, or a related disorder. MGUS is characterized by a serum M-protein concentration less than 3 grams per deciliter; fewer than 5 per cent plasma cells in the bone marrow; no or only small amounts of M-protein in the urine; absence of lytic bone lesions, anemia, hypercalcemia, and renal insufficiency; and, most important, the stability of the presence of the M-protein and the failure of other abnormalities to develop.

Incidence

During 1989, 764 patients with a serum M-protein were found at the Mayo Clinic. The most frequent clinical diagnosis was MGUS (benign monoclonal gammopathy), occurring in two thirds of patients (Fig. 151–3).

TABLE 151–1. CLASSIFICATION OF PLASMA CELL PROLIFERATIVE DISORDERS

I. Monoclonal gammopathies of undetermined significance (MGUS)
   A. Benign (IgG, IgA, IgD, IgM, and, rarely, free light chains)
   B. Associated neoplasms or other diseases not known to produce monoclonal proteins
   C. Biclonal gammopathies
   D. Idiopathic Bence Jones proteinuria
II. Malignant monoclonal gammopathies
   A. Multiple myeloma (IgG, IgA, IgD, IgE, and free light chains)
      1. Overt multiple myeloma
      2. Smoldering multiple myeloma
      3. Plasma cell leukemia
      4. Nonsecretory myeloma
      5. IgD myeloma
      6. Osteosclerotic myeloma
      7. Solitary plasmacytoma of bone
      8. Extramedullary plasmacytoma
   B. Waldenström's macroglobulinemia
      1. Other lymphoproliferative diseases
III. Heavy-chain diseases (HCD's)
   A. γ HCD
   B. α HCD
   C. μ HCD
IV. Cryoglobulinemia
V. Primary amyloidosis (AL)

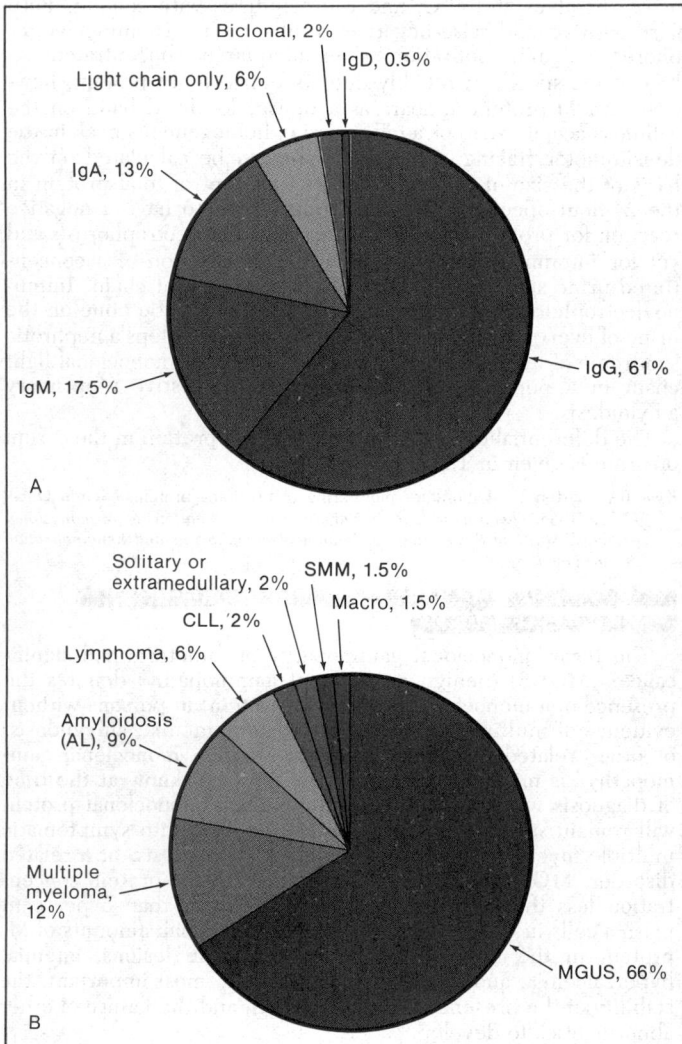

FIGURE 151–3. *A*, Distribution of monoclonal serum proteins in 764 patients seen at the Mayo Clinic during 1989. *B*, Diagnoses in 838 cases of monoclonal gammopathy seen at the Mayo Clinic during 1989.

The prevalence of MGUS is 1 per cent of patients older than 50 years and 3 per cent of those older than 70 years. Because of this high prevalence, it is of great importance for both the patient and the physician that it be determined whether the M-protein will remain benign or will evolve to multiple myeloma, amyloidosis, macroglobulinemia, or other lymphoproliferative disease.

Prognosis

At the Mayo Clinic, a long-term study of 241 patients with benign monoclonal gammopathy (i.e., patients in whom multiple myeloma, macroglobulinemia, amyloidosis, lymphoma, or related diseases were excluded) has been carried out. At the time when the M-protein was recognized, some of the characteristics of the patient group were as follows:

1. The median age was 64 years.
2. Approximately three fourths of the patients had other conditions seemingly unrelated to the monoclonal gammopathy that brought them to medical attention.
3. Anemia, leukopenia, leukocytosis, thrombocytopenia, renal insufficiency, and hypercalcemia, when present, were unrelated to the monoclonal protein.
4. Laboratory findings were as follows: The M-protein level ranged from 0.3 to 3.2 grams per deciliter (median, 1.7 grams per deciliter) and consisted of IgG (74 per cent), IgA (10 per cent), and IgM (16 per cent); an M-protein was found in the urine in only 15 patients; bone marrow plasma cells ranged from 1 to 10 per cent (median, 3.0 per cent).

TABLE 151–2. COURSE IN A SERIES OF 241 PATIENTS WITH BENIGN MONOCLONAL GAMMOPATHY*

Group	Status	Percentage of Patients
1	No significant increase of serum or urine M-protein (benign)	24
2	Increase of M-protein to >3 grams/dl	3
3	Died of unrelated cause	51
4	Developed myeloma (15%), macroglobulinemia (3%), amyloidosis (3%), or related diseases (1%)	22
Total		100

*During first 19 years (median) of follow-up.
 Modified from Kyle RA: Monoclonal gammopathy of undetermined significance and smoldering multiple myeloma. Eur J Haematol 43(Suppl 51):70, 1989.

At the time of current follow-up (median, 19 years; range, 11 to 32 years), the 241 patients can be divided into four groups (Table 151–2). Approximately one fourth of the patients have remained stable and can be classified as having benign monoclonal gammopathy, although they must continue to be observed because serious disease may still develop. No initial laboratory measurements or clinical factors were predictive of which patients would remain in this stable or benign group. In 3 per cent of the patients, the M-protein level increased to more than 3 grams per deciliter, but they did not develop symptomatic multiple myeloma, macroglobulinemia, or related disorders. Their condition remains clinically "benign," although with an M-protein that occasions concern. Approximately half of the patients died of seemingly unrelated causes without developing multiple myeloma, macroglobulinemia, or related disorders. Approximately one fourth of the patients (22 per cent) developed multiple myeloma (15 per cent), macroglobulinemia (3 per cent), amyloidosis (3 per cent), or related disorders (1 per cent) (Table 151–2), with an actuarial rate of 17 per cent at 10 years and 33 per cent at 20 years (Fig. 151–4). The interval from the time of recognition of the M-protein to the diagnosis of serious disease ranged from 2 to 22 years (median, 8 years).

Differentiation of MGUS from Multiple Myeloma and Macroglobulinemia

Differentiation of the patient with benign monoclonal gammopathy from one in whom multiple myeloma, macroglobulinemia, or a related disorder eventually develops is very difficult when the M-protein is first recognized. The size of the monoclonal protein is of some help—levels greater than 3 grams per deciliter usually indicate overt multiple myeloma or macroglobulinemia, but some exceptions, such as smoldering multiple myeloma (SMM), exist. Levels of immunoglobulin classes not associated with the M-protein (normal polyclonal or background immunoglobulins) are almost always reduced in multiple myeloma or

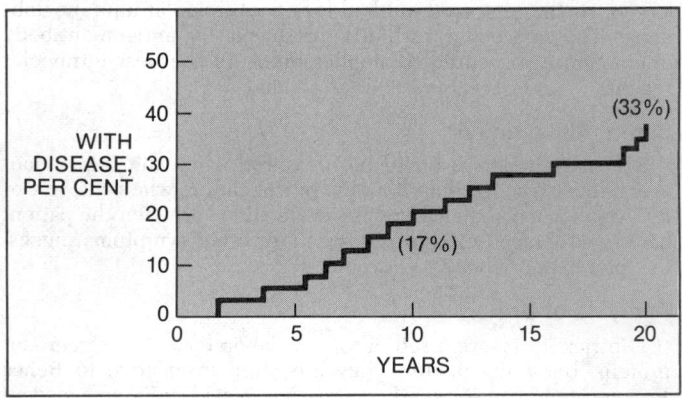

FIGURE 151–4. Incidence of multiple myeloma, macroglobulinemia, amyloidosis, or lymphoproliferative disease after recognition of monoclonal proteins. (From Kyle RA, Lust JA: The monoclonal gammopathies [paraproteins]. Adv Clin Chem, 28:145, 1990, with permission of Academic Press.)

Waldenström's macroglobulinemia, but a reduction may also occur in benign monoclonal gammopathy. The association of a monoclonal light chain (Bence Jones proteinuria) with a serum monoclonal gammopathy is suggestive of multiple myeloma or macroglobulinemia, but in many patients with small amounts of monoclonal light chain in the urine, the M-protein in the serum remains stable for many years. The presence of more than 10 per cent plasma cells in the bone marrow suggests multiple myeloma, but some patients with more plasma cells have remained stable for long periods. The presence of osteolytic lesions strongly suggests multiple myeloma, but metastatic carcinoma may produce lytic lesions as well as plasmacytosis and may be associated with an unrelated monoclonal gammopathy.

Certain research procedures show promise in differentiating the patient with MGUS or SMM from the patient with multiple myeloma. The plasma cell labeling index measures the synthesis of DNA, and when elevated it is good evidence that the patient has multiple myeloma or will soon have symptomatic disease. The use of a monoclonal antibody (BU-1) reactive with 5-bromo-2-deoxyuridine (BrdUrd) detects those cells synthesizing DNA, and the test can be performed in 4 to 5 hours.

In summary, no single technique reliably differentiates a patient with a benign monoclonal gammopathy from one who will subsequently have symptomatic multiple myeloma or other malignant disease. The M-protein level in the serum and urine should be serially measured, together with periodic re-evaluation of clinical and other laboratory features, to determine whether multiple myeloma or another related disorder is present.

If the serum M-protein is less than 2.0 grams per deciliter, electrophoresis should be repeated 6 months later, and if it is stable, it should be checked annually. If the serum M-protein is 2.0 grams per deciliter or more without evidence of myeloma or related disorders, electrophoresis should be repeated in 3 months, and if it is stable, the test should be repeated at 6 months. If there is no progression, electrophoresis should be performed annually thereafter. If an M-protein is present in the urine, the patient should be followed more closely.

Association of Monoclonal Gammopathies with Other Diseases

Monoclonal gammopathy frequently exists without other abnormalities, but certain diseases are associated with it, as would be expected in an older population. The association of two diseases depends on the frequency with which each occurs independently. Furthermore, an association may be biased because of differences in a referral pattern or in other selected patient groups. Of the myriads of associations that have been described, those listed below are the best established.

LYMPHOPROLIFERATIVE DISORDERS. An M-protein is found in 3 to 4 per cent of patients with a diffuse lymphoproliferative process but in fewer than 1 per cent of those with a nodular lymphoma. IgM monoclonal gammopathies are more common than IgG or IgA in lymphoproliferative diseases.

In a large series of patients in whom a serum IgM monoclonal gammopathy had been identified at the Mayo Clinic, more than half were originally considered to have MGUS (Table 151–3). During follow-up, 17 per cent of patients with MGUS of the IgM class developed a malignant lymphoid disease, most frequently Waldenström's macroglobulinemia.

An M-protein may be seen in angioimmunoblastic lymphadenopathy, angiofollicular lymph node hyperplasia (Castleman's disease), Sjögren's syndrome, and Kaposi's sarcoma.

LEUKEMIA. M-proteins occur in the sera of some patients with chronic lymphocytic leukemia (Table 151–3), but with no recognizable effect on the clinical course. M-proteins have also been recognized in hairy cell, adult T cell, chronic myelogenous, acute promyelocytic, and acute myelomonocytic leukemias, but without a documented increased incidence over that in the normal population.

NEUROLOGIC DISORDERS. Approximately 5 per cent of patients with sensorimotor peripheral neuropathy of unknown cause have an associated monoclonal gammopathy. In half of those with an IgM monoclonal gammopathy and peripheral neuropathy, the M-protein binds to myelin-associated glycoprotein (MAG). These patients have a slowly progressive sensorimotor neuropathy beginning in the distal extremities and extending proximally. Sensory involvement is more prominent than motor involvement. Cranial nerves and autonomic function are intact. The clinical and electrodiagnostic manifestations resemble those of chronic inflammatory demyelinating polyneuropathy. The relationship of the M-protein to the peripheral neuropathy is not clear.

DERMATOLOGIC DISEASES. Lichen myxedematosus (papular mucinosis, scleromyxedema) is characterized by papules, macules, and plaques infiltrating the skin and is associated with a cathodal IgG λ protein. Scleredema (Buschke's disease), pyoderma gangrenosum, and necrobiotic xanthogranuloma have also been associated with a monoclonal protein.

Monoclonal Gammopathies with Antibody Activity

In miscellaneous patients with MGUS, myeloma, or macroglobulinemia, the monoclonal protein has exhibited unusual specificity to one of various antigens. Examples include actin, dextran, antistreptolysin O, antinuclear activity, riboflavin, von Willebrand factor, thyroglobulin, insulin, double-stranded DNA, and apolipoprotein.

The binding of calcium by an M-protein may produce hypercalcemia without symptomatic or pathologic consequences. Affected patients should not be treated for hypercalcemia. Monoclonal proteins have also been found to bind to copper and to phosphate.

BICLONAL GAMMOPATHIES

Biclonal gammopathies occur in 2 to 3 per cent of patients with monoclonal gammopathies. Biclonal gammopathy of undetermined significance accounts for about two thirds of patients. The remainder have multiple myeloma, macroglobulinemia, or other lymphoproliferative diseases. Triclonal gammopathies may also occur.

IDIOPATHIC BENCE JONES PROTEINURIA

Bence Jones proteinuria is a recognized feature of multiple myeloma, primary amyloidosis, Waldenström's macroglobulinemia, and other malignant lymphoproliferative disorders. A benign Bence Jones proteinuria may also occur. Patients have been documented to have a stable serum level of M-protein and Bence Jones proteinuria for more than 15 years without developing multiple myeloma or related disorders.

Kyle RA, Lust JA: Monoclonal gammopathies of undetermined significance. Semin Hematol 26:176, 1989. *This is a comprehensive review of the pathogenesis of monoclonal gammopathies as well as the results of a long-term follow-up of benign monoclonal gammopathy. The association of monoclonal gammopathies with various diseases is emphasized.*

Merlini G, Farhangi M, Osserman EF: Monoclonal immunoglobulins with antibody activity in myeloma, macroglobulinemia and related plasma cell dyscrasias. Semin Oncol 13:350, 1986. *Monoclonal gammopathies with antibody activity are reviewed in detail. Many useful references are included.*

MULTIPLE MYELOMA

Multiple myeloma (myelomatosis, plasma cell myeloma, or Kahler's disease) is characterized by the neoplastic proliferation of a single clone of plasma cells engaged in the production of a monoclonal immunoglobulin. This clone of plasma cells proliferates in the bone marrow and frequently invades the adjacent bone, producing extensive skeletal destruction that results in

---

TABLE 151–3. CLASSIFICATION OF IgM MONOCLONAL GAMMOPATHIES AMONG 430 PATIENTS

Classification	Percentage of Patients
Monoclonal gammopathy of undetermined significance	56
Waldenström's macroglobulinemia	17
Lymphoma	7
Chronic lymphocytic leukemia	5
Primary amyloidosis (AL)	1
Lymphoproliferative disease	14
Total	100

From Kyle RA, Garton JP: The spectrum of IgM monoclonal gammopathy in 430 cases. Mayo Clin Proc 62:719, 1987; with permission of the Mayo Foundation, Rochester, MN.

bone pain and fractures. Anemia, hypercalcemia, and renal insufficiency are other important features.

Etiology

The cause of multiple myeloma is unknown. Radiation may play a role in some cases. The incidence of multiple myeloma increased modestly in atomic bomb survivors 20 years after exposure to more than 50 rads. Patients with ankylosing spondylitis who were given radiation therapy and workers exposed to radiation in nuclear plants have also exhibited modest increases in the incidence of this disease.

There is little evidence that chemicals cause myeloma. Increased risk of multiple myeloma has been reported in farmers, grain workers, furniture workers, and those exposed to pesticides, benzene, or asbestos. The number of cases is small, however, and more data are necessary. There is little evidence that repeated antigenic stimulation plays a role.

Multiple myeloma has occurred in familial clusters of two or more first-degree relatives as well as in monozygotic twins. Epstein-Barr virus (EBV) may be an etiologic agent in some cases. Myeloma has also been seen in patients with acquired immunodeficiency syndrome (AIDS).

Incidence and Epidemiology

Multiple myeloma accounts for 1 per cent of all malignant disease and slightly more than 10 per cent of hematologic malignancies in the United States. The annual incidence of multiple myeloma is 3 per 100,000. An apparent increase of incidence in recent years is probably related to increased availability and use of medical facilities. Multiple myeloma occurs in all races and all geographic locations. Its incidence in blacks is almost twice that in whites. Multiple myeloma is slightly more common in men than in women. The median age of patients at the time of diagnosis is 61 years; only 2 per cent of patients are younger than 40 years.

Biologic Aspects

T cells play an important role in normal B cell differentiation. When compared with normal controls, patients with multiple myeloma have a reduced percentage of CD4 cells and an increased percentage of CD8 cells.

An aneuploid myeloma cell population is found in approximately 80 per cent of cases. The pre-B common acute lymphoblastic leukemia antigen (CALLA) is expressed on some aneuploid myeloma cells. A myeloma pre-B–like malignant hybrid with coexpression of cytoplasmic μ, CALLA, terminal deoxynucleotidyl transferase (TDT), and plasma cell antigens (PCA-1 and PC-1) has been found in direct and cultured bone marrow specimens. Heavy- and light-chain immunoglobulin gene rearrangements demonstrated monoclonality of these cells, and double-labeling experiments (immunophenotype and labeling index) showed that the cells had a proliferative component exceeding that of myeloma, suggesting that they may represent the stem cell population of myeloma.

There is good evidence that plasma cell precursors of myeloma circulate in the peripheral blood. Several lymphoid growth factors are involved in the differentiation of normal B cells. Resting B cells enter into DNA synthesis stimulated by interleukin 4 (IL4), proliferate with IL5, and differentiate into plasma cells with IL6. Interleukin 6 appears to be an important growth factor for myeloma cells. Elevated levels of IL6 have been found in patients with progressive multiple myeloma, in contrast to those with MGUS. It has been postulated that expression of IL6 induces a polyclonal proliferation of plasma cells and that a second event, such as an altered oncogene expression, may transform the cells into a monoclonal process.

Cytogenetic Abnormalities

Chromosome abnormalities have been detected in about half of patients with multiple myeloma, but no specific abnormality has been demonstrated. Structural changes of chromosomes 1, 11, and 14, monosomies and trisomies, and translocations have been observed. Alterations in the expression of *c-myc* and *H-ras* have also been reported in myeloma.

TABLE 151–4. CLINICAL MANIFESTATIONS OF MULTIPLE MYELOMA

Skeletal involvement: pain, reduced height, pathologic fractures, hypercalcemia
Anemia: due mainly to decreased erythropoiesis; produces weakness and fatigue
Renal insufficiency: mainly due to "myeloma kidney" from light chains or hypercalcemia; rarely from amyloidosis
Recurrent infections: respiratory and urinary tract infections or septicemia due to gram-positive or gram-negative organisms
Bleeding diathesis: from thrombocytopenia or coating of platelets with M-protein
Amyloidosis: develops in 10% to 15%
Extramedullary plasmacytomas: occurs late in the disease
Cryoglobulinemia type I: rarely symptomatic

Clinical Manifestations (Table 151–4)

SYMPTOMS. Bone pain, particularly in the back or chest and less often in the extremities, is present at the time of diagnosis in more than two thirds of patients. The pain is usually induced by movement and does not occur at night except with change of position. The patient's height may be reduced by several inches because of vertebral collapse. Weakness and fatigue are common and often are associated with anemia. Fever is rare and, when present, is most often caused by an infection. The major symptoms may result from an acute infection, renal insufficiency, hypercalcemia, or amyloidosis.

PHYSICAL FINDINGS. Pallor is the most frequent physical finding. The liver is palpable in about 20 per cent of patients and the spleen in 5 per cent. Occasionally, extramedullary plasmacytomas may appear.

Laboratory Findings

A normocytic, normochromic anemia is present initially in two thirds of patients but eventually occurs in nearly every patient with multiple myeloma. The erythrocyte sedimentation rate is typically increased but is normal in 10 per cent of cases.

The serum protein electrophoretic pattern (cellulose acetate) shows a peak or localized band in 80 per cent of patients (see Fig. 151–1), hypogammaglobulinemia in almost 10 per cent, and no apparent abnormality in the remainder. IgG monoclonal protein is found in 50 per cent, IgA in 20 per cent, light chain only (Bence Jones proteinemia) in 17 per cent, IgD in 2 per cent, and biclonal gammopathy in 1 per cent, and 10 per cent have no serum M-protein at the time of diagnosis.

Immunoelectrophoresis or immunofixation of the urine reveals a monoclonal protein in approximately 80 per cent of patients. The κ/λ ratio is 2:1. Ninety-nine per cent of patients with multiple myeloma have an M-protein in the serum or urine at the time of diagnosis.

In the bone marrow of patients with multiple myeloma, plasma cells usually account for 10 per cent or more of all nucleated

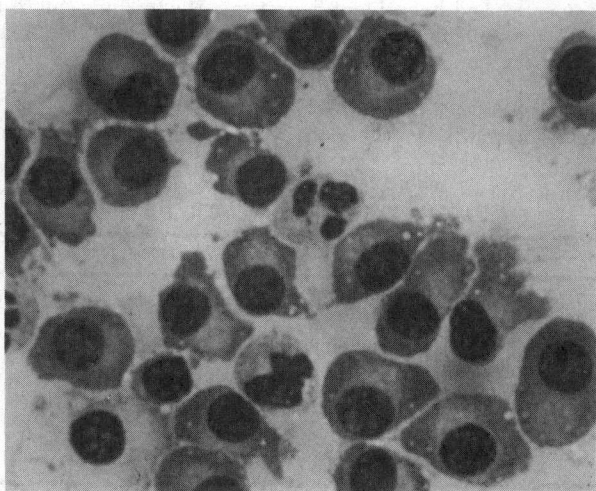

FIGURE 151–5. Bone marrow aspirate containing increased numbers of abnormal plasma cells.

cells, but they may range from less than 5 per cent to almost 100 per cent (Fig. 151–5) (see Color Plate 8H). Bone marrow involvement may be focal rather than diffuse, requiring repeated bone marrow examinations for diagnosis. Identification of a monoclonal immunoglobulin in the cytoplasm of plasma cells by immunoperoxidase staining is helpful for differentiating monoclonal plasma cell proliferation in multiple myeloma from reactive plasmacytosis (see Color Plate 6L) due to connective tissue disease, metastatic carcinoma, liver disease, and infections. The immunoperoxidase technique is also useful in recognizing neoplastic plasma cells that have atypical features.

Radiologic Findings

Conventional roentgenograms reveal abnormalities consisting of punched-out lytic lesions (Fig. 151–6), osteoporosis, or fractures in 80 per cent of patients at diagnosis. The vertebrae, skull, thoracic cage, pelvis, and proximal humeri and femora are the most frequent sites of involvement. Technetium-99m bone scanning is inferior to conventional roentgenography and should not be used. Computed tomography (CT) or magnetic resonance imaging (MRI) is helpful in patients who have skeletal pain but no abnormality on roentgenograms.

Diagnostic Criteria

Minimal criteria for the diagnosis of multiple myeloma are a bone marrow containing more than 10 per cent plasma cells or a plasmacytoma plus at least one of the following: (1) M-protein in the serum (usually greater than 3 grams per deciliter, (2) M-protein in the urine, and (3) lytic bone lesions. These findings must not be from metastatic carcinoma, connective tissue diseases, chronic infection, or lymphoma. Patients with multiple myeloma must be differentiated from those with MGUS and smoldering multiple myeloma.

Organ Involvement

RENAL. Proteinuria is present in almost 90 per cent of patients with multiple myeloma. Bence Jones proteinuria detected by immunoelectrophoresis or immunofixation is present in 80 per cent. The serum creatinine value is increased initially in almost half of patients.

The two major causes of renal insufficiency are "myeloma kidney" and hypercalcemia. Myeloma kidney is characterized by the presence of large, waxy, laminated casts in the distal and collecting tubules. The casts are composed mainly of precipitated monoclonal light chain. The extent of cast formation correlates directly with the amount of free urinary light chain and with the severity of renal insufficiency. With dehydration, acute renal failure may occur.

Hypercalcemia, which is present in 30 per cent of patients initially, is a major and treatable cause of renal insufficiency. Hyperuricemia may contribute to renal failure. Amyloidosis occurs in 10 to 15 per cent of patients and may produce a nephrotic syndrome or renal insufficiency or both. Acquired Fanconi's syndrome, characterized by proximal tubular dysfunction, results in glycosuria, phosphaturia, and aminoaciduria (see Ch. 82). Deposition of monoclonal light chains in the renal glomerulus (light-chain deposition disease) may produce renal insufficiency and the nephrotic syndrome.

NEUROLOGIC. Radiculopathy, the single most frequent neurologic complication, is usually in the thoracic or lumbosacral area and results from compression of the nerve by the vertebral lesion or by the collapsed bone itself. Compression of the spinal cord occurs in approximately 10 per cent of patients. Peripheral neuropathy is uncommon in multiple myeloma and, when present, is usually caused by amyloidosis. Rarely, myeloma cells diffusely infiltrate the meninges. Intracranial plasmacytomas almost always represent extensions of myelomatous lesions of the skull.

Other Systemic Involvement

Hepatomegaly from plasma cell infiltration is uncommon. Ascites is rare. Plasmacytomas of the ribs are common and present either as expanding bone lesions or as soft tissue masses. The incidence of infections is increased in multiple myeloma. *Diplococcus pneumoniae* and *Staphylococcus aureus* organisms have been the most frequent pathogens, but gram-negative organisms now account for more than half of all infections. Propensity to infection results from impairment of antibody response, deficiency of normal immunoglobulins, and neutropenia. Bleeding from coating of the platelets by the M-protein may occur. Occasionally, a tendency to thrombosis is present.

Treatment

Not all patients who fulfill the minimal criteria for the diagnosis of multiple myeloma should be treated. The patient's symptoms, physical findings, and all laboratory data must be considered. If there are doubts about whether to begin chemotherapy, treatment should be withheld and the patient re-evaluated in 2 or 3 months.

Chemotherapy is the preferred initial therapy for overt symptomatic multiple myeloma. Palliative irradiation should be limited to patients with disabling pain from a well-defined focal process that has not responded to chemotherapy. In most cases, analgesics together with chemotherapy control the pain.

The major controversy in chemotherapy is whether melphalan and prednisone or a combination of alkylating agents should be used. The oral administration of melphalan (L-phenylalanine mustard, Alkeran) and prednisone, a standard form of therapy, produces objective response in 50 to 60 per cent of patients. Melphalan may be given orally in a daily dose of 0.15 mg per kilogram for 7 days (8 to 10 mg per day), with 20 mg of prednisone given three times daily for the same period. Leukocyte and platelet levels should be determined at 3-week intervals, and the melphalan and prednisone therapy repeated in cycles every 6 weeks. The dose of melphalan should be adjusted until modest midcycle cytopenia occurs.

Many combinations of chemotherapeutic agents have been used. The best-known combination, the M2 protocol, includes melphalan, cyclophosphamide, carmustine (bischloroethylnitrosourea, or BCNU), vincristine, and prednisone. This regimen produces an objective response in 70 to 75 per cent of patients, but the median survival is approximately 2.5 years, which is not significantly different from that produced by melphalan and prednisone. The M2 and various other drug combinations have not clearly been shown to produce longer survival than does melphalan-prednisone.

The ideal duration of chemotherapy is unknown. Cessation of chemotherapy usually results in relapse, but continued chemotherapy may lead to the development of a myelodysplastic syndrome or acute leukemia. The peak incidence of acute leukemia occurs 3 to 5 years after initiation of therapy; the 5-year incidence is approximately 5 per cent, and the 10-year incidence is about 10 per cent in those who survive. Chemotherapy should be continued for 1 to 2 years and then discontinued if the M-protein levels in the serum and urine have been stable for at least 6 months and the patient has no other evidence of active disease. Patients should be followed closely, and the same chemotherapy should be reinstituted when relapse occurs.

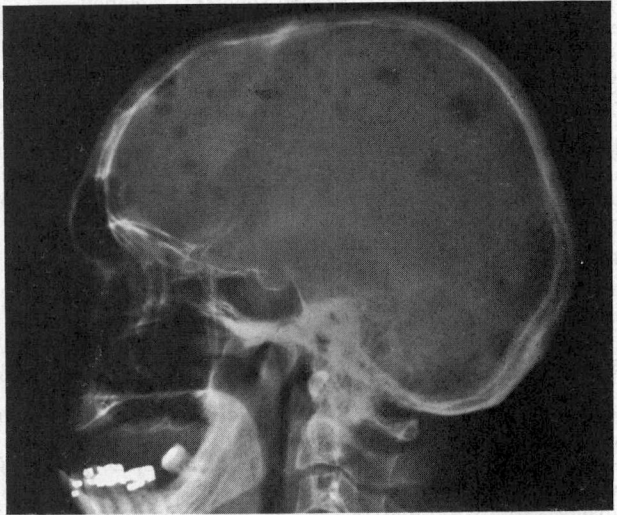

FIGURE 151–6. Skull roentgenogram showing multiple lytic lesions.

α_2-Interferon appears to be beneficial in prolonging the duration of remission in patients with multiple myeloma.

Treatment of Refractory Multiple Myeloma

Almost all patients with multiple myeloma who respond to chemotherapy eventually relapse. The highest response rates for patients with multiple myeloma resistant to alkylating agents have been with VAD (vincristine, Adriamycin [doxorubicin], and dexamethasone). VAD has induced remission in two thirds of patients who had relapse from a chemotherapeutic response. VBAP—vincristine, carmustine (BCNU), and doxorubicin (Adriamycin) on day 1 and prednisone daily for 5 days every 3 to 4 weeks—benefits approximately 40 per cent of patients. α_2-Interferon has been disappointing in the treatment of patients with multiple myeloma refractory to alkylating agents.

Management of Complications

HYPERCALCEMIA. Hypercalcemia, present in almost one third of patients at the time of diagnosis, should be suspected in the presence of anorexia, nausea, vomiting, polyuria, polydipsia, increased constipation, weakness, confusion, or stupor. If it is untreated, renal insufficiency usually develops. Hydration, preferably with isotonic saline plus prednisone (25 mg four times per day), relieves the hypercalcemia in most cases. The dosage of prednisone must be reduced and its use discontinued as soon as possible. If these measures fail, mithramycin, diphosphonates, calcitonin, or gallium nitrate may be beneficial. Patients with myeloma should be encouraged to be as active as possible because prolonged bed rest contributes to hypercalcemia. The manifestations and treatment of hypercalcemia are also discussed in Ch. 235.

RENAL INSUFFICIENCY. This occurs in half of patients with multiple myeloma and may develop insidiously or rapidly (acute renal failure). Hydration and prednisone are necessary if there is an accompanying hypercalcemia. Furosemide is helpful for maintaining a high urine flow rate (100 ml per hour). Hemodialysis is necessary in the event of symptomatic azotemia. Plasmapheresis may be helpful for regaining renal function, but patients with severe myeloma cast formation or other irreversible changes are unlikely to benefit from plasmapheresis. Allopurinol is necessary if hyperuricemia is present. For a more general discussion of renal insufficiency, see Ch. 76 and 77.

INFECTION. Prompt, appropriate therapy for bacterial infections is necessary. Prophylactic penicillin often benefits patients with recurrent gram-positive infections. Intravenously administered gamma globulin is helpful but expensive. Pneumococcal and influenza immunizations should be given to all patients (see Ch. 16).

SKELETAL LESIONS. Patients should be encouraged to be as active as possible but to avoid trauma. Fixation of fractures or impending fractures of long bones with an intramedullary rod and methyl methacrylate has produced good results.

MISCELLANEOUS COMPLICATIONS. Symptomatic hyperviscosity should be treated with plasmapheresis. The presence of an extradural plasmacytoma must be recognized and treated with radiation therapy and dexamethasone. If the neurologic deficit increases, surgical decompression is necessary.

Prognosis

Multiple myeloma has a progressive course, with a median survival of 6 months when no treatment is given. The serum β_2-microglobulin (β_2-M) level is the single most reliable prognostic factor in previously untreated multiple myeloma. The bone marrow plasma cell labeling index and age of the patient are also additional prognostic factors. Plasmablastic morphology, circulating myeloma cells in the peripheral blood, increased myeloma colony growth, and increased levels of IL6 are all associated with more aggressive disease. Patients who respond rapidly to chemotherapy and who have an elevated plasma cell labeling index have a shorter remission and survival.

Future Directions

A combination of alternating cycles of α_2-interferon with VBMCP (vincristine, BCNU, melphalan, cyclophosphamide, and prednisone) has produced an objective response in 80 per cent of previously untreated patients with myeloma. Forty per cent had a complete or nearly complete response. High-dose mel-

phalan produced a complete response in 27 per cent of previously untreated patients, but most have relapsed.

Bone marrow transplantation from an identical twin (syngeneic) or a human leukocyte antigen (HLA)–compatible donor (allogeneic) has been performed (see Ch. 153). Utilization of high-dose cyclophosphamide or melphalan plus total-body irradiation followed by autologous or allogeneic bone marrow transplantation for multiple myeloma refractory to chemotherapy has been described. Unfortunately, the relapse rate is high, and graft-versus-host reaction can be a serious problem in allogeneic transplantation.

Autologous bone marrow transplantation is potentially applicable to more patients. The two major problems are (1) eradication of multiple myeloma from the patient and (2) the removal of myeloma cells and their precursors from the autologous marrow. Purging of the marrow with monoclonal antibodies or chemotherapy is being investigated. The use of stem cells from autologous peripheral blood has successfully reconstituted the marrow of multiple myeloma patients treated with high-dose chemotherapy and total-body irradiation. The use of agents such as verapamil or quinine to reverse the resistance to doxorubicin is another interesting approach.

Anderson KC, Barut BA, Ritz J, et al.: Monoclonal antibody–purged autologous bone marrow transplantation therapy for multiple myeloma. Blood 77:712, 1991.

Barlogie B, Epstein J, Selvanayagam P, et al.: Plasma cell myeloma—new biological insights and advances in therapy. Blood 73:865, 1989. *This excellent review includes advances in the molecular biology and immunologic aspects of multiple myeloma.*

Bergsagel DE: Is aggressive chemotherapy more effective in the treatment of plasma cell myeloma? Eur J Cancer Clin Oncol 25:159, 1989. *This is a summary of prospective studies comparing single and multiple alkylating agents for the treatment of myeloma. The author concludes that aggressive chemotherapy does not significantly prolong survival when compared with single-agent therapy.*

Buzaid AC, Durie BGM: Management of refractory myeloma: A review. J Clin Oncol 6:889, 1988. *This is a comprehensive review of the therapy of refractory myeloma. The authors provide information on a wide variety of chemotherapeutic approaches to the refractory patient.*

Jagannath S, Barlogie B, Dicke K, et al.: Autologous bone marrow transplantation in multiple myeloma: Identification of prognostic factors. Blood 76:1860, 1990.

Kyle RA: Multiple myeloma: Review of 869 cases. Mayo Clin Proc 50:29, 1975. *The clinical and laboratory findings in a large series of multiple myeloma cases are presented. Results of long-term follow-up are emphasized.*

Kyle RA: Monoclonal gammopathies and the kidney. Ann Rev Med 40:53, 1989. *A review of the renal aspects of multiple myeloma, Waldenström's macroglobulinemia, acquired Fanconi's syndrome, light-chain deposition disease, and primary systemic amyloidosis is presented.*

Kyle RA, Greipp PR: Plasma cell dyscrasias: Current status. CRC Crit Rev Oncol Hematol 8:93, 1988. *This is a comprehensive review of monoclonal gammopathies with more than 450 references.*

Mandelli F, Avvisati G, Amadori S, et al.: Maintenance treatment with recombinant interferon alpha-2b in patients with multiple myeloma responding to conventional induction chemotherapy. N Eng J Med 322:1430, 1990.

VARIANT FORMS OF MULTIPLE MYELOMA
(Table 151–1)

Smoldering Myeloma

The diagnosis of smoldering multiple myeloma (SMM) depends on the presence of an M-protein level greater than 3 grams per deciliter in the serum and greater than 10 per cent plasma cells in the bone marrow, but no anemia, renal insufficiency, or skeletal lesions. Often, a small amount of M-protein is found in the urine, and the concentration of normal immunoglobulins in the serum is decreased. The plasma cell labeling index is low. Patients with SMM should be recognized because they must not be treated unless progression occurs. Biologically, patients with SMM have a benign monoclonal gammopathy (MGUS), but it is difficult to accept that diagnosis initially when the M-protein level is greater than 3 grams per deciliter and the bone marrow contains more than 10 per cent plasma cells.

Plasma Cell Leukemia

Patients with plasma cell leukemia (see Color Plate 8I, left) have greater than 20 per cent plasma cells in the peripheral blood and an absolute plasma cell count of at least 2000 per microliter. Plasma cell leukemia is classified as primary when it is diagnosed in the leukemic phase (60 per cent) or as secondary when there is leukemic transformation of a previously recognized multiple myeloma (40 per cent). Patients with primary plasma cell leukemia are younger and have a greater incidence of hepatosplenomegaly and lymphadenopathy, a higher platelet count, fewer bone lesions, a smaller serum M-protein component, and a longer survival (median, 6.8 versus 1.3 months) than patients with secondary plasma cell leukemia. Treatment of plasma cell leukemia is unsatisfactory, but partial responses do occur with melphalan and prednisone or with a combination of alkylating agents. Secondary plasma cell leukemia rarely responds to chemotherapy because the patients have already received chemotherapy and are resistant.

Nonsecretory Myeloma

Patients with nonsecretory myeloma have no M-protein in either the serum or the urine and account for only 1 per cent of patients with myeloma. For certainty of diagnosis, a monoclonal protein should be identified in the plasma cells by immunoperoxidase or immunofluorescence methods. More than a dozen patients in whom no monoclonal protein could be found within the myeloma cell have been described.

IgD Myeloma

The M-protein is smaller than in IgG and IgA myelomas, and Bence Jones proteinuria of the λ type is more common. Plasma cell leukemia, amyloidosis, and extramedullary plasmacytomas are more frequent with IgD myeloma. Survival is generally believed to be shorter than with other myeloma types, but IgD myeloma is often not diagnosed until later in its course.

Osteosclerotic Myeloma (POEMS Syndrome)

This syndrome is characterized by polyneuropathy, organomegaly, endocrinopathy, M-protein, and skin changes (POEMS). The major clinical features are a chronic inflammatory-demyelinating polyneuropathy with predominantly motor disability and sclerotic skeletal lesions. Except for the presence of papilledema, the cranial nerves are not involved. The autonomic nervous system is intact. Hepatomegaly occurs in almost one half of patients, but splenomegaly and lymphadenopathy occur in a minority. Hyperpigmentation and hypertrichosis are usually evident. Gynecomastia and atrophic testes as well as clubbing of the fingers and toes may be seen. In contrast to multiple myeloma, the hemoglobin level is usually normal or elevated, and thrombocytosis is common. The bone marrow usually contains fewer than 5 per cent plasma cells, and hypercalcemia and renal insufficiency rarely occur. Most patients have a λ M-protein. Evidence of Castleman's disease may be found. Diagnosis is confirmed by the identification of monoclonal plasma cells obtained at biopsy of an osteosclerotic lesion.

If the lesions are in a limited area, radiation therapy will produce substantial improvement of the neuropathy in more than half of the patients. If the patient has widespread osteosclerotic lesions, chemotherapy with melphalan and prednisone may be helpful.

Solitary Plasmacytoma (Solitary Myeloma) of Bone

The diagnosis of this disease is based on histologic evidence of a tumor consisting of monoclonal plasma cells identical to those seen in multiple myeloma. In addition, complete skeletal roentgenograms must show no other lesions of myeloma, the bone marrow aspirate must contain no evidence of multiple myeloma, and immunoelectrophoresis or immunofixation of the serum and concentrated urine should show no M-protein. Exceptions to the last-mentioned criterion occur, but therapy for the solitary lesion usually results in disappearance of the M-protein. Disease-free survival at 10 years ranges from 15 to 25 per cent. Almost 50 per cent of patients with solitary plasmacytoma are alive at 10 years. Treatment consists of radiation in the range of 4000 to 5000 rads (40 to 50 Gy). The most uncertain criterion for diagnosis is the length of observation necessary before it can be assured that the disease will not become generalized.

Extramedullary Plasmacytoma

Extramedullary plasmacytoma is a plasma cell tumor that arises outside the bone marrow. The tumor is found in the upper respiratory tract in approximately 85 per cent of cases, especially in the nasal cavity and sinuses, nasopharynx, and larynx. Extramedullary plasmacytomas may also occur in the gastrointestinal tract, central nervous system, urinary bladder, thyroid, breast, testes, parotid gland, and lymph nodes. The diagnosis is based on the finding of a plasma cell tumor in an extramedullary site and the absence of multiple myeloma on bone marrow examination, roentgenography, and appropriate studies of blood and urine. Treatment consists of tumoricidal irradiation. The plasmacytoma may occur locally, metastasize to regional nodes, or develop into multiple myeloma.

WALDENSTRÖM'S MACROGLOBULINEMIA (PRIMARY MACROGLOBULINEMIA)

Macroglobulinemia is the result of an uncontrolled proliferation of lymphocytes and plasma cells in which a large monoclonal IgM protein is produced. The cause is unknown, but it does occur more frequently in certain families. The median age of patients at the time of diagnosis is 60 years, and about 60 per cent are male.

Clinical Presentations

Weakness, fatigue, and bleeding (especially oozing from the oronasal area) are common presenting symptoms. Blurred or impaired vision, dyspnea, loss of weight, neurologic symptoms, recurrent infections, and congestive heart failure may occur. In contrast to multiple myeloma, lytic bone lesions, renal insufficiency, and amyloidosis are rare. Physical findings include pallor, hepatosplenomegaly, and lymphadenopathy. Retinal hemorrhages, exudates, and venous congestion with vascular segmentation ("sausage" formation) may occur. Sensorimotor peripheral neuropathy is common. Pulmonary involvement is manifested by diffuse pulmonary infiltrates and isolated masses. Pleural effusion may occur. Diarrhea and steatorrhea are uncommon.

Laboratory Evaluation

Almost all patients have moderate to severe normocytic, normochromic anemia. Coombs-positive hemolytic anemia is uncommon. The serum cholesterol value is often low. The serum electrophoretic pattern is characterized by a tall, narrow peak or dense band and is almost always of γ mobility. Seventy-five per cent of the IgM proteins have a κ light chain. Low molecular weight IgM (7S) is present and may account for a significant part of the elevated IgM level. A monoclonal light chain is present in the urine of 80 per cent of patients. The amount of urinary protein is usually modest.

The bone marrow aspirate is often hypocellular, but the biopsy is hypercellular and extensively infiltrated with lymphoid cells and plasma cells. The number of mast cells is frequently increased. Rouleaux formation is prominent, and the sedimentation rate is markedly increased unless gelation of the plasma occurs. About 10 per cent of macroglobulins have cryoproperties.

Diagnosis

The combination of typical symptoms and physical findings, the presence of a large monoclonal IgM protein (usually greater than 3 grams per deciliter), and lymphoid–plasma cell infiltration of the bone marrow provides the diagnosis. Multiple myeloma, chronic lymphocytic leukemia, and MGUS of the IgM type must be differentiated.

Treatment

Patients should not be treated unless they have anemia; constitutional symptoms such as weakness, fatigue, night sweats, or weight loss; hyperviscosity; or significant hepatosplenomegaly or lymphadenopathy. Chlorambucil (Leukeran) is usually given orally in a dosage of 6 to 8 mg per day and is reduced when the leukocyte or platelet value decreases. Patients should be treated for 2 years, and if the disease has reached a plateau state, the treatment can be discontinued and the patients followed closely. Chemotherapy should be reinstituted when the disease relapses. Combinations of alkylating agents, such as the M2 protocol (vincristine, BCNU, melphalan, cyclophosphamide, and prednisone), may be beneficial. α_2-Interferon may be of some use.

Transfusions of packed red blood cells should be given for symptomatic anemia. Spuriously low hemoglobin and hematocrit levels may occur because of the increased plasma volume from the large amount of M-protein. Consequently, transfusions should not be given solely on the basis of the hemoglobin or hematocrit value. Symptomatic hyperviscosity should be treated with plasmapheresis. The median survival in macroglobulinemia is 5 years.

HYPERVISCOSITY SYNDROME

Chronic nasal bleeding and oozing from the gums are frequent, but postsurgical or gastrointestinal bleeding may occur. Retinal hemorrhages are common, and papilledema may be seen. The patient occasionally complains of blurring or a loss of vision. Dizziness, headache, vertigo, nystagmus, decreased hearing, ataxia, paresthesias, diplopia, somnolence, and coma may occur. Hyperviscosity can precipitate or aggravate congestive heart failure. Most patients have symptoms when the relative viscosity is greater than 4 centipoises (cp), but the relationship between serum viscosity and clinical manifestations is not precise. Patients with symptomatic hyperviscosity should be treated with plasmapheresis. Plasma exchange of 3 to 4 liters should be performed daily until the patient is asymptomatic. The plasma should be replaced with albumin rather than plasma.

Fibbe WE, Jansen J: Prognostic factors in IgD myeloma: A study of 21 cases. Scand J Haematol 33:471, 1984. *Twenty-one patients with IgD myeloma from the Netherlands are described.*

Franchi F, Seminara P, Teodori L, et al.: The non-producer plasma cell myeloma: Report of a case and review of the literature. Blut 52:281, 1986. *The authors describe a case of nonsecretory (nonproducer) multiple myeloma and present an excellent review of the literature.*

Frassica DA, Frassica FJ, Schray MF, et al.: Solitary plasmacytoma of bone: Mayo Clinic experience. Int J Radiat Oncol Biol Phys 16:43, 1989. *This is a review of 46 cases of solitary plasmacytoma of bone. The presence of an M-protein did not significantly alter the survival or duration of disease-free survival.*

Jackson A, Scarffe JH: Prognostic significance of osteopenia and immunoparesis at presentation in patients with solitary myeloma of bone. Eur J Cancer 26:363, 1990.

Knowling MA, Harwood AR, Bergsagel DE: Comparison of extramedullary plasmacytomas with solitary and multiple plasma cell tumors of bone. J Clin Oncol 1:255, 1983. *This is a helpful review of extramedullary plasmacytomas and gives the reader a well-balanced report.*

Kyle RA, Garton JP: The spectrum of IgM monoclonal gammopathy in 430 cases. Mayo Clin Proc 62:719, 1987. *This study of 430 patients with an IgM monoclonal protein emphasizes the variable clinical patterns of disease. Sixty-three patients with Waldenström's macroglobulinemia are reviewed, and the clinical and laboratory features are provided.*

Kyle RA, Greipp PR: Smoldering multiple myeloma. N Engl J Med 302:1347, 1980. *This is a report of six patients who fulfilled the criteria for the diagnosis of multiple myeloma but whose conditions behaved like a benign monoclonal gammopathy. The authors emphasize that such patients must be recognized and not treated.*

Noel P, Kyle RA: Plasma cell leukemia: An evaluation of response to therapy. Am J Med 83:1062, 1987. *This review of 43 patients with plasma cell leukemia differentiates primary and secondary plasma cell leukemia. The short survival is emphasized.*

Takatsuki K, Sanada I: Plasma cell dyscrasia with polyneuropathy and endocrine disorder: Clinical and laboratory features of 109 reported cases. Jpn J Clin Oncol 13:543, 1983. *This provides an excellent picture of the clinical and laboratory features of a large number of patients with osteosclerotic myeloma (POEMS syndrome) from Japan.*

HEAVY-CHAIN DISEASES

The heavy-chain diseases (HCD's) are characterized by the presence of a monoclonal protein consisting of a portion of the immunoglobulin heavy chain in the serum or urine or both. These heavy chains are devoid of light chains and represent a lymphoplasma cell proliferative process. There are three major types: γ HCD, α HCD, and μ HCD.

Gamma Heavy-Chain Disease (γ HCD)

The abnormal protein consists of a γ chain with significant deletions of amino acids, including the C_{H1} domain of the constant region.

The median age of patients is approximately 60 years, although the condition has been noted in persons younger than 20 years. Patients with γ HCD often present with a lymphoma-like illness, but the clinical findings are diverse and range from an aggressive lymphoproliferative process to an asymptomatic state. Hepatosplenomegaly and lymphadenopathy occur in about 60 per cent of patients. Anemia is found in about 80 per cent of patients initially and in nearly all eventually. A few patients have had a Coombs-positive hemolytic anemia. The electrophoretic pattern often shows a broad-based band more suggestive of a polyclonal than a monoclonal protein. The urinary heavy-chain protein value ranges from a trace to 20 grams daily, but it is usually less than 1 gram per 24 hours.

Increased numbers of lymphocytes, plasma cells, or plasmacytoid lymphocytes are seen in the bone marrow and lymph nodes. The histologic pattern is variable and usually includes generalized or localized lymphoma or myeloma, but in some cases there is no evidence of a lymphoplasmacytic proliferative process.

Treatment is indicated only for symptomatic patients. Many different drugs have been used, but the results have been inconsistent and generally disappointing. Therapy with cyclophosphamide, vincristine, and prednisone is a reasonable choice. If there is no response to this regimen, doxorubicin should be added.

The prognosis of γ HCD is variable and ranges from a rapidly progressive downhill course of a few weeks' duration to the asymptomatic presence of a stable monoclonal heavy chain in the serum or urine.

Alpha Heavy-Chain Disease (α HCD)

This most common HCD occurs in patients from the Mediterranean region or Middle East, usually in the second or third decade of life. About 60 per cent are men. Most commonly, the gastrointestinal tract is involved, resulting in severe malabsorption with diarrhea, steatorrhea, and loss of weight. Plasma cell infiltration of the jejunal mucosa is the most frequent pathologic feature.

The serum protein electrophoretic pattern is normal in half the cases, and in the remainder an unimpressive broad band may appear in the α_2 or β regions. The diagnosis depends on the recognition of a monoclonal α heavy chain. The amount of α heavy chain in the urine is small, and Bence Jones proteinuria has never been reported.

Most often, α HCD is progressive and fatal, but response to melphalan or cyclophosphamide and prednisone may occur. Unexpectedly, antibiotics may also produce a remission.

Mu Heavy-Chain Disease (μ HCD)

This disease is characterized by the demonstration of a monoclonal μ chain fragment in the serum. The patient may present with chronic lymphocytic leukemia or lymphoma, but it is likely that the clinical spectrum will broaden when more cases are recognized.

The serum protein electrophoretic pattern is usually normal except for hypogammaglobulinemia. Bence Jones proteinuria has been found in two thirds of cases. The course of μ HCD is variable, and survival ranges from a few months to many years. Treatment with corticosteroids and alkylating agents has produced some benefit.

Brouet J-C, Seligmann M, Danon F, et al.: μ-Chain disease: Report of two new cases. Arch Intern Med 139:672, 1979. *This is a report of two cases of μ HCD and an excellent review of the literature.*

Haghighi P, Wolf PL: Alpha–heavy chain disease. Clin Lab Med 6:477, 1986. *This is a review of α HCD that emphasizes the histologic features.*

Kyle RA, Greipp PR, Banks PM: The diverse picture of gamma heavy-chain disease: Report of seven cases and review of literature. Mayo Clin Proc 56:439, 1981. *This report of seven cases of γ HCD from a single institution includes a detailed review of 49 cases from the literature. The clinical picture is emphasized.*

CRYOGLOBULINEMIA

Cryoglobulins are proteins that precipitate when cooled and dissolve when heated. They are designated as idiopathic or essential when they are not associated with any recognizable disease. Cryoglobulins are classified into three types: type I (monoclonal), type II (mixed), and type III (polyclonal).

Type I (monoclonal) cryoglobulinemia is most commonly of the IgM or IgG class, but IgA and Bence Jones cryoglobulins have been reported. Most patients, even with large amounts of type I cryoglobulin, are completely asymptomatic from this source. Others with monoclonal cryoglobulins in the range of 1 to 2 grams per deciliter may have pain, purpura, Raynaud's phenomenon, cyanosis, and even ulceration and sloughing of skin and subcutaneous tissue on exposure to the cold because their cryoglobulins precipitate at relatively high temperatures. Type I cryoglobulins are associated with macroglobulinemia, multiple myeloma, or MGUS.

Type II (mixed) cryoglobulinemia typically consists of a monoclonal IgM protein and polyclonal IgG, although monoclonal IgG or monoclonal IgA may also be seen with polyclonal IgM. Serum protein electrophoresis usually shows a normal pattern or a diffuse, polyclonal hypergammaglobulinemia pattern. The quantity of mixed cryoglobulin is usually less than 0.2 gram per deciliter. Vasculitis, glomerulonephritis, lymphoproliferative dis-

TABLE 151–5. CLINICAL CLASSIFICATION OF AMYLOIDOSIS

Amyloid Type	Classification	Major Protein Component
AL	Primary	κ or λ light chain
AA	Secondary	Protein A
AL	Localized	κ or λ light chain
AF	Familial	
	Neurologic	Transthyretin (prealbumin)
	Cardiopathic	Transthyretin (prealbumin)
	Nephropathic	
	Familial Mediterranean fever	Protein A
ASC₁	Senile cardiac amyloid	Transthyretin (prealbumin)
AB	Dialysis arthropathy	β_2-Microglobulin

ease, and chronic infectious processes are common. Purpura and polyarthralgias are frequently seen. Involvement of the joints is symmetric, but joint deformities rarely develop. Raynaud's phenomenon, necrosis of the skin, and neurologic involvement may be present. In almost 80 per cent of renal biopsy specimens, glomerular damage can be identified. Nephrotic syndrome may result, but severe renal insufficiency is uncommon. Hepatic dysfunction and serologic evidence of infection with hepatitis B virus are common.

Early administration of corticosteroids is the most frequent therapy. Cyclophosphamide, chlorambucil, or azathioprine should be used if there is no response. Plasmapheresis has been effective in some instances. α_2-Interferon has been of benefit.

Type III (polyclonal) cryoglobulinemia is not associated with a monoclonal component. Type III cryoglobulins are found in many patients with infections or inflammatory diseases and are of no clinical significance.

Montagnino G: Reappraisal of the clinical expression of mixed cryoglobulinemia. Springer Semin Immunopathol 10:1, 1988. *This is an important review summarizing the findings of four previous series of patients with type II cryoglobulinemia. Clinical features are emphasized, and therapy is described.*

PRIMARY AMYLOIDOSIS (AL) (see Ch. 197)

Amyloid (see Color Plate 8*I*, right), stained with Congo red, produces an apple-green birefringence under polarized light. It is a fibrous protein that consists of rigid, linear, nonbranching, aggregated fibrils of 7.5 to 10 nm width and of indefinite length. The type of amyloid cannot be differentiated by organ distribution or by electron microscopy. The amyloid fibrils in AL consist of the variable portion of a monoclonal light chain or, in some instances, the intact light chain (Table 151–5). The light-chain class is more frequently λ than κ (2:1), with a predominance of the λ_{VI} subclass. Patients with AL may have aberrant de novo synthesis or abnormal proteolytic processing of light chains. Amyloid P-component (AP) is a glycoprotein found in all types of amyloid, but its function is

unknown. The catabolism, or breakdown, of amyloid fibrils is a. important factor in pathogenesis.

Clinical Features

The median age at diagnosis is 61 years, and only 3 per cent of patients are younger than 40 years. Two thirds are male. Weakness or fatigue and loss of weight are the most frequent symptoms. Dyspnea, pedal edema, paresthesias, light-headedness, and syncope are frequently seen in patients with congestive heart failure or peripheral neuropathy. Hoarseness or change of voice as well as jaw claudication may occur.

The liver is palpable in 20 per cent of patients, but splenomegaly occurs in only 5 per cent. Macroglossia is present in 10 per cent of patients. Purpura often involves the neck, face, and eyes. Ankle edema is common.

Almost one third of patients have a nephrotic syndrome. Carpal tunnel syndrome, congestive heart failure, peripheral neuropathy, and orthostatic hypotension are other major presenting syndromes (Fig. 151–7). The presence of one of these syndromes and an M-protein in the serum or urine is a strong indication of AL, for which appropriate biopsy specimens must be taken for diagnosis.

Laboratory Findings

Anemia is not a prominent feature, but, when present, it is usually due to renal insufficiency, multiple myeloma, or gastrointestinal bleeding. Thrombocytosis occurs in 5 to 10 per cent of patients. Proteinuria is present initially in 80 per cent and renal insufficiency in almost 50 per cent of patients. Elevation of the serum alkaline phosphatase value is not uncommon. Hyperbilirubinemia is infrequent, but, when present, it is an ominous sign. Hypoalbuminemia and elevation of the cholesterol and triglyceride values are common with the nephrotic syndrome. The Factor X level is decreased in fewer than 5 per cent of patients and is rarely the cause of bleeding. The prothrombin time is increased in about 15 per cent of patients, and the thrombin time is prolonged in 60 per cent.

Immunoelectrophoresis or immunofixation reveals a monoclonal protein in the serum and in the urine of two thirds of patients. A monoclonal protein is found in the serum or urine in 85 per cent of patients.

Bone marrow plasma cells are usually only modestly increased. Only 15 per cent of patients have more than 20 per cent plasma cells in the marrow. Roentgenograms of the bones are normal unless the patient has multiple myeloma.

Organ System Involvement

CARDIAC AND CIRCULATORY. Congestive heart failure is present in approximately 25 per cent of patients at the time of diagnosis and develops during the course of the disease in an additional 10 per cent. The electrocardiogram frequently shows either low voltage in the limb leads or features consistent with

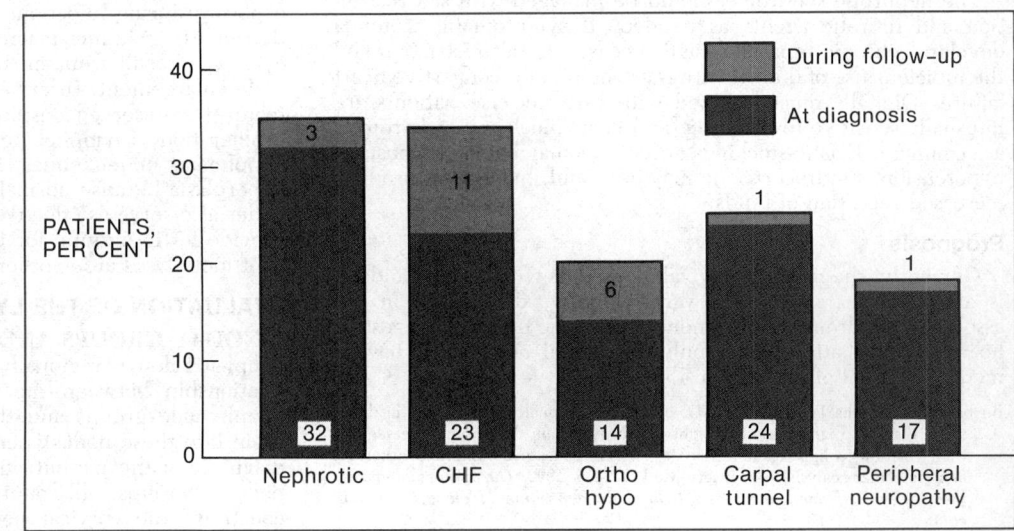

FIGURE 151–7. Syndromes seen at diagnosis and during follow-up of patients with primary amyloidosis (AL). Some patients had more than two syndromes at presentation. CHF = congestive heart failure; Ortho hypo = orthostatic hypotension. (Reprinted with permission from Kyle RA, Gertz MA: Systemic amyloidosis. CRC Crit Rev Oncol Hematol 10:49, 1990. Copyright CRC Press, Inc., Boca Raton, FL.)

an anteroseptal infarction (loss of anterior forces). Atrial fibrillation, atrial or junctional tachycardia, ventricular premature complexes, and heart block are common electrocardiographic features.

Echocardiography is a valuable technique for the evaluation of amyloid heart disease. Increased thickness of the ventricular wall and septum correlates with an increased incidence of congestive heart failure. Early cardiac amyloidosis is characterized by abnormal relaxation, whereas advanced involvement is characterized by restrictive hemodynamics. Intermittent claudication of the lower extremities, the upper extremities, or the jaw may be a prominent feature.

OTHER ORGANS. Nephrotic syndrome is present in one third of patients at the time of diagnosis. The degree of proteinuria does not correlate well with the extent of amyloid deposition in the kidney. Gross hematuria is rare. Other organ involvement includes the lungs and gastrointestinal tract, but it is asymptomatic in most instances. Sensorimotor peripheral neuropathy characterized by dysesthetic numbness involving the lower extremities occurs in one sixth of patients. Autonomic dysfunction may be a prominent feature and is usually manifested by orthostatic hypotension, diarrhea, or impotence. Amyloidosis can involve the periarticular structures and produce the shoulder pad syndrome. Rarely, osteolytic lesions from amyloid may occur. Pseudohypertrophy of skeletal muscles from amyloid deposition may be impressive. Petechiae, ecchymoses, papules, plaques, nodules, tumors, bullous lesions, thickening of the skin, and dystrophy of the nails may occur.

The diagnosis of amyloidosis depends on histologic proof. The initial diagnostic procedure should be abdominal fat aspiration, which is positive in more than 70 per cent of patients. A bone marrow aspiration and biopsy should be done to determine the degree of plasmacytosis, and results are positive for amyloid in about one half of patients. If the abdominal fat and bone marrow biopsy results are negative, a rectal biopsy specimen, including the submucosa, should be taken. If these sites yield negative findings, biopsy of the kidney, liver, carpal tunnel tissue, sural nerve, or endomyocardium should be performed.

Specific antisera are helpful for identifying the type of systemic amyloidosis. Antiserum to AP reacts with all amyloid types and is useful in demonstrating the presence of amyloid.

Treatment

Therapy of AL amyloidosis is not satisfactory. In a prospective study of treatment with melphalan and prednisone compared with colchicine, no significant difference in survival was noted (25 and 18 months, respectively). When the survival of patients who received only one regimen was analyzed, or when survival was determined from the time of entry into the study to the time of death or progression of disease, significant differences favoring melphalan and prednisone therapy were evident.

Supportive Measures

The nephrotic syndrome should be managed with salt restriction and diuretic agents as needed. If symptomatic azotemia develops, chronic renal dialysis is necessary. Salt restriction and the judicious use of diuretic drugs are helpful for congestive heart failure. Digitalis must be used with care because patients are unusually sensitive to the drug, and heart block and arrhythmias are common. Elastic stockings or leotards may benefit orthostatic hypotension. Fludrocortisone may be useful, but it does produce increased retention of fluids.

Prognosis

Currently, the median survival of patients with AL amyloidosis is almost 2 years. Survival varies greatly, depending on the associated syndrome; it is 6 months from the onset of congestive heart failure. Patients with only peripheral neuropathy have a median survival of more than 5 years.

Buxbaum JN, Chuba JV, Hellman GC, et al.: Monoclonal immunoglobulin deposition disease: Light chain and light and heavy chain deposition diseases and their relation to light chain amyloidosis: Clinical features, immunopathology, and molecular analysis. Ann Intern Med 112:455, 1990. *The authors emphasize the presence of amyloidosis and light-chain deposition of monoclonal light chains.*

Kyle RA, Gertz MA: Systemic amyloidosis. CRC Crit Rev Oncol Hematol 10:49, 1990. *This is a comprehensive review of primary, secondary, localized, hereditary, senile, and endocrine amyloidoses. More than 550 references are given.*

Kyle RA, Greipp PR: Amyloidosis (AL). Clinical and laboratory features in 229 cases. Mayo Clin Proc 58:665, 1983. *This is a review of the clinical and laboratory aspects of 229 patients with primary amyloidosis. Survival of the various syndromes is emphasized.*

Stone MJ: Amyloidosis: A final common pathway for protein deposition in tissues. Blood 75:531, 1990. *This is an excellent overview of systemic amyloidosis.*

152 Diseases of the Lymph Nodes and Spleen

Douglas V. Faller

PHYSIOLOGY AND FUNCTIONS OF THE LYMPH NODES

The lymph node is divided structurally into three primary areas: the cortex, paracortex, and medulla (Fig. 152–1). These areas are physically and functionally interlaced and surrounded by a series of sinuses. The *cortex* is the outermost portion of the lymph node, located immediately beneath the subcapsular sinus, and is the major site of B cell (antibody-producing lymphocyte) localization in the node. *Afferent lymphatic* drainage, carrying antigens and microorganisms, flows into this space and into immediate contact with lymphocytes, antigen-presenting non-phagocytic cells (histiocytes), and phagocytic cells (macrophages) of the cortex. Such immune stimulation results in enlargement of *lymphoid follicles* in the cortex, producing *germinal centers*, sites of intense B cell proliferation and antibody production. The *paracortex* lies between the cortex and medulla and is the primary site of localization of T cells. It additionally contains macrophages and histiocytes. The paracortex is also the site of lymphocyte trafficking, where recirculating T and B cells enter the lymphatics from the venous system. The *medulla* of the lymph node is made up of a tortuous network of endothelial cell–lined sinuses that coalesce at the hilus to form the *efferent lymphatic*. Antigens are effectively trapped during the slow percolation of lymphatic fluid through the node. In addition, the sinuses are decked with macrophages, which actively scavenge particulate matter and microorganisms.

The lymph node functions as the major site of interaction of antigen with cells of the immune system. Macrophages and histiocytes, which are capable of taking up and presenting antigen, are placed in intimate contact with helper T cells and B cells to facilitate lymphocyte stimulation and production of antibody. Antigen can reach the node in two ways. Antigen can flow in passively via the afferent lymphatics or be actively carried into the node by recirculating lymphocytes and macrophages.

Enlargement of lymph nodes (*lymphadenopathy*) can thus result from proliferation of resident lymphocytes following antigen exposure during infection. Hyperplasia of nonlymphoid cells in the nodes, including macrophages and circulating inflammatory cells, can result from inflammation or infection and also cause node enlargement. In either of these situations, the nodal architecture is preserved despite the cellular hyperplasia. Malignant proliferation of lymphocytes within the lymph node, as seen in lymphomas or leukemias, is easily distinguishable from benign hyperplasia because normal nodal structures are effaced. Lymph nodes also serve as effective traps for circulating tumor cells and provide fertile ground for their continued growth. Thus, malignant metastases are another cause of lymph node enlargement.

EVALUATION OF THE LYMPH NODES

NODAL GROUPS AND DRAINAGE PATTERNS. Because lymphatic flow is regionally distributed, an understanding of the relationship between the anatomic location of the superficial lymph node groups and the origin of afferent lymphatics that drain into these nodes is critical for examination and differential diagnosis of the patient with lymphadenopathy. Several lymph node subgroups, all draining structures in the head and neck, constitute the cervical nodes. The submental nodes, located

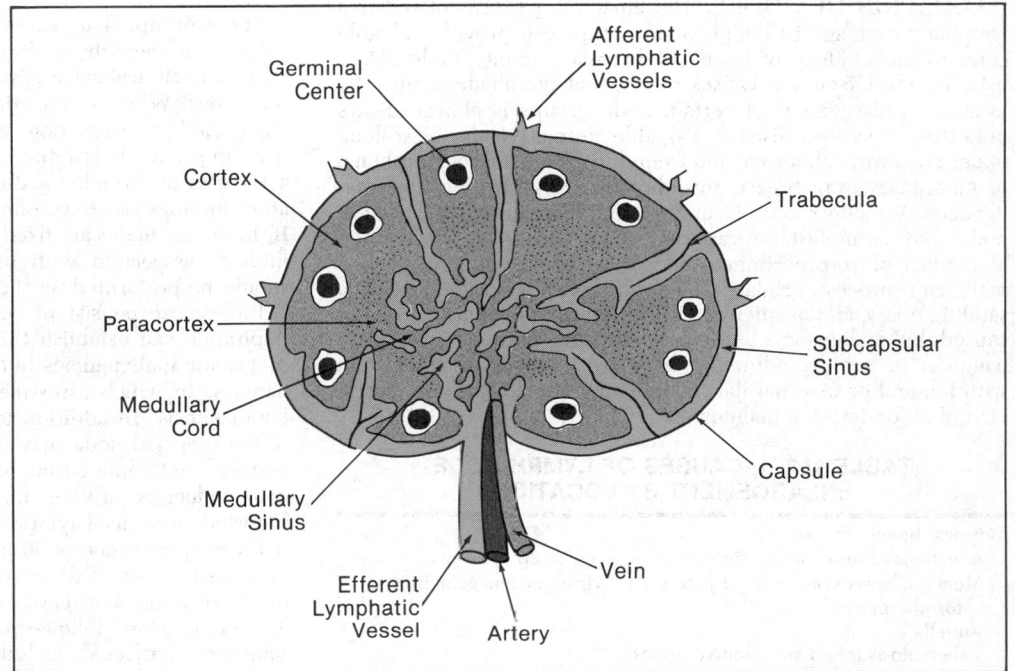

FIGURE 152–1. Diagrammatic representation of the structure of a lymph node.

under the chin, and the submandibular nodes, near the angles of the jaw, receive drainage from structures in the mouth and salivary glands. The jugular nodes, which lie along the anterior border of the sternocleidomastoid muscle, the supraclavicular nodes, found behind the midportion of the clavicle, and the suboccipital nodes, which lie in the posterior cervical triangle, receive lymphatics from many head and neck structures. In addition, the supraclavicular nodes also drain intrathoracic and intra-abdominal organ systems. Lymphatic flow from the eyes, the ears, and the scalp is directed toward the preauricular and postauricular node groups, which lie in front of and behind the ear, respectively. The central and lateral axillary node groups, which are located in the chest wall and along the upper humerus, respectively, receive drainage from the upper extremity, chest wall, breast, and intrathoracic structures. Other node groups with similar drainage patterns include the subscapular nodes, lying anterior to the latissimus dorsi muscle, the pectoral nodes, lying under the edge of the pectoralis major muscle, and the infraclavicular nodes, lying under the distal clavicle. The epitrochlear nodes, located just above the medial humeral epicondyle, receive lymphatic flow from the forearm and hand. The inguinal nodes lie along the inguinal ligament and drain the lower extremity and genitalia. The external iliac and femoral nodes, found in the femoral triangle, have a similar drainage pattern but also receive afferents from pelvic structures.

The deep node systems of the thorax and abdomen, including the hilar, mediastinal, abdominal, retroperitoneal, and pelvic nodes, receive afferent lymphatic flow directly from organs of the thorax, abdomen, and pelvis. In addition, they receive secondary drainage from the superficial node groups. Discovery of enlargement of these deep node groups is usually the result of a directed diagnostic workup or is occasionally made from surveillance roentgenography. However, the mass effect resulting from enlargement of deep node groups can result in distinctive symptoms that should suggest to the clinician a disease process producing internal adenopathy. Enlargement of thoracic nodes (hilar or mediastinal) can compress the trachea or mainstem bronchi (producing cough, dyspnea, or wheezing), the esophagus (resulting in dysphagia), the superior vena cava or subclavian vein (causing venous congestion in the face, neck, and arm), the phrenic nerve (causing paralysis of the diaphragm), or the recurrent laryngeal nerve (producing hoarseness). Because the abdomen and pelvis are less rigidly enclosed than the thorax, compression syndromes resulting from enlargement of deep node groups here are less common, but internal iliac or pelvic node enlargement can lead to venous or lymphatic congestion in the

leg or external genitalia. Extremely large abdominal and pelvic nodes are occasionally detectable by deep palpation.

SIGNIFICANCE OF LYMPH NODE ENLARGEMENT

Lymph node enlargement is a common finding on physical examination. Certain lymph nodes are palpable under normal circumstances. Submandibular nodes less than 1 cm in diameter are common in children and young adults, and inguinal nodes 0.5 to 2 cm in diameter are frequently found in healthy adults. The first component of an efficient approach to lymphadenopathy is evaluation of its significance. Assessment of three factors permits interpretation of the importance of the finding of lymphadenopathy and, in addition, begins to establish a differential diagnosis.

CLINICAL SETTING. The age of the patient is of major importance in evaluating lymphadenopathy, with lymph node enlargement more often reflecting serious disease in adults. Lymphadenopathy in patients less than 30 years of age is due to benign (and usually infectious) causes in at least 80 per cent of cases. In those more than 30 years of age, however, lymphadenopathy is due to a benign process only 40 per cent of the time. Clinical features and the setting frequently guide and direct the workup. For example, coexistence of fever and signs of localized or systemic infection, especially in a younger patient, usually suggests an infectious etiology. Alternatively, the presence of constitutional symptoms, such as weight loss, night sweats, or low-grade fevers, points to a malignant cause of localized adenopathy. The differential diagnosis of mediastinal adenopathy in a young patient from an endemic area must include histoplasmosis as well as lymphoma. Generalized lymphadenopathy in a homosexual, hemophiliac, or intravenous drug abuser suggests a human immunodeficiency virus (HIV)–related syndrome.

PHYSICAL CHARACTERISTICS. Palpation of lymph nodes is best performed with the fingertips, using a circular motion and gradually increasing pressure. Examination of enlarged lymph nodes reveals physical characteristics, such as firmness, mobility, and tenderness, that are helpful in narrowing the diagnostic choices. Because of rapid enlargement and stretching of the joint capsule, lymphadenopathy due to infectious processes is often tender. Nodes enlarged by infection can be matted or asymmetric, and the overlying skin may be inflamed and tender. The nodes may be suppurative, especially when the infectious agent is a mycobacterium or a pyogenic bacterium like staphylococcus. Metastatic tumor produces enlarged nodes that are firm, nontender, and frequently fixed to underlying tissue. Lymphomatous processes result in large, often symmetric lymph nodes that are firm, mobile, nontender, and rubbery.

LOCATION OF NODES. The anatomic patterns of regional lymphatic drainage to lymph node groups can provide valuable clues to the etiology of lymph node enlargement. Table 152–1 lists the most common causes of regional lymphadenopathy by location. Enlargement of certain node groups is almost always indicative of serious disease. Palpable supraclavicular or scalene nodes are always abnormal and frequently the result of lymphoma or metastases from breast, intrathoracic, or gastrointestinal malignancy. Virchow's node is an enlarged, firm left supraclavicular node due to metastatic gastrointestinal malignancy. Enlarged abdominal or retroperitoneal nodes are usually the result of a malignant process. Enlarged lymph nodes associated with a satellite mass and/or pleural or peritoneal effusions are often caused by malignancy. Although palpable inguinal nodes are common in healthy adults, progressive changes or association with femoral or external iliac adenopathy should raise the suspicion of an underlying malignancy.

TABLE 152–1. CAUSES OF LYMPH NODE ENLARGEMENT BY LOCATION

Cervical nodes
  Infections of head, neck, sinuses, ears, eyes, scalp, pharynx
  Mononucleosis syndromes (Epstein-Barr virus, cytomegalovirus, toxoplasmosis)
  Rubella
  Tuberculosis (often suppurative nodes)
  Lymphoma (often unilateral)
  Head and neck malignancy (often unilateral)
Scalene/supraclavicular nodes
  Lung, retroperitoneal, or gastrointestinal malignancy (e.g., Virchow's node)
  Lymphoma
  Thoracic or retroperitoneal bacterial or fungal infections
Axillary nodes
  Infections, bites, trauma to hands or arms
  Cat-scratch disease
  Lymphoma
  Breast carcinoma
  Brucellosis
  Melanoma
Epitrochlear nodes
  Infections of hand (unilateral)
  Lymphoma (unilateral)
  Sarcoidosis (bilateral)
  Tularemia (often unilateral)
  Secondary syphilis (bilateral)
Inguinal nodes
  Infections of leg or foot
  Lymphoma
  Pelvic malignancy
  Venereal diseases (lymphogranuloma venereum, syphilis)
  Pasteurella pestis
Hilar nodes
  Sarcoidosis
  Tuberculosis
  Systemic fungal infections
  Lung carcinoma (unilateral)
Mediastinal nodes
  Mononucleosis syndromes
  Sarcoidosis
  Tuberculosis
  Histoplasmosis
  Lung carcinoma
  Lymphoma
Abdominal/retroperitoneal nodes
  Mesenteric lymphadenitis (tuberculosis)
  Lymphoma
  Germ cell tumors/seminoma
  Prostatic carcinoma and other malignancies
Generalized lymphadenopathy (more than two separate sites)
  Infections (EBV, CMV, toxoplasmosis, tuberculosis, hepatitis, syphilis, HIV/AIDS, histoplasmosis)
  Malignancy (lymphoma, chronic myelogenous leukemia, chronic lymphocytic leukemia, acute leukemia)
  Drug reactions
  Systemic lymphadenopathy syndromes

DIAGNOSTIC APPROACH TO LYMPH NODE ENLARGEMENT

The workup of a patient presenting with newly discovered palpable adenopathy is directed by the factors mentioned previously: the clinical setting, physical characteristics, and location of the nodes. When an infectious cause is strongly suspected, a 14-day period of observation, with or without antimicrobial therapy, is appropriate. It is imperative to record the location and characteristics of the adenopathy carefully, including pertinent negative findings, so that follow-up observations can be validated. If, however, nodes are fixed or firm, or any of the aforementioned findings associated with malignancy are discovered, a biopsy should be performed on the node immediately.

Biopsy can consist of surgical excision or needle aspiration. Aspiration can establish the diagnosis in infectious processes or metastatic malignancies but is rarely helpful in lymphoid malignancies, in which assessment of nodal architecture is required for diagnosis. In addition to routine pathologic studies, analysis of the biopsied node may include (where appropriate) microbial cultures, antigenic typing of lymphocytes, chromosomal analysis, and molecular studies for gene rearrangements. Analysis of biopsied superficial lymph nodes in adults establishes the diagnosis in approximately 50 per cent of cases. One fourth of those patients in whom a diagnosis cannot be established by biopsy go on to develop a disease, usually a lymphoma, within a year. Therefore, close follow-up of patients with nondiagnostic first biopsies is indicated, including repeat biopsies if adenopathy and symptoms persist, as well as consultation with experienced hematopathologists.

Evaluation of deep lymph node groups for enlargement usually requires roentgenography or ultrasonography. Enlarged nodes deep in the axilla may be visualized by mammographic or xerographic techniques. Hilar and mediastinal nodes can be evaluated by standard chest radiographs or computed tomography (CT). Lymphangiography was formerly the standard for evaluation of pelvic, retroperitoneal and abdominal nodes but is being rapidly supplanted by CT.

DISEASE PROCESSES RESULTING IN LYMPHADENOPATHY

A number of mechanisms can produce enlargement of the lymph nodes: (1) hyperplasia of benign lymphocytes in response to infection and/or antigenic stimulation; (2) proliferation of circulating inflammatory and phagocytic cells in response to infection; (3) proliferation and infiltration of phagocytic cells in the lipid storage disorders; (4) neoplastic proliferation of malignant lymphocytes or phagocytes; and (5) infiltration by metastatic malignant cells.

Table 152–2 lists the most common diseases associated with lymphadenopathy and the pathophysiologic mechanism responsible for nodal enlargement. Infectious, inflammatory, and neoplastic disorders account for the vast majority of lymphadenopathy encountered in practice. In addition, there are a number of other uncommon diseases of unknown etiology that primarily involve the lymph nodes, or in which lymphadenopathy is prominent or even the cardinal manifestation of the disease.

Amyloidosis is a condition manifested by deposition of fibrillar material in various organs, including the lymph nodes (Ch. 197). The disease states associated with this deposition may be inflammatory, neoplastic, or hereditary. If the function of internal organs is not compromised by the deposited amyloid, lymphadenopathy, which is characteristically firm, nontender, and diffuse or localized may be the first manifestation of the condition. Analysis of sections from a biopsied node reveals the characteristic staining and ultrastructural properties of the amyloid material.

Sarcoidosis (Ch. 67) is a granulomatous disease of young adults involving multiple organ systems, most commonly the lungs, skin, eyes, and nervous system. Bilateral symmetric hilar adenopathy, often associated with paratracheal adenopathy in an asymptomatic patient, is characteristic of the disease. Peripheral lymphadenopathy is modest or absent. The differential diagnosis of hilar adenopathy must include lymphoma, lung carcinoma, histoplasmosis, and tuberculosis, although the symmetry of the

TABLE 152–2. CAUSES OF LYMPHADENOPATHY

Infection (lymphoid and/or phagocytic hyperplasia)
  Viral (herpesviruses [CMV, EBV, varicella zoster (V-Z)], rubella, HIV, hepatitis A, vaccinia)
  Bacterial (streptococcal, staphylococcal, *Brucella*, tularemia, *Listeria*, cat-scratch disease, *Pasteurella pestis, Haemophilus ducreyi*, syphilis, leptospirosis)
  Fungal (histoplasmosis, coccidioidomycosis)
  Mycobacterial (tuberculosis, leprosy)
  Chlamydial (trachoma, lymphogranuloma venereum)
  Parasitic (toxoplasmosis, trypanosomiasis, filariasis)

Inflammation (lymphoid hyperplasia)
  Rheumatoid arthritis, sarcoidosis, systemic lupus erythematosus, dermatomyositis, immune complex disease/serum sickness, angioimmunoblastic lymphadenopathy, drug reactions

Neoplasms
  Hematologic (myeloproliferative or lymphoproliferative): lymphomas, Hodgkin's disease, acute or chronic myeloid and lymphoid leukemias, malignant histiocytosis
  Metastatic (infiltrative): tumors of breast, lung, kidney, prostate, head and neck, and gastrointestinal tract; melanoma; germ cell tumors; seminoma; neuroblastoma; sarcoma

Infiltration
  Gaucher's disease, Niemann-Pick disease, amyloidosis

Endocrine (lymphoid hyperplasia)
  Hyperthyroidism

Disease of unknown cause with prominent lymphadenopathy
  Mucocutaneous lymph node syndrome
  Lymphomatoid granulomatosis
  Dermatopathic lymphadenitis
  Histiocytic disorder (Letterer-Siwe disease, erythrophagocytic lymphohistiocytosis, sinus histiocytosis, histiocytic medullary reticulosis, malignant histiocytosis)
  Giant follicular lymph node hyperplasia

adenopathy and frequent lack of associated symptoms in sarcoidosis are distinctive.

Mucocutaneous lymph node syndrome (Kawasaki's syndrome) is a disease of children and occasionally young adults, manifested by a distinctive erythematous and desquamative exanthem, conjunctivitis, and fever, with asymmetric cervical adenopathy found in 75 per cent of patients.

Lymphomatoid granulomatosis (Ch. 264) is an infiltration of blood vessel walls with atypical lymphoid and plasmacytoid cells that form granulomas. The vessels of the lung, skin, kidneys, and central nervous system are most often involved, and the intrathoracic lymph nodes are enlarged in 40 per cent of cases. The invading lymphocytes are most likely premalignant T cells, as up to half of patients will go on to develop a T cell lymphoma.

Angioimmunoblastic lymphadenopathy is characterized by a distinctive proliferation of immature and mature plasma cells in a setting of neovasculature. Hepatosplenomegaly and generalized lymphadenopathy are accompanied by a polyclonal hyperglobulinemia, hemolytic anemia, and systemic symptoms. Diagnosis can usually be established by lymph node biopsy, although the disease can be confused with the immunoblastic lymphadenopathy associated with drug reactions, especially phenytoin and allopurinol. One quarter to one half of patients with angioimmunoblastic lymphadenopathy go on to develop a B cell lymphoma (immunoblastic sarcoma).

HISTIOCYTIC DISORDERS

An array of diseases characterized by proliferation of normal or malignant histiocytes (antigen-presenting and antigen-processing mononuclear phagocytes) can manifest with lymphadenopathy as a prominent finding. The benign proliferative disorders can be subdivided according to whether or not the proliferating cell is a Langerhans (or Langerhans-like) histiocyte. The *Langerhans cell histiocytoses* (Ch. 149) occur most often in children with three overlapping presentations. In the past, they were collectively designated *histiocytosis X* (X for unknown etiology). The presentations include the following: (1) *eosinophilic granuloma* occurs in older children and adults and presents as solitary or multiple bone lesions; (2) *Hand-Schüller-Christian syndrome,* defined as the triad of lytic skull lesions, exophthalmos, and diabetes insipidus, usually affects young children; (3) *Letterer-Siwe disease,* a systemic histiocytosis disorder, occurs in infants and is manifested

by fever, eczematoid rash, otitis, lymphadenopathy, hepatosplenomegaly, and other visceral involvement.

The non–Langerhans cell histiocytoses are also nonmalignant proliferative disorders and can all result in regional or generalized lymphadenopathy. *Familial erythrophagocytic lymphohistiocytosis* and *infection-associated hemophagocytic syndrome* are both characterized by constitutional symptoms, pancytopenia, hepatosplenomegaly, lymphadenopathy, and the distinctive pathologic finding of phagocytosed erythrocytes in bone marrow or lymph node specimens. *Sinus histiocytosis* frequently manifests with massive cervical lymphadenopathy, fever, leukocytosis, and, less often, generalized lymphadenopathy. *Malignant histiocytosis (histiocytic medullary reticulosis)* is a progressive proliferation of atypical (but not clearly malignant) histiocytes and immature monocytoid cells, producing severe constitutional symptoms, generalized lymphadenopathy in 50 per cent of cases, hepatosplenomegaly, pancytopenia, and papulonodular skin lesions. True malignancies of histiocytes are rare. They include histiocytic sarcoma, true malignant histiocytosis, and monocytic leukemia, all of which produce prominent lymphadenopathy.

PHYSIOLOGY AND FUNCTIONS OF THE SPLEEN

The spleen, the largest lymphoid organ in the body, plays a major role in the cellular and humoral immune response to infection and inflammation. In addition, with its unique architecture and network of fixed phagocytic cells, the spleen is the primary filter for circulating senescent cells, antigens, and microorganisms in the blood. Unlike the lymph nodes, the spleen receives no direct lymphatic drainage. A spleen of average size (135 grams) receives a blood flow of 300 ml per minute. Splenic vessels from the hilus penetrate trabeculations formed by invaginations of the splenic capsule (Fig. 152–2). The central arterioles, surrounded by sheaths of lymphoid tissue, have branches (follicular arterioles) that take off at right angles, effectively skimming plasma and circulating antigens from the blood and delivering them directly to the splenic immune system. The terminal arterioles are open ended and dump the remaining concentrated blood cells into the splenic cords. Some cells are shunted rapidly into the venous collection system, but many percolate slowly through the open splenic cords for several minutes before squeezing through 0.5- to 2.5-μm slits between the endothelial cells and the discontinuous basement membrane of the venous sinusoids and re-entering the splenic venous system. The cut surface

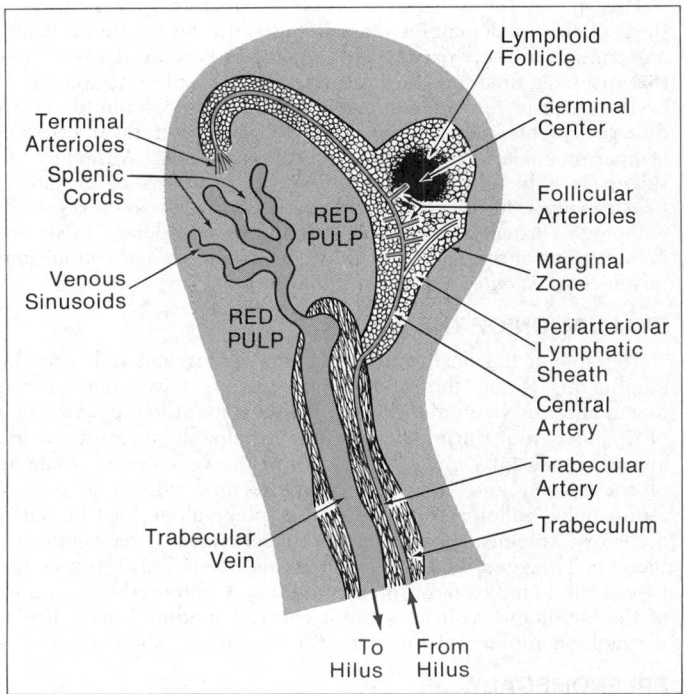

FIGURE 152–2. Diagrammatic representation of the structure of the spleen.

of the spleen displays a prominent red pulp, dotted with islands of white pulp, which serve to compartmentalize the filtrative and immunologic functions of the spleen, respectively.

THE WHITE PULP. The white pulp consists of periarteriolar lymphatic sheaths, with a mantle layer of small lymphocytes (predominantly T lymphocytes) surrounding lymphoid germinal centers, which contain B cells and plasmablasts. Blood-borne antigens and pathogens are concentrated and contact immune responder cells in the white pulp. Circulating particulate antigens and opsonized microorganisms are rapidly phagocytized by macrophages in both the white and the red pulp and are presented to the lymphocytes surrounding the germinal centers in the white pulp. Reactive plasmablasts secreting immunoglobulin M (IgM) appear, and the germinal centers enlarge within 24 hours. Consequently, the white pulp component of the spleen hypertrophies in response to infection and antigenic stimulation. The spleen is therefore important in mounting a response to new immune challenges and serves as the major source of IgM production in the body. The marginal zone of the spleen surrounds these periarteriolar lymphatic sheaths of the white pulp with a dense reticulum in which the terminal arterioles end. This marginal zone blends into the red pulp.

THE RED PULP. The splenic cords (of Billroth) make up the red pulp. Erythrocytes slowly traverse these nonendothelialized cords and are subjected to metabolic conditions (including hypoxia, glucose deprivation, and low pH) that stress senescent or even mildly damaged cells. Defective erythrocytes with abnormally stiff cytoplasm (as in the sickle cell hemoglobinopathies), deficient cellular membrane (as in the spherocytic hemolytic diseases), or excessive rigidity of membrane and cytoskeleton (as in the thalassemia syndromes) are then *culled* from this retarded microcirculation by the avidly phagocytic macrophages, reticular cells, and littoral cells that line the cords. *Pitting* of inclusions from erythrocytes is also performed by these phagocytes as the red cells are squeezed through narrow fenestrations into the venous sinuses. This pitting function removes Howell-Jolly bodies (nuclear remnants), Heinz bodies (denatured hemoglobin), and intraerythrocytic parasites, such as *Plasmodium* and *Bartonella*. New reticulocytes are *conditioned* in this environment, losing up to 30 per cent of their cell membrane and any remaining mitochondria. Iron from ingested red blood cells is stored by the splenic phagocytes and released to the plasma for *reutilization of iron*. In states of abnormal hemolysis, a buildup of hemosiderin occurs in these cells.

The spleen serves as a *reservoir* for platelets, with up to a third of the total platelet mass being sequestered there at any one time in a freely exchangeable pool. In certain disease states this reservoir function can be exaggerated. Acute entrapment of erythrocytes in the splenomegalic crisis of hemoglobin SC or SS disease (*splenic sequestration*) or the blackwater fever crisis of falciparum malaria can result in profound shock. Although the spleen is a blood-forming organ until 5 months of gestation, *hematopoiesis* in the adult spleen occurs only as a result of pathologic, usually neoplastic, conditions. Evidence exists for involvement of the spleen in the *regulation of blood volume* and in the *catabolism of low density lipoproteins*.

EVALUATION OF THE SPLEEN

The spleen lies against the posterior abdominal wall and the diaphragm. When the spleen enlarges, its lower pole moves down, anteriorly and to the right. It is best identified by detection of its movement during respiration. A palpable spleen is nearly always significantly enlarged, except in the very young. Imaging of the spleen and liver can be performed after injection of radiolabeled colloid. To visualize the spleen alone, or to identify accessory spleens, heat-damaged or chemically damaged red blood cells tagged with ^{51}Cr or ^{99m}Tc are used. This test can also be used as an indicator of splenic function. Computed tomography of the abdomen (with or without contrast medium) and ultrasonography complement the spleen scan as diagnostic studies.

SPLENOMEGALY

Five general mechanisms may enlarge the spleen: (1) reactive proliferation of lymphoid cells, (2) infiltration by neoplastic cells

TABLE 152–3. CAUSES OF SPLENOMEGALY

Infection (lymphoid hyperplasia)
  Viral, parasitic, bacterial, fungal
Inflammation (lymphoid hyperplasia)
  Rheumatoid arthritis, sarcoidosis, systemic lupus erythematosus, renal dialysis, beryllium, serum sickness
Neoplasms (infiltrative or myeloproliferative)
  Leukemia, lymphoma, polycythemia vera, myeloid metaplasia, Hodgkin's disease, metastatic tumors, primary tumors
Hemolytic diseases (phagocytic hyperplasia)
  Spherocytosis, thalassemia major, pyruvate kinase deficiency, paroxysmal nocturnal hemoglobinuria, hemoglobinopathies, immune cytopenias
Deficiency diseases
  Iron deficiency, pernicious anemia
Infiltration
  Gaucher's disease, Neimann-Pick disease, amyloidosis, extramedullary hematopoiesis
Splenic vein hypertension (vascular congestion)
  Cirrhosis, splenic or portal vein thrombosis, hepatic schistosomiasis, congestive heart failure
Endocrine
  Graves' disease, Hashimoto's thyroiditis
Hemophilia (subsequent to intensive therapy with clotting factor concentrate)
Other
  Cysts, angioimmunoblastic lymphadenopathy, histiocytoses, hyperlipidemias

or lipid-laden macrophages, (3) extramedullary hematopoiesis, (4) proliferation of phagocytic cells, and (5) vascular congestion. Diseases may cause splenomegaly by one or by a combination of these mechanisms (Table 152–3). The causes of massive splenomegaly (greater than 3000 grams) are somewhat more limited (Table 152–4). The myelodysplastic disorders and malignant lymphoid disorders are the most common causes of chronic massive splenomegaly in nontropical countries. Splenomegaly can be present as an isolated finding on physical examination, can exist in association with a systemic disorder, or can be discovered as a consequence of the secondary hematologic effects of splenic enlargement—the hypersplenism syndrome. Symptoms arising from splenomegaly may include pain from the stretched capsule of an acutely enlarged spleen or shock from atraumatic rupture of a tense capsule.

Evaluation of splenomegaly should include examination of the peripheral blood and frequently the bone marrow. A spleen scan is recommended to determine the size and shape of the spleen and to look for defects suggestive of tumors, cysts, or extrasplenic masses displacing the spleen. In general, diagnostic tests are not

TABLE 152–4. CAUSES OF MASSIVE SPLENOMEGALY

Acute
  Malaria (falciparum) with splenic sequestration crisis
  Sickle cell anemia with splenic sequestration crisis
Chronic
  Myelodysplastic
    Chronic myelogenous leukemia
    Myeloid metaplasia/myelofibrosis
    Polycythemia vera (end-stage)
    Primary thrombocythemia
  Neoplastic
    Lymphoma
    Malignant reticuloendotheliosis
    Hodgkin's disease
    Hairy cell leukemia
    Chronic lymphocytic leukemia
  Hematologic
    Thalassemia major
    Sickle cell anemia (rarely)
  Inflammatory-infiltrative
    Gaucher's disease
    Sarcoidosis
    Felty's syndrome
  Infectious
    Malaria
    Kala-azar

performed on the spleen itself; they are oriented toward the diagnosis of disease states producing splenomegaly. Chest radiography or liver function tests may reveal the etiology of the splenic enlargement. If lymphadenopathy is present, lymph node biopsy may yield a diagnosis. When systemic symptoms accompany splenomegaly but no lymphadenopathy is appreciated, a laparotomy with biopsies of liver, spleen, and lymph nodes is sometimes indicated. Such a study will produce a diagnosis of lymphoma in one third of cases, congestive splenomegaly in one quarter, and an inflammatory state in one fifth.

INFECTION. Systemic infections are the most common causes of moderate and transient splenomegaly. Splenic enlargement is the rule in mononucleosis due to Epstein-Barr virus infection but is less frequent in the heterophil-negative mononucleosis syndromes associated with cytomegalovirus, adenovirus, or acquired toxoplasmosis. Splenomegaly can be massive, however, in congenital toxoplasmosis or other infectious causes of the TORCH (toxoplasmosis, rubella, cytomegalovirus, and herpes simplex) syndrome. A palpable spleen is often detected in the course of viral hepatitis and influenza and less often in association with infectious lymphocytosis, pertussis, and roseola infantum. Bacterial infections causing splenomegaly include secondary syphilis, subacute bacterial endocarditis, and acute brucellosis. Hematogenous spread of tuberculosis or histoplasmosis can involve the spleen. Splenomegaly is common in tropical populations and is due to malaria, schistosomiasis, leishmaniasis (kala-azar), chronic worm infestation, and other disorders. Rickettsial infection can produce splenic enlargement, with a palpable spleen being noted in up to 40 per cent of patients with Rocky Mountain spotted fever. Modest splenomegaly is appreciated in 30 to 80 per cent of patients with the lymphadenopathy accompanying the HIV disease–related complex (ARC).

INFLAMMATION. Splenomegaly is found in systemic lupus erythematosus (20 per cent), rheumatoid arthritis (5 to 10 per cent), and Behçet's disease and frequently results in production of cytopenias by hypersplenism. Angioimmunoblastic lymphadenopathy, sometimes associated with anticonvulsant administration, is characterized by splenomegaly, autoimmune hemolytic anemia, and dysproteinemia. Regional ileitis is occasionally accompanied by a histiocytic infiltration of the spleen.

NEOPLASMS. The myelodysplastic disorders and leukemias (acute and chronic) commonly infiltrate the spleen, causing modest to massive enlargement. Splenic involvement is noted in 30 to 40 per cent of adult non-Hodgkin's lymphoma at presentation. Primary malignant tumors of the spleen are rare and include lymphangiosarcomas, hemangiosarcomas, fibrosarcomas, and leiomyosarcomas. They may present with local or systemic problems and are diagnosed by CT, spleen scan, and angiography. Metastatic tumor is a rare cause of splenomegaly.

STORAGE DISEASES. Previously undiagnosed Gaucher's disease is a cause of asymptomatic splenomegaly. Niemann-Pick disease and the sea-blue histiocyte syndrome can also present in this way. Diagnosis can often be made by bone marrow biopsy.

CHRONIC CONGESTIVE SPLENOMEGALY (BANTI'S SYNDROME). This complex is characterized by splenomegaly, pancytopenia as a consequence of hypersplenism, and gastrointestinal bleeding secondary to portal hypertension. The splenic vein hypertension is due to either intrahepatic disease (e.g., cirrhosis or schistosomiasis) or extrahepatic disease (such as portal or splenic vein thrombosis). Splenic vein thrombosis is most commonly caused by compression of the splenic vein by tumor or fibrosis. Pregnancy, trauma, or intravascular coagulation can predispose to portal vein thrombosis. The spleen is markedly enlarged and congested, with distended veins and venous sinuses. Periarteriolar hemorrhage, siderotic nodules, hyperplasia of the red pulp, and progressive fibrosis occur. Symptoms can range from vague gastrointestinal complaints to catastrophic bleeding from esophageal or gastric varices. Hematologic cytopenias may be severe but are rarely the major medical concern. Etiologic studies of congestive splenomegaly should include evaluation for alcoholism, liver function tests, liver-spleen scan, liver biopsy, and a search for varices. If no liver disease is found, venous obstruction should be considered and splenoportal venography performed. Splenic or hepatic vein thrombosis may be the initial presentation in an occult myeloproliferative disease, particularly polycythemia vera.

HYPERSPLENISM

Hypersplenism is an exaggeration of normal splenic function, with enhanced filtration and phagocytosis of the cellular elements of the blood. The hyperplastic spleen can sequester as much as 90 per cent of the total platelet pool or 45 per cent of the red cell mass. Four criteria support the diagnosis of hypersplenism: (1) cytopenia of one or more hematologic cell lines, (2) compensatory reactive marrow hyperplasia, (3) splenomegaly, and (4) correction of abnormalities by splenectomy.

Hypersplenism is frequently secondary to splenic enlargement. Splenomegaly due to infiltrative diseases (lymphoma, chronic leukemia, Gaucher's disease, amyloidosis) is not usually associated with the severe cytopenias of hypersplenism. Enlargement of the spleen due to hypertrophy of the phagocytic elements (inflammatory diseases) or secondary to congestive splenomegaly with slowing of the cellular transit time through the spleen, however, is frequently accompanied by anemia, thrombocytopenia, or granulocytopenia of varying degrees. The erythrostatic environment of hypersplenism is especially threatening to red blood cells with mild intrinsic abnormalities. The patient with well-compensated hereditary spherocytosis or elliptocytosis may experience acute, severe hemolysis from the transient splenic enlargement accompanying mononucleosis. Similarly, the anemia of chronic liver disease may worsen as the increasing pressure in the portal system causes stasis and destruction of acanthocytes in the spleen. The harsh metabolic environment of the splenic cords (hypoxia, low glucose levels, and low pH) is exaggerated in the enlarged and congested spleen. In addition, phagocytosis of red cells or platelets stimulates more reactive hyperplasia of splenic histiocytes, begetting more hypersplenism. This is the mechanism underlying *primary hypersplenism*, in which the spleen hypertrophies because of phagocytosis of defective red cells (hereditary spherocytosis), antibody-coated red cells (autoimmune hemolytic anemia), or antibody-coated platelets (autoimmune thrombocytopenia). Hypersplenism can be documented and quantified by demonstrating a decrease in the circulating half-life of labeled erythrocytes along with an increase in the spleen-liver uptake ratio.

INDICATIONS FOR SPLENECTOMY

Splenectomy may be indicated for either of two medical conditions: (1) to stage or control a basic disease process (Hodgkin's disease, hereditary spherocytosis, autoimmune cytopenias) or (2) to alleviate the consequences of hypersplenism secondary to other disease processes. In addition, the spleen may have to be removed because of traumatic or, rarely, spontaneous rupture causing intra-abdominal hemorrhage.

THROMBOCYTOPENIA. *Chronic autoimmune thrombocytopenia* (ITP) refractory to corticosteroid therapy usually improves (in 70 to 90 per cent of patients) after splenectomy, with the platelet count becoming normal in 60 per cent of patients. Those who do not respond completely can often be maintained on a lower corticosteroid dose. The thrombocytopenia accompanying *systemic* or *discoid lupus* responds poorly to splenectomy. *Thrombotic thrombocytopenic purpura* has been treated in the past with splenectomy and steroid therapy, but newer modalities, including plasmapheresis or plasma exchange, appear more promising (Ch. 154).

HEMOLYTIC ANEMIAS. *Autoimmune hemolytic anemia* caused by warm-reacting antibodies that does not resolve after 2 months of corticosteroid therapy may be treated by splenectomy. Two thirds of such patients have complete or partial remission, but the relapse rate is high. Splenectomy is a uniformly effective treatment for the anemia of *hereditary spherocytosis* (Ch. 134). Surgery should be delayed until the age of 5 years, if possible, to decrease the risk of overwhelming sepsis. Other congenital hemolytic anemias do not respond as consistently to splenectomy, and the decision to remove the spleen should be based on the severity of the anemia and lack of response to alternative treatments.

LEUKEMIAS. Splenectomy is routinely performed for symptomatic cytopenias or splenomegaly in *hairy cell leukemia* (leukemic reticuloendotheliosis). Improvement occurs in up to 85 per cent of patients, but recurrence of cytopenias is common.

Early splenectomy is no longer recommended, and the advent of alpha-interferon therapy for this disease may relegate splenectomy to a secondary role (Ch. 144). In the past, splenectomy was commonly carried out in patients with *chronic myelogenous leukemia* for relief of symptoms or prior to bone marrow transplantation. Any benefit is transient, however; survival is not affected, and the operation in this setting is associated with a high mortality. Splenectomy can provide useful palliation in patients with *prolymphocytic leukemia* and *chronic lymphocytic leukemia* who have symptomatic splenomegaly or autoimmune hemolytic anemia. Splenectomy improves the hematologic status and the quality of life in cases of severe *agnogenic myeloid metaplasia* (Ch. 143).

STORAGE DISEASES. Splenectomy can be performed in *Gaucher's disease* when splenomegaly produces mechanical or cytopenic problems. The spleen serves as a storage area for undigested cerebroside, so it is possible that splenectomy might accelerate the disease (Ch. 174).

FELTY'S SYNDROME. Neutropenia of variable degrees and splenomegaly, occasionally accompanied by thrombocytopenia or anemia, occur in about 1 per cent of patients with rheumatoid arthritis. The spleen appears to be both the source of the antibody coating the neutrophils and the means of their destruction. If the neutropenia is severe enough to cause frequent infections or skin ulcerations, splenectomy is beneficial in 60 to 80 per cent of patients.

THALASSEMIA MAJOR. In the setting of longstanding thalassemia, therapeutic splenectomy is often required. It appears, however, that aggressive transfusion regimens combined with iron chelation therapy may reduce the incidence of severe hypersplenism.

RENAL DIALYSIS HYPERSPLENISM. Up to 10 per cent of uremic patients undergoing long-term dialysis develop signs of hypersplenism. Splenectomy may decrease bleeding tendencies and transfusion requirements in this setting.

ALTERNATIVES TO SPLENECTOMY. Therapy with glucocorticoids inhibits phagocytosis and can provide a useful "chemical splenectomy" in short-term situations. Partial splenectomy is sometimes advocated in children to reduce the risk of postsplenectomy complications. Partial or complete embolization of the spleen using percutaneous catheterization is a relatively safe, effective, and noninvasive approach when surgery is contraindicated. Splenic irradiation (100 to 500 cGy) can provide transient therapy for hypersplenism or splenomegaly due to infiltrative diseases.

POSTSPLENECTOMY SYNDROMES AND HYPOSPLENISM

HEMATOLOGIC SEQUELAE. The hyposplenic or postsplenectomy state can often be diagnosed by examination of the peripheral blood smear (see Color Plate 6K). In the absence of splenic culling and pitting functions, nucleated red blood cells, Howell-Jolly and Heinz body inclusions, siderocytes, and acanthocytes are found in the circulation. Reticulocytes are no longer conditioned, and their redundant cell membrane produces target cells upon drying and staining.

A transient and modest increase in the leukocyte count occurs after splenectomy and lasts 1 to 2 weeks. The bulk of this *leukocytosis* is accounted for by early *neutrophilia*. Later, *lymphocytosis* and *monocytosis* become more prominent.

Splenectomy routinely results in prominent postoperative *thrombocytosis*, often producing platelet counts of 1 million or more per cubic millimeter for weeks to months following surgery. This elevation may persist in 40 per cent of patients. The risk of consequent thromboembolic phenomena after splenectomy is high only in the setting of myeloproliferative disease or paroxysmal nocturnal hemoglobinuria. Attempts should be made to decrease the platelet count with chemotherapy before surgery in such cases. Following surgery, therapy with anticoagulants and antiplatelet agents should be considered, especially if the patient is bedridden.

INFECTION. In the absence of the spleen, or in the setting of functional hyposplenism, certain inadequacies of immune function can be demonstrated. IgM levels fall, and complement-mediated opsonization is decreased. This is in part due to a fall in the levels of tuftsin and properdin, two opsonic proteins produced by the spleen. The ability to phagocytose circulating antigens is compromised, as is cell-mediated immunity.

The risk of *overwhelming sepsis* following splenectomy or in functional hyposplenism is especially high in children, up to 10 per cent per year in debilitated infants. The incidence falls to 1 per cent per year in older children and is rare, but reported, in adults. The etiologic organisms are encapsulated bacteria, predominantly pneumococcus and less commonly meningococcus or *Haemophilus influenzae*. These are poorly opsonized in the body, and the intact spleen, with its slow, tortuous blood flow past avid phagocytes, appears to be the primary site for clearance of these pathogens. All patients with decreased splenic function, whether due to functional hyposplenism or to splenectomy (traumatic or therapeutic), must be warned to take any febrile illness seriously. Prophylaxis with penicillin is recommended for all children with asplenia or splenic hypofunction (e.g., sickle cell anemia). Immunization with polyvalent vaccines to pneumococci, meningococci, and *H. influenzae* is advised for patients over the age of 3 years. Serologic response to these vaccines may not be normal in hyposplenia or asplenia. The optimal timing of vaccine administration (with respect to splenectomy) is not established, but vaccination should precede splenectomy and any chemotherapy, if possible. Serious infections with unusual organisms like *Babesia* or *Bartonella* also occur in hyposplenic individuals. A concurrent viral infection may predispose hyposplenic patients to fulminant bacteremias.

FUNCTIONAL HYPOSPLENISM. Repeated symptomatic or silent infarction of the spleen in the course of veno-occlusive diseases, like the sickle cell syndromes, results in substantial or total loss of splenic tissue (*autosplenectomy*). The spleen is shrunken and fibrosed. Circulating erythrocytes reflect the loss of the splenic filtration function and are found to contain mitochondrial remnants and inclusions of nuclear fragments (Howell-Jolly bodies) and denatured hemoglobin (Heinz bodies). Bizarrely shaped red cells, target cells, and large platelets are observed. Hyposplenism can occur even with a large or normal-sized spleen if splenic tissue has been replaced by sarcoid granulomas, amyloid, or multiple myeloma or if splenic phagocytes have been paralyzed by high-dose corticosteroid therapy. Other diseases linked with hyposplenism include ulcerative colitis, celiac disease, dermatitis herpetiformis, systemic lupus erythematosus, primary thrombocythemia, and Graves' disease. Such patients run the same risk of fulminant bacteremia as do those who have had their spleen surgically removed.

CONGENITAL ASPLENIA. This uncommon condition is associated with symmetric development of normally asymmetric organs or pairs of organs. Complex and multiple cardiovascular anomalies are the rule.

OTHER DISEASES OF THE SPLEEN

SPLENIC RUPTURE. Rupture of the capsule may be precipitated by trauma, by overly zealous palpation of an enlarged spleen (secondary to mononucleosis, sepsis, or leukemia), or rarely by dissection of a pancreatic pseudocyst into the spleen. The patient presents with left upper quadrant pain, sometimes radiating to the left scapular region, and abdominal guarding and rigidity, quickly progressing to hypovolemic shock. Usually, emergency splenectomy is indicated. In selected cases, nonoperative management or splenorrhaphy, including gluing or wrapping of the ruptured capsule ("hair netting"), is a treatment alternative to splenectomy.

SPLENIC INFARCTION. Infarction usually occurs in the setting of splenic enlargement secondary to myeloproliferative disease or vascular occlusive phenomena (sickle hemoglobinopathies, including SS, Sβ thalassemia, and SC diseases). These may be silent infarctions or present with severe left upper quadrant pain.

ARTERIAL ANEURYSMS. These lesions are most common in women beyond middle age. They may be asymptomatic or cause left upper quadrant pain or vague gastrointestinal complaints. The aneurysm of the spleen is sometimes palpable, and a bruit may be appreciated. Radiologic studies can reveal a calcified aneurysmal wall, and the diagnosis is made by sonography or angiography. Embolization of such aneurysms has been successful in situations in which surgery is contraindicated.

SPLENIC HEMANGIOMATOSIS. Diffuse cavernous hemangiomatosis of the spleen is rare, but the cavernous hemangioma is the most common benign tumor involving the spleen. The patient can present with splenic infarctions, splenomegaly, or thrombocytopenia secondary to platelet destruction within the hemangiomas, or the finding of hemangiomatosis may be incidental. The diagnosis can usually be made by CT or sonography.

SPLENIC CYSTS. Echinococcal infection should be suspected in a patient with an appropriate travel history, single or multiple splenic cysts with calcified walls, and eosinophilia. Serologic studies may be helpful in establishing the diagnosis. True splenic cysts (dermoids and mesenchymal inclusion cysts) are embryonic rests and may be diagnosed by CT, sonography, and angiography.

SPLENIC ABSCESS. An occult, deep-seated infection, splenic abscess usually follows a bacteremic episode. The source of the septicemia can be infected endocardium, lung (pneumonia, lung abscess, empyema), skin or soft tissue, pelvis (pelvic inflammatory disease or septic abortion), nasopharynx, or ear. Predisposing factors include previous splenic damage by infarction (secondary to sickle cell disease or leukemia), trauma, and infection (malaria, typhoid, ameba, cysts). Extension of an abscess into the spleen from adjacent perforated abdominal organs (stomach, transverse colon, tail of pancreas) can occur. In most series, streptococci are the most common etiologic agents, followed by staphylococci and, with increasing frequency, by gram-negative organisms (*Salmonella*, Enterobacteriaceae, *Pseudomonas, Serratia, Bacteroides*) and anaerobes. Presenting symptoms include fever, chills, and left upper quadrant pain, often accompanied by tenderness, muscle spasm, and subcutaneous edema over the spleen. Infection localized to the upper pole of the spleen can produce pleuritic pain and even left pleural effusion. An abscess in the lower pole may result in signs of peritoneal inflammation. A splenic friction rub may be appreciated. Splenic scan, sonography, and CT aid in the diagnosis. The differential diagnosis must include subphrenic abscess, pulmonary empyema, splenic infarction, perinephric abscess, neoplasms, and pancreatic pseudocyst. A combination of antibiotics and surgical intervention, usually splenectomy, is indicated. Single abscesses respond well, but multiple abscesses, often the result of generalized sepsis in a debilitated or immunocompromised patient, are associated with a high mortality.

Cahill CG, Wastell C: Splenic conservation. Surg Annu 22:379, 1990. *A comprehensive review of current surgical techniques aimed at preserving splenic function.*

Chaikof EL, McCabe CT: Fatal overwhelming postsplenectomy infection. Am J Surg 149:534, 1985. *A review of infection patterns in 776 splenectomized adults and children.*

Chun CH, Raff MJ, Contreras L, et al.: Splenic abscess. Medicine, 59:50, 1980. *Comprehensive review of this often fatal disease, discussing etiology, predisposing factors, diagnosis, and treatment.*

Hibberd PL, Rubin RH: Approach to immunization in the immunosuppressed host. Infect Dis Clin North Am 4:124, 1989. *A discussion of the roles of vaccines and adjunctive measures, such as antimicrobials and immunoglobulin, in the asplenic patient.*

Knecht H: Angioimmunoblastic lymphadenopathy: Ten years' experience and state of current knowledge. Semin Hematol 26:208, 1989. *A review of the idiopathic and drug-related forms of this disease and their natural history.*

Pochedly C, Sills RH, Schwartz AD (eds.): Disorders of the Spleen: Pathophysiology and Management. New York, Marcel Dekker, 1989. *Detailed description of splenic anatomy, physiology, and pathophysiology, with extensive discussion of the causes and sequelae of splenic hypofunction and hyperfunction.*

Shaw JH, Print CG: Postsplenectomy sepsis. Br J Surg 76:1074, 1989. *A review of the infectious consequences of elective and emergency splenectomy, with discussion of the role of immunization and prophylaxis.*

153 Bone Marrow Transplantation

Rainer Storb

PRINCIPLES OF MARROW TRANSPLANTATION

Transplantation of marrow from a donor identical with the recipient at the major histocompatibility complex reduces graft-versus-host disease (GVHD) and improves survival of the recipient. Successful human transplantation using allogeneic, human leukocyte antigen (HLA)–identical sibling donors was carried out first in children with immunodeficiency diseases and subsequently in patients with severe aplastic anemia and leukemia.

Marrow transplantation differs in several respects from transplantation of solid organs, in particular the kidney: (1) The host-versus-graft reaction can generally be abrogated by a single short course of high-dose immunosuppressive therapy given immediately before transplantation; (2) preceding blood transfusions are not beneficial but rather can interfere with subsequent marrow engraftment, particularly in patients with aplastic anemia; (3) until recently, donors have mostly been HLA-identical family members; (4) donors do not suffer a permanent organ loss, since the removed marrow is replaced within weeks; and (5) postgrafting immunosuppression of recipients can generally be terminated after 3 to 12 months.

To prepare for marrow transplantation, the recipient's immune system must first be destroyed. This is effectively accomplished by use of cyclophosphamide (CY), at 50 mg per kilogram per day for 4 days, or total body irradiation (TBI), at 800 to 1500 rads in midline tissue doses (4 to 25 rads per minute), either alone or combined with CY or other chemotherapeutic agents. An alternative has been to combine CY with busulfan. These programs not only set the stage for establishment of the allogeneic graft but also serve to kill leukemic cells, if that is the patient's basic disease.

After the conditioning regimen, 2 to 6 $\times$ 10^8 donor marrow cells per kilogram are infused intravenously. Most grafts are initially successful, so that within 2 to 4 weeks marrow cellularity increases and peripheral blood counts of donor origin rise. Over time, all hematopoietic and immune cells of the recipient are replaced by those from the marrow donor, including plasma cells and tissue macrophages.

COMPLICATIONS

Graft-versus-host disease may occur when genetically foreign, immunologically active lymphocytes are transferred into an immunosuppressed recipient incapable of rejecting the lymphocytes. This condition is found in all allogeneic marrow transplant recipients (donors are other than monozygous twins). Donor T lymphocytes present in the marrow inoculum recognize histocompatibility antigens of the host as foreign, become sensitized, proliferate, and attack recipient tissue, thereby producing the clinical syndrome of GVHD. The main targets of GVHD are skin, gastrointestinal tract, and liver. As perhaps the most effective immunosuppressive agent to prevent GVHD, methotrexate or cyclosporine is given within the first 3 to 12 months after grafting. The best results seem to be achieved when the drugs are combined. Once the drugs are discontinued, many patients do well with persisting graft-host tolerance. However, acute GVHD occurs in approximately 35 to 60 per cent of the patients, and as many as 40 per cent of afflicted patients die of associated infections. Xenogeneic antihuman thymocyte globulin (ATG), prednisone, or cyclosporine has been used to treat acute GVHD with some success. Better approaches to prevent or treat acute GVHD are necessary, such as the more imaginative use of known immunosuppressive agents, the use of "germ-free" isolation, or the removal of T lymphocytes from the marrow inoculum by antibodies to human T lymphocytes.

Chronic GVHD affects approximately 25 to 45 per cent of patients surviving more than 180 days. Most frequent in older patients and those who had acute GVHD, it may affect the same organs that are involved in acute GVHD and, additionally, mucous membranes. It resembles collagen vascular diseases and is characterized by severe immunodeficiency, impaired granulocyte chemotaxis, and recurrent, sometimes life-threatening bacterial infections. Combination therapy with prednisone and cyclosporine, azathioprine, CY, or procarbazine is effective in most patients with chronic GVHD.

Interstitial pneumonias, either of unknown etiology or associated with infectious agents such as cytomegalovirus, cause morbidity and fatality during the first 4 months after grafting. They are a major problem in patients who are treated with TBI and then receive transplants for leukemia, but a minor problem in

CY-treated patients receiving transplants for aplastic anemia. Probably these infections are the result of deficient immune reactivity of the compromised host, although radiation effects may also play a role. Effective methods of accelerating the immune reconstitution and/or the use of antiviral agents or hyperimmune globulin might be of value in eliminating the problem of interstitial pneumonia. Patients with cultures negative for cytomegalovirus should receive blood products from cytomegalovirus-negative donors.

CLINICAL RESULTS

SEVERE APLASTIC ANEMIA (Ch. 129). Aplastic anemia is most frequently attributable to a stem cell defect. In many cases, infusion of marrow from a monozygotic twin (syngeneic transplant) has been successful in reconstituting the marrow without immunosuppression of the recipient. Some syngeneic grafts have been successful only after preparation with CY and a second transplant, suggesting that these cases may involve other mechanisms, perhaps of autoimmune etiology, which can be overcome by CY. Allogeneic marrow transplantation (donors are HLA-identical family members) is often effective therapy for severe aplastic anemia, with significantly better survival.

Marrow graft rejection has been a major problem in aplastic anemia, most frequently caused by transfusion-induced sensitization. When transplantation is carried out in patients who have not received transfusions before transplantation, graft failure is the exception. Eighty-three per cent of our first 43 patients are alive between 6 and 16½ (median, 9) years after grafting (Fig. 153–1). We believe that the immunologic mechanisms involved in graft failure are, for the most part, iatrogenic (i.e., induced by previous blood transfusion).

Many programs are being carried out to avoid rejection in multiply transfused patients by using more intensive immunosuppressive conditioning regimens. In all programs, CY is used, but other features of the conditioning regimens vary. In Seattle, methotrexate and cyclosporine are used after grafting, and viable donor buffy coat cells have been infused together with the marrow inoculum. The donor's peripheral blood is a potential source of additional pluripotent hematopoietic stem cells and/or lymphoid cells capable of overcoming rejection. As a rule, the rejection rates have decreased and survival has increased. Of 65 Seattle patients with aplastic anemia who received marrow grafts from HLA-identical siblings following multiple transfusions, 70 per cent are alive after follow-up periods of 6 to 12½ years.

Most of the regimens have associated risks. The addition of buffy coat cells has led to an increased risk of chronic GVHD. Radiation regimens carry the potential risk for late malignant disease. A recent Seattle regimen combining CY and ATG appears effective in reducing the risk of graft rejection without the use of buffy coat cells. Nevertheless, emphasis should be placed on measures to prevent rather than to overcome the sensitization caused by blood transfusions. For this the physician should be aware of the possibility of marrow transplantation when aplastic anemia is first diagnosed. If an HLA-identical family member is available, early transplantation before transfusions is the therapy of choice. If transfusions are necessary, white blood cells should be removed as much as possible to reduce the chance of sensitization. Treatment of blood products with gamma radiation may prove effective in preventing sensitization.

LEUKEMIA (Ch. 144 and 145). Marrow grafting for leukemia presents the same general transplantation problems encountered with aplastic anemia. Graft rejection is rare, however. The unique problem is recurrence of leukemia. Formerly, marrow transplantation was carried out only after failure of all other therapies, when patients were undergoing advanced relapse. Of the first 100 patients with acute leukemia receiving grafts in Seattle after CY and TBI, 12 per cent are alive with the disease in remission between 12 and 18 years without any maintenance therapy. Approximately 75 per cent of all patients could be expected to have recurrent leukemia unless they died of other causes. Leukemic recurrence usually originated from host-type cells, indicating that it is difficult to kill every leukemic cell once the patient has reached the end stage of the disease. Currently, attempts are being made to reduce the rate of leukemic relapse and increase long-term survival in patients with leukemia receiving transplants in the end stage of their disease. Higher doses of TBI, by means of fractionating the radiation, and additional chemotherapeutic agents are being used. Most recently, monoclonal antibodies, to which short-lived high-energy beta-emitting radioactive isotopes have been coupled, have been used to increase the effect of the conditioning programs. These attempts may be doomed to failure, since, in an exponential cell kill process, it is difficult to kill the last leukemic cell. Some of the apparent cures may have occurred because of leukemic cell kill by immune mechanisms directed at non-HLA antigens expressed on leukemic cells. This theory is suggested by the observation of a graft-versus-leukemia effect in humans.

It is advisable to carry out marrow transplantation earlier in the course of leukemia while the disease is in remission. At this time, the number of leukemic cells in the body is small and the cells are not yet resistant to therapy. In addition, the patient is in a better clinical condition and therefore better able to tolerate the therapy. Accordingly, we began in 1976 to treat patients with acute nonlymphoblastic leukemia by marrow grafting when the disease was in first or subsequent remission and those with acute lymphoblastic leukemia when it was in second or subsequent remission after conditioning with CY and TBI.

Patients with acute nonlymphoblastic leukemia who receive chemotherapy have an approximate median duration of survival of 2 years. Only 15 to 20 per cent of patients who receive chemotherapy are alive at 5 years. Of the first 22 patients with acute nonlymphoblastic leukemia treated by marrow transplantation during first remission, 12 are alive with the disease in unmaintained remission between 10 and 12 years after transplantation. The survival curve shows a plateau at 55 per cent (Fig. 153–1).

Approximately 50 per cent of patients with acute lymphoblastic leukemia, especially children, can be cured by chemotherapy. Once relapse has occurred, another remission can often be induced with chemotherapy, but long-term survival of patients who have relapsed is poor, with very few alive at 2 years. Treatment of patients with acute lymphoblastic leukemia during second or subsequent remission by marrow transplantation seems justified in an attempt to change the otherwise grim outlook and perhaps "cure" some of these patients.

The survival curve of the first 22 patients with acute lymphoblastic leukemia in second or subsequent remission receiving marrow grafts in Seattle shows a plateau at 27 per cent, 11 to 12 years after transplantation (Fig. 153–1).

The results of marrow transplantation for the treatment of patients with chronic granulocytic leukemia in blast crisis have been similar to those in patients with leukemia in relapse. The projected survival is approximately 15 per cent (Fig. 153–2). The patients' marrows show absence of the Philadelphia chromosome, a unique result.

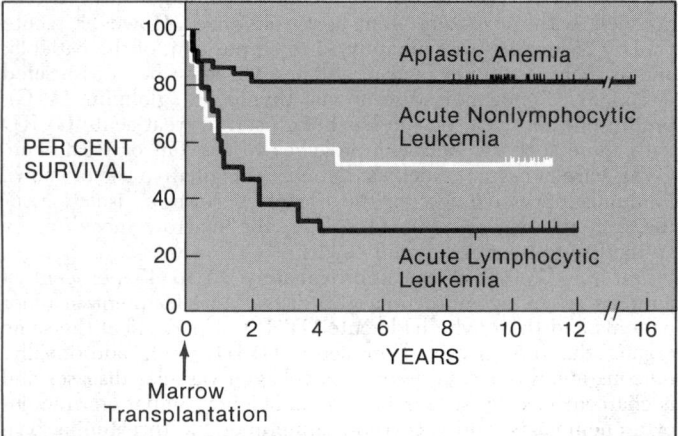

FIGURE 153–1. The survival of 43 untransfused patients with aplastic anemia, 22 patients with acute nonlymphoblastic leukemia having transplants in first remission, and 22 patients with acute lymphoblastic leukemia having transplants in second or subsequent remission after marrow grafts from HLA-identical family members. The surviving patients with leukemia remain in unmaintained remission. Day "0" is the day of marrow transplantation. The tick marks indicate living patients. Survival is as of May 1988.

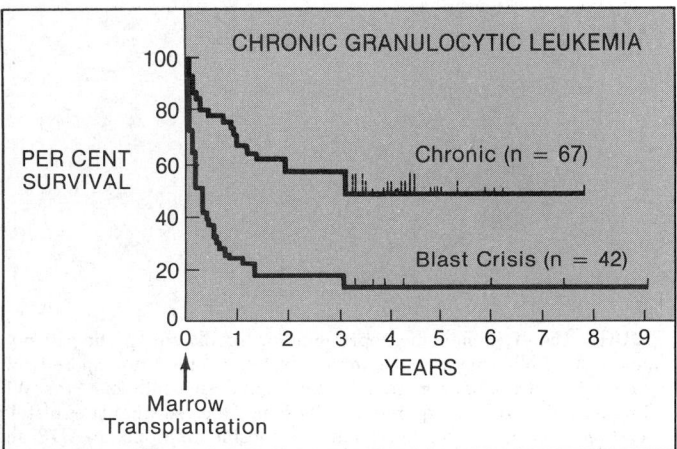

FIGURE 153–2. Survival after marrow grafting in patients with chronic granulocytic leukemia having transplants either in blast crisis or in chronic phase. The tick marks indicate living patients. Survival is as of March 1987.

Transplantation during the chronic phase of chronic granulocytic leukemia promises to improve these results. Although follow-up is still short, it appears that long-term disease-free survival will be on the order of 50 per cent (Fig. 153–2). Over the past 7 years, with the introduction of methotrexate and cyclosporine for GVHD prophylaxis, disease-free survival has increased to more than 70 per cent.

Marrow transplantation has now also been successfully applied to the treatment of patients with non-Hodgkin's lymphoma, myelofibrosis, multiple myeloma, preleukemia, and hairy cell leukemia.

Common to all results of marrow grafting for leukemia and lymphoma is the problem of recurrence of disease due to host cells that have survived the high-dose chemoradiation therapy. New treatment programs being explored in a number of centers are aimed at more effectively destroying the malignant cells, thereby increasing the success of marrow transplantation.

CONCLUSION

Marrow transplantation, once considered a desperate form of therapy in patients with end-stage disease, has now become increasingly successful when used early in the course of aplastic anemia or leukemia. The current success now obliges the physician to identify, soon after diagnosis, those patients who have suitable donors and who may be candidates for transplantation. Marrow grafting has now been extended to the therapy of patients with other hematologic malignant diseases and genetic disorders of hematopoiesis. In the longest survivor with malignant non-Hodgkin's lymphoma, the disease is now in unmaintained remission 16 years after marrow grafting. Cures of congenital Fanconi's anemia, paroxysmal nocturnal hemoglobinuria, thalassemia major, osteopetrosis, and certain genetic storage diseases have been achieved by marrow transplantation.

Many patients do not have HLA-identical siblings, and very few have monozygotic twins. To extend marrow transplantation to a larger number of patients, the use of less well matched family members has been explored, with remarkable success. Successful human transplants from unrelated donors for the treatment of patients with acute and chronic leukemias and aplastic anemia have been carried out. This work has been facilitated by the establishment of national bone marrow donor registries.

With the development of techniques to "purge" marrow from unwanted malignant cells and to cryopreserve marrow for indefinite periods, a renaissance of autologous marrow transplantation for the treatment of malignant diseases has occurred. Autologous marrow is an attractive option, since it avoids the problem of GVHD.

Ferrara JLM, Deeg HJ: Mechanisms of disease: Graft-versus-host disease. N Engl J Med 324:667, 1991. *This is a valuable, up-to-date, brief review of GVHD; with 55 references.*
Moller G (ed.): Graft-versus-host reaction. Immunol Rev 88:1, 1985. *Reviews by multiple authors of the pathophysiology, immunology, treatment, and prevention of acute and chronic GVHD in experimental animals and in humans.*
Storb R: Bone marrow transplantation. In DeVita VT Jr, Hellman S, Rosenberg SA (eds.): Cancer: Principles and Practice of Oncology. Vol. 2. 3rd ed. Philadelphia, JB Lippincott, 1989, pp 2474–2489. *Review of marrow transplantation as treatment for hematologic malignancies.*
Van Rood J, Zwaan F (eds.): Bone marrow transplantation. Semin Hematol 21:1, 1984. *Multiple-author reviews of marrow transplantation for malignant and nonmalignant hematologic diseases, including late complications and immune reconstitution.*

154 Hemorrhagic Disorders: Abnormalities of Platelet and Vascular Function

Marc Shuman

MECHANISMS OF HEMOSTASIS

Normal Hemostasis

Normally, blood clots in response to vascular damage to form a local seal. The mechanisms involved can be divided into three categories:

1. Vasoconstriction
2. Platelet adhesion and aggregation
3. Fibrin formation and stabilization

All three processes are intimately related and are initiated simultaneously. Once the clot is formed and tissue repair has started, digestion of the clot (fibrinolysis) begins, eventually leading to vascular patency. Blood coagulation and fibrinolysis are largely described in Ch. 155.

The normal sequence of events leading to clotting is initiated by trauma to the vessel, which constricts reflexly to reduce blood flow (Fig. 154–1). With damage to the vascular endothelium, platelets adhere to the subendothelial matrix (Fig. 154–2). Tissue factor, a protein-phospholipid complex, is exposed in the vessel wall and activates clotting by binding Factor VII.

The tissue factor–Factor VIIa complex activates coagulation Factor X ("extrinsic pathway") and Factor IX ("intrinsic pathway"). The intrinsic pathway can also be entrained by activation of coagulation Factor XII; however, it is unclear whether or how this is initiated in vivo, under physiologic conditions (Ch. 155).

After the first platelets adhere to the injured vessel, platelet aggregation begins, initiated probably through multifactorial mechanisms (Fig. 154–2). Collagen fibers bind to platelet surface receptors, which activate aggregation and stimulate secretion of intracellular granular contents, including adenosine diphosphate (ADP), prostaglandin G_2 (PGG_2), and thromboxane A_2. These secreted substances mediate and further amplify aggregation. Besides collagen, thrombin in minute concentrations ($\cong$ 1nM) aggregates platelets. Presumably, this is an additional stimulus to aggregation once the soluble clotting factors have been activated.

Platelets secrete serotonin and thromboxane A_2, which enhance vasoconstriction and expose surface sites that bind and accelerate the activation of Factors X and II (prothrombin) (Fig. 154–2). In addition to aggregating platelets, thrombin converts fibrinogen to fibrin, which becomes incorporated into the platelet plug. With crosslinking of fibrin strands by Factor XIIIa, a stable clot is formed.

Normally, activation of clotting and platelets is inhibited by an intact vascular endothelium and continuous blood flow (Fig. 154–3A). Endothelium makes PGI_2, which inhibits platelet activation and is vasodilatory. Thrombomodulin, an integral membrane endothelial protein, serves as a receptor for thrombin, which in this way activates protein C, a potent inhibitor of coagulation (Ch. 155). Activated protein C inactivates coagulation Factors Va and VIIIa. Endothelial cells also make tissue plasminogen activator, the primary activator of intravascular fibrinolysis. Platelets

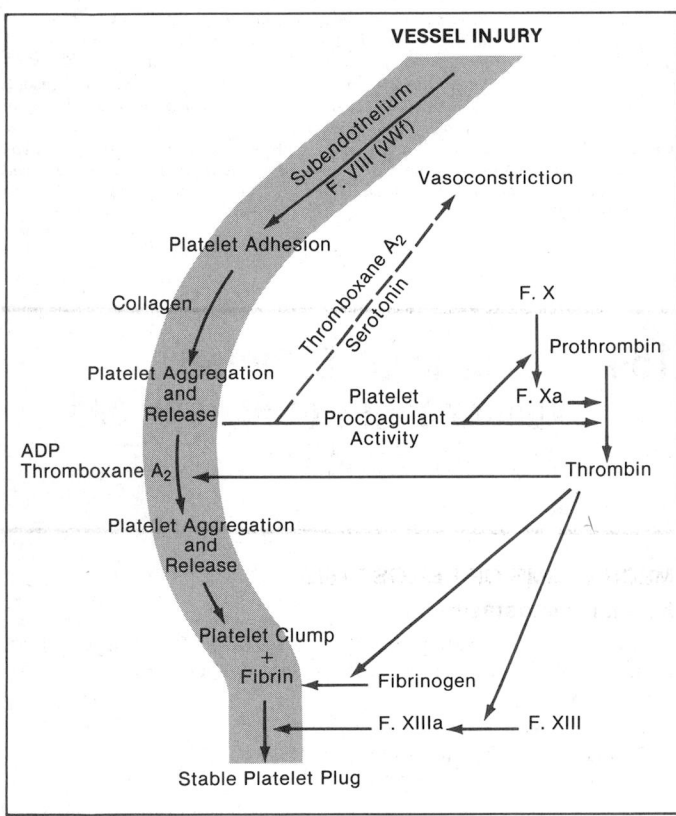

FIGURE 154–1. Schematic representation of platelet participation in hemostasis. Following vascular injury, platelets adhere to exposed subendothelial extracellular matrix. Under high shear conditions, von Willebrand factor (vWf) is required for adhesion. Collagen stimulates platelet secretion and aggregation. Secretion of adenosine diphosphate (ADP) and thromboxane A₂ further amplifies aggregation. Secretion of serotonin and thromboxane A₂ stimulates vasoconstriction. Factors IXa and VIIIa bind to specific platelet receptors, amplifying activation of Factor X. Factors Xa and Va bind to platelet receptors, amplifying thrombin formation. Thrombin aggregates platelets and converts Factor XIIIa and fibrinogen to fibrin. The end-product of these reactions is a crosslinked platelet-fibrin thrombus.

do not bind to the surface of normal endothelial cells. Vascular endothelium contains large amounts of heparan sulfate, a glycosaminoglycan, on its luminal surface. Antithrombin III binds with high affinity to heparan, thus providing a rapid and potent mechanism for inhibiting activated clotting factors. Clearly, the inner lining of blood vessels has a critical function in maintaining vascular patency by inhibiting activation of hemostasis.

Pathologic Hemostasis

Thrombi formed by platelets in the arterial system, called white thrombi, are composed primarily of fibrin and platelets. Red thrombi, found in the venous circulation, are composed of red blood cells trapped in the fibrin meshwork and usually contain few platelets. Clotting is activated pathologically in response to abnormalities in (1) the vessel wall, e.g., atherosclerosis; (2)

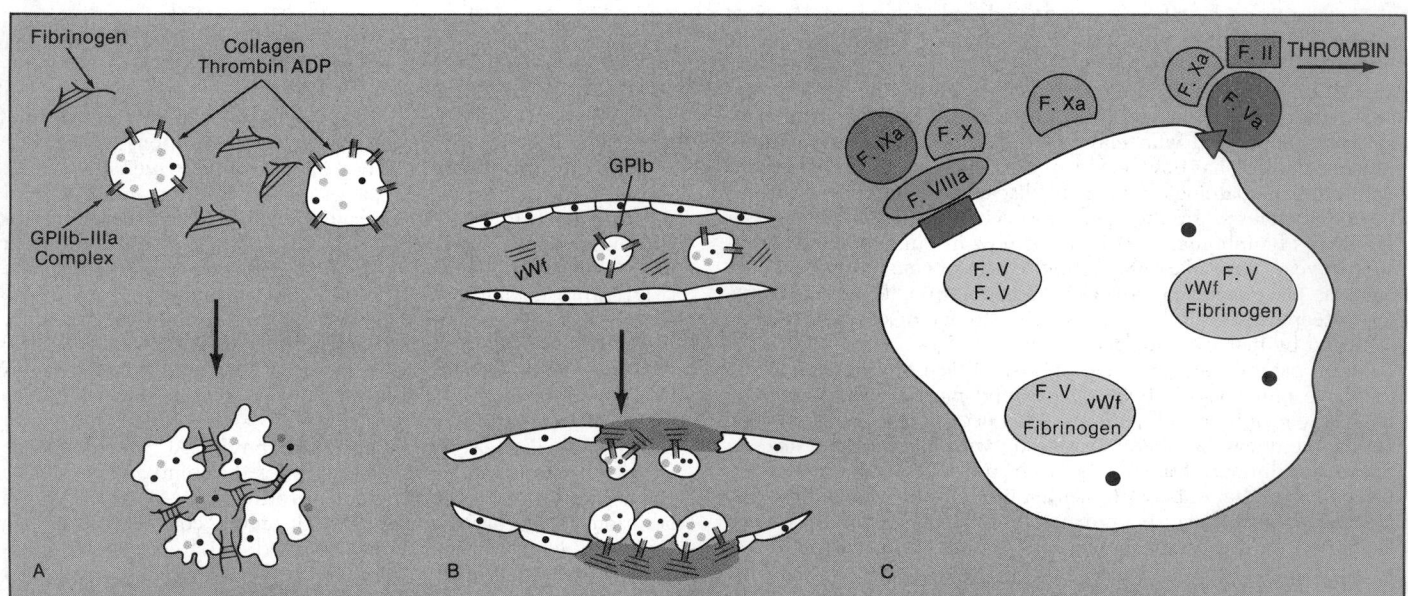

FIGURE 154–2. Platelet aggregation, adhesion, and enhancement of coagulation. *A*, Platelet aggregation. Several physiologic stimuli activate platelets, resulting in fibrinogen binding to specific receptors, GPIIb–IIIa. Binding of fibrinogen is followed by platelet aggregation. *B*, Platelet adhesion. Injury to the vascular endothelium results in exposure of extracellular matrix. Under high shear, von Willebrand factor binds to the platelet receptor GPIb. The platelet-vWf complex then binds to the subendothelium. *C*, Amplification of thrombin formation by platelets. Coagulation Factors IXa, VIIIa, and X form a Ca²⁺-dependent trimolecular complex on the platelet surface. Activation of Factor X is amplified several hundred thousand-fold. Coagulation Factors Xa, Va, and prothrombin form a Ca²⁺-dependent trimolecular complex on platelets. Thrombin formation is amplified several hundred thousand–fold.

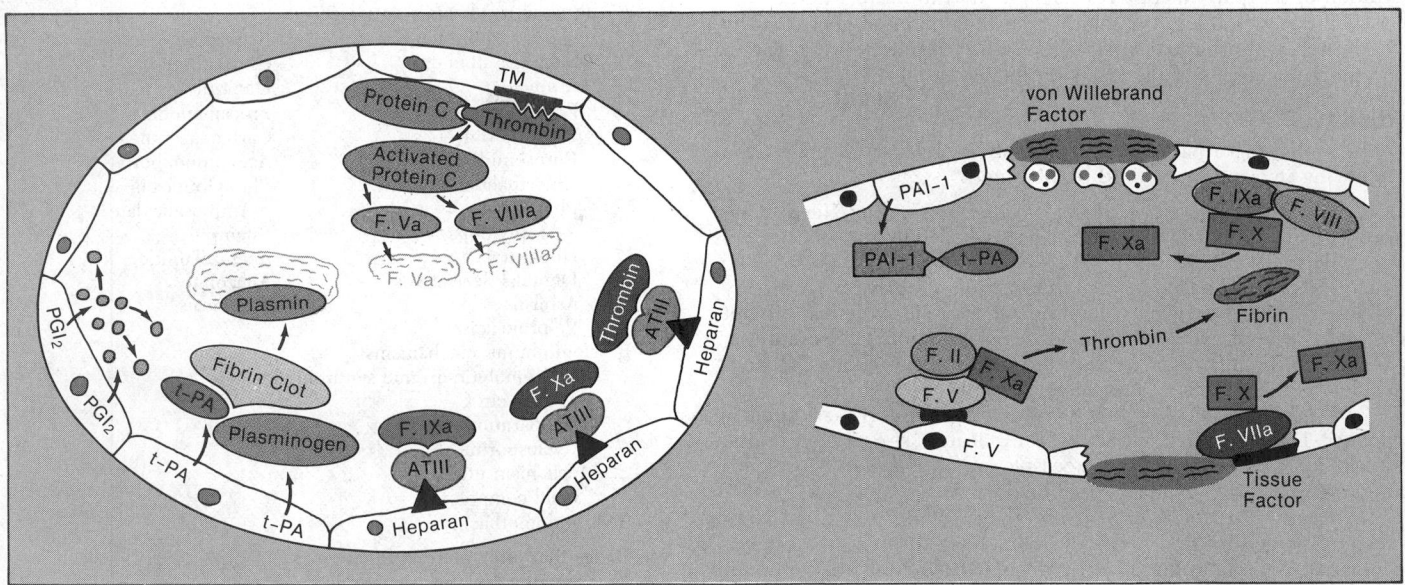

FIGURE 154-3. Regulation of coagulation by vascular endothelium. *Left,* Inhibition of activation of clotting by endothelium. Endothelial cells make substances that inhibit platelet secretion and aggregation and activate clotting factors. In addition, endothelium initiates degradation of the fibrin clot. *Right,* Activation of clotting by vascular endothelium. Injury to endothelium exposes tissue factor, which initiates the extrinsic pathway of clotting. Receptors for activation of Factor X and prothrombin amplify coagulation on the endothelial surface. Endothelium also secretes an inhibitor of clot lysis. PGI_2 = prostaglandin I_2; t-PA = tissue-plasminogen activator; PAI-1 = plasminogen activator inhibitor-1; TM = thrombomodulin; AT III = antithrombin III.

platelets, e.g., myeloproliferative disorders; and (3) the coagulation system, e.g., antithrombin III deficiency. Anatomic and/or biochemical alterations of the vascular intima are by far the most frequent causes of pathologic thrombosis. A variety of pathologic alterations of the vessel wall modify endothelial function in a prothrombotic fashion (Fig. 154-3B). At one extreme, the endothelial lining may be physically disrupted, with exposure of circulating blood to extracellular matrix and tissue factor. On the other hand, several substances may induce intact endothelium to promote thrombosis. Thus, interleukin 1, tumor necrosis factor, and endotoxin increase both endothelial plasminogen activator inhibitor-1, an inhibitor of fibrinolysis, and endothelial tissue factor. Moreover, endothelial cells express receptors for several of the coagulation factors, including Factors Va, IXa, Xa, so that once coagulation is initiated, it can be amplified on the endothelial cell surface. It is not difficult to imagine how rupture of an atherosclerotic plaque results in pathologic initiation of clotting, terminating in vascular occlusion. Thrombosis is clearly an important event in atherosclerotic vascular disease: (1) Platelet thrombi are found in the coronary circulation in fatal myocardial infarction; (2) fibrinolytic therapy can restore blood flow early in coronary occlusion; and (3) thrombin inhibitors prevent reocclusion of vessels after lysis of intracoronary thrombi (experimental studies in animals).

APPROACH TO THE PATIENT WITH A POSSIBLE BLEEDING DISORDER

When evaluating whether a bleeding disorder is present and, if so, its likely cause, very useful information may be obtained from the patient. The history may strongly suggest whether a bleeding diathesis is congenital or acquired and, if the latter, the most likely category into which it falls. Moreover, careful exam-

TABLE 154-1. DIFFERENTIAL DIAGNOSIS OF BLEEDING DISORDERS

	Hereditary			
	Hemophilia	*Von Willebrand's Disease*	*Qualitative Platelet Abnormalities*	*Blood Vessel Disorders*
Genetics	X-Linked recessive	Autosomal dominant	Autosomal dominant Autosomal recessive	Autosomal dominant
Type of Bleeding	Hemarthrosis Visceral CNS Soft tissues	Mucocutaneous	Mucocutaneous	Mucocutaneous Arterial rupture (Connective tissue disorders)
Onset of Bleeding	Delayed	Immediate	Immediate	Immediate
Physical Examination	Joint deformities Hematomas Ecchymoses	Ecchymoses	Petechiae Ecchymoses	Ecchymoses Telangiectasia (HHT) Skin, joint, and eye abnormalities (Connective tissue disorders)
Coagulation Tests	aPTT: Abn	aPTT: Abn/N	N	N
Bleeding Time	N	Abn	Abn	N/Abn
	Acquired			
	Coagulation	*Platelet*	*Blood Vessel Disorders*	
Type of Bleeding	Visceral Soft tissues	Mucocutaneous	Mucocutaneous	
Onset of Bleeding	Delayed	Immediate	Immediate	
Physical Examination	Hematomas Ecchymoses	Petechiae Ecchymoses	Ecchymoses Perifollicular hemorrhage (scurvy)	
Coagulation Tests	PT: Abn/N aPTT: Abn/N	N	N	
Bleeding Time	N	Abn	N/Abn	

CNS = central nervous system; HHT = hereditary hemorrhagic telangiectasia; N = normal; Abn = abnormal; aPTT = activated partial thromboplastin time; PT = prothrombin time.

ination of the patient may reveal signs that indicate whether the patient has a platelet, a vascular, or a coagulation defect. On the basis of this information, one can focus the laboratory investigation on particular types of disorders of hemostasis (Table 154–1).

History

In evaluating a patient with a putative bleeding disorder, the following information should be obtained:

1. *What is the duration of the bleeding tendency?* Has it been present since birth? Was there excessive bleeding at the time of circumcision?

2. *What are the frequency and duration of episodes?* A history of intermittent episodes (bleeding on some occasions, but not others) does not exclude the diagnosis of a hemorrhagic diathesis. Patients with mild von Willebrand's disease or Factor XI deficiency may give this type of history.

3. *What are the triggering events?* Is hemorrhage spontaneous? Has excessive bleeding complicated surgery or dental work? Is menstrual bleeding excessive (menorrhagia)? Was bleeding abnormal at the time of childbirth?

4. *What is the location of hemorrhage?* Skin, joints, gastrointestinal or genitourinary tracts? In platelet disorders, epistaxis, cutaneous bleeding, and excessive vaginal bleeding are common. Joint hemorrhage is common in hemophilia but rare in platelet disorders.

5. *What medication or medications is the patient taking?* (See Table 154–2.)

6. *What is the family history?* Are only males affected? Is there an X-linked recessive maternal pattern of transmission (hemophilia)?

Physical Examination

In platelet abnormalities or vascular defects, hemorrhage is usually mucosal and/or cutaneous. Bleeding from a clotting factor deficiency is often intramuscular or intra-articular. The presence of *petechiae,* small (<3 mm) hemorrhages in the skin or mucous membranes, indicates a platelet or vascular defect. Petechiae are not present in deficiencies of clotting factors. *Purpura,* larger cutaneous hemorrhages, are found more commonly in platelet than in blood clotting disorders. *Hematoma* refers to bleeding into tissues and occurs more commonly in coagulation disorders. Punctate *telangiectasia* on the tongue, nasal mucosa, lips, or fingertips is found in hereditary hemorrhagic telangiectasia.

The history and physical examination alone may strongly indicate into which category a bleeding diathesis falls (Table 154–1).

Laboratory Evaluation

Laboratory evaluation should be directed toward disorders suggested by the patient's history and physical examination. For example, a strong family history of a mild bleeding disorder affecting both sexes raises the possibility of von Willebrand's disease. The finding of petechiae suggests a platelet or blood vessel disorder. When the patient's history and physical examination are not helpful in focusing the investigation, the prothrombin time (PT), activated partial thromboplastin time (aPTT), and platelet count are helpful initial screening tests. An algorithm for proceeding with further evaluation, depending on some common patterns in the initial results, is shown in Figure 154–4.

BLOOD PLATELETS

Formation and Kinetics

Platelets are disc-shaped cells, 2 to 4 μm in diameter, normally found in the peripheral blood (150,000 to 300,000 per microliter). In Wright's-stained blood smears, they are identified by their blue-gray cytoplasm and red (lysosomal) granules and by lack of a nucleus (see Color Plate 5A). Their physiologic role in hemostasis has been described above (Fig. 154–2).

Platelets are formed in the bone marrow from giant polyploid cells called megakaryocytes. Megakaryocytes mature by a series of nuclear replications within a common cytoplasm (endomitosis), leading to four to six lobed nuclei, and by elaboration of specific granules in the cytoplasm. Following maturation, the megakaryocyte cytoplasm becomes demarcated into platelet subunits, and the platelets are released into the circulation through the marrow

TABLE 154–2. DRUGS THAT MAY ALTER HEMOSTASIS

I. Drugs reported to cause thrombocytopenia

A. Immune mechanism proposed*

Quinine/quinidine	Ranitidine
Sulfa compounds	Cimetidine
Ampicillin	Danazol
Penicillin	Procainamide
Thiazide diuretics	Carbamazepine
Furosemide	Acetaminophen
Chlorthalidone	Phenylbutazone
Phenytoin	*p*-Aminosalicylate
α-Methyldopa	Rifampin
Heparin	Acetazolamide
Digitalis derivatives	Anazoline
Aspirin	Arsenicals
Valproic acid	

B. Nonimmune mechanisms
(Hemolytic-uremic syndrome)
Mitomycin C
cis-Platinum
Cyclosporine

C. Mechanism undefined
Gold compounds
Indomethacin

II. Drugs that alter platelet function

A. Primary antiplatelet agents

Aspirin	Sulfinpyrazone
Dextran	Ticlopidine
Dipyridamole	

B. Drugs in which inhibition of platelet function is associated with prolongation of the bleeding time
Nonsteroidal anti-inflammatory agents
β-Lactam antibiotics
ε-Aminocaproic acid (>24 grams/day)
Heparin
Plasminogen activators (streptokinase, urokinase, tissue plasminogen activator)

III. Drugs that affect coagulation factors

A. Induction of antibodies inhibiting function
Lupus anticoagulant†‡
Phenothiazines
Procainamide
Factor VIII antibodies
Penicillin
Factor V antibodies
Aminoglycosides
Factor XIII antibodies
Isoniazid

B. Inhibitors of synthesis of vitamin K–dependent clotting factors (Factors II, VII, IX, X, proteins C and S)
Coumarin compounds
Moxalactam

C. Inhibitor of fibrinogen synthesis
L-Asparaginase‡

*List is limited to drugs for which there are multiple reports and there is in vitro or in vivo evidence for antiplatelet antibodies.

†Does not cause bleeding.

‡May cause thrombosis.

sinusoids. Two hematopoietic growth factors—interleukin 6 (IL6) and granulocyte/macrophage colony-stimulating factor—stimulate megakaryocyte maturation. Interleukin 6 also stimulates platelet production. Both growth factors also stimulate growth of other hematopoietic cells, however, and therefore are not specific.

Ordinarily, 1000 to 3000 platelets are produced from each megakaryocyte. Normally, 3 to 10 megakaryocytes are seen in bone marrow smears under low-power magnification, but none are seen in the peripheral blood smear. Platelets circulate for 9 to 10 days. Approximately one third reside in a splenic pool, which exchanges freely with the circulating pool. In diseases associated with platelet antibodies, the spleen is frequently the site of destruction. In addition, in disorders in which there is secondary splenic enlargement, thrombocytopenia may result from splenic sequestration (Ch. 152). Similarly, following splenectomy, the platelet count may increase to 1×10^6 per microliter.

An estimate of platelet number in the peripheral blood film (normal, increased, decreased) is quite useful in detecting patients with significantly low platelet counts. Normally, there are 3 to 10 platelets per high-power (oil immersion) field on the peripheral smear. Platelets are counted directly by phase microscopy using a counting chamber and a standard dilution of blood or by using an automated particle counter.

Platelet Function

Platelets contain three types of secretory granules: *lysosomes*, *α-granules*, and *dense bodies* (electron-dense organelles) (Fig. 154–5). Lysosomes in platelets, as in all other cells, contain acid hydrolases. α-Granules contain platelet-specific proteins: platelet Factor 4, which neutralizes heparin; β-thromboglobulin; and several growth factors, including platelet-derived growth factor (PDGF), endothelial cell growth factor (PD-ECGF), and transforming growth factor-β (TGF-β). (PDGF and PD-ECGF have also been identified in other tissues since their discovery in platelets.) α-Granules also contain several hemostatic proteins (fibrinogen, Factor V, and Factor VIII:vWf), but why these clotting factors are present in platelets in addition to plasma is unclear. Some of these proteins, such as fibrinogen, are endocytosed by megakaryocytes. Others (von Willebrand factor) are

synthesized by megakaryocytes. Dense bodies (δ-granules) contain adenosine triphosphate (ATP), ADP, Ca^{2+}, and serotonin.

In hemostasis, platelets (1) release potent vasoconstrictors—thromboxane A_2 and serotonin—from their intracellular granules, (2) aggregate and form a plug at the site of vessel injury, and (3) provide a surface for the activation of soluble coagulation factors (Fig. 154–2C).

At high shear rates, platelets require a plasma protein, von Willebrand factor, to adhere to subendothelial extracellular matrix (Fig. 154–2). Platelets aggregate and secrete their granular contents in response to a variety of substances. With striking morphologic changes, platelets discharge the contents of their secretory granules into the canalicular system and then extracellularly. At the same time, the platelet becomes irregularly spherical and develops multiple finger-like projections.

Platelets contain a membrane phospholipase C, which, upon stimulation by activating agents, hydrolyzes endogenous phosphatidylinositol to form a diglyceride. The diglyceride, in turn, is converted to arachidonic acid by a diglyceride lipase. Arachi-

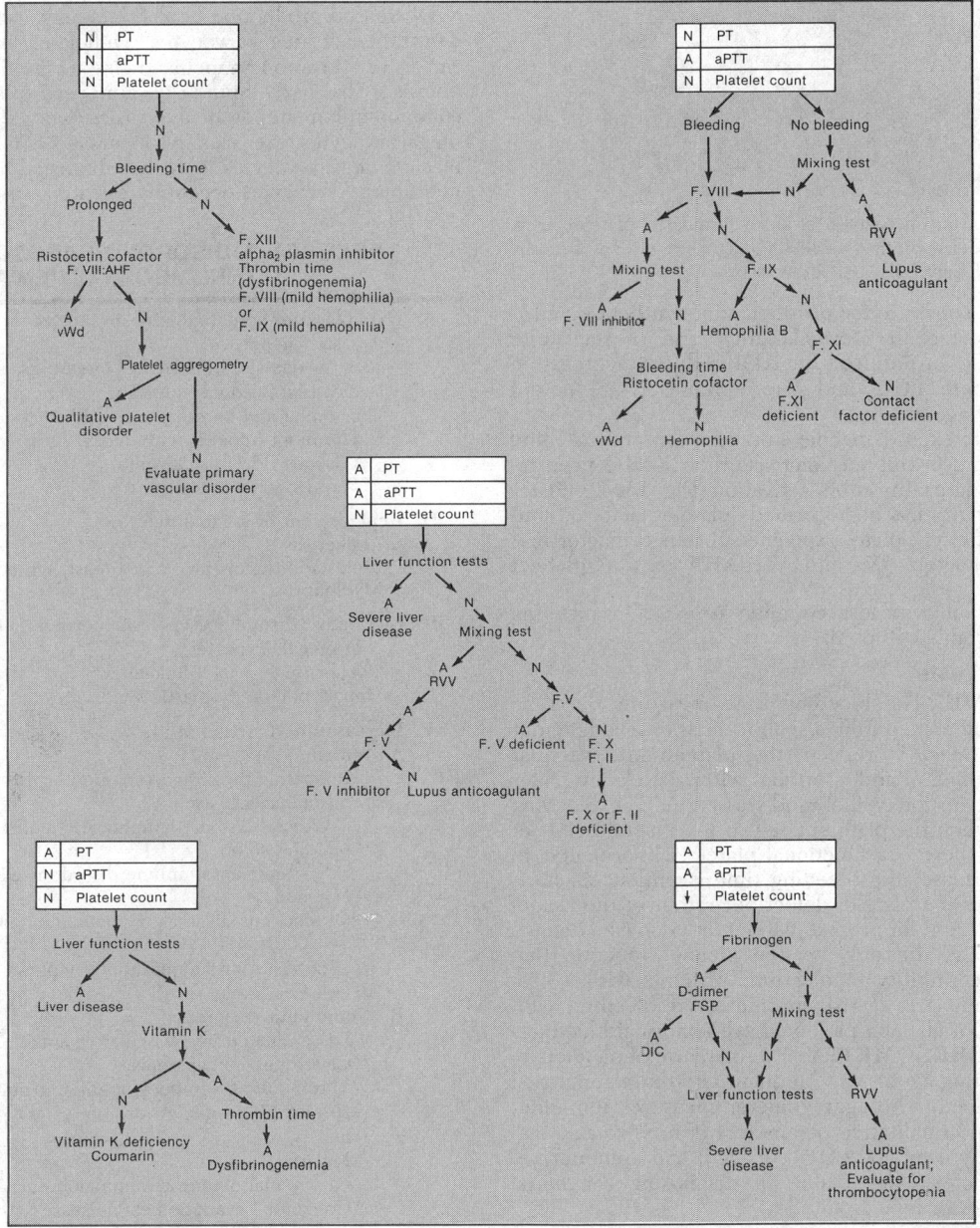

FIGURE 154–4. Algorithm for laboratory evaluation of bleeding disorders. vWd = von Willebrand's disease; A = abnormal; N = normal; RVV = Russell viper venom test; FSP = fibrin split products; PT = prothrombin time; aPTT = activated partial thromboplastin time; AHF = antihemophilic factor; DIC = disseminated intravascular coagulation.

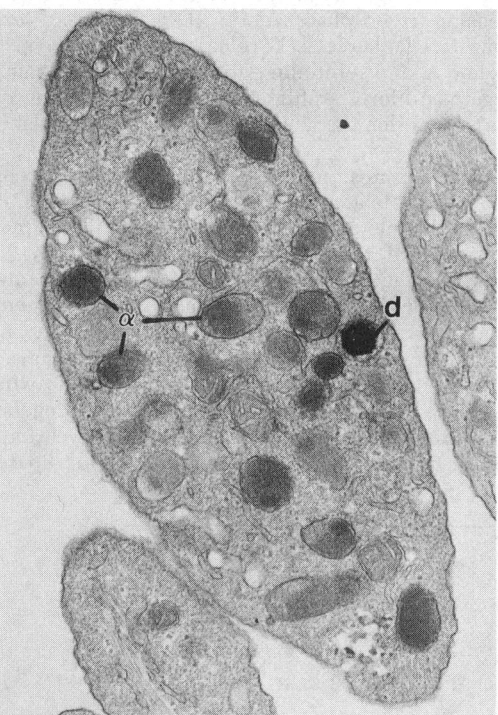

FIGURE 154–5. Electron micrograph of an unstimulated platelet. α = alpha granule; d = dense body (×24000). (Courtesy of Dr. Dorothy Bainton, University of California, San Francisco.)

donic acid acts as a substrate for prostaglandin synthetase and is subsequently converted to prostaglandins. The prostaglandin endoperoxide, PGG_2, is required for ADP-induced aggregation and release, and both PGG_2 and thromboxane A_2 are potent platelet aggregating agents.

Activated platelets expose specific surface receptors that bind Factor Xa and Va and in this way increase their local concentration, thus accelerating prothrombin activation (Fig. 154–2). Platelet procoagulant activity has been termed "platelet factor 3," but this refers to an activity, not to a specific substance. Factor X is also activated by Factors IXa and VIII:AHF on the platelet surface.

Platelet dysfunction is a less common cause of a bleeding diathesis than is thrombocytopenia.

Platelet Function Tests

BLEEDING TIME. The bleeding time measures the time required for bleeding to stop from a shallow incision, made under standardized conditions. It reflects the platelet and vascular components of coagulation and is normal with coagulation factor deficiencies (except in von Willebrand's disease). The bleeding time is prolonged when the platelet count is less than 90,000 per microliter or when there is a functional platelet abnormality. In von Willebrand's disease, the bleeding time is prolonged; however, this is not due to a platelet defect but rather to the lack of a plasma factor important for normal platelet function (see below). The bleeding time is the only test of platelet function that correlates with susceptibility to bleeding. Patients with a prolonged bleeding time are at risk for increased bleeding with surgery; however, not all such patients have abnormal bleeding.

PLATELET AGGREGOMETRY. The response of platelets to a variety of aggregating agents can be quantitated in platelet-rich plasma or whole blood. The aggregometer measures temporal, semiquantitative, and qualitative parameters of in vitro aggregation. Agents typically used are ADP, collagen, and epinephrine. This technique is of greatest value in diagnosing congenital qualitative platelet disorders.

ABNORMALITIES IN PLATELET COUNT

Thrombocytopenia

Low platelet counts (thrombocytopenia) can be caused by disturbances in production, in distribution, or in destruction.

The consequences of thrombocytopenia are entirely hemostatic. With normally functioning platelets, the following is expected:

1. Platelet count ≥ 100,000 per microliter—patients have no abnormal bleeding even with major surgery.
2. Platelet count, 50,000 to 100,000 per microliter—patients may bleed longer than normal with severe trauma.
3. Platelet count 20,000 to 50,000 per microliter—bleeding occurs with minor trauma, but spontaneous bleeding is unusual.
4. Platelet count < 20,000 per microliter—patients may have spontaneous bleeding.
5. Platelet count < 10,000 per microliter—patients are at high risk for severe bleeding.

DECREASED PRODUCTION OF PLATELETS

Hypoplasia of hematopoietic stem cells due to a variety of disorders may cause thrombocytopenia (Table 154–3); most of these disorders are discussed in other chapters. These include decreased numbers of megakaryoblasts and replacement of the bone marrow by abnormal tissue. Examination of the bone marrow reveals decreased numbers of megakaryocytes and either an overall decrease in cellularity or an infiltration by abnormal cells.

Decreased production of platelets may also be due to abnormal maturation of megakaryocytes. Deficiency of either B_{12} or folate can cause thrombocytopenia owing to ineffective thrombocytopoiesis (Ch. 132). Similarly, abnormal platelet production is common in hematopoietic dysplasias (Ch. 129). In both disorders, megakaryocytes are usually increased. In hematopoietic dysplasia, megakaryocytes may be abnormal in appearance, e.g., micromegakaryocytes occasionally with a single-lobed nucleus.

TABLE 154–3. DISORDERS ASSOCIATED WITH THROMBOCYTOPENIA

I. **Hypoplasia of hematopoietic stem cells**
   Aplastic anemia
   Marrow damage from drugs, chemicals, ionizing radiation, alcohol, infection
   Congenital and hereditary thrombocytopenias
      Thrombocytopenia with absent radii syndrome
      Wiskott-Aldrich syndrome
      May-Hegglin anomaly

II. **Replacement of normal marrow**
   Leukemias
   Metastatic tumor (prostate, breast, lymphoma)
   Myelofibrosis

III. **Ineffective thrombocytopoiesis (normal or increased numbers of megakaryocytes)**
   Cobalamin or folate deficiency
   Hematopoietic dysplastic syndromes

IV. **Increased destruction of platelets**
   A. Immune disorders
      Idiopathic thrombocytopenic purpura (ITP)
      Secondary causes:
         Cancer: chronic lymphocytic leukemia, lymphoma, and so on
         Systemic autoimmune disorders: SLE, polyarteritis nodosa
         Infectious diseases: infectious mononucleosis, CMV, HIV
         Drugs: quinine/quinidine, heparin, sulfa compounds (see Table 154–1)
   B. Nonimmune disorders
      Disseminated intravascular coagulation
      Cavernous hemangioma
      Thrombotic thrombocytopenic purpura
      Hemolytic-uremic syndrome
      Sepsis
      Malaria
      Paroxysmal nocturnal hemoglobinuria
      Congenital cyanotic heart disease
      Acute renal transplant rejection

V. **Disorders of distribution**
   Hypersplenism
VI. **Dilutional: secondary to transfusion**

IMMUNE DISORDERS. Three types of immunologic reactions result in the premature destruction of platelets: (1) the development of autoantibodies against platelet membrane antigens, (2) the binding of immune complexes to platelet Fc receptors, and (3) the lysis of platelets due to fixation of complement on their surface.

Idiopathic Thrombocytopenic Purpura (ITP). Idiopathic thrombocytopenic purpura is an autoimmune bleeding disorder characterized by the development of antibodies to one's own platelets, which are then destroyed by phagocytosis in the spleen and, to a lesser extent, the liver. Childhood ITP is usually acute and follows recovery from a viral infection. The incidence is equal in boys and girls. In adults, the onset is usually more gradual, without a preceding illness and with a chronic course. In a small percentage of adult cases, the disease has an acute onset. Ninety per cent of adults with ITP are under the age of 40, and the ratio of women to men is 3–4:1. In some patients' sera, antibodies against platelet glycoproteins IIb and IIIa have been observed. Patients develop petechiae, ecchymoses, and epistaxis. Women may develop menorrhagia. Death due to hemorrhage is unusual in chronic ITP, approximately 5 per cent of cases. Cerebral bleeding occurs in ~1 per cent of cases.

The diagnosis of ITP is usually one of exclusion of underlying systemic disorders that result in increased peripheral destruction or decreased production of platelets. On physical examination, the spleen is not enlarged, although it may be in childhood ITP as a consequence of viral infection. In ITP, the hemoglobin is normal unless the patient has significant bleeding. The peripheral blood smear reveals normochromic, normocytic red blood cells. Similarly, the leukocyte count and differential are normal, although these values may continue to reflect a preceding viral illness in children. Several assays for detecting antiplatelet antibodies on the platelet surface have been proposed. The value of these assays in diagnosing ITP, analogous to the direct Coombs test used to detect antibodies against red blood cells, is unclear. Most of these tests do not distinguish between autoantibodies and immune complexes that bind to the platelet Fc receptor. Furthermore, these assays do not differentiate between specific antiplatelet antibodies, and nonspecifically absorbed immunoglobulin G (IgG). In most cases of ITP, the diagnosis is clear-cut, and confirming the presence of antiplatelet antibodies is unnecessary. In complex cases, the antibody test may be helpful. The level of platelet-associated IgG does not correlate with the severity of thrombocytopenia. In more than 90 per cent of cases of chronic ITP, the antibody is IgG; most are IgG1.

If the general clinical evaluation and blood tests do not confirm the diagnosis of systemic disorders causing thrombocytopenia, the bone marrow should be examined. In ITP, the marrow is normal, although megakaryocytes may be increased in number (see Color Plate 8J).

In children, the disease is self-limited. Approximately 70 per cent recover within 4 to 6 weeks. In adults, indications for treatment depend on the severity of bleeding and the degree of thrombocytopenia. Asymptomatic patients with platelet counts above 40,000 per microliter can be observed with periodic evaluation to determine the natural fluctuations of their disease. On the other hand, patients with platelet counts below 20,000 per microliter are usually symptomatic and require treatment. Patients with platelet counts above 30,000 per microliter who have bleeding may have an acquired platelet function abnormality due to the antibody. Initially, bleeding associated with ITP is treated with prednisone or a similar corticosteroid at a dose of 1 to 2 mg per kilogram per day. Prednisone inhibits macrophage ingestion of antibody-coated platelets, in addition to suppressing antibody synthesis. Prednisone has also been shown to have a stabilizing effect on small blood vessels in thrombocytopenic animals. In 80 to 90 per cent of patients, the platelet count rises to hemostatic levels within 2 to 3 weeks. Failure to respond to steroids is indicated by a platelet count below 50,000 per microliter after 4 weeks of treatment. A subnormal platelet count after 6 weeks of treatment indicates steroid failure also. Once the platelet count has reached its apex and is stable, steroids should be tapered slowly. When the dose of prednisone is tapered, however, most patients (~90 per cent) exhibit a relapse of thrombocytopenia. Thus, the primary benefit of prednisone is in the acute management of bleeding.

Another effective approach to managing patients who are actively bleeding or for whom major surgery is necessary is the use of intravenous γ globulin. Immunoglobulin G concentrates raise the platelet count within 3 to 5 days in most patients and thus is the most rapidly active agent. Unfortunately, the therapeutic effect is usually transient, since the platelet count falls to baseline levels over the next month. In a few instances, repeated infusions of γ globulin lead to sustained remissions after discontinuation of therapy. It is proposed that IgG works by blocking Fc receptors on macrophages, thereby inhibiting phagocytosis. The dosage is 1 gram per kilogram per day on 2 successive days. In 80 per cent of patients, the platelet count rises above 50,000 per microliter with this therapy. Owing to the lack of a sustained remission in most patients with severe thrombocytopenia treated with steroids or IgG, a more definitive approach is necessary. Splenectomy results in improvement of the platelet count in ~70 per cent of patients and in sustained remission in approximately 60 per cent of patients with ITP, but there are no reliable tests to predict which patients will respond. The platelet count rises within a few days after splenectomy, or at most in 1 to 2 weeks. Benefit from splenectomy appears to be due to at least two mechanisms. As indicated, the spleen is the principal reticuloendothelial site of platelet destruction in ITP. In addition, the spleen appears to be the major site of synthesis of antibody production in ITP, with sufficient amounts made to account for the degree of thrombocytopenia seen.

A variety of other therapies have been shown to be efficacious in inducing partial or complete remissions in patients with chronic ITP in whom splenectomy has failed. Danazol, 200 mg three times per day, induces a remission in approximately 40 per cent of patients with chronic ITP. Response is delayed and takes anywhere from 4 to 6 weeks. The mechanism by which danazol induces a remission is unknown. Intravenous vincristine and vinblastine also raise the platelet count in ITP, usually within 1 to 2 weeks. Responses are transient, and remissions are not sustained.

Immunosuppressive agents—cyclophosphamide and azathioprine—have also been used to induce remissions in chronic ITP. Because of the small numbers of patients reported, the relative efficacy of these two drugs is unclear. Success in improving the platelet count has been reported in 20 to 30 per cent of cases. The potential benefit of these drugs must be weighed against the risks of toxicity, immunosuppression, suppression of hematopoiesis, and, in the case of cyclophosphamide, acute leukemia.

Management of ITP in pregnancy is complicated by the additional risk to the fetus of developing thrombocytopenia secondary to maternal antibodies. Intraventricular hemorrhage, gastrointestinal bleeding, and death have been reported in these newborns. Whether the mother had ITP prior to pregnancy is critical. When women first develop ITP during pregnancy, the risk of serious bleeding in the newborn is negligible. However, neonates born to women with a history of ITP preceding pregnancy have a 20 per cent risk of severe thrombocytopenia. Therefore, in addition to treating the underlying ITP, cesarean delivery is recommended to decrease the risk of intracranial bleeding in these newborns.

Berchtold P, McMillan R: Therapy of chronic idiopathic thrombocytopenic purpura in adults. Blood 74: 2309, 1989. *Reviews current experience with therapeutic options in ITP as well as experimental approaches.*

Platelet Antibodies Associated with Systemic Disorders. Antibodies directed against platelets and causing thrombocytopenia occur in several types of disorders, in all of which bone marrow megakaryocytes are normal or increased in number.

Immune Thrombocytopenia Due to Cancer. Antibody-mediated destruction of platelets occurs in lymphoproliferative disorders, such as chronic lymphocytic leukemia and lymphoma. Generally, thrombocytopenia improves with treatment of the underlying malignancy. Immune thrombocytopenia has also been associated with nonhematologic tumors, but it is unclear whether or not these have been chance associations. The platelet count improves with immunosuppressive therapy such as prednisone.

Thrombocytopenia Associated with Systemic Autoimmune Disorders. Immune thrombocytopenia is common in systemic lupus erythematosus (SLE) (Ch. 261). Whether this is due to specific antiplatelet antibodies, to antibodies against common antigens also found on platelets, or to immune complexes is unclear. The platelet count is usually mildly to moderately decreased. Treatment is usually directed at SLE, as other manifestations of the disease are present in most cases.

Occasionally, immune thrombocytopenia occurs in patients who have serologic evidence of lupus but who do not meet all of the criteria for the diagnosis of SLE. The decision to treat such patients with splenectomy is a difficult one, since other manifestations of SLE may appear subsequently. If the platelet count is severely decreased (less than 30,000 per microliter) and the patient has no other complications of SLE, splenectomy is a reasonable course of action. However, if the platelet count is moderately decreased (≥30,000 to 40,000 per microliter) and the patient does not have major bleeding problems, careful observation may be the best course.

Monthly intravenous cyclophosphamide, 0.75 to 1.0 gram per square meter of body surface area, has recently been shown to normalize platelet counts within 2 to 18 weeks in patients with SLE who were also taking prednisone. This therapy also allowed significant reduction in steroid dosage in these patients.

Immune thrombocytopenia occurs less commonly in other systemic autoimmune disorders.

Immune Thrombocytopenia with Viral Illnesses. Thrombocytopenia associated with antiplatelet antibodies has been reported in patients with infectious mononucleosis, with human immunodeficiency virus (HIV) infection, and with cytomegalovirus (CMV) infection. In the case of infectious mononucleosis and CMV infection, thrombocytopenia is usually self-limiting, with recovery in 3 to 4 weeks. In patients with severe thrombocytopenia, a short course of glucocorticoids may be indicated. The nature of the immune reaction has not been characterized.

HIV Thrombocytopenia (Ch. 419). Thrombocytopenia occurs frequently in patients infected with HIV, whether or not the illness has progressed to acquired immunodeficiency syndrome (AIDS). Patients are usually asymptomatic. Frequently, the causes are multifactorial: (1) infection causing increased platelet destruction and/or inhibition of platelet production due to granulomatous replacement of the bone marrow, (2) suppression of hematopoiesis by drugs used to treat AIDS or associated infections, and (3) immune destruction of the patient's own platelets. Antibodies associated with platelets have been demonstrated in these patients, although it is unclear whether thrombocytopenia is due to immune complexes bound to platelets or to specific antiplatelet antibodies. Treatment with prednisone is hazardous owing to the immunocompromised status of these patients. Similarly, splenectomy has the disadvantage of further compromising the immune system. Azidothymidine (AZT) treatment may raise the platelet count in some patients with mild to moderate thrombocytopenia. For acute bleeding, intravenous γ globulin raises the platelet count within a few days.

Immune Thrombocytopenia Due to Drug-Induced Antibodies (Table 154–2). More than 50 drugs have been reported to cause immune thrombocytopenia, but infrequently with conclusive in vitro confirmation. Quinine and quinidine often cause immune thrombocytopenia, and drug-dependent antibodies have been demonstrated conclusively. Sulfa compounds, including sulfisoxazole, sulfonamide, sulfamethoxypyridazine, and sulfamethazene, have also been demonstrated to cause immune thrombocytopenia. There are also multiple reports of immune thrombocytopenia caused by hydrochlorothiazide, phenytoin, methyldopa, heparin, and digitalis derivatives. In most instances, the drug must be present for antibody binding and thrombocytopenia to occur. Therefore, the platelet count returns to normal within a few days after discontinuation of the drug. Glucocorticoids do not accelerate recovery in drug-induced thrombocytopenia. Platelet antibody tests with and without the putative offending agent are useful in determining the cause of thrombocytopenia. Unfortunately, the test cannot be performed until the drug has been cleared from the plasma. In addition, a drug metabolite may be responsible for antibody formation and binding to platelets rather than the parent compound. Unless the metabolite is specifically tested, a negative result will be obtained.

Heparin-Induced Thrombocytopenia. The incidence of thrombocytopenia associated with heparin therapy appears to be 3 to 5 per cent, with a higher percentage of cases associated with bovine

TABLE 154–4. DIFFERENTIAL DIAGNOSIS OF ANEMIA AND THROMBOCYTOPENIA

Diagnostic Study	Autoimmune Disorders (Evans' Syndrome, Collagen-Vascular Disease)	Disseminated Intravascular Coagulation	Thrombotic Thrombocytopenic Purpura/Hemolytic-Uremic Syndrome
Peripheral blood smear	Microspherocytes	Schistocytes (+)	Schistocytes (+ + +)
Reticulocyte count	Increased (+ + +)	N/Increased (+)	Increased (+ + +)
Coombs' test	Positive	Negative	Negative
Coagulation tests	N	Abn (+ + +)	N/Abn (+)

N = normal; Abn = abnormal.

than with porcine preparations. The platelet count usually decreases after the first few days of treatment; the decline is gradual and is not usually associated with bleeding. The platelet count is rapidly corrected after heparin is discontinued. If the platelet count falls below 50,000 per microliter, heparin should be discontinued. Thrombocytopenia has been reported with the usual therapeutic doses as well as with the very low doses used for procedures such as hemodialysis.

NONIMMUNE DISORDERS ASSOCIATED WITH INCREASED CONSUMPTION OF PLATELETS. *Disseminated Intravascular Coagulation (DIC)* (Ch. 155). In this syndrome, discussed elsewhere, coagulation is pathologically activated, resulting in thrombin formation and the subsequent removal of platelets from the circulation.

Thrombotic Thrombocytopenic Purpura (TTP). This is a rare disease of unknown etiology, characterized by severe thrombocytopenia, microangiopathic hemolytic anemia (>96 per cent of patients), and neurologic abnormalities (>92 per cent of patients). Fever and renal involvement—proteinuria, hematuria, azotemia, and casts—are present in 98 per cent and 88 per cent of patients, respectively. Renal abnormalities are usually mild; the creatinine rarely exceeds 3.0 mg per deciliter. Azotemia is usually reversible, concomitant with remission, in contrast to the hemolytic-uremic syndrome (see below), in which renal failure is common and patients frequently have chronic renal insufficiency. In the involved organs, small vessels—i.e., arterioles and capillaries—are occluded by a hyaline material consisting principally of platelet thrombi. In addition, fibrin is detected in the vessel wall. Virtually any organ may be involved. Symptoms frequently wax and wane, presumably owing to aggregation and disaggregation of platelets. Thus, patients may have evanescent headache or aphasia or may be stuporous one moment and alert the next.

Thrombotic thrombocytopenic purpura must be considered when there is the acute onset of thrombocytopenia and anemia with microangiopathic changes of red blood cells on the peripheral blood smear in the absence of evidence of other disorders (Tables 154–4 and 154–5) (see Color Plate 6E, right). Although similar findings are present in DIC, patients with TTP have minimal changes in coagulation tests. Evans' syndrome, autoimmune hemolytic anemia and thrombocytopenia, is characterized by microspherocytes on peripheral smear, rather than by schistocytes, and by a positive Coombs test. Rarely, TTP has been reported to complicate SLE. More

TABLE 154–5. DISORDERS ASSOCIATED WITH THROMBOCYTOPENIA AND MICROANGIOPATHIC ANEMIA

Thrombotic thrombocytopenic purpura
Hemolytic-uremic syndrome
Disseminated intravascular coagulation
Malignant hypertension
Eclampsia
Vasculitis
  SLE
  Polyarteritis nodosa
Cavernous hemangioma
  (Kasabach-Merritt syndrome)
Disseminated carcinoma
Renal allograft rejection
Prosthetic heart valves
Malignant angioendotheliomatosis

commonly, patients with SLE have immune thrombocytopenia and anemia of chronic disease or immune hemolytic anemia (Ch. 261). Some patients with SLE, however, have microangiopathic hemolysis due to vasculitis. Thrombotic thrombocytopenic purpura has also been reported in association with oral contraceptives and pregnancy. In most cases, the diagnosis of TTP is straightforward. When the diagnosis is uncertain, gum, skin, or bone marrow biopsy may be helpful, with positive results reported in 40 to 60 per cent of cases. It is extremely important to establish the diagnosis and begin treatment rapidly, as delay in treatment can result in severe morbidity or in mortality. If untreated, most patients die within 3 months. Large-volume plasmapheresis, approximately two plasma volumes, with replacement infusion of normal plasma, is the treatment of choice for TTP, with a cure of approximately 70 per cent of patients. Infusion of large volumes of plasma without pheresis has induced remission in some patients also. However, not all patients respond to plasma infusion alone, and concomitant plasmapheresis becomes necessary. Since repeated courses of plasma infusion are usually necessary, the practical management of TTP is facilitated by plasmapheresis, which prevents excessive expansion of the blood volume and the subsequent risk of cardiovascular compromise. The best indication of the response to treatment is the platelet count, as a rise in platelets is the first sign of improvement. Plasmapheresis/plasma infusion should be continued until the platelet count is normal and stable. Complete correction of anemia and of neurologic signs and symptoms usually follows normalization of the platelet count. Why these treatments work is unknown. Approximately 10 per cent of patients have a chronic, relapsing form of TTP. In chronic TTP, abnormally large multimers of von Willebrand factor are present in the plasma of patients in remission.

Eisenstaedt RS, Colman RW, Marder VJ: Thrombotic thrombocytopenic purpura. In Colman RW, Hirsh J, Marder VJ, et al. (eds.): Hemostasis and Thrombosis: Basic Principles and Clinical Practice. 2nd ed. Philadelphia, JB Lippincott, 1987, pp 1016–1025. *A comprehensive review of the clinical manifestations; also includes current theories of pathogenesis and a review of therapeutic options.*

Hemolytic-Uremic Syndrome (HUS). Primarily a disorder of infants and young children, HUS rarely occurs in adults. Like those with TTP, patients with HUS have microangiopathic hemolytic anemia, but thrombocytopenia is mild to moderate and neurologic symptoms and signs are not present. In HUS, acute renal failure is a prominent feature, frequently requiring hemodialysis, while in TTP, the serum creatinine level is rarely higher than 2.5 mg per deciliter at presentation. Severe hypertension is a prominent feature also. Children typically present with gastrointestinal signs and symptoms, abdominal pain, and diarrhea. Hemolytic-uremic syndrome may occur in women who are in the postpartum period or who are taking oral contraceptives. In addition, HUS has been reported in patients with cancer who are receiving mitomycin C or *cis*-platinum chemotherapy.

Sepsis. In gram-negative (more commonly than gram-positive) sepsis, there is increased destruction of platelets apart from possible DIC. Binding of immune complexes of bacteria to the platelet may account for their accelerated destruction. Severe thrombocytopenia may occur.

DISORDERS OF DISTRIBUTION OF PLATELETS

With splenic enlargement, platelet pooling increases (e.g., Gaucher's disease, congestive splenomegaly, lymphoma) and may cause thrombocytopenia (Ch. 152). Platelet counts below 30,000 to 50,000 per microliter are unusual, however.

DILUTIONAL THROMBOCYTOPENIA

When packed erythrocytes or whole blood that is not fresh is transfused to replace blood loss, thrombocytopenia may occur. Approximately 35 to 40 per cent of platelets remain after replacement of one blood volume; microvascular bleeding due to thrombocytopenia occurs rarely after replacement of one to two blood volumes. Platelets should not be transfused unless thrombocytopenia and bleeding are documented. An algorithm for evaluating thrombocytopenia is shown in Figure 154–6.

Thrombocytosis

Elevation of the platelet count above the normal range is due to increased production and either is reactive or results from a myeloproliferative disorder. Most frequently, thrombocytosis is a secondary effect of an underlying disorder and not associated with complications. However, when it is due to a primary disorder of hematopoiesis, serious bleeding and/or thrombotic complications may result. Therefore, it is important to determine the cause of thrombocytosis.

ESSENTIAL THROMBOCYTHEMIA. Essential thrombocythemia is a myeloproliferative disorder in which the platelet count is elevated, frequently over 1×10^6 per microliter, and may be greater than 2×10^6 per microliter (see Color Plate 8K, right). In this disorder, platelet production is increased owing to a primary abnormality in megakaryocytopoiesis, with increased production of megakaryocytes and, consequently, of platelets. Complications may include thrombosis and/or bleeding. The former is the most common cause of death. In addition to increased numbers of platelets, abnormalities in platelet function have been demonstrated. Other myeloproliferative diseases, such as *agnogenic myeloid metaphasia* and *polycythemia vera*, are also associated with an elevated platelet count. The platelet count may be elevated in chronic myelogenous leukemia but rarely results in complications. Essential thrombocytopenia is discussed in detail in Ch. 143, which covers the myeloproliferative disorders.

REACTIVE THROMBOCYTOSIS. Elevated platelet counts occur secondarily in a number of unrelated disorders, but counts higher than 1×10^6 per microliter are unusual: *iron deficiency anemia; hemorrhage; post splenectomy* (Ch. 152); *inflammatory disorders, particularly inflammatory bowel disease; neoplasms (e.g., lung, gastrointestinal); leukemoid reaction* (Ch. 141).

No convincing evidence exists that reactive thrombocytosis increases the risk of thrombosis. Therefore, it should not be treated. With successful treatment of the primary disease, the count returns to normal.

Mitus AJ, Schafer AI: Thrombocytosis and thrombocythemia. In Colman RW, Rao AK (eds.): Platelets in health and disease. Hematol Clin North Am 4:157, 1990. *Complete discussion of the pathophysiology of thrombocytosis and its complications in myeloproliferative disorders as well as its differentiation from secondary causes.*

ABNORMALITIES IN PLATELET FUNCTION

Acquired Disorders of Platelet Function

DRUGS THAT INHIBIT PLATELET FUNCTION (Table 154–2). *Nonsteroidal anti-inflammatory agents* inhibit platelet function by blocking platelet synthesis of prostaglandins. Aspirin (acetylsalicylic acid, or ASA) irreversibly acetylates prostaglandin synthetase, and, as a result, platelet function is impaired for its lifespan. One ASA tablet (300 mg) is sufficient to cause this effect. Fortunately, in normal people, this does not result in excessive bleeding, but in patients with von Willebrand's disease or with severe coagulation factor deficiency (Factor VIII or IX), serious bleeding can result. For this reason, aspirin is contraindicated in these disorders.

High doses of the β-*lactam antibiotics*. i.e., penicillin and related compounds, induce a significant abnormality in platelet function that persists for 2 to 3 days after the drug is discontinued. The mechanism is unclear. The bleeding time is prolonged, and patients may have increased bleeding.

Renal Failure. Platelets function abnormally in patients with renal failure. The uremic metabolites responsible for this dysfunction are uncertain. Guanidinosuccinic acid and phenolic compounds that accumulate in uremia may inhibit platelet aggregation. Abnormal platelet adhesion and activation may occur in uremia as well as thrombocytopenia. The latter is usually mild and may be due to the underlying cause of renal disease.

Uremic bleeding is usually mucocutaneous and reflects abnormal platelet and/or vascular hemostatic functions. The bleeding time is commonly prolonged, but other causes of prolongation must be excluded (e.g., medication, congenital platelet disorders, and von Willebrand's disease). Moreover, a low hematocrit (<24 per cent) prolongs the bleeding time in uremia. Transfusion of packed red blood cells to a hematocrit above 26 per cent improves the bleeding time. Tests of coagulation are normal.

When a uremic patient is bleeding, the possibility of a structural lesion or other hemostatic abnormalities must be evaluated. When the hemostatic defect of renal failure is believed to be a significant contributing factor in bleeding, the patient should be dialyzed. Either peritoneal dialysis or hemodialysis is usually effective in reversing the hemostatic defect. If the bleeding time remains prolonged, and the patient is bleeding, other agents that have been reported to improve or correct the bleeding time can be tried: low-dose estrogens, 1-deamino-8-D-arginine vasopressin (DDAVP), or cryoprecipitate. The efficacy of these agents in managing uremic bleeding has not been firmly established. All three raise the plasma levels of Factor VIII:AHF/vWf, but uremic patients usually already have normal concentrations of these proteins. Because the abnormalities in renal disease are extracellular, i.e., in the plasma, platelet transfusion is not usually beneficial.

HEPATIC FAILURE (Ch. 123). Platelet function is sometimes abnormal in liver disease, but why this is so and the extent to which this dysfunction contributes to bleeding in these patients are unclear. The bleeding time may be prolonged in moderately severe liver disease when the platelet count is above 90,000 per microliter. DDAVP has been reported to improve the bleeding time in these circumstances. More commonly in hepatic failure, a bleeding diathesis is due to deficiencies of coagulation factors (Ch. 123).

PARAPROTEINEMIAS (Ch. 151). Abnormal platelet function occurs in a subset of patients with multiple myeloma, or Waldenström's macroglobulinemia. The bleeding time is usually prolonged in these patients, and bleeding can be moderately severe. If the level of the paraprotein is lowered by plasmapheresis and/or chemotherapy, the bleeding time and bleeding improve, suggesting a direct effect of the paraprotein on platelet function.

Paraproteins may impair platelet function by inhibiting platelet-fibrinogen interaction.

ACQUIRED STORAGE POOL DISEASE. Patients may develop mild platelet function abnormalities from loss of storage granules. Some of the situations or disorders in which this has been reported include cardiopulmonary bypass surgery, hairy cell leukemia, and disorders with antiplatelet autoantibodies. Platelet dysfunction following bypass surgery is transient and not of clinical importance once the first 24 hours after surgery have elapsed.

MYELOPROLIFERATIVE DISORDERS. Patients with essential thrombocythemia and, less commonly, agnogenic myeloid metaplasia, may have abnormalities of platelet function. In essential thrombocythemia, abnormalities usually occur at platelet counts greater than 1×10^6 per microliter and may lead to abnormal bleeding, thrombosis, or both. Although the functional abnormalities are not specific, a prolonged bleeding time indicates that the patient is at risk for bleeding. Treatment of bleeding patients with thrombocytosis should be directed at lowering the platelet count as rapidly as possible.

George JN, Shattil SJ: Medical progress: The clinical importance of acquired abnormalities of platelet function. N Engl J Med 324:27, 1991. *An excellent recent review of this important topic.*

Hereditary Disorders of Platelet Function

In general, the bleeding history is similar for these diseases: a lifelong history of easy bruising, epistaxis, and prolonged oozing after venipuncture, dental extractions, and other challenges to hemostasis. All hereditary platelet disorders are quite rare.

GLANZMANN'S THROMBASTHENIA. This autosomal re-

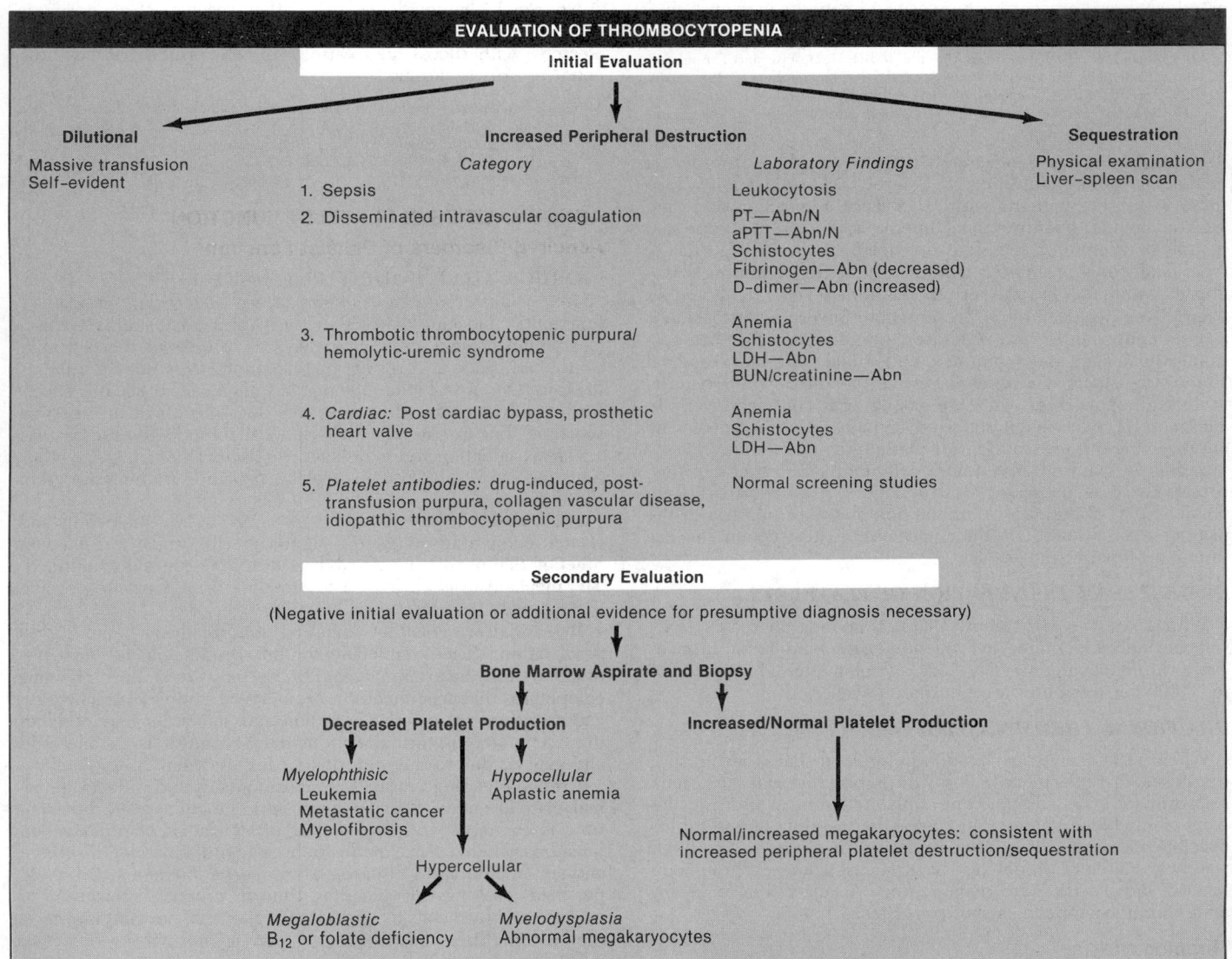

FIGURE 154–6. Evaluation of thrombocytopenia. Abn = abnormal; N = normal; PT = prothrombin time; aPTT = activated partial thromboplastin time; LDH = lactate dehydrogenase; BUN = blood urea nitrogen.

cessive bleeding disorder is characterized by a prolonged bleeding time and platelets that do not aggregate normally when stimulated with ADP, epinephrine, collagen, or thrombin. In Glanzmann's thrombocytopenia, two membrane glycoproteins (GPIIb-IIIa) that normally serve as the receptor for fibrinogen in activated platelets are markedly deficient (Fig. 154–2). Fibrinogen binding to platelets is required for normal platelet aggregation. The diagnosis is confirmed by demonstrating deficiency of platelet GPIIb-IIIa. The platelet count is always normal in this disease.

BERNARD-SOULIER SYNDROME. This autosomal recessive disorder is associated with "giant" platelets seen in the peripheral blood smear (see Color Plate 8K, left). Membrane protein abnormalities have also been demonstrated in this disease. Frequently, the platelet count is mildly decreased. In laboratory studies, platelets aggregate normally in response to ADP, collagen, or epinephrine but fail to aggregate in response to ristocetin. Physiologically, platelets fail to adhere normally to subendothelial connective tissue. This failure to adhere is due to defective binding of von Willebrand factor to a platelet membrane glycoprotein complex, GPIb-IX, which is deficient in this disease.

STORAGE POOL DISEASE (SPD). In this autosomal dominant disorder, platelet storage granules are decreased in number and/or content, presumably because of abnormal granule formation in megakaryocytes. The bleeding diathesis is mild and is found mostly in women. In SPD, with absent or decreased dense granules, platelets aggregate abnormally owing to inadequate secretion of ADP. Dense granule SPD is also associated with several other congenital disorders, including oculocutaneous albinism in both the Hermansky-Pudlak and Chédiak-Higashi syndromes, the Wiskott-Aldrich syndrome, and a syndrome in which there is thrombocytopenia and absent radii (TAR). Patients may also be deficient in α-granules, either in combination with dense granule deficiency or independently. The gray platelet syndrome refers to the latter situation, in which the absence of granule staining confers a gray color on the platelets. Mild thrombocytopenia may also be present in this disorder.

Bennett JS, Shattil SJ: Congenital qualitative platelet disorders. *In* Williams WJ, Beutler E, Erslev AJ, et al. (eds.): Hematology. 4th ed. New York, McGraw-Hill, 1990, pp 1407–1419.

VON WILLEBRAND'S DISEASE (see also Ch. 155). Von Willebrand's disease (vWd) is the most common congenital bleeding disorder, with an estimated incidence ranging from 0.1 to 2 per cent of the population in the United States. Several different types of vWd occur. Most commonly, vWd is an autosomal dominant disorder. Rarely, it is autosomal recessive, the most severe form. In the classic disorder, patients are deficient in both Factor VIII:AHF and vWf. The latter is a plasma glycoprotein necessary for adhesion of platelets to subendothelial connective tissue in blood flowing at high shear rates. Von Willebrand factor circulates in a noncovalent complex with Factor VIII:AHF. Unbound Factor VIII:AHF has a markedly shortened half-life; deficiency of vWf therefore results secondarily in Factor VIII:AHF deficiency. In vWd, Factor VIII:AHF levels are rarely below 5 per cent—hence the mild symptoms in this disorder, compared with hemophilia. The manifestations of this disease differ from hemophilia in that bleeding is predominantly in the skin and mucous membranes (epistaxis, bruising, and menorrhagia). The pattern of bleeding resembles that seen in platelet disorders rather than coagulation disorders. In contrast to hemophilia, hemarthrosis is rare. Von Willebrand's disease is discussed in detail in Ch. 155.

Acquired von Willebrand's Disease. Von Willebrand's disease secondary to SLE and lymphoproliferative disorders has been described. In some cases, deficiency of vWf is mediated by specific antibodies. Low levels of vWf have also been demonstrated in some patients with Wilms' tumor.

Pseudo von Willebrand's Disease. In this rare bleeding disorder, synthesis of plasma vWf is normal; however, because of a primary abnormality in the patients' platelets, high molecular weight vWf is bound spontaneously with high affinity. Consequently, plasma is depleted of high molecular weight multimers of vWf, resulting in an electrophoretic pattern similar to type II vWd. Addition of normal plasma to the patient's platelets results in spontaneous platelet aggregation in vitro. Moreover, patients are frequently thrombocytopenic owing to accelerated clearance of platelets bound with vWf. Transfusion of plasma or cryoprecipitate may result in worsening thrombocytopenia.

Ruggeri ZM, Zimmerman TS: Von Willebrand factor and von Willebrand disease. Blood 70:895, 1987. *A review of the disease and its pathogenesis.*

PLATELET TRANSFUSIONS

Indications

In general, when serious bleeding is a complication of thrombocytopenia, platelet transfusions are effective only when the cause is decreased production. When thrombocytopenia is due to increased peripheral destruction, or sequestration, the condition is usually refractory to platelet transfusion. Bleeding due to qualitative platelet disorders ordinarily responds to platelet transfusions except when it is secondary to uremia or hepatic failure or when an offending drug is still present in the circulation.

For patients with congenital platelet disorders, platelet transfusion must be given judiciously. With repeated transfusion, alloantibodies are formed. Eventually, it may become impossible to obtain a significant rise in the platelet count through transfusion. Therefore, platelet transfusions should be given only for serious bleeding or in preparation for surgery on patients with moderately severe platelet defects.

Platelet transfusions are indicated for patients who are bleeding actively and who have either a platelet count below ~50,000 per microliter or a qualitative platelet abnormality as manifested by a prolonged bleeding time. Platelet transfusions may also be indicated prophylactically before surgery or other invasive procedures. Prior to surgery, the platelet count should be above ~50,000 per microliter in most cases, and above 90,000 per microliter for surgery in which any abnormal bleeding will have unacceptable morbidity, as, for example, in surgery of the central nervous system or of the eye. For invasive procedures, such as kidney or liver biopsies, a platelet count above 50,000 per microliter is probably sufficient, but this recommendation assumes that platelet function is relatively normal.

Chronic Thrombocytopenia

For patients who are not bleeding, recommendations are based on the cause of thrombocytopenia. When thrombocytopenia is due to decreased production, the platelet count should be maintained above 10,000 to 20,000 per microliter. In patients with accelerated destruction of platelets, transfusion is generally not effective. In addition, in ITP, patients frequently tolerate low platelet counts with little bleeding.

Dosage

For patients who require platelet transfusions chronically, platelets should be obtained from a single donor for each transfusion (generally six to seven units) to reduce the risk of forming multiple alloantibodies (see below). In a 70-kg patient, one unit of platelets usually raises the platelet count by approximately 10,000 per microliter. The platelet count should be repeated 10 to 60 minutes after transfusion to assess the compatibility of the transfused platelets and to determine whether the desired platelet count has been achieved. In a patient who is actively bleeding, the platelet count should be maintained above ~50,000 per microliter.

Alloantibodies Against Platelets

In approximately 50 to 60 per cent of patients whose condition becomes refractory to random donor platelets, anti-HLA (human leukocyte antigen) antibodies appear to be responsible. The other presumed antigens have not yet been identified. In one rare form of alloimmunization, antibodies develop against the PL^{A1} antigen, an epitope on platelet glycoprotein IIIa. The difference between PL^{A1} positive and negative (PL^{A2}) is a single amino acid. Ninety-eight per cent of the normal population have PL^{A1}-positive platelets.

When PL^{A1}-negative patients are transfused with PL^{A1}-positive blood, they may develop anti-PL^{A1} antibodies. This syndrome, *posttransfusion purpura* (PTP), occurs primarily in women. Previous immunization is necessary, either by transfusion or by pregnancy. Why this syndrome is rare in spite of the frequency of PL^{A1}-minus in the population is unknown. Moreover, these patients not only rapidly clear transfused platelets from their circulation but also destroy their own platelets, becoming thrombocytopenic usually 5 to 10 days after transfusion. If patients with antibodies against the PL^A1 antigen become severely thrombocytopenic, treatment with plasmapheresis or exchange transfusion is necessary, as bleeding from thrombocytopenia can be life-threatening.

NEONATAL ALLOIMMUNE THROMBOCYTOPENIA. Thrombocytopenia due to maternal alloantibodies against fetal platelet antigens occurs in approximately 1 in 2000 to 1 in 4000 fetuses. Affected infants may have intracranial hemorrhages (estimated ranges between 10 and 30 per cent), and in families with an affected infant, the risk of recurrence is at least 75 per cent.

PL^A1 antibodies have been identified in most cases as being responsible for thrombocytopenia. Affected infants are treated by transfusion with washed maternal platelets. Women with a prior history of an affected infant should be delivered by cesarean section. Recently, in pregnant mothers with a prior affected infant, intravenous γ globulin was shown to raise fetal platelet counts with a reduction in the rate of intracranial hemorrhage.

Tomasulo PA, Petz LD: Platelet transfusion. *In* Petz LD, Swisher SN (eds.): Clinical Practice of Transfusion Medicine. 2nd ed. New York, Churchill Livingston 1989, pp 427–467. *Excellent review of specific indications for platelet transfusion and of managing alloimmunized patients.*

VASCULAR DISORDERS (Table 154–6)

Normal vascular function is necessary for effective hemostasis (Fig. 154–1). Alteration in the integrity or structure of blood vessels can lead to a bleeding diathesis, the symptoms and signs of which are indistinguishable from those of a platelet disorder.

Congenital Vascular Disorders Associated with Bleeding

HEREDITARY HEMORRHAGIC TELANGIECTASIA (RENDU-OSLER-WEBER DISEASE). This disorder, the most common genetic cause of vascular bleeding, is inherited as an autosomal dominant trait. The most common problem is spontaneous epistaxis. More than half of the patients have epistaxis by age 20 and 90 per cent by age 45. Telangiectasia occurs most frequently on the face in two thirds of patients, on the mouth in one half of patients, and on the cheeks, tongue, nose, and lower lip in approximately one third of patients. In about 40 per cent of patients, the hands and wrists are also involved. Beyond this cutaneous or mucosal involvement, the organ system affected most often is the gastrointestinal tract (~12 per cent). Death from intestinal bleeding occurs in 12 to 15 per cent of symptomatic patients. The liver, lungs, central nervous system, and urinary tract are involved in decreasing order of frequency. Pulmonary arteriovenous fistulas, present in ~5 per cent of patients, are manifested by cyanoses, dyspnea, clubbing, and thoracic murmurs. Hemoptysis is unusual. Surgical resection is successful in managing this complication in most patients. Stroke may occur in patients with central nervous system involvement, a complication that tends to occur in younger patients (mean age, 33). Careful inspection of the nose and mouth usually reveals the

TABLE 154–6. VASCULAR DISORDERS ASSOCIATED WITH BLEEDING

Congenital
  Hereditary hemorrhagic telangiectasia
  Cavernous hemangioma
  Connective tissue disorders
    Ehlers-Danlos syndrome
    Osteogenesis imperfecta
    Pseudoxanthoma elasticum
Acquired disorders affecting vascular hemostatic function
  Scurvy
  Immunoglobulin disorders
    Cryoglobulinemia
    Benign hyperglobulinemia
    Waldenström's macroglobulinemia
    Multiple myeloma
    Henoch-Schönlein purpura
  Glucocorticoid excess
    Cushing's syndrome
    Glucocorticoid therapy

diagnosis. In other cases, endoscopy or angiography may be necessary. Pathologic examination of involved tissue demonstrates dilated capillaries with loss of subendothelial structures.

Tests of platelet function and the bleeding time are normal. There is no consistently effective therapy, but the prognosis is relatively good.

CAVERNOUS HEMANGIOMA (KASABACH-MERRITT SYNDROME). Congenital subcutaneous and visceral hemangiomas may be associated with thrombocytopenia and bleeding in infants and children with this syndrome. Bleeding occurs at the site of the lesions or systemically owing to thrombocytopenia. Platelets are activated within the hemangioma and subsequently removed from the circulation. In addition, mild DIC may occur with consumption of fibrinogen. Thrombocytopenia is severer than the coagulation abnormalities. Spontaneous regression of hemangiomas may occur over a period of years. In cases in which thrombocytopenia is severe and tumors are few in number, surgery and/or radiation therapy may be effective. Intentional thrombosis of hemangiomas by administration of inhibitors of fibrinolysis, with or without cryoprecipitate, has been successful in managing thrombocytopenia in a few cases.

DISORDERS OF CONNECTIVE TISSUE. Genetic abnormalities in structural glycoproteins such as collagen can result in vascular fragility caused by weakening of the vessel wall. Bleeding may be limited to increased bruising or may manifest as internal hemorrhaging. Ehlers-Danlos syndrome, osteogenesis imperfecta, and pseudoxanthoma elasticum, discussed elsewhere in this book, are examples of inherited disorders of connective tissue that may be associated with a bleeding diathesis on this basis.

Acquired Disorders of Blood Vessels Causing Bleeding

SCURVY (Ch. 204). Severe vitamin C deficiency results in defective collagen formation in small blood vessels. Bleeding may occur in any tissue but is prominent in the lower extremities and is perifollicular in distribution. Other sites where bleeding is common include the gums, the subperiosteum in children, and into the muscles.

PURPURA ASSOCIATED WITH IMMUNOGLOBULIN DISORDERS. *Cryoglobulinemia* (Ch. 151). Patients with all three types of cryoglobulinemia have purpura as a complication of their disease. In type I cryoglobulinemia, bleeding may be due to obstruction of blood flow in the microcirculation at cold temperatures by cryoprecipitates, resulting in increased vascular fragility. In type II and III cryoglobulinemia, bleeding may be due to leukocytoclastic vasculitis associated with the immune complexes. Purpura occurs most commonly in the distal extremities.

Benign Hyperglobulinemia (Waldenström's Purpura). In this syndrome, patients have polyclonal hyperglobulinemia associated with purpura of the lower extremities. Leukocytoclastic involvement of the vessel wall may account for increased vascular fragility and bleeding. Commonly, the onset of purpura is preceded by a stinging sensation in areas of involvement. While there is generally no evidence of systemic vasculitis, this disorder may evolve into Sjögren's syndrome or SLE.

Amyloidosis (Ch. 197). Amyloid deposition in the skin and subcutaneous tissues alters the normal structural support for small blood vessels, resulting in increased vascular fragility (see Color Plate 8*I*, right). Purpura can occur at any site; but for unclear reasons, periorbital hemorrhage is a characteristic finding in systemic amyloidosis.

Waldenström's Macroglobulinemia and Multiple Myeloma (Ch. 151). Abnormalities in platelet function may occur with M proteins, as noted above. An additional contributing factor is hyperviscosity when it complicates these diseases. Slowing of blood flow and increased hydrostatic pressure may increase vascular fragility, leading to purpura.

Henoch-Schönlein Purpura. This childhood disorder is characterized by symmetric purpura and arthralgias of the lower extremities, abdominal pain, and melena. Rarely, adults are affected. Patients may give a history of a recent infectious illness. The disease has an acute onset with a maculopapular rash evolving into palpable purpura. Other complications include glomerulonephritis and hypertension (both of which are self-limiting) and intussusception. Involved tissues, including the skin, demonstrate vasculitis with immunoglobulin A (IgA) and complement deposition.

Henoch-Schönlein purpura usually remits spontaneously over a period of 1 to 2 months, although the course is often punctuated by flaring of symptoms and signs. Symptomatic improvement is obtained with glucocorticoids.

Miscellaneous Disorders

CUSHING'S SYNDROME. Cushing's disease or chronic administration of glucocorticoids results in increased bruising, particularly in the extremities. Abnormal bleeding probably results from alterations in the structure of the perivascular matrix, with loss of normal elasticity.

AUTOERYTHROCYTE SENSITIZATION (GARDNER-DIAMOND SYNDROME). This bizarre syndrome is charaterized by the development of purpura at any site on the body, preceded by pain and burning. It occurs almost exclusively in women. Usually, affected women have a history of severe stress and emotional problems. Tests for abnormalities in hemostasis are all normal.

The diagnostic test is the development of large ecchymoses within 24 to 48 hours at the site of subcutaneous injection of a small amount (~0.1 ml) of the patient's own blood or erythrocytes. Injection should be at sites inaccessible to the patient, and a concurrent control injection should be administered. The primary differential diagnosis is factitious purpura.

PURPURA SIMPLEX. Purpura simplex is the term used to describe the phenomenon commonly observed in young children and middle-aged women of easy bruisability, primarily of the lower extremities. Laboratory evaluation, including the bleeding time, is normal, and there is no evidence of vascular abnormalities. Other than bruising, affected women do not experience excessive bleeding with surgery and do not have internal bleeding.

155 Disorders of Blood Coagulation

Deane F. Mosher

Normal hemostasis requires interactions among blood vessels, the formed elements of blood, especially platelets and monocytes, and blood coagulation proteins. The general biology of hemostasis and the approach to a patient suspected of having a hemorrhagic diathesis have been discussed in Ch. 154, Hemorrhagic Disorders: Abnormalities of Platelet and Vascular Function. In the present chapter, attention is focused on hemorrhagic and thrombotic disorders that occur as a consequence of abnormalities of blood coagulation proteins.

REVIEW OF BLOOD COAGULATION

Blood coagulation, initiated by substances in injured tissues, is propagated by an interlocking network of enzymic events, the so-called coagulation cascade. These controlled reactions ensure that blood coagulation happens quickly and yet remains localized. Blood coagulation results in the formation of a protein scaffolding, the fibrin clot, that controls bleeding and serves as a nidus for subsequent cellular ingrowth and tissue repair. After several days the fibrin clot is lysed and replaced by a more permanent scaffolding of connective tissue matrix molecules. Abnormalities that result in delay of clot formation or in premature lysis of clots are associated with a bleeding tendency. Abnormalities that result in inappropriate activation or localization of blood coagulation are associated with thrombosis.

COAGULATION MOLECULES. Coagulation and fibrinolysis involve many blood plasma proteins (Table 155–1). This list grows longer as blood coagulation mechanisms are studied in greater depth. Structural and functional similarities allow one to put the proteins into one of several groups. Some are zymogens of serine proteinases and hence members of the serine proteinase family of proteins. Among the serine proteinase family are five proteins (Factors II, VII, IX, and X and protein C) that are modified by vitamin K–dependent posttranslational carboxylation of glutamic acid residues. A sixth plasma protein, protein S, is also modified

by this reaction. The modification allows the six proteins to bind Ca^{2+} and phospholipids and thereby participate efficiently in blood coagulation. Factors V and VIII function as helper proteins during blood coagulation and are homologous to each other and to ceruloplasmin, a Cu^{2+}-binding plasma protein. Other proteins are *serine proteinase inhibitors* and hence members of the "serpin" family of proteins. Most of the proteins listed in Table 155–1, including the vitamin K–dependent factors, are synthesized by hepatocytes. A number of the proteins, however, can also be synthesized by other cell types such as megakaryocytes, monocyte-macrophages, and endothelial cells.

There are also key molecules that are embedded in the external membrane of cells (tissue factor, thrombomodulin, urokinase receptor) or deposited in extracellular matrix (*e.g.*, heparan sulfate and dermatan sulfate). The molecules interact specifically with components of blood to initiate and modulate coagulation and fibrinolysis.

GENERAL MECHANISMS. Blood coagulation is activated, propagated, and controlled by mechanisms found in other proteolytic effector systems (e.g., complement). These mechanisms include the following:

1. Sequential activation by limited proteolytic cleavage
2. Amplification of the response by feedback loops
3. Use of binding or helper proteins to bring reactants together
4. Destruction of activated proteins by further proteolytic cleavage
5. Inhibition of activated proteinases by stoichiometric complex formation with specific inhibitor proteins, *i.e.*, the serpins

In addition, there is a mechanism that is, so far, unique to blood coagulation:

6. Formation of a five-part complex of an activated vitamin K–dependent factor, to-be-activated vitamin K–dependent zymogen, helper protein, Ca^{2+}, and phospholipid surface.

EXTRINSIC AND INTRINSIC PATHWAYS. Blood coagulation can be initiated by exposure of blood to tissue factor (the "extrinsic system") or by activation of contact factors of plasma (the "intrinsic system"). Both of these initiation pathways lead to a common pathway, which results in the elaboration of thrombin, the master coagulation enzyme. As shown in Figure 155–1A, the concept of the two initiation pathways and the common pathway is useful in understanding two major coagulation tests, the activated partial thromboplastin time (APTT), in which blood plasma is activated by the intrinsic pathway, and the prothrombin time (PT), in which tissue factor is added to plasma so that activation proceeds by the extrinsic pathway. It is unlikely that the two initiation pathways are so clearly delineated in vivo. Activation of Factor IX, an intrinsic factor, by Factor VII, an extrinsic factor, must be of considerable importance because deficiencies of Factors VII and IX, as well as the factors that follow Factor IX in the intrinsic and common pathways, *i.e.*, Factors VIII, X, V, II, and I, all are associated with a bleeding tendency. In contrast, deficiency of Factor XII, prekallikrein, or high molecular weight kininogen (HMWK) does not cause a bleeding problem, and Factor XI deficiency is associated with a bleeding tendency in only a minority of cases.

Tissue Factor and the Extrinsic Pathway. Factor VII is unique among coagulation factors because it circulates in an active configuration. To initiate coagulation, however, Factor VII requires tissue factor. Sites rich in tissue factor include brain, adventitia of blood vessels, organ capsules, epidermis, and mucosal epithelium. Therefore, tissue factor is not exposed to blood unless there is an anatomic disruption that allows blood access to the hemostatic envelope around blood vessels, organs, or the body itself. Tissue factor is present in many types of cells, including endothelial cells and monocytes. In response to a variety of stimuli, such as exposure to lymphokines or monokines, tissue factor becomes expressed on cell surfaces.

In the presence of tissue factor, phospholipid, and Ca^{2+}, Factor VII can activate Factors IX and X (Fig. 155–1B). Activated Factor X (X_a) then activates Factor II, and Factor II_a (thrombin) cleaves fibrinogen to fibrin. The time to clot formation after addition of tissue factor, phospholipid, and Ca^{2+} to citrated platelet-poor plasma is called the prothrombin time or PT, the single most important clotting test. When determined with an excess of tissue factor (as is generally done), the PT measures only factors of the extrinsic and common pathways and does not measure Factor IX.

Control of Factor VII/Tissue Factor by Extrinsic Pathway Inhibitor. Extrinsic pathway inhibitor (EPI) is a double-headed protease inhibitor of the pancreatic trypsin inhibitor class. One head of EPI binds to Factor X_a, and the second head inhibits Factor VII in association with tissue factor. Therefore, EPI extinguishes the Factor VII/tissue factor "match" that "ignites" blood coagulation (Fig. 155–1B). The "fuse" that propagates coagulation begins with Factor IX_a, not Factor X_a. This is why, when the concentration of tissue factor is low, most of Factor VII's clot-promoting activity is generated through Factor IX.

Contact Factors and the Intrinsic System. Activation of contact factors constitutes a second pathway for activating Factor X. Negatively charged surfaces, such as sulfatide micelles, glass, kaolin, and celite, bind Factor XII and HMWK. HMWK, in turn, binds prekallikrein and Factor XI. Binding to surfaces initiates a series of reciprocal cleavages of Factor XI and prekallikrein by activated Factor XII and of Factor XII by activated Factor XI and kallikrein (Fig. 155–1C). Activated Factor XI activates Factor IX in a reaction that requires Ca^{2+}. Kallikrein also releases bradykinin, a vasoactive and pain-causing octapeptide, from HMWK and low molecular weight kininogen. In the APTT, platelet-poor citrated plasma is allowed to incubate for 3 to 5 minutes with kaolin or ellagic acid to activate Factor XI optimally. Ca^{2+} and phospholipid are then added so that Factor XI_a can activate Factor IX, Factor IX_a can activate Factor X, and so on.

Amplification of Activation Pathways. Three analogous five-part propagating reactions take place (Fig. 155–1C): (1) Factor VII activates Factor X or IX in the presence of tissue factor, Ca^{2+}, and phospholipid; (2) Factor IX_a activates Factor X in the presence of Factor VIII, Ca^{2+}, and phospholipid; and (3) Factor X_a activates Factor II in the presence of Factor V, Ca^{2+}, and phospholipid. The phospholipid requirement for reaction 1 is

TABLE 155–1. PROTEINS INVOLVED IN BLOOD COAGULATION AND FIBRINOLYSIS

Protein	Synonym	Size in Kilodaltons*	Plasma Concentration in mg/dl (μM)*	Kind of Protein	Function†
Fibrinogen	Factor I	340	300(9)	Structural protein	Gels to form clot
Factor II	Prothrombin	72	15(2)	Vitamin K–dependent zymogen of serine proteinase	Activates I, V, VIII, XIII, protein C, and platelets
Factor V	Proaccelerin	350	2(0.05)	Ceruloplasmin-like binding protein	Supports X_a activation of II
Factor VII	Stable factor	50	0.01(0.002)	Vitamin K–dependent zymogen of serine proteinase	Activates IX and X
Factor VIII	Antihemophilic factor	350	0.01(0.0003)	Ceruloplasmin-like binding protein	Supports IX_a activation of X
Factor IX	Christmas factor	57	1(0.2)	Vitamin K–dependent zymogen of serine proteinase	Activates X
Factor X	Stuart-Prower factor	59	1(0.2)	Vitamin K–dependent zymogen of serine proteinase	Activates II
Factor XI	Plasma thromboplastin antecedent	160	0.5(0.03)	Zymogen of serine proteinase	Activates XII and prekallikrein
Factor XII	Hageman factor	75	2(0.2)	Zymogen of serine proteinase	Activates XI and prekallikrein
Factor XIII	Fibrin-stabilizing factor	320	3(0.08)	Zymogen of transglutaminase	Crosslinks fibrin and other proteins
von Willebrand factor	Factor VIII–related antigen	800–20,000	2(0.05)	Structural protein	Binds VIII, mediates platelet adhesion
Prekallikrein	—	88	2(0.3)	Zymogen of serine proteinase	Activates XII and prekallikrein, cleaves HMWK
High molecular weight kininogen (HMWK)	—	150	2(0.2)	Binding protein, unique	Supports reciprocal activation of XII, XI, and prekallikrein
Fibronectin	—	450	40(1)	Structural protein, unique	Mediates cell adhesion
Extrinsic pathway inhibitor	EPI, LACI	46	0.1(0.02)	Kunitz-type inhibitor	Inhibits VII/tissue factor in concert with X_a
Antithrombin III	Major antithrombin	60	20(2.5)	Serpin	Inhibits II_a, X_a, and other proteinases; cofactor for heparin
Heparin cofactor II	Minor antithrombin	55	5(0.6)	Serpin	Inhibits II_a, cofactor for heparin and dermatan sulfate
Protein C	—	62	0.4(0.06)	Vitamin K–dependent zymogen of serine proteinase	Inactivates V and VIII
Protein S	—	69	3(0.4)	Vitamin K–dependent binding protein	Cofactor for protein C_a, binds C4b-binding protein
Plasminogen	—	86	10(1.2)	Zymogen of serine proteinase	Lyses fibrin and other proteins
Alpha$_2$-antiplasmin	—	60	3(0.5)	Serpin	Inhibits plasmin
Prourokinase	—	50	tr	Zymogen of serine proteinase	Activates plasminogen
Tissue plasminogen activator	TPA	55	tr	Serine proteinase	Activates plasminogen
Plasminogen activator inhibitor 1	PAI1	52	tr	Serpin	Inactivates TPA and urokinase
Plasminogen activator inhibitor 2	PAI2	55	tr	Serpin	Inactivates TPA and urokinase

*For comparison, the size of albumin is 68 kilodaltons, and the plasma concentration of albumin is 3500 mg/dl (510 μM).
†For zymogens, the function after activation is given.
tr = trace.

satisfied by the surface of the tissue factor–containing cell. For the reactions involving Factor VIII or V, the phospholipid requirement is satisfied by platelet phospholipid.

The vitamin K–dependent factors (VII, IX, X, II) bind to the phospholipid surface in interactions that require gamma-carboxyl glutamic acid residues; the binding is Ca^{2+} dependent. Factors V and VIII contain domains for binding protease and zymogen, Ca^{2+}, and the phospholipid surface. Stimulated platelets contain discrete binding sites for Factor V. The accelerating role of platelets in the X_a-V-II reaction is called platelet factor 3 activity. Formation of the five-part complex dramatically increases the rate constant (K_{cat}) for activation of zymogen by protease. In the five-part complex, Factor V or VIII is most effective after it has been cleaved by Factor II_a (thrombin). Thus, thrombin is initially generated at a sluggish rate, but once a small amount of thrombin is generated so that it can cleave Factor V or VIII to a more active form, subsequent thrombin generation is "explosively" rapid and efficient, consuming almost all of the Factor II in plasma.

LOCALIZATION AND INHIBITION OF BLOOD COAGULATION. Blood coagulation is efficiently activated only on a phospholipid surface (Fig. 155–1C), and thus activation is localized to the area of injury. In addition to EPI described above, several mechanisms dampen activation by "snuffing out the fuse"

and thereby ensure that activated factors do not escape and cause thrombosis at a distant site (Fig. 155–1B).

Thrombin exhibits acquired altered specificity when complexed to thrombomodulin; rather than acting upon fibrinogen or Factors V and VIII, thrombin activates protein C (Fig. 155–1B). Activated protein C, in turn, inactivates thrombin-activated Factors V and VIII. In addition, activated protein C enhances fibrinolysis. Activation of protein C by thrombin-thrombomodulin complex, therefore, is a powerful anticoagulant event, just as the activation of Factors V and VIII by thrombin is a powerful procoagulant event. The cleavage of Factors V and VIII by activated protein C requires the sixth vitamin K–dependent protein of plasma, protein S. Protein S serves as a cofactor for activated protein C rather than acting as a proteinase. A portion of circulating protein S is complexed to C4 binding protein (C4bp).

Two antithrombins in plasma, called antithrombin III and heparin cofactor II, inhibit thrombin and other serine proteinases that are generated during blood coagulation. The antithrombins, members of the serpin family, are substrates for the proteinases. Upon cleavage the antithrombins undergo a structural rearrangement that allows them to form tight one-to-one complexes with the proteinases. As a result, the proteinases are irreversibly

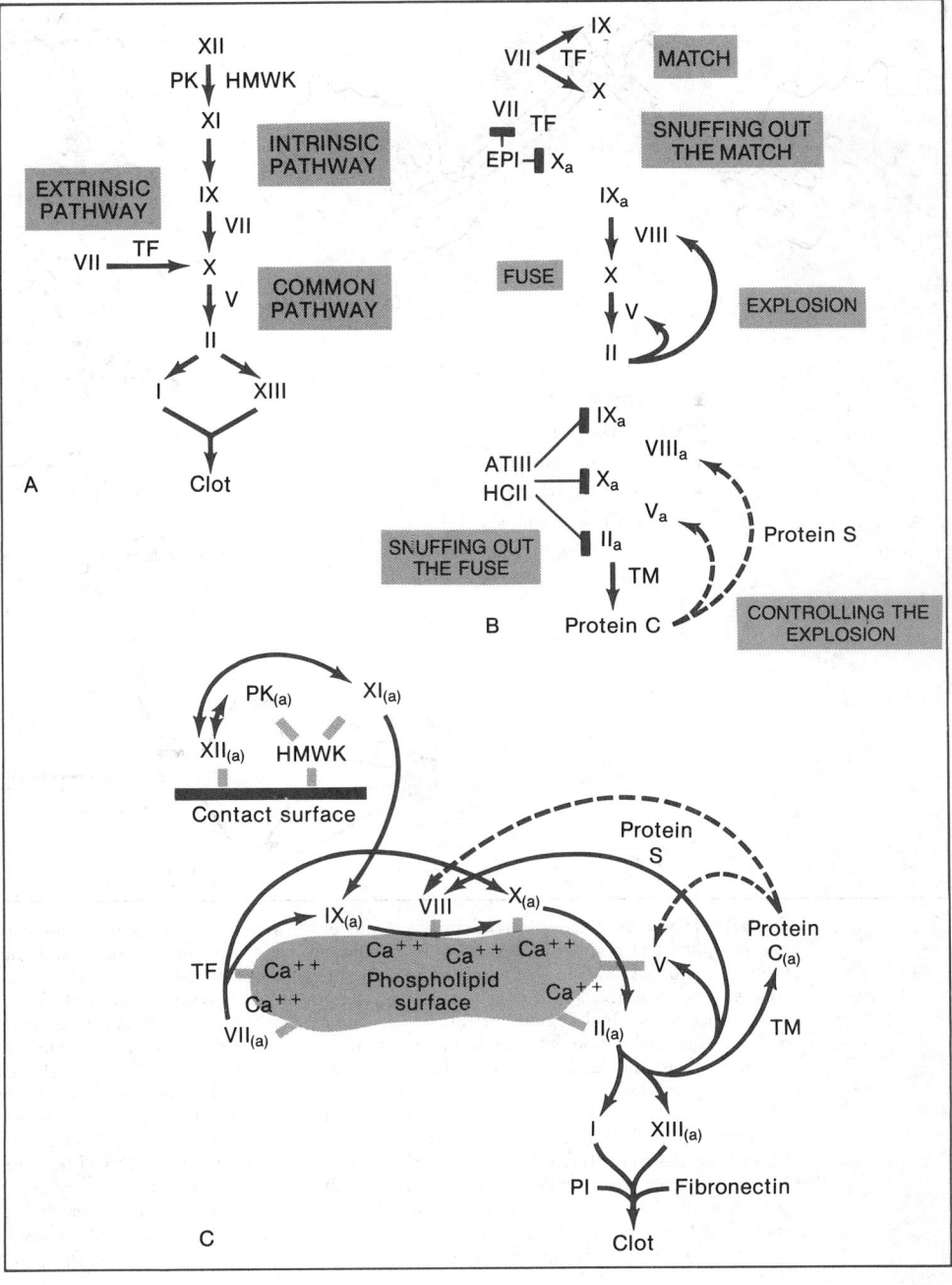

FIGURE 155–1. Diagrams of interactions among coagulation factors. *A* depicts the intrinsic, extrinsic, and common pathways in their simplest forms. *B* emphasizes critical stages in activation and control of blood coagulation. *C* is organized around the contact surface and the phospholipid surface. Solid lines with arrows indicate proteolytic activation. Broken lines with arrows indicate proteolytic inactivation. Solid lines with bars indicate complex formation and inactivation. The stippled patches indicate binding of proteins to surfaces or to one another. The subscript a indicates proteins that are zymogens and can be converted to active enzymes. PK = prekallikrein; HMWK = high molecular weight kininogen; TF = tissue factors; PI = alpha₂-antiplasmin; TM = thrombomodulin; EPI = extrinsic pathway inhibitor; ATIII = antithrombin III; HCII = heparin cofactor II.

inhibited. The rates at which both antithrombins combine with coagulation proteinases are accelerated many-fold by heparin and by heparan sulfate proteoglycan on the luminal surface of endothelial cells. The acceleration explains the anticoagulant action of heparin. The rate at which the heparin cofactor II combines with thrombin is accelerated by dermatan sulfate, a glycosaminoglycan found in the vessel wall.

As described in more detail below, inherited deficiency states of protein C, protein S, and antithrombin III have all been associated with thrombotic diatheses.

STRUCTURE OF FIBRINOGEN AND FIBRIN. Fibrinogen and fibrin monomer are extended trinodular molecules made up of pairs of three polypeptide chains (Fig. 155–2A). The three chains run through half of the molecule, that is, through half of the central E nodule and the whole of one of the two peripheral D nodules. The chains are thought to adopt a coiled-spring structure between the E and D nodules. This portion of the molecule is particularly susceptible to degradation by the principal fibrinolytic enzyme, plasmin. The nodules resist degradation

by plasmin. Thus the products of complete lysis of a clot by plasmin are one E nodule, two D nodules, and small fragments (Fig. 155–2B).

Thrombin cleaves negatively charged small peptides to convert fibrinogen to a clottable derivative called fibrin monomer. Fibrin monomer assembles to form an infinite branching network of fibrils (Fig. 155–2B). At physiologic fibrin concentrations, this network constitutes a strong gel and immobilizes blood. Fibrinogen is usually completely converted to fibrin during blood coagulation. Thus the concentration of fibrinogen antigen in serum is about 0.02 mg per deciliter, compared with 200 mg per deciliter in plasma. Fibrinogen, however, forms soluble complexes with fibrin monomer when the concentration of thrombin is low. The soluble complexes can escape from areas of active coagulation and be detected in the circulation.

The fibrin gel is modified by thrombin-activated Factor XIII. This enzyme, a transglutaminase, catalyzes covalent protein-protein crosslinking. Crosslinks are introduced between gamma chains of adjacent D domains, thus ligating the fibrin fibril end to end (Fig. 155–2B). Crosslinking of gamma chains renders the clot insoluble in protein denaturants such as 6M urea. The alpha

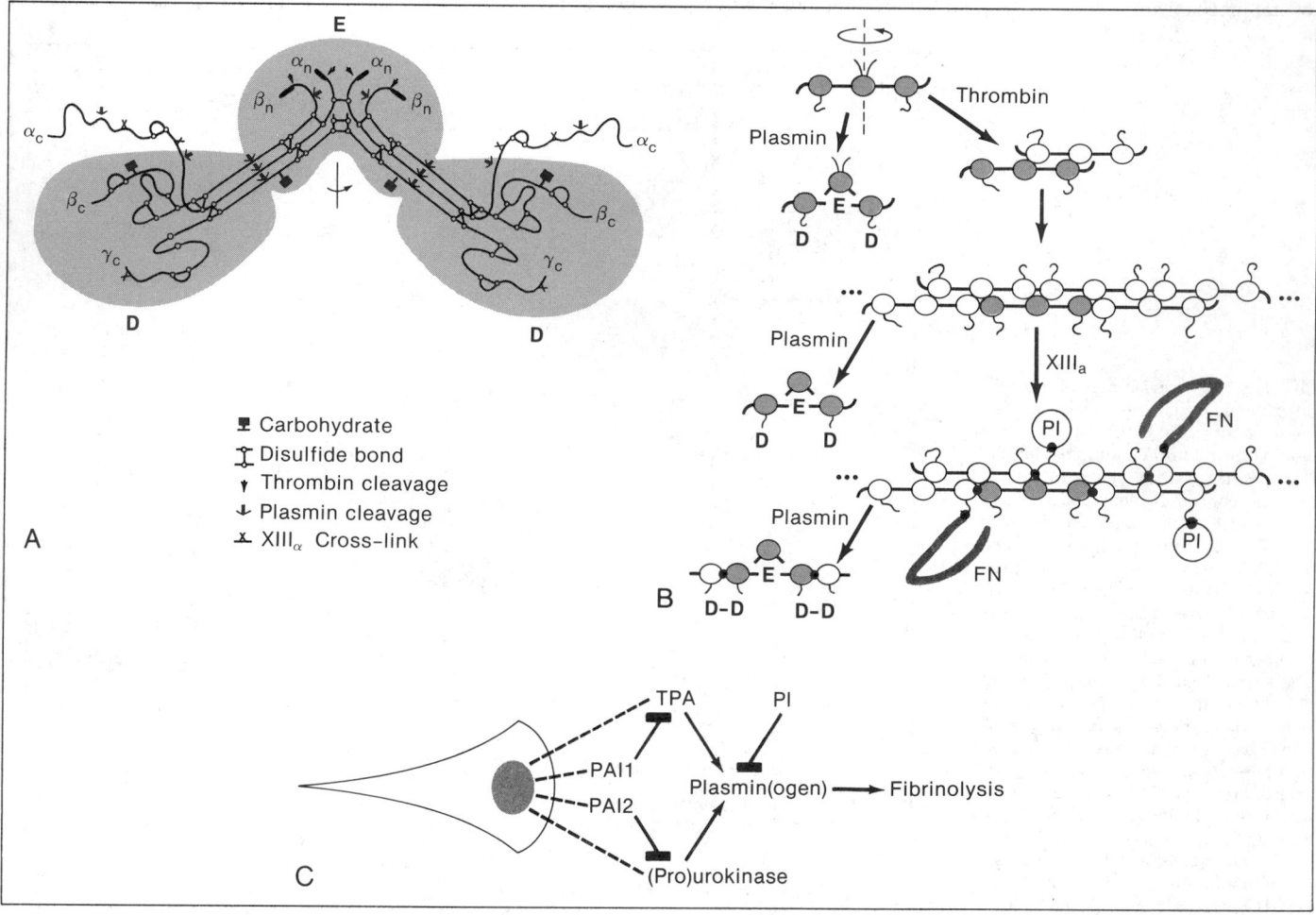

Carbohydrate
Disulfide bond
Thrombin cleavage
Plasmin cleavage
XIII$_\alpha$ Cross-link

FIGURE 155–2. *A,* Disposition of the six chains of fibrinogen. Fibrinogen is composed of a central E nodule and two peripheral D nodules. One set of three nonidentical chains—alpha, beta, and gamma—runs through half the molecule and is bound to the other set by disulfide linkages in the E domain, where the amino termini of all six chains come together. The strands connecting the peripheral nodules to the central nodule contain all three chains. The carboxyl terminal regions of the three chains constitute the globular D domain. In addition, the extreme carboxyl terminal region of the alpha chain extends out from the D domain. Thrombin releases acidic fibrinopeptides A and B from the E domain to yield fibrin; plasmin cleaves the molecule between E and D. *B,* Activation, assembly, crosslinking, and lysis of fibrinogen and fibrin. Fibrinogen and fibrin are both trinodular proteins. Clotting is initiated by release of the negatively charged fibrinopeptides from the E nodule. Assembly is driven by noncovalent E nodule–D nodule interaction. End-to-end covalent crosslinking occurs between gamma chains. Alpha$_2$-antiplasmin (PI) and fibronectin (FN) crosslink to the extended carboxyl terminal portion of the alpha chain. Plasmin cleaves this portion of the alpha chain and separates the D and E nodules. *C* depicts the proteolytic activation of plasminogen by its physiologic activators, urokinase and tissue plasminogen activator (TPA), and the control of the activation by plasminogen activator inhibitors (PAI1 and PAI2). These four molecules are secreted by cells. Plasmin is inhibited by alpha$_2$-antiplasmin (PI).

chains can ligate side to side among themselves or be crosslinked to fibronectin or alpha$_2$-antiplasmin. Both the "hardening" of the fibrin clot by crosslinking and the incorporation of other proteins into the clot are probably important. Deficiency of Factor XIII or of alpha$_2$-antiplasmin is associated with a bleeding tendency, and some patients with Factor XIII deficiency suffer from poor wound healing.

FIBRINOLYSIS. Cleavage of plasminogen to the active proteinase plasmin is carried out by two plasminogen activators: tissue plasminogen activator (TPA) and urokinase (Fig. 155–2C). TPA is secreted as an active serine proteinase, whereas urokinase can be activated from a somewhat active precursor, prourokinase. Among the activators of prourokinase is plasmin. TPA, plasminogen, and plasmin all bind to fibrin, and it is in a fibrin clot that TPA can activate plasminogen to plasmin most efficiently. Prourokinase does not bind to fibrin. However, small amounts of plasmin already bound to fibrin can activate prourokinase to urokinase, which then can activate more plasminogen to plasmin.

Localization of fibrinolysis to the fibrin clot is further ensured by binding of the activators, especially urokinase, to cells and an efficient array of inhibitors. Cells secrete specific inhibitors of TPA and urokinase, called plasminogen activator inhibitors 1 and 2, to regulate fibrinolysis in their local environment. Indeed, tightly controlled secretion of activator and inhibitor may allow a cell to localize plasminogen activation to volumes that are only nanometers across. Anti-TPA is present in the circulation in low concentrations. Also in the circulation is alpha$_2$-antiplasmin, which inhibits plasmin extremely rapidly and efficiently.

Plasmin degrades a variety of proteins in addition to fibrin, especially connective tissue proteins and undoubtedly has other physiologic functions besides lysis of fibrin clots. For instance, ovarian follicular cells secrete plasminogen activator in response to hormonal stimulation just prior to ovulation and thereby initiate degradation of the follicular wall.

Epsilon-aminocaproic acid (EACA) and its cyclic analogue, tranexamic acid, bind to plasminogen and plasmin and inhibit binding of these molecules to fibrin. As a result, the molecules are good inhibitors of plasminogen activation.

Streptokinase, a bacterial protein, forms a complex with plasminogen and causes a conformational change that opens up the active site of plasminogen. The streptokinase-plasminogen complex can degrade fibrin and activate free plasminogen to plasmin. The complex is not inhibited by alpha$_2$-antiplasmin.

Colman RW, Hirsh J, Marder VJ, et al. (eds.): Hemostasis and Thrombosis: Basic Principles and Clinical Practice. 2nd ed. Philadelphia, J. B. Lippincott Company, 1987. *Extensive information about the structure and function of blood coagulation proteins with earnest attempts to relate biochemical facts to clinical problems.*

Drake TA, Morrissey JH, Edgington TS: Selective cellular expression of tissue factor in human tissues. Am J Pathol 134:1087, 1989. *Immunohistochemical localization of the hemostatic envelope.*

Furie B, Furie BC: The molecular basis of blood coagulation. Cell 53:505, 1988. *Short review of mechanisms.*

APPROACH TO PATIENTS WITH COAGULATION DISORDERS

HISTORY AND PHYSICAL EXAMINATION. There are three components to effective hemostasis: the blood vessel, the platelets, and the network of soluble factors. Abnormal bleeding occurs with much greater frequency when two of the three components are compromised as, for example, in a hemophilic patient who suffers trauma or takes aspirin or in a patient with peptic ulcer and thrombocytopenia. Disorders of platelets or blood vessels often cause mucosal or superficial bleeding; deficiency of a coagulation factor results in a tendency to form soft tissue hematomas or to suffer from repeated hemarthroses. Thrombosis tends to occur when there is inflammation, abnormalities of the luminal surface of a large blood vessel, or stasis.

A personal history, family history, and physical examination are important parts of the evaluation of a possible coagulation problem. In taking a history, it is not enough simply to ask, "Do you or your close relatives bleed or clot abnormally?" One must also determine how the hemostatic system has been stressed: "Have you had any operations or tooth extractions? If so, did you bleed abnormally or require blood transfusions afterward? Are your menstrual periods heavy? Do you bruise easily? Do you take iron tablets? Have you ever had a limb immobilized?" And

so on. A formal family tree indicating how many family members are at risk and which ones have symptoms or laboratory evidence of a coagulation disorder should be constructed.

LABORATORY SCREENING TESTS. When a bleeding disorder is suspected, a group of reproducible and fairly inexpensive laboratory tests should detect most clinically significant abnormalities of platelets, blood vessels, and the coagulation factor network:

1. A complete blood count and examination of the blood smear screen for abnormalities in bone marrow function or platelet number and morphologic changes in red cells caused by intravascular thrombosis or microangiopathy.

2. A quantitative platelet count provides more definitive information about platelet number.

3. A template bleeding time screens for abnormalities of blood vessels and platelets.

4. The PT and APTT screen for abnormalities of the extrinsic and intrinsic coagulation pathways, respectively. Both tests are sensitive to abnormalities of the common pathway. The PT or APTT should be abnormally long if a single factor is below 20 to 40 per cent of its normal plasma concentration.

5. The solubility of the fibrin clot in concentrated (6M) urea detects clinically significant deficiency of Factor XIII. In the absence of Factor XIII, the clot is not covalently crosslinked and therefore is soluble.

Evaluation of a Prolonged PT or APTT. The first step is to perform mixing experiments of normal plasma and the abnormal plasma to decide whether the abnormal plasma is deficient in a coagulation factor or contains an inhibitor of coagulation. If the screening test of the mixture is normal, it is likely that the abnormal plasma is deficient in one or more factors, and specific factor assays can be done to identify the deficiency. If the screening test of the mixture is abnormal, it is likely that the abnormal plasma contains an inhibitor. Inhibitors may be of the so-called lupus type and directed against the phospholipid used in the assays or more rarely may be directed against a single coagulation factor. Lupus-type inhibitors rarely cause clinical bleeding. Indeed, as described below, some patients with lupus-type inhibitors suffer from repeated episodes of venous and arterial thrombosis. Inhibitors directed against single factors, especially VIII and IX, may cause serious bleeding.

SPECIFIC TESTS OF INDIVIDUAL PROTEINS. A plasma protein can be measured as the protein per se, usually with an immunoassay, or for protein activity. Plasma contains many different proteins, some of which influence the activity of the coagulation factor of interest and others of which may influence the endpoint of the assay. Activity assays for coagulation proteins are therefore less straightforward than many laboratory measurements. In general, there are two approaches for such activity assays: use of factor-deficient plasmas and use of chromogenic substrates.

Use of Factor-Deficient Plasmas. Normal plasma and the patient's plasma are compared for their ability to correct the PT or APTT of plasma from an individual severely deficient in the factor of interest. Thus Factor VIII can be measured, using plasma from an individual with severe classic hemophilia. If the patient has a Factor VIII deficiency, the patient's plasma should correct the APTT of the hemophilic patient's plasma less well than does normal plasma. By convention, the normal plasma is said to have 100 per cent, or 1 unit per milliliter, of activity. If a 1/10 dilution of the patient's plasma has the correcting power of a 1/100 dilution of normal plasma, the patient is said to have a Factor VIII activity of 10 per cent, or 0.1 unit per milliliter. Such an assay should be accurate to within 10 to 20 per cent of the reported value.

Use of Chromogenic Substrates. A chromogenic substrate is a small peptide that is cleaved by an activated proteinase to yield a colored product. The rate of cleavage can be measured with high precision in a spectrophotometer, using dilute solutions of plasma. As an example, plasminogen can be assayed by the addition of streptokinase to diluted plasma and quantification of cleavage of a chromogenic substrate by streptokinase-plasminogen complexes. Alternatively, antiplasmin can be assayed by addition of plasmin to diluted plasma and quantification of the loss of the ability of plasmin to cleave the same substrate due to formation of plasmin-inhibitor complexes. Such assays should be accurate to within 3 to 5 per cent of the reported value but may be subject to artifact. For instance, a patient with a recent streptococcal infection could have artifactually low apparent plasminogen activity because of neutralizing antibodies to streptokinase.

Indications for Specific Tests. When there is a suspicious bleeding history but normal screening tests, several specific assays should be considered. Mild Factor VIII or IX deficiency (10 to 40 per cent of normal) is clinically significant but may result in a screening APTT that is at the upper limits of normal but still within the normal range. Deficiency of plasma alpha$_2$-antiplasmin can be diagnosed only with a specific assay.

Evaluation of a possible thrombotic diathesis, at present, can be done only with specific assays for proteins C and S, antithrombin III, plasminogen, and perhaps other components of the fibrinolytic system.

Diagnosis of a 50 Per Cent Deficiency State. Laboratory studies of family members are often crucial to the evaluation, especially when the diagnosis centers on a heterozygous (50 per cent of normal) deficiency. The normal level (i.e., the value in 99 per cent of normal individuals) of a coagulation factor is typically 70 to 140 per cent; the level of the factor in individuals with heterozygous deficiency is typically 35 to 70 per cent; and the assay for the factor is accurate to within only 5 to 10 per cent of the reported value. The problem of distinguishing the 50 per cent deficiency state from normal is therefore a formidable one. If the apparent deficiency is found in other family members at risk, one can be much more confident that a true deficiency state exists. For example, a random woman with a 50 per cent Factor VIII level is probably not a carrier of classic hemophilia. If the sister of a hemophilic patient has a 50 per cent Factor VIII level, however, the sister has a 95 per cent chance of being a carrier. Heterozygous deficiency states associated with thrombosis (i.e., deficiency of antithrombin III, protein C, or protein S) present a similar problem. The most important facet of the care of a patient with heterozygote deficiency is appropriate counseling. Therefore, a physician should not be reluctant to arrange extensive family studies. To give an example, it would be much more efficient (and cost effective) to identify a patient with antithrombin deficiency as part of a family study and counsel that patient that he or she is at risk for thrombosis after surgery than to screen all patients prior to surgery with a specific assay for antithrombin. In the future it is likely that informative protein or restriction fragment length polymorphisms will be identified that will allow most deficiency states to be traced in families with more than 99 per cent confidence.

Suchman AL, Griner PF: Diagnostic uses of the activated partial thromboplastin time and prothrombin time. Ann Intern Med 104:810, 1986. *Critical evaluation of when these tests should be ordered and how the tests should be interpreted.*

INHERITED DISORDERS OF BLOOD COAGULATION

General Comments

The plasma protein coagulation factors that are named with Roman numerals, with the exception of Factor XII, were identified as a consequence of patients presenting with bleeding disorders that were eventually recognized as unique and familial. Bleeding may be due to a structural defect in a coagulation factor or to a lack of its synthesis. In the former situation there is immunologically cross-reacting material (CRM) present in the patient's plasma, and the patient is said to be CRM+. In the latter situation the patient is said to be CRM−.

GENETICS. Genetic material for the coagulation factors has been cloned, and considerable information about the exact genetic defects that underlie inherited bleeding disorders has been generated. Deficiencies of Factors VIII and IX are inherited as X-linked traits, with bleeding occurring in the male hemizygotes. Von Willebrand disease is usually an autosomal dominant disorder, although rare patients have severe autosomal recessive disease. Deficiencies of all of the other coagulation factors are transmitted as autosomal recessive traits, with clinically significant bleeding usually manifested only in patients with homozygous or double heterozygous deficiency. Heterozygous carriers may have

reduced plasma levels of a coagulation factor activity, but the deficiency seldom affects hemostasis. In the case of protein deficiencies associated with familial tendency to thrombosis, however, heterozygotes with 50 per cent of the normal level of the protein are at risk.

McKusick VA: Mendelian Inheritance in Man. 9th ed. Baltimore, The Johns Hopkins University Press, 1990. *Catalogs genetic defects.*

TREATMENT STRATEGIES. The most obvious treatment is replacement of the missing factor. Concentrates of Factors VIII and IX are readily available at a cost of 50 to 70 cents per unit. Because of its large size, Factor VIII distributes mainly in the blood plasma. There is approximately 40 ml of plasma per kilogram of body weight. Thus it would take 1400 units of Factor VIII to raise the plasma Factor VIII level of a 70-kg patient with severe classic hemophilia from less than 1 per cent (<0.01 unit per milliliter) to 50 per cent (0.5 unit per milliliter) as calculated by the following formula:

$$0.5 \text{ unit/ml} \times 40 \text{ ml/kg} \times 70 \text{ kg} = 1400 \text{ units}$$

Because of its smaller size, Factor IX is distributed in a volume 1½-fold to 2-fold greater than the plasma volume. Thus, proportionately more Factor IX than Factor VIII must be infused to achieve a similar response in a patient with hemophilia B. Because of its longer half-life in the body, however, Factor IX needs to be given less often than Factor VIII to maintain a therapeutic level.

The most important, indeed overriding, problem with purified factor concentrates is with contaminating viruses. Each batch of concentrate is made from thousands of units of plasma, some of which come from commercial plasmapheresis centers. There is a high likelihood that recipients are infected with hepatitis B, non-A, non-B hepatitis, and/or human immunodeficiency virus (HIV). This likelihood can be minimized by use of source plasma that does not contain antibodies to the viruses and has a normal level of transaminase. The infectivity of concentrates can be further decreased or eliminated by subjecting the concentrates to treatment (e.g., heating or extraction with an organic solvent) that will inactivate the viruses but preserve the activity of the factor of interest or by use of pure factor. In addition, products made by recombinant DNA techniques are coming on the market. These products, however, are significantly more expensive than former concentrates. Several treatment strategies do not require exposure to blood products at all (e.g., use of desmopressin to raise transiently the level of factor VIII and EACA to minimize mucosal bleeding).

When elective procedures that require prophylactic therapy to raise factor levels are contemplated, it is wise to test the proposed therapy prior to the procedure to be sure that target levels can be achieved.

HEMOPHILIA A (Factor VIII Deficiency)

Hemophilia A, the most frequently encountered serious inherited disorder of blood coagulation, occurs in 1 of 10,000 males. The majority of hemophilic patients give a positive family history with an X-linked inheritance pattern. In the remainder the mutation of the Factor VIII gene may be new. A hemophilic patient's daughters will all be carriers, but all his sons will be normal. A carrier woman has a 50 per cent chance of producing a hemophilic male or a female carrier. Because of random inactivation (lyonization) of the X chromosome, the carrier is a genetic mosaic with two populations of cells containing either a normal X chromosome or an abnormal X chromosome (bearing the hemophilic gene). Therefore, a carrier should have about 50 per cent of the normal level of Factor VIII activity. The range of Factor VIII levels in carriers is broad, probably because inactivation of one of the X chromosomes is often disproportionate. If extreme lyonization occurs, so that the preponderance of cells in the carrier female contains the X chromosome with the hemophilic gene, and the Factor VIII level is less than 40 per cent of normal, the woman may have clinical features of mild hemophilia.

CLINICAL MANIFESTATIONS. In general, the degree of Factor VIII deficiency correlates with the frequency of clinically significant bleeding. Furthermore, the degree of deficiency and bleeding severity tends to be similar in affected members of a given family. Hemophilia, therefore, is often classified as severe

(<1 per cent of normal activity), moderate (1 to 5 per cent of normal activity), or mild (5 to 25 per cent of normal activity).

Hematomas and Internal Hemorrhage. Bleeding from the umbilical cord is rare at birth. Soft tissue hematomas may develop in early infancy. More difficulties begin when the child becomes physically active, and these continue throughout life. Hematomas often occur in muscles and soft tissues. Considerable blood loss can occur into thigh muscles or the retroperitoneum; the extent of blood loss in these areas may be difficult to discern clinically and is frequently underestimated. The bleeding of hemophilia can involve virtually any anatomic area and give rise to secondary symptoms and signs caused by compression. If bleeding occurs in the pharynx or neck, airway obstruction can result. Severe bleeding may occur from peptic ulcerations. Partial intestinal obstruction may result from hemorrhage into the bowel wall. Mesenteric bleeding can lead to the development of bowel ischemia and necrosis. Hematuria can be painless or may manifest as ureteral colic produced by the formation of clots that obstruct the ureter. Subdural hematomas and other central nervous system hemorrhages are uncommon but represent a major cause of death and disability. Many bleeding episodes appear to develop spontaneously without a history of trauma or other provoking causes. Such spontaneous bleeding may occur during periods of stress, as before school examinations or following family dissension. When bleeding follows trauma, it may be delayed, since the primary hemostasis furnished by vessels and platelets is intact (see Ch. 154).

Hemarthroses. Bleeding occurs in joints, usually in the elbows, knees, and ankles and less often in the wrist and hand. In about half of hemophilic patients, repeated hemarthroses result in eventual deformity and crippling. These patients have Factor VIII activity levels well below 5 per cent of normal and usually less than 1 per cent of normal. The patient experiences considerable pain with bleeding into joints because of distention of the joint capsule. Movement is severely limited, causing disuse atrophy of the muscles about the joint. Pressure erodes the ends of long bones, causing periosteal pain, eventual necrosis, and pseudocyst formation. Hemarthrosis causes proliferation of the synovium. Thus a vicious circle is set into play in which a joint, once weakened, may experience hemorrhage again and again in a seemingly spontaneous manner.

Bleeding After Surgery. Major or minor surgery, including dental extractions, can result in marked blood loss in a hemophilic patient and therefore must be carried out in conjunction with Factor VIII replacement therapy to assure adequate hemostasis. Even those patients with mild hemophilia, Factor VIII levels of 5 to 25 per cent of normal, may develop clinically significant bleeding with surgery or trauma and require replacement therapy.

DIAGNOSIS. A history of joint and soft tissue bleeding, a family history compatible with X-linked inheritance, and the presence of arthropathy on physical examination all point to the diagnosis of X-linked hemophilia. Factor VIII deficiency is most likely, although Factor IX deficiency (hemophilia B) must also be considered. Laboratory screening tests should show a normal PT and prolonged APTT. The abnormal APTT should be corrected by all deficient plasmas except those from individuals with known Factor VIII deficiency. In particular, the abnormal APTT should be corrected by plasma from a patient with factor IX deficiency. If plasmas from patients with known deficiencies are not available, correction can be attempted with normal plasma absorbed with barium salts (which removes Factor IX but not Factor VIII) and serum (which contains Factor IX but not active Factor VIII). Absorbed plasma, but not serum, corrects the abnormal APTT of a patient with Factor VIII deficiency. A quantitative assay for Factor VIII can be done by testing the ability of dilutions of the patient's plasma to correct the defect in Factor VIII–deficient plasma.

Von Willebrand factor (see below) stabilizes Factor VIII in the circulation; severe deficiency of von Willebrand factor is therefore accompanied by severe deficiency of Factor VIII, and hemophilia A can be confused with von Willebrand disease. Unlike hemophilia, however, von Willebrand disease is inherited as an autosomal dominant trait, and the patient may present with a history of vascular-type bleeding. Upon screening, the bleeding time should be grossly prolonged in von Willebrand disease, whereas the bleeding time is usually at the upper limit of normal or only slightly prolonged in hemophilia. Further investigation should demonstrate deficiency or abnormality of von Willebrand factor and defective platelet aggregation mediated by the antibiotic ristocetin in von Willebrand disease but not in hemophilia. If the diagnosis remains in doubt, it may be helpful to perform laboratory tests on family members to determine the inheritance pattern of the deficiency.

TREATMENT. The patient and family must learn about the nature of hemophilia, the anticipated severity of the patient's disease, the recognition and management of various types of bleeding episodes, the difference the disorder may make in the patient's future lifestyle, and the genetics of its transmission.

General Considerations. A major goal of patient, family, and physician is to have the patient lead as normal a life as possible. This will entail some restrictions of activities for the affected child and limitations on career choices. The physician, guided by the medical history, the degree of physical impairment, the severity of bleeding in affected family members, and the plasma level of Factor VIII, should advise the patient to participate in activities commensurate with the severity of his disease. A hemophilic child should be reared in a protective environment until he understands the consequences of hemophilia and can take responsibility for his actions. The physician should be alert for denial mechanisms sometimes constructed by patient and parents about the disease. For example, the patient may develop a willingness and receive unconscious encouragement from the parents to participate in dangerous activities or to forgo needed treatments. With maturity, the patient usually accepts the constraints imposed by his disease. He should be encouraged to develop his education and interests as fully as possible and counseled to adopt a career that does not expose him to undue hazards, is compatible with his physical capabilities, and allows him access to adequate health insurance coverage.

To be free to develop as normal a life as possible, the patient must participate in a major way in his medical care. This has led to the widespread adoption of home care programs in which the patient treats himself at home with the backup of a primary physician, a nurse coordinator, and a multidisciplinary team of a hematologist, orthopedic surgeon, dentist, social worker, financial counselor, and so on. It is reasonable to expect a responsible patient in a home care program to work or go to school full time, to require a minimum of emergency room visits, and to be hospitalized only for major trauma, medical illness, or elective surgery. The major cost of such a program is replacement therapy: A patient may consume many thousands of dollars in blood products each year. Home care programs, however, are cost effective because bleeding episodes are treated when first symptomatic and do not proceed to the point at which hospitalization is required for aggressive replacement therapy and pain management. About 50 per cent of patients with hemophilia A have enough problems to make home care worthwhile.

Patients receiving long-term replacement therapy need regular evaluation at 6- to 12-month intervals. The clinic visit should include a physical examination, with special attention paid to joints, an inhibitor screen, a chemistry panel including tests of liver function, and tests for antibodies to hepatitis viruses and HIV.

Factor VIII Preparations. Bleeding episodes are managed primarily by administration of Factor VIII, either in the form of cryoprecipitate or as a commercially prepared lyophilized concentrate. The use of cryoprecipitate or Factor VIII concentrate avoids the complication of volume overload that would occur with the large amount of plasma that would be necessary to attain acceptable levels of Factor VIII activity.

Blood banks prepare cryoprecipitate by freezing individual bags of fresh normal plasma, each containing approximately 200 units of Factor VIII activity in 200 ml of plasma, at $-20°C$ and then thawing at 4°C. Approximately 50 per cent of the Factor VIII contained in the plasma remains as a precipitate, which is separated from the bulk of the plasma and stored frozen in individual bags containing approximately 100 units of Factor VIII activity in 20 to 40 ml of residual plasma. When needed, the appropriate number of bags is thawed at 37°C, and the contents are pooled and administered intravenously to the patient.

Lyophilized Factor VIII concentrate is available in vials containing different amounts of Factor VIII activity (exact amounts stated on the labels). The concentrates are readily soluble upon addition of diluent and thus can be prepared and administered intravenously within 30 minutes.

The major advantage of cryoprecipitate in the past is that it exposed the recipient to fewer donors and thus minimized the chance of blood-transmitted viral infection. Indeed, individuals have been supported from infancy to young adulthood with cryoprecipitate prepared from plasma donated sequentially by the same donor. The major disadvantages of cryoprecipitate are the inconvenience of thawing and pooling bags prior to administration and the need for the bags to stay frozen at −20°C until the time of administration.

The major advantages of lyophilized concentrates are stability on storage and convenience of administration. The current generation of concentrates have been processed to eliminate or inactivate HIV totally and possibly also hepatitis B and C.

Patients should be vaccinated against hepatitis B at the time of diagnosis and will be prime candidates for vaccines that may be developed in the future for non-A, non-B hepatitis viruses and HIV.

Replacement Therapy. Intensity of replacement therapy depends on the estimated plasma level of Factor VIII required to halt the bleeding and the disappearance rate of the infused Factor VIII. Very early hemarthrosis can be managed with a single infusion to attain a peak Factor VIII level of 25 to 50 per cent of normal. For more extensive hemorrhage or hematuria, Factor VIII infusions are usually continued for 2 days after cessation of symptoms or signs of bleeding. Muscle hematomas require a longer period of sustained Factor VIII levels, in the range of 40 to 60 per cent of normal for 4 to 6 days. Major trauma or surgery requires that the Factor VIII level be maintained at more than 70 per cent of normal until hemostasis is achieved and then in the range of 25 to 50 per cent of normal for 10 to 14 days. Plasma Factor VIII can be measured after administration of the calculated dose to document that the desired level has been achieved and prior to subsequent scheduled doses to determine whether desired levels have been sustained. If a low Factor VIII level persists despite replacement therapy, it may be that simply not enough Factor VIII is being given or that the patient has developed an inhibitor that neutralizes infused Factor VIII.

The amount of concentrate needed to achieve and maintain a desired level of Factor VIII activity can be estimated by knowing (1) that the patient's plasma volume is about 40 ml per kilogram of body weight, (2) the amount of Factor VIII activity in the average bag of cryoprecipitate (usually about 100 units) or in available vials of lyophilized concentrate Factor VIII activity, and (3) that Factor VIII has a half-life of about 10 to 12 hours in the circulation. Therefore, replacement therapy is ordinarily given three times a day when tight control of the level is needed and twice a day when deeper troughs in the level can be tolerated. Alternatively, a constant infusion of 1 to 2 units per kilogram per hour can be given after a loading dose.

Treatment of Hemarthroses. Joint bleeding is helped initially by immobilization of the affected limb and application of ice packs to diminish swelling and discomfort. Hemarthroses should not be aspirated unless such acute pain and tension are present that pressure necrosis is a major possibility. Aspiration should be performed only after administration of replacement Factor VIII. When pain and swelling have subsided, the patient should begin rehabilitation to regain motion and strength in conjunction with prophylactic replacement therapy. Patients with joint disease may benefit from periodic assessment by an orthopedic surgeon. In properly selected patients, synovectomy and artificial joint replacement have been very successful in improving the usefulness of severe chronic joint deformity.

Dental Care. The patient should be instructed about the importance of dental hygiene and should have frequent dental examinations. Bleeding in deep tissues of the oropharynx can be life threatening. Therefore, a local anesthetic should be administered by needle puncture only after prophylactic administration of Factor VIII concentrate. Extraction also requires prior administration of Factor VIII concentrate. For patients with mild or moderate hemophilia, it is likely that adequate levels of Factor VIII can be achieved with use of desmopressin, as described below for patients with von Willebrand disease. Administration of EACA by mouth, also described below, is useful in prevention of rebleeding after tooth extraction.

Use of Analgesics. Bleeding can cause extraordinary pain. Injudicious use of narcotics can lead to addiction in hemophilic patients. Aspirin must be avoided by the hemophilic because it decreases platelet aggregation and accentuates bleeding. Acetaminophen and codeine are recommended as the first choices of analgesics. In selected cases, ibuprofen can be given for chronic joint pain. The likelihood that ibuprofen will cause increased bleeding can be assessed by a template bleeding time after the patient has received the drug for several days. If the bleeding time is prolonged compared with the bleeding time before therapy, the drug should be discontinued.

Factor VIII Inhibitors. The possibility that the patient has acquired neutralizing antibodies to Factor VIII (Factor VIII inhibitor) should be of constant concern. An inhibitor may initially appear at almost any time in the life of a hemophilic patient and need not be associated with any obvious change in the clinical severity of the disorder. Patients with inhibitors present special problems. Much depends on the titer of the inhibitor, which is commonly expressed in Bethesda units: 1 Bethesda unit, by definition, inhibits 1 unit of Factor VIII, i.e., the Factor VIII in 1 ml of normal plasma. If one calculates the amount of Factor VIII required to neutralize the inhibitor and achieve a 50 per cent normal level of circulating Factor VIII in a patient who weighs 70 kg and has a plasma volume of 2800 ml and an inhibitor titer of 10 Bethesda units per milliliter, the amount is immense:

$$2800 \text{ ml} \times 10.5 \text{ units/ml} = 29,400 \text{ units}$$

Several strategies are available, all expensive and none totally adequate. Because some inhibitors take up to several hours to complex with and inhibit Factor VIII, it may be possible to maintain Factor VIII levels at a therapeutic level by constant infusion. If the inhibitor is of modest titer (1 to 10 Bethesda units per milliliter), it may be possible to remove enough inhibitor by plasmapheresis to make therapy feasible with lower amounts of Factor VIII. A patient receiving Factor VIII concentrate may have an anamnestic immune response with an increase in the titer and avidity of his inhibitor. Therefore, everything possible should be done to achieve permanent hemostasis in the 4- to 6-day "golden period" during which replacement therapy is possible. Patients with high titers of rapidly acting inhibitor can be given porcine Factor VIII concentrate or activated Factor IX concentrate that also contains activated Factor X and therefore "bypasses" Factor VIII in the coagulation cascade. Both concentrates are expensive, and the activated Factor IX concentrate has considerable thrombogenic potential.

ACQUIRED IMMUNODEFICIENCY SYNDROME (AIDS). Regardless of whether they have antibodies to HIV, patients who have used significant quantities of blood products in the 1980's must take proper precautions to protect their close contacts and loved ones. They can be assured that the virus is not transmitted by casual household contact. They must be taught safe disposal procedures for needles and other injection paraphernalia. It should be strongly recommended that condoms be used during all sexual intercourse. This raises an irreconcilable conflict for couples considering pregnancy. There is a high likelihood of transmission of HIV to the newborn of a virus-positive mother. Thus, wives of men with hemophilia who are considering pregnancy should receive specific education and counseling and be tested for antibodies to HIV before pregnancy occurs.

PROGNOSIS. The major long-term complications of moderate and severe hemophilia are (1) progressive joint deformity and crippling, (2) development of inhibitors to Factor VIII activity, (3) hepatitis and cirrhosis, and (4) AIDS.

Despite the availability of replacement therapy, many hemophiliacs, for a variety of reasons, are treated inadequately or haphazardly and become severely crippled and, ultimately, chronic invalids. The last three of the four complications listed above are seen more often in patients who receive frequent replacement therapy. Up to 15 per cent of hemophilic patients develop inhibitory antibodies to Factor VIII activity, usually in childhood. Most patients who have received Factor VIII concentrate in the past have been exposed to hepatitis viruses and HIV. The risks of chronic hepatitis and AIDS in exposed individuals are both high. Newer concentrates are much safer. On the whole, the availability of concentrates has been beneficial and has improved the prognosis of all forms of hemophilia A—mild, moderate, and severe. It is reasonable to hope that future cohorts of hemophiliacs will enjoy the benefits of replacement therapy without the complications.

CARRIER DETECTION. Women who have relatives with hemophilia frequently seek help to determine whether they may pass the disorder to their children. Daughters of men with the disorder, mothers of more than one hemophilic son, and mothers who have a hemophilic son and another hemophilic male relative in their pedigree are obligate carriers of the hemophilic gene. Only about 15 per cent of the instances of hemophilia arise because of spontaneous mutation. Determination of Factor VIII procoagulant activity is of limited usefulness in the identification of carrier women, because low-normal levels overlap with Factor VIII levels found in obligate heterozygotes. A major reason for scatter in Factor VIII levels is scatter in the levels of von Willebrand factor, which functions as a carrier protein for Factor VIII. Therefore, the overlap between normal persons and obligate carriers is decreased considerably if the Factor VIII level is corrected for the level of immunoreactive von Willebrand factor (sometimes called Factor VIII–related antigen). When the ratios of these two proteins are analyzed by logarithmic discriminant analysis, greater than 95 per cent of carriers can be identified. Such an analysis is best done by a laboratory that is highly experienced with the assays and has proved the validity of the analysis in an adequate number of obligate carriers.

Several restriction fragment length polymorphisms close to the gene for Factor VIII have been shown to be useful in tracing hemophilia A in families. In families in which the polymorphisms segregate with hemophilia, the polymorphisms can identify carriers with greater than 99 per cent confidence. The polymorphisms can also be used to diagnose hemophilia in fetuses in the first trimester, whereas assays of Factor VIII per se can be done only in the second trimester when the fetal circulation is accessible for blood sampling by fetoscopy.

Brettler DB, Forsberg AD, Levine PH, et al.: The use of porcine factor VIII concentrate (Hyate:C) in the treatment of patients with inhibitor antibodies to factor VIII. Arch Intern Med 149:1381, 1989. *Describes a favorable response when compared with other modalities.*

Levine PH: The clinical manifestations and therapy of hemophilias A and B. In Colman RW, Hirsh J, Marder VJ, et al. (eds.): Hemostasis and Thrombosis: Basic Principles and Clinical Practice. 2nd ed. Philadelphia, J. B. Lippincott Company, 1987, pp 97–111.

White GC II, Shoemaker CB: Factor VIII gene and hemophilia A. Blood 73:1, 1989. *Update on genetic defects and potential applications of new knowledge.*

VON WILLEBRAND DISEASE

This disorder is due to a deficiency or abnormality of a plasma protein, von Willebrand factor, that is required for the stabilization of Factor VIII in the circulation and for the normal adherence of platelets to sites of vascular injury. The gene for von Willebrand factor is on chromosome 12. The hallmarks of von Willebrand disease historically have been a low Factor VIII level, a long bleeding time, and autosomal inheritance. The last two characteristics distinguish von Willebrand disease from hemophilia A. With extensive characterization of von Willebrand factor over the past decade has come a broadening of the definition of von Willebrand disease, so that the name now encompasses a heterogeneous group of defects of von Willebrand factor.

FUNCTION OF VON WILLEBRAND FACTOR. Factor VIII and von Willebrand factor circulate in normal plasma as a complex. Endothelial cells and megakaryocytes-platelets synthesize, store, and secrete von Willebrand factor. Secretion increases when endothelial cells are stimulated or injured. Therefore the concentration of plasma von Willebrand factor is labile and can be increased by stimuli as innocuous as a vigorous Valsalva maneuver, and it is common to find levels of von Willebrand factor elevated 2-fold to 10-fold in ill patients. Von Willebrand factor exists as a series of multimers ranging in size from 850,000 to 12,000,000 daltons. The largest multimers, which have a half-life in the circulation of only several hours, are most active in mediation of platelet adhesion. Both large and small multimers complex with Factor VIII. Von Willebrand factor can interact with platelets in two different ways. It binds to platelet glycoprotein Ib in a reaction that is greatly enhanced by ristocetin (an

antibiotic that cannot be used because it causes thrombocytopenia). It also binds to platelet glycoprotein IIb-IIIa complex, but only when platelets are activated. Von Willebrand factor binds to collagen and other components of the vessel wall and thus mediates attachment and spreading of platelets to the subendothelium of damaged vessels. The role of von Willebrand factor in platelet adhesion is especially important when blood passes through the blood vessel at a high shear rate and the red blood cell count is normal or increased.

PATHOGENESIS OF VON WILLEBRAND DISEASE. In classic (type I) von Willebrand disease, patients have prolonged bleeding time, abnormal platelet aggregation in response to ristocetin, and parallel decreases in plasma Factor VIII activity, immunoreactive von Willebrand factor, and ristocetin cofactor activity. Patients with severe, usually homozygous, disease can have less than 1 per cent of normal von Willebrand factor in plasma and platelets and no detectable von Willebrand antigen in endothelial cells. Their Factor VIII levels may be less than 5 per cent of normal. Intravenous infusion of small amounts of normal plasma, hemophilic plasma, or normal serum into patients with severe von Willebrand disease results in a prolonged increase in Factor VIII that is out of proportion to the Factor VIII content of the transfused plasma or serum. This probably results from stabilization of the patients' endogenously produced factor VIII by infused von Willebrand factor.

A number of qualitative abnormalities of von Willebrand factor result in variant diseases called type IIA, type IIB, and so on. In type IIA disease the large and intermediate-sized multimers are not present in plasma or platelets. Von Willebrand factor function (e.g., ristocetin cofactor activity) is decreased more than von Willebrand factor antigen. These patients have abnormal platelet adhesion and long bleeding times, but normal Factor VIII activity. Abnormal multimer patterns can be ascertained by probing separated plasma proteins with antibodies to von Willebrand factors after agarose gel electrophoresis. Subtypes IIC, IID, etc., of von Willebrand disease have been identified, based on additional subtle abnormalities in the electrophoretic pattern of the multimers. In type IIB disease the largest multimers are missing from plasma but not from platelets, and the abnormal von Willebrand factor causes platelet aggregation at lower than usual ristocetin concentration. It is thought that the largest multimers are missing from plasma because the multimers bind spontaneously to platelets. In principle, such a spontaneous interaction could be due to defects in the patient's von Willebrand factor or in the patient's platelets ("pseudo von Willebrand disease"), and indeed patients have been identified in whom the defect is in the platelets (Ch. 154).

CLINICAL MANIFESTATIONS. Von Willebrand disease has a broad spectrum of clinical and laboratory features. It can range from a severe hemorrhagic disorder, in which the level of Factor VIII is low enough and the bleeding problems severe enough that the disease must be differentiated from classic hemophilia, to an asymptomatic condition that is a laboratory curiosity. The severity of symptoms due to von Willebrand disease can vary considerably even among afflicted family members, probably because there are a number of factors that control the synthesis and secretion of von Willebrand factor.

Patients with severe disease usually have inherited it from both parents, either as a true homozygous or as a double heterozygous disease. The principal bleeding problems are of the superficial type. Epistaxis is a frequent complaint, especially early in life, as is easy bruising. Hematuria and gastrointestinal bleeding occur less frequently, and hemarthroses are quite rare. Without adequate replacement therapy, postoperative bleeding is a major hazard. In patients with heterozygous type I or II disease, the hemorrhagic tendency usually becomes evident or troublesome only with trauma, surgery, or dental extractions. Women with the disorder commonly experience excessive menses and postpartum bleeding. In all forms of the disease, the frequency and severity of bleeding tend to lessen with age.

DIAGNOSIS. The classic findings in type I von Willebrand disease are prolonged bleeding time and a low level of Factor VIII. Confirmatory testing should reveal a low level of immunoreactive von Willebrand factor and absent or diminished platelet aggregation when ristocetin is added to the patient's platelet-rich plasma. The analysis using ristocetin can be made more sensitive and quantitative by testing the ability of dilutions of the patient's plasma to support agglutination of washed platelets; this is often called the ristocetin cofactor titer.

Electrophoretic analysis of the site distribution of von Willebrand factor multimers should be done in patients who are suspected of having type II von Willebrand disease on the basis of bleeding problems, prolonged bleeding time, and abnormal ristocetin-induced platelet aggregation but normal or only slightly decreased levels of von Willebrand factor and Factor VIII. In type IIA disease, the larger multimers are missing in both plasma and platelets. In type IIB disease (hypersensitivity to ristocetin), the larger multimers are missing in plasma but not in platelets.

It may be very difficult to know for sure whether someone with mild decreases in von Willebrand factor and Factor VIII, say, to 50 per cent of normal, has von Willebrand disease. A number of factors influence the plasma concentration of von Willebrand factor. People with type O blood have lower levels than do people with types A and B. Hypothyroidism causes the level of von Willebrand factor to fall. As mentioned above, endothelial cells can be stimulated to release von Willebrand factor. Thus, one must worry about both overdiagnosis and underdiagnosis. Serial studies of the same patient and studies of other family members can be helpful. Because symptoms in such patients are mild and tend to decrease with age, however, it may suffice to be honest with such patients about the ambiguities of the laboratory tests and counsel them to alert their physician about the possibility of von Willebrand disease in the event of trauma or major surgery.

TREATMENT. Indications for therapy in von Willebrand disease include surgery, severe epistaxis, severe menorrhagia, and recurrent gastrointestinal bleeding.

Replacement Therapy. Cryoprecipitate is equally rich in Factor VIII and von Willebrand factor and therefore corrects both the deficiency of Factor VIII and the long bleeding time of type I von Willebrand disease. Factor VIII concentrates are poor in von Willebrand factor and do not correct the bleeding time defect. Hence, replacement therapy in von Willebrand disease should be with cryoprecipitate rather than Factor VIII concentrate. Because the largest multimers of von Willebrand factor are cleared rapidly after infusion, the bleeding time is usually corrected only transiently. The smaller multimers allow the patient's own Factor VIII to circulate, and the Factor VIII level may remain elevated for considerably longer than would be predicted, based on the amount of infused Factor VIII. In the case of ongoing hemorrhage or major surgery, cryoprecipitate should be given, using the guidelines described above for Factor VIII replacement in hemophilia A. The infusion should be given immediately prior to maneuvers designed to achieve hemostasis. This practice will ensure that the bleeding time as well as the Factor VIII level is maximally corrected. It is not practical to give cryoprecipitate often enough to keep the bleeding time continuously corrected or to quantify the correction with serial bleeding times. Therefore, once hemostasis is achieved, therapy should be directed toward keeping the level of Factor VIII in the appropriate therapeutic ranges as described above for hemophilia A. This probably requires less cryoprecipitate than if one were treating a hemophiliac.

Desmopressin. Because there is not an effective virus-free purified concentrate of von Willebrand factor, considerable attention has been devoted to the therapeutic potential of desmopressin (1-deamino-8-D-arginine vasopressin, DDAVP), especially in patients with mild von Willebrand disease. Desmopressin causes release of von Willebrand factor and plasminogen activator from endothelial cells. EACA suppresses baseline and desmopressin-stimulated fibrinolysis and may be useful as an adjunctive therapy. Desmopressin, 0.3 µg per kilogram of body weight in 50 ml of saline, is given over 15 minutes. In type I disease, several-fold increases of both Factor VIII and von Willebrand protein occur 15 to 30 minutes after infusion, with a concomitant decrease in the bleeding time. The effect may last for several hours. The magnitude and duration of the response vary among individual patients, especially among those with type IIA disease. Desmopressin is contraindicated in type IIB disease because appearance of the large multimers in the circulation can cause thrombocytopenia.

To learn if the treatment is feasible in a given patient, one should quantify the response to a test dose of desmopressin at the time of diagnosis or 5 to 7 days prior to a planned procedure. For oral surgical procedures, EACA is given orally in a dosage of 75 mg per kilogram every 6 hours for 7 to 10 days beginning the evening before the procedure. It is controversial whether an antifibrinolytic agent should be given with major surgery.

Menstruation and Pregnancy. Excessive menstrual blood loss can be managed with hormonal suppression. Levels of Factor VIII, von Willebrand factor, and ristocetin cofactor activity may become normal during pregnancy. Therefore, these tests, along with determination of the bleeding time, should be repeated during the third trimester to plan for replacement therapy during delivery. Cryoprecipitate should be given if the Factor VIII level remains low. If the Factor VIII level is greater than 50 per cent, but the bleeding time remains long, cryoprecipitate should be on call, because postpartum blood loss is frequently severe enough to require replacement infusion.

Complications of Therapy. Chronic arthropathy is less common in von Willebrand disease than in hemophilia A. The complications of replacement therapy for severe von Willebrand disease are the same as those described above for hemophilia A. Rarely, antibodies that inhibit the activity of von Willebrand protein develop. Patients receiving blood products should be vaccinated against hepatitis B and monitored for the acquisition of hepatitis viruses and HIV.

Mannucci PM: Desmopressin. A nontransfusional form of treatment for congenital and acquired blood disorders. Blood 72:1449, 1988. *Review of therapeutic applications.*

Ruggeri ZM, Zimmerman TS: Von Willebrand factor and von Willebrand disease. Blood 70:895, 1987. *A review of the disease and its pathogenesis.*

HEMOPHILIA B (Factor IX Deficiency)

Factor IX deficiency is inherited as an X-linked disorder that presents with the historical and clinical features of classic hemophilia (hemophilia A). The severity of bleeding is usually similar in members of a single family. Factor IX–deficient patients have fewer symptoms than do patients with Factor VIII deficiency; patients with severe (<1 per cent of normal) Factor IX deficiency have the symptoms of patients with mild (1 to 5 per cent of normal) Factor VIII deficiency. Nevertheless, Factor IX deficiency causes serious bleeding problems. Patients with Factor IX deficiency can be more cavalier about their disease than can patients with Factor VIII deficiency, and therefore they are not as quick to seek medical attention when they need it—sometimes to their detriment.

CLINICAL MANIFESTATIONS. Many patients are asymptomatic until the hemostatic system is stressed by surgery or trauma. Patients with the most severe disease may develop muscle hematomas, gastrointestinal hemorrhage, and bleeding into large joints with progression to crippling joint deformities.

DIAGNOSIS. This disorder is suspected with the finding of a normal PT and prolonged APTT that can be corrected by normal serum but not by barium sulfate–adsorbed plasma. The inability of the patient's plasma to correct the prolonged APTT of plasma from a patient with known Factor IX deficiency establishes the diagnosis.

TREATMENT. The care and long-term goals of therapy for the patient with Factor IX deficiency are similar to those described above for the patient with hemophilia A. Most patients need less care than if they had hemophilia A, but they require the same intensity of education and counseling.

Replacement Therapy. Fresh frozen plasma is used to treat mild to moderate bleeding, especially in those patients who have hemorrhagic episodes infrequently. Ordinarily, transfusion of 500 ml of plasma twice daily is sufficient to maintain a level of Factor IX activity 10 to 12 per cent above baseline. EACA can be used as an adjunct to transfusions of plasma in patients with mucosal bleeding or dental work.

Patients with moderate to severe hemorrhage, such as large hemarthroses or muscle hematomas, and patients being prepared for surgery can be treated with commercially prepared Factor IX concentrate, aiming for levels that are approximately two thirds as high as those described above for Factor VIII replacement therapy. Because the volume of distribution and the half-life of Factor IX are both greater than for Factor VIII, a greater loading dose of Factor IX must be given than for Factor VIII, but subsequent doses can be given less frequently. The length of therapy is dependent on the severity of the hemorrhage and the patient's response. Therapy is generally continued for 2 days after bleeding and related symptoms have subsided.

Complications of Therapy. Currently available Factor IX concentrates are a mixture of all of the vitamin K–dependent factors—Factors II, VII, IX, and X and proteins C and S—and are heat treated. Factor IX stands up to heat treatment better than does Factor VIII, and therefore the concentrates are heated more vigorously and should be freer of infectious HIV than are Factor VIII concentrates. However, the concentrates are not free of infectious hepatitis viruses. Patients therefore should be immunized against hepatitis B.

Factor IX concentrates contain trace amounts of activated vitamin K–dependent factors and therefore are thrombogenic and carry a risk for thromboembolism, especially when used in high dosage in patients who have liver disease or are immobilized after surgery. EACA greatly enhances the risk of thromboembolism and should never be used as an adjunct to Factor IX concentrates. Indeed, some advocate that low-dosage heparin (5000 units every 12 hours) and plasma (as a source of antithrombins) be given to surgical patients receiving Factor IX concentrate. Because of these potential complications, it is advisable to reserve the use of Factor IX concentrates for patients who have acquired antibody to hepatitis B surface antigen as a result of prior exposure or immunization and for whom the benefits of treatment outweigh the risks of thromboembolism. In a situation in which levels greater than 10 to 15 per cent above baseline are desired but use of Factor IX concentrate is contraindicated, plasmapheresis can be used to prevent volume overload.

Antibody inhibitors to Factor IX occur in 5 to 10 per cent of treated patients.

CARRIER DETECTION. The normal range for Factor IX is narrower than the normal range for Factor VIII, and therefore carrier testing based on coagulation assays is better for hemophilia B than for hemophilia A. Nevertheless, laboratory definition of the carrier state is still an exercise in probabilities and is best done with genetic markers. The Factor IX gene exhibits considerable polymorphism, and informative genetic markers are found in most families. However, it is worthwhile doing Factor IX activity assays in known and potential carriers, because women who are carriers may have Factor IX levels that are sufficiently low to cause mild bleeding, especially after trauma or surgery.

Giannelli F, Green PM, High KA, et al.: Haemophilia B: Database of point mutations and short additions and deletions. Nucleic Acids Res 18:4053, 1990. *The only other specific group of inherited diseases with as many characterized mutations are the hemoglobinopathies.*

Thompson AR: Structure, function, and molecular defects of factor IX. Blood 67:565, 1986. *Comprehensive summary of information about Factor IX and hemophilia B.*

DEFICIENCIES OF CONTACT FACTORS

Deficiencies of Factor XII, prekallikrein, or HMWK are clinically benign, and deficiency of Factor XI may sometimes be benign. Patients with these abnormalities, however, have APTT's that are as prolonged as are those of patients with Factor VIII or IX deficiency. Therefore it is important to establish the correct diagnosis and to counsel the patient that he or she has a laboratory abnormality that carries little risk for bleeding.

Deficiency of Factor XII, Prekallikrein, or High Molecular Weight Kininogen

These autosomal recessive disorders are almost always asymptomatic and are usually identified as an abnormality in a routine APTT. The APTT of a mixture of patient's plasma and normal plasma should be normal, i.e., with no inhibitor demonstrable. The plasma concentrations of Factors VIII and IX should be normal. The coagulation defect can be identified by the inability of the patient's plasma to correct the APTT of the appropriately deficient plasma.

Deficiency of Factor XI

Factor XI deficiency is common among Ashkenazi Jews, and the prevalence of homozygous Factor XI deficiency in cities with a sizable Jewish population is comparable to the prevalence of hemophilia A. The defect is usually asymptomatic, but it is occasionally associated with bleeding. Major bleeding into mus-

cles or joints is rare. The inheritance pattern is autosomal recessive, so that the deficiency is found with equal frequency in men and women. The APTT is prolonged. The PT and bleeding time are normal. Normal serum or barium sulfate–adsorbed plasma both correct the APTT. Specific assays for Factors VIII and IX are normal. The diagnosis is established by demonstrating that the patient's plasma does not correct the APTT of Factor XI–deficient plasma.

Clinically significant bleeding usually occurs in association with trauma, surgery, or dental extractions. Fresh frozen plasma, 10 to 20 ml per kilogram, should be given as treatment of bleeding or as prophylaxis for surgery. One infusion should suffice, because Factor XI has a half-life of about 72 hours.

Silverberg M, Kaplan AP, Colman RW: Contact activation and its abnormalities. *In* Colman RW, Hirsh J, Marder VJ, et al. (eds.): Hemostasis and Thrombosis: Basic Principles and Clinical Practice. 2nd ed. Philadelphia, J. B. Lippincott Company, 1987, pp 18–38. *Well-referenced description of the biochemistry of Factor XI and the deficiency state.*

DEFICIENCIES OF THE EXTRINSIC AND COMMON PATHWAYS

Deficiencies of Factors VII, X, V, and II are all associated with clinically significant bleeding. The hemorrhagic diathesis is not as predictable or severe as in hemophilia A, but replacement therapy will probably be required at some point in a patient's lifetime, especially to control bleeding from mucous membranes, after dental extractions, or during menses.

Deficiency of Factor VII

CLINICAL MANIFESTATIONS. This is a rare autosomal recessive defect. Patients have a history of bleeding, usually beginning in infancy or early childhood. Bleeding, however, is frequently mild, even in patients with severe deficiency. Heterozygous relatives have no bleeding tendency. Mucous membrane bleeding, epistaxis, intramuscular hemorrhage, hemarthroses, and menorrhagia are the most common problems; gastrointestinal bleeding is less common, hematuria occurs only occasionally, and central nervous system bleeding is rare. Bleeding after dental extractions is predictable, and such extractions should be done with prophylactic replacement therapy. Clinical manifestations of bleeding can vary from mild to severe in the same patient. In fact, patients with impressive bleeding histories have undergone major surgery without accompanying hemorrhage. This phenomenon is unexplained and not consistent with the central role assigned to Factor VII in the physiologic initiation of blood coagulation. Also incongruent are observations of thromboembolism in Factor VII–deficient patients.

DIAGNOSIS. A diagnosis of Factor VII deficiency should be considered if the PT is prolonged whereas the APTT is normal. The coagulation time of the patient's plasma in response to Russell's viper venom, which directly activates Factor X, is normal. The diagnosis is established by the inability to correct the patient's PT with Factor VII–deficient plasma.

TREATMENT. Bleeding is treated with plasma, not necessarily fresh frozen, because Factor VII is very stable. The half-life of Factor VII is 2 to 6 hours, and therefore frequent treatment is needed during a bleeding episode. Levels of 15 to 20 per cent of normal can be obtained with a loading dose of plasma of 10 to 20 ml per kilogram followed by 3 to 6 ml per kilogram every 12 hours and should suffice to stop bleeding or as prophylaxis for surgery. Commercially available Factor IX concentrates, which contain Factors VII, IX, X, and II, can be used if it is essential to avoid any possibility of intravascular volume overload; such concentrates carry the risk of thromboembolism and hepatitis. Menorrhagia may require treatment with oral contraceptive agents.

Deficiency of Factor X

This deficiency is also a rare autosomal recessive disorder. Clinical symptoms include epistaxis; occasional mucous membrane, joint, and muscle hemorrhages; and gastrointestinal bleeding. Women may have severe, life-threatening menses and postpartum hemorrhage. The diagnosis is suspected when both the PT and APTT are prolonged. The abnormal tests are corrected with normal serum, but not with barium sulfate–adsorbed plasma. The clotting time of plasma in response to Russell's viper venom is usually prolonged, although an abnormal Factor X has been described that is activated normally by Russell's viper venom but not by the intrinsic or extrinsic systems of blood coagulation. The diagnosis is established by demonstration that the abnormal plasma does not correct Factor X–deficient plasma. Bleeding episodes are treated with plasma as described above for Factor VII deficiency; plasma needs to be given less often because the plasma half-life of Factor X is 24 to 48 hours.

Deficiency of Factor II (Prothrombin Deficiency)

Like deficiency of Factors VII and X, Factor II deficiency (hypoprothrombinemia) is a rare recessive disorder. Bleeding ranges from mild to severe and generally occurs only if the Factor II activity level is less than 20 per cent of normal. Symptoms include umbilical bleeding at birth, epistaxis, menorrhagia, postpartum hemorrhage, and bleeding after trauma or minor surgical procedures. The diagnosis is suspected if the PT and APTT are prolonged and the thrombin time is normal. Neither serum nor barium sulfate–adsorbed plasma corrects the abnormalities. A specific assay can be done based on the relative ability of the unknown to correct the PT of known factor II–deficient plasma. Alternatively, a test can be done in which clotting of plasma is initiated with Taipan viper venom, a specific activator of Factor II. Bleeding is treated with infusions of fresh frozen plasma, as described above for Factor VII deficiency. Infusions are necessary only every 2 days, since the half-life of Factor II is about 72 hours.

Global Deficiency of Vitamin K–Dependent Factors

These patients present as infants with bleeding, grossly prolonged PT and APTT, and low levels (<5 per cent of normal) of Factors II, VII, IX, and X, even though there is no evidence of liver disease, malabsorption, or ingestion of coumarin drugs. The levels of the vitamin K–dependent factors increase to 30 to 40 per cent of normal when the patients are given pharmacologic dosages (10 mg per day) of vitamin K, and the patients do well, with minimal symptoms. This syndrome is probably due to some abnormality of vitamin K metabolism, such as an abnormality of vitamin K epoxide reductase.

Deficiency of Factor V

CLINICAL MANIFESTATIONS. This disorder usually is inherited as an autosomal recessive trait. As with deficiencies of the other common pathway components, the severity of bleeding symptoms is variable, and hemorrhage most often involves the mucous membranes of the nose and oral cavity. Hemarthroses are unusual. Menorrhagia may be so severe as to be life threatening. Some women with Factor V deficiency, however, have normal menses or only mild menorrhagia. Obstetric deliveries may occur with little or no bleeding, but postpartum hemorrhage is frequent and requires replacement therapy.

DIAGNOSIS. Both the APTT and the PT are prolonged. The PT can be corrected by barium sulfate–adsorbed fresh plasma, but not by serum. Definitive diagnosis is established if the patient's plasma does not correct the deficiency of a patient known to lack Factor V activity. For unknown reasons, the bleeding time is prolonged in about one third of Factor V–deficient patients.

THERAPY. Factor V is an extremely labile protein. Treatment, therefore, should be with plasma that either is fresh or was frozen while fresh and has not been stored for more than several months. The therapeutic goal should be a Factor V activity level greater than 25 per cent of normal. Because Factor V is larger than the vitamin K–dependent factors, it should be possible to achieve such a level with the doses of plasma described above for Factor VII deficiency. The plasma half-life of Factor V activity is 12 to 36 hours. Cryoprecipitate and Factor VIII concentrate are not enriched in Factor V. Surgery should be done under the "cover" of prophylactic replacement therapy.

Platelets contain 10 to 20 per cent of the Factor V in blood, and therefore platelet concentrates are a good source of Factor

V. Several patients have responded well to platelet transfusion after developing neutralizing antibodies to Factor V.

Combined Deficiencies of Factors V and VIII

A number of patients have mild deficiencies of both Factors V and VIII inherited as an autosomal recessive trait. The basis of the syndrome is unknown, but it probably is related to some posttranslational modification of the two homologous proteins, which is necessary for their function. Therapy should be directed toward replacement of both proteins.

Roberts HR, Foster PA: Inherited disorders of prothrombin conversion. *In* Colman RW, Hirsh J, Marder VJ, et al. (eds.): Hemostasis and Thrombosis: Basic Principles and Clinical Practice. 2nd ed. Philadelphia, J. B. Lippincott Company, 1987, pp 162–181. *Thoroughly referenced, and an excellent source of more detailed information about the diagnosis and management of patients with rare but clinically important factor deficiencies.*

ABNORMALITIES IN CONVERSION OF FIBRINOGEN TO FIBRIN

Disorders of Fibrinogen

These disorders fall into two categories: absence (afibrinogenemia) or a low content (hypofibrinogenemia) of plasma fibrinogen and abnormally functioning plasma fibrinogen (dysfibrinogenemia). Afibrinogenemia and hypofibrinogenemia are autosomally recessive traits. Dysfibrinogenemia can be autosomally dominant or recessive.

AFIBRINOGENEMIA. In patients with absence of or low content of fibrinogen, the bleeding tendency may be noted at birth as continued oozing from the umbilical stump. The intensity and frequency of bleeding after trauma or surgery vary from mild to severe. Death from intracranial hemorrhage may occur in infancy or early childhood. It is not understood why some patients have a minimal bleeding tendency whereas others are very symptomatic. All assays that require formation of fibrin as an endpoint are abnormal. Plasma fibrinogen cannot be detected by immunologic or chemical (salting out) methods. The bleeding time may be markedly prolonged. Bleeding episodes should be treated with cryoprecipitate, which contains 8-fold to 10-fold more fibrinogen than does an equivalent amount of plasma. Plasma fibrinogen concentrations greater than 100 mg per deciliter are generally adequate and can be achieved by administration of one bag of cryoprecipitate for each 10 kg of body weight.

DYSFIBRINOGENEMIA. Dysfibrinogenemias are usually named after the cities in which they were discovered. The clinical features are very variable. Most individuals are asymptomatic. Some have mild to moderate bleeding tendencies, usually manifest only after surgery or trauma. Wound dehiscence is a problem in some. Some have a tendency for thrombosis. The abnormal proteins have a fascinating array of defects. For instance, several of the abnormal fibrinogens are poor substrates for thrombin, so that the fibrinopeptides are released slowly. Other abnormal fibrinogens, once converted to fibrin monomer by thrombin, display impaired aggregation into a fibrin gel. The diagnosis of these disorders should be suspected when delayed or poorly formed fibrin endpoints are observed in the PT, APTT, and thrombin time assays. The fibrinogen level, measured immunologically or chemically, is normal to low-normal. The majority of patients do not require treatment. In instances of bleeding or before surgical procedures on a patient known to have a propensity to bleed, replacement therapy in the form of cryoprecipitate should be given to attain a functioning plasma fibrinogen level of 100 to 150 mg per deciliter. Because the half-life of fibrinogen is 4 days, such infusions need to be given only once every several days. There are no absolute guidelines for how long therapy must be continued, but infusions of cryoprecipitate should be administered for 2 days after bleeding stops.

Deficiency of Factor XIII

Bleeding symptoms in Factor XIII deficiency occur in individuals with less than 1 to 2 per cent of normal plasma Factor XIII activity. The symptomatic deficiency state is an autosomal recessive trait. The bleeding diathesis is commonly apparent at birth as umbilical stump hemorrhage and continues throughout life. Wounds ooze slowly for days and heal poorly with scar formation. Intracranial hemorrhage after inapparent or only minor trauma is common. Males tend to be sterile, and women with the disorder have a high incidence of fetal loss unless they receive replacement therapy during pregnancy. Thrombin formation or conversion of fibrinogen to fibrin is not impaired. Consequently, the PT and APTT are normal. Platelet function tests are also normal. The laboratory diagnosis consists of demonstrating that a fibrin clot, made by recalcification of the patient's plasma, dissolves overnight at room temperature in 5M urea or 1 per cent monochloroacetic acid. Fibrin clots formed in the presence of greater than 1 to 2 per cent of the normal concentration of Factor XIII remain intact indefinitely in these solvents.

Treatment consists of giving fresh frozen plasma. Correction of the plasma concentration of Factor XIII to 5 to 10 per cent of normal provides normal hemostasis. The half-life of Factor XIII is approximately 12 days, and thus prophylactic replacement therapy is feasible. Because central nervous system hemorrhage is a major risk, Factor XIII–deficient patients are commonly given 5 to 10 ml per kilogram of fresh frozen plasma every 3 weeks. Extra plasma should be given in preparation for surgery or after head trauma. Development of inhibitory antibody to Factor XIII as a consequence of transfusion therapy is apparently rare.

Deficiency of Alpha₂-Antiplasmin

Congenital homozygous deficiency of alpha$_2$-antiplasmin is associated with a severe, hemophilia-like bleeding tendency. Heterozygous family members with plasma concentrations of the inhibitor 50 per cent of normal have a mild bleeding tendency characterized by postoperative bleeding, excessive bleeding after tooth extraction, and easy bruising after trauma. Levels of alpha$_2$-antiplasmin can be quantified with an activity assay. Patients with severe homozygous deficiency have fewer bleeding episodes when they receive long-term treatment with tranexamic acid. Heterozygotes would probably also benefit from treatment with tranexamic acid or EACA when symptomatic or when their antiplasmin level is depleted by stresses such as major surgery.

Leebeek FWG, Stibbe J, Knot EAR, et al.: Mild haemostatic problems associated with congenital heterozygous α$_2$-antiplasmin deficiency. Thromb Haemost 59:96, 1988. *Update on hemorrhagic diathesis associated with 50 per cent deficiency state.*

McDonagh J, Carrell N: Disorders of fibrinogen structure and function. *In* Colman RW, Hirsh J, Marder VJ, et al. (eds.): Hemostasis and Thrombosis: Basic Principles and Clinical Practice. 2nd ed. Philadelphia, J.B. Lippincott Company, 1987, pp 301–317. *Description of interesting and diverse set of disorders.*

INHERITED TENDENCIES TOWARD THROMBOSIS

There has been considerable progress in the biochemical definition of hypercoagulability. Quantitative or functional deficiencies of three plasma proteins—protein C, protein S, and antithrombin III—have been reported to be associated with a tendency toward thrombosis in affected families. Abnormalities of homocysteine metabolism have been shown to be associated with arterial thrombosis (Ch. 182). As more is learned about fibrinolysis, it is likely that genetic abnormalities of plasminogen, plasminogen activators, and plasminogen activator inhibitors that are associated with a thrombotic diathesis will be identified.

APPROACH TO THE PATIENT WITH A SUSPECTED THROMBOTIC TENDENCY. Patients with the recently described deficiency syndromes are fairly rare. It is therefore difficult to make firm guidelines about when or how to search for deficiency states and how to treat or counsel affected individuals. In general, it is worthwhile to evaluate the status of patients with family histories of thrombosis, young (<40 years old) patients, and patients with rare types of thrombosis (e.g., dural sinus or mesenteric vein thrombosis). Patients should be questioned and their status evaluated to ascertain whether they or family members have or have had conditions that would put them at risk for thrombosis (obesity, prolonged immobilization, injury to or abnormalities of vessels) or causes for secondary hypercoagulability (myeloproliferative syndrome, paroxysmal nocturnal hemoglobinuria, malignant disease, lupus anticoagulant). It has been estimated that of patients with "unexpected thrombosis," 1 to 2 per cent have deficiency of antithrombin III, 5 per cent have deficiency of protein C, and 5 per cent have deficiency of protein S. In my practice, the laboratory evaluation in individuals with a possible thrombotic diathesis includes activity assays of total antithrombin and plasminogen (readily available), activity and immunologic assays of protein C, and immunoassay of protein S

(available in coagulation reference laboratories). Plasma is also frozen at −70°C, with the anticipation that new tests may become available in the future. Patients with premature peripheral or cerebral occlusive arterial disease should be screened for excessive homocysteine accumulation after a standardized methionine-loading test.

Deficiency of Protein C

Two syndromes of hereditary protein C deficiency have been described: (1) heterozygous deficiency, in which half-normal concentrations of protein C are associated with an increased risk of venous thromboembolism, and (2) homozygous deficiency, in which total lack (<1 per cent of normal) of protein C is associated with neonatal purpura fulminans (ischemic necrosis of skin and digits) and massive venous thrombosis. Not all individuals with heterozygous deficiency have thrombosis. In families in which there is thrombosis, some family members with 50 per cent levels are asymptomatic, i.e., the phenotype displays autosomal dominance with incomplete penetrance. Heterozygous deficient individuals in other kindreds ascertained because of infants with homozygous deficiency do not seem at risk for thrombosis at all. It is likely, however, that homozygous deficiency is invariably associated with problems.

The diagnosis of protein C deficiency is based on decreased amounts of antigen or activity in plasma. For patients receiving long-term therapy with warfarin, other vitamin K–dependent proteins, e.g., Factors X and II, are also measured with an immunoassay to correct for the 35 to 50 per cent drop in the level of circulating vitamin K–dependent proteins caused by undercarboxylation. The antigenic measurements do not detect individuals with dysfunctional protein C.

Because not everyone with heterozygous protein C deficiency has thrombosis, long-term anticoagulation should be reserved for individuals who have had a thrombotic episode unless the family history is so striking that the physicians and affected members agree that prophylactic treatment is warranted. Asymptomatic family members should be counseled that they are at greater risk for thrombosis and advised about the dangers of prolonged immobilization of limbs, obesity, and smoking. When warfarin therapy is started in a patient with heterozygous deficiency, the anticoagulant effect should be achieved at a leisurely pace by daily administration of the predicted maintenance dose rather than by administration of a "loading dose" of drug. It is preferable to begin warfarin therapy while the patient is being treated with heparin. However, one should be aware that heparin induces thrombocytopenia and thrombosis in some patients, especially those who have received heparin for more than 10 days.

Infants with homozygous protein C deficiency respond acutely to administration of plasma or Factor IX concentrate, which is rich in protein C. Oral anticoagulants can be used to decrease the frequency of thrombotic events.

Deficiency of Protein S

Decreased levels of plasma protein S antigen or activity are associated with venous thrombosis. Correlation between antigen and activity is poor, because a fraction of protein S in plasma is complexed with C4b-binding protein, and only the fraction of protein S that is free has anticoagulant activity. The proportion of complexed and free protein S can be ascertained by crossed immunoelectrophoresis. The tendency toward thrombosis is inherited as an autosomal dominant trait with incomplete penetrance. Affected individuals tend to have levels of protein S that are 50 per cent of normal, i.e., they are heterozygous for the deficiency. The incidence of symptomatic heterozygous protein S deficiency is probably the same as the incidence of symptomatic protein C deficiency. Pending further information about this recently described syndrome, it seems reasonable to approach and treat heterozygous protein S deficiency using the guidelines described above for heterozygous protein C deficiency.

Deficiency of Antithrombin III

The average concentration of antithrombin III in deficient patients is approximately 50 per cent of normal. The most frequent manifestation of thromboembolism is lower extremity thrombophlebitis, often bilateral and recurrent and often with pulmonary embolism. Patients may develop venous insufficiency and chronic leg ulcers. Upper extremity thrombophlebitis and mesenteric vein thrombosis are less common. Rare patients may develop retinal or cerebral vein thrombosis, thrombosis of the renal vein or inferior vena cava, Budd-Chiari syndrome, priapism, or widespread clotting and defibrination syndrome. The cumulative incidences of thromboembolism are estimated to be 15 per cent by age 19, 50 per cent by age 29, and 85 per cent in individuals over 40 years. Complete, i.e., homozygous, lack of the major antithrombin has not been described. Patients homozygous for a dysfunctional antithrombin, however, have been reported.

Antithrombin deficiency can be ascertained by an activity assay in which diluted plasma and heparin are mixed with a known concentration of thrombin and the amount of uninhibited thrombin is quantified with a chromogenic substrate. Ongoing thrombosis and heparin therapy both lower the concentration of plasma antithrombin. Therefore, the diagnosis of antithrombin deficiency is best made after the patient has recovered from a thrombotic event.

A patient with acute thrombosis should be treated with heparin. Because of depletion of the major antithrombin, the level of antithrombin may become so low that the patient is resistant to heparin. In this case, a source of antithrombin should be infused, in the form of either fresh frozen plasma or, if available, antithrombin concentrate. The half-life of antithrombin is 16 to 24 hours. Administration of warfarin should be started promptly, and the patient probably should receive warfarin indefinitely.

Prophylactic use of anticoagulants should be considered in view of the spontaneous and unpredictable occurrence of thromboembolism with the potential for a fatal outcome. At the very least, affected individuals should be counseled about the risks of the disorder. Pregnancies should be managed in high-risk clinics prepared to cope with the difficult questions of how, when, or whether anticoagulants should be administered during the pregnancy.

Bovill EG, Bauer KA, Dickerman JD, et al.: The clinical spectrum of heterozygous protein C deficiency in a large New England kindred. Blood 73:712, 1989. Engesser L, Broekmans AW, Briët E, et al.: Hereditary protein S deficiency: Clinical manifestations. Ann Intern Med 106:677, 1987. *Good descriptions of the spectrum of clinical problems in these deficiency states.*
Menache D, O'Malley JP, Schorr JB, et al.: Evaluation of the safety, recovery, half-life, and clinical efficacy of antithrombin III (human) in patients with hereditary antithrombin III deficiency. Blood 75:33, 1990. *Phase I and II studies of a potentially valuable treatment modality.*

ACQUIRED ABNORMALITIES OF BLOOD COAGULATION

GENERAL COMMENTS. In a number of clinical situations, the APTT and/or PT become prolonged: use of heparin, use of fibrinolytic agents, vitamin K deficiency secondary to malabsorption or dietary deficiency, severe liver disease, use of coumarin anticoagulants to lower the activity of vitamin K–dependent factors, and consumption coagulopathy associated with severe illness. Rarer causes of acquired deficiencies include selective urinary loss of a coagulation factor in nephrotic syndrome, selective adsorption of a coagulation factor, especially Factor X, to amyloid, and selective neutralization or depletion of a clotting factor due to development of an antibody to the factor.

Heparin

Heparin is used commonly for its anticoagulant properties in the prevention of and therapy for thromboembolism and to keep blood fluid during extracorporeal circulation. By definition, 1 unit of heparin renders 1 ml of sheep blood incoagulable. The therapeutic concentration in a human (i.e., a patient with an APTT 1½ times longer than normal) is 0.1 to 0.3 units per milliliter.

Bleeding is the most common complication of heparin therapy. This can be minimized by (1) administration of the drug by continuous infusion rather than in boluses; (2) quantification of the anticoagulant effect at regular intervals by whole-blood clotting times or APTT; (3) selection of patients who do not have an

occult bleeding site or underlying bleeding diathesis; and (4) prohibition of aspirin and intramuscular injections. Despite this, purpura, ecchymoses, hematomas, gastrointestinal hemorrhage, hematuria, retroperitoneal bleeding, or bleeding at sites of invasive procedures may occur. Heparin is cleared from the circulation within 2 to 4 hours. Therefore, if bleeding is minimal and can be controlled by local measures, discontinuation of heparin may be all that is necessary. If bleeding is severe, the effects of heparin can be counteracted by giving 1 mg of protamine sulfate for each 100 units of heparin estimated to be in the patient's circulation.

After 7 to 10 days of heparin therapy, thrombocytopenia sometimes occurs, subsiding when heparin is discontinued. Mild thrombocytopenia is likely due to a direct effect of heparin on platelets. In some patients, the thrombocytopenia can be severe and associated with venous and/or arterial thrombosis and disseminated intravascular coagulation (DIC). In these patients the thrombocytopenia is probably immunologically mediated. It is important to be alert for such a patient, because one's tendency is to treat the thrombosis by increasing the dose of heparin, only to make the situation worse. Heparin therefore should be discontinued if the platelet count drops precipitously. Low molecular weight heparin holds the promise of providing anticoagulant activity without undesirable reactions with platelets and may be a therapeutic option in the future for patients with heparin-induced thrombocytopenia. For the present, however, the best defense is prophylactic, i.e., to initiate warfarin therapy early so that a stable anticoagulant effect is achieved during the first week of heparin therapy.

Several patients with neoplastic plasma cell disorders have had clinical bleeding caused by a circulating heparin-like proteoglycan that required the major antithrombin for its function and could be neutralized by protamine sulfate.

Turpie AGG, Levine MN, Hirsh J, et al.: A randomized controlled trial of a low-molecular-weight heparin (enoxaparin) to prevent deep-vein thrombosis in patients undergoing elective hip surgery. N Engl J Med 315:925, 1986. Salzman EW: Low-molecular-weight heparin: Is small beautiful? N Engl J Med 315:957, 1986. *Good update and review of trends in heparin therapy.*

Therapeutic Fibrinolysis (Thrombolysis)

Intravenous administration of streptokinase, urokinase, or tissue plasminogen activator is accepted useful therapy for deep vein thrombosis, pulmonary embolism, acute myocardial infarction, and peripheral arterial thromboembolism. These agents reestablish patency of vessels more quickly than does heparin. The dosage and method of administration of the agents are specific for the different conditions, and in some instances the agent is administered by selective catheterization of the involved vessel.

In the case of streptokinase or urokinase administered systemically, therapeutic effectiveness requires that systemic fibrinolysis be achieved, i.e., that the patients develop iatrogenic primary fibrinolysis. Prolongation of the thrombin time to twice normal is often taken as evidence that the desired effect has been achieved. Such patients also have decreased plasma fibrinogen, plasminogen, and alpha$_2$-antiplasmin. In the case of streptokinase administered locally or TPA administered systemically or locally, thrombi can be lysed with variable and sometimes minimal evidence of systemic fibrinolysis.

If the level of plasminogen falls to zero, the patient will be relatively resistant to further infusion of fibrinolytic agents. At that point, or at the end of the planned infusion, there is hypercoagulability, and anticoagulation with heparin should be carried out.

The main complication of fibrinolytic therapy is hemorrhage, usually in the form of continuous, slow oozing at sites of invasive procedures. If a pressure dressing does not control this bleeding, administration of the agent can be discontinued with the anticipation that fibrinolytic activity will subside within a few hours. Fresh frozen plasma can be given if the bleeding is severe.

Marder VJ, Bell WR: Fibrinolytic therapy. *In* Colman RW, Hirsh J, Marder VJ, et al. (eds.): Hemostasis and Thrombosis: Basic Principles and Clinical Practice. 2nd ed. Philadelphia, J. B. Lippincott Company, 1987, pp 1393–1437. *Comprehensive review of indications and strategies.*

Vitamin K Deficiency and Coumarin Anticoagulants

Metabolism and Function of Vitamin K. Vitamin K is required for the posttranslational gamma-carboxylation of specific glutamyl residues in Factors VII, IX, X, and II and of proteins C and S and certain other proteins, e.g., osteocalcin, which constitutes 1 per cent of the protein in bone. In vitamin K–deficient states, levels of the vitamin K–dependent plasma proteins are near normal; however, the functions of these proteins in reactions and assays (e.g., the PT) that require a phospholipid surface are severely impaired. As vitamin K deficiency develops, the activities of Factor VII and protein C decrease rapidly, followed by diminished activities of Factors IX, X, and II.

There are limited body stores of vitamin K. A normal diet containing green, leafy vegetables provides 300 to 500 μg of vitamin K, more than enough to meet the adult daily requirement of 1 μg per kilogram of body weight. In addition, vitamin K synthesized by normal gastrointestinal bacterial flora contributes to the daily requirement. Vitamin K is a fat-soluble vitamin, and solubilization of fat must occur before vitamin K can be absorbed (Ch. 102). Hence, vitamin K deficiency may occur in bile salt–deficient states, in all malabsorptive disorders, or with an inadequate dietary intake combined with gastrointestinal sterilization by orally administered antibiotics. Vitamin K occurs naturally in two forms, vitamin K_1 (phylloquinone) and vitamin K_2 (menaquinone), both of which require lipid for absorption. A synthetic water-soluble form, vitamin K_3 (menadione), is commercially available. Despite its ready absorption from intestine, menadione must be converted to vitamin K_2 by the liver and therefore is not as rapidly effective as vitamin K_1 in promoting the gamma-carboxylation reaction.

VITAMIN K DEFICIENCY OF THE NEWBORN. At birth, vitamin K levels are low, and production of vitamin K by intestinal bacteria is insufficient to meet an infant's requirements for production of normally functioning coagulation factors. The vitamin K–deficient state lasts for 3 to 5 days and may be the reason Israelites did not circumcise their babies until the eighth day (Leviticus 12:3). Cow's milk contains some vitamin K, but human milk contains essentially none (1 to 2 μg per liter). Unless vitamin K is given, the physiologic state of neonatal hypoprothrombinemia can lead to hemorrhagic disease of the newborn in the following high-risk groups: premature infants; breast-fed infants; infants of mothers who are receiving vitamin K antagonists, especially hydantoin anticonvulsants; and infants with malabsorption. If the PT is prolonged to greater than twice normal, it is common to encounter bleeding from the umbilicus, ecchymoses and hematomas, hematuria, and, most important, intracranial hemorrhage. Prophylactic intramuscular administration of a 1-mg dose of vitamin K_1 at delivery virtually eliminates the risk of subsequent hemorrhage. Excessive administration (5 mg or more) of vitamin K_3 may cause hemolytic anemia and kernicterus in the newborn and should be avoided.

MALABSORPTION SYNDROMES. Malabsorptive states (Ch. 102) with impaired absorption of fat, such as adult celiac disease, regional enteritis, use of cholestyramine or neomycin, or deficient intraluminal bile salts (obstruction of biliary ducts, cholestatic liver disease), are often associated with vitamin K deficiency. Similarly, various chronic diarrheas can cause vitamin K deficiency, presumably because of decreased transit time and relative malabsorption of fats. The hallmark of vitamin K deficiency is prolonged PT. If the PT is longer than twice normal, the patient likely will have ecchymoses, gingival bleeding, hematomas, hematuria, and/or melena. Daily oral administration of vitamin K_1 in supraphysiologic doses (2 to 10 mg) prevents the deficiency and should be routine in patients with malabsorption of fat. The bleeding tendency, once developed, is easily corrected by giving 10 to 25 mg of vitamin K_1 intramuscularly. In cases in which the bleeding diathesis is so severe that intramuscular injections are contraindicated, 20 to 40 mg of vitamin K_1 may be infused intravenously. It should be infused slowly at a rate of 1 mg per minute because the vehicle in which the vitamin is dissolved can cause an adverse reaction. If this does not correct the PT, it is unlikely that additional vitamin K will have any effect.

DEBILITATED PATIENTS WHO MAY BE RECEIVING ANTIBIOTICS. Patients who are without oral intake for more than several days and receiving antibiotics should be given parenteral vitamin K_1 at a dosage of 150 μg per day because they are likely to become vitamin K deficient. Patients with uremia or malignant disease are at special risk and may become vitamin K deficient on the basis of poor oral intake alone.

Some third-generation cephalosporins have a hypothrombi-nemic effect that is greater than would be expected from elimination of bowel flora. It has been suggested that the N-methyl-thiotetrazole side chain shared by cefamandole, moxalactam, and cefoperazone is cleaved from the antibiotic and interferes with the action of vitamin K, especially in patients who are borderline deficient in vitamin K.

COUMARIN ANTICOAGULANTS. Warfarin and other coumarin anticoagulants competitively inhibit the effects of vitamin K in the posttranslational gamma-carboxylation of vitamin K–dependent plasma proteins. Coumarin anticoagulants are administered for a long time for the prevention of recurrent thromboembolism in patients who have experienced deep vein thrombosis and pulmonary embolism or myocardial infarction. Patients should be reliable, able to be supervised, and without known potential sources of hemorrhage in the central nervous, gastrointestinal, or genitourinary systems.

Upon initiation of therapy, the activities of the proteins with the most rapid half-lives are lost first. Thus the activities of the vitamin K–dependent proteins become depressed in the following order: Factor VII and protein C, Factor IX, Factor X, and Factor II. The art of administration of warfarin involves balancing drug intake against vitamin K intake to prolong the PT about 1½ times as that of a normal control, e.g., 17 to 19 seconds compared with a control of 12 seconds. Ratios below this value are less effective in preventing thrombosis, whereas values twice normal or greater carry a high risk for hemorrhage. An adult receiving a normal diet usually needs 5 to 10 mg of warfarin per day to achieve the desired ratio. After initiation of therapy, it takes 3 to 4 days before the chosen dose of warfarin causes its maximal effect on the PT. The dose can then be altered to maintain the PT in the therapeutic range.

The syndrome of coumarin-induced skin necrosis recapitulates the syndrome of homozygous protein C deficiency. Upon initiation of warfarin therapy, the plasma concentration of protein C, which has a half-life of 6 hours, falls more quickly than the concentrations of Factors II, IX, and X, thus causing a hypercoagulable state. Therefore, therapy should be initiated with the predicted maintenance dose (rather than a "loading dose"), preferably while the patient is receiving heparin.

Once the PT is stabilized, it needs to be checked only every three to four weeks if the patient is on a stable diet and is in usual health. The therapeutic dose of warfarin may change dramatically if the diet is changed or if changes are made in the intake of one of the many drugs that enhance or depress the effect of warfarin (Table 155–2). Patients should wear a bracelet or neck tag stating that they are receiving an oral anticoagulant. They should not take aspirin in any of its forms.

It is not uncommon for patients to experience slight gingival bleeding, purpura with minimal trauma, or trace hematuria while receiving anticoagulants in the therapeutic range. These symptoms become more marked when there is overanticoagulation, and the patient is at risk for severe gastrointestinal or genitourinary hemorrhage, bleeding or hematoma formation after trauma, and intracranial bleeding. If the PT is prolonged and increased bleeding is not a clinical problem, warfarin, which has a half-life of 35 hours, can be omitted until the desired PT is obtained. When overanticoagulation results in clinically significant bleeding, the physician can give fresh frozen plasma, 10 to 20 ml per kilogram, as a source of normal vitamin K–dependent proteins, and/or give vitamin K, depending on the immediacy of the problem and whether continuation of warfarin is necessary. The effect of plasma on the PT is immediate but temporary. The use of Factor IX concentrates to treat warfarin overdose should be avoided because of occasional thrombotic complications and the risk of hepatitis. Oral or intramuscular vitamin K_1, 5 to 25 mg, should correct the PT within 8 to 24 hours. Slow intravenous infusion of vitamin K, 20 to 40 mg, should correct the PT in 4 to 6 hours. Administration of more than 5 mg of vitamin K makes the patient warfarin resistant and necessitates a round of re-anticoagulation. Therefore, the best strategy for the patient who needs continued anticoagulation is to give plasma and small doses (1 to 2 mg) of vitamin K while closely monitoring the PT and clinical state.

Patients occasionally present with bleeding complications after ingestion of a coumarin compound, either surreptitiously or as a

TABLE 155–2. DRUGS AND CONDITIONS THAT INFLUENCE RESPONSE TO WARFARIN

Increased Resistance to Warfarin

Hereditary warfarin resistance	Increased warfarin metabolism
Increase in dietary vitamin K	Barbiturates
Reduced drug absorption	Primidone
Malabsorption syndrome	Carbamazepine
Liquid paraffin laxatives	Ethchlorvynol
Cholestyramine resin	Glutethimide
Magnesium trisilicate	Meprobamate
	Griseofulvin
	Rifampin
	Nafcillin

Increased Sensitivity to Warfarin

Vitamin K deficiency	Synergism with warfarin
Malabsorption syndrome	Vitamin E
Wide-spectrum antibiotics	Anabolic steroids
Liquid paraffin	Danazol
Clofibrate	Blocking of warfarin metabolism
Displacement of albumin	Phenytoin sodium
binding	Chloramphenicol
Phenylbutazone	Clofibrate
Aspirin	Tricyclic antidepressants
Indomethacin	Erythromycin
Sulindac	Cimetidine
Mefenamic acid	Sulfamethoxazole-trimethoprim
Tolmetin	Sulfinpyrazone
Ibuprofen	Unknown mechanism
Naproxen	Quinine
Fenoprofen	Quinidine
Phenytoin sodium	Phenothiazine
Oral hypoglycemic agents	Disulfiram
Nalidixic acid	Sulfisoxazole
Estrogen	Amiodarone
Miconazole	

Adapted with permission from Peterson CE, Kwaan HC: Current concepts of warfarin therapy. Arch Intern Med 146:581, 1986. Copyright 1986, American Medical Association.

suicide attempt. Patients who take coumarins surreptitiously are usually depressed and receive gain from medical attention. They may belong to a health profession. The coumarin compounds in rat poisons are much more powerful than warfarin and can cause extreme resistance to vitamin K for weeks and even months.

Coumarin anticoagulants should not be given from the sixth to the twelfth week of gestation because of the high likelihood that characteristic facial and skeletal malformations, the so-called coumarin embryopathy, will be induced. Use of coumarin drugs in the second and third trimesters is associated with an increased incidence of central nervous system malformations presumed to be due to sporadic intracranial hemorrhages. If anticoagulation is needed during pregnancy, one approach is to switch to subcutaneous heparin between the sixth and twelfth week and after the thirty-eighth week.

Furie B, Furie BC: Molecular basis of vitamin K–dependent α-carboxylation. Blood 75:1753, 1990. *Update on the biochemistry of vitamin K action and the opposing effect of the coumarins.*

Hirsh J: Is the dose of warfarin prescribed by American physicians unnecessarily high? Arch Intern Med 147:769, 1987. *Recommendations on intensity of therapy in different situations. Good data in support of less intensive therapy.*

Iturbe-Alessio I, Fonseca MC, Mutchinik O, et al.: Risks of anticoagulant therapy in pregnant women with artificial heart valves. N Engl J Med 315:1390, 1986. *One group's approach to a difficult subject.*

Lipton RA, Klass EM: Human ingestion of a "superwarfarin" rodenticide resulting in a prolonged anticoagulant effect. JAMA 252:3004, 1984. Jones EC, Growe GH, Naiman SC: Prolonged anticoagulation in rat poisoning. JAMA 252:3005, 1984. *Illustrative case reports.*

O'Reilly RA: Vitamin K antagonists. *In* Colman RW, Hirsh J, Marder VJ, et al. (eds.): Hemostasis and Thrombosis: Basic Principles and Clinical Practice. 2nd ed. Philadelphia, J. B. Lippincott Company, 1987, pp 1367–1372.

Peterson CE, Kwaan HC: Current concepts of warfarin therapy. Arch Intern Med 146:581, 1986. *A concise review.*

Liver Disease

The liver is the major site of synthesis of fibrinogen, plasminogen, the vitamin K–dependent proteins, the antithrombins, and most other plasma proteins. The mechanisms by which steady-state concentrations of these proteins in plasma are regulated are obscure. As part of the "acute phase reaction" in response to interleukin 1, interleukin 6, and tumor necrosis factor, the synthesis of many plasma proteins, especially fibrinogen, increases at the expense of albumin synthesis. The normal liver seems to have a considerable reserve for production of fibrinogen but to be working at near-maximal capacity in the synthesis of vitamin K–dependent proteins.

Patients with liver disease occasionally develop petechiae, ecchymoses, prolonged bleeding after venipuncture, and/or gastrointestinal hemorrhage. Clinically significant bleeding may occur with biopsies and surgery. The causes of these problems are diverse.

In patients with alcoholic liver disease, bleeding can be secondary to dietary *vitamin K deficiency* and responds promptly to oral vitamin K. With more advanced disease, patients may become vitamin K deficient on the basis of fat malabsorption as well as poor nutrition, and parenteral vitamin K must be given. The synthesis of vitamin K–dependent factors becomes impaired as hepatocytes are lost, rendering the patient resistant to parenteral vitamin K. A poor prognosis is associated with a prolonged PT (greater than 1½ times normal) that does not become corrected after intravenous vitamin K. If the patient no longer responds to parenteral vitamin K, abnormal bleeding or correction of the PT prior to invasive procedures will require transfusions of fresh frozen plasma. In fulminant hepatocellular disease, *hypofibrinogenemia* can be profound enough to be considered the cause of bleeding; in such cases, both fresh frozen plasma and cryoprecipitate should be given.

Acquired dysfibrinogenemia, manifested by abnormal fibrin polymerization, has been observed in a number of patients having hepatic diseases such as alcoholic cirrhosis, postnecrotic cirrhosis of unknown cause, drug-induced hepatic failure, and hepatoma. The fibrinogen in these patients has an increased content of sialic acid. The clotting of these fibrinogens by thrombin is delayed in proportion to the increase of sialic acid. If the liver disease improves, the defect may disappear.

Patients with liver disease commonly have *increased fibrinolysis*, because of an inability to maintain normal levels of alpha$_2$-antiplasmin and/or decreased hepatic clearance of plasminogen activators. Enhanced fibrinolysis, however, is rarely the primary cause of bleeding. Occasionally, chronic, smoldering *disseminated intravascular coagulation* (DIC) may develop, in which case the platelet count is decreased and levels of several coagulation factors fall because of consumption. These patients do not require therapy unless they exhibit clinically significant bleeding, in which case the approach should be the same as for patients with other causes of diffuse intravascular coagulation (see below). Patients in whom LeVeen peritoneovenous shunts have been placed and women with acute fatty liver of pregnancy and marked deficiency of antithrombin III (<25 per cent of normal) are at particular risk of developing DIC.

Efforts should be made to normalize the PT, fibrinogen concentration, and platelet count in patients with liver disease prior to surgery, biopsy, or other invasive procedures. Factor IX concentrates are not recommended for prophylaxis in patients in whom the PT will not be corrected with parenteral vitamin K because such patients are likely to be deficient in plasma antithrombin, to have decreased hepatic clearance of activated clotting factors, and therefore to be at risk for thromboembolism. Platelet concentrates should be given if the platelet count is less than 75,000 per microliter. If hypersplenism is the cause of thrombocytopenia, however, it may be difficult to achieve a satisfactory platelet count.

Joist JH: Hemostatic abnormalities in liver disease. *In* Colman RW, Hirsh J, Marder VJ, et al. (eds.): Hemostasis and Thrombosis: Basic Principles and Clinical Practice. 2nd ed. Philadelphia, J. B. Lippincott Company, 1987, pp 861–872. *Review with good references.*

Renal Disease

Patients with uremia occasionally develop purpura, mucous membrane bleeding, gastrointestinal hemorrhage, and prolonged bleeding from venous and arterial needle puncture sites. Such patients usually have a prolonged bleeding time. The pathogenesis of the bleeding tendency is complex. The platelet count may be low. More important, platelet function is abnormal because of accumulation of a dialyzable substance in the circulation (Ch. 154). Anemia contributes to platelet dysfunction in vivo, because the stirring action of red cells causes a large increase in the diffusivity of platelets and allows platelets to be transported efficiently to areas where the vessel wall is injured. Erythropoietin therapy, therefore, normalizes the bleeding time. Daily infusion of cryoprecipitate has been useful in correcting the bleeding tendency in uremia. Although uncertain, the correction may be related to the high molecular weight von Willebrand factor multimers contained in cryoprecipitate. Desmopressin, which is effective in raising the plasma level of von Willebrand factor in patients with von Willebrand disease (see above), temporarily corrects the bleeding time in patients with uremia. Daily intravenous administration of conjugated estrogens may also correct the bleeding time over a period of days. Thus a number of therapeutic maneuvers can be tried in a symptomatic uremic patient: dialysis to restore platelet function; transfusion to normalize red cell and platelet number; and administration of cryoprecipitate, desmopressin, or conjugated estrogens.

Coagulation factors, especially vitamin K–dependent factors and Factor V, tend to be at low concentration in chronic renal disease, although not to levels that should cause bleeding. Some of these deficiencies probably result from hepatic insufficiency or from vitamin K deficiency secondary to oral antibiotic therapy, malabsorption caused by uremic enteritis, and diminished dietary intake. Very low plasma Factor IX levels (10 per cent of normal) have been observed in patients with severe nephrotic syndrome and preferential loss of Factor IX into the urine. Subclinical DIC occasionally occurs in patients with chronic renal disease, as evidenced by elevated amounts of fibrin degradation products in serum and urine. It has been suggested that loss of antithrombin III in nephrotic syndrome may cause renal vein thrombosis. There are no clear guidelines on when and how to treat such deficiencies. If the PT is long or the Factor IX level is low in a patient who is bleeding, fresh frozen plasma is the replacement product of choice, although it may be difficult to give enough to someone who cannot compensate for the large volume.

Di Minno G, Martinez J, McKean, M-L, et al.: Platelet dysfunction in uremia: Multifaceted defect partially corrected by dialysis. Am J Med 79:552, 1985. Castillo R, Lozano T, Escolar G, et al.: Defective platelet adhesion on vessel subendothelium in uremic patients. Blood 68:337, 1986. *Two studies of platelet function in uremic patients.*

Janson PA, Jubelirer SJ, Weinstein MJ, et al.: Treatment of the bleeding tendency in uremia with cryoprecipitate. N Engl J Med 303:1318, 1980. Mannucci PM, Remuzzi G, Pusineri F, et al.: Deamino-8-D-arginine vasopressin shortens the bleeding time in uremia. N Engl J Med 308:8, 1983. Livio M, Mannucci PM, Vigano G, et al.: Conjugated estrogens for the management of bleeding associated with renal failure. N Engl J Med 315:731, 1985. *Contain results of three different but possibly related approaches to improvement of the bleeding time in uremic patients. The mechanisms of the favorable clinical effects are enigmas.*

Van Geet C, Hauglustaine D, Verresen L, et al.: Haemostatic effects of recombinant human erythropoietin in chronic haemodialysis patients. Thromb Haemost 61:117, 1989. *Documents favorable effect of erythropoietin on the bleeding time.*

Factor VIII Inhibitors

An endogenously produced anticoagulant, usually referred to as a circulating anticoagulant or a circulating inhibitor, is an antibody that interacts with a clotting factor in a manner that neutralizes the functional activity of the factor. Production of such an antibody is pathologic and often results in hemorrhage. Factor VIII inhibitors are commonly observed in hemophilia A (Factor VIII deficiency) but are rare in nonhemophilic patients. Conditions in which sporadic Factor VIII inhibitors occur include the postpartum state, diseases of immunologic dysfunction, and old age. The sporadic inhibitors induce a hemophilia-like state, i.e., a significant bleeding diathesis, but are unlike the inhibitors of hemophilic patients in several ways. They tend to be of low titer (<1 to 20 Bethesda units) and to bind Factor VIII weakly. Titers often drop when patients are treated with cytoxan, 1 gram given intravenously, and prednisone, 80 mg per day, to be tapered once an effect is seen. Such a therapeutic response is rare in patients with hemophilia and an inhibitor. Acute bleeding episodes can be managed with variable success by continuous infusion of Factor VIII concentrate or cryoprecipitate.

When a Factor VIII inhibitor is present, the PT is normal but the APTT is prolonged. If the patient's plasma is incubated for several hours with an equal quantity of normal plasma, the APTT of the mixture should be prolonged. The Factor VIII level in the patient's plasma and in the mixture of patient's plasma and normal plasma should be low no matter what dilutions are tested, whereas the Factor IX level should be normal. These characteristics distinguish Factor VIII inhibitors from the antiphospholipid inhibitors associated with lupus erythematosus (lupus-type inhibitors). A lupus-type inhibitor may cause prolongation of the PT, especially when the test is done with diluted thromboplastin; does not require an incubation period to express inhibitory activity in mixtures of patient's and normal plasma; and may interfere with the assays for both Factors VIII and IX when the patient's plasma is tested at a 1:10 dilution but not when the patient's plasma is tested at a 1:200 or 1:500 dilution. The implications of having a Factor VIII inhibitor versus a lupus-type inhibitor are very different, and the physician and laboratory must be sure that the correct diagnosis is made, even though there is no single test with which to make the distinction.

Lian ECY, Larcada AF, Chiu AYZ: Combination immunosuppressive therapy after Factor VIII infusion for acquired factor VIII inhibitor. Ann Intern Med 110:774, 1989. *Description of 12 nonhemophilic patients with inhibitors.*

Lupus-Type Inhibitors

Patients with systemic lupus erythematosus sometimes develop a circulating anticoagulant unrelated to the severity or duration of disease. A similar inhibitor sometimes occurs in patients who do not have lupus. Patients who have the lupus-type inhibitor may also have anticardiolipin antibodies and thrombocytopenia. Only rarely is the inhibitor associated with clinically significant bleeding. When patients with the inhibitor do bleed, it is due to thrombocytopenia, platelet dysfunction, and/or acquired Factor II deficiency. Instead, patients with the lupus-type inhibitor are at increased risk of having recurrent thromboembolic events. Thrombosis can involve both veins and arteries. There is probably accelerated atherosclerosis. Women with the inhibitor have a greatly increased incidence of spontaneous abortion. Some patients have neurologic abnormalities that may be due to cerebral thrombosis or myelitis or both. In short, the problems associated with a lupus-like inhibitor can be devastating.

Inhibition of clotting tests is thought to be a consequence of binding of the inhibitor to the acidic phospholipids used in the PT and APTT. The prolongations of both assays can be very impressive. Presumably, platelet membranes, rather than phospholipid micelles, provide the surface for activation of Factors X and II, thus accounting for the fact that clinically significant bleeding does not occur. The pathogenesis of the thrombotic diathesis associated with lupus-type inhibitors is unknown. A reasonable hypothesis is that the lupus-type inhibitor and the anticardiolipin are members of a cross-reacting family of antiphospholipid antibodies, and within the family are antibodies that react in a noxious fashion with endothelial cells, e.g., to block prostacyclin production or to inhibit the cofactor activity of thrombomodulin in the protein C–protein S pathway.

Without knowledge of the pathogenesis of the thromboembolism, there is no rational approach to treatment. Anticoagulants should be given but may not be effective. It also is reasonable to try immunosuppressive therapy or plasmapheresis. Administration of corticosteroids and low-dose aspirin during pregnancy had favorable laboratory and clinical effects in a group of women with the inhibitor and impressive histories of spontaneous abortion.

Love PE, Santoro SA: Antiphospholipid antibodies: Anticardiolipin and the lupus anticoagulant in systemic lupus erythematosus (SLE) and non-SLE disorders. Ann Intern Med 112:682, 1990. *Illustrates well the dilemmas of lupus-type inhibitors.*

Miscellaneous Inhibitors of Clotting Factors

Approximately 5 per cent of patients with Factor IX deficiency (hemophilia B) develop inhibitors to Factor IX after repeated transfusion. Inhibitors to Factor V have been reported in about eight patients, only one of these being a Factor V–deficient patient. Acquired inhibitors to von Willebrand factor activity have developed in very few patients. An IgG inhibitor was found in a Factor XIII–deficient patient following transfusion. A few patients receiving isoniazid have developed an inhibitor directed toward the fibrin crosslinking sites; this results in defective fibrin polymerization.

Myeloma or macroglobulinemia may give rise to defective fibrin polymerization as a result of interference by high concentrations of immunoglobulin. If overt bleeding occurs, plasmapheresis may restore adequate hemostasis by reducing plasma protein concentration.

A very interesting inborn error of alpha₁-antiproteinase (alpha₁-antitrypsin) has been reported in which the mutant serpin is a rapid, specific inhibitor of thrombin, thus causing a severe hemorrhagic diathesis.

Sporadic Acquired Factor Deficiency

A number of patients with amyloidosis have Factor X deficiency because of its removal from the circulation through binding of zymogen Factor X to the amyloid deposits. Patients present with mild to severe bleeding, just as do individuals with the inherited form of Factor X deficiency. Replacement therapy can be given with plasma or factor concentrates. However, the in vivo half-life of Factor X is shortened.

Occasionally, a patient is seen with isolated factor deficiency but no evidence of a neutralizing antibody, e.g., when the patient's plasma is mixed 1:1 with normal plasma, the factor level in the mixture is 50 per cent. Such a patient with Factor II deficiency was studied in depth and shown to have a nonneutralizing antibody to Factor II. Administration of corticosteroids was associated with a rise in Factor II activity and cessation of bleeding, but circulating Factor II was bound to antibody. These observations suggested that nonneutralizing antibodies to Factor II cause plasma Factor II deficiency because of rapid clearance of the antigen-antibody complexes, which is slowed by corticosteroids. Demonstration of nonneutralizing antibodies requires special techniques and takes some time. Therefore, in a patient who is bleeding seriously, one may need to begin administration of corticosteroids, possibly supplemented with fresh frozen plasma, before the diagnosis is established.

Bajaj SP, Rapaport SI, Barclay S, et al.: Acquired hypoprothrombinemia due to nonneutralizing antibodies to prothrombin: Mechanism and management. Blood 65:1538, 1985. *Although this paper describes only one patient, it illustrates what may be a fairly common happening.*

Greipp PR, Kyle RA, Bowie EJ: Factor X deficiency in amyloidosis: A critical review. Am J Hematol 11:443, 1981. *Well-documented description of the cause of this deficiency.*

Syndromes of Disseminated Intravascular Coagulation (DIC)

GENERAL COMMENTS. In the following discussion, DIC is divided into four clinical syndromes: (1) *compensated DIC*, which may be associated with thrombosis but does not result in bleeding; (2) *defibrination syndrome*, in which the mechanisms that localize blood coagulation are overwhelmed by release of tissue factor, leading to massive utilization and depletion of fibrinogen, other clotting factors, and platelets and resultant thrombosis and/or bleeding; (3) *primary fibrinolysis*, in which the mechanisms that localize fibrinolysis are overwhelmed by release of plasminogen activators, leading to bleeding; and (4) *microangiopathic thrombocytopenia*, in which platelet microthrombi are widespread, leading to depletion of platelets, ischemic necrosis of tissues, and microangiopathic changes in red cells. The causes of DIC syndromes are many, and there is considerable overlap among syndromes. Patients with DIC often have multiple medical problems, including bone marrow failure, liver failure, renal failure, vitamin K deficiency, and the like, which may complicate the clinical and laboratory analysis in a given patient. Much of the controversy that surrounds DIC undoubtedly stems from attempts to lump diverse conditions and patients together. Despite its oversimplicity, the following scheme is useful because the treatments of the four paradigm syndromes are quite different. For many of the diseases associated with DIC, specific descriptions of the DIC and recommendations for treatment can be found under individual diseases elsewhere in this textbook.

COMPENSATED DIC. Patients with serious underlying diseases (trauma, infection, malignant tumor, and so on) usually have increased production and consumption of platelets, fibrinogen, and other coagulation proteins. Patients with traumatized or inflamed tissues manifest the "acute phase reaction," and a number of plasma alpha₁, alpha₂, and beta globulins, including alpha₂-antiplasmin and fibrinogen, increase in concentration, whereas other plasma proteins, including transferrin and albumin, decrease in concentration. In areas of trauma or inflammation, there is ongoing coagulation and fibrinolysis. Under such conditions, unclottable fibrin degradation products can be detected by immunoassay in serum. However, the PT is normal, the platelet count is normal or only minimally decreased, and plasma fibrinogen concentration is elevated. There is speculation that low-grade DIC is associated with microemboli and microthrombi that contribute to the organ failure commonly found in patients with severe illnesses. At this point, however, the only indication to use heparin or other anticoagulants in such patients is as prophylaxis or treatment of thrombosis in large vessels. An outstanding example of the need for anticoagulation is in the Trousseau syndrome of "migratory" venous thrombosis in patients with malignant disease (Ch. 159). Warfarin therapy is often ineffective in such patients, and they must instead be started on a long-term regimen of heparin therapy.

DEFIBRINATION SYNDROME. The prototype of defibrination syndrome is the rapid onset of generalized bleeding that occurs when tissue factor is released into the circulation after massive brain trauma or during amniotic fluid embolization. Laboratory tests in such patients demonstrate gross depletion of platelets and fibrinogen, increase in fibrin degradation products, prolongation of PT, and variable decreases in Factors V and VIII, Factor II and the other vitamin K–dependent factors, the antithrombins, and plasminogen. Defibrination syndrome occurs most frequently with shock, sepsis, cancer, burns, and obstetric complications. Patients with sepsis, especially due to meningococcus, may develop purpura fulminans or the Waterhouse-Friderichsen syndrome (hemorrhagic necrosis of vital organs, including the adrenals). The patient's hemostatic system must be supported while the patient is resuscitated and the underlying cause is treated. Thus the patient should receive platelet concentrates, cryoprecipitate as a source of fibrinogen, and fresh frozen plasma as a source of other plasma proteins, especially the antithrombins. An appropriate mix is 10 bags of cryoprecipitate for every 2 to 3 units of plasma. One's goals should be a platelet count of more than 50,000 per microliter, a fibrinogen concentration greater than 100 mg per deciliter, a PT that is within 2 to 3 seconds of normal, and a concentration of antithrombins that is greater than 40 per cent of normal. The role of heparin is controversial. It is my view that unless the patient improves quickly or active bleeding cannot be controlled, heparin should be infused in low dosages (10 to 15 units per kilogram per hour after a loading dose of 30 to 40 units per kilogram) with the goal of dampening further defibrination as the patient's clotting components are replenished with cryoprecipitate and plasma. If the patient has overt thrombosis, the dose of heparin can be increased. The low dose of heparin should not cause lengthening of the PT or APTT or exacerbate the bleeding diathesis. Patients who are severely ill and have defibrination syndrome are at high risk of becoming vitamin K deficient and therefore should receive parenteral vitamin K.

PRIMARY FIBRINOLYSIS. Primary fibrinolysis, in its pure form, results from massive release of plasminogen activator. Conditions associated with DIC that cause "primarily" fibrinolysis, if not primary fibrinolysis, include carcinoma of the prostate, acute promyelocytic leukemia, hemangiomas, and sustained release of plasminogen activator by endothelial cells produced by injection of venoms. A critical point is reached when enough plasmin is activated to deplete the circulation of alpha₂-antiplasmin. This allows plasmin to work unopposed on a variety of substrates in blood. Fibrinogen is lysed to fibrinogen degradation products. Because of the lack of fibrinogen and the inhibitory effect of degradation products on fibrin polymerization, the PT is prolonged. The platelet count, however, is appropriate for the state of the bone marrow, and antithrombin levels are normal. Ecchymoses, mucosal bleeding, and bleeding from needle puncture sites can be extensive. It is usually possible to give enough cryoprecipitate to keep plasma fibrinogen at a concentration greater than 100 mg per deciliter. There is, however, no concentrated source of alpha₂-antiplasmin. EACA, 1 gram per hour in an adult, may be effective in minimization of bleeding and should be given a therapeutic trial in a symptomatic patient if the activity of alpha$_2$-antiplasmin in plasma is less than 35 to 40 per cent of normal. If there is a worry about induction of thrombosis with EACA, heparin in a low dose can be infused simultaneously as described above.

MICROANGIOPATHIC THROMBOCYTOPENIA. The hallmarks of microangiopathic thrombocytopenia are a low platelet count and fragmented red cells on blood smear. Although the serum may contain fibrin degradation products, the PT is generally not elevated, and the fibrinogen concentration is normal or increased. Microangiopathic thrombocytopenia can be seen in patients with sepsis, malignant disease, immune complex disease, vasculitis, malignant hypertension, eclampsia, vascular malformations, and intravascular aspergillosis. The prototype conditions, however, are hemolytic-uremic syndrome (HUS) and thrombotic thrombocytopenic purpura (TTP) (Ch. 154). HUS involves mainly the vessels of the kidney, usually occurs in children, and ordinarily is self-limited. TTP involves many organs, including the brain, ordinarily occurs in adults, and usually causes death unless aggressively treated. Acute neurologic symptoms are the most striking feature of full-blown TTP. The pathogenesis of HUS and TTP is obscure. It has been suggested that patients lack prostacyclin; have von Willebrand factor multimers that are extra large and cause spontaneous platelet aggregation; have autoantibodies that damage endothelial cells; or have a circulating substance, possibly of microbial origin, that causes spontaneous platelet aggregation and that is neutralized by immunoglobulin present in normal plasma. There are intriguing instances in which HUS or TTP occurs in small clusters, is recurrent, or is familial. Whatever the cause (or causes), both HUS and TTP respond in the majority of cases to infusion of fresh frozen plasma. In some cases the requirement for plasma is so great that plasma exchange is necessary. In other cases, occasional infusion of 1 to 2 units of plasma suffices. If extensive plasmapheresis fails, therapeutic options include use of drugs that inhibit platelet aggregation, splenectomy, and use of vincristine.

SNAKE BITES. Venoms from various snakes, especially the vipers and rattlesnakes, contain proteins that can, depending on the species, clot fibrinogen, activate Factor II, Factor X, protein C, or platelets; or cause release of plasminogen activator from endothelial cells. Fortunately, the clinical problems associated with DIC syndromes from venoms are not as striking as the laboratory abnormalities displayed by the victims. Treatment in most instances can be conservative: administration of antivenoms, transfusion of platelets and/or plasma, and general supportive therapy. In some instances, hypofibrinogenemia and thrombocytopenia persist for weeks.

Williams EC, Mosher DF: Disseminated intravascular coagulation. *In* Benz E, Cohen H, Furie B, et al. (eds.): Hematology: Basic Principles and Practice. New York, Churchill Livingstone, 1990, pp 1394–1405. *More detailed exposition.*

PART XIII
ONCOLOGY

156 | Introduction

Bruce A. Chabner

HISTORICAL BACKGROUND AND DEFINITIONS

The term "cancer" is derived from *karkinos*, the Greek word for crab. Cancer as a clinical entity is described in the early writings of Greeks and Romans and has assumed a position of special significance as a much-feared disease and as an object of intensive biomedical investigation.

Peyton Rous, a Nobel laureate for his pioneering work on viral oncology, wrote, "Tumors destroy man in an unique and appalling way, as flesh of his own flesh, which had somehow been rendered proliferative, rampant, predatory and ungovernable."

About 1 million new cases of invasive cancer, excluding superficial skin cancers, are diagnosed each year, and half that number die each year of cancer. Cancer ranks second only to heart disease among the leading causes of death in the United States. Important trends have occurred in the incidence and mortality of cancer in the past two decades, with marked increases in deaths due to lung cancer in women and malignant melanoma, myeloma, brain tumors, and non-Hodgkin's lymphoma in men and women (Fig. 156–1). At the same time, mortality due to cancer has declined for the population less than 65 years of age, primarily as the result of improvements in treatment and early detection. There are also marked differences in the incidence rates of various cancers in different parts of the globe; esophageal, hepatocellular, and stomach cancer occur with much greater frequency in developing countries, undoubtedly as a function of exposure to hepatitis B and to carcinogens in the diet and the environment. Lung, breast, and colon cancer predominate in industrialized countries.

As a pathologic entity, cancer is defined by its properties of uncontrolled local proliferation of cells, with invasion of adjacent normal structure and by distant spread, or metastasis, via the bloodstream or lymphatics or within a body cavity. As a biologic entity, the malignant cell is defined by its ability to grow in tissue culture without the need for attachment to a firm surface and by its loss of responsiveness to growth regulatory signals that cause differentiation and suppress proliferation. Many malignant cells preserve the growth and antigenic properties characteristic of fetal cells, secrete proteins characteristic of fetal tissues (such as the α-fetoprotein of hepatocellular carcinomas and germ-cell tissues), and appear to be frozen in an early state of differentiation that recapitulates a specific stage in normal organ development.

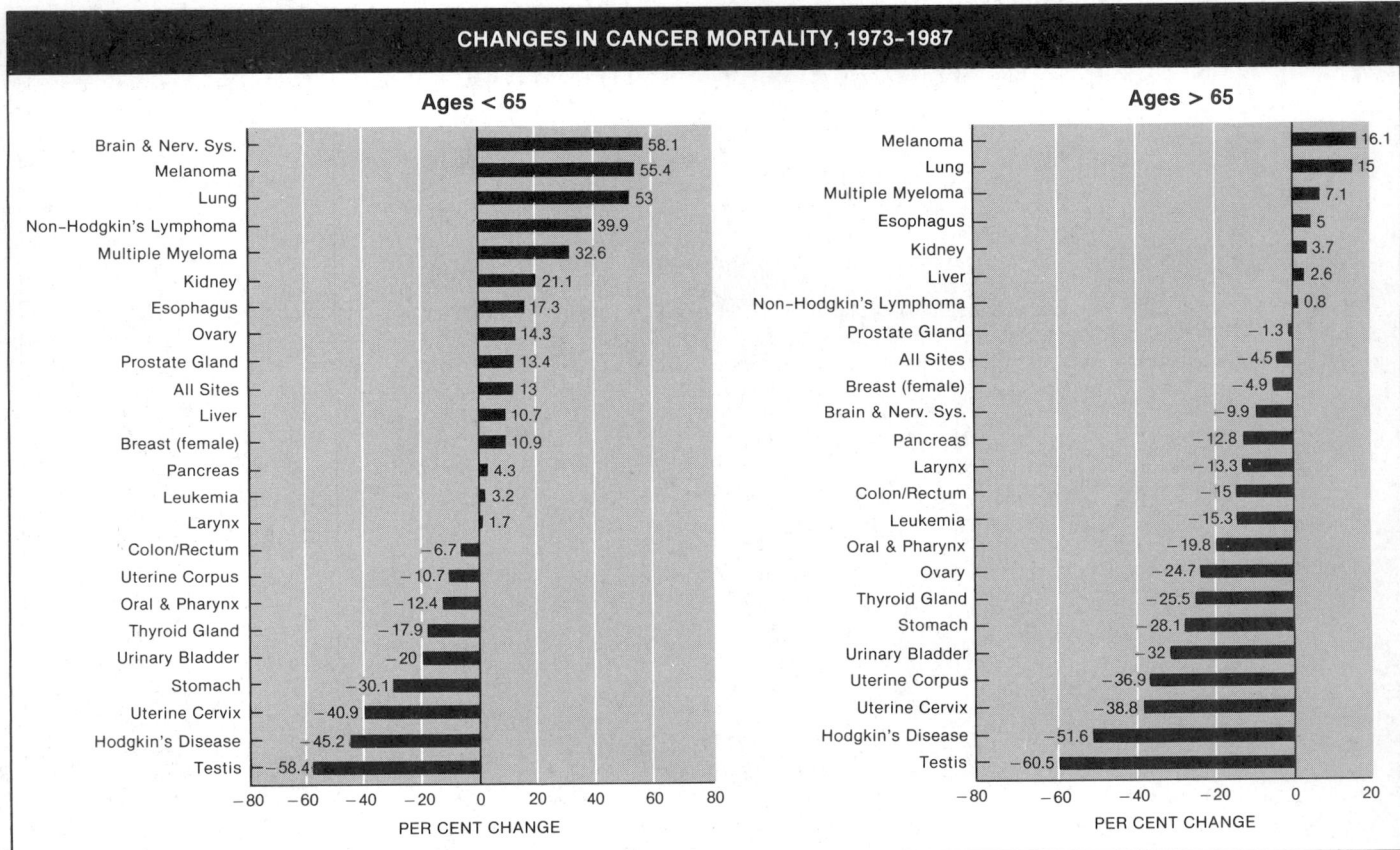

FIGURE 156–1. Changes in mortality rates for persons under and over 65 years of age. Note greater than 50 per cent increase in mortality due to cancers of the lung and bronchus and malignant melanoma in persons under 65. Also note the consistent decrease in mortality in most types of cancer affecting persons less than 65 years of age. (From Cancer Statistics Review: National Cancer Institute, Division of Cancer Prevention and Control, Surveillance Program. Bethesda, MD, National Institutes of Health, NIH Publ. No. 90-2789.)

TABLE 156–1. LYMPHOCYTIC LEUKEMIAS REFLECT PROGRESSIVE STAGES OF NORMAL LYMPHOID DIFFERENTIATION

Type of Leukemia	Phenotype and Molecular Features						
	Pan-B	Pan-T	TCR Re	CALLA	SIg	CIg	IgRe
Common type ALL:							
Early pre-B	+	–	–	+	–	–	H
Late pre-B	+	–	–	+	–	+	H
Mature B-cell ALL	+	–	–	+	+	+	H + L
B-cell CLL	+	–	–	+	+	+	H + L
Lymphoblastic ALL	–	+	β + γ	–	–	–	–
T-cell CLL	–	+	α, β, γ	–	–	–	–

ALL = acute lymphocytic leukemia; CLL = chronic lymphocytic leukemia; Pan-B = pan B-cell antigens; Pan-T = pan T-cell antigen; TCR Re = rearrangement of T-cell receptor genes (α, β, or γ chains) as indicated; CALLA = common ALL antigen (CD-10); SIg = surface immunoglobulin; CIg = cytoplasmic immunoglobulin; IgRe = immunoglobulin rearrangement, heavy (H) or light (L) chain. (From Greaves MF: Differentiation-linked leukemogenesis in lymphocytes. Science 234:697–704, 1986; with permission. Copyright 1987 by the American Association for the Advancement of Science.)

For example, malignancies arising from the lymphoid system reflect all stages and types of B- and T-lymphocyte development and preserve the same complex of immunoglobulin and T-cell receptor gene rearrangements and cell surface proteins (and in some cases potential for further differentiation) found in normal counterparts of the immune system (Table 156–1). These properties have become the basis for classification, diagnosis, and even treatment of tumors, as, for example, classification of lymphoid tumors based on reactivity with monoclonal antibodies. While the above characteristics are typical of most cancer cells, they are not universal. Some endocrine-related tumors, for example, not only maintain well-differentiated morphologic features of their tissue of origin but also retain endocrine function and produce bioactive hormonal substances typical of the mature tissue, as in pheochromocytomas.

Shimkin MB: Contrary to Nature. Washington, D.C., US Department of Health, Education and Welfare, 1977. *An outstanding and eminently readable work on the development of knowledge about cancer from earliest records to modern times. This well-illustrated book traces the impact of the scientists and institutions that have contributed to cancer research throughout the world.*

ETIOLOGY

A broad array of chemical, biologic, and physical agents can cause cancer either directly or indirectly. Most of the directly causative agents damage or alter DNA; these include chemicals—such as benzpyrene, benzene, aflatoxin, and nitrosamines—that form chemical adducts with DNA. Many such chemical carcinogens require activation by cytochrome P-450 enzymes found in liver and epithelial cells. DNA damage can also be caused by physical agents, such as ionizing radiation or ultraviolet light (see Ch. 158).

The precise manner in which these agents damage DNA and lead to cancer is under intensive investigation. One unifying hypothesis proposes that DNA damage results in breaks, translocations, or deletions that activate specific *oncogenes*, i.e., genes that have the potential to cause unrestrained growth if mutated in crucial ways. The biology underlying such mutation has been partially explained by studies of the transforming genes of certain animal RNA viruses (retroviruses) that produce tumors through activation of growth-factor receptors, G proteins, or other important regulatory steps. This topic is more fully discussed in Ch. 157. Analogous activation of oncogenes, such as of members of the *ras* and *myc* families, has been detected in human tumor cell lines and in tumors taken directly from patients with neuroblastoma, Burkitt's lymphoma, and colon cancer, but the precise cause of most human neoplasms remains uncertain at this time. Recently, certain viruses, such as the human T-cell leukemia virus, papilloma viruses, and the Epstein-Barr virus, have been implicated as the cause of human cancers, as have dietary factors such as saturated fats and the absence of fiber. The role of diet in cancer causation, although incompletely defined, is frequently the subject of patient inquiry and is discussed in further detail in Ch. 12.

Substances that are not themselves carcinogens may serve as tumor promoters when given in conjunction with or following exposure to specific carcinogens. These agents appear to work by promoting proliferation of cells already mutated by a primary carcinogen.

The major public health hazard relating to cancer in the United States is *tobacco. The incidence, time to occurrence, and site of cancer depend upon the frequency and mode of tobacco use (smoking, chewing), as well as on exposure to potentiating factors such as alcohol or asbestos.* About one third of cancers in the United States and Europe are related to the use of tobacco products, including those that occur in lung, esophagus, head and neck, and bladder. While specific dietary carcinogens have not been implicated as direct causes of common cancers in the United States, diets that contain high amounts of animal fat and are low in fiber and vegetables are associated with an increased risk of cancer of the colon and rectum. High alcohol intake increases esophageal and head and neck cancer. Sexual behavior patterns influence cancer risk, as reflected in the high incidence of cervical cancer (presumably due to papilloma virus) among women who have multiple sexual partners.

Some cancers are iatrogenic in origin, as in patients who develop acute leukemia or other cancers years after the use of cytotoxic chemotherapeutic drugs or radiotherapy, or in patients who receive immunosuppressive therapy following renal or cardiac transplantation. The most highly carcinogenic agents used in cancer chemotherapy are alkylating agents such as melphalan, cyclophosphamide, and chlorambucil, as well as certain drugs that form DNA adducts after metabolic activation, such as procarbazine.

In addition to environmental factors, *host susceptibility* is a critical determinant in the carcinogenic process. This is partly explained by genetic (or acquired) differences in the ability to metabolize a precursor to the proximate carcinogen, by differences in hormonal milieu and immunologic resistance, and by inherited or acquired mutation or deletion of specific genes, such as the retinoblastoma tumor suppressor gene, that protect against the development of cancer (so-called tumor suppressor genes). The high incidence of malignancy in certain kindreds, as observed in the inherited form of retinoblastoma, in familial polyposis, in the dysplastic nevus syndrome, and in kindreds with high incidence of various epithelial malignancies, is believed to result from inheritance of mutations in genes that protect normal cells against growth signals and proliferation (see Ch. 158). The alert clinician must always be attentive to clues of a predisposition to malignancy provided by a careful family and occupational history.

National Research Council: Diet and Health: Implications for reducing chronic disease risk. Washington, D.C., National Academy Press, 1989. *A definitive summary of the evidence for a relationship between diet and cancer.*

CANCER CELL GROWTH AND METASTASIS

A central concept in the understanding of cancer as a disease is its origin as a clonal proliferation of abnormal cells. Clonality of malignancies has been verified by chromosomal analysis and by molecular probes that identify unique DNA translocations or rearrangements in lymphomas, leukemias, and other tumors. Certain tumors, such as colon cancer, are believed to arise from pre-existing benign polyps, which are well-differentiated and noninvasive tumors confined to the mucosal surface; mutational events in these benign tumors lead to a site of malignant degeneration within the polyp and the emergence of a malignant, invasive tumor. These histologic events are paralleled by the acquisition of a sequence of specific genetic changes, such as loss of the p53 tumor suppressor gene on chromosome 17 and activation of the k-*ras* oncogene. Even after their establishment, malignant clones undergo further biologic evolution. Thus the clinically apparent tumors in man demonstrate multiple molecular and biochemical features, such as activation of oncogenes and deletion of suppressor genes, any one of which might be sufficient to cause malignant transformation. For example, small cell lung cancer in man is characterized by deletions of the 3p chromosome, activation of the l-*myc* oncogene, and deletion of the p53 and Rb tumor suppressor genes. Which of these events initiates the malignant transformation is uncertain, nor is the precise role of each abnormality in the final expression of the malignant phenotype understood.

Clonal evolution of malignancies is manifested in the natural history of many malignancies: (1) the transformation from the chronic to the acute phase (blastic crisis) of chronic granulocytic leukemia; (2) the transformation of nodular lymphomas to a diffuse histiocytic lymphoma; (3) the development of rapidly progressive metastases in a patient who had a slowly growing primary malignant melanoma; (4) the development of highly drug-resistant relapse in a patient with acute leukemia previously responsive to chemotherapy.

In general, clonal evolution proceeds along pathways that provide a growth advantage for the malignancy and allow for survival in a hostile environment. Thus, tumor cells elaborate autocrine (self-acting) growth factors and angiogenesis factors, secrete metalloproteinase and collagenases that digest basement membrane and allow invasion of adjacent structures, and express receptors that allow the attachment to laminin, a basement membrane protein. The digestion of collagen and basement membrane proteins allows tumor cells to invade through the walls of capillaries and lymphatics and thus to spread to distant sites. The ability to metastasize to distant sites is a consequence of these general properties, but in addition there is evidence that the ability to implant and survive in specific sites (such as lymph node, lung, or liver) results from the presence of additional biochemical factors elaborated by metastatic subclones. The pioneering work of Fidler and colleagues with the murine B-16 melanoma has demonstrated the existence of metastases that "home" and survive specifically in liver, lung, and other organs.

Although the survival and continuous proliferation of malignancy depend on the ability of a tumor cell to adapt to its milieu and to develop the specialized machinery for invasion and metastases, host factors play an important role in determining the fate of a malignant clone. Foremost among the host defenses is the immune system. Lymph nodes act as a barrier to metastases by filtering out tumor cells. For most malignancies, such as colon cancer and breast cancer, there is a finite, but small cure rate achieved by resection of a primary tumor and its draining lymph nodes when the nodes are involved with cancer, demonstrating that the lymph nodes represent a first line of defense. Several immune mechanisms are capable of killing tumor cells, including natural killer cells and the closely related lymphokine-activated killer cells (LAK cells) found in the mononuclear leukocyte fraction of the peripheral blood, T-lymphocyte–mediated cell killing as exemplified by tumor-infiltrating lymphocytes (TIL cells), and activated macrophages (see Ch. 159). The importance of an intact immune system in preventing cancer is graphically indicated by the high incidence of neoplasms in patients with primary immune deficiency states or in those receiving immunosuppressive therapy. These natural surveillance mechanisms are being exploited in new attempts to treat metastatic cancer.

Benign tumors may show a spectrum of variation from normal, and on occasion the distinction between a benign and a malignant lesion on the basis of histology alone may be subtle. A spectrum of morphologic findings may reflect progressive stages in neoplastic transformation. Dysplastic changes of bronchial epithelium or of the cervix are considered to be premalignant, although not necessarily destined to become cancerous, particularly if the inciting stimulus is removed. With the development of effective cancer-preventing agents, such as compounds of the retinoic acid class, the identification of dysplastic changes may allow early intervention to prevent progression to malignancy. As cells become more anaplastic in appearance, they may begin to show

microscopic invasion, progressing from carcinoma in situ to microscopic invasion and finally to overt invasive disease. *Dysplastic* changes in other organs also precede frank carcinomatous changes, but once malignant tumors are established they are programmed for continuing survival and growth except in rare cases of spontaneous regression.

CYTOGENETICS. Many types of cytogenetic abnormalities have been observed in leukemias and other cancers by study of metaphase preparations, by in situ hybridization with DNA probes, by high-resolution banding with the use of fluorescent acridine stains, and by other new techniques. The most common types of defects are inversions, deletions, and reciprocal translocations (exchanges of DNA between two chromosomes). Increasingly unique chromosomal abnormalities characteristic of particular tumors are being recognized, e.g., the Philadelphia chromosome (Ph[1]) in chronic myelogenous leukemia (CML), a translocation of a piece of chromosome 9, containing the c-*abl* oncogene, to the breakpoint cluster region (bcr) of chromosome 22. The Philadelphia chromosome is visibly detectable in karyotype preparations of 85 per cent of patients, and the translocation of the c-*abl* oncogene to the bcr of chromosome 22 is detectable by molecular techniques in most of the other 15 per cent of patients with clinical CML (see Ch. 144). The same clonal abnormalities also occur in myeloid, erythroid, and megakaryo-

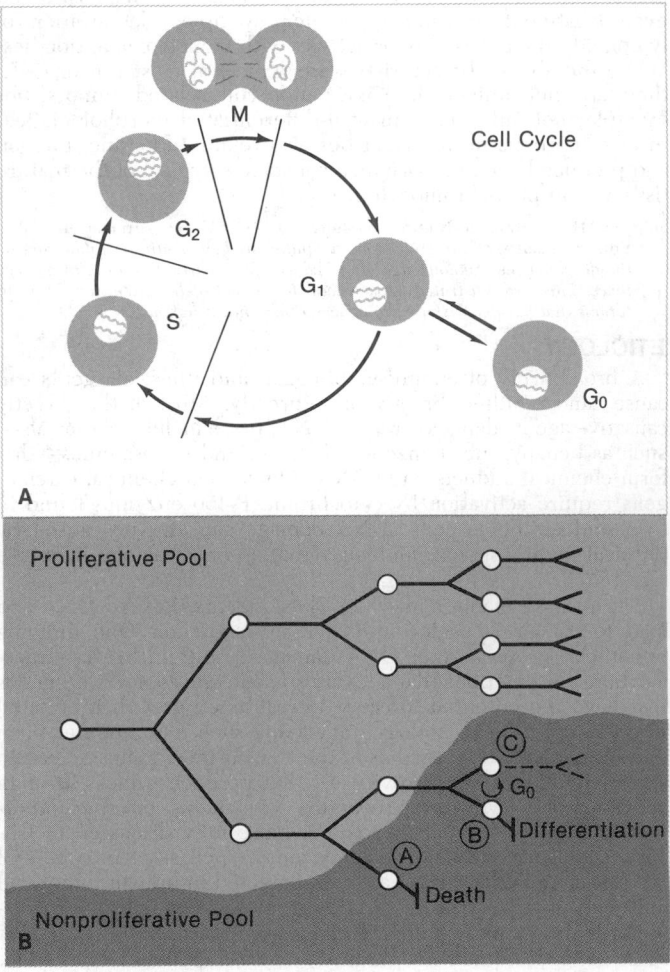

FIGURE 156–2. *A,* A diagrammatic representation of the events during the cell cycle. M is the period of mitosis—approximately 1 hour from prophase to cell division. G_1 reflects normal cell metabolism prior to DNA synthesis and usually constitutes more than half of the total cell generation time. Cells not actively undergoing replication are described as being G_0, where they may remain indefinitely or may be recruited back into the cycle. The DNA synthetic (S) phase is generally 6 to 12 hours. *B,* A schematic representation of tumor growth. As the cell population expands, a progressively higher percentage of cells leave the proliferative pool by death (A), by differentiation (B), or by entering resting phase G_0 (C), from which they may be recruited back into the proliferative pool if the population size is reduced.

cytic cells of CML patients, indicating an earlier common progenitor cell as the source of this clonal malignancy.

GROWTH KINETICS. Oncologists endeavor to quantify the growth rate of tumors as objectively as possible, using such parameters as the growth fraction of tumors, the duration of the cell cycle, the number of cells in the resting (G_o) phase, and the rate of cell death and removal (Fig. 156–2). The kinetics of tumor growth are crucial in determining prognosis and response to chemotherapy. "Doubling time" tends to be characteristic of particular tumors. *A tumor that has reached the size of clinical detectability (approximately 1 cm³) has already undergone approximately 30 doublings to reach 10^9 cells. Only 10 further doubling cycles are required to produce a tumor burden of approximately 1 kg, which is usually lethal.*

A simple exponential growth curve describes the early phase of growth of tumors (Fig. 156–3). As most tumors grow, the time required to complete a full cell cycle remains fairly constant, but an ever-increasing percentage of daughter cells enters a nonproliferating state, G_o, from which they may (potentially) be recruited back into cell cycle if the tumor cell population is reduced (see Fig. 156–2). The reasons for the progressive attenuation of proliferative rate are not completely understood but likely relate to progressive insufficiency of blood supply and hypoxia. For solid tumors, less than 30 per cent of the cells constituting the tumor mass are actively traversing the cell cycle by the time the tumor is detected; the remaining 70 per cent of cells are nonproliferating and are insensitive to most antimetabolites because they are not engaged in DNA synthesis. The progressive movement of cells into G_o and the increasing relative death rate of cells as the tumor grows larger combine to produce a slowing of the relative growth rate, reflected in a deviation of the growth curve away from a simple exponential function.

The later, clinical phases of tumor growth are best described by the Gompertz equation, which accommodates a continuous deceleration of the rate of increase in cell number with increase in tumor size. Tumors described by the Gompertz curve initially grow at a nearly exponential rate over a short span of observation, up to three or four doublings. Observation over a longer time span reveals the gradual slowing of relative growth rate (Fig. 156–3) to an eventual plateau level at which the rate of new cell production just equals the rate of cell loss. Such curves do not accommodate the heterogeneity of tumor cell population generated by mutations and the outgrowth of rapidly proliferating tumor subclones often observed in later stages of malignancy.

Strategies for cancer treatment are based on cell kinetic models (see Ch. 164). Both theoretical considerations and experimental evidence suggest that tumors are most susceptible to cytotoxic chemotherapy when their rate of proliferation is greatest, i.e., when the cell number is smallest (farthest to the left on the gompertzian curve in Fig. 156–3). Thus chemotherapy is most effective against rapidly proliferating tumors (lymphomas, leukemias, testicular cancers) and when used after surgical removal of the primary tumor, as in adjuvant chemotherapy of breast cancer and colon cancer. Bulk reduction of tumor by surgery or radiation therapy is followed by a wave of increased proliferation of residual tumor cells, creating opportunities for effective introduction of chemotherapeutic modalities. The fraction of cells killed by a given exposure to chemotherapy or radiation therapy is greatest when treatment is introduced at the earliest stages in the natural history of a malignancy, thus accounting for the cure of tumors in the adjuvant setting by a therapy ineffective against metastatic disease. Even in patients with overt metastatic cancer, surgical debulking is associated with an improved response to chemotherapy in some settings, as in patients with ovarian cancer.

DeVita VT, Hellman S, Rosenberg SA (eds.): Cancer: Principles and Practice of Oncology. Philadelphia, J. B. Lippincott Company, 1989. *The introductory chapters to this standard text contain very complete background information for the clinician on the general subjects of cancer etiology, biology, and metastases.*

Fidler JJ: Origin and biology of cancer metastasis. Cytometry 10:673–680, 1990. *Presents basic concepts of the clonal origin and organ predilection of cancer metastases.*

Franks LM, Teich N (eds.): Introduction to the Cellular and Molecular Biology of Cancer. New York, Oxford University Press, 1986. *Contains excellent chapters on lineages of hematologic malignancies, phenotypic markers of differentiation, and growth regulation in normal and malignant cells.*

Ruddon RW: Cancer Biology, 2nd ed. New York, Oxford University Press, 1987. *A very readable review of all aspects of cancer biology, including epidemiology, causation, genetics, and metastases.*

STAGING, CLASSIFICATION, MARKERS, AND PROGNOSIS

Staging and biologic characterization of clinical neoplasms are essential for providing prognostic information, guiding therapy, designing and evaluating clinical trials, and communicating information among physicians. The TNM system (Table 156–2) stages tumors according to three elements: size of the primary *tumor*, involvement of regional *nodes*, and presence or absence of *metastasis*. TNM staging is particularly useful in epithelial cancers such as cancer of the head and neck, breast cancer, and most types of lung cancer. In these tumors, the orderly progression of malignancy to involve lymph nodes and later distant sites lends itself to the TNM system. Other, more simplified systems are used for hematologic malignancies, sarcomas, and pediatric tumors, which lack the same orderly progression. There is no doubt that the complex TNM system, although difficult to use and remember, provides more specific prognostic information than do the simple staging systems often used in breast cancer (Ch. 227), colon cancer (Ch. 105), and prostate cancer.

In addition to anatomic extent of disease, other determinants affect prognosis and response to treatment. Thus, immunologic and molecular probes and karyotyping have defined subsets of

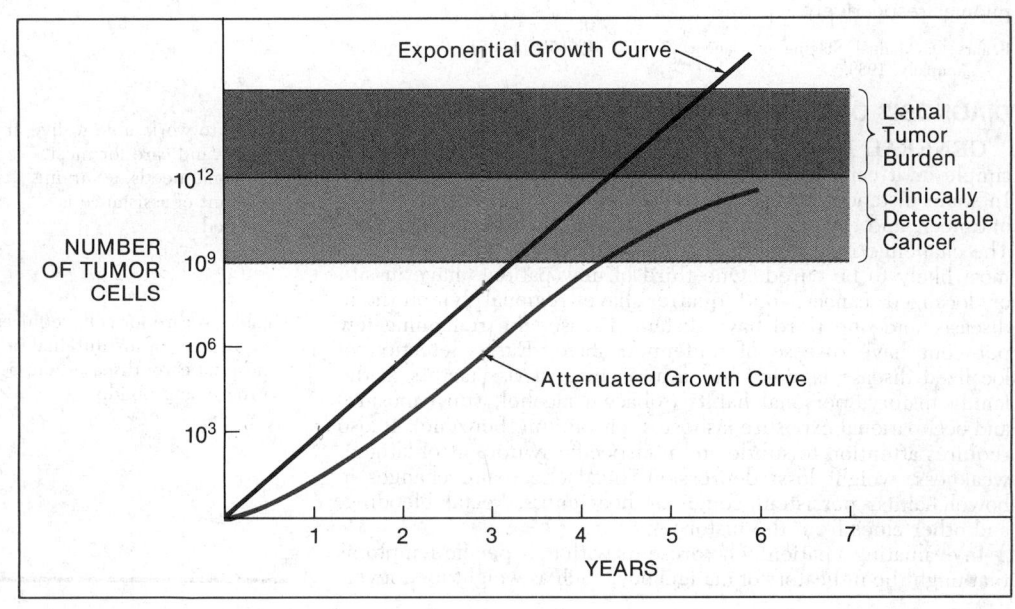

FIGURE 156–3. Schematic plot of exponential and attenuated (gompertzian) growth curves for hypothetical tumors. The clinical burden at the time of detection is probably 1 to 10 grams, depending on location and symptoms produced by the mass. The lethal body burden is also dependent on sites of involvement and impact on vital organ function. Note the slow period of tumor growth during the early preclinical phase, as the tumor establishes its blood supply and undergoes mutations that allow for unrestricted growth.

TABLE 156–2. THE TNM SYSTEM

Primary Tumor (T)

T_0	No evidence of primary tumor
T_{1b}	Carcinoma in situ
T_1, T_2, T_3, T_4	Progressive increase in tumor size and involvement, e.g., for breast cancer, 0–2 cm, 2–5, >5, any size plus skin or chest wall

Regional Lymph Nodes (N)

N_0	Regional nodes not demonstrable
N_{1a}, N_{1b}	Homolateral regional nodes (breast): metastases not suspected (a), suspected (b)
N_2, N_3	Homolateral regional nodes: fixed axillary (N_2), homolateral supraclavicular (N_3), or edema of arm; metastases suspected
N_x	Regional lymph nodes cannot be assessed clinically

Distant Metastasis (M)

M_0	No known distant metastasis
M_1	Distant metastasis present
Specific site_____	

The Manual for Staging of Cancer may be obtained free of charge from the American Joint Committee, 55 East Erie Street, Chicago, Ill. 60611.

patients with non-Hodgkin's lymphoma and with acute myelocytic leukemia who have unique clinical courses and responses to treatment. Immunophenotyping is now a standard step in defining prognosis and selecting therapy for childhood acute leukemia (Table 156–1). In breast cancer management, the clinician uses not only TNM information but also estrogen or progesterone receptor status and various measures of tumor proliferative capacity (Table 156–3) in defining prognosis and in selecting adjuvant therapy.

In addition to anatomic and biologic factors, the cancer patient's general condition influences prognosis and choice of therapy. The Karnofsky scale (Table 156–4) is the most widely used shorthand measure of a patient's performance status and, for many tumors, correlates closely with response to treatment and survival.

Other types of tumor markers may be useful in diagnosing or following the response to treatment of various cancers (see Ch. 160). Some of these are relatively specific markers such as the β-subunit of human chorionic gonadotropin and α-fetoprotein (germ-cell tumors of the testes and ovary), thyrocalcitonin (medullary carcinoma of the thyroid), serum acid phosphatase and prostate-specific antigen (prostate cancer), and monoclonal immunoglobulins (multiple myeloma). Others such as carcinoembryonic antigen (CEA) and serum lactate dehydrogenase (LDH) are less disease-specific but may nevertheless be useful indicators of disease progression for colon cancer and non-Hodgkin's lymphoma, respectively.

Beahrs O: Manual Staging of Cancer, 3rd ed. Philadelphia, J. B. Lippincott Company, 1988.

DIAGNOSIS OF CANCER AND ITS COMPLICATIONS

GENERAL EVALUATION. The diagnosis of cancer can be simple or it can challenge all the skills of clinical investigation. In some instances metastatic tumors may be the first indication of cancer, and the primary lesion may escape efforts at detection. The challenge is to detect cancer as early as possible, when it is most likely to be cured. One third of new patients have in situ or localized cancer, one quarter have regional lymph node disease, and one third have distant disease; the remaining few per cent have disease of undefined stage. Early detection of localized disease is aided by an awareness of risk factors in the family history, personal habits (tobacco, alcohol, sun exposure) and occupational exposure (asbestos, chromium, benzene). It also requires attention to subtle and nonspecific symptoms of fatigue, weakness, weight loss, depression, headache, pain, changes in bowel habits, persistent cough or hoarseness, rectal bleeding, and other clues from the history.

In evaluating a patient who presents with nonspecific symptoms that might be indicators of malignancy, such as weight loss, fever,

TABLE 156–3. TUMOR FEATURES PREDICTING HIGH RISK OF RELAPSE FOR PATIENTS WITH NODE-NEGATIVE BREAST CANCER*

		5-Year Recurrence Rate	
Factor	High-Risk Values	*Low Risk*	*High Risk*
Tumor size	> 2 cm	12%	20%
Hormonal status			
Estrogen receptor	< 10 fmol/mg protein	25%	34%
Nuclear grade	Qualitative	20%	36%
Proliferative rate			
S-phase fraction	> 7%	10%	29%
Protein expression			
Cathepsin D	Qualitative	29%	60%
Her-2/Neu	Qualitative	20%	60%

*Adapted from McGuire WL, Tandon AK, Allred DC, et al.: How to use prognostic factors in axillary node–negative breast cancer patients. J Natl Cancer Inst 82:1006, 1990.

or fatigue, the physician should carefully examine all mucosal surfaces, the sigmoid colon, and the rectum for masses or ulcerated lesions. In addition to elements of a routine examination, stool should be tested for occult blood. More subtle clues may be seen in the skin with findings such as petechiae, hyperpigmentation of skin folds (acanthosis nigricans), or atypical moles (dysplastic nevi). Attention should be paid to the presence of systemic cancer–associated effects, such as neuromyopathies (see Ch. 162 and 163). Leads from laboratory testing may be found in unexplained anemia, thrombocytopenia, hypercalcemia, or elevation of serum LDH and acid or alkaline phosphatase levels. Other frequent harbingers of cancer are pulmonary nodules or radiolucent bone lesions associated with new bone pain.

For the general internist, of equal importance is the strategy for early detection of occult malignancy in patients without complaints. Considerations of cost-effectiveness are still not resolved for many of the cancer screening tests, but their use undoubtedly saves lives. Those recommended for the average-risk individual are given in Table 156–5. For individuals from high-risk backgrounds, more frequent and earlier screening and additional tests may be indicated.

INITIAL DIAGNOSIS. Two major categories of diagnostic problems are associated with the management of cancer: obtaining the original diagnosis and correctly identifying the complications or intercurrent illnesses that may arise during the course of the

TABLE 156–4. "PERFORMANCE STATUS" (KARNOFSKY SCALE)

Criteria of Performance Status (PS)

Able to carry on normal activity; no special care is needed	100	Normal; no complaints; no evidence of disease
	90	Able to carry on normal activity; minor signs or symptoms of disease
	80	Normal activity with effort; some signs or symptoms of disease
Unable to work; able to live at home and care for most personal needs; a varying amount of assistance is needed	70	Cares for self; unable to carry on normal activity or to do active work
	60	Requires occasional assistance but is able to care for most needs
	50	Requires considerable assistance and frequent medical care
Unable to care for self; requires equivalent of institutional or hospital care; disease may be progressing rapidly	40	Disabled; requires special care and assistance
	30	Severely disabled; hospitalization is indicated although death not imminent
	20	Very sick; hospitalization necessary; active supportive treatment is necessary
	10	Moribund, fatal processes progressing rapidly
	0	Dead

TABLE 156–5. EARLY DETECTION OF OCCULT MALIGNANCY

Disease	Test Population	Screening Test	Frequency	Reduction in Cancer
Breast cancer	Women >50	Mammography	Yearly	20% reduction in deaths
Colon cancer	Men and women >50	Sigmoidoscopy Stool for occult blood	Every fifth year Yearly	Benefit unknown; 20% reduction in mortality is estimated*
Cervical cancer	Women >20	Pap smear	Yearly	>90% reduction in incidence

*See DeVita VT, Hellman S, Rosenberg SA (eds.): Cancer: Principles and Practice of Oncology. Philadelphia, J. B. Lippincott Company, 1989, pp 483–485; and Schottenfeld D, Fraumeni JF: Cancer Epidemiology and Prevention. Philadelphia, W. B. Saunders Company, 1982.

disease. A tissue diagnosis, usually from the primary site, is required in order to allow the patient and physician the certainty to embark on a plan of treatment. Although for most patients with lung, breast, or colon cancer the initial diagnosis is straightforward, some patients may present with metastatic disease but with no apparent primary lesion, or the primary mass may not be easily accessible to needle biopsy. In these patients, identification of the primary lesion and its biopsy are mandatory steps in patient management. *Indirect diagnostic techniques are not a substitute for a histologic or cytologic diagnosis of cancer.* Rarely it may not be possible to obtain tissue for histologic diagnosis, e.g., when there is a deep-seated brain tumor or when the patient's general condition is so poor that the malignancy has little bearing on prognosis.

Physicians often face the diagnostic dilemma posed by the discovery of a metastatic lesion of unknown primary site. In searching for the primary, two rules apply: *The clinician must consider the most common type of cancer in the given subject, taking into account age, sex, site of disease, and personal and family history, and must rule out the most treatable lesions, such as breast cancer in women and testicular cancer in young males.* Special immunohistologic or electron microscopic studies may be required to rule out malignant melanoma or lymphoma. The finding of mediastinal, retroperitoneal, or lymph node involvement and high human chorionic gonadotropin or α-fetoprotein levels are indicative of germ-cell tumors. Cisplatin-based chemotherapy programs may cure such patients.

DIAGNOSTIC PROBLEMS DURING CONTINUING CARE OF THE PATIENT WITH CANCER. The physician who undertakes the continuing care of a patient with cancer must be vigilant in promptly identifying complications arising from the progression of tumor and in detecting curable intercurrent illness that may be mistaken for manifestations of cancer itself. The patient with a known tumor who develops anorexia, weight loss, and jaundice may have cholecystitis and biliary obstruction rather than metastatic cancer and may die from that disorder unless the correct diagnosis is established. Furthermore, some potentially treatable conditions are actually caused by the cancer therapy— postoperative adhesions or radiation-induced strictures leading to bowel obstruction or chemotherapy-induced immunosuppression leading to an opportunistic fungal infection. Certain drugs may even produce complications that simulate paraneoplastic syndromes, such as inappropriate secretion of ADH, neuromyopathy, or cerebellar degeneration. Although errors in diagnosis of intercurrent medical and surgical illness sometimes seem almost inevitable, the best way to minimize these problems is to *assume that each new condition is due to a nonmalignant process, until it is proven otherwise. First recurrences of cancer must always be confirmed by biopsy because of their profound implications.*

PRINCIPLES OF MANAGEMENT OF THE PATIENT WITH CANCER

Subsequent chapters will outline strategies for the use of chemotherapy in patients with cancer, in addition to discussions of approaches to specific types of cancer. In this chapter, general principles of value in choosing therapies and in management of patients will be considered.

APPROACHES TO TREATMENT. A therapeutic strategy should be clearly defined for each patient with cancer, once the diagnosis has been firmly established, staging of the tumor has been carried out, and careful assessment has been made of the patient's overall physical, physiologic, and social situation. Such a strategy is often best devised by a multidisciplinary team,

including medical, surgical, and radiation oncologists who will weigh the possibilities of cure or significant palliation, consider the various treatment options and their expected untoward effects, and then define the best therapy for that patient. *Wherever possible, cancer treatment should be given according to standard protocols or as part of a peer-reviewed therapeutic trial, such as offered by the cooperative group program of the National Cancer Institute.* Detailed information about such trials and state-of-the-art therapies for specific types of cancer is available through the PDQ (Physicians Data Query) computer base, which is available at all medical school libraries and most tertiary-care hospitals in the United States. Trials information is also available through the National Cancer Institute's Cancer Information Service (1–800–4–CANCER). Improvisation, such as dosage attenuation, drug substitution, or changes in treatment schedule should not be undertaken unless there are compelling reasons for such changes.

Fortunately, the therapeutic horizons are constantly changing and improving. For example, patients with disseminated testicular cancer, acute lymphocytic leukemia, Ewing's sarcoma, Wilms' tumor, ovarian carcinoma, Hodgkin's disease, and histiocytic lymphoma now have an excellent chance for a cure. Cure is possible for a smaller fraction of patients with acute myelocytic leukemias, advanced ovarian cancer, and childhood sarcomas, and significantly palliative therapy is available for many additional patients with advanced cancer. Effective adjuvant therapies have been defined for early stages of breast cancer and colorectal cancer. Surgery or radiation therapy are the predominant forms of primary treatment. Although surgery is the sole initial treatment for over 50 per cent of patients with localized cancer, the use of adjuvant chemotherapy either before or after surgery is increasing. *Neoadjuvant chemotherapy*—defined as the use of drugs prior to surgery or radiotherapy to reduce the bulk of a primary tumor and thereby to render it more amenable to surgical removal or cure by radiotherapy—is being used with increasing frequency for head and neck, esophageal, and breast cancers. Combined-modality therapies reduce the extent of primary surgery required to cure limb sarcomas, bladder cancer, anal cancer, breast cancer, and head and neck cancer, thus preserving organ function and avoiding debilitation. The difficulty of attempting to predict tumor response to chemotherapy may one day be overcome through sensitivity tests in vitro, but for the present the selection process for drug regimens depends upon prior reports of clinical trials for particular types of cancer.

For patients with metastatic cancer, chemotherapy presents the only well-studied and well-understood alternative, although there is increasing experience with experimental biologic therapies. Chemotherapy should be administered only by physicians who have training and experience in its use and who are willing to use it with sufficient intensity to achieve optimal results. A thorough knowledge of the mechanisms of action, pharmacokinetics, routes of elimination, side effects, and interactions of the various chemotherapeutic drugs and irradiation is necessary to administer these agents with optimal safety and effectiveness. The risk of serious side effects may be much more acceptable to a patient who stands a good chance for a cure than to one who does not. After careful explanation by the physician of all options, the patient and his or her family must make the ultimate decisions about treatment. Therefore, good patient-doctor communication is essential for weighing treatment options.

One of the most difficult ethical dilemmas faced in cancer chemotherapy is the consideration of bone marrow transplantation, an expensive and dangerous procedure, in patients who have exhausted standard treatment alternatives. This decision requires a candid assessment of costs, likely therapeutic benefits, possible side effects, and the ability of the patient to withstand the emotional and physical stress of high-dose chemotherapy, the prolonged leukopenic interval, and in allogeneic transplants the immunosuppression required following transplant. No other setting in clinical practice more graphically poses the dilemma of a high-risk, potentially fatal, but possibly curative therapy as an alternative to a certain fatal outcome.

SUPPORTIVE CARE. In its broadest sense, "supportive care" refers to all types of medical care required to provide for the needs of the patient with cancer. Certain specific supportive-care programs for patients receiving aggressive chemotherapy for leukemia and other conditions have led to gratifying improvements in cure rates by anticipating and/or counteracting potentially fatal complications such as *infection* and *bleeding*. Early detection and vigorous antibacterial and antifungal treatment can be lifesaving for infected patients during periods of severe granulocytopenia. Similarly, platelet transfusions can minimize the risk of hemorrhage during periods of profound thrombocytopenia (platelet count less than 20,000 per cubic millimeter). These two advances, together with aggressive systemic and intrathecal chemotherapy, are responsible for the greater than 50 per cent cure rate that can now be achieved in childhood leukemia, for example. Most recently the availability of bone marrow colony-stimulating factors has allowed for abrogation of leukopenia and escalation of treatment dosage in conjunction with chemotherapy.

Severe *nausea* and *vomiting* induced by combination chemotherapy may be major, even limiting, factors in patient compliance because of the serious deterioration in the quality of life induced by these potent drugs. These side effects can largely be suppressed by newer antiemetics, such as the 5-hydroxytryptophan receptor antagonists. Anxiety, a very important part of the symptom complex, can be alleviated by benzodiazepines such as lorazepam.

General supportive care requires attention to nutritional, rehabilitative, psychosocial, and analgesic needs (see below). Anorexia and weight loss are almost invariably associated with advanced cancer; occasionally profound *cachexia* may occur in a patient with only a small and apparently localized lesion such as lung cancer. There are several potential explanations for nutritional problems—anatomic obstructions to chewing, swallowing, or digestion; liver disease; paraneoplastic syndromes; effects of chemotherapy; depression, or the release of peptides such as cachectin. In the individual patient it is often difficult to sort out the factors that contribute to anorexia and hypercatabolism. Regardless of etiology it is important to reverse this catabolic trend, since malnourished patients tolerate the usual courses of chemotherapy or radiation therapy very poorly and may die prematurely of complications related to treatment toxicity. Thus, in the case of a patient with recurrent cancer of the head and neck, improvement in nutrition is often a necessary prerequisite to the use of chemotherapeutic drugs. Increasingly, oncologists employ parenteral or tube feedings prior to major cancer surgery, radiation therapy, or chemotherapy. The dietitian familiar with the practical problems faced by these patients is an essential member of the team working with the patient and family.

The *psychosocial problems* that may be encountered by patients with cancer are profound and varied. Many of these are not unique to cancer and occur in age-matched patients with other types of chronic illness and shortened life expectancy. Shock, bereavement, anger, denial, withdrawal, and depression are common responses of people faced with such overwhelming problems. Disfigurement, feelings of shame and disgrace, loss of sexual activity, and job discrimination are problems that are more prevalent in patients with cancer than in those with many other illnesses. *The attitude of the physician and staff* is of key importance in helping the patient make the best possible adjustment, given all of the premorbid factors and limitations imposed by the illness. The physician who (verbally or nonverbally) conveys the impression that "There is nothing further that I can do" is sentencing his patient to untold misery or forcing him into the waiting arms of enthusiastic cancer quacks. All patients need help. Most patients respond positively to it, and they appreciate a gently supportive role that stresses honesty, trust, and a willingness simply to be available to help both patient and family with their fears and needs.

The *care of the patient who is dying of cancer* is the most sensitive issue for both patient and family. This is also commonly the period in which patients feel abandoned by physicians who themselves are frustrated by their inability to cure or cause remission of the illness and by the tragic human circumstances that often accompany such illnesses. Indeed, these take their toll on doctors and nurses as well as on relatives and friends, and busy cancer clinics recognize the need for support groups for their staff. (Indeed, unless there is an active self-renewing effort, oncology workers are subject to "burnout," an insidious syndrome difficult to recognize.) The physician must always prepare a reassuring setting so that when specific therapy is no longer warranted, patient comfort will be attended to in a considerate and thoughtful manner. In the final weeks of the illness, family members may require even more attention than the patient, and the team of doctor, nurse, social worker, and chaplain should provide the necessary support for all concerned, including staff.

Patients fear *pain* perhaps more than any other aspect of cancer, and there are many misconceptions about this subject by the public. Yet adequate techniques are available to control pain in most patients, if these are used in a timely and appropriate manner (see Ch. 8 and 26). Here, again, a careful history is an important initial step in diagnosis, for a patient with pain may have anything from cord compression to bone metastasis to a nonmalignant condition such as arthritis. Pain suppression is not a substitute for identification and treatment of a specific lesion. Relatively simple radiotherapy or neurosurgical procedures employed sufficiently early for localized pain and the *liberal use of narcotics for severe generalized pain* are usually successful in alleviating symptoms. One need not be concerned with potential narcotic addiction in dying patients. Patients themselves are often reluctant to take adequate doses of analgesics because of fears of addiction and should be encouraged to take them with sufficient frequency to alleviate pain *before* it becomes very severe.

Depending on the wishes of the family, it is often preferable to provide for the care of the dying patient in his or her own home. This can be done with a home care program supplemented by visiting nurses and volunteers. *Hospice programs* are rapidly developing in the United States, and these can provide the supportive ingredients for both the patient and family that others cannot supply. The patient is often much more comfortable in familiar surroundings near loved ones. Family and friends usually respond willingly to their duties when properly directed. Finally, the savings in costly hospitalizations can conserve already depleted financial resources. Indeed, careful curbing of unnecessary costly tests and interventions can make an enormous financial difference over the course of the illness.

Bonadonna G: Does chemotherapy fulfill its expectations in cancer treatment? Ann Oncol 1:11–21, 1990. *A thoughtful appraisal of the contributions of chemotherapy to cancer treatment by one of the pioneers of modern combination therapy regimens.*

Chabner BA, Collins JM (eds.): Cancer Chemotherapy, Principles and Practice. Philadelphia, J. B. Lippincott Company, 1990. *A detailed presentation of all pertinent aspects of anticancer drugs, including pharmacokinetics, dose adjustments for renal and hepatic dysfunction, drug interactions, and the rational design of protocols.*

McGuire WL, Tandon AK, Allred DC, et al.: How to use prognostic factors in axillary node–negative breast cancer patients. J Natl Cancer Inst 82:1006–1015, 1990. *A landmark paper summarizing the use of biochemical and molecular markers for prognosis in breast cancer.*

Physician Data Query (PDQ), National Cancer Institute: *PDQ is available to physicians at most medical libraries, at many hospitals, or through private computer software vendors* and contains information on state-of-the-art treatments for each pathologic type of cancer, as well as a listing of experimental protocols for each disease.*

---

*PDQ vendors for health professional inquiries as of November 1988: MEDLARS Management Section, National Library of Medicine, Bldg. 38, Rm 4N421, 8600 Rockville Pike, Bethesda, MD 20894, (301) 496–6193, (800) 638–8480; BRS/Saunders COLLEAGUE, 1350 Avenue of the Americas, Suite 1802, New York, NY 10019, 1–800–468–0908, in Pennsylvania or outside continental USA (215) 527–4155; Mead Data Central, MEDIS, 9333 Springboro Pike, Dayton, OH 45401, 1–800–277–4908; TELMED, Jakob Fugli Strasse 18, Postfach, CH-8048 Zurich, Switzerland; MEDIMATICA, Heemraadssingel, 3021 DM Rotterdam, The Netherlands.

157 Oncogenes

J. Michael Bishop

CANCER AS A GENETIC DISEASE

Astute observers have long nurtured the thought that cancer might be at its heart a genetic disease. The thought was at first vague and arose from seemingly disparate discoveries that included the existence of heritable diatheses to cancer, the presence of abnormal chromosomes in cancer cells, and the likelihood that many carcinogens act by inducing mutations in cellular DNA. Medical geneticists and epidemiologists first conceived the possibility of "cancer genes," prompted by occasional examples of human tumors whose occurrence seemed dictated by recessive or dominant inherited traits. Now the long-imagined cancer genes have been brought to view, first unearthed by two experimental strategies: the use of viruses that cause tumors in animals and the search for tumorigenic genes in the DNA of cancer cells. From these studies we have learned that the human genome contains a set of several dozen genes that may lie at the heart of every cancer. These genes take two forms. Some act in a dominant manner when mutated and are known as either proto-oncogenes or cellular oncogenes. Others are recessive when mutated and are known variously as tumor suppressor genes, recessive oncogenes, or (least desirably) anti-oncogenes. The discovery and isolation of these genes represent our present best hope of achieving an understanding of the molecular mechanisms by which cancer arises. We now have in view a keyboard on which many different carcinogens may play, the possible components of a final common pathway to neoplastic growth.

FIRST DESCRIPTIONS: VIRAL ONCOGENES

Documentation that specific genes can elicit cancerous growth emerged first from the study of viruses that cause tumors in animals. By the use of formal genetic analyses, and later of recombinant DNA, investigators were able to show that the tumorigenicity of many viruses can be attributed to viral germs now known as oncogenes.

The most decisive paradigm for the genetic origins of cancer came from the study of retroviruses, whose genes are carried in RNA but are copied into DNA by reverse transcriptase early in viral replication. The life cycle of retroviruses provides a microcosm of carcinogenesis (Fig. 157–1). The viral DNA produced by reverse transcriptase is inserted (or "integrated") into the chromosomal DNA of the host cell. Thereafter, the cell uses its own machinery to express the integrated viral genes. These events hold two possibilities for carcinogenesis.

First, the integration of viral DNA is potentially mutagenic: It can damage vital cellular genes, and it can influence their expression by bringing them under the sway of powerful viral signals. Virologists call this *insertional mutagenesis;* it may indeed be tumorigenic (see below), and the cellular genes perverted by viral DNA are candidate "proto-oncogenes."

Second, some (but not all) retroviruses carry oncogenes whose expression is sufficient to give rise to cancerous growth. The oncogenes of retroviruses make no apparent contribution to viral replication; therefore, their presence in viral genomes posed a puzzle. The puzzle was solved with the discovery that retroviral oncogenes are not viral genes at all, but wayward copies of cellular genes acquired during the course of viral replication by a process known formally as transduction, and carried as mere passengers in the viral genome. It is likely that transduction by retroviruses is a rare accident of nature, without design for the virus, and attributable to details of the curious means by which retroviruses replicate. There is no reason to believe that the transduction is limited to genes with tumorigenic potential. However, transduction of proto-oncogenes by retroviruses is of particular importance because it has brought to view cellular genes whose activities may be central to all forms of carcinogenesis.

THE PATHOGENIC MECHANISMS OF RETROVIRAL ONCOGENES

The study of viral oncogenes began with the hope that the mechanisms by which these genes act might help to reveal the

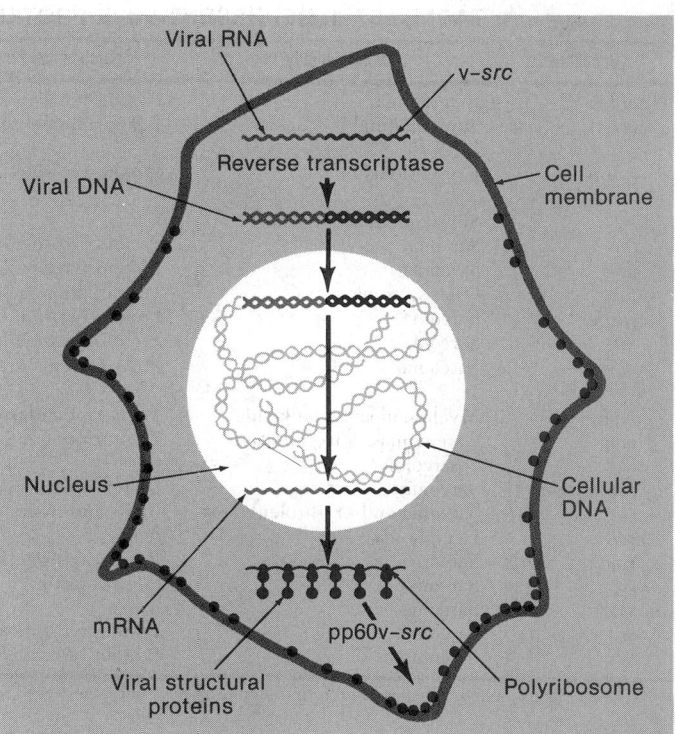

FIGURE 157–1. The molecular life cycle of retroviruses leads to insertion of viral genes into the chromosome of the host cell and the subsequent production of viral proteins that can transform the cell to neoplastic growth. In the example illustrated, the protein encoded by the *src* oncogene of the Rous sarcoma virus attaches to the inner surface of the plasma membrane and catalyzes phosphorylation of tyrosine residues in cellular proteins. (Modified from Bishop JM: Oncogenes and proto-oncogenes. Hosp Pract *18:*68, 1983, with permission from HP Publishing Co., Inc.)

inner workings of the cancer cell, to elucidate the biochemical abnormalities that prompt cancerous growth. This is now a burgeoning prospect because the number of retroviral oncogenes has grown to at least 20, each inducing specific forms of malignancy, each encoding a protein whose action apparently causes harm (Table 157–1). The first hint of how informative these genes might be came with the discovery that several retroviral oncogenes encode protein kinases, located on the plasma membrane of the cell and possessing a previously unencountered substrate specificity for tyrosine. Phosphorylation of tyrosine was discovered first through the study of retroviral oncogenes. But we now know that this same reaction is represented by hundreds, perhaps thousands, of enzymes within normal cells and that it plays a vital role in the governance of normal cellular phenotype. It would be difficult to envision a better explanation for neoplastic transformation: By phosphorylating numerous cellular proteins, a single enzyme could rapidly change myriad aspects of cellular structure and function. As the phosphorylated proteins are found (only a few have been, to date), doors are opened to the secrets of neoplastic growth.

Protein phosphorylation is not the only means by which retroviral oncogenes may act (Table 157–1). As more and more of the proteins encoded by oncogenes came into view, a provocative diversity emerged: Some of the proteins are protein kinases, others are GTP-binding proteins or transcription factors; some act in the nucleus of the cell, some in the cytoplasm, some at the plasma membrane (Fig. 157–2); and there is little correlation between what we now know of how oncogenes function and the character of their tumorigenicities. What does this diversity signify? The growth of cells is regulated by an interdigitating network that spans from the surface of the plasma membrane to the depths of the nucleus. If that network were to be touched at any point by an adverse influence and tilted out of balance, cancerous growth might ensue. It is now clear that the diverse means by which different oncogenes act mirror various components of the regulatory network, revealing how the network

TABLE 157–1. REPRESENTATIVE PROTEINS ENCODED BY RETROVIRAL ONCOGENES

Oncogenes	Tumorigenicity	Biochemical Properties	Subcellular Location	Cellular Homologue
abl	Lymphoma	Protein tyrosine kinase	Plasma membrane	
erb-A	Supplemental	Transcriptional repressor	Nucleus	Receptor for thyroid hormone
erb-B	Erythroleukemia	Protein tyrosine kinase	Intracellular and plasma membranes	Receptor for EGF
ets	Supplemental	?	Nucleus	
fgr	Sarcoma	Protein tyrosine kinase	Plasma membrane	
fims	Sarcoma	Protein tyrosine kinase	Plasma membrane	Receptor for CSF-1
fos	Osteosarcoma	Transcription factor	Nucleus	Transcription factor AP-1
fps/fes*	Sarcoma	Protein tyrosine kinase	Plasma membrane	
kit	Sarcoma	Protein tyrosine kinase	Plasma membrane	
mos	Sarcoma	Protein serine kinase	Cytoplasm	Embryonic cytostatic factor
myb	Myelomonocytic leukemia	Transcription factor	Nucleus	
myc	Carcinomas, leukemia and sarcoma	Transcription factor	Nucleus	
raf/mht/mil*	Sarcoma	Protein serine kinase	Membranes	
ras	Sarcoma and erythroleukemia	Binds and hydrolyzes GTP	Plasma membrane	GTPase regulatory proteins
rel	Lymphoma	?	?	
ros	Sarcoma	Protein tyrosine kinase	Plasma membrane	
sis	Sarcoma	Growth factor	Cytoplasm	Subunit β of PDGF
ski	Sarcoma	?	Nucleus	
src	Sarcoma	Protein tyrosine kinase	Plasma membrane	
yes	Sarcoma	Protein tyrosine kinase	Plasma membrane	

*Multiple names denote genes isolated from different species but later proved to be homologous.

performs its task. By studying oncogenes, we are learning of both cancerous and normal growth at one and the same time. It is an old adage of medical science that study of the abnormal can reveal the normal.

PROTO-ONCOGENES AND ONCOGENES

The cellular genes whose transduction engenders retroviral oncogenes provided the first glimpse and the first definition of proto-oncogenes. By all available criteria, these are cellular genes, not viral genes in disguise. They can be found in every member of every vertebrate species examined, probably in all metazoan organisms. Evolutionary conservation of this magnitude signifies that the proto-oncogenes serve essential functions for the species in which they are harbored. Proto-oncogenes are expressed in normal cells and tissues, and their expression can vary from one tissue to another, from one embryologic lineage to another, from one time in embryogenesis to another. It is widely assumed that, in their normal guise, proto-oncogenes help to control the growth and development of cells and organisms. This assumption has been strengthened by two discoveries. First, a number of proto-

oncogenes encode proteins known to participate in the regulation of cellular proliferation and differentiation, including platelet-derived growth factor (PDGF) and the receptors for epidermal growth factor (EGF) and colony-stimulating factor I (CSF-I) (Table 157–1). Second, mutations in the proto-oncogenes of fruit flies (*Drosophila melanogaster*) and laboratory mice cause profound disturbances of growth and development.

Why are the transduced forms of proto-oncogenes tumorigenic? What converts a proto-oncogene, a compliant member of the cellular citizenry, to an oncogene—an unruly and potentially lethal enemy? The possible answers to these questions have taken two general forms: Transduction may have unleashed the genes from their usual controls and inappropriate expression of otherwise normal genes might be the fatal flaw; alternatively, mutation during or after transduction could change the structure of the genes and the proteins they encode, giving rise to abnormal function. For the moment, it appears that either explanation may on occasion apply.

PROTO-ONCOGENES AS CANCER GENES

Do proto-oncogenes participate in many or all forms of tumorigenesis? Are they a common keyboard for all the players in carcinogenesis? Since these questions were first raised, the pertinent evidence has grown from a thin thread to a rich and provocative fabric of experimental observation.

1. Direct manipulation of proto-oncogenes isolated by molecular cloning has revealed that some (but not all) of these ostensibly normal genes can elicit neoplastic growth if they are first attached to viral signals that command vigorous gene expression and then inserted into cells in culture or used to create transgenic mice.

2. There is evidence that retroviruses without oncogenes of their own initiate tumorigenesis by the mutation of proto-oncogenes. The mutations may be of two sorts: those that enhance expression of a gene and those that change the structure of the protein(s) encoded by a gene.

3. Some human tumors (the exact number is not yet clear) display karyotypic evidence of gene amplification (double-minute chromosomes and homogeneously staining regions in marker chromosomes) and contain one or another proto-oncogene whose number has been multiplied as much as 200-fold over normal. As a consequence of amplification, the proto-oncogene is expressed in inordinately large amounts. Amplification of proto-oncogenes has been found in two patterns: as sporadic and occasional features of diverse tumors and as a common feature of particular tumors. The latter pattern gives promise of being

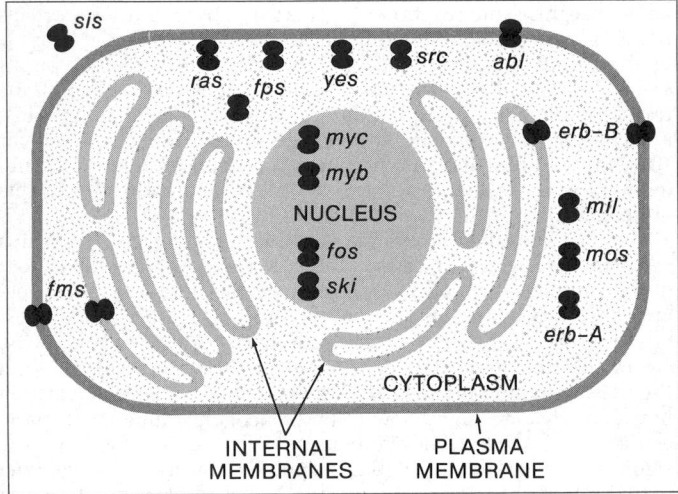

FIGURE 157–2. The products of oncogenes assume diverse locations within the cell, where they perform functions involved in the regulation of cellular growth and differentiation. (Modified from The Proteins of Oncogenes, by T. Hunter. Copyright © 1984 by Scientific American, Inc. All rights reserved.)

clinically useful. For example, amplification of the proto-oncogenes NMYC and NEU are common features of neuroblastoma and carcinoma of the breast, respectively, and apparently connote a poor prognosis.

4. At least several of the chromosomal translocations that typify a substantial variety of human tumors affect a proto-oncogene. As a consequence, expression of the proto-oncogene may be altered, or the gene may sustain mutations within the domain that encodes a protein. Representative examples include Burkitt's lymphoma (translocation of the proto-oncogene c-myc) and the Philadelphia chromosome (Ph¹) of chronic myelogenous leukemia (translocation of c-abl).

5. Application of DNA from a variety of human tumors to cells in culture can elicit neoplastic growth, as if the DNA contained oncogenes of the sort once found only in viruses. Approximately 20 per cent of all human tumors demonstrate activity of this type, no matter what their histopathology. The responsible genes have now been identified for a substantial variety of tumors. With remarkable frequency, they have proved to be one or another member of a family of proto-oncogenes known as ras genes and already familiar to us from the study of retroviruses. The ras genes have transforming activity because they have suffered mutations that change single amino acids in the protein products of the genes.

RECESSIVE GENETIC DAMAGE IN TUMORS

The oncogenes considered so far are thought to be genetically dominant: Their abnormalities have an impact even when a normal allele of the same gene is also present in the cell. But most if not all human tumors also bear lesions that are recessive, that make their presence known only when no normal counterpart is present. By inference from karyotypes and by the use of restriction endonucleases, substantial evidence has been obtained for the presence of recessive mutations in a variety of tumors. In each instance, the tumor is presumed to be entirely deficient in the function of at least one gene whose activity helps to regulate cellular proliferation. The examples of retinoblastoma and Wilms' tumor are the most celebrated, but other (and more common) examples are now also in view (Table 157–2). Four of the genes affected by recessive damage have been isolated to date: RB1, a gene first associated with the genesis and inheritance of retinoblastoma but now incriminated in a variety of other malignancies as well; a gene known as P53, named for the protein that it encodes and recessively damaged in a variety of human tumors; DCC, a gene deleted from a majority of adenocarcinomas of the colon; and WT1, a gene reputed to be involved in Wilms' tumor. Isolation of these "tumor suppressor genes" is a difficult endeavor and represents one form of medical research that would be greatly facilitated by having a complete physical map of the human genome—the first step in the controversial Human Genome Project.

Inheritance of recessive mutations can explain hereditary diatheses to several forms of neoplasm (again, retinoblastoma and Wilms' tumor are the seminal examples). By contrast, there is as yet no evidence to implicate any of the dominant oncogenes in the inheritance of cancer.

ONCOGENES AND THE MULTIPLE STEPS IN CARCINOGENESIS

The attribution of tumorigenesis to genetic damage seemed at first glance simplistic, since the genesis of tumors has long been described as a protracted and complex sequence of events. However, the identification of oncogenes and the proto-oncogenes from which they are derived has given us a tool with which to recognize several separate steps in tumorigenesis. Catalogues of genetic damage within individual tumors are taking shape, revealing how the malfunction of several different genes might combine to produce the malignant phenotype. For example, carcinomas of the colon contain no less than five different yet prevalent lesions—some genetically dominant, others recessive—and a similar plurality of lesions has emerged in carcinomas of the breast (five) and lung (four) and in neuroblastoma (three). It has even been possible to decipher the approximate order in which genetic lesions accumulate during the genesis of carcinoma of the colon. The phenomenon of tumor progression is moving rapidly from the realm of mystery to the realm of molecular

TABLE 157–2. REPRESENTATIVE RECESSIVE GENETIC LESIONS IN HUMAN CANCER

Tumor	Chromosomal Locus	Gene Incriminated
Retinoblastoma	13(q14)	RB1
Wilms' tumor	11(p13)	WT1
	11(p15)	?
Beckwith-Wiedemann syndrome (embryonal tumors)	11(p15)	?
Carcinoma of lung	3(p21)	?
	13(q14)	RB1
	17(p12–p13)	P53
Carcinoma of breast	3p	?
	11p	?
	13(q14)	RB1
Carcinoma of colon	5(q21–q22)	?
	17(p12–p13)	P53
	18(q21)	DCC
Neuroblastoma	1(p36.1)	?

reality. Moreover, detection of the lesions responsible for progression is likely to provide information useful for prognosis and therapeutic management.

THE FUTURE

By one means or another, more than a dozen genes have been implicated in the genesis of human tumors. In some instances, expression of the gene is enhanced or the structure of the gene product is changed, giving a dominant effect on function; in other instances, mutations eliminate the function of the gene in a recessive manner. Combinations of these events apparently lead to most if not all human tumors. These are remarkable conclusions, reached within a decade of the discovery of proto-oncogenes. However, the unknown still outweighs the known. How extensive is the role of proto-oncogenes in tumorigenesis? How are we to explain those human tumors that as yet offer no evidence of genetic lesions? How important are recessive genetic traits in tumorigenesis, how are they to be identified, and by what means do they act? What is the nature of heritable susceptibility to carcinogenesis and does this diathesis ever originate from proto-oncogenes? How do the proteins encoded by oncogenes conduct their nefarious business? Will we be able to parlay the growing information about oncogenes into devices for the prevention, diagnosis, and treatment of human cancer? It is too early to foretell how quickly the answers to these questions may come, but there now seems little reason to doubt that we have laid hold of cancer with a grip that should eventually extract the deadly secrets of the disease.

Bishop JM: The molecular biology of RNA tumor viruses: A physician's guide. N Engl J Med 303:675, 1980.
Bishop JM: Oncogenes. Sci Am 246(3):80, 1982.
Bishop JM: Trends in oncogenes. Trends Genet 1:245, 1985.
Bishop JM: The molecular genetics of cancer. Science 235:305, 1987.
Bishop JM: Oncogenes and clinical cancer. In Weinberg RA (ed.): Oncogenes and the Molecular Origins of Cancer. New York, Cold Spring Harbor Press, 1989, pp 327–358.
Hunter T: The proteins of oncogenes. Sci Am 251(2):70, 1984.
Sager R: Tumor suppressor genes: The puzzle and the promise. Science 246:1406, 1989.
Varmus HE: The molecular genetics of cellular oncogenes. Ann Rev Genet 18:553, 1984.
Weinberg RA: A molecular basis of cancer. Sci Am 249(5):126, 1983.
All of these references offer general reviews of this rapidly expanding area of medical research.

158 The Epidemiology of Cancer
William J. Blot

This chapter describes the distribution and causes of cancer in human populations. Through increased understanding of the patterns and determinants of the specific tumors, strategies can

TABLE 158–1. INTERNATIONAL VARIATION IN AGE-ADJUSTED INCIDENCE RATES FOR SELECTED CANCERS

Cancer Site	High-Rate Areas*	Rate†	Baseline Rate‡
Oral cavity	France, India	35–45	1–2
Nasopharynx	China, Hong Kong	30	<1
Esophagus	China, Iran	100+	1–2
Stomach	Japan	80	5
Colon/rectum	U.S., Australia	50–60	6
Liver	China	30	1
Pancreas	U.S. blacks	15	1
Larynx	Brazil	20	2
Lung	U.S. blacks	100	6
Skin melanoma	Australia	30	<1
Breast	U.S.	90	20
Uterine cervix	Brazil, Colombia, India	40–80	4
Ovary	Norway, Pacific Islands	15–25	4
Prostate	U.S. blacks	90	2
Bladder	U.S. whites, Spain	25–30	2
Non-Hodgkin's lymphoma	Switzerland	10	1
Hodgkin's disease	Canada	5	<1
Multiple myeloma	U.S. blacks	10	<1
Leukemia	Canada	12	2–3
Total	U.S. blacks	**400**	**100**

*Country in which high-rate areas occur is listed. The high rates do not necessarily persist throughout the country.

†Approximate age-adjusted (world standard) incidence rate per year per 100,000 population among males (except for breast, cervix, and ovarian cancers). Data collection periods vary by area but typically center on 1980.

‡Approximate age-adjusted incidence rate in typical low-rate area.

be developed to prevent cancer. Astute clinical observations can play a key role in this process, providing etiologic clues that can be evaluated by systematic epidemiologic investigations.

DESCRIPTIVE PATTERNS

THE GEOGRAPHY OF CANCER. Cancer affects all the world's populations, with about a threefold difference between areas with the highest and lowest age-adjusted rates. For certain cancers, the difference exceeds 100-fold (Table 158–1). Perhaps the most distinctive geographic patterns are seen for esophageal cancer. Pockets of exceptionally high mortality exist in areas of north central China, the Caspian littoral of Iran, and South Africa. In Linxian, China, for as yet unknown reasons, esophageal/gastric cardia cancer is the most common cause of death, causing over 30 per cent of all fatalities among adults. Clustering of elevated esophageal cancer rates has also been observed in parts of Europe and the United States. Heavy alcohol intake has been implicated in western populations, most recently in coastal South Carolina, where high rates of esophageal cancer among black men have been linked to consumption of moonshine whiskeys.

Geographic variation for other tumors is also noteworthy. Rates of oral cancer are highest in India and parts of south central Asia. Within the United States, elevated oral cancer mortality among females is found in the southern states, especially in rural areas. In both instances the cause is the same—high use of smokeless tobacco. Indeed, it was the observation of excess oral cancer mortality rates in several southern states, combined with clinical case descriptions, that led to epidemiologic investigations that in the early 1980's conclusively showed that snuff use can induce oral tumors. Among long-term users, risks of cancers of the gums and buccal mucosa, tissues in direct contact with the tobacco powder, were increased nearly 50-fold over those for tobacco abstainers.

In southeastern China, nasopharyngeal cancer is the most common malignancy. It is also a leading cancer among Alaskan Aleuts and Eskimos and occurs more frequently among Chinese than caucasian or black Americans. The primary cause of the cancer in southern China appears to be consumption of salted fish, especially during weaning and early childhood. The importance of early life events is also suggested by the up to threefold higher rates of nasopharyngeal cancer among Chinese-Americans

born and raised in China than among those born and raised in the United States. Similar migrant effects are seen for stomach cancer. Japanese-Americans born in Japan, where rates of stomach cancer are among the highest in the world, have a two- to threefold higher incidence of this cancer than Japanese-Americans born in the United States. American-born Japanese in turn experience more than twice the incidence of stomach cancer of white Americans. Such differences in rates suggest the strong influence of environmental factors.

The most common cancers in western countries, those of the lung, large bowel, and breast, also vary geographically. Within the United States, the highest rates of lung cancer are now found in the south. In the 1980's lung cancer mortality in southern rural counties surpassed that in northern cities, reversing a longstanding pattern. The shifts in lung cancer follow changes in cigarette smoking, now more prevalent in the south than elsewhere in the country. In addition, certain southern port and coastal areas still maintain excess lung cancer rates among males as a legacy of occupational exposures to asbestos in shipyards during World War II, when shipbuilding was the largest manufacturing industry in the United States. Colon and breast cancer show a contrasting pattern, with high rates in the northeast and low rates in the south, but the differentials are not large.

U.S. CANCER RATES AND TRENDS. It is estimated that in 1990 nearly 1,000,000 Americans developed and 500,000 died from cancer. Table 158–2 presents age-adjusted incidence rates during 1983 to 1987 (the most recent 5-year period for which complete data are available) for 28 cancers. The data derive from areas of the country participating in the SEER program of cancer registries (covering approximately 10 per cent of the U.S. population). Cancer, excluding basal and squamous cell skin cancers, was newly diagnosed in 429 of every 100,000 American males and 330 of every 100,000 American females each year during this period. The leading cancers among men are those of the prostate, lung, and colon/rectum, while among women the top three are breast, colon/rectum, and lung cancers. If mortality rather than incidence data are considered, the order shifts. Among males, lung cancer is by far the leading cause of cancer death (66.2 deaths per year per 100,000), followed by colon/rectum (24.1 per 100,000) and prostate (24.1 per 100,000) cancer. Among females, breast cancer death rates (27.4 per 100,000) were slightly higher than lung (26.0 per 100,000) and colon/rectum (17.0 per 100,000)

TABLE 158–2. AGE-ADJUSTED CANCER INCIDENCE RATES* IN THE UNITED STATES, 1983–1987, BY SEX

Cancer Site	Males	Females
Oral and pharynx	17.3	6.5
Esophagus	6.2	1.9
Stomach	12.1	5.4
Small intestine	1.3	0.8
Colon/rectum	61.2	43.4
Gallbladder and biliary	2.2	2.4
Pancreas	11.2	8.3
Larynx	8.4	1.6
Lung	84.2	35.6
Bone	1.0	0.7
Soft tissue	2.5	1.8
Skin melanoma	11.5	8.9
Breast	0.8	102.0
Uterine cervix	—	8.7
Uterus, corpus	—	21.9
Ovary	—	13.7
Prostate	89.3	—
Testis	4.1	—
Bladder	29.5	7.4
Kidney and renal pelvis	11.3	5.3
Eye	0.8	0.6
Brain and nervous system	7.1	5.0
Thyroid	2.5	6.0
Hodgkin's disease	3.3	2.3
Non-Hodgkin's lymphomas	15.3	10.4
Multiple myeloma	5.1	3.5
Leukemia	13.1	7.7
Total	**428.5**	**329.9**

*Age-adjusted (1970 U.S. population) incidence rates per year per 100,000 population.

cancer death rates during 1983 to 1987. However, by the late 1980's death rates from lung cancer had passed death rates from breast cancer among women in the United States.

For nearly all cancers, the incidence rates are higher among men than women, the exceptions being gallbladder and thyroid cancers. For some cancers, explanations for the male excess are evident (e.g., higher tobacco and alcohol intake account for most of the higher rates of oral, esophageal, laryngeal, and lung cancer among males), but for others (e.g., stomach cancer, leukemia) the reasons are enigmatic.

Rates of most cancers, particularly those deriving from epithelial tissue, rise steadily with advancing age, often exponentially. There are bimodal distributions for some cancers, however. Leukemia and nervous system tumors display an early childhood (age <5 years) peak, then rates decline before rising again in late middle age. Testis cancer occurs primarily between the ages of 20 and 40, while Hodgkin's disease incidence is highest at ages 20 to 30, declines somewhat, then rises again after age 50.

Racial differences in cancer occurrence are sometimes marked. Total cancer incidence during 1983 to 1987 was higher among black than white males by 22 per cent, while rates were higher among white than black females by 4 per cent. The black/white differences among males were particularly pronounced for esophageal, stomach, pancreas, lung, and prostate cancer and multiple myeloma, with age-adjusted incidence from 50 to 300 per cent higher among blacks than whites.

Rates of mortality of several cancers have been changing over the past decades (Fig. 158–1). Most notable has been the rise in lung cancer. Lung tumors were rarely diagnosed prior to the early 1900's, but incidence and mortality began a notable rise in the 1920's which has continued until today. The epidemic increase in lung cancer, almost entirely attributable to cigarette smoking, is beginning to end, however. Indeed, mortality from lung cancer between the mid 1970's and mid 1980's declined by nearly 30 per cent among white males below age 45, with smaller declines also noted for white females and nonwhites of both sexes. As younger Americans age and their more favorable lung cancer experience extends to older age groups, the overall rates of lung cancer should begin to decline. For white males the total age-adjusted rates have already plateaued, but the leveling off and subsequent decrease in lung cancer rates among females will not take place until after the year 2000. Rates of stomach and cervical cancers, the leading tumors early in this century, have declined in all groups, the former for reasons not yet fully understood, the latter at least in part due to cytologic screening for cervical pathology. The decreases in these tumors are beginning to end, however, and rates of gastric cardia cancer are now on the rise.

Although not shown in Figure 158–1, there has been nearly a doubling in incidence of melanoma and a 50 per cent rise in non-Hodgkin's lymphomas among whites since the early 1970's. In addition, the excess among blacks for certain cancers has been increasing over time. This is occurring for lung, oral, and laryngeal cancer but is particularly evident for esophageal cancer, rising rates of which have now made esophageal cancer the second leading cancer among black males below the age of 60. By contrast, rates of esophageal cancer have been stable or declining among whites. Reasons for the growing racial disparity are not entirely evident, although higher prevalences of cigarette smoking, heavy alcohol consumption, and nutritional disadvantages are suspect.

THE CAUSES OF CANCER

Cancer is believed to be a largely preventable disease. Clear knowledge now exists of the causes of most occurrences for several cancers, including those of the oral cavity and pharynx, esophagus, liver, larynx, lung, and uterine cervix. Agents influencing risk also have been identified for other cancers, but the search continues in order to clarify the etiologic factors that account for the bulk of malignancies in the United States and around the world. Most of the information currently available on risk factors for cancer has come from case-control studies assessing various characteristics and exposures of patients with individual cancers and from cohort studies determining rates of cancer among groups exposed to particular agents suspected of carcinogenic potential. Often the leads for these epidemiologic investigations were generated from descriptive studies of cancer rates and statistics and from alert clinical observations.

The striking variation in cancer rates within and between countries, the differing rates among migrants from one place to another, and the often marked trends over time suggest that most cancers are environmentally induced. Estimates of the per cent of cancer that is caused by environmental determinants are typically 75 per cent or higher, although it is likely that most tumors arise from the complex interplay of environmental and host, possibly genetic, factors. Those factors known to be related to the risk of cancer in humans are summarized below.

TOBACCO. Cigarette smoking is the dominant cause of the leading cancer (i.e., lung cancer) in the United States and many other western nations. The association was first suspected by clinical observation that new lung cancer patients were often smokers, then confirmed in the 1950's by case-control and cohort studies in the United States and Great Britain. In the years since the first U.S. Surgeon General's report on smoking in 1964, additional evidence has documented that risks of lung cancer rise in proportion to both duration of smoking and amount smoked per day, with risks of lung cancer more than 20 times greater among long-term heavy smokers than among nonsmokers. Lifelong filter smokers have experienced a somewhat smaller increase in risk than life-long nonfilter smokers, but the greatest protection comes from smoking cessation. Risks 10 years after quitting are typically only one third or less those of continuing cigarette smokers. Smoking affects all the major types of lung cancers, although squamous and small cell carcinomas more than adenocarcinomas. Cigarette smoking also increases risk of other cancers. It is a principal cause of cancers of the oral cavity and pharynx, esophagus, larynx, and renal pelvis; a major contributor to cancers of the pancreas, bladder, and kidney; and implicated to a moderate degree in cancers of the stomach and uterine cervix. In addition, smokeless tobacco is the predominant cause of buccal mucosa cancers in some populations. In total, tobacco use is thought to account for nearly one third of all cancers in the United States and thus is the largest single preventable cause of cancer.

While the effects of smoking are far greater for smokers themselves, the consensus of evidence from nearly 20 epidemiologic studies conducted around the world in the past decade is that long-term exposure to environmental tobacco smoke can also increase risk of lung cancer among nonsmokers. The excess risk of lung cancer among nonsmoking women married to smokers has averaged 30 per cent. Because of tobacco's harmful effects, efforts to induce smokers to quit and to encourage nonsmokers, particularly adolescents, not to start smoking must be continued. Smoking prevalence among adult men in the United States has declined from a peak of nearly 60 per cent in the 1950's to about 30 per cent today, but further reductions are attainable and critical to the nation's public health.

ALCOHOL. Alcohol combines with tobacco to cause cancers of the oral cavity and pharynx, esophagus, and larynx. Alcoholic beverages have also been implicated in the etiology of liver, rectal, and breast cancers, although the associations with the latter remain to be verified. In a large recent case-control study involving over 1100 oral and pharyngeal cancer patients in the United States, cancer risk was shown to increase progressively with increasing intake of alcoholic beverages among nonsmokers as well as smokers. Smoking and drinking tended to multiply the effects of each other, so that risk of oral cancer was increased over 35-fold among two-pack-a-day smokers who consumed more than four alcoholic drinks per day, compared with abstainers of both products. Similar tobacco-alcohol interactions have been observed for esophageal and laryngeal cancer. Ethanol has generally not been shown to be carcinogenic in experimental studies using animal models but seems likely to be the etiologic agent in humans, since all types of alcoholic beverages—beer, wine, dark and light spirits—have been linked with increased risk in epidemiologic studies.

OCCUPATIONAL HAZARDS. Occupational exposures have long been recognized as causes of cancer, beginning with the observation in the 1700's of scrotal cancer among chimney sweeps in London. Today at least 20 substances in the workplace have been associated with increased cancer risk (Table 158–3). About one half have been implicated in lung cancer, occasionally in an interactive manner with cigarette smoking. The exposure accounting for the largest number of occupational cancers is asbestos. Increased rates of lung cancer and mesothelioma have been found among asbestos miners and millers; factory workers handling asbestos textile and other products; shipyard, railroad, and construction workers; and other employees working in industries where asbestos was manufactured or used. Although exposure to asbestos can induce lung cancer among nonsmokers, smoking and asbestos combine in a multiplicative fashion to enhance lung cancer risk, so that removing either agent significantly lowers the cancer burden. Asbestos also has been associated with gastrointestinal and urinary (kidney) tumors.

Another potent occupational lung carcinogen is radon and its daughter products, found in high levels in underground mines throughout much of the world. Over 20-fold increases of lung

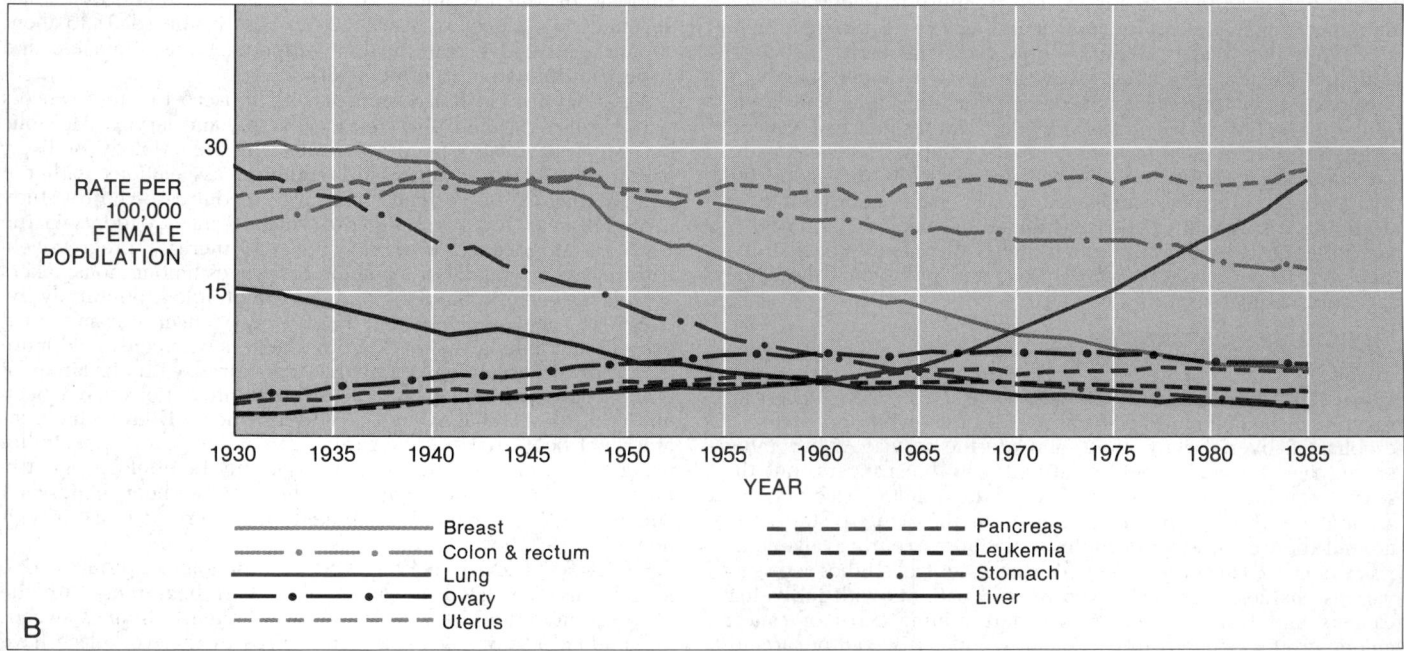

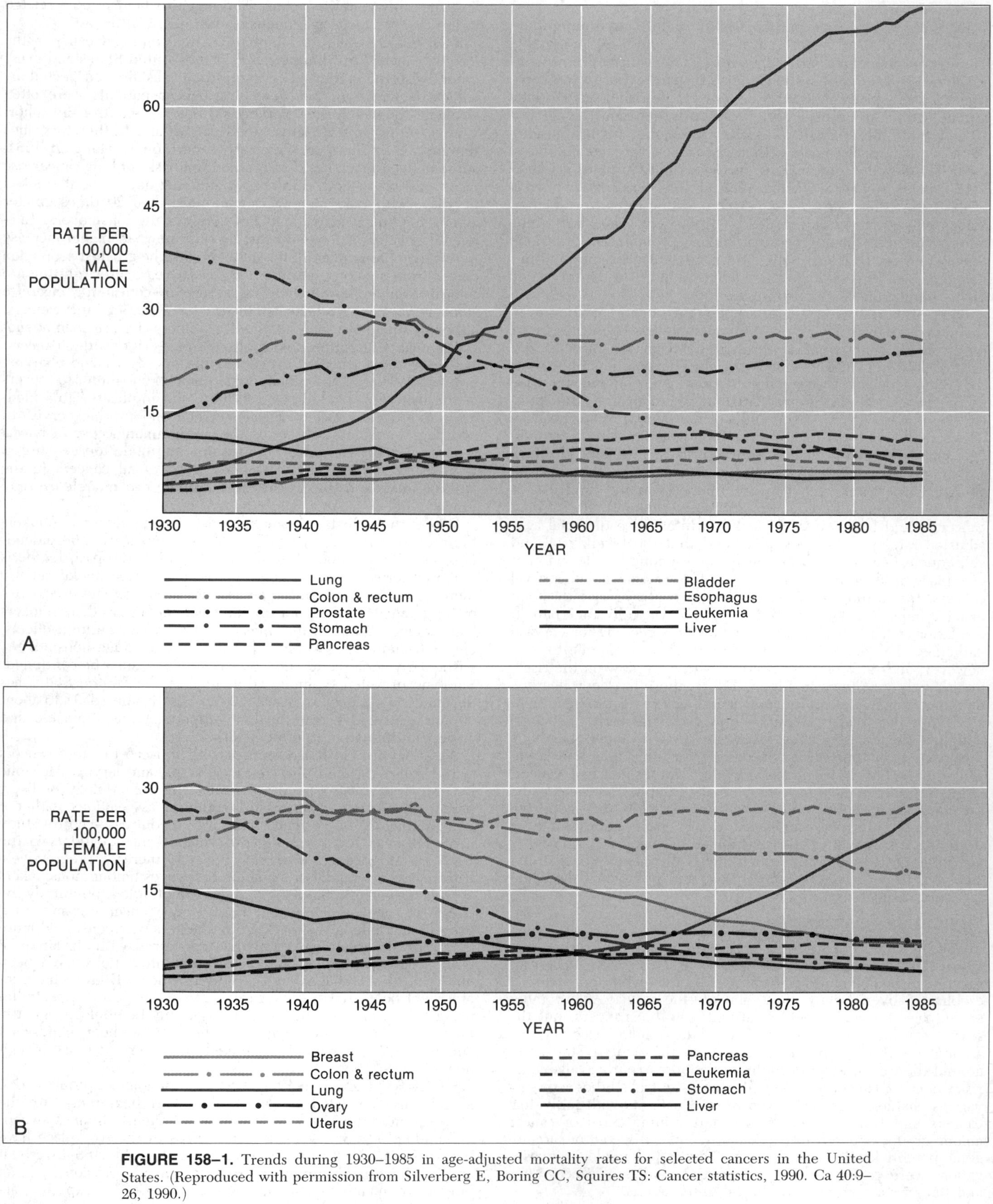

FIGURE 158–1. Trends during 1930–1985 in age-adjusted mortality rates for selected cancers in the United States. (Reproduced with permission from Silverberg E, Boring CC, Squires TS: Cancer statistics, 1990. Ca 40:9–26, 1990.)

TABLE 158–3. OCCUPATIONAL EXPOSURES RECOGNIZED AS HUMAN CARCINOGENS

Exposure	Site of Cancer
Aluminum production	Lung
4-Aminobiphenyl	Bladder
Arsenic	Lung, skin
Asbestos	Lung, pleura, peritoneum, GI tract, kidney
Auramine manufacture	Bladder
Benzene	Leukemia
Benzidine	Bladder
β-Naphthylamine	Bladder
Bischloromethylether	Lung
Boot and shoe manufacture	Bladder, nasal sinuses
Chromium (hexavalent) compounds	Lung
Coal gasification, coke production	Lung
Erionite	Mesothelioma
Isopropyl alcohol manufacture	Nasal sinuses
Magenta manufacture	Bladder
Mineral oils	Skin, other cancers
Mustard gas	Lung
Nickel compounds	Lung, nasal sinuses
Radon	Lung
Soots, tars, and oils (polycyclic hydrocarbons)	Lung, skin
Vinyl chloride	Liver
Wood dusts (furniture)	Nasal sinuses

cancer have been reported in some groups of radon-exposed miners, most of whom are also smokers, with the excesses most pronounced for small cell anaplastic carcinomas. Several chemicals, including inorganic arsenic, benzene, β-napthylamine and other aromatic amines, bischloromethyl ether, mustard gas, certain nickel compounds, and polycyclic hydrocarbons, have induced cancer in exposed workers (Table 158–3). Except for arsenic, there is confirmatory evidence of carcinogenicity from animal bioassays, often (but not always) with the carcinogen inducing similar tumors in the animals as in humans.

Among all cancers, those of the nasal cavity and sinuses and the urinary bladder have the highest proportion related to occupational exposures. In a nationwide survey of all nasal adenocarcinomas in Sweden over a recent 19-year period, nearly 25 per cent occurred among furniture makers as a result of wood dust exposures. It has been estimated that among American men up to 25 per cent of all bladder cancers are occupationally related. The percentages for other tumors are less, and for all cancers combined, it is generally thought that fewer than 5 per cent have been induced by workplace exposures.

ENVIRONMENTAL POLLUTION. Carcinogens have in some instances been identified in the air we breathe and water we drink. Quantifying the effects of air and water pollution has been extremely difficult, however, because of uncertainty over the amount and characteristics of exposures actually received by individuals. Air pollution, primarily from combustion products, earlier in this century was thought to be involved in the rise in lung cancer in Great Britain, the United States, and other countries, but now air pollution as found in most urban areas is considered to contribute to a small fraction (<10 per cent) of cases of this cancer. The percentage is higher in some areas of the world, including parts of China where excessive rates of lung cancer have been found among nonsmokers living in chimneyless houses and in homes heavily polluted by coal-burning heating systems. Increased risks of lung cancer have also been found among residents living near copper smelters, with industrial air emissions of inorganic arsenic suspected. Mesotheliomas have been diagnosed among women married to asbestos workers, presumably from handling clothing or otherwise being exposed to fibers brought home by their husbands. Since there are nearly linear dose-response relations between occupational asbestos exposure and mesothelioma and lung cancer, concern has arisen over possible health risks from lower levels of exposure that may occur in homes, schools, and other public places, although few such environmentally induced cancer cases have been documented. Pollutants in drinking water have also aroused concern.

Rates of bladder cancer have correlated with levels of halogenated compounds, some of which are carcinogenic in animal experiments, in some municipal water supplies. Recent laboratory tests also indicate an increased risk of osteogenic sarcomas following high levels of exposure to flouride in some subgroups of exposed animals, but epidemiologic investigations have found few or no unexpected changes in cancer rates following flouridation of water supplies.

MEDICINAL AGENTS. Among the chemicals considered to be causally associated with cancer in humans, nearly one half are medications (Table 158–4). These include drugs used in cancer treatment, especially alkylating agents, which have been found to induce acute nonlymphocytic leukemias and other cancers. The occurrence of second primary cancers in 5 to 10 per cent or more of those on therapy suggests that risks as well as benefits of chemotherapy with carcinogenic agents must be carefully assessed, particularly for patients whose long-term prognosis is otherwise highly favorable.

Exogenous estrogens have been implicated in cancer risk. Diethylstilbestrol (DES) taken during pregnancy has resulted in vaginal adenocarcinomas in offspring who were exposed in utero. The rising rates of endometrial cancer among American women in the 1970's were precipitated by use of conjugated estrogens for menopausal symptoms. Rates dropped abruptly following curtailment of use when the association with cancer became known. The link to breast cancer is less clear, although several investigations have found an increased risk among women receiving long-term estrogen replacement therapy for menopausal symptoms. Extended use of oral contraceptives prior to first pregnancy also has been reported to increase subsequent risk of breast cancer in some investigations, but as yet the widespread introduction of oral contraceptives in the 1960's has not been shown to have significantly influenced national rates of breast cancer in the United States. Combined (estrogen plus progestogen) oral contraceptives have been associated with a reduced risk of endometrial and ovarian cancer.

Certain immunosuppressive agents sharply increase risk of cancer. Indeed, among renal transplant recipients, the risk of subsequent lymphomas is increased over 30-fold, with the excesses occurring within months of immunosuppressive therapy—the fastest onset of any environmentally induced cancer.

RADIATION. Follow-up of survivors of the atomic bombs of Hiroshima and Nagasaki and of groups of patients receiving radiotherapy for ankylosing spondylitis, cancer, and certain other conditions provides conclusive evidence that ionizing radiation can induce cancer in humans as it does in lower animals. Leukemia is the initial carcinogenic consequence, occurring most frequently 5 to 10 years after exposure, with increased risks of a variety of solid tumors, particularly breast, thyroid, and lung cancers, following thereafter. Cancer risk tends to increase in proportion to radiation dose, in a linear fashion for some tumors

TABLE 158–4. MEDICINAL AGENTS RECOGNIZED AS HUMAN CARCINOGENS

Drug	Site of Cancer
Azathiopine	Lymphoma, skin, soft tissue sarcoma
Chlornaphazine	Bladder
1,4-Butanediol dimethanesulfonate (Myleran)	Leukemia
Combined chemotherapy for lymphoma, including MOPP*	Leukemia
Chlorambucil	Leukemia
Cyclophosphamide	Leukemia, bladder
Estrogens—conjugated	Endometrium
Estrogens—synthetic (DES)	Vagina, cervix
Estrogens—steroid contraceptives	Benign liver tumors
Melphalan	Leukemia
Methoxsalen with ultraviolet A therapy (PUVA)	Skin
Phenacetin-containing analgesics	Renal pelvis
Treosulphan	Leukemia

*MOPP: procarbazine, nitrogen mustard, vincristine, and prednisone

such as breast cancer, raising the possibility that some increase in risk may result from low-dose therapeutic or repeated diagnostic radiologic procedures. Significantly increased risks of breast cancer have been detected among atomic bomb survivors at doses somewhat below 50 rad, and head and neck tumors have followed less than 10 rad of scalp irradiation for tinea capitis in Israeli children. The findings suggest the need for prudence in the use of medical irradiation. Improvements in radiologic equipment, however, have resulted in lower radiation doses. Thus, for example, risks associated with mammography are now believed to be low enough to justify routine periodic screening for breast cancer among American women as young as age 40.

Ultraviolet radiation from sun exposure is the dominant cause of basal and squamous cell carcinoma and melanoma of the skin. The key to prevention is reduced solar exposure, even though there is uncertainty regarding variations in effect according to extent and timing of exposure. For melanoma, intermittent heavy sun exposures, particularly during childhood and adolescence, may carry the greatest risk.

DIET AND NUTRITION. Consistent evidence has arisen from around the world that diet and nutrition can influence cancer risk. Clearest are the inverse associations between risk of certain epithelial cancers, particularly oral, esophageal, stomach, and lung cancers, and intake of fresh fruits and vegetables. Risk of these cancers among persons in the highest quartile of consumption is lower, sometimes by more than one half, than among those in the lowest quartile of intake. Studies in experimental animals have shown that several compounds in these foods can inhibit carcinogenesis, but the ingredients responsible for the protective effects in people still remain to be clarified. Epidemiologic studies have shown that carotenoids, but not animal sources of vitamin A (retinols), are fairly consistently linked to reduced cancer risk, but vitamins C and E, which can inhibit the formation of carcinogenic N-nitroso compounds in vivo, and other possibly protective nutrients have also been identified. Recent studies in China and Italy suggest that garlic, onions, and other allium vegetables may significantly reduce the risk of stomach cancer, an intriguing finding because of the potent inhibitory properties of compounds in these vegetables documented in experimental animals. Some food contaminants, including aflatoxins sometimes found in moldy peanuts or grains, are also strong animal carcinogens. Rates of liver cancer tend to be high in parts of Asia and Africa where aflatoxin contamination is common.

Dietary fat, particularly saturated fat, and calories have been implicated in the risk of colon, breast, and other cancers, although the etiologic nature of the associations is still not well established. Dietary fiber has been reported to reduce the risk of colon cancer, but its role vis-à-vis that of other constituents in vegetables, grains, and other fiber-rich foods is not clear. Despite these uncertainties, it has been estimated that a high percentage of colorectal and breast cancers have a dietary etiology, in part because of the much higher rates of these cancers in western nations with high-fat, low-fiber diets. In total, some estimates suggest that one third or more of all cancers may be related to dietary and nutritional practices.

INFECTIOUS AGENTS. Several viral agents have been associated with human cancer, particularly cancers of the liver in endemic areas and of the uterine cervix worldwide. Hepatitis B virus (HBV) is the primary cause of hepatocellular carcinoma in China and other areas where infections are prevalent. Prospective follow-up studies show large increases in risk, with nearly all liver cancers arising among persons with prediagnosis HBV surface antigen positivity. The epidemiologic patterns of cervical cancer (with risks elevated among those with multiple sexual partners, early age at coitus) have long suggested a venereal component to etiology, but only recently have improvements in laboratory techniques enabled detection of human papillomavirus (HPV) as a likely etiologic agent in a high percentage of cases. Herpes simplex virus type 2 has also been associated with cervical cancer, but its independent or interactive role with HPV remains to be clarified. The Epstein-Barr virus has been implicated in both nasopharyngeal cancer and Burkitt's lymphoma, while certain human retroviruses have been associated with adult T-cell leukemias in Japan and the Caribbean. The human immunode-

ficiency virus, the cause of AIDS, is associated not only with Kaposi's sarcomas reported at the clinical diagnosis of nearly 5 per cent of AIDS patients, but also with increased risk of lymphoma among survivors of AIDS.

GENETIC SUSCEPTIBILITY. Risk of cancer is often increased when there is a history of cancer in the family. The increases for common cancers such as those of the lung, colon, and breast are typically on the order of two- to threefold. Shared environmental factors often may contribute to the familial clustering, but strong associations among subgroups with early age at onset of cancer or bilateral presentation of breast cancer indicate a genetic predisposition in some instances. The most marked genetic effects are seen for skin cancer, with tumors rarely appearing in persons inheriting darkly pigmented skin. A few cancers show mendelian inheritance patterns, including melanomas arising from familial dysplastic nevi and retinoblastomas. In addition, certain hereditary precancerous syndromes have been linked to increased cancer risk. Included are neurofibromatosis and other phacomatoses (associated with nervous system cancer), xeroderma pigmentosum and albinism (skin cancer), ataxia telangiectasia and certain other immunodeficiency syndromes (lymphoma, leukemia, and other cancers), Bloom's syndrome (lymphoma, leukemia, and other cancers), and Fanconi's anemia (leukemia). Investigations of families with unusually large numbers of members with the same or different cancers have provided insight into genetic patterns. In larger epidemiologic studies, increasing attention is being paid to systematic evaluations of genetic factors as reliable markers of host susceptibility become available. Lung cancer risk, for example, has recently been associated with the genetically controlled ability to metabolize the antihypertensive drug debrisoquine. Information on susceptibility factors will be crucial in understanding the mechanisms of carcinogenesis as well as delineating groups and individuals at high risk for targeted interventions.

International Agency for Research on Cancer: Overall Evaluations of Carcinogenicity: An updating of IARC Monographs Volumes 1 to 42. Monographs on the Evaluation of Carcinogenic Risks to Humans. Supplement 7. Lyon, World Health Organization, 1987. *A systematic review of epidemiologic and experimental evidence regarding carcinogenicity of over 150 substances.*

Ries LA, Hankey BF, Edwards BK (eds.): Cancer Statistics Review 1973–1987. Bethesda, MD, US Department of Health and Human Services, NIH Publication No. 90–2789, 1990. *Up-to-date listing of cancer incidence, mortality, and survival rates in the United States.*

Schottenfeld D, Fraumeni JF Jr (eds.): Cancer Epidemiology and Prevention. Philadelphia, W. B. Saunders Company, 1982. *A comprehensive review of cancer epidemiology, with individual chapters assessing 34 cancers and 16 causative agents, as well as basic concepts in cancer etiology and control.*

159 Paraneoplastic Syndromes

Paul A. Bunn, Jr.

The paraneoplastic syndromes are a heterogenous group of signs and symptoms indirectly caused by cancers at a distance from the primary tumor or its metastases. These "remote" or "biologic" effects of malignancy must be distinguished from direct effects of tumor or its metastases. The majority of paraneoplastic syndromes are caused by proteins secreted by these tumors. In some instances (e.g., endocrine paraneoplastic syndromes), the proteins (hormones) are well characterized, and the pathophysiology is well understood. These paraneoplastic syndromes invariably improve with effective antineoplastic therapy. In addition, drugs that interfere with the hormone action may be useful in severe cases or when the tumor fails to respond to therapy. An increasing number of paraneoplastic syndromes, especially those with neurologic manifestations, appear to be caused by immunologic reactions to tumor antigens that are shared with normal cells. These neurologic syndromes often do not improve even with effective antitumor therapy, perhaps because the nervous system cannot regenerate and damage is often permanent.

Recognizable paraneoplastic syndromes, other than wasting of the host or tumor cachexia, occur in a minority of cancer patients. They may be extremely important, however, in the early detection of the original cancer or may be the first sign of recurrence. They may also simulate metastatic disease and thus prevent patients from receiving curative therapy. Conversely, signs and symptoms of metastatic disease may be falsely ascribed to a paraneoplastic syndrome and thus lead to the withholding of systemic therapy. Paraneoplastic syndromes may be disabling but treatable with proper recognition. Thus, establishing a diagnosis is extremely important. True paraneoplastic syndromes must be distinguished from those caused by the primary tumor or its metastases, infections, toxicities of therapy, vascular abnormalities, obstruction caused by a tumor or its products, and fluid and electrolyte abnormalities. It is also important to understand which paraneoplastic syndromes respond to primary antitumor therapy. Alternative forms of therapy aimed at symptomatic control should be considered in those syndromes in which response to primary antitumor therapy is unlikely.

WASTING OF THE HOST. Wasting of the host, sometimes called tumor cachexia or the cachexia of malignant disease, is the most common of the paraneoplastic syndromes. The catabolic phase that usually accompanies malignant disease may be out of keeping with the size of the tumor and may be complex in its pathogenesis—decreased caloric intake (there is often a perverted sense of taste and smell with aversion to specific foods), malabsorption, loss of protein (e.g., hemorrhage or effusions), fever, and possibly a change in metabolic pathways. For example, increased anaerobic glycolysis with enhanced gluconeogenesis from amino acids and partial insulin resistance have been described. Possibly factors capable of distorting metabolism are secreted by the tumor, for example, tumor necrosis factor/ cachectin, a macrophage-derived factor that is capable of inhibiting the activity of certain lipogenic enzymes. Certainly the caloric expenditure tends to remain high, and the basal metabolic rate is increased, despite the reduced intake of calories, suggesting a deranged metabolism.

Treatment of the underlying tumor is the major approach to therapy. Replacement alimentation is reserved for patients undergoing surgical treatment or for patients with severe nutritional deficiency but for whom there is hope for significant remission or cure. Progestational hormones (e.g., Megace) may stimulate appetite and increase weight in patients.

ENDOCRINE PARANEOPLASTIC SYNDROMES. The original description of a paraneoplastic syndrome was that of ectopic Cushing's syndrome, as reported by Brown in 1928. The endocrine neoplastic syndromes are listed in Table 161–1 and are described in detail in Ch. 161, to which the reader is referred.

NEUROLOGIC PARANEOPLASTIC SYNDROMES (Table 159–1). Neurologic signs and symptoms appear frequently in cancer patients and are most often directly related to metastases, fluid and electrolyte abnormalities, vascular abnormalities, infections, or toxicity of therapy. True paraneoplastic syndromes are generally diagnosed by exclusion of these other conditions (Ch. 162). Subacute cerebellar degeneration, subacute motor neuropathy, sensory neuropathy, Eaton-Lambert syndrome, and dermatomyositis in older males are so strongly associated with cancer that their presence should lead to a search for a primary tumor when none is evident. Many of these syndromes are caused by immunologic reactions to cross-reacting antibodies, as mentioned above.

HEMATOLOGIC PARANEOPLASTIC SYNDROMES. Cancers may indirectly affect any of the hematopoietic cell lines, producing increases or decreases in either individual cell lineages or multiple lineages. Increased cell numbers are generally produced when the tumor secretes a stimulatory hormone/growth factor.

Erythrocytosis most often results from erythropoietin production by renal or liver tumors. In a large review, paraneoplastic erythrocytosis when found was most often associated with hypernephromas (35 per cent), benign renal abnormalities (14 per cent), hepatomas (19 per cent), cerebellar hemangioblastomas (15 per cent), uterine tumors (7 per cent), adrenal tumors and pheochromocytomas (3 per cent), and miscellaneous tumors (3 per cent). In rare cases, induction of local kidney or systemic hypoxia by tumors may also result in erythrocytosis.

Leukemoid reactions, granulocytosis, eosinophilia, and/or basophilia are most often produced when the tumor secretes a colony-stimulating factor (CSF) and thus are corrected by effective treatment of the primary tumor. Granulocytosis is most often

TABLE 159–1. PARANEOPLASTIC SYNDROMES

1. Wasting of the host—"tumor cachexia"
2. Endocrine/hormone—see Table 161–1
3. Neuromyopathies—see Table 162–1
4. Hematologic
   Erythrocytosis, granulocytosis, thrombocytosis
   Anemia (chronic disease, pure red cell aplasia, hypersplenic, autoimmune hemolytic anemia, microangiopathic hemolytic anemia)
   Granulocytopenia, thrombocytopenia
5. Thromboembolic
   Venous thrombosis (Trousseau's syndrome)
   Disseminated intravascular coagulation
   Nonbacterial thrombotic endocarditis (marantic endocarditis)
6. Renal
   Secondary to hormonal or metabolic effects
   Glomerulopathies—including the nephrotic syndrome
   Miscellaneous—myeloma kidney, amyloidosis, uric acid nephropathy, etc.
7. Dermatologic—see Table 163–4
8. Gastrointestinal
   Anorexia, nausea, vomiting
   Protein-losing enteropathy
   Malignant hepatopathy
9. Miscellaneous
   Lactic acidosis
   Clubbing/hypertrophic pulmonary osteoarthropathy
   Hyperlipidemia
   Hypertension—hypotension
   Hyperamylasemia
   Amyloidosis
   Arthritis

associated with lung, gastric, pancreatic, and brain cancers; melanomas; and Hodgkin's and non-Hodgkin's lymphomas. Eosinophilia is most often associated with lymphomas, especially Hodgkin's disease, and gastrointestinal carcinomas. These syndromes must be differentiated from chronic myelogenous leukemia and other causes of leukemoid reactions such as infection, inflammatory diseases, metabolic diseases, and certain drugs (Ch. 141).

Anemia is frequently associated with malignant disease, and granulocytopenia and thrombocytopenia may also be paraneoplastic in nature. *Autoimmune hemolytic anemia* is most often associated with B-cell lymphoproliferative neoplasms and less often with ovarian and lung cancers (Ch. 135). Successful treatment of the primary tumor often leads to improvement; corticosteroids are usually unsuccessful. *Pure red cell aplasia* is found in association with thymomas (50 per cent) and a variety of other cancers.

Microangiopathic hemolytic anemia, a rare cause of anemia in patients with cancer, is diagnosed by the presence of severe hemolytic anemia with fragmented erythrocytes seen in the blood smear and a negative Coombs test. Most often this syndrome is associated with mucin-producing adenocarcinomas, especially those from the stomach (55 per cent), breast (13 per cent), lung (7 per cent), and unknown primary site (10 per cent). It is often abrupt in onset and associated with thrombocytopenia and disseminated intravascular coagulation.

Granulocytopenia is usually the result of chemotherapy, radiation therapy, severe infection, or marrow involvement, but has been reported rarely in association with thymoma. A syndrome resembling *idiopathic thrombocytopenic purpura (ITP)* may occur in association with lymphomas (especially chronic lymphocytic leukemia, Hodgkin's disease, and immunoblastic lymphadenopathy) and less frequently with other malignant disorders.

THROMBOEMBOLIC PARANEOPLASTIC SYNDROMES. A *hypercoagulable* state is frequent in cancer patients and may manifest as (1) *migratory thrombophlebitis* (Trousseau's syndrome); (2) subacute or overt *disseminated intravascular coagulation* (DIC); and (3) *nonbacterial thrombotic endocarditis* (NBTE, marantic endocarditis); or (4) a combination of these three.

Thrombophlebitis occurs in as many as 1 to 11 per cent of cancer patients and is most often associated with mucin-producing adenocarcinomas of the gastrointestinal tract. It may also be seen with lung, breast, ovarian, and prostate cancers. The treatment of migratory thrombophlebitis is difficult; acute episodes require heparin. Long-term therapy with warfarin is generally unsuccessful, but long-term administration of subcutaneous heparin has had some limited success.

DIC may present as an acute hemorrhagic diathesis or be discovered incidentally as chronic laboratory abnormalities. Coagulation abnormalities by laboratory test may be seen in as many as 90 per cent of patients with cancer, but most of these never develop overt bleeding episodes. Acute episodes are most frequently associated with acute promyelocytic leukemia (APL) and adenocarcinomas (especially prostatic). Identification and treatment of all precipitating factors are the keystones to the management of DIC. This includes therapy for the primary tumor as well as for infection, acidosis, and other factors. Heparin is often used prophylactically in APL, although this is not mandatory if all coagulation parameters are normal and are monitored closely. For overt DIC, heparin appears to be superior to warfarin; spontaneous remission of DIC may occur in adenocarcinomas without any therapy.

NBTE is characterized by sterile verrucous lesions on the left-sided heart valves; these thrombi may embolize to the brain and other vital organs. These occur most often with mucin-producing adenocarcinomas. Therapy is directed to the primary tumor. The therapeutic role of heparin and warfarin is uncertain.

RENAL PARANEOPLASTIC SYNDROMES. Most renal abnormalities that occur in patients with cancer are due to metastases, obstruction, electrolyte and fluid imbalances, toxicity of therapy, or infection. The most common renal paraneoplastic syndrome, other than those linked to hormones (e.g., SIADH), is the nephrotic syndrome. In one report 10 per cent of patients with nephrotic syndrome had underlying malignant disease, with Hodgkin's disease being the most frequently associated disorder. Most of these patients have lipoid nephrosis (minimal change glomerulopathy). In contrast, patients with non-Hodgkin's lymphomas often have immunoglobulin deposits suggesting an immune complex etiology. In both instances the nephrotic syndrome resolves if there is a response to antitumor therapy. Patients with carcinomas most often have membranous glomerulonephritis with subepithelial electron-dense deposits. Other renal abnormalities associated with cancer include (1) the host of abnormalities associated with multiple myeloma and amyloidosis (Ch. 151); (2) the potassium wasting and hypokalemia syndrome caused by lysozyme secreted by patients with acute myelogenous leukemia (M4 or M5); (3) the syndrome of intrarenal obstruction preceded by mucoprotein secreted by patients with pancreatic carcinoma; and (4) the syndrome of nephrogenic diabetes insipidus found in some patients with leiomyosarcoma.

DERMATOLOGIC PARANEOPLASTIC SYNDROMES. This group of syndromes is summarized in Ch. 163. The strongest dermatologic associations with malignant disease are with acanthosis nigricans, erythema gyratum repens, tylosis, dermatomyositis in older males, flushing in the carcinoid syndrome and with the hereditary syndromes (Gardner's syndrome, Peutz-Jegher's syndrome, etc). Some of these syndromes may be caused by overexpression of epidermal growth factor.

GASTROINTESTINAL PARANEOPLASTIC SYNDROMES. *Protein-losing enteropathy* may be produced by inflammation and ulceration of the mucosa, obstruction of intestinal lymphatics (lymphomas), congestive heart failure (carcinoid, pericardial constriction), and undefined mechanisms. Although hypoalbuminemia is common in cancer patients, true protein-losing enteropathy is rare.

Malignant *hepatopathy* (Stauffer's syndrome) is characterized by biochemical abnormalities (increased alkaline phosphatase, hypercholesterolemia, prolonged prothrombin time) and hepatosplenomegaly in association with hypernephroma or malignant schwannoma without liver metastases. These abnormalities improve following resection of the primary tumor.

MISCELLANEOUS PARANEOPLASTIC SYNDROMES. *Fever* is a common finding in cancer patients and is often idiopathic. This is most common in lymphomas (where it is associated with a poor prognosis), hypernephromas, osteogenic sarcomas, and myxomas, although it may be found with other tumors. It almost always disappears with successful antitumor therapy. *Lactic acidosis* may be associated with acute leukemias and lymphomas and responds to successful antitumor therapy. *Hyperlipidemias* have been reported in association with multiple myeloma, hepatoma, and colon cancer.

Hypokalemia and hypertension with tumor production of renin have been reported with lung cancer, hypernephroma, and Wilms' tumor. *Hypotension* has been reported in association with a prostaglandin A-secreting hypernephroma and with intrathoracic tumors secondary to abnormal baroreceptor responses. *Hyperamylasemia* may be caused by lung cancers, especially adenocarcinomas, and is generally not associated with symptoms.

Hypertrophic pulmonary osteoarthropathy is characterized by clubbing, periostitis of the long bones, and occasionally polyarthritis. Involved bones include the distal ends of the tibia, fibula, humerus, radius, or ulna. It is associated most frequently with lung cancer (except small cell), mesothelioma (especially the benign form), and other cancers when they metastasize to the lungs or mediastinum. The abnormalities improve with successful treatment of the primary tumor. The etiology is unknown.

Amyloidosis occurs in association with multiple myeloma, lymphoma, or carcinomas (especially hypernephroma) in about 15 per cent of cases. The amyloidogenic protein is monoclonal light-chain (AL) in the case of B-cell tumors; other proteins (AA) are associated with other tumors (Ch. 197). Amyloidosis causes signs and symptoms by deposition in nerves, heart, kidney, and joints. Prognosis is poor, and there is no specific therapy. *Polyarthritis* has been reported in association with breast and other cancers. *Polymyalgia rheumatica* may precede development of several forms of cancer, and *systemic lupus erythematosus* (SLE) is associated with lymphomas, leukemias, thymomas, and testicular, lung, and ovarian cancers. Remission of SLE may occur with successful antitumor therapy.

Antman KH, Skarin AT, Mayer RJ, et al.: Microangiopathic hemolytic anemia and cancer: A review. Medicine 58:377, 1979. *Reviews the clinical manifestations and etiology of this syndrome.*

Barnes BE: Dermatomyositis and malignancy. A review of the literature. Ann Intern Med 84:68, 1976. *This review evaluates the association of dermatomyositis and malignant disease and shows the strong association in older males.*

Bunn PA Jr, Minna JD: Paraneoplastic syndromes. In DeVita VT, Hellman S, Rosenberg SA (eds.): The Principles and Practice of Oncology. Philadelphia, JB Lippincott Company, 1985, pp 1797–1842. *This chapter is an extensive review of all types of paraneoplastic syndromes with a complete bibliography.*

Crowthers D, Bateman CJT: Hematologic aspects of systemic disease—malignant disease. Clin Hematol 1:447, 1972. *This review discusses the various hematologic paraneoplastic syndromes in more detail.*

Furneaux HM, Rosenblum MK, Dalmau J, et al.: Selective expression of Purkinje-cell antigens in tumor tissue from patients with paraneoplastic cerebellar degeneration. N Engl J Med 322:1844, 1990. *Describes the mechanisms of neurologic paraneoplastic syndrome.*

Markham M: Response of paraneoplastic syndromes to antineoplastic therapy. West J Med 144:5, 1986. *A thorough review of the paraneoplastic syndromes that improve or disappear in response to effective antitumor therapy.*

McKinney TD (ed.): Renal Complications of Neoplasia. New York, Praeger, 1986. *A thorough review of all of the renal paraneoplastic syndromes.*

Rickles FR, Edwards RL: Activation of blood coagulation in cancer: Trousseau's syndrome revisited. Blood 63:14, 1983. *Reviews the possible causes of the hypercoagulable state in cancer.*

Sack GH, Levin J, Bell WR: Trousseau's syndrome and other manifestations of chronic disseminated coagulopathy in patients with neoplasms. Medicine 56:1, 1977. *A thorough review of the various manifestations of the hypercoagulable state associated with cancer.*

Torti FM, Dieckmann B, Beutler B, et al.: A macrophage factor inhibits adipocyte gene expression: An in vitro model of cachexia. Science 229:867, 1985.

Theologides A: Anorexins, asthenins, and cachectins in cancer. Am J Med 81:696, 1986. *These two articles suggest that "cachectin"—"tumor necrosis factor" and/or other monokines may play a role in the cachexia of malignant disease.*

Thirkill CE, Fitzgerald P, Sergott RC, et al.: Cancer associated retinopathy (CAR syndrome) with antibodies reacting with retinal, optic-nerve, and cancer cells. N Engl J Med 321:1589, 1989. *Describes the mechanisms of neurologic paraneoplastic syndrome.*

160 Tumor Markers

Paul A. Bunn, Jr.

In malignant disease there is aberrant expression of a number of genes. Many of the products of these genes, including hormones, enzymes, immunoglobulins, and a variety of other proteins, may be overexpressed on the cell surface of the cancer cell and are often secreted by the tumor cell. Cell surface antigens are usually assayed using monoclonal antibodies. Expression of specific antigens is useful for establishing a diagnosis and classification and providing prognostic information. Secreted proteins or biomarkers are potentially useful for (1) screening populations, (2) early detection of patients with suspected disease, (3) assessing tumor burden and prognosis, (4) assessing response to therapy, and (5) evaluating early recurrence. Currently available radioimmunoassays can often detect minute amounts (nanograms) of the marker substance. All of the marker proteins, however, are products of normal cells and may be present in small amounts in normal serum. Furthermore, the levels of some marker proteins may also increase with inflammation. Thus, to determine the clinical utility of each marker, the specificity, sensitivity, positive and negative predictive values, and accuracy must be considered. The sensitivity is defined as the number of positive tests divided by the number of true positives. The specificity is defined as the number of negative tests divided by the number of true negatives. The positive and negative predictive values are defined as the true positives divided by the true positives plus false positives and the true negatives divided by the true negatives plus false negatives, respectively. These reflect the confidence with which a positive test is correlated with malignancy or a negative test excludes malignancy. The accuracy (true positive plus true negative/number evaluated) gives an overall assessment of the marker's value. Very few tumor markers are sufficiently sensitive and specific to be useful for each of these purposes. The most established tumor markers include the β subunit of human chorionic gonadotropin (β-hCG), α fetoprotein (AFP), idiotypic immunoglobulins, and carcinoembryonic antigen (CEA).

CELL SURFACE ANTIGENS/TUMOR MARKERS

Evaluation of the expression of cell surface antigens is being used increasingly by pathologists to assist in securing a pathologic diagnosis and to provide prognostic information. Most often these tumor antigens are on the cell surface; however, cytoplasmic and nuclear antigens may also be assessed. Generally, monoclonal antibodies are used in immunohistochemical or immunocytochemical reactions to determine antigen expression. Flow cytometry and biologic assays may also be employed. Table 160–1 shows the most commonly employed antigens by tumor type. The panel of antigens screened for each tumor type is undergoing rapid evolution as new antigens are evaluated. The reader is referred to chapters on each specific malignancy for more information.

The non-Hodgkin's lymphomas always express panleukocyte antigens such as CD45 (T200, LCA). B-cell non-Hodgkin's lymphomas express cell surface immunoglobulin and B-cell antigens such as CD20, 21, and 22. Low-grade B-cell lymphomas usually express the CD5 antigen, which is generally present on mature T cells. Mycosis fungoides and the Sezary syndrome express mature helper T-cell antigens, including the T-cell receptor (CD3), sheep red blood cell receptor (CD2), and helper antigen (CD4), and lack CD8, IL-2 receptor (CD25), and CD7 antigens. Peripheral T-cell lymphomas usually express T-cell receptor antigens (e.g., CD3) and helper antigens (CD4) and have low expression of IL-2 receptors (CD25). By contrast, adult T-cell leukemia/lymphomas express IL-2 receptors (CD25) in addition to HTLV-1 viral antigens, T-cell receptors (CD3), and helper (CD4) antigens. Lymphoblastic lymphomas are of early T-cell lineage and therefore have rearranged T-cell receptor genes,

TABLE 160–1. CELL SURFACE TUMOR MARKERS

Tumor Type	Characteristic Cell Surface Antigens
Lymphomas	
B-cell	
Low grade	Idiotypic Ig, CD5, CD20-22, panleukocyte (CD45, T200, LCA)
Intermediate/high grade	Idiotypic Ig, CD20-22, panleukocyte (CD45, T200, LCA)
T-cell	
Mycosis fungoides/Sézary syndrome	TCR+, CD3+, CD4+, CD8−, CD25−, CD7−
Peripheral T-cell lymphoma	TCR+, CD4+, CD8−, CD3+, CD7−
Adult T-cell leukemia/lymphoma	TCR+, CD25+, CD4+, CD8−, HTLV-1+
Lymphoblastic lymphoma	TCR+, Tdt, CD2, CD7
Hodgkin's disease	Ki-1 (CD30), Leu M1 (CD15)
Leukemias	
Acute lymphoblastic leukemia (ALL)	
Common (80%)	Ig gene rearrangements, CALLA (CD10)
T-cell (15%)	CD7, CD2, TCR, Tdt
B-cell (5%)	Surface Ig, CD20-22
Acute nonlymphocytic leukemia (ANLL)	Myeloid (My) and monocyte (Mo) antigens
Chronic lymphocytic leukemia (CLL)	
B-cell (98%)	Surface Ig, CD20-22, CD5
T-cell (2%)	CD2, 3, 5 (CD4+8− or CD4−8+), TCR
Chronic myelogenous leukemia (CML)	LAP, B12, BCR/Abl
Myeloma	Cytoplasmic Ig, β₂ microglobulin, PCA-1
Carcinomas	
Lung cancers	
Non–small cell	CEA, Ca125, Ca19-9, blood group, HMFG
Small cell	NCAM, CKBB, NSE, GRP, chromogranin
Breast cancer	ER, PR, EGF receptors, cathepsin D, Her-2/neu oncogene
Gastrointestinal cancers	CEA, HMFG, other mucins, blood group antigens
Testicular cancer	β-hCG, AFP
Malignant melanoma	GD₂, GD₃, S100
Hepatoma	AFP
Sarcomas	Desmin, vimentin
Astrocytomas	Glial fibrillary proteins
Thyroid cancer	
Follicular/papillary	Thyroglobulin T₃, T₄
Medullary	Calcitonin, chromogranin, histaminase
Prostate cancer	PSA, PAP, NSE, HMFG's
Ovarian cancer	Ca125, Ca19-9
Pheochromocytoma	Calcitonin, chromogranin

Abbreviations: Ig = immunoglobulin; TcR = T-cell receptor gene rearrangements; LAP = leukocyte alkaline phosphatase; β-hCG = β subunit of human chorionic gonadotropin; AFP = α-fetoprotein; CEA = carcinoembryonic antigen; HMFG = human milk fat globulin; ER = estrogen receptor; PR = progesterone receptor; EGF = epidermal growth factor receptor; NCAM = neural cell adhesion molecule; CK-BB = creatine kinase BB isoenzyme; NSE = neuron-specific enolase; GRP = gastrin-releasing peptide (bombesin); PSA = prostate-specific antigen; PAP = prostatic acid phosphatase.

terminal deoxynucleotidyl transferase (Tdt), and CD2 and CD7 antigens. The cell of origin of Hodgkin's disease remains controversial, but these cells generally express LNFPIII (Leu-M1, CD15) and Ki-I (CD30).

The majority of patients with acute lymphoblastic leukemia have the "common" variety, which has characteristics of early B cells, including rearranged immunoglobulin genes and lack of surface Ig. These cells express the CALLA antigen (CD10). T-cell acute lymphoblastic leukemias, like the lymphoblastic lymphomas, are early T cells with rearranged T-cell receptor genes and the T-cell antigens (CD2 and CD7), and terminal deoxynucleotidyl transferase (Tdt). Myeloid markers are observed in about 25 per cent of ALL's. These biphenotypic cases may have a worse prognosis. ALL's with the Philadelphia chromosome and the BCR/Abl gene products also have a poor prognosis. B-cell ALL's express surface Ig and have a poor prognosis. Acute nonlymphocytic leukemias may express one or more myeloid (My) or monocyte (Mo) antigens depending on the FAB classification.

The vast majority of chronic lymphocytic leukemias (CLL) are of B-cell origin. These express surface immunoglobulin, CD20, 21, and 22 antigens, and the CD5 antigen (generally a T-cell marker). A few per cent of CLL's are of T-cell origin, expressing CD2 and CD3 antigens with rearranged T-cell receptor genes. These T-cell CLL's may have a helper (CD4+, CD8−) or a suppressor (CD4−, CD8+) phenotype. Chronic myelogenous leukemias have increased expression of leukocyte alkaline phosphatase and B12 and express the BCR/Abl oncogene product.

Multiple myeloma was initially thought to be a malignancy of mature plasma cells because of the large amount of cytoplasmic Ig. The finding of β_2 microglobulin and CALLA (CD10) in addition to Ig and TcR gene rearrangements in many cases suggests that the cell may be of primitive lymphoid origin.

Carcinomas nearly always express cytokeratins and lack pan-leukocyte and neural antigens. Non−small cell lung cancers often express CEA, human milk fat globule antigens, other glycolipid antigens, blood group antigens, the EGF receptor and abnormal *ras* protein. The latter may imply a poor prognosis in adenocarcinomas, although none of these is totally specific for lung cancer. Small cell lung cancers express a variety of neuroendocrine markers such as neural cell adhesion molecule (NCAM), neuron specific enolase (NSE), gastrin-releasing peptide (bombesin-like peptides), chromogranin, and the BB isoenzyme of creatine kinase.

Breast cancers may express estrogen (ER) or progesterone (PR) receptors, the Her2/neu oncogene product, epidermal growth factor receptors (EGF-R), and cathepsin D. Each of these has been reported to have prognostic implications.

Gastrointestinal adenocarcinomas (stomach, pancreas, colon, rectum) often express CEA, Ca125, Ca19-9, other HMFG, and mucin antigens. There are no site-specific antigens, and the clinical relevance of most antigens is undefined. Prostate cancers express prostate-specific antigen, which has a high sensitivity and specificity. NSE, CEA, and other mucin antigens may be expressed but are of less certain clinical relevance. Ovarian adenocarcinomas often express Ca125 and CA19-9, but these are not specific for ovarian cancer.

Testicular germ cell cancers express β-hCG and/or α-AFP in more than 90 per cent of cases. It is extremely important to look for these markers in cases of midline undifferentiated carcinomas, since these may be cured by chemotherapy.

Malignant melanomas nearly always express the S100 protein, although this may also be expressed in schwannomas, chordomas, and cartilaginous tumors. Melanomas usually express GD_2 and GD_3 antigens. Most primary hepatic carcinomas express AFP. Sarcomas express vimentin and dismin. Malignant astrocytomas express glial fibrillary proteins. Neuroblastomas express NCAM and other neural markers.

SERUM TUMOR MARKERS

A list of currently used markers is shown in Table 160–2.

HORMONES. Human chorionic gonadotropin (hCG) is a two-chain (α and β subunits) glycoprotein hormone secreted by the trophoblastic epithelium of the placenta. The β subunit is normally present in maternal serum during pregnancy, but its presence in males and nonpregnant females is indicative of cancer. Measurement of hCG has been used for the diagnosis and management of trophoblastic tumors (choriocarcinoma, hydatidiform mole) and certain germ cell tumors of the testes. Its level has prognostic importance. The rate of decline may be used to assess the effectiveness of therapy, and its reappearance is direct evidence of tumor recurrence. Extragonadal germ cell tumors often secrete β-hCG, and it can be used to help confirm the origin of undifferentiated mediastinal or retroperitoneal tumors. β-hCG may also be secreted by adenocarcinomas of the ovary, pancreas, stomach, and lung and by hepatomas.

A variety of other hormones may be useful tumor markers. Human placental lactogen is secreted by the majority of trophoblastic tumors and a minority of lung cancers, hepatomas, endocrine tumors, leukemias, and lymphomas.

Polypeptide hormones such as *adrenocorticotropic hormone (ACTH)* and *arginine vasopressin (AVP)* may be useful markers when produced by small cell lung cancer or other tumors with properties of amine precursor uptake and decarboxylation (APUD tumors). Similarly, *calcitonin* is used to predict medullary carcinoma of the thyroid in families or it can be used as a marker in APUD tumors that secrete it. *Gastrin-releasing peptide* (bombesin-like protein) is produced by the majority of small cell lung cancers. It is not an ideal tumor marker, however, because it is rapidly degraded in plasma. Elevated levels in the cerebrospinal fluid (CSF) may be useful for predicting leptomeningeal metastases.

TABLE 160–2. SERUM TUMOR CELL MARKERS

Marker	Tumor Types
Hormones	
β subunit of chorionic gonadotropin	Testicular cancers, choriocarcinoma, hydatidiform mole
AVP, ACTH	Small cell lung; APUD tumors
Calcitonin	Medullary thyroid carcinoma, small cell lung and APUD tumors
Gastrin-releasing peptide (bombesin)	Small cell lung cancer
Placental lactogen	Trophoblastic tumors, various carcinomas
Oncofetal Proteins	
α-Fetoprotein	Hepatoma, testicular cancers
Carcinoembryonic antigen (CEA)	Gastrointestinal tract, breast, lung, ovarian cancers
Enzymes	
L-dopa decarboxylase	Small cell lung cancer
Creatine phosphokinase (BB)	Prostate cancer, small cell lung cancer
Neuron-specific enolase	Prostate cancer, small cell lung cancer, others
Acid phosphatase (prostate specific)	Prostate cancer
Placental alkaline phosphatase	Uterus, ovary, breast, lung cancers
Lysozyme	Acute nonlymphatic leukemia (myelomonocytic and monocytic types)
Serum galactosyltransferase	Gastrointestinal carcinomas, breast and prostate cancers
Lactic dehydrogenase (LDH)	Lymphomas, Ewing's sarcoma, various carcinomas
Secreted Tumor Antigens	
CA 125	Ovarian cancer, other epithelial cancers
CA 19-9	Various carcinomas
Prostate-specific antigen	Prostate cancer
Other glycosphingolipids	Various carcinomas
β₂ microglobulin	Multiple myeloma
Miscellaneous	
Vitamin B₂–binding proteins	Acute or chronic myelogenous leukemia, myeloproliferative disease
Immunoglobulin	B-cell lymphoproliferative diseases
Polyamines	Various carcinomas
Chromogranin A	Small cell lung cancer; pheochromocytoma

ONCOFETAL PROTEINS. α-*Fetoprotein (AFP)* is normally secreted in large amounts during the twelfth through fifteenth weeks of gestation and then declines to low levels (<40 ng per milliliter) by the age of 1 year. Elevated levels occur in the majority (75 per cent) of patients with embryonal and teratocarcinomas of the testes and ovary, as well as in those with extragonadal germ cell tumors. Like β-hCG, the level has prognostic implications; the rate of decline predicts the effectiveness of therapy, and a rising titer is direct evidence of tumor progression. Elevated AFP levels are present in 70 to 95 per cent of hepatomas. The incidence is highest in areas where hepatoma is endemic. AFP is increased in a minority of patients with cancers of the pancreas, stomach, colon, and lung. Since AFP is produced by normal cells, there are instances of "false positives." AFP may be produced by benign liver tumors, by cirrhotic livers, or during hepatitis, although these entities usually produce levels less than 500 ng per milliliter. AFP may be increased in patients with ataxia-telangiectasia.

Carcinoembryonic antigen (CEA) is normally secreted during the second to sixth months of gestation. In nonsmoking adults, serum levels are less than 2.5 ng per milliliter, whereas smokers have normal levels up to 5 ng per milliliter. Serum levels of CEA may increase in a variety of inflammatory conditions (e.g., cirrhosis, pancreatitis, inflammatory bowel disease, and rectal polyps) as well as in a variety of human cancers.

Elevated levels of CEA are reported in patients with colon cancer (60 to 90 per cent), pancreatic cancer (80 per cent), gastric cancer (60 per cent), lung cancer (75 per cent), breast cancer (50 per cent), and many other malignant tumors in lower frequency. The frequency with which the level of CEA is elevated and the level attained are dependent on the extent of disease, the degree of differentiation (well-differentiated tumors produce more), and the presence of liver metastases. Because of the high false-positive rate in inflammatory diseases, the principal use of CEA is in monitoring response to therapy and disease progression, especially for carcinoma of the colon (Ch. 105). Elevated levels should return to normal following complete resection of the primary tumor. A persistent elevation or an increasing concentration is highly suggestive of residual or recurrent tumor. Surgical re-exploration in the face of increasing CEA without clinical evidence of disease may lead to discovery of surgically resectable recurrences. These resected patients may then have a long disease-free survival.

Radiolabeled antibodies to CEA and AFP are being evaluated for their ability to detect metastatic disease and for therapy. Preliminary studies show sensitivities in the range of 60 to 80 per cent.

ENZYMES. A variety of enzymes are also useful tumor markers in some settings. The key APUD enzyme, L-dopa decarboxylase, is often increased in patients with small cell lung cancer and other APUD tumors. The serum level of the BB isoenzyme of creatine phosphokinase is elevated in the majority of patients with small cell lung cancer or cancer of the prostate. Serum levels of neuron-specific enolase are often elevated in patients with these same tumors.

Prostatic epithelium also produces a specific *acid phosphatase* (*prostatic acid phosphatase*) whose serum level is elevated in about one third of patients with occult prostatic cancer and in 75 per cent of patients with more advanced prostatic cancers. *Placental alkaline phosphatase* is secreted by a minority of cancers of the female reproductive organs and breast and lung cancers. *Lysozyme*, a monocyte-derived enzyme, is frequently increased in patients with acute monocytic and myelomonocytic leukemia. An isoenzyme of *serum galactosyltransferase* is present in the serum of patients with gastrointestinal carcinomas (75 per cent), and breast cancer (78 per cent), as well as in a minority of patients with prostatic cancer and lymphoproliferative cancers. Serum lactic dehydrogenase (LDH) levels are elevated in a variety of malignant diseases, including lymphomas (especially Burkitt's), Ewing's sarcomas, and a variety of carcinomas. The extent of elevation may provide prognostic information as well as a useful measure of antitumor response.

SECRETED TUMOR ANTIGENS. The development of monoclonal antibody technology has led to recognition of many new glycoprotein and glycolipid antigens on tumor cells that may be secreted into the plasma. The antigen recognized by the monoclonal antibody *CA 125* is a useful marker for the majority of patients with ovarian cancer. *CA 19-9* recognizes an antigen secreted by many epithelial carcinomas, including colon cancer, but this marker is probably less useful than CEA. Many epithelial carcinomas, especially adenocarcinomas, secrete glycosphingolipids such as Lewis blood group antigens and human milk fat globule antigens. The value of these markers remains to be established. β_2 microglobulin, an HLA class I antigen, is present on the cell surface of most nucleated cells. It is secreted into the plasma in excess amounts in patients with multiple myeloma, where its level has prognostic value and may be useful in assessing response to therapy.

MISCELLANEOUS. *Vitamin B$_{12}$*-binding proteins are frequently increased in myeloproliferative disorders and occasionally in acute or chronic myelogenous leukemias. The idiotypic *immunoglobulins* produced by B-cell lymphoproliferative malignant disorders are excellent tumor markers and may be used to assess tumor burden as well as to follow response to therapy. More than 99 per cent of patients with multiple myelomas and Waldenström's macroglobulinemia secrete a heavy chain or a light chain (Ch. 151). Occasionally these tumors secrete globulins of more than one idiotype. Monoclonal antibodies to the idiotypic immunoglobulin are being evaluated as therapeutic agents. *Polyamines* are generally secreted in direct relation to the rate of proliferation. In many malignant diseases their quantitation has proven to be useful for prognosis and in assessing response. They are not sufficiently sensitive or specific for widespread use. *Chromogranin A* is a 68,000-dalton protein found in the neurosecretory granules of normal and malignant APUD cells. Serum measurement by radioimmunoassay may be a useful marker of small cell lung cancer disease activity and may be useful for the diagnosis of pheochromocytoma.

Aroney RS, Dermody WC, Aldernderfer P, et al.: Multiple sequential biomarkers in monitoring patients with carcinoma of the lung. Cancer Treat Rep 68:859, 1984. *Reviews the variety of proteins secreted by small cell lung cancers that can be used as tumor markers.*

Hakomori S: Glycosphingolipids. Sci Am 254(5):44, 1986. *This article reviews the various glycosphingolipid antigens present on cancer cells.*

Novis BH, Gluck E, Thomas P, et al.: Serial levels of CA 19-9 and CEA in colonic cancer. J Clin Oncol 4:987, 1986. *An article comparing the utility of these markers.*

Rosen SW, Weintraub BD, Vaitukaitus JL, et al.: Placental proteins and their subunits as tumor markers. Ann Intern Med 82:71, 1975. *A review of the value of placental proteins as tumor markers.*

Sobol RE, O'Connor DT, Addison J, et al.: Elevated serum chromogranin A concentrations in small cell lung cancer. Ann Intern Med 105:698, 1986. *This article is an example of one of several markers of neuroendocrine cells that are useful in following the course of small cell lung cancer patients.*

Wanebo HJ, Rao B, Pinsky CM, et al.: Preoperative carcinoembryonic antigen level as a prognostic indicator in colorectal cancer. N Engl J Med 299:448, 1978. *This article shows the value of oncofetal markers as prognostic indicators.*

161 Endocrine Manifestations of Tumors: "Ectopic" Hormone Production

Stephen B. Baylin

The clinical manifestations of cancer arise not only through the consequences of the invasive properties of primary and metastatic lesions, but also through the hormonal activity of proteins and small peptides secreted by tumor cells. Even though the tumor-associated production of these protein products is common, the incidence of paraneoplastic syndromes is less frequent. This is because these hormones are made, in tumors, either in amounts too small to result in a biologic response or in forms that are biologically inactive. For a given cancer, the spectrum of hormones produced often appears "foreign" with respect to the tissue of origin for the neoplasm. Hence, the term "ectopic" has been applied to this cancer-associated activity. In reality, studies over the past decade have increasingly demonstrated that such basic aspects of normal tissue development as cell lineage relationships and steps in embryogenesis and in cell differentiation during renewal of adult tissues often provide logical explanations for patterns of hormone production by specific cancer types. Also, the rapid elucidation of molecular events regulating gene expression is bringing further understanding of cellular relationships underlying hormonal production patterns in cancer.

Before considering individual endocrine syndromes associated with tumors, it is helpful to broadly classify cancer-associated hormone production patterns according to biologic concepts thought to underlie this phenomenon (Table 161–1). Much of this activity can be associated with the small polypeptide hormones normally secreted by cells that constitute classic endocrine tissues. Common neuroendocrine characteristics of these cells have been recognized and encompassed in the eponym *amine precursor uptake decarboxylase*, or "APUD" cells. Much of the "ectopic" hormone production by tumors involves the peptides from such cells, and the cancer most frequently represented— small cell lung carcinoma—has direct links to cells with APUD features. A common pattern of gene expression events in these cells during development may explain why APUD-associated tumors may often produce more than one small polypeptide hormone at a time.

A group of larger molecular weight glycoprotein hormones is more often produced by non–APUD-associated cancers (Table 161–1). Also, non-APUD tumors are more often associated with products of peptides which result in disorders of calcium homeostasis. The association of tumors and these gene expression events is much less well understood than that outlined above for APUD-cell tumors.

ECTOPIC ACTH PRODUCTION

Cushing's syndrome resulting from tumor cell production of ACTH is one of the first recognized and most common cancer-associated endocrine disorders. This disease is prototypical for the ectopic hormone syndromes associated with APUD cells and almost always occurs in tumors that arise from cells with endocrine features (Table 161–1). The cancer most commonly responsible for tumor-associated Cushing's syndrome is small cell lung carcinoma (SCLC), a common pulmonary neoplasm long recognized to have APUD features similar to those found in normal lung endocrine cells.

The expression of ACTH and related peptides by tumors, as was noted earlier for tumor-associated hormone production in general, is much more frequent than the actual occurrence of Cushing's syndrome. Thus, among all patients with SCLC, the incidence of clinical evidence of excess ACTH production is only 3 to 5 per cent. The biosynthetic events underlying production of biologically active ACTH are complex and involve a series of post-translational steps that cleave biologically active ACTH and other peptides from the precursor gene product, pro-opiomelanocortin (POMC). Normal pituitary cells contain all of the enzymes required for this processing. However, most cancer cells, even SCLC, cannot fully process the precursor POMC molecule even though they express, to variable levels, the POMC gene. In rare but well-documented situations, tumor-associated Cushing's syndrome can result from production of corticotropin-releasing factor (CRF) by cancer cells. The excess CRF then stimulates pituitary cells to release excess ACTH.

The symptoms of Cushing's syndrome in patients with cancer are much more varied and subtle than those in patients with pituitary-adrenal Cushing's disease (Ch. 217). The virulent behavior of the cancer most frequently involved, SCLC, means that the patients do not have time to develop the full spectrum of symptoms associated with Cushing's disease. The most prominent manifestations are therefore those associated with the early metabolic consequences of excessive glucocorticoid production, including generalized weakness, carbohydrate intolerance, and mental changes, and problems secondary to mineralocorticoid excess, including edema, hypertension, and hypokalemic alkalosis. Hypokalemia, especially, is more prominent in patients with tumor-associated ACTH excess than in patients with pituitary Cushing's disease. These symptoms and/or electrolyte changes in patients with cancer, and especially those with SCLC, should alert the physician to the possibility of ectopic Cushing's syndrome.

The diagnostic questions in ectopic Cushing's syndrome relate to documenting the source of excess ACTH secretion. A first clue for a nonpituitary tumor–related source is the finding of an extraordinarily high plasma ACTH value, much in excess of those found in pituitary Cushing's disease. Urinary free cortisol levels are always elevated and, unlike in Cushing's disease (Ch. 217), are usually *not* suppressible during a high-dose (8 mg per day) dexamethasone suppression test. Only in some patients with carcinoid tumors, and in the rare situation of tumors producing CRF, does this high-dose suppression test lower urinary cortisol in patients with "ectopic" Cushing's syndrome.

The treatment of tumor-associated Cushing's syndrome is often frustrating because of the aggressive nature of the cancers most frequently associated with this condition. An exception to this is

TABLE 161–1. HORMONE-SECRETING TUMORS

	Hormones Secreted
Tumors most frequently secreting APUD hormones	
Small cell lung carcinoma	ACTH,* CRF,* ADH,* calcitonin, GRP, GRF
Carcinoid tumors (lung, pancreas, GI tract, thymus, ovary)	ACTH,* GRF
Islet cell tumors of pancreas	ACTH,* GRF
Medullary thyroid carcinoma	ACTH,* GRF, GRP, somatostatin
Pheochromocytoma	ACTH,* GRF
Neural tumors (ganglioneuroma)	ACTH,* VIP,* GRF
Melanoma	ACTH*
Prostate	ACTH*
Tumors most frequently secreting large glycoprotein hormones	
Non–small cell lung carcinomas	hCG*
Testicular carcinomas (embryonal components)	hCG*
Sarcomas	hCG*
Tumors most frequently causing hormonally mediated hypercalcemia	
Squamous cell carcinoma (lung, head, and neck)	PTH RP*
Renal carcinomas	PTH RP*
Bladder carcinomas	PTH RP*
Adenocarcinomas	PTH RP*
Lymphomas	PTH RP*

*Responsible for producing a clinical syndrome.
ACTH = adrenocorticopic hormone
ADH = vasopressin
CRF = corticotropin-releasing factor
GRF = growth hormone–releasing factor
GRP = gastrin-releasing peptide
VIP = vasoactive intestinal polypeptide
hCG = human chorionic gonadotropin
PTH RP = parathyroid hormone–related peptide

carcinoid tumors, in which the clinical course is often protracted. The most efficacious therapy is primary eradication of the responsible neoplasm, either through chemotherapy or surgery. For SCLC, such complete tumor ablation is not usually possible. Alternatively, transient improvement may be obtained by using drugs, discussed in Ch. 217, which block steroid synthesis in the adrenal gland (such as metyrapone, aminoglutethimide, or ketoconazole).

CANCER-ASSOCIATED HYPERCALCEMIA

Hypercalcemia in patients with cancer is probably the most frequently seen paraneoplastic syndrome. In turn, cancer is the most commonly recognized cause of hypercalcemia in hospitalized patients. It is then imperative to rule out the presence of a tumor in any patient, especially one in the older age range, who has documented hypercalcemia.

The etiologies of tumor-associated hypercalcemia are varied. Direct effects of tumor metastases on bone resorption must always be considered, but it has become increasingly apparent that hormonal factors are more often involved. For many years, it was believed that parathyroid hormone (PTH), synthesized and secreted by tumor cells, was the etiologic agent. This hypothesis was based on detection of PTH immunoreactivity in sera of patients with tumors and hypercalcemia and presence of increased cyclic AMP levels in urine of such individuals.

However, during recent years, several groups have reported that a different small peptide, PTH-like peptide (PLP), which has partial homology to PTH only in the first 13 amino acids, is probably the humoral agent most frequently responsible for tumor-associated hypercalcemia. Interestingly, the gene for this hormone is normally ubiquitously expressed, and is not, as are other small polypeptide hormones, especially associated with normal cells having APUD endocrine features. Levels are especially high in normal keratinocytes, lactating mammary tissue, placenta, and other sites where the peptide appears to have a physiologic role. This distribution may explain why non-APUD tumors such as squamous cell, bladder, ovarian, and renal carcinomas have been most frequently associated to date with PLP secretion and hypercalcemia (Table 161–1).

Other humoral factors also play a variable role in producing hypercalcemia in patients with cancer. Growth factors, such as transforming growth factor (TGF-β), bone resorbing factors such as are found in hematologic malignancies, prostaglandins, and, occasionally, active vitamin D metabolites have all been documented as tumor products that can cause hypercalcemia. It is apparent, then, that multiple factors can be simultaneously active to cause the hypercalcemia associated with tumors.

The diagnosis of tumor-associated hypercalcemia should be suspected in any patient with hypercalcemia. The suspicion is obviously highest for a patient with known cancer who develops or presents with this metabolic abnormality. The most important alternative and treatable etiology for hypercalcemia is primary hyperparathyroidism (Ch. 235). Features favoring this latter condition include a longstanding history of hypercalcemia and presence of subperiosteal bone resorption and renal stones. High circulating PTH levels with high urinary cyclic AMP levels are characteristic of patients with primary hyperparathyroidism. In contrast, patients with cancer and hypercalcemia have relatively low PTH levels in conjunction with high urine cyclic AMP.

The treatment for tumor-associated hypercalcemia can be difficult because the cancers most frequently associated are often extensive and aggressive at the time of diagnosis. Direct ablation of, or reduction in, tumor mass is the optimal treatment when feasible. When this is not possible, treatment of the hypercalcemia depends upon its severity and consequences for the patient. The simplest therapeutic approaches employ combinations of hydration and diuretics. For more refractory and severe hypercalcemia, drugs such as mithramycin or diphosphonates may have to be added to this regimen. These treatments for hypercalcemia are discussed in more detail in Ch. 165.

TUMOR PRODUCTION OF HUMAN CHORIONIC GONADOTROPIN

The production by tumors of chorionic gonadotropin (hCG), a large molecular weight glycoprotein, is another example of hormonal activity most associated with the non-APUD group of cancers (Table 161–1). As for other hormones, asymptomatic production of hCG is far more frequent than the situation in which enough biologically active hCG is produced to cause symptoms in the patient. hCG is composed of α and β subunits, which are often discordantly produced by neoplasms. Production of the α subunit is particularly common, and elevated circulating levels of this peptide are often found in patients with multiple types of cancer. Production of intact hCG is common in tumors of trophoblastic origin (i.e., choriocarcinomas, testicular embryonal carcinomas, and seminomas), the normal source for hCG, and less often seen in cancers of the lung, pancreas, and other types.

The infrequent symptoms associated with tumor-associated secretion of hCG include precocious puberty in children and gynecomastia in adult males, usually associated with advanced tumors such as lung carcinoma. The treatment for these syndromes, especially in adults, is usually ineffective given the advanced nature of the tumors.

HYPOGLYCEMIA AND TUMORS

A long-recognized syndrome, most often associated with mesenchymal tumors (retroperitoneal fibrosarcomas, hemangiopericytomas and leiomyosarcomas, adrenocortical carcinomas, and hepatomas), is hormonally induced hypoglycemia. This metabolic disorder, first thought to be secondary to excess insulin produced by tumor cells, has subsequently been linked to production of insulin-like factors or so-called nonsuppressible insulin-like activity. Recently, the association of one such factor, insulin-like growth factor II (IGF-II), with tumor-related hypoglycemia has been strengthened by the demonstration of IGF-II mRNA and peptide in mesenchymal tumors associated with hypoglycemia. However, the physiologic role of IGF-II remains uncertain, since serum IGF-II levels in patients with these tumors have not been found to be uniformly elevated. The interpretation of these studies is made difficult by the presence of serum-binding proteins, and further studies are needed to establish convincingly the role of IGF-II in tumor hypoglycemia.

HYPONATREMIA, INAPPROPRIATE ANTIDIURETIC HORMONE SYNDROME (SIADH), AND CANCER

An important metabolic abnormality occurring in patients with cancer is hyponatremia. The classic syndrome is associated with the presence of hyponatremia, increased urine osmolality, increased urine sodium (>20 mEq per liter), and decreased serum osmolality (<275 mOsm per liter). A series of investigators over the years, using first biologic assays and later immunoassays, has established that these electrolyte imbalances result from production and secretion by tumor cells of a polypeptide hormone, vasopressin or antidiuretic hormone (ADH). As for other "ectopic" hormone syndromes associated with small polypeptide hormones, inappropriate secretion of ADH is most often associated with, but not restricted to, the APUD tumor, SCLC (Table 161–1). Such tumors most frequently have the cellular features necessary to synthesize a 20,000-dalton glycosylated prohormone, provasopressin, and to process this peptide to the smaller biologically active ADH molecule.

Recognition of SIADH is important because the symptoms of hyponatremia, such as lethargy and mental changes, can present severe problems for patients with cancer. Also, the hyponatremia can be successfully managed by fluid restriction, careful administration of saline solutions, and/or treatment with drugs such as demeclocycline.

OTHER TUMOR-ASSOCIATED HORMONE SYNDROMES

While the syndromes discussed above constitute the majority of cancer-related endocrine diseases, there are other less frequent tumor-associated hormonal states that are important for the clinician to recognize.

ONCOGENIC OSTEOMALACIA

A syndrome associated with bone pain and muscle weakness, together with the radiologic features of osteomalacia, can occur in patients with mesenchymal tumors such as benign osteoblastomas, giant cell osteosarcomas, hemangiomas, and occasionally epithelial tumors such as prostate and SCLC. Biochemical studies show hypophosphatemia and subnormal 1,25-dihydroxyvitamin D levels. The pathophysiology of this disorder is unclear but appears to involve a hormonally mediated and severe renal phosphate loss as the primary event. The tumor origin of the inciting factor is inferred from the observations that the syndrome can remit dramatically with irradiation of the neoplasm. When primary treatment of the tumor is not feasible, treatment with phosphorus replacement and vitamin D can provide substantial improvement of symptoms and hypophosphatemia.

POLYCYTHEMIA

Tumors such as hepatomas, hemangiomas, and renal carcinomas can cause polycythemia. Recently, such tumors have been shown to produce erythropoietin mRNA, and patients with this syndrome have been found to have elevated erythropoietin levels in their serum by immunoassay. In general, no treatment is required. However, intermittent phlebotomy is occasionally required to alleviate symptoms.

TROPHOBLASTIC HYPERTHYROIDISM

The thyrotropic activity inherent to the choriogonadotropin (hCG) molecule can occasionally account for appearance of a small goiter and mild hyperthyroidism in patients with choriocarcinomas or hydatidiform moles. Occasionally, the hyperthyroidism can be severe enough to require treatment with antithyroid drugs.

HYPERTENSION

Renin-secreting tumors must be considered in the differential diagnosis of hypertension and hypokalemia. Most commonly, these tumors arise in the juxtaglomerular cells, the normal source of renin. Extrarenal renin-secreting tumors are rare and include pancreatic, ovarian, and pulmonary tumors. In general, hypertension subsides upon removal of the tumors. However, extrarenal renin-secreting tumors are usually aggressive and quite advanced at the time of presentation. In these situations, angiotensin-converting enzyme inhibitors such as captopril may be required for treatment of hypertension.

ACROMEGALY

The production of growth hormone or, more rarely, growth hormone–releasing factor (GRF), has been documented in nonpituitary tumors such as carcinoids, pancreatic islet cell neoplasms, pulmonary carcinomas, and gastric, ovarian, and breast carcinomas. Uncommonly, this can produce the full manifestations of acromegaly. For production of GRF (Table 161–1), the associated tumors generally arise from endocrine cells. The treatment of tumor-associated acromegaly is, when feasible, removal of the causative neoplasm.

OTHER HORMONES PRODUCED BY TUMORS

A number of other hormones, often in the small polypeptide hormone category (some are shown in Table 161–1), may be found in tumor tissue and/or secreted by the tumor. Examples include calcitonin, somatostatin, and GRP in endocrine tumors. These hormones have not been associated with clinical syndromes in patients with these diseases but in some instances may be useful tumor markers to follow in monitoring disease course.

Baylin SB, Mendelsohn G: Ectopic (inappropriate) hormone production by tumors: Mechanisms involved and the biological and clinical implications. Endocr Rev 1:45, 1980. *This review concentrates on the biology of tumor-associated hormone production.*
de Bustros A, Baylin SB: Ectopic hormone production by tumors. *In* Moore WT, Eastman R (eds.): Diagnostic Endocrinology. Ontario, B.C. Decker, Inc., 1990, p 283. *This more recent review both discusses current concepts of the biology of tumor-associated hormone production and outlines the clinical syndromes that result.*
Odell WD: Humoral manifestations of cancer. *In* Williams RH (ed.): Textbook of Endocrinology, 7th ed. Philadelphia, W.B. Saunders Company, 1984.

Ectopic ACTH Production

Carey RM, Varma SK, Drake CR Jr, et al.: Ectopic secretion of corticotropin-releasing factor as a cause of Cushing's syndrome: A clinical, morphological and biochemical study. N Engl J Med 311:13, 1984. *This study provides an example of a patient with Cushing's syndrome caused by tumor production of CRF.*
Gerwirtz G, Yallow RS: Ectopic ACTH production in carcinoma of the lung. J Clin Invest 53:1022, 1974. *This paper is the classic first description of the presence of ACTH immunoreactivity, most in a biologically inactive form, in all lung carcinomas.*

Hypercalcemia and Cancer

Broadus AE, Mangin M, Insogna KL, et al.: Humoral hypercalcemia of cancer. N Engl J Med 319:556, 1988. *This is a good overall review of the biology and clinical aspects of the humorally mediated hypercalcemia of cancer.*
Burtis WJ, Brady TG, Orloff JJ, et al.: Immunochemical characterization of circulating parathyroid hormone–related protein in patients with humoral hypercalcemia of cancer. N Engl J Med 322:1106–1112, 1990. *This paper defines the incidence of increased circulating parathyroid hormone–related protein levels in patients with neoplasms.*

Chorionic Gonadotropin and Cancer

Braunstein GD, Vaitukaitis JL, Carbone PP, et al.: Ectopic production of human chorionic gonadotropin by neoplasms. Ann Intern Med 78:39, 1973. *This is a classic paper for defining the incidence of ectopic production of hCG.*

Hypoglycemia and Cancer

Gorden P, Hendricks CM, Kahn CR, et al.: Hypoglycemia associated with non-islet-cell tumor and insulin-like growth factors: A study of the tumor types. N Engl J Med 305:1452, 1981. *This paper reviews the tumor types associated with hormonally mediated hypoglycemia.*
Widmer V, Zapf J, Froesch ER: Is extrapancreatic tumor hypoglycemia associated with elevated levels of insulin-like growth factor II? J Clin Endocrinol Metab 55:833, 1982. *Some of the questions about the role of IGF-II in tumor-associated hypoglycemia are addressed.*

Vasopressin and Cancer

Amatruda TT Jr, Mulrow PJ, Gallagher JC, et al.: Carcinoma of the lung with inappropriate antidiuresis. Demonstration of antidiuretic-hormone–like activity in tumor extracts. N Engl J Med 269:544, 1963. *This paper is the classic description of ADH production by a lung carcinoma.*
Yamaji T, Ishibashi M, Katayama S, et al.: Neurophysin biosynthesis in vitro in oat cell carcinoma of the lung with ectopic vasopressin production. J Clin Invest 68:1441, 1981.

Osteomalacia and Cancer

Nuovo MA, Dorfman HD, Sun C-C, Chalew SA: Tumor-induced osteomalacia and rickets. Am J Surg Pathol 13:588, 1989. *This is a good overall review.*
Ryan EA, Reiss E: Oncogenous osteomalacia: Review of the world literature of 42 cases and report of two new cases. Am J Med 77:501, 1984. *This is another extensive review of this syndrome.*

Polycythemia and Cancer

DaSilva J-L, Lacombe C, Bruneval P, et al.: Tumor cells are the site of erythropoietin synthesis in human renal cancers associated with polycythemia. Blood 75:577, 1990. *This paper documents erythropoietin production from tumor cells.*
Hammond D, Winnick S: Paraneoplastic erythrocytosis and ectopic erythropoietins. Ann NY Acad Sci 230:219, 1974. *This paper reviews this association.*

Trophoblastic Hyperthyroidism

Nisula BC, Ketelslegers J-M: Thyroid-stimulating activity and chorionic gonadotropin. J Clin Invest 54:494, 1974.
Wilber JF, Spinella P: Identification of immunoreactive thyrotropin-releasing hormone in human neoplasia. J Clin Endocrinol Metab 59:432, 1984. *These above two papers describe the syndrome and the role of hCG.*

Hypertension and Cancer

Atlas SA, Hesson TE, Sealey JE, et al.: Characterization of inactive renin ("prorenin") from renin-secreting tumors of non-renal origin. J Clin Invest 73:437, 1984.
Ruddy MC, Atlas SA, Salerno FG: Hypertension associated with a renin-secreting adenocarcinoma of the pancreas. N Engl J Med 307:993, 1982.

Acromegaly and Cancer

Asa SI, Kovacs K, Thorner MO, et al.: Immunohistological localization of growth hormone-releasing hormone in human tumors. J Clin Endocrinol Metab 60:423, 1985.
Gubler U, Monahan JJ, Lomedico PT, et al.: Cloning and sequence analysis of cDNA for the precursor of human growth hormone-releasing factor, somatocrinin. Proc Natl Acad Sci USA 80:4311, 1983.
Mayo KE, Vale W, Rivier J, et al.: Expression-cloning and sequencing of a cDNA encoding human growth hormone-releasing factor. Nature 306:86, 1983. *This paper documents growth hormone "production" by tumors.*
Rivier J, Spiess J, Thorner M, et al.: Characterization of a growth hormone releasing factor from a human pancreatic islet tumor. Nature 300:276, 1982. *This paper documents GRF from neoplasms.*

162 Nonmetastatic Effects of Cancer on the Nervous System

Jerome B. Posner

When patients with systemic cancer develop nervous system dysfunction, metastasis is usually the cause. However, cancer can exert deleterious effects on the nervous system by mechanisms other than metastasis. Recognition of these nonmetastatic neurologic complications can prevent inappropriate and perhaps harmful therapy directed at a nonexistent metastasis. Sometimes nervous system symptoms precede the discovery of the cancer and can, if correctly interpreted, lead the physician to the diagnosis of an otherwise occult neoplasm.

An almost bewildering variety of neurologic disorders have been ascribed to effects of systemic cancer (Table 162–1). Most patients with nervous system dysfunction not caused by metastases are eventually found to be suffering from infection, vascular or metabolic disorders, or neurotoxicity of chemotherapy. This chapter discusses two other types of nervous system damage related to cancer not described elsewhere in this book: "remote effects" or paraneoplastic syndromes (Table 162–2) and radiation injury.

REMOTE EFFECTS

Remote effects of cancer on the nervous system (paraneoplastic syndromes) refer to neurologic disorders of unknown cause that occur at higher frequency in patients with cancer than in the general population. These syndromes are not common. Excluding patients with mild peripheral neuropathy or myopathy possibly associated with cachexia, remote effects of cancer affect less than 1 per cent of unselected patients with cancer. Lung cancer accounts for more than 50 per cent of cases; the incidence is greatest among patients with ovarian and small cell lung cancer and Hodgkin's disease. Because of its rarity, the diagnosis of paraneoplastic syndrome should never be accepted until a thorough evaluation has excluded metastatic or other nonmetastatic causes of neurologic dysfunction. In particular, infiltration of nerve roots by tumor in the leptomeninges may mimic paraneoplastic peripheral neuropathy.

Increasing evidence suggests that the etiology of most or all remote effects is autoimmune. Patients with the Lambert-Eaton myasthenic syndrome (see below) harbor an IgG antibody that reacts with voltage-gated calcium channels on the presynaptic neuromuscular junction. Complexing of these channels by the antibody prevents normal release of acetylcholine, which, in turn, causes the clinical symptoms of the disorder. About two thirds of patients with the Lambert-Eaton myasthenic syndrome have, or will shortly develop, evidence of small cell lung cancer. The tumors possess a protein antigen homologous with or identical to the calcium channels in the neuromuscular junction against which the antibody response is presumed to be directed.

TABLE 162–1. NONMETASTATIC EFFECTS OF CANCER ON THE NERVOUS SYSTEM

Remote effects or paraneoplastic syndromes (see Table 162–2)
Side effects of therapy
  Chemotherapy
  Radiation therapy (see Table 162–3)
Metabolic and nutritional abnormalities
  Destruction of vital organs (e.g., liver)
  Elaboration of hormonal substances by tumor
  Competition between tumor and brain for essential substrates (e.g., glucose)
  Malnutrition
Infections (usually associated with lymphomas)
  Parasites (e.g., toxoplasmosis)
  Fungi (e.g., cryptococcosis, aspergillosis, mucormycosis)
  Bacteria (e.g., *Listeria monocytogenes*)
  Viruses (e.g., herpes zoster)
Vascular disease
  Intracranial hemorrhage
  Cerebral infarction

TABLE 162–2. REMOTE EFFECTS OF CANCER ON THE NERVOUS SYSTEM (PARANEOPLASTIC SYNDROMES)

Brain and cranial nerves
  Dementia—limbic encephalitis
  Retinal degeneration
  Optic neuritis
  Opsoclonus-myoclonus
  Subacute cerebellar degeneration
  Brain stem encephalitis
Spinal cord
  Subacute motor neuronopathy
  Necrotizing myelopathy
  Myelitis
  Motor neuron disease
Dorsal root ganglia
  Subacute sensory neuronopathy
Peripheral nerve
  Subacute or chronic sensorimotor peripheral neuropathy
  Acute polyradiculoneuropathy (Guillain-Barré syndrome)
  Remitting and relapsing peripheral neuropathy
  Mononeuropathies
  Mononeuritis multiplex
  Brachial neuritis
  Autonomic neuropathy
  Peripheral neuropathy associated with paraproteinemia
Neuromuscular junction and muscle
  Lambert-Eaton myasthenic syndrome
  Myasthenia gravis
  Dermatomyositis, polymyositis
  Acute necrotizing myopathy
  Carcinoid myopathies
  Myotonia
  Cachectic myopathy
  "Neuromyopathy"

Removal of IgG from the serum of a patient with Lambert-Eaton myasthenic syndrome ameliorates the neuromuscular symptoms, and injection of that IgG into experimental animals reproduces the neurologic disorder. High titers of antibodies against other onconeural antigens (antigens shared between tumor and nervous system) are found in several other paraneoplastic syndromes (see below), suggesting a mechanism similar to that in the Lambert-Eaton syndrome. However, paraneoplastic syndromes may be a heterogeneous group of disorders in which other etiologies, such as opportunistic viral infections, competition between tumor in the nervous system for essential metabolites, and secretion by tumor of neurotoxins, may also play a role.

Paraneoplastic syndromes are usually classified by the anatomic site of neurologic disability (Table 162–2). However, it is common for more than one anatomic site to be involved (e.g., Lambert-Eaton syndrome and cerebellar degeneration, dementia and myelopathy, limbic encephalitis and sensory neuronopathy). When more than one symptom is present, the disorder can be called paraneoplastic encephalomyelitis or paraneoplastic encephalomyeloneuritis. Some of the more characteristic paraneoplastic syndromes are described in the paragraphs below.

Brain and Cranial Nerves

CEREBRUM. Cerebral remote effects are usually characterized by dementia with or without other neurologic findings. Loss of recent memory and affective alterations, either anxiety or depression, are the usual findings. Seizures are prominent in some patients; others have a fluctuating confusional state. When other abnormal neurologic signs are present, they usually point to the brain stem, cerebellum, or peripheral nerves (encephalomyelitis). The cerebrospinal fluid usually contains 10 to 40 lymphocytes per cubic milliliter, with a slight elevation of the protein concentration. Computed tomography (CT) and magnetic resonance imaging (MRI) are usually normal, but in occasional patients abnormalities can be found in the medial temporal areas. Antibodies reacting with neuronal nuclei can be found in patients with limbic encephalitis associated with small cell lung cancer.

Pathologically, there are two main groups: In some patients, no significant pathologic changes are found in the cerebrum despite clinical dementia. Other patients demonstrate widespread cerebral neuronal loss, gliosis, and perivascular collections of lymphocytes, particularly in the medial temporal lobes (limbic encephalitis) or the thalamus. In those patients who have anti-neuronal antibodies in blood and spinal fluid, the same antibodies can also be identified in the brain. The differential diagnosis includes brain or leptomeningeal metastases; fungal, parasitic, or viral infections (including multifocal leukoencephalopathy); and metabolic encephalopathy. Appropriate imaging, cerebrospinal fluid (CSF) examination, and other laboratory tests usually identify these disorders. The rapid onset of dementia in middle age accompanied by cerebellar, brain stem, or peripheral nerve dysfunction, but no other focal cerebral signs, suggests paraneo-plastic dementia as a remote effect of cancer. Degenerative dementias such as Alzheimer's disease usually are slower in onset and have a more protracted course. However, paraneoplastic dementia may be confused with Creutzfeldt-Jakob disease (see Ch. 478.6). There is no specific treatment for paraneoplastic dementias, but they occasionally improve with successful therapy of the cancer.

CEREBELLUM. Paraneoplastic cerebellar degeneration is clinically sufficiently characteristic to suggest cancer even when neurologic symptoms predate diagnosis of the tumor. Symptoms usually evolve over weeks, with bilateral and symmetric cerebellar dysfunction, the patient being equally ataxic in arms and legs. Severe dysarthria is usually present, vertigo and diplopia are common, but nystagmus may be absent. Some patients have neurologic signs pointing to disease outside the cerebellum (e.g., extensor plantar responses, diminished or exaggerated tendon reflexes, dementia). Early in the disorder there is a cerebrospinal fluid pleocytosis, and an elevated IgG content is common. The disease, which may be associated with any cancer, precedes the discovery of the neoplasm by a few weeks to 3 years in more than half the patients. Cerebellar atrophy may be seen on MR scan, particularly late in the course of the illness. In a subset of patients with gynecologic cancers (ovarian, uterine, fallopian tube, breast), an antibody reacting exclusively with cerebellar Purkinje cells and with the underlying tumor allows a definitive diagnosis to be made before the tumor is discovered. Other antibodies may be present in some other patients with nongynecologic tumors. The role of the antibody in the pathogenesis of the disease is not established.

Characteristic pathologic changes consist of diffuse or patchy loss of cerebellar Purkinje cells. There may be lymphocytic cuffs around blood vessels, particularly in the deep nuclei. The illness can be distinguished from cerebellar or leptomeningeal metastases by the symmetry of its signs and the absence of increased intracranial pressure as well as by MR and CSF examination. *Listeria* meningitis and progressive multifocal leukoencephalopathy may present with cerebellar signs also distinguishable by MR and CSF examination. In alcohol-nutritional cerebellar degeneration, truncal and lower extremity ataxia are prominent, but nystagmus, dysarthria, and upper extremity ataxia are mild or absent. Sporadic or familial cerebellar degenerative disorders are much slower in onset. Cerebellar dysfunction associated with viral infections (varicella, infectious mononucleosis) or with chemotherapy (5-fluorouracil, cytosine arabinoside) may mimic paraneoplastic cerebellar degeneration. Paraneoplastic cerebellar degeneration usually runs a subacute course and then stabilizes or, on rare occasions, improves with successful treatment of the tumor.

Cranial Nerves

Two rare but striking paraneoplastic syndromes affect the eyes. The first is characterized by rapid onset of blindness associated with retinal degeneration, usually of photoreceptors. In some such patients, antibodies that react with cells in the retina can be identified in the serum, suggesting that the disorder is an immune one. Optic neuritis, which does not differ clinically in any way from the idiopathic disorder, has also been described in some patients with underlying neoplasms. Opsoclonus (saccadic conjugate involuntary movement of the eyes), also called saccadomania, is often a paraneoplastic disorder. About 50 per cent of infants and children with opsoclonus have underlying neuroblastoma. In adults about 20 per cent of patients with opsoclonus

probably have an underlying cancer, usually breast cancer. The disorder in adults may be associated with an antibody different from that found in encephalomyelitis associated with small cell lung cancer. Except when the autoantibody is present, there is no way of clinically distinguishing paraneoplastic opsoclonus from opsoclonus caused by metabolic or structural abnormalities of the brain stem or cerebellum.

Spinal Cord

Two rare but distinct myelopathies complicate cancer: The first, *subacute motor neuronopathy*, affects anterior horn cells, usually in patients with Hodgkin's disease or other lymphomas. The course is subacute, with progressive painless asymmetric lower motor neuron weakness of legs and arms. Some patients complain of sensory symptoms, but sensory loss is mild or absent despite profound weakness. The major pathologic finding is degeneration of anterior horn cells. Sometimes there is inflammation in the anterior horns and demyelination in the white matter of the spinal cord. The clinical course is different from most remote effects in that many patients improve spontaneously, independently of the course of the underlying lymphoma. The etiology is unknown, but a similar disorder in mice harboring lymphomas appears to be caused by a retrovirus. Rarely, gray matter myelopathies with clinical courses resembling syringomyelia or autonomic insufficiency complicate systemic cancer.

The second condition is *subacute necrotic destruction of the spinal cord*, a myelopathy in which both gray and white matter are affected equally. Clinically, there is rapidly ascending sensory and motor loss, usually to midthoracic levels, the patient becoming paraplegic and incontinent within hours or days. The neurologic symptoms often precede the discovery of the neoplasm, and the illness is clinically and pathologically indistinguishable from idiopathic subacute necrotic myelopathy. Since epidural spinal cord compression from metastatic tumor or arteriovenous spinal cord anomalies may present similar clinical signs, a myelogram or MR scan is essential. Amyotrophic lateral sclerosis has been reported as a remote effect of cancer, but it is doubtful that it occurs in patients with cancer more often than in the general population.

Peripheral Nerves and Dorsal Root Ganglia

Four clinical peripheral nerve disorders occur in association with cancer. Characteristic of carcinoma is *subacute sensory neuronopathy* marked by loss of sensation with relative preservation of motor power. The illness usually precedes the appearance of the carcinoma and progresses over a few months, leaving the patient with moderate or severe disability. Cerebrospinal fluid pleocytosis and increased IgG content are common. Pathologically, there is destruction of posterior root ganglia with perivascular lymphocytic cuffing and wallerian degeneration of sensory nerves. Many of the patients have inflammatory and degenerative changes in brain and spinal cord as well (encephalomyelitis). The disorder, when associated with small cell carcinoma, is characterized by serum antibodies reacting against neuronal nuclei and small cell lung cancer cells. There is no treatment.

More common than sensory neuronopathy is a *distal sensorimotor polyneuropathy* characterized by motor weakness, sensory loss, and absence of distal reflexes in the extremities. The illness is pathologically characterized by either segmental demyelination or wallerian degeneration (or both) of sensory and motor peripheral nerves. Pathologically and clinically, the sensorimotor neuropathy is indistinguishable from polyneuropathies not associated with cancer. Indeed, some have suggested that late or terminal polyneuropathy may be due to nutritional deprivation associated with cancer. Its etiology, however, is not clear, and it does not respond to treatment with vitamins or other nutritional supplements.

A *polyneuritis* clinically and pathologically indistinguishable from acute postinfectious polyneuropathy (Guillain-Barré syndrome) also complicates cancers, particularly Hodgkin's disease. A few patients with *neuropathy limited to the autonomic nervous system* have been reported.

Neuromuscular Junction and Muscles

NEUROMUSCULAR JUNCTION. *Myasthenia gravis* is associated with thymomas but usually not other systemic tumors.

The Lambert-Eaton myasthenic syndrome is characterized by weakness and fatigability of proximal muscles, particularly of the pelvic girdle and thighs. The cranial nerves and respiratory muscles are usually spared. Patients often complain of dryness of the mouth, impotence, pain in the thighs, and peripheral paresthesias. On examination there is weakness of the proximal muscles, but strength increases over several seconds of sustained contraction. The deep tendon reflexes are diminished or absent. The diagnosis is made by electromyographic studies in which repeated nerve stimulations at rates above 10 per second cause a progressive *increase* in the size of the muscle action potential (the opposite of myasthenia gravis). About two thirds of patients with this syndrome either have or will develop cancer, usually small cell carcinoma of the lung. The neuromuscular defect in this illness is believed to be deficient release of acetylcholine. Similar findings have been produced in experimental animals by injection of either serum IgG or extract of tumor in patients with the disorder. Plasmapheresis and immunosuppressant drugs may relieve symptoms, as may successful treatment of the neoplasm. The illness responds poorly to anticholinesterase drugs but does respond to 3,4-diaminopyridine in doses up to 100 mg per day.

MUSCLE. Typical *dermatomyositis* or *polymyositis* may occur as a remote effect of cancer (see Ch. 268). Fewer than 10 per cent of patients with this disorder have cancer, but the figure is higher in older patients. The clinical picture of polymyositis associated with cancer (i.e., subacute development of weakness, particularly involving proximal muscles and sometimes bulbar muscles) is indistinguishable from that of dermatomyositis or polymyositis not associated with cancer. Pathologically, there may be two groups: one with the typical inflammatory lesions of polymyositis and one with little inflammation but severe muscle necrosis. The latter group may suffer an explosive clinical course. The patients respond somewhat less well to corticosteroid therapy than do those with dermatomyositis unaccompanied by cancer, although substantial improvement with steroid treatment does occur in some.

Muscle Weakness. Some patients with cancer complain of *weakness* and *fatigability* that seem worse than can be accounted for by their cancer alone. Cachexia and weight loss alone do not usually cause measurable muscle weakness. The weakness is usually proximal and produces particular difficulty climbing stairs or getting out of low chairs. Ankle reflexes may be diminished or absent. Further neurologic evaluation does not yield findings diagnostic of one of the remote effects of cancer described above. Brain and his colleagues have labeled this entity neuromyopathy because its exact anatomic locus is unclear, but others have suggested that it is a nonspecific accompaniment of cachexia and systemic illness. Specific (type II) muscle fiber atrophy develops early in patients with systemic cancer. The cause and treatment of the weakness are unknown.

Henson RA, Urich H: Cancer and the Nervous System. Oxford, Blackwell Scientific Publications Ltd., 1982. *Comprehensive clinical and pathologic descriptions of all the paraneoplastic disorders.*

Posner JB, Furneaux HM: Paraneoplastic syndromes. *In* Waksman BH (ed.): Immunologic Mechanisms in Neurologic and Psychiatric Disease. New York, Raven Press, 1990, pp 187–219. *A review of paraneoplastic syndromes, with emphasis on the evidence for autoimmune pathogenesis.*

NERVOUS SYSTEM INJURY FROM THERAPEUTIC RADIATION

Adverse effects of ionizing radiation on the nervous system (Table 162–3) are related to the total dose of radiation, the size of each fraction, the total duration over which the dose is received, and the volume of nervous system tissue irradiated. Other factors, such as underlying nervous system disease (e.g., brain tumor, cerebral edema), previous surgery, concomitant use of chemotherapeutic agents, and individual susceptibility, make it impossible to define precisely a safe dose of radiation therapy for a given individual. However, guidelines allow the radiation therapist to calculate generally safe nervous system doses. Adverse effects may involve any portion of the central or peripheral nervous system and may occur acutely or be delayed weeks to years following irradiation.

CLINICAL MANIFESTATIONS. *Acute encephalopathy* may follow large radiation doses to the brains of patients with increased intracranial pressure, particularly in the absence of corticosteroid prophylaxis. Immediately following treatment, susceptible patients develop headache, nausea and vomiting, somnolence, fever, and occasionally worsening of neurologic signs, rarely culminating in cerebral herniation and death. Acute encephalopathy usually follows the first radiation fraction and becomes progressively less severe with each ensuing fraction. This disorder is believed to result from increased intracranial pressure or brain edema from radiation-induced alteration of the blood-brain barrier. It responds to corticosteroids. Acute worsening of neurologic symptoms does not occur after spinal cord irradiation.

Early delayed reactions appear 6 to 16 weeks after therapy and persist for days to months. A transient, diffuse encephalopathy commonly follows prophylactic irradiation of the brain for leukemia in children and for small cell lung cancer in adults. The disorder is characterized by somnolence, often associated with headache, nausea, vomiting, and sometimes fever. The electroencephalogram may be slow, but there are no focal signs. Whole-brain irradiation for brain tumor sometimes causes lethargy and worsening of focal neurologic signs, simulating progression of the brain tumor. CT and MR scans may also suggest worsening. Both disorders usually respond to steroids, but resolve spontaneously even if untreated. Rarely, a brain stem disorder characterized by diplopia, ataxia, dysarthria, and dysphagia, and associated with foci of demyelination resembling acute multiple sclerosis, follows irradiation to the brain stem. *Early delayed myelopathy* follows radiation therapy to the neck or upper thorax and is characterized by Lhermitte's sign (an electric shock–like sensation radiating into various parts of the body when the neck is flexed). The symptoms resolve spontaneously. Early delayed radiation syndromes are believed to result from demyelination, possibly due to radiation-induced damage to oligodendroglia.

Late delayed radiation injury appears after months to years and may affect any part of the nervous system. In the brain, there are two clinical syndromes. The first follows whole-brain irradiation that has been administered either prophylactically or in some patients with primary and metastatic brain tumors. The disorder is characterized by dementia without focal signs. There is cerebral atrophy on CT or MR scan; pathologic changes are nonspecific, and there is no treatment. The second disorder affects patients who receive either focal brain irradiation during therapy of extracranial neoplasms or whole-brain irradiation for intracranial neoplasms. Neurologic signs suggest a tumor and include headache, focal or generalized seizures, and hemiparesis. MR or CT scans reveal a hypodense mass, sometimes with contrast enhancement. Neuropathologic features include coagulative necrosis of white matter, telangiectasia, fibrinoid necrosis

TABLE 162–3. RADIATION INJURY TO THE NERVOUS SYSTEM

Time After RT	Organ Affected	Clinical Findings
Primary injury		
Immediate (minutes to hours)	Brain	Acute encephalopathy
Early delayed (6 to 16 weeks)	Brain	Somnolence, focal signs
	Spinal cord	Lhermitte's sign
Late delayed (months to years)	Brain	Dementia, focal signs
	Spinal cord	Transverse myelopathy
	Peripheral nerves	Paralysis, sensory loss
Secondary injury (years)	Several	Brain, cranial and/or peripheral nerve sheath tumors
	Arteries (atherosclerosis)	Cerebral infarction
	Endocrine organs	Metabolic encephalopathy

of blood vessels with thrombus formation, glial proliferation, and bizarre multinucleated astrocytes. The clinical and imaging findings cannot be distinguished from those of brain tumor, and the diagnosis can be made only by biopsy. Positron emission tomography, using radiolabeled glucose, generally shows decreased metabolism in areas of radiation damage, whereas most tumors show increased metabolism. Corticosteroids sometimes ameliorate symptoms. Improvement in symptoms may be sustained even after corticosteroid withdrawal, but if symptoms recur, the treatment of the disorder, if focal, is surgical removal.

Late delayed myelopathy is characterized by progressive paralysis, sensory changes, and sometimes pain. A Brown-Séquard syndrome (weakness and loss of proprioception in the extremities of one side with loss of pain and temperature sensation on the other) is often present at onset. Patients occasionally respond transiently to steroids, and the disorder may stop progressing, but generally patients become paraplegic or quadriplegic. Pathologic changes include necrosis of the spinal cord. *Late delayed neuropathy* may affect any cranial or peripheral nerve. Common disorders are blindness from optic neuropathy and paralysis of an upper extremity from brachial plexopathy after therapy for lung or breast cancer. The pathogenesis is probably fibrosis and ischemia of the plexus. There is no treatment.

Radiation-induced tumors, including meningiomas, sarcomas, or, less commonly, gliomas, may appear years to decades after cranial irradiation and may follow low-dose irradiation. Malignant or atypical nerve sheath tumors may follow irradiation of the brachial, cervical, and lumbar plexuses. The central nervous system may also be damaged when radiation alters extraneural structures. Radiation therapy accelerates *atherosclerosis,* and cerebral infarction associated with carotid artery occlusion in the neck may occur many years after neck irradiation. *Endocrine* (pituitary, thyroid, parathyroid) dysfunction from radiation may be associated with neurologic signs. Hypothyroidism often presents as a neurologic disorder, and hyperthyroidism or hyperparathyroidism from radiation may also cause an encephalopathy.

Delattre JY, Posner JB: Neurologic complications of chemotherapy and radiation therapy. *In* Aminoff MJ (ed.): Neurology and General Medicine. New York, Churchill Livingston, Inc., 1989, pp 365–387. *A general review of common complications of cancer therapy.*

Gutin P, Leibel S, Sheline G (eds.): Radiation Injury to the Nervous System. New York, Raven Press, in press. *A comprehensive description of all of the nervous system side effects of therapeutic irradiation.*

Hildebrand J (ed.): Neurological Adverse Reactions to Anticancer Drugs. Berlin, Springer-Verlag, 1990. *Detailed descriptions of clinical findings and mechanisms of neurotoxicity of anticancer drugs.*

163 Cutaneous Manifestations of Internal Malignancy

Frank Parker

Cutaneous changes associated with internal malignant disease are diverse. Some skin alterations are clear indicators of underlying malignant disease. Others, less specific, arise in either the presence or absence of malignancy, but occur with sufficient frequency to arouse suspicion and the need to search for underlying carcinoma or lymphoma. These various skin findings may precede any signs associated with the internal malignant disease; they are therefore of crucial importance in early identification and cure of internal neoplasms.

Skin manifestations of internal malignant disease can be classified into two major groups: (1) those in which malignant cells can be found in the skin on biopsy (specific skin lesions) and (2) those in which malignant cells cannot be identified on a skin biopsy (nonspecific skin lesions). The specific lesions are diagnostic of the internal malignant disease, while the nonspecific skin alterations may or may not be associated with an internal neoplasm. Some of the nonspecific skin changes are clear indicators of underlying tumor; others merely arouse concern.

SPECIFIC SKIN LESIONS ASSOCIATED WITH INTERNAL MALIGNANT DISEASE

Carcinomas, leukemia, lymphoma, plasma cell dyscrasias, and sarcomas can all affect the skin specifically in clinically identifiable patterns. A biopsy of a suspicious skin lesion is helpful because the tissue of origin (primary underlying neoplasm) can often be identified.

Skin Metastases (Table 163–1 and Color Plate 16A)

Metastases to the skin are comparatively rare (approximately 1 to 5 per cent of internal malignancies), but when present are readily diagnosed by biopsy. Cutaneous metastases usually appear as flesh-colored to red-purple or brownish solitary papules or nodules, stony-hard to the touch, and often innocent in appearance. There is no relationship between site of origin and size, color, and consistency of the metastatic deposit. Lung cancer in men and breast cancer in women most commonly involve the skin; other sources include malignant tumors of the gastrointestinal tract, kidney, ovary, uterus, and urinary bladder and oral cavity carcinomas.

Clinical patterns of metastatic spread to skin depend on several factors such as the organ of origin and whether tumor is disseminated by lymphatics or blood. In general, those neoplasms that spread via lymphatics, such as breast and oral cavity carcinoma, localize in the skin late in the clinical course. Tumors that often embolize through venous channels, such as those arising in the lung, kidney, and ovary, can appear early in the skin and thus may be the first indication of the internal malignant disease.

Certain areas of the skin are predisposed to metastases, localizing near the site of the primary cancer (Table 163–1). Thus, abdominal wall metastases, especially around the umbilicus (Sister Mary Joseph's nodules), arise from neoplasms of the stomach, kidney, and ovary. The lower abdominal wall and external genitalia metastases arise from cancers of the genitourinary systems; face and neck skin metastases, from carcinomas of the oropharynx; and the scalp is a favorite site for metastases from breast, lung, and the genitourinary system.

Some patterns of metastatic disease are characteristic. For example, metastases to the scalp simulate wens or turban (pilar) tumors that may ulcerate. More distinctive is "alopecia neoplastica"—that is, areas of scarring alopecia in the scalp with induration and atrophy that simulate alopecia areata. Metastases from the breast and, less commonly, from the stomach, prostate, lung,

TABLE 163–1. INTERNAL MALIGNANCIES METASTATIC TO SKIN: CLINICAL FEATURES AND AREAS OF DISTRIBUTION

Primary Internal Malignancy	Cutaneous Clinical Features	Areas of Distribution
Breast	Papules, nodules—rock hard En cuirasse—scirrhous form Erysipelatoides—cellulitis form Alopecia neoplastica	Chest wall Trunk Scalp
Lung	Papules, nodules Scirrhous—morpheic form Erysipeloides—cellulitis form Alopecia neoplastica	Chest wall Scalp Face
Kidney	Angiomatous, pulsatile nodules Scirrhous—en cuirasse form Alopecia neoplastica	Abdominal wall, trunk Scalp Face External genitalia
Stomach, bowel, pancreas	Nodules Scirrhous—en cuirasse form Cellulitis—erysipelatoides	Anterior abdomen Periumbilical
Ovary, uterus	Nodules Cellulitis form—erysipelatoides	Umbilicus, abdomen
Oral cavity	Nodules	Face and neck
Thyroid	Pulsatile angiomatous nodules	Anywhere

uterus, and pancreas can produce dramatic changes in the chest wall: carcinoma en cuirasse. This scirrhous form of cutaneous metastatic spread produces extensive fibrosis of the dermis as a result of lymphatic involvement and obstruction by the cancer cells so that large areas of the chest are girdled by a thick, rigid encasement on which pink to flesh-colored papules and nodules evolve to form morphea-like plaques. The distinctive skin lesion of inflammatory carcinoma, or "carcinoma erysipeloides," is usually caused by breast cancer (less frequently by malignant tumors of the uterus, lung, and gastrointestinal tract) and simulates cellulitis over the ipsilateral chest wall anteriorly. Renal cell carcinoma and medullary and anaplastic forms of thyroid cancer, which are highly vascularized tumors, may simulate hemangiomatous nodules that pulsate on palpation when deposited in the skin. *Inflammatory oncotaxis* is a term describing the attraction of cancer cells to an area of tissue trauma resulting presumably because trauma (surgery and radiation) causes inflammation and capillary disruption, thus predisposing cancer cells to settle in these areas. For example, cutaneous metastases from colon, kidney, and cervix have been known to localize in abdominal wall surgical incisions.

Prognosis among patients with cutaneous metastases is poor, as they imply metastases elsewhere internally. If a cutaneous metastatic lesion is discovered years after the primary cancer is diagnosed, a second internal cancer should be ruled out, since only 10 per cent of internal cancers (mostly breast carcinoma) spread to the skin after 5 years' time. Clearly any skin nodule or papule of obscure origin and uncertain diagnosis should undergo biopsy, especially if there are reasons to suspect malignancy.

Lymphomas

Specific cutaneous involvement (neoplastic cellular proliferation in the skin) is seen less frequently in the lymphoma-leukemia group of neoplasms when compared with carcinomas. Rather, cutaneous manifestations are more often nonspecific (i.e., pruritus, petechiae, purpura, infections) in patients with leukemias and lymphomas, occurring in 25 to 40 per cent of such patients (see below, Nonspecific Skin Lesions Associated with Internal Malignant Disease). The specific skin lesions that are seen are similar in patients with lymphoma and leukemia, regardless of the various types of these neoplasms. Thus, skin lesions in all forms of lymphomas and leukemias appear as red, blue, and violaceous asymptomatic macules, nodules, and plaques that may ulcerate. Particularly suggestive are thickened, beefy-red arcuate lesions as well as poikilodermatous plaques (hyperpigmentation and hypopigmentation with telangiectasis throughout the thickened patches).

CUTANEOUS T-CELL LYMPHOMAS (Table 163–2)

These lymphomas are lymphoproliferative disorders of helper T lymphocytes with an affinity for skin (epidermotropism) in which atypical lymphocytes accumulate in clusters in the epidermis to form so-called Pautrier's abscesses. They represent at least three types of lymphoma: mycosis fungoides, Sézary syndrome, and adult T-cell lymphoma, each of which presents with variable clinical characteristics and biologic behavior.

Mycosis fungoides (see Color Plate 16B) usually follows a prolonged course, beginning with nonspecific skin lesions (so-called premycotic stage) that, after a variable number of years, evolve into histologically specific skin lesions (cutaneous patches, plaques—the mycotic stage) and then into ulcerative nodules and tumors (tumor stage).

Extracutaneous disseminated disease involves first lymph nodes and then, in advanced stages, liver and spleen and other internal organs. Less commonly the disease may begin with cutaneous nodules and tumors without evolving from patches and plaques. Several types of clinical lesions (patches, plaques, and tumors) may coexist in any one patient. The premycotic stage (biopsy of lesions is nonspecific) can persist from a few months to more than 40 years, the morphology of the skin lesions resembling a number of banal dermatoses: psoriasis or eczema or poikilodermatous telangiectatic, stippled pigmented patches. In the plaque stage the premycotic lesions become infiltrated, although indurated, red-purple plaques also arise from previously uninvolved skin. The lesions usually are oval to round, but they may also be arciform or annular or assume a horseshoe shape, or the entire

TABLE 163–2. CUTANEOUS T-CELL LYMPHOMAS

Lymphoma	Skin Lesions	Other Features
Mycosis fungoides	Erythematous patches, plaques, tumors, erythroderma	Late involvement of lymph nodes, internal organs
Sézary syndrome	Erythroderma with ectropion and leonine facies; often spares body folds	Sézary cells in blood with high WBC, hepatosplenomegaly, lymphadenopathy
Adult T-cell lymphoma	Erythroderma, papules, nodules	HTLV 1 virus antibodies, hepatosplenomegaly, osteolytic bone lesions, hypercalcemia
T immunoblastic lymphoma	Plaques, tumors	Arise from pre-existing mycosis fungoides or Sézary syndrome
Chronic lymphoblastic leukemia, T-cell type	Erythroderma, plaques, nodules	Prolonged course
T lymphoblastic lymphoma	Tumors of skin	Rapidly fatal with bone marrow and mediastinal involvement

integument may be infiltrated, producing a thickened, red hide (erythroderma). In the final stage, tumors develop from pre-existing plaques, erythroderma, or previously uninvolved skin. Tumors may be a few centimeters to 10 cm in size and often ulcerate. It is difficult to diagnose mycosis fungoides in the premycotic stage; it requires multiple skin biopsies over extended periods. However, the detection of rearranged T-cell receptor genes can be readily demonstrated in skin lesions of mycosis fungoides, and this may prove to be a sensitive and practical method for the early diagnosis of T-cell neoplasms (including mycosis fungoides, human T-cell lymphomas, and chronic lymphocytic leukemia). Clonal rearrangements for the β T-cell receptor genes are also found in lymph nodes removed from patients with mycosis fungoides and considered histologically to contain only benign lymphadenopathy.

The *Sézary syndrome* (see Color Plate 16C), the leukemic variant of mycosis fungoides, consists of generalized exfoliative dermatitis with edema, redness, and thickening of the skin associated with ectropion, leonine facies, keratoderma of the palms and soles, hepatosplenomegaly, and lymphadenopathy associated with large numbers of atypical T lymphocytes in the circulation. The latter, so-called Sézary cells, represent T cells with highly convoluted nuclei identical to the cells infiltrating the skin in mycosis fungoides. The immediate source of the circulating Sézary cells appears to be the skin, as the bone marrow is rarely involved. In many patients mycosis fungoides pursues a chronic course, and the patients die of unrelated causes; some experience rapid progression to cutaneous tumors and ulcerative lesions and disseminated disease (visceral involvement is frequently diffuse and resembles leukemic infiltrates). Sézary syndrome has a particularly poor prognosis. Staphylococcal or *Pseudomonas* septicemia is the most common terminal event, accounting for half of the deaths.

Adult T-cell lymphoma, which is associated with a retrovirus, human T-cell lymphoma virus (HTLV), occurs mainly in blacks in the United States. Cutaneous findings are prominent in 70 per cent of patients and may be the presenting feature. Flesh-colored papules, nodules, and tumors as well as generalized erythroderma may be present. The papules are diffusely disseminated over the trunk and coalesce to form plaques. Patients also display peripheral and mediastinal lymphadenopathy, and hepatosplenomegaly is found in half of the patients. A unique feature of this lymphoma is trabecular and bone marrow involvement with multiple "punched-out" osteolytic lesions in the axial skeleton and long bones associated with extreme hypercalcemia.

Several other forms of T-cell lymphomas occur with skin involvement and are outlined in Table 163–2.

NON-HODGKIN'S LYMPHOMAS AND CUTANEOUS B-CELL LYMPHOMAS (see Ch. 147)

Red, blue, or violaceous skin lesions occur in all forms of non-Hodgkin's lymphoma. They appear as papules, nodules, and plaques with occasional large, ulcerated tumors that evolve in the skin after lymph node involvement. Skin involvement can be seen as the initial presentation, or it may occur late in the course of the disease. It appears to have no impact on prognosis.

HODGKIN'S DISEASE (see Ch. 148)

The skin is not commonly involved in a specific way, but when it is, the erythematous papules, nodules, and plaques that often ulcerate are indistinguishable from the skin lesions found in non-Hodgkin's lymphoma. The site of predilection is the thoracic wall, spread being via retrograde lymphatic drainage pathways from massively enlarged axillary and cervical lymph nodes. Specific cutaneous involvement is seen in those patients with extensive and highly aggressive Hodgkin's disease.

Leukemias

Leukemia cutis usually develops months after the diagnosis of leukemia (55 per cent of patients) or at the time of diagnosis (38 per cent), but it can occasionally precede systemic disease and be the first sign of the underlying condition. Red to violaceous papules, nodules, and thickened plaques are the usual forms that leukemic infiltrates take, but rarely erythroderma is found. When chronic myelogenous leukemia (CML) enters the blast phase, greenish tumors may develop in the skin, forming chloromas or granulocytic sarcomas (see Ch. 144). Skin lesions in acute leukemias and chronic lymphocytic leukemia (CLL) are found on the face and extremities, while those associated with CML are more commonly seen on the trunk. In monocytic leukemia, widespread leukemia skin infiltrates occur, and oral mucosal involvement (gingival hyperplasia) is commonplace. In general, the histology of leukemic cells in skin for various forms of leukemia mimics that seen in the blood and bone marrow, but it is difficult to diagnose the type of leukemia from skin biopsies.

Plasma Cell Dyscrasias

Specific skin manifestations of multiple myeloma, extramedullary plasmacytoma, and Waldenström's macroglobulinemia consist of lymphoplasmacytoid cell infiltrates or deposition of monoclonal paraprotein immunoglobulins (see Ch. 151). Bluish red and flesh-colored nonulcerated nodules and plaques on the trunk are observed in 4 per cent of patients with multiple myeloma, representing in most instances extensions from underlying medullary plasma cell proliferation.

Cutaneous Histiocytic Malignant Tumors

Malignant tumors of histiocytes may be solitary or present as disseminated disease. Malignant histiocytosis (histiocytic medullary reticulosis), a systemic, progressive proliferation of atypical histiocytes, produces wasting, fever, lymphadenopathy, hepatosplenomegaly, pancytopenia, and skin lesions. Children and adults are affected, and skin lesions are an integral part of the disease, especially in children (up to 90 per cent have cutaneous changes). The reddish purple papulonodular and ulcerative plaques occur over the trunk and face early in the clinical course. Malignant histiocytosis is fatal in adults but is somewhat less aggressive in children.

Angioblastic Lymphadenopathy

Immunologically mediated, this often fatal disorder is characterized by proliferation of plasmacytoid immunoblasts and plasma cells. Fever, malaise, weight loss, hepatosplenomegaly, and generalized lymphadenopathy are accompanied in 40 per cent of cases by generalized, maculopapular, purpuric, and, at times, exfoliative erythroderma. Biopsy findings of involved lymph nodes are diagnostic (proliferation of plasma cells, arborizing vessels, and deposition of amorphous material), while skin biopsy reveals a lymphohistiocytic vasculitis composed of plasma and immunoblast-like cells.

Neuroblastoma

Neuroblastoma, a poorly differentiated tumor derived from primordial neural crest cells, arises within the sympathetic ganglion (cervical, thoracic, and pelvic tumors) and adrenal glands of children. It frequently metastasizes to bone, lymph nodes, liver, and skin. Bluish nodules appear over a wide area (causing these children to be called blueberry-muffin children). A helpful clinical sign occurs after rubbing these lesions: They blanch with a halo of surrounding erythema, probably related to the release of catechols contained in the cells of the tumors. Even though patients with neuroblastoma are not hypertensive, 85 per cent have increased urinary catecholamine metabolites.

Kaposi's Sarcoma (see Color Plates 12D and 16D)

Kaposi's sarcoma, a multifocal, vascular malignant tumor, can occur in four major clinical settings: African Kaposi's, classic Kaposi's in elderly Jewish or Mediterranean males, Kaposi's secondary to immunodeficiency conditions, and Kaposi's sarcoma occurring as a complication of acquired immunodeficiency syndrome (AIDS). In each instance the skin lesions are identical histologically and clinically; they present as purplish brown macules, plaques, papules, or nodules. The distribution and course of these sarcomatous lesions, however, vary according to the clinical setting (Table 163–3). Thus, classic Kaposi's sarcoma occurs in elderly males of Mediterranean background as purplish

TABLE 163–3. KAPOSI'S SARCOMA: COMPARISON OF VARIOUS FORMS

	Classic Form	African Form	Immunologic Deficiency State	AIDS Associated
Age	40–70 years	Middle age	Any age	20–50 years
Sex	M:F, 10–15:1	—	M or F	Mostly males
Social characteristics	Mediterranean or Jewish ancestry	Blacks in equatorial Africa	Patients taking immuno-suppressive drugs—renal transplant, etc.	Homosexuals, drug addicts, hemophiliacs
Occurrence	0.2% cancers in USA	10% of all malignant tumors in Africa	400% greater incidence than population at large	Increasing; 35% of AIDS patients
Clinical appearance of skin lesion	Multiple purple-brown macules, papules, plaques, nodules	Nodules, exophytic lesions, infiltrative, burrowing plaques	Papules, nodules	Multiple purple-brown macules, papules, nodules; follow cleavage lines of skin
Cutaneous location	Lower legs most often, occasionally arms	Extremities	Trunk, neck—widespread lesions	Widespread—upper body, face, neck
Mucosal involvement	Rare	Rare	—	Common
Node and systemic involvement	Rare—occasionally nodes, GI tract, liver in 10% of patients	Uncommon	—	Frequent; 75% with visceral involvement; 5% visceral lesions only
Course and prognosis	Indolent course, 15% mortality within 10 years	Indolent course	Good; may regress if immunosuppressive drugs can be stopped	Fulminant condition, poor prognosis
Response to therapy	Excellent	—	Good	Poor

macules that may progress to infiltrative plaques and nodules on the distal extremities, following an indolent course. The Kaposi's sarcoma occurring in young homosexuals and others with AIDS is characterized by widely distributed, red-brown macules, papules, and nodules over the upper body and progresses in a fulminant course. The Kaposi's lesions in AIDS often follow skin cleavage lines and frequently involve the oropharyngeal mucosa, appearing as purple hemorrhagic plaques. The importance of the immune status in the evolution of Kaposi's sarcoma is dramatically illustrated in renal transplant patients who are immunosuppressed. Kaposi's sarcoma develops after 9 to 16 months following transplantation and initiation of immunosuppressive drugs. Rapidly progressive, widespread, red to purple papules ensue, but they may regress when immunosuppressive therapy is withdrawn.

NONSPECIFIC SKIN LESIONS ASSOCIATED WITH INTERNAL MALIGNANT DISEASE (Table 163–4)

Malignant cells cannot be identified in the skin in a wide variety of cutaneous manifestations of internal malignant disease. The pathogenesis of these disparate skin reactions is obscure. Often the only evidence that malignancy and cutaneous changes are related is the observation that following removal of the tumor or treatment of the neoplasm the skin change subsides or disappears and may subsequently exacerbate if the neoplasm recurs. Skin manifestations may coincide with, antedate, or follow the clinical diagnosis of internal malignant disease.

Although nonspecific manifestations are often highly suggestive of underlying malignant disease, they are more frequently seen with other nonmalignant conditions. When these skin changes are observed, therefore, an internal neoplasm is only one of several possibilities in the differential diagnosis.

Nonspecific skin manifestations can be considered under two major headings: (1) skin changes common to many skin diseases, including internal malignancy and (2) syndromes and entities commonly associated with internal neoplasia.

Skin Changes Common to Many Skin Conditions, Including Internal Malignancy

Pruritus, unassociated with detectable abnormalities of the skin except for secondary lesions such as excoriations or prurigo-like papules, may be an important manifestation of various internal malignant diseases, including Hodgkin's disease, lymphocytic

TABLE 163–4. NONSPECIFIC SKIN LESIONS ASSOCIATED WITH INTERNAL MALIGNANCIES

I. Skin lesions common to many skin conditions, including internal malignancy
II. Syndromes and entities commonly associated with internal malignancy
  A. Nongenetic syndromes
    1. High incidence of association with internal malignancy
      Paget's disease
      Stewart-Treves syndrome
      Acanthosis nigricans
      Dermatomyositis
      Leser-Trélat syndrome
      Glucagonoma syndrome
      Bazex syndrome
      Pulmonary osteoarthropathy
      Carcinoid syndrome
    2. Low incidence of association with malignancy
      Sweet's syndrome
      Amyloid
      Urticaria pigmentosa and mastocytosis syndrome
      Bowen's disease
  B. Genetic syndromes
    1. High incidence of association with malignancy
      Torre's syndrome
      Gardner's syndrome
      Cowden's syndrome
      Multiple endocrine neoplasia 2b
      Ataxia-telangiectasia
    2. Low incidence of association with malignancy
      Neurofibroma
      Peutz-Jeghers syndrome
      Basal cell carcinoma nevus syndrome
      Bloom's syndrome

leukemia, carcinoid, polycythemia vera (in which pruritus often occurs after exposure to heat), and, less commonly, carcinoma. The itching may be mild or severe, localized or generalized, intermittent or constant. In Hodgkin's disease, itching is usually continuous and may be localized to the feet and lower part of the body, only later to become generalized. Up to 30 per cent of patients with Hodgkin's disease may itch. Pruritus of leukemia has a greater tendency to be generalized and may evolve into generalized erythroderma. Carcinomas of the gastrointestinal tract, lung, ovary, and prostate may also be associated with itching, which may precede recognition of these cancers by a year. Although dry skin (xerosis) is the most common cause of pruritus, other systemic causes of this bothersome symptom should be sought in addition to malignant disease, including drug reactions, cholestatic liver disease, uremia, diabetes, and thyroid disease.

Erythroderma, or exfoliative dermatitis, is a cutaneous reaction pattern with various causes. In 10 per cent of patients, total-body cutaneous redness, edema, scaling, and lichenification are associated with malignancy. In clinical practice the usual cause of exfoliative dermatitis is either a drug reaction or a generalized exacerbation of a pre-existing dermatosis such as atopic dermatitis, psoriasis, or contact dermatitis. When it is due to malignant disease, erythroderma is most pathognomonic of Hodgkin's disease, less frequently seen in lymphocytic leukemia, or rarely associated with underlying carcinoma. Erythroderma may be the first sign of Hodgkin's disease or leukemia. Skin biopsies do not reveal lymphomatous or leukemic infiltrates, although the patients clinically look similar to those with Sézary's syndrome (in which skin biopsies display diagnostic Sézary cells).

Figurate erythemas are red, gyrate, serpiginous, and annular bands that take on a pattern reminiscent of a wood grain and have been given descriptive names such as erythema gyratum repens and erythema annular centrifugum. These lesions are occasionally associated with neoplasia, especially breast and lung cancer.

Urticaria-like lesions, flesh-colored to red pruritic papules, nodules, and plaques, at times accompany leukemia, so-called leukemids. They may precede the development of leukemia by many months, and biopsy of the lesions does not show malignant cells. Treatment and control of leukemia often result in clearing.

Acquired hypertrichosis lanuginosa (malignant down), the sudden onset of excessive growth of fine, long, unpigmented fetal hair (lanugo) over the face, trunk, and limbs, has been associated with breast, uterine, pancreatic, pulmonary, and gastrointestinal carcinomas as well as lymphomas.

Herpes zoster is increased in incidence in patients with Hodgkin's disease and chronic lymphocytic leukemia as well as with a variety of neoplasms that are being managed with chemotherapy. This is evidence of the important role that impaired cellular immunity plays in activating viral replication. The painful, unilateral, grouped, clear, and often hemorrhagic umbilicated vesicles in a dermatomal distribution are readily recognized (see Ch. 374).

A number of miscellaneous dermatoses have occasionally been associated with internal malignant disease, but it is not entirely clear whether these associations are real or fortuitous. Table 163–5 lists some of these.

TABLE 163–5. DERMATOSES ASSOCIATED WITH INTERNAL MALIGNANT DISEASE

Dermatosis	Associated Cancer
Bullous lesions: pemphigoid, pemphigus, dermatitis herpetiformis	Rectal, breast, larynx, lymphoma
Tylosis: palmar hyperkeratosis	Esophagus
Acquired ichthyosis	GI leiomyosarcoma, lymphoma, multiple myeloma, lung, breast
Palmar fasciitis and polyarthritis: palmar fascial thickening with erythema, swelling of palms and dorsum of hands	Ovary

Syndromes and Entities Associated with Internal Neoplasia

A number of unique cutaneous syndromes, both genetic and nongenetic, are associated with internal neoplasms with sufficient frequency to alert the clinician to look for these potentially curable neoplasms early in their evolution. In some instances there is a high incidence of associated neoplasms, while in others this association is less clear.

NONGENETIC SYNDROMES AND ENTITIES ASSOCIATED WITH INTERNAL MALIGNANT DISEASE

HIGH INCIDENCE OF CUTANEOUS LESIONS ASSOCIATED WITH MALIGNANCY. *Paget's disease* of the breast is invariably found with an underlying intraductal mammary carcinoma. Erythematous scaling or weeping, sharply marginated patches on the nipple and areola of one breast should alert the clinician to examine the breast carefully. A breast mass may not be palpable or may not be definitely found with mammography, but in virtually every case an underlying carcinoma is present. Paget's disease can also occur in the anogenital region (extramammary Paget's disease). In this disorder, eczematous, pruritic, crusted, lichenified, well-demarcated patches may involve the lower abdominal wall, inguinal regions, genitalia, or perianal area. In up to 50 per cent of such patients, an underlying carcinoma of the rectum, prostate, urethra, other parts of the genitourinary tract, or apocrine gland is found. Biopsies taken from mammary and extramammary Paget's disease show the same diagnostic features, namely, large, round cells with clear cytoplasm in the epidermis (Paget's cells).

Stewart-Treves syndrome is the occasional occurrence of lymphoangiosarcoma as a complication of chronic lymphedema of the arm after radical mastectomy for carcinoma of the breast. Angiomatous, livid, or dusky red blebs and nodules exuding fluid may evolve from 2 to 20 years following mastectomy and the onset of the lymphedema. Angiosarcoma has also developed in congenital lymphedema as well as in lymphedema of the legs following surgery for cervical cancer.

Acanthosis nigricans (see Color Plate 16G) presents as soft, velvety, verrucous, brown hyperpigmentation of the body folds, especially those of the neck, axillae, and groin. When it occurs in patients over the age of 40 years, it is often a sign of an underlying malignant tumor, usually adenocarcinoma (most often stomach, gastrointestinal tract, and uterus; less commonly ovary, prostate, breast, and lung) and rarely lymphoma. Acanthosis nigricans involving the tongue and oral mucosa is highly suggestive of underlying malignancy. Acanthosis nigricans may appear before the malignant neoplasm 20 per cent of the time. Regression of the skin sign following therapy for the tumor and reappearance with reactivation of the tumor have been observed, suggesting that the underlying tumor secretes an as yet unidentified substance that is responsible for the verrucoid skin lesions. Acanthosis nigricans is more commonly found in individuals under 40 years of age, and then it is not usually associated with malignancy but rather with obesity or a variety of endocrinopathies (Cushing's disease, acromegaly, polycystic ovaries, hypothyroidism and hyperthyroidism, insulin-resistant diabetes). It also occurs on a familial basis. Special concern must be given to nonobese adults who have recently developed the verrucous areas in body folds. In 80 to 90 per cent of all instances the cancer arises in the stomach.

Dermatomyositis (see Color Plate 16H) developing in individuals over 40 years of age also calls for a careful search for underlying carcinoma (see Ch. 268). Although there is disagreement whether the incidence of internal malignant disease is increased in dermatomyositis, numerous cases have been reported with this association. Not uncommonly the dermatomyositis resolves upon removal of the carcinoma, but the syndrome recurs if the tumor reappears. In some instances the dermatomyositis precedes the cancer by several years. The search for neoplasm should be continued, therefore, even if the initial evaluation fails to find it, especially with (1) failure of the dermatomyositis to respond to conventional therapy (i.e., after systemic steroids), (2) a history of previous malignant disease, or (3) presence of atypical symptoms of the dermatomyositis. Malignant tumors of the breast and lung are those most commonly associated with dermatomyositis. Dermatomyositis is recognized by proximal muscle pain and weakness and a characteristic dermatitis that includes heliotrope rash (edematous, dusky, violaceous discoloration of the eyelids) along with a brilliant violaceous, erythematous telangiectatic scaling rash over the cheeks, forehead, V of the neck, elbows, and knees. Gottron's papules, slightly elevated red to violaceous papules or small plaques over the knuckles, are also an important finding in dermatomyositis.

The *Leser-Trélet sign*, the sudden appearance and growth of multiple seborrheic keratoses, occurs with underlying cancer in the elderly. This sign has been the subject of controversy, since seborrheic keratoses of the same histologic type are common in the elderly. Nevertheless, several case reports have described new and enlarging keratoses in association with cancer of the lung, adenocarcinoma of the bowel, mycosis fungoides, and Sézary's syndrome and, in some of these patients, the keratoses regressed when the malignant tumor was treated.

Necrolytic migratory erythema, associated with α-cell tumors of the pancreas and elevated glucagon levels, evolves as gradually enlarging erythematous patches with central, superficial blister formation progressing to central crusting and healing. Annular and figurate lesions result, with exudative, erosive, and crusting areas most pronounced in the perineum, groin, and perioral areas. Painful glossitis may be another prominent sign of the glucagonoma syndrome. The skin rash and stomatitis often resolve within a week after the tumor is removed. The pathogenesis of the skin and mucous membrane lesions is unclear. The glucagonoma syndrome is discussed more completely in Ch. 220. Similar skin lesions may be seen in association with severe zinc deficiency.

Bazex syndrome, or acrokeratosis paraneoplastica, is a unique cutaneous marker of carcinomas of the upper respiratory tract, especially seen with squamous cell carcinomas of the oral, pharyngeal, laryngeal, esophageal, and bronchial areas, primarily in males. When the tumor is asymptomatic, red to violaceous, scaling, psoriasis-like patches are found confined to the bridge of the nose, the fingers, toes, and margins of the ear helices. The nail folds are often red, scaling, and tender with grooving of the nails and onycholysis. Later the eruption on the acral areas becomes more extensive, spreading from the fingers to the palms and soles, which, in turn, become red and scaling and form a honeycomb-like thickening. The fingers and toes become violaceous and bulbous, and the rash evolves on the nose. In the last stage, if the tumor has not been treated and has progressed, new scaling lesions resembling psoriasis spread over the face, trunk, knees, arms, and scalp. Nail dystrophy (ridged, brittle, crumbling nails) is extensive.

Clubbing of the fingers is a well-known manifestation of bronchogenic carcinoma, mesothelioma, metastatic carcinoma to the thorax (from the colon, larynx, breast, or ovary) and occasionally Hodgkin's disease. *Hypertrophic pulmonary osteoarthropathy* is the term used when clubbing is accompanied by subperiosteal new bone formation along the shafts of the long bones of the extremities and digits. Joints of the ankle, knee, wrists, and hand may be painful and swollen. In some patients cutaneous thickening of the forearms and legs produces cylindric enlargement of the limbs, and the facial features become coarse with deep facial furrows simulating acromegaly. At times, deep confluent skin wrinkles evolve over the forehead and scalp, a condition termed *pachydermoperiostosis* when the skin changes accompany acromegaloid features.

Carcinoid, malignant tumor of the chromaffin cells of the gastrointestinal tract and, less frequently, the bronchus, may be associated with intermittent scarlet to violet red flushing of the head, neck, and upper part of the trunk. Eventually the erythema becomes permanent, and telangiectasis and tortuous veins evolve in the flushed areas. This syndrome and its cutaneous manifestations are described more fully in Ch. 230.

LOW INCIDENCE OF CUTANEOUS LESIONS ASSOCIATED WITH MALIGNANCY. *Amyloid deposits* in the skin may occur without obvious cause (cutaneous amyloidosis) as part of an inherited syndrome or secondary to plasma cell dyscrasias—either primary systemic amyloidosis or multiple myeloma. In the case of plasma cell dyscrasias, shiny, translucent, waxy, firm purpuric papules and plaques occur on the mucocutaneous junctions of the eyes, nose, and mouth along with macroglossia. Occasionally, infiltrated papules are not apparent, and only purpuric lesions evolve around the eyes ("raccoon eyes").

Urticaria pigmentosa consists of skin lesions that appear as numerous red-brown macules and papules on the trunk and extremities. Light stroking of the skin lesions causes urtication with edema and a red flare due to the release of histamine from the mast cells infiltrating the skin (Darier's sign). These skin lesions are sometimes associated with systemic mastocytosis (see Ch. 252) or, more rarely, with mast cell leukemia or myeloproliferative disorders (myelofibrosis, myeloid metaplasia, polycythemia, and granulocytic leukemia) with extensive infiltration of mature mast cells in the marrow and mast cells or basophils in the peripheral blood.

Bowen's disease of the skin consists of multiple superficial squamous cell cancers occurring in non–sun-exposed areas of the body, particularly in individuals with a history of long-term ingestion or exposure to arsenicals (drinking of well water, exposure to insecticides or industrial arsenicals). Bowen's skin lesions appear as discrete, red, scaling, flat to slightly raised patches that mimic eczematous or psoriatic patches. These skin lesions should be removed to prevent progression to invasive squamous cell carcinoma. The relationship of these lesions to internal malignancy is controversial, but a careful search for cancers of the larynx, lung, esophagus, liver, and bladder is warranted.

Sweet's syndrome (acute febrile neutrophilic dermatosis) is associated rarely with underlying chronic myelogenous leukemia. Red, tender, infiltrated plaques and annular lesions are distributed asymmetrically on the face, neck, and upper arms. The skin lesions consist of massive polymorphonuclear infiltration of the dermis, of unknown cause. Patients with Sweet's syndrome also suffer from fever, malaise, peripheral leukocytosis, arthralgias and arthritis, and conjunctivitis and episcleritis. Peripheral leukocyte counts generally range from 15,000 to 20,000 with 80 to 90 per cent mature polymorphonuclear leukocytes. Careful evaluation of the peripheral cells and occasionally of the bone marrow is indicated because of the possibility of coincident myelogenous leukemia.

GENETIC SYNDROMES ASSOCIATED WITH INTERNAL MALIGNANT DISEASE

HIGH INCIDENCE OF ASSOCIATION WITH INTERNAL MALIGNANCY. *Gardner's syndrome* consists of multiple epidermoid and sebaceous cysts of the face and scalp, fibrous tissue tumors of the skin (desmoid tumors, fibromas and fibrosarcomas), osteomas of the membranous bones of the face and head, and polyps of the colon and rectum (Ch. 105). No patients with this syndrome live beyond the seventh decade without developing adenocarcinoma of the bowel.

Cowden's disease, a condition in which there are numerous hamartomas of the skin, mucous membranes, and internal organs, is associated with malignant neoplasms of the breast and thyroid in a high percentage of patients. The hamartomas present on the skin as keratotic, warty papules and nodules on the central area of the face and on the hands and arms. Papular, cobblestone lesions may appear on the gingiva, palate, tongue, and larynx.

Torre's syndrome, another autosomal dominant condition, consists of multiple sebaceous gland tumors, sebaceous adenomas, sebaceous hyperplasia, and basal cell cancers with sebaceous differentiation. It is associated with cancers of the colon, duodenum, ampulla of Vater, uterus, and genitourinary tract. The skin tumors in this condition are yellowish or red papules and nodules.

Multiple Endocrine Neoplasia Type 2b (see Ch. 228). Medullary carcinoma of the thyroid and pheochromocytoma are found in association with a marfanoid habitus and multiple whitish to pink papular mucosal neuromas studding the lips, tip of the tongue, and, less often, the buccal mucosa, gingivae, palate, and pharynx. Neuromas also develop on the conjunctivae and corneas, and thickened corneal nerves may be found with slit-lamp examination.

Ataxia-telangiectasia, an autosomal recessive disorder associated with lymphomas, is recognized by telangiectasias over the ears, eyelids, nose, butterfly area of the face, and conjunctivae in association with progressive cerebellar ataxia, profound im-

munologic deficiency, and sinopulmonary infections (see Ch. 244). Hodgkin's disease, non-Hodgkin's lymphoma, or leukemia develops in 10 per cent of patients, with other malignant neoplasms such as ovarian dysgerminomas, gliomas, cerebellar medulloblastomas, and gastric adenocarcinomas occurring less frequently. Persons with *Wiskott-Aldrich syndrome* also display a propensity to malignant lymphomas (79 per cent) or leukemias (13 per cent) by the age of 10 years, probably related to widespread immunologic abnormalities of both the humoral and cell-mediated systems found in this condition. The skin changes are similar to atopic dermatitis (and are associated with petechiae due to thrombocytopenia).

LOW INCIDENCE OF ASSOCIATION WITH INTERNAL MALIGNANCY. Some dominant inherited conditions are associated with internal malignancy, but the relationship is not frequently found. Thus, patients with *neurofibromatosis* have café-au-lait spots, axillary freckles, and multiple neurofibromas. They are prone to develop pheochromocytomas (10 per cent of patients by the age of 60 years), acoustic neuromas, and neurofibrosarcomas.

Patients with the *Peutz-Jeghers syndrome* have numerous brown-black macules on the lips, perioral regions, hands, and feet in association with hamartomatous polyps of the small bowel, stomach, and, less commonly, colon (see Ch. 105). Malignancy occasionally develops in the polyps. *Nevoid basal cell carcinoma syndrome* is occasionally associated with the development of medulloblastoma or fibrosarcoma of the jaw.

Bloom's syndrome (telangiectatic redness of the skin in photoexposed areas and stunted growth) and the *Chédiak-Higashi syndrome* (light coloration of skin and hair) are autosomal recessive conditions associated with a propensity to develop leukemias and lymphomas.

Braverman IM: Skin Signs of Systemic Disease. Philadelphia, W. B. Saunders Company, 1981. *This classic book, on all skin signs associated with systemic disease, has many useful pictures of the cutaneous lesions related to internal malignant disease.*

Callen JP: Cutaneous Aspects of Internal Disease. Chicago, Year Book Medical Publishers, 1981. *This book, written by a number of authoritative authors, reviews in detail the varied manifestations of cutaneous signs of internal malignancy. Part 3 is especially useful in covering the hematologic and oncologic cutaneous signs of systemic lymphomas and carcinomas.*

Thiers BH, Maize C (eds.): Symposium on Cutaneous T Cell Lymphoma and Related Disorders. Dermatol Clin Vol. 3, No. 4, 1985. *A series of articles relating to the basic scientific and clinical features of cutaneous lymphomas by a number of authorities in the field.*

164 Principles of Cancer Therapy

Sydney E. Salmon

The treatment of hematologic malignancies and solid tumors is now an integral component of internal medicine. Over the past few decades the development of effective anticancer drugs has resulted in the progressive integration of medical management with surgery and radiotherapy into the initial multimodal treatment of cancer. The approaches to medical management have expanded with the development of new cytotoxic and endocrine agents and with the introduction of biologic therapy based on recombinant synthesis of interferons and cytokines. Medical management of complications of cancer represents an additional important aspect of the care of the cancer patient. It is therefore essential that the internist also be familiar with palliative aspects of cancer care, including management of pain syndromes (see Ch. 26) and treatment of life-threatening complications of cancer (see Ch. 165).

Although systemic therapy is currently curative in relatively few forms of metastatic cancer, it is now increasingly effective as a component of multimodal management of apparently localized cancers known to have a high frequency of occult micrometastatic spread. This approach has generally been predicted on the availability of specific systemic agents with antitumor activity in advanced cancers of the same histopathology. Not all patients are candidates for attempts at curative cancer therapy because of limitations in the available anticancer drugs and also because of comorbidity from other medical problems associated with increasing age. To a significant extent, cancer is a disease of the elderly, and treatment for many types of cancer in patients over the age of 65 remains quite difficult, perhaps owing to reduced host tolerance to the toxicities of many cancer chemotherapeutic agents. Thus it is important that the patient and his or her family be fully informed about the nature of the treatment planned, whether it is of curative or palliative intent. Inasmuch as prognosis for individual patients is currently based on statistical estimates, the physician must evaluate each patient individually in relation to relevant prognostic factors in attempting to establish prognosis and develop a treatment plan.

This chapter highlights the general principles, modalities, and therapeutic agents currently used in "comprehensive cancer management." At present, systemic therapy as the sole therapeutic approach is most effective against some of the hematologic malignancies and more rapidly proliferating solid tumors. For many types of cancer, current therapy other than surgery and/or radiotherapy is of only limited efficacy. However, identification and effective use of systemic agents accounts for most of the progress made in cancer treatment over the past two decades. The successes achieved provide impetus for additional basic and clinical cancer treatment research. At the basic science level there is increased understanding of the molecular abnormalities in cancer. As a result, a new era is beginning in which the

paradigms for cancer treatment are changing to more fully integrate fundamental understanding of cancer into approaches to both cancer treatment and cancer prevention.

DEVELOPMENT OF A TREATMENT PLAN

The major clinical features of cancer to be considered in developing a treatment plan include (1) specific histologic diagnosis of the neoplasm, (2) tumor burden (stage) and extent of specific organ involvement, and (3) biologic characteristics and other prognostic factors relevant to the specific type of cancer.

DIAGNOSIS. Accurate histologic diagnosis and staging critically influence treatment selection. Increasingly, immunohistochemical analysis is of help in subtyping lymphomas and in distinguishing among various morphologically "undifferentiated" neoplasms. In individual patients, undifferentiated or poorly differentiated tumors can be proven with immunohistochemistry to be lymphoma, melanoma, germ cell neoplasm, sarcoma, and so on (Fig. 164–1). Tumors of such diverse histogenesis can have markedly different prognosis and treatment. On occasion, electron microscopy is also helpful by identifying specific morphologic features such as melanosomes (in melanoma) or desmosomes (in carcinomas) that permit more specific classification. For some specific neoplasms, other distinctive biologic markers can be of value and identified with immunohistochemistry, hormone receptor expression, serum or urinary tumor markers (e.g., β-hCG, α-fetoprotein, carcinoembryonic antigen, CA-125, myeloma proteins, urinary 5-hydroxyindole acetic acid), karyotype, or molecular analysis. Increasingly, molecular biologic methods for DNA analysis are also playing a role in diagnosis by identifying characteristic gene rearrangements (e.g., Southern blots), gene dele-

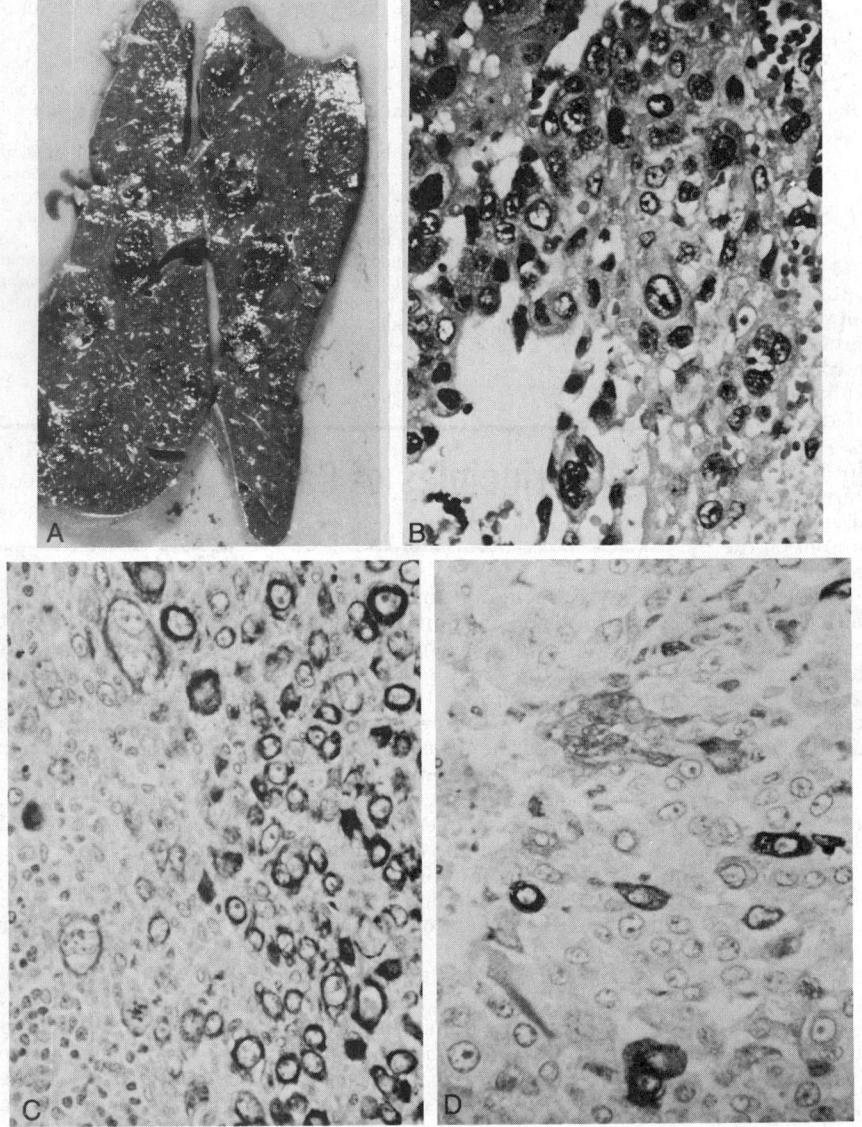

FIGURE 164–1. Example of the value of immunohistochemistry for cancer diagnosis. A 70-year-old man presented in shock with an acute abdomen. At emergency laparotomy he was found to have a ruptured spleen and hemoperitoneum as well as multiple metastatic lesions in the liver, spleen, and omentum. A, Gross appearance of spleen on cut section. B, By light microscopy the routine H & E–stained sections were interpreted as showing an undifferentiated large cell neoplasm. C, Positive immunoperoxidase stain for keratin established that the neoplasm was a carcinoma and excluded both large cell lymphoma and metastatic melanoma. Pertinent negative immunohistochemical findings (not shown) included stains for the S-100 antigen (melanoma) and leukocyte common antigen or anti-CD45 (lymphoma). D, Positive immunoperoxidase stain for β-hCG suggests the diagnosis of metastatic choriocarcinoma. The patient was then found to have a blood titer of 40,000 units per milliliter for β-hCG. Thus specialized testing changed the diagnosis from an undifferentiated cancer of unknown origin to a potentially treatable metastatic germ cell neoplasm. In this specific patient, clinical examination of the testes was negative for neoplasm. (Immunopathologic study by Dr. Raymond Nagle, University of Arizona College of Medicine, Tucson.)

TABLE 164–1. PROTO-ONCOGENE EXPRESSION OF IMPORTANCE IN PATHOGENESIS OF HUMAN NEOPLASMS

Neoplasm	Oncogene
Burkitt's lymphoma	c-myc
Follicular lymphoma	bcl-2
Chronic myelogenous leukemia	c-abl
Breast cancer	Her-2/neu
Ovarian cancer	Her-2/neu
Neuroblastoma	n-myc

tions, or oncogene expression. In recent years, cellular proto-oncogene amplification and expression have been linked to the pathogenesis of various neoplasms (Table 164–1).

In the leukemias and lymphomas, such information can prove important for selecting appropriate treatment approaches. For example, the approach to treatment of T-cell or B-cell lymphomas differs as a function of cell lineage, and this often cannot be identified with standard histologic approaches. Accordingly, it is important that the surgeon provide fresh tissue to the pathologist for cytogenetic or flow cytometric analysis; for touch preparations; or for cryopreservation for immunohistochemistry, receptor, or DNA analysis. Many of these specialized tests cannot be performed on tumor tissue that has been fixed. These specialized studies can in some instances provide evidence for a treatable or curable form of cancer that otherwise might go unrecognized. It is therefore very useful to obtain specialized pathologic studies prior to initiation of treatment.

STAGING. Assessment of the body burden of cancer by clinical means (staging) is important in developing the patient's treatment plan. Most staging systems assess the size of the primary tumor and define regional lymph node involvement, as well as the presence or absence of distant metastatic disease. It is important to distinguish between clinical and pathologic staging and to recognize that pathologic staging employing surgical biopsy is generally more accurate. Increasingly, staging can be accomplished by using noninvasive imaging procedures such as chest radiography and magnetic resonance imaging (MRI) or computerized tomography (CT) scanning. In the diagnostic workup of specific forms of cancer, such as breast or prostate cancer, a bone scan can be very useful when the tumor appears to be advanced but is of minimal use in early localized disease unless the patient has skeletal symptoms. For multiple myeloma, bone scans are of less use than skeletal radiographs. The temptation to use a variety of redundant and expensive tests such as CT, MRI, and ultrasonography for the same site in the same patient should be avoided. When invasive procedures such as staging laparotomy are considered, it is important to focus on the benefit-to-risk ratio of the procedure. In this appraisal the patient's age, performance status, concomitant medical problems, and histologic diagnosis all must be considered and the procedure carried out only if it appears likely to make a major and favorable improvement in the treatment plan. For patients who present with life-threatening local complications of cancer (e.g., spinal cord compression, upper airway obstruction, the superior vena cava syndrome, or obstructive jaundice), it is usually necessary first to treat the local complication on an urgent basis with irradiation, surgery, or chemotherapy before tumor staging can be completed.

OVERALL ASSESSMENT. Once diagnosis and staging have been performed, the information must be integrated to develop an optimal treatment plan for the individual patient. For patients with apparently localized cancers, multidisciplinary input is important, as a combined-modality approach to treatment may be indicated. The biologic characteristics of the specific cancer must also be considered. For many tumor types, histopathologic features such as grade of tumor cell differentiation are important, with a less differentiated or undifferentiated phenotype indicating a more aggressive neoplasm. For some sites, other biologic tests are of greater value than histologic grade. For example, in breast cancer, the presence or absence of estrogen or progesterone receptors and the DNA-index and ploidy status as determined by flow cytometry provide information that is useful in developing a treatment plan related to the aggressiveness of the neoplasm. Some patients with a minimal tumor burden (e.g., stage I) of currently incurable B-cell neoplasms (e.g., chronic lymphocytic

leukemia [CLL] and multiple myeloma) are best watched expectantly rather than treated. On the other hand, almost all patients with diffuse large cell (intermediate or high grade) lymphoma should be treated aggressively with curative intent irrespective of stage unless they are very elderly with other major medical problems. It is also important to recognize the severe limitations of current therapy for advanced or metastatic melanoma, pancreatic cancer, and non–small cell lung cancer.

Overall, the physician must synthesize a wide variety of pathologic, staging, and biologic information to reach a decision on therapy for the specific patient. In this context, it is important to decide whether curative therapy is available or not, and if so, whether the patient's age and overall medical condition permit a curative approach to be taken. If cure is not an option with available therapy, one must consider whether significant palliation with prolongation of survival (and relief of symptoms) can be achieved. For old and infirm patients a palliative approach may be preferable—particularly if there is significant morbidity associated with the treatment approach under consideration. On the other hand, some forms of cancer therapy are very effective and well tolerated even with advanced age (e.g., use of tamoxifen in adjuvant therapy of postmenopausal breast cancer or of chlorambucil for CLL). For many tumor types it is important to examine results of recent prospective clinical trials relevant to the patient's diagnosis and clinical setting.

THERAPEUTIC MODALITIES

There are currently three primary therapeutic approaches in the treatment of cancer: surgery, radiation therapy, and medical therapy.

Surgery

Cancer surgery is most useful to establish a tissue diagnosis, to excise the primary tumor with clear surgical margins free of tumor, and to determine the extent of cancer with surgical staging procedures. Surgery is a simple and safe means to remove solid tumors when the tumor is confined to a specific anatomic site of origin. However, in the case of some solid tumors, most patients already have metastatic disease at the time of presentation. In evaluating major surgery for an individual patient it is important to assess the operative risk-to-benefit ratio for the procedure in light of the patient's general health status, the extent of the tumor, and the likelihood that it can be completely removed. Additionally, the technical complexity of the surgical procedure, the type of anesthesia needed, and the experience of the personnel must also be considered. There are a number of specific roles that surgery can play in cancer treatment (Table 164–2).

With advances in both radiation and chemotherapy, the need for radical surgery has diminished. However, it remains a major primary approach to curative cancer therapy. For testicular cancer, even in the presence of limited metastatic disease, regional lymphadenectomy following radical orchiectomy can be curative and eliminate the need for chemotherapy in some patients who have metastases only to retroperitoneal lymph nodes. For many other sites, surgical resection of regional lymph nodes is carried out for diagnostic rather than therapeutic purposes, as involved regional nodes usually signify that the cancer has already disseminated. For example, in breast cancer, the presence or absence of axillary lymph node involvement is the

TABLE 164–2. APPLICATIONS OF SURGERY IN THE TREATMENT OF CANCER

1. Definitive treatment for primary cancer as a single modality
2. Use in combination with radiation and/or chemotherapy
3. Debulking residual disease (e.g., ovarian cancer) after resection of the primary
4. Resection of metastatic disease with curative intent (testicular cancer, pulmonary metastases in sarcoma)
5. Determining the extent of cancer, including regional node involvement (pathologic staging)
6. Treatment of emergency complications (e.g., obstructed viscus)
7. Palliation of symptoms and signs of locally invasive or metastatic cancer
8. Reconstruction and rehabilitation

single most important factor in evaluating the likelihood of distant recurrence, and this information is currently not obtainable by nonsurgical means. Similarly, surgical staging of nodal involvement in colorectal cancer plays an important role in deciding on whether adjuvant systemic chemotherapy is indicated.

Initial cancer therapy often requires a multimodal approach to maximize the chance of cure while simultaneously reducing the extent of surgery required and preventing the development of distant metastases. Multimodal approaches necessarily require close communication between the involved physicians prior to surgery. The opportunity for early communication is improved with histopathologic diagnosis by needle biopsy or local excision of the primary cancer before more extensive therapy. Two examples are of note in this regard: (1) the management of osteogenic sarcoma with limb salvage surgery, irradiation, and adjuvant chemotherapy and (2) the management of early breast cancer with lumpectomy, axillary staging followed by primary irradiation, and adjuvant systemic administration of cytotoxic or endocrine agents. In both instances, the combined approach yields a better cosmetic and functional outcome. With advances in breast conservation surgery, screening mammography is now more widely utilized, as a diagnosis of breast cancer is no longer tantamount to a subsequent mastectomy. The result is an increased ability to establish a diagnosis of breast cancer when the tumor is less extensive and when likelihood of cure is greater. Improved plastic surgical techniques have also made breast reconstruction possible for women who either require or prefer mastectomy.

In addition to its use in diagnosis, staging, and primary therapy, cancer surgery also plays an important role in the management of some patients with more extensive cancer. In ovarian cancer, when the gynecologic oncologist "debulks" peritoneal and omental spread to the status of minimal residual disease, patients become better candidates for systemic chemotherapy and have a better survival. Additionally, early resection of pulmonary metastases of soft tissue sarcomas, and of solitary brain metastases in melanoma, colon, or breast cancer, may provide marked palliation and improved survival of patients, albeit with only occasional cures.

Radiation Therapy

From the time of its initial development in the early 1900's, radiation therapy has made major strides in instrumentation, physics, radiobiology, treatment planning, and applications to curative and palliative cancer therapy. In general, the term "radiation" refers to ionizing radiation that is either electromagnetic or particulate (e.g., γ rays). Compared to surgery, there are distinct advantages in the use of radiotherapy in the locoregional treatment of cancer. Radiation causes less acute morbidity and can provide curative therapy for some specific sites while preserving organ or tissue structure and function. An excellent example is the use of radiation for the curative treatment of early-stage laryngeal cancer wherein vocal function can be preserved.

The basic unit of ionizing irradiation is the **gray** (Gy) which has superseded the rad (1 Gy = 100 rads). By interaction with molecular oxygen, radiation induces the formation of superoxide, hydrogen peroxide, or hydroxyl radicals that then damage or break cellular DNA, which is considered to be the critical target for radiation-induced cell death. Both single- and double-strand breaks of the DNA helix can be induced, with the latter constituting lethal damage. Single strand breaks, if not repaired by the cell, can also result in cell death. With high linear transfer (LET) radiation, direct damage to the molecular structure of DNA can be induced.

Radiation has limitations in treatment of bulky tumors. Large tumors frequently have poorly perfused and hypoxic zones in which radiation often fails to give rise to needed reactive intermediaries. Various forms of irradiation are used for differing therapeutic objectives. For example, electron beam irradiation deposits most of its energy in the skin and soft tissues and can be useful for superficial therapy in mycosis fungoides. Low energy (kilovoltage) x-rays expend most of their effects on the overlying tissues above a deep-seated tumor and therefore cause considerable normal tissue damage. By contrast, higher energy x-rays

(megavoltage) or γ-irradiation from a cobalt 60 source spare the skin and deposit their energy at greater depth and provide a better approach to treating deep-seated neoplasms. Use of radioactive implants can also be useful in some settings (e.g., cervical cancer). The use of multiple irradiation fields reduces the dose to normal tissue while increasing the dose to the tumor. The use of fractionated doses or radiation causes less cumulative damage to normal tissues than to the tumor, as the normal tissues are often able to repair sublethal damage more quickly. Additionally, as a tumor shrinks with therapy, its oxygenation can improve and thereby render it more radiosensitive. The selection of treatment is based on the relative radiosensitivity of the tumor and of the normal organs and tissues within the radiation field (Table 164–3).

The combined use of multiple fields, fractionated irradiation, and megavoltage radiation equipment is optimized by detailed treatment planning individualized to the patient's tumor. Although the major uses of radiotherapy involve local irradiation of sites of tumor involvement, total body irradiation is a valuable part of a preparative regimen together with high-dose chemotherapy for allogeneic or autologous bone marrow transplantation for leukemia or lymphoma. Total body irradiation in doses in the range of 10 Gy induces permanent aplasia of normal bone marrow and profound immunosuppression and is used only in conjunction with marrow transplantation.

Radiation therapy also has important palliative applications. One of these is for bone pain due to metastatic involvement of the skeleton. Irradiation can also cause sufficient cytoreduction of tumor in bone to permit healing of osteolytic lesions and thereby prevent pathologic fractures of weight-bearing bones. Other examples include tumor shrinkage to relieve postobstructive infection in lung cancer and to suppress bronchial or gastric bleeding secondary to cancer.

Although modern radiotherapy with megavoltage equipment has proven to be extremely useful, some even higher energy radiation approaches are currently in development. These include the use of higher LET sources of irradiation (e.g., neutrons, charged particles, heavy ions) which may also provide selective advantages for specific tumor sites and reduce the need for oxygenation of tumor tissue. Additionally, several classes of compounds are under study as **radiosensitizers** to enhance the cytotoxic effects of radiation on tumor cells. One class is the halopyrimidines, including bromodeoxyuridine, fluorouracil, and fluorodeoxyuridine, which sensitize DNA to strand breakage by radiation. A second class includes the nitroimidazoles (structural analogues of metronidazole [Flagyl]), which can enhance radiation damage to hypoxic cells by accepting free electrons and forming free radicals with oxygen. Several sulfhydryl compounds are also under investigation as potential radioprotective agents. Such compounds would need to exhibit selective uptake in normal cells in order to increase the therapeutic index of radiation for tumor cells, and this approach also remains experimental.

Although the term "radiation" normally refers to ionizing irradiation, there are also several other forms of radiation used in cancer treatment. These include hyperthermia and photodynamic therapy, both of which are still undergoing development. Some tumors show thermal sensitivity to temperatures in the range of 41 to 43°C and may be more sensitive than surrounding normal tissues. Hyperthermia appears to work best on bulky

TABLE 164–3. TOLERANCE OF NORMAL TISSUES TO IRRADIATION

Tissue	Toxic Effect	Limiting Dose (Gy)*
Bone marrow	Aplasia	2.5
Lung	Pneumonitis, fibrosis	15.0
Kidney	Nephrosclerosis	20.0
Liver	Hepatitis	25.0
Spinal cord	Infarction, necrosis	45.0
Intestine	Ulceration, fibrosis	45.0
Heart	Pericarditis, myocarditis	45.0
Brain	Infarction, necrosis	50.0
Skin	Dermatitis, sclerosis	55.0

*Radiation in 2.0-Gy fractions to the whole organ for 5 days weekly produces a 5 per cent incidence of the listed toxicities at the limiting doses listed.

TABLE 164–4. RESPONSIVENESS OF CANCER TO CHEMOTHERAPY*

Tumor Type	Useful Agents
A. Curable with chemotherapy in some patients and exhibiting improved survival in those not cured	
Choriocarcinoma (adjuvant, advanced)	MTX, VCR, Plat, Etop
Acute lymphocytic leukemia	VCR, Pred, Daun, MP, MTX
Acute nonlymphocytic leukemia	Ara-C, Daun, Mitox
Malignant lymphoma (Hodgkin's disease, diffuse high or intermediate grade non-Hodgkin's lymphoma)	Adr, Alk, VCR, Pred, Pro
Testicular carcinoma (advanced)	Plat, Etop, Bleo, VBL
Childhood sarcomas (adjuvant)	Adr, VCR, Alk, Act-D
Wilms' tumor (adjuvant)	VCR, Act-D
Osteosarcoma (adjuvant)	Adr, MTX, Alk, Plat
Rectal carcinoma (adjuvant)	FU, Mito, Nit
B. Improved survival after chemotherapy	
Breast carcinoma (adjuvant, advanced)	Alk, MTX, FU, Adr, Mito, VCR, Mitox, Tam
Ovarian carcinoma (adjuvant, advanced)	Plat, Alk
Multiple myeloma	Alk, Pred, VCR, Adr, IFN
Small cell lung carcinoma	Alk, Plat, Etop, Adr
Colon carcinoma (adjuvant)	FU, Lev
C. Useful palliation of symptoms of advanced cancer with chemotherapy but with limited or no improvement in survival	
Chronic myeloid leukemia	Alk, HU, IFN
Non-Hodgkin's lymphomas—low grade	Alk, Pred, IFN
Prostatic carcinoma	Endo, Sur
Thyroid carcinoma	Plat, FU, Adr
Soft tissue sarcomas	Adr, Dac
Head and neck carcinoma (combined modality)	Plat, FU
Bladder carcinoma	Plat, VBL, MTX, Adr
Esophageal (combined modality)	Plat, FU
D. Only occasionally responsive to current chemotherapy	
Primary brain tumors	Nit
Non–small cell lung carcinoma	Alk, Plat, Etop, MTX, FU, Adr
Melanoma	Dac, IFN
Gastric carcinoma	Plat, FU, Mito, Adr
Renal carcinoma	IFN, IL-2, VBL

*When indicated, favorable results obtained with adjuvant therapy are better than with surgery and/or radiation therapy. When annotated as "advanced," indicated results are obtained in the setting of overt metastatic cancer.

Act D = Actinomycin D; Adr = Adriamycin (doxorubicin); Alk = alkylating agent; Ara-C = cytarabine; Bleo = bleomycin; Dac = dacarbazine; Daun = daunorubicin; Endo = endocrine agent; Etop = Etoposide; FU = 5-fluorouracil; HU = hydroxyurea; IFN = interferon; IL-2 = interleukin-2; Lev = levamisole; Mito = mitomycin; Mitox = mitoxantrone; MP = 6-mercaptopurine; MTX = methotrexate; Nit = nitrogen mustard; Plat = platinum compound; Pred = prednisone; Pro = procarbazine; Sur = suramin; Tam = tamoxifen; VCR = vincristine; VBL = vinblastine.

tumors with poor blood supply in which the tumor cells are in an acidic environment. A variety of approaches is used to induce local or regional hyperthermia (e.g., ultrasonography, microwaves, regional perfusion) and may enhance the effects of ionizing irradiation or chemotherapy on local tumors.

Photodynamic therapy (PDT) is yet another form of nonionizing radiation therapy. PDT involves the preliminary systemic administration of a photosensitizing compound such as a hematoporphyrin derivative (e.g., dihematoporphyrin ether, Photofrin II). Such hematoporphyrins are concentrated in the vicinity of local tumors and can be activated with local exposure to visible red light (usually 630 nm), with a resulting preferential toxicity to cancer cells. The intense light used for PDT can be delivered via a fiberoptic probe, and therefore it can be used for various internal sites as well as on the skin. The mechanism of action of PDT is poorly understood but may involve vascular damage or a direct toxic effect on tumor cells. Side effects of photodynamic therapy include hypersensitivity to light (skin and eyes). Locally PDT induces transient sunburn and hyperpigmentation as well as local tumor necrosis. Tumor sites amenable to PDT include skin recurrences of breast cancer (e.g., chest wall) and malignant lesions in the endobronchus, peritoneal cavity, and bladder. Photodynamic therapy has not been approved by the Food and Drug Administration in the United States and therefore remains investigational.

Medical Therapy

As cancer may disseminate beyond its site of origin prior to diagnosis and because local treatment is frequently not curative, effective systemic drug therapy is needed. Limited clinical success with cytotoxic chemotherapy was first achieved about 40 years ago. Some of these early successes included findings that cytotoxic drugs could cure metastatic choriocarcinoma and induce complete remissions in children with acute leukemia. Subsequently, curative therapy was developed for a series of relatively uncommon neoplasms, and useful palliative therapy has been developed for some common forms of cancer (Table 164–4). With rare exceptions, effective therapy has utilized combinations of anticancer drugs. Increasingly, anticancer drugs are used in concert with surgery and/or irradiation.

Efforts to develop cytoxic and endocrine anticancer agents have been vigorous over the past two decades. Ideally, anticancer drugs should eradicate cancer without harming normal tissues; however, this goal has not been achieved, and most useful drugs have significant side effects. The introduction of anticancer drugs for clinical use has largely been predicted from animal tumor models. Perhaps because the initial murine models were for acute leukemia, many of the drugs that have been discovered are relatively general antiproliferative agents. Accordingly, they have greater efficacy in more rapidly proliferating tumors than in some of the more slowly growing solid tumors and are more toxic to rapidly growing tumors than to normal host tissues of the same histology. However, such generally antiproliferative agents can have significant toxic side effects on normal tissues that divide rapidly such as bone marrow, gastrointestinal mucosa, and skin.

CELL KINETICS AND RESPONSE TO CHEMOTHERAPY. A number of related factors, including total tumor burden, cell kinetics, and intrinsic sensitivity, influence the response to anticancer drugs. In both animal models and human tumors, growth occurs in accord with gompertzian kinetics. Initially growth occurs rapidly, and most tumor cells traverse the complete cell cycle. As the tumor burden grows larger, the rate of tumor cell doubling progressively slows (Fig. 164–2), and the fraction of cells traversing the cell cycle decreases as more and more cells remain "hung up" in a G_0 phase. Whereas the population doubling time may be in the range of 1 to 2 days at the subclinical phase (with less than 1 gram of tumor), by the time the tumor burden has reached 1 kg or more, the tumor cell population doubling time may be 3 to 6 months. A significant problem in the treatment of high tumor burden leukemias and metastatic solid tumors is that the tumor exhibits a significant degree of heterogeneity and subpopulations of cells exhibit differing biologic, kinetic, antigenic, and drug-sensitivity profiles.

Several important features related to cell kinetics and tumor burden are important with respect to drug dose, scheduling, and response to chemotherapy. Anticancer drugs can be classified as either cell cycle specific (CCS) or cell cycle nonspecific (CCNS) (Table 164–5). CCNS agents have greater effects on cycling than on noncycling cells but nonetheless can exert anticancer effects on noncycling cells, whereas CCS agents do not. Endocrine agents are also in a sense cycle-active, as they block the transition of tumor cells from G_1 to the S phase of the cell cycle. However, endocrine agents (e.g., prednisone, tamoxifen, progestins) are noncytotoxic and are considered to suppress growth rather than kill tumor cells. Endocrine agents are therefore often given for many years, whereas cytotoxic agents are usually given over a time course measured in months.

An important concept in cancer chemotherapy is that cellular killing with cytotoxic agents follows first-order kinetics, with a given dose of drug killing only a fraction of the tumor cells. This "fractional kill hypothesis" is particularly relevant to CCNS agents and predicts that the greater the dose of drug administered, the greater the "log kill" of tumor cells which will occur.

The concept of combination chemotherapy was developed to take advantage of the fact that many anticancer agents have

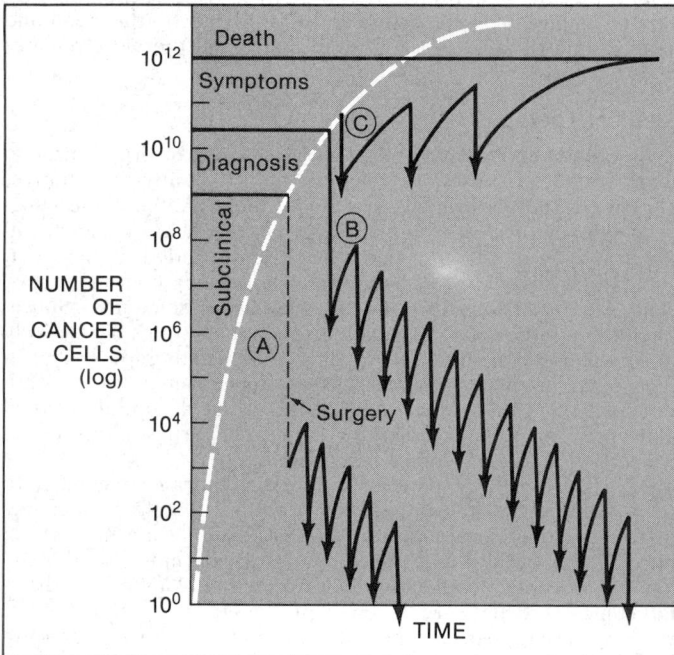

FIGURE 164–2. The relationship of tumor growth and tumor burden to treatment strategies and outcome with systemic chemotherapy. Human tumors grow in accord with the "Gompertz curve" *(dashed line)*, with a decreasing doubling time as tumor burden increases. Treatment interventions relate to tumor type and extent of disease. *A,* Surgery followed by pulse courses of adjuvant chemotherapy. *B,* Systemic chemotherapy for stage III Hodgkin's disease. *C,* Palliative chemotherapy for advanced non–small cell cancer. In *A,* combined modality has curative potential with the addition of chemotherapy after surgery. Cure is also possible in *B* with prolonged administration of combination chemotherapy. In *C,* the patient's tumor burden is too great and potency of the drugs for this specific form of cancer is inadequate. (Modified from Salmon SE, Sartorelli AC: Cancer chemotherapy. *In* Katzung BG (ed.): Basic and Clinical Pharmacology, 4th ed. Norwalk, CT, Appleton and Lange Co., 1989, p 685.)

differing mechanisms of action and side effects. This concept was based on the hypothesis that giving drugs with differing mechanisms of action may achieve synergistic antitumor effects while simultaneously retarding the rate of development of drug resistance. Additionally, by careful selection of drugs in a combination to include those with known single-agent activity against the tumor and different normal tissue toxicities, the side effects would be "spread" across different tissues and organs. The validity of this concept has been born out clinically, and optimal results for most tumor types sensitive to chemotherapy have been achieved with drug combinations, often employing CCNS and CCS agents with decidedly different mechanisms of action. For example, cisplatin has demonstrated clear-cut synergy with eto-

TABLE 164–5. RELATIONSHIP OF TUMOR CELL CYCLE TO ACTIVITY OF MAJOR CLASSES OF CYTOTOXIC ANTICANCER DRUGS

Cell Cycle–Specific (CCS) Agents	Cell Cycle–Nonspecific (CCNS) Agents
Antimetabolites (cytarabine, fluorouracil, methotrexate, mercaptopurine, hydroxyurea)	Alkylating agents (busulfan, cyclophosphamide, mechlorethamine, melphalan, thiotepa, chlorambucil)
Bleomycin	Antibiotics (dactinomycin, daunorubicin, doxorubicin, mitomycin)
Plant alkaloids (vincristine, vinblastine, etoposide, taxol)	Platinum compounds (cisplatin, carboplatin)
	Nitrosoureas (BCNU, CCNU)
	Dacarbazine
	Mitoxantrone
	L-Asparaginase

poside in testicular cancer and small cell lung cancer and with fluorouracil in both head and neck and esophageal cancer. The major potential toxicity for cisplatin is renal, whereas myelosuppression is the major side effect for both etoposide and fluorouracil.

New drugs entering clinical trials are normally first tested in patients with a large tumor burden of metastatic cancer who have relapsed from known effective chemotherapy regimens. Although this approach is ethically most acceptable, it nonetheless represents a significant obstacle to new drug development, as these patients have a lower probability of response to a new drug than those with a lower tumor burden or those who have not been previously treated. Additionally, some metastatic cells can gain access to pharmacologic sanctuaries (e.g., the central nervous system). The presence of the blood-brain barrier has been a major obstacle to the development of chemotherapy for primary or metastatic tumors in the brain. At present brain tumors are treated chiefly with surgery and radiation therapy.

DRUG RESISTANCE. For many of the drug-responsive tumor types listed in Table 164–3, major cytoreduction occurs with initial chemotherapy. However, some months to years thereafter, tumor regrowth occurs and continues even though therapy with the same drugs is reinstituted. This clinical observation usually reflects the acquisition of drug resistance by the tumor to the specific drugs used. In general, the development of drug resistance is considered to result from the high spontaneous mutation rate of cancer cells, which leads to the development of heterogeneous subpopulations, some of which exhibit resistance to various drugs. A variety of drug-resistance mechanisms has been identified in the laboratory, several of which have been documented to be clinically important. Perhaps the most important is a form of **multidrug resistance (MDR)**. MDR is mediated by a cell membrane glycoprotein (the **P-glycoprotein**), which functions as an energy-dependent efflux pump that actively extrudes a variety of cytotoxic agents from the cell (Fig. 164–3).

Drugs pumped out of the cancer cell by the P-glycoprotein include natural products such as plant alkaloids (vincas, podophyllotoxins), antibiotics (dactinomycin, doxorubicin, daunorubicin) and some synthetic agents (e.g., melphalan, mitoxantrone). The P-glycoprotein is normally expressed in tissues such as the gut and the kidney, perhaps to deal with toxic products in the environment. Cancer cells with mutations to "switch on" the expression of the gene responsible for encoding the P-glycoprotein show resistance to a wide variety of useful anticancer drugs. Techniques such as immunohistochemistry, Western blots, and

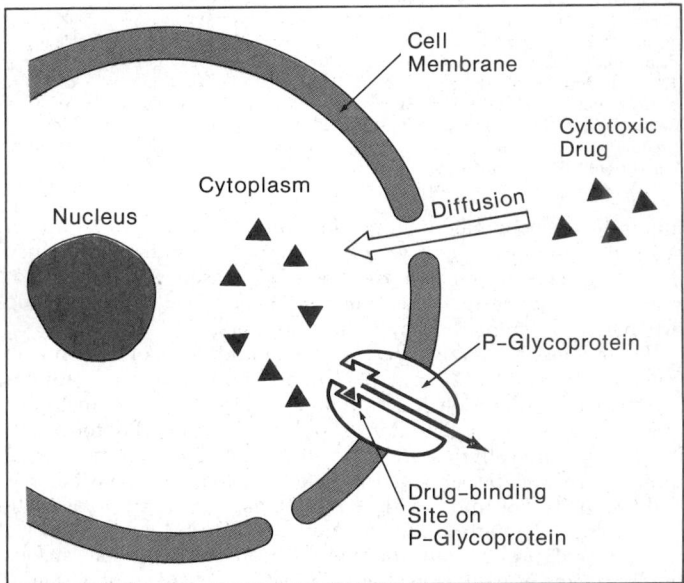

FIGURE 164–3. Model of cancer cell expressing P-glycoprotein. This transmembrane protein functions as an energy-dependent efflux pump or drug transporter. It has acceptor sites to which various natural product anticancer drugs bind, after which they are pumped out of the cell. Chemosensitizers such as verapamil also bind to the drug acceptor sites on P-glycoprotein and can competitively inhibit its function.

Northern blots can be used to detect the presence of P-glycoprotein in tumor tissues. Clinical studies suggest that patients whose tumors express P-glycoprotein have a poor prognosis. Culture studies performed on biopsy specimens in vitro have documented that P-glycoprotein–positive tumors usually exhibit resistance to doxorubicin. Tumor types such as sarcoma, neuroblastoma, malignant lymphoma, and myeloma are usually P-glycoprotein–negative at the time of diagnosis but are frequently positive for P-glycoprotein when the patient relapses from chemotherapy. A series of noncytotoxic drugs has been identified which are also subject to efflux by the P-glycoprotein (e.g., verapamil, cyclosporine, progestins). Such agents are now classified as **chemosensitizers** because they can competitively inhibit the function of P-glycoprotein in vitro by binding to the drug acceptor sites on the P-glycoprotein, inhibiting the efflux of the cytotoxic drug and thereby circumventing the drug resistance. In drug-resistant patients with malignant lymphoma and multiple myeloma, high doses of verapamil given simultaneously with vincristine and doxorubicin can reverse resistance to these agents, with some patients regaining remission. Although verapamil is not an ideal chemosensitizer (owing to its cardiovascular side effects), other potential chemosensitizers (quinidine, quinine, cyclosporine, nontoxic verapamil analogues) are now being tested in an effort to identify more effective and less toxic chemosensitizers. In the long run, such chemosensitizers may find their major use to prevent development of MDR expression.

An example of a more drug-specific mechanism of resistance has been identified for the antimetabolite methotrexate (MTX). MTX and its polyglutamated metabolites inhibit the function of the enzyme dihydrofolate reductase (DHFR). The normal function of DHRF in nucleic acid synthesis is to reduce inactive dihydrofolate to its active tetrahydrofolate form, which serves as a one-carbon donor for the synthesis of purine nucleotides and thymidylate. Some tumor cells that acquire MTX resistance have been found to have an increased number of DNA gene copies encoding for DHFR. This form of multiple gene reduplication is called **gene amplification.** The amplified DHFR genes in MTX-resistant cells produce a markedly increased number of copies of the DHFR enzyme, far exceeding the amount of MTX that can be delivered to the cell, and thereby allow tumor cell DNA synthesis and proliferation to continue. Gene amplification in mammalian cells has been observed only in tumor cells, but the phenomenon is not unique to MTX resistance.

PREDICTIVE TESTING IN VITRO. A variety of approaches has been developed to assess the probability of a patient's relapsing after primary therapy or responding to a given type or class of endocrine or cytotoxic agent. The goal of such efforts is to identify which patients might benefit from a planned treatment. The "S-phase" fraction of the tumor cell population undergoing DNA synthesis as well as DNA ploidy can be determined by flow cytometry. For several tumor types, patients with a high percentage of tumor cells in DNA synthesis and/or hyperdiploidy have a high likelihood of relapsing early after local primary cancer therapy. Taken with other prognostic characteristics, such flow cytometry assays may aid in identifying patients who should receive adjuvant chemotherapy. This approach is currently being applied in patients with stage I breast cancer in an effort to decide which patients are at higher risk for recurrence.

The results of S-phase and DNA ploidy analysis are often provided by diagnostic laboratories on breast cancer specimens along with the findings from estrogen and progesterone receptor testing. Estrogen and progesterone receptor assays in breast cancer have their primary use in identifying patients who are likely to respond to endocrine agents in either the adjuvant or recurrent cancer setting. These sex steroid hormone receptors are located in the cell nucleus and must bind the hormone and translocate it to cellular DNA to exert endocrine action via gene activation or suppression. Additionally, in the absence of adjuvant therapy, patients whose tumors are estrogen or progesterone receptor–positive have longer times to recurrence and a better overall prognosis than do patients whose tumors are receptor negative. Recent studies of another tumor cell constituent, the HER-2/neu oncogene, can be of prognostic value. Amplification of the number of copies of the HER-2/neu gene or increased expression of the gene product by RNA or protein analysis appears to predict a poor prognosis in both breast and ovarian cancer. The protein product of HER-2/neu is expressed on the surface of

tumor cells and structurally appears to be a hormone receptor analogous to the epidermal growth factor (EGF) receptor. However, the ligand for this presumed receptor has not yet been identified.

For specific anticancer drug testing, clonogenic and dye exclusion assays in vitro have been developed and applied with increasing success. Assays of this type are potentially of considerable value, because a critical factor regarding response to chemotherapy is the intrinsic sensitivity of the specific tumor to the agents being used for treatment. However, available techniques are labor intensive and must be applied to freshly biopsied and viable tumor specimens rapidly transferred to the testing laboratory. Chemosensitivity assays appear to be highly predictive of drug resistance but somewhat less accurate for predicting which drugs will be useful for an individual patient. Another type of testing for drug resistance that is now being applied to fresh frozen (and in some instances to fixed tissues) is immunohistochemical testing for P-glycoprotein expression.

PHARMACOKINETIC CONSIDERATIONS. Although intrinsic drug sensitivity appears to be the most critical determinant of response to chemotherapy, pharmacokinetic factors related to the route of administration, bioavailability, metabolism, and elimination are probably of greater importance in cancer therapy than in other areas of medicine. Many of the cytotoxic agents have a steep dose-response curve and a resulting narrow therapeutic index. Thus at too low an available dose level within the tumor, no response is seen. On the other hand, at higher doses, significant host toxicity supervenes and is usually dose-limiting. Because of the steep dose-response relationship, doses of most cytotoxic agents are calculated in relation to body surface area. This approach is more accurate than dose calculations based on body weight. The oral route of drug administration is often desired by patients but is not generally emphasized in cancer therapy, not only because of problems with compliance but also because of extremely marked variations in bioavailability in the blood after administration of oral formulations. For example, with the alkylating agent melphalan, more than a 10-fold variation in plasma levels has been documented after standard dosing. Unfortunately, plasma assays are not routinely available for most anticancer drugs, and the only semiquantitative indicator of bioavailability of cytotoxic agents is the occurrence of myelosuppression after drug administration. For patients presenting with hypercalcemia or other dire complications of myeloma, oral melphalan would therefore seem undesirable, as such patients need good drug bioavailability immediately. Similar difficulties are faced with oral administration of fluorouracil, methotrexate, and 6-mercaptopurine. On the other hand, for agents such as tamoxifen and cyclophosphamide, bioavailability is good after oral administration.

The intravenous route of drug administration is clearly preferable for most cytotoxic anticancer drugs, as it assures that adequate plasma levels can be achieved while minimizing problems with compliance. For some agents, continuous intravenous drug administration for 4 days or longer provides better results and less toxicity than do bolus or short-duration infusions. This is because tumor response for many agents can be related to the "area under the plasma disappearance curve (AUC)" for the drug, whereas toxicity generally relates more directly to peak plasma concentrations than to the AUC. With the advent of vascular access devices such as subcutaneous ports or external catheters and of sophisticated battery-powered infusion pumps, outpatient continuous infusion chemotherapy can now be used for stable drugs such as fluorinated pyrimidines, anthracyclines, and vinca alkaloids. Subcutaneous administration can be used effectively with drugs such as cytarabine, interferon-α, and erythropoietin. Subcutaneous dosing provides more sustained plasma levels than can be obtained with intravenous administration. Depot intramuscular formulations are available for a variety of endocrine agents used in treatment of breast or prostate cancer.

Regional administration of chemotherapy can also be used effectively for several tumor sites. One of these is metastatic colon cancer limited to the liver. Hepatic artery catheterization for arterial infusion of 5-fluorodeoxyuridine or 5-fluorouracil can be used effectively by connection of the catheter to an external pump or to an implantable perfusion pump. In either instance, arterial infusions are often administered for 14 days followed by a similar rest period. A relatively high objective response rate of metastatic colon cancer in the liver can be obtained by this means, but this route is ineffective for metastases outside the liver. Hepatic artery chemotherapy is expensive and associated with complications, including arterial thrombosis, biliary sclerosis, and chemical hepatitis. Nonetheless, it can induce sustained remissions for a year or more in selected patients with liver metastases. Regional infusion or isolated perfusion has been used with melanomas or sarcomas of the lower extremity. With intransit melanoma metastases of the lower extremity, melphalan or cisplatin has been administered in this fashion with or without regional hyperthermia.

Intracavitary drug administration has long been used in the bladder with instillation of a biologic agent such as BCG (bacille Calmette-Guérin) or interferon or a variety of cytotoxic agents (e.g., thiotepa, doxorubicin, mitomycin, cisplatin). Intraperitoneal drug administration has also gained increasing popularity and appears to show particular promise for patients with peritoneal carcinomatosis. It can induce remissions of established metastatic disease. In ovarian cancer intraperitoneal chemotherapy is being studied as a follow-up to cytoreductive surgery. Diffusion of intraperitoneally administered drugs is limited to a few millimeters of tumor tissue. Accordingly, intraperitoneal chemotherapy is seldom warranted in patients with bulky tumor masses. For optimal distribution, the drug is usually diluted in 2 liters of parenteral fluid for injection. Preferred drugs for intraperitoneal administration are those that tend to be largely limited to the peritoneal cavity and have good properties for tumor penetration. Mitoxantrone has these favorable characteristics, and cisplatin can also be quite useful. With both of these drugs, the intraperitoneal concentration of drug can be 1000-fold higher than measured in the systemic circulation. Other agents sometimes used in intraperitoneal administration include thiotepa, fluorouracil, and methotrexate. Intraperitoneal drug administration can be performed at repeated intervals with relative ease if a surgically implanted Tenkoff catheter is connected to a subcutaneous port. Mild to moderate chemical peritonitis and the development of peritoneal adhesions are common complications of intraperitoneal chemotherapy and limit repeated use.

The intrathecal route can be used to deliver therapy to the meninges. Both methotrexate and cytarabine can be given by this route for prevention of meningeal leukemia and for treatment of central nervous system leukemia or lymphoma. Intrathecal methotrexate has been used effectively for acute lymphoblastic leukemia as an adjuvant to initial systemic chemotherapy and has reduced the frequency of central nervous system relapse in patients in complete peripheral remission.

EVALUATION OF RESPONSE. Objective measurement of tumor shrinkage with medical or radiation therapy has prognostic importance. Subjective improvement alone is not evidence of response. Cure or significant prolongation of survival is seen in patients who achieve complete response (disappearance of all evidence of cancer). Whenever possible, confirmation of response should be obtained pathologically through the use of restaging procedures. Many patients achieve only a partial response, defined as a reduction of tumor burden by 50 per cent or more. Patients achieving partial responses generally have palliation of symptoms and usually have a prolonged period without tumor growth. Modest improvements in survival are seen in some patients with partial responses.

Tumor markers in the blood or urine can be useful in monitoring response to therapy (Table 164–6). Patients with testicular germ cell tumors and gestational choriocarcinoma cannot be considered potentially cured unless the titer of marker substance falls below the limit of detection. Tumor marker studies are also useful in judging responses in ovarian cancer, prostatic carcinoma, multiple myeloma, neuroblastoma, and the carcinoid syndrome. Markers of lesser predictive value are also available for colon and pancreatic cancer.

Response to adjuvant chemotherapy cannot be evaluated by these methods, as in this circumstance there is insufficient tumor present for assessment by physical or imaging studies or with tumor markers. However, in the neoadjuvant setting wherein chemotherapy is used prior to local surgery, the response to

TABLE 164–6. APPLICATIONS OF TUMOR MARKERS TO CANCER DIAGNOSIS AND THERAPY

Tumor Type	Marker*	Applications
Choriocarcinoma	hCG	Diagnosis, response
Testicular cancer	hCG, AFP	Diagnosis, response
Hepatoma	AFP	Diagnosis
Prostate cancer	PSA	Diagnosis, response
Multiple myeloma	M-proteins	Diagnosis, response
Carcinoid	5-HIAA	Diagnosis, response
Neuroblastoma	VMA	Diagnosis, response
Colon cancer	CEA	Response
Ovarian cancer	CA-125	Response
Pancreatic cancer	CA-19-9	Investigational

*hCG = human chorionic gonadotropin; AFP = α-fetoprotein; PSA = prostatic specific antigen; M-protein = monoclonal immunoglobulins; 5-HIAA = 5-hydroxyindoleacetic acid; VMA = vanillylmandelic acid; CEA = carcinoembryonic antigen.

chemotherapy provides an "in vivo sensitivity test" to determine whether the agents employed will be useful in adjuvant therapy after surgery. This approach has been used effectively in osteosarcoma even though calcified bone tumors do not shrink with therapy. This is because neovascularization, as detected by pre- and post-therapy angiography, regresses with effective chemotherapy. Furthermore, pathologic findings at the time of surgical resection after neoadjuvant chemotherapy can be important. In general, cure of osteosarcoma is achieved in patients whose tumors exhibit at least 90 per cent necrosis.

CYTOTOXIC ANTICANCER DRUGS. Safe and effective use of cytotoxic cancer chemotherapy requires considerable understanding of the pharmacology and toxicology of these drugs. This section provides a brief synopsis of some of the more important agents. The drug doses cited are for single-agent chemotherapy. When drugs are used in combinations, lower doses may be required for some agents. Therefore, it is generally wise to use effective and well-established combination protocols with known side-effect profiles rather than improvising combinations. The development of new combinations of standard drugs is best done in the research setting.

Alkylating Agents. The major clinically useful alkylating agents kill cells by binding to and crosslinking DNA via a bis(chloroethyl)amine, ethylenimine, or nitrosourea moiety. Although these agents likely kill cells by alkylating DNA (primarily at the N7 position of guanine), they also react chemically with sulfhydryl, amino, hydroxyl, and phosphate groups of all cellular nucleophilic (electron-rich) sites. The mechanism of action of alkylating agents involves intramolecular cyclization to form an ethylenimmonium ion that can transfer an alkyl group to a cellular target either directly or via formation of a carbonium ion. The interactions of alkylating agents with DNA can occur with one or both strands, as most alkylating agents contain two reactive groups. Alkylation of guanine can lead to abnormal base pairing with thymine or to depurination by excision of guanine residues. This effect results in DNA strand breakage. When crosslinking occurs between guanine residues on opposite strands, excision repair can disrupt the integrity of the DNA helix and result in a lethal mutation.

The initial alkylating agent introduced in clinical oncology was nitrogen mustard, an agent still used in treatment of Hodgkin's disease and mycosis fungoides. Nitrosoureas are a subset of alkylating agents that have an additional secondary mechanism of action involving carbamoylation of lysine residues of proteins by forming isocyanates. Alkylating agents are CCNS agents, but cells are most susceptible to alkylation in late G_1 and S phase, and the damage is manifest by a blockage in division after the G_2 phase. The mechanism of acquired resistance to alkylating agents may be a decreased retention of the alkylating agent, increased production of low molecular weight sulfhydryl compounds, and increased capacity to repair DNA damage. Although all alkylating agents have similar mechanisms of action, differences in their molecular structures reduce the degree of cross-resistance between various major subclasses. Alkylating agents also differ in the severity of early and late side effects. The major acute side effects are gastrointestinal (nausea and vomiting) and hematologic (myelosuppression). Most alkylating agents have strong vesicant action and can cause local tissue injury when infiltrated into the skin. All alkylating agents can potentially induce ovarian or testicular failure as well as acute leukemia. Agents such as melphalan and chlorambucil appear to be more leukemogenic than cyclophosphamide, whereas busulfan and the nitrosoureas cause more persistent damage to hemopoietic stem cells and more prolonged myelosuppression. The structures of some major alkylating agents are depicted in Figure 164–4.

Cyclophosphamide (Cytoxan) and Ifosfamide (Ifex). Cyclophosphamide is the most widely used alkylating agent and is effective in the treatment of both hematologic malignancies and solid tumors. It does not have significant vesicant effects, as it is a prodrug and must be biotransformed in the liver. Hepatic activation of cyclophosphamide via the microsomal P-450 mixed function oxidase system results in the generation of 4-hydroxcy-clophosphamide and aldophosphamide. Thereafter, in both normal and tumor tissue, aldophosphamide breaks down nonenzymatically to the active metabolite phosphoramide mustard plus acrolein. Cyclophosphamide is available in both intravenous and oral formulations and is well absorbed by the oral route. A commonly used single-agent dosage schedule for intravenous cyclophosphamide is 1.0 gram per square meter every 3 weeks. By either route cyclophosphamide produces a somewhat different and less severe pattern of myelosuppressive toxicity than other alkylating agents, as it appears to spare noncycling hematopoietic stem cells. Cyclophosphamide can cause severe neutropenia, but it is usually of relatively short duration. Thrombocytopenia is significantly less severe than with other alkylators, and this platelet-sparing effect is a useful feature. Other toxicities of cyclophosphamide include alopecia and immunosuppression. When high doses are used (e.g., for bone marrow transplantation), cyclophosphamide can also cause myocardial necrosis or inappropriate renal water retention. Although cyclophosphamide can cause acute nonlymphocytic leukemia and pulmonary fibrosis, these toxicities are more common with other alkylating agents. Both cyclophosphamide and a related analogue ifosfamide (Ifex) can cause hemorrhagic cystitis. Bladder toxicity can be blocked by administration of the uroprotective agent mesna (Mesnex), which is concentrated in the urine and neutralizes active moieties causing bladder toxicity. Mesna is particularly valuable with ifosfamide, which otherwise routinely causes bladder toxicity. Mesna is given with ifosfamide at 20 per cent of the ifosfamide dosage. Ifosfamide causes somewhat less hematologic toxicity than other alkylating agents. At present ifosfamide is used mostly for second-line therapy (e.g., for second-line therapy of testicular cancer or metastatic sarcomas).

Chlorambucil (Leukeran). Chlorambucil has antitumor activity similar to that of cyclophosphamide and is also well absorbed after oral administration. It is used primarily in the treatment of chronic lymphocytic leukemia, low-grade lymphomas, macroglob-

ulinemia, and polycythemia vera. Chlorambucil does not cause hemorrhagic cystitis or alopecia, and gastrointestinal side effects are mild. However, it is myelosuppressive. Acute nonlymphocytic leukemia has been reported in patients treated with chlorambucil for polycythemia vera or other disorders.

Melphalan (Alkeran). Melphalan is L-phenylalanine mustard and gains access to cells through an amino acid transport system. Unlike cyclophosphamide and chlorambucil, oral melphalan absorption can be erratic and affected by food intake, gastric acidity, and other factors. Melphalan is commonly given orally in a dosage of 10 mg per square meter per day for 4 days every 3 to 4 weeks. It is essential to follow serial CBC's closely, as some patients do not absorb the drug and the only clue to this is the absence of myelosuppression. If myelosuppression does not occur, melphalan dosage should be increased in subsequent courses until moderate myelosuppression is induced. Melphalan is commonly used in the treatment of multiple myeloma and ovarian cancer and occasionally for other tumor types. Melphalan induces acute nonlymphocytic leukemia in some patients treated for myeloma or ovarian cancer.

Busulfan (Myleran). Busulfan is a methane-sulfonate–based alkylating agent that has specificity for myeloid neoplasms and appears to have lesser antitumor activity in other forms of cancer. It is available only for oral administration and is used primarily for treatment of chronic myeloid leukemia (CML). Busulfan can produce protracted myelosuppression, and hematologic recovery should be complete before the next course is administered, or cumulative myelosuppressive toxicity may develop with severe or permanent bone marrow aplasia as a consequence. In addition to its myelosuppressive toxicity, myleran can cause pulmonary fibrosis, hyperpigmentation, weakness, and wasting. Although these last three features suggest adrenal insufficiency, adrenal function is normal.

Nitrosoureas. Carmustine **(BCNU)** and lomustine **(CCNU)** are the two FDA-approved nitrosoureas available for clinical use. Nitrosoureas are rapidly biotransformed via nonenzymatic hydrolysis to release moieties with alkylating and carbamoylating activities. Carmustine is available for intravenous use and lomustine for oral administration. The major toxicity of nitrosoureas at standard dosage levels is on hematopoietic stem cells, and prolonged myelosuppression can result. At high dosage (e.g., in preparative regimens for bone marrow transplantation) nitrosoureas can induce a chemical hepatitis or pneumonitis. Prolonged use of nitrosoureas with total doses greater than 1500 mg per square meter can also result in pulmonary fibrosis or renal failure. Because of their high lipid solubility and ability to cross the blood-brain barrier, the nitrosoureas have some activity against primary brain tumors. The nitrosoureas also are useful in the management of Hodgkin's disease and multiple myeloma and as part of combined modality therapy for cancers of the anal canal.

Platinum Compounds. Cisplatin and carboplatin are platinum-coordination compounds with broad-spectrum antitumor activity and synergistic interactions with a variety of other cytotoxic agents, including alkylating agents, antimetabolites, and natural products. Although the mechanism of action of the platinum compounds is not completely understood, they act similarly to alkylating agents in terms of their ability to bind to the N7 position of guanine and crosslink DNA. However, crosslinking with adenine and cytosine also occurs, as does binding to RNA and protein.

Cisplatin and carboplatin differ significantly in their toxicity profiles. Both drugs are administered intravenously. Cisplatin is commonly given in a dose of 100 mg per square meter every 3 weeks, whereas the dose of carboplatin is in the range of 450 mg per square meter at similar intervals, although larger doses may be tolerated. After intravenous infusion, the major acute toxicity for both cisplatin and carboplatin is nausea and vomiting. Satisfactory suppression of the gastrointestinal side effects of platinum compounds requires use of extremely potent antiemetic agents, often in combination. Cisplatin has the additional potentials of renal toxicity and a progressive neuropathy with large cumulative doses of drug. The nephropathy can be largely prevented if the patient is well hydrated with simultaneous saline infusions and diuretics are given with cisplatin. Myelosuppression is minimal with cisplatin but is dose-limiting with carboplatin. Although

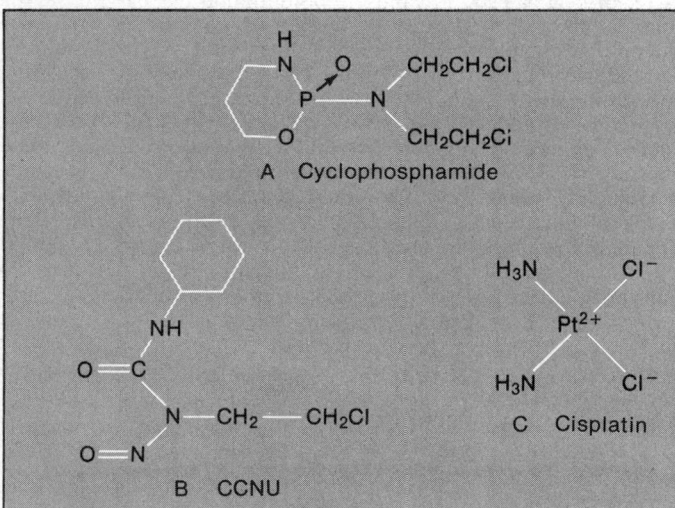

FIGURE 164–4. Alkylating agents. This figure depicts the structures of several prototypes representing subclasses within the general category of alkylating agents. *A*, Cyclophosphamide with bischlorethyl radical. *B*, CCNU, a nitrosourea. *C*, Cisplatin, one of the platinum-coordination complexes.

carboplatin is less toxic than cisplatin, its efficacy is equivalent. However, the lack of myelosuppression favors cisplatin for use in some drug combinations with myelosuppressive agents.

Antimetabolites. The antimetabolites are structural analogues of normal biochemical compounds, most of which are involved in DNA or RNA synthesis and generally function as CCS agents. Antimetabolites are classed in relation to their mechanisms of action. Structures of some major antimetabolites are shown in Figure 164–5.

Pyrimidine Antagonists. *Cytarabine (Cytosine Arabinoside, Cytosar-U, Ara-C).* Cytarabine is an S-phase–specific agent that is particularly useful in acute nonlymphocytic leukemia and to a lesser extent in other hematologic malignancies. Cytarabine is metabolized intracellularly to its active form, ara-CTP, which competitively inhibits DNA polymerase, blocking DNA synthesis. Ara-C is also incorporated into DNA, where it blocks chain elongation and ligation of fragments into newly synthesized DNA. Ara-C is given intravenously and has good CNS uptake into spinal fluid. It is administered either by continuous infusion in doses of at least 100 mg per square meter per day or in bolus doses of 50 to 100 mg every 8 to 12 hours by the intravenous or subcutaneous route for 5 to 7 days. In an alternative dosage schedule which exceeds the manufacturer's recommended maximum dose, high-dose ara-C is administered in doses of 1 to 3 grams every 12 hours for 5 to 6 days and causes higher response rates than do the standard dosage regimens. The duration of intracellular retention of ara-CTP appears to predict ara-C antileukemic effects, with best results in patients who have the longest ara-CTP retention times. The primary toxicity of both standard and high-dose ara-C is severe myelosuppression. With the high-dose regimen, chemical conjunctivitis is common and can be ameliorated with steroid ophthalmic drops. With rare exception, in order to achieve complete remissions in acute leukemia, ara-C must be administered with sufficient intensity to drive the bone marrow to severe hypocellularity and destroy the leukemic blast population. Thereafter the marrow is repopulated by residual normal progenitors that were suppressed by the leukemia. Ara-C is generally used in combination with daunorubicin in the treatment of acute nonlymphocytic leukemia but also acts synergistically with other drugs including cisplatin. Cytarabine can also be given intrathecally in doses of 75 to 100 mg as treatment for leukemic or carcinomatous meningitis.

Another structural analogue related to cytidine is 5-azacytidine (5-azaC). 5-AzaC is a second-line antileukemic agent that has yet to be approved in the United States by the Food and Drug Administration. 5-AzaC is metabolized intracellularly to 5-azaCTP and is incorporated into DNA and RNA, impairing protein synthesis. As with cytarabine, the primary toxicity of 5-azaC is prolonged myelosuppression, but protracted nausea and vomiting also occur. 5-AzaC is unstable and sensitive to light and to alkaline or neutral pH, leading to ring opening and inactivation. Therefore solutions of 5-azaC must be freshly mixed, preferably in Ringer's lactate, prior to administration.

Fluorouracil (5-FU) and Fluorodeoxyurine (5-FUDR). 5-FU is an important anticancer agent in the treatment of a variety of solid tumors, including cancers of the head and neck, breast, and colon. It acts synergistically with a variety of agents, including platinum compounds and radiation therapy. 5-FU undergoes biotransformation to ribosyl and deoxyribosyl nucleotide metabolites. 5-Fluorouridine triphosphate is incorporated into RNA and interferes with RNA processing and function. An additional metabolite, 5-fluorodeoxyuridine phosphate, forms a ternary complex that binds covalently to thymidylate synthetase and its cofactor, N5,10-methylenetetrahydrofolate. This in turn inhibits DNA synthesis, resulting in "thymineless death." 5-FU is usually given intravenously by bolus or infusion schedules but can also be used in intra-arterial, intracavitary, and topical therapy. An optimal schedule for 5-FU administration is a 5-day continuous infusion at a dose rate of 1.0 gram per square meter per day. This schedule causes some gastrointestinal toxicity but only a mild degree of myelosuppression. With this dosage schedule, full doses of cisplatin can be administered additionally, and this treatment program is very active in the neoadjuvant chemotherapy of head and neck and esophageal cancer. When 5-FU is administered on a weekly intravenous bolus schedule there is greater hematologic toxicity and mucositis with lower total doses. Less common toxicities observed with 5-FU include a neurologic syndrome associated with ataxia, chemical conjunctivitis, and a syndrome including chest pain and cardiac enzyme elevation consistent with myocardial ischemia. The bioavailability of 5-FU after oral administration is erratic, and the drug is metabolized mostly during its first pass through the liver.

Both the gastrointestinal toxicity and the antitumor activity of 5-FU can be enhanced by administration of leucovorin, which increases the binding of fluorodeoxyuridine phosphate to thymidylate synthetase. This combination appears to increase the antitumor activity of 5-FU in breast and colon cancer. Both interferon-α and levamisole also appear to enhance 5-FU activity in colorectal cancer. Levamisole potentiation has been observed only in the adjuvant setting. Both 5-FU and 5-FUDR can be given by hepatic artery infusion for patients with colorectal carcinoma metastatic to the liver. This approach is generally not warranted for patients who also have extrahepatic metastases. A commonly used schedule for hepatic artery 5-FUDR is 0.15 mg per kilogram per day for 14 days followed by a 14-day rest period during which saline infusions are administered. This schedule can induce tumor regression in the majority of patients with hepatic metastases of colorectal cancer if the anatomy of the arterial blood supply provides good drug delivery to the sites of metastasis as determined angiographically. With the use of a surgically placed vascular access catheter, outpatient hepatic artery infusions can be administered using either an internal or portable external pump. One limitation of this approach is that either 5-FU or 5-FUDR can induce a chemical hepatitis and biliary sclerosis with jaundice. Hepatic dysfunction can be most readily detected by obtaining liver chemistries on day 14 when 5-FU is to be discontinued.

Purine Antagonists. *6-Mercaptopurine and 6-Thioguanine.* The first thiopurine found to be a useful anticancer drug was **6-mercaptopurine** (Purinethol, 6-MP). A related agent, **6-thioguanine** (6-TG) is also in use. Both 6-MP and 6-TG are converted to nucleotide form by hypoxanthine-guanine phosphoribosyl transferase (HGPRT), and their metabolites inhibit a number of enzymes in the purine pathway. In contrast to 6-MP, some 6-TG metabolites are incorporated into both DNA and RNA. 6-TG has

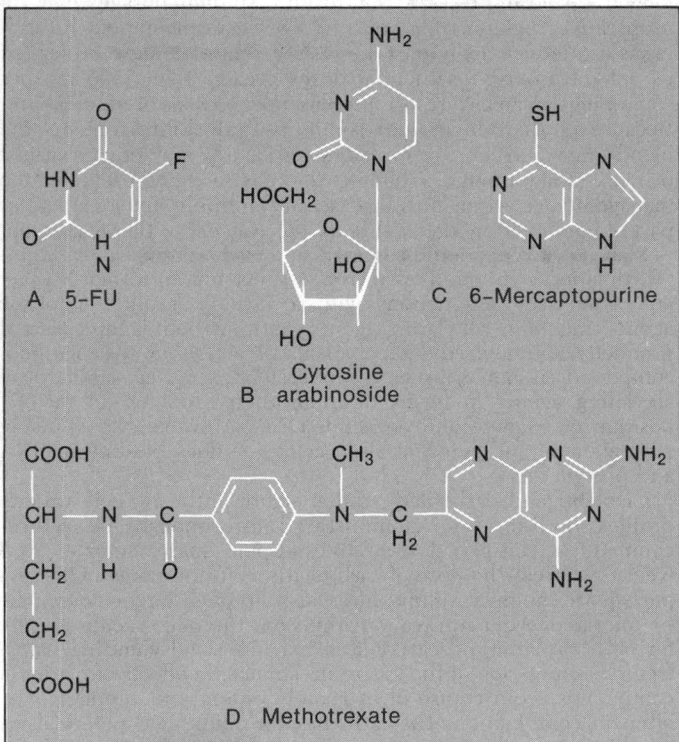

FIGURE 164–5. Antimetabolites. Depicted here are several antimetabolites that are structural analogues of molecules relevant to nucleic acid metabolism. *A,* 5-Fluorouracil. *B,* Cytarabine. *C,* 6-Mercaptopurine. *D,* Methotrexate.

some uses in acute nonlymphocytic leukemia in combination with cytarabine, whereas 6-MP is used primarily in acute lymphoblastic leukemia, particularly in childhood. Absorption of 6-MP is variable, and recent studies indicate that plasma monitoring of 6-MP concentration can identify poor absorbers who have a high likelihood of developing recurrent leukemia, presumably because of inadequate bioavailability of 6-MP. The 6-MP analogue azathioprine is a useful immunosuppressive agent. Because both 6-MP and azathioprine are catabolized by xanthine oxidase, patients must have their thiopurine doses reduced to 25 per cent of their standard doses if they are also receiving the xanthine oxidase inhibitor allopurinol. 6-TG is not catabolized by xanthine oxidase, and dose correction is not required for allopurinol.

Fludarabine (Fludara, 5-Fluoroadenosine Monophosphate). Fludarabine is an analogue of adenine which appears to act through inhibition of DNA polymerase and ribonuceotide reductase by its phosphorylated product fludarabine triphosphate and by incorporation into DNA. Fludarabine is the single most active agent available in the treatment of chronic lymphocytic leukemia and also exhibits some antitumor activity in other indolent lymphomas and macroglobulinemia. Fludarabine is often given intravenously in a dose of 30 mg per square meter per day over 30 minutes for 5 days every 4 weeks. The major toxicity is myelosuppression. In higher doses in early trials in patients with acute nonlymphocytic leukemia, it produced cortical blindness in some patients. In the lower-dosage schedule used in chronic lymphocytic leukemia and other lymphoid neoplasms, the side effects are usually mild and reversible. Fludarabine has not yet been approved by the Food and Drug Administration.

Additional purine antagonists are deoxycoformycin (DCF) and 2-chloroadenosine (2-CA). Both DCF and 2-CA are extremely active agents in the treatment of hairy cell leukemia and can produce prolonged complete remissions after a single course of treatment. Both agents also exhibit some antitumor activity in other lymphoid neoplasms (e.g., CLL). 2-CA and DCF have not been approved by the Food and Drug Administration and remain investigational.

Folic Acid Antagonists. The first antifol to be used clinically about 40 years ago was aminopterine, which was superseded by **methotrexate** (MTX). Both agents are structural analogues of folic acid. Other antifols have been developed (e.g., trimetrexate), but none has proven superior to MTX. Methotrexate can be administered orally, intramuscularly, or intravenously and is a useful agent primarily as a component of chemotherapy combinations for various types of cancer, including acute lymphoblastic leukemia, small cell lung cancer, and breast cancer. When used in high dosage with leucovorin rescue, it has definite antitumor activity in osteogenic sarcoma. MTX binds tightly to the catalytic site on dihydrofolate reductase (DHFR) and inhibits the synthesis of thymidylate and purine nucleotides, as well as of serine and methionine, by interfering with the ability of DHFR to be reduced and accept one-carbon units. Intracellular formation of polyglutamated forms of MTX is important to the action of MTX, as the polyglutamated forms have equivalent ability to inhibit DHFR action but have a longer intracellular retention time than MTX. The polyglutamates also inhibit other folate-dependent enzymes, including thymidylate synthetase. MTX is excreted unchanged in the urine within 12 hours of administration as long as hydration status and renal function are satisfactory.

The major toxicities of MTX are manifest in rapidly dividing tissues, including the bone marrow and the gastrointestinal mucosa, and to a lesser extent in the skin. At high dosages or in patients with impaired renal function, MTX can also induce renal toxicity. The toxic effects of MTX on the rapidly dividing tissues can be circumvented by administration of the reduced folate leucovorin (folinic acid) within 36 hours after MTX administration. Leucovorin rescue can also be used when methotrexate is intentionally administered in higher than manufacturer's recommended maximum dose (e.g., 1500 mg per square meter or more). When high-dose MTX is administered, leucovorin must be administered in dosage of 15 to 50 mg per square meter every 6 hours for 48 hours, with the duration of leucovorin rescue contingent on the serum methotrexate level. Increased leucovorin dosage and longer periods of rescue are needed in patients with impaired renal function. The high-dose MTX/leucovorin rescue regimen therefore requires good renal function.

NATURAL PRODUCT ANTICANCER DRUGS. The two main classes of natural antitumor products are plant alkaloids and antibiotics. Resistance to the natural products discussed below (with the exception of bleomycin) can be mediated by the P-glycoprotein multidrug resistance mechanism. Structures of some of the major natural product anticancer drugs are depicted in Figure 164–6.

***Plant Alkaloids.* Vincristine and Vinblastine.** The vinca alkaloids were isolated from the common periwinkle (*Vinca rosacea*). The major vincas in clinical use, vincristine (Oncovin) and vinblastine (Velban), result in precipitation of tubulin and disruption of cellular microtubules. Whereas the primary toxicity of vinblastine is hemopoietic, vincristine's major toxicity is to peripheral nerves, resulting in sensorimotor and autonomic neuropathies. Common symptoms of vincristine toxicity are paresthesias ("pins and needles sensation") in the digits and progressive muscular weakness, particularly in the lower extremities and associated with hyporeflexia. Foot drop can develop, as can occasional cranial, bladder, or bowel neuropathies. In general, individual bolus doses of greater than 2 mg are not recommended because of neurotoxicity. The neurotoxicity subsides slowly after the drug is discontinued, with improvement occurring over months. The lack of bone marrow toxicity of vincristine has made it useful for combination chemotherapy regimens. The vincas have vesicant effects and can be administered only intravenously. Both vincas have significant antitumor activity in leukemias and lymphomas as well as for selected solid tumors, including small cell lung cancer and breast cancer. Vincristine is used in various combinations, including "MOPP," "CHOP," "MACOP-B," and "M-BACOD" used in the treatment of lymphomas and "VMCP" and "VAD" used in the treatment of multiple myeloma. Vinblastine's most significant use has been in its incorporation into the "PVB" regimen for the treatment of nonseminomatous testicular cancers. Vinblastine is also used in combination with cisplatin in non–small cell lung cancer and with mitomycin in metastatic breast cancer.

Podophyllotoxins. Etoposide (VP-16, VePesid), a semisynthetic glucoside, is produced from extracts of the root of the mayapple or mandrake (*Podophyllum peltatum*). A closely related analogue, teniposide (VM-26) has not been approved in the United States by the Food and Drug Administration. The podophyllotoxins are CCS agents and block cells in the late S phase and early G_2 phase. Mechanistically, podophyllotoxins are thought to act as inhibitors of nuclear topoisomerase II, leading to DNA strand breaks. Additional effects include inhibition of nucleoside transport and mitochondrial electron transport. Etoposide is highly lipid soluble and water insoluble and requires a special formulation for intravenous administration. An oral formulation is also available. There is extensive protein binding of the drug, and good tissue distribution is achieved in all sites other than the brain. In one commonly used schedule, etoposide is administered intravenously for 3 days at a dose level of 150 to 200 mg per square meter per day. Etoposide is excreted primarily in the urine and to a lesser extent in the bile. Its dosage should be reduced by 50 per cent in patients with impaired renal function (serum creatinine greater than 2 mg per deciliter). The main side effect of etoposide is myelosuppression, although some gastrointestinal toxicity and alopecia are also associated with its use. Etoposide is used primarily in the treatment of metastatic testicular cancer in combination with cisplatin and bleomycin. In this combination etoposide is substituted for vinblastine, yielding a less toxic but equally effective regimen. Etoposide is also a potent agent in the treatment of small cell lung cancer, lymphomas, and monocytic leukemia.

Taxol. Taxol is a promising investigational anticancer agent derived from the bark of the western yew tree (*Taxus brevifolia*) but is not yet approved by the Food and Drug Administration and must be obtained through the National Cancer Institute. Taxol stabilizes cellular microtubules, thereby preventing cell division. It is water insoluble and is formulated for intravenous administration. The major toxicities are myelosuppressive and gastrointestinal. Taxol has confirmed activity in the treatment of refractory ovarian cancer and some activity against other tumor types as well. Because of the extremely low content of taxol in bark, efforts are now underway to develop a semisynthetic derivative.

ANTIBIOTICS. *Doxorubicin and Daunorubicin*. These two red anthracycline antibiotics were isolated from a variant of *Streptomyces peucetius* and are extremely useful in cancer chemotherapy. Daunorubicin (daunomycin) was the first agent in this class and is active in the treatment of acute leukemia. Its congener, doxorubicin (Adriamycin) has a broader spectrum of antitumor activity, including both hematologic malignancies and a variety of solid tumors such as carcinoma of the breast and thyroid, lymphoma, and myeloma, as well as osteogenic and soft tissue sarcomas. Daunorubicin is frequently used in combination with cytarabine in the treatment of acute leukemia, whereas doxorubicin is incorporated into regimens for solid tumors along with cyclophosphamide, fluorouracil, etoposide, vincristine, or cisplatin. Mechanistically, the anthracyclines intercalate with high affinity into DNA and inhibit the action of topoisomerase II, resulting in DNA strand breaks. Anthracycline cytotoxicity may also be related in part to the generation of free radicals. This appears to result from the chelation of divalent cations including Fe^{2+} and production of superoxide and other oxygen radicals. Both doxorubicin and daunorubicin must be administered intravenously by either bolus injection or prolonged infusion. Extravasation of anthracyclines can lead to severe tissue injury. Topical application of 1.5 ml of 99 per cent dimethylsulfoxide (DMSO)* has been reported to prevent the development of ulceration. For prolonged anthracycline infusions, use of a vascular access catheter is advisable to avoid drug extravasation. When ulceration and necrosis occur after an anthracycline extravasation, surgical debridement of the damaged tissues followed by skin grafting is usually required.

The most common acute toxicities of the anthracyclines include alopecia, nausea, vomiting, mucositis, and myelosuppression. A dose-dependent cardiomyopathy with reduced cardiac contractil-

---

* While commercially available, DMSO has not been approved for use by the United States Food and Drug Administration.

ity can develop as a delayed toxicity in patients who receive large cumulative doses of doxorubicin or daunorubicin. The cardiomyopathy can be serious and irreversible and is usually manifest as congestive heart failure. Acute cardiac arrhythmias are uncommon. The cardiac toxicity of anthracyclines is considered to result from the heart's lack of enzymes such as glutathione peroxidase which serve as free-radical scavengers. While various drugs have been tried in efforts to block free radical generation or to serve as free radical scavengers in the heart, there are currently no approved agents to block the development of anthracycline-induced cardiomyopathy. Several anthracycline analogues considered to have lesser cardiotoxicity have been evaluated clinically but have not yet shown sufficient advantage to be approved for licensure in the United States.

Monitoring for cardiac effects of anthracyclines is conducted serially by determining the left ventricular ejection fraction using radionuclide techniques. Endomyocardial biopsy can also be used. Periodic monitoring is normally initiated when a patient has received a total doxorubicin dose of 350 to 400 mg per square meter. Significant cardiac toxicity is uncommon with cumulative bolus doses of doxorubicin of less than 550 mg per square meter, above which the incidence rises progressively. Elderly patients and others with risk factors for cardiac disease (e.g., hypertension) are at somewhat higher risk for anthracycline cardiomyopathy. Use of anthracyclines is not recommended for patients who have major pre-existing heart disease. When doxorubicin is administered by continuous infusion (e.g., for 4 to 5 days), a significantly larger cumulative dose in the range of 1000 mg per square meter can usually be administered. However, regular monitoring of the ejection fraction is required, and doxorubicin should be discontinued if the left ventricular ejection fraction falls below 50 per cent.

***Bleomycin*.** Bleomycin (Blenoxane) comprises 11 closely related glycopeptide moieties produced by *Streptomyces verticillus*. The major components are bleomycins A2 and B2. The mechanism of bleomycin action involves its binding to DNA and generation of superoxide and other reactive oxygen species, including hydroxyl radicals. These reactive species induce both single- and double-

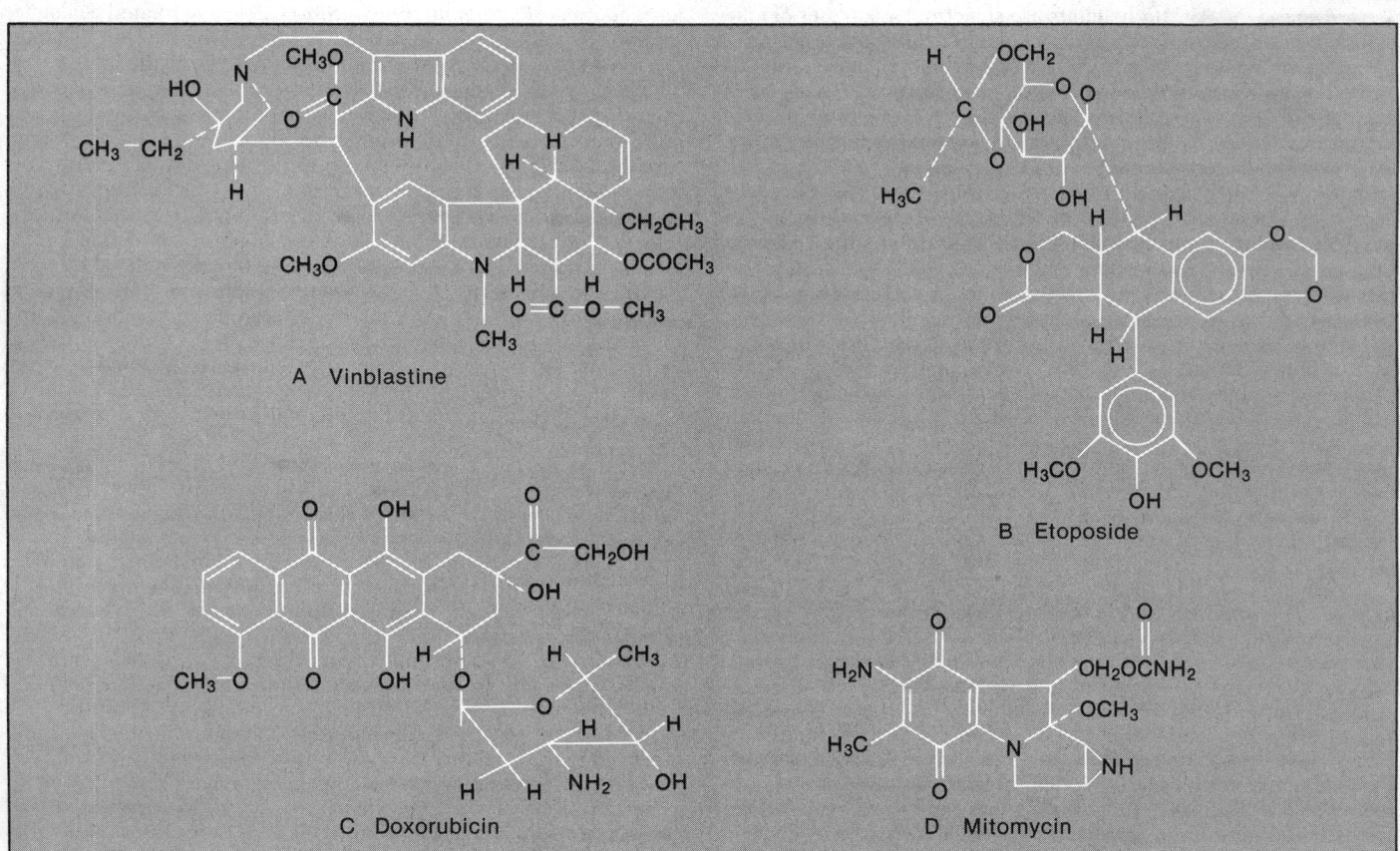

FIGURE 164–6. Natural product anticancer drugs. Commonly used plant alkaloids include *(A)* vinblastine (and its congener, vincristine) and *(B)* etoposide. Widely used antibiotics include *(C)* doxorubicin (and its congener, daunorubicin) and *(D)* mitomycin.

strand breaks. DNA fragmentation appears to result from the oxidation of a DNA-bleomycin-Fe^{2+} complex. Bleomycin's antitumor activity is schedule-dependent, and it is a CCS agent. It can be administered by subcutaneous, intramuscular, and intravenous routes. Bleomycin is synergistic with vinblastine or etoposide and with cisplatin, and its major uses are in carcinoma of the testis as well as squamous cell carcinomas of the head and neck, cervix, skin, penis, and rectum. It is also used in combination regimens for treatment of lymphomas.

One advantage of bleomycin is that it has minimal myelosuppressive effects and is useful in combination with drugs that cause leukopenia. Acute toxicities of bleomycin include anaphylactoid reactions and fever associated with hypotension and dehydration. Patients who have not previously been treated with bleomycin should receive a test dose (e.g., 1 to 2 mg) to see that they are not subject to this reaction. Individual therapeutic doses of bleomycin are usually in the range of 15 mg per square meter.

The most serious chronic reaction to bleomycin is pulmonary fibrosis related to the cumulative dose of drug and manifested by cough, dyspnea, and bilateral basilar infiltrates on chest radiography. It is possible to screen for earlier pulmonary abnormalities such as a decline in the diffusion capacity, which is usually detectable at total doses of bleomycin above 250 units. It is wise to discontinue use of bleomycin when the pulmonary diffusion capacity falls significantly. The incidence of pulmonary fibrosis rises at total doses above 450 units and is higher in patients with pre-existing pulmonary disease, after lung irradiation, and in the elderly. Unfortunately, there are no effective agents to reverse this toxicity and it is steroid insensitive. Other reactions to bleomycin include skin toxicity with blistering, desquamation, and hyperkeratosis of the palms and hyperpigmentation of skin creases.

Mitomycin. Mitomycin (Mutamycin, Mitocin-C, Mitomycin C) is isolated from *Streptomyces caespitosus*. The structure of this agent includes quinone, carbamate, and aziridine groups, which may play roles in its antitumor activity. Mitomycin functions as a CCNS alkylating agent after it has been activated in various tissues by the cytochrome P-450 system. Thereafter it can alkylate DNA to form intrastrand and interstrand crosslinks resulting in cell death. Mitomycin has "bioreductive" properties, with increased cytotoxic effects on poorly oxygenated tumor cells present in solid tumors. Mitomycin's clinical spectrum of antitumor activity includes breast, lung, gastrointestinal, genitourinary, and gynecologic cancers. Mitomycin has been incorporated into a variety of cytotoxic drug combinations for systemic administration, often in second-line therapy for patients who relapse from initial chemotherapy. It is usually administered intravenously, but it can be used for intravesical therapy of superficial bladder cancer. When used in combinations by the intravenous route, its normal dosage range is 10 to 15 mg per square meter.

The major toxicity of systemically administered mitomycin is myelosuppression, which is usually delayed until 4 to 6 weeks after injection. Mitomycin has a cumulative effect on bone marrow stem cells, which can lead to protracted marrow hypoplasia for 3 to 6 months after the drug has been discontinued. Nausea and vomiting and anorexia often occur at the time of drug administration but can usually be managed effectively with antiemetic agents. Occasionally, mitomycin can induce other serious reactions such as interstitial pneumonitis, nephrotoxicity, or hemolytic-uremic syndrome.

Actinomycin D. Actinomycin D (dactinomycin, Cosmegen) is the first effective antitumor antibiotic isolated from *Streptomyces*. It binds to the DNA helix by intercalation between adjacent guanine-cytosine base pairs and inhibits DNA-dependent RNA synthesis. It can also cause single-strand breaks. Actinomycin D has its greatest effect on ribosomal RNA synthesis, and this leads to cessation of most protein synthesis in sensitive cells. The drug is administered intravenously, and its major toxicity is myelosuppression, which is usually manifest in 7 to 10 days after injection. However, actinomycin D also causes significant gastrointestinal toxicity with abdominal cramps and diarrhea as well as mucositis. Actinomycin D commonly causes a radiation "recall" reaction wherein cutaneous erythema redevelops at a site of prior irradiation. The main clinical uses of actinomycin D are in pediatric oncology in combination chemotherapy for the treatment of Wilms' tumor, Ewing's sarcoma, and embryonal rhabdomyosarcoma. It also has some utility in adults in third-line

therapy of germ cell tumors of the testis or ovary, gestational choriocarcinoma, and soft tissue sarcomas.

Miscellaneous Agents

PROCARBAZINE. Procarbazine (Matulane) is an orally administered methylhydrazine derivative that has antitumor activity in Hodgkin's disease (as part of "MOPP" combination chemotherapy) and some use also in non-Hodgkin's lymphomas, lung cancer, and brain tumors. Procarbazine is usually given in a dose of 100 mg per square meter per day for 10 to 14 days in each chemotherapy cycle. Procarbazine is activated metabolically to provide a methyldiazonium ion that binds to nucleic acids and proteins as well as phospholipids and inhibits macromolecular synthesis. Its mechanism of cytotoxicity is thought to involve DNA strand scission, possibly via generation of H_2O_2. Procarbazine's principal toxicities are nausea, vomiting, and myelosuppression. One of procarbazine's metabolites is a monoamine oxidase (MAO) inhibitor that can cause toxicity when the patient is taking other MAO inhibitors. Patients taking procarbazine are potentially subject to hypertension if they ingest tyramine-rich foods such as ripe cheese, wine, and bananas. Disulfiram-like reactions are also seen, with sweating and headache after alcohol ingestion. Other infrequent reactions include hemolytic anemia and pulmonary reactions. Procarbazine is also known to be leukemogenic, carcinogenic, and mutagenic and is considered to play a significant role in the late leukemias and other second malignancies in patients with Hodgkin's disease. Procarbazine also produces azospermia and anovulation. As alternative combinations lacking procarbazine can be used in the treatment of Hodgkin's disease, the benefits versus risks of using this agent must be carefully considered.

DACARBAZINE. Dacarbazine (DTIC, dimethylimidazole carboxamide) is activated by oxidative *N*-demethylation. A methyl carbonium ion metabolite is thought to be the cytotoxic intermediate with alkylating activity. Dacarbazine is administered intravenously either in a single-day infusion schedule of 750 mg per square meter or in fractionated bolus doses over 5 days or more. DTIC causes severe nausea and vomiting, and potent antiemetic agents are required. Myelosuppression is relatively mild. Dacarbazine is used in combination chemotherapy for Hodgkin's disease ("ABVD"), for soft tissue sarcomas in combination with doxorubicin and other agents, and in single-agent chemotherapy for metastatic melanoma.

HEXAMETHYLMELAMINE (HMM). This investigational agent is available only in an oral formulation because of its sparing solubility. However, oral bioavailability of HMM is quite variable, and it produces nausea and vomiting as its dose-limiting toxicity. The severity of gastrointestinal toxicity increases with daily use, limiting the length of treatment courses (at doses of up to 12 mg per kilogram per day) to 2 to 3 weeks. Myelosuppression occurs, but it is mild. Additionally, hexamethylmelamine can induce both central and peripheral neurotoxicities, including altered mood, hallucinations, and peripheral neuropathy. HMM is thought to act as an alkylating agent, possibly via the enzymatic hydroxylation of its demethyl metabolites to cytotoxic methylol compounds. HMM exhibits antitumor activity in alkylating agent–resistant ovarian cancer and to a lesser extent in several other neoplasms (lung, breast cancer, lymphomas) but has not yet been approved for use in the United States by the Food and Drug Administration.

HYDROXYUREA (HYDREA, HU). Hydroxyurea acts as an inhibitor of ribonucleotide reductase, resulting in intracellular depletion of deoxynucleoside triphosphates and inhibition of DNA synthesis. It is available for clinical use in oral formulation. HU's major toxicity is to the bone marrow, and it causes transient dose-related myelosuppression. At high dosage, a megaloblastic anemia can develop which is nonresponsive to vitamin B_{12} or folic acid. Gastrointestinal side effects of nausea and vomiting are also common with high-dose therapy. HU is used as a secondary agent for palliative treatment of chronic myeloid leukemia, but it also has some use in head and neck cancer and metastatic melanoma.

MITOXANTRONE (NOVANTRONE). Mitoxantrone is an anthracenedione with a structure that appears analogous to that of the anthracyclines. It has been approved by the Food and Drug Administration as a second-line agent for treatment of acute leukemia in relapse but is also useful in the treatment of breast cancer and lymphoma. Mitoxantrone binds to DNA and causes strand breaks as well as inhibits DNA and RNA synthesis. In terms of cellular response by tumor cells, there is not complete cross-reactivity between mitoxantrone and the anthracyclines. Mitoxantrone dosage for acute leukemia is significantly higher than for solid tumors. Comparative studies in patients with advanced breast cancer suggest that it is slightly less active and less toxic than doxorubicin. Its major acute toxicity is myelosuppression. Gastrointestinal side effects, including nausea, vomiting, and mucositis as well as alopecia, are less severe than with the anthracyclines. Mitoxantrone can cause some cardiac toxicities, usually manifest by development of arrhythmia at the time of injection, and can exacerbate pre-existing anthracycline-induced cardiomyopathy. It can be used intraperitoneally in patients with ovarian cancer, as most of the drug remains in the peritoneal cavity. This reduces systemic toxicity, although it can induce chemical peritonitis with subsequent adhesions.

ASPARAGINASE (CRASNITIN, ELSPAR). L-Asparaginase is a bacterial enzyme that is isolated from *Escherichia coli* or *Erwinia carotovora*. Its major use is in the treatment of lymphoblastic leukemias and some lymphomas with a deficiency in asparagine synthetase and cellular dependence on exogenous asparagine. L-Asparagine is a nonessential amino acid, and most normal cells can synthesize their required asparagine. Therapeutically, L-asparaginase acts by depleting the plasma of asparagine by catalyzing its degradation to aspartic acid and ammonia. Blood glutamine levels are also reduced. Most patients develop fever and chills as well as nausea and vomiting after asparaginase administration, but these symptoms can usually be reduced or prevented by premedication with antiemetics and anti-inflammatory agents. Toxicities of asparaginase occur in the liver and result in abnormal liver function test results (SGOT, alkaline phosphatase, and bilirubin) as well as in hypoalbuminemia, and reductions in plasma levels of clotting factors and insulin. Other occasional toxicities include pancreatitis and central nervous system abnormalities, which can include confusion or coma. Repeated use of asparaginase leads to the development of antibodies to the bacterial enzyme that can inhibit its activity and accelerate its clearance as well as induce hypersensitivity reactions. Patients developing hypersensitivity after asparaginase administration may exhibit hypotension, laryngeal edema, bronchospasm, and urticaria. Switching to an asparaginase derived from a different bacterial species can bypass neutralizing antibodies that have developed in hypersensitive patients. The lack of myelosuppressive or gastrointestinal toxicity has facilitated incorporation of L-asparaginase into drug combinations for the treatment of acute lymphocytic leukemia.

Management of Toxicity

Most cytotoxic drugs have significant toxicities on host cells. Nonetheless, there are methods to reduce the toxicity for a variety of antitumor agents. Because of the steep dose-response curve of cytotoxic agents, it is desirable to administer them at the maximally tolerated doses.

DOSE ADJUSTMENTS FOR BONE MARROW TOXICITY. It is often necessary to make downward adjustments of myelosuppressive agents in order to avoid serious or life-threatening side effects such as granulocytopenic fever and thrombocytopenic bleeding. For most drugs, empiric schedules have been developed for drug administration with single agents or combinations of myelosuppressive drugs normally given every 3 to 4 weeks. The interval between treatments provides time for hematopoietic recovery of normal myeloid progenitors in the bone marrow and avoids cumulative myelosuppression. It is essential to check the patient's CBC, differential, and platelet count immediately prior to each course of myelosuppressive chemotherapy. During the first few cycles of chemotherapy, and at intervals thereafter, it is useful to check counts between treatment courses, particularly in order to determine the nadir of absolute granulocyte count (AGC). Nadir AGC's are determined by multiplying the total WBC by the percentage of granulocytes plus band forms. If the patient's AGC falls below 1000 per microliter, there is an increased risk of infection; AGC's below 500 are often associated with life-threatening infection. As hematopoietic recovery can occur rapidly after the nadir, the AGC immediately prior to the next course can be normal even though the nadir count may have been very low. For some drug combinations with low but brief AGC nadirs, prophylactic anti-infective agents (e.g., sulfamethoxazole-trimethoprim) are prescribed to bracket the AGC nadir to protect against infection secondary to neutropenia. In general, if the AGC immediately prior to the next course of chemotherapy is less than 2000 per microliter, the dose of myelosuppressive drugs should be reduced by 50 per cent. With an AGC of less than 1500 per microliter, the dosages should be reduced by 75 per cent. If the AGC is less than 1000, the dose of drug should be withheld until hematologic recovery has occurred. An additional approach to problems of myelosuppression involves the use of bone marrow growth factors as discussed below under "Biological Agents."

DOSE ADJUSTMENTS FOR IMPAIRED HEPATIC OR RENAL FUNCTION. The effects of altered hepatic or renal function on the clearance rates for anticancer drugs are not always predictable. Nonetheless, it is important to make downward dosage adjustments for specific drugs when altered hepatic or renal function plays a major role. The metabolism of doxorubicin depends upon good hepatobiliary function. Patients with a serum bilirubin of greater than 3.0 mg per deciliter should have their doxorubicin dose reduced by at least 50 per cent until drug tolerance is established.

Cisplatin, methotrexate, etoposide, hydroxyurea, and bleomycin are all cleared predominantly by renal excretion. In general, doses of these agents should be decreased in proportion to the decline in renal function as determined by creatinine clearance and reflected by the serum creatinine. These guidelines are at best approximate. It is very important to renormalize dosages if toxicity is not observed with myelosuppressive agents.

Endocrine Agents

Cancer cells often exhibit susceptibility to hormonal control mechanisms that regulate growth of the normal organ or tissue from which the neoplasm arose. Endocrine therapy appears generally to work through cytostatic rather than cytotoxic mechanisms and in most instances requires long-term suppression. Endocrine therapy includes the use of both hormones and "antihormones," which are either antagonists or partial agonists for a given endocrine mechanism. Inasmuch as the effects of hormones are receptor mediated, evaluation of receptors capable of binding hormones has played an important role in assessing both tumor types and individual patients for susceptibility to endocrine therapy. Dose schedules and applications of some major endocrine agents are summarized in Table 164–7.

STEROID HORMONES AND ANTIHORMONES. Cancers arising from endocrine organs and from the immune system show significant susceptibility to the effects of steroid hormones and steroid hormone antagonists and of hormone deprivation. The sex steroids and their antagonists represent major agents for the treatment of common cancers arising from the breast, prostate gland, and uterus. The role of endocrine ablation procedures (hypophysectomy, adrenalectomy, oophorectomy, orchiectomy) has diminished as systemic agents have been identified which can replace surgical procedures. Nonetheless, oophorectomy and orchiectomy are still useful in the treatment of endocrine-sensitive cancers of the breast and prostate, respectively.

Estrogens and Antiestrogens. Pharmacologic doses of estrogen have therapeutic effects in cancers of the prostate and the breast. Estrogen therapy remains a mainstay in the treatment of metastatic prostate cancer. Orchiectomy is an excellent alternative to estrogen therapy for prostate cancer, as it does not have feminizing side effects. Orchiectomy and estrogen therapy for prostate cancer are equally efficacious. There is no evidence to suggest an additive effect of the two.

For breast cancer, the use of the antiestrogen tamoxifen (Nolvadex) has largely replaced high-dose estrogen therapy because it is better tolerated. Tamoxifen improves survival of postmenopausal women with estrogen and/or progesterone receptor–positive breast cancer in both the adjuvant and metastatic settings. Some recent studies also suggest that tamoxifen may be a useful adjuvant drug for hormone receptor–negative cancers in postmenopausal women, but this finding is still controversial. In general, cytotoxic chemotherapy rather than endocrine therapy is recommended for women with hormone-receptor–negative breast cancer. Tamoxifen is available only in 10 mg tablets for oral administration, with a manufacturer's recommended dose of 10 mg twice daily. There is not a good scientific rationale for this schedule, because with chronic therapy, tamoxifen and its active metabolite dihydroxytamoxifen achieve a steady state with a large deep tissue reservoir. Accordingly, use of a single dose of 20 mg should be an acceptable alternative schedule with fewer problems with compliance. Serious or life-threatening toxicities of tamoxifen (thromboembolic disease, retinitis) are rare. Common side effects include hot flashes and weight gain, sometimes due to fluid retention. Mild nausea also occurs occasionally. In premenopausal women with hormone receptor–positive neoplasms and overt metastatic disease, both oophorectomy and antiestrogen therapy can be useful. However, in the adjuvant setting, the use of cytotoxic chemotherapy remains indicated irrespective of hormone receptor status, as it appears to have curative potential. The role of ovarian ablation or antiestrogen therapy added to chemotherapy in the adjuvant setting remains to be defined. Occasional palliative benefits have been reported for the use of tamoxifen in other neoplasms such as ovarian or endometrial cancer.

Androgens and Antiandrogens. Androgen therapy is contraindicated in prostate cancer because it is a growth stimulant. Virilizing androgens such as testosterone propionate, fluoxymesterone (Halotestin), and testosterone enanthate (Delatestryl) have all been used in the treatment of metastatic breast cancer with definite beneficial effects in hormone receptor–positive disease. However, androgen therapy has largely been replaced with antiestrogen therapy because the antiestrogen does not cause hirsutism, deepening of the voice, or changes in libido. Additionally, the oral halogenated androgens (e.g., fluoxymesterone) also can cause cholestatic jaundice. The antiandrogen flutamide (Eulexin) is a useful agent in the treatment of prostate cancer in combination with one of the gonadotropin-releasing hormone agonists (Lupron, Zoladex), and these combinations function as a "medical orchiectomy."

Progestins. Progestins are useful in palliative management of patients with metastatic breast or endometrial cancer and can cause tumor regression in patients with endocrine-sensitive disease. There is no evidence to suggest their utility in the adjuvant setting in either of these neoplasms. Occasional patients with prostate cancer also appear to benefit from progestational therapy. The most commonly used progestins include megestrol acetate (Megace), medroxyprogesterone (Provera), and hydroxyprogesterone caproate (Delalutin). Megestrol acetate is a useful oral progestin for second-line endocrine therapy for patients with metastatic breast cancer who show initial responsiveness to tamoxifen. In patients who experience disturbing side effects from tamoxifen (e.g., severe hot flashes), megestrol acetate may represent a reasonable alternative. In addition to its antitumor effects, megestrol acetate improves appetite in some patients with cancer-induced cachexia.

Glucocorticoids. Adrenal steroid hormones of the glucocorticoid class (e.g., prednisone, methylprednisolone, dexamethasone) are very useful anticancer agents in the treatment of lymphoid malignancies and may also potentiate the effects of cytotoxic agents in these tumor types as well as in breast cancer and perhaps other neoplasms. The glucocorticoids also play an important role in the treatment of complications of cancer (hypercalcemia, cerebral edema). Glucocorticoids are lympholytic and

TABLE 164–7. HORMONALLY ACTIVE AGENTS IN CANCER TREATMENT

Representative Agents	Dose (oral unless specified)	Toxicity A = Acute D = Delayed	Uses
Glucocorticoids			
Prednisone	20–100 mg/day or 50 mg qod (single dose)	A: Fluid retention, hyperglycemia, euphoria, depression, hypokalemia	Leukemia Lymphoma Myeloma Breast cancer Brain metastases
Dexamethasone	4–16 mg/day or 40 mg/day for 4-day pulses every 2–4 weeks	D: Osteoporosis, immunosuppression, gastrointestinal ulcers, cushingoid appearance, cataracts	
Estrogen			
Diethylstilbestrol	5 mg tid (breast) 1–3 mg qd (prostate)	A: Nausea, vomiting, fluid retention, hypercalcemia (flare reaction with bone metastases), uterine bleeding D: Feminization, accelerated coronary artery disease	Breast cancer Prostate cancer
Antiestrogen			
Tamoxifen	20 mg qd	A: Occasional nausea, fluid retention, hot flashes D: Retinal degeneration	Breast cancer
Aromatase Inhibitor			
Aminoglutethimide (plus hydrocortisone 20 mg bid)	250 mg bid (breast) 250 mg qid (prostate)	A: Dizziness D: Rash (transient)	Breast cancer Prostate cancer
Progestins			
Megestrol acetate	40 mg qid	A: Increased appetite (Megestrol), fluid retention	Breast cancer Endometrial cancer
Hydroxyprogesterone	1 gm IM biw	D: Weight gain, thromboembolism	Renal cancer
Androgens			
Fluoxymesterone	10–20 mg qd	A: Cholestatic jaundice (with oral drug)	Breast cancer
Testosterone	600 mg IM q 4–6 wks	D: Virilization	
Antiandrogen			
Flutamide	250 mg tid	D: Gynecomastia	Prostate cancer
Gonadotropin-releasing hormone agonists (depot formulations)			
Leuprolide acetate	7.5 mg SQ monthly	A: Transient flare of symptoms	Prostate cancer
Goserelin acetate	3.6 mg SQ monthly		Breast cancer (?)

nonmyelosuppressive and have therefore been incorporated into combination chemotherapy for acute and chronic lymphocytic leukemia, malignant lymphoma, and multiple myeloma.

AROMATASE INHIBITORS. Aminoglutethimide (Cytodren) inhibits the first step in adrenal steroid synthesis. Additionally, and probably more importantly, aminoglutethimide also inhibits the extra-adrenal conversion of the adrenal androgen androstenedione to estrone by the enzyme aromatase. Aromatase is found in body fat and some other tissues and provides an explanation for the presence of the weak estrogen estrone in the plasma of postmenopausal women. Aminoglutethimide is a useful agent in the palliative treatment of recurrent breast cancer in hormone receptor–positive patients. It is used in combination with hydrocortisone both to suppress endogenous steroid hormone synthesis (including androstenedione) as well as ACTH production and to slow the catabolism of aminoglutethimide. Aminoglutethimide is commonly administered in a dose of 250 mg twice daily along with 20 mg of hydrocortisone. Somewhat higher doses of aminoglutethimide have been employed for second-line endocrine therapy for metastatic prostate cancer. Patients receiving aminoglutethimide and hydrocortisone should be cautioned to avoid abrupt cessation of therapy to avoid symptoms of adrenal insufficiency.

GONADOTROPIN-RELEASING HORMONE (GnRH, LHRH) AGONISTS. Several synthetic analogues of natural GnRH (LHRH) are now clinically available. Both leuprolide acetate (Lupron) and goserelin acetate (Zoladex) are available in long-acting parenteral-depot formulations. These analogues are more potent than natural GnRH and function as GnRH agonists but also have an unusual effect on the pituitary, consisting of initial stimulation followed by long-term inhibition of the release of FSH and LH. This initial increase in gonadotropins can cause a transient increase in symptoms in patients with bone metastases. The inhibition of release of the gonadotropin reduces testicular androgen synthesis in males and ovarian estrogen production in women. The effects on testicular androgen production led to use of a GnRH agonist as an alternative to surgical orchiectomy in patients with prostate cancer. In comparative trials, GnRH agonists are as effective as estrogen therapy, and the two show comparable suppression of androgen synthesis and prostatic acid phosphatase. However, gynecomastia, nausea, vomiting, edema, and thromboembolic disease are not significant problems with the GnRH agonists. The effectiveness of GNRH agonists is enhanced by administration in combination with an antiandrogen (flutamide), and the combination has been reported to be more effective than a GnRH agonist alone in patients with Duke's D_2 metastatic prostate cancer. However, impotence results from this form of "medical orchiectomy," so it does not differ in that regard from surgical orchiectomy except that the effects of medical therapy are potentially reversible if treatment is discontinued. Medical orchiectomy is more expensive but acceptable to patients who decline surgical orchiectomy. GnRH agonists now show promise in combination with antiestrogens as endocrine therapy for premenopausal women with hormone receptor–positive breast cancer. The GnRH agonists are abortifacients in animals and should not be given to women who are or may become pregnant.

BIOLOGIC THERAPY

A major new form of cancer therapy, still early in its evolution, is the use of recombinant cytokines, growth factors, and monoclonal antibodies for the treatment of cancer. It is already clear that a number of biologic agents are directly useful as anticancer agents and that others play a supportive role. Thus, biologic therapy can now be considered the fourth major modality in cancer therapy. The term "biologic therapy" was developed to describe this heterogeneous group of agents that either are normal mammalian mediators or achieve antitumor effects through endogenous host defense mechanisms. Thus, the underlying concept is that the various biologic agents stimulate or participate in host immune defense mechanisms for the elimination of foreign molecules or cells, including transformed cells in neoplastic disease.

The biologic agents have also been termed "biologic response modifiers" (BRM's). Both the cellular and humoral limbs of

immunity can be exploited in cancer therapy. The cellular defenses include several classes of cytotoxic lymphocytes (natural killer [NK] cells), lymphokine-activated killer (LAK) cells, tumor infiltrating lymphoma (TIL), and cytotoxic T-lymphocytes (CTL), as well as antibody-dependent cytotoxic cells (ADCC). Additionally, the nonspecific cells of the reticuloendothelial system including activated macrophages may be important. Humoral agents with antitumor activities include cytokines such as interferons and interleukins as well as specific antibodies. Most of these humoral agents interact with specific immune effector cells in coordinated and synergistic fashion. The general availability of cytokines and growth factors has been facilitated by the development of recombinant DNA technology. Antibodies are highly specific and generally interact directly with their tumor targets when they are directed against cell surface constituents. Some humoral agents including the tumor necrosis factors α and β have potent local antitumor properties in preclinical models but have yet to be shown to be clinically useful.

Vaccines based on specific bacterial agents or extracts from bacteria can nonspecifically activate the host immune system. Using BCG, this approach has been applied successfully to intravesical therapy of in situ cancer of the urinary bladder. Specific cancer-associated antigen vaccines have been under active investigation for many years but have yet to be proven effective in cancer treatment. Approaches to biologic therapy of cancer are summarized in Table 164–8 and are discussed below.

INTERFERONS. The interferons (IFN's) are a family of antiviral proteins that differ in their cellular origin and polypeptide structure as well as in their clinical applications. The three major molecular species are IFN-α, -β, and -γ. IFN-α and -β mediate their action by binding to the same cell surface receptor, whereas a second cell surface receptor mediates the action of IFN-γ. IFN-α is the major IFN species for use in the treatment of hematologic malignancies and solid tumors. At present it is unclear whether IFN-β or -γ will have sufficient advantage over IFN-α in any specific cancer indication to gain regulatory approval. IFN-γ enhances granulocyte microbicidal function and macrophage activity and has definite value in the treatment of chronic granulomatous disease of children. IFN-γ may also prove useful in other infectious or inflammatory disorders as well.

Interferon-α. Recombinant IFN-α (IFN-α_2 Intron-A, Roferon) is a polypeptide cytokine with antiviral properties which is also useful for single-agent treatment of selected hematologic malignancies and solid tumors. The precise mechanism of antitumor action of IFN is still poorly understood, but it is known to activate the transcription of a number of cellular genes. IFN-inducible genes include those encoding for 2′,5′-oligoadenylate synthetases, RNase, and RNA-activated initiation factor 2 kinase, as well as for cellular proteins such as class I and II MHC antigens, β_2-microglobulin, metallothionein IIA, and Fc receptors. Additionally, IFN action inhibits the synthesis of a number of proteins in

TABLE 164–8. BIOLOGIC THERAPY OF CANCER: APPROACHES AND AGENTS

Approach	Agents
Active immunotherapy	
Nonspecific	Adjuvants: BCG, levamisole
	Cytokines: Interferons
	Interleukin-2
	Interleukin-4
	Tumor necrosis factors
Specific	Tumor cell vaccines
Passive serotherapy	
Antibodies	Polyclonal or monoclonal antibodies (alone or conjugated with drugs, radionuclides, or toxins)
Adoptive cellular therapy	Lymphokine-activated killer cells
	Tumor-infiltrating lymphocytes
Immunomodulators	Levamisole, thymic hormones
Bone marrow growth factors (see Table 164–10)	GCSF, GMCSF, MCSF, IL-3, EPO
Growth factor antagonists	Suramin
	Antibodies to growth factor receptors (e.g., EGF, HER-2/neu, IL-2 receptors)

sensitive tumor target cells including ornithine decarboxylase, a rate-limiting enzyme in polyamine metabolism. Although IFN-α also has antiviral and immunoregulatory properties that alter the biologic function of many cell types involved in humoral and cellular immunity, it is unclear whether these additional functions have any bearing on its antitumor properties above and beyond its direct receptor-mediated effects on sensitive tumor cells. The antitumor properties of IFN-α also appear to be schedule-dependent with a cytostatic mode of action. Most remissions induced by IFN are only partial.

IFN-α can be administered parenterally by intravenous, intramuscular, subcutaneous, and intracavitary routes. Its preferred route of systemic use is by subcutaneous administration, which provides the longest duration of action. The dosage schedules of IFN-α are quite variable, and higher dosages may be required for some tumor types than for others. The tumor type most sensitive to IFN-α is hairy cell leukemia (HCL). Usual dosages are in the range of 3 million IU administered subcutaneously three times weekly. At these low dosage levels, IFN usually causes only mild side effects such as fever and chills with the first few doses. On the other hand, for Kaposi's sarcoma, far more aggressive and toxic IFN schedules are required and can cause significant anorexia, weight loss, failure in concentration, and profound weakness. High-dose IFN can also induce occasional cardiac arrhythmias, nausea, vomiting, leukopenia, myalgias, proteinuria, and hepatic dysfunction ("transaminitis"). Dosages thus have been derived in relation to their effects on specific forms of cancer and individualized to patient tolerance. Optimal biologic and antitumor effects appear to be more related to tumor type and perhaps biologic response modification than to dose alone. At all dosage schedules examined, elderly patients appear to develop more marked side effects. Some of the major current uses and dosage levels for IFN-α are summarized in Table 164–9.

IFN-α is also useful in the treatment of chronic myeloid leukemia, multiple myeloma, and some of the low-grade non-Hodgkin's lymphomas, and in some patients with metastatic melanoma or renal cell carcinoma. In myeloma, IFN-α appears to play a valuable role in maintaining remissions induced by chemotherapy. Patients receiving recombinant IFN-α for HCL, CML, or renal cancer have developed neutralizing antibodies to the recombinant product at the time of disease progression after an IFN-induced remission. A limited number of patients with neutralizing antibodies have been successfully retreated by switching to nonrecombinant IFN-α. IFN-α has recently been incorporated into combination therapy with various cytotoxic and endocrine agents. At present, use of IFN-α in combination with 5-FU is being explored in the treatment of metastatic colorectal cancer based on encouraging preliminary reports with an active but toxic regimen. Although the clinical indications for IFN therapy continue to grow gradually, it clearly does not have the type of broad-spectrum anticancer effects that were initially envisioned.

INTERLEUKIN-2 (IL-2, PROLEUKIN). IL-2 is an immuno-modulatory cytokine that acts on T-cell progenitors to produce LAK cells that have cytotoxic effects in specific forms of cancer. Recombinant IL-2 has not yet been approved for therapeutic use by the United States Food and Drug Administration, although its use in renal cancer has been approved in some European countries. IL-2 has been used by direct intravenous infusion to induce LAK cells in the patient, or additionally after leukopheresis of the patient to obtain circulating lymphocytes that can then

be exposed to IL-2 in vitro for activation of lymphoid progenitors in tissue culture to form LAK cells. During the several days of culture in vitro there is marked cellular proliferation of activated LAK cells. The LAK cells are then reinfused into the patient over several days along with additional dosages of IL-2 as a form of "adoptive immunotherapy." After the initial reports of very high response rates to IL-2/LAK by investigators at the National Cancer Institute, a number of other investigators have explored the use of IL-2 alone or of IL-2 plus LAK cells. There is general agreement that either IL-2 or IL-2/LAK can induce tumor regression in 10 to 20 per cent of patients with renal carcinoma, melanoma, lymphoma, or other neoplasms.

Whereas the infusion of LAK cells causes relatively few side effects, IL-2 induces considerable toxicity. Patients receiving high-dose IL-2 must be in an intensive care unit with very close management of blood pressure, fluids, and electrolytes. The high-dose regimens are suitable only for younger patients without other significant disease or impairment of cardiac, pulmonary, hepatic, or renal function. Common side effects of high-dose LAK/IL-2 are probably due to lymphoid infiltrates in major organs and a capillary leak syndrome induced by IL-2. Shortly after initiation of high-dose IL-2 therapy, tachycardia develops, and a significant drop in arterial blood pressure occurs. As IL-2 administration continues, compensatory fluid retention occurs, and the patient develops significant weight gain as well as oliguria and azotemia. Vasopressors are often needed. However, weight gain and hepatic and renal dysfunction remain quite common with the high-dose IL-2 regimens. Even at lower doses that can be used in a conventional hospital or outpatient setting (e.g., 3 million IU per square meter daily by intravenous infusion for 2 weeks), hypotension and fluid retention are not uncommon.

Pulmonary metastases appear to be somewhat more sensitive to IL-2 or IL-2/LAK therapy than are other tumors. With the adoptive immunotherapy approach using IL-2/LAK, a small percentage of patients treated at the National Cancer Institute who had undergone prior removal of the primary tumor achieved complete remission with all evidence of metastatic disease disappearing for prolonged periods of time. Some controversy nonetheless remains as to whether the use of high-dose IL-2/LAK has any advantage over administration of IL-2 alone at a lower and better-tolerated dosage level.

The National Cancer Institute group has moved on from IL-2/LAK to the collection of another subset of T-lymphoid cells called tumor-infiltrating lymphocytes (TIL). These are obtained by extracting lymphocytes from tumor biopsies from the patient and activating them in vitro with IL-2. Subsequently they are reinfused along with IL-2. In the initial clinical studies, activated TIL cells appear to have greater antitumor activity (e.g., in melanoma) than LAK cells, with 50 per cent of patients responding to TIL/IL2 therapy. The findings with IL-2, IL-2/LAK, and IL-2/TIL provide the first clear indication that endogenous cells in the immune system are capable of being activated to manifest anticancer properties. Thus, the findings to date are perhaps less important as a specific treatment than as an indication that this approach to biologic therapy with cytokines may serve as the basis for even more effective immunologic approaches to treatment of cancer.

LEVAMISOLE (ERGAMISOLE). Levamisole is an anthelmintic agent that was found to have immunopotentiating properties.

TABLE 164–9. SOME CURRENT USES OF INTERFERON-α IN CLINICAL ONCOLOGY

Tumor Type	Dose (mU)	Response Rate (%)
Hairy cell leukemia	3/day or 3 times weekly	75–90
Chronic myeloid leukemia	5/m²/day	50–80
Multiple myeloma	3/m²/day or 3 times weekly	20–30*
Cutaneous T-cell lymphoma	10/day or 3 times weekly	45
Follicular (B-cell) lymphoma	5/day or 3 times weekly	30–50*
Kaposi's sarcoma	10/m²/day or 3 times weekly	30
Metastatic melanoma	5–10/m² 3 times weekly	10–20
Renal cell carcinoma	5–10/m² 3 times weekly	10–30
Carcinoid syndrome	5/m² 3 times weekly	20–30†

*Also being used for remission maintenance therapy.
†Reduction in symptomatology and 5-HIAA excretion.

Administration of levamisole to patients with Hodgkin's disease has been reported to enhance various tests of cell-mediated immunity but has not been shown to have a beneficial therapeutic effect in those patients. However, when combined with 5-FU, levamisole has recently been reported to play a significant role in adjuvant chemotherapy of patients with Duke's C colon cancer. With use of the combination after surgery the recurrence rate is one third less than with surgery alone. The mechanism of potentiation of 5-FU effectiveness remains obscure. In patients with overt metastatic colon cancer, the combination of 5-FU and levamisole does not appear to be any more useful than 5-FU alone.

ANTITUMOR ANTIBODY THERAPY. The use of antibodies as therapeutic agents for cancer has been a longstanding dream, as antibodies have the ability to home to tumor-associated antigens and to bind to tumor cells and lyse them either directly via complement fixation or through cooperative mechanisms also involving cellular immunity (e.g., ADCC). The selective binding of antibodies to tumor cells has led to their use as carriers for highly potent therapeutic agents. In addition, diagnostic uses have included radionuclide conjugates for tumor imaging. Within the past decade, considerable effort has been expended to evaluate polyclonal and monoclonal antibodies from different mammalian species as potential therapeutic agents for patients with cancer. Antibody therapy has incorporated both unconjugated and radionuclide-, drug-, and toxin-conjugated antibodies. A number of problems have beset the development of antibody therapy, the first of which has been to identify antigens that are expressed uniquely on malignant cells and either not at all or to a far lesser extent on normal host cells. At the present time, antibody-based therapy for cancer remains investigational and has not been approved by the Food and Drug Administration.

Antibody therapy has shown some encouraging results in malignant B-cell lymphoma (both Hodgkin's disease and non-Hodgkin's lymphomas as well as chronic lymphocytic leukemia) and perhaps in hepatocellular carcinoma. Objective tumor regressions have been observed after administration of unconjugated, radionuclide-conjugated, and toxin-conjugated antibodies directed at lymphoma cells. One of the most impressive pilot observations used murine anti-idiotypic antibodies to the cell surface Ig on neoplastic B cells, and at least one prolonged complete remission was achieved using this technique. However, development of anti-idiotypic antibodies has required preparing a specific antibody for each individual patient. More recently, increasing efforts in lymphoma have been focused on employing antibodies that recognize "shared idiotypes" or other lymphoid-associated antigens as targets for antibodies that can be developed through more conventional methods. For other tumor types, results with antibody-based therapy have been disappointing.

The logistics of heterologous murine antibody therapy remain difficult. For most tumor types studied in patients there is a relatively "narrow window" of 1 to 2 weeks of therapy before the recipient develops a vigorous human antimurine antibody (HAMA) response that renders further antibody administration difficult owing to rapid inactivation and clearance of the administered antibody. Attempts to block this HAMA reaction with immunosuppressive agents have thus far been unsuccessful. Perhaps in part because of associated defects in immunologic responsiveness, patients with monoclonal B-lymphoid neoplasms can sometimes be treated for a longer time before the HAMA response becomes significant. In efforts to minimize the HAMA reaction, molecular biologic techniques are now being used to either "chimerize" or "humanize" the murine antibodies so that the constant regions of their murine structural components are replaced with human immunoglobulin sequences. Another specialized application of antitumor antibodies has been for the purging ex vivo of tumor cells from the bone marrow to be reinfused into patients who are to receive high-dose chemotherapy and autologous bone marrow rescue. This application has been used with success in lymphoma, neuroblastoma, and some other tumor types.

GROWTH FACTOR ANTAGONISTS. The use of antagonists to polypeptide growth factors is in a sense an extension of endocrine therapy but represents a form of biologic therapy as well. One growth factor antagonist that has recently been rec-

ognized to have anticancer properties is suramin, which has been used since the 1920's for the treatment of African sleeping sickness. Suramin is a polysulfonated naphthylurea that binds tightly to heparin-binding growth factors such as fibroblast growth factor (FGF), platelet-derived growth factor (PDGF), and insulin-like growth factor (IGF-1). Exclusion of growth factors from their receptors can result in "programmed cell death." Suramin is active in the treatment of prostate cancer, presumably by blocking the action of FGF and other growth factors. However, suramin also inhibits the function of a variety of enzymes and other proteins, so its precise mechanism of antitumor action remains to be defined. The multiple actions of suramin also account for a broad range of toxicities, which can be severe or irreversible. One of these is adrenal insufficiency, which requires long-term adrenal steroid replacement. Frequent plasma monitoring of suramin concentrations is essential, because there is the potential for serious neuropathy when suramin concentrations exceed 300 μg per milliliter. The use of suramin in cancer therapy is currently investigational. Suramin represents the first member of a new class of investigational agents that are active as BRM's for cancer therapy. Another approach to growth factor receptor blockade involves use of monoclonal antibodies to epidermal growth factor (EGF) receptor and to the IL-2 receptor.

BONE MARROW GROWTH FACTORS. A new approach to supportive care for bone marrow failure associated with cancer and for maintaining adequate hematopoietic function between courses of myelosuppressive chemotherapy is to administer bone marrow growth factors to stimulate an increased rate of production of myeloid progenitors. The bone marrow growth factors are glycoproteins that function in overlapping and hierarchical fashion on bone marrow progenitors and not only result in cell proliferation but also activate differentiation and cell trafficking. The factors currently in clinical trials in cancer patients are summarized in Table 164–10. The major factors also potently stimulate the proliferation of myeloid precursors. Several of these recombinant proteins, including granulocyte colony–stimulating factor (GCSF), granulocyte-macrophage colony–stimulating factor (GMCSF), and erythropoietin (Epogen, EPO) (see Table 164–6), are now entering general use for cancer treatment. Both IL-3 and macrophage colony–stimulating factor are at an earlier stage of development and their role in supportive care is currently uncertain. GCSF and GMCSF are approaching approval by the Food and Drug Administration. EPO was recently approved for the anemia associated with renal failure. Clinical trials using subcutaneously administered GCSF or GMCSF have shown that use of either can shorten the duration of granulocytopenia, the frequency of infectious complications, and the duration of hospitalization after chemotherapy combinations that are normally given on an inpatient setting. With bone marrow transplantation (wherein high-dose chemotherapy and/or total body radiation is employed) both myelosuppressive and nonmyelosuppressive side effects can be diminished with the use of GCSF or GMCSF. Although IL-3 (multi-CSF) is only in early clinical trial, preliminary evidence suggests that this bone marrow growth factor can stimulate platelet and red blood cell as well as granulocyte production.

In preclinical studies, IL-3 also appears to act synergistically with GMCSF to produce more complete and rapid recovery of circulating granulocytes and platelets than can be obtained with either factor alone. The major toxicities of the growth factors that

TABLE 164–10. RECOMBINANT BONE MARROW GROWTH FACTORS OF POTENTIAL IMPORTANCE IN SUPPORTIVE CARE OF CANCER PATIENTS

Growth Factor*	Effects
GCSF	Stimulates granulocyte production
GMCSF	Stimulates granulocyte, macrophage, and eosinophil production
MCSF	Stimulates macrophage production and activation
IL-3	Stimulates granulocyte, macrophage, and platelet production
EPO	Stimulates production of RBC's

*GCSF = granulocyte colony–stimulating factor; GMCSF = granulocyte-macrophage colony–stimulating factor; MCSF = macrophage colony–stimulating factor; IL-3 = interleukin-3; EPO = erythropoietin.

stimulate white cell production include fever, myalgias, and occasional skin rashes. Pericarditis has been reported with high-dose GMCSF or GCSF. Recombinant erythropoietin is already in general clinical use for the anemia of renal failure. Preliminary studies also suggest that when used in pharmacologic doses, EPO can restore normal red blood cell counts in some patients with multiple myeloma and perhaps in some other hematologic malignancies as well. EPO also has promise for reducing the degree of anemia induced by cytotoxic chemotherapy.

SUMMARY

Medical management of cancer is a complex task that requires extensive knowledge and clinical experience. The requisite knowledge includes not only the pharmacology and toxicology of and indications for cytotoxic, endocrine, and biologic agents but also an appreciation of the important roles of surgery and radiation therapy. Increasingly, the medical specialist plays a role in the patient's primary treatment, and the major modalities must be combined effectively for success. The steep dose-response curves for cytotoxic drugs leave little margin for error, and effective doses are very close to toxic levels. The practitioner who reduces drug doses a priori in an attempt to reduce toxicities that occur with standard protocols markedly reduces the likelihood that treatment will be successful. It is particularly important that standard protocol dosage regimens be used in initial therapy for patients with tumor types listed in sections A and B of Table 164–4, as they have the most to lose if they receive reduced and ineffective dosage regimens. Physicians are encouraged to have their patients participate in formal clinical trials of cancer therapy that are conducted at major cancer centers or through the clinical trials cooperative groups. Current therapy for many forms of cancer is in need of improvement, and this goal requires active participation by oncologic specialists and patients in large-scale clinical research.

Chabner BA, Collins JM: Cancer Chemotherapy: Principles and Practice. Philadelphia, J.P. Lippincott Company, 1990. *An excellent reference on cancer chemotherapy, including detailed discussion of the pharmacology of anticancer drugs.*

DeVita VT, Hellman S, Rosenberg SA: Cancer: Principles and Practice of Oncology, 3rd ed. Philadelphia, J.B. Lippincott Company, 1989. *A comprehensive textbook covering clinical, diagnostic, and therapeutic approaches for all major forms of cancer. Major modalities of treatment as well as drug combination schedules are delineated in detail in relation to relevant tumor types.*

Salmon SE (ed.): Adjuvant Therapy of Cancer 6. Philadelphia, W.B. Saunders Company, 1990. *An up-to-date summary of results of the most recent clinical trials of adjuvant and neoadjuvant chemotherapy for most forms of cancer.*

165 Oncologic Emergencies

Stephen M. Hahn and Angelo Russo

The care of patients with cancer is an exercise in the management of chronic disease. However, when acute oncologic emergencies occur, rapid evaluation and institution of therapy are required. Since several cancer types are now routinely cured and there is a general increase in the quality of life and survival time in patients with cancer, the early recognition and treatment of oncologic emergencies have a definite role in medical management.

FEVER AND NEUTROPENIA

The most common emergency encountered in clinical oncology is fever (temperature greater than 38°C or 100.5°F) and neutropenia (absolute neutrophil count less than 1000 per cubic millimeter). Neutropenic cancer patients have an increased risk of systemic infection and rapid development of the septic syndrome. Empiric emergency antibiotic therapy is crucial.

Infection risk increases once the neutrophil count drops below 1000 per cubic millimeter. Disruption of the patient's other host defenses also predisposes to infection. Paramount among these is disruption of the gastrointestinal barrier with mucositis. Additional factors include the presence of indwelling catheters, invasive procedures, and abnormal cellular and humoral immunity.

The patient usually presents with few signs or symptoms other than fever. Localized infection may be present but not clinically apparent. A careful history and physical examination must be performed focusing on common sites of infection. The oral cavity should be inspected for evidence of mucositis. Lesions suggestive of anaerobic, viral (especially herpes simplex), and fungal (especially *Candida* species) infection may be present. Odynophagia strongly suggests esophagitis. Examination of soft tissue and skin, especially at catheter sites, may show early cellulitis or septic phlebitis. A perirectal abscess should be sought by careful palpation of the anorectal area for induration, fluctuance, or tenderness.

Cultures should be performed on all patients prior to the initiation of antibiotic therapy and routinely sent for isolation of bacteria and fungi. Blood cultures should be obtained both from the port of an indwelling central catheter and from peripheral veins. If an indwelling catheter is suspected to be the source of infection, it should be removed and the tip sent for Gram's stain and culture. Sputum examination by Gram's stain and culture is usually not helpful but should be obtained if sputum is produced. Gram's stain and bacterial, fungal, and viral cultures should be performed on all oral, skin, and soft tissue lesions. Biopsies of cutaneous lesions may be especially helpful in the diagnosis of systemic viral and fungal infections and can be safely performed in the neutropenic patient. Chest radiography, urinalysis with microscopy, and evaluation of ascites and pleural fluid should be performed. Although meningitis is not typically encountered in febrile neutropenic cancer patients, a lumbar puncture is indicated in those patients with suggestive clinical signs or symptoms.

Indwelling urinary tract catheters and unnecessary intravenous catheters are to be avoided. Strict handwashing by all hospital personnel is required. Aggressive prophylactic or therapeutic mouth care (suggested regimen: Nystatin suspension, benadryl/antacid/lidocaine mixture, and 5 per cent sodium bicarbonate solution, alternating each every 2 hours, administered as swish and spit) provides relief of symptoms and may improve the patient's course.

Once evaluated and hospitalized, the patient should be started without delay on broad-spectrum antibiotics that include coverage for *Pseudomonas* species and other gram-negative organisms. Based upon the isolate patterns at an individual institution, coverage for gram-positive organisms may be necessary. Suggested regimens are (1) a third-generation cephalosporin (ceftazidime, 1 gram every 4 hours intravenously) or (2) a semisynthetic penicillin (piperacillin or mezlocillin, 3 to 4 grams every 4 hours intravenously) plus an aminoglycoside (gentamicin or tobramycin, 2 mg per kilogram loading dose followed by one to three divided doses daily depending upon renal function). If a specific organism is suspected, appropriate antibiotics should be added to the initial regimen. For example, if infection of an indwelling catheter is likely, additional gram-positive coverage with vancomycin (500 mg every 6 hours intravenously) should be added for *Staphylococcus aureus* and *Staphylococcus epidermidis*. Anaerobic coverage with clindamycin (250 to 750 mg intravenously every 6 hours) is strongly recommended for patients with mucositis or periodontal infections.

If fever persists after the initiation of antibiotics, cultures and diagnostic studies should again be performed daily and broader gram-positive coverage should be added to the patient's regimen. Patients with prolonged neutropenia on broad-spectrum antibiotics are at high risk for fungal infection. Early institution of antifungal therapy may be life saving. If the patient remains febrile after 5 to 7 days, empiric antifungal therapy with amphotericin B should be started (0.5 to 1.0 mg per kilogram per day intravenously). In general, if the neutropenic patient remains febrile despite broad-spectrum therapy, one should consider the following diagnostic possibilities: a second bacterial isolate, abscess, anaerobic infection, gram-positive bacteria, atypical organisms, fungi, and viruses.

Approximately 50 per cent of patients with fever and neutropenia have a documented infection. If a causative organism or a specific infection is discovered, specific therapy should be initiated; however, broad-spectrum antibiotics should not be discontinued, since there is a 40 per cent chance of developing infection with a second isolate when antibiotic therapy is narrowed.

Patients with documented infections should be treated until the infection resolves (usually a 2-week course of antibiotic therapy). Antibiotics may be discontinued when the absolute neutrophil count exceeds 1000 per cubic millimeter if the patient is afebrile and no specific infection has been documented. Antibiotics should be continued in the patient who remains neutropenic even if he or she becomes afebrile. Clinical deterioration or the return of fever occurs in a significant proportion of these patients.

At one time, white cell transfusions were thought to be indicated in the patient with gram-negative infection and prolonged neutropenia. However, it is unclear whether this benefits the patient, and the risk of morbidity or mortality (infectious diseases, alloimmunization, and pulmonary toxicity) is significant. Therefore, white cell transfusions are not recommended as routine care of the febrile neutropenic patient. Prophylaxis with absorbable or nonabsorbable antibiotics is controversial and not routinely recommended. Prophylactic antibiotic regimens may actually prolong cytopenias or lead to the development of infection with resistant organisms. *Clostridium difficile* infection and vitamin K deficiency may occur in the setting of broad-spectrum antibiotic use.

SPINAL CORD COMPRESSION

Back or neck pain is a frequent complaint in the general population; in a cancer patient it can be a harbinger of neurologic disaster and merits immediate, careful evaluation. The pain is worsened by straining, sneezing, coughing, movement, and recumbency. Complaints may precede diagnosis by days to months; however, once neurologic signs are present, progression is usually rapid. Typically, back pain progresses to radicular pain followed by weakness, sensory loss, paralysis, and/or loss of sphincter control (manifested as urinary or fecal retention or incontinence). Early recognition is important, as ambulatory ability and maintenance of sphincter control at initiation of therapy are highly correlated with successful outcome. Less than 15 per cent of patients with paraplegia or loss of sphincter tone regain function. The site frequency of spinal cord involvement corresponds to the volume and number of vertebral bodies (thoracic>lumbar>cervical>sacral). Although any malignancy can metastasize to and encroach upon the epidural space, tumors of lung or breast, lymphoma, carcinoma of unknown primary, myeloma, sarcoma, carcinoma of the prostate or kidney, melanoma, and gastrointestinal and thyroid carcinomas are commonly associated with spinal cord compression.

Evaluation and treatment tempo are determined by physical examination (Fig. 165–1). The patient with signs of spinal compression deserves immediate treatment with dexamethasone (10 mg intravenously followed by 4 mg every 6 hours) and emergency evaluation. Patients with no neurologic findings may be expeditiously evaluated as outpatients. In two thirds of patients with spinal cord compression, plain film radiographs of the spine show erosion or loss of pedicles, partial or complete collapse of vertebral bodies, or paraspinous mass. Metrizamide myelography is the diagnostic gold standard. The test is quickly performed and more easily tolerated than magnetic resonance imaging (MRI). If after a lumbar injection, a myelographic block is identified, a C1-C2 puncture should be performed to visualize fully the extent of the block, as well as to define other rostral lesions (15 per cent). A computed tomography (CT) scan focused on the spinal block is often useful to further delineate the lesion. MRI is particularly helpful in delineating intramedullary, extramedullary, intradural, and extradural lesions. Encroachment (myeloma, lymphoma) on the cord through spinal foramina is particularly well demonstrated by MRI. Likewise, MRI avoids the risk (14 per cent) of neurologic deterioration with myelography in a patient having complete obstruction.

Although treatment should be individualized, radiation therapy is the treatment of choice in patients having radioresponsive tumors who have slowly evolving neurologic symptoms, incomplete block, cauda equina involvement, or widely metastatic disease. For the most part, treatment is considered palliative. Treatment is initiated with high-dose fractions, followed by lower-dose fractions. Steroids can be reduced judiciously as radiation therapy proceeds. The role of surgery in spinal cord compression

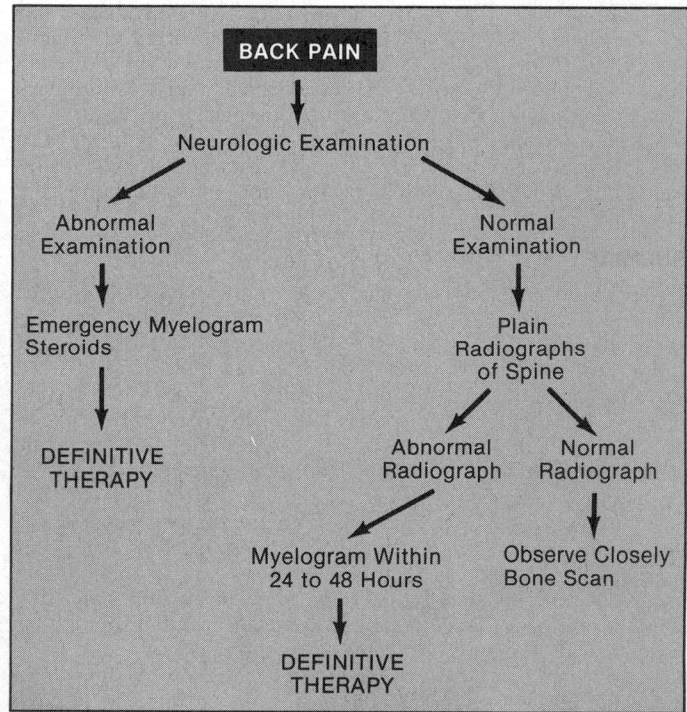

FIGURE 165–1. Flow diagram for evaluation of spinal cord compression in the cancer patient.

is evolving. Its use is recommended if a tissue diagnosis is needed, if neurologic dysfunction progresses during radiation treatment, if there is recurrent spinal cord compression in an area of previous radiation therapy, if there is spinal instability resulting from vertebral body collapse or bony protrusion into the spinal cord, or if the malignancy is considered radiation resistant (such as hypernephroma or melanoma). Simple laminectomy is not usually effective. The surgical procedure is dictated by tumor location and surgical experience and expertise. Radiation therapy should be used postoperatively. Chemotherapy for chemosensitive malignancies is used in addition to radiation or surgery.

INTRACRANIAL METASTASES

In the cancer patient, complaints of headache, altered mental status, and seizures may signal intracranial metastases. These processes are amenable to treatment and, if left untreated, could result in death. The differential diagnosis of altered mental status, seizures, and headache in a cancer patient includes iatrogenic causes (chemotherapy agents, narcotic analgesics, hypnotics, and antiemetics), metabolic disorders (hypercalcemia, hyponatremia, hypoglycemia, hypomagnesemia, hyperviscosity, hepatic encephalopathy), paraneoplastic syndromes (subacute cerebral degeneration, dementia, limbic encephalitis, optic neuritis, angioendotheliosis, progressive multifocal leukoencephalopathy), strokes (coagulation abnormalities, thrombocytopenia, Trousseau's syndrome), sepsis, and intracranial metastasis. Careful history and physical examination and laboratory evaluation are primary and should guide decision as to further workup. In the acutely ill cancer patient cranial CT should be done to define the presence and characteristics of the intracerebral lesion. MRI is more sensitive in defining metastatic lesions and differentiating between vascular and malignant lesions and should be considered if there is need to clarify CT scan findings. MRI requires more acquisition time, is highly sensitive to motion artifact, and is restricted to patients not requiring respiratory or cardiac monitoring and support. If no mass lesion is demonstrable, leptomeningeal carcinomatosis as the etiology of neurologic signs and symptoms is sought by examination of spinal fluid.

If there are signs of impending intracerebral herniation the patient should immediately have an endotracheal tube placed and be hyperventilated to maintain the P_{CO_2} between 25 and 30 mm Hg. Mannitol, up to 1.5 grams per kilogram, should be administered immediately and may be repeated every 6 hours. If there are signs of increased intracranial pressure without impending herniation, high-dose intravenous dexamethasone (10 mg every 6 hours) should be administered immediately to lessen cerebral edema. Status epilepticus requires immediate-acting drugs such as benzodiazepines and close attention to respiratory status. Seizures other than status epilepticus caused by intracranial metastasis are managed by phenytoin in an oral loading dose of 15 mg per kilogram followed by 300 mg per day. Drug levels should be monitored, since accompanying dexamethasone therapy can induce increased metabolism of phenytoin.

Radiation therapy for intracranial metastasis is usually palliative. A total dose of 30 Gy delivered over 10 to 15 fractions decreases motor deficits in approximately 33 per cent of patients and reduces or stops headaches in 50 per cent of patients. For patients with controlled or no evidence of systemic disease and a radioresponsive solitary intracranial metastasis in a site not amenable to surgery, radiation at higher doses (60 Gy) to the site of disease is justified to prolong survival. A surgically accessible solitary lesion in a patient with controlled systemic disease merits consideration of surgical removal of the tumor.

SUPERIOR VENA CAVA SYNDROME

Superior vena cava (SVC) syndrome is caused by either partial or complete obstruction of the superior vena cava. Obstruction results from extrinsic compression (90 per cent) or, less likely, fibrosis, thrombosis, or invasion. Both signs and symptoms can be subtle and evolve slowly (over 2 to 5 weeks). A spectrum of signs can be associated with the SVC syndrome, including cyanosis, edema, venous engorgement of the head, neck, arms, chest, and upper abdomen, varying degrees of airway obstruction, pleural and pericardial effusions, and tracheal edema. Nonpitting edema of the neck (Stokes' collar) can also be found. Symptoms, which frequently worsen when the patient lies down or leans forward, may include fullness or stuffiness in the ears or nose, eye disturbances, facial swelling, shortness of breath, cough, chest pain, voice changes (hoarseness), dysphagia, headache, stupor, seizures, and syncope. Back pain may herald simultaneous spinal cord compression by contiguously extending tumor. Upper extremity venography complements either CT scan or MRI with contrast in defining the obstruction.

In the past, malignancy-associated SVC syndrome was considered an oncologic emergency that merited immediate radiation treatment to avoid death from respiratory arrest or intracranial hemorrhage. Immediate therapy is indicated for impending airway obstruction (stridor) or increased intracranial pressure (stupor, seizure), particularly in a thrombocytopenic patient. Given the array of benign causes of SVC syndrome and the frequency of chemosensitive malignancies (small cell lung cancer and lymphomas), the etiology of SVC syndrome should be determined while judiciously managing the patient with diuretics and elevation of the head. Sputum cytology, bone marrow and lymph node biopsy, thoracentesis, bronchoscopy, and thoracotomy may confirm the etiology. The difference between a clotted and/or engorged vein with elevated pressures and a lymph node should be appreciated.

Once a neoplastic cause of SVC syndrome has been established, appropriate treatment should be initiated. In the majority of cases, radiation therapy remains the primary treatment with initial doses of 3 to 4 Gy per day followed by conventional doses of 1.5 to 2.0 Gy per day to a total dose of 30 to 50 Gy. The vast majority of patients (>85 per cent) experience relief within 3 weeks; however, symptoms usually recur. If small cell lung cancer, testicular cancer, or lymphoma is etiologic, appropriate chemotherapy should be administered through a lower extremity vein. Corticosteroids should be used for cerebral or laryngeal edema. The role of anticoagulants concurrent with radiation therapy remains undefined. As the use of indwelling, subclavian catheters for delivery of chemotherapy increases, the incidence of thrombosis as the etiology of SVC syndrome in cancer patients increases. Fibrinolytic therapy with urokinase (1000 U per square meter per hour during the first 24 hours; if no response, increase to 2000 U per square meter per hour for 48 hours) should be considered in those patients who have recently developed SVC syndrome and are not at high risk of dangerous bleeding. After successful fibrinolysis, heparin and subsequent coumadin therapy should be instituted to prevent recurrent SVC syndrome and to maintain the indwelling catheter.

CARDIAC TAMPONADE

Cardiac tamponade in a cancer patient may have a noncancerous etiology, may be the first manifestation of malignancy, or may signify disease progression. Diagnosis is necessary because tamponade is life threatening and successful treatment improves survival. Cardiac tamponade may result from primary tumors of the pericardium (mesothelioma, sarcoma, and teratoma) or more frequently from metastatic disease (carcinoma of the breast or lung, leukemia, lymphoma, melanoma, epidemic or nonepidemic Kaposi's sarcoma). When fluid pressure within the pericardial sac equals right atrial and ventricular diastolic pressure, cardiac tamponade occurs. As intrapericardial pressure increases, heart rate, myocardial contractility, and systemic resistance increase. If intrapericardial pressure increases rapidly, between 150 and 250 ml of fluid (normal volume <50 ml) may cause tamponade; however, if fluid accumulates slowly, more than 1 liter may be accommodated without decompensation. Symptoms are nonspecific and include shortness of breath, chest pain, cough, hoarseness, nausea, abdominal pain, hiccoughs, and distress. Signs associated with rapid effusion are a falling systolic pressure, elevated jugular venous pressure, a small, quiet heart (Beck's triad), and a narrowed arterial pulse pressure. If there has been chronic evolution of pericardial fluid, additional signs include percussion of an enlarged heart, most frequently on the left anteriorly but occasionally on the right in the fifth intercostal space (Rotch's sign), as well as a patch of dullness posteriorly below the angle of the left scapula (Ewart's sign) with bronchial breathing over this area. Pulsus paradoxicus is a classic but not constant sign of tamponade. The chest radiograph may show an enlarged globular (water bottle) heart and possibly pleural effusions. The pathognomonic finding on electrocardiogram of electrical alternans is rare; decreased voltage is frequently found. Two-dimensional echocardiography is the noninvasive, preferred diagnostic study and provides both anatomic and physiologic information. Right heart catheterization is the diagnostic gold standard and allows monitoring during therapeutic maneuvers (Fig. 165–2).

Pericardiocentesis provides immediate lifesaving treatment, allows fluid to be obtained for diagnosis, and, with insertion of a pigtail catheter, permits subsequent determination of the rate of fluid reaccumulation and instillation of drugs for treatment. Fluid can be serous, serosanguineous, or frankly hemorrhagic. In the case of hemorrhagic fluid, the absence of clot and a hematocrit lower than systemic levels weigh against the fluid resulting from

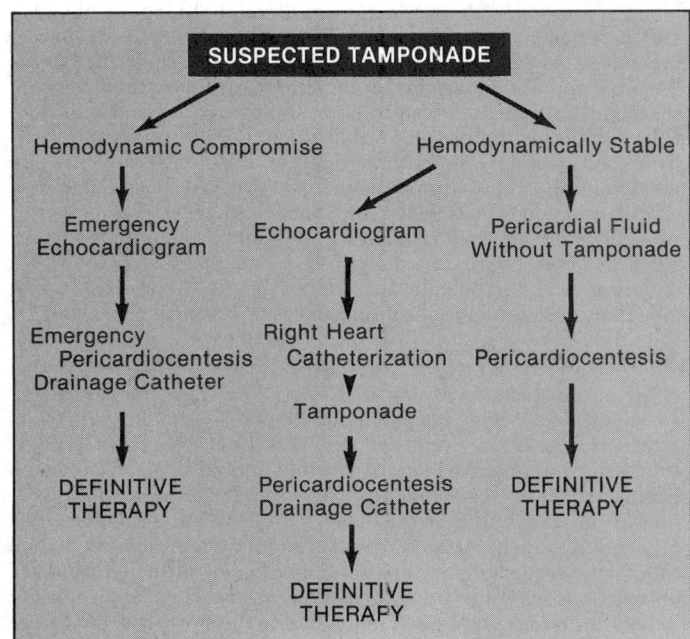

FIGURE 165–2. Flow diagram for evaluation of cardiac tamponade in the cancer patient.

puncture of the myocardium. Fluid should be sent for cultures and cytology. Once it has been established that the fluid is caused by a malignancy, there are three approaches to treatment: radiation, chemotherapy, and surgery. Radiation therapy up to 40 Gy is highly successful (approaching 100 per cent) in treating effusion caused by leukemias or lymphomas; however, unless all known disease can be encompassed within the radiation field, systemic chemotherapy is the treatment of choice for leukemic and lymphomatous pericardial effusions. Success rate for radiation control of melanoma, lung, and breast carcinoma is much lower. Surgical approaches to effusion include pericardiectomy, pleuro-pericardial window, and subxiphoid pericardiotomy. Pericardiectomy is the treatment of choice for radiation-induced constrictive pericarditis. Its use for malignant effusions is effective but carries more morbidity than either a window or subxiphoid pericardiotomy. A pleuropericardial window has a low complication rate (<5 per cent) and a relatively low recurrence rate. Subxiphoid pericardiotomy, unlike the window procedure, requires only local anesthesia and has virtually no complication or recurrence rate; however, there is an increased incidence of tumor cell dissemination. Drug instillation into the pericardial sac has been tried with various chemotherapeutic agents (thiotepa, methotrexate, nitrogen mustard), radioisotopes, and tetracycline. Tetracycline is highly effective in obliterating the pericardial space and eliminating fluid recurrence. However, there can be a period of transient fevers, arrhythmias, and chest pain. If tetracycline fails, surgical management is undertaken.

HEMOPTYSIS

The most common causes (tuberculosis, fungal infections, lung abscess, bronchiectasis, bronchial adenoma) of hemoptysis are not neoplastic; however, with increasing age, malignancies, especially of bronchogenic origin, are most common. Cancer patients who are immunocompromised and have underlying coagulation defects or thrombocytopenia and obstructing lung lesions are susceptible to infections that can cause hemoptysis. Greater than 600 ml of blood per 24 hours defines massive hemoptysis and is life threatening; however, because blood may be swallowed or aspirated, making volume determination difficult, hemoptysis associated with respiratory compromise should be considered an emergency.

Minor hemoptysis often presages massive hemoptysis; therefore, while the etiology of hemoptysis is pursued, observation, oxygen, and prevention of aspiration are prudent. The patient with massive hemoptysis is admitted to the intensive care unit. Correction of coagulopathy and thrombocytopenia, repletion of blood volume, and determination of site and etiology of bleeding are undertaken simultaneously. Bronchoscopy is the diagnostic procedure of choice for determination of site and etiology of bleeding and also allows direct therapeutic intervention. Surgical resection, if the patient can tolerate the procedure and if the site is localizable, is the procedure of choice. Other less ideal options have been used with varying degrees of success and include neodymium:yttrium-aluminum-garnet (Nd:YAG) laser-induced coagulation, endobronchial tamponade with a venous catheter, bronchial artery catheterization with embolization, and ice lavage. Nd:YAG laser is usually restricted to nonmassive hemoptysis; endobronchial tamponade should not be used for right upper lobe hemorrhages; embolization can result in spinal cord damage.

AIRWAY OBSTRUCTION

Airway obstruction by an intrinsic or extrinsic malignancy is an emergency, and management depends on the tempo of obstruction and the location, previous treatment, and type of tumor causing the obstruction. Steroids should be given to lessen edema and, in the case of lymphomas, begin treatment. Obstruction at or above the larynx and high tracheal region can be relieved by tracheostomy with subsequent definitive radiation therapy or surgery done in a nonemergency setting. More distal obstructions can be treated with surgery when indicated or radiation therapy (external and/or brachytherapy). Nd:YAG laser has found use in the care of high-grade, incomplete, centrally obstructing airway lesions. It is quick and safe and provides immediate relief. Restrictions to its use include lobar or segmental level lesions, extraluminal compression, total obstruction, upper lobe lesions, and tracheoesophageal fistula. The Nd:YAG laser treatment results in incomplete removal of tumor, and therefore high dose-rate brachytherapy (interstitial endobronchial radiation therapy) combined with laser treatment may be most useful. The use of visible light lasers and fiberoptics with photosensitizers (photodynamic therapy [PDT]) has also been used extensively for relief of obstructed airway lesions. In this case, even a lesion totally obstructing the airway can be completely removed because cylindric light-emitting fibers are used. Furthermore, PDT can be repeated. Repeat bronchoscopy 2 to 3 days following endobronchial PDT should be performed to remove necrotic tissue and evaluate the status of treatment.

HYPERCALCEMIA

Other than hyperparathyroidism, cancer is the second most frequent cause of hypercalcemia. It occurs in approximately 10 per cent of all cancer patients. Lung, particularly squamous cell, and breast cancers account for 40 to 60 per cent of all cases. Other primary malignancies frequently associated with hypercalcemia include multiple myeloma (approximately 50 per cent develop hypercalcemia at some time during disease), carcinoma of unknown primary, lymphoma (adult T-cell lymphoma), and gastrointestinal (cholangiocarcinoma and hepatoma), renal, head and neck, and prostate carcinomas. The metabolic disorder frequently occurs with metastases to bone but may occur without bone metastases. Calcium homeostasis is usually regulated between 9 and 10.6 mg per deciliter, 45 per cent of which is ionized (nonprotein bound) (see Ch. 232). In multiple myeloma associated with high immunoglobulin levels, the total serum calcium level can be exceedingly high, yet the ionized fraction can be within the normal range.

Malignancy-associated hypercalcemia can be caused by tumor secretion of parathyroid-like hormone, which results in increased bone and renal tubular calcium reabsorption. Likewise, osteolytic metastases can act directly on bone to cause calcium resorption or can secrete factors that result in bone resorption (prostaglandins) or activation of osteoclasts (osteoclast-activating factor).

The clinical manifestations may be manifold and nonspecific and depend in part on the general metabolic condition and associated illness of the patient, as well as the degree and rapidity of calcium elevation. Symptoms include polyuria, nocturia, polydipsia, anorexia, nausea, vomiting, abdominal pain, fatigue, lethargy, confusion, psychosis, agitation, stupor, obtundation, and coma. Laboratory values usually show an elevated serum calcium, commonly above 12 mg per deciliter. Electrocardiography may show narrowed QT, widened T wave, and elongated PR interval.

For patients who are symptomatic or who have serum calcium levels above 13 mg per deciliter, treatment should be immediate and aggressive. Because of the reversible defects of renal tubular absorption and subsequent loss of fluid coupled with decreased fluid intake, the patient is invariably volume depleted. Volume repletion followed by normal saline at a rate of 200 to 300 ml per hour results in calciuresis. Once rehydration is accomplished, urinary output should be maintained at 200 to 300 ml per hour. Saline-induced calciuresis can be augmented by furosemide. Electrolytes, including magnesium and phosphate, should be checked frequently and, when necessary, repleted. Salmon calcitonin (4 IU per kilogram every 12 hours increased to 8 IU per kilogram every 8 hours) can lower the serum calcium by 2 to 3 mg per deciliter within a few hours. Unfortunately, natriuresis and calcitonin are only temporizing measures. Once the patient is initially stabilized, the optimal choice is treatment of the underlying malignancy. Steroids can be effective in reducing hypercalcemia in multiple myeloma, lymphoma, and breast cancer. For chronic management of hypercalcemia, intravenous mithramycin (10 to 25 μg per kilogram) may be given every 48 hours up to three doses. The response to mithramycin may last up to 3 weeks. After the initial course, mithramycin may be administered up to twice weekly to maintain normocalcemia. Mithramycin can cause hypotension, hepatic and renal dysfunction, and bone marrow suppression, especially thrombocytopenia. Etidronate disodium is a diphosphonate that blocks osteoclast bone resorption and is approved for use in the United States. Initial administration is intravenous, 7.5 mg per kilogram per day for 3 days, and then orally, 20 mg per kilogram per day. In the future severe hypercalcemia may be treated with diphosphonates like aminohydroxypropylidene diphosphonate (APD). A single infusion of APD (45 mg) for severe malignant hypercalcemia has resulted in a response rate of 96 per cent, with normocalcemia achieved in 75 per cent of cases.

TUMOR LYSIS SYNDROME

Tumor lysis syndrome is a metabolic emergency that can be anticipated and prevented. Rapid tumor lysis is usually encountered upon initiation of chemotherapy in the setting of rapidly proliferating malignancies such as high-grade lymphomas or acute leukemias. Rarely it has been reported to occur in solid tumors. The syndrome can occur within 48 hours after arterial embolization of large tumors within the liver. Tumor lysis syndrome causes rapid and severe metabolic changes, including hyperkalemia, hyperuricemia, hyperphosphatemia, and hypocalcemia. End-organ dysfunction may also ensue. Hyperuricemia or hyperphosphatemia can cause renal failure secondary to uric acid or calcium phosphate crystallization in the tubules. Hypocalcemia caused by precipitation of calcium phosphate and lowered calcitriol levels can result in neuromuscular irritability, tetany, and obtundation. Hyperkalemia can be profound and cause cardiac arrhythmias and sudden death.

Treatment begins with identification of the patient at risk and prevention of the metabolic and end-organ changes. If a patient is likely to develop rapid tumor lysis associated with chemotherapy, hospital admission and initiation of measures to circumvent the syndrome are necessary. Volume status, electrolytes, blood urea nitrogen, creatinine, uric acid, phosphorus, and calcium serum levels are obtained before beginning chemotherapy. If the patient presents with evidence of tumor lysis syndrome prior to chemotherapy, every effort should be made to correct the metabolic abnormalities before starting chemotherapy. However, it is not always possible to postpone chemotherapy, and in such a setting, hemodialysis may be necessary. Hyperkalemia must be treated aggressively with sodium polystyrene sulfonate (Kayexalate) or if electrocardiographic changes are noted, calcium chloride, insulin, dextrose, and sodium bicarbonate. The next treatment priority is to avoid uric acid precipitation in the renal tubules. This is done by alkalinizing the urine with 0.25N sodium chloride containing two ampules (100 mEq) of sodium bicarbonate and maintaining a urinary output between 100 and 200 ml per hour. Additional bicarbonate is titrated to maintain urine pH greater than 7.0. Acetazolamide (250 mg by mouth once or twice daily) may be administered in the first days to further hasten urine alkalinization. Allopurinol (500 mg per square meter on day one and 300 mg by mouth on subsequent days) decreases uric acid production by inhibiting xanthine oxidase. Loop diuretics (furosemide) may be necessary to maintain urine flow. It should be noted that calcium phosphate crystal formation theoretically can be increased by alkalinization of the urine. However, practical considerations dictate that excretion of uric acid is of primary importance, and high-volume urinary output, even when alkaline, dilutes calcium phosphate in the urine and lessens the danger of phosphate crystalluria. Hypocalcemia occasionally requires therapy with intravenous calcium. Rarely, calcitriol replacement is necessary to obviate persistent hypocalcemia caused by low calcitriol levels. Hemodialysis is initiated when volume status, urinary output, acid-base status, and electrolyte changes signal its necessity.

HEMORRHAGIC CYSTITIS

Patients who have or are receiving cyclophosphamide or ifosfamide may present with a life-threatening urologic emergency, hemorrhagic cystitis. The cystitis results from metabolites (chlorethylazeridine, chloroacetic acid, and acrolein) of either chemotherapy agent. Because the metabolites are excreted by the kidney, high concentrations can accumulate in the bladder. If there is bladder outlet obstruction, ureteral hemorrhage may occur. The bladder grossly appears hyperemic and edematous with areas of punctate hemorrhage; mucosal erosions and sloughing are common. The best management entails prevention by maintaining a high urinary output to decrease the concentration of metabolites in the bladder and by correcting any coagulation defect. Systemic use of sodium 2-mercaptoethanesulfonate (Mesna) prevents mucosal irritation by detoxifying the metabolites

within the bladder. Once hemorrhagic cystitis occurs, conservative management with care to ensure excellent urinary output is often adequate. Blood product replacement may be necessary. The use of urethral catheters to remove metabolites and rest the bladder is controversial because catheters can provoke spasm and may prevent passage of clots. If conservative management is not effective, the bladder may be irrigated by N-acetylcysteine. If that fails, irrigation with 0.37 to 0.74 per cent formalin solution for 10 minutes frequently (85 per cent) stops bleeding after one treatment. To avoid ureteral reflux of formalin, the formalin-containing irrigation bag should not be elevated more than 15 cm above the pubis. If formalin fails to control hemorrhage, diversion of hypogastric arteries with ureteral diversion and cystectomy may be necessary.

HEMATOLOGIC EMERGENCIES

Thrombocytopenia is a common finding in patients who are undergoing chemotherapy. When the platelet count is 20,000 per cubic millimeter or less, platelets should be administered prophylactically. If the platelet count is less than 50,000 per cubic millimeter, platelets should be transfused for active bleeding or before surgery or an invasive procedure. When the patient is symptomatic or has a hemoglobin of less than 8.0 grams per deciliter, red blood cells should also be administered, but platelet infusion should underpin treatment.

Disseminated intravascular coagulation (DIC) is a coagulopathic state in which there is prolongation of prothrombin, thrombin, and partial thromboplastin times, an increase in fibrinogen degradation products, and a decrease in platelets, fibrinogen, and clotting factors. DIC resulting in life-threatening hemorrhage should be anticipated in patients with acute promyelocytic leukemia, and anticoagulation with heparin should be started before antineoplastic treatment is begun. For DIC associated with other underlying malignancies (gastrointestinal, lung, breast, and prostate), the treatment of choice is cytoreduction of the underlying cancer by appropriate antineoplastic treatment. If treatment of DIC is necessary before the underlying malignancy responds, then heparin administration should be titrated to control DIC. Coagulation factors should be administered and fibrinogen levels should be maintained well above 100 mg per deciliter by infusion of cryoprecipitate (titrate cryoprecipitate to keep plasma fibrinogen above 100 mg per deciliter).

Leukostasis may result when the white blood cell count exceeds 100,000 per cubic millimeter. An oncologic emergency is not defined by the degree of leukocytosis but rather by the symptoms associated with elevated white blood count. The problem is most often seen in all phases of chronic myelogenous leukemia as well as acute myelogenous leukemia. The dysfunction results from the lack of deformability of white blood cell blasts, with subsequent plugging of small vessels. The leukostasis syndrome manifests primarily in the central nervous system (stupor, dizziness, visual problems, ataxia, coma, intracranial hemorrhage, and sudden death) and pulmonary circuit (pulmonary infiltrates, hypoxia progressing to pulmonary failure with a scenario similar to that of the adult respiratory distress syndrome). Because extreme leukocytosis results in hyperviscosity, diuresis with volume contraction should be avoided. The primary goal of treatment is reduction of white blood cell count by leukapheresis (decrease white blood count by 20 to 60 per cent over 3 to 4 hours), followed by immediate effective therapy of the underlying leukemia. Because of the potential of leukemic cell lysis, measures should be instituted to prevent tumor lysis syndrome.

Cohen LF, Balow JE, Magrath IT, et al.: Acute tumor lysis syndrome: A review of 37 patients with Burkitt's lymphoma. Am J Med 68:486, 1980. *Description of the metabolic sequelae and management of acute tumor lysis.*

Delaney TF, Oldfield EH: Spinal cord compression. In DeVita VT, Hellman JS, Rosenberg SA (eds.): Cancer: Principles and Practice of Oncology. Philadelphia, J. B. Lippincott, 1989, pp 1978–1986. *A broad review of diagnosis and radiotherapy, surgical, and chemotherapy management of spinal cord compression.*

Kaufman D, Rosen N, Young RC: Clinical consequences and management of antineoplastic agents (pp 265–304) and Medical emergencies in patients with solid tumors (pp 481–498). In Parrillo JE, Masur H (eds.): The Critically Ill Immunosuppressed Patient—Diagnosis and Management. Rockville, Maryland, Aspen Publishers, Inc., 1987. *Excellent and practical discussions regarding the general topic of oncologic emergencies.*

Nieto AF, Doty DB: Superior vena cava obstruction: Clinical syndrome, etiology, and treatment. Curr Probl Cancer 10:443–484, 1986. *Classic review of the topic of SVC syndrome.*

Pizzo PA, Robichaud KJ, Gill FA, et al.: Duration of empiric antibiotic therapy in granulocytopenic patients with cancer. Am J Med 67:194, 1979. *Prospective study with diagnostic and treatment algorithms.*

166 Approach to the Patient with Metastatic Cancer, Primary Site Unknown

Daniel C. Ihde

DEFINITION

For a malignant neoplastic disease first to manifest itself by the appearance of visceral or nodal metastases, without any clue to the location of the primary cancer on initial assessment, is not an uncommon occurrence. Patients presenting in this fashion are said to have metastatic cancer, primary site unknown (MCPSU). Other terms employed to denote this clinical entity include cancer (or carcinoma) of unknown primary site and metastases of unknown origin. This syndrome has been heterogeneously defined both clinically and, as discussed later, pathologically. There is no consensus regarding the extent of evaluation required before the conclusion is reached that the site of primary cancer cannot be readily ascertained, but most authorities agree that complete history and physical examination, blood count and chemistry screening panel, tests of urine and stool for occult blood, chest radiograph, and routine histologic evaluation of the diagnostic pathologic specimen should be performed.

ETIOLOGY

The syndrome of MCPSU by definition results from occult but metastatic primary cancer, the etiology of which varies markedly depending upon the organ of origin of the malignant process. Interestingly, in a minority of patients the underlying primary site is not apparent even at autopsy. In 302 patients with MCPSU who eventually had postmortem examination, the primary site of cancer was identified in 27 per cent during life and in an additional 57 per cent at autopsy, with a residual 16 per cent in whom even autopsy did not disclose the primary neoplasm. If autopsy is not performed, the fraction of patients in whom the origin of cancer is not discovered is as high as 70 to 80 per cent.

INCIDENCE

Since there is no standard definition of the MCPSU syndrome, its incidence can only be estimated. Various authorities suggest that 2 to 12 per cent of all cancer patients present in this fashion, with the higher estimates generally based on case series from tertiary care centers. Since the incidence of malignant neoplasms in the United States is approximately 1,000,000 persons per year, it is likely that the MCPSU syndrome is diagnosed in as many as 50,000 to 60,000 patients annually.

PATHOGENESIS AND PATHOLOGY

The primary pathogenesis of the MCPSU syndrome is the sequence of events which led to the formation and dissemination of the primary cancer. This of course differs greatly depending upon the causative primary neoplasm. Why the primary cancer is not discovered by routine diagnostic evaluation is a question of major interest. The most common explanation is that the tumor is simply too small to be detected by physical examination and imaging studies. Other possibilities include prior surgical excision of the primary, as can occasionally be established in malignant melanoma presenting as MCPSU; hemorrhagic infarction with resultant necrosis and scarring, as is thought to occur in some testicular choriocarcinomas; and spontaneous regression, perhaps mediated by immunologic mechanisms.

Since pathologic confirmation of malignant neoplasm must be obtained and a search for the primary cancer by routine evaluation must be unrewarding before a tentative diagnosis of MCPSU is made, further scrutiny of the pathologic specimen assumes critical importance in the subsequent approach to the patient. Discussion between clinician and pathologist should always occur and may reveal that available pathologic material is inadequate for a more specific diagnosis because of suboptimal amount or preparation. This is more often the case with pathologically undifferentiated neoplasms or when the diagnosis of malignancy rests solely on cytologic material obtained by fine-needle aspiration, which provides little information on tissue architecture and is often insufficient for the detailed immunohistochemical or electron microscopic studies that can help elucidate the primary site or type of malignancy. If the pathologist believes examination of more tissue could be beneficial, careful communication among pathologist, clinician, and surgeon is essential to ensure that repeat biopsy yields sufficient, properly processed material.

Once an adequate pathologic specimen is available, routine light microscopic examination reveals adenocarcinoma in approximately 40 per cent of MCPSU patients, undifferentiated carcinoma or malignant neoplasm in 40 per cent, squamous carcinoma in 10 to 15 per cent, and, in fewer than 5 per cent each, melanoma, neuroblastoma, or other types of cancer. The pathologist must determine that the presumed metastasis is not the primary site of cancer. Carcinoma occurring in a setting of adjacent epithelial dysplasia suggests a primary neoplasm, whereas types of cells not normally present in the biopsy site, such as epithelial acinar structures in lymph nodes, confirm that the tumor is metastatic. Light microscopic examination can sometimes reveal structural features that suggest the origin of the cancer. For example, papillary adenocarcinoma most often arises in the thyroid, ovary, or lung, and signet ring adenocarcinoma in the gastrointestinal tract. Rosetting malignant cells are characteristic of neuroblastoma and psammoma bodies of thyroid or ovarian carcinoma.

More specialized studies are especially helpful in evaluating undifferentiated carcinomas or malignant neoplasms, which can prove to be poorly differentiated squamous cell carcinoma or adenocarcinoma, lymphoma, amelanotic melanoma, germ cell carcinoma, or undifferentiated sarcoma, and can also identify the organ of origin of some carcinomas. Immunohistochemical techniques are now more widely utilized than electron microscopy. Analysis with panels of monoclonal or polyclonal antibodies can suggest specific diagnoses, such as lymphoma with leukocyte common antigen positivity, melanoma or sarcoma with neuroectodermal S-100 antigen positivity, carcinoma with cytokeratin or epithelial membrane antigen positivity, prostatic carcinoma with prostate-specific antigen (PSA) positivity, thyroid carcinoma with thyroglobulin positivity, and germ cell carcinoma with reactivity to antibodies against human chorionic gonadotropin (hCG) or α-fetoprotein (AFP). However, it is not firmly established that the clinical behavior and response to therapy of malignancies, particularly undifferentiated neoplasms, diagnosed solely by immunohistochemical means are identical to the behavior and response of corresponding neoplasms diagnosed by light microscopy.

Electron microscopic findings may likewise be of value, particularly in undifferentiated neoplasms. Ultrastructural demonstration of microvilli is characteristic of adenocarcinoma, desmosomes of squamous carcinoma, premelanosomes or melanosomes of malignant melanoma, and cytoplasmic dense-core granules of neuroendocrine carcinomas such as small cell lung cancer.

Differing degrees of certainty which individual pathologists require to make a more specific diagnosis and differing numbers and types of specialized pathologic studies employed before the diagnosis of MCPSU is made account for the second major source of heterogeneity in patients reported to have the MCPSU syndrome.

CLINICAL MANIFESTATIONS

The first clinical manifestation and site of initial pathologic diagnosis of cancer in patients with MCPSU most often occurs in the lung or pleural space, liver, bone, or lymph nodes. Other presentations include cancer in the peritoneal space and pelvis, brain, epidural space, and skin. The distribution of metastases is clearly different in patients with MCPSU and those with an obvious primary site. For example, bone metastases are not common in overt pancreatic cancer but are frequent in pancreatic cancer presenting as MCPSU. Liver and lung metastases are uncommon in overt prostatic cancer but occur much more frequently in prostatic cancer with a clinically undetected primary site.

The most common eventually detected primary sites of cancer in MCPSU patients are the pancreas, lung, colon, and hepatobiliary structures. In MCPSU cases presenting above the diaphragm, the lung is the most common primary cancer site which is later discovered, while for infradiaphragmatic presentations, the pancreas is the most frequently documented primary site.

The distribution of eventually proven sites of cancer origin in patients with MCPSU is somewhat different from that of various cancers in the general population. Germ cell, adrenal, hepatobiliary, pancreatic, and renal cancers are relatively overrepresented among patients with the MCPSU syndrome, whereas malignancies of breast, uterus and uterine cervix, lung, and prostate are relatively underrepresented. Cancers in the latter group are more readily diagnosed by simple means such as physical examination and chest radiograph than are malignancies in the former group.

STAGING EVALUATION

The oncologic staging evaluation, or determination of the extent of tumor dissemination, is somewhat atypical in patients with MCPSU. With the presence of metastatic cancer already proven, considerable effort is often expended in attempting to document the site of the primary malignancy. However, this is frequently inappropriate, since most MCPSU patients prove to have advanced carcinoma refractory to therapy, and performing extensive testing to locate the primary tumor site could occupy a considerable fraction of the patient's life expectancy with only minimal prospects of affecting the ultimate outcome.

Identifying the primary tumor site benefits the patient in only three circumstances. First, tumor confined to a single peripheral lymph node region may be potentially completely eradicated, making control of the primary cancer in the area drained by affected nodes the dominant determinant of survival. An example is occult primary squamous carcinoma of the head and neck region presenting in cervical lymph nodes. Second, documenting that the primary tumor arises in an organ for cancers of which effective systemic treatment is available, such as breast cancer, strongly supports the administration of such therapy. Finally, localizing a primary tumor producing or about to produce disabling symptoms may allow institution of palliative therapy.

Identification of additional asymptomatic visceral metastatic sites of tumor is of no value in a patient with known visceral metastases. However, in patients whose MCPSU arises in a single peripheral lymph node region, discovery of visceral or distant nodal metastases may prevent unnecessarily radical locoregional therapy.

There is universal agreement that radiographic barium studies of the upper gastrointestinal tract and colon and intravenous pyelography are of no value in the absence of symptoms or signs suggestive of an occult primary cancer in the region being imaged, since false-positive studies occur more frequently than the uncommon true-positive result. Computed tomographic (CT) scans of the abdomen and chest probably have a higher yield, but in most cases detect only an untreatable primary malignancy, especially pancreatic and non–small cell lung cancer. In all patients with MCPSU, any imaging studies suggested by the comprehensive evaluation of the pathologic specimen which might support the diagnosis of a treatable malignancy, such as prostatic ultrasonography in an adenocarcinoma reacting with antibodies to PSA or CT scan to detect retroperitoneal lymphadenopathy in an undifferentiated neoplasm reacting with antibodies to leukocyte common antigen, should be performed. Imaging studies for evaluation of symptoms are always appropriate, since detection of a primary or metastatic tumor that requires palliative treatment, such as intestinal bypass for impending obstruction, may result.

Serum biochemical studies that may help diagnose a treatable neoplasm, such as hCG and AFP (germ cell carcinoma) and PSA and prostatic acid phosphatase (prostatic cancer), should be obtained in the appropriate clinical and pathologic setting. However, only markedly elevated values of these biomarkers are specific for germ cell (or hepatocellular in the case of AFP) carcinoma and prostatic cancer, respectively, since other cancers and benign conditions, such as liver disease and prostatic hypertrophy, are associated with more modest elevations. Moderate elevations do, however, support further evaluation for the specific treatable neoplasm in question. Estrogen receptor determinations can be performed on an appropriately prepared tumor biopsy, but only markedly elevated values strongly support the diagnosis of hormonally responsive breast or endometrial cancer, as many types of carcinoma can exhibit modestly elevated receptor protein levels.

The remainder of the staging evaluation in patients with MCPSU should be closely tailored to the specific clinical presentation. It is most useful to segregate patients into two groups, those with known tumor confined to lymph nodes and those with tumor in visceral site(s) with or without node involvement.

MCPSU CONFINED TO LYMPH NODES. Malignant melanoma and lymphoma can present as isolated lymphadenopathy in any node-bearing region, and, if neither is excluded by pathologic evaluation, a primary cutaneous melanoma (along with pathologic review of previously excised skin lesions) or other sites of adenopathy (and possibly evidence of bone marrow involvement), respectively, should be sought. Likely sites of origin of other primary cancers vary markedly by nodal area.

In patients with middle and upper cervical adenopathy in whom biopsy reveals squamous or poorly differentiated carcinoma, complete endoscopic examination with blind biopsies and CT scan to identify areas of submucosal thickening may disclose a primary cancer of the upper aerodigestive tract. Patients with supraclavicular adenopathy more often prove to have adenocarcinoma, which is likely to originate in the lung, breast, or (only in the left fossa) the gastrointestinal tract.

Adenocarcinoma presenting as isolated axillary adenopathy most likely originates in the breast in the female, with lung cancer another possibility in both sexes. Careful breast examination and mammography are always performed in this setting. With other pathologic diagnoses, lung and skin of the upper extremity should be considered as possible primary sites. Isolated inguinal malignant adenopathy may be either squamous cell carcinoma or adenocarcinoma, and the primary cancer often originates in the genitalia, skin of the lower extremity, and anorectal structures, which should be carefully examined. A fraction of MCPSU patients with poorly differentiated tumor confined to the mediastinal or retroperitoneal nodes prove to have germ cell carcinoma, and testicular examination and ultrasonography are appropriate.

MCPSU IN VISCERAL SITES. Approximately 85 per cent of MCPSU patients present with visceral metastases, and no reproducibly effective systemic therapy is currently available for the great majority. The clinician should focus on identifying neoplasms for which effective systemic treatment exists, specifically chemotherapy-responsive breast and ovarian cancer, pulmonary and extrapulmonary small cell carcinoma, germ cell carcinoma, and lymphoma; hormone-responsive prostatic, breast, and endometrial carcinoma; and papillary carcinoma of the thyroid, which is responsive to radioactive iodine administration. Unfortunately, no more than 10 per cent of MCPSU patients with visceral metastases are found to have one of these neoplasms.

In women, pelvic examination should be performed and mammography obtained if pathologic evaluation does not exclude breast cancer. Any suspicion of gynecologic neoplasm should lead to abdominal and pelvic CT scan or pelvic ultrasonography. Some women who present with malignant ascites revealing adenocarcinoma on cytologic examination and no evidence of metastases outside the peritoneal cavity have tumors with clinical behavior similar to that of ovarian carcinoma and may be candidates for exploratory laparotomy. The thyroid gland should be carefully palpated in both sexes.

In men, prostatic examination and perhaps ultrasonography should be performed, and blind prostatic biopsy may be appropriate if suspicion of prostate cancer is high. The possibility of an overlooked subareolar mass due to male breast cancer should not be forgotten. In younger men with predominant midline nodal presentations and minimal visceral tumor, especially confined to the lung, historical evidence of rapid tumor growth or response to previous therapy suggestive of the recently described and incompletely characterized syndrome of "poorly differentiated carcinoma of unknown primary site" should be sought, and testicular examination and ultrasonography performed.

TREATMENT

MCPSU CONFINED TO LYMPH NODES. Patients who, after the staging evaluation outlined above, have all known tumor confined to a single lymph-node bearing region should be approached aggressively, as a fraction of them will attain 5-year survival and even cure. Those with melanoma should undergo radical lymphadenectomy, with the expectation of 5-year survival of 15 to 35 per cent, depending upon the number and volume of nodal metastases, an outcome similar to Stage III melanoma managed with excision of the primary skin lesion and radical lymphadenectomy. If malignant lymphoma is the suspected diagnosis, combination chemotherapy appropriate for lymphoma followed by local irradiation is a reasonable approach.

Squamous and undifferentiated carcinoma in middle to upper cervical nodes is most often managed with radical neck dissection and irradiation, although irradiation alone may be sufficient for low-volume disease. The radiation field often includes the nasopharynx, oropharynx, and laryngopharynx to treat possible primary tumor sites. Five-year survival of 25 to 50 per cent can be anticipated, depending upon tumor volume. The outlook for patients with adenocarcinoma and supraclavicular node metastases is much more grim, with only occasional patients living 5 years after irradiation.

Isolated axillary adenopathy in women with biopsy-proven adenocarcinoma is often treated as breast cancer. Axillary node dissection and modified radical mastectomy are usually advocated in this setting and yield 5-year survival rates of 30 to 70 per cent, results as least as good as in overt Stage II breast cancer. Only half of mastectomy specimens reveal a primary tumor. More recently, similar survival has been reported in patients treated only with axillary dissection or excision, often in conjunction with breast irradiation. Since a fraction of patients clearly have breast cancer, systemic adjuvant therapy appropriate for Stage II breast cancer, either chemotherapy or tamoxifen depending upon the individual patient, should be considered. Men and women with squamous or undifferentiated carcinoma confined to axillary nodes should be evaluated for node dissection, since approximately 20 per cent will live 5 years after surgery. Although physical examination usually reveals the primary cancer in patients with malignancy in inguinal nodes, surgical extirpation or irradiation alone yields 5-year survival of approximately 25 per cent in patients without a documented primary site.

If MCPSU of undifferentiated pathology is confined to mediastinal or retroperitoneal nodes, a trial of aggressive combination chemotherapy, especially in younger patients, may be appropriate, since these nodal regions are common areas in which extragonadal germ cell tumors and lymphomas arise.

MCPSU IN VISCERAL SITES. Palliative or supportive care is often the major focus of management in MCPSU patients with visceral metastases, since most have widely disseminated cancer for which no effective systemic treatment is available. Occasionally, surgical resection of metastases may be beneficial, as in the case of a solitary brain metastasis or an obstructing intestinal lesion. Palliative irradiation, to brain or bone metastases, for example, is often effective. Chemotherapy (or in some instances hormonal therapy or radioactive iodine), which are the only

maneuvers that address the problem of distant metastatic disease, can be administered with realistic expectation of success in only a few subgroups of patients.

If either detailed review of the pathologic material or the staging evaluation raises reasonable suspicion of one of the primary cancers discussed above which might be expected to respond to systemic treatment, a trial of appropriate therapy should be initiated, provided that a favorable risk-benefit ratio is thought to exist in the individual patient.

Two other clinical settings also merit strong consideration of chemotherapy. In women with isolated malignant ascites, laparotomy with maximum feasible resection of tumor masses, provided they are confined to the peritoneal cavity, may be appropriate. Whether or not a primary ovarian tumor is identified, a recent study reports a relatively indolent clinical course in these patients, with some complete responses to chemotherapy regimens utilized in ovarian cancer.

The syndrome of "poorly differentiated carcinoma of unknown primary site" is not well defined but is of importance because a fraction of patients with some or all of the characteristics enumerated above have complete remissions, some of which are durable, with cisplatin-containing chemotherapy regimens utilized for testicular cancer. Originally these cases were thought to represent germ cell carcinomas in which a definitive pathologic diagnosis could not be rendered, but in one series of patients in whom more than one fourth completely responded to chemotherapy, even detailed retrospective pathologic review suggested that no more than 5 per cent of patients had initially unrecognized germ cell tumors. Thus, the pathogenesis of this syndrome remains obscure, and until therapeutic results are obtained after the prospective application of strict diagnostic criteria, utilized to select a group of patients that is then uniformly treated, the proportion that derives substantial benefit from chemotherapy will remain uncertain.

For the remaining patients with visceral MCPSU, there is no evidence that any treatment improves survival. Close observation with palliation of symptoms as they arise is an appropriate management strategy. Chemotherapy regimens for which responses in the MCPSU syndrome have been reported or investigational treatments may be given to fully ambulatory patients who understand the limitations of therapy but still desire it.

PROGNOSIS

The prognosis of most patients with MCPSU is poor. Median and 5-year survival in several large series of consecutive patients accrued in single institutions is approximately 5 to 6 months and 3 to 7 per cent, respectively. The most important prognostic features, as in most other cancers, are sites and volume of tumor involvement, ambulatory status, and degree of weight loss. Five-year survival is reported to be 25 to 50 per cent for patients whose tumor is confined to peripheral lymph nodes and less than 3 per cent for all other patients.

Greco FA, Vaughn WK, Hainsworth JD: Advanced poorly differentiated carcinoma of unknown primary site: Recognition of a treatable syndrome. Ann Intern Med 104:547, 1986. *The initial detailed description of the clinical characteristics and prognostic features of a subgroup of MCPSU patients surprisingly responsive to combination chemotherapy.*

Haskell CM, Cochran AJ, Barsky SH, et al.: Metastasis of unknown origin. Curr Probl Cancer 12:1, 1988. *A comprehensive and critical review of the MCPSU syndrome.*

Kirsten F, Chi CH, Leary JA, et al.: Metastatic adeno or undifferentiated carcinoma from an unknown primary site: Natural history and guidelines for identification of treatable subsets. Q J Med 62:143, 1987. *Analysis of a large consecutive series of MCPSU patients, with emphasis on identification of the small number of patients for whom potentially effective therapy is available.*

PART XIV
METABOLIC DISEASES

167 Introduction

James B. Wyngaarden

The term *metabolism* encompasses the numerous chemical transformations that occur within living organisms. These are often divided into two large categories. Those reactions or processes that are synthetic, and in general result in a larger molecule than any of the reactants, are called *anabolic*. Such reactions are usually energy requiring. Those reactions that are degradative and involve the breakdown of large molecules into smaller products are termed *catabolic*. Such processes are essentially energy yielding. The term *intermediary metabolism* refers to all changes that take place between the moment of entry of a nutrient into the organism and the discharge of all of the chemical products into the environment. It is customary to consider separately the intermediary metabolism of carbohydrates, lipids, and proteins, although no sharp lines can be drawn between the metabolic reactions of these three classes of compounds. The term *basal metabolism* refers to energy requirements for maintenance and conduct of cellular and tissue processes under conditions in which the effects of muscular activity and the work of digestion and metabolism of foodstuffs are minimal.

Part XIV of this textbook is concerned with metabolic diseases. A disorder is classified as a metabolic disease when the fundamental pathogenetic mechanism involves a chemical transformation or process. Many diseases of metabolism involve specific enzyme or other protein abnormalities. When these can be attributed to an underlying genetic abnormality, they are termed *inborn errors of metabolism* (see Ch. 31). There are now over 350 human genetic diseases whose biochemical defects have been defined. Most of these are described somewhere in this textbook or listed in Tables 31–1 and 176–1, but only a fraction has been collected into Part XIV. For example, hemolytic anemias attributable to specific enzyme defects are included with the other hemolytic anemias in Part XII, Hematologic Diseases, and adrenal hyperplasia attributable to specific enzyme defects is discussed in Part XVI, Endocrine and Reproductive Diseases. The disorders included in Part XIV are chiefly those whose manifestations are multisystemic or those in which the biochemical and genetic factors dominate the description.

PATHOGENESIS OF HEREDITARY METABOLIC DISEASES. The etiology of an inborn error of metabolism is a mutant gene. The alteration in DNA structure produces a disturbance in protein structure and function, which in turn affects cell and organ function. Hereditary metabolic diseases can be considered in terms of these three sequential levels.

Altered DNA Structure. The nature of mutations can be deduced from changes in amino acid sequences in the mutant proteins and the genetic codes (see Ch. 30). This approach has been applied most extensively in studies of variant hemoglobins and glucose-6-phosphate dehydrogenases. DNA restriction enzyme analyses and DNA sequencing techniques permit direct analysis of alterations in DNA structure. By these methods, point mutations, deletions, and insertions are readily identified, and hybrid proteins or prematurely terminated or aberrantly extended proteins explained in terms of genetic mechanisms. Restriction endonucleases identify many variations in gene structure as fragment-length polymorphisms. The latter approach provided the first clues to the genetic abnormality in cystic fibrosis and provided the starting point that eventually led to the identification of the abnormal gene and its product. With the availability of DNA cloning techniques it is possible to study directly the altered DNA sequence in many human mutations, even those that involve genes that code for quantitatively minor proteins, such as enzymes. These techniques also disclose mutations in noncoding regions of DNA that affect rate of synthesis, processing, or stability of specific messenger RNA's.

Altered Protein Function. Abnormalities in the synthesis or structure of a specific enzyme protein result in absence of or reduced or (occasionally) enhanced rates of a specific enzyme-catalyzed reaction. In many genetic enzyme deficiency states, a reduced but detectable level of enzymatic activity can be measured by sensitive assays. The residual enzyme activity can frequently be attributed to a catalytically abnormal enzyme, which may exhibit decreased affinity for substrates, cofactors, or inhibitors. In the most extensively studied series of enzyme defects, those involving glucose-6-phosphate dehydrogenase, most of the enzyme deficiencies reflect unstable enzymes whose activities decay as the erythrocyte ages. This is a common mechanism of enzyme deficiency in the anucleated red blood cell but has not been demonstrated to be an important cause of enzyme deficiency in disorders that affect primarily nucleated cells. The most interesting example of mutations leading to increased enzyme activities involves phosphoribosylpyrophosphate synthetase. Different mutations in an X-linked structural gene lead to four discrete subtypes exhibiting (1) reduced sensitivity to nucleotide regulators, (2) increased affinity for substrate, (3) increased specific activity per enzyme molecule, or (4) a combination of (1) and (3). Relatively few lesions, other than hemoglobinopathies, have been attributed to mutations in genes coding for nonenzymatic proteins. One example is the ZZ variant of alpha$_1$-antitrypsin deficiency, in which an altered protein is not susceptible to normal posttranslational processing (glycosylation), with the result that the defective glycoprotein cannot be secreted by the liver. In some nonenzymatic proteins, a structural abnormality leads to aggregation (e.g., sickle cell hemoglobin). In others, the mutation affects the affinity of a receptor for a specific ligand (e.g., the low density lipoprotein [LDL] receptor in familial hypercholesterolemia and the cytoplasmic androgen receptor in complete testicular feminization).

Disrupted Cell and Organ Function. Most genetic diseases first come to clinical attention because of disturbances at the level of cell and organ function. Several types of derangements occur:

1. Altered flux through metabolic pathways. This is the most frequent basis of recognition of an inborn error of metabolism. The product may be missing (albinism), or a precursor may accumulate (mucopolysaccharidoses) or be shunted into a toxic metabolite (phenylketonuria).

2. Disordered feedback regulation of synthetic pathways. Decreased synthesis of a regulatory end-product may result in faulty control of an early step of the pathway leading to excessive production of intermediates. The classic example is acute intermittent porphyria, in which a deficiency of porphobilinogen deaminase leads to diminished production of heme, a normal feedback inhibitor of porphyrin synthesis. Decreased production of heme leads to overactivity of δ-aminolevulinic acid synthetase, overproduction of nonheme porphyrins, and acute intermittent porphyria.

3. Disordered membrane function. This is the basis for a large group of genetic diseases in which there is impairment of a specific function of a plasma membrane protein. In one type, transmembrane transport of specific small molecules is defective, apparently because a membrane carrier protein is nonfunctional. The affected substrates can be amino acids (cystinuria), carbohydrates (renal glycosuria), or ions (renal tubular acidosis). In

another type, receptor-mediated endocytosis of a macromolecule is defective. In familial hypercholesterolemia a mutation in the gene that codes for a receptor results in defective uptake and degradation of LDL by body cells, resulting in accumulation of LDL and its cholesterol in plasma and arterial walls. Still another type involves a defect in a plasma membrane protein whose action is required for hormone action. In pseudohypoparathyroidism, the guanosine triphosphate (GTP)–sensitive N-protein is defective, and parathyroid hormone cannot stimulate adenylate cyclase in the target cell. The latter two types of defects are inherited as dominant traits, in contrast to those that involve transmembrane transport of small molecules, which behave like recessive traits.

4. Disordered intracellular compartmentation. A few examples of primary genetic defects in cell compartmentation are known. The ZZ variant of alpha$_1$-antitrypsin deficiency, discussed above, is one. Another is I-cell disease, in which there is a deficiency of a processing enzyme that is normally responsible for the occurrence of mannose-6-phosphate residues in lysosomal enzymes. In the absence of mannose-6-phosphate residues, enzymes do not bind to a specific receptor that directs them to the lysosome, and these enzymes pass through the cell into the plasma like a secretory protein. An additional example is a rare form of familial hypercholesterolemia in which there is an abnormal cell-surface receptor that can bind LDL but cannot transport it into the cell.

5. Distorted cell or tissue architecture. The distorted shapes of erythrocytes in sickle cell diseases and in hereditary spherocytosis are examples of this type. Another example is illustrated by the immotile cilia syndrome (Kartagener's syndrome), in which a structural protein of cilia, dynein, is defective. In consequence, the "dynein arms" that crosslink microtubules are missing, they cannot slide properly, and cilia cannot undulate. Still another type is exemplified by type VI Ehlers-Danlos syndrome, in which collagen is deficient in hydroxylysine and does not crosslink normally.

ACQUIRED METABOLIC DISEASES. There are many examples of metabolic diseases that are acquired rather than hereditary. Gout exists in primary and secondary varieties. The secondary types occur because of excessive nucleic acid turnover in myeloproliferative diseases or chronic hemolytic anemias, or because of impaired renal excretion of uric acid resulting from drug effects upon the kidney or acquired renal disease. Certain varieties of porphyria can be attributed to acquired intoxications. Hyperlipoproteinurias are common accompaniments of other diseases: hypothyroidism, the nephrotic syndrome, acute and chronic alcoholism, biliary obstruction. In many conditions there is a prominent interaction between hereditary and environmental factors: obesity and diabetes mellitus, ingestion of phenylalanine-containing proteins in phenylketonuria, ingestion of milk in galactosemia. Without the environmental stress, these conditions would remain silent.

Some of the diseases of metabolism are very common, such as diabetes, with a prevalence in the United States of about 2.5 per cent, and the hyperlipidemias. Others are quite rare, and a few are perhaps more properly regarded as biochemical anomalies rather than diseases—pentosuria, for example. The study of rare metabolic disorders has provided a better understanding of normal metabolic processes and, in some instances, has allowed early recognition of a disorder whose manifestations are preventable simply by adjustment of diet (galactosemia, phenylketonuria). The identification of specific enzyme defects has led to attempts at replacement therapy with inklings of success following enzyme infusion (Gaucher's disease, Fabry's disease) or organ transplantation (bone marrow in immunologic deficiency states; kidney in cystinosis, Fabry's disease, Gaucher's disease).

Becker KL: Principles and Practices of Endocrinology and Metabolism. Philadelphia, J.B. Lippincott, 1990.

Scriver CR, Beaudet AL, Sly WS, et al. (eds.): The Metabolic Basis of Inherited Disease. 6th ed. New York, McGraw-Hill, Inc., 1989. *An authoritative text that presents detailed discussions of various hereditary diseases of metabolism by recognized experts on each topic.*

DISORDERS OF CARBOHYDRATE METABOLISM

168 Galactosemia

Stanton Segal

The galactosemias are toxicity syndromes exhibited by patients with an inherited inability to metabolize the sugar galactose, which is a constituent of the disaccharide lactose found in milk and milk products. There are three disorders, each of which results from a deficiency of one of the enzymes that catalyze the normal conversion of galactose to glucose: galactokinase, galactose-1-phosphate uridyltransferase, and uridine diphosphate-4-epimerase. A defect in galactokinase is manifested primarily by cataract formation early in life. Uridyltransferase deficiency, which is the most prevalent and is commonly referred to as classic galactosemia, results in a syndrome of nutritional failure, liver disease, abnormal renal tubule function, cataracts, mental retardation, and ovarian abnormalities in affected females. A deficiency of epimerase activity clinically resembles transferase deficiency but may exist in a more benign form when the enzyme defect is limited to red blood cells. For all three disorders, the elevations of the level of galactose and its metabolites in blood, urine, and tissues can be corrected and the clinical manifestations alleviated by omission of dietary galactose.

ETIOLOGY. Galactokinase, galactose-1-phosphate uridyl-transferase, and uridine diphosphate-4-epimerase deficiencies are all autosomal recessive genetic disorders. The individual human genes have been located on chromosomes 17, 9, and 1, respectively. The tissues of obligate heterozygotes contain about 50 per cent of the normal enzyme activity, while homozygotes exhibit absence of or very little activity. Immunoelectrophoretic analysis has shown that patients with transferase deficiency produce a protein similar to the normal, but with severely reduced enzyme activity or reduced stability, suggesting single amino acid substitution defects in the majority rather than deletion mutations.

PREVALENCE. Uridyltransferase deficiency has a prevalence of 1 per 40,000 births and a carrier rate of about 1 per cent in the U.S. population. A gene known as the Duarte variant is allelic to the normal transferase and codes for a protein that is electrophoretically different and enzymatically less active. The gene frequency of the Duarte variant is about 0.05 per cent, and homozygotes for the Duarte variant have about 50 per cent of normal transferase activity in their red blood cells. Widespread neonatal screening has detected a number of babies with low red cell transferase activity who are compound heterozygotes with one gene for defective transferase and another for the Duarte variant. Such infants have only 10 to 25 per cent of red cell enzyme activity but rarely have impaired galactose utilization that requires treatment.

Galactokinase deficiency is quite rare, having a prevalence of 1 in 500,000 to 1 in 1 million births. Epimerase deficiency is also rare. The benign type has mainly been described in Swiss and Japanese populations, while only a few cases of symptomatic epimerase deficiency have been detected.

PATHOGENESIS. Galactose is converted to glucose by a unique series of three enzyme reactions. The first enzyme in the pathway, galactokinase, causes galactose to react with adenosine triphosphate (ATP) to form galactose-1-phosphate:

$$\text{Galactose} + \text{ATP} \rightarrow \text{Galactose-1-P}$$

Next, galactose-1-phosphate reacts with uridine diphosphate (UDP)–glucose to form UDP-galactose in a reaction catalyzed by uridyltransferase:

$$\text{Galactose-1-P} + \text{UDP-glucose} \rightleftharpoons \text{Glucose-1-P} + \text{UDP-galactose}$$

The third enzyme, epimerase, performs the spatial change of the hydroxyl group about the fourth carbon to convert galactose to glucose:

$$\text{UDP-galactose} \rightleftharpoons \text{UDP-glucose}$$

In the presence of pyrophosphate, UDP-glucose pyrophosphorylase cleaves UDP-glucose to glucose-1-phosphate, which is converted to glucose-6-phosphate by phosphoglucomutase and then enters various other pathways of glucose metabolism. Normally, this pathway functions efficiently. Galactose rapidly disappears from blood after intravenous infusion, even faster than a comparable amount of glucose. In normal individuals, liver extraction of galactose results in a rise in the level of blood glucose.

In each of the three forms of galactosemia, diminished enzyme activity produces an accumulation of the substrates proximal to the metabolic block: galactose in galactokinase deficiency, galactose and galactose-1-phosphate in transferase deficiency, and galactose, galactose-1-phosphate plus UDP-galactose in epimerase deficiency. When galactose is increased, alternative pathways form large amounts of otherwise trace metabolites. In one reaction galactose is reduced to form the sugar alcohol, galactitol, while in another, galactose is oxidized to galactonic acid. These metabolites accumulate in tissues and are excreted in considerable amounts in the urine.

Identification of accumulated metabolites and the elucidation of alternative pathways have provided insights into the relationship of biochemical toxicity and clinical manifestations of the disorders. In galactokinase deficiency, in which galactose and metabolites of alternative pathways are increased, the principal clinical finding is cataracts, without multiple organ involvement. These findings implicate galactose-1-phosphate as causing the severe multisystem disease of transferase deficiency and systemic epimerase deficiency. Cataract formation appears to be due to the formation of galactitol by lens aldose reductase. Galactitol, which cannot be further metabolized, accumulates in the lens and produces osmotic changes with imbibition of fluid, lens swelling, and protein precipitation. The exact biochemical alterations in target organs affected by transferase deficiency have not been defined. There are no structural alterations of the brain associated with mental retardation in cases of transferase deficiency, but liver dysfunction is accompanied by altered architecture of the liver characterized by pseudoacinar formation of hepatic cells. The ovaries of females afflicted with hypogonadism may be small, fibrotic, or streaked.

The fact that galactose-1-phosphate can be increased in red cells of transferase-deficient patients and that mental retardation and ovarian abnormalities can occur in patients with no exposure to galactose has fostered the concept that there is continuous self-intoxication in this disorder. This self-intoxication could occur as a result of the formation of UDP-galactose from UDP-glucose via epimerase activity and subsequent pyrophosphorolysis of UDP-galactose to liberate galactose-1-phosphate. The pyrophosphorylase plays a dual role in the process, since it is also responsible for the formation of UDP-glucose from uridine triphosphate and glucose-1-phosphate.

CLINICAL MANIFESTATIONS. Cataracts are the principal finding in patients with galactokinase deficiency, who otherwise are healthy. The cataracts are usually discovered in infants and children examined for other medical reasons. Pseudotumor cerebri has been described in some galactokinase-deficient patients as well as those with transferase deficiency. Cataracts have been observed in some heterozygous carriers, and patients under 40 years with cataracts frequently have lower than normal red cell galactokinase levels.

Uridyltransferase deficiency usually manifests itself shortly after birth or within the first few weeks of life with growth failure, vomiting, diarrhea, hepatomegaly, ascites, jaundice, hemolytic anemia, hypoglycemia, proteinuria, and a renal Fanconi syndrome. Cataracts may not be easily observed with an ophthalmoscope in young infants but are found on slit-lamp examination. Infants with this disease may die in the first few days of life from overwhelming *Escherichia coli* sepsis before other manifestations are evident. Without elimination of galactose from the diet, severely affected infants will die of inanition and liver failure. Occasionally, because of vomiting, the infant's formula is changed to one that is galactose free, with subsequent cessation of the toxicity syndrome. Later in childhood these patients have severe mental retardation and cataracts after milk is reintroduced into the diet. Mental retardation is frequent if therapy is not initiated within the first 2 to 3 months of life. Postpubertal females have a high incidence of hypergonadotropic hypogonadism expressed as either primary or secondary amenorrhea, but the testes of male patients are normal. There is no correlation of the clinical course with ovarian function, but the frequency of hypogonadism appears to correlate with undetectable red cell transferase activity.

Black patients with transferase deficiency may have a milder toxicity syndrome and in some cases have no symptoms. This has been called the Negro variant. Such patients have been found to metabolize some galactose because of the presence of 10 per cent of normal transferase activity in liver and intestinal mucosa. A toxicity syndrome resembling transferase deficiency occurs in cases of systemic epimerase deficiency.

DIAGNOSIS. Galactokinase deficiency should be suspected in any infant or child with cataracts and the diagnosis confirmed by assay of red blood cell or cultured fibroblast galactokinase. A presumptive diagnosis is possible by detection of reducing sugar in urine that is glucose oxidase negative (galactose) or by chromatographic analysis for galactitol in the urine. These urinary findings also obtain in transferase deficiency, whose definitive diagnosis requires the assay of red cell transferase activity. Since severely affected babies may be given blood transfusions before a diagnosis of galactosemia is considered, red cell transferase assay should be delayed until transfused blood has been replaced by the infant's own cells. However, assay of transferase in parents' red cells and the findings of 50 per cent of normal activity in both may be helpful in making a presumptive diagnosis in such infants or in those who may have died before specimens for assay were obtained.

In the differential diagnosis, hereditary fructose intolerance with hepatomegaly, liver dysfunction, hypoglycemia, renal Fanconi syndrome, and nonglucose reducing substance in the urine should be considered. Lactosuria, a common finding in a variety of gastrointestinal disorders, also causes a positive test result for reducing substance. However, many laboratories use glucose oxidase–based tests for blood and urinary sugar determination, and in such instances, galactosemia and galactosuria would go undetected. The greatest confusion in differential diagnosis is the distinction between transferase deficiency and primary liver disease. Because the liver is the major organ metabolizing galactose, any disruption of hepatocellular function may result in galactosemia and galactosuria. Red cell transferase assay should be employed to make the distinction. Patients with clinical findings resembling classic transferase deficiency galactosemia who have normal red cell transferase activity should also be tested for red cell epimerase activity.

Besides the quantitative assay of red cell transferase, the performance of starch gel electrophoresis or isoelectric focusing to determine isoenzyme banding may be useful in distinguishing the carrier for classic galactosemia, the homozygous Duarte variant, whose red cell enzyme activity is comparable to that of carriers for the classic disease, and mixed Duarte variant–classic galactosemia carriers, who have 10 to 25 per cent of normal activity, as well as the Rennes and Chicago variants of transferase deficiency. In addition to these variants with diminished red cell activity and electrophoretic abnormalities, there are other variant forms. The Indiana variant has typical symptoms of transferase deficiency galactosemia and unstable red cell activity, while clinical disease in the Münster variant is caused by abnormal inhibition of transferase by glucose-1-phosphate, the product of the reaction.

Many cases are currently diagnosed as a result of neonatal screening. More than one half of the states in the United States and several foreign countries test all newborns by analysis of heel-stick-blood spots on filter paper. All of the procedures used detect transferase deficiency. Some also detect galactokinase or epimerase deficiency. All positive test results require confirmation by quantitative assay of the individual enzymes. Such screening has resulted in delineation of the benign form of epimerase deficiency, in which galactose-1-phosphate appears to accumulate only in red blood cells. Subsequent studies have indicated that the epimerase in such cases is unstable because of increased requirement for cofactor NAD, which can be supplied by other cells but not red blood cells.

TREATMENT. The institution of a galactose-free diet is the cornerstone of treatment. With galactose elimination, early cataracts may regress. Liver dysfunction and renal tubule abnormalities disappear, and growth and development may be normal. Besides the banning of milk and all milk products, care should be taken to eliminate foods in which milk is used in cooking and baking or lactose has been added. There is no indication that the ability to metabolize galactose increases with age, so that dietary restrictions should not be relaxed in older children.

PROGNOSIS. Dietary galactose restriction does not ensure a normal outcome. Despite excellent treatment from birth, many patients with transferase deficiency have below average mental development with learning deficits, diminished attention span, visual perceptual difficulties, and speech abnormalities. Eighty per cent of affected females have hypergonadotropic hypogonadism. The outcome in patients without symptoms who are treated at birth does not differ from that in patients who are recognized within the first several weeks of life on the basis of the acute galactose toxicity syndrome caused by ingestion of galactose-containing feeds. Untreated infants, however, may not survive. Older patients may develop an ataxic neurologic syndrome while on galactose-restricted diets.

PREVENTION. The insufficiency of the galactose-restricted diet may be due to continuous self-intoxication with endogenously produced galactose metabolites, which may start in utero. Galactose restriction during pregnancy in cases in which the fetus is at risk has not altered the prognosis. Prenatal diagnosis can be performed by assay of transferase of a chorionic villus biopsy specimen or cultured amniotic cells or by determination of galactitol in amniotic fluid.

Fishler K, Koch R, Donnell GN, et al.: Developmental aspects of galactosemia from infancy to childhood. Clin Pediatr 19:38, 1980. *Data describing outcome of dietary treatment of uridyltransferase-deficient patients in relation to age at diagnosis reveal normal IQ but abnormal visual-perceptual status and electroencephalogram (EEG) in patients well treated before 3 months of age.*

Kaufman FR, Kogut MD, Donnell GN, et al.: Hypergonadotropic hypogonadism in female patients with galactosemia. N Engl J Med 304:944, 1981. *Describes amenorrhea and ovarian abnormalities in patients with uridyltransferase deficiency.*

Segal S: Disorders of galactose metabolism. *In* Scriver CH, Beaudet AL, Sly WS, et al. (eds.): The Metabolic Basis of Inherited Disease. 6th ed. New York, McGraw-Hill, 1989, pp 453–480. *Survey of outcome of more than 300 classic uridyltransferase-deficient patients reveals frequency of developmental delay, speech abnormalities, and ovarian dysfunction.*

Waggoner D, Buist NRM, Donnell GN: Long term prognosis in galactosemia: Results of a survey of 350 cases. J Inherited Metab Dis 13:802, 1990. *Most informative data yet published on long-term outcome, which indicate that dietary therapy, even when started at birth, does not necessarily prevent mental retardation or ovarian failure.*

169 The Glycogen Storage Diseases

Harry L. Greene

Glycogen is the storage form of glucose and is present in varying amounts in virtually all cells, although the liver is the primary organ for storage and subsequent release of glucose into

the circulation. Glycogen formation from glucose along with the release of glucose from glycogen is highly regulated, a process that aids in the maintenance of normal blood glucose concentrations during fasting. At least eight enzymes involved in glycogen synthesis and the hydrolysis to glucose are utilized in this control.

Glycogen storage diseases are characterized by an abnormal tissue concentration (>70 mg per gram of liver or >15 mg per gram of muscle) and/or an abnormal structure of the glycogen molecule. During the past 40 years, patients who have deficient activity in virtually every enzyme important in the normal synthesis or degradation of glycogen have been identified. With the exception of phosphorylase kinase deficiency, all are inherited in an autosomal recessive manner. Although the enzyme deficiency may vary among patients, the clinical expression of the disease can usually be traced to either the liver or the muscle.

HEPATIC FORMS OF GLYCOGENESIS

The various hepatic enzymatic deficiencies are expressed primarily as hypoglycemia and hepatomegaly, and three defects (branching enzyme, glycogen synthetase, and debranching enzyme) result in the accumulation of abnormally structured glycogen and may cause progressive hepatic cirrhosis and associated splenomegaly. Conversely, the accumulation of normally structured glycogen, as seen with deficiency of phosphorylase, phosphorylase b kinase, acid alpha-glucosidase, or glucose-6-phosphatase, is usually not associated with hepatic fibrosis and splenomegaly. Figure 169–1 summarizes the general location of enzymatic defects resulting in the hepatic forms of glycogenesis. With the exception of lysosomal acid glucosidase deficiency, hypoglycemia is a common presenting feature. Clinical and biochemical expressions of the various types of glycogen storage diseases are summarized in Table 169–1, and the more commonly diagnosed types are discussed below.

GLUCOSE-6-PHOSPHATASE DEFICIENCY (TYPE I GLYCOGEN STORAGE DISEASE). With the recent development of antibodies to several of the five components of glucose-6-phosphatase, this disorder has been subcategorized into types a, b, or c, with type a the most common; but all types have similar clinical features. As noted in Figure 169–1, all other enzymatic defects directly affect the formation or degradation of glycogen, with the exception of glucose-6-phosphatase. Similarly, the clinical expression of this defect is distinctly different from that of the other forms of glycogenosis. For example, fasting-induced

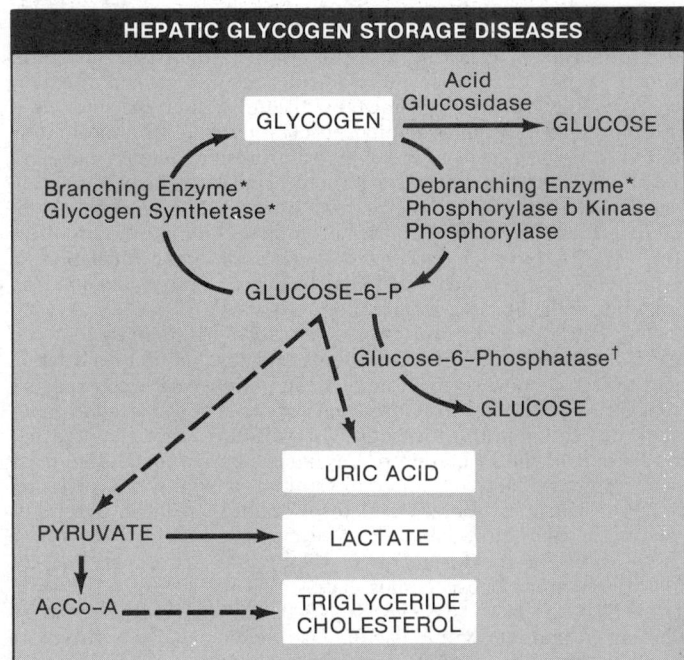

FIGURE 169–1. Mechanism for abnormalities in lipid, purine, and carbohydrate metabolism in the hepatic glycogen storage diseases. * = associated with hepatic cirrhosis. † = associated with elevated serum uric acid, lactate, and lipid levels and with hepatic adenoma.

hypoglycemia may be extreme, and, in combination with lactic acidosis, hyperlipidemia, and hyperuricemia, characterizes patients with type I. The mechanism for the striking abnormalities in lipid and purine metabolism as well as carbohydrate metabolism has been reviewed recently and results primarily from overproduction of substrate in response to a decline in blood glucose, as indicated in Figure 169–1. The documented reversal of these abnormalities by treatment that maintains the blood glucose level between 80 and 90 mg per deciliter supports the postulate that these changes are the result of hormonal responses to the hypoglycemia. Therapeutic intervention has been evaluated more extensively in patients with this defect than any other. As a result, it has been possible to devise reasonably effective dietary control for these patients that results in favorable development into adulthood.

Late Complications. As more patients have survived and developed into active, functioning adults, two subsequent, unexpected complications have become apparent: (1) single or multiple hepatic adenomas and (2) progressive glomerulosclerosis with renal failure. Adenomas usually develop in patients between 16 and 22 years of age, and it is unusual for a patient not to have adenomas by age 25 years. Since there is a tendency for subsequent malignant transformation of an adenoma, annual monitoring by ultrasound is recommended. Any rapidly expanding lesion should be considered potentially malignant and should undergo surgical biopsy, since serum alpha-fetoprotein measurements have been an unreliable marker for malignant transformation. There has been some indication that the adenomas could be prevented or reduced in younger children by more stringent dietary control; however, this hypothesis has not been substantiated in older individuals.

The development of progressive glomerulosclerosis, proteinuria, hypertension, and renal failure has been a recent observation and usually occurs in older patients (>18 years) who are less well managed and exhibit recurrent hypoglycemic episodes, chronic hypertriglyceridemia, and lactic acidosis. The mechanism causing the renal lesion is not defined, although some improvement in proteinuria has been seen following treatment with angiotensin-converting enzyme inhibitors.

DEBRANCHING ENZYME DEFICIENCY (TYPE III GLY-COGEN STORAGE DISEASE). This disease most often affects only the liver but may affect muscle as well. With muscle involvement, the serum creatine phosphokinase (CPK) level is elevated, and patients are usually classified as having type IIIb disease. Some patients may not show elevated CPK levels during early life, so evaluation during later childhood or adolescence should be performed. Hypoglycemia with fasting is less severe (usually 40 to 50 mg per deciliter) than in patients with type I, although hepatic enlargement may be substantially greater. Serum aspartate aminotransferase (AST) and alanine aminotransaminase (ALT) concentrations are commonly above 500 units per milliliter. Correspondingly, hepatic fibrosis of varying degrees is usually present during childhood and may be progressive. At least two adult patients (ages 43 and 55 years) presenting with "cryptogenic cirrhosis" and bleeding esophageal varices have been diagnosed as having debrancher enzyme deficiency.

Treatment of these patients has not been advocated, since the natural course of the disease has been thought to be benign. However, since growth retardation and cirrhosis may be serious complications, several patients have been treated with frequent feedings and raw cornstarch to maintain blood glucose levels between 75 and 100 mg per deciliter. Treated patients often show a significant reduction in serum transaminase levels and improvements in growth, and they may demonstrate improved muscle strength, although serum CPK activities remain elevated.

Clinical and laboratory features of the other, more unusual forms of hepatic glycogenoses are presented in Table 169–1.

MUSCULAR FORMS OF GLYCOGEN STORAGE

ACID ALPHA-GLUCOSIDASE DEFICIENCY (POMPE'S DISEASE, TYPE II GLYCOGEN STORAGE DISEASE). In this condition, virtually all tissues have an increased glycogen content. However, presenting clinical manifestations of the illness are cardiac enlargement, myocardial failure, and generalized muscle hypotonia without muscle wasting. The classic infantile form manifests during the first months of life, and few survive past the first year. The juvenile variant presents in later infancy or early childhood and progresses more slowly, with death in the

TABLE 169–1. CLASSIFICATION OF GLYCOGEN STORAGE DISEASES

Type	Enzyme Affected	Primary Organ Involved	Manifestations
O	Glycogen synthetase	Liver	Hypoglycemia, hyperketonia, FFT, early death
Ia	Glucose-6-phosphatase	Liver	Enlarged liver and kidney growth failure, fasting hypoglycemia, acidosis, thrombocyte dysfunction
Ib	Microsomal membrane G-6-P translocase	Liver	As in Ia; in addition, recurrent neutropenia, bacterial infections
Ic	Microsomal membrane P-transporter	Liver	As in Ia
II	Lysosomal acid glucosidase	Skeletal and cardiac muscle	*Infantile form:* early-onset, progressive muscle hypotonia, cardiac failure, death before 2 years *Juvenile form:* late-onset myopathy with variable cardiac involvement *Adult form:* limb-girdle muscular dystrophy–like feature
III	Amylo-1,6-glucosidase (debrancher enzyme)	Liver, skeletal muscle, heart	Fasting hypoglycemia, hepatomegaly in infancy; some have myopathic features, rarely clinical cardiac features
IV	Amylo-1,4-1,6-transglucosidase (brancher enzyme)	Liver, muscle	Hepatosplenomegaly, cirrhosis; may have late-onset myopathy
V	Muscle phosphorylase	Skeletal muscle	Exercise-induced muscular pain, cramps, and progressive weakness, sometimes with myoglobinuria; symptoms usually begin during adolescence or early adulthood
VI	Liver phosphorylase	Liver	Hepatomegaly, mild hypoglycemia, good prognosis
VII	Phosphofructokinase	Muscle, red blood cells	As in V; in addition, mild hemolytic anemia
Formerly VIb, VIII, or IX	Phosphorylase b kinase	Liver, leukocytes, (?) muscle	As in VI; X-linked inheritance
X	Cyclic AMP–dependent kinase	Liver, muscle	Hepatomegaly, mild hypoglycemia

second or third decade. The adult type manifests as a slowly developing adult-onset myopathy. In each case, the diagnosis is dependent on finding deficient activity of acid alpha-1, 4-glucosidase in muscle specimens or cultured fibroblasts. No treatment, including bone marrow transplantation and systemic enzyme infusion, has proved to be of long-term benefit to these patients.

MYOPHOSPHORYLASE DEFICIENCY (TYPE V GLYCOGEN STORAGE DISEASE, McARDLE'S DISEASE). Most of these patients are asymptomatic during early childhood and escape diagnosis until the second or third decade of life. Presentation with a history of muscle pain and cramps after exercise, signs of myoglobinuria, and painful cramping on an ischemic exercise test are characteristic. The diagnosis is suggested by an elevation in serum muscle CPK isoenzyme activity and by failure to elevate the serum lactate level with exercise. The diagnosis is established by documenting elevated muscle glycogen in the sarcolemmal regions and reduced muscle phosphorylase activity. Glucose or fructose ingestion prior to exercise is said to reduce the symptoms.

MUSCLE PHOSPHOFRUCTOKINASE DEFICIENCY (MUSCLE PHOSPHOGLYCERATE MUTASE DEFICIENCY, LACTATE DEHYDROGENASE [LDH-M] SUBUNIT DEFICIENCY, TYPE VII GLYCOGEN STORAGE DISEASE). These muscle glycogeneses are rare and clinically similar to myophosphorylase deficiency. Patients with phosphofructokinase deficiency may also show a mild hemolytic anemia. Diagnosis is dependent on muscle enzyme analysis. Treatment is aimed at avoiding strenuous exercise.

DIAGNOSIS AND PRENATAL DIAGNOSIS OF GLYCOGEN STORAGE DISEASE

Diagnostic enzyme analysis on hepatic or muscle tissue for all types of glycogen storage diseases is currently funded at Duke Medical Center, Division of Genetics. Prenatal diagnosis of three types of glycogen storage diseases (types II, III, and IV) is also possible and is performed on cultured amniotic cells in this laboratory.

Burchell A: Molecular pathology of glucose-6-phosphatase. FASEB J 4:2978, 1990. *This article provides the most up-to-date studies on the enzyme glucose-6-phosphatase and clears some of the confusion concerning the enzyme. It also describes a series of children with "partial" defects in the enzyme who experienced sudden infant death syndrome.*

Chen YT, Cornblath M, Sidbury JB: Cornstarch therapy in type I glycogen storage disease. N Engl J Med 310:171, 1984. *The usefulness of dietary raw cornstarch to maintain blood glucose concentrations is demonstrated.*

Ding JH, deBarsy T, Brown B, et al.: Immunoblot analyses of glycogen debranching enzyme in different subtypes of glycogen storage disease type III. J Pediatr 116:95, 1990. *This article provides newer insights into the molecular basis of type III glycogeneses.*

Folk CC, Greene HL: Dietary management of type I glycogen storage disease. J Am Diet Assoc 84:293, 1984. *This article provides a practical application of foods and food exchanges to management of glycogen storage diseases.*

Ghishan FK, Greene HL: Inborn errors of metabolism that lead to permanent liver injury. In Zakim D, Boyer TD (eds.): Hepatology: A Textbook of Liver Disease. 2nd ed. Philadelphia, W.B. Saunders Company, 1990. *An extensively referenced review that focuses on the altered metabolism treatment and outcome of the hepatic forms of glycogenesis.*

Hers HG, Van Hoof F, deBarsy T: The glycogen storage diseases. In Scriver CR, Beaudet AL, Sly WS, Valle D (eds.): The Metabolic Basis of Inherited Disease. 6th ed. New York, McGraw-Hill, 1989. *This is an extensively referenced article that provides information on the clinical and biochemical aspects of the glycogen storage diseases.*

170 Fructose Intolerance

Harry L. Greene

Fructose, a normal dietary constituent of fruits, vegetables, honey, and the disaccharide sucrose (table sugar), is present at a level of 50 to 100 grams in the average Western diet. It is rapidly absorbed in the proximal small intestine by a specific transport mechanism and extracted on first pass from the portal vein, with no appearance in the urine. Three defects in fructose metabolism

have been identified: (1) essential fructosuria, (2) hereditary fructose intolerance, and (3) fructose-1, 6-diphosphatase deficiency. The major pathway for fructose metabolism and the three defects in fructose metabolism are illustrated in Figure 170–1.

ESSENTIAL FRUCTOSURIA. This is a rare (about 1 in 130,000 births), asymptomatic autosomal recessive condition caused by deficient activity of fructokinase, the first reaction in fructose utilization. Since no pathologic condition results from the defect, the primary concern relates to the fact that fructose is a reducing sugar. Thus, the finding of a positive reaction with urinary Clinitest tablets may result in the erroneous suggestion of diabetes unless the glucose oxidase is determined with a dipstick.

HEREDITARY FRUCTOSE INTOLERANCE (HFI). This is a potentially life-threatening autosomal recessive disorder that can be very effectively treated by elimination of dietary fructose. It has a prevalence of 1 in 20,000 and is due to deficiency of fructose-1-phosphate aldolase (aldolase B). The enzyme is normally present in large amounts in liver, intestine, and renal cortex, and the excessive intake of fructose by patients with HFI adversely affects each of these organs. Patients with the disorder exhibit profoundly deficient activity of fructose-1-phosphate aldolase and a modest reduction in the activity of fructose-1, 6-diphosphate aldolase.

Symptoms develop only after ingestion of fructose, and since lactose is the carbohydrate source in mammalian milk, infants do not develop symptoms until the introduction of dietary fruits or other fructose-containing foods or medication, i.e., fruits, fruit juices, medicinal syrups, sucrose-containing infant formulas, and so forth. The primary symptoms are vomiting and symptoms of hypoglycemia within 20 to 30 minutes after fructose ingestion. Concomitant laboratory findings include an acute decrease in serum glucose and phosphate levels and an elevation in the uric acid level. With continued exposure to fructose, hyperbilirubinemia, lactic acidosis, hepatosplenomegaly, and liver failure develop in conjunction with renal tubular dysfunction (bicarbonaturia, aminoaciduria, phosphaturia). At this stage, liver biopsy shows fatty infiltration of histiocytes with cellular necrosis and mild bile duct proliferation with fibrosis. If exposure to fructose continues, progressive fibrosis, cirrhosis, and death from liver failure follow. The brain may also show diminished neurons.

The diagnosis is suggested by the presence of urinary reducing sugar that is detected by Clinitest tablets and that is not detectable by urinary dipstick, since this test is specific for glucose. Since similar clinical features may be present with galactosemia or tyrosinemia, confirmation of the diagnosis can be made by measurement of fructose-1-phosphate aldolase activity in liver or intestinal biopsy specimens. An intravenous fructose tolerance test (0.2 to 0.3 gram per kilogram in adults or 3 grams per square meter in children) after restriction of dietary fructose for several weeks has been used for confirmatory evidence of the illness but may cause hypoglycemia.

In spite of recurrent bouts of hypoglycemia and substantial liver disease, restriction of dietary fructose usually results in almost complete recovery during a 3- to 5-week period, and affected adults have normal intelligence. Older children and adults are protected from large dietary intakes of fructose by an aversion to sweets, although small amounts taken chronically may result in isolated, reversible somatic growth retardation.

FRUCTOSE-1, 6-DIPHOSPHATASE DEFICIENCY. This rare disorder was first described in 1970. Patients usually present before the age of 6 months with fasting-induced lactic acidosis, hypoglycemia, and hepatomegaly. The reaction to glycerol is similar to that with fructose ingestion but is less severe than in patients with HFI. The condition is due to a defect of hepatic fructose-1, 6-diphosphatase, a gluconeogenic enzyme (see Fig. 170–1). Thus, when hepatic glycogen stores are depleted, fasting hypoglycemia develops.

The diagnosis is suspected when, after some 12 to 16 hours of fasting, the blood sugar concentration falls and is not restored by glucagon administration, and acidosis (lactate) is present. Loading tests with fructose or glycerol may be dangerous because they lead to hypoglycemia and lactic acidosis. The diagnosis is confirmed by measurement of the enzyme in hepatic biopsy material.

Baker L, Winegrad AI: Fasting hypoglycemia and metabolic acidosis associated with deficiency of hepatic fructose-1, 6-diphosphatase activity. Lancet 2:13, 1970. *The first description of a patient with deficient fructose-1, 6-diphosphatase activity.*

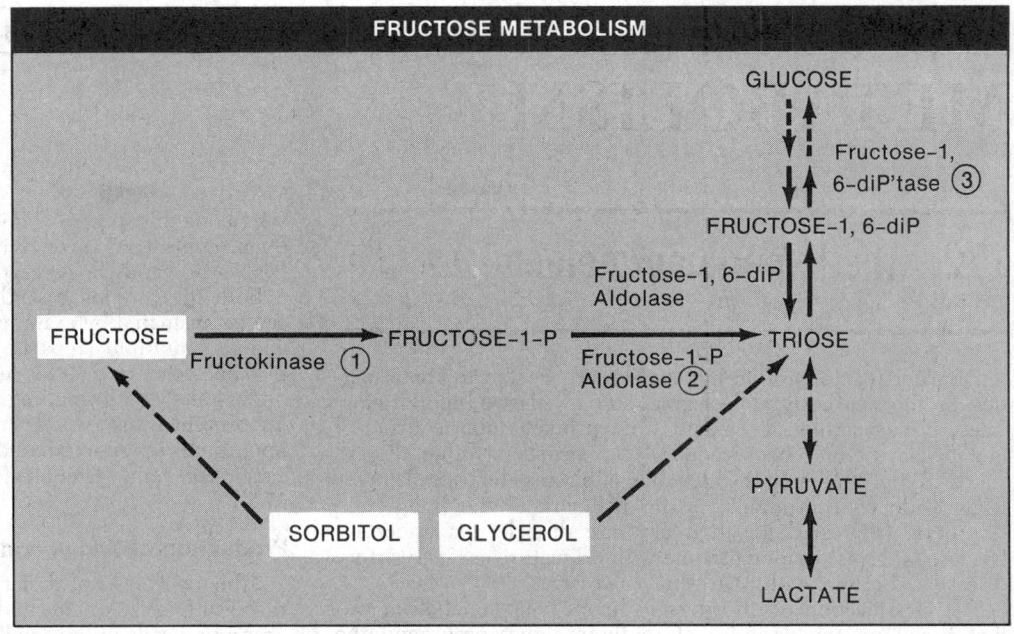

FIGURE 170–1. The major pathway for fructose metabolism and the three defects in fructose metabolism. 1 = Fructokinase deficiency results in asymptomatic fructosuria following ingestion of fructose or sorbitol. 2 = Fructose-1-phosphate aldolase deficiency results in hypoglycemia, lactic acidosis, and liver disease following ingestion of fructose or sorbitol. 3 = Fructose-1, 6-diphosphatase deficiency results in lactic acidosis and hypoglycemia with fasting, or hypoglycemia and acidosis following glycerol ingestion.

Ghishan FK, Greene HL: Inborn errors of metabolism that lead to permanent liver injury. *In* Zakim D, Boyer TD (eds): Hepatology: A Textbook of Liver Disease. 2nd ed. Philadelphia, W. B. Saunders Company, 1990. *An extensively referenced review that focuses on the altered metabolism, treatment, and outcome of patients with fructose intolerance.*

Odievre M, Gentil C, Gautier M, et al.: Hereditary fructose intolerance in childhood. Am J Dis Child 132:605, 1978. *This article is an excellent presentation of the clinical, hepatic, and biochemical changes that can be expected in children with HFI.*

Schulte MJ, Lenz W: Fatal sorbitol infusion in a patient with fructose-sorbitol intolerance. Lancet 2:188, 1977. *This paper illustrates the need to restrict sorbitol as well as fructose in patients with HFI.*

171 Primary Hyperoxaluria

Lloyd H. Smith, Jr.

Primary hyperoxaluria, a general term for two rare genetic disorders of glyoxylate metabolism, is characterized by excessive synthesis and urinary excretion of oxalic acid. Both disorders are transmitted as autosomal recessive traits. The diseases are usually clinically manifested in childhood by recurrent calcium oxalate nephrolithiasis or nephrocalcinosis, or both, leading to early renal failure. In addition to the usual clinical features of uremia, severe peripheral vascular insufficiency may complicate the course of the disease. At postmortem examination, calcium oxalate may be found widely deposited in extrarenal sites, a condition known as *oxalosis.* More rarely, milder forms of the disease may be found in adults. Although oxalate is an important constituent in approximately two thirds of all kidney stones, most adult patients with calcium oxalate nephrolithiasis excrete normal amounts of urinary oxalate (Ch. 88).

Primary hyperoxaluria type I (glycolic aciduria) represents a genetic defect in the activity of peroxisomal alanine: glyoxylate aminotransferase. As a result, glyoxylate accumulates and is excessively oxidized to oxalate and reduced to glycolate, both of which are excreted in increased amounts in the urine (more than 60 mg per 1.73 square meters per 24 hours each). In *primary hyperoxaluria type II* (L-glyceric aciduria), there is a defect in the enzyme D-glyceric dehydrogenase. Hydroxypyruvate accumulates and is reduced by lactate dehydrogenase (LDH) to L-glyceric acid, a compound that is undetectable in normal urine. The reduction of hydroxypyruvate to L-glycerate is probably coupled to the oxidation of glyoxylate to oxalate, both catalyzed by LDH. Each disease can be diagnosed by the characteristic pattern of metabolites in urine: type I, oxalate and glycolate; type II, oxalate and L-glycerate. Pyridoxine deficiency in laboratory animals and humans also leads to hyperoxaluria and even oxalosis with a urinary pattern similar to that of the genetic disease type I. With the onset of renal failure, the clearance of oxalate is reduced (its clearance is normally about 1.2 times that of creatinine), so that its urinary excretion may return to normal. The diagnosis may then be difficult to establish because measurements of serum oxalate are not readily available and, furthermore, serum oxalate levels rise in all forms of uremia.

No specific methods of treatment are now available. Efforts are directed toward reducing the amount of oxalate excreted and increasing its solubility. Large amounts of pyridoxine (200 to 400 mg per 24 hours) may decrease oxalate excretion in type I disease. More physiologic doses of pyridoxine (2 to 10 mg) may be effective in some patients. Dilute urine should be maintained by forcing fluids, and a phosphate or magnesium oxide supplement may offer partial protection against stone formation (Ch. 88). Renal homotransplantation has been disappointing because of rapid deposition of calcium oxalate in the transplanted kidney, but there have been some reports of success. Long-term dialysis and pyridoxine are therefore indicated when renal failure is severe. Recently, several patients have been successfully treated by combined renal and liver transplantations, which effectively reverse the metabolic abnormalities. Nitroglycerin may improve the peripheral vascular insufficiency associated with oxalosis. A search for an inhibitor of oxalate synthesis is highly indicated.

Increased urinary excretion of oxalate and stone diathesis (in the absence of glycolic aciduria or L-glyceric aciduria) occur in many patients who have small bowel disease and malabsorption (Ch. 102). Normally, oxalate and fatty acids of the small intestine compete for available calcium ion, and calcium oxalate is poorly absorbed. This important form of acquired hyperoxaluria results from excessive colonic absorption of dietary oxalate in the presence of significant steatorrhea. It can be controlled by a low-oxalate diet.

Danpure CJ, Jennings PR, Watts RWE: Enzymological diagnosis of primary hyperoxaluria type I by measurement of hepatic alanine: glyoxylate aminotransferase activity. Lancet 1:289, 1987. *This study established primary hyperoxaluria type I as a specific transaminase defect, a finding consistent with the therapeutic response to pyridoxine exhibited by some patients.*

Hillman RE: Primary hyperoxalurias. *In* Scriver CR, Beaudet AL, Sly WS, et al. (eds.): The Metabolic Basis of Inherited Disease. 6th ed. New York, McGraw-Hill, 1989, pp 933–944. *An excellent summary of oxalate metabolism and of current knowledge about the primary hyperoxalurias; 197 references are supplied.*

Yendt ER, Cohanim M: Response to a physiological dose of pyridoxine in Type I primary hyperoxaluria. N Engl J Med 312:953, 1985. *This article describes varying degrees of sensitivity in the reduction in oxalate excretion during pyridoxine therapy and raises the intriguing possibility that in some patients the diagnosis may be obscured by small amounts of the vitamin.*

DISORDERS OF LIPOPROTEIN METABOLISM

172 The Hyperlipoproteinemias

John D. Brunzell

Disorders of lipoprotein metabolism are related to abnormalities in the synthesis and degradation of plasma lipoproteins. These abnormalities may result from primary inborn errors of metabolism or may be secondary to a variety of other disease states. Hyperlipidemia, the elevation of plasma cholesterol and/or triglyceride concentrations, is the hallmark of the lipoprotein disorders. Clinical delineation of these disorders is important because of the association of some with premature coronary artery disease and others with recurrent pancreatitis.

The classification of disorders of lipoprotein metabolism was first based on the varieties of xanthomas that occur and the appearance of plasma turbidity caused by the accumulation of large, light-scattering lipoprotein particles in plasma. With the discovery of relatively discrete lipoprotein species, classification of these disorders was based on separation of lipoproteins by ultracentrifugation or by electrophoresis. Understanding of lipoprotein physiology has allowed classification of lipoprotein disorders according to pathophysiologic defects, with specific discrete apoprotein, enzyme, or receptor abnormalities identified in some disorders.

PHYSIOLOGY OF LIPOPROTEIN TRANSPORT

Structure and Function of Lipoproteins

The structure of the lipoprotein macromolecule is well suited for the solubilization of lipids in plasma. The nonpolar lipids—cholesteryl ester and triglyceride—are present in the lipoprotein core surrounded by a monolayer composed of specific proteins and the polar lipids, unesterified cholesterol and phospholipid. This monolayer allows the lipoprotein to remain miscible in plasma.

The lipoproteins function as an efficient vehicle for site-to-site transport of triglyceride and cholesterol of both exogenous and endogenous origin. Although caloric need is fairly constant throughout the day, food is ingested only periodically. The excess calories that enter the circulation with each meal are transported mainly as triglyceride to be stored in adipose tissue for future utilization between meals as free fatty acids. Ingested and synthesized cholesterol also needs to be transported to extrahepatic tissues to serve as a source of membrane cholesterol and as substrate for steroid hormone synthesis. The transport of triglyceride and cholesterol is accomplished by a spectrum of lipoproteins that have been classified by arbitrary operational boundaries according to either their density by ultracentrifugation or mobility by electrophoresis (Fig. 172–1). Fortunately, the lipoproteins, as separated by ultracentrifugation or electrophoresis, are so similar that the synonyms based on each of these methods of separation are essentially interchangeable.

The triglyceride-rich lipoproteins can enter the plasma as chylomicrons derived from dietary fat adsorbed from the gut or endogenously as triglyceride-rich very low density lipoprotein (VLDL) synthesized in the liver from glucose or circulating free fatty acids. After removal of some of their triglycerides and surface components, the remaining triglyceride-rich remnant of the chylomicron is taken up by the liver and degraded. The remnant of endogenous triglyceride-rich lipoprotein probably also requires the liver for further processing. In contrast to the chylomicron, however, only some components of VLDL are removed, resulting in formation of the low density cholesterol-rich lipoprotein.

This is likely to be an oversimplification, as there is a continuous spectrum of particles, and lipoproteins enter and exit at many sites along this spectrum of varying lipoprotein sizes. High density lipoproteins (HDL) interact with this system for transport of triglyceride and cholesteryl ester, as is noted later.

Both the physiology and the pathophysiology of lipoproteins can be evaluated by examining the sites of lipoprotein production and the multiple steps in lipoprotein catabolism. Most pathophysiologic abnormalities leading to hyperlipidemic states can be understood by examining four sites of regulation of plasma lipoprotein transport: (1) triglyceride-rich lipoprotein input, (2) lipoprotein lipase–mediated triglyceride catabolism, (3) remnant catabolism, and (4) cholesterol-rich lipoprotein catabolism (Fig. 172–2).

Production of Triglyceride-Rich Lipoproteins

After hydrolysis of dietary triglycerides in the small intestine, the resulting fatty acids and monoglycerides are taken up by the absorptive cells of the small intestine and incorporated into large triglyceride-rich lipoproteins with a specific form of apoprotein B (apo B-48), phospholipid, and a small amount of cholesterol. These chylomicrons are secreted from the absorptive cells into the lymphatics and subsequently enter the plasma via the thoracic duct. Chylomicron secretion and transport represent a system of high-capacity energy transport, allowing calories ingested at one time, over and above immediate needs, to be transferred to sites of storage for use between meals. The chylomicron remnant taken up and degraded by the liver suppresses synthesis of components of endogenous triglyceride-rich lipoproteins.

Input into plasma of triglyceride-rich lipoproteins also occurs from endogenous sources. During meals, plasma free fatty acids enter the liver, where they may be esterified with glycerol to form triglyceride. Between meals, free fatty acids are mobilized from adipose tissue triglyceride stores. These serve as a potential source for hepatic triglyceride synthesis. Lipogenesis, synthesis of fatty acids de novo from carbohydrate, also occurs in the liver. Fatty acids in the cytosol of the hepatocyte either can enter mitochondria, when oxidation occurs, or can remain in the cytosol, where they are esterified to form triglyceride. These processes appear to be regulated by changes in insulin and glucagon levels that occur with feeding: Glucagon enhances and insulin prevents mitochondrial fatty acid uptake by regulating long-chain acyl carnitine transferase. Insulin also induces lipogenic enzymes in the hepatocytes that regulate the synthesis of fatty acids.

Triglyceride synthesized in the liver, together with cholesteryl ester, is combined with the lipoprotein monolayer composed of phospholipid, unesterified cholesterol, and apoprotein B and is secreted into the hepatic venous outflow as triglyceride-rich VLDL. Hepatic apoprotein B (apo B-100) in VLDL has a larger molecular weight than does intestinal apoprotein B (apo B-48) found in chylomicrons.

In normal individuals, the majority of triglyceride input into the plasma is of dietary origin. Whereas the average American diet contains about 100 grams of triglyceride per day, less than 30 grams of triglyceride is secreted endogenously.

Lipoprotein Lipase–Mediated Triglyceride Catabolism

The triglyceride that enters the plasma in chylomicrons and endogenously synthesized triglyceride-rich lipoproteins is transported to adipose tissue for storage or to muscle for utilization. The enzyme in adipose tissue and muscle that catalyzes this triglyceride uptake is lipoprotein lipase (LPL). In adipose tissue the enzyme is synthesized in the fat cell, and following secretion and transport to the capillary endothelial cell, it hydrolyzes the triglyceride in these lipoproteins at the endothelial surface. At least two of the three fatty acids potentially releasable from triglyceride hydrolysis are then transported to the fat cell, where

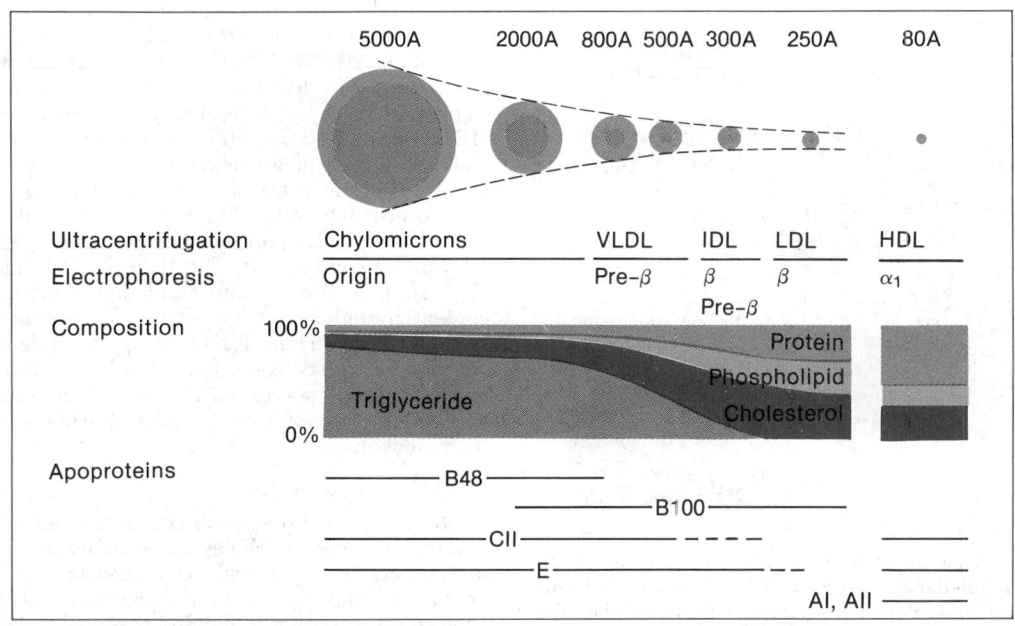

FIGURE 172–1. Classification of plasma lipoproteins by physical and chemical properties. (Modified from Bierman EL: Current Concepts: Hyperlipoproteinemia. The Upjohn Company, 1984.)

they are re-esterified with glycerol and stored as intracellular adipocyte triglyceride. The vast majority of the triglyceride in the adipocyte enters by this mechanism; little lipogenesis occurs de novo from glucose in adipose tissue in humans. The functional activity of LPL in adipose tissue is increased during and after meals. In humans, most of this increase in function is due to the increase in triglyceride-rich lipoproteins that serve as enzyme substrate. Although insulin is required to maintain LPL levels in adipose tissue, little change in enzyme levels occurs with normal

meals. Between meals, calories stored as triglyceride are released from the adipocyte as free fatty acids. This hydrolysis of intracellular adipocyte triglyceride is mediated by "hormone-sensitive" lipase of the fat cells. Between meals, when insulin levels are low and glucagon is increasing, hormone-sensitive lipase activity increases, and free fatty acids are released to be used for energy utilization by most tissues of the body.

The interaction of LPL with triglyceride in triglyceride-rich lipoproteins requires a cofactor, apoprotein CII. When secreted from the absorptive cell of the gut and from the liver, chylomicrons and VLDL do not contain this activator. Shortly after entering plasma these lipoproteins pick up apoprotein CII from a reservoir in circulating HDL. Thus the triglyceride-rich lipoproteins contain both substrate and activator for their hydrolysis by LPL. Following hydrolysis of the triglyceride in these lipoproteins, the apoprotein CII is released and again picked up by HDL. Thus, HDL appears to serve as a shuttle for apoprotein CII (as well as other lipoprotein components) (see below). Other apoproteins (CI and CIII) are transferred bidirectionally between triglyceride-rich lipoproteins and HDL and may play a role in LPL triglyceride hydrolysis, as well as other lipoprotein interactions.

Remnant Lipoprotein Catabolism

Following hydrolysis of the triglyceride in triglyceride-rich lipoproteins and the simultaneous removal of surface components, "remnant" lipoproteins are formed from chylomicrons and endogenous triglyceride-rich lipoproteins. The intermediate density lipoprotein fraction isolated by ultracentrifugation consists largely of remnant particles of VLDL. Those remnants formed from chylomicrons and large endogenous VLDL are often distributed, however, in the density range of small VLDL. Thus, remnants and endogenously synthesized triglyceride-rich lipoproteins cannot be separated completely by ultracentrifugation. Once formed, the remnant has a short half-life in plasma and appears to be taken up by the liver (Fig. 172–3). The endogenous triglyceride-rich lipoprotein remnant is further processed into the cholesterol-rich low density lipoprotein (LDL). During this catabolic process, further triglyceride and cholesterol as well as some surface proteins are removed. The remnant lipoprotein contains apoprotein B and several forms of apoprotein C and apoprotein E. The apoprotein E that accumulates as the remnant lipoproteins are formed appears to be important for hepatic uptake of those remnants. There is a complex interaction of hepatic receptors specific for apoprotein E and other receptors that bind both apoprotein B and apoprotein E, with the apoproteins in the

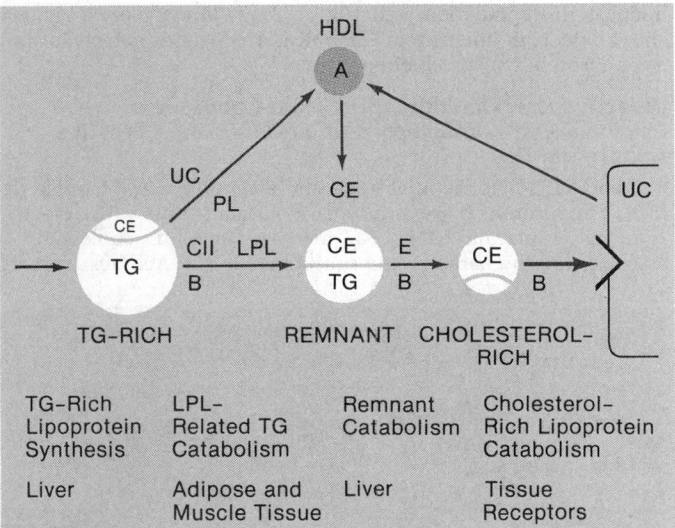

FIGURE 172–2. The triglyceride-rich very low density lipoprotein (VLDL) is synthesized in the liver and contains apo B, which remains with the particle through its subsequent catabolism. The triglyceride-rich lipoprotein core contains triglyceride (TG) and cholesteryl ester (CE) and surface unesterified cholesterol (UC) and phospholipid (PL). Upon entering plasma, acquired apo CII activates lipoprotein lipase (LPL) to catabolize TG core. The resulting remnant acquires apo E, which interacts with hepatic receptors to catabolize remnant to cholesterol-rich low density lipoprotein (LDL). The LDL binds to high-affinity receptor, with subsequent intracellular degradation of the lipoprotein. High density lipoproteins with apo AI and AII (A) acquire surface components of lipoproteins and plasma membranes of cells and form cholesteryl esters. These cholesteryl esters exchange with other lipoproteins or are delivered directly to the liver and may be the primary source of biliary cholesterol and bile acids.

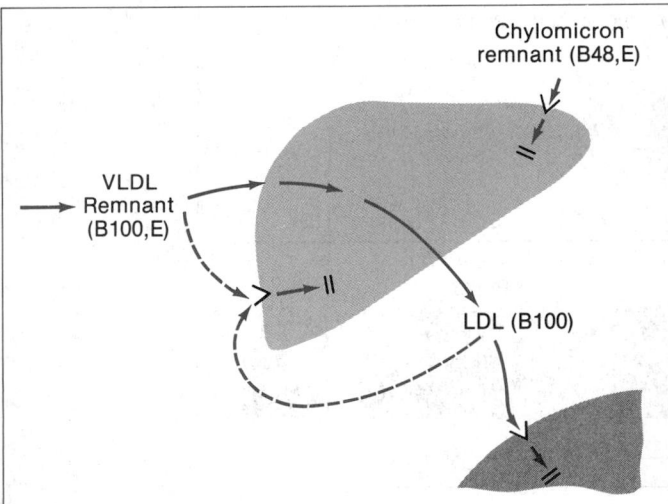

FIGURE 172–3. The liver is involved in the conversion of VLDL remnants containing apo B-100 and apo E to LDL, which are terminally catabolized via the LDL receptor in peripheral or hepatic tissue. The chylomicron remnant containing apo B-48 and apo E is processed completely in the liver via the apo E or chylomicron receptor.

remnant lipoproteins regulating their hepatic uptake. By the time the cholesterol-rich LDL has been formed, apoprotein B is the only apoprotein of the triglyceride-rich lipoproteins remaining.

Cholesterol-Rich Low Density Lipoprotein Catabolism

As the cholesterol-rich LDL normally arises from the remnant lipoprotein of VLDL, it contains the same amount of apoprotein B per lipoprotein particle as endogenous triglyceride-rich VLDL. Other apoproteins have been almost entirely removed, together with much of the phospholipid and some cholesterol. The cholesterol-rich lipoprotein can be removed from plasma by extrahepatic tissues, where it functions as the chief source of cholesterol for membrane synthesis or steroid hormone synthesis by these tissues. Alternatively, the lipoprotein may be taken up by the liver and degraded if not utilized peripherally. Apoprotein B in the cholesterol-rich lipoprotein appears to be recognized by a specific, high-affinity binding site in tissues (Fig. 172–4). Once bound, the lipoprotein is internalized by the cell in an endocytotic vesicle that fuses with a primary or pre-existing secondary lysosome. The protein moiety is degraded, and the cholesteryl ester is hydrolyzed to unesterified cholesterol by a lysosomal acid cholesteryl ester hydrolase. Hydrolysis of the triglyceride and phospholipid may also occur in the lysosome. The cell is able to regulate its own cholesterol content through a feedback control system in which intracellular free cholesterol suppresses endogenous cholesterol production by inhibiting the rate-limiting enzyme in cholesterol synthesis (HMG-CoA reductase). Furthermore, accumulation of intracellular free cholesterol limits the further uptake of cholesterol-rich lipoproteins by inhibiting synthesis of the lipoprotein receptor itself and stimulates its own re-esterification to cholesteryl ester by activating an acyl CoA:cholesterol transferase in the cytosol. Cholesterol content in the cell also is regulated by a receptor-mediated system involving HDL as a vehicle for cholesterol.

Apoprotein B containing lipoproteins may also be degraded by a scavenger system other than the high-affinity LDL receptor. This scavenger pathway involves the macrophage system and assumes greater importance in lipoprotein catabolism when defects in the LDL receptor or other abnormalities in lipoprotein catabolism exist.

Lipoprotein Surface Catabolism

Newly synthesized lipoproteins with their hydrophobic triglyceride and cholesteryl ester core are surrounded by a monolayer composed of protein, unesterified cholesterol, and phospholipid. As the core is removed and the lipoprotein decreases in size, several mechanisms process the resulting "excess" surface. The

catabolism of these surface components involves HDL and the enzyme lecithin-cholesterol acyl transferase (LCAT). The HDL synthesized by the liver and the intestine is composed of phospholipid and two major structural apoproteins, apoprotein AI and apoprotein AII. This HDL serves as an acceptor for the phospholipid (mainly lecithin) and unesterified cholesterol from the triglyceride-rich lipoprotein surface. The LCAT associated with HDL then removes a fatty acid from lecithin and transfers it to cholesterol, producing cholesteryl ester and lysolecithin. The cholesteryl ester is transferred from HDL to the liver directly or after transfer to other lipoproteins via lipid transfer protein, making the HDL apoproteins available to shuttle more lipoprotein surface components. The HDL, LCAT, and transfer proteins may also play a role in the regulation of intracellular cholesterol content by enhancing the efflux of free cholesterol from extrahepatic tissues. Thus, HDL may play a role in the transport of cholesterol from cells to liver, where it is ultimately excreted. In addition, HDL serves as the shuttle for apoprotein CII and apoprotein E to and from triglyceride-rich lipoproteins as part of their catabolism.

Cholesterol Excretion

Cholesterol and phospholipids are excreted as such in the bile, or after conversion of cholesterol into bile acid. A large proportion of the secreted bile acids is reabsorbed in the enterohepatic circulation and recycled. However, a net loss of bile acid, cholesterol, and phospholipid in the stool occurs by this pathway.

The definitive source of the cholesterol for output in the bile and for bile acid formation has not been determined. Cholesterol excreted into the bile may be synthesized directly in the liver. Alternatively, cholesterol may be secreted from the liver and gut in triglyceride-rich lipoproteins and may be esterified by the LCAT-HDL system, and it may re-enter the liver directly with HDL or via remnant lipoproteins.

INBORN ERRORS OF LIPOPROTEIN METABOLISM

The primary, or inborn, errors of lipoprotein metabolism leading to hyperlipidemia generally can be grouped into disorders associated with overproduction of triglyceride-rich lipoproteins or disorders due to defects in one of three catabolic steps in lipoprotein degradation (see Fig. 172–2). Much more is known about defects in lipoprotein catabolism than about defects leading to lipoprotein overproduction (Table 172–1).

Defective Low Density Lipoprotein Catabolism: Familial Hypercholesterolemia and Familial Defective Apoprotein B

DEFINITION. Familial hypercholesterolemia and familial defective apoprotein B are autosomal dominant traits with defective removal of plasma LDL. An increase in LDL cholesterol is associated with characteristic xanthomas in the Achilles tendons,

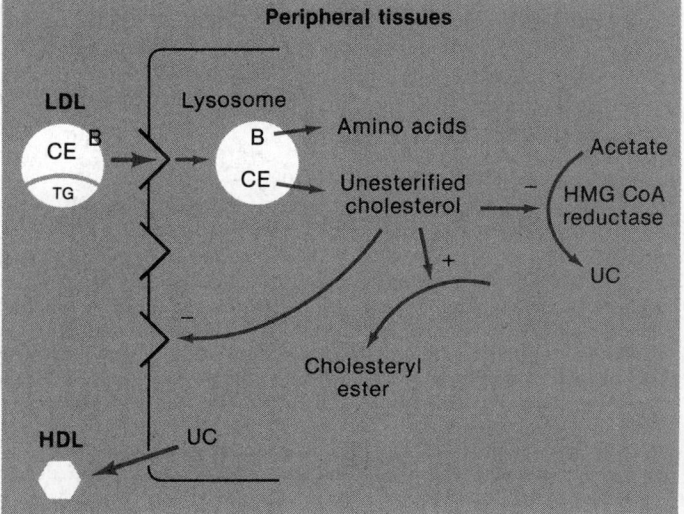

FIGURE 172–4. LDL containing apo B are removed from plasma by a high-affinity receptor and are processed in the lysosome. The resulting unesterified cholesterol regulates the cellular homeostatic mechanisms.

TABLE 172–1. INBORN ERRORS OF LIPOPROTEIN METABOLISM

Name	Prevalence	Physiologic Abnormality	Protein Abnormality	Lipoprotein Phenotype	Lipoproteins That Accumulate
Familial hypercholesterolemia	1/500	↓ LDL catabolism	Abnormal LDL receptor	IIA (IIB)	LDL ± VLDL
Familial dysbetalipoproteinemia	1/10,000	↓ Remnant catabolism	Abnormal apoprotein E	III	β VLDL
Lipoprotein lipase or apoprotein CII deficiency	Very rare	↓ TG catabolism	Absence of LPL or apoprotein CII	I (V)	Chylo ± VLDL
Familial hypertriglyceridemia	? 1/200	↑ VLDL-TG and bile acid synthesis	?	IV (V)	VLDL ± chylo
Familial combined hyperlipidemia	? 1/100	↑ Apoprotein B synthesis	Probably heterogeneous	IIA, IIB, IV	LDL and/or VLDL

Phenotypes based on World Health Organization recommendations.
Chylo = chylomicron; TG = triglyceride.

the patellar tendons, and the extensor tendons of the hands and with early coronary artery disease.

ETIOLOGY AND PATHOGENESIS. This disorder in LDL catabolism is caused by one of several alleles producing an abnormal LDL receptor or the ligand for that receptor, apoprotein B-100. One receptor allele is associated with the absence of LDL receptor synthesis and the others with the production of receptors of abnormal composition. These nonfunctional receptors are associated with decreased LDL catabolism and, in the heterozygote, with an approximate twofold increase in LDL levels. In the very rare homozygote, no receptor degradation occurs, and LDL is removed by a lower affinity "scavenger" pathway with a sixfold or greater increase of cholesterol-rich lipoproteins in plasma. In familial defective apoprotein B, amino acid 3500 of apoprotein B is mutated, impairing binding to the LDL receptor.

CLINICAL MANIFESTATIONS. This disorder often manifests as coronary artery disease in a young man, who then is noted to have elevated cholesterol levels. The mean age of the first myocardial infarction in men with heterozygous familial hypercholesterolemia who develop atherosclerosis is about 41 years. Affected women without additional risk factors may go through life without clinical manifestations of atherosclerosis. Low HDL cholesterol levels and cigarette smoking have marked effects on accelerating coronary artery disease and may be the major determinants of clinical disease in women. Peripheral vascular disease and cerebrovascular disease do not seem to be increased as much as coronary artery disease in this disorder. Lipid deposits in tendons are pathognomonic for this disorder. These xanthomas, usually bilateral, may be nodular irregularities in the Achilles tendons or extensor tendons of the hands but can extend to diffuse, generalized thickening. Corneal arcus and xanthelasma may occur but are found with other lipoprotein abnormalities as well.

DIAGNOSIS. Plasma cholesterol levels in familial hypercholesterolemia are in the upper 1 per cent of levels seen in the general population (e.g., 300 to 500 mg per deciliter). Since this disease seems to be present in 1 in 500 individuals, at least 1 person in 5 with such plasma cholesterol levels (and normal triglyceride levels) would be expected to have this disease. Patients with defective remnant removal and those with chylomicronemia may also have markedly elevated cholesterol levels, but they can be distinguished by the degree of coincident hypertriglyceridemia. Hypothyroidism and the nephrotic syndrome are also associated with elevated cholesterol levels. The increase in LDL in familial hypercholesterolemia uniquely is persistent, is almost always present in a parent, and is detectable at birth. The coexistence of tendon xanthomas and hypercholesterolemia is diagnostic of this disorder. Unilateral Achilles tendon thickening may be the result of injury.

TREATMENT. Discontinuation of smoking should be the first consideration for those who smoke. A diet low in saturated fat and cholesterol should be initiated in all affected individuals with this disorder, even though only a 5 to 15 per cent reduction in LDL levels occurs. Normalization of LDL levels may occur with the combination of a bile acid–binding resin (15 to 30 grams per day in divided doses with meals) combined with high-dose nicotinic acid with meals and at bedtime (1.0 to 4.0 grams per day). Compliance with each drug regimen has been poor. Fat-soluble vitamins should be given at bedtime, since the resins (colestipol or cholestyramine) prevent their absorption. Some recommend therapy with nicotinic acid and resins for all affected individuals. More conservatively, treatment can be restricted to postadolescent males and women with additional risk factors for coronary artery disease. Lovastatin, a drug that suppresses hepatic HMG-CoA reductase and hepatic cholesterol synthesis (at 20 to 80 mg per day), may be combined with a bile acid–binding resin for effective lowering of LDL levels.

Remnant Removal Disease: Dysbetalipoproteinemia

DEFINITION. This disorder is due to the interaction between (1) an autosomal recessive defect in apoprotein E with abnormal remnant catabolism and (2) independent overproduction of triglyceride-rich lipoproteins. This situation results in the accumulation of post-LPL remnants from both chylomicrons and endogenously synthesized VLDL that lead to xanthomas and coronary artery and peripheral vascular disease.

ETIOLOGY AND PATHOGENESIS. About 1 per cent of individuals have two genes leading to an abnormal apoprotein E. Multiple alleles exist for apoprotein E; those producing amino acid substitutions in a critical region of the apoprotein have abnormal apoprotein E binding to hepatic membranes. Affected individuals either have two identical abnormal genes or are compound heterozygotes with two different abnormal genes. Most of these individuals do not have hyperlipidemia but rather have low plasma cholesterol and LDL levels, presumably because of defective conversion of VLDL remnants to LDL. VLDL remnants that are cholesteryl ester enriched are present, but plasma triglyceride levels are usually normal. About 1 in 100 individuals with this abnormal apoprotein E has hyperlipidemia with remnant removal disease. These individuals appear to have an independent abnormality leading to hypertriglyceridemia in addition to the defect in apoprotein E, and they accumulate significant levels of chylomicron and VLDL remnants. Much rarer forms of remnant removal disease are caused by total absence of apoprotein E.

CLINICAL MANIFESTATIONS. This disorder may present initially as premature clinical atherosclerosis or as planar or tuberous xanthomas, or it may be detected as hyperlipidemia on routine laboratory screen. This disorder is usually not manifested as an abnormality in triglyceride or cholesterol levels in men until the third or fourth decade or in women until after menopause. The coexistent apoprotein E abnormality can be detected at birth. The onset of the xanthomas also is late. Planar xanthomas of the palmar crease and tuberous or tuberoeruptive xanthomas are highly suggestive of this disorder, although both can occur in severe, chronic obstructive liver disease with residual hepatocellular function. Atherosclerosis often is first noted in men around age 50 years. Peripheral vascular disease often predominates, but coronary artery disease is increased as well. In women, development of peripheral vascular and coronary artery disease after menopause is rapid compared with that in nonaffected females. The presence of estrogen in the premenopausal state seems to minimize the defect in remnant catabolism.

DIAGNOSIS. The presence of palmar or tuberous xanthomas in the absence of liver disease is diagnostic. Plasma cholesterol and triglyceride are increased to similar levels. A method for separation of VLDL from the remainder of the more dense lipoproteins is necessary to demonstrate that these VLDL are cholesteryl ester enriched and have beta mobility on electrophoresis ("beta VLDL") rather than the typical pre-beta mobility of

VLDL. An abnormal apoprotein E can usually be demonstrated by isoelectric focusing. The concentration of LDL is typically low, and HDL is often normal or slightly depressed. Hypothyroidism can aggravate this disorder or rarely can lead to remnant accumulation by itself.

TREATMENT. In obese individuals with this disorder, weight loss should be considered in lowering triglyceride and cholesterol levels. In postmenopausal women, low-dose ethinyl estradiol seems to normalize the defect in remnant removal and to correct the hypercholesterolemia. Clofibrate (1 gram twice a day) or gemfibrozil (0.6 gram twice a day) also is effective in decreasing lipid levels. Alternatively, high-dose nicotinic acid is considered by some investigators to be the drug of choice for treatment of this disorder. There is evidence that the form of atherosclerosis occurring with this disorder is partially reversible with treatment.

Defective Lipoprotein Lipase–Related Triglyceride Catabolism

DEFINITION. Familial LPL deficiency is a rare autosomal recessive trait characterized by complete absence of active enzyme protein in all tissues, leading to massive hypertriglyceridemia from birth and recurrent episodes of pancreatitis. Similar syndromes also are caused by inborn defects in other aspects of the LPL system.

ETIOLOGY AND PATHOGENESIS. Hydrolysis of triglyceride from chylomicrons and endogenous VLDL in vivo requires both LPL and its activator apoprotein CII. A defect of either of these proteins is associated with severely decreased triglyceride removal and massive hypertriglyceridemia. In infants and young children, the triglyceride accumulates primarily as chylomicron triglyceride of dietary origin. As the patient gets older, a defect in VLDL triglyceride removal becomes more apparent as well. Both LPL and apoprotein CII deficiency are autosomal recessive disorders; often consanguinity can be documented. A number of defects in the genes for LPL and apoprotein CII have been described. Individuals also exist who have LPL activity missing from only selected tissues or who have a familial inhibitor of LPL activity. These latter groups usually have less severe hypertriglyceridemia and become symptomatic later in life than in the classic form of LPL deficiency.

CLINICAL MANIFESTATIONS. Infants with LPL deficiency rapidly manifest intolerance to fatty foods. As these children grow, they learn to avoid certain high-fat foods, such as whole milk. Abdominal pain, often with pancreatitis, occurs in association with the high levels of chylomicron triglyceride. Eruptive xanthomas occur on extensor surfaces, notably the elbows, knees, and the buttocks, and are pathognomonic for chronic chylomicronemia. Hepatomegaly and occasionally splenomegaly occur because of the accumulation of lipid-laden foam cells. The hepatosplenomegaly rapidly diminishes on a fat-free diet, which clears the chylomicronemia. Eruptive xanthomas also disappear with time after lowering of chylomicron levels. Other signs and symptoms seen with chronic chylomicronemia may also occur (see below).

DIAGNOSIS. A young child with abdominal pain and milky, lactescent plasma should be studied for a genetic abnormality in LPL. Other causes of chylomicronemia before adulthood relate to the occurrence of a common form of hypertriglyceridemia with diabetes or glucocorticoid therapy. Absent or diminished activity of LPL can be demonstrated in adipose tissue or muscle tissue, or in plasma after administration of intravenous heparin. Apoprotein CII deficiency can be detected by radioimmunoassay or by gel electrophoresis of the protein components of lipoproteins or by testing the ability of the patient's plasma to activate purified LPL.

TREATMENT. In all the inborn errors of the LPL-related triglyceride removal system associated with chylomicronemia, a decrease in total dietary fat is absolutely indicated. A total of polyunsaturated and saturated fat as low as 10 to 20 per cent of calories is often required. Medium-chain triglycerides can be used to prepare some foods, since their fatty acids leave the gut unesterified via the portal vein rather than via the thoracic duct, as does chylomicron triglyceride. The goal is to decrease the amount of dietary fat to a level low enough to eliminate the occurrence of abdominal pain. These individuals can also be sensitive to agents that raise endogenous VLDL levels, such as alcohol or glucocorticoids, and to the effects of pregnancy.

Other Genetic Disorders with Mild to Moderate Hypertriglyceridemia

A number of less well characterized disorders associated with persistent or intermittent elevated VLDL levels exist. Some may be associated with increased hepatic secretion of VLDL, others with defective VLDL catabolism. It has been useful to classify those conditions into several relatively homogeneous groups on the basis of the existence of large, well-characterized families for each.

FAMILIAL HYPERTRIGLYCERIDEMIA. This apparently autosomal dominant trait may be quite common. Individuals with familial hypertriglyceridemia appear to have a defect leading to enhanced hepatic triglyceride synthesis with subsequent secretion of triglyceride-enriched, large VLDL. These individuals may also have increased cholesterol and cholic acid synthesis. LPL-related triglyceride removal and remnant lipoprotein catabolism appear to be normal. The LDL levels are normal, while HDL is triglyceride enriched with depletion of HDL cholesterol.

Most individuals with this disorder do not have an increased predisposition for coronary artery disease, remain asymptomatic, and are detected by routine lipid screen. Occasionally, with the onset of another disorder associated with elevated triglyceride levels, they develop the chylomicronemia syndrome (see below). These individuals develop no characteristic xanthomas. There is no increase in obesity in this disorder and no increase in the frequency of diabetes.

Persons with this disorder have persistent hypertriglyceridemia once they become adults. Below the age of 20, the abnormality usually is not manifested. Some of the increase in VLDL may persist after weight loss. Increased levels of LDL do not occur. One parent is characteristically affected, as are half of the siblings. These individuals appear to be quite sensitive to other factors that cause only mild hypertriglyceridemia in normal adults: obesity and alcohol, as well as estrogen, diuretic, beta-adrenergic blocker, and glucocorticoid therapy.

Treatment with clofibrate or gemfibrozil usually leads to significant decreases in VLDL levels. In families without evidence of increased atherosclerosis, no known benefit accrues from this therapy, and it should be discouraged. Drugs causing elevation of triglyceride levels should be avoided because they may precipitate massive chylomicronemia and pancreatitis.

FAMILIAL COMBINED HYPERLIPIDEMIA. It was first pointed out in 1973 that this disorder is very common in those with premature coronary artery disease, is inherited as an autosomal dominant trait, and is characterized by different "combinations" of hyperlipidemia: elevated cholesterol level alone, elevated triglyceride level alone, or elevations in levels of both lipids (familial multiple lipoprotein–type hyperlipidemia). It now appears that this disorder is better characterized as one with elevated plasma apoprotein B levels with variable lipid phenotype even in the same individual at different times, in contrast to familial hypercholesterolemia. The increase in apoprotein B, whether in VLDL or in LDL, appears to be caused by increased hepatic synthesis of the apoprotein. These individuals also have abnormalities in HDL, with a mild decrease in HDL cholesterol and apoprotein AI.

Men with this disorder have premature coronary artery disease with a mean age of infarct at about 40 years. Smoking has a marked effect on the prevalence of clinical heart disease. Individuals with this disorder are slightly more obese and may have more systemic hypertension. They have no characteristic xanthomas but occasionally have nonspecific xanthelasma.

OTHER FORMS OF HYPERTRIGLYCERIDEMIA. Individuals with chylomicronemia and triglyceride levels between 1000 and 2000 mg per deciliter are said to aggregate in families. In addition, there are individuals with primary hypertriglyceridemia who are noted to have a defect in VLDL removal not characterized by one of the above defects in the LPL system.

APPROACH TO THE PATIENT WITH MILD TO MODERATE HYPERTRIGLYCERIDEMIA. The major concern for the individual with hypertriglyceridemia relates to a possible increase in risk for atherosclerosis. When an individual is identified with elevated plasma triglyceride levels, acquired forms of hyperlipidemia should be identified and treated, and the primary forms of hypertriglyceridemia associated with defective remnant catabolism or LPL deficiency should be ruled out.

Elevations in plasma triglyceride levels often serve as a marker for associated abnormalities potentially related to atherosclerosis. A strong family history of early coronary artery disease in the father or mother's male relatives helps to identify such a hypertriglyceridemic individual at risk for early atherosclerosis.

The hypertriglyceridemic individuals who intermittently develop hypercholesterolemia caused by increased LDL levels as well as those who have elevated LDL apoprotein B levels with normal LDL cholesterol also seem to be ones at increased risk for atherosclerosis.

The level of HDL cholesterol is often low in the presence of hypertriglyceridemia. This situation can occur with familial LPL deficiency and with familial hypertriglyceridemia and does not seem to be associated with the increase in coronary risk seen with a low HDL cholesterol level in the absence of hypertriglyceridemia. However, a decrease in the level of the major apoprotein of HDL, apoprotein AI, seems to be a good predictor of risk, even in the presence of hypertriglyceridemia.

The aforementioned abnormalities characteristic of the hypertriglyceridemic subject at risk for atherosclerosis are similar to those in familial combined hyperlipidemia, which may account for a significant portion of this group.

While weight loss and clofibrate (or gemfibrozil) therapy lower VLDL levels, those at risk for early coronary artery disease may respond with an increase in LDL levels. Preferred therapy for the hypertriglyceridemic individual at risk, in particular the one with familial combined hyperlipidemia, may be like that used to treat elevated LDL levels in familial hypercholesterolemia: combined bile acid resin and high-dose nicotinic acid therapy, in addition to a diet low in saturated fat and cholesterol. Because of the uncertainty of the significance of elevated triglyceride levels and the unknown risks of lifelong drug therapy, many authorities have recommended diet therapy alone for hypertriglyceridemia.

ACQUIRED DISORDERS OF LIPOPROTEIN METABOLISM

Some disease states are associated with mild to moderate hyperlipidemia in the absence of primary forms of hyperlipidemia, while others seem to have a significant effect only in the presence of a familial form of hyperlipidemia. In general, these can be divided into conditions associated with increased levels of triglyceride-rich lipoproteins and those associated with multiple lipoprotein-type expression (acquired combined hyperlipidemia) (Table 172–2).

TABLE 172–2. ACQUIRED DISORDERS OF LIPOPROTEIN METABOLISM

A. Hypertriglyceridemia
  1. Mild to moderate hypertriglyceridemia
    a. Diabetes mellitus*
    b. Uremia and/or dialysis*
  2. Minimal hypertriglyceridemia alone
    a. Obesity
    b. Estrogen*
    c. Alcohol*
    d. Beta-adrenergic blocking agents*
  3. Rare forms of moderate to marked hypertriglyceridemia
    a. Systemic lupus erythematosus
    b. Dysgammaglobulinemias
    c. Glycogenosis type I
    d. Lipodystrophy
B. Combined hyperlipidemia
  1. Hypothyroidism*
  2. Nephrotic syndrome
  3. Glucocorticoid excess*
  4. Diuretics*
C. Hypercholesterolemia
  1. Acute intermittent porphyria
  2. Anorexia nervosa

*Can be associated with chylomicronemia syndrome when it occurs with the familial forms of hypertriglyceridemia.

Hypertriglyceridemia

DIABETES MELLITUS. Persons with untreated insulin-dependent diabetes and untreated symptomatic non–insulin-dependent diabetes have low adipose tissue or muscle LPL activity with a mild to moderate increase in triglyceride levels and decreased HDL cholesterol levels. With insulin resistance and milder degrees of insulin deficiency, hypertriglyceridemia is caused by excess free fatty acids mobilized from adipose tissue that are re-esterified in the liver and secreted as endogenous VLDL. Treatment with insulin or oral sulfonylurea agents will correct the abnormality in LPL over a period of weeks. In the treated diabetic, variability in free fatty acid mobilization and hepatic triglyceride synthesis, related to the degree of diabetic control, accounts for most of the variation in triglyceride levels.

CHRONIC UREMIA AND DIALYSIS. Many individuals with chronic uremia have elevated VLDL levels with hypertriglyceridemia and low HDL cholesterol levels. This condition persists after initiation of maintenance hemodialysis or peritoneal dialysis. These lipoprotein abnormalities appear to be related to defects in LPL-mediated triglyceride removal and, with smoking and hypertension, account for the marked atherosclerosis in the dialysis population.

OTHER. Obesity, estrogen use, and alcohol are associated with minimal to mild increases in triglyceride levels, usually not to levels considered abnormal, which appear to be caused by modest increases in hepatic VLDL secretion. Diuretic agents and beta-adrenergic blocking agents are also associated with small increases in triglyceride levels. The diuretics often raise LDL levels, while the beta-blocking agents decrease HDL.

Moderate to marked hypertriglyceridemia occurs extremely rarely in systemic lupus erythematosus or dysgammaglobulinemia caused by an immunoglobulin-lipoprotein interaction. Moderate hypertriglyceridemia can also occur in rare disorders such as glycogenosis (type I), lipodystrophy, and carnitine-palmitoyl transferase deficiency.

Combined Hyperlipidemia

HYPOTHYROIDISM. Thyroid hormone appears to be necessary for proper functioning of most steps in lipoprotein metabolism. Thyroxine is necessary for maintenance of the LDL receptor; in hypothyroidism LDL levels are elevated because of defective catabolism. Remnant removal is impaired, resulting in the accumulation of chylomicron with VLDL remnants, and finally the LPL level is low, resulting in hypertriglyceridemia. Thyroxine replacement corrects all of these defects.

NEPHROTIC SYNDROME. With urinary loss of albumin and the development of hypoalbuminemia, increases in the levels of VLDL or LDL or both occur. These lipoprotein abnormalities are associated with increased hepatic lipid synthesis and defective catabolism of triglyceride-rich lipoproteins. The latter defect may be related to the loss in the urine of cofactors required for LPL function.

GLUCOCORTICOID EXCESS. Excess glucocorticoid levels caused by Cushing's syndrome or exogenous steroid therapy are associated with elevated VLDL and/or LDL levels. The best studied situation is in the glucocorticoid-treated renal transplant subject, who in the absence of uremia or proteinuria has combined hyperlipidemia.

Hypercholesterolemia

Elevated LDL levels may occur in occasional individuals in response to high saturated fat and cholesterol feeding. Much of the hypercholesterolemia in the population has remained unexplained and has been termed multifactorial, suggesting that it is due to the interaction of multiple genes (polygenic) with the environment. Elevated LDL levels occur in acute intermittent porphyria and have been reported with hepatomas and in anorexia nervosa.

HYPERLIPIDEMIA AND ATHEROSCLEROTIC VASCULAR DISEASE

Although the etiology of atherosclerosis is multifactorial, the development of premature coronary artery disease and peripheral vascular disease is strongly dependent on abnormalities in plasma lipoprotein metabolism. Thus, coronary artery disease in men under the age of 60 years and in women of any age is more likely to occur in the presence of an inborn error or acquired form of hyperlipidemia. HDL may independently protect against atherosclerosis. Differences in HDL cholesterol levels between men and women may explain a large part of the sex difference in the risk for atherosclerosis.

Familial hypercholesterolemia is unequivocally associated with premature coronary artery disease, the expression of which is aggravated by cigarette smoking and low HDL cholesterol levels. Remnant removal disease is also associated with peripheral vascular and coronary artery disease. The increased atherosclerosis seen in patients with diabetes and in patients on long-term hemodialysis may also be related in part to abnormalities in lipoprotein metabolism. Nonetheless, all of these disorders still account for only a minor part of premature atherosclerosis. Mildly elevated levels of LDL, apoprotein B, or triglyceride, as well as low levels of HDL cholesterol and apoprotein AI, are likely to be present in the majority of patients with premature coronary artery disease. The frequency of familial combined hyperlipidemia or of other, as yet undefined, genetic forms of hyperlipidemia in this heterogeneous group of individuals has to be determined.

An increased risk for atherosclerosis that is independent of other lipoprotein abnormalties has been associated with elevated levels of lipoprotein (a) (Lp[a]). This lipoprotein consists of LDL with an additional large protein of varying molecular weight, apoprotein (a), attached to the apolipoprotein B. Lp(a) is higher than normal in familial hypercholesterolemia but is low or normal in homozygous LPL deficiency and remnant removal disease. This finding implies that the particle is not processed through the VLDL-LDL cascade and that it is removed via the LDL receptor. Increased lipoprotein (a) levels are associated with increased coronary artery disease, particularly in the presence of other risk factors for atherosclerosis. At present, no effective method lowers Lp(a) levels.

THE NATIONAL CHOLESTEROL EDUCATION PROGRAM

The National Cholesterol Education Program (NCEP) has devised a protocol based on total or LDL cholesterol levels for the detection, evaluation, and treatment of hyperlipidemia. Total cholesterol levels should be screened in young and middle-aged adults and in the children of high-risk families. This initial measurement may be made on a nonfasting plasma sample. The first decision is to determine which individuals are candidates for measurement of fasting plasma lipoproteins (Fig. 172–5). On the basis of data from the Multiple Risk Factor Intervention Trial (MRFIT) on one third of a million middle-aged men, a total cholesterol level above 240 mg per deciliter was arbitrarily called high and that below 200 per deciliter was regarded as desirable. The values between 200 and 240 mg per deciliter were termed borderline. By these criteria, about 15 per cent of the MRFIT men had high total cholesterol levels, 40 per cent had desirable levels, and the remaining 45 per cent had borderline levels. A major goal of the NCEP is to differentiate those borderline individuals who are at risk for premature atherosclerosis from those not at risk. Factors that were defined as indicating increased risk were male sex, a positive family history of premature atherosclerosis, cigarette smoking, hypertension, diabetes, truncal obesity, and an HDL cholesterol level below 35 mg per deciliter. Borderline individuals with two or more of these risk factors, individuals with pre-existing premature atherosclerosis, as well as those with high total cholesterol levels, are candidates for the measurement of fasting total cholesterol, HDL cholesterol, and triglyceride levels. To detect individuals with low HDL levels on a familial basis, individuals with desirable total cholesterol levels who have a strong family history of premature atherosclerosis should also be included.

The second NCEP decision, i.e., the identification of candidates for specific dietary therapy, is based on the LDL cholesterol level (Fig. 172–5). The LDL is calculated as follows:

$$\frac{LDL}{cholesterol} = \frac{total}{cholesterol} - \frac{HDL}{cholesterol} - \frac{triglyceride}{5}$$

Individuals with high LDL cholesterol levels (above 160 mg per deciliter) and those with borderline levels (130 to 160 mg per deciliter along with other atherosclerotic risk factors should be considered for the American Heart Association Step 1 or Step 2 diets, which restrict dietary saturated fat and cholesterol. While institution of the Step 1 diet can often be accomplished by the physician and staff through elimination of selected foods from the diet, the Step 2 diet usually needs the expertise of a nutrition specialist. The diet can be applied to a wide spectrum of age groups, from those as young as 2 years of age to the elderly, and often works best when based on the family unit. Individuals with desirable LDL levels or borderline levels without other risk factors for atherosclerosis require no specific dietary therapy. When a patient is considered for dietary therapy, the detection and subsequent treatment of causes of hyperlipidemia secondary to other diseases or drugs is essential, such as the replacement of diuretics and beta-adrenergic blocking agents with lipid-neutral medications, if possible.

The third NCEP decision, i.e., the initiation of drug therapy for elevated LDL cholesterol levels, can be considered after the patient has been on a diet low in saturated fat and cholesterol for 3 to 6 months (Fig. 172–5). The LDL level required before drug therapy should be considered is higher than that for dietary intervention. Because of biologic and laboratory variation in cholesterol levels, LDL cholesterol should be measured two or three times before drug therapy is initiated. Drug therapy should ideally be restricted to young and middle aged adults or to those who developed clinical atherosclerosis while middle aged. With rare exceptions, the use of drugs as a form of primary intervention in individuals over 65 years of age who do not have atherosclerosis is not recommended.

A young or middle-aged adult who has been on a diet low in saturated fat and cholesterol diet for 3 to 6 months and who continues to have an LDL cholesterol level higher than 190 mg per deciliter on several occasions is a candidate for drug therapy. Individuals with premature atherosclerosis or those who have high LDL cholesterol levels of 160 to 190 mg per deciliter with other risk factors as noted earlier are also candidates for drug therapy. If an individual has another disease that limits survival, drug therapy for hyperlipidemia should be questioned.

Once the decision has been made to initiate drug therapy, several protocols with single or combined drugs are possible. For milder increases in LDL cholesterol levels (perhaps in the range of 190 to 220 mg per deciliter), low-dose therapy with one to two scoops of bile acid–binding resin once or twice a day with major meals can be effective. Alternatively, 500 mg of crystalline nicotinic acid three times a day or 20 mg of lovastatin in the evening may be used. Higher doses of nicotinic acid (up to 1.0 gram four times a day) or lovastatin (up to 40 mg twice a day) can be used alone, or each can be combined with resin therapy in highly effective programs for lowering of LDL levels. Because of the high risk for muscle necrosis, lovastatin should not be combined with nicotinic acid, cyclosporine, erythromycin, or the fibric acids (clofibrate and gemfibrozil). When using nicotinic acid or lovastatin, it is recommended that liver function be monitored with serum glutamic-oxaloacetic transaminase (SGOT) levels every 6 to 12 weeks initially and then semiannually when treatment has been stabilized. Creatine kinase (CK) levels should be measured during lovastatin therapy. Contraindications to nicotinic acid therapy include liver disease, migraine headache, and insulin-resistant diabetes. The use of slow-release nicotinic acid should be discouraged because the incidence of hepatic dysfunction is high compared with that occurring when regular nicotinic acid is used. Another form of niacin, nicotinamide, does not affect lipid levels. The bile acid–binding resins also bind coumarin derivatives, digoxin, thyroxine, and possibly other drugs. In addition, the resins are contraindicated in patients in whom the increase in cholesterol is associated with triglyceride levels above 400 mg per deciliter, since resins markedly increase the plasma triglyceride toward levels that can cause pancreatitis.

The NCEP guidelines do not directly address the issue of hypertriglyceridemia. Most patients with mildly to moderately elevated triglyceride levels who are at risk for premature atherosclerosis can be treated under the NCEP guidelines by following estimated LDL cholesterol levels. This group of patients includes those with familial combined hyperlipidemia, those with remnant removal disease, and those at risk for atherosclerosis who have

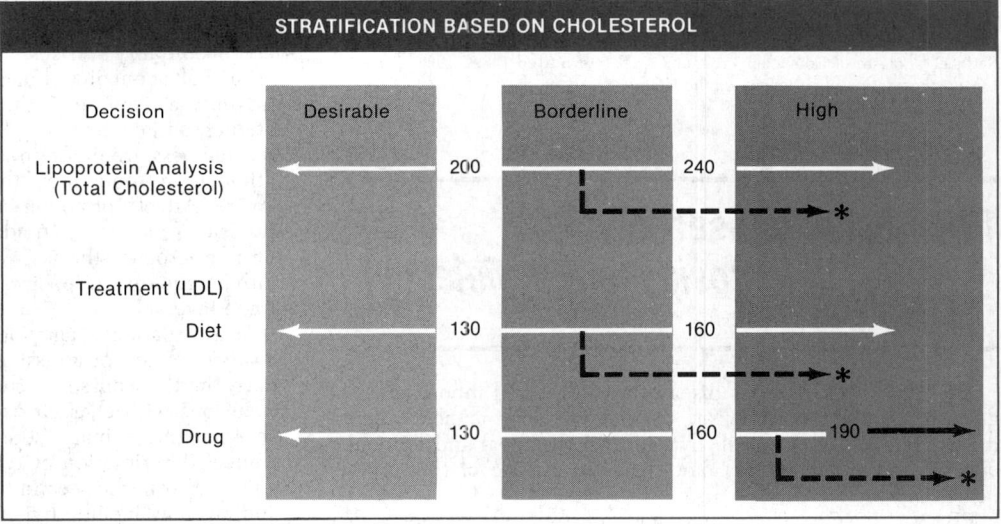

FIGURE 172–5. Stratification based on cholesterol for treatment of hyperlipidemia in patients at risk for premature atherosclerosis. The symbol * and dashed lines indicate high-risk patient; solid lines indicate cholesterol levels at which next step is considered.

other forms of hypertriglyceridemia. The fibric acid drugs (clofibrate and gemfibrozil) are drugs to be used for massive hypertriglyceridemia. They are also useful in remnant removal disease and in the treatment of selected individuals with milder hypertriglyceridemia, such as the patient who simultaneously has elevated triglyceride and LDL levels, as well as low HDL cholesterol levels (lipoprotein phenotype IIB with low HDL). The use of fibric acid drugs should be restricted to these three situations because of the limited benefit and the increased risk of gastrointestinal complications in other forms of hyperlipidemia.

This approach with drug therapy is conservative, focusing on those young to middle-aged men who are at very high risk for premature coronary artery disease due to hyperlipidemia. In North America, little evidence exists that total or LDL cholesterol levels are related to the development of new atherosclerosis in men after the age of 65 years, except at extreme levels, as seen in familial hypercholesterolemia. Therefore, we need to avoid aggressive use of either drug therapy or extremes of dietary modification because of the potential for harm. The majority of coronary artery disease becomes manifest after the age of 65, and we have yet to determine what role lipoproteins play in the risk of this disease in the elderly.

CHYLOMICRONEMIA SYNDROME

DEFINITION. Marked chylomicronemia with plasma triglyceride levels in excess of 2000 mg per deciliter is associated with a constellation of signs and symptoms called the chylomicronemia syndrome.

ETIOLOGY AND PATHOGENESIS. This syndrome can occur because of one of several inborn errors in the LPL system for plasma triglyceride removal as noted earlier. Much more commonly, the marked hypertriglyceridemia occurs as a result of the interaction of two common forms of hypertriglyceridemia, usually one genetic and one acquired. Untreated symptomatic diabetes mellitus in the presence of familial hypertriglyceridemia, familial combined hyperlipidemia, or, less commonly, remnant removal disease is a frequent cause of chylomicronemia. Commonly used drugs that interact with these inborn errors are the estrogens, diuretics, beta-adrenergic blocking agents, alcohol, and glucocorticoids. The effects of these drugs are often markedly exaggerated in patients with pre-existing hyperlipidemia. Hypothyroidism and uremia may also occasionally contribute.

CLINICAL MANIFESTATIONS. For unexplained reasons, some individuals are asymptomatic with plasma triglyceride levels as high as 29,000 mg per deciliter. More commonly, abdominal pain and/or pancreatitis or even chest pain is present. Impairment of recent memory can often be detected, and the patient may complain of paresthesias of the extremities, similar to the carpal tunnel syndrome. Lipemia retinalis can often be observed, hepatomegaly is common, splenomegaly can occur, and eruptive xanthomas are evidence of chronic chylomicronemia. All of these symptoms and signs clear when triglyceride levels are decreased

below 1000 or 2000 mg per deciliter. Marked hypertriglyceridemia may cause insulin resistance and impair control of diabetes. Also, many routine laboratory tests are invalid in the presence of milky plasma. Simple removal of chylomicrons from plasma by short-term ultracentrifugation helps to avoid this problem.

DIAGNOSIS. It is very simple to make a presumptive diagnosis of chylomicronemia syndrome by visual examination of the patient's plasma. Milky plasma always indicates the presence of chylomicrons, as does a plasma triglyceride level above 1000 mg per deciliter. In the presence of symptoms and signs of the chylomicronemia syndrome, a definitive diagnosis is made if these clear when the triglyceride level is lowered.

TREATMENT. With pancreatitis, the discontinuation of oral intake rapidly decreases triglyceride levels. With refeeding, fat must be avoided initially and replaced slowly. Often, mild to moderate abdominal pain can be treated by lowering dietary fat content and avoiding alcohol. The mainstay of treatment is to identify the causes of the elevation in triglyceride levels. A genetic form of hypertriglyceridemia is invariably present and may need to be treated with clofibrate, gemfibrozil, or nicotinic acid. The last drug is difficult to use in diabetic patients because it impairs insulin sensitivity. The acquired disease or agent contributing to the hypertriglyceridemia should be treated or removed, respectively. Slowly, the patient can be refed while the plasma is watched for turbidity and the patient's symptoms and signs are observed. With appropriate therapy, the chylomicronemia syndrome should rarely recur.

RARE DISORDERS OF LIPOPROTEIN METABOLISM

Several rare inherited disorders of lipoprotein metabolism are of considerable theoretical importance because they assist in the understanding of normal lipoprotein physiology. Each of these disorders is an autosomal recessive trait.

Abetalipoproteinemia presents in early childhood and is associated with the absence of apoprotein B–containing lipoproteins because of defective synthesis. Intestinal fat malabsorption, ataxia, neuropathy, retinitis pigmentosa, and acanthocytosis result. *Tangier disease* presents in childhood with absence of HDL and extremely low levels of apoproteins AI and AII. Cholesteryl esters are deposited in tonsils and other lymphoid tissues, and corneal opacities develop. *Lecithin-cholesterol acyl transferase deficiency* presents in the young adult as hemolytic anemia and renal failure. Although the free cholesterol level in plasma is variable, the cholesteryl ester level is very low. Other, even rarer disorders are described in recent reviews.

Diet and Health. Implications for Reducing Chronic Disease Risk. Committee on Diet and Health, Food and Nutrition Board, Commission on Life Sciences, National Research Council. Washington, D.C.. National Academy Press, 1989. *Well-referenced reviews concerning dietary therapy and atherosclerosis.*

LaRosa JC: Lipid disorders. Endocrinol Metab Clin North Am 19:211, Philadelphia, W. B. Saunders Company, 1990. *Twelve short clinical articles about hyperlipidemia and its complications.*

Lipoprotein and lipid metabolism disorders. *In* Scriver CR, Beaudet AL, Sly WS, et al. (eds.): The Metabolic Basis of Inherited Disease. 6th ed. New York, McGraw-Hill, 1989, pp 1129–1302. *Nine detailed, extensive reviews about inborn errors of lipoprotein metabolism.*

National Cholesterol Education Program. Arch Intern Med 148:3, 1988. *Extensive documentation of rationale for the NCEP.*

173 Fabry's Disease (α-Galactosidase A Deficiency)

Robert J. Desnick

DEFINITION. Fabry's disease is an X-linked inborn error of glycosphingolipid metabolism characterized by angiokeratomas (telangiectatic skin lesions), hypohidrosis, corneal and lenticular opacities, acroparesthesias, and vascular disease of the kidney, heart, and brain.

PREVALENCE. The disease has an estimated prevalence of 1 in 40,000 males.

ETIOLOGY AND PATHOGENESIS. Fabry's disease is an X-linked recessive trait that is manifested in affected males. Heterozygous females are usually asymptomatic or exhibit mild disease manifestations.

The disease results from the deficient activity of α-galactosidase A, a lysosomal enzyme encoded by a gene located on the long arm of the X chromosome (Xq21.33–Xq22). The enzymatic defect leads to the systemic accumulation of the neutral glycosphingolipid globotriaosylceramide, particularly in the plasma and lysosomes of vascular endothelial and smooth muscle cells. The progressive vascular glycosphingolipid deposition in affected males results in ischemia and infarction, leading to the major disease manifestations. Affected males who are in blood group B or AB have a more severe disease course, as these blood group substances also accumulate because of the enzyme deficiency. The complementary DNA (cDNA) and genomic sequences encoding α-galactosidase A have been isolated and characterized. Molecular studies have identified a variety of different mutations in the α-galactosidase A gene that are responsible for this lysosomal storage disease; these mutations include amino acid substitutions, gene rearrangements, and messenger RNA (mRNA) splicing defects.

PATHOLOGY. Fabry's disease is characterized by the marked deposition of globotriaosylceramide and related glycosphingolipids with terminal α-galactosyl moieties in the lysosomes of endothelial, perithelial, and smooth muscle cells of blood vessels. These glycosphingolipid deposits are also prominent in epithelial cells of the cornea, in glomeruli and tubules of the kidney, in muscle fibers of the heart, and in ganglion cells of the dorsal roots and autonomic nervous system. The skin lesions are telangiectases. Capillaries, venules, and arterioles show pathologic lipid storage, and there is marked dilatation of the capillaries of the dermal papillae just below the epidermis. The larger lesions are usually located in the upper dermis, where they may produce elevation, flattening, or hypertrophy of the epithelium, with keratosis—hence the term *angiokeratoma*. Ultrastructurally, the glycosphingolipid inclusions in lysosomes have a concentrically arranged lamellar or myelin-like structure.

CLINICAL MANIFESTATIONS. The angiokeratomas usually occur in childhood and may lead to early diagnosis. They increase in size and number with age and range from barely visible to several millimeters in diameter. The lesions are punctate, dark red to blue-black, and flat or slightly raised. They do not blanch with pressure, and the larger ones may show slight hyperkeratosis. Characteristically, the lesions are most dense between the umbilicus and knees, in the " bathing trunk area," but may occur anywhere, including the oral mucosa. The hips, thighs, buttocks, umbilicus, lower abdomen, scrotum, and glans penis are common sites, and there is a tendency toward bilateral symmetry. Variants without skin lesions have been described. Sweating is usually decreased or absent. Corneal opacities and characteristic lenticular lesions, observed on slit-lamp examination, are present in

affected males as well as in about 70 per cent of asymptomatic heterozygotes. Conjunctival and retinal vascular lesions are common and result from the systemic vascular involvement.

Pain is the most debilitating symptom in childhood and adolescence. Fabry's crises, lasting from minutes to several days, consist of agonizing, burning pain in the hands and feet and proximal extremities and are usually associated with exercise, fatigue, and/or fevers. These painful acroparesthesias usually become less frequent in the third and fourth decades of life, although in some men they may become more frequent and severe. Attacks of abdominal or flank pain may simulate appendicitis or renal colic. In addition, many affected men experience chronic acroparesthesias, which may occur daily, often associated with fatigue, exercise, stress, changes in the weather, and/or low-grade fevers.

As the patient's age increases, the major morbid symptoms result from the progressive involvement of the vascular system. Early in the course of the disease, casts, red cells, and lipid inclusions with characteristic birefringent "Maltese crosses" appear in the urinary sediment. Proteinuria, isothenuria, and gradual deterioration of renal function and development of azotemia occur in the second to fourth decades of life. Cardiovascular findings may include hypertension, left ventricular hypertrophy, anginal chest pain, myocardial ischemia or infarction, and congestive heart failure. Mitral insufficiency is the most common valvular lesion. Abnormal electrocardiographic and echocardiographic findings are common. Cerebrovascular manifestations result primarily from multifocal small vessel involvement. Other features may include chronic bronchitis and dyspnea, lymphedema of the legs without hypoproteinemia, episodic diarrhea, osteoporosis, retarded growth, and delayed puberty. Death most often results from uremia or vascular disease of the heart or brain. Prior to hemodialysis or renal transplantation, the mean age of death for affected men was 41 years. Atypical male variants with residual α-galactosidase A activity who are asymptomatic or mildly affected have been described.

DIAGNOSIS AND DIFFERENTIAL DIAGNOSIS. The diagnosis in affected males is most readily made from the history of painful acroparesthesias and hypohidrosis, the presence of characteristic skin lesions, and the observation of the corneal opacities and lenticular lesions. The disorder is often misdiagnosed as rheumatic fever, erythromelalgia, or neurosis. The skin lesions must be differentiated from the benign angiokeratomas of the scrotum in older men (Fordyce's disease) or from angiokeratoma circumscriptum. Angiokeratomas identical to those of Fabry's disease have been reported in fucosidosis, aspartylglycosaminuria, galactosialidosis, α-N-acetylgalactosaminidase deficiency, and sialidosis. The diagnosis is confirmed biochemically by the demonstration of markedly decreased α-galactosidase A activity in plasma, isolated leukocytes, or cultured fibroblasts or lymphoblasts.

Heterozygous females may have corneal opacities, isolated skin lesions, and intermediate activities of α-galactosidase A in plasma or cell sources. Rare female heterozygotes may have manifestations as severe as those in affected males. However, at-risk females in families affected by Fabry's disease who are asymptomatic should be studied by DNA diagnostic techniques, including the analysis of restriction fragment length polymorphisms (RFLP's) in and near the α-galactosidase A gene as well as the direct detection of the specific mutation in each family. Prenatal detection of affected males can be accomplished by the demonstration of deficient α-galactosidase A activity in chorionic villi obtained in the first trimester or in cultured amniocytes obtained by amniocentesis in the second trimester of pregnancy.

TREATMENT. Phenyltoin and carbamazepine have been shown to decrease the frequency and severity of the chronic acroparesthesias and the periodic crises of excruciating pain. Otherwise, treatment of the disease complications is supportive and nonspecific. Renal transplantation and chronic hemodialysis have become life-saving procedures. Replacement therapy using partially purified human enzyme has proved to be biochemically effective in pilot trials; however, sufficient enzyme has not been available to evaluate the clinical effectiveness of long-term replacement therapy. The recent availability of the cDNA encoding human α-galactosidase A should permit the future expression of sufficient quantities of recombinantly produced, active enzyme for further trials of enzyme replacement therapy.

Bernstein HS, Bishop DF, Astrin KH, et al.: Fabry disease: Six gene rearrangements and an exonic point mutation in the α-galactosidase A gene. J Clin Invest 83:1390, 1989. *Description of the first mutations in classic and variant cases.*

Desnick RJ, Bishop DF: Fabry disease: α-Galactosidase deficiency and Schindler disease: α-*N*-acetylgalactosaminidase deficiency. *In* Scriver CR, Beaudet AL, Sly WS, et al. (eds.): The Metabolic Basis of Inherited Disease. 6th ed. New York, McGraw-Hill, 1989. *A definitive chapter describing clinical, pathologic, biochemical, and molecular manifestations of Fabry's disease; more than 400 references.*

Desnick RJ, Dean KJ, Grabowski GA, et al.: Enzyme therapy XII: Enzyme therapy in Fabry disease: Differential *in vivo* plasma clearance and metabolic effectiveness of plasma and splenic α-galactosidase A isozymes. Proc Natl Acad Sci USA 76:5326, 1979. *Demonstration of the biochemical effectiveness and immunologic safety of enzyme replacement therapy.*

Sher NA, Letson RD, Desnick RJ: The ocular manifestations of Fabry's disease. Arch Ophthalmol 97:671, 1979. *A comprehensive and well-illustrated article on the ocular lesions in affected males and carrier females.*

Von Scheidt W, Eng CD, Fitzmaurice TF, et al.: An atypical variant of Fabry's disease confined to the heart. N Engl J Med 324:395, 1991. *A recently recognized mild variant of Fabry's disease with manifestations limited to the heart.*

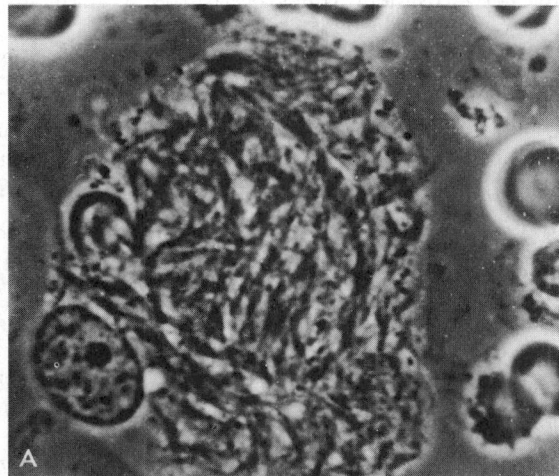
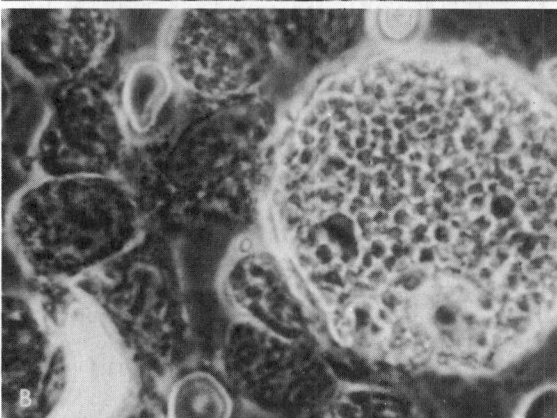

FIGURE 174–1. Appearance of the typical Gaucher cell (*A*) and a foam cell seen in Niemann-Pick disease (*B*). Both are viewed under phase microscopy in unstained smears of aspirated bone marrow. Magnification can be estimated from adjacent red cells.

174 Gaucher Disease

Edwin H. Kolodny

DEFINITION. This relatively common familial disorder results from progressive accumulation of glucocerebroside within phagocytic cells of the monocyte-macrophage system involving principally the liver, spleen, bone marrow, and lymph nodes. Three genetically distinct clinical types have been differentiated: type 1, a chronic nonneuronopathic or "adult" form that may appear at any age and is associated with hypersplenism and bone lesions; type 2, an acute neuronopathic or "infantile" form that presents in infancy with multiple brain stem signs; and type 3, a "juvenile" subacute neuronopathic form that presents in childhood and causes seizures, ataxia, and mental deterioration. The activity of glucocerebrosidase is deficient in all three types, but different mutations are responsible.

PATHOLOGIC PHYSIOLOGY AND PATHOGENESIS. Glucocerebroside contains equimolar amounts of sphingosine, fatty acid, and glucose. Considerable quantities of this compound are generated daily by the turnover of senescent red and white blood cells. In the central nervous system, glucocerebroside is produced in the course of ganglioside metabolism. A deacylated derivative, glucosylsphingosine, also accumulates in Gaucher disease. This highly cytotoxic compound is probably responsible for the nerve cell destruction that occurs in the neuropathic forms of the disease. Both of these glycolipids are degraded by the lysosomal enzyme glucosylceramide-β-D-glucosidase (glucocerebrosidase; E.C. 3.5.1.2.1). Its catalytic efficiency is increased by two low molecular weight, heat-stable proteins, SAP-2 and saposin A, that combine with the enzyme-lipid complex. Both the gene for active glucocerebrosidase and a pseudogene have been mapped to the q21→q31 region of chromosome 1.

Several mutations in the glucocerebrosidase gene have been characterized. The most common of these is a single base change in nucleotide 1226 of the complementary DNA (cDNA) causing an Asn[370] → Ser substitution. This mutation is present in about 70 per cent of Jewish patients and is associated with type 1 disease. Another mutation in nucleotide 1448 of the cDNA produces a Leu[444] → Pro change. This point mutation is found in all three forms of Gaucher disease and may be associated with other mutations in a complex allele resulting from recombination between the active gene and the pseudogene. Patients homoallelic for the nucleotide 1226 mutation have a milder phenotype than do those with a mixed 1226/1448 genotype. Homozygosity for the 1448 mutation results in neurologic forms of Gaucher disease.

A distinctive morphologic feature is the *Gaucher cell*, a large round or polyhedral phagocyte, 20 to 100 μm in diameter, containing one or more small eccentrically placed nuclei and a pale, striated cytoplasm resembling wrinkled tissue paper or crumpled silk (Fig. 174–1A). Under the electron microscope, this fibrillary network consists of numerous dilated saclike structures resembling lysosomes containing tubules; these are similar to the twisted bilayers characteristic of glucocerebroside deposits. The reaction of the Gaucher cell cytoplasm with the periodic acid–Schiff stain is strongly positive. Stains for iron and acid phosphatase are also positive, but the reaction with lipid stains is weak. The bone marrow of patients with chronic myelogenous leukemia often contains cells with a similar appearance; the deposits in these "pseudo-Gaucher" cells are linear rather than twisted.

Glucosylceramide is increased 2- to 3-fold in plasma and more than 200-fold in the spleen and liver. Gaucher cells are present in virtually all organs surrounding small blood vessels and as sheets infiltrating their parenchyma. The spleen may become massively enlarged and develop multiple infarcts and fibrosis. The red pulp of the spleen appears white because of lipid infiltration by Gaucher cells; foci of extramedullary hematopoiesis can occur. In most patients the liver is also enlarged, the Kupffer cells of their sinusoids transformed into Gaucher cells. Fibrosis is present, but there is no proliferation of the bile ducts, and liver failure is rare. Excretion of glucosylceramide into the bile probably prevents more massive accumulation within the liver. In some cases, portal hypertension develops.

Gaucher cells may completely fill the medullary cavity of bone and may cause thinning of the cortex, loss of its normal trabeculation, patchy myelosclerosis, bone infarcts, and osteonecrosis. The metaphyseal plate in the long bones is especially prone to damage. An *Erlenmeyer flask deformity* of the distal femur is an early radiographic sign of bone involvement. With progression of the disease, spontaneous fractures and painful lytic lesions are found. Diffuse pulmonary infiltration can occur, with direct involvement of the alveoli, pleura, and interstitium, resulting in dyspnea and cor pulmonale. Renal involvement with severe proteinuric nephropathy and glomerulonephritis occurs in a few cases.

Central nervous system pathology has been found in all three types. Perivascular collections of Gaucher cells, nerve cell loss, neuronophagia, and infiltration of microglia are the principal changes observed. The most affected areas in type 2 are the deeper layers of the frontal cortex and the nuclei of the basal ganglia, mid-brain, and brain stem. The high concentrations of glucosylsphingosine, a cytotoxic compound, present in the brain, liver, and spleen of type 2 patients probably contribute to the necrosis that occurs in these tissues.

The activity of tartrate-resistant acid phosphatase and angiotensin-converting enzyme and concentrations of several serum proteins, including the immunoglobulins, are increased, especially in type 1 patients. The increased acid phosphatase is the type 5 isozyme and therefore is of osteoclastic origin and indicative of bone involvement. Some older patients develop a monoclonal gammopathy with multiple myeloma. Leukemias and other forms of malignant neoplasms are also more frequent in elderly patients with type 1 disease.

CLINICAL MANIFESTATIONS. Type 1: Chronic Nonneuronopathic Type. This disease is transmitted as an autosomal recessive trait and affects both sexes equally. It has been observed in whites, blacks, and Asians, but more than one half of cases are found in Ashkenazic Jews. As many as 1 in 13 of this population is probably a carrier, so that it is not unusual for the disease to appear in two successive generations of the same family. Clinical symptoms in this so-called adult form may appear at any age, from the first year of life to the ninth decade. One third of all cases are diagnosed in the first decade; the majority of these patients are not of Jewish ancestry. They develop massive enlargement of the spleen and evidence a delay in somatic growth that may severely hamper their intellectual and social development. The condition in another 25 per cent of patients is not diagnosed until after age 30. These patients have a much more benign course. Only rarely do these individuals have serious hematologic or osseous complications.

The most common presenting symptom is excessive fatigue associated with a hypochromic anemia and splenomegaly. Frequently there is a long history of bleeding tendency, such as repeated epistaxis and ecchymoses, but this rarely attracts medical attention unless it is associated with significant hemorrhage, such as splenic rupture, bleeding from esophageal varices, subdural hematoma, or hemopericardium. The first indication in some patients may be the appearance of bone or joint pain or a pathologic fracture. Lytic lesions develop in the shafts of the long bones, vertebrae, ribs, and pelvis. This condition produces osteosclerosis and, in the most virulent cases, osteonecrosis and eventually collapse of bone. In the acute crises affecting bone or joints, there is severe, incapacitating pain, erythema, swelling, tenderness, and occasionally joint effusion. While only 20 per cent of all type 1 patients have significant clinical involvement of bone, more than one half have radiologic evidence of the Erlenmeyer flask deformity, with tapering of the midshaft of the femur and failure of normal trabeculation causing a widening of the distal end.

The clinical course is variable. In response to an acute infection, the size of the spleen may increase dramatically and then regress, but slowly progressive splenomegaly is the usual pattern. Anemia, thrombocytopenia, and leukemia are frequent but rarely cause significant morbidity. Bleeding may occur if the platelet count falls below 50,000 to 70,000 per cubic millimeter; however, the count usually rises again spontaneously within a few weeks. Hepatomegaly with a firm liver edge is common, and in a few severe cases liver failure and portal hypertension occur.

Type 2: Acute Neuronopathic Type. This form of the disease is much rarer than the adult type 1 variety. It is observed in infants of different ethnic groups and does not show any predilection for Jews. The disease usually presents a few months after birth with retroflexion of the head, strabismus, increasing muscular hypertonicity, and marked increase in the size of the liver and spleen. In some cases, developmental milestones are normal until the second or third year. The major central nervous system signs reflect brain stem and cranial nerve involvement. Extreme arching of the neck, retraction of the lips, trismus, laryngeal spasm with a chronic cough and stridor, and spastic rigidity of the extremities are present. Seizures and psychomotor retardation

also occur. Death results from respiratory infection within a few months to 2 years after signs appear.

Type 3: Juvenile Type. This includes a heterogeneous group of patients with signs of the chronic adult type combined with progressive neurologic disease that begins in childhood or adolescence. A subtype of this disease occurs in youngsters from the northern Swedish provinces Norbotten and Vsterbotten. Their growth is retarded, and there are hypersplenism and skeletal changes of the type that occurs in the chronic nonneuropathic form. In addition, they develop oculomotor apraxia, convergent squint, spasticity, clumsiness, seizures, and a decline in mental abilities. In splenectomized patients, white retinal infiltrates may appear, the infiltration of glucosylceramide into the central nervous system is accelerated, and the pace of mental deterioration is faster than in nonsplenectomized patients.

DIAGNOSIS. Gaucher disease should be suspected in any patient with unexplained splenomegaly and a bleeding tendency, bone or joint pains, or pathologic fractures. A radioisotope scan of the liver and spleen reveals the extent of the hepatosplenomegaly and the presence of infarcts. Radionuclide scintigraphy or magnetic resonance imaging (MRI) is useful for locating lytic changes in bone. The bone marrow may demonstrate Gaucher cells. The diagnosis is established by assaying the activity of glucosylceramide-β-D-glucosidase in leukocytes or cultured fibroblasts. The artificial fluorogenic substrate, 4-methylumbelliferyl-β-glucoside, is commonly employed as a substitute for the natural lipid substrate. The degree of enzyme deficiency is similar in all three clinical subtypes of Gaucher disease. Within the same family, expression of the disease may vary considerably, so that enzyme assays should be done on all close relatives of the patient, whether or not they are symptomatic. Heterozygotes have approximately one-half the normal enzyme activity; however, with current methods the range of values overlaps the normal range. Therefore, carrier detection cannot be done with 100 per cent certainty. Prenatal diagnosis is possible using cultured amniotic cells. DNA diagnosis is useful for predicting neurologic involvement in very young patients.

TREATMENT AND PROGNOSIS. Iron therapy may partially correct the anemia, but the persistent use of iron in the presence of adequate iron stores increases the risk of hemochromatosis. Splenectomy is performed for severe and persistent thrombocytopenia or when mechanical factors cause massive swelling, abdominal pain, or gastrointestinal dysfunction. Correction of the thrombocytopenia occurs immediately after the operation, with a less dramatic improvement noted in the anemia. In children, the growth curve usually improves. However, splenectomy may hasten the pace of lipid deposition into the liver and bones, and osteolytic lesions may appear within a few months after the operation. Therefore, the surgeon may elect to leave in place any accessory spleen tissue that is present or to perform a partial splenectomy. Acute lesions in bone and joints are initially treated with immobilization and the prevention of weight bearing. However, as soon as possible, a graduated program of exercises is introduced to maintain joint mobility and prevent further loss of bone. Fractures of the head and neck of the femur are usually treated by prosthetic hip replacement. A few attempts at bone marrow transplantation have been successful, but this procedure is still plagued by a high rate of complications. Enzyme replacement therapy using purified placental enzyme modified by the attachment of mannosyl residues has produced promising results. Weekly infusions of this commercially prepared experimental drug, known as Ceredase, have resulted in a decrease in liver and spleen size and an improvement in hematologic parameters in more than 12 type 1 patients. The prognosis in children with the early onset form of the type 1 disease is poor because of the severe lung, liver, and bone involvement in these cases. In milder cases of later onset, longevity is normal. Children with the infantile neuronopathic form do not survive beyond age 2 to 3 years, whereas those with the juvenile subacute neuronopathic variant may live into their third decade.

Barranger JA, Ginns EI: Glucosylceramide lipidoses: Gaucher disease. In Scriver CR, Beaudet AL, Sly WS, et al. (eds.): The Metabolic Basis of Inherited Disease. 6th ed. New York, McGraw-Hill, 1989. *A comprehensive review of the clinical and metabolic abnormalities in Gaucher disease.*

Eyal N, Wilder S, Horowitz M: Prevalent and rare mutations among Gaucher patients. Gene, in press. *Comprehensive review of mutations and methods for their identification.*

Hobbs JR, Hugh Jones K, Shaw PJ, et al.: Beneficial effect of pre-transplant splenectomy on displacement bone marrow transplantation for Gaucher's syndrome. Lancet 1:1111, 1987. *Result of bone marrow transplantation in six children are discussed.*

Rosenthal DI, Scott JA, Barranger J, et al.: Evaluation of Gaucher disease using magnetic resonance imaging. J Bone Joint Surg 68:802, 1986. *The sensitivity of MRI in detecting bone lesions is documented in this study of 24 patients.*

Rubin M, Yampolski I, Lambrozo R, et al.: Partial splenectomy in Gaucher's disease. J Pediatr Surg 21:125, 1986. *A review of the surgical outcome in 11 children with type 1 Gaucher disease.*

Stowens DW, Teitelbaum SL, Kahn AJ, et al.: Skeletal complications of Gaucher disease. Medicine 64:310, 1985. *Description of bone findings in 327 patients with Gaucher disease.*

175 Niemann-Pick Disease

Edwin H. Kolodny

DEFINITION. The eponym Niemann-Pick disease originally referred to the classic infantile form of lipid storage disease described by Albert Niemann and Ludwig Pick in the first two decades of this century. The lysosomal enzyme sphingomyelinase is absent in this disease; this causes widespread deposition of sphingomyelin, a ceramide phospholipid. Foam cells proliferate within the reticuloendothelial system, and there is nerve cell loss within the central nervous system. This acute neuronopathic form was subsequently designated type A to distinguish it from other variants of sphingomyelin lipidosis that have since been described (Table 175–1).

PATHOLOGY. Foam Cell. The cytoplasm of this large histiocyte contains numerous uniform-sized lipid-staining droplets that create a fine reticulated web resembling a honeycomb or mulberry (see Fig. 174–1B). Under the electron microscope, these cytosomes consist of both concentrically laminated membranous arrays and dense homogeneous bodies.

Sphingomyelin. The ceramide and phosphorylcholine portions of this lipid are linked by a phosphodiester bond that under normal circumstances is cleaved by sphingomyelinase. Sphingomyelin is increased 15- to 45-fold in the liver and spleen of patients with type A Niemann-Pick disease, and about half as much in type B patients. Sphingomyelin storage occurs in the brain of type A but not type B patients. The organs of type C patients exhibit a threefold to sixfold increase in sphingomyelin. In each variety of Niemann-Pick disease, bis (monoacylglycero) phosphate, unesterified cholesterol, glucosylceramide, and other neutral glycolipids also accumulate.

Sphingomyelinase. Patients with type A and type B Niemann-Pick disease are totally deficient in sphingomyelinase, the acid hydrolase that removes the phosphorylcholine moiety from sphingomyelin. Its complementary DNA (cDNA) has been isolated, and studies have been initiated to find the mutations responsible for types A and B Niemann-Pick disease. In type C patients, sphingomyelinase may be normal or partially deficient, but the principal finding is a defect in esterification and efflux of non-lipoprotein cholesterol from the lysosome. A low molecular weight protein, SAP-2, stimulates sphingomyelinase activity by binding to the enzyme, but no cases of Niemann-Pick disease with SAP-2 deficiency have thus far been reported.

CLINICAL MANIFESTATIONS. Type A. Hepatosplenomegaly, diffuse pulmonary infiltration, and developmental delay are noticeable as early as 1 to 2 months of age. Weight gain is poor partly because of vomiting associated with feedings. Lymphadenopathy, opisthotonic posturing, and seizures develop. Eye signs include periorbital puffiness, clouding of the corneas, yellowish discoloration of the lens, and cherry-red maculae. Inter-

mittent jaundice and anemia are present. The affected child becomes emaciated with very thin extremities, a protuberant abdomen, and ascites. Developmental milestones normal for a 1-year-old are never attained, and after the child lingers in a vegetative state for many months, death occurs, usually before the fourth year. Postmortem studies reveal a large yellow liver and atrophic brain with widespread nerve cell loss and gliosis. The cytoplasm of remaining neurons and of the glial cells is ballooned with lipid inclusions. A high percentage of patients with this rare autosomal recessive disorder are of Ashkenazic Jewish ancestry.

Type B. Severe early involvement of the lungs, liver, and spleen also characterizes type B Niemann-Pick disease, but mental development in this variant is normal. The chest radiograph reveals nodular densities throughout the lung fields and thickening of the interlobar fissures. Signs of hypersplenism, such as mild anemia, leukopenia, and thrombocytopenia with easy bruising, often occur. A few patients have been described with a brownish-red spot in the macula, and sea-blue histiocytes are sometimes found in the bone marrow. These cells contain ceroid, which confers on them a bluish cast when stained with Giemsa. Normal longevity is possible but may be limited by chronic pulmonary insufficiency and the mechanical effects of the enlarged spleen and liver on other abdominal organs.

Type C. This diagnosis has been applied to a heterogeneous group of patients with a variable age of onset. In some cases, neonatal jaundice is present during the first 3 months, but this generally subsides despite the progression of the disease. A liver biopsy in these instances may show chronic hepatitis with giant cells. The early-onset group of type C patients develop psychomotor delay during infancy, followed later by a supranuclear gaze palsy, blindness, spasticity, and dementia. The condition of these children deteriorates rapidly over a 2-year period, and they die at age 5 to 6 years. Other type C patients may not develop overt neurologic symptoms until early childhood. These consist of a decline in intellect, progressive impairment of vertical gaze, dysarthria, dysphagia, incoordination, seizures, and involuntary movements. A few have also developed cataplexy. These patients usually survive into adult life. Rarely, there is slower progression with onset in adolescence or adult life.

Type D. This designation is used for cases similar to type C occurring in descendents of an Acadian couple born in Yarmouth, Nova Scotia, in the 1600's.

DIAGNOSIS. Niemann-Pick disease should be suspected whenever vacuolated lymphocytes are present in the peripheral smear and foam cells are present in the bone marrow of a patient with hepatosplenomegaly. The infant of Ashkenazic Jewish heritage who develops slowly would suggest the type A variant. Early jaundice and a subsequent period of normal development might suggest a workup for type C Niemann-Pick disease. The foam cell, a lipid-laden histiocyte, should not be confused with the Gaucher cell, which also contains lipid, but of a different morphologic appearance. Vacuolated leukocytes and foam cells also occur in hypertriglyceridemia and certain other lysosomal storage diseases, such as fucosidosis, mannosidosis, G_{M1} gangliosidosis, Sandhoff disease, Wolman disease, and I-cell disease. In long-standing cases of type B disease, sea-blue histiocytes containing a ceroid-like material are also observed in the bone marrow. The definitive diagnosis of Niemann-Pick disease types A and B is based upon the assay of sphingomyelinase activity. Homogenates of cultured skin fibroblasts or leukocytes from these patients, when incubated with sphingomyelin labeled with ^{14}C in the choline portion of the molecule, have less than 5 per cent of control activity. Intermediate values are obtained for type A and type B heterozygotes. Type C homozygotes may exhibit a partial deficiency, but type C heterozygotes have normal sphingomye-

TABLE 175–1. THE SPHINGOMYELIN LIPIDOSES

Type	Descriptive Name	Racial and/or Geographic Predilection	Affects Brain	Deficiency
A	Acute neuronopathic	Ashkenazic Jewish	Yes	Sphingomyelinase
B	Chronic nonneuronopathic	No	No	Sphingomyelinase
C	Subacute neuronopathic or juvenile dystonic lipidosis	No	Yes	Cholesterol esterification
D	Nova Scotian	Yarmouth County, Nova Scotia	Yes	Unknown

linase activity. The defect in intracellular trafficking and efflux of cholesterol in type C patients and heterozygotes can be demonstrated in fibroblast culture by incubating the cells with low density lipoprotein (LDL) and ^{3}H-labeled oleate and then analyzing their content of unesterified and esterified cholesterol. The ultrastructural examination of skin biopsy specimens from type C patients has demonstrated lysosomes containing loosely arranged, dark, laminated structures within a clear matrix. Prenatal diagnosis of type A and type B Niemann-Pick disease is accomplished by determining the enzyme activity of cultured amniotic fluid cells. Fetuses with type C disease have been identified by studying the intracellular processing of LDL cholesterol in cultured chorionic villus cells.

TREATMENT. No specific treatment is available for any of the sphingomyelin storage diseases. In type B patients, splenectomy may be done to relieve mechanical pressure within the abdomen or to correct a thrombocytopenia with hemorrhagic diathesis. Neither replacement with exogenous enzyme nor organ transplants have been successful, but bone marrow transplanta-

tion has proved beneficial to one 3-year-old type B patient without central nervous system involvement. Type C patients may benefit from attempts to reduce intracellular cholesterol through dietary means and drugs. Animal models of Niemann-Pick disease are available for laboratory trials of these and other potential new therapies.

Fink JK, Filling-Katz MR, Sokol J, et al.: Clinical spectrum of Niemann-Pick disease type C. Neruology 39:1040, 1989. *Analysis of neurologic symptomatology in three phenotypes of Niemann-Pick disease type C.*

Levran O, Desnick RJ, Schuchman EH: Niemann-Pick disease: A frequent missense mutation in the gene encoding acid sphingomyelinase of Ashkenazi Jewish type A and B patients. Proc Natl Acad Sci (USA) 88, in press. *This is the first study to describe a mutation in the sphingomyelinase gene.*

Spence MW, Callahan JW: Sphingomyelin-cholesterol lipidoses: The Niemann-Pick group of diseases. *In* Scriver CR, Beaudet AL, Sly WS, et al. (eds.): The Metabolic Basis of Inherited Disease. 6th ed. New York, McGraw-Hill, 1989. *A comprehensive review of the different clinical forms of sphingomyelin lipidoses. Details of their pathology, metabolic disturbance, and enzymatic aspects are provided, as well as an extensive bibliography.*

Vanier MT, Rousson RM, Mandon G, et al.: Diagnosis of Niemann-Pick disease type C on chorionic villus cells. Lancet 1:1014, 1989. *Techniques for the prenatal diagnosis of Niemann-Pick disease type C are described, and references are provided for the defect in intracellular trafficking of cholesterol in this variant.*

INBORN ERRORS OF AMINO ACID METABOLISM

176 Hyperaminoaciduria (with a Classification of the Inborn and Developmental Errors of Amino Acid Metabolism)

Charles R. Scriver

Study of the appropriate inborn errors has improved our knowledge of amino acid metabolism, as well as the diagnosis and treatment of associated diseases. The inborn errors of renal amino acid transport reveal either a carrier or a metabolic process coupled to the transcellular flux that achieves normal reabsorption.

L-Aminoaciduria, representing less than 2 to 3 per cent of the total urinary nitrogen, is a normal phenomenon. Only 5 per cent

or less of the filtered amino acid load is not reabsorbed by the proximal portion of the renal tubule and is excreted in the urine. Efficiency of renal tubular transport of an amino acid is related to its chemical and steric structure, the amount in the glomerular filtrate, and the sex, age, and physiologic state of the subject. Abnormal aminoaciduria (hyperaminoaciduria) is a result of acquired or hereditary disturbances of cellular metabolism or transport. Table 176–1 shows the known hyperaminoacidurias. (The table includes several disorders of amino acid metabolism that do not show hyperaminoaciduria but affect organic acid and fatty acid derivatives; they can be detected in urine by gas chromatography.)

The hyperaminoacidurias are explained by several mechanisms acting on net reabsorption in the proximal tubule (Fig. 176–1):

1. *Saturation:* The concentration of amino acid in filtrate approaches or exceeds the capacity of the tubular system to reabsorb it (overflow or prerenal aminoaciduria).

2. *Competition:* One amino acid at elevated concentration competes with another sharing the transporter ("combined" aminoaciduria).

Text continued on page 1101

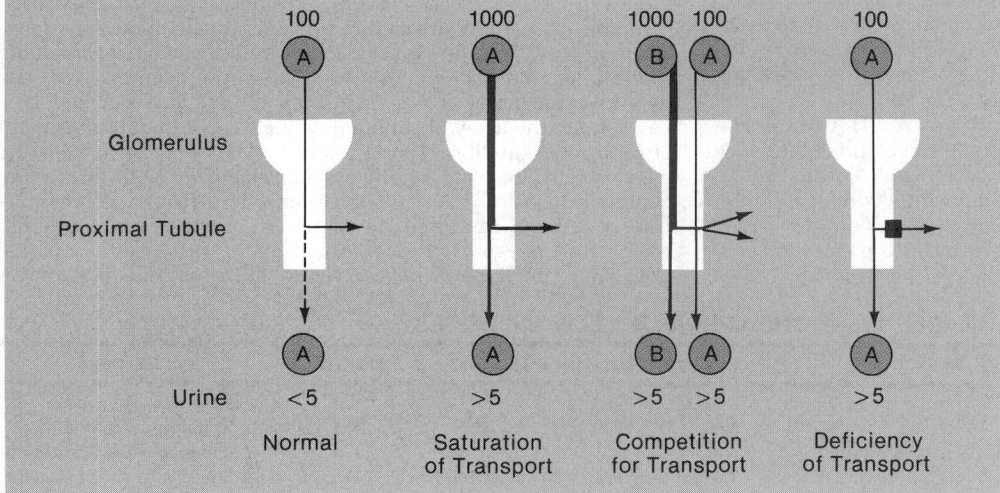

FIGURE 176–1. Mechanism of hyperaminoaciduria. *Panel 1:* Normal reabsorption reclaims more than 95 per cent of filtered amino acid molecules. Hyperaminoaciduria can occur if *(Panel 2)* filtered load increases (10× increase shown) and transport mechanism is saturated or if *(Panel 3)* amino acid (B) (in excess) competes with another (A) on a shared carrier or if *(Panel 4)* carrier is modified or coupling of energy to carrier is impaired.

TABLE 176–1. HEREDITARY AND ACQUIRED AMINOACIDOPATHIES

The aminoacidurias presented in this table are divided into acquired and inherited types. Disturbances related to perinatal adaptive phenomena of multifactorial origin are included. The classification recognizes physiologic factors affecting amino acid distribution between plasma and urine, and whether the disorder primarily affects catabolism or membrane transport of the amino acid(s).

Thus the disorders are grouped according to mechanism and preferred fluid for detection. The data refer to those conditions associated with perturbation of the normal content of ninhydrin-reactive metabolites in plasma or urine; some exceptions have been made to include ninhydrin-negative metabolites.

GROUP IA

The primary defect is in catabolism. There is a low renal clearance of amino acid but a hyperaminoaciduria by saturation of transepithelial transport. Detection in the plasma is preferable unless otherwise indicated, but the use of urine for screening (or diagnosis) is not precluded; assignment to this group implies primarily that diagnosis (or screening) of the condition is feasible by virtue of significant metabolite accumulation in blood (or plasma).

Amino Acid Affected:

↓ = decreased; ↑ = increased. Source of enzyme number is *Enzyme Commission.* IP = apparent inheritance pattern; AR = autosomal recessive; AD = autosomal dominant; (AR) = probably autosomal recessive; XL = X-linked. *Remarks:* CNS = central nervous system; CoA = coenzyme A; CSF = cerebrospinal fluid.

Condition or Disease	Amino Acid Affected	Enzyme Affected (Synonym) In Group A	IP	Remarks
Common Perinatal (Adaptive) Traits*				
Neonatal hyperphenylalani-nemia	Phenylalanine	Phenylalanine 4-mono-oxygenase (phenylalanine-hydroxylating system) [1.14.16.1]	—	Benign; may respond to folic acid; often occurs with tyrosinemia
Neonatal tyrosinemia	Tyrosine	4-Hydroxyphenylpyruvate dioxygenase (p-hydroxyphenyl pyruvic acid hydroxylase) [1.13.11.27]	—	Benign; responds to ascorbic acid and reduced protein intake
Hypermethioninemia	Methionine	? Methionine adenosyltransferase (ATP:L-methionine S-adenosyl-transferase) [2.5.1.6]	—	Benign; usually found with high protein intake
Hyperhistidinemia	Histidine	? L-Histidine ammonia-lyase [4.3.1.3]	—	Benign; related to high protein intake
Inherited Traits				
Hyperphenylalaninemia				
Classic phenylketonuria	Phenylalanine	Phenylalanine 4-mono-oxygenase (L-phenylalanine, tetrahydropteridine:oxygen oxidoreductase [4-hydroxylating]) [1.14.16.1]	AR	Plasma phenylalanine >16 mg/100 ml; causes mental retardation; when untreated, L-phenylalanine tolerance in diet is 250–500 mg/day
Atypical phenylketonuria	Phenylalanine	Same	(AR)	Plasma phenylalanine >16 mg/100 ml; similar to entry above, but dietary tolerance for L-phenylalanine is > 500 mg/day
Transient phenylketonuria	Phenylalanine	Same	(AR)	Plasma phenylalanine >16 mg/100 ml; change in status to that of next entry or normal, several months or years after birth
Benign hyperphenylalaninemia	Phenylalanine	Same	AR	Plasma phenylalanine <16 mg/100 ml on normal diet; benign trait
Dihydropteridine reductase deficiency	Phenylalanine	Dihydropteridine reductase [1.6.99.7]	AR	Deficient tetrahydrobiopterin cofactor also impairs biosynthesis of L-dopa and 5-hydroxytryptamine (5-HT) in CNS; low-phenylalanine diet does not correct this
Biopterin synthesis defects	Phenylalanine	Various enzymes in synthesis pathway	AR	See preceding entry
Hypertyrosinemias				
Tyrosinosis (Medes)	Tyrosine	Tyrosine aminotransferase (L-tyrosine:α-ketoglutarate aminotransferase) [2.6.1.5]	(AR)	One case known; myasthenia gravis probably incidental finding
Hypertyrosinemia I	Tyrosine (and methionine in acute stage)	Fumarylacetoacetate hydrolase [3.7.1.2]	AR	Hepatic cirrhosis and renal tubular failure; usually fatal in absence of tyrosine restriction
Hypertyrosinemia II	Tyrosine	Soluble (cytosol) tyrosine aminotransferase [2.6.15]	AR	Associated with developmental retardation; Richner-Hanhart syndrome in some patients
Hawkinsinuria	Tyrosine	4-Hydroxyphenyl pyruvate dioxygenase [1.13.11.27]	AD	Disease signs are variable and include failure to thrive; reflect formation of epoxides and adducts of glutathione

Table continued on following page

TABLE 176–1. HEREDITARY AND ACQUIRED AMINOACIDOPATHIES *Continued*

Condition or Disease	Amino Acid Affected	Enzyme Affected (Synonym) *In Group A*	IP	Remarks
Inherited Traits (Continued)				
Hyperhistidinemia†				
Classic form	Histidine (alanine in some cases)	L-Histidine ammonia-lyase [4.3.1.3]; liver, epidermis	AR	Harmless condition in majority
Branched-chain hyperaminoacidemia‡				
Classic maple syrup urine disease	Leucine, isoleucine, valine, al-loisoleucine	Branched-chain α-keto acid lipoate oxidoreductase (probably decarboxylase component) [1.2.4.3(4)]	AR	Postnatal collapse; mental retardation in survivors; diet therapy can be effective
Intermittent form	Leucine, isoleucine, valine, al-loisoleucine	Branched-chain α-keto acid oxidase(s)§ [1.2.4.3(4)]	(AR)	Intermittent symptoms; development may be otherwise normal
Mild form	Same	Same	(AR)	Unremitting; milder than classic form
Thiamine-responsive form	Same	Same	(AR)	Mild form; responsive to thiamine (vitamin B₁)
Multiple dehydrogenase form	Same (plus pyruvate and α-ketoglutarate)	Dihydrolipoamide dehydrogenase [1.8.1.4]	(AR)	Congenital lactic acidosis plus branched-chain amino-keto acid disorder
Hypervalinemia	Valine	Branched-chain amino-acid aminotransferase (valine aminotransferase) [2.6.1.66]	AR	Retarded development and vomiting; responds to diet
Type I hyperlysinemia	Lysine	Deficient "aminoadipic semialdehyde synthase" (bifunctional enzyme with lysine-ketoglutarate reductase [1.5.1.8] + saccharopine reductase [1.5.1.9] activities)	AR	Associated with mental retardation, hypotonia
Type 2 hyperlysinemia	Lysine, methionine and homocyst(e)ine	Only saccharopine reductase activity of bifunctional enzyme is deficient	AR	Same as above
Homocyst(e)inuria (methylene tetrahydrofolate [THF] reductase deficiency)	Methionine (low) and homocyst(e)ine (high)	5,10-Methylenetetrahydrofolate reductase [1.7.99.5]	AR	Defective remethylation of homocysteine to methionine; neurologic and behavioral symptoms associated
Homocyst(e)inuria (with methylmalonic aciduria)	Homocyst(e)ine (high), methionine (low): plus methylmalonate	Defective cobalamin coenzyme biosynthesis	AR	Defective remethylation of homocysteine and impaired methylmalonyl-CoA mutase (MMA mutase) activity; developmental delay
		Defective cobalamin transport (lysosomal)	(AR)	
Cystathioninuria†	Cystathionine	Cystathionine γ-lyase [4.4.1.1]	AR	Probably benign trait; vitamin B₆ corrects biochemical trait in most patients
Hyperglycinemias				
Ketotic form	Glycine and other glucogenic amino acids	Propionyl-CoA carboxylase (adenosine triphosphate [ATP]–hydrolyzing) propanoyl-CoA:carbon dioxide ligase (adenosine diphosphate [ADP]–forming) [6.4.1.3]	AR	Ketosis, neutropenia, mental retardation; often fatal; detectable in skin fibroblasts
Ibid.	Ibid.	Methylmalonyl-CoA mutase [5.4.99.2]	AR	Symptoms are those of methylmalonic aciduria with acidosis (some mutase-affected patients are responsive to vitamin B₁₂)
Ibid.	Ibid.	Acetyl-CoA acyltransferase (β-ketothiolase) [2.3.1.16] deficiency¶	AR	Signs are those of α-methyl-β-hydroxybutyric aciduria (with or without tiglic aciduria) and acidosis
Nonketotic form	Glycine	Glycine cleavage reaction (CO₂, NH₃, and hydroxymethyltetrahydrofolate formed) [1.4.4.2, 2.1.2.10]	AR	Severe CNS depression soon after birth; high CSF: plasma glycine ratio; benzoate decreases plasma glycine; no effect on CNS prognosis; strychnine improves seizures
Sarcosinemia†	Sarcosine	Sarcosine oxidase (sarcosine:oxygen oxidoreductase [demethylating]) [1.5.3.1]	AR	Benign trait
"Sarcosinemia" (glutaric aciduria, type II)	Sarcosine (glutaric acid and multiple fatty acids)	? Electron transfer flavoprotein (affecting multiple aryl-CoA dehydrogenases) [1.3.99.2–3]	AR	Postnatal lethargy, vomiting, coma, and acidosis; odor; multiple abnormalities of fatty acid oxidation

TABLE 176–1. HEREDITARY AND ACQUIRED AMINOACIDOPATHIES *Continued*

Condition or Disease	Amino Acid Affected	Enzyme Affected (Synonym) *In Group A*	IP	Remarks
Inherited Traits (Continued)				
Hyperprolinemias				
Type I	Proline	L-Proline dehydrogenase (oxidase) [1.5.99.8]	AR	Benign trait
Type II	Proline	1-Pyrroline dehydrogenase (△¹-pyrroline-5-nicotinamide carboxylate: adenine dinucleotide [NAD⁺] oxidoreductase) [1.5.1.12]	AR	△¹-Pyrroline-5-carboxylate and 3-hydroxy-1-pyrroline-5-carboxylate excreted in urine; associated convulsions?
Hyperhydroxyprolinemia	Hydroxyproline	4-Hydroxy-L-proline dehydrogenase (oxidase) [1.1.1.104]	AR	Benign trait
Hyperlysinemias, hypertryptophanemias, and related diseases				
Type I	Lysine (and glutamine)	Saccharopine dehydrogenase (nicotinamide-adenine dinucleotide phosphate [NADP⁺], lysine-forming) [1.5.1.8]	AR	Associated with mental retardation and hypotonia
Saccharopinuria†	Lysine, saccharopine, citrulline	? Saccharopine dehydrogenase (NADP⁺, L-glutamate–forming) (saccharopine dehydrogenase) [1.5.1.10]	AR	Associated with mental retardation
Pipecolic acidemia†	Pipecolic acid	L-Pipecolate dehydrogenase (pipecolate oxidase) [1.5.99.3]	AR	Hepatomegaly and mental retardation (peroxisomal disease)
α-Aminoadipic aciduria	α-Aminoadipic acid	?Mitochondrial α-aminoadipate amino transferase [2.6.1.39]	(AR)	Variable clinical features
α-Ketoadipic aciduria	α-Aminoadipic and α-ketoadipic acids	? α-Ketoadipic decarboxylase	(AR)	Mental retardation
Glutaric aciduria type I	Glutaric acid	? Glutaryl-CoA dehydrogenase [1.3.99.7]	(AR)	Mental retardation
Glutaric aciduria type II (multiple acyl-CoA dehydrogenase deficiency)	Glutaric acid, complex organic aciduria, sarcosine	Electron transport flavoprotein [1.3.99.2–3]	AR	Severe form, neonatal metabolic disease; adult form, recurrent hypoglycemia
Hydroxylysinemia	Free hydroxylsine	? Hydroxylysine kinase [2.7.1.81]	(AR)	Mental retardation
Tryptophanemia	Tryptophan (with indoleketonuria)	? Formamidase [3.5.1.9]	(AR)	Variable, probably benign
Hyperammonemias				
Carbamyl phosphate synthetase (CPS) deficiency	Glycine, glutamine	Carbamate kinase (ATP carbamate phosphotransferase) [2.7.2.2]	AR	Group of diseases with ammonia intoxication, protein intolerance, hepatomegaly, vomiting, and so on; argininosuccinicaciduria also has trichorrhexis nodosa
Ornithine transcarbamylase (OTC) deficiency	Glutamine	Ornithine carbamoyltransferase (carbamoylphosphate:L-ornithine carbamoyltransferase) [2.1.3.3]	XL	Same as above
Citrullinemia	Citrulline	Argininosuccinate synthetase (L-citrulline:L-aspartate ligase adenosine monophosphate [AMP]–forming) [6.3.4.5]	AR	Same as above
Argininosuccinicaciduria†	Argininosuccinic acid	Argininosuccinate lyase (L-argininosuccinate arginine-lyase) [4.3.2.1]	AR	Same as above
Hyperargininemia	Arginine	Arginase (L-arginine amidinohydrolase) [3.5.3.1]	AR	Deterioration of CNS function and IQ in childhood; hyperammonemia (inconstant) aggravated by protein
Hyperornithinemia	Ornithine	Unknown (mitochondrial ornithine transport system?)	AR	Associated with hyperammonemia and homocitrullinemia (HHH syndrome)
Hyperornithinemia (without hyperammonemia)	Ornithine	L-Ornithine; 2-oxoacid aminotransferase [2.6.1.13]	AR	Associated with gyrate atrophy of choroid and retina but no hyperammonemia
Hyperalaninemia	Alanine	Pyruvate dehydrogenase (lipoate) (pyruvate dehydrogenase) [1.2.4.1] deficiency	AR	Lactic acidosis
		Pyruvate carboxylase [6.4.1.1] deficiency, and other defects	AR	Intermittent lactic acidosis, intermittent hypoglycemia

Table continued on following page

TABLE 176–1. HEREDITARY AND ACQUIRED AMINOACIDOPATHIES *Continued*

Condition or Disease	Amino Acid Affected	Enzyme Affected (Synonym) In Group A	IP	Remarks
Inherited Traits (Continued)				
Aspartylglucosaminuria	Glycoasparagines	Aspartylglucosylaminase (2-acetamido-1[β¹-L-aspartamidol]-1,2-dideoxyglucose amidohydrolase) [3.5.1.26]	AR	Lysosomal disease; mental retardation
Glutathionemia†	Glutathione or related peptides	γ-Glutamyltransferase (γ-glutamyltranspeptidase) [2.3.2.2]	AR	Mental retardation associated with finding
Hyperthreoninemia	Threonine	Unknown	(AR)	Seizures
Other Conditions That May Affect Amino Acids in Plasma				
Protein-calorie malnutrition	Tryptophan/leucine/isoleucine/valine ↓; tyrosine/glycine/proline ↑	—	—	Severity of change related to severity of malnutrition
Prolonged fasting	Alanine ↓; threonine, glycine ↑	—	—	Early fasting does not show same pattern
Obesity	Leucine/isoleucine/valine/phenylalanine/tyrosine ↑; glycine ↓	—	—	Reflects insulin insensitivity
Hepatitis	Methionine/tyrosine ↑	—	—	Reflects severity of liver disease

*These conditions have been detected by screening methods applied in the newborn period of life. They should not be misdiagnosed as permanent disorders of amino acid metabolism also identifiable by screening.

†Urine screening is as efficient as, or even more reliable than, blood screening in these conditions.

‡A number of disorders of branched-chain amino acid catabolism cause accumulation of substances that are Ninhydrin negative. These compounds can usually be detected by gas-liquid chromatographic methods (see Goodman SI: Am J Hum Genet 32:781, 1980).

§Partial activity; more than 2 per cent of normal.

¶Hyperglycemia observed only in some patients with this enzyme deficiency.

GROUP IB

The primary defect is in catabolism. There is a high renal clearance of amino acid and a hyperaminoaciduria by saturation of transeptithelial transport. Detection in the urine is preferable.

Source of enzyme number is *Enzyme Commission*. IP = apparent inheritance pattern; AR = autosomal recessive; (AR) = probably autosomal recessive; AD = autosomal dominant.

Condition or Disease	Substance Affected (Synonym)	Enzyme Affected (Synonym) [Enzyme Commission No.]	IP	Remarks
Hypophosphatasia	Phosphoethanolamine	?Deficiency of ethanolaminephosphate phospho-lyase (O-phosphorylethanolamine phospho-lyase) [4.2.99.7]	AR	"Rickets" unresponsive to vitamin D; craniosynostosis; hypercalcemia; pyridoxal phosphate accumulation
Pseudohypophosphatasia	Phosphoethanolamine	? Same as above; activity present but altered	(AR)	Same as above
β-Aminoisobutyricaciduria	β-Aminoisobutyric acid	?	AD/AR	Benign polymorphic trait
4-Hydroxybutyricaciduria (γ-amino butyrate pathway)	γ-OH butyrate	Succinic semialdehyde dehydrogenase [1.2.1.24]	AR	Mental retardation, hypotonia; detectable by gas chromatographic analysis of urine, plasma, CSF
Hyper-β-alaninemia	β-Alanine	? β-Alanine-pyruvate aminotransferase (β-alanine transaminase) [2.6.1.18]		Seizures; somnolence; mental retardation
Carnosinemia	Carnosine	Aminoacyl-histidine dipeptidase (carnosinase) [3.4.13.3]	AR	Seizure and mental retardation; or benign possibly
Pyroglutamic aciduria*	L-Pyroglutamic acid (5-oxo-L-proline; pyrrolidone-2-carboxylic acid)	Glutathione synthetase [6.3.2.3]	AR	L-Pyroglutamic acid (5-oxo-L-proline) results from overproduction via modified γ-glutamyl cycle

*Urine screening is as efficient as, or even more reliable than, blood screening in these conditions.

TABLE 176–1. HEREDITARY AND ACQUIRED AMINOACIDOPATHIES *Continued*

GROUP II

There is a primary defect in catabolism and a secondary defect in transport. Hyperaminoaciduria is of combined origin—saturation and competition. Detection is possible in both plasma and urine.

| Disease | Amino Acids | | Remarks |
	Affected in Plasma	Present in Urine	
Hyperprolinemia, types I and II	Proline	Proline, + hydroxyproline and glycine	See entries in group 1A; competition occurs on iminoglycine transport system (see group III)
Hyper-β-alaninemia	β-Alanine	β-Alanine, + β-aminoisobutyric acid and taurine	See Hyper-β-alaninemia in group IB; competition occurs on β-amino transport system
Hyperlysinemia	Lysine	Lysine, + ornithine and arginine	See entries in group IA; competition occurs on "dibasic" transport system (see group III)
Hyperargininemia	Arginine	Ornithine and lysine and sometimes generalized hyperaminoaciduria	See Hyperargininemia in group IA; competition occurs on "diabasic" transport system (see group III); pathogenesis of generalized aminoaciduria unknown

GROUP III

The primary defect is in the renal membrane transport site. There is a high renal clearance of amino acid, and detection is possible only in the urine.

Activity Affected: Presumed gene product activity affected by mutant gene. IP = apparent inheritance pattern; AD = autosomal dominant; (AD) = probably autosomal dominant; AR = autosomal recessive; (AR) = probably autosomal recessive; XL = X-linked. *Remarks:* PTH = parathyroid hormone.

Trait	Substance Affected	Activity Affected	Other Tissues Affected	IP	Remarks
Common Perinatal (Adaptive) Traits					
Neonatal iminoglycinuria	Proline, hydroxyproline, glycine	Specific proline and specific glycine transport (probably)	—	—	Benign adaptive trait; prolinuria subsides at ~ 100 days, glycinuria at ~ 200 days after full-term birth
Neonatal cystine-lysinuria	Cystine and dibasic amino acids (lysine, ornithine, and arginine)	Specific dibasic transport system	—	—	Transient; evident in newborn period in some but not all infants
Inherited Hyperaminoacidurias					
Selective					
Hyperdibasic aminoaciduria type 2 (Lysinuric-protein intolerance)	Lysine, ornithine, arginine ("dibasic" group)	Shared "dibasic" amino acid transport system in basolateral membrane	Intestine (basolateral membrane, efflux defect); fibroblasts (plasma membrane; efflux defect on y+ system)	AR	Associated with protein intolerance, failure to thrive, hyperammonemia basolateral membrane defect; silent carrier
Hyperdibasic aminoaciduria type I	Lysine, ornithine, arginine	Shared "dibasic" amino acid transport system (brush-border membrane)	Intestine	AR/AD	Associated with mental retardation in one reported patient; carriers have hyperdibasic aminoaciduria
Isolated hyperlysinuria	Lysine	Lysine-specific system (brush border)	Intestine	AR	One proband reported
Classic cystinuria	Lysine, ornithine, arginine, and cystine	Shared system in brush-border membrane	Intestine	AR	"Negative" reabsorption of affected amino acid can occur; three alleles (? same locus), each causing different phenotypes: in type I carrier (vs. types II and III) no excess of amino acids in urine ("silent"); in type III patient, intestinal transport intact (or partial defect)
Hypercystinuria	Cyst(e)ine	Specific system for cyst(e)ine	?	(AR)	One pedigree only
Iminoglycinuria	Proline; hydroxyproline; glycine	Shared system for imino acids, glycine (and sarcosine)	Intestine	AR	Four alleles (? same locus); I and II are silent carriers; III and IV are hyperglycinuric carriers; I associated with intestinal defect; IV with K_m mutant
Hartnup disorder	Neutral amino acids (excluding imino acids, glycine, cyst(e)ine, and β-amino acids)	Shared system for large neutral amino acid group (luminal membrane)	Intestine	AR	Three alleles (? same locus); I, intestine affected; II, intestine normal; III, kidney normal; carrier "silent" in all

Table continued on following page

TABLE 176–1. HEREDITARY AND ACQUIRED AMINOACIDOPATHIES *Continued*

Trait	Substance Affected	Activity Affected	Other Tissues Affected	IP	Remarks
Inherited Hyperaminoacidurias (Continued)					
Hyperhistidinuria	Histidine	Specific sytem for histidine	Intestine	AR	Associated with mental retardation in siblings
Hyperdicarboxylic aminoaciduria (glutamate-aspartate transport defect)	Glutamic acid, aspartic acid	Shared dicarboxylic acid transport system (brush-border membrane)	Intestine ±	R	Benign
Idiopathic (primary genetic) Fanconi's syndrome	Generalized effect on all solutes and water	? Coupling of energy; ? tight junction integrity	Secondary to renal phenotype	AR (and AD)	Adult-onset and infantile-childhood forms are differentiated; basic defect unknown; probably several alleles
Secondary genetic forms of Fanconi's syndrome					
Cystinosis; type I, type II	Same as above (secondary response)	Cystine storage (lysosomal defect), with secondary damage to tubule and glomerulus (later)	Organ damage from cystine storage (thyroid, retina; CNS, and so on)	AR*	Several alleles; infantile (type I) and adolescent (type II) forms have differing rates for onset of nephropathy; "adult" form (type III) has no nephropathy
Hereditary fructose intolerance	Same as above, + fructose	Fructose-1-phosphate aldolase (fructose bisphosphate aldolase) (with secondary effects on cellular ATP)	Secondary to renal phenotype (hepatic cirrhosis)	AR	Nephropathy dependent on intact PTH-cAMP axis in kidney; responds to fructose withdrawal
Galactosemia	Same as above, + galactose	Galactose-1-phosphate uridyltransferase (with secondary effects on cellular ATP)	Secondary to renal phenotype (cataracts, CNS effects)	AR	Fanconi's syndrome responds to galactose withdrawal; "galactosemia" due to galactokinase deficiency does *not* include Fanconi's syndrome
Hereditary tyrosinemia	Same as above, + tyrosine metabolites	Unknown (with secondary effects on cellular ATP)	Secondary to renal phenotype (hepatic cirrhosis)	AR	Fanconi's syndrome responds to tyrosine restriction
Wilson's disease	Same as above, with proximal and distal renal tubular acidosis	Unknown (? secondary effects on cytochrome oxidase system)	Hepatolenticular degeneration	AR	Fanconi's syndrome responds to depletion of copper storage
Lowe's oculocerebrorenal syndrome	Generalized dysfunction with defective urinary NH_3 production	Unknown	An oculocerebro-intestinal-renal syndrome (? involving tissues with high γ-glutamyl cycle activity)	XL†	Basic defect still unknown: treatment for tubular reclamation defects does not improve mental retardation or the cataracts and hydrophthalmia
Vitamin D dependency (pseudodeficiency rickets)	Generalized defect (secondary response)	Type I: 25-Hydroxyvitamin D-1-α-hydroxylase Type II: defective binding of hormone	Deficiency of synthesis or AR binding affects intestinal absorption of calcium and initiates PTH response	AR	Nephropathy dependent on PTH excess and hypocalcemia (phenocopy occurs in vitamin D deficiency)
Miscellaneous					
Glycoglycinuria	Glucose and glycine	Unknown (the two solutes do *not* share a common carrier)	—	AD	Asymptomatic; normal T_m (maximal tubular reabsorptive capacity of kidneys) (type B) glucosuria; possibility that there is a heterozygous manifestation of a Fanconi-like tubulopathy merits consideration
Luder-Sheldon syndrome	Generalized amino acids, glucose, and phosphate	Unknown	—	AD	Symptoms of Fanconi's syndrome have occurred in probands
Rowley-Rosenberg syndrome	Generalized aminoaciduria	Unknown	—	AR	Associated components of syndrome; growth retardation, muscular hypoplasia, pulmonary involvement, and right ventricular hypertrophy

*For each type.
†Recessive.

Benson PF, Fensom AH: Genetic Biochemical Disorders. Oxford Monographs on the Medical Genetics No. 12. Oxford, Oxford Univesity Press, 1985. A "handbook," leaner than The Metabolic Basis of Inherited Disease (*the standard "encyclopedia"*), *that covers, in short essays, nearly all entries in Table 176–1.*

Scriver CT, Tenenhouse HS: Mendelian phenotypes as "probes" of renal transport systems for amino acids and phosphate. Handbook of Physiology (Renal Section), in press. *A review of the amino acid transport systems (in kidney and other tissues) delineated by mutations in humans and of their relative importance in metabolic homeostasis.*

Wellner D, Meister A: A survey of inborn errors of amino acid metabolism and transport in man. Annu Rev Biochem 50:911, 1981. *A crisp review of events in a field that now moves more slowly than it once did.*

3. Modification of transporter: The amino acid is not transported efficiently because its carrier is altered (renal aminoaciduria).

4. *Inhibition of substrate transfer:* The coupling of energy to the transporter is altered, and flux is impaired (renal aminoaciduria).

Renal transporters show preferences for either single free amino acids or specific groups of them. The transport systems identified in Table 176–1 (group III) were revealed through loss of function in the variant (mutant or developmental) state. Oligopeptides are transported on carriers different from those used by free amino acids.

Scriver CR, Beaudet A, Sly W, Valle D (eds.): The Metabolic Basis of Inherited Disease. 6th ed. New York, McGraw-Hill, 1989. *The Mendelian disorders of amino acid metabolism (catabolism or transport) are described, chapter by chapter, in detail.*

Scriver CR, Tenenhouse HS: Mendelian phenotypes as probes of renal transport systems for amino acids and phosphate. *In* Windhager E (ed.): Handbook of Physiology: Renal Physiology. 2nd ed. New York, Oxford University Press, in press. *An up-to-date review of the inborn errors of renal amino acid transport and associated transport systems.*

177 The Hyperphenylalaninemias

Charles R. Scriver

A widely accepted medical model of disease attributes manifestations (signs and symptoms) to a deviant underlying process (pathogenesis) that has its origins in both proximate and ultimate causes. According to this model, phenylketonuria, the best known form of hyperphenylalaninemia, is no longer a disease, although it continues to be a risk factor, because its principal manifestations (mental retardation, pigment dilution, mousy odor, neurotransmitter deficiency) occur only in rare cases escaping early diagnosis. This satisfactory turn of events came about because the pathogenesis of hyperphenylalaninemia (the risk factor) is offset by treatment. Genetic forms of hyperphenylalaninemia are described here; they are all autosomal recessive disorders. About 0.01 per cent of live births are affected.

PHENYLALANINE METABOLISM. Phenylalanine is an essential amino acid. The normal concentration in plasma is less than 0.1 mmole per liter (0.1 mM, 1.6 mg per deciliter). The balance between intake and utilization is largely controlled by a hydroxylation reaction (Fig. 177–1A). Impaired hydroxylation is the chief explanation for hyperphenylalaninemia. The reaction requires the apoenzyme *phenylalanine hydroxylase,* molecular oxygen, and *tetrahydrobiopterin* cofactor; the last-named is consumed in stoichiometric amounts to form tyrosine, the reaction product. The catalytic property of phenylalanine hydroxylase requires both moment to moment regeneration of tetrahydrobiopterin from dihydrobiopterin, a by-product of the hydroxylating reaction, and long-term renewal of the tetrahydrobiopterin pool by synthesis from precursors. The former is achieved by the enzyme *dihydropteridine reductase,* the latter by a *synthesis pathway* in which several enzymes act in sequence (Fig. 177–1B). Accordingly, there are several ways to impair phenylalanine hydroxylation. Failure to recognize the biologic heterogeneity of hyperphenylalaninemia may lead to erroneous counseling and ineffective (or unnecessary) treatment; all of its forms require special management of women during the reproductive period of life.

DISORDERS OF PHENYLALANINE HYDROXYLASE INTEGRITY. The phenylalanine hydroxylase enzyme is multimeric and homopolymeric. The polypeptide is encoded by a gene on chromosome 12, region q24.1, which is expressed only in liver in humans. Mutations at this locus cause either phenylketonuria (with plasma phenylalanine values above 1 mM on a normal diet) or nonphenylketonuric hyperphenylalaninemia (values below 1 mM, but greater than 0.125 mM). Phenylketonuria is typically associated with mental retardation in the untreated patient; the other form is not. The incidence of the phenylketonuric form varies by population (lower than 1 in 10,000 births in Ashkenazi Jews, Finns, and Blacks; higher in Scots, Irish, and Yemenite Jews).

The hydroxylation reaction accounts for about three quarters of the moment by moment outflow of phenylalanine; incorporation into protein is the other important route (Fig. 177–1A). If there is deficient hydroxylating activity, and dietary intake is not curtailed, phenylalanine accumulates in body fluids. Overflow into the alternative pathways generates excessive amounts of metabolites derived from phenylalanine, such as the pyruvic (causing phenylketonuria), lactic, and acetic acid derivatives (Fig. 177–1A). Overburden of phenylalanine and its by-products impairs brain development in ways still not fully understood.

Phenylketonuria was first described as a clinical entity in 1934 by Asjborn Fölling, who surmised that the disorder was autosomal recessive and an inborn error of metabolism. In the following three decades, phenylketonuria was seen as a paradigm for the biochemical basis of mental disease, of disease that could be prevented by deliberate restoration of normal metabolism, and of chemical individuality that could be used as the basis for a screening test and early diagnosis. Newborn screening for hyperphenylalaninemia is now one of the most widely applied "genetic" tests. The incidence of the risk factor has not changed, but the frequency of the associated disease is now trivial in screened populations. The practical issues for physicians are interpretation of a positive screening test result, accuracy of the test, and maternal hyperphenylalaninemia (all discussed below).

TETRAHYDROBIOPTERIN-DEFICIENT FORMS OF HYPERPHENYLALANINEMIA. Not every case of persistent hyperphenylalaninemia is explained by a primary hydroxylase deficiency. Tetrahydrobiopterin insufficiency impairs function of three hydroxylases (for phenylalanine, tryptophan and tyrosine) and synthesis of their products, notably 5-hydroxytryptophan (the precursor of serotinin) and L-dopa (the precursor of catecholamines) (Fig. 177–1B). The products function as neurotransmitters in brain, and deficiency of them gives rise to central nervous system disease (including retarded psychomotor development, basal ganglion dysfunction, and instability of body temperature). Regeneration of tetrahydrobiopterin is necessary to maintain catalytic function of the three hydroxylases. *Deficient activity of quininoid dihydropteridine reductase* (encoded by a gene on chromosome 4, region p15.3) blocks the cycle maintaining catalytic amounts of tetrahydrobiopterin. *Deficient activity of guanosine triphosphate, cyclohydrolase I, or 6-pyruvoyl tetrahydropterin synthase and "primapterinuria"* (due to an enzyme deficiency as yet uncharacterized) impair synthesis of tetrahydrobiopterin. The relevant genes have not yet been mapped or cloned in humans.

SCREENING AND DIAGNOSIS. Screening of newborn infants for hyperphenylalaninemia is normal practice. Capillary blood collected on filter paper from heel puncture is analyzed by the bacterial inhibition (Guthrie) assay, fluorimetric analysis, or other quantitative methods. Blood phenylalanine values above 2 mg per deciliter (0.125 mM) on the first day of life or thereafter are considered abnormal and require further investigation. The screening test is not infallible, and false-negative results do occur, some for biologic reasons. Urine screening for "phenylketones" is not reliable.

Every infant with persistent hyperphenylalaninemia is investigated to rule out disorders of tetrahydrobiopterin homeostasis. Urine pterin metabolites or blood cofactor levels are measured under special conditions; there are distinctive urine profiles as well as low blood levels in the disorders of tetrahydrobiopterin synthesis. The tests are done at established centers and require experienced interpretation. Measures of phenylalanine hydroxylase require liver biopsy and are seldom done. Dihydropteridine reductase can be measured in blood spots, fibroblasts, and amniocytes; the cyclohydrolase in phytohemagglutinin-stimulated leukocytes but not in fibroblasts; and the synthase in erythrocytes.

After exclusion of disorders of tetrahydropterin metabolism, hyperphenylalaninemia is classified as follows. About one half of cases with primary phenylalanine hydroxylase deficiency have "phenylketonuria," a generic term for severe hyperphenylalaninemia (>1 mM), low phenylalanine tolerance (<500 mg per day), and high risk of mental retardation in the absence of treatment. The remainder have nonphenylketonuric hyperphenylalaninemia

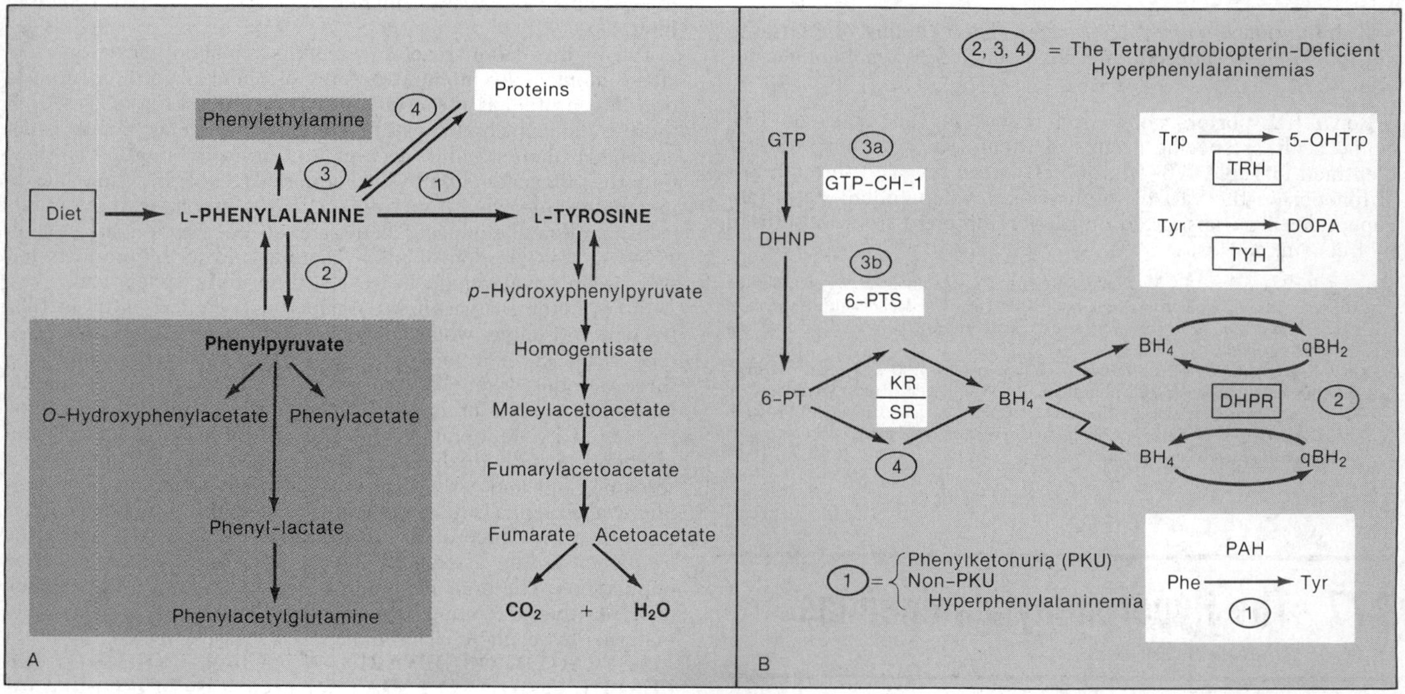

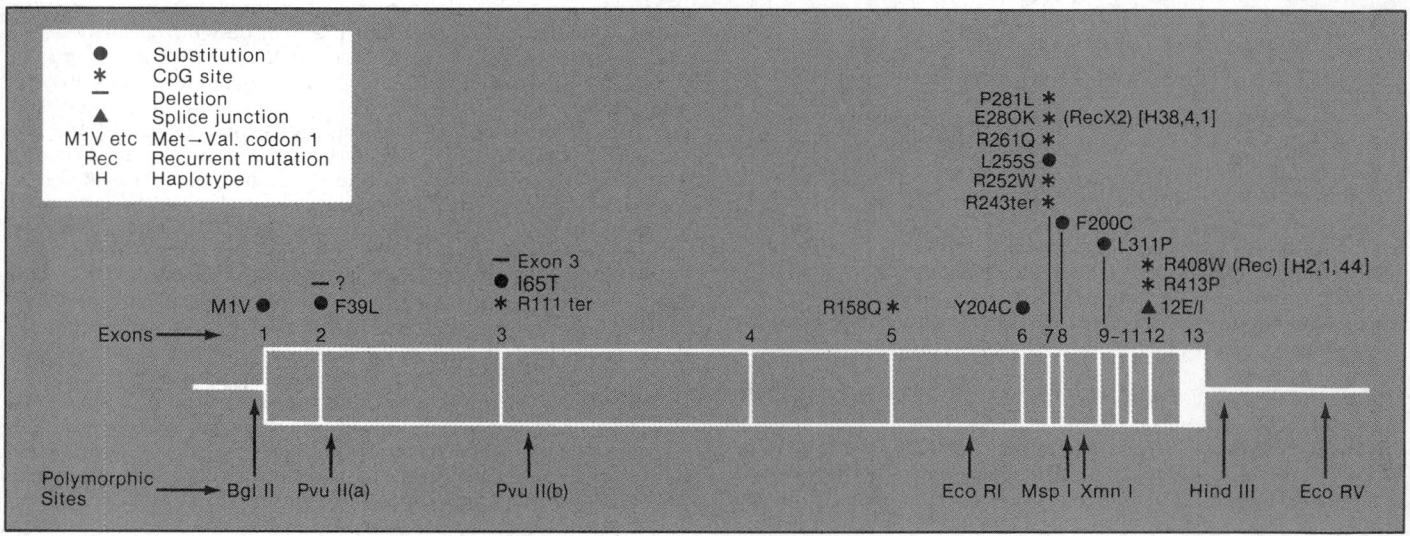

FIGURE 177–1. *A*, Intake of phenylalanine (an essential amino acid supplied only by diet) and its disposal by hydroxylation (1) (representing three quarters of normal runout), transamination (2), decarboxylation (3), and incorporation into proteins (4) (representing under a quarter of runout). *B*, Interrelations between phenylalanine hydroxylase (PAH), dihydropteridine reductase (DHPR), and the tetrahydrobiopterin (BH₄) biosynthesis pathway serving aromatic amino acid hydroxylation reactions. Mutations at the relevant chromosomal loci impair the hydroxylation reactions with effects on PAH activity only (1); DHPR activity (2); GTP-cyclohydrolase 1 (GTP-CH-1) activity (3); 6-pyruvoyltetrahydropterin synthase activity (6-PTS) (4); and "primapterin" metabolism (4). Disorders 2, 3a, 3b, and 4 impair function of three hydroxylases: PAH, tyrosine hydroxylase (TYH), and tryptophan hydroxylase (TRH). GTP = guanosine triphosphate; DHNP = dihydroneopterin triphosphate; 6-PT = 6-pyruvoyltetrahydropterin; KR = 2′-ketotetrahydropterin reductase; SR = sepiapterin reductase; qBH₂ = quinonoid dihydrobiopterin.

with lower blood phenylalanine values (<1mM), higher tolerance for dietary phenylalanine (>500 mg per day), and no elevated risk for mental retardation if not treated. There is a correlation between level of hepatic hydroxylase activity and clinical form; in broad terms, activity is less than 1 per cent of normal in phenylketonuria and more than 1 per cent of normal in nonphenylketonuric hyperphenylalaninemia.

DNA analysis (by polymerase chain reaction [PCR], nucleotide sequence analysis, Southern blot, and other methods) is useful in identifying mutations at the hydroxylase (Fig. 177–2) and the reductase loci. Interpretation of phenotype by mutation analysis is of increasing clinical relevance. Prenatal diagnosis by analysis of DNA in chorionic villus samples or amniocytes is now feasible for most (≈85 per cent) couples at risk.

FIGURE 177–2. Diagram of the phenylalanine hydroxylase (PAH) gene (≈90 kb, chromosome 12q24.1), showing exons *(vertical bars)*, polymorphic restriction sites *(arrows)*, and regions of over half the known mutations associated with phenylketonuria. The code (e.g., M1V) indicates normal residue, position in the PAH polypeptide, and replacement residue. One third of mutations involve hypermutable CpG dinucleotides; three mutations are "recurrent."

TREATMENT. The mainstay of treatment for primary phenylalanine hydroxylase deficiency is dietary restriction of the amino acid. There are several semisynthetic diet products ("orphan foods") for this purpose. Phenylketonuric patients can tolerate only 250 to 500 mg of phenylalanine per day to maintain the blood phenylalanine level well below 1 mM. Intake, blood levels of phenylalanine, and growth rate are monitored at frequent intervals to avoid undertreatment or overtreatment. Treatment into adult life is now recommended. Well-treated patients have normal or near-normal intellectual development.

The tetrahydrobiopterin-deficient forms require continuous replacement therapy of cofactor alone or in combination with neurotransmitter precursors and folinic acid is used in dihydropteridine reductase deficiency. Whether effective postnatal treatment of these disorders is feasible remains to be seen.

MATERNAL HYPERPHENYLALANINEMIA. This problem is relevant to all practitioners who counsel women about pregnancy. Intrauterine hyperphenylalaninemia places the fetus at risk of microcephaly, mental retardation, and organ malformations (notably cardiac). Accordingly, all females with hyperphenylalaninemia should be identified, followed (registries exist for this purpose), counselled about risk when they attain reproductive age, and treated with diet to maintain near-normal blood phenylalanine levels before conception and throughout the pregnancy. This treatment prevents harm to the fetus, but it is still under evaluation.

GENETICS. Mutant alleles (at all relevant loci) are recessive. Their aggregate frequency in the population is ≈ 0.01, meaning that 2 per cent of the population is heterozygous. Explanations for the high frequency of this "rare" phenotype and its genes include founder effects and genetic drift (observed in some populations), selective advantage in the heterozygote (unproved), hypermutability at the locus (observed), reproductive compensation (unlikely), and multiple loci involved in the trait (observed).

Levy HL: Maternal phenylketonuria. Prog Clin Biol 281:227, 1988. *A good up-to-date discussion of a major problem (maternal hyperphenylalaninemia).*

Scriver CR, Kaufman S, Woo SLC: The Hyperphenylalaninemias. *In* Scriver CR, Beaudet AL, Sly WS, et al. (eds.): The Metabolic Basis of Inherited Disease. 6th ed. New York, McGraw-Hill, 1989, pp 495–546. *A reference covering all major issues concerning the hyperphenylalaninemias.*

Trefz FK, Lichter-Konecki U, Konecki D: Phenylketonuria. Curr Opinion Pediatr 1:421, 1989. *A reference covering developments occurring after the preceding reference went to press.*

178 Alcaptonuria

James B. Wyngaarden

DEFINITION. Alcaptonuria is a rare hereditary disease in which homogentisic acid oxidase activity is missing. Homogentisic acid produced during the metabolism of phenylalanine and tyrosine accumulates and is excreted in the urine. It causes pigmentation of cartilage and other connective tissue (ochronosis) and in later years a degenerative arthritis of the spine and the larger peripheral joints. The disease has historical significance, for it was chiefly on the basis of study of families with alcaptonuria that Sir Archibald Garrod developed the concept of inborn errors of metabolism. The disease is inherited as an autosomal recessive trait. No method of detection of heterozygotes has been found.

INCIDENCE AND PREVALENCE. At least 600 cases have been reported, including one in an Egyptian mummy 3500 years old. A prevalence of three to five per million individuals was found in Northern Ireland.

PATHOGENESIS. The activity of homogentisic acid oxidase in the normal adult human liver is sufficient to metabolize over 1600 grams of homogentisic acid per day. Normally, no homogentisic acid can be detected in plasma or urine. In alcaptonuric individuals there is no detectable activity of this enzyme in liver or kidney tissue. Plasma levels of homogentisic acid rise to about 3 mg per deciliter, and the urinary excretion ranges from 4 to 8 grams per day. Mammalian tissue contains an enzyme called homogentisic acid polyphenoloxidase that catalyzes the oxidation of homogentisic acid to an ochronotic pigment, but pigment can also be produced nonenzymatically in the presence of oxygen and alkali, as, for example, in urine. The homogentisic acid polymer has a high affinity for cartilage and connective tissue macromolecules. The stained tissue is fragile and eventually may break down, leading to degenerative intervertebral disc or joint disease. Homogentisic acid may also have a direct effect upon collagen synthesis through inhibition of lysyl hydroxylase.

PATHOLOGY. In an adult alcaptonuric patient, cartilage in many areas, particularly the costal, laryngeal, and tracheal cartilage, is densely pigmented, sometimes being coal-black in appearance. Pigmentation is also present throughout the body in fibrous tissue, fibrocartilage, tendons, and ligaments. To a lesser degree, it is also found in the endocardium, in the intima of larger vessels, in various organs such as kidney and lung, and in the epidermis.

CLINICAL MANIFESTATIONS. Homogentisic acid is present in urine from birth, but urine is colorless when passed. Before the days of disposable diapers, the diagnosis was sometimes made when diapers turned brown in alkaline soaps. Pigment may appear in perspiration and stain clothing in the axillary and genital regions. Generally, the earliest change that can be detected externally is a slight pigmentation of the sclerae or the ears, beginning at 20 or 30 years of age. The cartilage of the ears may be slate blue or gray and feel irregular and thickened. Sometimes dusky discolorations of underlying tendons can be seen through the skin over the hands. In many patients, however, pigment is scarcely evident. The arthritis usually presents with limitation of motion of the hips, knee joints, or shoulders. There may be periods of acute inflammation, and later there is usually rather marked limitation of motion and ankylosis in the lumbosacral region. The arthritic complications are often severe and painful and may lead to extensive crippling. In addition, alcaptonuric patients appear to have a high incidence of cardiovascular disease, including generalized arteriosclerosis and chronic mitral and aortic valvulitis, with calcification of valves and annulus. At least one degenerated pigmented aortic valve has been replaced with a prosthesis. Myocardial infarction is a common cause of death. Other reported complications include ruptured intervertebral discs, prostatitis, and renal stones.

RADIOGRAPHIC CHANGES. These may be almost pathognomonic of alcaptonuria. The vertebral bodies of the lumbar spine show degeneration of the intervertebral discs with narrowing of the space and dense calcification of remaining disc material. There is variable fusion of vertebral bodies, but little osteophyte formation and minimal calcification of intervertebral ligaments. The degenerative changes of ochronotic arthritis are most severe in the hip, shoulder, and knee, and there may be calcific deposits in the tendons. The sacroiliac joints and smaller joints of the extremities usually show little or no abnormality. Ear cartilage may be calcified.

DIAGNOSIS AND DIFFERENTIAL DIAGNOSIS. The diagnosis is suggested by the history of pigmentary changes of urine, the presence of non-glucose reducing substance, the pigmentation of sclerae or cartilage, the arthritic episodes, and especially the typical radiographic changes of the lumbar spine. Specific identification of homogentisic acid in urine can be accomplished by chromatographic or enzymatic assays.

The ochronotic changes of skin and cartilage may be confused with pigmentary changes resulting from prolonged use of quinacrine hydrochloride (Atabrine) or from use of carbolic acid dressings for chronic cutaneous ulcers. The arthritis must be differentiated chiefly from rheumatoid arthritis, osteoarthritis, and gout.

TREATMENT. There is no effective treatment. Dietary restriction of phenylalanine and tyrosine of the degree necessary to reduce homogentisic aciduria is impractical and potentially deleterious. Large amounts of ascorbic acid have been given in an effort to reduce pigment formation. Ascorbic acid protects lysyl hydroxylase from inhibition by homogentisic acid in vitro. It does not alter the metabolic defect.

Justesen P, Anderson PE Jr: Radiologic manifestations in alcaptonuria. Skeletal Radiol 11:204, 1984. *Characteristic radiologic findings are demonstrated.*

La Du BN: Alcaptonuria. *In* Scriver CR, Beaudet AL, Sly WS, et al. (eds.): The Metabolic Basis of Inherited Disease. 6th ed. New York, McGraw-Hill, 1989, p 775. *A detailed discussion of the history, clinical features, and biochemical derangements of alcaptonuria and ochronosis.*

179 The Hyperprolinemias and Hydroxyprolinemia

Lloyd H. Smith, Jr.

The imino acids proline and hydroxyproline are nonessential; proline is readily synthesized in the body from glutamate and ornithine and hydroxyproline from proline. The synthesis of hydroxyproline occurs uniquely in peptide linkage largely as a constituent of collagen. Three rare genetic disorders of the degradative pathways of the acids have been described.

HYPERPROLINEMIAS. Two distinct disorders of proline metabolism, both transmitted as rare autosomal recessive traits, are associated with hyperprolinemia. In type I hyperprolinemia there is a block in the metabolism of proline to Δ'-pyrroline-5-carboxylate because of decreased activity of the enzyme proline oxidase. In type II hyperprolinemia, there is a block at the second step in the degradative pathway, the conversion of Δ'-pyrroline-5-carboxylate to L-glutamate, because of decreased activity of Δ'-pyrroline-5-carboxylate dehydrogenase. In both disorders the accumulation of proline in the blood leads to prolinuria and, through competition for a common renal tubular transport mechanism, to hydroxyprolinuria and glycinuria as well. In the type II disorder, there is also excessive urinary Δ'-pyrroline-5-carboxylate. The disorders can be diagnosed by finding the characteristic changes of hyperprolinemia and iminoaciduria as noted above. Although various forms of renal disease have been described with the type I disorder and neurologic abnormalities and seizures in some patients with either type I or type II hyperprolinemia, these may represent the bias of ascertainment. Since no clinical entity has been clearly established, there is no indicated therapy for either form of hyperprolinemia.

HYDROXYPROLINEMIA. An increased plasma level of free hydroxyproline associated with hydroxyprolinuria has been described in members of several families, but this disorder has not resulted in prolinuria or glycinuria. The disorder is assumed to be an autosomal recessive trait in which the homozygote has deficient activity of hydroxyproline oxidase. There is no associated abnormality of collagen metabolism, and the urinary excretion of peptide-bound hydroxyproline is normal. As in the case of the hyperprolinemias, no clinical entity has been demonstrated and no treatment is indicated.

180 Diseases of the Urea Cycle

Lloyd H. Smith, Jr.

Humans are ureotelic; they depend upon the synthesis of urea for nitrogen excretion. The only source of net urea formation is through the urea cycle (Fig. 180–1), which consists of five enzymes necessary for the sequential synthesis of carbamyl phosphate, citrulline, argininosuccinate, arginine, and urea. The pathway also serves for the de novo synthesis of arginine. When the function of this pathway is impaired, ammonia tends to accumulate. Genetic diseases associated with blocks at each of these five steps have been discovered and are described briefly below. In addition, one patient has been described with deficiency of N-acetylglutamate synthetase, which catalyzes the formation of acetylglutamate, which is required for the activation of carbamyl phosphate synthetase in step 1 (Fig. 180–1).

The associated clinical disorders resulting from the enzymatic defects prior to the synthesis of arginine are similar and can be described under two headings:

1. Neonatal presentation. After a normal pregnancy and delivery, the infant typically becomes symptomatic in 24 to 72 hours, with lethargy, vomiting, hypothermia, and hyperventilation. These symptoms rapidly progress to coma. The plasma ammonia level is high, and the blood urea nitrogen level is markedly reduced. A computed tomographic (CT) scan of the head reveals cerebral edema.

2. Late-onset presentation. These patients may present in later infancy or early childhood with recurrent episodes of hyperammonemia, characterized clinically by vomiting and central nervous system symptoms varying from lethargy, disorientation, and seizures to coma. These episodes may be precipitated by the stress of an infection or a change in diet or may appear with no evident precipitating cause. As in patients with neonatal presentation, respiratory alkalosis is common.

In all of the disorders of the urea cycle associated with hyperammonemia, ammonia itself appears to be the toxic metabolite, since the syndrome can be simulated in experimental animals by the infusion of ammonia. It is speculated that the central nervous system abnormalities can be attributed, at least in part, to the secondary intracellular accumulation of glutamine, with resulting increased osmolarity within the brain, particularly in astrocytes.

CARBAMYL PHOSPHATE SYNTHETASE (CPS) DEFICIENCY. Carbamyl phosphate (CAP) channeled for urea synthesis, in contrast to pyrimidine-channeled CAP, is synthesized in mitochondria from ammonia, bicarbonate, and ATP in a reaction catalyzed by CPS in the presence of N-acetylglutamate as an enzyme activator. Patients with deficiency of CPS usually present with hyperammonemia, protein intolerance, and neurologic symptoms as described above. The diagnosis is established by

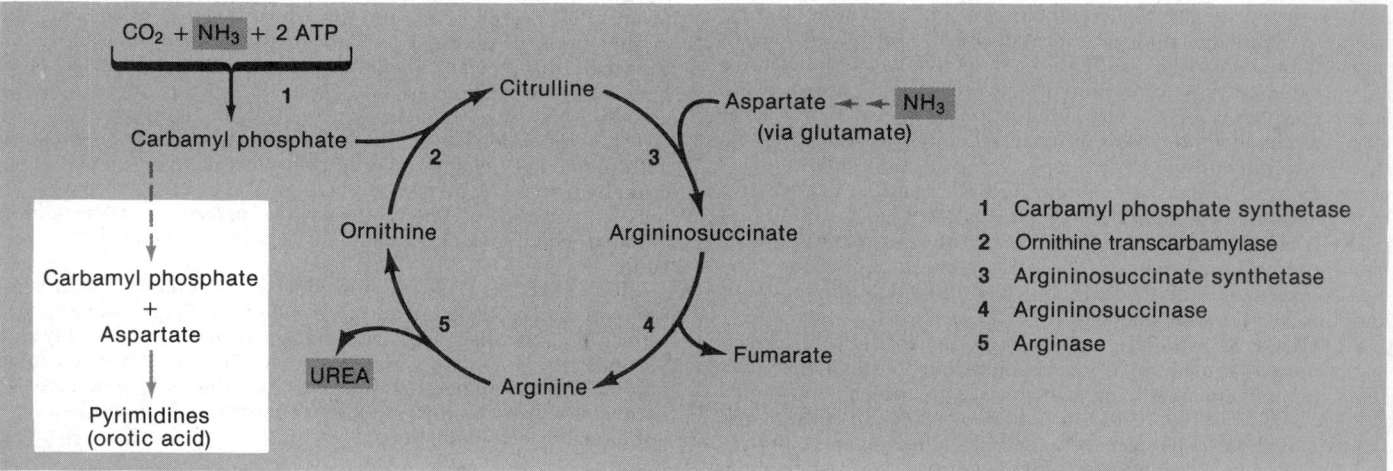

FIGURE 180–1. The urea cycle.

measuring carbamyl phosphate synthetase in a liver biopsy or in peripheral leukocytes. There are no characteristic changes in amino acids in blood or urine. Treatment is by protein restriction, the use of essential amino acids, and the administration of sodium benzoate or phenylacetate to enhance nitrogen excretion as hippurate or phenylacetylglutamine.

ORNITHINE TRANSCARBAMYLASE (OTC) DEFICIENCY. OTC, which catalyzes the mitochondrial carbamylation of ornithine by CAP to form citrulline, is coded for in band p 21.1 of the X chromosome. This most frequent genetic disorder of the urea cycle is therefore transmitted as an X-linked dominant trait, with hemizygous males rarely surviving the neonatal period; females manifest varying degrees of protein intolerance. The clinical onset can be acute and neonatal or late and intermittent, as noted above. As in the case of CPS deficiency, there are no detectable abnormalities of amino acid metabolism. Mitochondrial CAP accumulates, however, and spills over into the cytosol to drive pyrimidine synthesis (Fig. 180–1). This results in orotic aciduria as a constant finding. The enzyme defect can be shown in biopsy specimens from liver or intestinal mucosa or in leukocytes. Prenatal diagnosis of the disease is now possible using a gene-specific probe. The treatment is the same as that described above for CPS deficiency. In both CPS and OTC deficiencies, arginine becomes an essential amino acid. The addition of dietary citrulline as an arginine precursor is therefore recommended.

ARGININOSUCCINATE (ASA) SYNTHETASE DEFICIENCY (CITRULLINEMIA). Citrulline synthesized in mitochondria normally diffuses into the cytosol, where it is condensed with L-aspartic acid in the presence of ATP to form argininosuccinic acid. This reaction is catalyzed by ASA synthetase. Patients with neonatal citrullinemia have exhibited marked heterogeneity in the severity of their clinical and chemical manifestations. The associated hyperammonemia is, in general, less severe than in deficiency of CPS or OCT but does occur after protein ingestion. Citrulline is increased in blood and urine, sometimes more than 100-fold, but there is no evidence that it is toxic per se. Secondary orotic aciduria has been noted, presumably reflecting excess CAP. Patients with a late-onset form of presentation have been described, especially in Japan.

ARGININOSUCCINASE (ASase) DEFICIENCY (ARGININOSUCCINIC ACIDURIA). Cytosolic argininosuccinic acid undergoes reversible cleavage to arginine and fumarate catalyzed by ASase. Approximately 60 patients have been described with argininosuccinic aciduria. Clinical findings, which vary widely in severity, have included mental retardation, seizures, ataxia, hepatomegaly and hepatic fibrosis, and friable hair (trichorrhexis nodosa). In addition to large amounts of ASA in blood, urine, and cerebrospinal fluid (readily demonstrable by chromatography), patients with ASase deficiency may have citrullinemia. As part of dietary therapy, patients should receive supplementary arginine.

ARGINASE DEFICIENCY (HYPERARGININEMIA). Arginine is hydrolyzed to urea and ornithine, catalyzed by arginase, in the last step of the urea cycle. Patients with deficiency of arginase have exhibited mental retardation and spasticity. Arginine is increased in blood and urine and may occasionally cause secondary cystinuria owing to competitive inhibition of the renal tubular transport of dibasic amino acids. Hyperammonemia may be found after protein ingestion. The absence of arginase can be conveniently demonstrated in circulating erythrocytes.

181 Branched-Chain Aminoaciduria

Lloyd H. Smith, Jr.

Leucine, isoleucine, and valine are essential, so-called branched-chain amino acids that have certain structural resemblances and share some common metabolic pathways. Two rare genetic disorders in the degradative pathways of the branched-chain amino acids are described briefly.

MAPLE SYRUP URINE DISEASE. This disorder, also called *branched-chain ketonuria*, derives its name from the character-istic odor of the urine of affected infants. The disease is transmitted as a rare (1 in 68,000 to 290,000 births in large surveys) autosomal recessive trait in which the affected homozygote exhibits deficient activity in components of the branched-chain keto acid dehydrogenase multienzyme complex, which functions in the oxidative decarboxylation pathway of the keto acids of leucine, isoleucine, and valine. As a consequence, these three amino acids and their corresponding keto acids accumulate in excess in blood and urine and presumably throughout the body. A few patients have a variant disorder that responds in part to treatment with large amounts of thiamine (>150 mg thiamine per day), which may serve to stabilize the dehydrogenase multienzyme complex. The pathogenesis of the deleterious effects in maple syrup urine disease has not been firmly established and may be complex, but probably relates mostly to the accumulation of leucine.

In typical maple syrup urine disease, severe hypotonia, lethargy, feeding difficulties, and hypoglycemia develop in the first week in an infant who seemed normal at birth. Convulsions and decorticate rigidity may develop, and most patients die, commonly of intercurrent infection, within the first year of life (often within the first few weeks). Atypical cases with less severe or even intermittent clinical manifestations have been described. The diagnosis can usually be suspected from the characteristic odor of the urine and is confirmed by the abnormal pattern of amino acids and keto acids in blood and urine. The enzyme defect is demonstrable in leukocytes and fibroblasts.

Treatment—by careful dietary control of leucine, isoleucine, and valine—is simple in theory but difficult in practice because of the necessity to balance three individual essential amino acids that are not easily analyzed. In those few cases in which rigid dietary control with careful monitoring of plasma levels has been instituted early, the results have been gratifying. Thiamine therapy with pharmacological doses should be tried for at least several weeks in addition to dietary restrictions.

ISOVALERIC ACIDEMIA. This rare genetic disorder in the degradative pathway of leucine (>60 cases reported) is due to a block in the conversion of isovaleric acid to beta-methylcrotonic acid, which is catalyzed by isovaleryl-CoA (coenzyme A) dehydrogenase. Isovaleric acid accumulates in blood and urine and gives rise to an odor that has been described as being like sweaty feet. The pathogenesis of the associated clinical features has not been established. Symptoms, which usually begin in the first week of life, consist of attacks of vomiting, acidosis, tremors, lethargy, or even coma. Leukopenia, anemia, thrombocytopenia, and hyperammonemia have been observed during acute attacks. In addition to the acute neonatal form of isovaleric acidemia, a chronic intermittent form of intermediate severity may occur. As in the case of maple syrup urine disease, which it may clinically resemble, isovaleric acidemia may be suspected from the associated odor. The diagnosis is established by the demonstration of excess isovaleric acid in the serum by gas-liquid chromatography or of isovalerylglycine in the urine. Treatment is by strict control of dietary leucine. More recently, therapy with glycine and carnitine has shown promise by enhancing the removal of isovaleric acid as isovalerylglycine and isovalerylcarnitine, respectively.

Hyperprolinemia and Hydroxyprolinemia

Phang JM, Scriver CR: Disorders of proline and hydroxyproline metabolism. *In* Scriver CR, Beaudet A, Sly W, et al. (eds): The Metabolic Basis of Inherited Disease. 6th ed. New York, McGraw-Hill, 1989, pp 577–597. *An extensive analysis of the chemical derangements in these rare disorders.*

Diseases of the Urea Cycle

Beaudet AL, O'Brien WE, Bock H-GO, et al.: The human argininosuccinate synthetase locus and citrullinemia. Adv Hum Genet 15:161, 1986. *An excellent general review of this rare disorder, with particular emphasis on the molecular analysis of the defective gene.*

Brusilow SW, Horwich AL: Urea cycle enzymes. *In* Scriver CR, Beaudet A, Sly W, et al. (eds): The Metabolic Basis of Inherited Disease. 6th ed. New York, McGraw-Hill, 1989, pp 629–663. *A large number of disorders are associated with derangements in urea synthesis. This chapter gives a lucid summary of the biochemistry of urea synthesis and the pathogenesis of the various disorders associated with that pathway. As always in The Metabolic Basis of Inherited Disease, there is a large and useful bibliography (347 references).*

Rowe PC, Newman SL, Brusilow SW: Natural history of symptomatic partial ornithine transcarbamylase deficiency. N Engl J Med 314:541, 1986. *Studies of the disease in a series of symptomatic female heterozygotes with a description of clinical manifestations, therapy, and outcome.*

Branched-Chain Aminoaciduria

Danner DJ, Elsas LJ: Disorders of branched chain amino acid and keto acid metabolism. *In* Scriver CR, Beaudet A, Sly W, et al. (eds.): The Metabolic Basis of Inherited Disease. 6th ed. New York, McGraw-Hill, 1989, pp 671–692. *This is the most sophisticated general presentation of the pathogenesis of this group of disorders. Although the emphasis is on the biochemical basis, there is a useful clinical discussion and an extensive bibliography (268 references).*

182 Homocystinuria

S. Harvey Mudd

DEFINITION. The term *homocystinuria* designates a biochemical abnormality, not a disease entity. Several known genetic disorders lead to homocystinuria. Most common is cystathionine beta-synthase deficiency. In this condition ectopia lentis, mental retardation, bone abnormalities, osteoporosis, and thromboembolic phenomena are frequent.

PREVALENCE. More than 600 adequately documented cases of cystathionine beta-synthase deficiency have been reported. Screening of newborn infants indicates a *minimal* prevalence of 1 in 300,000 worldwide.

ETIOLOGY AND PATHOGENESIS. Cystathionine beta-synthase deficiency is inherited as an autosomal recessive trait. Deficient activity of this enzyme has been demonstrated in liver extracts, in brain, and in cultured skin fibroblasts and lymphocytes. The enzyme deficiency results in failure of homocysteine to react with serine to form cystathionine on the pathway to cysteine. Homocystine is the disulfide oxidation product formed from two molecules of homocysteine. Homocysteinyl moieties are currently detected in normal human plasma at total concentrations of 6 to 14 μM, depending upon the laboratory and method used. In vivo, some 75 to 80 per cent of these moieties are bound by disulfide linkage to proteins; the remainder are not protein bound. In cystathionine beta-synthase–deficient patients, fasting plasma concentrations up to 200 μM of non–protein-bound homocystine have been reported. The urine may contain up to 1 mmol of homocystine per day. Plasma methionine levels are also raised, and plasma cystine is low. Detailed studies, chiefly of cultured fibroblasts, suggest extensive heterogeneity in the genetic lesions producing deficient activity of cystathionine beta-synthase. An important manifestation of such genetic heterogeneity is pyridoxine responsiveness. In 40 to 50 per cent of cystathionine beta-synthase–deficient patients, administration of relatively large amounts of pyridoxine markedly reduces or eliminates homocystinuria, homocystinemia, hypermethionemia, and hypocystinemia. Within any one sibship, all affected sibs are either B_6 responsive or B_6 nonresponsive.

PATHOLOGY. There is breakage of the zonular fibers of the lens (possibly due to disruption of the highly disulfide-linked proteins of the microfibrillar system), with resulting subluxation. The skeleton is markedly osteoporotic, and the vertebrae show rarefaction with biconcave compression. Thrombi and emboli have been reported in almost every artery or vein. These result in brain infarcts, coronary occlusion and myocardial infarction, pulmonary infarcts, renal infarcts, and thrombophlebitis with pulmonary emboli. The pathogenesis of the thrombotic tendency is not clearly understood, but increase of plasma homocyst(e)ine, rather than plasma methionine, is likely to cause the thrombotic tendency.

CLINICAL MANIFESTATIONS. Among individuals with cystathionine beta-synthase deficiency, there is marked variation with regard to the major clinical features of this condition, their time of onset, and severity. Clinical manifestations tend to be less prevalent, slower in onset, or less marked among B_6-responsive patients than among nonresponsive ones. A survey of 629 patients showed that mental capabilities ranged from severely retarded to IQs as high as 130. Median IQ for B_6-responsive patients was 78; for B_6-nonresponsive patients, 56. Mental retardation, when present, most commonly becomes manifest during the first few years of life.

The incidence of dislocated optic lenses increases with age. By the age of 10 years, 55 per cent of B_6-responsive patients and 82 per cent of B_6-nonresponsive patients have dislocated lenses. Acute glaucoma and reduced visual acuity may result.

Thromboembolism is the life-threatening complication of cystathionine beta-synthase deficiency. By age 15, chances of having had a clinically detected thromboembolic event are 12 per cent among B_6 responders and 27 per cent among B_6 nonresponders. Large and small arteries and veins may be affected. Major cerebrovascular thrombosis may occur. Venous thrombosis with pulmonary emboli is common. By age 30 years, 4 per cent of B_6-responsive patients and 23 per cent of B_6-nonresponsive patients have died.

The spine is the most common site of osteoporosis, followed by the long bones. By age 15, chances of having radiologically detected spinal osteoporosis are 36 per cent among B_6 responders and 65 per cent among B_6 nonresponders. Scoliosis occurs in many individuals, although kyphosis is infrequent. Vertebral collapse and pathologic fractures of long bones may occur. The long bones are generally thin and excessively lengthened. Pectus carinatum or excavatum is common.

DIAGNOSIS AND DIFFERENTIAL DIAGNOSIS. The diagnosis is suggested by ectopia lentis and thromboembolic phenomena, together with other aforementioned features. On occasion, patients present with thrombotic disease and a paucity of other manifestations. The urinary cyanide-nitroprusside reaction is positive. Other disulfidurias—for example, cystinuria—also produce a positive cyanide-nitroprusside reaction, so homocystinemia and homocystinuria distinguish cystathionine beta-synthase deficiency from alternative forms of disulfiduria. Cystathionine beta-synthase deficiency is confirmed by demonstration of markedly reduced enzyme activity with cultured skin fibroblasts or phytohemagglutinin-stimulated lymphocytes or in a liver biopsy specimen.

Heterozygotes may be identified by assay of cystathionine beta-synthase activity in liver biopsy tissue. Cystathionine beta-synthase activities in cultured fibroblasts or phytohemagglutinin-stimulated lymphocytes from most heterozygotes are below the control range, but there is some overlap. For unequivocal identification, such studies are best accompanied by methionine loading tests. In some young adults, premature peripheral or cerebral occlusive arterial disease may be due to heterozygosity for cystathionine beta-synthase deficiency, and there is increasing evidence that mild homocysteinemia, whatever its cause, is an independent risk factor for vascular disease.

Rarer forms of homocystinuria are caused by decreased 5-methyltetrahydrofolate–dependent homocysteine methylation, owing either to decreased 5,10-methylenetetrahydrofolate reductase activity or to a variety of lesions that interfere with the ability to produce methylcobalamin. In all of these, plasma methionine levels are low. The condition is first noted in childhood. Homocystinuria also occurs following 6-azauridine triacetate administration.

TREATMENT. Management is directed toward the biochemical abnormality, with the aim of preventing or ameliorating clinical manifestations, and toward the clinical treatment of complications.

Newborns with cystathionine beta-synthase deficiency have almost always been treated with a low-methionine diet (usually accompanied by cystine supplementation). Such therapy prevents mental retardation and may decrease the rate of lens dislocations and reduce the incidence of seizures. It is too early to assess the effects on thromboembolic events, osteoporosis, or mortality. When the condition is diagnosed at later ages in B_6-responsive patients, pyridoxine treatment (doses up to 500 to 1000 mg per day) accompanied by folate repletion has been shown to produce a statistically significant reduction in the rate of initial thromboembolic events. When diagnosis is made at later ages in B_6-nonresponsive patients, strict methionine limitation, if accepted and carefully adhered to, may be beneficial in preventing thromboembolic events. In early studies of such patients, betaine, which lowers homocysteine by accelerating its methylation, has appeared useful. Antithrombotic therapy with aspirin and dipyridamole has also been advocated.

Cochran FB, Sweetman L, Schmidt K, et al.: Pyridoxine-unresponsive homocystinuria with an unusual clinical course. Am J Med Genet 35:519, 1990. *A patient presenting with asthma, pneumothoraces, and superior sagittal sinus thrombosis.*

Gibson MA, Kumaratilake JS, Cleary EG: The protein components of the 12-nanometer microfibrils of elastic and nonelastic tissues. J Biol Chem 264:4590, 1989. *Studies of the components that may be affected in the connective tissue disorders.*

Malinow MR, Kang SS, Taylor LM, et al.: Prevalence of hyperhomocyst(e)inemia in patients with peripheral arterial occlusive disease. Circulation 79:1180, 1989. *A useful summary of modern methods for analysis of plasma homocyst(e)ine and a review of studies implicating mild homocysteinemia as an independent risk factor for early vascular disease.*

McGill JJ, Mettler G, Rosenblatt DS, et al.: Detection of heterozygotes for recessive alleles. Homocyst(e)inemia: Paradigm of pitfalls in phenotypes. Am J Med Genet 36:45, 1990. *Critical discussion of problems in the identification of heterozygotes.*

Mitchell GA, Watkins D, Melancon SB, et al.: Clinical heterogeneity in cobalamin C variant of combined homocystinuria and methylmalonic aciduria. J Pediatr 108:410, 1986. *Contains a useful brief summary of other causes of homocystinuria.*

Mudd SH, Levy HL, Skovby F: Disorders of transsulfuration. In Scriver CS, Beaudet AL, Sly WS, et al. (eds.): The Metabolic Basis of Inherited Disease. 6th ed. New York, McGraw-Hill, 1989. *A detailed review of the clinical features of confirmed cases of cystathionine beta-synthase deficiency, with a discussion of metabolic factors in homocystinuria.*

Mudd SH, Skovby F, Levy HL, et al.: The natural history of homocystinuria due to cystathionine-β-synthase deficiency. Am J Hum Genet 37:1, 1985. *An international questionnaire study covering 629 patients. The natural history of the untreated disease is defined for the major clinical manifestations and the effects of therapies evaluated statistically.*

DISORDERS OF PURINE AND PYRIMIDINE METABOLISM

183 Gout

James B. Wyngaarden

Gout is a term representing a heterogeneous group of genetic and acquired diseases manifested by *hyperuricemia* and a characteristic *acute inflammatory arthritis* induced by *crystals* of monosodium urate monohydrate. Some patients develop aggregated deposits of these crystals (*tophi*) in and around the joints of the extremities that can lead to severe crippling. Many patients develop a *chronic interstitial nephropathy*. In addition, uric acid *urolithiasis* is common in gout.

These manifestations of gout can occur in different combinations. However, essential hyperuricemia alone, even when complicated by uric acid lithiasis, should not be called gout; gout signifies inflammatory arthritis or tophaceous disease.

A classification emphasizing the heterogeneity of gout is presented in Table 183–1.

PREVALENCE AND INCIDENCE. The prevalence of gout varies from about 0.13 to 0.37 per cent in Europe and the United States to 10 per cent in adult male Maori of New Zealand. Exceptionally high prevalences are also found in Filipinos in the United States and in natives of the Mariana Islands. During World Wars I and II, acute gouty arthritis was uncommon in Europe. When dietary protein again became plentiful, its frequency returned to prewar levels. Although formerly rare in Japan, gout has now become common in parallel with the increase in protein consumption in that country.

Primary gout is chiefly a disease of adult men; only about 5 per cent of cases are found in women, largely in the postmenopausal group. The frequency of gout is increased in patients taking diuretics, especially of the thiazide group; in certain nephropathies; and in polycythemia vera, myeloid metaplasia, or chronic hemolysis. Gout in all of its forms makes up about 5 per cent of arthritis cases.

GENETICS OF GOUT. A family history of clinical gout is generally found in 6 to 18 per cent of patients in the United States and Denmark. Figures of 40 to 80 per cent have been reported from England and also from the United States following tenacious family studies. About 25 per cent of first-degree relatives of gouty subjects are hyperuricemic, and about 20 per cent of these have symptomatic gout. Familial hyperuricemia is polygenic and multifactorial. Hyperuricemia is correlated with maleness, surface area, obesity, ponderal index, protein intake, social status, educational level, and alcohol ingestion. In primary gout associated with hypoxanthine-guanine phosphoribosyltransferase

(HPRT) deficiency and phosphoribosylpyrophosphate (PP-ribose-P) synthetase variants, the genetic transmissions are X linked. Glycogen storage disease type I, which is associated with a specific form of secondary gout, is an autosomal recessive trait.

PATHOGENESIS AND PATHOLOGY. The hallmark of gout is hyperuricemia. The risk of gout increases with the degree of hyperuricemia and also with age (Table 183–2). Virtually all patients with gout have serum urate values above 7.0 mg per deciliter. An occasional patient has a lower value at the time of attack, perhaps attributable to the urate diuresis that sometimes accompanies the inflammatory response. Repeat analyses show hyperuricemia during quiescent periods.

In normal prepubertal children, serum urate values average 3.6 mg per deciliter in both sexes. At puberty these levels increase. In the United States, the central 95 per cent segment of the distributions encompasses values of 2.2 to 7.5 mg per deciliter in adult males and 2.1 to 6.6 mg per deciliter in adult premenopausal females. After the menopause, mean values in women increase to approximate levels in men. Definitions of hyperuricemia based on distributions of serum urate are useful for epidemiologic studies. But statistical expressions are not adequate definitions of the pathophysiologic significance of hyperuricemia, for it is the *solubility* of urate in plasma and body fluids that is important. There is no evidence that urate in solution is toxic; all of the features of gout derive from responses to the urate crystal.

The solubility of urate in body fluids is strongly influenced by pH and temperature (Table 183–3). At pH 7.4 and 37°C, the solubility of urate in fluid having the sodium composition of plasma is 6.4 to 6.8 mg per deciliter. An additional 0.4 mg per deciliter is protein bound, chiefly to an alpha$_1$-alpha$_2$ globulin. Thus 7.0 mg per deciliter is about the solubility limit of urate in plasma at normal central body temperature and defines hyperuricemia in a physicochemical sense. But solubility is considerably less at the temperature of peripheral joints, which may be 32°C in the knee and 29°C in the ankle (Hollander, 1949).

Mechanisms of Hyperuricemia. The concentration of urate in plasma is determined by the balance between absorption and production of purines on the one hand and destruction and excretion on the other. Exogenous purines contribute substantially to body uric acid stores. Purine restriction leads to a reduction in the serum urate level of 0.6 to 1.8 mg per deciliter in normal subjects and in patients with idiopathic gout. Abnormalities of purine absorption have not been implicated as a cause of hyperuricemia.

Human beings lack uricase; therefore uric acid is the end-product of purine metabolism. In normal subjects approximately one third of the uric acid disposed of each day is degraded by bacteria in the gut, and two thirds is excreted unchanged by the

TABLE 183–1. CLASSIFICATION OF HYPERURICEMIA AND GOUT

Type	Disturbance in Uric Acid Metabolism	Inheritance
Primary		
I. Idiopathic (>99% of primary gout)		
A. Normal urinary excretion (80–90% of primary gout)	Decreased renal clearance ± overproduction	Polygenic
B. Increased urinary excretion (10–20% of primary gout)	Overproduction ± decreased renal clearance	Polygenic
II. Associated with specific enzyme or metabolic defects (<1% of primary gout)		
A. Increased activity of PP-ribose-P synthetase	Overproduction; increased synthesis of PP-ribose-P	X-linked
B. "Partial" deficiency of hypoxanthine-guanine phosphoribosyltransferase	Overproduction; increased PP-ribose-P concentration	X-linked
Secondary		
I. Associated with increased purine biosynthesis de novo		
A. "Complete" deficiency of hypoxanthine-guanine phosphoribosyltransferase	Overproduction; Lesch-Nyhan syndrome	X-linked
B. Glucose-6-phosphatase deficiency	Overproduction and decreased renal clearance; glycogen storage disease, type I (von Gierke)	Autosomal recessive
II. Associated with increased nucleic acid turnover	Overproduction, e.g., chronic hemolysis; polycythemia; myeloid metaplasia	—
III. Associated with decreased renal clearance of uric acid	Reduced renal functional mass; inhibition of secretion and/or enhanced reabsorption by drugs, toxins, or endogenous metabolic products	—

TABLE 183–3. SOLUBILITY OF URATE ION AS A FUNCTION OF TEMPERATURE IN THE PRESENCE OF 140 mM Na*

Temperature (°C)	Maximal Equilibrium Concentration of Urate in the Presence of 140 mM Na+ (mg/dl)
37	6.8
35	6.0
30	4.5
25	3.3
20	2.5
15	1.8
10	1.2

*From Loeb: Arthritis Rheum 15:189, 1972. Reprinted from Arthritis and Rheumatism Journal, copyright 1972. Used by permission of the American College of Rheumatology.

to 1000 mg per 24 hours. In men on a purine-restricted diet these values average 418 ± 70 mg per 24 hours. From 10 to 20 per cent of gouty subjects show basal values above the m + 2SD value. However, urinary urate measurements are insensitive in the assessment of purine production. With labeled uric acid, the miscible pool of uric acid in normal humans averages 1200 mg, and the daily rate of production averages 750 mg. One half to three fourths of the pool turns over each day. The difference between the rate of production and the rate of excretion of urate ranges from 100 to 365 mg per day and represents intestinal uricolysis. This method discloses an enlarged urate pool in all gouty subjects studied and increased turnover in most.

A second method of study of uric acid production involves measurement of incorporation of an isotopically labeled purine precursor, usually glycine, into urinary uric acid. The incorporation can be corrected for extrarenal disposal to give total incorporation values. By use of these methods, evidence of some degree of excessive production of uric acid has been obtained in about two thirds of gouty patients studied. The most extreme values are found in subjects with HPRT deficiency or PP-ribose-P synthetase variants, but these represent fewer than 1 per cent of gouty subjects. Many patients whose 24-hour urinary uric acid values fall within the normal range show modest increases in the rate of turnover of an enlarged uric acid pool and/or overincorporation of glycine into urate. Studies of the intramolecular distribution of ^{15}N in uric acid following administration of ^{15}N-glycine show excessive labeling of position 9, which is derived from the amide-N of glutamine and from ammonia. Thus many more gouty subjects show evidence of mild overproduction of purine than would have been deduced from urinary uric acid measurements alone.

The first unique reaction of purine biosynthesis and the site of metabolic regulation by purine ribonucleotide inhibitors is that which synthesizes phosphoribosylamine, catalyzed by amidophosphoribosyltransferase:

$$\text{Glutamine} + \text{PP-ribose-P} + H_2O \xrightarrow{Mg^{2+}}$$
$$\text{phosphoribosylamine} + \text{glutamic acid} + PPi$$

There are several possible mechanisms for loss of regulation at this site and acceleration of purine biosynthesis. These include (1) excessive concentrations of the substrates PP-ribose-P, glutamine, or both; (2) a structural alteration or increased amount of the enzyme, rendering it more active or less sensitive to inhibition by purine ribonucleotides; or (3) a reduced concentration of one of the regulatory nucleotides (adenosine monophosphate [AMP] or guanosine monophosphate [GMP]) that exert cooperative allosteric inhibition of enzyme activity. Intracellular levels of PP-ribose-P are strikingly raised in HPRT deficiency and also in PP-ribose-P synthetase overactivity. The increased concentration of PP-ribose-P drives purine biosynthesis both by furnishing more of the rate-limiting substrate and by allosteric activation of amidophosphoribosyltransferase. PP-ribose-P turnover is accelerated in gouty patients in whom uric acid is overproduced. However, erythrocyte PP-ribose-P levels are normal in gouty patients without specific enzyme defects. Plasma glutamate values are slightly raised in gouty subjects, both in the fasting state and after oral glutamate loads, but plasma glutamine levels are normal. Although reduced activities of glutaminase and of glutamic dehydrogenase have been postulated in gout, no direct

kidney. Decreased uricolysis has been excluded as a mechanism for hyperuricemia. In fact, with high urate concentrations in body fluids, enteric uricolysis is enhanced; with the onset of renal insufficiency, intestinal uricolysis assumes increased importance and in extreme instances may account for 80 per cent of daily urate disposition. By contrast, both increased purine biosynthesis and decreased renal excretion of uric acid play important roles in the pathogenesis of primary hyperuricemia.

Random urine samples in normal men commonly contain 500

TABLE 183–2. PREVALENCE OF GOUTY ARTHRITIS IN MEN IN RELATION TO SERUM URATE CONCENTRATION AND AGE

Serum Urate Level (mg/dl)	Mean Age 49 Years* (%)	Mean Age 58 Years† (%)
6.0–6.9	2	2
7.0–7.9	4	17
8.0–8.9	11	25
9.0–9.9	30	90
10 +	48	90

*Data from Zalokar et al.: J Chronic Dis 25:305, 1972.
†Data from Hall et al.: Am J Med 42:27, 1967.

evidence for such enzyme deficiencies exists. Any process that results in accelerated breakdown of intracellular adenyl nucleotides may lead to hyperuricemia by prompt degradation of daughter purine compounds to uric acid and to secondary acceleration of purine synthesis de novo through release of inhibition of amidophosphoribosyltransferase. This biphasic mechanism has been implicated in glycogen storage disease type I following fructose infusion, following alcohol ingestion, and in a gouty patient with a variant AMP deaminase that showed reduced sensitivity to guanosine triphosphate (GTP), its normal regulator. The last example has been proposed as a possible general mechanism in idiopathic gout. There are no examples of gout attributable to intrinsic alterations of the amidophosphoribosyltransferase itself.

In the normal turnover of nucleic acids and nucleotides, some are degraded to free purine bases, chiefly hypoxanthine and guanine. Nucleotides synthesized de novo in excess of nucleic acid requirements are promptly degraded to hypoxanthine. Guanine is deaminated to xanthine by guanase. Hypoxanthine and xanthine are oxidized to uric acid by xanthine oxidase (Fig. 183–1). Hepatic xanthine oxidase activity is increased in gouty overproducers, but this appears to be an induced rather than a primary change. Nevertheless, this is an additional factor contributing to accelerated uric acid synthesis in these patients.

In a substantial fraction of gouty subjects, the immediate pathogenetic mechanism of hyperuricemia appears to be a decreased renal tubular clearance of urate. Renal excretion of urate is a complex function of glomerular filtration, tubular reabsorption, and tubular secretion. Filtration of plasma urate is assumed to be complete, on the basis of micropuncture studies in animals and ultrafiltration studies of human plasma in vitro. Less than 5 per cent of plasma urate is protein bound in humans under physiologic conditions at 37°C. Filtered urate appears to be almost completely reabsorbed in the proximal tubule (presecretory reabsorption). Some of the secreted urate is also reabsorbed in the distal portion of the proximal tubule and to a lesser extent in the ascending portion of the loop of Henle and in the collecting ducts (postsecretory reabsorption). Excreted urate is thought to arise almost entirely by tubular secretion.

Studies in gouty patients have been interpreted as indicating reduced secretion of urate per nephron, but enhanced postsecretory reabsorption would also explain the data. The renal contribution to hyperuricemia is most marked in patients with normal 24-hour excretion values of urate, normal turnover values of the uric acid pool, and normal values of glycine incorporation into uric acid. But reduced renal urate clearances per nephron are not restricted to this group. With the exception of patients with HPRT deficiency or PP-ribose-P synthetase variants, overproducer gouty subjects as a group also show reduced renal urate clearance (Simkin). Thus, although some investigators have separated the large group of patients with an undefined biochemical lesion, *idiopathic gout*, into two discrete subgroups termed metabolic (overproducer) and renal gout, the evidence does not support such a categoric distinction, inasmuch as many subjects show both defects. Since chronic excessive alcohol consumption is common in gouty subjects and causes excessive turnover of adenine nucleotides and increased urate production and excretion, it is possible that some of the metabolic contributions to hyperuricemia in idiopathic gout are alcohol related.

The complexity of the pathogenesis of hyperuricemia is illustrated by two additional observations. The first is that asymptomatic hyperuricemia begins at puberty in the male as an exaggeration of the modest increase in serum urate concentration that normally occurs at that age and at the menopause in the female. Clearly, hormonal factors influence serum urate levels. The second is that both pathogenetic mechanisms may be reversible. Subjects with primary (idiopathic) gout are, on average, 15 to 30 per cent overweight, and 75 per cent or more show fasting hypertriglyceridemia. (Hyperuricemia is present in more than 80 per cent of all patients with hypertriglyceridemia.) In some gouty patients, weight reduction and abstinence from alcohol reverse hypertriglyceridemia, hyperuricemia, excessive urate excretion, and evidence of overproduction by isotopic studies, as well as evidence of impaired renal urate clearance.

The Acute Gouty Attack. In 1859, A. B. Garrod, in the second and fourth of his 10 propositions on the "The True Nature of Essence of Gout," wrote the following: "Investigations recently made in the morbid anatomy of gout, prove incontestably that true gouty inflammation is *always* accompanied with a deposition of urate of soda in the inflamed part. . . . The deposited urate of soda may be looked upon as the cause, and not the effect, of the gouty inflammation." The role of the urate crystal in acute gout was rediscovered in 1961 by McCarty and Hollander. In laboratory animals experimental gouty arthritis requires the presence of leukocytes. However, synovitis can also be produced experimentally by other crystals of similar size and shape, and it occurs in pseudogout caused by calcium pyrophosphate dihydrate crystals.

Although a number of cellular mechanisms are activated by the urate crystal, the exact sequence by which inflammation is initiated is uncertain. Hageman's factor, kallikrein, kinin-like peptides, and the complement system all participate in the response, but each has also been excluded as an obligatory factor. Urate crystals are leukotactic. Leukocytes and synovial lining cells ingest the urate crystals. Within minutes leukocytes release leukotriene B_4 (LTB_4) and a glycoprotein chemotactic factor (mw = 11,500). Production of these chemoattractants is blocked by colchicine. The acute inflammatory response to injected urate crystals is also blocked by prior treatment with colchicine, but the inflammatory response to purified crystal-induced chemotactic factor is not. Thus this factor and LTB_4 may be important mediators of the inflammatory reaction in gout. Monocytes are also stimulated by urate crystals in vitro, with release of interleukin 1. IL-1 may also contribute to initiation and amplification of gouty inflammation.

Crystal-cell interactions may be modulated by proteins adherent to the crystals. Crystals from patients with acute gout have surface coats of IgG and, to a lesser extent, of IgM, IgA, C3, and fibrinogen, but not of albumin. In studies in vitro, IgG coating enhances neutrophil responsiveness to urate crystals, whereas certain other proteins inhibit. Such modulating factors may account for the variable inflammatory responses to urate crystals in gouty subjects.

Phagocytosis of the crystal leads to rapid destruction of the phagolysosome membrane with release of hydrolytic enzymes into the cell. This results in cell necrosis and release of the crystal and lysosomal and cytoplasmic enzymes into the surrounding tissue.

The events leading to the putative burst of microcrystals of urate that initiates the acute attack are largely speculative. Three major theories have been advanced. The first postulates that trauma may result in shedding of crystals from pre-existing cartilaginous tophi into the synovial fluid. The second emphasizes the ability of organized proteoglycans of cartilage to absorb (solubilize) urate. Disruption and increased turnover of proteo-

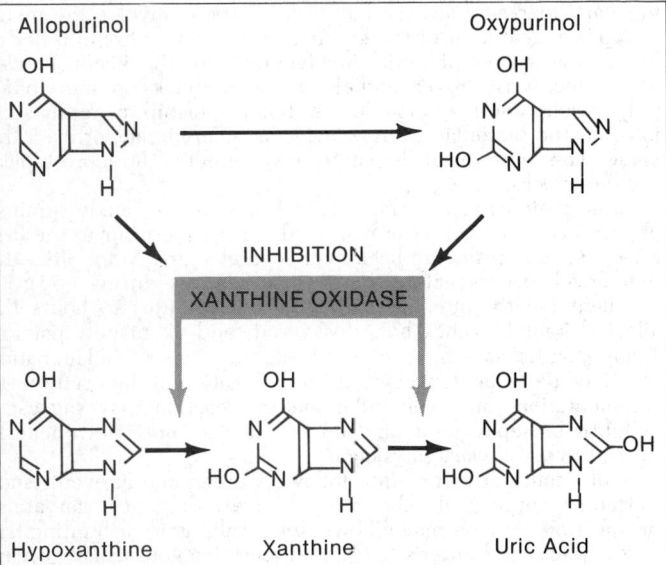

FIGURE 183–1. Pathway of uric acid synthesis catalyzed by xanthine oxidase and the site of action of allopurinol.

glycans are postulated to occur following trauma, with release of additional urate into the already supersaturated synovial fluid and resulting crystallization. The third postulates a joint effusion with trauma, followed by a more rapid rate of reabsorption of water than of solute, resulting in further supersaturation of synovial fluid with urate and precipitation of crystals. The first metatarsophalangeal joint is exposed to the greatest pressure per unit area of any joint in the body during walking, and it and other lower extremity joints, which are the joints predominantly involved in gout, are especially susceptible to trauma. In addition, the low temperature of peripheral leg joints favors crystallization of urate from supersaturated synovial fluid. Thus each of these theories, which are not mutually exclusive, has merit.

Tophi. The pathognomonic lesion of gout is the *tophus*, a deposit of fine acicular crystals of monosodium urate monohydrate, surrounded by a mononuclear reaction and a foreign body granuloma of epithelial and giant cells, some of which may be multinucleate. Urate crystals are water soluble, but when tissues are treated with nonaqueous fixatives (e.g., absolute alcohol), the crystals are preserved and are brilliantly anisotropic and negatively birefringent in compensated polarized light. Tophi are commonly found in articular and other cartilage, synovia, tendon sheaths and other periarticular structures, epiphyseal bone, the subcutaneous layers of the skin, and the interstitial areas of the kidney. The articular cartilages are the most common and at times the exclusive sites of urate deposition. The deposits, although superficial, are actually embedded in the intercellular matrix. In the joint, cartilaginous degeneration, synovial proliferation and pannus, destruction of subchondral bone, proliferation of marginal bone, and sometimes fibrous or bony ankylosis develop. The punched-out lesions of bone commonly seen on roentgenograms represent marrow tophus deposits, which may communicate with the urate crust on the articular surface through defects in the cartilage. In vertebral bodies, urate deposits involve the marrow spaces adjacent to the intervertebral discs, as well as the discs themselves.

All of these sites of urate deposition are rich in proteoglycans, and the postulated role of these substances in attracting and solubilizing urate when organized, and of releasing urate during metabolic turnover, cited above, may serve to explain both localization and occurrence of tophi. Curiously, the process in the tissues evokes only a minimal inflammatory response in comparison with the violence of the acute gouty attack brought about by crystals within the synovial space. Urate crystals stimulate mesenchymal cells of joints to produce collagenase and prostaglandin E_2, both of which may play roles in articular destruction.

The Gouty Kidney. The only distinctive histologic feature of the gouty kidney is the presence of sodium urate crystals in the medulla or pyramids and surrounding round cell and giant cell reaction. These are found in a high percentage of gouty patients at autopsy and are associated with acute and chronic interstitial inflammatory changes, fibrosis, tubular atrophy, glomerulosclerosis, and arteriolar nephrosclerosis. The earliest change in the kidney is an interstitial reaction, maximal near the loops of Henle, associated with tubular damage. In kidneys without tophi, the interstitial reaction tends to spare the medulla and juxtamedullary cortex. Although renal disease is common in gout, it is generally mild and only slowly progressive. The origin of the interstitial nephropathy is not known. It is not even certain that in the absence of crystalline deposits it is related to hyperuricemia. Other possibilities include nephrosclerosis, uric acid stone disease, urinary infection, aging, and lead poisoning. Crystalline deposits may occur within the distal tubules and collecting ducts and are probably composed of uric acid and related to the intratubular concentration of uric acid and the acid pH of the urine; they lead to dilatation and atrophy of the more proximal tubules. Deposits within the interstitium are composed of sodium urate and are believed to be related to the elevated urate concentration of plasma and interstitial fluid.

Uric Acid Urolithiasis. The overall incidence of renal stones in gout is about 20 per cent, about 200-fold higher than in the general population. In 84 per cent of gouty subjects, the stones are pure uric acid (not sodium urate); in 4 per cent, uric acid and calcium oxalate; and in 12 per cent, calcium oxalate or phosphate

alone. The incidence of stones rises with the degree of hyperuricemia and approximates 50 per cent at serum urate values above 12 mg per deciliter. Marked hyperuricemia probably influences stone formation primarily by increasing uric acid *excretion*. The incidence of stones rises above 20 per cent in gouty subjects when the uric acid excretion exceeds 700 mg per 24 hours, and reaches 50 per cent at values above 1100 mg per 24 hours. Patients with increased uricaciduria also have an increased incidence of calcium oxalate stones. Urate (not uric acid) can participate in "heterogeneous nucleation" with calcium oxalate.

Other factors in the pathogenesis of uric acid stones include the *concentration of uric acid in urine,* the *acidity* of urine, and possibly the availability of stone *matrix* and the level of *solubilizing substances* in the urine. The solubility of urate decreases with fall of pH because of the shift to free uric acid. The pKa of uric acid is 5.75. In plasma at pH 7.4, more than 99 per cent is present in ionized form (urate), whereas in urine at pH 5.0, about 85 per cent is un-ionized (uric acid). At this pH only 15 mg of uric acid per deciliter of urine is soluble at 37°C, so supersaturation is required to excrete an average uric acid load in a normal urine volume. The solubility increases more than 10-fold at pH 7.0 and more than 100-fold at pH 8.0 over pH 5.0.

Both gouty and nongouty uric acid stone formers exhibit unusually low urinary pH values when fasting and throughout the day. The persistently acid urine has been attributed to subnormal ammonium production with a compensatory increase in titratable acidity. There is debate whether these data reflect occult or measurable renal damage (e.g., interstitial nephropathy), aging, or an intrinsic renal defect. Regardless of the explanation, the tendency toward persistently acid urine favors uric acid stone formation.

CLINICAL MANIFESTATIONS. The clinical manifestations of gout are conveniently described in four categories: acute gouty arthritis, tophaceous gout, gouty nephropathy, and uric acid urolithiasis.

Clinical gout is extraordinarily rare before puberty, when males at risk for primary idiopathic gout first develop hyperuricemia. Exceptions occur in the juvenile gout of the Lesch-Nyhan syndrome or glycogen storage disease type I, in which marked hyperuricemia is present from infancy. Only about 20 per cent of hyperuricemic subjects ever develop acute gout, although this figure rises as the degree of hyperuricemia increases (Table 183–2). The peak age of onset of gout is about 45 years in men. Thus the usual gouty male is exposed to 30 years of hyperuricemia before an attack occurs. In women gout usually occurs some years after the menopause, when serum urate values rise to hyperuricemic levels in those genetically at risk for gout.

Acute Gouty Arthritis. When acute gouty arthritis develops, it often appears as a fulminating arthritic attack of incapacitating severity. Acute gout is predominantly a disease of the lower extremity. Seventy-five to 90 per cent of initial attacks are monoarticular, and at least half of first attacks involve the metatarsophalangeal joint of the great toe (podagra). Next in order of frequency as sites of initial involvement are the instep, ankle, heel, knee, wrist, finger, and elbow. Later attacks are more often polyarticular and may include the shoulder or hip, or rarely such joints as the sacroiliac, sternoclavicular, mandibular, or even the spine. The more distal the site of involvement, the more typical are the attacks.

Some patients report short, trivial episodes of "ankle sprains" or sore heels or twinges of pain in the great toe prior to the first attack, sometimes going back over several years. More often the first attack occurs with explosive suddenness during apparent excellent health, often at night. Within minutes to hours the affected joint becomes hot, dusky red, and exquisitely painful. Lymphangitis may be evident. Systemic signs of inflammation may include fever, leukocytosis, and elevation of the erythrocyte sedimentation rate. The inflammatory reaction may suggest a cellulitis or septic joint, and on occasion a joint is erroneously incised by an unwary physician.

Acute gouty arthritis often follows a precipitating event, such as trauma, surgery, alcohol or dietary overindulgence, starvation, or infection. Attacks may follow a long walk, golf, or hunting trip (e.g., "pheasant hunter's toe"). Postoperative gout usually occurs on the third to the fifth day. Alcohol intoxication and starvation increase serum urate levels by inhibition of renal excretion by the accompanying lactic acidosis and ketosis, respectively. Regular ingestion of alcohol also increases urate production by stimulating purine nucleotide catabolism. Thus the legendary association of gout with imbibition has a sound metabolic explanation. Experimentally, urate crystals coated with endotoxins are particularly inflammatory; a subthreshold dose of injected uncoated crystals becomes violently inflammatory when endotoxin is given intravenously. Perhaps these observations bear upon the role of infection in precipitating attacks. It is postulated that uricosuric agents and allopurinol may induce acute attacks by lowering synovial fluid urate levels and favoring shedding of synovial crystals during dissolution.

The course of an untreated attack is highly variable. Initial attacks are usually self-limited. Mild attacks may subside in several hours or a few days. Severe attacks may last many days to several weeks. As the attack subsides, the inflamed skin may desquamate. Once the attack has broken, recovery is generally rapid and complete. The patient then re-enters an asymptomatic phase, often termed *intercritical* gout. The subsequent course is difficult to predict. Some patients never have a second attack. Others never fully recover from the first episode and suffer a series of exacerbations leading directly to chronic gouty arthritis. More commonly, a pattern of recurrences develops. In an extensive series, 62 per cent of patients had recurrences within the first year, 16 per cent in 1 to 2 years, 11 per cent in 2 to 5 years, and 4 per cent in 5 to 10 years; 7 per cent had no recurrence during prolonged follow-up. In the untreated patient, the frequency of attacks often increases, and they may become more severe, last longer, and eventually resolve less completely, leading to permanent disability not responsive to measures usually effective in acute attacks.

Tophaceous Gout. Before effective control of hyperuricemia became possible, more than one half of gouty patients developed visible tophi. The incidence now ranges from 13 to 25 per cent. In noncompliant patients it still exceeds 50 per cent. Development of tophi is correlated with the degree of hyperuricemia, severity of renal involvement, and duration of disease. The time from initial attack to visible tophaceous involvement ranged from 3 to 42 years in one large series, with an average of 11.6 years. In 0.5 per cent of patients, tophi are present at the time of the initial attack; virtually all such patients have gout secondary to a myeloproliferative disease.

Chronic gouty arthritis is a consequence of the progressive inability to dispose of urate as rapidly as it is produced. Crystalline deposits of urate appear in and around joints. Destruction of tissue is particularly evident in cartilage and bone, leading to radiolucent "punched-out" lesions and to cortical erosions with characteristic "overhanging margins" (Fig. 183–2). A frequent site of tophaceous deposits is the external ear, especially the helix and antihelix. Subcutaneous deposits, especially of fingertips, palms, and soles, may be visible as yellowish-white infiltrates. Tophaceous deposits may produce irregular asymmetric tumescences over joints. The classic gout shoe has a window cut to accommodate a tender prominent joint, usually the first metatarsophalangeal. At later stages, fusiform or nodular enlargements of Achilles tendons, or saccular distentions of olecranon bursae, are common and characteristic.

The process of tophaceous deposition advances insidiously, and although the tophi themselves are relatively painless, often progressive stiffness and persistent aching limit the use of affected joints. Eventually, extensive destruction of joints and large subcutaneous tophi may lead to grotesque deformities and progressive crippling (Fig. 183–2). The tense, shiny, thin skin overlying

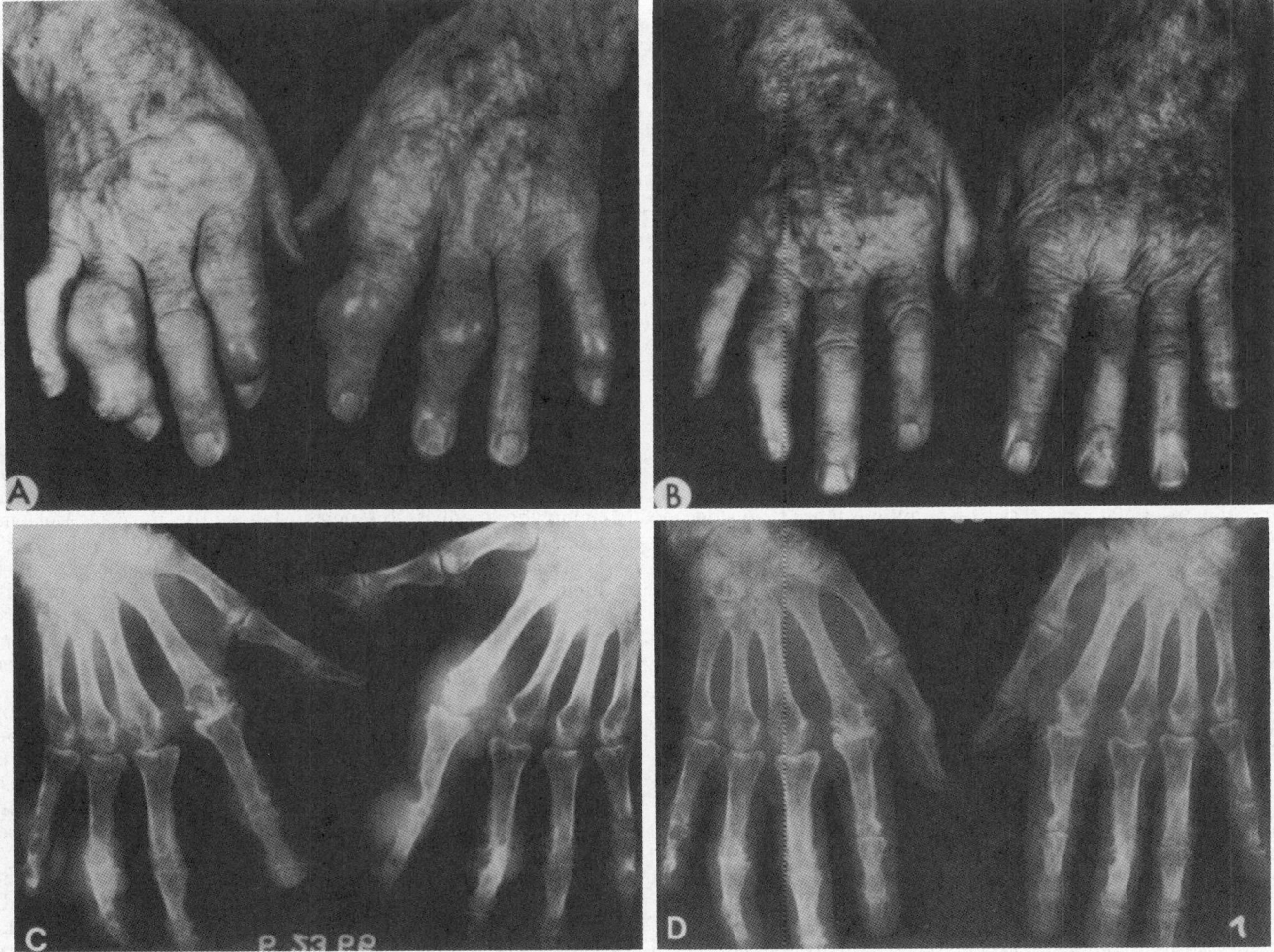

FIGURE 183–2. Chronic gouty arthritis (*A*) with tophaeceous destruction of bone and joints (*C*), and improvement after three years of treatment with allopurinol, prophylactic colchicine, and a moderately low purine diet (*B* and *D*). (Courtesy of R. Wayne Rundles, Duke University Medical Center.)

the tophus may ulcerate and extrude white chalky or pasty material composed of myriads of fine, needle-like crystals. The olecranon bursa may be massively distended with "urate milk." Rarely, tophi may involve the tongue, epiglottis, vocal cords, arytenoid cartilage, corpus cavernosum and prepuce of the penis, aorta, aortic or mitral valves, and cardiac conducting system, causing rhythm disturbances. They do not involve the liver, spleen, lungs, or central nervous system.

As chronic gouty changes and renal disease advance, acute attacks occur less frequently and are milder. No joint is exempt from chronic gouty involvement, although those of the lower extremity and hand are most commonly involved. The hip and spinal joints are rarely affected in the absence of extensive disease elsewhere. Radiographic changes of the sacroiliac joint and aseptic necrosis of the hip are sometimes attributable to gout.

Gouty Nephropathy. Renal disease is common in gout. One third of patients show isosthenuria and moderate proteinuria. The glomerular filtration rate is well preserved in many gouty subjects, but in others it gradually falls. Decline in renal function appears to be correlated with aging, renovascular disease and hypertension, renal calculi, pyelonephritis, or independently occurring nephropathy, including that of lead poisoning. Only occasionally is it ascribable to gout alone. Hyperuricemia alone had no deleterious effect upon renal function during follow-up studies of gouty subjects ranging up to 12 years (Berger and Yu). Renal dysfunction does not shorten life expectancy in the average gouty subject, even though uremia is the eventual cause of death in 17 to 25 per cent of subjects. The majority of gouty patients die of cardiac or cerebrovascular disease (60 per cent) or malignant disease, which occur in about the same incidence and at about the same time of life as in nongouty American men.

Hypertension is present in one third to one half of patients and may be severe (diastolic pressure >130 mm Hg) in 10 per cent. Arterial and arteriolar nephrosclerosis are frequently prominent post mortem. There are no characteristic clinical or laboratory features to distinguish gouty kidney from other causes of chronic renal failure. Renal failure from gouty nephropathy in the absence of gouty arthritis, tophi, or stones is extraordinarily rare; indeed, the entity is open to question.

Gouty nephropathy, sometimes referred to as *urate nephropathy* to emphasize the identity of the interstitial crystals, must be distinguished from *uric acid nephropathy*, an entirely different entity leading to acute renal failure from tubular obstruction by uric acid crystals (see Ch. 80).

Urolithiasis. The incidence of urolithiasis in gout is correlated with both the degree of hyperuricemia and the magnitude of the 24-hour uric acid excretion. Above serum levels of 12 to 13 mg per deciliter or excretion values of 1100 mg per 24 hours, the incidence is 50 per cent. Many of these subjects will have secondary gout, with a myeloproliferative disease such as polycythemia vera or myeloid metaplasia. The incidence of stones in such patients is 35 to 40 per cent. Of gouty subjects who pass stones, about one third have their first episode of urolithiasis before the onset of gouty arthritis, sometimes more than a decade earlier. Pure uric acid stones are radiolucent and are demonstrable in the body only by use of contrast media. Renal stones are reduced in frequency in gouty patients given allopurinol.

GOUT ASSOCIATED WITH SPECIFIC ENZYME DEFECTS. Gout occurring on the basis of specific enzyme defects has special clinical features. These forms of gout are rare, accounting for fewer than 1 per cent of cases.

Glycogen Storage Disease Type I (see Ch. 169). Over 50 cases of von Gierke's glycogen storage disease (glucose-6-phosphatase deficiency) and gout have been recorded. Gout does not complicate other forms of glycogen storage disease, although hyperuricemia has been reported in several forms with muscle involvement and attributed to excessive adenosine triphosphate (ATP) degradation following exercise. Subjects with glycogen storage disease type I may develop gouty arthritis by the end of the first decade of life. Chronic tophaceous gout and gouty nephropathy may account for a major portion of morbidity when these patients become adults. The sexes are involved equally. Avoidance of nocturnal hypoglycemia by a diet high in starch or by continuous intragastric feeding may markedly reduce or even correct hyperuricemia and ameliorate gout. The hyperuricemia also responds

to allopurinol, less well to uricosuric agents because of renal disease.

Hypoxanthine-Guanine Phosphoribosyltransferase Deficiency. Deficiency of HPRT gives rise to two different X-linked syndromes. A complete deficiency is associated with the Lesch-Nyhan syndrome (see Ch. 184). There is extreme exaggeration of uric acid production, and the greatly increased excretion leads to crystalluria, renal stones with ureteral colic, and sometimes uric acid nephropathy. Death from renal failure usually occurs by age 10; if allopurinol therapy is begun early, the patients may live into their 20's. A few of the more than 100 reported patients, all males, have had typical attacks of gouty arthritis.

An incomplete deficiency of HPRT is associated with renal stones and recurrent acute gouty arthritis. Erythrocytes show 0.2 to 50 per cent of normal HPRT activity; the disorder is heterogeneous. Fifteen per cent of patients show minimal to moderate neurologic dysfunction resembling spinocerebellar ataxis or cerebral palsy. A few have survived neonatal episodes of uric acid nephropathy. Gout usually begins in the second or third decade; tophi develop early. Three quarters of patients have renal stones, half of these before age 10. These subjects have more marked hyperuricemia (usually >10 mg per deciliter) and uricaciduria (usually >1 gram per 24 hours) than most gouty subjects. More than 100 cases—again, all males—have been described. HPRT normally catalyzes a reaction between hypoxanthine or guanine and PP-ribose-P in reconstituting ribonucleotides, often called a "salvage" reaction. In HPRT deficiency, intracellular PP-ribose-P levels are raised and drive the first reaction of purine biosynthesis to excess. The female heterozygous carriers of complete HPRT deficiency are not hyperuricemic, and their erythrocytes show normal HPRT assay values. Carriers of the partial defect may be hyperuricemic and may show intermediate levels of HPRT activity. Presumably, only cells possessing at least minimal HPRT activity survive lyonization. Heterozygotes for the partial defect may develop uric acid stones or typical gout, which may occur before the menopause. Partial HPRT deficiency should be considered in all women with gout or uric acid stones who exhibit raised urinary uric acid excretion values.

Phosphoribosylpyrophosphate Synthetase Variants. Patients with these variants resemble those with partial HPRT deficiency in showing marked hyperuricemia and uricaciduria and in developing uric acid stones or gout, and sometimes uric acid nephropathy, at an early age. They do not have neurologic abnormalities. Purine overproduction is prodigious. The enzyme abnormalities, of which there are four different types leading to increased activity (see Ch. 177), result in increased intracellular concentrations of PP-ribose-P and excessive purine biosynthesis. This, too, is an X-linked disorder, and all gouty patients are males. Fewer than 20 families with this disorder have been identified.

SECONDARY GOUT. Any acquired hyperuricemic state may be complicated by secondary gout. This disorder occurs in 5 to 10 per cent of patients with polycythemia vera or myeloid metaplasia, occasionally in secondary polycythemia complicating congenital heart disease or chronic pulmonary disease, in chronic myelogenous leukemia, in multiple myeloma, or in chronic hemolytic anemias. In such instances the mean age of onset is later (59 years), women are more commonly involved (16 per cent), and both serum and urinary uric acid values tend to be higher than in idiopathic primary gout. Acute gouty arthritis may occasionally antedate evidence of the myeloproliferative disorder by many months, or even by several years. A syndrome of coexisting sarcoidosis, psoriasis, and gout has been described but may represent fortuitous concurrence of common diseases.

In all the instances mentioned above, hyperuricemia appears to result from an increase in turnover of nucleic acid. Hyperuricemia may also result from reduced renal excretion of urate, either because of drug effects or because of parenchymal disease.

Hyperuricemia frequently follows the use of potent diuretic agents. Mean increases in serum urate concentrations are less than 2 mg per deciliter, but some subjects exhibit rises of 4 to 5 mg per deciliter. The hyperuricemic effect of diuretic agents results from salt and water loss, volume contraction, and avid solute reabsorption (including urate) in the proximal tubule. Typical gouty attacks may occur in patients receiving such drugs as hydrochlorothiazide, ethacrynic acid, or furosemide. In the 14-year study of the adult population of Framingham, Massachusetts, one half of the new cases of gout occurred in subjects taking potent diuretics. Ingestion of many other drugs may also lead to hyperuricemia. For example, patients with chronic renal failure treated with erythropoietin frequently develop hyperuricemia. Three to 5 per cent of patients with gout have diabetes, but this incidence is not far from that of diabetes in the population of equivalent age. In markedly obese patients, total caloric restriction may result in extreme hyperuricemia, which is correlated with serum levels of beta-hydroxybutyric acid and may be associated with severe attacks of acute gouty arthritis, especially of knees and ankles.

Chronic renal disease is a frequent cause of hyperuricemia, but only about 1 patient per 1000 develops gout. Uremia appears to interfere in some way with the inflammatory response to urate crystals. Gout continues to be found in patients who survive lead exposure early in life and go on to develop slowly progressive lead nephropathy. In addition, saturnine gout is particularly prevalent in the southeastern United States, where it is attributed to the chronic ingestion of moonshine whiskey of high lead content with resulting renal tubular damage. Lead nephropathy and polycystic renal disease predispose to gout more often than do other forms of chronic renal disease.

DIAGNOSIS. The diagnosis of acute gouty arthritis is not difficult when there is an explosive onset of a typical inflammatory attack of characteristic severity in a peripheral joint, especially of the lower extremity. The diagnosis is established by the demonstration of typical negatively birefringent needle-shaped crystals of sodium urate in the leukocytes of synovial fluid (Fig. 183–3). With proper technique, including the use of a polarizing microscope, intraleukocytic sodium urate crystals are found in over 95 per cent of aspirates from joints in acute gout. The leukocyte count may range from 1000 to more than 50,000, depending on the acuteness of the inflammation. A Gram stain should always be obtained to evaluate infection, which may coexist. In the rare event of failure to find crystals on the first attempt, a second aspirate obtained some hours later is usually positive. Urate crystals must be distinguished from calcium pyrophosphate dihydrate crystals of pseudogout. The latter are weakly positively birefringent under polarized light and usually more rectangular than urate crystals. A rapid response of pain and inflammation to the administration of colchicine is so characteristic as to be of diagnostic value as well. Responses of rheumatoid arthritis and sarcoid arthritis to colchicine are not so dramatic or complete as those in gout. The finding of hyperuricemia is anticipated and helpful, but since hyperuricemia is common (13 per cent of hospitalized male patients), it may coexist with other acute arthropathies. The presence of tophi or of typical roentgenographic findings of punched-out, destructive bone lesions helps establish the diagnosis of chronic tophaceous gout. In 70 per cent

of patients with crystal-proven gout, extracellular urate crystals are demonstrable in asymptomatic first metatarsophalangeal joints. Such crystals are rare (5 per cent) in hyperuricemic subjects who have never had clinical gout.

Each gouty patient should also have a determination of the 24-hour urinary excretion of uric acid. The sample should be collected after 3 days of moderate purine restriction, during an intercritical period. Values of greater than 600 mg per 1.72 square meters per day under these conditions probably indicate overproduction, and those of over 800 mg per day warrant additional studies for a specific subtype of primary gout, such as HPRT deficiency of PP-ribose-P synthetase overactivity, or of secondary gout, such as a myeloproliferative disorder. Elevated urinary uric acid values also signify that the patient is at higher risk for renal stone and represent an indication for allopurinol rather than uricosuric drug therapy for gout.

Chronic gouty arthritis may be diagnosed by the presence of urate deposits in or near the affected joints or bursae or of soft tissue deposits in the helix of the ear, the fingertips, the Achilles tendon, or other locations. The diagnosis may be confirmed by removal of the chalky contents of a tophus, by microscopic identification of sodium urate crystals by optical means, by chemical identification by the murexide test, or, preferably, by ultraviolet spectrophotometry and degradation by uricase.

DIFFERENTIAL DIAGNOSIS. Acute gout must be differentiated from acute rheumatic fever, rheumatoid arthritis, traumatic arthritis, osteoarthritis, pyogenic arthritis, sarcoid arthritis, cellulitis, bursitis, tendinitis, and thrombophlebitis. Podagra, the most common initial presentation of gout, can be mimicked by trauma, degenerative arthritis, acute sarcoidosis, psoriatic arthritis, pseudogout, palindromic rheumatism, Reiter's syndrome, or infection. Acute monoarticular arthritis of the great toe in the immediate postoperative period following parathyroidectomy can be caused by hydroxyapatite crystals. These various forms of "pseudopodagra" may be suggested by a negative examination of synovial fluid for urate crystals. Pseudogout (see Ch. 271), which is manifested by acute attacks of arthritis of knees and other joints, is usually accompanied by calcification of joint cartilage; the synovial fluid contains nonurate crystals of calcium pyrophosphate. However, gout and pseudogout may coexist, and both types of crystals will then be found in synovial fluid leukocytes.

Chronic gouty arthritis must chiefly be differentiated from rheumatoid arthritis, osteoarthritis, traumatic arthritis, and residua of pyogenic arthritis. The history of onset, progression, response to colchicine, and demonstration of hyperuricemia, asymmetric tumescences, typical roentgenographic changes, and tophi or crystals of urate in synovial fluid and leukocytes should establish the diagnosis.

TREATMENT. The therapeutic aims in gout are (1) to terminate the acute gouty attack as promptly and gently as possible, (2) to prevent recurrences of acute gouty arthritis, (3) to prevent or reverse complications of the disease resulting from deposition of sodium urate in joints and kidneys, and (4) to prevent formation of uric acid kidney stones. The therapeutic program differs according to the stage of the disease and the complications present. In the majority of patients it is possible to abort or prevent acute attacks, to control hyperuricemia, and to prevent chronic gouty arthritis, nephropathy, and stones.

Acute Attack. The affected joint should be placed at rest, and an anti-inflammatory agent administered promptly. Three types of agents are available: colchicine, nonsteroidal anti-inflammatory agents, and glucocorticoids (or adrenocorticotropic hormone [ACTH]). *Colchicine* is the only agent of specific diagnostic value in acute gout. It should be given as soon as the diagnosis is suspected. The initial dose of 0.6 to 1.2 mg of colchicine is followed by 0.6 mg every hour for 8 hours and then every 2 hours until pain is relieved or until nausea, vomiting, cramping, or diarrhea develops. Maximum tolerated doses range from 4 to 8 mg. In many patients dramatic relief of pain and onset of gastrointestinal side effects occur simultaneously. The diarrhea may be treated with paregoric, 4 ml, or Kaopectate, 30 ml, after each loose stool. Colchicine should be discontinued until gastrointestinal symptoms subside. Since the effective dose of colchicine varies, each patient should learn his or her own tolerance dose and stop just short of this in treatment of subsequent attacks. If

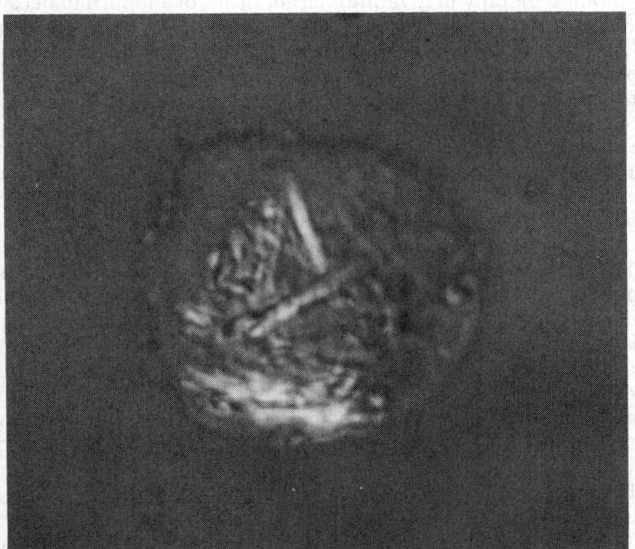

FIGURE 183–3. Sodium urate monohydrate crystals phagocytized by leukocyte in synovial fluid from acute gouty arthritis, examined by polarized light. (Courtesy of Edward W. Holmes, Duke University Medical Center.)

started promptly, colchicine affords relief over 90 per cent of the time; if treatment is delayed beyond 12 hours, only 75 per cent of patients will respond within 24 to 48 hours. Since colchicine is concentrated within cells and turns over with a half-life of about 30 hours, repeated courses of colchicine carry a higher risk of toxicity; treatment failures should be treated with a nonsteroidal anti-inflammatory drug (NSAID).

Colchicine may also be given intravenously (subcutaneous infiltration may result in tissue necrosis). The usual initial dose is 1 to 2 mg in 20 ml of saline solution given slowly, and if a single dose is not effective, the injection may be repeated once in 4 to 5 hours (maximum intravenous dose, 3 to 5 mg). Gastrointestinal symptoms are uncommon with intravenous administration, although occasionally nausea occurs.

Dose-related toxic responses to colchicine include alopecia (reversible), bone marrow suppression (leukopenia, thrombocytopenia, anemia), and hepatocellular damage. The drug should not be used in patients with advanced hepatic or renal disease.

NSAID's are equally effective in acute gout and are usually preferred to colchicine because they are so much milder for the patient. Indomethacin has been most widely used. It is given orally in initial doses of 50 mg three or four times a day. When pain is relieved, doses are tapered over another 48 to 72 hours. Other NSAID's, such as *naproxen* and *ibuprofen*, can also be used. With all NSAID's, renal function should be monitored, especially in hypertensive patients. *Phenylbutazone* and *oxyphenbutazone* (Tandearil) are also effective in acute gouty arthritis and may be preferred when the gouty attack has proceeded for some time or when the attack does not abate completely with colchicine or indomethacin. The initial dose is 400 mg orally, followed by 100 mg every 4 to 8 hours for 2 to 3 days. Bone marrow suppression may rarely occur, even after a short course of either drug.

If full doses of colchicine or NSAID's are contraindicated (e.g., in postoperative gout) or ineffective, *ACTH* may be employed by intravenous drip (40 units per day) or as intramuscular gel (40 to 80 units per day), or systemic glucocorticoids may be given for 2 to 3 days, rarely longer, following which the doses are reduced in stepwise fashion and discontinued. Unfortunately, rebound attacks of gout are rather common after such therapy. *Triamcinolone hexacetonide* in a dose of 5 to 20 mg injected intra-articularly into the involved joint is useful in treating acute gout limited to a single joint or bursa, particularly in patients in whom the standard drugs cannot be used, and relief from pain is usually prompt and complete within 24 to 36 hours. Steroid hormones are not recommended for parenteral use in acute gout, as the effects are inconsistent and rebound attacks frequent.

Uricosuric agents and allopurinol are of no value in treatment of the acute attack.

Interval Phase. The patient with gout should avoid high-purine foods so as to lessen the burden of uric acid excretion. A severe limitation of purine-containing foods is rarely indicated, unless renal function is poor. Gradual weight reduction is indicated if the patient is overweight and may of itself reduce hyperuricemia and the tendency to develop attacks of gout. Sudden weight reduction may precipitate gouty attacks and should be avoided. In general, diets of moderate protein content, somewhat low in fat, are preferred. Hypertension should be treated vigorously, even if antihypertensive agents worsen hyperuricemia; the result can be countered with appropriate antihyperuricemic drug therapy.

A high fluid intake is advisable to maintain a urinary output of 2000 ml per day to promote uric acid excretion. Beer, ale, and wine may precipitate attacks. Distilled alcoholic beverages in moderation generally have little influence on the gouty process. Illicit liquor (moonshine) should be prohibited. Excessive alcohol use in any form should be avoided, as it enhances purine production and also leads to hypertriglyceridemia.

Patients who recognize prodromal symptoms may abort acute attacks by prompt institution of colchicine, phenylbutazone, or indomethacin therapy; they frequently require only a few tablets to achieve success. The daily ingestion of 0.6 to 1.8 mg of colchicine is generally effective in reducing the number of acute gouty attacks in patients who are subject to frequent episodes. Toxicity is rare, but may include alopecia, bone marrow suppres-

sion, and hepatocellular damage. Maintenance colchicine therapy is particularly important during the first months or year after institution of uricosuric drugs or of allopurinol. Daily ingestion of indomethacin, 25 or 50 mg, has also been employed for this purpose and appears to be effective. The risks of renal and gastrointestinal toxicity make use of indomethacin undesirable as a prophylactic agent or as regular therapy for chronic gouty arthritis.

Chronic Gouty Arthritis. Use of a drug to lower the serum level of uric acid to 6 mg per 100 ml or less is indicated in all gouty patients with visible tophi, with roentgenographic evidence of urate deposits, or with a history of two or more major attacks of acute gouty arthritis. Allopurinol is the drug of choice unless the patient is already well managed with a uricosuric agent. With either type of agent the number of acute gouty attacks may be increased during the first few months unless maintenance colchicine therapy is given, whereas after 12 to 18 months the number may be decidedly reduced.

Allopurinol controls serum urate levels by inhibiting xanthine oxidase and thereby regulating production of uric acid (see Fig. 183–1). Allopurinol is converted to oxypurinol in the body, and the latter compound has a longer biologic half-life (28 hours), ultimately being largely excreted in the urine. Inhibition of conversion of hypoxanthine and xanthine to uric acid permits these precursors to be excreted instead. In gouty subjects other than those with HPRT deficiency, the increment in hypoxanthine plus xanthine excretion is only about two thirds of the decrement in uric acid excretion, presumably because of enhanced feedback inhibition of purine synthesis de novo by nucleotides reconstituted from hypoxanthine. The induced xanthinuria has not resulted in xanthine stone formation in the usual gouty subjects but has done so in a rare patient with HPRT deficiency and in patients being treated with antineoplastic agents. Use of allopurinol results in reduction of levels of uric acid in serum *and in urine*. The drug is effective even in the presence of renal failure, when uricosuric agents generally are not. Its action is not blocked by salicylates. The usual dose is 300 mg, given orally once a day. In the presence of moderate nitrogen retention, the dose of allopurinol should be reduced by one half or more (see Ch. 23), as the biologic half-life of the active metabolite, oxypurinol, is prolonged. Allopurinol is usually well tolerated but may cause gastric irritation, diarrhea, or skin rash or induce an attack of gout. Toxic hepatitis, epidermal necrolysis, and vasculitis may occasionally be severe, even fatal. Toxic effects are more frequent and more severe in the presence of renal failure. Intramuscular crystals of xanthine and oxypurinol have been described in patients receiving allopurinol, but their significance in terms of toxicity is not clear. Uricosuric agents may be used concurrently with allopurinol to hasten mobilization of urate deposits, but combined therapy may require larger doses of allopurinol because uricosuric drugs also enhance the excretion of oxypurinol. Since allopurinol decreases uric acid excretion, it is also very useful in controlling uric acid stone formation, especially in patients who are overproducers of uric acid. If the serum urate values can be controlled at levels below saturation of urate in body fluids, extensive resolution of soft tissue tophi and modest reduction in the size of bone erosions may be achieved, together with some recalcification of bone lesions (see Fig. 183–2). Joint mobility and comfort may be greatly improved.

Uricosuric drugs block tubular reabsorption of filtered urate. Those of use in gout are probenecid and sulfinpyrazone. These agents begin to lose effectiveness when the creatinine clearance falls below 80 ml per minute and are ineffective when the clearance falls below 30 ml per minute. *Probenecid* is given in doses of 0.5 gram to 3 grams daily in two or three evenly spaced doses (average dose, 1 to 1.5 grams). This drug may produce gastrointestinal upsets, headaches, or skin rash. *Sulfinpyrazone* may be given in doses of 100 to 600 mg daily in three or four divided doses (average dose, 300 mg). This drug is related to phenylbutazone and may cause untoward reactions but is generally somewhat better tolerated than probenecid. *Salicylates* block the uricosuric action of both probenecid and sulfinpyrazone and must not be used concurrently. Salicylates are uricosuric when given in high doses (4 to 6 grams daily), but few patients can tolerate these quantities.

With all uricosuric agents, the doses should be low initially to avoid sudden excretion of large quantities of urate and should be increased at weekly intervals to maintenance levels. Fluids should be forced to prevent formation of concentrated urine, especially during the late hours of the night. During the first days or weeks of therapy, the urine should be kept at pH 6 or above, by administration of sodium bicarbonate or sodium citrate–citric acid (Shohl's solution); this may be difficult to achieve, as acid urine tends to be produced in gouty patients. In patients in whom urate is being mobilized, and especially those in whom uric acid gravel is formed, alkalinization during the night, when fluid intake is reduced, is important. A single 250-mg tablet of acetazolamide (Diamox) taken at bedtime serves to keep the urine alkaline and dilute throughout the night.

In selected patients surgical removal of large extra-articular urate deposits, such as those in olecranon bursae, may be advisable. Occasionally, amputation of irreparably damaged digits, especially those containing draining sinuses, is indicated. Physical therapy and appropriate self-help devices are valuable in patients who are partially disabled.

Asymptomatic Hyperuricemia. Asymptomatic hyperuricemia is frequent in family members of patients with gout and in the general population. It usually requires no therapy, as only about one fifth of patients ever develop articular attacks, and adequate therapy can be instituted when these supervene. Exceptions may exist in patients with markedly elevated serum levels of uric acid, especially if urinary urate excretion is low and there is a family history of tophaceous disease. In such circumstances the asymptomatic subject should be treated with allopurinol before articular or renal complications develop. It is essential that the physician maintain frequent close observation of the patient.

Berger, L. Yu T-F: Renal function in gout: IV. An analysis of 524 gouty subjects including long-term follow-up studies. Am J Med 59:605, 1975. *An important study showing that deterioration of renal function in gout is largely associated with aging, renovascular disease, hypertension, renal calculi with pyelonephritis, or independently occurring nephropathy. Hyperuricemia alone had no deleterious effect on renal function over periods up to 12 years.*

Cherian PV, Schumacher HR Jr: Immunochemical and ultrastructural characterization of serum proteins associated with monosodium urate crystals (MSU) in synovial fluid cells from patients with gout. Ultrastruct Pathol 10:209, 1986. *Various proteins associated with intracellular urate crystals, IgG > IgM or IgA > C3 or fibrinogen, may influence the inflammatory properties of those crystals.*

Reibman J, Haines KA, Rich AM, et al.: Colchicine inhibits ionophore-induced formation of leukotriene B4 by human neutrophils: The role of microtubules. J Immunol 136:1027, 1986. *The mechanisms of colchicine action in inhibiting production of leukotriene B4 by neutrophils appears to depend upon its effect on the number and integrity of the microtubules.*

Simkin PS: Uric acid excretion in patients with gout. Arthritis Rheum 22:98, 1979. *An analysis of six published studies relating the rate of urate excretion to plasma urate levels in normal and gouty subjects. The kidneys of the average gouty person lag significantly behind the normal in their response to any concentration of plasma urate. The kidneys of overproducers (38 of 73 gouty subjects) were no less handicapped than those of other gouty subjects.*

Spillberg I, Mandell B, Mehta J, et al.: Mechanism of action of colchicine in acute urate crystal–induced arthritis. J Clin Invest 64:775, 1979. *Phagocytosis of urate crystals by neutrophils induces the synthesis and release of a glycoprotein that is chemotactic both in vitro and in vivo. Colchicine decreases production and release of this factor. Colchicine abrogates the acute arthritis produced by urate crystals in rabbits but has no effect upon the arthritis induced by injection of purified cell-derived chemotactic factor.*

Wyngaarden JB, Kelley WN: Gout. In Stanbury JB, Wyngaarden JB, Fredrickson DS, et al. (eds.): The Metabolic Basis of Inherited Disease. 5th ed. New York, McGraw-Hill Book Company, 1983. *A detailed account of purine metabolism and the pathogenesis of primary gout.*

Wyngaarden JB, Kelley WN: Gout and Hyperuricemia. New York, Grune & Stratton, 1976. *Everything you have always wanted to know about gout but never dared to ask, condensed into 500 pages.*

184 Other Disorders of Purine Metabolism

Edward W. Holmes

XANTHINURIA

Classic xanthinuria, which is inherited as an autosomal recessive trait, is the consequence of an isolated deficiency of xanthine oxidase. As a result of this enzyme deficiency, uric acid is replaced by xanthine and hypoxanthine as the end-products of purine metabolism. Serum urate concentrations in these patients range from 0 to 1.4 mg per deciliter, and urinary uric acid excretion ranges from 0 to 8 mg per day; serum oxypurine (xanthine plus hypoxanthine) concentrations and urine oxypurine excretion are increased in this disorder.

More than 50 patients with classic xanthinuria have been described, and the prevalence of this disorder is estimated to be approximately 1 in 45,000. Over 50 per cent of individuals with classic xanthinuria are asymptomatic, the diagnosis being suspected by the incidental finding of a very low serum urate concentration during evaluation of presumably unrelated medical problems. The diagnosis is virtually established by the demonstration of low serum and urinary uric acid levels in association with increased urinary oxypurine excretion, and it is confirmed by assaying liver or intestinal mucosa for xanthine oxidase activity. One third of patients develop radiolucent renal calculi composed of xanthine. Four adult patients have had myopathic symptoms characterized by muscle cramps following exercise, and crystalline deposits of xanthine and hypoxanthine have been found in skeletal muscle. Recurrent polyarthritis has been described in three patients, and it has been suggested, but not established, that this symptom may represent crystal-induced synovitis.

A subtype of xanthinuria has been described in which the deficiency of xanthine oxidase is associated with a deficiency of sulfite oxidase. Both of these enzymes require a molybdenum cofactor for catalytic activity, and absence of this cofactor has been demonstrated in the liver of a patient with this combined enzyme defect. Fifteen patients with an inherited deficiency of these two enzymes have been reported, and all presented in the first weeks of life with a severe neurologic disorder characteristic of isolated sulfite oxidase deficiency. Symptoms include feeding difficulties from birth, tonic-clonic seizures, nystagmus, enophthalmus, ocular lens dislocation, and Brushfield spots. As in isolated sulfite oxidase deficiency, urinary excretion of sulfate is low, while that of sulfite, thiosulfate, S-sulfocysteine, and taurine is increased. Characteristic biochemical findings of xanthinuria are also present.

An acquired phenocopy of the combined defect has been described in a 20-year-old male with short-bowel syndrome maintained for 18 months with total parenteral nutrition. In addition to hypouricemia and hypouricaciduria, urinary excretion of sulfite and thiosulfate was increased while excretion of sulfate was decreased. Following infusion of commercially available amino acid solutions the patient experienced headaches, night blindness, irritability, lethargy, and then coma.

The prognosis in classic xanthinuria is excellent, as shown by the high percentage of patients who are asymptomatic. Therapy for xanthine calculi includes high fluid intake, and on occasion allopurinol has been used in patients with residual xanthine oxidase activity to increase the excretion of hypoxanthine relative to xanthine, the former being more soluble than the latter. In patients with the inherited form of combined xanthine oxidase and sulfite oxidase deficiency, the neurologic symptoms have been refractory to therapy with a number of agents, including oral ammonium molybdate. With the acquired form of this combined disorder, treatment with ammonium molybdate reversed the biochemical abnormalities, and the neurologic symptoms were markedly ameliorated.

Holmes EW, Wyngaarden JB: Hereditary xanthinuria. In Scriver CR, Beaudet AL, Sly WS, et al. (eds.): The Metabolic Basis of Inherited Disease. 6th ed. New York, McGraw-Hill, 1989, pp 1085–1094. *A thorough coverage of the clinical and biochemical abnormalities found in classic xanthinuria.*

Johnson JL, Wadman SK: Molybdenum cofactor deficiency. In Scriver CR, Beaudet AL, Sly WS, et al. (eds.): The Metabolic Basis of Inherited Disease. 6th ed. New York, McGraw-Hill, 1989, pp 1463–1475. *Metabolic and clinical observations on 15 patients with this disorder.*

THE LESCH-NYHAN SYNDROME AND PARTIAL DEFICIENCY OF HYPOXANTHINE-GUANINE PHOSPHORIBOSYLTRANSFERASE

The Lesch-Nyhan syndrome, caused by a virtually complete deficiency of hypoxanthine-guanine phosphoribosyltransferase (HPRT) activity, is manifested clinically by hyperuricemia, excessive production of uric acid, and neurologic features, including self-mutilation, choreoathetosis, spasticity, and mental retardation. Partial deficiency of HPRT activity is associated with uric acid overproduction, severe gout, and occasionally neurologic abnormalities, but self-mutilation is absent. The Lesch-Nyhan syndrome occurs in about 1 in 100,000 births, and partial deficiency of HPRT is noted in less than 1 per cent of the gouty population.

ETIOLOGY AND PATHOGENESIS. The gene for HPRT is located on the X chromosome. Studies employing protein sequencing, RNA mapping, restriction fragment length polymorphism (RFLP), and DNA sequencing techniques have revealed a striking molecular heterogeneity as the basis for this disorder. Failure to reutilize hypoxanthine in the salvage pathway as a result of HPRT deficiency leads to increased oxidation of this purine base to uric acid. An increase in the intracellular concentration of phosphoribosyl-pyrophosphate, which also results from reduction in hypoxanthine reutilization, leads to an increase in the rate of purine biosynthesis de novo. The combined effect of these abnormalities is increased uric acid production resulting in hyperuricaciduria, which predisposes to uric acid crystal and stone formation, and hyperuricemia, which leads to gouty arthritis and tophaceous deposits. The biochemical basis for the unusual and devastating neurologic abnormalities seen in the Lesch-Nyhan syndrome is not clearly understood, but abnormalities in dopamine neuron function have been described. Positron-emission tomography has demonstrated a selective decrease in glucose utilization in the caudate nucleus.

CLINICAL MANIFESTATIONS. The deficiency of HPRT activity is fully expressed only in affected males. Females heterozygous for HPRT deficiency may have subtle abnormalities in purine metabolism, but they are generally asymptomatic.

Infants with the Lesch-Nyhan syndrome are normal at birth, and the earliest consistent abnormality is a delay in motor development noted at 3 to 4 months of age. Between 8 and 12 months, extrapyramidal signs develop, leading to choreoathetosis, and at about 1 year of age signs of pyramidal tract involvement, such as hyperreflexia, clonus, and scissoring of the legs, appear. Compulsive self-destructive behavior appears any time between early childhood and adolescence. This is the most distinctive neurologic feature of the syndrome and is manifested by biting of the fingers, lips, and buccal mucosa. Repeated attempts at self-injury, such as placing extremities in dangerous areas and self-inflicted head trauma, are also common. Sensation is intact in these children. Mental retardation is noted in most cases, but it is unclear whether the enzyme deficiency per se causes this or whether it is the result of poor performance on formal testing in children with dysarthria and choreoathetosis. Growth retardation is also a prominent feature of the syndrome. Uric acid crystalluria may be noted as orange crystals on the diaper during the first weeks of life and in untreated patients progresses to uric acid nephrolithiasis, obstructive uropathy, and azotemia. Hyperuricemia is usually present and may attain levels of 18 mg per deciliter, but the serum urate concentration may be normal, especially before puberty. Gout is unusual in the Lesch-Nyhan syndrome before 12 to 15 years of age. Death usually occurs in the second or third decade from infection or renal failure.

Patients with partial deficiency of HPRT develop uric acid crystalluria and renal calculi in childhood, and gouty arthritis often occurs before 20 years of age. Neurologic manifestations, including mental retardation, mild spastic quadriplegia, dysarthria, cerebellar ataxia, and seizures, are noted in 20 per cent of patients with partial HPRT deficiency, but self-mutilation does not develop. Patients with partial HPRT deficiency may seek medical attention with the only symptom being the passage of a renal calculus or an attack of gouty arthritis. Life expectancy is normal in these patients.

DIAGNOSIS. Self-destructive behavior is the most distinguishing clinical feature of the Lesch-Nyhan syndrome; whereas retarded children with other disorders will bite their fingers, mutilation to the point of tissue destruction is rare in any disorder other than the Lesch-Nyhan syndrome. Severe self-biting in other neurologic disorders is usually associated with a loss of pain sensation. As pointed out, hyperuricemia is usually present, but this is not an invariable finding. The diagnosis is established by demonstrating a virtual absence of HPRT activity in readily

accessible tissues such as erythrocytes. Analyses of erythrocyte lysates are not useful in identifying heterozygous female carriers, but this can be accomplished with cell culture of skin fibroblasts or through analysis of hair follicles.

Partial deficiency of HPRT should be suspected in male patients with the onset of gouty arthritis before 20 years of age and in young males with uric acid crystalluria or uric acid nephrolithiasis. Uric acid overexcretion is found invariably in patients with normal renal function, and the diagnosis is confirmed by enzyme assay. Patients with partial HPRT activity have erythrocyte lysate values that are usually in the range of 0.1 to 5 per cent of control values, rarely up 30 to 50 per cent of control values, while patients with the Lesch-Nyhan syndrome have values less than 0.01 per cent of control values.

TREATMENT. Uric acid stone formation, tophi, and gouty arthritis can be controlled in both the Lesch-Nyhan syndrome and partial deficiency of HPRT with drugs that inhibit xanthine oxidase activity. However, a few patients have developed xanthine stones with this therapy. No drugs have been found that correct the neurologic deficits, but supportive measures, such as restraints that reduce the tendency to self-mutilation, are well accepted by the patient. Drugs such as diazepam help control the movement disorder. Given the devastating neurologic complications of the Lesch-Nyhan syndrome, therapeutic abortion has been used as a preventive measure following heterozygote identification and intrauterine diagnosis.

Edwards NL, Recker D, Fox IH: Overproduction of uric acid in hypoxanthine-guanine phosphoribosyltransferase deficiency. J Clin Invest 63:922, 1979. *A careful analysis of the basis for uric acid overproduction in patients with HPRT deficiency.*

Stout JT, Caskey CT: Hypoxanthine phosphoribosyltransferase deficiency: The Lesch-Nyhan syndrome and gouty arthritis. *In* Scriver CR, Beaudet AL, Sly WS, et al. (eds.): The Metabolic Basis of Inherited Disease. 6th ed. New York, McGraw-Hill, 1989, pp 1007–1029. *A detailed description of the clinical and biochemical consequences of HPRT deficiency.*

Wilson JM, Stout JT, Palella TD, et al.: A molecular survey of hypoxanthine-guanine phosphoribosyltransferase deficiency in man. J Clin Invest 77:188, 1986. *A description of specific mutations at the molecular level in patients with HGPRT deficiency.*

2,8-DIHYDROXYADENINE RENAL STONES

Deficiency of adenine phosphoribosyltransferase (APRT), an enzyme in the salvage pathway of purine nucleotide synthesis, leads to the accumulation and increased urinary excretion of 2,8-dihydroxyadenine, the product of adenine oxidation by xanthine oxidase. Because of the insolubility of this purine, patients with this autosomal recessive disorder are predisposed to development of renal calculi composed of 2,8-dihydroxyadenine. More than 30 individuals homozygous for this enzyme deficiency have been identified; 6 presented with acute renal failure, and 3 of these patients suffered permanent renal damage. Renal colic may occur within the first months of life, as late as 40 years of age, or individuals with this disorder may be asymptomatic. 2,8-Dihydroxyadenine stones are usually radiolucent. The diagnosis is confirmed by analyzing the stone with ultraviolet, infrared, or mass spectrometry or x-ray crystallography or by demonstrating the absence of adenine phosphoribosyltransferase activity in erythrocyte lysates. Except for the excessive excretion of adenine and its metabolites, with the consequent development of renal calculi, no other biochemical or clinical abnormalities have been reported in individuals homozygous for this enzyme deficiency.

The prevalence of the homozygous state is not documented, but it is calculated to occur once in 35,000 to 250,000 births, since the prevalence of heterozygosity for adenine phosphoribosyltransferase deficiency varies from 0.4 to 1.1 per 100. Individuals heterozygous for the enzyme deficiency have no recognized clinical abnormalities.

Prognosis depends on renal function at the time of diagnosis. Therapy with dietary purine restriction, high fluid intake, and allopurinol—to prevent oxidation of adenine to 2,8-dihydroxyadenine—is effective in reducing stone formation and preserving renal function.

Simmonds A, Sahota AS, Van Acker KL: Adenine phosphoribosyltransferase deficiency. *In* Scriver CR, Beaudet AL, Sly WS, et al. (eds.): The Metabolic Basis of Inherited Disease. 6th ed. New York, McGraw-Hill, 1989, pp 1029–1044. *A detailed review of all known cases of complete APRT deficiency and discussion of the metabolic defect.*

Van Acker KJ, Simmonds A, Potter C, et al.: Complete deficiency of adenine phosphoribosyltransferase. Report of a family. N Engl J Med 297:127, 1977. *Adenine, 8-hydroxyadenine, and 2,8-dihydroxyadenine amounted to 25 per cent of urinary purines in two homozygous male children, one of whom had "pure uric acid stones" later correctly identified as 2,8-dihydroxyadenine.*

IMMUNE DYSFUNCTION ASSOCIATED WITH PURINE ENZYME DEFICIENCIES

Adenosine deaminase deficiency is an uncommon disorder, approximately 100 to 150 families having been identified, that leads to a clinical syndrome of severe combined immunodeficiency, i.e., a defect in both T cell and B cell function. About one fifth of patients with severe combined immunodeficiency, in which the disorder is inherited as an autosomal recessive condition, or more rarely as an X-linked recessive disorder, have this enzyme deficiency. Approximately 85 per cent of patients with adenosine deaminase (ADA) deficiency come to medical attention at 1 to 2 months of age with recurrent infections of the skin and the gastrointestinal and respiratory systems. Both ordinary and opportunistic pathogens are encountered, and candidiasis is almost invariably present. Diarrhea is common, as well as delayed physical growth and development. Physical findings are for the most part unremarkable except for the absence of lymph nodes and pharyngeal lymphoid tissue. A rachitic rosary, or prominence of the costochondral junctions, has been noted in some patients. Laboratory tests show absence of a thymic shadow, lymphopenia, negative skin test results for delayed hypersensitivity, attenuated lymphocyte responses to lectins and antigens in vitro, and hypogammaglobulinemia. The diagnosis is established by documenting ADA deficiency in erythrocyte lysates or other cell extracts. Approximately 15 per cent of individuals with this disorder have a milder disease with later age of onset and relative sparing of humoral immunity. In the severe form of this disorder, if untreated, overwhelming infection and sepsis lead to death before 2 years of age.

Current mechanisms favored to explain the immune defects observed in ADA deficiency are deoxy–adenosine triphosphate (ATP) accumulation leading to inhibition of ribonucleotide reductase with resultant decrease in DNA replication, and *S*-adenosylhomocysteine accumulation leading to inhibition of transmethylation reactions. Either or both of these proposed mechanisms could reduce lymphocyte proliferation and function.

Treatment of ADA deficiency by bone marrow transplantation has resulted in virtually complete immune reconstitution in some patients, and at present this is the preferred therapy if compatible donors are available. Enzyme replacement with PEG-ADA* has been documented to improve immune function, and this therapy is effective in long-term trials, i.e., more than 4 years of follow-up. Gene therapy has been approved for this disorder, and trials are under way at the present time.

Purine nucleoside phosphorylase (PNP) deficiency is less common than ADA deficiency, approximately 15 to 20 patients with this disorder having been recognized. PNP deficiency is also inherited as an autosomal recessive disorder, but it leads to a defect in cell-mediated immunity with little, if any, abnormality in humoral immunity. In patients with this disorder, diagnosis has been made as early as 4 months and as late as 9 years of age, with infections involving skin, lung, middle ear, mastoids, and urinary tract. Infections with nonbacterial agents have been most common, reflecting the primary defect in cellular immunity. Laboratory tests show lymphopenia, diminished number of circulating T cells, reduced lymphocyte response to antigens, and negative skin test results for delayed hypersensitivity. Immunoglobulin levels are normal, but several patients have exhibited signs of immunoregulatory abnormalities, as shown by autoimmune hemolytic anemia, antinuclear antibodies, and rheumatoid factor. In addition, patients with PNP deficiency have hypouricemia, a finding of no clinical consequence in itself, but one that suggests the diagnosis of this enzyme deficiency in a child with recurrent infections.

Confirmation of the diagnosis is obtained by assay of erythrocyte lysate or other cell extracts for purine nucleoside phosphorylase activity. It has been proposed that accumulation of deoxyguanosine triphosphate in T cells, with resultant inhibition of ribonucleotide reductase and DNA replication, is responsible for the immune defect in this disorder. The prognosis in purine

nucleoside phosphorylase deficiency is generally better than that for adenosine deaminase deficiency, but therapy with bone marrow transplantation and erythrocyte transfusion has been less successful.

Giblett ER: Adenosine deaminase and purine nucleoside phosphorylase deficiency: How they were discovered and what they may mean. *In* Elliot K, Whelan J (eds.): Enzyme Defects and Immune Dysfunction. Ciba Found Symp 68:3, 1979. *An interesting story about scientific serendipity and discovery of a new group of clinical disorders.*

Hershfield MS, Buckley RH, Greenberg ML, et al.: Treatment of adenosine deaminase deficiency with polyethylene glycol–modified adenosine deaminase. N Engl J Med 316:589, 1987. *Description of a novel form of enzyme replacement therapy that provides active enzyme with a prolonged half-life in the circulation.*

Kredich N, Hershfield MS: Immunodeficiency diseases caused by adenosine deaminase deficiency and purine nucleoside phosphorylase deficiency. *In* Scriver CR, Beaudet AL, Sly WS, et al. (eds.): The Metabolic Basis of Inherited Disease. 6th ed. New York, McGraw-Hill, 1989, pp 1045–1075. *An authoritative review of the clinical, laboratory, and biochemical abnormalities in these disorders. This chapter also includes a detailed discussion of purine nucleoside metabolism in normal and pathologic situations.*

MYOPATHY ASSOCIATED WITH MYOADENYLATE DEAMINASE DEFICIENCY

Deficiency of myoadenylate deaminase has been noted in approximately 2 per cent of muscle biopsies submitted for routine investigation in some centers. This isozyme of adenosine monophosphate (AMP) deaminase is found predominantly in skeletal muscle, and this is the only organ affected by this enzyme deficiency. In approximately half of the cases that have been carefully studied, AMP deaminase deficiency is not associated with other neuromuscular pathology, and in these individuals the enzyme deficiency is marked ($<$1 per cent of normal). In cases in which the residual enzyme activity is higher (1 to 10 per cent of normal), the patients have a broad spectrum of neuromuscular diseases. Three quarters of patients with primary myoadenylate deaminase deficiency report exercise-related symptoms of easy fatigability, cramps, and myalgias, usually beginning in childhood or young adulthood. Weakness without exercise is noted in fewer than one third of patients. Hypotonia has been described in two patients. Reduced AMP deaminase activity has occasionally been reported in patients with other neuromuscular disorders, but no definite association of this enzyme deficiency has been established with any symptom complex other than easy fatigability, cramps, and myalgias. Since a few individuals with myoadenylate deaminase deficiency have been reported to be asymptomatic, factors in addition to AMP deaminase deficiency may contribute to the exercise-related manifestations described above.

Serum creatine kinase activity is mildly and variably increased in about one half of patients with this disorder, and routine laboratory studies, including electromyography and histochemistry of muscle, are not diagnostic. In the patient with exercise-related symptoms, the specific diagnosis of myoadenylate deaminase deficiency is suggested by the finding of reduced NH_3 production in a forearm ischemic exercise test. Since all patients with reduced NH_3 production following ischemic forearm exercise do not have myoadenylate deaminase deficiency, the diagnosis needs to be confirmed by direct assay of AMP deaminase activity in skeletal muscle.

Adenosine monophosphate deaminase is one of the components of the purine nucleotide cycle, a series of reactions that is potentially important in energy production and utilization in skeletal muscle. Deficiency of myoadenylate deaminase activity may impair energy generation through diminished production of citric acid cycle intermediates, and it may adversely affect energy utilization through a reduction in the rate of adenosine triphosphate (ATP) hydrolysis by myofibrillar adenosine triphosphatase (ATPase).

The prognosis in myoadenylate deaminase deficiency is generally good. Present experience suggests that the symptoms are slowly progressive, and the disorder leads to mild disability in most cases, although there have been exceptions to these generalizations. No effective therapy is available at this time.

Fishbein WN: Myoadenylate deaminase deficiency: Inherited and acquired forms. Biochem Med 33:158, 1985. *Review of biochemical data supporting primary and secondary forms of AMP deaminase deficiency.*

Sabina RL, Swain JL, Holmes EW: Myoadenylate deaminase deficiency. *In* Scriver

---

*Polyethylene glycol–modified ADA.

CR, Beaudet AL, Sly WS, et al. (eds.): The Metabolic Basis of Inherited Disease. 6th ed. New York, McGraw-Hill, 1989, pp 1077–1084. *Discussion of the clinical and biochemical findings in 130 patients with myoadenylate deaminase deficiency, as well as a review of the role of the purine nucleotide cycle in skeletal muscle function.*

Sabina RL, Swain JL, Olanow CW, et al.: Myoadenylate deaminase deficiency: Functional and metabolic abnormalities associated with disruption of the purine nucleotide cycle. J Clin Invest 73:720, 1984.

185 Disorders of Pyrimidine Metabolism

Lloyd H. Smith, Jr.

Pyrimidine nucleotides share equally with purine nucleotides the chemical chore of transmitting genetic information for reproduction or for phenotypic expression within the cell. They also function in the intermediary metabolism of lipids and carbohydrates. Only a few disorders of pyrimidine metabolism have been recognized.

Hereditary orotic aciduria is a rare genetic disorder of pyrimidine metabolism characterized by megaloblastic anemia resistant to the usual hematinic agents, leukopenia, failure of normal growth and development, and the continued excessive urinary excretion of orotic acid. Patients also have impaired cellular immunity with intact humoral immunity. Orotic acid is highly insoluble and often forms a heavy sediment of urinary crystals that may on occasion result in ureteral or urethral obstruction. The disorder, which is transmitted as an autosomal recessive trait, is usually characterized by a reduction in two consecutive enzymatic activities in pyrimidine biosynthesis, orotate phosphoribosyltransferase (OPRT) and orotidine 5′-phosphate decarboxylase (ODC). Both enzymatic activities reside in a single multifunctional protein, uridine monophosphate (UMP) synthase, for which the gene is located on the long arm of chromosome 3. A single patient has been described with isolated deficiency of ODC. There is a prompt and sustained hematologic and general clinical response to oral uridine (2 to 4 grams per day), which must be continued indefinitely as replacement therapy. The

disease has attracted special attention because it represents a block in the de novo pathway of pyrimidine synthesis, is an example of a double defect in enzymatic activity (although now known to be attributable to a single protein), and produces a requirement for replacement of a normal metabolic intermediate, uridine.

Orotic aciduria, without the characteristic hematologic abnormalities, also occurs in *ornithine transcarbamylase deficiency*. It is presumed that this results from the overflow of carbamyl phosphate from urea synthesis (partially blocked in this disease) to pyrimidine synthesis. Orotic aciduria has also been found in purine nucleoside phosphorylase deficiency and in PP-ribose-P synthetase deficiency (see Ch. 184).

Excessive urinary excretion of orotic acid and orotidine occurs during treatment with *allopurinol* or *6-azauridine*.* Metabolic products of both compounds inhibit orotidine 5′-decarboxylase activity.

Pyrimidine 5′-nucleotidase deficiency is a rare form of hereditary hemolytic anemia, transmitted as an autosomal recessive trait. The erythrocytes exhibit prominent basophilic stippling owing to aggregates of undegraded ribosomes and on analysis contain very high concentrations of cytidine and uridine nucleotides. The mechanism by which the nucleotidase deficiency leads to hemolysis is unclear. Lead inhibits pyrimidine 5′-nucleotidase activity and leads to a similar anemia with basophilic stippling, possibly through this mechanism.

Dihydropyrimidine dehydrogenase deficiency is a rare disorder affecting an enzyme in the degradative pathway for the pyrimidine bases uracil and thymine. As a result, uracil and thymine accumulate in plasma and are excreted excessively in the urine. No distinctive clinical picture has been noted, although most cases have been found through screening studies for organic aciduria in patients with a variety of neurologic disorders.

Paglia DE, Fink K, Valentine WN: Additional data from two kindreds with genetically-induced deficiencies of erythrocyte pyrimidine nucleotidase. Acta Hematol 63:262, 1980. *This is the best description of clinical findings and the altered pyrimidine metabolism leading to hemolytic anemia in this rare but interesting genetic disease.*

Suttle DP, Becoft DMO, Webster DR: Orotic aciduria. *In* Scriver CR, Beaudet A, Sly W, et al. (eds.): The Metabolic Basis of Inherited Disease. 6th ed. New York, McGraw-Hill, 1989, pp 1095–1126. *This is the most complete description of normal pyrimidine metabolism in humans and the derangements that occur in hereditary orotic aciduria and in other disorders of pyrimidine metabolism.*

*Investigational drug.

INHERITED DISORDERS OF CONNECTIVE TISSUE

186 The Mucopolysaccharidoses

William S. Sly

The mucopolysaccharidoses (MPS) are a group of lysosomal storage diseases, each of which is produced by an inherited deficiency of an enzyme involved in degradation of acid mucopolysaccharides (now called glycosaminoglycans and abbreviated GAG's). They are clinically progressive and have many common features that result from accumulation of partially degraded GAG's in various tissues. They produce disability primarily from storage-related abnormalities of the connective tissue, the heart, the bony skeleton, and the central nervous system.

Delineation of this group of diseases on the basis of clinical features, radiologic findings, and biochemistry of the urinary

GAG's led to the famous classification of McKusick into MPS I to VI in 1966. Over the next 6 years, an exciting series of investigations from the laboratories of Neufeld and co-workers led to the discoveries that fibroblasts from patients with these disorders show storage abnormalities in culture, that fibroblasts from genetically different patients could "cross-correct" each other in culture, and that this "cross-correction" was due to secretion and recapture of lysosomal enzymes by the complementing fibroblast cell lines, each of which could secrete the enzyme the other was missing and take up the "corrective factor" for which it was deficient. These complementation studies served for nearly a decade as means for clinical diagnosis and for segregation of the disease into complementation groups (e.g., segregation of Hurler and Scheie syndromes into one complementation group, and separation of Sanfilippo syndrome into several complementing groups); they also guided the purification of the corrective factors, each of which was eventually identified as a specific GAG degradative enzyme. Although still useful in certain situations, the complementation assays have largely been replaced by direct assays for the enzymes listed in Table 186–1 as deficient for each of the disorders.

ETIOLOGY OF GLYCOSAMINOGLYCAN STORAGE. The GAG's are long linear polysaccharide molecules composed of repeating dimers, each of which contains a hexuronic acid (or galactose in the case of keratan sulfate) and an amino sugar. They are usually found in covalent linkage to a core protein on which they are synthesized and from which they branch like bristles from a brush. The individual GAG's differ from one another in the hexuronic acid-amino sugar combinations in the repeating dimers, in the linkages between these components, in the link-

TABLE 186–1. THE MUCOPOLYSACCHARIDOSES (MPS STORAGE DISEASES I TO VII)

Abbreviation	Eponym	Enzyme Deficiency	Major Storage Product	Urinary GAG's	Clinical Features
MPS U-H	Hurler	α-L-Iduronidase	DS ± HS	↑ 5–25X DS > HS	Onset 6–12 mo, coarse features, rhinorrhea, grunting respiration, corneal clouding, cardiac disease, visceromegaly, dwarfism, dysostosis multiplex, progressive mental retardation after the first year; death by 5–10 yr
MPS I-S (formerly MPS V)	Scheie	α-L-Iduronidase	DS + HS	↑ 5–25X DS > HS	Onset 5–15 yr, corneal clouding, stiff joints, clawhand, genu valgum, dysostosis multiplex, aortic valve disease; however, normal height, normal intelligence, and long survival (difficult to distinguish clinically from mild MPS VI)
MPS I-H/S	Hurler-Scheie	α-L-Iduronidase	DS + HS	↑ 5–25X DS > HS	Onset 2–4 yr, all findings of MPS-H but milder, slower progression, and survival into 20's
MPS II, severe	Hunter, severe form	L-Sulfoiduronate sulfatase	HS + DS	↑ 5–25X DS = HS	Onset 2–4 yr, clear corneas, deafness, all other features of MPS I-H, but milder; mental retardation progresses to profound state; death by 10–15 yr
MPS II, mild	Hunter, mild form	L-Sulfoiduronate sulfatase	HS + DS	↑ 5–25X DS = HS	Onset in first decade, short stature, clear corneas, joint stiffness, dysostosis multiplex, visceromegaly, cardiac disease, nerve entrapments, near-normal intelligence; survival to 30's–60's, depending on heart involvement
MPS III-A	Sanfilippo, type A	Heparan sulfate sulfamidase	HS	↑ 5–20X 85% HS	Onset 2–6 yr, large head, normal height; Hurler-like features, dysostosis multiplex, hepatomegaly are all mild; mental retardation is rapidly progressive and severe; death at end of puberty
MPS III-B	Sanfilippo, type B	N-acetyl-α-D-glucosaminidase	HS	↑ 5–20X 85% HS	Clinically indistinguishable from MPS III, type A
MPS III-C	Sanfilippo, type C	Acetyl CoA: α-glucosamide N-acetyltransferase	HS	↑ 5–20X 85% HS	Clinically indistinguishable from MPS III, type A
MPS III-D	Sanfilippo, type D	N-acetyl-α-D-glucosamine-6-sulfatase	HS	↑ 5–20X 85% HS	Clinically indistinguishable from MPS III, type A
MPS IV-A	Morquio, classic form	N-acetylgalactosamine-6-sulfatase (gal-6-sulfatase)	KS + Ch 6-S	↑ 3–5X KS + Ch-S	Characteristic facies, short-trunk dwarfism, deformed thorax, corneal clouding, hearing deficit, aortic valve disease, unstable neck, spinal cord transection; intelligence is normal; death usually in 20's from cardiorespiratory problems
MPS IV-B	Morquio-like syndrome	β-Galactosidase deficiency	KS + Ch 4-S	↑ 2–5X KS = Ch-S	Short stature, corneal clouding, mild dysostosis multiplex, prominence of lower face, pectus carinatum, hip deformity, normal intelligence
MPS VI	Maroteaux-Lamy, severe	N-acetylgalactosamine-4-sulfatase (arylsulfatase B)	DS + ?Ch 4-S	↑ 4–20X 70–90% DS	Onset 2–4 yr, growth failure from age 4 slowly progressive, joint stiffness, corneal clouding, aortic valve disease, and severe hip deformity; dysostosis multiplex, striking white cell inclusions; intelligence normal; death in 20's
	Maroteaux-Lamy, mild	N-acetylgalactosamine-4-sulfatase (arylsulfatase B)	DS + ?Ch 4-S	↑ 4–20X 70–90% DS	Onset 5–7 yr, short stature, severe osseous changes, especially in the hips; nerve entrapment, corneal clouding, aortic valve disease; normal intelligence, long survival; difficult to distinguish from MPS I-S
MPS VII	Sly	β-Glucuronidase	HS, DS, Ch-S	↑ 6–8X HS, DS Ch 4/6-S	Onset 1–2 yr, mild to moderate Hurler-like features, dysostosis multiplex, pectus carinatum, visceromegaly, cardiac murmurs, short stature, moderate mental retardation; slowly progressive after infancy; striking granulocyte inclusions; milder forms exist, as does a more severe form with neonatal ascites and death within 2 yr

DS = dermatan sulfate; HS = heparan sulfate; Ch-S = chondroitin sulfate; KS = keratan sulfate.

ages between repeating dimers, and in the degree to which individual sugar components are N-acetylated or N-sulfated. The major GAG's and their respective repeating dimers are chondroitin sulfate (glucuronic acid β1-3 N-acetylgalactosamine-4/6-sulfate); dermatan sulfate (iduronic acid α1-3 N-acetylgalactosamine-4-sulfate); heparan sulfate, which has both glucuronic acid and iduronic acid linked β1-4 and α1-3, respectively, to either N-acetylglucosamine or glucosamine N-sulfate; and keratan sulfate (galactose β1-4 N-acetylglucosamine-6-sulfate). The large proteoglycan molecules made up of protein cores and their GAG branches are secreted by cells and constitute a significant fraction of the extracellular matrix of connective tissue. Their turnover depends on their subsequent internalization by endocytosis, their delivery to lysosomes, and their digestion by lysosomal enzymes. Lysosomal proteases digest the core protein, endoglycosidases reduce the size of the GAG's to oligosaccharides of varying length, and many exoglycosidases act sequentially to degrade the GAG's to their monosaccharide components. Each lysosomal enzyme is specific for a specific linkage. An inherited deficiency for any enzyme involved disrupts the sequential degradative process and leads to accumulation in lysosomes of partially degraded GAG. The accumulation is progressive and eventually disrupts cellular architecture and disturbs cell function. The tissues and organs most affected and the severity depend on the degree of enzyme deficiency, i.e., whether partial or complete. Severity also depends on which enzyme is missing, since individual GAG's vary in their tissue distribution and their rate of turnover.

The causative enzyme deficiencies, the major storage products, and the clinical features of the mucopolysaccharidoses are summarized in Table 186–1. There is marked genetic heterogeneity within this group of disorders, with many different clinical phenotypes resulting from the different enzyme deficiencies (see MPS I–VII, Table 186–1). It is now clear also that quite different phenotypes can result from the same enzyme deficiency, depending on whether it is partial or complete (see MPS I-H, MPS I-S, and MPS I-H/S in Table 186–1).

GENETICS OF THE MUCOPOLYSACCHARIDOSES. Except for Hunter syndrome (MPS II), in which the missing enzyme is specified by a gene on the X chromosome and the inheritance is X linked, all of the mucopolysaccharidoses result from deficiencies of enzymes specified by autosomal genes. Thus the inheritance pattern is autosomal recessive. In most cases, affected offspring can be shown to be the products of heterozygous carrier parents, both of whom have about half-normal levels of the enzyme for which the affected patient is deficient. Even though the enzymes can now be measured for most of these disorders, the disorders are too rare to make screening for carriers practical. However, carrier status can be determined by enzyme assays in high-risk individuals, and prenatal diagnosis for most of these disorders is available to high-risk mothers, such as mothers of an affected offspring, who face a 25 per cent chance of another affected offspring in a subsequent pregnancy.

CLINICAL AND PATHOLOGIC CONSEQUENCES OF GLYCOSAMINOGLYCAN STORAGE. Connective tissue storage produces connective tissue laxity in most of these disorders, manifest by inguinal and umbilical hernias. Connective tissue thickening also occurs, owing in part to GAG storage and in part to excessive collagen deposition. This combination leads to coarse facial features, peripheral nerve entrapments, thickened meninges that may lead to cord compression and hydrocephalus, and thickened joint capsules. Connective tissue deposition in valve leaflets, the endocardium, and the myocardium produces symptomatic heart disease, a common cause of death in these patients, to which coronary vascular insufficiency also contributes. Most of these disorders produce short stature, partly because of impaired long-bone growth and partly because of vertebral abnormalities. These and many other changes in the bony skeleton are collectively referred to as *dysostosis multiplex*. Central nervous system storage may produce progressive mental retardation, especially in disorders involving impaired degradation of heparan sulfate (MPS I, II, and III). Corneal clouding and visual handicap result from storage of the partially degraded GAG's in the corneal stroma, especially in disorders involving impaired degradation of dermatan sulfate and keratan sulfate (MPS I, IV, and VI).

Hepatomegaly is common and may be massive but rarely is important clinically. Excessive urinary excretion of incompletely degraded GAG's (mucopolysacchariduria) is a constant finding of considerable diagnostic significance (Table 186–1) but has little pathologic significance.

HURLER SYNDROME (MPS I-H). Pathology. The basic defect is a deficiency of alpha-L-iduronidase, an enzyme that participates in degradation of dermatan sulfate and heparan sulfate. Accumulation of membrane-enclosed storage material in parenchymal and mesenchymal cells is the chief pathologic finding. It affects every organ. Vacuolated cells distended with storage material distort normal cell and tissue architecture. In most cells this storage material is granular and composed of GAG's. In neurons, lipids are also present, presumably because stored GAG's inhibit sphingolipid degradation.

Clinical Features. Although patients are thought to be normal until 6 months of age, they develop persistent nasal discharge, noisy breathing, frequent upper respiratory infections, stiff joints, a thoracolumbar gibbus, and some degree of chest deformity in the second half of the first year of life. Over the second year, the classic syndrome develops, with large head, coarse features, corneal clouding, hypertelorism, prominent eyebrows, thick lips, and broad, flat nose with depressed nasal bridge. The hands are short and stubby, and joint limitation produces a clawhand deformity. Abdominal protuberance results from hepatosplenomegaly and lax abdominal musculature, often with inguinal and umbilical hernias. Dwarfism is obvious by the end of the second year, by which time cardiac murmurs are present.

Developmental delay is obvious before 18 months of age, and mental retardation progresses slowly. Limitation of joint movement leads to contractures of the hands, the elbows, and the knees. Death usually occurs by the age of 10 from pneumonia or heart failure, after about 5 years of steady regression and nearly total loss of acquired skills. Hearing loss is usually moderate to severe, and coronary insufficiency and peripheral vascular insufficiency are important late findings.

Radiologic abnormalities of dysostosis multiplex are striking. The skull is large and scaphocephalic, and the calvarium is thickened. The sinuses are poorly developed. The sella is enlarged anteriorly and referred to as **J** shaped. The ribs are oar shaped, being narrow posteriorly and greatly expanded anteriorly. The medial third of the clavicle is thickened. The vertebrae are initially rounded and appear ovoid. One or two lower thoracic and upper lumbar vertebrae are often hypoplastic and wedge shaped, producing the gibbus deformity. The pelvis shows flared iliac wings, a small body of the ilium, and shallow oblique acetabula. The hips show coxa valga deformities. The metatarsals and phalanges are short and wide; the proximal ends of the metacarpals taper sharply, a classic finding called proximal pointing. The long tubular bones have expanded diaphyses. There is loss of normal angulation of the humerus at the shoulder. The radiologic changes are progressive, but the changes vary considerably from patient to patient at a given age. The lower extremities are generally more mildly affected than the upper extremities, except for the hips, which often show changes resembling aseptic necrosis of the femoral heads, changes that correlate with severe hip disability clinically.

Diagnosis. The diagnosis can be suspected on clinical and radiologic grounds, supported by demonstration of mucopolysacchariduria (dermatan sulfate [DS] > heparan sulfate [HS]), and established definitively by demonstration of the enzyme deficiency, using the commercially available phenyl-L-iduronide substrate. Enzyme activity can be measured in extracts of leukocytes or cultured fibroblasts.

Treatment. Only supportive and symptomatic treatment can be offered to patients, as no effective treatment for the storage abnormality is available.

SCHEIE SYNDROME (MPS I-S). This rare disorder is also due to a deficiency of alpha-L-iduronidase and is characterized by severe corneal clouding, deformity of the hands, and aortic valve disease. Symptoms appear between the ages of 5 and 15. The height is normal, as is the intelligence. The striking joint stiffness of the hands is similar to that seen in Hurler syndrome but is complicated by the carpal tunnel syndrome with median nerve entrapment. Aortic stenosis, regurgitation, or both are present but are usually not symptomatic in early life. Life expectancy may be nearly normal. Diagnosis depends on the same criteria as for Hurler syndrome. Corneal transplant and aortic valve replacement are reasonable, since intelligence is normal.

THE HURLER-SCHEIE COMPOUND (MPS I-H/S). Some patients with a phenotype that is intermediate between that of Hurler and that of Scheie syndromes are thought to represent compound heterozygotes, having inherited one Hurler and one Scheie gene from each parent.

HUNTER SYNDROME (MPS II). Hunter syndrome is distinguished from Hurler syndrome by three features: (1) slower progression with longer survival, (2) lack of corneal clouding, and (3) X-linked rather than autosomal recessive inheritance. A severe form and a mild form exist. The severe form has most of the features of Hurler syndrome, but they are slightly milder except for hearing impairment, which is more severe. The patients usually die by age 15. A much milder form has been reported with near-normal intelligence and near-normal survival. Diagnosis is made on the basis of the clinical findings, radiologic evidence of dysostosis multiplex, increased urinary GAG's, and demonstration of sulfoiduronate sulfatase deficiency on serum or on extracts of leukocytes or cultured fibroblasts. Carrier detection is still imperfect, but prenatal diagnostic tests are reliable.

SANFILIPPO SYNDROME (MPS III). This syndrome can be produced by a deficiency of at least four different enzymes, all of which participate in degradation of heparan sulfate (Table 186–1). Early development is normal but slows or halts between the ages of 2 and 6 years, after which mental deterioration is often rapid. Gait becomes unsteady, muscles atrophy, and the patient becomes bedridden. Death usually occurs by puberty. The head is large, the hair coarse, and hirsutism common. Visceromegaly is mild to absent. Cardiac involvement is rare. Height may be normal through the first decade and then falls behind. Skeletal findings of dysostosis multiplex are mild and include thickened calvarium, ovoid vertebral bodies, mild dysplasia of the pelvis, and mild rib changes. The clinical diagnosis may be suspected from the severe mental retardation, which appears disproportionate to relatively mild somatic and radiologic abnormalities, supported by the presence of heparan sulfaturia, and established definitively by demonstration of the specific enzyme deficiency.

MORQUIO SYNDROME, CLASSIC FORM (MPS IV-A). The predominant clinical features relate to skeletal abnormalities and to symptoms of spinal cord compression resulting from instability of the neck. Intelligence is normal. By the age of 2 years, pigeon chest deformity, genu valgum, and gait disturbance appear. Knees and wrists enlarge. The neck appears short, and the head seems to sit on the deformed thorax. Universal platyspondylisis, evident on radiogaphic examination, kyphoscoliosis, and contractures at the knees and hips all contribute to dwarfism. The face is unusual because of mid-face hypoplasia, depressed nasal bridge, flared nares, and prominence of the lower third of the face on side view. The teeth are widely spaced, and the dental enamel is thin. Corneal clouding is mild but slowly progressive. Long survival is rare, with death occurring between the ages of 20 and 40 from cardiopulmonary complications. The cardiac disease is valvular (aortic regurgitation). The respiratory problems arise from thoracic deformities and from neurotrophic myelopathy caused by atlantoaxial subluxation. Diagnosis depends on the clinical and radiologic features, which are characteristic; the finding of keratan sulfaturia (which may disappear in adolescence); and the deficiency of N-acetylgalactosamine-6-sulfatase, which is active on both GalNAc 6-S in chondroitin sulfate and Gal 6-S in keratan sulfate. The enzymatic assay is available in only a few laboratories. Treatment is symptomatic. Posterior cervical fusion should be done early in the disease to prevent spinal cord damage. Correction of the genu valgum requires a single operation at about 6 years.

THE MORQUIO-LIKE SYNDROME WITH BETA-GALACTOSIDASE DEFICIENCY (MPS IV-B). Short stature, mild pectus carinatum, corneal clouding, odontoid hypoplasia with cervical instability, mild dysostosis multiplex, moderate lumbar kyphosis, and mild genu valgum are all features that are found in this Morquio-like disease resulting from beta-galactosidase deficiency. Absent are hearing deficit, dental abnormalities, cardiac murmurs, hepatomegaly, and joint laxity. Keratan sulfaturia is present. The diagnosis is based on normal N-acetylgalactosamine-6-sulfatase levels and reduced beta-galactosidase levels. Presumably, this disorder reflects a mutation that impairs the

activity of the enzyme on galactose linkages in keratan sulfate but spares its activity on GM_1 ganglioside. Thus the findings of chondrodystrophy predominate, and the neurologic manifestations of GM_1 gangliosidosis are absent.

THE MAROTEAUX-LAMY SYNDROME, SEVERE AND MILD TYPES (MPS VI). Maroteaux and colleagues recognized a new form of mucopolysaccharidosis in 1963 that resembled Hurler syndrome but differed in that intelligence of the dwarfed, deformed patients was spared; the urinary GAG was almost exclusively dermatan sulfate; and the leukocytes exhibited striking metachromatic inclusions. Affected patients often die in their 20's from cardiac failure. Many suffer cervical cord compression and hydrocephalus resulting from thickened meninges. Since specific enzymatic assays have become available both for arylsulfatase B, missing in MPS VI, and alpha-L-iduronidase, missing in MPS I, it has become clear that many patients with milder forms of MPS VI exist who might previously have been thought to have Scheie syndrome. No specific treatment is available for the storage abnormality. However, shunting for hydrocephalus, spinal fusion for atlantoaxial subluxation, corneal transplants for visual handicap, and cardiac valve and hip replacement are all reasonable when required, because intelligence is preserved and patients with milder forms of the abnormality have the potential for long survival.

BETA-GLUCURONIDASE DEFICIENCY MUCOPOLYSACCHARIDOSIS (MPS VII). Most patients present by age 3 with a Hurler-like illness manifested by frequent upper respiratory infections, chest deformities, cardiac murmurs, hepatosplenomegaly, hernias, dysostosis multiplex, and mild to moderate mental retardation. Many develop corneal clouding. About 20 patients, showing a wide range of clinical severity, have been recognized. Most of the patients have shown slow progression in clinical abnormalities after the age of 6. The natural history beyond the teens is yet to be determined. Urinary GAG's have been increased, and heparan sulfate, dermatan sulfate, and chondroitin sulfate have all been reported to be increased in urine. Striking inclusions in leukocytes are typical, as in MPS VI. The diagnosis depends on the demonstration of the enzyme deficiency. Carrier detection and prenatal diagnosis are available.

OTHER DISORDERS RELATED TO THE MUCOPOLYSACCHARIDOSES. Mucolipidosis II (also called I-cell disease) and mucolipidosis III (also called pseudo-Hurler polydystrophy) are severe and milder forms, respectively, of a Hurler-like disease having many features in common with the mucopolysaccharidoses. However, these patients do not have mucopolysacchariduria.

These disorders result not from a deficiency of a single lysosomal enzyme, as do the mucopolysaccharidoses, but from a defect in the processing of N-acetylglucosaminyl phosphotransferase that normally targets acid hydrolases to lysosomes. Failure to add the phosphomannosyl recognition marker that normally directs their segregation into lysosomes allows acid hydrolases to be secreted instead. As a consequence, there is an intracellular deficiency of most of the enzymes involved in the degradation of GAG's (and an extracellular excess), which is part of a general pattern of deficiency involving nearly all lysosomal enzymes. The absence of mucopolysacchariduria, and the 10- to 50-fold elevations of levels of acid hydrolases in serum, distinguish these two disorders from the mucopolysaccharidoses with single-enzyme deficiency.

Another group of disorders, not classified with the mucopolysaccharidoses, may produce a Hurler-like picture, including mental retardation, visceromegaly, and dysostosis multiplex. These disorders result from single-enzyme deficiencies for enzymes involved in the catabolism of the oligosaccharide components of glycoproteins. Included are mannosidosis, fucosidosis, and the more recently delineated group of sialidoses (one of which has been described under the name mucolipidosis I). The sialidoses result from a deficiency of oligosaccharide N-acetylneuraminidase. The primary storage products in these disorders are oligosaccharides derived from glycoproteins. However, there is some storage of keratan sulfate as well. It appears that these enzymes are required for degradation of some oligosaccharide side chains on keratan sulfate. Impaired degradation of keratan sulfate may explain the dysostosis multiplex that mimics the skeletal findings of the mucopolysaccharidoses in these disorders.

Kelly TE: The mucopolysaccharidoses and mucolipidoses. Clin Orthop 114:116, 1976. *A nice summary of clinically relevant information.*

McKusick VA, Neufeld EF, Kelly TE: The mucopolysaccharide storage diseases. *In* Stanbury JB, Wyngaarden JB, Fredrickson DS, et al. (eds.): The Metabolic Basis of Inherited Disease. 5th ed. New York, McGraw-Hill, 1983. *A comprehensive chapter with good historical perspective.*

Neufeld EF, Muenzer J: The mucopolysaccharide storage diseases. *In* Scriver CR, Beaudet AL, Sly WS, et al. (eds.): The Metabolic Basis of Inherited Disease. 6th ed. New York, McGraw-Hill, 1989. *A current, comprehensive treatment of biochemical and genetic information.*

187 The Marfan Syndrome

Peter H. Byers

DEFINITION. The Marfan syndrome is a dominantly inherited connective tissue disorder characterized by musculoskeletal abnormalities (arachnodactyly, tall stature, scoliosis, pectus deformities, and ligamentous laxity), cardiovascular abnormalities (mitral valve prolapse and regurgitation, aortic valve insufficiency, and aortic dilatation, aneurysm, and dissection), lens dislocation, and myopia.

ETIOLOGY AND PATHOGENESIS. For most patients the molecular defect is not known. Recent studies have shown that monoclonal antibodies to fibrillin, a component of microfibrils of elastic fibers and of other microfibrils, stain the matrix of skin and the extracellular matrix of cultured fibroblasts from individuals with the Marfan syndrome poorly when compared with normal persons. Linkage studies using anonymous DNA markers indicate that the gene responsible for the Marfan syndrome is on the long arm of chromosome 15.

PREVALENCE. The Marfan syndrome affects about 1 in 15,000 individuals without racial or ethnic predilection.

PATHOLOGY. The mitral and aortic valves are characterized by "myxomatous degeneration" or the appearance of large pools of nonfibrous material that separate the normal cells of the valves. The valves may be thickened. In the absence of dissection there is accumulation of metachromatic material in the aortic media and disruption of the normal elastic laminae. Aortic dissection characteristically begins in the ascending aorta and may proceed in both directions. Death frequently results from cardiac tamponade due to hemopericardium, coronary occlusion, occlusion of the arteries to the brain, internal hemorrhage, or loss of perfusion of multiple abdominal organs.

CLINICAL MANIFESTATIONS. The Marfan syndrome is highly variable in its clinical manifestations, and affected members within the same family may differ in the degree to which they express the mutation; the differences between families may be explained, in part, by different mutations in a single connective tissue gene or mutations in different connective tissue genes. The diagnosis can be made occasionally in newborns because of lens dislocation, mitral valve prolapse, scoliosis, and tall stature with arachnodactyly. More commonly, affected infants may be tall, but cardiac findings are minimal. Many have mild to moderate scoliosis with pectus deformities (excavatum or carinatum); progression of scoliosis or pectus deformities may be rapid during the adolescent growth spurt. About half the patients with the Marfan syndrome have ocular lens dislocation, usually in a superior and nasal direction and generally nonprogressive after adolescence. Cataract formation and glaucoma are occasional complications of ectopia lentis. Mitral valve prolapse is seen in virtually all patients with the Marfan syndrome and in some progresses to symptomatic mitral regurgitation; associated rhythm disturbances may be symptomatic.

The major life-threatening complication of the Marfan syndrome is aortic dissection and rupture, and most deaths result from cardiovascular disease. The risk of dissection is well correlated with aortic diameter. In some children aortic root diameters, measured by echocardiography, are greater than normal, but, more commonly, aortic diameters do not exceed the normal range (20 to 37 mm) until adulthood and usually enlarge gradually, although the rate may vary. Aortic dissection in the Marfan syndrome is occasionally asymptomatic, but usually there is prolonged, severe substernal chest pain of a tearing or searing quality, often with radiation into the neck, back, and arms. It is often accompanied by diaphoresis, hypotension, and shock. Blood pressure in the two arms may differ. Rarely, pregnancy may be complicated by dissection, even in the presence of a normal aortic diameter.

DIFFERENTIAL DIAGNOSIS. The Marfan syndrome is one of several disorders in which the characteristic habitus is seen. *Contractural arachnodactyly* is a dominantly inherited disorder characterized by arachnodactyly, joint contracture, small, cup-shaped ears, pectus deformity, mild scoliosis, and mitral valve prolapse, but lens dislocation is absent and aortic dilatation is not a complication. *Homocystinuria* (see Ch. 182) is characterized by autosomal recessive inheritance, tight joints, peripheral vascular disease, thrombosis of arterial vessels, lens dislocation, osteoporosis, and, often, mild mental retardation. The diagnosis is confirmed by detection of excessive homocystine in the urine. In the *nonasthenic form* of the Marfan syndrome, body habitus is normal, but lens dislocation and mitral valve prolapse are common, and death from aortic aneurysm and dissection often establishes the diagnosis. Aortic dissection generally occurs in the fifth to seventh decades; the disorder is inherited in an autosomal dominant fashion. The *mitral valve prolapse syndrome* is commonly mistaken for the Marfan syndrome because of the presence of mitral valve prolapse, tall stature, and some of the mild skeletal features of the Marfan syndrome. The disorder is inherited in an autosomal dominant fashion; the absence of lens dislocation and progressive aortic root dilatation distinguishes it from the Marfan syndrome. Patients with the *Stickler syndrome* may have a marfanoid habitus, degenerative arthritis of multiple joints, cleft palate, and, generally, vitreal degeneration. The *marfanoid habitus* may be seen in some patients with sickle cell disease, the Klinefelter syndrome (the 47 XXY karyotype, see Ch. 222), and multiple endocrine adenomatosis type IIB (see Ch. 228).

TREATMENT. Treatment of the Marfan syndrome has several objectives: control of excessive height, prevention of glaucoma, regulation of blood pressure, and prevention of aortic dissection. Excessive height may be controlled by administration of testosterone (to boys) and estrogens (to girls) prior to puberty to hasten epiphyseal closure. Routine ophthalmologic examination is important to assure that dislocation of the lens into the anterior chamber does not occur and to treat any retinal detachment (the consequence of the high myopia that accompanies the syndrome). Rarely, the lenses must be removed because of recurrent anterior chamber displacement or because the lens edge is in the center of the visual field and adequate correction cannot be achieved. Blood pressure should always be maintained in the normal range. There is some indication that treatment with agents that decrease cardiac contractility (beta-adrenergic blockers, for example) may delay the rate of aortic progression, but this is an area of controversy, and appropriate controlled studies have not yet been published; nonetheless, in some centers such treatment is routine.

Recently, the advances in surgical technique have made replacement of diseased portions of the aorta a routine treatment that provides increased life expectancy. Replacement should be considered when aortic root diameter reaches approximately 55 mm and prior to decompensation of the left ventricle as a result of aortic valve insufficiency. A composite graft that includes an aortic valve is now used. In some patients, mitral valve function is compromised and the valve requires replacement or repair. Techniques for replacement of large portions of the aorta have also helped to prolong survival.

PROGNOSIS. The prognosis in the Marfan syndrome depends largely on the vascular complications. In one major study the mean age of death for all affected individuals was in the early 40's, and virtually all died of the cardiovascular complications. The judicious use of surgical replacement of the ascending aorta and, if needed, additional parts of the aorta appears to prolong survival. If the controlled studies of treatment with beta-adrenergic blockage demonstrate effectiveness, then another treatment of the cardiovascular complications will be available.

Patients with the Marfan syndrome should be observed yearly by an internist, a family physician, or a geneticist. Echocardiography should be performed yearly to follow aortic root diameter and the magnitude of mitral regurgitation and aortic insufficiency. Patients should see an ophthalmologist regularly and should consult with a cardiac surgeon as the aortic root diameter passes 50 to 55 mm.

Pregnancy usually is completed without complication, but women in whom the aortic diameter is greater than 40 mm (above the upper limits of normal) may be at greater risk for complications. All pregnancies should be followed in a high-risk center.

Prenatal diagnosis, the only form of prevention, is not currently available. Genetic counseling is important for all members of the proband's family to identify those who are affected.

Gott VL, Pyeritz RE, Magovern GJ Jr, et al.: Surgical treatment of aneurysms of the ascending aorta in the Marfan syndrome: Results of composite-graft repair in 50 patients. N Engl J Med 314:1070, 1986. *A review of the surgical approach to the patient with the Marfan syndrome: outcome, complications, criteria for selection, and longevity.*

Hollister DW, Godfrey M, Sakai LY, et al.: Immunohistologic abnormalities of the microfibrillar-fiber system in the Marfan syndrome. N Engl J Med 323:152, 1990. *Demonstration of defective staining of fibrillin and discussion of its presumed relevance in the Marfan syndrome.*

Kainulainen K, Pulkkinen L, Savolainen A, et al.: Location on chromosome of the gene defect causing Marfan syndrome. N Engl J Med 323:935, 1990. *Location of the Marfan gene using the techniques of "reverse genetics."*

Maumenee IH: The eye in the Marfan syndrome. Trans Am Ophthalmol Soc 79:684, 1981. *The most comprehensive review of the eye findings in the Marfan syndrome and their differential diagnosis.*

McKusick VA: Heritable Disorders of Connective Tissue. 4th ed. St. Louis, CV Mosby Company, 1972, pp 61–200. *Still the most comprehensive description of patients with the Marfan syndrome. Many case histories, easy and interesting to read; anecdotal.*

Pyeritz RE, McKusick VA: The Marfan syndrome: Diagnosis and management. N Engl J Med 300:772, 1979. *A more formal statistical compilation of the frequency of physical findings and complications in patients with the Marfan syndrome. Recommendations for management and follow-up.*

188 Ehlers-Danlos Syndrome

Peter H. Byers

DEFINITION. Ehlers-Danlos syndrome (EDS) is a group of more than 10 inherited connective tissue disorders characterized by abnormalities of the skin, ligaments, and internal organs. The clinical manifestations include skin fragility, abnormal scar formation, excessive bruising, joint laxity, and, in one variety, rupture of viscera and arteries (Table 188–1).

ETIOLOGY. Some forms of EDS result from defects in the synthesis and processing of types I and III collagens, the major proteins of skin, ligaments, tendons, blood vessels, and viscera. The molecular bases of EDS types I, II, III, V, and VIII are not known. The known defects include mutations affecting the structure, synthesis, processing, or stability of type III collagen (EDS type IV); deficient hydroxylation of lysyl residues in type I and type III collagen (EDS type VI); defective conversion of type I procollagen to collagen (EDS type VII); defective collagen crosslinking and abnormal cellular utilization of copper (EDS type IX); and a functional defect in fibronectin (EDS type X).

PREVALENCE. The prevalence of EDS is about 1 in 5000 births. EDS type III, benign familial hypermobility, accounts for most patients identified as having EDS; some forms are uncommon (EDS types IV, VI, VII, and VIII); others have been found in only a few families (EDS types IX and X). There is no racial or ethnic predisposition for any of the common types of EDS.

PATHOLOGY AND PATHOGENESIS. Dermal collagen fibrils in patients with EDS types I, II, III, and VI are larger than normal and irregular in outline when viewed by electron microscopy. In EDS type IV, skin is thin and collagen fibril diameter is frequently smaller than normal. Arterial wall thickness is usually less than normal, and tensile strength is diminished. Fibroblastic cells in dermis frequently have marked dilatation of the rough endoplasmic reticulum as a result of defective secretion of type III procollagen. There are no specific pathologic features of the other types of EDS.

CLINICAL MANIFESTATIONS. The clinical manifestations of each type of EDS are different (Table 188–1); it is important to identify patients with EDS type IV because of the grave consequences of the disease and to identify those with EDS types VI, V, and IX because of the risk of recurrence in their families.

EDS types I and II are characterized by marked joint laxity; soft, velvety, and hyperextensible skin; easy bruising; and "cigarette-paper" scars in areas of trauma. They differ in severity. Prematurity is common in EDS type I but rare in EDS type II. The major complications of both are recurrent joint dislocations, skin fragility, and early-onset osteoarthritis. The manifestations of joint laxity are more severe in childhood and decrease following puberty. At present the diagnosis depends on recognition of the appropriate clinical findings; electron microscopic studies of dermis may be confirmatory but are not specific. Patients with EDS type III are commonly seen by rheumatologists because of the joint discomfort and early onset of degenerative joint disease.

EDS type IV, the most severe form, usually results from dominant mutations in the genes of type III collagen; autosomal recessive inheritance has been described but is very rare. The diagnosis is confirmed by finding decreased amounts of type III collagen in skin, by identifying a defect in the structure, synthesis, or secretion of type III procollagen by cultured dermal fibroblasts, or by identifying a defect in gene structure. In the newborn

TABLE 188–1. CLINICAL FEATURES, MODE OF INHERITANCE, AND BIOCHEMICAL DISORDERS OF THE EHLERS-DANLOS SYNDROME

Type	Clinical Features	Inheritance*	Biochemical Disorders
I. Gravis	Soft, velvety, hyperextensible skin; easy bruising; "cigarette-paper" scars; hypermobile joints; varicose veins; prematurity	AD	Not known
II. Mitis	Similar to type I, but less severe	AD	Not known
III. Familial hypermobility	Soft skin, no scarring, marked large and small joint hypermobility	AD	Not known
IV. Arterial	Thin, translucent skin with visible veins; marked bruising; skin and joints have normal extensibility; arterial, bowel, and uterine rupture	AD (AR)	Abnormal type III collagen synthesis, secretion, or structure
V. X linked	Similar to type II	XLR	Not known
VI. Ocular	Soft, velvety, hyperextensible skin; hypermobile joints, scoliosis; ocular fragility and keratoconus	AR	Lysyl hydroxylase deficiency
VII. Arthrochalasis multiplex congenita	Congenital hip dislocation, joint hypermobility; soft skin with normal scarring	AD	Abnormal structure of the amino-terminal cleavage site in proα1(I) and proα2(I)
VIII. Periodontal	Generalized periodontitis; skin similar to type II	AD	Not known
IX. Cutis laxa, bladder diverticula	Soft, extensible, lax skin; bladder diverticula and rupture; short arms, limited pronation and supination; broad clavicles; occipital horns	XLR	Abnormal copper utilization with defect in lysyl oxidase
X. Fibronectin defect	Similar to type II	AR	Defect in fibronectin

* AD = Autosomal dominant; AR = autosomal resessive; XLR = X-linked recessive.

period some infants already have bruising, but most affected infants are difficult to identify. By adolescence the veins are readily visible on the trunk and extremities, and bruising is common. Vascular or bowel rupture is rare during childhood. Arterial fragility may manifest as sudden death, stroke, shock from retroperitoneal or intra-abdominal bleeding, or compartmental syndromes, depending on the site of vessel rupture. Prompt surgical intervention may be lifesaving, although tissue friability may make repairs difficult. Pregnancy may be complicated by arterial or uterine rupture, either of which is often fatal. Recurrent abdominal pain may result from repeated mural hemorrhage in the small intestine. Sigmoid rupture is common. Survival beyond the fifth decade is rare.

EDS type VI is an autosomal recessive disorder characterized by a marfanoid habitus, skin and joint findings similar to those in EDS type II, ocular fragility, and scoliosis. The diagnosis is made by finding decreased amounts of hydroxylysine in skin and confirmed by low levels of lysyl hydroxylase measured in cultured dermal fibroblasts. Late complications may include vascular rupture, as well as blindness from retinal detachment or globe rupture.

EDS type VII is often detected in the newborn period, because of bilateral congenital hip dislocation and marked joint laxity. The hips are often difficult to stabilize, and recurrent dislocation may continue at the hips and other joints. When suspected clinically the diagnosis can be confirmed in some patients by identifying intermediates in the conversion of type I procollagen to collagen in skin and confirming the defect in cultured dermal fibroblasts. The most common defect recognized is an abnormal structure of the proα2(I) chain caused by exon 6 skipping.

EDS type VIII is characterized by the combination of noninflammatory gingival loss (often leading to loss of teeth) and the cutaneous and joint signs of the EDS type II phenotype.

EDS type IX is noted in childhood with skin hyperextensibility and laxity, drooping facies, and minor skeletal anomalies. Evidence of bladder dysfunction may be present by the age of 6 years, and diverticula of the bladder and hydronephrosis may occur. Mild chronic diarrhea, orthostatic hypotension, short upper arms with limited pronation and supination, and the occipital inferior horns become apparent during adolescence. Intelligence is usually in the normal range; inheritance is X-linked recessive. The diagnosis is made by the low serum copper and ceruloplasmin levels and confirmed by low lysyl oxidase levels in cultured dermal fibroblasts. Maintenance of normal urinary drainage is important to prevent renal failure, and continuing bladder drainage may be essential to prevent rupture. There is some variation in severity among families.

DIFFERENTIAL DIAGNOSIS. The differential diagnosis is generally limited to the varieties of EDS, although some patients with the Marfan syndrome have marked joint laxity and others with forms of osteogenesis imperfecta have joint laxity and easy bruising. Patients with EDS type IV and EDS types I and II are often investigated for a bleeding diathesis before the correct diagnosis is made. Because of joint instability and laxity many patients with EDS types I, II, III, VI, and VII are investigated for developmental delay before it is recognized that they have a form of EDS.

TREATMENT. The gaping skin wounds that occur in some forms of EDS should be approximated carefully, and the removable sutures should be left in place for twice the usual time. Recurrent dislocations can often be repaired surgically, although further recurrence is more common than in unaffected individuals. Arterial rupture in patients with EDS type IV needs to be treated surgically unless bleeding is controlled by compartmental limitation (e.g., some retroperitoneal bleeding). The repair of affected arteries is often difficult because of extreme friability. If colon rupture recurs, the colon should be excised to prevent further episodes. Rupture of the small bowel is very rare. Some patients with EDS type VI respond to ascorbic acid (1 to 4 grams per day) with some symptomatic improvement and increased excretion of hydroxylysine in the urine. There is no metabolic treatment for other forms of EDS, and management is largely symptomatic.

PROGNOSIS. The prognosis in EDS depends on the specific type with which the patient is affected. Life expectancy is considerably shortened in EDS type IV because of organ and vessel rupture and may be decreased in EDS type VI; in all others, life expectancy is normal. With the exception of EDS type VI, no specific therapy is available that affects the natural history of the condition.

Prevention by prenatal diagnosis is feasible for some types of EDS. Heterozygosity for the EDS type VI mutation has been recognized by examination of amniotic fluid cells in a family at risk for recurrence. The structural mutations in EDS type VII and in EDS type IV should be recognizable by studies of collagens synthesized by chorionic villus cells in culture, but this approach has not yet been used. Analysis of copper uptake and distribution by amniotic fluid cells should facilitate prenatal diagnosis of EDS type IX. All families should have genetic counseling once a proband is identified.

Byers PH, Holbrook KA: Molecular basis of clinical heterogeneity in the Ehlers-Danlos syndrome. Ann NY Acad Sci 460:298, 1985. *The most comprehensive and up-to-date review of the molecular lesions in EDS.*

McKusick VA: Heritable Disorders of Connective Tissue. 4th ed. St Louis, C. V. Mosby Company, 1972, pp 292–371. *Although the classification is not up to date, the richness of clinical detail is unsurpassed. A delight to read because of the many case histories and the personal touch.*

189 Osteogenesis Imperfecta

David W. Rowe

Osteogenesis imperfecta (OI) is a heritable disorder of connective tissue that results primarily in fragile bones that break with minimal trauma. The disease may be limited to a few fractures in childhood, result in 50 to 100 fractures by adulthood with severe long-bone and chest deformity, or cause death in the newborn. The prevalence is 5 per 100,000 live births, and there is no known racial or ethnic predilection. A sufficiently large number of patients with varying degrees of bone disease have been characterized at the molecular level to develop molecular and clinical correlations. Thus it is now possible to predict with some degree of confidence the relative severity of bone disease that will result from a specific mutation within the type I collagen genes. Not only is it important for the internist to be aware of the genetic basis of classic forms of OI (Table 189–1), it will also be prudent to recognize those individuals with unusual forms of osteoporosis or those with a striking family history of osteopenic bone disease as potential candidates for mild OI due to a recognizable mutation in type I collagen genes.

PATHOGENESIS. The tissues that are abnormal in OI are composed primarily of type I collagen. This collagen type has a triple-helical conformation formed by two genetically distinct but related polypeptide chains in a ratio of two α1(I) and one α2(I) chains. The mildest form of OI (type I) appears to result from underproduction of type I collagen caused by reduced accumulation of α1(I) collagen messenger RNA (mRNA) within the

TABLE 189–1. CLINICAL CLASSIFICATION OF OSTEOGENESIS IMPERFECTA

Type	Description	Inheritance	Suspected Mutation
I	Mild, nondeforming	AD	Deficient amounts of α1(I) mRNA
II	Lethal in the perinatal period	NDM, GM (AR)	Mutations within helical domain of the α1(I) gene
III	Severe long-bone deformity and scoliosis	NDM, GM (AR)	Mutations within helical domain of either the α1(I) or the α2(I) gene
IV	Severity is intermediate between I and III with long-bone deformity	AD	Mutation within helical domain of the α2(I) gene

AD = autosomal dominant; GM (AR) = germinal mosaicism, which can appear as an autosomal recessive; NDM = new dominant mutation.

cytoplasm. In the more severe forms of OI (types II, III, and IV), there are mutations within the helical regions of either the α1(I) or the α2(I) chain. These changes result from either a partial gene deletion or a nucleotide point mutation that alters an amino acid essential to the helical conformation of the α chains. Molecules containing a mutant α chain do not form normal triple-helical molecules. Furthermore, molecules containing a mutant chain interfere with the interactions of adjacent normal molecules, thus weakening the entire structure. Such a mechanism accounts for the dominant inheritance of the disease. The severity of the clinical defect is probably related to the qualitative nature of the mutation and the extent to which the abnormal chains accumulate within specific tissues. Still unanswered is why bone is more severely affected in OI than are other tissues equally rich in type I collagen. Animal models of spontaneous or transgenically induced OI may provide a better understanding of the pathogenesis of bone fragility.

TYPE AND CLINICAL MANIFESTATIONS. The terms OI tarda and OI congenita have been replaced by a classification scheme based on relatively distinct syndromes that reflect fundamentally different defects in type I collagen biosynthesis (Table 189–1). Type I OI is the mildest form and is associated with nondeforming fractures during childhood, which cease after puberty. Fractures can reappear with trauma and in postmenopausal women. In most cases a dominant family history can be elicited, with the associated features of blue sclerae, joint laxity, and thin skin, findings that are less obvious in older affected individuals. More variable are hearing abnormalities, short stature, and dentinogenesis imperfecta. Sporadic cases occur and presumably reflect a new mutation. Fractures heal normally, and osteopenia is appreciated only on quantitative bone densitometry. By contrast, the most severe form of OI (type II) results in infants who do not survive the newborn period. Their bones have a crumpled appearance on roentgenography and are so weak that dismemberment may occur. The disorder is usually acquired as a sporadic new mutation, but recurrences clearly occur secondary to germinal mosaicism of one parent. In OI types III and IV, there are severe deformities of the long bones, marked short stature, and moderate joint laxity. Gray sclerae, impaired hearing, and dentinogenesis imperfecta are frequently present. Fractures and deformity are usually present at birth. A spectrum of severity makes prediction of outcome shortly after birth hazardous. Scoliosis can progress to a point of causing restrictive lung disease, and severe long-bone deformity can preclude ambulation. However, infants born with identical deformities can eventually ambulate with the assistance of external bracing or internal fixation of the long bones. The more severe outcome is classified as type III OI, while the milder form is type IV. Patients with type IV constitute the most heterogeneous group, and any individual case may have features of either type I or type III. Both dominant and recessive modes (germinal mosaicism) of inheritance are observed.

DIAGNOSIS. The diagnosis of each form of OI is based on the history, physical examination, family pedigree, and radiographic features. Only the milder forms of this disease should pose a diagnostic problem with other disorders that cause minimal bone deformity or fractures and osteopenia. The bowing and fractures associated with osteomalacia or rickets are differentiated by roentgenography and the biochemical measures of calcium, phosphorus, parathyroid hormone, and vitamin D. Juvenile, disuse, and steroid-induced osteoporosis can be distinguished by history. Other rare diagnoses to be considered are infantile cortical hyperostosis (Caffey's disease) and hypophosphatasia. Studies of collagen synthesis and collagen mRNA in cultured fibroblasts, plus analysis of restriction fragment length polymorphisms for the type I collagen genes, are beginning to provide the means for a specific diagnosis of the various forms of the disease. However, most of these methods remain experimental. Prenatal diagnosis by ultrasonography continues to be the primary technique for diagnosis of the severer forms (type II and type III) of the disease.

TREATMENT. The use of supplemental calcium, vitamin D, fluoride, anabolic steroids, calcitonin, growth hormone, and pyrophosphate has not been shown to provide a satisfactory response. Since many of these drugs were used in heterogeneous groups of patients with OI, there may be subgroups of patients who could benefit from certain medical regimens. At present, therapy primarily involves orthopedic treatment with external bracing and surgical straightening with intramedullary splinting (rodding) of the long-bone deformities. Use of lightweight plastic bracing will assume a greater role in promoting ambulation. However, attempts to halt the progression of scoliosis in OI, as well as maintenance of good muscle tone and range of motion, are crucial to the optimal use of the extremities. Creative use of physical therapy, especially in the form of swimming, may be the most useful preventive measure in this disorder.

Akeson WH, Bornstein P, Glimcher MJ: Symposium on Heritable Disorders of Connective Tissue. St. Louis, C. V. Mosby Company, 1982. *See Ch. 20 to 23 for a general review of clinical and morphologic aspects of OI.*

Albright JA, Millar EA: Osteogenesis imperfecta. Clin Orthop 159:2, 1981. *A collection of numerous articles on the pathology and treatment of this disease. Unfortunately, treatment strategies have not improved since this article was published.*

Rowe DW, Shapiro JR: Osteogenesis imperfecta. *In* Avioli L, Krane S (eds.): Metabolic Bone Disease. 2nd ed. Philadelphia, W.B. Saunders Company, 1990. *Contains detailed discussion on the molecular basis of each clinical type of OI. For the latest update of known mutations, see Sykes B: Nature 348:18, 1990.*

Smith R, Francis MJO, Houghton GP: The Brittle Bone Syndrome. London, Butterworth Company, 1982. *A comprehensive clinical review by one group of investigators having a large experience with OI. Chapter 7 contains a thorough differential diagnosis.*

190 Pseudoxanthoma Elasticum

Jouni Uitto

Pseudoxanthoma elasticum (PXE) (synonyms: Grönblad-Strandberg syndrome, systemic elastorrhexis) is a generalized progressive connective tissue disorder primarily affecting the elastic fibers. Clinically, PXE manifests as characteristic cutaneous lesions, ocular changes, and widespread vascular abnormalities. The relative severity of these changes results in a variety of clinical pictures. The onset of the disease may be in early childhood, and in most cases the cutaneous changes are evident before the age of 30 years. The exact incidence of PXE is not known, although estimates are about 1 in 160,000 persons. The male-female ratio is probably 1:1.

CLINICAL MANIFESTATIONS. *Skin.* The primary cutaneous lesions are relatively small (1 to 3 mm) yellowish papules that give the affected area a pebbly, "plucked chicken skin" appearance. The primary lesions tend to coalesce into larger plaques, and the skin of the involved areas becomes thickened and leathery (Fig. 190–1). Gradually, the affected skin becomes redundant, lax, and inelastic. The predilection sites are the face, neck, axillary folds, lower abdomen, and thighs. The nasolabial folds and chin creases may be strikingly accentuated. Yellowish lesions similar to those noted on the skin can also be seen on the mucous membranes.

Eye. The ocular changes are characterized by angioid streaks, i.e., grayish or brownish-red, poorly defined streaks radiating across the fundus of the eye. Their development usually starts later than that of the cutaneous lesions, often during the third or fourth decade. The ocular changes are commonly bilateral and include hemorrhages and exudates in Bruch's membrane, an elastin-rich structure located between the retina and the choroid. The degenerative changes of the eye frequently lead to impaired vision, and complete blindness, although rare, is one of the major complications of PXE. Angioid streaks may be present without noticeable cutaneous changes, but other accompanying observations, such as vascular changes, may lead to correct diagnosis of PXE. Angioid streaks can also be associated with other diseases—for example, Paget's disease of bone, sickle cell anemia, tumoral calcinosis, lead poisoning, and idiopathic thrombocytopenia.

Vascular Manifestations. The early manifestations of arterial involvement include hypertension, weak peripheral pulses, and, occasionally, intermittent claudication. The most devastating complications develop as a result of coronary occlusion or cerebral

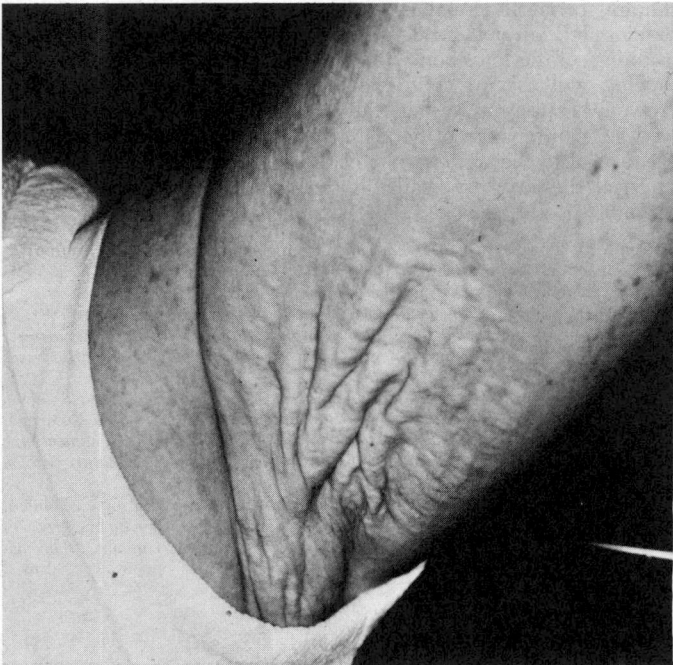

FIGURE 190–1. Typical cutaneous manifestations of pseudoxanthoma elasticum. The lesion demonstrates redundant and inelastic skin in the axillary fold.

hemorrhage; the most frequent complication is recurrent bleeding from the gastrointestinal tract. A common site of the gastrointestinal bleeding is the gastric mucosa, where the elastic fibers of the arteries are particularly affected. Bleeding from the urinary tract can also occur.

INHERITANCE. Most cases of PXE are inherited as an autosomal recessive disease. However, autosomal dominant inheritance has been documented in a few families, although delayed onset, incomplete expression, and lack of carrier detection complicate the genetic analysis.

In addition to the inherited forms, several cases with cutaneous findings consistent with PXE but without family history and without vascular or ocular involvement have been reported. In some of these cases, the development of skin lesions is related to external trauma, such as exposure to Norwegian saltpeter. Patients with an unusual perforating variant of cutaneous PXE have been described. In these patients the lesions are confined to the abdomen, most often in a periumbilical distribution. Periumbilical perforating PXE appears to be a distinct acquired form of the disease.

PATHOLOGY. Histopathologic examination of the involved skin demonstrates an accumulation of structures in the middle or lower dermis that stain positively with stains specific for elastic fibers, e.g., Verhoeff's stain. In contrast to the elastic fibers in normal skin, the elastic material in PXE appears irregularly clumped and fragmented. The accumulation of elastic fibers has also been quantitated by computerized morphometric analyses and by assay of desmosine, an elastin-specific crosslink compound. Characteristically, the fragmented elastic fibers contain calcium that appears bluish on routine hematoxylin-eosin stain and that can be demonstrated by calcium-specific stains. Electron microscopy of affected skin demonstrates that the amorphous elastin component has been replaced by bundles of granular material with staining properties different from those of normal elastin. Also, foci containing calcium hydroxyapatite crystals can be detected in the elastic fibers. These morphologic findings thus provide evidence for derangement in the organization of the elastic structures in PXE. Biochemical proof of the exact molecular defect in the structure or metabolism of elastin is, however, lacking, and it is unclear whether the calcification of elastic fibers is a primary or secondary event.

THERAPY. No specific treatment is available, and the primary prevention entails genetic counseling. Although treatment with vitamin E, vitamin C, or a low-calcium diet has been advocated in isolated case reports, no clinical proof of the efficacy of any of these therapies is available in the form of controlled clinical trials. In selected cases, plastic surgery may be helpful in improving the cosmetic appearance of the skin.

Neldner KH: Pseudoxanthoma elasticum. Clin Dermatol 6:1, 1988. *Extremely useful clinical account of PXE, based on the author's data on 100 patients followed over a 10-year period.*

Neldner KH, Martinez-Hernandez A: Localized acquired cutaneous pseudoxanthoma elasticum. J Am Acad Dermatol 1:523, 1979. *Clinical description of a distinct acquired form of pseudoxanthoma elasticum.*

Uitto J: Elastic fibers in cutaneous diseases. Curr Concepts Skin Dis 6:19, 1985. *A review of the molecular defects of elastin in heritable connective tissue diseases, including pseudoxanthoma elasticum.*

Uitto J, Paul JL, Brockley K, et al.: Elastic fibers in human skin: Quantitation of elastic fibers by computerized digital image analyses and determination of elastin by a radioimmunoassay of desmosine. Lab Invest 49:499, 1983. *Demonstration of increased elastin concentrations in the lesional skin in pseudoxanthoma elasticum.*

DISORDERS OF PORPHYRINS OR METALS

191 The Porphyrias

Karl E. Anderson

The porphyrias result from deficiencies of specific enzymes of the heme biosynthetic pathway, are usually inherited, and may be associated with striking accumulations of heme pathway intermediates. Porphyrias are more prevalent, and more often manifested in adults, than are most well-characterized inborn errors of major metabolic pathways. Clinical expression is variable and is influenced by factors such as hormones, drugs, and nutrition that have regulatory effects on the heme biosynthetic pathway. Different types of mutations of structural genes for heme pathway enzymes have been found for several types of porphyria. How-ever, genetic heterogeneity does not explain the variable clinical expression of these diseases.

Two major types of clinical manifestations are characteristic. First, cutaneous photosensitivity occurs in types of porphyria in which porphyrins accumulate. Tissue damage results from excitation of porphyrins by long-wave ultraviolet light. Second, neurologic effects occur in porphyrias characterized by accumulation of the porphyrin precursors δ-aminolevulinic acid (ALA) and porphobilinogen (PBG).

Because the porphyrias are uncommon and their symptoms are nonspecific, the diagnosis depends on a high index of suspicion. Confirmation by appropriate laboratory testing is essential. Porphyria must be differentiated from (1) "porphyrinuria," which can occur in various clinical conditions, and (2) minimal departures from reference ranges, both of which may have no clinical significance.

ENZYMES AND INTERMEDIATES OF THE HEME BIOSYNTHETIC PATHWAY IN THE PORPHYRIAS.

A type of porphyria has been associated with a deficiency of seven of the eight enzymes of the heme biosynthetic pathway (see Fig. 191–1). Heme is synthesized from glycine and succinyl CoA. Intermediates in the pathway include ALA, an amino acid; PBG, a pyrrole; and hydroxymethylbilane, a linear tetrapyrrole that undergoes spontaneous closure to form uroporphyrinogen I, which is not metabolized beyond coproporphyrinogen I. Uroporphyrinogen III cosynthase catalyzes inversion of one of the pyrroles of hydroxymethylbilane and closure of the molecule to form a porphyrin macrocycle, uroporphyrinogen III. The next two enzymes result in decarboxylation of six of the eight side chains of uroporphyrinogen, with sequential formation of 7-, 6-, and 5-carboxylate porphyrinogens, coproporphyrinogen, 3-carboxylate porphyrinogen, and protoporphyrinogen. The final two enzymes catalyze oxidation of protoporphyrinogen IX to protoporphyrin IX and insertion of ferrous iron in the porphyrin macrocycle to form heme.

Heme is synthesized in largest amounts in bone marrow and liver, where it is used primarily to make hemoglobin and cytochrome P450, respectively. Hepatic heme biosynthesis is regulated primarily by ALA synthase, which is under sensitive feedback control by cellular free heme content. ALA synthase is induced by many of the same drugs and steroids that induce hepatic cytochrome P450. Additional pathway enzymes and cellular uptake of iron are important in the regulation of heme synthesis in erythroid cells. Intracellular concentrations of intermediates, which are generally less than the Michaelis constant (K_m) values for heme pathway enzymes, may greatly influence reaction rates.

Heme pathway intermediates are utilized efficiently and excreted only in small amounts. Normally, ALA and PBG are excreted in much larger amounts than are porphyrins. Porphyrinogens undergo auto-oxidation outside cells and are excreted primarily as porphyrins. ALA, PBG, uroporphyrin, and 7-, 6-, and 5-carboxylate porphyrins are excreted mostly in urine, coproporphyrin in urine and bile, and harderoporphyrin (3-carboxylate porphyrin) and protoporphyrin in bile and feces. ALA, PBG, and porphyrinogens are colorless and nonfluorescent. Porphyrins are reddish and fluoresce when exposed to long-wave ultraviolet light.

CLASSIFICATION. Traditionally, porphyrias have been divided into erythropoietic and hepatic types, based on whether the excess production of intermediates takes place primarily in bone marrow or liver (Table 191–1). Some porphyrias have both erythroid and hepatic features. Porphyrias with neurovisceral symptoms are also termed "acute porphyrias." They share many clinical features and are similarly managed. Several "cutaneous porphyrias" manifest similar skin lesions, but treatment and prognosis differ considerably. Now that these disorders are better characterized, they are best classified in terms of their specific enzyme deficiencies.

PORPHYRIA WITH ALA-DEHYDRATASE DEFICIENCY (ALA-D PORPHYRIA).

In this very rare autosomal recessive disorder, ALA dehydratase is markedly reduced (1 to 2 per cent of normal), and urinary excretion of ALA and coproporphyrin III is increased. In this and other disorders in which ALA accumulates, coproporphyrin III may originate from excess ALA by metabolism to coproporphyrinogen III in tissues other than that in which the excess ALA originates. Symptoms resemble those of acute intermittent porphyria but may begin in childhood. Hemolysis may be present.

Other Conditions Associated with ALA-Dehydratase Deficiency. Lead poisoning and hereditary tyrosinemia can cause increased ALA and symptoms, including abdominal pain, ileus, and motor neuropathy, that are strikingly similar to those of the acute porphyrias. Lead concentrates in erythroid cells and inhibits ALA dehydratase. It also inhibits ferrochelatase, leading to excess erythrocyte protoporphyrin (complexed with zinc). Urinary coproporphyrin is increased.

In hereditary tyrosinemia, a deficiency of fumarylacetoacetase causes accumulation of succinylacetone (2,3-dioxoheptanoic acid), a structural analogue of ALA and a potent inhibitor of ALA dehydratase. Other heavy metals or styrene exposure can also inhibit ALA dehydratase.

ACUTE INTERMITTENT PORPHYRIA (AIP).

This is an autosomal dominant disorder that results from an approximately 50 per cent deficiency of PBG deaminase (formerly known as uroporphyrinogen I synthase). The enzyme is deficient in all individuals who inherit the mutant gene and remains fairly constant over time. Most persons with PBG deaminase deficiency remain asymptomatic.

Prevalence. AIP can occur in all races. Its prevalence in most countries has not been precisely estimated but may be most common (perhaps 5 per 100,000) in northern European populations. Prevalence in a chronic psychiatric population in the United States was estimated to be 210 per 100,000.

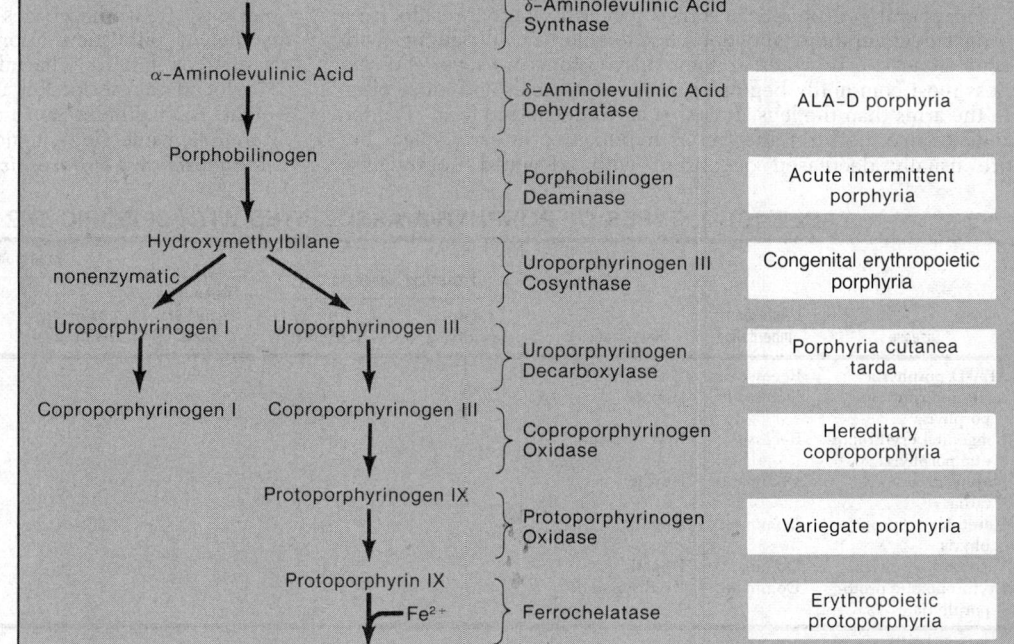

FIGURE 191–1. Intermediates and enzymes of the heme biosynthetic pathway, and diseases of porphyrin metabolism associated with deficiencies of specific enzymes. The initial and last three enzymes (in red) are mitochondrial, and the other four (in black) are cytosolic.

Etiology and Pathogenesis. In most patients with AIP, PBG deaminase is decreased in all tissues. However, the nature of the mutation at the PBG deaminase gene locus varies among AIP lineages. One type of mutation causes the enzyme to be deficient only in nonerythropoietic tissues.

Partial deficiency of PBG deaminase probably does not of itself greatly impair hepatic heme synthesis or induce ALA synthase. This fact is suggested by normal urinary ALA and PBG values and apparently normal cytochrome P450 content in most persons with clinically latent AIP. When the demand for hepatic heme is increased by drugs, hormones, or nutritional factors, induction of ALA synthase is accentuated by the presence of PBG deaminase deficiency. In clinically expressed AIP, hepatic cytochrome P450 may be reduced and can be restored by heme therapy.

Most drugs that are harmful in AIP induce hepatic ALA synthase and cytochrome P450. Sulfonamide antibiotics are not inducers and may inhibit PBG deaminase. Reduced caloric and carbohydrate intakes enhance induction of ALA synthase in animals and increase ALA and PBG levels and precipitate symptoms in AIP. Administration of carbohydrate can reduce hepatic ALA synthase and cytochrome P450.

The mechanism of neural damage in AIP is unknown, but porphyrias and related disorders associated with increased ALA have similar neurologic manifestations. ALA is structurally analogous to γ-aminobutyric acid (GABA) and can interact with GABA receptors. However, ALA and other products of the heme pathway have not been convincingly shown to be neurotoxic. The suggestion that heme deficiency may occur in nervous tissue in these disorders is also unproved.

Clinical Manifestations. Symptoms rarely occur before puberty and seldom, if ever, recur throughout adult life. Symptoms can begin after menopause. Characteristically, attacks last for several days or longer, often require hospitalization, and are followed by complete recovery. Abdominal pain is the most common symptom; it is usually steady and poorly localized but may be cramping. Other manifestations include nausea; vomiting; constipation; tachycardia; hypertension; mental symptoms; pain in the limbs, head, neck, or chest; muscle weakness; and sensory loss. Ileus, with distention and decreased bowel sounds, is common. However, increased bowel sounds and diarrhea may be present. Because the abdominal symptoms are neurologic rather than inflammatory, tenderness, fever, and leukocytosis are generally absent or mild. Tachycardia, hypertension, restlessness, fine tremors, and excess sweating may be due to sympathetic overactivity. Dysuria and bladder dysfunction may occur and require catheterization. Recurrent attacks tend to be similar in a given patient.

Peripheral neuropathy in AIP is primarily motor, results from axonal degeneration, and does not develop in all patients with acute attacks, even when abdominal symptoms are severe. Weakness most commonly begins in proximal muscles and more often in the arms than the legs. It can be asymmetric and focal. Tendon reflexes may be little affected or hyperactive in early stages but are usually decreased or absent with advanced neuropathy.

Cranial and sensory nerves can be affected. Progression to respiratory and bulbar paralysis and death seldom occurs unless porphyria is not recognized, harmful drugs are not discontinued, and appropriate treatment is not instituted. Sudden death, presumably the result of cardiac arrhythmia, may also occur.

The central nervous system can be involved. Anxiety, insomnia, depression, disorientation, hallucinations, and paranoia, which can be especially severe during acute attacks, may suggest a primary mental disorder or hysteria. Depression and other mental symptoms may be chronic. Seizures may occur as an acute neurologic manifestation of AIP itself or as a result of hyponatremia, or they can be due to causes unrelated to porphyria. Treatment of seizures is problematic because virtually all antiseizure drugs (except bromides) can exacerbate AIP. Hyponatremia may be due to hypothalamic involvement and inappropriate antidiuretic hormone (ADH) secretion or to vomiting, diarrhea, poor intake, or excessive renal sodium loss.

After several days, an attack may resolve quite rapidly; abdominal pain may disappear within a few hours and paresis within a few days. Even advanced neuropathy is potentially reversible. Repeated attacks may result in profound malnutrition.

Although liver function is generally well preserved, hepatic abnormalities may be more common in AIP than was previously recognized. AIP may predispose to chronic hypertension and may be associated with impaired renal function.

Precipitating Factors. Recognition of precipitating factors, which as a rule are multiple, is important in management. That endogenous steroid hormones are probably most important is indicated by the rarity of symptoms and excess ALA and PBG before puberty, more frequent clinical expression in women, premenstrual attacks in some women, and exacerbations after administration of sex steroid preparations. Progesterone and progesterone and androgen metabolites with a 5β-H configuration are potent inducers of hepatic ALA synthase. Cyclic attacks usually occur when progesterone levels are highest. Estrogens produce little or no induction of ALA synthase. However, administered estrogens may increase ALA and PBG excretion. Pregnancy is usually well tolerated. Attacks during pregnancy may result from hyperemesis gravidarum and reduced caloric intake.

Drugs remain important as causes of AIP attacks. Hormones and nutrition are often additive. Probably for this reason, (1) drugs may induce attacks in adults but are rarely reported to do so in children with PBG deaminase deficiency, (2) anticonvulsants do not induce attacks in some PBG deaminase–deficient subjects, and (3) barbiturate anesthetics more often exacerbate porphyria if symptoms were present before exposure to anesthetics. The major drugs known to be harmful or safe in the acute porphyrias are listed in Table 191–2. Barbiturates and sulfonamides are most notorious. Benzodiazepines are much less hazardous. There is insufficient published information to allow most drugs to be classified as definitely harmful or safe.

Reduced caloric intake, usually instituted in an effort to lose weight, is a common cause of attacks. They are also provoked by intercurrent infections, major surgery, and other conditions.

Diagnosis and Differential Diagnosis. The diagnosis of AIP is

TABLE 191–1. TYPES OF PORPHYRIA ASSOCIATED WITH SPECIFIC ENZYME DEFICIENCIES

Disease	Autosomal Inheritance	Classification	Presenting Symptoms		Excess Accumulations and Excretions				
			Photo-sensitivity	Neurologic	δ-Amino-levulinic Acid	Porpho-bilinogen	Uro-porphyrin	Copro-porphyrin	Proto-porphyrin
ALA-D porphyria	Recessive	—	−	+	+	−	−	+	+
Acute intermittent porphyria	Dominant	Hepatic	−	+	+	+	+	±	−
Congenital erythropoietic porphyria	Recessive	Erythropoietic	+	−	−	−	+*	+*	±
Porphyria cutanea tarda	Dominant†	Hepatic	+	−	−	−	+‡	+‡	−
Hereditary coproporphyria	Dominant†	Hepatic	+	+	+	+	±	+	−
Variegate porphyria	Dominant†	Hepatic	+	+	+	+	±	+	+
Erythropoietic protoporphyria	Dominant	Erythropoietic	+	−	−	−	−	−	+

*Mostly type I isomers.
†Homozygous forms of these disorders also occur.
‡Accompanied by 7-, 6-, and 5-carboxylate porphyrins and isocoproporphyrins.

TABLE 191–2. SOME SAFE AND UNSAFE DRUGS IN THE ACUTE PORPHYRIAS

Unsafe

Barbiturates	Succinimides
Sulfonamide antibiotics	Carbamazepine
Meprobamate	Valproic acid
Glutethimide	Pyrazolones
Methyprylon	Griseofulvin
Ethchlorvynol	Ergots
Phenytoin	Danazol
Mephenytoin	Alcohol
Chlorpropamide	Estrogens and progestins

Safe

Narcotic analgesics	Digoxin
Aspirin	Bromides
Acetaminophen	Insulin
Phenothiazines	Atropine
Penicillin and derivatives	Diazepam (small doses)
Streptomycin	Dicumarol
Glucocorticoids	Diphenhydramine
Propranolol	Ether
Guanethidine	Nitrous oxide
Neostigmine	Thiazides
Succinylcholine	Heparin

often delayed because symptoms are nonspecific and physical findings minimal. A high index of suspicion and demonstration of a marked increase in PBG are required. Assays for PBG employ Ehrlich's aldehyde (p-dimethylaminobenzaldehyde), which forms reddish-purple chromagens with PBG, urobilinogen, and other substances in urine. The Watson-Schwartz test is still widely used to screen for increased PBG but is subject to misinterpretation and false-positive reports, does not quantify PBG, and is less sensitive and only slightly more rapid than quantitative methods such as that Mauzerall and Granick described in 1956. Therefore, qualitative tests for PBG are not recommended. If used for screening, positive samples should be retested by a quantitative method. During an acute attack, PBG excretion generally is in the range of 50 to 200 mg per day (reference range, 0 to 4 mg per day), and ALA excretion is 20 to 100 mg per day (reference range, 0 to 7 mg per day). Such increases virtually assure a diagnosis of AIP, variegate porphyria (VP), or hereditary coproporphyria (HCP).

It is useful to follow ALA and PBG excretion because these values generally decrease with clinical improvement. Such reductions are particularly dramatic after heme therapy. After an attack, it is distinctly unusual for ALA and PBG to decrease to normal levels, except after prolonged periods of latency. In HCP and VP, excretion of ALA and PBG may decrease to normal levels more readily. Fecal porphyrins are usually normal or minimally increased, which distinguishes AIP from HCP and VP.

Decreased levels of PBG deaminase (most conveniently measured in erythrocytes) confirm the diagnosis of AIP. However, in some AIP lineages, the enzyme is deficient only in nonerythropoietic tissues. A wide normal range (up to threefold, which somewhat overlaps the AIP range) and increases in hemolytic disorders also impair interpretation of erythrocyte PBG deaminase results. Measurement of erythrocyte PBG deaminase is highly useful for analyzing pedigrees of known patients with AIP, but not for screening individual acutely ill patients. When family members are screened, the urinary PBG level should also be measured.

No single laboratory test fully excludes AIP, HCP, and VP. However, a normal result of a quantitative test for urinary PBG virtually excludes these disorders as a cause of current symptoms. Efforts to provoke increases in ALA and PBG for diagnostic purposes by glycine loading or administration of phenobarbital or estrogen may be dangerous and are not definitive.

Treatment. Acute attacks usually require hospitalization for treatment of severe pain, nausea, and vomiting and for administration of intravenous glucose and heme. Hospitalization also facilitates observation for neurologic complications, electrolyte imbalances, and nutritional status and investigation of precipitating factors. Narcotic analgesics are usually required for abdominal pain and small to moderate doses of a phenothiazine for nausea, vomiting, anxiety, and restlessness. Chloral hydrate can be

employed for insomnia. Diazepam in low doses is probably safe if a minor tranquilizer is required.

Carbohydrate can be given orally as sucrose, glucose polymers, or carbohydrate-rich foods. If oral intake is poorly tolerated or is contraindicated by distention and ileus, intravenous administration of glucose (at least 300 grams daily) is usually indicated. A central venous line facilitates more complete parenteral nutrition support and helps avoid excess fluid volumes.

Heme therapy is more effective than glucose in reducing ALA and PBG. Although glucose infusions may be employed first, heme therapy should probably be initiated early. Its effectiveness is reduced when treatment is delayed. A lyophilized hematin (hydroxy-heme) preparation is available in the United States. It is reconstituted with sterile water but is unstable and must be infused promptly. The usual recommended dosage is 3 to 4 mg per kilogram of body weight infused intravenously once or twice daily, but lower dosages (e.g., 1 to 1.5 mg per kilogram once daily) may be equally effective. More stable preparations of heme (heme arginate and heme albumin) are available in Europe. Heme therapy should be instituted only after the diagnosis of a porphyric attack is confirmed at least by a markedly increased urinary PBG value. Diagnosis is more difficult after heme administration, which can at least transiently normalize porphyrin precursor excretion.

Response to heme therapy depends on the degree of neuronal damage and may not be observed for at least 48 hours. Severe neurologic damage and subacute or chronic symptoms are unlikely to respond. Excessive dosages of hematin may induce acute renal tubular damage. Recommended doses of hematin commonly cause phlebitis at the site of infusion and a transient anticoagulant effect. Heme arginate seldom has these effects.

β-Adrenergic blocking agents may control tachycardia and hypertension in acute attacks of porphyria and are considered by some to hasten recovery. However, these agents may be hazardous in patients with hypovolemia, in whom increased catecholamine secretion may be an important compensatory mechanism. Many other therapies have been tried in this disease, without consistent success.

Treatment is facilitated by identifying and removing inciting factors, such as harmful drugs, and by nutritional restitution. Symptoms during the luteal phase of the menstrual cycle usually resolve with the onset of menses.

Prognosis. The outlook for persons with latent AIP is excellent and is further improved when precautions are taken to avoid attacks. Recurrent attacks of porphyria can be disabling but do not occur throughout adult life and during the past decade have only rarely been fatal. Most patients do well after the diagnosis is established and harmful factors are avoided.

Prevention. The diagnosis of AIP in utero is possible but is seldom indicated in view of the favorable outlook for most PBG deaminase–deficient patients. Although subjects with latent AIP are less sensitive to inducing factors than are patients with prior porphyric symptoms, they are advised to take similar precautions. Latent AIP should never be construed as a health risk that limits availability of health insurance.

Some specific measures help prevent the clinical expression of AIP:

1. Family members should be screened to detect latent cases.
2. Harmful drugs should be avoided.
3. "Crash diets" for weight reduction and even brief periods of starvation (e.g., during postoperative periods or intercurrent illnesses) should be avoided. Regimens for obesity should provide for gradual weight loss during periods of clinical remission of porphyria.
4. Investigational approaches for preventing frequent (especially cyclic) attacks include administration of gonadotropin-releasing hormone analogues or periodic heme infusions. Oophorectomy is an unacceptable option.

CONGENITAL ERYTHROPOIETIC PORPHYRIA (CEP). This is an autosomal recessive disorder that is caused by a deficiency of uroporphyrinogen III cosynthase, and only about 100 cases have been reported. CEP occurs in several animal species (including all fox squirrels).

Etiology and Pathogenesis. An approximately two-thirds reduction in uroporphyrinogen III cosynthase (intermediate reductions occur in heterozygotes) is found in erythrocytes and other tissues of patients with CEP. Type I porphyrin isomers are produced in greatest excess. Bone marrow production and excretion of type III isomers and formation of heme are also increased, reflecting a hemolytic state. Excess formation of uroporphyrinogen III and heme occurs at the expense of a considerable accumulation in bone marrow of hydroxymethylbilane, which is converted nonenzymatically to uroporphyrinogen I.

Hemolysis varies in degree and is an important influence on disease severity. Excess porphyrins in circulating erythrocytes may predispose to hemolysis. Erythroid cells in marrow are also destroyed and release porphyrins. Splenomegaly, which may be a response to the increased uptake of abnormal erythrocytes, can contribute to anemia and cause leukopenia and thrombocytopenia. Sunlight, other sources of ultraviolet light, and minor trauma to friable skin are other determinants of clinical expression. Drugs, steroids, and nutrition have little influence.

Clinical Manifestations. Reddish urine and severe cutaneous photosensitivity generally are noted in early infancy. However, the clinical expression is variable, and in at least five cases symptoms began in adult life. Bullae and vesicles on sun-exposed skin are prone to rupture and become infected. Areas of skin may be thickened, hypopigmented, or hyperpigmented and may manifest hypertrichosis. Loss of digits and facial features and corneal scarring can be severe. Porphyrins are deposited in the teeth (producing a reddish-brown color termed "erythrodontia") and in bone. Bone demineralization can be substantial. There are no neurologic manifestations. Hemolysis and splenomegaly are almost always present. Life expectancy is often shortened by infections or hematologic complications.

Diagnosis and Differential Diagnosis. Porphyrin excretion and concentrations in red cells and plasma are generally much greater in CEP than in other forms of porphyria. Porphyrins in urine are primarily uroporphyrin and coproporphyrin and in feces are mostly coproporphyrin. ALA and PBG values are normal. In most cases, uroporphyrin I predominates in erythrocytes. A predominance of protoporphyrin in red cells has been described in some cases of CEP and is characteristic of bovine CEP. Stimulation of erythropoiesis increases uroporphyrin and coproporphyrin. CEP is readily distinguished from erythropoietic protoporphyria (EPP) (see further on). *Hepatoerythropoietic porphyria* (homozygous familial porphyria cutanea tarda [PCT]) is clinically similar to CEP but is distinguished by excess isocoproporphyrin in feces and urine and decreased uroporphyrinogen decarboxylase activity in erythrocytes. Very rare homozygous cases of variegate porphyria and hereditary coproporphyria may also be characterized by photosensitivity in childhood and increased erythrocyte porphyrin levels.

Treatment and Prevention. Protection of the skin from sunlight and minor trauma and prompt treatment of secondary bacterial infections help prevent scarring and mutilation. Blood transfusions sufficient to suppress erythropoiesis may be the most effective treatment. Improvement may occur after splenectomy. Oral charcoal may be helpful by increasing fecal excretion of porphyrins. Because homozygotes can be detected in utero, affected families have options for preventing genetic transmission.

PORPHYRIA CUTANEA TARDA (PCT). This is the most common of the porphyrias and is due to a deficiency of uroporphyrinogen decarboxylase in the liver.

Etiology and Pathogenesis. Several forms of this disease have been identified:

1. In the "sporadic" form (type I), which appears to include most adult cases of PCT, the enzyme is deficient in liver but not in erythrocytes and may represent an acquired form of PCT or an underlying genetic trait that remains to be identified.
2. In a familial form (termed type II), uroporphyrinogen decarboxylase is deficient in erythrocytes and other tissues in addition to the liver. This autosomal dominant disorder has a high degree of variation in clinical expression and often no family history of photosensitivity.
3. Recently, a type III has been described, in which the enzyme is deficient in liver but not other tissues, and the

deficiency is clearly inherited. Types I to III are clinically similar and difficult to distinguish.
4. Hepatoerythropoietic porphyria, the homozygous form of familial PCT, resembles CEP clinically.
5. Examples of *toxic porphyria* have resembled PCT. Most notably, an extensive outbreak of porphyria occurred in eastern Turkey from 1955 to 1958 after seed wheat containing the fungicide hexachlorobenzene was used for food. Subsequently, hexachlorobenzene and several other chlorinated cyclic hydrocarbons, when administered to animals, caused decreased uroporphyrinogen decarboxylase (only in liver) and a pattern of excess porphyrins resembling that in PCT. Dichlorophenols and trichlorophenols and 2,3,7,8-tetrachlorodibenzo-*p*-dioxin (TCDD, dioxin) have been implicated in smaller outbreaks and single cases in humans. Patients with sporadic PCT seldom have a history of exposure to such chemicals.
6. A severe and intractable form of PCT occurs in some patients with advanced renal disease. Associations of PCT with systemic lupus erythematosus and the acquired immunodeficiency syndrome (AIDS) have also been described.

In liver, a massive accumulation of porphyrins, which may require many months, precedes the appearance of excess porphyrins in plasma and urine. Worsening of PCT by drugs (other than alcohol, estrogens, or iron) or other factors that induce heme synthesis is seldom reported. Hepatic ALA synthase may be little increased because amounts of porphyrins produced are small relative to rates of hepatic heme formation. By contrast, during attacks of the acute porphyrias, much larger amounts of intermediates are excreted (as porphyrin precursors) and ALA synthase is substantially induced.

Ferrous iron can inactivate normal uroporphyrinogen decarboxylase or the half-normal hepatic enzyme activity in familial PCT. Hepatic iron content is important in the clinical expression of PCT. Alcohol intake may promote iron absorption and stimulate hepatic heme and porphyrin synthesis. In some cases of PCT, a heterozygous state for hereditary hemochromatosis contributes to mild hepatic siderosis. Iron removal by therapeutic phlebotomy in PCT restores the enzyme after a prolonged remission, but not immediately.

The complex pattern of porphyrins in PCT is partly due to accumulation of type I and III isomers of uroporphyrin and the 7-, 6-, and 5-carboxylate porphyrins. In addition, 5-carboxylate porphyrinogen can be metabolized by coproporphyrinogen oxidase to a series of 4-carboxylate porphyrins termed isocoproporphyrins.

Biochemical findings in homozygous familial PCT are similar to those in adult heterozygous cases of PCT. Increased erythrocyte protoporphyrin in homozygotes may reflect an earlier accumulation of uroporphyrinogen, which, with cessation of hemoglobin synthesis, is metabolized to protoporphyrin. Similar explanations may account for increased erythrocyte protoporphyrin in other homozygous forms of porphyria.

Clinical Manifestations. PCT is most common in men but has become more frequent in women in association with alcohol and estrogen use. Cutaneous photosensitivity is the major clinical feature. Vesicles and bullae develop on the face, dorsa of the hands and feet, forearms, and legs. Sun-exposed skin also becomes friable. Minor trauma may precede the formation of bullae or cause denudation of the skin. Small white plaques ("milia") may precede or follow vesicle formation. Involved skin tends to heal slowly. Hypertrichosis and hyperpigmentation are sometimes present even in the absence of vesicles. Thickening, scarring, and calcification of affected skin ("pseudoscleroderma") may be striking. Neurologic effects are absent.

Porphyria cutanea tarda develops in some men treated with estrogens for prostate cancer and in some women treated with estrogens or oral contraceptives. Most patients with PCT have a history of moderate or heavy alcohol intake. Liver histopathology is usually nonspecific and not diagnostic of alcoholic liver disease. Cirrhosis and hepatocellular carcinomas are most common in older patients or at autopsy. Very rarely, hepatic tumors themselves contain and presumably produce excess porphyrins. Some of these cases have resembled PCT.

Diagnosis and Differential Diagnosis. Skin lesions in PCT, VP, and HCP are indistinguishable clinically and histologically, but it is important to differentiate these conditions before embarking on therapy. A predominance of uroporphyrin and 7-carboxylate porphyrin in urine and increased isocoproporphyrin in feces are diagnostic of PCT. In PCT, the urinary ALA level may be slightly increased; the PBG level is normal. Total fecal porphyrins are usually less increased in PCT than in other types of porphyria with photosensitivity. Plasma porphyrins are always increased in patients with porphyric skin lesions; their patterns can distinguish VP and EPP from PCT (see further on).

Treatment. PCT is the most readily treated form of porphyria. Patients are advised to discontinue alcohol, estrogens, iron supplements, or other contributing factors. Phlebotomies can gradually reduce hepatic iron stores and almost always produce remissions. Iron stores in PCT are seldom markedly increased and may be normal. Therefore, remission is sometimes achieved after only a few phlebotomies (an average of five to six in one series). About 500 ml of blood can be removed at intervals of 1 to 2 weeks, or longer as iron stores decrease. Ferritin and plasma or urinary porphyrin levels decrease before remission. These should be measured during a course of phlebotomies to avoid unnecessary depletion of iron stores and anemia. With remission, continued phlebotomies may not be needed even if ferritin levels later return to normal. Longstanding remissions may be achieved even after several relapses. Desferrioxamine may be effective in PCT but is much less efficient.

Courses of low-dose chloroquine (e.g., 125 mg twice weekly for several months, or as needed) or hydroxychloroquine are useful when repeated phlebotomies are contraindicated. Chloroquine concentrates in the liver, complexes to excess porphyrins, and promotes their removal. Chloroquine given in usual doses to patients with PCT may cause marked increases in photosensitivity and porphyrin excretion, as well as nausea, malaise, fever, and hepatocellular damage. Although these adverse effects are generally transient and are followed by complete remission, it is prudent to avoid them by using a low-dose regimen.

In patients with PCT and advanced renal disease, phlebotomy is usually contraindicated by anemia, and other treatments are not effective. Recent studies indicate that genetic recombinant erythropoietin can mobilize excess iron, support phlebotomy, and lead to remission of PCT; however, this treatment is still investigational.

HEREDITARY COPROPORPHYRIA (HCP) AND VARIEGATE PORPHYRIA (VP). These acute porphyrias are due to approximately 50 per cent deficiencies of coproporphyrinogen oxidase and protoporphyrinogen oxidase, respectively, and are autosomal dominant conditions. Both are much less common than AIP in most countries. VP is quite prevalent in South Africa, where most cases have been traced to a couple who emigrated from Holland in the late 1600's.

Etiology and Pathogenesis. Excess ALA and PBG levels during acute attacks of HCP and VP reflect induction of hepatic ALA synthase and the relatively low normal activity of PBG deaminase. Loss of coproporphyrinogen from the liver occurs more readily than loss of other porphyrinogens, and loss is even greater when heme synthesis is stimulated. In VP, protoporphyrinogen accumulates and is auto-oxidized to protoporphyrin. A functional association between protoporphyrinogen oxidase and coproporphyrinogen oxidase in mitochondria may help explain excretion of coproporphyrin in VP.

In *harderoporphyria*, a variant of HCP, a structurally altered enzyme with reduced substrate affinity results in accumulation of harderoporphyrin as well as coproporphyrin. *Dual porphyria* refers to kindreds and individual double heterozygotes with both VP and familial PCT.

Clinical Manifestations. Drugs, steroids, and nutritional factors that are detrimental in AIP provoke exacerbations of HCP and VP. Neurologic manifestations are identical to those in AIP. Skin manifestations are similar to those of PCT and usually occur apart from the neurovisceral symptoms. Impaired biliary excretion by concurrent liver diseases or use of drugs such as contraceptive steroids can cause porphyrin retention and worsen photosensitivity.

Diagnosis and Differential Diagnosis. Urinary levels of ALA, PBG, and uroporphyrin are increased during acute attacks. With resolution of symptoms, these levels normalize more readily than in AIP. The urinary coproporphyrin value is markedly increased in both HCP and VP. A marked, isolated increase in fecal coproporphyrin level is distinctive for HCP. Fecal coproporphy-

rin and protoporphyrin values are about equally increased in VP. The fluorescence spectrum of plasma porphyrins (at neutral pH) is characteristic and very useful for rapidly distinguishing VP from the other porphyrias. A different spectrum distinguishes EPP.

Treatment and Prognosis. Acute attacks of VP are treated like those in AIP. Striking decreases in attacks and deaths from VP in South Africa are attributed to identification of latent cases, avoiding harmful drugs, and better treatment during acute attacks. Measures that protect the skin from sunlight are helpful for photosensitivity. Cholestyramine may decrease photosensitivity occurring with liver dysfunction. Phlebotomies and chloroquine are not effective.

ERYTHROPOIETIC PROTOPORPHYRIA. This is an autosomal dominant condition caused by a deficiency of ferrochelatase. Although EPP was not clearly described until 1961, it is now perhaps the second most common form of porphyria.

Etiology and Pathogenesis. Excess protoporphyrin is found in erythroid cells, plasma, bile, and feces of patients in whom EPP is clinically expressed. Ferrochelatase is probably deficient in all tissues in EPP but becomes rate limiting for protoporphyrin metabolism primarily in bone marrow. Some obligate carriers have little or no increase in red cell protoporphyrin. Increases in plasma and fecal protoporphyrin are also variable. Such variations in clinical expression are not well explained.

Bone marrow reticulocytes are the primary source of protoporphyrin in EPP. Circulating erythrocytes and the liver contribute smaller amounts. In EPP, protoporphyrin in erythrocytes is not complexed with zinc and, compared with zinc protoporphyrin (found in lead poisoning, iron deficiency, and homozygous forms of porphyria), diffuses more readily into plasma. Zinc protoporphyrin dissociates less readily from hemoglobin-binding sites and persists in the red cell as long as it circulates. Disposition of the excess protoporphyrin in EPP depends on hepatic uptake, biliary excretion, and degree of enterohepatic circulation and is impaired by liver damage.

Clinical Manifestations. Cutaneous manifestations in EPP, which usually begin in childhood, are distinct from those of other porphyrias. Burning, itching, erythema, and swelling can occur within minutes of sun exposure. Diffuse edema of sun-exposed areas may resemble angioneurotic edema. Other characteristic skin changes include lichenification, leathery pseudovesicles, labial grooving, and nail changes. Scarring is rarely severe or deforming. Vesicles, pigment changes, friability, and hirsutism are unusual. There is no fluorescence of the teeth, and neuropathic manifestations are absent. Drugs that exacerbate hepatic porphyrias are not known to worsen EPP, although they are generally avoided as a precaution.

Hemolysis is uncommon or very mild in uncomplicated cases. Erythropoiesis and iron metabolism are generally normal. Mild anemia with hypochromia and microcytosis is noted in some cases and is unexplained. Gallstones composed at least partly of protoporphyrin may develop.

Liver function is usually normal in patients with EPP. Liver disease develops in only a minority of cases but can progress rapidly to liver failure and death. Excess protoporphyrin itself may have cholestatic effects and damage hepatocytes. Intercurrent factors such as viral hepatitis, alcohol, iron deficiency, fasting, and oral contraceptive steroids have sometimes contributed.

Diagnosis and Differential Diagnosis. Protoporphyrin is increased in bone marrow, circulating erythrocytes, plasma, bile, and feces. Urinary porphyrins and porphyrin precursors are at normal levels. Hepatic complications of EPP are often preceded by increasing levels of erythrocyte and plasma protoporphyrin, abnormal liver function findings, marked deposition of protoporphyrin in liver cells and bile canaliculi, and increased photosensitivity.

Treatment and Prognosis. β-Carotene has been developed and marketed primarily for treating EPP. Its clinical benefits have been substantiated in large series of patients. No side effects other than a mild and dose-related skin discoloration caused by carotenemia have been noted. Its mechanism of action may involve quenching of singlet oxygen or free radicals. Cholestyramine may reduce protoporphyrin levels by interrupting its enterohepatic circulation. Iron deficiency, caloric restriction, and drugs or hormone preparations that impair hepatic excretory function should be avoided.

Hepatic complications may resolve spontaneously if a reversible cause of liver dysfunction, such as viral hepatitis or alcohol, is contributing. Transfusions or intravenous hematin to suppress erythroid and hepatic protoporphyrin production, splenectomy, correction of iron deficiency, and cholestyramine or activated charcoal may be beneficial. Some patients have undergone liver transplantation. However, similar complications may develop in the transplanted liver.

Anderson KE: The porphyrias. In Williams WJ, Beutler E, Erslev AJ, et al. (eds.): Hematology. New York, McGraw-Hill, 1990, pp 722–742. One of several recent and detailed reviews on the genetic, biochemical, and clinical aspects of the porphyrias.

Anderson KE, Goeger DE, Carson RW, et al.: Erythropoietin for the treatment of porphyria cutanea tarda in a patient on long-term hemodialysis. N Engl J Med 322:315, 1990. Therapeutic approach to a previously intractable form of porphyria cutanea tarda.

Derooij F, Beaumont C, Wilson P, et al.: A point mutation G→A in exon-12 of the porphobilinogen deaminase gene results in exon skipping and is responsible for acute intermittent porphyria. Nucleic Acids Res 17:6637, 1989. Example of the recent advances in characterizing specific gene mutations in the porphyrias.

Held JL, Sassa S, Kappas A, et al.: Erythrocyte uroporphyrinogen decarboxylase activity in porphyria cutanea tarda—a study of 40 consecutive patients. J Invest Dermatol 93:332, 1989. Distinguishing types I to III of porphyria cutanea tarda in part by measuring erythrocyte uroporphyrinogen decarboxylase.

Mustajoki P, Tenhunen R, Pierach C, et al.: Heme in the treatment of porphyrias and hematological disorders. Semin Hematol 26:1, 1989. Review of heme therapy in the acute porphyrias.

Winkler MG, Anderson KE: Vampires, porphyria, and the media: The medicalization of a myth. Perspect Biol Med 33:598, 1990. How scientists and the media have distorted the image of a disease.

192 Wilson's Disease

Andrew Deiss

DEFINITION. Wilson's disease (hepatolenticular degeneration) is a hereditary disorder characterized by the accumulation of copper in the body, especially in the liver, brain, kidneys, and corneas. The excess copper leads to tissue injury and ultimately, if effective treatment is not instituted, to death.

ETIOLOGY AND PREVALENCE. Wilson's disease is inherited as an autosomal recessive trait. The gene responsible for the disturbance in copper metabolism is closely linked to the esterase D and retinoblastoma genes within chromosome 13q14–q21. The prevalence of the disease is approximately 30 per million.

PATHOGENESIS. Normally, loss of copper from the body occurs primarily through the bile. Much of biliary copper is secreted in a poorly absorbable form and thus is lost in the feces. Copper balance is normally maintained by this mechanism. In Wilson's disease biliary excretion of copper is impaired, and as a consequence total body copper is progressively increased. The specific nature of the metabolic abnormality that causes this defect is not known.

Positive copper balance begins in infancy in Wilson's disease and continues thereafter unless appropriate therapy is given. However, the distribution of copper changes as the disease progresses. Liver copper is actually greater in presymptomatic homozygotes than in symptomatic ones. Thus not only does net deposition of liver copper cease, but also a portion of previously deposited copper is lost from the liver and deposited elsewhere. This copper redistribution probably takes place when liver injury occurs. If this injury occurs abruptly in many hepatocytes, liver disease may be clinically manifested, and a large amount of copper may be released over a short period, creating the potential for acute erythrocyte injury and hemolytic anemia as well. However, if hepatocyte injury is more gradual, acute liver disease will not occur, and the patient will remain asymptomatic as the important site of copper deposition shifts to the brain. With the latter course, most patients present at a later time with neurologic

or psychiatric symptoms, usually with clinically inapparent cirrhosis.

The serum concentration of the copper-containing protein ceruloplasmin is low in 95 per cent of patients with Wilson's disease. The hypoceruloplasminemia is probably due in part to a decrease in ceruloplasmin gene transcription, but it is not believed to play a pathogenetic role in the disease.

PATHOLOGY. The diagnosis cannot be made on the basis of histologic sections of the liver. Fatty change and glycogen-filled nuclei are present early, followed later by piecemeal necrosis, lymphocytic infiltration, erosion of limiting plates, parenchymal collapse, and fibrosis. Ultimately, these abnormalities evolve into postnecrotic cirrhosis. Stains for copper are unreliable, being negative most frequently during the early stages of the disease, when diagnostic help is most needed.

In the brain, abnormal astrocytes and neuronal necrosis are widely distributed, and there is atrophy or cavitation of the basal ganglia and occasionally the cerebral cortex.

CLINICAL MANIFESTATIONS. Wilson's disease is a disorder of young persons. Although the disease may occur at any time from the age of 5 years into the sixth decade, two thirds of patients seek medical attention between the ages of 8 and 20. The physician should suspect the disorder in young people with signs of chronic or recurrent hepatic dysfunction or with characteristic neurologic abnormalities.

The hepatic symptoms are quite diverse. Commonly, a brief illness characterized by malaise, anorexia, jaundice, and increased aminotransferases is mistaken for viral hepatitis. Similar episodes may recur at intervals of months or years, or a latent period may occur during which the patient is asymptomatic until neurologic symptoms begin. If clinically overt hepatocyte injury persists over a longer period, a syndrome resembling chronic active hepatitis results. Occasionally, liver injury occurs precipitously; without rapid institution of appropriate treatment, death is likely in these patients and the need for prompt diagnosis is urgent. More commonly, however, hepatocyte injury is gradual and is not accompanied by symptoms of liver disease; nevertheless, cirrhosis develops ultimately in all patients. This liver injury may not be recognized until neurologic disease is evaluated.

Episodes of hemolytic anemia occur when massive release of copper from the liver takes place. Thus hemolysis is usually accompanied by overt liver disease; it occurs regularly in patients with fulminant hepatic failure. Hemolysis usually lasts only a short period and disappears spontaneously.

The neurologic signs at onset may take a variety of forms. Patients may start with a slightly dystonic facies in which the upper lip is drawn tightly over the teeth. Shortly afterwards they develop awkward, dystonic postures in the upper extremities and often an unsteady gait. Once recognized by prior experience, these particular neurologic manifestations are seldom mistaken. In other patients, tremor may be the initial sign, often a characteristic "wing-beating" rhythmic oscillating tremor of the upper extremities that in severe cases gradually extends to the trunk. Frequently, loss of coordination of fine movements, such as those required for handwriting, is the earliest neurologic sign. As the disease progresses, patients may develop combinations of these abnormalities. Dysarthria, rigidity, drooling, and titubation are late features. Seizures are infrequent and sensory abnormalities absent. The Kayser-Fleischer (K-F) ring, described below, is definitively diagnostic in the neurologic variety and nearly so in the hepatic form of the disease.

Psychological symptoms of Wilson's disease are prominent and consist of early development of intellectual deterioration, personality changes, and unstable behavior. Children begin to fail at school, and young adults may show difficulty in performing jobs once considered routine. Schizophreniform symptoms and other forms of bizarre behavior may appear, but the mental status examination always shows signs of organic dementia. Effective removal of excess copper often improves but usually fails to eliminate these symptoms completely.

Kayser-Fleischer rings are golden brown or greenish rings or arcs in Descemet's membrane at the limbus of the cornea. They are composed of copper-containing granules and develop primarily after redistribution of liver copper. They may be visible with the unaided eye, but slit-lamp examination should always be performed. K-F rings are present in all or nearly all patients in the neurologic or psychiatric stage of the disease but are not present in about one third of those with hepatic symptoms.

Rare symptoms ascribable to Wilson's disease include cholelithiasis, sunflower cataracts, arthropathy, renal calculi, heart disease, and the Fanconi syndrome.

DIAGNOSIS. The classic diagnostic features of K-F rings, low serum ceruloplasmin concentration (<20 mg per deciliter), and increased amounts of liver and urinary copper (>250 μg per gram of dry weight and >100 μg per 24 hours, respectively) are present in nearly all patients with fully evolved neurologic Wilson's disease, but only in about two thirds of those presenting with liver disease. In these patients, K-F rings often have not yet formed, and the serum ceruloplasmin concentration may be difficult to interpret. Even in Wilson's disease, serum ceruloplasmin increases during inflammation, estrogen administration, and pregnancy and may decrease during liver failure. Measurement of the copper content of the liver should resolve the problem. Hepatic copper is often greater than normal (50 μg per gram of dry weight) in a variety of chronic liver diseases, but it seldom reaches the concentration seen in most patients with Wilson's disease (>250 μg per gram of dry weight). In a patient with a disease clinically suggestive of Wilson's disease, hepatic copper of this magnitude is essentially diagnostic. If the diagnosis is still in doubt, incorporation of radioactive copper into ceruloplasmin can be measured; incorporation is negligible in Wilson's disease, normal in other liver disease, even with copper loading, and intermediate in 75 per cent of heterozygotes. All measurements of copper metabolism should be entrusted only to laboratories experienced with their determination, and the normal values of that laboratory should be used.

In primary biliary cirrhosis and chronic cholestasis, diseases with acquired abnormalities of copper excretion, liver copper may be greatly increased and K-F rings occur rarely. The age, symptoms, and laboratory abnormalities of patients with these diseases help distinguish them from those with Wilson's disease.

Early during the hemolytic anemia the urinary copper excretion is very great. The Coombs test result is negative. When hemolysis and acute liver disease occur concurrently in a young person, Wilson's disease is the most probable cause.

Examination of all siblings of patients with Wilson's disease is mandatory to identify presymptomatic homozygotes. K-F rings are usually absent. Serum ceruloplasmin concentration is reduced in 95 per cent of homozygotes and 20 per cent of heterozygotes. If it is low, liver copper content should be measured. Hepatic copper is slightly increased in most heterozygotes. If the copper is greater than 250 μg per gram of dry weight, Wilson's disease is present, and it should be treated as in symptomatic patients. Heterozygotes never become symptomatic and should not be treated. Some homozygotes will be missed by this evaluation, so continued follow-up is necessary.

TREATMENT. Without effective lifetime therapy, Wilson's disease is inevitably fatal. If treatment is begun early enough, symptomatic recovery usually is complete, and a life of normal length and quality can be expected. If treatment is begun too late, death may not be prevented, or recovery will be only partial.

Effective therapy depends upon establishing negative copper balance, thereby preventing deposition of more copper and mobilizing for excretion excess copper already deposited. Three agents are available that seem to be equally efficacious.

D-Penicillamine remains the drug of choice, at least until there is substantially more experience with the other agents. The usual dosage is 1 gram per day, given in divided doses 1 hour before meals and at bedtime. Response typically is quite slow, occurring over months, but it may occur more rapidly. A year or more is often required to obtain maximum improvement. At least 10 per cent of patients experience a worsening of their neurologic symptoms during the first month or two of treatment, and this phenomenon should not suggest that the diagnosis is in error. Compliance and the effectiveness of therapy must be monitored at 1- to 2-month intervals for the first year and twice yearly thereafter; monitoring consists of measurements of urinary copper, serum ceruloplasmin, and serum nonceruloplasmin copper (total serum copper minus ceruloplasmin copper). Nonceruloplasmin copper should decrease early and ceruloplasmin more gradually if treatment is adequate. Urinary copper levels increase at once to 1 to 5 mg per 24 hours during the first few months and then gradually decline as the excess of copper decreases.

Toxic effects are frequent. Rash, fever, adenopathy, neutropenia, or thrombocytopenia often occurs during the first 2 weeks of treatment. In such circumstances, penicillamine should be discontinued; when the symptoms have cleared, prednisone should be begun at a dose of 40 mg per day and penicillamine resumed at 250 mg per day and gradually increased to full dose over a period of a few weeks. The steroids can then be tapered and stopped. Side effects that occur later after initiation of penicillamine administration include proteinuria, nephrotic syndrome, systemic lupus erythematosus, Goodpasture's syndrome, and a variety of chronic skin diseases. These side effects can often be reversed by temporarily stopping penicillamine and resuming it after the symptoms have abated, sometimes with the addition of steroids. Suspension of treatment should never be permitted for more than a few months.

If penicillamine toxicity is not manageable, either trientine (250 mg 1 hour before meals and at bedtime) or zinc (50 mg of elemental zinc 1 hour before meals, preferably as the acetate) is an effective alternative. Experience is not extensive with either, but side effects have been minimal.

Some patients, especially those with fulminant hepatic failure, are so severely ill that the benefits of medical treatment cannot occur rapidly enough to prevent death. In these patients, liver transplantation, if successful, is curative.

Brewer GJ, Yuzbasiyan-Gurken V, Young AB: Treatment of Wilson's disease. Semin Neurol 7:209, 1987. *A thorough discussion of the details of treatment.*

Cartwright GE: Diagnosis of treatable Wilson's disease. N Engl J Med 298:1347, 1978. *An excellent description of the protean and often confusing clinical presentations of Wilson's disease and a few illustrations of what happens when the diagnosis is missed.*

Scheinberg IH, Sternlieb I: Wilson's Disease. Philadelphia, W. B. Saunders Company, 1984. *The authoritative monograph based on the authors' vast experience with all aspects of Wilson's disease.*

Walshe JM: Diagnosis and treatment of presymptomatic Wilson's disease. Lancet 2:435, 1988. *Criteria for identifying asymptomatic homozygotes in families of patients with Wilson's disease. Liver biopsies should be obtained for confirmation as the author recommends, and therefore more frequently than he has actually done.*

193 Hemochromatosis (Iron Storage Disease)

Arno G. Motulsky

DEFINITION. The most frequent cause of iron overload in persons of European origin is a common genetic disorder known as hemochromatosis. Massive iron deposits may develop after years of increased iron absorption, and functional organ impairment ensues. Secondary hemochromatosis with parenchymal cell involvement also occurs in a variety of anemias associated with ineffective erythropoiesis, increased iron absorption and multiple transfusions—most commonly in homozygous β-thalassemia.

ETIOLOGY, GENETICS, AND PATHOGENESIS. "Idiopathic" hemochromatosis results from an autosomal recessive gene that causes increased iron absorption in the gut. The nature of the basic defect remains unknown. Over many years, the excess iron is deposited in parenchymal cells of the liver and other organs. Clinical signs and symptoms develop when total body iron stores have reached levels of 15 to 40 grams, compared with normal total iron stores of 0.2 to 2.0 grams.

The gene for hemochromatosis is located on the short arm of chromosome 6 and is linked to the human leukocyte antigen (HLA) locus. The hemochromatosis gene is physically close to the HLA-A allele of the HLA complex. Clinically useful DNA markers are not yet available. About 70 per cent of hemochromatosis patients carry the HLA-A$_3$ allele, compared with 25 to 30 per cent of the general population.

Recombination between the hemochromatosis gene and the HLA-A allele is very rare. Since these genes are separate, hemochromatosis is not likely to be a direct effect of HLA-A gene action. An increased frequency of HLA-B$_7$ and HLA-B$_{14}$ is also observed and is caused by "hitchhiking" of each of these determinants with the closely linked hemochromatosis gene (linkage disequilibrium). The development of hemochromatosis requires a "double dose" of the mutant gene, and affected patients are homozygotes. Among sibships that include at least one homozygote whose condition has been definitely diagnosed, additional homozygotes as well as heterozygote carriers can often be defined by HLA testing using the principles of genetic linkage. Thus, the HLA status of the affected patient who has inherited a hemochromatosis gene from each of his or her parents is determined (Fig. 193–1). Sibs with both HLA haplotypes identical to that of the affected patient carry the linked hemochromatosis allele on the maternal as well as the paternal chromosome 6. Such persons are homozygous, are at high risk to develop iron overload, or may already be affected. Sibs who share only one HLA haplotype are heterozygotes, and sibs who share none are normal, not having inherited any hemochromatosis gene. No tests to detect heterozygotes in the general population exist. Detection of homozygotes in the population at large must utilize measures of iron status such as transferrin saturation and serum ferritin levels. HLA testing is of no value for population screening, nor is it useful for diagnosis in the absence of family testing.

The actual amount of stored iron at a given time depends upon factors such as age, sex, iron content of food, caloric intake, degree of alcohol ingestion, and unknown factors such as allelic heterogeneity. The amount of iron absorbed in younger persons is not enough to produce organ damage. Males generally eat larger quantities of food than females and therefore absorb more iron. Females lose iron periodically during menstruation and occasionally during pregnancy. Therefore, while the prevalence of homozygotes for the hemochromatosis gene is identical in both sexes, *clinically* apparent hemochromatosis occurs at least 10 times more frequently in males. Excessive alcohol intake further contributes to liver damage, and many patients give a history of excessive alcohol intake. Alcohol may stimulate iron absorption, and certain alcoholic beverages such as red wines contain increased amounts of iron.

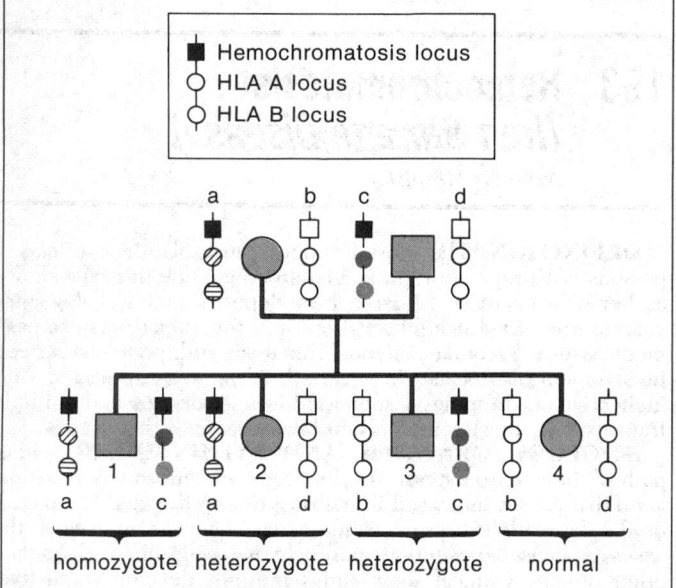

FIGURE 193–1. Hypothetical distribution of iron-loading alleles, each designated by an HLA haplotype, among family members of a patient (1) with fully developed idiopathic hemochromatosis. The "topographic" relationships between the gene (■) and the HLA loci (○) are diagrammatic approximations. The mother of the patient has two number 6 chromosomes, designated a and b, of which chromosome a carries the mutant allele of the hemochromatosis locus. In the father the mutant allele occurs on the sixth chromosome that is designated c. The patient inherited both mutant genes and is a homozygote. (From Bothwell TH, Charlton RW, Motulsky AG: Idiopathic hemochromatosis. *In* Stanbury JB, Wyngaarden JB, Fredrickson DS, et al. [eds.]: The Metabolic Basis of Inherited Disease. 5th ed. New York, McGraw-Hill Book Company, 1983.)

Excessive iron in various parenchymal organs is required before clinical manifestations develop. There is a fairly good correlation between the quantity of iron stored and the development of clinical signs and symptoms. Heterozygotes for the hemochromatosis gene may absorb somewhat increased amounts of iron, and minor, clinically benign iron overload may occur. However, test results of iron status in heterozygotes are closer to those found in normal individuals. It is conceivable that heterozygotes are at higher risk to develop iron overload under conditions in which normal persons would not be affected, as in porphyria cutanea tarda. However, iron overload in alcoholic liver disease appears *not* to be associated with the heterozygote state for hemochromatosis. Not all homozygotes develop clinical disease. In the fraction of those who do so, the development of disease depends upon the various circumstances affecting iron balance already discussed and upon unknown factors. It is clear that full-blown clinical findings are the "tip of the iceberg" and that many homozygotes have no symptoms or exhibit only mild, nonspecific findings.

PATHOLOGY. Although iron in reticuloendothelial cells is relatively harmless, parenchymal cell deposits are noxious. Iron in hemochromatosis is stored mostly in parenchymal cells as insoluble gold-brown aggregates known as hemosiderin. Normally, most iron is stored as ferritin, but with increasing iron overload the proportion of hemosiderin increases. With advancing hemosiderosis, fibrosis increases, and cirrhosis is frequent in fully developed cases.

Skin pigmentation is caused by epidermal melanin, while the slate-gray appearance is caused by hemosiderin. Pancreatic iron deposits are found in acinar cells and are not associated with clinically manifest exocrine deficiency. In the islets, B cells are selectively affected. Iron pigment is deposited in the sarcoplasm of cardiac myocytes and in synovial linings. The gonadotropic cells of the anterior pituitary gland may be heavily infiltrated with hemosiderin, leading to secondary testicular atrophy. Early cases exhibit significantly fewer pathologic findings.

PREVALENCE. Studies in Utah, Brittany (France), and Australia suggest homozygote frequencies varying between 1/200 and 1/600. This implies a high frequency of the heterozygote state for the disease, ranging from 8 to 13 per cent. The reasons for this high frequency are unknown. Hemochromatosis is one of the most common genetic diseases among Caucasoids. Since not all homozygotes develop typical findings, the frequency of the clinical disease is lower and was estimated to be roughly 1/5000 in the Pacific Northwest of the United States and 1/500 and 1/1000 in autopsy series in Scotland and southern Sweden, respectively. The frequency of hemochromatosis is much higher than usually suspected, since the majority of affected homozygotes do not exhibit classic symptoms.

CLINICAL MANIFESTATIONS IN THE FULL-BLOWN DISEASE. Because of the long time required to produce organ damage, the onset of clinical disease is usually, but not always, delayed to the age of 40 to 60. Males are more frequently and earlier affected than menstruating females. The most important clinical signs and symptoms in the fully developed disease include hepatomegaly, skin pigmentation, weakness and lethargy, chronic abdominal pain, diabetes, arthralgia, loss of libido, and impotence. However, more and more patients with few or no clinical findings are being discovered fortuitously.

Skin pigmentation is most pronounced in exposed areas and scars. With increasing hemosiderin deposits, the skin takes on a slate-gray appearance.

Hepatomegaly is the most common physical finding and may occur without symptoms and with normal liver function test results. Episodes of hepatic failure are rare but may be precipitated by blood loss or surgical procedures. *Splenomegaly* occurs. Chronic aching *abdominal pain* is common once cirrhosis has developed and may be the presenting symptom. Carcinoma of the liver is a relatively frequent late complication. Unfortunately, *once cirrhosis has developed, the risk of a malignant hepatoma appears undiminished by iron removal, emphasizing the importance of early case detection and initiation of iron-removing therapy* (see below). Other malignancies do not appear to occur more frequently. Atrial tachyarrhythmias and dilated cardiomyopathy with congestive heart failure are often observed.

Insulin-dependent diabetes is often seen. *Arthralgia* and *arthropathy* different from but often confused with rheumatoid arthritis or osteoarthritis are common. The second and third metacarpophalangeal joints are usually first involved. Knees, hips, shoulders, and lower back may be affected, and acute synovitis with pseudogout of the knees has been observed. Roentgenograms show chondrocalcinosis with small cysts characteristically affecting the second or third metacarpophalangeal joints. Osteoporosis is sometimes observed. *Loss of libido* and sexual impotence with testicular atrophy are common among men. Lethargy, increased sleep requirements, and inability to think clearly are frequent complaints. Infections with unusual organisms that grow better with excess iron may sometimes occur (*Yersinia enterocolitica*, *Pasteurella pseudotuberculosis*, and *Vibrio vulnificus*).

DIAGNOSIS. The clinical diagnosis of hemochromatosis requires a high index of suspicion and needs to be sought more frequently. Many patients are being detected fortuitously after discovery of abnormally saturated iron-binding capacity and high plasma ferritin levels. Iron overload should be considered among patients who present with any one or a combination of the following: hepatomegaly, weakness and lethargy, abnormal skin pigmentation, atypical arthritis, diabetes, impotence, unexplained chronic abdominal pain, or cardiomyopathy. Excessive alcohol intake increases the diagnostic probability. Diagnostic suspicions should be particularly high when the family history—particularly among sibs—is positive for clinical findings that might suggest hemochromatosis.

The diagnosis requires laboratory testing for iron overload. The most practical screening test is the determination of serum iron, of transferrin saturation, and of plasma ferritin. The serum iron value is elevated in patients with hemochromatosis, and there is increased iron saturation of transferrin, ranging between 60 and 100 per cent (normal is less than 50 per cent). However, abnormally high transferrin saturation can occur as a result of sample contamination, physiologic plasma iron fluctuation, iron therapy, liver disease, and red cell disorders. An abnormal value for transferrin saturation is seen early in the course of the disease and does not reflect the extent of iron storage. In contrast, a valuable noninvasive test to assess iron stores is the measurement of serum ferritin, which correlates reasonably well with the extent of iron storage in the absence of excessive alcohol consumption, inflammation, rheumatoid arthritis, neoplasia, and liver disease such as that induced by drugs or viral hepatitis. Without such complications, a level above 300 μg per liter in males and above 200 μg per liter in females suggests increased iron stores and requires further investigation. Ferritin levels ranging between 700 and several thousand micrograms per liter may be seen. The combination of testing for high transferrin saturation and for an elevated serum ferritin level gives the most reliable results. Rare families with significant iron overload and normal ferritin values have been described. Various imaging techniques such as hepatic computer tomography, magnetic resonance imaging, and magnetic susceptibility measurements promise to become useful for the assessment of hepatic iron stores.

Because of problems with specificity and sensitivity with all laboratory and imaging tests, and the absence of a test for the fundamental genetic defect, the "gold standard" test for hemochromatosis is a *liver biopsy*. Parenchymal hemosiderin deposits can be demonstrated histochemically, and the actual concentration of iron should be estimated biochemically. The extent of liver damage and cirrhosis will be apparent. Phlebotomies can be used as a therapeutic test to establish the diagnosis when a liver biopsy to assess the amount of iron biochemically is not available or not feasible. Weekly venesections of 500 ml (200 to 250 mg of Fe) deplete normal iron stores relatively rapidly. Patients with hemochromatosis require prolonged weekly venesections (2 to 3 years) until they are iron depleted (see below).

DIFFERENTIAL DIAGNOSIS. The most common differential diagnostic problem is raised by alcoholic liver disease not associated with HLA-linked hemochromatosis. Many such patients have an increased amount of stainable liver iron but no increased iron stores (usually less than 3 grams). Unlike genetic hemochromatosis, the iron in this disease is mostly located in reticuloendothelial cells. Liver function abnormalities are more severe than in hemochromatosis. Appropriate tests (including serum ferritin, liver biopsy, and sometimes a trial of phlebotomies—see above) can establish whether there is increased generalized iron storage. Iron overload due to chronic anemias (see below) rarely raises diagnostic problems.

FAMILY DETECTION FOR PREVENTION. Early treatment can remove increased iron stores that ultimately cause disease. Most important, treatment before the onset of cirrhosis appears to prevent the high frequency of hepatoma observed in hemochromatosis. All efforts should therefore be made to detect the disease *as early as possible*. Since the disease is an autosomal recessive trait, there is a 25 per cent chance that sibs of a patient are similarly affected. Testing for iron overload in sibs is therefore imperative. In addition, all family members should have a *single* determination of their HLA status to ascertain which sibs share all HLA determinants with the index case and therefore are homozygotes for the disease. If the characteristic abnormalities in iron metabolism are found, phlebotomies should be initiated after a liver biopsy has assessed the extent of iron storage. Sib testing should be begun at about puberty for males and after the age of 20 years for females. HLA-identical male sibs found to have a normal iron load should be restudied every 2 to 3 years, females somewhat less frequently. Frequent blood donations (three times a year) prevent potentially toxic iron accumulation and are recommended for HLA-identical sibs. Since the heterozygote frequency of hemochromatosis appears to be high among Causasians (~10 per cent), matings of homozygotes with heterozygote carriers are not uncommon, and one half of the offspring of such couples will be homozygotes (pseudodominant vertical transmission). Thus while parents and children of affected patients are usually obligate heterozygote carriers, some of these relatives may also be homozygotes. Family detection therefore should include the entire family.

Differentiation of heterozygotes from homozygotes with early disease may be difficult by serum ferritin and transferrin testing, since heterozygotes often have slightly abnormal values. Determination of HLA status may aid in such cases, since heterozygotes usually share only one-half their HLA haplotypes with their homozygote sibs. Treatment to remove iron is *not* required in heterozygotes.

TREATMENT. Excess iron can be removed by periodic venesections. The removal of one unit (approximately 500 ml) of blood depletes the body of 200 to 250 mg of iron. Weekly venesections are required for about 2 to 3 years to return iron stores to normal levels in patients with the full-blown disease and for lesser periods for those with early disease. Even though there is no medical contraindication to using blood from hemochromatic patients for blood transfusions, many blood banks discard such blood.

Phlebotomies should be monitored by frequent hematocrit determinations and plasma iron and ferritin levels 6 to 10 times per year (Fig. 193–2). After an initial fall, hematocrit levels stabilize at approximately 90 per cent of pretreatment levels. Indicators of iron status do not change until significant depletion of iron stores has occurred. After iron stores have been normalized as shown by ferritin and transferrin tests, venesections are required at 2- to 3-month intervals to prevent reaccumulation of iron. An iron-free diet is not necessary at any time during treatment. Treatment of hepatic, cardiac, endocrinologic, and metabolic complications is along conventional lines. Many manifestations of hemochromatosis *except* arthropathy, cirrhosis, and hepatoma are improved by phlebotomy therapy. Hypogonadism may also be irreversible, and diabetes may become milder but will not disappear.

PROGNOSIS. The 5-year survival rate after diagnosis in untreated patients with the fully developed disease was found to be 18 per cent and the 10-year survival rate, 6 per cent. The principal cause of death in such patients related to liver complications: hepatic failure and portal hypertension (30 per cent) and malignant hepatoma (30 per cent). An additional one third of patients died of cardiac failure.

Recently, 163 treated patients with relatively advanced signs and symptoms were studied in West Germany. There were 53 deaths. Cumulative survival was 92 per cent at 5 years, 76 per cent at 10 years, 59 per cent at 15 years, and 49 per cent at 20 years. Life expectancy was worse in patients who had cirrhosis or diabetes or who required more than 18 months of venesection for iron depletion. Death was due to cirrhosis in 25 per cent and to hepatoma in 25 per cent. By contrast, in *treated patients without cirrhosis, survival expectation was identical to that of*

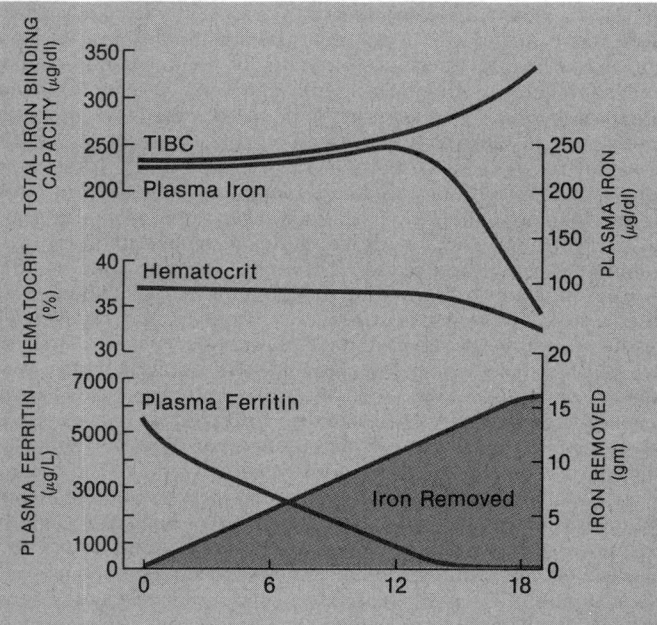

FIGURE 193–2. Serial changes in the hematocrit, plasma iron concentration, total iron-binding capacity, and plasma ferritin concentration in a subject with idiopathic hemochromatosis on repeated venesection therapy. (From Bothwell TH, Charlton RW, Cook JD, et al.: Idiopathic haemochromatosis. *In* Iron Metabolism in Man. Oxford, Blackwell Scientific Publications, 1979.)

the unaffected control population. It is noteworthy that hepatoma has never been reported in hemochromatosis without cirrhosis.

SECONDARY HEMOCHROMATOSIS. Excessive iron deposits in parenchymal cells can be observed in anemias associated with ineffective erythropoiesis, as in β-thalassemia major, in which severe iron loading already occurs before transfusion. Repeated transfusions produce further iron overload, and clinical symptoms of hemochromatosis occur early in life. Hepatic fibrosis is already common in children, as is retarded growth and delayed puberty. Cardiac death usually occurs in adolescence or early adulthood unless iron removal is carried out. Phlebotomies cannot be done, since these patients are severely anemic. Chelation therapy with desferrioxamine, together with frequent transfusions, has improved the prognosis markedly. Death due to complications of iron storage can be prevented if iron removal can be initiated before clinical signs and symptoms of iron overload appear.

Patients with hypoplastic anemias do not absorb increased amounts of iron but often require blood transfusions over prolonged periods. The transfused iron is largely stored in macrophages, and no clinical signs or symptoms are usually seen. Rarely, redistribution to parenchymal cells with development of hepatic cirrhosis or other typical organ involvement occurs.

Bothwell TH, Charlton RW, Motulsky AG: Hemochromatosis. *In* Scriver CR, Beaudet AL, Slye WS, et al. (eds.): The Metabolic Basis of Inherited Disease. 6th ed. New York, McGraw-Hill Book Company, 1989, pp 1433–1462. *A detailed discussion of all aspects of iron metabolism, genetics, and clinical findings in HLA-linked and secondary hemochromatosis.*

Edwards CQ, Griffen LM, Goldgar D, et al.: Prevalence of hemochromatosis among 11,065 presumably healthy blood donors. N Engl J Med 318:1355, 1988. *Attempts at screening for hemochromatosis in a general population.*

Fairbanks VG, Baldus WP: Hemochromatosis: The neglected diagnosis. Mayo Clin Proc 61:296, 1986. *A succinct summary of this underdiagnosed disease and practical advice regarding laboratory tests.*

Simon M, Fauchet R, LeGall JY, et al.: Immunogenetics of idiopathic hemochromatosis and secondary iron overload. *In* Immunogenetics of Endocrine Disorders. New York, Alan R. Liss, 1988. *Extensive discussion of iron overload with emphasis on HLA testing, but covering all aspects.*

Smith LH Jr: Overview of hemochromatosis. *In* Smith LH Jr (ed.): Cecil Textbook of Medicine. Update 1, pp 1–12. Philadelphia, W.B. Saunders Company, 1989. *An excellent referenced review of basic and clinical aspects of hemochromatosis.*

Strohmeyer G, Niederau C, Stremmel W: Survival and causes of death in hemochromatosis: Observations in 163 patients. Ann NY Acad Sci 526:245, 1988.

Recent data on natural history and survival of treated patients with fairly severe disease.

Weintraub LR, Edward CQ, Krikker M (eds.): Hemochromatosis. Proceedings of the First International Conference. Ann NY Acad Sci, Vol. 526, 1988. *The useful proceedings of an international conference on hemochromatosis that covered all basic and clinical aspects.*

194 Phosphorus Deficiency and Hypophosphatemia

Lloyd H. Smith, Jr.

Phosphorus is necessary for the structural and functional integrity of all living things. In hydroxyapatite it is a key constituent of bone; as a part of phospholipids (lecithin, sphingomyelin) it is necessary for the structure of all cell membranes, both external and internal (endoplasmic reticulum, lysosomes, nuclear membranes). It furnishes the backbone of nucleic acids, captures and stores metabolic energy ($\sim$P), serves as a second messenger in endocrinology (cyclic adenosine monophosphate [cAMP], cyclic guanosine monophosphate [cGMP]), regulates the release of O_2 by hemoglobin (2,3-diphosphoglycerate), and buffers urine. Even this partial list indicates that a severe deficiency of phosphorus would lead to widespread and serious consequences.

In an adult of average size there are approximately 700 to 800 grams (25 moles) of phosphorus, of which 80 to 85 per cent is in the skeleton and 10 per cent in muscle. Phosphate is the major anion of intracellular fluid (about 100 mM), where it is found mostly as phosphoproteins, phospholipids, or phosphosugars rather than as free orthophosphate. In extracellular fluid the normal concentration of phosphorus in adults is 2.7 to 4.5 mg per deciliter (0.9 to 1.5 mM), of which most is free; perhaps 10 per cent is protein bound. Serum phosphorus is normally higher in children (4.0 to 7.0 mg per deciliter). (It is conventional to express serum phosphate as the amount of elemental P, since pH influences the relative amounts of $H_2PO_4^-$ and HPO_4^- present.) The average American diet contains about 1000 mg of P, most of which is absorbed by active transport, increased by 1,25-dihydroxycholecalciferol. Approximately 90 per cent of that absorbed from the diet is excreted in the urine by a process involving filtration and partial renal tubular reabsorption. The tubular reabsorption of phosphate is diminished by parathyroid hormone (PTH), acting with cAMP as a second messenger. Through vitamin D, PTH, calcitonin, and the mineralization of osteoid, phosphate metabolism is closely linked with that of calcium. These interrelationships are discussed more completely in Ch. 232.

Hyperphosphatemia that is sustained occurs almost exclusively in three clinical conditions: (1) renal insufficiency (see Ch. 76), (2) hypoparathyroidism (including various types of pseudohypoparathyroidism) (see Ch. 235), and (3) acromegaly or gigantism (see Ch. 213). When severe, hyperphosphatemia may contribute to the acidosis of uremia, further reduce the extracellular fluid concentration of ionized calcium, or lead to metastatic calcification in extraosseous sites. Transient hyperphosphatemia may occur with acute tissue destruction, such as the tumor lysis syndrome or rhabdomyolysis.

CAUSES OF HYPOPHOSPHATEMIA. Hypophosphatemia (serum P < 2.7 mg per deciliter) may be associated with a normal total body phosphate (representing a transient intracellular shift) or with phosphate deficiency. The two most common causes of transient hypophosphatemia are (1) ingestion of carbohydrates, which deplete phosphate in extracellular fluid in the process of their intracellular transport and metabolism, and (2) acute respiratory alkalosis, which leads to an intracellular shift of phosphate through mechanisms not fully explained.

It is convenient to summarize the causes of hypophosphatemia as those that usually result in only moderate reductions in serum P (1.0 to 2.5 mg per deciliter) and those that may result in severe hypophosphatemia (P < 1.0 mg per deciliter) (Table 194–1).

Moderate hypophosphatemia may occur transiently during carbohydrate metabolism or alkalosis, as noted above, in the

I. Moderate hypophosphatemia (P 1.0 to 2.5 mg per deciliter)

Hyperparathyroidism—primary or secondary (in the absence of renal failure)

Osteomalacia (usually with hyperparathyroidism), malabsorption, deficiency of vitamin D, familial hypophosphatemic rickets, vitamin D–dependent rickets, oncogenic rickets

Carbohydrate administration or ingestion or enhanced metabolism—glucose, fructose, glycerol, lactate, insulin administration

Hypomagnesemia

Extracellular fluid (ECF) volume expansion

Acute alkalosis—bicarbonate infusion or moderate hyperventilation

Hemodialysis

II. Severe hypophosphatemia (P less than 1.0 mg per deciliter)

Chronic alcoholism and alcoholic withdrawal

Diabetic ketoacidosis, recovery phase

Enteric phosphate binding—excessive use of agents binding phosphate in the gut

Hyperalimentation

Nutritional recovery syndrome

Uptake by rapidly proliferating malignant tumors (rare)

*Modified from Knochel JP: Hypophosphatemia. West J Med 134:15, 1981.

absence of phosphate depletion. Increased PTH, associated with either primary or secondary hyperparathyroidism, reduces the renal tubular reabsorption of phosphate and leads to renal phosphate wasting. In familial hypophosphatemic rickets there may be a primary defect in the renal tubular reabsorption of phosphate. The association of hypophosphatemia with hyperparathyroidism and the various types of osteomalacia or rickets is discussed more fully in Ch. 234 and 235. In the various forms of the Fanconi syndrome, renal tubular dysfunction leads to phosphate wasting (Ch. 82). Hypomagnesemia and extracellular fluid volume expansion may result in reduced renal tubular reabsorption of phosphate and mild hypophosphatemia. Hemodialysis with equilibration against a dialysate deficient in phosphate may lead to overshoot hypophosphatemia. There are no well-defined acute metabolic consequences of moderate hypophosphatemia. Prolonged hypophosphatemia in this range may result in the defective mineralization of bone characteristic of osteomalacia or rickets.

Severe hypophosphatemia may cause serious metabolic consequences as described below. The most frequent cause of severe hypophosphatemia in clinical practice is *alcoholism*, especially during the withdrawal phase. The causes of phosphate depletion in alcoholics are complex and may include (1) poor dietary intake, (2) vomiting, (3) diarrhea, (4) the use of antacids that bind phosphate and reduce its absorption, (5) a possible phosphaturic effect of ethanol itself, (6) magnesium deficiency with phosphaturia, and (7) calcium deficiency with secondary hyperparathyroidism. The serum P level may be further reduced by the hyperventilation characteristic of alcohol withdrawal and by the therapeutic infusion of glucose. Patients with *uncontrolled diabetes mellitus* often become phosphate depleted through catabolism of intracellular organic phosphates and phosphaturia secondary to osmotic diuresis. Initial serum P levels are often normal or even high during diabetic ketoacidosis but rapidly fall to hypophosphatemic levels during the first 6 to 12 hours of treatment with volume expansion, glucose, and insulin. Hyperventilation with *marked respiratory alkalosis* can cause profound hypophosphatemia within minutes; metabolic alkalosis of the same degree causes only moderate hypophosphatemia. Excessive ingestion of *phosphate-binding antacids*, such as aluminum hydroxide, may inhibit phosphate absorption from the intestine sufficiently to cause chronic depletion, especially when combined with reduced dietary ingestion of phosphate. Excessive utilization of phosphate during tissue repletion may occasionally result in severe hypophosphatemia during *hyperalimentation* (without adequate supplementary P) and during the *nutritional recovery syndrome* of refeeding patients with protein-calorie malnutrition or starvation. Whatever its cause, severe hypophosphatemia requires early attention because of its potential consequences.

CONSEQUENCES OF SEVERE HYPOPHOSPHATEMIA (Table 194–2). The long-term consequences of severe hypophosphatemia are largely structural, those of metabolic bone disease (see Ch. 234). The short-term consequences may be considered to be metabolic, although the distinction is an arbitrary one.

Red cell dysfunction in severe hypophosphatemia may result from two biochemical abnormalities, depletion of intracellular 2,3-diphosphoglycerate (2,3-DPG) and of adenosine triphosphate (ATP). Phosphate is a cofactor for glyceraldehyde-3-phosphate dehydrogenase, an enzyme in the pathway of the synthesis of 2,3-DPG. When intracellular erythrocytic phosphate decreases, a block in the glycolytic pathway results, with accumulation of triose phosphates and depletion of 2,3-DPG. This molecule normally exercises a unique allosteric effect on the dissociation curve of oxyhemoglobin, shifting it "to the right" and thereby enhancing the tissue availability of oxygen (see Ch. 136.2). Reduction of erythrocytic 2,3-DPG, conversely, impairs effective oxygen delivery to the periphery. The same block in the glycolytic pathway reduces ATP synthesis. The degradation of AMP to inosine 5′-phosphate (IMP) by AMP deaminase is enhanced when the restraining influence of phosphate is reduced, further depleting the intracellular concentration of adenine nucleotides. As a result, the concentration of erythrocytic ATP tends to fall in parallel with the reduction of serum phosphorus. At a critical level of ATP (usually with serum $P < 0.5$ mg per deciliter), the energy metabolism of the erythrocyte may become inadequate to maintain the integrity of its membrane, and *hemolysis* may occur.

Leukocyte dysfunction has been demonstrated during phosphate depletion in experimental animals, characterized by impaired chemotaxis, phagocytosis, and bactericidal function. These defects presumably result from inadequate ATP for normal cellular functions, possibly including the synthesis of phospholipids in membranes. Similarly, *platelet dysfunction* occurs in experimental phosphate depletion, but no hemorrhagic diathesis has been attributed to phosphate deficiency in humans.

Many patients with severe hypophosphatemia complain of *weakness*. This is often nonspecific and difficult to delineate from that caused by the associated disorder, but improved diaphragmatic contractility has been noted following the treatment of hypophosphatemia in patients with respiratory failure. *Rhabdomyolysis* is an occasional complication of severe hypophosphatemia, perhaps being somewhat analogous to hemolytic anemia in its pathogenesis, i.e., related to deficiency of ATP. The severity of rhabdomyolysis varies from that manifested solely by an elevated serum level of "muscle enzymes" (aldolase and creatine phosphokinase) to a full-fledged syndrome of muscle weakness, pain, tenderness, and stiffness associated with myoglobinuria. Interestingly, the release of phosphate from the necrosis of muscle may suffice to return the serum P level to normal. A few patients with severe phosphate depletion have exhibited congestive cardiomyopathy, which has seemed to respond to phosphate repletion. These clinical observations are strengthened by the demonstration of decreased myocardial contractility during experimental phosphate depletion in dogs.

Severe hypophosphatemia may result in *central nervous system dysfunction* with a constellation of symptoms and signs designated as metabolic brain disease or metabolic encephalopathy (see Ch. 443). These abnormalities may vary from irritability, weakness, and paresthesias to obtundation, seizures, and coma. It is presumed that this central nervous system dysfunction results from

TABLE 194–2. CONSEQUENCES OF SEVERE HYPOPHOSPHATEMIA

I. Acute—"metabolic"

  Hematologic

   Red cell dysfunction and hemolysis

   Leukocyte dysfunction

   Platelet dysfunction

  Muscle

   Weakness

   Rhabdomyolysis

   Myocardial dysfunction

  Central nervous system dysfunction

  Peripheral neuropathy

  Hepatic dysfunction

II. Chronic—"structural"

  Osteomalacia or rickets (Ch. 234)

deranged energy metabolism of the brain secondary to ATP depletion. Observations have suggested that hepatic function is further impaired in alcoholics with severe hypophosphatemia, with early improvement during replacement therapy, but a clinical entity of *hypophosphatemic hepatic dysfunction* has not yet been well established.

TREATMENT OF HYPOPHOSPHATEMIA. The treatment of hypophosphatemia depends upon its cause, its acuteness, and its severity. Hypophosphatemia caused by acute respiratory alkalosis or the infusion of carbohydrates does not require replacement therapy. Chronic hypophosphatemia associated with aluminum hydroxide therapy, for example, may require reduction of the antacid and an oral source of supplemental phosphate such as milk (1 gram of P or 30 to 35 mmol per quart) or a balanced solution of phosphate salts (sodium or potassium salts, as in Fleet enema solution or Neutra-Phos). It is rare that hypophosphatemia is so acute and severe as to require parenteral replacement therapy. When such treatment is undertaken, it is well to remember that (1) it is unusual for hypophosphatemia to cause metabolic disturbances at concentrations greater than 1.0 mg per deciliter, so full parenteral replacement is neither necessary nor desirable; and (2) if hyperphosphatemia results, there is a danger of producing a decrease in ionized calcium (with tetany or convulsions) and/or metastatic calcification of soft tissues. It is usually safe and sufficient to administer intravenously 1 mmol of phosphate per kilogram of body weight evenly over a 24-hour period in the treatment of acute, severe hypophosphatemia associated with phosphate depletion. Since potassium depletion is so frequently associated with phosphate depletion both in alcoholics and in patients with diabetic ketoacidosis, it may be useful as a guideline to give half of parenterally administered potassium as its phosphate salt. Obviously, parenteral phosphate should not be given in the face of hyperphosphatemia.

Knochel JP: The clinical status of hypophosphatemia. N Engl J Med 313:447, 1985. *This useful editorial emphasizes the adverse effect of phosphate depletion on muscle function.*

Knochel JP, Jacobson HR: Renal handling of phosphorus, clinical hypophosphatemia, and phosphorus deficiency. *In* Brenner BM, Rector FC Jr (eds.): The Kidney. 3rd ed. Philadelphia, W. B. Saunders Company, 1986, pp 619–662. *This chapter in a major textbook offers an extensive discussion of the normal physiology of phosphate homeostasis and the causes and consequences of hypophosphatemia. There are 459 references.*

Rasmussen H, Tenenhouse HS: Hypophosphatemias. *In* Scriver CR, Beaudet AL, Sly WS, et al. (eds.): *The Metabolic Basis of Inherited Disease.* 6th ed. New York, McGraw-Hill, 1989, pp 2581–2609. *An authoritative discussion of phosphate homeostasis and the inherited syndrome of hypophosphatemic rickets caused by defects in renal tubular phosphate reabsorption.*

Yu GC, Lee DBN: Clinical disorders of phosphorus metabolism. West J Med 147:569, 1987. *This article gives an excellent general review of the clinical and pathophysiologic aspects of phosphate deficiency syndromes in humans.*

195 Disorders of Magnesium Metabolism

Lloyd H. Smith, Jr.

Magnesium is the fourth most common cation in the human body (after sodium, potassium, and calcium) and the cation in second highest concentration intracellularly. The average adult body contains about 25 grams (1000 mmol) of magnesium, of which 50 to 60 per cent is in bone. The normal serum magnesium concentration is 1.6 to 2.1 mEq per liter, approximately one fourth to one third being protein bound. The average American diet contains approximately 500 mg (20 mmol) of magnesium, much of this in chlorophyll. It has been estimated that about 0.15 mmol (3.5 to 4.5 mg) of dietary magnesium per kilogram per day is necessary to maintain a positive balance in adults. More is required in children. Magnesium is actively absorbed in the small intestine by a process that is enhanced by 1,25-dihydroxycholecalciferol, resulting in a net absorption of about 30 to 40 per cent of that ingested. This net absorption is balanced at equilibrium by renal excretion, which reflects filtration of the 65 to 75 per cent not protein bound followed by net renal tubular reabsorption of approximately 95 per cent. The kidney can control the excretion of magnesium over a wide range—from more than 250 mmol to less than 1 mmol per day. The factors that control the renal tubular reabsorption of magnesium are not completely understood but include sodium excretion, calcium excretion, parathyroid hormone, and extracellular fluid volume. Excretion is also increased by ethanol and by many diuretic agents.

Magnesium has a structural role in bone crystal. It also serves as an activator of a large number of specific enzymes. Of particular importance, it is a cofactor in all transphosphorylation reactions involving adenosine triphosphate (ATP), so that it is intimately involved in energy metabolism and the synthesis of macromolecules, for example. Perhaps even more basic in biology is its obligate role in the function of chlorophyll. By and large it has not been possible to correlate the signs or symptoms of magnesium deficiency or excess with any one of its specific biochemical functions.

HYPERMAGNESEMIA. Because of the ability of the normal kidney to excrete a magnesium load, significant hypermagnesemia is rarely seen in clinical practice. In the past, magnesium ion was occasionally infused as a hypotensive agent in the treatment of acute hypertension with the secondary production of symptomatic hypermagnesemia. In patients with renal insufficiency, the excessive use of magnesium, as in magnesium-containing antacids, may cause hypermagnesemia. The manifestations of hypermagnesemia are largely in the central nervous system and the cardiovascular system. Ionized magnesium is a sedative that depresses the function of the central nervous system and exerts a curare-like effect on the neuromuscular junction at high concentrations (>10 mEq per liter). The cardiovascular effects of hypermagnesemia are those of peripheral vasodilatation, resulting in hypotension, generalized depression of the cardiac conduction system, bradyrhythmias, and asystole with cardiac arrest in diastole. The cardiac effects of Mg^{2+} are usually manifested at serum concentrations greater than 10 mEq per liter, with asystole at levels greater than 25 mEq per liter, but a few patients have exhibited exceptional sensitivity with cardiotoxicity at levels of 4.5 to 5.5 mEq per liter. Factors that augment the cardiotoxicity of Mg^{2+} include hypocalcemia, hyperkalemia, acidosis, digitalis therapy, and renal insufficiency (beyond its effect on the serum Mg^{2+} level). Treatment of hypermagnesemia is usually limited to discontinuing its exogenous source. In severe hypermagnesemia, intravenous treatment with calcium may temporarily reverse many of the toxic effects because of the pharmacologic antagonism of ionized calcium and magnesium in the central nervous system.

HYPOMAGNESEMIA. Hypomagnesemia is a much more frequent metabolic derangement than hypermagnesemia and usually occurs as one component of a complex deficiency state, affecting many minerals, vitamins, and nutrients.

Causes of Hypomagnesemia. Magnesium deficiency and hypomagnesemia result from decreased absorption or from increased excretion (Table 195–1). Very rarely, hypomagnesemia may result from "loss" into bone during excessive osteogenesis, the "hungry bone syndrome," during the repair of osteitis fibrosa generalisata following the removal of a parathyroid tumor (see Ch. 235). Serum levels may also fall, as do those of calcium, during acute pancreatitis. In general, decreased absorption of magnesium occurs in the same circumstances as does decreased calcium absorption, especially that caused by dietary deficiency and malabsorption syndromes of whatever origin. Decreased absorption in uremia may result from deficiency of 1,25-dihydroxycholecalciferol. A few infants have been described with convulsions associated with hypocalcemia and hypomagnesemia in the absence of renal magnesium wasting. They have responded to continued high ingestion of magnesium, but not of calcium, and are thought to have a selective defect in gut absorption of magnesium. It is not clear whether ethanol diminishes magnesium absorption directly or only through diminished ingestion or vitamin D deficiency.

Increased loss of magnesium can occur from excessive vomiting, from diarrhea, or via the kidney. Rarely, patients may exhibit what appears to be an inherited renal tubular defect in magnesium reabsorption. These patients have tended to have potassium wasting as well and to present with hypokalemia, hypomagnesemia, and hypocalcemia (secondary to hypomagnesemia). In general, magnesium clearance tends to parallel that of sodium and calcium and may be increased by diuretics (osmotic, thiazides, ethacrynic acid, furosemide), by ionized calcium, and possibly by ethanol. Renal magnesium wasting also occurs as a result of the renal tubular effect of certain drugs, especially aminoglycosides, amphotericin B, and cisplatin. The magnesium wasting of uncontrolled diabetes mellitus probably results from tissue catabolism and osmotic diuresis. Lactation hypomagnesemia, well described in cattle, has been documented in two women.

Consequences of Hypomagnesemia. Hypomagnesemia rarely occurs as a single deficiency, so that it is not always possible to distinguish its signs and symptoms from those of associated deficiency states. Selective magnesium deficiency has been produced experimentally in humans, however, and it is based on these observations, together with clinical correlations in patients, that the spectrum of manifestations listed in Table 195–2 has been described. Patients with magnesium deficiency are lethargic, weak, and irritable with decreased attention span. They may have tetany with positive Chvostek's and Trousseau's signs because of associated hypocalcemia (see below). In experimental magnesium deficiency, muscles are weak and may show hyaline and vacuolar degeneration of myofibers, sometimes followed by leukocytic infiltration, segmental necrosis, and early calcification. Patients with hypomagnesemia are generally anorectic and may have nausea, vomiting, and poor intestinal motility. Hypomagnesemia may occur in congestive heart failure because of anorexia, malabsorption, and the excessive use of diuretic agents. Magnesium deficiency increases the sensitivity of the heart to digitalis glycosides, so that digitalis toxicity occurs at a lower serum level and also tends to persist longer. Hypomagnesemia has also been associated with cardiac arrhythmias independent of digoxin, including ventricular premature beats, ventricular tachycardia, and ventricular fibrillation. This association is often difficult to establish because other abnormalities generally coexist, especially hypokalemia.

Magnesium metabolism has a number of interesting interrelationships with that of calcium: (1) both are absorbed by the gut through mechanisms enhanced by vitamin D; (2) excess magnesium may inhibit calcium absorption, but not vice versa; (3) calcium and magnesium may compete for renal tubular reabsorption; (4) calcium and magnesium are physiologic antagonists in the central nervous system; and (5) magnesium is necessary for the normal secretion of parathyroid hormone (PTH) in response to hypocalcemia and also for the activity of PTH as a hormone at the site of its target organs. *Hypocalcemia* is one of the most consistent and important findings in magnesium deficiency with

TABLE 195–1. CAUSES OF HYPOMAGNESEMIA (SEEN MOST FREQUENTLY CLINICALLY IN ALCOHOLISM AND MALABSORPTION)

I. **Decreased absorption from dietary sources**
   Diet poor in magnesium
   Parenteral feeding without magnesium
   Ethanol effect on absorption
   Malabsorption syndromes
   Uremia
   Selective intestinal defect for magnesium absorption (rare)
II. **Increased loss of magnesium from the body**
   Gastrointestinal tract—diarrhea, fistulas, suction
   Kidney
     Primary renal tubular defects
     Secondary—diuretics, Ca^{2+}, ethanol, expansion of ECF, diabetes mellitus, treatment with gentamicin, cisplatin, or amphotericin B
   Breast—lactation hypomagnesemia (mostly in cattle, rarely in humans)
III. **Internal redistribution**
   Acute pancreatitis
   Increased loss into bone ("hungry bone syndrome")

TABLE 195–2. CONSEQUENCES OF MAGNESIUM DEFICIENCY

Neuromuscular
   Lethargy, weakness, fatigue, decreased mentation, paresthesias
   Neuromuscular irritability, in part due to associated hypocalcemia
   Hyaline and vacuolar degeneration of myofibers with segmental necrosis
Gastrointestinal
   Anorexia, nausea, vomiting
   Paralytic ileus
Cardiovascular
   Increased sensitivity to digitalis glycosides
   Cardiac arrhythmias
Metabolic
   Hypocalcemia—probably due to the combined result of decreased PTH secretion and decreased end-organ responsiveness to PTH
   Hypokalemia—tendency toward renal potassium wasting

hypomagnesemia. Hypocalcemia responds promptly to magnesium replacement and is accompanied by a rise in plasma PTH. A burst of PTH secretion occurs within minutes after the infusion of magnesium intravenously into patients with combined hypocalcemia and hypomagnesemia. Many of these patients show evidence of resistance to exogenous PTH as well. Hypomagnesemia therefore results in a complex combination of functional hypoparathyroidism and acquired pseudohypoparathyroidism. This entity should be suspected especially in alcoholics or patients with malabsorption who present with hypocalcemia. *Hypokalemia* is frequently found with hypomagnesemia. Although some of the conditions that cause magnesium depletion also produce potassium depletion, there is evidence that magnesium deficiency itself enhances renal excretion of potassium. This associated hypokalemia is usually resistant to potassium replacement unless magnesium is replaced first.

Treatment of Hypomagnesemia. The treatment of hypomagnesemia is rarely an acute emergency. When rapid replacement therapy is judged to be vital (convulsions, tachyrhythmias), 2 grams of $MgSO_4$ (16.3 mEq) can be given intravenously over several minutes. This can be followed by a constant intravenous infusion of approximately 1 mEq of magnesium per kilogram per 24 hours, which usually suffices for initial replacement therapy. Ampules often contain 1 gram of $MgSO_4 \cdot 7H_2O$, which is 8.1 mEq of Mg, so that initial replacement therapy usually requires 8 to 10 grams of $MgSO_4$ given either intravenously as above or intramuscularly as 2 grams every 4 hours for five doses. After the first day, approximately 0.5 mEq of Mg per kilogram per 24 hours should be given intravenously or intramuscularly for 2 to 5 days, based on the return of the serum magnesium level to normal. Parenteral replacement therapy is often preferable to oral therapy because of the tendency of magnesium salts to cause diarrhea. When renal function is impaired, the aforementioned schedules for magnesium replacement must be followed with extra caution and with careful monitoring of serum levels. When there is chronic loss of magnesium (renal wasting, for example), oral therapy is preferred and can be carried out with various preparations as tolerated without diarrhea—magnesium hydroxide tablets, magnesium acetate solution, or liquid milk of magnesia.

Shils ME: Magnesium in health and disease. Annu Rev Nutr 8:429, 1988. *This is an excellent general review of magnesium metabolism by an author who is an authority in the field. Extensive (203) references.*
Sjögren A, Edvinsson L, Fallgren B: Magnesium deficiency in coronary artery disease and cardiac arrhythmias. J Intern Med 226:213, 1989. *The authors give a useful analytic review of magnesium as a coronary dilator and its role in cardiac arrhythmias and in coronary artery disease.*
Whang R: Magnesium deficiency: Pathogenesis, prevalence, and clinical implications. Am J Med 82(Suppl 3A):24, 1987. *A succinct general review with a useful up-to-date list of 43 references.*

196 Familial Mediterranean Fever

Daniel G. Wright

DEFINITION. Familial Mediterranean fever (FMF) is an inherited, recurrent inflammatory disease of unknown cause. The disease is characterized by acute self-limited attacks of fever and peritonitis, sometimes accompanied by pleuritis, arthritis, and erythematous skin lesions. Among affected individuals in the Middle East and Europe, FMF is frequently complicated by amyloidosis and progressive renal failure. Familial Mediterranean fever has been given a number of other names: familial paroxysmal polyserositis, benign paroxysmal peritonitis, periodic peritonitis, and periodic disease. The first of these is descriptively accurate and an appropriate alternative name for the disease; the other terms, however, are misleading. Familial Mediterranean fever is not a benign condition, given the potentially lethal complication of amyloidosis. Moreover, attacks of acute serositis in FMF affect sites other than the peritoneum, and they recur at irregular, unpredictable intervals that do not reflect true periodicity.

INCIDENCE, PREVALENCE, AND GENETICS. Although FMF has been recognized in many parts of the world, it is largely restricted to ethnic groups originating in the eastern Mediterranean area. It is an uncommon disease, even in Israel, where the largest number of cases are seen. Half the reported cases of FMF are in patients of Sephardic Jewish ancestry; approximately 20 per cent of patients are Armenian, and another 20 per cent are of Turkish or Arabic descent. Most of the remaining patients are of Italian, Greek, or Ashkenazic Jewish ancestry. However, the disease has also been recognized rarely in individuals with Anglo-Saxon or northern European origins. The disease is familial, and in well-studied affected kindreds it appears to be inherited as an autosomal recessive trait. Nonetheless, nearly 50 per cent of patients do not give a positive family history for the disease. Among reported cases males predominate by a ratio of 3:2. Active efforts are under way to identify a genetic abnormality in this disease by genomic linkage studies of DNA from members of affected kindreds.

ETIOLOGY. Although many pathogenetic explanations have been suggested for the acute inflammatory episodes of FMF, the etiology of this disease remains unknown. Extensive studies have failed to establish an infectious or allergic basis for the disease, and no good evidence exists to support suggestions that FMF represents a hormonal or psychosomatic disturbance. Recently, it has been proposed that FMF might be caused by a genetically determined defect in the normal regulation of acute inflammatory responses. Abnormalities of suppressor T lymphocytes, altered metabolism of lipoxygenase products of arachidonic acid, and absence of a normal inhibitor of the complement-derived anaphylatoxin C5a have been described in FMF. However, the possible etiologic significance of these observations remains to be clarified and confirmed.

PATHOLOGY. Pathologic findings in FMF are those of nonspecific, acute inflammation. Neutrophilic infiltration predominates in exudates recovered from peritoneal, pleural, or joint spaces at the time of acute attacks. Serosal thickening and secondary adhesions may occur, which in the abdomen can lead to mechanical bowel obstruction. Amyloidosis is the most serious histopathologic finding in FMF. In affected individuals, amyloid is deposited in the intima and media of arterioles and in the subendothelium of venules in all major organs. There is also parenchymal deposition of amyloid, particularly in the renal glomeruli, adrenals, spleen, and alveolar septa of the lung, while the liver and heart are characteristically spared.

CLINICAL MANIFESTATIONS. In most patients the signs and symptoms of FMF begin during the first two decades of life, usually between the ages of 5 and 15 years. Rarely, however, the onset of the disease may occur in infancy or as late as the fifth or sixth decade. The duration and frequency of attacks vary considerably, even in the same patient. Acute attacks typically last 24 to 48 hours and recur once or twice a month. However, attacks may recur as frequently as several times a week or as infrequently as once a year, and symptoms may persist for as long as a week during individual episodes. Some patients experience spontaneous remission that persists for years, followed by recurrence of frequent attacks. Pregnancy is often associated with remission of attacks, which resume post partum. Some patients relate the occurrence of attacks to cold weather and find that they experience attacks more frequently during winter than summer. Recurrent attacks may also become less severe and/or less frequent as patients age or as they develop amyloidosis. Between attacks, patients typically feel entirely well.

Temperatures as high as 39° to 40°C accompany almost all attacks. Fevers may occur without concomitant evidence of serositis, but this is unusual. The rise in temperature is sometimes preceded by chills and typically peaks by 12 to 24 hours; diaphoresis frequently accompanies defervescence.

More than 95 per cent of patients experience abdominal pain and signs of peritonitis during acute attacks. Pain often begins in one quadrant and then becomes diffuse, sometimes with distention, rigidity, rebound tenderness, and ileus with nausea and vomiting. Pain may radiate to the back or to the shoulders, and upright abdominal roentgenograms may show small air-fluid levels and edema of the bowel. Although these signs and symptoms are self-limited, they can be indistinguishable from those of an acute abdominal emergency, and patients may undergo one or more exploratory laparotomies before the true nature of their disease is recognized. Potential uncertainties about the clinical management of acute abdominal episodes have led to the recommendation that elective appendectomy be carried out during a symptom-free period so that acute appendicitis does not confuse a patient's subsequent care.

Pleuritic pain occurs during acute attacks in 75 per cent of patients. Symptoms of pleuritis may sometimes precede abdominal pain, and a few patients experience pleuritic attacks without abdominal symptoms. Chest pain is usually one sided and may be associated with diminished breath sounds, a friction rub, plate atelectasis, and transient pleural effusion.

Nonspecific, mild arthralgia is a common feature of febrile attacks, and acute, monoarticular, or oligoarticular arthritis may occur. Although arthritis is unusual among patients in the United States, it is a frequently observed manifestation of FMF among Israeli patients. Arthritis usually affects large joints, the knee in particular, and effusions are common. Although arthritic episodes are typically short lived, joint symptoms may also be protracted and follow a course distinct from that of the acute abdominal and/or pleuritic attacks. Roentgenographic findings are nonspecific.

As many as a third of patients experience transient, erysipelas-like skin lesions that appear typically on the lower leg, ankle, or dorsum of the foot. These lesions are well-circumscribed, painful, erythematous areas of swelling, 5 to 20 cm in diameter, that subside spontaneously within 24 to 48 hours.

Self-limited pericarditis, conjunctivitis, aseptic meningitis, and other forms of serositis have been reported as manifestations of this disease but are unusual. Migraine-like headaches and emotional lability have also been observed during acute attacks, but it is unclear whether these are primary or secondary manifestations.

The most serious complication of FMF is systemic amyloidosis of the AA type. The natural history of amyloidosis in this disease is one of relentless progression to renal failure and death, which may occur in adolescence or even earlier. While a substantial proportion of Turkish and Israeli patients develop amyloidosis, this complication has been very unusual among patients in the United States and in several well-studied Armenian and Arabic kindreds. The genetic and/or environmental factors that explain these differences in the incidence of amyloidosis remain unclear.

In Israel, 90 per cent of patients who develop amyloidosis (particularly common in Sephardic Jews) do so after experiencing typical attacks of FMF (phenotype I); however, amyloidosis may occur in asymptomatic siblings of FMF patients, or it may precede the onset of typical FMF attacks (phenotype II).

Laboratory findings in FMF are nonspecific. During acute attacks, a prominent leukocytosis (up to 30,000 per cubic millimeter) is present, and the erythrocyte sedimentation rate and acute phase reactants are increased. These values return to normal between attacks. Elevated plasma dopamine beta-hydroxylase levels (which become normal during colchicine treatment) have been reported in patients with FMF, but confirmatory studies have yet to be done to determine whether this finding represents a specific diagnostic test for FMF. With amyloidosis, laboratory abnormalities reflect the associated nephrotic syndrome and renal failure.

DIAGNOSIS. The diagnosis of FMF is based primarily upon clinical presentation and history. In individuals of appropriate ethnic background with typical recurrent, self-limited attacks, diagnosis should not be difficult; in such individuals, delay in recognizing the disease is usually because the diagnosis is not considered. Nonetheless, when a patient is first seen or when attacks are infrequent, a variety of other acute febrile conditions must be considered and excluded by appropriate diagnostic studies and follow-up—in particular, appendicitis, pancreatitis, cholecystitis, and intestinal obstruction. Familial hyperlipidemia and porphyrias associated with abdominal symptoms must also be considered.

The diagnosis is usually most elusive when patients have a limited or atypical symptom complex. Isolated pleural attacks may closely mimic acute infections or pulmonary emboli. Arthritis, when it is a prominent manifestation, can at first be clinically indistinguishable from various infectious and noninfectious arthritides, and skin lesions on the lower legs may resemble cellulitis or superficial thrombophlebitis. Rare patients have febrile episodes without serositis, and these may require orderly evaluation to determine their origin. Recently, it has been reported that infusion of metaraminol diluted in normal saline provokes acute signs and symptoms of FMF with a high degree of specificity for the disease. However, the appropriate role of such a test in establishing the diagnosis remains unclear. At present, this procedure, which carries intrinsic risks from catecholamine effects and salt load, should be considered experimental and not for use in general practice.

Once FMF is diagnosed, a degree of diagnostic vigilance must be maintained, for patients are not immune to the more common acute illnesses that FMF mimics. Of note, these patients appear to be particularly prone to develop gallbladder disease.

TREATMENT. Colchicine treatment is effective in FMF. Several controlled clinical trials, together with extensive, uncontrolled clinical experience since the mid 1970's, have shown that prophylactic colchicine,* 0.6 mg orally two or three times a day, prevents or substantially reduces the acute attacks of FMF in 75 to 90 per cent of patients. Treatment failures are often associated with noncompliance and/or intolerance to the drug. Some patients can abort attacks with intermittent courses of colchicine, beginning at the onset of attacks (0.6 mg orally every hour for 4 hours, then every 2 hours for 4 hours, and then every 12 hours for 2 days). In general, patients who benefit from intermittent colchicine therapy are those who experience a recognizable prodrome before developing fever and clear-cut acute symptoms. Colchicine does not alter fully developed attacks. Patients who experience gastrointestinal intolerance to colchicine may benefit from reduced doses. Although definite chronic complications from colchicine have not become apparent with its long-term use in FMF, it is still recommended that a trial of intermittent colchicine therapy be attempted, particularly in young patients, before long-term colchicine prophylaxis is used. Azoospermia and chromosomal nondisjunctions have been associated with the use of this drug. This recommendation does not apply to individuals from ethnic groups and in geographic regions associated with a high risk of amyloidosis, for it is now evident that long-term colchicine therapy not only prevents the development of amyloidosis but may also arrest its progression in FMF.

* This use of colchicine is not listed in the manufacturer's directive.

Symptomatic and supportive treatment is indicated for patients who do not respond to colchicine. However, every effort should be made to avoid the use of narcotics. In the United States, addiction to narcotics has been a major long-term complication among FMF patients.

It has been estimated that patients with FMF and end-stage renal amyloidosis represent up to 6 per cent of the candidates for renal transplantation in Israel. Many such patients have received successful renal grafts. Of note, it has been suggested recently that these patients may be particularly susceptible to gastrointestinal and other side effects of the immunosuppressive drug cyclosporine.

PROGNOSIS. The prognosis for normal longevity for patients in the United States with FMF is excellent, and since the recognition of colchicine's efficacy in this disease, most patients can be maintained almost entirely symptom free. Except in very rare cases, this disease does not affect the physical growth and development of children. Long-term colchicine therapy has also clearly improved the prognosis of patients in the Middle East who are prone to develop amyloidosis, even those whose symptomatic attacks continue. However, among patients in whom amyloidosis has led to nephrotic syndrome or uremia and who are unable to receive a renal transplant or in whom renal transplantation has failed, the likelihood of eventual death from renal failure remains great.

Barakat MH, Karnik AM, Majeed HWA, et al.: Familial Mediterranean fever (recurrent hereditary polyserositis) in Arabs—a study of 175 patients and review of the literature. Q J Med 60:837, 1986. Meyerhoff J: Familial Mediterranean fever: Report of a large family, review of the literature, and discussion of the frequency of amyloidosis. Medicine 59:66, 1980. *These articles provide extensive reviews of the clinical and pathologic manifestations of FMF and describe differences in the incidence of amyloidosis.*
Dinarello CA, Wolff SM, Goldfinger SE, et al.: Colchicine therapy for familial Mediterranean fever. A double-blind trial. N Engl J Med 291:934, 1974. *One of several controlled trials that clearly established the efficacy of prophylactic colchicine therapy in preventing FMF attacks.*
Wright DG, Wolff SM, Fauci AS, et al.: Efficacy of intermittent colchicine therapy in familial Mediterranean fever. Ann Intern Med 86:162, 1977. *A double-blind study that shows intermittent courses of colchicine can successfully abort attacks in some patients with FMF.*
Zemer D, Pras M, Sohar E, et al.: Colchicine in the prevention and treatment of the amyloidosis of familial Mediterranean fever. N Engl J Med 314:1001, 1986. *A retrospective review of 1070 patients that provides convincing evidence that long-term colchicine therapy arrests the development of amyloidosis.*

197 The Amyloid Diseases

Joel N. Buxbaum

DEFINITION. The amyloid diseases constitute a group of conditions of diverse causes characterized by the accumulation of ultrastructurally fibrillar material in various tissues in quantities sufficient to compromise vital organ function. The associated disease states may be inflammatory, hereditary, or neoplastic, and the deposition can be local or systemic. The clinical outcome may be benign or as malignant as the most aggressive of neoplasms. In many senses, amyloid deposition is a symptom of an underlying disorder, much as anemia is a symptom of a variety of pathologic states. The symptoms of the amyloidoses depend upon the amount and localization of the deposits.

In tissue sections, with conventional staining techniques, all amyloid appears homogeneous and eosinophilic. All types bind Congo red and under polarized light emit an apple-green fluorescence when stained with this dye. With the electron microscope, amyloid is seen to contain two discrete structures: a major fibrillar component with a characteristic periodicity and a minor rodlike component that, when extracted and viewed on end, has the appearance of a pentagon with a hollow core (the P-component). The P-component appears to be physically and chemically identical in all amyloids and normally circulates as a soluble serum protein (SAP). Its role in the process of tissue infiltration has not been established.

The deposited fibril, regardless of its chemical nature, when isolated and analyzed has the x-ray diffraction pattern characteristic of a beta-pleated sheet. It is insoluble at physiologic salt concentrations but can be released from tissue deposits by extraction with distilled water. The latter observation, made in the early 1970's, allowed the chemical analysis of fibrils obtained from many preparations of amyloid from the tissues of individuals with different diseases. These studies have, in turn, permitted a more precise, chemically based, classification of the various amyloid syndromes (Table 197–1).

PATHOGENESIS

Amyloid A (AA) Amyloidosis. AA amyloid, so designated because it was the first nonimmunoglobulin amyloid fibril to be characterized chemically, is most frequently found when deposition takes place in the course of chronic inflammatory disease. In the past, chronic infectious processes, such as tuberculosis and osteomyelitis, were the usual precipitating causes. In recent years, the most commonly associated conditions have been the chronic noninfectious inflammatory disorders. Amyloid deposits have been found in up to 20 per cent of autopsies of patients with rheumatoid arthritis, but they are clinically significant in only 3 to 5 per cent of cases. For reasons that are unknown, the prevalence in juvenile rheumatoid disease varies considerably in different countries (e.g., 0.14 per cent in the United States to 10 per cent in Poland). Other inflammatory joint diseases, including the seronegative spondyloarthropathies, gout, and psoriasis, as well as inflammatory bowel disease, even without arthritis, have been associated with amyloid deposition. Some populations of drug abusers, particularly those using the subcutaneous injection route because of depleted vascular access, have been found to have a high frequency of AA disease. The chronic or recurrent skin abscesses found in these patients seem to be particularly effective in the induction of amyloidosis.

Renal deposition of the AA protein has been the ultimately fatal event in the course of some groups of patients with *familial Mediterranean fever* (FMF) (Ch. 196). In the past, 40 per cent or more of North African Sephardic Jews and 20 per cent or more of Turks with this disease succumbed to renal failure secondary to AA amyloid.

AA deposition is also seen in atrial myxomas, a variety of nonlymphoid tumors, and some non–immunoglobulin-producing lymphomas. Renal and gastric carcinomas and Hodgkin's disease have been the tumors most frequently associated with AA amyloid.

Kidneys, liver, and spleen are the most important sites of AA deposition. The nephropathy is characterized initially by proteinuria of the glomerular type. Early in the disease, the kidneys may be enlarged, but with time they shrink, and the course is one of progressive renal failure. A variety of tubular disorders have also been described, including renal tubular acidosis, because of impaired bicarbonate reabsorption, nephrogenic diabetes insipidus, glycosuria, and hyperkalemia produced by decreased renal potassium exchange. The liver disease is relatively nonspecific, usually resulting in only moderate hepatomegaly and liver function test abnormalities.

In the past, when chronic infections were the most frequent stimuli to amyloid deposition, a small number of cases were reported in which eradication of the infection resulted in arrest of progression, or actual regression, of the amyloidosis, as documented by biopsy. In general, even without treatment the course of AA disease is more chronic than that of AL amyloid (see below).

The deposited AA protein appears to be a discrete proteolytic product of its precursor apo-SAA that has a monomer molecular weight of 12,500 but circulates as a molecule of molecular weight 220,000 to 235,000 complexed to high density lipoprotein. It has also been found complexed to albumin. It behaves like an acute phase protein, rising rapidly in the course of inflammation (infectious or noninfectious), peaking, and then falling to normal levels with resolution of the episode. Serum levels are generally higher in the elderly. Its synthesis is stimulated by the monokine interleukin 6 (IL6), which, in turn, can be mediated by interleukin 1 and tumor necrosis factor. It appears that the predisposition to develop AA deposits resides in the production of an amyloidogenic isotypical form of SAA, the inability to degrade SAA completely, or both occurring in the same individual.

AL Amyloidosis. AL (or immunoglobulin [Ig] light chain–related) deposition is the most common form of amyloidosis currently seen in clinical practice. The proportion of the total number of cases that represent multiple myeloma or primary amyloid is difficult to judge, since marrow plasmacytosis may be

TABLE 197–1. CHEMICAL CLASSIFICATION OF THE AMYLOIDOSES

Clinical	Fibril Precursor	Fibril	Common Abbreviation
Systemic			
Primary or myeloma with amyloid	Ig light-chain or light-chain fragment	Light-chain fragment	AL
Secondary*	Serum amyloid A (SAA)	Amyloid A (AA)	AA
Dialysis associated	Beta$_2$-microglobulin (β_2m)	β_2m monomer or dimer	AB
Familial			
Neuropathic	Transthyretin (TTR)†	TTR variants	ATTR
	Apolipoprotein A1 (Apo-A1)	Apo-A1	AApoA1
	Gelsolin‡	Gelsolin peptides	AGel
Cardiomyopathic	TTR	TTR variants	ATTR
Nephropathic	SAA	AA	AA
Vascular			
HCHWA (Iceland)	Cystatin C§	Cystatin variant	ACys
HCHWA (Denmark)	Beta protein precursor	Beta protein	AB
Localized			
Senile			
Cardiac			
Atria	Atrial natriuretic factor (ANF)	ANF	AANF
Ventricles	TTR	TTR normal or variant	ATTR
Brain (Alzheimer's disease)	Beta protein precursor	Beta protein	AB
Pancreas	Islet-associated polypeptide (IAPP)‖	IAPP	AIAPP
Endocrine			
Medullary carcinoma thyroid	Procalcitonin	Procalcitonin, calcitonin	ACal
Islet cell tumor/insulinoma	IAPP	IAPP	AIAPP

*Inflammation associated.
†Transthyretin, formerly known as thyroxine-binding prealbumin, also carries retinol-binding protein.
‡Gelsolin is an actin-binding cytoskeletal protein.
§Cystatin C is a lysomal protease inhibitor also known as gamma trace.
‖The islet-associated polypeptide has also been called amylin.

significant in both and other diagnostic distinctions between the primary disease and myeloma may be blurred (Ch. 151). Functionally, both diseases are malignant. In myeloma, the outcome is related primarily to the proliferative capacity of the neoplastic clone. When AL deposition is present, it contributes to the poor prognosis. In primary amyloid, the growth of the dominant plasma cell clone appears to be limited, but the amyloidogenicity of its homogeneous product results in the ultimately fatal compromise of organ function, most commonly renal or cardiac.

AL deposition is more likely to occur in tongue, heart, lymph nodes, spleen, carpal ligaments, joints, peripheral nerves, and skin than in the AA type. Hence, macroglossia, cardiac failure, arrhythmias, carpal tunnel syndrome, peripheral neuropathy, and ecchymoses are more frequent in AL disease. A deficiency of Factor X has been reported with an attendant bleeding diathesis. There is evidence to suggest that some AL proteins may have affinity for the clotting factor, with resultant lowering of the plasma levels. Removal of an amyloid-laden spleen has reversed the deficiency in some patients. Blood vessels tend to be fragile in AL patients, since the amyloid is deposited in vessel walls. The deposits also decrease vascular compliance, thus contributing to the body's reduced capacity to respond to reflex-mediated changes in body position. The latter may lead to severe orthostatic hypotension as a major clinical problem. Coronary artery amyloid deposition can result in angina pectoris or myocardial infarction. Infiltration of the bowel wall or autonomic nerves may cause diarrhea, with or without malabsorption.

A large number of studies have documented that the deposited fibril protein is related to the excess monoclonal Ig light chain produced by the expanded plasma cell clone and found in the patient's serum, urine, or both. The actual tissue protein may represent the whole light chain or a fragment containing at least the variable region. Most consist of the entire variable and a portion of the light chain constant region. Amino acid sequence analyses of tissue AL protein and the light chain isolated from the same patient have demonstrated chemical identity.

Despite much careful investigation, it is still not clear what makes a given light chain amyloidogenic. Lambda chains are more frequently associated with amyloid deposition than kappa, and the $V\lambda_{VI}$ subgroup is heavily overrepresented. It has been suggested that tissue affinity could be charge related or that the interaction between light chain and tissues could represent that of an incomplete autoantibody with its antigen. Neither of these hypotheses has convincing experimental support. Further, it has not been established whether amyloidogenesis involves only the processing of intact light chains to fragments or whether some of the molecules are of synthetic origin and are predisposed to deposition without further processing. It is possible that both events occur.

Most AL patients, even those with primary amyloid, have a detectable monoclonal Ig (M-protein), usually free light chains of a single class, found in the serum or urine; however, up to 20 per cent have not had such proteins detectable. Analyses of a small number of the latter patients indicated that in short-term tissue culture their bone marrow cells synthesized an excess of free monoclonal light chains. Because of their low concentration in the serum and their presumably high affinity for tissues, they cannot be detected by conventional immunochemical techniques. In only one instance has an Ig heavy chain fragment been found to make up the fibril isolated from human amyloid tissue.

Individuals have been described in whom organ compromise has taken place because of the deposition of monoclonal light chains or light and heavy chain fragments, without discrete fibril formation. Some of the patients had clinical multiple myeloma; others did not. While the proteins have been identified in tissue deposits by immunofluorescence, only a few chemical studies of the tissue forms have been carried out; therefore, formal proof of their identity with a circulating precursor is lacking. The condition appeared to be analogous to AL amyloid, but with the deposited proteins not having the intrinsic properties necessary to form beta-pleated sheets of sufficient size and stability to make fibrils. More recently, individual patients with both fibrillar (amyloid) and nonfibrillar deposits of antigenically similar material have been described, making this simple explanation unlikely.

Senile Amyloidoses. The term *senile amyloid* has been used to describe Congo red–binding material found at autopsy in the tissues of elderly individuals. Such material is most commonly found in the heart but has also been noted in the pancreas, prostate, and brain. Recent data have shown that the fibrils are derived from a variety of tissue-specific proteins.

The cerebral plaques identified in Alzheimer's disease (Ch. 450) are Congophilic and appear to be critical in its pathogenesis. Techniques used to extract and characterize other forms of amyloid have been used to analyze material isolated from the plaques and from amyloid-containing cerebral vessels of these patients. It has been found to consist of a 4200-d polypeptide, the beta protein, which is a portion of a larger protein found in a variety of tissues, including the alpha granules of platelets, where it had previously been identified as a protease inhibitor, nexin 1.

Amyloid material has also been noted in the brain lesions of Creutzfeldt-Jakob patients (Ch. 478.6) and animals suffering from scrapie. Immunohistochemical and nucleotide sequence analyses have indicated that the Alzheimer and Creutzfeldt-Jakob proteins are separate entities.

While many individuals in their eighth and ninth decades have scattered atrial amyloid deposits, clinically significant cardiac disease, characterized by either congestive heart failure or arrhythmia, results from ventricular deposits, which occur less frequently. Once symptoms appear, the prognosis is poor. The presence of a chronic inflammatory disease (e.g., rheumatoid arthritis) or multiple myeloma does not increase the incidence of senile cardiac amyloid deposition, suggesting an independent pathogenesis for each of the three conditions.

The amyloid fibrils isolated from ventricular myocardium have an amino acid sequence identical to that of serum transthyretin (TTR), a normal molecule responsible for the transport of thyroxine and retinol-binding protein. Since TTR is not known to be synthesized by myocardial cells, its cardiac deposition suggests that the precursor is produced at a remote site and localizes at its target by an as yet unknown mechanism. Clinical studies have suggested that pulmonary involvement may be regularly associated with the cardiac deposition, implying that TTR fibrils may be more systemic than previously appreciated and that the disease should be called senile systemic amyloidosis (SSA). It is not yet clear whether the deposited TTR is normal or variant in its primary structure.

AL and AA disease and SSA make up the bulk of the amyloid diseases encountered in clinical practice; however, there are additional forms, the analyses of which have yielded insight into the general process of fibril deposition. One localized form has been found in approximately 40 per cent of medullary carcinomas of the thyroid, in which the fibrillar protein consists of procalcitonin and processed forms of calcitonin.

Structural analyses of the fibrils extracted from the Congo red–binding structures seen in the pancreas of elderly patients with type II diabetes mellitus, and insulinomas have shown that they are derived from a normal peptide product of the beta cell, which probably plays a role in normal glucose metabolism and is now known as islet amyloid polypeptide (IAPP), or amylin.

Hemodialysis-Associated Amyloidosis. During the past decade, a syndrome has been recognized in patients who have been maintained on long-term hemodialysis. It is characterized by carpal tunnel syndrome, i.e., compression of the median nerve by a thickened carpal ligament, and arthropathy, frequently severe enough to require joint replacement. Examination of the surgically excised ligaments and synovial and rectal biopsies from affected individuals have revealed amyloid. Chemical analysis of the fibrils shows that they consist of monomers and dimers of beta$_2$-microglobulin, the light chain of cell-surface major histocompatibility antigens A, B, and C. It has been suggested that the deposition is secondary to the accumulation of the normally totally excreted beta$_2$-microglobulin, which is retained by dialysis membranes with relatively small pore sizes.

Familial Amyloidosis. A growing number of genetically transmitted amyloid deposition diseases with characteristic clinical syndromes have been described; they are summarized in Table 197–2. The majority are primarily neuropathic with autosomal dominant inheritance. Other hereditary forms with nephropathic, cardiopathic, or cutaneous manifestations have also been delineated. Some of these, particularly those involving the heart, appear late in life and may be confused with AL heart disease. The

TABLE 197–2. FAMILIAL AMYLOID SYNDROMES*

Syndrome	Onset (yr)	Clinical Findings	Fibril
Neuropathic			
Portuguese-Japanese (I)†	20–40	Lower limbs, autonomic	ATTR Met 30†
Swedish (I)	30–50	Upper and lower extremities, pupillary abnormalities, renal disease, autonomic and central nervous system dysfunction	ATTR Met 30
Illinois-German (I)	>50	Lower limbs, bowel, renal	ATTR Tyr 77
Swiss-Indiana (II)	>40	Upper extremities, vitreous opacities	ATTR Ser 84
Maryland-German (II)	>40	Upper extremities	ATTR Leu 58
Appalachian	>40	Peripheral neuropathy, autonomic, cardiac	ATTR Ala 60
Israel	20's	Upper and lower extremities, autonomic dysfunction, vitreous opacities	ATTR Ile 33
Iowa (IV)	20–40	Upper and lower extremities, pupillary abnormalities and renal disease	AApoA1 Arg 26
Finland (V)	40's	Facial neuropathy, lattice corneal dystrophy	AGel Asn 187 (15)
Nonneuropathic			
Familial Mediterranean fever (FMF)	10–30	Inflammatory serositis, nephropathy	AA
Derbyshire	10–30	Deafness, urticaria, fever, renal disease	Not known
Polish	40–60	Splenomegaly, hypertension, renal disease	Not known
Irish-American-German (VIII)	40–60	Lung, renal disease	Not known
Iceland (VI)	20–40	Cerebral hemorrhage	ACys Gln 68
Denmark (III)	30–70	Cardiac failure	ATTR Met 111

*All appear to be autosomal dominant diseases except FMF, which is autosomal recessive.
†Roman numerals represent the clinical classification used when these were all called familial amyloidotic polyneuropathy.
‡Thyroxine-binding prealbumin or transthyretin; see Table 197–1.
§Position 49 substitution is not found in fibrils extracted from all tissues.

absence of an M-component and a firm or suggestive family history are more consistent with late-onset familial disease.

CLINICAL MANIFESTATIONS. Regardless of the type of protein, the clinical manifestations of amyloid deposition in a given organ are similar. The renal disease is manifested primarily by proteinuria, reflecting the glomerular localization of the deposition. Renal tubular defects have also been reported. Azotemia and renal failure usually occur late. The latter may be associated with vascular involvement. There is a 5 to 15 per cent incidence of renal vein thrombosis, particularly in patients with AA disease and the nephrotic syndrome. Amyloid renal disease may be associated with hypertension. The kidneys can be small, normal sized, or enlarged. Contraction of the kidneys is generally a late event.

The most characteristic cardiac presentation is that of a restrictive cardiomyopathy with congestive heart failure. Supraventricular arrhythmias are common, as are varying degrees of atrioventricular (AV) block. Echocardiographic studies usually show a thickened interventricular septum and posterior ventricular wall without a dilated ventricle and may reveal a "sparkling" of the myocardial echoes. In vitro studies have demonstrated binding of both calcium channel blocking drugs and digitalis glycosides to amyloid fibrils. It is likely that the sensitivity of some patients with myocardial amyloidosis to digoxin is due to the concentration in the myocardium by this mechanism, and these drugs are generally not used. Pulmonary involvement tends to mirror the cardiac disease both in frequency and in extent, but rarely it becomes the dominant clinical syndrome with impairment of both the mechanics of respiration and gas exchange. Localized upper and lower airway amyloid infiltration can present major mechanical problems requiring surgical intervention.

Gastrointestinal involvement is most frequently manifested by bleeding, although diarrhea and malabsorption due to either submucosal infiltration or autonomic neuropathy have been reported.

DIAGNOSIS. The diagnosis of amyloidosis is made by the demonstration of the typical tissue deposits. Over the years the choice of appropriate tissue for biopsy has widened. In patients in whom the diagnosis is suspected on clinical grounds, recent data suggested that subcutaneous fat aspiration yields Congo red–positive material in up to 85 per cent of cases of AL disease and two thirds of patients with AA deposits. Rectal biopsy in similar

patients yields positive results in 70 to 80 per cent if adequate mucosal and submucosal tissue is obtained. Some patients may have a positive rectal biopsy result and a negative subcutaneous fat aspirate, while others may show the reverse. Gingival tissue gives positive results in about one quarter of cases. Bone marrow biopsies have been positive in up to 40 to 50 per cent of patients with AL disease. These sites may be sampled with little chance of serious complications.

When there is evidence of involvement of a particular organ, diagnostic yields improve considerably. Operative specimens from carpal tunnel releases performed on patients with AL or hereditary neuropathic disease may show 95 per cent positivity. Renal biopsies in individuals with proteinuria have been reported to be positive in more than 90 per cent of patients. Liver biopsies also have a high yield; however, as with closed renal biopsies, significant, even fatal, bleeding has occurred. Hence these procedures are performed only after a thorough evaluation of clotting parameters. Liver biopsy is generally not carried out if a coagulopathy is present. Endomyocardial biopsy has become extremely useful in the diagnosis of the cardiac forms of amyloid deposition.

It has now become possible to distinguish the chemical types of amyloid in biopsy material. In the past a diagnosis of AL disease could be inferred by the presence in the serum and urine of monoclonal Ig's or light chains. Now diagnosis is facilitated by the use of antisera to the different light chain classes, AA proteins, beta$_2$-microglobulin, transthyretin, and gelsolin in the immunofluorescent or immunoperoxidase staining of biopsy samples. Since each of the deposited proteins arises from a different precursor, presumably in response to a different stimulus, it is reasonable to assume that these discriminatory methods will eventually have therapeutic implications.

As previously noted, all deposits, regardless of the origin of the fibril, contain P-component and stain with antibodies specific for that protein. Studies in experimental models of amyloid, as well as humans with the disease, have shown that exogenous P-component, administered intravenously, will home to amyloid deposits. Early results indicate that the procedure may be clinically useful in localizing and quantifying the extent of tissue deposition.

TREATMENT AND PROGNOSIS. AL deposition associated with multiple myeloma has been treated in the course of treating the neoplastic process. While 50 to 60 per cent of patients with myeloma respond to treatment with alkylating agents and prednisone with extension of survival, the disease has not yet been cured, nor has the amyloid deposition been reversed.

A number of patients with AL disease, but without overt myeloma, have been reported to show prolonged survival after therapy with protocols like those used for myeloma. As yet, no controlled study has shown enhanced survival with any treatment; nonetheless, it appears that some patients may respond to these regimens. There have also been occasional reports of improvement in AL disease during administration of the organic solvent dimethyl sulfoxide,* usually with concurrent alkylating agent therapy.

The most successful therapy of any form of amyloidosis has been the prophylactic use of colchicine* in patients with FMF (see Ch. 196). As a result of this experience and the observation that colchicine also prevents experimental casein-induced murine AA deposition, several groups have instituted large-scale trials of colchicine in both AA and AL disease. Apart from the FMF experience and the occasional AL patient, no regimen has been uniformly successful in the reversal of any form of amyloid deposition once it has become established; nonetheless, the increased efficacy of supportive care has resulted in longer survival with a better quality of life for many affected individuals. Both cardiac disease and renal disease have been managed more effectively with the judicious use of more potent diuretics. Some patients with AL disease and renal failure, whose monoclonal protein production has been stopped by alkylating agent therapy, have undergone successful renal transplantation. More potent antibiotics have improved the outcome of infectious episodes, and newer agents, such as somatostatin analogues to treat the diarrhea associated with amyloid bowel infiltration and autonomic neuropathy, have had a favorable impact on patient management.

Browning MJ, Banks RA, Tribe CR, et al.: Ten years' experience of an amyloid clinic. Q J Med 54:213, 1985. *The experience of a large British referral clinic, worth comparing with that of the Mayo Clinic (see Kyle reference, below).*

Buxbaum JN, Chuba JV, Hellman GC, et al.: Monoclonal immunoglobulin deposition disease: Light chain and light and heavy chain deposition diseases and their relation to light chain amyloidosis. Ann Intern Med 112:455, 1990. *Comparison of clinical and laboratory features of fibrillar and nonfibrillar Ig deposition (71 references).*

Castano EM, Frangione B: Human amyloidosis, Alzheimer disease and related disorders. Lab Invest 58:122, 1988. *A review of the human amyloidoses with emphasis on pathogenesis as related to the structure of the fibrils and their precursors (141 references).*

Isobe T, Araki S, Uchino F, et al.: Amyloid and Amyloidosis. New York, Plenum Press, 1988. *The proceedings of the Fifth International Symposium, summarizing current work and thinking in the field, including clinical, epidemiologic, and basic science reports covering all forms of amyloidosis.*

Johnson KH, O'Brien TD, Betsholtz C, et al.: Islet amyloid, islet amyloid polypeptide and diabetes mellitus. N Engl J Med 321:513, 1989. *A concise description of the structure of the fibril of pancreatic amyloid and its potential role as a mediator of the pathogenesis of type II diabetes mellitus (46 references).*

Kyle RA, Greipp PR: Amyloidosis (AL), clinical and laboratory features in 229 cases. Mayo Clin Proc 58:665, 1983. *The Mayo Clinic experience, with an excellent description of the relevant features of the most commonly encountered clinical form of amyloid (117 references).*

---

*This use is not listed in the manufacturer's directive.

---

198 Hereditary Syndromes Involving Multiple Organ Systems

Arno G. Motulsky

The emergence of clinical genetics as a specialty has led to the definition of a large number of previously undifferentiated birth defects and syndromes. In some of these diseases the origin is monogenic, and multiple organ involvement is caused by the action of the mutant gene in various tissues. In other cases, a detectable chromosomal error or a known teratogen (such as Dilantin) causes multiorgan birth defects. Most frequently, neither a specific genetic nor environmental cause can be identified. Clinical genetics has grown rapidly, and most physicians are unable to keep abreast of the many newly described syndromes.

While most of these conditions become manifest in infancy or childhood, adolescent and adult patients with such conditions often initially come to internists and primary care physicians, who should be aware of the various diagnostic, genetic, and management problems. A vague diagnosis of "multiple birth defects" or "genetic syndrome" usually is not sufficient. Optimal care often requires knowledge of the specific diagnosis and natural history of a given syndrome and appropriate genetic counseling must be based on a definite diagnosis. The reader is referred to various textbooks and compendia for orientation and diagnostic approaches. Because of phenotypic variability in most syndromes, diagnosis may be difficult and new syndromes continue to be described. A significant proportion of such cases remain undiagnosed, even by expert dysmorphologists. In this chapter a few selected syndromes are discussed briefly.

Buyse ML (ed.): Birth Defects Encyclopedia. New York, Mosby, 1990. *A massive multiauthored reference book listing all known birth defects regardless of etiology, with descriptions, illustrations, and references. For on-line search and retrieval, contact Maxwell Online, Inc., 8000 Westpark Drive, McLean, VA 22102 (telephone, 800-055-0906).*

de Grouchy J, Turlean J: Clinical Atlas of Human Chromosomes. 2nd ed. New York, John Wiley & Sons, 1984. *A good general reference volume for standard syndromes associated with cytogenetic abnormalities.*

Emery AEH, Rimoin DL: Principles and Practice of Medical Genetics. Vols. 1 and 2. New York, Churchill Livingstone, 1990. *The standard reference text in clinical genetics with full descriptions of disease entities and their genetics.*

Gorlin RJ, Pindborg JJ, Cohen MM Jr (eds.): Syndromes of the Head and Neck, 3rd ed. New York, Oxford University Press, 1990. *Helpful for reference and differential diagnosis.*

Jones KL: Smith's Recognizable Patterns of Human Malformation. 4th ed. Philadelphia, W. B. Saunders Company, 1988. *The short "bible" for description of malformation syndromes. Many photographs and accounts of many different types of defects. Practically useful.*

McKusick V: Mendelian Inheritance in Man. 9th ed. Baltimore, Johns Hopkins University Press, 1990. *Standard reference source listing definite and possible monogenic diseases, traits, and syndromes with short descriptions and literature citations. Continuously updated and also available with computer access. Contact OMIM User Support, Welch Medical Library, 1830 E. Monument Street, Baltimore, MD 21205 (telephone, 301-955-7058).*

Schinzel A: Catalogue of Unbalanced Chromosome Aberrations in Man. New York, W. de Gruyter, 1984. *The definitive detailed reference for unbalanced chromosomal aberrations.*

WERNER'S SYNDROME

Werner's syndrome is a rare disorder with some clinical features that resemble early aging. Onset of clinical findings is usually in the second or third decade. Affected patients are short because of absence of the adolescent growth spurt and have slender limbs. There is premature graying and then loss of hair. Atrophy and hyperkeratosis of the skin with ulcerations around the feet are often seen. A characteristic squeaky voice and atrophy of muscle, fat, and bone of the extremities are the rule. Soft tissue calcifications usually develop. Atherosclerosis is premature with coronary heart disease and medial calcification of peripheral vessels. Juvenile cataracts and osteoporosis are typical. Hypogonadism occurs in both sexes, and mild diabetes is common. Malignant tumors occur in about 10 per cent of cases, with an unusually high occurrence of meningiomas and sarcomas. Mean age of death is in the early 40's. The phenotype of Werner's syndrome has been considered a "caricature" of senescence rather than a true model of the normal aging process. The condition is inherited as an autosomal recessive trait. Fibroblasts from skin biopsies of patients with Werner's syndrome are difficult to culture. They grow more slowly, assume a senescent morphology more rapidly, and demonstrate a markedly reduced lifespan in vitro. DNA repair is normal. Karyotype preparations show a normal number of chromosomes, but spontaneously increased chromosome breakage and variable stable chromosomal rearrangements such as translocations involving several chromosomes (variegated translocation mosaicism) are seen. Werner's syndrome therefore can be classified among the group of chromosomal instability syndromes. No single enzymatic defect has been discovered yet to explain the multiple clinical, biochemical, and cytogenetic manifestations. Werner's syndrome is sometimes termed adult progeria, but it is entirely unrelated to the pediatric syndrome of progeria (Hutchinson-Gilford), in which death occurs in early adolescence from cardiac or cerebrovascular disease.

Epstein CJ, Martin GM, Schultz AL, et al.: The Werner's syndrome. Medicine 45:177, 1966. *A detailed summary of clinical and laboratory characteristics of 125 cases of Werner's syndrome.*

Salk W, Fujiwara Y, Martin GM (eds.): Werner's Syndrome and Human Aging. New York, Plenum Press, 1985. *Many articles dealing with more recent studies.*

SYNDROMES ASSOCIATED WITH HYPOGONADISM AND VARIOUS CONGENITAL ANOMALIES

LAURENCE-MOON-BARDET-BIEDL SYNDROME AND RELATED DISORDERS. The Laurence-Moon-Bardet-Biedl syndrome exhibits retinal dystrophy (usually pigmentary retinopathy), truncal obesity, hypogonadism, variable mild to severe mental retardation, and polydactyly. Renal structural or functional abnormalities are very common. Total blindness usually occurs after the age of 30 years. Hypogonadism is less frequently found in females, as are mental retardation and polydactyly. Interstitial nephritis may lead to renal failure.

Some investigators (the "splitters") distinguish between the Bardet-Biedl and the Laurence-Moon syndrome by the presence of spastic paraplegia and the absence of polydactyly and obesity in the latter condition. However, others (the "lumpers") believe that these distinctions relate to variable expression of a single disorder.

Alstrom's syndrome appears distinct and is also associated with retinal dystrophy and obesity. Affected patients are usually blind in early childhood and develop moderately severe deafness before age 10. Diabetes mellitus and slowly progressive chronic nephropathy in young adults are seen. Mental retardation and digital anomalies are not encountered.

Carpenter's syndrome (acrocephalopolysyndactyly) is a syndrome characterized by acrocephaly, syndactyly, and a characteristic facial appearance associated with polydactyly of the feet, obesity, mental retardation, and hypogonadism. The various characteristic skeletal findings should cause few diagnostic difficulties.

All these conditions (the syndromes of Laurence-Moon-Bardet-Biedl, Alstrom, Carpenter) are inherited as autosomal recessive traits.

PRADER-WILLI SYNDROME. In this not uncommon condition, infants are born with severe hypotonia and feeding difficulties. Boys exhibit a small penis and cryptorchidism. Thin, turned-down upper lips and up-slanting palpebral fissures are often seen. Skin and hair color tend to be fair and darken with age. Compulsive hyperphagia with development of severe central obesity occurs in later childhood. Hands and feet are characteristically small (acromicria). Young adults may present with pickwickian syndrome manifesting as cardiopulmonary compromise and somnolence. Severe obesity is the major cause of morbidity and mortality in this disorder. This syndrome is the most common syndromal cause of marked obesity. Affected patients are short, and there is hypogonadotrophic hypogonadism with sterility. Menstruation may be delayed or does not occur. Mild to severe mental retardation with behavioral and personality problems are the rule. Mild diabetes mellitus is often seen.

In many cases a chromosome abnormality affecting band q11-12 of the long arm of chromosome 15 has been detected by high-resolution methods. The defect usually is a small deletion in chromosome 15 transmitted from the clinically unaffected father. Although the syndrome usually occurs as a sporadic event, extremely rare familial cases have been reported. Parental chromosomes are usually normal or are balanced translocations. It is likely that an as yet undetectable chromosomal defect exists in those cases in which no visible chromosomal abnormality has been found. The relationship of the unique and specific chromosomal deletion to the pathogenesis of the syndrome remains unknown. An identical chromosome defect (15q11-12), if transmitted from the mother, causes the completely different Angelman (happy puppet) syndrome. These findings illustrate the important role of parental "imprinting" on chromosomal expression during development. The same defect has different effects, depending upon maternal or paternal origin.

NOONAN'S PHENOTYPE. This phenotype is often diagnosed, but its boundaries are not sharply defined because of marked clinical variability. Its frequency has been estimated as 1 in 1000 to 1 in 2500. There are no chromosomal abnormalities, in contrast to the Turner syndrome (XO) that it somewhat resembles ("male" Turner syndrome). However, females can be affected as well. Affected adolescents and adults have a triangular micrognathic facial appearance with frequent hypertelorism, occasional ptosis, and posteriorly angulated low-set ears with a thick helix. A short webbed neck is common. The simultaneous presence of superior pectus carinatum and inferior pectus excavatum is helpful diagnostically. Pulmonary valve stenosis is seen frequently and can be accompanied by other types of congenital heart defects. Mild mental retardation is occasionally found. Lymphatic dysplasia causing lymphedema and a mild bleeding tendency (Factor XI deficiency or von Willebrandt disease or thrombocytopenia) occur sometimes.

Autosomal dominant inheritance can be frequently documented, but many cases are sporadic and presumably caused by new mutations. Careful examination of first-degree relatives often shows minor signs of the condition.

Allanson JE: Noonan syndrome: Am J Med Genet 24:9, 1987. *A useful review.*

Butler MG: Prader-Willi syndrome: Current understanding of cause and diagnosis. Am J Med Genet 35:319, 1990. *Review of all aspects (including detailed cytogenetics) of the syndrome.*

Green JS, Parfrey PS, Harnett JD, et al.: The cardinal manifestations of Bardet-Biedl syndrome—a form of Lawrence-Moon-Biedl syndrome. N Engl J Med 321:1002, 1989. *Clinical findings of the syndrome among 32 patients in Newfoundland.*

Greenswag LR: Adults with Prader-Willi syndrome. A survey of 232 cases. Dev Med Child Neurol 29:145, 1987. *Review with special attention to adults.*

Ranke MB, Heidemann P, Kupfer C, et al.: Noonan syndrome, growth and clinical manifestations in 144 cases. Eur J Pediatr 148:220, 1988. *Review of clinical findings.*

Schachat AP, Maumenee IH: The Bardet-Biedl syndrome and related disorders. Arch Ophthalmol 100:285, 1982. *A critical assessment of these conditions.*

Index

Note: Page numbers in **boldface** indicate major discussions; page numbers in *italics* indicate illustrations; page numbers followed by t refer to tables.

The colophon on the front cover and spine is an abstraction which symbolizes the universal aspects of medicine. The circle represents the world. The stylized triangle in the upper area is the classic image of positive and negative forces—the Law of Life. The vertical line with the upper right staff suggests the staff of Æsculapius and Hermes, and the horizontal bar connects all three symbols into the total summation of medicine as Art and Science.

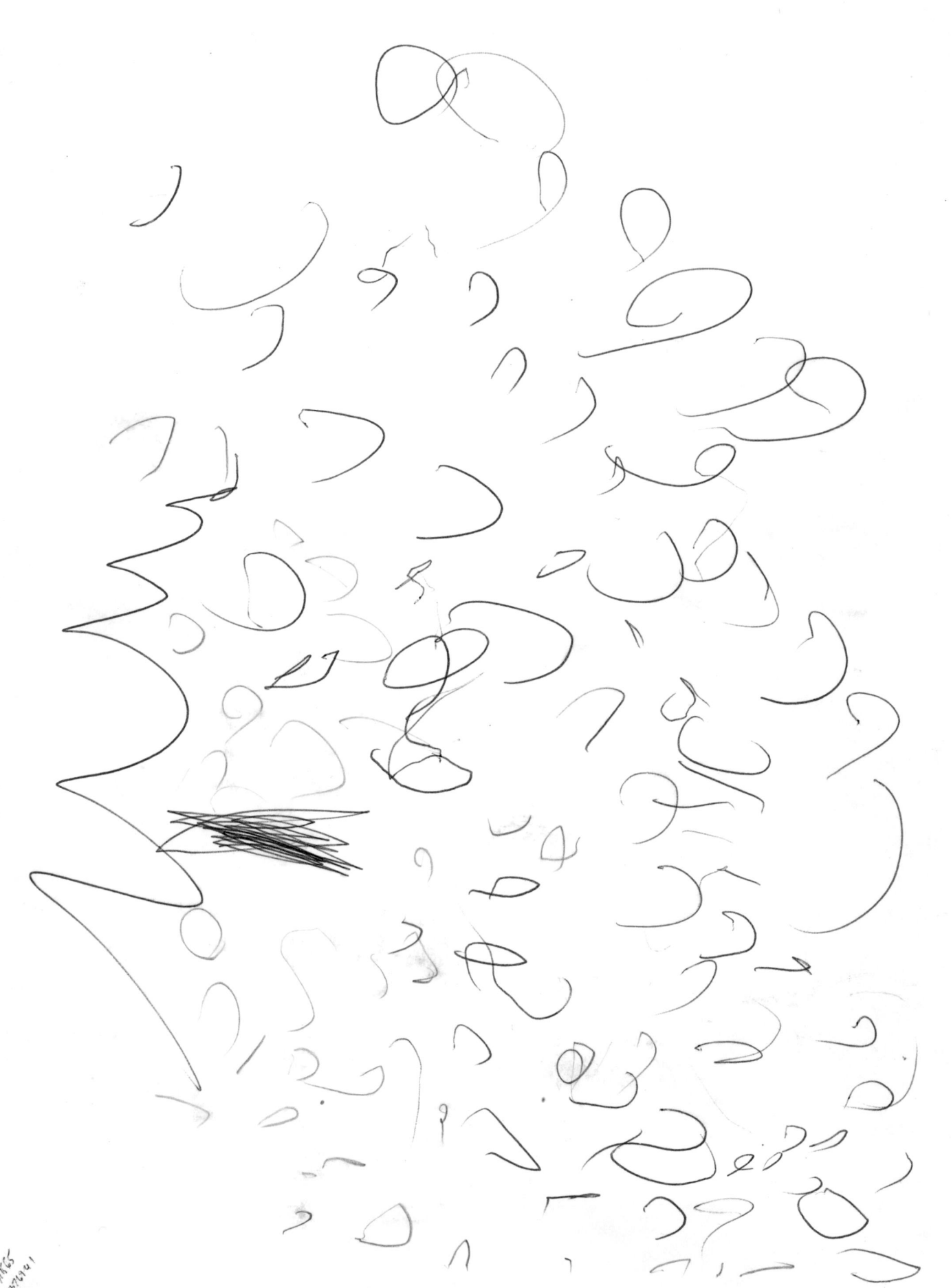